CLINICAL PHARMACY AND THERAPEUTICS

FIFTH EDITION

CLINICAL PHARMACY AND THERAPEUTICS

FIFTH EDITION

EDITORS

ERIC T. HERFINDAL, PHARM.D., M.P.H.

CHAIRMAN AND PROFESSOR, DIVISION OF CLINICAL PHARMACY
DIRECTOR, DEPARTMENT OF PHARMACEUTICAL SERVICES
SCHOOL OF PHARMACY
UNIVERSITY OF CALIFORNIA-SAN FRANCISCO
SAN FRANCISCO, CALIFORNIA

DICK R. GOURLEY, PHARM.D.

DEAN AND PROFESSOR OF CLINICAL PHARMACY
COLLEGE OF PHARMACY
UNIVERSITY OF TENNESSEE-MEMPHIS
MEMPHIS, TENNESSEE

LINDA LLOYD HART, PHARM.D.

PROFESSOR OF CLINICAL PHARMACY, DIVISION OF CLINICAL PHARMACY
DIRECTOR, DRUG INFORMATION ANALYSIS SERVICES
SCHOOL OF PHARMACY
UNIVERSITY OF CALIFORNIA-SAN FRANCISCO
SAN FRANCISCO, CALIFORNIA

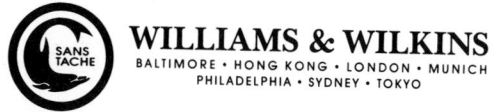

WILLIAMS & WILKINS
BALTIMORE · HONG KONG · LONDON · MUNICH
PHILADELPHIA · SYDNEY · TOKYO

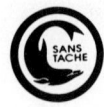

Editor: John P. Butler
Managing Editor: Linda Napora
Copy Editor: Anne K. Schwartz
Designer: Dan Pfisterer
Illustration Planner: Ray Lowman
Production Coordinator: Anne Stewart Seitz

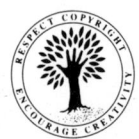
Accurate indications, adverse reactions, and dosage schedules for
drugs are provided in this book, but it is possible that they may
change. The reader is urged to review the package information data of
the manufacturers of the medications mentioned.

Printed in the United States of America

First Edition 1975
Second Edition 1979
Third Edition 1984
Fourth Edition 1988

Library of Congress Cataloging-in-Publication Data

Clinical pharmacy and therapeutics / editors, Eric T. Herfindal, Dick
    R. Gourley, Linda Lloyd Hart.—5th ed.
        p.   cm.
    Includes bibliographical references and index.
    ISBN 0-683-03966-0
    1. Chemotherapy.   2. Therapeutics.   I. Herfindal, Eric T.
II. Gourley, D. R. H., 1922–   .   III. Hart, Linda Lloyd.
    [DNLM: 1. Drug Therapy.   2. Therapeutics.   WB 330 C641]
RM262.C5   1992
615.5'8—dc20
DNLM/DLC
for Library of Congress   91-39787
                                                      CIP

PREFACE

The healthcare system continues to change at a dramatic rate. The factors that keep the healthcare system changing include: health manpower issues, an aging population, corporate influence on healthcare, government influence, economic pressures, and most of all Naisbitt's "High Tech." The biotechnologic development of drugs and the continued development of robotics and automation have been and will continue to be the major changes for the healthcare system and the profession of pharmacy. The future of the profession of pharmacy does not lie in dispensing of medications but in the provision of information and drug therapy recommendations to other healthcare providers and the patient concerning rational therapeutics. Because of these advances, the pharmacist must be prepared to meet the needs of the healthcare system and most importantly to provide pharmaceutical care to the patient. The relationship between practice and education continues to be as dynamic and intertwined as it was four years ago when the last edition of *Clinical Pharmacy and Therapeutics* was published. Clearly, the pharmacist's role in providing clinical services to the patient continues to expand. As the needs of the pharmacy student and practitioner have become much more sophisticated, so has Clinical Pharmacy and Therapeutics. This book addresses the needs of the student and practitioner by presenting contemporary drug therapy that can be used to prepare the pharmacy student or update the practitioner with unique skills and knowledge of drug therapy. We have expanded the book from 66 to 92 chapters to reflect advances in drug therapy. In addition, all laboratory values are listed with SI units as well as traditional values. There are now 20 sections and 92 chapters. Several chapters from the 4th edition were divided into two chapters to provide more in-depth coverage of the material. Those chapters that were divided include: General Nutrition—Vitamins and Minerals; Iron Deficiency and Megaloblastic Anemias—Other Anemias; Nausea and Vomiting; Diarrhea and Constipation; Rheumatoid Arthritis—Osteoarthritis; Alcoholism—Substance Abuse; and Upper Respiratory Tract Infections—Lower Respiratory Tract Infections. The new chapters are Clinical Pharmacokinetics, Drug Interactions, Clinical Laboratory Tests and Interpretation, Therapeutic Drug Monitoring and Patient Education, Biotechnology, Systemic L.E. and Other Autoimmune Joint Diseases, Osteoporosis and Osteomalacia, Burns, Common Eye Disorders, Common Ear Diseases, Sleep Disorders, Immunizations, AIDS, Bacteremia and Sepsis, Pancreatic Cancer, Gynecologic Cancer, Drugs in Pregnancy and Lactation, Critical Care Therapeutics, and Transplantation.

The companion case Workbook fulfills a need to help students develop skills in therapeutics. The Workbook allows the student to practice selecting, assessing, and monitoring drug therapy in a situation that cannot harm the patient. Students can use the cases to test their understanding and mastery of the material in the textbook. The Workbook has been expanded from 112 to 195 cases.

As in previous editions, the author selection was based on clinical experience and expertise in their area. The chapters are not mere distillations of the current literature but also include opinions based on clinical experience. It is our philosophy that pharmacists must make therapeutic judgments instead of merely serving as sources of information. We recognize that in some areas the information is conflicting and opinions vary; in those cases the authors present the various approaches in an unbiased manner, while sharing their clinical judgment. We recognize that a book alone cannot provide all the knowledge, skills, and judgment necessary to function effectively in the clinical environment. However, we believe that the combination of this textbook and the accompanying case workbook serves as an excellent starting point.

We wish to thank many individuals for their assistance in the publication of this edition. To the many contributors of the previous editions and other pharmacy educators and practitioners who responded to our survey, our grateful appreciation. To our colleagues at the University of California-San Francisco School of Pharmacy and the University of Tennessee College of Pharmacy who have worked with us as contributors, reviewers, and counselors, our thanks. Special thanks to our Administrative Assistants Sylvia Pass, Susan Heath, Eloise Muffatt, and Michelle Unterman as well as to our proof readers Sylvia Pass and Greta Gourley. Their support and devotion in meeting impossible deadlines have made our work possible. Our particular gratitude, however, goes to the contributing authors, without whose efforts there would not be a book.

E.T.H.
D.R.G.
L.L.H.

CONTRIBUTORS

DONALD P. ALEXANDER, Pharm.D.
B.S. Pharmacy, Ohio State University, Pharm.D., University of Utah, Associate Professor of Pharmacy, University of Iowa, Iowa City, Iowa

BRIAN K. ALLDREDGE, Pharm.D.
Associate Professor of Clinical Pharmacy and Neurology, Division of Clinical Pharmacy and Department of Neurology, University of California-San Francisco, San Francisco, California

ANN B. AMERSON, Pharm.D.
B.S., University of Kentucky, Pharm.D., University of Kentucky, Professor, Division of Pharmacy Practice and Science, College of Pharmacy, University of Kentucky, Lexington, Kentucky

ROBERT J. ANDERSON, Pharm.D.
B.S. Pharmacy, Purdue University, Pharm.D., University of Kentucky, Professor and Chairman, Department of Pharmacy Practice, Mercer University, Southern School of Pharmacy, Atlanta, Georgia

FRANCESCA T. AWEEKA, Pharm.D.
B.S. Biological Sciences, University of Southern California, Pharm.D., University of California–San Francisco, Assistant Clinical Professor of Pharmacy, Division of Clinical Pharmacy, University of California, San Francisco

JEFFREY N. BALDWIN, Pharm.D.
B.S. Pharmacy, SUNY at Buffalo, Pharm.D., University of Kentucky, Residency in Pediatric Pharmacy Practice, University of Kentucky, Associate Professor, Department of Pharmacy Practice, University of Nebraska Medical Center, Omaha, Nebraska

STEVEN L. BARRIERE, Pharm.D., F.C.C.P.
Pharm.D., University of California–San Francisco, Specialist in Infectious Diseases, Department of Pharmaceutical Services, Adjunct Professor of Medicine and Pharmacology, School of Medicine, UCLA Center for the Health Sciences, Los Angeles, California

RITA G. BATES, Pharm.D.
B.S. Pharmacy, University of Tennessee, Pharm.D., University of Tennessee, ASHP Residency in Hospital Pharmacy, Regional Medical Center at Memphis, Assistant Professor of Clinical Pharmacy, University of Tennessee, Clinical Pharmacist, Baptist Memorial Hospital, Memphis, Tennessee

CONSTANTINE G. BERBATIS, M.Sc., F.P.S.
M.Sc., University of Sydney, Deputy Administrator, Queen Victoria Medical Center, Melbourne, Australia

ROSEMARY R. BERARDI, Pharm.D.
B.S. Pharmacy, Ohio State University, Pharm.D., University of Michigan, Associate Professor of Pharmacy, College of Pharmacy, Clinical Pharmacist, Gastroenterology, University of Michigan Medical Center, University of Michigan, Ann Arbor, Michigan

KIMBERLY A. BERGSTROM, Pharm.D.
Pharm.D., University of California–San Francisco, Assistant Director of Pharmaceutical Services, Mount Zion Medical Center of the University of California, San Francisco, California

STANLEY J. BIRGE, M.D.
A.B., Amherst College, M.D., Washington University School of Medicine, Director, Program on Aging, Jewish Hospital of St. Louis, Associate Professor of Medicine, Washington University School of Medicine, St. Louis, Missouri

KATHRYN V. BLAKE, Pharm.D.
B.S. Zoology, University of North Carolina, Pharm.D., University of Florida, ASHP Accredited Clinical Pharmacy Residency, Shands Hospital, Gainesville, Florida, Clinical Research Scientist, Department of Medicine, Nemours Children's Clinic, Jacksonville, Florida

ERIC G. BOYCE, Pharm.D.
B.S. Pharmacy, University of Utah, Pharm.D., University of Utah, Associate Professor, Department of Clinical Pharmacy, Department of Pharmacy Practice and Pharmacy, Philadelphia College of Pharmacy and Science, Philadelphia, Pennsylvania

J. CHRIS BRADBERRY, Pharm.D.
B.S. Pharmacy, Northeast Louisiana University, M.S., Hospital Pharmacy, Northeast Louisiana University, Pharm.D., University of Tennessee, Professor and Head, Section of Pharmacy Practice, University of Oklahoma, College of Pharmacy, Oklahoma City, Oklahoma

REX O. BROWN, Pharm.D.
B.S. Pharmacy, Ferris State University, Pharm.D., University of Tennessee, Associate Professor, Department of Clinical Pharmacy, University of Tennessee, Memphis, Tennessee

KELLY J. BURCH, Pharm.D.
Pharm.D., University of Nebraska, Assistant Professor, Department of Clinical Pharmacy, University of Tennessee, Associate Director Clinical Pharmacy Services, Le Bonheur Children's Medical Center, Memphis, Tennessee

R. KEITH CAMPBELL, B.Pharm., M.B.A., F.A.P.P.
B.S. Pharmacy, Washington State University, M.B.A., Washington State University, Associate Dean, Professor of Pharmacy Practice, Certified Diabetes Educator, Department of Pharmacy Practice, Washington State University, Pullman, Washington

KIMBERLY A. CANTRAL, Pharm.D.
Pharm.D., Creighton University, Clinical Pharmacy Residency, University of Nebraska Medical Center, Assistant Professor, Department of Pharmacy Practice and Assistant Professor, Department of Family Medicine, University of Nebraska Medical Center, Omaha, Nebraska

JANNET M. CARMICHAEL, Pharm.D.
B.S. Pharmacy, University of Iowa, Pharm.D., University of Pacific, Associate Professor of Medicine, University of Nevada, School of Medicine, Reno, Nevada and Pharmacy Coordinator, VAMC, Reno, Nevada

BARRY L. CARTER, Pharm.D.
B.S. Pharmacy, University of Iowa, Pharm.D., Medical College of Virginia, Associate Professor and Assistant Head for Ambulatory Care, Department of Pharmacy Practice, College of Pharmacy, University of Illinois at Chicago, Chicago, Illinois

PEGGY L. CARVER, Pharm.D.
B.A. Biology, University of California–Los Angeles, Pharm.D., University of California–San Francisco, Clinical Residency, University of California–San Francisco, Postdoctoral Fellowship in Infectious Diseases, Hartford Hospital, Assistant Professor of Pharmacy/Clinical Pharmacist, Infectious Diseases, University of Michigan, College of Pharmacy and University of Michigan Medical Center, Ann Arbor, Michigan

BETTY J. CHAFFEE, Pharm.D.
B.S. Pharmacy, University of Toledo, Pharm.D., University of Iowa, Clinical Pharmacist in Hematology/Oncology, Clinical Assistant Professor, University of Michigan College of Pharmacy, Ann Arbor, Michigan

JUDY L. CHASE, Pharm.D.
Pharm.D., University of Arizona, Pharmacy Clinical Research Specialist, M.D. Anderson Cancer Center, Houston, Texas

MICHAEL L. CHRISTENSEN, Pharm.D.
B.S. Pharmacy, North Dakota State University, Pharm.D., University of Tennessee, Resident in Pediatrics, Le Bonheur Children's Medical Center and University of Tennessee, Fellow, Pharmacokinetics and Pharmacodynamics Section, St. Judge Children's Research Hospital, Assistant Professor, Department of Clinical Pharmacy, University of Tennessee, Memphis, Tennessee

LUELLA GRIGG CHRUCHWELL, M.D.
M.D., University of Tennessee, Residency, Internal Medicine, University of Tennessee, Resident, Department of Dermatology, University of Tennessee, Memphis, Tennessee

BRUCE D. CLAYTON, Pharm.D.
B.S. Pharmacy, University of Nebraska, Pharm.D., University of Michigan, Associate Dean and Professor of Pharmacy Practice, Butler University College of Pharmacy, Indianapolis, Indiana

EMILY B. COCHRAN, Pharm.D.
B.S. Pharmacy, University of Tennessee, Pharm.D., University of Tennessee, Assistant Professor, Department of Clinical Pharmacy, University of Tennessee, Memphis, Tennessee

WILLIAM R. CROM, Pharm.D.
B.S. Pharmacy, University of Nebraska, Pharm.D., University of Tennessee, Associate Member, Pharmaceutical Division, St. Jude's Children's Research Hospital, Associate Professor, Department of Clinical Pharmacy, University of Tennessee, Memphis, Memphis, Tennessee

JEAN K. DEVENPORT, Pharm.D.
Pharm.D., University of Southern California, Associate Professor of Pharmacy Practice, University of Utah, College of Pharmacy, Salt Lake City, Utah

BETTY J. DONG, Pharm.D.
Pharm.D., University of California–San Francisco, Clinical Professor of Pharmacy and Family and Community Medicine, University of California–San Francisco, Division of Clinical Pharmacy, San Francisco, California

ANTON C. DREYER, D.Sc.
B.S. (Pharm), D.Sc. Potchefstroom University for Christian Higher Education, Potchefstroom, South Africa, Professor, Department of Pharmacy Practice, Potchefstroom University for Christian Higher Education, Potchefstroom, South Africa

MICHAEL N. DUDLEY, Pharm.D.
Pharm.D., University of California–San Francisco, Associate Professor and Director, Antiinfective Pharmacology Research Unit, University of Rhode Island College of Pharmacy and Roger Williams General Hospital, Providence, Rhode Island

ROBERT E. DUPUIS, Pharm.D.
B.S. Pharmacy, Northeastern University, Pharm.D., State University of New York at Buffalo, Assistant Professor, Division of Pharmacy Practice, University of North Carolina, Chapel Hill, North Carolina

JAMES C. EOFF III, Pharm.D.
B.S. Pharmacy, University of Tennessee, Pharm.D., University of Tennessee, Professor of Clinical Pharmacy, University of Tennessee, Executive Associate Dean, University of Tennessee College of Pharmacy, Memphis, Tennessee

WILLIAM E. EVANS, Pharm.D.
B.S. Pharmacy, University of Tennessee, Pharm.D., University of Tennessee, Sabbatical, University of Basel, Biocenter, Department of Pharmacology, Basal, Switzerland, First Tennessee Chair of Excellence in Clinical Pharmacy, University of Tennessee College of Pharmacy and Chair Pharmaceutical Division, St. Jude Children's Research Hospital, Memphis, Tennessee

SUZANNE M. FIELDS, Pharm.D.
Oncology Research Fellow, Department of Clinical Pharmacy, University of Texas Health Science Center, San Antonio, Texas

REBECCA S. FINLEY, Pharm.D., M.S.
B.S., University of Cincinnati, Pharm.D., University of
Cincinnati, M.S. Institutional Pharmacy, University of
Maryland, Associate Professor, Department of Clinical
Pharmacy, University of Maryland, Baltimore, Maryland

CLARENCE L. FORTNER, M.S.
B.S. Pharmacy, University of Tennessee, M.S. Pharmacology,
University of Tennessee, Scientific and Medical Affairs
Executive, Adria Laboratories, Joppa, Maryland

REGINALD F. FRYE, Pharm.D.
B.S. Biology, Oglethorpe University, Pharm.D., Mercer
University, ASHP Clinical Pharmacokinetics Fellow, School of
Pharmacy, University of Pittsburgh, Pittsburgh, Pennsylvania

DARLENE F. FUJIMOTO, Pharm.D.
B.A. Biology, University of California–San Diego, Pharm.D.,
University of Southern California, Clinical Pharmacist,
Geriatrics, Department of Pharmacy, University of California,
Irvine Medical Center, Orange, California

STEPHEN H. FULLER, Pharm.D.
B.S. Pharmacy, Medical College of Virginia, Pharm.D.,
Medical College of Virginia, Assistant Professor, Department
of Pharmacy Practice, Campbell University, School of
Pharmacy, Fayetteville Area Health Education Center,
Fayetteville, North Carolina

MARK W. GARRISON, Pharm.D.
B.S. Pharmacy, University of Minnesota, Pharm.D., University
of Minnesota, Fellowship in Pharmacokinetics and Infectious
Diseases, University of Minnesota, Assistant Professor of
Pharmacy Practice, College of Pharmacy, Washington State
University, Spokane, Washington

MARK A. GILL, Pharm.D.
Pharm.D., University of California-San Francisco, Associate
Professor of Clinical Pharmacy, University of Southern
California, School of Pharmacy, Los Angeles, California

TRACEY L. GOLDSMITH, Pharm.D.
Pharm.D., University of Kentucky, Clinical Residency,
University of Kentucky, Clinical Manager-Critical Care,
Department of Pharmacy Services, Hermann Hospital,
Houston, Texas

EDGAR R. GONZALEZ, Pharm.D.
B.S. Pharmacy, Philadelphia College of Pharmacy, Pharm.D.,
University of Utah, Graduate Certificate in Gerontology,
University of Utah, Associate Professor of Pharmacy, Associate
Professor of Medicine, Clinical Coordinator, Critical Care
Pharmacy Services, Medical College of Virginia, Richmond,
Virginia

DICK R. GOURLEY, Pharm.D.
B.S. Pharmacy, University of Tennessee, Pharm.D., University
of Tennessee, Certificate in Health Systems Management,
Harvard University, Dean and Professor of Clinical Pharmacy,
University of Tennessee, College of Pharmacy, Memphis,
Tennessee

ANDRIES G. GOUS, Pharm.D.
B.Pharm., Potchefstroom University for Christian Higher
Education, Potchefstroom, South Africa, Pharm.D., University
of Tennessee, Clinical Pharmacist, Baragwanath Hospital,
Johannesburg, South Africa

HERMIEN GOUS, Pharm.D.
B.Pharm., Potchefstroom University for Christian Higher
Education, Potchefstroom, South Africa, Pharm.D., University
of Tennessee, Clinical Pharmacist, Baragwanath Hospital,
Johannesburg, South Africa

KATHLEEN K. GRAHAM, Pharm.D.
Clinical Assistant Professor, Antiinfective Pharmacology
Research Unit, University of Rhode Island, College of
Pharmacy, The Miriam Hospital, Providence, Rhode Island

DAVID J. HARPER, Pharm.D.
B.S. Pharmacy, University of Utah, Pharm.D., University of
Utah, Clinical Pharmacist, University of Utah Hospital, Salt
Lake City, Utah

LINDA LLOYD HART, Pharm.D.
B.S. Pharmacy, University of Kentucy, Pharm.D., University of
Kentucky, Professor of Clinical Pharmacy, Division of Clinical
Pharmacy, Director, Drug Information Analysis Services,
School of Pharmacy, University of California–San Francisco,
San Francisco, California

LEE HEADLEY, Pharm.D.
Pharm.D., University of California–San Francisco, Clinical
Pharmacist, University of California–Los Angeles Medical
Center, Los Angeles, California

DENNIS K. HELLING, Pharm.D., F.C.C.P.
B.S. Pharmacy, St. Louis College of Pharmacy, Pharm.D.,
University of Cincinnati College of Pharmacy, Professor and
Chairman, Department of Pharmacy Practice, University of
Houston, College of Pharmacy, Houston, Texas

RICHARD A. HELMS, Pharm.D.
B.S. Biology, Ohio State University, B.S. Pharmacy,
Massachusetts College of Pharmacy, Pharm.D., Duquesne
University, ASHP Accredited Residency in Hospital Pharmacy,
Mercy Hospital, Associate Professor and Vice Chair for
Clinical Programs, Department of Clinical Pharmacy,
Associate Professor, Department of Pediatrics, University of
Tennessee, Memphis, Tennessee

ERIC T. HERFINDAL, Pharm.D., M.P.H.
Pharm.D., University of California–San Francisco, M.P.H.,
University of California-Berkeley, Chairman and Professor,
Division of Clinical Pharmacy, Director, Department of
Pharmaceutical Services, School of Pharmacy, University of
California–San Francisco, San Francisco, California

JOHN W. HILL, Ph.D.
Ph.D. Learning Disabilities and Special Education, American
University, Foundation Professor, Special Education, Director,
Learning Disabilities Clinic, University of Nebraska at Omaha,
Omaha, Nebraska

JOHN D. HIRSH, Pharm.D.
Pharm.D., University of California–San Francisco, Director of
Pharmacy, Clinical Services and Education, University of
Pittsburgh Medical Center, Assistant Professor, Department of
Pharmacy and Therapeutics, School of Pharmacy, Pittsburgh,
Pennsylvania

VALERIE W. HOGUE, Pharm.D.
Pharm.D., Howard University, Clinical Residency, University
of California–San Francisco, Assistant Professor, Department
of Pharmacy Practice, Howard University College of Pharmacy
and Pharmacal Sciences, Washington, D.C.

JOHN M. HOLBROOK, Ph.D.
B.S. Pharmacy, Mercer University Southern School of
Pharmacy, Ph.D. in Pharmacology, University of Mississippi,
Professor of Pharmaceutical Sciences, Mercer University
Southern School of Pharmacy, Atlanta, Georgia

K. DALE HOOKER, Pharm.D.
B.A. Biology, Carson-Newman College, Pharm.D., Mercer
University Southern School of Pharmacy, Infectious Diseases
Clinical Residency, Medical University of South Carolina,
Postdoctoral Fellowship in Infectious Diseases, University of
Georgia and Medical College of Georgia, Assistant Professor
of Pharmacy and Medicine, University of Missouri–Kansas
City, Clinical Pharmacy Specialist, Infectious Diseases,
Veterans Affairs Medical Center, Kansas City, Missouri

CHRISTINE E. HULS, Pharm.D.
B.S. Pharmacy, Purdue University, Pharm.D., Purdue
University, Residency in Critical Care, Medical University of
South Carolina, Research Fellow in Infectious Diseases,
University of Houston, Research Fellow in Infectious
Diseases, University of Houston, College of Pharmacy, Texas
Medical Center, Houston, Texas

R. PETER IAFRATE, Pharm.D.
B.S., Northeastern University, Pharm.D., University of
Florida, Supervisor, Clinical Pharmacy Services, Assistant
Director, Department of Pharmacy, Shands Hospital, and
Assistant Clinical Professor, College of Pharmacy, The
University of Florida, Gainesville, Florida

MARIE WILKERSON JACKSON, Pharm.D.
B.S. Chemistry, Centre College of Kentucky, B.S. Pharmacy,
University of Kentucky, Pharm.D., University of Kentucky
Assistant Professor of Pharmacy Practice, Mercer University
Southern School of Pharmacy, Atlanta, Georgia and Area
Health Education Coordinator, The Medical Center of Central
Georgia, Macon, Georgia

MARTIN J. JINKS, Pharm.D.
Pharm.D., University of California–San Francisco, Professor
and Chair, Department of Pharmacy Practice, College of
Pharmacy, Washington State University, Pullman, Washington

MARTIN L. JOB, M.A., Pharm.D., M.A.
B.S. Pharmacy, Fordham University M.A. Health Science
Administration, New Jersey State College System, Pharm.D.,
Mercer University Southern School of Pharmacy, Professor,
Department of Pharmacy Practice, Mercer University School
of Pharmacy, Atlanta, Georgia and Assistant Director of
Pharmacy for Clinical Services and Education, DeKalb
Medical Center, Decatur, Georgia

ARCELIA M. JOHNSON-FANNIN, Pharm.D.
B.S. Chemistry, Dillard University, B.S. Pharmacy, Columbia
University, Pharm.D., Mercer University, Associate Professor
and Director, Academic Affairs, College of Pharmacy, Florida
A&M University, Tallahassee, Florida

PAUL M. JOST, M.D.
B.A., Tabor College, M.D., University of Kansas, Internal
Medicine Residency, St. Luke's Medical Center, Fellowship in
Infectious Diseases, Kansas City Department of Veterans
Affairs Medical Center, Kansas City, Missouri and the
University of Kansas School of Medicine, Kansas City, Kansas

STANLEY G. KAILIS, Ph.D., F.P.S.
Dip. Pharmacy, Perth Technical College, B.Sc. (Hons),
Western Australia University, Ph.D., Western Australia
University, Associate Professor of Pharmaceutical Biology and
Clinical Pharmacy, Curtin University of Technology, Perth,
Western Australia

DEBRA KALMAN, Pharm.D.
Pharm.D., University of Southern California, Fellow in
Infectious Diseases, Department of Pharmaceutical Services,
UCLA Medical Center, Los Angeles, California

JOAN E. KAPUSNIK-UNER, Pharm.D.
Pharm.D., University of California–San Francisco, Assistant
Clinical Professor of Pharmacy, Clinical Pharmacist, AIDS
Clinic, University of California–San Francisco and Clinical
Pharmacist in Infectious Diseases, San Francisco General
Hospital, San Francisco, California

STEVEN R. KAYSER, Pharm.D.
Pharm.D., University of California–San Francisco, Clinical
Professor of Pharmacy, University of California–San Francisco,
San Francisco, California

DONALD L. KENDZIERSKI, Pharm.D.
B.S., University of Wisconsin, Pharm.D., University of
Tennessee, Assistant Chief, Clinical Pharmacy Division,
Pharmacy Services, Edward Hines, Jr. VA Hospital, Hines,
Illinois

LOUISE KENDZIERSKI, Pharm.D.
B.S., University of Illinois, Pharm.D., University of Illinois,
Clinical Pharmacy Coordinator, Northwest Community
Hospital, Chicago, Illinois

WENDY KLEIN-SCHWARTZ, Pharm.D.
Pharm.D., University of Maryland, Associate Professor,
Clinical Pharmacy, University of Maryland, School of
Pharmacy, Director, Maryland Poison Center, Baltimore,
Maryland

JIM M. KOELLER, M.S.
Clinical Associate Professor, The University of Texas at Austin and Health Science Center, San Antonio, Texas

PETER J. S. KOO, Pharm.D.
B.S. Chemistry, University of Berkeley, Pharm.D., University of California–San Francisco, Associate Clinical Professor of Pharmacy, School of Pharmacy, University of California–San Francisco, San Francisco, California

WAYNE A. KRADJAN, Pharm.D.
Pharm.D., University of California–San Francisco, Professor and Chairman, Department of Pharmacy Practice, University of Washington, Seattle, Washington

S. CASEY LAIZURE, Pharm.D.
Pharm.D., University of North Carolina, Assistant Professor, Department of Clinical Pharmacy, University of Tennessee and The Memphis Neurosciences Center, Methodist Hospital, Memphis, Tennessee

VICTOR LAMPASONA, Pharm.D.
B.S. Pharmacy, St. John's University, Pharm.D., Medicial University of South Carolina, Associate Director for Clinical and Educational Programs, Emory University Hospital, Atlanta, Georgia

PHI-VAN T. LE, M.D.
M.D., University of Florida, Internship, University of Tennessee, Resident, Department of Dermatology, University of Tennessee, Memphis, Tennessee

RICHARD D. LEFF, Pharm.D., F.C.C.P.
B.S. Pharmacy, Creighton University, Pharm.D., University of Minnesota, Associate Professor of Pediatrics and Pharmacy, Department of Pediatrics and Pharmacy, Director, Pediatric Pharmacology, University of Kansas Medical Center, Kansas City, Kansas

ROBERT H. LEVIN, Pharm.D.
Pharm.D., University of California–San Francisco, Vice Chairman and Professor of Clinical Pharmacy, Professor of Family and Community Medicine, University of California–San Francisco, San Francisco General Hospital, San Francisco, California

DAVID R. LUKE, Pharm.D., F.A.C.A.
B.S. Pharmacy, University of Toronto, Pharm.D., Philadelphia College of Pharmacy and Sciences, Senior Clinical Research Scientist, Clinical Pharmacology Unit, Hoffmann-La Roche, Inc, New Newark, New Jersey

JANELLE M. MAHONEY, Pharm.D.
Pharm.D., University of Nebraska, Assistant Professor of Pharmacy Practice, St. Louis College of Pharmacy, Director of Geriatric Pharmacy Education, Program on Aging, Jewish Hospital at Washington University Medical Center, St. Louis, Missouri

PIERRE A. MALOLEY, Pharm.D.
Pharm.D., University of Nebraska, Assistant Professor, Department of Pharmacy Practice and Internal Medicine, University of Nebraska Medical Center, Omaha, Nebraska

HEWITT W. MATTHEWS, Ph.D.
B.S. Chemistry, Clark College, B.S. Pharmacy, Mercer University Southern School of Pharmacy, M.S., University of Wisconsin, Ph.D., Univerity of Winsconsin, Dean and Professor of Pharmaceutical Sciences, Mercer University Southern School of Pharmacy, Atlanta Georgia

GARY R. MATZKE, Pharm.D., F.C.P., F.C.C.P.
B.S. Pharmacy, University of Wisconsin, Pharm.D., University of Minnesota, Professor and Director, Clinical Scientist Program, School of Pharmacy, University of Pittsburgh, Pittsburgh, Pennsylvania

DIANE NYKAMP McCARTER, Pharm.D.
B.S. Pharmacy, Mercer University Southern School of Pharmacy, Pharm.D., Mercer University Southern School of Pharmacy, Associate Professor of Pharmacy Practice, Mercer University Southern School of Pharmacy, Atlanta, Georgia

WILLIAM J. McINTYRE, Pharm.D.
B.S. Pharmacy, Wayne State University, Hospital Residency, Providence Hospital, Pharm.D., Wayne State University, Clinical Residency, University of Kentucky, Fellow, Cancer Immunology, University of Texas Health Science Center, San Antonio, Texas

CONSTANCE A. McKENZIE, Pharm.D.
B.A. Sociology, University of Tennessee, Pharm.D., Mercer University Southern School of Pharmacy, Assistant Professor and Director, Drug Information, Campbell Univerity, Buies Creek, North Carolina

KELLIE D. McQUEEN, Pharm.D.
B.S., Pharm.D., Creighton University, Director, The Kapoor Center for Pediatric Drug Information, Denver, Colorado

GAIL W. McSWEENEY, Pharm.D.
B.S. Pharmacy, University of New Mexico, Pharm.D., University of Tennessee, Assistant Clinical Professor, Division of Clinical Pharmacy, School of Pharmacy, Univerity of California–San Francisco, San Francisco, California

DAVID MEYERS, M.D.
M.D., University of Iowa, Associate Professor of Medicine (Cardiology) and Preventive-Societal Medicine, University of Nebraska Medical Center, Omaha, Nebraska

ROBERT K. MIDDLETON, Pharm.D.
B.A. Biology, California State University–Fullerton, Pharm.D., University of California–San Francisco, Clinical Coordinator/Drug Utilization Manager, Alta Bates Medical Center, Berkeley, California

MIRTA MILLARES, Pharm.D.
Pharm.D., University of California–San Francisco, Ajunct Assistant Professor of Pharmacy Practice, University of Southern California, School of Pharmacy, Los Angeles, California, Pharmacist Specialist, Regional Drug Information Service, Kaiser Permanente Medical Care Program, Southern California Region, Downey, Califorina

SUSAN W. MILLER, Pharm.D
B.S. Pharmacy, Mercer University Southern School of
Pharmacy, Pharm.D., Mercer University Southen School of
Pharmacy, Associate Professor of Pharmacy Practice, Mercer
University Southern School of Pharmacy, Atlanta, Georgia

CHRISTINE A. MOWATT-LARSSEN, Pharm.D.
B.S. Pharmacy, Albany College of Pharmacy, Pharm.D.,
Medical University of South Carolina, Fellow, Department of
Clinical Pharmacy, University of Tennessee, Memphis,
Tennessee

TIMOTHY A. MULLENIX, Pharm.D., M.S.
B.S. Pharmacy, University of Iowa, M.S. Clinical Pharmacy,
University of Iowa, Pharm.D., University of South Carolina,
Assistant Professor, University of South Carolina, College of
Pharmacy, Columbia, South Carolina

JEAN K. NOGUCHI, Pharm.D.
Pharm.D., University of Southern California, Assistant
Professor of Clinical Pharmacy, University of Southern
California, School of Pharmacy, Los Angeles, California

PAUL E. NOLAN, Jr., Pharm.D.
B.S., Northeastern University, Pharm.D., University of
Kentucky, Associate Professor, Department of Pharmacy
Practice, Associate Clinical Scientist, University Heart Center,
University of Arizona, Tucson, Arizona

GARY M. ODERDA, Pharm.D., M.P.H.
Pharm.D., University of California–San Francisco, M.P.H.,
Johns Hopkins University, Professor and Chairman,
Department of Pharmacy Practice, University of Utah, College
of Pharmacy, Salt Lake City, Utah

MICHAEL A. OSZKO, Pharm.D.
B.S. Pharmacy, University of Pittsburgh, Pharm.D., University
of Cincinnati, Associate Professor, Department of Pharmacy
Practice, School of Pharmacy, The University of Kansas
Medical Center, Kansas City, Kansas

MICHAEL D. PARR, Pharm.D.
B.S. Biology, University of Nebraska, Pharm.D., University of
Nebraska, Residency, University of Kentucky, Assistant
Director, Department of Pharmacy, The University of
Hospital of Arkansas, Little Rock, Arkansas

STEPHANIE J. PHELPS, Pharm.D.
B.S. Pharmacy, Samford University, Pharm.D., University of
Tennessee, Associate Professor, Department of Clinical
Pharmacy, University of Tennessee, Director Therapeutic
Drug Monitoring Service, Le Bonheur Children's Medical
Center, Memphis, Tennessee

ROBERT W. PIEPHO, Ph.D., F.C.P.
B.S. Pharmacy, University of Illinois, Ph.D. Pharmacology,
Loyola University, Dean and Professor, University of
Missouri–Kansas City, Kansas City, Missouri

RANDALL A. PRINCE, Pharm.D.
B.S. Pharmacy, Philadelphia College of Pharmacy and
Science, Pharm.D., Philadelphia College of Pharmacy an
Science, Professor, University of Houston, College of
Pharmacy, Texas Medical Center, Houston, Texas

CYNTHIA L. RAEHL, Pharm.D.
B.S. Pharmacy, University of Wisconsin, Pharm.D., University
of Kentucky, Associate Professor, School of Pharmacy,
University of Wisconsin, Madison, Wisconsin

LORI A. REISNER-KELLER, Pharm.D.
B.S., California State Polytechnic University (cum laude),
Pharm.D., University of Southern California, Residency in
Clinical Pharmacy, University of California–San Francisco,
Fellowhip in Pharmacokinetics/Pharmacodynamics, University
of California–San Francisco, Clinical Pharmacist, UCSF Pain
Management Center, Division of Clinical Pharmacy,
University of California–San Francisco, San Francisco,
California

BETH H. RESMAN-TARGOFF, Pharm.D.
B.S. Pharmacy, State University of New York at Buffalo,
Pharm.D., State University of New York at Buffalo, Clinical
Assistant Professor, Section of Pharmacy Practice, University
of Oklahoma, College of Pharmacy, Oklahoma City, Oklahoma

RICHARD S. RHODES, Pharm.D.
B.S., Florida Agricultural and Mechanical University,
Pharm.D., Mercer University Southern School of Pharmacy,
Associate Professor, Pharmacy Practice, Idaho State Universty,
Pocatello, Idaho

TED L. RICE, B.S., M.S.
B.S. Pharmacy, University of the Pacific, M.S. Pharmacy,
University of North Carolina at Chapel Hill, Clinical
Pharmacist, Department of Pharmacy Services, University of
Michigan Medical Center, Clinical Assistant Professor,
University of Michigan, College of Pharmacy, Ann Arbor,
Michigan

DANIEL C. ROBINSON, Pharm.D.
B.A. Biology, California State University–Fullerton, Pharm.D.,
University of California–San Francisco, Associate Professor
and Chair of Clinical Pharmacy, Associate Professor of Clinical
Medicine, University of Southern California, Los Angeles,
California

KEVIN M. RODONDI, Pharm.D.
B.A. Biology, San Francisco State University, Pharm.D.,
University of California–San Francisco, Residency in Clinical
Pharmacy, University of California–San Francisco, Assistant
Clinical Professor of Pharmacy, School of Pharmacy, Division
of Clinical Pharmacy, University of California–San Francisco,
San Francisco, California

DIANE R. ROMAC, Pharm.D.
Pharm.D., University of the Pacific, Clinical Pharmacy
Residency, University of California–San Francisco, Assistant
Clinical Professor of Pharmacy, University of California–San
Francisco, Clinical Pharmacist, University of California–Davis,
Sacramento, California

RONALD J. RUGGIERO, Pharm.D.

B.S., University of San Francisco, Pharm.D., University of California–San Francisco, Associate Clinical Professor of Pharmacy, University of California–San Francisco, San Francisco, California

THERESA A. SALAZAR, Pharm.D.

Pharm.D., University of California–San Francisco, Assistant Clinical Professor of Pharmacy, Division of Clinical Pharmacy, University of California, San Francisco, California

P. RAVI SARMA, M.D., F.A.C.P.

M.B.B.S., Andhra Medical College, A.P., India. Residency in Internal Medicine, Cook County Hospital, Chicago; Fellowship in Hem-Onc, University of Illinois, Chicago and Emory University School of Medicine, Atlanta, GA

MICHAEL L. SCHMITZ, M.D.

B.A., Boston University, M.D., Boston University, Resident, Department of Orthopedics, Boston University School of Medicine, Boston, Massachusetts

MICHAEL A. SCHNEIDER, M.D.

M.D., University of Tennessee, Internship, Baptist Memorial Hospital, Memphis, Tennessee, Resident, Department of Dermatology, University of Tennesee, Memphis, Tennessee

ROWENA N. SCHWARTZ, Pharm.D.

B.S. Pharmacy, University of Illinois, Pharm.D., University of Texas, Assistance Professor of Pharmacy and Therapeutics, University of Pittsburgh, Coordinator of Pharmacy Services, Pittsburgh Cancer Institute, Pittsburgh, Pennsylvania

CHARLES F. SEIFERT, Pharm.D.

B.S. Pharmacy, North Dakota State University, Pharm.D., University of Texas, ASHP Clinical Pharmacy Residency, Truman Medical Center, Universty of Missouri–Kansas City, Associate Professor of Adult Medicine, Section of Pharmacy Practice, University of Oklahoma, College of Pharmacy, Oklahoma City, Oklahoma

MARK S. SHAEFER, Pharm.D.

B.A. Biology, University of California–San Diego, Pharm.D., University of California–San Francisco, Associate Professor, Pharmacy Practice, Assistant Professor, Surgery, University of Nebraska Medical Center, Omaha, Nebraska

SAM K. SHIMOMURA, Pharm.D.

Pharm.D., University of California–San Francisco, Professor of Clinical Pharmacy, University of California–San Francisco, San Francisco, California

ELIZABETH STUBITS SHLOM, Pharm.D.

B.S. Pharmacy, Philadelphia College of Pharmacy, Pharm.D., Philadelphia College of Pharmacy, Clinical Pharmacy Supervisor, St. Luke's/Roosevelt Hospital Center, New York, New York

CHARLES D. SINTEK, M.S.

B.S. Pharmacy, University of Nebraska, M.S. Clinical/Hospital Pharmacy, University of Iowa, ASHPAccredited Hospital/ Clinical Pharmacy Residency, Department of Veterans Affairs Medical Center, Iowa City, Iowa, Clinical Pharmacy Manager, Department of Veterans Affairs Medical Center, Adjoint Assistant Professor, University of Colorado School of Pharmacy, Denver, Colorado

ROBERT J. STAGG, Pharm.D.

Pharm.D., University of the Pacific, Assistant Clinical Professor of Pharmacy, University of California–San Francisco, San Franciso, California

GREGORY V. STAJICH, Pharm.D.

B.A. Natural Sciences, B.S. Medical Technology, University of South Florida, B.S. Pharmacy, Mercer University Southern School of Pharmacy, Pharm.D., Mercer University Southern School of Pharmacy, Associate Professor of Pharmacy Practice, Mercer University Southern School of Pharmacy, Atlanta, Georgia

CLINTON F. STEWART, Pharm.D.

B.S. Pharmacy, Auburn University, Pharm.D., University of Tennessee, Assistant Member, St. Jude Children's Research Hospital, Associate Professor, Department of Clinical Pharmacy, University of Tennessee, Memphis, Memphis, Tennessee

GLEN L. STIMMEL, Pharm.D., F.C.C.P.

Pharm.D., University of California–San Francisco, Professor of Clinical Pharmacy, Psychiatry and Behavioral Sciences, University of Southern California, Los Angeles, California

JANICE L. STUMPF, Pharm.D.

Pharm.D., University of California–San Francisco, Clinical Pharmacist, Department of Pharmacy Services, University of Michigan Medical Center, Clinical Assistant Professor, University of Michigan, College of Pharmacy, Ann Arbor, Michigan

KEN T. TAKEGAMI, M.D., M.P.H.

M.P.H., University of Hawaii School of Public Health, M.D., The Oho State University, Internship University of Tennessee, Resident, Department of Dermatology, University of Tennessee, Memphis, Tennessee

DAVID S. TATRO, Pharm.D.

B.A. Psychology, San Francisco State University, Pharm.D., University of California–San Francisco, Associate Director of Pharmacy, Director, Drug Information, Stanford University Hospital, Stanford, California

RICHARD E. THOMAS, Ph.D.

F.P.S., Sydney University, M.Sc., Sydney University, Ph.D., Sydney University, Associate Professor of Pharmacy Practice, Sydney University, Sydney, New South Wales, Australia

THEODORE G. TONG, Pharm.D.
B.S., University of Southern California, Pharm.D., University
of California–San Francisco, Professor of Pharmacy Practice,
Pharmacology and Toxicology, Associate Dean for Academic
Affairs, University of Arizona, Tucson, Arizona

KEVIN A. TOWNSEND, Pharm.D.
Pharm.D., University of Michigan, Clinical Pharmacist,
Department of Pharmacy Services, University of Michigan
Medical Center, Clinical Instructor, University of Michigan,
College of Pharmacy, Ann Arbor, Michigan

EARL S. WARD, Jr., Pharm.D., F.A.S.H.P.
B.S., University of Georgia, Pharm.D., Mercer University,
Associate Dean and Professor, Department of Pharmacy
Practice, Mercer University Southern School of Pharmacy,
Atlanta, Georgia

MARK D. WATANABE, Pharm.D., Ph.D.
Pharm.D., University of California–San Francisco, Ph.D.
Pharmaceutical Chemistry, University of California–San
Francisco, Assistant Professor of Pharmacy Practice, College
of Pharmacy, University of Illinois at Chicago, Chicago,
Illinois

ROBERT T. WEIBERT, Pharm.D.
Pharm.D., University of California–San Francisco, Clinical
Professor of Pharmacy (UCSF). UCSD Medical Center, San
Diego, California

LYNDA S. WELAGE, Pharm.D.
B.S. Pharmacy, University of Michigan, Pharm.D., State
University of New York at Buffalo, Postdoctoral Fellowship,
Clinical Pharmacokinetics Laboratory, Millard Filmore
Hospital, Assistant Professor of Pharmacy, College of
Pharmacy, Clinical Pharmacist-Surgery-Trauma/Burn,
University of Michigan Medical Center, University of
Michigan, Ann Arbor, Michigan

BARBARA G. WELLS, Pharm.D.
B.S. Pharmacy, University of Tennessee, Pharm.D., University
of Tennessee, Residency in Psychiatric Pharmacy, University
of Tennessee, Associate Professor and Vice Chair for
Educational Programs, Director Mental Health Pharmacy
Programs, Department of Clinical Pharmacy, University of
Tennessee, Memphis, Tennessee

JOHN R. WHITE, Jr., Pharm.D.
B.A. Zoology, University of Tennessee, Pharm.D., Mercer
University, Residency in Clinical Pharmacy, University of
California–San Francisco, Fellow in Pharmacokinetics,
University of California–San Francisco, Assistant Professor of
Pharmacy Practice, Washington State University College of
Pharmacy, Spokane, Washington

MICHAEL Z. WINCOR, Pharm.D.
B.S. Zoology, University of Chicago, Pharm.D., University of
Southern California, Assistant Professor of Clinical Pharmacy,
Psychiatry and the Behavioral Sciences, University of Southern
California, Los Angeles, California

THOMAS H. WISER, Pharm.D.
Professor and Assistant Dean, Department of Pharmacy
Practice, Purdue University, School of Pharmacy, West
Lafayette, Indiana

STACEY L. WOJTYSIAK, Pharm.D.
B.S. Pharmacy, University of Minnesota, Pharm. D.,
University of Minnesota, Residency in Nutrition Support,
University of Minnesota, Fellowship in Nutrition Support,
University of Tennessee, Assistant Professor of Pharmacy
Practice, Ferris State University, Big Rapids, Michigan

BRADLEY G. WULF, Pharm.D.
Pharm.D., University of Nebraska, Assistant Professor of
Pharmacy Practice, University of Nebraska Medical Center,
Omaha, Nebraska

CONTENTS

SECTION 15 : INFECTIOUS DISEASES

SECTION 16 : NEOPLASTIC DISORDERS

SECTION 17 : PEDIATRIC AND NEONATAL THERAPY

CHAPTER 1

CLINICAL PHARMACOKINETICS

S. CASEY LAIZURE, Pharm.D., and WILLIAM E. EVANS, Pharm.D.

Clinical pharmacokinetics is the application of pharmacokinetic principles in a patient care setting. Probably the most difficult aspect of clinical pharmacokinetics is understanding both the full potential and the practical limitations of using specific models of drug disposition to attain target concentrations based on only one or two measured serum drug concentrations (SDCs). While a good understanding of common pharmacokinetic models (e.g., first-order elimination and Michaelis-Menten kinetics) is crucial, the competent clinician will have knowledge of not only the mathematics of these models, but the principles, assumptions, and potential errors underlying their clinical application. Furthermore, a broad therapeutic knowledge is also necessary, as measured SDCs must be interpreted with respect to the clinical condition of the patient and the pharmacodynamics of the therapeutic agent. This chapter presents a pragmatic approach to clinical pharmacokinetics, focusing on the utilization of measured SDCs for the adjustment of patient drug therapy.

BASIC PHARMACOKINETIC PARAMETERS

The difficulty many clinicians have in understanding the three basic pharmacokinetic parameters of the one-compartment open model (volume of distribution (V), clearance (Cl), and half-life ($t_{1/2}$)) is due to the esoteric nature of their definitions and the difficulty of trying to build a foundation of basic concepts from terms that seem to contradict logic. For example, a drug that distributes in a volume greater than that of the human body or has a clearance that defines a volume of blood from which all drug is removed, have no apparent relationship to physiologic variables or anatomical structures associated with drug elimination from the body. This is not an attempt to refute the traditional definitions, but for the moment put them aside to concentrate on the pragmatic mathematical meanings, interrelationships, and how alterations in pharmacokinetic parameters affect the steady-state concentration after chronic dosing.

Volume of Distribution

The volume of distribution (V) is a proportionality constant that equates the SDC to the total amount of drug in the body (1). This concept is depicted in Figure 1.1 by using

drug distribution in a conical flask containing 70 ml of water and 30 ml of oil. In this example, the concentration of drug is measured only in the water phase, analogous to the measurement of drug in the blood (serum or plasma) of patients. The following examples are thus analogous to the common practice of measuring drug in serum and calculating the V based on the one-compartment open model, with the assumption of homogeneous distribution of drug throughout the body, equivalent to the measured serum concentration.

When drug is added to the flask, it partitions between the oil and water, depending on its lipophilicity. Hydrophilic compounds will tend to remain in the water phase, while lipophilic compounds will distribute more extensively into the oil phase. The *apparent* volume of distribution of drug in the flask is determined by measuring the concentration of drug in the water phase (drug in the oil phase does not contribute to the measured concentration in the water phase) and determining the volume that would be required to account for all the drug put in the flask. One hundred milligrams of a hydrophilic drug is put in one flask, and 90 mg distributes into the water and 10 mg into the oil. The measured concentration of hydrophilic drug in water is the total amount of drug in the water phase divided by the volume of water, i.e., 90 mg ÷ 70 ml = 1.29 mg/ml. Thus, accounting for all the drug in the flask, if it exists at the concentration measured in the water phase, is 100 mg ÷ 1.29 mg/ml = 78 ml (apparent volume of distribution). The apparent volume is close to the volume of water in the flask, because the hydrophilic drug distributes primarily into the water phase. In contrast, when 100 mg of a lipophilic drug is put into the other flask, 90 mg distributes into the oil phase and only 10 mg remains in the water phase. The measured concentration of lipophilic drug in the water is the total amount of drug in the water phase divided by the volume of water, i.e., 10 mg ÷ 70 ml = 0.14 mg/ml. Thus, accounting for all the drug in the flask, assuming it exists at the concentration measured in the water phase, is 100 mg ÷ 0.14 mg/ml = 714 ml (apparent volume of distribution). The apparent volume is much greater than the actual volume of the container, because most of the drug has distributed outside the water phase. Hence, the apparent volume is a function

Figure 1.1.

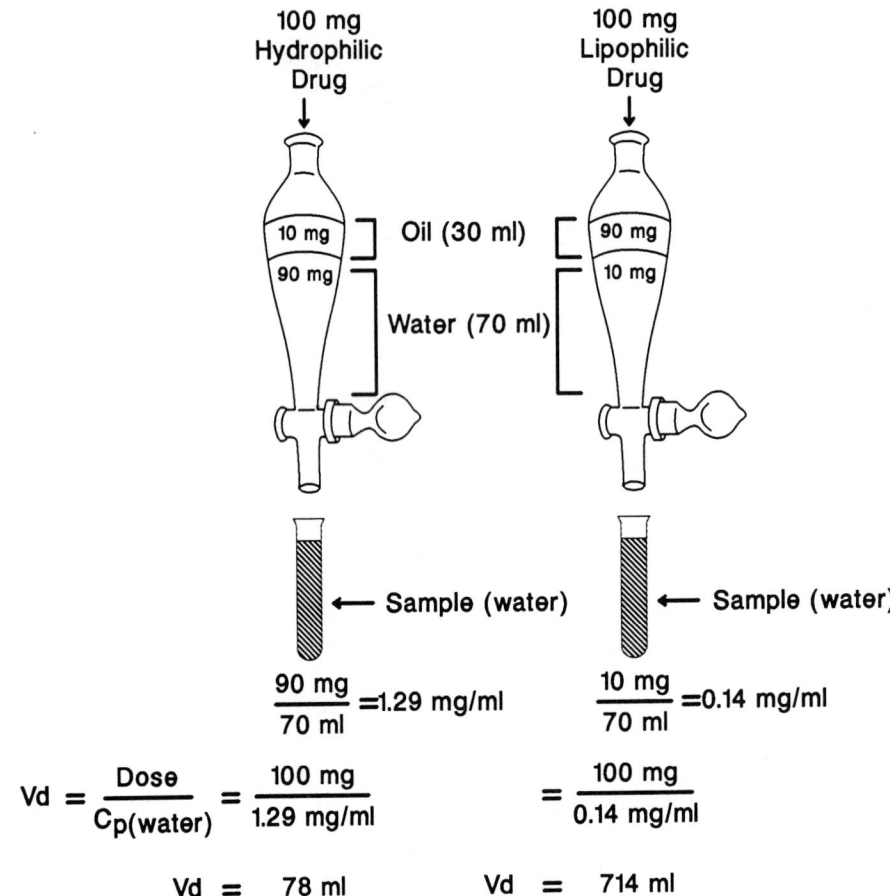

Vd = 78 ml   Vd = 714 ml

of the amount of drug put in the flask (or body) and the measured concentration of drug in the water phase (or serum), and is unrelated to any physical volume.

As can be appreciated from the above discussion, the V has no physiologic basis, and thus it is not related to the volume of serum, blood, total body water, etc. Theoretically, if V is determined experimentally from multiple SDCs after a single dose of a drug and the calculated V equals the volume of serum in the patient's body, then all the drug must be in the patient's serum, assuming a uniform concentration. When the V is greater than the serum volume, this means simply that to equate the SDC with the total amount of drug in the body, a value greater than the serum volume is required. A V greater than the serum volume indicates that some portion of the drug is located outside the serum. Though it is common to speculate on where a drug distributes, based on its V, technically such speculation is not valid. If a drug has a V of 0.7 liter/kg, it might be tempting to assume that the drug distributes in total body water, since total body water is approximately 70% of total body weight. However, the V could just as easily be increased because of distribution or binding to some other body tissue. The fact that the V is 0.7 liter/kg only indicates that the drug distributes outside the serum.

Determining where the drug goes when it leaves the serum compartment requires data other than V.

Assuming a one-compartment model and a single dose (X_o) of drug with first-order elimination (rate constant k), the total amount of the drug remaining ($X_{(t)}$) in the body after some time interval (t) can be converted to the serum concentration by dividing both sides of the following equation by V.

$$X_{(t)} = X_o e^{-kt} \qquad (1.1)$$

$$\frac{X_{(t)}}{V} = \frac{X_o e^{-kt}}{V} \qquad (1.2)$$

$$C_{(t)} = C_o e^{-kt} \qquad (1.3)$$

For a specific drug, if the V of the drug and an SDC are known, then the total amount of drug in the patient's body can be estimated. For example, if the measured SDC of theophylline is 12 mg/liter and the V is 35 liters, then the total amount of drug in the body can be estimated as follows:

$$\text{Amount} = (SDC)(V) \qquad (1.4)$$
$$= (12 \text{ mg/liter})(35 \text{ liter}) = 420 \text{ mg}$$

This same equation can also be used to calculate the loading dose necessary to achieve a specific peak SDC after a single dose. "Amount" in this case refers to the amount of the loading dose. Thus, the same equation can be used to calculate the loading dose necessary to achieve an initial theophylline SDC of 15 mg/liter in a patient with a V equal to 35 liters.

$$\text{Loading Dose} = (SDC_{TARGET})(V)$$
$$= (15 \text{ mg/liter})(35 \text{ liters}) \quad (1.5)$$
$$= 525 \text{ mg}$$

This equation assumes that the SDC of theophylline before the loading dose was zero. Patients with drug already in their body may only need a partial loading dose, e.g., a patient in status epilepticus with a phenytoin SDC of 5 mg/liter. If the desired target SDC is 20 mg/liter, then a loading dose that will raise the SDC from 5 to 20 mg/liter is needed. The following equation takes into account drug present in the patient when the loading dose is determined:

$$\text{Loading Dose} = \frac{(SDC_{TARGET} - SDC_{OBSERVED})(V)}{(S)(F)}$$
$$= \frac{(20 \text{ mg/liter} - 5 \text{ mg/liter})(70 \text{ liters})}{(0.92)(1.0)} = 1141 \text{ mg}$$
$$(1.6)$$

where $SDC_{OBSERVED}$ is the SDC before the partial loading dose is given, S is the fraction of active drug by weight in the salt formulation (parenteral phenytoin is phenytoin sodium that is 92% phenytoin), and F is the bioavailability ($F = 1$ for IV route). This latter equation is appropriate for calculating a partial or full loading dose for most drugs given by either the parenteral or oral route, when the V is known.

Clearance

Clearance is a proportionality constant that relates the rate of drug elimination to the SDC (1). Clearance should not be equated with the drug elimination rate, since Cl is a flow rate measured in units of volume per time (e.g., ml/min). However, if the Cl of a drug is known, then the rate of drug elimination can be calculated by multiplying the Cl by the SDC (assuming first-order drug elimination).

$$\text{Rate of drug elimination} = (SDC)(Cl) \quad (1.7)$$

The rate of drug elimination applies only to the SDC used in the calculation. If a different SDC value is used, a different rate of drug elimination will be calculated. Thus, the rate of drug elimination is constantly changing and directly proportional to the change in the SDC for a first-order process, i.e., as the SDC increases, the rate of drug elimination increases proportionately.

If a patient receives a drug by constant IV infusion, intermittent IV infusion, or oral dosing at regular intervals, the steady-state SDC is determined by the dose and the Cl. The steady-state SDC occurs when the rate of drug in (i.e., dose rate) is equivalent to the rate of drug out (i.e., *Rate of drug elimination*). The SDC at which the rate in equals the rate out is determined solely by the Cl parameter and dose.

CASE #1

L. L. presents to the emergency room diaphoretic and complaining of sharp substernal chest pain radiating to the left shoulder. The patient is admitted to rule out a myocardial infarction. L. L.'s physician begins a constant IV infusion of an antiarrhythmic drug at a rate of 4 mg/min. The following kinetic parameters are estimated from measured SDCs in this patient. Estimate the steady-state concentration that will occur with this dose.

$t_{1/2}$	1.5 hours
V	130 liters
Cl	1 liter/minute

The steady-state SDC is reached when the administration rate of the drug equals the rate of drug elimination (equation (1.7)) from the serum. Multiplying the SDC by the Cl gives the rate of drug elimination. The volume term (L) cancels out, leaving the units as mg/min, the same units as administration rate. When the SDC reaches 4 mg/liter, the rate of drug elimination equals the rate of drug administration (4 mg/min), and steady state is achieved.

SDC (mg/liter)		Cl (liter/min)	Rate of Drug Elimination (mg/min)
1	×	1	= 1
2	×	1	= 2
3	×	1	= 3
4	×	1	= 4 (steady state)

The steady-state SDC achieved with a constant IV infusion is calculated using the following equation:

$$C_{SS} = \frac{ko}{Cl} \quad (1.8)$$

where C_{SS} is the steady-state SDC, *ko* equals the rate of drug administration (amount/time), and Cl is the clearance. For a drug given by intermittent IV infusion or oral dosing, the mean steady-state SDC that will be achieved can be calculated using

$$\overline{C_{SS}} = \frac{(F)(D)}{(Cl)(\tau)} \quad (1.9)$$

where $\overline{C_{SS}}$ is the mean steady-state SDC, F is the bioavailability, D is the dose, Cl is the clearance, and τ is the dosing interval. Note that the mean steady-state concentration is defined as

$$\overline{C_{SS}} = \frac{AUC_\tau}{\tau} \qquad (1.10)$$

where AUC_τ is the area under the concentration-time curve for a single steady-state dosing interval and τ is the time duration of the dosing interval. The $\overline{C_{SS}}$ calculated from this equation is *not* equivalent to taking the average of the peak and trough from a dosing interval.

Half-Life

The half-life is the time required for the serum concentration to decrease by one-half (1). Half-life is a transformation of the elimination rate constant to a form more easily interpreted. Do not confuse k or $t_{1/2}$ with the drug elimination rate (equation (1.7)). The parameter k is a mathematical variable that defines a constant exponential rate of change. The k can be estimated from two measured SDCs (e.g., a measured peak and trough) drawn within the same dosing interval. Assuming a one-compartment model with first-order elimination, k is estimated by plotting the natural log (ln) of the concentration versus time, and determining the slope of the line passing through the peak and trough. The calculated slope will be equal to $-$k. The k may be calculated by taking the natural log of the quotient of the peak divided by the trough, and dividing by the time interval between the peak and trough. This solution to k can be derived from the standard calculation for the slope of a line from two points:

$$
\begin{aligned}
k &= -m \\
&= -\left[\frac{(\ln SDC_{TROUGH} - \ln SDC_{PEAK})}{(T_{TROUGH} - T_{PEAK})} \right] \\
&= -\left[\frac{\ln\left(\dfrac{SDC_{TROUGH}}{SDC_{PEAK}}\right)}{(T_{TROUGH} - T_{PEAK})} \right] \qquad (1.11) \\
&= \frac{\ln\left(\dfrac{SDC_{PEAK}}{SDC_{TROUGH}}\right)}{(T_{TROUGH} - T_{PEAK})}
\end{aligned}
$$

where m is the slope of the line of a semilog plot of the natural log of the SDCs versus time. The SDC_{PEAK} and SDC_{TROUGH} are Y values, and the T_{TROUGH} and T_{PEAK} are the corresponding times the trough and peak were collected, or the X values. Clinically, the last expression in equation (1.11) is used to calculate k. The penultimate expression differs from the last expression only in that the SDC_{PEAK} and SDC_{TROUGH} have been flipped, which only changes the sign of the answer from negative to positive. Obviously, there are limitations in estimating the slope of

a line from only two measured SDCs, as any error in the measured SDC or the time of collection will create error in the estimate of k (or $t_{1/2}$).

CASE #2

G. W. is a 55-year-old female patient receiving gentamicin, 80 mg every 8 hours. A peak SDC of 5.2 µg/ml is drawn 30 min after the end of a 30-min infusion and a trough SDC of 1.7 µg/ml is drawn seven hr after the end of the infusion. Calculate the half-life of gentamicin in this patient.

$$k = \frac{\ln\left(\dfrac{5.2\ \mu g/ml}{1.7\ \mu g/ml}\right)}{(7.5\ hr - 1.0\ hr)} = 0.172\ hr^{-1} \qquad (1.12)$$

To compute the half-life from k, divide the ln 2 (i.e., 0.693) by k.

$$t_{1/2} = \frac{\ln 2}{k} = \frac{0.693}{k} = \frac{0.693}{0.172\ hr^{-1}} = 4.0\ hours \qquad (1.13)$$

Measured peak and trough concentrations allow an estimation of $t_{1/2}$. The half-life provides information about specific aspects of the disposition of a drug, such as, how long it will take to reach steady-state once maintenance dosing is started and how long it will take for "all" the drug to be eliminated from the body once dosing is stopped (usually considered five half-lives). Also, once the k and an SDC are known, there are three calculations that will aid in the individualization of a patient's dosing regimen: (a) extrapolation, (b) back-extrapolation, and (c) determination of the time required for the concentration to decrease to some specified SDC. These functions are defined by solving for the appropriate variable in the following equation:

$$C_{(t)} = C_o e^{-kt} \qquad (1.14)$$

where $C_{(t)}$ is the concentration after t time has elapsed, C_o is a measured SDC, k is the elimination rate constant, and t is some specified time interval. In the previous gentamicin example ($SDC_{PEAK} = 5.2$ µg/ml; $SDC_{TROUGH} = 1.7$ µg/ml; $k = 0.172$ hr^{-1}; $\tau = 8$ hr), equation (1.14) can be used to calculate (a) the C_{MIN}, defined as the theoretical SDC at the end of the dosing interval (extrapolation), (b) the C_{MAX}, defined as the theoretical SDC at the instant the infusion is complete (back-extrapolation), and (c) determination of the time interval required for the concentration to fall from the C_{MAX} to some lower SDC (e.g., 0.5 µg/ml).

(a) The concentration at the end of the dosing interval is calculated by extrapolating from the SDC_{PEAK} to the end of the dosing interval (t = 7, 8 hr − 1 hr) using equation (1.14).

$$C_{(t)} = C_o e^{-kt}$$

$$= (5.2 \text{ μg/ml})e^{(-0.172\text{hr}^{-1})(7.0\text{hr})} \qquad (1.15)$$

$$= 1.5 \text{ μg/ml}$$

(b) Equation (1.14) can be rearranged to back-extrapolate, that is, determine the concentration that occurred at some earlier time. The theoretical peak concentration, C_{MAX}, which occurs at the instant the infusion is complete, is determined by back-extrapolating from the SDC_{PEAK} to the time the infusion ended (30 min).

$$C_{(t)} = \frac{C_o}{e^{-kt}} = \frac{5.2 \text{ μg/ml}}{e^{(-0.172\text{hr}^{-1})(0.5\text{hr})}} = 5.7 \text{ μg/ml} \qquad (1.16)$$

(c) The time interval for the concentration to drop from 5.7 μg/ml (C_{MAX}) to 0.5 μg/ml is determined by solving for t in equation (1.14).

$$t = \frac{\ln\left(\dfrac{C_o}{C_{(t)}}\right)}{k} = \frac{\ln\left(\dfrac{5.7 \text{ μg/ml}}{0.5 \text{ μg/ml}}\right)}{0.172 \text{ hr}^{-1}}$$

$$= 14.1 \text{ hours} \qquad (1.17)$$

The three pharmacokinetic parameters, Cl, V, and $t_{1/2}$ define specific characteristics of drug disposition that are well defined. Table 1.1 summarizes the clinical utility of each pharmacokinetic parameter.

RELATIONSHIP BETWEEN $t_{1/2}$, CLEARANCE, VOLUME, AND STEADY-STATE CONCENTRATION

Clearance and V are independent pharmacokinetic parameters. This means Cl may change without affecting V, and V may change without affecting Cl. Half-life is a dependent function whose value is dependent on Cl and V. If half-life changes then Cl, V, or both must have changed. An often inappropriately applied equation is

$$Cl = (k)(V) \qquad (1.18)$$

which is frequently interpreted to mean that Cl depends on V. A mathematical equation can be algebraically rearranged in many ways, but it should not be deduced that one parameter is dependent on another simply because of the way the equation is written. For example, if an experiment demonstrated that an increase in blood pressure (BP) correlates with increasing age, and a linear regression of BP (dependent variable) as a function of age (independent variable) is performed; an equation for the estimation of BP from age is derived:

$$BP = (Age)(m) + b \qquad (1.19)$$

where m is the slope of the regression line and b is the

Table 1.1.
Clinical Utility of the Three Basic Pharmacokinetic Parameters of the One-Compartment Open Model[a]

Parameter	Use	Equation
Volume of distribution, V (units: volume, e.g., liter)	Determine a loading dose	(1.6)
	Determine amount of drug in body	(1.4)
	Make qualitative assessment of distribution of drug in the body	
Clearance, Cl (units: volume/time, e.g., liter/hour)	Determine the steady-state concentration that will be achieved from a specific maintenance dose	(1.8) and (1.9)
Elimination rate constant, k (units: reciprocal time, e.g., hr^{-1})	Determine how long it will take to reach steady-state once maintenance dosing started	$5 \times t\frac{1}{2}$
Half-life, $t\frac{1}{2}$ (units: time, e.g., hours)	Determine how long it will take for the concentration to drop from some specified concentration to some lower concentration	(1.17)

[a] The three basic pharmacokinetic parameters of first-order elimination are clearance, volume, and half-life. These parameters have specific, well-defined clinical utility.

intercept. Equation (1.19) could be algebraically rearranged to give the following equation:

$$Age = \frac{BP - b}{m} \qquad (1.20)$$

It is obviously absurd to conclude from this equation that decreasing a patient's BP will decrease the patient's age. Thus, an equation does not necessarily define the interrelationships among the variables within the equation. This same situation exists for Cl = kV. The form of the equation that correctly reflects the interrelationship among the parameters is:

$$k = \frac{Cl}{V} \qquad (1.21)$$

Clearance and V are the primary pharmacokinetic parameters that determine drug disposition. Clearance can be thought of as representing the sum of all drug elimination processes in the body, while V represents the distribution of drug. The steady-state concentration of a drug achieved after constant IV infusion, or the mean steady-state concentration achieved after multiple oral or multiple intermittent IV infusions depends on Cl only (equations (1.8) and (1.9), respectively). Changes in the V have no effect on the steady-state or mean steady-state concentration. Intuitively it may seem that, for example, since a decrease in the V will mean that the same amount of drug is distributed in a smaller volume, the concentration must increase. However, the basic principle, which states that Cl and V are independent, would be violated, as the only way the steady-state concentration could increase is for the Cl to decrease (equations (1.8) and (1.9)). The logical deduction is that Cl is dependent on V, which is incorrect. The question then arises as to exactly what effect changes in the V have on drug disposition. The patient on the antiarrhythmic (Case #1) can be used to illustrate the consequence of a decrease in V.

CASE #1 (Revisited)

The patient is admitted to the hospital with chest pain. Subsequent clinical examination and laboratory data confirm a myocardial infarction (MI) complicated by congestive heart failure. The patient's condition improves over the next two days, the IV antiarrhythmic is discontinued, and an oral antiarrhythmic is prescribed. Two days later the patient again develops runs of premature ventricular depolarizations (PVDs) despite adequate oral antiarrhythmic therapy. The patient is put back on a continuous IV infusion of the same antiarrhythmic as before. However, the patient's congestive heart failure (CHF) has responded to therapy, which has lead to a diuresis of edematous fluid. The antiarrhythmic is distributed into total body water, with the result that the V of the antiarrhythmic has decreased by one-third. Clearance has remained unchanged. Describe how the drug disposition from the start of the 4 mg/min IV infusion to steady-state will be altered.

The Cl and V before and after CHF resolution are as follows:

	Before Treatment	After Treatment
Cl	1 liter/min	1 liter/min
V	130 liters	87 liters

The rate of drug elimination can be calculated by taking the present SDC and multiplying by the Cl (equation 1.7)). Though the V has decreased, the fact remains that at an SDC of 4 mg/liter and a Cl of 1 liter/min, the rate of drug elimination will be 4 mg/min (4 mg/min = 4 mg/liter × 1 liter/min). No matter how V changes, the rate of drug elimination at an SDC of 4 mg/liter will always be 4 mg/min as long as the Cl remains unchanged. On the other hand, k is a dependent function that will change with changes in Cl and V. How the k changes and what effect it has on drug disposition is more easily interpreted if k is expressed as $t_{1/2}$. Since k = Cl/V (equation (1.21)) and k = $0.693/t_{1/2}$ (rearrangement of equation (1.13)), then

$$\frac{0.693}{t_{1/2}} = \frac{Cl}{V} \tag{1.22}$$

Table 1.2.

The Effect of Changes in Clearance and Volume on Half-Life and Steady-State Concentration [a]

Independent Parameters		Dependent Parameters	
Clearance	Volume	Half-Life	C_{SS}
↑	↔	↓	↓
↓	↔	↑	↑
↔	↑	↑	↔
↔	↓	↓	↔
↑	↑	?	↓
↑	↓	↓	↓
↓	↑	↑	↑
↓	↓	?	↑

[a] Clearance and volume are independent parameters whose values determine the apparent elimination rate (or half-life) of drug from the serum and the steady-state concentration achieved after maintenance dosing. The half-life is affected by both the clearance (inversely proportional) and volume (directly proportional), as depicted in equation (1.23). The steady-state concentration is only affected by the clearance, as shown in equations (1.8) and (1.9). The "?" in the table indicates that the effect on half-life cannot be determined without knowing the specific changes in Cl and V.

Solving for $t_{1/2}$ gives the following:

$$t_{1/2} = \frac{0.693 \, V}{Cl} \tag{1.23}$$

This equation can be used to calculate the change in half-life when the V decreases from 130 to 87 liters.

$$t_{1/2_{130L}} = \frac{(0.693)(130 \text{ liters})}{1 \text{ liter/min}} = 90 \text{ min} \tag{1.24}$$

$$t_{1/2_{87L}} = \frac{(0.693)(87 \text{ liters})}{1 \text{ liter/min}} = 60 \text{ min} \tag{1.25}$$

The decrease in V results in a decrease in the $t_{1/2}$, with no change in the steady-state concentration. The time to reach steady-state will decrease from 7.5 hr (1.5 hr × 5) to 5.0 hours (1.0 hr × 5), but the steady-state concentration achieved will be unchanged. Table 1.2 gives the relative changes in $t_{1/2}$ and C_{SS} that occur when Cl and V change.

In the case of multiple intermittent IV infusions or oral dosing, the C_{SS} in Table 1.2 refers to the $\overline{C}_{SS}$ as defined in equation (1.10). Though it is true that changes in V do not alter the $\overline{C}_{SS}$, changes in V do affect the peak and trough concentrations within the dosing interval. Figure 1.2 compares and contrasts changes in Cl and V for a constant IV infusion and an intermittent IV infusion. As Figure 1.2**B** illustrates, a decrease in V for intermittent IV infusions leads to greater fluctuations between the peak and trough. It is possible that the increased fluctuation between the peak and trough could result in transient toxicities associated with high peaks or periods of subtherapeutic concentrations associated with low troughs. The ac-

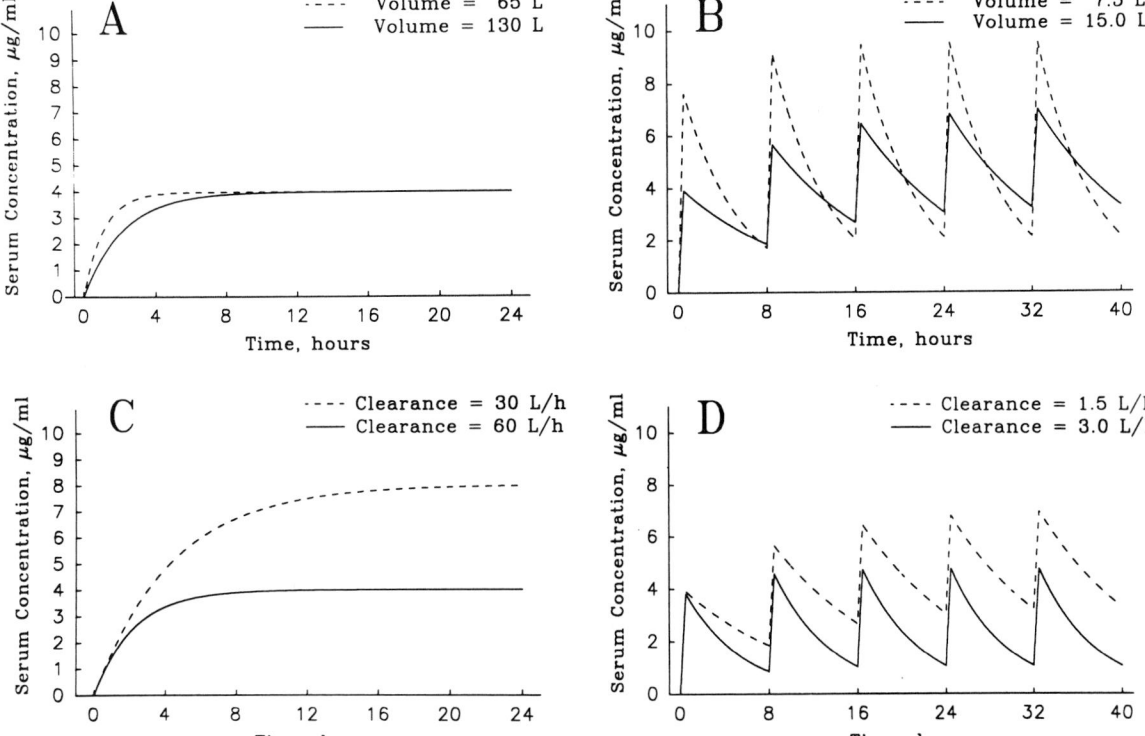

Figure 1.2. The effect of clearance and volume changes on the concentration-time profile of a continuous and intermittent IV drug infusion. **A** and **B** depict an IV constant infusion and an IV intermittent infusion, respectively. The *dashed line* represents the change in the concentration-time plot if the volume is decreased by one-half with no change in clearance. For both **A** and **B** the time to reach steady-state is decreased. For graph **A** the steady-state concentration is unchanged. For graph **B,** the mean steady-state concentration is unchanged, but the peak will be higher and the trough lower. **C** and **D** depict an IV constant infusion and an IV intermittent infusion, respectively. The *dashed line* represents the change in the concentration-time plot if the clearance decreases by one-half with no change in the volume. The time to reach steady-state is increased, and the steady-state concentration is doubled.

tual impact of alterations in V will depend on the degree of change in V and the pharmacodynamic characteristics of the particular drug in question.

USING SERUM DRUG CONCENTRATIONS FOR OPTIMIZATION OF DRUG THERAPY
Rationale for Therapeutic Drug Monitoring
Routine clinical monitoring utilizing SDCs is reserved for therapeutic agents that have a "defined" therapeutic range and a low therapeutic index. A "defined" therapeutic range is characterized by both upper and lower limits; where exceeding the upper limit is associated with a high probability of unacceptable toxicity, and falling short of the lower limit is associated with a low probability of achieving a clinical therapeutic benefit. A low therapeutic index indicates that the serum concentrations necessary to achieve the therapeutic effect are close to serum concentrations that result in significant clinical toxicity. The implication is that dosing patients on population-average pharmacokinetic parameters will result in an unacceptable frequency

of therapeutic failures or clinical toxicity directly attributable to low or high serum concentrations, respectively. The therapeutic ranges given in Table 1.3 are by no means supported by unequivocal evidence. Also, controversy surrounds the use of therapeutic ranges for drugs that have only a few well-controlled pharmacodynamic studies to establish such ranges. However, these ranges are generally accepted as an initial endpoint for therapy and represent the current standards of practice.

A therapeutic range must not be used as the primary determinant of a patient's drug regimen. It would be inappropriate to consider achievement of a specific serum concentration as the clinical endpoint of therapy. The endpoint of therapy is always defined by a clinical response. If the clinical response is achieved when the SDC is outside the commonly stated therapeutic range, the patient's clinical condition rather than the SDC should be considered. For example, if a patient taking digoxin for chronic atrial fibrillation did not respond when the steady-state trough SDC ($SDC_{SS\text{-}TROUGH}$) was below 2.0 ng/ml but is

Table 1.3.
Drugs Commonly Monitored in the Clinical Setting[a]

Drug	Therapeutic Range	Half-Life (hours)	Volume (liter/kg)	Clearance	SDC Type	Disposition	References
Digoxin	0.8–2.0 ng/ml	41	7.0	180 ml/min/1.73 m^2	$C_{SS\text{-}TROUGH}$	Two-compt	9, 10
Theophylline	5–20 μg/ml	8	0.5	0.65 ml/min/kg	$C_{SS\text{-}TROUGH}$	Two-compt	11
Lidocaine	1.5–5.0 μg/ml	2	1.2	15.6 ml/min/kg	C_{SS}	Two-compt	12, 13, 14
Procainamide	4–12 μg/ml	3.3	2.0	8.6 ml/min/kg	$C_{SS\text{-}TROUGH}$	Two-compt	15
Lithium[b]	0.6–1.4 mEq/liter	21	0.8	10–40 ml/min	$C_{SS\text{-}12\text{ hour}}$	Two-compt	16, 17
Quinidine	2–5 μg/ml	7	2.5	4.5 ml/min/kg	$C_{SS\text{-}TROUGH}$	Two-compt	18, 19
Gentamicin[c]	5–10 μg/ml peak	2	0.21	—	Zaske Eqn	One-compt	20, 21
Tobramycin[c]	<2 μg/ml trough	2.1	0.27	—	Zaske Eqn	One-compt	20
Amikacin[c]	20–30 μg/ml peak <5 μg/ml trough	2.2	0.25	—	Zaske Eqn	One-compt	21
Carbamazepine[d]	4–12 μg/ml	12.3	1.0	0.91 ml/min/kg	$C_{SS\text{-}TROUGH}$	—	22, 23
Phenobarbital	15–40 μg/ml	100	0.58	2.5 ml/min/m^2	$C_{SS\text{-}TROUGH}$	Two-compt	23, 24
Phenytoin	10–20 μg/ml	N/A[e]	0.7	N/A	$C_{SS\text{-}TROUGH}$	Nonlinear	25
Valproic acid	50–100 μg/ml	13	0.24	4–6 ml/min/m^2	$C_{SS\text{-}TROUGH}$	Two-compt	23, 26
Vancomycin	25–40 μg/ml peak 5–15 μg/ml trough	7	0.72	1.2 ml/min/kg	Zaske Eqn	Two-compt	27, 28

[a] This table is not all-inclusive, covering only the most commonly monitored drugs. The stated therapeutic ranges and the pharmacokinetic parameters are for patients with normal hepatic and renal function and have significant variability, as reported in the literature.
[b] Lithium clearance averages 20% of creatinine clearance.
[c] Aminoglycoside clearance is dependent on renal function. Half-life given assumes young patient with normal renal function.
[d] Carbamazepine parameter values after autoinduction.
[e] N/A = not applicable.

now responding with a SDC$_{SS\text{-}TROUGH}$ of 2.3 ng/ml (therapeutic range 0.8–2.0 ng/ml), as evidenced by an acceptable ventricular response and no drug toxicity, then this should be considered a clinically acceptable digoxin concentration with no need to change the dosage regimen.

Only a limited number of therapeutic agents are routinely monitored and doses adjusted by utilization of SDCs (Table 1.3). The methods by which dosing adjustments based on SDCs are made include

1. Collection of steady-state peak and trough SDCs after multiple intermittent IV infusions and application of Sawchuk/Zaske equations,
2. Collection of a single SDC at steady-state during a constant IV infusion,
3. Collection of a single trough SDC concentration at steady-state during multiple oral dosing,
4. Collection of two SDCs at two different steady-state concentrations achieved while on two different doses of a drug exhibiting Michaelis-Menten kinetics.

Sawchuk/Zaske Equations

The method proposed by Sawchuk and Zaske was originally used to adjust aminoglycoside doses in burn patients (2). However, this dosing adjustment method can be used for any drug that fulfills the following criteria:

1. Drug disposition can be adequately described by a one-compartment model,

2. The serum drug concentrations are determined after steady-state has been achieved,
3. Drug is given by an intermittent intravenous infusion,
4. Sufficient SDCs are available (minimum: one peak and one trough).

The first criterion should not be misconstrued to imply that the pharmacokinetic disposition must be monoexponential. The aminoglycosides are known to exhibit multicompartmental disposition, as does vancomycin, which may also be adjusted by this method. Multicompartment disposition does not preclude using the Sawchuk/Zaske method. However, if the disposition of the drug is complicated by a significant distribution phase or other multicompartment nature, then the clinical relevance of this simplification must be understood. The caveat to using Sawchuk/Zaske equations for dosage adjustment of drugs exhibiting multicompartment disposition is recognizing the possible errors involved. When applying this method, the distribution phase of a two-compartment drug such as vancomycin is ignored. This means that the predicted peak concentration will be lower than the actual peak concentration and indirectly implies that the actual peak during the distribution phase is not clinically important. Also, if a one-compartment model is assumed for a drug like vancomycin, then the peak concentration must not be collected in the distribution phase, as this will result in unacceptable error in the calculation of V and k (see Figure 1.3).

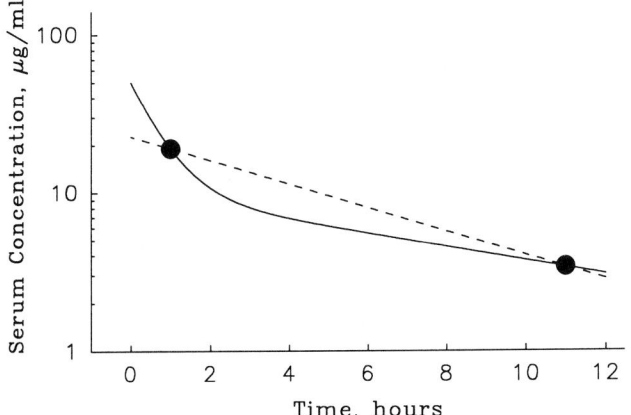

Figure 1.3. Consequence of sampling in the distribution phase and applying the Sawchuk/Zaske method of dosage adjustment. The *dashed* line illustrates the error incurred if the Sawchuk/Zaske equations are used to adjust dosage for a drug that exhibits two-compartment disposition and the peak SDC sample is collected in the distribution phase. The steeper slope calculated when the peak sample is collected in the α phase results in an overestimation of the terminal elimination rate constant, k (the estimated $t_{1/2}$ will be shorter than the actual $t_{1/2}$). The high peak and overestimated k will both contribute to underestimation of the volume. The error in clearance will be unpredictable as the underestimated volume and overestimated k will counteract each other. The larger the elevation of the peak, the greater the underestimation of the dose and τ, leading to low peaks and high troughs.

Application of the Sawchuk/Zaske method is often viewed as excessively complicated. However, a better description would be that this method is lengthy because the actual step-by-step process is straightforward.

1. Determine the amount and times of doses given to the patient and the values and times of the measured SDCs.
2. Calculate the elimination rate constant (half-life) from peak and trough.
3. Determine C_{MAX} (concentration at instant the infusion is completed).
4. Determine C_{MIN} (concentration at the end of the dosing interval).
5. Calculate the volume of distribution.
6. Decide the target peak and trough desired for patient's therapy.
7. Calculate τ.
8. Calculate dose.
9. Calculate the theoretical peak and trough that will be achieved from the dose and τ recommended.

CASE #3

Patient J. L. is a 55-year-old female with a suspected nosocomial acquired pneumonia. Gentamicin, 100 mg given as a 30-min infusion every 8 hr, is started. Peak and trough serum drug con-

centrations are determined around the third dose. The actual times of the doses and measured SDCs are as follows:

Time	
0810	Dose #1: 100 mg IV infusion over 30 min
1550	Dose #2: 100 mg IV infusion over 30 min
2355	Dose #3: 100 mg IV infusion over 30 min
2245	SDC #1: 1.8 μg/ml
0115	SDC #2: 5.1 μg/ml

For a nosocomial pneumonia a peak concentration of 8.0 μg/ml and a trough around 1.0 μg/ml is desired. Calculate the dose and τ that will achieve the desired peak and trough concentrations in this patient.

STEP 1

Time Line

0810	1550	2245	2355	0115
Dose #1	Dose #2	SDC #1	Dose #3	SDC #2

It is common practice to determine the trough and peak concentrations around the third aminoglycoside dose, as depicted on the time line above. The trough SDC sample is collected near the end of the second dosing interval, then the third dose is given and a peak SDC sample is collected 30 min after the end of a 30-min infusion. Since the trough and peak samples are collected during different dosing intervals, the time intervals between the peak and trough SDCs and the start of their respective dosing infusions are determined. Obtaining the trough and peak in this fashion is common practice. However, this method is not optimal, and good arguments can be made to collect samples for peak and trough determinations within the same dosing interval. The more extensively used former method is considered more efficient and generally considered adequate.

	Value	Time from Start of Last Infusion to the SDC
SDC #1 (trough)	1.8 μg/ml	1550 → 2245 = 6:55 (6.92 hr)
SDC #2 (peak)	5.1 μg/ml	2355 → 0115 = 1:20 (1.33 hr)

STEP 2

Because the SDCs are collected under steady-state conditions, they are treated as if they were collected within the same dosing interval. The time interval calculated above is based on the principle that at steady-state, dosing regimens are superimposable, such that, 6.92 hr after the start of each dosing infusion the SDC will be 1.8 μg/ml, and 1.33 hr after the start of the dosing infusion the SDC will be 5.1 μg/ml. Therefore, the time required for the concentration to decrease from 5.1 µg/ml to 1.8 µg/ml will be the time different between the two intervals, or 5.59 hr (6.92 hr − 1.33 hr). If a semilog plot of the natural log of the SDCs and the time intervals is constructed, the elimination rate constant (k) is defined as the negative slope of the line, or the k and $t_{1/2}$ may be calculated mathematically as previously discussed (equations (1.11), (1.12), and (1.13)):

$$k = \frac{\ln\left(\frac{SDC_{PEAK}}{SDC_{TROUGH}}\right)}{(T_{TROUGH} - T_{PEAK})}$$

$$= \frac{\ln\left(\frac{5.1\ \mu g/ml}{1.8\ \mu g/ml}\right)}{(6.92\ hr - 1.33\ hr)} = 0.186\ hr^{-1} \qquad (1.26)$$

$$t_{1/2} = \frac{\ln 2}{k} = \frac{0.693}{0.186\ hr^{-1}} = 3.73\ hr \approx 3.7\ hr \quad (1.27)$$

where SDC_{TROUGH} and SDC_{PEAK} are the measured trough and peak concentrations, and T_{TROUGH} and T_{PEAK} are the time intervals calculated in step 1. Do not confuse the time interval with the clock time that samples for the peak and trough determinations were collected.

STEP 3

The C_{MAX}, which is the theoretical peak concentration within the dosing interval occurring at the instant the infusion is complete, is calculated by back-extrapolation from the SDC_{PEAK} to the end of the infusion.

$$C_{MAX} = \frac{SDC_{PEAK}}{e^{(-k)(T_{PEAK} - T_{INFUSION})}}$$

$$= \frac{5.1\ \mu g/ml}{e^{(-0.186hr^{-1})(1.33hr - 0.5hr)}} = 5.95\ \mu g/ml$$

(1.28)

where T_{PEAK} is the time interval from the start of the dosing infusion to the time the peak samples was collected and $T_{INFUSION}$ is the length of the infusion.

STEP 4

The C_{MIN}, which is the theoretical trough concentration within the dosing interval occurring at the end of the dosing interval, is calculated by extrapolating from the C_{MAX} to the end of the dosing interval. The τ used in this equation is the scheduled dosing interval, which is not necessarily the actual dosing interval as documented in the patient's chart.

$$C_{MIN} = C_{MAX}e^{(-k)(\tau - T_{INFUSION})}$$

$$= 5.95\ \mu g/ml\ e^{(-0.186hr^{-1})(8hr - 0.5hr)} \quad (1.29)$$

$$= 1.47\ \mu g/ml$$

STEP 5

The calculation of V uses the C_{MAX} and C_{MIN} calculated previously.

$$V = \frac{\text{Dose}(1 - e^{-kT_{INFUSION}})}{(T_{INFUSION})(k)[C_{MAX} - (C_{MIN}e^{-kT_{INFUSION}})]}$$

$$= \frac{100\ mg(1 - e^{(0.186hr^{-1})(0.5hr)})}{(0.5\ hr)(0.186\ hr^{-1})}$$
$$\times (5.95\ mg/liter - 1.47\ mg/liter\,e^{(-0.186hr^{-1})(0.5hr)})$$

$$= 20.7\ \text{liters}$$

(1.30)

STEP 6

The target peak and trough are 8.0 µg/ml and 1.0 µg/ml, respectively.

STEP 7

A new dosing interval is calculated based on the desired steady-state peak and trough concentrations and the k calculated in step 2.

$$\tau = \frac{\ln\left(\frac{C_{MAX\text{-}TARGET}}{C_{MIN\text{-}TARGET}}\right)}{k} + T_{INFUSION}$$

(1.31)

$$= \frac{\ln\left(\frac{8.0\ \mu g/ml}{1.0\ \mu g/ml}\right)}{0.186\ hr^{-1}} + 0.5\ hr - 11.7\ hr$$

STEP 8

The new τ calculated in step 7 is rounded to a convenient dosing interval (12 hr) and used with the calculated k from step 2 and calculated V from step 5 to determine a new dose to achieve the desired peak and trough concentrations (step 6).

$$\text{Dose} = (T_{INFUSION})(k)(V)(C_{MAX\text{-}TARGET}) \quad (1.32)$$
$$\times \left(\frac{(1 - e^{-k\tau})}{(1 - e^{-kT_{INFUSION}})}\right)$$

$$\text{Dose} = (0.5\ hr)(0.186\ hr^{-1})(20.7\ \text{liters})(8.0\ mg/liter)$$

$$\times \left(\frac{(1 - e^{(-0.186hr^{-1})(12hr)})}{(1 - e^{(0.186hr^{-1})(0.5hr)})}\right)$$

$$= 155\ mg$$

(1.33)

Because our calculations represent an *estimation*, the dose should be rounded down to the nearest 10 mg interval, i.e., 150 mg.

STEP 9

Both the τ and the dose have been rounded to convenient values (recommendation is 150 mg q12h); therefore, the theoretical peak and trough SDCs at steady-state will be slightly different from the target values (from step 6).

$$C_{MAX\text{-}SS} = \frac{ko(1 - e^{-kT_{INFUSION}})}{(k)(V)(1 - e^{-k\tau})}$$

$$= \frac{\left(\dfrac{150 \text{ mg}}{0.5 \text{ hr}}\right)(1 - e^{(-0.186\text{hr}^{-1})(0.5\text{hr})})}{(0.186\text{hr}^{-1})(20.7 \text{ liter})(1 - e^{(-0.186\text{hr}^{-1})(12\text{hr})})}$$

$$= 7.8 \text{ μg/ml} \quad (1.35)$$

$$\begin{aligned}C_{MIN\text{-}SS} &= C_{MAX\text{-}SS}e^{(-k)(\tau - T_{INFUSION})} \\ &= (7.75 \text{ μg/ml})(e^{(-0.186\text{hr}^{-1})(12\text{hr} - 0.5\text{hr})}) \quad (1.35) \\ &= 0.9 \text{ μg/ml}\end{aligned}$$

Note that $C_{MAX\text{-}SS}$ and $C_{MIN\text{-}SS}$ are the concentrations occurring at the instant the infusion is complete and the end of the scheduled dosing interval, respectively. If the predicted clinical peak (30 min postinfusion) and trough (30 min preinfusion) are desired, they may be calculated by extrapolating 0.5 hr from the C_{MAX} and back-extrapolating 0.5 hr from the C_{MIN}, respectively.

Constant IV Infusions

From Table 1.3 there are two drugs commonly given by a continuous intravenous infusion, lidocaine and theophylline. The most appropriate time to draw a sample for SDC determination for estimation of the patient's clearance is after steady-state conditions have been achieved ($5 \times t_{1/2}$). A steady-state C_{SS} allows the calculation of Cl, which in turn allows the determination of the dose that must be given to achieve a specific target steady-state concentration (refer to Table 1.1 and equation 1.8)).

CASE #4

Patient K. N. has received several boluses of lidocaine, and a continuous IV infusion at a rate of 2 mg/min has been started. Ten hours after the start of the infusion an SDC is collected. K. N. has responded well to the lidocaine infusion but is still having occasional brief runs of PVDs (premature ventricular depolarizations). The SDC reported by the laboratory is 2.7 μg/ml. His physician wants to increase the infusion rate enough to achieve a steady-state concentration of 4.0 μg/ml. Calculate a new administration rate to achieve the desired steady-state concentration.

Equation (1.8) could be used to solve for clearance, and then using the calculated Cl and target C_{SS} a new ko could be calculated. However, this type of problem can also be solved more simply, without determining the Cl directly. First recognize that the ratio of the administration rate, ko, to the C_{SS} must be constant if the Cl is unchanged.

$$Cl = \frac{ko}{C_{SS}} \quad (1.36)$$

Thus, for any infusion rate the ko divided by the C_{SS} must equal the Cl. Given a known infusion rate and a measured steady-state SDC, a new infusion rate can be computed that will achieve a new target steady-state concentration ($C_{SS\text{-}TARGET}$):

$$\frac{ko_1}{SDC_{SS}} = \frac{ko_2}{C_{SS\text{-}TARGET}} \quad (1.37)$$

$$ko_2 = \frac{(ko_1)(C_{SS\text{-}TARGET})}{SDC_{SS}} \quad (1.38)$$

where ko_1 is the administration rate of the IV continuous infusion that achieved the measured steady-state concentration (SDC_{SS}), ko_2 is the new administration rate, and $C_{SS\text{-}TARGET}$ is the new estimated SDC achieved when ko_2 reaches steady-state conditions. Thus, for K. N. the new administration rate is calculated as follows:

$$\frac{2.0 \text{ mg/min}}{2.7 \text{ mg/liter}} = \frac{ko_2}{4.0 \text{ mg/liter}} \quad (1.39)$$

$$\begin{aligned}ko_2 &= \frac{(2.0 \text{ mg/min})(4.0 \text{ mg/liter})}{2.7 \text{ mg/liter}} \\ &= 2.96 \text{ mg/min} \approx 3.0 \text{ mg/min}\end{aligned} \quad (1.40)$$

This allows an easy and quick method for the adjustment of a continuous IV infusion, based on a steady-state SDC determination. However, the assumptions underlying this process, namely, that the measured SDC is a steady-state concentration, that the drug is eliminated by a first-order process, and that Cl has not changed, must always be remembered.

If an SDC is determined before steady-state conditions have been achieved, then its usefulness for dosage adjustment is much more limited, as the Cl cannot be calculated from an SDC that is not a steady-state concentration. It is possible to glean some information from a non-steady-state SDC, though the necessity of using a population-based rather than an individualized pharmacokinetic parameter makes specific dosage estimations much less reliable. The non-steady-state SDC can only be interpreted by assuming a value for the $t_{1/2}$. The $t_{1/2}$ is needed to estimate how close to steady-state conditions the SDC was drawn.

CASE #5

Patient D. E. is a 33-year-old nonsmoking female who has been on a theophylline constant IV infusion at a rate of 35 mg/hr for 12 hr. A theophylline SDC determined at this time (12 hr after the start of the infusion) is 16.2 μg/ml. Decide if the administration rate should be changed.

The real question being asked is, what will the serum concentration of theophylline be at steady-state? To answer this question the population value for $t_{1/2}$ will be assumed (Table 1.3, $t_{1/2} = 8$ hr). Remember that the $t_{1/2}$

determines how long it takes to reach steady-state (see Table 1.1). Usually this is considered to be $5 \times t_{1/2}$, thus steady-state would be achieved at 40 hr into the constant IV infusion. At 12 hr into the infusion, the SDC is between 50% ($t_{1/2} = 8$ hr) and 75% ($2 \times t_{1/2} = 16$ hr) of the steady-state concentration. The estimated fraction of the steady-state concentration the SDC at 12 hr represents is determined as follows:

$$\begin{aligned} \text{Fraction of } C_{SS} &= 1 - e^{-kt} \\ &= 1 - e^{(-0.087\text{hr}^{-1})(12\text{hr})} \quad (1.41) \\ &= 0.648 \end{aligned}$$

So, at 12 hr into the infusion, the SDC has accumulated to a concentration about 65% of what it will be when it reaches steady-state. To calculate the predicted concentration that will be achieved if the infusion is continued at the same rate to steady-state conditions the SDC is divided by the fraction of C_{SS}.

$$\begin{aligned} C_{SS} &= \frac{SDC_{(t)}}{1 - e^{-kt}} = \frac{16.2 \ \mu\text{g/ml}}{1 - e^{(-0.087\text{hr}^{-1})(12\text{hr})}} \quad (1.42) \\ &= 25.0 \ \mu\text{g/ml} \end{aligned}$$

where $SDC_{(t)}$ is the measured SDC at time t, and t is the time interval from the start of the IV infusion to collection of the sample. Thus, it would be prudent to reduce the administration rate to avoid accumulation of drug to concentrations associated with theophylline toxicity. The rate could be adjusted using equation (1.38), assuming the C_{SS} achieved at an administration rate of 35 mg/hr will be 25 μg/ml.

When applying the Sawchuk/Zaske equations to measured peak and trough SDCs or adjusting a constant IV infusion based on a single measured steady-state SDC, patient-specific pharmacokinetic parameters are estimated from the SDCs. In case #5 it is impossible to determine any patient-specific pharmacokinetic parameters, and thus, a population-based pharmacokinetic parameter must be used. This reduces the probability that the predicted steady-state concentration will be accurate; however, it is the best estimate that can be made from the available data.

Multiple Oral Dosing

The majority of therapeutic agents monitored by SDCs are drugs given by mouth. Unlike a drug administered by IV infusion, the Cl cannot be estimated based on a single measured SDC, nor can the Sawchuk/Zaske equations be applied to measured peak and trough concentrations. The amount of drug absorbed after oral administration (F) and the time of the C_{MAX} (T_{MAX}) are highly variable, which makes estimation of patient-specific pharmacokinetic parameters such as Cl and V infeasible. In this situation a measured steady-state trough concentration ($SDC_{SS\text{-}TROUGH}$) is used for dosage adjustment. For a drug that exhibits first-order elimination, dosage adjustment is based on an equation analogous to equation (1.37):

$$\frac{Dose_1}{SDC_{SS\text{-}TROUGH}} = \frac{Dose_2}{C_{SS\text{-}TROUGH}} \quad (1.43)$$

where $SDC_{SS\text{-}TROUGH}$ is the measured SDC corresponding to $Dose_1$, and $Dose_2$ is some new dose, with the corresponding $C_{SS\text{-}TROUGH}$ being the steady-state trough concentration that will be achieved given $Dose_2$. As in equation (1.37) the measured SDC is assumed to be a steady-state concentration, the drug is assumed to be eliminated by a first-order process, and the Cl is assumed to remain constant. Equation (1.43) also assumes that bioavailability (F) and the absorption rate (ka) remain constant, and that τ has not been changed.

CASE #6

Patient E. T. is a 55-year-old male who has been on 0.125 mg p.o. digoxin q.d. for the past month. E. T.'s physician would like the digoxin SDC to reach 1.6 ng/ml. An SDC sample drawn this morning was reported by the clinical chemistry laboratory as 0.8 ng/ml. The physician requests your assistance in adjusting E. T.'s regimen to achieve the desired target concentration of 1.6 ng/ml.

Using equation (1.43), a recommendation can be quickly determined.

$$\frac{0.125 \ \text{mg}}{0.8 \ \text{ng/ml}} = \frac{Dose_2}{1.6 \ \text{ng/ml}} \quad (1.44)$$

$$Dose_2 = \frac{(0.125 \ \text{ng/ml})(1.6 \ \text{ng/ml})}{0.8 \ \text{ng/ml}} = 0.25 \ \text{mg} \quad (1.45)$$

Thus, if the dose is increased to 0.25 mg every day, then the serum concentration should increase to 1.6 ng/ml. Caution should be exercised in applying this equation because of the number of assumptions necessary for the estimation to remain valid. Additionally, nothing is known about the peak concentration achieved within the dosing interval. If peak concentrations are unrelated to clinical efficacy and toxicity (digoxin), or if the half-life of the drug is extremely long, such that there is very little fluctuation between the peak and trough concentrations within a dosing interval (phenobarbital, phenytoin, lithium), then this assumption is reasonable. However, if the peak concentration is clinically important and $t_{1/2}$ is short relative to the dosing interval (theophylline, procainamide, carbamazepine, valproic acid), then careful consideration must be given to the possibility of high peak concentrations when increasing the dose based on measured trough SDCs.

CASE #7

Patient F. N. is an outpatient taking a generic brand of carbamazepine, 400 mg q8h. A measured steady-state trough concentration determined early this afternoon (7 hr after the last dose) was 6.3 µg/ml. The patient is complaining of transient headache, dizziness, and diplopia with an onset about 30 min after taking each dose and persisting for about 30 min to 1 hr. F. N. has been on this dosing schedule for the past month, and previous to this was taking 300 mg q8h. However, on this lower dosage the patient was having approximately two grand mal seizure episodes per month. The patient has not experienced any seizures on the higher dosing regimen.

In F. N. the peak concentration achieved is unknown, though the side effects experienced shortly after each dose would suggest that the peak concentration after each dose is causing transiently toxic concentrations. This would indicate a need to reduce the dose, but a lower dose may not control F. N.'s seizures. In fact, reducing the patient's dosage may not be appropriate in this circumstance, given the past history of seizure activity while on 300 mg q8h. Instead, the same daily dose of carbamazepine (1200 mg) could be given, but the dosage interval reduced from 8 to 6 hr, i.e., 300 mg q6h. This will reduce the peak concentration and increase the trough concentration, thereby reducing the fluctuation between the highest and lowest concentration within the dosing interval. The mean steady-state concentration should remain unchanged, as the total daily dose has not changed. The peak concentration will be reduced enough to ameliorate the transient concentration-dependent toxicities F. N. is experiencing.

Michaelis-Menten Kinetics (Phenytoin)

The pharmacokinetic parameters, Cl and $t_{1/2}$, and the methods of dosage adjustment discussed up to this point apply only to drugs that are eliminated by a first-order process. The individualization of phenytoin dosing in patients cannot be done with any of the three methods previously described because phenytoin obeys Michaelis-Menten kinetics (MMK) (3). The most significant clinical implication of MMK is that disproportionate changes in steady-state SDC occur with changes in dosage. Whereas, the ratio between the dose and C_{ss} is constant for first-order elimination processes for MMK the ratio of dose to C_{ss} decreases with increasing dose. Note that the V was not included in our list of pharmacokinetic parameters that are not applicable to MMK. This is because MMK pertains particularly to the elimination of drug from the body and not the distribution of drug in the body. The volume of distribution is not related (independent of Cl) to the elimination mechanisms of drug from the body, and the relationship of V to the total amount of drug in the body remains valid for drugs that obey MMK.

The best way to understand the concepts and clinical implications of MMK is to compare and contrast it with first-order elimination. For MMK the elimination rate of drug from the body is described by the following equation:

$$\text{Rate of Drug Elimination} = \frac{(V_{max})(C)}{K_m + C} \quad (1.46)$$

where C is the serum concentration (mg/liter), V_{max} is the maximum rate of drug elimination (mg/day), and K_m is the serum concentration at which the elimination rate is equal to one-half the maximum rate. Compare this equation with equation (1.7), the calculation of rate of drug elimination for a drug that obeys first-order elimination. The most important parameter determining the clinical importance of MMK is the K_m. If the normal therapeutic concentrations are much lower than the K_m, then equation (1.46) simplifies to a first-order process. As the K_m approaches the serum concentration, MMK become clinically important and must be considered. All drugs eliminated by liver metabolism must have some K_m and V_{max}, but fortunately the majority of drugs have K_m values that are much greater than the normal therapeutic concentrations. Table 1.4 compares the average value of K_m and V_{max} for phenytoin with a hypothetical drug for which K_m is much greater than the normal serum concentrations (approximating first-order elimination).

Table 1.4 shows that the Cl of phenytoin decreases as

Table 1.4.
Michaelis-Menten Kinetics: Dependence of Nonlinear Elimination on K_m[a]

SDC (mg/liter)	K_m (mg/liter)	V_{max} (mg/day)	Rate of Drug Elimination (mg/day)	Clearance (liter/day)
Drug A				
1	7	600	75	75
5			250	50
10			353	35
15			409	27
20			444	22
Drug B				
1	300	600	2	2.0
5			10	2.0
10			19	1.9
15			28	1.9
20			38	1.9

[a] Drug A is representative of K_m and V_{max} values within the normal range expected for phenytoin. Drug B represents a hypothetical drug whose V_{max} is identical to that of drug A, but for which the K_m is much greater. The rate of drug elimination is calculated using equation (1.46). The clearance is calculated by dividing the rate of drug elimination (mg/day) by the SDC (mg/liter), which is an algebraic rearrangement of equation (1.7). Drug B behaves in a first-order manner (clearance remains approximately constant), demonstrating that the most important parameter determining the extent of MMK seen in the therapeutic serum concentration range is the K_m. If for drug A and drug B the V_{max} were doubled to 1200 mg/day, then the rate of drug elimination would be doubled and the clearance would be doubled, but drug A would still obey MMK and drug B first-order kinetics.

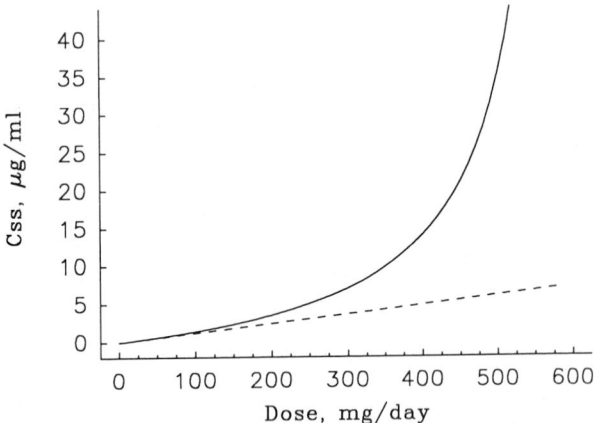

Figure 1.4. Relationship between dose and steady-state concentration for a drug exhibiting Michaelis-Menten kinetics. The relationship between steady-state concentration and dose for a drug that demonstrates Michaelis-Menten kinetics in the normal therapeutic serum concentration range ($K_m = 7$ μg/ml; $V_{max} = 600$ mg/day). At low concentrations ($Cp \ll K_m$) the drug obeys first-order elimination, as the concentration approaches and exceeds the K_m, there is a disproportionate increase in the steady-state concentration when the dose is increased. When the serum concentration is much greater than the K_m, the elimination approaches zero-order elimination. Zero-order is characterized by an infinitely increasing serum concentration, as such, steady-state concentrations will never occur.

the serum concentration increases. A decreasing Cl does not imply a decreasing rate of drug elimination; the rate of drug elimination increases with increasing serum concentration for drugs that obey MMK, but the increase in drug elimination is not proportional to the increase in the dose. This concept of a decreasing clearance with increasing serum concentration has two very important implications for dosage adjustment. An elimination rate constant, k, cannot be defined. Since Cl decreases as serum concentration increases, k decreases as the serum concentration increases (equation (1.21)). Thus, it is not possible to extrapolate or back-extrapolate if two SDCs are known, as the semilog plot of drug elimination is not linear. The ratio between a dose and its C_{ss} decreases as the dose increases. Again, this can be deduced by noting that the Cl decreases with increasing serum concentration and examining the effect of decreasing the Cl on equations (1.8) and (1.9) (Fig. 1.4).

Several methods have been proposed for adjusting phenytoin dosage based on steady-state SDCs. These methods require two SDCsss determined on samples collected while the patient is on two different maintenance doses. Mullen's method (4), often referred to as the direct-linear plot method, is preferable because it allows the new dosage to be read directly from the graph, without further calculation.

CASE #8

Patient C. W. has a long-standing seizure disorder controlled with phenytoin, 600 mg/day. However, at this dosage the patient experienced an unacceptable level of side effects, the most debilitating of which was ataxia. The steady-state concentration while the patient was on this regimen was 26 μg/ml. C. W. had been on 300 mg/day before the increase to 600 mg/day; however, on the lower dosage, which produced a steady-state concentration of 6 μg/ml, the patient experienced approximately one grand mal seizure episode per month. The patient's physician had hoped that the increase to 600 mg/day would produce a steady-state concentration around 16 μg/ml and result in good seizure control without unacceptable side effects. Recommend a dose to achieve a steady-state concentration of 16 μg/ml, using the Mullen method (direct-linear plot).

To estimate the dose required to achieve the target steady-state concentration of 16 μg/ml, a graph is constructed as illustrated in Figure 1.5. The steady-state SDC is plotted on the x-axis, and the daily dose is plotted on the y-axis. A line is drawn to connect each measured SDCss with its corresponding dose. Then a line is drawn

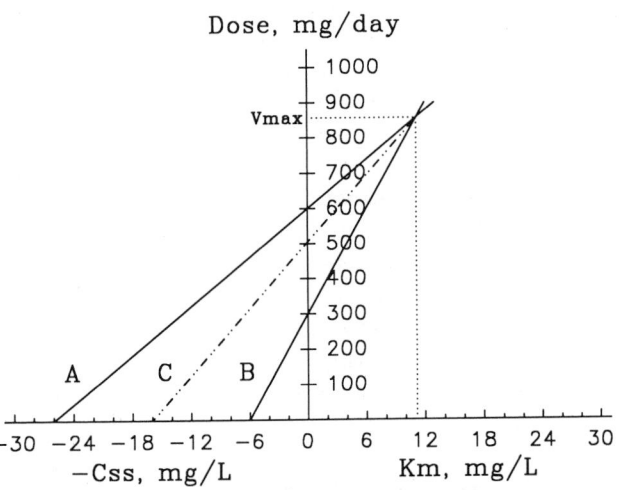

Figure 1.5. Direct-linear plot method for adjusting phenytoin dose. The direct-linear plot method for phenytoin dosage adjustment requires two steady-state SDCs obtained while the patient was on two different maintenance doses of phenytoin (route and formulation must be the same for both doses). In this illustration the patient had a measured SDCss of 26 μg/ml while on 600 mg/day (*line A*), and a measured SDCss of 6 μg/ml while on 300 mg/day (*line B*). *Lines A and B* are drawn from the SDCss achieved (x-axis) through the corresponding dose on the y-axis (y-intercept) to the point of intersection of *lines A and B*. The new dose is determined by drawing a line from this point of intersection back down to the desired steady-state concentration on the x-axis. The new daily dose is the y-intercept of this new line (*line C*). The V_{max} and K_m for this patient is read from the graph by drawing a line from the point of intersection of *lines A and B* to the y-axis and x-axis, respectively (*dotted lines*). If phenytoin sodium was the dosage form, then the K_m and V_{max} can be converted to phenytoin acid by dividing both by 0.92.

from the intersection of these two lines to the desired steady-state concentration on the x-axis. The dose to achieve the desired steady-state concentration is read where this line intersects the y-axis. Three assumptions underlying this method are:

1. Both SDCs were determined on samples collected under steady-state conditions;
2. The same dosage form (must be same brand name product) was administered;
3. Protein binding remains constant.

These assumptions must be followed strictly to avoid excessive error in the new dosage estimation. The clinical utility of this method is limited by the requirement for two SDCs determined on samples collected while the patient is on two different steady-state dosing regimens. In an inpatient setting, it is unlikely that two SDCs on two different steady-state dosing regimens will be available. This method is most likely to be used in a clinic for the adjustment of phenytoin in an ambulatory population. This introduces a fourth assumption, 100% patient compliance.

PHYSIOLOGIC VARIABLES AFFECTING DRUG CLEARANCE

Hepatic Drug Elimination

The disposition of drugs eliminated primarily by hepatic metabolism can be affected by alterations in protein binding, liver enzymes, and liver blood flow. It is important to understand the mechanism by which changes in protein binding, liver enzymes, or liver blood flow can affect drug disposition in order to predict when such changes may be of clinical importance in a specific patient. Compartmental mathematical models are inadequate for this purpose because they describe changes in total drug concentration, using hybrid parameters that do not correlate with the physiologic processes responsible for drug elimination. To evaluate changes in these determinants of hepatic drug clearance, a model that includes them as parameters and defines their mathematical relationship to clearance can be used. One such model is the venous equilibrium model (VEM). The VEM is an attempt to construct a pharmacokinetic model for drug clearance, using model parameters that correspond to specific physiologic determinants of drug elimination.

For drugs cleared predominantly by hepatic metabolic processes, the Cl of the drug from the body is approximately equivalent to the hepatic drug clearance (phenytoin, phenobarbital, theophylline, valproic acid, carbamazepine). In these cases, drug elimination is the difference between the amount of drug entering the liver and the amount of drug exiting the liver, as illustrated in Figure 1.6. C_{IN} is the concentration of drug in the blood entering the liver, C_{OUT} is the concentration of drug in the blood

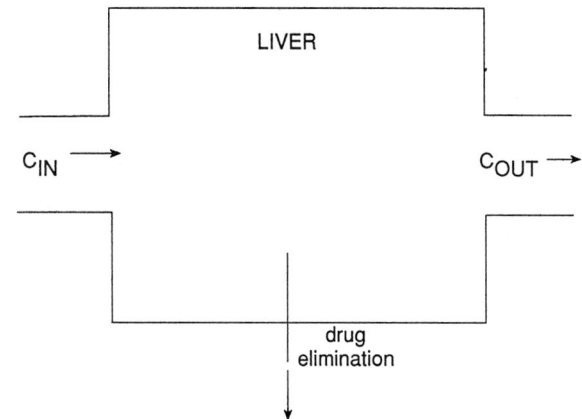

Figure 1.6. Venous equilibrium model of hepatic drug elimination. A hepatically eliminated drug enters the liver where it is metabolized. The difference between C_{IN} and C_{OUT} represents the amount of drug eliminated from the blood as it passes through the liver. From this simple scheme the concept of organ clearance is illustrated and used to explain the derivation of equations (1.47) and (1.48).

exiting the liver. Thus, the rate of drug elimination would be described by

$$\text{Rate of Drug Elimination} = (Q)(C_{IN}) - (Q)(C_{OUT})$$
$$(1.47)$$

where Q equals the liver blood flow (approximately 1.5 liter/min in humans), and C_{IN} and C_{OUT} are as previously defined. Since blood flow into the liver must be equivalent to blood flow out of the liver (it is within a closed system), equation (1.47) simplifies to $(Q)(C_{IN} - C_{OUT})$. This is the mg/min rate of drug eliminated by the liver. Dividing this by the mg/min rate of drug entering the liver gives a unitless parameter known as the extraction ratio (ER).

$$ER = \frac{(Q)(C_{IN} - C_{OUT})}{(Q)(C_{IN})} = \frac{C_{IN} - C_{OUT}}{C_{IN}} \quad (1.48)$$

The ER is an indicator of the efficiency of the processes responsible (e.g., metabolism) for eliminating drug from the blood as it passes through the liver. The ER can range from 0 to 1. An ER of 1 means 100% of the drug entering the liver is eliminated, while an ER of 0 means none of the drug entering the liver is eliminated. The hepatic clearance (Cl_H) of a drug is the liver blood flow multiplied by the ER, $Cl_H = (Q)(ER)$. The ER as defined in equation (1.48) assumes that the drug is not bound to any proteins in the blood. When protein binding is considered, the ER is best described by the following equation (5, 6):

$$ER = \frac{(f_U)(Cl_{INT})}{Q + (f_U)(Cl_{INT})} \quad (1.49)$$

where f_U is the fraction of the total drug in the blood that is unbound, Q is the liver blood flow, and Cl_{INT} is the intrinsic clearance of free drug. Cl_{INT} is the theoretical value for clearance of the drug by the liver if it is not protein bound, and is an indication of the liver's enzymatic capacity to eliminate a drug if access is not impeded by protein binding.

High-Clearance Drugs (Hepatic Elimination)

A high-clearance drug is one that has an extraction ratio greater than or equal to 0.7. For the purpose of qualitative prediction of the effect of changes in f_U, Cl_{INT}, and Q on $C_{SS-TOTAL}$ and $C_{SS-FREE}$, the extraction ratio is assumed to be 1.0. Thus, the Cl of the drug simplifies to $Cl_H = Q$, which means that the clearance is dependent on the rate of presentation of drug to the liver (i.e., the liver blood flow). For a high-extraction drug given by the IV route, alterations in protein binding and enzyme induction or inhibition have no effect on the clearance of drug by the liver. The elimination of drug by the liver is so efficient that protein-bound drug is stripped from its protein binding sites and metabolized. Concomitant administration of drugs that inhibit or induce hepatic enzymes also has little effect on drug elimination, because the metabolic capacity of the liver is so great that the small changes secondary to enzyme induction or inhibition are clinically irrelevant. Though protein-binding changes do not alter clearance of a high-extraction drug, they may alter the relationship between total drug concentration and therapeutic and toxic effects.

The free drug in the blood is the pharmacologically active portion of drug. Drug molecules bound to proteins are usually considered pharmacologically inactive, because the steric interference of the protein molecule inhibits binding of the drug molecule to the active receptor site, and protein-bound drug cannot easily diffuse from the blood compartment to the site of action. Thus, the therapeutic effect is more closely related to the free drug concentration than to the total drug concentration. The use of total concentration is strictly for purposes of feasibility, and in fact the underlying assumption is that the inter- and intraindividual variability in protein binding (or f_U) is relatively small. In the case of a high-extraction drug, a change in protein binding secondary to displacement from protein-binding sites (increase in f_U) or an increase in protein-binding receptor sites (decrease in f_U) will cause the free concentration of drug to increase or decrease, respectively, with no change in the total drug concentration; thus, altering the relationship between total concentration and therapeutic or toxic effects. Such alterations in f_U can lead to changes in the "therapeutic range," which is based on total SDC.

Low-Clearance Drugs

A low-clearance drug is one for which the hepatic elimination is restricted by the enzymatic capacity of the liver rather than by the liver blood flow. In this case, clearance is dependent on both the intrinsic free clearance of drug by the liver, Cl_{INT}, and the free fraction of drug in the blood, f_U, such that $Cl_H = f_U Cl_{INT}$. Alterations in liver blood flow, Q, have no effect on clearance of a low-extraction drug, as the rate of presentation of drug to the liver exceeds the ability of liver to eliminate the drug. Decreased protein binding will result in an increase in hepatic clearance, and an increase in protein binding will cause a decrease in hepatic clearance; while enzyme induction increases hepatic clearance and enzyme inhibition decreases hepatic clearance. Changes in f_U are particularly important because of the alteration in the total concentration-response relationship.

CASE #9

Patient E. W. is a 55-year-old male with a long-standing seizure disorder treated successfully with phenytoin, 200 mg b.i.d. Random levels in clinic have run between 12 and 19 μg/ml over the last 2 years. Six months ago E. W. was diagnosed with prostate cancer. The patient's prognosis remains good despite a weight loss of 35 pounds over the last 6 months. Today E. W. comes in to clinic with nystagmus upon lateral gaze and mild ataxia. A stat phenytoin is reported as 18.7 μg/ml. The only other clinically significant laboratory value is a low albumin, 2.9 mg/dl. E. W.'s physician says levels from past visits have been as high and even higher without any signs or symptoms of toxicity, and requests your expertise in speculating on the reason for this patient's apparent phenytoin toxicity.

Phenytoin is a highly protein-bound (90%), hepatically eliminated, low-extraction drug. The major plasma protein to which phenytoin binds is albumin. The effect of a low albumin level is fewer protein-binding sites in the plasma, which results in an increase in the f_U. Normally, phenytoin is 90% protein bound ($f_U = 0.10$), which is equivalent to a free phenytoin therapeutic range of 1.0 to 2.0 μg/ml. In the case of E. W., this would be equivalent to a free phenytoin concentration of 1.87 μg/ml. However, since the f_U is increased via a reduced number of albumin protein-binding sites in the plasma, the proportion of the measured total concentration that is free drug is increased such that the free concentration will be more than 10% of the measured total concentration.

A formula has been proposed for estimating the free concentration, based on the degree of hypoalbuminenia (7):

$$C_{FREE} = \frac{(SDC_{TOTAL})(0.1)}{(0.2)(\text{Alb}) + 0.1} \qquad (1.50)$$

where C_{FREE} is the estimated free concentration of phenytoin in the blood, SDC_{TOTAL} is the measured SDC, and Alb is the serum albumin level in mg/dl. For E. W., the estimated free concentration would be

$$C_{FREE} = \frac{(18.7 \text{ μg/ml})(0.1)}{(0.2)(2.9) + 0.1} = 2.8 \text{ μg/ml} \quad (1.51)$$

This estimate of the free phenytoin concentration would be equivalent to a total serum concentration of 27.5 μg/ml if the patient had a normal serum albumin. The f_U has increased from the presumed normal of 0.1 to 0.15

$$f_U = \frac{C_{FREE}}{C_{TOTAL}} = \frac{2.8\ \mu g/ml}{18.7\ \mu g/ml} = 0.15 \quad (1.52)$$

demonstrating that small increases in the f_U can have a significant effect on the relationship between the total measured phenytoin serum concentration and the free serum concentration. In the case of E. W., the phenytoin dose should be reduced, and free phenytoin concentrations measured instead of total concentrations, if available. Monitoring free phenytoin concentrations circumvents the need to apply equation (1.50), which should not be used for dosage adjustment because of the unreliability of this free concentration estimate.

The perturbations in drug disposition for high- and low-extraction drugs that are hepatically eliminated are summarized in Table 1.5. Protein-binding changes affect the f_U, alterations in intrinsic metabolic capacity through enzyme induction or inhibition affect the Cl_{INT}, and changes in blood flow secondary to hemodynamic instability are represented by changes in Q. This table only describes VEM predictions for high-extraction drugs given IV (lidocaine) and low-extraction drugs given by the IV or oral route (phenytoin, phenobarbital, valproic acid, carbamazepine, theophylline). For drugs with intermediate extraction ratios (between 0.3 and 0.7), simplification of these equations results in poor approximations, and since the parameters of the VEM are impractical to determine clinically, this physiologic model is not useful.

Renal Drug Elimination

The renal route of drug elimination is important for digoxin, procainamide, lithium, gentamicin, amikacin, tobramycin, and vancomycin. Unlike hepatic drug elimination, which cannot be quantitatively assessed, renal function can be estimated from a measured 24-hr urinary creatinine level or from a measured serum creatinine level using the Cockcroft-Gault equation (8):

$$CrCl = \frac{(140 - Age)(Weight)}{(72)(SCr)} \quad (1.53)$$

where CrCl is the estimated creatinine clearance in ml/minute, age is in years, weight is in kg (and refers to the lean body weight), and SCr is the serum creatinine level in mg/dl. Equation (1.53) is an estimation of creatinine clearance in males, based on serum creatinine level. If the patient is female, the same calculation is performed, but the answer is then multiplied by 0.85. The estimated creatinine clearance is an indication of the patient's kidney function and correlates with the renal elimination of drugs.

Table 1.5.

Venous Equilibrium Model: Effect of Changes in Q, f_U, and Cl_{INT} on Steady-State Free and Total Drug Concentration[a]

Independent Parameters			Dependent Parameters	
Q	f_U	Cl_{INT}	$C_{SS\text{-}TOTAL}$	$C_{SS\text{-}FREE}$
High-clearance drug (IV route only)				
↑	↔	↔	↓	↓
↓	↔	↔	↑	↑
↔	↑	↔	↔	↑
↔	↓	↔	↔	↓
↔	↔	↑	↔	↔
↔	↔	↓	↔	↔
Low-clearance drug (IV or p.o. route)				
↑	↔	↔	↔	↔
↓	↔	↔	↔	↔
↔	↑	↔	↓	↔
↔	↓	↔	↑	↔
↔	↔	↑	↓	↓
↔	↔	↓	↑	↑

[a] The parameters of the venous equilibrium model are liver blood flow (Q), fraction of drug unbound in the blood (f_U), and the free intrinsic clearance (Cl_{INT}). These three parameters determine the total steady-state concentration ($C_{SS\text{-}TOTAL}$) and the free or unbound steady-state concentration ($C_{SS\text{-}FREE}$) of drug in the blood. For a high-extraction drug (IV route), $C_{SS\text{-}TOTAL}$ and $C_{SS\text{-}FREE}$ are equally affected by changes in liver blood flow with f_U remaining constant; while changes in f_U are directly related to $C_{SS\text{-}FREE}$, but do not affect the $C_{SS\text{-}TOTAL}$. Changes in Cl_{INT} secondary to enzyme induction or inhibition do not affect $C_{SS\text{-}TOTAL}$ or $C_{SS\text{-}FREE}$. For a low-clearance drug, changes in liver blood flow do not affect $C_{SS\text{-}TOTAL}$ or $C_{SS\text{-}FREE}$; while changes in f_U are inversely related to changes in $C_{SS\text{-}TOTAL}$, but do not affect $C_{SS\text{-}FREE}$. Alterations in Cl_{INT} effect an inversely related change in $C_{SS\text{-}TOTAL}$ and $C_{SS\text{-}FREE}$ equally (f_U is unchanged). For both a high-extraction drug given IV and a low-extraction drug given IV or p.o., changes in f_U will alter the relationship between total serum drug concentration and free serum drug concentration at steady-state. This subsequently can result in a significant alteration in the relationship between total serum drug concentration at steady-state and the therapeutic and toxic effects, i.e., a change in the therapeutic range (e.g., case #9).

Assessment of a patient's renal function is particularly important for the initial maintenance dosing with drugs that are eliminated by the kidney. Once measured SDCs are available, the patient's drug therapy can be individualized, based on these SDCs, and serum creatinine determinations are used to assess the stability of renal function rather than for the adjustment of dosages. Various dosing nomograms developed based on the patient's estimated renal function are summarized in Table 1.6. Using a dosing nomogram that estimates dose based on renal function is subject to significant error and follow-up SDCs should be done.

CONCLUSION

The practice of clinical pharmacokinetics requires a broad therapeutic knowledge and a careful clinical assessment of the patient, in addition to a solid foundation in the pharmacokinetic principles. Too often, it is assumed that a measured SDC stands alone as an indicator of the adequacy

Table 1.6.
Maintenance Dosing Estimation for Drugs Primarily Eliminated by the Kidney[a,b]

Drug	Nomogram	References
Digoxin	$Cl_{DIGOXIN} = 1.07 \times CrCl + 28$	29
Aminoglycosides	Sarubbi-Hull nomogram	30, 31
Vancomycin	University of Alabama Hospital Vancomycin Dosing Nomogram[b] Loading dose = 15–20 mg/kg TBW (total body weight) Maintenance dose = 12–15 mg/kg TBW to be given each interval as determined from the CrCl[c]	32

CrCl	Dosing Interval
<10	d
10–15	96
16–25	72
26–35	48
36–40	36
41–50	30
51–65	24
66–85	18
86–120	12
>120	8

Drug	Nomogram	References
Lithium	None: SDCs should be monitored carefully when initiating therapy in patients with renal insufficiency	17, 33
Procainamide	None: NAPA[e] SDCs should be monitored in patients with renal insufficiency	15

[a] Reproduced with permission from University of Alabama Drug Resource Center.
[b] Drugs with significant renal elimination from Table 1.3 should have an initial maintenance dose estimate based on the patient's renal function. For most drugs that fall into this category there are many published nomograms of which one is listed above.
[c] CrCl = creatinine clearance based on a stable creatinine. If patient > 60 years old and Scr < 1.0, then use Scr of 1.0.
[d] Dosing in patients with CrCl < 10 use measured SDCs.
[e] N-acetylprocainamide.

or inadequacy of a patient's drug therapy. However, a SDC cannot be interpreted without a clinical assessment of the patient, including the disease state being treated, the clinical condition of the patient, a complete drug dosing history, the exact time the SDC sample was collected, pertinent laboratory data, and assessment of concomitant drug therapy (Table 1.7). Collection of this information is often difficult, and the clinical pharmacist must be prepared to perform a hands-on assessment, talk to the patient, and consult with physicians, nurses, and other health care providers associated with the patient's care.

The quality of pharmacokinetic assessment depends

Table 1.7.
Information Necessary for Clinical Interpretation of Measured SDCs[a]

Drug monitored	Dose Route of administration History: Length of time on this drug and length of time on present dosing regimen
Measured SDC	Exact time measured SDC sample collected Post dose time: Time interval between administration of last dose and collection of SDC. Reason for SDC determination
Patient information	Demographics: Age, sex, weight, height History of present illness Past medical history Laboratory data: SCr, liver function tests, any other abnormal lab values Pertinent clinical parameters: most common include heart rate, blood pressure, temperature, chest x-ray, nutritional status, mental status
Other drug therapy	Drug-drug interactions Drug-disease interactions Drug-food interactions

[a] The information needed to properly assess a patient's drug therapy will be highly variable and depend on the drug and clinical circumstances. This table is not all-inclusive, but represents a basic starting point.

first and foremost on the quality and integrity of patient-specific information and second, on understanding and proper application of the pharmacokinetic principles.

REFERENCES

1. Gibaldi M, Perrier D: Pharmacokinetics, ed. 2. New York: Marcel Dekker, Inc., 1982, ch 1–5.
2. Sawchuk RJ, Zaske DE: Pharmacokinetics of dosing regimens which utilize multiple intravenous infusions: gentamicin in burn patients. J Pharmacokinet Biopharm 4:183–195, 1976.
3. Martin E, Tozer TN, Sheiner LB, Riegelman S: The clinical pharmacokinetics of phenytoin. J Pharmacokinet Biopharm 5:579, 1977.
4. Mullen WM: Optimal phenytoin therapy: a new technique for individualizing dosage. Clin Pharmacol Ther 23:228–232, 1978.
5. Wilkinson GR, Shand DG: A physiologic approach to hepatic drug clearance. Clin Pharmacol Ther 18:377, 1975.
6. Shand DG, Cotham RH, Wilkinson GR: Perfusion-limited effects of plasma drug binding on hepatic drug extraction. Life Sci 19:125, 1976.
7. Sheiner LB, Tozer TN, Clinical pharmacokinetics: the use of plasma concentrations of drugs. In Melmon KL, Morrelli HF: Clinical Pharmacology: Basic Principles in Therapeutics. New York, Macmillan, 1978, pp 71–109.
8. Cockcroft D, Gault M: Prediction of creatinine clearance from serum creatinine. Nephron 16:31–34, 1976.
9. Keys PW, Digoxin. In Evans WE, Schentag JJ, Jusko WJ: Applied Pharmacokinetics, ed 1. Spokane, Applied Therapeutics Inc., 1980, p 319.
10. Reuning RH, Garaets DR, Digoxin. In Evans WE, Schentag JJ, Jusko

WJ: Applied Pharmacokinetics, ed 2. Spokane, Applied Therapeutics Inc., 1986, p 570.

11. Hendeles L, Massanari M, Weinberger M, Theophylline. In Evans WE, Schentag JJ, Jusko WJ: Applied Pharmacokinetics, ed 2. Spokane, Applied Therapeutics Inc., 1986, p 1105.

12. Benowitz NL, Meister W: Clinical pharmacokinetics of lignocaine. Clin Pharmacokinet 3:177–201, 1978.

13. Rowland M, Thomson PD, Guichard A, Melmon KL: Disposition of lignocaine in normal subjects. Ann NY Acad Sci 179:383–398, 1971.

14. Pieper JA, Rodman JH, Lidocaine. In Evans WE, Schentag JJ, Jusko WJ: Applied Pharmacokinetics, ed 2. Spokane, Applied Therapeutics Inc., 1986, p 639.

15. Coyle JD, Lima JJ, Procainamide. In Evans WE, Schentag JJ, Jusko WJ: Applied Pharmacokinetics, ed 2. Spokane, Applied Therapeutics Inc., 1986, p 698.

16. Nielsen-Kudsk F, Amdisen A: Analysis of the pharmacokinetics of lithium in man. Eur J Clin Pharmacol 16:271–277, 1979.

17. Amdisen A, Carson SW, Lithium. In Evans WE, Schentag JJ, Jusko WJ: Applied Pharmacokinetics, ed 2. Spokane, Applied Therapeutics Inc., 1986, p 978.

18. Ochs HR, Grub EE, Greenblatt DJ, Woo E, Bodem G: Intravenous quinidine: pharmacokinetic properties and effects on left ventricular performance in humans. Am Heart J 99:468–475, 1980.

19. Ueda CT, Quinidine. In Evans WE, Schentag JJ, Jusko WJ: Applied Pharmacokinetics, ed 2. Spokane, Applied Therapeutics Inc., 1986, p 712.

20. Schentag JJ, Aminoglycosides. In Evans WE, Schentag JJ, Jusko WJ: Applied Pharmacokinetics, ed 1. Spokane, Applied Therapeutics Inc., 1980, p 174.

21. Zaske D, Aminoglycosides. In Evans WE, Schentag JJ, Jusko WJ: Applied Pharmacokinetics, ed 2. Spokane, Applied Therapeutics Inc., 1986, p 331.

22. Bertilsson L, Tomson T: Clinical pharmacokinetics and pharmacological effects of carbamazepine and carbamazepine-10,11-epoxide. Clin Pharmacokinet 11:177–198, 1986.

23. Levy RH, Wilensky AJ, Friel PN, Other antiepileptic drugs. In Evans WE, Schentag JJ, Jusko WJ: Applied Pharmacokinetics, ed 2. Spokane, Applied Therapeutics Inc., 1986, p 540.

24. Wilensky AJ, Friel PN, Levy RH, Comfort CP, Kaluzny SP: Kinetics of phenobarbital in normal subjects and epileptic patients. Eur J Clin Pharmacol 23:87–92, 1982.

25. Winter ME, Tozer TN, Phenytoin. In Evans WE, Schentag JJ, Jusko WJ: Applied Pharmacokinetics, ed 2. Spokane, Applied Therapeutics Inc., 1986, p 493.

26. Klotz U, Antonin KH: Pharmacokinetics and bioavailability of sodium valproate. Clin Pharmacol Ther 21:736–743, 1977.

27. Matzke GR, McGory RW, Halstenson CE, Keane WF: Pharmacokinetics of vancomycin inpatients with various degrees of renal function. Antimicrob Agents Chemother 25:433–437, 1984.

28. Matzke GR, Vancomycin. In Evans WE, Schentag JJ, Jusko WJ: Applied Pharmacokinetics, ed 2. Spokane, Applied Therapeutics Inc., 1986, p 399.

29. Dobbs SM, Mawer GE, Rodgers EM, Woodcock BG, Lucas SB: Can digoxin dose requirements be predicted? Br J Clin Pharmacol 3:231–237, 1976.

30. Hull JH, Sarubbi FA: Gentamicin serum concentrations: pharmacokinetic predictions. Ann Intern Med 85:183–189, 1976.

31. Sarubbi FA, Hull JH: Amikacin serum concentrations: prediction of levels and dosage guidelines. Ann Intern Med 89:612–618, 1978.

32. Como JA, Farringer JA: Vancomycin dosing recommendations. Drug Information Bulletin 22:5, 1988.

33. DeVane CL: Fundamentals of Monitoring Psychoactive Drug Therapy. Baltimore: Williams & Wilkins, 1990, ch 2.

CHAPTER 2

ADVERSE DRUG REACTIONS AND DRUG-INDUCED DISEASES

ROBERT K. MIDDLETON, Pharm. D.

With the beneficial effect of drugs, there is an associated risk for developing an adverse drug reaction (ADR). Adverse drug reactions have a dramatic impact on every aspect of the healthcare system and society. For example, in 1987, 15,000 hospital admissions were the result of adverse drug reactions, and on average, 10% of all hospital admissions are caused by drugs; the range found in the literature is 2 to 18% (1). Similarly, the range of reported adverse reactions that occur during a hospitalization varies tremendously, from 1.5 to 43.5% (1). The occurrence of adverse reactions in nonhospitalized patients (i.e., outpatients) is less well documented, but available studies estimate that anywhere from 2 to 50% of this population may experience an adverse drug event (1). Lastly, in 1984, the estimate of ADRs was 15 reports per million prescriptions dispensed at retail pharmacies; this increased to 55 reports per million prescriptions dispensed for newly approved drugs (2).

COST OF ADRs

Adverse drug reactions result in tremendous costs to society, some of which are obvious, while others are more subtle, but no less important. Perhaps the most tangible impact is monetary. Studies have found that adverse drug reactions prolong hospitalization, thereby increasing healthcare costs. One study found that the length of stay may double because of ADRs (3); other investigators estimate that 1.5 to 11% of all patients have an extended hospitalization because of an adverse reaction (4, 5).

There is surprisingly scant documentation of the expense that drug-induced reactions add to healthcare, although a few studies have attempted to document these costs. One retrospective study reviewing the use of aminoglycosides found that 7.3% of patients receiving these agents developed nephrotoxicity, adding an additional $2500 per patient stay (6). One national estimate placed the cost of drug-induced morbidity at $7 billion annually (7).

The loss to society is also great. Projections as high as 140,000 deaths annually and perhaps 1 million hospitalizations yearly due to adverse drug effects have been made, although it is difficult to determine these figures precisely (8). The loss in terms of work force and productivity is immeasurable.

There is also a cost to society in terms of legal rami-fications, as the expense of rising malpractice and liability insurance is passed on to consumers. Several well-publicized law suits have resulted in companies removing medications or products from the market, e.g., A.H. Robbins and the Dalkon shield and Merrell-Dow and Bendectin®, a medication marketed to ameliorate morning sickness in pregnant women. In the former case, the manufacturer filed for bankruptcy (9).

Lastly, patients and consumers may lose faith not only in the healthcare system (i.e., physicians, pharmacists, hospitals) but also in the government on which they depend to screen and test drugs for toxicities before they reach the market.

PREMARKETING TRIALS AND THEIR LIMITATIONS

Although most drugs undergo extensive premarketing trials (known as phase I, II, and III clinical trials) to detect adverse effects and prove efficacy, these trials are limited in scope compared with the use of the drug in the general population. These limitations can be expressed as the "five too's" (10):

1. Too few. Before approval by the FDA, generally fewer than 2000 patients have received the drug. To put this into perspective, 16,000 patients must receive the drug to have only an 80% probability of detecting an ADR that occurred in one out of every 10,000 recipients.
2. Too simple. Since one goal of premarket testing is to show drug efficacy, premarketing trials often exclude patients with complicated medical histories or those who are receiving other drugs, since this may make establishing efficacy more difficult.
3. Too median. In general, premarketing trials exclude neonatal, pediatric, and geriatric patients. Furthermore, such trials seldom include pregnant or breast-feeding patients.
4. Too narrow. Premarketing trials generally investigate a drug for a single indication. Once approved, the drug maybe used to treat other diseases in differing populations with differing risks or predisposing factors.
5. Too brief. ADRs that occur only with chronic or long-term use cannot be detected in the short-term premarketing trials.

The need for effective postmarketing surveillance is clear.

POSTMARKETING SURVEILLANCE

Postmarketing surveillance refers to the monitoring of drug use after approval for the detection of unwanted effects and efficacy. The Food and Drug Administration (FDA) performs this function in the United States. The importance of postmarketing surveillance has increased in recent years, as the number of available drugs has dramatically increased and the number of new chemical entities (i.e., products not marketed in the U.S. as single entities or in combination with other drugs) approved each year has increased. For example, in 1961, only 656 drugs were available in the U.S.; by 1989, this number had swelled to approximately 8000 (1). From 1975 through 1985, an average of 21 new drugs were approved each year (1). In both 1989 and 1990, 23 new drugs entered the U.S. market (11, 12). A study of domestic ADR reports to the FDA by health professionals in 1987 underscores the prominence of newly approved drugs in ADR reporting. This review found that new chemical entities accounted for almost 20% of the total reports received, 22% of serious reports, and 24% of the lethal reports (13). A review of national adverse drug reaction reporting from 1984 through 1989 confirmed this finding, with 21% of all reports involving a new chemical entity (14).

Coincident with the increasing number of drug approvals, steps have been taken in the last few years to shorten the length of time required for drug testing prior to approval and for the approval process itself (15–19). Zidovudine, for example, underwent clinical trials, FDA review, and approval only 2 years after early in vitro testing began (20). By contrast, drugs approved in 1985 and 1986 required an average of 2.6 years for FDA review *alone* (21). Furthermore, investigational drugs are more readily accessible to patients through a variety of mechanisms (16, 22).

BACKGROUND

As stated above, postmarketing surveillance in the United States falls under the jurisdiction of the FDA. The cornerstone of this surveillance program is the ADR monitoring system, also known as the spontaneous reporting system (SRS). The spontaneous reporting system was established in 1961 as a companion program to an American Medical Association (AMA) sponsored national ADR registry. With the termination of the AMA registry in 1970, the SRS, under the auspices of the Division of Epidemiology and Surveillance (DES) within the Center for Drug Evaluation and Research at the FDA, remains the sole means by which adverse drug events can be reported (23). The FDA began computerizing ADR reports in the mid-1960s. Currently over 500,000 such reports are retrievable, dating from 1969 to the present[1] (24).

---

[1] Much of this information can be obtained through the Freedom of Information Act by writing to the Freedom of Information (FOI) Office (HFI-35), Food and Drug Administration, 5600 Fishers Lane, Rockville, MD 20857. Information about the scientific reviews for newly approved drugs and summaries of the basis for drug approval, which often contain information on ADRs discovered during premarketing testing, can also be obtained through the Freedom of Information Act.

Table 2.1.
Definitions of Adverse Drug Reactions and Their Sources

Food and Drug Administration (FDA)[23]	World Health Organization (WHO)[25]	Karsch and Lasagna[25]
Any experience associated with the use of a drug, whether or not considered drug-related, and includes any side effect, injury, toxicity, or sensitivity reaction, or significant failure of expected pharmacological action	Any response to a drug which is noxious and unintended, and which occurs at doses used in man for prophylaxis, diagnosis, or treatment	Any response to a drug which is noxious and unintended, and which occurs at doses used in man for prophylaxis, diagnosis, or treatment, excluding failure to accomplish its intended purpose

GOALS OF THE SRS

The goal of the SRS is to identify potential adverse effects from medications. It does this by detecting trends about possibly serious and/or previously unknown adverse drug events, especially regarding newly approved drugs. Such "signals" may take the form of clusters of reactions occurring at approximately the same time or in a single population (23).

The definition of an adverse drug reaction differs depending on the source. Table 2.1 provides the FDA's definition, with definitions from other sources commonly encountered in the literature (25, 26).

WHO REPORTS ADRs TO THE FDA

The Kefauver-Harris Amendments, passed in 1962, legally require drug manufacturers to report any adverse reactions brought to their attention for drugs marketed with a New Drug Application (NDA) or Abbreviated New Drug Application (ANDA); thus, pharmaceutical companies are the major source of ADRs received by the FDA. At least 90% of all reports received by the FDA each year come from pharmaceutical manufacturers (23, 27). Manufacturers, in turn, obtain their reports from a variety of sources including health professionals, consumers, sales representatives, the medical literature, and ADRs detected during clinical trials. In addition, as of 1985, manufacturers are required to submit all data relating to adverse reactions from foreign affiliates (23).

Health professionals and consumers voluntarily submit the remaining 10% of reports received by the FDA; pharmacists account for nearly one-third of these reports (26). In 1987, health professionals submitted 4000 ADRs directly to the FDA, while in 1986 consumers submitted over 5000 reports (23).

"Fold in thirds, tape & mail - DO NOT STAPLE FORM"

NO POSTAGE
NECESSARY
IF MAILED
IN THE
UNITED STATES
OR APO/FPO

BUSINESS REPLY MAIL

FIRST CLASS MAIL   PERMIT NO. 1895 ROCKVILLE, MD

POSTAGE WILL BE PAID BY ADDRESSEE

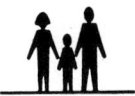

VAERS

c/o ERC BioServices Corporation

A Division of Ogden Biomedical Services Group

1055 First Street, Suite 130

Rockville MD 20850-9788

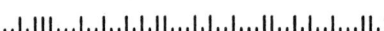

DIRECTIONS FOR COMPLETING FORM

(Additional pages may be attached if more space is needed.)

GENERAL

- Use a separate form for each patient. Complete the form to the best of your abilities. Items 3, 4, 7, 8, 10, 11, and 13 are considered essential and should be completed whenever possible. Parents/Guardians may need to consult the facility where the vaccine was administered for some of the information (such as manufacturer, lot number or laboratory data.)

- Refer to the Vaccine Injury Table (VIT) for events mandated for reporting by law. Reporting for other serious events felt to be related but not on the VIT is encouraged.

- Health care providers other than the vaccine administrator (VA) treating a patient for a suspected adverse event should notify the VA and provide the information about the adverse event to allow the VA to complete the form to meet the VA's legal responsibility.

- These data will be used to increase understanding of adverse events following vaccination and will become part of CDC Privacy Act System 09-20-0136, "Epidemiologic Studies and Surveillance of Disease Problems". Information identifying the person who received the vaccine or that person's legal representative will not be made available to the public, but may be available to the vaccinee or legal representative.

SPECIFIC INSTRUCTIONS

Form Completed By: To be used by parents/guardians, vaccine manufacturers/distributors, vaccine administrators, and/or the person completing the form on behalf of the patient or the health professional who administered the vaccine.

Item 7:   Describe the suspected adverse event. Such things as temperature, local and general signs and symptoms, time course, duration of symptoms diagnosis, treatment and recovery should be noted.

Item 9:   Check "YES" if the patient's health condition is the same as it was prior to the vaccine, "NO" if the patient has not returned to the pre-vaccination state of health, or "UNKNOWN" if the patient's condition is not known.

Item 10: Give dates and times as specifically as you can remember. If you do not know the exact time, please
and 11:   indicate "AM" or "PM" when possible if this information is known. If more than one adverse event, give the onset date and time for the most serious event.

Item 12: Include "negative" or "normal" results of any relevant tests performed as well as abnormal findings.

Item 13: List ONLY those vaccines given on the day listed in Item 10.

Item 14: List ANY OTHER vaccines the patient received within four weeks of the date listed in Item 10.

Item 16: This section refers to how the person who gave the vaccine purchased it, not to the patient's insurance.

Item
Item 17: List any prescription or non-prescription medications the patient was taking when the vaccine(s) was given.

Item 18: List any short term illnesses the patient had on the date the vaccine(s) was given (i.e., cold, flu, ear infection).

Item 19: List any pre-existing physician-diagnosed allergies, birth defects, medical conditions (including developmental and/or neurologic disorders) the patient has.

Item 21: List any suspected adverse events the patient, or the patient's brothers or sisters, may have had to previous vaccinations. If more than one brother or sister, or if the patient has reacted to more than one prior vaccine, use additional pages to explain completely. For the onset age of a patient, provide the age in months if less than two years old.

Item 26: This space is for manufactures' use only.

Figure 2.1.   Form FDA 1639 for reporting adverse drug reactions (sides 1 and 2).

DEPARTMENT OF HEALTH AND HUMAN SERVICES
PUBLIC HEALTH SERVICE
FOOD AND DRUG ADMINISTRATION (HFN-730)
ROCKVILLE, MD 20857

ADVERSE REACTION REPORT
(Drugs and Biologics)

Form Approved: OMB No. 0910-0230.

FDA
CONTROL NO

ACCESSION
NO.

I.	REACTION INFORMATION

1. PATIENT ID/INITIALS (In Confidence)	2. AGE YRS.	3. SEX	4-6. REACTION ONSET			8.-12. CHECK ALL APPROPRIATE:
			MO.	DA.	YR.	

7. DESCRIBE REACTION(S)

□ PATIENT DIED

□ REACTION TREATED WITH Rx DRUG

□ RESULTED IN, OR PROLONGED, INPATIENT HOSPITALIZATION

13. RELEVANT TESTS/LABORATORY DATA

□ RESULTED IN PERMANENT DISABILITY

□ NONE OF THE ABOVE

II.	SUSPECT DRUG(S) INFORMATION

14. SUSPECT DRUG(S) (Give manufacturer and lot no. for vaccines/biologics)

20. DID REACTION ABATE AFTER STOPPING DRUG?

15. DAILY DOSE	16 ROUTE OF ADMINISTRATION

□ YES   □ NO   □ NA

17. INDICATION(S) FOR USE

21. DID REACTION REAPPEAR AFTER REINTRODUCTION?

18. DATES OF ADMINISTRATION (From/To)	19 DURATION OF ADMINISTRATION

□ YES   □ NO   □ NA

III.	CONCOMITANT DRUGS AND HISTORY

22. CONCOMITANT DRUGS AND DATES OF ADMINISTRATION (Exclude those used to treat reaction)

23. OTHER RELEVANT HISTORY (e.g. diagnoses, allergies, pregnancy with LMP, etc.)

IV. ONLY FOR REPORTS SUBMITTED BY MANUFACTURER	V. INITIAL REPORTER (In confidence)
24. NAME AND ADDRESS OF MANUFACTURER (Include Zip Code)	26.-26a. NAME AND ADDRESS OF REPORTER (Include Zip Code)

24a. IND/NDA. NO. FOR SUSPECT DRUG	24b MFR. CONTROL NO.	26b. TELEPHONE NO. (Include area code)

24c. DATE RECEIVED BY MANUFACTURER	24d. REPORT SOURCE (Check all that apply) □FOREIGN □ STUDY □LITERATURE □HEALTH PROFESSIONAL □CONSUMER	26c. HAVE YOU ALSO REPORTED THIS REACTION TO THE MANUFACTURER? □ YES □ NO

25 15 DAY REPORT? □ YES □ NO	25a REPORT TYPE □ INITIAL □ FOLLOWUP	26d ARE YOU A HEALTH PROFESSIONAL? □ YES □ NO	Submission of a report does not necessarily constitute an admission that the drug caused the adverse reaction.

NOTE: Required of manufacturers by 21 CFR 314.80

FORM FDA 1639 (7/86)   PREVIOUS EDITION MAY BE USED

Figure 2.1. *(Continued)*

REPORTING ADRs

Manufacturers

Manufacturers must submit three types of ADR reports on Form FDA 1639 (Fig. 2.1). The first type of report deals with any serious reaction not listed in the current product labeling, as well as any reports of drug overdose, cancer, or congenital defects. These reports, called 15-Day Reports, must be submitted within 15 working days of detection or notification. Submission of 15-Day Reports allows the FDA to focus on reactions that may potentially have greater impact on consumers.

The second type of submission, the periodic report, contains descriptions of serious labeled reactions and all nonserious reactions, any actions taken by the manufacturer during the reporting period, and a copy of the current product labeling for the drug in question. For newly approved drugs, such periodic reports must be submitted quarterly for the first 3 years after approval and annually thereafter. All approved drugs, therefore, require at least annual submission of a periodic report.

Lastly, manufacturers must submit an increased frequency report upon discovery of growing numbers of serious, labeled reactions and deaths, beyond what might be expected from increased drug use alone. These reports also must be submitted within 15 working days (23, 26).

Health Professionals and Consumers

Healthcare providers and the lay public can submit ADR reports directly to the FDA on Form FDA 1639 or Form FDA 1639a (Fig. 2.1). These forms can be obtained from a variety of sources, including medical and pharmacy journals (e.g., *Clinical Pharmacy, American Journal of Hospital Pharmacy (AJHP)*, drug references (e.g., American Hospital Formulary Service Drug Information, *Physicians' Desk Reference* (PDR)), FDA publications (*FDA Medical Bulletin*), and directly from the FDA. Except for the section to be completed by the manufacturer on Form 1639, both forms request similar information, including patient characteristics, suspected drug(s) and manufacturer(s), suspected reaction(s), outcome, concurrent medications, concurrent diseases, and reporter identity[2] (23, 26).

The FDA has found ADR submissions directly from health professionals to be superior to those received from pharmaceutical companies (14, 27). For example, the delay between occurrence of the ADR and receipt of the report is generally shorter with practitioners than with manufacturers. Even with 15-Day Reports, manufacturers must internally process all ADRs they receive, which can lead to delays in submission. Obviously, reports sent directly to the FDA by health providers or consumers require no such

processing. In addition, since clinicians have better access to medical records and laboratory data and have usually witnessed the reaction firsthand, the quality of the reports submitted by health practitioners is generally superior to those received by manufacturers.

The impact of ADRs received from clinicians is greater than might be expected, given the small number of submissions compared with those from manufacturers. For example, in 1970, direct reporting by health professionals accounted for only 1% of reports received by the FDA; however this represented 24% of the labeling changes found in the 1980 *Physicians' Desk Reference* (27).

What Should Be Reported

The question of what constitutes a reportable adverse drug event can be answered by examining the FDA's definition of an ADR and the types of reactions the FDA is most interested in (Tables 2.1 and 2.2) (23, 24, 28). With the increasing speed of drug approval, the FDA has become increasingly committed to monitoring reactions involving new chemical entities. Thus, any reaction to a "new" drug (i.e., a drug on the market 3 years or less), whether it is included in the product labeling and despite its severity, should be reported. The FDA places particular emphasis on *unexpected* reactions (i.e., a reaction not listed in the current product labeling) and *serious* reactions (i.e., the reaction causes hospitalization or increases the length of hospitalization, results in permanent disability or death, is life-threatening, or results in cancer, congenital anomaly, or overdose). Reactions of this degree should be reported for any medications, not only newly approved ones (2, 23). Also, while the emphasis of reporting is for "drugs," the FDA also oversees ADR reporting for biologicals (e.g., vaccines) as well as devices, and any reactions for these agents or products should be reported as well.

Table 2.2.
Reportable Adverse Drug Reactions[a]

New and unexpected reactions[b], particularly from new chemical entities[c,d]

All serious reactions[e], particularly from new chemical entities[c,d]

Unusual increases in the frequency or severity of reactions

Reports of therapeutic failure which may suggest bioavailability problems

[a] Modified from Baum C, Anello C, The spontaneous reporting system in the United States. In Strom BL: Pharmaco-epidemiology. New York, Churchill Livingstone, 1989, pp ;107–118; and Johnson JM: Contributing to drug safety (editorial). Am J Hosp Pharm 47:1280, 1990.

[b] Unexpected reactions are those not found in the current product labeling.

[c] New chemical entities are products not previously marketed in the US either as single agents or in combination products.

[d] Emphasis should be placed on *newly approved* new chemical entities, i.e., those marketed for 3 years or less.

[e] Any reaction that causes hospitalization or significant or permanent disability, is life-threatening or fatal, or results in cancer, congenital anomaly, or overdose is considered serious.

---

[2] It is important to note that although the information contained in these reports is available through the Freedom of Information Act, the reporter and patient identities are kept confidential.

The Department of Health and Human Services has established a new system for reporting adverse events associated with administration of certain vaccines, which went into effect November 1, 1990. The new system, called the Vaccine Adverse Event Reporting System (VAERS) (Fig. 2.2), replaces two separate surveillance programs maintained by the FDA for publicly purchased vaccines and the Centers for Disease Control (CDC) for privately purchased vaccines, respectively. Adverse events that should be reported to the VAERS are outlined in Table 2.3. Besides these events, any reaction to a vaccine should be reported if the health professional feels it is warranted (29).

One reason often cited for not reporting an adverse drug experience is the uncertainty that the drug in question was in fact responsible for the reaction. However, absolute certainty of a cause-and-effect relationship is not necessary; included on both FDA form 1639 and 1639a is the statement "Submission of a report does not necessarily constitute an admission that the drug caused the

Table 2.3.
Reportable Events following Vaccination[a]

Vaccine/Toxoid	Event	Interval from Vaccination
DTP, P, DTP/polio combined	A. Anaphylaxis or anaphylactic shock	24 hours
	B. Encephalopathy (or encephalitis)[b]	7 days
	C. Shock-collapse or hypotonic-hyporesponsive collapse[b]	7 days
	D. Residual seizure disorder[b]	
	E. Any acute complication or sequela (including death) of above events	No limit
	F. Events in vaccinees described in manufacturer's package insert as contraindication to additional doses of vaccine[c] (such as convulsions)	See package insert
Measles, mumps and rubella; DT, Td, tetanus toxoid	A. Anaphylaxis or anaphylactic shock	24 hours
	B. Encephalopathy (or encephalitis)[b]	15 days for measles, mumps, and rubella vaccines; 7 days for DT, Td, and T toxoids
	C. Residual seizure disorder[b]	
	D. Any acute complication or sequela (including death) of above events	No limit
	E. Events in vaccinees described in manufacturer's package insert as contraindication to additional doses of vaccine[c]	See package insert
Oral polio vaccine	A. Paralytic poliomyelitis in:	
	a nonimmunodeficient recipient	30 days
	an immunodeficient recipient	6 months
	a vaccine-associated community case	No limit
	B. Any acute complication or sequela (including death) of above events	No limit
	C. Events in vaccinees described in manufacturer's package insert as contraindication to additional doses of vaccine[c]	See package insert
Inactivated polio vaccine	A. Anaphylaxis or anaphylactic shock	24 hours
	B. Any acute complication or sequela (including death) of above event	No limit
	C. Events in vaccinees described in manufacturer's package insert as contraindication to additional doses of vaccine[c]	See package insert

[a] From Anon: New vaccine adverse event reporting system. FDA Drug Bull 20:7–8, 13–14, 1990.

[b] Shock-collapse or hypotonic-hyporesponsive collapse may be evidenced by signs or symptoms such as decrease in or loss of muscle tone, paralysis (partial or complete), hemiplegia, hemiparesis, loss of color or turning pale white or blue, unresponsiveness to environmental stimuli, depression or loss of consciousness, prolonged sleeping with difficulty arousing, or cardiovascular or respiratory arrest.

Residual seizure disorder may be considered to have occurred if no other seizure or convulsion unaccompanied by fever or accompanied by a fever of less than 102°F occurred before the first seizure after the administration of the vaccine involved, AND, if in the case of measles-, mumps-, or rubella-containing vaccines, the first seizure occurred within 15 days after vaccination, OR in the case of any other vaccine, the first seizure occurred within 3 days after vaccination, AND, if two or more seizures unaccompanied by a fever of <102°F occurred within 1 year after vaccination.

The terms seizure and convulsion include grand mal, petit mal, absence, myoclonic, tonic-clonic, and focal motor seizures and signs.

Encephalopathy means any significant acquired abnormality of, injury to, or impairment of function of the brain. Among the frequent manifestations of encephalopathy are focal and diffuse neurologic signs, increased intracranial pressure, or changes lasting at least 6 hours in level of consciousness, with or without convulsions. The neurologic signs and symptoms of encephalopathy may be temporary with complete recovery, or they may result in various degrees of permanent impairment. Signs and symptoms such as high-pitched and unusual screaming, persistent unconsolable crying, and bulging fontanel are compatible with an encephalopathy, but in and of themselves are not conclusive evidence of encephalopathy. Encephalopathy usually can be documented by slow wave activity on an electroencephalogram.

[c] The health care provider must refer to the CONTRAINDICATION section of the manufacturer's package insert for each vaccine.

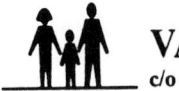
DIRECTIONS FOR COMPLETING FORM

(Additional pages may be attached if more space is needed.)

GENERAL

- Use a separate form for each patient. Complete the form to the best of your abilities. Items 3, 4, 7, 8, 10, 11, and 13 are considered essential and should be completed whenever possible. Parents/Guardians may need to consult the facility where the vaccine was administered for some of the information (such as manufacturer, lot number or laboratory data.)
- Refer to the Vaccine Injury Table (VIT) for events mandated for reporting by law. Reporting for other serious events felt to be related but not on the VIT is encouraged.
- Health care providers other than the vaccine administrator (VA) treating a patient for a suspected adverse event should notify the VA and provide the information about the adverse event to allow the VA to complete the form to meet the VA's legal responsibility.
- These data will be used to increase understanding of adverse events following vaccination and will become part of CDC Privacy Act System 09-20-0136, "Epidemiologic Studies and Surveillance of Disease Problems". Information identifying the person who received the vaccine or that person's legal representative will not be made available to the public, but may be available to the vaccinee or legal representative.

SPECIFIC INSTRUCTIONS

Form Completed By: To be used by parents/guardians, vaccine manufacturers/distributors, vaccine administrators, and/or the person completing the form on behalf of the patient or the health professional who administered the vaccine.

Item 7: Describe the suspected adverse event. Such things as temperature, local and general signs and symptoms, time course, duration of symptoms diagnosis, treatment and recovery should be noted.

Item 9: Check "YES" if the patient's health condition is the same as it was prior to the vaccine, "NO" if the patient has not returned to the pre-vaccination state of health, or "UNKNOWN" if the patient's condition is not known.

Item 10: Give dates and times as specifically as you can remember. If you do not know the exact time, please
and 11: indicate "AM" or "PM" when possible if this information is known. If more than one adverse event, give the onset date and time for the most serious event.

Item 12: Include "negative" or "normal" results of any relevant tests performed as well as abnormal findings.

Item 13: List ONLY those vaccines given on the day listed in Item 10.

Item 14: List ANY OTHER vaccines the patient received within four weeks of the date listed in Item 10.

Item 16: This section refers to how the person who gave the vaccine purchased it, not to the patient's insurance.

Item 17: List any prescription or non-prescription medications the patient was taking when the vaccine(s) was given.

Item 18: List any short term illnesses the patient had on the date the vaccine(s) was given (i.e., cold, flu, ear infection).

Item 19: List any pre-existing physician-diagnosed allergies, birth defects, medical conditions (including developmental and/or neurologic disorders) the patient has.

Item 21: List any suspected adverse events the patient, or the patient's brothers or sisters, may have had to previous vaccinations. If more than one brother or sister, or if the patient has reacted to more than one prior vaccine, use additional pages to explain completely. For the onset age of a patient, provide the age in months if less than two years old.

Item 26: This space is for manufacturers' use only.

Figure 2.2. Form for reporting adverse vaccine reactions—VAERS (sides 1 and 2).

VACCINE ADVERSE EVENT REPORTING SYSTEM
24 Hour Toll-free information line 1-800-822-7967

VAERS

Patient identity kept confidential

For CDC/FDA Use Only
VAERS Number _____
Date Received _____

Patient Name: _____

Last   First   M.I.

Address
_____
_____
_____

City   State   Zip

Telephone no. (_____)_____

Vaccine administered by (Name): _____

Responsible
Physician _____
Facility Name/Address
_____
_____
_____

City   State   Zip

Telephone no. (_____)_____

Form completed by (Name): _____

Relation to ☐ Vaccine Provider   ☐ Patient/Parent
Patient   ☐ Manufacturer   ☐ Other
Address *(if different from patient or provider)*
_____
_____
_____

City   State   Zip

Telephone no. (_____)_____

1. State	2. County where administered	3. Date of birth ___/___/___ mm dd yy	4. Patient age	5. Sex ☐M ☐F	6. Date form completed ___/___/___ mm dd yy

7. Describe adverse event(s) (symptoms, signs, time course) and treatment, if any

8. Check all appropriate:
☐ Patient died   (date ___/___/___)
                         mm   dd   yy
☐ Life threatening illness
☐ Required emergency room/doctor visit
☐ Required hospitalization (_____days)
☐ Resulted in prolongation of hospitalization
☐ Resulted in permanent disability
☐ None of the above

9. Patient recovered ☐ YES ☐ NO ☐ UNKNOWN

10. Date of vaccination ___/___/___ mm dd yy AM
Time _____ PM

11. Adverse event onset ___/___/___ mm dd yy AM
Time _____ PM

12. Relevant diagnostic tests/laboratory data

13. Enter all vaccines given on date listed in no. 10

	Vaccine (type)	Manufacturer	Lot number	Route/Site	No. Previous doses
a.					
b.					
c.					
d.					

14. Any other vaccinations within 4 weeks of date listed in no. 10

	Vaccine (type)	Manufacturer	Lot number	Route/Site	No. Previous doses	Date given
a.						
b.						

15. Vaccinated at:
☐ Private doctor's office/hospital   ☐ Military clinic/hospital
☐ Public health clinic/hospital   ☐ Other/unknown

16. Vaccine purchased with:
☐ Private funds   ☐ Military funds
☐ Public funds   ☐ Other /unknown

17. Other medications

18. Illness at time of vaccination (specify)

19. Pre-existing physician-diagnosed allergies, birth defects, medical conditions (specify)

20. Have you reported this adverse event previously?
☐ No
☐ To doctor
☐ To health department
☐ To manufacturer

Only for children 5 and under

22. Birth weight _____ lb. _____ oz.

23. No. of brothers and sisters

21. Adverse event following prior vaccination (check all applicable, specify)

	Adverse Event	Onset Age	Type Vaccine	Dose no. in series
☐ In patient				
☐ In brother or sister				

Only for reports submitted by manufacturer/immunization project

24. Mfr. / imm. proj. report no.

25. Date received by mfr. / imm. proj.

26. 15 day report?
☐ Yes ☐ No

27. Report type
☐ Initial   ☐ Follow-Up

Health care providers and manufacturers are required by law (42 USC 300aa-25) to report reactions to vaccines listed in the Vaccine Injury Table.
Reports for reactions to other vaccines are voluntary except when required as a condition of immunization grant awards.

Form VAERS -1

Figure 2.2. *(Continued)*

adverse reaction." Thus the reporter need not be absolutely certain that the drug did cause the ADR; only a suspicion is needed to submit a report to the FDA. This is a key element of the spontaneous reporting system that allows it to be effective.

FOLLOWING A REPORT THROUGH THE FDA

A brief description of the FDA's processing of ADR reports is important to understand how information is retrieved and how each report is evaluated (30, 31). Reports are initially separated according to the source. Manufacturers submit periodic reports in duplicate; one copy goes to the DES and one copy to the division within the FDA responsible for monitoring the drug or biologic in question. Direct reports from health professionals and all 15-Day Reports are sent directly to the DES for individual review and evaluation.

In order for these reports to be placed into the FDA's computerized data base, the reaction must be uniformly coded, which allows data to be rapidly retrieved for evaluation. A "dictionary" of standard terms, called the coding thesaurus of standardized reaction terms (COSTART), serves this purpose. Each reaction can receive up to four COSTART terms, with the reaction assigned the most serious terms in the COSTART thesaurus. The COSTART terms are then further classified into one of 12 body systems for additional ease of retrieval. After coding, the reports are entered into the data base unevaluated. Each computer-entered case may contain up to five drugs for each ADR, entered according to the degree of suspicion attributed by the person submitting the report.

All 15-Day Reports and direct reports are individually evaluated. Professionals analyze each report, examining the temporal relationship between the reaction and the drug, whether there was a positive dechallenge and rechallenge, the seriousness of the reaction, whether the current product labeling lists the reaction, and whether the reaction is reported in the medical literature. Reactions to new chemical entities and all unexpected or serious reactions receive priority. If necessary, additional information may be solicited from the manufacturer or the individual submitting the report.

If similar cases are found, the report becomes a monitored adverse reaction (MAR), signaling an important adverse drug reaction. MARs are evaluated by a team of epidemiologists, professional reviewers, statisticians, and data base specialists in terms of population exposure, concurring medical literature, reactions to drugs within the same pharmacologic class, the degree of documentation, and the availability of additional epidemiological data bases for further investigation. Each MAR is presented at monthly safety conferences within the FDA that involve the reviewing team, the division that originally approved the new drug application, and other FDA officials, for further discussion and agreement on a course of action. MARs may be assigned either Annual or Signal status. Annual MARs are followed for 1 year, then reevaluated as described. If no additional reports are received, the MAR may be concluded. Signal MARs are scrutinized in more detail, including a review of premarketing data, current marketing information, and the feasibility for implementing formal epidemiological studies.

RESULTS OF SRS

The SRS has successfully monitored several thousand drugs annually and detected many significant adverse drug reactions (Table 2.4) (32–34). It has been estimated that 50 to 100 investigations of "signals" and 20 to 30 labeling changes occur annually as a result of the SRS (14). Once an adverse reaction to a drug is detected by the SRS, several options are available to the FDA to deal with the event (33). The most drastic measure is removal of the drug from the market as was the case with several drugs (Table 2.4). The FDA may remove a drug from the market, yet make it available as an investigational drug, as it did with phenformin, an oral hypoglycemic agent that caused lactic acidosis. Phenformin is available from the FDA only under an investigational new drug (IND) exemption for a select subset of patients with adult-onset diabetes mellitus or the dermatological conditions atrophie blanche or livedo vasculitis (35). Removal of a drug from the market because of an adverse reaction is not always permanent. For example, bupropion, which caused seizures in bulimic patients, was removed from the U.S. market in 1986, only to be reintroduced in 1989 with guidelines for minimizing the risk of seizures (36, 37).

Other actions are available to the FDA to ensure public safety. For example, the FDA will commonly request changes in product labeling that alert prescribers and consumers to the potential hazards of that medication or will institute restrictions on the availability of the drug. These changes may be "boxed" or "highlighted" warnings, restrictions on indications for use or availability, newly added monitoring parameters, changes in dosing guidelines, or restrictions on the use of excipients in the formulation of products (33).

After a significant adverse drug reaction is detected and a decision on a course of action determined, the information must be communicated rapidly and systematically. To accomplish this, the FDA frequently requires manufacturers to mail "Dear Doctor" letters to prescribers, describing the adverse reaction, the FDA's evaluation, the company's response, and other pertinent information. Such letters are also frequently sent to pharmacists. This information is also often published in a variety of sources, for example, medical, pharmacy, or nursing journals, the FDA's publication the *FDA Medical Bulletin* (formerly the *FDA Drug Bulletin*), and trade newsletters (e.g., *FDC Re-*

Table 2.4.
Results of ADR Monitoring by the FDA[a]

Drug	Therapeutic Class	Reaction	FDA Action
Aminoglutethimide	Anticonvulsant	Endocrine disorder	Withdrawn; later reintroduced for the management of hormone-dependent malignant tumors
Aminopyrine/dipyrone	Analgesic, antipyretic, antiinflammatory	Bone marrow suppression	Withdrawn
Benoxaprofen	Nonsteroidal antiinflammatory	Hepatotoxicity, skin rash, photosensitivity	Withdrawn
Bupropion	Antidepressant	Seizures	Withdrawn; reintroduced with labeling changes
Clindamycin/lincomycin	Antibiotic	Colitis	Labeling changes
Clozapine	Antipsychotic	Granulocytopenia	Delayed marketing in the U.S.
Diethylstilbesterol	Oral contraceptive	Vaginal carcinoma in daughters	Restricted use
Imipenem/cilastatin	Antibiotic	Seizures	Labeling changes
Isotretinoin	Oral acne product	Teratogenicity	Labeling changes; "Boxed Warning"
Midazolam	Benzodiazepine	Respiratory depression and/or arrest	Labeling changes; "Boxed Warning"
Nomifensene	Antidepressant	Hemolytic anemia	Withdrawn
Phenformin	Oral hypoglycemic	Lactic acidosis	Withdrawn; available under IND exemption
Phenylbutazone	Analgesic, antipyretic, antiinflammatory	Agranulocytosis, aplastic anemia	Labeling changes; "Boxed Warning"
Pyrimethamine/sulfadoxine	Antimalarial	Toxic epidermal necrolysis	Changes in indication; "Boxed Warning"
Suprofen	Nonsteroidal antiinflammatory	Renal failure/flank pain	Withdrawn
Terfenadine	Antihistamine	Cardiotoxicity	Labeling changes
Ticrynafen	Diuretic	Hepatotoxicity	Withdrawn
Vancomycin	Antibiotic	Peritonitis with intraperitoneal administration	"Dear Doctor" letter sent by FDA
Zomepirac	Nonsteroidal antiinflammatory	Anaphylaxis, renal failure	Withdrawn

[a] Adapted from McQueen K: ADR monitoring: rationale, impact and cost issues. Calif J Hosp Pharm 2:5–7, 1990; Bakke OM, Wardell WM, Lasagna L: Drug discontinuation in the United Kingdom and the United States, 1964 to 1983: issues of safety. Clin Pharmacol Ther 35:559–567, 1984; and Hoffman RP: Drug Death. A Danger of Hospitalization. Springfield: Charles C Thomas, 1989, ch 5.

ports. *Prescription and OTC Pharmaceuticals*, the "Pink Sheets"). FDA-requested drug recalls are given high priority, and all pharmacies are directly contacted. The FDA continues to monitor closely drugs on which action has been taken.

NATIONAL REPORTING

From 1981 through 1987, the FDA received an average of 36,000 adverse reaction reports each year. When the reports from 1984 through 1989 are examined, the number jumps to approximately 52,300 annually, largely as a result of changes in manufacturer reporting requirements that occurred in 1985 and 1987 (14, 23). While these numbers may initially appear impressive, they represent only a small fraction of the ADRs assumed to be occurring. Studies have placed the prevalence of an adverse drug event at 2 to 50%, depending on the type of setting described, the type of medical specialty, and the age of the patient (1). In 1987 there were approximately 36 million admissions to short-term hospitals in the United States. If, on average 10% of hospitalized patients experience a drug-induced illness, this would mean 3.6 million ADRs[38] Thus, 52,000 reports represent less than 1.5% of the ADRs that occurred. Put another way, a 1988 survey found that on average a physician in the U.S. sees one serious and seven moderate ADRs each year, although the FDA received only 12 reports of any severity per 100 physicians in 1986 (39).

Although underreporting of adverse drug reactions is not unique to the United States (40), the U.S. lags behind many other countries in reporting. Results of a survey of 15 countries, published in 1986, found that the United States ranked ninth in the average rate of reporting per million population per annum. The top-ranked country, Denmark, with a population of 5.12 million, received an average of 260 reports per million population, compared with the U.S., with a population of 226.54 million, which received an average of 62.5 reports per million population (41). The same trend was seen when the data were examined in terms of the number of reports received per 1000 practitioners. However, these countries and others may have vastly different monitoring systems from that used in the U.S. For example, the national registries in Denmark, Finland, the Netherlands, Sweden, and the United Kingdom exclude pharmacists from reporting adverse drug reactions, while in Japan, ADR reports are accepted only from designated university, national, and municipal hospitals, thus excluding healthcare workers practicing outside these settings (41). In addition, the healthcare system in many of these countries also differs greatly from that in the United States; thus, the obligations, both legal and ethical, of health professionals to report adverse reactions also may be very different from those in the U.S.

Reasons for Poor Reporting

A survey of 3000 physicians, published in 1988, sought to assess their perceptions, opinions, and reporting behavior regarding the FDA ADR reporting system (42). An alarming 43% of the 1121 respondents were unaware of the FDA reporting system, suggesting lack of knowledge as the biggest reason for low U.S. reporting rates. Perhaps even more distressing was that of the 418 respondents aware of the SRS who had detected an adverse reaction, only 76 (18%) reported the reaction to either the FDA or the manufacturer of the drug; only 21 practitioners reported the reaction directly to the FDA. Table 2.5 lists the reasons for not reporting a detected adverse drug reaction. Other studies in the U.S. and abroad have reached similar conclusions about poor reporting rates (43, 44).

Improving Reporting in the U.S.

Recognizing the need to stimulate direct reporting of ADRs, the FDA initiated pilot projects in Mississippi, Rhode Island, Colorado, and Massachusetts designed to simplify the reporting process and enhance awareness of the SRS through a variety of means, including establishing telephone lines for direct reporting of ADRs, in some in-

Table 2.5.
Reasons for Poor Reporting of Adverse Drug Reactions[a]

Unaware of the Spontaneous Reporting System
Lack of reporting forms
Reaction already documented
Too busy
Felt reporting the reaction was not important
Reporting form too much trouble to complete
Minor or expected reaction
Dislike interacting with the government
Concern over liability
Unfamiliar with how to report the reaction

[a] Adapted from Rogers AS, Israel E, Smith CR, et al.: Physician knowledge, attitudes, and behavior related to reporting adverse drug events. Arch Intern Med 148:1596–1600, 1988.

stances to pharmacist-staffed drug information centers; reporting of ADRs to the Department of Health (rather than directly to the FDA), which then forwarded reports to Washington, D.C.; establishing newsletters devoted to state-specific ADR reporting; educational campaigns consisting of presentations and articles in local medical journals and hospital newsletters; and direct contact with emergency room and hospital pharmacy staffs (42, 45, 46). Results of the Rhode Island Adverse Drug Reaction Reporting Project have been described in detail, and after 3 years show overwhelming success (47). From 1981 to 1985 (preproject years), Rhode Island averaged 11.6 direct reports per year to the FDA. By 1988, this number had risen to 201, a greater than 17-fold increase. In addition, 85% of responding physicians surveyed in Rhode Island were familiar with the FDA/Rhode Island Department of Health reporting system, and 69% of respondents were familiar with the reporting forms and the guidelines of the system, compared with 55% of respondents and 39% of respondents, respectively, before the project was initiated. Reporting rates have increased fourfold in Maryland and Mississippi (42). It has yet to be determined whether similar projects will be initiated in other states.

Both hospital and community pharmacists represent a relatively untapped source of adverse reaction reporting, and calls to increase direct pharmacist reporting of adverse reactions have been made (2, 28, 48).

Community pharmacists can play a key role in monitoring adverse reactions to over-the-counter (OTC) medications, a class of drugs often ignored in ADR monitoring, as well as direct patients to their physicians if an ADR is suspected.

In the past several years, hospital pharmacists have played an increasingly large role in reporting adverse drug reactions (see below). Hospitalized patients experience approximately 700 million drug exposures annually, and of the almost 25 new drugs approved each year, nearly 30% are used chiefly in hospitals; thus hospital pharmacists are presented with ample opportunity to report ADRs. In 1989, approximately 2500 reports were received directly from pharmacists (28).

In 1987, a unique network of pharmacists was formed to enhance postmarketing surveillance of drugs, with three objectives: (a) to determine the association between drug exposure and outcome(s); (b) to document known or suspected drug-associated risks in specific populations; and (c) to detect previously unknown serious adverse drug reaction (49). At its inception, the program involved over 380 clinical pharmacists from throughout the United States and Canada, practicing in a variety of settings, including hospital medical and surgical services, nursing homes, drug information centers, community pharmacies, ambulatory care clinics, home health services, pharmacy administration settings, and clinical pharmacokinetic services. A 3-month pilot project monitored over 2000 patients receiving antibiotics nationwide and found the overall incidence of adverse reactions to be 7.5% (50).

STRENGTHS AND WEAKNESSES OF THE SRS

An observational approach to ADR monitoring, such as the SRS, has several advantages (2, 23, 41, 51, 52). Perhaps most importantly, it is comprehensive, covering the entire United States, all healthcare settings, and all drugs, and it potentially enlists the aid of all healthcare providers as well as consumers in reporting adverse reactions. Additionally, because it monitors large populations over long periods of time, the spontaneous reporting system can detect rare reactions that would not be discovered in small premarketing trials. Descriptive experience of drug use in populations excluded from premarketing trials (e.g., children and pregnant women) can also be obtained. Lastly, it is inexpensive to operate relative to other postmarketing surveillance techniques.

The SRS is not without its drawbacks, however. Chief among these is the inability to obtain incidence rates for adverse drug reactions. To provide such information, two figures must be known: the number of people experiencing the reaction and the total number of people exposed to the drug. Unfortunately, it is impossible to know accurately the number of patients experiencing a given adverse reaction since ADRs are so underreported.

Several secular factors influence the reporting of ADRs to the FDA and affect the climate of reporting. Media attention or exposure in professional journals, for example, may artificially stimulate reporting, not only by health providers, but potentially by consumers as well. The acuteness and severity of the reaction also affect reporting rates. Prescribers are more likely to report a reaction that occurs shortly after initiating therapy rather than one after long-term use. Likewise, severe reactions are more often reported than mild or moderate reactions. Furthermore, reporting of adverse events is related to the duration of time on the market, with reporting generally peaking after 2 or 3 years of marketing, followed by a decline in the number of reports (the "Weber curve" or "Weber effect"). In the United States, for example, approximately 700 adverse reaction reports were received for piroxicam after its second year of marketing; this declined to approximately 200 reports by the end of its fifth year (52). The size of a manufacturer's sales force and the amount of time drug representatives interact with prescribers may also impact on the number of reports manufacturers submit to the FDA; a more highly detailed and promoted product would be expected to accrue more adverse drug reaction reports than less advertised or highlighted products. This may be one explanation for the Weber curve. Further, the design and quality of a manufacturer's ADR tracking program and the effort devoted to reporting will affect re-

porting rates. Lastly, the SRS is subject to underascertainment (i.e., not recognizing an adverse event is drug related) and overascertainment (i.e., attributing an outcome to a drug, when it was not the true cause of the event).

Currently it is not possible to determine accurately the number of patients exposed to a drug over a given period (i.e., the denominator needed to establish ADR incidence rates). Although it is possible to obtain prescription data on drugs (e.g., the number of new prescriptions written in 1 year), this does not indicate actual drug *exposure*. What is available through the SRS are *reporting rates*, for example, the number of ADR reports per million prescriptions, rather than true incidence rates. Thus the information provided by spontaneous reports cannot be used to quantify the degree of risk a drug poses to the public and cannot be used to compare the degree of risk between drugs (23).

In summary, the strengths and limitations of the SRS define it as a system for signal detection and hypothesis generation regarding potential adverse drug events. Such signals or trends can then be analyzed using formal epidemiologic studies and databases.

PHARMACOEPIDEMIOLOGY

Postmarketing surveillance, including the SRS used by the FDA, is a component of the larger discipline of pharmacoepidemiology, the study of drug use and its effects, both beneficial and adverse, in large populations (53). By using formal epidemiologic techniques, the signals generated by the SRS can be further investigated in smaller, better defined populations to clarify populations at risk, the incidence of the reaction, possible risk factors, etc. Currently several resources or data bases are used to supplement the SRS. The reader is referred to several excellent resources on this increasingly important area (54–57).

INTERNATIONAL ADR REPORTING (WHO PROJECT)

The FDA is a member of the World Health Organization (WHO) Collaborating Center for International Drug Monitoring, and as such contributes and receives information from the program regularly. Currently 28 countries participate in the program, which was established in 1968 with the goal of increasing early recognition of new and unexpected adverse reactions (58). Reviewing pooled data from the diverse geographic, social, and medical populations enhances the ability to identify rare adverse events. The WHO data base currently contains more than 660,000 records and receives 60,000 to 70,000 new reports annually. Interested readers are referred to more detailed descriptions of the program (59–61). Given that the WHO program relies on spontaneous submissions from participating countries, it is subject to the same strengths and weaknesses of any spontaneous reporting system, as described above for the SRS in the United States.

Product Quality Assurance

Two voluntary programs in the United States monitor drug product quality, one operated by the FDA (FDA Drug Quality Reporting System, FDA-DQRS) and the other operated by the United States Pharmacopeia (USP Drug Product Problem Reporting Program, USP-DPPR). Both programs share the goal of ensuring public safety by monitoring and improving the quality of prescription and nonprescription drugs. Examples of reported problems include defects in containers, precipitation of liquids, erroneous package inserts, poor tablet or capsule quality, and discolored or mottled products, any of which may contribute to an adverse reaction or failure of the expected action of the drug.[3] Pharmacists have actively participated in both programs and thus have helped to ensure the quality of the nation's drug supply. The FDA-DQRS also serves as a national center on the status of drugs that are unavailable or thought to be in short supply (62, 63).

HOSPITAL-BASED ADVERSE DRUG REACTION MONITORING

The role of hospitals in detecting and reporting adverse drug reactions is becoming increasingly important. This is reflected by the emphasis the Joint Committee on Accreditation of Healthcare Organizations (JCAHO, an independent hospital accrediting body) has placed on this area in recent years and the recognition by the FDA that hospitals can play an important role in postmarketing surveillance (28, 64). Although adverse reaction monitoring is the joint responsibility of the medical and pharmacy staffs, it often becomes the obligation of the pharmacy department to develop, initiate, and manage the ADR reporting.

To be effective, an ADR program must have four fundamental components: (*a*) a definition of an ADR that clearly describes what is a reportable adverse drug reaction; (*b*) a concurrent method of monitoring and reporting adverse drug events; (*c*) a system for evaluating ADRs for severity and causality (probability); and (*d*) a system for using the results of the ADR program. Since JCAHO requires hospitals to follow written procedures in reporting ADRs (65) (Table 2.6), each of these components should be reviewed and approved by the Pharmacy and Therapeutics (P&T) Committee prior to initiating the program.

As mentioned previously, there is some variation in

---

[3] Drug quality problems may be reported directly to the USP at 1-800-638-6725 or to the FDA at 1-800-FDA-1088; reporting forms may also be obtained by calling these numbers. All reports received by the USP are communicated to the FDA-DQRS.

Table 2.6.
JCAHO Requirements for Hospital Adverse Drug Reaction Monitoring[a]

1. Medication errors and adverse drug reactions are reported immediately in accordance with written procedures.
2. This requirement includes notification of the practitioner who ordered the drug.
3. An entry of the medication administered and/or the drug reaction is properly recorded in the patient's chart.
4. Hospitals are encouraged to report any unexpected or significant adverse reactions promptly to the Food and Drug Administration and to the manufacturer.

---

[a] Adapted from Joint Commission on Accreditation of Healthcare Organizations: Accreditation Manual for Hospitals, 1989. 875 North Michigan Avenue, Chicago, IL 60611.

what constitutes an adverse drug reaction (Table 2.1). Each hospital should define what is and is not a reportable adverse reaction for that institution and use that definition consistently. Only then can in-house comparisons of reporting rates be made accurately. Since hospitals may define an ADR differently, between-hospital comparisons of reporting rates may not always be valid. For example, hospitals that choose to include poisonings in their definition have a higher incidence of ADRs than those hospitals that do not. Other situations that may or may not be included in an ADR definition are reactions from investigational drugs, reports of intentional drug overdoses, and reactions resulting from failure to take a prescribed medication.

Several methods for detecting ADRs have been described in the literature. These include retrospective chart review, concurrent (during drug therapy) surveillance, and prospective (before drug therapy) monitoring (66). JCAHO requires hospitals to have a concurrent monitoring system in place, while the American Society of Hospital Pharmacists (ASHP) recommends both concurrent and prospective monitoring programs (65, 67).

Using retrospective chart review, a pharmacist can select a single drug and review the medical records of patients who have received the targeted drug for adverse reactions. This may be particularly useful for tracking ADRs from newly released products. Unfortunately this method is unreliable, as there is no way of knowing whether a patient experienced a reaction to the drug in question prior to reviewing the chart. It is also time consuming and does not allow a prompt response to trends that may be discovered. This method of identifying ADRs should be used only as a supplement to the other two means.

A concurrent monitoring system relies on the medical staff to voluntarily report ADRs as they happen, thus allowing timely evaluation. The information gained by using a concurrent monitoring system is generally more complete and accurate than that obtained by retrospective

Table 2.7.
Alerting Orders[a]

Type of Alerting Order	Example
One-time stat doses	Sub-cutaneous (applies only to epinephrine) epinephrine, nalaxone, corticosteroids, dextrose 50%, sodium polystyrene sulfate
PRN orders	Antihistamines, topical corticosteroids
Short-course therapy	Oral corticosteroids (e.g., 20 mg prednisone p.o. × 7 days); parenteral corticosteroids (e.g., 60 mg IV methylprednisolone × 3 days)
Abrupt discontinuation of medication	Aminoglycosides, antiarrhythmic agents, anticonvulsants
Abrupt decrease in dose followed by a stat serum level	Theophylline, phenytoin, aminoglycosides, drug interactions (e.g., digoxin-verapamil, cimetidine-theophylline)
Stat laboratory tests	Stool guiac, prothrombin time

[a] Adapted from Miwa LJ, Randall RJ: Adverse drug reaction program using pharmacist and nurse monitors. Hosp Formul 21:1140–1146, 1986; and Tse CST, Madura AJ: An adverse drug reaction reporting program in a community hospital. QRB 13:336–340, 1988.

chart review and can include the impressions of the physicians and nurses involved, as well as descriptions of the reaction by patients themselves. Ideally, all health professionals should report ADRs in a concurrent system as they are detected. The reality, however, is that the reporting rate is often very low. Thus, many programs have been developed that rely almost exclusively upon nurses and/or pharmacists for reporting adverse drug events (68–70).

An example of prospective adverse reaction detection involves reviewing chart orders for "alerting orders" (Table 2.7) that may signal that an ADR has occurred (69–71). When one of these orders is received, the chart can then be reviewed or the physician contacted directly to determine whether an ADR has taken place. Another form of prospective ADR monitoring involves identifying patients at risk for adverse reactions (e.g., elderly patients) or patients receiving drugs associated with a high incidence of ADRs (e.g., amiodarone). Patients falling into either of these categories can then be monitored during their hospitalization for any reactions that may develop.

A problem faced by many hospitals is how to stimulate reporting of adverse drug reactions, particularly by the medical staff. In the previously discussed study by Rogers et al. (42), almost one-half of the respondents were unaware of the federal ADR reporting program. If this is any reflection of physician knowledge of ADR reporting on a local level, education of hospital staff is essential to increasing the numbers of ADR reports. Another way to enhance ADR reporting is to make it simple. Rogers et al. found that the main reason physicians failed to report adverse drug reactions was the poor availability of reporting

forms. Many physicians also felt the forms were too much trouble to complete. This clearly suggests two ways ADR reporting might be increased: design a reporting form that is easy to complete, requesting only essential information, and make it widely available (e.g., by placing them on each nursing station and in each satellite pharmacy as well as providing them directly to the medical and nursing staff). Additionally, allowing ADRs to be reported directly to the pharmacy or drug information service (if available) would facilitate reporting. These methods have been shown to increase the number of ADR reports (70, 72).

Once an ADR is identified, a report is completed, often forwarded to the pharmacy, and the reaction is evaluated for its severity and causality. Many pharmacies, because of manpower shortages and/or time constraints, are unable to evaluate each ADR immediately. Adverse reactions that should receive priority are those that are of greatest interest to the FDA, as discussed earlier.

Determining the causality of a drug reaction (i.e., the probability that the drug in question is the cause of the reaction) is somewhat arbitrary as there are no standardized guidelines. Often pharmacists must rely on their clinical judgment, their review of the literature, and communication with the manufacturer. Several algorithms have been devised, some complex, to assist the pharmacist in assessment (73–76). Despite the scheme, assessing causality focuses primarily on 4 elements: (a) the temporal relationship between drug administration and the appearance of the reaction, (b) whether the patient was dechallenged or rechallenged (Table 2.8), (c) whether the reaction has been previously reported, and (d) whether the event could be explained by an existing condition or another agent. Many algorithms use a weighted scoring system, allocating points for responses to questions about each of these areas. Although not well studied, a numeric scoring system seems to give the most reproducible results (77). Recently, computerized systems using Bayesian analysis to assess causality of adverse reactions have been developed. Although currently too complex for routine use,

Table 2.8.
Dechallenge/Rechallenge

	Positive	Negative
Dechallenge	Reaction subsides or resolves when the suspect drug is withdrawn	Reaction continues or worsens, despite withdrawal of the suspect drug
Rechallenge	Reaction recurs upon restarting the suspect drug in a patient with a positive dechallenge	Reaction does not recur, despite restarting the suspect drug, in a patient with a positive dechallenge

Table 2.9.
Severity of an Adverse Drug Reaction[a]

Minor—no antidote, therapy, or prolongation of hospitalization required
Moderate—a change in drug therapy, specific treatment, or an increase in hospitalization by at least 1 day
Severe—potentially life-threatening, caused permanent damage, or required intensive medical care
Lethal—directly or indirectly contributed to the death of the patient

[a] Adapted from Anon: ASHP guidelines on adverse drug reaction monitoring and reporting. Am J Hosp Pharm 46:336–337, 1989; and Miwa LJ, Randall RJ: Adverse drug reaction program using pharmacist and nurse monitors. Hosp Formul 21:1140–1146, 1986.

once refined, such systems will eliminate much of the bias incorporated into ADR causality assessment (78, 79).

Table 2.9 provides some guidelines for determining the severity of an adverse reaction (69). Although there may be slight variations, many ADR programs follow similar guidelines.

While an individual pharmacist is often the one evaluating the adverse reaction, many programs use an ADR team consisting of pharmacists, nurses, and physicians to jointly evaluate ADRs (70, 80). Such a group may be a subcommittee of the P&T Committee and has the advantage of drawing on expertise from several different areas.

An effective ADR program can provide information that affects the entire hospital. Frequent review of ADR reports will allow pharmacists to identify trends within the hospital, in a sense mirroring the FDA spontaneous reporting system. For example, reactions to a drug might be identified on a single medical ward or service, perhaps indicating that the drug is being used inappropriately or excessively. This can lay the groundwork for a drug utilization evaluation, which may be organized by the quality assurance program. Similarly, by monitoring and detecting medication errors, an ADR program can assist in ongoing quality assurance and risk management activities.

Regular nursing, physician, and pharmacist education about the progress of the program and new or important reactions can make them aware of the effects of the new drug and increase their level of awareness of the ADR program. This can take the form of inservices or articles in a pharmacy newsletter. In addition, all ADRs should be reported to the P&T Committee on a regular basis of review, discussion, and distribution to the representative medical and nursing services. Through the P&T Committee, changes in prescribing practices can be instituted and drugs can be removed from the formulary or restricted to specialized clinics or situations, based on information gathered from the ADR program.

CONCLUSION

Adverse drug reactions are an important cause of morbidity and mortality worldwide. The FDA performs post-marketing surveillance of all drugs in the United States through the spontaneous reporting system and monitors drug product quality along with the United States Pharmacopeia. Although an effective means of detecting rare, unexpected adverse drug events, the SRS lacks the ability to produce adverse reaction incidence rates. Formal pharmacoepidemiologic methods are used to supplement the SRS in this regard. Adverse reactions are highly underreported, and pharmacists can play a leadership role in fostering reporting to the FDA, particularly in hospitals where several successful programs have documented the impact of clinical pharmacy in this area.

REFERENCES

1. Manase HR Jr: Medication use in an imperfect world: drug misadventuring as an issue of public policy, part 1. Am J Hosp Pharm 46:929–944, 1989.
2. Edlavitch SA: Adverse drug event reporting. Improving the low US reporting rates (editorial). Arch Intern Med 148:1499–1503, 1988.
3. Melmon KL: Preventable drug reactions—causes and cures. N Engl J Med 284:1361–1368, 1974.
4. Miller RR: Drug surveillance utilizing epidemiologic methods: a report from the Boston Collaborative Drug Suveillance Program. Am J Hosp Pharm 30:584–592, 1973.
5. Gardner P, Watson LJ: Adverse drug reactions: a pharmacist-based monitoring system. Clin Pharmacol Ther 11:802–807, 1970.
6. Eisenberg JM, Koffer H, Glick HA, et al.: What is the cost of nephrotoxicity associated with aminoglycosides? Ann Intern Med 107:900–909, 1987.
7. Southwick K: A prescription for trouble: drugs to counteract drugs. Health Week 2:1, 12, 1988.
8. Talley RB, Laventurier MF: Drug-induced illness (letter). JAMA 229:1043, 1974.
9. Willig SH, A view from the US court room. In Strom BL: Pharmacoepidemiology. New York, Churchill Livingstone, 1989, pp 85–103.
10. Rogers AS: Adverse drug events: identification and attribution. Drug Intell Clin Pharm 21:915–920, 1987.
11. Anon: Approval times for 1989 NMEs. FDC Reports Prescription and OTC Pharmaceuticals 52:3–6, 1990.
12. Anon: FDA approves 23 new molecular entities in 1990. FDC Reports Prescription and OTC Pharmaceuticals 53:9–11, 1991.
13. Kennedy DL, Goetsch RA, Dries MW: Use and reported adverse effects of new chemical entities. Am J Hosp Pharm 46:558–565, 1989.
14. Faich GA: National adverse drug reaction reporting. 1984–1989. Arch Intern Med 151:1645–1647, 1991.
15. Gershon D: Fast track for AIDS and cancer drugs. Nature 346:685, 1990.
16. Nightengale SL: New procedures to expedite the approval of drugs for life-threatening and severely debilitating illnesses. JAMA 260:2980, 1988.
17. Marwick C: FDA seeks swifter approval of drugs for some life-threatening or debilitating diseases. JAMA 260:2976, 1988.
18. Miller HI, Young FE: The drug approval process at the Food and Drug Administration. New biotechnology as a paradigm of a science-based activist approach. Arch Intern Med 149:655–657, 1989.
19. Mariner WK: New FDA drug approval policies and HIV vaccine development. Am J Public Health 80:336–341, 1990.
20. Young FE: The role of the FDA in the effort against AIDS. Pub Health Rep 103:242–245, 1988.

21. Kaitin KI, Richard BW, Lasagna L: Trends in drug development: the 1985–86 new drug approvals. J Clin Pharmacol 27:542–548, 1987.

22. Goyan JE. Drug regulation: quo vadis? (editorial). JAMA 260:3052–3053, 1988.

23. Baum C, Anello C. The spontaneous reporting system in the United States. In Strom BL: Pharmacoepidemiology. New York, Churchill Livingstone, 1989, pp 107–118.

24. Anon. Brief description with caveats of system. Standard reply letter to request for information on adverse drug reaction reporting, US Food and Drug Administration, December, 1988.

25. Karch FE, Lasagna L: Adverse drug reactions. A critical review. JAMA 234:1236–1241, 1975.

26. Sills JM, Tanner LA, Milstein JB. Food and Drug Administration monitoring of adverse drug reactions. Am J Hosp Pharm 43:2764–2770, 1986.

27. Rossi AC, Knapp DE: Discovery of new adverse drug reactions. A review of the Food and Drug Administration's Spontaneous Reporting System. JAMA 252:1030–1033, 1986.

28. Johnson JM: Contributing to drug safety (editorial). Am J Hosp Pharm 47:1280, 1990.

29. Anon: New vaccine adverse event reporting system. FDA Drug Bull 20:7–8, 13–14, 1990.

30. Turner WM, Milstein JB, Faich GA, Armstrong GD: The processing of adverse reaction reports at FDA. Drug Inf J 20:147–150, 1986.

31. Gelberg A, Armstrong GD, Dreis MW, Anello C: Technological developments with the FDA adverse drug reaction file system. Drug Inf J 25:19–28, 1991.

32. McQueen K: ADR monitoring: rationale, impact and cost issues. Calif J Hosp Pharm 2:5–7, 1990.

33. Bakke OM, Wardell WM, Lasagna L: Drug discontinuation in the United Kingdom and the United States, 1964 to 1983: issues of safety. Clin Pharmacol Ther 35:559–567, 1984.

34. Hoffman RP: Drug Death. A Danger of Hospitalization. Springfield: Charles C Thomas, 1989, ch 5.

35. Anon: Facts and Comparisons Drug Information. St. Louis, JB Lippincott, 1978, p 769.

36. Anon: Bupropion for depression. Med Lett Drugs Ther 31:97–98, 1989.

37. Davidson J: Seizures and bupropion: a review. J Clin Psychiatry 50:256–261, 1989.

38. Hoffman RP: Drug Death. A Danger of Hospitalization. Springfield: Charles C Thomas, 1989, ch 2.

39. Faich GA, Dreis M, Tomita D: National adverse drug reaction surveillance 1986. Arch Intern Med 148:785–787, 1988.

40. Lumley CE, Walker SR, Hall GC, et al.: The under-reporting of adverse drug reactions seen in general practice. Pharmaceut Med 1:205–212, 1986.

41. Griffin JP. Survey of the spontaneous adverse drug reaction reporting schemes in fifteen countries. Br J Clin Pharmacol 22:83S–100S, 1986.

42. Rogers AS, Israel E, Smith CR, et al.: Physician knowledge, attitudes, and behavior related to reporting adverse drug events. Arch Intern Med 148:1596–1600, 1988.

43. Milstien JB, Faich GA, Hsu JP, et al.: Factors affecting physician reporting of adverse drug reactions. Drug Info J 20:157–164, 1986.

44. Walker SR, Lumley CE: The attitudes of general practitioners to monitoring and reporting adverse drug reactions. Pharmaceut Med 1:195–203, 1986.

45. Fincham JE: Pilot projects to stimulate adverse drug reaction reporting. J Clin Pharm Ther 12:243–247, 1987.

46. Scott HD, Thacher A, Rosenbaum SE, et al.: Adverse drug reaction reporting systems: the United Kingdom and the United States. Rhode Island Med J 71:179–184, 1988.

47. Scott HD, Thacher-Renshaw A, Rosenbaum SE, et al.: Physician reporting of adverse drug reactions. Results of the Rhode Island Adverse Drug Reaction Reporting Project. JAMA 263:1785–1788, 1990.

48. Fincham JE: Adverse drug reaction reporting and pharmacists. J Clin Pharm Ther 14:79–81, 1989.

49. Grasela TH, Schentag JJ: A clinical pharmacy-oriented drug surveillance network: I. Program description. Drug Intell Clin Pharm 21:902–908, 1987.

50. Grasela TH, Edwards BA, Raebel MA, et al.: A clinical pharmacy-oriented drug surveillance network: II. Results of a pilot project. Drug Intell Clin Pharm 21:909–914, 1987.

51. Faich GA: Adverse drug reaction monitoring. N Engl J Med 314:1589–1592, 1986.

52. Sachs RM, Bortnichak EA: An evaluation of spontaneous adverse drug reaction monitoring systems. Am J Med 81 (suppl 5B):49–55, 1986.

53. Strom BL, Tugwell P: Pharmacoepidemiology: current status, prospects, and problems (editorial). Ann Intern Med 113:179–181, 1990.

54. Jones JK, Inpatient data bases. In Strom BL: Pharmacoepidemiology. New York, Churchill Livingstone, 1989, pp 213–227.

55. Lawson DH, Beard K, Intensive hospital-based cohort studies. In Strom BL: Pharmacoepidemiology. New York, Churchill Livingstone, 1989, pp 135–148.

56. Serradell J, Bjornson DC, Hartzema AG: Drug utilization study methodologies: national and international perspectives. Drug Intell Clin Pharm 21:994–1001, 1987.

57. Stewart RB: Pharmacoepidemiology. Drug Intell Clin Pharm 21:121–124, 1987.

58. Strandberg K, International drug monitoring. In Dukes MNG, Beeley L: Side Effects of Drugs Annual 14. Amsterdam, Elsevier, 1990, pp 459–465.

59. Olsson S: International reporting of adverse drug reactions: the WHO program. Sem Derm 8:72–74, 1988.

60. Faich GA, Castle W, Banlowski Z, CIOMS ADR Working Group: International reporting on adverse drug reactions: the CIOMS project. Int J Clin Pharmacol Ther Toxicol 28:133–138, 1990.

61. Edwards IR, Lindquist M, Wiholm BE, Napke E: Quality criteria for early signals of possible adverse drug reactions. Lancet 336:156–158, 1990.

62. Anon: USP DPPR notes anniversary. White Sheet 25:4, 1991.

63. Anon: Fact sheet on the FDA Drug Quality Reporting System (FDA-DQRS), US Food and Drug Administration Drug Quality Reporting System, November, 1988.

64. Hoffman RP: Adverse drug reactions revisited—JCAHO. Hosp Pharm 23:685–686, 1988.

65. Joint Commission on Accreditation of Healthcare Organizations: Accreditation Manual for Hospitals, 1989. 875 North Michigan Avenue, Chicago, IL 60611.

66. Koch KE: Use of standardized screening procedures to identify adverse drug reactions. Am J Hosp Pharm 47:1314–1320, 1990.

67. Anon: ASHP guidelines on adverse drug reaction monitoring and reporting. Am J Hosp Pharm 46:336–337, 1989.

68. Kilarski DJ, Ziegler B, Coarse J, Buchanan C: Adverse drug reaction reporting system: developing a well-monitored program. Hosp Formul 21:949–952, 1986.

69. Miwa LJ, Randall RJ: Adverse drug reaction program using pharmacist and nurse monitors. Hosp Formul 21:1140–1146, 1986.

70. Kimelblatt BJ, Young SH, Heywood PM, et al.: Improved reporting of adverse drug reactions. Am J Hosp Pharm 45:1086–1089, 1988.

71. Tse CST, Madura AJ: An adverse drug reaction reporting program in a community hospital. QRB 13:336–340, 1988.

72. Vorce-West T, Barstow L, Butcher B: System for voluntary reporting of adverse drug reactions in a university hospital. Am J Hosp Pharm 46:2300–2303, 1989.

73. Naranjo CA, Busto U, Sellers M, et al.: A method for estimating the probability of adverse drug reactions. Clin Pharm Ther 30:239–245, 1981.
74. Blanc S, Leuenberger P, Berger JP, et al.: Judgements of trained observers on adverse drug reactions. Clin Pharm Ther 25:493–498, 1979.
75. Jones JK: Adverse drug reactions in the community health setting: approaches to recognizing, counseling, and reporting. Fam Community Health 5:58–67, 1982.
76. Kramer MS, Leventhal JM, Hutchinson TA, Feinstein AR: An algorithm for the operational assessment of adverse drug reactions: I. Background, description, and instructions for use. JAMA 242:623–632, 1979.
77. Michel DJ, Knodel LC: Comparison of three algorithms used to evaluate adverse drug reactions. Am J Hosp Pharm 43:1709–1714, 1986.
78. Lane DA, Kramer MS, Hutchinson TA, et al.: The causality assessment of adverse drug reactions using a Bayesian approach. Pharmaceut Med 2:265–283, 1987.
79. Naranjo C, Lanctôt KL: Microcomputer-assisted Bayesian differential diagnosis of severe adverse reactions to new drugs: a 4-year experience. Drug Info J 25:243–250, 1991.
80. Prosser TR, Kamysz PL: Multidisciplinary adverse drug reaction surveillance program. Am J Hosp Pharm 47:1334–1339, 1990.

CHAPTER 3

DRUG INTERACTIONS

DAVID S. TATRO, Pharm. D.

A drug interaction can be defined as the modification of the effects of one drug (i.e., the object drug) by the prior or concomitant administration of another (i.e., the precipitant drug) (1). Adverse drug interactions can cause a loss in therapeutic effect, toxicity, or unexpected increases in pharmacologic activity. The basic definition of a drug interaction should focus on patient outcomes that are of potential clinical importance and not on additive or beneficial effects occurring with simultaneous drug administration. Thus, one should be seeking a response that is greater than the sum of the independent actions of the drugs (i.e., potentiation) or an action that is less than expected (i.e., antagonism).

This chapter does not consider physical or chemical interactions (i.e., intravenous incompatibilities) or beneficial interactions (i.e., clinically useful or intended interactions such as coadministration of probenecid and penicillin).

In a study involving 9,900 patients with 83,200 drug exposures, 234 (6.5%) of 3,600 adverse drug reactions were attributed to drug interactions (2). The incidence of potential drug interactions has been observed to be 17% in surgical patients, 22% in patients on medical wards, 19% in nursing home patients, and 23% in outpatient clinics (3–6). In a prospective study involving 2,422 patients, of 113 patients taking potentially interacting drugs, only 7 patients developed clinical evidence of a drug interaction (0.3%) (7). This does not preclude the more frequent occurrence of certain clinically significant drug interactions (8).

Knowledge of drug interactions may allow early recognition and prevention of adverse consequences. The most comprehensive understanding of clinically significant drug interactions can be achieved by combining knowledge of the mechanism(s) of drug interactions with the recognition of high-risk patients and the identification of drugs with a narrow therapeutic index (9).

MECHANISMS OF DRUG INTERACTIONS

Understanding the pharmacology of a drug and the mechanism by which a drug may interact can assist in predicting or allowing early recognition of a drug interaction. In a drug interaction, the drug whose effect is altered (either increased or decreased) is referred to as the object drug, while the drug that induces the interaction is the precipitant drug.

Drug interactions are frequently characterized as either pharmacokinetic or pharmacodynamic. Pharmacokinetic interactions influence the disposition of a drug in the body and involve the effects of one drug on the absorption, distribution, metabolism, and excretion of another. Due to large inter- and intrapatient variability in drug disposition, pharmacokinetic interactions seldom produce serious clinical consequences. Pharmacokinetic interactions are frequently associated with changes in plasma drug concentrations, and when feasible, observing the clinical status of the patient as well as monitoring serum drug levels may provide useful information about potential interactions. Pharmacodynamic interactions are related to the pharmacologic activity of the interacting drugs are more frequent. Mechanisms of pharmacodynamic interactions include synergism, antagonism, altered cellular transport, and effects on receptor sites.

Pharmacokinetic Interactions

Pharmacokinetic interactions are characterized by changes in the kinetics of the object drug, including absorption, distribution, metabolism, and excretion.

ALTERED GASTROINTESTINAL (GI) ABSORPTION

Changes in drug absorption from the GI tract can result from various mechanisms, including altered pH, altered bacterial flora, formation of drug chelates or complexes, drug-induced mucosal damage, and altered gastrointestinal motility. These changes may produce either a decrease or increase in drug absorption. The former is the most common. Frequently interactions affecting absorption require the simultaneous presence of both drugs in the stomach; therefore, separating the administration times of the two agents by at least 2 hours will often prevent these interactions. Drug interactions affecting the absorption rate of a drug are most important clinically when the drug has a short half-life or when a rapid peak plasma level is needed to achieve a therapeutic effect (9). In the latter instance, a decrease in the rate of absorption of the object drug may produce subtherapeutic concentrations. Unless the bioavailability of a drug is significantly altered, interactions changing the absorption rate of a drug with a long half-life will usually be of little clinical consequence. Cancer patients receiving chemotherapy may experience drug-induced mucosal damage, decreasing the bioavailability of poorly absorbed medications (9).

Altered pH. The nonionized form of a drug is more lipid-soluble and more readily absorbed from the gastrointestinal tract into the systemic circulation than the ionized form. Most drugs are weak acids or bases. Acidic drugs that have dissolved tend to be absorbed in the upper portion of the GI tract where they are in an acidic medium. The opposite is true of weak bases. Drugs such as antacids that increase the gastric pH may delay the absorption of certain drugs (e.g., ciprofloxacin).

Clinical Consideration. Clinically important interactions occurring by this mechanism are rare. This interaction may be avoided by adjusting the administration times of the two agents. Separating the administration times by at least 2 hours will often prevent these interactions.

Clinically Important Examples. The administration of an aluminum-magnesium hydroxide antacid with ciprofloxacin may decrease the absorption of the antibiotic, resulting in a decrease in the pharmacologic effect (10–12). If antacids are administered during ciprofloxacin therapy, the antacid should be given at least 6 hours before or 2 hours after the antibiotic dose (12). In addition to antacids, H_2 antagonists may significantly alter gastric pH.

Altered Intestinal Bacterial Flora. Antibiotic administration may decrease the number of bacteria in the GI tract. The greatest numbers of bacteria are found in the large intestine. Some drugs have been shown to be affected by changes in the intestinal flora (13).

Clinical Considerations. This mechanism of interaction appears to be rare. Drug interactions resulting from changes in the intestinal bacterial flora tend to involve drugs that are either incompletely absorbed from the upper GI tract or undergo enterohepatic recirculation (13). The onset and reversal of this interaction are delayed, requiring up to several weeks. Thus, adjusting the administration times of the two drugs would not alter interactions occurring by this mechanism.

Clinically Important Example. In approximately 10% of patients receiving digoxin, 40% or more of an orally administered dose of the drug is metabolized by gastrointestinal flora to inactive digoxin reduction products (10, 14, 15). Erythromycin appears to reverse this process by altering GI bacteria, allowing more digoxin to be absorbed. Digoxin toxicity may occur (15). The effects of this interaction may persist for weeks to months after erythromycin is discontinued.

Complexation or Chelation. Certain drugs (e.g., tetracycline) can combine with other drugs (e.g., iron preparations) or food (e.g., milk) in the GI tract to form poorly absorbed complexes.

Clinical Considerations. Although different mechanisms may cause changes in the absorption of the object drug from the GI tract, clinically important interactions are uncommon. Administration of the object drug in the absence of the precipitant will minimize the occurrence of this interaction. Therefore, it may be necessary to lengthen the interval between administration of the two drugs as much as possible, preferably by 2 to 4 hours.

Clinically Important Examples. Tetracycline forms an insoluble chelate with iron salts, decreasing absorption and serum levels of both drugs (10). The antiinfective response may be decreased. A similar mechanism has been proposed for the decreased absorption of ciprofloxacin and norfloxacin occurring during concomitant administration of sucralfate (16–18). The binding resin cholestyramine decreases the absorption of exogenously administered thyroid by binding thyroid hormone in the GI tract (18). Other agents that can interfere with drug absorption by binding to the object drug or by forming complexes or chelates with the object drug include activated charcoal, antacids, colestipol, and various polyvalent cations (e.g., iron salts).

Drug-induced Mucosal Damage. Drugs that damage the GI mucosa may reduce the absorption of certain drugs (9, 19).

Clinical Considerations. Antineoplastic agents are most frequently implicated. This mechanism remains to be confirmed.

Clinically Important Example. Reduced GI absorption of certain digoxin preparations has been attributed to alterations in the intestinal mucosa induced by chemotherapy regimens (e.g., cyclophosphamide, vincristine, procarbazine, plus prednisone) (20, 21). The effects of this interaction appear to be minimized by administration of digoxin capsules or digitoxin (21, 22).

Altered Motility. Increased absorption can occur when the drug is retained at the site of optimal absorption for a prolonged period of time. Because of the large absorptive area of the small intestine, it is the primary site of drug absorption from the gastrointestinal tract. Changes in GI motility may increase or decrease absorption. Increasing GI motility decreases absorption by reducing the length of time that an orally administered drug is in contact with the absorbing surface (19). A decrease in bioavailability may be seen as a result of slowing dissolution or delaying gastric emptying.

Clinical Considerations. Clinically important interactions from this mechanism are rare. Interactions occurring as a result of altered GI motility result from systemic administration of the precipitant drug. Therefore, separating the administration times of the interacting drugs would not circumvent this interaction.

Clinically Important Examples. The increase in cyclosporine absorption occurring with concurrent administration of metoclopramide has been attributed to an increase in stomach emptying time. This may result in an increase in the immunologic and toxic effects of cyclosporine (23). Conversely, by increasing GI motility, metoclopramide may decrease the absorption of orally administered digoxin

(24). This interaction may not occur with digoxin formulations that have high bioavailability (e.g., digoxin capsules or elixir) (25). Anticholinergic drugs are an example of a class of drugs that slow gastrointestinal transit time.

DISPLACED PROTEIN BINDING

Many drugs are reversibly bound to plasma proteins. Concurrent administration of more than one drug bound to the same protein fraction may displace either agent from its binding site, increasing the free concentration of the displaced drug. The drug with the highest affinity (i.e., association constant) for the binding site will displace the drug with the lower association constant (26). Following displacement from the protein-binding site, there is immediate redistribution to the tissues. Subsequently, a compensatory increase in metabolism or excretion results in a steady-state free plasma level similar to the level that existed prior to the displacement (19). Drugs bound to plasma protein are pharmacologically inactive, since they are not available to extravascular receptor sites. In addition, the bound form is not available for metabolism or excretion. Thus, once the object drug is displaced from the protein-binding site, not only is more drug free to exert its pharmacologic action, but additional drug becomes available for metabolism, excretion, and redistribution to other tissues.

The absolute concentration of unbound drug is referred to as the free concentration, while the fraction of the total concentration of unbound drug is the free fraction (26). The total plasma concentration of drug is the sum of the bound form and the free (unbound) drug. When drug is released from plasma protein, the increase in free drug concentration is transient. As the free fraction increases, it becomes available for metabolism, and the total drug concentration will decrease. Because drugs that are highly bound to plasma protein tend to remain in the vascular space, the volume of distribution of these drugs is frequently small (26). An equilibrium is maintained between the free drug in the circulation and the protein-bound drug, and as the drug is metabolized and excreted, the agent is released from its protein-binding site.

The fact that one drug displaces another is not sufficient to predict the pharmacologic outcome of a potential interaction. The overall pharmacologic effect of protein displacement is usually minimal. Clinically important interactions may result from protein displacement if displacement is accompanied by enzyme inhibition or if the displaced drug has a small apparent volume of distribution, a narrow therapeutic index, and a rapid onset of action (9).

Plasma proteins serve as a storage site or reservoir, limiting extravascular distribution. Examples of protein-binding sites are listed in Table 3.1 (26).

The systemic clearance of certain drugs (e.g., lido-

Table 3.1.
Drug Protein Binding Sites

Binding Site	Drug
Plasma Protein	
Albumin	Warfarin
Alpha-l-acid glycoprotein	Amitriptyline
	Disopyramide
	Lidocaine
	Propranolol
Lipoprotein	Cyclosporine
Transcortin	Corticosteroids
Tissue	
Sodium-potassium ATPase	Digoxin

caine, propranolol) is independent of protein binding. Since both the bound and unbound forms of these drugs are removed from the plasma, their clearance is determined by hepatic blood flow. Thus, changes in protein binding will not affect the clearance of these drugs.

Clinical Considerations. Clinically important drug interactions involving displacement from protein binding are uncommon because an object drug displaced from plasma protein is rapidly cleared from the body (8). Important interactions occur when displacement is accompanied by enzyme inhibition, as occurs during coadministration of warfarin and phenylbutazone.

Clinically Important Examples. Examples of drugs that are highly protein bound include phenytoin (90%), tolbutamide (96%), and warfarin (99%) (8). Common precipitant drugs include sulfonamides (e.g., sulfisoxazole), aspirin, and phenylbutazone (8). The metabolite of chloral hydrate, trichloroacetic acid, displaces warfarin from its protein-binding site, increasing the hypoprothrombinemic effect of warfarin (27, 28). However, the effect is slight and transient. With continued coadministration of the drugs, the free warfarin levels return to the concentrations that existed prior to the interaction. Although phenylbutazone displaces warfarin from plasma protein, it also inhibits the metabolism of the more potent S (−) warfarin enantiomorph, increasing the anticoagulant response to warfarin (29, 30).

ALTERED METABOLISM

The effects of one drug on the metabolism of a second are well documented. The concurrent administration of one drug with another may lead to an increase or decrease in the metabolic rate. These modifications may affect both the intensity and duration of activity. The major site of drug metabolism is the liver; however, other tissues, including white blood cells, skin, lung, and GI tract, are involved in drug metabolism. Drug-metabolizing enzymes primarily convert lipophilic drugs into water-soluble metabolites, which may be more readily excreted.

Drug metabolism may be divided into two types, phase I, which includes hydroxylation, oxidation, and reduction, and phase II, which includes glucuronide, glycine, and sulfate conjugation. Phase II metabolism is frequently preceded by phase I, preparing the drug for conjugation (31). The major hepatic enzyme system consists of the microsomal P-450 mixed-function oxygenases; however, there are numerous forms of cytochrome P-450 (9). Drug interactions involving this enzyme system occur only if both drugs bind to the active site of the same form of the enzyme. Because of inter- and intrapatient variability, it is difficult to anticipate the clinical importance of potential interactions that occur by alterations in metabolism.

Increased Metabolism (Enzyme Induction). This interaction mechanism results from increased production of drug-metabolizing enzymes (i.e., enzyme binding sites) and primarily involves phase I metabolism (31). Since protein synthesis is involved, this interaction typically has a slow onset and may require up to 3 weeks before the maximum effect is observed. Although the precipitant drug usually induces the enzymes that enhance the metabolism of the object drug, some drugs (e.g., carbamazepine) increase their own metabolism. When the drug responsible for enzyme induction (i.e., the precipitant drug) is discontinued, the process will reverse. However, reversal of enzyme induction is frequently a slower process than the onset. As the number of enzymes decrease, the serum concentration of the object drug will gradually increase if the dose is not decreased. Thus, for example, in patients receiving warfarin and phenytoin concurrently, bleeding could occur if the enzyme inducer, phenytoin, is discontinued without adjusting the anticoagulant dose.

Clinical Considerations. This mechanism of interaction has a slow onset because protein synthesis is involved and may take up to several weeks before the maximum effect is seen. If an interaction occurs, the serum levels of the object drug may be reduced, producing a decrease in therapeutic activity. To compensate for this interaction, when practical, monitor serum drug levels and observe the patient for loss of therapeutic effects. It is frequently necessary to increase the dose of the object drug or select a noninteracting alternative. When a patient is stabilized on both drugs, if the precipitant drug is discontinued or the dose is decreased, serum levels of the object drug may increase and toxicity could occur. Dissipation of the effects of the interaction after discontinuation of the precipitant drug is also slow. Once again, patients should be monitored for changes in clinical response.

Clinically Important Examples. Phenytoin increases the hepatic metabolism of mexiletine, producing a decrease in steady-state plasma mexiletine levels and a reduction in efficacy (32). Similarly, theophylline and phenytoin appear to increase the metabolism of each other. When both drugs are administered concomitantly, serum drug concentrations may decrease, and loss of seizure control or an exacerbation of pulmonary symptoms may result (10). Other drugs that induce hepatic enzymes include barbiturates (e.g., phenobarbital), carbamazepine, chronic ingestion of ethanol, griseofulvin, phenytoin, primidone, and rifampin (8), while environmental agents include cigarette smoke and diet.

Decreased Metabolism (Enzyme Inhibition). As occurs with enzyme induction, enzyme inhibition usually involves the liver and results from competition between the precipitant and object drugs for binding sites on the enzyme. However, since this mechanism involves direct competition, the onset of interactions is more rapid than with enzyme induction, frequently occurring within hours. Unless the precipitant drug has a long half-life, enzyme inhibition will reach a maximum effect within 24 hours (33). Less commonly, a noncompetitive mechanism, which suspends the metabolic activity of an enzyme, may be involved (34).

Drug interactions involving enzyme inhibition often result in clinical effects that are protracted or intensified as the object drug reaches a steady-state plasma level. The enzymes most frequently involved are monooxygenases (9). When metabolism of the object drug is inhibited, new steady-state serum levels are achieved in approximately five half-lives. However, the inhibitory effect of the precipitant drug on the metabolism of the object drug is usually maximal within three half-lives. Upon discontinuing the enzyme-inhibiting drug (i.e., precipitant drug), plasma concentrations of the object drug will decrease, resulting in loss of efficacy unless appropriate action is taken. The time frame for reversal of the interaction is dependent on the half-life of the object drug, but it usually occurs within 24 hr. As with most pharmacokinetic interactions, enzyme inhibition appears to be dose-related, with higher doses producing greater inhibition.

Clinical Considerations. Enzyme induction is one of the most common mechanisms of drug interactions. The onset and reversal of this interaction often occur within 24 hours. This interaction usually produces an increase in serum drug concentration, resulting in a possible augmentation of both the pharmacologic and toxic effects of the object drug. Clinically important interactions are most frequent with those drugs that have a narrow therapeutic index and when the serum level is near the upper end of the therapeutic range. When a hepatic microsomal enzyme-inducing drug (e.g., carbamazepine) is coadministered with an enzyme inhibitor (e.g., verapamil), the effect of the inhibitor appears to predominate and the effect of the inducer is attenuated. Stereospecific drug interactions involving warfarin metabolism are the most clinically important when the greatest effect occurs with the more potent S($-$) enantiomer (8).

Clinically Important Examples. Omeprazole appears to inhibit the oxidative metabolism of diazepam, resulting in increased serum levels of the benzodiazepine and producing an increase in the pharmacologic effect (35). Similarly, isoniazid inhibits the hepatic metabolism of phenytoin, producing an increase in serum phenytoin levels and a corresponding increase in the pharmacologic and toxic effects of the drug (36, 37). Phenytoin toxicity appears to be most important in patients who are slow acetylators of isoniazid (37). Other drugs that significantly inhibit metabolic enzymes include allopurinol, amiodarone, chloramphenicol, cimetidine, ciprofloxacin, diltiazem, erythromycin, isoniazid, ketoconazole, metronidazole, monoamine oxidase inhibitors, omeprazole, phenylbutazone, quinidine, and verapamil.

First-Pass Metabolism. Some drugs are metabolized extensively during the first pass through the wall of the gastrointestinal tract and liver (9, 19). In this instance, relatively small amounts of a drug will reach the systemic circulation (e.g., 10% of an orally administered dose of propranolol). Thus, drugs that increase or decrease liver blood flow may have profound effects on the bioavailability of the object drug. In addition, drugs with a high first-pass metabolism tend to compete for metabolic enzyme sites, enhancing each other's bioavailability (19). In other instances oral bioavailability may be decreased due to increased first-pass metabolism in the presence of enzyme induction.

Clinical Considerations. The object drug must be given orally. A clinically important interaction will be seen when the precipitant drug is either an enzyme inducer or inhibitor.

Clinically Important Examples. Propafenone increases plasma levels of both metoprolol and propranolol by decreasing first-pass metabolism and reducing systemic clearance. Propafenone and the β-blockers are metabolized by the hepatic cytochrome P-450 oxidase system, and propafenone appears to inhibit metoprolol and propranolol metabolism (38, 39). The pharmacologic and toxic effects of these β-blockers may be increased. Rifampin lowers serum verapamil levels by increasing first-pass hepatic metabolism of verapamil (40, 41). In addition, rifampin appears to induce the hepatic microsomal enzymes responsible for the metabolism of verapamil.

RENAL EXCRETION

The renal excretion of one drug may be increased or decreased by the coadministration of another drug. Most lipid-soluble drugs are metabolized by the liver to inactive, water-soluble metabolites prior to renal excretion. Various mechanisms may be involved with interactions affecting renal elimination, including competition for active tubular secretion and pH-dependent renal tubular transport.

Active Tubular Secretion. Active tubular secretion of drug molecules occurs in the proximal portion of the renal tubule. In order for the drug to pass from the systemic circulation to the tubular lumen, the drug is transported, by combining with a protein, through the basolateral and brush border membranes. Although each protein has a unique affinity for an anion or cation, drugs that use a similar system for transport appear to interact by competitive inhibition of transport proteins (42). Saturation of the transport system by the precipitant drug may decrease the tubular secretion of the object drug.

Clinical Considerations. Interaction resulting from this mechanism tends to occur rapidly. Plasma levels of the object drug may be increased, producing an increase in therapeutic and toxic effects.

Clinically Important Examples. Probenecid appears to impair the tubular secretion of methotrexate. Methotrexate serum levels have been reported to be increased three- to fourfold during concurrent administration of probenecid (43). Quinidine reduces the renal and biliary clearance of digoxin by 30 to 40%, increasing serum digoxin levels in approximately 90% of the patients receiving both drugs (10, 44).

Passive Tubular Reabsorption. Excretion and reabsorption of many drugs from the renal tubules occur by passive diffusion, which is regulated by the concentration and lipid solubility of the drug on both sides of the cell membrane (42). Nonionized drug molecules are reabsorbed preferentially over ionized drugs, with the ratio being determined by the pH and pK_a of the drug (42). Although strongly acidic and basic drugs tend to be ionized in the usual range of urinary pH (i.e., 5 to 8), the degree of ionization of weak acids and bases varies with the pH of the urine. Therefore, an increased amount of weakly acidic drug will be reabsorbed from an acidic urine, while basic drugs will be excreted. The opposite is true in an alkaline urine (1).

Clinical Considerations. Interference with renal elimination may be clinically important if the fraction of unmetabolized drug is large and if the drug has a narrow therapeutic index (e.g., thiazide diuretics decrease renal lithium clearance, producing toxicity).

Clinically Important Examples. Administration of sodium bicarbonate, 245 mEq administered over 5 hours, has been reported to increase renal lithium clearance, possibly decreasing the clinical effectiveness of lithium (45). Chronic antacid therapy with a magnesium and aluminum hydroxide combination has been associated with increased salicylate clearance and a 30 to 70% decrease in serum salicylate levels (10).

Pharmacodynamic Interactions

In contrast to pharmacokinetic interactions, pharmacodynamic interactions have not been amply studied or reported. Pharmacodynamic interactions involve changes in the response of the patient to a drug combination, without alterations in the serum concentration or pharmacokinetics of the object drug. Inasmuch as pharmacologic responses to a drug may be difficult to assess, pharmacodynamic studies are difficult to perform (46). Investigations are further complicated because pharmacokinetic and pharmacodynamic drug interactions may occur simultaneously. Since pharmacodynamic interactions often involve drugs with similar or opposing pharmacologic activity, many of these interactions can be anticipated by an understanding of the pharmacology of each of the drugs (1). Frequently, observing patients for changes in their clinical condition and making the appropriate dosage adjustment will correct the situation.

Synergistic and Antagonistic Effects. When a drug interaction involves synergistic or antagonistic effects, the therapeutic or toxic effects of two concurrently administered agents are greater or less, respectively, than the sum or the difference of their individual activities. These interactions frequently involve drugs acting on the same organ system (e.g., central nervous system) or site.

Clinical Considerations. Synergism is probably the most common mechanism by which drug interactions occur.

Clinically Important Examples. Synergism: Propranolol and verapamil have synergistic or additive cardiovascular effects (10). Both drugs have direct negative inotropic and chronotropic effects. Propranolol does not affect verapamil kinetics, and verapamil has only minimal effects on propranolol concentration. The pharmacologic as well as toxic effects of propranolol and verapamil may be enhanced. Aminoglycosides have been reported to stabilize the postjunctional membrane and impair prejunctional calcium influx and acetylcholine output, thereby potentiating the neuromuscular effects of succinylcholine (10).

Antagonism: The capacity of warfarin to interfere with the activation of the vitamin K–dependent clotting factors is reversed by vitamin K administration, allowing possible thrombus formation.

Altered Transport System and Effects at Receptor Sites. These drug interactions involve interference with physiological transport systems, limiting the access of certain drugs into cells.

Clinical Considerations. The serum level of the drugs will be unchanged unless a pharmacokinetic interaction occurs simultaneously.

Clinically Important Examples. Both phenothiazines (e.g., chlorpromazine) and tricyclic antidepressants (e.g., amitriptyline) inhibit the neuronal uptake of guanethidine, preventing the antihypertensive activity of guanethidine (10).

HIGH-RISK DRUGS

Drugs having the highest risk of being involved in a clinically important drug interaction frequently have a narrow therapeutic index, a steep dose-response curve, and potent pharmacologic effects (1, 7, 9). When a drug has a narrow therapeutic index, the toxic dose may be only slightly greater than the therapeutic dose. Similarly, when a drug has a steep dose-response curve, a small change in dose may result in a large increase in clinical effect. Therefore, a small increase in the serum concentration of drugs with these characteristics may produce an exaggerated pharmacologic response or toxicity.

Patients receiving drugs with a narrow therapeutic index should be monitored routinely for possible drug interactions. Examples of drugs with a narrow therapeutic index include aminoglycoside antibiotics, digoxin, hypoglycemic agents, lithium, phenytoin, theophylline, and warfarin (8, 9). Conversely, a slight decrease in the plasma level of drugs with a steep dose-response curve may result in significant loss of therapeutic effects. Examples include corticosteroids, carbamazepine, quinidine, oral contraceptives, and rifampin (9). Drugs with a wider therapeutic index are less likely to be involved in clinically important interactions.

HIGH-RISK PATIENTS

Drugs interactions that would be of minor clinical importance in most patients with less severe forms of a disease could cause significant exacerbation of the clinical condition in patients with more severe forms of the disease, such as cardiac arrhythmias, severe epilepsy, brittle diabetes, status asthmaticus, hypoxia, hypothyroidism, aplastic anemia, or hepatic precoma (9, 47). Loss of therapeutic activity can be particularly important in situations that could result in an unwanted outcome (e.g., pregnancy) or where a serious pathological condition is being suppressed, (e.g., connective tissue disorder or a malignancy) (9). Since the risk of experiencing a drug interaction increases with the number of drugs a patient receives, severely ill or the elderly who are taking multiple drugs may also be at an increased risk for drug interactions (9).

Additionally, patients being treated for certain diseases appear to be at an increased risk of experiencing a drug interaction because of the drug therapy prescribed for their disorder (48). Patients being treated for cardiovascular disease, connective tissue disorders, gastrointestinal disease, infection, metabolic disorders, psychiatric illness, respiratory ailments, or seizures frequently receive agents that are involved in drug interactions (47, 48).

ONSET

The time of onset of drug interactions varies considerably, ranging from seconds to weeks (49). Knowledge of the onset can help minimize the adverse effects of interactions by enabling the clinician to select the most appropriate monitoring parameters. Interactions that occur with the administration of the first dose or within 24 hours of administration of the precipitant drug may require immediate attention. Since protein synthesis is involved in enzyme induction, it may be 2 weeks or more before the full potential for a clinically important interaction is evident. Thus, an interaction would not be expected to occur by this mechanism in a patients receiving 1 or 2 days treatment with an enzyme-inducing drug (49). Conversely, enzyme inhibition results from competition between two drugs for the same enzyme site and may occur rapidly after administration of the precipitant drug. Patients should be monitored for changes in their clinical status soon after initiation of an interacting combination.

The time of onset of an interaction may be affected by the half-lives of the respective drugs. When the precipitant drug has a long half-life, it may take several days for plasma levels to reach steady state, delaying the onset of the interaction. The half-life of the object drug may also influence the onset of the interaction. Drug interactions occurring by similar mechanisms may have a more rapid onset when the object drug has a shorter half-life, since new steady-state plasma levels will be achieved faster. For example, cimetidine inhibits the metabolism of warfarin and theophylline. The latter drug has a considerably shorter half-life than the former. Therefore, a clinically important interaction may occur within a few days of adding cimetidine to the drug regimen of a patient stabilized on theophylline but may require a week or longer for a patient receiving warfarin.

The mechanism by which a drug interaction occurs can influence the onset of clinical effects. When relevant, the effect of the mechanism on the onset of an interaction was described in the clinical considerations section for the specific mechanism of interaction (see "Mechanisms of Drug Interaction").

CIRCUMVENTING AN INTERACTION

Many drug interactions can be avoided if adequate precautions are taken. Monitoring therapy and making appropriate adjustments in the drug regimen may circumvent a potentially serious drug interaction. Patients receiving drugs with a narrow therapeutic index should be monitored routinely for possible drug interactions. Drug interactions in this category may be life-threatening or have serious clinical consequences. Hospitalized patients are frequently given warfarin with an interacting agent without clinical consequences. In the hospital setting, patients' prothrombin times are monitored daily and appropriate adjustments are made in the warfarin dose whether or not a potential drug interaction is suspected. No symptoms of an interaction are observed. However, in order to avoid possible bleeding or the risk of exacerbating the condition being treated, adjustments in the warfarin dose are necessary if the interacting drug is discontinued after the patient is discharged from the hospital.

DRUG INTERACTION RESOURCES

It is not surprising that the administration of one drug may modify the action of another drug given simultaneously. Whenever a patient receives multiple drug therapy, the possibility of a drug-drug interaction exists. In addition, as the number of drugs a patient receives increases, so does the potential for a drug interaction. Fortunately, those interactions with the greatest clinical importance are infrequent.

It would be impractical for pharmacists or physicians to be aware of all possible drug interactions. However, over the past two decades, drug interactions have received considerable attention. The medical literature is replete with anecdotal case reports, controlled clinical trials, and review articles on this subject. In addition, new interactions are constantly being reported. Comprehensive textbooks have been written on drug interactions, detailing the clinical effects, mechanisms, and management of potential drug interactions (10, 50). Computer systems have been developed for storage and retrieval of drug interaction information and for patient monitoring (51, 52). Other available sources of drug interaction information include meetings, continuing education programs, and professional seminars. Even the manufacturer's package brochure contains a section on known and suspected drug interactions.

It is frequently difficult to interpret the relevance of much of the drug interaction data since they are derived from animal or in vitro studies, investigations involving healthy volunteers given a single dose of a drug, and anecdotal case reports (9). In addition, studies may illustrate and emphasize pharmacokinetic findings without demonstrating clinically important changes in patient outcome.

PROBLEMS ASSOCIATED WITH USING THE MEDICAL LITERATURE TO DETERMINE CLINICAL IMPORTANCE (10, 53–55)

Animal Studies. It may not be possible to extrapolate interactions based on animal studies to humans. Animals frequently receive much higher doses on a mg/kg basis than would be administered to humans.

Anecdotal Case Reports. Drug interactions based on a single case report require additional controlled studies to determine their clinical importance. One must rule out other alternative explanations for the observed event (e.g., natural progression of the disease being treated).

Healthy Volunteers. Results of studies involving healthy volunteers or a small number of patients may not allow adequate evaluation of a potential interaction. Some pharmacokinetic interactions may be determined in normal, healthy volunteers but may not be clinically important when observed in patients. In other instances, healthy volunteers may not exhibit an interaction that is observed in patients. For example, the ability of erythromycin to reduce warfarin clearance is significantly more pronounced in patients than in healthy subjects.

Magnitude of Effect. A study may fail to identify or accurately describe a potential drug interaction because of the magnitude of the effect of that interaction. Factors that may interfere with assessing the degree of effect are discussed below.

1. *Order of administration*: Treatment with the object drug is started after the patient is stabilized on the precipitant drug. No interaction may be observed in this instance until the precipitant drug is discontinued. Thus, in a patient receiving chronic cimetidine treatment prior to the initiation of warfarin therapy, no interaction would be observed. However, if cimetidine was discontinued after the warfarin dosage was stabilized, a higher dose of anticoagulant might be required. Clinically important interactions are more likely to occur when the precipitant drug is added to the regimen of a patient stabilized on the object drug.

2. *Duration of treatment*: An interaction with a delayed onset may not be observed if the study is not conducted for an adequate period of time. Neurotoxicity occurring with concurrent administration of lithium and carbamazepine may only be observed after the drug combination is given for several days.

3. *Adequate dose*: Most drug interactions are dose-related. Larger doses of the precipitant drug tend to produce greater effects in the object drug. If an adequate dose of the drug is not administered, one may fail to observe an interaction. Thus, while high-dose salicylates (e.g., aspirin >3 g/day) antagonize the uricosuric action of probenecid, occasional low doses do not.

4. *Dosage form*: It is necessary, for example, to consider the effects of food on theophylline absorption on an individual product basis. Although food can be ingested with many theophylline preparations without the occurrence of an interaction, *Theo-24* taken less than 1 hr before a high-fat meal may cause a significant increase in both theophylline absorption and peak serum levels.

5. *Presence of multiple drugs*: In a preliminary investigation, the presence of propylene glycol in IV nitroglycerin preparations was reported to interfere with the anticoagulant effect of heparin. Subsequent studies have demonstrated that the effect on heparin is due to the nitroglycerin.

Extrapolation to Chemically or Pharmacologically Related Drugs. Based upon pharmacokinetic (e.g., elimination) or pharmacodynamic differences, not all members of a drug class may interact in the same manner. Cimetidine inhibits the hepatic microsomal enzymes involved in the metabolism of diazepam; however, famotidine does not appear to affect diazepam metabolism. In addition, cimetidine does not alter oxazepam metabolism.

Mean Values. For drug interactions that occur in a small number of patients, no statistically significant difference in response may be observed between the control group and the study group. However, if one analyzes the results for individual subjects, there may be a clinically important change in a small number of patients. For example, some patients exhibit a fivefold increase in serum digoxin levels during concurrent administration of quinidine, while in others the effect is minimal.

Variability in Patient Response. In well-controlled drug interaction studies, it is not unusual to find a wide variation in the response of patients to the same drug regimen. Thus, while one patient may experience a life-threatening reaction, a second patient may not experience any adverse effects. Frequently it is not possible to explain these differences; however, the factors listed below account for some of the variability.

1. *Age*: The very young and the elderly may be at increased risk of experiencing drug interactions. Studies have indicated that elderly patients receive approximately 25% of all prescription drugs dispensed. In addition, this age group uses over-the-counter medications extensively. Furthermore, elderly patients may have other chronic diseases or decreased renal or hepatic function, necessitating careful monitoring of drug therapy. However, irrespective of age, drug therapy should be closely monitored in any patient with decreased organ function. Drug interactions involving enzyme induction may occur less frequently in elderly patients (56).

2. *Genetic factors*: Certain drug interactions may be more important in some patients because of genetic factors. For example, the toxicity resulting from the inhibitory effect of isoniazid on phenytoin metabolism appears to be more significant in slow acetylators of isoniazid than in patients who metabolize the drug more rapidly.

3. *Disease states*: Various diseases, such as impaired renal function, hepatic dysfunction, hypoalbuminemia, may adversely influence the response to various drugs used concurrently. In addition, patients with certain disease states, including cardiovascular, connective tissue, GI, lipid, infectious, psychiatric, respiratory, or seizure disorders, may be at an increased risk of experiencing moderate-to-severe drug interactions (48). This may be related either to changes in the disposition of the drug as a result of the disease or, more commonly, to the types of drugs used in the treatment of the disease.

4. *Alcohol consumption*: Acute alcohol intolerance (disulfiram reaction) may occur in patients consuming alcohol while taking other drugs, including cefamandole, cefoperazone, cefotetan, and moxalactam.

5. *Smoking*: Smoking has been shown to increase the activity of drug-metabolizing enzymes in the liver. Smoking stimulates the metabolism of theophylline and mexiletine. Compared with nonsmokers, smokers may require larger doses of these drugs to maintain therapeutic serum levels. In addition, an enzyme-inducing drug may not have as important an effect on the object drug as might occur in a nonsmoking patient receiving the same drug combination. There is evidence indicating that the effects of administering multiple enzyme-inducing drugs to the same patient are less than additive (57).

When evaluating the medical literature for a drug interaction, be aware of the type of documentation supporting the proposed interaction, i.e., case report, animal study, or controlled study. With a controlled study, one must evaluate the study design, including sample size, route of drug administration, duration of therapy, and type of subjects (e.g., normal volunteers vs. clinical patients).

CONCLUSION

It is important to understand the clinical significance of potentially interacting drug combinations. Although one does not want the choice of therapy to be detrimental to the patient, it is equally important not to deprive a patient of worthwhile treatment by overreacting to a potential interaction that lacks clinical significance or that can be easily circumvented. Most interacting drug combinations can be administered concurrently if the patient is monitored appropriately and corresponding adjustments are made in the drug dose, dosing interval, or route of administration. Understanding the mechanisms by which drugs interact as well as a knowledge of those drugs and patients at increased risk of experiencing potentially important drug interactions will allow one to anticipate and prevent clinically significant problems. Careful attention should be given to those interactions involving drugs that have a narrow therapeutic index (e.g., digoxin, phenytoin, theophylline, warfarin). When a patient's clinical condition changes unexpectedly, all drug treatment should be reviewed. When possible, a suspected interaction should be placed in clinical perspective, and one should be prepared to offer recommendations for minimizing possible consequences.

Factors that will help minimize the occurrence of drug interactions include (a) knowing the over-the-counter drugs that the patient may take; (b) avoiding unnecessary therapy; (c) observing the patient for unexpected changes in clinical response; and (d) monitoring serum drug levels, particularly for drugs with a narrow therapeutic index.

Educating patients about potential drug interactions that may be associated with their treatment regimens is important. Patient knowledge of unexpected reactions that could occur with coadministration of their current medications with other prescription and over-the-counter drugs could lead to the early detection or prevention of possibly important drug interactions.

REFERENCES

1. Berkow R (ed): The Merck Manual of Diagnosis and Therapy, ed 15. New Jersey: Merck Sharp & Dohme Research Laboratories, 1987, pp 2456–2461.
2. Boston Collaborative Drug Surveillance Program: Adverse drug interactions. JAMA 220:1238–1239, 1972.
3. Durrence CW, DiPiro JT, May JR, et al.: Potential drug interactions in surgical patients. Am J Hosp Pharm 42:1553–1555, 1985.
4. Borda IT, Slone D, Jick H: Assessment of adverse reactions within a drug surveillance program. JAMA 205:645–647, 1968.
5. Blaschke TF, Cohen SN, Tatro DS, Drug-drug interactions and aging. In Jarvik LF, Greenblatt DJ, Harman D (eds): Clinical Pharmacology in the Aged Patient. New York, Raven Press, 1981, vol 16, pp 11–26.
6. Stanaszek WF, Franklin CE: Survey of potential drug interaction incidence in an outpatient clinic population. Hosp Pharm 13:255–263, 1978.
7. Puckett WH, Visconti JA: An epidemiological study of the clinical significance of drug-drug interactions in a private community hospital. Am J Hosp Pharm 28:247–253, 1971.
8. Aronson JK, Grahame-Smith DG: Adverse drug interactions. Br Med J 282:288–291, 1981.
9. McInnes GT, Brodie MJ: Drug interactions that matter: a critical reappraisal. Drugs 36:83–110, 1988.
10. Tatro DS (ed): Drug Interaction Facts. St. Louis: Facts and Comparisons, (Quarterly) 1990, pp 110, 164, 281, 290, 353, 365, 615, 627, 691, 735.
11. Hoffken G, Borner K, Glatzel PD, et al.: Reduced enteral absorption of ciprofloxacin in the presence of antacids. Eur J Clin Microbiol 4:345, 1985.
12. Nix DE, Watson WA, Lener ME, et al.: Effects of aluminum and magnesium antacids and ranitidine on the absorption of ciprofloxacin. Clin Pharmacol Ther 46:700–705, 1989.
13. Hansten PD, Horn JR: Drug interactions during absorption from the gastro-intestinal tract. Drug Interactions Newsletter 9:475–480A, 1989.
14. Lindenbaum J, Rund DG, Butler VP, et al.: Inactivation of digoxin by the gut flora: reversal by antibiotic therapy. N Engl J Med 305:789–794, 1981.
15. Morton MR, Cooper JW: Erythromycin-induced digoxin toxicity. DICP, Ann Pharmacother 23:668–670, 1989.
16. Parpia SH, Nix DE, Hejmanowski LG, et al.: Sucralfate reduces the gastrointestinal absorption of norfloxacin. Antimicrob Agents Chemother 33:99–102, 1989.
17. Nix DE, Watson WA, Handy L, et al.: The effect of sucralfate pretreatment on the pharmacokinetics of ciprofloxacin. Pharmacotherapy 9:377–380, 1989.
18. Garrelts JC, Godley RJ, Peterie JD, et al.: Sucralfate significantly reduces ciprofloxacin concentrations in serum. Antimicrob Agents Chemother 34:931–933, 1990.
19. Brodie MJ, Feely J: Adverse drug interactions. Br Med J 296:845–849, 1988.
20. Kuhlman J, Zilly W, Wilke J: Effects of cytotoxic drugs on plasma level and renal excretion of beta-acetyldigoxin. Clin Pharmacol Ther 30:518–527, 1981.
21. Kuhlman J, Wilke J, Rietbrock N: Cytostatic drugs are without significant effect on digitoxin plasma level and renal excretion. Clin Pharmacol Ther 32:646–651, 1982.
22. Bjornsson TD, Huang AT, Roth P, et al.: Effects of high-dose cancer chemotherapy on the absorption of digoxin in two different formulations. Clin Pharmacol Ther 39:25–28, 1986.
23. Wadhwa NK, Schroeder TJ, O'Flaherty E, et al.: The effect of oral metoclopramide on the absorption of cyclosporine. Transplant Proc 19:1730–1733, 1987.
24. Manninen V, Melin J, Apajalahti A, et al.: Altered absorption of digoxin in patients given propantheline and metoclopramide. Lancet 1:398–399, 1973.
25. Johnson BF, Bustrack JA, Urbach DR, et al.: Effect of metoclopramide on digoxin absorption from tablets and capsules. Clin Pharmacol Ther 36:724–730, 1984.
26. Hansten PD, Horn JR: Mechanisms of drug interactions: protein binding displacement. Drug Interactions Newsletter 9:449–456, 1989.
27. Boston Collaborative Drug Surveillance Program: Interaction between chloral hydrate and warfarin. N Engl J Med 286:53–55, 1972.

28. Udall JA. Warfarin–chloral hydrate interaction: pharmacological activity and clinical significance. Ann Intern Med 81:341–344, 1974.

29. Banfield C, O'Reilly R, Chan E, et al.: Phenylbutazone-warfarin interaction in man: Further stereochemical and metabolic considerations. Br J Clin Pharmacol 16:669–675, 1983.

30. O'Reilly RA, Trager WF, Motley CH, et al.: Stereoselective interaction of phenylbutazone with [^{12}C/^{13}C]warfarin pseudracemates in man. J Clin Invest 65:746–753, 1980.

31. Hansten PD, Horn JR: Drug interaction mechanism: enzyme induction. Drug Interactions Newsletter 10:519–525, 1990.

32. Begg EJ, Chinwah PM, Webb C, et al.: Enhanced metabolism of mexiletine after phenytoin administration. Br J Clin Pharmacol 14:219–223, 1982.

33. Dossing M, Pilsgaard H, Rasmussen B, et al.: Time course of phenobarbital and cimetidine mediated changes in hepatic drug metabolism. Eur J Clin Pharmacol. 25:215–222, 1983.

34. Hansten PD, Horn JR: Drug interaction mechanisms: enzyme inhibition. Drug Interaction Newsletter 10:541–547, 1990.

35. Gugler R, Jensen JC: Omeprazole inhibits oxidative drug metabolism. Gastroenterology 89:1235–1241, 1985.

36. Murray FJ: Outbreak of unexpected reactions among epileptics taking isoniazid. Am Rev Respir Dis 86:729–732, 1962.

37. Brennan RW, Dehejia H, Kutt H, et al.: Diphenylhydantoin intoxication attendant to slow inactivation of isoniazid. Neurology 20:687–693, 1970.

38. Wagner F, Kalusche D, Trenk D, et al.: Drug interaction between propafenone and metoprolol. Br J Clin Pharmac 24:213–220, 1987.

39. Kowey PR, Kirsten EB, Fu CHJ, et al.: Interaction between propranolol and propafenone in healthy volunteers. J Clin Pharmacol 29:512–517, 1989.

40. Mooy J, Bohm R, van Baak M, et al.: The influence of antituberculosis drugs on plasma level of verapamil. Eur J Clin Pharmacol 32:107–109, 1987.

41. Barbarash RA, Bauman JL, Fischer JH, et al.: Near-total reduction in verapamil bioavailability by rifampin: electrocardiographic correlates. Chest 94:954–959, 1988.

42. Hansten PD, Horn JR: Interactions associated with modified drug excretion. Drug Interactions Newsletter 9:497–503, 1989.

43. Aherne GW, Piall E, Marks V, et al.: Prolongation and enhancement of serum methotrexate concentrations by probenecid. Br Med J 1:1097–1099, 1978.

44. Hedman A, Angelin B, Arvidsson A, et al.: Interactions in the renal and biliary elimination of digoxin: stereoselective differences between quinine and quinidine. Clin Pharmacol Ther 47:20–26, 1990.

45. Thomsen K, Schou M: Renal lithium excretion in man. Am J Physiol 215:823–827, 1968.

46. Bauer LA: Pharmacodynamic drug interactions. Drug Interactions Newsletter 10:563–571, 1990.

47. Tatro DS: Drugs interfering with control of the diabetic patient: Hypoglycemic drug-drug interactions. Rev Drug Interaction 1:3–34, 1974.

48. Hansten PD, Horn JR: Patients at increased risk for adverse drug interactions. Drug Interactions Newsletter 10:589–595, 1990.

49. Hansten PD, Horn JR: The time course of drug interactions. Drug Interaction Newsletter 9:429–434, 1989.

50. Hansten PD: Drug Interactions. Philadelphia: Lea & Febiger, 1985.

51. Tatro DS, Briggs RL, Chavez-Pardo R, et al.: Detection and prevention of drug interactions utilizing an online computer system. Drug Info J 9:10–17, 1975.

52. Tatro DS, Briggs RL, Chavez-Pardo R, et al.: Online drug interaction surveillance. Am J Hosp Pharm 32:417–420, 1975.

53. Hansten PD, Horn JR: Pitfalls in the evaluation of drug interaction literature. Drug Interactions Newsletter 7:27–30, 1987.

54. Hansten PD, Horn JR: The assessment of risk in the clinical outcome of drug interactions. Drug Interactions Newsletter 6:21–26, 1986.

55. Tatro DS: Understanding drug interactions. Facts and Comparisons Drug Newsletter 7:57–59, 1988.

56. Salem SAM, Rejjayabun P, Shepherd AMM, et al.: Reduced induction of drug metabolism in the elderly. Age Ageing 7:68–73, 1978.

57. Perucca E, Hedges A, Makki A, et al.: A comparative study of the relative enzyme-inducing properties of anticonvulsant drugs in epileptic patients. Br J Clin Pharmacol 18:401–410, 1984.

CHAPTER 4

CLINICAL TOXICOLOGY

GARY M. ODERDA, Pharm.D., M.P.H., and WENDY KLEIN-SCHWARTZ, Pharm.D.

Clinical toxicology deals with the assessment and medical management of persons exposed acutely or chronically to potentially harmful agents. Because of the diverse nature of the substances involved in poisonings as well as the wide range of clinical manifestations and their treatment, optimal management of the poisoned patient is achieved through an interdisciplinary approach to patient care.

GENERAL INFORMATION

Poisoning is a serious problem in the United States today. The American Association of Poison Control Centers (AAPCC) data collection system reported 1,581,540 human poison exposures in 1989 (1). This figure does not reflect the actual number reported to poison centers nationally, since reporting is voluntary and there are no legal reporting requirements for poisonings. Although it is difficult to be certain of the true magnitude of the problem, it is estimated that each year 2.1 to 4.6 million poison exposures occur nationally, with accidental poisoning accounting for 5315 deaths in 1987 (1, 2).

Poisoning is a common pediatric medical emergency. Sixty-one percent of poisonings occur in children under 6 years of age (1). Most childhood poisonings are accidental and occur via the oral route. Children's natural curiosity can at times have disastrous consequences. The most common substances involved in poison exposures in children under 6 years of age are drugs, household products, personal care products, and plants. The drugs most commonly involved are analgesics and antipyretics, antihistamines, cough and cold products, vitamins, and topical preparations.

Thirty years ago aspirin was the leading cause of accidental poisonings and poisoning deaths in children under 5 years of age. There has been a progressive decline in both ingestions and deaths from aspirin since the mid-1960s (3). The percentage of ingestions of aspirin in those under 5 years of age decreased steadily from about 25% in 1966 to 3.9% in 1979 (4). In 1989, AAPCC data showed that ingestions of aspirin alone in children 5 years of age and under accounted for 0.52% of exposures (1). Many factors are responsible for this decrease, including an increased awareness on the part of the general public of the dangers of aspirin. The child-resistant container (CRC) requirement for all products containing aspirin and all liquid preparations containing methylsalicylate played a major role in the decline. One hopes that CRCs will further decrease the number of intoxications from other products on which these closures are now required. The limit of 36 tablets (81 mg each) per bottle of children's aspirin has helped reduce the severity of the ingestions that still occur.

Approximately 18% of poisonings occur in adults 17 years of age or older. They are often intentional (suicide or drug abuse) but may also be accidental (e.g., industrial exposure). Although poison prevention activities may decrease the number of pediatric exposures and minimize the severity of childhood intoxications, these efforts generally have little impact on unintentional poisonings in adults. One possible exception is poisoning in the elderly. Many of these ingestions are accidental and are amenable to poison prevention efforts (5). Poisonings in adults are generally responsible for more significant morbidity and mortality than those in children.

ROLE AND STATUS OF POISON CENTERS

The first poison center was established in Chicago in 1953. Today, poison centers exist in most major U.S. metropolitan areas. During the 1970s the concept of regionalization of poison centers developed in an attempt to more efficiently and effectively meet the needs of the poisoned patient. Many large centers serve as regional centers and provide information to a large population or geographic area. This may involve a major metropolitan area, a portion of a large state, an entire state, or several states. It is not unusual for these regional centers to handle 15,000 to 30,000 or more calls per year. Fifty to 100 regional poison centers could adequately serve the entire United States. In this way duplication of information sources and staff would be avoided. Poison centers receive calls relating to drugs, substance abuse, chemicals, household products, personal care products, plants, animal toxins, fish toxins, food poisoning, and others. Approximately 40% of calls involve exposures to drugs. The majority of calls to the poison center come from the general public and can be managed without admission to a healthcare facility.

The American Association of Poison Control Centers, which developed standards for regional poison centers, also certifies regional centers. According to a survey conducted in 1989, there are 104 poison centers in the United States, of which 35 are certified as regional poison centers by the American Association of Poison Control Centers.

A regional poison center provides telephone information 24 hours a day, using comprehensive information sources and management protocols, and has access to regional treatment facilities for patient referral and transport. Additional services include a regional system for providing poisoning care, public and health-professional education programs, and a regional data collection and reporting system.

Clinical pharmacists or nurses often administer the day-to-day operation of the center as well as provide professional input into the management of the poisoned patient. Specialists in poison information, usually pharmacists or nurses, are responsible for providing primary telephone consultations.

Poison information and drug information centers differ in several respects. Poison centers usually provide services to both professionals and the general public, whereas drug information centers usually provide information only to health professionals. Poison centers usually get more calls than drug information centers. Rapid retrieval of information is necessary in poison centers because of the potential emergency nature of calls. Therefore, the information sources used for handling most cases are secondary resources. Often the assessment and recommendations are provided during the initial call to the center. As a result, the depth of research performed in a poison center is less than that in a drug information center.

POISON PREVENTION

A major component of poison center activity is poison prevention education.

All prescription drugs should be dispensed in CRCs unless specifically excluded by law. In those few instances in which a patient requires a non-CRC, the pharmacist should warn the patient to store the container properly to avoid an accidental poisoning. Elderly patients who request non-CRCs may not have young children of their own, but many have grandchildren who come to visit.

Pharmacists should promote the distribution of syrup of ipecac by providing information and urging families to purchase 1 ounce of ipecac syrup for each young child. Parents should be cautioned to contact their poison center, physician, or pharmacist before giving the ipecac, so that the situation can be evaluated to determine the appropriateness of administering an emetic. If syrup of ipecac is indicated, the health professional can review dosing with the caller, follow up to determine if the person has vomited, and provide additional instructions about the side effects of ipecac or symptoms to watch for that might indicate the need for additional evaluation and treatment. If ipecac is not indicated, the health professional can discourage its use and recommend other treatment if necessary.

ANALYSIS OF A POISONING SITUATION—TYPES OF QUESTIONS ASKED

In many poisoning calls, the caller does not volunteer enough information initially for the pharmacist to assess the situation. The fact that an overdose has occurred is not always obvious. Occasionally a poisoning situation can be uncovered only by persistent questioning. Inquiries about tablet identification or other general information may involve a poisoning, and this information can be elicited by determining why the caller needs the information.

In addition, poisoning should be considered in the differential diagnosis whenever there is an abrupt onset of illness with multiple organ system involvement, especially if the patient is a child under 3 years of age or has a history of a previous ingestion (8).

When a poisoning is suspected, the following information must be obtained to "analyze" a poisoning situation:

1. Substance. This information should include ingredients and their percentages. Examples of situations where the substance involved may be unknown include patients who are unable to give a history (e.g., patient is comatose), those who ingest tables or capsules from an unmarked container, and those who ingest an unidentified plant.
2. Amount. If an accurate determination of the amount ingested is impossible and the product is potentially toxic, one must assume that a potentially toxic amount was ingested or that the total amount originally in the container was ingested.
3. Time since exposure. By knowing the onset and duration of action of the substance, one can determine whether the symptoms are consistent with the history of the amount and the time since exposure. In addition, treatment recommendations, such as whether or not to empty the stomach, may be influenced by the length of time since ingestion.
4. Symptoms. Determine whether symptoms are consistent with the substance involved. If not, determine what other substances or medical conditions may be responsible for these symptoms. Severe signs and symptoms, such as respiratory and cardiovascular collapse, may necessitate immediate treatment. Some treatment modalities are contraindicated when certain signs or symptoms are present (e.g., emetics in the comatose patient).
5. Age and weight of patient. These are important considerations in determining both the toxicity of the substance and possible antidotes.
6. Past medical history and prior therapy. The patient's medical history may influence the severity of the intoxication or treatment. Some home remedies may complicate therapy, whereas other prior treatment may influence subsequent recommendations.

INFORMATION SOURCES

After obtaining the poisoning history and the patient's current clinical status, one must consult appropriate information sources. The major toxicologic information sources are secondary sources designed to allow rapid retrieval of toxicity and management information. The current primary literature should be consulted in some cases.

The following references are strictly toxicology-oriented and do not include other important references such as pharmacology or drug interaction texts that are available in both pharmacies and poison centers.

Poisindex

The Poisindex (B. Rumack, editor; published by Micromedex, Englewood, CO; new edition published 4 times yearly) is a computer-generated system with information on most commercial products and other agents that are commonly ingested, including biologicals such as plants and venomous animals. It is usually used as a computer-accessible data base, either as a compact disk (CD-ROM) system or a multiuser mainframe computer system. It also is available on microfiche. The editorial board is comprised of individuals actively involved with poisoning and poison centers throughout the United States.

For each product, the manufacturer's name, the type of product, ingredients, percentages (if available), and tablet imprint (if applicable) are listed. Specific toxicity information may also be included. The user is referred to the appropriate managements for all agents.

Managements are preceded by "overviews" that contain summaries of emergency treatment and toxicity information eliminating the need to scan many screens of information initially. The overview is followed by the complete management, which includes information on available forms, pharmacology, clinical effects, kinetics, range of toxicity, laboratory values (blood levels, etc.), treatment, and major references.

The major advantages of this system are (a) ease of use; (b) storage of a large amount of data in a small space; (c) up-to-date information; (d) detailed management protocols; (e) information on drugs, chemicals, household products, food poisoning, mushrooms, snakes, and drug imprint codes; and (f) cross-referenced product information. It is an essential resource for poison centers and is also useful for other healthcare providers.

Textbooks

CLINICAL TOXICOLOGY OF COMMERCIAL PRODUCTS

Clinical Toxicology of Commercial Products, ed. 5 (Gosselin, R. E., Smith, R. P., Hodge, H. C., (eds). Baltimore: Williams & Wilkins, 1984) is divided into seven sections: "First Aid and General Emergency Treatment," "Ingredients Index," "Therapeutics Index," "Supportive Treatment," "Trade Name Index," "General Formulations," and "Manufacturers Names and Addresses." Most commonly one looks up the name of a product in the trade name index, which lists the ingredients and their percentages. One then looks up each ingredient in the ingredients index for specific toxicity information. The therapeutics index has detailed toxicity and treatment information on general categories such as antihistamines. The general formulations index is very useful in those sit-

uations where a brand name is unavailable. If, for example, one is dealing with a child who drank an unknown brand of furniture polish, one could find the ingredients usually found in furniture polishes.

TOXICOLOGY OF THE EYE

Toxicology of the Eye, ed. 3 (Grant, W. G., Springfield, IL: Charles C. Thomas, 1986) is an excellent resource that covers the effects of various agents upon contact with the eye. In addition, those agents for which systemic intoxication produces ocular effects (e.g., methanol) are included. Specific human information is discussed where available. A separate treatment section is included.

INDUSTRIAL HYGIENE AND TOXICOLOGY

Industrial Hygiene and Toxicology, ed. 3 (Patty, F. A. (ed), New York: Interscience Publishers, 1981) is a series published in three volumes. Volume I discusses general principles, volumes IIA, IIB, and IIC specific toxicology information, and volume III, industrial hygiene practice. Poison centers find volumes IIA, IIB, and IIC the most useful. Both chronic and acute exposures to industrial chemicals are described. For each chemical the following information is provided: (a) source, use, and industrial exposure; (b) physical and chemical properties; (c) determination in the atmosphere; (d) physiologic response; (e) hygiene standard of permissible exposure; (f) flammability; and (g) odor and warning properties.

Medical Toxicology. Diagnosis and Treatment of Human Poisoning (Ellenhorn, M. J., Barceloux, D. G., New York: Elsevier, 1988), *Clinical Management of Poisoning and Drug Overdose*, ed. 2 (Haddad, L. M., Winchester, J. F. (eds), Philadelphia: W. B. Saunders, 1990), and *Goldfrank's Toxicology Emergencies*, ed. 4 (Goldfrank, L. W., Flomenbaum, N. E., Lewin, N. A., et al. (eds), Norwalk, CT: Appleton and Lange, 1990) are textbooks of clinical toxicology that provide brief reviews of poisoning by drugs, chemicals, and biologicals and their management.

DECREASING ABSORPTION

The toxic potential of an ingestion can be decreased by minimizing the absorption of the ingested agent from the gastrointestinal tract. Emptying the stomach, administering an adsorbent, and inducing catharsis are potential treatments that should be considered when a sufficient amount of a potentially toxic substance has been ingested within a reasonable time period. For most substances, this time period is within the previous 4 hr. Drugs for which gastrointestinal (GI) emptying may be warranted up to 10 to 12 hr after ingestion include salicylates, which delay gastric emptying; anticholinergics, which decrease GI motility; and phenytoin, which is absorbed slowly and erratically from the GI tract.

Table 4.1.
Utilization of GI Decontamination Procedures (1989 AAPCC National Data Collection System)[a]

	Number	%
Total poison exposures	1,581,540	100.0
Ipecac syrup	110,800	7.3
Gastric lavage	41,056	2.7
Activated charcoal	101,525	6.7
Cathartics	85,016	5.6

[a] Data from Litovitz TL, Schmitz BF, Bailey KM: 1989 Annual Report of the American Association of Poison Control Centers National Data Collection System. Am J Emerg Med 8:394–442, 1990.

Activated charcoal has become the primary treatment to prevent absorption from the GI tract in emergency room–treated patients. The use of ipecac syrup or gastric lavage may be appropriate in some of these patients. For example, patients who have taken agents not adsorbed by activated charcoal may benefit from ipecac or lavage. The major role of ipecac syrup is for use in the home to remove toxic agents from the GI tract and prevent absorption. A summary of the use of GI decontamination procedures as reported to the AAPCC is shown in Table 4.1.

The efficacy of ipecac syrup–induced emesis was evaluated in 20 children between 12 and 20 months of age who had ingested salicylates (16). Lavage was performed and emesis induced in each patient, and the amount of salicylates returned by each method was measured. Approximately one-half of the patients were lavaged first, and the other half were given syrup of ipecac first. Overall, ipecac removed significantly more salicylate than lavage, even when emesis was induced after lavage was completed. The study concluded that ipecac-induced emesis is superior to gastric lavage for emptying the stomach and it leaves little or no salicylate that could potentially be removed by lavage.

Goldstein (17) reported two acute overdoses in adults seen 10 to 15 min after ingestion. Each patient was lavaged with 3 liters of normal saline through a 20 French tube. Both patients were then given ipecac, and they vomited successfully. In one case 25 tablets were found in the vomitus, and in the other 10 to 15 tablets.

In many of these studies, either the size of the lavage tube is not mentioned or it is smaller than is currently recommended. The smaller tubes, including Levine tubes, are clearly too small to remove large tablet particles, whole tables, or groups of tablets clumped together. Lavage with a large Ewald tube, 28 to 36 French, or larger, should empty the stomach more efficiently and be as effective as emesis. A prospective study of 88 patients seen in an emergency department for drug overdose found gastric lavage to be superior to ipecac-induced emesis when thiamine

was used as a marker of recovery of gastric samples (18). A controlled study in 18 fasting normal adult volunteers who ingested 25 100-μg cyanocobalamin tablets on two separate occasions reported a mean return of 28% with ipecac-induced emesis compared with 45% after gastric lavage with a modified 32 French orogastric tube (19). Potential methodologic biases leave this issue unresolved (20).

Another important clinical consideration is the low percentage return with both emesis and lavage. In 14 humans given magnesium hydroxide and then ipecac, a mean return of 28 ± 7.0% was found, with a range of 0 to 78% (21). Arnold et al. (15) found that under optimal conditions dogs given sodium salicylate returned 38% (range 2 to 69%) after lavage and 45% (range 7 to 75%) after ipecac-induced emesis. When the administration of ipecac was delayed until 30 min after ingestion and lavage was not performed until 1 hr after ingestion, only 13% (range 0 to 40%) was removed by lavage and 39% (range 5 to 74%) by emesis (15). A small 16 French tube was used for lavage. A similar study in dogs utilizing barium sulfate, found that 29 ± 10% (range 10 to 62%) was returned with gastric lavage, 19 ± 9% (range 2 to 31%) with ipecac, and 74 ± 5% (range 54 to 87%) with apomorphine (22).

In situations where gastric emptying is warranted, emesis with syrup of ipecac should routinely be the procedure of first choice in children. Either emesis or lavage can be considered in adults. In those cases where emetics are contraindicated (e.g., the CNS-depressed patient), lavage is preferred. Lavage should also be performed if induction of emesis with ipecac fails.

Although induction of emesis or gastric lavage has been considered standard procedure for gastric emptying, their role in gastrointestinal decontamination has recently been questioned. Several studies comparing ipecac and/or lavage with activated charcoal treatment have found activated charcoal superior (23–25). A crossover study in 12 adult volunteers given 24 81-mg aspirin tablets and randomly assigned to a control group (no further treatment), ipecac group, activated charcoal/cathartic group, or ipecac/activated charcoal/cathartic group found that aspirin absorption was decreased in both the ipecac group and the activated charcoal/cathartic group (23). Analysis of the effectiveness of ipecac/activated charcoal/cathartic was not possible, since 8 of 10 volunteers vomited up the charcoal and cathartic. However, activated charcoal/cathartic was significantly more effective than ipecac, and it was concluded that activated charcoal/cathartic used alone is superior to other treatment. Similarly, a randomized crossover study in six healthy adult volunteers comparing ipecac with activated charcoal following therapeutic doses of acetaminophen, tetracycline, and aminophylline found activated charcoal to be significantly more effective than ipecac in reducing drug absorption (24). In both these studies therapeutic or subtoxic doses were given, so extrapolation of these results to the overdosed patient may not be appropriate.

Tennenbein and others compared prevention of ampicillin absorption in human volunteers. Each volunteer was given 5 grams of ampicillin and then gastric lavage, ipecac, or activated charcoal and a cathartic in a crossover design with a washout period between each phase. The amount absorbed was compared with a control phase that utilized no procedures to limit absorption. Charcoal and cathartic was most effective, preventing absorption of 57%, followed by ipecac (38%), and gastric lavage (32%).

Two studies have attempted to evaluate the outcomes of overdosed patients given different GI decontamination procedures. Kulig et al. performed a prospective randomized study of ipecac or lavage plus activated charcoal and a cathartic versus activated charcoal and a cathartic in 592 acute oral drug overdose patients (25). There were no differences in number of hospital days, number of days in the intensive care unit, clinical deterioration, or morbidity and mortality between the two groups.

Albertson compared ipecac syrup and activated charcoal with activated charcoal alone in 200 overdosed patients (26). The only statistically significant difference was in the mean time the patients spent in the emergency room, with a mean of 6.8 hr in the ipecac and charcoal group and 6.0 hr in the activated charcoal alone group. There was no difference in the percentage hospitalized, the percentage admitted to an ICU, or the number of hospital or ICU days. A difference was seen in the percentage of patients developing complications, with 5.4% in the ipecac and charcoal group, as compared with 0.9% in the charcoal alone group. It is unclear what role ipecac played in some of the adverse effects.

Overall, these data suggest that GI decontamination with activated charcoal and a cathartic is as effective as or superior to gastric emptying with ipecac or lavage. Some poison centers have adopted protocols that recommend activated charcoal and a cathartic only for GI decontamination in hospital-treated patients. Ipecac syrup continues to have a significant role in patients who do not require treatment in a healthcare facility. It is important to remember that data evaluating GI decontamination procedures are preliminary, and the standard regimen of lavage followed by activated charcoal and a cathartic is still considered an appropriate course of therapy.

Emetics

Emetics are agents that induce vomiting. Although emetics can act logically on the GI tract or centrally through stimulation of the chemoreceptor trigger zone and the vomiting center, vomiting occurs only if the medullary centers are still responsive. Emetics are absolutely contraindicated in the following situations:

1. Patients with CNS depression manifested by severe lethargy, loss of the gag reflex, or unconsciousness. The risk of aspiration of the vomitus into the lungs, a potentially severe complication, is significant.
2. Patients who are seizing or in whom seizures are imminent. Aspiration is an important risk in these patients.
3. Patients who have ingested a caustic. Strong acids and bases may produce severe burns of the mucous membranes of the mouth and esophagus. By inducing emesis these tissues will be reexposed to the caustic, and further damage may occur. In addition, the force of vomiting may cause perforation of the damaged esophagus.

There has been some concern that emetics may be ineffective in patients who have overdosed on drugs with antiemetic properties. Two studies concluded that antiemetics do not significantly interfere with the effectiveness of emetics (27, 28). However, both studies failed to address such issues as the amount of antiemetic ingested and the time between ingestion and emesis or to document through laboratory analysis whether a sufficient quantity of the ingested agent was present to produce an antiemetic effect. Three cases of serious toxicity related to ipecac administration involved patients who ingested a phenothiazine, failed to vomit with ipecac, and developed cardiac toxicity (29, 30). Therefore, caution may be warranted in phenothiazine ingestions, and ipecac should be reserved for asymptomatic patients who have ingested the antiemetic within the hour.

Another controversial issue involves the use of emetics in hydrocarbon (e.g., kerosene, gasoline) exposures. Because of their low viscosity, low surface tension, and high volatility, hydrocarbons are likely to be aspirated and produce severe pulmonary toxicity. When aliphatic hydrocarbons are ingested, emptying the stomach is unnecessary, since absorption from the GI tract does not appear to be responsible for production of toxicity. Ingestions of aromatic hydrocarbons, halogenated hydrocarbons, or potentially dangerous chemicals such as pesticides in a hydrocarbon solvent may require gastric emptying. Two retrospective studies have concluded that ipecac-induced emesis does not increase the risk of aspiration of hydrocarbons (31, 32). Based on these studies and recent clinical experience, syrup of ipecac can be safely administered under medical supervision following the ingestion of a systemically toxic hydrocarbon.

Syrup of ipecac is considered the emetic of choice both in the home and in hospital settings. It is a local and centrally acting emetic and is available without prescription in 15- and 30-ml containers. Analysis of reports from various sources suggests that syrup of ipecac is almost 100% effective in producing emesis when 15 ml or more are given (33, 34). Although the use of ipecac syrup at home in children under 1 year of age has been questioned, several recent studies have demonstrated that ipecac syrup is

Table 4.2.
Development of Side Effects Possibly Related to Ipecac Administration[a]

Side Effect	Patients with Side Effect (%)	
	6–11 Months	12–35 Months
Diarrhea	25.7	25.8
Drowsiness	19.0	19.5
Irritability/hyperactivity	5.7	2.6
Coughing/choking	2.9	3.6
Diaphoresis/flushing	1.0	0.0
Fever	4.8	0.7

[a] Modified from MacLean W: A comparison of ipecac syrup and apomorphine in the immediate treatment of ingestion of protein. J Pediatr 82:121, 1973.

effective at inducing vomiting and safe in this age group (35–37).

Vomiting usually occurs about 18 min after administration of a 15- to 30-ml dose (33). The dose of syrup of ipecac is 10 ml in children under 1 year of age, 15 ml in older children, and 30 ml in adolescents and adults. Fluid administration is important, since induction of vomiting may not be successful if the stomach is nearly empty. Although milk delays vomiting from syrup of ipecac in adult volunteers (38), a recent study failed to demonstrate a delay in clinical situations involving children (39). At least 6 to 8 oz of fluid are recommended in children and 12 to 16 oz in adults. If vomiting does not occur in 15 to 20 min, the initial dose may be repeated one time. If vomiting still does not occur, the decision to lavage is based primarily on the condition of the patient and the potential danger of the ingested agent, not on the fact that the ipecac remains in the stomach.

The most common side effects of therapeutic doses of ipecac are diarrhea and mild drowsiness. The latter may be secondary to vomiting and not a direct pharmacologic effect. The adverse effects in children between 6 and 11 months of age and 12 and 35 months of age who were given ipecac syrup for a potentially toxic ingestion are summarized in Table 4.2 (35).

Protracted vomiting (persistent vomiting for longer than 3 hr after the initial episode) was seen in 4.2% of all patients. This is of concern since persistent vomiting may delay the administration of activated charcoal.

Toxic reactions with large doses of syrup of ipecac or the inadvertent use of the fluid extract of ipecac (which is 14 times stronger than ipecac syrup) have been reported. The most frequent complications are GI and cardiovascular. In large doses, ipecac is a cardiotoxin and has been shown to cause reversible depression of T waves, bradycardia, atrial fibrillation, and hypotension. Death has been reported following ingestion of as little as 10 ml of the fluid extract in a 4-year-old child (40). A 14-month-old child died following a therapeutic dose of ipecac syrup, but death was attributed to an anatomic defect (41). A fatal intracerebral hemorrhage has been reported in an 84-year-old female given ipecac syrup and activated charcoal following a nontoxic amount of boric acid (42). Fatalities have also been reported in adults with bulimia or anorexia nervosa who take large amounts chronically to lose weight (43).

Many other potential emetics could be considered for emptying the stomach in a poisoning. The majority of these agents are not recommended, however, because of lack of effectiveness or toxicity. Although subcutaneous apomorphine acts within 3 to 5 min and results in a more efficient evacuation of stomach contents than ipecac, apomorphine can produce protracted vomiting as well as CNS, respiratory, and cardiovascular depression that may not respond to naloxone (21, 44). Direct irritation of the gastric mucosa by copper and zinc sulfate produces emesis within 5 to 10 min; however, gastric emptying is not reliable, and gradual absorption from the bowel could potentially cause widespread capillary damage and kidney and liver injury. Salt water is unreliable, unpalatable, and can produce hypernatremia, convulsions, and death (45–48). Mustard water is unpalatable and ineffective. Mechanically induced emesis or gagging by stroking the pharynx with either a blunt object or a finger is considered ineffective since the percentage of people who vomit after this procedure is quite low and the mean volume of vomitus is low (49).

Children frequently vomit following the ingestion of liquid dishwashing detergents. An evaluation of liquid dishwashing detergents as emetics found them to be effective in producing vomiting (50). However, poor palatability resulted in a high rate of refusal to drink the solution; 6 of 15 patients refused it or drank only half of it, and only one of these people vomited. The use of liquid dishwashing detergent as an emetic should be limited to home-managed situations where syrup of ipecac can not be obtained within 30 min.

Gastric Lavage

Gastric lavage is a procedure in which a tube is inserted into the stomach through the nose or the mouth. The patient should be in the left lateral decubitus position with the head forward and down. The contents of the stomach are first aspirated through this tube. Fluid is instilled into the tube, allowed to mix with gastric contents, and then removed via the same tube. The process is repeated until the gastric washings are clear. The procedure usually takes 20 to 30 min to complete. Unlike emesis induction, lavage is limited to the hospital setting.

Lavage may be performed in comatose patients. The patient's airway should be protected by prior insertion of a cuffed endotracheal tube to prevent aspiration. Patients with convulsions may be lavaged after their seizures have been controlled. Lavage is contraindicated in caustic ingestions, since the lavage tube may produce additional esophageal and gastric damage as it is being passed. Initial management of a caustic ingestion is limited to dilution with milk or water followed by an evaluation of the extent and degree of burns.

The size of the lavage tube is one of the most important factors determining the effectiveness with which the stomach will be emptied. Optimally a 36 French (12 mm or about ½ inch in diameter) or larger Ewald or Lavacuator tube should be used by the oral route in adults. Nasogastric tubes usually are smaller and therefore less effective. Smaller tubes (16 to 18 French) must be used in children, markedly limiting the effectiveness of the procedure.

The lavage solution is usually tap water or a normal saline solution. In children, however, it is safer to use normal or one-half normal saline instead of water because of the child's limited tolerance for electrolyte-free solutions. Water intoxication, tonic and clonic seizures, and coma can result from a 5% increase in body water from absorption of electrolyte-free solutions. Each wash is approximately 200 to 300 ml in adults or 10 ml/kg (usually 50 to 100 ml) in children. The procedure usually requires several liters of fluid in adults.

Activated Charcoal

As the only modality to decrease GI absorption, or following emesis or lavage, activated charcoal adsorbs any of the ingested agent remaining in the GI tract. Activated charcoal is an odorless, tasteless, fine black powder that is an effective nonspecific adsorbent of a wide variety of drugs and chemicals. Two characteristics are necessary for activated charcoal to be effective: (a) small particle size and large surface area and (b) low mineral content (vegetable origin). For these reasons neither burnt toast nor charcoal tablets are effective. Activated charcoal products with higher surface areas have been developed (51). Activated charcoal has been shown to be relatively ineffective for cyanide, ethanol, methanol, caustic alkalis, and mineral acids (52).

The dose of charcoal is approximately 10 times the amount of the ingested agent. Since this does not allow for binding of tablet excipients or food to the charcoal, which decreases its adsorptive capacity, it is a good idea to give an excess of charcoal. The usual doses of activated charcoal are 60 to 100 g in adults or 15 to 30 g in children. One level measuring tablespoonful of activated charcoal contains between 5 and 6 g. If commercially packaged charcoal products are not used, the pharmacy should prepackage weighed charcoal, since the density of charcoal products may vary. Activated charcoal should be stored in tightly sealed glass or metal containers. Prolonged exposure to the atmosphere will decrease adsorptive capability.

Activated charcoal is mixed with water to the consistency of a slurry and is administered either orally or by lavage tube. Charcoal does not mix well with water and must be shaken vigorously. This is not as big a problem with commercially packaged products that contain sorbitol or a suspending agent.

Since activated charcoal adsorbs ipecac effectively, the activated charcoal must be given after vomiting from ipecac has occurred. Otherwise, vomiting may not occur and the adsorptive capacity of charcoal will be reduced.

Although generally only one dose of a cathartic is recommended, in some cases the activated charcoal is repeated. It is critically important to know whether a cathartic is present in a commercial activated charcoal product. A 55-year-old salicylate-poisoned patient inadvertently received 30 g of magnesium sulfate every 6 hr for four doses, 120 cc of 70% sorbitol for two doses, and an activated charcoal preparation containing 70% sorbitol for four doses (53). She developed an acute abdomen and died. Autopsy revealed a profoundly dilated bowel containing fluid and activated charcoal, with a perforation at the hepatic flexure. This case illustrates that when multiple doses of activated charcoal are given it is essential that an activated charcoal preparation that does not contain a cathartic be available.

Cathartics

Cathartics are used in conjunction with activated charcoal to further decrease the absorption of the ingested agent from the GI tract. By speeding the travel of gastric contents, the likelihood of absorption is decreased. A study in rats demonstrated that sodium sulfate enhanced the effect of activated charcoal in preventing the absorption of the drugs tested (54). There are no clinical studies in overdose patients to document the efficacy of cathartics, and studies in human volunteers have shown conflicting findings. Two studies in human volunteers found that cathartics had no effect on aspirin absorption when used with activated charcoal (55, 56). A study utilizing sorbitol as the cathartic demonstrated that activated charcoal and sorbitol significantly reduced aspirin absorption, compared with activated charcoal alone (57). An additional effect of cathartics has been demonstrated when the ingested agent is a sustained-release product (58).

Saline cathartics, such as magnesium sulfate and magnesium citrate, or hyperosmotic cathartics, such as sorbitol, are the agents of choice. Irritant cathartics, such as aloes or cascara, and oil-based cathartics, such as castor oil, are generally not recommended.

Magnesium sulfate is administered orally in approximately a 10% concentration at 250 mg/kg or 15 to 20 g in an adult. Magnesium sulfate is more generally available as Epsom salts or as a sterile 10 or 50% solution. Magnesium citrate is used in a dose of 200 ml in adolescents and adults or 5 ml/kg in children. The adult dose of sorbitol is usually

1 to 3 g/kg as a 35 to 70% solution, and the children's dose is 1 to 1.5 g/kg as a 35% solution.

Cathartics are administered orally or via lavage tube. If charcoal has been administered, the appearance of a charcoal stool indicates that the charcoal (and hopefully the toxic agent) has passed through the GI tract. A study in human volunteers demonstrated that sorbitol enhanced gastrointestinal transit of charcoal to a greater extent than did magnesium citrate or magnesium sulfate (59). The onset time of sorbitol is most rapid, followed by magnesium citrate, and then magnesium sulfate. These cathartics are generally considered safe. However, the patient's hydration and electrolyte balance should be monitored, especially if repeated doses of the cathartic are administered. Magnesium-containing cathartics should not be used in patients with decreased renal function, since absorbed magnesium may accumulate and produce toxicity. Hypermagnesemia has been reported following a single 17.5-g dose of magnesium citrate in a 77-year-old theophylline-intoxicated woman with poor renal function (60).

HASTENING EXCRETION

If a poison has been absorbed in potentially dangerous quantities, multiple-dose activated charcoal, forced diuresis, alteration of urine pH, dialysis, and hemoperfusion can be considered. These procedures are not warranted in most poisoned patients and do not replace good supportive care.

Multiple-Dose Activated Charcoal

Elimination via the GI tract can be augmented for drugs that are secreted into the stomach or undergo biliary secretion. The use of multiple doses of activated charcoal has also been termed "gastrointestinal dialysis." Multiple doses of activated charcoal appears to have the most promise with theophylline and phenobarbital. The excretion half-life for theophylline has been reported to increase between 50 and 75% following multiple doses of activated charcoal (61, 62). A randomized trial in patients with phenobarbital overdose demonstrated a reduction in phenobarbital half-life in the multiple-dose versus single-dose charcoal groups but found no differences in the time course or patient outcome (63). With the cyclic antidepressants, which undergo enterohepatic recycling, the effectiveness of multiple-dose charcoal has not been demonstrated convincingly (64–67).

The Poisindex system suggests multiple-dose activated charcoal for the following agents:

Amitriptyline	Cyclosporine
Atrazine	Dapsone
Carbamazepine	Desmethyldiazepam
Chlorpropamide	Dextropropoxyphene
Diazepam	Phenobarbital
Digitoxin	Phenylbutazone
Digoxin	Phenytoin
Doxepin	Prioxicam
Glutethimide	Porphyrins
Imipramine	Proscillaridin
Meprobamate	Quinine
Methotrexate	Salicylates
Nadolol	Sotalol
Nortriptyline	Theophylline

Inclusion in the above list does not necessarily imply that multiple-dose activated charcoal significantly enhances excretion, is necessary to treat poisonings with these agents, or has been adequately studied. Multiple-dose activated charcoal may play an important role for some poisonings. To evaluate its role appropriately, further study must demonstrate a positive effect in enhancing elimination of the agent and a positive effect on outcome.

In multiple-dose activated charcoal regimens, activated charcoal is administered every 4 to 6 hr. A cathartic is administered with the first dose but is generally not administered with subsequent doses. When multiple doses of cathartics have been administered, fluid and electrolyte problems, including hypernatremia and hypermagnesemia, have been reported (60, 68–71).

Alteration of Urine pH

Therapeutic maneuvers to enhance the renal elimination of drugs can be considered when managing the poisoned patient. Despite the theoretical advantages of removing the drug from the body more quickly, there are no controlled trials documenting changes in medical outcome.

Only the nonionized forms of weak acids and bases are capable of crossing membranes and being reabsorbed. For some drugs, adjusting the pH of the tubular filtrate will increase the amount of drug in the ionized form, thereby decreasing tubular reabsorption. The effectiveness of urine pH alteration will depend on the pK_a of the drug and the extent of renal elimination of active drug.

Urine alkalinization increases the renal elimination of phenobarbital (not short-acting barbiturates, such as pentobarbital and secobarbital) and salicylate. Sodium bicarbonate is administered (usually in adults 88 mEq is added to the first liter of intravenous fluid, with subsequent doses of 1 to 2 mEq/kg as needed; 2 mEq/kg is added to initial intravenous fluids in the pediatric patient and infused over 1 hr) with a goal of a urine pH of 7.0 to 8.0. An alkaline urine may be difficult to achieve in severely salicylate-poisoned children and is not recommended by some clinicians for this group (72). Tromethamine and acetazolamide are no longer recommended as alkalinizing agents because their potential toxicities may worsen the course of the intoxication.

Urine acidification increases the renal elimination of

amphetamines, phencylidine, and strychnine; however, it is no longer recommended. Overdoses with these drugs, especially phencyclidine, can produce muscle injury resulting in rhabdomyolysis and myoglobinuria, which, in the presence of an acid urine, can precipitate in the tubules, leading to acute renal failure.

Dialysis and Hemoperfusion

In the severely intoxicated patient, hemodialysis or hemoperfusion may be considered for rapid removal of certain toxins from the blood. Hemodialysis removes drugs from the blood by diffusion across a synthetic semipermeable membrane. The dialysate is replaced, continuously or intermittently, with fresh solution of carefully defined composition. This specialized technique is not available at all hospitals.

The use of dialysis in poisoning cases is limited. To be considered, the ingested agent must be dialyzable, distributed in or rapidly equilibrated with plasma water, and removed at a rate significantly higher than that of normal metabolism and renal excretion. Because a drug is dialyzable does not mean that dialysis is indicated.

Dialysis may be considered in patients who are severely intoxicated with a dialyzable drug and are not responding to conservative therapy. Dialysis may be indicated for severe intoxications with ethanol, isopropanol, lithium, phenobarbital, theophylline, and salicylates. Occasionally dialysis is considered when the ingested agent is not dialyzable but the procedure will correct hyperosmolarity or severe acid-base or electrolyte abnormalities not responding to fluid therapy.

Two examples where dialysis may be indicated before significant toxicity develops are methanol and ethylene glycol ingestion. In both cases these agents are metabolized to compounds more toxic than the originally ingested agent. Methanol is metabolized to formaldehyde and formic acid; ethylene glycol is metabolized to glyoxylate, lactate, and oxalic acid. If the methanol and ethylene glycol can be removed by dialysis before metabolism, toxicity will be reduced.

Hemoperfusion involves pumping blood from the patient through a cartridge containing coated activated charcoal, uncoated activated charcoal in a fixed bed system, or a resin. To be effective, not only must the toxin be adsorbed by the material in the column but the amount removed by hemoperfusion must significantly reduce the total body burden of the ingested agent. For some drugs that are effectively adsorbed, such as the cyclic antidepressants, a large volume of distribution results in a relatively small proportion of the total body burden being eliminated, even if the blood is completely cleared of the drug after passing through the column. Theophylline is an example of a drug for which hemoperfusion has been found to be extremely effective, producing a marked drop in blood levels and a rapid improvement in the clinical picture (73). Potential complications include bleeding, destruction of blood cells (including a significant drop in the platelet count immediately following the procedure), removal of plasma proteins, and hypothermia (74).

As with dialysis, hemoperfusion should be limited to severely intoxicated patients who have ingested a hemoperfusable drug and are not responding to conservative therapy. In most situations, aggressive supportive care should be adequate to maintain patients until their own bodies can detoxify and eliminate the toxin.

SYSTEMIC ANTIDOTES

Systemic antidotes are available for only a few commonly ingested agents. Antidotes act by a variety of mechanisms to antagonize the effects of a systemically absorbed toxin.

Antidotes do not replace supportive measures such as emptying the stomach. If an antidote is available for a particular intoxicant, specific indications should be considered before its use.

Table 4.3 lists major systemic antidotes. Naloxone, deferoxamine, digoxin immune Fab, and N-acetylcysteine are also discussed below.

NALOXONE

Naloxone is a pure opiate antagonist without opiate agonist properties. The use of nalorphine and levallorphan has been abandoned because they have both opiate agonist and antagonist properties.

Naloxone competes directly with the opiate for the receptor site, reversing CNS and respiratory depression. The antagonistic effects can be as short as 30 min but may last as long as 1 to 4 hr. It is important to note that the antagonistic action of naloxone may be shorter than the duration of action of the ingested agent, especially with methadone and diphenoxylate. It is very important that these patients be watched carefully and that naloxone boluses be readministered or a naloxone infusion be used if indicated.

Naloxone antagonizes naturally occurring and synthetic opiates, including heroin, morphine, codeine, meperidine, propoxyphene, pentazocine, diphenoxylate, and dextromethorphan. For some opiates, particularly propoxyphene, larger than usual doses of naloxone may be required. Naloxone is indicated in opiate intoxications with CNS and respiratory depression. It should also be used diagnostically along with glucose and thiamin in all comatose patients presenting to an emergency treatment facility. If given at a high enough dose, naloxone rapidly reverses any opiate-induced symptoms. Since naloxone has no opiate agonist activity, administration to patients in whom the coma is not opiate-induced will produce no adverse effects.

Table 4.3.
Major Systemic Antidotes

Antidote	Poison	Usual Dosage and Route	Comments
Atropine	Carbamate insecticides Organophosphate insecticides Other anticholinesterase	Test dose of 2 mg IV in an adult and 0.05 mg/kg in a child up to 2mg; anticholinergic symptoms will be seen only if poisoning is not present. Doses are repeated as needed (up to 2000 mg/day in severe cases), with the end point being cessation of secretions.	In severe organophosphate ingestions usually given in combination with pralidoxime.
BAL	Arsenic, gold, mercury, lead	Given by deep i.m. Dosage variable depending on the agent being chelated and severity of intoxication. Usually 3–5 mg/kg/dose.	Contraindicated in iron, cadmium, or selenium since complex is toxic. For lead, used in combination with other agents.
Cyanide antidote kit (amyl nitrite, sodium nitrite, sodium thiosulfate)	Cyanide	Amyl nitrite—breathe 30 sec of each 60 sec until sodium nitrite is ready. For adults 300 mg of sodium nitrite (10 ml) is usually given IV followed by 12.5 g of sodium thiosulfate IV. If symptoms persist, one-half the above dosage of sodium nitrite is repeated. The dose for children depends on the hemoglobin level and is included in the package literature.	Overzealous administration of sodium nitrite especially in children can produce severe methemoglobinemia.
Deferoxamine	Iron	90 mg/kg IV every 8 hours at a rate not to generally exceed 15 mg/kg/hr IV (see text). Test dose prior to obtaining serum iron level in asymptomatic patients = 90 mg/kg up to 1 g i.m. A maximum of 6.0 g in either children or adults/24 hr should not be exceeded.	Indications: serum iron ≥ 63 μmol/liter (350 μg/dl) and/or symptomatic patients. Pink-red urine indicates the presence of the deferoxamine-iron chelate; urine color change is not always present.
Digoxin immune Fab (Digibird)	Digoxin Digitoxin	Administered IV. Dose = body load (mg)/0.6 (mg per vial). See package insert for dosing. Tables based on amount ingested or levels.	Only indicated in severe cases unresponsive to standard antiarrhythmics (see text).
Diphenhydramine	Phenothiazine-induced extrapyramidal symptoms	Adults: 50 mg IV. Children: 1–2 mg/kg up to a total of 50 mg IV.	
d-Penicillamine	Copper, gold, mercury, lead, arsenic	Children: 20–100 mg/kg/day (depends on the metal being chelated). Adults: 1–1.5 g/day.	Avoid in patients with penicillin allergy. Inhibits enzymes that are pyridoxal dependent, thus pyridoxine usually given concurrently (10–25 mg/day).
Ca-EDTA	Lead, zinc, cadmium, manganese, copper	75 mg/kg/day IV or i.m. given in 3–6 divided doses for up to 5 days. May repeat course after at least 2 days.	May produce renal tubular necrosis. If decreased renal function present dialysis may be necessary to remove chelate.
Ethanol	Ethylene glycol, methanol	Ethanol is given to maintain a 22 mmol/liter (100 mg/dl) blood level. Loading dose (oral) is 0.8 ml/kg of 95% ethanol given over 30 min followed by an average maintenance dose of 0.15 ml/kg/hr p.o. Loading dose (IV) of 10% ethanol is 7.6 ml/kg IV over 30–60 min followed by an average maintenance dose of 1.4 ml/kg/hr IV. Monitor blood levels of ethanol and adjust dose accordingly.	Chronic drinkers may require higher doses and nondrinkers may require lower doses. Dose must be adjusted if dialysis is used. Glucose usually simultaneously administered.
Methylene blue	Nitrates and nitrites	0.2 ml/kg IV of a 1% solution over 5 min	
N-Acetylcysteine	Acetaminophen	140 mg/kg orally diluted 1:3 with Coke, Fresca, grapefruit juice, or water as a loading dose. Then 70 mg/kg every 4 hours for a total of 17 maintenance doses.	Intravenous use is investigational (see text).
Naloxone	Opiates	0.1 mg/kg/dose IV in children; 2–4 mg in adults (see text).	Should be given several times if no effect before ruling out opiates as the cause of symptoms. Short duration of action.
Physostigmine	Anticholinergics	Children: 0.5 mg slow IV. If no response and no cholinergic symptoms, give 0.5 mg every 5 min until a response is seen or 2 mg is reached. Repeat lowest effective trial dose if severe symptoms recur. Adults: 1–2 mg slow IV. May repeat up to 4 mg total if no response and no cholinergic symptoms. 1–4 mg may be repeated as needed for severe symptoms.	Short duration of action. Atropine should be available to reverse cholinergic effects should they occur. Must be given slowly. Of limited usefulness.
Pralidoxime	Organophosphates, severe carbamate ingestions, but not carbaryl	Adults: 1 g IV over 2 min. Children: 25–50 mg/kg slow IV. Either dose may be repeated every 8–12 hours as needed.	Given in combination with atropine. Little benefit if administered more than 36 hours after poisoning.

The usual adult dose is 0.4 to 2 mg intravenously. Doses of 0.1 mg/kg or 0.4 to 2 mg have been recommended in children. If no response is seen, the dose should be repeated. At least 10 mg total of naloxone should be administered before ruling out opiates as the cause of toxicity. A continuous infusion of naloxone can be considered after the initial bolus dose of naloxone reverses the narcotic effects if (a) long-acting agents such as methadone or diphenoxylate have been taken, (b) poorly antagonized agents such as propoxyphene have been taken, (c) large doses of naloxone were required to reverse the initial opiate effects, or (d) the naloxone must be repeated frequently to reverse recurring opiate effects. The infusion is initiated at $\frac{2}{3}$ of the naloxone bolus dose per hour. At 15 min after initiation of the infusion, half of the bolus dose should be readministered. The infusion rate is titrated against the patient's response. If the patient becomes symptomatic at a given infusion rate, symptoms should be reversed with a naloxone bolus and the infusion rate should be increased. In adults, the naloxone concentration in D_5W is adjusted to deliver the required dose in 100 ml of solution per hour.

DEFEROXAMINE

Deferoxamine is a chelating agent that binds with ferric iron. The iron-deferoxamine complex (ferrioxamine) is less toxic and more easily excreted than iron alone. Ferrioxamine produces a pink-red colored urine in some patients. A color change indicates that free iron was present and chelated. Since false negatives are possible, the absence of a urine color change does not rule out iron poisoning.

Deferoxamine should be given in iron intoxications when free iron is present in the serum. This usually occurs at serum iron levels of 63 to 90 μmol/liter (350 to 500 μg/dl) or greater. In iron-intoxicated patients whose clinical status suggests a severe iron intoxication (severe vomiting, coma, hypotension, acidosis), deferoxamine use should be considered before laboratory results are available.

Deferoxamine is generally given intravenously at a dose of 90 mg/kg every 8 hr, at a rate of 15 mg/kg/hr. At higher infusion rates hypotension may occur. Preliminary evidence suggests that higher infusion rates can be used safely if necessary in severe iron poisonings (75). In those cases where hypotension occurred, it responded to a decrease in infusion rate. Prior to obtaining laboratory results, asymptomatic patients with a history of ingestion of $\geq$60 mg/kg of elemental iron can be given a test dose of deferoxamine intramuscularly. The test dose is 90 mg/kg, up to 1 g. The maximum recommended dose is 6 g/day, although there is no evidence to support this limitation.

The most common adverse reactions to deferoxamine include generalized erythema, urticaria, and hypotension.

DIGOXIN IMMUNE Fab

Digoxin immune Fab (Digibind) can be lifesaving in digitalis glycoside poisoning (77). Digoxin immune Fab has a high binding affinity for digoxin, and the complex is excreted renally. Although digoxin immune Fab will bind digitoxin, its affinity for digitoxin is approximately $\frac{1}{10}$th that for digoxin.

Digoxin immune Fab should be considered in life-threatening digoxin or digitoxin poisoning from either acute or chronic exposure. Although serum concentrations of digoxin may be helpful in evaluating digoxin-poisoned patients, determination of whether digoxin immune Fab should be used is based on the patient's clinical status. Digoxin immune Fab is indicated in patients with life-threatening arrhythmias (e.g., ventricular arrhythmias), conduction defects or progressive bradyarrhythmias (e.g., severe sinus bradycardia), or third-degree heart block or in severe hyperkalemia resistant to treatment. Life-threatening digitalis toxicity was reversed in 21 of 26 patients in one series and 52 of 56 patients in another series with digoxin immune Fab administration (77, 78). The failures were the result of inadequate supply of digoxin immune Fab ($n = 2$), refractory low cardiac output ($n = 5$), anoxic CNS damage ($n = 1$) or multiple-drug overdose with uncertain diagnosis of digitalis toxicity ($n = 1$). A potential complication of digoxin immune Fab is heart failure in patients with intrinsically poor cardiac function who depend on the inotropic effect of digoxin.

Each vial of digoxin immune Fab contains 40 mg, which will bind 0.6 mg of digoxin or digitoxin. The dose can be determined either from the amount of digoxin or digitoxin ingested in acute poisonings or by the serum level in chronic intoxications. In general, the number of vials required equals the body load (in milligrams) divided by 0.6 (mg per vial). Tables to determine the dose in children and adults, based on either the amount ingested or the serum concentration, are included in the package insert. The total serum digoxin level will increase markedly after administration of digoxin immune Fab, but the digoxin is bound to the Fab fragment and is not toxic. The serum potassium level will drop.

N-ACETYLCYSTEINE

N-acetylcysteine is indicated for the treatment of acetaminophen poisoning. The major toxic effect of acetaminophen overdose is hepatic necrosis, which results from saturation of the enzymes in the nontoxic sulfate and glucuronide conjugation pathways and increased formation of the toxic metabolite by the cytochrome P_{450} mixed-function oxidase system. Glutathione, which detoxifies the toxic metabolite in therapeutic doses, is depleted in overdoses. The protective effect of N-acetylcysteine relates to its activity as a glutathione substitute or precursor or to enhancement of the activity of the sulfate-conjugation pathway.

N-acetylcysteine therapy should be initiated in adults with a history of ingesting ≥7.5 g of acetaminophen, in children with ≥200 mg/kg of acetaminophen, or in any patient in whom the amount ingested in unknown. N-acetylcysteine therapy can be initiated up to 24 hr postingestion but is most effective if started early. A study of 2540 patients with acetaminophen overdoses treated with oral N-acetylcysteine found that N-acetylcysteine therapy is most efficacious if initiated within 8 hr of the ingestion but that an effect on liver enzyme elevations could be demonstrated up to 24 hr postingestion (79). A plasma acetaminophen concentration should be obtained at ≥4 hr postingestion and interpreted with the modified Matthew-Rumack nomogram to determine whether to continue N-acetylcysteine. The nomogram, a semilogarithmic plot of plasma acetaminophen level vs. time, has two lines, which define the plasma acetaminophen level as "no hepatic toxicity" (below the lower line), "possible hepatic toxicity" (between the two lines), and probable hepatic toxicity (above the upper line). A 4-hr plasma acetaminophen concentration of 992 μmol/liter (150 μg/ml) is considered to be possibly hepatotoxic. A plasma acetaminophen concentration that falls at or above the lower line is an indication for the full course of N-acetylcysteine, even if the level subsequently falls below the lower line. If the initial plasma acetaminophen concentration is below the lower line, N-acetylcysteine is not necessary.

N-acetylcysteine is approved for use in the United States in an oral dosing regimen consisting of a loading dose of 140 mg/kg followed by 17 maintenance doses of 70 mg/kg. Available in a 10% or 20% concentration, the solution should be diluted to a 5% solution before the patient drinks it or it is put down a nasogastric tube.

The main side effects of N-acetylcysteine are nausea and vomiting. Patients may have difficulty retaining N-acetylcysteine, which should be readministered if the patient vomits within 1 hr of the dose. Another important consideration is the potential interaction between oral N-acetylcysteine and activated charcoal. Since in vitro and human volunteer studies on charcoal adsorption of N-acetylcysteine have reported conflicting results, the clinical importance of the interaction is unclear. Ekins found a 39% decrease in the plasma N-acetylcysteine area-under-the-curve when 140 mg/kg of N-acetylcysteine was administered 30 minutes after 100 grams of activated charcoal (80). By increasing the N-acetylcysteine dose by 40%, to compensate for its adsorption by concomitantly administered charcoal, the bioavailability of N-acetylcysteine could be assured in eight volunteers (81). These findings are preliminary. Until further data are available, 2 hr after the activated charcoal is administered, the remaining charcoal should be removed by lavage prior to administration of the loading dose of N-acetylcysteine.

In Europe and Canada, intravenous administration of N-acetylcysteine is standard, with a dosage regimen consisting of 300 mg/kg over a 20-hour period. Investigations of a 20-hr intravenous protocol and a 48-hr intravenous protocol have been conducted in the United States, but an intravenous preparation is not yet available (82).

CONCLUSION

Clinical toxicology provides a challenging opportunity for pharmacist involvement in patient care. To function effectively as an information resource, it is essential to remain up to date on new developments in this growing field. Management of the poisoned patient may involve providing supportive care, terminating the exposure, hastening excretion of the toxin, and administering antidotes. A thorough evaluation of the patient and application of these general treatment principles to the specific poisoning situation are essential for definitive treatment.

REFERENCES

1. Litovitz TL, Schmitz BF, Bailey KM: 1989 Annual Report of the American Association of Poison Control Centers National Data Collection System. Am J Emerg Med 8:394–442, 1990.
2. Anon: Vital Statistics of the United States 2(part A):298, 1990.
3. Done AK: Aspirin overdosage: incidence, diagnosis and management. Pediatrics 62(suppl):890, 1978.
4. Anon: Tabulation of 1979 Reports. Natl Clgh Poison Control Cent Bull 25:1, 1981.
5. Klein-Schwartz W, Oderda GM, Booze L: Poisoning in the elderly. J Am Geriatr Soc 31:195, 1983.
6. Manoguerra T: The status of poison control centers in the United States—1989; A report from the AAPCC. Vet Hum Toxicol 33:131–150, 1991.
7. Kinnard W: The role of the pharmacist in the control of acute poisoning. Clin Toxicol 4:659, 1971.
8. Mofenson HC, Greensher J: The unknown poison. Pediatrics 54:336, 1974.
9. Morelli HF, Rational therapy of poisoning. In Melmon KL, Morelli HF (eds): Clinical Pharmacology: Basic Principles and Therapeutics, ed. 2, New York, Macmillan, 1978, pp 1028–1051.
10. Done AK: Pharmacologic principles in the treatment of poisoning. Pharmacol Physicians 3:1, 1969.
11. Benowitz NL, Rosenberg J, Becker CE: Cardiopulmonary catastrophes in drug-overdosed patients. Med Clin North Am 63:267, 1979.
12. Lovejoy FH: Aspirin and acetaminophen: a comparative view of their antipyretic and analgesic activity. Pediatrics 62(suppl):904, 1978.
13. Yaffe SJ, Sjoquist F, Alvan G: Pharmacologic principles in the management of accidental poisoning. Pediatr Clin North Am 17:495, 1970.
14. Abdallah AH, Tye A: A comparison of the efficacy of emetics and stomach lavage. Am J Dis Child 113:471, 1967.
15. Arnold FJ Jr, Hodges JF Jr, Barta RA Jr: Evaluation of the efficacy of lavage and induced emesis in treatment of salicylate poisoning. Pediatrics 23:286, 1959.
16. Boxer L, Anderson FP, Rowe DS: Comparison of ipecac-induced emesis with gastric lavage in the treatment of acute salicylate ingestion. J Pediatr 74:800, 1969.

17. Goldstein L: Emesis vs. lavage for drug ingestion. JAMA 208:2162, 1969.

18. Auerbach PS, Osterloh J, Braun O, et al.: Efficacy of gastric emptying: gastric lavage versus emesis induced with ipecac. Ann Emerg Med 15:692, 1986.

19. Tandberg D, Diven BG, McLeod JW: Ipecac-induced emesis versus gastric lavage: a controlled study in normal adults. Am J Emerg Med 4:205, 1986.

20. Litovitz TL: Emesis versus lavage for poisoning victims. Am J Emerg Med 4:294, 1986.

21. Corby D, Decker W, Moran M, et al.: Clinical comparison of pharmacologic emetics in children. Pediatrics 42:361, 1968.

22. Corby D, Lisciandro R, Lehman R, et al.: The efficacy of methods used to evacuate the stomach after acute ingestions. Pediatrics 40:871, 1967.

23. Curtis RA, Barone J, Giacona N: Efficacy of ipecac and activated charcoal/cathartic. Prevention of salicylate absorption in a simulated overdose. Arch Intern Med 144:48, 1984.

24. Neuvonen PJ, Vartiainen M, Tokola O: Comparison of activated charcoal and ipecac syrup in prevention of drug absorption. Eur J Clin Pharmacol 24:557, 1983.

25. Kulig K, Bar-Or D, Cnatrill SV, et al.: Management of acutely poisoned patients without gastric emptying. Ann Emerg Med 14:562, 1985.

26. Albertson TE, Derlet RW, Foulke GE, et al.: Superiority of activated charcoal alone compared with ipecac and activated charcoal in the treatment of acute toxic ingestions. Ann Emerg Med 18:56–59, 1989.

27. Thomas M, Verhulst H: Ipecac syrup in antiemetic ingestions. JAMA 195:147, 1966.

28. Manoguerra AS, Krenzelok EP: Rapid emesis from high-dose ipecac syrup in adults and children intoxicated with antiemetics and other drugs. Am J Hosp Pharm 35:1360, 1978.

29. Bourianoff G: No time for ipecac. Emerg Med 3:5, 1971.

30. MacLeod J: Ipecac intoxication—use of a cardiac pacemaker in management. N Engl J Med 268:146, 1963.

31. Molinas S: A note on the use of syrup of ipecac by poison control centers. Natl Clgh Poison Control Cent Bull (March-April):4–6, 1966.

32. Ng R, Darwish H, Stewart D: Emergency treatment of petroleum distillate and turpentine ingestion. Can Med Assoc J 111:537, 1974.

33. Robertson W: Syrup of ipecac—a slow or fast emetic? Am J Dis Child 103:136, 1962.

34. MacLeon W: A comparison of ipecac syrup and apomorphine in the immediate treatment of ingestion of poison. J Pediatr 82:121, 1973.

35. Litovitz TL, Klein-Schwartz W, Oderda GM, et al.: Safety and efficacy of ipecac administration in children younger than one year of age. Pediatrics 76:761, 1985.

36. McCray EA, Bonfiglio JF, Sigell LT: Home administration of syrup of ipecac to infants. Drug Intel Clin Pharm 18:792, 1984.

37. Gaudreault P, McCormick MA, Lacouture PG, et al.: Poisoning exposures and use of ipecac in children less than 1 year old. Ann Emerg Med 15:808, 1986.

38. Varipapa RJ, Oderda GM: Effect of milk on ipecac induced emesis. N Engl J Med 296:112, 1977.

39. Grbcich PA, Lacouture PG, Lewander WJ, et al.: Does milk delay the onset of ipecac induced emesis? (abstract). Vet Hum Toxicol 28:499, 1986.

40. Bates B, Grunwaldt E: Ipecac poisoning. Am J Dis Child 103:1, 1962.

41. Robertson WO: Syrup of ipecac associated fatality: a case report. Vet Human Toxicol 21:87, 1979.

42. Klein-Schwartz W, Gorman RL, Oderda GM, et al.: Ipecac use in the elderly: the unanswered question. Ann Emerg Med 13:1152, 1984.

43. Adler AG, Walinsky P, Krall RA, et al.: Death resulting from ipecac syrup, JAMA 243:1927, 1980.

44. Schofferman J: A clinical comparison of syrup of ipecac and apomorphine use in adults. J Am Coll Emerg Physicians 5:22, 1976.

45. Laurence B, Hopkins B: Hypernatremia following a saline emetic. Med J Aust 1:1301, 1969.

46. DeGenaro F, Nyhan W: Salt—a dangerous antidote. Pediatrics 78:1048, 1971.

47. Barer J, Hill L, Hill R, et al.: Fatal poisoning from salt used as an emetic. Am J Dis Child 125:889, 1973.

48. Robertson W: A further warning on the use of salt as an emetic agent. J Pediatr 79:877, 1971.

49. Dabbous IA, Bergman AB, Robertson WO: The ineffectiveness of mechanically induced vomiting. J Pediatr 66:952, 1965.

50. Geiseker DR, Troutman WG: Emergency induction of emesis using liquid detergent product: a report of 15 cases. Clin Toxicol 18:283, 1981.

51. Cooney DO: A "superactive" charcoal for antidotal use in poisonings. Clin Toxicol 11:387, 1977.

52. Picchioni AL: Charcoal and saline laxatives for treatment of poison ingestion. Vet Hum Toxicol 21:132, 1979.

53. Brent J, Kulig K, Rumack BH. Iatrogenic death from sorbitol and magnesium sulfate during treatment for salicylism. Vet and Hum Tox 31:334, 1989 (abstract).

54. Chin L, Picchioni AL: Charcoal and saline laxatives for treatment of poison ingestion. Vet Hum Toxicol 21:132, 1979.

55. Sketris IS, Mowry JB, Czajka PA, et al.: Saline catharsis: effect on aspirin bioavailability in combination with activated charcoal. J Clin Pharmacol 22:59, 1982.

56. Easom JM, Caraccio TR, Lovejoy FH: Evaluation of activated charcoal and magnesium citrate in the prevention of aspirin absorption in humans. Clin Pharm 1:154, 1982.

57. Krenzelok EP, Heller MB: Comparison of activated charcoal and activated charcoal with sorbitol in human volunteers (abstract). Vet Hum Toxicol 28:498, 1986.

58. Goldberg MJ, Spector R, Park GD, et al.: The effect of sorbitol and activated charcoal on serum theophylline concentrations after slow-release theophylline. Clin Pharmacol Ther 41:108, 1987.

59. Krenzelok EP, Keller R, Stewart RD: Gastrointestinal transit times of cathartics combined with charcoal. Ann Emerg Med 14:1152, 1985.

60. Weber WA, Santiago R, Hypermagnesemia: a potential complication during treatment of theophylline intoxication with oral activated charcoal and magnesium-containing cathartics. Chest 95:56, 1989.

61. Berlinger WG, Spector R, Goldberg MJ, et al.: Enhancement of theophylline clearance by oral activated charcoal. Clin Pharmacol Ther 33:351, 1983.

62. Ohning BL, Reed MD, Blumer JL: Continuous nasogastric administration of activated charcoal for the treatment of theophylline intoxication. Pediatric Pharmacol 5:241, 1986.

63. Pond SM, Olson KR, Osterloh JD, et al.: Randomized study of the treatment of phenobarbital overdose with repeated doses of activated charcoal. JAMA 251:3104, 1984.

64. Goldberg MJ, Park GD, Spector R, et al.: Lack of effect of oral activated charcoal on imipramine clearance. Clin Pharmacol Ther 38:350–353, 1985.

65. Karkkainen S, Neuvonen PJ: Pharmacokinetics of amitriptyline influenced by oral charcoal and urine pH. Int J Clin Pharmacol Ther Toxicol 24:326–332, 1986.

66. Scheinin M, Virtanen R, Iisalo E: Effect of single and repeated doses of activated charcoal on the pharmacokinetics repeated doses of activated charcoal on the pharmacokinetics of doxepin. Int J Clin Pharmacol Ther Toxicol 23:38–42, 1985.

67. Swartz CM, Sherman A: The treatment of tricyclic antidepressant

overdose with repeated charcoal. J Clin Pyschopharmacol 4:336–340, 1984.

68. Caldwell JW, Nowa AJ, Dehaass DD: Hypernatremia associated with cathartics in overdose management. West J Med 147:593–596, 1987.

69. Garrelts JC, Watson WA, Sweet DE, et al.: Magnesium toxicity secondary to catharsis during management of theophylline poisoning. Am J Emerg Med 7:34–37, 1989.

70. Grean J, Woolf A: Hypermagnesemia associated with catharsis in a salicylate-intoxicated patient with anorexia nervosa. Ann Emerg Med 18:200–203, 1989.

71. McCord MM: Toxicity of sorbitol-charcoal suspension. J Pediatr III:307–308, 1987.

72. Elenbaas RM: Critical review of forced alkaline diuresis in acute salicylism. Crit Care Q 4:89, 1982.

73. Russo M: Management of theophylline intoxication with charcoal-column hemoperfusion. N Engl J Med 300:24, 1979.

74. Pond S, Rosenberg J, Benowitz NL, et al.: Pharmacokinetics of hemoperfusion for drug overdose. Clin Pharmacokinet 4:329, 1979.

75. Boehnert M, Lacouture PG, Guttmacher A, et al.: Massive iron overdose treated with high-dose deferoxamine infusion (abstract). Vet Hum Toxicol 27:291, 1985.

76. Brashares Z, Conley W: Physostigmine in drug overdoses. J Am Coll Emerg Physicians 4:46, 1975.

77. Smith TW, Butler VP, Habert E, et al.: Treatment of life-threatening digitalis intoxication with digoxin-specific Fab antibody fragments. Experience in 26 cases. N Engl J Med 307:1357, 1982.

78. Wenger TL, Butler VP, Haber E, Smith TW: Treatment of 63 severely digitalis-toxic patients with digoxin-specific antibody fragments. J Amer Coll Cardiol 5:118A–123A, 1984.

79. Smilkstein MJ, Knapp GL, Kulig KW, Rumack BH: Efficacy of oral N-acetylcysteine in the treatment of acetaminophen overdose. Analysis of the national multicenter study (1976 to 1985). N Engl J Med 319:1557, 1988.

80. Ekin BR, Ford DC, Thompson MIB, Bridges RR, Rollins DE, Jenkins RD: The effect of activated charcoal on N-acetylcysteine absorption in normal subjects. Am J Emerg Med 5:483, 1987.

81. Chamberlain JM, Gorman RL, Oderda GM, Klein-Schwartz W, Klein BL: The use of activated charcoal in a simulated poisoning with acetaminophen: a new loading dose for N-acetylcysteine. Vet Hum Toxicol 32:346, 1990 (abstract).

82. Rumack BH (ed): Poisindex Information System, Micromedex, Acetaminophen management. (1990), 66.

CHAPTER 5

CLINICAL LABORATORY TESTS AND INTERPRETATION

CHARLES F. SEIFERT, Pharm.D., J. CHRIS BRADBERRY, Pharm.D., and BETH H. RESMAN-TARGOFF, Pharm.D.

This chapter reviews routinely encountered laboratory tests not thoroughly covered in other parts of this text. Sodium, potassium, chloride, carbon dioxide content, calcium, magnesium, phosphate, and urinalysis are more than adequately covered in the chapters on fluid and electrolytes, acid-base disorders, and renal diseases. The coverage of other laboratory tests supplements the major chapters discussing their clinical application.

Patient evaluation based on information obtained through laboratory data should support a good history and physical examination. If the laboratory data do not match the history and physical examination, they should be suspect and the tests repeated. Several steps are involved in the collection, evaluation, and reporting of laboratory data. These multiple steps allow an increased chance of error. Therapeutic and management decisions may be made daily based solely on a misleading laboratory value. Examples of this error include estimations of creatinine clearances based on non-steady-state serum creatinine values, normal hematocrits in dehydrated patients, and the evaluation of total phenytoin concentrations in hypoalbuminemic patients. This chapter discusses the routinely utilized laboratory tests, including their regulation, critical ranges, clinical applications, and drug interference.

GENERAL PRINCIPLES

Specimen Collection

Blood and urine are by far the body fluids most frequently used for analytic purposes. Phlebotomists should be familiar with the test being performed and know the appropriate container for collection and how the procedure for collection affects the results. Verification that computer-printed labels match requisitions at the nurses' station and the patient's wrist band is essential. Specimens should never be drawn without first identifying the patient. Proper techniques help avoid hemolysis and bacterial contamination. Particular attention should be paid to tests where timing is important (e.g., in relation to ingestion of food or drugs). Special precautions are necessary for blood cultures and specimens obtained from indwelling catheters, especially central venous access catheters. Urine collection must also follow a very strict procedure to insure valid results. A freshly obtained specimen is crucial when testing for bilirubin, red cells, and white cells in the urine, as these undergo decomposition when standing at room temperature. Unpreserved urine specimens are also predisposed to microbial overgrowth at room temperature. A good rule for all specimens is to either deliver them to the laboratory within 1 hour of collection or refrigerate them. Proper techniques for performing each method of collection can be found in Henry J. B. (ed) *Clinical Diagnosis and Management by Laboratory Methods* (1) or other textbooks on laboratory methods.

Methods of Analysis

Several methods are available in the clinical laboratory to assay substances in body fluids. Two commonly employed techniques are chromatography and immunoassays. The type of compound to be measured determines which assay is used. Certain methods are used for qualitative measurements and others for quantitative measurements. Qualitative measurements detect only whether the substance is present and not the quantity of substance. A urine toxicology screen is an example of a qualitative test in which knowing if a substance is present is usually more important than knowing its amount.

Sensitivity and specificity are important determinants of a clinical laboratory test. Sensitivity is commonly defined as the lowest detectable value of a substance, and specificity as the ability to accurately quantitate the substance of interest in the presence of other interfering substances. Sensitivity and specificity are calculated by the formulas below.

$$\text{Sensitivity} = \frac{\text{True positives}}{\text{True positives} + \text{False negatives}} \times 100$$

$$\text{Specificity} = \frac{\text{True negatives}}{\text{True negatives} + \text{False positives}} \times 100$$

Ideally, sensitivity and specificity should each be at least 95%. The ideal analytical method depends upon several factors, including sample requirements, analysis time, sensitivity, specificity, accuracy, precision, ease of operation, versatility, and cost. Most clinical laboratories have strict performance criteria for their assay techniques. These criteria vary widely between institutions and can greatly affect the accuracy of individual patient determinations. Most clinical laboratories use the most accurate method with the best automation at a reasonable cost. For each individual clinical laboratory, particular attention to accuracy, precision, and quality control are essential for reliable reproducible results. If laboratory values do not fit with the clinical picture, laboratory personnel should check and verify these variables.

Reference Values

Normal ranges are provided as a guideline, but individual laboratories may vary considerably. Critical or treatment values are stressed throughout the chapter whenever possible. Values outside the quoted normal range may be considered abnormal but not important, whereas certain values in the normal range with a particular disease state are actually abnormal (e.g., normal hemoglobin in a patient with chronic obstructive airway disease). Laboratories may evaluate substances with different assays, which are more or less precise. Certain tests are time-dependent, and the time the sample is drawn is crucial in determining if the patient sample is truly within the reference range. This is especially true for most serum drug concentrations. Most of the normal reference ranges quoted in this chapter are taken from Wallach J.: *Interpretation of Diagnostic Tests* (2).

Drug Interference

Medications affect laboratory test results in two major ways. Because of a drug's intrinsic pharmacokinetic, pharmacologic, or toxicologic properties, it may alter the formation, regulation, release, or elimination of the substance being tested (e.g., hydrochlorothiazide blocking the tubular secretion of uric acid, exogenous insulin effects on serum glucose, or toxic acetaminophen concentrations on serum transaminases). The medication may also interfere directly with the assay used to detect the substance (e.g., ascorbic acid causing a false-negative result with urine glucose determination by the glucose oxidase method). Each laboratory test discussion in this chapter includes a brief section on common medications that affect the test results.

Système Internationale d'Unités (SI units)

Since 1975, when the U.S. Congress passed the metric conversion act, this country has been very gradually converting from conventional units to SI units. The impetus to convert all measurements of substances in body fluids to a molar concentration unit was based on the fact that substances in the body interact on a molar basis. It would also standardize units internationally. Several societies, including the American Medical Association and the American College of Physicians, and their official journals (*JAMA* and *Annals of Internal Medicine*) have adopted SI units as their sole reference standard. Other journals still accept both sets of units. Reference laboratories in most hospitals and most clinicians in the United States have not accepted this change willingly and still use the old conventional reference standards. For each laboratory test in this chapter, both conventional units and SI units with conversion factors will be given.

LABORATORY TESTS

SERUM CREATININE, SCr

(males = 0.6–1.3 mg/dl, females 0.1 mg/dl lower; SI = 50–110 μmol/liter, conversion factor [CF] = 88.40)

Creatinine is an amino acid formed as a waste product of creatine, an important energy storage substance in muscle metabolism. Creatinine is an anhydride of creatine and is not utilized in the body (3). Formation of creatinine is relatively constant, with about 1 to 2% of creatine transformed to creatinine each 24 hours (Fig. 5.1). This in turn depends on the total muscle content of creatine and creatine phosphate. The serum concentration of creatinine is also relatively constant, and urinary excretion is the result of glomerular filtration, with only a small amount excreted by active tubular secretion.

Factors that affect creatine levels, such as diet, fever, and muscle damage, do not readily influence the serum creatinine level. Since serum creatinine production is relatively constant and excretion is primarily by glomerular filtration, the serum creatinine level is a good index of renal function and is a more reliable indicator of renal function than the blood urea nitrogen (BUN).

Serum creatinine concentration increases in the presence of impaired renal function. Since up to 50% of renal function is lost before the serum creatinine level becomes abnormally elevated, it is not a good indicator of early renal dysfunction. Creatinine clearance based on 24-hour urinary excretion of creatinine is the most reliable clinically available test to evaluate glomerular filtration. Several methods exist for the rapid estimation of creatinine clearance, based on the patient's age, ideal body weight, and serum creatinine level. The methods are discussed in more detail in the Chapters 19, "Renal Diseases" and 1, "Clinical Pharmacokinetics." A steady-state serum creatinine level is necessary for an accurate estimation. Certain methods are more inaccurate in the elderly and in patients with decreased muscle mass (4). Other causes of increased serum creatinine concentration include ingestion of creatinine in the diet, muscle disease, acromegaly, and pre- and postrenal azotemia. Decreases in serum creatinine concentration are usually not clinically significant, but they can occur as an artifact when the serum bilirubin is markedly elevated.

Drugs that may cause an increased serum creatinine level by interference with tubular secretion of creatinine are acetohexamide, cephalosporins, cimetidine, salicylates, and trimethoprim. Drugs such as ascorbic acid, levodopa,

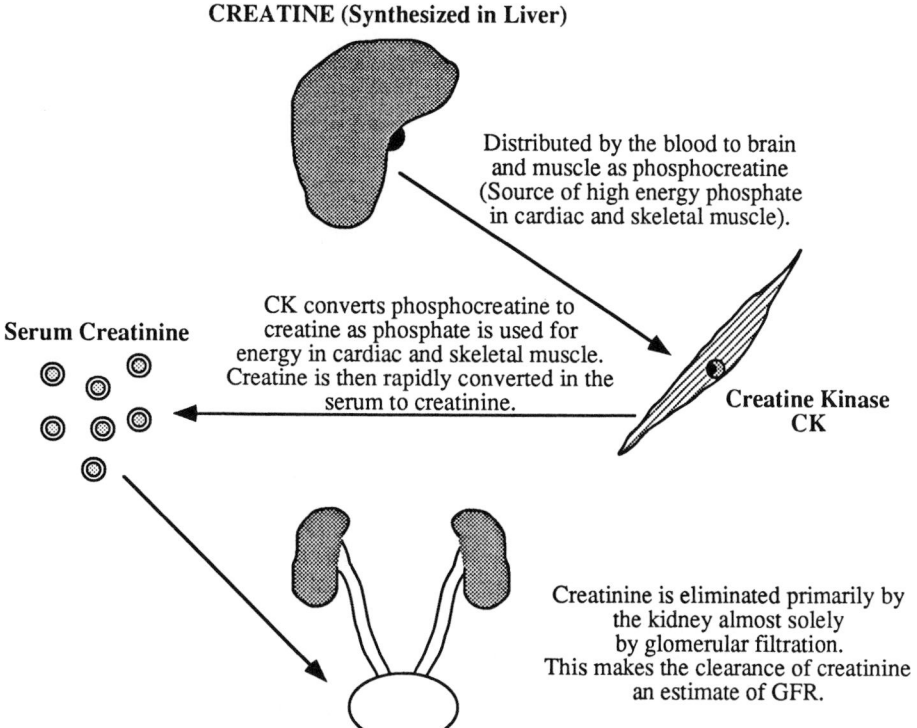

CREATINE (Synthesized in Liver)

Distributed by the blood to brain
and muscle as phosphocreatine
(Source of high energy phosphate
in cardiac and skeletal muscle).

Serum Creatinine

CK converts phosphocreatine to
creatine as phosphate is used for
energy in cardiac and skeletal muscle.
Creatine is then rapidly converted in the
serum to creatinine.

**Creatine Kinase
CK**

Creatinine is eliminated primarily by
the kidney almost solely
by glomerular filtration.
This makes the clearance of creatinine
an estimate of GFR.

Figure 5.1. Creatinine production.

p-aminohippurate, and PSP may cause increases by interference with the analytical methodology of the serum creatinine determination (2).

BLOOD UREA NITROGEN, BUN
(5–25 mg/dl; SI = 1.8–8.9 mmol/liter; CF = 0.357)

Urea is the predominant end product of protein and amino acid catabolism and is made in the liver through the urea cycle. It is the main nonprotein nitrogen (NPN) constituent in the blood. Other NPN substances include amino acids, uric acid, creatinine, and ammonia. Total NPN determinations are no longer used clinically. Urea is distributed to all intra- and extracellular fluids and is freely diffusible across most cell membranes (3). Urea is excreted mostly by the kidneys, with only small amounts excreted in sweat and in the intestines.

When there is a large increase of nonprotein compounds such as urea in the blood, the condition of azotemia is present. Azotemia can be categorized as prerenal, renal, or postrenal. Prerenal azotemia is the result of inadequate perfusion of kidneys with otherwise normal renal function. Causes of prerenal azotemia include dehydration, decreased blood volume, shock, and heart failure. Renal azotemia refers to decreased glomerular filtration as a result of acute or chronic renal disease. Postrenal azotemia is most commonly the result of urinary tract obstruction. There are two analytical procedures for the determination

of urea nitrogen, a direct colorimetric method and an indirect enzymatic procedure. The enzymatic method is used today on most automated analyzers (3).

BUN can be used as a rough guide to renal function. As with creatinine levels, a clinically important elevation will not be observed until glomerular filtration is decreased by at least 50%. A decreased BUN is usually not clinically important; however, a few conditions may cause a decrease. These include poor nutrition, high fluid intake, and severe liver disease where urea synthesis is decreased. Drugs that may increase BUN by methodologic interference are chloral hydrate, chloramphenicol, ammonium salts, aminophenol, asparagine, acetohexamide, and sulfonylureas, and those that decrease it are chloramphenicol, and streptomycin (2).

BUN and serum creatinine concentrations may be evaluated simultaneously. To give more information than either alone, the BUN is divided by the SCr. This is termed the BUN:creatinine ratio; the normal ratio ranges from 40 to 60:1. Table 5.1 indicates clinical causes of elevated BUN and serum creatinine with increased or normal BUN:creatinine ratios.

PLASMA GLUCOSE

(fasting 60–100 mg/dl; SI units = 3.3–5.6 mmol/liter; however normal ranges depend on the method; CF = 0.05551)

Table 5.1.
BUN:Creatinine Ratio in Clinical Conditions with Elevated BUN and Serum Creatinine

≥60:1	Prerenal azotemia (e.g., heart failure, dehydration)
	Postrenal azotemia (e.g., obstructive uropathy)
	Impaired renal function plus excess protein intake or tissue breakdown
	Drugs such as tetracycline and glucocorticosteroids
<60:1	Prerenal azotemia in hepatic cirrhosis
	Renal dialysis
	Renal failure in muscular patients
	Decreased urea production (e.g., low protein intake, severe diarrhea or vomiting)

Laboratory determinations of glucose level are usually performed on venous plasma specimens. Whole blood determinations are used only for capillary blood in fingerstick devices. Serum and plasma glucose concentrations are identical and are 10 to 15% higher than whole blood measurements. Glucose is one of the clinically important carbohydrates along with fructose and galactose. Disorders of carbohydrate metabolism such as diabetes are evaluated in part by measurement of plasma glucose in either the fasting state or after suppression or stimulation. The concentration of glucose in the blood is regulated within narrow limits by hormones produced by the pancreas as well as through other mechanisms mediated by the adrenergic and cholinergic nervous systems (5). Glucose is a major source of energy for brain, muscle, and fat. The brain is the only tissue not requiring insulin for glucose utilization. If glucose is not available exogenously (fasting state), the body, through hormonal mechanisms (counter-regulatory hormones: glucagon, epinephrine, cortisol, and somatostatin), will form its own glucose by tissue and hepatic gluconeogenesis and hepatic glycogenolysis. Glucose is therefore carefully regulated by glucagon and insulin secretion, which compensate for food ingestion and fasting. (Please refer to Chapter 17, "Diabetes Mellitus" for a detailed discussion of carbohydrate metabolism in normal and diabetic patients.)

Methods for clinical determination of glucose are either chemical or enzymatic. Chemical analysis is based on the reducing properties of glucose and utilizes a color change reaction that is measured spectrophotometrically. The enzymatic method is based on the reaction of glucose and glucose oxidase. This is a very specific method and is generally inexpensive. Ascorbic acid can interfere with this method and produce decreased values.

Elevated plasma glucose concentrations, or hyperglycemia, can be caused by a number of syndromes and diseases. The classification of hyperglycemia is shown in Table 5.2 (5). A fasting plasma glucose of 7.7 mmol/liter (140 mg/ml) or greater is considered abnormal.

Hypoglycemia is a syndrome of low plasma glucose with related symptoms. In the adult an overnight fasting plasma glucose below 2.5 mmol/liter (45 mg/dl) is considered abnormal, and one above 3.0 mmol/liter (55 mg/dl) is considered normal. In neonates less than 1.9 mmol/liter (35 mg/dl) is abnormal, and in infants and children less than 2.5 mmol/liter (45 mg/l) is abnormal. Table 5.3 shows the classification of common causes of hypoglycemia (5).

URIC ACID

(males = 4.0–8.5 mg/dl, SI units = 240–510 μmol/liter; females = 3.0–7.5 mg/dl, SI units = 180–450 μmol/liter; CF = 59.48) (See Chapter 30 "Gout and Hyperuricemia.")

Uric acid is the end product of purine metabolism. The major rate-limiting step in the synthesis of uric acid is the intracellular concentration of 5-phosphoribosyl-1-pyrophosphate (PRPP). Uric acid serves no biologic func-

Table 5.2.
Classification of Hyperglycemia

Primary
  Insulin-dependent diabetes mellitus
  Non-insulin-dependent diabetes mellitus
Secondary
  Hyperglycemia resulting from disease of the pancreas
    Inflammation
      Acute pancreatitis (rare)
      Chronic pancreatitis
      Pancreatitis due to mumps
      ? Cell damage due to coxsackievirus B_4 infection
      ? Autoimmune disease
    Pancreatectomy
    Pancreatic infiltration
      Hemochromatosis
      Tumors
    Trauma to pancreas (rare)
  Hyperglycemia related to other major endocrine diseases
    Acromegaly
    Cushing's syndrome
    Thyrotoxicosis
    Pheochromocytoma
    Hyperaldosteronism
    Glucagonoma
    Somatostatinoma
  Hyperglycemia caused by drugs
    Steroids
    Thiazide diuretics, β-blockers, phenytoin, and diazoxide
    Oral contraceptives
    Alloxan and streptozotocin
  Hyperglycemia related to other major disease states
    Chronic renal failure
    Chronic liver disease
    Infection
  Miscellaneous hyperglycemia
    Pregnancy
    Related to insulin-receptor antibodies (acanthosis nigricans)

Table 5.3.
Classification of Common Causes of Hypoglycemia

No anatomic lesion present
  Fasting plasma glucose normal
    Reactive hypoglycemia
      Functional hypoglycemia
      Alimentary hypoglycemia
      Diabetic and impaired glucose tolerance
  Fasting plasma glucose low
    Drug-induced hypoglycemia
      Sulfonylureas
      Phenformin
      Insulin
      Ethanol
      Salicylates
      Combinations of the above
    Factitious—fasting glucose normal or low
Anatomic lesion present
  Insulinoma
  Extrapancreatic neoplasms
  Adrenocortical insufficiency
  Hypopituitarism
  Massive liver disease

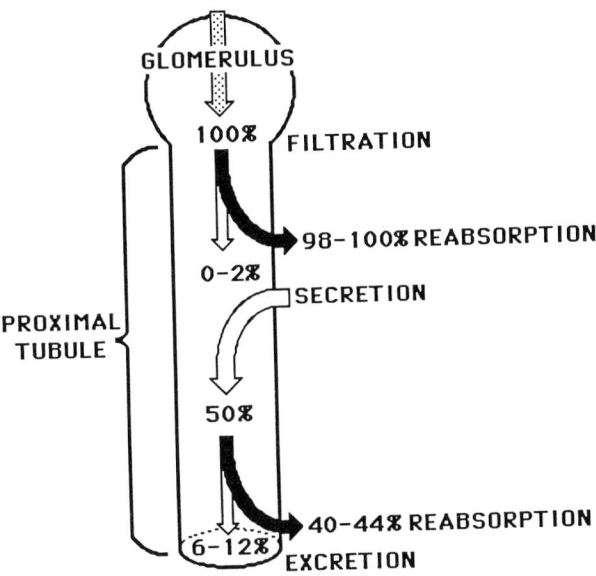

Figure 5.2.   Uric acid excretion.

tion. Approximately two-thirds of uric acid is excreted renally and one-third through the gastrointestinal tract. Assuming that the uric acid filtered through the glomerulus equates to 100%, 98 to 100% of this glomerular filtrate is reabsorbed in the proximal portion of the proximal convoluted tubule (Fig. 5.2) (6). Fifty percent of the original amount is secreted into the distal portion of the proximal convoluted tubule but 40 to 44% is subsequently reab-

sorbed, and 6 to 12% of the original glomerular filtrate eventually excreted.

Hyperuricemia is due to either an overproduction of uric acid (increased destruction of nucleoproteins, high protein diets, or inborn enzymatic defects) or an underexcretion (renal defect). Since the serum is saturated with urate at a concentration of 416 μmol/liter (7 mg/dl), as serum urate concentrations exceed this saturation point, monosodium urate crystals deposit in and around the joints and cartilage and in the kidneys, sometimes eliciting the disease known as gout. As urinary pH is increased, the solubility of uric acid is increased; decreasing urinary pH may precipitate urate nephrolithiasis in patients with high urine uric acid concentrations. Asymptomatic hyperuricemia is classified as an elevated serum uric acid without symptoms of acute gouty arthritis (6). With increasing uric acid levels, there is an increased risk of developing acute gout. There is a 2.0 to 4.1% 5-year cumulative incidence of gouty arthritis in adult males with prior serum urate levels ranging from 416 to 529 μmol/liter (7.0 to 8.9 mg/dl) as compared with a 5-year cumulative incidence of 0.5 to 0.6% with prior serum urate levels of $\leq$410 μmol/liter ($\leq$6.9 mg/dl). The incidence of gouty arthritis increases tremendously as urate levels rise above 535 μmol/liter (9.0 mg/dl). The 5-year cumulative incidence for adult males with prior serum urate levels of 535 to 589 μmol/liter (9.0 to 9.9 mg/dl) and $\geq$595 μmol/liter ($\geq$10.0 mg/dl) were 19.8% and 30.5%, respectively (7). After one attack of gout, a patient may never have another or may have a recurrence from 3 to 42 years later (mean = 11.4 years) (7).

Agents that have a cytotoxic effect causing an increased turnover of nucleic acids may increase uric acid concentrations (e.g., antimetabolite and chemotherapeutic agents used to treat neoplastic diseases, such as methotrexate, busulfan, vincristine, prednisone, and azathioprine) (2). Agents that decrease the renal clearance or block tubular secretion may cause a substantial elevation in serum urate concentrations (e.g., thiazide and loop diuretics, pyrazinamide, and ethambutol). Diuretic-induced hyperuricemia accounts for 95% of acute attacks of gout in women over 60 years of age and 56% of men (8). Some agents, such as salicylates, probenecid, sulfinpyrazone, and phenylbutazone, inhibit the tubular secretion of urate at low doses, but at high doses also inhibit tubular reabsorption, inducing a marked uricosuric effect (3). Allopurinol therapeutically lowers serum uric acid by inhibiting xanthine oxidase (enzyme that converts xanthine to uric acid in purine metabolism), while uricosuric agents such as probenecid are also used therapeutically to lower serum uric acid by blocking proximal tubular reabsorption. Ascorbic acid, glucose, levodopa, methyldopa, and theophylline may interfere with the analytical technique and cause false high results (2, 3).

Enzymes

Enzymes are located all body tissues and are responsible for the organic catalytic conversion of chemicals throughout the body. When enzymatically active cells are lysed or destroyed, certain enzymes are released into the serum. These enzymes are measured to assess which tissue is damaged. Only active cells release high quantities of enzymes in the serum. The more acute and extensive tissue injury is, the greater the rise in enzymes released from that tissue. Chronic smoldering damage causes moderate release of similar enzymes, with patterns usually different than those in acute injury.

Isoenzymes are proteins with different amino acid sequences, arising primarily from different tissues, which have the same enzymatic action. Clinically these isoenzyme fractions are used to determine which tissue is damaged, and through their particular patterns clinical diagnoses are made. Isoenzymes are usually separated by gel electrophoresis. For example, creatine kinase has two enzymatic subunits, MM and BB. BB is found predominantly in brain and travels very rapidly to the anode, whereas MM, which is predominantly found in skeletal muscle, moves very slowly toward the anode (9). Even though the two isoenzymes have the same enzymatic activity, they are of different sizes and electronegativity and predominate in different tissues.

Enzymatic units are determined on a micromolar catalytic basis. One international unit (IU) is the amount of enzyme that catalyzes the conversion of one micromole of substrate per minute. The SI unit for enzymatic activity is known as the katal (kat). One katal is equal to one mole catalyzed per second (9). One μkat is equal to one micromole of substrate catalyzed per second, therefore, one μkat = 60 IU.

CREATINE KINASE, CK

(0–130 IU/liter, SI = 0–2.17 μkat/liter, however, normal ranges vary considerably with method, CF = 0.0167)

Creatine kinase (CK), formerly known as creatine phosphokinase, catalyzes the conversion of phosphocreatine to creatine, releasing high-energy phosphate to skeletal and cardiac muscle (Fig. 5.1). Creatine is an unstable molecule and is converted very rapidly to creatinine. CK is a dimer consisting of two subunits, M and B. Brain tissue yields approximately 90% BB (CK_1) and 10% MM (CK_3), cardiac tissue yields approximately 40% MB (CK_2) and 60% MM, whereas normal serum contains virtually 100% MM as does skeletal muscle. Clinical conditions causing elevated serum CK primarily involve skeletal muscle or cardiac tissue. The brain fraction is almost never observed in serum, even after a cerebrovascular accident, since the enzyme does not readily cross the blood-brain barrier (9).

Almost any damage to skeletal muscle will cause an elevation in serum CK. Severe acute rhabdomyolysis secondary to trauma, prolonged coma, or overdoses of various drugs may cause dramatic rises in CK, ranging from 167 to 1670 μkat/liter (10,000 to 100,000 IU/liter) (10). Other conditions damaging skeletal muscle, such as progressive muscular dystrophy, polymyositis/dermatomyositis, delirium tremens, seizures, or hypothyroidism, may cause significant elevations in CK.

CK is the first enzyme to increase in an acute myocardial infarction (MI). Serum concentrations begin to rise approximately 4 to 8 hours after the acute event, peak at 12 to 24 hours, and may persist throughout the initial 72-hour period (11). An MB fraction greater than 6% of the total is indicative of myocardial injury (12). Several studies have shown that patients with a history of angina compatible with acute MI in whom total peak CK serum concentrations were normal, but MB isoenzyme fractions were greater than 6% of the total had true acute microinfarctions (13–18).

Intramuscular injections of medications may cause a variable increase in CK of two to six times the normal concentration. These elevations return to normal within 48 hours after cessation of the injections. CK rises in over 50% of patients receiving countershock or defibrillation but usually returns to normal in 48 to 72 hours (2). Several medications have been reported to cause rhabdomyolysis in therapeutic and overdose situations, including opiates, cocaine, phencyclidine, amphetamines, theophylline, antihistamines, fibric acid derivatives, barbiturates, aminocaproic acid, certain antibiotics, chloroquine, colchicine, corticosteroids, and vincristine (10). Patients receiving therapeutic doses of neuroleptics may rarely experience the neuroleptic malignant syndrome, which may cause severe elevations in CK (19). Lovastatin has also been reported to cause severe rhabdomyolysis alone (0.5%) or in combination with gemfibrozil (5%), niacin, cyclosporin (as high as 30%), and erythromycin (20).

LACTATE DEHYDROGENASE, LDH

(100–190 IU/liter, SI units = 1.67–3.17 μkat/liter, CF = 0.0167)

Lactate dehydrogenase (LDH) catalyzes the conversion of pyruvate to lactate anaerobically to generate ATP (21). LDH is in high concentration in cardiac and skeletal muscle, liver, kidney, lung parenchyma, and erythrocytes. It is essential to have prompt analysis of the sample, which has to be hemolysis-free for an accurate LDH measurement. LDH can be separated into five distinct components. The five LDH isoenzymes are all approximately the same molecular weight but have different charges. LDH_5 has the greatest mobility and LDH_1 the least. Table 5.4 lists the LDH isoenzymes and their relative activity in each tissue (9).

Serum LDH concentration almost always increases after an acute MI. The serum LDH level begins to rise

Table 5.4.
Lactate Dehydrogenase (LDH) Isoenzymes Nomenclature[a]

Nomenclature of Isoenzyme Starting with Most Anodic	Composition: Proportion of Monomers[b] in Each Isoenzyme	Relative Content[c] of Isoenzyme						
		Lung	Myocardium	Liver	Skeletal Muscle	Brain	Kidney	RBC
1	HHHH	+	+ + + +	±	±	+ +	+	+ + +
2	HHHM	+ + +	+ + + +	±	±	+ +	+	+ + +
3	HHMM	+ + + +	+	+	+	+ +	+ +	+
4	HMMM	±	±	+ +	+ +	+ +	+ +	±
5	MMMM	±	±	+ + + +	+ + +	±	+ +	±

[a] From Zimmerman HJ, Henry JB, Clinical enzymology. In Henry JB: Clinical Diagnosis and Management by Laboratory Methods, ed. 17. Philadelphia, WB Saunders, 1984, pp 251–282.
[b] Monomer H (myocardial); monomer M (skeletal muscle).
[c] Content graded from ±, which represents almost no activity, to + + + +, which represents high activity.

10 to 12 hours after the acute event, reaching a peak in 48 to 72 hours, with prolonged elevation for up to 10 to 14 days (2). An increased serum LDH level, with LDH_1 greater than LDH_2 (flipped enzymes), occurs in acute myocardial infarction in approximately 80% of patients, but also occurs in acute renal infarction, pernicious anemia, and hemolysis (2). In a large myocardial infarction with biventricular failure, LDH_5 levels may also be elevated because of liver congestion.

LDH_5 levels may be markedly increased in hepatitis and may also be increased in other hepatic disorders. LDH elevations may occur 50% of the time in malignant tumors, usually with a nonspecific isoenzyme pattern. LDH is elevated in approximately 60% of patients with lymphomas and 90% of patients with leukemias. Marked increases in LDH_5 levels are seen in patients with skeletal muscle damage, including extensive burns and trauma. Pulmonary embolus and infarction may cause elevations in LDH_2 and LDH_3; if cor pulmonale is present, LDH_5 will also rise. In nephrotic syndrome, LDH_4 and LDH_5 will rise, but in nephritis and renal infarction LDH_1 and LDH_2 rise. All forms of hemolysis, including sickle cell crisis and drug-induced hemolysis, will cause elevations in LDH_1 and LDH_2 levels (22, 23).

All drugs causing damage to the above-mentioned tissues cause elevations in LDH. Hepatotoxic agents and agents inducing hemolysis will increase serum LDH concentrations (23, 24).

ASPARTATE AMINOTRANSFERASE, AST

(males = 8–46 IU/liter, SI units = 0.13–0.77 μkat/liter; females = 7–34 IU/liter, SI units = 0.12–0.57 μkat/liter; CF = 0.0167)

Aspartate aminotransferase (AST), formerly known as serum glutamic oxaloacetic transaminase (SGOT), is one of several transaminases responsible for transfer of amino groups in gluconeogenesis. AST is responsible for transferring an amino group from aspartate to α,β-glutaric acid, forming glutamate and oxaloacetate (21). The highest concentrations of AST are located in cardiac and hepatic tissues.

AST is the second enzyme to increase after an acute MI, usually appearing within 6 to 8 hours after onset, peaking in 24 hours, and returning to baseline in 4 to 6 days (2). AST levels rise in virtually all types of hepatic diseases. Its peak concentration and ratio to other enzymes reflect the type of hepatic damage. These differences will be discussed later, under hyperbilirubinemia.

Several medications may cause elevations in AST levels because of either direct hepatocellular damage or cholestasis (24). Anticholinergics and opioids cause elevation of transaminase levels because of spasm of the sphincter of Oddi (25). Several agents (commonly isoniazid and rifampin) may cause transient elevations in transaminase levels (24, 26, 27). Initially, dye-binding techniques were used to assay for transaminases, which accounted for several drug interferences including isoniazid, but with newer ultraviolet techniques very little interacts with the assay (25).

ALANINE AMINOTRANSFERASE, ALT

(males = 7–46 IU/liter, SI units = 0.12–0.77 μkat/liter; females = 4–34 IU/liter, SI units = 0.07–0.58 μkat/liter; CF = 0.0167)

Alanine aminotransferase (ALT), formerly known as serum glutamate pyruvate transaminase (SGPT), transfers an amino group from alanine to α-ketoglutarate, forming glutamate and pyruvate (21). ALT is very specific for hepatic tissue and is almost always absent in acute myocardial infarction. It is much more sensitive to hepatic damage, and levels rise faster and higher than those of AST in most types of hepatocellular damage.

γ-GLUTAMYL TRANSPEPTIDASE, GGTP

(males = 9–69 IU/liter, SI units = 0.15–1.15 μkat/liter; females = 3–33 IU/liter, SI units = 0.05–0.55 μkat/liter; CF = 0.0167) γ-Glutamyl transpeptidase (GGTP) catalyzes the transfer of a γ-glutamyl group from one peptide to another (21). The kidneys, liver, and pancreas contain large quantities of GGTP. Several isoenzymes of GGTP have been isolated, but to date, no clinical utility for them has been found (9).

The elevation of GGTP level parallels that of alkaline phosphatase and rises higher in cholestatic and obstructive diseases than in acute hepatocellular diseases. It is always elevated in acute pancreatitis, and its rise is faster and greater than that of alkaline phosphatase in obstructive jaundice. GGTP is the most sensitive biochemical indicator of alcohol exposure, since elevation exceeds that of other commonly monitored liver enzymes. In alcoholic hepatitis, GGTP is usually the enzyme that increases fastest and has the highest peaks. Agents such as phenytoin and phenobarbital which induce the cytochrome P-450 enzyme system may cause increases in GGTP (2).

PHOSPHATASES

Phosphatases are primarily responsible for catalyzing cleavage of monophosphate esters and may be acid or alkaline (21). Acid phosphatases have optimal enzymatic activity at a pH of 5, and alkaline phosphatases have an optimal enzymatic activity at a pH of 9 (9). Acid phosphatase (0.2–11.0 IU/liter, SI units = 3–183 μkat/liter; CF = 16.67) is primarily found in prostate, erythrocytes, and platelets. Approximately 60–75% of men with prostate cancer have elevated acid phosphatase concentrations (2).

Alkaline phosphatase (ALP), (25–100 IU/liter, SI units = 0.4–1.7 μkat/liter; CF = 0.0167) is found in most tissues but is derived predominantly from hepatic, osseous, and intestinal cells (2). The placenta produces high concentrations of ALP in the third trimester as a result of high fetal osteoblastic activity. Children in the active growth phase produce ALP at two to five times adult rates. Serum isoenzymes may be separated through electrophoresis on acrylamide gel, however, this technique is not widely available clinically, and separation of osseous and hepatic isoenzymes is still difficult with this technique (9). Heating serum to 56°C will inactivate 90% of the osseous isoenzyme, and separation of the hepatic and osseous isoenzymes is readily achieved clinically by this method.

ALP is increased in most disorders of bone involving osteoblastic activity. Metastatic disease to bone may cause substantial elevations in ALP levels. ALP is also increased in acute fractures, hyperparathyroidism, osteogenic sarcoma, and Paget's disease (9).

ALP is secreted into bile, and an elevation in enzyme level may be the first clue to intra- and extrahepatic cholestasis (12, 28). Intra- and extrahepatic disease cannot be separated by the peak height of the serum ALP concentration (28). When biliary obstruction is complete, ALP serum concentrations are almost always three to eight times normal; whereas, in incomplete obstruction, concentrations are only two to three times normal (29).

AMYLASE

(60–160 Somogyi units/dl; 111–296 IU/liter; SI units = 1.86–4.96 μkat/liter; CF: Somogyi to IU = 1.85, Somogyi to SI = 0.031)

Amylase enzymatically cleaves large polysaccharides into oligo- and monosaccharides in the gastrointestinal tract, through salivary and pancreatic stimulation. Amylase is present as α-, β-, and γ-amylase, but only α-amylase is of clinical interest. Amylase is present in a variety of human tissues including the pancreas, salivary glands, muscle, adipose tissue, kidney, brain, lung, fallopian tubes, intestine, spleen, and heart (30). Normal serum amylase is composed of approximately 40% pancreatic isoenzyme (P-type isoamylase) and 60% salivary isoenzyme (S-type isoamylase) (31). This percentage changes with age, so that after the age of 70, P-type isoamylase comprises only 20% of total serum amylase (30).

Serum amylase concentration rises within 6 to 48 hours after the onset of acute pancreatitis in over 80% of patients (31). Values over four times the upper limit of normal are highly suggestive of the diagnosis (30). This is a sensitive measure of acute pancreatitis, but it is not highly specific, since several other conditions may present with acute abdominal pain and elevated serum amylase levels, including biliary colic, perforated peptic ulcer, and mesenteric infarction (31). In acute pancreatitis, the urinary clearance of amylase is increased, possibly because of altered renal tubular function. A urinary amylase to creatinine ratio greater than 0.04 suggests acute pancreatitis; however, this method is unreliable, since elevated ratios may also be seen with other conditions, such as burns, renal insufficiency, and ketoacidosis (30, 31). The usefulness of isoenzyme separation is limited because other intestinal sources also account for P-type isoamylase. Patients with acute alcoholic pancreatitis have normal serum amylase levels approximately 30% of the time (31).

Parotitis and mumps cause increases of S-type isoamylase. Chronic alcohol consumption may also increase S-type isoamylase. This is an important consideration because alcohol is the most common cause of acute pancreatitis. Macroamylase is a circulating complex of normal amylase bound to either IgG or IgA (30). Analysis of macroamylase reveals variable amounts of both P-type and S-type isoamylase. Macroamylasemia is an acquired benign condition that must be separated from other causes of hyperamylasemia.

Medications that cause spasm of the sphincter of Oddi, such as narcotics and cholinergic agents, may cause increases in serum amylase (2). Agents that precipitate acute pancreatitis include azathioprine, estrogens, thiazide diuretics, furosemide, sulfonamides, and tetracycline. With all of these agents, acute pancreatitis occurred within approximately 2 weeks to 4 months after initiating therapy (32). Certain pancreatic enzyme preparations contain amylase and lipase, which may elevate serum amylase and lipase values (2).

LIPASE

(0–1.5 Cherry-Crandal units/ml; 0–417 IU/liter; SI units = 0–6.95 μkat/liter; CF: Cherry-Crandal to IU = 278, Cherry-Crandal to SI = 4.63)

Lipase hydrolyzes glycerol esters of long-chain fatty acids at the 1 and 3 positions, producing β-monoglyceride and two moles of free fatty acid. Serum lipase should not be confused with lipoprotein lipase; these are entirely different enzymes. Lipase is located in stomach, intestine, leukocytes, fat cells, and milk but predominates in the pancreas (30). Serum lipase concentrations are usually elevated in patients with acute pancreatitis and are more predictive than amylase, but technical difficulty in measurement because of the long incubation period limits widespread clinical use (30, 31). Serum lipase increases at approximately the same time as amylase in acute pancreatitis, but the elevations in concentration may persist for

much longer than those of serum amylase. Serum lipase concentrations may also be elevated in other acute abdominal illnesses (31). Medications that may elevate serum lipase concentrations are very similar to those that elevate serum amylase.

Bilirubin

(Total <1.5 mg/dl, direct <0.5 mg/dl; SI units = total <26 μmole/liter, direct <8.6 μmole/liter, CF = 17.1)

Bilirubin is a metabolic byproduct of the lysis of erythrocytes by the reticuloendothelial system (Fig. 5.3). The reticuloendothelial system catabolizes hemoglobin into free iron, globin, and biliverdin, which is rapidly converted to bilirubin. Unconjugated bilirubin is poorly soluble in serum, therefore it is transported to the liver bound to albumin. This unconjugated form is also known as indirect or prehepatic bilirubin. In the liver, glucuronyl transferase conjugates bilirubin with two molecules of glucuronic acid, forming bilirubin diglucuronide (29). This form of bilirubin is highly soluble in serum and is known as direct or hepatic bilirubin. Direct bilirubin is transported through the biliary tree with bile acids and stored in the gall bladder as bile. When bile is released during the digestive process,

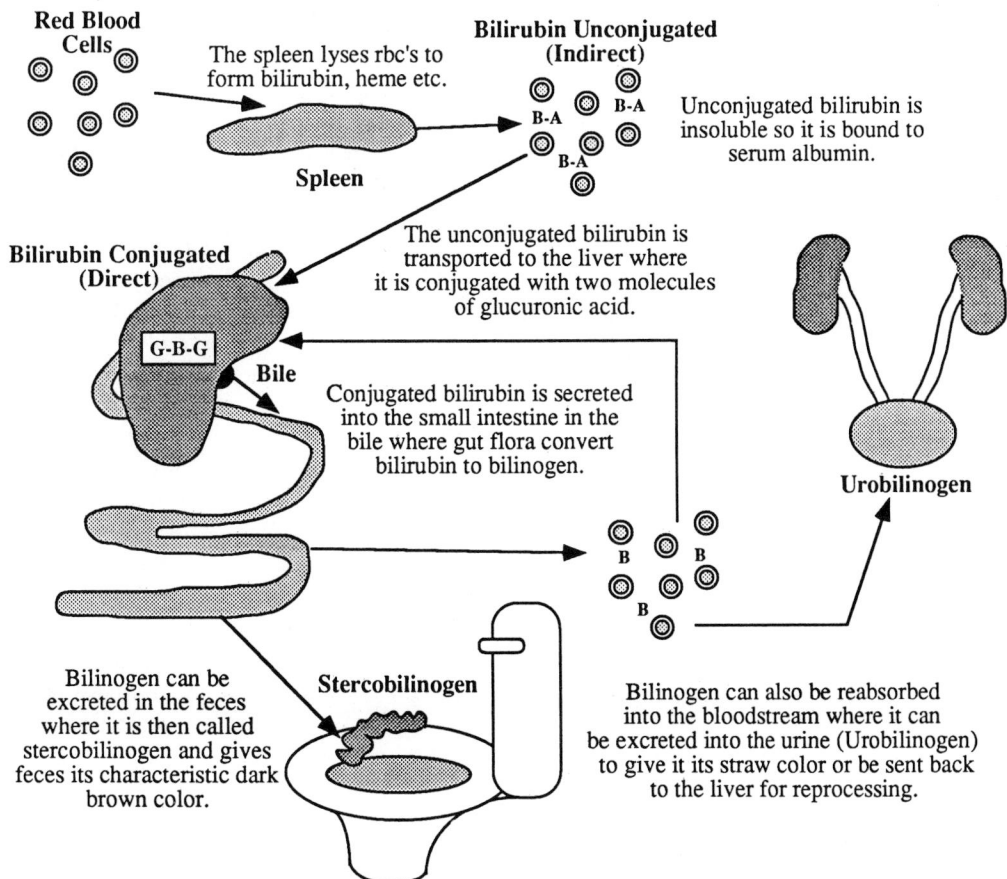

Figure 5.3. Bilirubin formation, metabolism, and excretion.

intestinal bacteria convert bilirubin into several compounds, collectively referred to as bilinogen. An estimated 10% of bilinogen is reabsorbed from the intestine into the bloodstream and resecreted by the liver. Small amounts of bilinogen are then excreted in the urine (urobilinogen), accounting for the urine's straw color. Most bilinogen, however, is directly eliminated in the feces (stercobilinogen), accounting for their characteristic dark brown color. Small portions of bilinogen are converted to bilins by intestinal flora and are also eliminated in the feces. The presence of bilirubin in the urine implies direct bilirubin, since indirect bilirubin is bound to serum albumin, which should normally not be filtered by the glomerulus (28). δ-Bilirubin is a protein-bound pigment that may falsely raise total bilirubin measurements during hepatobiliary disease.

Causes of hyperbilirubinemia can be classified into three broad categories: (*a*) prehepatic (hemolysis), (*b*) hepatic (defective removal of bilirubin from the blood or defective conjugation), and (*c*) posthepatic (obstruction of the extrahepatic biliary tree), also referred to as cholestatic or obstructive (29). As serum bilirubin concentrations rise above approximately 34 μmol/liter classic scleral icterus and jaundice develop. Table 5.5 summarizes the enzymatic patterns of the common etiologies of hyperbilirubinemia.

Hemolytic jaundice results from the rapid destruction of erythrocytes overwhelming the ability of the liver to process excess bilirubin. Tissue hematomas or collection of blood in body cavities may increase the serum bilirubin concentration. Severe sepsis or malignancy-induced disseminated intravascular coagulation, sickle cell crisis, or certain medications may induce hemolytic anemia. Drug-induced hemolytic anemia may be immune-mediated (23) (methyldopa, penicillins, cephalosporins, quinidine, ibuprofen, and triamterene); hemoglobin oxidation–mediated (33) (dapsone, antimalarials, sulfonamides, aspirin, nitrates, methylene blue, and ascorbic acid); megaloblastic-mediated (34) (antineoplastics, anticonvulsants, and al-

cohol); or sideroblastic-mediated with bone marrow suppression (35) (chloramphenicol, alcohol, lead, and antituberculous agents).

Hepatocellular injury from viral hepatitis, alcoholic hepatitis, toxin-mediated hepatitis, or cirrhosis may elevate serum bilirubin concentrations. Viral hepatitis usually causes elevations in direct bilirubin levels. Viral hepatitis may cause extreme elevations in transaminase levels (167 to 334 μkat/liter, 10,000 to 20,000 IU/liter), with ALT levels usually greater than those of AST. Medications commonly reported to cause direct hepatocellular damage include acetaminophen, halothane, tetracycline, valproic acid, isoniazid, rifampin, methyldopa, and labetalol (24, 36). Drug-induced hepatocellular damage may be indistinguishable from acute viral hepatitis. Alcoholic hepatitis presents in patients with either acute or chronic alcohol ingestion. Transaminase level elevations are only a fraction of those seen in viral or toxin-induced hepatitis. AST concentration is usually greater than that of ALT, but GGTP levels may be markedly elevated because of the effects of alcohol on GGTP release.

Patients with obstructive jaundice usually present with light clay-colored stools and dark cola-colored urine because of reabsorption of conjugated bilirubin from the biliary ducts, with redistribution to the urine and lack of bilinogen in the stool. The lack of bile acids in the gastrointestinal tract because of obstruction may cause steatorrhea. Transaminase levels are usually only mildly elevated unless severe obstruction occurs causing hepatocellular damage. ALP and GGTP concentrations are usually quite high. The most common cause of biliary obstruction is choledocholithiasis (gallstones) obstructing the common bile duct. Obese, middle-aged women are highly predisposed to choledocholithiasis; however, it may occur in both sexes at any age. Other causes of obstructive jaundice include carcinoma of the head of the pancreas, pancreatitis, and other neoplastic invasion of the papilla

Table 5.5.
Usual Enzymatic Patterns in Hyperbilirubinemia

	Fecal Bilinogen	Urine Bilirubin	Direct Bili (% total)	AST	ALT	ALP	GGTP	LDH
Hemolysis	↑	−	<20	nl	nl	nl	nl	↑ ↑ ↑ LDH$_1$ > LDH$_2$
Hepatocellular damage (viral or toxin)	↓	+	>40	↑ ↑ ↑ ↑	↑ ↑ ↑ ↑ ↑	↑ ↑	↑ ↑	↑ ↑ LDH$_5$
Alcoholic hepatitis	↓	+	<30	↑ ↑	↑	↑	↑ ↑ ↑	nl
Obstructive or cholestatic jaundice	↓	+	>50	↑	↑	↑ ↑ ↑	↑ ↑ ↑	↑ LDH$_5$
Alcoholic cirrhosis	nl	±	<30	↑ ↑ nl (25%)	↑ nl (50%)	↑	↑	nl

of Vater. Cholestatic changes may be due to an intrahepatic defect of the transport of bilirubin into hepatic canaliculi (29). Cholestatic jaundice closely resembles posthepatic biliary obstruction, except that the stools are only somewhat lighter than normal because of less exclusion of bilirubin from the duodenum. Common medications that induce obstructive or cholestatic jaundice include C-17 alkyl steroids, estrogens, chlorpromazine, and erythromycin estolate. Other medications may cause a mixed picture of hepatic injury through an atypical (phenytoin) or granulomatous pattern (quinidine, allopurinol) (24).

Common pitfalls in the application of liver function tests in the etiology of hyperbilirubinemia include (a) dependence on single tests rather than patterns of abnormality; (b) normal results, implying no disease (cirrhosis has normal AST in 25% and ALT in 50%), (c) abnormal liver function tests, suggesting only liver disease, (d) failure to recognize hepatocellular disease with low transaminase and high ALP levels or failure to recognize cholestasis or obstruction with high transaminase and low ALP levels; and (e) failure to repeat tests that did not correlate with clinical results (29).

Serum Proteins

TOTAL PROTEIN

(6.0–8.0 g/dl; SI units = 60–80 g/liter; CF = 10)

Serum proteins are separated by serum protein electrophoresis into prealbumin, albumin, and globulin fractions.

ALBUMIN

(3.5–5.5 g/dl; SI units = 35–55 gm/liter; CF = 10)

Albumin is by far the most abundant serum protein. Albumin is synthesized in the liver and accounts for up to 65% of total protein. Albumin has three major functions:

(a) controlling oncotic pressure in the plasma, (b) transporting amino acids synthesized in the liver to other tissues, and (c) transporting poorly soluble organic and inorganic ligands (37).

Albumin accounts for 80% of the oncotic pressure of the plasma. Capillary hemodynamics are controlled by four major forces, including intravascular oncotic pressure, interstitial oncotic pressure, capillary hydrostatic pressure, and interstitial hydrostatic pressure (Fig. 5.4). Intravascular oncotic pressure and interstitial hydrostatic pressure are the forces holding fluid in the intravascular space, while capillary hydrostatic pressure and interstitial oncotic pressure force fluid into tissue spaces. Normally, intravascular oncotic pressure overrides capillary hydrostatic pressure having a net hemodynamic flow into the vasculature. These forces may be disrupted, causing local edema, ascites, or anasarca. Malnutrition, malignancy, severe trauma, or burns cause a net catabolic state, decreasing serum albumin concentration and oncotic pressure. In hepatic cirrhosis there is decreased synthesis of albumin and increased portal capillary pressure resulting in ascites. In severe sepsis, toxin-mediated increases in capillary permeability allow intravascular albumin to escape into the interstitial tissues, accounting for increases in interstitial oncotic pressure. Nephrotic syndrome and protein-losing enteropathies cause increased losses of serum albumin, resulting in anasarca. Congestive heart failure alters pulmonary capillary hydrostatic pressure, resulting in pulmonary edema. Table 5.6 summarizes changes in capillary hemodynamics, resulting from various disease states. Dehydration and hemodilution may increase or decrease serum albumin concentrations.

Albumin acts as a carrier protein for both organic and inorganic molecules, which may bind ionically or covalently (37, 38). Several common medications that are highly insoluble in serum bind over 90% to albumin, in-

Figure 5.4. Capillary hemodynamic forces.

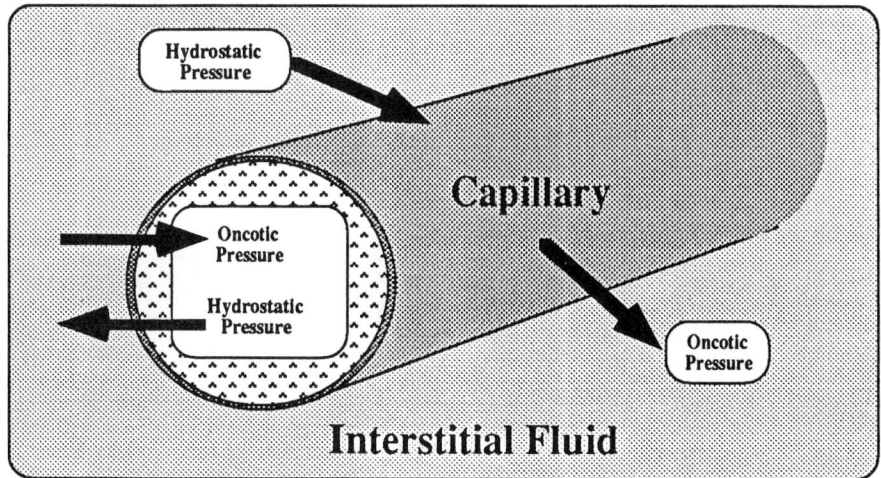

Table 5.6.
Common Disease States Resulting in Altered Capillary Hemodynamics

Disease	Mechanism	Serum Albumin	Capillary Hydrostatic Pressure	Interstitial Oncotic Pressure
Malnutrition	Decreased protein synthesis; increased protein catabolism	↓ ↓ ↓ [a]	nl	nl
Malignancy	Increased protein catabolism	↓ ↓	↓ ↑	nl
Burns	Increased protein catabolism; altered skin capillary permeability	↓ ↓ ↓	nl	↑ ↑, Skin
Hepatic cirrhosis	Decreased albumin synthesis; increased portal capillary hydrostatic pressure	↓ ↓ ↓	↑ ↑ ↑, Portal	↓ ↑
Sepsis	Toxin-altered capillary permeability	↓ ↓ ↓	nl	↑ ↑ ↑
Congestive heart failure	Increased pulmonary and systemic capillary hydrostatic pressure due to biventricular failure	↓ ↑	↑ ↑ ↑, Pulmonary and Systemic	nl
Nephrotic syndrome	Loss of albumin into the urine due to glomerular damage and leakage	↓ ↓ ↓	nl	nl

[a] Symbols: ↓ ↑ = may be decreased or increased, nl = normal, ↓ ↓ ↓ = dramatically decreased, ↑ ↑ ↑ = dramatically increased.

cluding phenytoin, salicylates, phenylbutazone, first-generation sulfonylureas, valproic acid, warfarin, and certain sulfonamides (38, 39). Since free drug is thought to be the active portion, changes in serum albumin concentrations may have a large influence on drug distribution and pharmacologic effect (40).

GLOBULIN

(2.3–3.5 gm/dl; SI units = 23–35 gm/liter; CF = 10)

The globulin fraction is composed of four major components: α_1- α_2- β-, and γ- (37). Important proteins located in the α_1 zone are α-1-antitrypsin, which is a scavenger enzyme for lysosomal proteases, and α_1 acid glycoprotein (AAG). Young patients with homozygous α-1-antitrypsin deficiency develop severe pulmonary emphysema because of protein lysis by elastase. AAG is an acute-phase reactant that acts as a carrier protein for certain poorly soluble medications. AAG is increased transiently in a variety of clinical conditions, including burns, chronic pain, enzyme induction, rheumatoid arthritis, morbid obesity, myocardial infarction, malignancy, surgery, or trauma. Several common medications bind to AAG, including amitriptyline, chlorpromazine, dipyridamole, disopyramide, erythromycin, imipramine, lidocaine, meperidine, methadone, nortriptyline, phencyclidine, propranolol, and quinidine (38). The transient elevations in AAG levels during the previously mentioned conditions may cause important changes in the binding and pharmacologic effect of these medications.

The α_2 portion consists primarily of α_2-macroglobulin, haptoglobin, and ceruloplasmin. α_2Macroglobulin is another major protease inhibitor; haptoglobin is a carrier protein for hemoglobin; and ceruloplasmin is a copper-binding protein. The β portion is composed of low-density lipoprotein (LDL), transferrin, C_3, and fibrinogen (37). LDL is the major transport protein for cholesterol to tis-

sues; transferrin transports ferric iron stores to bone marrow for erythropoiesis; C_3 is a major component of the complement system; and fibrinogen is a coagulation precursor for fibrin. The gamma globulin portion is composed of antibody immunoglobulins IgA, IgE, IgG, and IgM. IgA is responsible for surface immunity; IgE binds to mast cells and is responsible for hypersensitivity reactions; IgM is responsible for initial humoral immunity and IgG for sustained humoral immunity (37). The primary disorder associated with hypergammaglobulinemia is multiple myeloma.

Complete Blood Count with Differential, CBC with Diff

The complete blood count (CBC) provides information about the erythrocytes, leukocytes, and platelets. The number of parameters provided with a CBC depends on the type of machine used for the analysis. Any other desired tests may be ordered separately (41).

In the normal adult, blood cells are made predominantly in the bone marrow of the sternum, ribs, vertebral bodies, pelvic bones, and the proximal portions of the humerus and femur. The pathways of hematopoiesis from the uncommitted stem cell and the relationship between the different cell lines are shown in Figure 5.5 (42).

ERYTHROCYTES, Ercs

(males = $5.4 \pm 0.8 \times 10^6/mm^3$, SI units = $5.4 \pm 0.8 \times 10^{12}/liter$; females = $4.8 \pm 0.6 \times 10^6/mm^3$, SI units = $4.8 \pm 0.6 \times 10^{12}/liter$; CF = 1)

The main function of erythrocytes, or red blood cells, is to carry oxygen from the lungs to the tissues. Anemia occurs when the hemoglobin level, hematocrit, and/or erythrocyte count are below the normal range. This can be a result of impaired erythrocyte production, increased

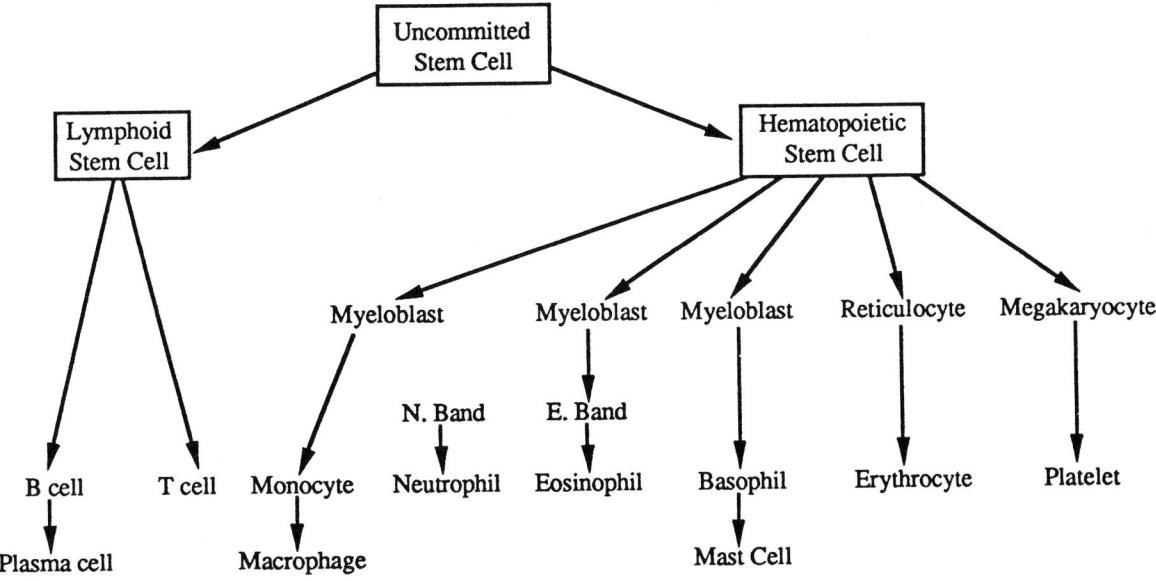

Figure 5.5. Hematopoiesis.

erythrocyte destruction, or blood loss. The extent of anemia is generally described by the hemoglobin or hematocrit values. The red blood cell indices may be used to further characterize the anemia by cell morphology or color. Normal-sized Ercs are called normocytes, small ones are microcytes, and large Ercs are macrocytes. If there is abnormal variation in size, the patient is said to have anisocytosis, which is a feature of most anemias (41). Those with normal amounts of hemoglobin are said to be normochromic; those with decreased, hypochromic; and those with increased hemoglobin levels, hyperchromic (43). Abnormally shaped cells are poikilocytes. Polycythemia means "many blood cells" but usually refers to an increased red blood cell mass (41).

Red cell production is regulated by tissue oxygenation (43). Tissues receive inadequate oxygen if there is an insufficient supply in inspired air, impaired oxygen transport from the alveoli into the blood stream, inadequate hemoglobin to carry oxygen, abnormal blood flow, or a failure of hemoglobin to release bound oxygen at tissue sites (41). These can occur in diseases such as anemia, in cardiac or pulmonary disease, or with decreased oxygen tension in the air, such as occurs at high altitudes (42). Smokers tend to have a mild stimulation of erythrocyte production (41). Hypoxia or decreased oxygenation stimulates the production of erythropoietin, primarily by the kidneys (42). About 10 to 15% of erythropoietin is produced by the liver. Erythropoietin stimulates and accelerates all aspects of Erc production and release. Erythropoietin increases in most anemias, but not those associated with chronic diseases (43). If tissue oxygen concentrations are perceived as inadequate, erythrocyte production continues, regardless of the erythrocyte count or hemoglobin concentration, and secondary or reactive polycythemia can occur (41).

The life span of erythrocytes in circulation is 120 days. They are removed by the reticuloendothelial system of the bone marrow, spleen, and liver. With an abnormally large spleen, there is increased destruction of normal cells. The spleen may be enlarged in conditions such as liver disease, congestive heart failure, leukemias, lymphomas, and protozoal infections. There can be accelerated destruction of erythrocytes by a normal spleen when they contain abnormal hemoglobin or have abnormal membranes or enzymes. Increased destruction can also occur with abnormal physical, chemical, microbiologic, or immunologic conditions (43).

Hemolysis refers to the disruption of the mature erythrocyte membrane and release of hemoglobin before the end of the usual life span. It can take place in the spleen or vasculature. This accelerated destruction of cells can occur in response to physical trauma or massive exertion, severe burns, infections such as malaria, or toxic insults such as *Clostridium* infections or brown recluse spider bites. Hemolysis can also occur with drugs and chemicals such as arsine gas or copper salts. With oxidizing drugs such as nitrites or nitrates, methemoglobin can be formed and lead to severe cases of erythrocyte destruction (43).

Destruction of erythrocytes may be mediated by antibodies. Various types of antibody-mediated hemolysis are associated with drugs (e.g., methyldopa, penicillin). The erythrocytes may also be destroyed as "innocent bystanders." Drug-antibody complexes can settle on the surface of erythrocytes and attract complement, which hemolyzes the cells. This has been reported with quinine derivatives, *p*-aminosalicylic acid, phenacetin, sulfonamides, and insecticides (43).

Patients with chronic diseases such as infections, renal or liver disease, various endocrine disorders, rheumatoid arthritis, or neoplasms often have anemia (44). Aplastic anemia involves a pancytopenia or a depression of erythrocytes, leukocytes, and platelets. It can occur secondary to infections, neoplasms, or drugs such as chloramphenicol, gold, colchicine, aspirin, phenylbutazone, sulfonamides, phenytoin, folate antagonists, or purine or pyrimidine analogs. Up to 50% of cases are primary or idiopathic, where there is no known predisposing cause. This may lead to leukemia or other myeloproliferative diseases. Polycythemia vera is a myeloproliferative syndrome in which there is a spontaneous increase in erythrocytes. The predominant picture is one of erythrocyte proliferation, but other elements of the blood are also hyperactive. It usually occurs in older adults and is slightly more common in men than in women. Thrombosis and hemorrhage are common complications (43).

HEMOGLOBIN, Hb

(males = 16.0 ± 2.0 g/dl, SI units = 9.9 ± 1.2 mmol/liter; females = 14.0 ± 2.0 g/dl, SI units = 8.7 ± 1.2 mmol/liter; CF = 0.6206)

Hemoglobin, the primary component of erythrocytes, transports oxygen and carbon dioxide. Hemoglobinopathies occur when genes code for abnormal amino acid sequences. The most common abnormal hemoglobin is sickle hemoglobin. Thalassemias result from defects in the manufacturing process (43).

The preferred assay for hemoglobin is the cyanmethemoglobin method. Errors in venipuncture technique can lead to hemoconcentration, which results in falsely elevated values for hemoglobin and cell counts. The difference in the normal range between men and women is thought to result mainly from androgen stimulation of erythropoiesis and its effect on the marrow. Estrogen probably has a slight suppressive effect on erythrocyte production. Menstrual blood loss is also a contributing factor. In older men, the hemoglobin level tends to fall. This occurs to a lesser extent in women, who may even have a slight increase in the value. As a result, there is a less than 0.39 mmol/liter (1 g/dl) sex difference in hemoglobin in older individuals. There is a diurnal variation of approximately 8 to 9% in hemoglobin concentrations, with the highest value occurring in the morning and the lowest in the evening (41). Hemoglobin values are approximately 0.39 mmol/liter (1 g/dl) lower in blacks than in whites. Some attribute this to a higher incidence of iron deficiency anemia in blacks (45).

HEMATOCRIT, Hct

(males = 47.0 ± 5.0%, SI units = 0.47 ± 0.05; females = 42.0 ± 5.0%, SI units = 0.42 ± 0.05; CF = 0.01)

The hematocrit is the ratio of the volume of erythrocytes to that of whole blood or the packed erythrocyte volume. It increases when more fluid is lost than erythrocytes and dehydration occurs, as occurs in patients with vomiting, diarrhea, or prolonged fever. An inappropriate polycythemia occurs with renal cancer, hepatomas, pheochromocytomas, or aldosterone-secreting adrenal adenomas with increased erythropoietin and increased hematocrit (43). The hematocrit is unreliable for patient assessment immediately after blood loss or transfusion (41).

RETICULOCYTES

(0.5–1.5% erythrocytes; SI units = 0.005–0.015; CF = 0.01)

Reticulocytes are immature erythrocytes. Generally, the absolute reticulocyte count is more useful than the percentage of erythrocytes. Reticulocytes provide an estimate of erythrocyte production; however, as the hematocrit drops, increasingly immature reticulocytes are released into the blood. These cells take longer to mature in circulation as indicated below:

Hct (%)	Reticulocyte Maturation Time (days)
0.45 (45)	1.0
0.35 (35)	1.5
0.25 (25)	2.0
0.15 (15)	2.5

To estimate erythrocyte production in response to anemia accurately, a correction factor must be used to account for this longer maturation time and avoid overestimating the erythropoietic response. The corrected reticulocyte count can be calculated by

$$\text{Corrected count} = \text{Reticulocyte count (\%)} \times \frac{\text{Patient's Hct}}{\text{Normal Hct}} \div \text{Maturation time}$$

This value can then be compared to the average normal reticulocyte count of 0.01 (1%) to estimate how much Erc production has actually increased (42). The reticulocytes are most markedly increased in patients with hemolysis or acute blood loss (41). They also increase when iron or vitamin B_{12} is administered to a deficient patient (41). If the reticulocyte count is normal, but the hemoglobin level low, there is an inadequate response to anemia, such as may be seen in iron deficiency. If the reticulocytes are increased, but the hemoglobin level is normal, there is probably some destruction or loss of erythrocytes occurring, and the body is compensating appropriately for the loss (43).

ERYTHROCYTE INDICES

The size and hemoglobin content of erythrocytes can be quantitated by the red blood cell indices. They are similar in men and women.

The mean corpuscular volume (MCV) is the average volume of erythrocytes. It can be measured by machines or calculated by the formula MCV = Hct/Ercs. The normal range is 87 ± 5 femtoliters (fl) in SI units (a femtoliter is 10^{-15} liter) or 87 ± 5 μm^3/cell (2). The MCV is decreased in microcytic anemia and increased in macrocytic anemia (41). Young erythrocytes and reticulocytes are larger than mature cells, so when there is rapid red cell production, the MCV will be increased. This type of macrocytosis can be observed in compensated hemolytic conditions or when a patient is recovering from acute blood loss. Megaloblastic changes can occur when DNA production is impaired but RNA production is normal (43). This causes nuclear maturation to lag behind cytoplasmic maturation (42). This change occurs in all cells, but it is most dramatic and can be most easily diagnosed in erythrocyte precursors. The most common causes of megaloblastosis are deficiencies of vitamin B_{12} or folic acid, which are required for DNA synthesis. Drugs that interfere with DNA synthesis such as folate antagonists (e.g., methotrexate, trimethoprim, or sulfonamides) or inhibitors of purine or pyrimidine synthesis may also cause megaloblastosis. It may also result from drugs that decrease folate absorption, such as oral contraceptives, phenytoin, and cycloserine. Alcohol can impair folic acid, absorption and interfere with folate-dependent enzymatic reactions. Megaloblastic anemia can also be associated with myxedema, multiple myeloma, widespread neoplastic disease, and enzyme defects such as occur in Lesch-Nyhan syndrome. A microcytic anemia is associated with iron deficiency anemia, thalassemias, and anemia of chronic disease (43).

The mean corpuscular hemoglobin (MCH) is the weight of the hemoglobin in the average red blood cell. It is calculated by MCH = Hb/Ercs (41). The normal range is 29 ± 2 picograms (pg) or 1.8 ± 0.1 fmol in SI units (CF = 0.06205) (2). In microcytic anemia it is decreased, and in macrocytic anemia, increased (41). Hypochromic cells are associated with iron deficiency anemia, thalassemias, and anemia of chronic disease (43).

The mean corpuscular hemoglobin concentration (MCHC) is the average concentration of hemoglobin in a given volume of packed erythrocytes and is described by MCHC = Hb/Hct (41). The normal range is 34 ± 2 g/dl or 21 ± 1 mmol/liter in SI units (CF = 0.6205) (2). In microcytic anemia, it is decreased. In macrocytic anemia, it may be normal or decreased. In hypochromic anemias, both the MCH and the MCHC are decreased (41).

The red cell distribution width (RDW) is an estimate of erythrocyte anisocytosis and is simply a coefficient of variation for the size of erythrocytes. The reference value is 11.5 to 14.5 (2). It may be calculated by RDW = (standard deviation of Erc size)/MCV.

ERYTHROCYTE SEDIMENTATION RATE, ESR

(males = 0–13 mm/h; females = 0–20 mm/h, Westergren technique)

The erythrocyte sedimentation rate is the length of fall of the top of a column of erythrocytes in anticoagulated blood in a given period of time. It is directly proportional to the weight of the cell aggregates and inversely proportional to the surface area. Microcytes settle more slowly than macrocytes. The ESR generally increases in anemia and following an injury, and decreases if there are abnormal or irregularly shaped erythrocytes. The ESR increases gradually with age and increases modestly during pregnancy. The ESR is used mainly as an indicator of active inflammatory diseases (e.g., rheumatoid arthritis), chronic infection (e.g., tuberculosis), collagen disease, or neoplastic disease (e.g., multiple myeloma) and may be used to monitor the disease course. The Westergren technique is widely used as the standard for determining ESR, but some laboratories still use the Wintrobe method or the Zeta Sedimentation Rate (41).

LEUKOCYTES, Lkcs

($4.5–11.0 \times 10^3$/mm^3; SI units = $4.5–11.0 \times 10^9$/liter; CF = 1)

There are six normal types of leukocytes or white blood cells: neutrophils, bands, lymphocytes, monocytes, eosinophils, and basophils. The differential white count indicates the fraction of the total leukocyte count that is accounted for by each type (addition of the differential should total 1.00). The white cell and differential counts can change within minutes to hours of stimulation (43). Cigarette smokers have a higher average leukocyte count. It is about 30% higher in heavy smokers who inhale, with an increase in neutrophils, lymphocytes, and monocytes. In leukocytosis, the total Lkc count is increased above the normal range. Exercise can lead to a leukocytosis with an increase in neutrophils due to shifting of cells and lymphocyte drainage into blood (41). The leukocyte count tends to be lower in blacks than in whites (45).

The leukocyte count and/or the differential count may be abnormal in patients with sepsis, but this is not always the case, and normal values would not rule out an infection. False results may occur with hemorrhage, hemolysis, trauma, diabetic ketoacidosis, and sickle cell crisis. The differential count is often abnormal after surgery (45).

Leukemias are malignant diseases characterized by abnormal leukocytes, which may be greatly increased in number, although the number may also be decreased. A massive increase in leukocytes in response to a nonhematologic condition is called a "leukemoid reaction" because the hematologic picture strongly resembles that seen in chronic leukemia. Different cell lines may predominate depending on the etiology (43, 46).

GRANULOCYTES

Granulocytes are leukocytes with granules in their cytoplasm. They develop from the same precursor cell as monocytes in the bone marrow (Fig. 5.5). Their synthesis is stimulated by the hormone colony-stimulating factor for granulocytes (G-CSF) and monocytes (GM-CSF) (42). Unlike erythrocytes, granulocytes retain their nuclei. Mature cells remain in the marrow and serve as a "storage pool." The cells can be released within minutes of a stimulus. Granulocytes have a life span of about 9 to 15 days, but they usually spend only about one day in circulating blood. Their primary site of activity is in tissues. There are three main types of granulocytes: neutrophils (including bands), eosinophils, and basophils (43).

NEUTROPHILS

$(1.1–7.0 \times 10^3/\text{mm}^3$, SI units = $1.1–7.0 \times 10^9/\text{liter}$; CF = 1)

In normal adults, about 0.51 ± 0.15 of leukocytes are neutrophils (2), also called polymorphonuclear (meaning many forms of nuclei) leukocytes, PMNs, polys, segmented neutrophilic granulocytes, or segs. The lower limit of the normal range is $1.5 \times 10^9/\text{liter}$ ($1.1 \times 10^3/\text{mm}^3$) for white adults and $1.1 \times 10^9/\text{liter}$ ($1.1 \times 10^3/\text{mm}^3$) for blacks. There is some diurnal variation in neutrophils, with higher values occurring in the afternoon and lower in the morning. The nuclei of neutrophils have two to five lobes connected by thin filaments (41). Their cytoplasm is packed with enzyme-containing granules that react with both acidic and basic stains.

When tissue is damaged or foreign material enters the body, substances are released that stimulate neutrophils to move to that area. This is called chemotaxis. Chemotaxis can be abnormal in some diseases, such as Hodgkin's disease, cirrhosis, rheumatoid arthritis, and diabetes mellitus. The neutrophils then phagocytize and destroy microorganisms and other materials at the site enzymatically. The neutrophils must attach to the particles before they can engulf them. This attachment is enhanced by the presence of antibodies or by complement coating the surface of the particles. It is decreased by exposure to alcohol, aspirin, or corticosteroids (43). This action of neutrophils is important in host defense against infection, but it may also play a part in causing tissue damage to the host in other diseases (47).

Neutrophils are stored in the bone marrow and in the marginal granulocyte pool along blood vessel walls or in capillary beds. In response to stress, they can be released from these sites into the circulating pool, resulting in a neutrophilia. In an acute infection, the neutrophils leave the circulation and migrate into the tissues. Production of neutrophils will also increase, in which case, more immature forms will be seen. If supply cannot keep up with demand, a neutropenia may occur. A toxic suppression of the bone marrow may also be involved in this process (46).

An increase in neutrophils is associated with some infections (especially bacterial), various inflammatory diseases (e.g., rheumatoid arthritis, vasculitis), tissue necrosis (e.g., as in myocardial infarction or crush injuries), metabolic disorders (e.g., uremia, diabetic ketoacidosis, thyroid storm), and malignant tumors. Endogenous or exogenous adrenal corticosteroids cause lymphocytes and eosinophils to disappear from circulation within 4 to 8 hr, with circulating granulocytes increasing later (43). Prolonged use of corticosteroids can lead to chronic neutrophilia by decreasing the rate at which neutrophils leave the circulation (46). Epinephrine can cause granulocytosis within minutes and probably is the mediator of neutrophilic leukocytosis associated with physiologic stimuli such as exercise, emotional stress, or exposure to extreme temperatures. Other drugs that can stimulate neutrophilia include lithium, histamine, heparin, digitalis, and many toxins, venoms, and heavy metals (e.g., lead, mercury) (43).

Neutropenia is a result of impaired production, increased destruction, or altered distribution of neutrophils. It occurs when the absolute neutrophil count is below the normal range and is associated with certain bacterial (typhoid, tularemia, brucellosis), viral, and protozoal (especially malaria) infections, or an overwhelming infection of any kind. It can be caused by drugs interfering with DNA synthesis (e.g., phenothiazines, phenytoin, antibiotics, sulfonamides), idiosyncratic drug reactions (e.g., chloramphenicol, gold salts, propylthiouracil, phenylbutazone, quinidine), or treatment with cytotoxic drugs or radiation (43, 46). There can be increased destruction of neutrophils through immunologic mechanisms in patients receiving drugs such as aminopyrine, phenylbutazone, or sulfapyridine (46). Neutropenia is also seen with hypersplenism from liver or storage diseases, some collagen-vascular diseases (e.g., lupus erythematosus), and folic acid or vitamin B_{12} deficiency. A more severe form of neutropenia is agranulocytosis, where the granulocytes suddenly disappear. Often, other blood elements are also affected (43). When the absolute neutrophil count is below $1.0 \times 10^9/\text{liter}$ ($1.0 \times 10^3/\text{mm}^3$), there is an increased risk of infection, and when it is less than $0.5 \times 10^9/\text{liter}$ ($0.5 \times 10^3/\text{mm}^3$), this risk is very high (46).

BANDS

$(0.1–2.0 \times 10^3/\text{mm}^3$; SI units = $0.1–2.0 \times 10^9/\text{liter}$; CF = 1)

Bands or stabs are the immature form of neutrophils. They have thicker strands connecting their nuclear lobes or U-shaped nuclei (41). Band neutrophils normally average 0.08 ± 0.03 of leukocytes (2). A "shift to the left" means there is an increase in bands and other immature neutrophils in the blood (41). The term is derived from a time when the differential count was reported on a grid that listed the immature forms on the left and the mature neutrophils on the right (43).

EOSINOPHILS

$(0-0.7 \times 10^3/mm^3$; SI units $= 0-0.7 \times 10^9/liter$; CF $= 1$)

Eosinophils are structurally similar to neutrophils, but their cytoplasm contains larger round or oval granules that contain enzymes and have a strong affinity for acid (red) stains. Their nuclei usually contain two connected segments (41). Eosinophils normally average 0.027 of leukocytes (2). The count is higher in allergic individuals (41). Eosinophils are capable of phagocytosis but are not bactericidal. They modulate activities associated with immunologically mediated inflammation and can damage the larvae of some helminth parasites. Eosinophils are increased in allergic diseases (e.g., asthma, hay fever), parasitic infections (e.g., trichinosis), certain skin disorders (e.g., atopic dermatitis, eczema, pemphigus), neoplastic diseases, collagen vascular diseases, adrenal cortical hypofunction, ulcerative colitis, and "hypereosinophilic" syndromes (43, 46). Eosinophils are decreased during acute stress or other conditions with increased epinephrine secretion or elevated levels of adrenal corticosteroids and in acute inflammatory states (46).

BASOPHILS

$(0-0.15 \times 10^3/mm^3$; SI units $= 0-0.15 \times 10^9/liter$; CF $= 1$)

Basophils resemble neutrophils except their nuclei are less segmented and their cytoplasmic granules are larger and have a strong affinity for basic (blue) stains (41). They average about 0.005 of total leukocytes (2). They show diurnal variation with levels highest during the night and lowest in the morning (46). Tissue basophils are called mast cells and have immunoglobulin E antibodies on their cell membranes. They react with allergens and cause release of histamine and other substances from the basophil granules, producing allergic reactions. Basophils may be increased in chronic hypersensitivity states in the absence of the specific allergen, in myeloproliferative disorders, and hypothyroidism (43, 46). They may be decreased with chronic corticosteroid therapy, acute infection or stress, or in patients with hyperthyroidism (46).

LYMPHOCYTES

$(1.5-4 \times 10^3/mm^3$; SI units $= 1.5-4 \times 10^9/liter$; CF $= 1$)

Lymphocytes are mononuclear cells without cytoplasmic granules (41). They average 0.34 ± 0.10 of leukocytes in adults (2). They may form plasma cells, which are not normally present in blood (41). Plasma cells may be found in patients with neoplasms (e.g., multiple myeloma), chronic infections, and allergic states (46). Lymphocytes and plasma cells are important for the immune defenses of the body. Normally, about 75 to 80% of circulating lymphocytes are T cells, which are responsible for cell-mediated immunity including delayed hypersensitivity, graft rejection, graft-versus-host reactions, defense against intracellular organisms, and probably defense against neoplasms. They have a life span of months to years. They are named for the thymus gland, where they differentiate (42).

B lymphocytes account for 10 to 15% of circulating lymphocytes and are responsible for humoral immunity (43). They are named for the bursa of Fabricius, where they develop in birds. In humans, the bursal equivalent is thought to be in fetal liver and bone marrow, with further differentiation occurring in secondary lymphoid organs. These organs, important for postnatal lymphocyte production, include the spleen, lymph nodes, and intestine-associated lymphoid tissue. B cells have a life span of days and can differentiate into antibody-producing plasma cells (42).

There are also "null" lymphocytes, which cannot be classified. Although lymphocytes can be found in circulation, they concentrate mainly in lymph nodes, spleen, the mucosa of the alimentary and respiratory tracts, bone marrow, liver, skin, and chronically inflamed tissue.

Changes in the proportion of lymphocytes in the total leukocyte count usually reflect changes in numbers of granulocytes. An absolute or relative increase in lymphocytes occurs with some viral or other infections (e.g., tuberculosis, infectious mononucleosis, cytomegalovirus, pertussis, toxoplasmosis), inflammatory or immunologic diseases, and hypersensitivity reactions to drugs (e.g., phenytoin, p-aminosalicylic acid). When the number of lymphocytes is decreased abnormally (lymphopenia) or function is impaired, the patient suffers from immunodeficiency. This can be an inherited disorder or may be associated with immunodeficiency syndromes (e.g., AIDs), diseases such as congestive heart failure, renal failure, malnutrition, or advanced tuberculosis, and with defects of lymphatic circulation (43). Lymphopenia can also occur after administration of antineoplastic drugs or high-dose corticosteroids and after irradiation (46).

MONOCYTES

$(0.2-0.9 \times 10^3/mm^3$; SI units $= 0.2-0.9 \times 10^9/liter$; CF $= 1$)

Monocytes are the largest cells in normal blood, with a diameter two to three times that of erythrocytes. They have a single nucleus that is partly lobulated and may appear round or oval. Their cytoplasm contains fine granules (43). Monocytes average 0.04 of leukocytes (2). After circulating briefly, they enter the tissues, transform into the larger macrophages, and remain for several months. Macrophages are capable of motility, phagocytosis, enzyme secretion, particle recognition, and interactions with the immune system (43). They have important functions in host defense and the control of hematopoiesis. They remove old or defective blood cells in the marrow and inhaled particles in the lungs (42). They are increased in some infectious diseases (e.g., mycotic, rickettsial, protozoal, viral infections; tuberculosis, subacute bacterial endocarditis, hepatitis), and granulomatous, collagen-vascular, and neoplastic diseases (43, 46). The circulating monocytes and tissue macrophages together compose the mononuclear phagocyte or reticuloendothelial system (42).

PLATELETS
(200–350 × 10^3/mm^3; SI units = 200–350 × 10^9/liter; CF = 1)

Platelets maintain the integrity of blood vessels and play a key role in hemostasis. The precursors of platelets are megakaryocytes (Fig. 5.5) (43). Their proliferation and maturation are controlled by megakaryocyte colony-stimulating factor (Mk-CSF) and thrombopoietin. Normally, about two-thirds of platelets are in circulation and one-third are in the spleen. When the spleen is enlarged, however, up to 80 to 90% may be sequestered there. In patients without a spleen, all are in circulation. Platelets circulate for about 8 to 11 days (42).

The major site for destruction of platelets is the spleen. Antibodies may also destroy platelets. They may be directed against the platelets, or the platelets may be "innocent bystanders" that are destroyed when an immune complex attaches to them. This may occur with exposure to drugs such as quinine, quinidine, or heparin (43).

Thrombocytopenia, a reduced number of circulating platelets, can occur as a congenital or acquired disorder. It may result from decreased production, abnormal distribution or dilution, or increased destruction of platelets. These may be associated with factors such as neoplasms, immune processes, infections, metabolic disorders, exposure to drugs, chemicals, or toxins, or an enlarged spleen, and may be combined with abnormalities of other blood elements (as in aplastic anemia). Thrombocytosis, an increased number of circulating platelets, can be part of a reactive process or a myeloproliferative disorder (48). Half of patients with an otherwise unexplained increase in platelets are found to have a malignancy (2).

Platelets are activated at times of vascular injury by exposure to substances such as collagen and thrombin. They adhere to exposed surfaces and aggregate in the presence of calcium (48). They release adenosine diphosphate (ADP), which promotes further aggregation and platelet plug formation (43). Aggregation is also stimulated by thromboxane A_2 from platelets and inhibited by prostacyclin (prostaglandin I_2) from vascular endothelium. Both are products of platelet arachidonic acid metabolism mediated by cyclooxygenase (Fig. 5.6). Platelets also release various substances that activate or allow progression of the clotting cascade. These actions lead to the formation of thrombi. Overall platelet function may be assessed by the bleeding time, and various in vitro techniques employing activator substances used to assess platelet aggregation. Platelet contraction within thrombi is responsible for clot retraction (48).

If the count is less than 30 to 40 ·× 10^9/liter (30 × 10^3 to 40 × 10^3/mm^3), the patient is at a high risk for bleeding, and if it is less than 10 × 10^9/liter (10 × 10^3/mm^3), bleeding usually occurs (49). Platelet function is impaired in various diseases such as severe uremia or liver disease or when there are high levels of abnormal serum proteins. Numerous drugs can also interfere with platelet function (43). Most affect the arachidonic pathway shown in Figure 5.6 (50). Aspirin irreversibly acetylates platelet cyclooxygenase, thus inhibiting aggregation for the life of the platelet by decreasing formation of thromboxane A_2. This effect is observed for up to 10 days following ingestion of aspirin. Most other nonsteroidal antiinflammatory drugs also affect platelet cyclooxygenase, but it is a reversible effect observed only while the drug is present. Other drugs inhibit platelet effects by activating adenylate cyclase (e.g., prostanoids) or inhibiting phosphodiesterase (e.g., dipyridamole), both of which result in increased cyclic-AMP (48). Ticlopidine is a drug that inhibits the ADP pathway (51). Examples of additional drugs that may inhibit aggregation include dextran, antimicrobial agents, membrane-stabilizing agents, and sympathetic blocking agents (48). Synthesis of platelets is inhibited by many antineoplastic agents. Ethyl alcohol can inhibit both synthesis and function of platelets (43).

Coagulation Tests
CLOTTING CASCADE

The clotting cascade involves the progressive activation of clotting factors, with the end result of a fibrin clot. Platelets and other substances help or accelerate this progression. A simplified diagram of the traditional clotting cascade is shown in Figure 5.7. The process is actually much more complex, with additional points of factor interaction. The clotting factors are identified by Roman numerals, although they also have other names (43). Each factor must be activated before it can in turn activate other factors in the sequence. The active forms of most factors are serine proteases, except V and VIII, which act as cofactors. Factors II, VII, IX, and X require vitamin K for their synthesis (52). The main source of phospholipid is platelets (43). Ionized calcium is required for some of the steps to proceed. The intrinsic pathway is initiated by contact activation within the blood vessels. The extrinsic pathway is

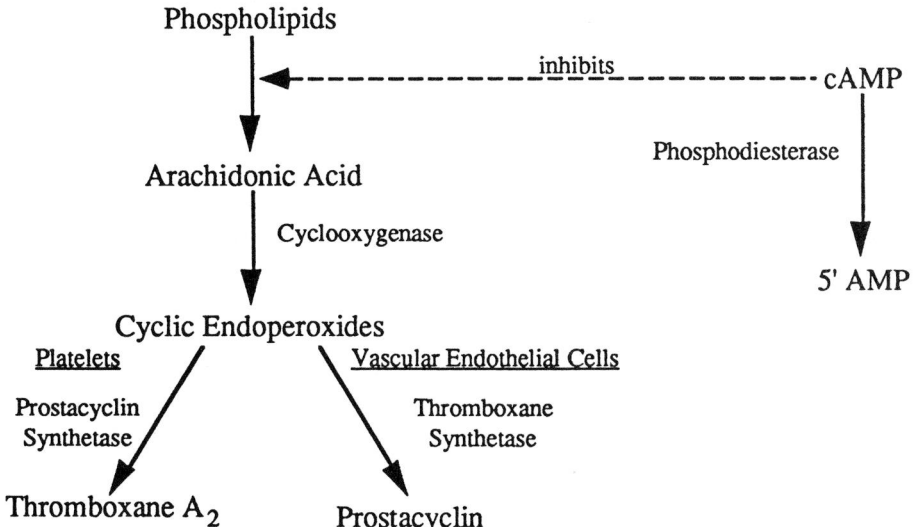

Figure 5.6. Arachidonic acid pathway.

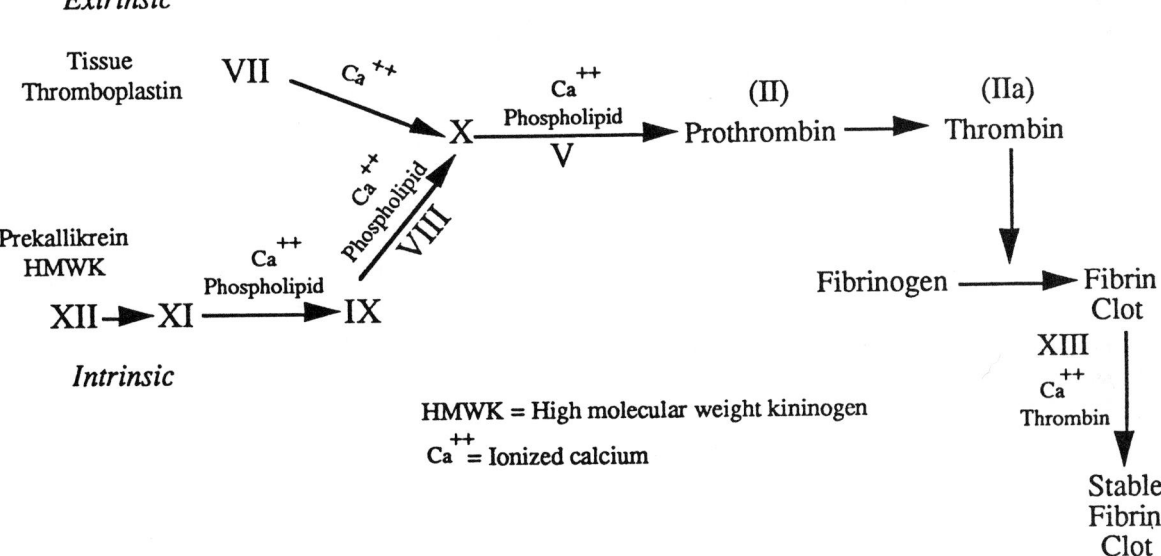

Figure 5.7. Clotting cascade.

stimulated by tissue factors from outside the vessels. The two pathways come together at factor X to form the common pathway.

Different tests are used to assess the body's ability to form a clot, by evaluating the function of different parts of the pathways, and they are also used to monitor drug therapy. For most coagulation tests, the blood is centrifuged to remove platelets, and citrate is added to bind calcium and thus prevent the cascade from progressing (52). Clotting factor concentrations that are 20 to 25% of normal may produce normal clotting tests but are not sufficient to meet a severe hemostatic challenge. Artifactually abnormal tests may be observed in patients with severe

anemia, hyperlipidemia, or polycythemia (43). Patients with defective or deficient clotting factors can experience bleeding. This may be a congenital disorder such as hemophilia, where there is a deficiency of factor VIII or IX, an acquired disorder such as the impaired factor synthesis seen in liver disease, or an effect of drugs (52).

ACTIVATED PARTIAL THROMBOPLASTIN TIME, aPTT
(25–37 sec)

The aPTT is used to assess the integrity of the intrinsic and common coagulation pathways. It is performed by adding a contact activating agent (e.g., kaolin, ellagic acid, or celite), phospholipid, and calcium to citrated plasma, then measuring the time required for a clot to form. It will be prolonged if there is a deficiency of factor XII, XI, IX, VIII, X, V, or II, or fibrinogen, prekallikrein, or high molecular weight kininogen, or if an inhibitor of one of these is present. It is not affected by abnormal factor VII. It is usually prolonged when the concentration of the clotting factors is less than 30% of normal. It is also abnormal in patients with a lupus-like anticoagulant and sometimes in those with liver failure, since many clotting factors are manufactured in the liver. It may be shortened in an active coagulopathy or malignancy. It is the main test used to monitor heparin therapy and will be prolonged in the presence of thrombolytic drugs or coumarin derivatives (52).

PROTHROMBIN TIME, PT
(11–16 sec)

The PT is used to evaluate the extrinsic and common pathways. Tissue thromboplastin (e.g., brain or lung extract) and calcium are added to citrated plasma, and the time to clot formation is measured. In the U.S., rabbit brain thromboplastin is commonly used, which is much less sensitive to changes in clotting factor concentrations than the human brain thromboplastin used in other countries (53). The PT is prolonged by a deficiency of factor VII, X, V, or II, or fibrinogen, or the presence of an inhibitor to one of those factors. It is not affected by abnormal factor VIII or IX (52). The PT is sometimes expressed as the International Normalized Ratio (INR). This is calculated by the formula INR = R^c, where R is the ratio of patient's PT : mean control PT, and c is the International Sensitivity Index (ISI), which relates an individual batch of thromboplastin to the World Health Organization international reference preparation (53). For example, a quoted therapeutic range for warfarin in the treatment of deep venous thrombosis in this country (rabbit brain thromboplastin) would be 1.3 to 1.5 times the control value; the corresponding INR would be 2.0 to 3.0. The PT is prolonged in liver disease, in patients with a vitamin K deficiency, and in widespread intravascular coagulation or fibrinolysis. It is used to monitor coumarin (e.g., warfarin) treatment but may be prolonged by the presence of heparin or a thrombolytic drug (43). An extensive discussion of drugs that affect the clotting tests is found in Chapter 40 "Thromboembolic Diseases."

THROMBIN TIME, TT
(10–15 sec)

The TT is used to appraise the body's ability to convert fibrinogen to fibrin. Thrombin is added to citrated plasma, and the time for clotting is measured. The time is prolonged if there is a deficiency or abnormality of fibrinogen, if an inhibitor is present, or if heparin or fibrin degradation products are present (52). It may be used in monitoring thrombolytic therapy (e.g., streptokinase, urokinase, alteplase, or anistreplase).

BLEEDING TIME
(180–240 sec)

The bleeding time is an imprecise test used to assess platelet function. It is performed by making a uniform incision on the arm. Blood that beads up is removed by filter paper, with care taken not to touch the wound and disturb platelet plugs. The blood is removed to prevent fibrin from forming and stopping the bleeding. The end point of the test is when there is no longer a spot on the filter paper after blotting. The test is prolonged when there is platelet dysfunction, when the number of platelets is less than 100×10^9/liter (100×10^3/mm^3), or when a platelet-inhibiting drug is present. The bleeding time with reduced platelets may be calculated by

$$\text{Bleeding time} = (30.5 - \text{Platelet count/mm}^3)/3850.$$

If the time is longer than that calculated, platelet dysfunction may also be a factor. If it is shorter, many young, active platelets may be present (43).

CONCLUSION

This chapter has reviewed commonly encountered clinical laboratory tests including serum creatinine, blood urea nitrogen, plasma glucose, uric acid, enzymes, bilirubin, serum proteins, clotting tests, and complete blood count with differential. Reliable measurements are an integral component in the management of any patient. Laboratory values that do not correlate with a patient's clinical picture should be suspect and repeated. Reference values should be taken from the clinical laboratory in which the test was performed. Critical or treatment values for a given test in a clinical situation should be used rather than just normal or abnormal values. Drugs may alter a particular laboratory test, and medication histories and administration profiles should be reviewed thoroughly for potential drug causes of these alterations. Clinical laboratory tests are a major component of the diagnosis and treatment of patients today. Understanding their regulation, critical ranges, clinical applications, and limitations is vital.

REFERENCES

1. Linke EG, Henry JB, Clinical pathology/laboratory medicine purposes and practice. In Henry JB: Clinical Diagnosis and Management by Laboratory Methods, ed. 17. Philadelphia, WB Saunders, 1984, pp 2–23.
2. Wallach J: Interpretation of Diagnostic Tests. A Synopsis of Laboratory Medicine, ed. 4. Boston: Little, Brown, 1986.
3. Woo J, Cannon DC, Metabolic intermediates and inorganic ions. In Henry JB: Clinical Diagnosis and Management by Laboratory Methods, ed. 17. Philadelphia, WB Saunders, 1984, pp 133–164.
4. Smith CL, Hampton EM: Using estimated creatinine clearance for individualizing drug therapy: a reassessment. DICP Ann Pharmacother 24:1185–1190, 1990.
5. Howanitz PJ, Howanitz JH, Carbohydrates. In Henry JB: Clinical Diagnosis and Management by Laboratory Methods, ed. 17. Philadelphia, WB Saunders, 1984, pp 165–179.

6. Stanaszek WF, Seifert CF: Arthritis in the elderly: presentation, treatment and monitoring aspects. J Geriatr Drug Ther 3:5–89, 1989.

7. Campion EW, Clynn RJ, DeLabry LO: Asymptomatic hyperuricemia. Risks and consequences in the normative aging study. Am J Med 82:421–426, 1987.

8. Borg EJT, Rasker JJ: Gout in the elderly. A separate entity? Ann Rheum Dis 46:72–76, 1987.

9. Zimmerman HJ, Henry JB, Clinical enzymology. In Henry JB: Clinical Diagnosis and Management by Laboratory Methods, ed. 17. Philadelphia, WB Saunders, 1984, pp 251–282.

10. Koppel C: Clinical features, pathogenesis and management of drug-induced rhabdomyolysis. Med Toxicol Adv Drug Exp 4:108–126, 1989.

11. Zeller FP, Bauman JL: Current concepts in clinical therapeutics: acute myocardial infarction. Clin Pharm 5:553–572, 1986.

12. Young LY, Smith GH, Interpretation of clinical laboratory tests. In Young LY, Koda-Kimble MA: Applied Therapeutics. The Clinical Use of Drugs, ed. 4. Vancouver, Applied Therapeutics, 1988, pp 29–48.

13. Heller GV, Blaustein AS, Wei JY, Geer D: Implications of increased myocardial isoenzyme level in the presence of normal serum creatine kinase activity. Am J Cardiol 51:24–27, 1983.

14. Ingwall JS, Kramer MF, Fifer MA, et al.: The creatine kinase system in normal and diseased human myocardium. N Engl J Med 313:1050–1054, 1985.

15. White RD, Grande P, Califf L, Palmeri ST, Califf RM, Wagner GS: Diagnostic and prognostic significance of minimally elevated creatine kinase-MB in suspected acute myocardial infarction. Am J Cardiol 55:1478–1484, 1985.

16. Hong RA, Licht JD, Wei JY, Heller GV, Blaustein AS, Pasternak RC: Elevated CK-MB with normal total creatine kinase in suspected myocardial infarction: associated clinical findings and early prognosis. Am Heart J 111:1041–1047, 1986.

17. Lee TH, Weisberg MC, Cook F, Daley K, Brand DA, Goldman L: Evaluation of creatine kinase and creatine kinase-MB for diagnosing myocardial infarction. Clinical impact in the emergency room. Arch Intern Med 147:115–121, 1987.

18. Yusuf S, Collins R, Lin L, Sterry H, Pearson M, Sleight P: Significance of elevated MB isoenzyme with normal creatine kinase in acute myocardial infarction. Am J Cardiol 59:245–250, 1987.

19. Pearlman CA: Neuroleptic malignant syndrome: a review of the literature. J Clin Psychopharmacol 6:257–273, 1986.

20. Henwood JM, Heel RC: Lovastatin. A preliminary review of its pharmacodynamic properties and therapeutic use in hyperlipidaemia. Drugs 36:429–454, 1988.

21. Montgomery R, Dryer RL, Conway TW, Spector AA: Biochemistry. A Case-Oriented Approach, ed. 2. Saint Louis: CV Mosby, 1977.

22. Diggs LW: Sickle cell crises. Am J Clin Pathol 44:1–19, 1965.

23. Petz LD: Drug-induced immune haemolytic anaemia. Clin Haematol 9:455–483, 1980.

24. Kaplowitz N, Aw TY, Simon FR, Stolz A: Drug-induced hepatotoxicity. Ann Intern Med 104:826–839, 1986.

25. Sher PP: Drug interferences with clinical laboratory tests. Drugs 24:24–63, 1982.

26. Girling DJ: The hepatic toxicity of antituberculosis regimens containing isoniazid, rifampicin, and pyrazinamide. Tubercle 59:13–32, 1978.

27. Mitchell JR, Zimmerman HJ, Ishak KG, et al.: Isoniazid liver injury: clinical spectrum, pathology, and probable pathogenesis. Ann Intern Med 84:181–192, 1976.

28. Chopra S, Griffin PH: Laboratory tests and diagnostic procedures in evaluation of liver disease. Am J Med 79:221–230, 1985.

29. Zimmerman HJ, Function and integrity of the liver. In Henry JB: Clinical Diagnosis and Management by Laboratory Methods, ed. 17. Philadelphia, WB Saunders, 1990, pp 217–250.

30. Wu WT, Kao YS, Exocrine pancreatic function. In Henry JB: Clinical Diagnosis and Management by Laboratory Methods, ed. 17. Philadelphia, WB Saunders, 1984, pp 537–549.

31. Geokas MC, Baltaxe HA, Banks PA, Silva J, Frey CF: Acute pancreatitis. Ann Intern Med 103:86–100, 1985.

32. Mallory A, Kern F: Drug-induced pancreatitis: a critical review. Gastroenterology 78:813–820, 1980.

33. Gordon-Smith EC: Drug-induced oxidative haemolysis. Clin Haematol 9:557–586, 1980.

34. Scott JM, Weir DG: Drug-induced megaloblastic change. Clin Haematol 9:587–619, 1980.

35. Yunis AA, Salem Z: Drug-induced mitochondrial damage and sideroblastic change. Clin Haematol 9:607–619, 1980.

36. Clark JA, Zimmerman HJ, Tanner LA: Labetalol hepatotoxicity. Ann Intern Med 113:210–213, 1990.

37. McPherson RA, Specific proteins. In Henry JB: Clinical Diagnosis and Management by Laboratory Methods, ed. 17. Philadelphia, WB Saunders, 1984, pp 204–216.

38. Svensson CK, Woodruff MN, Lalka D, Influence of protein binding and use of unbound (free) drug concentrations. In Evans WE, Schentag JJ, Jusko WJ: Applied Pharmacokinetics. Principles of Therapeutic Drug Monitoring, ed. 2. Spokane, Applied Therapeutics, 1986, pp 187–219.

39. Oellerich M, Influence of protein binding commentary. In Evans WE, Schentag JJ, Jusko WJ: Applied Pharmacokinetics. Principles of Therapeutic Drug Monitoring, ed. 2. Spokane, Applied Therapeutics, 1986, pp 220–228.

40. Zini R, Riant P, Barre J, Tillement JP: Disease-induced variations in plasma protein levels. Implications for drug dosage regimens (Part I). Clin Pharmacokinet 19:147–159, 1990.

41. Nelson DA, Morris MW, Basic methodology. In Henry JB: Clinical Diagnosis and Management by Laboratory Methods, ed. 17. Philadelphia, WB Saunders, 1984, pp 578–625.

42. Nelson DA, Davey FR, Hematopoiesis. In Henry JB: Clinical Diagnosis and Management by Laboratory Methods, ed. 17. Philadelphia, WB Saunders, 1984, pp 626–651.

43. Widmann FK: Clinical Interpretation of Laboratory Tests, ed. 9. Philadelphia, FA Davis, 1983.

44. Nelson DA, Davey FR, Erythrocytic disorders. In Henry JB: Clinical Diagnosis and Management by Laboratory Methods, ed. 17. Philadelphia, WB Saunders, 1984, pp 652–703.

45. Shapiro MF, Greenfield S: The complete blood count and leukocyte differential count. An approach to their rational application. Ann Intern Med 106:65–74, 1987.

46. Davey FR, Nelson DA, Leukocytic disorders. In Henry JB: Clinical Diagnosis and Management by Laboratory Methods, ed. 17. Philadelphia, WB Saunders, 1984, pp 704–748.

47. Malech HL, Gallin JI: Neutrophils in human diseases. N Engl J Med 317:687–694, 1987.

48. Miller JL, Blood platelets. In Henry JB: Clinical Diagnosis and Management by Laboratory Methods, ed. 17. Philadelphia, WB Saunders, 1984, pp 749–764.

49. Firkin F, Chesterman C, Penington D, Rush B: deGruchy's Clinical Haematology in Medical Practice, ed. 5. Oxford: Blackwell Scientific Publications, 1989.

50. Kessler CM: Anticoagulation and thrombolytic therapy: practical considerations. Chest 95(suppl):245s–256s, 1989.

51. Hass WK, Easton JD, Adams HP, et al.: A randomized trial comparing ticlopidine hydrochloride with aspirin for the prevention of stroke in high-risk patients. N Engl J Med 321:501–507, 1989.

52. Miller JL, Blood coagulation and fibrinolysis. In Henry JB: Clinical Diagnosis and Management by Laboratory Methods, ed. 17. Philadelphia, WB Saunders, 1984, pp 765–787.

53. Hirsh J, Poller L, Deykin D, Levine M, Dalen JE: Optimal therapeutic range for oral anticoagulants. Chest 95(suppl):5s–11s, 1989.

CHAPTER 6

PATIENT EDUCATION AND CHRONIC DISEASE MONITORING

BARRY L. CARTER, Pharm.D., F.C.C.P. and DENNIS K. HELLING, Pharm.D., F.C.C.P.

Statistics on adverse drug reactions, hospitalizations because of adverse drug effects, and the associated morbidity and mortality are staggering (1–3). Many factors contribute to these drug-related problems, including lack of awareness by the patient, drug interactions, and noncompliance (4–10). Many preventable problems could be avoided by better patient information and improved monitoring (6–10). For example, these problems could be minimized if pharmacists took responsibility for educating patients about their medications and took an active role in monitoring for adverse drug reactions, drug interactions, and noncompliance (1–3, 11). While patients frequently misinterpret prescription directions, many patients are intentionally noncompliant (4, 5).

Patient education and chronic disease monitoring are two of the most important functions performed by pharmacists. The pharmacist must approach each patient in an organized manner, obtain information from the patient, and present useful patient education and/or monitoring plans.

The information presented in this chapter can be used in any setting in which pharmacy is practiced. The most common settings are hospital education and discharge counseling programs, community pharmacies, ambulatory hospital clinics, and family practice programs.

PATIENT EDUCATION

Patient education, as it relates to pharmacy practice, may be defined as an intervention designed to improve patient drug knowledge, medication compliance, and therapeutic outcome. Patient counseling may be defined as a one-on-one, interactive session designed to modify patient knowledge or behavior. Patient counseling typically provides extensive individualized information in order to overcome barriers to appropriate therapy. Patient counseling is most effective when the patient actively participates, when appropriate, in some of the decision making.

In recent years there has been a major increase in consumer demand for medical and prescription information. While patients typically rank the physician as their most important source of prescription information, 50 to 80% also identify the pharmacist as an important source (12). In the past, pharmacists' responsibility for patient counseling has not been clear in practice standards and law. However, recent legal cases are precedent-setting and have resulted in new standards for patient counseling (13). Several state boards of pharmacy have mandated patient counseling, and the National Association of Boards of Pharmacy (NABP) recently suggested that state pharmacy practice acts be revised to include the following elements (14):

1. That each pharmacy maintain a current copy of an approved text that contains information for the pharmacist and an approved source of information for the patient;
2. That institutional pharmacies have adequate information sources available to patients within the institution and at discharge;
3. That the pharmacist, upon dispensing a medication, be available for oral consultation with the patient and inquire as to the patient's understanding of the use of the medication; and
4. That each pharmacy have a private area for consultations with patients.

The NABP also strongly encouraged state boards to require by law or regulation patient profiles, drug-use review, and patient counseling. These recommendations would apply to any ambulatory setting, including institutional outpatient services and community pharmacies.

Most hospitals, HMOs, and many ambulatory clinics and family practice offices have patient education committees. The pharmacist should be an active participant in the activities of this committee. These committees usually have interdisciplinary involvement, with members contributing their own expertise. The committee determines the types of educational interventions that will be offered by the institution. The pharmacist should assist with development of written education materials, protocols for discharge counseling, and protocols for ambulatory medication instruction (15, 16). Studies have found that discharge counseling can reduce medication administration errors and readmission (6, 8).

The major emphasis that is placed on patient education and monitoring requires that pharmacists in all patient-care settings have an in-depth knowledge of patient education, counseling, and monitoring techniques. Patient education and monitoring can be provided to institutional patients during their stay, inpatients at discharge, and ambulatory patients in outpatient clinics, community pharmacies, health maintenance organizations, or in the home.

This chapter addresses patient education, counseling and monitoring techniques, the preferences of consumers, and chronic disease monitoring in the various patient-care settings.

DETERMINING PATIENT INFORMATION NEEDS

The desires of the patient must be assessed initially for each encounter in which the pharmacist will provide patient education. This is not to suggest that patients who feel they need no information may not require education. The approach must be tailored to the patients so that they will be receptive to the educational intervention. Identifying various information-seeking behaviors may assist the pharmacist in developing a patient-specific approach to counseling.

Morris and colleagues published the results of a telephone survey examining the prescription information-seeking behavior of 835 individuals (12). The four distinct types of behavior described in their study were uninformed (34%), physician-reliant (40%), pharmacist-reliant (19%), and questioners (7%). The "uninformed" group, who were the oldest and least likely to have received physician or pharmacist counseling (written or verbal), may not recognize the consequences of improper drug use. The "physician-reliant" group (those who received prescription information from the physician) were generally passive recipients of physician information and were the most likely to obtain prescriptions from chain pharmacies. The "pharmacist-reliant" people were the youngest, were more likely to obtain prescriptions from independent pharmacies, received more counseling at the pharmacy, and perceived few barriers to receiving information. The fourth group, classified as "questioners," included those who were more likely to receive their information from books or magazines. This group required clear information that answered specific questions and appeared to be the most difficult group to satisfy.

This interesting study suggests that patients gravitate to the information source they feel is most appropriate or with which they feel most comfortable. The study also suggests that pharmacists must develop a campaign to proactively seek patients to counsel, in order to inform them of the value of pharmacist consultation. While community pharmacists are often willing to provide counseling when requested by the patient (17, 18), this may be insufficient, because many patients who need counseling do not ask for assistance. This is especially true for the "uninformed" or "physician-reliant" patients who do not perceive the need for or value of pharmacist counseling.

Schondelmeyer and Trinca studied consumer demand and their willingness to pay for a counseling service in chain pharmacies (19). Patients were allocated to groups of either no charge, $1, $2, or $3, and they could either accept or refuse the service. The study found that 88% of patients accepted the service at no charge, 25% accepted and paid $1, 36% accepted and paid $2, and 17% paid $3 per prescription. The vast majority of patients were willing to use the service again. Interestingly, only 25% of those who refused the service did so because of cost. Many refused the service because they did not want more information, did not have time, or were not feeling well. These results contradict data that show that chain pharmacy patrons are more price-sensitive and less likely to value pharmacist counseling (as they are more physician-reliant).

Various studies have found discrepancies between the information that clinicians perceive as important and what patients desire. Physicians and pharmacists have been reluctant to volunteer in-depth discussions of rare or serious side effects for fear of frightening patients, which could decrease their compliance with treatment (20). However, Quaid found that seizure patients wanted to receive specific information on potentially serious side effects associated with carbamazepine (20). While the patients perceived the drug to be risky, no patient refused treatment, and there was no evidence for a negative effect of giving patients extensive information. The authors also concluded that patients given more information may be better able to correctly recognize side effects should they occur.

These studies suggest that patients are becoming sophisticated consumers of health education. While a large group are passive recipients, the majority of patients seek information from a variety of sources. In many cases these sources are not health professionals, but rather, books, magazines, friends, or relatives. By recognizing these behaviors and patient-specific needs, the pharmacist can tailor the educational approach to the individual patient.

PATIENT LEARNING AND BEHAVIOR

One of the most important aspects of patient education is an understanding of how patients learn. However, demonstration of learning and knowledge does not guarantee that a patient will follow directions or alter behavior. Patients are faced with numerous choices each day, which may cause them to miss doses, not follow a diet, or continue smoking. These choices may be influenced by social, attitudinal, or financial factors, which may take precedent over the patient's proven knowledge and ability to manage a treatment regiment (21, 22). Therefore, health professionals must provide all of the needed information, identify barriers, and develop methods to overcome them.

Factors that must be considered when providing patient education include the attitudes and health beliefs of patients (21–24). Patients must perceive that they have a disease and that it is potentially harmful. They must believe that the therapy will be of value to them and that the value will be greater than the cost, side effects, and other barriers. For instance, if patients are not convinced of their diagnosis of hypertension or deny the medical problem, they may never fill the prescription. These beliefs and attitudes are probably responsible for the large percentage of prescriptions that are never filled (up to 25% in some studies) and the 30 to 80% of patients who fail to adhere to the treatment regimen.

The sequence of steps involved in learning has been described in several ways but has common features (21, 25). The pharmacist must recognize the complexity of counseling in order to design the most appropriate approach to a given patient. Once a message is sent, it must be received and comprehended by the patient. The patient must then retain and be able to recall this information. Patients must also be motivated to accept the message so that they can perform the desired function or comply with the treatment regimen.

Most studies have found that adherence to a medication regimen can not be predicted by patient demographics such as age, gender, education, or race (22, 23). While lack of knowledge may lead to noncompliance, many patients who do not take medication appropriately understand the treatment plan but choose to alter or discontinue therapy. Factors that predict difficulties with compliance include increasing the number of daily doses, longer duration of therapy, asymptomatic disease, and cost. One common reason for discontinuation is a fear that side effects might occur. Dissatisfaction with the physician, pharmacist, or waiting time may also contribute to noncompliance (22, 24).

Clearly, therapeutic regimens require that patients modify their behavior in order to take their medication appropriately. In addition to improving knowledge, patient education must motivate patients to recognize the importance of the prescribed therapy. Patient education cannot be a one-way dispensing of information; pharmacists must respect the patient's right to choose. Patients will not comply just because *we* (as health professionals) know that it is important or because they are told to comply. The most successful education occurs when patients participate in some of the decision making so that they can make informed decisions (21).

COMPONENTS OF PATIENT EDUCATION

Mullen et al. identified several critical features of effective patient education techniques (Table 6.1) (26).

Relevance means that the program should be tailored to the individual needs of the patient, including knowledge, reading ability, beliefs, and experiences. In addition, the method and pace of the program must be *individualized*, acknowledging the differences in the way people learn and the rate at which they learn (21). Different teaching skills may be needed at different times for the same patient. A well-rounded educational intervention may not

Table 6.1.
Components of High-Quality Patient Education Interventions[a]

Relevance	Program should be tailored to the knowledge, reading level, visual acuity, beliefs, circumstances, and prior experience of the learners
Individualization	Learning is an individual process; program more effective if questions are answered when they arise and when education is paced appropriately for the learner
Feedback	Facilitates learning by showing patients the extent of their progress; used to assess the degree of learning by the patient
Reinforcement	Provides rewards for desired behavior, often by praise or congratulations
Facilitation	Methods used to reduce barriers to the regimen; may include special containers, adjustment of the regimen around the patient's activities, or reducing costs
Combination	Combinations of the above are more effective than single interventions; can accommodate learning abilities or preferences, increase retention of information, and promote reinforcement

[a] From Mullen PD, Green LW, Persinger GS: Clinical trials of patient education for chronic conditions: a comparative meta-analysis of intervention types. Prev Med 14:753–781, 1985.

be able to meet all of its objectives on the first visit (e.g., with a new prescription). Often, components of the intervention must occur at follow-up visits or when medications are refilled. A continuous assessment of patient attitudes, beliefs, knowledge, and skills is required (21).

Feedback is very important and can be of two types. Feedback may be provided to patients concerning their progress (e.g., changes in blood sugar values or blood pressure). Feedback solicited from the patients helps you determine their level of understanding. This can be done when a new medication is dispensed. Feedback can also be obtained periodically during chronic therapy, in order to sustain a specific behavior. For instance, the patient can be questioned about compliance and knowledge when refills are obtained. Caring, empathetic questioning can reinforce the importance of the behavior and show the patient the importance the pharmacist places on it.

Reinforcement provides rewards for a given behavior and may be positive and negative (27). Verbal praise or congratulations for good compliance or a change in behavior may be the most effective. Negative reinforcement or fear-arousing may be effective, but it must be used cautiously (27). Negative reinforcement might include a discussion of the physical consequences of smoking or of untreated hypertension. However, the patient may block out the entire message if it produces too much fear. Continuous reinforcement is essential. It cannot be assumed that a history of excellent adherence will continue. This is particularly true for patients with chronic, asymptomatic conditions (7).

Facilitation can be accomplished with a new prescription or with refills. For new prescriptions, the patient should be questioned about meal patterns, work schedules, and daily activities. All potential barriers to adherence must be explored. The medication regimen can then be tailored to the patient, with specific administration times suggested. Facilitation should also occur when the pharmacist identifies adverse reactions or problems with compliance that may be associated with improper administration. This may involve suggesting to take a drug with food, providing alternative administration times, or providing the patient with special containers. It may also require suggesting alternative drugs to the physician, which may decrease adverse reactions, improve compliance, or reduce cost.

Combinations of these techniques are most useful. A thorough patient education program will incorporate all of these concepts and modify them to the specific needs of the individual. For patients with chronic, asymptomatic diseases it is important to continue to provide education, feedback, and reinforcement because information retention declines with time, and compliance may diminish (7, 18, 27).

TYPES OF PATIENT EDUCATION

Patient education may be verbal, written, or audiovisual (15, 19, 20, 28, 29). *Verbal* education can be one-on-one counseling, or it may be provided to small groups of patients with similar conditions. *Written* information can include special labels for prescription bottles, patient package inserts (PPIs), single-page materials that are developed by individual pharmacists or organizations, and booklets. *Audiovisual* programs have generally used slide-tape programs or videocassettes. All of these methods (with the possible exception of PPIs) have been shown to improve knowledge and information retention (26, 27). A combination of verbal and written or the use of verbal counseling along with audiovisual aids is generally superior to the use of traditional written material only (27, 28). Most patients prefer a combination of written and verbal information, and studies have found this approach to be most effective in improving knowledge (30). Providing only written information, especially when it is in the form of an auxiliary label or PPI, is generally insufficient patient education.

When comparing efficacy, volume, logistics, and cost, the preferred method is to provide both written and verbal information. This is especially important for new prescriptions (30). The presentation should be individualized to the patient as discussed above. The pharmacist must highlight important aspects in the written material for patient review. The patient should be given opportunity to ask

Table 6.2.

Required Elements of Pharmacist-Conducted Patient Counseling[a,b]

Using suitable verbal, written, or audiovisual communication techniques, the pharmacist should inform, educate, and counsel patients (or their representatives) about the following:

Drug name (generic and brand name)

Intended use and expected action

Route, dosage form, dosage, and administration schedule

Special directions for preparation

Special directions for administration

Precautions to be observed during administration

Common side effects that may be encountered, avoidance and action required if they occur

Techniques for self-monitoring of drug therapy

Proper storage

Potential drug-drug or drug-food interactions or other therapeutic contraindications

Prescription refill information

Action to be taken in the event of a missed dose

Other information peculiar to the specific patient or drug

[a] From Statement on pharmacist-conducted patient counseling: official statement of the American Society of Hospital Pharmacists. J Hosp Pharm 41:331, 1984.
[b] These 13 points are applicable to both prescription and nonprescription drugs. The pharmacist must also counsel patients in the proper selection of nonprescription drugs as well as when and if they should be used.

questions and encouraged to contact the pharmacist if problems or other questions arise. The information that patients should understand about each of their prescription and nonprescription drugs is displayed in Tables 6.2 and 6.3 (31, 32).

Preprinted medication instructions are available from manufacturers, pharmacy or medical associations, the United States Pharmacopeia, or private companies. With the advent of word processing and desk-top publishing, the pharmacist can create high-quality materials, tailor them to specific patients, and modify content when necessary. When reviewing these materials, the pharmacist should consider the important elements of written education techniques. In addition to the content areas listed in Table 6.2, particular attention should be paid to the elements for designing written medication instructions displayed in Table 6.4 (33–35). Pharmacists who design their own materials should include the name of the pharmacy, the name of the patient's pharmacist, and a telephone number to call if questions or problems arise.

The most readable written education materials are on no more than one page, front and back. They can be short and succinct (Fig. 6.1) or more comprehensive, such as those found in the USPDI, "Advice for the patient" (19, 36). The goals of the handout should be stated in the material. The material should be in lists rather than in paragraphs. Key items or warnings should be highlighted with bullets or icons. Terms should be concrete and familiar to

Table 6.3.
Required Elements of Pharmacist-Conducted Patient Counseling for Nonprescription Drugs[a]

Using suitable verbal, written, or audiovisual communication techniques, the pharmacist should
  Obtain relevant data and inform, educate, and counsel patients (or their representatives) about
    Onset of symptoms
    Duration of symptoms
    Severity of symptoms
    Description of symptoms
    Location of symptoms
    Other associated symptoms
    Factors that provide relief of symptoms
    Self-treatment history
    Other medical problems, drug therapy, allergies, and sensitivities
  Perform physical assessment (if indicated)
  Determine the patient's condition and/or need for referral
  Recommend either no treatment, a nonprescription product, or physician referral (depending on the nature and severity of the problem)
  Educate the patient about proper use, dosage, and precautions of the drug treatment (see Table 6.2)
  Answer the patient's questions
  Arrange for follow-up on the patient's response
  Make a complete entry of all of the above into the patient's pharmacy record

[a] Adapted from Guidelines for pharmacist's communications. Texas State Board of Pharmacy Newsletter (April–June):7, 1990.

Table 6.4.
Rules for Designing Written Medication Instructions

Begin with a title that names the goal and expand the title by describing the goal in the first sentence.
Use list format, with each action or warning numbered and presented on a separate line.
Include a medication schedule and warning icons.
Mention actions in the order in which they will be performed.
Explicitly signal which information is important.
Use common names for medication and anchor medication schedules to routine activities such as meals and bedtime. When possible, state an exact time that corresponds to the patient's work (school), meal, and sleep schedule.
Print in at least 14-point font size for the elderly and visually impaired.
Use common concrete words.
Use single-clause, active, affirmative sentences (except for negatively worded warnings).
Have no greater than a fourth-grade readability score.
Describe medication schedules with explicit words and phrases.
Include the name of pharmacy, name of pharmacist, and telephone number(s).

Adapted from Morrow D, Leirer V, Sheik J: Adherence and medication instructions: review and recommendations. J Am Geriatr Soc 36:1147–1160, 1988.

the patient. The print size should be at least 14 point if the material will be used by the elderly.

If only one handout will be prepared for all patients receiving a given drug, the readability should be below the eight-grade level, and preferably at the fourth-grade level (33). Alternatively, two or three handouts at different readability levels could be prepared for each drug. Methods are available for determining readability (34, 37). In some communities, handouts may be needed in several languages.

Audiovisual (AV) materials might be reserved for common conditions with lengthy or complex instructions. Some AV materials are available from pharmaceutical manufacturers for products that have complicated applications, mixing, or administration features. The patient should be allowed time to view the material in a private or semiprivate area. The pharmacist should then reinforce important concepts and give the patient an opportunity to ask questions. In the hospital, an audiovisual program can be provided on the hospital's closed-circuit television system. After the patient has viewed the program, information can be reinforced by the pharmacist with discharge counseling (29).

TECHNIQUES OF PROVIDING PATIENT COUNSELING

Comprehensive sources are available which discuss communication and counseling skills (38, 39). When interviewing a patient or conducting a counseling session, the pharmacist must always be aware of the patient's verbal and nonverbal messages and barriers to effective communication. We must also be aware of our own verbal and nonverbal messages.

When we send a message, we develop the words based upon our understanding, past experiences, and culture. The receivers must decode our message. They may not receive the intended message if their experiences, first language, or culture is different from our own. We can ensure that the message was correctly received by using feedback. Feedback may be nonverbal (e.g., a confused expression) or verbal. In addition to volunteered verbal feedback, we can check the level of understanding by asking the receiver questions. For instance, "Mrs. Jones, I have given you a lot of information about your captopril. Would you please tell me how, and at what times, you plan to take it?"

Barriers

The prescription counter or a desk between the counselor and the patient can be a significant barrier to effective communication with patients. In addition, the raised platform in many pharmacies causes the pharmacist to be much higher than the patient and can cause intimidation.

CAPTOPRIL (KAP-toe-pril)
CAPOTEN (Common Brand Name)

Captopril is a drug used to treat high blood pressure. It may also be used to help control fluid in the heart and lungs.

Some people who take this drug may have:

     ---dizziness
     ---fainting or lightheadedness
     ---a loss of taste for the first 2-3 months

These usually go away once your body gets used to the medication.

Call your doctor if you have any:

     ---fever or sore throat
     ---skin rash
     ---chest pain
     ---increased dizziness or lightheadedness
     ---fast or irregular heart beat

Your dose of captopril is: _____

Take your medication: _____

Your doctor's name and phone number is: _____

_____

DO NOT STOP TAKING YOUR MEDICATION WITHOUT TALKING TO YOUR DOCTOR!! TELL ALL YOUR DOCTORS THAT YOU ARE TAKING THIS MEDICATION!! ASK YOUR DOCTOR ABOUT THE NEED FOR FOLLOW-UP TESTS WHILE TAKING THIS MEDICATION? SOME PEOPLE HAVE OTHER SIDE EFFECTS!! CALL YOUR DOCTOR WITH ANY QUESTIONS!!

THOMAS JEFFERSON UNIVERSITY HOSPITAL | DEPARTMENT OF NURSING
DEPARTMENT OF PHARMACY

Figure 6.1. Example of medication teaching card for captopril. (From McGinty MK, Chase SL, Mercer ME: Pharmacy-nursing discharge counseling program for cardiac patients. Am J Hosp Pharm 45:1546, 1988, with permission.)

Clerks or technicians are also barriers to good communication if the patient perceives that the pharmacist is inaccessible. Other patients within hearing distance are another important barrier that should be avoided. Finally, noise (telephones, typewriters, music) is a significant barrier, especially for the hearing-impaired patient. In addition to auditory deficits, patients may have other functional barriers including visual or psychological disturbances (e.g., anxiety, depression, memory impairment).

There are many pharmacist-related barriers to good communication. The two most significant communication barriers for pharmacists are time and low priority for counseling. Pharmacists must recognize that patient education and physician communication are two of their most important functions. Each pharmacy setting must be examined so that activities and functions can be arranged to allow maximal time for patient counseling. In many cases,

counseling and drug therapy monitoring are ongoing activities with individual patients. When extended discussions are necessary, the pharmacist should attempt to schedule patients to return for counseling at a mutually convenient time. Technicians, maximally utilized, increase the pharmacist's efficiency and time for counseling and monitoring. Other pharmacist barriers include shyness and/or lack of confidence. Communication and counseling skills are not innate. They must be learned and practiced in order to reduce apprehension.

THE COUNSELING SESSION

Good counseling requires appropriate nonverbal behavior. In addition to watching nonverbal cues from the patient, pharmacists must be constantly aware of the nonverbal messages they are sending the patient. Casual dress or leaning back in a chair with arms crossed suggests an un-caring, disinterested, less-than-professional pharmacist.

The pharmacist should be at eye level with the patient. Ideally, both should be seated at an appropriate distance, approximately 2 to 3 feet in western cultures, although a closer distance is expected in some cultures. The counselor should face the patient directly (frontal appearance), in an open posture. The pharmacist should not cross the arms or legs, should sit erect with a slight forward lean (attending to the patient), and should use good eye contact with the patient. This will suggest confidence and help the pharmacist to detect nonverbal cues. Eye contact should be varied, with occasional glances down or to the side to avoid staring. In some cultures, strong eye contact is not used.

When initiating an interview or counseling session, the pharmacist must establish rapport by introducing himself and shaking the patient's hand. Patients should be addressed as Mr., Ms., or Mrs., not by their first names. This may not be essential for children, but it is certainly important when the patient is older than the interviewer.

The pharmacist should have a plan for the session, including questions to pursue in order to identify problems. The patient should also understand the goals of the session. This can be accomplished by briefly telling the patient what will be covered, "First, I would like to describe briefly how this medicine works, then we will talk about the appropriate times and methods of taking it. Finally, I want to mention some side effects that are not common, but that you should be aware of and report to me and your doctor, in the unlikely event that they occur." After this discussion, the important information should be summarized at the end of the session (39).

The pharmacist should attempt to keep the session on track, but not appear rude when refocusing the patient's attention. A combination of open- and closed-ended questions should be used, but open-ended questions are preferred. A closed-ended question can be answered yes or no (e.g., "Are you taking your medication?"), but this often results in a loss of information. A patient may answer "yes" because he has not stopped taking it, even though he has missed many doses. A better question is "How many times in the last week or month have you missed a dose of this medication?"

Counseling hearing-impaired patients requires special attention. Hearing difficulties in elderly patients are generally not related to vocal volume. Elderly people often lose the ability to hear or distinguish high-frequency tones (female voices) and consonants. Background conversations or noise can significantly impair their understanding of the spoken word. These individuals frequently use some lip reading for assistance. Therefore, the pharmacist should face the patient and speak slowly, with good enunciation,

without covering his mouth. The pharmacist should not shout at the patient.

When the session is concluded, the pharmacist should determine the level of understanding by eliciting feedback. This is done by asking the patients to describe their level of understanding of all aspects of the therapy. The pharmacist can then correct misunderstandings and fill in missing information. Finally, the pharmacist should give the patient one last opportunity to ask questions. The patient should be informed that the pharmacist is always available to answer questions. The pharmacist should then conclude the interview, give the patient a business card with a telephone number, and shake the patient's hand.

MONITORING

Drug therapy monitoring by pharmacists implies the assessment of pharmacotherapeutic regimens for efficacy, adverse effects, drug interactions, and noncompliance. Numerous studies have demonstrated the value of clinical pharmacy services in the chronic management of hypertensive, diabetic, and anticoagulated patients (7, 40–52).

In a study based in a hospital ambulatory clinic, physicians referred patients to a clinical pharmacist and a nurse clinician (43). Patients were evaluated during a control period, and a clinical pharmacist was introduced into the clinic to monitor and counsel patients. Compared to the control period, study patients were more compliant (72% vs. 20%) and blood pressure control was better (69% vs. 29%). These results were statistically significant, and the benefit remained after 4 years of follow-up. The cost savings due to reduced duplication of drugs, reduced office visits, and improved care greatly exceeded the cost of providing the service.

The value that patient education and monitoring services have on patient knowledge, compliance, and blood pressure control was reported by McKenney et al. in 1973 (7). Hypertensive patients were divided into a control group and a study group. The study group received comprehensive education and monitoring when they received prescriptions from the pharmacist. The community pharmacist interacted frequently with the physicians in a nearby urban health center in order to modify therapy when problems with compliance or adverse effects arose. Both compliance and blood pressure control were better in the study group. When these services were discontinued, compliance and blood pressure control in the study group returned to preintervention levels.

This type of drug therapy monitoring can be used in many ambulatory pharmacy environments. Pharmacist-directed anticoagulation, hypertension, lipid, and general medicine assessment clinics are now common. In these settings, physicians refer patients for interim care, which is provided by pharmacists. The pharmacist is responsible for reviewing the medical record and the treatment plan designed by the physician. The pharmacist then conducts an interview, which includes the medication history, signs or symptoms of disease, or adverse reactions. In many of these clinics, the pharmacist performs limited assessments in order to evaluate drug efficacy or potential toxicity. These include obtaining vital signs, performing limited physical assessment, ordering laboratory tests, and when appropriate, ordering serum drug level determinations. In some of these clinics, the pharmacist will then consult with the physician in order to modify therapy, develop more intensive diagnostic plans, or schedule follow-up visits. It is also common for the pharmacists to use protocols that allow them to make all treatment modifications. In this case, the physician is available when significant problems are identified.

While the above drug therapy monitoring functions have typically been confined to institutional-based ambulatory practice and the Indian Health Service, many community pharmacies have designed extensive monitoring services. Typically, these are initiated with the cooperation and support of selected physicians who have a good working relationship with the pharmacist. These services have frequently been expanded later to broader groups of patients.

On large inpatient services or in busy ambulatory clinics it may not be possible to interact during each prescribing event. Therefore, pharmacists may want to direct their efforts to high-risk patients, to those on certain drug regimens (e.g., drugs with narrow therapeutic indices) or to the elderly. Koecheler and co-workers identified six prognostic indicators that could be used to identify ambulatory patients with a high risk of adverse outcomes (53). These include patients with:

Five or more medications in the drug regimen;
Twelve or more medication doses per day;
Medication regimen changed four or more times during the previous 12 months;
More than three concurrent disease states present;
History of noncompliance;
Drugs that require therapeutic drug monitoring.

The pharmacist in a very busy practice might focus monitoring efforts on patients who meet these criteria.

Monitoring in the Community Pharmacy

In the community pharmacy setting, the pharmacist could select patients meeting the above criteria or identity other patients requiring more intensive monitoring. These may include patients with specific chronic diseases (e.g., hypertension, diabetes) or those taking potentially toxic drugs (e.g., theophylline, warfarin, or anticonvulsants). Alternatively, the pharmacist may focus on elderly patients receiving multiple medications. Eventually the service must be explained so that all of these high-risk patients receive drug therapy monitoring by the pharmacist.

In addition to conducting a thorough interview for disease control and signs and symptoms of adverse drug reactions, the pharmacist should assess vital signs, when appropriate, for the specific drug(s) in the regimen. Laboratory testing is not typically available to the community pharmacist, but serum glucose monitoring is invaluable when caring for diabetic patients. In some cases it is possible to perform serum drug level assessments (e.g., theophylline) using only blood from a finger stick. It is likely that additional rapid laboratory and drug analysis tests will be available to the community pharmacist. Pharmacokinetic monitoring may be necessary to ensure adequate control or prevent adverse reactions (see Chapter 1). While pharmacokinetic monitoring is usually considered an inpatient service, it can be adapted easily to community or ambulatory settings (54).

With prior approval from the patient's physician, it may be appropriate to make modifications in the patient's regimen. Obviously, this level of drug therapy monitoring can only be performed when there is extensive communication between the pharmacist and the physician. The pharmacist should document all subjective and objective information

Table 6.5.
Key Patient Education and Monitoring Functions Provided by Pharmacists[a]

1. Conduct a patient interview and interpret its result.
2. List and explain the monitoring parameters and therapeutic end points for the safe and efficacious use of each drug in the regimen.
3. Monitor drug therapy prospectively for potential drug-drug, drug–laboratory test, drug-diet, drug-disease, and drug-condition interactions, and recommend modifications in drug therapy, when appropriate, to minimize such interactions.
4. Use interviews, physical assessment, and interpretation of laboratory test results to monitor therapy for adverse and therapeutic effects.
5. Take a medication history, assess the patient's attitude toward compliance, and evaluate the influence of these factors on therapeutic response. Initiate strategies to correct noncompliant behavior.
6. Counsel patients on drug use.
7. Serve on a healthcare team providing primary or consultative care.
8. Formulate individualized drug regimens prospectively, based on the purpose of the medication(s), concurrent disease(s) and drug therapies, pharmacokinetic parameters of the drug(s), and the patient's clinical condition.
9. Devise individualized drug regimens and recommend adjustments based on therapeutic response.
10. Describe the clinical manifestations of potential toxicities associated with a patient's medication, assess the significance of the toxicity, and recommend an appropriate course of action.
11. Communicate effectively with patients, physicians, nurses, other health professionals and peers.
12. Manage a patient's drug therapy by
    a. designing a drug therapy treatment plan and advising prescribers on its implementation.
    b. using established therapeutic protocols, or
    c. independently prescribing or adjusting drug therapy in instances where supportive legislation exists.

[a] Adapted from ASHP supplemental standard and learning objectives for residency training in primary care pharmacy practice. Am J Hosp Pharm 47:1851–1854, 1990.

and all recommendations that are provided to the patient. The physician should be provided with a written summary or consultation letter following each encounter with the patient. This letter should include all pertinent subjective and objective information, recommendations, and changes in therapy, if applicable.

Standards of practice have been developed which describe the interviewing, monitoring, and patient education activities that are essential for clinical pharmacists (55) and for pharmacotherapy specialists (56). The types of pharmaceutical services may differ slightly from one setting to another. The new learning objectives for ASHP-accredited primary-care residencies provide a general description of the monitoring functions that should be performed in am-

bulatory settings (55). In order to provide effective drug therapy monitoring, the pharmacist must understand which monitoring parameters and therapeutic end points are important for each regimen. Potential problems may be limited by prospective monitoring of drug therapy for drug-drug or drug-disease interactions. The functions that relate to patient education and monitoring are displayed in Table 6.5.

DOCUMENTATION OF PATIENT EDUCATION AND MONITORING
Organized Healthcare Settings

Optimally, whenever the pharmacist has interviewed a patient, provided education, or obtained monitoring infor-

Figure 6.2. Pharmacist monitoring and assessment guidelines for digoxin. (From McKenney JM, Wyant SL, Atkins D, et al.: Drug therapy assessments by pharmacists. Am J Hosp Pharm 37:825, 1980, with permission.)

Monitoring Elements	Action
Disease Related	
Congestive heart failure: Shortness of breath, orthopnea, dyspnea on exertion, paroxysmal nocturnal dyspnea, nocturia, dependent edema, rales, tachycardia, weight gain, jugular vein distention, gallop rhythm, hepatomegally.	Diet assessment Blood pressure EKG, rhythm strip Chest X-ray Renal function tests Dose change Regimen change Referral
Atrial fibrilliation: Dizziness, weakness, palpitations, ventricular rate > 120, irregularly irregular pulse, symptoms of congestive heart failure, pulmonary and peripheral embolism.	
Drug Related	
Toxicity: Palpitations, irregular pulse, bradycardia (pulse < 60), anorexia, nausea, vomiting, diarrhea, visual changes-blurred vision, color changes halos, weakness, fatigue, confusion, headache, delirium.	Digoxin level EKG Thyroid function tests SMA 6-60 or 12-60 Patient education Compliance-improving strategies Dose change Regimen change Discontinuation Referral
Other: Electrolytes, renal status, thyuuroid function, hypoxia	
Compliance/inappropriate drug use	
Patient Disposition	

1. **Renew therapy. Drug may be continued if above signs or symptoms** are absent or stable.
2. **Refer patient if (a) there is evidence of worsening congestive failure** or atrial fibrilliation or (b) digoxin toxicity is detected or suspected.
3. **Consult physician to achieve (a) alteration in dose to control con-** gestive heart failure or atrial fibrilliation or (b) addition or deletion from regimen to control congestive heart failure or atrial fibrillation.

mation, the findings should be documented in the patient's medical record (hospital, nursing home, or ambulatory clinic). The pharmacist must determine the most effective means to document the information in the medical record. In an organized healthcare setting, the pharmacist should obtain the privilege of recording this information into the patient's medical record. This information must be obtained and recorded in a logical and consistent manner. Figure 6.2 displays an example of monitoring and assessment guidelines for digoxin, used by a pharmacist-operated assessment clinic (57).

The pharmacist should document the data in a problem-oriented approach, addressing issues in the order: subjective, objective, assessment, and plan (SOAP). An extensive discussion of this topic appears in the accompanying workbook. Information volunteered by the patient or obtained by questioning the patient (including methods of drug administration, adverse reactions, and compliance) should appear in the subjective section. Specific monitoring performed by the pharmacist, physician, or laboratory should be included in the objective section. This includes data such as vital signs, blood glucose determinations, serum drug levels, or physical signs of an adverse effect. The assessment should include drug-related problems or issues identified by the pharmacist. The plan should include all recommendations made to the patient or physician by the pharmacist. These might include patient education recommendations or suggestions for modifications in the therapeutic regimen.

Community Pharmacy

Pharmacists who provide extensive counseling should maintain their own records, containing all data collected, as described above. If significant problems such as adverse drug reactions or interactions are detected, they must be communicated directly to the physician (rather than to other office personnel). The pharmacist should be prepared to suggest alternative recommendations to the physician.

In community pharmacies where patients are seen for drug therapy monitoring, the pharmacist should routinely evaluate the patients' drug therapy. Ongoing patient counseling and patient education should ensure compliance and encourage the patient to volunteer potential adverse reactions and misunderstandings. Community pharmacists who provide this advanced-level service should be in frequent contact with the physician. The pharmacist should talk to the physician when problems are identified and send patient-specific summaries (subjective and objective data) periodically. This is important in community pharmacies because the pharmacist may not be able to make notations directly in the physician's medical record, and the physician should have access to this valuable information.

SUMMARY

Some of the most important functions provided by the pharmacist include patient education and drug therapy monitoring. The pharmacist must understand not only the critical components of communication and counseling but also the needs and demands of patients. Each pharmacist should have a structured approach for obtaining information from the patient and for providing patient education. A detailed plan for evaluating therapeutic efficacy or toxicity should be established by the pharmacist for each disease or drug category. Most importantly, the pharmacist should document the data in the patient's medical record and/or communicate this information to the physician.

REFERENCES

1. Manasse HR Jr: Medication use in an imperfect world: drug misadventuring as an issue of public policy. Part 1. Am J Hosp Pharm 46:929–944, 1989.
2. Manasse HR Jr: Medication use in an imperfect world: drug misadventuring as an issue of public policy. Part 2. Am J Hosp Pharm 46:1141–1152, 1989.
3. Hepler CD, Strand LM: Opportunities and responsibilities in pharmaceutical care. Am J Hosp Pharm 47:533–543, 1990.
4. Mazzullo JM, Lasagna L, Griner PF: Variations in interpretation of prescription instructions: the need for improved prescribing habits. JAMA 227:929–931, 1974.
5. Covington TR, Porter ME: Improper prescription instructions: a factor in patient compliance. Patient Counseling and Health Education (Winter/Spring):97–100, 1979.
6. Markey BT, Igou JF: Medication discharge planning for the elderly. Patient Education and Counseling 9:241–249, 1987.
7. McKenney JM, Slining JM, Henderson HR, Devins D, Barr M: The effect of clinical pharmacy services on patients with essential hypertension. Circulation 48:1104–1111, 1973.
8. Cole P, Emmanuel S: Drug consultation: its significance to the discharged hospital patient and its relevance as a role for the pharmacist. Am J Hosp Pharm 28:954–960, 1971.
9. Maronde RF, Chan LS, Larsen FJ, et al.: Underutilization of antihypertensive drugs and associated hospitalization. Med Care 27:1159–1166, 1989.
10. McKenney JM, Harrison WL: Drug-related hospital admissions. Am J Hosp Pharm 33:792–795, 1976.
11. McKenney JM, Wasserman AJ: Effect of advanced pharmaceutical services on the incidence of adverse drug reactions. Am J Hosp Pharm 36:1691–1697, 1979.
12. Morris LA, Grossman R, Barkdoll G, Gordon E: A segmentational analysis of prescription drug information seeking. Med Care 25:953–964, 1987.
13. Simonsmeier LM, Brushwood DB: Drug counseling by pharmacists: the need for legal recognition. Patient Education and Counseling 13:43–52, 1989.
14. Anon: NABP approves resolutions on patient counseling, model rules for regulation of out-of-state pharmacies. Am J Hosp Pharm 46:1512–1514, 1989.
15. McGinty MK, Chase SL, Mercer ME: Pharmacy-nursing discharge counseling program for cardiac patients. Am J Hosp Pharm 45:1545–1548, 1988.
16. Hladik WB, White SJ: Evaluation of written reinforcements used in counseling cardiovascular patients. Am J Hosp Pharm 33:1277–1280, 1976.
17. Ascione FJ, Kirking DM, Duzey OM, Waenzloff NJ: A survey of

patient education activities of community pharmacists. Patient Education and Counseling 7:359–366, 1985.

18. Carroll NV, Gagnon JP: The relationship between patient variables and frequency of pharmacist counseling. Drug Intell Clin Pharm 17:648–652, 1983.

19. Schondelmeyer SW, Trinca CE: Consumer demand for a pharmacist-conducted prescription counseling service. Am Pharm NS23:321–324, 1983.

20. Quaid KA, Faden RR, Vining EP, Freeman JM: Informed consent for a prescription drug: impact of disclosed information on patient understanding and medical outcomes. Patient Education and Counseling 15:249–259, 1990.

21. Rankin SH, Stallings KD: Patient Education, ed. 2. Philadelphia: JB Lippincott, 1990.

22. Smith DL: Patient compliance with medication regimens. Drug Intell Clin Pharm 10:386–393, 1976.

23. Boyd JR, Covington TR, Stanaszek WF, Coussons RT: Drug defaulting. Am J Hosp Pharm 31:362–367,485–491, 1974.

24. Becker MH, Maiman LA: Sociobehavioral determinants of compliance with health and medical care recommendations. Med Care 13:10–24, 1975.

25. Leventhal H, Cameron L: Behavioral theories and the problem of compliance. Patient Education and Counseling 10:117–138, 1987.

26. Mullen PD, Green LW, Persinger GS: Clinical trials of patient education for chronic conditions: a comparative meta-analysis of intervention types. Prev Med 14:753–781, 1985.

27. Morris RW, Burkhart VD, Lamy PP: Technical and theoretical aspects of patient counseling using audiovisual aids. Drug Intell Clin Pharm 9:485–488, 1975.

28. Crichton EF, Smith DL, Demanuele F: Patient recall of information. Drug Intell Clin Pharm. 12:591–599, 1978.

29. Burkle WS, Lucarotti RL: Videotaped patient medication instruction program using closed-circuit television. Am J Hosp Pharm 41:105–107, 1984.

30. Culbertson VL, Arthur TG, Rhodes PJ, Rhodes RS: Consumer preferences for verbal and written medication information. Drug Intell Clin Pharm 22:390–396, 1988.

31. Anon: Statement on pharmacist-conducted patient counseling: official statement of the American Society of Hospital Pharmacists. Am J Hosp Pharm 41:331, 1984.

32. Anon: Guidelines for pharmacist's communications. Texas State Board of Pharmacy Newsletter (April-June):7, 1990.

33. Morrow D, Leirer V, Sheikh J: Adherence and medication instructions: review and recommendations. J Am Geriatr Soc 36:1147–1160, 1988.

34. Miller A: When is the time ripe for teaching? Am J Nurs July:801–804, 1985.

35. Solinsky D, Gross SM, Seutsch T, et al.: Application of psychological principles to the design of written patient information. Am J Hosp Pharm 40:266–271, 1983.

36. Anon: Advice for the patient: drug information in lay language. In: USP DI, vol II, ed. 10. The United States Pharmacopeial Convention, Inc., 1990.

37. Pichert JW, Elam P: Readability formulas may mislead you. Patient Education and Counseling 7:181–191, 1985.

38. Tindall WN, Beardsley RS, Kimberlin CL: Communication Skills in Pharmacy Practice: A Practical Guide for Students and Practitioners, ed. 2. Philadelphia: Lea & Febiger, 1989.

39. Riccardi VM, Kurtz SM: Communication and Counseling in Health Care. Springfield, Illinois: Charles C Thomas, 1983.

40. Morton WA, Bridges ME: Pharmaceutical services in a medical screening clinic. Am J Hosp Pharm 35:574–578, 1978.

41. Tiggelar JM: Protocols for the treatment of essential hypertension and type II diabetes mellitus by pharmacists in ambulatory care clinics. Drug Intell Clin Pharm 21:521–529, 1987.

42. Monson R, Bond CA, Schuna A: Role of the clinical pharmacist in improving drug therapy: clinical pharmacists in outpatient therapy. Arch Intern Med 141:1441–1444, 1981.

43. Bond CA, Monson R: Sustained improvement in drug documentation, compliance, and disease control: a four-year analysis of an ambulatory care model. Arch Intern Med 144:1159–1162, 1984.

44. D'Achille KM, Swanson LN, Hill WT Jr: Pharmacist-managed patient assessment and medication refill clinic. Am J Hosp Pharm 35:66–70, 1978.

45. McKenney JM, Witherspoon JM, Pierpaoli PG: Initial experiences with a pharmacy clinic in a hospital-based group medical practice. Am J Hosp Pharm 38:1154–1158, 1981.

46. McKenney JM, Witherspoon JM: The impact of outpatient hospital pharmacists on patients receiving antihypertensive and anticoagulant therapy. Hosp Pharm 20:406–415, 1985.

47. Reinders TP, Steinke WE: Pharmacist management of anticoagulant therapy in ambulant patients. Am J Hosp Pharm 36:645–648, 1979.

48. Nappi JM. Measuring the effectiveness of an anticoagulation clinic managed by a pharmacist. Wisc Pharm 6:164–168, 1980.

49. Garabedian-Ruffalo SM, Gray DR, Sax MJ, et al.: Retrospective evaluation of a pharmacist-managed warfarin anticoagulation clinic. Am J Hosp Pharm 42:304–308, 1985.

50. Sczupak CA, Conrad WF: Relationship between patient-oriented pharmaceutical services and therapeutic outcomes of ambulatory patients with diabetes mellitus. Am J Hosp Pharm 34:1238–1242, 1977.

51. Hawkins DW, Fiedler FP, Douglas HL, et al.: Evaluation of a clinical pharmacist in caring for hypertensive and diabetic patients. Am J Hosp Pharm 36:1321–1325, 1979.

52. Morse GD, Douglas JB, Upton JH, et al.: Effect of pharmacist intervention on control of resistant hypertension. Am J Hosp Pharm 43:905–909, 1986.

53. Koecheler JA, Abramowitz PW, Daniels CE: Indicators for the selection of ambulatory patients who warrant pharmacist monitoring. Am J Hosp Pharm 46:729–732, 1989.

54. Robinson JD, Lopez LM, Stewart WL: How to establish a pharmacokinetics consulting service for ambulatory patients. Am J Hosp Pharm 41:2048–2056, 1984.

55. Anon: ASHP supplemental standard and learning objectives for residency training in primary care pharmacy practice. Am J Hosp Pharm 47:1851–1854, 1990.

56. Practice Guidelines for Pharmacotherapy Specialists: A position statement of the American College of Clinical Pharmacy, the ACCP Clinical Practice Affairs Committee, 1989–1990. Pharmacotherapy 10:308–311, 1990.

57. McKenney JM, Wyant SL, Atkins D, Davis L, Carasiti ME: Drug therapy assessments by pharmacists. Am J Hosp Pharm 37:824–828, 1980.

CHAPTER 7

BIOTECHNOLOGY

KIMBERLY BERGSTROM, Pharm.D.

Although major advances in our understanding of the immune system have occurred in the last decade, much remains to be learned. Undoubtedly the acquired immune deficiency syndrome (AIDS) epidemic has been responsible for the increased focus on the immune system. This attention has yielded virtually daily breakthroughs that are exposing new pieces of a very complex and important puzzle. It is clear that many diseases, including cancer, infections, and genetic diseases, are influenced by the immune system. Concomitantly, recombinant DNA technology has enabled us to produce commercially viable quantities of immune factors identical to those found in humans, which can effectively alter the immune response.

The primary function of the immune system is to defend the host from foreign substances. The immune system must first recognize the foreign substance as "nonself" and then proceed to destroy or neutralize it (1). The immune system has two functional divisions of defense against foreign substances: specific and nonspecific.

NONSPECIFIC IMMUNE RESPONSE

The nonspecific (innate) immune response is stimulated the first time a foreign substance (antigen) enters the host (1). Components of the nonspecific response perform functions that provide both physical and biochemical defenses (2). Physical defenses are provided by the skin, mucous membranes, and cilia of the respiratory tract. The biochemical defenses include the process of inflammation, release of lysozyme, and the initiation of the complement cascade (2). *Inflammation* is a complex series of events that occur when tissue is injured. Vasoactive substances such as histamine are released, which stimulates neutrophil and macrophage migration to the area of tissue injury to ingest (phagocytose) the antigen responsible (2).

Complement is set in motion by either the recognition of an antigen-antibody complex or bacteria or viruses. The cascading effect of activated proteins stimulates biological activities including chemotaxis of monocytes, neutrophils, basophils and eosinophils; the release of hydrolytic enzymes; and ultimately the destruction or inactivation of the invading antigen (2). Lysozyme (a bactericidal substance) is also released from nasal mucosa, saliva, and tears in high concentrations in response to bacterial invasion.

Nonspecific cellular components of the innate system include granulocytes (neutrophils, 60–70% of WBCs; basophils, <1% of WBCs; eosinophils, 1–3% of WBCs) and mononuclear phagocytes (monocytes and macrophages). Eosinophils ingest immune complexes (antigen-antibody complexes) and clear parasitic organisms (2). Basophils help to mediate immune responses by releasing substances such as histamine in response to antigen-antibody complexes. Macrophages and neutrophils are primarily responsible for the ingestion of particles—a process termed phagocytosis.

Phagocytosis is an important component of the nonspecific immune response. Macrophages (phagocytes) envelop the antigen and expose it to internal enzymes that degrade and inactivate the antigen. The antigen is then either completely digested by degradative enzymes or it appears on the surface of the macrophage where T lymphocytes (from the specific immune system) can recognize the antigen and react to it (3).

SPECIFIC IMMUNE RESPONSE

The specific immune system recognizes and eliminates antigens with specialized and sophisticated cells, primarily macrophages and T and B lymphocytes. T lymphocytes are primarily responsible for cell-mediated immunity, delayed hypersensitivity, transplant rejection, and tumor surveillance (Fig. 7.1). B lymphocytes are responsible for humoral, or antibody-mediated, immunity.

There are four types of T lymphocytes: T-helper, T-suppressor, cytotoxic T cells, and memory T cells. T-helper cells regulate the cell-mediated response to antigens. When macrophages of the nonspecific immune system present antigen to the T-helper cell, a series of events is set into motion: the T-helper cells release interleukin-2 (IL-2) and γ-interferon, which in turn stimulate other helper T cells and natural killer T cells, respectively. IL-2 also stimulates *cytotoxic T cells*, which attack the antigen-presenting cells, causing cellular lysis and death, by boring holes through the cell membrane and releasing lysing enzymes (2).

Suppressor T cells have the opposite effect on cells. They act on cytotoxic cells and plasma cells to inhibit their proliferation and the production of antibodies. Suppressor T cells play a critical role in the development of tolerance, which is particularly important in cases of autoimmune disease or some types of drug therapy.

Memory T cells are integrally involved in delayed hypersensitivity reactions. They secrete macrophage-chemotactic factor, which stimulates chemotaxis of monocytes

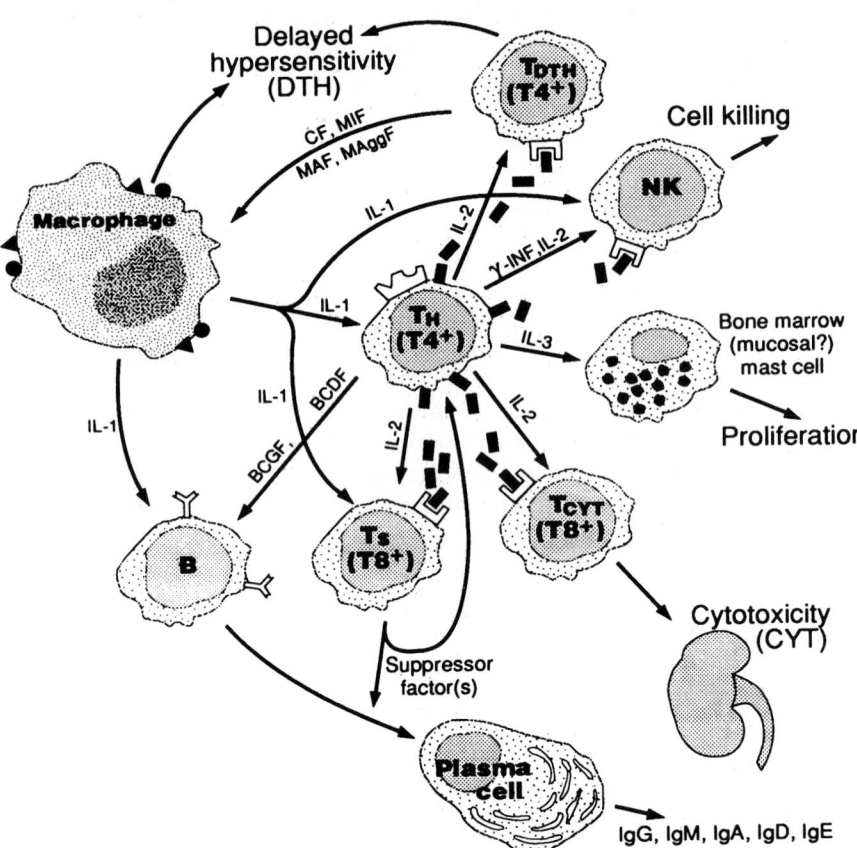

Figure 7.1. Cellular events of cell-mediated immunity and response. (From Bellanti JA, Rocklin RE: Cell-mediated immune reactions. In Immunology III. Philadelphia, WB Saunders, 1985, p 181, with permission.)

and macrophages to the antigen contact site, and macrophage inhibitory factor, which helps to keep macrophages in the area. The delayed hypersensitivity reaction occurs 24 to 48 hr after initial contact, because of the time required to accumulate these cells.

B lymphocytes are responsible for antibody-mediated or humoral immunity. Each mature B lymphocyte carries on its surface an antibody that is specific for one particular antigen (1). If a mature B lymphocyte comes in contact with its specific antigen, it will be stimulated to differentiate into an antibody-producing cell called a plasma cell. Plasma cells that encounter T-helper cells may differentiate further into memory cells, which have a long lifespan. Upon future encounters with that specific antigen, memory cells can more quickly mount a heightened immune response (1). Antibody production is the primary responsibility of the B lymphocyte.

Antibodies are made up of four polypeptide chains, two light chains and two heavy chains. The basic structure of an antibody is similar to a "Y" (Fig. 7.2). The top portion binds to a specific antigen and is known as the Fab portion (fragment of antigen binding). The base of the antibody, called the Fc (crystallizable fragment), is the portion that determines the biological function of the antibody, such as complement activation and opsonization (2). Opsoni-

zation is the ability of antibodies to increase their adherence to foreign antigens to facilitate phagocytosis. Antibodies are generally divided into five distinct classes: IgG, IgM, IgA, IgE, and IgD. Each class of antibody has its own specific function and response to antigen (Table 7.1).

A third type of lymphoid cells that is important to the specific immune system are killer cells and natural killer (NK) cells. Killer cells recognize and destroy antigen bound to antibodies (antibody-dependent cell-mediated cytotoxicity). Natural killer cells also have the ability to recognize and destroy tumor and other foreign antigens. This cytotoxicity is independent of antibody-antigen binding.

Antibody-dependent cell-mediated cytotoxicity requires the orchestration of many substances including lymphokines, monokines, colony-stimulating factors, interleukins, and others to communicate between cells and to elicit the checks and balances of the immune system. In the absence of a normally functioning immune system, the host is susceptible to infection, tumors, and eventually death.

RECOMBINANT DNA TECHNOLOGY

Many of the cellular mediators of the immune system can now be produced in clinically useful quantities by recom-

Table 7.1.
Characteristics of the Five Classes of Human Immunoglobulins[a]

Variable	Immunoglobulin Class				
	IgG	IgM	IgA	IgE	IgD
Heavy chain	γ	μ	α	ε	δ
Subclasses	γ 1, 2, 3, 4	μ 1, 2	α 1, 2	None	None
Extra chains	None	Joining	Joining & secretory	None	None
Serum conc. (mg/100 ml)	1,000	100	250	0.01	3
Plasma half-life (days)	21	5	6	2	3
Molecular weight	150,000	900,000 (polymer)	350,000 (polymer)	190,000	180,000
Major function	Primary or secondary response	Primary response	Secretory response	Allergic response	Membrane receptor (?)

[a] Reprinted with permission from Tami JA, Parr M, Thompson JS: The immune system. Am J Hosp Pharm 43:2485, 1986.

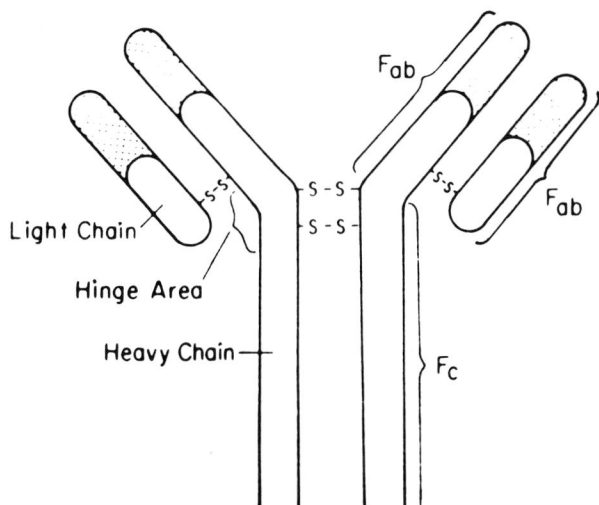

Figure 7.2. Basic structure of an antibody. (From Campion J: A basic review of the immune system. US Pharmacist 15(8):19–26, 1990, with permission.)

binant DNA technology. With this technology, the natural genetic processes that take place in mammalian, bacterial, and yeast cells can be manipulated to produce human proteins, such as erythropoietin, in large enough quantities to be useful in the treatment of human disease.

Recombinant DNA technology entails isolating the gene (i.e., a specific segment of DNA) that contains the genetic code for a desired protein and inserting it into a cell that can reproduce that protein rapidly. The result is large quantities of human protein.

Yeast cells, *Escherichia coli* bacteria, and mammalian cells (Chinese hamster ovary cells, human myeloma cells) are used most commonly to reproduce human proteins. These cell types are used because they can be genetically manipulated easily and quickly, they multiply and divide rapidly, and they provide large quantities of protein (4).

E. coli and yeast cells are genetically simple and well-understood cell types, which makes them ideal host cells for recombinant DNA molecules. However, they cannot perform some of the more complicated processes of fine-tuning proteins, such as glycosylation, that the more advanced mammalian cells can perform. If glycosylation is not necessary, as with interferons, *E. coli* is a less expensive and simpler choice for a host cell (4).

In order to produce a specific protein, the corresponding gene from the DNA strand must be isolated. A gene can be isolated easily if the amino acid sequence of the desired protein is known. If not, a DNA probe may be used to isolate the specific gene. The desired gene is then cut precisely from the DNA molecule by restriction enzymes.

The isolated gene is then inserted into the host cell, with a plasmid, to produce the desired protein (Fig. 7.3). A plasmid is a circular strand of DNA that can replicate freely inside a host cell. Plasmids are found in *E. coli*, where they are isolated and cut open (4). The human gene is then spliced to the plasmid by DNA ligase to form the recombinant DNA molecule. The DNA molecule is inserted into the host cell through a process called transformation (the uptake of foreign DNA into a cell) (4). As host cell division and replication takes place, the plasmid-containing human gene is also replicated. The host cell replicates into millions of genetically identical cells capable of producing the desired protein. The protein is secreted, harvested, purified, and formulated into the final commercial product (4).

Among the commercially available pharmaceuticals that have been developed through recombinant DNA technology are human insulin, human growth hormone, interferons (α-, β-, γ-), tissue plasminogen activator, hep-

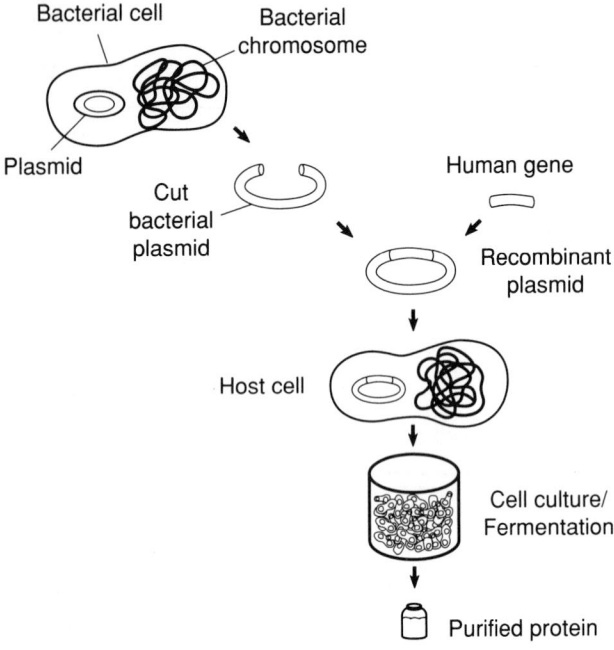

Figure 7.3. Summary of the steps typically involved in the formation of a recombinant DNA molecule. (Reprinted with permission from Anon: An Introduction to Pharmaceutical Biotechnology. Regents of the University of Wisconsin System, 1990.)

atitis B vaccine, and hematopoietic growth factors (granulocyte-colony-stimulating factor, granulocyte-macrophage-colony-stimulating factor, erythropoietin). Many more are in clinical trials (Table 7.2).

IMMUNOTHERAPEUTICS
Immunization

When an antigen enters an organism, the specific immune system stimulates antibody production against that specific antigen. It retains memory of that antigen exposure, so that upon reexposure to the antigens, it can mount a rapid and complete immune response. *Active immunization* uses this basic principle to help develop a complete and long-lasting immunity to certain diseases by exposing the body to a harmless portion of the antigens. (See Chapter 59, "Immunization Therapy") for a more complete discussion of active and passive immunization.

Recombinant Vaccines

With recombinant DNA technology, a vaccine that is devoid of both pathogenic potential and extraneous material can be produced. Recombinant DNA technology has also made it possible to develop vaccines from organisms that are difficult to grow, such as cancer cells and the AIDS virus. One example of a biotechnologically produced recombinant vaccine is the hepatitis B (HB) vaccine. The

gene encoding the hepatitis B surface antigen polypeptide has been incorporated into a plasmid and cloned in yeast, *E. coli*, and mammalian cells. The ability of the recombinant hepatitis B vaccine to confer immunity is similar to that of the plasma-derived vaccine. Other recombinant vaccines that have been produced and are being studied include malaria, cholera, typhoid fever, influenza, and rabies (2).

Biological Response Modifiers

Cytokines are responsible for the growth and differentiation of the cells of the immune system (Fig. 7.4). Cytokines that are products of monocytes and macrophages are termed monokines, while those derived from lymphocytes

Table 7.2.
Recombinant DNA Pharmaceutical Products in the Pipeline[a]

Product	Potential Use
Atrial natriuretic factor—ANF	Regulates blood pressure, water and salt excretion
Epidermal growth factor	Wound healing, cataract surgery
β-Interferon	Kaposi's sarcoma, glioma
Interleukins 1, 2, 3, 4, 6	Cell differentiation and growth, applications in cancers, AIDS, other immunodeficiencies
Lymphokine-activated killer cells	Cancers (in combination with IL-2)
Macrophage colony-stimulating factor	Infectious diseases
Monoclonal antibodies	
HA1A	Septic shock
CD5	Graft vs. host disease
E5	Gram-negative sepsis
CR103	Colorectal CA
Platelet-derived growth factor	Production of platelets, applications in leukemias, bone marrow transplantation, aplastic anemia, thrombocytopenia, AIDS
Stem cell growth factor	Stimulate production of all blood cell lines, applications in leukemias, aplastic anemias, AIDS
Superoxide dismutase (SOD)	Prevents damage from superoxide free radicals, applications in cardiac treatment and organ transplants.
Tumor necrosis factor	Antitumor and antiviral applications

[a] Adapted from Conlan M: Biotechnology: are you ready for it? Drug Topics 134(10):34–41, 1990; Anon: Increasing number of biotechnology products near marketing, PMA survey shows. Clin Pharm 9:408, 1990; and Anon: Biotechnol Monitor 1:1–12, 1991.

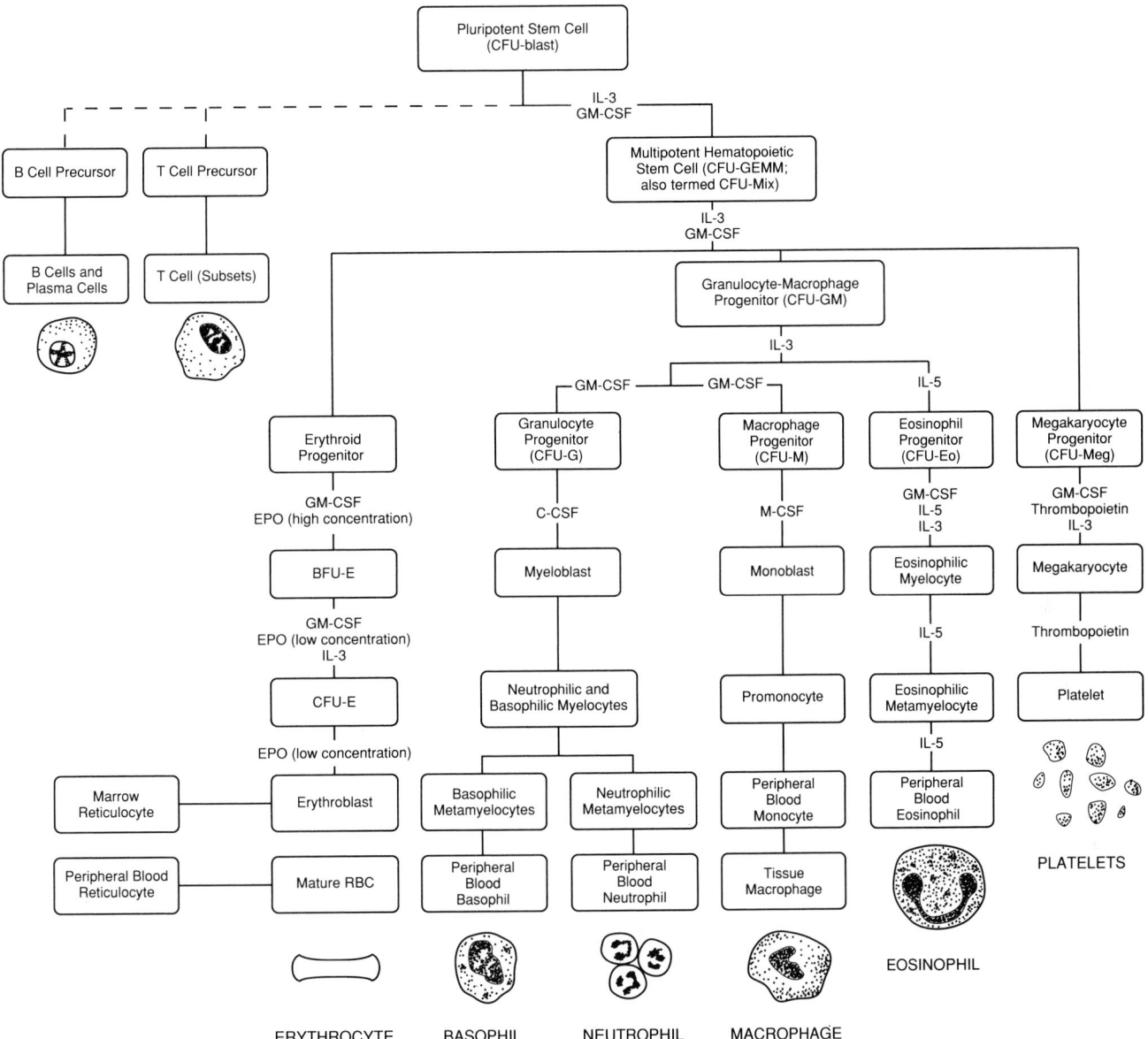

Figure 7.4. Differentiation of the hematopoietic stem cell from the pluripotent form to the highly differentiated macrophages, lymphocytes, erythrocytes, and granulocytes and the growth factors that are responsible for their differentiation.

(From Shriner, DA: Colony-stimulating factors: clinical trials in humans. Highlights on Antineoplastic Drugs 8:6–14, 1990, with permission.)

are termed lymphokines. Cytokines have a broad range of overlapping immunological, inflammatory, and physiological properties. The cytokines that have been produced through recombinant DNA technology are broadly termed *biological-response modifiers*. They include interleukins, colony-stimulating factors, and interferons. These immunomodulators may be specific (e.g., target identifiable tumor antigens) or nonspecific (alter the response and function of the immune system against a stimulus without reference to a specific antigen).

INTERLEUKINS

The interleukins have been called the "hormones of the immune system." They are the molecular mediators of immune system cells and induce replication and differentiation of those cells and activate the expression of certain functions. At least 15 different interleukins have been identified, each with its own cell targets and functions. Some of the interleukins have been cloned through recombinant DNA technology and are undergoing clinical trials to determine their clinical usefulness.

IL-1. Interleukin 1 is a prominent regulator of the immune system with potent immunomodulatory activity. It is produced by a number of cells, including mononuclear phagocytes, fibroblasts, natural killer cells, endothelial cells, vascular smooth muscle cells, epithelial cells, and T lymphocytes (5, 6). IL-1 production can be induced by bacterial lipopolysaccharide, IL-2, tumor necrosis factor, leukotrienes, and IL-1 itself. It is responsible for stimulating the proliferation of T and B lymphocytes, IL-2, and IL-3, and it is thought to increase interferon production and IL-2–induced cytotoxicity (5). It is being studied to determine its ability to differentiate early progenitor cells into functional cell lines.

IL-2. Also known as T cell growth factor, IL-2 has been shown to increase the proliferation of a subset of T lymphocytes called lymphocyte-activated killer cells (LAK cells), which can lyse a broad range of tumor targets (5). IL-2 given alone to 115 patients with a variety of tumor types showed 9 partial responses (24%) in patients with melanoma and 4 complete and 7 partial (21%) responses in patients with renal cell carcinoma (7). The four complete responders remained free of disease from 15 to 24 months. Six of the seven partial-response renal cell patients remained stable with no disease progression, 15 months after the trial (7). IL-2 given in combination with LAK cells has shown similar clinical results. The combination of IL-2 and LAK cells is termed adoptive immunotherapy, which means the transfer of active immunologic reagents (LAK cells stimulated by IL-2) to a tumor-bearing host. The goal of adoptive immunotherapy is to have tumor-targeted immunologic agents destroy the tumor specifically.

The drawback to IL-2 therapy is its toxicity. IL-2 patients participating in clinical trials required intensive care to undergo IL-2 and LAK cell therapy. IL-2 produces a severe capillary leak syndrome that leads to fluid retention, prerenal azotemia, respiratory distress, and interstitial edema (5, 7). A marked lymphocyte infiltration into critical organs may also lead to temporary organ dysfunction.

IL-2 has been shown to activate macrophages, enhance their tumoricidal activity, and increase tumor necrosis factor (TNF) production. Combinations of IL-2 and TNF are currently being studied.

IL-3. IL-3 has been called multi-colony-stimulating factor because of its ability to stimulate the proliferation and activity of every member of the hematopoietic cell line (5). IL-3 acts directly on progenitor stem cells to amplify their response to the more lineage-specific factors (granulocyte colony stimulating factor (G-CSF), macrophage colony-stimulating factor (M-CSF), erythropoietin), resulting in erythroid, granulocytic, monocytic, and megakaryocytic proliferation. A recombinant IL-3 product is now in clinical trials in combination with other colony-stimulating factors (CSFs) (8). A preliminary report in 14 adults (receiving subcutaneous IL-3 in doses of 60 to 500 μg/m² for 15 days for various cancers) showed that the nine patients who could be evaluated had a marked increase in neutrophils, eosinophils, monocytes, reticulocytes, and platelets. IL-3 may be one of the most important lymphokines of the future for the treatment of these cytopenias.

IL-4. IL-4 has been characterized as a B cell growth factor. In addition, IL-4 has been shown to enhance myeloid (monocyte) colony formation and eosinophil growth and differentiation. IL-4 is produced by a subset of activated T cells and has been shown to inhibit the induction of both lymphokine-activated killer (LAK) cells and natural killer (NK) cells in vitro.

IL-5. IL-5 is also derived from a T cell subset and is known as T cell replacing factor, B cell growth factor II, and eosinophil differentiation factor (5). IL-5 acts primarily on B cells to stimulate the production of IgA. Since IgA is responsible for inducing a secretory response to gastrointestinal or respiratory pathogens, IL-5 may play an important role in mucosal immunity (5), one of the first defense mechanisms of the nonspecific immune system.

IL-6. IL-6 is produced primarily by leukocytes and is known as B cell stimulating factor, T cell stimulating factor, and β-2-interferon (5). It is similar to IL-3 and IL-1 in that it stimulates early progenitor cells (pre–T cells) to respond to the more lineage-specific colony-stimulating factors.

IL-7. IL-7 has just recently been characterized (9). It is produced by the stromal cells of the bone marrow and is responsible for early lymphocyte proliferation.

COLONY-STIMULATING FACTORS

The colony-stimulating factors (granulocyte-macrophage colony-stimulating factor (GM-CSF), granulocyte colony-stimulating factor (G-CSF), macrophage colony-stimulating factor (M-CSF), and erythropoietin (EPO)) are the most promising of the cytokines because of their broad range of clinical applications (10). These glycoproteins have been cloned through DNA technology and three (G-CSF, GM-CSF, and EPO) have been approved by the FDA for clinical use. Colony-stimulating factors help regulate the growth and differentiation of hematopoietic cells. There are two main classes of colony stimulating factors. Class 1 CSFs such as IL-3 or GM-CSF act at the partially committed stem cell level to cause differentiation and proliferation of multiple cell lines (monocytes, granulocytes, eosinophils, etc.). Class 2 CSFs such as G-CSF, M-CSF, and erythropoietin act on already differentiated cell lines to stimulate proliferation of more specific cell types (11).

Granulocyte-macrophage colony-stimulating factor has been approved for use in patients with non-Hodgkin's lymphoma, acute lymphoblastic leukemia (ALL), and Hodgkin's disease undergoing bone marrow transplantation (BMT) to help accelerate myeloid recovery. Because of its effect on partially committed stem cells, it has been shown to induce the proliferation of macrophages and granulocytes. GM-CSF is also capable of activating mature granulocytes and macrophages.

There have been three randomized, double-blind, placebo-controlled trials that have evaluated the safety and efficacy of GM-CSF following bone marrow transplantation (9, 12). GM-CSF at a dose of 250 $\mu g/m^2$ or placebo were given as IV infusions over 2 hr, beginning within 2 to 4 days of transplantation and continued for 21 consecutive days in 128 patients. Sixty-eight percent (68%) of the patients had non-Hodgkins lymphoma, 13% had acute lymphocytic leukemia (ALL), 18% had Hodgkin's lymphoma, and one patient had acute myelogenous leukemia (AML). The patients with non-Hodgkins lymphoma and ALL given GM-CSF reached an absolute neutrophil count of >500, 6 days earlier than placebo-treated patients did, and the median duration of hospitalization was 6 days shorter for these patients. There were also fewer days of infectious episodes and antibiotic administration in the GM-CSF-treated group (8). In patients with Hodgkin's disease, there was only a trend noted toward earlier engraftment in the GM-CSF-treated group (vs. placebo).

GM-CSF has also been used to accelerate myeloid recovery in patients undergoing chemotherapy for AML (13, 14). In one uncontrolled trial, GM-CSF reduced the median recovery time of neutrophils by 4 days in patients receiving 6-thioguanine, standard dose cytarabine, and daunorubicin, and by 9 days in patients receiving high-dose cytarabine and mitoxantrone (14).

GM-CSF has been studied in phase 1 trials in 16 severely leukopenic, immunocompromised AIDS patients (12, 15–17). An IV bolus dose followed 2 days later by 14 days of continuous infusion produced normal or above normal neutrophil counts within 7 days. There was a variable and inconsistent rise in monocytes and lymphocytes as well, but the majority of cells produced were leukocytes, specifically neutrophils and bands (immature neutrophils). After the 14-day infusion, there was a precipitous drop in leukocyte count back to baseline.

Small studies have been conducted with GM-CSF in myelodysplastic and aplastic anemia patients (8, 12, 15, 17, 18). In 3 of 8 myelodysplastic patients treated with GM-CSF, there was a multilineage effect seen, with proliferation of WBCs, platelets, and RBCs. With repeated cycles, a priming effect was noted (i.e., a half-dose during a subsequent cycle was as effective as the full dose in the first cycle). This priming effect may be due to GM-CSF binding to stromal cells in the bone marrow and then slowly being released in a sustained manner. Of 10 GM-CSF–treated aplastic anemia patients, 9 showed significant increases in WBCs and granulocytes, but not in RBCs and platelets. Further studies are needed to substantiate the use of GM-CSF in these patient populations.

The most commonly reported adverse effects of GM-CSF in early trials included fever, nausea, vomiting, diarrhea, malaise, myalgia, rash, peripheral edema, and weight gain (11). The higher doses used in these early trials contributed to these side effects. With currently recommended doses, these side effects are not often seen. Other less commonly seen but more severe adverse effects include renal and hepatic dysfunction in patients with preexisting dysfunction, and respiratory distress. At higher doses, 16 to 32 $\mu g/kg/day$, a large vessel thrombosis has occurred in one patient (19), and a capillary leak syndrome has been seen in conjunction with adult respiratory distress syndrome (ARDS). Other side effects noted with higher doses include renal failure and hypotension.

Granulocyte Colony-stimulating Factor. G-CSF is a cell-lineage–specific colony-stimulating factor that stimulates granulocyte progenitor cells to differentiate into granulocytes. G-CSF has recently been approved for neutropenia in patients with nonmyeloid malignancies receiving myelosuppressive chemotherapy. Studies have consistently shown a significantly shorter duration of leukopenia than in placebo controls (12, 19, 20). Small studies of G-CSF have shown reductions in infection, mucositis, and fever and greater adherence to scheduled chemotherapy regimens (12, 21).

G-CSF has also been studied prospectively in a chemotherapy dose-intensification trial in patients with relapsed or refractory acute leukemia (22). One hundred eight patients were randomized to receive G-CSF (200 $\mu g/day$) or placebo after intensive induction chemotherapy with mitoxantrone, etoposide, and enocitabine (not available in the U.S.). Additional mitoxantrone or etoposide was given until the bone marrow became hypoplastic with leukocyte counts of <1000. Therapy with G-CSF or placebo continued until peripheral counts exceeded 1500/mm^3. Recovery of neutrophils to 500 mm^3 and 1000 mm^3 was significantly faster with G-CSF than without.

The most important side effect seen with G-CSF has been bone pain (20, 23). Other side effects include fatigue, myalgia, and inflammation at the site of injection. More severe reactions have been reported rarely and include increasing alkaline phosphatase levels, increasing urate levels, and cutaneous necrotizing vasculitis (11).

Macrophage Colony-stimulating Factor. Macrophage colony-stimulating factor, also called CSF-1, selectively stimulates the proliferation and differentiation of the macrophage cell line. Although it is more specific to the macrophage cell line, its ability to stimulate macrophage proliferation is weaker than that of either GM-CSF or IL-3. M-CSF is currently in clinical trials.

TUMOR NECROSIS FACTOR AND LYMPHOTOXIN

There are two types of tumor necrosis factor (TNF): α and β. TNF-α, or cachectin, is produced by a number of cell types including monocytes, neutrophils, NK cells, and T and B lymphocytes (5). It is thought to cause tissue wasting (cancer cachexia). TNF-β, or lymphotoxin (LT), is a cytotoxic protein produced by activated T cells. TNF-α and TNF-β bind to the same receptor on cell surfaces with the same affinity.

Preliminary work has begun in humans because animal studies have shown marked tumor regression in high tumor burden mouse sarcomas. Phase I clinical trials in 27 patients with advanced solid tumors, primarily colorectal and soft tissue sarcoma, show tumor regression and confirm the feasability of progressing to phase II and III clinical trials. Toxicity has been serious, depending upon the dose used. Side effects include fever, rigors (occasionally with hypertension), nausea, vomiting, fatigue, headache, and hypotension.

TNF has also been found to play a major role in Gram-negative shock. Endotoxin produced by infecting Gram-negative organisms stimulates monocytes to release TNF, which in turn is responsible for the fever, metabolic acidosis, diarrhea, hypotension, disseminated intravascular coagulation, and death that can accompany Gram-negative shock.

ERYTHROPOIETIN

Erythropoietin is the primary regulator of red blood cell production and thus is an important cytokine for the erythroid cell line. Recombinant human erythropoietin alpha (rHEPO) is produced through recombinant DNA technology and is approved for use in the treatment of anemia associated with chronic renal failure in patients on dialysis as well as in predialysis patients and severe anemia associated with zidovudine (AZT) therapy in AIDS.

Erythropoietin was the first of the biotechnologically produced stimulating factors to be approved for use in humans, and many trials have confirmed its benefit in transfusion-dependent patients. While the use of erythropoietin in anemia in renal failure patients and AIDS patients is discussed in their respective chapters (see Chapter 13, "Other Anemias," and Chapter 70, "Acquired Immunodeficiency Syndrome (AIDS)"), it is important to be aware of the studies regarding its use in the anemia of cancer patients.

Several small clinical trials have evaluated the usefulness of erythropoietin in patients with various malignancy-induced or chemotherapy-induced anemias. In one study, 13 patients with multiple myeloma–associated anemia were given erythropoietin (150 μg/kg subcutaneously, three times weekly) for 3 weeks, and if no response was seen, the dose was increased by 50 μg/kg/dose every 3 weeks to a maximum of 250 μg/kg/dose. Doses of erythropoietin were adjusted to maintain hemoglobin levels in the range of 120 to 140 g/liter. Eleven of 13 patients responded with an increase in hemoglobin level greater than

or equal to 20 g/liter (2 g/dl). No adverse effects were noted, and most patients reported a subjective improvement in quality of life, with correspondingly fewer signs or symptoms of anemia (24).

Similar reports have been confirmed in small numbers of patients with non-Hodgkins lymphoma and in a single case report of a patient with metastatic testicular cancer. The common adverse effects associated with erythropoietin therapy are mild and include hypertension, rash, headache, arthralgias, and nausea and vomiting.

A rapid rise in red blood cell count can induce severe hypertension, thrombosis, and seizures.

INTERFERONS

The interferons are a group of 20 or more glycoproteins produced by a variety of cell types in response to viral infections (25). They have antiproliferative and differentiation effects on tumor cells and can act as immunoregulatory agents that induce effector cell functions such as macrophage cytotoxic activity, NK cell activity and T lymphocyte cytotoxic activity (Table 7.3) (26). Interferons also boost antibody-dependent cell-mediated cytotoxicity by enhancing cell surface antigen expression of major histocompatibility antigens and tumor-associated antigens. Three different types of interferons have been characterized, based upon their cells of origin. α-Interferon is produced by leukocytes, β-interferon is produced by fibroblasts, epithelial cells, and macrophages; and γ-interferon is produced by T lymphocytes. While naturally occurring interferons are glycosylated, recombinant interferons produced in E. coli are not. However, activity does not seem to be diminished by their unglycosylated state. α- and β-interferon are similar in structure, receptor interactions and biologic effects; however γ-interferon is distinct in structure and receptor site and appears to have greater antitumor, immunosuppressive, and cytolytic effects (27).

An important clinical phenomenon in the course of

Table 7.3.
Immunomodulatory Activities of the Interferons[a]

Enhance (low dose) or suppress (high dose) natural killer activity
Augment antibody-dependent cellular cytotoxicity (ADCC)
Enhance tumoricidal activity of macrophages
Regulate antibody production in B cells
Enhance cytotoxic phase of mixed lymphocyte culture (MLC)
Depress lymphoproliferative phase of mixed lymphocyte culture
Increase expression of cell-surface antigens, HLA-A, B, C, DR, and B2 microglobulin[b]

[a] From Roth, M.S., Foon, K.A.: Current Status of Interferon Therapy in Oncology, Progress in Hematology, 15:19–33, 1987, with permission.
[b] Only IFN-γ has consistently increased expression of HLA-DR, and IFN-γ, unlike α- or β-, is able to increase expression of HLA-A, B, and C proteins on the cell surface at concentrations that are considerably lower than those necessary to induce an antiviral effect.

Table 7.4.
Incidence (%) of Adverse Experiences[a]

Adverse Effect	All Patients ($n = 1403$)	
	Any Severity	Grades III, IV
Flu-like symptoms	96	37
Nausea/vomiting	42	5
Other gastrointestinal symptoms	24	2
Central nervous system	33	7
Cardiovascular	12	2
Skin	13	1
Respiratory	6	1
Alopecia	6	<1
Weight loss	5	1
Hepatic	<1	0

[a] From Spiegel RJ: The alpha interferons: clinical overview. Semin Oncol 14: 1–12, 1987, with permission.

treatment with interferons is the production in some patients of antiinterferon antibodies (28). Although there is no documented relationship between antibody development and the response rate to certain tumors or overall survival, the detection of antibodies has been shown to coincide with termination of response and amelioration of interferon side effects. Studies suggest that the α-2a preparation is more immunogenic that α-2b and that antiinterferon antibodies are seen more often in certain subsets of patients, particularly those with renal cell cancer and Kaposi's sarcoma (29). Determination of antibody development is important, so that dosage adjustments can be made to insure continued response in those patients.

α-Interferon. α-Interferon was the first of the interferons approved for clinical use, and there are at least 20 different subtypes (25). Two of the recombinantly produced interferons are α-2a and α-2b, which differ by one amino acid. Both have been approved for use in the treatment of hairy cell leukemia (mean response rate, 75% (29)), Kaposi's sarcoma (mean response rate, 33% (28, 29)), genital warts, and most recently, hepatitis C (formerly non-A non-B hepatitis). In a clinical trial, 166 patients with chronic hepatitis C were randomized to receive α-interferon, 3 million units, or 1 million units three times weekly for 24 weeks, or no treatment (30). Forty-six percent of patients treated with 3 million units had either a complete or a near-complete remission, while 28% of patients given 1 million units had a complete or near-complete response. Eight percent of untreated patients had at least a partial response. The probability of relapse for both treatment groups approached 50% at 6 months. In a review of α-interferon, Spiegel (29) reported the incidence of adverse effects in 1403 patients (Table 7.4).

β-Interferon. β-Interferon appears to be better tolerated, but does not appear to possess the same immuno-

modulatory or antiviral effects as α-interferon (27). In clinical trials, the activity against solid tumor types (renal cell, melanoma, and colorectal cancers) has been modest (27). Likewise, in hairy cell leukemia, chronic myelogenous leukemia, or non-Hodgkins lymphoma, it does not seem to offer any advantage over α-interferon. The best clinical responses to β-interferon have been seen in Kaposi's sarcoma (31), with a 40 to 50% response rate, and glioma brain tumors, where a 10 to 20% response rate has been reported (27).

γ-Interferon. γ-Interferon has been approved to reduce infectious complications in patients with chronic granulomatous disease, an inherited immunodeficiency syndrome. A study of 128 patients who received either γ-interferon or placebo (subcutaneously three times a week for 1 year) had two study end points. The first was the time to serious infection (defined as a clinical event leading to hospitalization and parenteral antibiotic administration), and the second end point was the number of serious infections, length of hospitalization, and effect on existing infection. After 1 year, 77% of patients treated with γ-interferon were infection-free versus 30% in the placebo-treated group. There was also a twofold reduction in the number of serious infections in the γ-interferon group (vs. placebo). γ-Interferon is projected to have far-reaching applications in both tumor and viral indications as well as in collagen vascular disorders.

The toxicities of γ-interferon appear to be similar to those of α- and β-interferon, although headaches appear to be more severe and may be dose-limiting. γ-Interferon has also been shown to increase serum triglyceride levels by inhibiting lipoprotein lipase.

MONOCLONAL ANTIBODIES

Monoclonal antibodies can be used to target and destroy tumor cells and specific molecules required for tumor growth and differentiation, and may be used to deliver antitumor agents to specific tumor sites (32). In theory their applications seem endless, but developing these applications has been slow, partly because of the difficulties inherent in monoclonal antibody production.

Monoclonal antibody production begins with the identification of the B lymphocyte responsible for the production of a specific antibody to a specific antigen (33). Antigen to which the desired antibody will respond is first injected into a mouse (Fig. 7.5). The antigen in turn stimulates B lymphocytes, which produce antibody against that antigen. B lymphocytes are then recovered from the spleen of the mouse. Only a few of the B lymphocytes recovered from the mouse spleen actually secrete the desired antibody. Those B lymphocytes are then mixed with myeloma cells (an immortal cell line that can live forever in culture) in polyethylene glycol, resulting in the membranes of the two cell types being fused together. This fused myeloma

Immunization and fusion

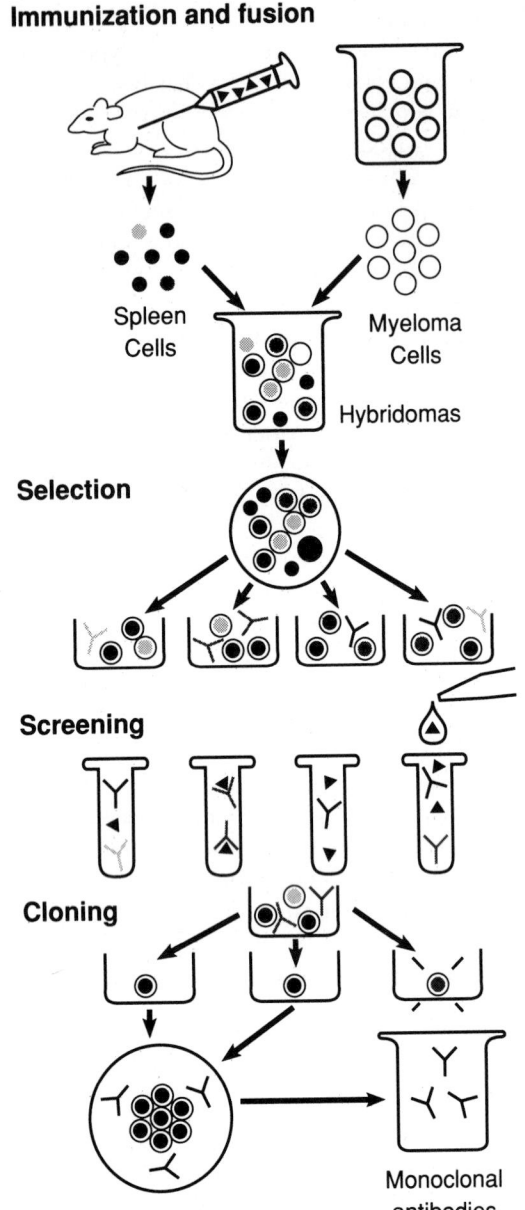

Figure 7.5. Summary of the steps involved in the production of monoclonal antibodies. (Reprinted with permission from Chisholm R: On the trail of the magic bullet. High Technology Business 3:57–63, 1983.)

and B lymphocyte is called a hybridoma. The hybridomas are then allowed to grow for several weeks. Either the ELISA or RIA method is then used to select the appropriate antibody-secreting hybridoma. The target antigen is chemically bound to the bottom of a testing tray in wells, and hybridoma cells are added to each of the wells. Specific antibodies produced inside the wells will bind to the antigen at the bottom of the wells. Radioactive or enzyme-labeled secondary antibodies specific for the primary an-

tibodies are then added to the wells and the mixture is incubated and rewashed. The wells that show radioactivity or a color reaction caused by the enzyme contain the desired antibody. Once identified, the hybridomas containing the desired antibody can be cloned.

Once a specific antibody to a tumor cell antigen has been cloned, it has many applications in cancer therapy (Fig. 7.6). Monoclonal antibodies directed at specific tumor cells can affect antibody-dependent cell-mediated cytotoxicity. As with the regular immune system, when an antibody attaches to an antigen, effector cells such as monocytes, macrophages, granulocytes, and some lymphocytes can bind to the Fc portion of the antibody and cause enzymatic puncture of the tumor cell membrane, resulting in cell death.

Monoclonal antibodies can also be targeted against molecules that are critical to that tumor's growth or differentiation. For example, monoclonal antibodies have been prepared against epidermal growth factor to inhibit growth of epidermal carcinomas. Antibodies against bombesin, an autocrine growth factor for small cell lung cancer, have helped to inhibit tumor growth in this cancer.

Monoclonal antibodies have also been developed against leukemias, lymphomas, melanoma, and GI cancers. Doses of antibodies used in these trials ranged from 1 to 500 mg per patient, given as a single dose three times weekly or daily for 1 week (32). Doses exceeding 5 to 10 mg/hr have resulted in dyspnea and wheezing due to leukoagglutination and the trapping of white cells in the lungs. Frequently seen side effects include chills, fevers, flushing, urticaria, headache, rigors, myalgias, pruritus, dyspnea, wheezing, nausea, vomiting, diarrhea, hypotension, and

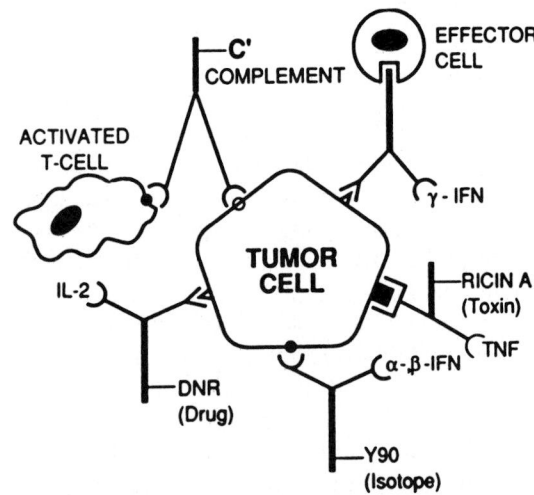

Figure 7.6. Various uses of monoclonal antibodies. (From Dillman R: Monoclonal antibodies for treating cancer. Ann Intern Med 111:592–603, 1989, with permission.)

facial edema. Rare toxicities include anaphylactic reactions, serum sickness, and facial palsy.

Monoclonal antibodies have been used to deliver antitumor agents, including radioisotopes, toxins, chemotherapeutic agents, and drug-filled liposomes, to specifically targeted tumor cells. Specific antitumor effects have been seen with iodine-131–labeled monoclonal antibodies directed against B and T lymphomas, while iodine-131–labeled antimelanoma monoclonal antibodies have produced poor results. The theoretical advantage of radioconjugates is that the radioisotope does not have to enter the cell to induce a killing effect, it merely needs to get into the area of the tumor (the field effect) (33). Nearby healthy tissue (especially in areas where the conjugate may be detained, such as the liver and spleen of the reticuloendothelial system) may be injured (32). The toxicity seen with this type of therapy has been primarily thrombocytopenia and granulocytopenia.

Monoclonal antibodies can be fused with whole or parts of plant or bacterial toxins to form what are called immunotoxins (33). Studies have shown some clinical responses using antimelanoma antibodies coupled to ricin–A chain, a plant toxin (32). Dose-related toxicities include decreases in serum proteins, weight gain, and edema. Monoclonal antibodies are also being developed against specific bacterial endotoxins to help prevent endotoxemia, Gram-negative sepsis, and septic shock (34, 35).

The safety and efficacy of the HA1A monoclonal antibody used in reducing mortality from Gram-negative bacteremia has been evaluated in a double-blind, placebo-controlled trial. The HA1A antibody is directed against endotoxin, the lipopolysaccharide component of the cell wall of Gram-negative bacteria. Endotoxin is responsible for many serious adverse systemic effects associated with Gram-negative bacteremia. Two hundred patients with Gram-negative bacteremia were randomized to groups receiving either placebo or 100 mg of HA1A antibody. A 49% mortality rate was seen in the placebo-treated population after 28 days, versus 30% in the HA1A-treated group. Thus a 39% reduction in mortality was seen with the HA1A monoclonal antibody (34). Adverse effects noted with the HA1A antibody were mild and infrequent and included one case of localized hives at the HA1A injection site and one patient who developed facial flushing and mild hypotension (34). Larger randomized trials comparing the HA1A antibody to placebo or conventional treatment for Gram-negative bacteremia, sepsis, and septic shock will be important in determining where this product will fit into our antimicrobial armamentarium.

Antineoplastic-monoclonal antibody conjugates can also be used to deliver antineoplastics to specific areas of the body (33). This improves the therapeutic-to-toxic ratio seen with systemic chemotherapy. In one study, a small number of patients with advanced colorectal or ovarian cancer, were treated with an antibody-vindesine conjugate. Although no therapeutic responses were seen, the conjugate was given safely. Liposome-carrying drugs conjugated to monoclonal antibodies show promise. The liposomes concentrate the drug in cells of the reticuloendothelial system, liver, and spleen and thus reduce drug uptake by other critical organs such as the heart, kidney, and GI tract. Liposome-containing doxorubicin has been developed to reduce the potential for cardiotoxicity of this drug.

There are still problems that need to be solved before the monoclonal conjugates are commercially available. There is a limit to the absolute quantity of monoclonal antibodies that can be produced, but as techniques are refined, this issue will become less important. The specificity and binding of monoclonal antibodies to antigens is not absolute, and administered monoclonal antibodies do not always concentrate in the targeted tissues. Finally, our own immune system produces antibodies to the mouse monoclonal antibody conjugates and can illicit an immune response (32).

CONCLUSIONS

A thorough knowledge of the immune system is a prerequisite to the understanding of many human diseases. With the availability of new knowledge about the regulation of the immune system coupled with the powerful tools offered by recombinant DNA technology, a new era in the diagnosis and treatment of many diseases that have eluded effective intervention is beginning. Although only a handful of products are currently commercially available, many more are in development, and they will undoubtedly alter significantly the way we treat many diseases.

REFERENCES

1. Tami JA, Parr M, Thompson J: The immune system. Am J Hosp Pharm 43:2483–2493, 1986.
2. Keoller J, Tami J: Concepts in Immunology and Immunotherapeutics. Bethesda, MD: ASHP Publication, 1990.
3. Campion J: A basic review of the immune system. US Pharmacist 15(8):19–26, 1990.
4. An Introduction to Pharmaceutical Biotechnology. Regents of the University of Wisconsin System. 1990.
5. Staren E, Esner R, Economou J: Overview of biological response modifiers. Semin Surg Oncol 5:379–384, 1989.
6. Kirkpatrick C: Biological response modifiers. Interferons, interleukins, and transfer factor. Ann Allergy 62:170–176, 1989.
7. Chang A, Rosenberg S: Overview of interleukin-2 as an immunotherapeutic agent. Semin Surg Oncol 5:385–390, 1989.
8. Goldstone A, Khwaja A: The role of haemopoietic growth factors in bone marrow transplantation. Leuk Res 14:721–729, 1990.
9. Starr C: Growth factors fortify immune systems of cancer patients. Drug Topics 134(8):18–20, 1990.
10. Gabrilove J: Introduction and overview of hematopoietic growth factors. Semin Hematol 26:1–4, 1989.
11. Yee GC: Focus on GM-CSF and G-CSF: promising biotherapeutics for use in hematology and oncology. Hosp Formul 25:943–948, 1990.

12. Appelbaum FR: The clinical use of hematopoietic growth factors. Semin Hematol 26:7–14, 1989.

13. Bettelheim P, Muhm M, Valent P, et al.: GM-CSF in combination with cytotoxic chemotherapy in AML patients. Bone Marrow Transplantation 1:127–130, 1990.

14. Buechner T, Hiddemann W, Koenigsmann M, et al.: Recombinant human GM-CSF following chemotherapy in high-risk AML. Bone Marrow Transplant 1:131–133, 1990.

15. Shriner DA: Colony-Stimulating factors: clinic trials in humans. Highlights on Antineoplastic Drugs 8:6–14, 1990.

16. Groopman J: New directions in hematologic biotherapy. Semin Hematol 26:1–6, 1989.

17. Groopman J: Clinical applications of colony-stimulating factors. Semin Oncol 15:27–33, 1988.

18. Gutterman J: Clinical studies of granulocyte-macrophage colony stimulating factor. Semin Oncol 15:52–53, 1988.

19. Moore M: Hematopoietic growth factors in cancer. Cancer 65:836–844, 1990.

20. Morstyn G, Lieschke G, Sheridan W, et al.: Clinical experience with recombinant human granulocyte colony-stimulating factor and granulocyte macrophage colony-stimulating factor. Semin Hematol 26:9–13, 1989.

21. Glaspy J, Golde D: Clinical applications of the myeloid growth factors. Semin Hematol 26:14–17, 1989.

22. Ohno R, Tomonaga M, Kobuyashi T, et al.: Effect of granulocyte colony-stimulating factor after intensive induction therapy in relapsed or refractory acute leukemia. N Engl J Med 323:871–877, 1990.

23. Glaspy J, Golde D: The colony-stimulating factors: biology and clinical use. Oncology 4:25–33, 1990.

24. Adamson J: The promise of recombinant human erythropoietin. Semin Hematol 26:5–8, 1989.

25. Nelson B, Borden E: Interferons: biological and clinical effects. Semin Surg Oncol 5:391–401, 1989.

26. Borden E, Sondel P: Lymphokines and cytokines as cancer treatment. Cancer 65:800–814, 1990.

27. McManus Balmer C: Clinical use of biologic response modifiers in cancer treatment. DICP, Ann Pharmacother 24:761–767, 1990.

28. Figlin RA: Biotherapy in clinical practice. Semin Hematol 26:15–24, 1989.

29. Spiegel RJ: The alpha interferons: clinical overview. Semin Oncol 14:1–12, 1987.

30. Davis G, Balart L, Schiff E, et al.: Treatment of chronic hepatitis C with recombinant interferon alfa. N Engl J Med 321:1501–1506, 1989.

31. Triozzi P, Rinehart J: The role of IFN-β in cancer therapy. Cancer Surv 8:799–807, 1989.

32. Dillman R: Monoclonal antibodies for treating cancer. Ann Intern Med 111:592–603, 1989.

33. Vaickus L: Antitumor antibodies as therapeutic reagents. P&T 15(12):143–161, 1990.

34. Ziegler MD, Fisher C, Sprung C, et al.: Treatment of gram-negative bacteremia and septic shock with HA-1A human monoclonal antibody against endotoxin. N Engl J Med 324:429–436, 1991.

35. Baumgartner JD, McCutchan J, Van Melle G, et al.: Prevention of gram-negative shock and death in surgical patients by antibody to endotoxin core glycolipid. Lancet pp 59–63, July 13, 1985.

36. Conlan M: Biotechnology: are you ready for it? Drug Topics 134(10):34–41, 1990.

37. Anon: Increasing number of biotechnology products near marketing, PMA survey shows. Clin Pharm 9:408, 1990.

38. Anon: Biotechnology Monitor 1:1–12, 1991.

39. Roth MS, Foon KA: Current status of interferon therapy in oncology. Prog Hematol 15:19–33, 1987.

40. Spiegel R: Alpha interferons: a clinical overview. Urology 34:75–79, 1989.

41. Bellanti JA, Rocklin RE: Cell-mediated immune reactions. Immunology III. Philadelphia: WB Saunders, 1985, p 181.

42. Chisholm R. On the trail of the magic bullet. High Technology Business 3:57–63, 1983.

CHAPTER 8

FLUID AND ELECTROLYTE THERAPY AND ACID-BASE BALANCE

GAIL W. McSWEENEY, Pharm.D.

The body maintains its internal environment by balancing fluids, electrolytes, acids, and bases. Body weight is approximately 60% water; within this are dissolved or suspended the elements and formed substances required to metabolize nutrients and drugs, generate energy, maintain and manufacture body components, and eliminate waste. These processes can be done efficiently only within the very narrow limits of size, composition, and pH of the internal fluid. Disorders of body water, salts, and pH are not diseases, they are alterations in homeostasis, during which the body cannot continue to function normally or protect and repair itself.

PHYSIOLOGY OF BODY WATER BALANCE (1–3)

Body water is divided into 3 compartments: intracellular, interstitial, and vascular. The interstitial and vascular compartments taken together are referred to as the extracellular fluid (ECF). In the nonobese, well-conditioned 70-kg man, water inside the cells (intracellular fluid, ICF) comprises 40 to 45% (30 liters) of body weight. Interstitial water, that between cells, accounts for 11 to 15% (10 liters), and vascular water, that inside the walls of the blood vessels, is approximately 5% (3.5 liters).

The actual amount of body water varies according to age, sex, and body muscle/fat content; when estimating body water in an individual, these factors must be taken into consideration. At birth, the newborn is approximately 75% water; the slight weight loss seen shortly after birth is actually water loss as the infant adjusts to an air environment. By the end of the first year of life, the total body water (TBW) is about 60%. Men usually have a higher water content than women of the same age, height, and weight, because of their greater muscle mass. This difference is estimated to be about 5%. Obese people are less than 60% water as fat has negligible intracellular water, the absolute decrease being a function of the degree of obesity. For practical purposes, estimations of TBW in obese patients are made using ideal rather than actual body weight. Many elderly individuals are also below 60% water. Because of decreases in endogenous anabolic sex hor-

mones and exercise, they are less muscular than younger people of the same body size.

Body water is constantly being circulated in the vascular system, with the connections between the three compartments occurring at the capillary level. Under usual conditions, the volume of each compartment remains constant, but a continuous interchange of individual molecules occurs across the water-permeable cell membranes. This is regulated by hydrostatic and protein (oncotic) pressures. Cardiac output and arterial tone determine the intravascular or "blood" pressure. At the level of the arterial capillary, this hydrostatic pressure is approximately 17 mm Hg, and it forces solute-free water into the interstitial or "third" space. Proteins, primarily albumin, in the third space simultaneously pull water from the vascular system. On the venule side of the capillary bed, intravascular oncotic pressure pulls 95% of the water back into the vascular compartment. The remaining 5% is eventually returned by the action of the lymphatic collecting ducts (Fig. 8.1).

The volume of the 3 compartments will remain normal only as long as these hydrostatic and oncotic forces remain normal *relative* to each other. In assessing the appropriateness of body water content, it is crucial to evaluate not only the total volume but also the distribution among the 3 body spaces.

Dehydration refers to the state in which the water volume, but usually not the amount of solute, is low in all 3 compartments. Hypovolemia is the state in which the intravascular volume is low; it does not define in any way the volumes of the interstitial and intracellular spaces. "Total body water overload" is an often used but imprecise term; it means only that TBW is greater than 60% and does not describe specifically the volume of any individual compartment.

If blood (hydrostatic) pressure is normal but oncotic pressure is low, as is the case with low levels of albumin, fluid will accumulate in the interstitial space; a condition called edema. The volume of the third space gradually expands at the expense of the vascular space. In the most severe cases, death results from too low a circulating blood volume (hypovolemia) in the presence of total body edema

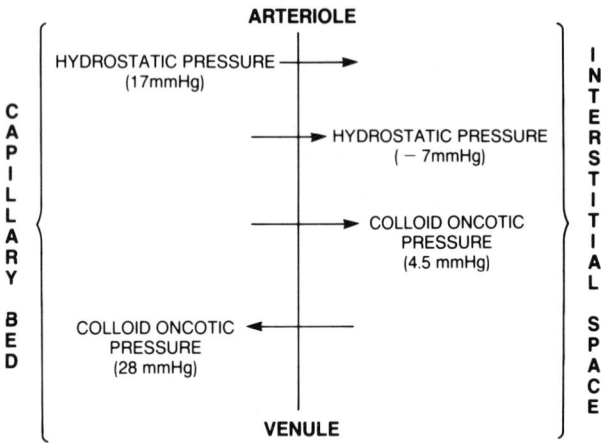

Figure 8.1. Forces regulating water movement in the extracellular fluid.

Table 8.1.
Approximate Composition of Body Fluid (mmol/liter)

	Plasma (total = 300)	Interstitium (total = 304)	Cell (total = 300)
Na	141	144	16
K	4	4	150
Ca	2.5	2.5	—
Mg	2	2	34
Cl	100	114	—
HCO₃	25	30	10
PO₄/SO₄	1	1.5	50
Protein/acid	25	6	40

(interstital space overload) and a TBW of greater than 60%. When the term "TBW overload" is used, the real distribution of water must be determined before appropriate action can be taken. In the example given, the action to maintain life is to give more fluid to support the circulating vascular volume, even if the edema worsens and the TBW continues to rise.

PHYSIOLOGY OF BODY SOLUTE BALANCE (2, 4)

Osmotic pressure keeps the volume of the three body fluid compartments constant. Only solute-free water can move freely across cell membranes. The concentration of dissolved ions (electrolytes) in each compartment creates the osmotic pressure to hold water in each space. These ions and their distribution are listed in Table 8.1. The normal serum osmolality (osmotic concentration) is 280 to 300 mmoles/kg (280 to 300 mOsm/liter). Sodium and chloride are the main ions in the ECF, and potassium and phosphate are those of the ICF. There are other ions present, but they are at concentrations too low to contribute much to the osmotic gradient. Other osmotically active substances present are glucose, urea, phospholipids, choles-

terol, and neutral fats. Osmolality is determined by all the particles mentioned, but the nonelectrolytes contribute little. The effective osmolality is very close to twice the serum sodium in the ECF and twice the potassium in the ICF (Table 8.1).

The equation used to determine osmolality is

$$\text{Osmolality (mmol/kg)} = 2 \times \text{Na (mmol/liter)}$$
$$+ \text{glucose(mmol/liter)}/18 + \text{urea(mmol/liter)}/3$$

A molecule of glucose has $\frac{1}{18}$th and urea has $\frac{1}{3}$rd the osmotic activity of an atom of an electrolyte. Body processes function best within a serum osmolality of 280 to 300 mmol/kg, so the kidneys will attempt to maintain this value and increase the excretion of glucose and urea when concentrations rise. If this is not possible, they will increase the excretion of sodium. In the physiologic sense, the need (biologic priority) to maintain a normal osmolality is greater than the need to maintain a normal sodium level.

When the concentration of ions in any compartment changes, water migrates across cell membranes to reestablish osmotic equilibrium. If the serum sodium concentration rises, the osmolality of the vascular space will be higher than that of the interstitial and intracellular spaces. Water will move from these two areas into the vascular space until the correct relative osmolalities of all three are reestablished. The result is a decrease in the size of the interstitial and intracellular spaces and an increase toward normal of the volume of the vascular space. The clinical condition with an equal percentage decrease in TBW distributed throughout all water compartments is called dehydration. If the serum sodium concentration falls, the opposite happens and the size of the interstitial and intracellular compartments increases.

MAINTENANCE FLUID AND ELECTROLYTE REQUIREMENTS

Salt and water balance in the body is maintained primarily by the equilibrium between oral intake of fluid and electrolytes, evaporation of solute-free water across the skin and lungs, and controlled renal excretion of water and electrolytes. The amount of water that evaporates (insensible loss) is a function of body surface area and respiratory rate. In a 70-kg man, the amount is approximately 1 liter/day and remains constant. The kidneys increase or decrease their output by the action of antidiuretic hormone (ADH) and aldosterone, which compensates for daily variations in oral fluid and electrolyte intake.

ADH regulates the amount of water reabsorbed in the distal tubule of the kidney, by assessing the osmolality of the ECF. If the osmolality of the ECF is higher than normal, ADH will be released and water will be reabsorbed in the renal tubules. If the osmolality is low, the converse will be true. Aldosterone acts to increase sodium reabsorption, and release of the hormone is stimulated by a low circulating blood volume and a low total body sodium concentration. These hormones, along with stimulation of thirst centers in the brain, enable the body to maintain TBW and total body sodium levels within 1% of normal over wide variations in daily intake. In the case of an extremely low circulating plasma volume, these two hormones acting together can cause the kidneys to reabsorb essentially all salt and water. ADH, also known as vasopressin, will increase vascular tone and cause constriction of blood vessels, especially those leading to the kidneys. This is the mechanism for acute tubular necrosis and renal failure seen in hypovolemic shock. Renal failure can be reversed if the vascular volume is restored before permanent injury to the kidneys occurs.

The amount of water and electrolytes needed to replace insensible loss and to maintain a urine output sufficient to excrete metabolic waste varies according to body size in a nonlinear way. The first 10 kg of body weight require 100 ml/kg, the next 10 kg require 50 ml/kg, and each kg beyond 20 requires 20 ml/kg. A 50-kg man has a water requirement of 2100 ml/day (1000 ml for his first 10 kg of weight, 500 ml for the next 10 kg, and 600 ml for the remaining 30 kg). Calculation of requirements in children follows the same rule; a 15-kg child has a water requirement of 1500 ml/day. "Ideal" weight should be used in obese individuals. Insensible loss of free water increases in febrile patients. A patient requires an extra 10% of the calculated need for water for each 1°C elevation in body temperature.

The amounts of electrolytes needed to maintain normal total body levels vary because the kidneys constantly adjust excretion. This adjustment is centered around increasing or decreasing sodium excretion to maintain a normal circulating vascular volume and composition. When necessary, the kidney can reduce sodium loss to zero by increasing potassium and hydrogen excretion (Fig. 8.2). For practical purposes, the electrolyte levels needed to maintain homeostasis without stimulating inordinate amounts of ADH and aldosterone are linearly related to the water requirement. The values used to determine daily maintenance fluid and electrolyte needs are listed in Table 8.2.

Oral or intravenous replacement of maintenance needs should always include sodium and potassium. Deficiencies of the other electrolytes develop more slowly, and they are not always given during short-term therapy. For a 50-kg woman with normal TBW and electrolytes, an appropriate maintenance IV solution is D5 1/2NS with KCl, 20 mmol/liter, infused at 85 ml/hr. This provides 2040 ml of fluid, 70 mmol of sodium, and 41 mmol of potassium, almost exactly the amounts calculated using Table 8.2. This patient will also receive Cl, 115 mmol. Cations must be given with an equal number of anions to maintain electrical

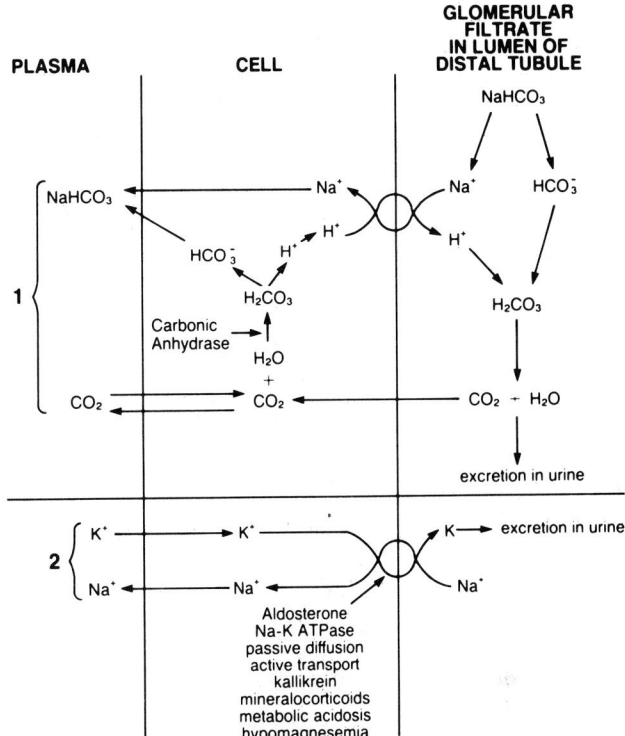

Figure 8.2. Mechanisms of Na-K exchange in the distal renal tubule.

Table 8.2.
Maintenance Requirements per 24 Hours[a]

Water		
	0–10 kg	100 ml/kg
	10–20 kg	50 ml/kg
	>20 kg	20 ml/kg
Electrolytes		
Na	3 mmol/100 ml H_2O requirement	
K	2 mmol/100 ml H_2O requirement	
Cl	2 mmol/100 ml H_2O requirement	
Ca	0.05–0.1 mmol/kg	
Mg	0.05 mmol/kg	
PO_4	0.1 mmol/kg	

[a] Use ideal body weight in obese patients.

neutrality, but hyperchloremia rarely occurs in patients with adequate renal function. Acetate salts of sodium and potassium are available and can be used if chloride anions must be avoided. Acetate is converted to bicarbonate in the body. Bicarbonate salts are not added routinely to IV solutions because they raise pH and may cause precipitation of electrolytes or drugs.

DISORDERS OF BODY WATER AND SOLUTE (5–13)

Sodium

Serum sodium is the major determinant of the intravascular volume because it is the osmotically active substance in greatest concentration in the compartment. Abnormalities in water and salt intake or excretion alter the sodium concentration. This impacts on the volume of the interstitial space because its major osmotic substance is also sodium and the two compartments are in equilibrium with each other.

The usual concentration of sodium in the serum is 135 to 147 mmol/liter (135 to 147 mEq/liter). Levels above or below this are referred to, respectively, as hyper- or hyponatremia. The terms are somewhat imprecise in that they refer to concentration and do not stipulate whether the abnormality is the result of alterations in the total body amounts of sodium, water, or both.

Hypernatremia is almost always the result of a free water deficit, but a true high total body sodium concentration can result from an excessive intake of salt. This is, however, almost impossible to do if renal function is adequate. Clinically important symptoms of hypernatremia do not generally appear until the serum level is greater than 160 mmol/liter and are the result of dehydration in the central nervous system (Table 8.3). The treatment for hypernatremia depends on whether the cause is too little water or too much sodium.

Hypernatremia from water loss indicates a decrease in total body water, not just intravascular volume. As the gradient across the three compartments is always in osmotic equilibrium, the interstitial sodium concentration and the intracellular potassium concentration will be essentially the same as that of intravascular sodium. The amount of free water needed to return all three values to normal is calculated, based on the TBW, by use of the following equation:

$$\text{Water deficit (liters)} \doteq$$

$$[1 - 140/\text{measured serum Na(mmol/liter)}]$$

$$\times \text{ body weight (kg)} \times 0.06$$

Replacement of the deficit is done with electrolyte-free oral or intravenous solutions, such as D5W, given over 18 to 24 hours in addition to calculated maintenance fluid and electrolyte needs. Treatment for sodium overload is directed at removal of sodium from the body and involves the use of diuretics and D5W to increase renal elimination while maintaining a normal total body water.

Hyponatremia describes a serum sodium concentration less than 135 mmol/liter (135 mEq/liter) but clinically important symptoms do not usually appear until the level is below 120 mmol/liter (120 mEq/liter) (Table 8.3) and are the result of CNS water intoxication. As with hypernatremia, the cause must be determined before treatment is begun. Hyponatremia can result from dilution or depletion, or be factitious.

Dilutional hyponatremia is a condition in which the total body sodium is increased but TBW is increased to a greater degree. The result is a low serum sodium concentration. It occurs in conditions such as cirrhosis and congestive heart failure when effective cardiac output reaching the kidneys is diminished. This, along with the low sodium concentration, is a stimulus for ADH and aldosterone secretion. The result is further salt and water retention, and the affected individuals are usually edematous. Diuretics are not a primary treatment and may be contraindicated because this condition is caused by decreased renal blood flow and delivery of sodium to the distal tubule. Salt and water restriction, bed rest (to increase venous return to the heart), and correction of the primary disorder are the initial treatments. These measures must not, however, be so aggressive as to compromise intravascular volume or further decrease renal blood flow.

Hyponatremia from depletion is a true decrease in the total body sodium, with or without a water deficit. It most commonly results from gastrointestinal losses from vomiting, excessive diuretic therapy, adrenal insufficiency, and replacement of losses from perspiration with electrolyte-free fluid. Patients show signs of dehydration (dry mucous membranes, skin tenting, lethargy) and, in extreme cases,

Table 8.3.
Sodium

Serum level > 147 mmol/liter	Serum level < 135 mmol/liter
Etiology	
Decreased water intake	Low-sodium diet with diuretics
Fever	Diuretics
Excessive salt intake	Congestive heart failure
Diabetes insipidus	Cirrhosis
Hyperventilation	Replacement of body secretion loss with electrolyte-free solutions
	Adrenal insufficiency
	Osmotic diuresis
Signs and symptoms	
Thirst	Apathy/agitation
Dry mucous membranes	Fatigue
	Anorexia/nausea
Decreased skin turgor	Headache
Acute weight loss	Muscle cramps
Confusion	Tachycardia
Hallucinations	Oliguria/anuria
Intracranial hemorrhage	Confusion
	Seizures
Coma	Coma
	Shock

hypovolemia. The amount of sodium needed to replace the deficit is calculated by use of the following equation:

$$\text{Sodium deficit (mmol)} =$$
$$[140 - \text{measured serum Na(mmol/liter)}]$$
$$\times \text{body weight (kg)} \times 0.6$$

Appropriate solutions to replace the sodium deficit are 0.9% saline (155 mmol of Na and Cl/liter) or 3% saline (500 mmol of Na and Cl/liter) given in addition to daily maintenance fluids and electrolytes. As hyponatremia does not usually occur acutely, replacement of the deficit may be made over a period of several days if necessary to avoid intravascular volume overload, pulmonary edema, or congestive heart failure.

Factitious hyponatremia is the result of accumulation of osmotically active substances, such as glucose and lipids, in the intravascular space. Sodium is diluted as water moves from the interstitial to the vascular space to normalize the osmotic pressure. The degree of hyponatremia seen is usually mild. Serum Na will fall only 1.6 mmol/liter for every 5.3 mmol/liter (100 mg/dl) increase in blood glucose, and treatment consists of correcting the underlying disorder.

Alterations in Fluid Compartment Integrity (14–16)

Trauma, tissue ischemia, endotoxemia, hypoalbuminemia, and decreased cardiac output result in hypovolemia by damaging capillary membranes or by disrupting the hydrostatic and oncotic forces governing fluid movement through them. The symptoms of hypovolemia are tachycardia, low central venous pressure (CVP), low pulmonary wedge pressure, and decreased urine output. Blood pressure is not a good measure of this condition, as increases in sympathetic tone can maintain the blood pressure near normal in the presence of a decreased circulating volume.

In trauma, ischemia, and endotoxemia, capillary pore size increases (capillary leak syndrome) and water, solute, and plasma proteins, primarily albumin, flow into the interstitial (third) space. This leak can be localized to an area of injury or ischemia (surgery, trauma) or generalized throughout the body (endotoxemic shock from Gram-negative sepsis). The amount of fluid lost from the intravascular space varies with the degree of injury, but it can be enough to cause cardiovascular collapse and death if circulating volume is not maintained.

Treatment consists of correcting the underlying disorder to normalize capillary permeability and replacement of the lost intravascular fluid. The solutions chosen must have the composition of the lost fluid. Blood has no role in this therapy, as the formed elements of the intravascular fluid are not being lost to the third space.

The two categories of replacement solutions are crystalloid and colloid. Crystalloid is a general term for any solution containing electrolytes. Normal (0.9%) saline or lactated Ringer's solution are used most commonly for treatment of hypovolemia, as they are isotonic with the ECF and are most effective in maintaining the circulating volume.

Colloid is a general term for a solution containing plasma proteins or other colloidal molecules. There are three types available. Plasma protein fraction (PPF) is approximately 85% albumin and 15% globulin; it is available as a 5% solution. Albumin is available as a 5% or 25% solution, and hetastarch as a 6% solution. All three also contain 130 to 160 mmol of Na and Cl/liter. Hetastarch is a mixture of ethoxylated amylopectin molecules (average molecular weight, 450,000) which exert the same hemodynamic effect as albumin. Hetastarch is not extracted from pooled human plasma and is much less expensive than PPF or albumin.

The use of colloid infusions remains controversial. While some albumin does leak into the third space, it is proportionately less than the amount of salt and water, and serum protein levels do not fall appreciably. Colloid will temporarily decrease the rate at which fluid migrates into the third space, but it may exacerbate hypovolemia later as it goes into the interstitial space itself. Unless the actual serum albumin is below the level needed to maintain the venule oncotic pressure gradient [20 to 25 g/liter (2 to 2.5 g/dl)] or aggressive crystalloid therapy is not restoring intravascular volume, the routine use of colloid solutions is not recommended.

The rate of fluid administration into the vascular space must meet or exceed the rate of loss, to maintain tissue perfusion. It can exceed one liter/hr in extreme cases. Urine output should be kept at a minimum of 0.5 ml/kg/hr, the level at which a circulating volume sufficient to perfuse body tissues is present. Normalization of heart rate and CVP also indicate normal intravascular volume and should be monitored hourly along with urine output. During the resuscitation process, IV fluid administration is adjusted hourly to maintain an adequate intravascular volume. It is important to remember that while edema can appear during this process, it is not the resuscitation process itself that is causing the edema. When healing begins, this extra fluid and solute will be returned to the vascular compartment and excreted. Diuretics have no role in the correction of edema caused by capillary leak syndromes, and their use can further deplete the intravascular volume.

Hypoalbuminemia without a concurrent capillary leak can result in hypovolemia with edema. Venule capillary oncotic pressure is low, and fluid that moved into the interstitial space on the arterial side of the capillary bed is not returned to the vascular system. Treatment for this condition consists of intravenous albumin or hetastarch in sufficient amounts to normalize the arteriovenous capillary oncotic pressure. Edema will resolve when this is done.

Table 8.4.
Approximate Concentrations of Ions in Body Secretions (mmol/liter)

Secretion	Na	K	Cl	HCO$_3$
Saliva	10	25	10	15
Stomach	60	10	85	—
Bile	150	5	100	40
Pancreas	140	5	80	120
Small bowel	110	5	105	30
Terminal ileum	117	5	105	—
Sweat	45	5	60	—
Cerebrospinal fluid	140	3	130	—

Hypovolemia due to a decreased cardiac output (congestive heart failure, cardiomyopathy, myocardial infarction) cannot be corrected by giving fluids. In these conditions, hypovolemia exists on the arterial side of the heart due to "pump failure"; the venous side of the circulatory system may be overloaded, and the patient is edematous. Treatment options are confined to drugs that will improve cardiac output, such as inotropes. If hypovolemia is the result of blood loss, then whole blood or packed red blood cells with normal saline (NS) or lactated Ringer's (LR) are indicated to reestablish the hematocrit above 0.25 (25%) along with a normal circulating volume.

Losses of Body Water and Solute

In prolonged vomiting, diarrhea, or losses through perforations in organs or the gastrointestinal tract leading to the skin (fistulas), water and solute are lost from the body. The composition of these fluids depends on the area affected (Table 8.4). When the exact site of origin of the fluid is not known, laboratory analysis of it will help in the selection of an appropriate replacement solution. This analysis is often necessary in the case of enterocutaneous (communication between the GI tract and the skin) fistulas. As they can make a circuitous tract through the body before reaching the skin, the organ nearest the exit site to the skin is not necessarily the one from which the fluid is draining. Diarrhea is most often of distal small bowel or colonic origin, but in cases of secretory diarrhea, such as in giardiasis or acquired immunodeficiency syndrome (AIDS), the fluid may arise from the duodenum or jejunum. In all cases of abnormal loss, the composition of the fluid should be determined. Appropriate replacement solutions, in addition to maintenance needs, are given at a rate to restore and maintain normal body water and solute.

ACID-BASE BALANCE (17–23)

For physiologic processes to occur at a normal rate, body pH must remain within a narrow range. It varies slightly among body compartments (the ICF has a pH of approximately 6.9, and some subcellular components, such as the mitochondria, have normal levels even lower), but a normal total body acid-base balance is defined as an arterial pH between 7.35 and 7.45.

Cellular metabolism, energy generation, and protein metabolism add large amounts of acid to the body daily. It is predominately in the form of carbon dioxide (CO_2), but some hydrogen ions and weak organic and inorganic nonvolatile acids are also generated. Almost no alkaline substances result from body processes, so acid-base homeostatic mechanisms are directed at buffering or eliminating acids. Hemoglobin, proteins, and phosphate are important systems but buffer only nonvolatile acids. Their capacity is also fixed. No adjustment can be made if the amount of acid in the body increases. Quantitatively these systems contribute little to the overall buffering capacity of the body, so they will not be discussed in detail.

The bicarbonate-carbonic acid system buffers CO_2 and can adjust quickly to changes in the daily acid load. It keeps body pH in the normal range by maintaining the correct ratio between the concentrations of bicarbonate (HCO_3) and carbonic acid (H_2CO_3) in the blood. This relationship is described by the Henderson-Hasselbalch equation:

$$pH = pKcarbonic\ acid + log\ (HCO_3/H_2CO_3)$$

When the HCO_3/H_2CO_3 (24 mmol/1.2 mmol) concentrations are at a ratio of 20:1, the pH will be 7.4, as the pKcarbonic acid is fixed at 6.1. Carbonic acid concentrations are not obtained in the clinical setting. A 40 mm Hg partial pressure of carbon dioxide (pCO_2) corresponds to an H_2CO_3 concentration of 1.2 mmol. The pCO_2 is maintained within the normal range by its diffusion and elimination across the lungs. The rate is adjustable to the amount of CO_2 generated by cellular metabolism. The capacity of the lungs to excrete CO_2 is so great that it can only be saturated in cases of severe pulmonary disease.

The kidneys are responsible for reabsorbing bicarbonate ions from the glomerular filtrate and for the generation of new HCO_3 ions in renal tubular cells. This is accomplished by the action of the enzyme carbonic anhydrase on carbon dioxide and water to form carbonic acid. Carbonic acid dissociates into H and HCO_3; the H ion is secreted into the urine and the HCO_3 transported into the vascular system. This reaction cannot be saturated if renal function is normal (Fig. 8.2).

Acid-base disturbances begin as changes in CO_2 or HCO_3 concentration. If the problem begins with CO_2, the resultant change in pH is referred to as being of respiratory origin; if it is with HCO_3, the change is of metabolic origin. A plasma pH below 7.35 is called acidosis and can be of respiratory or metabolic origin. A plasma pH above 7.45 is called alkalosis and is also from respiratory or metabolic causes. When the plasma pH goes outside the normal range, the lungs and the kidneys begin to compensate. If the respiratory center in the medulla oblongata perceives a change in pH, it causes the lungs to adjust the pCO_2 by instantaneously increasing or decreasing the respiratory rate. While very fast, this compensatory mechanism can only respond to minor changes in HCO_3 concentration. It is limited by the individual's mechanical ability to breathe in and out and by the capacity of the intracellular hemoglobin and phosphate buffering systems. The kidneys may take several days to compensate for primary changes in CO_2 concentration, but they have a greater ability to normalize the HCO_3/pCO_2 ratio.

It cannot be overemphasized that it is the ratio between CO_2 and HCO_3, not the absolute numbers, that determines pH. The body has a greater physiologic need to have a normal pH than it does to have normal levels of CO_2 and HCO_3. A high plasma HCO_3 level is not synonymous with metabolic alkalosis; it will also be seen in compensated respiratory acidosis. The alteration in one may well be the appropriate response to a change in the other. The result is a normal pH. No attempt, other than to determine and correct the primary problem, should be made to correct an isolated abnormal level. The only exceptions are when the plasma pH is above 7.6 or below 7.1, as death may be imminent. It is appropriate at these points to give bicarbonate or hydrochloric acid to normalize the pH of the body, without regard to the etiology of the disturbance.

Primary Acid-Base Disturbances
METABOLIC ACIDOSIS

Metabolic acidosis is the condition in which the plasma pH is below 7.35 as a result of a low bicarbonate concentration in the blood. As the bicarbonate concentration falls, the lungs attempt to lower the pCO_2 and maintain a normal pH by increasing the depth and rate of respiration (Kussmaul breathing). The symptoms of metabolic acidosis are in the cardiopulmonary or central nervous system, but they are not usually clinically important at a pH above 7.1 (Table 8.5).

Table 8.5.
Metabolic Acidosis (pH < 7.35, HCO_3 < 22 mmol/liter)

Etiology	Signs and Symptoms
Ketoacidosis	Kussmaul breathing
Renal failure	Hyperkalemia
Hypoxia/anoxia	Ventricular arrhythmias
Diarrhea	Lethargy
Salicylates	Stupor
Methanol	Coma
Chloride loading	

A low serum bicarbonate level results from increased losses from the body, decreased renal regeneration of HCO_3, or increased amounts of acid added to the body by metabolic processes or ingestion. With the addition of acid, the fall in HCO_3 is actually an appropriate compensatory response to maintain the electrical neutrality of the blood (a condition with an even higher physiologic priority than maintenance of a normal pH). The number of positively charged ions in the body must always equal the number of those negatively charged. In the plasma, neutrality is achieved with dissolved electrolytes and proteins in the following relationship:

$$Na = Cl + HCO_3 + \text{``unmeasured anions''}$$

Unmeasured anions consist of plasma proteins and small amounts of other negatively charged substances, such as SO_4 and PO_4, not "measured" by the laboratory tests used clinically. The usual amounts of these anions in the blood have a combined ionic strength of 8 to 16 mmol/liter (8 to 16 mEq/liter). This value is referred to as the "anion gap" and rarely changes. Assuming that Na remains constant, a change in the number of any one of the anions will necessitate a change in one or both of the others to maintain electrical neutrality. As the number of unmeasured anions is usually fixed, it is the Cl or HCO_3 that will change. Metabolic acidosis occurs when and because the HCO_3 goes down and the HCO_3/CO_2 ratio becomes abnormal. If it is the Cl anion that is decreased, the pH remains normal because HCO_3 remains normal.

Metabolic acidosis is divided into non- and positive anion gap varieties. In non–anion gap acidosis, the number of unmeasured anions is unchanged, so hyperchloremia secondary to chloride loading, an actual loss of bicarbonate, or decreased bicarbonate generation is decreasing the serum bicarbonate level. In positive anion gap acidosis, the number of unmeasured anions has increased, and the HCO_3 and Cl levels must drop to maintain electrical neutrality. The cause of a positive anion gap acidosis is the contribution of nonvolatile acids to the blood. This can be from abnormal metabolic processes, such as those seen in diabetic ketoacidosis and hypoxia, or in poisonings by substances that dissociate at plasma pH. Salicylate and methanol overdoses commonly cause this kind of metabolic acidosis. It is important to make the distinction between the two types of metabolic acidosis before determining a treatment regimen.

TREATMENT OF NON–ANION GAP METABOLIC ACIDOSIS

Loss of bicarbonate (prolonged diarrhea, gastrointestinal fistulas), inability to generate bicarbonate (renal failure), or chloride loading (normal saline infusions, NaCl overdoses) are the three causes of this type of metabolic acidosis. Treatment consists of correcting the underlying cause and replacing the bicarbonate deficit. Except in cases of renal failure, the kidneys will generate sufficient bicarbonate and normalize the pH when the cause of the acidosis has been eliminated. Acute replacement of HCO_3 is only necessary when the plasma pH is 7.1 or when the patient is exhibiting life-threatening symptoms of acidosis. The goal of bicarbonate replacement therapy is to achieve a plasma pH of 7.2, not necessarily to normalize it.

Since the onset of acidosis has usually been gradual, the CNS has slowly equilibrated to a low pH. Rapidly changing the plasma pH, relative to the CNS pH, can cause seizures and death. As the plasma pH normalizes over hours or days by renal bicarbonate generation, the CNS pH will equilibrate at a tolerable rate and complications will be avoided. The risk of inducing alkalosis or hypernatremia from the administration of $NaHCO_3$ often outweighs the benefit of quickly normalizing the pH.

Non–anion gap acidosis in renal failure is the result of the inability of the kidneys to generate bicarbonate. It is usually chronic and mild, and most patients are asymptomatic. Renal failure severe enough to cause acidosis almost always necessitates hemodialysis, because of low or no urine output. Modifications in the composition of the dialysate are routinely used to adjust HCO_3 concentrations and pH. Sodium bicarbonate is not routinely given (except as emergency therapy) because these patients are also chronically sodium- and water-overloaded.

If the pH is at or below 7.1, bicarbonate must be given. The bicarbonate deficit can be determined by use of the following equation:

$$HCO_3 \text{ deficit (mmol)} = [24$$
$$- \text{ measured } HCO_3 \text{ (mmol/liter)}] \times \text{ body weight (kg)}$$
$$\times 0.5$$

The volume of distribution of HCO_3 is estimated to be 10% less than the total body water, so the factor used is 0.5 rather than 0.6. One-half the calculated dose is given (this amount will usually change the pH by 0.2). The goal of therapy is to correct existing cardiac or CNS disturbances without creating new ones. In cases of diarrheal or fistula outputs that have exceeded the ability of the kidneys to replace HCO_3, it is also necessary to give bicarbonate. This is usually done with sodium or potassium salts of acetate, for reasons stated previously, but sodium bicarbonate can be used. The composition of the fluid being lost should be determined by laboratory analysis, and the amount of base given should correct the initial deficit and then match daily loss.

POSITIVE ANION GAP METABOLIC ACIDOSIS

Positive anion gap acidosis is the result of a rise in the number of unmeasured anions (nonvolatile acids) in the plasma, with a resultant drop in HCO_3 concentration. These acids can be the by-products of metabolic processes seen in diabetes and prolonged starvation (ketosis), anaerobic carbohydrate metabolism, or accumulation of ingested acids or of acids normally produced which cannot be eliminated, as in renal failure. With intracellular hypoglycemia, fat becomes the sole substrate for energy generation in the body. This quickly results in the production of ketone bodies. In diabetes, the low intracellular glucose level is caused by a lack of insulin, which prevents glucose transport from the blood to cells. In starvation, an absence of glucose from the body has occurred, which forces a change to fat metabolism. Ketone bodies dissociate and contribute hydrogen ions and the anion β-hydroxybutyrate. In cases of tissue hypoxia, insufficient oxygen to support the action of the Krebs cycle results in the activation of an alternative pathway for energy generation. This is the Cori cycle, which has lactic acid as its metabolic by-product. Hydrogen ions and the anion lactate accumulate, and acidosis results.

The treatment for anion gap acidosis is always correction of the underlying problem. Intravenous insulin is given in the case of diabetes. In lactic acidosis, restoration of an appropriate circulating volume or plasma oxygen carrying capacity is indicated. In poisonings, hemodialysis or gastric lavage may be necessary to remove toxic substances from the body. To reiterate, HCO_3 is given only if the pH is at or below 7.1 or if there are clinically important symptoms of acidosis.

METABOLIC ALKALOSIS

Metabolic alkalosis is defined as a plasma pH above 7.45 because of a high bicarbonate concentration in the blood. The anion gap is not affected by this condition. As the HCO_3 rises, the lungs compensate by lowering the depth and rate of respiration (Cheyne-Stokes breathing) to increase the pCO_2 and normalize the plasma pH, but generally, important symptoms do not appear at a pH below 7.6 (Table 8.6).

The most common causes of metabolic alkalosis are loss of chloride ion (nasogastric suction, loop diuretics,

Table 8.6.
Metabolic Alkalosis (pH > 7.45, HCO_3 > 28 mmol/liter)

Etiology	Signs and Symptoms
Liver failure	Cheyne-Stokes breathing
Diuretics	Hypokalemia
Nasogastric suction	Muscle cramping
Hyponatremia	Seizures
Hyperaldosteronism	
Corticosteroids	

mineralocorticoid excess) or ECF depletion. Diuretics and mineralocorticoids stimulate exchange of hydrogen and potassium ions for sodium in the renal tubules. This induces both hypokalemia and alkalosis (Fig. 8.2). Diuretics cause volume depletion and hyponatremia, which further stimulate H and K loss.

Volume depletion itself leads to alkalosis, as the concentration of HCO_3 molecules occupying a smaller plasma space increases. This condition is referred to as contraction alkalosis. As the body generates almost no basic substances during metabolism and base ingestion is uncommon, alkalosis from other causes is rare.

TREATMENT OF METABOLIC ALKALOSIS

Metabolic alkalosis as the result of sodium and chloride loss with volume contraction is referred to as "saline-responsive." Replacement of sodium will stop aldosterone-stimulated exchange of H for Na in the renal tubules. Replacement of chloride ions will stop the generation of HCO_3 to maintain electrical neutrality, and volume expansion will reduce HCO_3 concentration in the vascular space. Normal saline is the treatment of choice in this condition because it is slightly higher in sodium (155 mmol/liter) and much higher in chloride (155 mmol/liter) than the ECF. The amount of this solution that restores the TBW deficit should normalize sodium and chloride levels. Some patients with metabolic alkalosis have TBW overload and may not be able to tolerate a sodium load. The alkalosis can be treated with an infusion of hydrochloric acid or arginine hydrochloride. HCl is preferred, as these patients commonly have severe hepatic dysfunction. Administration of arginine can precipitate hepatic coma. The dose of HCl to replace the hydrogen and chloride deficits can be determined by the use of the following equation:

$$HCl \ (mmol) = [103 - measured \ Cl \ (mmol/liter)] \times body \ weight \ (kg) \times 0.2$$

The volume of distribution of chloride is 33% of TBW, so the multiplication factor is 0.2. Giving one-half the HCl deficit over 12 to 24 hr should lower the plasma pH by 0.2 and not cause a significant CNS pH gradient. Hydrochloric acid solutions for intravenous use are not commercially available; extemporaneous compounding of a 0.1 to 0.2 N solution (10 to 20 mmol HCl/liter) will be necessary. Infusion into a central venous catheter rather than a peripheral IV line is recommended, to reduce the risk of phlebitis.

Metabolic alkalosis can be the result of hypokalemia secondary to ICF/ECF exchange of hydrogen for potassium ions and from mineralocorticoid excess. These types of alkalosis are "saline-resistant," and treatment consists of potassium replacement. The decreased aldosterone deg-

Table 8.7.
Respiratory Acidosis (pH < 7.35, pCO_2 > 40 mm Hg)

Etiology	Signs and Symptoms
Emphysema	Anxiety
Airway obstruction	Disorientation
Bronchoconstriction	Vasodilation
Pneumonia	Increased cardiac output
Respiratory depression	Coma

radation (secondary hyperaldosteronism) seen in severe hepatic disease may respond to spironolactone. Patients with mineralocorticoid-producing tumors of the adrenal or pituitary glands will require aminoglutethimide or surgery.

RESPIRATORY ACIDOSIS

Respiratory acidosis is a plasma pH lower than 7.35 as the result of a pCO_2 higher than 40 mm Hg. The hemoglobin buffering system is activated in acute respiratory acidosis and sequesters hydrogen ions inside red blood cells. It is, however, a weak system and can only raise the HCO_3 by 1 mmol/liter for every 10 mm Hg rise in pCO_2. To correct the plasma pH, a 5 mmol/liter increase in HCO_3 is needed for every 10 mm Hg rise in pCO_2. The slow generation of HCO_3 in the kidney will eventually raise the plasma HCO_3 concentration enough to compensate for the respiratory acidosis and normalize the pH.

Since the CO_2 excretion capacity of normal lungs is always greater than the metabolic production, respiratory acidosis occurs only as a result of severe pulmonary disease (Table 8.7).

TREATMENT OF RESPIRATORY ACIDOSIS

Treatment always consists of correcting the underlying pulmonary disorder and may include antibiotics, bronchodilators, and steroids. Intubation and mechanical ventilation may be required if respiratory depression accompanies the acidosis. Rapid correction of the pH should be avoided, and administration of bicarbonate is indicated only if plasma pH is at or below 7.1. Chronic respiratory acidosis with emphysema and chronic obstructive pulmonary disease (COPD) develop slowly and rarely require treatment. The stimulus for respiration in these patients may still be an elevated CO_2, but many have adapted to hypoxia as the respiratory drive. Lowering the pCO_2 and raising the pO_2 acutely may precipitate apnea.

RESPIRATORY ALKALOSIS

Respiratory alkalosis is a pCO_2 lower than 40 mm Hg, causing a plasma pH higher than 7.45. The defense against

Table 8.8.
Respiratory Alkalosis (pH > 7.45, pCO₂ < 40 mm Hg)

Etiology	Signs and Symptoms
Hyperventilation	Confusion
Respiratory stimulants	Tetany
Hypoxemia	Syncope

this type of alkalosis is the movement of hydrogen ions (H_2PO_4 goes to HPO_4) from the intracellular to the vascular space. The phosphate buffering system, like hemoglobin, is small in capacity and will not normalize the pH in severe respiratory alkalosis. It can only lower the HCO_3 concentration by 3.5 mmol/liter for every 10 mm Hg drop in pCO_2 (Table 8.8).

TREATMENT OF RESPIRATORY ALKALOSIS

As voluntary hyperventilation, mechanical ventilation, and hypoxemia are the causes of respiratory alkalosis, correction of the disorder involves normalizing the pCO_2 by raising the CO_2 concentration of inspired air. This can be done by adjusting the concentration of inspired CO_2 delivered by a ventilator or respirator or by having the patient breathe into a paper bag.

Compensatory Responses to Acid-Base Disturbances

All acid-base disturbances will engender a compensatory response, e.g., primary metabolic acidosis will result in a drop in pCO_2 (compensating respiratory alkalosis). It can be difficult to determine the primary disturbance if the plasma pH has been returned to normal. It is also possible for two primary acid-base problems to occur together. The only exception is that respiratory acidosis and respiratory alkalosis cannot occur simultaneously. Correct diagnosis and a medication history are essential to establish the cause(s) and initiate treatment. No simple calculation using the arterial blood gases and serum electrolyte levels is possible, given the complexity of the body buffering and compensatory mechanisms. Excellent nomograms by Arbus (18) and Cogan and Rector (19) (Fig. 8.3) aid the clinician in determining (within 95% confidence limits) the etiology of an acid-base disturbance. This determination, combined with the history, guides treatment decisions.

ELECTROLYTES

The major electrolytes in the body are sodium, potassium, chloride, bicarbonate, calcium, magnesium, and phosphate. Normal serum levels are listed in Table 8.1. Sodium concentration is linked to body water (maintenance of normal body levels and correction of abnormalities have been discussed above). Chloride serves as the major anion to sodium in the ECF; it has no intrinsic physiologic function. Bicarbonate is linked to the acid-base homeostatic system and has also been discussed above. The remaining electrolytes are required to maintain membrane potentials for nerve conduction and muscle contraction (K, Ca, Mg), to generate the energy needed to maintain these potentials, and to do the work of body functions and movement (PO_4). The reservoirs of these ions are the intracellular space and bone.

Serum levels fall slowly when intake goes down, as numerous hormonal and homeostatic mechanisms keep serum levels within the normal range. The intravascular concentrations of these electrolytes are low relative to sodium and to their own intracellular concentrations. It is, however, the intravascular concentrations that govern physiologic activities. Serum levels must be kept within a narrow range or serious difficulties (such as cardiac arrhythmias, seizures, and tetany) will result.

Potassium (24–31)

The amount of potassium in the vascular space accounts for only 0.4% of the total amount in the body. In normal serum concentration ranging from 3.5 to 5.0 mmol/liter (3.5 to 5 mEq/liter), potassium has major functions in impulse transmission, cardiac contractility, and aldosterone secretion. The major route of excretion of this ion is the kidney, and elimination can be increased if intake is high. The kidneys are unable to conserve potassium, and a deficiency will develop rapidly if intake drops. Hyponatremia

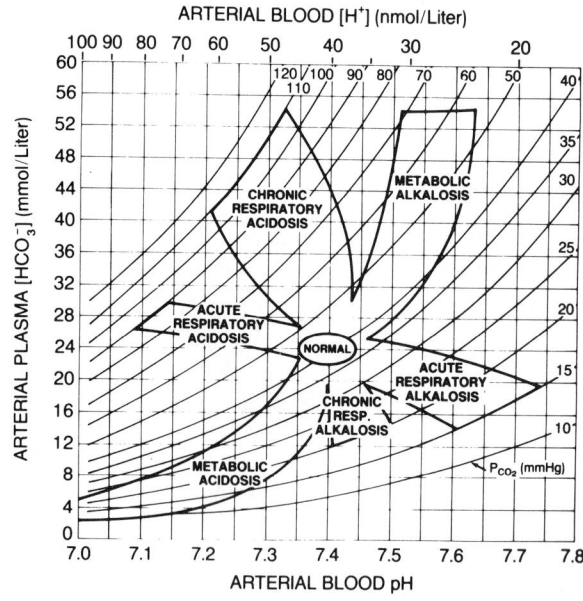

Figure 8.3. Acid-base nomogram. (From Cogan MG, Rector FC, Acid-base disorders. In Brenner BM, Rector FC (eds): The Kidney, ed 3. Philadelphia, WB Saunders, 1986, pp 457–518).

will also increase renal potassium loss via mechanisms discussed above (Fig. 8.2).

Serum potassium levels do not completely depend on the relationship between intake and output and sodium homeostasis. The large intracellular pool of potassium is a source of ions for the intravascular compartment. A low serum level usually represents not just a low circulating amount of K but also an intracellular deficit that can approach several hundred millimoles. Changes in acid-base status alter the location of potassium ions in the body. In acidosis, potassium is exchanged for hydrogen ions in the attempt by the body to buffer protons (acid) in the intracellular space and maintain a normal pH. The converse is true in alkalosis. The serum potassium level will rise (acidosis) or fall (alkalosis) by 0.6 mmol/liter for every 0.1 change in pH from the value of 7.4.

HYPERKALEMIA

A high serum potassium concentration can be a true medical emergency that almost always manifests itself as the sudden appearance of cardiac arrhythmias. This most commonly occurs at serum levels above 6 mmol/liter. The symptoms and causes of hyperkalemia are listed in Table 8.9. Total body potassium can be high, normal, or (occasionally) low. Only the intravascular concentration causes the cardiac disorders seen clinically. Any exogenous sources of potassium (e.g., IV fluids or drugs containing

Table 8.9.
Potassium

Serum Level > 5 mmol/liter	Serum Level < 3.5 mmol/liter
Etiology	
Renal failure	Amphotericin B
Acidosis	Diuretics
Crush injury	Diarrhea
Red cell hemolysis	Decreased intake
Potassium-sparing diuretics	Corticosteroids
Excess ingestion of potassium	Renal tubular acidosis
(salt substitutes)	Alkalosis
Adrenal insufficiency	Vomiting
Hypoaldosteronism	Fanconi's syndrome
	Hyperaldosteronism
	Licorice
Signs and symptoms	
ECG findings	ECG findings
Peaked T waves	Flat or inverted T waves
Depressed S-T segment	Depressed S-T segment
Disappearance of P wave	Muscle weakness
Widened QRS complex	Diminished reflexes
Muscle weakness	Paralysis
Paresthesias	Weak pulse
GI hypermotility	Ileus
Flaccid paralysis	Depression
	Confusion
	Hypotension

K) should be discontinued immediately. The life-threatening potential of the cardiac abnormality determines the type, complexity, and sequence of treatment given. Measures used to correct hyperkalemia either normalize neuromuscular membrane potential, shift ions back into the intracellular space, or remove potassium from the body. Muscular contractility is determined by the relative concentrations of potassium, calcium, and magnesium on the cell membrane. If the arrhythmia is immediately life-threatening, 2.5 to 5 mmol (5 to 10 mEq) of calcium is given over several minutes to temporarily correct the cardiac problem. Other measures aimed at normalizing the serum potassium must be initiated simultaneously. If necessary to maintain cardiac function, a constant IV infusion of calcium at a rate determined by simultaneous ECG monitoring is indicated. This therapy should not continue for long periods, as hypercalcemia will become a problem. Calcium gluconate (2.3 mmol/g) or calcium chloride (6.8 mmol/g) are the products used.

Another treatment approach shifts potassium ions from the vascular to the intracellular space. Sodium bicarbonate administration produces a temporary alkalosis and lowers serum potassium levels by 0.6 mmol/liter for every 0.1 elevation in pH. This therapy, like calcium infusion, should not be continued for long periods, as sodium overload and problematic metabolic alkalosis can result. Fifty-milliliter vials and preloaded syringes of 8.4% (1 mmol/liter) and 500-ml containers of 5% (0.6 mmol/liter) sodium bicarbonate are commercially available.

Glucose/insulin infusions are another possible treatment. Potassium ions move with glucose across cell membranes, when stimulated by insulin. A ratio of 2 to 3 g glucose per unit of insulin is needed to maintain a normal blood glucose level (25 to 30 units of regular insulin per liter of 10% dextrose solution or 10 units in 50 ml of 50% dextrose are commonly administered solutions). Although this is a temporizing measure (as potassium is not removed from the body), it can be continued without significant complication for longer periods of time than calcium or sodium bicarbonate infusions.

The final two therapies remove potassium from the body but act slowly. While they should be initiated as soon as possible, they will not correct cardiac arrhythmias in a timely fashion and cannot be considered acute treatments for hyperkalemia. The cationic-anionic exchange resin sodium polystyrene sulfonate, given orally or rectally, binds potassium to itself by exchange with sodium in the GI tract. One gram of resin will remove 1 mmol of potassium and add 2 to 3 mmol of sodium. The resin is very constipating, so it is given with sorbitol (an osmotic cathartic) and water to prevent fecal impaction. The oral route is preferred over rectal administration because the contact time with the GI mucosa is longer. The initial dose is 30 to 60 g of resin in 120 to 240 ml of 20% sorbitol; if indicated, it can be repeated every 1 to 2 hours. Sodium overload can occur, so monitoring for CHF, edema, and pulmonary edema is required. Patients will complain about this therapy, because the resin has the consistency of sand and an unpleasant taste. As a last resort, peritoneal- or hemodialysis can be used to remove potassium from the body.

HYPOKALEMIA

Hypokalemia can be a medical emergency, with cardiac abnormalities appearing at serum levels below 3 mmol/liter. Fortunately, the patient may exhibit muscle weakness and malaise first, which allows the clinician to identify and correct the condition before ECG changes appear. The symptoms and etiologies of hypokalemia are listed in Table 8.9. Correction of underlying diseases or discontinuation of drug therapy contributing to hypokalemia is a basic part of the initial treatment.

Hypokalemia secondary to hyponatremia is almost always accompanied by hypochloremic alkalosis because the renal sodium conservation mechanisms attempt to reabsorb sodium by secreting potassium and hydrogen ions. For every 3 mmol Na reabsorbed, 2 mmol of K and 1 mmol of H are lost. The hydrogen ion needed for this exchange is generated from water and CO_2. Carbonic anhydrase causes the formation of carbonic acid (H_2CO_3) in renal tubular cells, which then dissociates into H and HCO_3. Hydrogen ion is secreted into the urine and bicarbonate resorbed into the blood. HCO_3 ions accumulate, and alkalosis results.

Correction of concomitent hyponatremia and alkalosis must accompany treatment of hypokalemia for the treatment to be successful because continuing renal excretion and intracellular shifting of potassium will prevent replacement (Fig. 8.2). Administration of the chloride salt of potassium is the treatment of choice because correction of alkalosis is necessary. As chloride-loading proceeds, bicarbonate excretion by the kidneys increases proportionately and the alkalosis will resolve.

An intracellular deficit of potassium almost always accompanies the intravascular deficit. Large amounts of potassium may be required to normalize the serum level. Oral or intravenously administered potassium shifts slowly into the ICF to correct this deficit, so the rate of KCl infusion must not be so rapid as to cause hyperkalemia in the interim. Under most conditions, intravenous KCl at 10 mmol/hr will not cause hyperkalemia in a patient with a serum level below 3.5 mmol/liter. Infusion into a peripheral vein at a rate greater than 10 mmol/hr can also cause intolerable pain and phlebitis at the IV site. A 30 to 40 mmol dose given over 3 to 4 hr in D5W is the usual rate of potassium replacement. The serum potassium is checked 1 to 2 hr later, and the treatment is repeated until the level is 3.8 to 4.0 mmol/liter.

Oral administration of KCl can correct hypokalemia, but many patients will experience considerable GI irritation and vomiting when given more than 20 mmol/dose or 60 mmol/day. They will also often refuse therapy because of the bad taste of liquid KCl preparations, even though the solutions are highly flavored. Wax-matrix tablets (rather than 10% KCl solutions) have reduced these problems, but attempts to replace large potassium deficits by mouth are often unsuccessful.

Chloride (4)

Chloride is the major anion in the ECF. It has no intrinsic physiologic function and usually goes up or down in concentration with total body sodium. A change in chloride concentration causes a problem because it affects the serum HCO_3 concentration. The effect can be acidosis or alkalosis as a function of the resultant abnormality in the HCO_3 to pCO_2 ratio. Disorders of total body chloride are the result of loss from the body (vomiting, diuretics), hypernatremia, chloride loading (normal saline infusion), or changes in acid-base balance. In acidosis and alkalosis, the change in the serum chloride concentration is almost always a compensation for the change in the bicarbonate level. The serum chloride concentration will not normalize, nor should there be an effort made to alter it by giving or withholding chloride, until the acid-base abnormality is corrected. Then the chloride concentration will be normalized automatically by renal homeostatic mechanisms.

HYPERCHLOREMIA

A serum level greater than 105 mmol/liter is considered abnormal. As it is the result of metabolic acidosis, hypernatremia, or chloride loading, treatment is aimed at correcting the underlying disorder. The composition of oral or intravenous fluids should be determined and adjustments made if they appear to be the cause of the problem. Changing a normal saline infusion to lactated Ringer's or 0.5 N saline or replacing NaCl with Na acetate may solve the problem. If the hyperchloremia is caused by metabolic acidosis or respiratory alkalosis, correction of these disturbances is the only treatment.

HYPOCHLOREMIA

A serum chloride concentration below 95 mmol/liter is considered to be hypochloremia. Because the ECF chloride level changes with that of ECF sodium, hyponatremia results in hypochloremia. This is an appropriate compensatory mechanism to maintain electrical neutrality, and the chloride concentration will normalize with correction of the ECF sodium concentration.

The most common causes of hypochloremia are nasogastric (NG) suction, vomiting, and diuretic therapy. Large amounts of chloride and acid are lost with stomach fluid so therapy consists of replacement of the volume of the NG aspirate or vomiting with high-chloride-containing solutions such as NS or LR. Diuretics cause hypochloremia by mechanisms discussed in the section on hyponatremia. Therapy consists of liberalizing NaCl intake, reducing the diuretic dose, or correcting hyponatremia and hypokalemia.

Calcium (32–42)

The major repository of calcium in the body is bone. Only 1% of the total amount in the body is in the fluid spaces. The normal serum concentration is 2.2 to 2.6 mmol/liter (8.8 to 10.3 mg/dl), but only 50% is available to exert its physiologic effect. The other 50% is bound to albumin and other proteins. Serum calcium concentration, like that of the other intracellular ions, does not depend entirely on daily intake and excretion. The synchronous activity of parathyroid hormone, vitamin D, and calcitonin regulates GI absorption, renal excretion, and skeletal deposition or resorption of calcium. These hormones establish and maintain a normal serum calcium level. There is also an inverse relationship between serum calcium and phosphate (i.e., if one goes up or down, the other will change in the opposite direction).

Calcium has a variety of specific physiologic functions in the body. It is essential to neuromuscular conduction by stabilizing cell membrane permeability and excitability, it inhibits some enzymes in the Krebs cycle, stimulates gastrin, reduces renal blood flow, and is active in the blood coagulation cascade as factor IV. The normal concentration range is narrow, and most laboratories measure total serum calcium, not just the active, ionized 50%.

This presents a problem in determining the amount of physiologically active ion in the serum. Since 50% is bound, primarily to albumin, a low serum albumin level results in a low laboratory value, which does not necessarily mean that there is a simultaneously low ionized level. For each 10 g/liter change in the serum albumin concentration, total serum calcium will change 0.2 mmol/liter in the same direction. For example, a patient with an albumin level of 20 g/liter has a reported total calcium of 1.95 mmol/liter. Although this value is below normal, it does not represent a low ionized (free) level. Mathematically correcting the albumin to a normal of 40 g/liter raises the total calcium to 2.3 mmol/liter. It can be assumed from this correction that the free calcium level is normal and that physiologic hypocalcemia is not present. If only the ionized calcium concentration is reported, this correction need not be made.

Acid-base disturbances affect the ionized/bound calcium ratio but not total serum calcium. Some hydrogen ions circulate in the blood, bound to albumin. In acidosis, additional H ions are bound to albumin as the body attempts to buffer acid and normalize the plasma pH. This displaces calcium ions from their binding sites, and the amount of free calcium in the blood rises. The converse is true in alkalosis. For each 0.1 change in pH, the ionized calcium concentration changes 0.42 mmol/liter in the opposite direction.

HYPERCALCEMIA

Hypercalcemia is defined as a corrected total serum calcium concentration above 2.6 mmol/liter (10.3 mg/dl) or an ionized value above 1.15 mmol/liter. The symptoms and causes are listed in Table 8.10. Any sources of exogenous calcium should be immediately discontinued. Mental aberrations seen with hypercalcemia can be profound and not necessarily related in a linear fashion to the degree of hypercalcemia. Any evaluation of an apparently mentally ill or comatose patient should include a determination of the serum calcium level.

The therapies for hypercalcemia involve shifting ions back into the bone or removing calcium from the body. The removal therapies are given first because they work faster and are generally more effective in an acute situation. Loop diuretics, such as furosemide, increase renal excretion of calcium along with sodium. The initial dose of furosemide is 1 mg/kg given with an amount of normal saline to achieve a urine output of 200 to 500 ml/hr and

Table 8.10.
Calcium

Serum Level > 2.6 mmol/liter (total, corrected) 1.2 mmol/liter (ionized)	Serum Level < 2.2 mmol/liter (total, corrected) 1.0 mmol/liter (ionized)
Etiology	
Bone neoplasms	Renal failure
Hyperparathyroidism	Hypoparathyroidism
Hypervitaminosis D	Vitamin D deficiency
Prolonged immobilization	Diuretics
Sarcoidosis	Mithramycin
Paget's disease	Transfusion with citrated blood
Lithium	Pancreatitis
Adrenal insufficiency	Hyperphosphatemia
Acidosis	Alkalosis
Idiopathic hypercalcemia of infancy	Colchicine
Hypervitaminosis A	Hypomagnesemia
Aluminum osteodystrophy	Fluoride poisoning
Signs and symptoms	
Muscle weakness	Numbness/tingling of fingertips and around mouth
Anorexia	
Fatigue	Hyperactive reflexes
Nausea	Chvostek's sign
Lethargy	Trousseau's sign
Depression	Tetany
Psychosis	Lethargy
Stupor	Depression
Coma	Psychosis
	Stupor
	Coma

maintain a normal body water and sodium concentration. Potassium must be added to avoid hypokalemia. The therapy is adjusted to normalize the serum calcium, and it may be required for extended periods if the cause of the hypercalcemia cannot be corrected.

Treatments that shift calcium back into bone are hormonal, slow, and often become ineffective because of tachyphylaxis. Calcitonin is used because it increases bone uptake of calcium. Salmon and human preparations are available. While the hypocalcemic effect of calcitonin is rapid, it is of short duration, and tachyphylaxis usually develops within days. The starting dose for treatment of hypercalcemia is 4 IU/kg of salmon calcitonin given every 12 hours by subcutaneous or intramuscular injection. This can be increased to a maximum dose of 8 IU/kg given every 6 hr, but additional hypocalcemic effect may not result. Human calcitonin is approved for use only in Paget's disease, and equivalent dose ranges and intervals for the treatment of hypercalcemia have not been determined. Intranasal salmon calcitonin has been evaluated in the treatment of osteoporosis and in pain associated with osteoporotic vertebral fractures but not in the treatment of hypercalcemia. There is no intranasal preparation of calcitonin currently available in the United States.

Intravenous gallium nitrate has recently become available for use. In comparisons with salmon calcitonin in patients with the hypercalcemia of malignancy, it more effectively reduced serum calcium levels and had a longer duration of action. The mechanism of action is not well understood, but gallium appears to inhibit bone turnover. It is given by continuous infusion in doses of 100 to 200 mg/m^2 for 5 days. As it can be nephrotoxic, adequate patient hydration is essential, and other potentially nephrotoxic agents should be avoided during the treatment period.

Etidronate disodium is a diphosphonate that inhibits osteoclastic bone resorption by binding hydroxyapatite. Initial treatment is with 7.5 mg/kg/day given intravenously once daily for 3 days. The infusion time must be at least 2 hr. Therapy has been continued for as long as 7 days, but there is a risk of causing hypocalcemia. Once the serum calcium level has been controlled, oral therapy with 20 mg/kg/day can be given if the hypercalcemia is expected to recur (e.g., bone metastases in cancer patients). Pamidronate, a diphosphonate similar to etidronate, is currently under investigation. It may have quicker onset and longer duration of action than etidronate, without the disadvantage of inhibiting bone mineralization at high doses.

Steroids, such as prednisone, are useful in the management of chronic mild hypercalcemia. The initial dose of prednisone varies between 15 and 100 mg/day, with an onset of action of 3 to 10 days. Steroids work by antagonizing activation of vitamin D in the liver and by reducing

bone resorption. Thus, they are not effective in hypercalcemia secondary to hyperparathyroidism.

Oral phosphate is a treatment option in hypercalcemia that is the result of hypophosphatemia (a rare occurrence). The ordinary reciprocal relationship between serum calcium and phosphate levels has not been maintained in hypercalcemia from other causes, so the degree to which the serum calcium will fall with phosphate treatment is usually small. The risk of soft tissue calcification often makes this therapy unacceptable. Raising the serum phosphate will raise the calcium phosphate product if the serum calcium does not fall proportionately. This can result in precipitation of insoluble $CaPO_4$ complexes in tissue when the product exceeds 5 (serum calcium is multiplied by serum phosphate to get this value). In the rare instances when hypophosphatemia is the cause, administration of 30 to 100 mmol/day (1 to 3 g) of phosphorus should solve the problem. Replacement products available are Phospho-Soda (solution, 25 mmol (800 mg) P/5 ml) and Neutra-Phos (capsules, 8 mmol (250 mg) P; solution 32 mmol (1 g) P/300 ml). These products contain considerable amounts of sodium and potassium as the obligate cations, and caution must be exercised with their use.

An effective but potentially toxic therapy is mithramycin, indicated only when other therapies fail. It is a cancer chemotherapeutic agent that acts in hypercalcemia by inhibiting DNA-dependent bone osteoclast RNA synthesis. This slows or stops bone resorption. The initial dose is 25 µg/kg up to a weekly maximum of 150 µg/kg. The onset of action is 12 to 48 hr and the duration, 3 to 7 days. While these doses are considerably smaller than those used in cancer treatment, the risk of hematologic and gastrointestinal toxicity remains.

HYPOCALCEMIA

Hypocalcemia is defined as a corrected serum level below 2.20 mmol/liter (8.8 mg/dl) or an ionized level below 1 mmol/liter. The symptoms and causes are listed in Table 8.10. Acute treatment involves intravenous administration of calcium. The chloride salt contains 6.8 mmol/g (13.5 mEq Ca/g) and the gluconate and gluceptate salts, 2.3 mmol/g (4.6 mEq Ca/g). The initial dose is 2.5 to 5 mmol of Ca followed by an infusion of 0.075–0.1 mmol Ca/kg/hr. Calcium level, blood pressure, and ECG should be monitored during this process, to evaluate cardiac function and avoid hypercalcemia. Patients whose symptoms of hypocalcemia do not resolve with calcium replacement should be evaluated for hypomagnesemia because the abnormalities can mimic each other and often appear together.

Treatment of chronic hypocalcemia is directed at correcting the underlying cause. Most commonly, chronic hypocalcemia is caused by a low level of biologically active vitamin D. This occurs in advanced hepatic or renal disease because of decreased transformation of cholecalciferol (D_3) by these organs to the active form, 1,25-dihydroxy-cholecalciferol (1,25-DHC). The serum calcium level will not normalize until the level of 1,25-DHC is normal. Therapy usually involves calcium and vitamin D supplementation. Ergocalciferol (D_2) in a dose of 1.25 to 5 mg (50,000–200,000 IU/day) or dihydrotachysterol (DHT) in a dose of 0.25 to 1 mg/day (equivalent to 30,000 to 120,000 IU of D_2) are most commonly used. The onset of action can be several weeks, and the effect is prolonged because of the long half-life of vitamin D.

Activated forms of vitamin D can be given. 25-Hydroxycholecalciferol (calcifediol) in doses of 25 to 200 µg/day or 1,25-DHC (calcitriol) in doses of 0.25 to 1 µg/day are available. The active forms of vitamin D have an onset of action of 3 to 7 days and have shorter half-lives than D_2. They are preferred in treatment because the risk of hypercalcemia is less. Calcium supplementation in doses of 25 to 100 mmol/day (1 to 4 g) is begun simultaneously. Several salts of calcium are available for oral therapy. Calcium carbonate contains the highest amount of elemental calcium, 10.2 mmol (400 mg) per 1000 mg $CaCO_3$. Calcium lactate is 1.5 mmol (60 mg) per 300 mg, calcium gluceptate contains 2.2 (80 mg) per 1000 mg, and calcium gluconate, 2.3 mmol (90 mg) per 1000 mg. Calcium carbonate is the preferred preparation as the number of tablets the patient must take is lower than with the other salts. Liquid $CaCO_3$ and Ca gluceptate are available for use in patients with achlorhydria or those receiving H_2 antagonist therapy, since tablet dissolution in the GI tract may be incomplete without gastric acid. When hypocalcemia is due to hypoparathyroidism, parathyroid hormone replacement is indicated and is the only therapy that will raise the serum calcium concentration.

Magnesium (43–44)

The average adult body contains approximately 1000 mmol (2000 mEq) of magnesium, 99% of which is in bone and the intracellular compartment. Of the 1% remaining in the vascular space, 25% is bound to proteins; it is the ionized 75% that exerts the physiologic effect. Serum magnesium is maintained in the normal range of 0.8 to 1.2 mmol/liter (1.6–2.4 mEq/liter) by efficient renal conservation/excretion mechanisms and by drawing on the intracellular space for "new" ions when intake falls. With calcium and potassium, magnesium regulates neuromuscular excitability and conduction on the cell membrane. It also has a role in the release of parathyroid hormone. Deviations from a normal serum magnesium level rarely appear as an isolated electrolyte disturbance. Most often, calcium, potassium, and phosphate levels are also abnormal, indicating a generalized abnormality in the intracellular compartment. This can be seen in prolonged starvation.

Table 8.11.
Magnesium

Serum Level > 1.2 mmol/liter	Serum Level < 0.8 mmol/liter
Etiology	
Renal failure	Amphotericin B
Hyperparathyroidism	cis-Platinum
Hypoaldosteronism	Diuretics
Adrenal insufficiency	Diarrhea
Lithium	Hypervitaminosis D
	Vitamin D deficiency
	Vomiting
	Hyperaldosteronism
	Aminoglycosides
Signs and symptoms	
Weakness	Tremor
Nausea/vomiting	Hyperactive reflexes
Hypotension	Confusion
Respiratory depression	Seizures
Coma	

HYPERMAGNESEMIA

Hypermagnesemia is defined as a serum level above 1.2 mmol/liter (2.4 mEq/liter), but serious symptoms do not usually occur until the level is above 2.4. The symptoms and causes of hypermagnesemia are listed in Table 8.11. Since large loads of magnesium can be excreted easily by the kidneys, hypermagnesemia is rarely seen without attendant severe renal dysfunction. Magnesium-containing antacids are often a contributing factor, and all sources of exogenous magnesium should be discontinued.

The treatments for an elevated magnesium involve eliminating it from the body or shifting it back into the intracellular space. Glucose and insulin can be used, as in the treatment of hyperkalemia. Renal function is almost always severely impaired in patients with hypermagnesemia, so the only effective means of removing it from the body are peritoneal- and hemodialysis.

HYPOMAGNESEMIA

Hypomagnesemia is defined as a serum level below 0.8 mmol/liter (1.6 mEq/liter). Symptoms can appear at levels below 0.6. The symptoms and causes of hypomagnesemia are found in Table 8.11. Hypomagnesemia usually appears with hypokalemia, -calcemia, and -phosphatemia. Levels of these electrolytes should be measured when low levels of magnesium are found. As with the other intracellular electrolytes, there is almost always a generalized deficit. The total body deficit of magnesium may be as much as 25 mmol before the serum level begins to fall.

Therapy is with the sulfate or oxide salts of magnesium. The available product for intravenous administration is magnesium sulfate. Each gram of the 50% solution contains 4 mmol (8 mEq) of magnesium. The initial dose is 0.25 mmol/kg/day if the serum level is less than 0.6 mmol/

liter, and 0.15 mmol/kg/day if it is between 0.7 and 1.2. This amount should be given over 1 to 4 hr and the serum level checked 1 to 2 hr later. The delay before measuring allows time for intracellular shifting, as an exact replacement dose cannot be determined from the serum level alone. Oral replacement of large deficits can be difficult because magnesium is a saline cathartic and may produce diarrhea. If this route of administration is chosen, up to 20 mmol/day given in divided doses will usually be tolerated. Magnesium oxide capsules are given most commonly (6.2 mmol/250 mg MgO), but solutions of $MgSO_4$ are also available for oral administration.

Phosphorus (45–47)

Of the total body phosphate, 99.99% is contained in bone and the intracellular space. The normal serum level is 0.8 to 1.6 mmol/liter (2.5 to 5 mg/dl). The equilibrium between serum calcium (reciprocal with PO_4), intracellular stores, parathyroid hormone, vitamin D, renal conservation/excretion mechanisms, and oral intake maintains a normal serum level. The specific physiologic function of phosphate in the body is to form high-energy phosphate bonds of adenosine di- and triphosphate in glycolysis (anaerobic metabolism) and the Krebs cycle. Release of oxygen from hemoglobin is facilitated by 2,3-diphosphoglycerate in red blood cells.

HYPERPHOSPHATEMIA

Hyperphosphatemia is defined as a serum level above 1.6 mmol/liter and almost always results from decreased excretion in the presence of severe renal dysfunction. Symptoms and causes of hyperphosphatemia are listed in Table 8.12. The only available treatments are minimizing intake, decreasing absorption from the GI tract by precipitation with aluminum or calcium, and glucose-insulin infusions. Peritoneal- or hemodialysis is used to lower serum phosphate levels, but neither is very efficient.

HYPOPHOSPHATEMIA

Hypophosphatemia is defined as a serum level below 0.8 mmol/liter, but symptoms rarely appear if it is above 0.3. The abnormality is usually simultaneous with deficits in other intracellular ions. Symptoms and causes are listed in Table 8.12. Therapy consists of replacement with the sodium or potassium salts of phosphate. Repletion must be slow because calcium-phosphate precipitation in soft tissue, renal failure, and hyperphosphatemia can result from aggressive therapy. The initial dose is 0.3 to 0.6 mmol/kg/day if the serum level is below 0.3 and 0.2 to 0.3 mmol/kg/day if it is between 0.4 and 0.8. This therapy should be given over at least 12 hr, to allow for intracellular shifting, and the serum level should be checked 3 to 4 hr later. Oral replacement can be given with Phospho-Soda or Neu-

Table 8.12.
Phosphorus

Serum Level > 1.6 mmol/liter	Serum Level < 0.8 mmol/liter
Etiology	
Renal failure	Aluminum antacids
Hyperparathyroidism	Prolonged starvation
	Nutritional repletion
	Diuretics
	Vitamin D deficiency
	Hyperaldosteronism
	Corticosteroids
	Alkalosis
	Renal tubular defects
	SIADH
Signs and symptoms	
Renal osteodystrophy	Muscle weakness
$CaPO_4$ complex deposition in	Bone pain
soft tissue	Paresthesias
	Irritability
	Respiratory insufficiency
	Hemolytic anemia
	Rhabdomyolysis
	Proximal muscle atrophy
	Cardiomyopathy
	Seizures
	Coma

tra-Phos in divided doses (refer to the section on hypercalcemia for the phosphate content of these products).

CONCLUSION

Identification and correction of disorders in fluids and electrolytes and in acid-base balance can be difficult. The internal environment is dynamic and continuously reacting to internal and external forces that disturb homeostasis. Normal serum electrolyte levels do not always reflect normal body water or pH status. Abnormal values may be appropriate compensatory responses to maintain homeostasis. Normal body functions continue only within narrow ranges of ionic composition, pH, and intravascular volume and pressure. When evaluating a patient, a hemodynamic status sufficient to perfuse and oxygenate cells is the first priority, and action must be taken immediately if the patient is to survive. With the exception of exsanguination (acute, massive blood loss), changes in fluids, electrolytes, and pH occur slowly, and some compensatory mechanisms are operating. Treatment should not be so aggressive as to complicate a situation that may already be life-threatening. It must be given in a way and at a rate that will reestablish and maintain homeostasis without iatrogenic (treatment-induced) complications.

REFERENCES

1. Robertson GL, Berl T, Pathophysiology of water metabolism. In Brenner BM, Rector RC (eds): The Kidney, ed 3. Philadelphia, WB Saunders, 1986, pp 385–423.

2. Moore FD, McMurray JD: Total body water and electrolytes: intravascular and extravascular phase volumes. Metabolism 5:447, 1956.

3. Cohn SH, Vaswani A: Changes in body chemical composition with age measured by total-body neutron activation. Metabolism 25:85, 1976.

4. Earley LE, Daugharty TM: Sodium metabolism. N Engl J Med 281:72–86, 1969.

5. Feig PU, McCurdy DK: The hypertonic state. N Engl J Med 297:1444–1454, 1957.

6. Weitzman RE, Kleeman CR: The water depletion syndrome (hyperosmolar) and water excess (hyposmolar) syndromes. West J Med 132:16–38, 1980.

7. Hierholzer K, Wiederholt M: Some aspects of distal tubular solute and water transport. Kidney Int 9:198–218, 1976.

8. Bartter FE, Schwartz WB: The syndrome of inappropriate secretion of anti-diuretic hormone. Am J Med 42:790, 1967.

9. Narins RG, Joned ER: Diagnostic strategies in disorders of fluid, electrolyte and acid-base homeostasis. Am J Med 72:496, 1982.

10. Giebisch G, Stanton B: Potassium transport in the nephron. Annu Rev Physiol 41:241–256, 1979.

11. Chonko AM, Bay W: The role of renin and aldosterone in the salt retention of edema. Am J Med 63:881–889, 1977.

12. Espiner EA, Tucci JR: Effect of saline infusions on aldosterone secretion and electrolyte excretion in normal subjects and patients with primary hyperaldosteronism. N Engl J Med 277:1–7, 1977.

13. Good DW, Velazquez H: Luminal effects on potassium excretion: low sodium concentration. Am J Physiol 246:F46–F55, 1982.

14. Ross AD, Angaran DM: Colloids and crystalloids—a continuing controversy. Drug Intell Clin Pharm 18:202–212, 1984.

15. Lewis RT: Albumin: role and discriminative use in surgery. Can J Surg 23:322–333, 1980.

16. Hulse JD, Yacobi A: Hetastarch: an overview of the colloid and its metabolism. Drug Intell Clin Pharm 17:334–341, 1983.

17. Hyneck ML: Simple acid-base disorders. Am J Hosp Pharm 42:1992–2006, 1985.

18. Arbus GS: An in-vivo acid-base nomogram for clinical use. Can Med Assoc J 109:291, 1973.

19. Cogan MG, Rector FC, Acid-base disorders. In Brenner BM, Rector FC (eds): The Kidney, ed 3. Philadelphia, WB Saunders, 1986, pp 457–518.

20. Emmett M, Narins RG: Clinical use of the anion gap. Medicine 56:38, 1977.

21. Narins RG, Emmett M: Simple and mixed acid-base disorders: a practical approach. Medicine 59:161, 1980.

22. Adroque HJ, Madias NE: Changes in plasma potassium concentration during acute acid-base disturbances. Am J Med 71:456, 1981.

23. Weber JN: Treatment of metabolic alkalosis with intravenous administration of hydrochloric acid. CSHP Voice 13:1–3, 1986.

24. Brater DC: Serum electrolyte abnormalities caused by drugs. Prog Drug Res 30:9, 1986.

25. Surawicz B: Relationship between the ECG and electrolytes. Am Heart J 73:814, 1967.

26. Knochel JP: Neuromuscular manifestations of electrolyte disorders. Am J Med 72:521, 1982.

27. Pearson E, Fish H: Potassium content of selected medicines, foods and salt substitutes. Hosp Pharm 6(9):6–9, 1971.

28. Stanszek WF: Current approaches to management of potassium deficiency. Drug Intell Clin Pharm 19:176, 1985.

29. Cox M: Potassium homeostasis. Med Clin North Am 65:67–73, 1981.

30. Hollifield JW, Slaton PE: Thiazide diuretics, hypokalemia and cardiac arrhythmias. Acta Med Scand (suppl) 647:67–73, 1981.

31. DeFronzo RA, Bias M: Clinical disorders of hyperkalemia. Annu Rev Med 33:521, 1982.

32. Pederson KO: The effect of bicarbonate, CO_2 and pH on serum calcium fractions. Scand J Clin Lab Invest 27:145, 1971.

33. Suki WN, Rouse D: Hormonal regulation of calcium transport in the thick ascending limb renal tubules. Am J Physiol 241:F171, 1981.

34. Bell NH: Hypercalcemic and hypocalcemic disorders: diagnosis and treatment. Nephron 23:147, 1979.

35. Massry SG, Coburn JW: Role of serum Ca, parathyroid hormone, and NaCl infusion on renal Ca and Na clearance. Am J Physiol 214:1403, 1968.

36. Ryzen E, Martodam RR: Intravenous etidronate in the management of malignant hypercalcemia. Arch Intern Med 145:449–452, 1985.

37. Bordier P: The effect of 1(OH)D3 and 1,25(OH)2D3 on the bone of patients with renal osteodystrophy. Am J Med 64:101–107, 1978.

38. Kanis J: Vitamin D metabolism and its clinical application. J Bone Joint Surg 64B:542–557, 1982.

39. Bilezikian JP: Calcium and bone metabolism, part IV. In Becker KL (ed): Principles and Practice of Endocrinology and Metabolism. Philadelphia, JP Lippincott, 1990.

40. Austin LA, Heath H: Calcitonin. N Engl J Med 304:269–280, 1981.

41. Pun KK, Chan LWL: Analgesic effect of intranasal salmon calcitonin in the treatment of osteoporotic vertebral fractures. Clin Ther 2:205–208, 1989.

42. Warrell JP, Israel R: Gallium nitrate for acute treatment of cancer-related hypercalcemia. A randomized, double-blind comparison to calcitonin. Ann Intern Med 108:669–674, 1988.

43. Massry SG, Seelig MS: Hypomagnesemia and hypermagnesemia. Clin Nephrol 7:147, 1977.

44. Dickerson RN: Treating hypomagnesemia. Hosp Pharm 20:761–763, 1985.

45. Chernow B, Rainey TG: Iatrogenic hyperphosphatemia: a metabolic consideration in critical care medicine. Crit Care Med 9:772, 1981.

46. Vannatta JB, Whang R: Efficacy of intravenous phosphate therapy in the severely hypophosphatemic patient. Arch Intern Med 141:885, 1981.

47. Dickerson RN: Treating hypophosphatemia. Hosp Pharm 20:920–925, 1985.

CHAPTER 9

GENERAL NUTRITION

JOHN M. HOLBROOK, Ph.D. and DIANE NYKAMP McCARTER, Pharm.D.

In addition to the vitamins and minerals discussed in Chapter 10, other nutrients that are essential for normal body function include lipids, carbohydrates, proteins, and water. These nutrients are termed "essential" because they are required to sustain life and because they must be obtained from exogenous sources. Some authorities also include fiber as an essential nutrient because of its role in preventing cancer of the gastrointestinal tract.

ENERGY SOURCES

The oxidative metabolism of carbohydrates, lipids, and proteins provides energy for the body. This energy is expressed in units of heat, kilocalories or simply calories. One calorie of energy is the amount of heat required to raise the temperature of one kilogram of water at room temperature one degree Celsius (1°C). In the metric system, this amount of energy is expressed in joules. One kilocalorie is equal to 4.184 kilojoules (1).

The energy values (physiologic fuel values) of these nutrients are

Carbohydrates—4 kcal/g;
Lipids—9 kcal/g;
Protein—4 kcal/g.

The metabolism of lipids provides more than twice the amount of energy produced by the metabolism of protein or carbohydrate. The metabolism of one teaspoon of sugar (4 g) provides 16 kcal of energy, while the metabolism of 4 grams of lipid provides 36 kcal. Since many foods contain large amounts of water, which provides no calories, their caloric value by weight would not correspond to their pure caloric value. For example, a protein source such as chicken, which contains a large amount of water, would provide fewer than 4 kcal per gram.

Carbohydrates

Carbohydrates occur in nature in simple and complex forms. The category of simple carbohydrates (simple sugars) includes monosaccharides and disaccharides. Monosaccharides such as glucose are the only sugars that can be absorbed directly from the gastrointestinal tract into the blood stream. They are the most rapidly available sources of energy and are the only sugars capable of being used directly to produce energy for the body. Disaccharides such as sucrose, maltose, and lactose are the most abundant sugars found in foods. They must be digested into simple sugars prior to being absorbed. Sucrose and maltose are found in many foods, but the only natural source for lactose is milk. Lactose is catabolized into glucose and galactose by the enzyme lactase. An individual who is deficient in lactase will obtain fewer calories from milk than an individual with normal lactase function. It is estimated that 60 to 90% of adult American blacks and Orientals have some degree of lactose malabsorption compared with 5 to 15% of white American adults (2).

The category of complex carbohydrates (polysaccharides) includes starch (most prevalent), dextrin, inulin, and fiber. Complex carbohydrates are digested in the gastrointestinal tract more slowly than simple carbohydrates, thus the glucose they provide is made available more slowly. Foods high in complex carbohydrates are often recommended for individuals requiring weight loss or control. Such foods alleviate hunger while providing less readily available glucose and fewer calories than are obtained from the simple sugars.

Lipids

Lipids are structurally heterogeneous compounds that are soluble in organic solvents. They are the body's major form of stored energy and also serve as structural components of membranes. Lipids are categorized as simple lipids (fats), compound lipids such as phospholipids, and derived lipids such as cholesterol and fatty acids.

Triglycerides are composed of glycerol and fatty acids and are the most abundant lipids found in nature. They are also the major form of stored lipids in mammals and are found primarily in subcutaneous deposits and in skeletal muscle. Fatty acids are aliphatic carboxylic acids that do not occur in nature but are part of the structure of most major lipids.

Cholesterol is required by the body for the synthesis of bile acids and steroid hormones. However, its essential nature is often overshadowed by concerns related to its role in the incidence of atherosclerotic heart disease. It is found in the diet as a component of saturated fats but is also synthesized in the body, chiefly by the liver, but also in the intestines and the endocrine glands. The synthesis of cholesterol by the liver is partially controlled by an inhibitory feedback mechanism related to dietary cholesterol intake. This mechanism does not inhibit the production of cholesterol in the intestine or endocrine glands. Although dietary cholesterol can suppress hepatic cholesterol synthesis, the ingestion of even large amounts will not reduce its synthesis by more than 40% (3).

Proteins

Proteins are complex molecules composed of amino acids. They are found in the body as independent structures as well as in combination with other substances such as in mucoproteins and lipoproteins. Prior to their absorption, proteins are broken down into their individual amino acid units. Once absorbed, these amino acids are used primarily for the production of new body protein. They may also be used as an energy source when other energy sources have been depleted. When the diet contains excessive amounts of protein, these amino acids may be used for energy or stored in the form of triglycerides.

Not all types of protein are equal in their ability to support body growth, provide for maintenance of body tissue, and provide necessary components for the repair of damaged body tissue. The most highly functional proteins are termed complete proteins or proteins of high biologic value. They have a protein efficiency ratio (PER) of 2.5 or higher. Proteins capable of supporting life but not growth have a PER value between 0.5 and 2.5. Proteins that can support neither life nor growth are termed incomplete proteins and have a PER value of less than 0.5. The difference between the PER values of proteins is based on their amino acid content. Of the amino acids, 8 are considered to be essential for adults, and 9 are considered to be essential for infants. Essential amino acids must be provided in the diet in amounts appropriate to sustain life. The remaining amino acids are considered to be nonessential and can be synthesized in sufficient quantities to meet the needs of the body.

Protein sources with the highest PER values supply large amounts of all of the essential amino acids. These proteins sources include milk, oatmeal, dairy products, fish, and meat. Often the protein needs of the body are met using combinations of incomplete proteins, especially when the incomplete proteins are lower in calories or undesirable nutrients (e.g., lipids) than are complete proteins. Table 9.1 lists the amino acids and Table 9.2 lists various protein sources with their PERs.

WATER

Water is the most abundant body element and accounts for 50 to 70% of total body weight. This percentage decreases with age and varies inversely with the percentage of body fat (4). The minimal daily requirement for water is highly variable and is dependent on obligatory water losses such as urinary output, perspiration, water exhaled as vapor, and loss via feces. Certain disease states and injuries may also increase water loss (e.g., burns).

The daily water intake of an individual should meet or

Table 9.1.
Amino Acids

Essential Amino Acids	Nonessential Amino Acids
Isoleucine	Alanine
Leucine	Asparagine
Lysine	Aspartic acid
Methionine	Cysteine
Phenylalanine	Glutamic acid
Threonine	Glutamine
Tryptophan	Hydroxyproline
Valine	Hydroxylysine
Histidine[a]	Proline
	Serine
	Tyrosine

[a] Essential for infants.

Table 9.2.
Protein Efficiency Ratios (PER)

Complete Proteins or Proteins with High Biologic Value (PER ≥2.5)		Protein Capable of Supporting Life but Not Growth (PER = 0.5–2.5)	
Food	PER	Food	PER
Egg	3.92	Meat	2.30
Fish	3.55	Oats	2.19
Milk	3.09	Peanuts	1.65
		Peas	1.57
		Whole wheat	1.53

exceed expected water loss which, for an adult, is approximately 2500 ml. The intake of slightly more water is highly recommended to facilitate normal function of the gastrointestinal tract and kidney.

FIBER

Fiber and roughage are terms used to designate a group of carbohydrates that are not digested, absorbed, or used by the human body to provide energy or build tissue. The fiber content of foods was once reported as crude fiber, which is defined as the residue remaining after a food has been treated with solvents, hot acid, and hot alkali. The term dietary fiber is currently used to describe the total fiber content of foods. Examples of dietary fiber include cellulose, hemicellulose, lignin, pectin, gums, mucilages, and some oligosaccharides and polysaccharides. The source of most fiber is the structural material of plants such as whole grains, vegetables, fruits, and nuts.

Until the initial reports of Burkitt regarding "fiber deficiency diseases" (4), the nutritional value of fiber was largely overlooked. It has been suggested more recently that daily fiber intake may actually promote health (5) and provide protection against colon cancer by decreasing the length of time that feces containing potential carcinogens remain in the colon, by diluting intestinal contents, and by absorbing and/or influencing the metabolism of cancer-promoting substances (6).

NUTRITIONAL REQUIREMENTS

To provide the body with the appropriate amount of energy, the diet should be "balanced" with regard to the intake of lipids, carbohydrates, and protein. The amount of energy sources needed depends on body size and the amount of physical activity in which the individual engages. Individual nutritional requirements are rarely, if ever, static, because a number of factors may alter nutritional needs. Some of these factors are environmental, physical, and emotional stress, changes in lifestyle, and aging. The body is extremely adaptable, but for positive adaptive processes to occur, it must be supplied with the necessary nutrients in appropriate quantities to meet changing needs. The relationship of appropriate nutrient intake and maintenance of a healthy lifestyle to the prevention and alleviation of a number of diseases has been well documented; however, the optimal amounts of nutrients required for an individual remains unknown.

Adult recommended dietary allowances (RDAs) have been established for essential vitamins and minerals as discussed in Chapter 8. The RDA for protein has been established at 0.8 g/kg. RDAs have not been established for lipids and carbohydrates because energy requirements change constantly.

Specific changes in nutrient intake may be required as part of therapy for some individuals. These changes may include reduction in the intake of sodium, lipids, or carbohydrates or increased intake of vitamins and minerals.

Energy (calorie) requirements for an individual are often estimated from body weight. This method is obviously not entirely accurate, since genetic makeup and other factors previously mentioned play a role in determining the rate of calorie utilization. Ideally, calorie intake should equal calorie use. Unfortunately for many individuals, changes in lifestyle and aging occur without appropriate changes in dietary habits. In such situations, energy is stored as lipids and excessive weight gain may occur.

Even moderately excessive calorie intake or decreased use of energy result in an increase in the amount of stored fat and a decrease in skeletal muscle mass. This is not an uncommon situation in the United States, where an increasingly large number of individuals are involved in lifestyles that require little or no physical exercise. The individual's health may be compromised by excessive body fat as well as the increased potential for the development of cardiovascular disease.

IDEAL BODY WEIGHT

The ideal body weight (IBW) for an individual is that weight most conducive to performing daily activities and maintaining an optimal state of health. This weight is related to the individual's height, bone structure, and muscle mass. Based on compiled statistics, the best estimate of the weight to maintain throughout life is that which is proper for one's height and body structure at the age of 25. Weight-height correlation tables have frequently been used to estimate the "normal" body weight for one's height and body frame size. However, many individuals have found false security in the use of these tables as indicators of general good health, because they are only averages and have little relationship to the optimal weight or nutritional status of an individual. As the average weight of the population has increased over the years, weights listed in these tables have also increased.

Although many physicians still rely on these tables, other practitioners have begun to use the fat content of the body as a more appropriate indicator of health and fitness. An appropriate percentage of body fat for median-age adult males is 15%, and for females is 22% (7). The appropriate percentage of body fat is expected to increase to some extent with aging. Trained athletes and individuals engaged in strenuous physical activity may maintain much lower body fat percentages than these.

Body fat content has been estimated by several anthropometric methods. These methods differ in degree of exactness as well as in ease of performance. The most highly accurate method for determining body fat content involves measurement of body density by comparing the weight of the individual in air to that when totally submerged in water. This method is expensive as well as time consuming, and difficulties may arise in submerging some patients.

Since most clinicians have neither the facilities nor the time to use this method, body fat content is frequently determined by caliper measurements of the thickness of the layer of fat (skinfold) located at selected subcutaneous sites. Body density is calculated from these skinfold thicknesses, and body fat content is estimated from body density. Body fat percentage is determined using the following equation (8):

$$\text{Body fat percentage} = (4.95/\text{Body density} - 4.42) \times 100$$

Several equations have been developed to determine body density. The following is one of the more frequently used equations for males. It uses skinfold measurements at the abdomen, chest, and thigh (9).

$$\text{Body density} = 1.1093800$$
$$- 0.0008267 \,(\text{Sum of three skinfolds})$$
$$+ 0.0000016 \,(\text{Sum of three skinfolds})^2$$
$$- 0.0002574 \,(\text{Age})$$

For women, body density may be determined using

the following equation, which also uses three skinfold measurements (triceps, abdomen, and suprailiac)

$$Body\ density = 1.089733$$
$$- .0009245\ (Sum\ of\ three\ skinfolds)$$
$$+ 0.0000025\ (Sum\ of\ three\ skinfolds)^2$$
$$- 0.0000979\ (Age).$$

Other anthropometric measurements help assess the state of an individual's health. These include measurement of arm muscle mass as an estimate of total body muscle mass (skeletal muscle protein reserve), and measurement of the circumference of the chest, waist, and hips for comparison with standardized tables for estimation of body fat content. Estimated body fat content may also be used to assess growth rate, weight change, available fat stores, state of health, cardiovascular risk and nutritional requirements in hospitalized patients.

At one time, it was recommended that 35 to 40% of total calories be obtained from fat, 35 to 40% from carbohydrate, and 20 to 30% from protein. However, with increased knowledge about the energy needs of the body has come an awareness of the health risks associated with certain types of dietary intake, such as the excessive intake of dietary lipids. The American Medical Association and the American Dietetics Association have recently recommended a dietary intake much lower in lipids. Their current recommendation is that calories should be provided in the following manner: 20% from fat, 30% from protein, and 50% from carbohydrate. Fat intake for the sedentary individual should perhaps be even lower. The increased emphasis on lowering fat intake is directly related to an increasing body of information that correlates the occurrence of cardiovascular disease with excessive plasma cholesterol levels. However, decreasing fat intake below 20% is difficult if the diet is to be varied and provide other essential nutrients.

Maintenance of ideal body weight and weight reduction in general have become almost an obsession of the U.S. population in recent years. This preoccupation with weight loss has led many individuals to experiment with "quick weight loss" diets, which cause rapid weight loss by extreme caloric restriction or other alterations in diet. The use of such diets may result in adverse health consequences to the individual. For example, concern has been expressed recently that weight reduction diets favor the development of cholesterol gallstones through a marked reduction in bile acid secretion (10).

DIETARY GOALS

Between 1975 and 1977, the Senate Select Committee on Nutrition and Human Needs (which has since been disbanded) released reports documenting that certain dietary

Table 9.3.

Relationship between Dietary Intake and Diseases/Conditions[a]

Dietary Intake	Disease
High ethanol intake	Cirrhosis, hypertension, stroke
High sugar intake	Tooth decay
High sodium intake	Hypertension, stroke
High calorie intake (excessive)	Hypertension, stroke, coronary heart disease, adult-onset diabetes mellitus
High saturated fat and cholesterol intake	Coronary heart disease
High-fat diet	Cancer of breast, colon, and prostate gland
Low-fiber diet	Diverticulosis, colon cancer

[a] Adapted from Suitor CJW, Crowley MF: Nutrition Principles and Application in Health Promotion, ed. 2. Philadelphia: JB Lippincott, 1984.

Table 9.4.

U.S. Dietary Goals[a]

1. To avoid overweight, consume only a much energy (calories) as is expended; if overweight, decrease energy intake and increase energy expenditure.
2. Increase the consumption of complex carbohydrates and "naturally occurring" sugars from about 28% of energy intake to about 48% of energy intake.
3. Reduce the consumption of refined and processed sugars by about 45% to account for about 10% of energy intake.
4. Reduce overall fat consumption from approximately 40% to about 30% of energy intake.
5. Reduce saturated fat consumption to account for about 10% of total energy intake and balance that with polyunsaturated and monounsaturated fats, which should account for about 10% of energy intake each.
6. Reduce cholesterol consumption to about 300 mg per day.
7. Limit the intake of sodium by reducing the intake of salt to about 5 grams per day.

[a] Adapted from U.S. Senate Select Committee on Nutrition and Human Needs: Dietary Goals for the United States, ed. 2. Washington: U.S. GPO, December, 1977.

practices contribute substantially to the incidence of heart disease, cancer, stroke, hypertension, diabetes mellitus, arteriosclerosis, and hepatic cirrhosis (11, 12). These reports also related other widespread conditions such as tooth decay and diverticulosis to the American "diet-style." A listing of these dietary practices and related conditions is presented in Table 9.3 As a result of these reports, this committee, with input from other interested organizations, published "Dietary Goals for the United States," whose purpose was to provide practical guidelines to the consumer as well as set national dietary goals. This publication was revised and the second edition was released in December 1977 (13). The goals are presented in Table 9.4.

The publication of these goals has met with mixed reviews. Some reviewers considered these goals to be unrealistic because of the substantial changes in eating practices which would be required. In 1980, "Nutrition and Your Health, Dietary Guidelines for Americans" (14) was released. This publication provided information similar to that provided earlier by the Senate Committee and stressed the importance of appropriate dietary habits in the maintenance and improvement of health. Today we are becoming increasingly aware of the importance of the information provided by these guidelines in health maintenance. Most recently, the American Medical Association has further strengthened these recommendations by stating that sodium intake should be reduced to one gram per 1000 calories and that cholesterol intake should be limited to 100 milligrams per 1000 calories (14), thus directly relating the intake of these nutrients to caloric intake.

SPECIAL CONSIDERATIONS
Nutrition and Aging

The geriatric population is the fastest-growing segment of our society. It has been projected that the nation's population aged 65 and over will exceed 31.8 million by the year 2000 (15).

While it is known that nutritional status plays a significant role in the quality of life of the elderly, the assessment of their nutritional needs and the identification of appropriate dietary goals to insure their health has just begun.

With increasing age, lean body mass, metabolic rate, and physical activity decline, and protein tissue is gradually replaced with fat, even though the individual may not become overweight. The decrease in physical activity and metabolic rate mandate a lowering of caloric intake to prevent excessive weight gain. For men, energy expenditure decreases by 21% between ages 20 and 74 and by another 31% between ages 75 and 99. The National Research Council has suggested that caloric intake be reduced by 5% per decade after the age of 55 (16). This caloric reduction should be effected by reducing fat and carbohydrate intake, since protein requirements are at least as great in the elderly as in younger age groups.

Over half the population over the age of 65 years has hypertension and/or diabetes (17). Dietary recommendations for the elderly to reduce or control these conditions include the reduction of fat, sugar, and sodium intake. Dietary fat should consist of roughly equal quantities of saturated, monounsaturated, and polyunsaturated types to reduce cholesterol intake. Sugar intake should be decreased to reduce overall caloric intake and also because sugar may synergize the hypertensive effect of sodium (18). Controversy exists over the degree to which sodium intake should be restricted in the elderly, although it is generally acknowledged that sodium restriction should be considered adjunctive to the management of hypertension in this population.

Diabetes in the elderly is frequently associated with excess body weight, which is, in turn, associated with an imbalance between caloric intake and energy expenditure. Control of these diabetic patients requires great care to insure a diet that supplies the essential nutrients without excess calories. The goal of such a diet is to supply adequate protein, vitamin, mineral, and fiber intake while reducing carbohydrate and fat intake to effect a gradual weight loss.

A continuous loss of bone calcium begins around the age of 40, and at approximately 60 years of age, calcium absorption from the gastrointestinal tract begins to decline substantially. For the elderly, decreased absorption of calcium may be compounded by an inadequate dietary intake of calcium-rich foods such as dairy products, by a deficiency of lactase, with the resultant excess lactose interfering with calcium absorption, and by hypovitaminosis D. These effects contribute significantly to the high incidence of osteoporosis that occurs in this population. To offset the effects of reduced calcium absorption, it has been suggested that a calcium intake of 1000 mg or more per day and a vitamin D intake of 600 to 800 IU per day should be provided, either by dietary adjustment or supplementation (19).

Other substantive changes encountered during aging include a reduced production of saliva (which makes food less palatable), reduction in taste and smell acuity, impaired digestion (especially of fats and lactose), and loss of teeth or poorly fitting dentures. The combination of these effects may lead to decreased appetite and deficiencies of essential nutrients.

Anemia is also often seen among the elderly. This has been related to deficiencies of iron, folic acid, and/or vitamin B_{12}, but it may also be related to a higher requirement for these nutrients during the aging process.

Vitamin Supplementation

In many third world countries where malnutrition is common, much of the population would benefit greatly from a vitamin supplement in addition to their limited dietary intake. However, in the U.S., where overnutrition is more common, the need for vitamin supplementation in the general population is much lower. In some clinical situations vitamin supplementation is advantageous, such as in pregnancy and lactation, blood coagulation disorders, and chronic renal failure, where greater than normal amounts of vitamins are required to meet specific needs or where vitamin deficiencies may be present. Recent studies have demonstrated the beneficial effects of pyridoxine in the treatment of premenstrual syndrome and rebound scurvy, although it is not known whether these symptoms are directly related to a pyridoxine deficiency. An overview of vitamin use in clinical practice is provided in Table 9.5 (20–24).

Both the healthy consumer and the patient are often

Table 9.5.
Clinical Uses of Vitamin Supplements[a]

Conditions	Types of Patients	Supplement
Increased metabolic requirements	Pregnant/lactating females	Vitamin A, B-complex, iron, Ca, C, folic acid
	Menstruating females	B-complex, iron, Ca, C, folic acid
	Infants/children	Multivitamin
	Hyperparathyroid	Multivitamin
	Hyperthyroid	Multivitamin
	Stress/fever	Multivitamin
	Smokers	Vitamin C
Malabsorption syndromes	Chronic diarrhea	B-complex
	Chemotherapy	A, D, E, folic acid
	Postsurgical	A, D, E, folic acid
	Liver disease	A, D, E, folic acid
	Genetic abnormalities	A, D, E, folic acid
	Laxative users	A, D, E, folic acid
Inadequate dietary intake	Vegetarians	B-12
	Affective disorders	Multivitamin
	Hospitalized	Multivitamin
	Elderly	Multivitamin + iron and Ca
	Alcoholic	Multivitamin
	Nausea and vomiting	Multivitamin
Anemia	General iron deficiency	Iron
	Pernicious anemia	B-12
	Megaloblastic anemia	Folic acid
Osteoporosis	Postmenopausal females	1.5–2.0 g calcium carbonate (40% elemental calcium) daily use may reduce cortical bone loss; 60–75 mg daily of sodium fluoride with 1.5 g elemental calcium (do not give simultaneously); exercise regularly to maximize peak adult bone mass
Renal disease/hemodialysis	Dialysis patients	Sodium potassium, and phosphorus restriction; active vitamin D and/or calcium supplements; dialysis removes water-soluble vitamins, especially pyridoxine; supplement to meet RDA for: thiamin, niacin, pantothenic acid, biotin, 1 mg folic acid, and 100 mg ascorbic acid; a prenatal vitamin is usually sufficient; ferrous sulfate 325 mg–650 mg may also be supplemented
Physiologic stress due to infections, fever, surgery, burns, or trauma	Postsurgical Hospitalized patients	Recommended daily allowances—established in 1952 by the National Academy of Sciences for the stressed patient are:

Vitamin C	500%
Vitamin B$_1$	667%
Vitamin B$_2$	588%
Vitamin B$_6$	100%
Vitamin B$_{12}$	61%
Folic acid	375%
Panothenic acid	200%

[a] Adapted from Woolf AD, Dixon ASJ: Osteoporosis—an update on management. Drugs 28:565–576, 1984; Riggs BL, Melton LJ III: Involutional osteoporosis. N Engl J Med 314:1676–1686, 1986; Dixon ASJ: Non-hormonal treatment of osteoporosis. Br Med J 2:999–1000, 1983; Liddle VR, Nutrition for the patient with end stage renal disease. In Lancaster LE: The Patient with End Stage Renal Disease, ed. 2. New York, John Wiley & Sons, 1984; and Bolinger AM, Korman NER, Anemias. In Young LY, Koda-Kimble MA (eds): Applied Therapeutics, ed. 4. Vancouver, Applied Therapeutics, 1988.

confused about vitamin supplements. Questions arise about the actual need for a supplement as well as the type of vitamin preparation that should be used. Vitamin preparations include dietary supplements, such as the OTC vitamin preparations that contain 50 to 150% of RDAs, therapeutic supplements that contain more than 150% of RDAs, and prenatal vitamin preparations that supply extra amounts of the nutrients essential for the development of the fetus, such as B complex, iron, calcium, folic acid, and vitamins A and C. Prenatal vitamins are also used for renal

failure patients, in whom loss of nutrients during the dialysis procedure and altered metabolic status is commonly seen. In the highly competitive vitamin supplement market, many preparations are also targeted at specific populations such as the elderly and children. While various factors in the life of the individual may result in a need for a supplement, there is no strong evidence that supplementation is required for the healthy individual if dietary intake is adequate.

While it would be expected that most individuals

would be able to obtain an adequate vitamin intake from their diet, the Food and Drug Administration estimates that 40% of the U.S. adult population uses a daily vitamin supplement (25). Perhaps the prevalence of vitamin supplements leads many individuals to believe that a supplement of some type is necessary. Not only are the products prevalent as multivitamin preparations, they are also available in a variety of strengths of single entity vitamins and minerals.

Quantities of vitamins in excess of ten times the RDA are termed megadoses. Many healthy individuals engage in megadose vitamin intake in the belief that these massive doses will enhance or maintain their health. Megadoses of vitamins may be justified in the treatment of certain conditions, but in many instances, the excessive doses are unwarranted and may actually pose a health problem. Some conditions, such as psychiatric disorders and loss of libido, have been treated with megadoses of vitamins without clinical evidence to support their use. Unfortunately, the possibility of developing toxicity, including psychiatric complications, is often not considered by the public, who may be uninformed and consider vitamins to be generally nontoxic.

Information about the rational use of vitamins is often not provided with OTC multivitamin or single entity supplements. In addition, news media often provide information about the use of vitamins for special conditions without providing essential information on the hazards of large doses. The pharmacist must provide counseling and answer questions about the use of vitamins.

Premenstrual Syndrome

Premenstrual syndrome (PMS) is characterized by symptoms such as irritability, depression, headaches, weight gain, mood swings, and extreme anger. While the etiology of PMS is not well understood, nutritional therapy has been found to be of benefit in the management of these symptoms in some individuals. Dietary changes that have been reported to be beneficial include elimination of caffeine and alcohol intake, reduction of refined sugar and salt intake, increased protein intake (six high-protein meals daily), and increased pyridoxine intake, up to 200 mg per day. In addition, cessation of smoking, reduction of excessive body weight, and regular exercise have been found to be important to the management of severe PMS (26–29).

Nutrient-Drug Interactions

Interactions between nutrients and drugs may occur via a variety of mechanisms and may be either beneficial or detrimental to the patient with regard to both therapeutic outcome and nutritional status. A knowledge of potential interactions is essential in safeguarding the health of the patient, in minimizing the risk of malnutrition, and, when possible, in using the interaction beneficially.

While the number of potential nutrient-drug interactions continues to increase, their significance in the clinical setting and for the general population remains difficult to evaluate. Most of these interactions are considered to be nonspecific, although some specific interactions have been documented. Table 9.6, lists the vitamin-drug interactions of fat- and water-soluble vitamins.

Nutrient-drug interactions may be divided into two general categories:

Interactions that occur because of food in the gastrointestinal (GI) tract altering the rate or extent of drug absorption;
Interactions that occur because of drugs in the GI tract altering the absorption or utilization of nutrients.

Food in the GI tract may alter the rate or extent of drug absorption by

Acting as a physical barrier to absorbing surfaces
Altering GI tract motility and/or secretions
Reacting chemically with drugs

Food in the GI tract will generally alter the rate but not the extent of drug absorption. This type of interaction is of concern when obtaining a rapid therapeutic effect or achieving the highest possible blood level is critical. Rapid absorption is least critical when drugs are administered chronically. When the rate of absorption is of primary concern, the drug should be administered on an empty stomach, either 1 hr before or 3 hr after a meal. Notable exceptions to this generalization occur with griseofulvin, trichloroethylene, and calcium salts, whose absorption is improved when they are administered with a fatty meal (30–32). Care should be taken to limit the amount of fat in meals or to lower the dose of these drugs to prevent this interaction.

Both the presence of food and the anticipation of eating alter motility and secretions of the GI tract. Large meals and meals that contain large quantities of fat decrease the rate of movement of food through the GI tract. This action may enhance the absorption of drugs administered with the meal by increasing the length of time that the drug is in contact with absorbing surfaces. Conversely, small quantities of food are propelled more rapidly through the GI tract, resulting in a decrease in the length of time that the drug is in contact with absorbing surfaces.

The anticipation of eating stimulates the secretion of gastric acid, which lowers stomach pH and facilitates the absorption of acidic drugs. This increased acidity also results in a more rapid destruction of acid-labile drugs such as some antibiotics.

Some nutrients alter the absorption of drugs by mechanisms other than by affecting the environment. Dairy products and other foods that contain calcium or iron de-

Table 9.6.
Vitamin-Drug Interactions

Vitamin	Drug	Interaction/Effect
Fat-soluble vitamins		
Vitamin A	Aluminum hydroxide	Decreased absorption of vitamin A
	Anticoagulants, oral	Increased anticoagulant effect with large dose of vitamin A
	Isotretinoin	Avoid supplements containing vitamin A
	Oral contraceptives	May increase serum concentration of vitamin A
Vitamin D	Digitalis	May cause hypercalcemia induced cardiac arrhythmias
	Phenobarbital	Decreased activity of vitamin D
	Phenytoin	Decreased activity of vitamin D
	Verapamil	May cause hypercalcemia-induced arrhythmias
Vitamin E	Anticoagulants, oral	Increased anticoagulant effect
	Vitamin A	Increased serum concentration of vitamin A
Vitamin K	Anticoagulants, oral	Decreased anticoagulant effect
	Antimicrobial/antiinfective agents	Decreased vitamin K synthesis
	Moxalactam disodium	Disturbances in vitamin K dependent clotting function (decreased prothrombin) may result in increased bleeding time
All fat-soluble vitamins	Cholestyramine	Decreased vitamin absorption
	Mineral oil	Decreased vitamin absorption
	Neomycin	Decreased vitamin absorption
	Laxatives (bisacodyl, cascara, phenolphthalein)	Decreased vitamin absorption
	Antimicrobial/antiinfective agents	Decreased vitamin, fat, cholesterol absorption
Water-soluble vitamins		
Ascorbic acid	Anticoagulants, oral	May decrease anticoagulant effect
	Clinitest	Produces a false-positive result with 1–3 g/day of vitamin C
	Ethinyl estradiol	May increase serum concentration of ethinyl estradiol
	Hemocult home-test kit	Produces a false-positive result with 3 g/day of vitamin C; urinary ascorbic acid will interfere with detection of occult blood in urine
	Iron	May increase absorption of iron
	Oral contraceptives	May increase serum concentration of oral contraceptives
	Phenothiazines	Decreased phenothiazine effect after vitamin C deficiency corrected
	Salicylates	May increase absorption of salicylates with 2 g/day of vitamin C
	Testape	Produces a false-negative result with 1–3 g/day of vitamin C
	Tricylic antidepressants	Decreased therapeutic response of tricyclic with 2 g/day of vitamin C
Cyanacobalamin	Chloramphenicol	Decreased cyanocobalamin effect
	Cholestyramine	Decreases absorption of cyanocobalamin
	Cimetidine	Decreased absorption of cyanocobalamin
	Colchicine	Decreased absorption of cyanocobalamin
	Potassium time-released	Decreased absorption of cyanocobalamin
Folic acid	Oral contraceptives	May produce folate depletion
	Phenytoin and phenobarbital	Decreased phenytoin/phenobarbital effects
	Sulfasalazine	Decreased dietary folate absorption
	Triamterene	May decrease folate absorption
	Trimethoprin	May decrease folate absorption
Niacin	Adrenergic blockers	May cause an additive, vasodilation effect resulting in postural hypotension
	Isoniazid	Niacin requirement may be increased
Pyridoxine	Barbiturates	Decreased barbiturate effect
	Hydralazine	May increase pyridoxine requirement
	Isoniazid	May increase pyridoxine requirement
	Levodopa	Decreased levodopa effect (but not with carbidopa)
	Oral contraceptives	May increase pyridoxine requirement
	Phenytoin	Decreased phenytoin effect

[a] Adapted from Anon: Vitamin supplements. Med Lett Drugs Ther 27:66–67, 1985.

crease the absorption of tetracycline antibiotics by chelation. Dairy products may also produce an alkaline environment in the stomach and decrease the absorption of acidic drugs. In addition, this alkaline environment dissolves the enteric coating of certain drugs (e.g., bisacodyl), resulting in premature release of the drug into the stomach, where it may be destroyed and produce irritation, rather than into the small intestine where it would be absorbed.

Nutrients may also alter the response to drugs by affecting metabolism and/or excretion of the drug or by producing a pharmacologic effect in the patient.

Drug metabolism may be increased by food contaminants (such as pesticide residues) and food additives that induce hepatic microsomal enzymes and increase the rate of drug metabolism.

Drug excretion may be enhanced or inhibited by nutrients that alter urinary pH. Acid ash diet components such as meats, cheese, eggs, baked goods, and acidic fruits produce an acidic urine and favor the reabsorption of acidic drugs such as aspirin and phenobarbital. Alkaline ash diet components such as dairy products and most vegetables and fruits produce an alkaline urine that enhances the reabsorption of basic drugs such as amphetamine. Antacids may enhance the effects of alkaline ash diets on the reabsorption of drugs.

A variety of nutrients and food additives have been reported to possess pharmacologic activity that may produce adverse drug interactions. One of the more potentially dangerous of these interactions involves monoamine oxidase inhibitors such as phenelzine, procarbazine, and furazolidone with foods containing tyramine or other agents that possess sympathomimetic activity. Monoamine oxidase is an enzyme found in the GI tract, liver, and adrenergic nerve endings. It is responsible for the metabolism of these naturally occurring sympathomimetic agents before they can be absorbed. Inhibition of monoamine oxidase allows these sympathomimetic agents to be absorbed in significant amounts, which may result in a hypertensive crisis (33).

Drugs may alter the absorption or use of nutrients by both specific and nonspecific mechanisms. The most frequently documented specific interactions in this category are malabsorption syndromes. These syndromes may be related to (a) direct toxic effects of the drug to the intestinal mucosa, (b) inhibition of enzymes, (c) binding of bile and fatty acids, (d) alteration of dietary ions and (e) alteration of pH. Some of these interactions and their effects on absorption are listed in Table 9.6.

Oral contraceptives and anticonvulsants such as phenytoin have been reported to decrease folic acid absorption by interference with polyglutamate conjugase, the enzyme responsible for converting folate to free folic acid (34). Anticonvulsants also block the 25-hydroxylation of vitamin

D by hepatic enzymes. During chronic anticonvulsant therapy, this interaction may result in evidence of bone disease, such as elevated alkaline phosphatase levels and decreased bone density.

Antacids such as aluminum hydroxide decrease the absorption of phosphate and may be used as phosphate binders in renal dialysis patients. They may also decrease the absorption of iron and vitamin A by chelation and alteration of the pH of the small intestine. These effects would be expected to occur only after chronic, high-dose therapy, although some cases of osteomalacia related to antacid therapy have been reported (35).

Hypocholesteremic agents decrease the absorption of vitamin B_{12}, the fat-soluble vitamins (and other lipids), iron, and sugars by decreasing the intestinal pH and by binding with bile (36). Chronic use of cholestyramine has also been reported to induce a vitamin K deficiency by an unknown mechanism (37).

The chronic use of irritant laxatives such as phenolphthalein may inhibit nutrient absorption by increasing motility and altering the structural integrity of the small intestine (37). Lubricating laxatives such as mineral oil act as a physical barrier to nutrient absorption, inhibit the formation of lipid micelles, and solubilize the fat-soluble vitamins. Rickets and osteomalacia may occur following the prolonged and excessive use of mineral oil (38).

Colchicine decreases the absorption of lipids, carotine, sodium, potassium, lactose, and cyanocobalamin by producing mitotic arrest, structural defects in the mucosa, and enzyme damage (39). Sulfasalazine, an agent used in colitis and enteritis therapy, may produce a significant folate deficiency by mucosal blockade of folate uptake (39).

Ethanol has been reported to produce a deficiency of a number of nutrients including folic acid, cyanocobalamin, niacin, thiamine, and magnesium by inhibition of intestinal absorption or by increasing their rate of excretion. Ethanol also decreases the production of pyridoxal phosphate from pyridoxine and impairs the conversion of retinol to retinal. This latter effect may result in the occurrence of night blindness (39).

Drugs may also affect taste acuity, alter taste, and/or alter appetite. Griseofulvin, penicillamine, clofibrate, lincomycin, and certain tranquilizers have been reported to decrease taste acuity or alter taste (40). Chloral hydrate, paraldehyde, and other unpleasant-tasting drugs may leave an aversive aftertaste that will decrease appetite. These drugs should not be taken before meals.

Central nervous system (CNS) stimulants such as the amphetamines and methylphenidate are used for the treatment of hyperkinesis, narcolepsy, and certain seizure disorders. They suppress appetite and should be administered only with or after meals. Other psychoactive drugs such as neuroleptics, antidepressants, and antianxiety agents stimulate appetite in some individuals and suppress appetite in others. In patients whose appetite is stimulated, the effect may be secondary to improvement in mood or mental status and may result in excessive weight gain. Appetite suppression may be related to nonspecific depression of the CNS and may resolve as tolerance to the drug's effects develop.

Drugs that affect autonomic nervous system function may alter motility and secretions of the GI tract. For example, cholinergic drugs increase GI tract tone and motility and gastric acid secretion. Increased motility may increase the rate at which nutrients pass through the alimentary tract and decrease their absorption. Anticholinergic drugs decrease motility of the gastrointestinal tract and allow more nutrients to be absorbed; however, they also produce dry mouth and constipation, which may significantly alter eating behaviors (41).

While our understanding of the mechanisms by which drugs and nutrients interact is increasing rapidly, remember that most of the interactions that have been mentioned here are likely to occur in only a small portion of patients. However, they may occur in and be of significance to any patient, and this potential should always be kept in mind. Some of the interactions mentioned may be used to the advantage of the patient, especially in decreasing the adverse effects of drugs, in maintaining optimal blood levels, and in preventing the destruction of drugs in the GI tract.

CONCLUSION

Lipids, carbohydrates, and protein are essential nutrients because they are used by the body to produce energy. To maintain an appropriate (ideal) body weight, energy sources should be ingested in amounts that are approximately equal to energy expenditure. For most healthy individuals, the relative quantities of energy sources in the diet should be 50% carbohydrate, 20% lipid, and 30% protein. Appropriate quantities of fiber should be included in the diet to promote health and provide protection against certain types of cancer such as cancer of the colon and breast.

Nutritional considerations in the geriatric population are especially important. As aging occurs, physical activity usually decreases, necessitating a decrease in caloric intake to prevent weight gain. Dietary restriction or enhancement may be necessary to control hypertension and diabetes, to prevent or decrease the occurrence of osteoporosis, and to prevent anemia.

Vitamin supplementation may play an important role in the treatment of specific disease states. However, for most of the population of the U.S., there is little, if any, justification for the use of vitamin supplementation.

Vitamin supplements are used during pregnancy and lactation, in blood coagulation disorders, and in renal failure where greater than normal amounts of vitamins are needed. For most healthy individuals, megadoses of vitamins may actually pose a health problem.

A number of nutrient-drug interactions have been documented. Such interactions may occur because of food in the GI tract altering drug absorption or because of drugs in the GI tract altering nutrient absorption or use. While many such interactions have been reported, their significance in many instances is still unknown.

REFERENCES

1. Suitor CJW, Crowley MF: Nutrition Principles and Application in Health Promotion, ed. 2. Philadelphia: JB Lippincott, 1984, p 33.
2. Anderson L, Dibble MV, Tukki PR, et al.: Nutrition in Health and Disease, ed. 17. Philadelphia: JB Lippincott, 1982, p 441.
3. Hunt SM, Grof JL, Holbrook JM: Nutrition Principles and Clinical Practice. New York: John Wiley Sons, 1980, p 92.
4. Burkitt DP, Walter ARP, Painter NS: Dietary fiber and disease. JAMA 229:1068, 1974.
5. Kromhout D, Bosschieter EB, de Lezenne Coulader C: Dietary fiber and 10-year mortality from coronary heart disease, cancer and all causes. Lancet 2:518–521, 1982.
6. Suitor CJW, Crowley MF: Nutrition Principles and Application in Health Promotion, ed. 2. Philadelphia: JB Lippincott, 1984, p 519.
7. Bailey C: Fat or Fit? Boston: Houghton Mifflin, 1977, p 8.
8. Pollock ML, Wilmore JH, Fox SM: Exercise in Health and Disease. Philadelphia: WB Saunders, 1984, p 67.
9. Jackson AS, Pollock ML: Practical assessment of body composition. Physician Sportsmed 13:76–90, 1985.
10. Liddle RA, Goldstein RB, Saxton J: Gallstone formation during weight-reduction. Arch Intern Med 143:1750–1753, 1989.
11. U.S. Senate Select Committee on Nutrition and Human Needs: Nutrition and Health. Washington: U.S. GPO, December, 1975.
12. U.S. Senate Select Committee on Nutrition and Human Needs: Diet Related to Killer Diseases. Washington: U.S. GPO, July 27, 28, 1976.
13. U.S. Senate Select Committee on Nutrition and Human Needs: Dietary Goals for the United States, ed. 2. Washington: U.S. GPO, December, 1977.
14. USDA and DHEW: Nutrition and Your Health: Dietary Guidelines for Americans. Washington: U.S. GPO, 1979.
15. Young EA: Nutrition, aging and the aged. Med Clin North Am 67:295–313, 1983.
16. Lamy PP: Nutrition and the elderly. Drug Intell Clin Pharm 15:887–891, 1981.
17. Greene J: Nutritional care considerations of older Americans. J Natl Med Assoc 71:791–793, 1979.
18. Srinivasan SR, Berenson GS, Radhakrishnamurthy B, Dalferes ER, Underwood D, Foster TA: Effects of dietary sodium and sucrose on the induction of hypertension in spider monkeys. Am J Clin Nutr 33:561–569, 1980.
19. Hearney RP, Gallagher JC, Johnston CC: Calcium nutrition and bone health in elderly. Am J Clin Nutr 36:986–1013, 1982.
20. Woolf AD, Dixon ASJ: Osteoporosis—an update on management. Drugs 28:565–576, 1984.
21. Riggs BL, Melton LJ III: Involutional osteoporosis. N Engl J Med 314:1676–1686, 1986.
22. Dixon ASJ: Non-hormonal treatment of osteoporosis. Br Med J 2:999–1000, 1983.
23. Liddle VR, Nutrition for the patient with end stage renal disease. In Lancaster LE: The Patient with End Stage Renal Disease, ed. 2. New York, John Wiley & Sons, 1984, pp 98–100.
24. Bolinger AM, Korman NER, Anemias. In Young LY, Koda-Kimble MA (eds): Applied Therapeutics, ed 4. Vancouver, Applied Therapeutics, 1988, pp 1051–1068.

25. Anon: Vitamin supplements. Med Lett Drugs Ther 27:66–67, 1985.

26. Pariser SF, Stern SL, Shank ML, Falko MJ, et al.: Premenstrual syndrome: concerns, controversies and treatment. Am J Obstet Gynecol 153:59–604, 1985.

27. Chakmakjian ZH: A critical assessment of therapy for the premenstrual tension syndrome. J Reprod Med 28:532–538, 1983.

28. Lyon K, Lyon M: The premenstrual syndrome: a survey of current treatment practices. J Reprod Med 29:705–711, 1984.

29. True BL, Goodner SM, Burns EA: Review of the etiology and treatment of premenstrual syndrome. Drug Intel Clin Pharm 19:714–721, 1985.

30. Lehmann P: Food and drug interactions. FDA Consumer, HEW Publication No. (FDA) 78-3070, U.S. GPO, March, 1978.

31. Pierpaoli PG: Drug therapy and diet. Drug Intel Clin Pharm 6:89–99, 1972.

32. Cooper JW: Food-drug interactions. U.S. Pharm 1:17–28, 1976.

33. Colosanti BK, Antidepressant therapy. In Craig CR, Stitzel RE: Modern Pharmacology, ed. 2. Boston, Little, Brown & Co, 1976, p 525.

34. Longstrieth GF, Neucome AD: Drug-induced malabsorption. Mayo Clin Proc 50:284–293, 1975.

35. Bloom WL, Finchum D: Osteomalasia with pseudofractures caused by ingestion of aluminum hydroxide. JAMA 174:1327–1330, 1960.

36. Roe DA: Drug-Induced Nutritional Deficiencies. Westport, CN: AVI Publishing, 1976, chap 5.

37. Visintine RE: Xanthomatous biliary cirrhosis treated with cholstyramine, a bile-aid-absorbing resin. Lancet 2:341–343, 1961.

38. Sinclair L: Rickets from liquid paraffin. Lancet 1:792, 1967.

39. Barone S, Vitamins. In Craig CR, Stitzel RE: Modern Pharmacology, ed. 3. Boston: Little, Brown & Co, 1990, pp 993–1002.

40. Fagan L: Griseofulvin and dysgeusia: implications? (letters). Ann Intern Med 74:795–796, 1971.

41. Piper DW, de Carlo DJ, Doe WF, et al.: Gastrointestinal and hepatic diseases. In Speight TM (ed): Avery's Drug Treatment, ed. 3. New York, Adis Press, 1987, p 744.

CHAPTER 10

VITAMINS AND MINERALS

DIANE NYKAMP McCARTER, Pharm.D. and JOHN HOLBROOK, Ph.D.

For several decades, the relationships between dietary insufficiencies and the occurrence of diseases such as scurvy, pellagra, and beriberi have been well-known. More recently, researchers have discovered a relationship between maintenance of optimal health and good nutritional practices. Proper nourishment improves the ability to learn, concentrate, participate in physical activities, and resist or overcome injury and disease. It is also critical to the prevention and management of heart disease, diabetes, hypertension, obesity, and other disorders.

The literature (both technical and lay) abounds with information about the use of nutrients to prevent or treat disorders. The public has become more concerned with nutrition, especially how good nutrition relates to self-care and wellness. The public is also concerned with the amount of food consumed and the use of nutritional supplements.

This chapter focuses on the basic nutrients that the body requires for life.

VITAMINS

Vitamins are non-energy-producing organic substances that are essential in small amounts for the maintenance of normal metabolic functions. With the exception of vitamins D and K, vitamins are not synthesized by the body and must be supplied in the diet (1). Vitamins are categorized into two groups: the fat-soluble vitamins A, D, E, and K and the water-soluble vitamins, B complex and C. Vitamins are derived from natural sources (plants, animals, and microorganisms) or synthetic sources, and there are no structural or therapeutic differences between the two kinds of vitamins. Vitamin K and biotin are synthesized by microorganisms in the intestinal tract. Unlike biotin, enough vitamin K is synthesized to meet the daily requirement without dietary supplementation. Vitamin D is synthesized in the skin from endogenous or dietary cholesterol.

Vitamin Requirements

The recommended dietary allowance (RDA) is the nutritional standard that specifies the amounts and kinds of nutrients necessary to maintain a positive state of health. It is determined by the Food and Nutrition Board of the National Academy of Science National Research Council (NAS/NRC). The RDA has replaced the minimum daily requirement (MDR) because individual requirements vary according to sex, age, and physical condition (2). The RDA is believed to be adequate for known nutritional needs of healthy individuals. RDAs are not intended to cover therapeutic nutritional requirements in disease or other abnormal states. For example, extra allowances are needed for women during pregnancy and lactation, and allowances vary for age and sex as well.

The "official" listings of United States Recommended Daily Allowances (US-RDAs) differ from the RDA. US-RDAs serve as legal standards for nutritional labeling of products controlled by the United States Food and Drug Administration. Generally, they represent the higher value of the male or female RDA and are grouped into only four age categories instead of the usual six found with the RDAs. Table 10.1 lists vitamin and mineral RDA values for all age groups.

Vitamin Stability

In general, fat-soluble vitamins are not destroyed at usual cooking temperatures. However, water-soluble vitamins are dissolved easily in cooking water and may be destroyed through heating. Ascorbic acid suffers the greatest loss in nutritive value through cooking. Riboflavin is only sparingly soluble and is not removed as quickly as the other water-soluble vitamins. When meats are broiled or roasted, thiamin losses are 25% or less (3). Constant low-temperature cooking improves palatability of meat but decreases the nutritive value. The wilting of vegetables or dehydration of foods results in considerable vitamin loss. Dicing or cutting and failure to store properly also cause vitamin loss from foods. To retain the maximum vitamin content, consume raw fruit or vegetables or cook them in a small quantity of water in a covered container for a short period of time. Other appropriate cooking methods include steaming and microwaving, as compared with conventional cooking. This is especially beneficial for vegetables containing thiamin, riboflavin, pyridoxine, folic acid, and ascorbic acid. Microwave cooking requires a shorter cooking time and less water and generally results in greater retention of heat-labile nutrients (4).

Fat-soluble Vitamins

Vitamins A, D, E, and K are classified as fat-soluble vitamins. Absorption of these vitamins is facilitated by bile salts or dietary fat, and they are stored in moderate amounts in the body. Vitamins A and D function like hor-

Table 10.1.
Recommended Dietary Allowances[a]

	Age (years)	Weight (kg)	Weight (lbs)	Vitamin A (IU)	Vitamin D (IU)	Vitamin E (IU)	Ascorbic Acid (C) mg	Folacin mcg	Niacin (B3) mg	Riboflavin (B2) mg	Thiamin (B1) mg	Pyridoxine HCl (B6) mg	Cyanocobalamin (B12) µg	Calcium mg	Phosphorus mg	Iodine mcg	Iron mg	Magnesium mg	Zinc mg
Infants	0.0–0.5	6	13	2100	400	4	35	30	6	0.4	0.3	0.3	0.5	360	240	40	10	50	3
	0.5–1.0	9	20	2000	400	6	35	45	8	0.6	0.5	0.6	1.5	540	360	50	15	70	5
Children	1–3	13	29	2000	400	7	45	100	9	0.8	0.7	0.9	2.0	800	800	70	15	150	10
	4–6	20	44	2500	400	9	45	200	11	1.0	0.9	1.3	2.5	800	800	90	10	200	10
	7–10	28	62	3500	400	10	45	300	16	1.4	1.2	1.6	3.0	800	800	120	10	250	10
Males	11–14	45	99	5000	400	12	50	400	18	1.6	1.4	1.8	3.0	1200	1200	150	18	350	15
	15–18	66	145	5000	400	15	60	400	18	1.7	1.4	2.0	3.0	1200	1200	150	18	400	15
	19–22	70	154	5000	300	15	60	400	19	1.7	1.5	2.2	3.0	800	800	150	10	350	15
	23–50	70	154	5000	200	15	60	400	18	1.6	1.4	2.2	3.0	800	800	150	10	350	15
	51+	70	154	5000	200	15	60	400	16	1.4	1.2	2.2	3.0	800	800	150	10	350	15
Females	11–14	46	101	4000	400	12	50	400	15	1.3	1.1	1.8	3.0	1200	1200	150	18	300	15
	15–18	55	120	4000	400	12	60	400	14	1.3	1.1	2.0	3.0	1200	1200	150	18	300	15
	19–22	55	120	4000	300	12	60	400	14	1.3	1.1	2.0	3.0	800	800	150	18	300	15
	23–50	55	120	4000	200	12	60	400	13	1.2	1.0	2.0	3.0	800	800	150	18	300	15
	51+	55	120	4000	200	12	60	400	13	1.2	1.0	2.0	3.0	800	800	150	10	300	15
	Pregnancy			+1000	+200	+3	+20	+400	+2	+0.3	+0.4	+0.6	+1.0	+400	+400	+25	b	+150	+5
	Lactation			+2000	+200	+4	+40	+100	+5	+0.5	+0.5	+0.5	+1.0	+400	+400	+50	c	+150	+10

[a] Reproduced from Recommended Dietary Allowances, ed. 9 with the permission of the National Academy of Sciences, Washington, D.C., 1980.
[b] This increased requirement cannot be met by ordinary diets; therefore, the use of 30 to 60 mg of supplemental iron is recommended.
[c] Same requirement as for nonpregnant women, but continue supplementation for 2 to 3 months after parturition.

mones, interacting with specific intracellular receptors in their target tissues. Toxicity associated with the fat-soluble vitamins is due to a relatively low urinary excretion. The characteristics of fat-soluble vitamins are found in Table 10.2.

VITAMIN A

Functions

Vitamin A is essential for vision, for dental development, and for growth and reproduction. Vitamin A is also necessary for the synthesis of hydrocortisone and for the regulation and differentiation of epithelial tissue. The integrity of the mucous membranes of the eyes, skin, mouth, gastrointestinal tract, and genitourinary tract is maintained by this vitamin, which is required for the production of mucus (5).

Properties

Vitamin A includes three natural compounds found in animal sources (retinol, retinal, and retinoic acid) and three provitamins found in plants (α-, β-, and γ-carotene). Retinol is apparently responsible for the actions of the vitamin in the reproductive process, and retinal is the functional compound of the visual cycle. Retinoic acid, the active form of vitamin A, is associated with growth and cell differentiation. Retinoic acid cannot replace retinal in the visual cycle and is not able to support reproduction (6). β-Carotene, the most abundant plant source, does not possess inherent vitamin A activity but yields retinol after absorption and metabolism. One international unit (IU) of vitamin A is equal to 0.3 μg retinal or 0.6 μg β-carotene. Large amounts of β-carotene can be ingested over a long period of time without development of toxic effects (other than skin pigmentation), since only one-half of absorbed carotene is converted to retinol (7, 8).

When the amount of retinol ingested is similar to the RDA, absorption is complete. When ingested in excess, some retinol is excreted.

Deficiency

A deficiency of vitamin A is usually due to fat malabsorption syndromes or malnutrition. Deficiency produces a variety of symptoms that include nyctalopia (night blindness), diminished production of corticosteroids, xerophthalmia (drying of the cornea), keratinization of the skin, growth failure, and fetal malformations. A deficiency of vitamin A can impair resistance to infections because of breakdown of mucous membrane (9).

Toxicity

Acute and chronic vitamin A toxicity are well-recognized conditions in adults. Acute poisoning may occur after a single dose in excess of 1,000,000 units. Chronic toxicity is mainly determined by the dose and duration of therapy. Usually a dose of more than 100,000 units daily for several months causes hypervitaminosis A (10). Prolonged use of vitamin A in daily doses of 25,000 units causes a hypervitaminosis, a syndrome that generally manifests as a cirrhotic-like liver syndrome. Symptoms from chronic use of vitamin A include fatigue, vomiting, cheilosis (cracking lips), dizziness, nausea, and irritability, followed by generalized skin desquamation. Pruritus, dry scaly skin, bone pain, changes in texture of hair and nails, increased cerebrospinal fluid pressure, and hypercalcemia may also occur. Concern about an excess intake of vitamin A during pregnancy has increased in recent years because of its structural and metabolic relationship to other vitamin A analogs (retinoids) especially 13-*cis*-retinoic acid (isotretinoin), which causes teratogenic effects. A daily dose lower than 10,000 IU is not thought to be teratogenic (11).

Therapeutic Uses

Vitamin A analogs (retinoids) have been developed to improve the therapeutic index of vitamin A. Isotretinoin and etretinate (12) were developed as less toxic and more effective agents. They have, however, caused embryopathy (13). Retinoids have had a major impact on the practice of dermatology and are under investigation in oncology (14, 15). Retinoids may play a role in cancer prophylaxis (16, 17) and in the treatment of skin lesions (18). Retinol supplements may reduce the risk of development of lung cancer in smokers and may also protect against cervical cancer (19). Also, a consistent relationship has been found with an above average intake of β-carotene and a lowered incidence of cancer, especially when β-carotene is used in combination with vitamins E and C (17, 20).

Until further research is conducted, advice to vitamin A users is understandably conservative. Doses higher than 10,000 units should not be recommended, instead consumers should rely on dietary intake of foods containing β-carotene. Excess use of retinol supplements may cause serious adverse reactions. However, increasing one's natural retinol dietary intake by eating more green and yellow vegetables may be beneficial, while avoiding adverse reactions. β-Carotene is a precursor for vitamin A and does not produce vitamin toxicity because only 20 to 30% of a given dose of β-carotene is absorbed from the gastrointestinal tract, and it is metabolized at a rate approximately 50 to 60% of normal. No definitive statement can be made at this time about the use of vitamin A in wound healing. Studies have indicated a beneficial effect, but more clinical trials are needed to justify the use of vitamin A in wound healing.

VITAMIN D

Functions

Vitamin D is considered a hormone rather than a vitamin, although it is not a natural hormone. Vitamin D, in con-

Table 10.2.
Summary of Fat-soluble Vitamins[a]

Vitamin	Function	Deficiency	Large Doses	Therapeutic Uses	Sources
Vitamin A Retinol Retinal Retinoic acid β-Carotene	Growth Vision Dental development Reproduction Synthesis of hydrocortisone Epithelial tissue differentiation Maintenance of mucous membranes	Nyctalopia Xerophthalmia Faulty bone and tooth development Keratinization Fetal malformation Decreased production of cortical steroids Impaired resistance to infection	Acute Fatigue Cheilitis Dizziness Nausea and vomiting Irritability Desquamation Chronic Hypercalcemia Dry scaly skin Bone pain Changes in texture of hair and nails Increased cerebrospinal pressure Pruritus	Dermatology Oncology	Liver Milk Butter or margarine Dark-green leafy vegetables Carrots Sweet potatoes
Vitamin D Ergocalciferol—D_2 Cholecalciferol—D_3	Bone mineralization Maintenance of normal neuromuscular activity Maintenance of serum calcium and phosphorus levels	Associated with inadequate calcium and phosphorus Ricketts (children) Osteomalacia (adults) Secondary hyperparathyroidism	Hypercalcemia (weakness anorexia, vomiting, diarrhea, polydipsia, polyuria & mental changes) Constipation Proteinuria Vague aches Metallic or bad taste Renal failure Hypertension	Renal osteodystrophy Hypoparathyroidism	Sunlight Butter Egg yolk Fatty fish Liver Fortified milk and bread
Vitamin E dl-α-Tocopherol (α-TE) (1 mg = 1.49 IU)	Antioxidant, maintains integrity of cell membrane Enhance vitamin A utilization Inhibition of prostaglandin production Cofactor in steroid metabolism Related to action of selenium	Neurologic syndrome (ataxia, muscle weakness, nystagmus, loss of touch/pain) Anemia in premature infants Hemolysis of red blood	Increase the effects of oral anticoagulants	Intermittent claudication Retrolental fibroplasia	Wheat germ oil Nuts Green leafy vegetables
Vitamin K Phylloquionone—K_1 Menaquinone—K_2 Analog:Menadione—K_3	Coagulation Formation of prothrombin and other clotting proteins	Prolonged clotting time Symptoms of deficiency can be produced by coumarin anticoagulants and by antibiotic therapy	Vomiting Toxicity can be induced by water-soluble analogues Neonatal jaundice Dietary supplements can block the effect or oral anticoagulant	Coagulation disorders Anticoagulant-induced prothrombin deficiency	Green leaves (spinach, cabbage) Liver Synthesis in intestine by bacteria Cheese, egg yolk

[a] Adapted from Williams SR (ed): Nutrition and Diet Therapy. St. Louis: Times Mirror/Mosby, College Publishing, 1985; Luke B (ed): Principles of Nutrition and Diet Therapy. Boston: Little, Brown & Co., 1984; and Robinson CH, Lawler MR, Chenoweth WL, Garwick AE (eds): Normal and Therapeutic Nutrition, ed. 17. New York: Macmillan, 1986.

junction with parathyroid hormone (PTH) and calcitonin, is needed for calcium and phosphate absorption. This in turn supports normal mineralization of bone and neuromuscular activity.

Properties

Vitamin D refers to both D_2 (calciferol, ergocalciferol) and D_3 (cholecalciferol). D_2 and D_3 occur naturally and are equipotent. Either of them may supply the body's daily requirements. These forms have an onset of action time of 10 to 24 hr and may be stored in the body for prolonged periods.

Dihydrotachysterol (DHT) is the synthetic vitamin D analog activated in the liver, and it does not require renal hydroxylation. DHT has a rapid onset of action (2 hr), a shorter half-life, and a greater effect on mobilization of bone salts than does vitamin D (21).

Ninety percent of dietary vitamin D is absorbed from the small intestine. Vitamin D_3 may be absorbed more rapidly and completely than vitamin D_2.

The supply of vitamin D depends on ultraviolet light radiation for conversion of plant ergosterol to vitamin D_2 or for conversion of skin 7-dehydrocholesterol to vitamin D_3. Vitamins D_2 and D_3 require activation by both the liver and the kidney. Vitamin D_3 is absorbed into the circulation and converted by hepatic microsomal enzymes to 25-hydroxycholecalciferol, which in turn is hydroxylated in the kidney to its active metabolite, 1,25-dihydroxycholecalciferol (calcitrol). Calcitrol has pharmacologic activity that lasts from 3 to 5 days. The production rate of calcitrol is closely regulated by plasma calcium and parathyroid hormone. The active form of D_3 is responsible for promoting intestinal calcium absorption and mobilization of calcium from bone. Paradoxically, vitamin D mobilizes calcium from the bone to maintain proper plasma levels (22, 23).

Deficiency

Vitamin D deficiency may be induced by renal disease, malabsorption syndromes (colitis, sprue), short bowel syndrome, hypoparathyroidism, and long-term anticonvulsant therapy. Vitamin D deficiency leads to inadequate absorption of calcium and phosphorus from the intestinal tract. This leads to faulty mineralization of bone and teeth, resulting in rickets in children and osteomalacia in adults. Also, increased parathyroid hormone secretion is seen due to a decreased serum calcium level, resulting in secondary hyperparathyroidism.

Toxicity

Large doses of vitamin D, 50,000 to 100,000 IU per day, may result in toxicity, although tolerance to vitamin D varies widely. Initial manifestations of toxicity result from hypercalcemia and include weakness, anorexia, vomiting, diarrhea, polydipsia, polyuria, mental changes, and proteinuria. Prolonged hypercalcemia may result in soft-tissue calcification including heart, blood vessels, renal tubules, and lungs. Death can result from cardiovascular or renal failure.

Therapeutic Uses

A vitamin D–resistant state exists in chronic renal failure. Renal osteodystrophy is characterized by a decreased ability of the kidney to convert 25-hydroxycholecalciferol to 1,25-dihydroxycholecalciferol. Active vitamin D (calcitrol) or dihydrotachysterol must be supplemented to lower the concentration of PTH and raise the concentration of calcium in the plasma (24). Vitamin D supplementation is also needed in hypoparathyroidism that is characterized by hypocalcemia and hyperphosphatemia. If a patient has an inadequate diet and little exposure to sunlight, a vitamin D supplement should be given.

An anticonvulsant-induced hypocalcemia is thought to be due to induction of hepatic microsomal P-450 enzyme system and is treated with vitamin D, 25-hydroxycholecalciferol and possibly calcium. Combination therapy is required because vitamin D obtained from the diet, supplements, or sun exposure is converted to inactive metabolites with prolonged anticonvulsant use. A favorable response is seen with a combination of vitamin D and 25-hydroxycholecalciferol.

VITAMIN E
Functions

Many of the actions of vitamin E are related to its antioxidant properties. Vitamin E stabilizes the lipid portion of a cell membrane by preventing oxidation of polyunsaturated phospholipids, thereby maintaining the integrity of the cell membrane (25). Other functions of vitamin E include enhancement of vitamin A utilization, inhibition of prostaglandin production, and stimulation of an essential cofactor in steroid metabolism. Selenium acts synergistically with vitamin E to protect cell membranes from oxidative damage.

Properties

α-Tocopherol is the most active and abundant form of vitamin E, occurring naturally as wheat germ oil. Vitamin E is 20 to 40% absorbed from the gastrointestinal tract and is distributed to all tissues via the lymphatic system.

Deficiency

Vitamin E deficiency occurs primarily in premature infants and in patients with severe malabsorptive disease, such as cystic fibrosis. The neurological syndrome of ataxia, muscle weakness, nystagmus, and loss of the sense of touch/pain has been attributed to vitamin E deficiency (26–28). Vitamin E deficiency may also lower the age of onset or increase the rate of progression in patients predisposed to Alzheimer's disease (29).

Toxicity

Current literature includes little evidence that vitamin E produces any harmful effects. A daily intake of 200 to 600 mg (1 mg/dl α-tocopherol = 1.49 IU) appears to be innocuous in most people. The most commonly recurring complaint with large doses (300 to 3200 IU/day) is gastrointestinal upset (nausea, flatulence, or diarrhea), weakness, or fatigue (30). Large doses of vitamin E may increase the incidence of sepsis and necrotizing enterocolitis when serum vitamin E levels are maintained at 5 mg/dl (normal range 1.0 to 3.0 mg/dl) in low-birth-weight infants and have been associated with a high mortality rate when given intravenously (31, 32). Vitamin E can also increase the effects of oral anticoagulants (33, 34).

Therapeutic Uses

Some therapeutic uses for vitamin E that have been proposed include treatment of cancer, aging, circulatory conditions, arthritis, cataracts, and strenuous exercise. However, its benefits in the healthy population are not known. Oral vitamin E has been associated with a decrease in the number of irreversibly sickled cells in sickle cell anemia, but studies fail to show a therapeutic role for vitamin E (35). Prolonged vitamin E therapy of 400 mg/day for at least 3 months has been shown to be beneficial to some patients with intermittant claudication (30, 36). Administration of 100 mg/kg/day appears to be effective in preventing retrolential fibroplasia in premature infants receiving oxygen therapy (37). Vitamin E supplements no longer appear to be necessary in premature infants for the treatment of hemolytic anemia because commercial infant formulas now contain less iron and the appropriate ratio of vitamin E to fatty acids to prevent the development of hemolytic anemia (38).

Vitamin E is reported to be beneficial in a wide range of conditions. Scientists now believe that vitamin E serves with selenium as a cellular antioxidant, protecting cell membranes from peroxidase damage. However, there is no scientific basis for vitamin E supplementation in a host of conditions including infertility, cancer, angina, muscular dystrophy, diabetes, premenstrual syndrome, nocturnal leg cramps, and enhancement of athletic performance.

VITAMIN K
Functions

The only rational use of vitamin K is for the correction of bleeding tendencies caused by its deficiency. Such a deficiency is unlikely to occur because of intestinal bacterial synthesis of the vitamin. For this reason, there are no dietary recommended allowances.

Properties

Vitamin K is essential for the hepatic synthesis of prothrombin and other clotting proteins. Vitamin K compounds are chemically referred to as quinones and include phylloquinone (K_1) and menaquinone (K_2), which are synthesized by intestinal flora, and menadione (K_3), the water-soluble analog.

Deficiency

Vitamin K deficiency, clinically resulting in hemorrhage, may occur following destruction of intestinal flora associated with antibiotic use, especially with prolonged poor dietary intake as may be seen during hospitalization (39). The role of antibiotics, especially select third-generation cephalosporins, in producing hypoprothrobinemia is thought to be due to a common sturctural side chain that inhibits a vitamin K–dependent step in the synthesis of prothrombin in the liver. Prothrombin time should be monitored, and in many instances a prophylactic dose of vitamin K is given (40, 41). Also, large amounts of vitamins A and E interfere with absorption of vitamin K (42). Advanced liver damage, when caused by cancer and cirrhosis, results in a deficiency of clotting factors that can not be alleviated by the administration of vitamin K. However increased prothrombin time as a result of vitamin K deficiency will respond.

Infants are unable to synthesize vitamin K because they have a sterile intestinal tract at birth. A single prophylactic dose of 0.5 to 1 mg, intramuscularly or subcutaneously, of vitamin K should be given to infants to protect them until vitamin K synthesis begins and to supplement dietary vitamin K. Phylloquinone (phytonadione) is the agent of choice to prevent bleeding tendencies (43), but caution is required with IV use. The prophylatic dose is especially important to breast-fed infants because human milk has low concentrations of vitamin K. Thus breast-fed babies have an increased frequency of hemorrhagic disease (44).

Toxicity

Vitamin K is relatively nontoxic, even in massive doses. Too rapid an intravenous injection of phylloquinone may result in flushing and cause a sense of construction in the chest. Menadione in doses of more than 10 mg parentally may produce hemolysis, hyperbilirubinemia, and kernicterus in premature newborns. Large daily intakes of vitamin K (i.e., 250 mg of dietary vitamin K found in approximately 8 ounces of cauliflower, lettuce, spinach, or broccoli) may antagonize the hypoprothrombionic effect of oral anticoagulants.

WATER-SOLUBLE VITAMINS

The B complex vitamins and vitamin C are the water-soluble vitamins. The vitamin B complex group includes thiamin, riboflavin, nicotinic acid, pyridoxine, pantothenic acid, biotin, folic acid, and cyanocobalamin.

Water-soluble vitamins serve as cofactors for specific enzyme systems in the body. Many water-soluble vitamins are not active until phosphorylation occurs after ingestion (thiamin, riboflavin, niacin, and pyridoxine) or until coupled to specific nucleotides (riboflavin, niacin).

Water-soluble vitamins are stored to a limited extent only, so a day-to-day supply is desirable. When excessive amounts are ingested, the unneeded portion is generally excreted, resulting in a minimal toxicity. However, even water-soluble vitamins can be toxic, especially when large amounts are ingested for prolonged periods.

Certain conditions may deplete the supply of water-soluble vitamins, resulting in a deficiency state. Fever may accelerate metabolism of these vitamins. The stress of injury or surgery, hyperthyroidism, and diarrhea may also cause a deficiency.

Deficiencies of water-soluble vitamins may begin as a depletion of body stores without evidence of clinical symptoms such as abnormal laboratory indices. Initial clinical symptoms include loss of appetite, weight loss, headache, apathy, insomnia, or excitability. In severe deficiency states, specific clinical syndromes such as beri-beri or pellegra occur. Characteristics of the water-soluble vitamins can be found in Table 10.3.

THIAMIN

The principle role of thiamin (B_1) is as a coenzyme in the form of thiamin pyrophosphate. This coenzyme plays a vital role in the intermediate metabolism of carbohydrates in decarboxylation (removal of carbon dioxide) and in transketolation (transfer of carbon units), such as the conversion of pyruvic acid into acetyl-CoA and the synthesis of acetylcholine. Individual requirements for thiamin are related to metabolic rate and are greatest when carbohydrates are the primary source of calories. Thiamin is also necessary for the transmission of nerve impulses.

Thiamin deficiency results in beri-beri, characterized by peripheral neuritis. The symptoms of peripheral neuritis include sensory disturbances in the extremities, loss of muscle strength, poor memory, depression, muscle wasting (dry beri-beri), edema (wet beri-beri), tachycardia, and an enlarged heart.

In the United States, the most common cause of thiamin deficiency is alcoholism. Excessive alcohol intake is frequently associated with poor dietary habits, decreased absorption of nutrients, and decreased activation of thiamin pyrophosphate. The Wernicke-Korsakoff syndrome, characterized by paralysis of eye muscles and nystagmus and associated with excess alcohol intake, is primarily due to a thiamin deficiency (45).

NIACIN

Niacin, vitamin B_3, is a component of the coenzymes nicotinamide adenine dinucleotide (NAD) and nicotinamide adenine dinucleotide phosphate (NADP). These two coenzymes are important in the oxidation-reduction reactions essential for tissue respiration. Niacin (nicotinic acid) is essential for converting food to energy, fat synthesis, growth, and healthy skin. Niacin may be converted in the body to niacinamide (nicotinamide), but either form can be used by the body.

Both alcoholism and protein-calorie malnutrition may lead to the niacin deficiency state known as pellagra, with initial symptoms of an erythematous eruption resembling sunburn. Later the "three Ds" of dermatitis, diarrhea, and dementia occur, followed by death if the deficiency is not corrected.

Therapeutic Uses

Niacin (but not niacinamide) is a peripheral vasodilator. It causes the release of histamine, resulting in a transient flushing of the skin as well as a tingling sensation, dizziness, nausea, gastrointestinal upset, and activation of peptic ulcer disease (46). The flushing sensation generally begins 20 min after ingestion and lasts 30 to 60 min. After 3 to 6 weeks of therapy, the flushing side effect usually decreases markedly (47). The adverse effects of niacin may be diminished by increasing the dose slowly (100 mg, three times a day each week), administering with food or milk, or administering 60 min after a 325-mg dose of aspirin.

Nicotinic acid is also effective in lowering total cholesterol and low-density lipoprotein (LDL) levels, while concurrently increasing high-density lipoprotein (HDL) levels. Nicotinic acid is used in treatment of lipid disorders, with doses from 3 to 6 g each day. Nicotinic acid is available at a relatively low cost, but it is not free of serious side effects. (See Chapter 18, "Hyperlipidemia.") Niacin may cause reversible hepatitis, glucose intolerance, and hyperuricemia. Fasting blood glucose levels, liver function values, and uric acid levels should be monitored during chronic therapy (48, 49).

Sustained-release nicotinic acid formulations have been used in the treatment of hyperlipidemia, because it was thought that the gradual absorption of niacin would minimize adverse reactions and increase compliance. However, sustained-release formulations have not been proven to be successful. Flushing is not decreased, only delayed. Sustained formulations have also been shown to increase the incidence of gastrointestinal adverse effects (nausea, vomiting, and diarrhea). Niacin-induced elevated

Table 10.3.
Water-soluble Vitamins[a]

Vitamin	Function	Deficiency	Large Doses	Sources
Thiamin 　Vitamin B_1	Metabolism of 　carbohydrates Normal growth Functioning of nervous 　system Synthesis of acetylcholine	Beriberi Peripheral neuritis Loss of memory Depression Muscle wasting Edema Tachycardia Enlarged heart	Nontoxic even in very large 　doses of 100–500 mg 　parenterally	Milk Pork Liver Nuts Whole grains Enriched flour & 　cereals
Riboflavin 　Vitamin B_2 　Flavin 　　mononucleotide 　Flavin adenine 　　dinucleotide	Building and maintaining 　body tissues	Cheilosis 　Glossitis Seborrheic dermatitis Burning & itching eyes Achlorhydria	No toxicity	Milk Eggs Meat Liver Green leafy vegetables
Niacin 　Nicotinic acid 　Nicotinamide	Enzymes that convert food 　to energy Tissue respiration Fat synthesis Growth Healthy skin	Pellagra 　Erythematous eruptions 　Dermatitis 　Diarrhea 　Dementia	Transient flushing of skin 　and tingling sensation 　(vasodilation) Dizziness Nausea Gastrointestinal upset Peptic ulcer disease Liver toxicity Hyperuricemia Glucose intolerance Lower serum lipids with 3– 　6 g cholesterol and 　triglycerides	Lean meats Fish Whole grains Green vegetables
Pyridoxine 　Vitamin B_6 　Pyridines; pyridoxine; 　　pyridoxamine; 　　pyridoxal	Transformation of amino 　acids Metabolism of tryptophan 　to serotonin Modify action of steroid 　hormones	Seborrheic-like skin 　Glossitis Stomatitis Peripheral neuropathy Anemia Drugs: hydralazine, 　penicilliamine, isoniazid, 　cycloserine, and estrogen	Peripheral sensory 　neuropathy Ataxia	Wheat Corn Meat Potatoes
Ascorbic Acid 　Vitamin C	Synthesis of collagen— 　important for wound 　healing and stress due to 　injury and infection Synthesis of epinephrine 　from adrenal glands Conversion of folic acid to 　folinic acid Absorption of iron	Defect in collagen 　formation—poor wound 　healing, aching joints, 　weakened cartilage and 　capillary walls Scurvy	Possible kidney stones Diarrhea with 4–15 g/day Gout Lower serum cholesterol Rebound scurvy Increased absorption of iron Interference with oral 　anticoagulants Treatment of pressure sores Impaired bacterial activity	Citrus fruits Tomatoes Leafy vegetables Melons
Pantothenic acid	Metabolism of 　carbohydrates Gluconeogenesis Synthesis and degradation 　of fatty acids Synthesis of sterols Synthesis of steroid 　hormones Synthesis of porphyrins ·	Usually only seen with 　severe, multiple, B 　complex deficits	Essentially nontoxic in 　humans	Meat Poultry Fish Cereals Fruits, vegetables Milk
Biotin	Carbohydrate metabolism Fat metabolism	Seborrheic dermatitis Algesia	Essentially nontoxic in 　humans	Liver Egg yolk Synthesized by 　intestinal bacteria
Folic acid	Maturation of red blood 　cells Interrelated with B_{12}	Megaloblastic anemia Pregnancy	Essentially nontoxic in 　humans	Liver Green leafy vegetables
Cobalamin B_{12}	Synthesis of DNA Formation of red blood 　cells	Pernicious anemia Peripheral neuropathy Macrocytic anemia	Essentially nontoxic in 　humans	Liver, meat, milk, egg, 　cheese

[a] Adapted from: Marcus R, Coulston AM: Water-soluble vitamins. In Gilman AG, Goodman LS, Rall TW, Murad F (eds): The Pharmacologic Basis of Therapeutics, ed. 7. New York, Macmillan, 1985; Tuckerman, MM, Truco SJ (eds): Human Nutrition. Philadelphia: Lea & Febiger, 1983; and Luke B (ed): Principles of Nutrition and Diet Therapy. Boston: Little, Brown & Co., 1984.

liver enzyme levels may be associated especially with extended-release forms because of the 1.5 g/day dosage regimen used rather than the dosage of regular niacin over a 6-week period. The efficacy of extended-release niacin in reducing seum low-density lipoprotein and total cholesterol and in elevating high-density lipoproteins is presently being studied (50, 51).

PYRIDOXINE

Vitamin B$_6$ consists of a group of related compounds known as the pyridines, which include pyridoxine, pyridoxamine, and pyridoxal. The pyridines are converted to the active form of vitamin B$_6$, pyridoxal phosphate, in the gastrointestinal tract (52).

Pyridoxal phosphate is a coenzyme involved in the metabolism of protein, carbohydrates, and fat. In protein metabolism, vitamin B$_6$ participates in the decarboxylation of amino acids and in the conversion of tryptophan to niacin or serotonin. Pyridoxine may also modify the actions of steroid hormones by interacting with steroid receptor complexes (53).

Vitamin B$_6$ deficiency due to dietary restriction is seldom seen in adults, although deficiency in the alcoholic population may be as high as 30%. Symptoms of pyridoxine deficiency includes seborrhea-like skin lesions on the face, glossitis, stomatitis, peripheral neuropathy, and anemia. Drug-induced deficiencies have been observed with vitamin B$_6$ antagonists such as hydralazine, penicillamine, isoniazid, cycloserine, and estrogen. Pyridoxine has been reported to decrease phenobarbital and phenytoin serum levels when daily doses of 200 mg are administered for 4 weeks. Pyridoxine antagonizes the therapeutic action of levodopa as it facilitates the conversion of levodopa to dopamine outside the CNS. Patients on levodopa should avoid supplemental B$_6$. Concurrent B$_6$ does not adversely affect the levodopa/carbidopa combination, as carbidopa is a peripheral dopa decarboxylase inhibitor.

Large daily doses of 0.2 to 6 g/day for 2 months to 3 years may result in toxic symptoms of peripheral sensory neuropathies, with associated ataxia and numbness and clumsiness of the hands and feet (54, 55).

Pyridoxine supplementation has been reported to be beneficial in several clinical situations. Women who report symptoms of depression while taking oral contraceptives may be deficient in pyridoxine. Some studies suggest that these women may respond favorably to a daily supplement of 50 mg (56–58). Vitamin B$_6$ may be prescribed for women who have decreased pyridoxine plasma level.

In doses up to 100 mg administered 3 times daily, pyridoxine may relieve paresthesia and pain in hands of patients with carpal tunnel syndrome. As an alternative to surgery, vitamin B$_6$ may be used in the treatment of carpal tunnel syndrome. However, at high dosages the patient must be monitored for toxic symptoms.

Pyridoxine may also be used to alleviate symptoms of premenstrual syndrome (PMS), such as depression, irritability, tension, breast tenderness, edema, headache, and acne, which may be related to abnormal tryptophan metabolism produced by pyridoxal phosphate deficiency. Side effects associated with pyridoxine, 25 to 100 mg twice daily are minimal (59). Pyrodoxine appears to be safe and effective in the majority of females studied for treatment of premenstrual syndrome (PMS) (60–63).

VITAMIN C

Ascorbic acid is involved in a variety of metabolic functions, including direct stimulation of peptide synthesis and hydroxylation of proline and lysine in the formation of collagen, synthesis of epinephrine, and conversion of folic acid to folinic acid. Also, vitamin C facilitates the gastrointestinal absorption of iron.

The adrenal cortex, leukocytes, and platelets contain high concentrations of vitamin C. The amount found in the leukocytes is less susceptable to depletion than that present in plasma (64).

A deficiency of ascorbic acid results in defective collagen synthesis. Joint pain, anemia, poor wound healing, and increased susceptibility to infection are among the signs of deficiency. The severe form of vitamin C deficiency is scurvy. The clinical findings of scurvy include ecchymoses, petechial hemorrhages, easy bruising, loosening of the teeth secondary to gum inflammation, muscle weakness, and joint pains. Plasma levels of vitamin C may be lowered in cigarette smokers and women taking oral contraceptives (65, 66).

Large daily doses of 1 to 3 g of ascorbic acid may result in formation of kidney stones because of excessive excretion of oxalate produced from the metabolism of ascorbic acid (67). Severe diarrhea and precipitation of gout as the result of excretion of uric acid in predisposed people may also occur (68).

Rebound scurvy may be seen in both infants and adults following the use of megadoses of vitamin C (69). An infant born to a mother taking large amounts of vitamin C can metabolize the vitamin at a more rapid rate than normal. Adults who abruptly stop high-dose therapy experience loosened teeth and bleeding gums. In both instances, an increased rate of vitamin C elimination results in a relative deficiency when large quantities are no longer available. Therefore, patients should be advised to taper the dose of vitamin C instead of suddenly discontinuing therapy.

Other adverse effects that have been reported with intake of megadoses of vitamin C include absorption of excessive amounts of iron (70), uricosuria with resultant stone formation (71), gastrointestinal disturbances, interference with anticoagulants, destruction of red blood cells (72), and impaired bactericidal activity of leukocytes (73, 74).

Ingestion of 1 to 3 g of vitamin C has been advocated by Pauling as a protective factor against the common cold. Some studies show a decrease in frequency and severity of symptoms of the common cold (75), while others have found this not to be true (76–78). The claims of vitamin C for prevention of the common cold remain unsubstantiated by randomized, well-designed, double-blind clinical studies.

Well-designed studies have proven that megadose vitamin C therapy is of no benefit in the survival of patients with terminal cancer.

PANTOTHENIC ACID

Pantothenic acid, a constituent of coenzyme A, is needed for enzyme-catalyzed reactions such as the metabolism of carbohydrates; gluconeogensis; synthesis and metabolism of fatty acids, and synthesis of sterols, steroid hormones, and porphyrins. Since pantothenic acid is widely distributed in the diet, a deficiency is rare and would be expected to occur only in a malnourished individual.

BIOTIN

Biotin is important in carbohydrate and fat metabolism. Biotin is available in a wide variety of foods and is also synthesized by bacteria in the intestinal tract. A deficiency is rare but may occur due to inadequate synthesis. Exfoliative dermatitis is the primary deficiency symptom. Biotin-deficient infants (due to malabsorption syndrome) exhibit Leiner's disease and can receive biotin intravenously by Roche under compassionate investigational new drug (IND).

VITAMIN B_{12}

Vitamin B_{12} participates as a coenzyme in DNA synthesis, cell reproduction, red blood cell formation, and nerve tissue maintenance. It may also be required for the incorporation of folic acid into cells.

Vitamin B_{12} also occurs in several forms designated as cobalamins. Commercially available cyanocobalamin is the most stable form.

Intrinsic factor is secreted by parietal cells in the stomach and regulates the amount of vitamin B_{12} absorbed in the terminal ileum. Because vitamin B_{12} is so well conserved by the body through enterohepatic cycling, signs of deficiency may not be seen for 3 to 5 years after absorption has ceased. Because cyanocobalamin is important in cell production, the signs and symptoms of deficiency are manifested in organ systems with rapidly replicating cells. A deficiency results in megaloblastic anemia characterized by mature cells that lack oxygen-carrying capacity. Megaloblastic anemia may also occur following surgical removal of the stomach portion that produces intrinsic factor or part of the ileum where absorption of the vitamin occurs.

Pernicious anemia, a genetic disorder, occurs when intrinsic factor is not produced, and consequently, vitamin B_{12} is not absorbed. In pernicious anemia, mature red blood cells are not produced because of a lack of DNA. The characteristic symptoms of the disorder include pallor, anorexia, dyspnea, prolonged bleeding time, weight loss, glossitis, and neurologic disturbances including depression and unsteady gait (see Chapters 12–13).

A vitamin B_{12} deficiency may exist in the geriatric patient, without the classic laboratory, hematologic, or clinical manifestations. This vitamin B_{12} deficiency appears to be due to an inability to absorb protein-bound vitamin B_{12}, despite a lack of gastric abnormalities. This vitamin B_{12} deficiency manifests itself by neurologic and psychiatric abnormalities without the classic hematologic abnormalities. Geriatric patients with a serum B_{12} level of <200 pg/ml should be treated initially with 1 mg per day of B_{12} until the serum B_{12} concentration is raised to >300 pg/ml or B_{12} intramuscularly (100 μg i.m./day for 2 weeks, then 1000 μg i.m./month for life) if the serum B_{12} concentration does not come up to >300 pg/ml (79, 80). Vitamin B_{12} is available as oral tablets, parenteral intramuscular injection, and intranasal gel. The gel is reported by the manufacturer to have greater bioavailability than oral tablets and is easier to administer than an intramuscular injection.

Cyanocobalamin has no therapeutic value beyond that of correcting deficiencies. The use of vitamin B_{12} to boost energy is of no value.

FOLIC ACID

Folic acid is functionally related to cyanocobalamin because they are both essential for DNA synthesis. Folic acid is also important in cell reproduction, including red blood cell formation and protein synthesis.

Folacin is the generic term for folic acid (pteroylglutamic acid). Approximately 25% of the folacin found in food is in the active (tetrahydrofolic acid) form and is readily absorbed and stored in the liver. Ascorbic acid prevents its oxidation.

The usual causes of folic acid deficiency are similar to those previously discussed for other B vitamins. In addition, a deficiency may occur during pregnancy, with oral contraceptive use, in the elderly as the result of a poor diet, and in infants whose formulas lack folic acid or vitamin C.

The anemia that results from folic acid deficiency is characterized by a reduction in the number of red blood cells, the release of large nucleated cells (macrocytic, megoblastic), low hemoglobin levels with a high color content in RBCs, and lowered leukocyte and platelet counts.

Folic acid therapy corrects the anemia associated with vitamin B_{12} deficiency, but it does not prevent or correct

Table 10.4.
Vitamin-like Compounds

Compound	Function (Probable)	Comment	Sources

Bioflavanoids
  Rutin
  Hesperidin
	Maintain normally capillary permeability & fragility; reported to be used in conditions such as vascular hypertension, arthritis, & cancer	Found in citrin (rind of green citrus fruits)	Leafy vegetables, citrus, fruits, beer, wine, tea

Choline	Lipotropic effect, resulting in a decreasing rate of fat deposition in the liver & acceleration of its removal; precursor of acetylcholine	Component of the phospholipid lecithin; causes fishy odor of the breath and body; reported to cause clinical depression	Meats, grains, egg yolks, liver, vegetables
Inositol	Isomer of glucose	Component in cell membrane phospholipids & plasma lipoproteins	Grains, nuts, fruits, vegetables, yeast, milk
β-Aminobenzoic acid PABA	Necessary for bacterial synthesis of folic acid; reported to be used in preventing or causing a regression of fibrosis	Sulfonamides are inhibited by PABA and therefore should not be taken concomitantly	Yeast, liver, rice, bran, whole wheat

neurologic disturbances associated with vitamin B_{12} deficiency (see Chapter 13).

VITAMIN-LIKE COMPOUNDS

Compounds that may be found on the vitamin shelf include bioflavonoids, choline, insoitol, and p-aminobenzoic acid. These compounds, however, can not be called vitamins, as they have not been demonstrated to be essential in the diet of humans. Information regarding the vitamin-like compounds can be found in Table 10.4.

MINERALS

Minerals are inorganic substances that are classed as either macro- or micronutrients. Macronutrients are required daily in amounts of 100 mg or more, whereas micronutrients are required in amounts of less than 100 mg daily. A list of these minerals is included in Table 10.5. Other minerals are found widely in nature and in the human body, but their functions are uncertain, and many are considered to be contaminants. With all minerals, a narrow therapeutic index exists between general requirements and toxic levels.

Sources of minerals vary according to the composition of the soil in which they are found. In regions where the soil has been depleted of minerals, the population may experience marginal deficiencies. Deficiencies may also occur because of chronic ingestion of highly refined foods (flour and cereals) unless they have been fortified with the minerals lost during processing. Whole-grain foods are preferred to refined foods because of their high content of zinc, copper, and iron as well as pyridoxine, pantothenic acid, biotin, folic acid, and vitamin E.

In this chapter, emphasis is placed on a discussion of calcium, iron, and zinc because of their well-understood functions. Information about other minerals is summa-

Table 10.5.
Minerals

Macronutrients	Micronutrients (trace elements)
Calcium	Iron
Phosphorus	Zinc
Magnesium	Iodine
Sodium	Copper
Potassium	Fluorine
Chloride	Manganese
Sulfur	Selenium
	Chromium
	Cobalt

rized in Table 10.6. Table 10.7 lists the interactions that involve minerals.

CALCIUM

Calcium is essential for the functional integrity of the nervous and muscular systems, for normal cardiac function, for conversion of prothrombin into thrombin, and as the major component of bone.

Ninety-nine percent of total body calcium is found in bone, and 1% is present in serum. Of the serum calcium, 45% is bound to plasma proteins and inactive. The calcium in bone serves as a reservoir to maintain normal plasma calcium levels (81). The interaction of PTH, vitamin D, and calcitonin is responsible for maintaining a normal calcium level of 2.12 to 2.62 mmol/liter (8.5 to 10.5 mg/dl).

Calcium absorption occurs in the small intestine at a relatively steady rate of 30% of intake, increasing to approximately 50% during growth periods, pregnancy, and lactation.

An acute calcium deficiency resulting in a plasma level below 8.0 mg/dl results in tetany (82, 83). Chronic calcium deficiency, usually caused by inadequate dietary intake,

Table 10.6.
Summary of Minerals[a]

Minerals	Physiological Functions	Deficiency	Clinical Applications
Chlorine (chloride), major anion of the extracellular fluid	Required for fluid-electrolyte balance, acid-base balance, gastric acidity	Deficiency of chloride alone is rare	Losses occur in GI disorders, vomiting, diarrhea, and the tube drainage
Chromium	Favors normal glucose tolerance	Impaired glucose clearance; peripheral neuropathy; ataxia	Required for normal glucose utilization; role in management of diabetes remains controversial; required for carbohydrate and lipid metabolism; lowers serum cholesterol and LDL; increases HDL
Cobalt	Integral part of B_{12}	Pernicious anemia	Excess leads to polycythemia
Copper 30% absorbed from diet; inversely related to zinc; essential for proper iron utilization	Synthesis of melanin, collagen, hemoglobin, and connective tissue	Decreased red blood cell production and poor wound healing	Menke's kinky hair syndrome; absorption disorder; toxicity; Wilson's disease
Fluoride	Contributes to structure of teeth and soft tissues	Dental carries	May be useful in osteoporosis, toxicity: fluorosis, mottled enamel
Iodine	Synthesis thyroxine and tridothyronine	Creatinism; goiter; myxedema	Regulation of basal metabolic rate growth, reproduction, cellular metabolism
Magnesium 25–65% absorbed primarily in small intestine. Efficiently absorbed and highly conserved: a person on a high magnesium diet will absorb only about 1/4 of the intake, but on a low magnesium diet more than 3/4 of the intake will be absorbed	Nerve cell function; enzyme activator; synthesis of skeleton	Occurs in alcoholics, diabetics and with malabsorption syndrome; symptoms: tremor, spasm, irritability, lack of coordination, convulsions; excretion enhanced by mineral-corticoids, hypercalcemia, phosphate, depletion, alcohol ingestions	Uses in therapy include: magnesium sulfate IV as anticonvulsant, electrolyte replenisher, uterine relaxant; magnesium gluconate for oral supplementation; magnesium citrate or sulfate as laxative; magnesium carbonate, oxide, hydroxide, trisilicate as antacid; hypermagnesemia is rare except in renal failure; excess may cause diarrhea
Manganese Substitute for magnesium in come reactions	Cofactor for enzyme systems involved in bone formation; required for formation of mucopolysaccharides	Has not been observed in humans	
Molybdenum	Cofactor for xanthine oxidase	Has not been observed in humans	
Phosphorus 70% absorbed from jenunum, maintained by renal resorption; normal plasma concentration: 3.0 mg/dl to 4.5 mg/dl	Skeletal synthesis; component of vitamins and essential for coenzyme formation; contributes to structure of teeth and soft tissue	Occurs if prolonged excessive use of alcohol or nonabsorbable antacids, prolonged vomiting, liver disease, hyperparathyroidism.	Dibasic calcium phosphate is used orally; hyperphosphatemia is associated with chronic renal disease, hypoparathyroidism, tetany
Potassium Major cation of intracellular fluid; normal range: 3.5–5.0 mEq/liter 3–4.5 mg/dl	Required fluid-electrolyte balance, acid-base balance, muscle activity, carbohydrate metabolism, protein synthesis	Produces, sore, weak, or painful muscles	Losses occur in GI disorders and diarrhea; used in treatment of diabetic acidosis; required for fluid balance
Selenium 90% absorbed	Acts synergistically with vitamin E to protect cell membranes from oxidative damage	Thigh tenderness, deficiency due to TPN, malnutrition	Incidence of cancer maybe due to low intake of selenium; marginal deficiency when soil content is low
Sodium Major cation of extracellular fluid; normal range: 136–145 mEq//liter; under hormonal control of aldosterone	Required for fluid balance, acidbase balance, cell permeability, normal muscle irritability	Losses occur in GI disorders and diarrhea; weakness, mental confusion, nausea, lethargy, and muscle cramping may result	Fluid balance, blood pressure membrane permeability, neuromuscular function may be altered due to depletion or retention
Sulfur Obtained from protein	Structure of skin and cartilage; component of vitamins; important coenzyme formation		

[a] Adapted from: Tuckerman MM, Turco SJ (eds): Human Nutrition. Philadelphia: Lea & Febiger, 1983; and Williams SR (ed): Nutrition and Diet Therapy. St Louis: Times Mirror/Mosby College Publishing, 1985.

Table 10.7.
Mineral Interactions

Mineral	Drug/Agent	Interaction/Effect
Calcium	Corticosteroids	Decreased calcium absorption
	Fiber	Decreased calcium absorption
	Iron	Decreased iron absorption
	Oxalic acid (found in rhubarb & spinach)	Decreased calcium absorption
	Phenytoin	Decreased absorption of phenytoin
	Phosphorus (found in dairy products)	Decreased calcium absorption
	Phytic acid (found in bran & cereals)	Decreased calcium absorption
	Quinidine	Decreased quinidine renal excretion and increased pharmacologic effects
	Salicylates	Increased salicylic acid renal excretion and decreased pharmacologic effects
	Tetracycline	Decreased serum levels of tetracycline
	Thiazide diuretics	Increased absorption of calcium
	Vitamin D	Increased absorption of calcium
Copper	Penicillamine	Copper deficiency
Iodine	Lithium	Additive or synergistic effect in inhibiting thyroid function
Iron	Antacids	Decreased iron absorption
	Ascorbic acid	200 mg ascorbic acid per 30 mg iron increases absorption of iron
	Caffeine	Decreased absorption of iron
	Dairy products	Decreased absorption of iron
	Oxalic acid (found in rhubarb & spinach)	Decreased absorption of iron
	Phosphorus (found in dairy products)	Decreased absorption of iron
	Phytic acid (found in bran & cereals)	Decreased absorption of iron
Magnesium	Alcohol	Decreased absorption of magnesium
	Calcium	Decreased absorption of magnesium
	Diuretics	Increased absorption of magnesium
	Phosphorus	Decreased absorption of magnesium
Phosphorus	Antacids (Al or Mg)	Decreased absorption of phosphorus
	Calcium	Decreased absorption of phosphorus
	Iron	Decreased absorption of phosphorus
Zinc	Alcohol	Decreased serum zinc levels
	Bran or diary products	Decreased zinc absorption
	Copper	An excess of either may cause a decreased absorption of the other
	Diuretics	Increased zinc excretion
	Penicillamine	Zinc deficiency
	Phytic acid	Decreased zinc absorption
	Phosphorus	Decreased zinc absorption
	Tetracycline	Decreased tetracycline absorption

results in osteoporosis or osteomalacia in adults and rickets in children.

A chronic excess intake of calcium may cause adverse effects. One to 2 g of calcium per day is unlikely to cause problems, but patients sometimes decide that more is better. The adverse effects of excess calcium ingestion range from minor to life-threatening and are clearly dose-related. Possible adverse effects include nausea, bloating, constipation (which may be prevented by increased fiber and water consumption), and flatulence (especially with oral intake of calcium carbonate) (84). Symptoms of hypercalcemia generally occur with ingestion of more than 4 to 5 g/day (85). Signs and symptoms of hypercalcemia include nausea, vomiting, anorexia, headache, muscle weakness, depression, apathy, fatigue, hypertension, nervousness, insomnia, and urolithiasis (86, 87).

Calcium supplements are suggested for prevention or control of osteoporosis (88–90), hypertension (91, 92) and colon cancer (93), but the only confirmed use is for correction of dietary deficiency. Of commercially available supplements, calcium carbonate (oyster shell) provides the greatest amount of elemental calcium (40%). In patients with achlorhydria (especially geriatric patients), calcium carbonate is not absorbed to a great extent on an empty stomach, but it is well absorbed with meals. Calcium citrate (21% elemental calcium), when compared with calcium carbonate, has been shown to have better solubility and absorption, particularly in patients with impaired acid secretion.

Two natural sources of calcium, bone meal and dolomite, should be avoided because of the risk of leaf contamination. The risk of poisoning is especially great for pregnant/lactating women, infants, children, and possibly the elderly.

IRON

Iron is essential in the functioning of all biological systems because it is the oxygen carrier in hemoglobin and myoglobin. It also functions in the respiratory chain.

Iron in the body is either functional or stored. Functional iron is found in hemoglobin and myoglobin, whereas stored iron is found in association with transferrin, ferritin, and hemosiderin. The storage sites of ferritin and hemosiderin are the liver, spleen, and bone marrow.

Dietary iron absorption is highly variable, ranging from 2 to 35%, depending on the type and source. Heme iron and nonheme iron are the two forms of dietary iron. Heme iron is obtained from animal protein sources and is 15 to 35% absorbed (94). Meat may facilitate the absorption of heme iron by stimulating production of gastric acid (95). Nonheme iron constitutes most dietary iron found in grain products, vegetables, and dairy products and has an absorption rate of 2 to 20%. Absorption of nonheme iron is influenced by the levels of iron stores and by concomitantly consumed dietary components. Factors such as ascorbic acid and meat, fish, or poultry may increase the bioavailability of nonheme iron.

Iron deficiency is the most commonly recognized nutritional deficiency in the United States and is by far the major cause of anemia (96, 97). Iron deficiency usually occurs in high-risk groups that include infants, children, adolescents, women of childbearing age, frequent blood donors, and chronic aspirin users. Iron deficiency in these groups is usually treated or prevented with supplements. (See chapter on iron deficiency anemia.)

ZINC

Zinc is important in the growth and maintenance of healthy skin and in development and continued functioning of the male sex organs. It is also necessary for the synthesis of DNA, RNA (98), and connective tissue and bone. It is necessary for the uptake of insulin by adipose tissue (99), normal sense of taste, increased oxygen-carrying capacity in normal and sickle red blood cells (100), spermatogensis, ova formation, and the mobilization and transport of vitamin A from the liver.

Ten to 40% of dietary zinc is absorbed from the small intestine. The absorption of zinc, like that of iron, appears to be associated with the nutritional status of the individual (101). Decreased absorption of zinc has been associated with the formation of insoluble complexes with phytate (cereals), calcium, vitamin D, protein, and fiber. An increased copper intake can also suppress zinc absorption by competition for albumin binding sites (102). Zinc salts, acetate or sulfate, appear to have the highest degree of

bioavailability (103). Zinc sulfate can be irritating to the gastrointestinal tract.

Increased urinary excretion of zinc may be associated with surgery, diabetes, fever, alcohol consumption, and therapy with corticosteroids, estrogens, and thiazide diuretics. A zinc deficiency has also been associated with hypogonadal dwarfism (104). Clinical manifestations of zinc deficiency also include loss of taste (hypogeusia) or smell (105), dermatitis, macular degeneration, and poor wound healing (106). Acrodermatitis enteropathica is the human genetic deficiency.

Zinc therapy may be of value in facilitating wound healing and in treating hypogeusia in zinc-deficient patients in dosages of 220 mg, two to three times daily.

Reported signs of zinc toxicity in humans include anorexia, nausea, lethargy, dizziness, and diarrhea. Vomiting may occur after ingestion of more than a 2-g dose (107). Moderate doses of zinc (150 mg administered twice daily for 6 weeks) have been reported to increase the LDL/HDL ratio (108) and to impair cell-mediated immunity (109).

CHROMIUM

Chromium is an essential component of glucose tolerance factor, a compound containing glycine, glutamic acid, cysteine, and niacin, and is associated with glucose and lipid metabolism and insulin activity. Although the therapeutic role of chromium in the treatment of diabetes remains unknown, chromium is essential for the efficient use of insulin, by facilitating the binding of insulin to the cell membrane, and is also required for normal glucose metabolism. Patients receiving total nutrition who develop glucose intolerance, insulin resistance, and central and peripheral nervous system disorders, have regained normal function after chromium (not insulin) administration. Limited findings suggest a reduction in total serum cholesterol with chromium supplements. Chromium may also lower LDL-cholesterol and increase HDL-cholesterol. A deficiency in chromium is exhibited by hyperglycemia, glucosuria, peripheral neuropathy, and ataxia.

SELENIUM

Selenium, an antioxidant, is a component of the enzyme glutathione peroxidase, which is thought to deactivate lipid peroxidase. Lipid peroxidases are strong oxidizing agents that cause cell injury. The relationship between dietary selenium intake and incidence of cancer is being investigated. Limited epidemiologic evidence suggests that the risk of certain types of cancer, especially breast cancer, is inversely related to selenium intake. Because of the potential for toxicity, unsupervised use of selenium for cancer prevention should be discouraged. Selenium is being used (although claims remain to be unfounded) in heart disease, arthritis, heavy metal poisoning, sexual dysfunction, and aging. Selenium toxicity includes loss of hair, brittle fingernails, fatigue, irritability, and garlic odor or breath. No evidence suggests a deficiency of selenium in humans, and supplementation is not recommended.

CONCLUSION

Vitamins are organic compounds that are essential for the body's biochemical processes. Vitamins, or their precursors, must be consumed from the diet, since they generally are not manufactured by the body, and under certain circumstances, are insufficiently produced. A positive relationship exists between the maintenance of optimal health and a good nutritional diet. Vitamin supplementation should not be a substitute for a well-balanced diet. For the normal population, the recommended number of daily servings from the five basic food groups (meats, vegetables, fruits, dairy products, and grains) provide the needed recommended dietary allowances. However, certain groups in the general population, with increased metabolic requirements, malabsorption syndromes, inadequate dietary intake, or stress, require additional nutrients.

The fat-soluble vitamins A, D, E, and K are stored in the body for months. Therefore, toxicity due to fat-soluble vitamins is related to accumulation and low urinary excretion. The water-soluble vitamins, vitamin B complex and C, have very small reserves maintained in the body, and a day-to-day supply is desired. Water-soluble vitamins can cause adverse effects, such as when large quantities of specific compounds are ingested for prolonged periods.

Consumers often have questions about compounds that are not considered to be "true" or "real" vitamins. To protect the health as well as the finances of the consumer, the pharmacist must be knowledgeable and provide the necessary information about vitamin-like substances.

Minerals are inorganic substances. Several of these elements, particularly calcium, iron, and zinc, have been found to be important catalysts in various enzymatic activities or play a role in hormonal metabolism. The importance of these elements must not be overlooked while investigators attempt to understand the nutritional importance of other minerals.

REFERENCES

1. Anon: Federal Register 44:16139, 1979.
2. Anon: Food and Drug Administration Drug Bulletin 13:27, 1983.
3. Robinson CH, Lawler MR, Chenoweth WL, Garwick AE (eds): Normal and Therapeutic Nutrition, ed. 17. New York: Macmillan, 1986, pp 180–183.
4. Hoffman CJ, Zabik ME: Effects of microwave cooking/reheating on nutrients and food systems: a review of recent studies. J Am Diet Assoc 85:922–926, 1985.
5. Williams SR (ed): Nutrition and Diet Therapy. St Louis: Times Mirror/Mosby College Publishing, 1985, pp 120–123.
6. Robinson CH, Lawler MR, Chenoweth WL, Garwick AE (eds): Normal and Therapeutic Nutrition, ed. 17. New York: Macmillan, 1986, p 159.
7. Luke B (ed): Principles of Nutrition and Diet Therapy. Boston: Little, Brown Co, 1984, p 137.
8. Stirling HF, Laing SC, Barr DG: Hypercarotenemia and vitamin A overdosage from proprietary baby food. Lancet 1:1089, 1986.
9. Sommer A, Djunaedi E, Loeden AA, Tarwotjo R: Impact of vitamin A supplementation on childhood mortality. Lancet 1:1169–1173, 1986.
10. Anon: Toxic effects of vitamin overdosage. Med Lett 26:73–74, 1984.
11. Kizer KW, Fan AM, Bankowska J, et al.: Vitamin A—a pregnancy hazard alert. West J Med 152:78–81, 1990.
12. Ballag W: Vitamin A and retinoids: from nutrition to pharmacotherapy in dermatology and oncology. Lancet 1:860–863, 1983.
13. Lammer EJ, Chen DT, Hoar RM, Agnish ND, et al.: Retinoic acid embryopathy. N Engl J Med 313:837–841, 1985.
14. Goodman DS: Vitamin A and the retinoids in health and disease. N Engl J Med 310:1023–1031, 1984.
15. Willett WC, Polk BF, Underwood BA, Stampfer MJ, et al.: Relation of serum vitamins A and E and carotenoids to the risk of cancer. N Engl J Med 310:430–434, 1984.
16. Wald N, Idle M, Boreham J, Bailey A: Low serum-vitamin-A and subsequent risk of cancer: preliminary results of a prospective study. Lancet 2:813–815, 1980.
17. Anon: Vitamin A and cancer. Lancet 2:325–326, 1984.
18. Kessler JF, Levine N, Meyskens FL Jr, Lynch PJ, et al.: Treatment of cutaneous T-cell lymphoma (mycosis fungoides) with 13-cis-retinoic acid. Lancet 1:1345–1347, 1983.
19. Walker AR: Cancer of the cervix. Some aspects of epidemiology, screening, risk factors and survival. S Afr Med J 68(5):316–320, 1985.
20. Shekelle RB, Lepper M, Lius S, et al.: Dietary vitamin A and risk of cancer in the Western Electric study. Lancet 2:1185–1190, 1981.
21. Haynes RC Jr, Murad F, Agents affecting calcification: calcium, parathyroid hormone, calcitonin, vitamin D, and other compounds. In Gilman AG, Goodman AS: The Pharmacological Basis of Therapeutics, ed. 7. New York, Macmillan, 1985, pp 1536–1538.
22. Haussler MR, McCain TA: Basic and clinical concepts related to vitamin D metabolism and action. N Engl J Med 18:974–983, 1977.
23. Deluca HF: Recent advances in metabolism of vitamin D. Annu Rev Physiol 43:199–209, 1981.
24. Johnson C, Acute and chronic renal failure. In Young LY, Koda-Kimble MA (eds): Applied Therapeutics, ed. 4. Vancouver, Applied Therapeutics, 1988, p 561.
25. Robinson CH, Lawler MR, Chenoweth WL, Garwick AE (eds): Normal and Therapeutic Nutrition, ed. 7. New York: Macmillan, 1986, p 167.
26. Muller DPR, Lloyd JK, Wolff OH: Vitamin E and neurological function. Lancet 1:227, 1983.
27. Sokol RJ, Guggenheim MA, Iannaccone ST, et al.: Improved neurologic function after longterm correction of vitamin E deficiency in children with chronic cholestasis. N Engl J Med 313:1580–1586, 1985.
28. Satel SL, Riely CA: Vitamin E deficiency and neurologic dysfunction in children. N Engl J Med 314F:1389–1390, 1985.
29. Burns A, Holland T: Vitamin E deficiency. Lancet 1:805–806, 1986.
30. Bendich A, Machlin LJ: Safety of oral intake of vitamin E. Am J Clin Nutr 48:612–619, 1988.
31. Johnson B, Bowen FW Jr, Abbasi S, et al.: Relationship of prolonged pharmacologic serum levels of vitamin E to incidence of sepsis and necrotizing enterocolitis in infants with birth weight 1,500 grams or less. Pediatrics 75:619–638, 1985.
32. Lorch V, Murphy D, Hoerstern LR, Harris E, Fitzgerald J, Sinha

SN: Unusual syndrome among premature infants associated with a new intravenous vitamin E product. Pediatrics 75:598–602, 1985.

33. Corrigan JJ, Marcus PI: Coagulaopathy associated with vitamin E ingestion. JAMA 230:1300, 1974.

34. Evans CDH, Lacy JH: Toxicity of vitamins: complications of a health movement. Br Med J 292:510, 1986.

35. Natta CL, Machlin LJ, Brin M: A decrease in irreversibly sickled erythrocytes in sickle cell anemia patients given vitamin E. Am J Clin Nutr 33:968–971, 1980.

36. Haeger K: Long-time treatment of intermittent claudication with vitamin E. Am J Clin Nutr 27:1179–1181, 1974.

37. Hittner HM, Gadio LB, Rudolph AJ, et al.: Retrolental fibroplasia: efficacy of vitamin E in a double-blind clinical study of preterm infants. N Engl J Med 305:1365, 1981.

38. Ehrenkranz RA: Vitamin E and the neonate. Am J Dis Child 134:1157–1166, 1980.

39. Lampe KF, McVeigh S, Rodgers BJ (eds): Drug Evaluations, ed. 6. Chicago, American Medical Association, 1986, p 850.

40. Ne UHC. Adverse effects of new cephalosporins (letter). Ann Intern Med 98:415–416, 1983.

41. Lipsky JJ. N-methyl-thio-tetrazole inhibition of the gamma carboxylation of glutamic acid: possible mechanism for antibiotic associated hypoprothrombinaemia. Lancet 2:192–193, 1983.

42. Robinson CH, Lawler Mr, Chenoweth WL, Garwick AE (eds): Normal and Therapeutic Nutrition, ed. 7. New York: Macmillan, 1986, p 170.

43. Mandel HG, Cohn VH, Fat-soluble vitamins. In Gilman AG, Goodman LS: The Pharmacological Basis of Therapeutics, ed. 7. New York, Macmillan, 1985, p 1586.

44. O'Connor ME, Livingstone DS, Wilkins D: Vitamin K deficiency and breast-feeding. Am J Dis Child 137:601–602, 1983.

45. Hoyumpa AM: Mechanisms of thiamine deficiency in chronic alcoholism. Am J Clin Nutr 33:2750, 1980.

46. Marcus R, Coulston AM, Water-soluble vitamins. The vitamin B complex and ascorbic acid. In Gilman AG, Goodman LS, Rall TW, Murad F (eds), The Pharmacological Basis of Therapeutics, ed. 7. New York, Macmillan, 1985, p 1558.

47. Hoeg JM, Gregg RE, Brewer HB: An approach to the management of hyperlipoproteinemia. JAMA 255:512–521, 1986.

48. Grimm RH, Hunninghake OM: Lipids and hypertension. Implications of new guidelines for cholesterol management in the treatment of hypertension. Am J Med 80:56–62, 1986.

49. Figge HL, Figge J, Souney PF: Nicotinic acid: a review of its clinical use in the treatment of lipid disorders. Pharmcotherapy 8(5):287–294, 1988.

50. Simpson T: Extended-release niacin not problem free (letter). Am J Hosp Pharm 48:237–239, 1991.

51. Knapp T, Middleton RK: Adverse effects of sustained release niacin (letter). DICP 25:253–254, 1991.

52. Robinson CH, Lawler MR, Chenoweth WL, Garwick AE (eds): Normal and Therapeutic Nutrition, ed. 7. New York, Macmillan, 1986, p 188.

53. Marcus R, Coultston AM, Water-soluble vitamins. The vitamin B complex and ascorbic acid. In Gilman AG, Goodman LS, Rall TW, Murad F (eds): The Pharmacological Basis of Therapeutics, ed. 7. New York, Macmillan, 1985, pp 1560–1561.

54. Schaumburg H, Kaplan J, Windebank A, Vick N, et al.: Sensory neuropathy with low dose pyridoxine abuse. A new megavitamin syndrome. N Engl J Med 310:445–448, 1983.

55. Parry G, Bredesen DE: Sensory neuropathy with low-dose pyridoxine. Neurology 35:1466, 1985.

56. Adams PW, Wynn V, Rose DP, Seed M, Folkard J, et al.: Effect of pyridoxine hydrochloride (vitamin B_6) upon depression with oral contraception. Lancet 1:897–904, 1973.

57. Adams PW, Wynn V, Seed M, et al.: Vitamin B_6, depression, and oral contraception. Lancet 2:516–517, 1974.

58. Miller LT: Do oral contraceptive agents affect nutrient requirements—Vitamin B_6? J Nutr 116(7):1344–1345, 1986.

59. Williams MT, Harris RI, Dean BC: Management of premenstrual syndrome. J Int Med Res 13:174–179, 1985.

60. Abraham GE, Hargrove JT: Effect of vitamin B_6 on premenstrual symptomatology in women with premenstrual tension syndromes: a double-blind crossover study. Infertility 3:155–165, 1980.

61. Brush MG, Perry M: Pyridoxine and the premenstrual syndrome (letter). Lancet 1:1399, 1985.

62. Williams MJ, Harris RI, Dean BC: Controlled trial of pyridoxine in the premenstrual syndrome. J Int Med Res 13:174–179, 1985.

63. Brush MG, Bennett T, Hansen K: Pyridoxine in the treatment of premenstrual syndrome. Br J Clin Pract 42(11):448–452, 1988.

64. Matthews HW, Wells K: Vitamins, part IV: water soluble. J Natl Pharmaceut Assoc 27:8–13, 1982.

65. Kallner AB, Hartmann D, Hornig DH: On the requirements of ascorbic acid in man: steady-state turnover and body pool in smokers. Am J Clin Nutr 34:1347–1355, 1981.

66. Rivers JM: Oral contraceptives and ascorbic acid. Am J Clin Nutr 28:550–554, 1975.

67. Schmidt KH, Hagmaier V, Horning DH, Vuilleumier J, Ratishauser G: Urinary oxalate excretion after large intakes of ascorbic acid in man. Am J Clin Nutr 34:305–311, 1981.

68. Stein HB, Hasan A, Fox IH: Ascorbic acid-induced uricosuria: a consequence of megavitamin therapy. Ann Intern Med 84:385–388, 1976.

69. Tuckerman MM, Turco SJ (eds): Human Nutrition. Philadelphia: Lea & Febiger, 1983, p 99.

70. Cook J, Monser ER: Vitamin C and the common cold and iron absorption. Am J Clin Nutr 30:235–241, 1977.

71. Stein HB, Fox IH: Ascorbic acid-induced uricosuria—a consequence of megavitamin therapy. Ann Intern Med 84:385–388, 1976.

72. Alhadeff L, Gualtieri CT, Lipton M: Toxic effects of water-soluble vitamins. Nutr Rev 42:33–40, 1984.

73. Shilotri PG, Bhat KS: Effect of megadoses of vitamin C on bactericidal activity of leukocytes. Am J Clin Nutr 30:1077–1081, 1977.

74. Luke B (ed): Principles of Nutrition on Diet Therapy, Boston, Little, Brown & Co, 1984, p 156.

75. Baird IM, Hughes RE, Wilson HK, Davies JEW, Howard AN: The effects of ascorbic acid and flavonoids on the occurrence of symptoms normally associated with a common cold. Am J Clin Nutr 32:1686–1690, 1979.

76. Pitt HA, Costrini AM: Vitamin C prophylaxis in Marine recruits. JAMA 241:908–911, 1979.

77. Sperber SJ, Hayden FG: Chemotherapy of rhinovirus colds. Antimicrob Agents Chemother 32(4):409–419, 1988.

78. Coulehan JL: Ascorbic acid and the common cold: an evaluation of the evidence. Postgrad Med 66:153–160, 1979.

79. McRae TD, Freedman ML: Why vitamin B_{12} deficiency should be treated aggressively. Geriatrics 44(11):70–79, 1989.

80. Carethers M: Diagnosing vitamin B_{12} deficiency, a common geriatric disorder. Geriatrics 43(3):89–112, 1988.

81. Kesler D, Peterson CD: Oral calcium supplements. Postgrad Med 78(5):123–125, 1985.

82. Haynes RD Jr, Murad F, Agents affecting calcification: calcium, parathyroid hormone, calcitonin, vitamin D, and other compounds. In Gilman AG, Goodman AS, Rall TW, Murad F (eds): The Pharmacological Basis of Therapeutics, ed. 7. New York, Macmillan, 1985, pp 1517–1518.

83. Lutwak L, Singer FR, Urist MR: Current concepts of bone metabolism. Ann Intern Med 80:630, 1974.

84. Precup AV (ed): United States Pharmacopeia Drug Information Advice for the Patient. Vol 2, ed. 9, p 104.

85. Orwoll ES: The milk-alkali syndrome: current concepts. Ann Intern Med 97:242–248, 1982.

86. Randall RE, Strauss MB, McNeely WF: The milk-alkali syndrome. Arch Intern Med 107:163, 1961.

87. Hunter H III, Callaway CW: Calcium tablets for hypertension (editorial). Ann Intern Med 103:946–947, 1985.

88. Nordin BEC, Heaney RP: Calcium supplementation on the diet: justified by present evidence. Br Med J 300:1056–1560, 1990.

89. Trachtenbarg DE: Treatment of osteoporosis. Postgraduate ed 87(4):263–270, 1990.

90. Kanis JA, Passmore R: Calcium supplementation of the diet. Part II. Br Med J 298:205–208, 1989.

91. Grobbee DE, Waal-Manning: The role of calcium supplementation in the treatment of hypertension. Drugs 39(1):7–18, 1990.

92. Henry HJ, McCarron DA, Morris CD, Parrott-Garcia M: Increasing calcium intake lowers blood pressure: the literature reviewed. J Am Diet Assoc 85:182–185, 1985.

93. Lipkin M, Newmark H: Effect of added dietary calcium on idonic epithelia-cell proliferation in subjects at high risk for familiar colonic cancer. N Engl J Med 313:1381–1384, 1985.

94. Monsen ER: Iron nutrition and absorption: dietary factors which impact iron bioavailability. J Am Diet Assoc 88(7):786–790, 1990.

95. Monsen ER, Hallberg L, Laurisse M, Hegsted M, Cook JD, et al.: Estimation of available dietary iron. Am J Clin Nutr 31:131–141, 1978.

96. Dallman PR: Iron deficiency: diagnosis and treatment. West J Med 134:496–504, 1981.

97. Ivey M, Elmer G, Nutritional supplement mineral and vitamin products. In Handbook of Non-prescription Drugs, ed. 8. Washington, D.C., American Pharmaceutical Association, 1986, pp 221–223.

98. Taylor KB, Anthony LE: Clinical Nutrition. New York, McGraw-Hill, 1983, p 518.

99. Kutsky RJ: Handbook of Vitamins, Minerals and Hormones. New York, Van Nostrand Reinhold, 1981, vol I, p 66.

100. Prasad AS, Cossack ZT: Zinc supplementation and growth in sickle cell disease. Ann Intern Med 100:367–371, 1984.

101. Taylor KB, Anthony LE: Clinical Nutrition. New York, McGraw-Hill, 1983, p 517.

102. Sandstead HH: Copper bioavailability and requirements. Am J Clin Nutr 35:809–813, 1982.

103. Prasad AS: Zinc deficiency in man. In Hambidge KM, Nichols BL Jr (eds): Zinc and Copper in Clinical Medicine. New York, SP Medical and Scientific Books, 1978, p 11.

104. Halsted JA, Smith JC Jr, Irwin MI: A conspectus of research on zinc requirements of man. J Nutr 104:345, 1974.

105. Prasad AS: Clinical, biochemical and nutritional spectrum of zinc deficiency in human subjects: an update. Nutr Rev 41:197–208, 1983.

106. Pories WJ, Henzel JH, Rob CG, Stain WH: Acceleration of wound healing in man with zinc sulfate given by mouth. Lancet 1:121–124, 1967.

107. Prasad AS, Zinc deficiency and toxicity. In Prasad AS, Oberleas D (eds): Trace Elements in Human Health and Disease. New York, Academic Press, 1976, pp 15–16.

108. Fosmire GJ: Zinc toxicity. Am J Clin Nutr 51:225–227, 1990.

109. Chandra RK: Excessive intake of zinc impairs immune response. JAMA 252:1443–1446, 1984.

110. Williams SR (ed): Nutrition and Diet Therapy. St. Louis: Times Mirror/Mosby, College Publishing, 1985, p 132.

111. Luke B (ed): Principles of Nutrition and Diet Therapy. Boston: Little, Brown & Co, 1984, p 141.

112. Robinson CH, Lawler MR, Chenoweth WL, Garwick AE (eds): Normal and Therapeutic Nutrition, ed. 17. New York: Macmillan, 1986, p 169.

113. Marcus R, Coulston AM, Water-soluble vitamins. In Gilman AG, Goodman LS, Rall TW, Murad F (eds): The Pharmacological Basis of Therapeutics, ed. 7. New York, Macmillan, 1985, pp 1551–1572.

114. Tuckerman MM, Turco SJ (eds): Human Nutrition. Philadelphia: Lea & Febiger, 1983, pp 91–123.

115. Luke B (ed): Principles of Nutrition and Diet Therapy. Boston: Little, Brown & Co, 1984, pp 158–159.

116. Tuckerman MM, Turco SJ (eds): Human Nutrition. Philadelphia: Lea & Febiger, 1983, pp 27, 34–36, 141–155.

117. Williams SR (ed): Nutrition and Diet Therapy. St. Louis: Times Mirror/Mosby College Publishing, 1985, pp 180–181.

CHAPTER 11

PARENTERAL AND ENTERAL NUTRITION

REX O. BROWN, Pharm.D. and STACEY L. WOJTYSIAK, Pharm.D.

Specialized nutrition support includes parenteral and enteral nutrition. The practice of providing specialized nutrition support to patients is a relatively young discipline compared with other medical specialities. In 1968, Dudrick et al. reported that growth and development could be sustained with long-term parenteral nutrition in an infant who could not be fed via the gastrointestinal tract (1). Most practitioners consider this the beginning of modern clinical nutrition. During the last 25 years, many advances have been made to allow safe and efficacious delivery of parenteral and enteral nutrients.

Since the original report of Dudrick et al., the prevalence and complications of malnutrition have become more appreciated. Clearly, 30 to 50% of hospitalized patients in the United States have some malnutrition. Patients with malnutrition have poor wound healing, depressed immunocompetence, and an increased prevalence of septic and other postoperative complications.

Parenteral and enteral nutrition are powerful and relatively expensive interventions; however, they are not without complications. This has led to the development of nutrition support teams that assist in making specialized nutrition support safe and efficacious. Traditionally, the nutrition support team has consisted of multidisciplinary healthcare practitioners including a physician, pharmacist, nurse, and dietitian. The pharmacist's role has ranged from ensuring provision of a properly compounded parenteral nutrition solution to being the director of the team. Most commonly, the pharmacist provides assistance in prescribing the parenteral or enteral nutrient formula, monitors the patient for metabolic complications, educates other practitioners about compatibilities and drug-nutrient interactions, and assists the institution in developing a cost-effective formulary of nutrition products. In some institutions, the pharmacist is the director or coordinator of the nutrition support team with complete or nearly complete responsibility for parenteral and enteral nutrition administration.

NUTRITIONAL ASSESSMENT

Nutritional assessment evaluates a patient's nutritional status (2), and can be used to detect and quantitate malnutrition in a variety of diseases. Nutritional assessment includes both science and art in interpreting the different tests and measurements available. The correct clinical interpretation of these measurements requires a thorough understanding of the particular disease process. Only then can the nutritional status be diagnosed correctly. Delayed wound healing, impaired collagen formation, and decreased resistance to infection have all been associated with undernutrition (i.e., a depressed body cell mass). Patients with undernutrition can have this wasting process halted or reversed by specialized nutrition support. It is not known whether improvement in nutritional status can improve patient outcome (3).

Nutritional assessment has traditionally been divided into four parts: history and physical examination, anthropometric measurement, biochemical assessment of serum proteins, and evaluation of immune status.

History and Physical Examination

The history and physical examination should be used as a screening mechanism to identify patients who require a more thorough assessment. A history of unintentional weight loss, either chronic or acute, is usually a sign of suboptimal nutritional intake or altered metabolism. Chronic disease, gastrointestinal disease, certain social factors, or an abnormal metabolic state all may be risk factors for developing malnutrition (Table 11.1). Physical signs suggestive of malnutrition include edema, decubitus ulcers, muscle wasting, poor would healing, and glossitis. Patients with documented unintentional weight loss, chronic disease, or physical signs as described above should have a thorough nutritional assessment.

Anthropometric Measurements

The anthropometric measurements are used to assess fat and somatic protein stores. The somatic protein stores include skeletal muscle and the visceral organs and are also referred to as the body cell mass. Subcutaneous fat is often assessed by a series of skinfold measurements with an instrument called a Lange caliper. The most popular sites for skinfold measurement in the institutionalized patient are the triceps and subscapular area. These areas are usually available in a cooperative patient. Normal values exist for each measurement individually or as a sum in adult patients from ages 18 to 55 years. A value below the 40th percentile suggests some fat depletion. This method is attractive because it is relatively noninvasive and inexpensive. The assessment of skinfold measurements can be erroneous, however, if a patient has edema, if the equipment is not standardized, or if several observers are used. Also,

Table 11.1.
Risk Factors for Undernutrition That Can Be Detected in a Patient History and Physical Examination

Chronic disease
    Renal failure
    Liver failure
    Chronic obstructive pulmonary disease
    Congestive heart failure
    Diabetes
Gastrointestinal disease
    Peptic ulcer disease
    Inflammatory bowel disease
    Pancreatitis
    Short bowel syndrome
Social factors
    Alcohol abuse
    Drug abuse
Abnormal metabolic state
    Cancer
    Sepsis
    Trauma or thermal injury

Table 11.2.
Formulas for Ideal Body Weight

Male	50 kg + 2.3 kg for each inch above 60 inches
Female	45.5 kg + 2.3 kg for each inch above 60 inches

some individuals may have very little subcutaneous fat and yet be in excellent physical condition (e.g., trained athletes such as runners or body builders).

The somatic protein compartment may be assessed indirectly by using body weight, midarm muscle circumference (MAMC), or arm muscle area (AMA). Chronic assessment of body weight is a relatively good marker of nutritional status in most patients. As mentioned earlier, acute or chronic weight loss is a harbinger of poor nutritional intake or altered metabolism. Fluid-overload or edema results in a body weight greater than the patient's usual weight, which could mask impending undernutrition, especially in the critical care setting where these are relatively common. Overhydrated patients often lose substantial weight during specialized nutrition support administration. This is actually desirable when excess fluid is mobilized. Conversely, other patients may retain excessive fluid and salt during specialized nutrition support intervention and gain weight very rapidly. Obviously weight fluctuations must be interpreted very carefully in all patients. Another way to assess body weight is to compare the patients' weight with their ideal body weight (Table 11.2) or with the Metropolitan Life Insurance Company Tables of 1984.

Somatic protein stores can also be assessed by calcu-

lation of the MAMC or AMA. The MAMC is calculated from the triceps skinfold (TSF) and midarm circumference (MAC) as follows:

$$\text{MAMC (in cm)} = \text{MAC (in cm)} - \pi \, \text{TSF (in mm)}/10$$

The AMA is calculated from the MAMC as follows:

$$\text{AMA (in cm}^2) = (\text{MAMC in cm})^2/4 \, \pi$$

Both of these methods are relatively easy, inexpensive, and noninvasive. The problems with skinfold measurements also exist with these assessments of somatic protein stores (edema, variation among observers).

Biochemical Assessment of Serum Proteins

Serum concentrations of several visceral proteins have been used initially and serially during specialized nutrition support intervention to assess nutritional status. Unfortunately, other factors such as metabolic stress, hydration status, and hepatic function may influence these serum concentration measurements. Although these serum markers lack sensitivity and specificity, some of them serve as very good prognostic indicators of patient outcome and therefore continue to be the subject of intense study. Albumin, transferrin, and prealbumin are constitutive proteins used most frequently. Other serum proteins are being studied, but their role in nutritional assessment has not yet been determined.

Albumin is a protein with a half-life of 21 days and a large body pool compared with other secretory proteins. The normal serum concentration of albumin is 35 to 50 g/liter (3.5 to 5.0 g/dl) in adults. A decrease in the serum concentration of albumin suggests inadequate protein intake, especially when the serum concentration is chronically depressed. An albumin concentration of 30 to 34 g/liter (3.0 to 3.4 g/dl) suggests mild protein depletion; 25 to 29 (2.5 to 2.9), moderate depletion; and <25 (2.5), severe depletion. Bed rest, overhydration, and metabolic stress such as sepsis can all depress the serum concentration of albumin. Regardless of the cause, a depressed serum albumin concentration is associated with increased hospital morbidity and mortality. Therefore, many practitioners consider the serum albumin concentration to be very important. Because albumin has a long half-life and large body pool, it responds very slowly to specialized nutrition support intervention. In fact, some patients demonstrate a decrease in the serum albumin concentration during specialized nutrition support, presumably due to an increase in extracellular water and salt (4). Often, these patients have an ongoing septic process that increases aldosterone and antidiuretic hormone activity. Because other factors (mentioned above) can lower the serum concentration of albumin, the use of it as a nutritional marker must be interpreted cautiously. Its use as a prognostic indicator, however, cannot be ignored.

Transferrin is a secretory protein with a half-life of 8 days which serves as a carrier for iron. It has a much smaller body pool than albumin and its normal serum concentration is 2 to 3.5 g/liter (200 to 350 mg/dl). Some investigators have suggested calculating serum transferrin from total iron-binding capacity; however, direct measurement is much more accurate. A serum concentration of transferrin of 1.5 to 2 g/liter (150 to 200 mg/dl) suggests mild protein depletion; 1 to 1.5 g/liter (100 to 150 mg/dl), moderate depletion; and <1g/liter (<100 mg/dl), severe depletion. Because transferrin has a smaller body pool and shorter half-life than albumin, it is much more sensitive to protein-calorie deprivation or nutritional repletion. Therefore, it is used frequently in serial monitoring of patients receiving specialized nutrition support. Serum transferrin concentrations are attractive because they respond to nutritional repletion rather quickly (e.g., with weekly monitoring), are easy to measure, and are becoming available in many institutions. Iron deficiency anemia increases the transferrin serum concentration, while injury and sepsis depress it.

Prealbumin, also called thyroxine-binding prealbumin, has a normal serum concentration of 15 to 40 mg/dl. It is the major carrier protein for thyroxine and retinol-binding protein and has a half-life of 2 days. Because of the short half-life and relatively small body pool, prealbumin is quite sensitive to nutritional deprivation and repletion. Many institutions have added this laboratory test because it is inexpensive and relatively easy to perform. The serum concentration of prealbumin rises during nutrition support, even when the nitrogen balance remains negative. The correlation between improvement in nitrogen balance and increase in serum prealbumin concentration is highly significant; however, other events besides nutritional intake influence the prealbumin concentration. Acutely stressful events such as trauma or sepsis are known to depress the prealbumin serum concentration.

Several other serum protein concentrations are being studied for their role in documenting nutritional repletion. Retinol-binding protein, fibronectin, and insulin-like growth factor I have all been studied recently. Retinol-binding protein serum concentration is influenced by vitamin A status and the glomerular filtration rate. Its very short half-life of 12 hr may make it too sensitive to nutritional deprivation or intake. It may reflect the composition of the last meal instead of nutritional intake over a few days or weeks. Fibronectin is a glycoprotein nonspecific opsonin. It has a half-life of about 24 hr and is synthesized by the liver. Although fibronectin appears to respond positively during nutrition support, many other factors can alter its serum concentration (e.g., sepsis, trauma, shock). Insulin-like growth factor-I is a growth hormone–dependent protein that possesses broad anabolic activity. The concentration correlates very well with nitrogen balance and increases during nutritional repletion

(5). Clinical trials using human growth hormone and insulin-like growth factor-I as adjunct therapy to nutrition support are currently being conducted in the United States.

There are several acute-phase proteins (e.g., C-reactive protein) that increase markedly during stressful events and decrease during recovery. The role of these proteins in nutrition support intervention is unclear; however, some of them are included in the Prognostic Inflammatory and Nutritional Index (6). This index includes the acute-phase proteins, α-1 acid glycoprotein and C-reactive protein, and the constitutive proteins, albumin and prealbumin. Other investigators have attempted to predict postoperative morbidity and mortality from preoperative nutritional status. One example of this is the Prognostic Nutritional Index, which includes serum albumin and transferrin concentrations, triceps skinfold, and cell-mediated immunity (7).

Evaluation of Immune Status

The relationship between malnutrition, depressed immune status, and infection has been appreciated for years. Many of these observations have been done in third-world countries where the prevalence of undernutrition is relatively high in the general population. Traditionally, an assessment of immune stores (total lymphocyte count) and immune function (cell-mediated immunity) has been done in hospitalized patients who require specialized nutrition. Immune stores are usually assessed by determination of the total lymphocyte count (TLC), which includes predominantly thymus-derived lymphocytes (T cells). The total lymphocyte count is calculated from the product of peripheral white blood cell count (WBC) and the percentage of lymphocytes.

TLC (cells/liter) (cells/mm^3)

= WBC (cells/liter) (cells/mm^3) $\times$ % lymphocytes/100

A TLC $>2 \times 10^9$/liter (>2000/mm^3) suggests adequate immune stores. A TLC of 1.2 to 2.0 $\times$ 10^9/liter (1200 to 2000/mm^3) suggests mild depletion; 0.8 to 1.2 $\times$ 10^9/liter (800 to 1200/mm^3), moderate depletion; and <0.8 $\times$ 10^9/liter (<800/mm^3), severe depletion of immune reserves.

Immune function is usually assessed by measuring the response to common antigens through skin testing. Antigens that have been used in this procedure include *Candida albicans*, mumps, streptokinase/streptodornase, tetanus, and *Trichophyton*. One product that is produced commercially includes seven antigens and a placebo that can be placed simultaneously (CMI Multitest, Merrieux). Most patients that have intact immune function will respond to both *Candida* and mumps skin tests; therefore these are most commonly used. A positive test result is at least a 5-mm area of induration at the site of application within 24 to 48 hr. Geriatric patients may react slowly and not demonstrate a positive response until 74 hr after application. Many other factors, such as drug therapy (e.g., steroids, histamine antagonists) and certain disease states (e.g., cancer) can interfere with the body's response to cell-mediated immunity. Also, results can be questionable if standardized methods of application and observation are not used. A review of the use of skin testing seriously questioned the role of this assessment method in specialized nutrition support (8). Since then, immunology has experienced a resurgence, undoubtedly due to the AIDS epidemic and successful solid organ transplantation, and this renewed interest has been carried over to specialized nutrition support. Several clinical trials are currently being conducted to identify specific nutrients that improve immune function. Some compounds that show particular promise include arginine, omega-3 fatty acids, β-carotene, and nucleotides.

Types of Malnutrition

Patients with malnutrition can usually be categorized by using the above methods of nutritional assessment. Marasmus is a form of undernutrition that results from a chronic deprivation of protein and calories. Patients with this disorder are relatively easy to identify as they have considerable wasting of somatic protein and fat. Their serum protein concentrations and immune status are often intact. This disorder is seen in patients who suffer from chronic disease and ingest a suboptimal amount of nutrition over a relatively long period of time (i.e., semistarvation). Table 11.3 contrasts the various types of malnutrition.

Kwashiorkor is traditionally classified as protein deficiency. Patients with kwashiorkor typically have adequate or excess caloric stores, as evidenced by sufficient body fat (Table 11.3). These patients often have a weight-for-height value that exceeds normal. Kwashiorkor patients have depressed serum concentrations of most proteins and often have depressed immune function. The most common cause of this disorder is severe metabolic stress (e.g., trauma, sepsis, thermal injury). Less common are patients who ingest adequate calories and a low-protein diet over

a long period of time. Kwashiorkor is often difficult to diagnose at the bedside because these patients appear to be well nourished.

Kwashiorkor-marasmus mix results when a patient with marasmus is subjected to high metabolic stress. These patients have deficits in all categories of the nutritional assessment and have the highest risk for hospital morbidity and mortality (Table 11.3).

Patients with excess body weight secondary to fat are classified as obese if they are >20% above their ideal body weight. Obesity is a type of malnutrition that usually results from a prolonged increase in calories over what is needed or used. If subjected to metabolic stress, these patients can quickly develop kwashiorkor.

Nutritional assessment is used frequently to document malnutrition in the hospital and in outpatients. An adequate history and physical examination in concert with the assessment of fat stores, somatic protein stores, serum protein concentrations, and immune function, enable the practitioner to effectively identify patients at nutritional risk. Some investigators have suggested that clinical judgement during the history and physical examination is as effective as the complete nutritional assessment (9). Perhaps these practitioners need special training to be able to correctly identify the patients at nutritional risk (10).

Because no one nutritional-assessment marker effectively identifies all patients at nutritional risk and because many nonnutritional factors alter the currently used tests, investigators continue to evaluate new methods of nutritional assessment. Some of the methods currently under investigation include bioelectric impedance analysis, underwater weighing, muscle-strength testing, neutron-activation analysis, and radioisotope analysis. Some of these methods will be too expensive or invasive for general clinical use; however, others such as bioelectric impedance analysis and muscle-strength testing show particular promise.

ENERGY AND PROTEIN REQUIREMENTS

After completion of the nutritional assessment in a patient who is going to receive specialized nutrition support, the nonprotein energy and protein goals must be determined. These goals will be different for each patient, based on the nutritional-assessment results, the purpose for initiating specialized nutrition support, and the size of the patient.

Energy

The energy requirements for an individual patient may be predicted by several different methods. The degree of metabolic stress and any chronic disease afflicting the patient also determine energy requirements. The most widely used method is the calculation of the basal energy

Table 11.3.
Types of Malnutrition

Characteristic	Marasmus	Kwashiorkor	Kwashiorkor-Marasmus Mix	Obesity ↓
Weight for height	↓	normal or ↑	↓	↑
Fat stores	↓	↑	↓	↑
Somatic protein stores	↓	normal or ↑	↓	↑
Serum protein concentrations	normal	↓	↓	normal
Immune function	normal	↓	↓	normal

expenditure (BEE) using the Harris-Benedict equations developed in 1919 (11). The BEE was developed by measuring oxygen consumption using direct calorimetry in 239 healthy male and female subjects. The two equations use the patient's gender, weight, height, and age.

Males: BEE = 66.4730 + 13.7516 Wt

+ 5.0033 Ht + 6.7550 Age

Females: BEE = 655.0950 + 9.5630 Wt

+ 1.8496 Ht + 4.6756 Age

BEE is in kilocalories per day, Wt is in kilograms, Ht is in centimeters, and Age is in years. BEE reflects the number of kilocalories expended during a 24-hr period in a subject at bedrest in a fasted state in a semidark room. This value can be multiplied by a correction factor that accounts for physical activity or stress to determine an energy goal (12). Examples of these correction factors appear in Table 11.4.

In certain circumstances, all of the information required to calculate the BEE may not be available, so an alternative method may be used to determine the energy requirements. If the patient's weight is known, an estimated nonprotein energy goal may be calculated. A range of 25 to 35 kcal/kg/day is generally accepted for most patients (13). An energy goal of 25 kcal/kg/day would be used for an elective surgical patient who is otherwise healthy, whereas a septic or trauma patient would require at least 35 kcal/kg/day. A severely burned patient may require as much as 45 kcal/kg/day initially.

By using the Harris-Benedict equations with correction factors, patients receive energy based on their primary disease state or injuries. However, multiple stress factors may alter the energy requirement for a particular patient. Factors such as pulmonary toilet (pounding on the back to break up lung secretions) and pain can raise energy requirements, while sedation and immobilization may lower them. Thus, the ideal way to determine an individual patient's energy requirement is to measure the resting energy expenditure (REE) of that patient. Indirect calori-

metry may be used. This involves using a mobile metabolic cart and measuring the concentration of oxygen consumed (VO_2) and carbon dioxide produced (VCO_2) over time. After measuring VO_2 and VCO_2, the complete Weir formula can be used to calculate the patient's REE (15).

REE = (3.941 VO2 + 1.106 VCO2)1.44 − 2.14 UUN

REE is in kilocalories per day, VO2 is in milliliters per minute, VCO2 is in milliliters per minute, and UUN is urinary urea nitrogen in grams per 24 hours. If a 24-hr urine sample is obtained the same day indirect calorimetry is performed, the nitrogen data are used in the calculation. The difference in the REE obtained from the complete Weir formula and the abbreviated Weir equation (without the UUN term) is less than 2% (15). Thus a 24-hr urine specimen is not required for each REE determination by indirect calorimetry. Many practitioners add 10 to 30% to the REE to allow for movement and patient interventions during the day (14, 16). Information may also be gained about net substrate oxidation by using the respiratory quotient (RQ). RQ is the ratio of VCO_2 to VO_2. Carbohydrate is oxidized at an RQ of 1.0 (i.e., for every mole of oxygen consumed, one mole of carbon dioxide is produced), while fat is oxidized at an RQ of 0.7 (less carbon dioxide is produced for the oxygen consumed). In between these two quotients is the "theoretical" desired RQ of 0.85, where "mixed substrate" oxidation exists, or the mutual oxidation of carbohydrate and fat. Although protein can be oxidized for fuel (RQ = 0.8), the body proteins are not intended as energy sources because they are structural elements of functioning organs.

Protein

Protein requirements for an individual depend on many factors. In health, the recommended daily allowance (RDA) for protein for an adult person is 0.8 g/kg/day (17). In a hospital environment patients are generally stressed and thus may require higher doses of protein. Depending on the clinical status of the patient, the protein requirement may range from the RDA to >2.0 g/kg/day. As metabolic stress increases, the protein required to maintain adequate protein stores increases. An elective operative procedure such as cholecystectomy results in mild stress and a modest increase in protein requirements (Table 11.5). Patients with infections or malignancy have a moderate degree of stress, while those who experience a traumatic injury or are septic may be severely stressed (18). Severe thermal injury may require protein doses >2.0 g/kg/day in selected situations.

Although the doses presented in Table 11.5 are reasonable goals, each patient should be monitored closely to determine whether the desired response is achieved (e.g., nutritional repletion, wound healing). During periods of metabolic stress, protein turnover is markedly increased,

Table 11.4.
BEE Correction Factors for Activity and Injury[a]

Condition	% by which to increase BEE
Confined to bed	↑ 20%
Elective surgery	↑ 20%
Ambulatory	↑ 30%
Traumatic injury	↑ 35%
Major septic episode	↑ 60%
Severe thermal injury	↑ 110%

[a] From Long CL, Blakemare WS: Energy and protein requirements in the hospitalized patient. J Parenter Enter Nutr 3:69–71, 1979.

Table 11.5.
Protein Requirements for Hospitalized Adult Patients

Condition	Protein Dose (g/kg/day)
Maintenance	1.0
Mild stress	1.2
Moderate stress or repletion	1.5
Severe stress	2.0

Table 11.6.
Calculation of Nitrogen Balance

Nitrogen balance $= N_{IN} - N_{OUT}$

$$N_{IN} = \frac{\text{Protein intake (g)}}{6.25}$$

$N_{OUT} = \text{UUN (g/liter)} \times \text{24-hr urine volume (liters)} + 4 \text{ g}$

and urinary excretion of urea nitrogen is elevated, which can lead to rapid erosion of the lean body mass if adequate protein is not administered. The "gold standard" to measure protein nutriture is nitrogen balance, with the obvious goal of achieving nitrogen equilibrium or a positive balance. This measurement is obtained by subtracting nitrogen output from nitrogen input during a 24-hr period (Table 11.6). Nitrogen input is calculated by dividing protein intake for 24 hr by 6.25 (protein is approximately 16% nitrogen). Nitrogen output is calculated by adding 4 g to the grams of urea nitrogen excreted by the kidneys during a 24-hr period. The 4 g represents nonmeasurable nitrogen losses such as stool losses, skin losses, and nonurea nitrogen losses in the urine. A nitrogen balance of 2 to 6 g/day suggests adequate intake of nonprotein energy and protein. A nitrogen balance between -2 and 2 g/day suggests that nitrogen equilibrium has been attained. A nitrogen balance below -2 g/day suggests more protein, more calories, or both are needed. Once the energy and protein requirements have been calculated and the nutrient formula has been prescribed, many practitioners calculate the nonprotein calorie (energy) to nitrogen ratio (NPC:N). Unstressed patients generally require a NPC:N of 150:1, while stressed patients require a ratio of 100:1. This reflects the increased protein needs of patients who are infected or injured (19).

PARENTERAL NUTRITION

Clinicians and investigators have long recognized the need for intravenous nutrition support in various patient populations. This is especially important in patients without a functional gastrointestinal tract. Over 100 years ago, six major dietary components were recognized: water, salt, vitamins, carbohydrates, fat, and protein. The landmark experiments conducted by Dr. Stanley Dudrick and colleagues in beagle puppies and later in humans in the late 1960s changed the medical world's perspective on parenteral nutrition support (1). They demonstrated successful administration of parenteral nutrition over a period of several weeks by documenting growth and improved nutritional status (1). Today, industry and clinical investigators continue to discover new parenteral nutrition products that improve upon existing ones targeted to benefit specific patient populations.

Generally, parenteral nutrition should be reserved for patients who require specialized nutrition support and who do not have a functional or accessible gastrointestinal tract. With the multitude of available parenteral nutrient products, the practitioner needs sound guidelines so patients may receive this therapy in a safe and efficacious way. Indications for the use of parenteral nutrition have been developed by the American Society for Parenteral and Enteral Nutrition (20). These indications are summarized in Table 11.7.

Types of Parenteral Nutrition

Parenteral nutrition may be given via a central or peripheral vein. Although central parenteral nutrition is more commonly used, peripheral parenteral nutrition is used by some institutions in certain patients.

Peripheral parenteral nutrition can be used in patients that are being weaned from central parenteral nutrition to a normal diet, or as an adjunct to an oral or enteral diet. Generally, 900 mOsm/liter is the maximum concentration tolerated by peripheral veins (21). Actually, a solution of 600 mOsm/liter is better tolerated and may lower the risk

Table 11.7.
Summary of A.S.P.E.N. Guidelines for Parenteral Nutrition[a]

Parenteral nutrition should be used
  Massive small bowel resection
  Chronic radiation enteritis
  Severe vomiting or diarrhea
  Patients unable to consume oral intake due to chemotherapy, radiation therapy, organ transplantation
  Severe pancreatitis
  Undernutrition with inability to absorb enteral nutrients
  Catabolic state associated with inability to use enteral route for >5 days
Parenteral nutrition would be helpful
  Enterocutaneous fistulae
  Undernutrition with major abdominal surgical procedure
  Inability to use enteral route within 7–10 days of hospitalization
  Small-bowel obstruction secondary to adhesions
  High-dose chemotherapy
  Inflammatory bowel disease

[a] From: Guidelines for use of total parenteral nutrition in the hospitalized adult patient. J Parenter Enter Nutr 10:441–445, 1986.

of phlebitis. Subtherapeutic doses of heparin or hydrocortisone, or concurrent infusion of fat emulsion with peripheral parenteral nutrition have been used in attempts to decrease the risk of phlebitis. Peripheral parenteral nutrition is intended to be used for short periods of time (e.g., 5 to 7 days) as adjunctive therapy. Dilute nutrient solutions must be used to maintain the osmolality of the solution within limits that the peripheral vein can tolerate. A solution with a final protein concentration of 3 to 5% and a dextrose concentration of 5 to 10% is commonly used for this type of therapy. It is extremely difficult, if not impossible, to meet a patient's nutritional requirements, because of the large volumes of fluid required. Also, the administration of peripheral parenteral nutrition has not demonstrated a significant benefit over 5% dextrose alone, which makes this therapy questionable (22).

Most patients receive parenteral nutrition via a large central vein. The superior vena cava is used most often after percutaneous catheterization of the subclavian, internal, or external jugular veins. The catheter may be placed in the operating room or at the patient's bedside using sterile technique and radiographic verification. A double or triple lumen catheter is used most often because patients who require parenteral nutrition often receive other intravenous medications or blood products. This provides access for the additional intravenous infusions without interrupting the administration of the parenteral nutrition. By having the catheter tip placed into the superior vena cava, very concentrated substrates may be infused because of the high rate of blood flow in this vein. Thus, required nutrients may be delivered in relatively small volumes without causing thrombophlebitis. This method is particularly effective in patients who have large energy and protein requirements or who require fluid restriction. If the catheter is properly cared for, it can be used indefinitely. The disadvantages of central parenteral nutrition include the increased prevalence of mechanical and metabolic complications (addressed in a later section).

Parenteral Nutrition Formula Components

PROTEIN

The initial protein products used in parenteral nutrition solutions were hydrolysates of naturally occurring proteins (fibrin, casein). Today, commercially available forms of parenteral protein are provided as crystalline amino acids. Generally, the protein in a parenteral nutrition solution is not included in the energy intake, because ideally it should be used for protein synthesis. However, if protein is oxidized for energy, it will yield 4 kcal/g. Patients undergoing severe metabolic stress may require large doses of protein and actually use it as a preferential calorie source.

Currently marketed amino acid products in the United States are provided as standard or modified amino acids.

Table 11.8.
Parenteral Amino Acid Categories with Examples

Patient Category	Example of Amino Acid Product
Normal (normal organ function)	Aminosyn, FreAmine III, Travasol
Fluid-restricted	Novamine 15%
Liver failure	HepatAmine
Renal failure	Aminosyn RF, NephrAmine, RenAmin
Metabolic stress	FreAmine HBC, Branchamin, Aminosyn-HBC

Standard amino acid products are used for patients with normal organ function and relatively normal nutritional needs. The modified amino acid formulations are marketed for patients with hepatic failure, renal failure, fluid restriction, or high metabolic stress. Currently available amino acid products for parenteral nutrition are listed in Table 11.8.

The standard amino acid formulas are composed of physiologic mixtures of essential and nonessential amino acids. Although these products are commercially available in several concentrations, many institutions are now stocking only the 10% concentrations, because lower concentrations can be made by adding sterile water with an automated compounder. These products are marketed with or without maintenance electrolytes.

Patients with severe liver failure develop many metabolic abnormalities, including disturbances in electrolyte and amino acid homeostasis (23). Some of these patients develop hepatic encephalopathy associated with decreased concentrations of branched-chain amino acids (BCAA) and elevated concentrations of aromatic amino acids (AAA) and methionine. The BCAAs include leucine, isoleucine, and valine, and the AAAs are phenylalanine, tyrosine, and tryptophan. In the absence of encephalopathy, liver failure patients who require parenteral nutrition may be maintained on standard amino acids. However, when hepatic encephalopathy is severe, the modified amino acid formula for hepatic failure may be used. Generally, patients should meet one of the following criteria to receive the modified amino acid: hepatic encephalopathy ≥grade 2, abnormal aminogram with a plasma molar ratio of BCAA:AAA of 2 or less, or hepatic encephalopathy associated with parenteral nutrition solutions containing standard amino acid solutions in doses needed for nutritional support. The modified amino acid formula contains high concentrations of BCAAs and low concentrations of AAAs and methionine. Parenteral nutrition with this product will normalize the amino acid profile. Some patients have demonstrated improvement in hepatic encephalopathy and a lower prevalence of mortality after receiving this formulation (24).

Patients with severe renal failure also have several metabolic changes, including electrolyte alterations and protein intolerance. Those who are not being dialyzed should have their daily protein dose restricted to 0.5 g/kg/day. Acute renal failure patients undergoing hemodialysis may be given 1.0 to 1.2 g protein/kg/day, while peritoneal dialysis patients may receive 1.2 to 1.5 g protein/kg/day. Modified amino acids for renal failure, which contain primarily essential amino acids, are more expensive than standard amino acids. Prospective, randomized controlled studies have demonstrated that standard amino acids are as effective as modified amino acids in renal failure patients who require parenteral nutrition (25). Thus, patients with severe renal failure should be given standard amino acids as part of parenteral nutrition in most clinical situations (26).

Some critically ill patients who require parenteral nutrition are markedly fluid-overloaded. In these patients, it is usually beneficial to use the smallest possible volume. The commercially available 15% amino acid product can be used to concentrate the parenteral nutrition formula in patients with overhydration or edema. Currently, this product is very expensive, so it should be reserved for patients who need severe fluid restriction.

Patients who are highly stressed have altered energy and protein metabolism. These patients take up BCAAs into skeletal muscle for energy. This has led to development of modified amino acid products with enhanced concentrations of the BCAAs. These products have been proposed to stimulate protein synthesis, decrease protein catabolism, and serve as a preferential fuel source. The many clinical trials using amino acids with an enhanced branched-chain content have produced equivocal results. Some suggest that patients receiving these modified amino acids have decreased skeletal muscle catabolism and enhanced protein synthesis (27). In contrast, other studies have found a lack of clinical benefit when BCAA-enriched solutions were compared with standard amino acids (28). Given the expense of the products and the equivocal results of clinical trials, careful evaluation is needed when using these products.

CARBOHYDRATE

The nonprotein energy source in parenteral nutrition solutions may be carbohydrate or fat. The carbohydrate component of the nutrient solutions is usually dextrose. Other carbohydrates such as xylitol, fructose, or sorbitol have been studied, but have not gained wide acceptance in the United States. Each gram of hydrated dextrose provides 3.4 kilocalories. Dextrose stock solutions of 5 to 70% are available for use in parenteral nutrition solutions. Many institutions are stocking primarily the 70% dextrose solutions because dilutions can be made using an automated compounder and sterile water. Final concentrations equal to or less than 10% dextrose in parenteral nutrition solutions may be infused peripherally. Solutions with higher concentrations should be administered through a large central vein.

Generally, dextrose infusion should not exceed 5 mg/kg/min (25 kcal/kg/day) during parenteral nutrition (29). This appears to be the maximum rate of dextrose utilization by the human body. Rates above 5 mg/kg/min are associated with lipogenesis, resulting in increased carbon dioxide production and hepatic steatosis.

Hospitalized patients receiving parenteral nutrition who have normal organ function often receive dextrose at a final concentration of 25% (Table 11.9). Therefore, a 70-kg patient would only receive 2 liters of parenteral nutrition if the dextrose infusion was held at 5 mg/kg/day as suggested above. Patients who are metabolically stressed may not tolerate this dose of carbohydrate, and yet they have large requirements for protein. They often need to receive less dextrose, such as 15% dextrose in the parenteral nutrition solution. Fluid-restricted patients (e.g., patients with congestive heart failure or liver failure) may receive smaller volumes of parenteral nutrition solutions when concentration dextrose is used. Patients with oliguric acute renal failure who are not undergoing dialysis often require fluid and protein restriction. High-calorie, low-protein parenteral nutrition formulas in small volumes are desired in these type of patients (Table 11.9).

FAT

The first fat emulsion introduced into the United States contained cottonseed oil, but it was removed from the U.S. market in 1965 because of severe adverse reactions. Today, commercially available fat emulsions contain soybean oil or combinations of soybean and safflower oils. Unless contraindicated, fat emulsions should be given as part of a patient's parenteral nutrition regimen to prevent essential fatty acid deficiency or to serve as a calorie source (30). Essential fatty acid deficiency has both biochemical and clinical signs. Biochemical evidence usually becomes apparent within 1 to 3 weeks after fat-free parenteral nutrition is started. Biochemical evidence includes increased serum concentrations of saturated fatty acids, decreased concentrations of essential fatty acids, and a triene:tetraene ratio greater than 0.4. This ratio is the concentration of 5,8,11-eicosatrienoic acid (a fatty acid that appears in essential fatty acid deficiency) divided by the concentration of arachidonic acid. Clinical evidence of essential fatty acid deficiency does not usually appear until several weeks of glucose-based parenteral nutrition has been given. Manifestations of essential fatty acid deficiency include thrombocytopenia, delayed wound healing, fatty liver, alopecia, and dry, thick, desquamating skin.

Intravenous fat emulsions provide a concentrated source of calories (9 kcal/g of fat) and correct or prevent essential fatty acid deficiency. Absolute contraindications to the administration of fat emulsions include pathologic

Table 11.9.

Examples of Some Parenteral Nutrition Solution Bases[a]

	Standard	Stress	Liver Failure	Acute Renal Failure
Components	500 ml D^{50}W	500 ml D^{30}W[b]	500 ml D^{70}W	500 ml D^{70}W
	500 ml AA 10%	500 ml AA 10%	500 ml AA 8%[c]	250 ml AA 10%[d]
Dextrose (%)	25	15	35	47
Amino acids (%)	5	5	4	3.3
Nonprotein energy (kcal/unit)	850	510	1190	1190
Protein (g/unit)	50	50	40	25

[a] Each patient's parenteral nutrition solution must be individualized, based on the metabolic state, fluid and electrolyte status, and size of the patient.

[b] Intravenous fat is generally used to supply some of the nonprotein energy.

[c] Hepatamine is often used if the patient has severe hepatic encephalopathy.

[d] When dialysis is instituted, the protein can often be liberalized to 500 ml of 5% AA.

Table 11.10.

Intravenous Fat Emulsion Products

Product	Lipid Source	Linoleic Acid (%)	Linolenic Acid (%)
Intralipid	100% soybean	50	9
Soyacal	100% soybean	49–60	6–9
Liposyn II	50% soybean/ 50% safflower	65.8	4.2
Liposyn III	100% soybean	54.5	8.3

Table 11.11.

An Example of Adult Electrolyte Concentrations Used in Parenteral Nutrition Solutions of Patients with Normal Electrolyte Concentrations and Normal Organ Function

Sodium	50 mEq/liter
Potassium	40 mEq/liter
Chloride	60 mEq/liter
Acetate	74 mEq/liter
Phosphorous	15 mM/liter
Calcium	5 mEq/liter
Magnesium	12 mEq/liter

hyperlipemia, lipoid nephrosis, severe egg allergy, and acute pancreatitis associated with hyperlipidemia. Patients with acute pancreatitis who do not have hyperlipidemia may receive fat emulsions. Fat emulsions should be used cautiously in patients with severe liver disease, acute respiratory distress syndrome, high metabolic stress, or blood coagulation disorders. Most clinicians administer 10 to 40% (maximum of 60%) of the nonprotein calories as fat, with the remainder being given as carbohydrate. The usual adult daily dose of fat is 0.5 to 1 g/kg/day, with the maximum dose being 2.5 g/kg/day. Table 11.10 lists commercially available fat emulsions, which are marketed in concentrations of 10% (1.1 kcal/ml) or 20% (2.0 kcal/ml). Currently, most clinicians infuse the daily dose of fat over a 24-hr period as a continuous infusion (e.g., 250 ml of 20% lipid infused at 10 ml/hr) or as a component of a total nutrient admixture. The 10% and 20% products can be infused at a maximum rate of 125 ml/hr and 60 ml/hr respectively; however, this is rarely done now. The lipid emulsions contain varying amounts of the essential fatty acids, linoleic and linolenic acid, and also contain egg yolk phospholipid as an emulsifying agent and glycerin, which makes the product isotonic.

If administered in the recommended doses, intravenous fat emulsions are very safe. Most side effects are due to the administration of excessive doses of fat emulsions

or excessive rates of infusion. Adverse reactions include nausea and vomiting, headache, fever, chills, chest or back pain, and irritation at the infusion site. Reactions that may be associated with long-term use include hepatomegaly, jaundice, splenomegaly, and thrombocytopenia. Fat-overload syndrome, reported with doses exceeding 4 g/kg/day, includes focal seizures, fever, leukocytosis, and shock. Fat emulsions have also been reported to suppress immune function when relatively large doses of these products are infused. Currently, fat emulsion products are being developed that contain different fatty acid profiles, designed for better utilization of fat. Fat emulsions containing medium-chain triglycerides, short-chain triglycerides, or carnitine may become available after clinical trials are completed. Most likely, these new products will be marketed as combinations of the different triglycerides (e.g., long-chain triglyceride, 25%, and medium-chain triglyceride, 75%).

ELECTROLYTES

Electrolytes in maintenance or therapeutic doses must be added to the parenteral nutrition daily to maintain electrolyte homeostasis (Table 11.11). Requirements for individual electrolytes vary, depending on many factors in a patient's clinical course. Electrolyte imbalance may arise from insufficient intake, extraordinary losses, or a combination of both. Patients may have large renal or extrarenal losses of electrolytes and fluid. Occasionally these may need to be quantified by collecting the appropriate fluids and analyzing their electrolyte content. Extrarenal electrolyte losses may include losses from diarrhea, vomiting, fistulae, or nasogastric suctioning. In addition, various pharmacotherapeutic interventions may decrease or increase individual electrolyte requirements. For example, sodium ticarcillin administration delivers a substantial amount of sodium to the patient and causes renal potassium wasting. Amphotericin B therapy increases magnesium and potassium renal losses. Relative electrolyte deficiencies may develop as a result of intracellular shifts of electrolytes from the extracellular fluid compartments. For instance, intracellular shifts of potassium occur during metabolic alkalosis because intracellular hydrogen ions are exchanged for extracellular potassium ions. Also, refeeding chronically starved patients results in an intracellular shift of potassium, phosphorus, and magnesium.

Electrolytes are available as single- or multiple-entity products. When calculating individual electrolyte requirements, the clinician must take into account the obligate electrolyte content of the particular amino acid solution chosen for parenteral nutrition. For example, most amino acid products contain substantial amounts of chloride and acetate salts. Once the phosphorus has been added, the remaining cations are given as chloride or acetate salts. Patients with metabolic acidosis should have the majority of electrolytes added as acetate salts, while patients with metabolic alkalosis should have most salts added as chlorides.

VITAMINS/TRACE ELEMENTS

Vitamins are an essential component of a patient's daily parenteral nutrition regimen, as they are necessary for normal metabolism and cellular function. There are four fat-soluble and nine water-soluble vitamins recognized as essential. The American Medical Association Nutrition Advisory Group established guidelines for daily parenteral administration of vitamins during parenteral nutrition (31). These amounts are shown for 12 of the vitamins in Table 11.12. These 12 vitamins are available in the suggested amounts from several commercial manufacturers as a multiple-entity product that is added to the parenteral nutrition solutions daily. Vitamin K is usually not included in adult, commercially available multiple-vitamin formulations, to avoid complications in patients receiving warfarin. Patients not receiving anticoagulants may receive vitamin K, 1 mg/day or 5 to 10 mg per week, during parenteral nutrition. Many of the vitamins are available as single-entity products that can be used for patients with documented vitamin deficiencies.

Trace elements are also a necessary part of a daily

Table 11.12.
Recommended Adult Intravenous Doses of Vitamins[a]

Vitamin	Daily Intravenous Doses
Fat-soluble vitamins	
A	3,300 I.U.[b]
D	200 I.U.
E	10 I.U.
Water-soluble vitamins	
B_1 (thiamin)	3.0 mg
B_2 (riboflavin)	3.6 mg
B_3 (pantothenic acid)	15.0 mg
B_5 (niacin)	40.0 mg
B_6 (pyridoxine)	4.0 mg
B_{12} (cyanocobalamin)	5.0 μg
C (ascorbic acid)	100.0 mg
Folic acid	400.0 μg
Biotin	60.0 μg

[a] Doses do not include requirements for pregnancy and lactation.
[b] I.U. = International Units.

Table 11.13.
Recommended Adult Intravenous Doses of Trace Elements

Element	Daily Intravenous Dose
Zinc[a]	2.5–4.0 mg
Copper	0.5–1.5 mg
Chromium[b]	10–15 μg
Manganese	0.15–0.8 mg
Selenium	40–120 μg

[a] Acute catabolic state, additional 2.0 mg.
[b] Intestinal losses, increase daily dose to 20 μg.

parenteral nutrition solution. Trace elements are metabolic cofactors essential to the proper functioning of several enzyme systems in the body. The American Medical Association Nutrition Advisory Group has also published guidelines for four trace elements known to be important in human nutrition (32): zinc, copper, manganese, and chromium. The suggested amounts are shown in Table 11.13. Since the original recommendations, substantial evidence for the essentiality of selenium has accumulated, and many clinicians now add this trace element to the parenteral nutrition on a daily basis. Zinc requirements are increased in metabolic stress or with large gastrointestinal losses. Zinc, chromium, and selenium are excreted by the kidneys, while manganese and copper are excreted through the biliary tract. Therefore, patients with cholestatic liver disease should have copper and manganese restricted or withheld from the parenteral nutrition solution. Selenium stores are depleted in patients with thermal injury, AIDS, and liver failure. Therefore, patients with these diseases should have selenium added initially to the parenteral nutrition solution. The trace elements are available as single- or multiple-entity products for admixture into parenteral nutrition solutions. Parenteral guidelines for molybdenum and iodine have not been established; however, these trace elements are available commercially.

Total Nutrient Admixtures

Traditionally, parenteral nutrition solutions consisted of an admixture of dextrose and protein (two-in-one), however intravenous fat is being added to these solutions at some institutions. The intravenous admixture of dextrose, amino acids, and fat emulsion is known as a three-in-one or total nutrient admixture (33). Intravenous fat is an water-in-oil emulsion stabilized by the anionic emulsifier, egg yolk phospholipid. When properly prepared, the total nutrient admixture is stable for at least 48 hr.

The use of total nutrient admixtures is increasing because it has several advantages. It may decrease the risk of infection because fewer central-line manipulations are involved. It also decreases the time spent by the nursing staff in parenteral nutrition administration. In addition, lipids mixed with dextrose and amino acids do not support bacterial growth as well as the fat emulsion alone. By giving the fat emulsion slowly and continuously over a 24-hr period, there is improved oxidation of the lipids and less potential for immunosuppression due to the long chain triglycerides.

Despite these advantages, there are some concerns about the total nutrient admixture system. It is not possible to detect particulate matter in a total nutrient admixture. Also, because the fat particles are fairly large, the total nutrient admixture cannot be filtered with a 0.22-micron filter. Furthermore, only a few medications are known to be compatible with and can be added to the total nutrient admixture. Those drugs that are known to be compatible include cimetidine, ranitidine, famotidine, heparin, and insulin. There is also potential for increased wastage using this method of parenteral nutrition administration because most pharmacies prepare one bag for each 24-hr period.

The order in which the three macronutrient substrates are admixed is important to ensure stability. The dextrose and amino acids should be mixed first, and then the fat emulsion should be added. Electrolytes, vitamins, and trace elements may be added before or after the fat emulsion is added, as long as they are not added directly to the fat emulsion. Creaming and coalescence of the fat emulsion results when electrolytes are added directly to it. The anionic emulsifier in the fat emulsion may be adversely affected by divalent cations and acidifying agents. Therefore, limitations exist on the doses of divalent cations that may be added to the total nutrient admixture. Adding these electrolytes beyond the recommended amounts will neutralize the negative potential at the surface of the emulsion and cause the admixture to coalesce.

Complications of Parenteral Nutrition Support

The complications of parenteral nutrition support may be divided into three broad categories: infectious, technical, and metabolic. Catheter-related sepsis, the most common infectious complication, may occur as a result of contamination during line placement or poor catheter care. Catheter sepsis can be minimized by a strict protocol for line placement and catheter care. Many institutions have nutrition support nurses who assist in line placement and perform the central catheter dressing changes.

Technical complications, such as pneumothorax, hydrothorax, and arterial puncture, may occur during placement of the catheter. Proper training and careful technique minimize the chance of a technical complication.

Several metabolic complications may occur. Fluid overload may occur because patients receiving parenteral nutrition often require several other intravenous fluids. The macronutrient substrates are available in several concentrations; thus, the parenteral nutrition solution may be concentrated to decrease the volume of fluid administered when fluid problems exist or are anticipated. Metabolic acidosis or metabolic alkalosis occur with relative frequency in patients who receive parenteral nutrition. Metabolic acidosis may be treated by minimizing the chloride salts and maximizing the acetate salts in the parenteral nutrition solution. Metabolic alkalosis may be treated by maximizing the chloride salts and restricting the acetate salts. Metabolic complications related to the carbohydrate component of parenteral nutrition include hyperglycemia, hyperosmolar coma, and adverse effects of overfeeding. Hyperglycemia is usually identified by frequent monitoring of serum glucose concentrations. This complication may be managed by the addition of insulin, by decreasing the dextrose concentration in the parenteral nutrition solution, or by decreasing the infusion rate. Carbohydrate overfeeding may cause excess carbon dioxide production leading to respiratory acidosis, elevations of liver function test results, and hepatic steatosis. These problems can usually be avoided by a dextrose infusion rate equal to or less than 5 mg/kg/min (25 kcal/kg/day). Disorders may occur with virtually all of the electrolytes. Malnourished patients who begin parenteral nutrition often experience hypokalemia and hypophosphatemia secondary to the intracellular shift of those ions, induced by dextrose. Vitamin and trace element disorders may also occur (e.g., vitamin A toxicity during parenteral nutrition in patients with renal failure and decreased serum zinc concentrations in severe metabolic stress). The doses of these micronutrients may be increased or decreased as necessary to alleviate metabolic complications.

Table 11.14.
Guidelines for Monitoring the Patient Receiving Parenteral Nutrition Support

1. Check q6h. If >250 mg/dl, draw stat serum glucose and potassium samples
2. Measure total fluid intake and output daily
3. Weigh patient two times per week
4. Sliding scale with regular human insulin
5. Draw samples for prealbumin or transferrin tests q. week
6. Draw samples for SMA-24 at least q. week, SMA-7 daily in ICU patient[a]
7. Draw samples for magnesium, phosphorus determinations two times per week
8. Collect 24-hour urine for nitrogen balance determination q. week

[a] The frequency of laboratory measurements will be dictated by the severity of the patient's illness.

Monitoring of Parenteral Nutrition Support Patients

Because many metabolic complications may occur in patients receiving parenteral nutrition support, the patients should be monitored daily. Table 11.14 lists some guidelines for monitoring patients on parenteral nutrition.

Drug Compatibility Considerations in Parenteral Nutrition Support

By using the parenteral nutrition solution as a drug vehicle, the overall amount of fluid administered and the number of line manipulations are decreased. Patients who are fluid restricted, receive home parenteral nutrition, or have limited venous access may benefit from receiving their medications in the parenteral nutrition solution.

Drugs that are added to the parenteral nutrition solution must be physically and chemically stable in it. It is not wise to add a drug to these solutions when frequent dosage changes are anticipated. When no dosage changes are anticipated and the drug is physically compatible, it could be added. Amino acid concentration, pH of the solution, and ambient room temperature all may affect the stability of the drug added to the parenteral nutrition solution. Also, drugs added to the parenteral nutrition solution may have an adverse effect on selected nutrients.

Numerous studies have been conducted on calcium and phosphorous compatibility in parenteral nutrition solutions. Excessive concentrations of these nutrients yield a precipitate of calcium phosphate. The results of the studies concerning maximum concentrations of calcium and phosphorous are equivocal. Generally, solutions with amino acid concentrations >2.5% and a pH of less than 6.0 favor solubility of calcium and phosphorous. Some studies have reported incompatibilities between iron and fat. Also, adding human albumin to a total nutrient admixture is not recommended; however, it is compatible in a two-in-one solution. Whenever a question of compatibility arises, it is best to obtain information from a text on intravenous admixtures. If no data exist on a particular combination, the safest approach is to not add the medication to the parenteral nutrition solution.

ENTERAL NUTRITION

The use of enteral nutrition dates back to the ancient Egyptians, who used nutritional enemas to preserve health. Enteral nutrition by tube has been mentioned and used over the subsequent centuries; however, only during the last 20 years has it been used extensively in the hospital and home. Most practitioners feel that if the gastrointestinal tract is functional and accessible, it should be used for the delivery of specialized nutrition support. The development of new feeding tubes, modern equipment for administration, surgically placed enterostomies, and sophisticated enteral formulas have greatly improved this method of administering nutrients. A recent focus on the "gut" during critical illness has changed the role of enteral feeding. Stressful events such as major trauma, thermal injury, or sepsis appear to allow gastrointestinal bacteria to translocate across the gut lumen (34). In animal models, these bacteria are taken up by the mesenteric lymph nodes, spleen, and liver. This translocation of gut organisms is thought to lead to sepsis and multiple organ failure syndrome. Enteral feeding by tube is thought to preserve the gastrointestinal mass and prevent this translocation, resulting in fewer infections (35). Consequently, practitioners in specialized nutrition support are making extraordinary effects to deliver enteral nutrients to the critically ill patient. Traditionally, pharmacists have not been involved extensively in this method of specialized nutrition support. This is changing because of the issues mentioned above, an appreciation of the many drug-nutrient interactions that occur in patients receiving enteral nutrition support, and the many hospital pharmacies that are becoming involved in the preparation and delivery of the enteral nutrient formulas (36).

The American Society for Parenteral and Enteral Nutrition has published guidelines for the rational use of enteral nutrition support (37). A summary of these recommendations appear in Table 11.15. Enteral nutrition should not be used when the gastrointestinal tract is not functional (e.g., postoperative ileus) or when enteral nutrients are undesirable (e.g., severe acute pancreatitis).

Types of Enteral Feeding Delivery

There are many ways to deliver enteral nutrients into the gastrointestinal tract, and enteral nutrition support can be delivered safely and efficaciously in most patients, as either short- or long-term therapy.

Nasogastric or nasoduodenal feeding tubes are used for patients who need enteral access for a short-term pe-

Table 11.15.
Summary of the A.S.P.E.N. Guidelines for Enteral Nutrition[a]

Enteral nutrition should be used
    Undernutrition with inadequate oral intake of nutrients for 5 consecutive days
    Normal nutrition status with <50% of required nutrients taken orally for 7–10 days
    Severe dysphagia
    Major thermal injury
    Low-output enterocutaneous fistulas
    Massive small-bowel resection (50–90%)
Enteral nutrition would be helpful
    Major trauma
    Radiation therapy
    Mild chemotherapy
    Liver failure and severe renal dysfunction

From: Guidelines for the use of enteral nutrition in the adult patient. J Parenter Enter Nutr 11:435–439, 1987.

Table 11.16.
Types of Administration Devices for Enteral Feeding

Nasogastric and nasoduodenal tubes
    Flexiflo (Ross)
    Kangaroo (Cheeseborough-Ponds)
    Dobbhoff (Biosearch)
    Corpak (Corpak)
    Entriflex (Biosearch)
    ENtube (ENtech)
Gastrostomy
    Stamm gastrostomy
    Percutaneous endoscopic gastrostomy (PEG)
Jejunostomy
    Tube jejunostomy
    Needle catheter jejunostomy (NCJ)

riod (e.g., a few weeks). These soft, small-bore tubes have virtually replaced the large nasogastric tube, which is now only used for nasogastric suction. These tubes, made of polyurethane or silicone, have several advantages over the large nasogastric tubes. Many of them have a tungsten tip, which facilitates transpyloric passage of the tube into the small bowel. Irritation to the nose, pharynx, and esophagus is decreased when these smaller tubes are used. Also, patients may eat food and swallow without difficulty when these softer tubes are used. These tubes are usually packaged with a stylet, which aids in proper placement during intubation. Several examples of these tubes are listed in Table 11.16.

A surgical gastrostomy provides the enteral route for a long-term period (months to years) (38). The nutrients are infused directly into the stomach via the gastrostomy tube, bypassing the mouth, pharynx, and esophagus. The Stamm gastrostomy and percutaneous endoscopic gas-

trostomy (PEG) are the two most common types of gastrostomies for long-term use. The Stamm gastrostomy is usually done by a general surgeon in the operating room, using general anesthesia. PEGs are done by general surgeons or gastroenterologists in a surgical suite or at the bedside, using local anesthesia.

Jejunostomies for enteral feeding administration are done for both short-term and long-term access (39). A tube jejunostomy is placed during a laparotomy and can be used for long-term enteral access. This type of jejunostomy is particularly effective in a patient who has severe, chronic gastroparesis (e.g., some diabetics). The chance of aspiration of nutrients is decreased, because both the pyloric and the lower esophageal sphincter protect the airway when feedings are delivered into the jejunum. The needle catheter jejunostomy (NCJ) is also placed surgically at the time of laparotomy, but this is used for short-term enteral access. Patients with an NCJ can be fed immediately after placement. When supplemental enteral feedings are no longer needed and the patient is taking adequate nutrients by mouth, the NCJ can be removed at the bedside without surgical intervention.

Enteral Nutrition Products

Currently, more than 150 enteral products are marketed in the United States. Most organized healthcare settings (hospitals, nursing homes) that are involved in the administration of these products develop formularies by creating several categories and stocking one product in each one. (Table 11.17 lists 13 categories of enteral formulas and some examples in each category.) Patients with normal fluid requirements, normal nutritional needs, and normal electrolyte status can usually be treated with isotonic, nutritionally complete formulas. Several institutions use products with added dietary fiber as their standard enteral formula in the conditions above, presumably for improved gastrointestinal tolerance. Patients who are eating part of their diet orally can often be supplemented by ingestion of 16 to 32 ounces of an oral enteral supplement. This obviates placement of an enteral feeding tube. Fluid-restricted enteral formulas are reserved for patients who have a problem with overhydration (e.g., congestive heart failure). These products are extremely low in free water and are potentially dangerous in a patient who does not need severe fluid restriction. When gastrointestinal digestive capabilities are compromised, a chemically defined enteral formula is often used because most of the nutrients are in elemental or predigested form. Several products are marketed for patients with renal failure, liver failure, respiratory failure, diabetes, compromised immune function, and severe metabolic stress. When a patient's specific needs cannot be met with commercially available enteral formulas, specific macronutrients (carbohydrate, fat, pro-

Table 11.17.
Enteral Formula Categories with Examples

Isotonic tube feeding	(Isocal, Osmolite)
Oral supplement	(Ensure, Ensure Plus, Sustacal)
Fluid-restricted tube feeding	(MagnaCal, Two Cal-HN, Isocal-HCN)
Chemically defined tube feeding	(Vital-HN, Criticare-HN, Vivonex-TEN)
Fiber-containing tube feeding	(Enrich, Ultracal, Jevity Compleat B Modified)
Low-protein, low-electrolyte, or electrolyte-free tube feeding[a]	(AminAid, Travasorb-Renal, Replena)
Modified protein, electrolyte-free tube feeding[b]	(HepaticAid, Travasorb-Hepatic)
Low-carbohydrate, high-fat tube feeding[c]	(Pulmocare, Glucerna)
High-protein tube feeding[d]	(Stresstein, Traumacal, Replete)
Immune stimulant feeding[e]	(Impact)
Protein module	(Promod, Promix-RD)
Fat module	(Microlipid)
Carbohydrate module	(Polycose, Sumacal)

[a] Used occasionally in acute renal failure.
[b] Used in liver failure with hepatic encephalopathy.
[c] Used occasionally in respiratory failure or diabetes.
[d] Used occasionally in trauma or sepsis.
[e] Clinically efficacy under investigation.

tein) can be added to these formulas to meet special needs. Several of these are listed in Table 11.17.

Administration of Enteral Feedings

There are essentially three ways to administer enteral feeding to institutionalized or home-bound patients: continuous, intermittent, and bolus. Continuous feeding, used preferentially in the institutionalized patient, involves an enteral pump so that the formula can be infused at a constant rate. The advantages of this method are less risk of aspiration, less nursing time, decreased gastrointestinal distention, and decreased diarrhea. Continuous feeding is more sophisticated and more expensive than the other methods. Intermittent feeding is used in the home setting and in some extended-care facilities. The desired volume of formula (usually 240 to 480 ml) is infused over a short period of time (e.g., 1 hr), several times each day. Bolus feeding consists of rapid administration of the desired volume of formula into the patient's ostomy tube. This method is most often used in the home-bound or nursing-home patient who has a gastrostomy tube in place. When bolus feedings are administered into the stomach, the risk of aspiration, gastric distention, and diarrhea is higher. The bolus method is, however, the simplest method of administering enteral nutrients, making it attractive in the home setting when an enteral pump is not provided.

Enteral nutrition support is usually started at a slow rate and increased gradually over time to the desired goal.

Most patients can tolerate an initial rate of 25 to 50 ml/hr. The isotonic formulas can often be started at 50 ml/hr, while the more concentrated formulas (2 kcal/ml) are started at 25 ml/hr. Patients who are slowly regaining bowel function should be started at a more conservative rate (e.g., 25 ml/hr). Many institutions advance the infusion rate of the enteral nutrition formula by 25 ml/hr/day when gastrointestinal tolerance and fluid/electrolyte status are acceptable. This gets most patients to the desired rate within 3 to 4 days. It has been suggested that hyperosmolar enteral formulas be diluted when enteral tube feeding is initiated, to improve gastrointestinal tolerance, but this is not supported by published studies. In fact, in one study, patients who received a undiluted hyperosmolar enteral formula received more calories and protein without any increase in gastrointestinal side effects than groups receiving diluted hyperosmolar formulas or isotonic formulas (40). Therefore, many institutions discourage the use of diluted enteral formulas (e.g., half-strength) to achieve better tolerance.

Complications of Enteral Nutrition Support

The complications of enteral nutrition support can be divided conveniently into four categories: pulmonary, gastrointestinal, mechanical, and metabolic. Aspiration of enteral nutrition formula into the lungs is the most serious complication of this type of therapy. It occurs in the patient who has developed vomiting or impaired gastric emptying. This serious complication often results in pneumonia, requiring mechanical ventilation in an intensive care unit. Frequent examination of the abdomen and meticulous checking of gastric residuals aspirated through the feeding tube may help to identify patients who are at risk for aspiration. Prokinetic drugs such as metoclopramide and erythromycin have been used with some success in patients who have poor gastric emptying of enteral nutrition formulas. Diabetics and patients who have a septic process are particularly prone to delayed gastric emptying.

Gastrointestinal complications include vomiting and diarrhea. Vomiting can usually be prevented by advancing the enteral feeding rate slowly, as described earlier, and checking the patient's abdomen often. Most institutions elevate the head of the patient's bed at least 30°. Diarrhea is a frequent problem in patients who receive enteral nutrition support; however, its cause is often elusive. Patients who have their enteral nutrient rate decreased by $\frac{1}{3}$ to $\frac{1}{2}$ often demonstrate decreased diarrhea. The rate may then be gradually increased to the desired goal, as tolerated. Suggested causes of diarrhea in association with enteral tube feeding include antibiotic administration, hypoalbuminemia, hyperosmolar formulas, lactase deficiency, and lack of a nutrition support team. The authors of an excellent report carefully examined diarrhea in tube-fed patients and found hyperosmolar drug solutions (e.g., theophylline) to be the most likely cause (41). Therefore, all drugs administered via the gastrointestinal tract should be inspected in patients who have diarrhea associated with enteral tube feeding. Some patients demonstrate decreased stool volume and frequency when they are switched from a standard enteral formula to a chemically defined formula. Pharmacologic agents should be used as a last resort in treating diarrhea.

Mechanical complications include a feeding tube that has become kinked or occluded. A kinked tube can be made functional by slowly withdrawing the tube until it straightens out. This should be done without the enteral formula infusing. Slow irrigation of the tube lumen with warm water administered by a 10-ml syringe will open some occluded feeding tubes. Cranberry juice, cola syrup, and pancreatic enzymes in water have also been used with some success. Occasionally, an occluded tube can be saved by passing the stylet back into the lumen of the tube. This may remove or "break up" any concretion formed within the lumen. This should be done by a physician and only in tubes that do not let the stylet exit through it.

Virtually all of the metabolic complications that happen with parenteral nutrition can occur with enteral nutrition. Hyperglycemia is usually not as severe with enteral nutrition support because the nutrients are being infused into the gastrointestinal tract rather than into a large vein. Some institutions where the pharmacy department prepares and dispenses the enteral formulas have programs that allow the addition of electrolytes (e.g., KCl, Fleet Phosphosoda) to help treat or prevent metabolic complications.

Monitoring of the Enteral Nutrition Support Patient

Patients who receive enteral nutrition support should be monitored frequently to insure safety and efficacy. Many of the complications described above can be averted with meticulous patient monitoring. Some enteral tube feeding guidelines for monitoring are listed in Table 11.18.

Table 11.18.
Monitoring the Patient Receiving Enteral Nutrition Support

1. Raise head of bed to at least 30° at all times
2. Check gastric residuals q6h. If >150 ml, hold feedings for 4 hours and recheck: if <150 ml, restart, or if still >150 ml, hold feedings
3. Check for glucose q6h. If >250 mg/dl, draw stat serum glucose and potassium samples
4. Draw samples for SMA-24, magnesium determination as needed[a]
5. Draw sample for prealbumin determination q. week
6. Collect 24-hour urine for nitrogen balance q. week

[a] The frequency of laboratory measurements is dictated by the severity of the patient's illness.

Drug Compatibility Considerations in Enteral Nutrition Support

In many patients receiving enteral nutrition support, the feeding tube may be the only way to administer drugs. Therefore, any incompatibilities between drug and enteral formula or tube are of paramount importance. Phenytoin and warfarin have been reported to be altered during enteral nutrition administration. Patients who received both phenytoin (300 mg per day as the suspension) and enteral tube feeding were reported to have subtherapeutic serum concentrations, compared with patients who received the drug without enteral feedings (42). Interestingly, there does not appear to be a problem with this drug administered as a capsule to normal subjects who take oral enteral supplements concurrently (43). It is unclear what effect the difference in subjects (patients vs. normal subjects) or the effect of administering the drug through a tube has on this interaction. Difficulty has been reported in attaining a therapeutic prothrombin time with warfarin administration during concurrent enteral feeding. Initially this was thought to be caused by the large vitamin K content of some commercially available enteral formulas. The manufacturers have decreased the vitamin K content of most enteral formulas over the last 10 years; however, the problem with warfarin bioavailability and enteral formulas still exists. One study demonstrated reduced recovery of warfarin mixed with an enteral formula compared with it mixed with distilled water (44).

HOME CARE
Home Nutrition Therapy

Although most hospitalized patients on parenteral or enteral nutrition can be changed to an oral diet before discharge, some require continued specialized nutrition support at home. The hospital nutrition support team members work with one of the several home health care companies or a hospital-based home health service. The team devises a specialized nutrition support prescription that will meet the patient's nutritional requirements and an administration schedule that will be compatible with the patient's lifestyle. Parenteral or enteral nutrition formulations are often given as a nocturnal continuous drip over a 10- to 18-hr period. This allows patients to hold employment or participate in other activities during the day. Some patients on enteral nutrition, however, prefer periodic bolus feedings during the day. The home health service will compound the enteral or parenteral formula and provide the patient with the necessary equipment for its administration. Approximately 5 to 7 days prior to hospital discharge, clinicians from the home health service or nutrition support team will begin training the patient and family to administer the nutrition regimen. The patient and family are also trained to detect adverse effects that may occur during administration. In addition, the home health service works with the patient's physician to ensure that the patient is monitored between office visits. The home health service will visit the patient at home whenever necessary to solve any mechanical problems that might arise.

The patient and family must be willing and able to assume the added responsibility involved with home nutrition support for the therapy to be successful. This type of therapy is often cost-prohibitive to many patients; however, partial or complete reimbursement by third-parties is frequently available. Provision of specialized nutrition support in the home setting remains costly, yet, it is much more economical than keeping the patient hospitalized for extended periods of time. Specific guidelines have been developed to help identify those who may benefit from specialized nutrition support in the home (45). Examples include patients with extensive small bowel resection (short bowel syndrome), chronic enteritis from radiation therapy, or severe Crohn's disease. These patients receive parenteral nutrition via a permanent, centrally placed catheter (e.g., Hickman catheter). Patients who receive home enteral nutrition can absorb nutrients via the gastrointestinal tract, but are unable to consume adequate nutrients by mouth. Examples of patients who receive home enteral nutrition include patients with severe ulcerative colitis, colon cancer, cerebral trauma, or head and neck cancer. The administration route chosen for enteral feeding will depend on the patient's diagnosis and the estimated duration of enteral nutrition support. Surgical gastrostomy or jejunostomy is often used in these patients. Home nutrition programs have increased the quality of life for many patients who require these therapies and have allowed many to return to nearly normal lifestyles.

PHARMACOKINETIC/PHARMACODYNAMIC CONSIDERATIONS

Altered disposition of drugs has been demonstrated with both malnutrition and changes in macronutrient intake (46). Much of this research has been performed in animal models, however, more clinical studies in patients are being conducted. In general, the systemic clearance of many drugs is decreased significantly in patients in an undernourished state, compared with that in well-nourished patients. One study demonstrated that elderly patients (usually with a reduced body weight) are given doses of drugs that are 30 to 45% higher than younger patients, when the doses were normalized for weight (47). This is of particular concern since many elderly patients have a decreased creatinine clearance that makes them particularly susceptible to drug toxicity. Other drugs have increased clearance when they are given concurrently with aggressive doses of macronutrients (e.g., protein). Clearances of theophylline in children (48) and gentamicin in normal adult subjects (49) increased significantly when

they were given with relatively high protein diets. This may be clinically important, as there is a trend to give higher doses of protein to patients who require specialized nutrition support, especially in the critical care setting.

CONCLUSION

The pharmacist is an integral member of the nutrition support team and should be involved in the care of patients who receive specialized nutrition support. The Board of Pharmaceutical Specialties has recently approved a petition recognizing Nutritional Support Pharmacy Practice as a specialty. Certification by written examination became available in 1992.

Parenteral nutrition solutions are prepared in the pharmacy, using sterile technique. Because of this requirement, pharmacists will always be involved with the administration of parenteral nutrition, and more than likely, in the clinical monitoring of the patient receiving this therapy. The pharmacist must become more involved in enteral nutrition. Many data connect the gastrointestinal tract and enteral nutrition to the multiple organ failure syndrome. It will be unfortunate if the pharmacist is not involved with this therapy as more data become available. Most likely an increased number of patients will receive enteral nutrition support and fewer, parenteral nutrition over the next few years.

The delivery of specialized nutrition support continues to be a ripe area of specialized practice for the pharmacist. A sound base in sterile technique, nutrient metabolism, fluid and electrolytes, acid-base, and drug-nutrient interactions is needed to be effective in this area.

REFERENCES

1. Dudrick SJ, Wilmore DW, Vars HM, Rhoads JE: Long-term parenteral nutrition with growth, development, and positive nitrogen balance. Surgery 64:134–142, 1968.
2. Blackburn GL, Bistrian BR, Maini BS, Schlamm HT, Smith MF: Nutritional and metabolic assessment of the hospitalized patient. J Parenter Enter Nutr 1:11–22, 1977.
3. Dempsey DT, Mullen JL, Buzby GP: The link between nutritional status and clinical outcome: can nutritional intervention modify it? Am J Clin Nutr 47:352–356, 1988.
4. Starker PM, Gump FE, Askanazi J, Elwyn DH, Kinney JM: Serum albumin levels as an index of nutritional support. Surgery 91:194–199, 1982.
5. Donahue SP, Phillips LS: Response of IGF-1 to nutritional support in malnourished hospital patients: a possible indicator of short-term changes in nutritional status. Am J Clin Nutr 50:962–969, 1989.
6. Ingenbleek Y, Carpentier YA: A prognostic inflammatory and nutritional index scoring critically ill patients. Int J Vitam Nutr Res 55:91–101, 1985.
7. Buzby GP, Mullen JL, Matthews DC, Hobbs CL, Rosato EF: Prognostic nutritional index in gastrointestinal surgery. Am J Surg 139:160–166, 1980.
8. Twomey P, Rombeau J: Utility of skin testing in nutritional assessment: a critical review. J Parenter Enter Nutr 6:50–58, 1982.
9. Baker JP, Detsky AS, Wesson DE, Wolman SL, Stewart S, Whitewell

J, Langer B, Jeejeebhoy KN: Nutritional assessment: a comparison of clinical judgment and objective measurements. N Engl J Med 306:969–972, 1982.

10. Roubenoff R, Roubenoff RA, Preto J, Balke CW: Malnutrition among hospitalized patients: a problem of physician awareness. Arch Intern Med 147:1462–1465, 1987.

11. Harris JA, Benedict FG: A biometric study of basal metabolism. Carnegie Institute of Washington, publ no 279, Washington, D.C., 1919.

12. Long CL, Schaffel N, Geiger JW, et al.: Metabolic response and injury and illness: estimation of energy and protein needs from indirect calormetry and nitrogen balance. J Parenter Enter Nutr 3(6):452–456, 1979.

13. Long CL, Blakemare WS: Energy and protein requirements in the hospitalized patient. J Parenter Enter Nutr 3:69–71, 1979.

14. Feurer I, Mullen JL: Bedside measurement of resting energy expenditure and respiratory quotient via indirect calorimetry. Nutr Clin Pract 2:43–49, 1986.

15. Weir JB de V: New methods for calculating metabolic rate with special reference to protein metabolism. J Physiol (London) 109:1–9, 1949.

16. Swinamer DL, Phang PT, Jones RL, et al.: Twenty-four hour energy expenditure in critically ill patients. Crit Care Med 15:637–643, 1987.

17. Hegsted DM: Assessment of nitrogen requirements. Am J Clin Nutr 31:1669–1677, 1978.

18. Shaw JHF, Wildbore M, Wolfe RR: Whole body protein kinetics in severely septic patients: the response to glucose infusion and total parenteral nutrition. Ann Surg 205:288–294, 1987.

19. Smith MF, Blackburn BL, Bistrian BR, et al.: Beneficial effects of high nitrogen-calorie (N:CAL) rations in intravenous hyperalimentation (IVH). Surg Forum 28:63–64, 1977.

20. Anon: Guidelines for use of total parenteral nutrition in the hospitalized adult patient. J Parenter Enter Nutr 10:441–445, 1986.

21. Daly JM, Masser E, Hansen L, et al.: Peripheral vein infusion of dextrose amino acid solutions ±2% fat emulsion. J Parenter Enter Nutr 9:296–299, 1985.

22. Figueras-Felip J, Rafecas-Renau A, Sitges-Serra A, et al.: Does peripheral hypocaloric parenteral nutrition benefit the postoperative patient? Results of a multicenter randomized trial. Clin Nutr 5:117–121, 1986.

23. Blackburn GL, O'Keefe SJD: Nutrition in liver failure. Gastroenterology 97:1049–1051, 1989.

24. Cerra FB, Cheung NK, Fischer JF, et al.: Disease-specific amino acid infusion (F080) in hepatic encephalopathy: a prospective, mixed double-blind, controlled trial. J Parenter Enter Nutr 9:288–295, 1985.

25. Feinstein EI, Blumenkrantz MJ, Healy M, et al.: Clinical and metabolic responses to parenteral nutrition in acute renal failure. Medicine 60:124–137, 1981.

26. Mirtallo JM, Schneider PS, Marko, et al.: A comparison of essential and general amino acid infusions in the nutritional support of patients with compromised renal function. J Parenter Enter Nutr 6:109–113, 1982.

27. Oki JC, Cuddy PG: Branched-chain amino acid support of stressed patients. DICP Ann Pharmacother 23:399–410, 1989.

28. von Meyenfeldt MF, Soeters PB, Vente JP, et al.: Effect of branched chain amino acid enrichment of total parenteral nutrition on nitrogen

sparing and clinical outcome of sepsis and trauma. A prospective randomized double-blind trial. Br J Surg 77:924–929, 1990.

29. Burke JF, Wolfe RR, Mullancy CJ, et al.: Glucose requirements following burn injury: parameters of optimal glucose infusion and possible hepatic and respiratory abnormalities following excessive glucose intake. Ann Surg 190:275–285, 1979.

30. Roesner M, Grant JP: Intravenous fat emulsions. Nutr Clin Pract 2:96–107, 1987.

31. Anon: Multivitamin preparations for parenteral use—a statement by the Nutrition Advisory Group. J Parenter Enter Nutr 3:253–262, 1979.

32. Anon: Guidelines for essential trace element preparations for parenteral use—A statement by the Nutrition Advisory Group. J Parenter Enter Nutr 3:263–267, 1979.

33. Driscoll DF: Clinical issues regarding the use of total nutrient admixtures. DICP, Ann Pharmacother 24:296–303, 1990.

34. Wilmore DW, Smith RJ, O'Dwyer ST, Jacobs DO, Ziegler TR, Wang XD: The gut: a central organ after surgical stress. Surgery 104:917–923, 1988.

35. Moore FA, Moore EE, Jones TN, McCroskey BL, Peterson VM: TEN versus TPN following major abdominal trauma—reduced septic morbidity. J Trauma 29:916–922, 1989.

36. Vanderveen TW: Pharmacy involvement in enteral nutrition. Am J Hosp Pharm 40:857–859, 1983.

37. Anon: Guidelines for the use of enteral nutrition in the adult patient. J Parenter Enter Nutr 11:435–439, 1987.

38. Shellito PC, Malt RA: Tube gastrostomy. Ann Surg 201:180–185, 1985.

39. Sarr MG, Mayo S: Needle catheter jejunostomy: an unappreciated and misunderstood advance in the care of patients after major abdominal operations. Mayo Clin Proc 63:565–572, 1988.

40. Keohane PP, Attrill H, Love M, Frost P, Silk DB: Relation between osmolality of diet and gastrointestinal side effects in enteral nutrition. Br Med J 288:678–680, 1984.

41. Edes TE, Walk BE, Austin JL: Diarrhea in tube-fed patients: feeding formula not necessarily the cause. Am J Med 88:91–93, 1990.

42. Bauer LA: Interference of oral phenytoin absorption by continuous nasogastric feedings. Neurology 32:570–572, 1982.

43. Nishimura LY, Armstrong EP, Plezia PM, Oacono RP: Influence of enteral feedings on phenytoin sodium absorption from capsules. Drug Intell Clin Pharm 22:130–133, 1988.

44. Anon: Guidelines for use of home total parenteral nutrition. J Parenter Enter Nutr 11:342–344, 1987.

45. Kuhn TA, Garnett WR, Wells BK, Karnes HT: Recovery of warfarin from an enteral nutrient formula. Am J Hosp Pharm 46:1395–1399, 1989.

46. Anderson KE: Influences of diet and nutrition on clinical pharmacokinetics. Clin Pharmacokinet 14:325–346, 1988.

47. Campion EW, Avorn J, Reder VA, Olins NJ: Overmedication of the low-weight elderly. Arch Intern Med 147:945–947, 1987.

48. Feldman CH, Hutchinson VE, Sher TH, Feldman BR, Davis WJ: Interaction between nutrition and theophylline metabolism in children. Ther Drug Monit 4:69–76, 1982.

49. Dickson CJ, Schwartzman MS, Bertino JS: Factors affecting aminoglycoside disposition: effects of circadian rhythm and dietary protein intake on gentamicin pharmacokinetics. Clin Pharmacol Ther 39:325–328, 1986.

CHAPTER 12

IRON DEFICIENCY AND MEGALOBLASTIC ANEMIAS

STANLEY G. KAILIS, Ph.D., F.P.S. and CONSTANTINE G. BERBATIS, M.Sc., F.P.S., M.S.

Anemia is a hematologic condition in which there is quantitative deficiency of circulating hemoglobin, often accompanied by a reduced number of erythrocytes, causing pallor, weakness, and breathlessness. Causes of anemia are blood loss, impaired erythropoiesis, or abnormal erythrocyte destruction.

Iron deficiency anemia and the megaloblastic anemias result from a lack of nutrients essential for erythropoiesis. A lack of iron can lead to iron deficiency, and in severe cases, iron deficiency anemia; whereas, a lack of either vitamin B_{12} (B_{12}) or folic acid can result in megaloblastic anemia. Subclinical deficiency states can occur without the development of anemia. In most cases, these anemias are either preventable or treatable by providing the appropriate nutrient. For the effective treatment of these anemias: the deficiency state must be documented; it must be confirmed that the anemia is due to the deficiency; the pathologic state responsible for the deficiency must be identified and where possible rectified; and the sufferer must comply with the treatment.

Anemia is not a single disease entity but a sign of disease, which has many causes. Regardless of the cause, anemia is associated with a reduction in circulating hemoglobin because of reduced numbers of erythrocytes, less hemoglobin per erythrocyte or a combination of both.

The number of erythrocytes in normal individuals varies with age, gender, and atmospheric pressure. Persons living at high altitudes have more erythrocytes to compensate for the reduced oxygen in the air. At sea level, the average normal adult male has 5.5×10^{12} erythrocytes/1 liter ($5.5 \times 10^6/mm^3$). The erythrocytes occupy 47% of the blood, and this value is termed the packed cell volume (PCV) or hematocrit (Table 12.1). Blood from healthy adult males contains approximately 160 g/liter (16 g/dl) of hemoglobin. All these parameters are lower for healthy adult women. Values for neonates, which show no gender differences, are higher at birth, but after several weeks they decrease to below those of adult women. Thereafter the values rise gradually, and at puberty male/female differences appear.

The physiologic importance of low circulating hemo-globin is the reduced capacity for blood to carry oxygen. Consequently less oxygen is available to tissues, including those of the heart, brain, and muscles, leading to the clinical manifestations of anemia. The hemoglobin levels below which anemia is likely are 110 g/liter for children 6 months to 6 years of age, 120 g/liter (12 g/dl) from 6 years to 14 years of age, 130 g/liter (13 g/dl) for adult men, 120 g/liter (12 g/dl) for adult women, and 110 g/liter (11 g/dl) in pregnancy.

GENERAL FEATURES OF ANEMIAS

The term anemia denotes a complex of signs and symptoms that indicate an underlying disorder. Regardless of the cause of anemia, the clinical features are due to the tissue hypoxia and the associated cardiovascular-pulmonary compensatory responses. Overt signs of anemia are pallor of the skin, mucous membranes (particularly the conjunctiva), and nail beds. Symptoms include faintness, malaise, dizziness, ease of fatigue, lack of concentration, irritability, headache, intermittent claudication, palpitations, ankle edema, and angina. Cardiomegaly and high-output heart failure are also possible in severe cases.

Even though the symptoms of anemia are distinctive, they can also be manifestations of other disorders. A comprehensive history and physical examination are important in the assessment of the anemic patient. More specifically, dietary habits, drug histories, and occupation should be documented. Close questioning about blood loss, menses, gastrointestinal symptoms, and the number of pregnancies provides useful information.

DIAGNOSIS OF ANEMIAS

Hematologic and biochemical tests, including a full blood screen, are essential for identifying the type of anemia and in many cases directing the treatment. In most cases the full blood screen will reveal anemia (low hemoglobin), microcytosis, macrocytosis, and poikilocytosis (abnormal shaped) or whether anisocytosis (variably sized erythrocytes) are present. Routine blood screens may reveal unsuspected hematologic abnormalities.

Table 12.1.
Selected Hematologic and Biochemical Parameters

Component	Specimen[a]		Conventional	SI
			Reference Range	
Hematocrit	B	Male	45–52%	0.42–0.52
		Female	37–48%	0.37–0.48
Hemoglobin	B	Male	13–18 g/dl	8.1–11.2 mmol/liter
		Female	12–16 g/dl	7.4–9.9 mmol/liter
Erythrocyte count	B		$4.2–5.9 \times 10^6/mm^3$	$4.2–5.9 \times 10^{12}/liter$
Mean corpuscular volume (MCV)	Ery		80–94 fmol	80–94 fmol
Mean corpuscular hemoglobin (MCH)	Ery		27–32 pg	1.7–2.0 fmol
Mean corpuscular hemoglobin concentration (MCHC)	Ery		32–36 g/dl	19–22.8 mmol/liter
Iron	S	Male	80–180 µg/dl	14–32 µmol/liter
		Female	60–160 µg/dl	11–29 µmol/liter
Transferrin	S		170–370 mg/dl	1.7–3.7 g/liter
Total iron-binding capacity (TIBC)	S		250–410 g/ml	45–72 µmol/liter
Reticulocyte count	B		0.5–1.5%	
			Red cells	
Ferritin	S	Males > females	2–20 µg/dl	20–200 µg/liter
Folate (as pteroglutamic acid)				
Normal	S		2–10 ng/ml	4–22 nmol/liter
Borderline	S		1–1.9 ng/ml	2.5–4 nmol/liter
	Ery		150–800 ng/ml	
Vitamin B$_{12}$	S		200–1000 pg/ml	150–750 pmol/liter

[a] S, serum; B, whole blood; Ery, erythrocyte.

Traditionally, the first step in identifying the cause of anemia is a careful examination of a peripheral blood smear. Additional tests can confirm the diagnosis. Future developments in automatic chemistry may reduce the need for the peripheral blood smear (1).

Many aspects of the cellular elements of blood can be quantified by automated blood analyzers, including blood hemoglobin concentration, cell counts, and the mean corpuscular volume (MCV). From these primary measurements, the hematocrit, mean corpuscular hemoglobin (MCH), and the mean corpuscular hemoglobin concentration (MCHC) are automatically calculated. The MCV, MCH, and MCHC are also collectively known as the erythrocyte indices. The MCV is particularly valuable in differentiating microcytic anemias, which have a reduced MCV (<80 fl), from macrocytic anemias which have a greater than normal MCV (>95 fl). Hypochromic anemias such as iron deficiency anemia have a low MCHC, indicating lower than normal hemoglobin concentrations. A recently introduced parameter, the red blood cell distribution width (RDW), which is expressed as the *coefficient of variation of the volume of distribution width*, gives an indication of the variation in erythrocyte size in a blood sample. A characteristic of iron deficiency anemia is an increased RDW, reflecting the anisocytosis seen in blood smears. Selected laboratory characteristics of iron deficiency anemia and megaloblastic anemias are summarized in Table 12.2.

Other hematologic investigations involve reticulocyte counts, differential white cell count, platelet count, and microscopic examination of peripheral blood smears and bone marrow aspirates. The normal life span of an erythrocyte is 120 days. As old erythrocytes are removed from the circulation by reticuloendothelial cells, they are replaced by young erythrocytes from the bone marrow. These immature cells, called reticulocytes, make up 1 to 1.5% of the total erythrocyte population in a normal individual. Reticulocyte identification and counting involves staining techniques that visualize endoplasmic reticular material, which is absent in mature erythrocytes. As reticulocytes represent a young population of red blood cells, they are an important marker of bone marrow activity. Reticulocytosis, an increase in reticulocyte numbers, indicates increased bone marrow activity. Transient reticulocytosis often occurs in response to iron, B$_{12}$, or folic acid therapy for the respective deficiency states.

Biochemical tests for assessing anemias include measurement of serum iron, ferritin, transferrin, and transferrin saturation. Other specific tests can be directed toward the identification of a particular deficiency state or anemia. Serum B$_{12}$ or folate as well as erythrocyte folate levels can be measured. However reduced levels of these nutrients must be addressed in conjunction with hematologic tests and the patient's clinical status.

GENERAL MANAGEMENT OF DEFICIENCY ANEMIAS

When the deficiency or anemia has been defined, treatment is directed toward reducing the severity of symptoms,

Table 12.2.
Selected Laboratory Characteristics of Iron Deficiency Anemia and Megaloblastic Anemias

Type	MCV[a]	RDW	Peripheral Smear	Additional Investigations
Iron deficiency	L[b]	H	Hypochromic, microcytic	↓ Fe, ↓ ferritin, ↑ transferrin, Bone marrow iron stain
Vitamin B$_{12}$ deficiency[c]	H	H	Macrocytic	↓ S-vitamin B$_{12}$, achlorhydria, ↑ antiparietal antibodies
Folate deficiency	H	H	Macrocytic	↓ S-folate[d], ↓ erythrocyte folate[e]
Chronic disease	L	H	Hypochromic, microcytic	↓ Fe, ↓ transferrin
	N	N	Normochromic, normocytic	
Blood loss	N	N	Normochromic, normocytic	Clinical evidence, occult blood test

[a] N, normal; L, low; H, high.
[b] Normal in early iron deficiency.
[c] Includes pernicious anemia.
[d] Varies with diet.
[e] Provides a measure of tissue stores.

or where possible, toward eliminating the cause. This may involve restoring missing nutrients, restoring blood volume by transfusions, or treating the cause by medical or surgical methods. Careful assessment of the patient's drug history may help identify possible pharmacotherapeutic agents that could be involved in the etiology. As deficiency states of iron, vitamin B$_{12}$, or folic acid often require long-term or lifelong therapy, patients must be counseled appropriately.

IRON DEFICIENCY ANEMIA

Iron deficiency occurs when the body iron is insufficient for the normal formation of hemoglobin, iron-containing enzymes, and other functional iron compounds such as myoglobin and those of the cytochrome system. Iron deficiency exists when body iron is reduced to the extent that overt anemia occurs (2).

Hematologic characteristics of severe iron deficiency are hypochromic and microcytic erythrocytes that have a low MCHC and MCV. Other conditions with similar hematologic characteristics such as thalassemia, sideroblastic anemia, and the anemia of chronic disease can be differentiated from iron deficiency anemia by assessing iron stores. Erythrocytes of persons with mild iron deficiency often appear to be normal (i.e., normocytic).

Occurrence of Iron Deficiency

Iron deficiency, estimated to occur in over 500 million persons throughout the world, is the most common cause of anemia (3, 4). Data from the second Nutritional Health and Nutrition Examination Survey (NHANES II) in the United States indicated that the prevalence of iron deficiency was 0.2% for men, 2.6% for premenopausal women, and 1.9% for postmenopausal women (5). Iron deficiency is most frequently seen in infants and menstruating and pregnant women.

Physiologic Importance of Iron

Iron is an essential element for many physiologic processes including erythropoiesis, tissue respiration, and several en-

zyme-catalyzed reactions. Iron deficiency, in addition to its hematologic effects, may also be associated with diverse problems such as; impaired work performance in adults (6); low birth weight, prematurity, and increased perinatal mortality (7); impaired psychomotor behavior and cognitive function in infants and young children (8); and abnormalities of epidermal structures, heat production, catecholamine turnover, mentation, and resistance to infection (9). Oxidative metabolism by tissues is more effective when iron stores are normal (10). Behavioral effects associated with iron deficiency, best described in children, include decreased academic achievement, which can be reversed by giving iron (11).

Iron, one of the transition metals which exists in more than one oxidation state, forms stable complexes with some proteins. The average adult body contains 3 to 5 g of elemental iron. Functional iron exists predominantly as hemoglobin (2.5 g) in circulating erythrocytes, with lesser amounts in myoglobin (130 mg) and tissue enzymes (8 mg). Circulating transferrin, the iron-binding protein that supplies iron to all tissues, contains 4 mg of iron in the ferric form (Table 12.3).

Hemoglobin, a hemoprotein, is the oxygen-binding protein in erythrocytes of veterbrates which transports oxygen absorbed from the lungs to the tissues. Each hemoglobin molecule consists of four heme groups surrounding a globin group forming a tetrahedral structure. Heme accounts for 4% by weight of the molecule and contains all the iron. Hemoglobin forms an unstable, reversible bond with oxygen, allowing for oxygen release at lower oxygen tension, as is encountered in the tissues. Globin consists of linked pairs of polypeptide chains. The composition of these chains in adults differs from those in the fetus as well as in individuals with genetically determined disorders such as thalassemia and sickle cell anemia. (See Chapter 13, "Other Anemias.") In the fetus and newborn, hemoglobin has two alpha and two gamma globin chains. Erythrocytes have a finite life span and as they are replenished the hemoglobin of new cells have beta chains

Table 12.3.
Iron Distribution in the Body and Its Function

	Site	Amount[a]	Function
Functional			
Hemoglobin	Erythrocytes	2–2.5 g	Oxygen transport in blood
Myoglobin	Muscle	140 mg	Oxygen transport in muscle
Cytochromes	Mitochondria		Electron transport system
Enzymes	Various		Various[b]
Transferrin	Circulation	4 mg	Transport
Storage			
Ferritin and hemosiderin	Reticuloendothelial cells of the liver, spleen, and bone marrow	1 g (males) 100–400 mg (females)	Iron stores

[a] Total body iron is 3–5 g.
[b] See text for details.

replacing the gamma chains. The normal human adult has two alpha and two beta chains. In iron deficiency anemia, as well as other chronic anemias, hemoglobin has a reduced affinity for oxygen. This allows oxygen to transfer more readily from the erythrocytes than in normal states, resulting in more tolerable tissue oxygenation.

Myoglobin, a hemoprotein in muscle, accepts oxygen from hemoglobin in the peripheries and acts as an oxygen store in muscle. If oxygen supply is limited, myoglobin releases its oxygen to cytochrome oxidase, the terminal enzyme in the mitochondrial respiratory chain, which has a higher affinity for oxygen than myoglobin and so allows oxidative phosphorylation to occur.

Transferrin a β-globulin synthesized by the liver, is a specific iron-binding protein in blood which transports iron through the plasma and extravascular spaces. Each molecule of transferrin can bind two molecules of iron in the ferric state. In normal circumstances, it is only 30 to 50% saturated. The ability of transferrin to bind iron is called the iron-binding capacity. The total iron-binding capacity (TIBC), which reflects serum transferrin concentrations, is a well-recognized value in the investigation of anemias. It represents the amount of iron that can bind to transferrin to give 100% saturation of the binding sites. The TIBC is increased in iron deficiency and reduced in iron overload. Most cells obtain their iron from transferrin. In the case of reticulocytes and developing erythrocytes in the bone marrow, most of the iron taken up is used for hemoglobin synthesis.

Storage iron (1 g), in the form of ferritin and hemosiderin, located mainly in the parenchymal cells of the liver and the reticuloendothelial cells of the bone marrow, spleen, and liver, replenishes functional iron. Iron stores account for one-third of body iron in healthy adult males. Iron stores are more variable and one generally lower or absent in children and menstruating females. Low iron stores do not indicate iron deficiency and are not associated with abnormalities.

Table 12.4.
Daily Iron Requirements[a]

Infant	
0–4 months	0.5 mg
5–12 months	1.0 mg
Children	1.0 mg
Adolescent male	1.8 mg
Adolescent female	2.4 mg
Menstruating female	2.8 mg
Adult male	1.0 mg
Postmenopausal female	1.0 mg
During pregnancy	3–4 mg

[a] Values represent actual iron absorbed.

Iron Requirements

Body iron is usually kept constant by a delicate balance between the amounts lost and absorbed. There is no physiologic mechanism for excreting iron in humans; the quantity of iron lost daily is similar to that absorbed. Consequently, there is only a limited ability to compensate for excessive loss or absorption of iron. Iron balance is a conservative system, and in the normal adult, even if iron intake is negligible, it takes at least 2 to 3 years to develop iron deficiency.

Iron requirements are determined by total losses from the body. Daily iron requirements vary according to age and gender, requirements are higher for menstruating women and during pregnancy, whereas normal men and postmenopausal women require only 1 mg each day (Table 12.4). Iron losses in normal women are higher than those in men because of menstruation and pregnancy. Total daily iron loss amounts to 1 mg/day (14 μg/kg/day) (12) in males. Losses by postmenopausal or nonmenstruating women are similar to those of men. Iron losses occur from the gastrointestinal tract by sloughing of iron-containing mucosal cells and extravasation of erythrocytes; by exfoliation of skin; and by shedding urinary tract epithelial cells. Loss of iron through sweat is minimal, so manual laborers working in humid conditions are not at risk.

Blood loss in menstruating women varies, and if in excess of 80 ml, it can lead to iron deficiency. Average iron losses due to menstruation are about 0.6 mg/day; however, over 30% of menstruating women lose between 0.9 and 1.4 mg/day of iron. Daily iron loss for most menstruating women, which includes obligatory losses, is 1.5 to 2 mg/day. Menstrual iron losses are reduced by 50% in women taking oral contraceptives but increased by up to 100% if they are using an intrauterine device (13, 14).

Iron requirements increase to 3 to 4 mg/day during pregnancy because both maternal and fetal iron requirements must be met by the mother. Even though menstruation ceases, iron losses by the mother are still greater than in the nonpregnant state. Iron is needed for obligatory losses, for the expanded maternal erythrocyte mass that occurs in pregnancy, and for the placenta and fetus. Elemental iron requirements for a well-nourished 55-kg woman during pregnancy are at least 1000 mg (20 mg/kg). At term, 270 to 450 mg of this iron is in the fetus. Iron requirements are greatest in the second and third trimester (5 to 6 mg/day) when the highest fetal erythrocyte requirements occur. Some of the iron incorporated in the expanded maternal erythrocyte mass returns to the iron pool after pregnancy, but peripartum blood loss partially nullifies this contribution. Because menstruation does not start until several weeks after delivery, iron losses are reduced. However, breast-feeding offsets some of the gain.

Human breast milk is low in iron, falling from 0.5 mg/liter to 0.3 mg/liter within 6 min of delivery. Maternal iron loss, estimated to be about 0.3 mg/day by the third month after delivery, should not pose a major problem to mothers, except for those in developing countries who continue to breast-feed well after menstruation has commenced.

The need for iron is high in the first year of life and subsequent childhood years because of rapid growth and erythropoiesis during this period. Normal full-term infants need to absorb a minimum of 0.3 mg of iron daily in the first year of life. Premature infants can need up 1 mg/day. With increasing age, the requirements for children increase progressively to 0.5 to 0.8 mg/day. The growth spurt of adolescence results in a daily iron requirement of about 1.6 mg/day. The RDAs for iron, to meet these levels of uptake, are summarized in Table 12.5. Normal infants need 1 mg/kg/day of dietary iron, and for low-birthweight infants 2 mg/kg/day is required. As the usual infant diet cannot provide this amount of iron, iron supplementation of 10 mg/day is necessary during the first year of life. For adolescent males and females during their growth spurt, 12 mg/day and 15 mg/day, respectively, are recommended. It is advised that women continue this supplementation throughout the reproductive years (15). Because the iron requirements of pregnancy, particularly during the second

Table 12.5.

Recommended Daily Allowances for Iron, Folic Acid and Vitamin B_{12}[a]

Category	Age (yr)	Iron (mg)	Age (yr)	Folic Acid (μg)	Age (yr)	Vitamin B_{12} (μg)
Infants	0–0.5	6	0–0.5	25	0–0.5	0.3
	0.5–1	10	0.5–1	35	0.5–1	0.5
Children	1–10	10	1–3	50	1–3	0.7
			4–6	75	4–6	1
			7–10	100	7–10	1.4
Males	11–18[b]	12	11–14[b]	150	11+	2
	19+	10	15+	200		
Females	11–50	15	11–14[b]	200	11+	2
	51+	10	15+	180		
Pregnant		30		400		2.2
Lactating		15		260–280		2.6

[a] Values determined by the Food and Nutrition Board of the National Research Council. RDA provides adequate nutrition in most healthy persons under usual environmental stresses and are not minimum requirements. (See reference 26.)
[b] Adolescents.

and third trimesters, cannot be met from dietary sources, 30 mg/day of elemental iron should be taken. The daily iron requirement of 10 mg/day for adult men and postmenopausal women can usually met from dietary sources.

Food Iron Absorption (12)

Iron is present in a wide variety of foodstuffs, particularly red meats, poultry, brewer's yeast, wheat germ, some dried beans, and some vegetables. The iron content of food and its bioavailability determines whether the diet can meet physiologic requirements. Milk is a relatively poor source of iron as is a diet high in cereal content and low in animal protein. An average Western diet contains 10 to 20 mg of iron/day, which can deliver 1 to 2 mg of iron to the body. The diet of poorer populations includes little animal meat and so contains very low amounts of iron.

The main sites of iron absorption are the duodenum and proximal jejunum, the upper parts of the small intestine. Only part of dietary iron is actually absorbed (12). This depends on a number of factors including; the amount of iron in the diet, the physiologic status of the small bowel where iron is absorbed; the composition of the diet; and the erythropoiesis rate. Adults with normal iron stores absorb 5 to 10% of dietary iron (1 to 2 mg/day). Iron absorption increases with decreasing levels of iron stores, and in those with severely depleted stores, may rise to 50% of the total intake.

Food iron, generally organically bound, is present as two major pools, nonheme iron and heme iron. Nonheme iron is the major source of dietary iron. For dietary iron to be absorbed, it must be released from the organically bound forms in food. Ingested organic nonheme iron complexes and heme compounds are broken down in the acid environment in the stomach to ferric ions and heme molecules, respectively. The fate of the ferric ions includes reduction to the ferrous state and release from complexes by gastric secretions; chelation with ligands associated with molecules in the stomach contents; and binding to gastroferrin, a specific iron-binding protein released by the stomach. Only soluble iron in the form of heme, or nonheme iron as a low molecular weight chelate or bound to gastroferrin is readily absorbed by the luminal cells. Iron absorbed by these cells is incorporated into an iron-carrier pool, most of which is deposited as ferritin or used by the mitochondria for enzyme synthesis. It is then lost by sloughing during the usual intestinal cell turnover. A smaller proportion of the iron from the carrier pool is transferred to the plasma, where the ferric form binds tightly to transferrin.

Heme iron is highly available (20 to 40%) in the iron-depleted patient because it is absorbed within the porphyrin ring and so not exposed to inhibitory ligands in the diet. It is absorbed via specific, high-affinity, brush border binding sites. When the heme is absorbed, iron is released to the mucosal cell, where it enters the general iron pool. However heme iron represents only a small fraction of dietary iron, particularly in poorer populations. Iron from heme alone is poorly absorbed, but when it is associated with hemoglobin, meat, protein, or soy proteins, absorption increases. Baking and prolonged frying significantly reduce heme iron absorption. Iron absorption from ferritin, hemosiderin, and ferric oxides is less than that from the nonheme dietary pool.

When iron stores are low or depleted, a higher proportion of available iron is absorbed. Absorption is reduced when the stores are replete. The serum ferritin concentration, which reflects body iron stores, is inversely related to iron absorption. Malabsorption of iron, associated with mucosal abnormalities, has been reported for persons living on and around the Indian subcontinent and Haiti. In some clinical states such as primary hemochromatosis, thalassemia, and sideroblastic anemia, iron absorption remains normal and even raised, despite increased iron stores. Giving additional iron to sufferers of these conditions is therefore inappropriate and potentially dangerous.

A number of factors can inhibit, or promote the absorption of nonheme iron (Table 12.6). Foods that can reduce iron absorption by forming less-soluble complexes include coffee, tea, milk and milk products, eggs, whole grain breads and cereals, and any food containing bicarbonates, carbonates, oxalates, or phosphates.

Commercial processing or enhancers can improve nonabsorption from food in some cases. Enhancers of nonheme iron absorption include meat, and food acids such as citric, lactic, or ascorbic acids. Ascorbic acid, the most powerful promoter, has a dose-related effect on nonheme

Table 12.6.
Factors Associated with Iron Absorption

Factor	Associations
Favoring absorption	
Inorganic iron	Ionic iron, particularly in the ferrous form, is better absorbed than ferric iron and organically bound iron
Ascorbic acid	Probably by assisting the conversion of ferric iron to ferrous iron
Acid	Gastric HCl promotes the release and conversion of dietary iron to the ferrous form
Chelates	Iron chelated to low molecular weight substances such as sugars (fructose and sucrose), amino acids, and succinate facilitates binding of iron to the intestinal mucosa
Clinical states	Iron deficiency, increased erythropoiesis, pregnancy, anoxia, pyridoxine deficiency
Reducing absorption	
Alkaline	Alkaline pancreatic secretions containing phosphate probably convert iron to insoluble ferric hydroxide, antacids
Dietary	Dietary phosphates and phytates in cereals, tannins in tea (probably complex iron)
Clinical states	Chronic diarrhea, steatorrhea, adequate iron stores, decreased erythropoiesis, acute or chronic inflammation

iron absorption. In its presence, ferric iron is converted to the ferrous state, maintaining the solubility of the iron in the alkaline environment of the duodenum and upper jejunum. Ascorbic acid also forms an alkaline-stable chelate with ferric chloride in the stomach. Meat itself a rich source of iron, promotes absorption of nonheme iron. Quantitatively 1 g of meat enhances nonheme iron absorption to the about the same extent as 1 mg of ascorbic acid. Citric acid, a common food additive and a less powerful promoter of iron absorption, has an additive effect to ascorbic acid.

Etiology of Iron Deficiency (1, 2, 16–20)

The primary cause of iron deficiency in adults is blood loss or pregnancy (Table 12.7). Blood loss from any body site is the major cause of iron deficiency in adult males and nonmenstruating females. Bleeding may be occult or overt. A common site of blood loss is the gastrointestinal tract. Iron deficiency anemia should be treated as a warning signal of gastrointestinal cancer and should not be passed off as a nutritional deficiency without adequate investigation. Where bleeding is not obvious, a test for occult blood in the stool may give the first indication of blood loss. Common sources of blood loss in the gastrointestinal tract are peptic ulcers and esophageal varices. Nonsteroi-

Table 12.7.
Factors Associated with Iron Deficiency

Factor	Associations
Dietary	Starvation, poverty, vegetarianism, religious practice, food faddism
Blood loss	
Females	Menorrhagia, postmenopausal bleeding, pregnancy
General	Esophageal varices, peptic ucler, drug-induced gastritis, carcinomas of stomach and colon, ulcerative colitis, hemorrhoids, renal or bladder lesions (hematuria), hookworm infestation, other organ bleeding (hemoptysis); widespread bleeding disorders
Malabsorption	Celiac disease (gluten-induced enteropathy); partial and total gastrectomy, chronic inflammation
Increased requirements	Rapid growth such as in childhood and adolescence, frequent pregnancies

dal antiinflammatory agents such as aspirin and indomethacin are frequently responsible for gastrointestinal bleeding, especially if taken with warfarin. In the absence of upper gastrointestinal symptoms, investigations should be directed to the lower gastrointestinal tract. Bleeding hemorrhoids rarely result in anemia, but neoplasms are a common cause of bleeding, particularly in the elderly. Colonic cancer, which can cause bleeding, increases 40-fold between the ages of 40 and 80 years. Other causes of gastrointestinal blood loss include hookworm infestation, Meckel's diverticulum and ulcerative colitis. Hookworm is a major cause of iron deficiency anemia in tropical areas.

Adolescent females are susceptible to iron deficiency because of the growth spurt associated with adolescence and the menarche. Menorrhagia, heavy menstrual bleeding, is the chief cause of iron deficiency in fertile women.

Sports anemia, particularly in marathon runners and other endurance athletes, is a newly recognized type of iron deficiency anemia (21–22). Blood loss is believed to result from ischemia of the gastrointestinal tract, as blood is shunted to muscles during prolonged exercise. Marathon runners can lose at least 3 mg of iron daily for several days after a marathon race. Another short-term anemia related to sport is the dilutional anemia that can result from plasma volume expansion in the early weeks of conditioning.

Poor nutrition, defective intake, or decreased assimilation of iron rarely causes iron deficiency in persons living in Western countries. Iron deficiency due to inadequate dietary iron intake is predominantly a problem of infants and children. In some populations however, where the diet is mainly of vegetable origin with little meat, women are likely to suffer from nutritional iron deficiency. Malabsorption of iron may occasionally cause iron deficiency. It is rarely an important cause unless the iron stores are low or there are other contributing factors such as blood loss,

pregnancy, increased gastrointestinal blood loss, or poor nutrition. The two most common conditions in which iron absorption is a problem are gluten enteropathy (celiac disease) and gastrectomy. Other conditions associated with iron deficiency anemia include pernicious anemia (PA), pica syndrome, and chronic inflammatory disease such as rheumatoid arthritis.

Clinical Findings and Manifestations

Iron deficiency precedes the manifestations of anemia. Most individuals with iron deficiency have minimal anemia and are asymptomatic. Progression of iron deficiency anemia is often insidious, with symptoms becoming evident when the blood hemoglobin concentration falls below 100 g/liter (10 g/dl). Mildly lowered hemoglobin concentrations, however, are always associated with a decreased work capacity.

The usual signs and symptoms of anemias are often present (Table 12.8). Other problems due to the gross epithelial changes associated with chronic iron deficiency include brittle or spoon shaped nails, angular stomatitis, atrophic tongue, and pharyngeal and esophageal webs causing dysphagia and atrophic gastric mucosa.

Half the sufferers of iron deficiency anemia experience pica, a condition in which the individual craves unnatural foods (such as chalk or clay) or has an unusual craving for a single food. Pagophagia or habitual ice eating is a common form of pica in some communities. Others consume earth and particles of clay cooking pots. Such ingestions have lead to metabolic problems including heavy metal poisoning (23).

Table 12.8.
Features of Patients with Iron Deficiency

Clinical manifestations	
Appearance	Tired, listless, lifeless appearance
Skin and hair	Pale skin, inelastic and often dry; dry and often scanty hair
Mouth	Papillary atrophy and erythema of the tongue, angular stomatitis
Eye	Pearly white sclerae
Nails	Flattened, longitudinally rigid, concave (koilonychia)
Cardiovascular system	Slight cardiomegaly, tachycardia, functional systolic murmur, cardiomegaly, ankle edema
Neurologic	Generally normal
Blood picture	
Hemoglobin	5–10 g/100 ml (moderate to severe)
MCV	Decreased
MCHC	Decreased
Marrow iron stores	Depleted
Serum iron	Reduced
Serum ferritin	Reduced
Serum transferrin	Increased

Hematologic Changes in Iron Deficiency (1, 2)

In iron deficiency anemia, hematologic changes are evident only after all body iron stores have been depleted, when there is insufficient iron to maintain normal erythrocyte morphology and mass. Blood hemoglobin concentrations and erythrocyte numbers are normal in mild cases. With increasing severity, the MCV and erythrocyte count decrease markedly, and the RDW increases.

In severe cases, blood hemoglobin concentrations of 70 g/liter (7 g/dl) for females and 90 g/liter (9 g/dl) for males, microscopic examination of peripheral blood smears shows hypochromia and poikilocytosis. The proportion of reticulocytes is usually normal, but transient increases may follow acute hemorrhage or treatment with iron. The white cell count can be normal, and the platelet count often increases. Examination of bone marrow aspirates shows moderate erythroid hypoplasia, and many of the erythroid precursors, such as normoblasts, have little cytoplasm.

Diagnosis of Iron Deficiency Anemia (1, 2, 16, 18)

Identification of most cases of iron deficiency anemia is made on the basis of a full blood count and peripheral smears. The ultimate proof of iron deficiency is the absence of stainable iron in bone marrow aspirates. Since bone marrow aspiration is painful and expensive, it is not used routinely. It is useful in investigating mixed anemias. Severe iron deficiency anemia (Fig. 12.1) is characterized by microcytosis (low MCV), reduced erythrocyte numbers, and cells of uneven size and shape (high RDW). Serum iron and ferritin concentrations are usually low, whereas

serum TIBC and transferrin saturation are high and low, respectively.

Once a microcytic anemia is detected in the differentiation, a number of potential causes must be explored. An elevated erythrocyte count and a normal RDW (as seen in thalassemia and hemoglobin E) excludes iron deficiency. Similarly, a peripheral blood smear showing hypochromia, erythrocyte targeting, and basophilic stipling is characteristic of thalassemia minor. Some cases of anemia of chronic disease are mildly microcytic, but generally these have a normal RWD. Sideroblastic anemia has both normal and hypochromic erythrocytes as well as an elevated RWD. Anemia due to acute blood loss is characterized by erythrocytes with a normal MCV and RDW.

Serum ferritin levels are an indirect but accurate index of body iron stores and are very useful in establishing the type of anemia. Ferritin concentrations fall in iron deficiency states and increase abnormally in iron storage conditions. Ferritin, measured by immunologic means, is an intracellular iron-storage protein, traces of which enter the plasma compartment. Serum ferritin concentrations of less than 15 µg/liter (0.15 µg/dl) (normal, 20 to 200 µg/liter) (2 to 20 µg/dl) are diagnostic for iron deficiency in adults. Iron deficiency can be differentiated from anemia of chronic diseases by a low serum ferritin level and/or absence of stainable iron in the bone marrow.

Determination of serum iron levels and the TIBC are traditional methods for evaluating body iron stores. However these are less sensitive than ferritin determinations. A low serum iron and high TIBC level is generally characteristic of iron deficiency. Low serum iron levels with a

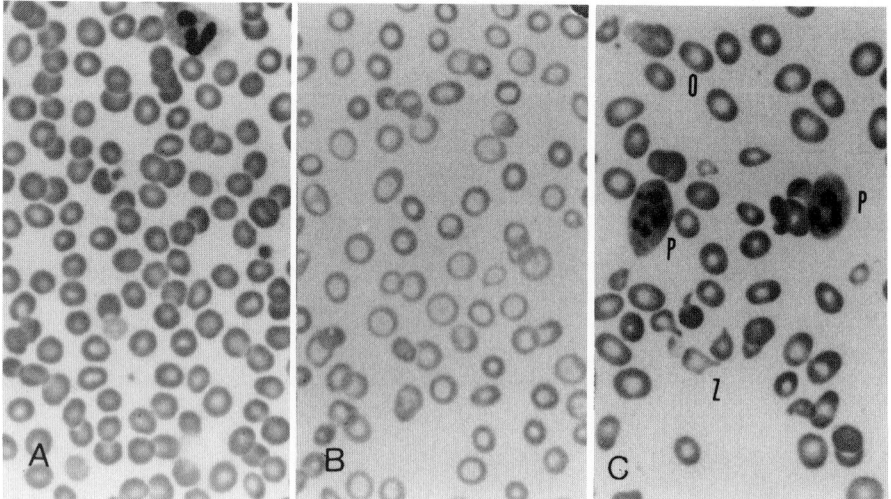

Figure 12.1. Photomicrographs of low-power views of peripheral blood showing **A,** normal erythrocytes, **B,** microcytosis and hypochromia typical of iron deficiency anemia, and **C,** macrocytosis typical of megaloblastic anemia due to either vitamin B_{12} or folic acid deficiency. **B,** All cells depicted are erythrocytes and anisocytosis is obvious. **C,** Oval (O) and bizarre (Z) shaped erythrocytes (poikilocytosis) can be seen. Hypersegmented or multilobed neutrophilic granulocytes (P) cells characteristic of megaloblastic anemia can also be seen.

high TIBC are associated with anemias of chronic disease. Serum iron levels are normal or high in thalassemia, hemoglobinopathies, and sideroblastic anemia. Transferrin saturation, another indicator of body iron stores, is below 16% in most cases of iron deficiency anemia. Transferrin saturation levels below 5% are found only in iron deficiency. However there is considerable overlap with anemias of chronic disease.

Interpretation of serum ferritin levels requires further discussion. Generally levels are about 100 μg/liter (10 μg/dl). A serum ferritin level below 12 μg/liter (1.2 μg/dl) indicates the absence of iron stores. Ferritin is an acute-phase reactant to inflammatory diseases such as rheumatoid arthritis. In these diseases, serum ferritin concentrations increase, with the lower level of normal increasing to 50 μg/liter (5 μg/dl). Subjects with levels between 12 μg/liter and 50 μg/liter should be investigated further for iron deficiency anemia. An abnormal release of ferritin from hepatocytes can also occur with acute hepatic necrosis or inflammation. To rule out iron deficiency anemia, serum ferritin levels in persons with liver disease, especially hepatitis, should be on the order of 200 μg/liter (20 μg/dl) (24, 25).

Medical disorders can modify the clinical features of iron deficiency anemia. Persons with polycythemia rubra vera, chronic obstructive airways disease, or those that smoke tobacco heavily are predisposed to elevated blood hemoglobin concentrations. If also iron deficient, they have the typical features of iron deficiency anemia, except their erythrocyte count is often above 6×10^{12}/liter, and blood hemoglobin concentrations are within the normal range. In polycythemia, iron is lost through gastrointestinal bleeding and as a consequence of phlebotomy, a recognized treatment for this condition. In contrast, iron deficiency anemia in patients with chronic renal failure may have a normocytic picture, because the shortage of erythropoietin allows the developing erythrocytes a longer maturation time in the bone marrow.

In the absence of a specialized hematology facility, a tentative diagnosis of iron deficiency can be made by giving a trial of iron therapy and monitoring hemoglobin concentrations and reticulocyte counts. Significant reticulocytosis occurs 7 to 10 days after the start of treatment, and the hemoglobin concentrations increase at a rate of 2 g/liter/day (0.2 g/dl/day) over a period of 3 to 4 weeks. Inflammatory disease may retard reticulocytosis.

Prevention and Management of Iron Deficiency (16, 18, 19)

Management is directed toward the cause. It may involve giving pharmacologic agents such as cimetidine or ranitidine for bleeding stomach ulcers, surgery for neoplasms, or removing precipitants such as gluten in celiac disease. Prophylactic or therapeutic doses of iron are used, as ap-

propriate. As iron stores are replenished slowly, therapy is continued for at least a year. Some cases require transfusion.

Prophylaxis

In addition to ensuring a diet adequate in fish, meat, and vegetables, women with heavy menstrual periods or repeated pregnancies usually require iron supplementation. Fruit and vegetables that enhance iron bioavailability include lemons, oranges, tomatoes, beets, broccoli, cauliflower, pumpkin, and turnips.

In pregnancy, a routine measurement of blood hemoglobin concentration at the first prenatal visit can guide the need for iron prophylaxis or therapy. Active prophylaxis with oral iron should be used during the second trimester, because even an iron-rich diet usually cannot provide sufficient iron. This will avert a negative iron balance during pregnancy. Ferrous sulfate is the least expensive form of iron therapy and the best salt for iron delivery. Daily prophylactic doses containing 50 to 100 mg of elemental iron, equivalent to 250 to 500 mg of ferrous sulfate, are given. If iron deficiency anemia occurs during pregnancy it should be treated in the usual way.

To reduce the likelihood of iron deficiency in breast-fed babies, suitable iron-rich foods can be given from the age of 4 to 6 months. Low-birth-weight infants may be given liquid iron supplements from 3 months on. The usual prophylactic dose of ferrous sulfate oral solution is 5 mg/kg body weight.

In societies where the diet lacks iron-rich food, iron supplementation as a public health measure, although controversial, is the only practical approach to the prevention and treatment of iron deficiency anemia (3, 4). This may be accomplished by either iron fortification of essential foods such as flour, sugar, salt, milk, and eggs, ascorbic acid–fortified juices, or the daily ingestion of iron in solid or liquid dosage forms.

Treatment of Iron Deficiency (26–29)

Iron deficiency can be corrected by the administration of either oral or parenteral iron, but indiscriminate administration of iron may delay the diagnosis of underlying causes. Most iron therapy is given by the oral route, with few situations justifying the use of parenteral iron. If the diagnosis is correct, hemoglobin levels improve within a few weeks, and the patient feels better. Adequate iron must be supplied in the early stages of treatment so that the response is optimal.

Oral Iron Therapy (26)

Solid and liquid oral dosage forms contain one of a variety of iron compounds, which vary in iron equivalence, cost, and effectiveness. Iron absorption from ferrous salts is con-

Table 12.9.
Common Iron Preparations

Proprietary Name	Active Ingredient	Elemental Iron	Iron (%)
Tablets			
Ferrous sulfate, USP (generic)	Ferrous sulfate heptahydrate	60 mg/300 mg	20
Feosal (initial formulation)	Ferrous sulfate dried	60 mg/200 mg	30
Fergon	Ferrous gluconate	39 mg/325 mg	11.5
Ferrous fumarate	Ferrous fumarate	66 mg/200 mg	33
Liquids			
Mol-Iron liquid	Ferrous sulfate	10 mg/ml	
Mol-Iron drops	Ferrous sulfate	25 mg/ml	
Feosol elixir	Ferrous sulfate	8 mg/ml	
Fer-In-Sol syrup	Ferrous sulfate	6 mg/ml	
Fer-In-Sol drops	Ferrous sulfate	25 mg/ml	
Fergon elixir	Ferrous gluconate	7 mg/ml	
Feostat suspension	Ferrous fumarate	6.6 mg/ml	
Feostat drops	Ferrous fumarate	25 mg/ml	

sidered better than that from ferric salts. Sustained-release, slow-release, or enteric-coated (30) preparations of iron, although useful for prophylaxis, are relatively ineffective in treating iron deficiency and so should be avoided. Preparations of iron salts in combination with other minerals or vitamins is a wasteful way to treat iron deficiency. A therapeutic dose of 200 mg ferrous sulfate, three times a day, is commonly used, but although very effective, such doses have been criticized as being too high, because the amount of elemental iron is likely to exceed the bone marrow capacity for hemoglobin synthesis (31). Another disadvantage of high doses is gastric irritation, which is thought to be due to free iron released in the stomach. This problem can be alleviated by either reducing the dose, taking the iron with food (at the expense of lower absorption), or changing to another salt (such as ferrous gluconate, which contains less iron). The therapeutic dose of an oral ferrous sulfate solution is 10 mg/kg body weight. When switching from one form of iron to another, care must be taken in calculating the doses of different salts (Table 12.9).

Maximum absorption of iron occurs if it is given before or between meals. Large doses are more likely to cause gastric irritation, diarrhea, or constipation. Some patients may also notice black stools during iron therapy, which should not be confused with darkened tarry stools, or melena, that occur with gastrointestinal bleeding.

Drug Interactions and Related Problems with Oral Iron (26)

Tetracyclines, pancrelipase, and antacids, particularly those containing carbonates or magnesium trisilicate, lower the bioavailability of iron. If these agents must be taken concurrently, dosing times should be separated by 1 to 2 hours.

Ascorbic acid in doses of 200 mg can increase iron absorption from 10% to 20 to 30%. Its routine use in such a high dose is usually unwarranted, as it is often possible to increase the dose of iron. This is also less expensive. Adding ascorbic acid may be beneficial in malabsorption states. High alcohol and ferric iron consumption for prolonged periods increases both iron absorption and hepatic storage of iron, resulting in iron toxicity. As foods can reduce iron absorption, oral iron supplements should be given 1 hour before or 2 hours after ingestion of food.

Parenteral Iron Therapy (26)

As the response to parenteral iron therapy is like that to oral therapy, there are few indications for its use. It also carries a number of risks, including local skin reactions and rare anaphylactic reactions. Additional problems reported with i.m. use of iron dextran include generalized aches and pains and painful local lymphadenopathy that may occur many hours after injection. Selected cases in which parenteral iron administration may be indicated include severe iron malabsorption, noncompliance with oral iron (e.g., mentally defective patients and persons in poor societies), severe intolerance that cannot be controlled by altering the dose or form of oral iron, excessive iron loss (e.g., bleeding hereditary hemorrhagic telangiectasia), and inflammatory bowel disease. Parenteral iron is available as iron dextran and iron sorbitex, two colloidal, nonionic forms complexed to carbohydrate compounds. Patients taking oral iron should stop such therapy for at least 1 week before parenteral iron therapy is commenced.

IRON DEXTRAN

Iron dextran is a high molecular weight complex of ferric hydroxide and dextran. In addition to the above indications, it has been used (a) to treat iron deficiency refractory to oral iron treatment and some cases of anemia associated with rheumatoid arthritis; (b) when normal serum iron and iron stores must be rapidly achieved, such as in emergency surgery in iron-deficient patients; (c) when iron deficiency is diagnosed in pregnancy; and (d) in iron-deficient premature infants.

The usual method of administration is by deep i.m. injection into the ventrolateral aspect of the upper and outer quadrant of the buttock. The correct technique for i.m. injections must be used. A study using computer tomography scans suggested that i.m. injections are often delivered accidentally into the subcutaneous, intralipomatous region. In the case of iron dextran, a Z-track injection avoids leakage through the needle track and staining of the skin. Necrotic skin ulcerations have occurred after multiple i.m. iron dextran injections (32).

It is claimed that absorption of iron dextran from the injection site is virtually complete and that maximum serum levels are reached within 1 or 2 days, but variable amounts do bind locally for several months. Iron dextran is transported from the muscle by the lymphatic circulation to the blood, and then to the liver, where it is taken up by the reticuloendothelial cells. These cells release iron, which is taken up by transferrin. The iron is utilized by the body or stored as ferritin or hemosiderin for later use. Some of the iron dextran remains trapped inside the reticuloendothelial cells, but it is gradually released. During the first week or so after injection the iron present in the plasma is largely iron dextran and unrelated to transferrin-bound iron.

The initial dose of iron dextran is usually 1 ml of an injection (50 mg Fe) on the first day, then 2 ml/day, or at longer intervals, according to the hemoglobin response. The total volume of iron dextran injection required to restore hemoglobin levels to normal and replenish iron body stores can be calculated from the following formula.

$$\text{Volume of iron dextran injection} = 0.66 \times \frac{(W)(D)}{50}$$

where W = body weight in kilograms and D = percentage hemoglobin deficiency, which is calculated using the formula:

Percentage hemoglobin deficiency (D)

$$= 100 - \frac{\text{patients Hb(g/dl)} \times 100}{14.8}$$

This formula does not take into account iron losses and iron bioavailability. Therefore higher doses are probably required to give an increase in the whole blood hemoglobin of 2 g/liter/day).

An alternative method is giving periodic i.m. injections until the hemoglobin level has returned to a desired level. One milliliter is needed for each 1% decrease in hemogloblin for a 70-kg adult. On this basis, maximum doses for children are 0.5 ml for those weighing under 4 kg, 1 ml for those 4 to 10 kg, and 2 ml for those over 10 kg.

IV iron dextran use avoids deposition in skeletal muscle and local reactions. It is useful in patients who have gastrointestinal problems that prevent adequate iron absorption. Giving it by this route carries about a 10% prevalence of serious adverse effects including anaphylactic and other allergic reactions. Care must be exercised. The regimen involves several IV injections or an infusion or iron dextran in 0.9% sodium chloride solution or in 5% dextrose solution given over 6 to 8 hr. Local phlebitis is less likely to occur if 0.9% sodium chloride is used as the diluent rather than dextrose.

Iron dextran injections should not be given to patients with severe liver disease or acute kidney infections because of the risk of iron toxicity. Patients with a history of allergy should receive a trial of small doses followed by a gradual increase in the dose. Single large doses should not be administered to persons with rheumatoid arthritis because this may exacerbate the disease.

Contraindications to Iron Therapy and Iron Toxicity

The absolute indication for iron is iron deficiency anemia, which should be confirmed by laboratory test. Iron preparations should not be used in conditions such as hemochromatosis and hemosiderosis, which already signify iron overload. In thalassemias as well as anemic conditions with chronic inflammatory disease such as rheumatoid arthritis, iron is contraindicated, as these conditions have normal to excess iron stores because of impaired utilization of iron. Care must be exercised in giving iron to alcoholic subjects because increased iron store, with or without hemochromatosis, can occur in this group. Those with alcoholic liver disease such as cirrhosis generally do not suffer from hemochromatosis, but those with marked increases in iron deposition and body stores are likely to have genetically determined hemochromatosis. Iron should be used carefully in enteritis, diverticulitis, colitis, and ulcerative colitis because of local effects. Persons receiving repeated blood transfusions generally become iron overloaded because of the high erythrocytic iron content.

Iron toxicity can be either acute, such as in overdosage and accidental poisoning, or chronic, as in overload that occurs in hemochromatosis and hemosiderosis, and thalassemia. An iron-overloaded person usually has more than 4 g of body iron. Iron ordinarily stored in reticuloendothelial cells is deposited as ferritin and hemosiderin into hepatocytes of the liver and eventually other tissues and organs. Hemochromatosis is associated with severe iron overload. Recently, noninvasive methods such as computed tomography and magnetic resonance imaging have been used to determine hepatic iron content.

Increased Iron Absorption

The pathogenesis of iron overload is associated with either increased mucosal iron absorption, the parenteral administration of iron as blood transfusions, or injections of therapeutic iron preparations. Diet is unlikely to cause iron overload unless other factors or problems are present. Normal individuals absorb the usual amounts of iron, even when the dietary iron load is increased 5 to 10 times. Amounts of 300 to 500 mg/day can be tolerated. There are some exceptions. Worldwide, the consumption of alcoholic beverages is considered to be a common cause of iron overload. Another potential cause of iron overload is the controversial practice in some developed countries of fortifying food with iron. Although this addition may be useful for women, it may lead to a grossly excessive intake of iron by men. The prevalence of hemochromatosis is 0.5%, which is higher than that of iron deficiency in men. Indiscriminate use of iron supplements can be harmful. Intrinsic metabolic abnormalities may account for increased iron absorption from the small intestine. Such abnormalities occur in primary idiopathic hemochromatosis (hereditary hemochromatosis) and in some anemias.

Iron overload secondary to anemias can be divided into two classes: that in patients with hypoplastic bone marrow, where the main source of iron is blood transfusion (e.g., aplastic anemia) and that in patients with hyperplastic bone marrow, where the iron excess results from increased iron absorption secondary to ineffective erythropoiesis (e.g., thalassemia major, sideroblastic anemia, and some hemolytic anemias).

Monitoring Iron Therapy

Laboratory tests are especially useful in monitoring the response to iron therapy, including blood hemoglobin concentrations, reticulocyte counts, serum ferritin concentration, and if necessary, serum iron level and the TIBC. In many centers parameters of the hemograms are used as therapeutic indicators.

The initial aim of treatment of iron deficiency is to reverse the anemia. With treatment this should be achieved in the first 2 to 3 months. Once the hemoglobin reaches 100 g/liter, the urgency for correcting the anemia decreases. Serial blood hemoglobin measurements should indicate a rise of 2 to 10 g/liter/week (0.2–1 g/dl/day). A speedy recovery generally indicates that the cause of iron loss is no longer present. Weekly reticulocyte counts give some idea of bone marrow activity, because in the early stages of treatment, reticulocytosis occurs. The rate of rise in blood hemoglobin concentration also depends on the severity of the anemia and on the usual range for an individual. The rate of rise for a male with a usual blood hemoglobin of 160 g/liter (16 g/dl) will be faster than that for a pregnant subject who would normally have a blood hemoglobin of about 105 g/liter (10.5 g/dl). Early in the treatment and depending upon the severity of the deficiency, larger doses of iron should be used. Following a good hemoglobin response, doses can be reduced.

A second objective in instituting iron therapy is to replenish iron stores. Generally this is a nonurgent phase of treatment, and iron replacement can be undertaken over 3 to 6 months. Serum ferritin concentration and iron saturation can be used as guides for this stage of therapy. Some patients will require long-term iron therapy because of blood loss or malabsorption problems. Doses of iron for these patients should be adjusted to the losses. Periodic serum ferritin determinations should be used as a guide to the patient's iron status.

Failure to respond to iron therapy can be due to a number of factors, including noncompliance, chronic disease, incorrect diagnosis, or an inadequate iron formulation.

MEGALOBLASTIC ANEMIAS (18–20)

Megaloblastic anemia is characterized by a lowered blood hemoglobin mass because of reduced erythropoiesis due to defective DNA synthesis in the developing erythroid cells of the bone marrow. Other rapidly dividing tissue can also be affected, particularly the mucosal epithelium of the gastrointestinal tract. Because RNA synthesis continues in the developing erythroid cells, there is an increase in cytoplasmic mass. The resulting megaloblasts are characterized by an abnormal nucleus because of greater cytoplasmic (rather than nuclear) maturity. Cells released into the circulation are larger than normal (i.e., macrocytic). These erythrocytes have a reduced life span, so megaloblastic anemias have some of the features of hemolytic anemias, such as hyperbilirubinemia. In addition to the erythroid changes, similar effects on other hemopoietic cell lines in the bone marrow can lead to leukopenia, thrombocytopenia, or pancytopenia. Morphologic changes observed in the peripheral smear include macroovalocyte erythrocytes and multilobed neutrophilic granulocytes. Mitotic figures in developing erythroid cells in the bone marrow are another feature of megaloblastic anemias (Fig. 12.2).

Either B_{12} or folic acid is required for the synthesis of purine and pyrimidine nucleotides, precursors of DNA synthesis. Reduced availability or absence of one-carbon-unit coenzymes, such as methylcobalamin (active B_{12}) or formyltetrahydrofolic acid (active folic acid), results in impaired DNA synthesis in developing erythroid cells. These cells do not divide normally, and fewer, large but well-hemoglobinized cells (megaloblasts) form in the bone marrow. When these cells lose their nuclei (the usual process going from nucleated erythroid precursors to the nonnucleated erythrocyte), they are released into the circulation as macrocytes (MCV >120 fl). The result is a macrocytic, normochromic anemia.

Causes of megaloblastic anemia include a dietary deficiency or impaired utilization of B_{12} or folic acid (Table 12.10). Worldwide, folic acid dietary deficiency is believed to be the most common cause of vitamin deficiency. Drug ingestion is the second most common cause of megaloblastic anemia. This can follow the use of cytotoxins such as antineoplastics and immunosuppressive agents that disrupt DNA synthesis rather than by interfering directly with vitamin B_{12} or folic acid metabolism. For example, 5-fluorouracil inhibits thymidylate synthesis, hydroxyurea reduces dATP and dGTP by inhibiting ribonucleotide reductase, and cytosine arabinose competes with dTMP for binding sites on DNA polymerase. Antimitotic agents (e.g., vincristine) and alkylating agents (e.g., chlorambucil, cy-

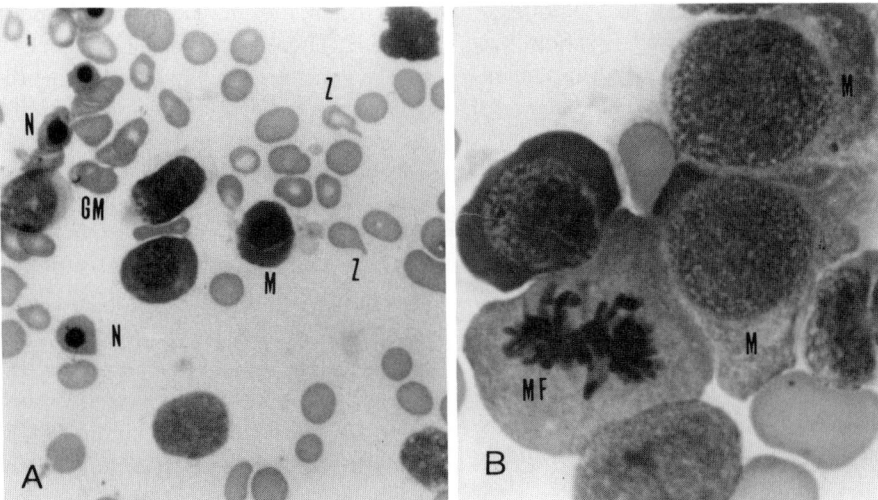

Figure 12.2. Photomicrographs of medium (**A**) and high-power (**B**) views of megaloblastic bone marrow. The nonnucleated erythrocytes are of abnormal shapes (Z), including some with a teardrop appearance. Megaloblasts (M) and a developing erythroid cell with mitotic figures (MF) characteristic of megaloblastic anemias are prominent. Other cells present include nucleated erythrocytes (N) and a giant metamyelocyte (GM).

Table 12.10.
Causes of Vitamin B_{12} and Folic Acid Deficiencies

Vitamin B_{12} deficiency	
Dietary	Inadequate intake
Malabsorption	Inadequate production of intrinsic factor, competition for vitamin B_{12}, disorders of terminal ileum, drug-related
Impaired transport	Transcobalamin II deficiency
Folic acid deficiency	
Dietary	Inadequate intake, unbalanced diet, excessive cooking
Malabsorption	Intestinal mucosal changes
Increased requirements	Pregnancy, infancy, malignancy, increased hematopoiesis
Impaired metabolism	Drug-related, enzyme deficiencies

clophosphamide, or busulfan) do not cause megaloblastic anemia.

General Management of Megaloblastic Anemias (18, 19)

Megaloblastic anemias exhibit the usual features of anemia. Before instituting therapy, the cause and pathophysiologic mechanism must be identified. The common megaloblastic anemias are corrected by replacement therapy (discussed in detail below). The leukopenia associated with megaloblastic anemia is rarely severe enough to predispose the patient to infection. Marked thrombocytopenia may occasionally result in life-threatening hemorrhage, which should be treated with platelet transfusions. Other manifestations include glossitis, dysphagia, anorexia, diminished levels of circulating immunoglobulins, and reduced lymphocyte reactivity.

Vitamin B_{12} Absorption and Metabolism (33, 34)

Vitamin B_{12}, also known as cobalamin, is not a single substance and occurs in both synthetic and biologically active forms. It is a cobalt-containing vitamin that cannot be synthesized by mammalian tissue but only by microorganisms. Therefore, it must be present in the diet. Some bacterial synthesis of B_{12} occurs in the large bowel and the cecum, but there is no absorption at these sites. This is, however, a source for coprophagous mammals (i.e., those that eat feces). Unlike many vitamins, it is not formed by higher plants. Vitamin B_{12} is synthesized by bacteria in the rumina of sheep and cattle, as long as there are traces of cobalt in the fodder. Methylcobalamin, deoxyadenosylcobalamin, and hydroxocobalamin are the major forms in foods. Cyanocobalamin, commonly used for therapeutic purposes, does not occur in the natural state, but is an artifact of the isolation procedure.

For humans, dietary B_{12} is present in most foods of animal origin, complexed to protein. Sources include fresh liver (the richest source) as well as eggs, meat, kidney, milk, dairy products, fish, and shellfish. Fruits, vegetables, and grains lack the vitamin. Nonanimal sources, which contain relatively small amounts of the vitamin, include fermented soy products and yeasts. Because B_{12} is water soluble and relatively heat stable, it is bioavailable from cooked food.

The daily requirement for humans is only 0.5 to 1.0 mg, and the total body stores amount to only 2 to 5 mg. The average diet in the United States supplies 15 mg/day, but there is a wide variation, from 1 to 100 mg/day. Some unusual diets, such as vegan-vegetarian, macrobiotic, or reducing diets that drastically restrict food selection, may not supply the minimum daily requirements. Supplementation is required for patients receiving total parenteral nutrition, those with malnutrition, or those undergoing weight loss, because of insufficient dietary intake.

Vitamin B_{12} uptake and transport is by an orderly sequence of events involving three different binding proteins, intrinsic factor (IF), R proteins, and transcobalamin II. IF, a specific B_{12}-binding glycoprotein, is synthesized and secreted by the parietal cells of the stomach. Secretion of IF parallels the secretion of hydrochloric acid. The R proteins are a group of high-affinity, B_{12}-binding glycoproteins, produced by leukocytes (and probably other tissues), present in a variety of biological secretions including gastric fluid, plasma, saliva, tears, milk, and bile. Their function is not fully understood, but they appear to act as storage sites for the vitamin as well as providing a means of disposal for excess and unwanted vitamin B_{12} analogs. Transcobalamin II is the plasma acceptor protein for recently absorbed B_{12}.

Vitamin B_{12}, particularly at the usual low levels in foods, is well absorbed from the gastrointestinal tract by a process involving interaction between the B_{12} bound to IF and the mucosal cells of the distal ileum. The vitamin, which is protein-bound in foods, is released during gastric digestion. Although cobalamins can bind to R proteins or to IF, at the low gastric pH, binding to gastric R protein is favored. The relative binding of the vitamin may also depend upon the dose, as well as the amounts of R protein and IF secreted. The cobalamins remain bound to R protein in the upper small intestine until pancreatic proteases such as trypsin partially degrade the complex, releasing B_{12}, which then binds to IF. Persons with pancreatic insufficiency could become B_{12} deficient; however, few cases of megaloblastic anemia due to such a deficiency have been reported. The IF-B_{12} complex, which is highly resistant to proteolysis, passes down the small intestine to the distal ileum, where it attaches to specific receptors on the luminal side of the mucosal cells (enterocytes). The attachment is non-energy-dependent, however extracellular calcium and a pH greater than 5.4 are required. How cobalamins are transported across the enterocyte and the fate of IF is poorly understood. One possibility is that IF is released at the cell surface and the vitamin is taken up by the enterocyte. Recent animal studies support receptor-mediated endocytosis. Vitamin B_{12} passes from the mucosa into the capillary circulation, but no IF passes into the blood.

A second mechanism for B_{12} absorption, involving diffusion and not IF, provides small quantities of the vitamin. This mechanism is only biologically important when large amounts are ingested.

Once in the circulation, cobalamins bind to transcobalamin II. There is increasing evidence that transcobalamin II plays an active role in transporting the vitamin from the enterocyte either by entering the cell or by attaching to its plasma membrane. Even though transcobalamin II accepts the newly absorbed vitamin, most circulating cobalamins are bound to transcobalamin I. An explanation for this is that B_{12} bound to transcobalamin II is quickly cleared from the blood ($t_{1/2}$ = 1 hr), whereas it takes several days to clear it from transcobalamin I.

The daily cellular requirements for B_{12} are low, and much of that ingested is stored in the liver. The amount in the liver is 2 to 5 mg, which represents 40 to 50% of the total body content. Vitamin B_{12} is conserved in the body by enterohepatic recycling. Biliary excretion of B_{12} is much higher than excretion in urine or feces. Vitamin B_{12} and its analogs in bile are excreted bound to biliary R protein. When the complex comes into contact with pancreatic enzymes in the upper small intestine, B_{12} and its analogs are released because of biliary R protein degradation. Only B_{12} binds to fresh intrinsic factor; the analogs are excreted in the feces. Bile, as well as being the major route of B_{12} analog excretion, possibly plays a role in enhancing B_{12} absorption. When the diet contains little or no B_{12}, as may be the case for strict vegans, biliary cobalamin is conserved to the extent that clinical deficiency may take up to 20 years to develop. When malabsorption occurs, such as in pernicious anemia (PA), endogenous as well as dietary B_{12} is lost and deficiency develops within 3 to 6 years. This accounts for the slow and insidious course of PA.

Vitamin B_{12} Deficiency

Deficiency occurs when the serum concentration of B_{12} is less than 150 pmol/liter (200 pg/ml). Reduced erythropoiesis due to B_{12} deficiency also results in impaired utilization of iron and folic acid, leading to elevations in serum iron concentration, transferrin saturation, and ferritin and folate levels. Thus, normal-to-elevated levels of serum folate and iron saturation in the presence of B_{12} deficiency strongly indicate accompanying deficiencies. The stages of B_{12} deficiency are outlined in Table 12.11.

Etiology of Vitamin B_{12} Deficiency (18, 33, 34)

Causes of B_{12} deficiency include inadequate intake, malabsorption, B_{12} degradation, and increased requirement. Most cases of deficiency are secondary to malabsorption associated with addisonian pernicious anemia (PA), gastric lesions, gastrectomy, and a number of small bowel disorders. PA is the most common specific type of B_{12} malabsorption in North America.

Table 12.11.
Stages of Vitamin B_{12} Deficiency

Stage	B_{12} Status	Comment
1	Normal	
2	Negative balance	Decreased TCII-bound B_{12}
3	Depletion	Serum B_{12} <150 μg/liter
4	Biochemical deficit	Abnormal dUST and/or hypersegmentation of netrophil nuclei and possibly increased serum methylmalonic acid
5	Overt clinical deficiency	Macroovalocytes develop, blood hemoglobin falls

a Modified from Jandl JH, The hypochromic anemias and other disorders of iron metabolism. In Blood: Text Book of Hematology. Boston, Little, Brown & Co, ch 6, 1987.

Nutritional Deficiency of Vitamin B_{12}

Dietary causes are rare and are possibly only important in strict vegans, breast-fed babies of vegan mothers, and persons living in countries where poor nutrition is widespread. Vegans are strict vegetarians who do not consume foods of animal origin, including milk, cheese, and eggs. A number of years on a restricted unbalanced diet can result in deficiency. Deficiency is less likely in vegans who ingest sufficient calories from a wide selection of food. Here microbial contamination of foods can provide trace amounts of B_{12}. The elderly are also susceptible, particularly if they are living on tea and cereal, toast, or biscuits for financial reasons or because of unavailability of food or lack of interest in preparing meals. PA is also common in the elderly. Vegetarians have serum B_{12} levels of 200 to 250 pmol/liter (260–330 pg/ml), which on average are lower than those of omnivores.

Gastric Disorders

Gastric disorders, most commonly gastrectomy, are the second most common cause of vitamin B_{12} malabsorption. Some abnormalities of the stomach, in the presence of an adequate diet, prevent the release of the vitamin from foods. These include atrophic gastritis, achlorhydria, vagotomy, partial gastrectomy, and the use of H2-receptor antagonists. A point worth noting is that the remaining amount of IF still can promote absorption of synthetic crystalline cyanocobalamin. Complete gastrectomy results in an absolute deficiency of IF and megaloblastic anemia develops 3 to 6 years after surgery unless supplementation is given. Partial gastrectomy is a variable cause of B_{12} deficiency. Deficiency is also possible if sufficient gastric mucosa has been destroyed by ingestion of corrosive chemicals, by tumors or by chronic gastritis.

Intestinal Problems

Small intestine disorders are the third most common cause of B_{12} deficiency. A number of abnormal situations leading to malabsorption range from impaired transfer of the vitamin from R protein to competition for luminal B_{12} or a low pH in the ileum.

Absorption of B_{12}, as indicated by the Schilling test, is impaired in 50 to 70% of patients with pancreatic insufficiency. Defective absorption can be partially corrected by giving oral pancreatic preparations and/or sodium bicarbonate. B_{12} malabsorption also occurs in the Zollinger-Ellison syndrome if the associated hypersecretion of gastric acid is left uncontrolled. The associated lowering of pH in the duodenum inactivates pancreatic proteolytic enzymes.

Surgical resection or bypass of the ileum also increases the likelihood of malabsorption. Most persons who have lost more than 5 cm of distal ilium have abnormal Schilling test results. Even in the presence of IF, B_{12} malabsorption occurs in conditions such as tropical sprue, Crohn's disease, celiac disease, lymphomas, and Whipple's disease, where alteration or destruction of the ileal absorptive surface occurs. In the recessive disorder, Imerslund-Grasbeck's disease, selective malabsorption of B_{12} by a poorly understood mechanism, occurs in association with proteinuria.

Bacterial overgrowth, particularly by *Bacteroides* and coliforms, in blind loops or diverticula result in B_{12} malabsorption. Absorption returns to normal when patients are given tetracycline, lincomycin, or metronidazole. The mechanism of B_{12} uptake by bacteria is unclear. Most intestinal bacteria avidly absorb the unbound vitamin, but only small amounts are taken up when it is bound to IF. Infestation by the tapeworm *Diphyllobothrium latum* (from eating undercooked freshwater fish), resulting in competition for the vitamin, is a potential problem in Scandinavian countries, Japan, and the USSR. Possibly the parasite releases B_{12} from its IF complex.

Drug-induced Vitamin B_{12} Deficiency

Drug-induced B_{12} deficiency has been associated with a number of pharmacotherapeutic agents including colchicine, *p*-aminosalicylic acid, and the biguanide hypoglycemic agents. The latter are thought to affect transcellular transport of B_{12}. Other agents implicated include ethanol and cholestyramine, which reduce B_{12} absorption in the ileum.

Persons exposed to nitrous oxide gas for prolonged periods of time show megaloblastic marrow changes that can be corrected by B_{12} administration. Nitrous oxide may block the homocysteine-methionine reaction in cells of the bone marrow, nervous system, and other tissues. Peripheral neuropathy has also been reported in dentists chronically exposed to nitrous oxide. Alcoholics are particularly vulnerable to B_{12} deficiency because of chronic gastritis, poor diet, folate deficiency, and pancreatic insufficiency.

Pernicious Anemia (33)

Pernicious anemia (PA) is due to B_{12} malabsorption because of a lack of IF and hydrochloric acid secretion. The term pernicious is used because the anemia develops insidiously and progressively. Two types of PA have been described. The adult type, by far the more common of the two, occurs with a prevalence of 0.2 to 0.6%. It rarely occurs before 30 years of age, and between 45 and 60 years affects women more frequently than men. There is a distinctive racial and geographic distribution of PA, which is far more common in temperate regions such as North America and northern Europe than in tropical countries. The disease also afflicts blacks, especially women, more than was once believed. Juvenile PA is less common, and patients often develop clinical features of B_{12} deficiency during the second decade of life. Inherited conditions leading to PA in infancy or early childhood may be due to a lack of IF or the production of abnormal IF by an otherwise normal stomach.

Current evidence suggests that PA is caused by an autoimmune reaction against gastric parietal cells. PA has been linked with other immunologic problems. PA occurs more commonly in persons with diseases afflicting the immune system such as Grave's disease, myxedema, thyroiditis, idiopathic adrenocortical insufficiency, vitiligo, and hypoparathyroidism. Relatives of patients with PA also show a higher incidence of the disease. Most sufferers have increased levels of circulating antibodies, particularly those directed against antiparietal cells and IF. The latter antibodies are generally characteristic of PA.

Clinical Manifestations (34–37)

Many clinical manifestations are common to all forms of B_{12} deficiency, all of which are likely to occur in severe deficiency (Table 12.12). Clinical manifestations reflect anormalities of the blood, gastrointestinal tract, and nervous system. In severe cases the peripheral blood film exhibits severe macrocytic anemia, leukopenia with hypersegmentation of the polymorphonuclear cells, and thrombocytopenia. The diagnostic triad of symptoms are weakness, painful tongue, and numbness and tingling of extremities. In many instances, at least two of these symptoms are encountered.

The onset of PA is insidious, and most patients present with signs and symptoms of anemia. Patients are generally well nourished, although they may have lost weight. The mucous membranes are usually pale, and in Caucasians the skin is pale and yellow-tinted because of the anemia and the mild jaundice of ineffective erythropoiesis.

Nonspecific symptoms related to coexisting anemia and neurologic involvement include apathy, weakness, fatigue, palpitations, and breathlessness. In elderly patients, the deficiency may manifest initially as postural hypotension or congestive heart failure. Other symptoms may com-

Table 12.12.
Clinical Features of Pernicious Anemia

Symptoms and physical appearance[a]
  Pallor, slight jaundice and faint icterus of the sclera
  Anorexia accompanied by a mild degree of weight loss; a flabby rather than a wasted appearance; diarrhea
  Dyspnea, palpitations, sensation of extra heartbeats, weakness, vertigo, tinnitus, precordial pain and heart murmurs
  Paraesthesiae, difficulty in walking, loss of vibratory sense, incoordination of movements
  Disturbed mentation, such as irritability, memory disturbances and mild depression; serious mental symptoms may develop
  Mild pyrexia
  Difficulty in urination
Organ involvement
  Atrophic glossitis
  Mild hepatosplenomegaly
  Enlarged heart
  Nervous system—spinal cord and peripheral nerve degeneration
  Achylia gastrica
  Gastric cancer

[a] Similar features occur in all types of vitamin B_{12} deficiency.

plicate the picture, suggesting primary involvement of the gastrointestinal, cardiovascular, or genitourinary systems. Neurologic manifestations involving the spinal cord can develop before the anemia. Sometimes these are so advanced that primary neurologic disease is suspected. Because PA usually occurs in the elderly, it can be difficult to determine to what extent age-related changes contribute to the clinical findings. The laboratory findings in PA are outlined in (Table 12.13).

Gastrointestinal manifestations such as atrophic glossitis (sore and abnormally smooth tongue), anorexia, indigestion, and diarrhea occur because the normally rapidly proliferating epithelium is deprived of adequate amounts of B_{12}.

A long-standing lack of B_{12} results in distinct changes in the nervous system, beginning with demyelination of nerves and leading to neurologic abnormalities. Peripheral nerve damage results in symmetrical parasthesias (numbness and tingling of the extremities) and reduction of pain and temperature sensation. The most serious problem, subacute degeneration of the spinal cord, is associated with loss of position and vibration sense, resulting in ataxia and weakness. Lateral column disruption leads to weakness and spasticity, exemplified by myoclonus, hyperreflexia, and a positive Babinski's sign. If the condition remains untreated, instability of gait and virtual paralysis result.

Psychiatric manifestations include impaired mentation, delirium, paranoia, psychosis, irritability, depression, and personality changes. Psychiatric symptoms may occur in the absence of hematologic abnormalities or signs of neuropathy. The mechanism is unknown but could be secondary to folic acid deficiency.

183

Table 12.13.
Laboratory Findings in Pernicious Anemia

Parameter	Comments
Hematocrit	Normal to decreased
Peripheral smear	Macrocytic, occasional nucleated cells and a reticulocyte index well below 1
Erythrocytes	Oval-shaped variations in size, some bizarre-shaped poikilocytes); mean corpuscular volume (MCV) greater than normal (100–160 fl)' mean corpuscular hemoglobulin (MCH) is increased, which results in a normal mean corpuscular hemoglobulin concentration (MCHC); increased hemolysis
Leukocytes	Hypersegmentation of polymorphonuclear cell nuclei is a consistent finding; if more than 3 cells have 5 lobes or a single cell has 6 lobes, this is presumptive diagnosis of a megaloblastic anemia; there can be mild to moderate neutropenia
Platelets	Reduced in number and bizarre in appearance on occasion
Serum B_{12}	Decreased
Serum folate	Normal; sometimes elevated because of folate metabolic trap
Gastric secretion	Achlorhydria (histamine-fast achlorhydria found in most patients); total volume of the gastric secretion and its enzyme content are markedly reduced; increased serum gastrin
Antibodies	Antiparietal and anti–intrinsic factor antibodies present
Others	Methylmalonic acid excretion is enhanced; plasma unconjugated bilirubin and lactic acid dehydrogenase (type 1) increased because of enhanced intramedullary destruction of erythrocytes; iron kinetics data are abnormal

Megaloblastosis and Neurologic Manifestations

In humans, B_{12} deficiency causes megaloblastic anemia indistinguishable from that found in folate deficiency, as well as subacute combined degeneration of the spinal cord related to the B_{12} deficiency. Although controversial, the most widely accepted view on the underlying biochemical mechanisms for these pathologies is an intracellular methylfolate trap due to reduced cellular methionine (Fig. 12.3). Methylcobalamin is an essential cofactor in the conversion of homocysteine to methionine. Impairment of this reaction results in deranged folate metabolism, thought to underly defective DNA synthesis and the megaloblastosis in persons deficient in B_{12}. It is proposed that in B_{12} deficiency states, unconjugated N-5-methyltetrahydrofolate taken up by cells from the plasma is a poor substrate for conversion to other forms, such as N-5, 10-methylenetetrahydrofolate. Useful metabolites are utilized by cells for the most essential methylation reactions, at the expense of DNA and protein synthesis and cell division. This in part explains why partial remission of the hematologic

manifestations occurs if patients consume large quantities of folic acid. Although flooding the DNA synthetic pathways allows the bone marrow to return to normal, neurologic lesions do not respond readily in the short or long term. Without adequate treatment with B_{12}, the methylating capacity of cells is ultimately reduced, resulting in subacute degeneration of the spinal cord.

Impaired conversion of homocysteine to methionine may in part cause the neurologic lesions of B_{12} deficiency. Methionine is required for the synthesis of choline and choline-containing phospholipids and for methylation of myelin proteins. Additionally, a lack of adenosylcobalamin, required for the conversion of methylmalonyl-CoA to succinyl-CoA, leads to accumulation of methylmalonyl CoA- and propionyl-CoA. This leads to the synthesis of nonphysiologic odd-numbered fatty acids, which are subsequently incorporated into neuronal lipids.

During folate deficiency, cellular methionine synthesis is also diminished, which diverts folate from DNA synthesis and megaloblastosis develops. Because folate is used selectively to conserve methionine and nerve tissue concentrates folate, subacute degeneration is absent in folate deficiency.

Diagnosis of Vitamin B_{12} Deficiency (34, 38, 39)

The triad of anti-IF antibodies, low serum B_{12} level, and megaloblastic anemia is diagnostic for PA. Macrocytic anemia, peripheral neuropathy, and dementia also suggests B_{12} deficiency. Clinical diagnosis can be confirmed by a complete blood count, serum B_{12} and folate measurements, and a reticulocyte count. The etiology can be determined by the Schilling test. Serum B_{12} levels can be used for routine screening.

Hematologic tests revealing macrocytosis must be followed up with other tests to determine the cause. Macrocytosis may be an incidental finding when patients are being investigated for other problems, such as alcoholism or respiratory problems. Macrocytosis is also possible in association with liver disease, myxedema, acute myelogenous leukemia, acquired sideroblastic anemia, aplastic anemia, hemolytic anemia, posthemorrhagic states and splenectomy, and is seen in the aged.

Macrocytosis is not always present in B_{12} deficiency (40). It may be blocked by concurrent iron deficiency or anemia of chronic disease. Concurrent α thalassemia, a problem of particular relevance to American blacks, can also mask macrocytosis (41). Laboratory tests used for the differential diagnosis include serum B_{12} and folate determinations, erythrocyte folate determination, the Schilling test, and a test for IF antibodies. In PA, serum concentrations of B_{12} are low, but the serum folate is within the normal range.

A number of independent factors can influence B_{12} test results. Falsely low values can occur in folic acid de-

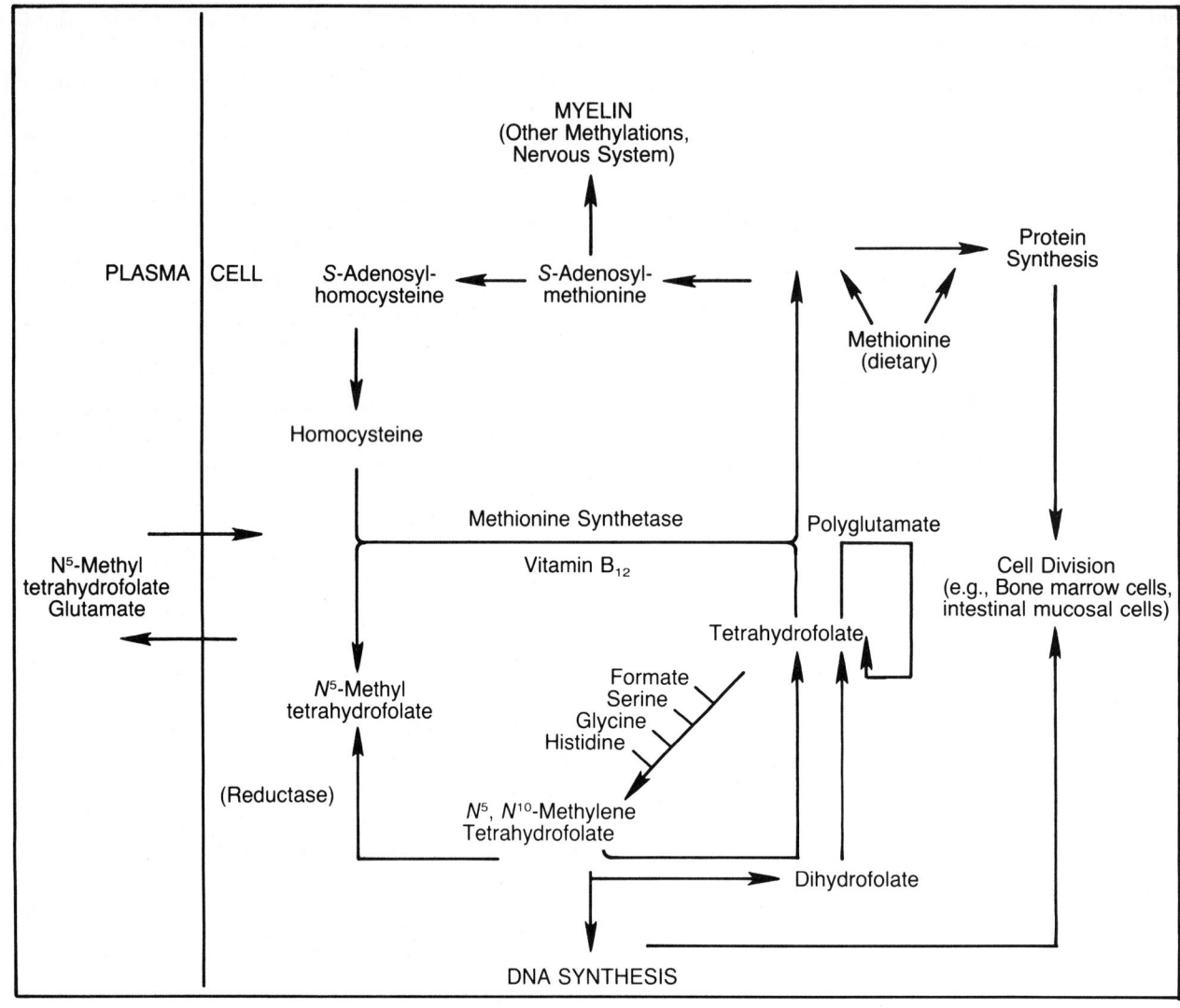

Figure 12.3.   Normal vitamin B_{12} and folate metabolism in mammalian cells.

ficiency. Excluding laboratory errors and dietary factors, low results are obtained with the radioimmunoassay if radiopharmaceuticals have also been used in the patient for investigations such as bone scanning, erythrocyte mass testing, thyroid function evaluation, or cardiac testing. Antibiotic therapy can falsely lower measurements obtained by the microbiologic method. In vitro decomposition of B_{12} is also possible if subjects have consumed high doses of ascorbic acid.

Lower B_{12} levels have also been observed in the elderly. However this may not represent a true deficiency state, since most had a positive Schilling test. A greater heterogenity in results has also been observed in the elderly (42). Elderly subjects with low serum B_{12} levels should be further evaluated. Low serum levels are also common in pregnancy. Reduced synthesis of transcobalamin I in many patients with multiple myeloma also leads

to low levels. A Schilling test (with or without IF) should be performed in all cases of suspected B_{12} malabsorption to determine whether there is a lack of IF or an ileal defect. Several types of Schilling tests are available (34, 38). The standard test is divided into three stages. In stage I, an oral dose of 1 μg of ^{57}Co-labeled B_{12} is given, followed by a 1 mg i.m. flushing dose of unlabeled B_{12}, and the 24-hr urine excretion of the label is measured (Table 12.14). The large i.m. dose of B_{12} saturates its binding proteins in the blood. Consequently there are fewer binding sites for ^{57}Co-labeled B_{12}, and a substantial proportion is excreted in the urine. B_{12} absorption is considered to be impaired if less than 10% of the label is excreted in the urine. If less than 5% is excreted, the diagnosis is consistent with PA. Note that this test depends on renal function and a complete 24-hr urine collection.

Stage II of the test distinguishes between the possible

Table 12.14.
Summary of Schilling Test Results in Vitamin B$_{12}$ Deficiency

Condition	Stage I	Stage II	Stage III
Normal	Normal		
Inadequate diet	Normal		
Pernicious anemia	Low	Normal	
Bacterial overgrowth	Low	Low	Normal
Ileal defect	Low	Low	Low

causes of the malabsorption (e.g., PA, lack of ileal absorptive sites, or bacterial overgrowth proximal to the terminal ileum). This is performed by giving 10 mg of hog IF with the radiolabeled B$_{12}$ and measuring excretion of the radiolabel. Previous exposure to hog IF (e.g., consumption of IF in some OTC vitamin preparations) may give low results. In these cases malabsorption can be detected by using normal human gastric juice rather than hog IF. If the results are inconclusive, stage III of the test is performed, which involves giving the patient antibiotics, usually tetracycline 250 mg p.o. q.i.d., for 10 to 14 days, and then repeating the stage I test.

Vitamin B$_{12}$ replacement therapy should be given for several weeks before repeating the Schilling test, to allow any intestinal megaloblastosis that accompanies deficiency states to resolve. Although this reversal may take several weeks, it is probably corrected in most patients over one cycle of intestinal epithelial cells. Megaloblastosis of the mucosal epithelium cells may cause secondary malabsorption and possibly a false-positive Schilling test. If malabsorption is not reversed with added IF, other causes should be explored.

Care must be taken when interpreting the Schilling test results for patients also taking H2 antagonists such as cimetidine, ranitidine or famotidine. Such agents may cause falsely abnormal results by preventing the degradation of R protein and decreasing the secretion of endogenous intrinsic factor. Reduced hydrochloric acid production caused by H2 antagonists as well as other situations in which acid and intrinsic factor secretion is reduced, such as achlorhydria, vagotomy, or partial gastrectomy, can give falsely normal Schilling test results (43, 44). The problem here is that the aqueous, crystalline B$_{12}$ used in the test differs in bioavailability from the usually food-bound vitamin that must be released to participate in the uptake process. A modified Schilling test, (PBAT), using protein-bound B$_{12}$, more closely resembles the physiologic state.

Serum anti-IF antibodies should also be measured. This test has positive results in 50% of patients with PA and combined with a low serum B$_{12}$ is useful in the differential diagnosis. A disadvantage is that positive results can be associated with other autoimmune disorders. Less commonly used tests include thymidine uptake (dUST test) by bone marrow cells and serum methylmalonic acid or homocysteine measurements (43, 44).

Management of Vitamin B$_{12}$ Deficiency (34, 35, 45)

Depending on the cause, either oral or parenteral B$_{12}$ replacement therapy is used. A diagnosis of B$_{12}$ deficiency should be confirmed by laboratory investigations before beginning therapy, although in seriously ill patients it may be necessary to administer both B$_{12}$ and folic acid while awaiting confirmation.

The aims of treatment are hematologic remission, reversal or retardation of the nervous system complications, and replenishment of B$_{12}$ stores. "Shotgun" treatments with hematinic combinations and the use of parenteral B$_{12}$ injections as placebo injections should be discouraged, because there is no rational basis for their use. Dietary deficiencies can be treated with oral cyanocobalamin, but for malabsorption in PA, i.m. or deep s.c. injections of cyanocobalamin or hydroxocobalamin are used (45). Small amounts of cyanocobalamin are sometimes included in TPN solutions.

In severe cases of PA, the patient should be confined to bed until the hemoglobin has increased to about 70 g/liter. The diet should be light, easily digested, and contain protein, iron, and ascorbic acid. Blood transfusions are rarely indicated, but they have been used cautiously in patients who are dyspneic at rest, those who have not responded to B$_{12}$, and those who have a 20 to 30 g/liter (2 to 3 g/dl) very low hemoglobin level. Packed cells (rather than whole blood) are used to prevent fluid overload and cardiovascular crisis.

Persons with serum B$_{12}$ levels of <150 pmol/liter (200 pg/ml) should be treated, even in the absence of macrocytosis or a normal Schilling test result. A potential problem exists; therapeutic doses given before a diagnosis is made can mask some of the clinical manifestations of subacute degeneration of the spinal cord. Those with a normal Schilling test result and a serum B$_{12}$ level of <150 pmol/liter (200 pg/ml) should be given oral B$_{12}$ (1 mg/day) until serum levels are raised to >250 pmol/liter 330 pg/ml. If this response is not achieved or results of a Schilling test are abnormal, the patient should be treated for PA.

A number of different parenteral B$_{12}$ regimens are in use. Because of the relative safety of these agents, large doses of 1000 μg of either cyanocobalamin or hydroxocobalamin can be given weekly, followed by monthly injections for a year to replenish stores. After this, injections (up to 3 months apart, based on the patient's response) are given for life, to maintain remission. When patients with untreated PA are given 1000 μg of cyanocobalamin, the serum concentration of the vitamin remains in the normal range for at least 1 week. The megaloblastosis can be transformed in a few hours, and the soreness of the tongue and affective disturbances recede in 1 day. Reversal of neurologic manifestations and dementia takes longer and may be incomplete. Although similar doses are used to treat both hematologic and neurologic problems, higher doses have been suggested for the latter.

Alternative lower dosing regimens can also be used. Single 80-µg doses completely reverse a megaloblastic bone marrow. However, doses under 15 µg are generally insufficient to completely correct the abnormality. If a low-dose regimen is used, more frequent administration is required. A suitable low-dose regimen for cyanocobalamin in the initial treatment of deficiency states is 100 µg/day for 6 to 7 days, followed by 100 µg/day every other day for 7 doses if clinical improvement and reticulocyte response occurs. Then 100 µg/day is given every 3 to 4 days for another 2 to 3 weeks. Maintenance therapy is usually 100 to 200 µg/month. The regimen for hydroxocobalamin is similar. In PA or after total gastrectomy or extensive ileal resection, parenteral therapy is required for life. The initial dose is low for children, but the maintenance dose is the same as that for adults. For children with intracellular defects of B_{12} metabolism, hydroxocobalamin is more effective for treatment than cyanocobalamin and usually requires high doses, of the order of 500 to 1000 µg/day. For children with transcobalamin II deficiency, oral cyanocobalamin is the preferred treatment.

Hypokalemia is a potential problem of B_{12} therapy related to the rapid conversion of bone marrow from megaloblastic to normoblastic, particularly in patients with marked anemia, thrombocytopenia, and neutropenia. Sudden death is possible due to the increased potassium requirements for erythropoiesis.

It has been emphasized in the past that oral cyanocobalamin may be an effective way to treat B_{12} deficiency, including PA (31). In dietary deficiency or in vegans where absorption is normal, this is the preferred route. The oral dose of dietary cyanocobalamin for dietary supplementation is 1 µg/day and up to 25 µg/day for persons with increased requirements. Because approximately 1% of an oral dose of B_{12} can be absorbed by a nonspecific process, even in the absence of IF, PA can be treated by giving 1000 µg/day p.o. for 1 month, followed by 1000 µg/week p.o. to maintain remission. Such therapy may be erratic, so it should be assessed frequently.

Oral cyanocobalamin may be justified for patients with bleeding disorders or for those allergic to parenterally administered B_{12} (rare). Oral administration means less frequent visits for injections, but careful compliance counseling about the importance of lifelong therapy is important. Before the availability of the crystalline forms of B_{12}, PA was managed adequately with daily doses of liver containing 240 µg of B_{12}. Oral B_{12} is not useful in small bowel disease, in malabsorption syndromes, or following gastric or ileal resection.

Monitoring Therapy

The patient's progress should be monitored clinically and by appropriate laboratory testing (e.g., a full hemogram and reticulocyte count). Reticulocytosis with a maximum reticulocyte count occurs by about the 4th to 7th day after treatment has commenced. The neutrophil count also increases by this time, although the hypersegmented polymorphonuclear neutrophils will persist for 10 to 14 days. Macrocytosis may persist for several months after treatment is started because of the long half-life of erythrocytes. The serum iron concentration, which may be within the reference range or elevated before treatment, decreases to deficient levels within 24 hr of starting treatment. Some patients show a pause in the response to B_{12} 2 to 3 weeks after beginning therapy, and the hemoglobin fails to rise over 100 to 110 g/liter (10–11 g/dl). This is probably due to a depletion of iron stores, resulting from the accelerated erythropoiesis, and it responds to oral ferrous sulfate, 200 mg three times a day.

Because of the potential for life-threatening hypokalemia associated with rapid erythropoiesis, serum potassium concentrations should be monitored during the first 48 hr of treatment, particularly if potassium-depleting diuretics are also being used.

Synthetic Vitamin B_{12} (45)

The two synthetic forms of B_{12} incorporated into pharmaceuticals are cyanocobalamin and hydroxocobalamin. Indications for both of these agents are similar, although hydroxocobalamin may be preferred for treating B_{12} deficiencies because optic neuropathies may degenerate with the administration of cyanocobalamin. A disadvantage of hydroxocobalamin is that in rare cases some persons may develop antibodies to the transcobalamin-hydroxocobalamin complex and therefore it must be discontinued.

Oral cyanocobalamin is well absorbed, with peak serum levels being reached 8 to 12 hr after oral ingestion. In contrast, peak serum levels following i.m. injection are reached in 1 hr. Following absorption, regardless of the route of administration, both forms of the vitamin are highly protein bound to the transcobalamins. Both are metabolized in the liver, followed by biliary and urinary excretion. Doses beyond the daily needs ar excreted, largely unchanged, via the urine. Cyanocobalamin i.m. is excreted more rapidly than is hydroxocobalamin, which is more highly protein bound than the former. The half-life of synthetic B_{12} is about 6 days; its half-life in the liver is 400 days. With impaired liver or kidney function, more frequent dosing is necessary.

Synthetic B_{12} is usually well tolerated, and allergic reactions are rare. Medical attention should be sought if a rash or wheezing develops. Although anaphylactic reactions can occur after parenteral administration, they are rare. An intradermal test dose is recommended for patients with a history of suspected allergic reactions to B_{12}. Subjects intolerant to naturally occurring B_{12} in foods may be intolerant to the synthetic forms also. Other symptoms, such as mild diarrhea and transient itching, only require medical attention if they continue and worry the patient. A potential problem is that B_{12} therapy can mask the signs of polycythemia vera.

No adverse effects have been documented when the normal daily requirements for these agents has been administered during pregnancy. B_{12} crosses the placenta, and at birth the neonatal level can be 2 to 5 times that of the mother. Cyanocobalamin injection containing benzyl alcohol should not be used in neonates or immature infants because of possible toxicity of this preservative. B_{12} is excreted in breast milk, and no problems have been reported for humans taking the normal daily requirements. No geriatric problems have been reported.

Many pharmacologic agents can reduce the absorption of B_{12} from the gastrointestinal tract and thus increase the requirements. These include excessive consumption of ethanol for longer than 2 weeks, prolonged use of cholestyramine, colchicine, and in particular aminoglycoside antibiotics. Concurrent use of chloramphenicol may antagonize the hemopoietic response, so hematologic monitoring is necessary and (if possible) an alternative antibiotic should be used. As large doses of ascorbic acid may destroy B_{12}, patients should avoid such ingestion within 1 hr of taking oral B_{12}. Large doses of folic acid may also reduce B_{12} concentrations in the blood.

Finally, megadoses of B_{12}, 10 times or more the RDA, have no proven value and should be discouraged. Cyanocobalamin has no proven value in the treatment of acute viral hepatitis, allergies, amblyopia, delayed growth, malnutrition or tardy appetite, fatigue, mental disorders, multiple sclerosis, sterility, trigeminal neuralgia, or other neurologic conditions or in retarding the aging process.

Prognosis (35)

If correctly diagnosed and treated, cases of B_{12} deficiency and especially PA have an excellent prognosis. Anemia can be reversed, and early vigorous treatment is required to slow and reverse neurologic complications and neuropsychiatric manifestations.

FOLIC ACID DEFICIENCY (19–21)

Folate deficiency, like B_{12} deficiency, results in megaloblastic anemia and other hematologic abnormalities. Malnourishment however is more of a problem with folate deficiency. Folic acid is an important factor in cell division, and without it, division stops at metaphase. Adequate folic acid is required for normal erythropoiesis, including the maturation of megaloblasts into normoblasts in the bone marrow.

Absorption and Metabolism of Folic Acid (46)

Folic acid is present in many plant and animal foods, either as free folic acid or as polyglutamates, with the folic acid conjugated to glutamic acid. The best sources of folic acid include green leafy vegetables, fruits, and organ meats such as liver and kidney. Because heat destroys 50 to 90% of folic acid in foods, canned or overcooked food may be devoid of the vitamin.

The human requirement for folic acid, which depends on metabolic and cell turnover rates, varies from 50 μg/day in infancy to up to 100 μg/day in adults. Healthy persons have total body folic acid stores of 5 to 10 mg; half of which is stored in the liver as N-5-methyltetrahydrofolate. More than 2% is degraded daily, so a continuous dietary supply is essential.

Active absorption of folic acid occurs mainly in the proximal part of the small intestine. Conjugated folic acid (such as in foods) is absorbed to a lesser degree than free folic acid; however a conjugase in the epithelial cells converts the polyglutamates into absorbable monoglutamates. During absorption, the folic acid is reduced and methylated to N-5-methyltetrahydrofolate. However in malabsorption syndromes, absorption of folic acid from food is impaired. In contrast, folic acid from pharmaceutical products is almost completely absorbed in the upper duodenum, even in the presence of malabsorption. The principal circulating form of folic acid, N-5-methyltetrahydrofolate, is extensively bound to plasma proteins. There is no specific transport protein. Plasma levels vary from 3 to 21 ng/ml and closely reflect the dietary intake. Erythrocyte folate levels, 160 to 640 ng/ml of whole blood standardized to a hematocrit of 45%, are a better indicator of folate status than are the serum levels. Some enterohepatic cycling of folic acid occurs, although significant amounts are not reabsorbed from the bile.

Folic acid is excreted almost entirely as metabolites by the kidney. Amounts beyond the daily requirement are excreted, largely unchanged, in the urine. Because folic acid is removed by hemodialysis, dialysis patients should be given increased amounts (100 to 300% of the RDA).

Etiology of Folate Deficiency (18–20)

Folate deficiency is one of the common causes of nutritional anemias. Inadequate diet, alcoholism, pregnancy, and malabsorption syndromes are the most frequent causes of folate deficiency. Other causes include increased requirements, enhanced metabolism, and interference in the metabolism or clearance by other pharmacotherapeutic agents (47, 48). The patient's diet, ethanol intake, or signs and symptoms associated with malabsorption may indicate the cause of folate deficiency.

Folic acid intake may be reduced if insufficient attention is paid to the diet and folic acid–rich foods are excluded or if food is poorly prepared or overheated. Persons at risk include alcoholics whose main caloric intake is in the form of ethanol; narcotic addicts who have a poor diet; the elderly, who often do not feel like eating or who eat commercially prepared foods; institutionalized persons who have no control over their diet; adolescents and teenagers, who may skip meals and eat junk foods; and some infants. Megaloblastic anemia due to simple dietary deficiency of folic acid is common and sometimes severe among people living in the tropics or in underdeveloped countries. It is less common in more prosperous countries.

Several reasons have been suggested for folate deficiency in alcoholics. These include reduced dietary intake, inactivation of folate conjugase, impaired enterohepatic cycling, and depletion of liver folate stores. Malabsorption of folate is frequently a problem in persons with tropical sprue, a condition in which there is chronic inflammation of the bowel. Tropical sprue responds to either folic acid or oral antibiotic therapy. Regional ileitis, celiac disease, and resection of the small intestine may also lead to folic acid malabsorption.

Drugs are the most common cause of megaloblastic anemia after folate or B_{12} deficiency. Interference, either directly or indirectly, with DNA synthesis in developing erythroid cells is the most common effect of these drugs. Signs of folate deficiency often appear in epileptics, but these are due to dietary habits as much as to therapy. These agents, especially phenytoin and primidone, which possibly reduce intestinal absorption of the vitamin, rarely induce megaloblastic anemia. As the CNS effect of phenytoin may decrease with concurrent use of folic acid, an increase in the phenytoin dose may be necessary. The importance of the interaction can be determined by monitoring serum phenytoin levels.

Oral contraceptives and estrogen preparations may impair folate absorption in some women. Folate requirements are increased in long-term users of corticosteroids or analgesics. Antibiotics can interfere with the microbiologic assay of folate, giving falsely low results. Also, folic acid supplements should be taken 1 hr before or 4 to 6 hr after cholestyramine ingestion, to avoid reduced absorption of the vitamin.

Chemotherapeutic agents such as 6-thioguanine, azathioprine, and 6-mercaptopurine, which are the purine analogs, act as direct inhibitors of DNA synthesis, resulting in drug-induced megaloblastic anemia. Similar effects occur with the pyrimidine analogs, 5-fluorouracil and cytosine arabinoside; and hydroxyurea and procarbazine. Methotrexate and to a lesser extent pentamidine, pyrimethamine, and trimethoprim, when used for prolonged periods or at high doses, impair DNA synthesis by inhibiting dihydrofolate reductase. Giving leucovorin calcium (a folinic acid compound), particularly when methotrexate is being used, reduces the risk of megaloblastic anemia. Although oral sulfonamide agents can reduce the intestinal

absorption of folic acid, supplementation is not generally given with the usual antibiotic courses. Patients taking sulfasalazine chronically may require supplementation.

An increased requirement for folic acid occurs during pregnancy, infancy, malignancy, increased erythropoiesis, and when there is a rapid cell turnover. During pregnancy, a large increase in nucleic acid synthesis is associated with growth of the fetus, placenta, and uterus, and the increased maternal erythrocyte mass. Folate requirements may increase threefold during pregnancy, and if supplements are not taken, particularly in the last trimester, megaloblastic anemia may develop in the mother. Other problems that can affect folate status in the mother during pregnancy are urinary tract infections and nausea and vomiting, which may restrict food intake.

Folate deficiency is extremely common in myeloproliferative disorders such as chronic myeloid leukemia and myelofibrosis, often leading to thrombocytopenia or anemia. The increased folate requirements in chronic hemolytic anemia, exfoliative dermatitis, generalized psoriasis, or extensive burns can also lead to folate deficiency. In these cases adequate supplementation is required. Anemia is more likely to occur if several contributing factors are present.

Clinical Features

Signs and symptoms of folate deficiency are similar to those of other megaloblastic anemias. Specifically these include megaloblastosis, glossitis, diarrhea, weight loss, and neurologic manifestations. The disease progresses slowly, and the hemoglobin level may fall to an ominously low 20 to 30 g/liter.

Diagnosis

In all patients with macrocytosis and where megaloblastosis is suspected, peripheral blood smears, both serum folate and B_{12} concentrations, and erythrocyte folate levels should be measured. Megaloblastosis possibly due to folic acid deficiency must be interpreted in the light of B_{12} status because of similar findings in B_{12} deficiency. Another problem is that some patients with PA have low serum folate levels secondary to megaloblastosis of the intestinal epithelial cells. The diagnosis of megaloblastic anemia due to folate deficiency requires showing reduced folate tissue levels, as reflected by erythrocyte folate concentrations. Anemia occurs only when tissue levels are depleted. A normal serum folate concentration does not exclude deficiency. Serum folate levels have the disadvantage of being sensitive to dynamic changes in folate metabolism, such as reflecting folate absorbed from a recent meal.

Bone marrow studies should be undertaken when a myeloproliferative disease or hemolytic anemia is suspected, to confirm the megaloblastosis. Also, because serum iron, iron saturation and ferritin studies are unreliable in patients with folate or B_{12} deficiency, bone marrow studies are required to determine iron stores, particularly in cases of malabsorption.

Management of Folic Acid Deficiency (18, 19)

Folic acid is indicated for the prevention and treatment of folic acid deficiencies. Dietary improvement is preferred over supplementation with pharmaceutical preparations. Where possible, folic acid should not be given until B_{12} deficiency or PA has been excluded. The danger here is that large doses of folic acid (e.g., >1 mg/day) can reverse the hematologic aspects of PA but not the spinal cord degeneration, which can worsen. If it is essential to give some folic acid, doses of 100 μg/day are enough to meet the patient's minimal requirements but not enough to convert the megaloblastic marrow in PA.

Although folate levels are readily restored by 5 mg of folic acid daily, in practice much lower doses can be used. Where absorption is normal, as little as 50 to 100 μg/day may suffice. In long-standing folate deficiency, secondary malabsorption due to megaloblastosis of intestinal epithelial cells increase requirements, and here 250 to 500 μg/day is usually sufficient. Severely ill patients with hemoglobin levels of less than 50 g/liter need blood transfusions until folic acid therapy has increased erythropoiesis. To replenish depleted folate stores, a daily dose of 1 to 2 mg/day for 2 to 3 weeks should suffice.

The duration of therapy depends upon the underlying cause. It can take 3 to 4 months to clear folate-deficient erythrocytes from the blood. Replacement therapy should be continued until the underlying problem has been corrected. If this is impossible, lifelong therapy is required. B_{12} studies should also be undertaken in this latter group and prophylactic doses of B_{12} given if required. Long-term therapy may be required in chronic hemolytic states, myelofibrosis, and refractory malabsorption. Postgastrectomy states, prolonged stress or infection, chronic fever, and persistent diarrhea may also increase requirements. Supplementation is required in patients receiving TPN or undergoing rapid weight loss or in those with malnutrition. Low doses of folic acid, 500 μg/day, can be given to patients with megaloblastic anemia due to antiepileptic agents, without stopping the antiepileptic therapy. Higher doses of folic acid rarely increase the risk of seizures. Use of folic acid in preventing mental disorders is of unproven benefit.

Prophylactic folate therapy during pregnancy, particularly in women with poor diets, multiple pregnancies, or thalassemia minor, is useful in preventing megaloblastic anemia. Folate deficiency is rare in well-nourished women with normal pregnancy. As the greatest risk is in the latter part of the pregnancy, prophylaxis is achieved by giving 300 μg/day in the last trimester. This is generally given as a combination iron/folate preparation. Some authorities frown on giving this combination during the whole pregnancy. Subclinical maternal folate deficiency during pregnancy can result in underweight, premature infants and less than optimal health for the mother. Supplementation may be necessary for infants receiving unfortified formulas (e.g., evaporated milk), those being breast-fed by mothers with folic acid deficiency, or those with a low birth weight.

Monitoring Therapy

Response to treatment can be monitored by following the reticulocyte count, which peaks 5 to 8 days after commencing treatment. A rise in the erythrocyte count and blood hemoglobin level and a concurrent fall in the MCV are important monitoring signs. Measuring erythrocyte folate levels several months during the treatment can confirm replenishment of tissue stores. In patients with severe megaloblastic anemia, potassium levels should be monitored during the early stages of treatment.

Folic Acid

The common pharmaceutical form of folic acid is dihydrofolate, available as either the acid or the sodium salt. Both oral and parenteral forms are available. Parenteral administration is indicated when oral administration is unacceptable (preoperatively, postoperatively, or if nausea or vomiting is a problem) or not possible (malabsorption syndromes or following gastric resection).

No major side effects have been reported with folic acid administration, even when 10 times the RDA was taken for 1 month. Megadoses of folic acid taken for long periods should be discouraged unless some benefit is observed because zinc deficiency may occur. Rare side effects associated with allergic reactions include fever and rashes.

CONCLUSION

Anemia due to a deficiency of iron, B_{12}, or folic acid can usually be treated simply and effectively. Determining the primary cause and its subsequent management may be more difficult. Where possible, dietary manipulation should be used as a maintenance strategy. In some cases, particularly with PA, lifelong therapy is necessary. Compliance can be a major problem after the hemoglobin levels rise and the patient begins to feel better.

REFERENCES

1. Djulbegovic B, Hadley T, Pasic R: A new algorithm for diagnosis of anemia. Postgrad Med 85:119–130, 1989.
2. Cook JD, Skikne BS: Iron deficiency: definition and diagnosis. J Int Med 226:349–355, 1989.
3. Jacobs A: Iron deficiency and iron overload. CRC Crit Rev Oncol/Hematol 3:143–186, 1985.
4. Mayer E, Adieles-Tegman M: The prevalence of anemia in the world. World Health Stat Q 38:302–316, 1985.

5. Cook JD, Skikne BS, Lynch SR, et al.: Estimates of iron sufficiency in the US population. Blood 68:726–731, 1986.
6. Dallman PR: Manifestations of iron deficiency. Semin Hematol 19:19–30, 1982.
7. Murphy JF, O'Riordan J, Newcombe RG, Coles EC: Relation of hemoglobin levels in first and second trimesters to outcome of pregnancy. Lancet 1:992–994, 1986.
8. Lozoff B: Behavioural alterations in iron deficiency. Adv Pediatr 35:331–319, 1988.
9. Dalman PR: Iron deficiency and the immune response. Am J Clin Nutr 46:329–334, 1987.
10. Dalman PR: Biochemical basis for manifestations of iron deficiency. Annu Rev Nut 6:13–40, 1988.
11. Soemantri AG, Pollitt E, Kim I: Iron deficiency anaemia and educational achievement. Am J Clin Nutr 42:1221–1228, 1986.
12. Bothwell TH, Baynes RD, Macfarlane BJ, MacPhail APM: Nutritional iron requirements and food iron absorption. J Int Med 226:357–365, 1989.
13. Cole SK, Billeweca WZ, Thomson AM: Sources of blood loss in menstrual blood loss. J Obstet Gynaecol Br Comm 78:933–939, 1971.
14. Nilsson L, Solvel L: Clinical studies on oral contraceptives—randomised double blind crossover study of four different populations. Acta Obstet Gynaecol Scand 46(suppl. 8):1–31, 1967.
15. Herbert V: Recommended dietary intakes (RDI) of iron in humans. Am J Clin Nutr 45:679–686, 1987.
16. Beutler E: The common anemias. JAMA 359:2433–2437, 1988.
17. Finch C: Minisymposium. Introduction: knights of the oval table. J Int Med 226:345–348, 1989.
18. McGrath K: Treatment of anaemia caused by iron, vitamin B_{12} or folate deficiency. Med J Aust 151:695–697, 1989.
19. Stander PE: Anemia in the elderly: symptoms, causes, and therapies. Postgrad Med 85(2):85–96, 1989.
20. Beddall A: Anemias. Practitioner 234:714–715, 1990.
21. Newhouse IJ, Clement DB: Iron status in athletes: an update. Sports Med 5(6):337–352, 1988.
22. Nickerson HJ, Holubets MC, Weiler BR, et al.: Causes of iron deficiency in adolescent athletes. J Pediatr 114:657–658, 1989.
23. Sayetta RB: Pica: an overview. Am Fam Physician 33(5):181–185, 1986.
24. Cook JD: Clinical evaluation of iron deficiency. Semin Hematol 19(1):6–18, 1982.
25. Jandl JH: The hypochromic anemias and other disorders of iron metabolism. In Blood: Text Book of Hematology. Boston, Little, Brown & Co, ch 6, pp 181–235, 1987.
26. United States Pharmacopeial Convention Inc: Iron supplements (systemic) in USP DI. Drug information for the health care professional, ed 11th, Rockville: United States Pharmacopeial Convention Inc., 1991 IB: pp 1555–1565.
27. Paparella P, Papadia LS, Brizio AM, Mancuso S: Effects of routine iron supplementation in pregnancy. Curr Ther Res 48:348–355, 1990.
28. Heese HD, Smith S, Watermeyer S, et al.: Prevention of iron deficiency in preterm neonates during infancy. S Afr Med J 77:339–345, 1990.
29. Hibbard BM: Iron and folate supplements during pregnancy: supplementation is only valuable in some patients. Br Med J 197:1324–1325, 1988.
30. Rudinskas L, Paton WP, Walker SE, et al.: Case report: poor clinical response to enteric-coated iron preparations. Can Med Assoc J 141:565–566, 1989.
31. Crosby WH: Overtreating the deficiency anemias. Arch Intern Med 146:779, 1986.
32. Fuller JD, Williams JW, McRorie TI: Necrotic bilateral buttocks ulcerations occurring after multiple intramuscular iron dextran injections. Arch Dermatol 124:1722–1723, 1988.
33. Schjonsby H: Vitamin B_{12} absorption and malabsorption. Gut 30:1686–1691, 1989.
34. Carethers M: Diagnosing vitamin B_{12} deficiency, a common geriatric disorder. Geriatrics 43(3):89–112, 1989.
35. McRae TD, Freedman ML: Why vitamin B_{12} deficiency should be managed aggressively. Geriatrics 44(11):70–79, 1989.
36. Martin DC: B_{12} and folate deficiency dementia. Clin Geriatr Med 4(4):841–853, 1988.
37. Hector M, Burton JR: What are the psychiatric manifestations of vitamin B_{12} deficiency? J Am Geriatr Soc 36:1105–1112, 1988.
38. Nickoloff E: Schilling test: physiologic basis and use as a diagnostic test. CRC Crit Rev Clin Lab Sci 26:263–276, 1988.
39. Bunting RW, Bitzer AM, Kenney RM, Ellman L: Prevalence of antibodies and vitamin B_{12} malabsorption in older patients admitted to a rehabilitation hospital. J Am Geriatr Soc 38:743–747, 1990.
40. Thompson WG, Babitz L, Casino C, et al.: Evaluation of criteria used to measure vitamin B_{12} levels. Am J Med 82:291–294, 1987.
41. Green R, Khul W, Jacobsen R, et al.: Masking of macrocytosis by alpha-thalassemia in blacks with pernicious anemia. N Engl J Med 307(21):1322–1323, 1982.
42. Schneider EL, Vining EM, Hadley EC, Farnham SA: Recommended dietary allowances and the health of the elderly. N Engl J Med 313:157–160, 1986.
43. Doscherholmen A, Swain WR: Impaired assimilation of egg Co57 vitamin B_{12} in patients with hypochlorhydria and achlorhydria and after gastric resection. Gastroenterology 64:913–919, 1973.
44. Salom IL, Silvis SE, Doscherholmen A: Effect of cimetidine on the absorption of vitamin B_{12}. Scand J Gastroenterol 17:129–131, 1982.
45. United States Pharmacopeial Convention Inc: Folic Acid (Systemic) in USP DI. Drug information for the health care professional, ed 11th, Rockville: United States Pharmacopeial Convention Inc., 1991 IA: pp 1359–1361.
46. United States Pharmacopeial Convention Inc: Vitamin B_{12} (Systemic) in USP DI. Drug information for the health care professional, ed 11th, Rockville: United States Pharmacopeial Convention Inc., 1991 IB: pp 1586–2589.
47. Butterworth CE, Tamura T: Folic acid safety and toxicity: a brief review. Am J Clin Nutr 50:353–358, 1989.
48. Khot T, Pettit-Young N: Folic acid supplementation and long term therapy with co-trimoxazole. Aust J Hosp Pharm 19:364–365, 1989.

CHAPTER 13

OTHER ANEMIAS

JANICE L. STUMPF, Pharm.D. and KEVIN A. TOWNSEND, Pharm.D.

Although the clinical features of anemias resulting from many causes are often similar, treatment modalities and prognosis are quite distinct. In this chapter, a variety of anemias are discussed, including the anemias of chronic disease and renal failure, aplastic anemia, sickle cell anemia, thalassemia, and hemolytic anemia.

ANEMIA OF CHRONIC DISEASE

The anemia of chronic disease is a mild, often asymptomatic condition that occurs in conjunction with a variety of infectious, inflammatory, and neoplastic disorders. The anemia develops 1 to 2 months after the onset of diseases such as chronic osteomyelitis, tuberculosis, rheumatoid arthritis, systemic lupus erythematosis, vasculitides, and carcinomas including Hodgkin's disease and solid tumors. Although renal insufficiency is also a chronic disease, the associated anemia manifests differently, and therefore, it will be discussed separately.

The common pathology of anemia of chronic disease appears to be a defect in iron transport from the reticuloendothelial system, hepatocytes, and intestinal epithelial cells to the plasma and erythroid precursor cells (1). In addition, a moderate shortening of red blood cell lifespan may be noted, which is unaccompanied by increased erythrocyte production, In fact, erythropoietin concentrations may be low relative to the measured hematocrit.

Although the reasons for these abnormalities are not presently known, it has been suggested that the endogenous pyrogen interleukin-1 may be the primary mediator of the pathology that presents as anemia of chronic disease (1). Interleukin-1 stimulates the elaboration of high concentrations of lactoferrin from leukocytes at sites of inflammation. This protein preferentially binds iron and prevents its mobilization to the plasma. Macrophages then take up the iron-lactoferrin complex, resulting in accumulation of iron in the cells of the reticuloendothelial system. Alternatively, interleukin-1 may induce the synthesis of ferritin, allowing increased iron storage and restricting the amount of iron available to the bone marrow.

Because it is associated with many diseases and a unifying pathogenesis has not yet been elucidated, anemia of chronic disease remains a diagnosis of exclusion. The erythrocytes are typically normochromic and normocytic, but they may be microcytic. The hematocrit concentration rarely falls below 0.30; if it does, other causes of anemia should be thoroughly investigated. The reticulocyte count is low or within normal limits, and serum iron levels and iron-binding protein saturation are reduced. However, in contrast to the picture of iron deficiency anemia, ferritin levels are increased in the anemia of chronic disease. These and other manifestations, including elevations in haptoglobin and fibrinogen levels and erythrocyte sedimentation rate, are known collectively as the "acute phase" reaction, a response to inflammation that may persist with chronic conditions.

Because the anemia of chronic disease is generally mild, no specific therapy is necessary in most cases. The degree of anemia correlates well with the severity of the associated disease state, and reversal of the underlying disorder will correct the anemia. If, however, the patient becomes symptomatic, blood transfusions may be beneficial (2). Iron replacement regimens have been attempted, but they have been uniformly ineffective and may place the patient at risk of iron toxicity. Iron should not be prescribed.

ANEMIA OF RENAL FAILURE

The anemia that complicates end-stage renal disease is generally more severe than that associated with other chronic diseases. The severity of anemia appears to correlate with the extent of the uremia, but not with the etiology of the underlying renal disease. Most patients with serum creatinine concentrations over 310 μmol/liter (3.5 mg/dl) and 97% of those on maintenance dialysis are affected. The cells are normochromic and normocytic, but frequently irregular in shape. Although hematocrit levels may fall to 0.20 to 0.30 or less, not all patients become symptomatic. This tolerance of such low hematocrit concentrations may be explained by the compensatory reduction in oxygen-hemoglobin affinity, allowing improved delivery of oxygen to the tissues. Despite this adaptation, an estimated 25% of patients receiving dialysis required treatment with blood transfusions before the widespread use of recombinant erythropoietin (3). In addition to the commonly known symptoms of anemia such as fatigue, increasing angina, and shortness of breath, vague complaints of generalized coldness, anorexia, insomnia, and depression, which were not associated with anemia until recently, may be improved with adequate therapy.

Pathogenesis

The anemia of renal failure is a multifactorial process, but it is primarily the result of reduced secretion of erythropoietin by the diseased kidneys. This hormone stimulates the proliferation and maturation of erythrocytes and is released when the availability of oxygen to the organs is diminished. Although synthesized to some extent extrarenally in the liver, serum erythropoietin concentrations in uremic patients are markedly lower than those measured in patients with similar degrees of anemia and normal renal function.

Other factors that contribute to the anemia are the accumulation of inhibitors of erythropoiesis, reduced red blood cell life-span, and chronic blood loss. In support of the presence of suppressive substances, erythropoietin-induced stimulation of erythroid progenitors is blunted in vitro by uremic serum. In addition, while erythropoietin levels remain stable, the anemia improves following dialysis, perhaps indicating removal of these substances. Parathyroid hormone and the polyamine spermine have both been implicated in reducing marrow responsiveness to erythropoietin; however data are conflicting and the identity of the inhibitory substances remains unknown.

Erythrocyte survival is decreased due to a mild, chronic hemolysis to an average of one-half normal in uremia. The cause of red cell destruction is unclear, but hypersplenism or increases in erythrocyte fragility induced by parathyroid hormone may contribute. This abnormality may not be corrected by dialysis, yet it does not appear to be a defect in the red cells. A similar reduction in erythrocyte life-span is noted after transfusion of blood products from nonuremic donors to renal failure patients.

Chronic blood loss from a gastrointestinal source and during hemodialysis may contribute to the anemia. Due to defects in platelet function, uremic patients have an elevated risk of bleeding; occult blood loss is reported in over 20% of dialysis patients (4). An estimated 2 g of iron is lost annually during hemodialysis, increasing the likelihood of a concurrent iron deficiency anemia. In addition, the intestinal absorption of iron may be compromised by the chronic use of iron-cheating antacids. Other factors that may aggravate the anemia of end-stage renal disease include folic acid deficiency due to losses to the dialysate, the accumulation of the fat-soluble vitamin A, aluminum toxicity due to long-term hemodialysis and the use of aluminum-containing phosphate bindings, and osteitis fibrosa, a complication of hyperparathyroidism in which myelofibrosis reduces viable erythroid cellular mass.

Treatment

Prior to the initiation of therapy aimed at the primary abnormality, other potential causes of anemia should be identified and addressed. Iron and folate supplementation should be provided as necessary and blood loss and the use of aluminum-containing antacids minimized whenever possible. The treatment for acute symptoms of hypoxia consists of the transfusion of red blood cells. However,

although transfusions may readily correct the anemia, they carry the risk of hypersensitivity reactions and the transmission of viral hepatitis. In addition, bone marrow suppression and iron overload requiring deferoxamine therapy may occur after multiple, chronic transfusions.

ANDROGENS

Traditionally, the administration of androgens has been recommended for treatment of anemia in selected patients with end-stage renal disease. These agents stimulate the synthesis of erythropoietin and/or the production of red blood cells in the bone marrow. However, they are not universally effective and rarely fully correct the anemia. Elevations in hematocrit concentrations of 0.05 or more compared to baseline were documented in 50% of patients able to tolerate the drugs in a 6-month controlled, crossover trial (5). Therapy with the injectable formulations nandrolone decanoate and testosterone enanthate resulted in significantly greater improvements in hematocrit levels than did the two oral androgens studied, fluoxymesterone and oxymetholone. Transfusion requirements were not reduced during androgen therapy. Patients with lower pretreatment hematocrit concentrations, bilateral nephrectomies, or intact parathyroid glands had poorer response rates. Based on these results and the propensity for virilization effects such as hirsuitism, changes in external genitalia, amenorrhea, acne, and voice deepening, the usefulness of androgens for this indication is limited. Injectable androgens are recommended over oral agents, and nandrolone decanoate is preferred in females because of its greater ratio of anabolic to androgenic activities. Nandrolone decanoate and testosterone enanthate are administered as weekly intramuscular injections of 1.5 to 2.5 mg/kg and 4 to 7 mg/kg, respectively. If an adequate response is not achieved after a 6-month trial, the agent should be discontinued. Therapy with oral androgens (fluoxymesterone 10 to 30 mg daily) may then be attempted. However, in addition to the adverse effects associated with the injectable agents, the oral androgens may also induce liver dysfunction and hepatic cancer.

RECOMBINANT HUMAN ERYTHROPOIETIN

Advances in recombinant technology have made possible the production of human erythropoietin (rHuEpo, epoetin alfa), a peptide whose 166-amino-acid structure is identical to that of the native hormone. The availability of rHuEpo has revolutionized the therapy of anemia associated with end-stage renal disease and all but eliminated the use of androgen therapy.

In a multicenter study of the efficacy of rHuEpo, intravenous doses of 150 or 300 U/kg were administered to 333 anemic patients three times weekly after hemodialysis (6). Target hematocrit concentrations of 0.35 or 0.06 in-

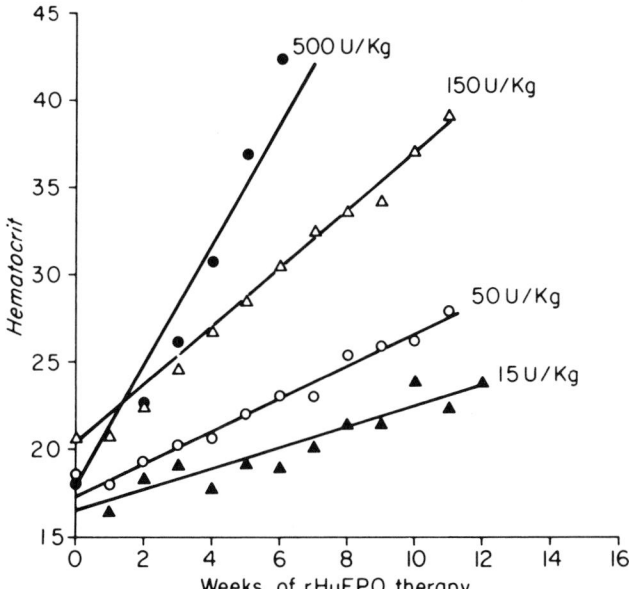

Figure 13.1. The rates at which hematocrit increases with various doses of rHuEpo. (From Eschenbach JW, Egrie JC, Downing MR, et al.: Correction of the anemia of end-stage renal disease with recombinant human erythropoietin. N Engl J Med 316:73–78, 1987, with permission.)

creases from baseline were achieved, in over 97% of patients within 12 weeks. In addition, the need for routine red cell transfusions was eliminated within 2 months. Quality of life was enhanced, as evidenced by increased energy and activity levels, cold tolerance, and appetite. A median dosage of 75 U/kg maintained these effects. Lack of response in the remaining patients was attributed to other causes of anemia, such as myelofibrosis and blood loss. Antibodies to rHuEpo were not detected in any patient.

Patients with end-stage renal disease with hematocrit levels under 0.30 may be considered candidates for rHuEpo treatment. Dose-dependent rises in hematocrit and reticulocyte counts are seen after 2 to 6 weeks of therapy (Fig. 13.1) (7). Initial doses of 50 to 100 U/kg three times weekly are currently recommended. Hematocrit concentrations should be determined weekly. If the hematocrit has not increased to the target range or by 5 or 6 points after 8 weeks of therapy, the dose should be increased. Once a hematocrit of 0.30 is attained, the dose should be reduced and titrated to maintain hematocrit concentrations of 0.35 (8). Although commonly given as an intravenous bolus following hemodialysis, rHuEpo may also be administered subcutaneously and has been used in both predialysis and continuous ambulatory peritoneal dialysis patients. Preliminary data indicate that peak serum concentrations are prolonged after subcutaneous administration and that this route may provide similar responses following lower doses. The efficacy of intraperitoneal ad-

ministration is the focus of current investigation. Although the elimination route of rHuEpo remains unclear, hepatic metabolism has been suggested. The half-life after intravenous doses ranges from 4 to 13 hours in renal failure patients, allowing intermittent dosing. The necessity of thrice weekly dosing regimens has not yet been confirmed.

Adverse effects associated with rHuEpo therapy include myalgias, headache, flank pain, hypertension, and seizures. Increases in blood pressure appear to be a hemodynamic consequence of the rising hematocrit. As the anemia is corrected, compensatory vasodilation decreases and peripheral vascular resistance (and blood pressure) increases. Diastolic blood pressure elevations exceed 10 mm Hg or require the institution or upward adjustment of antihypertensive medications in 35% of patients within 3 months of rHuEpo initiation. Seizures may accompany uncontrolled hypertension. Therefore, close monitoring and control of blood pressure levels are essential.

Increases in predialysis concentrations of serum creatinine, potassium, and phosphate have also been documented. The reduced effectiveness of dialysis noted with higher hematocrit levels and decreased dietary intake may account for these changes. In addition, clotting of arteriovenous access sites has occurred, although at an incidence no greater than that of a historical control hemodialysis population not receiving rHuEpo.

During the acute erythroid response, iron may be used more rapidly than it is released to transferrin from the reticuloendothelial system. A functional as well as an absolute iron deficiency may therefore develop, which may compromise further response to rHuEpo. Patients with pretreatment iron overload have experienced beneficial 39% reductions in serum ferritin levels within 6 months. Ferritin levels and transferrin saturation should be determined at baseline and monthly until the goal hematocrit is achieved. Iron stores should be measured at 2- to 3-month intervals thereafter (8). If the ferritin concentration or transferrin saturation falls below 100 µg/liter or 20%, respectively, intravenous or oral iron supplementation should be initiated.

The availability of rHuEpo offers clinicians the means to correct the anemia of renal disease on a long-term basis in both dialysis and predialysis patients. The high response rate indicates that the predominant cause of the anemia is erythropoietin deficiency. Other pathogenetic mechanisms, such as the presence of inhibitors of erythropoiesis, may also be operative, yet they may be overwhelmed clinically by an excess of exogenous erythropoietin. The high cost of rHuEpo should be considered in the context of savings resulting from reductions in other interventions. Routine blood transfusions, androgen therapy, and hospitalizations due to complications of these modalities may be completely eliminated. In addition, improvements in quality-of-life parameters may represent a greater reha-

SECTION 3 : DISEASES OF THE BLOOD

bilitation potential and a return to productive lives for more patients with end-stage renal disease.

APLASTIC ANEMIA

Aplastic anemia is distinguished by hypocellularity of the bone marrow and subsequent pancytopenia that is unrelated to malignancy or myeloproliferative disease. The characteristic anemia, neutropenia and thrombocytopenia result from failure of the pluripotential stem cell due to congenital or acquired processes. Although the causative mechanisms remain unknown, advances in therapy have greatly improved the overall prognosis.

Pathogenesis

In normal hematopoiesis, three cell lines originate from the pluripotential stem cell, producing erythrocytes, granulocytes, and platelets. Both cellular and humoral factors regulate the stem cells to maintain a balance between self-replication and differentiation into particular cell types. Aplastic anemia develops when hematopoiesis is interrupted because of deficient or defective stem cells. In addition to reduced number of progenitor cells, suggested pathophysiologic mechanisms include immune-mediated suppression of stem cell function, disturbances in the bone marrow microenvironment, and alterations in the cellular or humoral interactions that normally sustain hematopoiesis (9). Current research and the success of a variety of treatment modalities support the concept of aplastic anemia as a condition consisting of several pathogenetic abnormalities.

Etiology

Although numerous etiologies have been identified, 70% of causes of aplastic anemia are classified as idiopathic. Myelosuppression is a component of several congenital diseases, but it is more commonly acquired after exposure to drugs, chemicals, ionizing radiation, or viruses (Table 13.1).

Bone marrow suppression resulting from drugs or chemicals is often dose- and duration-dependent and may result from direct or immune-mediated stem cell toxicity. Chloramphenicol is the best-documented cause of drug-induced aplastic anemia. Reversible erythroid suppression is noted in approximately 50% of those receiving over 1 week of high-dose systemic therapy, but it has been reported following even ophthalmic administration of the antibiotic. In contrast, rare idiosyncratic marrow suppression manifesting weeks to months after exposure is also associated with chloramphenicol. Before the availability of bone marrow transplantation and alternative treatments, this reaction was fatal in 90% of cases, often within 1 year of clinical presentation (9).

Aplastic anemia may also arise concurrently with or

Table 13.1.
Etiologies of Aplastic Anemia

Acquired
  Drugs and chemicals
    Acetazolamide
    Anticonvulsants
      Carbamazepine
      Phenytoin
      Primidone
    Arsenic
    Benzene
    Chloramphenicol
    Chlorpromazine
    Ethanol
    Gold salts
    Insecticides
    Phenylbutazone
    Quinacrine hydrochloride
    Sulfa drugs
  Viral
    Cytomegalovirus
    Epstein-Barr virus
    Hepatitis
    Herpes varicella-zoster
    Influenza
    Rubella
  Other
    Ionizing radiation
    Paroxysmal nocturnal hemoglobinuria
    Pregnancy
    Thymoma
Congenital
  Dyskeratosis congenita
  Fanconi's anemia
  Schwarchman-Diamond syndrome

following viral infection. Hepatitis, most often non-A, non-B, precedes up to 5% of cases of aplastic anemia; however the severity of the infection does not predict the subsequent development of bone marrow suppression. Myelosuppression is usually noted within 6 months of the onset of hepatitis.

Clinical Presentation

Stem cell dysfunction may be incomplete and result in unequal effects on each cell type. Therefore, the earliest clinical signs are determined by the cell line affected to the greatest degree. Often, features of a mild anemia, such as pallor and fatigue, will be reported initially and may be more pronounced if accompanied by bleeding due to thrombocytopenia. Ecchymoses and petechiae also indicate a low platelet count. Less commonly, infection caused by the underlying neutropenia is the presenting manifestation of aplastic anemia. Signs of infection such as fever should be monitored closely as the neutropenia progresses, since inflammation may not be apparent.

Decreased numbers of morphologically normal cells

are observed in the peripheral blood. The erythrocytes are normochromic and normocytic or slightly macrocytic. The corrected reticulocyte count is markedly reduced, as is the absolute granulocyte count. Bone marrow biopsy reveals extensive areas of hypocellularity interspersed with small patches of hematopoietic cells.

Epidemiology and Prognosis

The annual incidence of aplastic anemia in Western nations is estimated to be 5 to 10 per million population (9). The prevalence of disease is higher in Korea and Japan, perhaps reflecting increased exposure to viral hepatitis and environmental toxins. Two peaks are evident in the distribution of ages of onset; approximately 25% of those affected are younger than 15 years whereas another third are over 60 years of age.

Annual deaths attributed to aplastic anemia in 1984 averaged nearly 9 per million population in the United States (10). With supportive care alone, 80% of patients with severe pancytopenia as assessed by the International Aplastic Anemia Study Group Criteria (Table 13.2) die within 1 to 2 years, with median survival of 6 months (11). Advances in bone marrow transplantation have dramatically improved this outcome; currently, long-term disease-free survival (up to 16 years) after transplantation in 65 to 80% (12, 13). Immunosuppressive therapy is generally less successful, with survival rates of 35 to 65% (14).

Treatment

The management of patients with aplastic anemia includes removal of potential etiologic agents, supportive care, and the restoration of normal hematopoiesis with pharmacologic therapy or bone marrow transplantation (12). In mild cases, supportive care should be provided in anticipation of spontaneous recovery. Blood transfusions, preferably leukocyte-depleted products, should be reserved for patients with symptomatic anemia, to delay sensitization to alloantigens. Blood products from family members should

Table 13.2.
International Aplastic Anemia Study Group Criteria for Severe Aplastic Anemia[a,b]

Site	Findings	
Peripheral blood	Neutrophils	$<0.5 \times 10^9$/liter
	Platelets	$<20 \times 10^9$/liter
	Reticulocytes	<0.01[c]
Bone marrow	Severe hypocellularity	
	Moderate hypocellularity with <30% of residual cells hematopoietic	

[a] From Camitta BM, Storb R, Thomas ED: Aplastic anemia: pathogenesis, diagnosis, treatment and prognosis (part 2). N Engl J Med 306:712–718, 1982, with permission.
[b] Defined by any two or three blood criteria and either marrow criterion.
[c] Corrected for hematocrit.

not be used in candidates for marrow transplantation because of the development of antibodies to histocompatibility antigens of the donor, increasing the risk of graft rejection. Overall, nontransfused patients fare better after bone marrow transplantation than their transfused counterparts.

Antiplatelet antibodies that reduce platelet function and life-span also develop after 1 to 2 months of repeated transfusions. Patients often become refractory to subsequent transfusions, although a dose-response relationship has not been established. Platelets should be administered to maintain the platelet count over 20×10^9/liter (20,000/mm^3) and to treat active bleeding.

Because of the risk of hematoma, intramuscular injections should be avoided whenever possible in patients with thrombocytopenia as should aspirin, nonsteroidal antiinflammatory drugs, and other agents with antiplatelet properties. Menses should be hormonally suppressed to prevent menorrhagia in females with aplastic anemia.

Prompt recognition and treatment of infection is vital in the aplastic anemia patient with severe neutropenia. Broad-spectrum antibiotics should be initiated in any patient with fever of unknown origin. If a pathogen is not identified and the patient continues to be febrile after 48 to 72 hours of treatment, empiric antifungal therapy with amphotericin B should be considered.

BONE MARROW TRANSPLANTATION

Bone marrow transplantation has become the treatment of choice for severe aplastic anemia, with greatest success achieved in younger patients undergoing the procedure soon after diagnosis (9, 12, 13). Initially, an HLA-compatible donor must be identified. There is a 25% chance that a sibling will be HLA-identical. Graft rejection may develop because of minor antigenic differences between donor and recipient marrow and previous sensitization by blood transfusions. Therefore, a course of immunosuppressive therapy is administered immediately prior to transplantation. Most commonly, this "conditioning" regimen consists of intravenous cyclophosphamide (50 mg/kg daily for 4 days) alone or combined with total body or total lymphoid irradiation. These protocols have reduced graft rejection to 3 to 5% in some series (12). Two to 6 weeks after intravenous infusion of marrow cells, the donor cells have engrafted, and blood cells begin to be produced.

The interval between transplantation and the return of hematopoiesis and normal immune function poses the greatest threat to the patient. Supportive care should include isolation in a sterile environment, transfusions of blood products as required, and close monitoring for signs of infection. Prophylactic antifungal therapy and bowel sterilization with nonabsorbable oral antibiotics may be undertaken in attempts to reduce the frequency of systemic infections. Interstitial pneumonitis may complicate transplantation within the first 3 months, and before the availability of antiviral agents such as acyclovir and ganciclovir, was associated with a mortality rate of over 40% (15). In over 30 to 70% of cases, cytomegalovirus was implicated, however infection with *Aspergillus, Candida, Pneumocystis carinii*, herpes simplex virus, and herpes varicella-zoster virus has also been reported. Trimethoprim-sulfamethoxazole and acyclovir prophylaxis are now frequently administered to inhibit activation of *Pneumocystis* and herpes viruses, respectively. In addition, the use of immune globulin to prevent cytomegalovirus activation is advocated at some centers.

Acute graft versus host disease (GVHD), in which donor lymphocytes attack the host tissue, occurs in 30 to 60% of patients within 2 months after transplantation, despite prophylactic immunosuppression (12). Regimens of methotrexate or cyclosporine alone or in combination are used to prevent GVHD, and the addition of prednisone may further improve outcome (13). Initial presenting signs of acute GVHD include rash and diarrhea. Elevations in liver function test values and severe immunodeficiency may also develop. Once established, GVHD may be managed with antithymocyte globulin, prednisone or cyclosporine, yet response is variable.

Chronic GVHD manifests 6 to 12 months posttransplantation in 20 to 30% of surviving patients (9). The reaction is similar to a systemic autoimmune disease (e.g., systemic lupus erythematosis) with skin, gastrointestinal, hepatic, lymphoid, lung, and ophthalmic involvement. Eighty percent of afflicted patients recover following treatment regimens of prednisone and cyclophosphamide or azathioprine (9). The risk of acquiring and the severity of GVHD are directly correlated to the age of the patient. Therefore, most bone marrow transplants are performed in patients under the age of 40 years.

IMMUNOSUPPRESSION

Immunosuppressive therapy is generally reserved for older patients with aplastic anemia or those without an HLA-matched marrow donor. A variety of agents, both alone and in combination, have been used to treat the disease, including antithymocyte globulin (ATG), antilymphocyte globulin (ALG), corticosteroids, and cyclosporine (12, 14).

ATG and ALG are investigational agents that are prepared in animals and react against human thymocytes and lymphocytes, respectively. The mechanism by which these agents positively affect aplastic anemia is unknown, but, presumably, they inactivate cytotoxic lymphocytes responsible for suppression of hematopoiesis. The overall efficacy of ATG/ALG is difficult to assess from current research, because of variations in preparations, treatment protocols, and severity of illness in the study populations. However, complete responses, in which blood counts are restored to normal values, are elicited in 10 to 25% of treated patients, whereas 20 to 45% will have partial improvements in indices and no longer require blood transfusions (12).

In a typical treatment protocol, a test dose is administered and in the absence of anaphylaxis, is followed by an 8- to 10-day course of 15 mg/kg/day ATG or ALG infused intravenously over 4 to 12 hours. Response is usually observed within 1 to 3 months after therapy. A second course may be effective in those who fail initial therapy and in the 25 to 30% of patients who relapse.

Adverse effects of ATG/ALG include fever, chills, rash, headache, and hypotension. Serum sickness, manifesting with fever, rash, and arthralgias, may be evident 1 to 2 weeks after therapy; however symptoms may be alleviated by concurrent corticosteroid therapy. Transient reductions in white blood cell and platelet counts are also reported. Hematologic complications such as myelodysplasia, leukemia, and paroxysmal nocturnal hemoglobinuria, develop in 30 to 50% of patients, with the prevalence increasing with time.

Data on the usefulness of high-dose methylprednisolone in conjunction with ATG/ALG are conflicting, yet response rates of 73% have been documented (12). Steroids are frequently added to the regimen to control antiserum-induced toxicities. The efficacy of high-dose corticosteroids alone for the treatment of aplastic anemia has not been conclusively demonstrated.

In a preliminary report, the combination of ALG with methylprednisolone and cyclosporine produced complete responses in 39% of patients. Furthermore, sole therapy with cyclosporine has yielded response rates similar to those of ATG (12, 14). Effects are usually observed after 2 to 10 weeks of treatment. Long-term maintenance therapy with cyclosporine is often required, increasing the risk of renal toxicity and other adverse effects. Although at present cyclosporine appears to be a potential alternative to ATG or ALG treatment, more controlled studies are necessary to establish its place in therapy.

ANDROGENS

Androgens were once used widely for the treatment of aplastic anemia because of their stimulatory effects on hematopoiesis (predominantly red cell production) (12). However, in patients with severe disease, oral oxymetholone and intramuscular nandrolone decanoate produced responses similar to those following supportive care alone. In addition, androgens do not potentiate the effects of ATG or ALG therapy. Although androgens have no apparent role in the management of severe forms of the disease, those with mild aplastic anemia or Fanconi's anemia not amenable to marrow transplantation may benefit from treatment. Initial responses are detected after 3 to 6 months of therapy, however adverse effects such as virilization and hepatotoxicity may limit the prolonged courses required to achieve effects in all cells lines.

FUTURE DIRECTIONS: RECOMBINANT GROWTH FACTORS

Recombinant human granulocyte-macrophage colony-stimulating factor (GM-CSF) is a newly available growth factor that stimulates the proliferation of progenitor cells and thus may have applications to many hypoplastic disorders (16). Continuous intravenous infusion of GM-CSF administered to small numbers of aplastic anemia patients has produced marked elevations in leukocyte counts, primarily due to increases in neutrophils. Improvements in red cell and platelet counts were rare. In general, response was inversely related to the severity of disease, and the effects did not persist after GM-CSF discontinuation.

Transient, but inconsistent, increases in reticulocyte, platelet, and leukocyte counts have also been demonstrated following daily subcutaneous injections of recombinant human interleukin-3 in a phase I/II trial (17). Large-scale prospective clinical studies in aplastic anemia populations are necessary to determine optimal protocols for therapy with recombinant hematopoietic growth factors, both alone and in combination with other treatment modalities.

SICKLE CELL ANEMIA

The term sickle cell disease encompasses a variety of hemoglobinopathies, including sickle cell anemia, sickle hemoglobulin C (SC) disease, and sickle cell thalassemia. Although the clinical presentation of these disorders is often similar, the manifestions of sickle cell anemia are more severe and are therefore the focus of the following discussion.

Pathophysiology

The hemoglobin molecule is a tetramer comprised of four polypeptides linked to iron-carrying heme groups. Nearly 400 different types of hemoglobin have been distinguished, including hemoglobins A_1, A_2, C, F, and S. Only three variants are considered to be normal, hemoglobin A_1 (Hb A_1), hemoglobin A_1 (Hb A_2), and fetal hemoglobin (Hb F). Fetal hemoglobin accounts for 70 to 80% of the hemoglobin in the red cells of newborns. A gradual conversion occurs until the eighth postnatal month when the normal adult pattern of 97% Hb A_1, 2 to 3% Hb A_2, and 1% Hb F is represented (9).

The Hb A_1 tetramer consists of two pairs of globin chains, alpha and beta, which have distinct primary structures. Sickle cell anemia is a homozygous condition that results from the substitution of valine for glutamic acid in both of the beta chains. Because each parent contributes a single beta chain gene, the heterozygous genotype AS is also possible and is expressed as the sickle cell trait phenotype.

Deoxygenation in the capillaries induces rapid polymerization of the sickling hemoglobin, Hb S, and results in the formation of helical strands of parallel fibers. The elongated, crescent-shaped cells characteristic of sickle cell anemia are thereby produced. The affected erythrocytes are rigid and are unable to pass through the microvasculature, leading to vaso-occlusion with subsequent painful ischemia and chronic organ damage. In general, the sickling is reversible upon reexposure to oxygen, however, repeated sickling episodes will eventually damage the cell membrane. The sickled conformation will be sustained and the cells subject to hemolysis and removal by the liver or spleen.

The rate of Hb S polymerization depends upon its concentration in the erythrocyte. The copolymerization of Hb S with Hb F inhibits further polymer growth; intracellular Hb F concentrations are inversely correlated with disease severity.

Epidemiology

The Hb S gene confers protection against *Plasmodium falciparum* infection in infancy. Therefore, populations residing in or originating from areas wherein malaria is endemic have the highest frequency of the AS and SS genotypes. The distribution of sickle disease is no longer restricted to Africa, Saudi Arabia, and India, however areas of concentration remain. Up to 50% of individuals in west central Africa possess the Hb S gene. Among blacks in the United States, 0.14% have sickle cell anemia, whereas 8.6% have the sickle trait (18).

Diagnosis

The diagnosis of sickle cell diseases depends upon hemoglobin electrophoresis, which reveals the types and proportion of hemoglobins present (9, 19). This rapid, inexpensive screening test establishes the genotype of the individual, enabling appropriate genetic counseling and education. If both parents have the AS genotype, there is a 1 in 4 chance that their child will have homozygous SS disease. Prenatal diagnosis is also possible. Genotyping may be performed in the fifteenth week of gestation, using fetal cells obtained from amniocentesis.

Clinical Presentation

Sickle cell anemia presents with constitutional, hematologic and vaso-occlusive manifestations (Table 13.3) late in the first postnatal year, after levels of the protective fetal hemoglobin have diminished. Skeletal growth and sexual maturation are impaired, although catch-up growth is apparent by adulthood.

Because of recurrent microinfarcts, the spleen is initially enlarged, and then completely fibrosed by 6 years of age. This functional "autosplenectomy" and defects in other host defenses greatly increase the likelihood of infection, especially with *Streptococcus pneumoniae* and *Haemophilus influenzae*.

Table 13.3.
Complications of Sickle Cell Anemia

Constitutional
  Impaired growth and development
  Increased risk of infection
    Meningitis
    Osteomyelitis
    Pneumonia
    Pyelonephritis
    Septicemia
Hematologic
  Hemolytic anemia
  Aplastic crises
  Splenic sequestration crises
Vaso-occlusive
  Cardiovascular
    Cardiac enlargement
    Systolic murmur
  Gastrointestinal
    Autosplenectomy
    Gallstones/cholecystitis
    Hepatic crises/RUQ syndrome
    Hepatic insufficiency
    Intrahepatic cholelithiasis
  Genitourinary
    Hematuria
    Impotence
    Priapism
    Renal insufficiency
  Neurologic
    Cerebral thrombosis
    Intracerebral hemorrhage
    Seizures
    Subarachnoid hemorrhage
  Ocular
    Retinopathy
    Secondary glaucoma
  Painful crises
  Pulmonary
    Chronic obstructive disease
    Infarction
  Skin/skeletal
    Arthropathy
    Aseptic necrosis
    Dactylitis
    Leg ulcers

Hemolysis accompanied by inadequate erythropoiesis results in a normochromic, normocytic anemia, with hematocrit levels ranging from 0.18 to 0.30. The chronic anemia leads to a hyperdynamic circulatory system and subsequent cardiac hypertrophy and systolic ejection murmurs. The anemia is aggravated during aplastic crises, when erythropoiesis is further suppressed by acute infection or folate deficiency.

Painful vaso-occlusive crises produced by sludging of sickled cells in the microcirculation are the most common reason for hospitalization. The frequency and severity of painful crises vary greatly between individuals. Approxi-

mately 5% of those with sickle cell anemia require inpatient pain management over 40 times each year, whereas another 30% are rarely or never affected by severe pain (19). The episodes are sudden in onset and last for an average of 5 to 7 days. Pain is most often reported in the long bones, spine, pelvis, chest, and abdomen and must be differentiated from infection and other acute processes. Factors that may precipitate vaso-occlusive crises include acidosis, heat or exercise (dehydration), cold vasoconstriction), infection, stress, menses, and high altitudes.

Recurrent sickling and subsequent infarction cause chronic damage to many organ systems. Hematuria and an inability to concentrate urine progress in some patients to renal failure. Neurologic complications such as cerebrovascular accidents and seizures develop in 25% of patients. Chronic obstructive pulmonary disease and intrahepatic fibrosis are also reported. Impotence occurs in 25% of males with the disease, usually after multiple episodes of priapism.

In addition to indices or anemia, laboratory abnormalities include elevations in platelet count and leukocytosis due to demargination of granulocytes from vessel walls into the circulation. Irreversibly sickled cells are seen in the blood smear.

Individuals with sickle cell trait are generally asymptomatic, although sickling manifestations may occur at extreme levels of hypoxia or acidosis. Transient hematuria, renal papillary necrosis, pulmonary embolism, and splenic infarction have been rarely associated with the AS phenotype. Life expectancy is normal in sickle trait patients, in contrast to those with sickle cell anemia. However, sickle cell anemia patients may now survive well into adulthood with rapid recognition and management of complications.

Management of Major Complications
ANEMIA

Physiologic adaptations such as low Hb S–oxygen affinity allow patients with sickle cell anemia to tolerate relatively low hematocrit levels. Therefore, therapy is supportive, with blood transfusions reversed for acute, symptomatic exacerbations in the anemia. High folate utilization arising from continuously elevated red cell production may lead to folate deficiency and induce an aplastic crisis. Folate supplementation (1 mg p.o. daily) is recommended to maintain adequate stores. Aplastic crises may also develop from viral or bacterial infections, necessitating prompt diagnosis and treatment. Recovery of erythropoiesis generally occurs within 5 to 10 days, as the underlying infection resolves.

INFECTION

Bacterial infection is the leading cause of death in patients with sickle cell anemia. Therefore, a thorough search for an infectious source should be undertaken in any patients presenting with a painful crisis and fever.

Pneumonia may be treated empirically with parenteral cefuroxime, as its spectrum of activity includes the most likely pathogens, *S. pneumoniae* and *H. influenzae*. If a clinical response is not apparent after 24 to 48 hours, infection with *Mycoplasma pneumoniae* should be suspected and erythromycin added to the antibiotic regimen.

Children over the age of 2 years should be immunized with polyvalent pneumococcal vaccine and a booster dose given after 3 to 5 years to children younger than 10 years at the time of revaccination. Although a 50% reduction in the incidence of pneumococcal infection has been demonstrated after immunization, the vaccine protects against a limited number of pneumococcal serotypes. Therefore, long-term prophylactic administration of oral penicillin may be advisable. *H. influenzae* vaccination should also be administered.

Salmonella species are isolated in up to 80% of sickle cell disease patients with osteomyelitis. A 4- to 6-week course of treatment with ampicillin or a cephalosporin is required. Leg ulcers should receive local care and be monitored closely for potential progression to osteomyelitis.

PAINFUL CRISES

The goals of therapy for painful vaso-occlusive crises are to provide supportive care and effective analgesia, while eliminating potential precipitating factors (19, 20). Vigorous enteral or parenteral hydration should be initiated and oxygen administered if hypoxia from pulmonary involvement is evident. Both nonnarcotic and narcotic analgesics were used, depending upon the severity of pain.

Those with mild-to-moderate painful crises should be managed as outpatients. Oral hydration with 3 to 5 liters (100 ml/kg for children) of fluid daily should be encouraged and the pain treated with acetaminophen, aspirin, or nonsteroidal antiinflammatory drugs. Pain unresponsive to these agents may be controlled by codeine or oxycodone, as single agents or in combination with acetaminophen.

Inpatient management with parenteral hydration and narcotic analgesics is necessary for severe painful crises. Scheduled, around-the-clock narcotic administration is preferred over "prn" regimens. The pain-anxiety cycle is thereby diminished and relief is often achieved with lower total doses (20). Oral narcotic protocols have been used (21), yet are not universally accepted by patients, especially if nausea and vomiting are present. Frequent intramuscular or subcutaneous injections cause local pain and promote the formation of abscesses and subsequent infection. In addition, drug absorption may be erratic. Peak effects associated with intravenous bolus administration may lead to excessive central nervous system depression. Continuous intravenous infusions are ideal for initial therapy, as a dosage range may be specified, allowing safe titration to

pain control. Success with patient-controlled analgesia has been reported (22).

Because narcotics have similar effects at equianalgesic doses, various regimens will alleviate symptoms. Agents with mixed agonist-antagonist properties (e.g., pentazocine, buprenorphine) are not recommended for patients with histories of outpatient narcotic use, since withdrawal may be precipitated. Although widely used, meperidine should be avoided, as its metabolite, normeperidine, accumulates after repeated high doses and may induce seizures, especially in the presence of renal insufficiency or underlying neurologic disease. The relatively short duration of action of meperidine of 2 to 4 hours also makes administration less practical. Morphine sulfate is the narcotic of choice. In patients unable to tolerate morphine because of nausea, vomiting, or pruritis, hydromorphone may be substituted. Adjuvant therapy with hydroxyzine may promote analgesia and reduce narcotic requirements. However, adverse effects may also be potentiated, and therefore, combinations remain controversial.

Doses must be individualized and based upon the degree of outpatient narcotic use and previous inpatient needs. The development of tolerance to narcotic analgesic effects after chronic administration may dramatically increase parenteral requirements. Although patients may appear manipulative and exhibit drug-seeking behavior, adequate analgesia should be provided. Placebos should not be given.

A continuous intravenous infusion of morphine (100 mg/100 ml 5% dextrose) at a rate of 0.05 to 0.10 mg/kg/hr may be used for the first 24 to 48 hours (20). Alternatively, 0.10 to 0.15 mg/kg morphine doses may be administered as intravenous boluses every 2 to 3 hours. Adverse effects such as respiratory depression, oversedation, and blood pressure reductions should be monitored, and the dose decreased if indicated. As the pain subsides, the continuous infusion should be discontinued and the total daily morphine requirement divided into 4 to 6 intravenous bolus doses. The dose should be tapered by 20 to 30% daily while the interval is maintained. Once the daily intravenous dose is 50% of that initially required, conversion to an equianalgesic dose of an oral narcotic can be made.

Because of the addictive potential, chronic oral narcotic use should be discouraged, although some feel that severe painful crises may be aborted by early treatment (20). Unfortunately, many become both psychologically and physically dependent on these agents. Continuity of care and communication between providers is therefore essential to eliminate the possibility of multiple sources of narcotic prescriptions. Psychosocial support and nonpharmacologic coping techniques, such as relaxation therapy, behavior modification, and self-hypnosis, should be thoroughly explored.

Management of the Sickle Cell Disease

Partial exchange transfusions, in which over 50% of the patient's erythrocytes are replaced by donor red cells, prevent vaso-occlusive crises. Hypertransfusion, until the hematocrit level has doubled, temporarily halts erythroid Hb S production and also inhibits sickling. Because of the inherent risks of hepatitis transmission and iron overload, however, transfusions are generally reserved for the management of acute complications such as strokes and priapism and for prophylaxis preoperatively and in late pregnancy.

Pharmacologic therapy directed against the sickling abnormality has yielded minimal clinical benefit, in part because of limiting adverse effects (9, 19). Inhibitors of Hb S polymerization (e.g., sodium cyanate and urea) are not dependably effective. In addition, sodium cyanate is associated with neurologic toxicity. Studies of cetiedil, a peripheral vasodilator that alters fluid and electrolyte transport across the red cell membrane, are underway. Cetiedil-induced increases in red cell volume functionally decrease intracellular Hb S concentrations and thereby reduce the polymerization rate. Pentoxifylline may prevent vaso-occlusive crises by increasing red cell deformability and decreasing blood viscosity. These effects improve blood flow through the microvasculature in peripheral vascular occlusive diseases. However further studies are required to establish this agent's role in sickle cell anemia.

The antineoplastics 5-azacytidine and cytarabine enhance production of the protective fetal hemoglobin. However, bone marrow suppression produced by these agents is problematic and long-term efficacy uncertain. More promising are the results of recent clinical studies of hydroxyurea (23, 24). After treatment with hydroxyurea, the proportion of Hb F and the number of cells containing Hb F were increased, resulting in prolonged red cell survival. Clinical efficacy, as measured by changes in the frequency of painful crises and hospitalization for sickling complications, has yet to be demonstrated.

Bone marrow transplantation from a sibling donor converted a leukemic homozygous SS patient to the AS phenotype (25). Overall, the risk of this procedure greatly outweighs the benefit in sickle cell anemia. In the future, however, advances in genetic engineering may "cure" the disease by transferring normal hemoglobin genes into sickle cell patients.

THALASSEMIAS

The thalassemias are a group of hereditary disorders of hemoglobin synthesis characterized by impaired production of one or more of the normal polypeptide chains of globin. Any of the four definitive polypeptides that occur in normal hemoglobin may be involved (α, β, γ, δ). However, the most prevalent thalassemia syndromes are those that involve diminished or absent synthesis of either the alpha (α-thalassemia) or beta (β-thalassemia) globin chains of Hb A_1 (9, 26).

Pathogenesis

The imbalance in polypeptide chain production secondary to impaired synthesis of either the α chain or the β chain of globin is the underlying factor that accounts for the pathogenesis of all the clinically severe thalassemia syndromes. Reduced production of the normal $\alpha_2\beta_2$ tetramer of Hb A_1 results in the production of smaller erythrocytes with a low hemoglobin content. The synthesis and accumulation of normal globin chains within the red cell leads to the formation of unstable aggregates that may precipitate and cause cell membrane damage. These deformed cells undergo premature destruction, either in the bone marrow (intramedullary hemolysis) or the peripheral circulation (27). Chronic hemolysis is a primary complication of the clinically important α- and β-thalassemia syndromes (e.g., Hb H disease and β-thalassemia major). The "ineffective erythropoiesis" and microcytic, hypochromic anemia described above is associated with a compensatory increased absorption of dietary iron, which may contribute to iron overload in patients receiving blood transfusions. There is also an increase in erythropoietic activity in the bone marrow and in extramedullary sites (i.e., liver, spleen, and lymph nodes). In severe cases (e.g., β-thalassemia major) excessive erythropoiesis results in bone marrow hypertrophy, lymphadenopathy, and hepatosplenomegaly (27).

Epidemiology

The thalassemia syndromes are collectively one of the most common genetic disorders in humans. An estimated 190 million people throughout the world carry a hemoglobinopathy gene (i.e., 4% of the world's population), and more than half of these are thalassemia genes (28). Populations that are the most affected include Asians, Africans, Eastern Indians, and Mediterranean cultures (9, 29). Since the geographic distribution of this disorder is similar to that of malaria, it is thought that certain types of thalassemia may offer protection from *Plasmodium falciparum* infection (26). α-Thalassemia is more common in Southeast Asia, China, and certain areas of Africa, while β-thalassemia syndromes are concentrated in Mediterranean countries such as Greece and Italy. In North America, β-thalassemia is found primarily in people of Greek, Italian, and African ancestry. Genetic analysis studies indicate that approximately 30% of black Americans are "silent carriers" of α-thalassemia (9).

Because of their similar geographic distributions, coinheritance of sickle cell anemia and thalassemia is not uncommon. Detailed discussion of various sickle cell–thalassemia syndromes can be found elsewhere (9).

Table 13.4.
Comparison of α-Thalassemia Syndromes

Syndrome	Genotypes	RBC Morphology	Clinical Manifestations
Silent carrier	$-\alpha/\alpha\alpha$	Normal	None
α-Thalassemia trait	$-\alpha/-\alpha$ or $--/\alpha\alpha$	Microcytic	Mild anemia
Hb H disease	$--/-\alpha$	Microcytic; deformed	Chronic hemolysis; splenomegaly
Hydrops fetalis	$--/--$	Nucleated RBC	In utero or neonatal death

α-Thalassemia

There are four genes involved in the production of α globin chains, with one pair occurring on each DNA strand (α α/ α α). The most common forms of α-thalassemia result from deletion of one or more of these genes. Four such syndromes have been identified (Table 13-4).

The deletion of a single a α gene is classified as a "silent carrier state" and is the most common single gene abnormality in the world. Up to 2% Hb Bart's, an abnormal hemoglobin containing a γ_4 polypeptide tetramer, can be isolated in cord blood of these individuals at birth. Hb Bart's disappears within the first year of life. Fortunately, there are virtually no clinical manifestations of the silent carrier state, and laboratory values such as hemoglobin concentration and mean corpuscular volume (MCV) are usually within normal limits (30). These individuals do not require treatment.

The deletion of two α genes is classified as "α-thalassemia trait" or "α-thalassemia minor." The most common genotype for this disorder is a homozygous α gene deletion ($-\alpha/-\alpha$). Individuals with α-thalassemia trait experience a mild microcytic, hypochromic anemia without hemolysis (30). In Southeast Asians, however, both α gene deletions frequently occur on the same chromosome ($--/\alpha\alpha$). This genotype is associated with a more pronounced microcytosis [MCV in the 70 to 80 fl (70 to 80 μm_2) range] and mild hemolysis. In α-thalassemia trait, Hb Bart's (γ_4) constitutes 2 to 10% of hemoglobin in cord blood and disappears within the first year of life (9). Hemoglobin concentrations of adults with α-thalassemia trait are usually normal or only slightly decreased (30). Not surprisingly, this disorder is often identified in patients by chance during routine laboratory blood tests. Diagnosis is typically done through a DNA electrophoretic analysis technique known as Southern mapping (30). Because most patients are asymptomatic, treatment is seldom warranted.

Another α-thalassemia syndrome, more common in Asian populations, is Hb H disease. This disorder is associated with the deletion of three of the four α genes ($--/-\alpha$). Hemoglobin H is an unstable tetramer of β globin chains (β_4) that is formed when there is a marked reduction of α globin production yielding a substantial surplus of β globin chains. This hemoglobin variant constitutes 5 to 30% of total circulating hemoglobin in affected adults. In patients with Hb H disease, Hb Bart's represents 10 to 40% of the hemoglobin pool at birth and is found in trace amounts during adulthood (9). The unstable β_4-containing Hb H gradually undergoes oxidation and precipitates within the cell. These deformed cells are removed and hemolyzed primarily by the spleen.

Clinically manifestations associated with Hb H disease include microcytosis, mild to moderate chronic hemolytic anemia, mild jaundice, and splenomegaly (30). Enlargement of the spleen results both from the trapping of deformed red cells and from extramedullary erythropoiesis in that organ. In most patients, Hb H disease is not severe enough to impair routine activities, interfere with reproductive function, or reduce longevity (30). However, circumstances such as infection, pregnancy, or exposure to oxidant drugs can precipitate severe exacerbations of the hemolytic anemia.

In certain patients with Hb H disease, especially those with severe splenomegaly, splenectomy is often beneficial in reducing symptoms and slowing the rate of hemolysis. In rare instances, patients with severe forms of Hb H disease are blood transfusion–dependent (30).

Deletion of all four α genes is classified as "Hb Bart's hydrops fetalis" and is incompatible with life (30). An affected fetus is either prematurely stillborn in the second or third trimester or will expire within hours after birth. Hemoglobin in an affected fetus will be > 80% Hb Bart's. Physical findings include massive edema (hydrops), ascites, and hepatomegaly, while peripheral blood examination reveals immature nucleated erythrocytes (erythroblasts), target cells, reticulocytosis, and hypochromia.

Since most α-thalassemia syndromes are associated with a relatively benign clinical course, prenatal diagnosis is usually not critical. An exception to this is situations where couples are at risk of a hydrops pregnancy (e.g., Southeast Asians, Chinese, or prior α-thalassemic hydrops pregnancy). Prenatal diagnosis of the fetus involves gene mapping of DNA acquired by chorionic villus sampling (first trimester) or by amniocentesis (second trimester) (30). A positive diagnosis of Hb Bart's hydrops fetalis allows the option of early termination of the pregnancy, which may protect the health of the mother by avoiding such problems as toxemia and peripartum hemorrhage.

β-Thalassemia

In contrast to α-thalassemia where gene deletion is the mechanism, β-thalassemia syndromes usually result from faulty mRNA transcription of the β gene (9). Since α and δ chain production is usually unaffected, increased levels of Hb A_2 ($\alpha_2 \delta_2$) are common to most of the β-thalassemias.

Table 13.5.
Comparison of β-Thalassemia Syndromes

Syndrome	Hb[a]	Clinical Manifestations	Conventional Treatment
Heterozygous			
Minima	Normal	None	None
Minor	>100	Mild anemia	Genetic/medical counseling
Homozygous			
Intermedia	70–100	Moderate-severe anemia; impaired growth and splenomegaly in severe cases	Intermittent blood transfusion and chelation therapy (deferoxamine)
Major	20–70	Severe anemia; abnormal skeletal growth; splenomegaly; iron overload complications	Chronic blood transfusion and chelation therapy (deferoxamine)

[a] Typical hemoglobin concentrations (g/liter).

Despite the multitude of genetic variations that cause β-thalassemia, patients can be classified as either heterozygous or homozygous for the "β-thal" gene. Further distinction is then made, based on clinical manifestions and severity (i.e., phenotype) of the syndrome (Table 13.5).

Heterozygous β-thalassemia is much less severe than homozygous forms of the disease. Patients have either a clinically undetectable disorder ("β-thalassemia minima") or one that results in only mild anemia ("β-thalassemia minor" or "β-thalassemia trait"). In general, patients with β-thalassemia minima are asymptomatic, have laboratory blood values (i.e., hemoglobin concentration and MCV) within normal limits, and require no treatment. Definitive diagnosis can be made by measuring the relative synthetic rates of β and α chains (9).

Patients with β-thalassemia minor usually have a mild hypochromic, microcytic anemia. Hemoglobin concentration in these individuals is generally not less than 100 g/liter (10 g/dl). Microcytosis is more pronounced, with MCV values of approximately 60 fl (60 μm^3). Clinical manifestions such as splenomegaly and hyperplastic marrow are usually absent. Nutritional deficiencies, infection, and pregnancy may exacerbate anemia in patients with β-thalassemia minor. However, since these individuals are predisposed to iron overload because of enhanced absorption of dietary iron, long-term iron supplementation and routine blood transfusions during pregnancy should be avoided, if possible. Medical care for these individuals should also involve genetic counseling (9). Screening patients for β-thalassemia minor is often done through quantification of Hb A_2. Ranges of Hb A_2 levels in normal patients and those with β-thalassemia minor are 2 to 3% and 3.5 to 8%, respectively (9).

Homozygous forms of β-thalassemia can be classified as either "β-thalassemia intermedia" or "β-thalassemia major." The intermedia form is associated with moderate anemia and may require intermittent treatment with blood transfusions. Hemoglobin concentrations in patients with β-thalassemia intermedia usually range from 70 to 100 g/liter (7 to 10 g/dl). In contrast, β-thalassemia major (also known as Cooley's anemia) is associated with severe anemia and requires intensive chronic treatment. Hemoglobin concentration and MCV in these patients usually range from 20 to 70 g/liter (2 to 7 g/dl) and 50 to 60 fl (50 to 60 μm^3), respectively (9, 31).

CLINICAL PRESENTATION OF β-THALASSEMIA MAJOR

Excessive erythropoiesis (secondary to severe anemia) in the bone marrow and extramedullary sites is a primary complication of untreated patients with β-thalassemia major. Bone marrow hypertrophy with subsequent abnormal skeletal growth usually develops in children from the second year of life through 10 years of age. Abnormal skeletal changes are most apparent in the craniofacial bones, because of maxillary overgrowth, protrusion of teeth, and separation of orbits. Cortical thinning of weight-bearing bones may lead to recurrent fractures in these patients. Fortunately, skeletal abnormalities are almost completely prevented if adequate blood transfusion therapy is initiated early in life. Excessive extramedullary erythropoiesis leads to lymphadenopathy and hepatosplenogaly (27).

Red cell damage and subsequent chronic hemolysis that occurs in β-thalassemia major is due to precipitated intracellular aggregates of excess α chains. Removal of these deformed red cells by the spleen contributes to splenomegaly, which if uncorrected by splenectomy, can signify increase the blood transfusion requirements of patients. Chronic hemolysis is also associated with gallstone formation, which is present in 70% of thalassemic children over 15 years of age (27, 31).

TREATMENT

Currently, the standard treatment in patients with β-thalassemia major is supportive therapy, with the main goals being to avoid or reduce major complications of the disease. Therapies that have been introduced recently (e.g., bone marrow transplantation) and other approaches that are still being developed (e.g., gene therapy) are directed more toward actually "curing" the underlying disease.

Transfusion and Chelation. The primary approach to treatment of patients with β-thalassemia major is chronic blood transfusions in conjunction with intensive iron chelation therapy. The goals of transfusion therapy are to suppress excessive erythropoiesis and prevent anemia. This can be accomplished by initiating "high-transfusion" programs prior to 4 years of age. It is generally accepted that high-transfusion programs (i.e., maintaining hemoglobin above 100 g/liter) are clinically superior to low-transfusion programs (i.e., maintaining hemoglobin above 70 g/liter). Important advantages of the high-transfusion approach include fewer skeletal abnormalities, normal or nearly normal growth prior to adolescence, less severe hepatosplenomegaly, and decreased incidence of cardiomegaly due to anemia. There is no evidence that iron accumulation and toxicity develop earlier in patients who receive high-transfusion therapy as compared with those who receive low-transfusion therapy (27).

Although some variations exist between institutions, a typical high-transfusion program involves transfusing 12 to 15 ml/kg of packed red blood cells (PRBCs) over 4 to 5 hours every 3 to 4 weeks on an outpatient basis. Longer intervals between transfusions (i.e., every 5 to 6 weeks) have been shown to increase iron accumulation and, therefore, should be avoided. This will usually cycle a patient's hemoglobin between 100 to 120 g/liter (10 to 12 g/dl) and 150 to 170 g/liter (15 to 17 g/dl). The adequacy of a given transfusion regimen is best evaluated by monitoring the patient's growth rate (27, 31, 32).

Important complications associated with chronic blood transfusions include sensitization reactions, transmission of viral infection, and iron overload. Febrile and urticarial reactions to PRBCs, caused by sensitization to leukocyte surface antigens, may occur. However, the incidence of these reactions has been greatly reduced through improved typing and matching techniques. Many institutions administer leukocyte-depleted RBC products to thalassemic patients to avoid this complication (27, 31, 32). A more hazardous problem of chronic blood transfusions is the transmission of viral infections. Careful screening of donors and donated blood products has reduced the risk of human immunodeficiency virus (HIV) transmission to 1 per 150,000 units transfused. Hepatitis B, in contrast, may be prevented through proper vaccination of uninfected thalassemic patients who are initiating or being maintained on chronic transfusion programs. Hepatitis C (i.e., non-A non-B hepatitis) transmission remains a relatively common threat to transfused patients, with an incidence of 6 to 8%. The recent development of screening techniques for donors infected with hepatitis C should reduce the transmission of this disease in the future (27, 31).

The primary cause of morbidity and mortality in patients with β-thalassemia major is iron overload associated with the intensive administration of blood products. Each unit of PRBCs (450 ml) contains 200 to 250 mg of elemental iron; the normal iron content of the body is 2 g. By 12 years of age, a properly transfused thalassemic has likely received 55 to 60 g of iron, and there is no natural mechanism by which excess amounts may be excreted. Iron overload and subsequent toxicity occurs when the capacity of the storage proteins (ferritin and hemosiderin) and the transport protein (transferrin) is exceeded. The molecular mechanism of toxicity is thought to be the accumulation of unbound iron both intracellularly and in the circulation acting as a catalyst in Haber-Weiss and Fenton reactions, which produce reactive oxygen species that oxidize membrane lipids and damage cells (27, 31, 32).

The clinical effects of iron overload are most pronounced in the liver, pancreas, and heart. Normal growth may be impaired by an excess iron burden. In transfused thalassemic children, hepatic fibrosis usually develops by 7 years of age, and older patients will often have histologic evidence of cirrhosis. Other than mild prolongations of clotting time, clinical problems associated with hepatic dysfunction in these individuals are uncommon. Diabetes mellitus secondary to the effects of hemochromatosis on the pancreas may occur and can be managed by standard insulin replacement therapy. The manifestions of iron overload on the heart include pericarditis, atrial and ventricular arrhythmias, and congestive heart failure. In underchelated patients, cardiac dysfunction is the primary cause of death (27, 31). Growth and development failure associated with thalassemia is probably due to a combination of the chronic disease process and the accumulation of iron associated with blood transfusion programs (27). For these reasons chronic iron chelation therapy must accompany standard blood transfusion regimens.

The only agent currently available for chelating and removing excess iron is deferoxamine, a polyhydroxamic acid introduced in 1961. Following parenteral administration, deferoxamine penetrates cell membranes and combines with free intracellular iron to form the complex ferrioxamine. Liver parenchymal cells serve as a large source of chelatable iron. Ferrioxamine is then transported extracellularly and is readily excreted in the urine and the bile. The general goal of treatment with deferoxamine is to create a "negative iron balance," where measured urinary iron excretion exceeds the amount of iron administered during transfusions. It may be necessary to provide enough deferoxamine to chelate all free intracellular and extracellular iron, to avoid iron-related organ damage (27, 31, 33).

Chelation therapy is usually initiated in transfusion-dependent patients by 3 to 4 years of age. Due to poor oral absorption, deferoxamine must be given parenterally. The subcutaneous and intravenous routes are superior at promoting urinary iron excretion as compared with the intramuscular route. Furthermore, the half-life of deferoxamine in the blood following intravenous injection is very short (5 to 10 minutes). Therefore, continuous infusion is used to maximize exposure time between the drug and excess iron. A typical deferoxamine dosing regimen is 40 mg/kg/day infused subcutaneously over 8 to 10 hours, 5 to 7 days a week. Larger doses of deferoxamine (e.g.,

120 mg/kg over 8 hours) are generally administered intravenously on days of transfusion therapy. Treatment is usually administered with a portable infusion pump, at night, while the patient is sleeping. Monitoring total body iron burden and chelation therapy efficacy should include the measurement of serum ferritin concentrations [normal: 18 to 300 μg/liter (18 to 300 ng/ml)] and urinary iron excretion. However, urinary iron excretion may significantly underestimate the amount of iron being removed from the body when biliary excretion is high (27, 32, 33).

For patients who are poorly compliant, are extremely iron overloaded [i.e., serum ferritin > 5000 μg/liter (>5000 ng/ml)], or have iron-induced cardiac disease prior to chelation therapy, high-dose intravenous deferoxamine therapy is used. Experience with doses of 6 to 12 g daily for up to 41 months has been reported. Because rapid intravenous infusion may cause hypotension, the rate of administration should not exceed 15 mg/kg/hr. Because of the large amounts of deferoxamine being administered in this type of protocol, annual drug costs may range from $30,000 to $60,000 (32, 34).

The clinical benefits of regular chelation therapy initiated at an early age include reduced iron stores and the avoidance of iron-induced organ damage. Patients who are compliant with a chelation program are less likely to develop cardiac disease (i.e., congestive heart failure and arrhythmias) than those who are not compliant and can avoid the lethal complications of iron overload for at least 20 years. In a limited number of patients, high-dose deferoxamine has been associated with dramatic improvements in cardiac function, while iron-induced endocrine disorders have not responded as well.

Deferoxamine used in conventional doses is a relatively safe drug. Common side effects during subcutaneous infusion programs are mild and include local irritation and urticaria at the injection site and abdominal discomfort. Several recent reports, however, have associated deferoxamine with a variety of adverse visual and auditory effects. The mechanism of this toxicity is not well understood, yet patients on deferoxamine should receive regular vision and hearing evaluations. Patients with minimal iron burdens and patients receiving high doses of deferoxamine are likely to be at greater risk for toxicity (31, 34).

Because of the inconvenience, high cost, and frequent noncompliance with parenteral deferoxamine therapy, research efforts have focused on the development of a safe, effective, and inexpensive oral medication for iron chelation. The most promising compounds to date are those of the hydroxypyridone family. However, more clinical testing of these agents must be done to show adequate safety and efficacy.

In thalassemic patients with iron overload, leukocyte ascorbic acid levels frequently indicate deficiency. When these individuals receive vitamin C supplementation in conjunction with chelation treatment, urinary iron excretion has been demonstrated to increase from 20 to 250%. Caution must be used, however, as cardiac toxicity has been reported in patients receiving 500 mg of vitamin C concurrently with deferoxamine. A proposed mechanism for this toxicity involves ascorbic acid combining with released iron to generate free radicals that oxidize membrane lipids and cause cell damage. Therefore, if vitamin C supplementation is used, only low doses (such as 100 mg at the time of deferoxamine infusion) should be given (27, 32).

Patients with β-thalassemia intermedia are often not blood transfusion–dependent. However, in severe forms of this syndrome, ineffective erythropoiesis and anemia are sometimes severe enough to inhibit growth and development. In these cases, patients with β-thalassemia intermedia should be treated with intermittent courses of transfusion and chelation therapy (as described above) to induce healing of bones and promote proper growth (31).

Splenectomy. Due to increased erythropoietic activity and trapping of red cells by the spleen, patients with β-thalassemia major develop splenomegaly. Proper transfusion therapy may slow the process, but gradual enlargement of the spleen usually occurs. In patients who receive chronic transfusion therapy, enlargement of the spleen is associated with increased transfusion requirements to maintain an adequate hemoglobin concentration. The administration of greater volumes of blood products increases the amount of iron a patient receives and makes successful chelation therapy more difficult. Therefore, when blood transfusion requirements reach approximately 250 ml/kg/year, splenectomy is indicated. Following spleen removal, requirements generally return to baseline. Since splenectomized patients, especially young children, are predisposed to bacterial sepsis, removal of the spleen should be avoided until the age of 4 or 5 years, if possible. Prophylactic oral penicillin therapy (e.g., 250 mg twice daily) in splenectomized young children is appropriate. All splenectomized patients should be vaccinated against *Haemophilus influenzae* type b, pneumococcus, and meningococcus at the earliest appropriate age (27, 31, 32).

Alternative Therapeutic Options. Considerable experience has now been gained with bone marrow transplantation (BMT) in patients with β-thalassemia major. The survival rate and disease-free survival rate reported from a group of 139 patients receiving BMT for thalassemia were 73% and 58%, respectively (35). Therefore, assuming that an HLA-compatible donor exists, BMT offers thalassemic patients a good chance to be "cured" of their disease. Unfortunately, the incidence of graft failure and early mortality associated with this procedure is high (15% to 25% in most centers). In contrast, conventional transfusion and chelation therapy is associated with a high rate of survival and a good quality of life for the first two decades.

Thalassemic patients for whom medical therapy is unavailable or not complied with and who have a histocompatible donor may be candidates for BMT (31, 35).

Another approach to treating patients with β-thalassemia major is to reduce transfusion requirements by increasing Hb F synthesis. Agents currently available that increase Hb F synthesis include 5-azacytidine and cytarabine. However, the adverse effects (bone marrow suppression, mutagenicity) and unknown long-term efficacy of these agents have limited their use in the treatment of thalassemia.

Genetic engineering is another treatment approach that holds great potential for curing patients with thalassemia. Current limitations in the use of this therapy for the treatment of thalassemia include inefficient gene expression and regulation.

Prenatal Diagnosis. Prevention is another approach in dealing with β-thalassemia major. The use of prenatal diagnostic techniques has led to a significant reduction in the incidence of this disease in areas where prenatal detection programs have been implemented. Using tissue specimens obtained by amniocentesis and DNA analysis techniques, a safe and accurate diagnosis can be made at 8 to 14 weeks gestation (31).

PROGNOSIS

Prior to the implementation and modification of adequate transfusion and chelation programs, children with β-thalassemia major suffered from progressive enlargement of the liver and spleen, congestive heart failure, and recurrent infections. More than 80% of these patients died within the first 5 years of life. The introduction and widespread use of high-transfusion programs along with chelation therapy has led to a significant improvement in the quality and duration of life for thalassemic patients, and survival through the first and second decades of life is very common.

HEMOLYTIC ANEMIAS

Hemolytic anemias are due to an increased rate of red blood cell (RBC) destruction. The anemia is of clinical concern when the rate of red cell destruction exceeds that of erythropoiesis. The hemolytic process may occur chronically or manifest as an acute episode, depending on the etiologic mechanism. Acute hemolysis is generally a more clinically threatening event. Many anemias have a hemolytic component because of the production of defective or damaged red blood cells (e.g., megaloblastic anemias, thalassemias) (9). As there are many causes of hemolytic anemia, this section focuses on those amenable to specific medical treatment and those that are drug-induced.

Etiology and Classification

Hemolytic anemias can be categorized as either inherited or acquired disorders. Inherited hemolytic anemias in-

Table 13.6.
Classification of Hemolytic Anemias

Inherited
  Globin synthesis defect
    Sickle cell anemia
    Thalassemia
    Unstable hemoglobin disease
  Erythrocyte membrane defect
    Hereditary spherocytosis
    Hereditary elliptocytosis
    Hereditary stomatocytosis
  Erythrocyte enzyme defect
    Hexose-monophosphate shunt defect (e.g., glucose-6-phosphate dehydrogenase)
    Glycolytic (Embden-Meyerhof) enzyme defect (e.g., pyruvate kinase)
    Other enzyme defect (e.g., adenylate kinase)
Acquired
  Immune-mediated
    Warm-reacting antibody (IgG)
      Secondary (e.g., collagen vascular disease, lymphoproliferative disorders)
      Drug-induced
      Idiopathic
    Cold agglutinin disease (IgM)
      Acute (e.g., mycoplasma pneumonia, infectious mononucleosis)
      Chronic (e.g., lymphoid neoplasms, idiopathic)
    Transfusion reactions
    Hemolytic disease of newborns
  Microangiopathic and traumatic
    Disseminated intravascular coagulation
    Hemolytic-uremic syndrome
    Thrombotic thrombocytopenic purpura
    Prosthetic or diseased heart valves
  Infection
  Exogenous substances
  Other
    Paroxysmal nocturnal hemoglobinuria
    Liver disease
    Hypophosphatemia

clude defective globin synthesis, erythrocyte membrane defects, and erythrocyte enzyme deficiencies. Acquired hemolytic disorders are caused by some extrinsic event and do not involve a genetic component. Typically, the acquired hemolytic anemias are either immune-mediated, due to physical stress on the red cell, or are induced by certain infections (Table 13.6).

Epidemiology

The prevalence and distribution of sickle cell anemia and thalassemia have been discussed previously. With respect to other inherited hemolytic disorders, the incidence of hereditary spherocytosis and hereditary elliptocytosis in the United States is approximately 220 and 400 per million, respectively. Glucose-6-phosphate dehydrogenase (G6PD) deficiency is the most common inherited erythrocyte enzyme disorder worldwide, affecting over 100 million people, but not all patients with G6PD deficiency are significantly predisposed to oxidative hemolysis (9, 35).

Most acquired hemolytic anemias are idiopathic. Many are due to immune reactions, collagen vascular disease, or malignancy. Drugs are the causative agents in less than 10% of cases.

Pathophysiology

The average RBC life-span is 120 days. During severe hemolytic episodes this can be reduced to as low as 5 to 20 days. Red cells are either hemolyzed within the circulation (intravascular hemolysis) or taken up by the reticuloendothelial system (RES) and destroyed (extravascular hemolysis). Intravascular hemolysis may be caused by trauma to the RBC, complement fixation to the RBC (immune-mediated), or by exposure to exogenous substances. Under normal circumstances, however, most RBC catabolism occurs extravascularly by the RES in the liver and spleen. Specific drug-induced mechanisms of RBC hemolysis are discussed later in the context of G6PD deficiency and immune-mediated hemolysis.

Following lysis of the RBC, hemoglobin is released into the blood where it is bound by the plasma protein haptoglobin. Free heme molecules are bound by the plasma protein hemopexin. The hemoglobin-haptoglobin complex is rapidly cleared from the circulation by the RES, and the heme component is metabolized to unconjugated (indirect) bilirubin. In the liver, this is linked with glucuronic acid, forming conjugated (direct) bilirubin, which passes from the bile duct into the intestine. Fecal bacteria metabolize conjugated bilirubin to urobilinogen, which is primarily excreted in the feces. Iron from heme catabolism is stored as ferritin or hemosiderin.

During hemolysis, if the haptoglobin binding capacity is exceeded, unbound hemoglobin levels increase resulting in hemoglobinemia. In this case, free hemoglobin is filtered through the glomerulus and is usually reabsorbed by the proximal tubules. In severe intravascular hemolysis, the reabsorptive capacity is exceeded, causing hemoglobinuria. Also during severe intravascular hemolysis, some heme molecules in the circulation are transferred from hemopexin to albumin, forming methemalbumin. When the conjugating capacity of the liver is exceeded during moderate or severe hemolysis, unconjugated bilirubin serum levels increase.

Diagnosis

The primary diagnostic features of hemolytic anemia are a marked reticulocytosis with jaundice (including scleral icterus) due to hyperbilirubinemia. A corrected reticulocyte count greater than 0.025 (2.5%) is a typical response to hemolysis. The severity of the anemia may also be judged by the extent to which the hematocrit is decreased.

Table 13.7.
Common Diagnostic Features of Hemolytic Anemia

	Moderate Hemolysis	Severe Hemolysis
Physical findings		
Jaundice	+	+
Hemoglobinuria	0	+
Laboratory indices—plasma/serum		
Reticulocytosis	+	+ +
Plasma hemoglobin	+	+ +
RBC hemoglobin	Decreased	Decreased
Hematocrit	Decreased	Decreased
Bilirubin (unconjugated)	+	+ +
Haptoglobin	Decreased	Decreased or absent
Hemopexin	Normal or decreased	Decreased or absent
Methemalbumin	0	+
Lactate dehydrogenase	+ (Variable)	+ + (Variable)
Laboratory indices—urine		
Hemoglobin	0	+
Hemosiderin	0	+

The enzyme lactate dehydrogenase is released from the RBC during hemolysis, and plasma levels may be elevated. Red cells frequently undergo morphologic changes during hemolytic episodes, with spherocytosis being the most common abnormality. Splenomegaly is usually present in cases of chronic hemolysis. A summary of important findings in hemolytic anemia is presented in Table 13.7.

With respect to immune-mediated hemolysis, diagnostic evaluation includes the direct Coomb's antiglobulin test, which detects IgG or C3 (complement) on the surface of a patient's RBCs. The indirect Coomb's test detects antibodies against RBCs in the serum rather than on the surface of the RBC itself. During oxidative hemolytic anemias, denatured hemoglobin precipitates within the RBC, forming Heinz bodies which are visible during microscopic examination.

Inherited Hemolytic Anemias

Hereditary spherocytosis, elliptocytosis, and stomatocytosis are all genetic disorders inherited in an autosomal dominant fashion and associated with altered RBC morphology. Hemolysis and clinical sequelae tend to be more pronounced with hereditary spherocytosis than with the other two. Splenectomy usually corrects anemia in these individuals. Supplemental folic acid therapy (1 mg daily) is also recommended.

G6PD DEFICIENCY

The most prevalent inherited RBC enzyme defect is G6PD deficiency, a sex-linked (X-chromosome) disorder. Females are predominantly heterozygous and have both nor-

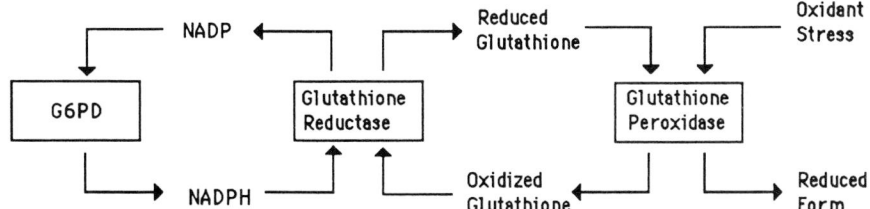

Figure 13.2. Antioxidant mechanism of G6PD. *NADP* = nicotinamide adenine dinucleotide phosphate.

mal and G6PD-deficiency RBCs. They are fairly resistant to RBC hemolysis. Men and homozygous women, however, have predominantly G6PD-deficient RBCs and are predisposed to more severe hemolytic episodes. Cultural distribution of this disorder is similar to that of thalassemia. It occurs frequently in blacks and people of Mediterranean cultures. The "A-" variant of G6PD is found primarily in blacks. Enzyme activity in these individuals is 8% to 20% of normal. In the United States, approximately 13% of black males and 3% of black females are affected. The Mediterranean-type variant of G6PD has 0% to 4% of normal enzyme activity. Consequently, these individuals are generally at greater risk of developing hemolytic anemia, and the associated clinical manifestations are more pronounced.

Hemolytic Mechanism. The G6PD enzyme, in conjunction with glutathione and nicotinamide adenine dinucleotide phosphate (NADPH), serves as a protective antioxidant for RBCs against external oxidative stresses (Fig. 13.2). In G6PD deficiency, oxidative stresses on the RBC, such as drugs, infection, or acidosis, can lead to denaturation of the globin chains. Denatured globin precipitates intracellularly onto the cell membrane as Heinz bodies, and premature hemolysis occurs (36, 37). This type of disorder is frequently referred to as "oxidative hemolysis."

Many drugs have been associated with hemolytic anemia in G6PD-deficient individuals. More commonly used drugs and other substances that have been reported are listed in Table 13.8. A patient's susceptibility to oxidative stress from a particular drug varies according to several factors. The type of G6PD genetic variant present (i.e., type A- or Mediterranean-type) is a major determinant. Other factors include patient age, other sources of oxidant stress, dose of an offending drug, patient metabolism of an offending drug, and patient elimination of an offending drug (37).

Treatment. Withdrawing any potentially oxidant drugs or other substances is the initial step. In patients with A-variant G6PD deficiency, hemolysis is usually mild and self-limited, and therapy is seldom required. In Mediterranean-type deficiency, splenectomy is usually not beneficial and blood transfusions are rarely necessary. Patients who develop severe hemolytic anemia with hemoglobi-

Table 13.8.
Common Drugs and Substances Associated with Hemolytic Anemia in G6PD Deficiency

Antimalarials	Antibacterials
Chloroquine	Chloramphenicol
Hydroxychloroquine	Sulfamethoxazole
Primaquine	Sulfacetamide
Quinacrine	Nalidixic acid
Quinine	Nitrofurantoin
Analgesics	Nitrofurazone
Phenacetin	*p*-Aminosalicylic acid
Aspirin	Miscellaneous
Probenecid	Dapsone
	Naphthalene
	Aqueous vitamin K
	Methylene blue
	Fava beans

nuria may require intravenous hydration to maintain adequate urine output.

The primary approach to caring for patients who have documented G6PD deficiency or those who may be at risk (e.g., family history, ethnic background) is prevention. Several factors should be considered prior to initiating such patients on a potentially hemolyzing drug, including patient age, renal function, type of G6PD variant that may be present, availability of alternative drugs, and severity of primary illness. A specific quantitative assay of G6PD is available for screening patients who may be deficient.

Acquired Hemolytic Anemias

Acquired hemolytic anemias are made up of a diverse group of disorders (Table 13.6). Microangiopathic hemolytic anemias, including disseminated intravascular coagulation, hemolytic-uremic syndrome, and thrombotic thrombocytopenic purpura, are generally caused by alterations such as fibrin deposition or narrowing of the microvasculature. Therapy for these disorders involves treatment of the underlying disease. Acquired hemolytic anemias secondary to red blood cell trauma occur in up to 10% of patients with prosthetic or diseased heart valves, because of pressure gradient stresses placed on the RBC membrane. Beneficial treatment in these patients includes correcting iron deficiency and limiting exertional activity. Valve replacement may be necessary when less invasive measures fail.

AUTOIMMUNE HEMOLYSIS

Autoimmune hemolytic anemia results from the production of anti-RBC antibodies by the patient's own immune system. These disorders are classified according to the temperature at which the antibodies have the greatest affinity for an interaction with red cells.

Cold Agglutinin Disease. Cold agglutinin disorders involve the binding of IgM antibodies to RBCs at low temperatures ($<37°C$). This agglutination process is quickly reversed during warming. Most cold agglutinins do not appreciably shorten red cell survival. Acute cold agglutinin disease is frequently associated with mycoplasma pneumonia or infectious mononucleosis. The chronic form often occurs spontaneously in elderly patients and results in poor peripheral circulation. Treatment of cold agglutinin disease involves avoiding cold environments. Occasionally patients may respond to plasmapheresis or cytotoxic agents such as cyclophosphamide or chlorambucil. Transfusions, splenectomy, or corticosteroids are of little or no value.

Warm-Antibody Type. Warm-reacting antibodies have the greatest affinity for red cells at room temperature ($37°C$) and are usually of the IgG or (occasionally) IgA type. This type of immunohemolytic anemia may be idiopathic, secondary to an underlying disease that affects the immune system (e.g., chronic lymphocytic leukemia, non-Hodgkin's lymphoma, or systemic lupus erythematosus) or secondary to certain drugs. Many of these patients have a chronic mild anemia and splenomegaly, but the clinical presentation of these patients varies widely. The direct Coomb's test is positive for IgG but usually not for C3. The indirect Coomb's test is usually negative.

Treatment of Warm-Antibody Immunohemolytic Anemia. Prior to treating patients with immunohemolytic anemia, drugs that have been associated with this condition (discussed below) should be excluded as the cause. Therapy should be guided by the severity of the anemia. Patients with mild hemolysis usually do not require therapy. When hemolysis is clinically important, corticosteroid therapy is usually effective. The mechanism of steroid action in immunohemolytic anemia is thought to involve a reduction in the clearance of IgG-coated red cells from the circulation and an inhibition of antibody synthesis. Typically, prednisone is administered in a dose of 1 mg/kg/day and continued until hemoglobin levels have normalized. Hemoglobin concentration usually begins to increase within 3 to 4 days after prednisone is initiated. Once hemoglobin has returned to baseline, prednisone therapy is tapered slowly over a period of several months. Up to

Table 13.9.
Drugs Associated with Immunohemolytic Anemia

Autoimmune (Methyldopa Type)	Drug Adsorption (Hapten Type)	Immune Complex Adsorption (Innocent Bystander Type)
Methyldopa	Penicillins	Quinidine
Levodopa	Cephalosporins	Quinine
Mefenamic acid	Tetracycline	Phenacetin
Cimetidine		Acetaminophen
Procainamide		

75% of patients treated in this manner will have a sustained suppression of hemolysis. However, half of these patients will relapse as steroids are tapered or once they are withdrawn. Splenectomy is indicated in patients who fail steroid therapy, cannot tolerate steroids, or would require excessive doses.

Drug-Induced Immunohemolytic Anemias. Drugs that have been associated with immunohemolytic anemias are listed in Table 13.9. There are three proposed mechanisms by which drugs may initiate this condition.

Autoimmune (Methyldopa Type). Up to 10% of patients receiving methyldopa in doses of 2 g daily develop a positive direct Coomb's test. Only a small percentage of these patients ($<1\%$) will develop an extravascular hemolysis. The patient's red blood cells are coated with IgG. The mechanism of this condition is not well understood but may involve the inhibition of suppressor T cells. Hemolysis gradually subsides over a period of weeks, but patients may remain Coomb's positive for more than a year.

Drug Adsorption (Hapten Type). In patients receiving large doses of penicillins (e.g., 15 to 20 million units per day) or cephalosporins, drug adsorbs to the RBC membrane, forming a hapten complex. Antibodies are then formed against this complex, resulting in extravascular hemolysis within 7 to 14 days after initiation of the drug. Red cells are Coomb's positive for IgG during therapy. Hemolysis subsides immediately after the drug is withdrawn.

Immune Complex Adsorption (Innocent Bystander Type). In this type of drug-induced immunohemolytic anemia, the offending agent induces the production of either IgG or IgM antibodies. A drug-antibody complex forms, which then adheres nonspecifically to the red cell membrane. Complacent (C3) is activated and fixes to the membrane surface. The drug-antibody complex dissociates from the RBC, and only C3 is detected by a Coomb's test. The hemolytic process may occur either extravascularly or intravascularly and may be associated with hemoglobinemia, hemoglobinuria, and acute renal failure.

A fourth type of process may occur secondary to the administration of high-dose cephalosporins. In this case, the drug binds to the red cell membrane, causing it to be modified, which results in the nonspecific adsorption of serum proteins. This process is not immune-mediated nor does hemolysis occur.

CONCLUSION

Anemia is a reduction in the concentration of viable erythrocytes or hemoglobin in the circulation, resulting in a reduced oxygen-carrying capacity of blood. There are several basic mechanisms by which this may occur including impaired or absent erythropoiesis (e.g., aplastic anemia, anemia of renal failure), impaired hemoglobin synthesis (e.g., sickle cell anemia, thalassemia), and premature red cell destruction (e.g., hemolytic anemia). These mechanisms may coexist. Diseases or conditions that are frequently the primary cause of anemia include chronic infection or inflammation, neoplastic diseases, renal disease, exposure to certain pathogens or chemicals, exposure to certain drugs, inherited abnormalities, and autoimmune processes.

Anemia has many potential etiologies and is actually a symptom of an underlying condition. The treatment of patients should focus not only on correcting the anemia and its associated symptoms but also on identifying and correcting underlying causes, when possible.

REFERENCES

1. Lee GR: The anemia of chronic disease. Semin Hematol 20:61–80, 1983.
2. Beutler E: The common anemias. JAMA 259:2433–2437, 1988.
3. Eshbach JW: The anemia of chronic renal failure: pathophysiology and the effects of recombinant erythropoietin. Kidney Int 35:134–148, 1989.
4. Neff MS, Goldberg J, Slifkin RF, et al.: Anemia in chronic renal failure. Acta Endocrinol Suppl (Copenh) 271:80–85, 1985.
5. Neff MS, Goldberg J, Slifkin RF, et al: A comparison of androgens for anemia in patients on hemodialysis. N Engl J Med 304:871–875, 1981.
6. Eschbach JW, Abdulhadi MH, Browne JK, et al.: Recombinant human erythropoietin in anemic patients with end-stage renal disease. Ann Intern Med 111:992–1000, 1989.
7. Eschbach JW, Egrie JC, Downing MR, et al.: Correction of the anemia of end-stage renal disease with recombinant human erythropoietin. N Engl J Med 316:73–78, 1987.
8. Ad Hoc Committee for the National Kidney Foundation: Statement on the clinical use of recombinant erythropoietin in anemia of end-stage renal disease. Am J Kidney Dis 14:163–169, 1989.
9. Jandl JH: Blood: Textbook of Hematology. Boston: Little, Brown & Co. 1987.
10. Hine LK, Gerstman BB, Wise RP, et al.: Mortality resulting from blood dyscrasias in the United States, 1984. Am J Med 88:151–153, 1990.
11. Camitta BM, Storb R, Thomas ED: Aplastic anemia: pathogenesis, diagnosis, treatment and prognosis (part 2). N Engl J Med 306:712–718, 1982.
12. Katsanis E, Ramsay NKC: Treatment of acquired severe aplastic anemia. Am J Pediatr Hematol Oncol 11:360–367, 1989.
13. Storb R, Buckner CD: Human bone marrow transplantation. Eur J Clin Invest 20:119–132, 1990.
14. Loughran TP, Storb R: Treatment of aplastic anemia. Hematol Oncol Clin North Am 4:559–575, 1990.
15. Weiner RS, Bortin MM, Gale RP, et al.: Interstitial penumonitis after bone marrow transplantation. Ann Intern Med 104:168–175, 1986.
16. Jimenez JJ, Vargas-Cuba R, Temple JD: The role of recombinant hematopoietic growth factors in blood diseases. Adv Intern Med 35:393–414, 1990.
17. Ganser A, Lindemann A, Seipelt G, et al.: Effects of recombinant human interleukin-3 in aplastic anemia. Blood 76:1287–1292, 1990.
18. Schneider RG, Hightower B, Hosty TS, et al.: Abnormal hemoglobins in a quarter million people. Blood 48:629–637, 1976.
19. Galloway SJ, Harwood-Nuss AL: Sickle-cell anemia—A review. J Emerg Med 6:213–226, 1988.
20. Shapiro BS: The management of pain in sickle cell disease. Pediatr Clin North Am 36:1029–1045, 1989.
21. Friedman EW, Webber AB, Osborn HH, et al.: Oral analgesia for treatment of painful cirsis in sickle cell anemia. Ann Emerg Med 15:787–791, 1986.
22. Schechter NL, Berrien FB, Katz SM: The use of patient-controlled analgesia in adolescents with sickle cell pain crisis: A preliminary report. J Pain Symtpom Manage 3:109–139, 1988.
23. Rodgers GP, Dover GJ, Noguchi CT, et al.: Hematologic responses of patients with sickle cell disease to treatment with hydroxyurea. N Engl J Med 322:1037–1045, 1990.
24. Goldberg MA, Brugnara C, Dover GJ, et al.: Treatment of sickle cell anemia with hydroxyurea and erythropoietin. N Engl J Med 323:366–372, 1990.
25. Johnson FL, Look AT, Gockerman J, et al.: Bone-marrow transplantation in a patient with sickle cell anemia. N Engl J Med 311:780–783, 1984.
26. Steinberg MH: Thalassemia: molecular pathology and management. Am J Med Sci 296:308–321, 1988.
27. Festa RS: Modern management of thalassemia. Pediatr Ann 14:597–606, 1985.
28. Wonke B: Prospects of β-thalassemia major. Indian Pediatr 24:969–975, 1987.
29.. Huisman TH: Frequencies of common β-thalassemia alleles among different populations: variations in clinical severity. Br J Haematol 75:454–457, 1990.
30. Liebhaber SA: α-Thalassemia. Hemoglobin 13:685–721, 1989.
31. Fosburg MT, Nathan DG: Treatment of Cooley's anemia. Blood 76:435–444, 1990.
32. Lerner N: Medical management of β-thalassemia. Prog Clin Biol Res 309:14–22, 1989.
33. Pippard MJ: Iron overload and iron chelation therapy in thalassemia and sickle cell haemoglobinopathies. Acta Haematol 78:206–211, 1987.
34. Cohen A: Current status of iron chelation therapy with deferoxamine. Semin Hematol 27:86–90, 1990.
35. Barrett AJ, Lucarelli G, Gale RP, et al.: Bone marrow transplantation for thalassemia—a preliminary report from the international bone marrow transplant registry. Prog Clin Biol Res 309:173–185, 1989.
36. Valentine WN, Tanaka KR, Paglia DE: Hemolytic anemia and erythrocyte enzymopathies. Ann Intern Med 103:245–257, 1985.
37. Gordon-Smith EC: Drug-induced oxidative haemolysis. Clin Haemotol 9:557–586, 1980.

CHAPTER 14

CLOTTING DISORDERS

CHARLES D. SINTEK, M.S. and RICHARD S. RHODES, Pharm.D.

HEMOSTASIS

Definitions and Components

Normal hemostatic mechanisms maintain blood in the fluid state within the vasculature. These complex and highly integrated mechanisms also protect the organism from traumatic blood loss and arrest hemorrhage at the site of injury. Blood vessels, platelets, coagulation factors, natural inhibitors, and the fibrinolytic system play roles (1). Normal hemostasis involves three responses: the vascular response, the formation of a platelet plug, and the formation of a fibrin clot. In addition, naturally occurring plasma inhibitors inhibit the activity of activated clotting factors in an attempt to limit and localize the site of thrombosis, fibrinolysis, and inflammation. The fibrinolytic system also dissolves and removes excess fibrin deposits to preserve vascular patency.

The normal vascular response to trauma is vasoconstriction, which shunts blood away from the damaged area. In small vessels this response can assist the hemostatic process. Traumatic disruption of the endothelial lining of the blood vessel triggers formation of the platelet plug, the primary hemostatic mechanism. The secondary hemostatic mechanism controls the formation of a fibrin clot from the ordered interaction of a series of tissue and blood components or factors. Primary and secondary hemostasis operate simultaneously. During this time, inhibitor systems also operate to prevent propagation of the clot, and fibrinolysis is activated for eventual removal of the clot.

Platelet Physiology and Function

Platelets play a dominant role in the spontaneous prevention of blood loss from damaged blood vessels. Immediately following tissue injury, platelets clump together to stop the flow of blood and maintain the integrity of the vascular system. They play a major part in a series of steps that lead to the formation of a permanent insoluble fibrin clot, which is essential for long-term effectiveness.

Platelets, or thrombocytes, anucleate granular structures approximately 2 to 3 microns in diameter, are fragments of megakaryocytes, which are large stem cells formed in the bone marrow. These giant stem cells disintegrate into platelets, which are released into the blood. The normal platelet concentration is 150,000 to 400,000/mm^3 of blood, and platelet production appears to be directly proportional to demand. This allows for the repair of minor ruptures that occur routinely in everyday

life. Although formed in the bone marrow, approximately 20 to 30% of platelets are in the spleen and the remainder in the circulation. The average life-span of platelets is 10 days, and younger platelets are more active physiologically than older cells (2).

The initial response to vascular injury, transient vasoconstriction, is caused by contraction of the vessel wall smooth muscle and instantaneously diminishes blood flow from the rupture. This external vascular trauma disrupts the endothelium, causing platelets to come into contact with exposed subendothelial connective tissue and collagen fibers, elastin, adenosine diphosphate (ADP), epinephrine, and other substances of the vessel wall. Platelets do not adhere to intact endothelium.

Within seconds after tissue insult, the hemostatic plug is formed in a series of steps.

1. Adhesion. When platelets come into contact with exposed vessel subendothelium, they attach to this site of vascular injury. Factor VIII and von Willebrand factor, proteins that circulate in plasma as a large complex, are required for normal platelet adhesion. A deficiency in this protein complex leads to serious defects in platelet adhesiveness.
2. Release reaction. Adhered platelets release the contents of their granules, including ADP, vasoactive amines, platelet factor IV, calcium, lysosomal enzymes, prostaglandins, thromboxane A$_2$ (a platelet-derived growth factor), and platelet-specific proteins. This release attracts more platelets to the injured area. Thrombin, ADP, and epinephrine promote the accumulation of additional platelets to the growing platelet plug.
3. Aggregation. The initial adhesion of platelets to extruded substances of the injured vessel and the release of ADP stimulate platelet aggregation. The platelets become sticky, adhere, and recruit other passing platelets. Platelet aggregation can occur in response to a variety of other substances, such as thrombin, epinephrine, and collagen.

Arachidonic acid, which is stored in platelet phospholipids, plays an important role in the development of the normal hemostatic plug. Adhesion to collagen causes the cleaving of arachidonic acid from phospholipids by cyclooxygenase. This platelet enzyme converts free arachidonic acid into prostaglandin endoperoxides, which are converted into thromboxane A$_2$. Thromboxane A$_2$, a more potent stimulator of platelet release and aggregation than ADP, may help prolong the vasospasm needed for normal hemostasis because of its arterial vasoconstrictor activity. Another prostaglandin metabolite of arachidonic acid, prostacyclin, is synthesized by cyclo-oxygenase from the walls of arteries and veins. In contrast to thromboxane A_2, prostacyclin is a potent inhibitor of platelet aggregation and causes vasodilation. Its action may aid in localizing the hemostatic plug to the immediate area of tissue damage.

Formation of the platelet plug can rapidly stop bleeding, but reinforcement by fibrin is needed to produce a stable insoluble thrombus. Only through stimulation of the coagulation cascade, involving the extrinsic and intrinsic blood clotting systems, can the loose aggregation of platelets be transformed into a permanent hemostatic plug.

Coagulation

The nomenclature and characteristics of factors involved in the coagulation cascade are summarized in Table 14.1. The Roman numeral designations for clotting factors correspond generally to their order of discovery. Many clotting factors fall into one of two major groups, based on their biochemical properties. Factors XI, XII, prekallikrein, and high-molecular-weight (HMW) kininogen are known as contact activation factors because they initiate the contact phase of coagulation pathway. Factors II, VII, IX, and X are vitamin K–dependent coagulation factors synthesized by the liver. Vitamin K is an essential cofactor for liver carboxylation of glutamic acid residues in their polypeptide structure. The γ-carboxylglutamic acid residues allow the calcium binding essential for normal clotting activity. Vitamin K–deficient individuals continue to produce factors II, VII, IX, and X, but in inactive forms. Factor III (tissue factor) is found in many tissues, factor IV (calcium) comes from diet and bone. Hepatic biosynthesis provides the other factors listed in Table 14.1 (3).

Coagulation results from a series of discrete reactions, each resulting from a reaction complex composed of an enzyme, a substrate, and a reaction accelerator. These components are assembled on specific lipid surfaces and are held together by calcium ions. Most coagulation factors are present as zymogens (inert precursor forms) and must be converted to their active enzymatic forms during coagulation (e.g., factor Va is the activated form of factor V).

Table 14.1.
Characteristics of Coagulation Factors[a]

Factor	Synonym(s)	Plasma Half-Life (hr)	Plasma Concentration (mg/dl)	Coagulation Pathway (E, I, C)[b]	Biochemical Group
Procoagulants					
I	Fibrinogen	100–150	200–400	C	
II	Prothrombin, prethrombin	50–80	10	C	Vitamin K dependent
III	Tissue factor, tissue thromboplastin	—	0	E	
IV	Calcium ion	—	9–10	E, I, C	
V	Proaccelerin, labile factor	24	1	C	
VII	Proconvertin, SPCA, stable factor	6	0.05	E	Vitamin K dependent
VIII	Antihemophilic factor (AHF) Antihemophilic globulin Antihemophilic factor A Platelet cofactor I	12	0.01	I	
vWf	von Willebrand factor	24	1		
IX	Christmas factor Antihemophilic factor B Plasma thromboplastin component Platelet cofactor II	24	0.3	I	Vitamin K dependent
X	Stuart-Prower factor	25–60	1	C	Vitamin K dependent
XI	Plasma thromboplastin antecedent Antihemophilic factor C	40–80	0.5	I	Contact factor
XII	Hageman factor	50–70	3	I	Contact factor
XIII	Fibrin stabilizing factor	150	1–2	C	
Prekallikrein	Fletcher factor	35	5	I	Contact factor
HMW kininogen	Contact activation factor	150	6	I	Contact factor
Inhibitors/fibrinolysis					
Antithrombin III		24–36	18–30	I	Vitamin K dependent
Protein C		16	0.4	I, C	Vitamin K dependent
Protein S		42	2.3	I, C	Vitamin K dependent
Plasminogen		48	20–40	C	

[a] Adapted from Saito H, Normal hemostatic mechanisms, pp 18–49, and Bauer KA, Rosenberg RD, The hypercoagulable state, pp 267–291, in Ratnoff OD, Forbes CD (eds): Disorders of Hemostasis; Philadelphia, WB Saunders, 1991; and Comp PC, Production of plasma coagulation factors; in Williams WJ, Beutler E, Erslev AJ, et al. (eds):Hematology, ed. 4; New York, McGraw-Hill, 1983, p 293.

The goal of coagulation is the generation of a fibrin clot, which is accomplished by the conversion of the soluble plasma protein fibrinogen to the insoluble fibrous protein fibrin. The critical step in this process is the generation of thrombin. Thrombin circulates in the plasma as the inactive prothrombin. Thrombin is cleaved from prothrombin by activated factor X (Xa). Factors V and Va accelerate the cleavage of prothrombin by factor Xa. There are two classic pathways that lead to the generation of factor Xa. The first is designated the extrinsic coagulation pathway because one component (tissue factor) is not a normal constituent of the blood. The second is the intrinsic pathway and all of its components are normal blood constituents.

The extrinsic pathway is initiated by release into the circulation of a lipoprotein (factor III, tissue factor) from damaged tissue. Factor III forms a calcium-dependent complex with factor VII that converts circulating factors IX and X to their active forms (1).

Contact of blood with an abnormal surface initiates the intrinsic pathway. This pathway uses components from the blood plasma in a series of proteolytic reactions, with each reaction forming the enzyme for the next. The first reaction involves formation of factor XIa through the interaction of factor XII, factor XI, prekallikrein, kallikrein, and HMW kininogen. This is the contact phase of the intrinsic coagulation pathway. It is initiated by the contact of factor XII with collagen fibers that are exposed in the subendothelial layer of traumatized blood vessels. Generation of factor XIa initiates the remainder of the intrinsic pathway. Factor XIa then cleaves factor IX, forming factor IXa. Factor IXa then activates factor X. Factor VIII serves to accelerate the activation of factor X (1).

The intrinsic and extrinsic pathways of coagulation differ in how factor X is activated. Once factor X is activated, both follow the common pathway. Factor Xa cleaves prothrombin, forming thrombin. Thrombin in turn cleaves fibrinogen to give fibrin monomer. Factor XIII then catalyzes the polymerization of fibrin monomer to fibrin, a highly cross-linked insoluble network that holds the platelet plug firmly in place.

Several control mechanisms limit the coagulation process to the site of vascular injury and maintain and/or restore blood flow (1, 4). Blood flow itself washes away and/or dilutes active coagulation factors generated locally at the site of injury. The liver and/or reticuloendothelial system remove activated coagulants, fibrin, and plasminogen activators from the circulation. Feedback inhibition mechanisms in both the intrinsic and extrinsic coagulation pathways limit and control their activity.

Naturally occurring plasma inhibitors such as antithrombin III and protein C inhibit the activity of activated clotting factors. Antithrombin III neutralizes thrombin, kallikrein, and factors IXa, Xa, XIa, and XIIa. Activated protein C inhibits factors Va and VIIIa. Protein S is a cofactor in the action of protein C.

Fibrinolysis is initiated with the formation of a fibrin clot, in an effort to remove the clot and restore blood flow. Fibrinolysis is mediated by the enzyme plasmin. Plasmin circulates in the inactive form plasminogen and in this form binds to polymerizing fibrin. Tissue plasminogen activators present in endothelial cells and other tissue activate plasminogen to form plasmin. Plasmin can cleave many proteins, including fibrinogen, fibrin, factor V, and factor VIII. These control mechanisms help maintain fluid circulation during clotting, which prevents the massive thrombosis that would result if the clotting process were left unopposed.

PLATELET DISORDERS
Thrombocytopenia

Thrombocytopenia is defined as a decrease in the number of blood platelets and characterized by a prolonged bleeding time with a normal coagulation time. It is one of the most common causes of abnormal bleeding. A platelet count below 150,000/mm^3 is generally considered thrombocytopenia, although clinical manifestations do not occur until the platelet count is below 50,000/mm^3. When platelet counts are between 10,000 and 20,000/mm^3, spontaneous bleeding can occur, including petechiae and purpura as well as mucosal, deep tissue, and intracranial bleeding.

Thrombocytopenia has many causes, which must be distinguished or isolated so the appropriate therapeutic approach can be used. A decrease in the platelet count may occur from (a) a decrease in production; (b) altered distribution (sequestration); or (c) increased destruction of platelets.

A decrease in platelet production can occur from conditions that affect normal thrombopoiesis and decrease the number of marrow megakaryocytes. Examples include marrow injury (e.g., myelosuppressive drugs, chemicals, radiation, infection); marrow failure (e.g., aplastic anemia, hereditary disorders); or marrow replacement (e.g., tumor, fibrosis) (5). Ineffective thrombopoiesis, caused by vitamin B$_{12}$ or folate deficiency, is characterized by a normal or increased number of megakaryocytes in the bone marrow, but inadequate availability of platelets in the circulation.

Altered distribution of platelets can result from any disorder that causes splenomegaly (e.g., myeloproliferative diseases, hepatic cirrhosis, and lymphomas). Normally, the spleen stores approximately one-third of the circulating platelets and removes nonfunctional platelets. During splenic enlargement, the spleen can contain up to 80% of the circulating thrombocytes, causing thrombocytopenia by sequestering platelets and increasing the rate of destruction.

Increased destruction of platelets can result from increased platelet utilization, severe blood loss, and immunologic mechanisms. Disseminated intravascular coagulation (DIC) is an example of a condition that causes increased platelet consumption. DIC occurs from widespread activation of the clotting mechanisms. Depletion of platelets and other clotting factors as a result of continuous intravascular clotting is caused by a number of disorders (e.g., shock, burns, transfusions, obstetric complications) (6). Immunologic causes of thrombocytopenia include drug-induced immune thrombocytopenias (e.g., quinidine, gold, quinine, heparin), autoantibody production (e.g., systemic lupus erythematosus, idiopathic thrombocytopenic purpura), and alloantibody-produced thrombocytopenias (e.g., placental transfer, transfusions). Other causes of thrombocytopenia of a nonimmunologic nature are thrombotic thrombocytopenic purpura (TTP) and prosthetic heart valves.

Idiopathic Thrombocytopenic Purpura

Idiopathic thrombocytopenic purpura (ITP) is characterized by decreased numbers of circulating platelets (shortened platelet survival), normal or increased numbers of megakaryocytes in the bone marrow, and major clinical signs and symptoms related to bleeding abnormalities secondary to the reduced platelet count. It occurs in the absence of diseases or toxins that decrease platelet levels. The word *idiopathic* refers to a disease of unknown origin, which is actually a misnomer since most research has indicated an autoimmune mechanism in the pathogenesis of ITP (7). Because most cases of ITP involve immune-mediated platelet destruction by antiplatelet autoantibodies, the term autoimmune thrombocytopenic purpura (ATP) is also used to describe this syndrome. Nevertheless, although the mechanism of platelet destruction is known, the etiology of the immunologic involvement is still in question.

EPIDEMIOLOGY

ITP often occurs without other immunologic manifestations. Clinically, ITP is divided into two forms, acute and chronic. The acute form most commonly occurs in children 2 to 7 years of age and affects both sexes equally. It also occurs in the adult population; is often preceded by viral infections or immunizations; and resolves within 6 months. A previous upper respiratory viral infection several weeks before onset is found in 80% of cases. The annual incidence of the clinical syndrome is approximately 4:100,000 children, although many cases are undiagnosed because of its transient and self-limiting nature. The chronic form occurs more often in females, between 20 and 40 years of age, with a female:male ratio of 3:1 (8). Chronic ITP, which undergoes remissions and exacerbations, is a more persistent disease, lasting for more than 6 months. It has

an insidious onset, and although the incidence is unknown, is a common problem.

Human immunodeficiency virus (HIV)-associated thrombocytopenia is one of the most common hematologic complications of the infection and is becoming part of the clinical spectrum of the acquired immunodeficiency syndrome (AIDS) (9). Thrombocytopenia in patients with AIDS or AIDS-related complex (ARC) resembles ITP in clinical presentation (9). Patients have normal megakaryocytes with no evidence of splenomegaly and respond to corticosteroids, high-dose intravenous immunoglobulins, and splenectomy.

PATHOGENESIS

ITP appears to be immunologically mediated. Most researchers believe that an antiplatelet IgG antibody bound to the platelet surface reacts with host platelets, which causes rapid destruction of the reticuloendothelial organs, especially the spleen and liver. There are two main reasons for this line of thought: (a) levels of platelet-associated IgG antibodies increase in more than 90% of patients with ITP, and (b) normal individuals develop thrombocytopenia when injected with plasma from patients with ITP (10, 11).

The pathologic mechanism of thrombocytopenia in AIDS patients remains unclear. In addition to the high levels of IgG antibodies found on platelet surfaces, there appears to be platelet surface deposition of immune complexes and complement (12, 13). Platelet levels may also drop with marrow replacement with tumors or fungi or mycobacteria infiltration (12).

SIGNS AND SYMPTOMS

Clinically, signs and symptoms are related to extensive hemorrhagic abnormalities associated with a low platelet count. Purplish discoloration seen through the epidermis (purpura) and small punctate hemorrhages (petechiae) are the classic signs of ITP. These can occur anywhere on the external surface of the skin, as well as internally, with the gastrointestinal tract being the most common site. Mucosal bleeding of the nasal, buccal, and vaginal areas; easy bruising; conjunctival hemorrhage; epistaxis; and menorrhagia are common. Hematuria, retinal hemorrhage, and joint bleeding are less common, and although rare, central nervous system (CNS) hemorrhage can occur. Intracranial bleeding normally arises early in the acute form of ITP, occurs in less than 1% of cases, and is considered the most serious risk in ITP. It is usually associated with a high mortality.

DIAGNOSIS AND CLINICAL FINDINGS

Diagnosis is usually a process of eliminating other disorders that are related to thrombocytopenia. This is especially true in children with signs and symptoms of acute ITP. Although the number of tests required in children is debated, a bone marrow examination is usually performed to rule out more life-threatening diseases such as leukemia, marrow hypoplasia, consumption coagulopathy, and aplastic anemia (14). Other conditions that must be excluded are DIC, sepsis, thyroid disease, transfusions, tuberculosis, and autoimmune diseases such as systemic lupus erythematosus (SLE), lymphoproliferative diseases, and Hodgkin's disease. Drug-induced thrombocytopenia should also be ruled out, and any drug capable of causing thrombocytopenia should be discontinued. If platelet levels do not return to normal within a few weeks, drug-induced thrombocytopenia can be ruled out. Splenomegaly, adenopathy, fever, and malaise are uncommon and may suggest other disorders.

Laboratory testing is most useful for diagnosing ITP. A complete blood examination shows a decreased number of platelets associated with a normal blood count. The platelets are usually larger in size and appear to be less mature than normal. Bleeding time is prolonged, whereas the whole blood clotting time, prothrombin time, partial thromboplastin time, and erythrocyte sedimentation rate usually remain normal. Chronic gastrointestinal hemorrhage may cause an iron-deficiency anemia that is directly related to the amount of blood lost. Bone marrow examination shows normal or increased numbers of megakaryocytes, although larger and immature. Tests that detect the presence of platelet-bound IgG antibodies are probably the most useful diagnostic tool, since the platelet-associated immunoglobulins are present in over 90% of patients with ITP (11).

Since immunologic thrombocytopenia has become a common finding in patients with AIDS, HIV infection should be considered in the differential diagnosis of thrombocytopenia in patients who fit into high-risk categories (homosexuals, intravenous drug abusers, hemophiliacs) (15).

TREATMENT

The major goals in the treatment of ITP are to decrease the risk of hemorrhage and obtain complete remission of the disease. Traditionally these ends are met either by decreasing the production of platelet-associated antibodies or by inhibiting platelet destruction.

Because more than 80% of patients with acute ITP will recover within 6 months regardless of therapy, much controversy has arisen about whether to treat the disease or let it run its course. Intracranial hemorrhage is usually the primary concern of clinicians who prefer the initial use of steroids. Others choose not to use steroids because of the risk of side effects, the low frequency of CNS bleeding, and the reality that hemorrhagic signs and symptoms will most likely diminish in days and platelet count will increase

in a few weeks without therapy. Regardless, prednisone is usually considered to be the first line of therapy for the acute and chronic forms of ITP. Prednisone increases the life-span of platelets by suppressing phagocytosis of the platelet-antibody complex, and it may inhibit IgG antibody production. The platelet count should improve or return to normal within 1 to 2 weeks in approximately 60 to 70% of patients (16). In acute ITP, children usually receive 1 mg/kg/day and adults 40 to 60 mg/day. If platelet counts do not respond in 2 to 3 weeks or if massive doses of steroids are required to maintain platelet levels, alternate therapy should be considered. Precautionary measures include avoiding drugs that inhibit platelet function, such as aspirin, and limiting the amount of patient activity.

Therapy for chronic ITP is usually initiated with 1 mg/kg/day of prednisone, although 2 mg/kg/day has been used in severe cases. A positive response should be seen in 3 to 7 days, although 2 to 4 weeks may be needed for maximal response of the platelet count (7). Once the platelet count is above 100,000/mm^3, the dose of prednisone should be tapered slowly and reduced to an alternate-day schedule. If a therapeutic response is obtained and the patient can tolerate the drug, prednisone is given on a long-term basis, because the disease is recurrent and spontaneous remission is not common. The response rate to steroid therapy is approximately 40 to 50%, but only 20 to 30% of all patients can be maintained on corticosteroids because of adverse reactions (17).

Effects of corticosteroids in HIV-associated thrombocytopenia are highly variable. One study reports moderate to excellent initial response in 16 of 17 homosexual patients taking 60 to 100 mg/day of prednisone. However, when the dose was decreased, the platelet counts of 13 patients decreased to pretreatment values (18). Many other studies reported the same initial response and failure to maintain platelet counts once prednisone was decreased or withdrawn. The high rate of steroid-induced adverse effects, the low rate of sustained response, and the possibility of opportunistic infections must all be considered before using corticosteroid therapy in patients with HIV-associated thrombocytopenia.

In patients refractory to steroid treatment or in cases of life-threatening hemorrhage, splenectomy is usually considered next. Because the spleen is a major site of platelet-associated antibody production and platelet destruction, its removal is associated with a high success rate. A complete remission of ITP has been reported in up to 80% of patients following splenectomy, with the most favorable results occurring in those who have responded to corticosteroids (11). The risk of sepsis in children under 6 years of age and in immunosuppressed patients often precludes splenectomy as a therapeutic option. Patients who have previously responded favorably to corticosteroids appear to have improved immediate and long-term response to splenectomy (19). The efficacy of splenectomy in patients with HIV-associated thrombocytopenia is currently unknown. The literature reports effects ranging from increased platelet counts of 12 months duration to patients who show no response. Splenectomy, like glucocorticoid therapy, may increase the susceptibility to opportunistic infections in patient with HIV-induced thrombocytopenia.

Intravenous high-dose gammaglobulins offer a new therapeutic approach to ITP management. They are believed to saturate macrophage receptors, which prevents or slows loss of antibody-coated platelets by inhibiting Fc receptor–mediated reticuloendothelial system function (20). A dose of 0.4 g/kg/day for 5 days or 1 g/kg/day for 2 days usually results in a rapid but transient rise in platelet count in both children and adults. The advantages of intravenous gammaglobulin treatment are its ability to raise platelet counts rapidly and its lack of serious side effects. Disadvantages include a long infusion time of 4 to 8 hours to minimize side effects and high cost (more than $1000/daily dose for a 20-kg child) (14). Nevertheless, high-dose intravenous gammaglobulin therapy may be of value when a temporary but rapid rise in platelets is necessary (e.g., for surgery or the prevention of internal hemorrhage).

The use of intravenous immune globulin in the treatment of HIV-associated thrombocytopenia shows a high initial response rate, ranging from 70 to 100% (21, 22). Because it does not increase susceptibility to opportunistic infections, intravenous gammaglobulin therapy may be the treatment of choice for HIV-associated thrombocytopenia (9).

Immunosuppressive therapy is usually reserved for those cases that are refractory to glucocorticoids and splenectomy. Azathioprine, cyclophosphamide, and the vinca alkaloids (vincristine and vinblastine) are the most commonly used cytotoxic agents.

Azathioprine, which is cytotoxic for macrophages, is given in a dose of 1 to 3 mg/kg/day (or between 100 and 200 mg/day). It is usually given in conjunction with steroids, and the dose is reduced if the patient becomes leukopenic (16). Approximately one-half of patients show an adequate platelet response over a number of months. Continued therapy is usually needed to maintain platelet levels, since complete remission is rare (8). Side effects are usually less serious than those with cyclophosphamide, with bone marrow suppression being the most important. Azathioprine is usually considered the safest agent for long-term therapy.

Cyclophosphamide appears to be more effective than azathioprine, with several studies showing complete remission of refractory cases in 30 to 40% of patients (8). It is given in an oral dose of 2 to 3 mg/kg/m^2 per day or 300 to 600 mg/m^2 intravenously every 3 weeks (8). Improvement is usually seen in 2 to 6 weeks, with a maximum response in platelet count seen in 8 weeks. Treatment is usually continued for 4 to 6 weeks after an adequate platelet count is achieved. Serious side effects include bone marrow suppression, hemorrhagic cystitis, and bladder fibrosis.

Vinca alkaloids have been reported to be beneficial in more than 50% of patients refractory to steroids and splenectomy. Maintenance therapy is normally needed since complete remission is unusual (23). Vincristine (0.25 mg/kg with a maximum dose of 2 mg) and vinblastine (0.125 mg/kg with a maximum dose of 10 mg) are given intravenously every 7 to 10 days (11). Response occurs more rapidly than the azathioprine or cyclophosphamide, but relapses usually occur in 3 to 4 weeks. These agents are believed to decrease the rate of destruction of platelets by inhibiting phagocytosis and decreasing antibody levels. Vincristine and vinblastine have been loaded onto platelets in an attempt to deliver them selectively to macrophages responsible for platelet destruction, but results have been variable to date. Side effects of vincristine include transient malaise, fever after injection, temporary jaw pain, alopecia, and a variety of neuropathies. Leukopenia, abdominal pain, and headache are associated with vinblastine.

Although androgens, such a testosterone enanthate, have been used for years to decrease corticosteroid requirements and adverse effects, their lack of effectiveness and masculinization properties restrict their usefulness. Danazol, a nonvirilizing androgen, reportedly has raised platelet counts. It is thought to be caused by decreased phagocytosis of platelets by decreasing the number of phagocytic cell IgG Fc-receptors (24). Doses are usually between 400 and 800 mg/day, although low doses (50 mg) have been effective (25, 26). Clinical response is normally seen within 8 weeks, although low-dose therapy may require 6 months. Response rates of 20% have been reported in patient with refractory ITP (19). The frequency of side effects is low, but danazol is contraindicated during pregnancy. Colchicine can inhibit microtubule function and phagocytosis, and has shown some initial benefit in the treatment of ITP, although its long-term effect is unknown. Plasma transfusion and plasma exchange have been used in the treatment of ITP, and may have some merit, especially in life-threatening emergencies, but for chronic ITP they are of little value.

Anti-Rh(D) immunoglobulin has been used with moderate success in the treatment of autoimmune thrombocytopenia purpura and in a few cases of refractory HIV-associated thrombocytopenia. The mechanism of action appears to be inhibition of reticuloendothelial system function, however, it does not appear to be effective in Rhesus-negative patients (16). Use of anti-Rh (D) immunoglobulin for HIV-associated autoimmune thrombocytopenia significantly increased platelet counts in two studies. However, as with non-HIV-related autoimmune thrombocytopenia, this effect seems to be of short duration and this therapy must be considered experimental (27–29). Another experimental approach is the use of zidovudine for the treatment of HIV-associated thrombocytopenia in patients without AIDS (13). This small study showed some potential for zidovudine in increasing platelet counts, however, larger studies must be performed.

PROGNOSIS

The prognosis for the acute form of ITP is excellent, with more than 80% of patients showing spontaneous remission within 6 months of diagnosis. The major concern for the clinician is whether or not to treat a disease that is generally benign and self-limiting. The chief concern is CNS bleeding, regardless of its low frequency of occurrence. Generally, a platelet count under 20,000/mm^3 associated with active bleeding is reason to institute therapy to decrease the likelihood of intracranial hemorrhage (10). In this case, prednisone or intravenous immunoglobulins are the therapies of choice. In patients who are resistant and show persistent thrombocytopenia of the chronic form of ITP, a splenectomy is then considered.

Although complete remission of the chronic form of ITP is rare, the long-term prognosis is usually favorable. Corticosteroids are considered first-line therapy, followed by splenectomy for those who are resistant. The objective of therapy in chronic ITP is to maintain the patient hemostatically safe, not necessarily to obtain a complete remission. Prednisone and/or splenectomy will achieve this in most patients. Immunosuppressant therapy is usually reserved for patients who relapse or show no benefit from splenectomy. Newer, unconventional and experimental forms of therapy may be justified in patients who fail to respond to more traditional management. High-dose gammaglobulin and plasma exchange appear to be useful in emergency situations where a rapid rise in platelet count is needed.

Thrombotic Thrombocytopenic Purpura (Moschcowitz' Disease)

Thrombotic thrombocytopenic purpura (TTP) is an uncommon but devastating disorder that appears to be a clinical syndrome of widespread multisystem involvement instead of a single disease entity. The original triad of clinical characteristics consisting of thrombocytopenic purpura, microangiopathic hemolytic anemia, and neurologic abnormalities has been expanded to a pentad with the addition of fever and renal dysfunction. Extensive widespread occlusive hyaline microthrombi formation in the capillaries, venules, and arterioles of nearly all organs is the hallmark of the disease and is responsible for the high mortality associated with the disorder.

ETIOLOGY

Despite many theories on the cause of TTP, the primary etiology remains unknown. Immunologic abnormalities have been suspected because of the hemolytic anemia and thrombocytopenic purpura associated with the disease and because TTP has occurred in other diseases of an immune nature, such as systemic lupus erythematosus (SLE), scleroderma, Sjögren's syndrome, and rheumatoid arthritis. Bacteria, viruses, toxins, and drugs have also been suggested as causative factors.

EPIDEMIOLOGY

Although TTP has been reported in all age groups, ranging from infants to the very old, it most commonly occurs between the ages of 30 and 40. It is found in both genders, with most studies showing females having a slightly higher occurrence. The overall incidence in the population is not known, but it is believed to be small.

PATHOGENESIS

The pathogenesis of the disorder is unknown. Many believe that the diffuse microvascular thrombi are associated with abnormal platelet aggregation, adhesion, and release on the microarterial endothelial surfaces. The resultant occlusive hyaline microthrombi in arterioles and capillaries are composed of fibrin and platelets and occur most commonly in the brain, heart, spleen, adrenals, kidney, and pancreas (30). Evidence suggests a number of mechanisms in the pathogenesis of TTP. Fibrinolytic activity appears to be absent in the area of microvascular thrombi but is normal in the circulating blood. This suggests that certain defects at the site of occurrence are part of the pathogenesis (30). Also, a deficiency of prostacyclin-stimulating factor in the plasma of patients with TTP has been shown (30). This factor stimulates prostacyclin, which causes vasodilation and is a natural inhibitor of platelet aggregation and adhesion. The lack of this factor would favor excessive platelet thrombi formation.

Because of the reported success rates of plasma exchange and blood transfusion, much research is now centered on the possibility that serum factors hold the key to the pathogenesis of the disorder. The numerous defects in patients with TTP suggest that more than one etiologic factor plays a role in its pathogenesis.

SIGNS AND SYMPTOMS

Presenting signs and symptoms of TTP are variable and nonspecific, including complaints of malaise, weakness, fatigue, abdominal pain, nausea and vomiting, arthralgia, fever, and hemorrhages. Neurologic symptoms such as headache, syncope, vertigo, ataxia, aphasia, mental status changes, and seizures are the most frequent complaints. Signs of hemorrhage, including petechiae and purpura, are the next most common.

DIAGNOSIS AND CLINICAL FINDINGS

TTP should be suspected in patients with the symptoms mentioned above. The diagnosis can usually be confirmed by the subendothelial and intraluminal occlusive accumulation in arterioles and capillaries of hyaline material consisting of fragmented platelets and fibrin deposits (31). Hematologic findings show severe hemolytic anemia associated with a negative Coomb's test in the majority of patients. Bilirubin and lactate dehydrogenase levels are elevated. Peripheral blood smears reveal odd-shaped fragmented and frequently nucleated red blood cells. Severe thrombocytopenia is invariably present, with bone marrow and platelet studies showing megakaryocyte hyperplasia and shortened platelet survival. Platelet counts are normally below 50,000/mm^3. Renal involvement is present in most patients, with laboratory tests showing proteinuria, microscopic hematuria, and elevated blood urea nitrogen and serum creatinine levels. Hematologic, neurologic, renal, cardiovascular, gastrointestinal, and pulmonary abnormalities appear to be secondary to microthrombi occlusion in blood vessels. In more than 90% of cases where the disease terminates in death, neurological symptoms are present (32).

TREATMENT

Because of the multisystem involvement of TTP, many forms of therapy have been tried. Success is unpredictable, with each approach showing some benefit in certain individuals but little benefit in most. Treatments have included corticosteroids, splenectomy, antiplatelet agents, heparin, dextran, immunosuppressive agents, and combinations of these. Because of the low success rate and the high mortality associated with these regimens, therapy was usually empiric. In the past, TTP was fatal in most cases, but in the last 10 years researchers have had remarkable success in treating TTP with plasma infusions, exchange transfusions, and plasmapheresis.

The efficacy of steroids, antiplatelet agents, splenectomy, and combinations of these has been hard to assess. Generally these approaches have been unsatisfactory, showing only occasional remissions. Although steroids have been reported to cause remission in a few individuals with TTP, the overall response rate when used alone is approximately 11% (33). Success rates appear to be a little higher when used in conjunction with other therapeutic regiments, but not enough to alter the poor prognosis. Because the occlusive microthrombi in TTP are composed of fibrin and platelets, antiplatelet agents such as aspirin, dipyridamole, sulfinpyrazone, and dextran are used. In combination with exchange plasmapheresis, the antiplatelet agents have shown great promise; when used alone their efficacy appears to be minimal.

Plasma exchange transfusions with fresh frozen plasma have produced a response in 76% of patients with TTP (34). One study showed complete remission in 10 of 13 (77%) patients, using a combination of exchange plasmapheresis and antiplatelet agents (35). Other investigators show similar results. The therapeutic rationale for plasma exchange is the removal of toxic substances and immune complexes from the plasma of TTP patients (34). Infusions of fresh frozen plasma have also shown great promise in the treatment of TTP. The basis for this therapy is either the replacement of a plasma factor that is responsible for platelet aggregation inhibition or the replacement of factors responsible for the stimulation of prostacyclin. The overall response rate for plasma infusions is in the 60% range (34). Because many patients have experienced complete remissions and others were sustained with intermittent plasma infusions, plasma infusions, plasmapheresis, or both are now the treatment of choice for TTP (12). Infusions of prostacyclin have received much attention, since deficiencies of this platelet aggregation inhibitor have been demonstrated in patients with TTP. To date, the effectiveness of this modality has been questionable, and results have been disappointing.

Guidelines for the management of TTP have been variable and scarce. Machin has suggested the following sequence of therapy for the treatment of TTP (36). Initially, infusions of fresh frozen plasma should be instituted after the diagnosis is confirmed and a baseline plasma sample has been collected. The amount infused and the duration of the infusion vary widely among individual patients. Most patients will respond within 48 to 72 hours after 6 to 8 units of fresh frozen plasma daily (36). Volume overload must be considered during plasma infusion. Patients who relapse require further infusion and/or maintenance infusion. Plasma exchange and replacement with fresh frozen plasma are usually the next step for those patients who are unresponsive to 2 days of plasma infusion alone (36). Maintenance therapy with antiplatelet agents (300 mg of aspirin twice weekly and 400 to 600 mg of dipyridamole daily) is started after remission and continued for several months because of the small number of relapses that occur after an initial remission (20).

PROGNOSIS

Prior to 1965, TTP was considered an infrequent, complicated, progressive, and nearly always fatal disease. The mortality rate for untreated cases was 80% within 3 months, and the prognosis for treated individuals was not much better. Plasma therapy has greatly improved survival rates, with the greatest improvement (60 to 75%) noted with exchange transfusion or plasmapheresis, so most treatment and research is centered here (32). Until the etiology of TTP is known, it will be hard to establish exact therapeutic guidelines, because of the sporadic nature of the disease and variable individual response rates.

Drug-Induced Platelet Disorders

In the last decade an increasingly large number of drugs has been found to impair platelet function, with over 70 drugs being implicated in causing thrombocytopenic purpura alone (12). Although many of these agents have been used clinically for their antithrombotic effect, all have other therapeutic indications. The clinician must recognize drugs that affect platelets adversely, to permit close monitoring of platelet counts in patients with hemorrhagic disorders who are taking these drugs or avoiding their use entirely. Familiarity with these agents also aids assessment of drugs as the causative factor in patients with platelet abnormalities.

Although many drugs adversely affect platelet activity, the literature must be evaluated carefully before an "antiplatelet" label is placed on a therapeutic agent that only rarely produces drug-induced platelet dysfunction. Other therapeutic agents or diseases must be eliminated as causative factors, and the clinical importance of the event, as well as the risk/benefit potential, must be established.

The effect of aspirin (acetylsalicylic acid) on platelets is due to its ability to inhibit platelet synthesis of cyclic endoperoxides and thromboxane A_2 by irreversibly acetylating platelet cyclo-oxygenase, which causes a corresponding decrease in prostacyclin production. Platelets can no longer synthesize cyclo-oxygenase, but endothelial cells can produce new cyclo-oxygenase, and thus prostacyclin synthesis resumes after the drug is metabolized. The peak effect of a single dose of aspirin occurs in 2 to 4 hours, but because its effects on platelets are irreversible, its pharmacologic activity may last up to 10 days, or the life of the platelet.

Other nonsteroidal antiinflammatory agents, such as phenylbutazone, indomethacin, ibuprofen, and fenoprofen, also prevent thromboxane A_2 generation by inhibiting platelet cyclo-oxygenase. However this enzyme inhibition is reversible, and the bleeding time is only slightly prolonged.

Heparin-associated thrombocytopenia should be suspected in patients who have a decreased platelet count while on heparin therapy. This drug-induced thrombocytopenia appears to be caused by the production of heparin-generated antibodies directed at unknown platelet antigens (37). The sequence of events results in platelet aggregation and platelet thrombus formation followed by severe thrombocytopenia. Heparin-associated thrombocytopenia normally occurs within 1 week of administration and is not dose dependent.

Dipyridamole is used therapeutically for its antithrombotic activity, usually in combination with aspirin. The mode of action is believed to be the prevention of cyclic AMP breakdown by inhibition of phosphodiesterase activity. The increase in platelet cyclic AMP levels inhibits platelet aggregation and release. Since prostacyclin inhibits platelet aggregation by raising intracellular levels of cyclic AMP, many researchers believe that the antiplatelet effect of dipyridamole involves potentiation of the antiaggregatory activity of prostacyclin. Unlike aspirin, dipyridamole does not prolong bleeding time or platelet survival.

Penicillin and related compounds also prolong bleeding time and have clinically important effects on platelet function. High doses of carbenicillin decrease the affinity of membrane receptors for platelet agonists such as ADP and epinephrine, with a resultant decrease in platelet aggregation. Penicillin G, ampicillin, ticarcillin, and methicillin have all been implicated as having similar effects, although their antiplatelet activity is not as well documented.

Sulfinpyrazone, like aspirin and dipyridamole, is used clinically for its antithrombotic activity. This drug, which is used primarily as a uricosuric agent, inhibits platelet function in a number of ways. The parent drug and its metabolites inhibit platelet cyclo-oxygenase, platelet adhesion to collagen and to subendothelial structures, and the synthesis of prostaglandins. Unlike aspirin, sulfinpyrazone prolongs platelet survival, has no effect on bleeding time, and reversibly inhibits cyclo-oxygenase.

Dextran, a partially hydrolyzed polymer of glucose, is used as a plasma volume expander in certain types of shock, impaired renal function, and other conditions where improved circulation is critical. It also has therapeutic use in the prophylaxis of venous thrombosis and pulmonary thromboembolism. The mechanism of the antiplatelet activity of dextran is uncertain, but may involve platelet aggregation inhibition and decreased platelet agonist activity. Because dextran prolongs bleeding time, impairs the polymerization of fibrin, decreases the viscosity of blood, and alters platelet function, it should be used with caution in the presence of a decreased platelet count.

Alcohol is another agent that impairs platelet function or primary hemostasis. Alcoholism is associated with many factors that cause platelet dysfunction. Large quantities of ethanol can decrease thromboxane A_2 production by inhibiting prostaglandin endoperoxide synthesis, causing a decrease in platelet aggregation and release. Alcoholism can also decrease ADP storage pools and platelet agonist (ADP, epinephrine) activity. The effect on platelets can occur in the absence of liver disease and is reversible.

Clofibrate, an antilipemic agent, has been used therapeutically for its antithrombotic action, although its effectiveness to date is questionable. Its antiplatelet activity is caused by inhibition of collagen and ADP-induced platelet aggregation and reduced platelet adhesiveness. Clofibrate has also been shown to prolong platelet survival.

Drug-induced immune thrombocytopenia is a relatively uncommon platelet disorder that is caused by a very small number of drugs. Although the mechanism remains unclear, most research identifies IgG as the causative immunoglobulin. A popular hypothesis suggests formation of a immunoglobulin-drug immune complex that attaches to and destroys the platelet. Previous exposure to the drug, rapid clinical onset, severe thrombocytopenia on reexposure, and reversal of thrombocytopenia upon discontinuation of the drug are characteristic of drug-induced immune thrombocytopenia (38). Heparin, gold, methyldopa, quinidine, quinine, and valproic acid are a few of the more commonly used drugs that have been implicated in drug-induced immune platelet destruction.

Cytotoxic agents can cause thrombocytopenia because of their myelosuppressive action on the hematopoietic system, although some of these agents affect platelets more than others. As opposed to drug-induced thrombocytopenia, which occurs after platelets have reached the circulation, antineoplastic agents cause a dose-dependent bone marrow reduction in platelets before they are released. The clinician must know the dose of each agent that affects thrombocytes so that effective, safe, tolerable dosage regimens can be selected.

Because thrombocytopenia is caused by a wide variety of drugs, much attention has been placed on the mechanisms that cause this disorder. These mechanisms are not completely understood in many instances because of the difficulty in excluding other causes of decreased platelet counts. Table 14.2 lists some commonly used drugs that cause thrombocytopenia, although the mechanisms are not known in many cases.

COAGULATION DISORDERS
Hemophilia and von Willebrand's Disease

Hemophilia and von Willebrand's disease (vWd) are rare, inherited, coagulation factor–deficiency disorders that result in lifelong impaired hemostasis and hemorrhagic tendency (39, 40). Although heterogeneous, they usually involve a defect in a single coagulation protein. Hemophilia A (classic hemophilia) and hemophilia B (Christmas disease) are caused by a functional deficiency in coagulation factors VIII and IX, respectively. Both are inherited as X-linked, recessive disorders and are seen almost exclusively in males. Von Willebrand's disease is the result of a quantitative or qualitative abnormality in von Willebrand factor (vWf), a protein necessary for normal platelet function and coagulation. A deficiency in factor VIII is often secondarily present in vWd. Classic vWd is inherited as an autosomal dominant trait, with males and females both affected.

Factor VIII and vWf are large and distinct proteins that exist in the plasma as a complex linked by noncovalent bonds (Table 14.3). The liver appears to be a major site of factor VIII synthesis (3). Factor VIII is unstable in the absence of vWf. The plasma half-life of factor VIII is approximately 12 hours and it is consumed during the clotting process (1, 41). Factor VIII functions as a procoag-

Table 14.2.
Drugs That Cause Thrombocytopenia

Amrinone (8)[a]	Ethanol (7)[a]
Antiinflammatory agents (1, 2, 3)[a]	Estrogens (7)[a]
Aspirin	Furosemide (1, 5)[a]
Fenoprofen	Gold salts (2)[a]
Indomethacin	Heparin (2)[a]
Phenylbutazone	Histamine H_2 antagonists (8)[a]
Piroxicam	Cimetidine
Tolmetin	Ranitidine
β-Blockers (3, 4, 8)[a]	Methyldopa (2)[a]
Alprenolol	Penicillins (3, 5, 8)[a]
Oxprenolol	Ampicillin
Propranolol	Carbenicillin
Carbamazepine (2, 8)[a]	Methicillin
Clofibrate (3)[a]	Penicillin G
Cytotoxic agents (7)[a]	Ticarcillin
Busulfan	Penicillamine (2, 8)[a]
Cytarabine	Phenytoin (2)[a]
Daunorubicin	Quinidine (2)[a]
Flucytosine	Quinine (2)[a]
Fluorouracil	Rifampin (8)[a]
Mechlorethamine	Sulfinpyrazone (1, 4)[a]
Mercaptopurine	Thiazide diuretics (8)[a]
Methotrexate	Chlorothiazide
Mithramycin	Hydrochlorothiazide
Mitomycin	Tocainide (8)[a]
Dextran (4, 8)[a]	
Digitoxin (2)[a]	Trimethoprim (8)[a]
Dipyridamole (3, 5, 6)[a]	Valproic acid (2)[a]

[a] Numbers in parentheses indicate confirmed and suspected mechanisms of thrombocytopenia: 1, Inhibits cyclo-oxygenase; 2, Drug-induced immune; 3, Inhibits aggregation; 4, Inhibits adhesion; 5, Inhibits release reaction; 6, Inhibits phosphodiesterase; 7, Myelosuppression; 8, Mechanism not documented.

ulant in the intrinsic pathway of blood coagulation, enhancing the rate of factor X activation. The coagulant activity of factor VIII (VIII:C) is measured by an assay using pooled plasma as the reference standard. A value of 1.0 international unit (IU)/ml (100% of normal) is assigned to the reference standard. Normal factor VIII coagulant activity ranges from 0.5 to 2.0 IU/ml (42). The severity of hemophilia A is related to the VIII:C level. A person with a VIII:C of 3% has 0.03 IU of factor VIII per ml of plasma. Table 14.4 lists the classifications of hemophilia according to severity, factor level, and hemorrhagic tendency.

Von Willebrand's factor (vWf) is an adhesive glycoprotein composed of protein subunits linked by disulfide bonds. It exists as a series of multimers ranging from 500,000 to 20 million in molecular weight. The larger multimers appear to have the greater hemostatic capacity. Normal plasma levels of vWf range from 5 to 10 μg/ml (40). Synthesis of vWf occurs in megakaryocytes and endothelial cells. It forms a complex with and serves as a carrier protein for factor VIII in the normal blood. Von Willebrand factor stabilizes factor VIII, protects it from degradation, and localizes it to bleeding sites, where

Table 14.3.
Nomenclature of Factor VIII and von Willebrand Factor[a]

Nomenclature	Abbreviation	Description
Factor VIII	VIII	Factor VIII protein that exists in plasma as a complex with von Willebrand factor; measured in standard coagulation assays; decreased or absent in hemophilia A
Factor VIII antigen	VIII:Ag	Antigenic component(s) of factor VIII measured by immunoassay
Factor VIII coagulant activity	VIII:C	Clot-promoting activity of factor VIII; term sometimes used interchangeably with factor VIII; decreased or absent in hemophilia A, may be decreased in von Willebrand's disease
von Willebrand factor	vWf	Large multimeric glycoprotein that exists in plasma as a complex with factor VIII; appears to stabilize factor VIII and localize it to sites where it can be activated and thereby promote coagulation; necessary for a normal bleeding time
von Willebrand factor antigen	vWf:Ag	Antigenic component(s) of vWf measured by immunoassay; normal in hemophilia A but may be normal, decreased, or absent in vWd; formerly called factor VIII-related antigen (VIIIR:Ag)
Ristocetin cofactor activity		Property of normal plasma that supports ristocetin-induced platelet aggregation; normal in hemophilia; reduced or absent in most cases of vWd

[a] Adapted from Gralnick HR, von Willebrand's disease. In Ratnoff OD, Forbes CD (eds): Disorders of Hemostasis. Philadelphia, WB Saunders, 1991, pp 203–244.

Table 14.4.
Classification of Hemophilia A and B according to Severity, Factor Level, and Hemorrhagic Tendency[a]

Severity	Factor VIII/IX Level	Hemorrhagic Tendency
Severe	<1% of normal (<0.01 IU/ml)	Spontaneous bleeding in early infancy; frequent spontaneous hemarthroses and deep tissue bleeding requiring treatment
Moderate	1–5% of normal (0.01–0.05 IU/ml)	Bleeding following mild to moderate trauma; rare spontaneous bleeding; occasional spontaneous hemarthrosis
Mild	6–60% of normal (0.06–0.60 IU/ml)	Bleeding following moderate to severe trauma or surgery; rare spontaneous bleeding

[a] Adapted from Roberts HR, Jones MR, Hemophilia and related conditions—congenital deficiencies of prothrombin (factor II), factor V, and factors VII to XII. In Williams WJ, Beutler E, Erslev AJ, et al. (eds): Hematology, ed. 4. New York, McGraw-Hill, 1990, pp 1290–1294.

needed activation and blood coagulation can proceed. The factor VIII/vWf complex mediates the adhesion of platelets to exposed vascular subendothelial surface when blood vessels are traumatized. Factor VIII localized to the site then participates in secondary hemostasis. Von Willebrand's disease (vWd) manifests abnormal platelet function and impaired blood coagulation as a result of quantitative and qualitative abnormalities in vWf.

Factor IX is one of four clotting factors dependent on vitamin K for functional activity. It is synthesized in the liver and once activated acts enzymatically in the intrinsic pathway of coagulation to convert factor X to its active form. Factor VIII, calcium, and platelet phospholipid serve as cofactors in the activation of factor X by factor

IX. Unlike factor VIII, factor IX is not consumed during the clotting process. The plasma half-life of factor IX is about 24 hours (1, 41). Hemophilia B, also known as Christmas disease, is caused by a congenital deficiency in factor IX activity. This disorder appears to be more heterogenous than hemophilia A. Families studied manifest both structural defects and variable decreases in levels of the protein (43–45). As in hemophilia A, the severity and hemorrhagic tendency of hemophilia B is related to factor levels (Table 14.4). The two diseases are indistinguishable based on clinical presentation alone.

PATHOGENESIS AND CLASSIFICATION OF DISEASE

The coagulation abnormality in hemophilia A is due to reduced levels of factor VIII coagulant activity (VIII:C) or a molecular defect in the procoagulant portion of the factor VIII molecule. The level of factor VIII antigen (VIII:Ag) is usually normal or increased, despite low levels of VIII:C (46, 46). Measurement of VIII:Ag levels will help to determine whether the patient has a reduced level of factor VIII (CRM−, cross-reacting-material–negative) or has produced an altered molecule (CRM+) (46).

The defect in hemophilia B is a functional deficiency in factor IX. In most cases there is a proportional reduction in both factor IX antigen (IX:Ag) and factor IX coagulant activity (IX:C), with a mean ratio of IX:Ag to IX:C that is similar to normal. This type of defect is quantitative and designated CRM−. In rare cases the defect is qualitative (CRM+) due to synthesis of an abnormal factor IX. In this case the levels of IX:Ag are disproportionately higher than those of IX:C and are accompanied by higher than normal ratio of IX:Ag to IX:C (45).

Hemophilia A and B are transmitted as X-linked recessive disorders, and thus males are almost exclusively affected. All sons of a hemophiliac father and normal mother are normal, and all daughters are obligate carriers of the disorder. A carrier mother and a normal father will have sons and daughters with a 50% chance of having the disorder and being carriers, respectively. Hemophilia is very rare but can occur in females (e.g., the daughter of an affected male and a female carrier or in cases of spontaneous mutation to the disorder (39, 45). More than 60% of hemophiliacs have a positive family history for the disorder; other cases may involve mutation of the maternal or fetal gene (45).

Carriers of hemophilia A may be detected by evaluation of the relative levels of VIII:Ag and VIII:C in conjunction with family history. Females who are obligatory carriers have VIII:Ag levels that are normal or slightly higher than normal, with a relative decrease in VIII:C. Normal females have VIII:C that is proportional to the level of VIII:Ag (45). Assay of IX:C is sometimes helpful in the detection of hemophilia B carriers, since the mean level in carriers is about 50% of normal (39, 44). Purification of the factor VIII and IX molecules and identification of their gene structures and locations on the X chromosome have resulted in the recent availability of DNA probes capable of identifying carriers (1, 45). The ability to detect the carrier state allows appropriate genetic counseling of carrier females.

Von Willebrand's disease is a heterogeneous disorder with both autosomal dominant and autosomal recessive patterns of inheritance (40). Autosomal dominant inheritance is more common. In contrast to hemophilia, which occurs in males and skips generations, vWd occurs in both sexes and in each generation. Approximately 33% of individuals who carry the gene have no symptoms, and most affected individuals are only moderately symptomatic. The chance of an affected individual transmitting the gene to his or her child is 50% for any pregnancy. However, due to variable penetrance, only about 33% of offspring are clinically affected.

The defect in vWd is a quantitative or qualitative abnormality of vWf. Patients with vWd characteristically exhibit a normal platelet count and prolonged bleeding time. Von Willebrand's disease results in failure of platelets to adhere properly to subendothelial surfaces. Most patients have mild to moderate forms of the disease, with bleeding mainly superficial, involving the skin and mucous membranes. There can be spontaneous cessation of such bleeding. Types I, II and III vWd are the three major variants of vWd, based on inheritance, laboratory, and clinical findings (40, 44).

Overall, the most common form of vWd is autosomal dominant type I disease. Type I vWd accounts for 70% of patients and varies significantly in severity of bleeding manifestations and laboratory abnormalities. Three subtypes of type I vWd have been identified. Type IA vWd, the most common form, has vWf multimers normal in quality and distribution but decreased in number, as evidenced by a decreased concentration of vWf:Ag. Factor VIII:C, vWf:Ag, and ristocetin cofactor activity are all decreased to the same relative extent in type IA disease. Type IB is similar to type IA except there is a relative decrease in the level of large vWf multimers. In type IC disease, all the plasma vWf multimers are present, but a structural abnormality exists (40).

Type II vWd, usually transmitted by autosomal dominant inheritance, is characterized by a decrease in the largest or both the largest and the intermediate molecular weight multimers of vWf. There are several subtypes of type II vWd (40). In type IIA vWd the large and intermediate multimers of vWf are absent from the plasma and platelets, while plasma VIII:C and vWf:Ag are usually normal. In addition, ristocetin-induced platelet aggregation of the patient's platelet-rich plasma and ristocetin cofactor activity are both markedly reduced or absent. Type IIB vWd differs from type IIA in that ristocetin-induced platelet aggregation of the patient's platelet-rich plasma is enhanced in the presence of decreased ristocetin cofactor activity. In this case the large multimers of vWf are absent from the plasma, while the platelet vWf multimers and plasma VIII:C are normal. Type IIB vWd is unique in that some patients also exhibit transient or persistent thrombocytopenia. Type IIC vWd is rare and is inherited as an autosomal recessive trait. The larger vWf multimers are missing from both the plasma and platelets, but the small multimers are increased. Five additional subtypes (D-H) of type II vWd have also been characterized.

Type III vWd, clinically and biologically the most severe form of the disease, is inherited as an autosomal recessive trait. VIII:C is markedly reduced, and vWf is undetectable in platelets and plasma. Patients may experience severe clinical bleeding such as hemarthrosis and intramuscular hemorrhage. Therapy for these patients may be complicated by the development of anti-vWf antibodies after infusion of plasma products (40).

Platelet- or pseudo-type vWd is a platelet defect that mimics type IIB vWd (40). There is also an acquired form of vWd that may occur in individuals who have recent onset bleeding with no bleeding history or family history of vWd. Such individuals will have a prolonged bleeding time, decreased ristocetin cofactor activity, and variable levels of VIII:C and vWf:Ag (40). Usually the development of acquired vWd is related to autoimmune, lymphoproliferative, or myeloproliferative disorders. Such patients sometimes have a circulating inhibitor (anti-VIII:vWf antibody) that decreases ristocetin cofactor activity, presumably by binding and accelerating removal of the VIII:vWf complex from the plasma.

Identification of the specific variants and subtypes of vWd can be useful in making therapeutic decisions (40, 44). Patients with type I vWd usually have an excellent response to desmopressin (DDAVP). DDAVP is not useful in type III vWd because of the absence of vWf in the patient's endothelial cells. Patients with type IIA vWd respond variably to DDAVP. DDAVP is usually contraindicated in type IIB and platelet/pseudo vWd since an abnormally high vWf-platelet reactivity may cause thrombocytopenia.

OCCURRENCE

Hemophilia A has been reported in all ethnic groups and in many animal species (44, 45). In the United States, this disorder appears less common among Americans of African descent. The incidence of the hemophilias (both A and B) is estimated at 20:100,000 males; 10:100,000 of the whole population. Factor IX deficiency accounts for 10 to 15% of cases, with factor VIII deficiency accounting for the remainder. Among Americans, the Amish of Ohio and Pennsylvania have a relatively higher incidence of hemophilia B, perhaps for geographic or social reasons. The Japanese appear to have a significantly lower incidence of hemophilia B.

The true incidence of von Willebrand's disease is difficult to establish because of the great variability in clinical and laboratory manifestations of the disorder. Unlike hemophilia, it is most commonly diagnosed in adult life, and mild cases may never be diagnosed. Thus, although its exact incidence is unknown, it may be the most common inherited disease, possibly involving as much as 10% of the population (47). One center reported that among their diagnosed cases, vWd occurs at a frequency about one-half that of hemophilia A (i.e., about 3 to 4 cases per 100,000 population) (44). Type I vWd is the most commonly diagnosed form of the disorder, accounting for 70% of patients (40). Type II vWd is found in 10 to 12%, and type III vWd in 20 to 25% of patients.

SIGNS AND SYMPTOMS

The clinical presentations of hemophilia A and B are identical and vary according to the magnitude of the coagulation factor deficiency. About 60 to 70% of patients with hemophilia A and 50% of those with hemophilia B have the severe form of the disease, with levels of factor VIII or IX less than 1% of normal (43, 44). Such patients are subject to frequent episodes of spontaneous bleeding.

Except for skin bruises, hemarthrosis is the most frequent manifestation of hemophilia (48). The knees are most commonly affected, followed by the elbows, ankles, and wrists (45). Acute hemarthrosis is accompanied by pain, swelling, and limitation of movement. Patients can sometimes sense the bleeding and report a feeling of warmth or prickling before objective signs of hemarthrosis are present. Recurrent episodes of hemarthrosis result in chronic hemophilic arthritis and associated disability.

Chronic hemophilic arthritis is characterized by pain, loss of movement, atrophy of associated muscles, synovitis, and cartilage destruction, which may result in a need for mobility aids or confinement to a wheel chair (45).

Intramuscular bleeding and hematomas are also common causes of morbidity in patients with hemophilia. Bleeding into muscle can occur spontaneously and has been reported to occur in association with emotional stress (45). Skin bruising will also be evident if the onset is related to trauma. Affected muscles will be tender and swollen. Continued bleeding results in spasm, restricted movement, and severe pain. Large muscle hematomas can compress adjacent nerves and cause associated neuropathy. Peripheral neuropathy has been reported in 5 to 15% of hemophiliacs (45). Compression of blood vessels by hematomas can result in ischemia or gangrene.

Gastrointestinal bleeding occurs in 10 to 20% of hemophiliacs but is a rare cause of mortality (45). Retroperitoneal hemorrhage is potentially life-threatening, because of large loss of blood volume and associated severe hypotension (44). Hematuria is seen in about 25% of hemophiliacs. Most cases are not due to trauma and tend to resolve spontaneously after 2 to 3 days (45). Intracranial bleeding is a common cause of morbidity and mortality in hemophiliacs. Death occurs in 30 to 40% of those who experience intracranial bleeding (45). Such patients may present with seizures, persistent headache, or unexplained neurologic signs.

Other complications include bleeding into the vertebral canal, retropharyngeal bleeding, and pseudotumors (hemophilic blood cysts) (44, 45). Hemorrhage into the vertebral canal is rare and presents dramatically with acute onset of pain and progressive paralysis. Retropharyngeal bleeding may accompany pharyngitis. Affected patients complain of inability to swallow their saliva. Pseudotumors are rare, progressive, cystic swellings involving muscle. They are produced by recurrent hemorrhage and accompanied by radiographic evidence of bone involvement (45). Pseudotumors present as painless masses that enlarge over a period of months to years. Pain may occur in conjunction with fracture of adjacent bone or with nerve involvement. Ulceration can occur if the overlying skin is involved.

Patients with moderately severe hemophilia (factor levels of 1 to 5% of normal) can have spontaneous bleeding; however, bleeding usually begins after some identifiable trauma. Their signs and symptoms are then similar to those of severe hemophilia. Patients with mild hemophilia (factor levels >5% of normal) generally must suffer moderate to severe trauma before hemorrhage occurs.

Mild hemophilia often is not diagnosed until late childhood or adulthood, when the patient exhibits excessive bleeding postoperatively, after dental extractions, or after joint or muscle trauma. Patients may also be diagnosed during routine blood screening tests prior to elective surgery. In this situation a prolonged activated partial thromboplastin time (APTT) is discovered, which leads to further evaluation and diagnosis of the clotting disorder.

Bleeding in vWd is mainly superficial, involving the skin and mucous membranes, and rarely causes death. Bleeding from vWd tends to be easier to control than the bleeding of hemophilia. The most common clinical presentations of patients with vWd are epistaxis, easy bruising, hematomas, menorrhagia, gingival bleeding, gastrointestinal bleeding, prolonged bleeding with cuts or trauma, bleeding after tooth extractions, and postpartum or postoperative hemorrhage. Spontaneous bleeding into joints or muscle is unusual, except in severe forms of the disease. Hemorrhage-related deaths are usually associated with the gastrointestinal tract (45).

DIAGNOSIS AND CLINICAL FINDINGS

A clotting disorder should be suspected in any patient who exhibits or reports unusual bleeding. A careful history can provide much valuable information and important clues to the diagnosis. In addition to hemophilia and vWd, the differential diagnoses for bleeding include various acquired coagulation factor deficiencies or platelet abnormalities such as those found in starvation, vitamin K deficiency, liver disease, disseminated intravascular coagulation, renal failure, and cancer. In addition, circulating anticoagulants (acquired antibodies that inhibit specific coagulation factors) may be present in patients with systemic lupus erythematosus, collagen diseases, malignancies, and drug-induced lupus (42). Unlike hemophilia and vWd, these disorders may involve multiple clotting factors and patients who are more acutely ill. The onset, location, and pattern of bleeding should help determine whether to suspect a disorder of platelets (vWd) or coagulation factors (hemophilia).

The diagnosis of hemophilia is most commonly made in infancy, and nearly all are diagnosed by 3 to 4 years of age. Circumstances in which the diagnosis is commonly made include prolonged bleeding after circumcision, palpable ecchymoses over a bony prominence, large hematomas after deep i.m. injections, and slow, constant bleeding for days from the oral mucous membranes in association with seemingly trivial lacerations. At about 2 years of age the child may start to show large soft tissue and periarticular hemorrhages that can cause limping and pseudoparalysis of the affected extremity. Bleeding into muscles and joints usually begins to cause problems at about 3 to 4 years of age. Musculoskeletal bleeding is the major source of morbidity during mid-childhood and adolescence.

Mild to moderate vWd is commonly diagnosed in adult life, while the severe forms of the disease are usually diagnosed in early childhood. Mucocutaneous bleeding such as epistaxis, easy bruising and hematomas, menorrhagia,

gingival bleeding, and bleeding from the gastrointestinal tract are the most common clinical symptoms of vWd (40). Patients with hemophilia have normal platelet function and therefore tend not to exhibit petechiae, a pattern of bleeding associated with the platelet dysfunction of vWd. Spontaneous hemarthrosis is possible in patients with severe forms of vWd.

Posttraumatic bleeding is excessive and prolonged in both hemophilia and vWd. Such bleeding is frequently noted with dental extractions, after trauma or cuts, and in the postpartum and postoperative setting.

A detailed history to look for similar problems in parents, siblings, children, aunts, uncles, grandparents, and cousins will help to identify any patterns of inheritance that may be clues to the diagnosis. Physical examination is useful in defining and evaluating the nature and extent of any current hemorrhage as well as potential complications of the disorder. For example, a patient with acute hemarthrosis will have a warm-to-hot and swollen joint. Repeated episodes of hemarthrosis can lead to chronic hemophilic arthritis, with degenerative lesions of the joints resulting in limitation of range of motion and gross deformity.

Laboratory tests can be used to screen for clotting disorders and to confirm the diagnosis. Several diagnostic screening tests are useful for the initial evaluation of the blood coagulation system. The bleeding time is the time required for blood flow to cease after a standardized cut is made in the skin of the ear lobe (Duke technique) or the forearm (Ivy technique). The Ivy technique is the more popular and standardized measure of bleeding time. Factors that prolong the bleeding time include a decrease in platelet number and/or activity, vWf deficiency, and antiplatelet drugs such as aspirin. The bleeding time is usually normal in hemophilia and prolonged in vWd (42).

The prothrombin time (PT) is a screening test that measures clot formation via the extrinsic coagulation pathway. The test is performed by adding a "complete" thromboplastin (equivalent to tissue thromboplastin) to citrated blood and measuring the coagulation time after addition of calcium. A prolonged PT indicates a deficiency in one or more of factors II (prothrombin), V, VII, and X, a significant decrease in fibrinogen, or the presence of an inhibitor. The PT is normal in hemophilia and vWd (42).

The partial thromboplastin time (PTT) measures fibrin formation via the intrinsic coagulation pathway. A "partial" thromboplastin such as cephalin is added to citrated plasma, and the clotting time is measured at 37°C after the addition of calcium. An activated partial thromboplastin time (APTT) is a PTT modified to eliminate the variable of contact activation. The APTT is performed by adding an activating agent such as kaolin, Celite, powdered glass, or ellagic acid to the plasma before adding the partial thromboplastin. A decrease in one or more of clotting factors V, VIII, IX, X, XI, XII, or prothrombin will prolong the PTT and APTT. Presence of a clotting factor inhibitor or heparin will also prolong these tests. The PTT (or APTT) is prolonged in most patients with hemophilia and vWd (42). However, the test result may be normal in patients with mild disease who have nearly normal VIII:C (≥40% of normal) (40, 42). The platelet count is normal in hemophilia and vWd (42).

Bleeding disorders suspected on the basis of history, physical examination, and screening laboratory tests must be confirmed by more specific tests of clotting function performed by an experienced coagulation laboratory. The diagnosis of hemophilia may be confirmed using specific assays of the clot-promoting activity of factors VIII and IX (VIII:C, IX:C). These tests mix patient plasma with plasma known to be deficient in the clotting factor in question and measure the degree of correction of the APTT, as compared with normal plasma. The VIII:C is decreased in both hemophilia A and vWd. Specific tests for vWd assess vWf:Ag levels, ristocetin-induced platelet aggregation, ristocetin cofactor activity, and the multimeric structure of vWf. Results of these tests are normal in hemophilia. The pattern of abnormality in these screening and specific tests is useful in differentiating between hemophilia and vWd and in distinguishing among the different types of vWd (40, 42).

MANAGEMENT OF HEMOPHILIA AND VON WILLEBRAND'S DISEASE

Prompt replacement of the deficiency clotting factor is of prime importance in the treatment of hemorrhage in hemophilia and vWd. Blood products available in the United States for the treatment of hemophilia A include fresh frozen plasma, cryoprecipitate, factor VIII concentrate, factor IX complex (also known as prothrombin complex concentrate, PCC), and antiinhibitor coagulant complex (also known as activated prothrombin complex concentrate, APCC). For hemophilia B, fresh frozen plasma, factor IX complex (PCC), and antiinhibitor coagulant complex (APCC) are available. In some cases, such as dental surgery, tranexamic acid or ε-aminocaproic acid and desmopressin (DDAVP) may be used in conjunction with or as a replacement for blood component therapy in hemophilia A and von Willebrand's disease. Tranexamic acid and ε-aminocaproic acid but not DDAVP may be similarly useful in hemophilia B. The choice of therapy depends upon the exact nature and severity of the bleeding disorder.

Fresh Frozen Plasma. One unit of donated blood has a volume of about 450 ml, of which 175 to 250 ml is plasma. Fresh frozen plasma (FFP) is the fluid portion from a single unit of fresh whole blood which has been centrifuged, separated, and frozen solid at ≤ −18°C within 6 hours of collection (49). It contains all clotting factors and

all multimers of vWf normally present in fresh whole blood. The properly prepared product contains between 100 and 200 IU of factor VIII and IX per bag or vial. FFP requires thawing in a water bath at 37°C just before use. Thawing takes about 20 minutes. FFP should be infused as soon after thawing as possible, to avoid significant degradation of clotting factors. The FFP used must be blood group–specific and administered through a transfusion set with a blood filter. To ensure hemostasis in an adult with hemophilia, a volume of 1.5 to 2.0 liters may be required, which may be repeated in 24 hours (45). Maximum, safe, single doses are limited to 10 to 20 ml/kg because of the potential for fluid overload and congestive heart failure. Healthy adult patients can tolerate up to 20 ml/kg over a short period. Such doses are unlikely to achieve a level of greater than 20 to 30% for VIII:C and 15 to 20% for IX:C (44). The volume of FFP necessary to achieve hemostasis has limited its usefulness in hemophilia and vWd.

Until about 1964, FFP was the mainstay of replacement therapy for hemophilia A and B and vWd. FFP is now rarely used in these conditions, replaced by cryoprecipitate and clotting factor concentrates. Current indications for the use of FFP include emergency reversal of warfarin therapy, antithrombin III deficiency, thrombotic thrombocytopenic purpura, inherited single coagulation factor deficiencies other than hemophilia or vWd, multiple coagulation factor deficiencies, and immediate therapy while awaiting the diagnosis of a bleeding disorder. FFP may also be used in mild cases of hemophilia where replacement therapy is only rarely required and no other clotting factor replacement product is available (45, 49, 50).

In addition to intravascular volume overload, the risks associated with administration of FFP include transfusion reactions, allergic and anaphylactoid reactions, Rh alloimmunization, and disease transmission. Acute hemolytic transfusion reactions occur in about 1:100,000 patients receiving blood product transfusions (51). Urticaria and fatal noncardiogenic pulmonary edema have been reported as allergic or anaphylactoid reactions. Urticaria is most likely due to the recipient reacting to plasma proteins in the transfused FFP. If urticaria is the only adverse effect and a more serious type of reaction can be excluded, treatment with diphenhydramine will usually allow the recipient to receive the remainder of the FFP (51). Noncardiogenic pulmonary edema may be related to antileukocyte antibodies in donor plasma. Patients show chills, fever, cough, and increasing respiratory distress. Treatment is supportive, based on blood gasses and hemodynamic monitoring (50).

Alloimmunization occurs when the recipient produces antibodies against antigens in donor blood products. Disease occurs when the recipient is then rechallenged with the offending antigen. Rh alloimmunization secondary to

FFP is probably due to small amounts of contaminating red blood cells (50, 51). This can result in hemolytic disease in a newborn if the fetal blood contains antigens that are detected by maternal antibodies (51). Alloimmunization can also result in fever or allergic reactions (51).

The potential for transfusion-transmitted viral disease from FFP is similar to that from whole blood, red blood cells, or platelets (50). However, FFP is prepared from single donors and therefore carries less risk of hepatitis and human immunodeficiency virus (HIV) transmission than factor concentrates from pooled plasma (44). The risk of hepatitis following multiple transfusions is probably between 3 and 10% (49). The risk of acquired immunodeficiency syndrome (AIDS) in association with the transfusion of FFP plasma is apparently extremely low. Virtually all cases of AIDS in hemophiliacs are related to treatment with clotting factor concentrates or cryoprecipitate (50, 52).

Cryoprecipitate. Cryoprecipitate is the protein that precipitates when single donor units of FFP are thawed at 4°C. The protein precipitate is then separated by centrifugation. The final product contains 50 to 80% of the starting factor VIII (between 80 and 150 IU of factor VIII) in a volume of about 10 ml. When stored below −20°C the product has a shelf life of 6 to 12 months (43). Prior to administration, the product must be thawed at 37°C and if desired may be further diluted with small amounts of normal saline. After gentle agitation, the cryoprecipitate is administered at a rate of about 10 ml/min, using a transfusion set with a blood filter. Individual units or pools of several individual units of blood group–specific cryoprecipitate should be administered shortly after thawing, to avoid loss of factor VIII activity. An average concentration of 100 IU of factor VIII/bag is recommended for purposes of dosage calculation (44).

Cryoprecipitate is a rich source of VIII:C and all multimers of vWf. It is also rich in fibrinogen and factor XIII and contains trace amounts of albumin and globulin (45). It is the least expensive form of concentrated factor replacement useful in the treatment of hemophilia A and vWd. Cryoprecipitate has about 8 to 10 times the factor VIII activity found in FFP. It does not contain factor IX and is not useful in the treatment of hemophilia B.

The factor VIII concentration in cryoprecipitate can be increased by administration of DDAVP to donors just before donation. DDAVP-stimulated donors can provide a factor VIII yield of about 3000 to 4000 IU/donation (compared to 1400 IU/donation for unstimulated donors) (53). Concern about the risk of HIV infection and hepatitis has resulted in the use of carefully screened DDAVP-stimulated donors to provide a safe and relatively low cost form of factor replacement therapy (45). One DDAVP-stimulated donor may, in some cases, be able to provide for the entire yearly cryoprecipitate needs of a patient with mild hemophilia A or vWd. Such a case may require donations every 2 to 3 weeks. This frequency of donation appears to be safe for the donor.

Cryoprecipitate was the primary therapy for vWd prior to the availability of DDAVP. It is the only product that will regularly improve and correct the bleeding time, and it is still the product most frequently used in severe vWd (54). Cryoprecipitate is also the most frequently used blood product when sustained levels of VIII:C and vWf are needed in surgical and posttraumatic cases of vWd and hemophilia A. The treatment of choice for mild hemophilia A patients who require infrequent infusions, have not been exposed to plasma products, and have no immunity against the hepatitis viruses is also cryoprecipitate (45).

Advantages of cryoprecipitate include simplicity of preparation, ease of administration, relatively low cost, and (because of the single, carefully screened donors) a significantly decreased risk of hepatitis and HIV infection (45). Disadvantages are the variability of the preparation from one unit to another and the potential for alloimmunization, allergic, and anaphylactoid reactions related to contamination with antigenic red blood cells and red blood cell fragments (45).

Factor VIII Concentrate. Human factor VIII concentrate is used in the treatment of severe hemophilia A. One product (Humate P, Armour) appears to contain all the vWf multimers and may thus be useful in the treatment of types I and II-A vWd resistant to DDAVP and of type III vWd (40, 55). Other factor VIII concentrates essentially lack vWf. Factor VIII concentrate is available as a lyophilized powder prepared from cryoprecipitate obtained from large pools of plasma donors by various purifying and concentrating techniques. Individual vials are assayed and labeled with the actual factor VIII contents, which may vary from 250 to 1500 IU/vial. The lyophilized powder is stable until expiration, when stored at 2° to 8°C. Prior to reconstitution both powder and diluent should be warmed to 37°C. The reconstituted product is then drawn up into a plastic syringe through a filter needle. After reconstitution the product is not refrigerated and should be administered within 3 hours. Blood group–specific factor VIII is administered to the patient by slow IV injection or by IV infusion at a rate not to exceed 10 ml/min. Products available include Hemofil M (Hyland Therapeutic), Profilate HP (Alpha Therapeutic), Profilate SD (Alpha Therapeutic), Koate-HS (Cutter), Koate-HT (Cutter), Humate P (Armour) and Monoclate (Armour).

Factor VIII concentrate is prepared by purification of pooled cryoprecipitate using chemical or monoclonal antibody techniques (44, 56). A factor VIII product produced by recombinant DNA techniques is currently undergoing trials in the U.S. and Europe and may be available soon. One method of preparation of factor VIII concentrate involves chemical processes that remove protein contaminants and vitamin K–dependent clotting factors. Products resulting from this process are also rich in fibrinogen. The more steps in the purification process the lower the final yield of factor VIII. Final products will also contain α- and β-globulin, blood group alloantibodies, and trace amounts of some chemicals used in the purification process (e.g., aluminum or polyethylene glycol). Monoclonal antibody techniques use antibody against vWf or factor VIII to absorb the factor VIII:vWf complex or factor VIII, respectively, from cryoprecipitate. The adsorbed product is eluted through an affinity column and subjected to ion-exchange chromatography. With each method, viral inactivation precedes final formulation in albumin (56).

Preparation of factor VIII concentrate by recombinant DNA techniques was made possible by the identification of the gene for factor VIII and its cloning into Chinese hamster ovary cell lines (56). The cloned cells synthesize and excrete factor VIII into the culture medium. Monoclonal antibody techniques are then used to purify the product. Initial experience indicates that this product will be safe and effective with few side effects, but further study and long-term experience are still needed.

Advantages of factor VIII concentrate include higher purity (compared with cryoprecipitate); ease of storage, reconstitution, and administration; and the ability to administer large, known amounts of factor VIII in small volumes. This product is thus suitable for use in the hospital and outpatient clinics and in home therapy as well. Disadvantages include high cost and the risk of hepatitis and HIV infection caused by the large pool (2,000 to 20,000) of donors required (45).

The problem of viral disease (hepatitis and HIV) transmission has been addressed by careful donor screening procedures to inactivate and kill the viruses, such as dry heating of concentrate, pasteurization, heating in solution, and extraction with detergents and organic solvents (45, 56). These procedures appear to have significantly reduced the transmission of viral disease, but whether it has been eliminated is still unclear, and surveillance studies continue (45). Recombinant DNA technology may make it possible to treat hemophilia A with a virus-free concentrate (45). Adverse reactions to factor VIII concentrate include allergic reactions, fever, chills, stinging at the site of injection, and hemolytic anemia caused by blood group isoagglutinins (50). Massive doses may increase the risk of bleeding because of hyperfibrinogenemia.

A porcine factor VIII concentrate (Hyate:C, Speywood Laboratories) prepared by polyelectrolyte fractionation techniques is also available. This product is of higher purity than human-derived products. Its use is limited to the treatment of patients with inhibitors to human factor VIII who have life- or limb-threatening bleeding episodes or who require essential surgery. It is used when alternatives have been exhausted or are likely to be ineffective (45, 50,

57). Most inhibitors in hemophiliacs react less strongly with porcine factor VIII than with human factor VIII (57). In addition, pigs are not known to carry the human HIV or hepatitis viruses, so there is no risk of transmission of these infections (45). The animal protein is antigenic, and response to treatment can diminish with continued use if antibodies develop.

Adverse reactions to porcine factor VIII include transfusion reactions, allergic reactions, and thrombocytopenia. The platelet count should be monitored during therapy. Other reactions (e.g., fever, chills, rashes, nausea, and headache) are rare and respond to hydrocortisone or antihistamine administration (45). Porcine factor VIII is supplied in vials containing 400 to 700 IU of VIII:C and should be stored at −15 to −20°C.

Factor IX Complex (Prothrombin Complex Concentrate). Factor IX complex is made from pooled plasma, in a process like that used for factor VIII concentrates, starting with the supernatant from cryoprecipitate. The final product is lyophilized and then heat-treated to eliminate viral contamination. It contains from 400 to 600 IU of factor IX per bottle or vial (actual factor IX content is indicated on each label). Factor IX complex is also known as prothrombin complex concentrate (PCC) since it also contains prothrombin (factor II), factor VII, and factor X. Only small amounts of factor VII are present, but factors II, IX, and X are present in approximately equal numbers of units (45). Products currently available are Konyne-HT (Cutter), Profilnine Heat-Treated (Alpha Therapeutic) and Proplex T (Hyland). The lyophilized powder is stable for 2 years at 2° to 8°C.

Factor IX complex is indicated for the prevention or treatment of bleeding in patients with moderate to severe hemophilia B. Prior to the availability of factor IX complex, fresh frozen plasma was the mainstay of therapy for hemophilia B. FFP is now used for treatment of minor bleeding or when factor IX complex is not available. Factor IX complex is also used to treat bleeding in patients with hemophilia A and B who have inhibitors to factors VIII and IX, respectively (50, 58). How factor IX complex can bypass the inhibited factors is unknown, but the product contains activated factors VII, IX, and X, phospholipid and phospholipid-bound factor VIII coagulant activity (59). Factor IX complex may be used to treat patients with deficiencies of factors II, VII, and X, when treatment with FFP is not possible or not effective (50).

Factor IX complex is reconstituted like factor VIII concentrate is and administered by slow intravenous infusion at a rate of approximately 100 IU/min, not to exceed 3 ml/min. Some patients develop fever, chills, headache, flushing, tingling, or changes in pulse or blood pressure with factor IX complex infusion. These symptoms may subside if the infusion is stopped and then restarted at a slower rate.

Patients treated with factor IX complex are at risk of disseminated intravascular coagulation (DIC), venous and arterial thrombosis, and sudden death from myocardial infarction (39, 44, 45, 50). Factor IX complex contains thrombogenic materials such as the activated forms of factors IX and X (44). In addition, factor IX complex may generate coagulant or kinin activity when left in solution for longer than a few hours (39). Administration by continuous intravenous infusion is therefore not recommended. The risk of thrombosis and DIC is greater in patients with significant liver dysfunction, crush injuries, extensive soft tissue bleeding, and those who have undergone orthopaedic surgery (58). Myocardial infarctions have occurred in younger patients with inhibitors who received repeated large doses of factor IX complex (58). Clinical monitoring for signs and symptoms of thrombosis, DIC, and myocardial infarction is recommended. In addition, serial measurement of antithrombin III levels may be helpful, since they may decline significantly in acute thrombosis and DIC (4, 50). Because of the risk of thrombosis and myocardial infarction, some clinicians recommend the addition of 100 units of heparin for each 500 IU of factor IX (50). The diluent supplied with Proplex T (Hyland) contains heparin. The antifibrinolytic agents, tranexamic acid and ε-aminocaproic acid, should not be administered concomitantly with factor IX complex because of the increased risk of thrombotic complications (50). Large, repetitive doses of factor IX complex should be avoided because of the risk of thrombosis. In addition, it is unlikely that additional doses will be beneficial if a bleeding episode fails to respond to 2 or 3 doses of factor IX complex (58).

Because of the risk of virus transmission, only factor IX complex that has been heat-treated or otherwise sterilized should be used. The risk of viral transmission has been reduced by heat-treating products and screening donors for hepatitis and HIV, but it has not been eliminated (50, 60). Virtually all patients who have received multiple transfusions of factor IX complex have been exposed to hepatitis B and non-A, non-B hepatitis (39, 45). Previously untreated patients exposed to single infusions of factor IX complex been reported to have a 5% to 42% risk of developing non-A, non-B posttransfusion hepatitis (50). The majority of these patients are actually infected with the recently identified hepatitis C virus. Virus removal or inactivation and product purification methods used in the preparation of factor IX complex are not as advanced as those used with factor VIII concentrates. Heat treatment is currently the only method licensed in the U.S. for viral inactivation. It appears to remove HIV infectivity, but non-A, non-B hepatitis still appears to be a problem (60). Solvent/detergent-treated products being developed and studied may have improved virus inactivation and be less thrombogenic (60). The future holds the possibility of a factor IX product that is pure and virus-free, thanks to recombinant DNA technology (60).

Antiinhibitor Coagulant Complex (Activated Prothrombin Complex Concentrate). Antiinhibitor coagulant complex is an activated prothrombin complex concentrate (APCC) prepared from pooled human plasma that contains variable amounts of activated and precursor clotting factors in concentrated form. It also contains factors from the kinin-generating system. These products are much more costly than factor IX complex (nonactivated prothrombin complex concentrate). APCC may be indicated in patients with factor VIII or IX inhibitors whose bleeding is not controlled by factor IX complex. APCC should be reserved for patients inadequately treated or controlled with factor IX complex, since it is much more costly, and at best, only marginally more effective (58, 59).

APCC products available are Autoplex T (Hyland) and Feiba VH Immuno (Immuno-U.S.). Autoplex T is labeled in units of factor VIII correctional activity. Feiba VH Immuno is labeled in units of factor VIII inhibitor bypassing activity. One unit is the amount of APCC which, upon addition to an equal volume of factor VIII deficient or inhibitor plasma, will correct the clotting time to normal. Autoplex T is heat-treated and Feiba VH Immuno is vapor-heated to reduce viral transmission. Autoplex T contains heparin and polyethylene glycol as stabilizing agents. The unreconstituted products should be refrigerated at 2 to 8°C. APCC is administered by IV infusion at a rate not to exceed 10 ml/min. Doses vary, depending on the severity of hemorrhage, but are generally in the range of 25 to 100 units/kg at 6 to 12 hour intervals, with a maximum of 200 units/kg/day. Reconstituted products should not be refrigerated, and administration should be completed within 1 hour (Autoplex T) and 3 hours (Feiba VH Immuno) after reconstitution. The concomitant use of antifibrinolytic agents is not recommended. APCC is contraindicated in patients with signs of fibrinolysis or in the presence of disseminated intravascular coagulation. Adverse effects and viral transmission risks are the same as those described above for factor IX complex (39, 44, 45, 50, 58, 59).

Antifibrinolytic Agents. ε-Aminocaproic acid (6-aminohexanoic acid, EACA, Amicar) and tranexamic acid (4-aminomethylcyclohexane, AMCA, Cyclokapron) are potent inhibitors of the fibrinolytic system. Fibrinolysis accelerates the destruction of blood clots and can result in clot lysis and recurrent bleeding, especially in patients with hemophilia and vWd. Fibrinolysis occurs when tissue-type plasminogen activator is released from endothelial cells and converts plasminogen to plasmin in the presence of fibrin. Plasmin then breaks down the fibrin clot. Plasmin and plasminogen both bind to fibrin through their lysine-binding sites. The antifibrinolytic agents are lysine analogs that act by saturating lysine-binding sites on plasminogen and plasmin, decreasing their attachment to fibrin, and delaying fibrinolysis. The fibrin matrix is preserved, and both collagen synthesis and the tensile strength of the granulation tissue increase. Inhibition of fibrinolysis by EACA or AMCA may allow more normal clot formation and dissolution in patients with hemophilia and vWd.

The antifibrinolytic agents, alone or in combination with cryoprecipitate, are valuable in the prevention and treatment of mucous membrane bleeding such as epistaxis, oral bleeding, gastrointestinal bleeding, and menorrhagia in patients with vWd (55). These drugs are particularly useful in the prevention of delayed bleeding after dental extractions or oral surgery in patients with both hemophilia and vWd, as is evidenced by significant decreases in (a) need for cryoprecipitate, factor VIII, or factor IX concentrates; (b) blood loss from the dental socket; (c) transfusion reactions; (d) transfusion requirements; (e) days spent in the hospital; (f) fall in hemoglobin; (g) blood loss; and (h) cost of dental extractions (45, 61–63). Minimizing the use of factor replacement therapy during dental extractions lowers the risk of transmission of viral hepatitis and HIV infection. However, currently no data justify the use of fibrinolytic agents for the prevention of spontaneous bleeding in patients with hemophilia and vWd (45).

The primary uses of antifibrinolytic agents in hemophilia have been in the treatment of oral mucous membrane bleeding and in the prevention of bleeding during dental extractions (oral surgery). EACA or AMCA alone is effective in most cases of mild hemophilia. In moderate to severe hemophilia they are used in conjunction with an initial infusion factor VIII or IX (44, 45). An oral regimen of 50 mg/kg of EACA every 6 hours, from 24 hours before dental extraction to 7 to 10 days after it, appears to achieve localized hemostasis (44, 63). For example, the hemophiliac will receive a dose of factor VIII or IX concentrate to raise the level to 50% (0.5 IU/ml) just before surgery and is started on EACA 50 mg/kg by mouth every 6 hours or AMCA 25 mg/kg by mouth every 6 to 8 hours and continuing for 2 to 10 days (45, 61, 62). An adult intravenous (IV) loading dose of EACA of 10 g followed by an intravenous infusion of 1 g/hr has also been used. The IV regimen for tranexamic acid is a 10 mg/kg loading dose followed by 10 mg/kg IV three to four times daily. A combination of an IV loading dose just prior to oral surgery followed by oral therapy is also used for both agents. If used alone, oral EACA or AMCA is started the day before dental surgery (44, 62). Both EACA and AMCA provide a beneficial local antifibrinolytic effect when administered topically as a mouth rinse (64).

Oral doses of EACA are rapidly and almost completely absorbed, producing peak plasma concentrations at about 2 hours. A dose of 100 mg/kg produces a peak plasma concentration of 30 μg/ml with an elimination half-life of 1 to 2 hr (61). An intravenous dose of 100 mg/kg produces an initial serum concentration of 1500 μg/ml which de-

clines to 35 μg/ml within 3 to 4 hr (61). Plasma levels of 130 μg/ml inhibit systemic fibrinolysis (63). EACA is excreted unchanged via the kidneys, with clearance of 80% of the drug in 12 hr (oral administration) and 90% excreted in the urine within 4 to 6 hr (intravenous administration) (61). Urine levels reach 50 to 100 times those found in the plasma. Due to rapid excretion, an intravenous loading dose followed by a continuous intravenous infusion is recommended to maintain a systemic effect, while oral administration is adequate for a localized effect (61, 63).

Tranexamic acid (AMCA) is 7 to 10 times more potent than EACA, with no greater toxicity, and AMCA has now largely replaced EACA as the agent of choice (61). Thirty to 50% of an oral dose is absorbed from the gastrointestinal tract, reaching peak levels in 2 to 3 hr. The serum half-life is about 2 hr, but therapeutic levels remain in the serum for 7 hr and in some tissues for up to 17 hr (62). The therapeutic serum level is 5 to 10 μg/ml (61). A 1 g oral dose produced a peak plasma concentration of 8 μg/ml at 3 hr after dosing. Food has no influence on absorption. AMCA is excreted unchanged by the kidneys, with about 40% of an oral dose recovered in the urine within 24 hr (61, 62). Intravenous administration of a 10-mg/kg dose of AMCA resulted in plasma concentrations of 18, 10, and 5 μg/ml at 1, 3, and 5 hr, respectively (61). About 45% of the intravenous dose is recovered in the urine after 3 hr, and about 90% after 24 hr. AMCA is widely distributed and results in greater and more sustained antifibrinolytic activity in the tissues than EACA. It can cross the blood-brain barrier and diffuse into joint fluid and the synovial membrane. Dosage interval adjustment is recommended for patients with decreased renal function. Patients with a glomerular filtration rate (GFR) of >50 ml/min need no dosage adjustment. Patients with a GFR of 10 to 50 ml/min or <10 ml/min should have the usual dose given at intervals of 24 and 48 hours, respectively (65).

Adverse effects of EACA include anorexia, nausea, vomiting, diarrhea, hypotension, syncope, impotence, and rashes. EACA doses above 30 g/day are not recommended. Muscle weakness and myonecrosis have been reported with large doses and long-term administration (45). Nausea, vomiting, diarrhea, and orthostatic hypotension have been reported with AMCA. Retinal degeneration has been detected in animals given high doses of AMCA, but no retinal change have been observed in humans (62). Some patients have complained of changes in color vision. AMCA should not be used in patients with impaired color vision, and ophthalmologic examination is recommended for patients who receive the drug for longer than several days.

Extravascular blood clots formed during therapy with EACA and AMCA may be resistant to physiologic fibrinolysis (62). Patients with hematuria are at risk for intrarenal obstruction from thrombosis in the renal pelvis or bladder. A few patients have developed intracranial thrombosis as well. EACA and AMCA should not be used in patients with hematuria or subarachnoid hemorrhage, because of the risk of renal thrombosis and cerebral edema or infarction (62). EACA and AMCA should not be used in the treatment of hemarthrosis or bleeding into sites where rapid resorption of clotted blood is essential. Clots formed with EACA absorbed to fibrin strands may take months to dissolve and may contribute to fibrosis and further joint destruction (44). Likewise, these drugs should not be used in patients with disseminated intravascular coagulation (DIC). Use in combination with factor IX complex (PCC) or antiinhibitor coagulant complex (APCC) increases the risk of thrombosis and should be avoided if possible. When combination use is necessary, some hematologists recommend delaying the antifibrinolytic agent until 8 hours after after PCC or APCC injection. Concurrent use of estrogens with EACA or AMCA may also increase the risk of thrombosis. Patients with atherosclerosis should not receive EACA or AMCA because of the risk of thrombosis (70).

Danazol. Danazol (Danocrine), a testosterone derivative anabolic steroid with mild androgenic activity, was reported to increase factor VIII and IX levels in moderately and severely affected hemophiliacs when used in a dosage of 600 mg/day orally for 14 days (66). The increase in factor VIII levels was associated with a decrease in transfusion requirements. However, the experience of others and double-blind crossover controlled studies of danazol therapy in hemophilia A and B have found no significant benefit (67–69). It has proven to be a disappointment in the treatment of vWd as well (55). Danazol is associated with numerous adverse effects including weight gain, irritability, drowsiness, myalgia, muscle cramps, skin eruptions, hepatic dysfunction, hepatosplenic peliosis, and increased fibrinolysis with associated bleeding (44, 67–69). Danazol is therefore not a first-line drug for the treatment of hemophilia, and some have concluded that its risks outweigh its benefits and it should not be used.

Desmopressin. Desmopressin (1-desamino-8-D-arginine-vasopressin acetate trihydrate, DDAVP) is a synthetic analog of vasopressin, the natural antidiuretic hormone secreted by the posterior pituitary. Unlike vasopressin, DDAVP has no vasopressor activity but has increased antidiuretic activity. Intravenous infusion of DDAVP causes a transient but marked increase in factor VIII:C and vWf in patients with mild to moderate hemophilia A and vWd (40, 45, 54, 70). In vWd, ristocetin cofactor activity is increased and bleeding time shortened. By increasing the factor VIII:C, DDAVP also shortens the prolonged APTT. DDAVP is thought to act centrally to cause release of a second messenger that in turn stimulates release of factor VIII and vWf from endothelial storage sites (44). Many of the vWf multimers released by DDAVP are larger than

normal, but the half-life of the newly released factor VIII is similar to that seen after infusions of plasma, cryoprecipitate, or factor VIII (40, 70, 71). DDAVP also enhances fibrinolysis through the release of tissue plasminogen activator. Routine coadministration of antifibrinolytic agents, used frequently in dental surgery, is not needed in all patients (70). DDAVP has been used to treat mild to moderately severe acute bleeding and as prophylaxis for surgical procedures. It allows many patients to avoid or markedly reduce their need for prophylactic or therapeutic blood products (69).

DDAVP is available as an injection (4 μg/ml) and a nasal solution (100 μg/ml). Intravenous administration results in a greater and more predictable increase in factor VIII:C and vWf than intranasal or subcutaneous administration (45, 70). The DDAVP available in the U.S. for intranasal use, while adequate for treatment of diabetes insipidus, is not concentrated enough to provide the dose (0.2 to 0.4 μg/kg) needed for hemophilia and vWd in a volume suitable for nasal administration (70). The dosage for subcutaneous injection is the same as that for intravenous infusion. The injection currently available in the U.S. is not concentrated enough to allow comfortable administration of the volume needed per dose as a subcutaneous injection. More concentrated forms of DDAVP are available in Europe. When they become available in the U.S., DDAVP may become practicable for self-administration at home as prophylaxis for soft tissue bleeding or to avoid excessive bleeding during menstruation (40).

The response to intravenous DDAVP appears to be dose-related up to a dose of about 0.3 μg/kg (45). Increases in VIII:C and vWf appear as early as 30 min after DDAVP infusion, peak at 300 to 400% of baseline in 30 min to 2 hr, and persist for 6 to 12 hr (54, 70). The recommended intravenous dose of desmopressin is 0.3 to 0.4 μg/kg diluted in 50 ml of normal saline for adults (10 ml for children who weigh less than 10 kg) and infused slowly over 15 to 30 min (44, 70). The efficacy of DDAVP in hemophilia A is related to its ability to increase VIII:C to levels adequate to provide hemostasis for bleeding episodes and surgery (70). Factor VIII:C levels of 30 to 50% of normal are adequate for minor surgery, while levels above 50% of normal are needed for major surgery. Increases in VIII:C and ristocetin cofactor activity and shortened bleeding time indicate DDAVP response in vWd. The range of individual responses is wide and variable. A test dose of 0.3 μg/kg is recommended to document that the patient will respond with an adequate increase in VIII:C before DDAVP is used in surgery (45, 70). Patients with baseline levels of factor VIII:C of at least 4 to 5% are more likely to have an adequate response to DDAVP (44, 72).

Some patients who receive repeated doses of DDAVP at 12- to 24-hr intervals may develop a decrease in response. This tachyphylaxis, from presumed depletion of tissue stores of factor VIII and vWf, may result if intravenous infusions are spaced too closely (40, 44, 70). Because the onset of tachyphylaxis is variable, the efficacy of repeated infusions must be assessed in each individual patient. Depleted stores of factor VIII and vWf will probably be replenished if the interval between doses is 48 hours or more (44, 70). In many cases 1 to 4 infusions of DDAVP alone may control bleeding, while other patients may require supplementation with factor VIII concentrate or cryoprecipitate (73). Patients who require elevated levels of factor VIII:C for longer periods of time, such as a 2-week recovery period following major surgery, may be effectively treated with DDAVP infusions alternating with infusions of plasma, cryoprecipitate, or factor VIII concentrate (44). For elective surgery it may be possible to use DDAVP-stimulated factor VIII–rich cryoprecipitate or plasma that has been obtained beforehand from the patient or designated donors (44, 45).

The most common side effect of DDAVP is cutaneous vasodilation, which causes a transient feeling of heat and facial flushing. Other side effects include headache, a slight increase in heart rate, a slight decrease in blood pressure, nausea, mild abdominal pain, and vulval pain (40, 70, 72). Many of these side effects respond to slowing the rate of infusion (72). Rare major adverse effects are hyponatremia and seizures, myocardial infarction, cerebral infarction, venous thrombosis, and unstable angina (40, 70). Water retention has not been a problem for most patients when normal fluid intake is maintained. Patients receiving intravenous fluids or those with a tendency to retain water should be carefully monitored for fluid intake and output (44). Because DDAVP can also cause the release of tissue plasminogen activator, some clinicians given EACA or AMCA concurrently with desmopressin to prevent fibrinolysis, especially after dental procedures (72, 73).

Clinical Use of Clotting Factor Products in Hemophilia. The appropriate dose and dosing interval for factor VIII and IX replacement depends on the baseline level of factor activity; the site of bleeding or surgery; the severity of injury or bleeding or the extent of surgery; the factor level necessary to achieve and maintain hemostasis; the presence or absence of inhibitors; the plasma volume of the patient; and the biological properties (half-life and distribution) of the deficient factor. By definition, 1 international unit (IU) of factor VIII or IX is that amount of clotting factor activity found in 1 ml of fresh normal pooled plasma. One IU is equal to 100% clotting factor activity (44). An intravenous dose of 1 IU/kg produces an increase of approximately 2% for factor VIII:C and 1% for IX:C (39, 45, 50).

The plasma half-life of factor VIII is 8 to 15 hr, and it is distributed within the intravascular space (44, 45). A 12 hr dosing interval is commonly used for factor VIII. Factor IX is distributed outside the vascular space as well,

and the shorter half-life seen with the initial infusion is presumably due to initial distribution and saturation of the extravascular compartment (41, 45). The initial half-life of factor IX may be 4 to 6 hours, while the steady-state half-life after repeated infusions is 18 to 30 hours. A 24-hr dosing interval is commonly used with factor IX.

Producing and maintaining a minimum factor VIII level of 50% in a patient with a baseline level close to zero and without an inhibitor requires an initial dose calculated to produce a level of 100% (50 IU/kg or 3500 IU for a 70-kg man) and subsequent doses of 25 IU/kg (1750 IU for a 70-kg man) given approximately every 12 hr). An initial dose of 100 IU/kg and subsequent doses of 50 IU/kg given every 24 hr should accomplish the same goal if factor IX were the deficient factor. The dose and dosing interval should always be adjusted and individualized, based on actual measurements of pre- and postdose factor levels.

An alternative method for estimating factor VIII doses is based on plasma volume (39). Plasma volume is approximately 5% of body weight in kg. A 70-kg man thus has a plasma volume of 3.5 kg, or approximately 3500 ml. A factor VIII dose of 3500 IU should produce a 100% level, and a maintenance dose of 1750 IU every 12 hr should maintain that level above 50%. Factor levels are measured before and 15 minutes after the end of an infusion, to assess the adequacy of the dosage regimens.

Superficial cuts will usually respond to pressure application. Larger wounds, bleeding into areas of prior pathology, or major surgery require replacement therapy (50). Bleeding episodes in hemophilia can be divided for purposes of management into minor and major, depending on whether or not they are a threat to function or life. Minor bleeding episodes can usually be controlled by one or two infusions of factor to a level of 20 to 40% (45, 50, 74). Major bleeding episodes generally require treatment with higher levels of factor replacement for longer periods of time, as discussed below. Factor VIII replacement to a level of approximately 30% was reported to result in cessation of bleeding in 70 to 90% of patients and in 85–95% of patients in whom factor levels of 30–50% were actually achieved (50). Factor IX levels of 30 to 40% usually provide effective hemostasis (50).

Minor hemorrhages may include hemarthrosis, skin and subcutaneous bleeding, muscle hemorrhage, nontraumatic hematuria, epistaxis, and mouth bleeding. Such bleeding episodes generally respond to a single infusion of factor to a minimum level of 20 to 40% (45, 50, 74). Joint or muscle hemorrhage after significant trauma or in a chronically affected joint may require replacement to levels of 30 to 50%, maintained for 2 to 3 days (39, 43). Prompt therapy, ideally initiated in the home, is necessary to prevent the chronic crippling arthropathy seen after repeated episodes of hemarthrosis. Most subcutaneous hemorrhages and minor cuts do not require treatment.

Patients with deep cuts requiring suturing may need a second infusion at the time of suture removal. Hematuria unrelated to trauma is common, seldom causes significant blood loss, and may not require treatment if mild and lasting less than 24 hours (74). Nosebleeds may be no more common in hemophiliacs than in normal individuals (74). They usually require no treatment unless they become troublesome or involve major blood loss, when a single infusion to a level of 30 to 50% is frequently all that is required (39, 74). Bleeding from the mouth or oropharynx can usually be successfully treated with a single infusion to a factor level of 30 to 50% in conjunction with EACA or AMCA. Oral mucous membrane bleeding after small lacerations or in association with tooth extractions can usually be controlled with a single infusion to 50 to 75% with concomitant EACA or AMCA. Additional infusions are generally not required if an antifibrinolytic agent is used (74). Topical thrombin applied with a cotton-tipped applicator to the bleeding site may also be helpful.

Major bleeding episodes may include intracranial hemorrhage, muscle hemorrhage, hemorrhage threatening an airway, hematuria, gastrointestinal hemorrhage, retroperitoneal hemorrhage, and retropharyngeal hemorrhage (39, 45, 74). Factor IX doses for life- or limb-threatening bleeding should produce levels of 50 to 80% initially, then 30 to 40% for at least a few days (50).

Intracranial bleeding, either spontaneous or after trauma, is a common cause of morbidity and mortality among hemophiliacs. It is more common in children and young adults than in older hemophiliacs. Former mortality rates of about 75% decreased to 30 to 40% with the availability of factor VIII concentrate (45). Fifty per cent of survivors are likely to have neurological impairment. Seizures, persistent headache, and neurologic signs may be presenting features. Seizures may occur with the acute bleeding or weeks to months later, presumably from fibrosis associated with the healing process. For this reason many patients receive prophylactic anticonvulsants for several months after a seizure associated with intracranial bleeding (45). High blood pressure is a risk factor for intracranial bleeding and it should be controlled. Treatment requires massive infusions to maintain factor VIII levels at 75 to 100% with appropriate neurosurgical management until resolved, which frequently requires 7 to 10 days of therapy (39, 45). Several weeks of treatment may be required (44).

Spontaneous or traumatic bleeding into muscle is common and occurs in up to 75% of severe hemophiliacs (45). Painful and expanding intramuscular lesions are usually seen. Traumatic intramuscular bleeding is usually associated with superficial bruising as well. Intramuscular bleeding can occur after intramuscular injections, which are therefore contraindicated in hemophilia. Bleeding into a tight muscle compartment can produce compression of nerves, blood vessels, and other adjacent structures. Compression of a nerve can result in loss of function. Compression of an artery can produce ischemia and gangrene. Superficial intramuscular hematomas are treated with factor VIII replacement to 30 to 50% for 1 to 2 days (39). Iliopsoas muscle hemorrhage is frequent, very painful, and can lead to compression of the femoral nerve with associated neurological findings. Patients frequently present with acute, severe abdominal and groin pain. Factor VIII should be replaced to an initial level of 70% and maintained at 30% until pain, swelling, and tenderness are gone. Infusions are then discontinued until a 50% replacement is given on the first day of ambulation (74). A similar treatment regimen is recommended for other frequent sites of intramuscular hemorrhage (forearm, arm, calf, thigh) and for hemorrhage threatening an airway (74). Intramuscular hematomas should not be aspirated because of the risk of introducing an infection or creating a chronic sinus tract (45).

Hematuria is common in hemophiliacs, and up to 25% of patients will have hematuria at first presentation (45). Most cases of hematuria are spontaneous, short-lived, (2 to 3 days) and resolve without treatment. In rare cases hematuria causes clot formation in the urinary tract, which can lead to renal colic or obstruction. Treatment with antifibrinolytic agents (EACA or AMCA) theoretically increases the risk of such clots and is not recommended for patients with hematuria. Treatment of hematuria consists of high fluid intake to dilute and flush out clots. Factor replacement therapy may be needed to control the bleeding. Factor VIII replacement to 30 to 100% until the hemorrhage is resolved is recommended for hematuria associated with hemorrhage that is severe, prolonged, or painful (39, 43). EACA or AMCA are sometimes used when bleeding continues despite adequate hemostasis with factor VIII replacement (45). High-dose corticosteroids may be useful when hematuria does not respond to conventional treatment (45). How they stop hematuria is unknown, but they do affect capillary permeability. Corticosteroids have little effect on the level of factor VIII or its duration of action.

Upper gastrointestinal bleeding is common in hemophilia, occurring in 13 to 20% of adult patients (45). Prior to the availability of factor VIII concentrate, it accounted for up to 33% of deaths in hemophilia (45). Therapy with factor VIII is usually effective. Duodenal ulcers are frequently diagnosed at the time of bleeding. Fungal esophagitis may result in upper gastrointestinal bleeding in HIV-positive hemophiliacs. Patients with gastrointestinal bleeding should be managed the same way as patients with normal coagulation mechanisms after the coagulation problem has been corrected. Factor replacement should maintain a factor VIII level of 50 to 100% for 7 to 10 days and at least until the ulceration is healed (39, 45, 74). Patients with duodenal ulcers are then treated with H_2-receptor antagonists (45).

Retroperitoneal and retropharyngeal hemorrhage requires initial factor VIII replacement to 100% and maintenance levels of 50% until resolution, which usually takes at least 7 to 10 days (39, 44, 74).

Surgical coverage with factor replacement permits even complex major surgery in hemophiliacs without inhibitors. An inhibitor assay is recommended at least twice yearly and prior to surgery (45). If the assay is negative, the surgery may proceed. Major surgery is best done at a hemophilia center. Major surgery patients should receive 80 to 100% factor VIII replacement just before surgery, maintenance of a 30 to 60% level for 4 to 7 days, and a minimum of 20 to 40% level for an additional 4 to 10 days or until all drains and sutures are removed (44, 50). For major surgery in hemophilia B patients, a factor IX level of 60 to 80% just before surgery is recommended, then levels above 30% for 5 to 7 days, and above 15 to 20% for an additional 7 to 10 days (50). Orthopaedic surgery requires an presurgery factor VIII level of 100% followed by an 80% level for 4 days, and a 40% level for another 4 days. If the patient is casted, the factor replacement may be be discontinued until the rehabilitation program is begun. A level above 10% should be maintained during the rehabilitation program, which usually lasts about 3 weeks. If the patient was not casted, a level of 20% should be maintained for ambulation (44). Patients should be monitored carefully for hemorrhage during postoperative physical therapy. Factor replacement may be required for several weeks after orthopaedic surgery (50).

Dental extractions can often be done on an outpatient basis with a single factor infusion calculated to give a factor VIII level of 30 to 50% just before the procedure. A repeat dose of factor replacement may be needed in 3 days if the procedure is extensive. DDAVP is preferred for increasing factor VIII levels in dental surgery if a test dose indicates it will work (50). EACA or AMCA should be given concomitantly, starting at least 4 hours before the procedure and continuing for 2 to 10 days after dental surgery (45, 50, 61, 62). DDAVP is not effective for patients with hemophilia B. They should receive factor IX replacement to a level of 30 to 40% (50). Antifibrinolytic agents should be avoided before the factor IX infusion but may be started at least 3 to 4 hours afterward (50). Prophylactic antibiotics are recommended to prevent infection in the socket (45).

A factor VIII replacement dose of 100%, 1 hour before the procedure, with maintenance of a 60% plasma level for 4 days and a 20% level for an additional 4 days has been recommended for other minor surgeries (44). All surgical replacement regimens except outpatient dental extractions should involve daily assay of factor level before a dose.

Hemophilia is rare in females since they are usually unaffected carriers. Female carriers of hemophilia A have a mean factor VIII level of 50%, which tends to increase during pregnancy (45). In some rare cases the level is low enough to result in bleeding. Such cases usually emerge after surgery or trauma or in association with menstruation or childbirth. Pregnant female carriers should have their factor VIII levels monitored during antenatal visits. Factor replacement at delivery, if needed, is given after separation of the placenta, to avoid any risk of transmission of viral infection to the infant. Bleeding is more common in female carriers of hemophilia B (45). If needed, pregnant carriers receive fresh frozen plasma at delivery but after placental separation.

While factor replacement is definitive therapy for hemorrhage, other helpful measures must not be overlooked. Appropriate diagnostic tests and examinations should be conducted to monitor the patient's clinical status and response to therapy. Ancillary measures such as immobilization and cold applications may help decrease the amount of pain and bleeding. While acetaminophen and narcotic analgesia may be necessary in some patients, aspirin and other nonsteroidal antiinflammatory agents that impair platelet function will increase the risk of gastrointestinal bleeding. All patients should be warned against taking such medications (45). The recovery period should involve exercises and physical therapy, occupational therapy, and speech therapy as needed to allow as full a return of function as possible.

Treatment of von Willebrand's Disease. The product of choice for prophylaxis or treatment of bleeding in vWd depends on the severity and type of vWd and the clinical setting. The goals of therapy are to normalize the VIII:C and bleeding time (40). In most cases cryoprecipitate is the therapy of choice for severe hemorrhages and major surgery. If cryoprecipitate is not available, fresh frozen plasma (FFP) may be substituted. Humate-P (Armour), a factor VIII concentrate, contains the full complement of vWf multimers and can also be used in the treatment of vWd. Cryoprecipitate and FFP contain all of the components of the factor VIII molecule, including factor VIII:C, all multimers of vWf, and the factor VIII/von Willebrand factor complex. After administration of cryoprecipitate most patients with vWd exhibit an immediate increase in VIII:C, which peaks in 6 to 8 hours. Some increase in VIII:C may be noted for 24 to 48 hr after the infusion. The bleeding time may be significantly shortened or completely normalized for up to 4 hours after cryoprecipitate infusion. Some improvement in bleeding time may be noted up to 20 hr after the infusion. Dosing of cryoprecipitate is empiric. One bag/10 kg body weight/day has been recommended (40). Cryoprecipitate should be administered twice daily if it is critical to maintain normal hemoastsis at all times. Bleeding time, VIII:C, and platelet counts should be monitored regularly.

For major surgery in vWd, a VIII:C level of at least 40 to 70% is recommended during the operation and the first postoperative day. Levels of 30 to 40% should be maintained until the 7th day, and 10 to 15% until healed (75). Minor surgery requires a level of 20 to 50% during operation and then about 15% for 6 to 8 days (75). The recommended levels are 20 to 50% and 15 to 20% for severe hemorrhagic conditions and minor bleeding episodes, respectively (75). The required duration of factor replacement is less clear in vWd than it is for hemophilia but is probably shorter (74). Either DDAVP (if there is an adequate response) or cryoprecipitate may be used for hemostasis in mild hemorrhages, minor surgery, and oral surgery in patients with type I and type IIA vWd. DDAVP causes release of tissue plasminogen activator and therefore carries some risk of enhanced fibrinolysis. Some centers routinely use EACA or AMCA in conjunction with DDAVP for this reason (40). Other centers may limit use of the antifibrinolytic agents to oral surgery procedures. EACA and AMCA are useful with cryoprecipitate or DDAVP for oral surgery procedures in all types of vWd.

Patients with type I vWd have an excellent response to DDAVP, with a 3- to 5-fold increase in VIII:C, vWf, and ristocetin cofactor activity, as well as a shortening of the bleeding time (40). Type I vWd patients may maintain adequate hemostasis with DDAVP administration every 12 hours, without cryoprecipitate. Others may require cryoprecipitate supplementation. Patients with type IIA vWd respond more variably to DDAVP, with a partial correction in the bleeding time and some increase in the VIII:C, but they frequently require cryoprecipitate for adequate hemostasis (40, 44, 45).

DDAVP is contraindicated in type IIB vWd because of the rapid development of transient, severe thrombocytopenia (40, 44, 45). Cryoprecipitate or cryoprecipitate in conjunction with EACA or AMCA (in the case of oral surgery) are useful in type IIB vWd. Patients with types IIC, IID, IIF, IIG, and IIH vWd probably do not respond to DDAVP, but they should be evaluated for its potential usefulness (40). DDAVP is ineffective in patients with type III vWd (40, 44). For these patients cryoprecipitate should be used for the treatment of hemorrhage and in both minor and major surgical procedures. Both DDAVP and cryoprecipitate may cause thrombocytopenia in platelet- or pseudo-vWd. Transfusions of normal platelets with low-dose cryoprecipitate or the use of Humate-P may be tried in these patients (40). Patients with acquired vWd appear to have a shorter duration of response to DDAVP. High-dose intravenous gamma globulin may be useful in patients with acquired vWd who are refractory to DDAVP (70).

Pregnancy is associated with significant increases in VIII:C, vWf antigen, and ristocetin cofactor activity but the bleeding time usually remains prolonged during pregnancy (40). These increases sometimes allow patients with type I vWd to deliver without hemostatic support. Patients with severe (type III) vWd or variants will probably require prophylactic cryoprecipitate during delivery. All patients are particularly at risk for hemorrhage during the first few days and for the month after delivery. The time frame for increased risk of hemorrhage may be related to the rapid decline in VIII:C, vWf, and ristocetin cofactor activity to nonpregnancy levels (40). Estrogens and oral contraceptives are sometimes used empirically to prevent or treat menorrhagia in females with vWd (40). Short-term treatment with EACA or AMCA or prophylaxis with cryoprecipitate are sometimes necessary for patients with menorrhagia (45). Long-term use of antifibrinolytic agents is not recommended because of the risk of rhabdomyolysis.

Management of Patients with Inhibitors. About 10 to 15% of patients with hemophilia A and 1 to 4% of patients with hemophilia B develop inhibitors (IgG antibodies) that destroy the functional activity of factor VIII or IX (58). Inhibitors occur unpredictably, have a variable natural history, and are associated with increased morbidity and mortality in hemophilia patients. The main goal of therapy for hemophiliacs with inhibitors is to control bleeding episodes. A second goal for many patients is the induction of tolerance to factor administration, so the patient can be treated with and respond to doses normally used in patients without inhibitors (45). A shortened factor half-life and failure to respond to factor replacement infusions indicate the presence of an inhibitor.

Patients with inhibitors can be divided into "high responders" and "low responders." High responders have a strong anamnestic response to factor administration and low responders have little or no anamnestic response (76). First administration of factor to a high responder results in an increase in antibody that gradually declines over a period of weeks to months. Subsequent exposures to even minute amounts of factor result in a rapid increase in inhibitor, which peaks in about 12 weeks (45). Bleeding episodes in high responders can be extremely difficult to manage.

The Bethesda method is the most widely used assay for the presence of inhibitors. One Bethesda unit (BU) denotes the ability of the patient's plasma to inactivate 50% of the factor activity in an equal volume of normal plasma. Low responders have inhibitor titers that remain below 10 BU/ml, even after challenge with factor VIII or IX (77). Low responders may convert to high responders unpredictably. There is currently no way to predict which low responder patients are likely to convert (45). High responders usually have inhibitor titers above 10 BU/ml, which often increase to levels above 100 BU/ml after administration of factor VIII or IX. About two-thirds of hemophilia A patients with inhibitors are high responders (58).

Effective treatment of acute bleeding in low responders is frequently possible with factor administration (45). Some centers avoid administration of factor except in serious or life-threatening bleeding. Others treat low responders like patients without inhibitors and hope that inhibitor levels do not rise. Such patients may require higher than normal doses of factor at intervals of 1 to 4 hours or by continuous infusion (45, 78). High responders may respond to factor administration initially when inhibitor levels are low. However, both low and high responders with inhibitor levels greater than 3 to 6 BU/ml require massive factor doses to overcome the inhibitor and establish hemostasis (78). These doses may not be logistically and economically possible.

Alternatives to factor VIII concentrate or factor IX complex for treatment of hemophilia with inhibitors include PCC, APCC, or porcine factor VIII. PCC and APCC are currently recommended for treatment of patients with factor VIII or IX inhibitors with joint or muscle hemorrhage (58). The dose for both is 75 to 100 IU/kg repeated one to two times at 8- to 12-hour intervals (58, 78). Single doses are effective in about 50% of patients with hemarthroses (58). More than 2 to 3 doses are associated with increased risk of thromboembolism and disseminated intravascular coagulation. If the bleeding does not respond after 2 to 3 doses it is unlikely to respond to additional doses (58). If adequate levels of VIII:C or IX:C can be maintained for 2 to 4 days, it is usually possible to achieve hemostasis (78). APCC was initially thought to be superior to PCC in efficacy. However, no clear advantage has been demonstrated and APCC is usually tried after PCC.

Porcine factor VIII concentrate is an alternative for treatment of hemophilia A patients with inhibitors. The cross-reactivity of human factor VIII inhibitors with porcine factor VIII is variable but averages 15–25% (79). The dose of porcine factor VIII is empiric in a range of 10 to 100 IU/kg, depending on the severity of the clinical indication and the patient's inhibitor history (57). Most patients with a human inhibitor level of less than 50 BU/ml (or porcine inhibitor level of less than 15 BU/ml) respond favorably to porcine factor VIII. If the human inhibitor level is over 100 BU/ml, a response is less likely unless massive doses are used. Efficacy is followed clinically and with 10-min postinfusion VIII:C levels. Porcine factor VIII is preferable to PCC or APCC if there is an adequate response. Porcine factor VIII has been used in the prophylaxis of hemorrhage and home therapy as well as in treatment of acute hemorrhage (79).

Repeated plasmapheresis, to reduce inhibitor titer, and immediate factor replacement may allow emergency surgery or successful treatment of life-threatening hemorrhage in a high responder (44, 45). Inhibitors reappear rapidly after plasmapheresis. Extracorporeal adsorption of inhibitor from plasma run through a protein A–Sepharose column and then returned to the patient has also been used to reduce factor VIII or IX inhibitor levels (45). However, this procedure is rarely available and very expensive. Elective surgery is generally avoided in inhibitor patients except in low responders with an obvious indication for surgery or those in whom immune tolerance has been induced. Dental extractions can sometimes be performed with antifibrinolytic therapy alone (44).

Induction of immune tolerance to reduce or eliminate antifactor antibodies is a major therapeutic advance in the treatment of hemophilia (77). Immune tolerance is defined as the elimination of the inhibitor, the normalization of the half-life of the infused factor, and the absence of anamnestic response to factor administration (76). Induction of immune tolerance in low-responder hemophilia A patients can frequently be accomplished with daily administration of low doses (25 to 50 IU/kg) of factor VIII over a period of months until inhibitor levels are undetectable. Tolerance is maintained with lower doses of factor VIII administered intermittently, usually 1 to 3 times weekly (80). The mechanism of induction of tolerance is unknown, but it may be related to antigen blockade of responsive B lymphocytes or to the persistent exposure to factor VIII antigen or factor VIII:inhibitor complex resulting in suppression of the antibody response.

The Bonn protocol uses high-dose factor VIII with APCC to induce immune tolerance, and lower doses of factor VIII to maintain it (80). Factor VIII, 100 IU/kg, and APCC (FEIBA), 40 to 60 IU/kg, are administered every 12 hours initially, followed by factor VIII alone in a daily dose of 150 IU/kg until the inhibitor is undetectable and the half-life of factor VIII is normal. Patients are then continued on low-dose factor VIII several times weekly to maintain tolerance and prevent bleeding. This regimen, although effective, is very expensive and demanding of patients and providers. Others have reported success in inducing tolerance with high-dose factor VIII alone, administered over a period of months (80).

The Malmö treatment model uses high-dose gamma globulin and cyclophosphamide in combination with factor VIII or IX for induction of immune tolerance in high responders (76, 81). In this case, tolerance to the clotting factor is facilitated by gamma globulin and cyclophosphamide. Factor VIII or IX is initially infused in a dose estimated to neutralize the inhibitor and raise the factor VIII:C/IX:C to 40 to 100 IU/dl. Factor administration is then continued at intervals of 8 to 12 hours to maintain the VIII:C/IX:C at 30 to 80 IU/dl. Intravenous cyclophosphamide is given in a dose of 12 to 15 mg/kg for the first 2 days, then continued orally at a daily dose of 2 to 3 mg/kg for 8 to 10 additional days. Intravenous gamma globulin, 0.4 g/kg is given for 5 days, starting on day four. After disappearance of the inhibitor, regular factor VIII or IX is administered at a dose of 30 IU/kg two to three times weekly to maintain tolerance. If the initial inhibitor levels are ≥10 Bethesda IU, adsorption to a protein A–Sepharose column is used to reduce or remove the inhibitor before beginning the induction regimen.

Induction of immune tolerance offers the following benefits: (a) reliable and effective treatment with doses of concentrate comparable to those used in patients without inhibitors; (b) absence of anamnestic response after treatment with concentrate; (c) elective surgery risks similar to those of noninhibitor patients; (d) fewer and better-controlled hemorrhages; (e) more successful physical rehabilitation; (f) decreased pain; (g) increased productivity; and (h) overall improvement in quality of life (80). Risks include the potential for uncontrolled hemorrhage during times of peak inhibitor levels and the transmission of viral infection from prolonged continuous exposure to pooled plasma products. The high costs of this treatment may be offset by fewer or shorter hospitalizations and improved patient productivity and quality of life.

Approximately 10% of patients with severe (type III) vWd develop antibodies to vWf after receiving blood products containing vWf (40). These patients may have an anamnestic increase in this inhibitor in association with an anaphylactoid reaction after administration of FFP or cryoprecipitate. Use of hydrocortisone or antihistamines before these infusions is recommended to decrease the severity of the anaphylactoid reactions (40). Plasmapheresis, extracorporeal adsorption onto a protein A-Sepharose column, and high-dose intravenous gamma globulin (1 g/kg on 2 successive days) have been successfully used to decrease the inhibitor and allow successful FFP or cryoprecipitate treatment of severe or life-threatening hemorrhage.

COMPLICATIONS OF THERAPY

Almost all moderately or severely affected hemophiliacs who have had multiple transfusions have chronic active hepatitis or chronic persistent hepatitis (39). Non-A, non-B hepatitis, hepatitis B, and δ hepatitis are most commonly encountered. Antibody to hepatitis B surface antigen is present in about 90% of hemophiliacs, and at least 10% are positive for hepatitis B surface antigen (HBsAg). Over 50% of hemophiliacs have slight abnormalities in liver transaminases. Most patients are asymptomatic, but some go on to develop cirrhosis. Hemophiliacs who test negative for HBsAg and anti-HBsAg antibody should be immunized with hepatitis B vaccine (44, 46). HBsAg-positive patients frequently have a superimposed δ agent infection, which can lead to severe active hepatitis, cirrhosis, and an increased risk of hepatocellular carcinoma (39). Use of cryoprecipitate or FFP (single donor products) instead of concentrates whenever possible decreases the risk of hepatitis (74).

About 90% of severe hemophiliacs and 60 to 80% of all hemophiliacs exposed to plasma concentrates are HIV-antibody positive, indicating exposure to the AIDS virus (39, 45). Many hundreds of hemophiliacs have already died of AIDS. Use of cryoprecipitate or FFP instead of concentrate whenever possible should decrease the risk of acquiring AIDS (44). Use of heat or chemically sterilized factor VIII concentrate and PCC reduces the risk of transmission of AIDS, but not hepatitis (45). Porcine factor VIII is not associated with hepatitis or HIV virus transmission. Patients who are HIV-antibody negative should be retested at 6- to 12-month intervals. Patients who are hepatitis or HIV positive should be educated on how to protect their intimate family contacts from possible infection (46). In the future the availability of factor VIII or IX products prepared using recombinant DNA technology may allow treatment with a virus-free product.

Disseminated intravascular coagulation (DIC) and thrombosis, including pulmonary thromboembolism and myocardial infarction, have been reported with the use of PCC and APCC. Significant liver disease, high doses, prolonged therapy, rapid infusion and concurrent EACA or AMCA therapy may increase the risk (39, 44, 45, 50). Patients receiving PCC or APCC should be monitored for DIC and thrombosis. Infusions should be given at a rate of about 15 min/vial. Heparin should be added to PCC used for treatment of hemophilia B (74). If possible, the use of antifibrinolytic agents concurrently with PCC or APCC should be avoided. The risk versus benefit of administration of PCC or APCC to patients with liver dysfunction should be carefully considered. Prolonged therapy should be avoided. FFP should not be overlooked as a potential substitute for PCC in patients with hemophilia B, especially during the last days of a treatment course.

Patients with types A, B, or AB blood may develop severe immune hemolysis, especially during prolonged therapy, if treated with factor concentrate containing high levels of anti-A or anti-B isohemagglutinins (69, 74). Concentrates with low titers of these isohemagglutinins are preferable for prolonged therapy and in patients who have developed immune hemolysis. Blood type–specific single-donor products may be used safely to treat these patients. Some concentrates with increased amounts of fibrinogen may cause paradoxical bleeding, so products low in fibrinogen are preferred for extended treatment (74).

SELF-TREATMENT AND PROPHYLAXIS IN HEMOPHILIA

The availability of effective and stable factor concentrates has made possible programs for home self-treatment and prophylaxis of bleeding in hemophilia. With a properly motivated and educated parent or family member being responsible, most hemophilia patients over 3 years old can receive factor therapy in the home (39, 45). Patients 6 years or older can usually be taught to self-administer factor concentrate in the correct doses for the appropriate length of time (39). Home therapy is taught at regional comprehensive hemophilia diagnostic and treatment centers. The education program used in preparing patients for self-administration of factor concentrate in the home includes: (a) early signs and symptoms of bleeding into various organs, (b) venipuncture, (c) storage of concentrate and supplies in the home or office, (d) reconstitution procedures, (e) technical aspects and aseptic technique for preparation of the concentrate for infusion, (f) how to infuse the concentrate, (g) maintenance of records or diaries with dates administered, volumes, units, lot numbers, and effects of infusions, and (h) disposal of used syringes and needles (45).

Self-administration in the home has several advantages. Early initiation of factor replacement can result in more rapid recovery from acute bleeding episodes (74). Self-therapy may result in a decrease in the morbidity associated with chronic hemophilic arthropathy (82). In addition, self-treatment results in fewer severe bleeding episodes, shorter duration of immobilization and pain, less frequent interruption of family life for emergency room and clinic visits, fewer days missed from school and work, lower unemployment, fewer hospital admissions, fewer hospital inpatient days/year, less out-of-pocket expense/patient/year, lower overall cost of care/patient/year, and the psychological benefits of self-sufficiency and self-esteem (45, 74, 83).

The cost of clotting factor may actually increase with home therapy. Currently, studies are under way to determine the minimum effective doses of concentrates for control of early bleeding in hemophiliacs on home therapy. Some patients self-administer concentrate as prophylaxis prior to engaging in activities known to precipitate bleeding. Despite the risk of HIV infection and hepatitis, self-treatment in the home is a key component of comprehensive hemophilia care (39).

PROGNOSIS AND CONCLUSIONS

The prognosis for vWd is usually quite good. Most patients have mild forms of the disease and effective blood product therapies are available for those rare patients with severe disease. DDAVP and antifibrinolytic agents are useful for many patients, allowing effective prophylaxis and treatment of bleeding while avoiding the risks associated with receiving blood product transfusions. More concentrated forms of injectable and intranasal DDAVP are needed in the U.S. if patients are to benefit from self-administration of this agent for prophylaxis and treatment of bleeding.

The past 10 years have been associated with great progress and continuing problems in the care of hemophilia patients. Carrier detection and 1st trimester prenatal diagnosis using DNA analysis of factor VIII and IX genes can now be performed accurately. Factor concentrates, available since the early 1980s, have greatly improved the prognosis for hemophilia patients suffering from acute

hemorrhage. The availability of home therapy has resulted in further improvement in their prognosis and quality of life. Clinicians, patients, and their families can all benefit from taking advantage of information available from the local and national hemophilia societies and the World Federation of Hemophilia. This information and support can be of great assistance in understanding, managing, and coping with this disease.

Hemophilia patients with inhibitors continue to be a major therapeutic problem and are at higher risk of morbidity and mortality from hemorrhage. Disability from repeated hemarthroses remains an important problem in the management and rehabilitation of patients with severe hemophilia. Actual or potential infection with hepatitis and HIV are major problems facing all hemophilia patients requiring repeated blood product transfusions. The application of physical and chemical virucidal procedures to the manufacturing process has reduced but not eliminated the risk of hepatitis and HIV infection. All healthcare workers dealing with hemophilia must be familiar with hepatitis and AIDS. Factor VIII concentrate prepared using recombinant DNA technology is now undergoing clinical trials and holds promise as a form of therapy free of the risk of transmitting infection.

Disseminated Intravascular Coagulation

PATHOGENESIS

Disseminated intravascular coagulation (DIC) is a dynamic clinicopathologic syndrome that can occur as a complication of a variety of disease processes (Table 14.5). It may be characterized by either thrombosis or hemorrhage, since it involves activation of both the coagulation and fibrinolytic systems. The clinical manifestations of bleeding or thrombosis are extremely variable and depend on the underlying disease process and the balance between coagulation and fibrinolysis in the individual patient. Although the pathogenic mechanism is poorly understood, DIC is thought to be triggered by acute activation of the hemostatic mechanisms resulting in thrombin generation and intravascular consumption of blood coagulation factors. The stronger the triggering process and the longer the process continues, the more severe the associated DIC (84). Aggregation and removal of platelets from the circulation follows the initiation of the DIC process by thrombin. The triggering event for DIC is the release of foreign procoagulant material into the circulation, secondary to tissue or vascular endothelial injury (85). Malignant neoplasms, for example, may be associated with tissue injury, while septicemia may cause injury to the vascular endothelium. The enhanced hemostasis leads to fibrin deposition in the vascular beds, which can result in ischemia and eventual necrosis of vital tissues and organs. Hemorrhage may follow as continuation of the clotting process depletes the blood of fibrinogen, platelets, and various

Table 14.5.
Diseases or Pathological States Associated with DIC[a]

Bacterial infections: Legionnaires' disease, *Bacteroides*, *Haemophilus* meningitis, typhoid fever, *Shigella*, *Clostridium welchii*, Gram-negative sepsis, Gram-positive septicemia

Fungal infections: Aspergillosis, candidiasis, histoplasmosis

Viral infections: Chicken pox, measles, dengue fever, Korean fever, herpes simplex, influenza, yellow fever, congenital rubella

Other infections: Mycoplasma pneumonia, psittacosis, Rocky Mountain spotted fever, tuberculosis, malaria

Carcinomas: Breast, colon, esophagus, gallbladder, kidney, larynx, lung, pancreas, prostate, ovary, stomach, uterus

Leukemias: Acute promyelocytic, acute myelocytic, chronic myelocytic, T cell acute lymphoblastic, eosinophilic, hairy cell

Other malignancies: Melanoma, pheochromocytoma, neuroblastoma, sarcoma, histiocytosis X, polycythemia vera

Trauma: Burns, multiple injury, head injury, snake bite, fresh-water submersion, fat embolism, hypothermia

Surgery: Extracorporeal circulation, transurethral prostatectomy

Obstetrics: Missed abortion, hydatiform mole, septic abortion, preeclamptic toxemia, eclampsia, dead fetus syndrome, abruptio placenta, amniotic fluid embolism, acute fatty liver of pregnancy

Immune complex: Incompatible transfusion reaction, systemic lupus erythematosus, anaphylaxis, renal transplant

Hematologic: Thalassemia major, sickle cell crisis, paroxysmal nocturnal hemoglobinuria

Others: Necrotizing enterocolitis, intravenous pyelogram, diabetic ketoacidosis, sarcoidosis, hereditary telangiectasis, Kasabach-Merritt syndrome, malignant hypertension, postcardiac arrest, aortic aneurysm, pulmonary embolism, aspirin poisoning, organic solvent poisoning, heat stroke

[a] Adapted from Carr ME: Disseminated intravascular coagulation: pathogenesis, diagnosis, and therapy. J Emerg Med 5:311–322, 1987.

other blood clotting factors. In an effort to maintain homeostasis in the face of fibrin deposition, the fibrinolytic system is activated with digestion of fibrin by plasmin. Fibrin degradation products (FDP), also known as fibrin split products (FSP), accumulate in the circulation as a result of degradation of both fibrin and fibrinogen. FDP, by inhibiting further polymerization of fibrin, act as anticoagulants themselves and contribute to the bleeding problem. Consumption and degradation of clotting factors, thrombocytopenia, and inhibition of coagulation by FDP result in a bleeding diathesis (84). Thus both bleeding and thrombosis may be encountered in DIC, depending on the balance of coagulation and fibrinolysis.

CLINICAL PRESENTATION AND DIAGNOSIS

The diagnosis of DIC requires a high index of suspicion and aggressive laboratory testing. Signs and symptoms of DIC can be variable and confusing. The clinical presentation of a given patient reflects both the DIC and the underlying disorder and will depend on the tissues and organs involved and the severity of the DIC and disease processes. In general, there are two distinct modes of presentation of DIC: acute and chronic.

Chronic DIC is characterized by intermittently abnormal coagulation accompanying chronic disease (84). The clinical findings of chronic DIC tend to be less florid and the laboratory abnormalities more subtle. Laboratory findings suggestive of chronic DIC include decreased, low, or borderline-low fibrinogen levels and platelet counts and increased FDP (85). Over time these patients may develop overt clinical problems, especially thrombotic complications such as thrombophlebitis, nonbacterial thrombotic endocarditis, or pulmonary embolism (84, 86). Patients with metastatic malignancies often manifest DIC as a "hypercoagulable syndrome" with recurrent thrombotic events. Trousseau's syndrome, with a migratory superficial thrombophlebitis, is a variant of this syndrome (86). Successful antineoplastic therapy may eliminate both the clinical symptoms and the laboratory abnormalities of DIC in these patients. If treatment of the underlying cancer is inadequate, chronic subcutaneous heparin may be required to prevent recurrent thrombosis (85). Long-term oral anticoagulation is ineffective, and antiplatelet drugs have no documented clinical benefit in the prevention of thrombosis in chronic DIC (84, 86). Patients with mild chronic DIC may experience abnormal bleeding under significant hemostatic stress, such as surgery or invasive procedures.

In acute DIC, the clinical and laboratory features develop rapidly, over a few hours to days. The patient is critically ill from the underlying disease as well as the DIC. Most causes of DIC induce the acute form of the disorder. Acute DIC usually presents with both thrombosis and bleeding. Areas of trauma, invasive procedures, or pathology will tend to bleed, since even small wounds lack normal hemostasis (85). Bleeding from multiple sites is usually seen, with surgical wound bleeding, oozing from venipuncture sites, hematuria in catheterized patients, gastrointestinal oozing, and blood-tinged secretions from endotracheal tubes common. In the skin, microvascular thrombosis of end-arterioles with associated bleeding results in petechiae, purpura, spreading hematomas, hemorrhagic bullae, acral cyanosis, and even gangrene of the digits, nose, ear lobes, and other areas of end circulation. End-organ dysfunction secondary to microvascular thrombosis is also common. The most commonly affected organs include the lung, the kidneys, and the central nervous system. End-organ damage may also be due to the underlying disease itself. Patients may manifest hematuria, oliguria, acute renal failure, diarrhea, abdominal distress, ileus, vomiting, respiratory distress, deterioration of consciousness, convulsions, and coma (87). Pallor and jaundice secondary to hemolytic anemia and vascular collapse and shock due to hypotension may also occur. Adult respiratory distress syndrome (ARDS) appears to be a common terminal event in patients with acute DIC (85).

Laboratory findings associated with acute DIC are a

decreased platelet count, a decreased fibrinogen level, increased amounts of fibrin degradation products (FDP), and a prolonged prothrombin time (85). Thrombocytopenia is a cardinal finding, and platelet counts are below 50,000/mm³ in about 50% of cases. The plasma fibrinogen level (normally 200 to 400 mg/dl) is less than 150 mg/dl in 70 to 80% of patients with DIC, because of fibrinogen consumption in clotting and plasmin-induced fibrinogenolysis (85, 87). A normal fibrinogen level may be observed in DIC associated with pregnancy, sepsis, and malignancy, since the fibrinogen level may be elevated in these conditions by themselves (85, 86). FDP levels (normally under 10 μg/ml) are elevated above 40 μg/ml as a result of fibrinogen degradation by plasmin or breakdown of fibrin by fibrinolysis (85). The prothrombin time (PT) is prolonged more than 3 seconds in 90% of patients with DIC, secondary to consumption of factors II, V, X and fibrinogen during the clotting process (84, 85). The diagnosis of DIC is established by the combination of a prolonged prothrombin time, thrombocytopenia, and a low fibrinogen level (if liver disease is absent) (84, 85). An increase in FDP level is very useful but nonspecific, since numerous disease processes can result in FDP elevation (84, 88).

Other laboratory tests that are sometimes used in the screening and evaluation of patients with suspected acute DIC include the activated partial thromboplastin time (APTT), thrombin time (TT), antithrombin III level, D-dimer, euglobulin clot lysis time, fibrin monomer, fibrinopeptide A, and protein C levels (42, 84–86). The APTT is prolonged in DIC, but it is not as useful as the PT because of the wider range of normal values. The TT is prolonged by low plasma fibrinogen levels, as well as by heparin and FDP. The levels of antithrombin III, an important inhibitor of blood coagulation, are decreased in DIC and in the coagulopathy of liver failure. D-dimer is a specific cross-linked product specific for fibrin degradation by plasmin. Its presence in the plasma is helpful in the diagnosis of DIC. The euglobulin clot lysis time may be shortened in DIC by plasminogen activators in the plasma. Fibrin monomer in the plasma shows that thrombin has cleaved the fibrinogen molecule. Fibrinopeptide A is a peptide cleaved from fibrinogen by the action of thrombin and present in increased amounts in the plasma in DIC. Protein C, a natural anticoagulant, is decreased in DIC secondary to it consumption.

MANAGEMENT OF DISSEMINATED INTRAVASCULAR COAGULATION

Some patients show classic laboratory evidence of DIC, but remain asymptomatic without bleeding or thrombosis (85). Only careful observation and follow-up are appropriate for such patients, especially if the underlying disorder is being treated. It is important to be aware that these patients can deteriorate and develop florid DIC when subjected to physiologic stresses such as surgery, invasive procedures, or disease progression (85, 86).

Other patients develop acute severe DIC with life-threatening hemorrhage and thrombosis requiring complex management and monitoring. The cornerstone of effective management is prompt and aggressive treatment to control or remove the underlying disease, or the stimulus for DIC will continue. Aggressive antibiotic therapy for sepsis is an example of successful treatment of the underlying disorder resolving the hemostatic abnormality. Patients require vigorous supportive therapy to manage factors that aggravate the DIC. Such factors as acidosis, fluid and electrolyte disturbances, hypoxia, and hypovolemia must be effectively managed while treating the underlying disorder (86). If treatment of the underlying disease and supportive therapy are successful, the need for DIC management should be transient.

Treatment of DIC involves replacement of the depleted coagulation factors and platelets, and in some cases treatment to interrupt the process itself (84–87). Frequent clinical and laboratory monitoring is essential. Intramuscular medications should be avoided and venipunctures kept to a minimum to avoid creating additional sites of oozing, bleeding, and hematoma formation.

Clotting factor and/or platelet replacement therapy is probably unnecessary if there is laboratory evidence of DIC but no active bleeding (86). Replacement therapy with platelets, fresh frozen plasma, or cryoprecipitate will probably be required if the patient is actively bleeding or requires an invasive procedure or surgery. If the hemorrhage has been severe enough to cause anemia, it will also be necessary to administer blood. Factor VIII concentrates are not appropriate, because DIC depletes multiple coagulation factors. Prothrombin complex concentrates (PCC or APCC) may actually worsen or induce DIC. The argument that replacement therapy may "fuel the fire" and cause thrombosis in patients with DIC is theoretically possible and may rarely occur, but it has not been substantiated in clinical practice (85, 86). Replacement therapy is not indicated in chronic DIC or cases of DIC associated with gross thrombosis (85). Replacement therapy (see below) has been shown to decrease hemorrhage in acute DIC (86). Objective measures of successful management include decreased transfusion requirements, cessation of bleeding, an increase in platelet count and plasma fibrinogen concentration, a decrease in FDP, and a return of the PT and APTT to normal.

Depending on the need, replacement therapy is usually accomplished with platelet concentrates, cryoprecipitate, and/or fresh frozen plasma. Vitamin K deficiency may exist in DIC patients, especially intensive-care patients with the effects of inadequate nutrition and receiving broad-spectrum antibiotics. Such patients should receive vitamin K supplementation to help correct levels of vitamin K–dependent clotting factors.

Platelet transfusions are indicated for marked thrombocytopenia (platelet count $<20,000/mm^3$) or for ongoing hemorrhage (84, 86). Each unit of platelets should increase the platelet count by about 50,000 to $10,000/mm^3$ (86). At least 10 units of platelet concentrate are given in the presence of thrombocytopenia and serious bleeding (89). One or two units of fresh frozen plasma or 15 units of cryoprecipitate usually improve factor deficiencies, unless the clotting process is severe (89). Cryoprecipitate transfusion is indicated for fibrinogen levels less than 50 mg/dl or fibrinogen levels less than 100 mg/dl with bleeding (84). Each unit of cryoprecipitate should result in a fibrinogen increment of about 5 to 10 mg/dl (86). Platelet and fibrinogen levels should be determined 30 to 60 min after a transfusion and every 6 hr thereafter. Subsequent doses will depend on response and half-life of the platelets and clotting factors. The bone marrow usually takes several days to replenish circulating platelets. With effective therapy the platelet count should stabilize and then increase. FDP level will decrease with effective therapy, but it may take 24 to 48 hours for a decrease to be noticeable (85). The plasma fibrinogen concentration may be the most useful test for following these patients. It will stabilize and increase with effective therapy. Changes in the balance between fibrinogen synthesis and consumption can be seen within hours, while platelet and FDP levels may take days to show meaningful trends (85).

In patients with DIC and clinical evidence of fibrin deposition (e.g., dermal necrosis, acral or dermal ischemia, or venous thromboembolism) heparin is clearly indicated and has been associated with a decrease in mortality (86). Patients with DIC should therefore be monitored for evidence of thromboembolism and dermal or acral ischemia or cyanosis. Such patients may exhibit a bluish to purple discoloration of the feet, hands, nose, and cheeks accompanied by generalized sweating and cold, mottled fingers and toes. They require immediate heparin therapy if necrosis or gangrene is to be prevented.

The use of heparin in the treatment of patients with DIC and hemorrhage is controversial. Since the bleeding of DIC is due to thrombin-initiated coagulation and subsequent depletion of clotting factors and platelets, it seems reasonable to interrupt this process by using heparin to inhibit thrombin. However heparin is also a potent anticoagulant and carries its own risk. Prospective, randomized studies of the effects of heparin in DIC are lacking and impractical to perform because of the great variability in the patients susceptible to DIC and the disorders that may trigger the disorder. Anecdotal evidence suggests that some patients benefit in terms of hemorrhage control and survival (85). The indication for heparin in active acute DIC is bleeding unresponsive to or inadequately responsive to treatment of the underlying disease and/or replacement therapy (86). In these cases it must be used in conjunction with replacement of hemostatic factors. In addition, there are several specific clinical situations accompanied by DIC where heparin therapy appears to be beneficial, including amniotic fluid embolism, severe incompatible transfusion reaction, dead fetus syndrome, purpura fulminans, septic abortion, heat stroke, septicemia, thrombotic complications of chronic DIC of malignancy, and prevention of chemotherapy-induced DIC in acute promyelocytic leukemia (84).

The dosing of heparin in acute DIC is also controversial (86). Many investigators recommend full-dose heparin with a loading dose followed by continuous infusion of 15 to 20 units/kg/hr. Others recommend continuous administration of lower doses (5 to 10 units/kg/hr) without a loading dose. Most patients with DIC may already be bleeding and already have an abnormal APTT. The APTT is then useless for monitoring and adjusting heparin therapy. Feinstein has recommended using a 1:1 mixture of patient plasma and normal control plasma for assessing the APTT in this situation, with the goal of an APTT 1.5 times the normal control (86). If available, heparin levels might be useful for dosage adjustment. Although no specific therapeutic range has been defined for DIC, levels of 0.2 to 0.4 units/ml (using an activated factor X–based assay) and 0.5 to 2.0 units/ml (using a protamine sulfate neutralization assay) have been offered as general guidelines in certain cases of venous thromboembolism (90, 91). Fibrinogen levels and platelet counts are also useful in monitoring the effectiveness of heparin therapy for DIC. Attainment and maintenance of adequate fibrinogen levels and platelet counts is an indication of appropriate heparin dosing. Inability to achieve those levels can indicate a need to increase the heparin dose (86). In general, heparin should be continued until fibrinogen levels are above 100 mg/dl and platelet counts above $100,000/mm^3$ (87). The in vivo activity of heparin requires adequate functional antithrombin III, which may be low in patients with DIC (86). Patients who fail to respond to heparin may have low antithrombin III levels and require replacement of antithrombin III by transfusion with FFP or antithrombin III concentrate. Heparin is probably contraindicated when excessive bleeding occurs in a closed space where vital functions might be compromised (86). Therefore heparin should be avoided in DIC with intracranial, intraspinal, pericardial, or peritracheal hemorrhage. Rarely, heparin in conjunction with eternal drainage might be necessary in such cases.

Antifibrinolytic therapy (EACA or AMCA) is not recommended for most patients with DIC because it may cause widespread fibrin deposition in the microcirculation and ischemic organ damage or failure (86). If the DIC patient has life-threatening bleeding and evidence of extensive secondary fibrinolysis, antifibrinolytic therapy may be helpful (86). Antifibrinolytic agents should not be used in DIC without concomitant heparin therapy.

Exchange transfusions are sometimes used in the treatment of DIC. Their usefulness may be related to removal of FDP, activated clotting factors, and toxins, all of which aggravate bleeding (85, 87).

PROGNOSIS AND CONCLUSIONS

Some patients with chronic DIC may be asymptomatic with only laboratory evidence of the disorder. Others may have recurrent episodes of thromboembolism requiring long-term subcutaneous heparin for prophylaxis. Patients with chronic DIC may convert to acute DIC and hemorrhage under severe physiologic stress such as major surgery.

Acute DIC may be an incidental preterminal event occurring in a variety of acute catastrophic illnesses. It may be brief and end promptly with effective treatment of the underlying disorder. Alternatively, patients may die from hemorrhage and progression of the underlying disorder. Mortality rates for patients with acute DIC, reported to be 50 to 85%, may in fact reflect the mortality rates of the underlying disorders (87). The prognosis is unlikely to improve until better methods of prevention and treatment of the underlying disorders become available.

Drug-induced Coagulopathy

ANTIBIOTIC-ASSOCIATED HYPOPROTHROMBINEMIA

Hypoprothrombinemia with or without bleeding is occasionally seen in hospitalized patients treated with antibiotics, especially cephalosporins (92). The newer, broad spectrum antibiotics moxalactam, cefamandole, cefoperazone, and cefoxitin appear to be implicated more frequently than older, more narrow spectrum agents. Hypoprothrombinemia has been reported in association with penicillins, carbenicillin, cefotetan, ceftizoxime, cefotaxime, chloramphenicol, sulfonamides, tetracycline, and tobramycin plus clindamycin (92–95).

Several mechanisms may be involved in the development of antibiotic-associated hypoprothrombinemia and bleeding. First, broad spectrum antibiotics may destroy bowel flora that synthesize vitamin K. Second the parent antibiotic may inhibit the activity of vitamin K–dependent clotting factors. Third, the NMTT (N-methylthiotetrazole) side chain on moxalactam, cefamandole, cefoperazone, cefotetan, and cefmetazole may inhibit the liver γ-carboxylation of vitamin K–dependent clotting factors I, VII, IX, and X. Lastly, the β-lactam antibiotics azlocillin, carbenicillin, ticarcillin, mezlocillin, piperacillin, and moxalactam, may impair platelet aggregation in some patients. Impaired platelet aggregation may be an additional factor in the risk of bleeding in patients who receive broad spectrum antibiotic therapy (93, 94).

It has been estimated that hypoprothrombinemia occurs in 0.05 to 0.08% of hospitalized patients and that over 80% of those who develop coagulopathy had received antibiotics (92). The frequency of antibiotic-associated hypoprothrombinemia appears to be greater in patients with risk factors other than antibiotic therapy, since not all patients who receive these agents experience drug-associated coagulopathy. The following appear to be predisposing factors to antibiotic-associated coagulopathy: (a) critical illness; (b) malnutrition or decreased dietary intake of vitamin K; (c) impaired intestinal absorption of vitamin K, as may occur with gastric suctioning of bile acids, with the impaired intestinal transport seen with ileus, peritonitis, or bowel obstruction, or with intestinal mucosa damage caused by chemotherapy; (d) impaired renal function, which may increase antibiotic or NMTT plasma levels; (e) severe hepatic dysfunction that results in impaired synthesis of coagulation factors; and (f) impairment of hepatic synthesis of clotting factors by cimetidine therapy in patients with sever liver disease (92, 93).

The diagnosis and treatment of antibiotic-associated coagulopathy are relatively simple. The prothrombin time is useful in monitoring and assessing patients at risk for antibiotic-associated hypoprothrombinemia. This coagulopathy is readily reversed by vitamin K (phytonadione), 10 mg parenterally over 12 hr for 1 to 2 doses (92, 93). It is also appropriate to administer vitamin K prophylactically to patients at risk of acquiring hypoprothrombinemia secondary to vitamin K deficiency. A prophylactic dose of 10 mg of phytonadione, orally or parenterally, once or twice weekly has been suggested.

Careful monitoring for coagulation defects is important for all seriously ill patients. Patients at risk for vitamin K deficiency receiving drugs that also impair coagulation (heparin, warfarin) or impair platelet function (moxalactam, broad-spectrum penicillins, aspirin, NSAID) are particularly at risk for bleeding. While phytonadione administration will prevent or correct the vitamin K deficiency, discontinuation of the offending drug and platelet transfusions may be required to reverse the platelet defects.

DRUG-INDUCED INHIBITORS OF COAGULATION

There have been very rare reports of coagulation factor inhibitors (antibodies) in association with drug therapy (59, 78, 94). Patients on long-term chlorpromazine have been reported to have an inhibitor that may prolong the PT and APTT. An inhibitor directed at prothrombin has been reported in a patient taking procainamide. Isoniazid therapy has been reported to result in development of an inhibitor to factor XIII, factor V, and fibrinogen. A factor V inhibitor has also been noted in patients receiving streptomycin and cephalothin. Allergic reactions to penicillin, sulfonamides, and phenytoin have been associated with the development of inhibitors to factor VIII.

CONCLUSION

Reports of antibiotic-associated hypoprothrombinemia began to appear more frequently in conjunction with the availability of the extended spectrum cephalosporins. These occurrences have increased the general awareness of the potential dangers of drug-induced coagulopathies. There appear to be several mechanisms involved in the development of clinically important hypoprothrombinemia in hospitalized patients. However, cephalosporins containing the NMTT side chain may be associated with a higher risk of hypoprothrombinemia than other antibiotics. Drug-induced platelet dysfunction may predispose these patients to bleeding.

Rare reports implicate some drugs in the development of inhibitors to coagulation factors. Complications such as thromboembolism or bleeding may occur in these patients as well. The clinician must consider drugs as a possible contributing factor in the development of bleeding or thromboembolism. It may then be possible to prevent some of these problems and to detect and treat them more promptly and appropriately when they occur.

CONCLUSIONS

Normal hemostasis results from the ordered interaction of vascular tissue, platelets, and plasma coagulation factors. Disorders of hemostasis commonly involve platelets, coagulation factors, or both. Thrombocytopenia occurs when there is either decreased platelet production or increased peripheral platelet destruction or sequestration. Coagulation factor deficiencies may be inherited or acquired. Hemophilia A and B and von Willebrand's disease constitute more than 90% of severe inherited coagulation deficiencies. Acquired coagulation factor deficiencies may be due to vitamin K deficiency, liver disease, DIC, or the adverse effects of drug administration. The clinical presentation common to all these hemostatic disorders is unexpected, unusual, or excessive bleeding. A thorough history, physical examination, and laboratory evaluation of the patient will usually allow an accurate diagnosis. Treatment may be complex and expensive, requiring a multidisciplinary approach in which the pharmacist assists other caregivers in the efficient provision of effective drug therapy, in the avoidance of complications and adverse effects, and in the education of patient and family members.

REFERENCES

1. Saito H: Normal hemostatic mechanisms. In Ratnoff OD, Forbes CD (eds): Disorders of Hemostasis. Philadelphia, WB Saunders, 1991, pp. 18–47.
2. Nossel HL: Bleeding. In Petersdorf RG, Adams RD, Braunwald E, et al. (eds): Harrison's Principles of Internal Medicine, ed. 10. New York, McGraw-Hill, 1983, p. 293.
3. Comp PC: Production of plasma coagulation factors. In Williams WJ, Beutler E, Erslev AJ, et al. (eds): Hematology, ed. 4. New York, McGraw-Hill, 1990. pp 1285–1294.
4. Bauer KA, Rosenberg RD: The hypercoagulable state. In Ratnoff OD, Forbes CD (eds): Disorders of Hemostasis. Philadelphia, WB Saunders, 1991, pp 267–291.
5. Nossel HI: Platelet disorders. In Petersdorf RG, Adams RD, Braunwald E, et al. (eds): Harrison's Principles of Internal Medicine, ed. 10. New York, McGraw-Hill, 1983, p 1895.
6. Cline MJ, Territo MC: Hematopoietic disorders. In Melmon KL, Morrelli HF (eds): Clinical Pharmacology, ed. 2. New York, Macmillan, 1978, p 649.
7. McVerry BA: Management of idiopathic thrombocytopenic purpura. Br J Haematol 59:203–208, 1985.
8. Burns TR, Saleem A: Idiopathic thrombocytopenic purpura. Am J Med 75:1001–1007, 1983.
9. Hoffman DM, Caruso RF, Mirando T: Human immunodeficiency virus–associated thrombocytopenia. Drug Intell Clin Pharm 23:157–160, 1989.
10. Bussel JB: Management of idiopathic thrombocytopenic purpura in childhood. NY Sate J Med 85:499–501, 1985.
11. McMillan R: Chronic idiopathic thrombocytopenic purpura. N Engl J Med 304:1135–1147, 1981.
12. Marcus AJ: Hemorrhagic disorders: abnormalities of platelet and vascular function. In Wyngaarden JB, Smith LH (eds): Cecil Textbook of Medicine, ed. 18. Philadelphia, WB Saunders, 1988, pp 1042–1060.
13. Hirschel B: Zidovudine for the treatment of thrombocytopenia associated with human immunodeficiency virus (HIV). Ann Intern Med 109:718–721, 1988.
14. Buchanan GR: Childhood acute idiopathic thrombocytopenic purpura: how many tests and how much treatment required. J Pediatr 106:928–930, 1985.
15. Handin RI: Clotting disorders. In Wilson JD, Braunwald E, Isselbacher KJ, et al. (eds): Harrison's Principles of Internal Medicine, ed. 12. New York, McGraw-Hill, 1991, pp 1500–1505.
16. Warkentin TE, Kelton JG: Current concepts in the treatment of immune thrombocytopenia. Drugs 40:531–542, 1990.
17. Rosse WF, Logue GL: Immune thrombocytopenia and granulocytopenia. In Isselbacher KJ, Adams RD, Braunwald E, et al. (eds): Harrison's Principles of Internal Medicine, Update II. New York, McGraw-Hill, 1982, p 86.
18. Walsh C, Krigel R, Lenette E, Karpatkin S: Prognosis, response to therapy and prevalence of antibody to the retrovirus associated with the acquired immunodeficiency syndrome. Ann Intern Med 103:542–545, 1985.
19. Brannan DP, Guthrie TH: Idiopathic thrombocytopenic purpura in adults. South Med J 81:75–80, 1988.
20. Saleh M, Court W, Huster W, et al.: Effect of commercial immunoglobulin G preparations on human monocyte Fc-receptor dependent binding of antibody coated platelets. Br J Haematol 68:47–51, 1988.
21. Oksenhandler E, Bierling P, Farcet JP, et al.: Response to therapy in 37 patients with HIV-related thrombocytopenic purpura. Br J Haematol 66:491–495, 1987.
22. Tertian G, Risler W, Lebras P, et al.: Intravenous gammaglobulin treatment for thrombocytopenic purpura in patients with HIV infection. Eur J Hematol 39:180–181, 1987.
23. Harrington WJ, Ahn YS, Byrnes JJ, et al.: Treatment of idiopathic thrombocytopenic purpura. Hosp Pract 18:205–220, 1983.
24. Schreiber AD, Chien P, Tomaski A, et al.: Effect of danazol in immune thrombocytopenic purpura. N Engl J Med 316:503–508, 1987.
25. Ahn YS, Mylvaganam R, Garcia RO, et al.: Low-dose danazol therapy in idiopathic thrombocytopenic purpura. Ann Intern Med 111:177–181, 1987.
26. Ahn YS, Rocha R, Myvaganam R, et al: Long-term danazol therapy in autoimmune thrombocytopenia: unmaintained remission and age-dependent response in women. Ann Intern Med 111:723–729, 1989.

27. Biniek R, Malessa R, Brockmeyer NH, et al.: Anti-Rh (D) immunoglobulin for AIDS-related thrombocytopenia. Lancet 2:627, 1986.

28. Durand JM, Harle JR, Verdot JJ, et al.: Anti-Rh (D) immunoglobulin for immune thrombocytopenic purpura. Lancet 1:49–50, 1986.

29. Boughton BJ, Chakraverty R, Baglin TP, et al.: The treatment of chronic idiopathic thrombocytopenia with anti-D (Rho) immunoglobulin: its effectiveness, safety and mechanism of action. Clin Haematol 10:275–284, 1988.

30. Kwaan HC: The pathogenesis of thrombotic thrombocytopenic purpura. Semin Thromb Hemost 5:184–198, 1979.

31. Myers TJ, Wakem CJ, Ball ED, et al.: Thrombotic thrombocytopenic purpura: combined treatment with plasmapheresis and antiplatelet agents. Ann Intern Med 92:149–155, 1980.

32. Cooper RA, Bunn FH: Hemolytic anemias. In Wilson JD, Braunwald E, Isselbacher KJ, et al. (eds): Harrison's Principles of Internal Medicine, ed. 12. New York, McGraw-Hill, 1991, pp 1531–1543.

33. Bukowski RM, Hewlett JS, Reimer RR, et al.: Therapy of thrombotic thrombocytopenic purpura: an overview. Semin Thromb Hemost 7:1–8, 1981.

34. Bukowski RM: Thrombotic thrombocytopenic purpura: a review. Prog Hemost Thromb 6:287–337, 1982.

35. Myers TJ: Treatment of thrombotic thrombocytopenic purpura with combined exchange plasmapheresis and anti-platelet agents. Semin Thromb Hemost 5:199–215, 1979.

36. Machin SJ: Thrombotic thrombocytopenic purpura. Br J Haematol 56:191–197, 1984.

37. Schafer AI: The hypercoagulable states. Ann Intern Med 102:814–828, 1985.

38. Hackett T, Kelton JG, Powers P: Drug-induced platelet destruction. Semin Thromb Hemost 8:116–137, 1982.

39. Roberts HR, Jones MR: Hemophilia and related conditions—congenital deficiencies of prothrombin (factor II), factor V, and factors VII to XII. In Williams WJ, Beutler E, Erslev AJ, et al. (eds): Hematology, ed. 4. New York, McGraw-Hill, 1990, pp 1453–1473.

40. Gralnick HR: Von Willebrand's disease. In Ratnoff OD, Forbes CD (eds): Disorders of Hemostasis. Philadelphia, WB Saunders, 1991, pp 203–244.

41. Comp PC: Life-span of plasma coagulation factors. In Williams WJ, Beutler E, Erslev AJ, et al. (eds): Hematology, ed. 4. New York, McGraw-Hill, 1990, pp 1290–1294.

42. Walter Bowie EJ, Owen CA: Clinical and laboratory diagnosis of hemorrhagic disorders. In Ratnoff OD, Forbes CD (eds): Disorders of Hemostasis. Philadelphia, WB Saunders, 1991, pp 48–74.

43. Buchanan GB: Hemophilia. Pediatr Clin North Am 27:309–326, 1980.

44. Karayalcin G: Current concepts in the management of hemophilia. Pediatr Ann 14:640–659, 1985.

45. Forbes CD, Madhok R: Genetic disorders of blood coagulation: clinical presentation and management. In Ratnoff OD, Forbes CD (eds): Disorders of Hemostasis. Philadelphia, WB Saunders, 1991, pp 141–202.

46. Kasper CK, Graham JB, Kernoff PBA, et al.: Hemophilia: state of the art in hematologic care 1988. Vox Sang 56:141–144, 1989.

47. Johnson RS, Heldt LV, Keaton WM: Diagnosis and treatment of von Willebrand's disease. J Oral Maxillofac Surg 45:608–612, 1987.

48. Pelligra SJ: Hemophilia: pathophysiology and musculoskeletal complications. South Med J 80:1148–1152, 1987.

49. Anon: Fresh-frozen plasma: Indications and risks. JAMA 253:551–553, 1985.

50. Menitove JE: Preparation and clinical use of plasma and plasma fractions. In Williams WJ, Beutler E, Erslev AJ, et al. (eds): Hematology, ed. 4. New York, McGraw-Hill, 1990, pp 1659–1673.

51. Tarnower A, Clark D: Blood component therapy. New guidelines for avoiding complications. Postgrad Med 86(8):48,50–51,55–56,58,65, 1989.

52. Ragni MV, Tegtmeier GE, Levy JA, et al.: AIDS retrovirus antibodies in hemophiliacs treated with factor VIII or factor IX concentrates, cryoprecipitate, or fresh frozen plasma: prevalence, seroconversion rate, and clinical correlations. Blood 67:592–595, 1986.

53. McLeod BC, Scott JP: Plasma exchange donation of cryoprecipitate after DDAVP stimulation: an alternative source of factor VIII. In Kasper CK (ed): Recent Advances in Hemophilia Care. New York, Alan R Liss, 1990, pp 189–198.

54. Berry EW: Use of DDAVP and cryoprecipitate in mild to moderate haemophilia A and von Willebrand's disease. In Kasper CK (ed): Recent Advances in Hemophilia Care. New York, Alan R Liss, 1990, pp 269–278.

55. Logan LJ: Management of von Willebrand's disease. In Kasper CK (ed): Recent Advances in Hemophilia Care. New York, Alan R Liss, 1990, pp 279–290.

56. Roberts H: Highly purified factor VIII concentrates. In Kasper CK (ed): Recent Advances in Hemophilia Care. New York, Alan R Liss, 1990, pp 167–176.

57. Kernoff PB: The clinical use of porcine factor VIII. In Kasper CK (ed): Recent Advances in Hemophilia Care. New York, Alan R Liss, 1990, pp 47–56.

58. Lusher JM: Strategies to promote hemostasis in patients with F VIII inhibitors. In Kasper CK (ed): Recent Advances in Hemophilia Care. New York, Alan R Liss, 1990, pp 39–46.

59. Shapiro SS, Siegel JE: Hemorrhagic disorders associated with circulating inhibitors. In Ratnoff OD, Forbes CD (eds): Disorders of Hemostasis. Philadelphia, WB Saunders, 1991, pp 245–266.

60. Menache D: New concentrates of factors VII, IX and X. In Kasper CK (ed): Recent Advances in Hemophilia Care. New York, Alan R Liss, 1990, pp 177–187.

61. Verstraete M: Clinical application of inhibitors of fibrinolysis. Drugs 29:236–261, 1985.

62. Anon: Tranexamic acid. Med Lett Drug Ther 29:89–90, 1987.

63. Shira RB: Epsilon aminocaproic acid in hemophiliacs undergoing dental extractions: a concise review. Oral Surg 51:115–120, 1981.

64. Sindet-Pedersen S, Stenbjerg S: Effect of local antifibrinolytic treatment with tranexamic acid in hemophiliacs undergoing oral surgery. J Oral Maxillofac Surg 44:703–706, 1986.

65. Bennett WM, Aranoff GR, Golper TA, et al.: Drug Prescribing in Renal Failure. Dosing Guidelines for Adults. Philadelphia, American College of Physicians, 1987, p 66.

66. Gralnick HR, Rick ME: Danazol increases factor VIII and factor IX in classic hemophilia and Christmas disease. N Engl J Med 308:1393–1395, 1983.

67. Garewal HS, Corrigan JJ, Durie BGM, et al.: Effect of danazol on coagulation parameters and bleeding in hemophilia. JAMA 253:1154–1156, 1985.

68. Hathaway W: Danazol and hemophilia. JAMA 253:1167, 1985.

69. Spero JA: Complications of the treatment of hemostatic disorders. In Ratnoff OD, Forbes CD (eds): Disorders of Hemostasis. Philadelphia, WB Saunders, 1991, pp 555–575.

70. Bolan CD, Alving BM: Pharmacologic agents in the management of bleeding disorders. Transfusion 30:541–551, 1990.

71. Kasper CK: Desmopresssin acetate (DDAVP). Good news. JAMA 251:2464–2565, 1984.

72. Anon: Desmopressin for hemophilia and other coagulation disorders. Med Lett Drugs Ther 26:82, 1984.

73. Beatriz F, Kasper CK, Rickles FR, et al.: Response of patients with mild and moderate hemophilia A and von Willebrand's disease to treatment with desmopressin. Ann Int Med 103:6–14, 1985.

74. Gill FM: Congenital bleeding disorders: hemophilia and von Willebrand's disease. Med Clin North Am 68:601–615, 1984.

75. Coller BS: Von Willebrand's disease. In Ratnoff OD, Forbes CD (eds): Disorders of Hemostasis. Orlando, Grune & Stratton, 1984, pp 241–269.

76. Nilsson IM, Berntorp I, Zettervall O: Induction of immune tolerance in patients with hemophilia and antibodies to factor VIII by combined treatment with intravenous IgG, cyclophosphamide, and factor VIII. N Engl J Med 318:947–950, 1988.

77. Roberts HR: Induction of immune tolerance to factor VIII: a plea for caution. JAMA 259:84–85, 1988.

78. Furie B: Acquired anticoagulants. In Williams WJ, Beutler E, Erslev AJ, et al. (eds): Hematology, ed. 4. New York, McGraw-Hill, 1990, pp 1514–1522.

79. Hay CRM, Laurian Y, Verrroust F, et al.: Induction of immune tolerance in patients with hemophilia A and inhibitors treated with porcine VIIIC by home therapy. Blood 76:882–886, 1990.

80. Ewing NP: Induction of immune tolerance with factor VIII concentrate in patients with hemophilia A and inhibitors. In Kasper CK (ed): Recent Advances in Hemophilia Care. New York, Alan R Liss, 1990, pp 59–68.

81. Nilsson IM, Berntorp E: Induction of immune tolerance in patients with hemophilia and antibodies to factor VIII by combined treatment with intravenous IgG, cyclophosphamide, and factor VIII or IX. In Kasper CK (ed): Recent Advances in Hemophilia Care. New York, Alan R Liss, 1990, pp 69–78.

82. Levine PH: Efficacy of self-therapy in hemophilia. A study of 72 patients with hemophilia A and B. N Engl J Med 291:1381–1384, 1974.

83. Anon: Hemophilia, beaten on one front, is beset on others. JAMA 256:3200, 1986.

84. Carr ME: Disseminated intravascular coagulation: pathogenesis, diagnosis, and therapy. J Emerg Med 5:311–322, 1987.

85. Colman RW, Rubin RN: Disseminated intravascular coagulation due to malignancy. Semin Oncol 17:172–186, 1990.

86. Feinstein DI: Treatment of disseminated intravascular coagulation. Semin Thromb Hemost 14:351–362, 1988.

87. Choudhry VP, Thavaraj V, Saraya AK: Disseminated intravascular coagulation: diagnosis and current therapy. Indian Pediatr 27:280–288, 1990.

88. Marder VJ, Francis CW: Clinical aspects of fibrinolysis. In Williams WJ, Beutler E, Erslev AJ, et al. (eds): Hematology, ed. 4. New York, McGraw-Hill, 1990, pp 1543–1558.

89. Casciato DA, Lowitz BB: Hematologic complications. In Manual of Bedside Oncology. Boston, Little, Brown & Co, 1983, pp 611–622.

90. Ockelford P: Heparin 1986. Indications and effectiveness. Drugs 31:81–92, 1986.

91. Letsky EA, Swiet M De: Thromboembolism in pregnancy and its management. Br J Haematol 57:543–552, 1984.

92. Schentag JJ, Welage LS, Grasela TH Jr, Adelman MH: Determinants of antibiotic-associated hypoprothrombinemia. Pharmacotherapy 7:80–86, 1987.

93. Sattler FR, Weitekamp MR, Sayegh A, Ballard JO: Impaired hemostasis caused by beta-lactam antibiotics. Am J Surg 155(5A):30–39, 1988.

94. Ey FS, Goodnight SH: Bleeding disorders in cancer. Semin Oncol 17:187–197, 1990.

95. Wurtz RM, Sande MA: Cefotetan and coagulopathy. J Infect Dis 160:555–556, 1989.

CHAPTER 15

ADRENOCORTICAL DYSFUNCTION AND CLINICAL USE OF STEROIDS

ELIZABETH STUBITS SHLOM, Pharm. D.

Cortisol (hydrocortisone) is the prototype of the group of steroids referred to as glucocorticoids. Glucocorticoids maintain the body's homeostasis by regulating physiologic functions involved in stress as well as normal daily living. Cortisol and other steroid hormones such as androgens, aldosterone, and estrogens are manufactured and secreted from the cortex of the adrenal glands. These glands function on their own to provide the body with basal levels of steroid hormones and also respond to adrenocorticotropic hormone (ACTH) and the hypothalamic-pituitary-adrenocortical (HPA) feedback system. During nonstressful times, cortisol aids in the management of glucose and metabolic functioning. Cortisol also helps maintain adequate fluid and electrolyte balance. When the body is exposed to stresses such as pain, trauma, or infection, glucocorticoids modulate inflammatory processes, immune reactions, and neurochemical imbalances.

Cortisol disorders involve either too much or too little cortisol in the body. When the adrenal cortex manufactures and secretes excess cortisol the condition and symptom complex are called Cushing's syndrome. This usually occurs in response to pituitary microadenomas causing excess ACTH production (Cushing's disease), but it can be independent of ACTH, such as when there are cortisol-producing tumors of the adrenal cortex. Addison's disease, or hypocortisolism, is often idiopathic and results either from insufficient ACTH or destruction of the adrenal gland itself. If not identified and treated early, both these disorders are associated with a high mortality rate.

PHYSIOLOGY

The adrenal glands are triangular-shaped organs that weigh approximately 4 g each, located directly above the poles of the kidneys. The adrenal gland is composed of two physiologically distinct organs—the adrenal medulla and the adrenal cortex. Both of these endocrine organs are responsible for producing substances that aid the body in coping with stress. The adrenal medulla, which makes up the innermost portion of the adrenal gland, manufactures and secretes epinephrine and norepinephrine, hormones referred to as catecholamines. Secretion of catecholamines is under the control of the sympathetic nervous system.

The adrenal cortex is located on the outer portion and makes up 90% of the adrenal gland. The adrenal cortex is subdivided into three zones: the outer zona glomerulosa, the medial zona fasciculata, and the inner zona reticularis. The zona fasciculata makes up 75% of the cortex, while the zona glomerulosa and zona reticularis make up 15% and 10%, respectively. The zona fasciculata and zona reticularis are responsible for glucocorticoid and androgen synthesis, while the zona glomerulosa manufactures aldosterone. Estrogen synthesis also occurs to a small degree in the zona fasciculata and zona reticularis. All adrenocortical hormones are derived from esterified cholesterol.

The activities of glucocorticoids provide energy in times of stress. Glucocorticoids inhibit the uptake of glucose by most body organs, except the liver, heart, and brain. Cortisol increases hepatic gluconeogenesis and blunts the action of insulin. Lipolysis is also inhibited by glucocorticoids. All these actions contribute to hyperglycemia and hyperlipidemia when there are excess glucocorticoids. In a starved individual glucocorticoids thus help preserve vital body functions.

Glucocorticoids influence inflammation and immunologic responses. When cortisol levels are elevated, the body's response to an infectious agent or physical trauma is blunted. Although the exact mechanisms are unclear, glucocorticoids are thought to inhibit cellular mediators of the inflammatory response, inhibit antigen processing, and decrease serum lymphocyte levels.

Glucocorticoids also affect the body in other ways. Cortisol enters the central nervous system by crossing the blood-brain barrier and effects mood changes. Cortisol decreases serum calcium levels in hypercalcemia. Glucocorticoids enhance gastric acid secretion when predisposing factors exist. Lastly, excess glucocorticoids inhibit growth. These glucocorticoid actions help to explain the symptoms and clinical manifestations seen with cortisol excess and deficiency.

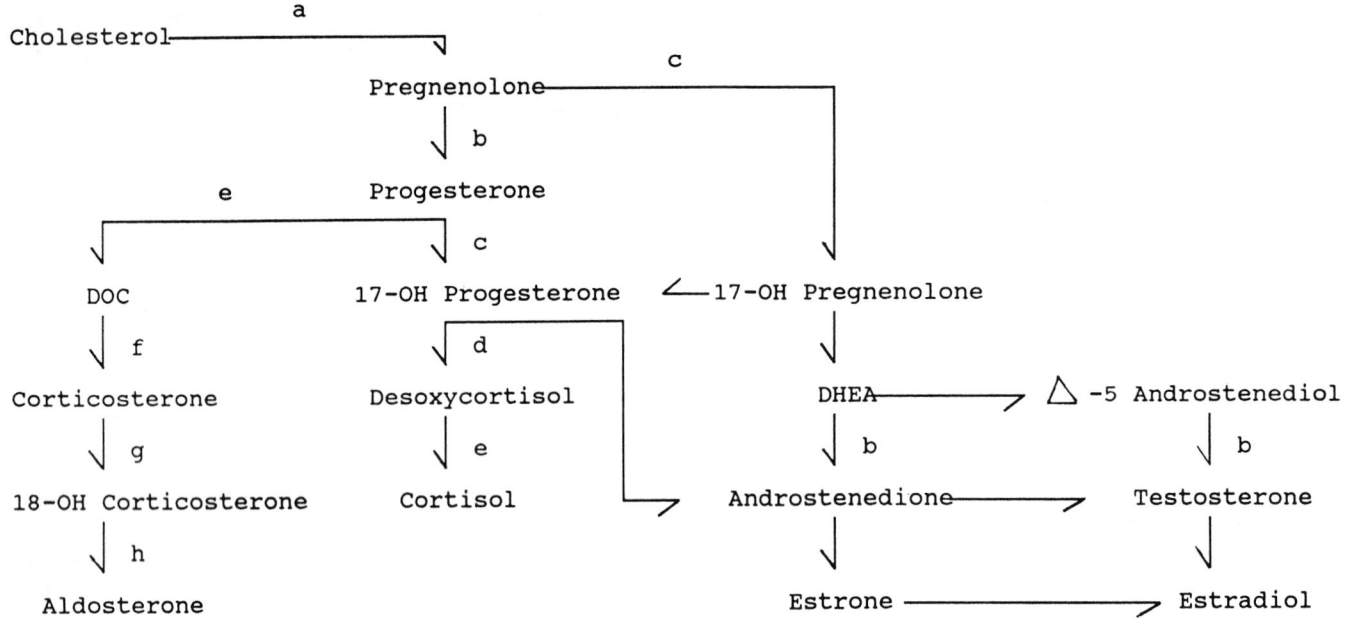

Figure 15.1. Adrenal corticosteroid synthesis. *a*, Cholesterol side-chain cleavage; *b*, 3-β-hydroxysteroid dehydrogenease; *c*, 17-α-hydroxylase; *d*, 21 hydroxylase; *e*, 11-β-hydroxylase; *f*, hy-droxylase; *g*, corticosterone methyl oxidase; *h*, 18-OH dehydro-genase. *DHEA*, dehydroepiandrosterone; *DOC*, 11-desoxycor-ticosterone.

Table 15.1.
Conditions That Stimulate ACTH and Cortisol Secretion[a]

Cold exposure	Hypoglycemia
Pain	Infection
Anxiety	Trauma
Hemorrhage	Toxins
Exercise	Depression
Starvation	Alcoholism

[a] Adapted from Tepperman J, Tepperman HM, ACTH and adrenal glucocorticoids. In Tepperman J, Tepperman HM: Metabolic and Endocrine Physiology. Chicago, Year Book Publishers, 1987, p 183.

HYPOTHALAMIC-PITUITARY-ADRENAL FEEDBACK SYSTEM

For cortisol to be produced and released into plasma by the adrenal cortex during stress, plasma ACTH must be increased. ACTH, also called corticotropin or adrenocor-ticotropin, is secreted by the anterior pituitary gland under the regulatory control of corticotropin-releasing factor (CRF), which is secreted by the hypothalamus. Cate-cholamines and vasopressin have also been shown to stim-ulate the release of ACTH (1). In stressful situations (Table 15.1), ACTH secretion increases to many times the basal rate, which increases cortisol production and secretion.

The major effect of ACTH on cortisol production is to stimulate the conversion of cholesterol to pregnenolone.

This is accomplished by an increase in cholesterol binding to mitochondrial cytochrome P-450 in adrenal cortex cells. Cytochrome P-450 catalyzes the conversion of this rate-limiting step in steroid hormone production. Once cho-lesterol is converted to pregnenolone, further enzyme-mediated conversions occur before the adrenocortical hor-mones are produced (Fig. 15-1).

As cortisol levels increase in response to ACTH stim-ulation, CRF release from the hypothalamus is stopped. The decrease in CRF leads to a reduction in further ACTH and cortisol secretion. This complete chain of events is called the hypothalamic-pituitary-adrenal axis.

CIRCADIAN RHYTHM

In addition to stress-induced release of cortisol, another factor influences cortisol secretion—the daily circadian rhythm. The circadian, or diurnal, rhythm is the cyclic release of cortisol occurring throughout a 24-hour period as a result of intrinsic endocrine function.

By the age of 3 years an individual's circadian rhythm is usually established. Minimal secretion of cortisol occurs just before and in the initial hours of sleep, while maximal secretion of cortisol occurs just before and in the initial hours of wakefulness (Fig. 15.2). During the rest of the day intermittent secretion of cortisol occurs. This cyclic pattern is influenced most by feeding patterns, but it can also be affected by changes in sleep patterns of at least 2 to 3 weeks duration (3).

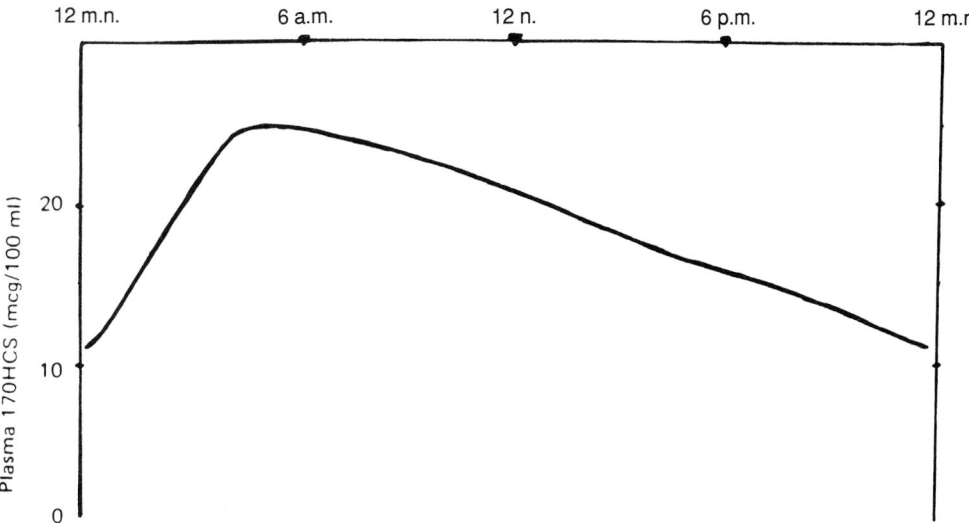

Figure 15.2. Diurnal variation in plasma cortisol. (Reprinted with permission from Pincus G, Nakao T, Tait JF, (eds): Symposium on the Dynamics of Steroid Hormones. New York, Academic Press, 1965, p 387.)

CORTISOL PHARMACOKINETICS

As described, serum levels of cortisol vary throughout the day because of the circadian rhythm and a variety of stresses. The basal secretion of cortisol by the adrenal cortex ranges from 8 to 37.5 mg/day in an unstressed individual, and can be as high as 200 to 500 mg/day when stress is present (3, 4).

When a serum level of cortisol is measured in an individual patient, it is compared with what would be considered a normal level at that particular time during the circadian rhythm. Highest serum cortisol levels occur early in the morning (around 0800) in reaction to peak ACTH levels a few hours earlier. Morning serum cortisol levels are normally within the range of 83 to 552 nmol/liter (3 to 20 μg/dl) when measured by radioimmunoassay (RIA) using a competitive-protein-binding technique (3). When using a fluorimetric assay, the slightly higher range of 138 to 690 nmol/liter (5 to 25 μg/dl) is considered normal (3). Both serum cortisol and ACTH levels decrease progressively throughout the day, with a nadir around 2000 to 2400. The serum cortisol level at 2000 is usually one-half to one-third the 0800 level, and always less than 276 nmol/liter (10 μg/dl) (5). Cortisol is 90% protein-bound in the serum, with 75% bound to corticosteroid-binding-globulin (CBG), also known as transcortin, and 15% bound to serum albumin. Unbound cortisol is the active component that provides feedback to the HPA system and regulates the secretion of ACTH.

Cortisol clearance occurs in the liver, where it is conjugated with glucuronide or sulfate groups (3). This increases the water solubility of the compound, necessary for renal excretion. The plasma half-life of cortisol is 70 to 90 min, with less than 1% of unchanged cortisol excreted by the kidneys over 24 hr. Clearance of cortisol is decreased in liver disease, hypothyroidism, starvation, pregnancy, infancy, and old age. Clearance is increased in high-estrogen states, neonates, and severe chronic illness. Medications that induce hepatic microsomal enzymes also increase cortisol clearance. These medications include phenytoin, phenobarbital, secobarbital, aminoglutethimide, and rifampin. On the other hand, cortisol clearance is decreased by ketoconazole, an hepatic enzyme inhibitor.

When analyzing serum cortisol levels, the RIA assay is preferred over the fluorimetric assay because the fluorimetric assay produces false serum cortisol results with concurrent use of certain medications (spironolactone, quinacrine, niacin, quinidine, benzyl alcohol), in uremia, and in hyperbilirubinemia (3, 5). Although medications do not interfere with the RIA method, false serum cortisol results may occur with pregnancy, congenital adrenal hyperplasia, and adrenal cancer.

CUSHING'S SYNDROME
Definition and Etiology

Cushing's syndrome is the clinical manifestation of a chronic and inappropriate elevation of serum cortisol levels. The syndrome was first described by Harvey Cushing in 1932 in the Johns Hopkins Medical Journal (6). Dr. Cushing noted that 12 patients with adenomas of the pituitary gland had similar clinical findings: increased adipose tissue in the face, neck, and trunk; hypertrichosis in females and prepubertal males; amenorrhea; striae; hypertension; easy fatiguability; weakness; and, spinal deformities. Cushing was unable to identify the underlying hormonal imbalance and multiple etiologies of hypercortisolism. This was accomplished later by other endocrinologists who expanded on Cushing's original findings.

Ever since the corticosteroids have been available for therapeutic use, the primary cause of Cushing's syndrome has been iatrogenic. However, spontaneous Cushing's syndrome has many different etiologies, nearly all of which result in excess cortisol secretion by the adrenal gland.

The causes of cortisol hypersecretion are classified as either ACTH-dependent or ACTH-independent (Fig. 15-3). ACTH-dependent etiologies, based on a chronic hypersecretion of ACTH, account for approximately 83% of all cases of spontaneous Cushing's syndrome. Elevated ACTH levels lead to overstimulation of the adrenal zona fasciculata and zona reticularis, and therefore, increased secretion of cortisol and androgens. ACTH-dependent causes include:

1. Pituitary microadenomas resulting in an increased release of ACTH (Cushing's disease);
2. Ectopic, malignant ACTH-secreting tumors (e.g., oat cell carcinoma of the lung, islet cell tumor, thymoma and bronchial adenoma);
3. Ectopic CRF-secreting tumors.

Of these etiologies, only Cushing's disease is responsive to the HPA feedback system (7).

ACTH-independent etiologies involve cortisol-secreting tumors, which lead to elevated serum cortisol levels and secondarily suppressed ACTH release. Accounting for less than 20% of patients with Cushing's syndrome, ACTH-independent causes include

1. Nodular hyperplasia of the adrenal cortex,
2. Adrenal cortical tumors;
3. Ectopic production of cortisol.

The overall incidence of Cushing's syndrome is only 1 in 1000, with females at a 3.5 times higher risk than males, and having a propensity to developing pituitary microadenomas (Cushing's disease) as the cause of Cushing's syndrome. Over 50% of people who develop spontaneous Cushing's syndrome are between 20 and 40 years of age. The 5-year mortality rate for untreated Cushing's syndrome exceeds 50%.

Clinical Manifestations

The clinical manifestations of Cushing's syndrome are usually insidious in onset and encompass many different organ

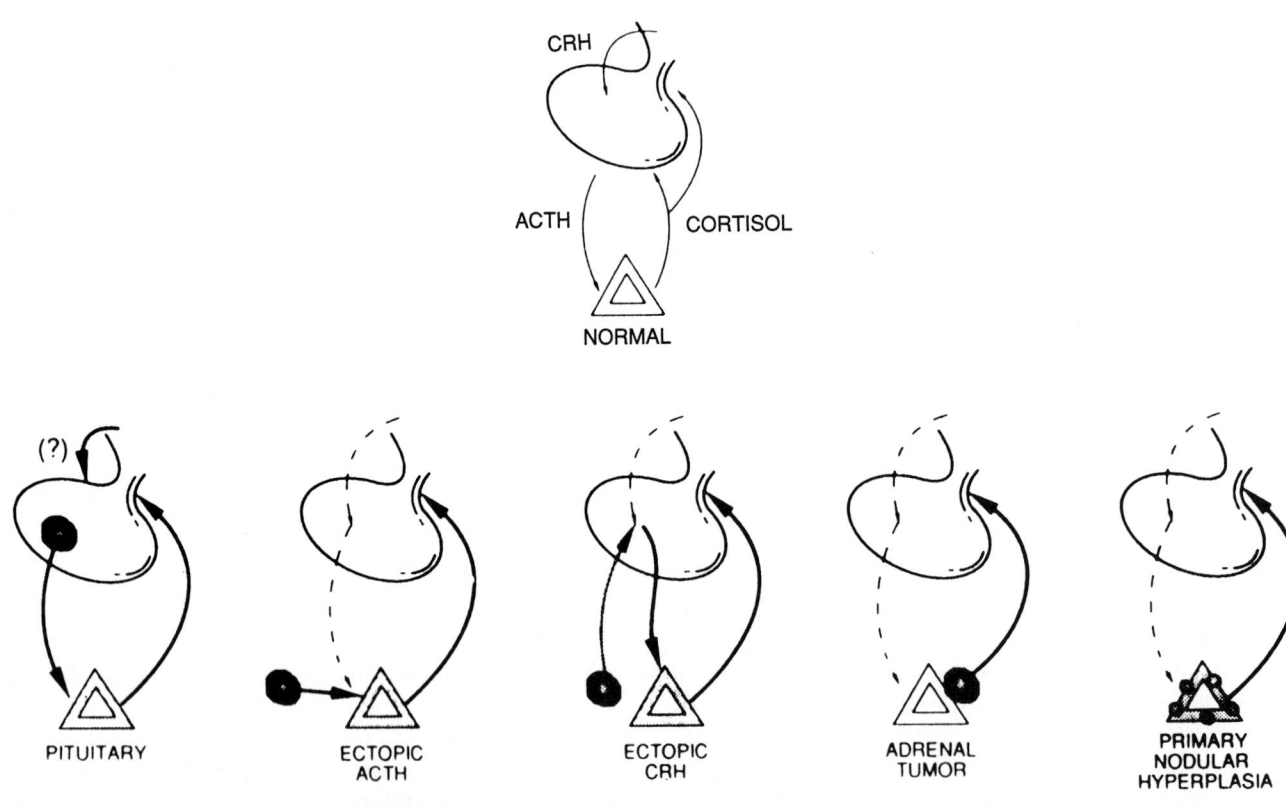

Figure 15.3.   Etiologies of Cushing's syndrome. (Reprinted with permission from Schteingart DE: Cushing's syndrome. Endocrinol Metab Clin North Am 18:311–338, 1989.)

Table 15.2.
Presenting Signs and Symptoms in Cushing's Syndrome

Sign or Symptom	(N = 601) %	(N = 50) %
Obesity	88	84
Generalized		60
Truncal		40
Moonface	75	84
Menstrual irregularities	60	76
Muscular weakness	61	58
Bruising	42	36
Psychological difficulties	42	
Acne	45	
Hirsutism	65	82
Backache	40	
Striae		52
Osteoporosis on x-ray		46
Hypertension		
BP 140/90		72
BP 100 diastolic		54
Renal calculi		16
Cholelithiasis		10

Reprinted with permission from Kishi DT, Romac DR, Adrenocortical dysfunction. In Herfindal ET, Gourley DR, Hart LL: Clianical Pharmacy and Therapeutics, Baltimore, William & Wilkins, 1988, p 114.

systems (Table 15.2). Often the clinical signs are vague, and the patient will see many different specialists before the syndrome is finally diagnosed.

An overall change in appearance and increased total body fat are classic initial findings. Obesity is common, and fat is redistributed to central areas of the body, which results in truncal or centripetal obesity with a protuberant abdomen and wasted extremities. Rounding of the face ("moon facies") and increased dorsicervical fat pads ("buffalo hump") are also classic findings.

The skin of a patient with Cushing's syndrome is fine and translucent, because of atrophy of the epidermal layer and connective tissue beneath it. Facial plethora, vascular striae, easy bruising, and poor wound healing are often present. Hyperpigmentation from the stimulatory action of cortisol on melanocytes may be seen. The growth of fine lanugo facial hair is also a common result of cortisol hypersecretion.

An increase in androgen levels may accompany hypercortisolism. This is manifested in female patients as the abnormal growth of body hair (hirsutism). Androgen excess also contributes to acne, seborrhea, and amenorrhea in women. Male patients with Cushing's syndrome experience a decrease in libido, a decrease in body hair, and testicular atrophy.

Muscle wasting and myopathy are common in Cushing's syndrome because of the catabolic effects of cortisol on muscle tissue. Proximal muscle weakness, primarily of the lower extremities, is often exhibited as difficulty in climbing stairs and standing up from a sitting position.

Hypercortisolism has many effects on the metabolic functions of bone. Inhibition of osteoblasts by cortisol may cause osteopenia and ultimately osteoporosis (8). Hypercalciuria is also promoted by increased cortisol levels and frequently results in kidney stone formation. In adults, bone pain and fractures are commonly seen as a result of hypercortisolism. Children with Cushing's syndrome have premature closure of the long bone epiphyses, leading to stunted growth and short stature.

Diastolic hypertension is another frequent finding in Cushing's syndrome. The elevated blood pressure is thought to result from mineralocorticoid excess or a direct inhibitory effect of cortisol on prostacyclin, a potent vasodilator (8). Mineralocorticoid excess also contributes to the hypokalemia, hypernatremia, and edema seen in Cushing's syndrome.

Psychiatric disturbances are common in patients with Cushing's syndrome. Manifestations range from mild irritability to mania, depression, and suicide. Common symptoms include mood lability, euphoria, increased anxiety, crying, insomnia, and decreases in memory and concentration.

Immunosuppression occurs with hypercortisolism. This leads to a predisposition for bacterial and opportunistic infections ranging in severity from fungal skin infections to *Pneumocystis carinii* pneumonia and cryptococcal meningitis. These complications contribute significantly to the morbidity of Cushing's syndrome. Immunosuppression also results in anergic responses to skin tests in patients with Cushing's syndrome.

Certain laboratory test findings are specific to patients with Cushing's syndrome. Electrolyte abnormalities include hypokalemia and alkalosis. Clinically unimportant hypernatremia may be found. Renal function tests may be altered secondary to nephrocalcinosis, hypertension, or repeated infections. Hypercalciuria and hypophosphatemia are common. Hyperglycemia and glycosuria are frequent. Plasma lipoproteins and cholesterol levels are often elevated. Patients may have elevated hemoglobin, hematocrit, and red blood cell counts (polycythemia). The total white blood cell count may be elevated, with granulocytosis and lymphopenia.

Diagnosis

A preliminary clinical diagnosis of Cushing's syndrome must be evaluated through various laboratory tests. These are referred to as "dynamic" tests because they test the functional status of the HPA system. Initial tests determine the presence of Cushing's syndrome, and further tests determine the underlying etiology. An algorithm for the diagnosis of Cushing's syndrome can be found in Figure 15.4.

SCREENING TESTS

Screening tests for Cushing's syndrome include measurement of serum cortisol levels and 24-hr urinary free cortisol.

Sequential serum cortisol levels are often determined in patients with suspected Cushing's syndrome. These patients typically demonstrate little or no fluctuation in a constantly normal or elevated serum cortisol level. This lack of diurnal variation usually occurs months or years before frank elevation of serum cortisol levels is observed. However, since cortisol is highly bound to corticosteroid-binding globulin (CBG) in the serum, the measurement of serum cortisol levels may lead to misleading and false-positive results in patients with elevated CBG levels. This may occur in pregnancy, diabetes mellitus, hyperthyroidism, estrogen therapy, and obesity (10). In any case, serum cortisol levels are not diagnostic in up to 30% of patients with Cushing's syndrome and are rarely used for this purpose today.

On the other hand, 24-hr urinary free cortisol is consistently elevated in Cushing's syndrome. This test measures unbound cortisol excreted by the kidney over a 24-hr period, which is proportional to the unbound fraction of cortisol in the plasma. Normal basal urinary free cortisol ranges from 20 to 100 µg/24 hr, and when it is above 100 to 125 µg/24 hr, Cushing's syndrome is likely (11). The sensitivity and specificity of this test in identifying true hypercortisolism is close to 96% (12). False-positive results are seen in patients under stress, with endogenous depression, or receiving exogenous hydrocortisone or cortisone acetate (12, 13).

The 24-hr urinary free cortisol test has replaced a previous urine test that measured the glucocorticoid metabolite, 17-hydroxycorticosteroid (17-OHCS). The urine test for 17-OHCS was associated with a higher false-positive rate than is urinary free cortisol, particularly in obese patients (8, 11). Currently, the urinary free cortisol test is considered the best screening test for Cushing's syndrome.

DEXAMETHASONE SUPPRESSION TESTS

After a screening test for hypercortisolism gives positive results, a dexamethasone suppression test (DST) is employed as the next step in the diagnosis of Cushing's syndrome. Dexamethasone, when administered exogenously, inhibits ACTH secretion and suppresses cortisol serum levels in a normal individual. However, dexamethasone does not interfere with laboratory readings of serum cortisol. For this reason, dexamethasone is preferred over other glucocorticoids when testing the HPA feedback system.

Three DSTs are commonly used:

1. the overnight test (which may also be used as a screening test);
2. the low-dose 2-day test;
3. the high-dose 2-day test.

Usually two or all three of these tests are used in succession.

For the overnight test the patient takes 1 mg of dexamethasone at 2300, with serum cortisol measured at 0800 the next day. Normal suppression of the HPA feedback system produces a morning cortisol level under 138 nmol/liter (5 µg/dl) (8, 11). If the serum cortisol level is higher or if the results are in question, the suppression tests are continued.

For the 2-day low-dose DST the patient is administered 0.5 mg dexamethasone orally every 6 hours for 2 days (eight doses). Serum cortisol level is checked at 0800 on the third day. A normal response results in a morning cortisol suppression to less than 138 nmol/liter (5 µg/dl). If the serum cortisol level is elevated, then Cushing's syndrome is likely and the third DST is conducted.

During the 2-day high-dose DST the patient takes 2 mg of dexamethasone orally every 6 hours for 2 days (eight doses). Originally, the high-dose DST was conducted by comparing two 24-hr urine collections measuring the cortisol metabolite 17-OHCS. Currently, this test is performed by comparing serum cortisol levels. The serum cortisol level is measured as a baseline prior to dexamethasone administration and at 1600 on the second day (8, 14) or at 0800 on the third day (15). At this point, if the serum cortisol level is less than 138 nmol/liter (5 µg/dl), or 50% of the baseline value, then a presumptive diagnosis of pituitary microadenoma (Cushing's disease) is made (8). This is because pituitary microadenomas are HPA-responsive at very high glucocorticoid serum levels. Conversely, if the serum cortisol level is greater than 138 nmol/liter (5 µg/dl), then Cushing's syndrome is most likely due to an ACTH-independent etiology or to ectopic ACTH production (8).

A variation on this high-dose 2-day DST was described by Tyrrell et al. in 1986 (15). Their high-dose DST is conducted by obtaining a baseline serum cortisol at 0800, administering a single dose of dexamethasone 8 mg orally at 2300, and measuring serum cortisol at 0800 the next day. The predictive power of this test in diagnosing the etiology of Cushing's syndrome is similar to that of the high-dose 2-day DST.

False-positive results are common in the DST and occur most often with obesity or when CBG levels are elevated by high-estrogen states seen with pregnancy or oral contraceptive use. False-positive results also occur

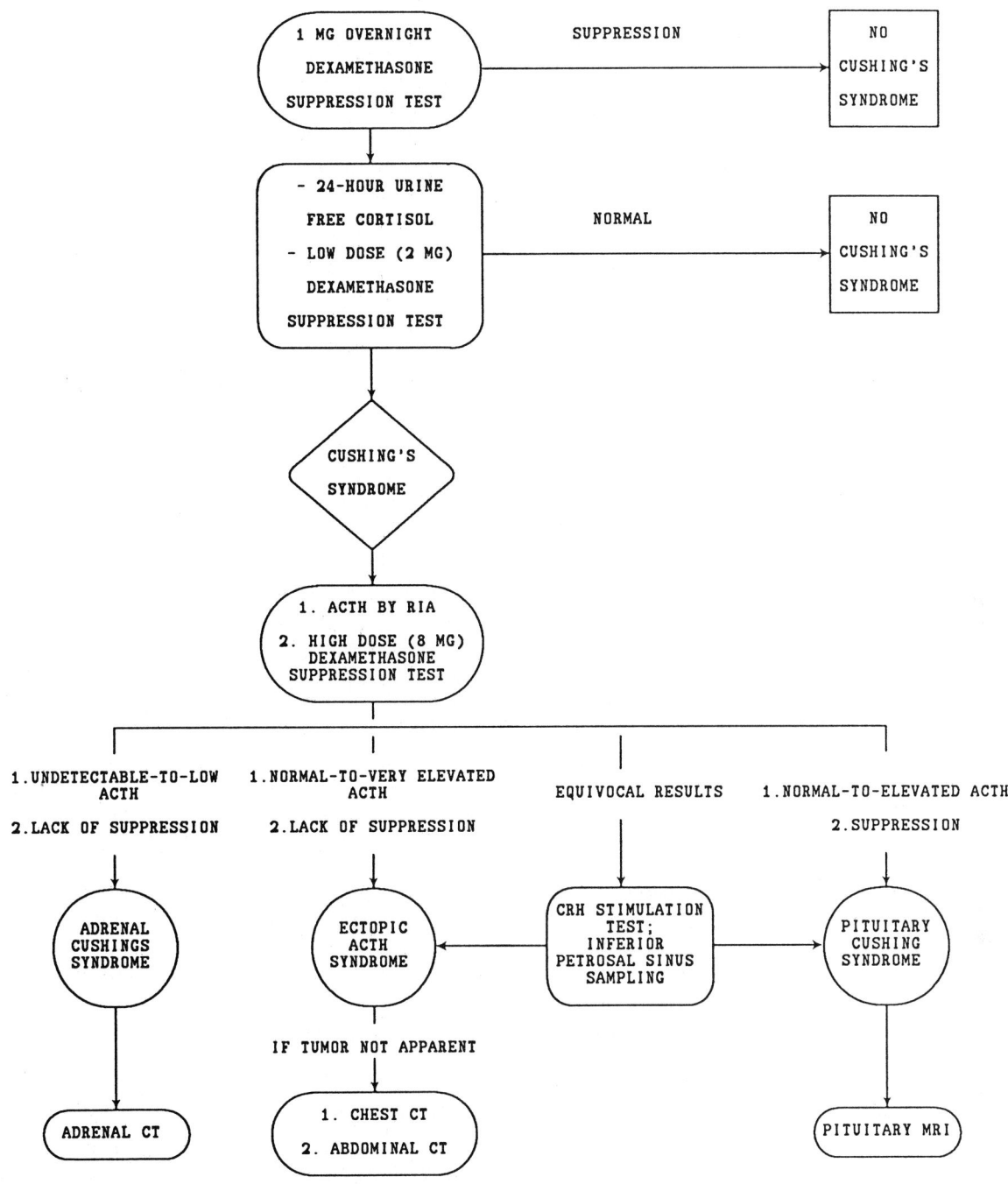

Figure 15.4. An algorithm for the diagnosis of Cushing's syndrome. (Adapted from Kaye TB, Crapo L: The Cushing's syndrome: an update on diagnostic tests. Ann Intern Med 112:434–444, 1990, with permission.)

when serum cortisol levels are elevated by stresses, such as depression, anxiety, alcohol abuse, and uremia (11). In addition, false positives can occur if the metabolism of dexamethasone is increased by hepatic microsomal enzyme inducers such as phenytoin or phenobarbital. (See Table 15.3 for a complete list of drug interactions with glucocorticoids.)

LOCALIZATION TESTS

After a diagnosis of Cushing's syndrome is made, localization studies are conducted to further determine the etiology of the syndrome and the treatment. If a pituitary source is suspected (e.g., Cushing's disease) a CAT (computerized axial tomography) scan or MR (magnetic resonance) scan of the brain is conducted (7, 9, 18).

Table 15.3.
Drug Interactions with Glucocorticoids

Increased metabolism of glucocorticoids
  Barbiturates, phenytoin, rifampin, carbamazepine, aminoglutethimide, ketoconazole
Decreased metabolism of glucocorticoids
  Cyclosporine, troleandomycin, erythromycin, estrogens, oral contraceptives, ketoconazole
Exacerbation of glucocorticoid-induced hypokalemia
  Amphotericin B, ethacrynic acid, furosemide, hydrochlorothiazide
Exacerbation of glucocorticoid-induced gastritis
  Aspirin, indomethacin, other nonsteroidal antiinflammatory agents, alcohol
Glucocorticoid-induced reduction in efficacy
  Insulin, oral antidiabetic agents, vaccines, warfarin, salicylates

Adapted from Hansten PD, Horn JR: Drug Interactions, ed. 6; Philadelphia, Lea & Febiger, 1989; and Tatro DS: Drug Interaction Facts; St. Louis, JB Lippincott, 1990.

Measurement of serum ACTH levels by RIA technology will help determine whether ACTH is being secreted at a rate that is higher than normal. Plasma ACTH normally ranges between 4 and 22 pmol/liter (20 to 100 pg/ml) in the morning (5). With Cushing's syndrome due to adrenal tumors, ACTH is suppressed to less than 4 pmol/liter (20 pg/ml). With Cushing's disease due to pituitary microadenomas, plasma ACTH is normal or increased slightly to 9 to 44 pmol/liter (40 to 200 pg/ml). Ectopic ACTH syndromes lead to highly elevated ACTH levels of 22 to 440 pmol/liter (100 to 2000 pg/ml) (5).

Although measurement of plasma ACTH provides valuable information in the diagnosis of Cushing's syndrome, many problems accompany this test. ACTH levels vary significantly during the day, and ACTH has a very short half-life in the serum (approximately 15 to 25 min). In addition, ACTH samples are very unstable and require special handling. Samples should be drawn into prechilled tubes, immediately put on ice, and spun down as soon as they are removed from the ice. Finally, ACTH assays are not available at many institutions.

If an adrenal source of Cushing's syndrome is suspected, a CAT scan of the abdomen should be conducted to rule out adrenal adenoma or carcinoma. Alternatively, an adrenal scan using a radioiodinated contrast agent can be used.

A new test, not yet widely available, is the synthetic ovine CRH stimulation test (8, 9, 11). This test can be used to diagnose pituitary microadenomas (Cushing's disease) as the underlying cause of hypercortisolism. To conduct this test, 1 μg/kg or 100 μg of CRH is administered. Blood is drawn at baseline and at 15, 30, 60, 90, and 120 minutes after administration of CRH to measure both ACTH and serum cortisol levels. In Cushing's disease (pituitary microadenoma), CRH administration elicits an increased release of ACTH and cortisol. ACTH is usually increased by 50% or more, and cortisol is increased by 20% or more. With other etiologies, ACTH levels show no response to CRH administration, either because ACTH is maximally suppressed (e.g., primary adrenal tumors) or because of an ectopic ACTH syndrome. The CRH stimulation test is, therefore, another means of diagnosing Cushing's syndrome due to a pituitary cause.

Surgical Treatment

The treatment of Cushing's syndrome depends upon the underlying etiology, and in most cases, surgery is the treatment of choice. Where a pituitary microadenoma is the cause, microsurgery with a transphenoidal approach is used. This usually successfully obliterates ACTH hypersecretion. However, in some situations pituitary irradiation may be necessary, in which case remission is delayed for up to 6 to 18 months (11).

With benign tumors such as adrenal adenoma or adrenocortical nodular hyperplasia, unilateral adrenalectomy is the primary treatment. Malignant adrenal carcinoma and ectopic ACTH-producing tumors are treated by surgical resection whenever possible. If metastases are present, palliative treatment with steroid-inhibiting medications (e.g., ketoconazole, mitotane) will decrease the cushingoid symptoms and may even decrease tumor size. However, medical treatment has not been shown to prolong survival in these patients.

In rare cases bilateral adrenalectomy is performed. However, this is a last resort, since both adrenal cortices are removed and the patient will require replacement therapy permanently.

In all cases where surgery is used to remove the cause of hypercortisolism, high-dose glucocorticoid therapy is needed in the immediate postoperative period, usually with a rapid taper (e.g., total course of less than 10 days) once the patient is stabilized. This ensures adequate replacement while the HPA feedback system is undergoing recovery.

Medical Treatment

Medical treatment of Cushing's syndrome is reserved for intractable cases or situations with a delay in surgery. Two types of medications are used:

1. Medications that inhibit the pituitary secretion of ACTH;
2. Medications that inhibit the adrenocortical secretion of cortisol.

ACTH-dependent syndromes benefit most from the first type of medication, which includes cyproheptadine and bromocriptine. The second type of medication includes aminoglutethimide, metyrapone, ketoconazole, and mitotane. Table 15.4 provides a summary of medications used in the treatment of Cushing's syndrome.

Table 15.4.
Medications Used to Treat Cushing's Syndrome

Name	Mechanism	Dose[a]	Response Time	HC[b] Replacement	Adverse Effects
Cyproheptadine	Inhibits ACTH secretion	Initially: 8 mg p.o. q.d. MD: up to 24 mg p.o. q.d.	4–6 weeks	Not necessary	Appetite stimulation, weight gain, sedation
Bromocriptine	Inhibits ACTH secretion	10–20 mg/day	NA[c]	NA	Nausea, hypotension, headaches
Aminoglutethimide	Inhibits cortisol synthesis by blocking cholesterol conversion to pregnenolone	Initially: 250 mg p.o. q.i.d. MD: 500–2000 mg/day divided q.i.d.	NA	Necessary	Drowsiness, lethargy, reversible blood dyscrasias, nausea, anorexia, dizziness, headaches, skin rash, hypotension, tachycardia
Metyrapone	Inhibits cortisol by blocking final step in cortisol synthesis	Initially: 250 mg p.o. b.i.d. MD: up to 1000 mg p.o. q.i.d.	4 months	Necessary	Dizziness, sedation, skin rash, hirsutism, hypertension
Mitotane	Destruction of adrenocortical cells that synthesize cortisol	Initially: 500 mg p.o. b.i.d. MD: 3–12 g/day divided t.i.d.-q.i.d. (doses can be tapered with long-term treatment)	2 weeks–6 months	Necessary	Anorexia, nausea, vomiting, diarrhea, lethargy, impaired memory, hepatotoxicity
Ketoconazole	Inhibits cortisol synthesis by blocking cholesterol conversion to pregnenolone	Initially: 800–1200 mg/day MD: 600–800 mg/day	4–6 weeks	Not necessary	Nausea, vomiting, fatigue, pruritis, gynecomastia, hepatotoxicity

[a] MD = maintenance dose
[b] HC = hydrocortisone.
[c] NA = information not available.

CYPROHEPTADINE

Cyproheptadine (Periactin), an antihistamine and serotonin-antagonist, was first reported in 1975 by Krieger et al. to be effective in the treatment of Cushing's disease in three patients (19). After 4 to 6 weeks of therapy each patient had a marked improvement in cushingoid symptoms, as well as a normalization of response to a low-dose DST. However, serum cortisol levels did not revert to a normal circadian rhythm. Subsequent reports have been contradictory about the efficacy of cyproheptadine in Cushing's syndrome (20, 21). Krieger reviewed cyproheptadine treatment in 1976 and reported a 60% success rate (22).

The mechanism of action of cyproheptadine is thought to be an antiserotonin effect on the hypothalamus, resulting in the inhibition of ACTH secretion (7). A maximum dose of 24 mg/day is used, with a decrease in cushingoid manifestations as early as a month after beginning treatment. The clinical effects usually last as long as the medication is continued. Adverse effects are common and include increased appetite, weight gain, and sedation.

BROMOCRIPTINE

Bromocriptine (Parlodel), an ergot alkaloid derivative, is a dopamine receptor agonist and prolactin inhibitor that has been used experimentally to induce a temporary remission of ACTH-dependent Cushing's syndrome (23, 24). Bromocriptine is FDA-approved for use in syndromes associated with excess prolactin secretion from the anterior pituitary, such as galactorrhea, amenorrhea, and female infertility. It has also been used to decrease the tumor size of pituitary adenomas. In Cushing's syndrome, bromocriptine may decrease excess ACTH secretion from pituitary microadenomas, but it is inconsistently effective.

Large doses of 10 to 20 mg/day of bromocriptine have been used in Cushing's syndrome. These are higher than the doses used to treat elevated prolactin levels (7.5 to 10 mg/day). When treating Cushing's syndrome, adverse effects included nausea in 50% of patients, headaches, and hypotension during the first few days of treatment.

At this time, the use of bromocriptine in Cushing's syndrome must be evaluated further before it can be generally recommended.

AMINOGLUTETHIMIDE

Aminoglutethimide (Cytadren) was originally marketed as an anticonvulsant when it was noted to significantly inhibit the synthesis of cortisol, aldosterone, and estrogens. Since then it has been used to treat Cushing's syndrome (ACTH-dependent) and as a secondary agent in estrogen-receptor-positive breast cancer.

In Cushing's syndrome, aminoglutethimide acts by blocking the first step in the synthesis of cortisol—the conversion of cholesterol to pregnenolone. The effects of aminoglutethimide are short-lived, however, due to a compensatory rise in ACTH levels. The pituitary increases the output of ACTH in response to low cortisol levels, which overrides the effect of aminoglutethimide to decrease cortisol output. The result is a rebound in cortisol synthesis and secretion, which can occur as early as a few days after treatment initiation.

Clinical effects of aminoglutethimide are usually longer-acting in patients with cortisol-secreting adrenal carcinoma or when used concomitantly with metyrapone or pituitary irradiation (25). Because of the complete cessation of cortisol synthesis, exogeneous steroid replacement therapy with hydrocortisone should be prescribed to prevent adrenocortical insufficiency.

Doses of aminoglutethimide in Cushing's syndrome are usually 500 to 2000 mg per day. There are many adverse effects with aminoglutethimide including drowsiness, lethargy, reversible blood dyscrasias (e.g., neutropenia, aplastic anemia), nausea, anorexia, dizziness, headaches, hypotension, and tachycardia. Skin rashes are common and will usually abate over time if therapy is continued. Aminoglutethimide has been shown to increase the hepatic metabolism of dexamethasone and warfarin, but not hydrocortisone.

METYRAPONE

Metyrapone (Metopirone) is an 11-β-hydroxylase inhibitor that blocks the final step in the adrenal synthesis of cortisol. In the past, metyrapone was used in Cushing's syndrome as a testing agent, to differentiate pituitary from adrenal causes. More recently it has been recommended for the treatment of Cushing's syndrome as an adjunctive agent in combination with aminoglutethimide (26). Serum ACTH levels usually increase during metyrapone treatment, but unlike the situation with aminoglutethimide, these levels are insufficient to overcome the adrenal blockade.

The dosing range of metyrapone is 250 mg orally twice a day up to 1000 mg orally four times a day. Because of its high cost, it is usually prescribed for short-term treatment only. Adverse effects are primarily gastrointestinal, but also commonly include dizziness, hypotension, sedation, and skin rash. Because of the accumulation of adrenal androgens and mineralocorticoid precursors with metyrapone, adverse effects may also include hirsutism in women and hypertension.

MITOTANE

Mitotane (o,p-DDD, Lysodren) is an antineoplastic agent that was first used to treat adrenal carcinoma, and later used for Cushing's syndrome by Southern et al. in 1961 (27). It acts by inhibiting cortisol synthesis and also destroys the adrenocortical cells that secrete cortisol. The zona reticularis is most sensitive to the action of mitotane and the zona glomerulosa is least sensitive (7, 11, 27). Mitotane also partially suppresses ACTH levels (28), and it can be used alone or in conjunction with pituitary irradiation.

The usual dose of mitotane is 3 to 12 g/day orally, in 3 or 4 divided doses. Treatment is initiated with a dose of 500 mg orally twice a day and increased to 1 g orally four times a day, as required to suppress cortisol levels. Response to treatment occurs within 4 to 12 months. In most patients, treatment must be continued on a long-term basis or combined with pituitary irradiation because of a high rate of relapse with a single treatment period (29). Doses can be tapered to as low as 500 mg orally twice weekly and continue to maintain a state of remission (28). Hydrocortisone replacement therapy should be initiated within 2 to 4 weeks of mitotane therapy and should also include replacement mineralocorticoid therapy (29).

The most common adverse effects of mitotane include anorexia, nausea, lethargy, and impaired memory. Hepatotoxic effects may lead to increased serum alkaline phosphatase levels. Decreased serum thyroxine levels may also occur, as a function of decreased plasma binding. Intolerable adverse effects can be managed by discontinuing the medication for a few days and restarting at a lower dose.

KETOCONAZOLE

Ketoconazole (Nizoral) is an imidazole derivative used primarily as an antifungal agent. It inhibits the synthesis of ergosterol in fungi and cholesterol in mammalian cell walls.

At high doses, ketoconazole also inhibits adrenocortical cytochrome P-450 (which is where cholesterol side-chain cleavage occurs) blocking the formation of pregnenolone and further cortisol precursors (7, 30). By this mechanism, ketoconazole has been discovered to be a potent, but reversible, inhibitor of abnormal adrenal cortisol synthesis.

Patients with Cushing's syndrome have responded to high-dose ketoconazole treatment within 4 to 6 weeks of treatment (7, 31). In addition, when doses are managed properly, some synthesis of cortisol still occurs, which makes replacement hydrocortisone unnecessary (30, 31). Usual initial doses are 800 to 1200 mg/day, with maintenance doses slightly lower, at 600 to 800 mg/day.

Adverse effects include nausea, vomiting, fatigue, pruritus, gynecomastia in males, and hepatotoxicity. The use of ketoconazole warrants regular monitoring of liver function tests, and the drug should be discontinued if transaminase abnormalities persist or worsen (32). Ketoconazole is highly bound to plasma proteins and is metabolized by hepatic microsomal enzymes.

Many drug interactions with ketoconazole have been identified. Ketoconazole requires an acidic gastric environment for optimal absorption. Antacids and cimetidine decrease the absorption of ketoconazole, and their administration should be separated by at least 2 hours. By another mechanism, isoniazid combined with rifampin has been shown to decrease ketoconazole levels during simultaneous administration of all three medications. This decrease in ketoconazole levels is thought to be due to increased hepatic metabolism. For this reason, it is recommended that ketoconazole be administered 8 to 12 hours after isoniazid and rifampin.

Due to ketoconazole-induced hepatic enzyme inhibition, cyclosporine serum levels have been shown to increase when given with ketoconazole. An increase in warfarin activity may also be seen with ketoconazole therapy, because of plasma protein binding displacement. When ketoconazole is used concomitantly with cyclosporine or warfarin, monitoring parameters of these medications (i.e., cyclosporine levels, serum creatinine levels, and prothrombin times with warfarin) should be followed closely.

Conclusion

Cushing's syndrome can lead to significant morbidity and early mortality if left untreated. Cushing's syndrome is most commonly caused by excess administration of exogenous corticosteroids. Endogenous, or spontaneous, Cushing's syndrome is usually of pituitary origin, but it may also be due to an ectopic or adrenal tumor. Irrespective of the cause, hypercortisolism leads to a constellation of symptoms and the 5-7 year mortality rate for untreated Cushing's syndrome is over 50%. Infections and cardiovascular complications (e.g., stroke, myocardial infarction, congestive heart failure) are usual causes of death in patients with untreated hypercortisolism.

Surgical removal of the cause of hypercortisolism, without removing the adrenal glands themselves, is the primary treatment. As a temporary measure, medical treatment with or without irradiation can be palliative. When medical treatment is used, cyproheptadine is the medication of choice in treating ACTH-dependent etiologies. In ACTH-independent etiologies, mitotane remains the preferred agent, however ketoconazole also provides effective treatment and does not require glucocorticoid replacement. The use of aminoglutethimide in conjunction with metyrapone should be reserved for the short-term only.

Although the mortality rate for patients with treated Cushing's syndrome still remains high at four times that of the normal population, early intervention and treatment can improve the morbidity and prognosis for these patients.

ADDISON'S DISEASE
Definition and Etiology

Adrenocortical insufficiency is an insidious illness that can lead to rapid mortality if untreated. It results from primary or secondary causes. Primary adrenocortical insufficiency, also known as Addison's disease, results from destruction of the adrenal cortex. Secondary adrenocortical insufficiency is due to deficient pituitary ACTH secretion causing atrophy of the adrenal cortex.

Tuberculosis used to be the most frequent cause of Addison's disease, but it is much less common today in developed countries, because of the decreased incidence of tuberculosis. Approximately 80% of primary adrenocortical insufficiency is now idiopathic. The remaining 20% of Addison's disease occurs as a complication of tuberculosis or in rare situations is due to cancer, infections, trauma, hemorrhagic disorders, AIDS, or congenital adrenal hypoplasia. The most common cause of secondary adrenocortical insufficiency is steroid withdrawal in a patient with adrenal atrophy due to exogeneous glucocorticoid therapy.

Overall, Addison's disease is an uncommon disorder with an incidence of 50 cases per million persons (33). It is usually diagnosed in the third to fifth decades of life. A sexual predisposition is observed, with females developing idiopathic Addison's disease two and one-half times more often than males. When adrenocortical insufficiency is due to tuberculosis, it is more common in males over the age of 40 years. Before corticosteroids were introduced in the late 1940s, patients with chronic adrenal insufficiency had a mortality rate of 80% within 3 years of diagnosis. Today, the overall mortality rate is 1.4 per million.

Drug-induced Addison's Disease

Medications have been implicated as the cause of Addison's disease in certain situations. Enzyme inhibitors used in Cushing's syndrome and adrenal cancers, such as metyrapone and aminoglutethimide, decrease cortisol secretion and may precipitate Addison's disease. The potential for this to occur is greatest when patients are not given exogenous steroid replacement therapy. Ketoconazole also decreases cortisol secretion and has been known to cause adrenocortical insufficiency at high doses. Adrenal radiation and mitotane are both adrenocortical toxins that can culminate in adrenocortical insufficiency.

Anticoagulants such as heparin and warfarin have been reported to cause Addison's disease as a result of adrenal hemorrhage. Waterhouse-Friderichsen syndrome develops when adrenocortical hemorrhage results from anticoagulant use, sepsis, or trauma and is accompanied by fulminant septicemia. Lastly, rifampin and other hepatic enzyme inducers may increase the metabolism of cortisol and precipitate adrenocortical insufficiency in patients with preexisting partial adrenal insufficiency (34).

Pathogenesis

In addition to primary or secondary causes, adrenocortical insufficiency can also be acute or chronic. When Addison's disease occurs as a result of gradual destruction of the adrenal gland, chronic adrenal insufficiency is manifested. Patients with chronic adrenocortical insufficiency often have normal basal cortisol secretion, but may have difficulty in increasing cortisol secretion with stress. Over time, even basal cortisol secretion becomes inadequate, and clinical manifestations of adrenocortical insufficiency become evident. However, without an acute stressful event, chronic adrenal insufficiency usually will go unnoticed because of the vague symptoms of the disease.

Approximately 25% of patients who are diagnosed as having Addison's disease are in active or impending adrenal crisis. Acute adrenocortical insufficiency is manifested when steroid need, generated by stress of surgery, trauma, or infection, exceeds the capacity of the adrenal gland for cortisol production. In these patients, the acute stressful event precipitates an addisonian crisis. This generally occurs when 90% or more of the adrenal cortex is nonfunctioning, and it is usually accompanied by elevated ACTH levels.

Clinical Manifestations

Signs and symptoms of chronic Addison's disease may be present for months to years without being diagnosed. Nonspecific symptoms that occur in most patients with Addison's disease include anorexia, weakness, fatigue, and weight loss (3, 5). Both mineralocorticoid and glucocorticoid deficiencies contribute to symptoms of salt craving, dizziness, and low systolic blood pressure.

Hyperpigmentation of the skin and mucous membranes is usually the hallmark characteristic that prompts the physician to test for adrenal insufficiency. It is most pronounced in sun-exposed areas of the body and at pressure points, but also occurs on palmar creases, nail beds, the tongue, nipples, naval, and perivaginal and perianal mucosa. Hyperpigmentation, present in 92% of patients, is caused by increased melanocyte-stimulating hormone (MSH) and β-lipotropin serum levels that accompany increased ACTH levels (35, 36). Areas of unpigmented skin (vitiligo) also occur but at a much lower incidence of approximately 4 to 17%.

Prolonged gastrointestinal symptoms such as nausea, abdominal discomfort, diarrhea, and vomiting are warning signs that may signal progressive adrenal insufficiency and impending crisis (37).

ADDISONIAN CRISIS

Acute addisonian crisis results when a patient with undiagnosed Addison's disease becomes stressed or is exposed to a stressful event such as trauma or hemorrhage. The signs and symptoms of addisonian crisis are more profound than those of chronic insufficiency and demand immediate diagnosis and treatment. Significant anorexia develops and is accompanied by nausea and vomiting. This leads to severe dehydration and hemodynamic instability. Fever, with or without a concurrent infection, is often present. Abdominal pain and tenderness may confuse the diagnosis as one of an acute abdominal event. Weakness, fatigue, and confusion become profound, and without appropriate treatment, coma and shock are likely to develop.

Hyperpigmentation may exist in patients with previous chronic adrenocortical insufficiency, and if present, is again the distinctive finding that suggests the diagnosis. Laboratory abnormalities such as hyponatremia, hyperkalemia, eosinophilia, lymphocytosis, hypoglycemia, and increased blood urea nitrogen (BUN) levels are all seen in adrenal crisis. Hypoglycemia, due to a decrease in hepatic gluconeogenesis, is otherwise a rare finding in a patient with shock and is highly suggestive of addisonian crisis.

Diagnosis

Clinical and laboratory findings should alert the clinician to the possibility of acute adrenocortical insufficiency in a hospitalized, acutely ill patient. Once an addisonian crisis is suspected, treatment should be instituted at the same time or before beginning a series of diagnostic tests. Failure to treat these patients promptly could lead to rapid deterioration and death. Figure 15.5 provides an algorithm for the diagnosis of chronic or acute Addison's disease.

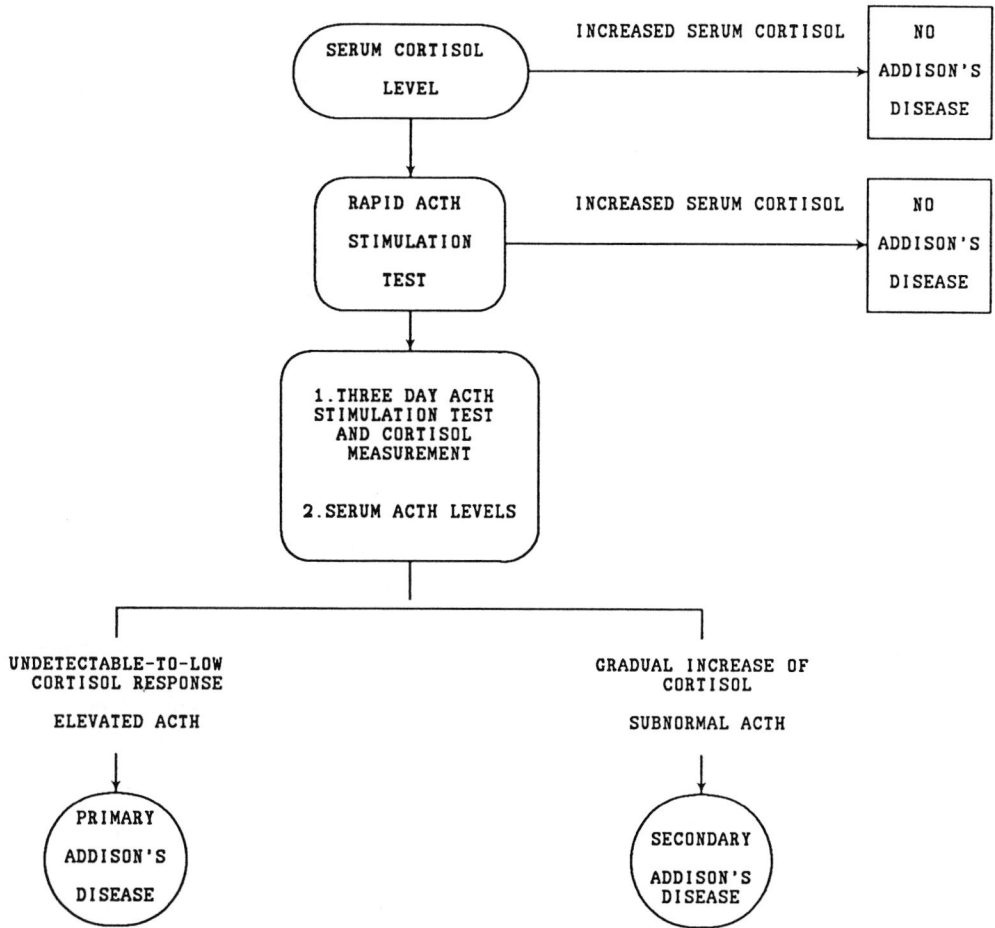

Figure 15.5. An algorithm for the diagnosis of Addison's disease.

SCREENING TESTS

Diagnosis of primary adrenocortical insufficiency is based on dynamic laboratory tests that show a failure of the adrenal cortex to respond to ACTH stimulation. Although plasma cortisol levels are usually low to absent, random measurement of serum cortisol levels rarely provides confirmation of impaired cortisol production. For this reason, serum cortisol levels alone are not recommended as a method of screening for Addison's disease. However, if a serum cortisol level is low and a simultaneously drawn serum ACTH level is high, a presumptive diagnosis of Addison's disease can be made. Further diagnosis of Addison's disease is based on ACTH stimulation tests used to test for adrenal reserve.

ACTH STIMULATION TESTS

The rapid ACTH stimulation test is the method of choice for initial assessment of the patient (3, 36). Either 25 units of ACTH or 0.25 mg of cosyntropin (synthetic ACTH) is administered by the intramuscular or intravenous route.

Samples for serum cortisol levels are obtained just before the injection as a baseline, and once or twice at 30 to 120 min after ACTH is given (35, 36). A normal response includes an increase in serum cortisol to 690 nmol/liter (25 μg/ml) or more at any time during the test or an increase of at least 193 to 276 nmol/liter (7 to 10 μg/ml) over the baseline serum cortisol level (36). A subnormal response signifies either primary adrenocrotical insufficiency or lack of adrenocortical response due to atrophy resulting from secondary adrenocortical insufficiency. A subnormal response may also occur in normal, but stressed, individuals whose adrenal cortex is already functioning at full capacity.

A 3-day ACTH-stimulation test may be conducted to confirm the diagnosis of Addison's disease. This 3-day test is conducted by administering 25 units of ACTH gel (Acthar-gel) intramuscularly or 0.25 mg of cosyntropin in 500 to 1000 ml of normal saline over 6 to 8 hours. This is done once a day in conjunction with 24-hr urine collections for 17-hydroxycorticosteroid (17-OHCS), or urinary free cortisol, or by measuring serum cortisol levels. In Addison's disease, the increase in serum or urine cortisol or urinary 17-OHCS is expected to be absent or minimal. In secondary adrenocortical insufficiency due to reduced ACTH stimulation, the expected cortisol rise is slow but progressive. In this manner both the diagnosis and etiology of adrenocortical insufficiency can be delineated.

PLASMA ACTH LEVELS

Plasma ACTH levels can be measured as an alternative to the cumbersome 3-day ACTH-stimulation test. ACTH levels are usually elevated to more than 55 pmol/liter (250 pg/ml) in patients with primary adrenocortical insufficiency. With secondary adrenocortical insufficiency, plasma ACTH levels are between 0 and 11 pmol/liter (0 to 50 pg/ml), which is considerably lower than expected with low serum cortisol levels (3). Serum ACTH levels are difficult to measure, and not all institutions provide serum ACTH level interpretations.

Treatment

ADDISONIAN CRISIS

Treatment of adrenocortical insufficiency is based on glucocorticoid replacement, with or without additional mineralocorticoid replacement. High doses of glucocorticoids are required in acute addisonian crisis. Hydrocortisone is the preferred corticosteroid, since it has sufficient mineralocorticoid activity (Table 15.5). It is administered initially as 100 mg intravenously every 6 hr. Usually patients will stabilize within 24 hr, and at that time the dose can be decreased to 50 mg intravenously every 6 hr. The hydrocortisone dose can be further reduced to a maintenance regimen of 20 to 30 mg/day after approximately 4 or 5 days (3, 5, 35, 38). Severely ill patients may require increased doses of hydrocortisone until the other complications (e.g., sepsis) have subsided.

A mineralocorticoid such as fludrocortisone may be added to therapy when the dose of hydrocortisone is less than or equal to 50 to 60 mg/day (3, 5). Intravenous dexamethasone or prednisolone may be used in place of hydrocortisone in patients with congestive heart failure or renal failure, to minimize fluid retention.

The administration of intravenous saline and glucose is recommended to treat dehydration, shock, and hypoglycemia. However, the correction of metabolic abnormalities is secondary and will not occur until glucocorticoids are administered (39).

MAINTENANCE THERAPY

Addison's disease is a life-long illness without a cure, which requires chronic corticosteroid replacement. Although hydrocortisone is the most natural replacement corticosteroid, cortisone acetate, prednisone, and prednisolone may also be used. Dexamethasone should be avoided for chronic maintenance therapy, however, because of a higher incidence of adverse effects and a lack of mineralocorticoid effects.

Hydrocortisone is usually administered as 15 to 30 mg/day, divided into a twice or three times daily regimen, with a larger portion of the dose administered in the morning. When cortisone acetate is used in place of hydrocortisone, the dosage is approximately 20% higher, because of the need for conversion of cortisone acetate to hydrocortisone in the liver. Prednisone (which is converted in the liver to prednisolone) is another alternative, at 5 to 7.5 mg/day.

When a mineralocorticoid is necessary (e.g., with orthostatic hypotension or electrolyte abnormalities), fludrocortisone (Florinef) is used. Doses should be titrated to the patient's need and often range from 0.05 to 0.1 mg daily or every other day. In patients with cardiac or renal

Table 15.5.
Comparison of Glucocorticoid Medications

Name	Biologic Half-Life (hr)	Equivalent Dose (mg)	Relative Potency		Physiologic Replacement Dose (mg)
			Glucocorticoid	Mineralocorticoid	
Short-acting					
Hydrocortisone (cortisol)	8–12	20	1.0	1.0	30
Cortisone acetate	8–12	25	0.8	0.8	37.5
Intermediate-acting					
Prednisone	18–36	5	3.5–4	0.8	7.5
Prednisolone	18–36	5	4.0	0.8	7.5
Methylprednisolone	18–36	4	5.0	0.5	6
Triamcinolone	18–36	4	5.0	0	6
Long-acting					
Dexamethasone	36–54	0.75	25–30	0	0.75–1.0
Betamethasone	36–54	0.60	25–30	0	0.75–1.0
(Fludrocortisone			10	125–400	0.5–1.0)

disease, the salt and water retention related to mineralo-corticoid use must be closely monitored.

Surgical Prophylaxis

Any patient being prepared for surgery who had been maintained on corticosteroid treatment within the past 12 months should be considered for perioperative corticosteroid prophylaxis. Regimens for perioperative corticosteroids are discussed in the section "Clinical Use of Steroids."

Conclusion

Adrenocortical insufficiency can be either primary or secondary, acute or chronic. Primary adrenal insufficiency, Addison's disease, is usually idiopathic, while secondary adrenal insufficiency is largely due to the use of exogenous corticosteroids. Chronic Addison's disease is very difficult to recognize because of the nonspecific symptoms such as anorexia, weight loss, and fatigue. Acute addisonian crisis is also difficult to recognize, but it requires prompt treatment, even before laboratory diagnosis is complete.

Before exogeneous corticosteroids were available as a treatment modality, adrenal insufficiency associated with stress was usually fatal. At the same time, chronic adrenal insufficiency was associated with an 80% mortality within 3 years. Today, adrenal insufficiency can be treated effectively with corticosteroids, when diagnosed on a timely basis.

PATIENT EDUCATION

Patients with Cushing's syndrome or Addison's disease should be advised to always carry an identification card or bracelet that states their need for hydrocortisone in the event of trauma or severe stress. They should also be instructed to maintain a diet with adequate salt and potassium. If they are taking oral corticosteroid replacement but are experiencing continuous vomiting or diarrhea or are unable to take their medications, they should seek parenteral replacement. Lastly, if they are experiencing a high fever, they should contact their physician if symptoms do not resolve within 24 to 48 hours.

CLINICAL USE OF STEROIDS

Each year over 5 million people in the U.S. will use corticosteroids. Exogenous corticosteroids have been found to be useful in the treatment of many disease states (Table 15.6). These range from short-term, self-limited conditions such as allergic rhinitis to life-threatening diseases such as leukemia and idiopathic thrombocytopenic purpura (ITP). Corticosteroids are used by all age groups—to treat respiratory distress syndrome in neonates, and rheumatoid arthritis in the elderly. New uses for corticosteroids are

Table 15.6.
Disease States in Which Glucocorticoids Are Used

Primary or secondary adrenocortical insufficiency
Rheumatic disorders
    Acute gouty arthritis
    Rheumatoid arthritis
    Osteoarthritis
Renal diseases
    Glomerulonephritis
    Nephrotic syndrome
Collagen disorders
    Systemic lupus erythematosus
    Polymyositis
    Wegener's granulomatosis
    Giant-cell arteritis
Allergic disorders
    Angioedema
    Urticardia
    Contact or atopic dermatitis
    Allergic rhinitis
    Erythema multiforme (Stevens-Johnson syndrome)
Respiratory diseases
    Bronchial asthma
    Fulminating or disseminated tuberculosis
    Aspiration pneumonitis
    Neonatal respiratory distress syndrome
Dermatologic diseases
    Pemphigus
    Bullous dermatitis herpetiformis
    Severe psoriasis
Gastrointestinal diseases
    Ulcerative colitis
    Crohn's disease
    Sprue
Malignancies
    Breast cancer
    Leukemia
    Lymphoma
    Chemotherapy-induced emesis
Hepatic diseases
    Chronic active hepatitis
    Subacute hepatic necrosis
    Alcoholic hepatitis
Miscellaneous
    Septic shock
    Hypercalcemia
    Organ transplantation
    Sarcoidosis
    Idiopathic thrombocytopenic purpura (ITP)
    Hemolytic anemia
    Multiple sclerosis
    Cerebral edema

being discovered constantly, for example the use of steroids in preventing transplant rejection.

Mechanism of Action

Corticosteroids are composed of 21-carbon molecules. The biological activity of the corticosteroid depends upon the presence of a hydroxyl group at the 11-carbon site. Glucocorticoids that rely on conversion to the active form in the liver do not have biologic activity before this conversion. Examples include cortisone and prednisone, which are converted in the liver to hydrocortisone and prednisolone, respectively. For this reason, cortisone and prednisone are only available for systemic treatment. To have clinical activity, a corticosteroid used for topical treatment must already be in the active, 11-β-hydroxyl form.

The primary pharmacologic actions of glucocorticoids are thought to require binding of the steroid to intracellular receptors. Once binding occurs, the net effect of the steroid is an alteration of gene transcription and protein synthesis (40). Glucocorticoids also are thought to have various degrees of binding to mineralocorticoid receptors in the kidney and brain (41), which explains the mineralocorticoid activity of some glucocorticoids. Cortisol (hydrocortisone) has equal affinity for both glucocorticoid and mineralocorticoid receptors. Dexamethasone has the lowest affinity for the mineralocorticoid receptor compared to cortisol, followed by betamethasone and prednisolone. Fludrocortisone, on the other hand, has an affinity almost 12 times higher than that of cortisol (40).

Response to a glucocorticoid is tissue-specific. In addition, tissues that do not contain glucocorticoid receptors may be affected because of mediators produced by primary tissue responses. The primary activity of glucocorticoids shields the body from its own defense mechanisms that are activated in stressful situations. If uncontrolled, the body's defense mechanisms can go too far and cause injury. The defense mechanisms that glucocorticoids appear to "dampen" include (a) insulin release; (b) inflammatory processes involving bradykinin, histamine, eicosanoids, serotonin, or plasminogen activator; (c) neurochemical release (CRF, ACTH, β-endorphins); (d) immune reactions (particularly cellular responses); and (e) antidiuretic hormone release. When using a corticosteroid clinically only one or two of these effects may be desired. Unfortunately, at this time there is no steroid that mediates one system preferentially.

Other effects of glucocorticoids do not appear to be related to immunosuppression or antiinflammatory activity. For example, glucocorticoids tend to reverse hypercalcemia associated with sarcoidosis, probably by inhibition of the conversion of 25-hydroxycholecalciferol to 1-α, 25-dihydroxycholecalciferol (42). Another example is the reduction in brain edema by corticosteroids in postoperative or posttraumatic settings.

Pharmacokinetics

The systemic effects of glucocorticoids depend upon three factors:

1. The amount of active drug delivered to the systemic circulation;

2. The potency or interaction of the steroid at the receptor site;
3. The length of time the steroid remains at the receptor site.

Pharmacokinetic principles aid us in understanding these three factors.

BIOAVAILABILITY

The bioavailability of oral corticosteroids depends upon the rate of dissolution of the oral preparation in the gastrointestinal tract and its absorption into the systemic circulation. For corticosteroids that are converted in the liver to the active form (e.g., prednisone to prednisolone), bioavailability refers to the active component available in the systemic circulation.

When oral prednisone or hydrocortisone is administered to healthy volunteers, bioavailability ranges from 50 to 100%, with the time to peak prednisolone levels occurring at approximately 1.3 to 3 hr (43). Fluctuation in availability is primarily due to variable rates of tablet dissolution. Enteric coating of oral steroid products, such as prednisolone, has been shown to decrease the rate but not the extent of absorption (43). Also, food does not decrease the bioavailability of oral prednisolone, but when enteric-coated prednisolone tablets are taken with food, a significant decrease in bioavailability is seen (44). For this reason, enteric-coated steroid preparations should not be taken with food.

Absorption of corticosteroids from other routes of administration has also been studied. Corticosteroids are administered as retention enemas, skin creams and ointments, preparations for inhalation, and ophthalmic liquids. Systemic absorption will occur to some degree with each of these. Approximately 30 to 90% of a hydrocortisone retention enema will be absorbed (44, 45). A daily dose of 400 μg of beclomethasone (2 puffs every 6 hr) is physiologically equivalent to a dose of 7.5 mg of prednisone daily (45).

Absorption of steroid preparations applied to the skin is increased by young age, administration after a bath (4 to 5 times increased absorption), plastic occlusion (10 times increased absorption), thin skin (e.g., eyelids, scrotum, forehead), and damaged skin (46). High potency and ointment preparations also have increased absorption. Overall, it is prudent to use the lowest effective topical corticosteroid concentration for the shortest possible time, to minimize absorption and effects on the HPA-axis.

DISTRIBUTION

Corticosteroids are primarily lipophilic compounds that distribute widely throughout the body. The apparent volume of distribution of prednisolone, however, is only 0.35 to 0.7 liter/kg (43). This relatively low volume of distribution is caused primarily by high protein binding in the serum. Steroids are bound in the serum to two proteins, albumin and transcortin (corticosteroid-binding globulin or CBG). At low concentrations, hydrocortisone and prednisolone are 80 to 90% protein bound. However, protein binding decreases to approximately 60 to 70% at high steroid concentrations because of a saturation of transcortin binding sites (43, 47). At high concentrations, plasma protein binding is decreased and free drug is available to diffuse more readily into peripheral tissues. This is reflected in a higher volume of distribution of the drug and increased risk for adverse reactions. Similar effects occur in patients with hypoalbuminemia, both serum albumin and transcortin levels are reduced and the free fraction of corticosteroids is increased. In these patients, a reduction in corticosteroid dose is recommended.

Clearance

Clearance of corticosteroids occurs primarily via the liver by metabolic hydroxylation and conjugation. Less than 15% of a corticosteroid dose is eliminated unchanged in the urine. Along with changes in volume of distribution with increasing serum concentrations, total body clearance also increases. After a low dose of prednisolone, the clearance is approximately 7 liter/hr. When a higher dose of prednisolone is administered, the mean clearance increases to 12 liter/hr (43). This alteration in total body clearance occurs primarily with prednisolone doses below 70 mg/day (44).

Factors that decrease the hepatic clearance of corticosteroids include liver or renal failure, age over 65 years, and concomitant ketoconazole or oral contraceptive use. An increase in clearance occurs with long-term use of corticosteroids (i.e., enzyme induction may occur), in hyperthyroidism, and with enzyme-inducing medications such as phenytoin, rifampin, and barbiturates (Table 15.3).

HALF-LIFE

Half-life reflects both the volume of distribution and the clearance of a compound. When these two parameters increase with increasing corticosteroid dose, no change in half-life is expected. This has been shown to be true with prednisolone. The half-life of prednisolone ranges from 2.6 to 5 hours and is constant with increasing doses (43, 47). Hydrocortisone, however, appears to have a dose-dependent increase in half-life. Even considering this dose-dependent change, the half-life range for hydrocortisone is only 1.2 to 1.8 hours (43). The clinical significance of this increase in half-life is minimal.

The half-lives of the glucocorticoids are relatively similar, but marked differences have been observed in the physiologic effects of the different agents. The corticosteroids can be divided into 3 groups, based on their biologic half-life (45, 48, 49). Short-acting agents such as hydrocortisone and cortisone suppress ACTH activity for 8 to 12 hours. Intermediate-acting agents such as prednisone, prednisolone, methylprednisolone, and triamcinolone suppress ACTH activity for 18 to 36 hours. The longest acting corticosteroids suppress ACTH for 36 to 54 hours and include dexamethasone and betamethasone. The duration of ACTH suppression is also prolonged as the dose of any agent is increased. The pharmacodynamic differences exhibited appear to be related to differences in receptor activity and cannot be explained by the individual agent's pharmacokinetic properties.

Adverse Effects

The adverse effects associated with high-dose corticosteroids are similar to those exhibited with endogenous hypercortisolism (as discussed in "Cushing's Syndrome" earlier in this chapter). Endogenous hypercortisolism usually involves an increase in ACTH levels, which leads to increased cortisol, aldosterone, and adrenal androgen production. For this reason, Cushing's syndrome is usually accompanied by edema, hypertension, and hirsutism. With iatrogenic hypercortisolism, cortisol levels are elevated, but ACTH levels are suppressed and fewer mineralocorticoid and androgenic effects are seen. This will also depend on which corticosteroid is being administered; for example, hydrocortisone has more mineralocorticoid effects than prednisone or dexamethasone.

In addition to the effects seen with endogenous hypercortisolism, certain adverse effects are seen almost exclusively with iatrogenic hypercortisolism. These include euphoria, intracranial hypertension, vasculitis, pancreatitis, gastritis, glaucoma, cataracts, and ischemic bone necrosis. When therapy with corticosteroids is begun, these severe adverse effects should be considered. Prospective monitoring for these complications and correct dosing will help reduce morbidity and mortality associated with long-term corticosteroid treatment.

OSTEOPOROSIS

Osteoporosis is a significant obstacle to corticosteroid treatment. Steroids lead to a decrease in bone formation and an increase in bone resorption (50). Bone loss is more prominent in trabecular bones (e.g., ribs and vertebrae) than in the long bones of the body (50). Steroid-induced osteoporosis occurs at a higher rate in post-menopausal women, alcoholics, and patients with altered vitamin D absorption or metabolism.

The cause of steroid-induced bone loss is multifactorial. Gastrointestinal absorption of calcium is decreased, and renal elimination of calcium is increased. This leads to decreased serum calcium levels, which induces secondary hyperparathyroidism. This further leads to an increase in osteoclast activity, which increases serum calcium levels and results in osteomalacia.

Information on the treatment of this condition is limited. Although lowering the dose of the glucocorticoid is recommended, alternate-day regimens have not been shown to affect bone loss. Treatment of steroid-induced osteoporosis with exercise, vitamin D, and calcium supplements may be helpful (50). Another treatment modality is the use of hydrochlorothiazide when hypercalciuria is present (50). The use of estrogen replacement in postmenopausal women has also been suggested. The efficacy of these treatment regimens in steroid-induced osteoporosis has not yet been adequately studied.

INFECTIONS

Infections are common in steroid-treated patients and include those of bacterial, fungal, viral and parasitic origin. Gram-negative bacteria and fungi such as *Candida albicans* and *Cryptococcus* are particularly troublesome in patients on long-term corticosteroids. Reactivation of tuberculosis is another concern in patients with a previously positive tuberculin skin test. However, the literature does not show an increased incidence of primary tuberculosis in these patients (40).

In addition to being more susceptible to infectious complications, detection of an infectious process in a patient treated with steroids may be difficult. This is due to the immunosuppressant activity of corticosteroids, which blunts the typical manifestations of an infection such as an elevated white blood cell count and inflammation. For this reason, any slight deterioration in well-being should be accompanied by an aggressive search for and treatment of an infectious etiology.

PEPTIC ULCER DISEASE

Gastritis and peptic ulcer disease are controversial complications associated with glucocorticoid administration. The incidence of these complications has been reported as significantly higher than with placebo, but still at a fairly low incidence of 1.8% in a study that pooled data from 71 previously reported trials of 3064 total patients (52). However, steroid-induced peptic ulcer disease may lead to severe complications such as perforation and death, as was reported by Dayton and Kleckner in 1987 (53). In their retrospective chart review they found that patients over 50 years of age had an 85% mortality rate when they developed perforation of a gastric ulcer due to corticosteroid use.

Gastritis and peptic ulcer disease associated with corticosteroids occur as both acute and chronic complications and are more common in the stomach than in the duodenum. This adverse effect tends to be independent of the type of corticosteroid and dose; however pulse-dosing is more highly associated with perforation (53). Monitoring for this complication should include baseline and follow-up endoscopy.

Table 15.7.
Adverse Effects of Topical Steroids

Skin atrophy and fibrosis
Ichthyosis-like changes
Flushing
Telangiectasia
Abnormal pigmentation
Superficial infections (bacterial, fungal, parasitic)
Acne
Rosacea-like dermatitis
Perioral dermatitis
Purpura
Delayed skin healing
Glaucoma
Cataracts
Photosensitivity
False scars

Adapted from Takeda K, Arase S, Takahashi S: Side effects of topical corticosteroids and their prevetion. Drugs 36 (suppl 15):15–23, 1988.

Subjective complaints with steroid-induced peptic ulcer disease are not necessarily correlated with endoscopic findings but should be managed with antacid regimens. The use of prophylactic antacids is also recommended in patients on intermittent high doses of corticosteroids (pulse-dosing) and those over the age of 50 years. Although prophylactic use of histamine-2 antagonists such as cimetidine and randitidine is commonly employed, this practice should be limited to patients with additional risk factors for developing peptic ulcer disease (e.g., previous history of peptic ulcer disease, concomitant use of aspirin). The use of nonsteroidal antiinflammatory agents and other medications that irritate the gastrointestinal mucosa should be curtailed as much as possible.

TOPICAL GLUCOCORTICOIDS

Topical corticosteroids exhibit adverse effects unique to their mode of application. Prolonged use of fluorinated glucocorticoids (e.g., triamcinolone, betamethasone, dexamethasone) on the face causes steroid-induced acne. A list of complications can be found in Table 15.7.

Glucocorticoid Selection

Glucocorticoid preparations differ in their duration of action, mineralocorticoid effects, route of administration, and cost. Hydrocortisone and cortisone acetate are the glucocorticoids that most closely approximate the body's natural glucocorticoid, cortisol. These agents have both glucocorticoid and mineralocorticoid activity and are the preparations of choice in adrenocortical insufficiency. Dexamethasone is a synthetic glucocorticoid that has minimal mineralocorticoid activity and is a particularly useful agent in patients with brain edema, congestive heart failure, or renal failure. Prednisone is an effective, inexpensive glucocorticoid that must be monitored for its mineralocorticoid effects.

Dosing of Corticosteroids

When dosing corticosteroids the best approach is to use the lowest dose for the shortest time possible, and to administer doses in the morning. When corticosteroid therapy is initiated, the dose should be individualized, based on the agent being used and the condition being treated. High doses are used initially to achieve antiinflammatory or immunosuppressant effects. Once the clinical response is achieved, the steroid can either be discontinued abruptly, tapered then discontinued, or tapered for long-term replacement or immunosuppressive treatment. Alternate-day dosing is preferred for chronic corticosteroid treatment, since this is associated with fewer adverse effects and less HPA suppression.

HPA SUPPRESSION

When exogenous corticosteroids are administered, secretion of CRF (corticotropin releasing factor) and ACTH (adrenocorticotropic hormone) is suppressed. The degree of HPA suppression is influenced by factors that include dose, dosing interval, time of administration, length of therapy, and route of administration (45, 55). When glucocorticoids with long half-lives are used (e.g., dexamethasone), serum levels are sustained and the circadian rhythm is disrupted. For this reason, dexamethasone produces more HPA suppression than does a short-acting glucocorticoid such as prednisone. Glucocorticoids administered as a single morning dose produce less HPA suppression than a regimen of divided doses throughout the day. This is because the dosing follows the body's natural circadian rhythm, with high cortisol levels in the morning and low levels in the evening. Although the exact time course required for initiation of HPA suppression is not known, the degree of HPA suppression increases as corticosteroid therapy is continued.

Variations in onset of HPA suppression have been seen between different patients and different studies. Overall, any patient receiving physiologic prednisone doses of 20 to 30 mg/day for more than 7 days, or lower doses of prednisone such as 5 to 20 mg/day for 1 month or longer, should be considered to have HPA suppression. In these patients, discontinuation of therapy requires a slow tapering process, and elevated doses of corticosteroids are required with surgery or stress for up to 1 year after steroids are discontinued.

ALTERNATE-DAY THERAPY

Dosing of glucocorticoids on an alternate-day basis can minimize HPA suppression and adverse effects, while still providing effective treatment of many disease processes.

Alternate-day dosing should be considered for any patient requiring corticosteroid therapy that will last longer than several weeks. Conditions that can be managed effectively by alternate-day administration include ulcerative colitis, renal transplant rejection, chronic dermatoses, myasthenia gravis, and asthma (40). Conditions that show a less favorable response to alternate-day dosing include rheumatoid arthritis, systemic lupus erythematosus, and giant cell arteritis (56).

Short- or intermediate-acting corticosteroids are appropriate for alternate-day dosing. These preparations allow a partial recovery of the HPA axis on the days when the glucocorticoid is not administered. In addition, cushingoid adverse effects such as moon facies, obesity, striae, carbohydrate intolerance, myopathy, infections, and growth inhibition in children are less likely to develop with alternate-day dosing (57).

Daily dosing of glucocorticoids is used initially, and when the disease state is under control, dosing is switched over to alternate days. This change should be made as early in treatment as possible, before the HPA axis has been suppressed significantly. However, a conservative approach should be considered when converting to alternate-day dosing. This is recommended for three reasons (57):

1. HPA suppression may have already occurred;
2. Even with normal HPA function, steroid withdrawal symptoms may occur;
3. The underlying disease may be exacerbated.

The conversion schedule chosen depends upon the underlying disease, duration of therapy, patient's acceptance of alternate-day dosing, and the use of adjunctive therapy (57). First, the daily dose may need to be decreased to 15 to 20 mg/day of prednisone equivalent, and then converted to a single morning dose. Next, a very gradual switch to alternate-day dosing can be started. This is accomplished by reducing 1 day's dose by approximately 10 to 20% and adding the same amount to the next day's dose. This dose should then be continued for at least three cycles before the next reduction in dose is made. An example of a conversion to alternate-day dosing is shown in Table 15.8.

During the conversion period, the patient should be monitored closely for adrenocortical insufficiency and exacerbation of the primary disease. Steroid withdrawal may occur and is usually manifested by fatigue, weakness, arthralgia, nausea, hypotension, and dizziness. This is usually managed by restarting small glucocorticoid doses on the off-day or by reinstituting the initial dosing regimen used before the tapering process began (40). Exacerbation of the primary disease should be managed with agents other than steroids when possible.

Discontinuation of Glucocorticoids

Short-term, low-dose (i.e., < 20 mg of prednisone per day) glucocorticoid treatment of up to approximately 3 weeks

Table 15.8.
Scheme for Conversion to an Alternate-Day Regimen for Glucocorticoids (Initial dose prednisone 60 mg/day)

Day	Dose (mg)	Day	Dose (mg)
A. Reduce dosage by 5 mg every 3 days until a dose of prednisone 20 mg is reached:			
1	55	13	35
2	55	14	35
3	55	15	35
4	50	16	30
5	50	17	30
6	50	18	30
7	45	19	25
8	45	20	25
9	45	21	25
10	40	22	20
11	40	23	20
12	40	24	20
B. Reduce dosage by 2.5 mg on alternate days every three cycles until no prednisone on alternate days:			
25	20	49	20
26	17.5	50	7.5
27	20	51	20
28	17.5	52	7.5
29	20	53	20
30	17.5	54	7.5
31	20	55	20
32	15	56	5
33	20	57	20
34	15	58	5
35	20	59	20
36	15	60	5
37	20	61	20
38	12.5	62	2.5
39	20	63	20
40	12.5	64	2.5
41	20	65	20
42	12.5	66	2.5
43	20	67	20
44	10	68	0
45	20	69	20
46	10	70	0
47	20	71	20
48	10	72	0

duration can usually be discontinued abruptly with few steroid withdrawal effects (45). The discontinuation of chronic glucocorticoid treatment, however, can be a lengthy and frustrating process. As with the conversion of divided daily doses, exacerbation of the underlying disease can occur with or without steroid withdrawal reactions. One method of tapering chronic glucocorticoid doses for discontinuation of therapy is shown in Table 15.9.

Perioperative or Stress Doses

High-dose, intravenous glucocorticoids are required for surgery or stress in patients with HPA suppression. This includes patients maintained on chronic supraphysiologic doses (i.e., > 7.5 mg of prednisone per day) and patients who recently (up to 1 year) discontinued glucocorticoid treatment. Stress doses are used to replace exogenously the maximum output of cortisol by the adrenal cortex, which is approximately 200 to 500 mg/day.

For major surgical procedures, the dose of hydrocor-

Table 15.9.
Scheme for the Gradual Reduction and Discontinuation of Glucocorticoids (Initial dose prednisone 40 mg/day)

Day	Dose (mg)	Day	Dose (mg)
A. Reduce dosage by 5 mg on alternate days until a dose of prednisone 10 mg is reached:			
1	40	7	40
2	35	8	20
3	40	9	40
4	30	10	15
5	40	11	40
6	25	12	10
B. Reduce by 2.5 mg on alternate days every 3 cycles until no prednisone on alternate days			
13	40	25	40
14	7.5	26	2.5
15	40	27	40
16	7.5	28	2.5
17	40	29	40
18	7.5	30	2.5
19	40	31	40
20	5	32	0
21	40	33	40
22	5	34	0
23	40	35	40
24	5	36	0
C. If the patient remains stable, reduce by 5 mg on alterante days until a dose of 10 mg every other day is reached:			
37	35	43	20
38	0	44	0
39	30	45	15
40	0	46	0
41	25	47	10
42	0	48	0
D. Reduce by 2.5 mg on alternate days every three cycles until a dose of 2.5 mg every other day is reached:			
49	7.5	58	0
50	0	59	5
51	7.5	60	0
52	0	61	2.5
53	7.5	62	0
54	0	63	2.5
55	5	64	0
56	0	65	2.5
57	5	66	0
E. Drop to 1 mg on alternate days for 1 week			
F. Stop all glucocorticoids.			

Reprinted, with permission, from Helfer EL, Rose LI: Corticosteroids and adrenal suppression. Characterizing and avoiding the problem. Drugs 38:838–845, 1989.

tisone employed is usually above 200 mg/day (4). Intramuscular or intravenous hydrocortisone, as the phosphate or hemisuccinate salt, is administered at a dose of 100 mg every 6 to 8 hr beginning just prior to surgery. Intravenous hydrocortisone is continued at the same dose or decreased by 50% each day for 3 days. The patient is then converted to oral hydrocortisone therapy at a dose of 20 mg twice a day and may be continued on this dose until the seventh day after surgery (4).

With minor surgery a similar regimen is used. Hydrocortisone is administered at a dose of 100 mg intravenously every 6 hr for the first 24 hr. After the first day, therapy is converted to oral hydrocortisone and tapered rapidly over a few days.

With other types of stress, such as acute asthmatic attacks, intravenous hydrocortisone is administered at a dose of 50 to 100 mg every 6 to 8 hr until the stress has abated (4). The glucocorticoid dose can then be tapered rapidly to the previous maintenance regimen.

In each of these regimens, patient response must be monitored. Perioperative complications may lead to sustained stress after surgery, and intravenous hydrocortisone may need to be continued. The continued use of high-dose corticosteroids may also be deleterious, increasing the patient's susceptibility to infection, altering fluid and electrolyte status, and impairing surgical healing. Patient assessment is essential to optimizing the use of perioperative or stress doses of corticosteroids.

CONCLUSION

Adrenocortical steroid hormones are necessary to maintain metabolic homeostasis of the human body for normal daily living and during times of severe stress. When the normal production and secretion of cortisol, the body's major glucocorticoid hormone, are disturbed, serious clinical diseases result. Sustained hypercortisolism produces Cushing's syndrome, while chronic adrenocortical insufficiency results in Addison's disease. When cortisol is not available to aid the body in dealing with an acute stressful event, rapidly fatal addisonian crisis results. Each of these conditions can be managed effectively once the diagnosis is known.

Exogenous corticosteroids have been used to treat a variety of illnesses. Efficacy is greatest in illnesses with an inflammatory or immunologic basis. However, the long-term use of systemic corticosteroids is associated with many adverse effects, including electrolyte abnormalities, susceptibility to infections, osteoporosis, gastritis, and peptic ulcer disease. For this reason, the smallest dose should be used for the shortest period of time or on alternate days to minimize adrenal atrophy. Discontinuation of corticosteroids must be done very slowly if HPA suppression has occurred. While the drug is being gradually discontinued, the patient should be monitored for disease recurrence or

the steroid withdrawal syndrome. Doses of corticosteroids in response to stress (e.g., surgery) will be required for up to 1 year after steroid withdrawal in patients who have HPA suppression.

REFERENCES

1. Axelrod J, Reisine TD: Stress hormones: their interaction and regulation. Science 224:452–459, 1984.
2. Tepperman J, Tepperman HM, ACTH and adrenal glucocorticoids. In Tepperman J, Tepperman HM: Metabolic and Endocrine Physiology. Chicago, Year Book Publishers, 1987, p 183.
3. Baxter JD, Tyrrell JB, The adrenal cortex. In Felig P, Baxter JD, Broadus AE, Frohman LA: Endocrinology and Metabolism. New York, McGraw-Hill, 1987, p 511.
4. Byyny BL: Preventing adrenal insufficiency during surgery. Postgrad Med 67(5):219–226, 1980.
5. Tyrrell JB, Forsham PH, Glucocorticoids and adrenal androgens. In Greenspan FS, Forsham PH: Basic and Clinical Endocrinology. East Norwalk, CT,Lange, 1986, p 272.
6. Cushing HC: The basophil adenomas of the pituitary body and their clinical manifestations (pituitary basophilism). Bull Johns Hopkins Hosp 1(3):137–195, 1932.
7. Schteingart DE: Cushing's syndrome. Endocrinol Metab Clin North Am 18(2):311–338, 1989.
8. Felicetta JV. Cushing's syndrome: How to pinpoint and treat the underlying cause. Postgrad Med 86(8):79–90, 1989.
9. Kaye TB, Crapo L: The Cushing syndrome: an update on diagnostic tests. Ann Intern Med 112:434–444, 1990.
10. Tyrrell JB, Laboratory evaluation of adrenocortical function. In Wyngaarden JB, Smith LH: Cecil Textbook of Medicine. Philadelphia, WB Saunders, 1988, p 1348.
11. Aron DC: Cushing's syndrome: current concepts in diagnosis and treatment. Compr Ther 13(12):37–44, 1987.
12. Trecan GV, Laudet MH, Thomopoulos P, Luton JP, Bricaire H: Urinary free corticoids: an evaluation of their usefulness in the diagnosis of Cushing's syndrome. Acta Endocrinol 103:110–115, 1983.
13. Aron DC, Findling JW, Tyrrell JB: Cushing's disease. Endocrinol Metab Clin North Am 16(3):705–730, 1987.
14. Ashcraft MW, van Herle AJ, Vener SL, Geffner DL: Serum cortisol levels in Cushing's syndrome after low- and high-dose dexamethasone suppression. Ann Intern Med 97:21–26, 1982.
15. Tyrrell JB, Findling JW, Aron DC, Fitzgerald PA, Forsham PH: An overnight high dose dexamethasone suppression test for rapid differential diagnosis of Cushing's syndrome. Ann Intern Med 104:180–186, 1986.
16. Hansten PD, Horn JR: Drug Interactions, ed. 6. Philadelphia, Lea & Febiger, 1989.
17. Tatro DS: Drug Interaction Facts. St. Louis, JB Lippincott, 1990.
18. Carpenter PC: Diagnostic evaluation of Cushing's syndrome. Endocrinol Metabol Clin North Am 17(3):445–472, 1988.
19. Krieger DT, Amorosa L, Linick F: Cyproheptadine-induced remission of Cushing's disease. N Engl J Med 293(18):893–896, 1975.
20. Hsu TH, Gann DS, Tsan KW, Russell RP: Cyproheptadine in the control of Cushing's disease. Johns Hopkins Med J 149:77–83, 1981.
21. Tyrrell JB, Brooks RM, Forsham PH: More on cyproheptadine. N Engl J Med 295(7):1137–1138, 1976.
22. Krieger DT: Cyproheptadine for pituitary disorders. N Engl J Med 295(7):394–395, 1976.
23. McKenna MJ, Linares M, Mellinger RC: Prolonged remission of Cushing's disease following bromocriptine therapy. Henry Ford Hosp Med J 35(4):188–191, 1987.
24. Jeffcoate WJ: Treating Cushing's disease. Br Med J 296(6617):227–228, 1988.

25. Thoren M, Adamson U, Sjoberg HE: Aminoglutethimide and metyrapone in the management of Cushing's syndrome. Acta Endocrinol 109:451–457, 1985.

26. Orth DN: Metyrapone is useful only as adjunctive therapy in Cushing's disease. Ann Intern Med 89(1):128–130, 1978.

27. Southren AL, Weisenfeld S, Laufer A, et al: Effect of O,p'DDD in a patient with Cushing's syndrome. J Clin Endocrinol Metab 21:201–208, 1961.

28. Schteingart DE, Tsao HS, Taylor CI, McKenzie A, Victoria R, Therrien BA: Sustained remission of Cushing's disease with mitotane and pituitary irradiation. Ann Intern Med 92:613–619, 1980.

29. Luton JP, Mahoudeau JA, Bouchard P, et al.: Treatment of Cushing's disease by O,p'DDD. N Engl J Med 300(9):459–464, 1979.

30. Oates JA, Wood AJJ: The use of ketoconazole as an inhibitor of steroid production. N Engl J Med 317(13):812–818, 1987.

31. Sonino N, Boscaro M, Merola G, Mantero F: Prolonged treatment of Cushing's disease by ketoconazole. J Clin Endocrinol Metab 61:718–722, 1985.

32. McCance DR, Hadden DR, Kennedy L, Sheridan B, Atkinson AB: Clinical experience with ketoconazole as a therapy for patients with Cushing's syndrome. Clin Endocrinol 27:593–599, 1987.

33. Baxter JD, Adrenocortical hypofunction. In Wyngaarden JB, Smith LH: Cecil Textbook of Medicine. Philadelphia, WB Saunders, 1988, p 1351.

34. Wilkins EGL, Hnizdo E, Cope A: Addisonian crisis induced by treatment with rifampicin. Tubercle 70:69–73, 1989.

35. Burke CW: Adrenocortical insufficiency. Clin Endocrinol Metab 14(4):947–976, 1985.

36. Kannan CR: Diseases of the adrenal cortex. Dis Mon 34(10):601–674, 1988.

37. Tobin MV, Aldridge SA, Morris AI, Belchetz PE, Gilmore IT: Gastrointestinal manifestations of Addison's disease. Am J Gastroenterol 84(10):1302–1305, 1989.

38. Bayliss RIS: Adrenal cortex. Clin Endocrinol Metab 9(3):477–486, 1980.

39. Waise A, Young RJ: Pitfalls in the management of acute adrenocortical insufficiency: discussion paper. J R Soc Med 82(12):741–742, 1989.

40. Tyrrell JB, Baxter JD, Glucocorticoid therapy. In Felig P, Baxter JD, Broadus AE, Frohman LA: Endocrinology and Metabolism. New York, McGraw-Hill, 1987, p 787.

41. Munck A, Mendel DB, Smith LI, Orti E: Glucocorticoid receptors and actions. Am Rev Respir Dis 141:S2–S9, 1990.

42. Frame B, Parfitt AM: Corticosteroid-responsive hypercalcemia with elevated 1-alpha, 25-dihydroxyvitamin D. Ann Intern Med 93:449–451, 1980.

43. Begg EJ, Atkinson HC, Gianarakis N: The pharmacokinetics of corticosteroid agents. Med J Aust 146:37–41, 1987.

44. Frey BM, Frey FJ: Clinical pharmacokinetics of prednisone and prednisolone. Clin Pharmacokinet 19(2):126–146, 1990.

45. Helfer EL, Rose LI: Corticosteroids and adrenal suppression. Characterizing and avoiding the problem. Drugs 38(5):838–845, 1989.

46. Giannotti B: Current treatment guidelines for topical corticosteroids. Drugs 36(suppl 5):9–14, 1988.

47. Pickup ME: Clinical pharmacokinetics of prednisone and prednisolone. Clin Pharmacokinet 4:111–128, 1979.

48. Harter JG: Corticosteroids: their physiologic use in allergic disease. N Y State J Med 66:827–834, 1966.

49. Haynes RC, Murad F, Adrenocorticotropic hormone: adrenocortical steroids and their synthetic analogs: inhibitors of adrenocortical steroid biosynthesis. In Gilman AG, Goodman LS, Rall TW, Murad F: Goodman and Gilman's The Pharmacological Basis of Therapeutics. New York, MacMillan, 1985, p 1459.

50. Baylink DJ: Glucocorticoid-induced osteoporosis. N Engl J Med 309(5):306–308, 1983.

51. Bollett AJ: Minimizing side effects in the use of corticosteroids. Res Staff Physician 34(4):17–20, 1988.

52. Messer J, Reitman D, Sacks HS, Smith H, Chalmers TC: Association of adrenocorticosteroid therapy and peptic-ulcer disease. N Engl J Med 309:21–24, 1983.

53. Dayton MT, Kleckner SC, Brown DK: Peptic ulcer perforation associated with steroid use. Arch Surg 122:376–380, 1987.

54. Takeda K, Arase S, Takahashi S: Side effects of topical corticosteroids and their prevention. Drugs 36(suppl 5):15–23, 1988.

55. Byyny RL: Withdrawal from glucocorticoid therapy. N Engl J Med 295(1):30–32, 1976.

56. Hunder GG, Sheps SG, Allen GL, Joyce JW: Daily and alternate day corticosteroid regimen in treatment of giant cell arteritis. Ann Intern Med 82:613–618, 1975.

57. Axelrod L: Glucocorticoid therapy. Medicine 55(1):39–65, 1976.

CHAPTER 16

THYROID AND PARATHYROID DISORDERS

BETTY J. DONG, Pharm.D.

THYROID DISORDERS

Hypothyroidism, hyperthyroidism, and thyroid nodules are well-known disorders of the thyroid gland which affect a large proportion of the population. Since drugs constitute a major form of medical management, the practitioner should have a basic understanding of the physiology; pathophysiology, and hormone biosynthesis of the thyroid; the laboratory and clinical manifestations of each disease; and the numerous pharmacological and medical interventions available.

Physiology

Regulation of Thyroid Function. The thyroid gland, a highly vascular organ lying on top of the trachea, consists of two lobes connected by a middle lobe known as the isthmus. The gland synthesizes, stores, and releases two major metabolically active hormones: triiodothyronine (T_3) and thyroxine (T_4). T_3 is considered the more active of the two thyroid hormones because the thyroid receptor protein within the cell nucleus has about a 10-fold higher affinity for T_3 than for T_4. Regulation of hormone synthesis is achieved via an intricate negative feedback mechanism involving the gland, the hypothalamic-pituitary axis (Fig. 16.1), and autoregulation of iodide uptake. Physiologic factors such as dopamine and stress are also known to influence the hypothalamic-pituitary axis.

Low circulating levels of thyroid hormone initiate the release of thyroid-stimulating hormone (TSH) from the pituitary and the secretion of thyrotropin-releasing factor (TRF) from the hypothalamus. Rising TSH levels increase iodide trapping by the gland, causing a subsequent increase in hormone synthesis and circulating hormone levels. Higher circulating hormone levels then feed back to the pituitary and hypothalamic centers to shut off TRF, TSH, and further hormone biosynthesis. As the hormone levels drop, the hypothalamic-pituitary centers once again become responsive to release of TSH and TRF. Loss of this negative feedback mechanism can produce hypothyroidism or hyperthyroidism.

The gland also has an inherent ability to regulate its uptake of iodide and prevent excessive thyroid hormone production if a large iodide load is ingested (i.e., radiographic iodine dye). This autoregulation, known as the Wolff-Chaikoff block, is not overcome by TSH stimulation and occurs when a critical intrathyroid iodide concentration is established within the gland. The normal gland escapes from the block within 7 to 14 days, which prevents subsequent development of hypothyroidism and goiter. Escape occurs by a decrease in iodide transport or by an iodide leak, both of which tend to decrease the intrathyroid iodide concentration and remove the block to further hormone synthesis. In certain thyroid disorders, (e.g., Hashimoto's disease) the gland cannot escape from the Wolff-Chaikoff block, causing hypothyroidism (1). Conversely, hyperthyroidism results if this critical block does not occur (e.g., Jod-Basedow disease).

Hormone Synthesis/Transport/Metabolism. Both T_4 and T_3 are synthesized within the gland. However, most T_3 production results from peripheral conversion of T_4 to T_3. About 35 to 40% of the secreted T_4 is peripherally monodeiodinated to active T_3, and about 40% is converted to inactive reverse T_3 (rT_3), which has little or no thyroid activity. Extrathyroidal conversion of T_4 to T_3 accounts for about 80% of the total daily production of T_3. However, the peripheral conversion of T_4 to active T_3 is decreased and the conversion to inactive rT_3 is increased in many acute and chronic disorders (see "Euthyroid Sick Syndrome").

Dietary inorganic iodide trapped by the gland is promptly oxidized by peroxidase to iodine before its incorporation with tyrosine molecules to form monoiodotyrosine (MIT) and diiodotyrosine (DIT). Subsequently, T_4 formation occurs through the coupling of two diiodotyrosyl residues, and that of T_3 by coupling a diiodotyrosyl and monoiodotyrosyl residue. The synthesized hormones are then stored within thyroglobulin until they are released into the circulation by enzymatic cleavage.

In the circulation, the hormones exist in both the active, free and the inactive, or protein-bound, forms. Thyroxine is 99.89% bound; only 0.02% is free. This high affinity for the plasma proteins (thyroxine-binding globulin (TBG), 80%; thyroxine-binding prealbumin (TBPA), 10 to 15%; and albumin 4 to 5%) accounts for the high serum concentration and the slow metabolic degradation ($t_{1/2}$ = 7 days) of thyroxine. T_3 is three times more potent metabolically than T_4, but its biologic activity is similar because the lower affinity of T_3 for the plasma proteins results in a lower serum concentration and greater clearance ($t_{1/2}$ = 1.5 days). About 0.2% of T_3 is free and active.

Overview of Thyroid Assessment

Assessment of thyroid disorders includes

1. A history of any symptoms of either thyroid excess or deficiency;

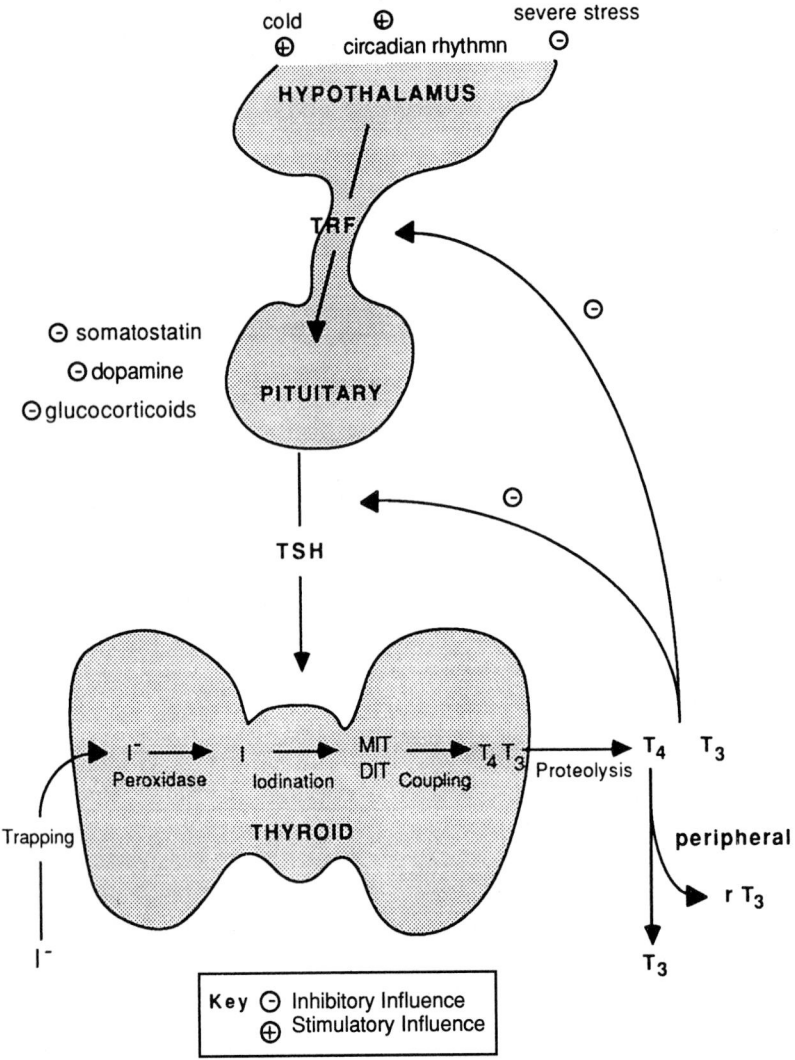

Figure 16.1. Hormone synthesis via negative-feedback control on the hypothalamic-pituitary-thyroid axis.

2. A history of any neck or thyroid symptoms (e.g., pain, tenderness, difficulty swallowing or breathing);
3. A history of any familial thyroid abnormalities;
4. A history of any upper chest or neck irradiation as a child;
5. An examination of the thyroid for enlargement, consistency, and nodularity;
6. An examination for thyroid hormone effects on target systems;
7. A complete medication history for any thyroid or antithyroid drugs;
8. Appropriate thyroid function tests.

THYROID FUNCTION TESTS

Several laboratory tests are used to assess thyroid homeostasis and metabolic function (2). These tests evaluate circulating hormone levels, glandular activity, hypothalamic-pituitary function, autoimmunity, and measurements of various nonspecific metabolic indices (Table 16.1). Normal ranges depend on the laboratory and the assay used. Initial screening tests for thyroid disorders

should include a free thyroxine by equilibrium dialysis (FT_4D) (or a free thyroxine index (FT_4I)) and a thyrotropin-stimulating hormone (TSH) level. Thyroid antibodies (TgATA, AMA) confirm the presence of an autoimmune thyroid disorder if a goiter and/or clinical symptoms are present. The total and bound T_3 (TT_3) and the TRH (thyrotrophin-releasing hormone test) are most useful in the diagnosis of hyperthyroidism. The thyroid uptake (RAIU), thyroid scan, fine-needle aspiration (FNA), and serum thyroglobulin test offer information in the evaluation of nodular disease and malignancy.

Circulating Hormone Levels. Tests of circulating hormone levels measure (either directly or indirectly) the total free and protein-bound concentrations of T_4 and T_3. Direct measurements of circulating hormone levels include the FT_4D, TT_4, and TT_3. Indirect measurements include the free thyroxine index (FT_4I), the resin T_3 uptake (RT_3U), the T_4 uptake (T_4U), and the free T_3 index (FT_3I).

Table 16.1.
Thyroid Function Tests

Test	Normal Values	Measures	Hyperthyroidism	Hypothyroidism	Comments
TT$_4$ (total thyroxine)	64–142 mmol/liter (5–11 μg/dl)	Total T$_4$ both free and bound	↑	↓	Altered by changes in thyroxine-binding globulin (TBG)
FT$_4$D (free thyroxine)	12–26 pmol/liter (0.8–2.0 ng/dl)	Free T$_4$ measured by equilibrium dialysis	↑	↓	Accurate measure of direct free T$_4$
FT$_4$I (free thyroxine index) calculated using RT$_3$U	(16–50 mmol/liter (1.3–4.2)	Product of RT$_3$U × TT$_4$; estimate of active free T$_4$ levels	↑	↓	Compensates for changes in TBG concentration; usually reflects true thyroid status except in euthyroid sick syndrome
FT$_4$I (calculated using T$_4$U)	107–118 mmol/liter (6.5–12.5)	Division of total T$_4$ by T uptake result	↑	↓	Compensates for changes in TBG, prealbumin, and albumin
RT$_3$U (resin T$_3$ uptake)	0.25–0.37 (25–37%)	Indirect measure of degree of saturation of TBG sites by T$_4$	↑	↓	Altered by changes in TBG
T$_4$ uptake	0.6–1.2 uptake units	Available binding sites on TBG, prealbumin, and albumin	↑	↓	Altered by changes in TBG, prealbumin, and albumin
TT$_3$ (total T$_3$)	1.46–2.92 mmol/liter (95–190 ng/dl)	Total T$_3$ both free and bound	↑	↓	Altered by changes in TBG
FT$_3$I (free T$_3$ index)	0.37–1.08 nmol/liter (24–70 ng/dl)	Product of RT$_3$U × T$_3$; estimate of active free T$_3$ levels			See comments for FT$_4$I
RAIU (^{123}I radioactive-iodine uptake)	At 5 hr—5–15% At 24 hr—10–35%	Iodine trapping ability of gland without regard to ultimate fate of iodine	↑	↓ ↑ in early gland failure	Normals vary depending on the degree of dietary iodide intake and on geographical locale; interfered by iodine intake
TSH (thyrotropin-stimulating hormone)	0.4–4.8 mU/liter (0.4–4.8 μu/ml)	Pituitary TSH	↓	↑	Most sensitive indicator of adequate circulating thyroid levels
Antibodies					
ATgA (thyroglobulin)	0–8%	Autoimmune process, (i.e., Hashimoto's, Graves' disease)	Often +	Often +	Microsomal more sensitive, elevated even with remission
AMA (microsomal)	<1:100 titer		Often +	Often +	
TSI	Negative	Thyroid-stimulating immunoglobulin	+ (Graves')	−	Confirmatory for Graves' disease
TRH test (thyrotropin-releasing hormone test)	2 to 5-fold rise in serum TSH 30 min after injection 400 μg TRH IV	Ability of pituitary to respond appropriately to TRH and to endogenous thyroid levels	No response	Exaggerated response if primary hypothyroidism; no response in pituitary	Very sensitive test to determine hyperthyroid state if other tests not confirmatory
Thyroid scan	Isotopes scan with ^{123}I or ^{99}TcO$_4$	Areas of hypofunctioning (cold), areas of hyperfunctioning (hot), and size of gland	Diffusely enlarged; can have hot areas	Cold areas with Hashimoto's disease	Not usually done unless discrete nodules are felt on physical examination

Free Thyroxine (FT₄D). The FT_4D by equilibrium dialysis is a measure of the actual free thyroxine. This method is much more reliable than the widely available analog measurements of the free thyroxine or the commonly used calculated FT_4I. If the FT_4D by equilibrium dialysis is available, it can replace the TT_4 and FT_4I tests. Similarly, free T_3 (FT_3) can also be measured by equilibrium dialysis; however, this test is not yet readily available.

Free Thyroxine Index, Free T3 Index. The FT_4I and the FT_3I are indirect calculated estimates of the free T_4 and T_3, as derived from TT_4 and TT_3 measurements. Because the TT_4 and the TT_3 depend upon TBG, any change in the amount of TBG or the degree of TBG saturation will influence these results (Table 16.2). These fluctuations in TBG do not accurately reflect the active-free hormone levels, which remain unchanged in a euthyroid state. The FT_4I and FT_3I correct for these TBG changes. An exception is in the euthyroid sick syndrome, where the FT_4I or FT_3I can be falsely low. For example, if TBG levels are increased in a euthyroid patient (e.g., pregnancy or estrogen-containing oral contraceptives), the increased number of binding sites will produce a falsely elevated TT_4 and TT_3. However, the free T_4 levels and free T_3 levels remain normal, as indicated by the FT_4I and FT_3I. Conversely, if TBG levels and therefore TBG binding sites are decreased in a euthyroid patient (e.g., androgen therapy, nephrosis, cirrhosis), a falsely depressed TT_4 and TT_3 will be seen. Drugs that displace T_4 and T_3 from TBG, e.g., large doses of salicylates (levels >15 mg/100 ml), will also produce a falsely low TT_4 and TT_3, because the binding sites are occupied by salicylates. In these latter situations, both the FT_4I and FT_3I index are normal in the euthyroid individual.

Two methods can be used to calculate the index, and the one selected depends on the laboratory performing the assays. An older method used to calculate the FT_4I and FT_3I index is the product of either the TT_4 or TT_3 and the resin T_3 uptake test (RT_3U). A newer method uses the T_4 uptake.

Resin T₃ Uptake. The resin T_3 uptake (RT_3U) is an indirect assessment of the concentration and saturation of TBG by T_4. In this test, a fixed amount of labeled T_3 and a resin sponge are added to the serum and allowed to equilibrate. At equilibrium, the radioactive T_3 will bind to the unoccupied sites on the patient's circulating TBG, and the remaining unbound radioactive T_3 will be picked up by the resin sponge.

The amount of radioactivity remaining in the sponge will be inversely proportional to the number of unbound sites on the TBG. Therefore, the radioactivity on the resin is higher if most sites on the patient's TBG are occupied (i.e., hyperthyroidism) or if fewer sites are available e.g., androgens (increased RT_3U). Conversely, when there are more unoccupied TBG sites (e.g., hypothyrodisim) or

more available sites (e.g., pregnancy), most of the labeled T_3 will bind to the patient's TBG and a smaller proportion will be removed by the resin (decreased RT_3U).

A popular modification of the RT_3U test, used in over 50% of hospitals, is the fluorescein-labeled T_4 uptake test. This method uses T_4 instead of radioactive T_3 and allows not only an estimate of TBG binding sites but also an estimate of prealbumin and albumin sites, without the additional risk of radioactivity. The patient's serum is incubated with labeled T_4. Binding of the fluorescein-labeled T_4 to T_4-binding proteins in the patient's serum increases the polarization of fluorescent light emitted by the fluorescein-labeled T_4. The increase in fluorescence polarization is directly proportional to the amount of protein binding of fluorescein-labeled T_4. Usually T_4 uptake results are not reported by laboratories. Most report only the FT_4I, which gives quite different normal values than those obtained using the RT_3U method. Using this method, the FT_4I and FT_3I are calculated by *dividing* the TT_4 or TT_3 by the T_4 uptake test result. For example, if TT_4 is 10 μg/dl and RT_3U is 30%, the FT_4I will be 3.0. If the index is calculated using the T_4 uptake of 1.0, a normal FT_4I of 10 will be reported.

Glandular Activity. The radioactive iodine uptake test (RAIU) measures only the iodine-trapping ability of the gland, without regard to the ultimate fate of the iodine. After a tracer dose of radioactive iodine, the percentage iodine uptake is measured at 5 and at 24 hours. An elevated uptake (>35% at 24 hr) typically occurs in hyperthyroidism, whereas a depressed uptake (<30% in 24 hr) is seen in hypothyroidism. However, elevated uptake can also occur in early hypothyroidism, indicating an attempt by the failing gland to increase iodine uptake and subsequent hormone synthesis. A thyroid scan is usually obtained concurrently. The scan, a picture of the gland, detects hypofunctioning, non-iodine-concentrating, "cold" areas or hyperfunctioning, hyper-iodine-concentrating, "hot" areas in parts of or the whole gland. A scan and uptake should be obtained if discrete thyroid nodules or irregularities are palpable, if there is a history of prior neck irradiation, or if ablative radioactive iodine therapy is indicated. Difficulty with accurate interpretation of the RAIU dictates that it be used as an adjunct rather than a primary diagnostic tool. Fluctuations in the total iodide pool, through either dietary or therapeutic maneuvers, will falsely alter the true value of the RAIU (Table 16.2).

Hypothalamic-Pituitary Function. The integrity of the negative-feedback hypothalamic-pituitary axis is measured by the serum thyrotropin (TSH) and the thyrotropin-releasing hormone (TRH) tests (Table 16.1).

TSH Levels. The sensitive assay for TSH is the most accurate indicator of hypothyroidism and adequate hormone replacement therapy. It may also be used to detect hyperthyroidism or overreplacement therapy. Serum TSH

Table 16.2.
Summary of Laboratory Alterations by Drug/Disease States[a]

Drugs/Disease	Mechanism	TT_4	RT_3U	FT_4I/FT_4D	TT_3	^{131}I Uptake	TSH	Comment
Estrogens, oral contraceptives, clofibrate, heroin addicts, methadone maintenance, genetic, pregnancy, acute and chronic active hepatitis	Increase serum TBG concentrations	↑	↓	No change	↑	No change	No change	FT_4I/FT_4D corrects alterations in TBG; reflects true thyroid status
Androgens, anabolic steroids, danazol, glucocorticoids, L-asparaginase, nephrotic syndrome, cirrhosis, genetic	Decrease serum TBG concentration	↓	↑	No change	↓	No change	No change	FT_4I/FT_4D corrects alterations in TBG; reflects true thyroid status
Phenytoin in vitro, high dose furosemide, high-dose salicylates (4–5 g/day) phenylbutazone, Fenoclofenac, Halofenate, mitotane, chloral hydrate, 5-fluorouracil	Displacement of T_4, T_3 from TBG	↓	↑ or little to no change	No change	↓	No change ^{131}I with phenyl butazone	No change	FT_4I/FT_4D corrects alterations in TBG; reflects true thyroid status
Iodide-containing compounds, contrast medium, Providone-iodine, kelp, tincture iodine, saturated solution potassium iodide (SSKI), Lugol's solution	Dilution of total body iodide pools	No change if test done by radioimmuno assay	No change	No change	No change	↓	No change	No change in thyroid status
Strong diuresis by furosemide, ethacrynic acid; iodine deficiency	Decrease total body iodide pools	No change	No change	No change	No change	Variable	No change	No change in thyroid status
Phenytoin carbamazepine	Alter cellular uptake and metabolism of T_4	↓	↑ or no change		No change	No change	No change	No change in thyroid status
Phenobarbital	Hepatic enzyme inducer of T_4 metabolism	↓ in hypothyroid patients, no change in euthyroid						

(continued)

Table 16.2. (Continued)

Drugs/Disease	Mechanism	TT$_4$	RT$_3$U	FT$_4$I/FT$_4$D	TT$_3$	^{131}I Uptake	TSH	Comment
Propranolol, glucocorticoids, old age, fasting, malnutrition, acute and chronic systemic illness	Impair peripheral conversion of T$_4$ to T$_3$; ↑ rT$_3$	Normal or ↓	Normal or ↑	Normal or ↓	↓	No change	No change	Patient is clinically euthyroid. Free T$_4$ is normal or slightly elevated in severe illness; T$_4$ binding to TBG is impaired
Amiodarone, iopodate, iopanoate	Impair peripheral and pituitary conversion of T$_4$ to T$_3$	↑		↑	↓	↓ Iodide release from iodinated contrast	Transient ↑ with aminodarone	Patient is clinically euthyroid; but can cause hyper- or hypothyroidism in patient with underlying thyroid disorders

^{a} See Table 16.1 for abbreviations.

elevations often occur before other overt clinical and laboratory manifestations of hypothyroidism. Therefore, the TSH can be elevated despite a normal FT$_4$D or TT$_4$ and FT$_4$I, indicating early subclinical hypothyroidism or insufficient hormone replacement. Likewise, in hyperthyroidism or in overreplacement therapy, the TSH is suppressed into the subnormal range, even though circulating hormone levels are within the normal range. The TSH can also be used to differentiate primary thyroid failure (elevated TSH) from diminished secondary pituitary deficiency (absent or low normal TSH). Lastly, the TSH is invaluable in excluding secondary thyroid failure in patients with the euthyroid sick syndrome. The sensitive TSH assays are not perturbed by high levels of human chorionic gonadotropins (HCG) in pregnancy. However, factors that influence dopamine, which physiologically controls TSH secretion, may alter the level. Dopamine agonists (e.g., dopamine, levodopa, bromocriptine) and corticosteroids can falsely lower TSH secretion, and dopamine antagonists (e.g., metoclopramide) can falsely increase TSH secretion (2).

Thyrotropin-releasing Hormone (TRH) Test. The TRH stimulation test is an easy and safe test that can be performed on an outpatient basis to confirm the diagnosis of hyperthyroidism. Rarely, reversible hypotension and shock are reported. The TRH test is only indicated in the diagnosis of thyrotoxicosis when other clinical and laboratory indices are not confirmatory (e.g., Graves' ophthalmopathy or borderline high FT$_4$I and FT$_3$I, and suppressed TSH (2).

Protirelin (synthetic TRH), 200 to 400 μg IV, should produce a 2- to 4-fold increase from baseline TSH levels in euthyroid patients after 30 to 45 min. In thyrotoxic patients, a flat, blunted TSH response is expected because relatively high circulating thyroid hormone levels block further elevations of TSH after TRH administration. However, a blunted TSH response [<2mU/liter (2 μu/ml)] may also occur in euthyroid patients with renal failure, depression, and starvation; in patients >40 years old; and in those receiving adequate thyroid hormone suppression therapy, chronic glucocorticoid therapy, dopamine infusions, or L-dopa therapy (2).

Tests of Autoimmunity: Antibodies. TgATA; AMA. Two main antigens are identified in the thyroid gland: thyroglobulin and the microsomal component. The presence of antithyroglobulin (TgATA) and antimicrosomal (AMA) antibodies suggests an autoimmune process such as Graves' disease and/or Hashimoto's thyroiditis. However, because antibodies can occur in asymptomatic patients or in patients with collagen vascular disorders, their presence is not diagnostic of thyroid illness. The levels of TgATA and AMA are consistently high during the acute phases of autoimmune thyroid disease and decline during remission and after therapy. The AMA is the more sensitive of the two antibodies because levels remain detectable after remission, whereas TgATA titers revert to normal.

Thyroid-stimulating Immunoglobulin (TSI). An IgG immunoglobulin capable of stimulating the thyroid gland is commonly present in 90% of patients with Graves' disease. There is no need to run a TSI test on a patient with a classic Graves' presentation because the test is expensive (approximately $100) and offers no additional therapeutic or diagnostic information. However, it may confirm the diagnosis of Graves' disease in patients with an atypical presentation. The TSI should be done in the pregnant female with a history of Graves' disease. A high maternal TSI titer provides predictive information about the risk of neonatal Graves' disease. Lastly, the presence or absence of TSI in the serum of treated patients with Graves' disease may act as a prognostic indicator of the potential for relapse and remission.

Nonspecific Indices

A number of nonspecific indices may result from changes in thyroid function. Serum cholesterol, carotene, SGOT, creatine phosphokinase (CPK), and LDH levels may be elevated in hypothyroidism. The opposite occurs in hyperthyroidism.

Euthyroid Sick Syndrome

Many acute and chronic nonthyroid disorders (e.g., starvation, acute depression and other psychiatric disorders, acute infection, chronic cardiac, pulmonary, renal, hepatic, and neoplastic disorders, and AIDS) are associated with impaired peripheral conversion of T_4 to T_3, leading to abnormal and confusing thyroid function test results, despite euthyroidism (3–6). This euthyroid sick syndrome, most common in hospitalized patients, requires appropriate recognition to eliminate dangerous and unnecessary hormone replacement. Abnormalities in thyroid function test results vary, but often include a decreased TT_4, TT_3, decreased calculated free T_4 and T_3 index, normal or elevated FT_4D, and usually, a normal or slightly elevated TSH (<10 mU/liter (10 μU/ml), indicating euthyroidism. The slight elevations in TSH concentrations tend to be transient and indicate a recovery phase. Less frequently, hyperthyroxinemia (e.g., psychiatric illness) occurs instead. An abnormal binding inhibitor in the sera of sick patients probably accounts for some of the abnormal alterations seen. Reversal of the thyroid abnormalities is a good prognostic indicator of recovery and decreased mortality (6). Thyroid hormone supplementation is dangerous, unnecessary, and may impair normal recovery of thyroid homeostasis (3).

HYPERTHYROIDISM/THYROTOXICOSIS
Symptoms

Hyperthyroidism or thyrotoxicosis is a syndrome characterized by increased metabolism of all body systems as a result of excessive quantities of thyroid hormone. The clinical symptoms (listed in Table 16.3) reflect increased adrenergic activity, primarily cardiovascular and neurological. Not all manifestations are present in the same patient. Exogenous ingestion of sympathomimetics or agents with sympathomimetic-like activity will accentuate the hyperthyroid symptoms.

Thyrotoxicosis-induced increases in heart rate (HR), stroke volume (SV), and cardiac output may mimic new-onset or worsening angina, atrial fibrillation, extrasystoles, or congestive heart failure (high output) and are usually resistant to conventional treatment until euthyroidism is achieved. Clinically, a rapid bounding pulse, an elevated systolic blood pressure, a wide pulse pressure, cardiomegaly, and a systolic murmur are seen. Tachycardia, increased voltage, and a prolonged P-R interval are seen on an electrocardiogram (ECG). It is important to eliminate thyrotoxicosis as causing or exacerbating the cardiac disease, especially in the elderly, because definitive pharmacologic therapy (i.e., digitalis) is altered (see section on drug kinetics).

Occasionally, a severely toxic patient may have none of the classic hyperthyroid symptoms. This apathetic or masked hyperthyroidism is typical of the elderly patient (7). The presenting symptoms of fatigue, apathy, listlessness, dull eyes, extreme weakness, congestive heart failure, delayed speech and mentation, and low-grade fever are confusing and obscure the diagnosis. Likewise, premature atrial contractions, atrial fibrillation, or tremor may be the only clue to occult hyperthyroidism in the elderly. Untreated, coma and death are assured. Therefore, the onset of any new cardiac, neurologic, or "failure-to-thrive" symptoms in the elderly demands an evaluation for underlying thyroid disease. Occult thyrotoxicosis is easily confirmed by standard laboratory tests.

Etiology

Thyrotoxicosis has many causes. The primary causes of hyperthyroidism are listed in Table16.4. Rarely, thyrotoxicosis results from thyrotropin-secreting pituitary tumors, from ectopic thyroid tissue (e.g., struma ovarii), from TSH-like substances produced by hydatidiform moles and choriocarcinomas, from self-administration of thyroid (factitious hyperthyroidism), from posttraumatic or radiation injury to the thyroid, and from the initial transient stages of Hashimoto's thyroiditis (hashitoxicosis).

Graves' Disease

Graves' disease, the most common cause of hyperthyroidism, is characterized by symptoms of thyrotoxicosis, a diffusely enlarged goiter, infiltrative ophthalmopathy, and dermopathy. Not all of these findings are required for the diagnoses. The diagnosis of Graves' disease is confirmed

Table 16.3.
Signs and Symptoms of Hyperthyroidism and Hypothyroidism

Body System	Hyperthyroidism	Hypothyroidism
General	Heat intolerance; weight loss despite increased appetite; increased sweating; weight gain due to increased appetite.	Cold intolerance; weight gain despite decreased appetite; hoarseness and lowering of the voice pitch; decreased sweating, easy fatigability
Head	Thinning of the hair; fine texture	Dry, brittle, and sparse hair; thinning of the lateral aspects of the eyebrows; puffy facies, large tongue
Eyes	Prominence of the eyes, lid lag, lid retraction, can proceed to loss of visual acuity	Edematous eyelids; ptosis
Neck	Soft diffusely enlarged goiter with or without bruits/thrills	Goiter in primary hypothyroidism none found in pituitary disorders
Cardiac	Palpitations; high output failure; edema; increased pulse and systolic pressure; wide pulse pressure; presence of systolic murmurs	Cardiac enlargement; poor heart sounds; precordial pain; low output failure; dyspnea
Gastrointestinal	Diarrhea, loose bowels, or hyperdefecation	Constipation
Genitourinary	Amenorrhea or decreased in length of menstrual flow	Menorrhagia, dysmenorrhea
Extremities	Pretibial myxedema; Plummer's nails; hot, flushed and moist skin; palmar erythema	Broad hands and feet; pretibial myxedema; cold and dry skin; brittle nails, yellowish
Neuromuscular	Fatigue, weakness, tremor, rapid deep tendon reflexes	Muscle pain and weakness, paresthesias; delayed deep tendon reflexes
Emotional	Nervousness, irritability, emotional liability; insomnia or shortened sleep cycles	Emotional instability, depression, lethargy, decreased energy and increased sleep requirements; mental sluggishness

Table 16.4.
Etiology of Hyperthyroidism

Graves' disease	Toxic diffuse goiter
Toxic nodules	Single and multinodular
Jod-Basedow disease	Iodine-induced
Factitious	Self-administration
Tumors	Secretion of thyroid-stimulating substance
Subacute thyroiditis	Viral inflammatory condition
Hashitoxicosis	Early phase of Hashimoto's disease
T_3-toxicosis	Often precedes onset of T_4-toxicosis

Table 16.5.
Characteristics of Graves' Disease

Triad of hyperthyroidism, goiter, and ophthalmopathy
Laboratory findings:
    Elevated TT_4, FT_{4D}, FT_4I, TT_3
    Positive ATgA, AMA, TSI
    Flat TRH response curve
    Suppressed TSH
Family history

by abnormally high levels of TT_4, FT_4I or FT_4D, and TT_3, a suppressed TSH, a positive TSI, positive antibodies (TgATA and AMA) in 80% of patients, and a blunted TSH response to TRH (Table 16.5). The RAIU is elevated and a diffusely enlarged "hot" gland is seen on a scan.

The etiology of the disease is unknown. It is predom-inantly a disease of females (5:1 ratio), with its peak onset occurring between the ages of 30 to 40 years. It has a strong familial predisposition, although the mode of genetic transmission is not known. Precipitation of the disease has been associated with trauma, severe emotional stress, weight reduction involving strict diet restriction, stimulants, thyroid hormone, and administration of iodides (Jod-Basedow disease) (1, 8).

Graves' disease, like Hashimoto's thyroiditis, appears to have an autoimmune basis related to disorders of the regulatory suppressor T lymphocytes. The major subsets of T lymphocytes are helper and suppressor T lymphocytes. Normally, helper T lymphocytes interact with B lymphocytes to produce appropriate immunoglobulins, while suppressor T lymphocytes exercise immunological surveillance by preventing T lymphocytes from inappropriately producing immunoglobulins. In Graves' disease, a defect in suppressor T lymphocytes may be responsible for formation of the abnormal thyroid-stimulating immunoglobulin (TSI) found in the blood of patients with active disease (9, 10). The presence of lymphocytic infiltration of the thyroid gland, IgG immunoglobulins, and antibodies directed against both thyroglobulin and microsomal tissue strongly support an autoimmune basis for Graves' disease.

The thyroid gland in Graves' disease is usually diffusely enlarged and symmetrical, with a firm and rubbery consistency. Thrills and bruits may be present in a hyperfunctioning goiter. A thrill, which is less common, is likely to be felt in the region of the superior thyroid arteries. Bruits are usually audible over the entire thyroid gland. Both will disappear in euthyroidism.

Ophthalmopathy. The ocular manifestations consist of noninfiltrative and the characteristic infiltrative ophthalmopathy (11–14). Noninfiltrative ocular abnormalities result from hyperactivity of the sympathetic nervous system and can be found in any thyrotoxic condition. Increased sympathetic tone on Muller's superior palpebral muscle results in spasm and retraction of the upper lid, widening the palpebral fissure to give the characteristic stare or frightened expression. Lid lag is present when the eyelid movement lags behind eye movement, and a narrow white rim of sclera becomes visible between the upper lid and the cornea. These ocular changes are reversible with control of the thyrotoxicosis.

The infiltrative ocular findings are the most striking abnormalities of Graves' disease. They may appear before thyrotoxicosis, during the acute phases of the disease, or even years after successful therapy of the thyrotoxicosis. The ocular involvement may be unilateral or bilateral and may not reverse with achievement of euthyroidism. The most severe forms are often encountered in patients who are euthyroid or hypothyroid after radioactive iodine ablation (11–14). Exacerbations of the eye symptoms may also occur abruptly after RAI therapy (13). It is not known why the eyes and associated muscles are attached while other organ systems are spared. Histological examination reveals lymphocytic infiltration and deposition of mucopolysaccharides, fat, and water in all retrobulbar tissues.

Mild eye symptoms are found in 50% of patients; the most severe forms occur in less than 5%. Various degrees of the following signs and symptoms occur:

1. Edema and swelling of the lids and periorbital tissue, resulting in chemosis, excessive tearing, photophobia, and conjunctivitis.
2. Proptosis (protrusion of the cornea more than the normal 18 to 20 mm beyond the lateral margin of the orbit) results from an increase in orbital contents. This often results in a wide-eyed staring expression. The globes are firmer and harder than normal. Increased tearing and irritation may occur from the exposed conjunctiva. Corneal scarring and ulceration result if the proptosis causes the lid to remain open, exposing and drying out the eye during sleep.
3. Limitation of extraocular eye movements as a result of paralysis of the extraocular muscles. Loss of upward gaze and loss of convergence occur commonly. Diplopia may result.
4. Blindness may occur from venous congestion and hemorrhage of the retina and optic nerve.

Dermopathy. The dermopathy of Graves' disease, also known as pretibial myxedema, can occur with the infiltrative ophthalmopathy. Mucopolysaccharide infiltration of the skin causes the cutaneous thickening and hyperpigmentation usually seen over the tibial aspects of the leg. Similar lesions can appear on the dorsa of the feet and hands. Pretibial myxedema is usually asymptomatic, but can be painful or pruritic. Like the infiltrative ocular symptoms, pretibial myxedema can occur at any time in the course of the disease. If necessary, the clinical diagnosis can be confirmed by tissue biopsy. Treatment with topical corticosteroids and Saran wrap is often effective.

Toxic/Multinodular Disease

Toxic nodule (Plummer's disease) is characterized by a single autonomous hyperfunctioning nodule in an otherwise normal gland. The nodule, usually 3 to 5 cm in diameter, is not under TSH regulation, and can produce normal or supraphysiological amounts of thyroid hormone, causing suppression of existing normal thyroid tissue. Patients can be either euthyroid or toxic. A "hot" nodule appears on scans as an area of increased iodine concentration, but the rest of the thyroid may not be visible if it is suppressed by the nodule. A toxic nodule is the least common of the three major causes of hyperthyroidism.

New onset of thyrotoxicosis in patients in their 5th or 6th decade of life usually results from toxic multinodular goiters. These patients often have a history of a large, firm, multinodular goiter (multiple nodules) without any symptoms of hypothyroidism or hyperthyroidism for many years. However, many of the nodules function autonomously and activate in later years. This is the most common cause of thyrotoxicosis in the elderly.

Subacute Thyroiditis

Subacute thyroiditis (de Quervain's thyroiditis) is a spontaneous, remitting, inflammatory thyroid condition that is believed to have a viral etiology. Clinical features include the acute onset of diffuse or localized swelling of the gland, tenderness or pain with swallowing, a recent history of flu-like symptoms, fever, malaise, and symptoms of either hyper- or hypothyroidism. Laboratory abnormalities include an elevated erythrocyte sedimentation rate (ESR), a low or undetectable RAIU, leukocytosis, and changes in thyroid hormone levels. Elevations in T_4 levels and clinical hyperthyroidism occur from leakage of hormones and iodoproteins from the inflamed gland in the early stages of the disease. Hypothyroidism can result if long-standing inflammation of the gland prevents further hormone synthesis after the initial hormone stores are depleted.

The disease is self-limiting, and spontaneous recovery is common. Treatment is symptomatic and consists of heat, rest, analgesics, and antithyroid agents, if necessary to control the hyperthyroidism. Corticosteroids are indicated for severe inflammation if analgesics are ineffective. In the hypothyroid phase, transient thyroid replacement may be required to suppress further TSH stimulation to the damaged gland.

T3-Toxicosis

T3 thyrotoxicosis is characterized by normal levels of T_4 and elevated levels of T_3. T_3 toxicosis is seen in Graves' disease, toxic goiters and carcinomas, and is reported in children. Preferential T_3 secretion, producing toxicity, is more prevalent in iodine-deficient areas. Elevated T_3 levels often precede the onset of frank T_4 toxicosis after withdrawal of antithyroid medications in asymptomatic patients with a history of Graves' disease. Therefore, the T_3 level is a good monitoring parameter of relapse in these patients.

Drug-induced Thyrotoxicosis

Iodine-induced thyrotoxicosis (Jod-Basedow disease) was first described in the 1800s in residents of iodine-deficient areas who became symptomatic after adequate iodine supplementation. Most cases occurred in patients with multinodular goiters and autonomous functioning nodules that were activated by the increased iodine supplements (1, 8). Iodides do not cause the underlying thyroid disease; they produce thyrotoxicosis in abnormal thyroid glands that have lost the protective Wolff-Chaikoff block. Thyrotoxicosis has also been reported following injections of radiocontrast material or iodinated topical preparations (1, 8, 15).

Paradoxically, lithium is also associated with the development of hyperthyroidism (16). Since lithium acts like iodides in preventing hormone release, lithium is probably suppressing frank hyperthyroidism that became evident after its withdrawal. Lithium has thus been advocated in the treatment of hyperthyroidism if other options are not feasible.

Amiodarone, which contains 37.2% iodine by weight, is implicated in numerous reports of hyperthyroidism (17–19). The prevalence ranges from 1 to 5% and is more common in areas of endemic iodine deficiency. Probably, this complication is due to its high iodine content rather than to a direct pharmacological effect. Because euthyroid patients on amiodarone normally have hyperthyroxinemia, actual thyrotoxicosis must be documented with serum TT_3 levels, TSH, TRH, and clinical symptoms.

Treatment of Thyrotoxicosis

The major treatment modalities for the management of thyrotoxicosis are the thioamides, radioactive iodine (RAI), and surgery (Table 16.6). Each has its own advantages and limitations, so treatment must be individualized. In most cases, all three treatment modalities are appropriate and effective. The type of hyperthyroidism, its severity, the patient's age, the existence of thyroid and nonthyroid complications, as well as social and economic issues should be considered in treatment selection. For example, uncomplicated patients with Graves' disease may be managed medically with thioamides until remission occurs. However, elderly patients with toxic multinodular disease are best managed with definitive treatment such as radioactive iodine or surgery because spontaneous remission is unlikely. Likewise, women with Graves' disease who plan on future pregnancies should have their thyrotoxicosis permanently controlled prior to pregnancy with either surgery or radioactive iodine to prevent disease flares and relapse during pregnancy and the postpartum period (20–21). If RAI or surgery is selected, most elderly patients and all severely thyrotoxic patients should be pretreated with thioamides. Pretreatment depletes the gland of stored hormones, reduces the hypermetabolic rate, and prevents leakage of hormone from the gland after RAI or during surgery, preventing thyroid storm (22–23). However, the final decision in the uncomplicated patient is often empiric, depending upon available resources and the physician's experience; and it should be a joint patient-physician decision after discussion of the benefits and risks of each method. Interestingly, a survey of practicing thyroidologists also showed considerable variation in the selected treatment methods (24).

Pharmacologic Management

THIOAMIDES

The thioamides, propylthiouracil (PTU), and methimazole, prevent thyroid hormone synthesis by inhibiting the oxidation binding of iodide and its coupling to tyrosine residues. PTU (but no methimazole) inhibits the peripheral deiodination of T_4 to T_3, so serum T_3 levels decline 20 to 30% more rapidly in thyrotoxic patients. An immunosuppressive mechanism is also postulated (25, 26).

Theoretically, thioamides are preferred over radioactive iodine and surgery to treat the uncomplicated hyperthyroid patient because they do not destroy the gland and control the disease until remission occurs. Therefore, chronic thyroid replacement, which is likely with RAI or surgery, may not be necessary. This advantage of thioamides may be irrelevant because the natural history of Graves' disease appears to be eventual hypothyroidism even if no glandular destruction occurs.

Thioamide selection is based largely on personal preference, although certain pharmacological differences may dictate the choice. Generally, PTU is preferred over methimazole in severely toxic patients or those with thyroid storm because it blocks the peripheral conversion of T_4 to T_3 and therefore has faster onset. PTU is also the thioamide of choice in pregnancy and in the lactating mother (see section on pregnancy). Although PTU is more commonly prescribed, methimazole is preferable because it can be given as a single daily dose; is more potent and requires fewer tablets; is cheaper; is better tolerated; and at low

Table 16.6.
Management of Thyrotoxicosis

Method	Drug	Dose	Mechanism of Action	Toxicity	Comments
Thioamides	Propylthiouracil (PTU) 50 mg tablets	100–200 mg every 6 hr initially, maintenance of 50–150 mg daily; can be formulated for rectal administration	Blocks organification of hormone synthesis, also inhibits peripheral conversion of T_4 to T_3; immunosuppressive?	Skin rashes, agranulocytosis, gastrointestinal symptoms, hepatitis	Poor remission rate of 20–30%; onset of action approximately 2–4 weeks; DOC in pregnancy and during lactation
	Methimazole (Tapazole) 5- and 10-mg tablets	30–40 mg once daily initially, maintenance of 5–10 mg daily; can be formulated for rectal administration	Blocks organification of hormone synthesis; immunosuppressive?	Same as PTU; secreted in breast milk; tetratogenic scalp defects	Appears to have no cross sensitivity to PTU with regard to rashes; Longer duration of action than PTU; DOC for single daily dosing
Iodides	Lugol's solution 8 mg iodide/drop; Saturated solution of potassium iodide (SSKI) 50 mg/drop	6 mg iodide/day although larger doses are given	Blocks release of hormone from the gland; decreases the vascularity of the gland and increases firmness which facilitates easier removal of the gland during surgery	Hypersensitivity reactions—rashes, rhinorrhea, parotid and submaxillary swelling	Can be used for symptomatic control of hyperthyroidism in patients on Thioamides, in thyroid storm and as a preoperative adjunct; DO NOT USE PRIOR TO RAI
Adrenergic antagonist	Propranolol (Inderal) 10-, 20-, 40-, 60-, 80-, 90-mg tablets, 1 mg/ml IV	20–40 mg orally every 6 hr	Blocks the peripheral action of thyroid hormone, no effect on underlying disease state. Blocks T_4 to T_3 conversion peripherally	Bradycardia, congestive heart failure, asthma, inhibits hyperglycemic response to hypoglycemia	Acute onset provides symptomatic relief while awaiting onset of action of thioamides, RAI, or surgery
	Diltiazem (Cardizem) 30-, 60-, 90-, 120-mg tablets, 90-, 120-mg SR-release tablets	60 mg p.o. q.i.d. or 120 mg t.i.d.		Hypotension, bradycardia, pedal edema	Alternative to patients unable to use β-blockers (e.g., asthma, diabetes)
Radioactive Iodine	^{131}I	80 to 100 μCi/g thyroid tissue	Destruction of the gland	Hypothyroidism, fear of malignancy, leukemia, and genetic damage	Slow onset of action approximately 2–4 weeks, full effects seen within 3–6 months
Surgery	Iodides, thioamides or propranolol preoperative to induce relief of symptoms	5–10 drops/day of iodides for 10–14 days prior to surgery; see above doses for propranolol and thioamides	Subtotal removal of the gland is surgical procedure of choice	Hypothyroidism, hypoparathyroidism, complications of surgery and anesthesia	Incidence of hypothyroidism indirectly proportional to gland remnant left
Iodinated contrast media	Ipodate, Iopanoic acid	500 mg–1 g q.d. or 3 g q 3rd day	Blocks $T_4 \rightarrow T_3$ conversion; release of iodides. See iodides	Similar to iodides	Rapid onset of action; not for chronic use because effects not sustained

doses, is less toxic than PTU (27). Therefore, methimazole is recommended except in those identified situations where PTU is preferable and in patients unable to tolerate PTU.

Biopharmaceutics. Although methimazole is 10 times more potent than PTU (100 mg of PTU = 10 mg of methimazole), they are equally effective if given in equipotent doses. Both drugs are absorbed rapidly from the gastrointestinal tract, and peak plasma concentrations are reached within 30 minutes of ingestion. The serum half-lives of 4 to 6 hours for methimazole and 1 to 2 hours for PTU do not change as the thyroid status changes. However, the duration of action depends upon the intrathyroid half-life and not on the short plasma half-lives. The duration of action of methimazole is 24 to 36 hours, allowing once-daily administration (28). The intrathyroid duration of PTU is much shorter, requiring dosing every 6 to 8 hours to be effective.

Dosing Regimens. Depending on the severity of the thyrotoxicosis, therapy is initiated with either 30 to 40 mg/day orally of methimazole, given as a single daily dose or in three divided doses, or 400 to 600 mg/day of PTU, given in four divided doses. Although initial single-dose regimens have been used successfully with PTU, the best results are obtained by achieving euthyroidism by multiple dosing, then changing to a maintenance single-dose regimen. Severely toxic or "storm" patients may require doses as high as 1200 mg/day of PTU or its equivalent, given in divided doses. Both drugs can be formulated for rectal administration (29–30). Once the patient is euthyroid, usually after 6 to 8 weeks (dependent on elimination of existing thyroid stores; $t_{1/2}$ = 7 days), the initial dose can be reduced gradually on a monthly basis by $\frac{1}{3}$ until a daily maintenance dose of 5 to 10 mg of methimazole or 50 to 150 mg/day of PTU is reached. Tapering should not start until symptoms are reduced and circulating thyroxine levels are normal. If symptoms do not resolve within the specified time, patient noncompliance, incomplete blockage of synthesis by insufficient dosage, or an inadequate dosing interval should be considered as causes of failure. Drug failures are more likely to occur with PTU than with methimazole. Some clinicians advocate the concomitant use of exogenous thyroxine during antithyroid therapy to prevent hypothyroidism and suppress goiter formation from excessive PTU or methimazole administration. However, proper dosing of thioamides should alleviate this problem, so concomitant thyroxine therapy is only recommended when proper titration is difficult.

Prior to the administration of thioamides, a baseline TT$_4$ and FT$_4$I or FT$_4$D, TSH, and white blood cell count (WBC) with differential should be obtained to help monitor therapy. A baseline WBC with differential is used to ascertain the development of agranulocytosis, because hyperthyroidism per se can be associated with a relative reduction in the neutrophil count. The above thyroid function tests should be normalized within 6 to 8 weeks after the onset of therapy, paralleling the clinical response. The FT$_4$D or TT$_4$ and FT$_4$I, and TSH should be monitored a minimum of 6 weeks after the onset of therapy and 6 weeks after any change in the dosing regimen. Once a stable thioamide maintenance dose is reached, thyroid function tests can be routinely monitored every 3 to 6 months.

Duration of Therapy. The duration of thioamide therapy for Graves' disease is empiric, generally 12 to 18 months. Shorter courses of 3 to 6 months have been advocated, but they yielded remission rates of 20–40% (31, 32). Conversely, several studies suggest that the remission rate increases with the duration of therapy (32–34). An 18-month treatment period yielded higher remission rates (61.8%) than therapy for 6 months (41.7%). A study in children noted a 25% increase in the remission rate when the duration was increased by 1 year (34). Therefore, a minimum treatment duration of 12 months is recommended to increase the remission rate. Longer treatment durations may be used if there are no adverse effects.

Hyperthyroid patients on thioamides can be managed effectively by the pharmacist using a treatment algorithm (Fig. 16.2).

Prognosis. Disappointing remission rates of 30 to 40% after discontinuation of thioamide therapy has led to progressive disenchantment with antithyroid drugs as a definitive therapy for Graves' disease. It is unclear why some patients remain in remission while others relapse. Concomitant autoimmune thyroiditis may cause the permanent remission. Besides extending the duration of therapy, better remission rates may result from the administration of high thioamide blocking doses (i.e., 600 to 800 mg of PTU) throughout treatment (35). The higher doses and the longer duration of thioamide treatment may produce successful remission by suppressing TSI.

Several factors may be predictive of remission and justify a longer trial of thioamide administration. The best predictor for remission is a reduction in goiter size to normal during therapy. Patients with small goiters, with mild and short-duration symptoms and illness, and disappearance of TSI during therapy also have a better chance of remission (32–34). Analysis of HLA specificities (HLA-B8 and DW3) in conjunction with IgG immunoglobulin levels may be highly predictive of remission or relapse after withdrawal of thioamides.

Adverse Reactions

Toxic reactions to PTU and methimazole occur in 1 to 5% of patients.

A pruritic maculopapular skin rash, without other systemic manifestations, is the most frequently encountered adverse effect. In mild cases, the rash may disappear spontaneously despite continued therapy. If the rash persists,

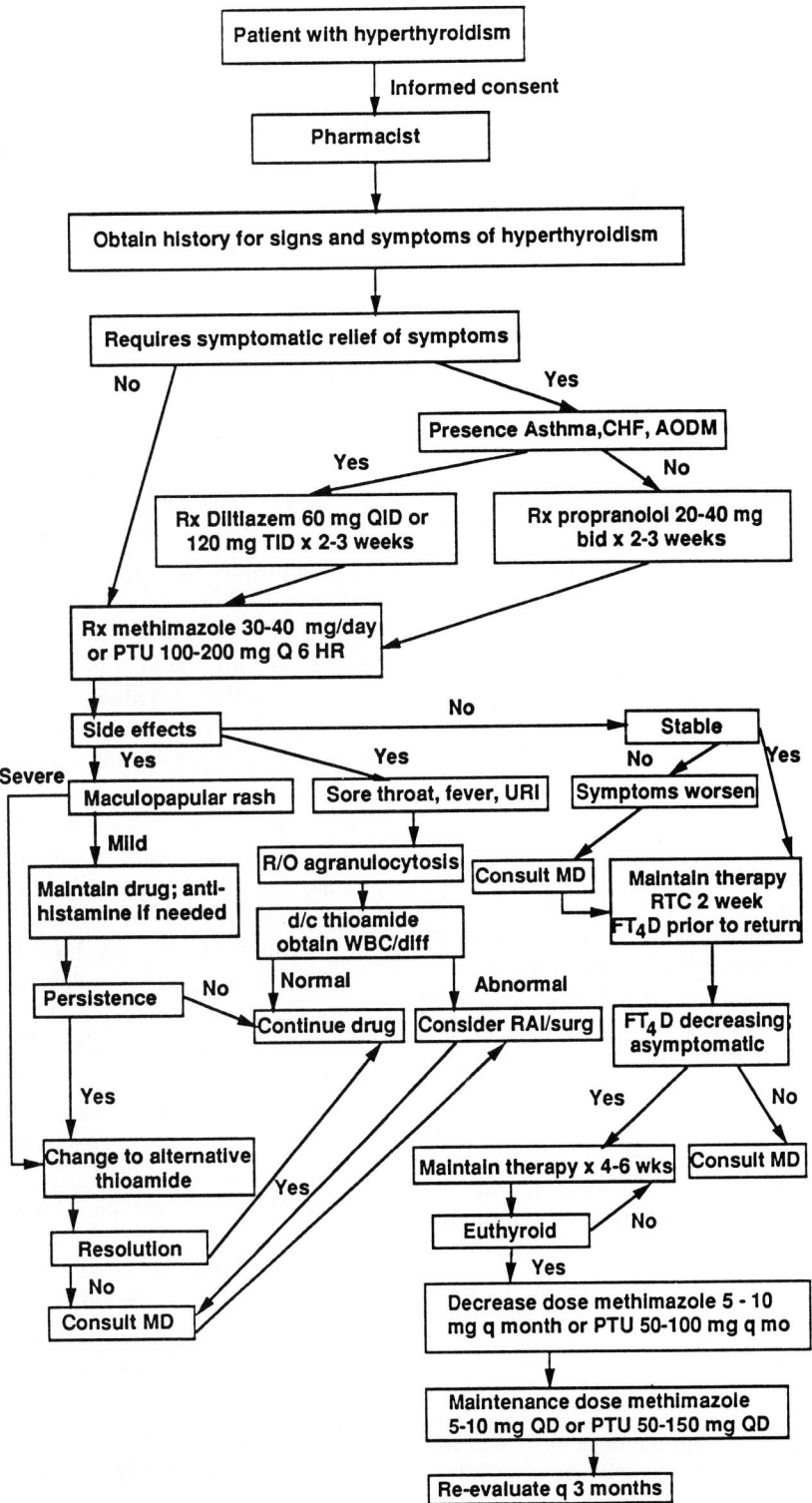

Figure 16.2. Treatment algorithm for hyperthyroidism.

another thioamide can be substituted because little cross-sensitivity appears to exist. However, if the rash is associated with concomitant systemic symptoms (i.e., fever, arthralgias) or if angioneurotic edema, hives, or other anaphylactoid reactions occur, substitution with another thioamide is not recommended.

Hepatitis may be more common than previously recognized (35–36). Hepatocellular and obstructive hepatitis have been reported from both agents; however, hepatocellular damage is most prevalent with PTU, and obstructive jaundice with methimazole. This idiosyncratic reaction typically occurs during the initial phases of therapy, although delayed reactions have been noted. Reversals may occur with early detection; however, fatalities have been reported. Because of the severity of the reaction and the potential for cross-sensitivity, substitution with the alternative thioamide is not recommended.

Rarely, hypoprothrombinemia (PTU), serological abnormalities (lupus erythematosus (LE), antinuclear antibody (ANA)), lupus, and lupus-like syndromes have also been reported. Recovery occurs after withdrawal of the drug or institution of steroids.

Agranulocytosis (<500 PMNs) is the most serious (but infrequent) adverse reaction to the thioamides. The prevalence is between 0.5 and 6%. The onset of fever, malaise, gingivitis, and sore throat is so abrupt that routine WBC counts are not indicated. All patients should be instructed to immediately report the onset of such symptoms to a pharmacist or physician. Older patients (age >40 years) and those on high-dose methimazole (more than 40 mg/day) therapy appear to be at greater risk for developing this toxic reaction, although it is not necessarily dose-related. Low doses (<30 mg/day) of methimazole may be safer than any dose of PTU (37). Sex is not a predictive factor. This reaction is more likely to occur during the first 6 weeks of therapy although it can occur at any time in the course of treatment. Fortunately, complete symptom reversal and return of granulocytes is often seen within a few days to 3 weeks after discontinuation of the thioamides. If infection occurs, antibiotics, adrenal steroids, and possibly hospitalization (bacteria-free room) are indicated. Rechallenge with the same drug or a alternative thioamide is not recommended because the risk of recurrent agranulocytosis outweighs the benefits of therapy. The degree of cross-sensitivity is not known.

Monovalent Anions

Potassium perchlorate is the only monovalent anion with sufficient antithyroid activity to be clinically useful. In doses of 1 g/day, perchlorate is concentrated by the gland, where it interferes with iodide binding and causes the discharge of nonorganified iodide. Since perchlorate is a competitive inhibitor of iodide, its antithyroid effect can be overcome by iodine administration. The severe toxicity of irreversible aplastic anemia and nephrotic syndrome has limited the usefulness of the monovalent anions.

Iodides

Although iodides have been known to relieve the symptoms of thyrotoxicosis since the 1920s, their clinical use has largely been superseded by the thioamides and the β-blockers. Several actions are recognized when iodides are administered: inhibition of organification (Wolff-Chaikoff effect), inhibition of hormone release, and a decrease in gland size and vascularity (1). The rapid relief of thyrotoxic symptoms after 2 to 7 days of iodide administration suggests that inhibition of hormone release is the predominant mechanism of action; a block in organification would not be apparent for several weeks. This rapid response is beneficial for patients in thyroid storm and for those awaiting the onset of thioamide therapy. However, iodides should not be used prior to RAI therapy (or if RAI is to be eventually considered as therapy) because iodides can block effective RAI retention by the gland for several weeks after use.

Iodides are routinely given 10 to 14 days before surgery to decrease the vascularity and increase the firmness of the hyperplastic gland, which facilitates surgical removal. Preoperatively, the combination of propranolol and iodides can also be used, although the established regimen of thioamides and iodides is preferable.

Stable iodine is available as either Lugol's solution (5% iodine and 10% potassium iodide), containing 8 mg of iodide per drop, or as the more palatable saturated solution of potassium iodide (SSKI), containing 50 mg/drop.

The major adverse effects of iodides are hypersensitivity reactions, including rashes, drug fever, sialadenitis, conjunctivitis, rhinitis, and collagen vascular disorders. In individuals with underlying thyroid disorders, iodides can either induce hyperthyroidism (e.g., multinodular goiter) from failure of the Wolff-Chaikoff block or precipitate goiter and hypothyroidism (i.e., Hishimoto's thyroiditis) in patients unable to escape from the Wolff-Chaikoff block (1, 8, 15).

Avantages of iodide therapy include simplicity, low cost, low toxicity, and no gland destruction. Limitations of treatment includes escape, treatment relapse, allergic reactions, and interference with subsequent RAI therapy.

Lithium

Lithium, which acts like iodides in inhibiting hormone release, has been recommended in doses of 800 to 1200 mg/day for the treatment of thyrotoxicosis (16). Lithium serum levels must be maintained within therapeutic levels to avoid side effects: tremor, ataxia, dizziness, confusion, coma, nausea, vomiting, diarrhea, cardiac arrhythmias, and circulatory collapse. Hyponatremia or sodium depletion from diuretics can potentiate lithium toxicity and should be avoided. Lithium should not be considered a first-line agent but should be reserved for special situations when iodides and β-blockers are contraindicated.

Adrenergic Antagonists

Because many of the signs and symptoms of thyrotoxicosis are mediated through the sympathetic nervous system, drugs that deplete or block the effects of thyroid hormones on tissue catecholamines can provide symptomatic relief before thioamides, RAI, or surgery. These agents do not affect the underlying disease process so they should not be used as primary therapy. Reserpine (0.25 mg to 4.0 mg p.o. or i.m.) and guanethidine (80 mg/day p.o.) can be used. However, their slow onset (up to several weeks) and frequent side effects (especially marked hypotension) have resulted in their replacement by safer and more effective agents, the β-blockers.

Propranolol is the β-blocker most widely used and studied in the treatment of thyrotoxicosis, and therefore the standard against which others are judged. When propranolol is given orally in doses of 20 to 40 mg three to four times a day as necessary, symptomatic relief of palpitations, anxiety, sweating, tremor, and diarrhea occurs; weight loss, however, remains unaffected (38). Severely toxic patients may require as much as 240 to 480 mg of propranolol a day to achieve symptomatic relief. Propranolol is also surprisingly effective in controlling the neuromuscular manifestations, especially periodic paralysis. It can be used as an adjunct to thioamides and RAI during therapy of neonatal thyrotoxicosis, pregnancy, or thyroid storm, and as a preoperative medication prior to surgery. Although β-blockers have been used successfully as sole agents preoperatively (39), they are not recommended in the severely toxic patient because inadequate control of severe thyrotoxicosis has resulted in storm (40).

All the selective and nonselective β-blockers (e.g., naldolol, atenolol, metoprolol) appear equally effective in the symptomatic relief of hyperthyroidism, although larger doses of metoprolol may be needed in hyperthyroidism because of hyperthyroid-increased hepatic clearance (38). β-Blockers possessing intrinsic sympathomimetic activity (e.g., pindolol) may not reduce the heart rate as much as β-blockers without it. The calcium-channel blockers, particularly diltiazem, may be a useful alternative when β-blockers are contraindicated (e.g., in patients with asthma, congestive heart failure (CHF), or insulin-dependent diabetes). Diltiazem (120 mg/t.i.d. or 60 mg q.i.d. orally) is well tolerated and appears to be as effective as propranolol in suppressing the symptoms of thyrotoxicosis (41). However, verapamil has produced detrimental effects in thy-

rotoxicosis. The potential synergistic benefits of calcium blockers and β-blockers in the management of thyrotoxicosis is unknown.

The kinetics and blood levels of propranolol in toxic patients are subject to large interindividual variation. This is attributed to a significant first-pass effect seen with oral doses, altered hepatic function in hyperthyroidism, and the presence of an active metabolite, 4-hydroxypropranolol. Data on the kinetics of propranolol in thyroid disease are subject to criticism because little information is available about the metabolite. Nevertheless, the clearance of propranolol in thyrotoxicosis may be increased as much as 50% because of enhanced liver blood flow and increased activity of drug-metabolizing enzymes (38). Because of the increased volume of distribution, the elimination half-life is unchanged. Although the lower propranolol levels reported in hyperthyroidism may be due to individual variations, data suggest that higher propranolol doses are necessary acutely in toxic patients because of the increased clearance rate. The clearance of metoprolol is similarly enhanced in hyperthyroidism. The converse is true in hypothyroidism. The clearance of β-blockers such as atenolol and nadolol that are excreted renally is unaltered in hyperthyroidism.

Radioactive Iodine (RAI)

Radioactive iodine therapy is indicated for hyperthyroidism in patients past adolescence, those with a history of prior thyroid surgery, those who are poor surgical risks because of complicating nonthyroid illness, those with Graves' ophthalmopathy, and those who fail thioamides or experience thioamide toxicity. RAI is absolutely contraindicated in pregnancy because the RAI crosses the placenta and destroys the fetal thyroid. It is also the treatment of choice in elderly patients with cardiac disease and in those with toxic multinodular goiters.

^{131}I, which has a half-life of 8 days and delivers high energy beta radiation to a maximal depth of 2 mm, is the isotope commonly used. ^{125}I, which has less tissue penetration and a half-life of 60 days, has not resulted in the lower incidence of hypothyroidism that was initially hoped for. Because ^{125}I emits gamma rays that penetrate only a few microns, larger therapeutic doses are required, which considerably increases the total body radiation without altering the incidence of hypothyroidism.

The dose of RAI administered is determined with a formula that incorporates an estimate of the gland size, the amount of RAIU at 24 hours, and the standard microcurie of iodine given per gram of thyroid tissue. At the University of California San Francisco, patients receive approximately 80 to 100 microcurie per gram of thyroid tissue. Despite the formula, the proper dose of RAI is difficult to calculate or predict. The optimal dose is one that prevents recurrent hyperthyroidism as well as hypothyroidism.

$$\text{Millicuries (mCi) of } I^{131} \text{ given}$$

$$= \text{estimated gland weight (g)} \times 100 \text{ microcurie/g}$$

$$\times\ 100\ \%\ \text{24-hr RAI}$$

Pretreatment with thioamides for 1 month or with propranolol prior to and after RAI therapy is necessary to prevent exacerbations of thyrotoxicosis in the elderly, in patients with severe heart disease, or in those with large intraglandular stores of hormones. Iodides should not be used before RAI therapy because ^{131}I uptake will be significantly impaired. Thioamides should be discontinued 1 week before and after RAI therapy to facilitate optimal ^{131}I uptake and retention. Propranolol can be used without compromising RAI therapy.

Resolution of the hyperthyroidism is slow after RAI treatment. Improvement of symptoms becomes apparent 2 to 3 weeks after RAI; however, maximum effects do not occur until 2 to 3 months after an ablative dose. Because of this delayed onset, iodides, ipodate, thioamides, or propranolol may be necessary for symptomatic control after RAI is given. If a second dose is required, a larger dose of RAI must be given to optimize gland uptake, exposing the body to greater radiation.

The lowest appropriate age limit for radioactive iodine therapy is controversial. However, after more than 25 years of extensive clinical experience, RAI is generally accepted as safe for most adult patients under 35 years of age (42). Adolescents have also been treated safely with RAI, although it is not recommended in this age group.

The major concerns about RAI therapy include carcinogenesis, leukemia, and genetic damage. So far, none of these hazards is documented and surveillance is ongoing. The radiation dose to the gonads in patients treated with ^{131}I is generally less than 3 rads, which is not significantly different from gonadal irradiation received from commonly used diagnostic tests such as barium enemas or pyelograms. The major complication of RAI is hypothyroidism, which is most common the first year after therapy and increases at a constant rate of 2.5%/year thereafter, accounting for a 20-year prevlence of 30 to 70%. Immediate side effects of ^{131}I therapy are minimal and may include mild thyroid pain and tenderness, temporary thinning of the hair, and (rarely) dysphagia. Aggravation and worsening of Graves' ophthalomopathy may occur, leading to recommendations to institute prophylactic corticosteroids (13). Generally, RAI therapy is effective, quick, easy, painless, and relatively nontoxic.

Ipodate/Iodinated Contrast Media
An unlabeled use for iodinated contrast dye is in the acute management of hyperthyroidism (43–44). When ipodate

is administered in a dose of 500 mg to 1 g orally daily or 3 g every 3rd day to thyrotoxic patients, dramatic improvement in both subjective and objective symptoms parallels a rapid fall in the thyroid hormone levels. The changes in serum T_4, serum T_3, and reverse T_3 (rT_3) levels are consistent with the inhibition of the peripheral deiodination of T_4 to T_3. Reductions in serum T_3 levels are apparent within 6 hr of ipodate administration, declining to 50% of baseline at 24 hr, and 70% of baseline (nadir) at 48 hr. T_3 levels remained suppressed for 3 to 5 days after a single administration. Similarly, T_4 levels reached their nadir 3 days after administration and remained depressed for as long as 6 days after the last dose. When compared with propylthiouracil, ipodate produced earlier symptomatic and objective improvement and more rapid declines in T_3 hormone levels. The prolonged suppression of T_3 and T_4 levels suggests that inhibition of hormone secretion, resulting from the iodine released, may be an additional mechanism of action for ipodate. Although similar inhibition of peripheral T_3 production is seen with most iodinated contrast media, such as iopanoic acid (Telepaque), ipodate (Oragrafin), which contains 61.4% iodine, is the most potent.

Because ipodate is relatively nontoxic, it provides a useful addition to the acute treatment of thyrotoxicosis. Ipodate is recommended as an adjunct to thioamides in the severely toxic or storm patient and as an alternative in patients allergic to thioamides. It may also be an effective preoperative preparation in lieu of iodides, but experience is very limited. Another potential use is in patients who may eventually be treated with radioactive iodine therapy because ipodate does not appear to interfere with RAI retention as much as iodides. These agents are not indicated for chronic therapy because the reductions in hormone levels seen within the first month of therapy are not sustained in most hyperthyroid patients (43–44).

Surgery
Thyroidectomy is an effective method of therapy for patients in whom RAI or thioamides are contraindicated; for those with large goiters, causing cosmetic disfigurement, respiratory embarrassment, or swallowing difficulties; for those with suspected malignancies; and for selected pregnant and pediatric patients. Prior thyroid surgery should be considered a strong deterrent to further surgery because reoperation increases the hazards of vocal cord paralysis and hypoparathyroidism, 10-fold and 30-fold, respectively. Other poor surgical candidates are patients with severe cardiac, respiratory, or debilitating diseases and patients in the third trimester of pregnancy (because of the risk of precipitating spontaneous labor).

The ideal surgical end point is a 3 to 8 g remnant of thyroid tissue, left after surgery that results in neither a recurrence of the thyrotoxicosis nor hypothyroidism (45).

The risk of recurrent thyrotoxicosis is directly proportional to the amount of thyroid remnant left. Increasing the remnant gland size by 1 g decreases the risk of postoperative hypothyroidism by 10%; conversely, increasing the remnant size above 10 g increases the risk of recurrent disease without changing the risk of hypothyroidism. Although permanent euthyroidism may not always be feasible, one series reported a 94% euthyroid success rate using a modified subtotal thyroidectomy. A subtotal thyroidectomy is the most popular form of surgery performed for hyperthyroidism because it offers the best chance of euthyroidism. Others advocate a total thyroidectomy, despite the risk of hypothyroidism, to ensure complete resolution of the hyperthyroidism. Since the natural course of Graves' disease in approximately 15 to 20% of patients is progression to hypothyroidism, regardless of the treatment selected, the type of surgical procedure may be irrelevant.

Surgery appears to be as safe as nonsurgical treatments for hyperthyroidism if it is performed by experienced hands on patients adequately prepared by the standard combination of thioamides, iodides, or propranolol. In adequately prepared patients, operative mortality and development of thyroid storm is low. Vocal cord paralysis and permanent hypoparathyroidism occurred in fewer than 1% of patients following a subtotal thyroidectomy. Because of the catastrophic nature of these complications, only surgeons experienced in thyroid surgery should perform such operations.

The major complication is hypothyroidism, which occurs in the first 6 months to 3 years postoperatively, but can develop insidiously as late as 10 years postoperatively. Prevalences of 5 to 75% are reported. The prevalence of hypothyroidism is inversely proportional to the remnant of thyroid tissue left; remnants of 2 to 4 g result in an prevalence of 70%.

The disadvantages of surgery include expense, need for hospitalization, risks of anesthesia, postoperative complications, and the patient's fear of surgery. These disadvantages may outweigh the advantages of rapid definitive surgical intervention.

SPECIAL TREATMENT CONSIDERATIONS
Pregnancy

The combination of pregnancy and thyrotoxicosis is a rare occurrence (0.02 to 1.4% of the pregnant population) because most hyperthyroid patients are relatively infertile. Usually the thyrotoxicosis and treatment antedate the pregnancy. Nevertheless, because management of hyperthyroidism in pregnancy is difficult, pregnancy is best avoided until the hyperthyroidism is permanently controlled. Hyperthyroidism may be difficult to monitor during pregnancy because similar symptoms are inherent to both conditions. Also, pregnancy appears to transiently ameliorate the symptoms of thyrotoxicosis, inducing a spontaneous remission, and a relapse during delivery or 3 to 4 months after delivery (20–21). The basis for this improvement may be the fall in both the concentrations of thyroid-stimulating immunoglobulins (TSI) and the titers of thyroid antibodies in pregnancy. However, untreated maternal thyrotoxicosis can result in abortion, perinatal death, and prematurity, so proper treatment is crucial.

Pregnancy and hyperthyroidism create special management problems because the fetal thyroid, which begins functioning during the 12th to the 14th week, is also at risk. Radioactive iodine is absolutely contraindicated because transplacental passage of ^{131}I will destroy the fetal thyroid. Chronic iodide administration should also be avoided because ingestion of as little as 12 mg of iodine throughout pregnancy has resulted in fetal goiter and asphyxiation. Vaginal povidone or topical iodine can produce high serum concentrations of iodine and should also be avoided (46).

Surgery can be performed safely in the second trimester after suitable preparation with thioamides or short-term administration of iodides. During the last trimester, surgery is not recommended because of the risk of precipitating spontaneous abortion (20).

Thioamides, which cross the placenta, can be used throughout pregnancy if certain precautions are followed. PTU, and not methimazole, is generally considered the drug of choice in pregnancy because maternal use of methimazole is associated with congenital skin defects i.e. aplasia cutis (20). However, some have concluded that the association between methimazole and congenital skin defects is not supported sufficiently to preclude the use of this drug during pregnancy (47–48). If no other therapeutic options are available, one must balance the dangers of untreated maternal hyperthyroidism against the risks of methimazole toxicity. The dangers of fetal goiter and hypothyroidism are reduced if initial doses of PTU are maintained below 300 mg/day (given in divided doses) and maintenance doses of 50 to 100 mg/day are employed throughout pregnancy (20, 48). Clinically, the mother should be maintained in a comfortable mildly hyperthyroid state with the FT$_4$I or FT$_4$D in the upper ranges to prevent fetal thyroid suppression. The appearance of an enlarged maternal goiter during therapy is alarming because it implies the development of maternal and fetal hypothyroidism. The concomitant use of thyroid hormone is not helpful because thyroid does not cross the placenta and may make maternal management more difficult.

Fortunately, the intellectual development of offspring exposed to antithyroid drugs in utero appears to be no different than that of siblings not exposed (49). PTU is also preferred over methimazole in the breast-feeding mother because insignificant amounts of PTU are excreted in the milk, whereas 7 to 16% of a methimazole dose is detected in breast milk (50).

Propranolol or another β-blocker is a reasonable short-term adjunct to PTU during pregnancy. Chronic administration of β-blockers should be avoided during pregnancy, particularly in the last trimester, because of the risk of fetal respiratory depression, small placenta, intrauterine growth retardation, impaired responses to anoxic stress, and postnatal bradycardia and hypoglycemia. Propranolol is also excreted in breast milk and should be avoided during lactation. Such findings indicate that propranolol, like iodides, should be used only on a short-term basis in pregnancy.

Exophthalamos/Ophthalmologic Complications

Because the pathogenesis and progression of the ocular symptoms are not well understood, symptomatic and empiric treatment is recommended until euthyroidism occurs. The treatment of choice in patients with Graves' exophthalmos is thyroid ablation, using either RAI or surgery, because the eye symptoms may progress in those continuing to receive thioamides (11–14).

Periorbital edema and chemosis (inflammation of the conjunctiva) respond to elevation of the head of the bed to promote diuresis. Protective glasses, methylcellulose, hydrocortisone drops, and avoidance of smoke and dust may alleviate photophobia and external irritation. With patients whose eyes do not completely close while sleeping, taping the eyelids shut at night is necessary to prevent corneal scarring and drying (11).

Systemic corticosteroids are indicated for progressive inflammatory exophthalmos and decreasing visual acuity (13). Prednisone, 80 to 120 mg/day administered in divided dose for 1 to 2 weeks, often produces dramatic resolution of the eye symptoms. When symptoms resolve, the dose can be tapered over 2 weeks and then gradually withdrawn. In addition to their antiinflammatory action, corticosteroids suppress TSI levels and decrease T_3 levels by impairing the peripheral conversion of T_4 to T_3. Immunosuppressive agents, such as cyclophosphamide and azathioprine, have not been as effective as steroids (14). External orbital radiation therapy, which achieves similar results, may be used in patients with contraindications to steroids.

After euthyroidism is achieved and the eye symptoms are stable, lid or orbital surgery can provide cosmetic or visual corrections.

Neonatal Thyrotoxicosis

Neonatal thyrotoxicosis results from stimulation of the fetal thyroid by transplacental passage of TSI from the maternal circulation. The infants are extremely ill and require supportive measures including sedation, cooling, oxygen, fluid, and electrolyte replacement, in addition to management of the thyrotoxicosis by thioamides, iodides, or propranolol. Fortunately, the disease is self-limiting, and symptoms disappear in 1 to 2 months as the level of TSI declines. Antithyroid drugs should be withdrawn at this time. High levels of maternal TSI (>60) help to predict the risk of neonatal thyrotoxicosis, and TSI levels should be monitored in all pregnant females with a history of Graves' disease.

Pediatrics

Hyperthyroidism in children is rare, accounting for about 1 to 5% of cases. It is unusual in the first 5 years of life; the peak incidence occurs between the ages of 10 and 12 years. Similarities to the adult form include a preponderance of females over males and a history of precipitation of the disease by acute infection, trauma, and stress. The presenting signs and symptoms are similar to those seen in the adult in most respects, i.e., nervousness, weight loss, tremor, eye signs but with the notable exception of cardiovascular manifestations. Excessive thirst, behavioral manifestations of restlessness, and inability to concentrate bring on difficulties in school and in family relationships.

Optimal management of the disease in children is controversial, although all three methods: surgery, RAI, and thioamides have been used (51).

Radioactive iodine is usually not recommended because of the high risk of hypothyroidism and the fear of genetic damage, leukemia, and carcinogenesis, although these are unsubstantiated (42, 51). External radiation to the head and neck of children is associated with a high risk of subsequent thyroid carcinoma and dysfunction, although similar results have not been shown with internal RAI radiation (51).

The usual treatment choices include the thioamides and subtotal thyroidectomy. The risks of surgery (mortality, scaring, recurrence of thyrotoxicosis, hypothyroidism, laryngeal and parathyroid damage) must be weighed against the benefits of speedy correction of the thyrotoxicosis and the lack of need for compliance to the rigid dosing schedules of the thioamides.

Thioamide use in children is similar to the regimen used in adults. Thioamides are the method of choice in patients with small goiters and mild disease, where a high remission rate is likely. The limitations of medical management include noncompliance, strict parental and physician supervision, the low remission success rates, and the risks of adverse reaction. The advantages of treatment include the potential for remission without damage to the gland.

The appropriate method depends upon the circumstances and individuals involved.

Thyroid Storm

Thyroid storm is a medical emergency characterized by

1. Acute onset of high fever (sine qua non);

2. Cardiovascular symptoms: tachycardia, tachypnea, shock, congestive heart failure, and arrhythmia;
3. Gastrointestinal symptoms: diarrhea, vomiting, abdominal pain, and liver enlargement;
4. Central nervous system involvement: agitation and psychosis progressing to apathy, stupor, and coma.

The pathogenesis of storm is not well understood but appears to be an exaggerated form of thyrotoxicosis. Storm can be precipitated by childbirth, stress, infection, trauma, diabetic acidosis, RAI treatment, and the abrupt discontinuation of antithyroid medication (22–23).

Prompt recognition and immediate treatment can decrease the 100% mortality rate to 7% or better. Treatment is directed at five major areas:

1. Support of vital functions is by sedation, oxygen, fluids, use of antipyretics, treatment of infection, correction of electrolyte abnormalities, and the routine use of corticosteroids (hydrocortisone 100 to 200 mg IV every 6 hours) in case of underlying hypoadrenalism. T_3 levels are also reduced by corticosteroid administration.
2. Use of thioamides and iodides blocks synthesis and release of hormones. Preferably, large doses of PTU 200 to 300 mg every 6 hours (600 to 1200 mg/day) or of methimazole 30 to 60 mg every 6 hours should be given. Theoretically, iodides should be given 1 hr after thioamide administration so as to not interfere with the latter's effect and prevent iodizing existing hormone stores which will aggravate existing storm. Iodides (e.g., Lugol's solution 30 to 60 drops p.o. daily) and the combination of thioamides often relieve symptoms within 1 day. Lithium, which is similar in effect to iodides, can be used in doses of 500 to 1500 mg/day, but has no advantage over iodides.
3. Blockage of the metabolic effects is accomplished by propranolol 20 to 80 mg p.o. every 6 hr or 0.5 to 2 mg IV every 4 hr or diltiazem 60 to 120 mg p.o. t.i.d-q.i.d. Reserpine 1 to 3 mg i.m. every 8 hr and guanethidine 20 to 50 mg p.o. every 8 hr can also be used, but they have slow onsets of action.
4. Eliminate and correct precipitating factors.
5. Remove circulating hormone by plasmapheresis, exchange transfusion, and dialysis when routine measures fail.

HYPOTHYROIDISM

Hypothyroidism or myxedema is a syndrome characterized by a slowing down of all body processes because of a deficiency of thyroid hormone. Thyroid hormone stimulates oxygen consumption and is essential for normal growth, maturation, and regulation of all organ systems.

Clinical Features

The signs and symptoms of hypothyroidism are listed in Table 16.3. Typical symptoms include weakness, fatigue, lethargy, cold intolerance, and weight gain (which often precede the late physical findings). Marked physical changes include a puffy and masklike facies, edematous eyelids, myxedematous skin changes (especially over the pretibial aspects of the leg), loss of hair from the lateral aspects of the eyebrows, a large tongue, cardiomegaly, and a yellowish tint to the skin. Myxedematous cachexia is characterized by intensification of all hypothyroid signs and symptoms and often precedes the onset of myxedema coma. The exception is the elderly patient, whose symptoms may be nonspecific, atypical, and easily missed unless considered in the differential diagnosis (52).

The cardiovascular manifestations of hypothyroidism can mimic or exacerbate preexisting low-output congestive heart failure. Angina typically becomes quiescent; rarely, the severity and frequency of attacks increase. Hypothyroidism-increased levels of cholesterol may accelerate atherosclerotic changes. Clinical findings include cardiomegaly resulting from loss of muscle tone and mucopolysaccharide deposition, dyspnea, edema and pleural effusions due to impaired cardiac output, decreased stroke volume, and decreased myocardial contractility. Characteristic ECG changes resembling ischemia are seen: slow rate and low voltage, flattened or inverted T waves, and, occasionally, increased P-R interval and widened QRS complex. Although glomerular filtration rate (GFR) and renal plasma flow (RPF) are reduced because of decreased cardiac output and blood volume, overt evidence of renal failure does not occur. In severe myxedema, delayed water excretion leading to edema results from changes in GFR or inappropriate antidiuretic hormone (ADH) secretion.

Course

The onset of naturally occurring hypothyroidism (most commonly Hashimoto's thyroiditis) is a gradual, insidious, and nonspecific process that may go unnoticed by the patient or be attributed to normal aging. It may occur with amazing placidity over several months to years before the appearance of a terminal myxedematous state. In contrast, the symptoms occurring from iatrogenic hypothyroidism (i.e., from RAI therapy or surgery) occur rapidly and rarely go unrecognized by the patient.

Laboratory Parameters

Pertinent diagnostic laboratory parameters include a decreased TT_4 and FT_4I or FT_4D and an elevated TSH level, unless a pituitary etiology exists. The presence of antibodies suggests an autoimmune etiology. An RAIU is not necessary for diagnosis of hypothyroidism; it is usually decreased but an elevated uptake may occur in the early stages of hypothyroidism. Elevations of serum AST, LDH, CPK, cholesterol and triglyceride levels occur from delayed metabolism of enzymes.

Etiology

Primary hypothyroidism, a disorder of the gland, can be classified as either nongoitrous (no goiter) or goitrous. Goitrous forms include Hashimoto's thyroiditis, drug-induced, dyshormonogenesis, endemic, and multinodular goiters. Nongoitrous forms include cretinism (congenital hypothyroidism), iatrogenic, idiopathic atrophy, and secondary hypothyroidism, either of pituitary or hypothalamic origin.

A goiter (enlargement of the thyroid) should be considered an abnormal finding. Goiters result from TSH stimulation, usually in response to low levels of circulating hormone. However, some patients with a goiter can be euthyroid because the increased TSH secretion causing the goiter, also is capable of transiently maintaining normal hormone levels.

Secondary Hypothyroidism. Secondary hypothyroidism can be of either pituitary or hypothalamic etiology. Hypothalamic hypothyroidism arising from inadequate secretion of thyrotropin-releasing factor (TRF) is rare. Low or absent levels of TSH suggest a pituitary etiology, which can occur from postpartum hemorrhage (Sheehan's syndrome), head injury, pituitary tumors, or idiopathic atrophy of the hypophysis. Concomitant disorders of the adrenals and gonads (Simmond's disease or panhypopituitarism) may also occur. Primary, pituitary, and hypothalamic hypothyroidism can be differentiated by the TRF and TSH tests.

Iatrogenic. Iatrogenic hypothyroidism resulting from radioactive iodine and surgery is one of the most common forms. As previously discussed, virtually all patients receiving radioactive iodine and about 50 to 75% of patients undergoing thyroidectomies will become myxedematous (42, 45). Therefore, all patients with a prior history of RAI or surgery should be monitored routinely for development of hypothyroidism.

Idiopathic Atrophy. Idiopathic atrophy of the thyroid and destruction of the gland represent the end stages of Hashimoto's thyroiditis. Antibodies (indicating a destructive immune process) are frequently found.

Cretinism (Congenital Hypothyroidism). Congenital nongoitrous hypothyroidism produced by a deficiency of thyroid hormone in utero or in the neonate may result from defective hormone synthesis, from pituitary or hypothalamic dysfunction, and from incomplete growth of the gland (agenesis). Ectopic thyroid tissue, destruction of the gland by maternal autoantibodies, or destruction by RAI therapy are other possible causes of agenesis. Neonatal goitrous hypothyroidism has been reported after maternal ingestion of iodides and after thioamide therapy (20, 46).

The clinical presentation depends on the severity, the age of onset, and the etiology of thyroid deficiency. Early recognition of congenital hypothyroidism is now possible by cord TSH levels determined at time of delivery. This extremely important because the clinical symptoms are subtle and not recognized until the child is older and irreversible damage results. The earliest manifestations are

a heavy expression, a pig-like appearance of the eyes, hypothermia, prolonged jaundice, umbilical hernia, hoarseness, thick tongue, protuberant abdomen, constipation, and drooling. Delayed developmental characteristics, failure to thrive, poor appetite, and cretinoid facies may not be recognized until the infant is 3 to 6 months old and neurological damage is irreversible (53). Growth retardation, delayed physical development, and hypothyroid symptoms similar to those seen in a adult are of concern. Radiologic evidence of epiphyseal dysgenesis is pathognomonic of neonatal hypothyroidism.

Endemic Hypothyroidism. Endemic goiter is a descriptive term for thyroid enlargement resulting from iodine deficiency during the growth years. Females are affected more often than males, as occurs with other thyroidal disorders. The amount of dietary iodine deficiency determines the degree of nodularity and gland enlargement. Patients may be clinically and chemically euthyroid or hypothyroid. Nevertheless, thyroxine suppression therapy is often indicated to prevent further gland enlargement. Laboratory findings include a normal or low FT_4D or TT_4 and FT_4I, and a normal or elevated TSH level.

Dyshormonogenesis. Dyshormonogenesis refers to a specific group of familial thyroid disorders resulting from abnormalities in the synthesis, delivery, or peripheral action of thyroid hormones. Impaired hormone synthesis can occur from defects in iodine accumulation, from iodide organification resulting from dehalogenase deficiency, and from a coupling abnormality. Patients with impaired thyroglobulin synthesis, release of abnormal iodopeptides, and peripheral tissue resistance to thyroid have also been described.

Because specific tests are not available, diagnosis depends on elimination of other goitrous causes of hypothyroidism. Laboratory manifestations include low or normal circulating hormone levels, increased TSH levels, and absence of antibodies. A defect in organification can be detected by the potassium perchlorate discharge test.

Drug-induced. Goiters can result from the use of certain drugs with antithyroid activity. (See Table 16.7) The thioamides and the monovalent anions, which are used therapeutically in the treatment of hyperthyroidism, can produce goiter if excessive doses are used (goitrogenic).

Iodides and iodide-containing compounds (e.g., povidone iodine, amiodarone) can produce hypothyroidism and goiter in patients with unrecognized thyroid disorders (1, 17–19). Each 200-mg tablet of amiodarone contains 75 mg of organic iodide. The prevalence of amiodarone-induced hypothyroidism has been reported to range from a low of 1.0% to a high of 9.8%. These patients are inordinately sensitive to iodides and unable to escape normally from the Wolff-Chaikoff block and resume hormone synthesis. High-risk patients include those with cystic fibrosis, untreated Hashimoto's thyroiditis, and patients with

Table 16.7.
Drug-induced Thyroid Disease

Drug	Mechanism	Laboratory	Comments
Cholestyramine, Colestipol	Binds T_4 in gut, decreases absorption of T_4	$\downarrow T_4$, $\downarrow$ free T_4, $\uparrow$ TSH in hypothyroidism	Administer at least 4–5 hr apart
Nitroprusside	Metabolized to thiocyanate, an anion inhibitor	$\downarrow T_4$, $\downarrow$ free T_4, $\uparrow$ TSH	Increased risk with renal failure
Lithium	Inhibits hormone release	$\downarrow T_4$, $\downarrow$ free T_4, $\uparrow$ TSH	Usually in patients with underlying thyroid disease
Iodides, amiodarone, ipodate	Inhibits organification Decreases release T_4, T_3	$\downarrow T_4$, $\downarrow$ free T_4, $\uparrow$ TSH	Usually in patients with underlying Hashimoto's disease or with Graves' disease previously treated with RAI or surgery
	Provides substrate to iodide-deficient autonomous thyroid tissue; loss of Wolff-Chaikoff control	$\uparrow T_4$, $\uparrow$ free T_4, $\uparrow T_3$, $\downarrow$ TSH	Usually in nontoxic multinodular goiters with autonomous function (Jod-Basedow disease)
Sulfonylureas, sulfonamides, PAS, resorcinol, phenylbutazone	Inhibits organic binding and organification	$\downarrow T_4$, $\downarrow$ free T_4, $\uparrow$ TSH	Rare
Natural goitrogens cabbage, etc.	Contains thiocyanate and other goitrogens	$\downarrow T_4$, $\downarrow$ free T_4, $\uparrow$ TSH	Rare, need large consumption of raw vegetables

Graves' disease previously treated with RAI or surgery. Older patients and those on long-term amiodarone also appear to be at greater risk of amiodarone-induced hypothyroidism. Unfortunately, the goiter or hypothyroidism may not always be reversible after discontinuation of the iodides or amiodarone. Thyroxine can be given concomitantly, if necessary, to treat the hypothyroidism and goiter.

Lithium is also associated with the development of hypothyroidism and goiter in up to 10% of patients (16). Most patients have a positive family history of thyroid illness, positive thyroid antibodies, abnormal gland findings, and undiagnosed underlying thyroid illness. Lithium's antithyroid effect is similar to that of the iodides and was first demonstrated in patients with bipolar disorder as a side effect of lithium therapy. The onset of a nontender, diffuse goiter with or without hypothyroidism is variable and may appear after 5 months to 2 years of treatment. The goiters are responsive to T_4 therapy or discontinuation of lithium.

Thiocyanate is a well-known inhibitor of iodide trapping, particularly if high blood concentrations are present. Thiocyanate-induced hypothyroidism may result from long-term use of nitroprusside in patients with renal insufficiency. Plants such as rutabagas, cabbage, and turnips, contain thioglucosides, which are metabolized in the body to thiocyanates. These dietary goitrogens do not produce significant hypothyroidism unless large amounts are ingested raw over a long time period.

Multinodular Goiter. Multinodular goiter describes an enlarged thyroid gland containing many hypofunctioning or "cold" and autonomously functioning "hot" nodules. It is a common disorder, affecting women more than men

and occurring in about 4% of all adults beyond age 30. The possibility of malignancy must be eliminated, especially if a history of irradiation is present. Otherwise, cold nodules in a multinodular goiter are rarely malignant. The pathogenesis is not well understood, but is related to iodide deficiency, dietary goitrogens, and enzymatic defects. Clinically, patients can be euthyroid but often develop hyper-, or hypothyroidism in their later years. Pressure symptoms or a choking sensation from compression of the trachea or esophagus, respectively, by the enlarged gland is an indication for surgical removal. Otherwise, thyroxine therapy is indicated to decrease and prevent further growth of the gland. However, therapy usually does not shrink the gland back to normal size. A clinically euthyroid patient with a suppressed TSH level should be the goal of therapy.

Hashimoto's Thyroiditis. Hashimoto's thyroiditis, the most common cause of goiter and/or hypothyroidism, is similar to Graves' disease in prevalence (3 to 6/10,000/year). Like other thyroid disorders, it is 15 to 20 times more common in females than males and has a strong familial predisposition. Its peak occurrence is in the middle years, although any age group is at risk. It is commonly characterized by diffuse enlargement and lymphocytic infiltration of the gland, an immunologic disturbance, and hypothyroidism. Hashimoto's thyroiditis is a graded disease with many different clinical presentations. Patients can present with either thyrotoxicosis in the early stages, (Hashitoxicosis), euthyroidism and goiter, hypothyroidism and goiter, or hypothyroidism without goiter in the late stages of the disease. Euthyroidism occurs if the gland is able to compensate by increasing hormone synthesis in response to TSH stimulation. Asymptomatic thyroiditis, characterized by euthyroidism, absence of goiter, normal levels of circulating hormones, and positive antithyroid antibodies, may precede the clinical manifestations of overt goiter and hypothyroidism.

Pathophysiology. An autoimmune process, resulting from defects in suppressor T lymphocytes, is responsible for Hashimoto's thyroiditis (9). Antibodies directed against thyroglobulin, a microsomal component, and a colloid component, as well as cell-mediated immunity against thyroid antigens are present. Hashimoto's thyroiditis often coexists with other autoimmune disorders including Graves' disease, rheumatoid arthritis, and other collagen vascular diseases. Pernicious anemia, resulting from gastric antibodies directed against intrinsic factor, can be found in about half of the patients with Hashimoto's disease and vice versa. Some postulate that Graves' and Hashimoto's thyroiditis are actually the same disease at different ends of the spectrum because mild thyrotoxicosis may precede the onset of hypothyroidism; similarly, hypothyroidism is the end result of Graves' disease.

As previously discussed, the Hashimoto's gland is unable to bind iodide effectively and is inordinately sensitive to the antithyroid effects of exogenous iodides. This ineffective utilization of iodides results in the formation and release of inactive nonhormonal iodoproteins into the circulation, causing further increases in TSH secretion and goiter formation. If the gland can maintain hormone synthesis in response to TSH stimulation, then euthyroidism is maintained. However, the gland eventually fails to keep up with metabolic demands, resulting in goiter and hypothyroidism. Laboratory findings include a low or normal FT_4D or TT_4 and FT_4I, normal or elevated TSH level, and positive antithyroglobulin and antimicrosomal antibodies.

Treatment of Hypothyroidism

Thyroid Dose Regimens. The administration of thyroid hormones provides adequate replacement therapy for hypothyroidism and shrinkage of any existing goiter through suppression of TSH production (Fig. 16.1). The average replacement dose is often quoted as 100 to 200 μg daily of thyroxine, which parallels the normal thyroid production. However, this simplistic approach is inappropriate and dangerous. Dosing requirements depend on many factors that include an evaluation of the patient's age and weight, the severity and duration of the illness, the presence or absence of cardiac disease, and the bioavailability of the hormone preparation.

The average daily maintenance dose for uncomplicated hypothyroidism is 100 to 150 μg/day of levothyroxine, which is about 1.6 to 1.7 μg/kg body weight or about 0.7 to 0.8 μg/lb (54, 55). In the elderly, lower levothyroxine doses, 100 μg or less daily (<1.6 μg/kg/day), may be

needed to maintain euthyroidism (56). These recommended hormone replacement doses are based on branded levothyroxine products with an FDA-recommended thyroxine tablet content and an average bioavailability of 80% (55). The branded preparations are similar but not necessarily bioequivalent (57). Caution should be employed in extrapolating these dosage guidelines to generic preparations with an unknown bioavailability and potentially different tablet thyroxine content from that stated on the label (55, 58). However, as more manufacturers adopt the use of HPLC assay to standardize the tablet content of thyroxine products, the difference between branded and generic products may be minimal.

Patients receiving chronic levothyroxine replacement therapy should be evaluated at yearly intervals to ensure that the current levothyroxine dosage is still warranted (59). Because of the availability of more potent products and the advent of the sensitive TSH assay, many patients on chronic replacement therapy will require a reduction in their original levothyroxine dosage. A reduction in levothyroxine dosage is also necessary as the patient ages. Optimally, both the FT_4D or FT_4I and TSH levels should be maintained within the normal range. Suppression of the TSH level into undetectable ranges should be avoided in replacement therapy to minimize overreplacement and subclinical signs of hyperthyroidism (59, 60). Supraphysiologic doses may also predispose patients to decreased bone density and increase the risk of bone loss and osteoporosis (60–62).

The initial dose of T4 administered depends on the patient's age, on the severity and duration of the hypothyroidism, and on the coexistence of underlying cardiac disease. In young, healthy patients with disease of short duration, levothyroxine can be administered in close-to-full replacement doses (e.g., 100 to 150 μg daily) without fear of precipitating toxicity. This dose can then be adjusted as necessary, using the patient's symptoms and laboratory values obtained at steady state (i.e., after 4 to 6 weeks of therapy). However, in patients with long-standing and severe myxedema, in elderly patients, and in patients with cardiac disease (e.g., angina, CHF) who are likely to be extremely sensitive to the metabolic effects of thyroid hormone, therapy must be instituted with minute doses of thyroxine to avoid cardiovascular complications of failure, angina, tachycardia, and myocardial infarction. These complications can occur with subtherapeutic doses, so careful monitoring is critical. Control of any angina should occur before attempting thyroxine therapy (63, 64). If necessary, coronary bypass surgery can be performed in hypothyroid patients, with minor complications. Successful and safe replacement of thyroxine is often achieved after coronary bypass. In the high-risk patient, initial doses should not exceed 12.5 to 25 μg of T_4 daily. The patient should be told to report any cardiac symptoms immediately. If

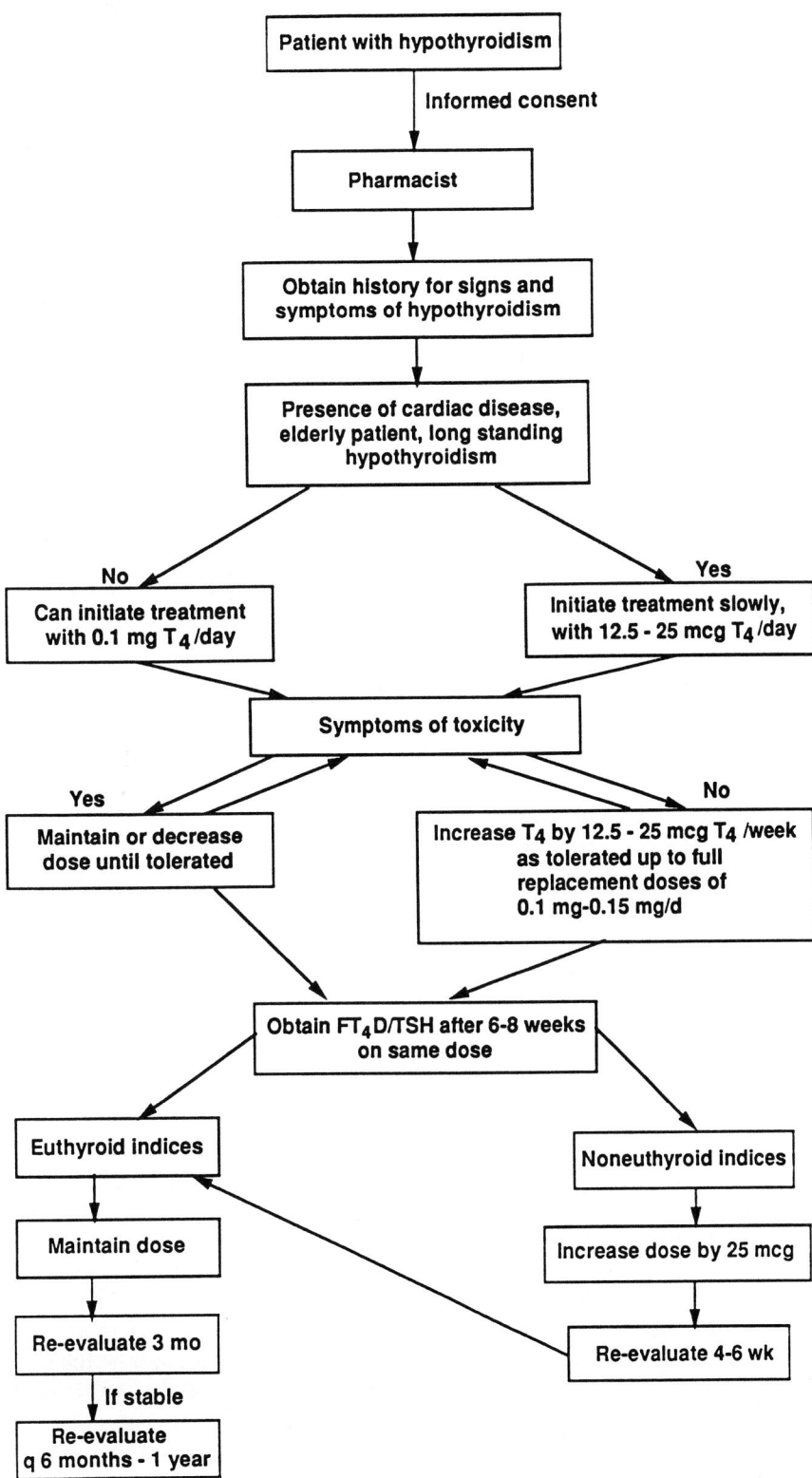

Figure 16.3. Treatment algorithm for hypothyroidism.

well tolerated after 1 week, the dose can be increased by similar increments every 1 to 2 weeks until therapeutic levels are achieved. It is not necessary to monitor thyroid function tests until the patient has maintained a therapeutic dose for a minimum period of 6 to 8 weeks. Complete euthyroidism may never be achieved in high-risk individuals without further compromising the cardiac status (63).

Hypothyroid patients on levothyroxine can be managed effectively by the pharmacist using a treatment algorithm (Fig. 16.3).

T_3 has been recommended as the drug of choice in patients with cardiovascular problems because its effects lapse quickly (i.e., 3 to 5 days) as a result of its short half-life (as opposed to 7 to 10 days for T_4). However, the greater potential for cardiotoxicity with T_3 outweighs its advantage of rapid elimination, so its use can not be recommended.

Management of Congenital Hypothyroidism. Normal growth and physical and mental development is determined by the age that treatment is instituted and by how well euthyroidism is maintained (53). The earlier that treatment is initiated, the better the prognosis for normal growth and mental development. Maenpaa reported normal intellectual development in 81% of patients if treatment was started prior to age 3 months (65). Mean IQ was higher in those receiving treatment before 3 months than in those treated after 3 months. If treatment was delayed until 6 months to 1 year, mental development was impaired despite subsequent treatment. Despite early therapy, neurologic deficits also occurred if replacement was inadequate to increase the serum $TT_4 > 103$ mmol/liter (8 μg/dl) and suppress the TSH into the normal range after 3 to 4 months of therapy. Dwarfism did not occur if therapy was delayed until 5 years old. Infants born athyreotic may have a worse prognosis or normal mental development because of late detection, compared with those born with an abnormal or ectopic thyroid gland.

The preparation of choice for hormone replacement is levothyroxine. Thyroxine tablets can be crushed and mixed with either breast milk or formula; suspensions should not be used because of questionable stability. T_3 can be used, but is not recommended for the reasons outlined below (see section on thyroid preparations). The appropriate replacement dose of T_4 depends on the age of the infant and the presence of risk factors (53, 66). (Table 16.8) Full replacement doses can be started in the uncomplicated infant without cardiac disease. However, the infant with long-standing and severe myxedema will be extremely sensitive to minute doses of thyroid, necessitating initiation with very small doses of thyroxine to prevent toxicity (i.e., hyperactivity and irritability). In these infants, initial doses of T_4 should not exceed 25 to 33% of the normal recommended dose. If no toxicity occurs after

Table 16.8.
Dose of T4 for Infants and Children[a]

Age	T_4 Dosage μg/kg/day
0–3 months	10–15
3–6 months	6–8
6–12 months	5–7
1–10 years	3–6
10–16 years	2–4

[a] Information from LaFranchi S: Diagnosis and treatment of hypothyroidism in children. Compr Ther 13:20–30, 1987; and Fisher DA, Foley BL: Early treatment of congenital hypothyroidism. Pediatrics 83:785–789, 1989.

1 to 2 weeks, doses can be gradually increased by similar increments every 1 to 2 weeks until full replacement doses are achieved or until the dose is limited by toxicity.

The optimal replacement dose is determined by normal physical and mental development and reversal of other hypothyroid signs and symptoms. Adequate replacement is achieved when the serum TT_4 level reaches 129 to 154 mmol/liter (10 to 12 μg/dl) (53, 66). Normalization of the TSH level should not be used as the sole criterion because the hypothalamic-pituitary system is relatively unresponsive to the negative feedback effect of thyroid hormone, causing TSH levels to remain elevated for months, despite proper or excessive hormone replacement. TSH levels should normalize within 3 to 4 months after the start of therapy; attempts to normalize TSH levels earlier may result in overreplacement, producing symptoms of overmetabolism, irritability, brain dysfunction, and premature craniosynostosis.

THYROID PREPARATIONS

All of the commercially available preparations of thyroid hormones are effective (Table 16.9). However, levothyroxine is considered the replacement hormone of choice (see discussion below).

Desiccated thyroid (USP) is usually obtained from hog thyroids, although beef and sheep are also used. Because this preparation is standardized only by iodine content (0.17 to 0.23% iodine), the hormone ratio of T_4 to T_3 may vary from a 2:1 (hog) to 3:1 with beef or sheep. Therefore, variability in potency may result from changes in the ratio of the two hormones or from the quantity of organic iodine present. Desiccated thyroid suffers from problems inherent to all T_3-containing preparations (see T_3, below). Improper or prolonged tablet storage, causing a loss of potency, can also contribute to an unpredictable response. Desiccated thyroid tablets appear to be stable for 5 years or longer if they are kept dry. Inactive preparations containing small amounts of T_4 and T_3 or iodinated casein and

Table 16.9.
Thyroid Preparations in Treatment of Hypothyroidism

Preparation[a]	Content	Advantages	Disadvantages	Effect on Thyroid Tests	Comments
Desiccated thyroid USP ¼, ½, 1, 1½, 2, 3, 4, 5 grains	Defatted, dried pig thyroid powder, containing 0.17–.23% iodine	Inexpensive	Poor standardization with variable hormonal content and T_4/T_3 ratios; deterioration with storage	Normal FT_4D/FT_4I, RT_3U, TSH	Potency may vary from batch to batch; problems inherent to all T_3 containing products; see T_3 comments.
Thyroglobulin ½, 1, 1½, 2, 3, grains	Partially purified pig thyroglobulin	Standardized biologically	More expensive than desiccated thyroid	Normal range for thyroid function tests	No real advantage over thyroid extract
Sodium L-thyroxine[a] 0.025, 0.05, 0.075, 0.088, 0.1, 0.125, 0.15, 0.175, 0.2, 0.3 mg Inj 100, 200, 500 μg	Synthetic, pure T_4	Stable, smooth action, relatively inexpensive; long half-life ($t_{1/2}$ = 7 days)	Slow onset of action, cumulative effects; generics and branded products do not differ in tablet content	Normal thyroid function tests; TSH in normal range	May be more potent than desiccated thyroid, should lower the T_4 dose by ½ gr to avoid toxicity when changing from desiccated thyroid to L-thyroxine
Sodium L-thyronine, 5, 25, 50 μg	Synthetic, pure T_3	Uniform absorption, fast onset of action	Expensive, short half-life (1.5 days) difficult to monitor—must use T_3 and TSH levels	Low TT_4, normal TT_3 and RT_3U, normal TSH	Requires multiple daily dosing schedule; not DOC for hormone replacement; supraphysiologic T_3 levels occur
Liotrix	Contains T_4 and T_3 in a ratio of 4:1 (mimics natural secretion of hormone	Both short- and long-acting effects	Expensive	Normal thyroid function values	No real need for Liotrix since T_4 is peripherally converted to T_3

[a] Dose equivalence: 1 grain desiccated thyroid = 1 grain thyroglobulin = 0.1 mg L-thyroxine = 37.5 μg L-thyronine = liotrix-1 (See "Comments" column)

tablets containing excessive biological activity have been observed (67). Allergic reactions to the protein component may also occur. During therapy, laboratory parameters of TT_4 and FT_4I or FT_4D, TT_3, and TSH should remain ideally within normal limits. For these reasons, desiccated thyroid should be an obsolete preparation. However, because this preparation is inexpensive, therapy may be continued if cost is an issue and the person is reluctant to change. Otherwise, all patients should be changed to levothyroxine. Because desiccated preparations may be subpotent, an equivalent dosage of levothyroxine may not be reasonable, and dosage titration is recommended. Theoretically, 60 mg of desiccated thyroid is equivalent to 100 μg of levothyroxine.

Thyroglobulin is a purified hog extract, standardized biologically to give a $T_4:T_3$ ratio of 2.5:1. It has no advantages over desiccated thyroid but is slightly more expensive. One grain of thyroglobulin is equivalent to one grain of thyroid USP.

Triiodothyronine or T_3 is a chemically pure agent with predictable potency, excellent bioavailability, and a half-life of 1.5 days. T_3 is not recommended for routine thyroid replacement therapy because of its high cost, the need for multiple daily dosing to ensure a uniform response, its greater potential for cardiotoxicity, and greater difficulty in monitoring therapeutic and toxic responses. Because of its rapid absorption, supraphysiologic levels of T_3 occur after ingestion, producing symptoms of mild toxicity in susceptible individuals. Furthermore, T_3 administration does not change pretreatment TT_4, FT_4I, and FT_4D levels, which if not properly recognized, causes therapeutic confusion despite adequate hormone replacement. T_3 administration is best monitored by TSH, TT_3 and FT_3 levels. T_3 is primarily used as a diagnostic agent in the T_3 suppression test and when short-term hormone replacement therapy is indicated. T_3 is commonly given as short-term hormone replacement therapy following total thyroidectomy for thyroid cancer, to patients who need repeat scans and RAIU. The thyroid hormones must be eliminated completely before the scan. Because T_3 has a short half-life, it is rapidly eliminated after discontinuation, producing a short period of tolerable hypothyroidism prior to RAIU and scan. T_3 has also been recommended as the drug of choice for myxedema coma because of its rapid onset of action (1 to 3 days). Its routine use in this condition is limited by the lack of a commercial intravenous preparation and its greater cardiotoxic risk. Generally, a dose of 25 to 37.5 μg of T_3 is equivalent to 0.1 mg of L-thyroxine. Patients should not receive T_3 as routine hormone replacement therapy.

L-Thyroxine, the most commonly prescribed synthetic thyroid preparation, is the preparation of choice for hormone replacement. Its popularity stems from its uniform potency, its relatively low cost, and its lack of foreign protein antigenicity. L-Thyroxine is relatively stable but does lose about 6% of its potency per year (68). Its long half-life of 7 days makes it amenable to once-a-day dosing, increasing patient compliance and allowing more convenient dosing schedules. The average bioavailability of branded thyroxine preparations is 80%; the bioavailability of generic preparations is unknown (55). This should be considered when changing from p.o. to IV or i.m. dosing regimens. Levothyroxine preparations manufactured after 1985 are consistent and standardized by HPLC assay for tablet levothyroxine content (55, 57). Previously, generic preparations did not contain the thyroxine content stated on the label (58), and therefore, were not recommended in the treatment of hypothyroidism. Although 0.1 mg of L-thyroxine is, theoretically, equivalent to 1 grain of desiccated thyroid, such equivalents may not be valid if dosage titrations were initially based on inactive desiccated thyroid preparations. In one study, only 60 μg of L-thyroxine was equivalent to desiccated thyroid1 grain (69). This disparity in equivalence should be noted especially when changing to L-thyroxine in patients requiring more than 2 grains/day of desiccated thyroid. Adequate replacement therapy is indicated by normalization of TSH, and FT_4D or FT_4I levels. L-Thyroxine replacement may produce TT_4 levels in the hyperthyroid ranges in about 20% of individuals; however, no adjustment in L-thyroxine dosage is necessary if the TSH levels are normal and the patients are clinically euthyroid. T_3 levels are often within the normal range (70).

Liotrix is a combination of synthetic T_4 and T_3 in a 4:1 ratio that mimics the natural secretion of hormones. It is available commercially as Euthroid and Thyrolar. Because these preparations approximate the normal thyroid production, they were considered the agents of choice, before it was recognized that a significant amount of T_4 is converted peripherally to T_3. These products are stable, are chemically pure, have predictable potency, and produce laboratory values similar to those seen with T_4 administration. In Euthroid-1, 60 μg of T_4 and 14 μg of T_3 are equivalent to 1 grain of thyroid, while in Thyrolar-1, 50 μg of T_4 and 12.5 μg of T_3 represent the same equivalency. Because Euthroid is 20% more potent than Thyrolar, substitution with the alternative product may alter the patient's response. Because of its high cost, problems inherent to all T_3 containing preparations, and lack of therapeutic rationale, there is no advantage or need for administration of Liotrix.

SPECIAL CONSIDERATIONS

Pregnancy

Maternal myxedema is associated with congenital defects, abnormal fetal development resulting from poor placenta maturation, spontaneous abortions, stillbirths, and mental retardation. The exact effect of the maternal thyroid function on the fetus is unclear because normal offspring have been reported in women who remained hypothyroid throughout pregnancy. The greatest dangers to the fetus from inadequate maternal replacement therapy are poor placental development and poor maintenance of the pregnancy. The most critical period is the first trimester. The fetal thyroid begins functioning by the 12th to 14th week of pregnancy and does not depend on the maternal thyroid hormones, which do not cross the placenta. Pregnant hypothyroid patients often need a 20% increase from their baseline replacement dose during the pregnancy (70). Therefore, the FT_4I or FT_4D, and TSH levels should be monitored at least every month for the first 3 months to insure adequate thyroxine replacement. If hormone replacement therapy is adequate and maternal euthyroidism is maintained, as evidenced by normal TSH and FT_4I, or FT_4D levels, a normal pregnancy is likely. TT_4 levels will be elevated because of pregnancy-induced TBG levels.

Myxedema Coma

Myxedema coma is the end stage of long-standing uncorrected hypothyroidism. The clinical symptoms include hypothermia, advanced hypothyroid symptoms, markedly delayed or absent deep tendon reflexes, and altered sensorium, ranging from stupor to coma. Other significant findings include carbon dioxide narcosis, hyponatremia, hypoglycemia, shock, and paranoid psychosis (23).

Coma can be precipitated by cold weather (hypothermia), stress (surgery), infection, trauma, acid-base disturbances, and by unrecognized concomitant illness (e.g., diabetes, arteriosclerotic cardiovascular disease (ASCVD)). Respiratory depressants of any kind, which are metabolized slowly in the hypothyroid patient (e.g., anesthetics, narcotics, phenothiazines, sedative-hypnotics) can precipitate coma by aggravating preexisting hypothermia and carbon dioxide retention. Immediate and aggressive therapy is required to prevent the high mortality rate of 60 to 70%.

Treatment is directed at three main areas. Replacement therapy with large doses of L-thyroxine, 400 μg IV stat, should be given to saturate the TBG. This dose can be reduced, if necessary, if there are cardiac risk factors. T_3, 20 to 50 μg IV every 8 hours, although not commercially available, can also be administered. Maintenance doses of 50 μg T_4 IV or 5 μg T_3 daily should be started as soon as possible. Hydrocortisone 50 to 100 mg IV every 6 hours must be given concomitantly because of undetected hypopituitarism masquerading as myxedema.

Supportive measures include assisted ventilation, glucose infusions for hypoglycemia, restriction of fluids because of hyponatremia, and use of plasma expanders for shock and circulatory collapse. Cooling blankets may further aggravate shock by vasodilation and are not recommended. Lastly, precipitating factors should be eliminated or corrected. If the proper treatment and support are provided, consciousness, restoration of normal vital functions, and normalization of TSH levels occur within 24 hours.

Thyroid Nodules

The discovery of asymptomatic single or multiple nodules in a normal or enlarged thyroid gland is a very common occurrence. Thyroid function tests are often normal and patients are euthyroid. The possibility of malignancy must be eliminated. It is often difficult to determine clinically, if any nodule is cancerous. In general, 10 to 20% of cold nodules in a thyroid scan may be cancerous, while hot nodules are rarely carcinogenic.

A high index of suspicion for thyroid carcinoma requires surgical intervention. A fine-needle biopsy of the nodule, performed in the outpatient setting, may provide supporting information for or against surgery. Significant risk factors are listed in Table 16.10 (71). In euthyroid, nonirradiated patients with a low index of suspicion for cancer, TSH suppression therapy with L-thyroxine 0.15 to 0.2 mg daily is recommended to decrease further stimulation and growth of the nodule (72). If significant regression of the nodule(s) occurs after 3 to 6 months of therapy, treatment is continued indefinitely. Any growth of the nodule during thyroid suppression therapy is alarming and requires rebiopsy or surgical removal because of the risk of malignancy.

A significant increase in thyroid abnormalities (20 to 33%) and thyroid cancers (6 to 9%) is observed in adults who received external irradiation to the thyroid 20 to 25 years earlier (71). Patients with a prior history of external irradiation to the thymus, tonsils, adenoids, or upper head and neck region are at increased risk and require further thyroid evaluation. Benign abnormalities reported in irradiated glands include focal hyperplasia, Hashimoto's thyroiditis, adenomas, Graves' disease, and colloid nodules. Papillary, mixed papillary-follicular, and follicular malignancies are reported. Because these tumors are slow growing, the prognosis is good if no metastases are involved. Therefore, all patients with a history of childhood irradiation should be evaluated by a physician skilled in thyroid examinations. A physical examination of the thyroid, baseline TT_4 and FT_4I or FT_4D levels, and antibody levels

Table 16.10.
Risk Factors for Thyroid Cancers[a]

Evidence	Low Index of Suspicion	High Index of Suspicion
History	Familial history of thyroid disease or endemic goiter	Previous history of neck or head irradiation
Patient characteristics	Older women; soft nodule; multinodular goiter	Children, young adults, males; solitary firm dominant nodule; vocal cord paralysis; enlarged lymph nodes; hoarseness
Laboratory characteristics	High levels of antithyroid antibodies; hot nodules on scan; cystic lesion on echo; negative thin-needle biopsy (although does not rule out malignancy)	Elevated thyroglobulin; elevated serum calcitonin; cold nodule on scan; solid lesion on echo; positive thin-needle biopsy
Thyroxine therapy (not recommended in patients with history of irradiation)	Regression after 0.2–0.3 mg/day for 3–6 months	No regression

[a] Adapted from Rojeski MT, Gharib H: Nodular thyroid disease. Evaluation and management. N Engl J Med 313:428–436, 1985.

should be obtained, even if the patient is asymptomatic. Unpalpable cancers have been found during surgery. If no abnormalities are found, routine yearly examinations are recommended. The administration of thyroid hormone suppression therapy for patients with a history of irradiation and no detectable thyroid abnormalities is probably not harmful, but it does not appear to prevent the appearance of new thyroid abnormalities in the first 4 to 5 years of therapy (71). The presence of any palpable nodules is a strong indications for surgery; a fine-needle biopsy may provide confirmatory information.

Drug Interactions (Drug Kinetics and Thyroid Function)

A number of drugs and disease entitites can alter laboratory values and make interpretation of thyroid status difficult (Table 16.2). Conversely, thyroid dysfunction can affect the metabolism and clinical effectiveness of several therapeutic agents (Table 16.11) (38, 73).

Digitalis. Hyperthyroid patients tend to be clinically resistant to the glycosides, whereas hypothyroid patients are very sensitive. This observation is consistent with alteration

Table 16.11.
Effect of Thyroid Status on Drug Action

Drug	Thyroid Status	Mechanism of Action	Clinical Effect as Compared to Euthyroidism
Sympathomimetics, (asthma and cold preparations)	Hyperthyroidism	Increased sensitivity to catecholamines	Exacerbation of thyrotoxic symptoms, especially cardiac
Digitalis	Hyperthyroidism	Increased volume of distribution; ? increased renal clearance of digitalis	More resistant to digitalis effect; may necessitate increased doses to achieve therapeutic effect
	Hypothyroidism	Decreased volume of distribution of digitalis, ? decreased renal clearance	Increased sensitivity to digitalis effect; requires less digitalis to achieve therapeutic effect
Insulin	Hyperthyroidism	Increased renal clearance/metabolism of insulin	May need more insulin to control diabetes
	Hypothyroidism	Delayed turnover	Need less insulin to control diabetes
Coumadin	Hyperthyroidism	Increased metabolism of clotting factors—decreased half-life of clotting factors	Require less coumadin to achieve anticoagulation
	Hypothyroidism	Delayed turnover of clotting factors—increased half-life of clotting factors	Require more coumadin to achieve anticoagulation
Respiratory depressants (barbiturates, phenothiazines, narcotics)	Hypothyroidism	Increased sensitivity to the respiratory depressant effects of these agents	Increased CO_2 retention, may precipitate myxedema coma
Propranolol Metoprolol	Hyperthyroidism	Increased metabolic clearance	May require higher doses to achieve clinical response
Theophylline	Hypothyroidism	Decreased metabolic clearance	May require less drug to achieve clinical response.

of digitalis kinetics in thyroid dysfunction. Both the volume of distribution (Vd) and the clearance are decreased in hypothyroidism; an increased Vd and clearance occurs in hyperthyroidism. The half-life is not changed. Because the Vd determines the loading dose, and the clearance the maintenance dose, both the loading and the maintenance dose should be lower in hypothyroidism. Likewise, larger loading and maintenance digoxin doses are required for thyrotoxicosis. The dose of digoxin must be adjusted as euthyroidism occurs, to prevent toxicity and maintain maximal therapeutic effects.

Warfarin. Warfarin therapy is also altered by thyroid dysfunction. In thyrotoxicosis, both the synthesis and the catabolism of vitamin K–dependent clotting factors are increased, producing no net change in the level of clotting factors. However, an enhanced anticoagulant response occurs, because the warfarin-induced decrease in clotting factor synthesis is combined with hyperthyroidism-induced increases in factor catabolism. The opposite occurs in hypothyroidism; the anticoagulant response is less because of delayed catabolism of clotting factors. Therefore, thyrotoxic patients need less warfarin and myxedematous patients require more warfarin to achieve the same hypoprothrombinemic response. As the thyroid status cor-

rects, appropriate dosage adjustments are necessary to maintain therapeutic effectiveness and prevent toxicity.

Hormone. The kinetics of many hormones, including thyroid, are influenced by changes in thyroid status. This results from alterations in hepatic blood flow and metabolism. T_4 has a normal half-life of 6 to 7 days. In hyperthyroidism, the half-life is shortened to 3 to 4 days, and in hypothyroidism, the half-life is prolonged to 9 to 10 days. Similar changes are described for T_3.

The half-life, secretion, and metabolism of cortisol are similarly affected. Infused cortisol has a half-life of 110 minutes in euthyroid patients, 155 minutes in hypothyroid patients, and 50 minutes in thyrotoxic patients. Although, the clearance of cortisol changes as the thyroid status changes, the plasma levels remain constant because of compensatory changes in secretion rates to maintain homeostasis.

The metabolism of the sex hormones in thyroid dysfunction is opposite to that expected. Higher plasma levels of testosterone, estrogens, and androgens are found in hyperthyroidism; the converse is true in hypothyroidism. It appears that the higher plasma levels found in thyrotoxic patients result from changes in protein binding and slower elimination.

Insulin kinetics and glucose metabolism also appear to be altered by changes in thyroid status. Glucose intolerance is often observed because of increased insulin degradation rates in patients with hyperthyroidism. Clinically, hypoglycemia is more common in hypothyroidism, suggesting a delay in insulin degradation rates. Catecholamine levels are unchanged by thyroid dysfunction, although many of the thyrotoxic symptoms mimic catecholamine excess and hypothyroid symptoms mimic catecholamine deficiency.

There is definite evidence of hepatic enzyme induction in thyrotoxicosis and delayed metabolism in hypothyroidism (73). The clearance of antipyrine, a drug widely used as an marker of hepatic microsomal function, is increased in hyperthyroidism and decreased in hypothyroidism. Similar results occur with theophylline (73). Nevertheless, it is not possible to extrapolate such changes to the metabolism of other drugs cleared by the liver. Phenytoin is one example. Even though phenytoin can induce hepatic microsomal enzyme metabolism of thyroid hormones, changes in thyroid function do not appear to affect its metabolism. On the other hand, hypothyroid patients are inordinately sensitive to the effects of respiratory depressants, such as anesthetics, narcotics, phenothiazines, and sedative hypnotics, all of which undergo hepatic metabolism.

Absorption of agents such as riboflavin, ethanol, and acetaminophen appear to be increased in thyrotoxicosis and delayed in hypothyroidism. The significance of this is not clear because most of the data were obtained through animal studies.

PARATHYROID DISORDERS

To understand the treatment of common parathyroid disorders, the effects of parathyroid hormone, the consequences of excessive secretion or lack of end organ response, and its relationship to calcium metabolism must first be understood (Fig. 16.4).

Parathyroid hormone (PTH), the principal regulator of extracellular ionic calcium, is released from the parathyroid glands via a negative feedback system responsive to plasma calcium levels. Normal plasma ionic calcium is maintained through the action of PTH on kidney, bone, and intestine. Most of the total body calcium is found in bone, and only a small fraction of the calcium circulates in the bloodstream as the active (ionized) or inactive (bound) forms. Approximately 40% of the total serum calcium is bound, primarily to albumin, 15% is complexed with phosphate or other anions, and 45% is the ionized active form. Therefore, reductions in serum albumin will alter the concentration of protein-bound calcium and increase the free ionized fraction proportionally. The normal total serum calcium concentration is approximately 2.12

to 2.62 mmol/liter (8.5 to 10.5 mg/dl), depending on the laboratory. In patients with hypoalbuminemia, the serum calcium can be adjusted by adding 0.2 mmol/liter (0.8 mg/dl) for each 10 g/liter (1 g/dl) of albumin below a normal level of 40 g/liter (4 g/dl) to the measured serum calcium. This formula may not completely correct for albumin, and direct determination of ionized calcium levels may be useful.

PTH protects against hypocalcemia by the following mechanisms:

1. Increasing release of calcium and phosphate from bone resorption.
2. Increasing reabsorption of calcium and magnesium by the kidney.
3. Increasing intestinal absorption of calcium indirectly via vitamin D.
4. Increasing conversion of the metabolite 25-hydroxycholecalciferol to active vitamin D_3 (1,25-dihydroxycholecalciferol or $1,25(OH)_2D_3$ or calcitriol) through stimulating the activity of renal tubular 25-OH-1-α-hydroxylase.
5. Increasing the renal excretion of bicarbonate (bicarbonaturia), producing an acidosis that decreases the ability of circulating albumin to bind calcium, thus increasing calcium by physiochemical means. PTH also acts on the kidney to increase phosphate excretion (hyperphosphaturia) and prevent elevations in plasma phosphate levels from increased bone resorption.

Thus, a reciprocal relationship between calcium and phosphate exists. In hyperparathyroidism, serum calcium is elevated and hypophosphatemia occurs. Conversely, in hypoparathyroidism, hypocalcemia and hyperphosphatemia are seen.

Hyperparathyroidism

Primary hyperparathyroidism is an endocrine disorder characterized by excessive uncontrolled release of parathyroid hormone (PTH) from adenomatous (single-gland involvement, 80%), hyperplastic (multiple-gland involvement, 20%), or malignant (<2%) parathyroid glands. Hyperparathyroidism, associated with multiple endocrine neoplasia syndromes (MEN), is almost always due to multiple-gland involvement. The hallmark of this disorder is hypercalcemia because of the failure of the negative feedback cycle to suppress further PTH secretion. The etiology of this disorder is unknown, although inheritance via an autosomal dominant trait is described.

Prevalence. Hyperparathyroidism may be more common than previously recognized. Earlier detection of asymptomatic disease has resulted from the widespread use of routine serum calcium measurements. Various studies prior to 1969 indicate an prevalence of 10 to 20 cases per 100,000. In a careful population-based study, an incidence of 7.8 cases/100,000 jumped to 42 cases/100,000 after the introduction of routine calcium measurements. This in-

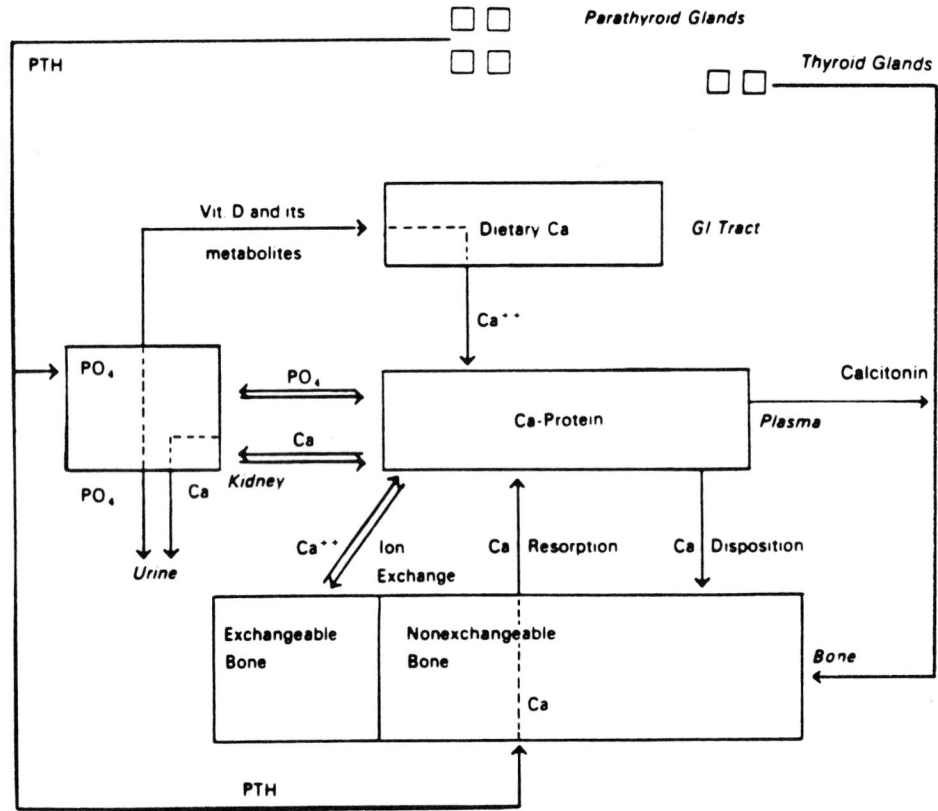

Figure 16.4. Simplified diagram of some of the normal relationships of parathyroid hormone (PTH) and calcium metabolism (From Ivey MF, Parathyroid disorders. In Herfindal ET,

Hirschman JL (eds): Clinical Pharmacy and Therapeutics, ed. 2. Baltimore, Williams & Wilkins, 1979, p 470.)

creased prevalence of hyperparathyroidism is concentrated in persons 40 years old or older and is 2 to 4 times more common in women than in men. The annual incidence is about 277 per million people (74).

Patient Characteristic	Prevalence
Both sexes ≤ 39 years	10:100,000
Both sexes ≥ 40 years	50:100,000
Female ≥ 60 years	188:100,000
Male ≥ 60 years	91:100,000

Pathogenesis. Excessive release of PTH causes hypercalcemia and hypophosphatemia via the mechanisms previously described. Mild to moderate hyperchloremic acidosis may exist from PTH-induced bicarbonaturia. Hypercalciuria results when the renal threshold for reabsorbing calcium is exceeded; serum calcium is usually greater than 2.99 mmol/liter (12 mg/dl). Complications of nephrolithiasis occur from prolonged hypercalciuria in an alkaline medium (bicarbonaturia). Other extraskeletal metastatic calcifications may produce rheumatologic complaints of calcific tendinitis and chondrocalcinosis. Osteomalacia and osteitis fibrosa cystica result from depletion of vitamin D, because of prolonged PTH renal conversion of 25-OH-D_3 to active 1,25$(OH)_2D_3$.

Diagnosis. Because the patient is frequently asymptomatic, the diagnosis is made in 80 to 90% of cases by finding an elevated serum calcium level (usually >2.62 mmol/liter (10.5 mg/dl) and an elevated PTH level. The intact PTH level using an IRMA assay, is the more sensitive of the PTH assays and should be used to confirm the diagnosis of hyperparathyroidism. Total serum calcium levels should be elevated in three separate measurements before hypercalcemia is established.

Other abnormal laboratory findings include hypophosphatemia, hyperphosphaturia, hypercalciuria, low serum bicarbonate concentration, elevated serum chloride levels, and elevations in alkaline phosphatase activity with bony involvements. Radiographic manifestations of osteitis fibrosa cystica, nephrolithiasis, or other extraskeletal calcifications can be present. Other causes of hypercalcemia should be eliminated (Table 16.12).

Clinical Presentations; Signs and Symptoms

Before the routine use of serum calcium measurements, patients typically presented with symptoms resulting from severe hypercalcemia and bone and renal involvement. Serum calcium levels <2.99 mmol/liter (12 mg/dl), com-

Table 16.12.
Some Causes of Hypercalcemia

Hyperparathyroidism
    Primary: parathyroid adenomas, hyperplasia, or carcinoma
    Secondary: compensatory increase in PTH due to low calcium levels
       (renal failure, osteomalacia, intestinal malabsorption)
Granulomatous disease (sarcoidosis, tuberculosis)
Drugs
    Vitamin D, vitamin A, or calcium intoxification
    Milk-alkali syndrome
    Thiazide diuretics
    Lithium
Malignancies
    Nonhematologic (breast, bronchus)
    Hematologic (myeloma, leukemia, lymphoma)
Endocrine (Addison's disease, thyrotoxicosis, acromegaly, pheochromo-
    cytoma)
Immobilization
Bone disorders (Paget's osteoporosis)
Idiopathic hypercalcemia of infancy
Familial hypocalciuric hypercalcemia
Miscellaneous: renal transplant, hemodialysis

monly produce gastrointestinal symptoms (e.g., anorexia, nausea, and vomiting) and neurologic manifestations of weakness, delayed deep tendon reflexes, and altered mental status. Rarely, patients are asymptomatic. The high-risk, elderly female may show confusion and dehydration. However, earlier detection of the disease has changed the clinical presentation. Most patients now are relatively asymptomatic or have nonspecific complaints of weakness and easy fatigability.

The clinical spectrum and complications of primary hyperparathyroidism are presented in Table 16.13. The severity of the clinical manifestations, especially the degree of hypercalcemia, is generally proportional to the degree of hyperfunctioning tissue and the level of PTH elevation.

Treatment of Hyperparathyroidism

Asymptomatic. National Institutes of Health Consensus Development panel has concluded that the diagnosis of hyperparathyroidism in an asymptomatic patient does not always mandate surgery. In patients with uncomplicated or asymptomatic rises in serum calcium, no previous episodes of life-threatening hypercalcemia, and normal renal and bone status, the indications for surgery are less clear because the true progression of the disease is unknown (75). There are no objective criteria to predict which patients will eventually require surgery and which patients can be managed medically. Generally, long-term follow-up studies indicate a benign course with stable hypercalcemia, and rarely, progressive loss of renal function. In a 5-year prospective study of 134 patients with mild asymptomatic hyperparathyroidism, only 20% required surgical

intervention because of progression of their disease, and 58% had no deterioration in their clinical status (76). Likewise, in a 10-year follow-up, 88% of patients had minimal progression of their disease (77). However, evaluation of long-term follow-up was complicated by poor patient compliance with medical visits and the high number of patients lost to follow-up over the 10-year period. In this asymptomatic group, it appears that the risks and costs of surgery must be weighed against the presumed benefits. Nevertheless, many studies tend to favor early surgical intervention to normalize serum calcium levels, prevent further bone loss, and increase bone density, even though surgery may be less effective in patients with mild disease and difficult-to-locate PTH abnormalities. If medical observation is selected, then patients should be monitored closely at 3- to 6-month intervals by ionized serum calcium and phosphorous levels, renal function tests, and skeletal x-rays. Patients should be told to restrict dairy products, vitamin D–containing preparations, and excessive sunlight exposure. If progression of the disease occurs, then surgical intervention is indicated.

Surgery. Surgical exploration of the neck and removal of adenomatous, hyperplastic, or malignant tissue is the definitive treatment of choice for symptomatic primary hyperparathyroidism (78). Surgery is absolutely indicated in patients with (*a*) serum calcium levels >2.74 mmol/liter (11 mg/dl); (*b*) evidence of bony involvement; (*c*) evidence of renal involvement; (*d*) complications from hyperparathyroidism; and (*e*) coexisting disease states that may be exacerbated by elevations in serum calcium levels (e.g., hypertension).

Most critical to the surgical treatment of primary hyperparathyroidism is an experienced and skilled surgeon. In competent hands, the evidence of postoperative complications (i.e., vocal cord paralysis) is minimal and the cure rate high.

Postoperatively, serum calcium levels normalize or fall below normal within 24 to 48 hours. Hypocalcemia is usually mild and transient, although tetany and permanent hypoparathyroidism can occur. Patients at high risk for the latter include those with evidence of bone demineralization, those with renal involvement, those with steatorrhea, those undergoing total parathyroidectomy, and those undergoing multiple neck explorations. Serum calcium levels should be monitored daily until levels stabilize, around the 5th to 6th postoperative day. Symptoms of tetany or pretetany should be treated intravenously with 10 to 20 ml of 10% calcium gluconate, given slowly until symptoms are relieved. Modest degrees of hypocalcemia postoperatively need not be treated except by ensuring an adequate calcium intake. A small percentage of patients will develop permanent hypoparathyroidism, requiring treatment with vitamin D (see "Hypoparathyroidism").

Medical Management. There is no pharmacological sub-

Table 16.13.
Signs and Symptoms of Hypercalcemia and Hyperparathyroidism

System	Symptoms	Complications	Laboratory Tests
Gastrointestinal	Nausea, vomiting, anorexia, constipation, abdominal pain, weight loss	Peptic ulcer disease 10–15%, chronic pancreatitis, fecal impaction/intestinal obstruction	↑ Amylase
Genitourinary	Polyuria, nocturia, polydipsia, dehydration, symptoms of uremia, renal colic pain	Nephrocalcinosis 20–30%, renal failure, pyleonephritis	Hematuria, inability to concentrate urine, pyuria ↓ Na, ↓ K, ↓ Mg
Skeletal	Vague aches and pains, arthralgias, localized swellings	Osteitis fibrosa cystica, pathologic fractures, bone cysts; calcium depositions leading to gout, pseudogout	Radiologic → subperiosteal bone resorption
Neurologic	Emotional lability, slow mentation, poor memory, weakness, easy fatigability, drowsiness, coma, ataxia, altered mental status, hallucinations	Depression, psychoses; headaches, myopathy (proximal), coma	Hyperactive deep tendon reflexes
Cardiovascular	Bradycardia	Hypertension 20–60%, cardiac arrest, bundle branch block, heart block	ECG: ↓ Q-T interval, ↑ P-R, ↑ QRS
Metabolic	Dehydration	Hyperchloremic acidosis	HCO_3 ↓ Cl ↑
Others	Pruritus due to ectopic calcifications in skin; ectopic calcifications in lungs, kidneys, etc.; red eyes	Anemia, band keratopathy, thrombosis	

stitute for the surgical management of hyperparathyroidism. However, medical management of hypercalcemia is necessary in patients who refuse surgery, in symptomatic patients prior to surgery, in those with life-threatening hypercalcemia, in those with resistant or recurrent hyperparathyroidism despite previous neck surgery, and in poor surgical candidates.

Several therapeutic options are available (79–86), although not all are useful in the treatment of hypercalcemia from primary hyperparathyroidism (see Table 16.14). In general, hypercalcemia is corrected by inhibiting bone resorption, increasing calcium excretion, or decreasing calcium absorption. Many of these options are very effective and should lower serum calcium in virtually all patients. A single agent or a combination of agents may be required, depending on the severity of the hypercalcemia, the degree of dehydration, and the etiology of the hypercalcemia. Supportive therapeutic measures should also include restriction of dietary calcium intake, mobilization, and avoidance of thiazide diuretics, which decrease urinary calcium excretion.

Hydration with normal saline is the initial treatment of choice for hypercalcemia >2.99 mmol/liter (12 mg/dl) from any etiology (79, 80). Because hypercalcemia often causes vomiting and polyuria (resulting in dehydration, hypokalemia, and hypomagnesemia) adequate electrolyte replacement and volume expansion are critical. Rehydration should occur at a rate determined by the degree of volume depletion and sufficient to maintain adequate urine output. Adequate hydration should reverse mild hypercalcemic symptoms, restore glomerular filtration rate, in-

crease calcium excretion, and improve serum calcium levels elevated by dehydration, but it is usually not sufficient alone to normalize severe hypercalcemia. Serum calcium levels often decrease by 0.25 to 0.50 mmol/liter (1 to 2 mg/dl) within 6 to 12 hours. Nevertheless, hydration should be used cautiously in patients who are unable to tolerate large fluid volumes (e.g., in CHF, RF).

In emergent hypercalcemic crisis, aggressive treatment with istonic normal saline, loop diuretics, and plicamycin (mithramycin) is required to prevent coma and death. Forced diuresis with loop diuretics to maintain urinary flow rates of >150 ml/hr often lower calcium levels within 6 to 12 hours. Higher doses of furosemide, 80 to 100 mg every 2 hr, may be required. Forced diuresis should not be used in patients with renal failure or those not adequately hydrated.

Plicamycin (mithramycin) is often successful if forced diuresis and hydration fail (79, 80). It acts by inhibiting bone resorption and is very effective in treating hypercalcemia from hyperparathyroidism, malignancy, vitamin D intoxification, and sarcoidosis. A normocalcemic effect can be expected within 12 to 72 hours after a single dose of 25 μg/kg/day, given slowly in 1 liter of fluid over 4 to 6 hours to minimize gastrointestinal toxicity. Because maximum reductions in calcium levels may not occur for 2 to 5 days, it is advisable to wait at least 48 hours before administering additional doses to avoid hypocalcemia. Repeated daily doses for 3 to 4 doses may be necessary. The duration of action is highly variable, ranging from 5 to 15 days. Reduced doses of 12.5 μg/kg/day may be tried in patients with preexisting hepatic or renal dysfunction.

Table 16.14.
Treatment of Hypercalcemia/Hyperparathyroidism

Method	Mechanism of Action	Dose	Onset of Calcium-lowering Effect	Toxicity	Effective in Primary Hyperparathyroidism	Comments
Hydration, replacement of depleted electrolytes	Increase in calcium excretion	4–5 liters of normal saline for 1 day, then 3 liters/day as needed to replace dehydration	6–12 hr	Volume overload, congestive heart failure	Yes	Cautious administration in patients with CHF, RF, SIADH; careful monitoring of fluid status and electrolytes is crucial
Forced diuresis with loop diuretics, e.g., furosemide	Increase in calcium excretion	As much as needed to maintain urinary flow rates of >150 ms/hr, e.g., furosemide 80–100 mg q 1–2 hr	6–12 hr	Volume overload, side effects of diuretics	Yes	Treatment of choice for life-threatening hypercalcemia if hydration is ineffective, and for comatose patients if renal function is adequate; avoid in dehydration; avoid thiazides which decrease calcium excretion
Sodium phosphates	Decreases calcium by raising calcium phosphate ion product above the solubility product and precipitating calcium phosphate complexes within soft tissue	p.o./rectal elemental phosphorous 2–3 g/day given in 4 divided doses; IV 25–50 mmoles inorganic phosphorous infused over 6–8 hr	IV: minutes up to 1 week Oral/rectal: delayed	IV can cause tetany, convulsions, metastatic calcifications associated with hypocalcemia, renal failure & death; oral/rectal can cause diarrhea, nausea, vomiting	Yes	Useful in chronic management of mild disease (serum calcium <11 mg/dl) with no renal abnormality; IV route not recommended for acute hypercalcemic crisis due to high risk of toxicity
Mithramycin	Inhibits bone resorption by direct effect on osteoclast	25 µg/kg/day IV q.d. × 3–4 doses; 12.5 µg/kg/day if preexisting hepatic/renal dysfunction	12–72 hrs; maximum decline in 2–5 days	Nausea, vomiting, ↓ platelets, hemorrhage; renal and hepatic damage most common after repeated doses in debilitated patients	Yes	Effective in hypercalcemia of any etiology; toxicity increases with doses >30 µg/kg/day or with consecutive doses; close monitoring of platelet counts, PT, renal, and hepatic function necessary
Calcitonin	Inhibits bone resorption	4 IU/kg s.q. or i.m. q 12 hr; maximum of 8 IU/kg q 6 hr	Maximum effect in 6–9 hr; duration of 24 hr	Allergic reactions	Yes	Relatively free of toxicity; less effective than mithramycin; refractoriness decreased with steroids; combinations of mithramycin and calcitonin may produce unwanted hypocalcemia
Estrogens, progestins	Inhibits bone resorption	0.625–1.25 mg Premarin q.d. p.o.; norethindrone 5 mg daily	Maximum effect 2 months	Nausea, vomiting, risks of estrogen/progestin therapy	Yes	Effective option in postmenopausal women with hyperparathyroidism
Glucocorticoids	Inhibits activity of osteoclasts and osteoblasts; decreases calcium absorption	Prednisone 30–100 mg/day p.o. or equivalent initially, then decrease to effective maintenance dose	48–72 hr; maximum onset of 1 week	Cushingoid symptoms, muscle wasting, osteoporosis	Rarely effective	Most effective in malignant disorders, vitamin D intoxification, sarcoidosis
Indomethacin	Inhibits prostaglandins which exhibit PTH-like hormone effect	25 mg q 6 hr p.o.	3 days, maximal effects within 11 days	Nausea, vomiting, diarrhea, GI irritation, GI bleeding, headache, dizziness, renal failure	No	Especially effective in patients with liver metastasis because of high levels of prostaglandins produced
Dialysis	Removal of calcium	Hemodialysis or peritoneal	Immediately	Complications of dialysis	Yes	Temporary hypocalcemic effect with the calcium rebounding rapidly after cessation of dialysis
Mobilization	Inhibits bone resorption	Daily ambulation	Long-term effect	None	Yes	Improve hypercalcemia by ↑ weight-bearing stress on skeletal muscle

(continued)

Table 16.14. (*Continued*)

Method	Mechanism of Action	Dose	Onset of Calcium-lowering Effect	Toxicity	Effective in Primary Hyperparathyroidism	Comments
β-Blockers	Catecholamines ↑ PTH secretion	Propranolol 40–80 mg/day p.o. in divided doses, maximum 320 mg/day	3–5 months	Effects of β-blockade	Possibly not effective	Abnormal parathyroids tend to lose their responsiveness to catecholamines
Cimetidine	Histamine stimulates release of PTH	300 mg p.o./IV q.i.d.	24–48 hrs after IV administration; variable effect with p.o. administration	Toxicity of H_2 blockers	Possibly effective if given IV	Larger than normal therapeutic doses for treatment of ulcer disease may be necessary
Bisphosphonates (diphosphonates)	Impairs function of osteoclast; ↓ bone resorption	Investigational APD 15–30 mg IV daily.	Chronic treatment average 1–3 months	?	Yes	No FDA approval
Etidronate disodium		5–10 mg/kg/day given once daily IV (over 4 hr)	1–3 months	Hyperphosphatemia, diarrhea, nausea, paradoxical ↑ in bone pain in Paget's disease	No	Indicated for treatment of Paget's disease and malignancy Less potent inhibitor of bone resorption than the newer biphosphonates

However, its cumulative toxicity generally limits its repeated usage in patients with renal failure, hepatic disease, bone marrow suppression, thrombocytopenia, or bleeding disorders.

Calcitonin is a reasonable alternative for patients in whom forced diuresis or mithramycin is contraindicated or ineffective (79, 80). Synthetic salmon and human calcitonins are now available; most experience is with the more potent and longer-acting salmon calcitonin. Calcitonin inhibits bone resorption and enhances urinary calcium excretion. Calcitonin is not usually the agent of choice because its hypocalcemic effect is modest, less consistent, and less prolonged than that of mithramycin. Calcium levels will decrease within 6 to 9 hr and peak within 24 to 48 hr after administration of 4 MRC IU/kg i.m. or s.q. every 12 hr; maximum daily doses of 32 MRC units have been used. The duration of action is transient and variable. However, loss of efficacy can occur after 2 to 6 days because of an escape phenomenon, causing serum calcium levels to rise despite continued administration. The concomitant use of steroids (e.g., prednisone 30 to 60 mg daily) may antagonize the escape and prolong the action of calcitonin in patients who become refractory. Calcitonin is well tolerated; transient nausea and vomiting are the most common toxicity. Because of its potential for anaphylactoid reactions, the manufacturer recommends initial skin testing with 1 IU/0.1 ml cutaneously, especially in atopic individuals or those with a history of hypersensitivity to calcitonin.

Intravenous phosphates are not recommended in the management of acute hypercalcemia because of the risk of metastatic soft tissue calcifications, renal failure, and even death (79, 80). Phosphates lower serum calcium levels by raising the calcium phosphate ion product above the solubility product (approximately 58 when calculated using mg/dl) and precipitating calcium phosphate complexes within the body, primarily in soft tissues. The primary use of oral phosphates is in the outpatient management of patients with hypophosphatemia and mild hypercalcemia. Normalization of serum calcium levels is not the goal because of the risk of soft tissue calcifications. Oral neutral phosphates in a dose of 1 to 2 g q.i.d. have been used chronically to treat mild hyperparathyroidism. Sodium or potassium phosphate capsules, containing 250 mg (8 mmol) of phosphate, are administered by emptying the capsules and diluting the contents with 75 mL of water. Diarrhea is the rate-limiting toxicity.

Chronic oral administration of estrogens (e.g., conjugated estrogens 1.25 mg q.d., ethinyl estradiol 30 µg daily) and progestogens (e.g., norethindrone 5 mg daily) has been shown to reduce serum calcium levels and calciuria and to decrease bone turnover in postmenopausal women with primary hyperparathyroidism (81, 82). Estrogens and progestins block the PTH-resorptive effects. Normalization of serum calcium levels is more likely with estrogens than with progestins; therefore, estrogens are the agents of choice unless contraindications exist. The reductions in serum calcium are variable and modest; some women do not respond, and the decline in others may be less than 0.25 mmol/liter (1 mg/dl). Bone mass may also increase. This mode of chronic therapy could protect against chronic PTH-bone resorption in postmenopausal women who refuse or fail surgery.

Corticosteroids are not recommended for the treatment of hypercalcemia in primary hyperparathyroidism because of the poor response (79, 80).

Several pharmacological agents have been investigated in hopes of finding a medical treatment for the hypercalcemia of hyperparthyroidism (79, 83–86). The most promising include the biphosphonates and WR-2721 (79, 86). These have included the following:

Propranolol. β-Blockers have been recommended because β-adrenergic catecholamines have been shown to stimulate PTH secretion. However, most studies with propranolol have been disappointing, suggesting that abnormal parathyroid glands may lose their normal responsiveness to catecholamines (83).

Cimetidine. Because histamine stimulates release of PTH in vitro and in vivo, the use of cimetidine has been recommended (84). Initial favorable reports have not been confirmed, and conflicting results have been reported. For cimetidine to be effective, larger doses than those used for peptic ulcer, and required.

WR-2721. This radioprotector agent has many effects on calcium metabolism (80). WR-2721 inhibits PTH secretion, inhibits bone resorption, and blocks renal reabsorption of calcium. However, reductions in serum calcium after administration appear modest and too transient to be useful.

Gallium Nitrate. Gallium nitrate is an antitumor drug that inhibits bone resorption. Although gallium nitrate appears to be effective in the acute management of malignancy-related hypercalcemia, long-term efficacy or toxicity studies have yet to be done (80).

Biphosphonates. The biphosphonates (diphosphonates) have been shown to be potent inhibitors of PTH-mediated bone resorption both in vivo and in vitro (79, 86). Most biphosphonates are poorly absorbed orally and must be given intravenously to obtain a prompt antiresorptive effect. Etidronate, the first biphosphonate available in the United States, has been disappointing in the management of hyperparathyroidism (85). It has weak hypocalcemic activity when given orally and when compared with other biphosphonates. Aminohydroxypropylidene biphosphonate (APD), a promising investigational agent, is a more potent inhibitor of bone resorption than is etidronate. Several reports attest to the efficacy of intravenous and possibly oral aminohydroxypropylidene in the management of acute hypercalcemia from hyperparathyroidism and malignancies (86). Another potent biphosphonate, dichloromethylene biphosphonate, is no longer available for clinical use because leukemia developed in patients in clinical trials.

Therefore, no medical management of hyperparathyroidism is available. Further investigations are necessary to find an effective medical treatment for primary hyperparathyroidism. Until such time, surgery remains the treatment of choice.

Prognosis

Surgical resection of benign parathyroid lesions is generally curative in primary hyperparathyroidism. Recurrences are common when multiple glands are involved and rare when a single gland is involved.

Hypoparathyroidism

Hypoparathyroidism is an endocrine disorder characterized by a deficiency of parathyroid hormone, hypocalcemia, and hyperphosphatemia.

Etiology/Prevalence. The most common cause of hypoparathyroidism is surgical excision or exploration of the anterior neck. In experienced surgical hands, the prevalence of permanent hypoparathyroidism is less than 1% for all thyroid and parathyroid surgeries (45, 78). This risk is increased significantly after subtotal parathyroidectomy for parathyroid hyperplasia (multiple-gland involvement) or after repeated neck surgery for recurrent disease.

Other rare causes include idiopathic hypoparathyroidism (unknown etiology), neonatal hypoparathyroidism, destruction of the parathyroid glands by radiation or metastatic disease, inactive parathyroid hormone, and target organ resistance to PTH (pseudohypoparathyroidism). Functional hypoparathyroidism occurs from severe hypomagnesemia and reverses with magnesium replacement. Because magnesium is required for normal release of PTH and for the action of PTH peripherally, hypocalcemia may persist until the hypomagnesemia is corrected. Some causes of hypomagnesemia include starvation, prolonged intravenous feeding, malabsorption, chronic alcoholism, diuretics, aminoglycosides, and *cis*-platinum therapy.

Pathogenesis. Deficiency of PTH hormone produces (*a*) decreased bone resorption, (*b*) hyperphosphatemia and hypophosphaturia, (*c*) decreased intestinal absorption of calcium, (*d*) decreased levels of active 1,25-OH-D$_3$, (*e*) hypocalcemia and hypercalciuria, and (*f*) metabolic alkalosis from decreased bicarbonate excretion.

Diagnosis. Hypoparathyroidism should be suspected with hypocalcemia, hyperphosphatemia, undetectable levels of PTH, and a history of previous neck surgery. Serum phosphate concentrations may not always be elevated because of dietary restrictions, use of aluminum-containing phosphate binders, or increased mineral uptake by bone. Normal or elevated PTH levels and hypocalcemia excludes the diagnosis of hypoparathyroidism and strongly suggests end organ resistance to PTH (pseudohypoparathyroidism). Serum magnesium levels should be checked to exclude the diagnosis of functional hypoparathyroidism. Other types of hypocalcemia, including drug-induced should be excluded (Table 16.15).

The long-term use of anticonvulsants such as phenytoin, phenobarbital, and structurally related compounds increases the hepatic conversion of vitamin D$_3$ and 25-OH-D$_3$ to biologically inactive metabolites, causing decreased concentrations of active 25-OH-D$_3$, malabsorption of calcium, hypocalcemia, and osteomalacia. This risk is greater in patients on long-term combination anticon-

Table 16.15.
Causes of Hypocalcemia

Hypoparathyroidism
    Surgical: postthyroidectomy, postparathyroidectomy, post neck explo-
      ration
    Idiopathic (unknown)
    Neonatal
    Destruction of parathyroids (tumor, radiation)
    Pseudohypoparathyroidism (end-organ resistance to PTH)
    Inactive PTH hormone
Magnesium deficiency (functional hypoparathyroidism)
Acute pancreatitis/malabsorption
Renal failure—secondary hypoparathyroidism
Osteomalacia
Drugs: phenytoin, phenobarbital, cholestyramine (see text); laxative
    abuse with phosphate enemas; aminoglycoside nephrotoxicity
Hyperphosphatemic states—rhabdomyolysis, EDTA, phosphate enema
Vitamin D deficiency
Hyperalimentation

vulsant therapy, those with low dietary calcium intake, those with little sunlight exposure, those with diseases predisposing to vitamin D malabsorption, and in blacks because of their greater resistance to the irradiating effects of sunlight. Changes in serum calcium, alkaline phosphatase and phosphate levels and the bony changes of osteomalacia should be closely monitored in these patients. Fortunately, anticonvulsant-induced hypocalcemia and osteomalacia are responsive to vitamin D therapy (87, 88).

Another iatrogenic cause of hypocalcemia and osteomalacia is the long-term administration of cholestyramine, which binds the bile acids necessary for vitamin D absorption from the intestine. Therapy with higher doses of vitamin D is necessary to overcome the gut inhibitory effects of cholestyramine on vitamin D absorption.

Clinical Findings

The clinical manifestations of hypoparathyroidism are related to the severity and the chronicity of hypocalcemia. Abrupt declines in serum calcium level (e.g., within the first 48 hours after parathyroidectomy) are much more likely to produce hypocalcemic symptoms than are gradual reductions of calcium levels. Changes in acid-base status also affect the symptoms. Alkalosis worsens the hypocalcemia by increasing the plasma protein binding of calcium and decreasing the free ionized fraction. Conversely, acidosis improves the hypocalemia by increasing the free, active, and ionized calcium levels.

The signs and symptoms of hypocalcemia and hypoparathyroidism are presented in Table 16.16.

Treatment of Hypoparathyroidism

Theoretically, the most appropriate therapy for hypoparathyroidism is the administration of PTH. However, no suitable oral preparation is available. An effective alternative to PTH therapy is the administration of calcium supplements and vitamin D to increase intestinal calcium absorption.

A daily intake of 1 to 2 g of elemental calcium and phosphate restriction via aluminum hydroxide–binding gels will usually maintain calcium homeostasis in patients with mild hypoparathyroidism. Symptomatic patients with serum calcium levels below 1.87 mmol/liter (7.5 mg/dl) often require concomitant therapy with vitamin D to maintain eucalcemia.

If dietary intake is inadequate, calcium supplementation can be provided effectively through various calcium-containing salts. Calcium gluconate, containing small amounts of calcium, is not very palatable because large numbers of tablets must be administered to attain a therapeutic dose. Similarly, calcium chloride is not the best choice because of gastric irritation occurring from its high calcium content. Calcium carbonate is usually preferred because it is well tolerated, requires fewer tablets to be administered, and is more effective than are supplements containing small amounts of calcium (gluconate, lactate). However calcium carbonate may not be the drug of choice for elderly patients because of their impaired calcium absorption due to achlorhydria (89). The best-tolerated calcium carbonate preparation (and the most expensive) is Os-Cal, which contains 250 to 500 mg of elemental calcium per tablet. Other calcium preparations include Tums (200 mg), Calcimax (325 mg), and Caltrate (600 mg). One gram of calcium is provided by the following salts:

Calcium carbonate	2.5 g	(40% calcium)
Calcium chloride	3.7 g	(27% calcium)
Calcium gluconate	12.0 g	(9% calcium)
Calcium lactate	9.0 g	(11% calcium)

Constipation is a potential problem with all calcium supplements and should be managed.

Vitamin D should be started for hypocalcemic symptoms as soon as possible. The selection of an appropriate vitamin D preparation depends on the etiology of the hypocalcemia, cost, onset of action, metabolism, and duration of toxicity after discontinuation (Table 16.17) (87, 88). The newer vitamin D_3 preparations are biologically active and superior to vitamin D_2 in rapidity of onset and offset of action, but they are also more expensive. They should be reserved for difficult-to-manage patients and those with low serum levels of $1,25(OH)_2D_3$ (i.e., those with hypoparathyroidism or renal osteodystrophy).

A review of vitamin D metabolism is depicted in Fig. 16.5. The generic term vitamin D refers to dietary ergocalciferol (vitamin D_2) and cholecalciferol (vitamin D_3). Cholecalciferol is produced in the skin after ultraviolet sunlight exposure. Ergocalciferol is absorbed from the jejunum from dietary sources and undergoes metabolism like cholecalciferol. One milligram of vitamin D_2 is equal

Table 16.16.
Clinical Features of Hypocalcemia/Hypoparathyroidism

System	Signs/Symptoms	Complications/Sequelae	Comments
Musculoskeletal	Circumoral and distal numbness and tingling, muscle twitching; hyperreflexia, positive Chvostek's and Trousseau's signs	Tetany: carpopedal spasm, laryngeal stridor, convulsions	Requires emergency treatment with intravenous calcium
Neurologic	Papilledema, increased CSF pressure; basal ganglia calcifications extrapyramidal symptoms; abnormal EEG	Epilepsy; parkinsonism: complication in 20% of patients with hypoparathyroidism	Improves with eucalcemia, increased sensitivity to dystonic reaction of phenothiazines
Psychiatric	Irritability	Depression, psychosis, mental retardation in 20% of children	May improve with eucalcemia
Integument	Dry scaly skin, coarse friable dry hair, longitudinal ridges on nails	Exfoliative dermatitis, atopic eczema, psoriasis, increased candida infection	May improve with eucalcemia
Ocular	Visual impairment and opacities of the lens	Lenticular cataracts most common sequelae of hypoparathyroidism	Eucalcemia halts progression of cataracts
Cardiac	Symptoms of heart failure, irregular rhythm, EKG: ↑ Q-T interval	Cardiac dilation	Improves with eucalcemia
Others	Impaired dental development; intestinal malabsorption with steatorrhea		Improves with eucalcemia
Laboratory results	Increased CPK, LDH; ↓ calcium, ↑ phosphate, urinary phosphate low, urinary calcium low to absent, PTH low		

to 40,000 IU (87). The active form of vitamin D is 1,25-dihydroxycholecalciferol ($1,25(OH)_2D_3$), which is activated in the kidney by the 1-α-hydroxylase enzyme after hepatic 25-hydroxylation. Because parathyroid hormone and hypophosphatemia stimulate activity of this renal hydroxylase enzyme, a suitable vitamin D preparation for patients with hypoparathyroidism already possesses the 1-α-hydroxyl group (i.e., DHT, calcitriol). Conversely, in anticonvulsant-induced vitamin D deficiency where there is a decrease in circulating 25-hydroxycholecalciferol ($25-(OH)D_3$) but normal levels of active 1,25-dihydroxycholecalciferol, the most appropriate preparation is calcifediol.

Vitamin D_2 is commonly used in the treatment of hypoparathyroidism because it is the least expensive of all the preparations. However, it may be less effective than DHT or calcitriol for the reasons stated above. Furthermore, it has a slow onset of action and a prolonged period of toxicity after discontinuation. Vitamin D therapy can be initiated with 25,000 to 50,000 units/day and gradually increased to maintenance doses of 50,000 to 100,000 units/day, after checking calcium levels. Maximal effects on serum calcium are achieved in 4 to 6 weeks. DHT is often preferred over vitamin D_2 because of its more rapid onset of action and its more rapid dissipation in cases of inadvertent overdose. The initial dose of DHT is 0.8 to 2.4 mg daily for several days, then a maintenance dose of 0.2 to 1 mg daily. Calcitriol is also highly effective in doses of 0.25 μg/day initially, increased as necessary to a maintenance dose of 1 to 3 μg daily (Table 16.17). Doses of all preparations should be increased gradually only after maximal effects are achieved, to avoid hypercalcemia. Ideally, serum calcium levels should be maintained between 2.12

and 2.25 mmol/liter (8.5 and 9 mg/dl), leaving a margin for fluctuations. Serum calcium and phosphorous levels should be checked at least monthly until stable, and then every 6 months to a year thereafter.

The main toxicity of all vitamin D preparations is hypercalcemia, which can be prevented by close monthly monitoring of serum calcium, phosphorus, and alkaline phosphatase levels. Availability of $25(OH)D_3$ and $1,25(OH)_2D_3$ assays in more specialized centers may help prevent toxicity from hypercalcemia. Corticosteroids are effective antidotes in vitamin D intoxification. Calcitriol may also be associated with deterioration of renal function in patients with previously stable renal function.

Severe hypocalcemia complicated by tetany requires emergency treatment with 5 to 10 ml of intravenous calcium gluconate 10% given slowly until symptoms are relieved or until the serum calcium level increases above 1.87 mmol/liter (7.5 mg/dl). A continuous effect can be maintained by infusing 10 to 50 ml of 10% calcium gluconate in 1 liter of normal saline over 24 hr. Too vigorous treatment of the tetany can cause irreversible tissue calcifications. Hypomagnesemia should be corrected, and oral calcium and vitamin D supplements started immediately. Drugs that exacerbate hypocalcemia (i.e., loop diuretics) should be avoided. Phenothiazines should be used cautiously because dystonic reactions may occur. Also, inadvertent hypercalcemia may increase the risk of digitalis toxicity in patients receiving digoxin.

Prognosis

The prognosis is excellent. Improvement of most symptoms can be expected with restoration of normal serum calcium levels.

Table 16.17.
Comparison of Vitamin D Preparations

Vitamin D Preparation	Abbreviation	Brand Name	Dose	Kinetic

Calciferol
Ergocalciferol
Caps 10,000 units
     25,000 units
     50,000 units
Liquid 8,000 IU/ml
	Vitamin D$_2$	Calciferol Drisdol	50–400,000 units/day
			1 mg = 40,000 U
			3 mg = 120,000 U
				Onset approximately 2 weeks (4–12 weeks range); long t$_{1/2}$ (half-life); highly protein bound; slow elimination: duration 3–6 months

Dihydrotachysterol
Caps 125 µg
     200 µg
     400 µg
Solution 0.25 mg/ml
	DHT	Hytakerol	Initial 0.2–2.5 mg/day
			Maintenance 0.5–1 mg/day
				Rapid onset within 2 hr; maximal onset 7–15 days

Calcifediol (25-hydroxy-vitamin D$_3$) Caps 20, 50 µg	25(OH)D$_3$	Calderol	50–100 µg/day	More rapid onset than with vitamin D$_2$ but slower than with DHT, onset 15 days
Calcitriol (1,25-dihydroxyl-vitamin D$_3$) Caps 0.25 µg Caps 0.50 µg	1,25(OH)$_2$D$_3$	Rocaltrol	0.25 µg daily initially; then 0.5–3 µg/day	Rapid onset: 1–3 days; t$_{1/2}$ = 2–3 hr
Alfacalcidol	1-(OH)D$_3$	Not commercially available in U.S.	1–2 µg	Similar to calcitriol

Activity	Time for Reversal of Toxic Effects after Discontinuation	Comments
Biologically inactive; requires activation by hepatic 25-hydroxylation and by renal 1-α-hydroxylase.	16–18 weeks	Least expensive; requires bile salts for complete absorption in gut; poor shelf-life stability
Requires only hepatic 25-hydroxylation for activation; contains 1α-hydroxyl group so no kidney activation necessary	3–9 days	Three times more potent than vitamin D; main action is to increase calcium absorption; calcium supplementation recommended; more effective in CRF and hypoparathyroidism than vitamin D$_2$
Requires kidney for bioactivation	4 weeks	1.5 times as potent as vitamin D$_2$; preparation of choice in deficiency associated with anticonvulsant therapy, intestinal malabsorption, and hepatobiliary disease; also effective in renal osteodystrophy; therapeutic blood level monitoring available
Active	2–10 days	Most potent & most expensive preparation available; requires calcium supplementation in hypoparathyroidism; major advantage is rapid onset/offset of effect
Rapid conversion to 1,25(OH)$_2$D$_3$	5–10 days	Similar to calcitrol

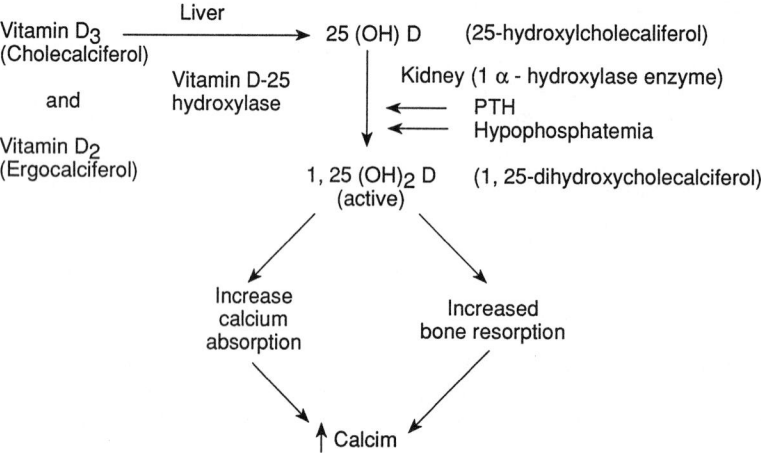

Figure 16.5.   Activity and metabolism of vitamin D.

REFERENCES

1. Silva JE: Effects of iodine and iodine-containing compounds on thyroid function. Med Clin North Am 69:881–898, 1985.
2. Surks MI, Chopra IJ, Mariash CN, et al.: American Thyroid Association guidelines for use of laboratory tests in thyroid disorders. JAMA 263:1529–1532, 1990.
3. Brent GA, Hershman JM: Thyroxine therapy in patients with severe nonthyroidal illnesses and low serum thyroxine concentrations. J Clin Endocrinol Metab 63:1–7, 1986.
4. Wartofsky L, Burman KD: Alterations in thyroid function in patients with systemic illness: the "euthyroid sick syndrome." Endocr Rev 3:164–217, 1982.
5. LoPresti JS, Fried JC, Spencer CA, et al.: Unique alterations of thyroid hormone indices in the acquired immunodeficiency syndrome (AIDS). Ann Intern Med 110:970–975, 1989.
6. Slag MF, Morley JE, Elson MK, et al.: Hypothyroxinemia in critically ill patients as a predictor of high mortality. JAMA 245:43–45, 1981.
7. Tibaldi JM, Barzel US, Albin J, et al.: Thyrotoxicosis in the very old. Am J Med 81:619–621, 1986.
8. Fradkin JE, Wolff J: Iodide-induced thyrotoxicosis. Medicine 62:1–20, 1983.
9. Volpe R: Autoimmunity causing thyroid dysfunction. Endocrinol Metab Clin North Am 20:565–587, 1991.
10. Ishikawa N, Eguchi K, Otsubo T, et al.: Reduction in the suppressor-inducer T cell subset and increase in the helper T cell subset in thyroid tissue from patients with Graves' disease. J Clin Endocrinol Metab. 65:17–23, 1987.
11. Jacobsen DH, Gorman CA: Diagnosis and management of endocrine ophthalmopathy. Med Clin North Am 69:973–988, 1985.
12. Sridama V, DeGroot LJ: Treatment of Graves' disease and the course of ophthalmopathy. Am J Med 87:70–73, 1989.
13. Bartalena L, Marcocci C, Bogazzi F, et al.: Use of corticosteroids to prevent progression of Graves' ophthalmopathy after radioiodine therapy for hyperthyroidism. N Engl J Med. 321:1349–1352, 1989.
14. Bahn RS, Gorman CA: Choice of therapy and criteria for assessing treatment outcome in thyroid-associated ophthalmopathy. Endocrinol Metab Clin North Am 16:391–407, 1987.
15. Vorherr H, Vorherr UF, Mehta P, et al.: Vaginal absorption of povidone-iodine. JAMA 244:2628–2629, 1980.
16. Salata S, Klein I: Effects of lithium on the endocrine system: a review. J Lab Clin Med 110:130–136, 1987.
17. Albert S, Alves LE, Rose E: Thyroid dysfunction during chronic amiodarone therapy. J Am Coll Cardiol 9:175–183, 1987.
18. Borowski GD, Garofano CD, Rose LI: Effect of long-term amiodarone therapy on thyroid hormone levels and thyroid function. Am J Med 78:443–450, 1985.
19. Nademanee K, Piwonka RW, Singh BN, et al.: Amiodarone and thyroid function. Progr Cardiovasc Dis 6:427–437, 1989.
20. Burrow GN. The management of thyrotoxicosis in pregnancy. N Engl J Med 313:562–565, 1985.
21. Walfish PG, Chan JYC: Post-partum hyperthyroidism. Clin Endocrinol Metab 14:417–447, 1985.
22. McDermott MT, Kidd GS, Dodson LE, et al.: Radioiodine-induced thyroid storm: case report and literature review. Am J Med 75:353–359, 1983.
23. Nicoloff JT: Thyroid storm and myxedema coma. Med Clin North Am 69:1005–1017, 1985.
24. Solomon B, Glinoer D, Lagasse R, et al.: Current trends in the management of Graves' disease. J Clin Endocrinol Metab 70:1518–1524, 1990.
25. McGregor AM, Smith BR, Hall R, et al.: Specificity of the immunosuppressive action of carbimazole in Graves' disease. Br Med J 284:1750–1751, 1982.
26. Ludgate ME, McGregor AM, Weetman AP, et al.: Analysis of the T cell subsets in Graves' disease: alterations associated with carbimazole. Br J Med 228:526–530, 1984.
27. Cooper DS. Which antithyroid drug? Am J Med 80:1165–1168, 1986.
28. Roti E, Gardini E, Minelli R, et al.: Methimazole and serum thyroid hormone concentrations in hyperthyroid patients: effects of single and multiple daily doses. Ann Intern Med 111:181–182, 1989.
29. Walter RM, Bartle W: Rectal administration of propylthiouracil in the treatment of Graves' disease. Am J Med 88:69–70, 1990.
30. Nabil N, Miner DJ, Amatruda JM. Methimazole: an alternative route of administration. J Clin Endocrinol Metab 54:180–181, 1982.
31. Bouma DJ, Kammer H, Greer MA. Follow-up comprison of short-term versus 1-year antithyroid drug therapy for the thyrotoxicosis of Graves' disease. J Clin Endocrinol Metab 55:1138–1142, 1982.
32. Allannic H, Fauchet R, Orgiazzi J, etal.: Antithyroid drugs and Graves' disease: a prospective randomized evaluation of the efficacy of treatment duration. J Clin Endocriol Metab 70:675–679, 1990.
33. Tamai H, Nakagawa T, Fukino O, et al.: Thionamide therapy in Graves' disease: relation of relapse rate to duration of therapy. Ann Intern Med 92:488–490, 1980.
34. Lippe BM, Landaw EM, Kaplan SA: Hyperthyroidism in children treated with long term medical therapy: twenty-five percent remission every two years. J Clin Endocrinol Metab 64:1241–1245, 1987.
35. Romaldini JH, Bromberg N, Werner RS, et al.: Comparison of effects of high and low dosage regimens of antithyroid drugs in the management of Graves' hyperthyroidism. J Clin Endocrinol Metab 57:563–570, 1983.
36. Vitug AC, Goldman JM. Hepatotoxicity from antithyroid drugs. Horm Res 21:229–234, 1985.
37. Cooper DS, Goldminz D, Levin AA, et al.: Agranulocytosis associated with antithyroid drugs. Effects of patient age and drug dose. Ann Intern Med 98:26–29, 1983.
38. Feely J, Peden N: Use of β-adrenoreceptor blocking drugs in hyperthyroidism. Drugs 27:425–446, 1984.
39. Adlerberth A, Stenstrom G, Hasselgren P: The selective β_1-blocking agent metoprolol compared with antithyroid drug and thyroxine as preoperative treatment of patients with hyperthyroidism. Results from a prospective, randomized study. Ann Surg 205:182–188, 1987.
40. Feely J, Crooks J, Forrest AL, et al.: Propranolol in the surgical treatment of hyperthyroidism including severely thyrotoxic patients. Br J Surg 68:865–869, 1981.
41. Milner MR, Gelman KM, Phillips RA, et al.: Double-blind crossover trial of diltiazem versus propranolol in the management of thyrotoxic symptoms. Pharmacotherapy 10:100–106, 1990.
42. Graham GD, Burman KD: Radioiodine treatment of Graves' disease. An assessment of its potential risks. Ann Intern Med 105:900–905, 1986.
43. Noguchi K, Suzuki H, Nakahata M, et al.: Prolonged treatment of hyperthyroidism with sodium tyropanoate, an oral cholecystographic agent: an re-evaluation of its clinical utility. Clin Endocrinol 25:293–301, 1986.
44. Wang YS, Tsou CT, Lin WH, et al.: Long term treatment of Graves' disease with iopanoic acid (Telepaque). J Clin Endocrinol Metab 65:679–682, 1987.
45. Weber CA, Clark OH: Surgery for thyroid disease. Med Clin North Am 69:1097–1115, 1985.
46. l'Allemand D, Gruters A, Heidemann P, et al.: Iodine-induced alterations of thyroid function in newborn infants after prenatal and perinatal exposure to povidone iodine. J Pediatr 102:935–938, 1983.
47. Van Dijke CP, Heydendael RJ, De Kleine MJ: Methimazole, carbimazole, and congenital skin defects. Ann Intern Med 106:60–61, 1987.
48. Momotani N, Noh J, Oyanagi H, et al.: Antithyroid drug therapy for Graves' disease during pregnancy. Optimal regimen for fetal thyroid status. N Engl J Med 315:24–28, 1986.

49. Burrow GN, Klatskin EH, Genel M: Intellectual development in children whose mothers received propylthiouracil during pregnancy. Yale J Biol Med 51:151–156, 1978.

50. Kampmann JP, Johansen K, Hansen JM, et al.: Propylthiouracil in human milk. Lancet 1:736–738, 1980.

51. Hamburger J: Management of hyperthyroidism in children and adolescents. J Clin Endocrinol Metab 60:1019–1024, 1985.

52. Rosenthal MJ, Sanchez CJ: Thyroid disease in the elderly—missed diagnosis or overdiagnosis? West J Med 143:6453–647, 1985.

53. LaFranchi S: Diagnosis and treatment of hypothyroidism in children. Compr Ther 13:20–30, 1987.

54. Hennessey JV, Evaul JE, Tseng Y-C, et al.: L-Thyroxine dosage: a re-evaluation of therapy with contemporary preparations. Ann Intern Med 105:11–15, 1986.

55. Fish LH, Schwartz HL, Cavanaugh J: Replacement dose, metabolism, and bioavailability of levothyroxine in the treatment of hypothyroidism. N Engl J Med 316:764–770, 1987.

56. Griffin JE: Hypothyroidism in the elderly. Am J Med Sci 299:334–345, 1990.

57. Hennessey JV, Burman KD, Wartofsky L: The equivalency of two L-thyroxine preparations. Ann Intern Med 102:770–773, 1985.

58. Stoffer SS, Szunpar WE: Potency of current levothyroxine preparations evaluated by high performance liquid chromatography. Henry Ford Hosp Med J 36:64–65, 1988.

59. Helfand M, Crapo LM: Monitoring therapy in patients taking levothyroxine. Ann Intern Med 113:450–454, 1990.

60. Ross DS: Subclinical hyperthyroidism. Possible danger of overzealous thyroxine replacement therapy. Mayo Clin Proc 63:1223–1229, 1988.

61. Paul TL, Kerrigan J, Kelly AM, et al.: Long-term L-thyroxine therapy is associated with decreased hip bone density in premenopausal women. JAMA 259:3137–3141, 1988.

62. Stall GM, Harris S, Sokoll LJ, et al.: Accelerated bone loss in hypothyroid patients overtreated with L-thyroxine. Ann Intern Med 113:265–269, 1990.

63. Levine HD: Compromise therapy in the patient with angina pectoris and hypothyroidism. Am J Med 69:411–418, 1980.

64. Myerowitz D, Kamienski RW, Swanson DK, et al.: Diagnosis and management of the hypothyroid patient with chest pain. J Thorac Cardiovasc Surg 86:57–60, 1983.

65. Maenpaa J: Congenital hypothyroidism. Aetiological and clinical aspects. Arch Dis Child 47:914–923, 1972.

66. Fisher DA, Foley BL: Early treatment of congenital hypothyroidism. Pediatrics 83:785–789, 1989.

67. Rees-Jones RW, Rolla AR, Larsen PR: Hormonal content of thyroid replacement preparations. JAMA 243:549–550, 1980.

68. Stoffer SS, Szpnunar WE: Levothyroxine loses potency with age (letter). JAMA 255:1881–1882, 1986.

69. Sawin CT, Hershman JM, Fernandez-Garcia R, et al.: A comparison of thyroxine and desiccated thyroid in patients with primary hypothyroidism. Metabolism 27:1518–1525, 1978.

70. Mandel SJ, Larsen PR, Seely EW, et al.: Increased need for thyroxine during pregnancy in women with primary hypothyroidism. N Engl J Med 323:91–96, 1990.

71. Rojeski MT, Gharib H: Nodular thyroid disease. Evaluation and management. N Engl J Med 313:428–436, 1985.

72. Berghout A, Wiersinga WM, Drexhage HA, et al.: Comparison of placebo with L-thyroxine alone or with carbimazole for treatment of sporadic non-toxic goitre. Lancet 336:193–197, 1990.

73. O'Connor P, Feely J: Clinical pharmacokinetics and endocrine disorders. Therapeutic implications. Clin Pharmacokinet 13:345–364, 1987.

74. Heath DA: Primary hyperparathyroidism. Clinical presentation and factors influencing clinical management. Endocrinol Metab Clin North Am 18:631–645, 1989.

75. Consensus Development Conference Panel: Diagnosis and management of asymptomatic primary hyperparathyroidism: consensus development conference statement. Ann Intern Med 114:593–597, 1991.

76. Scholz DA, Purcell DC: Asymptomatic primary hyperparathyroidism. A ten year prospective study. Mayo Clin Proc 56:473–478, 1981.

77. Gaz RD, Wang C: Management of asymptomatic hyperparathyroidism. Am J Surg 147:498–502, 1984.

78. Clark OH, Duh QY: Primary hyperparathyroidism. A surgical perspective. Endocrinol Metab Clin North Am 18:701–713, 1989.

79. Attie MF: Treatment of hypercalcemia. Endocrinol Metab Clin North Am 18:807–828, 1989.

80. Schaiff RAB, Hall TG, Bar RS: Medical treatment of hypercalcemia. Clin Pharm 8:108–121, 1989.

81. Marcus R: Estrogens and progestins in the management of primary hyperparathyroidism. Endocrinol Metab Clin North Am 18:715–722, 1989.

82. Wishart J, Horowitz M, Need AG, et al.: Treatment of postmenopausal hyperparathyroidism with norethindrone. Long term effects on forearm mineral content. Arch Intern Med 150:1951–1953, 1990.

83. Vora NM, Kukreja SC, Williams GA, et al.: Parathyroid hormone secretion: effect of β-adrenergic blockade before and after surgery for primary hyperparathyroidism. J Clin Endocrinol Metab 53:599–601, 1981.

84. Sherwood JK, Garcia M, Ackroyd FW, et al.: Hyperparathyroid crisis reviewed: a role for parenteral cimetidine? Am Surg 52:320–332, 1986.

85. Licata AA, O'Hanlon O: Treatment of hyperparathyroidism with etidronate disodium. JAMA 249:2063–2064, 1983.

86. Schmidli RS, Wilson I, Espiner A, et al.: Aminopropylidine diphosphonate (APD) in mild primary hyperparathyroidism: effect on clinical status. Clin Endocrinology 32:293–300, 1990.

87. Kumar R, Riggs BL: Series on pharmacology in practice. 11. Vitamin D in the therapy of disorders of calcium and phosphorus metabolism. Mayo Clin Proc 56:327–333, 1981.

88. Haussler MR, Cordy PE: Metabolites and analogues of vitamin D. Which for what? JAMA 247:841–844, 1982.

89. Recker RR. Calcium absorption and achlorhydria. N Engl J Med 313:70–73, 1985.

90. Adams JS: Vitamin D–metabolite-mediated hypercalcemia. Endocrinol Metab Clin North Am 18:765–778, 1989.

CHAPTER 17

DIABETES

JOHN R. WHITE, JR., Pharm.D. and R. KEITH CAMPBELL, B. Pharm., M.B.A.

Diabetes mellitus was recognized as early as 1500 BC by Egyptian physicians who described a disease associated with "the passage of much urine." The term diabetes (diabetes = siphon) was coined by the Greek physician Aretaeus the Cappadocian around 2 AD. Aretaeus noticed that patients with diabetes had a disease that caused the siphoning of the structural components of the body into the urine ("a melting down of the flesh and limbs into urine"). Although it had been known for centuries that the urine of patients with diabetes was sweet, it was not until 1674 that a physician named Willis coined the term diabetes mellitus (mellitus = honey).

Diabetes mellitus (DM) is a complex condition that affects multiple organ systems. There is still much to be learned about diabetes mellitus; however, recent advances have enhanced the understanding and treatment of DM. The impact of these changes on the diabetic patient has been dramatic. Self-monitoring of blood glucose in combination with better education programs and new treatment protocols has been the most significant change in the treatment of diabetes since the discovery of insulin. Other advances in the treatment of the disease include

A new classification system for diabetes;
Increased evidence to support "tight" control of blood glucose;
Funding and initiation of a long-term study to review the benefits of tight control;
New methods of monitoring control;
Greater emphasis on patient self-monitoring;
Diabetes education program recognition standards;
Diabetes educator certification;
Purer insulins;
Widespread production of biosynthetic human insulin;
New treatment methods, including internal and external insulin infusion devices.

A thorough, positive education program for the diabetic patient about the disease, medication, blood and urine testing, and hygiene is a major component of diabetic management. Poor control of diabetes is often the result of medication error, misinterpretation of test results, and ignorance of the disease (1). The diabetic needs a complete educational program with input from the entire health team. The physician must diagnose the condition accurately, classify the type of diabetes, and stimulate the patient to learn to control and monitor the condition. The dietitian explains the importance of diet control and the food exchange system. The nurse helps the patient develop a positive attitude, learn how to perform tests to monitor control, inject insulin, and keep records of the factors that affect diabetic control. The pharmacist's easy access to the patient offers a unique opportunity to help the patient maintain a proper therapeutic regimen. The pharmacist can answer patient questions about the disease, blood testing, urine testing, drug therapy, diet products, and foot care, and can reinforce the information provided by other members of the team. The pharmacist also can monitor the course of diabetic patients. Since diabetic patients see pharmacists more often than any other health professional, the pharmacist is in a unique position to have a significant effect on the treatment of diabetic patients. Pharmacists who want to help their diabetic patients must not only understand pharmacological facts but also become competent in selecting, initiating, and individualizing drug therapy for the various types of diabetic patients. Thus, the pharmacist performs three significant functions: referral, monitoring of therapy, and education.

DEFINITION

Diabetes mellitus is difficult to define because it is a spectrum of conditions that display hyperglycemia as a common symptom. Until recently, diabetes was considered to be a single disease. It is clear now that diabetes is a heterogeneous group of disorders caused by various genetic predispositions and precipitating factors. Not only does insulin-dependent (type I) diabetes differ from non-insulin-dependent (type II) diabetes, but there appears to be heterogeneity within each of these two types (2). Diabetes is a chronic disease characterized by disorders in carbohydrate (and associated fat and protein) metabolism because of an absolute or relative deficiency in the action of insulin and possibly abnormally high amounts of glucagon and other insulin-antagonizing substances such as growth hormone, sympathomimetic amines, and corticosteroids (the so-called counter-regulatory hormones). Insulin secretion in diabetes may be normal or totally deficient.

Properly classifying the diabetic into one of several categories with hyperglycemia as a clinical finding is critical in developing a patient-specific treatment regimen. In the past, patients with diabetes have been classified in numerous ways, including: degree of glucose tolerance; age of onset (juvenile or adult); body weight; degree of hyperglycemia, glucosuria, or both; susceptibility to ketoacidosis; insulin dependency; degree of severity and stability;

treatment priority; presence or absence of hypertension; lipid profile variance; and the presence or absence of large and small blood vessel lesions.

A classification of diabetes and other categories of glucose intolerance based on contemporary knowledge of this heterogeneous syndrome was developed by the National Diabetes Data Group in 1980 to assure consistency in treatment (3). Table 17.1 summarizes the new classification system, compares it with old methods, and gives therapy recommended for each classification.

The two major clinical presentations of diabetes are type II maturity-onset and type I juvenile-onset. Eighty percent of diabetics are identified after the age of 35 years and are of the obese, maturity-onset type (4). They retain some pancreatic function and may be controlled by diet, or diet plus an oral hypoglycemic agent. Insulin may be required in 20 to 30% of cases, although these patients rarely develop ketoacidosis (4). Many type II diabetics have normal or high levels of insulin, and it is possible that sluggish insulin secretion in response to glucose and a relative tissue resistance to insulin because of a low number of insulin receptors may be responsible for the symptoms.

Ten percent of type II diabetics are stable, non-obese, maturity-onset types; while 5% have brittle, adult-onset diabetes that more closely resembles the juvenile-onset presentation. Insulin-dependent (type I) diabetes accounts for only 15 to 20% of diabetes cases (4). These patients have no pancreatic function and require insulin to sustain life. The blood glucose levels of type I diabetics may fluctuate widely despite treatment, and they are more prone to ketosis than are the type II diabetics. Table 17.2 compares the distinguishing features of the two major clinical types of diabetes.

PREVALENCE

Diabetes mellitus and its complications are now the third leading cause of death in the United States, accounting for 300,000 lives each year (5). Almost 6% of Americans may have diabetes, and the incidence is increasing by 600,000 new cases yearly or at a rate of approximately 6%. Seven to 8% of hospital admissions are due to diabetes. A new diabetic is diagnosed every 60 seconds, and the chance of developing diabetes doubles with every 20% excess weight and every decade of life.

Table 17.1.
Classification and Therapy of Diabetes

Current Terminology	Others	Diet	Exercise	Insulin	Oral Hypoglycemic	Education
Type I: insulin-dependent diabetes mellitus (IDDM)	Juvenile onset (JOD) Youth onset (YOD) Ketosis prone Brittle	1. Regular meal schedule 2. Restrict "simple sugars" 3. No restriction of total carbohydrate (i.e., 50–60% of total calories) 4. Limited fats (i.e., 22% of total calories) 5. Avoid fad diets 6. Increase fiber	Yes	Yes	No	Yes
Type II: non-insulin-dependent diabetes mellitus (NIDDM) A. Obese B. Normal weight	Adult onset (AOD) Maturity onset (MOD) Ketosis resistant	Obese: 1. Hypocaloric intake 2. Limit fats Nonobese: 1. Eucaloric intake 2. Restrict "simple sugars" 3. Limit fats 4. Increase fiber 5. Beware of "dietetic"	Yes	Not usually	Individualize	Yes
Diabetes associated with other conditions Secondary diabetes	Hyperglycemia secondary to pancreatic disease, endocrine disease, drug or chemicals, certain genetic syndromes	Change if underlying condition necessitates	Yes	Adjust to correct hyperglycemia	Individualize	Yes
Gestational diabetes (GDM)	Gestational diabetes	1. Avoid simple sugars 2. Avoid excessive weight gain	Yes	Use to tightly control diabetes	No	Yes
Impaired glucose tolerance (IGT)	Asymptomatic diabetes Chemical diabetes Borderline diabetes Latent diabetes	Avoid extra calories; hypocaloric intake if overweight, or usual diabetic diet	Yes	Not usually	No	No

Table 17.2.
Distinguishing Features of Two Major Types of Diabetes Mellitus

	Insulin-Dependent Type I (IDDM)	Non-Insulin-Dependent Type II (NIDDM)
Age of onset	Usually, but not always, during childhood or puberty	Frequently over 35
Type of onset	Abrupt	Usually gradual
Prevalence	0.5%	5–6%
Incidence	<10–15%	>75%
Family history of diabetes	Infrequently positive	Commonly positive
Primary cause	Pancreatic β cell deficiency	End organ (insulin receptors) unresponsiveness to insulin action
Nutritional status at time of onset	Usually undernourished	Usually obese
Postglucose plasma or serum insulin[a]	Absent	>100 μU/ml at 2 hr
Symptoms	Polydipsia, polyphagia, and polyuria	Maybe none
Heptomegaly	Rather common	Uncommon
Stability	Blood sugar fluctuates widely in response to small changes in insulin dose, exercise, and infection	Blood sugar fluctuations are less marked
Etiology	Unknown; possible factors include *Inheritance:* associated with specific HLA tissue types, but only 40–50% concordance in twins *Autoimmune disease:* 50–80% circulating islet cell antibodies *Viral infections:* Coxsackie, mumps, influenza	Unknown; possible factors include *Inheritance:* 95–100% concordance in twins, but not associated with specific HLA tissue types *Autoimmune disease:* negative <10% circulating islet cell antibodies No evidence for viral infections
Proneness to ketosis	Frequent, especially if treatment program is insufficient in food and/or insulin	Uncommon except in the presence of unusual stress or moderate to severe sepsis
Insulin defect	Defect in secretion; secretion is impaired early in disease; secretion may be totally absent late in disease	*Insulin deficiency:* most patients show failure of insulin secretion to keep pace with inordinate demands engendered by obesity; may appear initially as failure to respond to glucose alone, suggesting an impairment in the glucoreceptor of the pancreatic β cell *Insulin resistance:* some patients have a defect in tissue responsiveness to insulin and evidence of hyperinsulinemia; in such patients, insulin resistance may be mediated by decreased number of insulin receptors in target cells
Plasma insulin (endogenous)	Negligible to zero	Plasma insulin response may be either adequate but delayed, so that postprandial hypoglycemia may be present when diabetes is discovered, or diminished but not absent
Vascular complications of diabetes and degenerative changes	Infrequent until diabetes has been present for >5 years	Frequent
Usual causes of death	Degenerative complications in target organs (e.g., renal failure due to diabetic nephropathy)	Accelerated atherosclerosis (e.g., myocardial infarction); to lesser extent, microangiopathic changes in target tissues (e.g., renal failure)
Diet	Mandatory in all patients	If diet is utilized fully, hypoglycemic drug therapy may not be needed
Insulin	Necessary for all patients	Necessary for 20–30% of patients
Oral agents	Rarely efficacious	Efficacious

[a] Normal response is between 50 and 135 μU ml at 60 min and less than 100 μU ml at 120 min after 100 g of oral glucose.

Diabetes is the leading cause of new cases of blindness; diabetics are 25 times more prone to blindness than non-diabetics. Diabetics are 17 times more prone to kidney disease, and approximately half of insulin-dependent diabetics will succumb to end-stage renal disease (ESRD) (5). Diabetes is the leading cause of ESRD requiring chronic hemodialysis and renal transplantations. Microangiopathy (small blood vessel disease) occurs prematurely and progresses at an accelerated rate in patients with diabetes (responsible for 75% of deaths of non-insulin-dependent diabetics). Diabetics are twice as prone to heart disease and stroke as nondiabetics and are 25 times more prone to developing gangrene. Diabetes is the leading cause of nontraumatic amputations in the U.S. Up to 50%

of men with diabetes of long duration are sexually impotent.

The economic cost of diabetes is greater than $14 billion annually and is growing. The average diabetic generated costs of $3200 in 1984 (6). More than a billion dollars are expended for diabetics with renal problems annually. The economic costs for insulin-dependent diabetics are approximately 13% higher than for type II diabetics.

ETIOLOGY

Numerous factors have been associated with the development of diabetes. Table 17.3 summarizes some of the factors that have been linked to the development of diabetes. Understanding of the etiology of diabetes is far from complete.

One factor that seems to be common to all types of diabetics is stress. Emotional and physiologic stress may contribute as precipitating factors in the development of diabetes. With this in mind it is interesting to note that more initial presentations of the disease are observed in North America during the winter months.

Type I diabetics have a defect in pancreatic B cell function, which may be attributed to several causes. Genetic defects in production of certain macromolecules may interfere with proper insulin synthesis, packaging, or release, or the B cells may not recognize glucose signals or replicate normally. Extrinsic factors that affect B cell function include damage caused by viruses such as mumps or Coxsackie B4, by destructive cytotoxins and antibodies released by sensitized lymphocytes, or by autodigestion in the course of an inflammatory disorder involving the adjacent exocrine pancreas.

Genetic susceptibility to insulin-dependent diabetes appears to be linked to two genes on chromosome 6. These genes control the production of human lymphocyte antigens (HLA) DR3, and DR4 (4, 7). Individuals with either or both of these antigens have a greater chance of developing diabetes than the individual without the antigen/s.

Table 17.3.
Etiologic Factors Associated with Diabetes Mellitus

Obesity
Increasing age
Heredity
Emotional stress
Autoimmune B cell damage
Endocrine diseases; e.g., Cushing's disease
Viral stress decreasing B cells
Vasculitis in tissue highly perfused with capillaries (eye, kidney, etc.)
Insulin receptor defects
Drugs (e.g., cortisone, estrogen, thyroid, phenytoin, diazoxide, thiazide diuretics)
Post insulin-receptor defects

Ninety-five percent of patients with type I diabetes have one or both of these antigens. However, 40% of patients without diabetes possess one or both of these antigens.

The reaction of these predisposed individuals to certain environmental stimuli (B cell cytotoxic virus or chemicals) is abnormal and leads to B cell destruction either directly through autoimmune mechanisms or because of lack of regeneration of the B cell after damage (7). The above hypothesis is being studied vigorously. Someday perhaps individuals susceptible to diabetes can be identified and preventive steps taken.

Many type II diabetics secrete excess insulin and are obese. The hyperinsulinism and insulin-resistance may be correlated with a decrease in insulin receptors. Studies have also shown that the tissues of type II patients exhibit reduced insulin binding. A reduced number of insulin receptors and the problem of insulin binding are major factors in the etiology of non-insulin-dependent diabetes (8).

Blood glucose levels can be elevated by a variety of mechanisms. Some diabetic patients may have elevated blood glucose because of an excess of glucagon. Others have a defect in somatostatin or an excess of growth hormone, cortisol, epinephrine, or other hormones that influence the regulation of blood glucose. Numerous drugs have been implicated in increasing blood glucose levels, including chlorthalidone, corticosteroids, diazoxide, phenytoin, glucagon, caffeine, cyclophosphamide, lithium, epinephrine and other catecholamines, estrogens, ethacrynic acid, furosemide, lithium, nicotinic acid, thiazide diuretics, thyroid preparations, and sugar-containing medications (9). Other drugs may cause lower-than-normal blood glucose levels, including anabolic steroids, sulfonylureas, disopyramide, ethanol, fenfluramine, monoamine oxidase inhibitors, propranolol, and large doses of salicylates (9).

In summary, an individual's blood glucose level can be elevated via numerous mechanisms. There can be a decrease in the amount of insulin produced or released, a defect in the ability to sense glucose and respond by releasing insulin, or a genetic mutation in the structure of insulin. Insulin antibodies can reduce the effectiveness of insulin. There can be decreased insulin receptor affinity, as well as a decrease in the actual number of receptors, a post-insulin-receptor defect, and many hormones and chemicals can affect blood glucose levels.

PATHOPHYSIOLOGY AND SYMPTOMS

A great deal must be learned about the specific cellular biochemical mechanisms that are involved in the pathophysiology of diabetes. However, the consequences of a lack of insulin or a lack of effect of insulin are well known. The sequelae of high blood glucose levels may be subcategorized into acute and chronic effects. Symptoms and consequences differ between type I and type II diabetes. The complex cellular effects of insulin provide numerous clues to the type of intervention that should be made to improve the prognosis of a diabetic patient.

NORMAL INSULIN PRODUCTION AND EFFECTS

Insulin is a polypeptide composed of 51 amino acids in two chains (A and B) connected by two disulfide bonds. Insulin is synthesized and stored in the β-cells of the islets of Langerhans, located in the pancreas. The pancreas produces a parent protein called preproinsulin. Preproinsulin is cleaved to form a smaller protein, proinsulin. Proinsulin is cleaved to form equimolar amounts of C-peptide and insulin (4). The normal human pancreas contains approximately 200 units of insulin. A basal amount of insulin is secreted continuously at a rate of approximately 0.5 to 1.0 units/hr. Insulin is also released in response to blood glucose levels of 100 mg/dl or more. The average daily insulin secretory rate in the adult is 25 to 50 units per day. Insulin is cleared metabolically by the liver, peripheral tissues, and the kidney. Insulin follows first-order elimination kinetics. The serum half-life of insulin is approximately 4 to 5 min.

The important metabolic sites that are sensitive to insulin include the liver, where glycogen is synthesized, stored, and broken down; skeletal muscle, where glucose oxidation produces energy; and adipose tissue, where glucose may be converted to fatty acids, glyceryl phosphate, and triglycerides. Insulin affects the metabolism of carbohydrates, protein, and lipids (10).

CARBOHYDRATE METABOLISM

In the nondiabetic, insulin in concert with glucagon, somatostatin, growth hormone, corticosteroids, epinephrine, and parasympathetic intervention maintains the blood glucose between 40 and 160 mg/dl at all times. At least three types of cells have been identified in the islets of Langerhans of the normal human pancreas. The α-cells produce glucagon, which acts to increase blood glucose levels. The β-cells are responsible for producing, storing, and releasing insulin. The δ-cells produce a tetradecapeptide called somatostatin. Somatostatin inhibits both insulin and glucagon secretion and suppresses growth hormone (10). Its primary effect is to suppress glucagon, which results in a fall in blood glucose levels. Unfortunately, this effect persists for only 60 to 120 min.

These three cell types work together to maintain control of glucose. Ingestion of a carbohydrate in a nondiabetic results in a prompt increase in the amount of insulin released into the blood. At the same time, there is a decrease in plasma glucagon. Glucagon is released in response to low blood glucose levels and the ingestion of protein. The release of glucagon stimulates insulin secretion, and insulin in turn inhibits the release of glucagon.

The presence of insulin favors the uptake and utilization of glucose by insulin-sensitive sites. In the skeletal muscle, glucose uptake and subsequent energy production is increased. In the liver, glucose uptake and the formation of glycogen is increased in the presence of insulin.

A minimum blood glucose level of 40 mg/dl is required to provide adequate fuel for the brain, which can use only glucose as an energy source and does not depend upon insulin for its utilization. Glucose spills into the urine, resulting in energy and water loss, when blood glucose levels exceed the renal threshold of the kidneys (180 mg/dl) in persons with normal renal function.

PROTEIN METABOLISM

The presence of insulin favors the production of structural proteins from constituent amino acids. When glucose is present intracellularly in sufficient quantities for needed energy production, most structural proteins will retain their integrity. In the absence of insulin, the production of structural proteins is not favored and intracellular glucose levels cannot match energy demands. To produce energy, skeletal muscle will convert its structural proteins to constituent amino acids. The liberated amino acids are transported to the liver where they are converted to glucose via gluconeogenesis. Hepatic glucose enters the blood but is not taken up by needed tissue because of an insulin deficiency. Thus, hyperglycemia is escalated and structural proteins are wasted.

FAT METABOLISM

The presence of insulin favors the production of triglycerides from free fatty acids. When insulin deficiency causes an energy deficit, free fatty acids are liberated from storage as triglycerides. The free fatty acids are oxidized to form β-hydroxybutyric acid, acetoacetic acid, and acetone. β-Hydroxybutyric acid may be used as an energy source, but in the absence of insulin the production of these keto acids will eventually be greater than their metabolism and excretion. If insulin is not given to the patient, metabolic ketoacidosis will ensue. The keto acids will cause the pH to decline, and the diuresis secondary to the elimination of ketones and glucose will cause dehydration. The body's neutralizing factors will eventually be depleted, and the patient will deteriorate to coma and possibly death. Figure 17.1 shows the clinical manifestations in an untreated type I diabetic who is insulinopenic.

METABOLISM IN TYPE II PATIENTS

In type II diabetics, the problem is not a lack of insulin, but the insulin is not effective (11). Usually glucose utilization is sufficient to avoid ketoacidosis. However, glucose does accumulate in the blood and can reach very high levels, resulting in a syndrome called diabetic nonketotic hyperosmolar coma. Both ketoacidosis and hyperosmolar coma are treated by first determining the cause of the

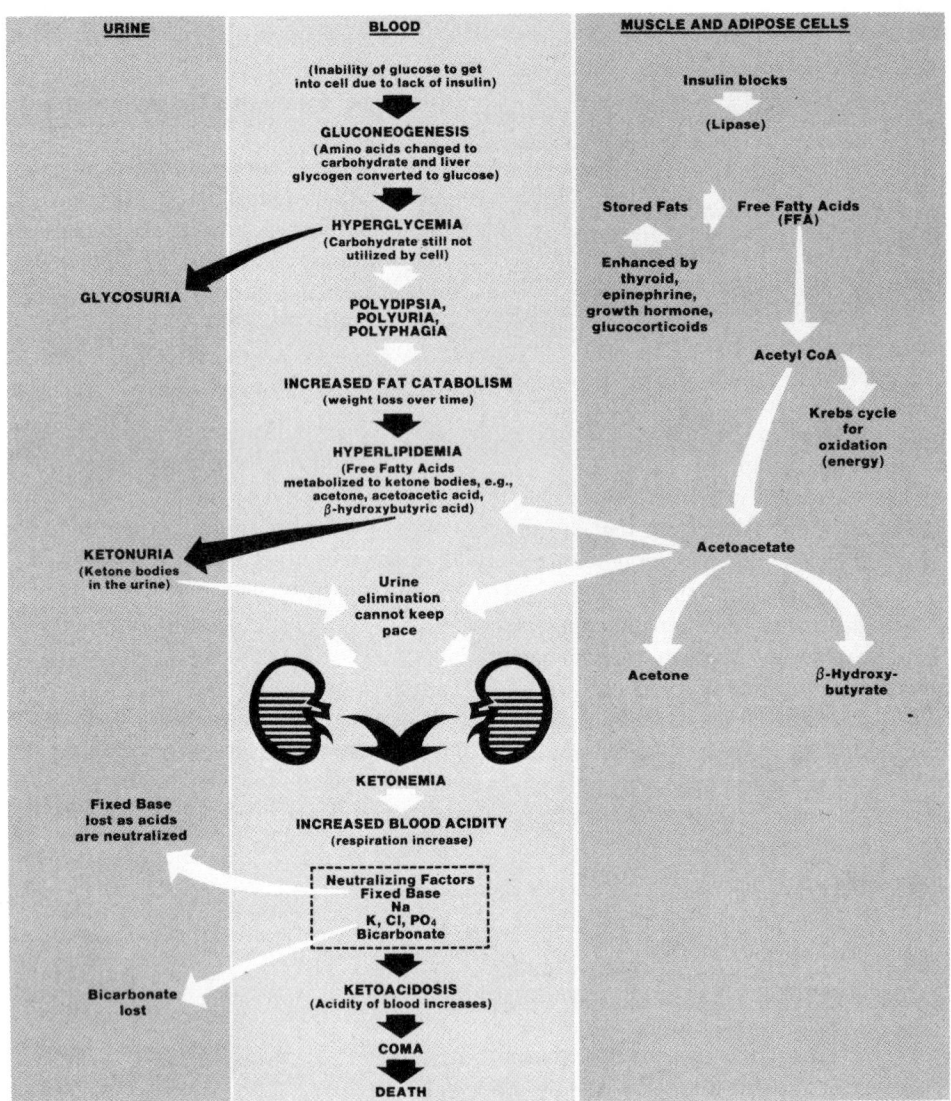

Figure 17.1. Clinical manifestations of a complete lack of insulin.

problem, then giving fluids and electrolytes and low doses of insulin either intravenously or intramuscularly. Close monitoring of electrolytes, pH, acid-base balance and glucose levels is required to avoid complications.

In summary, in the "fed" state, a high insulin level is necessary for incorporation of glucose into liver and muscle glycogen; for muscle to consume glucose for energy needs; for both liver and adipose tissue to make fatty acids from glucose; for amino acids to be incorporated into muscle protein; for circulating chylomicrons to discharge their fatty acids into adipose tissue; and for these in turn to be reesterified and incorporated into the triglyceride storage droplet in the middle of the cell (10). Thus, in patients who are insulinopenic (type I), the acute problems affect fat, protein, and carbohydrate metabolism, resulting in high blood glucose and ketone levels. In patients who have ineffective insulin (type II), enough insulin gets into cells

to meet the patient's energy requirements, but glucose accumulates in the blood, causing hyperglycemia with relatively minor acute symptoms.

To complicate the picture even further, many other factors cause an increase in blood glucose, including Cushing's disease, pheochromocytoma, aldosteronism, hyperthyroidism, pancreatitis, cirrhosis, pregnancy, emotional stress, infections, and miscellaneous drugs (mentioned earlier). Many factors can decrease blood glucose levels, such as an exogenous insulin excess, nonfasting reactive hypoglycemia, fasting hypoglycemia, and several medications (12).

SYMPTOMS

Type I diabetes typically presents with the usual signs of polyuria, polyphagia, polydipsia, weakness, weight loss, dry skin, and often ketoacidosis (30% of all cases of diabetic ketoacidosis occurs in previously undiagnosed patients) (13). Type II diabetes frequently has no symptoms and is often discovered when glucose is discovered in the urine or when elevated blood sugar levels are noticed during a routine examination. Careful study of these older, obese diabetics sometimes reveals glucosuria, proteinuria, postprandial hyperglycemia, microaneurysms, and even retinal exudates.

Other symptoms of hyperglycemia associated with diabetes include blurred vision, tingling, numbness in the feet, slow-healing skin infections, itching, drowsiness, and irritability. Patients with the above symptoms and those with a family history of diabetes or who are overweight and in the 40- to 65-year-old age group, should be screened closely for hyperglycemia. Monilial infections of the vagina and anus and a history of complications during pregnancy are warning signs to test for diabetes. The earlier diabetes is diagnosed, the more easily it can be brought under control and the better the long-term prognosis.

LONG-TERM EFFECTS OF HYPERGLYCEMIA

Diabetics often develop kidney failure (nephropathy), lesions of the eye (retinopathy), and atrophy of the peripheral nerves (neuropathy). Generally, these processes occur because the walls of the capillaries that supply these tissues with blood and nutrients thicken. The molecular mechanisms leading to these late complications of diabetes have not been established conclusively (14, 15). Over the years there has been considerable debate on whether the lesions that develop within the diabetic's retina, kidneys, nerves, and vascular system are due to a disorder in the structure and function of blood vessels or whether they are a consequence of prolonged hyperglycemia caused by inadequate metabolic control. Few diabetologists believe that microvascular complications occur independently of hyperglycemia and insulin deficiency or that glycemic control is not a factor. A long-term, multicentered study to review this premise is currently under way at 21 centers in the U.S. and Canada. The study is known as the Diabetes Control and Complications Trial (DCCT) and is being conducted in four phases. Diabetic retinopathy is the primary outcome being assessed, with secondary outcomes including neuropathy, nephropathy, and neurobehavioral and cardiovascular complications. This study and others will hopefully resolve this debate. Substantial evidence supports the concept that the microvascular complications of diabetes are decreased by reduction in blood glucose concentrations (14, 15). Because of these findings there is a renewed emphasis on strict, but reasonable, control to prevent severe chronic diabetic complications. Patients are being taught to normalize their blood glucose levels through multiple injections of insulins or the use of insulin infusion pumps in conjunction with self-blood-glucose monitoring and a strict diet and exercise program. The

Table 17.4.
Harmful Effects of Hyperglycemia

Increased capillary basement membrane thickening
Glucose metabolized via polyol pathway, increased sorbitol
Faulty lipid metabolism, atherosclerosis
Abnormal minor (glycosylated) hemoglobins
Impairment of phagocytosis (ability to fight infection)
Increased platelet adhesiveness
Red blood cell inflexibility
Increased neonatal morbidity and mortality

acute effects of hyperglycemia are summarized in Table 17.4.

Data on the link between hyperglycemia and chronic complications are being evaluated. It is generally agreed that the better the glycemic control, the more promising the long-term outcome. However, a small percentage of patients may be relatively resistant to long-term complications, even with poor glycemic control, while another small subgroup may suffer multiple chronic complications while being treated intensively. Table 17.5 summarizes the complications of diabetes mellitus and the treatment recommendations for each complication.

Major advances have been made in the treatment of some specific complications of diabetes. Retinopathy can be successfully treated by laser photocoagulation. If the patient suffers a retinal vitreous hemorrhage, surgical vitrectomy can help restore the patient's vision (16). Strict blood glucose control before and during pregnancy has greatly reduced the incidence of perinatal mortality in infants of diabetic mothers (11). Neuropathies and diabetic cataracts improve with strict glycemic control and have also recently been treated experimentally with aldose reductase inhibitors. Two such agents, sorbinil and tolrestat, are currently in clinical trials. Furthermore, diabetic impotency can be treated surgically by inserting a penile prostheses (17) or use of new ErectAid-type devices. Training the diabetic to monitor foot care and treat any foot problems vigorously can reduce the incidence of gangrene in the extremities. Tight metabolic control can also reduce the thickness of basement membranes and improve the lipid blood levels in diabetic patients. Diabetics who normalize their blood glucose and glycosylated hemoglobin levels have a decreased frequency of severe infections (11).

Type I diabetic patients are predisposed to the development of diabetic nephropathy. The basement membrane of the capillaries in the glomerulus thickens and progresses to a nodular pattern (Kimmelstiel-Wilson syndrome). Nephropathy usually occurs in diabetics 10 to 15 years after diagnosis. Proteinuria is the first clinical manifestation with progression to hypertension, azotemia, hypoalbuminemia, and edema. Treatment is initiated to control the complications of nephropathy, and dialysis or transplantation may be necessary for patients who have

Table 17.5.
Complications of Diabetes Mellitus and Their Treatment

Body Location	Description	Treatment
Eyes	Retinopathy, cataract formation, glaucoma, and periodic visual disturbances; leading cause of new blindness	Strict control of blood glucose to avoid need for treatment via laser photocoagulation, vitrectomy
Mouth	Gingivitis, increased incidence of dental cavities and periodontal disease	Strict control and daily hygiene, see dentist, floss, brush, and Water-Pik often
Reproductive system (pregnancy)	Increased incidence of large babies, stillbirths, miscarriages, neonatal deaths, and congenital defects	Strict control before and during pregnancy
Nervous system	Motor, sensory and autonomic neuropathy leading to impotency, neurogenic bladder, parathesias, gangrene	Strict control, daily foot care, surgery, tricyclic antidepressants and phenothiazines
Vascular system	Large vessel disease and microangiopathy	Strict blood glucose control, artery bypass surgery
Skin	Numerous infections and specific lesions due to small vessel disease, increased lipids in blood, and pruritus	Strict control, daily hygiene
Kidneys	Diabetic glomerulosclerosis causing nephropathy	Strict control, eventually diet low in proteins, prednisone, dialysis and renal transplantation
Reticuloendothelial system (infections)	Diabetics have a higher incidence of cystitis, tuberculosis, skin infections; more difficult time overcoming infections, moniliasis common in diabetic women	Strict control and aggressive antiinfective therapy

progressive renal disease. Strict blood glucose control is necessary to reduce, or possibly prevent, pathological changes caused by hyperglycemia. Angiotensin-converting enzyme (ACE) inhibitors have been evaluated for use in the prevention and treatment of diabetic nephropathy. Currently it appears that ACE inhibitors may be more useful in the prevention of diabetic nephropathy than in its treatment. Additionally, other antihypertensives such as the calcium-channel blockers may be as effective as the ACE inhibitors (18).

Because of the high incidence of gangrene in diabetic patients, foot care is a major topic in the educational process of diabetes. This complication results from a combination of factors including atherosclerosis, decreased pain sensation due to neuropathy, decreased responsiveness of leukocytes, and trauma. The reduced blood flow results in ischemic tissue changes. The diabetic, due to neuropathy, does not detect areas of injury or infection, and the progression to gangrene can be rapid. Diabetics should thus be instructed to monitor foot care on a daily basis, never go barefoot, strictly control their blood glucose, and avoid trauma to the feet by properly cutting toenails and selecting shoes that fit properly (12).

DIAGNOSTIC TESTS

Most currently used diagnostic tests measure an individual's ability to handle a glucose load. Type I diabetics are usually easy to diagnose because they have all the classic symptoms of diabetes and high amounts of glucose in the urine and blood. Type II diabetics are more of a challenge because they often do not have the classic symptoms. Furthermore, many of these patients are borderline, and tests do not give a clear indication whether or not the patient is a diabetic. Table 17.6 summarizes the criteria developed by the National Diabetes Data Group and adopted by the American Diabetes Association. These criteria are now

Table 17.6.
Criteria for Diagnosis of Diabetes and Impaired Glucose Tolerance

1. Diabetes—adult
   a. Unequivocal elevation of plasma glucose level and classic symptoms (polyuria, polydipsia, weight loss)
   b. Fasting plasma glucose (FPG) 7.8 mmol/liter (140 mg/dl) on more than one occasion
   c. Oral glucose tolerance test (OGTT) with FPG 7.8 mmol/liter (140 mg/dl), 2-hr PG 11.1 mmol/liter (200 mg/dl), one intervening PG 11.1 mmol/liter (200 mg/dl)
2. Diabetes—children
   a. Plasma glucose 11.1 mmol/liter (200 mg/dl) with classic symptoms
   b. OGTT (1.75 g glucose/kg body weight up to maximum of 75 g) with FPG 7.8 mmol/liter (140 mg/dl), 2-hr PG 11.1 mmol/liter (200 mg/dl), one intervening PG 11.1 mmol/liter (200 mg/dl)
3. Gestational diabetes
   Two or more of the following plasma glucose concentrations exceeded with a 100-g glucose dose: FPG 5.8 mmol/liter (105 mg/dl); 1-hr postdose 10.5 mmol/liter (190 mg/dl); 2-hr postdose 9.2 mmol/liter (165 mg/dl); 3-hr postdose 8.0 mmol/liter (145 mg/dl)
4. Impaired glucose tolerance
   OGTT with FPG 7.8 mmol/liter (140 mg/dl), 2-hr PG 7.8 mmol/liter (140 mg/dl) and 11.1 mmol/liter (200 mg/dl), one intervening value 11.1 mmol/liter (200 mg/dl)
5. Normal glucose values—nonpregnant adults OGTT with FPG 6.4 mmol/liter (115 mg/dl), 2-hr PG 7.8 mmol/liter (140 mg/dl), intervening PG 11.1 mmol/liter (200 mg/dl)

recommended for use in the diagnosis of diabetes and impaired glucose tolerance.

Oral Glucose Tolerance Test (OGTT)

This diagnostic test measures a person's ability to handle a glucose load over a period of time, and although controversial, it is a quite reliable test for diabetes. Following an overnight fast, a sample is drawn for a morning fasting blood sugar determination, and a 75-g glucose load is ingested by the patient, followed by blood samples drawn at ½ hr intervals for 2 hr, and a 3 hr (19). Urine samples are often taken at the same time and tested for glucose to estimate the renal threshold for glucose. In normal subjects the blood glucose returns to normal in less than 2 hours. In diabetics, the glucose peak is higher, occurs much later, and declines at a slower rate. A normal OGTT result occurs when the fasting plasma glucose is less than 6.4 mmol/liter (115 mg/dl), the 2-hr plasma glucose is less than 7.8 mmol/liter (140 mg/dl), and the intervening glucose values are below 11.1 mmol/liter (200 mg/dl). Because of the criterion that accepts the random or fasting glucose levels as diagnostic, many clinicians have questioned the need for this test. Several other factors including infections, stress, pregnancy, metabolic abnormalities and certain drugs can impair glucose tolerance and produce abnormal results. One should screen for these factors when using the OGTT.

Fasting Plasma Glucose (FPG)

Various blood or plasma tests for glucose are used in establishing the diagnosis of diabetes. The simplest test is the FPG which uses blood drawn from the patient (usually after an overnight fast). A normal fasting plasma glucose result depends upon the particular laboratory, but it is usually set between 3.6 mmol/liter (65 mg/dl) and 6.1 mmol/liter (110 mg/dl). The diagnosis of diabetes may be confirmed in the patient with two or more fasting plasma glucose levels that are elevated above 7.8 mmol/liter (140 mg/dl). However, a normal fasting plasma glucose does not rule out diabetes. This test is used in nonpregnant adult patients who are neither receiving drugs nor have other diseases that could be responsible for the abnormal results (19).

2-Hour Postprandial (2HPP) Blood Glucose

The 2HPP is used as a screening test. A sample is drawn for a blood glucose level determination 2 hours after a 100-g glucose load. In nondiabetics, blood glucose levels return to normal in less than 2 hours following a glucose challenge, whereas hyperglycemia persists in a diabetic. Although this test is often used to evaluate diabetes control, it can be manipulated easily by the diabetic patient.

Note that each of the blood glucose tests can be manipulated by diabetic patients that improve their blood glucose control several days before the test. Furthermore, blood glucose test results may be elevated by emotional stress, physical exertion, and stimulants such as tobacco and caffeine. Other causes of elevated blood glucose levels include acute stress such as fever, trauma, major operations, myocardial infarctions, or cerebral vascular accident (12). Chronic illness that causes prolonged physical inactivity, starvation and malnutrition can result in abnormally low fasting blood glucose levels. Potassium depletion from any cause can result in fasting hyperglycemia (12). Another cause of pseudohyperglycemia is chronic renal disease with uremia. Do not label a patient as diabetic unless it is certain that the disease exists. A false diagnosis leads to personal frustrations, including insurance "riders," driver's license limitations in some states, and possible limitations in employment opportunities (12). Pharmacists monitoring elderly patients should realize that tolerance to glucose decreases with age. Some elderly patients are labeled as diabetics and placed on medications that are probably unnecessary.

Glycosylated Hemoglobin (Hemoglobin A_{1c})

Glycosylation of hemoglobin is a postsynthesis, nonenzymatic chemical reaction between glucose and phosphorylated sugar (glucose-6-phosphate) and the N-terminal valine of the β chain of the hemoglobin molecule (4). Since hemoglobin is exposed to the ambient glucose concentration in the blood, a higher concentration of glucose results in more glycohemoglobin formation. This hemoglobin becomes an important index of the long-term control of diabetes and may be a more reliable index than the degree of hyperglycemia or glucosuria. In the nondiabetic, glycosylated hemoglobin is between 3 and 8% of all hemoglobin, whereas in patients with poorly controlled diabetes it may range between 8 and 20%. Glycohemoglobin is a clinically useful gauge of glycemic control. Glycohemoglobin concentration correlates with the level of glycemic control for the previous 60 days, or when the red blood cells are about half-way through their 120-day cycle. The major subcategory of the glycohemoglobins is hemoglobin A_{1c}. Some laboratories test specifically for hemoglobin A_{1c}, while others test for all glycosylated hemoglobins. It is important to know which test a laboratory is using and what their specific normal range is. Many recent studies have shown that when a relatively uncontrolled diabetics bring their blood glucose levels under strict control, there is a dramatic improvement in glycosylated hemoglobins (4, 20). Studies are in progress to determine whether long-term hemoglobin A_{1c} values will correlate positively with diabetic microangiopathy. This test may be particularly useful for patients with poor compliance in record-keeping or those who make an extra effort to achieve acceptable plasma glucose levels only at the time of physician visits. The test can be taken at any time and is not affected by recent meals or physical activities. It is not a test done frequently, but rather 2 to 3 times a year. Some clinicians are studying this test for use as a screening or diagnostic test. Additional tests are being evaluated to determine if specific glycoproteins such as glycoalbumin correlate well with diabetes control.

Self-monitoring of Blood Glucose

Since 1980, there has been a trend to teach diabetic patients to self-monitor blood glucose. This procedure has received increasing medical acceptance, and annual sales of glucose-monitoring products have grown rapidly. This movement is continuing to gain momentum and may soon result in blood glucose monitoring by all patients with diabetes. The objective of diabetes treatment is to achieve blood glucose levels as close to normal as possible through a program of education, diet, exercise, and medications. Achieving the objective requires active and routine patient involvement.

Besides the possibility of decreasing complications, strict blood glucose control can also decrease depression and avoid some of the problems inherent in urine testing. Urine tests are inconvenient, messy and affected by a wide variety of medications, and they do not reflect the current blood glucose levels because of differences in patients' renal thresholds and residual urine left in the bladder (20).

Self-monitoring of blood glucose is feasible, practical, and acceptable to patients. It allows the patient to better understand the factors that affect blood glucose levels; gives an accurate reflection of the blood glucose after exercise, before and after meals, and when the patient is placed on medications or is ill; helps the patient better understand diabetes and the objectives of therapy; assists in detecting and therefore avoiding hypoglycemia; helps the patient understand the symptoms of hypo- and hyperglycemia; improves the relationship between the healthcare professional and the patient; and helps the patient to become a more active, intelligent participant in managing diabetes.

The disadvantages of self-monitoring glucose, which include the increased expense and the annoyance of obtaining a drop of blood, are greatly outweighed by the many advantages. Several devices are now available to help the patient obtain a drop of blood easily and almost painlessly (21).

Several methods of determining blood glucose levels are available to diabetic patients. Selection of a specific product should be made on the basis of cost, ability to perform the test accurately, accuracy of the method, flexibility of the system (is a meter required?), convenience to the patient, and motivation of the patient to achieve strict control. Since maintenance of blood sugar control is impossible without measurement and since it is convenient and less costly for the patient to self-monitor, self-monitoring of blood glucose levels is highly recommended for all types of diabetic patients. Pregnant diabetics, patients with altered or shifting renal thresholds, labile patients who have difficulty bringing their diabetes under control, patients with frequent hypoglycemia, those who have difficulty using a urine test, and those who prefer monitoring their own blood glucose levels are all excellent candidates for self-monitoring blood glucose. Blood glucose monitoring is a necessity for patients who are using continuous subcutaneous insulin infusion.

Most of the tests available for use by patients involves the glucose oxidase/peroxidase reaction to detect the glucose. Some of the tests use a reflectance photometer to read the strip and give a digital readout of the blood glucose values. Other methods have a color reaction on the strip which is compared to a chart on the side of the bottle. A relatively new meter, the Direct 30/30 Glucose Sensor (CPI/Lilly), does not require the use of test strips.

Chemstrip bG and Glucostix test strips, some of the most commonly used strips, provide a manual readout or may be used in combination with a glucose meter. The meters are calibrated in various manners and ranges. Some of the meters can evaluate glucose concentrations as high as 333 mmol/liter (600 mg/100 ml). A drop of blood is applied to the test strip for 30 to 90 seconds, depending upon the strip, which is wiped off and inserted into the meter for the reading. Accurate timing is essential to the success of these systems. Since each system is different, it is important to make sure that the patient understands the specific characteristics of the system that has been prescribed.

The visually read strips are less expensive and very portable. The meter-read monitoring of blood glucose gives a more accurate determination of blood glucose concentration. Both systems greatly improve the patient's ability to understand the factors that affect blood glucose levels and therefore improve blood glucose control.

Urine Tests

Patient-performed tests are available for the evaluation of urine glucose, urine ketones, and urine protein.

Glucosuria is observed with many conditions (e.g., pregnancy or impaired renal function) and is not a persistent finding in diabetes. It does occur when the mean blood glucose level is 10 mmol/liter (180 mg/dl) or higher, but rarely when the level is below 7.2 mmol/liter (130 mg/dl). The major exception occurs when the renal threshold for glucose is increased by age; therefore older diabetics may "spill" no glucose at all despite a high blood glucose level. Thus one of the major disadvantages of using urine testing to monitor diabetes is the fact that renal thresholds for glucose differ from patient to patient. Also, residual urine is left in the bladder, even when the patient double-voids. This means that any urine test could be affected by the blood glucose levels for the previous 2 to 3 hours.

Even though blood glucose monitoring by patients is gaining momentum, many relatively stable diabetics must continue to use urine tests to monitor their diabetes. The two types of tests available are the glucose oxidase method (Tes-Tape, Clinistix, and Diastix, Chemstrip uG and uGK), which is specific for glucose, and the copper reduction method (Clinitest), which may be affected by reducing substances in the urine (22). Many people use urine tests to augment the information from self-read glucose mon-

Table 17.7.
Substances That May Cause False-Positive Glucosuria by Copper Reduction Method

	Nalidixic acid
Ascorbic acid (large quantities)	p-Aminosalicylic acid
Cephalothin, other cephalosporins	Penicillin (massive doses)
Chloral hydrate	Probenecid
Isoniazid	Salicylates
L-Dopa	Streptomycin
Metaxalone	Sugars (galactose, lactose,
Methyldopa	fructose)

itoring—usually achieving better control than would have been possible with either method alone.

The glucose oxidase method is specific for glucose and the simplest to perform, but it is not the best method for monitoring insulin therapy because it is qualitative. Figures appear on many of the product labels, but glucose oxidase tests are quantitative only when the amount of glucose in the urine is less than 0.25%. Larger amounts (2, 3 and 4%) were misinterpreted as 0.5% or less in 502 out of 804 tests (23). This high rate of error makes control of hyperglycemia difficult. Diastix is the only glucose oxidase product that makes quantitative claims; however, false low readings are common with high concentrations of glucose (greater than 1.5%) or moderate to large amounts of ketones. For this reason, difficult-to-control diabetics should be on a self-monitoring blood glucose program. Ascorbic acid in high doses (1 to 2 g) interferes with the glucose oxidase test, resulting in a false-negative reading. Other false-negative results have been reported in the presence of methyldopa, levodopa, and high levels of ketones. These reactions are less common than the ascorbic acid reactions. Switching to a copper reduction test eliminates this problem.

Some cautionary notes apply to the copper reduction method. Whether double voiding should be a requirement for urine testing is being questioned (24). The Clinitest tablet generates its own heat and anaerobic environment by the production of foam. The test tube should not be agitated during the reaction. Also, the patient should observe the reaction while it is occurring, since a very high glucose content results in the so-called pass-through phenomenon, which is a fleeting bright-orange color that appears during "boiling" and fades to a greenish-brown when the reaction stops. This color may be interpreted falsely as 0.75 to 1%, when there is actually more than 2% glucose in the urine. The pass-through phenomenon can be eliminated by using 2 drops of urine instead of 5 drops. Patients using Clinitest who spill more than 2% glucose should also test their urine for acetone. Many drugs cause a false-positive result with the copper reduction test (22) (Table 17.7). Clinitest tablets disintegrate in the presence of mois-

ture and light, so they should not be stored in the bathroom. The tablets change from a normal speckled robin's egg blue to white with splotches of dark blue when exposed to moisture and light. Clinitest tablest are poisonous and caustic; the lid should be kept on tight, and the bottle kept out of the reach of small children. Should ingestion occur, vomiting should *not* be induced.

Labile patients should not use urine tests and should be encouraged to self-monitor for blood glucose instead. More stable patients can test their urine from 1 to 4 times per day. Some very stable patients need to test only 2 to 3 times a week. At the first sign of stress, infection, or change in control, the patient should be encouraged to test the urine or blood more often.

Available urine ketone tests include Acetest, Chemstrip K, Ketostix, and others. Urine ketone testing should be encouraged for the diabetic patient during acute illness, stress, or when blood glucose levels are not well controlled.

Lastly, urine tests are available for the evaluation of urine proteins. Constant routine monitoring of urine protein is usually not warranted. Urine protein tests are used primarily as a screening tool for diabetic nephropathy. Diabetic patients who test negative with standard dipstick methods may be further evaluated with an in-office microalbumin screening test (Micro-bumintest), or by 24-hr urine collections analyzed via RIA. These methods are much more sensitive than the standard dipstick method. Patients who have had type I diabetes for more than 5 years should be screened annually, while patients with type II diabetes should be screened annually from the time of diagnosis (25).

GENERAL PRINCIPLES IN THE TREATMENT OF DIABETES

The treatment objectives for diabetics are summarized in Table 17.8. In achieving the objectives, one must remember that diabetes is a heterogeneous condition and that

Table 17.8.
Treatment Objectives for Diabetes Mellitus

Normalize glucose metabolism
    Normalize glycosylated hemoglobin
    Urine glucose and ketones negative
    Fasting blood glucose: 3.9–8.3 mmol/liter (70–150 mg/dl)
    2-Hr postprandial glucose level less than 10 mmol/liter (180 mg/dl)
    Urinary excretion of glucose less than 5% in 24 hr
Avoid symptoms of diabetes mellitus
Avoid frequent hypoglycemia
Normalize nutrition and achieve ideal body weight
Achieve normal growth and development
Minimize or prevent complications
Accept diabetes with a realistic but positive attitude
Enjoy normal and flexible lifestyle
Promote emotional well-being; have patient take charge of condition

there is tremendous variance among patients. The treatment protocol must be individualized and can be developed only after the type of diabetes has been categorized. In general, glucose metabolism is normalized in diabetic patients who achieve excellent control. There is very strong evidence to suggest that excellent control does decrease the severity of the complications and very possibly postpones their onset. Excellent control will significantly improve the quality of life by producing a relative degree of healthiness. The most challenging diabetic patients to control are the type I insulin-dependent diabetics who have wide daily fluctuations of blood glucose.

Achieving these objectives combines a program of weight loss and diet with an individualized exercise program and the use of medications, either insulin for the type I diabetic or possibly insulin or oral agents for the type II diabetic. Diet, exercise, and medications are greatly enhanced by a program of education and weight reduction.

Education

The *Guidelines for Diabetes Care* (26) published by the American Diabetes Association contains a summary of specific guidelines for education of individuals with diabetes in both acute care and ambulatory care facilities. It specifically lists the steps that should be followed in teaching diabetic patients to care for themselves. Diabetics spend 365 days a year caring for themselves and monitoring the results of their efforts. Thus each diabetic must understand diabetes and be taught to follow the specific steps necessary to care for the condition and to evaluate whether or not the treatment protocol is achieving its objectives.

The educational process requires a health team that includes a physician, a nurse, a dietitian, a pharmacist, and possibly a social worker and exercise physiologist. The diabetic must be continually educated and should participate with other diabetic patients. This can be achieved by active involvement in the Juvenile Diabetes Foundation or the American Diabetes Association local affiliate. The educational process must be well organized and assesses each individual patient's needs. Patients must be evaluated periodically for their competence in performing urine or blood tests, mixing and injecting insulin, rotating injection sites, using the diet exchange system, and following an exercise prescription. Table 17.9 lists some statistics that show a strong need for diabetic patient education (5) Basically, education for a diabetic should be broken down into a least three areas:

1. Initial management of the diabetes provides information necessary to bring the patient under control and gives the patient some time to adjust to the condition. This level of education is based upon the limitations of the individual and family in accepting and/or assimilating all they must know about diabetes at the time of diagnosis and the limitations of some settings in providing additional education.

Table 17.9.
Need for Patient Education

3 of 5 patients make errors in insulin measurement
65–90% of patients have major deficits in selecting and using foods according to prescribed diet
Less than 10% of diabetics were following a "minimally adequate regimen"
35% of patients lack any formal training
17% were placed on insulin without instructions
50% who had been trained could not demonstrate skills in any of the major areas of self-care

2. Home management of diabetes emphasizes increasing knowledge and flexibility as some experience is gained in living with diabetes. This level is essential for every individual, but it must be tailored to each person's needs and capacity. It is offered preferably in a nonhospital, as-close-to-home-as-possible environment.
3. Improvement of lifestyle is the third area in which educational guidelines should be developed. It deals with advanced learning and is viewed as enriching the individual's life with flexibility, insight, and self-determination. Many diabetics are forced to discover this information by trial and error.

At each level of education information is provided about nutrition, medication, self-monitoring, what to do with hypoglycemia, how to handle hyperglycemic episodes and illness, what activities should be practiced on a daily basis, specific steps in developing good hygiene, and a routine schedule. Assessing psychological adjustment is a method of determining whether or not the patient is accepting the educational process.

Exercise

Although exercise is nearly always recommended by physicians as part of the treatment of diabetes, it is seldom prescribed. Now more physicians understand the improvement that exercise brings to the control of diabetes, and programs are being developed to specifically prescribe exercise treatment on a daily basis for diabetic patients (27, 28). Exercise does improve insulin sensitivity, or the ability of insulin to be used to drive glucose into the cell. Exercise lowers blood glucose by allowing glucose to penetrate the muscle cell and be metabolized without the assistance of insulin. Glucose may be used to varying extents without insulin in all types of cells. Exercise improves circulatory function, an important factor in diabetic management. Exercise also helps maintain normal body weight and aids in breathing, digestion, and metabolism. An exercise log may help the patient maintain a regular daily schedule. Patients who monitor their own blood glucose become motivated to exercise because they see the beneficial effects of exercise on maintaining good blood sugar and control.

An exercise program should be prescribed for both

type I and type II diabetics. Diabetics should be evaluated before the exercise prescription is determined. The person's health, interests, and motivation should be considered in developing a specific method of exercising. If blood glucose levels are above 16.6 mmol/liter (300 mg/dl), exercise can result in an excessive rise in counterregulatory hormones, with inadequate insulin availability, these hormones can cause decreased muscle glucose uptake and increased liver glucose production that actually causes blood glucose levels to increase further. Type I diabetics should know their blood glucose level before beginning exercise. If the blood glucose level is under 16.6 mmol/liter (300 mg/dl), injected insulin that has been absorbed subcutaneously can possibly be absorbed more rapidly, resulting in excessive insulin, which in combination with the exercise, can cause a serious drop in blood glucose. Diabetic patients over 40 years of age and those who have had diabetes for more than 25 years should have an exercise stress test and then have an individualized graded exercise program prescribed. Diabetics with peripheral sensory neuropathy and/or vascular insufficiency should avoid exercise that may cause trauma to the feet (e.g., jogging). Diabetics with proliferative diabetic retinopathy should avoid strenuous exercise that might induce hemorrhage. Another problem is preventing hypoglycemia during exercise. Hypoglycemia can be prevented by ingesting additional carbohydrates before exercise begins (approximately 15 g 30 min before exercising). Patients should also inject insulin at a nonexercise site (e.g., in the abdomen if they are going to be running. Patients should log their exercise and monitor its effect on their blood glucose control; this encourages regular exercising. If hypoglycemia occurs repeatedly during regularly scheduled exercise, it may require a decrease in the insulin dose. Patients should be warned to wear an identification bracelet or necklace when exercising, in case they do become hypoglycemic. Diabetics should also carry a quick source of sugar when exercising, in case of an insulin reaction.

Diet

Diet is the cornerstone of treatment of both type I and type II diabetics. It is the first line of treatment in type II diabetics, and in combination with exercise and insulin, is a necessary component of treatment regimens for type I diabetics. Table 7.10 provides a quick overview of diabetes diet therapy.

Patients should be taught to read labels carefully, because many sugarless and dietetic products actually contain a large number of calories and are not effective in helping the diabetic patient achieve or maintain an ideal body weight. Diabetics should also avoid quick-acting simple sugars because they cause a rapid rise in blood glucose levels. The new guidelines from the American Diabetes Association Task Force on Nutrition do state that a pru-

Table 17.10.
Diabetes Diet Therapy

Diet compliance is critical
Avoid fad diets and prolonged fasting
Note that "dietetic" does not equal "diabetic," read labels carefully
Avoid quick-acting (simple) sugars
Decrease consumption of animal (saturated) fats
Control calories, attempt to achieve an ideal body weight
Increase amount of fiber in the diet
Try to avoid alcohol
Avoid smoking
Take vitamin-mineral supplements
Understand and use the diabetic diet system & the glycemic index

dent amount of simple sugar may be ingested. Ingestion of animal (saturated) fats should be minimized because of the increased incidence of atherosclerotic disease in diabetic patients. The main factor in diabetes diet therapy is to control calories. Some excellent studies have shown the importance of increasing fiber in the diet of diabetics. However, patients must see how they respond to the various types of fibers. Some of the fibers that have a high degree of pectin can cause constipation, while other fiber products, because of their bulk, can cause flatulence and diarrhea (29). To achieve the objectives of diet therapy, the patient must spend some time with a dietitian to work out specifically the number of calories to be ingested each day and the percentage of those calories that should be carbohydrates, fat, and protein. Patients must learn the relatively simple "diabetic diet exchange system." The diet exchange system allows patients to have a large variety of foods, and if the patient follows the diet, weight can be lost and ideal body weight can be achieved. Remember, about 80% of diabetic patients are of the obese, non-insulin-dependent type. If weight loss can be achieved in this group, often the diabetes will disappear. Table 17.11 gives dietary recommendations for type I and type II diabetics (30). Diet therapy in type II diabetics has a high degree of failure and often creates feelings of frustration, pessimism, failure, and anger, which in turn result in poorly informed and inadequately motivated patients. The failure rate can also cause frustration and a negative attitude on the part of the physician who treats the patient. Successful diet programs require behavior modification on the part of the patient. Patients should be encouraged to join groups such as Weight Watchers and to keep a diet log similar to an exercise log. For a period of 4 to 10 days patients should record each time they eat, how much they eat and why they eat—whether food ingested was due to social pressure, loneliness, depression, nervousness, or the time of day, or whether the patient truly needed nourishment. If patients use smaller plates, take only one helping of food, and are conscious of why they eat, it is possible to change their dietary behavior. Diet support groups can be of assistance in modifying behavior (19).

Table 17.11.
Dietary Strategies for Two Types of Patients with Diabetes

Strategy	Obese, Non-Insulin-Dependent	Nonobese, Insulin-Dependent
Decrease calories	Yes	No
Protect or improve pancreatic β cell function	Very urgent priority	Seldom important because β cells are usually extinct
Increase frequency and number of feedings	Usually no	Yes
Maintain day-to-day consistency of intake of calories	Not crucial if average caloric intake remains in low range	Desirable
Maintain day-to-day consistency of ratios of carbohydrates, protein, and fat for each of the feedings	Not crucial	Desirable
Time meals consistently	Not crucial	Very important
Allow extra food for unusual exercise	Not usually appropriate	Usually appropriate
Use food to treat, abort, or prevent hypoglycemia	Yes	Important
During complicating illness, provide small frequent feedings or give carbohydrate intravenously to prevent starvation ketosis	Often not necessary because of resistance to ketosis	Important

One reason for diet therapy failure in diabetics is that physicians or dietitians prescribe changes in diet without first adjusting the dose of insulin or oral agents. The first step in diet therapy should be to prescribe an exercise program, lower the medication dose, and put the patient on a diet containing fewer calories. Insulin overtreatment is probably one of the most common causes of inadequate diabetic control and weight gain. In one group of diabetic patients, 75% needed a reduction in insulin dose of at least 10%; 35% of the overtreated patients had large appetites, and 30% had hepatomegaly and headaches (28). Diabetic patients should learn to determine whether or not they have involved themselves in a vicious cycle of taking too much insulin and then eating up to that level of insulin. Note also that type II diabetic patients have too much insulin to begin with, and even after eating a large meal they will still feel hungry, possibly because of their excess insulin levels.

Alcohol Use in the Diabetic

In general, alcohol use is discouraged in diabetic patients, but each individual diabetic should be assessed to determine if the advantages of alcohol (e.g., reducing emotional tension, relieving anxiety, and stimulating appetite) outweigh the potential effects on blood glucose control.

Either hyper- or hypoglycemia may develop in diabetics who ingest alcohol. Hypoglycemia is the most common effect. The hypoglycemic effect of alcohol is believed to be due to either increased early endogenous insulin response to glucose or to inhibition of hepatic gluconeogenesis. Relatively small quantities of alcohol (48 ml of 100-proof) may cause this effect. Thus, if a diabetic patient is fasting and consumes alcohol, hypoglycemia may be severe, leading to coma or death. If the person has adequate amounts of glucose in the blood, then alcohol has a less serious effect.

Patients who consume alcoholic beverages must consider the caloric content of the beverage and should be encouraged to choose "light" drinks over standard brews. The sugar content of wines and mixed drinks must also be considered. Alcohol in combination with sugar in a patient who is fed can add to the hyperglycemic state.

The additive hypoglycemic effects of alcohol and insulin have produced severe hypoglycemia resulting in coma, brain damage, and even death. Tolbutamide and chlorpropamide have been reported to interact with alcohol, resulting in a "disulfiram-like" reaction. An advantage of the 2nd generation sulfonylureas is that they do not cause a disulfiram reaction when taken with alcohol.

Patients who do choose to consume ethanol should be counseled to do so only in small quantities (1 to 2 oz/day), slowly, and in combination with food.

MEDICATIONS IN THE TREATMENT OF DIABETES MELLITUS

The medications used to treat diabetes can be categorized into two broad areas: oral hypoglycemic agents and insulin. The oral agents are effective only in type II (non-insulin-dependent) diabetics. Insulin is used for all type I diabetics and in approximately 30% of type II diabetics. Insulin is also used in all diabetics during times of stress, such as infection, surgery, ketoacidosis, or hyperosmolar coma.

Sulfonylureas

Drug therapy should not be considered for the patient with mild, well-tolerated type II diabetes until after treatment with diet for an appropriate length of time (3 to 4 months).

If diet therapy fails, then a trial of sulfonylureas is indicated. Before 1970, when the University Group Diabetes Program (UGDP) published its very controversial report, most non-insulin-dependent diabetics were placed on sulfonylureas. The UGDP was a prospective study initiated in 1961 to evaluate the effectiveness of antidiabetic therapy in preventing vascular and late complications of diabetes. Eight hundred patients from 12 different diabetic clinics were included in the study. These newly diagnosed type II diabetics who should have been treated with diet alone were assigned at random to one of five treatment programs; tolbutamide in fixed doses of 1.5 g, placebo or diet alone, insulin in a fixed dose, insulin in variable doses, and phenformin. The study was interrupted because of an unexpected higher incidence of cardiovascular deaths in the tolbutamide and phenformin-treated groups. Controversy surrounding the study is still not settled, and many emotional editorials have appeared in the literature about the faults of the study and the conclusions that were made. Even though subsequent studies failed to substantiate the findings of the UGDP (31, 32), the oral hypoglycemic agents were less frequently used until the late seventies, and currently the FDA still requires that tolbutamide package inserts contain reference to "an increased risk of cardiovascular mortality." In 1984 two, new, more potent agents were approved for use in the United States. The marketing of these products stimulated the use of oral antidiabetic agents. Currently, oral hypoglycemic agents account for approximately 1% of all prescriptions written in the United States (33). Seventy-five percent of this market is controlled by three agents, glyburide, glipizide, and chlorpropamide. It is estimated that 40% of all type II patients are treated with oral hypoglycemic agents.

Sulfonylureas have demonstrated both pancreatic and extrapancreatic effects, but are useful only in patients with intact viable β-cells (type II patients) (34, 35). In the absence of other secretagogues, sulfonylureas in vitro directly stimulate the release of insulin. In vivo sulfonylureas sensitize β-cells to glucose, increasing insulin secretion indirectly. Additionally, glucagon release from the pancreas is inhibited by sulfonylureas. Sulfonylureas may affect glucose levels by several extrapancreatic mechanisms such as increasing insulin receptor binding affinity, increasing insulin's effect by a postreceptor action, and decreasing hepatic insulin extraction. The relative clinical importance of each of these mechanisms is still a subject of research and debate.

The following patient characteristics are sometimes predictive of a positive clinical response to sulfonylureas:

1. Patients who are not diagnosed as diabetics until after the age of 40;
2. Duration of diabetes less than 5 years;
3. Patients who are close to their ideal body weight;
4. No prior insulin treatment, or control of disease with less than 40 units per day;
5. Fasting blood glucose <10 mmol/liter (180 mg/dl).

After a firm diagnosis of diabetes (by the oral glucose tolerance test) has been made, diet has been given an adequate trial, and the criteria for the use of oral hypoglycemics have been met, an appropriate drug can be selected. The products that are available in the United States are summarized in Table 17.12. Efficacy, potency, and toxicity are major factors to consider in the selection of a drug. The differences in metabolism of each sulfonylurea account for clinical differences in the onset, duration of action, and sometimes side effects. Tolbutamide and chlorpropamide are the oldest drugs and are therefore the best studied. Long-term studies of these agents indicate a primary failure rate of from 3 to 30%, an overall success rate of 20%, and an incidence of adverse effects less than 5%. In general, the incidence of adverse effects reported for chlorpropamide is higher than that for the other products—approximately 9% for chlorpropamide versus 1 to 3% for tolbutamide. The severity of many of these side effects can be correlated with differences in the half-life, metabolism, and excretion, of the drugs. Note that chlorpropamide has the longest half-life and also has the highest incidence of side effects of a serious nature. For this reason, some clinicans favor tolbutamide because of its short half-life and lesser toxicity. The side effects of sulfonylureas are summarized in Table 17.13. Patient counseling guidelines for the sulfonylureas are summarized in Table 17.14.

The sulfonylureas that are metabolized to inactive or weakly active metabolites (i.e., tolbutamide, tolazamide, glipizide, and glyburide) are safer for patients with renal failure. The most common side effect of the sulfonylureas is hypoglycemia. Glyburide and glipizide, the second-generation agents, have been marketed with specific claims differentiating them from the previously marketed first-generation products. The substitution on the aryl-sulfonylurea nucleus are large nonpolar groups. This results in a marked increase in the hypoglycemic activity. The second-generation drugs are 50 to 100 times more potent on a weight basis. Glyburide and glipizide also produce fewer drug interactions from protein binding displacement than do first-generation agents, because they are present physiologically at much lower concentrations than their first-generation counterparts and because they bind nonionically. Frequent drug-drug interactions in first-generation drugs result in enhanced hypogycemia and occur with alcohol, anabolic steroids, β-adrenergic blocking agents, dicoumarol, monoamine oxidase inhibitors, phenylbutazone, salicylates, and sulfonamides (9). Drugs that may interfere with diabetes control by causing hyperglycemia include asparaginase, clonidine, corticosteroids, diazoxide, estro-

Table 17.12.
Biopharmaceutics and Pharmacokinetics of the Oral Hypoglycemic Agents

Drug	Total Daily Dose (mg)	Doses/Day	Half-Life (hr)	Dosage Forms (mg)	Onset of Action (hr)	Duration (hr)	Metabolism and Excretion	Comments
Tolbutamide (Orinase)	500–3000	2–3	5–6	250, 500	1	6–12	Hepatic metabolism to hydroxy- and carboxytolbutamide which are weakly active and inactive, respectively; metabolites are excreted via kidneys	Most benign, least potent, short t1/2, good choice in renal failure
Acetohexamide (Dymelor)	250–1500	1–2	5	250, 500	1	12–18	Metabolized to hydroxyhexamide (greater activity than parent compound) and inactive metabolites; metabolites excreted via kidney	Avoid in patients with renal failure; significant uricosuric effects
Tolazamide (Tolinase)	100–1000	1–2	7	100, 250, 500	4–6	16–24	Multiple metabolites; hydroxytolazamide moderately active, other metabolites inactive; metabolites excreted via kidney	Absorbed slowly, possible choice in patients with renal failure
Chloropropamide (Diabenense)	100–500	1	35	100, 250	1	24–72	80% metabolized to weakly active and inactive metabolites excreted via kidney, 20% of parent compound excreted unchanged	Antabuse-like reaction, highest incidence of hypoglycemia; avoid in elderly and in patients with renal failure
Glyburide (Diabeta, Micronase)	1.25–20	1–2	3–5	1.25, 2.5, 5.0	1.5	18–24	Metabolized to moderately active and inactive metabolites; metabolites excreted 50% via fecal route, 50% via renal route	Potent agent, dose should be divided if >10 mg/day; may require dosage adjustment if Clcr is <30 ml/min
Glipizide (Glucotrol)	2.5–40	1–2	3–7	5.0, 10.0	1	16–24	Metabolized to inactive compounds excreted via renal (88%) and fecal (12%) routes	Potent agent, dose should be divided if >15 mg/day; good choice in renal failure patients; patients should be instructed to take on an empty stomach

° 30A (Gerich)

Table 7.13.
Side Effects of Sulfonylureas

GI: less than 5%—take with meals (except glipizide)
Skin: less than 2%
Antabuse effect: approximately 4%, especially with chlorpropamide
Hepatotoxicity: rare, greater than 500 mg Diabinese daily
Hematological: Very rare—cause and effect is questionable
SIADH: 4% with chlorpropamide (if on a diuretic, incidence increases)—
    does not occur with 2nd-generation drugs
Hypoglycemia: especially in elderly and patients with renal insufficiency

Table 17.14.
What the Pharmacist Should Tell the Diabetic Taking Sulfonylureas

Name, purpose, directions for use
Can be taken with food (except glipizide)
Take regularly, exactly as physician prescribed
Contact M.D. if fever, sore throat, or mouth lesions
Exercise caution when using alcohol
Use drug in conjunction with diet
Use of other drugs should be physician or pharmacist approved
Carry sugar source for hypoglycemia

gens, ethacrynic acid, furosemide, glucagon, lithium, niacin (high doses), phenytoin, sympathomimetic amines, and thiazide diuretics (9).

Chlorpropamide causes an increased sensitivity to circulating levels of antidiuretic hormone in approximately 4% of patients. The chlorpropamide-induced inappropriate antidiuretic hormone activity is reversible. Improvement occurs within a week after the medication is discontinued.

Conditions in which the sulfonylureas are usually contraindicated include acidosis, severe infections accompanying diabetic onset, major surgery (during and after), sulfa sensitivity, and pregnancy. Sulfonylureas also are possible teratogens. They should not be used early in pregnancy, and are absolutely contraindicated late in gestation since they may cause prolonged and severe hypoglycemia in the newborn. Approximately 40% of type II diabetics do not achieve satisfactory control with the oral agents. Secondary failures occur in patients who respond initially to oral agents then fail to be adequately controlled. The secondary failure rate ranges from 3 to 30%. The failure rate tends to increase year after year for patients experiencing initial satisfactory control. Patients who fail to respond to the first-generation drugs should be started on one of the second-generation products.

Dosing of Sulfonylureas

Sulfonylurea therapy should be initiated with a low dose of the chosen agent and may be increased weekly on the basis of blood glucose control, urine glucose levels, and symptoms. Use of low doses initially is particularly important in the elderly because their poor eating habits and decreased renal function predispose them to hypoglycemic reactions. Lower doses are given once daily before breakfast, while higher doses are split and given two or more times during the day, depending upon the half-life of the drug.

Doses of any given agent should be pushed to maximal levels before a decision to abandon therapy is made. Increasing the doses above maximum levels results in an increased frequency of adverse effects without producing any further decrease in blood glucose and is not recommended. Treatment with any given agent should continue for 1 month before a change in therapy is warranted. Lack of response to the sulfonylureas after this trial period is called "primary failure." In these patients, either a trial of another oral agent or insulin therapy is indicated. Patients treated with insulin may later be given a trial of oral agents. Patients who do not respond to either insulin or oral agents, or type II patients who are extremely insulin resistant may be treated with a combination of insulin and oral agents.

Insulin

Type I diabetics with absolute insulin deficiency must be treated with exogenous insulin. Generally persons who require insulin initially tend to be under 30 years old, lean, prone to developing ketoacidosis, and markedly hyperglycemic even in the fasting state. Insulin is indicated for type II diabetics who do not respond to diet therapy, either alone or combined with oral hypoglycemic drugs. Occasionally type II diabetics need doses of 10 to 20 units of intermediate-acting insulins to bring hyperglycemia under control. Insulin therapy is also necessary for some type II diabetics who are subjected to the stress of infection, pregnancy, or surgery.

Diabetic children should begin giving their own injections at around age 8 to 9 years, although parents should administer one or two injections per week to stay in practice and should inject into areas difficult for the child to reach. By combining the appropriate diet modification, exercise, and variable mixtures of short- and longer-acting insulins, it has been possible to achieve acceptable but not excellent control of blood glucose. All patients using insulin should be strongly encouraged to self-monitor blood glucose levels.

CHOICE OF INSULINS

Choice of insulin must be governed by such factors as time-action profile, effects of mixing, species, strength and purity (Table 17.15). Several manufacturers of insulin on the United States market offer over 30 different brand names

Table 17.15.
Factors Considered in Comparing Insulins

Kinetic formulation, time-action profile
Species source (human versus pork versus beef)
Strength (U-40 vs. U-100 vs. U-500)
Methods of achieving long action (e.g., protein, such as protamine; Zn
   content)
Purity
Mixability
Cost, manufacture dependability, availability

of insulin. Selection of insulin must be made after consideration of all the mentioned factors. Choice of an insulin product based purely on cost is inappropriate. Table 17.16 summarizes the insulins available in the United States and compares their onsets and durations of action as well as the species source, and strength.

Time-Action Profiles

Insulins may be categorized into three groups, based on their time-action profiles; short-acting, intermediate-acting, and long-acting. While general parameters such as time of onset, time to peak, and duration of action of these various groups of insulin are cited in Figure 17.2, these numbers are only guidelines and should not be substituted for documentation of individual patient response. A number of factors such as species, site of injection, depth of injection, ambient temperature, individual patient characteristics, and exercise may alter the time-action profiles of insulins (Table 17.17).

The short-acting insulins include *semilente*, *regular*, and *regular buffered* insulins (4). Regular and buffered regular insulin formulations are clear and contain solubilized crystalline insulin. Regular insulins are the *only* insulin products that may be administered by the intravenous route, because all other insulin formulations are suspensions. Buffered regular is the insulin of choice for external insulin infusion pumps. It is buffered with diphosphates rather than acetates, which makes the insulin more stable in insulin catheters, preventing crystallization. Semilente is an amorphous precipitate of insulin and zinc in the form of a suspension, with a slightly delayed onset and peak and a longer duration of action than regular insulin.

Intermediate-acting insulins include *NPH* and *lente* insulins. Some clinicians consider human ultralente to be an intermediate-acting formulation since its time-action profile falls between that observed with classic intermediate-acting insulins and the long-acting insulins. NPH (neutral protamine Hagedorn) preparations contain a suspension of zinc-insulin crystals and protamine. Protamine is a protein derived from fish sperm, which causes an allergic response in a small number of patients. Lente insulin is a suspension composed of a 30:70 mixture of semilente and

Table 17.16.
Insulins Available in the United States

Product	Manufacturer	Strength
Short-acting		
Beef		
Iletin II regular	Lilly	U-100
Semilente	Novo Nordisk	U-100
Pork		
Iletin II regular	Lilly	U-100, -500
Regular	Novo Nordisk	U-100
Purified pork regular	Novo Nordisk	U-100
Velosulin	Novo Nordisk	U-100
Beef/Pork		
Iletin I regular	Lilly	U-40, -100
Iletin I semilente	Lilly	U-40, -100
Human		
Humulin regular	Lilly	U-100
Humulin BR	Lilly	U-100
Novolin R	Novo Nordisk	U-100
Velosulin human R	Novo Nordisk	U-100
Intermediate-acting		
Beef		
Iletin II lente	Lilly	U-100
Ilente II NPH	Lilly	U-100
Lente	Novo Nordisk	U-100
NPH	Novo Nordisk	U-100
Pork		
Iletin II lente	Lilly	U-100
Iletin II NPH	Lilly	U-100
Purified pork lente	Novo Nordisk	U-100
Purified pork NPH	Novo Nordisk	U-100
Insulated NPH	Novo Nordisk	U-100
Beef/Pork		
Iletin II NPH	Lilly	U-40, -100
Iletin II lente	Lilly	U-40, -100
Human		
Humulin L (lente)	Lilly	U-100
Humulin N (NPH)	Lilly	U-100
Novolin L (lente)	Novo Nordisk	U-100
Novolin N (NPH)	Novo Nordisk	U-100
Insulatard NPH human	Novo Nordisk	U-100
Long-acting		
Beef		
Ultralente	Novo Nordisk	U-100
Beef/Pork		
Iletin I ultralente	Lilly	U-40, -100
Human		
Humulin U (ultralente)	Lilly	U-100
Fixed combinations		
(all are U-100 insulins)		
		NPH/REG
Pork		
Mixtard	Novo Nordisk	70/30
Human		
Humulin 70/30	Lilly	70/30
Novolin 70/30	Novo Nordisk	70/30
Mixtard human 70/30	Novo Nordisk	70/30

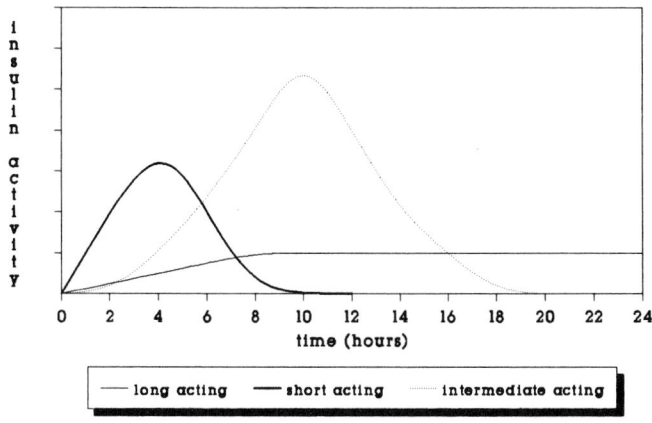

Insulin Time Action Profiles
short vs. intermediate vs. long acting

Insulin Type	onset	peak	duration
Short-acting	.5-1 hr	2-4 hrs	6-8 hrs
Intermediate-acting	1-4 hrs	6-10 hrs	16-24 hrs
Long-acting	4-6 hrs	18 hrs	24-36 hrs

Figure 17.2. Time-activity relationships.

Table 17.17.
Factors Affecting Serum Insulin Concentrations

1. Site of injection—abdominal vs. arm vs. leg vs. thigh
2. Exercise enhances absorption
3. Depth of injection
4. Concentration of insulin—in 40–100 U range—not significant
5. Increase in ambient temperature, increased absorption
6. Massage of site increases absorption
7. Insulin antibodies attract and hold insulin
8. Variance in degrading enzymes at site yields day-to-day variation
9. Insulins react with receptors

ultralente. The lente insulins are produced from various forms of the zinc-insulin complex and are very useful in the patient with a sensitivity to protamine.

The long-acting insulins previously included protamine zinc (PZI) and ultralente insulins. PZI is no longer marketed in the U.S. The long-acting insulins, with the possible exception of human ultralente, are not usually associated with a peak effect but instead provide a sustained, relatively consistent insulin activity.

Strength

In March 1980 the Food and Drug Administration decertified U-80 insulin. Thus at the present time there are two stengths of insulins available for use: U-40 and U-100. U-500 insulin may be special-ordered from Eli Lilly and Company but is available only with a prescription. In foreign countries, patients are required to have a prescription from a physician to get insulin, and U-40 insulin is often the only strength available.

Insulin vials and syringes from some manufacturers are color-coded to decrease errors and aid in the identification of the product. U-40 insulin vials and syringes designed to be used with U-40 insulins are color-coded red; U-100 insulin vials and syringes are color-coded orange with black lettering.

Species Source

The *species source of insulin* can influence the effect of the insulin on blood glucose control and insulin resistance and sensitivity. Commercially available species sources of insulin include beef, pork, beef/pork mixtures, biosynthetic human, and semisynthetic human. Structurally, beef and pork insulin differ from human insulin by three and one amino acids, respectively (4). Degree of antigenicity paralles structural similarity, pork being less antigenic than beef, but more antigenic then human insulin. About 80% of patients with persistent local allergy to mixed beef-pork insulin improve if treated with pure pork insulin or human insulin (4). Initial data indicate that insulin antibody formation occurs at a slower rate in patients receiving synthetic human insulin than in those using purified pork or beef insulin. It is predicted that purified pork insulin will not be of much use in the future, since it costs more than the human insulin and has no advantages over it.

Human insulin is the least antigenic of the available insulins. However, its solubility is greater than the animal-source insulins. This increased solubility results in more rapid absorption and a shorter duration of action. Therefore a patient being switched from one source of insulin to another source of insulin should be monitored very closely.

The two forms of human insulin, biosynthetic–recombant DNA origin and semisynthetic may be therapeutically equivalent, but they are not generically equivalent. Recombinant insulin is produced by the insertion of the

Table 17.18.

Recommendations for Dosing Insulin When Changing from Beef to Human or Conventional to Purified

Highly variable from patient to patient to patient—MONITOR PATIENT CLOSELY

Decrease of 9–20% reported

Recommend 10% dose decrease if normal doses

Recommend 20% decrease if patient receiving more than 50 units/day

Table 17.19.

Patients Who Should Use Human Insulin

Patients with insulin resistance (using more than 100–200 units/day)

Patients with insulin allergy (local cutaneous reactions, rashes, etc.)

Patients with lipoatrophy or lipohypertrophy

All type II diabetics using insulin for a short period of time (e.g., during surgery, infections)

Any patient using insulin intermittantly (e.g., gestational diabetics, TPN patients)

All newly diagnosed type I patients

Pregnant diabetics, antibodies are passed to fetus

human gene for proinsulin into the *Escherichia coli* genome via plasmids. The genetically altered *E. coli* are fermented in a medium conducive to the production of proinsulin. The bacteria are heat killed, the proinsulin is harvested, enzymatically altered to form insulin, and purified. Semisynthetic human insulin is produced by enzymatic transpeptidation of pork insulin at position 30 of the B chain, substituting threonine for alanine.

The recommendations for dosing insulin when changing from beef to pork or from conventional to purified insulin are summarized in Table 17.18. Human insulin is indicated in the patient types listed in Table 17.19. Patients who suffer from insulin allergy (local cutaneous reactions, rashes) should definitely be placed on human insulin. A small percentage of patients are allergic to pork insulin and may be treated with human or purified beef insulin. If the local reactions continue, however, they may be treated by mixing an antihistamine such as diphenhydramine with the insulin before injection. Oftentimes, if the patient continues to use the insulin despite the mild local cutaneous reaction, the patient will become desensitized and the problem will disppear after several weeks. Also, desensitization kits can be obtained from Eli Lilly & Co.

Purity

Another factor that may affect insulin choice is purity. New analytic techniques using chromatography and electrophoresis to separate and isolate protein have made purer forms of insulin readily available. The average content of such minor components of insulin as proinsulin, glucagon, and somatostatin has been decreased, resulting in fewer insulin-sensitivity reactions. All insulins listed in the table are now classified as highly purified insulins, because they have fewer than 10 parts per million of proinsulin. High purification of human insulin is clinically important because it may result in reduced insulin doses, decreased frequency of lipoatrophy (subcutaneous concavities caused by wasting of the lipid tissue), and a decreased insulin antibody titer.

INSULIN DOSING

A number of dosing regimens are used in the administration of insulin (Fig. 17.3). Commonly used methods include

1. Single daily injection of intermediate-acting insulin;
2. Two daily injections of intermediate-acting insulin;
3. Two daily injections of 70/30 intermediate/short-acting, premixed insulin;
4. Two daily injections of split and mixed intermediate and short-acting insulin;
5. Three daily injections of short-acting insulin in combination with a single injection of long-acting insulin;
6. Continuous subcutaneous insulin infusion (insulin infusion pump);
7. Sliding scale (multiple daily injections of short-acting insulin).

Choice of regimen depends on patient and practitioner motivation, the patient's ability to monitor control and adjust doses, and the level of control desired. Initial goals at the time of diagnosis are to eliminate the threat of ketoacidosis, obviate overt signs and symptoms of the disease, replete body mass, and rebalance fluid and electrolyte status. Some practitioners prefer to achieve this goal initially with method 1, while others feel that the psychologic acceptance of two or more injections is greater if introduced soon after diagnosis.

Daily Insulin Requirements. Most patients require between 0.5 and 1.0 units of insulin per kg per day. This total daily dose may be given as one injection (method 1) or may be divided into several doses to more closely mimic physiologic insulin secretion. Premeal doses of insulin are adjusted approximately 1 to 2 units of insulin for each 2.8 mmol/liter (50 mg/dl) of desired fall in blood glucose levels.

Method 1. A single injection of intermediate-acting insulin is not sufficient to control blood glucose levels for a 24-hr period. This regimen usually results in hyperglycemia before the next dose and may cause hypoglycemia that coincides with peak levels about 8 hours after the dose. A dose high enough to cover the patient for 24 hours is usually also high enough to cause hypoglycemia at the peak. This regimen may circumvent ketoacidosis in most patients, but it results in erratic blood glucose swings. Unfortunately, many patients are treated with this regimen. The level of control afforded by this method is minimal. Patients treated with this regimen can be expected to have

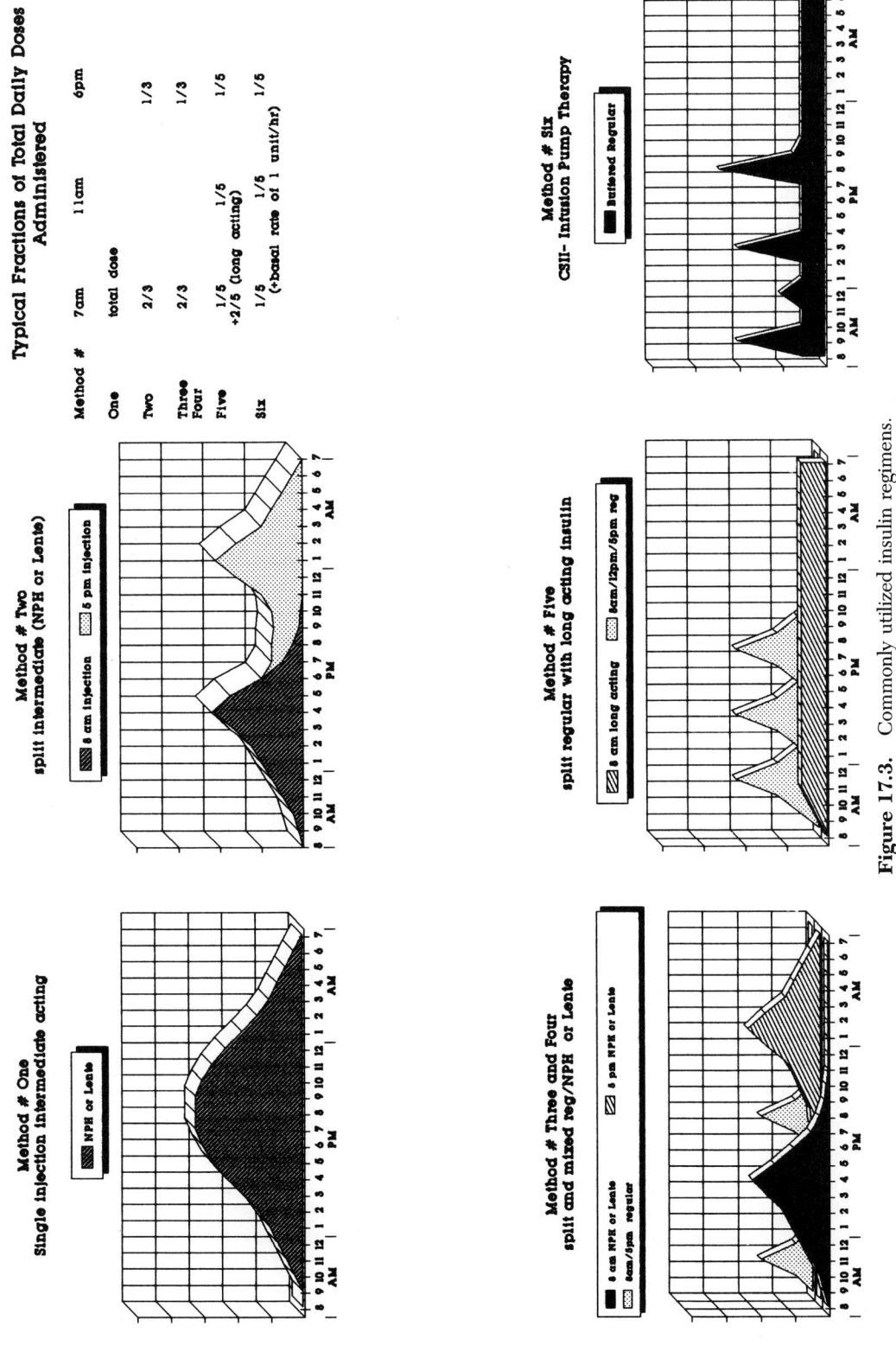

Figure 17.3. Commonly utilized insulin regimens.

HbA$_{1c}$ levels of approximately 11 to 13%, with blood glucose levels commonly above 16.6 mmol/liter (300 mg/dl) and they sometimes complain of symptoms.

Method 2. Glycemic control by method 2 is slightly greater than that with method 1. With method 2, ⅔ the total daily insulin requirements is injected before breakfast, and ⅓ is injected just before the evening meal. Both doses are intermediate-acting formulations. The chance of experiencing hypoglycemia is lower with this method than it is with method 1. The level of control afforded by this method is marginal to average, with HbA$_{1c}$ and blood glucose levels slightly lower than with the above regimen.

Methods 3 and 4. These two methods provide average to above average control with two injections per day. The only difference between them is that with method 3 the patient can increase or decrease the individual doses but cannot alter the ratio of short-acting to intermediate-acting insulin. The patient usually takes ⅔ the total daily dose before breakfast, and ⅓ the total daily dose before the evening meal. The split and mixed regimen is initiated with a 70/30 mixture of intermediate/short acting insulin, but this ratio may be altered according to insulin needs. With these methods, the patient should monitor blood glucose levels before meals and at bedtime, and alter the appropriate insulin dose accordingly. Of the two methods, method 4 is preferred, however method 3 is significantly more effective than methods 1 or 2. A common variation of method 3 is to administer a mixed (intermediate and short-acting) dose before breakfast, a dose of short-acting insulin before the evening meal, and a dose of intermediate-acting insulin at bedtime. Glycemic control expected with this method may range from average to good, with HbA$_{1c}$ levels from 7 to 9%, premeal blood glucose levels from 6.7 to 8.9 mmol/liter (120 to 160 mg/dl), and very little evidence of symptoms.

Method 5. This multidose method uses doses of short-acting insulin before each meal in combination with one or two daily doses of long-acting insulin that provide basal insulin. Variations of this method include the administration of regular insulin before each meal, with a dose of intermediate-acting insulin at bedtime. This regimen requires much patient motivation, but it provides excellent glycemic coverage and allows the patient a great deal of latitude in meals (the patient may increase or decrease the dose of compensate for anticipated meals).

Method 6. Continuous subcutaneous insulin infusion (CSII) is an excellent method of insulin administration. Initially it requires intensive patient training, but the latitude in lifestyle afforded by the pump is unparalleled by other dosage regimens. CSII provides the patient with a continuous basal amount of insulin ($\approx$ 1 unit/hr) in combination with pulsatile doses to cover meals. Pumps currently available are about the size of a deck of cards and weigh only a few onces. Insulin reaches the patient via a

Table 17.20.
Criteria for Selecting Insulin Pump Patients

1. Pregnant diabetics
2. Diabetics with early complications
3. Diabetics who have had a renal transplant
4. Brittle (difficult-to-control) diabetics
5. Motivated type I diabetics
6. At present, type II and children are not being encouraged
7. All patients must be:
   a. Willing and highly motivated
   b. Capable of being educated
   c. Responsible for keeping records and following specific procedures
   d. Willing to perform and log blood tests daily
   e. Willing to be hospitalized for 2–4 days if necessary

small plastic catheter and through a subcutaneous needle. Table 17.20 summarizes the criteria used for selecting insulin pump patients (38). Numerous products are in the developmental stage. The pumps can be compared on the bases of insulin-dilution requirements, size, ease of use, type and completeness of alarm system, supplemental dose features, whether or not they indicate the total amount of insulin given over a 1-day period, and cost. Numerous auxiliary items must be purchased by pump patients. Glycemic control with methods 5 and 6 will in most cases be very good. HbA$_{1c}$ levels may approach normal (6 to 7%), and preprandial blood glucose levels of between 4.4 and 6.7 mmol/liter (80 and 120 mg/dl) may be expected.

Method 7. The sliding-scale method described here is reserved for hospitalized patients who undergo frequent blood glucose monitoring. Insulin dosage adjustments with some of the other methods are based on patient-specific sliding scales. The sliding-scale method may be used for a diabetic patient who is acutely ill and requires more insulin than normal, or it may be used initially after diagnosis to determine daily insulin requirements. Basic sliding scales vary from institution to institution and with various patient responses. The following is an example of a sliding scale using regular insulin for an adult:

(mmol/liter)	Blood Glucose (mg/100 ml)	Subcutaneous Insulin Dose (units)
<7.8	<140	0
7.8–11.1	140–200	2
11.1–16.6	201–300	5
16.6–22.2	301–400	10
>22.2	>400	12

The scale is adjusted, based on patient response to various doses of insulin.

Interpretation of Blood Glucose Levels

Several problems may be encountered with self-monitoring of blood glucose. Proper patient technique and understanding of the individual method should always be ascertained before insulin dose adjustments. Patients being treated with methods 3 through 6 should routinely check blood glucose levels at least four times daily, before meals and at bedtime. Additionally, early morning (3 to 4 AM), and postprandial levels may be checked on a non-routine as-needed basis. Patients who use method 1 should also be taught to check blood glucose levels. However, it is difficult to target particular out-of-range levels, since only one dose is administered daily.

Generally, an increase in insulin dose of 1 unit can be expected to decrease the blood glucose level by approximately 2.8 mmol/liter (50 mg/dl). Some patients adjust doses daily, based on the previous days response. This approach may be reasonable for some, however it is probably more prudent to alter doses only after a trend has been identified.

Several problems have been observed with the interpretation of morning fasting blood glucose levels. The first is called the *dawn phenomenon* (36). This effect results from a rise in blood glucose levels that increases insulin need starting at about 5 AM and continuing until about 9 AM. The early morning glucose rise can be caused by insufficient treatment; but in studies on patients with continuous subcutaneous insulin infusion, the dawn phenomenon still occurred. Food ingestion could influence the early morning rise. Yet in studies of fasting patients, blood glucose levels increased in the early morning. Although the condition is not fully understood and the prevalence of the phenomenon is not known, it is a cause for concern to patients trying to achieve strict control. The most logical explanation for the dawn phenomenon is an increased glucose production or decreased glucose utilization because of the morning rise of cortisol levels and/or other circadian factors.

Another problem requiring dosage adjustments is the *Somogyi phenomenon*, early morning hyperglycemia that is secondary to hypoglycemia. In simpler terms, during sleep, a diabetic patient suffers an episode of hypoglycemia that releases hormones that increase blood glucose levels such as cortisol, glucagon, and epinephrine. These hormones cause blood glucose levels to increase, and when the patient arises in the morning, tests of blood or urine glucose show elevated levels. Since the precipitating problem in the Somogyi phenomenon is hypoglycemia, the necessary step in treatment is to decrease the insulin dose.

The assessment of morning hyperglycemia must include an early morning (3 to 4 AM) blood glucose determination. If hypoglycemia is observed then, the bedtime or evening insulin dose should be decreased. If the level is within normal limits or high, a slight increase in the evening insulin dose is warranted.

MIXING AND STORING INSULIN

Because of improved purity, insulins are more stable and may be stored at room temperature for up to 1 month.

Insulin should be injected at room temperature. If insulin is purchased in bulk, however, the vials that are not in use can be kept in the refrigerator. Insulin should be protected from extreme temperatures, and caution should be exercised by patients traveling in very hot or very cold climates.

The increased use of split and mixed regimens has increased interest in the question of insulin stability in mixtures. Regular and NPH insulin are stable when mixed together in any ratio and is considered the mixture of choice when short- and intermediate-acting insulins are required (37). Premixed NPH and regular is available in Europe in the following ratios: 90:10, 80:20, 70:30, 60:40, and 50:50. Patients should be instructed to adhere to the following sequence when mixing NPH and regular insulin:

1. Inject the appropriate quantity of air into the NPH vial;
2. Inject the appropriate quantity of air into the regular vial;
3. Withdraw the dose of regular;
4. Withdraw the dose of NPH.

Regular and lente (also ultralente) insulin interact when mixed, which blunts the effects of the short-acting insulin (37). Patients should either inject immediately after mixing or consistently inject after a measured period of time. The reaction between lente and regular continues for 24 hours, so the response from an injection taken immediately after mixing may differ significantly from response to an injection taken 24 hours after mixing. Patients may require a higher ratio of lente/regular than would be required with NPH/regular. Velosulin regular and Humulin BR should not be mixed with lente insulins. The phosphate buffers precipitate the zinc from these formulations and increase the activity of short-acting insulin.

Lente insulins may be mixed with each other in any ratio without affecting the time-action profile of the components. These mixtures remain stable up to 18 months.

Regular and PZI insulins are not stable when mixed and should be injected separately.

ADVERSE REACTIONS TO INSULIN

The major complications of insulin therapy (38) are summarized in Table 17.21. These adverse effects may be categorized as immunologically mediated and pharmacologically mediated. Hormones and drugs that influence the insulin requirements are given in Table 17.22.

HYPOGLYCEMIA

A special effort should be made to teach the diabetic patient about the symptoms and treatment of hypoglycemia. Factors predisposing the patient to insulin reactions (hypoglycemia) include insufficient food intake (skipping meals, vomiting, or diarrhea), excessive exercise, inaccurate measurement of insulin, concomitant intake of hypoglycemic drugs, or termination of diabetogenic conditions.

Table 17.21.
Complications of Insulin Therapy

Related to insulin purity and/or species source
  Insulin lipoatrophy
  Insulin allergy (local, 5–10%; systemic less than 1%)
  Insulin antibody formation (100%, including immunologic resistance)
Unrelated to insulin purity and/or species source
  Hypoglycemia (100%)
  Insulin edema
  Insulin lipohypertrophy
  Complications of diabetes secondary to inadequate control by conventional forms of insulin therapy

Table 17.22.
Hormones and Drugs Influencing the Requirements of Insulin

Increasing Requirement	Decreasing Requirement
Cortisol	Tetracycline
Prednisone	Salicylates
Glucagon	Alcohol
Growth hormone	Biguanides
Catecholamines	Sulfonylureas
Thyroxine	Propranolol
Oral contraceptives	
Diuretics	
Phenytoin	

Symptoms include a parasympathetic response (nausea, hunger, or flatulence), diminished cerebral function (confusion, agitation, lethargy, or personality changes), sympathetic responses (tachycardia, sweating, or tremor), coma, and convulsions. Ataxia and blurred vision are also common. In elderly patients with decreased nerve function, diabetics with advanced neuropathy, patients with long-standing diabetes, or patients receiving β-blockers, the symptoms of hypoglycemia are sometimes lacking, and the reaction may go undetected and untreated. All manifestations of hypoglycemia are relieved rapidly by glucose administration. In unconscious patients, injections of glucagon or IV glucose or dextrose may be required.

Because of the potential danger of insulin reactions, the diabetic patient should always carry packets of table sugar or candy for use at the onset of hypoglycemic symptoms. Note also that if a hypoglycemic person is mistakenly thought to be hyperglycemic and given insulin, severe hypoglycemia and subsequent brain damage may result. Thus, when there is doubt about whether a diabetic is hypo- or hyperglycemic, sugar should be given initially until the condition can be evaluated accurately. Spouses or care givers of patients with diabetes should be trained to administer glucagon in the event of hypoglycemia-induced unconsciousness. Glucagon should be administered in a dose of 1 mg given subcutaneously or intramuscularly.

Virtually every patient who is treated with insulin will experience hypoglycemia at some time. Ten percent of insulin-treated patients experience at least one episode of severe hypoglycemia requiring assistance per year. Mortality secondary to hypoglycemia in insulin-treated patients may be as high as 3% (39).

LIPOHYPERTROPHY

Lipohypertrophy is encountered in patients who do not rotate injection sites. With repeated use, a single injection site becomes anesthetized, which encourages the use of that site. These fatty tumorous formations usually resolve after the patient begins to rotate injection sites and use proper injection technique. There is no evidence to suggest that this problem is of immuologic origin, therefore switching to more highly purified products will have little effect.

INSULIN RESISTANCE

Insulin resistance, a state requiring more than 200 units of insulin per day for more than 2 days in the absence of ketoacidosis or acute infection, occurs only in about 0.0001% of diabetic patients. These patients almost invariably have high titers of insulin-neutralizing antibodies or are very obese. These patients should first be switched to a human insulin, and if necessary, placed on glucocorticoids (prednisone in a dose of 5 to 80 mg/day) (4).

LIPOATROPHY

Lipoatrophy, or the wasting away of fatty tissue, appears to be an immunologically mediated phenomenon. The loss of fat is observed more commonly at the injection site, but it may occur distant from it. This adverse effect is more common in females than in males. The treatment of choice for insulin lipoatrophy is human insulin, which should be injected directly into the atrophied area until the site has filled in. After resolution of the problem, the patient should be instructed to continue to inject the area every 2 to 3 weeks to prevent reoccurrence (40).

DIABETIC KETOACIDOSIS

The physiologic events leading to diabetic ketoacidosis (DKA) are described in Figure 17.1. DKA is a life-threatening condition that occurs secondary to an insulin deficit. DKA may occur in diabetic patients who also have an active infection, in diabetic patients who discontinue insulin therapy, or in diabetic patients subjected to other forms of stress (e.g., myocardial infarction, stroke). Twenty to 30% of DKA cases occur in persons previously undiagnosed as diabetics (13).

Signs and symptoms of DKA include polydipsia, polyuria, weakness, fruity breath, dry mucous membranes, tachycardia, and hypotension. Level of consciousness may range from almost normal to frankly comatose. Laboratory signs include elevated serum glucose, creatinine, and blood urea nitrogen levels. Hyponatremia is common, along with glucosuria and ketonuria.

Treatment of DKA consists of insulin, fluids, and electrolytes. Insulin is usually administered initially with a bolus IV dose of between 0.1 and 0.2 units/kg, followed by a continuous infusion of 0.1 unit/kg/hr. Normal saline is administered at a rate of 0.5 to 1 liter/hr until blood pressure and pulse have been stabilized, at which point 0.45% sodium chloride may be substituted. Some practitioners recommend the use of either dextran, or 5% albumin initially in the presence of shock. When blood glucose levels begin to approach normal limits, D5 0.45% sodium choloride may be used. If potassium levels are elevated initially, no potassium should be administered until the level reaches the normal range. Patients with potassium levels within the normal range should be given 10 to 20 mEq/hr; hypokalemic patients may be given much larger doses. Phosphate use in DKA is controversial, but phosphate is usually administered to patients with low levels at a rate of 5 to 10 mmol/hr. Bicarbonate should only be administered to patients with arterial pH levels <7.1, and in doses of 44 mEq c/hr (13, 41).

PROGNOSIS

The outlook for the diabetic patient has never been more positive. More and more government funds are being allocated for diabetes research to better understand the condition and to develop treatments to normalize blood glucose levels and decrease long-term complications. Many states have funds through the Centers for Disease Control to develop diabetes control projects to reduce the morbidity and mortality of diabetes. Much research is also being done on transplantation of pancreas or islet tissues. Much work is being done to develop a miniaturized closed-loop system that could be implanted in diabetic patients to determine their blood glucose levels and automatically inject insulin to maintain blood glucose at a preset level. With the massive amount of work being done in diabetes, it is expected that within 10 years there will either be a device that makes living with diabetes so easy that the patient is virtually unaware of being diabetic, or there will be a surgical transplantation technique that will cure the condition. The new approach to educating patients and giving them responsibility for self-monitoring should also produce positive results and decrease complications, while prolonging the diabetic's life-span and improving the quality of life. The DCCT study project previously noted is underway and appears to have the experimental controls necessary to achieve its goal—a valid, quality assessment of the effect of tight glycemic control on chronic complications. The new oral hypoglycemic agents and human insulins add further potential flexibility to diabetes therapy.

CONCLUSION

Diabetes is a complex, heterogenous disorder that requires a health team effort if treatment objectives are to be achieved. A combination of diet, exercise, medications, and education that results in the patient "taking charge" of the condition, improves the outlook for the diabetic. There is still much information needed if diabetes is to be conquered.

The role of the pharmacist in the treatment of diabetes has been overlooked too long. The pharmacist can have a significant effect in educating the patient and in monitoring the diabetic condition. Pharmacists have a unique opportunity, because of their position in the healthcare system, to have an impact upon the treatment of diabetes. The few pharmacists who have taken an active interest in the diabetic patient have achieved a great deal of positive professional feedback and increased income. One step that pharmacists can take to improve the care of the diabetic is to develop a diabetes care center within a community pharmacy. The pharmacist must become involved in a sincere effort. The pharmacist must communicate with other members of the health team and reinforce the information they provide to the diabetic patient. The pharmacist must also participate actively in diabetes associations; keep up on the various educational methods and programs on diabetes; and become active in the American Association of Diabetes Educators. Last, the pharmacist must carry a complete line of diabetes care products for diabetic patients. The opportunity for pharmacists in the care of diabetes is great, and those who participate will find that the rewards are even greater.

REFERENCES

1. Watkins JD, Robers DE, Williams TF, et al.: Observation of medication errors made by diabetic patients at home. Diabetes 16:883, 1967.
2. Salans LB: Diabetes mellitus, a disease that is coming into focus. JAMA 247:590, 1982.
3. National Diabetes Data Group: Diabetes 28:1039, 1979.
4. Galloway JA, Potvin JH, Shuman CR (eds): Diabetes Mellitus, ed. 9. Indianapolis: Lilly Research Laboratories, 1988.
5. Podolsky S: Clinical Diabetes: Modern Management. New York: Appleton-Century-Crofts, 1980, p 17.
6. Bonheim R: Brother can you spare $14 billion? Diabetes Forecast 38(3):32–35, 1985.
7. Zimmet P, King H, Serjeantson S, Kirk R: The genetics of diabetes mellitus. Aust NZ J Med 16:419–424, 1986.
8. Davidson MB: Review: pathogenesis of type 2 diabetes mellitus: an interpretation of current data. Am J Med Sci 29(7):35–39, 1986.
9. Hansten PD: Drug Interactions, ed 5. Philadelphia: Lea & Febiger, 1985, pp 150–169.
10. Cahill GF Jr, Disorders of carbohydrate metabolism: diabetes mellitus. In Wyngaarden JB, Smith LH Jr: Cecil Textbook of Medicine, ed 16. Philadelphia, WB Saunders, 1982, vol 1, pp 1054–1056.

11. Kaplan SA: Diabetes mellitus. UCLA conference. Ann Intern Med 96:635–649, 1982.

12. Olson OC: Diagnosis and Management of Diabetes Mellitus. Philadelphia: Lea & Febiger, 1981, pp 10–17.

13. Sanson TH, Levine SN: Management of diabetic ketoacidosis. Drugs 38(2):289–300, 1989.

14. Prevention & Treatment of Five Complications of Diabetes: A Guide for Primary Care Practitioners, developed by the National Diabetes Advisory Board, U.S. Dept. of Health and Human Services (HHS83-8392), 1983.

15. Raskin R, Rosenstock J: Blood glucose control and diabetic complications. Ann Intern Med 105:254–263, 1986.

16. Campbell RK, Klein OG: Eye care for the diabetic patient. JAMA 245:2087, 1981.

17. Bohannon NJ, Zilbergeld B, Bullard DG, et al.: Treatable impotence in diabetic patients. West J Med 136:6–10, 1982.

18. Reddi AS, Camerini-Davalos RA: Diabetic nephropathy. Arch Intern Med 150:31–43, 1990.

19. Rifkin H (ed): The Physician's Guide to Type II Diabetes (NIDDM): Diagnosis and Treatment. New York: American Diabetes Association, 1984.

20. Jovanovic L, Peterson CM: The clinical utility of glycosylated hemoglobin. Am J Med 70:331, 1981.

21. Campbell RK: Diabetes and the Pharmacist, ed 2. Elkhart, IN: The Ames Co. 1986.

22. Campbell RK, Diabetes care products. In Handbook of Nonprescription Drugs, ed 8. Washington, D.C.: American Pharmaceutical Association, 1986.

23. Leonards JR: Evaluation of enzyme tests for urinary glucose. JAMA 163:260, 1957.

24. Guthrie DW, Hinnen D, Guthrie RA: Single-voided vs. double-voided urine testing. Diabetes Care 2:269–271, 1979.

25. Roenstock J: Management of early diabetic nephropathy. Drug Ther 12:61–68, 1989.

26. Guidelines for Diabetes Care: American Association of Diabetes Educators, Pitman, N.J./American Diabetes Association, New York, 1981.

27. Brownless, Vlassara H: Exercise and the diabetic patient. Drug Ther 12:66, 1982.

28. Richter EA, Ruderman NB, Schneider SH: Diabetes and exercise. Am J Med 70:201, 1981.

29. Kurtzman P: Role of food fiber in health. US Pharm 7:63, 1982.

30. West KM, Recent trends in dietary management. In Podolsky S: Clinical Diabetes: Modern Management. New York, Appleton-Century-Croft, 1980, p 70.

31. Paasikivi J, Wahlberg F. Preventative tolbutamide treatment and arterial disease in mild hyperglycemia. Diabetologia 7:323–327, 1971.

32. Ohneda A, Maruhama Y, Itabashi H, et al.: Vascular complications and long term administration of oral hypoglycemic agents in patients with diabetes mellitus. Tohoku J Exp Med 124:205–222, 1978.

33. Kennedy DL, Piper JM, Baum C: Trends in use of oral hypoglycemic agents, 1964–1986. Diabetes Care 11:558–62, 1988.

34. Gerich JE: Oral hypoglycemic agents. N Engl J Med 321:1232–1245, 1989.

35. Skillman TG, Feldman JM: The pharmacology of the sulfonylureas. Am J Med 70:361, 1981.

36. Schmidt MI: The dawn phenomenon. Infusion 1:1, 1982.

37. Anderson JH, Campbell RK: Mixing insulins in 1990. The Diabetes Educator 16:380–387, 1990.

38. Galloway JA, DeShazo RD, The clinical use of insulin and the complications of insulin therapy. In Ellenberg M. Rifkin H: Diabetes Mellitus: Theory and Practice, ed 3. Garden City, NY, Medical Exam Publishing, 1982.

39. Gerich JE: Glucose counterregulation and its impact on diabetes mellitus. Diabetes 37:1608–1617, 1988.

40. Valenta LJ, Elias AN: Insulin-induced lipodystrophy in diabetic patients resolved by treatment with human insulin. Ann Intern Med 102:790–791, 1985.

41. Androgue HJ, Barrero J, Ryan J, et al.: Diabetic ketoacidosis: A practical approach. Hosp Pract Feb 15, 1989, pp 83–112.

CHAPTER 18

HYPERLIPIDEMIA

KEVIN M. RODONDI, Pharm.D.

Coronary heart disease (CHD) is one of the leading causes of morbidity and mortality in the United States and other industrialized nations. Three of the treatable risk factors for CHD are hypertension, cigarette smoking, and hypercholesterolemia (1, 2). Public health efforts, as well as an increasing health consciousness of the average American, have focused attention on these treatable risk factors, and particularly, on cholesterol. The consumer is continuously bombarded with information on the dangers of elevated cholesterol levels. Commercial interests have taken advantage of increasing concerns to market the latest food or products to lower cholesterol levels in the blood. The result can lead to misconceptions and an unnecessary concern about cholesterol by the layman.

Hyperlipidemia is defined as an abnormal elevation in blood cholesterol, cholesterol esters, triglycerides, or phospholipids. The clinical importance of hyperlipidemia depends on which of these lipids are elevated and to what extent. Studies have demonstrated that elevated cholesterol levels are an independent and significant risk factor for CHD (1, 3). Hypertriglyceridemia has not been established as an independent risk factor for CHD and is only considered a marker for other underlying lipoprotein disorders (1, 4).

Although the association between elevated cholesterol and CHD is established, the benefit of interventions to lower cholesterol levels is controversial (5–8). Clinical studies conducted to assess the benefits of cholesterol reduction have been criticized for biased reporting methods that can overemphasize the benefit of lowering cholesterol levels. The extrapolation of benefits in specific study patient populations to the public at large has also been questioned. Clinicians still disagree whether and when to treat elevated cholesterol levels. Concensus statements have been developed by several groups outlining current recommendations for the treatment of hypercholesterolemia and hypertriglyceridemia (1, 2, 4, 9, 10). These position papers agree that (a) there is overwhelming evidence that elevated cholesterol increases the risk of CHD; (b) evidence indicates that lowering serum cholesterol levels is beneficial in reducing the risk of CHD; (c) a balanced approach to the patient must address all risk factors for CHD; (d) a sustained commitment on the part of the clinician and the patient is necessary to make any intervention worthwhile in reducing the risk of CHD; (e) dietary intervention is the cornerstone of therapy; and (d) drug therapy should only be used in patients who fail dietary therapy or who have significantly elevated cholesterol levels.

LIPIDS AND LIPID TRANSPORT

Cholesterol is a lipid precursor of bile acids and steroid hormones and a primary component of cell membranes. The amount of cholesterol required for normal life functions is manufactured by the body. In the average person, cholesterol levels in the blood reflect about 40 to 60% endogenous cholesterol, with the remainder coming from the diet (11). Triglycerides are composed of free fatty acids that are used as an energy source. Triglycerides in the body are provided by fats in the diet and the conversion of carbohydrates in the liver.

Cholesterol and triglycerides, as well as other lipids, are transported through the bloodstream in spherical particles called lipoproteins. They have been divided into five major categories depending on their composition: (a) chylomicrons, composed of exogenous or dietary triglycerides; (b) very low density lipoproteins (VLDL), composed primarily of triglycerides; (c) remnant particles or intermediate-density lipoproteins (IDL), composed of cholesterol esters and triglycerides; (d) low-density lipoproteins (LDL) composed primarily of cholesterol; and (e) high-density lipoproteins (HDL), composed of cholesterol. LDL accounts for 60 to 70% of total serum cholesterol and is the major artherogenic class of lipoproteins. HDL is 20 to 30% and VLDL is about 10 to 15% of total serum cholesterol (1, 12).

Cholesterol and triglycerides in the diet enter into the exogenous pathway of lipid transport (Fig. 18.1). Cholesterol and triglycerides form chylomicrons in the intestinal endothelium, which then enter the lymphatic system where they are transported into the general circulation. Once in the bloodstream, the chylomicrons interact with the enzyme lipoprotein lipase on the vascular endothelium, which hydrolyzes the triglycerides into free fatty acids and monoglycerides that are absorbed by muscle and adipose tissue. The fatty acids are oxidized as an energy source or converted back into triglycerides. This process converts the chylomicron into a cholesterol-rich remnant particle. This remnant particle is taken up by the liver, which converts the cholesterol into bile salts or redistributes it to other body tissues. Bile salts are excreted by the

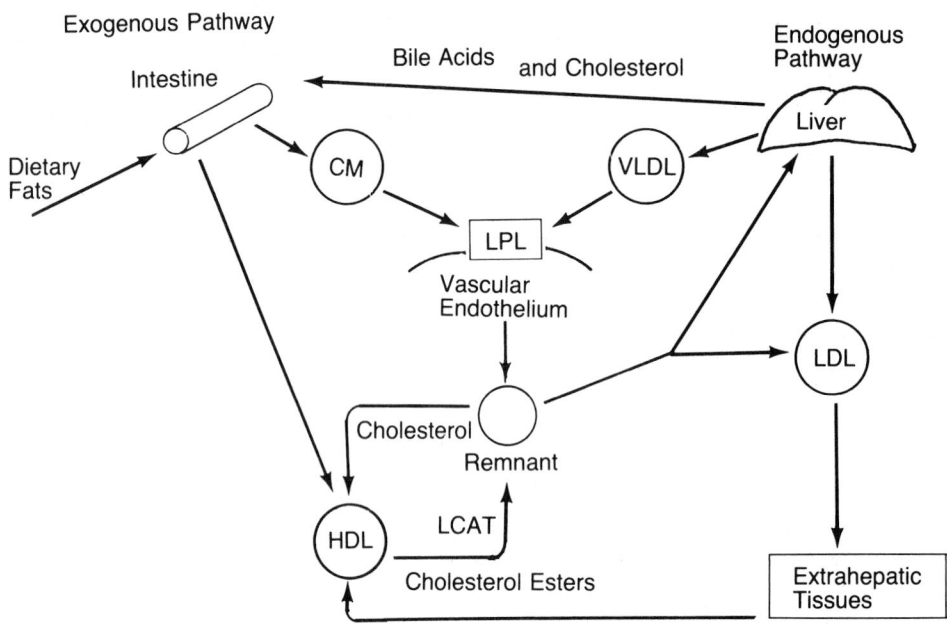

Figure 18.1. Lipid Transport. Schematic of exogenous and endogenous lipid pathways. *CM*, chylomicron; *VLDL*, very low density lipoprotein; *LPL*, lipoprotein lipase; *LDL*, low-density lipoprotein; *HDL*, high-density lipoprotein; *LCAT*, lecithin cholesterol acyltransferase.

liver into the intestine where they solubilize dietary fats to increase their absorption (12).

Lipids produced by the body are transported through the endogenous pathway. Triglycerides can be synthesized by the liver, especially in the presence of excess carbohydrates. The liver secretes the triglycerides into the bloodstream as VLDL. Like chylomicrons, VLDL is converted into a VLDL remnant by interacting with lipoprotein lipase on the vascular endothelium. Approximately one-half of these remnants are metabolized by the liver. The remainder undergo further transformation into LDL, where most of the triglycerides are removed and replaced with cholesterol esters. LDL transports cholesterol to various body tissues where it interacts with LDL receptors on cell membranes. The LDL particles are taken up by the cells, and the cholesterol is used for steroid synthesis or as part of cell membranes. Excessive circulating LDL cholesterol will cause cholesterol to be deposited outside the cell, causing artherogenic plaques to form in the vascular endothelium. Some LDL particles are degraded and eliminated through a scavenger pathway (12).

High-density lipoproteins are synthesized by the liver and the intestine. The HDL particle serves as a receptacle for circulating free cholesterol in the tissues and is returned to the liver and kidney to be catabolized. An individual with abnormally low HDL levels (less than 0.9 mmol/liter (35 mg/dl)) appears to be at an increased risk of CHD, presumably by the decreased ability to remove excess circulating cholesterol (1).

ETIOLOGY OF HYPERLIPIDEMIA

Hyperlipidemia can be caused by genetic predisposition, through secondary causes (e.g., underlying disease states, drugs, or lifestyle), or both. The most severe forms of hyperlipidemia occur in individuals with specific inherited traits that have resulted in defects in lipid metabolism or transport (e.g., absence of LDL receptors). Patients with hereditary (primary) disease usually require medication and intensive intervention to prevent morbidity associated with the condition. Mild or moderate hyperlipidemia is most commonly caused by some degree of inherited predisposition in combination with one or more secondary causes (1).

Concomitant diseases, lifestyle, and medications are the three main secondary causes of hyperlipidemia. Hypothyroidism, nephrotic syndrome, and diets high in saturated fats and cholesterol can contribute to hypercholesterolemia (1, 13). A high intake of fats, carbohydrates, total calories and alcohol, as well as a sedentary lifestyle increases triglyceride levels. Type II diabetes mellitus is a common cause of hypertriglyceridemia that is aggravated by the associated obesity (1, 4).

Some medications, especially antihypertensives (14, 15), can cause unintended changes in lipid levels. Thiazide diuretics, loop diuretics, and β-blockers without intrinsic sympathomimetic activity have been found to increase total cholesterol, LDL cholesterol, and triglyceride levels, and to lower HDL levels. Prazosin, clonodine, and to a lesser extent, calcium-channel blockers may improve the lipid profile by reducing total cholesterol, LDL choles-terol, and triglyceride levels while causing an increase in HDL levels. Estrogens and isotretinoin (16) may unfavorably alter lipid levels. Chronic amiodarone administration has been reported to cause a dose-dependent increase in cholesterol levels independent of its effect on thyroid function (17).

CLINICAL IMPLICATIONS OF HYPERLIPIDEMIA

Although increased serum cholesterol levels have been linked directly to the risk of CHD, it is LDL cholesterol that is more closely associated with the risk and extent of disease. The association of cholesterol levels with the risk of CHD is not a linear relationship. Patients with cholesterol levels above the 95th percentile of the population have a disproportionately higher risk of developing CHD (1, 9).

A number of clinical trials have studied the effect of dietary or pharmacologic interventions for cholesterol reduction in altering CHD risk. Some of the more recent and widely cited studies include the Lipid Research Clinics Coronary Primary Prevention Trial (LRC-CPPT) (18, 19) and the Helsinki Heart Study (20). Both studies showed a reduction in CHD morbidity and mortality after cholesterol reduction by dietary and pharmacological intervention in large populations of asymptomatic middle-aged men with mean plasma cholesterol levels of 7.5 mmol/liter (290 mg/dl) (desirable levels <5.2 mmol/liter (200 mg/dl)) who where followed for more than 5 years. However, study critics contend that the absolute benefit of cholesterol reduction demonstrated in these studies was reported in a biased fashion that has led professionals and layman into ascribing greater benefits to cholesterol reduction than actually occur (5–8). In addition, most clinical research has been in a narrow study population of middle-aged men

Table 18.1.
Conversion Table for Lipids[a]

Cholesterol		Triglycerides	
mg/dl[c]	mmol/liter	mg/dl[d]	mmol/liter
35	0.9	250	2.8
130	3.4	400	4.5
160	4.1	500	5.6
190	4.9	1000	11.3
200	5.2		
240	6.2		

[a] Modified from The Expert Panel: Report of the National Cholesterol Education Program expert panel on detection, evaluation, and treatment of high blood cholesterol in adults. Arch Intern Med 148:36–69, 1988.
[b] To convert serum cholesterol to plasma levels multiply by 0.97.
[c] To convert cholesterol levels in mg/dl to mmol/liter multiply by 0.02586.
[d] To convert triglyceride levels in mg/dl to mmol/liter multiply by 0.01129.

Table 18.2.
Classification of Cholesterol Levels Based on NCEP Guidelines[a]

	Total Cholesterol[b] (mmol/liter)	LDL Cholesterol[c] (mmol/liter)
Desirable	<5.2	<3.4
Borderline high	≥5.2 or <6.2	≥3.4 or <4.1
High	≥6.2	≥4.1

[a] From The Expert Panel: Report of the National Cholesterol Education Program expert panel on detection, evaluation, and treatment of high blood cholesterol in adults. Arch Intern Med 148:36–69, 1988.
[b] LDL cholesterol is considered a more accurate predictor of CHD than total cholesterol. Because LDL cholesterol is a calculated value and total cholesterol is a good predictor of LDL cholesterol, total cholesterol can be used to monitor patient progress.
[c] LDL cholesterol is calculated from fasting levels of total cholesterol, HDL cholesterol, and triglycerides as follows: LDL cholesterol = total cholesterol − HDL cholesterol − (triglycerides/5).

with elevated cholesterol levels, and the results may not be applicable to the population at large.

Despite the controversy surrounding the clinical research, most clinicians agree that the apparent benefit of cholesterol reduction in study patients at risk for CHD warrants interventions in the general population for those at increased risk (1). This position is strengthened by recent studies in patients with coronary artery disease or previous myocardial infarction where interventions to lower lipid levels halted progression of coronary lesions, reduced the incidence of cardiac events, and also resulted in the regression of measurable coronary lesions (21–23). Several groups have published position papers outlining recommendations for the treatment of hypercholesterolemia including the American Heart Association (9), and more recently, the National Cholesterol Education Program (NCEP) (1).

The NCEP has established a classification scheme for total cholesterol and LDL cholesterol levels that is outlined in Table 18.2. The NCEP classification scheme of total and LDL cholesterol offers guidelines that can be used in making treatment decisions. According to NCEP criteria, desirable cholesterol levels have been defined as less than 5.2 mmol/liter (200 mg/dl). Lower cholesterol levels may require interventions if other CHD risk factors are present. Table 18.3 describes recommended actions for the desirable, borderline high, and high cholesterol levels. Other risk factors for CHD that must be considered in treatment decisions are described in Table 18.4.

Although triglycerides have not been linked to CHD risk, hypertriglyceridemia may be a sign of underlying lipid abnormalities, since patients in this classification often have elevated LDL cholesterol and decreased HDL cholesterol levels. The National Institutes of Health (NIH) conference (4) has defined serum triglyceride levels above 5.6 mmol/liter (500 mg/dl) as "distinct hypertriglyceride-

Table 18.3.
Recommended Actions and Follow-up after Cholesterol Screening[a]

Classification	Action
Desirable cholesterol level	Repeat cholesterol level in 5 years
Borderline high cholesterol level and no other CHD risk factors	Dietary information; recheck cholesterol level annually
Borderline high cholesterol level in high risk patient or High cholesterol level	Further lipoprotein analysis; treatment decision based on LDL level

[a] From The Expert Panel: Report of the National Cholesterol Education Program expert panel on detection, evaluation, and treatment of high blood cholesterol in adults. Arch Intern Med 148:36–69, 1988.

Table 18.4.
CHD Risk Factors Based on Factors Other Than Cholesterol[a]

A patient is at high risk for CHD if he or she has
1. Definite CHD by clinical or objective findings of
   • Definite prior myocardial infarction
   • Definite myocardial ischemia (e.g., angina)

OR

2. Two CHD risk factors:
   • Male sex
   • Family history of premature CHD (definite MI or sudden death before age 55 in parent or sibling)
   • Cigarette smoking (>10 per day)
   • Hypertension
   • Low HDL cholesterol concentration (<0.9 mmol/liter, confirmed by repeat measurement)
   • Diabetes mellitus
   • History of definite cerebrovascular or occlusive peripheral vascular disease
   • Severe obesity (≥30% over ideal weight)

[a] From The Expert Panel: Report of the National Cholesterol Education Program expert panel on detection, evaluation, and treatment of high blood cholesterol in adults. Arch Intern Med 148:36–69, 1988.

mia" and levels above 2.8 mmol/liter (250 mg/dl) as "borderline hypertriglyceridemia." Fasting triglyceride levels above 11.3 mmol/liter (1000 mg/dl) require treatment because of associated complications including acute pancreatitis, lipemia retinalis, and eruptive skin xanthomas. There is disagreement on whether triglyceride levels over 5.6 mmol/liter (500 mg/dl) should be treated because of a possible increase in CHD risk, especially if there are no other CHD risk factors. Because of the diffuclty in assessing risk, nonpharmacologic interventions to reduce triglyceride levels are appropriate and may include dietary intervention, exercise, smoking cessation, reducing alcohol intake, and evaluating medications that may increase triglyceride levels. Patients with borderline hypertriglyceridemia usually

do not require treatment unless they have elevated cholesterol levels or significant risk factors for CHD. Triglyceride levels below 2.8 mmol/liter (250 mg/dl) can be considered normal in the absence of other CHD risk factors (1, 4).

PATIENT EVALUATION

NCEP guidelines recommend screening all adults for elevated cholesterol levels every 5 years. Interventions based on the total cholesterol level are listed in Table 18.5. Patients with moderate elevations in total cholesterol without other risk factors should get dietary counseling and return for annual screening. Patients with significant elevations in total cholesterol levels or moderate increases of cholesterol levels in the presence of other risk factors, require further assessment of LDL cholesterol levels. This is accomplished by taking a fasting total cholesterol level, HDL cholesterol level, and triglyceride level. The LDL is then calculated by the following formula:

$$\text{LDL cholesterol} = \text{total cholesterol} - \text{HDL cholesterol} - \text{triglycerides}/5.$$

The LDL cholesterol level is then classified as desirable, borderline high or high (Table 18.2). LDL cholesterol levels should be determined on two or more separate occasions and the results averaged to determine the patient's risk category. Significant interlaboratory variability in cholesterol level determinations has been well documented, therefore the clinician should be confident that results used to classify a patient's risk have been determined accurately (24). Patients with LDL cholesterol levels above 4.1 mmol/liter (160 mg/dl) or 3.4 mmol/liter (130 mg/dl) in the presence of definite CHD or 2 or more risk factors

Table 18.5.
NCEP-Recommended Interventions Based on LDL Cholesterol[a]

Intervention	Initiate Treatment if LDL-Cholesterol (mmol/liter)	Minimal Goal of LDL Cholesterol Level to Achieve (mmol/liter)[b]
Dietary treatment		
No risk factors	≥4.1	<4.1
High risk	≥3.4	<4.1
Diet and drug treatment		
No risk factors	≥4.9	<4.1
High risk	≥4.1	≤3.4

[a] From The Expert Panel: Report of the National Cholesterol Education Program expert panel on detection, evaluation, and treatment of high blood cholesterol in adults. Arch Intern Med 148:36–69, 1988.
[b] Because LDL-cholesterol is a calculated value, and total cholesterol is a good predictor of LDL-cholesterol, total cholesterol can be used to monitor patient progress. Total cholesterol levels of 5.2 mmol/liter and 6.2 mmol/liter, approximate LDL-cholesterol levels of 3.4 mmol/liter and 4.1 mmol/liter, respectively.

are considered to be at increased risk for CHD and require intervention. The patient assessment should include a thorough evaluation to determine any secondary causes of hyperlipidemia and other risk factors of CHD (1).

TREATMENT

A comprehensive treatment plan must address all the risk factors for CHD. Secondary hyperlipidemia may resolve by treating underlying causes including hypothyroidism, diabetes mellitus, diet, and drugs. Most triglyceride levels in the range of 2.8 to 8.5 mmol/liter (250 to 750 mg/dl) result from a secondary cause that can be treated (1). Initial treatment should also include smoking cessation and control of hypertension when appropriate. The patient's lifestyle should be assessed, and simple methods of reducing cholesterol levels and risk of coronary heart disease such as moderate exercise (20 minutes of aerobic exercise three times weekly) and weight control should be part of the overall treatment plan.

Diet

Diet is the cornerstone of therapy for the treatment of hyperlipidemia. Three dietary habits can significantly add to cholesterol levels: (a) a high intake of saturated fats; (b) a high intake of cholesterol; and (c) caloric intake in excess of requirements, leading to obesity (1, 25). Several dietary protocols have been developed, and most follow the recommendations of the American Heart Association (25) and the more recent National Cholesterol Education Program (1) recommendations. These diets all have the goals of reducing total fat intake to less than 30% of calories, reducing saturated fat intake while increasing polyunsaturated and monosaturated fats, reducing cholesterol consumption, keeping daily total caloric intake at levels required to reach and maintain an ideal weight, and providing carbohydrate and protein at appropriate ratios for a balanced diet. NCEP dietary guidelines are summarized in Table 18.6.

Step 1 of the NCEP diet is a balanced approach recommended for all individuals as a public health effort and is also part of the initial treatment program of patients being treated for hypercholesterolemia. Step 2 is used for patients with severe forms of hypercholesterolemia or those who do not receive adequate control of cholesterol using the step 1 diet. Low fat diets are difficult to maintain, since most easily obtained or prepared foods in industrialized nations are high in fats and total calories. Most patients require intensive and sustained dietary counseling to maintain the dietary plan, because it usually results in a change in how they and their families prepare and eat their food. In addition, fats add flavor to the diet and increase satiety, so reducing fat consumption makes the diet less pleasing.

All patients being screened for cholesterol levels should receive dietary information modeled after the NCEP or similar dietary protocols. Patients with CHD risk factors and/or cholesterol levels requiring intervention should be given thorough dietary counseling to help them adhere to the NCEP diet as part of their treatment. Patients usually understand the concept behind a dietary treatment plan, but often do not understand how to apply the concept to their daily eating habits.

Patients should be instructed on which foods to choose or avoid (Tables 18.7 and 18.8). In general, packaged, highly processed foods and most snack products are high in calories and fat. Patients should be reminded that foods low in cholesterol may not necessarily be low in fats. Nutritional labeling included on most foods can serve as a check for calories, fat and cholesterol content. A conversion of fat content in grams to calories will determine if it represents over 30% of calories for a product, which is not desirable. Total grams of fat multiplied by 9 kcal/g yields calories from fat.

Recent studies have documented a cholesterol-lowering benefit from increasing fiber in the diet, particularly with oat bran (26, 27). It is unclear if this is through a direct effect or by taking the place of fats in the diet (28).

Table 18.6.
Dietary Therapy of High Blood Cholesterol Level[a]

Nutrient	Step 1 Diet	Step 2 Diet
Total fat	Less than 30% of total calories	Less than 30% of total calories
Saturated fatty acids	Less than 10% of total calories	Less than 7% of total calories
Polyunsaturated fatty acids	Up to 10% of total calories	Up to 10% of total calories
Monosaturated fatty acids	10 to 15% of total calories	10 to 15% of total calories
Carbohydrates	50 to 60% of total calories	50 to 60% of total calories
Protein	10 to 20% of total calories	10 to 20% of total calories
Cholesterol	Less than 300 mg/day	Less than 200 mg/day
Total calories	To achieve and maintain desirable weight	To achieve and maintain desirable weight

[a] From The Expert Panel: Report of the National Cholesterol Education Program expert panel on detection, evaluation, and treatment of high blood cholesterol in adults. Arch Intern Med 148:36–69, 1988.

Table 18.7.
Recommended Diet Modifications to Lower Blood Cholesterol (The NCEP Step 1 Diet)[a]

Category	Choose	Decrease
Fish, chicken, turkey, and lean meats	Fish, poultry without skin, lean cuts of beef, lamb, pork or veal, shellfish	Fatty cuts of beef, lamb, pork; spare ribs, organ meats, regular cold cuts, sausage, hot dogs, bacon, sardines, roe
Skim and low-fat milk, cheese, yogurt, and dairy substitutes	Skim or 1% fat milk (liquid, powdered, evaporated), buttermilk	Whole milk (4% fat; regular, evaporated, condensed; cream, half-and-half, 2% milk, imitation milk products, most nondairy creamers, whipped toppings
	Nonfat (0% fat) or low-fat yogurt	Whole-milk yogurt
	Low-fat cottage cheese (1% or 2% fat)	Whole-milk cottage cheese (4% fat)
	Low-fat cheeses, farmer or pot cheeses (all of these should be labeled no more than 2 to 6 g of fat per ounce)	All natural cheeses (e.g., blue, Roquefort, Camembert, cheddar, Swiss), low-fat or light cream cheese, low-fat or light sour cream, cream cheeses, sour cream
	Sherbet, sorbet	Ice cream
Eggs	Egg whites (2 egg whites equal 1 egg in recipes), cholesterol-free egg substitutes	Egg yolks
Fruits and vegetables	Fresh, frozen, canned, or dried fruits and vegetables	Vegetables prepared in butter, creams, or other sauces
Bread and cereals	Homemade baked goods using unsaturated oils sparingly, angel food cake, low-fat crackers, low-fat cookies	Commercial baked goods: pies, cakes, doughnuts, croissants, pastries, muffins, biscuits, high-fat crackers, high-fat cookies
	Rice, pasta	Egg noodles
	Whole-grain breads and cereals (oatmeal, whole wheat, rye, bran, multigrain, etc.)	Breads in which eggs are a major ingredient
Fats and oils	Baking cocoa	Chocolate
	Unsaturated vegetable oils: corn, olive, rapeseed, (canola oil), safflower, sesame, soybean, sunflower	Butter, coconut oil, palm oil, lard, bacon fat
	Margarine or shortenings made from one of the unsaturated oils listed above, diet margarine	
	Mayonnaise, salad dressings made with unsaturated oils listed above, low-fat dressings	Dressings made with egg yolk
	Seeds and nuts	Coconut

[a] From The Expert Panel: Report of the National Cholesterol Education Program expert panel on detection, evaluation, and treatment of high blood cholesterol in adults. Arch Intern Med 148:36–69, 1988.

Table 18.8.
Fatty Acid Composition of Vegetable Oils and Animal Fats[a]

High in saturated fats		
Coconut oil	Palm kernel oil	Butterfat
Cocoa butter	Palm oil	Beef tallow
High in monosaturated fats, low in saturated fats		
Olive oil	Peanut oil	Rapeseed (Canola) oil
High in polyunsaturated fats, low in saturated fats		
Soybean oil	Corn oil	Sunflower oil
Safflower oil		

[a] Information taken from American Medical Association Council on Scientific Affairs: Saturated fatty acids in vegetable oils. JAMA 263:693–695, 1990.

Commercial interests, particularly manufacturers of breakfast cereals, have capitalized on these findings and sometimes make bold claims about the healthful effects of their bran-laden products. Since there is no negative effect from moderate increases of bran in the diet, patients should not be discouraged from this practice. However, they should be cautioned about commercially available bran products that may be high in sugar or fats to increase their palatability. Excessive bran consumption should be avoided because of the potential for constipation, impaction, or other complications.

Diet alone can reduce cholesterol levels by 5 to 10% or more in compliant patients, and intervention should be given a 6-month trial before determining its effectiveness in lowering cholesterol levels. Patients are less likely to succeed on dietary therapy without ongoing counseling and follow-up. Drug therapy must be considered if an adequate trial of dietary therapy does not achieve the desired goal. An algorithm summarizing diet therapy is outlined in Figure 18.2.

Drug Therapy
Drug therapy must be sustained to reduce the risk of CHD effectively. All nondrug approaches to reduce cholesterol or triglycerides must be given an adequate trial before exposing the patient to the risks associated with drug therapy. Patients with LDL cholesterol levels between 4.1 and 4.9 mmol/liter (160 to 190 mg/dl) may still be able to reach their goal by maximizing nondrug treatment (Fig. 18.2). However, patients with LDL cholesterol levels above 4.9 mmol/liter (190 mg/dl) or above 4.1 mmol/liter (160 mg/dl) with CHD or 2 CHD risk factors will probably require drug therapy if dietary intervention fails.

The appropriate drug should be selected by considering (a) the type of hyperlipidemia; (b) the effectiveness

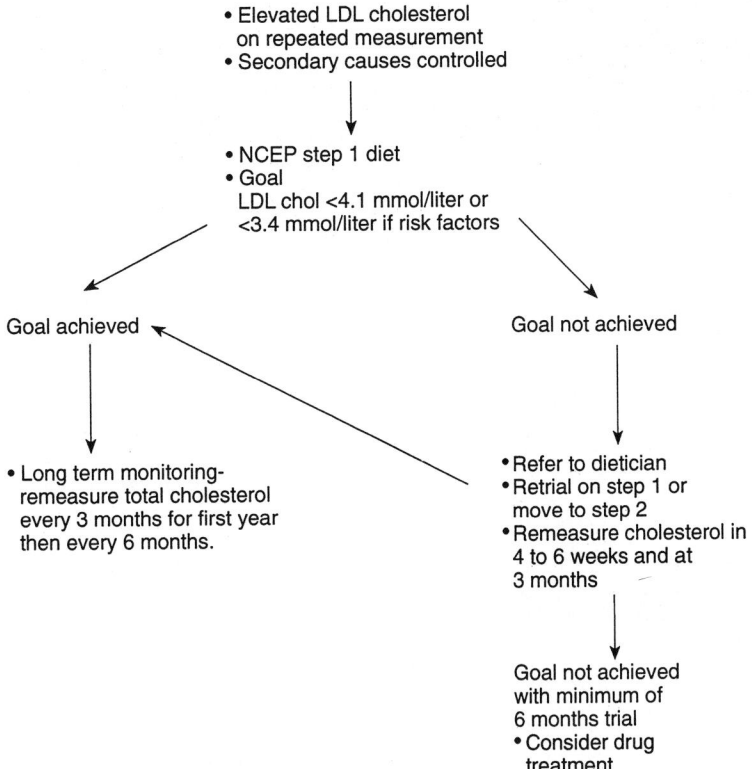

- Elevated LDL cholesterol
  on repeated measurement
- Secondary causes controlled

- NCEP step 1 diet
- Goal
  LDL chol <4.1 mmol/liter or
  <3.4 mmol/liter if risk factors

Goal achieved

Goal not achieved

- Long term monitoring-
  remeasure total cholesterol
  every 3 months for first year
  then every 6 months.

- Refer to dietician
- Retrial on step 1 or
  move to step 2
- Remeasure cholesterol in
  4 to 6 weeks and at
  3 months

Goal not achieved
with minimum of
6 months trial
- Consider drug
  treatment

Figure 18.2. Diet therapy algorithm.

of the drug (Table 18.9); (*c*) the adverse-effect profile of the drug; (*d*) the patient's compliance history; and (*e*) the cost of therapy (Table 18.10). Nonpharmacologic therapy should be continued while a single drug is added to the treatment plan. The dose should be increased until the goal is achieved, the maximum dose is reached, or the patient cannot tolerate the side effects. If the goal is not achieved after an adequate trial, a more effective agent should be considered, or a second drug with a different mechanism of action can be added to the regimen. A drug therapy algorithm is summarized in Figure 18.3

BILE ACID–BINDING RESINS

Cholestyramine and colestipol are bile acid–binding resins that are indicated for the treatment of hypercholesterolemia. Following oral administration, bile acid–binding resins form a nonabsorbable complex with bile acids in the intestine, which removes the bile acids from the enterohepatic circulation. The resins may also increase LDL catabolism in the liver by causing an increase in LDL receptors, resulting in a decrease in the LDL cholesterol level of 15 to 20%. There may be a slight, compensatory increase in VLDL production, causing an increase in triglyceride levels. Although the increase is usually small, and may be transient, it should be considered in patients with a mixed hyperlipidemia with both cholesterol and triglyceride.

The major side effects of the bile acid–binding resins are constipation, bloating, abdominal pain, gas, and nausea. Constipation, which occurs in about 20% of patients, can be reduced with stool softeners and increased dietary fiber. Side effects may become more tolerable with prolonged therapy. Bile acid–binding resins have been reported to interfere with the absorption of fat-soluble vitamins when doses over 24 g daily are given. Although rare, vitamin A, D, and K deficiencies have been reported with the use of binding resins.

Bile acid–binding resins may bind to numerous drugs and interfere with their absorption when given concomitantly. The binding resins can decrease the absorption of digoxin, warfarin, iron salts, thiazides, antibiotics, thyroid hormones, and phenobarbital. Patients should be instructed to take other medications 1 hr before or 4 hr after taking cholestyramine or colestipol, to avoid potential interactions.

The bile acid–binding resins should be given in at least 4 oz of a beverage or soup or sprinkled on a highly pulpy fruit like applesauce. The dose should be sprinkled on top of the desired liquid to allow hydration before mixing. The drug should not be taken dry, to reduce the risk of esophageal irritation or blockage. Colestipol beads are odorless

Table 18.9.
Drugs Used in the Treatment of Hyperlipidemia

Drug	Effects on Lipids	Mechanism of Action	Usual Daily Dose	Side Effects	Comments
Cholestyramine	↓ Cholesterol	↑ LDL metabolism	12–24 g in 2–4 divided doses	Constipation, bloating, abdominal pain, gas	Taste and side effects may limit compliance, binds many drugs
Colestipol			15–30 g in 2–4 divided doses		
Niacin	↓ Triglycerides and cholesterol	↑ LDL catabolism	2–3 g t.i.d.	GI, flushing, pruritus, hepatotoxicity	Side effects limit compliance
Neomycin	↓ Cholesterol	↓ Cholesterol absorption	1 g b.i.d.	Abdominal cramping, diarrhea	Not FDA approved, potential ototoxicity and nephrotoxicity
Dextrothyroxine	↓ Cholesterol	↑ LDL catabolism	6 mg in a single dose	↑ Metabolism, angina, arrhythmias, thyroid suppression	Cardiac toxicity limits usefulness
Probucol	↓ Cholesterol	↑ LDL clearance	500 mg b.i.d.	Diarrhea, abdominal pain, HA, dizziness, paresthesias	Can decrease HDL
Lovastatin	↓ Cholesterol	↓ Cholesterol synthesis, ↑ LDL catabolism	20–80 mg in 1 or 2 doses	GI, myalgias, myositis, lens opacities, elevated liver enzymes	Newest agent, long term effects unknown; prodrug
Simvastatin	↓ Cholesterol and triglycerides		40–80 mg in 2 doses	Similar to lovastatin	Pending FDA approval; prodrug
Pravastatin	↓ Cholesterol		40 mg in 1 to 2 doses	Similar to lovastatin	Pending FDA approval
Clofibrate	↓ Triglyceride and cholesterol	↑ VLDL catabolism	0.5–1 g b.i.d.	GI, myositis, elevated liver enzymes, cholilithiasis	Possible long-term toxicity
Gamfibrozil	↓ Triglyceride and cholesterol	↑ VLDL catabolism	600 mg b.i.d.	GI, myalgias, increased liver enzymes	Similar to clofibrate with potentially fewer side effects

Table 18.10.
Cost Comparison for Drugs Used to Treat Hyperlipidemia

Generic Name	Trade Name	Unit	Wholesale Cost/Unit[a] (dollars)	Average Daily Dose	Daily Cost Average Regimen (dollars)
Cholestyramine	(Questran)	Bulk	4 g	0.57	24 g	3.42
		Packet		0.91		5.46
	(Cholybar)	Bar		0.99		5.94
Colestipol	(Colestid)	Bulk	5 g	0.51	30 g	3.06
		Packet		0.75		4.50
Niacin	(Various)	Tablet	500 mg	0.10	6 g	1.20
	(Nicobid)	Sustained release		0.55		6.60
Neomycin	(Various)	Tablet	500 mg	0.25	2 g	1.00
Dextrothyroxine	(Cholixin)	Tablet	2 mg	0.92	6 mg	2.76
Probucol	(Lorelco)	Tablet	500 mg	0.81	1 g	1.62
Lovastatin	(Mevacor)	Tablet	40 mg	2.73	40 mg	2.73
Clofibrate	(Various)	Capsule	500 mg	0.15	2 g	0.60
Gemfibrozil	(Lopid)	Tablet	600 mg	0.75	1200 mg	1.50

[a] Wholesale costs May 1991. Median dollars used for generic products available from multiple manufacturers. Costs may vary by region.

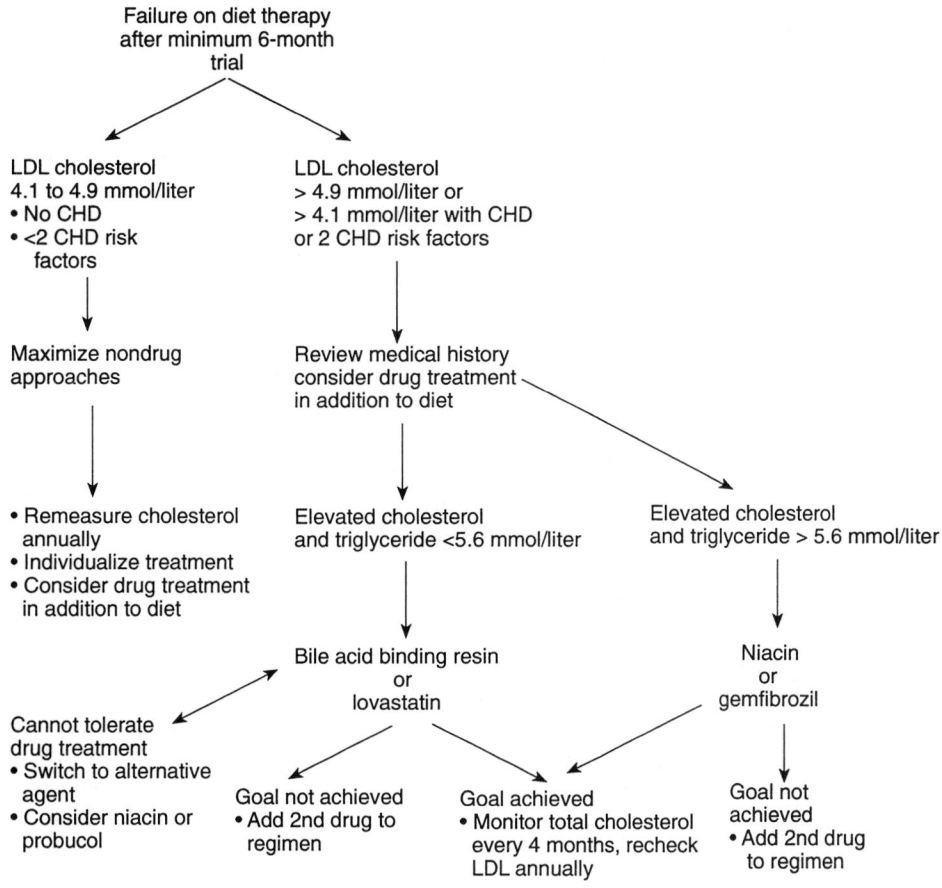

Figure 18.3. Drug therapy algorithm.

and tasteless, as compared with cholestyramine powder, and may be preferable to some patients. A bar containing 4 g cholestyramine is also available and should be thoroughly chewed before swallowing and followed by plenty of fluids.

The usual daily doses of cholestyramine and colestipol are 24 g and 30 g, respectively, given in four divided doses. The daily dose can also be given in two divided doses without a loss in efficacy. A common regimen is to divide the total daily dose by the number of meals the patient routinely eats in a day. The dose is then given with each of the patient's meals. The taste and side effects make the bile acid–binding resin difficult to tolerate for the lifelong regimen required for the treatment of hypercholesterolemia. This should be considered in patients with a history of noncompliance.

NIACIN (NICOTINIC ACID)

Niacin reduces both triglyceride and cholesterol levels and is indicated for the treatment of hypertriglyceridemia, hypercholesterolemia, or mixed hyperlipidemias. Nicotinamide, which shares the vitamin properties of niacin, does not share the lipid-lowering properties. Niacin acts by de-creasing VLDL synthesis by the liver, with a concomitant drop in LDL production. Niacin may also cause a rise in HDL levels by reducing their catabolism. Niacin generally decreases VLDL triglyceride levels by 40%, LDL cholesterol levels by 40%, and increases HDL levels by 20%.

The most prominent side effect of niacin is a prostaglandin-mediated reaction causing acute flushing and pruritus. This side effect is usually seen at the beginning of therapy, with subsequent dosing changes, and with resuming therapy after missed doses. Tolerance to this adverse effect develops quickly with continued dosing. Flushing and pruritus can be prevented by giving 325 mg of aspirin 30 min before each dose and by giving niacin with food.

Niacin can cause abdominal pain and discomfort, and some clinicians avoid niacin in patients with a history of peptic ulcer disease (PUD) because of concern over aggravating PUD or interfering with the clinical presentation. The gastrointestinal upset can be reduced by administering all doses with food. Sustained release preparations are available that may reduce GI discomfort, although this is not well documented. Adverse effects include a dose-dependent increase in aspartate aminotransferase and alkaline phosphatase levels, jaundice, and chronic liver damage. Elevations in liver enzyme levels usually occur if the niacin dose is increased by more than 2.5 g/month. Although these changes may resolve with continued dosing, liver enzymes should be monitored periodically. Some clinicans believe that the sustained-release niacin preparations are associated with a higher incidence of liver function abnormalities (29). Niacin can cause hyperuricemia and glucose intolerance, but this is usually not a problem unless the patient has preexisting gout or diabetes.

The usual dose of niacin ranges from 3 to 6 g daily in divided doses, but amounts as high as 9 g daily have been used. Therapy should be initiated slowly to minimize the risk of liver toxicity and so the patient can become tolerant to the flushing and GI distress associated with the drug. The starting dose is 100 mg given 3 times daily; the daily dose is gradually increased by 300 mg each week until the desired effect is achieved or the maximum dose is reached.

NEOMYCIN SULFATE

Although several studies have documented the cholesterol-lowering ability of the aminoglycoside, neomycin (30, 31), the drug is not FDA-approved for the treatment of hyperlipidemia. The exact mechanism of action is unknown; however, the drug may reduce the absorption of cholesterol from the gut. Neomycin has not gained favor as a lipid-lowering agent because of concerns over potential nephro- and ototoxicity. The drug is poorly absorbed from the gastrointestinal tract, and the risk of toxicity is low unless the patient has preexisting renal dysfunction. Neomycin can cause a 15 to 25% reduction in total cholesterol levels, primarily by a reduction in LDL.

The most common adverse effects include abdominal cramping and diarrhea, which occurs in 50% of patients and may subside with continued therapy. Increased monilial infections, staphylococcal colitis, and resistant coliform bacteria have also been reported. Neomycin may interfere with the absorption of digoxin. The usual dose of neomycin is 2 g daily given as two divided doses.

DEXTROTHYROXINE SODIUM

Levothyroxine can increase the number of LDL receptors and increase LDL catabolism. In addition, it can increase the enzymatic conversion of cholesterol. Dextrothyroxine, the dextro isomer of thyroxine, was synthesized in the hopes of retaining the lipid-lowering properties while avoiding the metabolic and cardiac side effects associated with levothyroxine. Unfortunately, these side effects persist and can limit the usefulness of this drug.

Adverse effects include increased metabolism, precipitation of arrhythmias, aggravation of angina, and suppression of thyroid function. Therefore, dextrothyroxine is contraindicated in patients with a history of heart disease or arrhythmias. Dextrothyroxine may potentiate the anticoagulant effect of warfarin.

Dextrothyroxine is best tolerated in young adults with no preexisting heart disease. Therapy is started with a single daily dose of 1 to 2 mg. The dose can be increased slowly every 4 to 6 weeks by 1 to 2 mg increments to a maximum of 8 mg daily or as tolerated by the patient.

PROBUCOL

Probucol can cause a 10 to 21% reduction in total cholesterol levels, which includes a reduction in both LDL and HDL cholesterol levels. Its effect on triglycerides is variable. The clinical significance of lowering HDL levels is unclear, but because of the higher incidence of CHD associated with low HDL levels, the effect is undesirable.

The adverse effects of probucol tend to be minor and transient. They include diarrhea in about 10% of patients, flatulence, abdominal pain, nausea, and vomiting. Headache, dizziness, and parasthesias have also been reported.

The usual adult dose is 500 mg twice a day, given with the morning and evening meals. The total daily dose should not exceed 1 g.

HMG-CoA REDUCTASE INHIBITORS

The HMG-CoA reductase inhibitors are a new class of drugs for the treatment of hyperlipidemia. Lovastatin (mevinolin) is the first commercially available agent in this class. These agents inhibit the enzyme 3-hydroxyl-3-methylglutaryl-coenzyme A (HMG-CoA) reductase, which is responsible for the conversion of HMG-CoA to mevalonate early in the synthetic pathway for endogenous cholesterol production. Lovastatin causes a significant reduction in serum LDL cholesterol levels, apparently by an increase in LDL receptors in response to decreased cholesterol production. The increased LDL receptors further decrease circulating free cholesterol levels. Lovastatin can decrease total and LDL cholesterol levels as much as 30% and 40%, respectively. Lovastatin may also cause a decrease in triglyceride levels and an increase in HDL levels. The cholesterol-lowering effect of lovastatin is increased when it is given with another cholesterol-lowering agent (11, 32). Adverse effects of lovastatin include diarrhea, abdominal cramps, constipation, and myalgias. Myositis (myalgias with a marked increase in serum creatine phosphokinase) can also occur and is more common when lovastatin is given in combination with gemfibrozil and cyclosporine. Reversible lens opacities that do not impair vision have been reported with lovastatin. For this reason, annual eye examinations are recommended for those on lovastatin therapy. Elevations in serum transaminase levels may require discontinuing therapy in some patients. These elevations can occur 3 to 12 months after therapy begins and usually reverse when therapy is discontinued. Liver function tests should be performed periodically, and lovastatin should be discountinued if liver enzyme levels are three times normal values.

Lovastatin is most effective in lowering cholesterol levels when given in a twice daily dosing regimen. A once daily dosing regimen given at night is also effective, since it takes effect during the peak of cholesterol synthesis in the early morning hours. The least effective dosing regimen is once every morning. Dosing starts at 20 mg given with the evening meal. The dose can be increased every 4 weeks by 20-mg increments until the desired effect is achieved or a maximum dose of 80 mg is reached. Doses of 20 to 40 mg daily are usually sufficient for patients with a moderately increased cholesterol. Lovastatin should be administered with meals because this increases the bioavailability by about 50%.

Pravastatin and simvastatin, two other agents in this class, are currently undergoing clinical trials and are pending approval by the US Food and Drug Administration. Simvastatin is an analog of lovastatin, and in doses of 20 to 80 mg daily it can significantly lower LDL cholesterol and total cholesterol and can decrease triglyceride levels (33, 34). Lovastatin and simvastatin are both prodrugs that require conversion to an active metabolite in the liver. A third agent, pravastatin, is administered in its active form and is metabolized to inactive components. Pravastatin also can effectively lower cholesterol levels at doses of 20 to 40 mg daily (35, 36).

HMG-CoA reductase inhibitors are much easier for patients to tolerate than standard first-line drug therapy for hypercholesterolemia, and therefore better accepted. However, since this class of drugs is relatively new, long-term effects have not been well described. Studies to document the effect of HMG-CoA reductase inhibitors on CHD risk are currently underway. It is reasonable to expect a benefit because of their documented ability to reduce cholesterol levels. As more experience is gained with the HMG-CoA reductase inhibitors, they may take the place of current first-line agents because of increased patient acceptance.

CLOFIBRATE

Clofibrate was the first drug approved by the FDA for the treatment of hyperlipidemia. Clofibrate increases VLDL catabolism by increasing lipoprotein lipase activity, reduces cholesterol production in the liver, and increases LDL catabolism. The result is a decrease in VLDL and triglyceride levels, and a minor decrease in total and LDL cholesterol levels. Clofibrate is indicated in the treatment of hypertriglyceridemia.

The Coronary Drug Project (37) demonstrated a high incidence of noncardiovascular mortality and a higher incidence of cholelithiasis requiring surgery or causing complications with clofibrate. As a result, clofibrate is no longer considered an agent of first choice. The most frequent adverse effects of the drug are nausea, diarrhea, and gastrointestinal distress, which usually decrease with contin-

ued use. Clofibrate can also cause an increase in aspartate aminotransferase levels and has been associated with a flu-like syndrome accompanied by a rise in creatine phosphokinase levels. Clofibrate can potentiate the effect of warfarin, causing an increase in the prothrombin time. The usual dose is 2 g given daily in two to four divided doses.

GEMFIBROZIL

Gemfibrozil is similar to clofibrate and also decreases plasma triglyceride levels by increasing VLDL catabolism via lipoprotein lipase. In addition, gemfibrozil may reduce the synthesis and excretion of VLDL. Gemfibrozil can reduce triglyceride and VLDL concentrations by 40 to 60%. LDL levels may decrease or increase, but HDL levels usually increase by 17 to 31% (20).

Adverse effects of gemfibrozil are similar to those of clofibrate, although less severe. The most common side effects are gastrointestinal, and include abdominal and epigastric pain, diarrhea, nausea, vomiting, and flatulence. Other side effects include rashes, headache, blurred vision, dizziness, leucopenia, muscle pains, and liver function test abnormalities.

The dose of gemfibrozil ranges from 900 to 1500 mg daily in two divided doses given 30 minutes before the morning and evening meals. The usual dose is 1200 mg daily. Gemfibrozil can be used to treat hypertriglyceridemia as well as some mixed hyperlipidemias.

FISH OIL

Recent evidence suggests that diets that include a large amount of fish can reduce the incidence of coronary thrombosis and reduce the mortality of CHD. The fat in fish is rich in highly unsaturated omega-3 fatty acids, mainly eicosapentaenoic acid (EPA) and docosahexaenoic acid (DHA). The effect of these fatty acids on lipids is equivocal. Studies have shown both increases and decreases in LDL cholesterol levels, decreases in triglyceride levels, and no change or an increase in HDL cholesterol level. These studies used diets rich in fish or fish oil or doses of omega-3 fatty acids of up to 30 grams/day (38, 39).

Adverse effects include diarrhea, increases in bleeding time, and decreases in platelet aggregation. Fish oil capsules available on the market recommend doses of 3 g/day or less, which may have no substantial effect on serum lipids. There is no acceptable evidence that fish oil can prevent heart disease (38).

SUMMARY

The association between hypercholesterolemia and CHD risk has been established, although the link between hypertriglyceridemia and CHD is not apparent. Although hyperlipidemia must be treated in specific patient groups, the benefit of interventions in the general public is controversial. An estimated 36% of American adults between the ages of 20 and 74 years are candidates for intervention for hypercholesterolemia using NCEP criteria (40). The cost of medical therapy is substantial, and cost-benefit models estimate that interventions are most cost effective in high-risk groups (41). Medical therapy for smoking cessation and the control of hypertension is less costly and can result in a greater reduction in CHD risk than controlling cholesterol levels (42). This emphasizes the need for a balanced approach to each patient at risk for CHD, which addresses all risk factors as part of the treatment plan.

A multidisciplinary approach to treatment must reinforce lifestyle changes and compliance to therapy. Nonpharmacologic interventions must be emphasized, even after a decision is made to use drug therapy. The decision to begin drug therapy for hyperlipidemia should be patient-specific and should address the potential risks and benefits for that patient.

REFERENCES

1. The Expert Panel: Report of the National Cholesterol Education Program Expert Panel on Detection, Evaluation, and Treatment of High Blood Cholesterol in Adults. Arch Intern Med 148:36–69, 1988.
2. Working Group on Management of Patients with Hypertension and High Blood Cholesterol: National education programs working group report on the management of patients with hypertension and high blood cholesterol. Ann Intern Med 114:224–237, 1991.
3. Pekkanen J, Linn S, Heiss G, et al.: Ten-year mortality from cardiovascular disease in relation to cholesterol level among men with and without preexisting cardiovascular disease. N Engl J Med 322:1700–1707, 1990.
4. National Institutes of Health Office of Medical Applications of Research: Treatment of hypertriglyceridemia. JAMA 251:1196–1200, 1984.
5. Brett AS: Treating hypercholesterolemia; how should practicing physicians interpret the published data for patients? N Engl J Med 321:676–680, 1989.
6. Labreche DG: Reassessment of the value of lowering serum cholesterol: questioning the wisdom of widespread intervention. Clin Pharm 7:592–603, 1988.
7. Leaf A: Management of hypercholesterolemia; are preventive interventions advisable? N Engl J Med 321:680–684, 1989.
8. Olson RE: A critique of the report of the National Institutes of Health expert panel on detection, evaluation, and treatment of high blood cholesterol. Arch Intern Med 149:1501–1503, 1989.
9. Gotto AM, Bierman EL, Connor WE, et al.: Recommendations for treatment of hyperlipidemia in adults. Circulation 69:1065A–1090A, 1984.
10. National Institutes of Health Office of Medical Applications of Research: Lowering blood cholesterol to prevent heart disease. JAMA 253:2080–2086, 1985.
11. McKenny JM: Lovastatin: a new cholesterol lowering agent. Clin Pharm 7:21–36, 1988.
12. Schaefer EJ, Levy R: Pathogenesis and management of lipoprotein disorders. N Engl J Med 312:1300–1310, 1985.
13. Joven J, Villabona C, Vilella E, et al.: Abnormalities of lipoprotein metabolism in patients with the nephrotic syndrome. N Engl J Med 323:579–584, 1990.
14. Weinberger MH: Antihypertensive therapy and lipids. Arch Intern Med 145:1102–1105, 1985.
15. Flamenbaum W: Metabolic consequences of antihypertensive therapy. Ann Intern Med 98:875–880, 1983.
16. Marsden J: Hyperlipidemia due to isotretinoin and etretinate: possible mechanism and consequences. Br Med J 114:401–407, 1986.
17. Wiersinga WM, Trip MD, Van Beeren MH, et al.: An increase in plasma cholesterol independent of thyroid function during long term amiodarone therapy. Ann Intern Med 114:128–132, 1991.
18. Lipid Research Clinics Program: The lipid research clinics coronary primary preventions trial results. I. Reductions in incidence of coronary heart disease. JAMA 251:351–364, 1984.
19. Lipid Research Clinics Program: The lipid research clinics coronary primary preventions trial results. II. The relationship of reduction in incidence of coronary heart disease to cholesterol lowering. JAMA 251:365–374, 1984.
20. Frick MH, Elo O, Haapa K, et al.: Helsinki heart study: primary-prevention trial with gemfibrozil in middle aged men with dyslipidemia. N Engl J Med 317:1237–1245, 1987.
21. Brown G, Albers JJ, Fisher LD, et al.: Regressions of coronary artery disease as a result of intensive lipid-lowering therapy in men with high levels of apolipoprotein B. N Engl J Med 323:1289–1298, 1990.
22. Buchwald H, Varco RL, Matts JP, et al.: Effect of partial ileal bypass surgery on mortality and morbidity from coronary heart disease in patients with hypercholesterolemia. N Engl J Med 323:946–955, 1990.
23. Rossouw JE, Lewis B, Rifkind BM: The value of lowering cholesterol after myocardial infarction. N Engl J Med 323:1112–1119, 1990.
24. Garber A, Sox HC, Littenberg B: Screening asymptomatic adults for cardiac risk factors: the serum cholesterol level. Ann Intern Med 110:622–639, 1989.
25. American Heart Association Nutrition Committee: Dietary guidelines for healthy American adults. Circulation 77:721A–724A, 1988.
26. Van Horn LV, Liu K, Parker D, et al.: Serum response to oat product intake with a fat modified diet. J Am Diet Assoc 86:759–764, 1986.
27. Anderson JW, Story L, Sieling B, et al.: Hypocholesterolemic effects of oat bran or bean intake for hypercholesterolemic men. Am J Clin Nutr 40:1146–1155, 1984.
28. Swain JF, Rouse IL, Curley CB, Sacks FM: Comparison of the effects of oat bran and low-fiber wheat on serum lipoprotein levels and blood pressure. N Engl J Med 322:147–152, 1990.
29. Etchason JA: Niacin-induced hepatitis: a potential side effect with low-dose time release niacin. Mayo Clin Proc 66:23–28, 1991.
30. Hoeg JM, Schaefer EF, Romano CA, et al.: Neomycin and plasma lipoproteins in type II hyperlipoproteinemia. Clin Pharmacol Ther 36:555–565, 1984.
31. Miettenen T: Effects of neomycin alone and in combination with cholestyramine on serum cholesterol and fecal steroids in hypercholesterolemic subjects. J Clin Invest 301:595–597, 1979.
32. Sitori CR: Pharmacology and mechanism of action of the new HMG-CoA reductase inhibitors. Pharmacol Res 22:555–563, 1990.
33. Stuyt PM, Mol MJ, Stalenhoef AF, et al.: Simvastatin in the effective reduction of plasma lipoprotein levels in familial dysbetalipoproteinemia. Am J Med 88:42–45, 1990.
34. Hagemaenas FC, Pappu AS, Illingworth DR: The effect of simvastatin on plasma lipoproteins and cholesterol homeostasis in patients with heterozygous familial hypercholesterolemia. Eur J Clin Invest 20:150–157, 1990.
35. Pan HY, DeVault C, Vilella E, et al.: Pharmacokinetics and pharmacodynamics of pravastatin alone and with cholestyramine in hypercholesterolemia. Clin Pharmacol Ther 48:201–207, 1990.
36. Wiklund O, Angelin B, Fager G, et al.: Treatment of familial hy-

percholesterolemia: a controlled trial of the effects of pravastatin or cholestyramine therapy on lipoprotein and apolipoprotein levels. J Intern Med 228:241–247, 1990.

37. Coronary Drug Project Research Group: Clofibrate and niacin in coronary heart disease. JAMA 231:360–381, 1975.

38. Anon: Fish oil for the heart. Med Lett 29:7–9, 1987.

39. Mueller BA, Talbert RL: Biological mechanisms and cardiovascular effects of omega-3 fatty acids. Clin Pharm 7:795–807, 1988.

40. Semps C, Robinson F, Haines C, et al.: The prevalence of high blood cholesterol levels among adults in the United States. JAMA 262:45–52, 1989.

41. Kinosian BP, Eisenberg JM: Cutting into cholesterol; cost-effective alternatives for treating hypercholesterolemia. JAMA 259:2249–2254, 1988.

42. Taylor WC, Pass, TM, Shepard DS, Komaroff AL: Cholesterol reduction and life expectancy. Ann Intern Med 106:605–614, 1987.

43. American Medical Association Council on Scientific Affairs: Saturated fatty acids in vegetable oils. JAMA 263:693–695, 1990.

CHAPTER 19

ACUTE AND CHRONIC RENAL DISEASES

DANIEL C. ROBINSON, Pharm.D. and MIRTA MILLARES, Pharm.D.

The prognosis of patients with renal disease has improved dramatically over the past three decades because of technological advances in the treatment and prevention of renal failure. The therapeutic use of dialysis and transplantation in renal disease patients is discussed in Chapter 20. As of October 1990, approximately 120,000 patients with chronic renal failure were receiving maintenance hemodialysis in the United States (1). Additionally, several million patients in the United States have some form of renal disease not requiring dialysis. A thorough understanding of renal disease and its complications is essential to the management of any heterogenous patient population.

Renal diseases are broadly classified as being either acute or chronic depending on their onset, clinical course, and prognosis. Many etiologies are involved with renal insufficiency and resultant multiple organ dysfunction. Complications of renal disease reflect impairment of the normal physiologic function of the kidney, primarily regulation of water and electrolyte balance, arterial blood pressure, erythrocyte production, vitamin D activity, and excretion of metabolic waste products and foreign chemicals. In chronic renal failure, many complications can be managed using drug therapy. The impact of renal failure on drug clearance and elimination must be considered in drug selection, doses, and dosing intervals in patients with any renal insufficiency. Furthermore, many pharmacologic agents are nephrotoxic and can worsen or cause renal dysfunction.

Patients with renal failure frequently have other major medical problems requiring aggressive drug therapy. In the medical management of these patients, the clinician must be able to assess the degree of renal insufficiency, recognize pharmacologic agents that can worsen renal function, and perform pharmacokinetic adjustments of drug dosing.

ASSESSMENT OF RENAL FUNCTION

Laboratory tests used to assess renal function do so through their ability to reflect the glomerular filtration rate (GFR). An ideal substance should be freely filtered, not reabsorbed or secreted by the renal tubules; have no effect on filtration rate; and be easily quantified in plasma and urine. Unfortunately the three tests used clinically—blood urea nitrogen (BUN), creatinine, and creatinine clearance—are less than ideal (2, 3).

Inulin, a fructose polysaccharide, is recognized as the substance whose clearance most accurately reflects GFR. Inulin clearance has had limited application in clinical medicine, since it is an exogenous compound that must be given by continuous infusion, and most laboratories do not measure inulin.

Blood urea nitrogen is derived through hepatic deamination of amino acids, causing liberation of ammonia that combines with available CO_2. Urea, which is eliminated primarily by the kidney through glomerular filtration, undergoes reabsorption in the proximal tubule. The extent of reabsorption depends upon the urine flow rate, so that 40% of the filtered urea is reabsorbed with diuresis and 60% is reabsorbed with antidiuresis. The normal values for BUN are 4 to 5.4 mmol/liter (10 to 15 mg/dl) and may increase to over 54 mmol/liter (150 mg/dl) with severe renal failure. The BUN is less accurate than either serum creatinine levels or creatinine clearance in assessing renal function. The major limitations are related to a number of factors that can alter BUN without changes in renal function (3). Urea production depends on protein catabolism and is therefore altered by changes in dietary intake, liver disease, blood in the gastrointestinal tract, steroid-induced catabolism, and the antianabolic effect of tetracyclines, doxycycline being the only exception (4). Since the amount of urea reabsorbed is inversely proportional to the urine flow rate, low-flow states will elevate BUN disproportionately to changes in serum creatinine concentration. Any factors that lower the absolute or effective blood volume (and hence renal blood flow) will increase BUN. Table 19.1 lists factors responsible for an elevation of BUN in the absence of renal impairment (5, 6).

Creatinine production is a function of muscle metabolism, which under normal conditions is relatively constant from day to day. As a function of muscle mass, creatinine production depends on body size (surface area) and age. Because creatinine is filtered by the glomerulus and is secreted only slightly by the renal tubule, its clearance closely approximates the GFR. The normal values for serum creatinine are 70 to 115 μmol/liter (0.8 to 1.3 mg/

Table 19.1.
Factors Elevating BUN without Renal Impairment

High-protein diet
Febrile illness with catabolism
Gastrointestinal bleeding
Hyperthyroidism
Hypovolemia
  Diuretic-induced
  Hemorrhage
  Vomiting and diarrhea
Decreased cardiac output
  Congestive heart failure
  Myocardial infarction
Steroids—catabolic effect
Tetracyclines—antianabolic effect

dl) for males and 50 to 90 μmol/liter (0.6 to 1.0 mg/dl) for females. Factors other than a decreased GFR can alter the serum creatinine level and must be considered when assessing renal function. Hypercatabolic states, myositis, muscle trauma, extreme exercise, and prolonged motor seizures can increase serum creatinine concentration (6). Patients with decreased muscle mass as a result of old age or cachexia will have a decreased creatinine production, and therefore, a low or normal serum creatinine level even though their renal function may be impaired.

A normal creatinine clearance rate is 1.67 to 2.33 ml/sec (97 to 140 ml/min) for males and 1.42 to 2.08 ml/sec (85 to 125 ml/min) for females. Creatinine clearance is a derived term that requires a timed (usually 24 hr) and measured urine collection:

$$Cl_{cr} = (U_{cr}/P_{cr}) \times V \qquad (19.1)$$

where Cl_{cr} = creatinine clearance in milliliters per minute, U_{cr} = urine creatinine concentration in milligrams per deciliter, P_{cr} = plasma creatinine concentration in milligrams per deciliter measured at the midpoint of the collection period, and V = urine volume per unit time (i.e., total urine volume collected divided by total time of collection, expressed in milliliters per minute). The renal clearance of any measurable substance can be calculated in precisely the same way. A major disadvantage in determining creatinine clearance in this manner is the time and personnel required for its collection. A patient or care giver will, on occasion, accidentally omit or discard a urine specimen without adding it to the total collection. Any such error, in addition to incomplete bladder emptying, results in underestimation of the patient's actual creatinine clearance. One method of estimating whether the creatinine clearance is valid is to compare the collected creatinine in milligrams with the estimated creatinine production. If the patient's renal function is stable, creatinine production equals creatinine excretion. Based on data from 936 males

and 219 females the rate (mg/kg/24 hr) of creatinine production (R_{cr}) can be calculated (7) for males:

$$R_{cr} = 27 - (0.173 \times age) \qquad (19.2)$$

and for females:

$$R_{cr} = 25 - (0.175 \times age) \qquad (19.3)$$

For example, using the above formula, a 45-year-old, 70-kg man with stable renal function produces 1345 mg of creatinine per day. If the amount of measured creatinine collected in the urine is significantly less, the collection was probably incomplete, and a repeat test should be performed.

Laboratory determination of the serum creatinine concentration is based on the alkaline picrate method of Jaffe, with minor modifications to accommodate automation and increased specificity. Since this is a colorimetic test, other noncreatinine chromogens can result in overestimation of serum creatinine. Some of these agents are reported in Table 19.2 (5, 8–10). Large elevations in serum creatinine levels without appreciable changes in the BUN should alert the clinician to possible laboratory interference.

Although a timed and measured urine collection is required for accurate determination of creatinine clearance, a number of formulas are available for calculating the creatinine clearance from serum creatinine levels; these are discussed in the section on dosing modification in renal failure.

Urinalysis

A urinalysis is usually performed on a random sample of urine and provides useful information about the presence of renal disease. A urinalysis consists of the following major components.

Table 19.2.
Agents Causing a False Elevation in Serum Creatinine by the Jaffe Method[a]

Acebutolol	Fluorescein
Acetohexamide	Fructose
Acetoacetate	Glucose
Acetone	Levodopa
Aminohippuric acid	Methyldopa
Ascorbic acid	Moxalactam
Cephalothin	Nitrofurantoin
Cefamandole	Phenolsulfonphthalein
Cefoperazone	Pyruvate
Cefoxitin	Sulfobromophthalein

[a] Adapted from Siest, G, Galteau M-M: Drug Effects on Laboratory Test Results. Analytic Interferences and Pharmacological Effects. St Louis, Yearbook Medical Publishers, 1988; Ross DL, Neely AE: Textbook of Urinalysis and Body Fluids. Norwalk, CT: Appleton-Century-Crofts, 1983, pp 68–122; and Young DS: Effects of Drugs on Clinical Laboratory Tests, ed.3. Washington, D.C.: The American Association of Clinical Chemistry, 1990.

APPEARANCE

The urine should be clear, not turbid, and usually light yellow in color. Agents that may cause urine to change color are shown in Table 19.3. Increasing amounts of bilirubin produce colors ranging from yellow-brown to deep olive green. Urine containing old blood, hemosiderin, or myoglobin is brown to black. Small amounts of red blood cells produce a characteristic smokey appearance. Patients with porphyria may void a normal-colored urine, but the sample may develop a deep purple or brownish color on

Table 19.3.
Drugs Causing Changes in Urine Color Not Related to Disease

Color	Drug
Darkening on standing	Cascara
	Chloroquine
	Levodopa
	Methocarbamol
	Methyldopa
	Metronidazole
	Nitrofurantoin
	Phenytoin
Red	Anthraquinone
	Daunorubicin
	Deferoxamine
	Doxorubicin
	Ibuprofen
	Phenolsulfonphthalein
	Phenolphthalein
	Phenothiazines
	Phensuximide
	Rifampin
	Senna
	Sulfabromophthalein
Orange-brown	Cascara
	Chloroquine
	Chlorzoxazone
	Furazolidone
	Ibuprofen
	Iron sorbitex
	Phenazopyridine
	Phenytoin
	Primaquine
	Quinine
	Senna
	Sulfamethoxazole
	Sulfasalazine
Blue-green	Amitriptyline
	Doan's Pills
	Indigo blue
	Methylene blue
	Resorcinol
	Triamterene
Deep yellow	Cascara
	Fluorescein
	Quinacrine
	Riboflavin

Table 19.4.
Conditions Associated with Persistent Changes in Urine pH[a]

Persistently acid urine (pH <7.0)
  Metabolic acidosis
  Respiratory acidosis
  Pyrexia
  Phenylketonuria
  Alkaptonuria
Persistently alkaline urine (pH >7.0)
  Urinary tract infection with urea-splitting organisms
  Metabolic alkalosis
  Carbonic anhydrase inhibitors
  Hyperaldosteronism
  Cystinosis

[a] Adapted from Friedman RB, Young DS: Effects of Disease on Clinical Laboratory Tests, ed. 2. Washington, D.C.: The American Association of Clinical Chemistry, 1990; Ross DL, Neely AE: Textbook of Urinalysis and Body Fluids. Norwalk, CT: Appleton-Century-Crofts, 1983, pp 68–122; and Kark RM, Lawrence JR, Pollak VE, et al.: A Primer of Urinalysis, ed. 2. New York: Harper & Row, 1963.

standing. Food pigments, such as the pigment in beets, can color the urine red (6, 8, 9).

pH

The pH of the urine varies between 4.5 and 8 in patients with healthy kidneys. The pooled daily specimen is usually acid (pH 6). Decreased pulmonary ventilation during sleep causes respiratory acidosis and the development of a highly acid urine. Following meals, the urine becomes alkaline for a few hours. Thus, pH varies widely depending on the time of collection. Highly concentrated urine is usually strongly acidic and may be irritating. When urine stands, it becomes alkaline as urea is broken down to ammonia. Tests for pH should therefore always be done on freshly voided urine [8,9].

Urine that is persistently acid or alkaline may suggest the presence of systemic or urinary tract disease. Conditions associated with persistently acid urine and persistently alkaline urine are listed in Table 19.4 (6,8,9). Some agents that are known to alter urine pH are listed in Table 19.5 (10).

CONCENTRATING ABILITY

Specific gravity is the most convenient way of measuring the amount of dissolved solids in the urine, principally urea, sodium, and chloride. In health the specific gravity may range from 1.003 to 1.030. Concentration and dilution of the urine refer to specific gravities greater than or less than 1.010, respectively.

The measurement of osmolality, although not a bedside procedure, is more accurate and less influenced by large dense molecules such as protein and radiographic contrast media. To test concentrating ability, the patient

Table 19.5.
Agents Causing a Change in Urine pH

Increase urine pH
  Acetohexamide
  Amiloride
  Amphotericin B
  Cimetidine
  Citrates (potassium or sodium citrate)
  Epinephrine
  Niacinamide
  Ranitidine
  Sodium bicarbonate
  Triamterene
Decrease urine pH
  Ammonium chloride
  Ascorbic acid
  Corticotropin
  Diazoxide
  Glucose
  Methenamine mandelate
  Metolazone
  Niacin
  Sucrose

is either deprived of water for a number of hours or given vasopressin 10 USP units subcutaneously. Failure to concentrate urine to more than 800 mOsm/kg or 1.020 specific gravity demonstrates decreased concentrating ability. When renal function approaches 20% of normal, the specific gravity and osmolality become fixed and stabilize at 1.010 and 300 mOsm/kg, respectively. The term "isosthenuria" is used to describe urine that is consistently at 1.010 or 300 mOsm/kg (8, 9).

PROTEIN CONTENT

Less than 0.15 g of protein is normally excreted in the urine per day. Proteinuria is an important indicator of renal disease. Its evaluation requires a knowledge of factors that cause proteinuria without renal pathology. Nonpathologic or functional proteinuria is transient in nature and usually occurs in young adults. Proteinuria can occur with excessive exercise, exposure to cold, postural changes such as standing from a recumbent position, and pregnancy. Proteinuria associated with renal disease occurs as a consequence of numerous disorders, listed in Table 19.6 (9, 11). Proteinuria associated with the nephrotic syndrome is discussed in a later section.

Protein in the urine is measured by sulfosalicylic acid, heat and acetic acid, or dipstick methods. Because of its simplicity, the dipstick method is frequently used as a screening test for proteinuria. Various commercially available urine dipstick products detect protein in the urine. Drugs may cause false-positive results with the sulfosalicylic acid and the heat and acetic acid methods but not with the dipstick method (Table 19.7). A list of test prod-

ucts with their measured urine constituents is included in Table 19.8.

GLUCOSE AND KETONES

Since glucose and ketones are of primary interest in diabetes mellitus the reader is referred to Chapter 17. Causes of glycosuria other than diabetes include gastrectomy; familial renal glycosuria, Fanconi's syndrome, nephrotic syndrome, Cushing's syndrome, or infection; the injection or endogenous liberation of epinephrine; and pregnancy.

CELLS AND CASTS

Normal urine contains a small number of red blood cells, white blood cells, and hyaline casts. Casts are cylindrical elements with parallel sides that derive their shape and

Table 19.6.
Diseases Associated with Proteinuria[a]

Infectious disease
  Poststreptococcal glomerulonephritis
  Infective endocarditis
  Syphilis
Neoplastic disease
  Lymphoma
  Leukemia
  Carcinoma: colon, lung, breast, stomach, kidney
Multisystem and connective tissue diseases
  Systemic lupus erythematosus
  Polyarteritis
  Sarcoidosis
  Sjogren's syndrome
  Amyloidosis
  Diabetes mellitus
Miscellaneous conditions
  Allergic reactions: bee stings, serum sickness
  Chronic allograft rejection
  Preeclampsia

[a] Adapted from Hutt MP, Kelleher SP, Proteinuria and the nephrotic syndrome. In Schrier RW (ed): Renal and Electrolyte Disorders, ed. 3. Boston, Little, Brown & Co, 1986, pp 565–589.

Table 19.7.
Causes of False Reactions in Urine Protein Tests

Conditions or Drugs	Methods[a]		
	Heat and Acetic Acid	Sulfosalicylic Acid	Dipstick Methods
Highly alkaline urine	−	−	−
p-Aminosalicylate	+	+	0
Contrast media	+	+	0
Penicillin (high dose)	+	+	0
Sulfonamides	0	+	0
Tolbutamide metabolites	+	+	0

[a] (+), False-positive; (−), false-negative; (0), not affected.

Table 19.8.
Multiple Urine Test Products

Product	Glucose	Protein	pH	Blood	Ketones	Bilirubin	Urobilirubin	Specific Gravity
Chemstrip GP	X	X						
Uristix	X	X						
Combistix	X	X	X					
Hema-Combistix	X	X	X	X				
Chemstrip 5L	X	X	X	X	X			
Labstix	X	X	X	X	X			
Bili-Labstix	X	X	X	X	X	X		
Chemstrip 6L	X	X	X	X	X	X		
Multistix	X	X	X	X	X	X	X	
Multistix SG	X	X	X	X	X	X	X	X
Chemstrip 7L	X	X	X	X	X	X	X	
N-Multistix	X	X	X	X	X	X	X	
N-Multistix-C	X	X	X	X	X	X	X	
N-Multistix SG	X	X	X	X	X	X	X	X

Table 19.9.
Cells Found in Urine

Cell	Normal Values	Clinical Importance
Red cell	0–2/HPF[a]	Genitourinary (GU) tract lesions, acute tubulointerstitital disease, anticoagulants, systemic disease resulting in coagulation disorders
White cell	0–5/HPF	Urinary tract infection, GU inflammation
Renal epithelial cell (nonsquamous)	0–2/HPF	Tubular damage
Bacteria	None	Urinary tract infection (criteria for infection depends on method of urine collection)
Oval fat bodies[b]	None	Nephrotic syndrome, diabetic glomerulosclerosis, major skeletal trauma

[a] HPF, high-power field.
[b] Renal tubular epithelial cells containing fat droplets.

Table 19.10.
Casts Found in Urine

Hyaline	Normal finding, particularly in dehydration
Granular	Renal parenchymal disease, dehydration
Fatty	Nephrotic syndrome, diabetic glomerulosclerosis
Red cell	Glomerulonephritis, systemic lupus erythematosus, bacterial endocarditis
White cell	Pyelonephritis
Epithelial cell	Tubular damage

CHRONIC RENAL FAILURE

Chronic renal failure (CRF) is defined as a progressive deterioration in renal function as evidenced by a rise in BUN and serum creatinine levels, a decline in creatinine clearance, and the development of uremic symptoms. Uremia refers to the symptom complex associated with severe renal impairment, which may take from months to years to develop. A list of complications of chronic renal failure is provided in Table 19.11. Although the concentration of urea can be correlated with the degree of renal impairment, no specific uremic toxins have been identified as being responsible for all the complications of the uremic syndrome. Other uremic toxins that have been identified include ammonia, guanidine, guanidinosuccinic acid, methyl guanidine, and myoinositol (12–14).

Etiology

Chronic renal failure has many causes, which can be divided into those originating in the kidney, those caused by systemic disease, and those caused by drugs or chemicals. For a complete listing see Table 19.12 and Table 19.13. In general, kidney damage that leads to chronic renal failure is irreversible. Many patients with CRF progress over

size from the tubular segment in which they were formed. They are formed from Tamm-Horsfall mucoprotein, a product of the renal tubules. Factors favoring cast formation are an acid pH, highly concentrated urine, proteinuria, and stasis within the tubules. The transparent hyaline casts are composed entirely of protein. Cellular casts represent red blood cells, white blood cells, or renal epithelial cells trapped within the protein matrix. Granular casts represent degraded cellular casts and usually indicate renal parenchymal damage. Tables 19.9 and 19.10 list the cells and casts that may be found in urine and their importance (8, 9).

Table 19.11.
Complications of Renal Failure

Sodium and water imbalance
Acid-base imbalance
Potassium imbalance
Anemia
Hemostatic defects
Calcium and phosphate abnormalities
Hyperuricemia
Carbohydrate intolerance
Hypertension
Gastrointestinal disturbances
Neuromuscular disturbances
Renal osteodystrophy
Dermatological disorders
Psychological disorders

Table 19.12.
Etiology of Chronic Renal Failure

Renal
 Glomerulonephritis
  Acute
  Chronic
  Rapidly progressive
 Interstitial nephritis
 Ischemic renal disease
  Bilaterial renal artery stenosis
  Bilateral fibromuscular hyperplasia
  Urinary tract infection (pyelonephritis)
 Congenital anomalies
  Polycystic kidney disease
  Medullary cystic disease
  Hypoplastic kidneys
Systemic diseases
 Diabetes
 Hypertension
 Systemic lupus erythematosus
 Polyarteritis nodosa
 Amyloidosis
 Chronic hypercalcemia
 Chronic hypokalemia
 Hyperuricemia
Drugs and chemicals
 See "Drug-induced Nephropathies" in text

time to end-stage renal disease requiring dialysis or transplantation. Therefore, potentially reversible factors that further compromise kidney function must be sought and corrected. Some of these reversible factors are listed in Table 19.14.

Complications and Treatment

Of the numerous complications of chronic renal failure listed in Table 19.11, only the most common and clinically relevant factors are discussed here. Most patients with

more than 25% of normal renal function have few if any symptoms because of the tremendous adaptive abilities of the failing kidney.

Management of patients is aimed at controlling complications of CRF and can usually be accomplished with drug therapy. However, patients with uncontrollable complications or severe symptoms despite therapy may require

Table 19.13.
Drugs Associated with Nephrotoxicity

Acute tubular necrosis	Mefanamic acid
Antibiotics	Phenylbutazone
Aminoglycosides	Tolmetin
Amphotericin B	Metals
Bacitracin	Bismuth
Cephalosporins	Gold
Polymixins	Miscellaneous
Sulfonamides	Allopurinol
Metals	Azathioprine
Antimony	Captopril
Bismuth	Cimetidine
Mercurials	Clofibrate
Platinum	Furosemide
Chelates	Phenytoin
Dimercaprol	Thiazides
EDTA	Glomerulonephritis
Contrast media	Allopurinol
Miscellaneous agents	Ampicillin
Acetaminophen	Captopril
Aminocaproic acid	Cocaine
Carbamazepine	Cyclophosphamide
Cisplatin	Daunorubicin
Cyclosporine	Fenoprofen
Methotrexate	Gold
Methoxyflurane	Heroin
Phenazopyridine	Hydralazine
Streptozocin	Methicillin
Acute tubulointerstital disease	Penicillamine
Penicillins	Penicillin
Amoxicillin	Rifampin
Ampicillin	Sodium diatrizoate
Carbenicillin	Sulfonamides
Methicillin	Thiazides
Nafcillin	Trimethadione
Oxacillin	Chronic tubulointerstitial disease
Penicillin	Acetaminophen
Other antibiotics	Aspirin
Cephalosporins	Lithium
Cotrimoxazole	Methyl-CCNU
Erythromycin	Phenacetin
p-aminosalicylate	Miscellaneous mechanisms
Polymixins	Prerenal azotemia
Rifampin	NSAIDs
Sulfonamides	Renal tubular acidosis &
NSAIDs	concentration defects
Fenoprofen	Lithium
Ibuprofen	Amphotericin B
Indomethacin	Postrenal obstruction
	Methysergide

**Table 19.14.
Reversible Factors Causing Renal
Function Impairment**

Hypovolemia
    Diarrhea
    Vomiting
    Excessive diuretic use
    Excessive sodium restriction
Urinary obstruction
Urinary tract infection
Low cardiac output
    Congestive heart failure
    Arrhythmias
Hypertension
Hypercalcemia
Hyperuricemia
Hypokalemia
Drugs
    Diuretics
    Antihypertensives
    Nephrotoxins

temporary dialysis. When uremic symptoms develop that can no longer be managed, maintenance dialysis or transplantation may be indicated (see Chapter 20).

SODIUM AND WATER IMBALANCE

When creatinine clearance falls to less than 0.42 ml/sec (25 ml/min) the ability of the kidney to handle wide fluctuations in sodium and water intake is lost. If placed on a low-sodium diet, most patients are unable to reduce sodium excretion to match sodium intake, resulting in hyponatremia. Some patients, usually those with interstitial nephritis or medullary or polycystic kidney disease, may require a large sodium intake to maintain sodium balance.

Most patients with significant renal impairment have an impaired ability to concentrate and dilute their urine. Nocturia is an early indicator of renal impairment, because the ability of the kidney to concentrate urine in response to the normal diurnal variation in antidiuretic hormone secretion is lost. A normal daily solute load of 600 mOsm can be excreted in 500 ml of urine if the urine can concentrate to 1200 mOsm/liter. The patient with renal impairment who is unable to concentrate urine to greater than 300 mOsm/liter would require 2 liters of urine to excrete the same osmolar load. Fluid restriction in such a patient would result in retention of normally excreted solutes such as urea and creatinine.

ACID-BASE IMBALANCE

Metabolic acidosis is a common finding in advanced renal failure. Normal kidneys are responsible for excreting 60 to 70 mEq of hydrogen daily. The renal failure patient excretes 30 to 40 mEq/day, resulting in a positive hydrogen ion balance, most of which is probably buffered by bone salts. Since hydrogen is a product of metabolism, little can be done to control the daily load. Metabolic acidosis in CRF is usually well tolerated unless serum bicarbonate levels are below 15 mmol/liter (mEq/liter). Treatment consists of administering sodium citrate daily. Sodium bicarbonate is available in 325 mg and 650 mg tablets. Each 325 mg tablet provides 4 mEq of bicarbonate. Bicitra solution is a combination of sodium citrate and citric acid and provides 1 mEq bicarbonate equivalent/ml of solution. Usual doses range from 20 to 200 mEq of bicarbonate/day (0.5 to 3 mEq/kg/day). Potassium citrate is avoided because of the potential of hyperkalemia.

POTASSIUM IMBALANCE

Even though potassium is excreted almost exclusively in the urine, hyperkalemia rarely occurs in patients who have GFR above 0.08 ml/sec (5 ml/min) in the absence of acute changes in potassium intake. This balance is maintained by increased potassium secretion in the distal renal tubule and increased fecal potassium losses. Factors that jeopardize this balance include the administration of potassium-sparing diuretics such as spironolactone, triamterene, or amiloride; increased potassium intake; and acidosis, which shifts potassium extracellularly from the intracellular compartment.

Treatment of hyperkalemia (discussed in Chapter 8 "Fluid & Electroytes Therapy and Acid-Base Balance") depends on the serum potassium level and the absence or presence of electrocardiographic changes consistent with hyperkalemia. If peaked T waves, widened QRS complexes, prolonged P-R intervals, or absent P waves are noted, therapy is begun with 5 to 10 ml of 10% calcium chloride infused over 1 to 2 min. The intravenous injection can be repeated in 5 to 10 min in order to provide 1 to 2 hr of protection from the electrical consequences of hyperkalemia. Since calcium does not affect serum potassium levels, other measures must be instituted.

Sodium bicarbonate 50 mEq injected intravenously will increase serum pH, favoring the intracellular movement of potassium. This may be repeated as needed to maintain a slightly alkaline serum pH.

A solution containing 2 g of glucose for every unit of regular insulin will also cause an intracellular shift of potassium. A typical solution might consist of 500 ml of 10% glucose with 25 units of insulin to run over 4 hr. Sodium bicarbonate may be added to this solution for continuous infusion. Careful monitoring is needed to avoid fluid and sodium overload with these regimens.

Since the above regimens have no effect on the total body potassium and their effects are transient, a cation-exchange resin (sodium polystyrene sulfonate) is often

Table 19.15.
Phosphate-binding Capacity of Selected Antacids[a]

Product	Content	Aluminum Content (g/30 ml)	Phosphate Bound (mg) per 5 ml Antacid	
			pH 2.0	pH 8.0
Amphogel	Aluminum hydroxide	0.664	13.4	11.6
Alternagel	Aluminum hydroxide	1.2	19.8	4.8
Aludrox	Aluminum & magnesium hydroxide	0.637	26.2	13.3
Basaljel Extra Strength	Aluminum carbonate	1.0	24.2	6.0
Gelusil	Aluminum & magnesium hydroxide	0.2	27.5	5.6
Gelusil II	Aluminum & magnesium hydroxide	0.4	31.0	10.4
Mylanta	Aluminum & magnesium hydroxide	0.415	17.9	4.6
Mylanta II	Aluminum hydroxide	0.830	5.4	0.9
Riopan	Aluminum & magnesium hydroxide	0.276	18.1	15.0

[a] Adapted from Balasa RW, Murray RL, Kondelis NP, et al.: Phosphate-binding properties and electrolyte content of aluminum hydroxide antacids. Nephron 45:16–21, 1987.

needed to provide a sustained effect. Sodium polystyrene sulfonate can be given orally as a suspension or as a retention enema. The enema contains 30 g in 120 ml of sorbitol and must be retained for 30 to 60 min. The oral suspension can be given in a dose of 15 to 60 g. The enema or oral dose is repeated as needed.

CALCIUM AND PHOSPHORUS ABNORMALITIES

At a creatinine clearance below 0.42 ml/sec (25 ml/min) urinary phosphorus excretion diminishes slightly. The modest elevation in serum phosphorus concentration causes a reduction in ionized calcium, which stimulates parathyroid hormone (PTH) production. An increase in PTH tends to normalize serum calcium concentrations by promoting calcium resorption from bone. In addition, PTH enhances renal tubular phosphorus excretion. The net effect is a relative normalization of phosphorus and calcium levels with a slight but significant increase in circulating PTH. As renal function declines further, the ability of the kidney to increase phosphorus excretion is impaired. A sustained elevation in serum phosphorus concentration inhibits the renal conversion of 25-hydroxycholecalciferol (25-HCC) to 1,25-dihydroxycholecalciferol (1,25-DHCC), which results in impaired intestinal calcium absorption and bone resistance to PTH.

Numerous skeletal abnormalities result from disturbances in calcium and phosphorus metabolism secondary to chronic renal failure. These bone abnormalities can be referred to collectively as renal osteodystrophy. Management of renal osteodystrophy is aimed at keeping serum calcium and phosphorus levels near normal, suppressing PTH secretion, and improving skeletal metabolism. Early conservative management consists of restricting dietary phosphorus through reduction of high-phosphorus-containing foods such as meat, milk, legumes, and carbonated beverages or the use of phosphate-binding antacids. The

Table 19.16.
Oral Calcium Preparations

	% Calcium	Strength	Elemental Calcium Content
Liquid			
Calcium glubionate	6.5	1800 mg/5 ml	115 mg/5 ml
Tablets			
Calcium gluconate	9	500 mg	45 mg
		650 mg	58.5 mg
		1000 mg	90 mg
Calcium lactate	13	325 mg	42.3 mg
		650 mg	84.5 mg
Calcium carbonate	40	625 mg[a]	250 mg
		650 mg	260 mg
		667 mg	266.8 mg
		750 mg	300 mg
		1250 mg	500 mg
		1500 mg[a]	600 mg

[a] Chewable.

phosphate-binding capacity of antacids depends on their aluminum content and the local pH (Table 19.15) (15). Given with or immediately after meals and at bedtime, they complex dietary phosphorus contained in gastrointestinal secretions, preventing absorption. Periodic measurement of phosphorus is necessary to titrate antacid administration and prevent hypophosphatemia. Aluminum toxicity can occur in patients with chronic renal failure requiring dialysis. In these patients, monitoring of serum aluminum levels may be indicated.

Hypocalcemia may be treated with oral calcium supplements. One to 1.5 g of elemental calcium is given daily in two to four divided doses. The calcium salts available and their elemental calcium content are listed in Table 19.16. Therapy should not be instituted unless serum phos-

Table 19.17.
Oral Vitamin D Preparations

Drug Name	Abbreviated Chemical Name	Brand Name	Strength[a]	Daily Dose
Calcifediol	25-OHD$_3$	Calderol	10 μg (cap)	25–100 μg
			50 μg (cap)	
Calcitriol	1,25-(OH)$_2$D$_3$	Rocaltrol	0.25 μg (cap)	0.25–1 μg
			0.5 μg (cap)	
Dihydrotachysterol	Synthetic D$_4$	Hytakerol	0.125 mg (cap)	
			0.25 mg/ml (oil)	
			0.125 mg (tab)	
			0.2 mg (tab)	
			0.4 mg (tab)	
		DHT	0.125 mg (tab)	0.25–2 mg
			0.2 mg/5ml (soln)	
Ergocalciferol	Synthetic D$_2$	Vitamin D	25,000 IU (cap)	50,000–500,000 IU
			50,000 IU (cap)	
		Drisdol	50,000 IU (cap)	
			8,000 IU/ml (drops)	
		Calciferol	50,000 IU (cap)	
			8,000 IU/ml (drops)	

[a] 50,000 IU = 1.25 mg.

phorus concentration is under 1.75 to 1.95 mmol/liter (5.5 to 6 mg/dl). A calcium-phosphorus product (Ca × P) greater than 5.63 SI (70) must be prevented to avoid soft tissue calcification.

If serum calcium and PTH cannot be normalized with more conservative regimens, a trial of vitamin D is warranted (Table 19.17). Of the many vitamin D congeners available, calcitriol offers an advantage over ergocalciferol (vitamin D$_2$) and cholecalciferol (vitamin D$_3$) in that it has a shorter onset and duration of action. The potential for vitamin D intoxication and sustained hypercalcemia, which may require weeks for resolution, is a major hazard associated with pharmacologic doses of vitamins D$_2$ and D$_3$. If vitamin D intoxication occurs with the use of 1,25-(OH)$_2$D$_3$ it is rapidly corrected upon discontinuing therapy.

PLATELET AND BLEEDING ABNORMALITIES (See also Chapter 14 "Clotting Disorders")

Bleeding is a frequent complication of uremia manifested by ecchymosis, purpura, gastrointestinal bleeding, and epistaxis. Capillary fragility and coagulation factor defects do not appear to play a major role. Quantitative and qualitative platelet abnormalities are presumed to be causative in most patients. Although severe thrombocytopena <50 × 10^9/liter (less than 50,000/mm^3) is rare, minor deficiencies <150 × 10^9/liter (less than 150,000/mm^3) have been noted in over half the patients studied. Platelet factor 3 is reduced and platelet aggregation is inhibited in advanced renal failure, resulting in prolonged bleeding times and poor clot retraction. Uremic toxins may be responsible

Table 19.18.
Causes of the Anemia of Chronic Renal Failure

Decreased erythopoietin activity
Shortened red blood cell life-span
Gastrointestinal blood loss
Dialysis
    Iron deficiency from dialyzer blood loss
    Folic acid deficiency from dialyzer blood loss
    Red cell destruction from hemolysis
    Splenic sequestration

for these abnormalities. Treatment for severe bleeding requires the administration of fresh platelet concentrates. Deamino-8-arginine (DDAVP) has also been used to improve bleeding times through a mechanism that does not affect platelets (16). Prevention depends on adequate treatment of the uremic state with hemodialysis or peritoneal dialysis. Patients are told to avoid all drugs having antiplatelet activity, particularly aspirin.

ANEMIA (See also Chapter 13 "Other Anemias")

Anemia develops in virtually all patients with chronic renal failure. The anemia is normochromic and normocytic, and rarely does the hematocrit fall below 20%. In the absence of congestive heart failure and angina, the anemia is usually well tolerated. The anemia is caused by a number of factors that are listed in Table 19.18. The earliest clinical signs are pallor and fatigue, which occur when serum creatinine exceeds 265 μmol/liter (3 mg/dl) (17). The primary cause of the anemia of CRF is a decrease in erythropoietin activity. Natural erythropoietin is produced and secreted primarily by the kidney in response to hypoxia. Erythropoietin (EPO) enhances erythropoiesis by stimulating bone marrow production of erythroid cells. In patients with normal renal function, serum EPO levels rise to 10 to 100 times the normal level, in response to anemia. In patients with CRF, maximal EPO production is blunted in response to hypoxia, indicating an impaired ability to produce EPO by the kidneys (18).

A recombinant human erythropoietin (epoetin) became available in the U.S. in late 1989 for the treatment of anemia associated with CRF, which was a major advance. The need for red blood cell transfusions or anabolic steroids and their concomitant risks may be eliminated or decreased. Epoetin is administered either intravenously or subcutaneously. The usual starting dose ranges from 50 to 100 units per kg three times a week. It is important to evaluate and adequately control hypertension prior to initiating therapy. Hypertension occurs in approximately 25% of patients receiving epoetin, perhaps related to too fast a rate of rise in the hematocrit. Although rare, seizures have occurred in patients receiving epoetin and also may be related to a fast rise in the hematocrit. It is therefore important to monitor the hematocrit and reduce the dose, usually in increments of 25 u/kg per dose, if the hematocrit increases more than 0.04 (4) points in 2-week period (19).

Initiation of epoetin therapy requires adequate iron stores. Transferrin saturation should be at least 20% and ferritin concentration at least 100 μg/liter (mg/ml) before initiating therapy. Patients may require supplemental iron therapy while receiving epoetin (19).

Once the hematocrit reaches the target range of 0.30 to 0.33 (30 to 33%), the dose is reduced. Maintenance doses of epoetin must be individualized to maintain the hematocrit within the therapeutic range. In patients with CRF not on dialysis, the usual maintenance dose needed is around 75 to 150 units per kg administered once weekly. Many patients are able to self-administer the dose at home. CRF patients who are on dialysis often require doses around 75 units/kg three times weekly (19).

Treatment of any existing deficiencies such as iron deficiency or folic acid deficiency is instituted with replacement therapy. Iron deficiency may be secondary to chronic blood loss due to uremia, blood loss due to dialysis, or malabsorption of iron. Iron deficiency should be treated with oral ferrous sulfate, 300 mg three times daily, or parenteral iron in patients with gastrointestinal intolerance. Aluminum-containing antacids can chelate iron and prevent absorption. Patients receiving these antacids for control of hyperphosphatemia are instructed to take the antacid at least 1 hr before or 2 hr after an iron dose to avoid this interaction. Folic acid is removed during dialysis,

which can result in folic acid deficiency. Daily supplementation of folic acid is then necessary. A regular dialysis schedule will improve the anemia of uremia, often circumventing the need for blood transfusions.

Anabolic steroids cause an increase in erythropoiesis and are therefore useful in patients who remain symptomatic despite efforts at correcting deficiencies. Three classes of anabolic steroids are available: the testosterone esters, 17-methylated compounds, and 19-nortestosterone. The testosterone esters, testosterone enanthate (Delatestryl) or cypionate (Depo-testosterone) are given intramuscularly, 300 mg every week. These agents have the highest androgenic activity and cause side effects such as hirsutism that are particularly intolerable to female patients. Fluoxymesterone (Halotestin), a 17-methylated compound, can be given orally in doses of 15 to 30 mg daily. These agents have a greater anabolic/androgenic ratio and are therefore better tolerated by female patients. The major disadvantage of these agents is a greater risk for hepatotoxicity and an association with hepatocellular carcinoma from chronic use. 19-Nortestosterone (nandrolone decanoate) has several advantages over the other anabolic steroids. Nandrolone decanoate (Deca-durabolin) has the greatest anabolic/androgenic ratio and therefore produces the fewest masculinizing effects. It is also less hepatotoxic than the 17-methylated compounds. Nandrolone decanoate is administered intramuscularly, 100 to 200 mg weekly. Side effects common to all anabolic steroids mentioned include hyperlipidemia, fluid retention, varying degrees of virilization, and acne. Swelling and hematoma formation can result after intramuscular administration. The need for anabolic steroids has been reduced greatly by the availability of epoetin.

CARBOHYDRATE ABNORMALITIES

In chronic renal failure patients, the degradation and secretion of insulin and the tissue sensitivity of insulin are all abnormal. Approximately 70% of chronic renal failure patients have varying degrees of glucose intolerance, as evidenced by elevated postprandial blood glucose levels, even though fasting glucose levels are often normal. The major mechanism appears to be peripheral resistance to circulating insulin (20, 21).

The kidney plays a major role in the metabolism and excretion of insulin. Thirty to 40% of the insulin reaching the kidneys is cleared by this organ. In severe renal failure the insulin half-life is prolonged, and the insulin requirements of uremic diabetics may be decreased. Insulin, however, remains the treatment of choice in the management of diabetes associated with chronic renal failure. In the rare event that oral hypoglycemic agents must be used, tolbutamide is the drug of choice. It has a relatively short half-life that is not increased with renal failure, and no active metabolites (20, 21).

HYPERURICEMIA (See also Chapter 30 "Gout and Hyperuricemia")

An elevated serum uric acid is observed commonly in chronic renal failure as a result of impaired renal excretion. The degree of hyperuricemia correlates with the severity of renal dysfunction. Serum uric acid levels are usually maintained within normal limits until the creatinine clearance falls below 0.5 ml/sec (30 ml/min). Potential complications from hyperuricemia are gouty attacks, uric acid kidney stones, and urate nephropathy. For unknown reasons, chronic renal failure patients rarely develop gout unless they have a history of primary gout. The association between hyperuricemia and progressive renal disease due to urate deposition is also unclear. There is little evidence that deterioration of renal function occurs more rapidly in hyperuricemic patients than in nonhyperuricemic patients.

HYPERTENSION (22–24) (See also Chapter 35 "Hypertension")

The kidney plays a major role in the control of blood pressure, through regulation of the extracellular fluid volume and the renin-angiotensin system. In an individual patient, it is often difficult to determine whether the hypertension or the renal failure came first. In any event, the aggressive treatment of hypertension can improve long-term survival by limiting renal vascular injury.

In renal vascular disease, hypertension usually results from an increase in the activity of the renin-angiotensin system. Hypertension in renal disease affecting the glomeruli, renal tubules, or interstitium is due largely to sodium retention with increased extracellular fluid volume. However, in most patients with CRF, both renin excess and increased fluid volume contribute to hypertension.

Since extracellular volume expansion is a major cause of hypertension in patients with impaired renal function, sodium restriction and diuretics are often used initially. Because thiazide diuretics are ineffective at a creatinine clearance rate of less than 0.33 to 0.5 ml/sec (20 to 30 ml/min), furosemide is the preferred agent. The dose can range from 40 to over 200 mg/day. Although metolazone is a thiazide diuretic, it is effective in conjunction with furosemide in advanced renal failure because of its inhibition of proximal sodium and chloride reabsorption. Usual doses required are 2.5 to 5 mg daily. Metolazone used in conjunction with furosemide can cause severe electrolyte abnormalities, primarily hypokalemia, and therefore it should be restricted to refractory cases. The potassium-sparing diuretics spironolactone, triamterene, and amiloride should be avoided in renal failure because of the potential for severe hyperkalemia. Questions have been raised about the initial use of diuretics, which lack renal protective effects because of stimulation of the renin-angiotensin system and maintenance of a high glomerular capillary pressure (24).

The most useful agents in renal failure are those that affect the renin-angiotensin system, and do not adversely affect renal perfusion. β-Blockers decrease blood pressure by inhibiting renin release in addition to their β-blocking and central effects. Propranolol has been shown to decrease GFR and renal blood flow in some studies. Nadolol and atenolol are excreted to a large extent by the kidneys and require dosage modification at creatinine clearances below 0.83 ml/sec (50 ml/min).

The central-acting agents methyldopa and clonidine are both useful in reducing blood pressure with no decrease in renal blood flow. Because methyldopa and its active metabolite accumulate with decreased renal function, dosing adjustments are necessary. Clonidine requires dosing adjustments at clearances below 0.83 ml/sec (50 ml/min).

The peripheral vasodilators, hydralazine and minoxidil, are not used alone in the hypertension of renal failure because of compensatory mechanisms causing increased renin release, sodium retention, and tachycardia, which occur as a result of decreased peripheral vascular resistance. However, in combination with agents that decrease volume and renin, they are effective in the management of uncontrolled hypertension. These agents do not require dosing modifications in renal failure because of their high hepatic clearance. The α-adrenergic blockers prazosin, terazosin, and doxazosin reduce blood pressure by producing venous and arterial vasodilation. They are useful in treating patients with renal failure, do not adversely affect renal function, and do not require dosing modifications with decreased creatinine clearance.

Captopril, enalapril, and lisinopril are oral angiotensin-converting enzyme (ACE) inhibitors that exhibit greatest blood pressure control in patients with high renin activity. The ACE inhibitors lower blood pressure primarily by decreasing peripheral resistance. In patients with renal impairment, some studies have shown a beneficial effect of ACE inhibitors on glomerular filtration rate and renal plasma blood flow. The ACE inhibitors may be useful in renal vascular hypertension; however, caution must be exercised in the presence of renal artery stenosis because of the possibility of precipitating acute tubular necrosis (see "Drug-induced Nephropathies," below). The ACE inhibitors may be used alone or in combination with other classes of antihypertensives. Although captopril, at the higher doses of the drug used initially, was found to cause proteinuria, newer studies have found that the ACE inhibitors may be beneficial in reducing proteinuria, especially in patients with concomitant diabetes and in hypertension associated with chronic glomerular disease. Most ACE inhibitors are excreted renally and thus require dosage modification in patients with renal impairment (23).

GASTROINTESTINAL DISORDERS

Patients with advanced renal failure commonly have gastrointestinal complications such as anorexia, nausea, and vomiting. They complain frequently of a metallic or salty taste and their breath smells of ammonia. They may develop stomatitis, parotitis, erosive gastritis, uremic colitis, and mucosal and submucosal ulcerations.

Uremics have high urea concentrations in salivary secretions, which undergoes conversion to ammonia in the presence of bacterial ureases. Many symptoms are due to the irritative effects of ammonia on the gastrointestinal tract.

Frequently antacids are administered to patients with gastrointestinal irritation. When the creatinine clearance falls to below 0.5 ml/sec (30 ml/min) magnesium-containing antacids should be restricted. If magnesium-containing antacids are given in chronic renal failure, serum magnesium levels may rise above 3.0 mmol/liter (6 mEq/liter), causing depression of the central nervous system, lethargy, somnolence, and loss of deep tendon reflexes. Dialysis removes magnesium effectively and may be indicated if severe toxicity develops.

Nephrotic Syndrome

Nephrotic syndrome is the metabolic and clinical consequence of continued heavy proteinuria, usually greater than 3 g of protein/day. In addition to proteinuria this syndrome is characterized by hypoalbuminemia, edema, hyperlipidemia, and hypercoagulability. A large number of glomerular lesions can be associated with sufficient proteinuria to produce nephrotic syndrome. Factors causing glomerulonephropathies that result in nephrotic syndrome include systemic, metabolic, and endocrine diseases; allergens; microorganisms; drugs; and toxins (Table 19.6).

Increased glomerular permeability to plasma protein leads to each of the clinical and metabolic derangements associated with nephrotic syndrome. Hypoalbuminemia is the direct result of albumin loss in the urine, which accounts for 60 to 90% of urinary protein. Loss of larger molecular weight proteins including immunoglobulins is associated with abnormalities in immune response and increased susceptibility to serious infections. Enhanced hepatic synthesis of lipoproteins appears to result from hypoalbuminemia and a reduction in colloid osmotic pressure. The associated hyperlipidemia may cause an increased risk of ischemic heart disease. Edema is due to sodium retention by the kidney and a reduction in intravascular colloid osmotic pressure. Edema seen with nephrotic syndrome is marked by a distribution pattern that

includes the face and periorbital region, particularly in the morning. Edema of the lower extremities can be seen as the day progresses. Numerous defects in clotting factors, the fibrinolytic system, and platelet function are responsible for the hypercoagulable state. Low levels of antithrombin III seem to correlate with the clotting defects.

Treatment is aimed at reducing risk factors and symptoms associated with nephrotic syndrome. Hypoalbuminemia is managed by maintaining an adequate dietary protein intake to insure optimal hepatic albumin synthesis. Growing children require 3 to 5 g per kilogram per day. Adults require 1 to 1.2 g per kilogram per day. Edema calls for dietary sodium restriction of 1 to 2 g per day. Nonsteroidal antiinflammatory drugs such as indomethacin 150 mg daily or angiotensin-converting enzyme inhibitors have been shown to reduce proteinuria and reduce the tendency for edema formation. Hyperlipidemia is treated with dietary control of saturated fat and cholesterol intake. Lipid-lowering agents may be used if LDL-cholesterol levels remain elevated. Efforts should also be directed toward reducing other atherosclerotic risk factors such as smoking and hypertension and adding a mild exercise program. Treatment of the hypercoagulable state is directed toward prevention of embolic events. Patients should avoid prolonged immobilization. Prophylactic anticoagulation is necessary with unavoidable immobilization or in patients with a previous history of thromboembolism (75).

Because of the large variety of glomerular diseases associated with nephrotic syndrome, histologic evaluation is often necessary to determine the specific lesion. Treatment depends on the histologic findings or the presence of signs or symptoms suggestive of a systemic disease. Idiopathic nephrotic syndrome, that arising from an unknown cause, is usually treated with steroids. Steroid therapy with oral prednisone 60 mg/m²/day in divided doses for 4 to 8 weeks is used to achieve remission, particularly in children. Steroids are then used primarily to minimize the frequency and complications of relapse. Short courses of intermittent steroid therapy, 40 mg/m² in a single dose on alternate days for 4 weeks have been used to prevent relapse and minimize steroid toxicity. Cytotoxic therapy has been used in frequently relapsing patients who develop steroid toxicity. Cyclophosphamide (2 to 3 mg/kg/day) and chlorambucil (0.2 mg/kg/day) induce prolonged remission. The reader is referred to disease-specific treatment protocols for other types of glomerulonephropathy (11, 22, 76).

ACUTE RENAL FAILURE
Definition

Acute renal failure is defined as a sudden decline in renal function accompanied by an accumulation of nitrogenous wastes normally excreted by the kidney. It is caused by a process within the kidney itself and is not reversed by correction of extrarenal factors. Urine volume may vary over a wide range. A urine volume under 50 ml/day constitutes anuria. If the urine volume is below 400 ml but above 50 ml/day, it is described as oliguria. Urine volumes that exceed 400 ml/day are referred to as nonoliguria or high-output acute renal failure. Up to 50% of drug-induced acute renal failure is nonoliguric. "Acute renal failure" should be distinguished from "acute tubular necrosis." Acute tubular necrosis is a histologic finding signifying necrotic damage to the renal tubules, and not all patients developing acute renal failure exhibit tubular necrosis on renal biopsy. Unfortunately, these terms are often used interchangeably.

Etiology

Prerenal azotemia is caused by any event that results in decreased renal perfusion or intense renal vasoconstriction. The causes of prerenal azotemia are listed in Table 19.19. Postrenal azotemia is simply an accumulation of nitrogenous wastes secondary to obstruction of urine flow in the urinary tract. The causes of postrenal azotemia are listed in Table 19.20. Acute renal failure has been associated with numerous surgical and medical insults. A list of causes is provided in Table 19.21. Some specific drug-induced nephropathies are discussed separately.

With a patient who suddenly develops oliguria with rising BUN and serum creatinine concentrations, it is important to distinguish among (a) acute renal failure, (b) prerenal azotemia, and (c) postrenal azotemia. Initial efforts should be directed toward ruling out urinary tract obstruction. Factors suggesting obstruction include a normal urinalysis, rapid changes in urine output, and residual urine on postvoiding catheterization. If renal calculi are

Table 19.19.
Causes of Prerenal Azotemia

Hypovolemia
    Blood loss
    Vomiting, diarrhea
    Diuretic overuse
    Burns
Peripheral vasodilation
    Bacteremia
    Antihypertensive drugs
Decreased cardiac output
    Myocardial infarction
    Congestive heart failure
    Pulmonary embolism
    Pericardial tamponade
Increased renal vascular resistance
    Anesthesia
    Surgery

Table 19.20.
Causes of Postrenal Azotemia

Bilateral ureteral obstruction
    Intraureteral
        Blood clots
        Stones
        Crystals
    Papillary necrosis
        Acute pyelonephtritis
    Extraureteral
        Tumor
        Retroperitoneal fibrosis
Bladder neck obstruction
    Mechanical
        Bladder infection
        Prostatic hypertrophy
        Bladder carcinoma
    Functional
        Autonomic insufficiency
        Ganglionic blocking agents
        Anticholinergics
Urethral obstruction

Table 19.21.
Causes of Acute Renal Failure

Sequelae of prolonged prerenal azotemia
Nephrotoxins
Ischemic events
    Massive hemorrhage
    Crush injury
    Transfusion reaction
    Septic shock
    Pregnancy
Glomerulus and small blood vessel disease
    Poststreptococcal glomerulonephritis
    Bacterial endocarditis
    Malignant hypertension
    Systemic lupus erythematosus
    Drug-induced vasculitis
Other causes
Hyperuricemia
Hypercalcemia

present, a radiograph of the abdomen will detect the 90% that are radiopaque.

In the absence of obstruction the urinary indices provide the most reliable method of distinguishing prerenal azotemia from acute renal failure. Table 19.22 will help in distinguishing reversible prerenal failure from acute renal failure, but its usefulness is limited following the administration of diuretics or in those patients with underlying chronic renal failure.

Treatment

The treatment of acute renal failure consists of the prevention of associated complications. Infection and gastro-

Table 19.22.
Urinary Findings in Prerenal Azotemia and Other Forms of Acute Renal Failure[a]

	Prerenal Azotemia	Acute Renal Failure
Urine sodium	<20	>40
Urine osmolality	>500	<400
Urine plasma creatinine (U/PCr)	>40	<20
Renal failure index:	<1	>2
$\quad$ Urine sodium		
$\quad$ $\overline{\text{U/P Cr}}$		
Fractional sodium excretion:	<1	>1
$\quad$ U/P sodium × 100		
$\quad$ $\overline{\text{U/P Cr}}$		
Urine sediment	Normal	Granular casts, cellular debris

[a] Adapted from Schrier RW, Conger JD, Acute renal failure: pathogenesis, diagnosis and management. In Schrier RW (ed): Renal and Electrolyte Disorders, ed. 3. Boston, Little, Brown & Co, 1986, pp 423–460.

intestinal bleeding are complications that frequently plague the very ill patient in an acute care setting. Careful maintenance of intravenous lines, minimal use of indwelling bladder catheters, and early recognition and treatment of wound and other infections is necessary. Surveillance for signs of blood loss, such as testing stools for occult blood, monitoring the hematocrit, and control of gastric pH with H_2-antagonists or antacids, will minimize the morbidity associated with bleeding.

Patients with nonoliguric renal failure have a better prognosis, with fewer complications, fewer requirements for dialysis, and shorter hospital courses than those with oliguric renal failure. Although no carefully controlled studies exist, some evidence shows that early conversion of oliguric to nonoliguric renal failure with furosemide and/or mannitol will improve the patient's outcome. The combined effects of increased cardiac output and renal blood flow with dopamine administration may benefit patients unresponsive to diuretics alone. Dopaminergic effects predominate at doses 1 to 5 μg/kg/min and result in increased renal flow because of renal artery vasodilation. At higher doses, however, α-receptor effects predominate and cause renal artery vasoconstriction.

The early use of dialysis in the management of acute renal failure has been associated with increased survial. A small prospective study of casualties during the Vietnam War demonstrated that patients whose BUN was maintained below 18 mmol/liter (50 mg/dl) and whose serum creatinine concentration was maintained below 442 μmol/liter (5 mg/dl) had a mortality rate of 37%, whereas those given dialysis for a BUN above 43 mmol/liter (120 mg/dl) and serum creatinine concentration above 884 μmol/liter

(10 mg/dl) had a mortality rate of 80%. It is postulated that early dialysis provides a better biochemical environment for fighting infections and for wound healing. For the same reason, maintenance of adequate nutrition during acute renal failure has been advocated.

Most patients developing acute renal failure have a complete clinical recovery if early supportive therapy is provided. Some, however, may regain only a fraction of their previous renal function, and a few may go on to chronic end-stage renal failure.

DRUG-INDUCED NEPHROPATHIES

The kidneys are uniquely vulnerable to toxic injury because of their high blood flow, large endothelial surface area, concentrating ability, and metabolic activity. Representing only 0.4% of total body weight, the kidneys receive 20 to 25% of the cardiac output. Relative to their weight, the kidneys have the largest endothelial surface area of any organ. Concentration of potential nephrotoxins occurs within the renal tubules, through secretion and reabsorption, thus exposing the tubular lumen and peritubular cells to high concentrations of potential toxins. Renal medullary and papillary tissues are vulnerable to toxic damage because of a combination of low blood flow and extremely high solute concentration. Finally, the kidneys are highly active metabolic organs capable of transforming relatively innocuous substances, such as acetaminophen, into highly reactive metabolites.

The lesions associated with drug-induced nephropathy can be divided into four major categories: acute tubular necrosis (ATN), acute tubulointerstitial disease (ATID), chronic tubulointerstitial disease (CTID), and glomerulonephritis (GN). A list of drugs and chemicals associated with each of these lesions is provided in Table 19.13.

Acute tubular necrosis is a nonspecific response to either ischemia or direct toxic insult. Acute renal failure results from cellular by-products of tubular necrosis obstructing the proximal tubule. As intratubular pressure increases and glomerular filtration is reduced, filtered wastes regain access to the circulation by leaking across transtubular membranes (33–35). The type of cellular injury associated with acute tubular necrosis varies with the type of renal insult. In a study of 121 patients who developed acute tubular necrosis, the following renal insults were found: hypotension (74%), dehydration (35%), sepsis (31%), toxins (25%), and pigmenturia (22%). More than one acute insult was identified in 65% of these patients (36).

Acute tubulointerstitial disease, also known as acute interstitial nephritis, is characterized by interstitial edema and renal cellular infiltrates made up of monocytes, large and small lymphocytes, and plasma cells. Eosinophils may or may not be present. Tubular damage is suggested by the presence of cellular infiltrates located along the tubular basement membrane or between tubular epithelial cells (37). Drug-induced acute tubulointerstitial disease appears to be a hypersensitivity reaction and often is associated with systemic signs of an allergic reaction such as fever, skin rash, eosinophilia, and arthralgia. Hypersensitivity is further suggested by the small number of patients developing the reaction, the lack of dose-related effect, and a sudden recurrence with reinstitution of therapy (38, 39).

The renal lesions associated with chronic tubulointerstitial disease are deep within the medulla, close to the tip of the renal papilla. Capillary sclerosis and necrosis of these medullary structures can extend to include degeneration of the loops of Henle. Interstitial fibrosis can cause tubular compression, resulting in functional impairment of the tubules. Clinical symptoms consist of progressive renal insufficiency, varying degrees of hypertension, hematuria, leukocyturia, and proteinuria. Analgesic nephropathy, the most widely known form of this disease, is responsible for more chronic renal failure worldwide than any other drug-induced nephropathy.

Glomerulonephritis may be caused by several different mechanisms. In some cases there is a direct dose-dependent effect on glomerular structures; in the majority, however, the glomerulus is involved through immunologic reactions. Drugs may act as haptens or antigens that either produce circulating antigen-antibody complexes or cause complex formation within the glomerulus. Damage to or alteration of the glomerular basement membrane produces proteinuria, a hallmark of this disease. The most common drug-induced lesion has been membranous glomerulonephritis with proteinuria and nephrotic syndrome. Nephrotic syndrome consists of heavy proteinuria (>3.5 g/day), hypoalbuminemia <30 g/liter (3.0 g/dl), edema, and hyperlipidemia (11).

Selected Nephrotoxic Drugs

AMINOGLYCOSIDES

Aminoglycosides are avidly concentrated within the renal cortex. Following initial binding to tubular brush border membranes, they are vacuolized and taken up by the proximal tubular cells. Once within the cell, they are transported to the lysosomes. Continued uptake results in lysosomal dysfunction and eventual degeneration, allowing lysosomal enzymes to act on other cell organelles. Tubular cell necrosis may result from continued exposure. The initial manifestations of nephrotoxicity include release of brush border and lysosomal enzymes, glycosuria, aminoaciduria, and tubular proteinura. Defects in proximal tubular transport may be detected by the presence of β_2-microglobulin. Hypokalemia, hypomagnesemia, and loss of concentrating ability may also be seen. Patients who develop aminoglycoside nephrotoxicity are most often non-

oliguric. The occurrence of toxicity is most closely related to the duration of therapy and is usually seen between the 7th and 10th days. Observers have implicated from 6 to 12 additional risk factors for the development of nephrotoxicity, including age, dose, high trough serum concentrations, and initial renal function; however, each of these has been discounted in well-controlled studies. Proper patient selection based on culture and sensitivity data, early withdrawal of unnecessary therapy, and dose adjustment to ensure therapeutic levels seems to be the most prudent way of minimizing toxicity (40–46).

AMPHOTERICIN B

Interaction of amphotericin B with membrane sterols results in disruption of cell membranes. The possibility of direct vasoconstriction of the renal vasculature has also been suggested. Toxicity is dose-related and is seen in up to 80% of patients treated with a cumulative dose of 2 to 3 g. Early manifestations of amphotericin B nephrotoxicity include renal-concentrating defects, distal renal tubular acidosis with potassium wasting, and modest proteinuria. The occurrence of renal failure is usually associated with proximal tubular necrosis. Since nephrotoxicity often limits a full course of therapy, many attempts to limit toxicity have been tried. To date, no regimen or manipulation in therapy has been found to attenuate the toxicity consistently, although encouraging results have been seen with sodium supplementation of 150 mEq/day. Alternate-day therapy may be used when toxicity is recognized, and discontinuation is recommended when the BUN exceeds 18 mmol/liter (50 mg/dl) (40, 47, 48).

CYCLOSPORINE

Cyclosporine has achieved a major role in the prevention of allograft rejection. The most common side effect is a dose-dependent decline in GFR with reversible increases in serum creatinine and BUN concentrations. This toxicity can complicate the management of renal transplant recipients since distinguishing between graft rejection and cyclosporine toxicity is difficult, even with the use of decision algorithms (49). In a review of 122 biopsies from 60 consecutive allograph recipients receiving cyclosporine, it was considered that a diagnosis of rejection could only be made with the finding of diffuse interstitial infiltrates or arteritis (50). Enhanced toxicity may occur with the simultaneous use of acyclovir, ketoconazole, amphotericin B, aminoglycosides, and cotrimoxazole. Reduction in toxicity has been attempted with transdermal clonidine and thromboxane synthetase inhibitors (51, 52). Attempts have been made to monitor plasma levels of cyclosporine to maintain trough concentrations at 100 to 250 ng/ml. In vitro data suggest that there is little immunosuppression in mixed lymphocyte cultures at concentrations below 100 ng/ml. The search for a therapeutic window between toxic and subtherapeutic concentrations will continue, and the use of pharmacokinetic monitoring will be an important function at transplantation centers (53–55). (See Chapter 20 "Dialysis & Renal Transplantation.")

RADIOGRAPHIC CONTRAST MEDIA

The increased use of contrast media associated with intravenous pyelography, angiography, and computed tomography has led to greater recognition of this class of agents as an important cause of acute renal failure. The diagnosis must be considered when one of these agents is used in a high-risk patient who subsequently develops any degree of renal failure. Mild nonoliguric renal failure may be transient, with serum creatinine reaching a peak in 3 to 5 days with a return to baseline within 10 to 14 days. Severe oliguric renal failure may occur within 24 hr of the contrast study, with either a return to baseline within 3 weeks, residual renal impairment, or renal failure requiring dialysis. High-risk patients include those with diabetes mellitus, preexisting renal disease, multiple myeloma, advanced age, coexisting liver disease, peripheral vascular disease, hypertension, dehydration, and prior exposure to contrast media. On urinalysis the urine may be isosmolar; however, the specific gravity is extremely high. Urinary sodium concentration is low, and fractional sodium excretion (FE_{Na}) is extremely low, when compared with that in other forms of renal failure. The precise mechanism of nephrotoxicity in unknown but may include impaired renal perfusion, glomerular injury, tubular injury, and tubular obstruction. Prevention is aimed at avoidance of unnecessary procedures; vigorous hydration, particularly in high-risk patients; using low doses of contrast media; and avoidance of multiple contrast procedures. The use of hyperosmolar (1500 mOsm/kg) or less hyperosmolar (750 mOsm/kg) contrast agents does not seem to influence the risk for developing nephrotoxicity. Extracellular volume expansion with 800 ml/hr of normal saline during the procedure and liberal oral or parenteral fluids both before and after the procedure have minimized toxicity dramatically, even in high-risk patients (40, 56–58).

ANGIOTENSIN-CONVERTING ENZYME INHIBITORS

Acute reversible nonoliguric renal failure has been observed during initiation of captopril and enalapril therapy. This complication is most often seen in patients with bilateral renovascular disease or renal artery stenosis. Renal failure has also been described in patients with a low cardiac output and decreased effective renal blood flow. The underlying mechanism appears to be interference with the normal compensatory process in such patients. Low renal perfusion pressures result in activation of the renin-angiotensin system to maintain sufficient arterial pressures to reestablish renal blood flow. Inhibition of the angio-tensin-converting enzyme can thus produce an acute decline in renal perfusion, resulting in ATN. An immunologic mechanism may be responsible for renal impairment in some patients, because of associated symptoms such as fever, rash, and eosinophilia. Proteinuria with nephrotic syndrome is a rare complication of captopril therapy. More commonly, a reversible mild proteinuria has been seen that may improve even with continued therapy (59–61).

CHRONIC ANALGESIC ABUSE

The two renal lesions seen with chronic analgesic abuse are papillary necrosis and cortical interstitial nephritis. Together they represent the syndrome identified as chronic tubulointerstitial disease (CTID). Ischemia is an important factor in the development of papillary necrosis, since the oxygen tension near the papillae is about 20 mm Hg. Local production of prostaglandins probably promotes dilation of medullary blood vessels and maintains local blood flow. Prostaglandin inhibitors therefore have a role in the development of chronic toxicity. In addition, the kidney is capable of converting phenacetin and acetaminophen to highly reactive intermediates in the presence of salicylates. Combination analgesic therapy seems always to be a feature in this disease. Other clinical features of this disease include nocturia, hematuria, renal colic, and the occasional finding of necrotic tissue in the urine. Of patients who develop this form of chronic renal failure, approximately 23% have continued deterioration of renal function and 12% either die or receive maintenance dialysis within 6 months of diagnosis. Healthcare practitioners can play a critical role in recognizing analgesic abusers. Reformulation of essentially all combination analgesic products that once contained phenacetin has not caused a significant reduction in this disease (62–65).

CISPLATIN

Cisplatin is highly concentrated in the proximal tubular cells. Intracellular transformation of the chloride ligands on the molecule into a highly reactive aquated compound is thought to occur because of the low intracellular chloride concentration. This transformed molecule is then able to alkylate purine and pyrimidine bases of DNA. ATN occurs because cellular degeneration results in a proximal tubular obstruction from cellular debris. The incidence and severity of renal toxicity is both dose- and duration-dependent. A rise in serum creatinine and BUN levels may be preceded by proteinuria, tubular casts, enzymuria, and the presence of β_2-microglobulin in the urine. Cisplatin nephrotoxicity has been reduced with predose hydration of a saline solution. One such approach has been the administration of 5% dextrose in 0.45 to 0.9% sodium chloride at a rate of 250 ml/hr beginning 2 hr prior to cisplatin. The dose of cisplatin is administered in 250 ml of a 3%

sodium chloride solution. Mannitol 12.5 g is given as a bolus immediately prior to cisplatin and then infused at the rate of 10 g/hr for 3 hr. This technique provides adequate chloride to prevent the aquation reaction within the cisplatin container and provides an osmotic diuresis to minimize exposure to proximal tubular cells (40, 66, 67).

DOSING MODIFICATION IN RENAL DISEASE (See Chapter 1 "Clinical Pharmacokinetics")

Drugs that are largely dependent on the kidney for elimination are expected to require major dosing modification in states of impaired renal function. Since drug clearance by the kidneys is closely related to their ability to clear endogenous creatinine, estimations of creatinine clearance are commonly performed to facilitate dosing in this patient population.

Many formulas have been derived that relate serum creatinine (cr) to an estimated creatinine clearance (Cl_{cr}):

$$Cl_{cr}(\text{ml/min}) = \frac{(140 - \text{age}) \times \text{wt (kg)}}{72\, cr\,(\text{mg/dl})} \quad (19.4)$$

$$Cl_{cr}(\text{ml/min/72 kg}) = \frac{(140 - \text{age})}{cr\,(\text{mg/dl})} \quad (19.5)$$

$$Cl_{cr}(\text{ml/min/1.73 m}^2) = \frac{98 - 0.8\,(\text{age} - 20)}{cr\,(\text{mg/dl})} \quad (19.6)$$

For equations (19.4) and (19.5), the creatinine clearance for females is 85% of the calculated value (68). For equation (19.6), the creatinine clearance for females is 90% of the calculated value (69). The choice between equations (19.4) and (19.5) depends upon the intended application of the result. If creatinine clearance is being estimated to provide an accurate reflection of actual glomerular filtration rate, then equation (19.4) is preferred. However, if the result is going to be compared with a normal creatinine clearance to determine the fraction of normal renal function for dosing adjustment, equation (19.5) is preferred. Both equations (19.5) and (19.6) allow comparison of clearance, adjusted for either weight or body surface area, with estimates of renal function in persons without renal impairment.

Both drug clearance (Cl) and the rate constant for elimination (k) depend upon the sum of all processes of clearance or elimination; for example

$$Cl = Cl(\text{renal}) + Cl(\text{hepatic}) + Cl(\text{other})$$

$$k = k(\text{renal}) + k(\text{hepatic}) + k(\text{other})$$

In the current discussion the elimination rate constant (k) is defined as:

$$k = k(\text{renal}) + k(\text{nonrenal}) \quad (19.7)$$

Since the fraction excreted unchanged term (f) describes the fraction of total drug that is eliminated by the kidneys, the following relationship is established:

$$k(\text{renal}) = k(f) \quad \text{and} \quad k(\text{nonrenal}) = k(1 - f)$$

Substitution into equation (19.7) yields

$$k = k(f) + k(1 - f)$$

Since nonrenal elimination is assumed to be unchanged in renal impairment, multiplication of the $k(f)$ term by a patient's fractional renal function (Fx) provides an estimate of the elimination rate constant in failure (k_{fail} described by equation (19.9) (below). Thus,

$$Fx = \frac{Cl_{cr}(\text{patient})}{Cl_{cr}(\text{normal})} \quad (19.8)$$

and

$$k_{fail} = k(f)Fx + k(1 - f)$$

which can be simplified to

$$k_{fail} = k[f(Fx - 1) + 1] \quad (19.9)$$

where k is the normal elimination rate constant ($k = .693/t_{1/2}$), f is the fraction excreted unchanged, and Fx is the fraction of normal renal function, as described previously. The normal creatinine clearance [$Cl_{cr}(\text{normal})$] is assumed to be 100 ml/min/1.73 m^2 (or 72 kg).

Once k_{fail} has been determined, dosing adjustments can be made for any first-order drug in patients with renal impairment. Table 19.23 provides normal kinetic parameters for a selected group of drugs.

By selecting target plasma concentrations for peak and trough levels, as in the case of intermittent dosing, a suitable dosing interval can be established. Equation (19.10) relates two plasma concentrations to the first-order decay process:

$$Cp_t = Cp_o e^{-k_{fail}} \quad (19.10)$$

where Cp_o is the initial concentration and Cp_t the concentration at time t. Solving for t in equation (19.10) determines the time required to reduce the plasma concentration from Cp_o to Cp_t

$$t = \frac{\ln(Cp_o/Cp_t)}{k_{fail}} \quad (19.11)$$

Since the calculated time t from peak to trough plasma concentration does not always represent a reasonable dosing interval, an acceptable dosing interval (τ) will be chosen (e.g., 4, 6, 8, 12, 24, or 48 hr). The peak and/or trough plasma concentrations will be modified slightly, depending on how close t was to the selected τ.

The amount of drug lost with each dosing interval is the dose that needs to be replaced to maintain the desired peak and trough concentrations. Just as equation (19.10)

Table 19.23.
Pharmacokinetic Parameters[a]

Drug	Oral Bioavailability (%)	Half-Life (hr)	Volume of Distribution (liter/kg)	Fraction Excreted Unchanged	Plasma Protein Binding (%)
Acebutolol	37	2.7	1.2	0.4	26
Acecainide	83	9.5	1.4	0.85	11
Acetaminophen	80	2	1	0.03	15
Acetazolamide	95	4.1	0.2	0.8	92
Acetohexamide[b]	c	2	0.2	0.1	80
Acetohydroxamic	55	8	0.55	0.55	0
Acyclovir	23	2.5	0.6	0.75	15
Alfentanil		1.6	1	0.01	90
Allorpurinol[b]	85	5	0.6	0.3	0
Alprazolam	92	10.6	0.72	0.2	71
Alprenolol[b]	9	2.5	3.4	0.01	85
Amantadine	70	16	6.6	0.7	67
Amdinocillin		1.1	0.22	0.59	10
Amikacin		2.3	0.27	0.98	5
Amiloride		21	17	0.49	40
Aminoglutethimide	100	10	0.74	0.2	24
Amiodarone	35	600	66	0.01	99
Amitriptyline[b]	48	16	14	0.02	94
Amoxicillin	93	1	0.41	0.52	18
Amphetamine	98	12	4.1	0.4	15
Amphotericin-B		18	0.76	0.03	95
Ampicillin	50	1.3	0.37	0.9	18
Amrinone	93	3.6	1.2	0.25	40
Aprindine[b]	90	30	4	0.01	90
Aspirin[d]	68	5	0.21	0.4	85
Atenolol	55	6.3	0.7	0.8	5
Atropine	50	4.3	1.7	0.57	18
Auranofin	20	480	0.05	0.15	60
Azathioprine	60	0.2	0.81	0.02	30
Azlocillin		1	0.22	0.65	28
Aztreonam		1.6	0.18	0.67	56
Betamethasone	72	5.6	1.4	0.05	64
Betaxolol	0	15	7.4	0.16	53
Bleomycin		3.1	0.27	0.68	0
Bretylium	23	9	5.9	0.8	4
Bumetanide	90	1	0.15	0.55	95
Busulfan	unknown	2.6	0.99	0.01	unknown
Caffeine	100	4.9	0.61	0.01	36
Captopril	65	1.9	0.81	0.38	27
Carbamazepine[b]	80	15	1.4	0.01	74
Carbamazepine-epoxide	90	7.4	1.1	0.01	50
Carbenicillin	5	1	0.18	0.8	50
Cefaclor	90	0.8	0.24	0.6	25
Cefadroxil		1.3	0.15	0.93	5
Cefamandole		0.8	0.16	0.96	74
Cefazolin		1.8	0.12	0.85	79
Cefonicid		5	0.11	0.88	98
Cefoperazone		1.8	0.1	0.28	90
Ceforanide		2.8	0.14	0.84	80
Cefotaxime		1.2	0.24	0.65	40
Cefotetan		3.7	0.19	0.65	84
Cefoxitin		0.7	0.31	0.78	73
Cefsulodin		1.6	0.26	0.7	22
Ceftazidime		1.8	0.25	0.88	17
Ceftizoxime		1.8	0.36	0.93	28
Ceftriaxone		8	0.15	0.6	90
Cefuroxime		1.7	0.198	0.96	35
Cephalexin	90	0.9	0.25	0.96	14

(continued)

Table 19.23. (*Continued*)

Drug	Oral Bioavailability (%)	Half-Life (hr)	Volume of Distribution (liter/kg)	Fraction Excreted Unchanged	Plasma Protein Binding (%)
Cephalothin	52	0.6	0.25	0.52	71
Cephapirin[b]		1.2	0.13	0.48	62
Cephradine	95	0.77	0.25	0.84	12
Chlorambucil	87	1.3	0.29	0.01	99
Chloramphenicol	85	2.7	0.91	0.25	53
Chlordiazepoxide[b]	100	10	0.3	0.01	96
Chloroquine[d]	89	1030	115	0.61	61
Chlorothiazide	30	1.5	0.2	0.92	94
Chlorpheniramine	35	13	2.5	0.2	72
Chlorpromazine[b]	32	30	20	0.01	96
Chlorpropamide	90	33	0.1	0.2	87
Chlorthalidone	64	44	3.9	0.65	76
Cilastatin		0.8	0.2	0.7	35
Cimetidine	62	2	0.81	0.6	20
Cinoxacin		2.1	0.33	0.7	63
Ciprofloxacin	83	3.5	2	0.35	30
Cisplatin		0.53	0.28	0.23	
Clavulanic acid	75	0.9	0.21	0.43	9
Clindamycin	85	2.7	0.65	0.12	94
Clofibrate	95	8.6	0.12	0.06	96
Clonazepam	98	23	3.2	0.01	86
Clonidine	95	8.5	2.1	0.62	20
Cloxacillin[e]	49	0.6	0.1	0.75	93
Cocaine	57	0.8	2	0.02	91
Codeine	50	2.9	2.6	0.01	7
Cyclophosphamide	74	6.5	0.64	0.07	13
Cyclosporine	23	5.6	1.2	0.01	93
Cytarabine	20	2.6	3	0.11	13
Dapsone	90	22	1	0.15	73
Demeclocycline	70	12	1.8	0.45	80
Desipramine	38	22	20	0.02	82
Desmethyldiazepam	99	73	0.78	0.01	97
Dexamethasone	78	3	0.82	0.03	68
Diazepam[b]	100	40	1.1	0.01	98
Diazoxide	90	48	0.21	0.4	94
Diclofenac	54	1.1	0.17	0.01	99
Dicloxacillin[e]	70	0.8	0.08	0.6	94
Diflunisal	90	11	0.1	0.06	99
Digitoxin	90	160	0.54	0.32	97
Digoxin	65	39	4.5	0.6	25
Diltiazem	44	3.2	5.3	0.04	80
Diphenhydramine	51	4.1	6.5	0.02	78
Disopyramide	83	6	0.59	0.55	28
Doxepin[b]	30	16	20	0.01	0
Doxorubicin	5	36	25	0.15	82
Doxycycline	93	16	0.75	0.4	86
Enalapril	41	11	1.7	88	50
Encainide[b,f]	30	2.3	3.6	0.05	70
Enoxacin	79	5		0.6	0
Erythromycin	36	1.6	0.71	0.13	84
Esmolol		0.13	1.9	0.01	55
Ethambutol	77	3.1	1.5	0.79	25
Ethanol	80	0.24	0.54	0.03	0
Ethosuximide	100	45	0.72	0.25	0
Etoposide	55	7.5	0.24	0.37	94
Famotidine	41	3.2	1.25	0.67	18
Fenoprofen	0	3	0.15	0.03	99
Fentanyl		3.7	4	0.08	80
Flecainide	95	20	1.5	0.25	40

(*continued*)

Table 19.23. (*Continued*)

Drug	Oral Bioavailability (%)	Half-Life (hr)	Volume of Distribution (liter/kg)	Fraction Excreted Unchanged	Plasma Protein Binding (%)
Flucloxacillin	49	0.8	0.11	0.41	96
Flucytosine	84	4.2	0.68	0.98	4
Flunitrazepam	85	15	3.3	0.01	78
Fluorouracil	28	0.16	0.25	0.02	10
Fluxetine	60	53	35	0.02	94
Flurazepam (desalkyl)		74	22	0.01	97
Furosemide	63	1.5	0.12	0.66	98
Gentamicin		2	0.25	0.95	5
Glipizide	90	2.8	0.16	0.08	96
Glyburide	90	1.6	0.12	0.01	99
Gold thiomalate		600	0.26	0.75	95
Griseofulvin	45	14	1.6	0.01	0
Guanadrel	90	12		0.45	20
Guanethidine	35	120	60	0.43	0
Halperidol	70	17	17	0.01	92
Hexobarbital	90	3.7	1.2	0.01	48
Hydralazine	25	1	1.6	0.1	12
Hydrochlorothiazide	71	2.5	0.83	0.95	64
Ibuprofen	85	2	0.15	0.03	95
Imipenem		0.9	0.23	0.69	17
Imipramine[b]	27	18	23	0.01	95
Indomethacin	98	2.4	0.26	0.15	90
Isoniazid	95	2	0.67	0.18	0
Isosorbide dinitrate	22	0.8	1.5	0.01	28
Isotretinoin		14	7	0.01	99
Kanamycin		2	0.26	0.9	1
Ketaconazole	unknown	3.3	2.4	0.01	99
Ketamine	20	2.3	1.8	0.04	12
Ketoprofen	90	1.5	0.11	0.01	99
Labetalol	18	4.9	9.4	0.03	50
Lidocaine[b]	35	1.8	1.1	0.02	35
Lincomycin	100	5	0.44	0.2	72
Lithium	100	22	0.8	0.95	0
Lorazepam	93	14	1.3	0.01	91
Lorcainide	40	7.6	6.4	0.02	83
Melphalan	71	1.4	0.62	0.12	0
Meperidine[b]	60	3.5	4.5	0.05	55
Meprobamate	0	10	0.75	0.15	10
Mercaptopurine	12	0.9	0.56	0.22	19
Methadone	92	35	3.8	0.24	89
Methicillin		0.9	0.42	0.88	40
Methohexital		3.9	2.2	0.01	0
Methotrexate	65	7.2	0.55	0.48	34
Methyldopa	25	1.8	0.37	0.28	8
Methylprednisolone	82	2.5	0.84	0.05	50
Metoclopramide	70	5	3.4	0.2	40
Metocurine		4.7	0.35	0.5	35
Metoprolol	38	3.2	4.2	0.1	13
Metronidazole	99	9	0.74	0.1	10
Mexiletine	90	9.2	6	0.1	63
Mezlocillin[d]		1	0.2	0.73	30
Miconazole	27	22	21	0.05	91
Midazolam	44	1.9	1.1	56	95
Minocycline	100	18	1.3	0.11	76
Minoxidil	95	3.1	2.7	0.2	0
Moricizine	38	4	4.3	0.01	95
Morphine	26	1.9	3.2	0.08	35
Moxalactam		2.1	0.25	0.76	50
Nadolol	34	18	2.1	0.73	20
Nafcillin	36	1	0.35	0.25	86

(*continued*)

Table 19.23. (*Continued*)

Drug	Oral Bioavailability (%)	Half-Life (hr)	Volume of Distribution (liter/kg)	Fraction Excreted Unchanged	Plasma Protein Binding (%)
Nalidixic acid	100	2	0.4	0.02	93
Naltrexone	20	2.7	19	0.01	20
Naproxen	99	14	0.16	0.01	99
Netilmicin		2.2	0.2	0.85	5
Nicardipine	25	1.3	1.1	0.01	95
Nicotine	30	2	2.6	0.16	5
Nifedipine	50	1.8	0.78	0.01	96
Nitrazepam	78	26	1.9	0.01	84
Nizatidine	90	1.3	1.2	0.61	35
Nomifensine[b]	unknown	3	8	0.01	70
Norfloxacin	35	5	3.2	0.29	15
Nortriptyline	51	31	18	0.02	94
Oxacillin[e]	33	0.5	0.33	0.46	93
Oxazepam	97	6.8	0.6	0.01	98
Oxytetracycline	60	9	1.4	0.7	30
Pancuronium		2.3	0.26	0.67	29
Penbutolol	95	21	0.52	0.05	90
Penicillin-G	22	0.6	0.2	0.7	60
Pentamidine		6.2	16	0.03	
Pentazocine	47	4.6	7.1	0.15	65
Pentoxifylline	19	1.6	2.4	0	0
Phenobarbital	98	100	0.54	0.24	55
Phenylbutazone[b]	90	56	0.1	0.03	96
Phenylethylmalonamide	91	16	0.69	0.79	8
Phenytoin[c]	98	22	0.6	0.02	90
Pindolol	75	3.6	2.3	0.54	51
Piperacillin		1	0.16	0.71	21
Piroxicam	0	48	0.15	0.04	99
Practolol	95	7	1.6	0.9	10
Prazosin	68	2.9	0.6	0.01	95
Prednisolone	82	2.2	1.5	0.15	93
Prednisone[b]	80	3.6	0.97	0.03	75
Primidone[b]	92	8	0.59	0.42	19
Probenecid	100	7	0.13	0.01	89
Procainamide[b]	89	3.5	1.9	0.67	15
Propranolol[b]	26	3.9	4.3	0.01	87
Protriptyline	84	78	22	0.01	92
Pyridostigmine	14	1.9	1.1	0.85	0
Pyrimethamine	0	83	2.9	0.65	87
Quinidine[b]	75	6.2	3	0.18	87
Quinine	90	11	1.8	0.12	93
Ranitidine	52	2.1	1.3	0.69	15
Reserpine	unknown	60	1.7	0.01	40
Rifampin	c	3.5	0.97	0.07	89
Sisomicin		3	0.19	0.45	10
Sotalol	60	9	0.7	0.6	54
Spironolactone	25	1.6	14	0.01	90
Streptomycin		2.6	0.25	0.6	48
Sufentanil		2.7	1.7	0.06	93
Sulfadiazine	100	9.9	0.29	0.57	54
Sulfamethoxazole	100	10.1	0.21	0.14	62
Sulfinpyrazone	100	4	0.74	0.39	98
Sulfisoxazole	96	6.6	0.15	0.49	90
Sulindac		15	2	0.01	99
Suprofen	90	2.5	0.17	0.15	99
Suramin		1152	0.57	0.6	99
Temazepam[b]	85	13	1.06	0.01	97
Terazosin	90	12	0.8	0.12	92
Terbutaline	14	14	1.8	0.56	20
Tetracycline	77	9.9	1.4	0.58	65

(*continued*)

Table 19.23. (*Continued*)

Drug	Oral Bioavailability (%)	Half-Life (hr)	Volume of Distribution (liter/kg)	Fraction Excreted Unchanged	Plasma Protein Binding (%)
Tetrahydrocannabinol	8	32	8.9	0.01	95
Theophylline	96	9	0.5	0.18	56
Thiopental		9	2.3	0.01	85
Ticarcillin		1.3	0.21	0.92	65
Timolol	50	4.1	2.1	0.15	10
Tobramycin		2.2	0.28	0.95	5
Tocainide	89	13	3	0.4	10
Tolbutamide	93	5.9	0.1	0.01	96
Tolmetin	90	4.9	0.54	0.07	99
Trazodone	81	5.9	1	0.01	93
Triamterene	54	4.2	13.4	0.52	61
Triazolam	44	2.9	1.1	0.02	90
Trimethoprim	100	11	1.8	0.69	44
Tubocurarine		2	0.39	0.63	50
Valproic acid	100	14	0.22	0.02	93
Vancomycin		5.6	0.39	0.79	30
Vecuronium		1.5	0.21	0.18	30
Verapamil[b]	22	4	5	0.03	90
Warfarin	93	37	0.14	0.02	99
Zidovudine	63	1.1	1.4	0.18	22

[a] The values in this table are representative of the literature and do not reflect the large veriability that may be present with certain drugs or parameters. Adapted principally from Benet LZ, Williams RL, Design and optimization of dosage regimens; pharmacokinetic data. In Gilman AG, Rall TW, Nies AS, Taylor P (eds): The Pharmacologic Basis of Therapeutics, ed. 8., New York, Pergamon Press, 1990, pp 1650–1735; and Benet LZ, Massoud N, Pharmacokinetic Basis for Drug Treatment. New York, Raven Press, 1984, pp 1–28.

[b] Drug with active metabolite(s). Adapted from Gambertoglio JG, Effects of renal disease: altered pharmacokinetics. In Benet LZ, Massoud N, Gambertoglio JG (eds): Pharmacokinetic Basis for Drug Treatment. New York, Raven Press, 1984, pp 149–171.

[c] Drug is well absorbed, although not extensively studied.

[d] Drugs displaying saturation kinetics. Values for half-life are dose dependent and should not be applied to general populations.

[e] Drugs that do not require modification in renal failure becuase of increased nonrenal elimination.

[f] Data are representative of extensive metabolizers (approximately 90% of population).

relates plasma concentrations, equation (19.12) relates two amounts of drug in the body to the first-order decay process:

$$A_t = A_o e^{-kt} \qquad (19.12)$$

where A_t = the amount of drug present at the time of measurement and A_o = the initial amount of drug. The amount lost with each dosing interval is $A_o - A_t$. By substituting equation (19.12) into this simple relationship:

$$\text{amount lost} = A_o - A_o e^{-kt}$$

or

$$\text{amount lost} = A_o(1 - e^{-kt})$$

Since the amount of drug (*A*) in the body at any time is equal to the product of the plasma concentration (*Cp*) and the volume of distribution (V_d)

$$\text{dose} = Cp_o V_d (1 - e^{k_{fail}\tau}) \qquad (19.13)$$

A stepwise approach to dosing adjustment for renal impairment is given below.

Step	Equation
1. Estimate the patient's creatinine clearance.	(19.5) or (19.6)
2. Determine fractional renal function (*Fx*).	(19.13)
3. Obtain normal pharmacokinetic parameters from Table 19.23 or other sources	
4. Determine k_{fail}.	(19.9)
5. Selected desired peak and trough concentrations, and calculate a dosing interval. *Note:* If concentrations are unknown, the peak is estimated by dividing a normal dose by the volume of distribution found in Table 19.23. The trough is estimated by using equation (19.10), where *t* equals a normal dosing interval.	(19.11)
6. Calculate the dose.	(19.3)

Equation (19.13) assumes that the dose is given as a bolus and that no drug is lost during the infusion period. This may, in fact, be a reasonable assumption, since we are dealing with patients who have real impairment and delayed drug elimination. The amount of drug lost during

Table 19.24.
Relative Error in Assuming Negligible Elimination during an Infusion[a]

$$(n = t_{1/2}/t')^2$$

n	% Relative Error
1	27.8
2	15.5
3	10.7
4	8.2
5	6.6
6	5.6
7	4.8
8	4.2
16	2.1
32	1.1

[a] From Robinson DC, Principles of pharmacokinetics. In Maronde RF (ed): Topics in Clinical Pharmacology and Therapeutics. New York, Springer-Verlag, 1986, pp 1–12, with permission.

an infusion period depends on the relationship between half-life ($t_{1/2}$) and time of infusion (t'). Table 19.24 predicts the error that occurs by assuming negligible drug elimination during an infusion. For example, a postdose plasma concentration for a drug with an estimated $t_{1/2}$ of 4 hr that was infused over 30 min would be overestimated by 4.2% if the bolus equation were used. For intermittent infusion kinetics the reader is referred to other sources (73, 74).

CONCLUSION

The normally functioning kidney is a marvelous organ that regulates and maintains the body's internal environment. Although it is highly susceptible to a variety of injuries, the kidney can recover from most of the iatrogenic misadventures it encounters. On the other hand, a large number of patients have progressive renal disease secondary to systemic disorders such as diabetes and hypertension and require aggressive management of the underlying condition to halt the progression of disease. A third type of renal disease results from intrinsic disorders of the kidney, for which little can be done to halt disease progression. The goals of therapy are the symptomatic support and normalization of the internal environment through dietary control, judicious use of drugs, and dialysis. In each case outcome is improved with early recognition and effective therapeutic management of renal disease.

REFERENCES

1. Personal communication: National Kidney Foundation, 1990.
2. Kampmann JP, Hansen JM: Glomerular filtration rate and creatinine clearance. Br J Clin Pharmacol 12:7–14, 1981.
3. Baum N, Dichoso CC, Carlton CE: Blood urea nitrogen and serum creatinine: physiology and interpretations. Urology 5:583–588, 1975.
4. Neu HC: A symposium on the tetracyclines: a major appraisal. Bull NY Acad Med 54:141–155, 1978.
5. Siest G, Galteau M-M: Drug Effects on Laboratory Test Results. Analytical Interferences and Pharmacological Effects. St. Louis, Year Book Medical Publishers, 1988.
6. Friedman RB, Young DS: Effects of Disease on Clinical Laboratory Tests, ed. 2. Washington D.C.: The American Association of Clinical Chemistry, 1990.
7. Bjornsson TD: Use of serum creatinine concentrations to determine renal function. Clin Pharmacokinet 4:200–222, 1979.
8. Ross DL, Neely AE: Textbook of Urinalysis and Body Fluids. Norwalk, CT: Appleton-Century-Crofts, 1983, pp 68–122.
9. Kark RM, Lawrence JR, Pollak VE, et al.: A Primer of Urinalysis, ed. 2. New York: Harper & Row, 1963.
10. Young DS: Effects of Drugs on Clinical Laboratory Tests, ed 3. Washington D.C.: The American Association of Clinical Chemistry, 1990.
11. Hutt MP, Kelleher SP: Proteinuria and the nephrotic syndrome. In Schrier RW (ed): Renal and Electrolyte Disorders, ed. 3. Boston, Little, Brown & Co, 1986, pp 565–589.
12. Alfrey AC: Chronic renal failure: manifestations and pathogenesis. In Schrier RW (ed): Renal and Electrolyte Disorders, ed 3. Boston, Little, Brown & Co, 1986, pp 461–494.
13. Levey AS, Madaio MP, Perrone RD: Laboratory assessment of renal disease: clearance, urinalysis, and renal biopsy. In Brenner BM, Rector FC (eds): The Kidney, ed 4. Philadelphia, WB Saunders, 1991, pp 919–968.
14. Tsochope W, Ritz E: The management of renal insufficiency. In Suki WN, Massry SG (eds): Therapy of Renal Diseases and Related Disorders. Boston, Martinus Nijhoff, 1984, pp 495–504.
15. Balasa RW, Murray RL, Kondelis NP, et al.: Phosphate-binding properties and electrolyte content of aluminum hydroxide antacids. Nephron 45:16–21, 1987.
16. Watson AJS, Keogh JAB: 1-Deamino-8-D-arginine vasopressin on prolonged bleeding time in chronic renal failure. Nephron 32:49–52, 1982.
17. Fried W, Hematological aspects of uremia. In Nissenson AR, Fine RN, Gentile DE (eds): Clinical Dialysis, ed 2. Norwalk, CT, Appleton-Crofts, 1990, pp 391–408.
18. Paganni EP: Overview of anemia associated with chronic renal disease: primary and secondary mechanisms. Semin Nephrol 9(suppl 1):3–8, 1989.
19. Schwenk MA, Halstenson CE: Recombinant human erythropoietin. DICP, Ann Pharmacother 23:528–536, 1989.
20. Rabkin R, Simon NM, Steiner S, Calwell JA: Effect of renal disease on renal uptake and excretion of insulin in man. N Engl J Med 282:182–186, 1970.
21. Smith JD, DeFronzo RA: Endocrine dysfunction in chronic renal failure. In Nissenson AR, Fine RN, Gentile DE (eds): Clinical Dialysis, ed 2. Norwalk, CT, Appleton-Crofts, 1990, pp 458–493.
22. Eknoyan G: Noninflammatory vascular diseases of the kidney. In Suki WN, Massry SG (eds): Therapy of Renal Diseases and Related Disorders. Boston, Martinus Nijhoff, 1984, pp 283–288.
23. Mason NA: Angiotensin-converting enzyme inhibitors and renal function. DICP, Ann Pharmacother 24:496–505, 1990.
24. Bauer JH, Reams GP: Antihypertensive drugs. In Brenner BM, Rector FC (eds): The Kidney, ed 4. Philadelphia, WB Saunders Co, 1991, pp 2148–2173.
25. Border WA, Glassock RJ: The management of nephrotic syndrome. In Suki WN, Massry SG (eds): Therapy of Renal Diseases and Related Disorders. Boston, Martinus Nijhoff, 1984, pp 195–208.

26. Schrier RW, Conger JD: Acute renal failure: pathogenesis, diagnosis and management. In Schrier RW (ed): Renal and Electrolyte Disorders, ed. 3. Boston, Little, Brown & Co, 1986, pp 423–460.

27. Dixon BS, Anderson RJ: Nonoliguric acute renal failure. Am J Kidney Dis 6:71–80, 1985.

28. Wilkes BM, Mailloux LU: Acute renal failure: pathogenesis and prevention. Am J Med 80:1129–1136, 1986.

29. Brezis M, Rosen S, Epstein FH, Acute renal failure. In Brenner BM, Rector FC (eds): The Kidney, ed. 4. Philadelphia, WB Saunders, 1991, pp 993–1061.

30. Hyneck ML: Current concepts in clinical therapeutics: drug therapy in acute renal failure. Clin Pharm 5:892–910, 1986.

31. Man HJ, Fuhs DW, Hemstrom CA: Acute renal failure. Drug Intell Clin Pharm 20:421–438, 1986.

32. Hou SH, Bushinsky DA, Wish JB, et al.: Hospital-acquired renal insufficiency: a prospective study. Am J Med 74:243–248, 1983.

33. Myers BD, Moran SM: Hemodynamically mediated acute renal failure. N Engl J Med 314:97–105, 1986.

34. Stein JH, Fried TA: Experimental models of nephrotoxic acute renal failure. Transplant Proc 17:72–80, 1985.

35. Solez K, Racusen LC, Olsen S: The pathology of drug nephrotoxicity. J Clin Pharmacol 23:484–490, 1983.

36. Rasmussen HH, Ibels LS: Acute renal failure: multivariate analysis of causes and risk factors. Am J Med 73:211–218, 1982.

37. Antonovych TT: Drug-induced nephropathies. In Sommers SC, Rosen PP (eds): Pathol Annu 19(part 2):165–196, 1984.

38. Laberke HG: Drug-associated nephropathy part II: tubulointerstitial lesions. In Berry CL et al. (eds): Current Topics in Pathology. New York, Springer-Verlag. 1980, pp 183–215.

39. Revert L, Montoliu J: Acute interstitial nephritis. Semin Nephrol 8:82–88, 1988.

40. Bennett WM, Elzinga LW, Porter GA: Tubulointerstitial disease and toxic nephropathy. In Brenner BM, Rector FC (eds): The Kidney, ed 4. Philadelphia, WB Saunders, 1991, pp 1430–1496.

41. Matzke GR, Lucarotti RL, Shapiro HS: Controlled comparison of gentamicin and tobramycin nephrotoxicity. Am J Nephrol 3:11–17, 1983.

42. Sawyers CL, Moore RD, Lerner SA, et al.: A model for predicting nephrotoxicity in patients treated with aminoglycosides. J Infect Dis 153:1062–1068, 1986.

43. Williams PJ, Hull JH, Sarubbi FA, et al.: Factors associated with nephrotoxicity and clinical outcome in patients receiving amikacin. J Clin Pharmacol 26:79–86, 1986.

44. Johnson MW, Mitch WE, Heller AH, et al.: The impact of an educational program on gentamicin use in a teaching hospital. Am J Med 73:9–14, 1982.

45. Garrison MW, Rotschafer JC: Clinical assessment of a published model to predict aminoglycoside-induced nephrotoxicity. Ther Drug Monit 11:171–175, 1989.

46. Contreras AM, Gamba G, Cortes J, et al.: Serial trough and peak amikacin levels in plasma as predictors of nephrotoxicity. Antimicrob Agents Chemother 33:973–976, 1989.

47. Heidemann HTH, Gerkens JF, Spickard WA, et al.: Amphotericin B nephrotoxicity in humans decreased by salt repletion. Am J Med 75:476–481, 1983.

48. Sacks P, Fellner SK: Recurrent reversible acute renal failure from amphotericin. Arch Intern Med 147:593–595, 1987.

49. Kahan BD: Clinical summation. An algorithm for the management of patients with cyclosporine-induced renal dysfunction. Transplant Proc 17:303–308, 1985.

50. Neild GH, Taube HE, Hartley RB, et al.: Morphological differentiation between rejection and cyclosporin nephrotoxicity in renal allografts. J Clin Pathol 39:152–159, 1986.

51. Luke J, Luke DR, Williams LA, et al.: Prevention of cyclosporine-induced nephrotoxicity with transdermal clonidine. Clin Pharm 9:49–53, 1990.

52. Smeesters C, Chaland P, Giroux L, et al.: Prevention of acute cyclosporine A nephrotoxicity by a thromboxane synthetase inhibitor. Transplant Proc 20(suppl 2):658–564, 1988.

53. Luke RG, Greifer I: Posttransplant risks of cyclosporine: nephrotoxicity. Am J Kidney Dis 5:342–343, 1985.

54. Whiting PH, Simpson JG: The enhancement of cyclosporine A included nephrotoxicity by gentamicin. Biochem Pharmacol 32:2025–2028, 1983.

55. Burckart GJ, Canafax DM, Yee GC: Cyclosporine monitoring. Drug Intell Clin Pharm 20:649–652, 1986.

56. Mission RT, Cutler RE: Radiocontrast-induced renal failure. West J Med 142:657–664, 1985.

57. Dawson P: Contrast agent nephrotoxicity. An appraisal. Br J Radiol 58:121–124, 1985.

58. Parfrey PS, Griffiths SM, Barrett BJ, et al.: Contrast material-induced renal failure in patients with diabetes mellitus, renal insufficiency, or both. N Engl J Med 320:143–149, 1989.

59. Textor SC, Gephardt GN, Bravo EL, et al.: Membranous glomerulopathy associated with captopril therapy. Am J Med 74:705–711, 1983.

60. Peirpont GL, Francis GS, Cohn JN: Effect of captopril on renal function in patients with congestive heart failure. Br Heart J 46:522–527, 1981.

61. Packer M: Identification of risk factors predisposing to the development of functional renal insufficiency during treatment with converting-enzyme inhibitors in chronic heart failure. Cardiology 76(suppl 1):50–55, 1989.

62. Knapp M, Avioli LV: Analgesic nephropathy. Arch Intern Med 142:1197–1199, 1982.

63. Schreiner GE, McAnally JF, Winchester JF: Clinical analgesic nephropathy. Arch Intern Med 141:349–357, 1981.

64. Nanra RS: Renal effects of antipyretic analgesics. Am J Med 75(suppl):70–81, 1983.

65. Goldberg M: Analgesic nephropathy historical and epidemiological overview. In Bertani T (ed): Drugs and Kidney. New York, Raven Press, 1986, pp 193–201.

66. Litterst CL: Alterations in the toxicity of cis-dichlorodiamine-platinum-II and in tissue localization of platinum as a function of NaCl concentration in the vehicle of administration. Toxicol Appl Pharmacol 61:99–108, 1981.

67. Finley RS, Fortner CL, Grove WR: Cisplatin nephrotoxicity: a summary of preventative interventions. Drug Intell Clin Pharm 19:362–367, 1985.

68. Cockcroft DW, Gault MH: Predictions of creatinine clearance from serum creatinine. Nephron 15:31–41, 1976.

69. Jelliffe RW: Estimation of creatinine clearance when urine cannot be collected. Lancet 1:975–976, 1971.

70. Benet LZ, Williams RL: Design and optimization of dosage regimens; pharmacokinetic data. In Gilman AG, Rall TW, Nies AS, Taylor P (eds): The Pharmacologic Basis of Therapeutics, ed. 8. New York, Pergamon Press, 1990, pp 1650–1735.

71. Benet LZ, Massoud N: Pharmacokinetics. In Benet LZ, Massoud N, Gambertoglio JG (eds): Pharmacokinetic Basis for Drug Treatment. New York, Raven Press, 1984, pp 1–28.

72. Gambertoglio JG: Effects of renal disease: altered pharmacokinetics. In Benet LZ, Massoud N, Gambertoglio JG (eds): Pharmacokinetic Basis for Drug Treatment. New York, Raven Press, 1984, pp 149–171.

73. Robinson DC, Principles of pharmacokinetics. In Maronde RF (ed):

Topics in Clinical Pharmacology and Therapeutics. New York, Springer-Verlag, 1986, pp 1–12.

74. Gibaldi M, Perrier D (eds): Pharmacokinetics. New York, Marcel Dekker, 1982.

75. Bernard DB, Salant DJ: Clinical approach to the patient with proteinuria and the nephrotic syndrome. In Jacobson HR, Striker GE, Klahr S (eds): The Principles and Practice of Nephrology. Philadelphia, BC Decker, 1991, pp 250–261.

76. Sherbotle JR, Hoyer JR: Idiopathic nephrotic syndrome: minimal-change disease and focal segmental glomerulosclerosis. In Jacobson HR, Striker GE, Klahr S (eds): The Principles and Practice of Nephrology. Philadelphia, BC Decker, 1991, pp 288–292.

CHAPTER 20

DIALYSIS AND RENAL TRANSPLANTATION

GARY R. MATZKE, Pharm.D., F.C.P., F.C.C.P, DAVID R. LUKE, Pharm.D., F.A.C.A.,
ROBERT DUPUIS, Pharm.D., and REGINALD F. FRYE, Pharm.D.

Renal failure may be due to glomerular or tubular damage of the kidney by prerenal factors, such as dehydration or decreased cardiac output, or postrenal factors, such as ureteral obstruction or neoplasm (1). Renal failure may also develop secondary to systemic diseases (e.g., diabetes mellitus) or result from exposure to toxic substances. Progressive renal disease ultimately results in disturbances of electrolyte and water balance and in the accumulation of nitrogenous waste products, such as creatinine and urea nitrogen (2). The effects of renal failure extend beyond the kidney and are seen in other organ systems. Cardiovascular, pulmonary, neuromuscular, and central nervous system disturbances are common in patients with renal failure (2, 3).

The principal purpose of dialysis is to serve as an "artificial kidney" and restore to normal the concentrations of electrolytes and waste products within the bloodstream. Although dialysis can mimic the filtration function of the kidney, it does not replace the renal tubular reabsorptive or secretive functions that have been lost. Furthermore, dialysis does not compensate in any way for the endocrinologic and metabolic activities of the kidney, which appear to decline in parallel with the loss of filtration capacity (4). Despite these limitations, the maintenance of life after the development of end-stage renal disease can be achieved by the use of dialysis therapy. Dialysis therapy can be divided into two main types: (a) that done by the bloodstream (i.e., hemodialysis), and (b) that done by the peritoneal cavity (i.e., peritoneal dialysis).

Long-term hemodialysis treatment of chronic renal failure was first initiated in the 1960s after the introduction of the Scribner shunt, an external-access device that provided permanent access to the bloodstream (3, 5). The ends of this shunt are implanted into an artery and a vein and connected to the hemodialysis system outside of the body (5). In 1966, Brescia and Cimino developed a surgical technique to create an internal-access device (6). Anastomosis of an artery and a vein forms an arteriovenous (AV) fistula that allows access to the circulation by skin puncture. These advances in blood access ushered in the current era of hemodialysis.

Although the first human use of peritoneal dialysis was reported by Ganter in 1923, the broad utilization of this mode of therapy was limited by the availability of a suitable access device for chronic therapy (3). However, the development of this type of device in the late 1960s did not greatly enhance the use of peritoneal dialysis (7). The principle reasons for this were the high rate of adverse effects, especially peritonitis and bowel perforation, and the lack of patient acceptance. This lack of patient acceptance was in part due to the severe limitations on the patient's lifestyle. Specifically, the dialysis process often required 10 to 12 hours per treatment and three or four treatments a week.

In 1978, continuous ambulatory peritoneal dialysis (CAPD) was developed and freed patients from most of these lifestyle limitations (8). As the name implies, CAPD is a continuous dialysis process that allows the patient a more normal ambulatory lifestyle. The peritoneal cavity is continuously filled with dialysis fluid that the patient exchanges three to six times per day. Exchanges are performed by gravity, and no machinery is required for the filling and draining procedures.

Hemodialysis and peritoneal dialysis are thus relatively new treatment modalities for renal insufficiency. Furthermore, due to frequent modifications in dialyzer membranes, delivery systems for blood and dialysate, and peritoneal dialysis techniques, the state of the art is rapidly changing.

PRINCIPLES OF DIALYSIS

Despite continual modifications in the biotechnology of dialysis, the basic principles of hemodialysis and peritoneal dialysis have remained unchanged since the introduction of these modes of therapy over 50 years ago. Fundamentally, hemodialysis consists of the perfusion of heparinized blood and physiologic salt solution on opposite sides of a semipermeable membrane. The waste products of protein metabolism move from the blood into the dialysate by passive diffusion along concentration gradients (1) (Fig. 20.1). Inversely, if a substance is in the physiologic salt solution (i.e., dialysate) in a higher concentration than that in the blood, this solute will diffuse from the dialysate into the systemic circulation.

The second process that occurs during dialysis is ultrafiltration, the extraction of water from the blood by a hydrostatic pressure gradient. This is the primary mode for removal of excess body fluids. Ultrafiltration (expressed as ml/hr/mm Hg) can be maximized by increasing the hydrostatic pressure gradient (mm Hg) across the dialysis membrane. Total separation of diffusion and ultrafiltration does not occur in standard hemodialysis situations. However, these two processes may be performed in sequence in some selected patients. This form of "sequential" hemodialysis therapy is particularly beneficial for patients with fluid overload between dialysis periods as well as for patients with poor cardiac function who are unable to tolerate simultaneous, extensive ultrafiltration. With sequential dialysis, some patients may tolerate removal of as much as 4 liters of fluid/hr (9). The primary problem of long-term sequential dialysis treatment is that the reduced diffusion time may not allow adequate removal of uremic waste products.

As with hemodialysis, dialysis across the peritoneal membrane also consists of diffusion and ultrafiltration (10). Diffusion occurs from the blood to the dialysate or from the dialysate to the blood depending upon the concentration gradient for the particular substance (Fig. 20.2). The degree of diffusion is influenced critically by the thickness of the peritoneal membrane, the effective surface area of the membrane that is exposed to the dialysate, the peritoneal capillary blood flow, the dialysate flow rate, the volume of instilled dialysate, and the temperature of the dialysate (10).

Unlike hemodialysis, where the membrane that separates the blood from the dialysate compartment can be selected to obtain the optimal diffusion and ultrafiltration, with peritoneal dialysis only one membrane is available per patient. Ultrafiltration during peritoneal dialysis can be accomplished by changing the dextrose concentration in the dialysate. An increase in dextrose concentration will result in an increase in the amount of fluid removed.

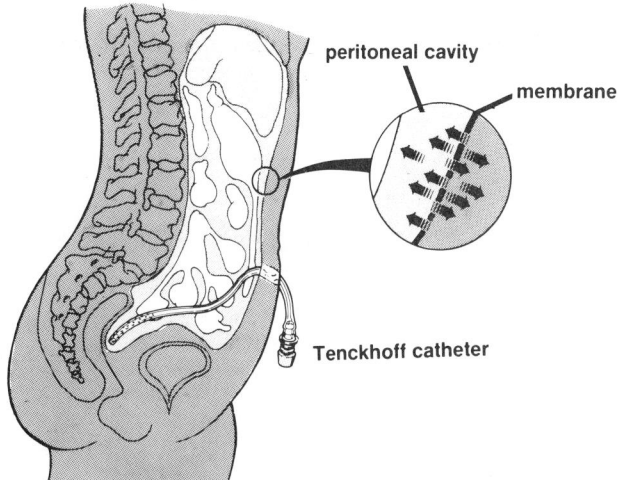

Figure 20.2. Diffusion and ultrafiltration occur across the peritoneal membrane and are depicted in the expanded insert of this figure. These processes are bidirectional, that is, solutes and water can be absorbed from the peritoneal cavity or drawn into the cavity. The rate-limiting process is the concentration of a particular solute and dextrose in the dialysis fluid.

DIALYSIS ACCESS

Dialysis access can be achieved at the bedside by insertion of a catheter into the femoral or subclavian vein for hemodialysis or via the insertion of a stylocath (single-use catheter) into the peritoneal cavity for peritoneal dialysis. Significant problems can occur with these initial temporary access devices, including venous thrombosis, emboli, and infection (9).

Permanent access to the bloodstream for hemodialysis (11) or the peritoneal cavity for peritoneal dialysis (12) may be accomplished by several techniques. The simple AV fistula has the longest survival of all blood-access devices, with the lowest rate of complications. Bovine grafts and polytetrafluoroethylene (PTFE) grafts have also been used for chronic dialysis access. The choice of a blood-access device depends primarily on how soon the patient will require dialysis and the adequacy of the patient's vascular system.

The first catheter developed for long-term peritoneal dialysis was described by Tenckhoff in 1968 (7, 12). The present version of this catheter has a low rate of abdominal discomfort during dialysis and may be used immediately for initiation of dialysis. Several other catheters for long-term peritoneal dialysis have been introduced in the last few years (12). The relative advantages and disadvantages of these access devices remain theoretical.

DIALYZERS

In recent years numerous new hemodialysis filters have become available (13, 14). Two basic forms of dialyzers,

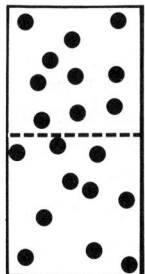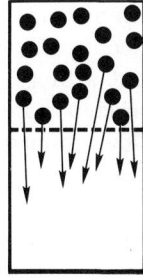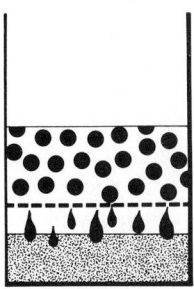

Diffusion   **Ultrafiltration**

Figure 20.1. Diffusion of endogenous solutes from the blood to the dialysate (*left panel*) is limited by the pore size of the membrane (*shown as a dashed line*), the molecular size of the solute, and the time that the dialysate fluid is in contact with the blood. Ultrafiltration (*right panel*) is the removal of plasma water with or without the accompaniment of solute. The limiting processes for water removal are the amount of pressure the membrane can tolerate without rupturing and the pressure difference that is created across the membrane.

Table 20.1.
Characteristics of Frequently Used Dialysis Filters[a]

Filter	Composition	Urea (ml/min) (BFR[b] = 200)	Clearance (ml/min) (BFR = 300)	Ultrafiltration Coefficient (ml/hr/mm HG)
Hollow fiber				
Asashi				
AM-100L	Cuprammonium rayon	155	184	2.4
AM-300M	Cuprammonium rayon	183	235	6.4
Baxter				
CA 50	Cellulose acetate	127	144	2.4
CA 110	Cellulose acetate	176	215	5.3
CA 210	Cellulose acetate	192	266	10.1
CF 12.11	Cuprophan	160	192	2.9
CF 15.11	Cuprophan	169	205	4.1
CD Medical				
3500	Cellulose acetate	130	155	3.5
4000-R	Cellulose acetate	157	174	3.8
Fresenius				
F-60	Polysulfone	180	225	5.8
F-80	Polysulfone	185	235	7.6
Terumo				
TAF 8	New regenerated cellulose	160	196	4.0
TAF 12	New regenerated cellulose	180	232	6.1
Toray				
B2-0.5	Polymethylmethacrylate	123	NA	2.5
B2-1.6	Polymethylmethacrylate	183	NA	4.2
Flat plate				
Gambro				
10-3N	Cellulose	152	190	3.5
10-5N	Cellulose	175	210	4.8

[a] Adapted from Nolph KD, Peritoneal anatomy and transport physiology; and Tawa NE, Tilney NL, Angioaccess in the renal failure patient. In Maher JF (ed): Replacement of Renal Function by Dialysis, ed. 3. Dordrecht, Holland, Kluwer Academic Publishers, 1989.
[b] BFR, blood flow rate.

the flat plate and the hollow fiber dialyzer, now predominate) (Table 20.1). Most dialysis centers use several types of dialyzers and select the optimal dialysis filter for the individual patient. For stable young patients without cardiac or bleeding problems, the dialyzer with the highest clearance of urea and creatinine, the two primary uremic waste products, should be selected. With older patients, very small individuals, and those with multiple medical complications, greater attention and individualization is required (9).

TECHNIQUE

In essence, the process of hemodialysis consists of pumping the patient's heparinized blood through the blood compartment of the dialysis filter at a rate of 200 to 500 ml/min (15). (Fig. 20.3) Generally anticoagulation is achieved by infusing heparin either continuously or intermittently throughout dialysis into the blood line of the dialyzer. The dialysate fluid is prepared from a commercially available concentrated liquid or dried salts and treated water. This fluid is warmed to body temperature and then perfused through the dialysate compartment of the dialysis filter. Although several types of hemodialysis machines may still be available in different clinical settings, most of the current generation of dialysis machines are single-pass systems. That is, the dialysate flows through the system one time and is not recycled. This process results in greater efficiency of diffusion since there is no accumulation of endogenous solutes within the dialysate compartment.

The duration of dialysis therapy has steadily decreased during the last 20 years from approximately 12 hours three times a week to 4 hours three times a week (4). Recent advances in dialysis technology, including the use of highly permeable membranes and precise volumetric control systems, have made "high flux" or short dialysis a practical form of treatment (16). With this mode of dialysis, it may be possible to reduce dialysis time by approximately 30 to 40% while maintaining adequate solute and fluid removal.

Shortening of the duration of dialysis is not without complications (17). Indeed the use of "short" (i.e., less

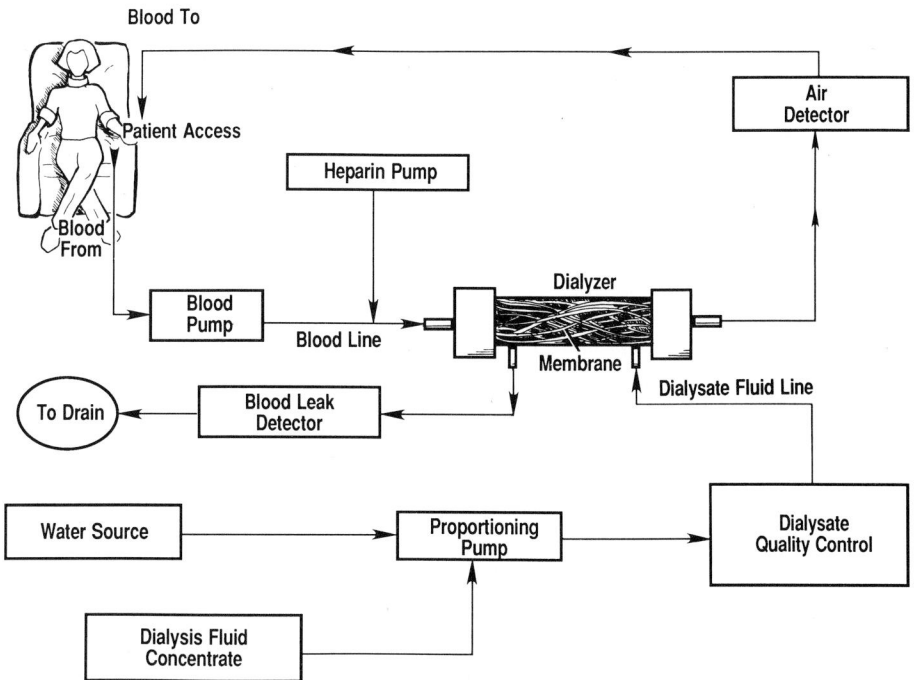

Figure 20.3. Outline of the blood flow and dialysate flow pathways during hemodialysis. Blood flows from the patient via the blood pump at a rate of 200 to 500 ml/min through the dialyzer and back to the patient. Heparin is administered into the blood line to prevent blood clotting in the dialyzer. The dialysate is prepared via the combination of dialysis fluid concentrate with water then pumped at a rate of 500 to 800 ml/min through the dialysate side of the dialyzer.

than 3½ hr) dialysis treatments has been associated with an increased risk of morbidity and mortality, which may be due in part to insufficient removal of urea and other endogenous waste products and/or nonoptimal variance in the patient's interdialytic weights. Maintenance of an appropriate interdialytic weight requires that a certain volume of fluid be removed each dialysis session. If the dialysis period is shortened, fluid must be removed more rapidly, which may produce symptomatic hypotension in some patients. Conversely, if less than the optimal amount of water is removed during dialysis, hypertension may result secondary to the interdialytic weight (fluid) gain (18).

Peritoneal dialysis has also undergone several modifications over the years. Currently, three types of peritoneal dialysis procedures are in use. Chronic ambulatory peritoneal dialysis is by far the most frequently used technique. With this dialysis technique, the patient instills 1 to 3 liters of dialysate into the abdominal cavity, folds up the dialysate bag (which is still attached to the peritoneal catheter) and continues with normal daily activities (8). The patient usually performs four exchanges per day. This allows approximately 4 to 5 hr during the day and 8 hr for the overnight dwell of the fluid in the peritoneal cavity. After each equilibration period of 5 to 8 hr, the peritoneal cavity is drained and the fluid discarded. Using sterile tech-

niques, the patient refills the peritoneal cavity with fresh fluid. The other two modes of dialysis—intermittent dialysis performed with automated equipment or a cycler, and continuous cycler peritoneal dialysis—are not used frequently for long-term therapy of renal insufficiency (9). They are the predominant routes of peritoneal dialysis in the acute care environment.

COMPLICATIONS

Complications of dialysis can be divided into those related to the dialysis access, those related to the dialysis procedure itself, and those general medical problems that may or may not be specifically related to dialysis. The predominant complications that may occur secondary to hemodialysis access are clotting of the access, infection, ischemia and/or gangrene, and high-output congestive heart failure (9, 19). Complications of peritoneal access include catheter site infection, peritoneal fluid leakage, and inflow or outflow obstruction, which may occur because of kinking or constriction or may be secondary to catheter malposition or intraluminal obstruction by fibrin plugs (9, 20).

Complications related to the hemodialysis procedure include disequilibrium syndrome, hypotension, and air embolism, as well as muscle cramps and pruritus (4, 9). Of these, hypotension is probably the most common complication and may occur in as many as 10% of all hemodialysis procedures. Peritonitis is by far the major complication associated with chronic peritoneal dialysis therapy (21, 22).

The incidence of peritonitis is approximately 1.3 episodes per patient per year (22). The most frequently isolated organisms are Gram-positive, with *Staphylococcus epidermidis* being the most prevalent, followed by *Staphylococcus aureus* and *Streptococcus* species. The most common Gram-negative organisms isolated include *Escherichia coli, Klebsiella, Enterobacter*, and *Pseudomonas*. Fungi are isolated in less than 5% of cases and culture-negative peritonitis represents 3 to 10% of cases (21, 23). Empiric therapy generally includes vancomycin or a first-generation cephalosporin such as cefazolin, with or without an aminoglycoside. The third-generation cephalosporin ceftazidime has been shown to be an effective and less toxic alternative to aminoglycosides (24). The recent publication of a series of algorithmic approaches to the initiation and evaluation of an infective therapy should standardize and optimize the treatment of CAPD peritonitis (22). The other potential complications of peritoneal dialysis include abdominal wall hernias, backache, hyperglycemia, and hypertension.

DIALYSIS PRESCRIPTION

Determination of the optimal dialysis prescription for a given patient in terms of the method of dialysis, choice of dialysis filter if hemodialysis is used, dialysis time, and the frequency of the dialysis procedure is an individualized process. The dialysis therapy prescription is devised to provide adequate solute (diffusional component) and fluid removal (ultrafiltration). Urea kinetic modeling can be used to assess small solute removal and is based on the following relationship between dialysis filter urea clearance (K), time on dialysis (t), and urea volume of distribution (Vdu);

$$\text{Dialysis Index (DI)} = (K \cdot t)/Vdu \qquad (20.1)$$

DI is a unitless parameter that functions as an index of the adequacy of dialysis. Values of 1.8 for twice-weekly and 1 for thrice-weekly dialysis have been recommended (25). Although the use of this index is controversial, inadequate dialysis, i.e., Kt/Vdu under 0.8, has been associated with a higher rate of morbidity and dialysis failure (26). Once the desired DI is determined, the patient's dialysis prescription (i.e., filter selection and blood flow rate, BFR) can be calculated.

Since the time on dialysis is often dictated by the dialysis center, based on patient load and equipment availability, and the urea volume of distribution is approximately 60% of the patient's total body weight (25), the primary variable in this relationship is the dialysis filter

urea clearance. Therefore, if an 80-kg patient is to be dialyzed for 240 min three times weekly to achieve a DI of 1.0, the first component of the dialysis prescription can be calculated as:

$$Vdu = (0.60 \text{ liter/kg})(80 \text{ kg}) = 48 \text{ liter}$$
$$K = (Vdu \cdot DI)/t \qquad (20.2)$$
$$K = (48 \text{ liter} \cdot 1)/240 \text{ min}$$
$$K = 0.193 \text{ liter/min} = 193 \text{ ml/min}$$

Two dialysis filters that provide a K of this magnitude are the Baxter CA 210 (filter 1) at a BFR of 200 ml/min and the CF 1211 (filter 2) at a BFR of 300 ml/min. The urea clearance of a dialysis filter is blood flow rate–dependent, so an increase in blood flow rate increases urea clearance. Patients blood flow through their vascular access is another determinant in the dialysis filter selection process. The Baxter CF 12.11 at a BFR of 300 ml/min has the same urea clearance as the Baxter CA 210 at 200 ml/min BFR. The choice between these two filters depends also on the second part of the dialysis prescription, i.e., the patient's fluid removal requirement.

The fluid removal component of the dialysis prescription is calculated using the ultrafiltration coefficient (Kuf) of the dialysis filter (Table 20.1). Through trial and error a postdialysis target weight is determined for every patient; typically 0 to 5 kg will be removed during each dialysis session (27). If 4 kg or 4 liters are to be removed from the patient during the four-hr dialysis, the required transmembrane pressure (TMPt) to provide sufficient fluid removal is calculated as follows:

$$TMP_t = FRR/Kuf \qquad (20.3)$$

where *FRR* is the desired fluid removal rate in ml/hr (in this example, 1000 ml/hr).

$$TMP_t^{CA210} = (1000 \text{ ml/hr})/(10.1 \text{ ml/hr/mm Hg})$$
$$= 99 \text{ mm Hg}$$
$$TMP_t^{CF1211} = (1000 \text{ ml/hr})/(2.9 \text{ ml/hr/mm Hg})$$
$$= 345 \text{ mm Hg}$$

The second step in the process is calculating the dialyzer compartment pressure (DCP) needed to achieve the desired weight loss:

$$DCP = TMP_t - BCP \qquad (20.4)$$

where *BCP* equals mean arterial pressure minus oncotic pressure and *DCP* is a function of the dialysis filter's Kuf and the desired rate of fluid removal from the patient.

Assuming the BCP equals 75 mm Hg (i.e., mean arterial pressure of 100 minus oncotic pressure of 25) the required DCP for the CA210 and CF1211 filters can be calculated as follows:

$$DCP^{CA210} = 99 \text{ mm Hg} - 75 \text{ mm Hg}$$
$$= 24 \text{ mm Hg}$$
$$DCP^{CF1211} = 345 \text{ mm Hg} - 75 \text{ mm Hg}$$
$$= 270 \text{ mm Hg}$$

If filters with equivalent urea clearance values are available, filter selection can be made on the basis of Kuf. If a patient requires a large amount of fluid removal during each dialysis session, the dialysis filter with the larger ultrafiltration coefficient is most appropriate. This allows greater fluid removal than the filter with the lower Kuf at the same TMP value. If the patient requires little fluid removal, the dialysis filter with the smaller Kuf would be more suitable. Although these mathematical modeling approaches are helpful, the patient's well-being and freedom from complications remain the predominant guide to the adequacy of dialysis (26).

THERAPEUTIC CONSIDERATIONS FOR THE DIALYSIS PATIENT

Patients receiving chronic dialysis therapy require modification of the dose of almost all commonly used medications (28, 29). The disposition of drugs that depend largely on the kidney for elimination (i.e., the fraction excreted unchanged by the kidney exceeds 60%) may be influenced greatly by changes in renal function. Furthermore, recent evidence indicates that the pharmacokinetics of many drugs that are predominantly eliminated by hepatic routes may also be markedly affected by the development of severe renal insufficiency (30). Thus all new drugs should be evaluated in patients with renal insufficiency during the development process. This information can then form the basis for individualization of drug therapy regimens for dialysis patients. In addition to these changes in renal and nonrenal clearance, alterations in protein binding and volume of distribution may alter the serum concentration time of a drug in dialysis patients markedly, relative to subjects with normal renal function (31).

The effects of the hemodialysis or peritoneal dialysis procedure itself on the pharmacokinetic characteristics of a drug (and thus its serum concentration time profile) are complex (32, 33). Since multiple dialysis filters are available and several techniques are currently in use for the delivery of hemodialysis therapy, use of yes-or-no information in terms of dialyzability is totally inappropriate. Rather, references that provide quantitative estimates of the effect of hemodialysis or peritoneal dialysis on the elimination half-life or total body clearance of a drug

should be used (32–34). A compilation of data for many commonly used antibiotics is given in Table 20.2. These data, coupled with specific information about the type of dialysis procedure that was used, can be extrapolated to individual patient situations. This clearance information together with the estimated patient-specific pharmacokinetic parameters can be used to design a dosing regimen for a given drug in a patient receiving dialysis.

For the patient on dialysis, the clearance of the drug from the plasma (Cl_d) can be defined as the sum of the residual renal clearance (Cl_{pt}), the nonrenal clearance (Cl_{nr}), and the dialysis clearance (Cl_{hd}):

$$Cl_d = Cl_{pt} + Cl_{nr} + Cl_{hd} \qquad (20.5)$$

The characteristics of a drug that have the most favorable impact upon its dialyzability include a low molecular weight, low protein binding, a small volume of distribution, a rapid rate of equilibration between tissue binding sites and blood, and a limited amount of nonrenal metabolism and excretion. The additional effect of dialysis clearance is not usually considered important unless the procedure increases overall plasma clearance by at least 30% (33) and/or the fractional drug removal exceeds 0.30 (35).

The actual amount of drug removed by hemodialysis is the product of the concentration of drug in the recovered dialysate and the dialysate volume. This value divided by the total body stores of the drug prior to dialysis (product of predialysis concentration and volume of distribution) yields the actual fraction of drug removed by dialysis (aFDR). It is often not clinically feasible or analytically practical to measure dialysate drug concentrations, and several methods to predict the FDR have been proposed (35). It is important prior to using these formulae to differentiate clearance by dialysis (Cl_{hd}) from the clearance during dialysis (Cl_d); the latter equals the sum of the patient's residual endogenous clearance ($Cl_{pt} + Cl_{nr}$) and Cl_{hd}. The fractional drug removal by dialysis may be calculated as follows:

$$FDR = (Cl_{hd}/Cl_d) \cdot [1 - e^{-[Cl_d/V_d]t}] \qquad (20.6)$$

where V_d is the volume of distribution of the drug and t is the time of dialysis.

Alternatively, FDR may be estimated using the off-dialysis and during-dialysis elimination rate constants. Again, the overall elimination rate constant, K_d, must be differentiated from the dialysis elimination rate constant, K_{hd}, and the patient's residual elimination rate constant, K_{pt}. The half-life off-dialysis divided into 0.693 yields K_{pt} and 0.693 divided by the half-life during-dialysis yields K_d. The dialysis elimination rate constant $K_{hd} = K_d - K_{pt}$. Therefore, FDR may also be calculated as follows:

$$FDR = (K_{hd}/K_d) \cdot [1 - e^{-(K_d t)}] \qquad (20.7)$$

Table 20.2.
Effect of Hemodialysis and Intermittent Peritoneal Dialysis on the Clearance and Half-Life of Selected Drugs[a]

Drug	$t_{1/2}$ (hr)		Effect of Dialysis			
	Normal	ESRD[b]	$t_{1/2\ HD}$	Cl_{HD}	$t_{1/2\ PD}$	CL_{PD}
Amikacin	1.6	39	3.8–5.5	30–36	18–26	6.7
Ampicillin	1.3	10–20	2.9–5.0	30–154	ND	ND
Azlocillin	0.9	5.1	2.2	ND	2.5	ND
Aztreonam	2.0	7.0	2.7	43	7.0	2.1
Carbenicillin	1.0	18.2	4.3	39.6	ND	ND
Cefaclor	0.7	2.5	1.6	75	ND	ND
Cefazolin	2.2	28.0	2.6–5.0	NR	32	NR
Cefamandole	1.0	10.4	4–7	29	7.2	10.2
Cefmetazole	1.3	29.4	1.5–3.3	86	ND	ND
Cefonicid	4.4	67.0	3.4	NR	ND	ND
Cefotetan	3.0	13.1	9.4/5.7	NR	ND	ND
Cefoxitin	0.8	13–25	4	NR	NR	1.5
Cefuroxime	1.3	15–22	3.5	NR	11.8	4.7
Cefoperazone	1.8	2.3	reduced	NR	ND	ND
Cefotaxime	0.9	2.5	1.9–3.4	14–40	2.9–4.4	NR
Ceftazidime	1.8	26.0	2.8	27–50	8.7	8.5
Ceftizoxime	1.6	28.1	5.3	45	ND	ND
Ceftriaxone	8.0	15.0	16	31	ND	ND
Cephalexin	0.8	19.0	4.5	25	ND	ND
Chloramphenicol	3.4	5.3	3.2	21–54	ND	ND
Cinoxacin	2.1	9.0	ND	ND	ND	ND
Ciprofloxacin	4.4	8.4–12	3–5.5	29.6–47	ND	ND
Clavulanic acid	1.0	4.3	NR	141	ND	ND
Clindamycin	2.2–3.3	1.9–3.4	1.6–3.1	NR	ND	ND
Cloxacillin	0.6	2.0	NR	NR	ND	ND
Dicloxacillin	0.7	2.2	NR	NR	ND	ND
Erythromycin	2.1	4.0	0.8	28.5	ND	ND
Gentamicin	2.2	53	5.2–11.3	24–47	8.5	12.5
Imipenem	0.9	2.9	1.0	84	ND	ND
Metronidazole	7.9	7.7	2.8	58–125	5.6	15.8
Mezlocillin	1.0	4.3	2.0	28.7	2.1	7.4
Nafcillin	1.0	2.1	NR	0	ND	ND
Netilmicin	2.1	42	3.7–5.2	38–65	ND	ND
Norfloxacin	3.1–7.4	6.5–9.0	ND	ND	ND	ND
Ofloxacin	5–8	28–38	NR	116	ND	ND
Penicillin G	0.7	4.1	2.3	37.5	ND	ND
Piperacillin	1.2	3.9	1.3–2.4	74	ND	ND
Sulfamethoxazole	10	13.3	3.2–11.1	21–84	13–18	1.2
Sulfisoxazole	6.0	11.0	6.0	ND	ND	ND
Ticarcillin	1.2	14.8	3.4	33	10.6	7.2
Tobramycin	2.5	58	4.3–6.7	31–70	25	4.7
Trimethoprim	14	26–40	5–9.4	29–66	17–24	5.1
Vancomycin	6.9	161	NR	16.1	30–43	2.3–14.2

[a] $t_{1/2}$, terminal half-life; $t_{1/2\ HD}$, half-life during hemodialysis (hr); Cl_{HD}, hemodialyzer clearance (ml/min); $t_{1/2\ HD}$, half-life during peritoneal dialysis (hr); Cl_{PD}, peritoneal dialysis clearance (ml/min); ND, no data; NR, not reported.
[b] ESRD, end-stage renal disease.

FDR assessment may help optimize individualized drug therapy for hemodialysis patients. For several drugs, the clearance and half-life on and off dialysis has been determined (Table 20.2). If, for example, a dialysis patient received 1 g of cefmetazole intravenously just prior to 3 hours of dialysis, the FDR, using literature values for clearance (Table 20.2) and steady state volume of distribution (14 liters or 0.19 liter/kg (36), could be calculated as

Cefmetazole clearance off dialysis, Cl_{pt}, is 0.38 liter/hr.
Cefmetazole clearance by dialysis, Cl_{hd}, is 5.17 liter/hr.

$$
\begin{aligned}
Cl_d &= Cl_{pt} + Cl_{hd} \\
&= 0.38 \text{ liter/hr} + 5.17 \text{ liter/hr} \\
&= 5.55 \text{ liter/hr} \\
FDR &= (5.17/5.55) \cdot [1 - e^{-[5.55/14] \cdot 3}] \\
&= (0.932)(0.696) \\
&= 0.648
\end{aligned}
\tag{20.8}
$$

The FDR can also be calculated using elimination rate constants, as follows:

Cefmetazole half-life off dialysis is 29.4 hr.

$$
\begin{aligned}
K_{pt} &= 0.693/t_{1/2} \\
K_{pt} &= 0.693/29.4 \\
&= 0.0236 \text{ hr}^{-1}
\end{aligned}
\tag{20.9}
$$

Cefmetazole half-life during dialysis is 2.1 hr.

$$
Kd = 0.693/2.1 - 0.33 \text{ hr}^{-1}
$$

Thus,

$$
\begin{aligned}
K_{hd} + K_d - K_{pt} \\
&= 0.33 - 0.0236 \\
&= 0.306 \text{ hr}^{-1} \\
FDR &= (0.306/0.33)[1 - e^{-(0.33 \cdot 3)}] \\
&= 0.583
\end{aligned}
\tag{20.10}
$$

The FDR can serve as an index of the relative dialyzability of various drugs and determine whether or not an adjustment must be made to optimize a patient's dosage regimen.

Endogenous clearance of a drug during the period between dialyses may also affect drug regimen design. Knowledge of the amount of drug removed both during and between dialysis treatments is often necessary to design an optimal therapeutic regimen. Patients may require postdialysis or interdialytic dosing when the maintenance of serum concentrations within a narrow range is necessary to maximize efficacy or minimize toxicity. Unfortunately, accurate information on the dialysis kinetics of many drugs is not readily available (38). However, if one assumes that drug removal by dialysis and during the interdialytic period follows first-order kinetics—that is, the drug concentration declines monoexponentially depending upon the clearance, the volume of distribution, and the time between observations—then the serum concentration time profile and dosing regimen for an individual patient may be predicted, as is demonstrated in the following case example.

CASE STUDY

A.L. is a 70-kg nonsmoking female who has been maintained on hemodialysis for 2 years. Because of an acute exacerbation of her asthmatic condition, intravenous theophylline therapy with a desired goal of peak and trough concentrations of 19 and 11 mg/liter, respectively, is to be initiated.

What is the initial dose that should be administered to achieve a peak concentration of 19 mg/liter?

The first step is to calculate the patient's volume of distribution (V_d):

$$
V_d = V_d^a \times \text{total body weight}
\tag{20.11}
$$

where V_d^a is the average value for dialysis patients, derived from the literature, expressed in liters/kg. The initial dose (ID) can then be calculated as:

$$
ID = C_{max} \times V_d
\tag{20.12}
$$

where C_{max} is the desired peak concentration. Pharmacokinetic data from the literature indicate that the mean theophylline volume of distribution is 0.5 liters/kg and the desired C_{max} is 19 mg/liter. Thus the V_d is 35 liters and the ID is 665 mg.

What maintenance dose and dosing interval are required to maintain the desired peak and trough concentrations if this patient is not dialyzed?

The dosing interval (τ) can be calculated as follows, where C_{min} is the desired trough concentration and Cl_p is the total body clearance (approximately 1.4 liter/hr) during the interdialytic period:

$$
\tau = [\ln C_{max} - \ln C_{min}]/(Cl_{pt}/V_d)
\tag{20.13}
$$

The maintenance dose (MD) can be calculated as:

$$
MD = [C_{max} \times V_d][1 - e^{-(CL_{pt}/Vd)\tau}]
\tag{20.14}
$$

The values calculated for τ and *MD* must be rounded off to clinically feasible values. For this example, the calculated τ is 13.7 hr, which should be rounded to 12 hours. This value is used to calculate the MD which is thus 252.7 mg every 12 hours. This is not feasible clinically; thus 250 mg every 12 hours is the most practical dosing regimen during the interdialytic period. Since τ and MD have been altered from the values calculated using the desired C_{max}

and C_{min}, the C_{max} and C_{min} associated with the new (250 mg every 12 hr) regimen can be calculated as:

$$C_{max} = MD/V_d[1 - e^{-(Clpt/Vd)\tau}] \quad (20.15)$$

$$C_{min} = C_{max}(e^{-(Clpt/Vd)\tau}) \quad (20.16)$$

Substitution of this patient's pharmacokinetic parameters into these two equations results in a C_{max} of 18.8 mg/liter and C_{min} of 11.9 mg/liter.

What is this patient's theophylline serum concentration before dialysis?

The concentration before dialysis (CbD) depends on the C_{max} that is attained as well as the Cl_{pt}, V_d, and the time from attainment of C_{max} to the start of dialysis (t). If dialysis is initiated 4 hr after intravenous drug administration, the CbD is approximately 16.0 mg/liter, whereas if dialysis is initiated at the end of the dosing interval (i.e., 11.5 hr after the attainment of C_{max}), the CbD is approximately 11.9 mg/liter. If this patient is to start dialysis 4 hr after the administration of theophylline, the CbD is:

$$CbD = C_{max}e^{-[Clpt/Vd]t}$$

$$= (18.8 \text{ mg/liter}) \, e^{-[(1.4 \text{ liters/hr})/(35 \text{ liters})]4 \text{ hr}} \quad (20.17)$$

$$= 18.8 \text{ mg/liter} \times 0.85$$

$$= 16 \text{ mg/liter}$$

To know how much drug, if any, to give as a supplemental dose, the effect of dialysis on the plasma concentration time profile must be determined. The most critical new piece of information required to calculate this value is the dialysis clearance of theophylline, which has been reported to vary from approximately 20 to 100 ml/min (35). Thus it is critical to know the type of dialysis filter to be used, the clearance of theophylline by this filter, and the duration of dialysis (tD).

What will the postdialysis theophylline concentration (CaD) be?

The clearance by dialysis (Cl_{hd}) is approximately 90 ml/min or 5.4 liters/hr, and the duration of dialysis is 4 hr. Therefore, the total clearance during dialysis (Cl_d) is approximately 6.8 liter/hr. Substitution of this value into equation (20.8) results in the prediction that the serum concentration of theophylline after dialysis will be 46% of the concentration at the start of dialysis.

$$CaD = CbD \times [e^{-[(Clhd + Clpt)/Vd]tD}]$$

$$= 16 \text{ mg/liter} \times [e^{-[(5.4 + 1.4)/35]4}] \quad (20.18)$$

$$= 16 \text{ mg/liter} \times 0.46$$

$$= 7.4 \text{ mg/liter}$$

All the data necessary to calculate the supplemental dose needed to maintain the desired serum concentration time profile are now available. There are three options in terms of the desired concentration time profile (Fig. 20.4). The optimal choice depends upon the patient's clinical

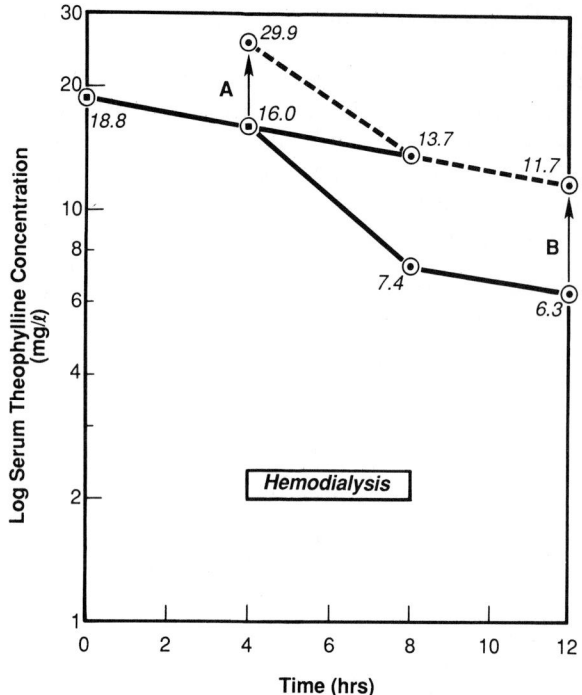

Figure 20.4. The serum concentration time profile of theophylline in patient A.L. in the predialysis, dialysis, and postdialysis periods. If it is desired to maintain the same C_{min}, then the serum concentration immediately after administration of the dose bD (A) would increase to 29.9 mg/liter. If it is desired to maintain the same C_{max}, the serum concentration will decrease to 7.4 mg/liter at the end of dialysis and the C_{min} will thus be 6.3 mg/liter. A dose aD of 437 mg would then be required to reachieve the C_{max}, an increase of 187 mg above the usual maintenance dose (B).

status and the relationship of response to specific serum concentrations. The first option is to allow the plasma concentration to decline below the desired C_{min} for the duration of the dialysis procedure and to give a larger dose than the usual maintenance dose (dose aD) to reachieve the desired maximum concentration.

How is dose aD calculated?

$$\text{Dose aD} = V_d(C_{max} - C\tau D) \quad (20.19)$$

where $C\tau D$ is the concentration at the end of the dosing interval on the dialysis day:

$$C\tau D = CaD \, e^{-(Clpt/Vd)taD} \quad (20.20)$$

where taD is the time from the end of dialysis to the end of the dosing interval. In this example, taD is 4 hours. Thus

$$C\tau D = 7.4 \text{ mg/liter} \times 0.85$$

$$= 6.3 \text{ mg/liter}$$

$$\text{Dose aD} = 35 \text{ liters} (18.8 - 6.3 \text{ mg/liter})$$

$$= 35 \text{ liters} (12.5 \text{ mg/liter})$$

$$= 437.5 \text{ mg}$$

This value must be rounded to a clinically useful value of 400 to 450 mg.

Alternatively, a dose can be administered before dialysis (dose bD), to maintain the same minimum serum concentration as on a nondialysis day. What method estimates the dose bD?

$$\text{Dose bD} = [\{(C_{min}\, e^{-(Clpt/Vd)taD})V_d\}$$
$$/(e^{-\{(Clhd\,+\,Clpt)/Vd\}tD})] - (CbD\, V_d)$$
$$= [\{(11.7/0.85)35L\}/0.46] - 560$$
$$= [480/0.46] - 560 \qquad\qquad (20.21)$$
$$= 1045 - 560$$
$$= 485\, mg$$

To accomplish this, one must accept the potential adverse effects resulting from a higher serum concentration early in dialysis. In this case, the C_{max} after this dose would be approximately 30 mg/liter.

The last alternative is for individuals receiving a continuous infusion of theophylline. In this situation, one can calculate the continuous infusion rate (dose C) needed during the dialysis period to maintain the desired steady-state average serum concentration (Css). *What is the infusion rate that would be required to maintain a Css of 14.9 mg/liter in this patient?*

$$\text{Dose C} = Css \times (Clpt + Clhd) \qquad (20.22)$$

In this example, the dose C required during dialysis is

$$\text{Dose C} = (14.9\ mg/liter) \times (6.8\ liters/hr)$$
$$= 101\ mg/hr$$

This value is approximately five times the infusion rate of 21 mg/hr that is required to maintain the Css of 14.9 mg/liter during the interdialytic period.

Unfortunately, few clinicians have the patients to endure exercises like this. It is often easier to follow standard general guidelines for dosing, hence the widespread use of tables and nomograms. In the future, however, it is likely that the availability of therapeutic-drug-concentration monitoring coupled with more specific data on the dialyzability of drugs will take clinical drug dosing in the dialysis patient out of the realm of "best guess."

RENAL TRANSPLANTATION

Renal transplantation has become the ultimate and preferred treatment for end-stage renal disease over the last two decades. Approximately 9000 kidney transplants are currently performed each year in the United States, and far more would be done if the donor organ supply were not limited. Five-year graft survival rates have increased from 50% in the early 1970s to 80 to 90% in the 1990s. This has been associated with a reduction in patient mor-

bidity and mortality. The initial enhanced success in allograft and patient survival was primarily due to the introduction of potent immunosuppressants such as prednisone, azathioprine, antilymphocyte globulin, and cyclosporine. Improved patient care prior to and following transplantation, more judicious use of immunosuppressants with appropriate therapeutic drug monitoring, improved methods of organ preservation, and a decreased incidence of surgical complications have contributed to the reduced patient morbidity and mortality during the last 5 to 10 years (39, 40). The long-term outcome of renal transplantation in patients with functioning allografts for 10 years or more has similarly been improved, with many patients resuming relatively normal lives. These improvements have been achieved despite the fact that patients previously declared "high-risk," such as the elderly, diabetics, and patients requiring a second graft, are now routinely transplanted.

The therapeutic principles that guide the use of immunosuppressant agents are applicable to many transplantation situations including liver, heart, pancreas, lung, bone marrow, and multiple organ systems. Moreover, immunosuppressants are used in a number of other clinical syndromes, including cancer, rheumatoid arthritis, and inflammatory bowel disease, as well as experimentally in the treatment of some autoimmune disorders. Thus, the pharmacology, adverse effects, drug interactions, and pharmacokinetics of the drugs discussed in this chapter may be applicable in many other clinical situations.

Patient Selection and Risk Factors

Although transplantation appears to solve many of the problems of chronic organ failure, this procedure may not be the optimal therapy for all patients. Multiple factors are considered in the evaluation of a patient's candidacy for treatment. In the 1970s and early 1980s, elderly patients were not routinely transplanted, principally because of a perceived unfavorable risk/benefit ratio. However, patients older than 60 years of age are now transplanted routinely in some centers, and little, if any, difference in patient morbidity and graft survival (compared with younger populations) has been observed (41). In contrast, the age of the cadaveric donor of the transplanted organ has been shown to markedly alter allograft survival. Transplantation of a kidney from an older cadaver donor (>50 years old) is associated with a significantly lower 3-year graft survival rate, compared with younger cadaveric kidneys (<10 years old; 55 versus 66%) (42). Obese subjects also have a greater risk of posttransplant complications, mortality, and immediate graft rejection, compared with nonobese patients (43). Furthermore, since the disposition of cyclosporine and other immunosuppressants may be altered in obese subjects, these patients may have a higher risk of adverse events, including insufficient immunosuppression (44).

In the past, preexisting diabetes mellitus was a contraindication to transplantation, mostly because of increased infection rates and worsening of the diabetes by immunosuppressant therapy. However, in a recent study, graft atherosclerosis, rejection, and lethal infections were not significantly different between diabetic and nondiabetic heart transplantation recipients (45). It was concluded that insulin-dependent diabetic patients can be transplanted with careful patient selection and close monitoring of their drug therapy. Indeed, combined kidney and pancreas transplantation has been highly effective in patients with diabetic nephropathy. Patient and kidney survival rates have exceeded 90%, and the pancreas has remained functional in almost all patients for up to 28 months following transplantation (46).

Pretransplantation Procedures

HISTOCOMPATIBILITY TESTING

The donor kidney (allograft) contains antigens that will be recognized as foreign to the recipient of the allograft. One method of coding the antigenic capabilities of the allograft is via human leukocyte antigen (HLA)–typing of the donor kidney and the recipient. The response to these antigens is an important determinant of allograft survival. Four HLA loci (A, B, C, and D) are divided into two classes defined by their structure, tissue distribution, and function. The principle antigens (class I), determined by the A, B, and C loci, are distributed in almost all tissues; the antigen determined by the D locus (class II) is located primarily on some B and T lymphocytes, monocytes, and endothelial cells. Class I antigens promote the formation of antibody-producing B cells and cytotoxic T lymphocytes. Class II antigens also trigger B cell generation and signal proliferation of helper T cells, which in turn stimulate the B cells to produce immunoglobulins G and M. The value of HLA typing is evidenced by the fact that graft survival is greater when the HLA match is better for both living-related and cadaveric donor transplants (47). This is particularly important since the number of cadaveric transplants performed each year has consistently exceeded living related transplants by a factor of six (40).

Matching is also performed for ABO blood group compatibility. Preformed reacting antibodies of the recipient can quickly destroy any ABO-incompatible donor cells and trigger an immune response, leading to hyperacute rejection. Therefore, ABO compatibility is essential for transplant success. Preformed antibodies secondary to exposure to various antigenic stimuli such as blood transfusions, pregnancy, and previous transplant may occur in potential recipients. These are tested for with a series of cell panels, referred to as panel-reactive antibodies (PRA). These represent a group of known HLA specificities. A potential recipient with high PRA may be considered a poor candidate for transplantation (48). Histocompatibility testing has dramatically diminished the occurrence of hyperacute rejection. It has improved long-term graft survival and facilitated the increase in cadaveric and nonrelated living donor transplants.

BLOOD TRANSFUSIONS

In addition to histocompatability testing, the most common procedure performed prior to transplantation is the administration of blood transfusions. In the 1970s and early 1980s, it was recognized that blood transfusions prior to renal transplant increased graft survival by 15 to 20% in patients receiving azathioprine and steroids (49). The mechanism for this beneficial effect is unknown. Since the introduction of cyclosporine this beneficial effect of blood transfusions appears to be no longer evident (50). Although the role of blood transfusions has been questioned, many programs still use this procedure prior to transplant. Irrespective of the immunosuppressive era, blood transfusions appear to be detrimental for patients who have been pregnant or previously transplanted, because of sensitization or induction of lymphocytotoxic antibodies (51).

Rejection

Following transplantation, circulating macrophages recognize the transplanted organ as a foreign body. These circulating macrophages release interleukins that attract specific T lymphocytes to the area. These T cells form receptors for interleukin-1 and interleukin-2, as well as insulin and transferrin. Interleukin-1, which is released by the activated macrophage, attaches to the receptor on the T cell and prompts the release of interleukin-2. Other T cells, macrophages, and B cells are summoned to the site of the transplanted organ by interleukin-2, to mount an attack against the allograft. Immunosuppressants such as cyclosporine, steroids, and azathioprine are targeted against one or more of these immune response mediators (Fig. 20.5).

Four types of allograft rejection have been reported: hyperacute, accelerated, acute, and chronic (52). Hyperacute rejection, occurring within minutes to hours following transplantation, may be related to the preservation techniques of the allograft, and little to no success has been reported with pharmacologic treatment. An increased incidence of this form of rejection is usually associated with prolonged organ ischemia (53). Also, antibodies in the circulation of the patient may rapidly attack the transplanted organ, resulting in irreversible damage and ultimate graft failure. Minimization of the histocompatibility mismatching of patient serum with donor tissue prior to transplantation usually prevents hyperacute rejection (54). Accelerated rejection generally occurs within 2 to 5 days following transplantation. The mechanism of this form of rejection is unclear but may also be related to a poor his-

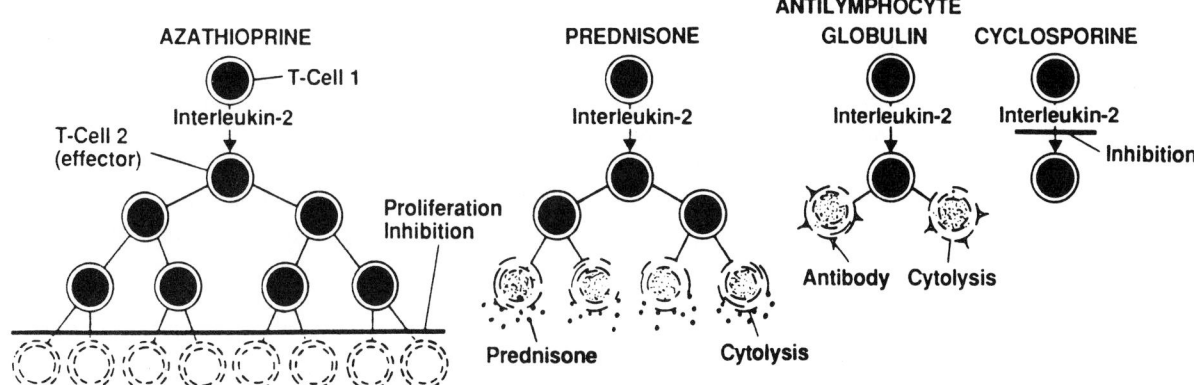

Figure 20.5. The mechanism of action of the various immunosuppressive agents. Azathioprine inhibits proliferation of effector lymphocytes; prednisone is cytolytic; antilymphocyte globulin is directed against B and T cells; and cyclosporine inhibits the production and/or activity of interleukin-2, which results in an inhibition of T cell proliferation.

Table 20.3.
Immunosuppressive Regimens for Prophylaxis and Acute Treatment of Rejection[a,b]

Immunosuppressive	Duration of Use	Prophylactic Regimen	Acute Rejection Regimen
Azathioprine	Initial	1–3 mg/kg IV/p.o. q.d.	
	Maintenance	1–3 mg/kg p.o. q.d.	
Cyclosporine	Initial	2.5–5.0 mg/kg IV q.d. or	
		8–15 mg/kg p.o. q.d.	
	Maintenance	4–6 mg/kg p.o. q.d.	
Methylprednisolone	Initial	125–1000 mg IV × 3 days	125–1000mg IV × 3 days
Prednisone	Initial	2–3 mg/kg p.o. q.d.	2–3 mg/kg p.o. q.d. × 3 days
	Maintenance	0.1–0.2 mg/kg p.o. q.d.	0.1–0.2 mg/kg p.o. q.d.
ALG or ATG	Initial	10–20 mg/kg IV q.d. × 7–14 days	10–20 mg/kg IV q.d. × 7–14 days
Muromonab-CD3	Initial	5 mg IV q.d. × 10–14 days	5 mg IV q.d. × 10–14 days

[a] Adapted from Walker AM (d): Transplant Protocols. Chestnut Hill, MA: Epidemiology Resources Inc., 1990.

[b] Refers to adult renal transplant patients only.

[c] Prophylactic regimen usually maintained, but may be reduced because of the addition of other immunosuppressive agents.

tocompatibility match between donor and recipient. Like hyperacute rejection, accelerated rejection is difficult to treat and usually results in organ failure.

Acute and chronic rejection processes are most frequently encountered, 10 to 60 days and over 3 months after transplantation, respectively. In both cases, immunosuppressant therapy with cyclosporine, steroids, and antilymphocyte globulin has reduced the incidence and extent of rejection (55). Clinical manifestations of acute rejection include fever, hypertension, oliguria, graft tenderness, and impaired renal function occasionally requiring temporary dialysis (56). The acute process can be reversed in approximately 75% of patients who are treated with high pulse doses of steroids, antilymphocyte globulin (ALG or ATG), or Muromonab-CD3 (OKT3) (Table 20.3) (57). Chronic rejection is associated with fibrotic and lipoid changes that are usually not responsive to pulse immu-

nosuppressive regimens. Thus, chronic rejection often results in an insidious loss in organ function. Fortunately, long-term studies have demonstrated that the use of cyclosporine, steroids, and azathioprine, usually in combination, has significantly reduced the development of this form of rejection.

Immunosuppressant Therapy

In the 1960s, when nonspecific agents such as azathioprine and steroids were utilized, 1-year graft survival rates of cadaveric renal transplants averaged 50%. In the 1970s, antilymphocyte globulin was introduced, and its addition to this regimen resulted in an improvement in graft survival (58). Cyclosporine was first used in renal transplantation in 1978, in combination with azathioprine and steroids. Since its introduction, 1-year graft survival has increased dramatically and now averages 80 to 90% for cadaveric transplants (58) and >90% for living related transplant recipients (59). Cyclosporine and the monoclonal antibody muromonab-CD3 target-selected pathways of the immune system, thus inhibiting the rejection processes following transplantation while preserving other immune functions. The incidence and extent of adverse effects are thus reduced when these immunosuppressants that attack single components of the host immune system are used.

Patient and graft survival statistics are often confounded by factors other than the use of specific immunosuppressive agents. Since the ultimate failure of the recipient's original organ may be due to a vascular disorder (e.g., diabetes mellitus), the transplanted organ is also likely to be susceptible to a similar fate. Accelerated atherosclerotic lesions have indeed been found in kidney transplants within 1 year following transplantation (60). In many cases, these lesions have been responsible for transplantation failures. Importantly, apart from pancreatic transplantation in diabetic patients, renal transplantation rarely corrects the underlying disease state. Thus, a chronic disease process may continue to affect other organ systems, and result in patient morbidity and death. An example of this is underlying cardiovascular disease and renal transplantation. The patient may never develop rejection and yet die from heart disease unrelated to the graft (61). Although survival rates of transplantation patients are not significantly different from those of patients maintained on chronic hemodialysis therapy, their quality of life improves significantly following renal transplantation (62). Moreover, because of refinements in immunosuppressive regimens, healthcare costs associated with transplantation (i.e., drug costs and length of hospitalization) are reduced markedly following transplantation, compared with those of chronic dialysis therapy (63).

The goal of immunosuppression is to maximize transplant organ function and patient survival while minimizing drug-related toxicity. The diversity of protocols used to achieve this goal is impressive (Table 20.3). They include monotherapy with cyclosporine; dual therapy with cyclosporine and steroids or azathioprine; triple therapy with cyclosporine, azathioprine, and steroids, and quadruple therapy with the addition of antilymphocyte globulin or muromonab-CD3 to the triple-drug regimen. Combination therapy is used predominantly to take advantage of the synergistic immunosuppressive effects and to minimize drug-related toxicities. Other regimens involve the initial use of antilymphocyte globulin or muromonab-CD3, azathioprine, and steroids and the later introduction of cyclosporine, to avoid any early nephrotoxic effects of cyclosporine (64, 65). This appears to decrease the duration of delayed graft function and improve graft survival. Other immunosuppressants, such as antilymphocyte globulin and muromonab-CD3, have been used in conjunction with conventional immunosuppressants for the treatment of acute rejection. While the actual number of immunosuppressive agents is relatively small compared with other therapeutic areas, the protocols for their use are diverse, and they depend on the transplant program (66).

STEROIDS

Adrenal corticosteroids, such as prednisone and methylprednisolone, are a mainstay of immunosuppression after kidney transplantation. Their primary mechanism of action is via blocking macrophage release of interleukin-1, which in turn prevents the activation of T and B lymphocytes and other macrophages (Fig. 20.5).

Pharmacokinetics. The bioavailability of prednisone tablets is complete in transplant patients and similar to that in healthy subjects (67). However the absorption of enteric-coated prednisolone preparations is erratic in kidney transplant recipients (68). Prednisone, the most commonly prescribed oral steroid, is converted to its active form, prednisolone. Both inhibition and induction of steroid metabolism have been reported in the transplant population. A 50 to 100% reduction in prednisolone concentrations has been reported with the concomitant use of phenytoin, barbiturates, carbamazepine, and rifampin (69). Inhibition of metabolism, with a resultant increase in prednisolone concentrations, has been reported with ketoconazole (70). Prednisolone clearance and volume of distribution are similar in children and adults (71). However, elderly subjects have a lower total body clearance of prednisolone, as compared with younger adults (72). Since guidelines for the dosing of corticosteroids are highly variable, the significance of these pharmacokinetic changes remain unclear (Table 20.4).

Toxicity. The long-term therapeutic usefulness of corticosteroids is hampered by a complex toxicity profile precipitated by either chronic administration or acute withdrawal of therapy. Steroids increase protein catabolism, which can raise the blood urea nitrogen (BUN) level. Since an elevated BUN level is usually one of the first signs of rejection after kidney transplantation, the steroid-induced rise in levels may confound interpretation of allograft function. Additionally, demargination of lymphocytes lining the blood vessels by steroids may confound the diagnosis of an acute infectious process. Although still debatable, steroids may also accelerate atherosclerotic changes in heart and kidney transplant patients (73). Avascular necrosis has been reported in approximately 10% of all transplanted patients and may be related to chronic steroid use (74).

A reduction in the total daily dose or a change to alternate-day therapy generally minimizes toxicity while preserving immunosuppressive activity. In one study of 189 renal transplant patients (75), low-dose steroid therapy coupled with azathioprine was equally efficacious and carried reduced risk, when compared with the high-dose steroid regimen. Pediatric nephrologists have reported that

Table 20.4.
Pharmacokinetic Parameters of Cyclosporine, Prednisolone and Azathioprine in Renal Transplant Recipients[a,b]

Immunosuppressive	F (%)	Half-Life (hr)	Clearance (ml/min/kg)	Vd$_{ss}$ (liter/kg)
Cyclosporine[c]				
Adults	27.6	10.7	5.7	4.5
	(21.2)	(4.3–53.4)[d]	(0.6–23.9)[d]	(3.6)
Children	30.8	7.4	11.8	4.7
	(10.2)	(8.1–16.5)[d]	(9.8–15.5)[d]	(1.5)
Prednisolone	86.1 (P)			
	(9.1)			
	93.6 (PN)	3.3	2.3	0.68
	(9.2)	(0.5)	(0.46)	(0.08)
Azathioprine (MP)	60	1.0	57.3	0.81
	(31)	(.40)	(31.0)	(0.7)

[a] Adapted from Venkataramanan R, Harbucky K, Burckart G, Ptachinski RJ: Clinical pharmacodynamics in organ transplant patients. Clin Pharmacokinet 16:134–161, 1989.

[b] Mean (SD), abbreviations: MP, 6-mercaptopurine; P, prednisone; PN, prednisolone.

[c] Cyclosporine measured by an HPLC whole blood technique.

[d] Range of reported individual values.

alternate-day steroid administration results in less growth retardation in children with a renal transplant. Also, with the advent of newer immunosuppressants such as cyclosporine, it has been suggested that much lower doses of steroids may be used without loss in allograft survival (76, 77).

Dosing Guidelines. The maintenance dose of corticosteroids which has been used varies markedly and depends on the steroid that is used and the transplant program. Initially, a transplant recipient may receive intravenous methylprednisolone 125 to 1000 mg preoperatively or intraoperatively and then be converted to oral prednisone, postoperatively. For example, one oral prednisone dosage regimen consists of 1 to 1.5 mg/kg/day for 3 days immediately following transplantation, tapering quickly to 0.2 to 0.3 mg/kg/day over 2 weeks. This dose is then maintained for a 6-month period. Another prednisone regimen consists of a taper from 200 mg on day 1 to 20 mg by day 7 and ultimately a maintenance of 10 to 30 mg daily or every other day. For acute rejection, high-dose IV methylprednisolone, usually 250 to 1000 mg daily for 3 days is used as first-line therapy, or oral prednisone, 2 to 3 mg/kg/day (66).

The pharmacist should stress the need for continuous dosing with steroids. Since exogenous administration of corticosteroids signals the adrenal gland to halt the production of endogenous cortisol, acute cessation of therapy will result in adrenal insufficiency. This syndrome is rarely fatal, but symptoms include arthralgia, fever, malaise, and myalgia; thus, dose changes should be performed over a long time to allow the adrenal gland to adjust. (See Chapter 15, "Adrenocortical Dysfunction and Clinical Use of Steroids.")

AZATHIOPRINE

Azathioprine, a prodrug of 6-mercaptopurine, induces the synthesis of abnormal purine ribonucleotides, which are falsely incorporated into nucleic acid building blocks. Thus, T and B lymphocyte differentiation and growth are inhibited, and the response of activated T cells to the antigenic transplanted organ is blocked. Azathioprine also blocks bone marrow production of lymphocytes, thus suppressing host defenses against infections as well as the cellular immunity response to the foreign allograft (Fig. 20.5). Azathioprine therapy need not follow an antigenic response and may be used prior to transplantation. Azathioprine therapy is generally initiated 2 days prior to live-related transplants or on the day of cadaver transplant.

Azathioprine has been used predominantly in conjunction with low-dose cyclosporine and corticosteroids (77, 78). In one trial of 209 renal transplantations, the effects of cyclosporine (15 mg/kg/day) and steroids were compared with those of oral cyclosporine at a lower dose (10 mg/kg/day), azathioprine 2 mg/kg/day orally, and a prednisone taper to 0.15 mg/kg/day by 90 days after transplantation (77). Although the 2-year graft and patient survival rates were not significantly different in the two groups, hypertension was more common in those given triple-drug therapy than in patients given only cyclosporine and steroids. This study is the first to question critically the need to include azathioprine in immunosuppressive regimens of renal transplantation patients. Other studies have demonstrated excellent long-term graft and patient survival with azathioprine (79).

Pharmacokinetics. Early investigations indicated that the oral absorption of azathioprine was complete (80). More recently, carefully designed studies have shown that the oral absorption of azathioprine is slow and erratic, resulting in a bioavailability of 6-mercaptopurine of approximately 60% in kidney transplant patients (81). Azathioprine is 30% bound to albumin in the plasma and is rapidly converted to 6-mercaptopurine (Table 20.4). Since azathioprine undergoes extensive hepatic metabolism to active metabolites, metabolic inhibitors and inducers may affect its disposition and pharmacologic activity profoundly. Blockade of the formation of the inactive metabolite, 6-thiouric acid, by xanthine oxidase inhibitors such as allopurinol will result in accumulation of the parent compound, 6-mercaptopurine. Therefore, the dose of azathioprine should be reduced by 75% when used in conjunction with allopurinol. Although only a small fraction of the dose is excreted by the kidneys, clearance of the metabolites largely depends on renal function. Thus, the dosing interval may need to be prolonged in patients with reduced renal function.

Toxicity. Bone marrow suppression, particularly leukopenia, is the primary marker of the pharmacologic activity of azathioprine, although depression of white blood cell counts is not linked directly efficacy. Patients receiving chronic azathioprine therapy should be followed closely with weekly blood counts, at least initially. It appears that these toxicities are dose-dependent and either temporary withdrawal or dose reduction promotes reversal. Although a drop in lymphocytes is expected, platelet and erythrocyte counts will also decrease, predisposing the patient to bleeding disorders and anemia. Furthermore, loss of bone marrow function increases the susceptibility to opportunistic infections, particularly with viral and bacterial organisms. In addition, hepatotoxicity and pancreatitis have been reported with chronic administration (82).

Dosing Guidelines. The intravenous formulation can be infused over 30 min to 8 hr, depending on the clinical situation. Despite data indicating poor bioavailability, most protocols maintain the oral dose at the same dose level as the intravenous form, with periodic (at least weekly, initially) monitoring of white blood cell counts. Maintenance doses of azathioprine range between 1 and 3 mg/kg/day (Table 20.3) (66).

CYCLOSPORINE

Cyclosporine is a novel T cell–specific immunosuppressant that is used widely to prevent rejection following transplantation, as well as for the treatment of other disorders including psoriasis (83) and rheumatoid arthritis (84). Cyclosporine specifically and reversibly inhibits the release of interleukin-2, thereby preventing activation of T and B lymphocytes, as well as macrophages and other immunomodulating cells (85) (Fig. 20.5). In contrast to nonspecific immunosuppressants such as azathioprine, myelosuppression does not occur with cyclosporine. The immunosuppressive activity of cyclosporine is only effective after the recipient has been exposed to the antigen. Therefore, cyclosporine is not indicated for aggressive treatment after a rejection process has commenced. In these situations, other agents such as antilymphocyte globulin, steroids, and muromonab-CD3 are effective. Clinical trials with cyclosporine have consistently demonstrated its efficacy in prevention of rejection in renal, bone marrow, cardiac, heart, and liver transplantations (86).

Pharmacokinetics. The pharmacokinetics of cyclosporine have been studied extensively in various types of transplant recipients, including those who have received kidneys (Table 20.4) (87–89). The absorption of cyclosporine is often erratic, resulting in an absolute bioavailability of the oral solution ranging from 10 to 80% with a mean of 30% (88). The oral capsule formulation demonstrates similar relative bioavailability (90). Food, particularly a high-fat meal, can increase the absolute bioavailability of cyclosporine (91).

The binding of cyclosporine is extensive in the vascular space, with more than 50% of the drug bound to erythrocytes and other cellular components. More than 90% of the drug remaining in the plasma compartment is bound to lipoproteins. The partitioning of drug between blood and tissue compartments is affected by changes in hematocrit and lipoprotein concentrations; thus, anemia and lipid disorders may alter cyclosporine pharmacokinetics and effect dramatically (89, 92). The blood concentrations of cyclosporine are generally twice those of the plasma. Cyclosporine is metabolized extensively. At least 25 metabolites that are excreted primarily via the biliary tract have been identified. Pediatric renal transplants have a twofold higher clearance than adult transplants (93). The activity of most of these metabolites remain unclear. The hydroxylated metabolite M-17 does possess 10 to 20% of the immunosuppressant activity of cyclosporine, while the demethylated metabolite M-21 appears to have toxic potential (94). Urinary excretion of cyclosporine and metabolites is relatively minimal, accounting for less than 6% of the total amount of drug after 4 days (95).

Toxicity. Although once thought to be the ideal maintenance drug for patients receiving transplants, use of cyclosporine is complicated by an extensive toxicity profile, with nephrotoxicity considered the most significant adverse effect. The incidence of nephrotoxicity and the other frequently reported adverse events in transplant patients (including hypertension, hyperuricemia, neurotoxicity, and hepatotoxicity are depicted in Figure 20.6 (96, 97). Cyclosporine causes hypertrichosis and acne in 50% of patients. This cosmetic problem can lead to noncompliance with teenagers and female patients. Although the incidence of nephrotoxicity ranges from 30 to 74%, cyclosporine produces a 20 to 30% decrease in glomerular filtration in almost all patients (97). Acute nephrotoxicity may appear early in the course of CSA therapy, immediately or within the first week after transplant, as the result of hemodynamic changes associated with vascular lesions that may resolve with continued therapy or secondary to a direct toxic effect of the vehicle cremophor in the intravenous formulation (98). The intravenous formulation is associated with an 8-fold increase in acute renal functional changes, compared with the oral formulation (99). Prolonged infusion rates and administration of drug with Intralipid have reduced the extent of acute nephrotoxicity. Other investigational formulations for intravenous use, such as liposomal cyclosporine, have reduced the extent of nephrotoxicity while targeting the drug against cytotoxic T lymphocytes (100).

Subacute nephrotoxicity may occur within the first few months after transplantation. This occurs in approximately 30% of patients and must be distinguished from rejection.

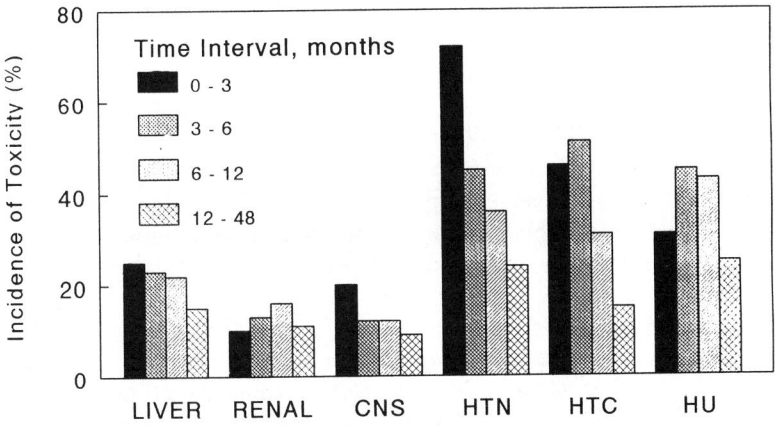

Figure 20.6. The more common toxicities found with chronic cyclosporine and prednisone use in kidney transplant recipients followed 1 to 4 years posttransplant ($N = 402$). HTN, hypertension; CNS, neurologic; HTC, hypertrichosis; HU, hyperuricemia.

It is concentration-related and responds to dosage adjustment. Chronic nephrotoxicity occurs in approximately 15% of renal transplants (96); the mechanism is somewhat unclear. Attempts to ameliorate toxicity have included concomitant use of centrally acting vasodilators, calcium-channel blockers, and vascular decongestants (101–103). However, the high incidence of chronic nephropathy currently limits the usefulness of the drug in the presence of preexisting renal dysfunction. Furthermore, the primary diagnosis of kidney allograft rejection may be confounded by the possibility of interstitial fibrosis caused by the chronic administration of cyclosporine. Generally, the dose of cyclosporine should be lowered or discontinued when more than a 2-fold increase in the baseline serum creatinine level is observed and other causes of renal dysfunction have been eliminated.

Drug Interactions. Many drug interactions have been reported with cyclosporine (104, 105). Most are single-case reports of a change in cyclosporine concentrations and/or clinical toxicity or loss of immunosuppressive activity (Table 20.5). Thus, it is difficult to determine the frequency and magnitude of many of these interactions.

Erythromycin and ketoconazole appear to cause the greatest increase in cyclosporine concentrations. This occurs rapidly upon introduction of these agents, i.e., within 24 to 48 hours. If not appropriately managed, cyclosporine toxicity can occur (104). The primary mechanism is thought to be inhibition of hepatic metabolism. However, since P450 enzymes are also found in human intestinal mucosa, inhibition may also occur at this site and result in an increase in cyclosporine absorption. The calcium antagonists are often used in the transplant population for control of hypertension. Diltiazem, verapamil, and nicardipine have been reported to increase cyclosporine concentrations significantly (105). Diltiazem and ketoconazole have been used intentionally, along with cyclosporine, to decrease cyclosporine dosage requirements and its associated cost (106, 107). The impact of this approach on long-term outcome has not been assessed. Nifedipine, on the

Table 20.5.
Drug Interactions Reported with Cyclosporine (CSA)

Increased CSA Levels	Decreased CSA Levels
Acetazolamide	Carbamazepine
Colchicine	Methylprednisolone[b]
Danazol	Nafcillin
Diltiazem	Octreotide
Erythromycin	Phenobarbital
Ethanol	Phenytoin
Fluconazole	Rifampin
Imipenim/Cilastatin	Sulfonamides
Itraconazole	Trimethoprim
Ketoconazole	
Methylprednisolone[a]	
Metoclopramide	
Nicardipine	
Nifedipine	
Norethisterone	
Oral contraceptives	
Sulindac	
Verapamil	

[a] Increased cyclosporine levels, measured by nonspecific RIA.
[b] Decreased cyclosporine levels, measured by HPLC.

other hand, has no effect on cyclosporine. Classic metabolic inhibitors, such as ciprofloxacin and cimetidine also have no effect. In contrast, metabolic inducers such as phenytoin, phenobarbital, carbamazepine, and rifampin increase cyclosporine dose requirements. These interactions can lead to loss of effect and rejection (105).

Antimicrobials such as aminoglycosides and amphotericin B have additive nephrotoxic effects unrelated to any alteration in cyclosporine disposition. Finally, cyclosporine appears to inhibit the metabolism of the antilipidemic agent, lovastatin. This combination has been reported to result in rhabdomyolysis and acute renal failure (108). In view of the potential for clinically significant interactions, whenever other agents are added or discontinued, cyclosporine concentrations and clinical response should be carefully monitored.

Dosing and Monitoring Guidelines. The dose of cyclosporine has been reduced markedly since its introduction to the U.S. market. Intravenous maintenance doses, which are typically begun 12 to 24 hr after the transplant, range from 2.5 to 5.0 mg/kg/day intravenously every 12 hr infused over a minimum of 2 hr or continuously throughout a 24-hr period (Table 20.3). The initial oral dose is generally 8 to 15 mg/kg/body weight/day. This is generally reduced to an oral maintenance regimen of 4 to 6 mg/kg/day by 6 months. The oral formulation is initiated as soon as the patient can tolerate oral medications.

The oral solution has an unpleasant aftertaste that can be partially masked with chocolate milk, milk, or fruit juice. The solution should be ingested immediately after mixing, since the stability of the diluted form has not been studied. The oral capsule formation is an alternative for those who cannot tolerate the unpleasant taste or the inconvenience of the solution. The undiluted oral solution is stable for 2 months after opening. Most patients take the oral dose as a single daily dose with breakfast. Some patients with rapid clearance, especially children, may require more frequent administration with higher doses.

Because of its narrow therapeutic index, wide variability in absorption and metabolism, and potential for a significant number of drug interactions, monitoring of cyclosporine concentrations is important. The therapeutic range associated with maximum efficacy and minimum toxicity depends on whether the concentrations are measured in whole blood or plasma, the transplant type and protocol, and the assay methodology.

The consensus panel on cyclosporine monitoring recommended whole blood as the optimal biologic fluid, in part because plasma concentrations depend on hemocrit and the temperature at which it is separated from the red blood cells. They also recommended that a specific method that measures cyclosporine only should be used (109). Multiple specific (HPLC, RIA, FPIA, EMIT) and nonspecific (RIA, FPIA) assays have been developed. The nonspecific methods have variable degrees of crossreactivity with several metabolites of cyclosporine and thus represent a measure of cyclosporine and some or all of its metabolites. These data may be of some utility clinically, but clearly they would not be appropriate for characterization of cyclosporine disposition.

Although no uniformly accepted guidelines for the desired range of cyclosporine concentrations have been adopted, trough whole blood concentrations above 600 ng/ml and below 100 ng/ml have been associated with toxicity and rejection, respectively. Cyclosporine dosage should therefore be adjusted to maintain steady-state whole blood concentrations within the range of 100 to 400 ng/ml. Excellent graft survival rates may be achieved with cyclo-sporine whole blood levels under 200 ng/ml, especially when cyclosporine is used in combination with other immunosuppressive agents (110).

OTHER AGENTS

Antilymphocyte or antithymocyte globulin (ALG or ATG, respectively), the purified polyclonal globulin extract from goat, rabbit, or horse serum sensitized to human lymphocytes, is effective in removing circulating T lymphocytes and blocking their formation. Several protocols have been proposed for their routine use in the initial posttransplant period (Table 20.4). As with other animal products, a test dose of ALG or ATG must be administered prior to full dosing and the patient monitored for an immunologic reaction. Furthermore, ALG or ATG should be infused into a large central vein to prevent thrombophlebitis. Dosing of ALG or ATG is based on the patient weight, white blood cell count, and platelet count. ALG or ATG is also used for the treatment of acute rejection following transplantation. The primary adverse events associated with ALG or ATG are fever, chills, myalgias, urticaria, nausea, vomiting, leukopenia, and thrombocytopenia (111).

Biotechnology has provided a number of new therapeutic agents for the prevention or treatment of rejection following transplantation. Monoclonal antibodies, such as muromonab-CD3 (orthoclone, OKT3), have been used for the treatment of acute renal allograft rejection, with or without concomitant immunosuppressive therapy (112). This is a murine antibody that is directed against the CD3 (T3) antigen on the surface of human T lymphocytes and inhibits both established cytotoxic T cell activity and the induction of new cytotoxic T cells. The drawbacks to its use include expense, rapid antigen modulation, and a lack of sustained immunosuppressive activity, most likely because of the development of neutralizing antibodies directed against the murine component. For the treatment of acute rejection, the recommended dose is 5 mg IV once daily for adults and 2.5 mg a day for pediatric patients, for 10 to 14 days. The major side effects associated with the first few doses included fever, chills, headache, hypertension or hypotension, and pruritus. This can be accompanied by nausea, vomiting, and diarrhea (111). This appears to occur secondary to release of interleukins, tumor necrosis factor, and interferon from T lymphocytes. The use of methylprednisolone, just prior and 2 to 6 hr after the first and second dose appears to reduce the severity of this reaction (114). Muromonab-CD3 should be administered to patients whose body weight has increased >3% during the week prior to muromonab-CD3, since this is a risk factor for pulmonary edema.

Antibodies to muromonab-CD3 develop often, usually within 7 days of initial administration, and decrease the responsiveness to this agent (115). Administration of other immunosuppressives at reduced doses decreases the incidence and degree of antibody production (116). When retreatment with this agent is considered, the patient should have an antibody titer determined prior to treatment. Patients with very high titers ($\geq 1:1000$) should not be treated until this decreases to $\leq 1:100$ (115). Muromonab-CD3 administration has also been associated with a higher incidence of cytomegalovirus infections (117) and possibly the development of lymphomas (118).

The interleukin-2 receptor on activated T lymphocytes is composed of two chains, an alpha chain (P55) and a beta chain (P75), with differing affinities for the interleukin-2 molecule. The prophylactic effects of a murine IgG_{2a} monoclonal antibody to the human P55 chain (33B3.1) were compared with those of ATG in 100 renal transplant recipients (119). Whereas the number of rejection episodes and patient and graft survival rates were similar between the groups, those given ATG had significantly more episodes of infection. Development of antibodies to 33B3.1 reduced the circulating levels of 33B3.1 markedly and predisposed the patients to acute graft-rejection episodes. Recently, a chimeric monoclonal IgG_1 antibody to the P55 chain (anti-Tac; Hoffman-La Roche) has been developed for the prophylaxis of transplantation rejection (120). Antibodies to both the alpha and beta chains, as well as the linking of toxins to the monoclonals (e.g., interleukin-2 toxin) have been proposed to selectively deplete certain types of cells (121).

Preliminary studies of other novel immunosuppressants, FK506, 15-deoxyspergualin, and mizoribine, have shown promise in animal and patient studies. Deoxyspergualin is an analog of the antibiotic spergualin. It appears to have a completely different mechanism of action than ALG, OKT3, and cyclosporine. Initial clinical trials indicate its efficacy for acute rejection. Its toxicity profile consists of gastrointestinal and hematologic effects (122). FK506 is a macrolide antibiotic with immunosuppressive properties like those of cyclosporine. Initial use indicates potential benefit in transplant recipients intolerant or refractory to other immunosuppressives, including cyclosporine (123). Its side effect profile is similar to that of cyclosporine, except for hypertrichosis and gingival hyperplasia. Mizoribine is an imidazole that blocks the response to interleukin-2. It has been used in combination with cyclosporine and prednisone with good success (124).

Role of the Pharmacist

Pharmacists have many avenues for interaction with transplant patients such as patient education, pharmacokinetic dosage individualization, and evaluation of the pharmacoeconomics of transplantation, as well as participation members of the patient care/research team. In a retrospective study of 538 renal, 50 heart, and 13 liver transplant recipients, more than 90% of those who were noncompliant with their medications and follow-up care either lost their allografts or died. An increased incidence of noncompliance was found in patients under 20 years of age, compared with those over 40 years (125). Similarly, noncompliance was greater in Hispanics and blacks than in Caucasian patients. The pharmacist should be able to devise creative methods to enhance compliance in the transplant patient, particularly in the populations at greatest risk for rejection. Increased education of patients, simplification of their medication regimens, and individualized, personalized approaches to follow-up care may ultimately decrease the incidence of noncompliance and thereby, graft rejection.

The pharmacist can also play a significant role in public education about organ procurement programs. Although medical technology for prevention of the rejection process has grown exponentially in the last decade, procurement of organs remains slow. Thus, the rate-limiting step in transplantation is not patient or transplanted organ survival but availability of donor organs. In the United States, one of five patients initiated on hemodialysis is transplanted with a donor kidney; the low kidney supply is largely responsible for the other four patients not being transplanted. Further emphasis on community awareness programs for donor organs is required to optimize the potential of transplantation.

REFERENCES

1. Rose BD: Pathophysiology of Renal Disease, ed. 2. New York: McGraw-Hill, 1987.
2. May RC, Kelly RA, Mitch WE: The pathophysiology of uremia. In Brenner BM, Rector FC (eds): The Kidney, ed. 4. Philadelphia, WB Saunders, 1991, pp 1997–2019.
3. Drukker W: Hemodialysis: a historical review. In Maher JF (ed): Replacement of Renal Function by Dialysis, ed. 3. Dordrecht, Holland, Kluwer Academic Publishers, 1989, pp 21–86.
4. Lazarus JM, Hakim RM: Medical aspects of hemodialysis. In Brenner BM, Rector FM (eds): The Kidney, ed. 4. Philadelphia, WB Saunders, 1991, pp 2223–2299.
5. Quinton W, Dillard D, Scribner BH: Cannulation of blood vessels for prolonged hemodialysis. Trans Am Soc Artif Intern Organs 6:104, 1960.
6. Brescia MJ, Cimino JE, Appel K, Hurwich BJ: Chronic hemodialysis using venapuncture and a surgically created arteriovenous fistula. N Engl J Med 275:1089, 1966.
7. Oreopoulous DG: Chronic peritoneal dialysis. Clin Nephrol 9:166–173, 1978.
8. Popovich RP, Moncrief JW, Nolph KD, Ghods AJ, Twardowski ZJ, Pyle WK: Continuous ambulatory peritoneal dialysis. Ann Intern Med 88:449, 1978.
9. Comty CM, Collins AJ: Dialytic therapy in the management of chronic renal failure. Med Clin North Am 68(2):399–425, 1984.
10. Nolph KD: Peritoneal anatomy and transport physiology. In Maher JF (ed): Replacement of Renal Function by Dialysis, ed. 3. Dordrecht, Holland, Kluwer Academic Publishers, 1989, pp 516–537.
11. Tawa NE, Tilney NL: Angioaccess in the renal failure patient. In Maher JF (ed): Replacement of Renal Function by Dialysis, ed. 3. Dordrecht, Holland, Kluwer Academic Publishers, 1989, pp 218–229.
12. Ash SR, Carr DJ, Diaz-Buxo JA: Peritoneal access devices. Hy-

draulic function and biocompatibility. In Nissenson AR, Fine RN, Gentile DE (eds): Clinical Dialysis, ed. 2. Norwalk, CT, Appleton and Lange, 1990, pp 212–239.

13. Sigdell JE: Operating characteristics of hollow-fiber dialyzers. In Nissenson AR, Fine RN, Gentile DE (eds): Clinical Dialysis, ed. 2. Norwalk, CT, Appleton and Lange, 1990, pp 97–117.

14. Sigdell JE: Parallel-plate dialyzers. In Nissenson AR, Fine RN (eds): Dialysis Therapy. Philadelphia, Hanley and Belfus, 1986, pp 82–85.

15. Colton CK, Lowrie EG: Hemodialysis: physical principles and technical considerations. In Brenner BM, Rector FC (eds): The Kidney, ed. 2. Philadelphia, WB Saunders, 1981, pp 2425–2489.

16. Anon: Shortened dialysis. Dial Transplant 15:553–563, 1986.

17. Held PJ, Levin NW, Boubjerg RR, Pauly MV, Diamond LH: Mortality and duration of hemodialysis treatment. JAMA 265(7):871–875, 1991.

18. Wizemann V, Kramer W: Short-term dialysis—long-term complications. Blood Purif 5:193–201, 1987.

19. Golding AL: Complications of vascular access for chronic hemodialysis. In Nissenson AR, Fine RN (eds): Dialysis Therapy. Philadelphia, Hanley and Belfus, 1986, pp 9–13.

20. Hamburger RL: Complications of acute peritoneal catheter insertion. In Nissenson AR, Fine RN (eds): Dialysis Therapy. Philadelphia, Hanley and Belfus, 1986, pp 114–116.

21. Vas SI: Peritonitis in patients on peritoneal dialysis. In Nissenson AR, Fine RN (eds): Dialysis Therapy. Philadelphia, Hanley and Belfus, 1986, pp 126–129.

22. Keane WF, Everett ED, Fine RN, Golper TA, Vas S, Peterson PK, Gokal R, Matzke GR: Continuous ambulatory peritoneal dialysis (CAPD) peritonitis treatment recommendations: 1989 update. Peri Dial Inter 9:247–256, 1989.

23. Walshe JJ, Morse GD: Infectious complications of peritoneal dialysis. In Nissenson AR, Fine RN, Gentile DE (eds): Clinical Dialysis. Norwalk, CT, Appleton and Lange, 1990, pp 301–318.

24. Millikin SP, Matzke GR, Keane WF: Antimicrobial treatment of peritonitis associated with continuous ambulatory peritoneal dialysis. Perit Dial Inter 11:252–260, 1991.

25. Gotch FA: Kinetic modeling in hemodialysis. In Nissenson AR, Fine RN, Gentile DE (eds): Clinical Dialysis. Norwalk, CT, Appleton and Lange, 1990, pp 118–147.

26. Gotch FA, Yarian S, Keen M: A kinetic survey of U.S. hemodialysis prescriptions. Am J Kidney Dis 15:511–515, 1990.

27. Daugirdas JT, Dumer F, Zasuwa GA, Levin NW: Chronic hemodialysis prescription. In Daugirdas JT, Ing TS (eds): Handbook of Dialysis. Boston, Little, Brown and Co, 1988, pp 72–86.

28. Schrier RW, Gambertoglio JG (eds): Handbook of Drug Therapy in Liver and Kidney Disease. Boston, Little, Brown and Co, 1991.

29. Bennett WM, Aronoff GR, Golper TA, et al.: Drug prescribing in renal failure: dosing guidelines for adults. Philadelphia, Am Coll Physicians, 1987.

30. Gibson TP: Renal disease and drug metabolism: an overview. Am J Kidney Dis 8:7–17, 1976.

31. Reidenberg MM, Drayer DE: Alteration of drug protein binding in renal disease. Clin Pharmacokinet 9(suppl 1):18–26, 1984.

32. Paton TW, Cornish WR, Manual MA, Hardy BG: Drug therapy in patients undergoing peritoneal dialysis: clinical pharmacokinetic considerations. Clin Pharmacokinet 10:404–425, 1985.

33. Lee CC, Marbury TC: Drug therapy in patients undergoing haemodialysis: clinical pharmacokinetic considerations. Clin Pharmacokinet 9:42–66, 1984.

34. Matzke GR, Keane WF: The use of antibiotics in patients with renal insufficiency. In Peterson PK, Verhoef J (eds): Antimicrobial Agents Annual 1. New York, Elsevier, 1986, pp 472–488.

35. Lee CC: The assessment of fractional drug removal by extracorporeal dialysis. Biopharm Drug Disposition 3:163–173, 1982.

36. Halstenson CE, Guay DRP, Opsahl JA, et al.: Disposition of cefmetazole in healthy volunteers and patients with impaired renal function. Antimicrob Agents Chemother 34:519–523, 1990.

37. Van Stone JC: Hemodialysis apparatus. In Daugirdas JT, Ing TS (eds): Handbook of Dialysis. Boston, Little, Brown and Co, 1988, pp 72–86.

38. Gibson TP: Problems in designing hemodialysis drug studies. Pharmacotherapy 5:23–29, 1985.

39. Slavis SA, Novick AC, Steinmuller DR, Streem SB, Braun WE, Staffon RA, Mastroianni B, Graneto D: Outcome of renal transplantation in patients with a functioning graft for 20 years or more. J Urol 144:20–22, 1990.

40. Alexander JW: The cutting edge. A look to the future in transplantation. Transplantation 49:237–240, 1990.

41. Cardella CJ, Oreopoulos DG, Honey J, Cook G, deVeber GA: Renal transplantation in patients 60 years of age or older. Transplant Proc 18:151–152, 1986.

42. Rao KV, Kasiske BI, Odlund MD, Neu AL, Anderson RC: Influence of cadaveric donor age on post-transplant renal function and graft outcome. Transplantation 49:91–95, 1990.

43. Holley JL, Shapiro R, Lopatin WB, Tzakis AG, Hakala TR, Starzl TE: Obesity as a risk factor following cadaveric renal transplantation. Transplantation 49:387–389, 1990.

44. Yee GC, Lennon TP, Ginuen DJ, Chency CL, Oeser D, Deeg HJ: Effect of obesity on cyclosporine disposition. Transplantation 45:649–651, 1989.

45. Ladowski JS, Kormos RL, Uretsky BF, Griffith BP, Armitage JM, Hardesty RL: Heart transplantation in diabetic recipients. Transplantation 49:303–305, 1990.

46. Schylack JA, Mayes JT, Hricik DE: Combined kidney and pancreas transplantation. A safe and effective treatment for diabetic nephropathy. Arch Surg 135:881–885, 1990.

47. Opelz G: The Collaborative Transplant Study: The benefit of exchanging donor kidneys among transplant centers. N Engl J Med 318:1289–1291, 1988.

48. Mason DW: Effector mechanisms in allograft rejection. Annu Rev Immunol 4:119–145, 1986.

49. Opelz G: Current relevance of the transfusion effect in renal transplantation. Transplant Proc 17:1015–1022, 1985.

50. Opelz G: HLA antigen sensitization: a problem in graft survival. Transplant Proc 21(suppl 2):39–41, 1989.

51. Pfaff WW, Howard RJ, Schornik JC: Incidental and purposeful random donor blood transfusion. Sensitization and transplantation. Transplantation 47:130–133, 1989.

52. Rao KV: Mechanism, pathophysiology, diagnosis, and management of renal transplant rejection. Med Clin North Am 74:1039–1057, 1990.

53. Finn WF: Prevention of ischemic injury in renal transplantation. Kidney Int 37:171–182, 1990.

54. Gilks WR, Gore SM, Bradley BA: Renal transplant rejection. Transient immunodominance of HLA mismatches. Transplantation 50:141–146, 1990.

55. Grino JM, Alsina J, Sabater R, Castelao AM, Gilvernet S, Andres E, Sabate I, Mestre M, Seron D, Diaz C: Antilymphoblast globulin, cyclosporine, and steroids in cadaveric renal transplantation. Transplantation 49:1114–1117, 1990.

56. Keown PA, Stiller CR, Wallace AC. Effect of cyclosporine on the kidney. J Pediatr 111:1029–1033, 1987.

57. Ortho Multicenter Transplant Study Group: A randomized clinical trial of OKT3 monoclonal antibody for acute rejection of cadaveric renal transplants. N Engl J Med 313:337–342, 1985.

58. Sutherland DE, Fryd DS, Strand MH: Results of the Minnesota randomized prospective trial of cyclosporine vs. azathioprine—antilymphocyte globulin for immunosuppression in renal allograft patients. Am J Kidney Dis 5:318–327, 1985.

59. Chan GLC, Canafax DM, Ascher NL, Payne WA, Fryd DS, Noreen H, Sutherland DER, Simmons RL, Najarian JS: HLA-identical renal transplant: no rejections with a cyclosporine-azathioprine-prednisone protocol. Clin Transplant 2:9–14, 1988.

60. Kasiske BL, Umen AJ: Persistent hyperlipidemia in renal transplant patients. Medicine 66:309–315, 1987.

61. Dunn J, Golden D, VanBuren CT, Lewis RM, Lauren J, Kahan BO: Causes of graft loss beyond two years in the cyclosporine era. Transplantation 49:349–353, 1990.

62. Simmons RG, Abress L, Anderson CR: Quality of life after kidney transplantation. Transplantation 45:415–421, 1988.

63. Canafax DM, Gruber SA, Chan GLC, Miles CJ, Matas AJ, Najarian JS, Cipolle RJ: The pharmacoeconomics of renal transplantation: increased drug costs with decreased hospitalization costs. Pharmacotherapy 10:205–210, 1990.

64. Michael HJ, Francos GC, Burke JF: A comparison of the effects of cyclosporine vs. antilymphocyte globulin on delayed graft function in cadaver renal transplant recipients. Transplantation 48:805–808, 1989.

65. Benvenisz AI, Cohen D, Stegall MD, Hardy MA: Improved results using OKT3 as induction immunosuppression in renal allograft recipient with delayed graft function. Transplantation 49:321–327, 1990.

66. Walker AM (ed): Transplant Protocols. Chestnut Hill, MA: Epidemiology Resources Inc., 1990.

67. Haynes RC, Murad F: Adrenocorticotropic hormone: adrenocorticosteroids and their synthetic analogs. In Goodman AG, Goodman LS, Rall TW, Murad F (eds): The Pharmacological Basis of Therapeutics, ed. 8. New York, MacMillan, 1990, pp 1431–1462.

68. Henderson RG, Wheatley T, English J, Chakraborty J, Marks V: Variation in plasma prednisolone concentrations in renal transplant recipients given enteric-coated prednisolone. Br Med J 1:1534–1536, 1979.

69. Frey BM, Frey FJ: Clinical pharmacokinetics of prednisone and prednisolone. Clinical Pharmacokinet 19:126–146, 1990.

70. Zuchery RM, Frey BM, Frey FJ: Impact of ketoconazole on the metabolism of prednisolone. Clin Pharmacol Ther 45:366–372, 1989.

71. Rose IG, Nichelson JA, Ellis EF: Prednisolone disposition in steroid dependent asthmatic children. J Allergy Clin Immunol 67:188–193, 1981.

72. Stuch AE, Frey BM, Frey FJ: Kinetics of prednisolone and endogenous cortisol suppression in the elderly. Clin Pharmacol Ther 43:354–361, 1988.

73. Ekstrand A, Ahonen J, Gronhagen-Riska C, Groop L: Mechanisms of insulin-resistance after kidney transplantation. Transplantation 48:563–568, 1990.

74. Braun WE: Long-term complications of renal transplantation. Kidney Int 37:1363–1378, 1990.

75. d'Apice AJF, Bucher GJ, Kincaid-Smith P: Low-dose vs. high-dose steroids: a prospective trial for interaction of steroid and azathioprine dosages. Transplant Proc 16:1000, 1984.

76. Sterioff S, Engen DE, Zincke H: Current status of renal transplantation—1986. Mayo Clin Proc 61:573–578, 1986.

77. Brinker KR, Dickerman RM, Gonwa TA, Hull AR, Langley JW, Long DL, Nesser DA, Trevino G, Velez RL, Vergne-Narini PJ: A randomized trial comparing double-drug and triple-drug therapy in primary cadaveric renal transplants. Transplantation 50:43–49, 1990.

78. Canafax DM, Simmons RL, Sutherland DE, Fryd DS, Strand MH, Ascher NL, Payne WD, Najarian JS: Early and late effects of two immunosuppressive drug protocols on recipients of renal allografts: results of the Minnesota randomized trial comparing cyclosporine vs. antilymphocyte globulin-azathioprine. Transplant Proc 18:192–196, 1986.

79. Halloron P, Ludwin D, Bear R, Aprile M, McQuarrie B, Poolr R, White N: Intermodal immunosuppression for cadaver renal transplantation: results using antilymphocyte globulin, azathioprine, cyclosporine, and prednisone. Transplant Proc 19:1931–1932, 1987.

80. Elion GB: Significance of azathioprine metabolites. Proc R Soc Med 64:257–259, 1972.

81. Ding TL, Gambertoglio JG, Ammond J: Azathioprine (AZA) bioavailability and pharmacokinetics in kidney transplant patients. Clin Pharmacol Ther 27:250, 1990.

82. Chan GLC, Canafax DM, Johnson CA: The therapeutic use of azathioprine in renal transplantation. Pharmacotherapy 7:165–177, 1987.

83. Ellis CN, Fradin MS, Messana JM: Cyclosporine for plaque-type psoriasis. Results of a multi-dose, double-blind trial. N Engl J Med 324:277–284, 1991.

84. Tugwell P, Bombardier C, Gent M: Low-dose cyclosporine vs. placebo in patients with rheumatoid arthritis. Lancet 335:1051–1055, 1990.

85. Foxwell BMJ, Ruffel B: The mechanisms of action of cyclosporine. Immunol Allergy Clin North Am 9:79–93, 1989.

86. Kahan BD: Cyclosporine. N Engl J Med 321:1725–1738, 1989.

87. Wilms HWF, Staeten V, Lison AE: Different pharmacokinetics of cyclosporine A early and late after renal transplantation. Transplant Proc 20:481–484, 1988.

88. Venkataramanan R, Harbucky K, Burckart G, Ptachinski RJ: Clinical pharmacokinetics in organ transplant patients. Clin Pharmacokinet 16:134–161, 1989.

89. Awni WM, Kasiske BL, Heim-Duthoy K, Rao KV: Long-term cyclosporine pharmacokinetic changes in renal transplant recipients: effects of binding and metabolism. Clin Pharmacol Ther 45:41–44, 1989.

90. Nashan B, Black J, Wonigert K: Effect of the application form of cyclosporine on blood levels: comparison of oral solution and capsules. Transplant Proc 20:637–639, 1988.

91. Gupta SK, Benet LV: Food increases the bioavailability of cyclosporine in healthy volunteers. Clin Pharmacol Ther 45;148, 1989.

92. Luke DR, Beck JE, Vadiei K, Yousefpour M, LeMaistre CF, Yau JC: Longitudinal study of cyclosporine and lipids in patients undergoing bone marrow transplantation. J Clin Pharmacol 30:163–169, 1990.

93. Ptachinski RJ, Burkart GJ, Rosenthal JT, Venkataramanan R, Howie DL, Taylor RJ, Avner ED, Ellis D, Hakala TR: Cyclosporine pharmacokinetics in children following cadaveric renal transplantation. Transplant Proc 18:766–767, 1986.

94. Copeland KR, Yatscoff RW: Immunosuppressive activity and toxicity of cyclosporine metabolites characterized by mass spectroscopy and nuclear magnetic resonance. Transplant Proc 22:1146–1149, 1990.

95. Beveridge T, Gratwohl A, Michol F: Cyclosporine A: pharmacokinetics after a single dose in man and serum levels after multiple dosing in recipients of allogenic bone marrow grafts. Curr Ther Res 30:5–18, 1981.

96. Kahan BD, Flechner SM, Lorber MI, Golden D, Conley S, Van Buren CT: Complications of cyclosporine-prednisone immunosuppression in 402 renal allograft recipients exclusively followed at a single center from one to five years. Transplantation 43:197–204, 1987.

97. Kahan BD: Cyclosporine nephrotoxicity: pathogenesis, prophylaxis, therapy and prognosis. Am J Kidney Dis 8:323–331, 1986.

98. Luke DR, Kasiske BL, Matzke GR, Awni WM, Keane WF: Effects of cyclosporine on the isolated perfused rat kidney. Transplantation 43:795–799, 1985.

99. Williams GM, Irwin B, Burdick J, Pennington L: Intravenous cyclosporine and kidney function: the Johns Hopkins experience. Transplant Proc 18:66–69, 1986.

100. Venkataramanan S, Awni WM, Jordan K, Rahman YE: Pharmacokinetics of two alternative dosage forms of cyclosporine: liposomes and intralipid. J Pharm Sci 79:216–219, 1990.

101. Luke J, Luke DR, Williams LA, LeMaistre CF, Yau JC: Prevention of cyclosporine-induced nephrotoxicity with transdermal clonidine. Clin Pharm 9:49–54, 1990.

102. Brunner LJ, Vladiei K, Lyer LV, Luke DR: Prevention of cyclosporine-induced nephrotoxicity with pentoxifylline. Renal Fail 11:97–104, 1989.

103. Wagner K, Neumayer HH: Influence of the calcium antagonist diltiazem on delayed graft function in cadaveric kidney transplantation: results of a 6-month follow-up. Transplant Proc 29:1353–1357, 1987.

104. Yee GC, McGuire TR: Pharmacokinetic drug interactions with cyclosporine (part I). Clin Pharmacokinet 19:319–322, 1990.

105. Yee GC, McGuire TR: Pharmacokinetic drug interactions with cyclosporine (part II). Clin Pharmacokinet 19:400–415, 1990.

106. McCauley J, Ptachinski RJ, Shapiro R: The cyclosporine-sparing effects of diltiazem in renal transplantation. Transplant Proc 21:3955–3957, 1989.

107. Butman SM, Wilk J, Nolan P, Fagan T, Machle M: Cyclosporine and concomitant ketoconazole after cardiac transplantation: intermediate term findings and potential savings. J Am Coll Cardiol 13(suppl A):62A, 1989.

108. Norman DJ, Illinworth DR, Mimson J, Hosinpond J: Myolysis and acute renal failure in a heart transplant recipient receiving lovastatin. N Engl J Med 318:46–47, 1988.

109. Shaw LM: Critical issues in cyclosporine monitoring: report of the task force on cyclosporine monitoring. Clin Chem 33:1269–1288, 1987.

110. Lindholm A, Dahlquist R, Groth CG: A prospective study of cyclosporine concentration in relation to its therapeutic effect and toxicity after renal transplantation. Br J Clin Pharmacol 30:443–452, 1990.

111. Condie RM, Washosky BL, Hall O: Efficacy of Minnesota antilymphoblast globulin in renal transplantation: a multicenter, placebo-controlled, prospective, randomized double-blind study. Transplant Proc 17:1304–1311, 1985.

112. Delmonico FL, Cosimi AB: Monoclonal antibody treatment of human allograft recipients. Surg Gynecol Obstet 166:89–98, 1988.

113. Thistlewaite JR, Stuart JK, Mayes JT: Complications and monitoring of OKT3 therapy. Am J Kidney Dis 11:112–119, 1988.

114. Goldman M, Abamosicz D, De Pauiu LD, Alegne ML, Widem I, Venestacten P, Kisnaert P: OKT3-induced cytokine release attenuation by high-dose methylprednisolone. Lancet 1:802–803, 1989.

115. Schroeder TJ, First MR, Mansour ME, Hurtubise PE, Harikaran S, Rychman FC, Munder R, Melvin DB, Renn I, Ballistriec WF, Alexander JW: Autoimmune antibody formation following OKT3 therapy. Transplantation 49:48–51, 1990.

116. Hricik DE, Mayes JT, Schulah JA: Inhibition of anti-OKT3 antibody generation by cyclosporine-results of a prospective randomized trial. Transplantation 50:237–240, 1990.

117. Singh N, Drummer JS, Kusni S: Infection with cytomegalovirus and other herpes viruses in 121 liver transplant recipients: transmission by donated organ and effect of OKT3 antibodies. J Infect Dis 158:124–131, 1988.

118. Swinnen LJ, Contanzo-Nordin MR, Fisher SG: Increased incidence of lymphoproliferative disorder after immunosuppression with the monoclonal antibody OKT3 in cardiac-transplant recipients. N Engl J Med 323:1723–1728, 1990.

119. Soulillus J-P, Cantarovich D, Le Mauff B, Giral M, Robillard N, Houmant M, Him M, Jacques Y: Randomized controlled trial of a monoclonal antibody against the interleukin-2 receptor (33B3.1) allografts. N Engl J Med 322:1175–1182, 1990.

120. Kinkman RH, Shaprio ME, Carpenter CB, Millford ED, Ramos EL, Tilney NL, Waldmann TA, Zimmerman CE, Strom TB: Early experience with anti-TAC in clinical renal transplantation. Transplant Proc 21:1766–1768, 1989.

121. Kirkman RL, Bacha P, Barrett LV, Forte S, Murphy JR, Strom TB: Prolongation of cardiac allograft survival in murine recipients treated with a diptheria toxin-related interleukin-2 fusion protein. Transplantation 47:327–330, 1989.

122. Amimiya H, Suzuki S, Ota K, Takahashi K, Sonoda T, Ishibashi M, Omoto R, Koyama I, Dohik, Fukuda Y, Futeau K: A novel rescue drug, 15-deoxyspergulin; first clinical trials for recurrent graft rejection in renal patients. Transplantation 49:337–343, 1990.

123. Macleod AM, Thomson AW: FK506: an immunosuppressant for the 1990s? Lancet 337:25–27, 1991.

124. Kokado Y, Ishibashi M, Jiang H, Takahara S, Sonoda T: A new triple-drug induction therapy with low-dose cyclosporine, mizoribine and prednisolone in renal transplantation. Transplant Proc 21:1575–1578, 1989.

125. Schweizer RT, Rovelli M, Palmeri D, Vossler E, Hull D, Bartus S: Noncompliance in organ transplant recipients. Transplantation 49:374–377, 1990.

CHAPTER 21

ACID PEPTIC DISORDERS

EARL S. WARD, Pharm.D. and MARIE W. JACKSON, Pharm.D.

Peptic ulcer disease includes ulceration anywhere in the gastrointestinal tract where parietal cells secrete hydrochloric acid (HCl). The Barrett ulcer of the esophagus, gastric ulcer, duodenal ulcer, postbulbar ulcer, some cases of Meckel's diverticulum, and stomal or jejunal ulcers following surgery for peptic ulceration are all classified as peptic ulcer diseases. Peptic ulcer disease results when there is an inbalance between aggressive factors (acid secretion) and protective factors (mucosal defense) (Table 21.1) (1, 2).

Most estimates suggest that between 5 and 10% of the general population will develop a peptic ulcer during their lifetime. Duodenal ulcers are four times more common than gastric ulcers. Peptic ulcer is a recurrent disease, and most clinical studies have shown that more than 50% of patients will have a recurrence within 1 year of diagnosis. Duodenal ulcers are almost never malignant, but 5% of gastric ulcers are cancerous. For this reason, careful evaluation of the patient and follow-up are extremely important with gastric ulcer disease.

GASTRIC SECRETION

The secretion of gastric HCl is intimately related to peptic ulcer disease. A peptic ulcer does not develop when there is no acid secretion. Three pathways stimulate gastric acid secretion. The endocrine pathway causes the release of gastrin, while the neurocrine and paracrine pathways cause the release of acetylcholine and histamine, respectively (3).

Acetylcholine is released at parietal cells by local nerves, stimulation of the vagus, and distention of the stomach that is mediated through receptors in the gastric wall. These cholinergic reflexes can be blocked by atropine. Acetylcholine also sensitizes parietal cells to other stimuli, such as gastrin and histamine, and plays a role in the cholinergic release of gastrin from the antral G cell in man (4).

Gastrin has several known physiological actions. It is a potent stimulant of gastric acid and pepsinogen secretion, and also stimulates hepatic bile flow, insulin release from the pancreas, and pancreatic secretions. In addition, gastrin stimulates gastric and intestinal motility, and increases lower esophageal sphincter pressure, which promotes closure of the sphincter.

Gastrin may be measured accurately in the blood by radioimmunoassay; the normal gastrin level is less than 200 pg/ml. A gastrin assay is necessary for the diagnosis of the gastrin-producing pancreatic adenoma (Zollinger-Ellison syndrome) in which fasting blood gastrin levels are extremely high. Gastrin levels are not elevated in chronic peptic ulcer disease. In pernicious anemia with its achlorhydria, serum gastrin levels are elevated because the stimulus to the "turning off" of gastrin (i.e., acid production) is absent.

Histamine is present in many of the tissues of the body, including the gastric mucosa. For many years the physiologic role of histamine in gastric secretion was controversial. The discovery by Black and co-workers of a new class of antihistaminic drugs, the H_2-receptor antagonists, identified the important physiologic role of histamine in gastric acid secretion. H_2-receptor antagonists both block the receptor for histamine on the parietal cell and inhibit acid secretion stimulated by gastrin and acetylcholine.

Gastric secretion occurs continuously, and is termed interdigestive "basal" when no stimuli are present. Stimulated gastric secretion can be divided into three phases: cephalic, gastric, and intestinal.

The cephalic phase begins in response to thought, sight, taste, smell, or chewing of food. Vagal stimulation causes the release of acetylcholine, which causes the parietal cell to secrete hydrochloric acid. Gastrin is also released from the antrum. The gastric phase is mediated by both gastrin and cholinergic nerves. Food causes distention of the stomach, leading to stimulation of the vagus nerve. Chemicals in amino acids and peptides cause further release of acid through the release of gastrin. As the gastric pH decreases, gastrin output in response to amino acids is decreased.

The intestinal phase begins when food enters the proximal portion of the small intestine. Gastric acid is secreted in response to intestinal gastrin.

The normal gastric mucosa is protected from ulceration by several mechanisms. Secretion of mucus and bicarbonate helps to protect the epithelial cells of the stomach from damage. The epithelial cells serve as a barrier to hydrogen ion back-diffusion across the gastric mucosa. These cells turn over rapidly and allow the gastric mucosa to heal itself. Gastric mucosal blood flow also plays a very important role in removing hydrogen ions that cross the gastric mucosa. If this blood flow is decreased, the risk of mucosal damage is increased. Prostaglandins stimulate the secretion of bicarbonate and mucus as well as regulate gastric mucosal blood flow. Normal pyloric function allows stomach emptying.

Table 21.1.
Factors That Influence Development of Peptic Ulcer Disease

Aggressive Factors	Protective Factors
HCl, pepsin	Secretion of mucus
Ulcerogenic drugs (ASA, NSAID, corticosteroids)	Gastric mucosal blood flow
	Bicarbonate secretion
Alcohol, nicotine	Rapid gastric epithelial cell
Gastric mucosal ischemia	turnover
Helicobacter pylori	Normal pyloric function

DUODENAL ULCER

A duodenal ulcer is a benign ulcer in the wall of the duodenum, extending into the muscularis mucosa. The true cause of duodenal ulcers is unknown, although it has been assumed for years that they are related to excessive secretion of HCl by the parietal cells of the stomach (5). Only one-third to one-half of patients with duodenal ulcers exhibit basal gastric hypersecretion and show evidence of an increased parietal cell mass by a markedly increased peak acid secretion on gastric analysis testing.

Duodenal ulcer disease is both chronic and recurrent. Duodenal ulcers probably represent a stage in a disease process that begins with acute inflammation of the duodenal mucosa and progresses through more severe stages of duodenitis until an ulcer develops. The ulcer usually persists for 4 to 6 weeks, but may on occasion heal rapidly. The whole process may repeat itself at some later point, depending upon as yet unknown stimuli. Certain risk factors such as cigarette smoking, chronic use of aspirin, nonsteroidal antiinflammatory drugs, or alcohol contribute to increased risk. Smokers have earlier and more frequent recurrence, with increased mortality (6). Patients who experience gastrointestinal bleeding also have a higher incidence of recurrence. Psychosomatic factors probably do not play an important role in the development of the ulcer, and a relationship to a variety of stress situations seems at best only vaguely associated with the development of new ulcers. A recurrent ulcer may or may not develop in the same location as the previous one.

BENIGN GASTRIC ULCER

In the United States, gastric ulcer occurs about one-fourth as frequently as duodenal ulcer. Like duodenal ulcer, it is more common in men than in women. The incidence increases after 50 years of age, and it is unusual in the younger age population.

Unlike duodenal ulcer, which is thought to be a disorder of gastric acid hypersecretion, gastric ulcers tend to be associated with lower rates of acid secretion, when compared with normal subjects. A gastric ulcer is most com-

mon at the junction between the antrum and the fundus of the stomach, on the lesser curvature.

Within the last 10 years, various investigators have shown that gastric ulcers, although an acid peptic disease like other ulcers, may be primarily caused by the breakdown of the mucosal barrier and to back-diffusion of acid across the gastric mucosa. Normally, less than one-tenth of the gastric HCl secreted by the parietal cells is reabsorbed through the gastric mucosal by back-diffusion. In patients with gastric ulcers, the figure tends to be much higher. The healing of a gastric ulcer does not result in normalization of the gastric mucosal barrier to back-diffusion. Back-diffusion remains high, even if the ulcer has disappeared. Furthermore, a gastric ulcer does not necessarily recur at the site of the previous ulcer, suggesting that the defect in the mucosal barrier is generalized, rather than localized (7).

The mucosal barrier consists of the plasma membrane of the surface epithelial cells, which, because of the high phospholipid content and the tight junctions between cells, is impermeable to ionized material. A number of agents can damage the mucosal barrier. Salicylates, fatty acids, ethanol, lysolecithin, and bile salts all disrupt the normal mucosal barrier. This allows rapid back-diffusion of hydrogen ion from the lumen into the mucosa, causing cellular destruction and increased capillary permeability within the damaged mucosa. This in turn results in extravasation of plasma proteins, producing mucosal edema. The rapid cell turnover of the gastric mucosa is also disrupted, leading to desquamation and loss of gastric epithelial cells in the area.

HELICOBACTER PYLORI

Many patients with peptic ulcer disease have colonization of the gastric mucosa with *Helicobacter pylori* (*H. pylori*) (8). In one study, *H. pylori* was isolated from antral biopsy specimens in 98% of patients with duodenal or gastric ulcer, 70% of patients with nonulcer dyspepsia, and 20% of normal volunteers (9). The role of this organism in the development or recurrence of peptic ulcer disease is controversial. Some experts believe the *H. pylori* causes an increase in acid and gastrin secretion in response to a meal (10). In addition the organism may cause inflammation of the gastric mucosa, which disrupts the normal mucosal defense system and allows the development of an ulcer.

CLINICAL FINDINGS

The symptoms of peptic ulcer disease are quite varied. The slight differences between duodenal ulcer and gastric ulcer are so subtle that the differentiation cannot be made on symptoms alone. Burning pain in the epigastric area is most common. Less commonly it radiates to other areas, such as the back or lower abdomen. Duodenal ulcers often exhibit a cycle of pain-food-relief. Food may worsen the pain in gastric ulcer (5).

RADIOLOGY AND ENDOSCOPY

Fiberoptic endoscopes permit direct examination of the esophagus, stomach, and first and second portions of the duodenum. Thus, most areas in which upper GI disease occur are readily accessible to direct visualization and biopsy. Equivocal lesions can be biopsied with relative ease, and one can obtain adequate visualization of superficial erosions not readily visible radiographically. Endoscopy has become the primary method of diagnosing sources of upper GI bleeding. Additionally, endoscopy should be the preferred procedure in evaluating upper GI problems in pregnant women, in whom radiation is to be avoided. The diagnostic accuracy rate of endoscopy in ulcer disease is in the 95% range.

An upper GI series may be useful in the initial examination of the patient with ulcer pain or dyspepsia. However 15 to 30% of lesions may be missed in the standard upper GI series.

TREATMENT

The goals of treatment in peptic ulcer disease are to relieve pain, heal the ulcer, prevent complications such as GI bleeding or perforation, and prevent recurrence of the ulcer. Antacids, H_2-receptor antagonists, sucralfate, and acid-pump inhibitors are used in the treatment of peptic ulcer disease.

Antacids

Antacids provide symptomatic relief and heal peptic ulcers. While they are as effective as H_2-receptor antagonists and sucralfate, antacids have a greater frequency of side effects and require more frequent dosing.

Antacids heal duodenal ulcers by neutralizing gastric acid. In order to buffer the acid that the stomach constantly produces, the antacid must be present in the stomach. The rate of gastric emptying limits the amount of antacid in the stomach. The fasting stomach empties its contents into the duodenum as often as every 30 min to 1 hr. Frequent administration of antacid is necessary to buffer the constant secretion of acid. A more practical regimen, however, is hourly or every-other-hour administration. A regimen that administers antacids several times between meals to take advantage of the buffering ability of the meals is a popular dosage schedule. Fordtran showed that administration of 30 ml of a high-potency antacid 1 hr after a meal caused neutralization of the acid secreted in response to the meal for 3 hr (11). The Fordtran regimen is to give the antacid 1 hr and 3 hr after a meal and again at bedtime, for a total of seven administrations of antacid per day. This is the regimen most commonly used in the treatment of duodenal ulcer. The efficacy has been shown repeatedly in numerous studies. Petersen and associates gave the equivalent of 30 ml of Mylanta II (without simethicone) seven times daily, 1 and 3 hr after meals, and at bedtime (12). Patients were randomized between this regimen and a placebo. Both groups were instructed to take 30 ml of an antacid if they had pain. If diarrhea developed, an equivalent dose of an aluminum-containing antacid or placebo was given. The total daily acid-neutralizing ability of this regimen exceeds 1000 mEq. Pain relief, antacid use, and ulcer healing (as demonstrated by endoscopy) were all measured. There was ulcer healing in 78% of the patients receiving antacids and 45% of those receiving placebo. There was no correlation between ulcer healing and pain relief in this study. Two-thirds of the antacid group developed diarrhea requiring the addition of an aluminum-containing antacid.

Lower dosages of antacids (15 ml, 6 times daily) have also proven to be effective and may be more conducive to patient compliance (13). Since antacids must be present in the stomach to work, the patient may be awakened at night with pain caused by nocturnal acid secretion. A treatment period of 4 to 6 weeks is necessary to heal 70 to 80% of duodenal ulcers. Treatment for longer than 6 weeks does not offer any advantage, except possibly in smokers. Antacid efficacy studies in patients with gastric ulcers have produced variable results (14).

Side effects include diarrhea (magnesium-containing antacids) or constipation (aluminum-containing antacids). There is some concern over the long-term safety of aluminum-containing antacids. Aluminum binds phosphate, which may lead to bone problems (15).

Antacids may also cause drug interactions. Interactions have been reported with ketoconazole, tetracycline, ferrous sulfate, and isoniazid.

H_2-Receptor Antagonists

The development of the first H_2-receptor antagonist, cimetidine, has changed the way that patients with peptic ulcer disease are treated.

H_2-receptor antagonists are the most frequently used agents for the treatment of peptic ulcer disease. Currently four drugs are available in this country, cimetidine, ranitidine, famotidine, and nizatidine. They differ in potency, chemical structure, adverse effects, and ability to cause drug interactions. Famotidine is the most potent, followed by nizatidine, ranitidine, and cimetidine (16, 17).

H_2-receptor antagonists competitively block the H_2 receptor on the parietal cells, causing inhibition of gastric acid secretion. This effect on gastric acid secretion is dose-dependent and reversible.

H_2-receptor antagonists are more effective than placebo in healing duodenal and gastric ulcers. Agents are of equal efficacy with 80% of duodenal ulcers healed in 4

Table 21.2.
Dosage Schedule for Peptic Ulcer Disease

	Initial	Maintenance
Cimetidine	300 mg q.i.d. 400 mg b.i.d. 800 mg h.s.	400 mg h.s.
Ranitidine	150 mg b.i.d. 300 mg h.s.	150 mg h.s.
Famotidine	20 mg b.i.d. 40 mg h.s.	20 mg h.s.
Nizatidine	150 mg b.i.d. 300 mg h.s.	150 mg h.s.
Sulcralfate	1 g q.i.d. 2 g b.i.d.	1 g b.i.d.
Omeprazole	20 mg q.d.	

Table 21.3.
Factors Associated with Peptic Ulcer Recurrence

Smoking (>10 cigarettes/day)	ASA or NSAID ingestion
Gastric acid hypersecretion	History of ulcers
Male sex	Low-fiber diet
Age	Poor compliance
H. pylori gastritis	

weeks and more than 90% healed in 8 weeks. Gastric ulcers may take longer to heal and usually require at least 8 weeks of treatment.

H_2-receptor antagonists may be given in divided daily doses or at bedtime as a single dose for acute initial therapy of duodenal and gastric ulcers. The dosage regimens are equivalent and may be administered for up to 8 weeks (Table 21.2). Maintenance therapy for duodenal ulcer should be given as a single dose at bedtime.

Duodenal ulcer recurrence is reported to range between 20 and 80% within 12 months following cessation of therapy (18). Risk factors associated with recurrence of peptic ulcers are listed in Table 21.3. Full-dose H_2-receptor therapy (Table 21.2) may be given intermittently to patients at low risk if there is evidence of ulcer recurrence. Patients with risk factors should receive daily maintenance H_2-receptor antagonist therapy after the ulcer is healed initially. Treatment may be needed indefinitely. Both cimetidine and ranitidine have good long-term safety data, with no increased risk of gastric cancer (19, 20).

CIMETIDINE

Cimetidine is approved for active and maintenance therapy of duodenal ulcer, active benign gastric ulcer hypersecretory conditions, and gastroesophageal reflux disease (21). Cimetidine is well-absorbed following oral administration, with peak levels produced within 1 hr of administration. Cimetidine is metabolized in the liver and has a

half-life of about 2 hr in patients with normal renal function. The half-life increases as renal function diminishes.

Cimetidine, like the other H_2-receptor antagonists, has very few major side effects. Diarrhea, usually mild and transient, dizziness, and headache have been reported, with a prevalence under 1%. Mental status alteration (confusion, agitation, anxiety, etc.) may occur, especially in severely ill patients (renal/hepatic impairment) and in the elderly, if the dose is not adjusted appropriately. Gynecomastia has been reported in about 4% of patients receiving high-dose cimetidine for long-term treatment of Zollinger-Ellison syndrome. Cimetidine has been reported to cause mild transient increases in several laboratory test results (AST, serum creatinine levels, etc.), which are not usually clinically important. Cimetidine inhibits the cytochrome P-450 enzyme system in the liver and may cause several drug interactions with warfarin, phenytoin, propranolol, and theophylline. Cimetidine has also been reported to potentiate the myelosuppressive effects of certain oncology agents. Signs and symptoms of toxicity should be monitored carefully in patients receiving these drugs concomitantly, or other H_2-receptor antagonists that do not exhibit these drug interactions should be used. H_2-receptor antagonists have also been shown to potentiate the effect of ethanol (22).

The oral dose of cimetidine may be found in Table 21.2. Cimetidine may also be administered i.m. or IV in doses of 300 mg every 6 to 8 hr. Dosage should be reduced in patients with a creatinine clearance of less than 30 ml/min.

RANITIDINE

Ranitidine is approved for the active and maintenance therapy of duodenal ulcer, active benign gastric ulcer, hypersecretory conditions, and gastroesophageal reflux disease (21).

Ranitidine is well-absorbed after oral administration with peak serum levels occurring in 2 to 3 hr. The elimination half-life of ranitidine averages 1.7 to 3.2 hr. Ranitidine is metabolized in the liver and excreted in the urine. The elimination of ranitidine is prolonged in patients with renal impairment.

Adverse effects of ranitidine are similar to those of cimetidine with the exception of headache, which occurs in approximately 3% of patients.

Ranitidine does not interact with the hepatic cytochrome P-450 system in the same manner as cimetidine. It only minimally inhibits hepatic metabolism of drugs such as coumadin, theophylline, diazepam, and propranolol. This may produce variable effects with the interacting drugs. These interactions do not appear to be as important as those experienced with cimetidine.

The dose of ranitidine for peptic ulcer disease may be found in Table 21.2. Ranitidine may be administered in i.m. or IV dosages of 50 mg every 6 to 8 hr. Dosage reduction should be made in patients with creatinine clearances less than 50 ml/minute.

FAMOTIDINE

Famotidine is indicated for active and maintenance therapy for duodenal ulcer, active benign gastric ulcer, and hypersecretory conditions (21). Famotidine is absorbed incompletely from the GI tract following oral administration, and peak plasma concentrations occur in 1 to 4 hr. Famotidine has the longest half-life of the H_2-receptor antagonists, with an average elimination half-life of 2.5 to 4 hr. The half-life is increased in patients with renal impairment. Famotidine is metabolized in the liver and excreted in the urine. Side effects of famotidine are similar to those of the other H_2-receptor antagonists. However it does not appear to exhibit antiandrogenic activity or affect the hepatic clearance of other drugs. Some evidence indicates that famotidine may have a negative inotropic effect, but further study is needed to confirm the clinical importance of this.

The dosage of famotidine for peptic ulcer disease is given in Table 21.2. Famotidine may be given by slow IV injection in doses of 20 mg every 12 hr. Dosage adjustment should be made in adults with creatinine clearances less than 30 ml/minute.

NIZATIDINE

Nizatidine, the newest H_2-receptor antagonist, is indicated for active and maintenance therapy for duodenal ulcer and treatment of gastroesophageal reflux disease (21). Nizatidine is well-absorbed orally from the gastrointestinal tract, with peak plasma concentrations occurring within 0.5 to 3 hr. Nizatidine is metabolized in the liver and excreted in the urine. The elimination half-life is 1 to 2 hr in normal patients and is increased in patients with renal impairment.

The adverse effects seen with nizatidine are similar to those of other H_2-receptor antagonists. There is no evidence of antiandrogen effects, and no serious effects on central nervous system have been reported. Hepatitis has been reported more frequently than with the other H_2-receptor antagonist. However more data are needed to confirm the comparative incidence. There is no effect on the cytochromic P-450 enzyme system, making nizatidine a favorable choice when other drugs that might interact with other H_2-receptor antagonists are administered.

The dosage for nizatidine in peptic ulcer disease may be found in Table 21.2. It is only available for oral administration.

Other Agents

SUCRALFATE

Sucralfate, a complex of sulfated sucrose and aluminum hydroxide, is indicated for short-term treatment and maintenance therapy of duodenal ulcer (21). It has a unique mechanism of action since it neither buffers nor inhibits acid production. Sucralfate does have antipeptic activity, which is strongest at the acid pH values expected in the stomach. Sucralfate also binds to free proteins, which suggests that the concentration of sucralfate at the ulcer site is higher than that in adjacent normal tissue (23).

In several studies, sucralfate 1 g given 30 to 60 min before meals and at bedtime (4 times daily) has been shown to heal about 80% of duodenal ulcers in 4 to 6 weeks. This is comparable to H_2-receptor antagonists. Relapse rates in duodenal ulcer patients treated with sucralfate appear to be similar to those observed with H_2-receptor antagonists. Sucralfate appears to be effective in healing gastric ulcers as well. About 80% of patients treated for 6 to 8 weeks appear to heal, compared with 40% of patients receiving placebo (24). Sucralfate is not FDA-approved for gastric ulcer treatment.

Side effects are minimal, since the drug is very poorly absorbed. Constipation is the most frequent adverse effect. Other minor complaints include diarrhea, nausea, indigestion, dry mouth, and dizziness. Drug-associated laboratory abnormalities have not been observed.

The dosage of sucralfate is 1 g four times a day on an empty stomach. A dosage of 2 g bid has also been shown to be effective. The tablets should not be chewed. Antacids should not be taken 30 min before or after sucralfate.

ACID-PUMP INHIBITORS

Omeprazole is in a new class of acid-pump inhibitors. Omeprazole binds irreversibly to the acid (proton) pump of the parietal cell and inhibits acid secretion (25).

Omeprazole is indicated for the management of hypersecretory states such as Zollinger-Ellison syndrome, gastroesophageal reflux (GERD), and severe erosive esophagitis, and for short-term treatment of active duodenal ulcer.

Omeprazole absorption is variable and increases with increasing dosage. It undergoes extensive metabolism in the liver and has an elimination half-life of 0.5 to 1.5 hr. Omeprazole reduces peak acid output by 80%, causing serum gastrin levels to increase significantly. The effect on gastric acid secretion may persist for 24 to 72 hr following a dose.

Adverse effects of omeprazole are similar to those with ranitidine and include headache, diarrhea, abdominal pain, and nausea in less than 5% of patients. Because of its potent acid suppression, development of gastric carcinoid tumors is a concern. Tumors have been reported in rats, but not in humans. In 40 patients with Zollinger-Ellison syndrome treated with 82 ± 31 mg per day there was no evidence of the development of these tumors for up to 4 years (6 to 51 months) (26). Omeprazole interacts with the cytochrome P-450 system and may cause important drug interactions like those seen with cimetidine.

Omeprazole 20 mg once daily has been shown to be effective for short-term (4 weeks) treatment of active duodenal ulcer. Some patients may require an additional 4 weeks. Omeprazole is not indicated for maintenance therapy. In one study comparing 20 mg and 40 mg once daily of omeprazole with 150 mg twice daily of ranitidine, the healing rate at 4 weeks was 97%, 100%, and 82%, respectively (27). There was no significant difference in healing between 20 mg and 40 mg of omeprazole. These was also no significant difference in relapse rates (60% at 6 months). The pain relief with omeprazole was faster (2 days) than with ranitidine (7 days).

ANTICHOLINERGICS

Anticholinergics are decreasing in importance in the treatment of duodenal ulcers. Although they are effective antagonists of acid secretion, the magnitude of their acid secretory reduction is of the order of 30 to 35% rather than the 85 to 90% reduction achieved with H_2-receptor antagonists. Anticholinergics may be used with antacids to help prevent stomach emptying and to prolong the buffering activity of antacids. Anticholinergics have no place in the treatment of patients with gastric ulcers. The minor antisecretory activity of this class of drugs is offset by the ability to reduce the motility of the GI tract. This causes retention of acid and pepsin in the stomach.

Treatment of *H. pylori*

The treatment of *H. pylori* infection remains controversial, and no regimen is currently FDA-approved. One regimen, reported to be effective in eradicating the organism for up to 12 months in 75% of patients, is bismuth plus metronidazole 250 mg three times a day for 4 weeks (28). Bismuth is available in the United States as Pepto-Bismol (bismuth subsalicylate). The effective dosage of bismuth is 525 mg four times a day (8). Further studies in larger patient populations are needed to evaluate the above regimen and alternative antibiotics in the event that *H. pylori* is resistant to metronidazole.

Summary

The H_2-receptor antagonists appear to be equal in effect in their treatment of duodenal and gastric ulcer. Use of these products should be determined by potential for adverse effects, drug interactions, and cost. Sucralfate may be used as an alternative to H_2-receptor antagonists, but there is not convincing evidence that the combination of sucralfate with an H_2-receptor antagonist is any more beneficial than either agent alone. Omeprazole has demonstrated improved healing of duodenal ulcers in a shorter time period (4 weeks) and faster onset of pain relief, compared with H_2 receptor blockers.

ZOLLINGER-ELLISON (GASTRINOMA) SYNDROME

Zollinger-Ellison syndrome occurs in less than 1% of patients with peptic ulcer disease. It is caused by a gastrin-producing adenoma of the pancreas and (sometimes) other endocrine glands that cause continuous secretions of HCl. The range of basal gastrin concentration in patients with duodenal ulcer disease without gastrinoma is usually from 0 to 120 pg/ml, depending on the sensitivity of the assay being used. A serum gastrin concentration above 1000 pg/ml with compatible clinical findings supports the diagnosis of Zollinger-Ellison syndrome (29).

Characteristically there are severe, often unremitting and numerous recurrences of peptic ulcers. These may be either gastric or duodenal and are often multiple, occurring in unusual locations such as the third part of the duodenum or even the jejunum. The patient has persistent ulcer pain and diarrhea. Zollinger-Ellison syndrome occurs in adults of both sexes with equal frequency and rarely in children.

Treatment

H_2-RECEPTOR ANTAGONISTS

H_2-receptor antagonists may be used in higher doses for the treatment of Zollinger-Ellison syndrome. The usual dosage of these agents are: cimetidine 300 mg four times a day; ranitidine 150 mg twice daily; and famotidine 20 mg every 6 hours (21).

OMEPRAZOLE

The initial dosage for patients with Zollinger-Ellison syndrome is 60 mg daily. In patients unresponsive to the usual dose, 60 mg twice daily may be effective (26).

Summary

Omeprazole may be considered the drug of choice in treating this disorder. Patients have been safely treated for up to 4 years with no major adverse effects. However, further evaluation of long-term safety is essential.

GASTROESOPHAGEAL REFLUX DISEASE (GERD)

Gastroesophageal reflux disease is the syndrome produced by retrograde flow of gastric contents into the esophagus, which may lead to esophageal injury. The syndrome is caused by a malfunctioning lower esophageal sphincter (LES). This relaxation of the lower esophageal sphincter may be transient. The decrease in lower esophageal sphincter tone allows the refluxed gastric contents to enter the esophagus and irritate the mucosal tissue. If the esophageal mucosal tissue is not efficient in clearing the acid, injury may occur. The role of gastric emptying in the development of this condition is not clear. There may be no difference in gastric emptying between patients with

Table 21.4.
Drugs That Decrease LES Pressure

α-Adrenergic antagonists	Progesterone
β-Adrenergic antagonists	Nitrates
Anticholinergics	Calcium-channel blockers
Theophylline	Dopamine
Benzodiazepines	Prostaglandins E_1, E_2, A_2
Narcotics	

GERD and normal persons (30, 31). The classic clinical symptom of GERD is heartburn, which most often occurs as substernal burning after a meal. Other symptoms include regurgitation, belching, and dysphagia. Approximately 40% of the population experiences heartburn at least monthly. If the symptoms become severe or the condition recurs more frequently, treatment may be required.

Diagnosis is based on patient history, including diet. Foods such as onions, chocolate, peppermint, and high-fat foods, may contribute to decreased LES tone. Drugs may also decrease LES tone (Table 21.4). Endoscopy is often done to determine the extent of esophageal damage. Twenty-four-hour ambulatory pH monitoring of the esophagus is used to determine the pattern of daytime and nocturnal reflux.

Treatment

The nondrug treatment for GERD includes modification of the diet to eliminate foods that precipitate an attack, cessation of smoking, and elevation of the head of the bed with blocks. If this does not reduce symptoms, antacids may be added for their ability to neutralize acid and bind bile salts. Antacids should be used hourly in the acute phase until symptoms lessen, and then 1 and 3 hr after meals and at bedtime. Alginic acid may be just as effective as antacids at controlling symptoms. If antacids or alginic acid do not control symptoms adequately, either H_2-receptor antagonists or omeprazole should be added to the regimen.

H_2-receptor antagonists may be used to treat GERD. Ranitidine should be used in a dosage of 150 mg twice daily. Ranitidine has been shown to be significantly more effective than placebo treatment in decreasing the frequency and severity of heartburn (32). Other H_2-receptor antagonists have been used as follows: cimetidine 400 to 800 mg twice daily, famotidine 20 to 40 mg twice daily, and nizatidine 150 to 300 mg twice daily.

Omeprazole 20 to 40 mg daily has been used in the management of GERD and esophagitis. One study reported that 20 mg daily is superior to ranitidine and resulted in 85% healing of esophageal ulcerations, versus 50% healing in the ranitidine group (33). More rapid relief of symptoms occurred in the omeprazole group. Another study compared ranitidine 300 mg twice daily and ome-

prazole 20 mg once daily in the treatment of moderate to severe esophagitis. Both drugs reduced the exposure of esophageal mucosa to acid over a 24-hr period and decreased the number of reflux episodes (34).

Sucralfate 1 g four times a day has also been used in the treatment of GERD. One study showed no difference between sucralfate 1 g four times a day and ranitidine 150 mg twice a day (35).

Sometimes prokinetic drugs such as metoclopramide must be added to the regimen. Metoclopramide increases LES pressure and increases gastric emptying. Dosages of 10 mg four times a day 30 min before meals and at bedtime may be used with an H_2-receptor antagonist or omeprazole. Side effects include depression, lethargy, restlessness, insomnia, skin rashes, blurred vision, and dry mouth (21).

GERD is a chronic condition, with up to 90% of patients having a recurrence within 6 months. This may necessitate continued treatment. The H_2-receptor antagonists have been shown to be safe for long-term therapy, but omeprazole therapy must be limited to 8 weeks. Up to 90% of patients will have a recurrence of GERD within 6 months. Approximately 5 to 10% of patients will be refractory to treatment and require surgery (36).

Summary

Management of GERD requires both nondrug and drug therapy in most patients. Patients should be tried on a regimen of antacids combined with either H_2-receptor antagonists or omeprazole for initial therapy.

STRESS-RELATED ULCERATION

Stress ulceration can be defined as superficial gastroduodenal erosions of the gastric mucosa that develop when severe physiologic demands are placed upon a critically ill individual (37). This type of ulceration differs from traditional peptic ulcer disease in several ways (Table 21.5). With stress ulceration the lesions are small and numerous versus the single lesion seen in PUD. The lesions are superficial instead of deep or penetrating and are located in

Table 21.5.
Comparison between Stress Ulcer and Chronic Peptic Ulcer[a]

Stress Ulcer	Chronic Peptic Ulcer
Multiple lesions	Single lesions
Superficial	Deep
Duodenal bulb and gastric antrum	Acid-producing areas of stomach
Asymptomatic	Symptomatic
Superficial capillaries	Single vessel

[a] From Friedman G: Peptic ulcer disease. Clin Symp 40:2–28, 1988, with permission.

the duodenal bulb and gastric antrum rather than the acid-producing areas. These ulcerations tend to be asymptomatic versus symptomatic (38). Furthermore, stress ulcerations are more closely associated with an acute process, versus the chronic inflammatory process regularly associated with peptic ulcer disease. Virtually all untreated seriously ill patients develop stress ulceration, with 5 to 20% of all ICU patients developing serious upper gastrointestinal hemorrhage. The mortality associated with hemorrhage ranges from 50 to 80% (38, 39). The incidence of stress ulceration and associated complications has decreased over the past 20 years because of better supportive measures including better ventilatory support, nutritional support, hemodynamic monitoring, and administration of prophylactic agents (40). However, much effort continues to be expended toward prevention and treatment.

Risk Factors

All seriously ill patients are at risk for stress ulceration (Table 21.6). Specific complications and factors have been identified as placing a patient at higher risk. As early as the mid-1800s, patients with severe burns (> 35% body surface area) and those who had undergone major surgery were considered to be at high risk for gastrointestinal bleeding (38). Patients with prolonged stays in intensive care settings or prolonged mechanical ventilation are also at increased risk for ulceration. Other factors include severe head injury, coma, multiple trauma, kidney transplantation, and multiple-organ system failure (40, 41). Critically ill patients developing sepsis, hypotension, or jaundice have an even higher risk for bleeding (40). The more severe the underlying problem and the greater number of risk factors, the greater the chance of ulceration and bleeding.

Pathogenesis

Although the pathophysiologic mechanisms of stress ulcerations are not completely defined, many theories have implicated changes in gastric acidity and ischemic changes in gastric mucosa (Table 21.7). Acid appears to be necessary for the development of mucosal damage, since ulceration does not occur at the gastric pH >7 (38, 42).

Table 21.6.
Risk Factors for Stress Ulcer Bleeding[a]

Hypotension	Sepsis
Burn >30% BSA	Respiratory failure
Multiple trauma	Closed head injury
Jaundice	Hepatic failure
NSAIDs	Uremia

[a] From Friedman G: Peptic ulcer disease. Clin Symp 40:2–28, 1988, with permission.

Table 21.7.
Factors in the Pathogenesis of Stress Ulcers[a]

Gastric acidity
Mucosal ischemia
Mucus production
Bicarbonate secretion
Mucosal prostaglandins
Epithelial cell removal

[a] From Friedman G: Peptic ulcer disease. Clin Symp 40:2–28, 1988, with permission.

Although some patients (e.g., those with severe head injuries) may secrete excess acid, other patients may secrete normal or below normal amounts of acid. Consequently, it is not the amount of acid that makes the patient vulnerable to stress ulceration, but the way the gastric mucosa responds to the acidic conditions (37). Gastric mucosal cells have high energy requirements, and gastric mucosal blood flow is necessary for the maintenance and integrity of the gastric mucosal barrier (38). A decrease in mucosal blood flow decreases the energy supply to the cells and allows mucosal damage and necrosis to occur. Mucosal ischemia prevents the gastric mucosa from controlling back-diffusion of hydrogen ions. It is theorized that the activity of hydrogen ion back-diffusion leads to ulceration and finally hemorrhage. Damage to mucosal cells also leads to a decrease in mucus production and bicarbonate secretion, allowing more acid-induced injury. Inhibition of mucosal prostaglandin synthesis adds to the gastric mucosa susceptibility. Prostaglandins assist in the resistance of gastric mucosa to noxious stimuli by suppressing acid secretion, maintaining mucosal blood flow, and stimulating mucus formation and bicarbonate secretion (37). Inhibition of prostaglandins increases mucosal susceptibility to acid injury. Finally, alterations in gastric epithelial cell regeneration, the reparative cell process for mucosal integrity, may also contribute to ulcerations during prolonged periods of stress.

Diagnosis

Since most high-risk ICU patients have nasogastric (NG) tubes in place, observation of frank blood from NG aspirate is a quick method of detecting GI bleeding. Not all bleeding can be detected in this way. Methods for detection of microscopic blood loss include guaiac and Hemoccult tests (40). Only a few of the positive test results disclose conditions resulting in serious bleeding. The only definitive mechanism for diagnosing acute gastric mucosal injury is upper GI endoscopy. Routine use of this procedure without prior indication of ulceration or bleeding may be unwarranted.

Treatment

The question of providing stress ulceration prophylaxis to all intensive care patients continues to be raised. Many studies have been performed to provide a solution to this dilemma. One recent study examined the effects of prophylaxis with H2-antagonists and antacids versus no treatment in critically ill neurosurgical patients (43). No significant difference was detected between the two groups in terms of endoscopic findings or overt GI bleeding. Another study compared cimetidine and placebo in the prevention of stress-related gastric mucosal damage in patients in intensive care units (44). From this multicenter study, one (2%) of 54 patients receiving continuous infusion of cimetidine (50 mg/hr) experienced upper gastrointestinal hemorrhage, in comparison with seven (21%) of 33 patients receiving placebo. The risk of bleeding for patients receiving cimetidine was decrease by 9.4%. Continuous-infusion cimetidine was well-tolerated and resulted in minor, reversible side effects in 4% of patients receiving treatment.

Although the issue of treatment remains unresolved, the consensus is that stress ulceration prophylaxis should be provided to critically ill patients since mortality associated with upper GI bleeding remains high (45).

Antacids were the agents used first for prophylaxis of stress ulcerations. Today, they are used continually for maintenance of gastric pH >4. As previously mentioned, a reduction of gastric acid levels and an increase in gastric pH help prevent stress ulceration. Studies comparing H2-receptor antagonists with antacids have shown antacids to be equally effective in maintaining pH > 4 and in preventing overt bleeding (38, 42). A study in which antacids and H2-antagonists were administered both as intermittent boluses and as continuous infusions concluded that significantly fewer patients bleed while receiving either continuous infusion regimen (38).

Current antacid therapy includes doses of 30 to 90 ml of a highly potent magnesium/aluminum antacid such as Mylanta II or Maalox TC. Initially a 30-ml dose is administered every 1 to 2 hr via the nasogastric tube (42). The tube may or may not be clamped for 30 min after antacid administration. Frequently, the pH of the NG aspirate is monitored to ensure that the goal of therapy is being met. If the pH remains below the therapeutic goal, the dose of the antacid may be doubled. Doses can be increased until the goal pH is maintained. Continuous infusions of antacids (60 ml/hr) have also been used and were effective in preventing gastric bleeding (38). Although effective agents in preventing gastric bleeding, antacids have some disadvantages. When compared with other drugs such as sucralfate and H2-antagonists, antacids are associated with a higher frequency of nosocomial pneumonias (42). These results suggest that acid inhibition by antacids may promote intragastric bacterial growth, which then may be aspirated into the lungs of critically ill patients.

Table 21.8.
Continuous Infusion Doses for Stress Ulceration Prophylaxis

Drug	Dose (mg/hr)
Cimetidine	37.5–100
Ranitidine	6.25–12.5
Famotidine	3.2–4.0

H2-antagonists are considered to be the gold standard for stress ulceration prophylaxis (45). Originally, treatment consisted of administration of intermittent doses of these agents. However, GI pH was not maintained above 4 consistently (45). In contrast, continuous infusion of H2-antagonists resulted in better control of GI pH $\geq$ 4 as well as more sustained antisecretory concentrations of the drug (Fig. 21.1) (44–47). Consequently, more ICU patients are receiving H2-antagonists via continuous infusion. Studies have used continuous infusion doses from 37.5 to 100 mg/hr with cimetidine (44, 46), 6.25 to 12.5 mg/hr with ranitidine (45), and 3.2 to 4 mg/hr with famotidine (Table 21.8) (45).

Sucralfate has also been reviewed for efficacy in the prevention of stress-related gastric mucosal damage (38, 42). Sucralfate tablets can be swallowed whole, or when dissolved in a small amount of water to form a slurry, poured down nasogastric or other feeding tubes. Sucralfate 1 g q4h is as effective as antacids administered every 2 hr and H2-antagonists given via continuous infusion for the prevention of gastric bleeding. Use of these cytoprotective agents requires nasogastric tubes or oral administration (47).

The gastric mucosal protective effects of prostaglandin analogs have also been studied in critically ill patients (39, 41, 42, 48). Misoprostol, the only prostaglandin E1 analog on the market, appears to facilitate regeneration of the mucosa after injury by NSAIDs and may aid in the prevention of stress ulcerations. Comparisons with misoprostol and antacids have shown equal efficacy in maintaining GI pH and in preventing GI bleeding. The prostaglandin analog appears to have no therapeutic advantage over antacids.

DRUG-INDUCED ULCERATION

The use of medications frequently leads to adverse effects, and a large percentage of them are gastrointestinal. Although agents such as erythromycin, iron salts, corticosteroids, and potassium chloride (49) may be linked to gastroduodenal damage, the agents most frequently associated with GI insult are aspirin and the nonsteroidal

Figure 21.1. Effect of cimetidine bolus (*light line*) versus primed infusion (*bold line*) on gastric pH in the "typical patient." (With permission, from Ostro MJ, Russell JA, Soldin SJ, et al.: Control of gastric pH with cimetidine: boluses versus primed infusions. Gastroenterology 89:532–537, 1985.)

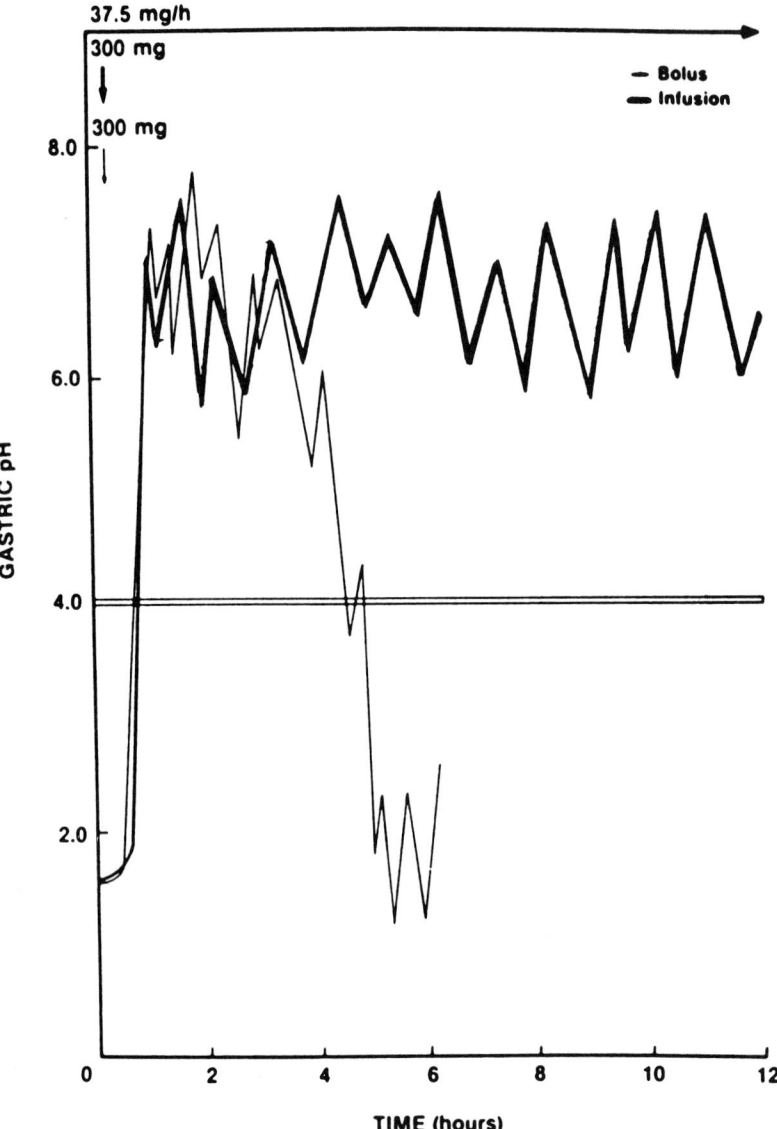

antiinflammatory drugs (NSAIDs). Even with short-term administration, ibuprofen, naproxen, tolmetin, indomethacin, phenylbutazone, and salicylates cause both gastric and duodenal mucosal damage. Elderly patients with rheumatoid- and osteoarthritis appear to be at increased risk of ulceration and overt hemorrhage. In one retrospective study, users of NSAIDs were found to be four times more likely to die from peptic ulcer disease or upper gastrointestinal bleeding than nonusers (50).

Cigarette use increases the risk of ulceration and its complications in persons taking NSAIDs (51). Individuals who smoke have impaired healing and recurrence of ulcers. Smoking also increases the likelihood that surgery will be required for ulcer repair.

Pathogenesis

NSAIDs are thought to induce damage of the gastric mucosa via two mechanisms: (*a*) by direct effects of the acidic agent on the gastric mucosa, and (*b*) by inhibiting the production of protective prostaglandins (Fig. 21.2) (52, 53). Gastric mucus provides a barrier that protects the stomach epithelium from gastric contents through several mechanisms: (*a*) the mucosa secretes bicarbonate, via receptor-mediated active transport, which buffers acidic contents, (*b*) the mucus layer thickens in response to epithelial injury, allowing rapid epithelialization to take place after insults from agents such as aspirin and ethanol, and (*c*) gastric blood flow helps to protect the mucosa from injury. If the mucous barrier is disrupted, a compensatory in-

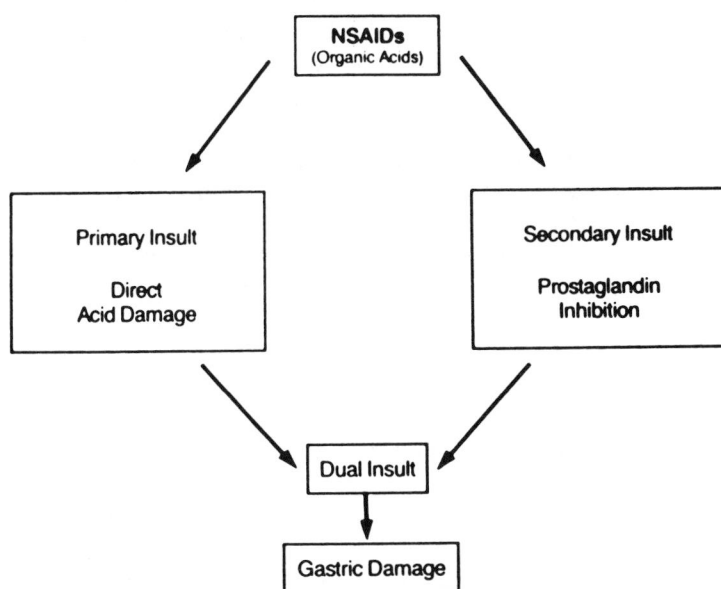

Figure 21.2. NSAID dual-insult hypothesis. (With permission, from Schoen RT, Vender RJ: Mechanisms of nonsteroidal anti-inflammatory drug-induced gastric damage. Am J Med 86:449–458, 1989.)

crease in blood flow helps to remove the H + ions that can damage the mucosa. When the blood flow does not increase, cell death follows.

Prostaglandins are stimulated by stress or trauma to the cell membranes (52). These protective substances have an antisecretory effect on gastric acid production and defend the stomach against acid and other noxious substances. Prostaglandins further aid the gastric defense by stimulating bicarbonate secretion and synthesis of mucus.

NSAIDs act as weak organic acids that can increase basal levels of gastric acid secretion (52). They also alter and disrupt cell membranes, thus allowing back-diffusion of H + ions to occur. Once these weak acids disrupt cell membranes, they become trapped within the mucosal cells. Extreme morphological alterations occur in the exposed mucosal cells. NSAIDs also inhibit prostaglandin synthesis, further disrupting mucosal defense mechanisms.

Treatment

Aspirin and other nonsteroidals are effective as analgesics and antiinflammatory agents and will continue to be used in the treatment of rheumatoid- and osteoarthritis. Consequently, availability of effective treatment for the management and prevention of NSAID-induced ulcerations is important. Limited studies conclude that H2-antagonists accelerate healing, when compared with placebo (51). Conflicting studies have shown cimetidine to offer no significant benefit for patients who receive chronic therapy with NSAIDs (53). In a placebo-controlled study, 104 rheumatoid arthritis patients who required NSAID therapy were placed on either cimetidine or placebo for the treatment of NSAID-induced gastropathy. Cimetidine was shown to be no more effective than placebo in healing

NSAID-induced ulceration. However, once NSAID therapy was discontinued, cimetidine was shown to be significantly more effective than placebo in healing the gastric ulceration induced by NSAIDs. In another study, omeprazole was more effective in healing ulcers than ranitidine in the presence of continuous NSAID treatment (51). Continued use of NSAIDs impaired healing in the patients treated with ranitidine but not in the patients receiving omeprazole 40 mg a day.

Recently, prostaglandin E1 analogs have been studied for efficacy in protecting the gastric mucosa against ulcerogenic agents (54). Since prostaglandins appear to facilitate regeneration of the mucosa after injury by NSAIDs, misoprostol, the only prostaglandin E1 analog on the market, should be effective in the healing and prevention of such mucosal damage. Misoprostol aids in mucosal defense by enhancing secretion of mucus, increasing bicarbonate outflow, and increasing mucosal blood flow (51). Misoprostol also has some antisecretory effect, but this is considered to contribute minimally, since the more potent antisecretory H2-antagonists failed to prevent NSAID-induced ulceration (54).

Several studies have compared misoprostol with placebo in the treatment or prevention of NSAID-induced gastroduodenal injury (53, 54). In one study misoprostol 200 μg administered four times daily was determined to be significantly more effective than placebo in treatment of gastric and duodenal mucosal injury (53). In a similar study, participants in treatment groups with misoprostol 100 μg and 200 μg had significantly fewer gastric ulcers than did those in the placebo group (54). Differences were detected between the 100-μg and 200-μg treatment groups in the prevalence of NSAID-induced ulceration

(4.2% versus 0.7%). Although not statistically significant, the percentage of patients who were free from NSAID-induced abdominal pain was higher in the misoprostol groups. Few studies compare misoprostol to active treatment regimens in the treatment of NSAID-induced mucosal damage. In one study conducted in healthy adults, misoprostol was determined to be significantly more effective than cimetidine in preventing gastroduodenal damage from the administration of tolmetin (53). In studies of critically ill patients, misoprostol has been compared with antacids for the treatment of stress ulceration (39, 41). The agents were equally effective in preventing upper gastrointestinal lesions (41).

Misoprostol is indicated for the prevention of NSAID-induced gastric ulceration in patients at high risk of complications from gastric ulcers (i.e., elderly patients, patients with concomitant diseases, or patients with a history of peptic ulceration) (55). Misoprostol has not been shown to prevent duodenal ulceration in patients taking NSAIDs. This agent is rapidly and extensively absorbed and converted to the active free acid by rapid esterification. The plasma protein binding of misoprostol is less than 90%. It does not affect the cytochrome P-450 enzyme system and does not require dosage alteration in the presence of renal dysfunction. Plasma concentrations of misoprostol are decreased when the dose is administered with food, and concomitant use of antacids decreases total bioavailability. The recommended dose of misoprostol is 200 μg four times daily with meals. Doses of 50 to 200 μg inhibit basal and nocturnal secretion as well as acid secretion produced from meals, histamine, pentagastrin, and coffee. Only the 200-μg dose had substantial effects on nocturnal secretion and histamine- and meal-stimulated secretion (55). A dosage of 100 μg four times daily is suggested for patients who do not tolerate the higher dose.

The most commonly reported adverse effects of misoprostol are gastrointestinal. Diarrhea, abdominal pain, dyspepsia, flatulence, and nausea appear to be the most troublesome effects (54). These adverse effects are similar to the symptoms seen with gastric ulceration. The diarrhea may be dose-related and occurs early in the course of therapy (55). It may be self-limited but may require discontinuation of the drug in some patients. Abdominal cramping, spotting, and menstrual disturbances may occur. Due to its abortifacient properties, misoprostol is contraindicated during pregnancy. Women in their child-bearing years must not be pregnant when therapy is initiated and are advised to use effective contraception while on misoprostol therapy. If pregnancy occurs while on misoprostol therapy, the patient is encouraged to discontinue therapy and contact her physician immediately.

The therapeutic efficacy of aspirin in the treatment of rheumatoid arthritis is not affected by misoprostol (53). Studies of misoprostol with ibuprofen or diclofenac have

concluded that misoprostol does not affect the pharmacokinetics of the other agents.

Currently, misoprostol is the only agent indicated for the prevention of NSAID-induced gastric ulceration. Numerous studies compare misoprostol with placebo, but few studies have evaluated the efficacy of misoprostol in comparison with active treatment regimens. More studies should evaluate therapeutic efficacy of misoprostol in comparison with H2-antagonists, omeprazole, sucralfate, and antacids. Since the price of medications continue to rise, cost effectiveness also must be addressed.

CONCLUSION

Acid peptic disorders continue to challenge the medical profession. As more therapeutic agents come onto the market, treatment decisions will become more complex. All healthcare professionals must evaluate each individual case carefully and to scrutinize the medical literature closely to determine the most appropriate form of therapy for each case.

REFERENCES

1. Ohning G, Soll A: Medical treatment of peptic ulcer disease. Am Fam Physician 39:257–270, 1989.
2. Hurwitz A, Carter CA: The pharmacology of anti-ulcer drugs. DICP Ann Pharmacother 23:S10–16, 1989.
3. Wolfe MM, Soll AH: The physiology of gastric acid secretion. N Engl J Med 319:1707–1715, 1988.
4. Guyton AC: Textbook of Medical Physiology. Philadelphia: WB Saunders, 1991, ch 64.
5. McGuigan JE, Braunwald E, Isselbacher KJ, et al. Harrison's Principles of Internal Medicine. New York: McGraw-Hill, 1987, ch 235.
6. Korman MG, Hansky J, Eaves ER, et al.: Influence of cigarette smoking on healing and relapse in duodenal ulcer disease. Gastroenterology 89:871–874, 1983.
7. Davenport HW: The gastric mucosal barrier. Digestion 5:162, 1972.
8. Peterson WL: *Helicobacter pylori* and peptic ulcer disease. N Engl J Med 324:1043–1048, 1991.
9. Rauwse AJ, Langenberg W, Houthoff HJ, et al.: *Campylobacter* pyloridis-associated chronic active antral gastritis. Gastroenterology 94:33–40, 1988.
10. Levi A, Beardshall K, Swift I, et al.: Antral *Helicobacter pylori*, hypergastrinaemia and duodenal ulcers: effect of eradicating the organism. Br Med J 299:1504–1505, 1989.
11. Fordtran JS, Morawski S, Richardson C: In-vitro and in-vivo evaluation of antacids. N Engl J Med 288:923, 1973.
12. Petersen WL, Sturdevant R, Fordtran J: Healing of duodenal ulcer with an antacid regimen. N Engl J Med 297:341–344, 1977.
13. Weberg R, Aubert E, Dahlberg O, et al.: Low dose antacids for duodenal ulcer. Gastroenterology 95:1465–1469, 1988.
14. Isenberg JI, Petersen WL, Elashoff JD, et al.: Healing of benign gastric ulcer with low dose antacid or cimetidine: a double-blind, randomized, placebo controlled trial. N Engl J Med 308:1319–1324, 1982.
15. Spencer H, Lender M: Adverse effects of aluminum-containing antacids on mineral metabolism. Gastroenterology 76:603–606, 1979.
16. Feldman M, Burton ME: Histamine₂-receptor antagonists (part one). N Engl J Med 323:1672–1680, 1990.
17. Feldman M, Burton ME: Histamine₂-receptor antagonists (part two). N Engl J Med 323:1749–1755, 1990.

18. Berardi RR, Savitsky ME, Nostrent TT: Maintenance therapy for prevention of recurrent peptic ulcers. Drug Intell Clin Pharm 21:493–501, 1987.

19. Freston JW: Mechanisms of relapse in peptic ulcer disease. J Clin Gastroenterol 11(suppl 1):S34–38, 1989.

20. Freston JW: H$_2$-Receptor antagonists and duodenal ulcer recurrence: analysis of efficacy and commentary on safety, cost and patient selection. Am J Gastroenterol 82:1242–1247, 1987.

21. Anon: Miscellaneous GI drugs. AHFS 90, American Society of Hospital Pharmacists, 1990, pp 1666–1696.

22. Holt S. Alcohol and H$_2$ receptor antagonists: over the counter and under the table. Am J Gastroenterol 85:516–517, 1990.

23. Nagashima R: Developments in characteristics of sucralfate. J Clin Gastroenterol 3(suppl 2):103–110, 1981.

24. Marks IN, Lucke W, Wright JP, et al.: Ulcer healing and relapse rates after initial treatment with cimetidine or sucralfate. J Clin Gastroenterol 3(suppl 2):163–165, 1981.

25. Lampkin TA, Ouellet D, Hak LJ, et al.: Omeprazole: a novel antisecretory agent for the treatment of acid-peptic disorders. DICP Ann Pharmocother 24:393–402, 1990.

26. Maton PN, Vinayer R, Furcht H, et al.: Long-term efficacy and safety of omeprazole in patients with Zollinger-Ellison syndrome: a prospective study. Gastroenterology 97:827–836, 1989.

27. Bardhan KD, Porro GB, Bose K, et al.: A comparison of two different doses of omeprazole versus ranitidine in treatment of duodenal ulcers. J Clin Gastroenterol 8(4):408–413, 1986.

28. Weil J, Bell GD, Powell K, et al.: *Helicobacter pylori* infection treated with a tripotassium dicitrato bismuthate and metronidazole combination. Aliment Pharmacol Ther 7:651–657, 1990.

29. Friedman G: Peptic ulcer disease. Clin Symp 40:2–28, 1988.

30. Ogorek CP, Fisher RS: Detection and treatment of gastroesophageal reflux disease. Gastroenterol Clin North Am 18:293–313, 1989.

31. Vantrappen G, Janssens J: Gastroesophageal reflux disease, an important cause of angina-like chest pain. Scand J Gastroenterol 24(suppl 168):73–79, 1989.

32. Sontag S, Robinson M, McCallum RW, et al.: Ranitidine therapy for gastroesophageal reflux disease. Arch Intern Med 147:1485–1491, 1987.

33. Sandmark S, Carlsson R, Fausa O, et al.: Omeprazole or ranitidine in the treatment of reflux esophagitis. Results of a double-blind, randomized Scandinavian multi-center study. Scan J Gastroenterol 23:625–632, 1988.

34. Fiorucci S, Santucci, L, Morelli A: Effect of omeprazole and high doses of ranitidine on gastric acidity and gastroesophageal reflux in patients with moderate-severe esophagitis. Am J Gastroenterol 85:1458–1462, 1990.

35. Simon B, Muller P: Comparison of the effect of sucralfate and ranitidine in reflux esophagitis. Am J Med 83(suppl 3B):43–47, 1987.

36. Richter JE: A critical review of current medical gastroesophageal reflux disease. J Clin Gastroenterol 8(suppl 1):72–80, 1986.

37. Gonzalez ER: Pathophysiological changes in the critically ill patient: risk factors for ulceration and altered drug metabolism. DICP Ann Pharmocother 24(suppl):S5–7, 1990.

38. Kleinam RL, Adair CG, Ephgrave KS: Stress ulcers: current understanding of pathogenesis and prophylaxis. DICP Ann Pharmacother 22:452–460, 1988.

39. Zinner MJ, Rypins EB, Martin LR, et al.: Misoprostol versus antacid titration for preventing stress ulcers in postoperative surgical ICU patients. Ann Surg 210(5):590–95, 1989.

40. Stannard VA, Farquhar IK, Morris DL: Stress ulceration and gastric function in the critically ill patient. Dig Dis Sci 8:80–88, 1990.

41. Alijani MR, Benjamin SB, Collen MJ, et al.: Misoprostol: a prostaglandin E1 analogue versus antacid in the prevention of stress ulcers in kidney transplant patients. Transplant Proc 21(1):2145–2146, 1989.

42. Siepler JK, Mowers RM, Alexander CL: Prevention of stress-related mucosal bleeding. U.S. Pharm March:H-29–38, 1990.

43. Reusser P, Gyr K, Scheidegger D, et al.: Prospective endoscopic study of stress erosions and ulcers in critically ill neurosurgical patients: current incidence and effect of acid-reducing prophylaxis. Crit Care Med 18(3):270–274, 1990.

44. Karlstadt RG, Iberti TJ, Silverstein J, et al.: Comparison of cimetidine and placebo for the prophylaxis of upper gastrointestinal bleeding due to stress-related gastric mucosal damage in the intensive care unit. J Intensive Care Med 5(1):26–32, 1990.

45. Moore JG: Achieving pH control in the critically ill patient: the role of continuous infusion of H2-receptor antagonists. DICP Ann Pharmacotherapy 24:S28–30, 1990.

46. Ostro MJ, Russell JA, Soldin SJ, et al.: Control of gastric pH with cimetidine: boluses versus primed infusions. Gastroenterology 89:532–537, 1985.

47. Dellinger RP: Pathophysiology, monitoring, and management of the ventilator-dependent patient: considerations for drug therapy, emphasis on stress ulcer prophylaxis. DICP Ann Pharmacotherapy 24:S8–11, 1990.

48. Earnest DL: Controlling gastric pH: the impact of newer agents on the critically ill patient. DICP Ann Pharmacotherapy 24:S31–34, 1990.

49. Lewis JH: Gastrointestinal injury due to medicinal agents. Am J Gastroenterol. 81:819, 1986.

50. Griffin MR, Ray WA, Shaffner W. Nonsteroidal antiinflammatory drug use and death from peptic ulcer in elderly persons. Ann Intern Med 109:359–363, 1988.

51. Flier JA, Underhill LH: Pathogenesis of peptic ulcer and implications for therapy. N Engl J Med 322(13):909–916, 1990.

52. Schoen RT, Vender RJ: Mechanisms of nonsteroidal antiinflammatory drug-induced gastric damage. Am J Med 86:449–458, 1989.

53. Roth S, Agrawal N, Mahowald M, et al.: Misoprostol heals gastroduodenal injury in patients with rheumatoid arthritis receiving aspirin. Arch Intern Med 149:775–779, 1989.

54. Graham DY, Agrawal NM, Roth SH: Prevention of NSAID-induced gastric ulcer with misoprostol: multicentre, double-blind, placebo-controlled trial. Lancet 1277–1280, 1988.

55. Anon: Misoprostol—Facts and Comparisons. St. Louis: Facts and Comparisons, 1989, pp 305g–i.

CHAPTER 22

INFLAMMATORY BOWEL DISEASE

ROSEMARY R. BERARDI, Pharm.D.

Inflammatory bowel disease (IBD) is a general term used to describe two chronic, nonspecific inflammatory disorders of the gastrointestinal (GI) tract, the etiology of which remain unknown. Inflammatory bowel diseases can be divided into ulcerative colitis (UC) and Crohn's disease (CD). Ulcerative colitis is usually limited to the colon and rectum; it may affect the rectum alone, only the descending and sigmoid colon and rectum, or the entire colon (Fig. 22.1). Crohn's disease may affect any part of the GI tract from mouth to anus. The disease may involve only the terminal ileum, be restricted to regions of the small intestine (regional enteritis), involve the colon alone, or affect both the small and large intestine (Fig. 22.1). This anatomic classification is important, since the response to therapy may vary, depending on the site of involvement. Both disorders are characterized by recurrent inflammatory episodes and remissions. However, their clinical features and underlying pathophysiologic differences usually permit an accurate diagnosis in most patients.

It is estimated that IBD afflicts approximately 2 million Americans, usually before the age of 40. In the United States, complications of these diseases are estimated to claim 1000 lives a year (1–5). Despite years of research, cures have not been found.

EPIDEMIOLOGY

The epidemiologies of UC and CD share many features. In general, the diseases are more common in western populations and in urban rather than rural societies (1, 2). There is a higher rate among Jewish people born in the U.S. and Europe than in Israeli-born Jews (1, 4, 5). Both diseases are more common in whites than in nonwhites. Ulcerative colitis and CD appear to affect both sexes equally, with a slight increase in women reported in some series (1, 4, 5). The diseases tend to occur in the same family, with reports of both disorders occurring in different members of the same family (1, 3). Although UC and CD can occur at any age, the peak age of incidence of both diseases is in the teens or early twenties. A second peak may occur again during the late fifties, but this remains controversial (1, 4, 5).

The incidences and prevalences of CD and UC are similar. However, in recent years, the occurrence of CD has increased in the U.S., especially in women and blacks (1, 5). Although changing rates may imply genetic and environmental factors, epidemiologic studies have not yet resolved this question.

ETIOLOGY AND PATHOGENESIS

The causes of UC and CD are not known. It is possible that infectious agents, genetic factors, biochemical abnormalities, or the environment trigger the onset of disease and that the immune system mediates the inflammatory response and tissue damage (4–6). Chronicity may result from an inappropriate or incomplete response by the immune system. Many of the similarities between UC and CD suggest that they might be heterogeneous disorders with distinctly different trigger factors. Alternatively, tissue damage may be indirect, nonspecific, or an "innocent bystander" effect caused by a local mucosal immunoregulatory defect (4–6). Exogenous factors such as smoking, drugs, stress, and diet may modify disease activity by interacting with the mucosal immune system. (1, 7–9). No one agent has been identified as a trigger of either disease.

Infectious Agents

The chronic inflammatory nature of IBD has always suggested an infectious etiology, but attempts at culturing bacterial pathogens have been largely unsuccessful. The bacterial overgrowth often seen in CD, reflects a favorable environment for bacterial growth, but is not related to the pathogenesis. The similarity of CD to tuberculosis suggests that the disease might be caused by an atypical mycobacterium, however, this theory remains unproven. It seems unlikely that *Clostridium difficile* or *Helicobacter jejuni* are etiological agents in either CD or UC, but a coexisting infection may influence disease exacerbation. The role of gut anaerobes, viruses, and defective cell-wall bacterial variants remains uncertain (4, 5). Although no conclusive evidence implicates a specific pathogen in IBD, host immune and genetic factors may be required to initiate the infectious process.

Genetic Influences

The increased frequency of IBD in whites, Jews, and family members suggests a genetic predisposition to the disease. In addition, the disease has appeared in monozygotic twins (3–5). However, since no specific genetic marker has been confirmed for IBD, it is difficult to sort out the genetic from the environmental factors.

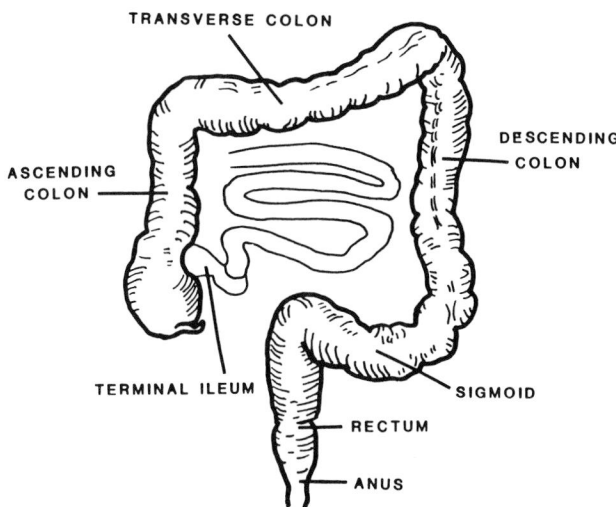

Figure 22.1. Anatomic location of various segments of the bowel.

Immunologic Mechanisms

Altered immunologic findings have been reported in patients with IBD, many of which appear with the active inflammatory process and subside with its quiescence. Theories of pathogenesis include: impaired cellular immune mechanisms, lymphocyte-mediated cytotoxicity, immediate hypersensitivity reactions in the intestine, autoimmune antibody-mediated damage to intestinal epithelial cells, the formation of antigen-antibody complexes, and an allergic reaction to cow's milk in the diet (4, 5). Abnormalities in humoral and cell-mediated immunity may represent a secondary phenomenon. The facts that these diseases may be accompanied by extraintestinal manifestations, that treatment with corticosteroids or immunosuppressive agents is usually associated with a favorable therapeutic response, and that removal of diseased bowel is often followed by disappearance of immunological components, suggest an autoimmune mechanism (4, 5).

Endogenous mediators of inflammation, such as prostaglandins, interleukins, mast cell products, neuropeptides, and various metabolites of arachidonic acid including leukotrienes and lipoxins, frequently correlate with disease activity and provide a rationale for drug therapy. The inflammatory process may also be related to ischemic injury involving the release of reactive oxygen free radicals (6). It is likely that the immune system plays an important role in the pathogenesis of IBD and in mediating tissue injury. However, no consistent immunologic abnormality has been established as the primary defect in UC or CD.

Abnormalities of Mucin

There is evidence to suggest that a single species of colonic mucin is reduced in patients with UC but not in patients with other forms of colitis. It is unknown whether these alterations are related to the pathogenesis of the disease.

Psychologic Factors

Emotional and psychologic factors have been implicated in the etiology of IBD, but there is no evidence that stress is causative and that psychotherapy is effective (4, 5). Psychologic factors may influence the clinical course of the disease and the patient's response to therapy, since acute flares of activity often occur in association with stressful events. Thus, it is possible that the nervous system has a regulatory effect on the immune system. Management of IBD should include the realization that the symptoms of IBD, such as diarrhea, pain, and rectal bleeding, are in themselves likely to cause various psychologic responses to the disease.

Dietary Factors

Inflammatory bowel disease has been linked to chemical food additives, milk, increased consumption of refined sugars, and reduced intake of dietary fiber. However, no firm epidemiologic or experimental evidence implicates dietary or other environmental factors in IBD (1, 4, 5).

Smoking

Extensive evidence implicates cigarette smoking as a risk factor for the development of CD (1). Following surgery, patients with CD who smoke appear to have an increased risk of recurrence, when compared to nonsmokers (7). In contrast, there tends to be a decreased risk of UC among cigarette smokers (1).

Drugs

Nonsteroidal antiinflammatory drugs (NSAIDS) can cause inflammatory changes in the ileum and colon and should be avoided in patients with known UC or CD. NSAIDS have been linked to colitis in patients without previous IBD, and they may also activate quiescent IBD (1, 8). There is conflicting evidence about oral contraceptive use and UC, although a recent report suggests no association (1, 9).

ANATOMIC, PATHOLOGIC AND CLINICAL FEATURES

The distinction between the anatomic and pathologic features of UC and CD can assist in understanding the clinical features of the diseases. A summary of some of the most important anatomic, pathologic, and clinical features is presented in Table 22.1.

Anatomic and Pathologic Features
ULCERATIVE COLITIS

Ulcerative colitis affects primarily the mucosa and submucosa of the rectum and the left colon, with the rectum

Table 22.1.

Important Anatomic, Pathologic, and Clinical Features of Ulcerative Colitis and Crohn's Disease[a]

Feature	Ulcerative Colitis	Crohn's Disease
Anatomic		
Small bowel only	0	+ +
Small bowel and colon	0	+ + +
Colon only	+	+ +
Anorectal only	+ + +	0
Diffuse, continuous involvement	+ + +	+
Cobblestoning	0	+ + +
Pathologic		
Transmural	0	+ + +
Fissures and fistulas	+	+ +
Crypt abscesses	+ + +	+
Strictures	0	+ +
Shortening of the colon	+ +	0
Pseudopolyps	+ +	0
Clinical		
Rectal bleeding	+ + +	+
Diarrhea	+ + +	+ + +
Abdominal pain	+	+ + +
Malaise, fever	+	+ + +
Weight loss	+ +	+ + +
Extraintestinal manifestations	+	+
Perianal disease	+	+ +
Intestinal obstruction	0	+ +
Toxic megacolon	+ +	+
Risk of malignancy	+ +	+

[a] Frequencies represent estimates and are categorized as being consistent (+ + +), frequent (+ +), infrequent (+), or rare (0). None of the features is always present or always absent.

involved histologically in >90% of the cases. Distal ulcerative colitis may be differentiated into proctitis and protosigmoiditis, depending on the location of mucosal inflammation. Lesions usually develop in the rectum and spread proximally; however, initial disease may involve the entire colon (Fig. 22.1). The disease extends to the total colon (universal or pancolitis) in 5 to 10% of patients and may involve a minimal portion of the terminal ileum (backwash ileitis). In severe forms of UC, such as toxic megacolin, deeper layers of the colon may be involved.

Unlike CD, the inflammatory process in UC is continuous, with no intervening areas of normal mucosa, and deeper layers of the bowel are not usually involved. Chronic recurrent mucosal inflammation with concomitant tissue repair may lead to characteristic findings that include formation of crypt abscesses, pseudopolyps, shortening of the colon (foreshortening), and a "lead-pipe" appearance of the colon. Dysplasia in colonic biopsies may represent a premalignant change and a risk of carcinoma (4).

CROHN'S DISEASE

The term "Crohn's disease" is preferred to "granulomatous enteritis" or "regional enteritis," since not all patients with CD have accompanying granulomas and the disease can affect any part of the GI tract from mouth to anus, not just a specific region. The distal ileum and right colon (ileocolitis) are the most common sites of involvement, accounting for more than two-thirds of cases affecting the small bowel. Although the terminal ileum is generally involved, other areas of the small intestine can be affected, either alone or with the colon. The colon is involved in about two-thirds of patients, with about 15 to 20% having only colonic involvement. In most patients with CD of the colon, the rectum is spared. Sections of bowel that appear normal by radiology or colonoscopy can have histologic features of CD (5).

In contrast to UC, CD is characterized by chronic inflammation extending through all layers of the bowel wall as well as the mesentary and regional lymph nodes. Mesenteric nodes are enlarged and are often matted together to form an abdominal mass. The transmural process can lead to the formation of fissures and fistulas, and a thickened, edematous bowel, which can result in stenosis with possible obstruction. The disease is distinguished from UC in that it often involves segments of the bowel separated by normal-appearing bowel, called "skip lesions." In advanced cases, the mucosa has a nodular or "cobblestoned" appearance. Although certain anatomic and pathologic features enable CD of the colon to be distinguished from UC, this distinction is not possible in about 20% of cases (5).

Clinical Features

ULCERATIVE COLITIS

The clinical features of UC vary with the severity of the disease and are presented in Table 22.2. Categorizing the disease as mild, moderate, or severe is important, since therapy and prognosis are related to disease classification. Clinically mild UC is the most common form of the disease and afflicts about 60% of all patients. In these individuals, the disease usually involves just the sigmoid and rectum. Neither bleeding nor diarrhea is severe, and systemic symptoms are usually absent. Moderate disease affects about 25% of all patients, and diarrhea with varying degrees of rectal bleeding is a major symptom. Abdominal cramping is more prominent and usually relieved by defecation. Severe UC occurs in 10 to 15% of all patients, and the onset of symptoms is usually sudden. Diarrhea is profuse, and rectal bleeding and abdominal cramps are severe. The patient is usually febrile, dehydrated, and profoundly weak. Blood loss can result in a rapid pulse, low blood pressure, and anemia. Death may occur during the acute attack (4).

CROHN'S DISEASE

The clinical features of CD vary from patient to patient, but usually reflect the anatomic location of the disease.

Table 22.2.
Clinical Features of Ulcerative Colitis Based on Disease Severity

	Mild	Moderate	Severe
Frequency	60%	20–25%	10–15%
Location	Rectum and distal colon	Rectum and $\frac{1}{3}$–$\frac{1}{2}$ of colon	Rectum and entire colon
Weight loss	Uncommon	<10 lb	>10 lb
Fever	Uncommon	Intermittent	Persistent
Abdominal pain	Uncommon	Common	Severe
Bowel sounds	Normal	Normal	Absent
Diarrhea	3–5 stools/day	>5 stools/day	Hourly
Rectal bleeding	Intermittent	Common	Severe
Tachycardia	Uncommon	Frequently	Common
Anemia	Uncommon	Hct >0.30 (30%)	Hct <0.30 (30%)
Leukocytosis	Uncommon	Common	Common
Albumin	Normal	Normal	Reduced
Extraintestinal manifestations	Uncommon	Common	Severe
Risk of malignancy	Not increased	Increased after 10 yr (2%)	Increased after 10 yr (5–10%)
Mortality (acute attack)	<0.5%	2%	10–25%

The major symptoms are diarrhea (>90%) and abdominal pain (>80%). A low-grade fever (>50%) occurs in the absence of any complications. Malabsorption and nutritional deficiencies frequently result in weight loss (>80%). The abdominal pain tends to be steady and localized to the right lower quadrant. A colicky or cramping pain, usually associated with bowel movements, may be superimposed upon the steady pain. When the disease is confined to the small bowel, diarrhea tends to be less severe and often occurs without bleeding. With colonic involvement, diarrhea is more frequent and rectal bleeding is present in about half of the patients. Most patients have recurrent episodes of diarrhea, abdominal pain, and fever lasting from a few days to several months. Perianal fissures, fistulas, and abscesses may be the presenting feature. The disease may be mild, moderate, or severe depending upon the extent of involvement (5).

NUTRITIONAL ASPECTS

In general, patients with severe UC or CD are prone to losses of extracellular fluid volume and electrolytes, anemia, and hypoalbuminemia. Nutritional deficiencies are frequent and complex in CD because of the problem of food avoidance and the many mechanisms responsible for malabsorption and malnutrition. Some of these mechanisms include inadequate food intake; inflammatory involvement of the small intestine resulting in decreased absorption of nutrients, lactase deficiency, and protein-losing enteropathy; small bowel bacterial overgrowth with associated malabsorption of cobalamin and altered bile salt metabolism; intestinal surgery; and the catabolic effects of chronic inflammation (5). Prolonged periods of poor nutrition and underlying disease can result in protein-calorie malnutrition, dehydration, acid-base and electrolyte dis-

Table 22.3.
Extraintestinal Manifestations of Inflammatory Bowel Disease[a]

Manifestation	Incidence (%)
Arthritis/arthralgias	25–30
Skin lesions	3–5
Aphthous mouth ulcers	5–10
Iritis	5–10
Ankylosing spondylityis	10–15
Abnormal liver transaminase levels	30–50
Liver disease	1–3
Cholelithiasis°	20–30
Nephrolithiasis°	25–35
Renal disease°	1–3

[a] In general, the extraintestinal manifestations in ulcerative colitis and Crohn's disease are similar in type and prevalence. Asterisk (°) indicates manifestations seen primarily in Crohn's disease.

turbances, and deficiencies of vitamins D, K, B_{12}, and folic acid (10). The consequences of these nutritional disorders can be especially serious in children with CD and may lead to growth retardation and delayed sexual maturation.

EXTRAINTESTINAL MANIFESTATIONS OF INFLAMMATORY BOWEL DISEASE

Many extraintestinal manifestations are associated with IBD, and these may precede or accompany the underlying intestinal disorder (Table 22.3). Systemic manifestations occur in 10 to 20% of patients with IBD and appear to be related primarily to the clinical activity of the inflammatory process and its anatomic location, or to the disordered physiology of the small intestine (4, 5, 11). In most instances, the prevalence of the arthritic, skin, and eye manifestations is similar in patients with UC and CD with colonic involvement. Disturbances in the physiology of the small intestine, mainly in CD, may give rise to additional systemic manifestations. Unfortunately, there is no definitive explanation for the pathogenesis, association, or manifestation of many of these symptoms.

Musculoskeletal

Arthritis and arthralgias are the most common extraintestinal manifestations of both UC and CD and may present as a migrating arthritis of the large peripheral joints, mostly affecting the joints of the lower extremity, or as ankylosing spondylitis. The erythrocyte sedimentation rate is elevated and the antinuclear factor and rheumatoid factor are negative. In most patients, the migrating arthritis tends to parallel the activity and severity of the bowel disease, subsiding with therapy, colectomy, or spontaneous remission. In contrast, the ankylosing spondylitis may appear years before bowel symptoms and run a course independent of the intestinal disease (4, 5, 11).

Skin and Mucous Membranes

Inflammatory disorders of the skin and mucous membranes also occur in patients with IBD. The major skin manifestations; erythema nodosum and pyoderma gangrenosum occur primarily in patients with UC. Aphthous ulcers of the mouth and tongue occur often and tend to parallel the intestinal disease activity.

Ocular

Ocular manifestations occur in about 4% of patients with IBD and include conjunctivitis, iritis/uveitis, blepharitis, and episcleritis. Iritis/uveitis is the most common lesion and is bilateral in half the cases.

Hepatobiliary

Minor abnormalities in hepatic transaminases occur commonly in patients with IBD; however clinically important liver disease is uncommon (4, 5, 11). Cirrhosis, chronic hepatitis, and sclerosing cholangitis, although infrequent, tend to occur more often in UC. Fatty infiltration of the liver is common and may reflect malnutrition and protein depletion. The increased prevalence of cholelithiasis in CD with ileal involvement or resection results from diminished bile salt reabsorption, which is conducive to cholesterol gallstone formation (4, 5, 11).

Genitourinary and Renal

Genitourinary complications include urinary tract infections and urinary obstruction and are associated primarily with CD (5, 11). Nephrolithiasis occurs most often in ileal CD and frequently results from dehydration, inactivity, and changes in the composition of the urine (i.e., increased oxalate absorption from the colon due to decreased avail-

able calcium in the gut lumen secondary to malabsorption of fatty acids). Renal amyloid may cause nephrotic syndrome and renal failure in CD (5, 11).

Hematologic and Thromboembolic

The most common hematologic complication in IBD is iron-deficiency anemia secondary to blood loss, although chronic anorexia and malabsorption can lead to other complex anemias (4, 5, 11). A small number of patients may develop an idiopathic hemolytic anemia or a drug-related hemolytic anemia associated with the administration of sulfasalazine. Thromboembolic events resulting from abnormalities of clotting factors during active episodes may complicate the courses of both diseases. Therapy involves the risk of colonic bleeding during anticoagulation.

LOCAL COMPLICATIONS

Local complications arise from the intestinal component of IBD and may be classified as minor (not life-threatening) and major (potentially life-threatening). Minor complications include pseudopolyps, anal fissures and fistulas, perianal abscesses, and rectal prolapse. Major complications include intestinal obstruction, toxic megacolon, colonic perforation, cancer of the colon, and massive hemorrhage (4, 5).

Fistula Formation

The incidence of fistula formation is much higher in CD than in UC and may be the initial indication of the disease (5). Fistulas occur most commonly in the perianal and perirectal areas, with enterocutaneous, enterovaginal, and enteroenteric fistulas occurring less often.

Intestinal Obstruction

Intestinal obstruction as a result of inflammatory activity is rarely a problem in UC. Alternatively, small bowel obstruction is a frequent complication of CD and may be due to the inflammation and edema of the involved intestine or to the fixed narrowing of the bowel secondary to scar formation (5).

Perforation

Intestinal perforation is uncommon in CD. However, it may complicate toxic megacolon or occur in UC in the absence of toxic dilation. The risk of perforation is usually greatest in severe colitis and during an initial severe attack. Approximately one-third of all deaths related to UC result from colonic perforation and peritonitis (4, 12).

Cancer of the Colon

The risk of malignancy is greater in patients with IBD than in the general population, with a higher incidence observed in UC than in CD (4, 5, 13). Development of colonic cancer in UC increases when the duration of the disease is more than 10 years, when the disease involves the entire colon, and when there has been a chronic continuous course rather than intermittent disease (4, 13). Because cancer of the colon arising from UC is extremely virulent, efforts are made to detect early malignant changes. A yearly colonoscopy with multiple mucosal biopsies looking for severe dysplasia is recommended for patients at risk. More frequent examinations may be required, depending on the degree of risk and histologic findings. Although a prophylactic total colectomy can cure UC and prevent colonic cancer, the risks of carcinoma and severe colitis must be weighted against the risks of surgery and the inconvenience of an ileostomy.

Massive Hemorrhage

Although rectal bleeding is common in CD and UC, massive hemorrhage occurs infrequently, and then usually in patients with severe disease. Most patients can be managed medically with blood transfusions, but occasionally surgery is required to control the bleeding.

Toxic Megacolon

Toxic megacolon may occur in CD of the colon but is more common in UC (4, 12). This serious local complication is usually preceded by a rapidly deteriorating clinical course and is associated with a high mortality. It is characterized by acute dilation of all or part or the colon to a diameter greater than 6 cm, with systemic toxicity (4, 12). The pathogenesis of toxic megacolon is not well understood, but it is thought that the deep inflammatory process that involves all layers of the colon accounts for both the systemic toxicity and the loss of colonic muscular tone. Although factors that contribute to increased luminal pressure or decreased colonic muscular tone may contribute to colonic dilation, none of these factors appears to be causitive. Thus excessive use of anticholinergic drugs, opiates, and other antimotility agents used to treat diarrhea in these patients may precipitate this complication. In addition, severe electrolyte abnormalities, particularly hypokalemia, have been reported to contribute to colonic dilation.

Clinically, the patient is severely ill with a high fever, profound weakness, tachycardia, volume depletion, electrolyte imbalance, leukocytosis, abdominal pain, distention, and tenderness. A decrease in stool frequency may reflect colonic atony rather than improvement of colitis. Toxic megacolon can occur at any time in the natural course of the disease and may be complicated by colonic perforation and peritonitis. Because the risk of spontaneous perforation is high, barium enema examination and colonoscopy should be postponed until the disease is less active.

Toxic megacolon is considered a medical emergency that requires rapid and intensive therapy. Treatment consists of fluid and electrolyte replacement, blood transfusions if indicated, and large doses of corticosteroids (prednisolone 100 to 200 mg/day or an equivalent dose of other steroids) given intravenously in divided doses in an effort to resolve the inflammatory process in the colon. Because of the fear of perforation and the likelihood of bacteremia, intravenous therapy with broad-spectrum antibiotics directed at enteric Gram-negative, enterococci, and anaerobic pathogens should be instituted. Nasogastric suction is begun to remove swallowed air and to reduce the passage of fluid into the colon. Medications that decrease intestinal motility should be withdrawn. The initial 24 to 48 hr of treatment are crucial and determine the future management of the patient. If significant improvement does not occur and if perforation seems imminent, an emergency colectomy should be performed. The overall mortality in medically and surgically treated patients is between 10 and 30%. If perforation occurs, the mortality rate approaches 50% (4, 12).

DIAGNOSIS AND CLINICAL COURSE

The diagnosis of IBD should be considered in all patients who present with persistent abdominal pain and diarrhea or bloody diarrhea. On occasion, fever, weight loss, or one of the extraintestinal manifestations of UC may overshadow the intestinal symptoms. Since UC and CD are "nonspecific" diseases, the diagnosis is usually made by exclusion and depends on the course of the illness, the clinical manifestations, and the sites of bowel involvement. The diagnosis may be supported by sigmoidoscopy, barium enema, colonoscopy, negative stool findings, and mucosal biopsy. Once the diagnosis of IBD is established, the distinction between UC and CD of the colon is usually possible.

Laboratory Tests

In general, laboratory tests are usually nonspecific and do not establish a diagnosis. Leukocytosis and an elevated erythrocyte sedimentation rate tend to reflect the inflammatory process, and electrolyte abnormalities exist when there is severe diarrhea. Anemia may be present with chronic blood loss, and the serum albumin level provides an indication of the patient's nutritional status and overall clinical condition. Laboratory features of malabsorption such as prolonged prothrombin time or macrocytosis may be present when CD involves the small intestine. Elevations of hepatic transaminase levels may reflect a coexisting liver disease.

Radiography, Sigmoidoscopy, and Colonoscopy

Sigmoidoscopic examination of the bowel is often the initial diagnostic procedure and is most important in establishing mucosal inflammation in both UC and CD of the distal colon. A rectal biopsy usually confirms the presence of an abnormal and inflamed mucosa. Radiologic findings also provide essential information in the diagnosis of suspected IBD. In both UC and CD, the barium enema may reveal the extent of the disease. A plain film of the abdomen frequently provides important information, especially in those patients in whom the barium enema may be contraindicated. When CD involves the small bowel, upper intestinal x-rays are usually indicated. Colonoscopy assists in the differential diagnosis of UC and CD, especially in those patients whose disease extends beyond the reach of the sigmoidoscope. It is often used for follow-up to disease progression, for cancer surveillance, and to observe for signs of recurrent CD after surgical resection. Mucosal biopsies are not always helpful in the differential diagnosis of IBD, but they may reveal dysplastic changes in patients with long-standing disease.

Clinical Course

ULCERATIVE COLITIS

The onset of UC is relatively abrupt, and symptoms range from small amounts of rectal bleeding to colonic hemorrhage with fulminant diarrhea. Most patients (60 to 75%) will have highly variable (mild to severe) intermittent attacks with varying intervals of asymptomatic remissions. A smaller number (5 to 15%) may be troubled by continuous symptoms, with intermittent flares of disease activity. The severity of the disease has important therapeutic and prognostic implications. Patients with mild disease have a prognosis similar to that of the general population, with the development of colonic cancer being rare. About 5% of patients will die within 1 year of the onset of symptoms. The risk of death is greatest when the initial onset of symptoms is rapid, colonic involvement is extensive and severe and when the patient is over 60 years of age. Most of those with an initial moderate attack will have subsequent attacks of moderate severity. About 25% of all patients will require a colectomy within 5 to 10 years after onset of the disease, usually for continuous disease, toxic megacolon, perforation, or stricture (4). An increased risk of colon cancer is related to the extent and duration of the colitis (4, 13).

CROHN'S DISEASE

The clinical course of CD varies greatly from one patient to another and is often unpredictable. In most patients, the onset is insidious. The course is characterized by recurrent attacks of diarrhea, abdominal pain, and low-grade fever, resulting in gradual deterioration over a period of years, with shorter and shorter asymptomatic intervals. Blood loss and poor nutrition leads to anemia, weight loss, malnutrition, and fatigue. Approximately 10 to 20% of patients with CD will remain symptom-free for as long as 20 years after the initial episode. Perianal or perirectal disease develops in about 50% of patients at some time. Partial or complete obstruction constitutes the most frequent indication for surgery and occurs more rapidly in patients with ileocolitis than in those with only small bowel or only colonic involvement (5). Severe disease usually requires surgery, but it is associated with a high recurrence rate. Death occurs in 10 to 20% of patients as a result of disease progression or complications, and is higher during the first few years after the diagnosis and again after the disease has been present for about 15 years (5).

MANAGEMENT

The treatment of IBD remains empirical and depends on the clinical status of the patient. Acute exerbations, quiescent symptom-free periods, and chronic symptomatic periods constitute the phases of IBD, which must be identified in order to determine the goals of therapy. Treatment is directed at terminating an acute attack and inducing remission, preventing relapse, and controlling chronic symptoms. The approach to management should be individualized and includes general supportive measures, drug treatment against the disease process itself, management of the patient's nutritional status, and surgical intervention, if necessary.

Supportive Measures

When symptoms of active disease are present, the patient should be placed on bed rest and the severity of the disease assessed. Moderate to severe disease usually requires hospitalization. It is advisable to eliminate oral intake during an acute attack and to correct fluid and electrolyte losses intravenously. Blood transfusions may be required when there is continued active bleeding. Agents to control diarrhea are often effective in mild to moderate disease, but should be used with extreme caution for fear of precipitating toxic megacolon. When fever, leukocytosis, and rebound abdominal tenderness exist, broad-spectrum antibiotic coverage should be initiated after appropriate cultures for infection have been obtained. Iron, folic acid, and B_{12} deficiencies should be identified and treated with appropriate replacement. Because oral iron therapy may aggravate IBD, it may be preferable to give iron parenterally or as a blood transfusion. Fat malabsorption in patients with CD is accompanied by malabsorption of vitamins A, D, and K, and replacement of these vitamins may be necessary. Additionally, patients with small intestinal CD may present with deficiencies of calcium, magnesium, B complex vitamins, and vitamin C and require appropriate replacement. The decision to institute nutritional therapy should be based on the patient's nutritional status and anticipated clinical course. Supportive psychiatric care may assist in the treatment of relapse and in the prevention of recurrent disease.

Table 22.4.
Drugs Used in the Treatment of
Inflammatory Bowel Disease

Antiinflammatory agents
  Sulfasalazine
  5-Aminosalicylic acid (5-ASA)
    Mesalamine
    Olsalazine
    Balsalazide
    Ipsalazide
  Adrenocorticosteroids
    Hydrocortisone
    Prednisone
    Prednisolone
    Methylprednisolone
    Tixocortol pivalate
    Beclomethasone dipropionate
    Budesonide
  Corticotrophin (ACTH)
Immunosuppressives/immunomodulators
  Azathioprine
  6-Mercaptopurine (6-MP)
  Cyclosporine A
  Methotrexate
  Interferon
  Levamisole
  Chloroquine
Antibiotics
  Metronidazole
Antidiarrheals/antispasmotics
  Diphenoxylate
  Loperamide
  Codeine phosphate
  Tincture of opium
  Tincture of belladonna
  Cholestyramine
  Hydrophilic compounds
  Octreotide
  Clonidine
Lipoxygenase inhibitors
  Eicosapentanoic acid (fish oil)
Oxygen-derived free radical scavengers
  Superoxide dismutase
  D-Penicillamine
  α-Tocopherol
Antituberculous agents
  Streptomycin
  Rifabutin
  Ethambutal
Mast cell stabilizers
  Cromoglycate sodium
Cytoprotective agents
  Sucralfate

Drug Treatment

Although drug treatment of UC and CD shares certain common principles, the response to therapy may differ. Since CD involves deeper layers of the bowel wall, affects the small intestine and/or the colon, often recurs after surgical resection, and is associated with fistulas and per-

irectal abscesses, medical therapy is less effective and healing tends to occur over a longer period of time. The principal drugs used to treat IBD are sulfasalazine and corticosteroids (Table 22.4).

SULFASALAZINE

Sulfasalazine (salicylazosulfapyridine, SASP) is the most commonly prescribed medication used in the treatment of UC and CD. It is a conjugate of 5-aminosalicylic acid (5-ASA) and sulfapyridine (SP) linked by a diazo bond (Fig. 22.2). When administered orally, about 20% of the SASP dose is absorbed, some of which is excreted in the bile. The remainder of the parent drug passes unchanged into the colon where colonic bacteria cleave the diazo bond to form 5-ASA and SP. Most of the liberated 5-ASA remains in the colon and is excreted in the feces. The SP is absorbed, metabolized in part by acetylation in the liver, and excreted in the urine (14, 15). Since both 5-ASA and SP are absorbed readily when given orally, the diazo linkage provides a delivery system by which 5-ASA can reach the diseased intestinal sites in higher concentrations.

The exact mechanism by which SASP acts is uncertain, since its antibacterial activity is unlikely to account for its clinical activity in patients with IBD. 5-ASA, the primary active moiety, is thought to act by interfering with arachidonic acid metabolism. (14–18). It is possible that 5-ASA inhibits the lipoxygenase pathway and decreases chemotactically active leukotrienes (inflammatory mediators) within the intestinal mucosa (Fig. 22.3). It was once thought that 5-ASA inhibited the cyclooxygenase pathway, thereby lowering intestinal prostaglandin levels, but this theory is unlikely because NSAIDS appear to exacerbate IBD. 5-ASA may act through other mechanisms, e.g., as a scavenger of oxygen-derived free radicals or by interference with immunoregulation (6, 15–18).

Increased intestinal transit (diarrhea) and concomitant antibiotic administration may result in reduced breakdown of SASP and decreased liberation of 5-ASA. In some patients, bacterial overgrowth may permit the metabolism of

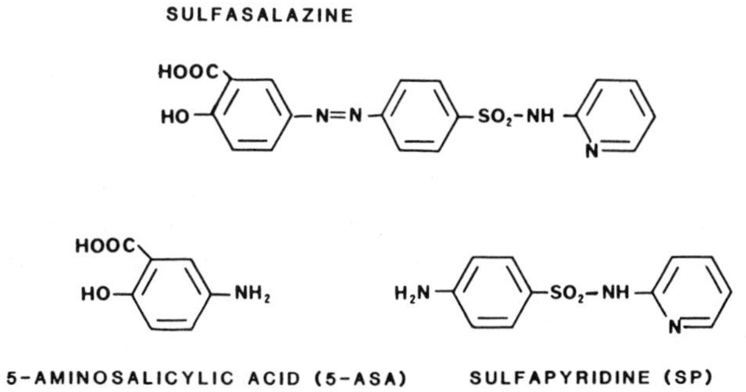

Figure 22.2. Structures of sulfasalazine, 5-aminosalicylic acid, and sulfapyridine.

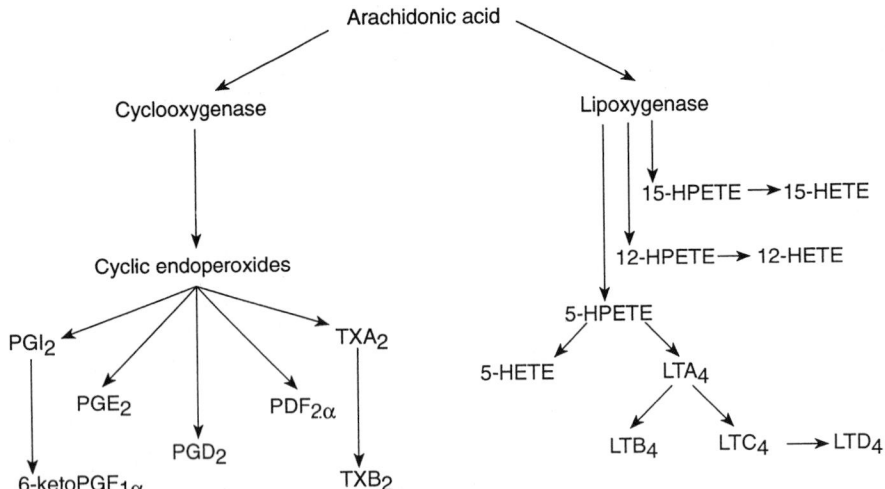

Figure 22.3. Arachidonic acid metabolism.

SASP in the small intestine with delivery of 5-ASA to more proximal portions of the bowel.

Use in Ulcerative Colitis. The efficacy of SASP in the treatment of severe acute UC is uncertain and is considered to be inferior to corticosteroids (4, 16–19). This may be due, in part, to the diminished metabolism of SASP in the colon as a result of severe diarrhea. Although studies have shown the drug to be effective in mild to moderate attacks of UC, steroids produce more frequent remissions and a more rapid response (4, 16–19). The oral dose of SASP used for acute mild or moderate disease is usually 2 to 4 g/day given in four divided doses. Although higher doses (6 to 8 g/day) have been employed, they are often intolerable, and there is no evidence that they are more effective. Because of dose-dependent adverse effects, therapy is initiated with a lower dose (500 mg twice a day) and gradually increased by 500 mg every 2 to 3 days.

Once remission is induced, 1 to 2 g/day of SASP is effective in decreasing the frequency of relapse in most patients (4, 16–19). Although the relapse rate appears to vary inversely with the daily dose, higher doses of 4 g/day are associated with increased adverse effects. In most patients, the optimum maintenance dose is 2 g/day. If this dose causes troublesome adverse effects, a daily dose of 1 g is better than no maintenance treatment. Alternatively, if flare-ups occur while on 2 g/day, a larger dose is worth trying. The duration of maintenance therapy remains unresolved, but most clinicians favor prolonged or indefinite treatment if the drug is well tolerated.

Use in Crohn's Disease. Sulfasalazine is also effective in the treatment of symptomatic mild or moderately active CD (5, 16, 17). The drug appears to be more effective in patients with colonic involvement than in those with only small bowel disease. Formation of 5-ASA in the colon may be responsible for this difference in efficacy. Patients unresponsive to steroid therapy tend to not respond to SASP. A dose of 3 to 4 g/day of SASP is usually used to treat the active phase of the disease, although some patients may require higher doses (4 to 6 g/day). As in active UC, response to sulfasalazine requires 3 to 4 weeks of treatment.

Patients with quiescent CD are often treated with lower doses of SASP to maintain remission. However, controlled clinical trials have found SASP to be no more effective than placebo in preventing recurrent attacks (5, 16, 17). Other studies have shown SASP to be ineffective in preventing postoperative recurrence of CD after resection (5, 16, 17). Therefore, SASP cannot be recommended as maintenance therapy in CD patients treated either medically or surgically.

Sulfasalazine is often used in combination with local or systemic corticosteroids in CD, on the assumption that the effects of the two drugs are additive and/or SASP produces a steroid-sparing effect. Combining SASP with oral corticosteroids may result in faster initial improvement than with SASP alone, but differences in efficacy are not apparent with continued therapy (20). Combination therapy offers no clear steroid-sparing effect.

Adverse Effects. The frequency of adverse effects reported with SASP varies from 10 to 45%. They appear to be of two types: a dose-related toxicity and a hypersensitivity reaction (16, 18). Many patients complain of one or more of the following symptoms, especially during the initial 6 to 8 weeks of therapy: nausea, malaise, headache, anorexia, vomiting, or dyspepsia. These symptoms often can be relieved by lowering the dose or temporarily discontinuing the drug. The frequency of these adverse effects appears to correlate with SP levels in the serum, especially when the dose of SASP exceeds 4 g/day. Intolerance to the gastrointestinal symptoms may be overcome by beginning with a dose of 500 mg/day and gradually increasing it or by administering the drug with meals. An increased frequency of adverse effects may occur in patients who are slow acetylators (16, 18).

Sulfasalazine may cause a number of hematologic

changes, some of which are thought to be dose-related. Sulfapyridine levels >50 µg/ml been associated with anemia and leukopenia, both of which can be managed with a reduction in SASP dose (16, 18). Hemolysis has been noted in patients with glucose-6-phosphatase deficiency. Other less common hematologic effects that are typical of the sulfonamides, in general, include agranulocytosis, thrombocytopenia, sulfhemoglobinemia, and methemoglobinemia.

In addition to the above hematologic effects, SASP has been associated with other hypersensitivity reactions typical of the sulfonamides. Skin rashes occur commonly, and in 2 to 3% of patients progress to a point that requires discontinuation of the drug. The drug may also cause reversible male infertility (16, 18). Fever, pulmonary infiltrates, parathesia, hepatitis, pancreatitis, polyneuritis, a serum sickness–type reaction, hair loss, and a lupus-like syndrome with polyarthritis and vasculitis have been reported with this agent.

Desensitization. The dose-related adverse effects of SASP may be minimized by briefly withholding the drug and reinstituting it at a lower dose. Alternatively, hypersensitivity reactions may require permanent withdrawal of the drug in a patient who is otherwise receiving therapeutic benefit. In patients with less serious reactions (fever and/or rash), a desensitization program can be undertaken by first discontinuing the drug and withholding it until the side effects subside (18). The drug can then be restarted using an extremely low dose. The dose is increased progressively in small increments over a prolonged time period until adequate therapeutic doses are achieved. Desensitization is particularly important in patients with UC because of the established value of SASP in preventing relapses and because treatment can be maintained without the need for corticosteroids.

Drug Interactions. The concurrent administration of antibiotics may alter the therapeutic activity of SASP, since the metabolism of the drug depends on normal intestinal flora. Because SASP inhibits folic acid absorption and/or interferes with hepatic metabolism, folate deficiency may occur in patients receiving long-term SASP therapy (18). Interaction between SASP and other highly protein-bound drug, such as warfarin, may lead to displacement of these drugs from their protein binding sites. Sulfasalazine may decrease serum digoxin concentrations. The concurrent administration of iron and SASP appears to result in chelation and possibly in decreased blood levels of both drugs. The clinical importance of these drug interactions is uncertain.

5-AMINOSALICYLIC ACID

The active moiety of SASP appears to be 5-ASA (mesalamine). SP, the moiety is responsible for the toxicity of the drug, acts as a carrier for the active component. When given by mouth, 5-ASA is absorbed rapidly from the prox-

imal gastrointestinal tract and metabolized to acetyl-5-aminosalicylic acid (Ac-5-ASA), which is eliminated renally (14–16). For 5-ASA to provide a topical effect in the distal small intestine and colon, it must be protected from oral absorption or be given rectally. Thus, a number of new oral and topical dosage formulations have been developed to circumvent these problems.

Oral Preparations. Several strategies have been employed to create an SP-free oral preparation that can deliver high concentrations of 5-ASA to the inflamed bowel. In general, oral agents are preferable to enemas or suppositories for long-term use because of their ability to deliver medication beyond the splenic flexure of the colon. These second-generation formulations include the use of coupling agents other than SP, pH-dependent enteric-coated tablets, and sustained-release dosage forms (18, 21–23).

Olsalazine consists of two salicylate moieties linked by a diazo bond. The drug remains intact until it is acted upon by colonic bacteria, which split the bond and release two molecules of 5-ASA. On a molar basis, olsalazine delivers twice as much 5-ASA as SASP without the sulfa-related adverse effects (21, 22). Olsalazine, in a dose of 500 mg twice a day, is indicated for the maintenance of remission of UC in patients intolerant of SASP. Higher doses (1.5 to 3 g/day) appear to be effective in treating mild to moderately active UC (24). Balsalazide and ipsalazide, investigational drugs similar to olsalazine, join 5-ASA to an unabsorbed inert vehicle (16–18, 22).

Asacol, a delayed-release product, contains 400 mg of 5-ASA coated with an acrylic resin (Eudragit-S) that dissolves at pH >7, the intraluminal pH of the distal ileum and colon (16–18, 21–23). Pentasa, a slow-release dosage form of 250 mg of 5-ASA microgranules encapsulated in ethylcellulose, dissolves gradually in the small intestine and colon (16–18, 21–23). Other oral aminosalicylates undergoing investigation include Rowasa, Salofalk, Claversal, and 4-ASA (16–18, 21–23).

The oral formulations of 5-ASA are as effective as topical 5-ASA and SASP for active and maintenance treatment of UC; however, the response rate appears to be related to the dosage of 5-ASA administered. Preliminary results suggest that oral 5-ASA is also effective in treating active CD, but its use as maintenance therapy in quiescent CD remains equivoal (18, 22, 25). The most frequently reported adverse effect with olsalazine is a dose-dependent secretory diarrhea, which occurs in 17% of patients receiving 1 g/day. Patients should be informed of the high incidence of diarrhea, since it is often difficult to distinguish from the underlying disease. About 80 to 90% of patients intolerant to SASP will tolerate 5-ASA; however, patients allergic to aspirin should avoid 5-ASA. Approximately 10 to 20% of patients will experience a rash or fever with 5-ASA, indicating a possible sensitivity to 5-ASA (16–18, 21–23). The possibility of analgesic nephropathy due to absorbed 5-ASA or Ac-5-ASA exists in patients on 5-ASA-liberating medications for prolonged periods of time.

Topical Preparations. Rectal administration of 5-ASA exerts a topical antiinflammatory effect in the distal colon and rectum (16–18, 23–27). Less than 15% of the drug is absorbed and excreted in the urine as Ac-5-ASA metabolites (23, 26). The 5-ASA rectal suspension (4 g/60 ml retention enema at bedtime) is indicated for the treatment of mild to moderate active UC, proctosigmoiditis, or proctitis. Improvement occurs within a week, but the usual course of therapy is 3 to 6 weeks, depending on symptoms and sigmoidoscopic findings. In patients with mild to moderate UC, the 5-ASA enema is as effective as oral SASP or hydrocortisone enema. Additionally, patients refractory to oral SASP and oral or rectal hydrocortisone may respond to rectal 5-ASA (16–18, 23, 26). Rectal suppositories (500 mg twice/day), indicated for distal ulcerative proctitis, should be retained at least 1 to 3 hours or longer to achieve maximum benefit (23, 27). Lower daily doses of the enema (1 to 2 g/day) or the suppository (250 to 500 mg/day) and alternate-day dosing have been investigated for maintenance therapy for UC, but the optimal regimen has not been determined (26, 27). Rectal 5-ASA appears to be less effective in CD; however, clinical trials are limited.

Adverse effects of rectal 5-ASA occur in 1 to 10% of patients and include headache, flatulence, abdominal pain, diarrhea, dizziness, and fatigue, many of which are indistinguishable from the underlying disease. Anal irritation or a hypersensitivity reaction to 5-ASA or the sulfite contained in the rectal suspension may occur. Most patients intolerant of SASP will tolerate the 5-ASA enema or suppository. The monthly cost of 5-ASA enemas should be considered when other less costly treatment alternatives are acceptable.

ADRENOCORTICOSTEROIDS

The adrenocorticosteroids remain the drugs of choice in the treatment of acute moderate to severe attacks and exacerbations of IBD. When compared with SASP in the treatment of moderate disease, they provide a more immediate response, with clinical improvement usually seen within a few days to a week. The exact mechanism by which steroids suppress intestinal inflammation is unknown, but theories include interaction with the immune system, inhibition of prostaglandins, stabilization of lysosomal membranes, and blocking of kinin release (4, 5, 28).

The adrenocorticosteroids most widely used to treat UC and CD include hydrocortisone, prednisone, prednisolone, and methylprednisolone. Steroids are usually given intravenously in the acutely ill patient and later replaced by oral therapy once the disease subsides. Various rectal dosage forms are available for topical use in patients with mild to moderate disease limited to the distal colon and/or rectum. The potential adverse effects of adrenocorti-

costeroids (see Chapter 15 "Adrenocortical Dysfunction and Clinical Use of Steroids") limit their usefulness in the prolonged treatment of IBD.

Use in Ulcerative Colitis. The efficacy of adrenocorticosteroids in treating active UC is well documented (4, 28). The dose and route (parenteral, oral, or topical) of steroid administration varies with disease severity and activity.

Parenteral. The continuous or intermittent intravenous administration of methylprednisolone in divided doses of 40 to 80 mg/24 hr is preferred in the very ill patient. Equipotent doses of intravenous prednisolone, betamethasone, dexamethasone, or hydrocortisone may also be used; however, hydrocortisone is associated with increased mineralocorticoid activity. Once clinical improvement occurs, parenteral therapy should be discontinued and oral steroids instituted. However, if the patient deteriorates or if no real progress occurs with the administration of parenteral steroids after 7 to 10 days, the patient should be considered for colectomy (4). Pulsed intravenous methylprednisolone therapy of 1 g/24 hr is no more effective than traditional parenteral dosing regimens for the treatment of severe active UC (28, 29).

In most severely ill patients, intravenous steroids are considered superior to ACTH because they do not depend on adrenal responsiveness and they have fewer adverse effects. However, evidence suggests that in patients with new-onset severe UC or patients who have not received recent corticosteroid therapy, parenteral ACTH (120 units/24 hr) is the drug of choice (16, 17, 28).

Oral. Most patients with mild to moderately active UC will respond favorably to oral steroids. For moderate disease, prednisone 20 to 40 mg/day produces improvement or remission in several weeks. The optimum oral prednisone dose is 40 mg/day, providing the maximal response with a minimum of adverse effects (4, 28). Other steroids of equivalent activity (prednisolone, hydrocortisone, or methylprednisolone) may be used.

In an attempt to mimic the natural diurnal rhythm of adrenocorticosteroid secretion and to minimize side effects, single morning doses and alternate daily dosing is advocated. However, when prednisone is used to treat active disease, the daily dose is often divided. Once remission is achieved, the dose should be changed to a single morning dose or the largest portion of the dose should be given in the morning. Because the decrease in side effects seen with alternate-day steroids is frequently paralleled by a diminution in the therapeutic effect in patients with UC, this form of therapy is generally not advisable. However, growth-stunted children who require maintenance steroids may benefit from this regimen.

Topical. Patients with mild attacks of UC, especially those with disease limited to the distal colon and rectum, frequently respond to rectal instillation of steroids (4, 16, 17, 28). The beneficial effect of rectal steroids may result from both local and systemic antiinflammatory effects, since variable quantities of the rectal dose are absorbed (4, 17, 28). Although rectal steroid preparations may result in up to 50% of the rectal drug being absorbed, the degree of adrenal suppression and adverse effects appear to be less than is observed with oral administration of the equivalent dose of the same drug (4, 28). A number of factors may account for variation in systemically absorbed steroids. These include the volume and composition of the fluid vehicle, the nature and dose of the steroid compound, and the dwell time in the colon. Acute intestinal inflammation does not appear to alter the amount of drug absorbed. Doses of 100 mg of hydrocortisone or 40 mg of methylprednisolone are usually administered by rectal instillation.

Retention enemas should be administered at bedtime to permit overnight contact with the inflamed mucosa. An additional dose may be administered in the morning after the first bowel movement. Once remission occurs, usually within 2 to 3 weeks, an alternate-night schedule may be used for an additional 2 weeks. Patients should be instructed to instill the enema in the supine position and then change to the left, right and prone positions for at least 20 min each, to facilitate maximal topical coverage. Although rectal steroid enemas can spread as far proximally as the hepatic flexure, they appear to be most effective in UC patients with left-sided colitis or protosigmoiditis.

New topical steroids such as becomethasone diprionate, tixocortal pivalate, and budesonide retain their local antiinflammatory effects, but appear to be devoid of systemic effects (17, 28, 30). The lack of systemic adverse effects is related to their extensive first-pass metabolism in the liver and in the blood by erythrocytes (17, 28, 30). Although these agents are currently under investigation, none has been approved for use in the U.S.

Rectal foam preparations may be useful in patients who are unable to retain enemas because of local inflammation, tenemus, or diarrhea. A foam preparation is more easily retained than a liquid enema; however, it usually does not spread beyond the sigmoid colon (28). although foams offer the added advantage of convenience and compliance, they are most effective in patients whose disease is confined to the sigmoid or rectum.

Once remission of UC occurs, oral steroids should be gradually tapered. The reduction of the steroid dose should be based on the duration of steroid therapy and prevention of exacerbations. Although controversial, the concensus is that oral steroids have no value in the maintenance of remission and that prolonged steroid therapy can be harmful (4, 16). Maintenance of quiescent UC can be accomplished successfully in most patients with oral SASP, and if necessary, occasional steroid enemas (4, 16).

If a patient requires more than 15 mg/day of oral prednisone, either for maintenance or to control extraintestinal manifestations, alternate forms of therapy or elective colectomy should be considered.

Use in Crohn's Disease. The use and doses of steroids in the treatment of CD are similar to those described for UC. Steroids are beneficial in relieving the symptoms of active CD, particularly during an acute attack, although the results are not always as dramatic as those in UC (5, 17). Therapy is usually initiated with daily doses of 40 to 60 mg of prednisone or steroid equivalent, and in severe cases the corticosteroid should be administered intravenously. If improvement occurs, the oral steroid dose should be tapered and eventually withdrawn.

Unfortunately, the response to steroid therapy in CD is often less successful than that in UC, and it is usually more difficult to achieve a remission. Sometimes patients remain symptomatic when the prednisone dose is reduced below 15 to 20 mg/day. Steroids should be used with caution in CD patients, especially in the presence of fistula, abscess, and malnutrition, because of the increased risk of infection as well as fluid and electrolyte disturbances. Because of this, the decision to begin treatment with corticosteroids should be made only after the risks and benefits have been carefully evaluated for an individual patient. Even when the clinical response to steroid therapy appears to be satisfactory, the disease tends to progress (5).

The efficacy of steroid therapy in CD depends on disease location. Patients with disease of the small intestine only and those with both small bowel and colonic involvement appear to respond more favorably to steroids than those with colonic CD, although clinical experience suggests that steroid enemas are effective in left-sided Crohn's colitis (5, 16). As in UC, continuing steroid therapy after remission induction generally does not alter the frequency of recurrence. Although controversial, recent evidence suggests that alternate-day prednisone is a reasonable treatment and maintenance option for patients with CD unresponsive to SASP (16, 31). Steroids do not appear to alter the frequency of relapse after surgery (5). When symptoms persist or recur despite surgical resection, immunosuppressive therapy should be considered.

IMMUNOSUPPRESSIVE THERAPY

The evidence that immune factors play a probable etiologic role in IBD has led to the use of immunosuppressive agents. These agents are usually considered third-line therapy for patients unresponsive or intolerant to SASP and corticosteroids.

Azathioprine and 6-Mercaptopurine. The specific mechanism by which azathioprine (AZA) and 6-mercaptopurine (6-MP) act in the treatment of IBD is uncertain, but it is probably related to immunomodulating and their effect on mediators of the inflammatory process. Since 6-

MP is the active metabolite of AZA, the two drugs probably have similar therapeutic and toxic effects (16, 17, 28, 32–35).

Early clinical trials failed to confirm the efficacy of AZA (2 mg/kg/day) or 6-MP (1.5 mg/kg/day) when used as single agents to treat IBD refractory to SASP, steroids, or metronidazole. Recent evidence suggests that both drugs have a steroid-sparing effect in CD and UC when added to the patient's steroid regimen; however, experience in treating UC is very limited (32–35). In addition, when AZA or 6-MP are continued after the steroid is withdrawn, remission is usually sustained. Unfortunately, there is a high relapse rate when attempting to taper or stop the immunosuppressive agent (33–35). Azathioprine and 6-MP are also effective in relieving some of the extraintestinal symptoms and in healing CD fistulas. Since response to AZA or 6-MP may require 3 to 6 months or longer therapy is often discontinued prematurely or changed because of the concern about potential adverse effects.

The long-term use of AZA and 6-MP has been associated with toxic adverse effects such as bone marrow depression, pancreatitis, and malignancy, as well as the development of serious infections. However, recent studies suggest a lower incidence of these adverse effects when AZA and 6-MP are used in reduced doses to treat IBD (33–36). Despite an improved safety profile, patients on long-term immunosuppressive therapy should be monitored closely with frequent blood counts and checked for signs of infection.

In patients with refractory UC, a bowel resection can be curative; however, some patients may wish to avoid colectomy. In Crohn's patients, the use of AZA or 6-MP should be restricted to those with refractory disease whose clinical condition or extent of intestinal involvement preclude bowel surgery. In these patients, it seems reasonable to begin with an initial dose of 50 mg of either AZA or 6-MP, with subsequent increases to a dose not exceeding 1.5 mg/kg/day. The immunosuppressant should be added to the drug regimen in an attempt to taper or withdraw steroid therapy.

Cyclosporine A. A limited number of studies suggest that cyclosporine A (CP), a suppressor of cell-mediated immunity, may have a role in the treatment of CD or UC patients refractory to the usual treatment modalities (16, 17, 28, 37). Results of one controlled trial indicate that an oral dose of 5 to 7.5 mg/kg/day has a beneficial therapeutic effect in patients resistant to or intolerant of corticosteroids (37). Improvement was higher among patients who received CP and corticosteroids than among those who received CP alone. Response to CP usually occurred within several weeks, but recurrence was reported when the drug was withdrawn. Lower maintenance doses of 2 mg/kg/day do not appear to protect against relapse of CD

(38). The potential advantages of CP therapy must be balanced against the risk of nephropathy and other potentially serious adverse effects. Although the results of these studies are encouraging, the use of CP in the treatment of refractory IBD, should be limited to controlled clinical trials until the drug's efficacy can be substantiated and the toxicities assessed.

Methotrexate. Methotrexate, a folic acid antagonist, is currently under investigation for the treatment of refractory IBD (39, 40). In an open-labeled trial, preliminary results suggest that the drug may have a more rapid response than AZA or 6-MP and that it may be more effective in CD than in UC (39). Of major concern are the potential teratogenic and hepatotoxic effects associated with the drug. Additional clinical studies are needed to elucidate the dose, efficacy, and safety of methotrexate in IBD.

METRONIDAZOLE

Metronidazole (MTZ) appears to be effective in the treatment of active CD, but its therapeutic benefit in active UC is unresolved (17, 40, 41). The mode of action of MTZ in IBD is unclear, but is presumed to be related to its antibacterial and immunosuppressive properties. When used as primary therapy, MTZ appears to be similar to SASP in treating active CD. In addition, nonresponders who fail SASP therapy, may respond to MTZ. There is sufficient evidence to suggest that the drug may be more effective in patients with colonic CD, fistula, or perineal disease (17, 41). Effective doses range from 10 to 20 mg/kg/day, and response to treatment usually requires several months. Higher doses may be required in patients with refractory perineal disease (17, 40). Most patients with mild to moderate Crohn's colitis or ileocolitis will respond to 250 mg of MTZ four times daily. Attempts to reduce or discontinue the MTZ dose have been associated with worsening disease activity. The usefulness of MTZ in the prevention of recurrent CD is not well studied. However, a dose of 600 mg/day has been reported to be effective in the maintenance of remission in patients with UC (42).

Many adverse effects, including nausea, metallic taste, dark urine, and parathesia have been reported with the short-term use of MTZ. The most troublesome of these is parathesia, which has been reported to occur in up to 50% of patients and appears to be dose-dependent (17, 40). Although the drug has not been proven to be mutagenic, teratogenic, or carcinogenic in humans, results of animal and laboratory tests have caused concern about these possibilities. Therefore, the drug should be discontinued after several months if ineffective, and should be tapered after 3 to 4 months, if possible, when the disease is controlled. At present, MTZ should be reserved for those CD patients with fistula and colonic or perineal involvement who do not respond to SASP.

ANTIDIARRHEAL AND ANTISPASMOTIC AGENTS

Antidiarrheal and antispasmotic drugs such as diphenoxylate, loperamide, codeine, belladonna, and tincture of opium are an effective and useful adjunct to first-line therapy in patients with mild chronic IBD and in those who have diarrhea resulting from bowel resection. Symptomatic treatment of diarrhea may permit a reduction in the dosage of other drugs, thereby reducing the incidence of adverse effects. However, they are ineffective in the severe forms of IBD, since diarrhea results from a loss of colonic absorptive capacity because of widespread destruction of the colonic mucosa (43). Furthermore, they may contribute to the development of ileus or toxic megacolon.

Cholestyramine is the treatment of choice for patients with bile salt–induced diarrhea resulting from resection of the terminal ileal. The formation of oxalate kidney stones and steatorrhea may also be prevented with cholestryamine. Clonidine or octreotide may prove to be effective in enhancing fluid and electrolyte absorption in refractory diarrhea, but their utility is limited because of the many adverse effects associated with their use (43).

PAIN MANAGEMENT

Intestinal inflammation commonly leads to severe cramping abdominal pain, especially in patients with CD. Pain management should be aimed at treatment of the underlying disease. Opiates may be used to supplement treatment, but they should not become the mainstay of chronic pain control. In severe pain, narcotics should be dosed on a scheduled basis rather than P.R.N. (44). Unfortunately, iatrogenic drug addiction has become a common problem among Crohn's patients, which can best be prevented by having only one physician prescribe and manage pain medications.

POTENTIAL NEW DRUGS

Many other agents have been proposed for use in treating IBD, including interferon, chloroquine, levamisole, and mast cell stabilizers such as cromoglycate sodium (16, 17, 40, 45). Controlled trials of antituberculous agents are needed to confirm their role in the treatment of CD (17). The use of inhibitors of leukotriene synthesis, such as eicosapentanoic acid derived from fish oil and other omega-3 fatty acids, suggest that dietary supplementation may be effective in the treatment of UC (17, 40, 45). The use of oxygen-derived free radical scavengers (superoxide dismutase) looks promising, and it is possible that α-tocopherol and penicillamine work by this mechanism (17, 40). It is unlikely that topical sucralfate is useful in treating distal colitis (17). Theoretically, inhibitors of complement activation and neuropeptides such as substance P, may have a role in the treatment of IBD (40). Although results obtained from clinical trials with several of the agents appear promising, their efficacy has not been established, and their role, if any, in the management of IBD is unknown.

Recommendations

The goal of medical therapy in IBD is to induce remission and to prevent symptomatic recurrence. Selection of a drug, dose, and the route of administration is determined by the location, extent, and severity of intestinal involvement (Figs. 22.4 & 22.5)

ULCERATIVE COLITIS

Patients with acute severe UC will usually require intravenous steroids equivalent to 40 to 80 mg/day of methylprednisolone. If the patient improves progressively during the next 7 to 10 days, oral steroids should replace the parenteral form. Once remission has been induced with steroids, they should be gradually withdrawn, and maintenance SASP therapy instituted at 1 to 2 g/day. Since both efficacy and adverse effects are dose-related, the SASP dose should be adjusted to produce minimal undesirable side effects while maintaining remission.

Acute moderate disease may respond to oral doses of 2 to 4 g/day of SASP. Lower doses may be attempted initially and increased gradually as tolerance to the adverse effects develops. However, it may take 3 to 4 weeks for improvement of symptoms. Nightly steroid enemas may provide additional therapeutic benefit. If a more immediate response is required or if response to SASP is inadequate, it should be discontinued and oral prednisone instituted in doses of 20 to 40 mg/day. Steroids should be tapered over 2 to 3 weeks and 1 to 2 g/day SASP begun as maintenance therapy. If the patient remains steroid-dependent, addition of AZA or 6-MP may permit withdrawal of the steroid in those individuals wishing to avoid a colectomy.

Patients with mild active UC or those in whom the disease involves only the rectum usually respond to either 2 to 4 g/day of oral SASP or rectal steroid retention enemas. Although 5-ASA enemas and suppositories are effective, the cost of a course of therapy is many times that of SASP or steroid enemas. Thus, their use is often reserved for individuals with mild to moderate active disease of the distal colon who do not respond to corticosteroids or SASP. Frequent relapses may require maintenance therapy with low-dose SASP. Olsalazine should be used in individuals intolerant to SASP.

CROHN'S DISEASE

Patients with severe CD usually require intravenous steroids in doses similar to those used in UC. Steroids should

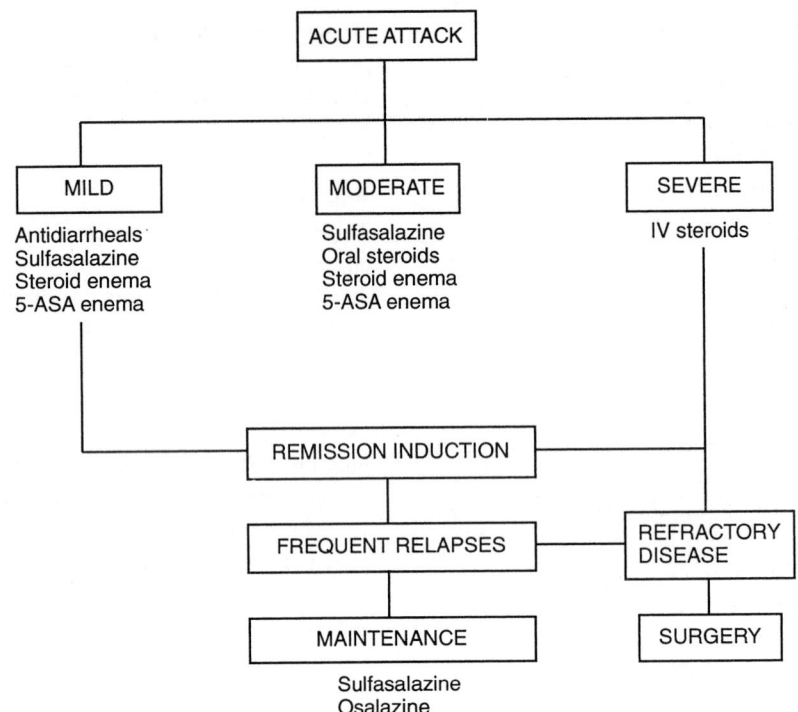

Figure 22.4. Recommended therapy for ulcerative colitis.

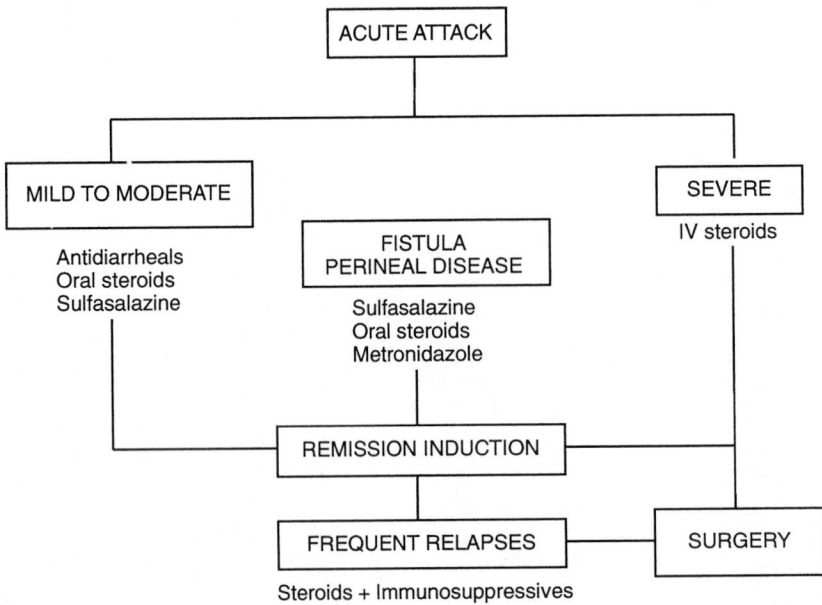

Figure 22.5. Recommended therapy for Crohn's disease.

be continued until symptomatic relief is observed, and then tapered. In patients whose symptoms worsen when steroids are withdrawn, alternatives to continuous steroid therapy should be considered.

Therapy for patients with mild to moderate ileitis or ileocolitis should be initiated with 40 to 60 mg/day of oral prednisone. Sulfasalazine, in doses of 3 to 4 g/day should be tried for 4 to 6 weeks in mild to moderate active CD that involves the colon. If the response to SASP is inadequate, oral prednisone should be instituted. Since neither corticosteroids nor SASP prevent relapses in CD, they should be discontinued after a remission has been achieved.

For patients with chronic active CD that require >15 mg/day of prednisone to control symptoms, consideration should be given to the addition of either AZA or 6-MP to the regimen in an attempt to withdraw or reduce the steroid dose. Metronidazole, in a maximum dose of 20 mg/kg/day, may be useful in patients with Crohn's colitis, fistula, or severe perianal disease.

Treatment During Pregnancy

Management of IBD in pregnancy is of concern because the disease occurs frequently in young adults and many of the drugs (or their metabolites) used in treatment cross the placental barrier and are secreted into breast milk (46, 47). Sulfasalazine and adrenocorticosteroids do not appear to affect the fetus (46). There is little evidence to support the fact that the SASP causes kernicterus or is teratogenic. Alternatively, MTZ and the immunosuppressants should be avoided; however, recent evidence suggests that AZA is not harmful to the fetus (46, 47). In most patients, pregnancy does not affect the course of IBD, nor is the outcome of pregnancy affected. In addition, IBD does not adversely affect fertility, but male patients should be informed that SASP may reversibly inhibit spermatogenesis. Although it is always best to avoid medication during pregnancy, the risk to benefit ratio must be carefully evaluated in each individual.

Treatment of Children

When IBD begins in childhood, the clinical course is similar to that observed when the onset occurs later in life, except for more severe growth retardation, which is more common in the patient with CD. Since malnutrition is thought to be the primary cause of growth failure, nutritional supplementation must be pursued aggressively. Medications used in the treatment of IBD in children are similar to those used to treat adult patients. However, prolonged use of high-dose steroids may suppress growth and cause other steroid-related adverse effects. Although MTZ and the immunosuppressants have been used in children, they should be used with caution because of the potentially serious complications related to these drugs (48).

Nutritional Therapy

Maintenance of adequate nutrition is difficult in patients with IBD, especially those who have undergone extensive small bowel resection. In general, patients with CD are at greater risk of developing malnutrition than those with UC. Specific replacement of vitamins, minerals, and other nutrients is indicated whenever there is clinical or laboratory evidence of deficiency (10). Total parenteral nutrition (TPN) should be used only in the event of failure or the impossibility of enteral nutrition (49, 50).

The nutritional status of debilitated patients with severe active IBD improves clinically when they are receiving TPN. While parenteral nutrition is considered to be a valuable adjunct to therapy in both severe UC and CD, there is little evidence that the overall course of either of these diseases is altered by bowel rest and adequate nutrition (50). However, more rapid healing of fistulas and improvement in perineal disease has been reported in Crohn's patients receiving TPN (50). In addition, prolonged home TPN has been effective in maintaining Crohn's patients with extensive small bowel resection. Until more definitive information is obtained from controlled studies, TPN should be used primarily to improve the nutritional status of severely ill patients with IBD who cannot be fed interally and in those selected Crohn's patients in whom bowel rest may be of value.

Surgical Treatment

Surgery in IBD is indicated only after failure of all reasonable attempts at medical therapy or for actual and impending complications. The decision to operate must be balanced against the disabilities of the disease and the long-term side effects of drug therapy.

Surgery is eventually required for 20 to 25% of patients with UC (4). In contrast to CD, removal of the colon in UC removes the primary focus of the disease and usually rids the patients of systemic complications. Generally accepted indications for surgical intervention in patients with UC include failure of medical management, toxic megacolon, colonic perforation or hemorrhage, anal complications, and the risk of developing colonic cancer. Prophylactic colectomy has been recommended in children and in adults with universal (pan)colitis who have had the disease for at least 10 years. However, the most reasonable guidelines for most patients with long-standing disease are once-yearly evaluations that include colonoscopy with accompanying histologic examination of biopsies for precancerous changes. Total proctocolectomy with establishment of a permanent ileostomy is the operative procedure of choice, and it may be carried out in a single stage or a two-staged procedure (4). The rectum must always be removed because of the continuing risk of neoplasia. Postoperative mortality is 3% in elective colectomy, 10 to 15%

in patients undergoing emergency surgery for acute severe disease, and 50% in those with colonic perforation (4).

The indications for surgery in CD are influenced in part by the site of involvement and the fact that the surgery is not curative. Possible indications include failure of medical management, intestinal obstruction, strictures, fistulas, abscess formation, perforation, and hemorrhage. Approximately 75% of patients will require surgery within 20 years of initial symptoms, with the rate of recurrence after intestinal resection reported to be as high as 90 to 95% (5). In view of the high recurrence rate following resection, the procedure of choice is usually conservative intestinal resection of diseased bowel with primary bowel anastomosis. The most controversy occurs when CD involves only the colon. Increasing losses of the small bowel through resection and disease may eventually limit its absorptive surface resulting in malabsorptive syndromes and malnutrition.

PROGNOSIS

The prognosis of IBD is favorably affected by the use of SASP, 5-ASA analogs, corticosteroids, and immunosuppressive agents, as well as supportive measures such as TPN. In spite of the chronicity of these diseases, the tendency to relapse, and numerous complications, most patients respond favorably to long-term medical management.

In acute UC, 90% of patients will respond to medical management with successful induction of a remission. The overall mortality of an acute initial attack is about 5%, which is increased when there is total colonic involvement, when onset occurs over age 60, and when toxic megacolon develops. Left-sided colitis and ulcerative proctitis respond well to current drug therapy and have favorable prognoses. The prognosis for long-standing, universal colitis depends on the development of carcinoma, but it can be improved with colectomy or yearly colonoscopy with biopsy.

The long-term prognosis of CD is not as favorable as that for UC, because of the variable nature of the disease and the less than optimal response to medical therapy. Many patients will require surgery at some point; however, surgery is often followed by disease recurrence. In contrast to UC, the mortality increases with the duration of the disease and ranges from 5 to 10%. Most deaths appear to be related to peritonitis and sepsis.

SUMMARY

Despite the limitations of present medical and surgical treatment, most patients with IBD can adjust to the exacerbations and complications of their chronic illness and manage to lead productive lives. Management must be individualized and should involve emotional support by the family and members of the healthcare team. Until the etiology of IBD is understood, definitive drug therapy is probably beyond the reach of medicine. Fortunately, a few drugs offer most patients some assistance. Promising new agents await confirmation of their efficacy in the treatment of IBD.

REFERENCES

1. Langman MJS, Epidemiology of inflammatory bowel disease. In Allan RN, Keighley MRB, Alexander-Williams J, Hawkins C (eds): Inflammatory Bowel Diseases. New York, Churchill Livingstone, 1990, p 25.
2. Sonnenberg A, McCarty DJ, Jacobsen SJ: Geographic variation of inflammatory bowel disease within the United States. Gastroenterology 100:143–149, 1991.
3. Orholm M, Munkholm P, Langholz E et al.: Familial occurrence of inflammatory bowel disease. N Engl J Med 324:84–88, 1991.
4. Cello JP, Schneiderman DJ, Ulcerative colitis. In Sleissenger MH, Fordtran JS (eds): Gastrointestinal Disease: Pathophysiology, Diagnosis, Management. Philadelphia, WB Saunders, 1989, p 1435.
5. Donaldson RM, Crohn's disease. In Sleissenger MH, Fordtran JS (eds): Gastrointestinal Disease: Pathophysiology, Diagnosis, Management. Philadelphia, WB Saunders, 1989, p 1327.
6. Zipser RD (ed): Mediators of inflammatory bowel disease: proceedings of a symposium. Dig Dis Sci 33(suppl):4S–84S, 1988.
7. Sutherland LR, Ramcharan S, Bryant H, et al.: Effect of cigarette smoking on recurrence of Crohn's disease. Gastroenterology 98:1123–1128, 1990.
8. Kaufmann HJ, Taubin HL: Nonsteroidal anti-inflammatory drugs activate quiescent inflammatory bowel disease. Ann Intern Med 107:513–516, 1987.
9. Lashner BA, Kane SV, Hanauer SB: Lack of association between oral contraceptive use and ulcerative colitis. Gastroenterology 99:1032–1036, 1990.
10. Fernandez-Banares F, Abad-Lacruz A, Xiol S, et al.: Vitamin status in patients with inflammatory bowel disease. Am J Gastroenterol 84:744–748, 1989.
11. Mayer L, Janowitz HD, Extra-intestinal manifestations. In Allan RN, Keighley MRB, Alexander-Williams J, Hawkins C (eds): Inflammatory Bowel Diseases. New York, Churchill Livingstone, 1990, p 501.
12. Fazio VW, Toxic megacolon: natural history and management. In Jagelman DC (ed): Mucosal Ulcerative Colitis. Mount Kisco, NY, Futura, 1986, pp 159–175.
13. Ekbom E, Helmick C, Zack M, et al.: Ulcerative colitis and colorectal cancer. N Engl J Med 323:1228–1233, 1990.
14. Lauritsen K, Laursen LS, Rask-Madsen JR: Clinical pharmacokinetics of drugs used in the treatment of gastrointestinal diseases (part II). Clin Pharmacokinet 19:94–125, 1990.
15. Klotz U, Maier KE: Pharmacology and pharmacokinetics of 5-aminosalicylic acid. Dig Dis Sci 32(suppl):46S–50S, 1987.
16. Scottile RF, Quandt CM, Present DH, et al.: Medical management of inflammatory bowel disease. DICP 23:963–973, 1989.
17. Peppercorn MA: Advances in drug therapy for inflammatory bowel disease. Ann Intern Med 112:50–60, 1990.
18. Dew MJ, Sulphasalazine and aminosalicylates in treatment. In Allan RN, Keighley MRB, Alexander-Williams J, Hawkins C (eds): Inflammatory Bowel Diseases. New York, Churchill Livingstone, 1990, p 365.
19. Margolin ML, Krumholz MP, Fochios SE, et al.: Clinical trials in

ulcerative colitis: historical review. Am J Gastroenterol 83:227–243, 1988.

20. Rijk MCM, van Hogezand RA, van Lier HJJ, et al.: Sulphasalazine and prednisone compared with sulphasalazine for treating active Crohn disease. Ann Intern Med 114:445–450, 1991.

21. Robertson MG: New oral salilcylates in the therapy of chronic idiopathic inflammatory bowel disease. Gastroenterol Clin North Am 18:43–50, 1989.

22. Martin F: Oral 5-aminosalicylic acid preparations in treatment of inflammatory bowel disease. Dig Dis Sci 32(suppl):57S–63S, 1987.

23. Fitzgerald JM, Marsh TD: Mesalamine in ulcerative colitis. DICP 25:140–145, 1991.

24. Zinberg J, Molinas S, Das KM: Double-blind placebo-controlled study of olsalazine in the treatment of ulcerative colitis. Am J Gastroenterol 85:562–566, 1990.

25. Hanauer SB: The role of mesalazine in Crohn's disease. Scand J Gastroenterol 25(suppl 172):56–59, 1990.

26. Compieri M, Gionchetti P, Belluzzi , et al.: Role of rectal formulations: enemas. Scand J Gastroenterol 25(suppl 172):63–65, 1990.

27. Williams CN: Role of rectal formulations: suppositories. Scand J Gastroenterol 25(suppl 172):60–62, 1990.

28. Leonard-Jones JE, Corticosteroids and immunosuppressive drugs. In Allan RN, Keighley MRB, Alexander-Williams J, Hawkins C (eds): Inflammatory Bowel Diseases. New York, Churchill Livingstone, 1990, p 373.

29. Rosenberg W, Ireland A, Jewell DP: High-dose methylprednisolone in the treatment of acute ulcerative colitis. J Clin Gastroenterol 12:40–41, 1990.

30. Halpern Z, Sold O, Baratz M, et al.: A controlled trial of beclomethasone versus betamethasone enemas in distal ulcerative colitis. J Clin Gastroenterol 13:38–41, 1991.

31. Bello C, Goldstein F, Thornton JJ: Alternate-day prednisone treatment and treatment maintenance in Crohn's disease. Am J Gastroenterol 86:460–466, 1991.

32. Present DH, Meltzer SJ, Krumholz MP, et al.: 6-Mercaptopurine in the management of inflammatory bowel disease. Ann Intern Med 111:641–649, 1989.

33. Steinhart AH, Baker JP, Brzezinski A, et al.: Azathioprine therapy in chronic ulcerative colitis. J Clin Gastroenterol 12:271–275, 1990.

34. Adler DJ, Lorelitz BL: The therapeutic efficacy of 6-mercaptopurine in refractory ulcerative colitis. Am J Gastroenterol 85:717–722, 1990.

35. O'Brien JJ, Bayless TM, Bayless JA: Use of azathioprine or 6-mercaptopurine in the treatment of Crohn's disease. Gastroenterology 101:39–46, 1991.

36. Present DH, Meitzer SJ, Krumholz MP, et al.: 6-Mercaptopurine in the management of inflammatory bowel diseases: short- and long-term toxicity. Ann Intern Med 111:641–649, 1989.

37. Brynskov J, Freund L, Rasmussen SN, et al.: A placebo-controlled, double-blind, randomized trial of cyclosporine therapy in active chronic Crohn's disease. N Engl J Med 321:845–850, 1989.

38. Lobo AJ, Joby LD, Rothwell J, et al.: Long-term treatment of Crohn's disease with cyclosporine: the effect of a very low dose on maintenance of remission. J Clin Gastroenterol 13:42–45, 1991.

39. Kozarek RA, Patterson DJ, Gelfand MD, et al.: Methotrexate induces clinical and histologic remission in patients with refractory inflammatory bowel disease. Ann Intern Med 110:353–356, 1989.

40. Hanauer SB: Inflammatory bowel disease revisited: newer drugs. Scand J Gastroenterol 25(suppl):97–106, 1990.

41. Babb RR: Editorial: the use of metronidazole (Flagyl) in Crohn's disease. J Cln Gastroenterol 10:479–481, 1988.

42. Gilat T, Leichtman G, Delpr G, et al.: A comparison of metronidazole and sulfasalazine in the maintenance of remission in patients with ulcerative colitis. J Clin Gastroenterol 11:392–395, 1989.

43. Barrett KE, Dharmsathaphorn K: Pharmacological aspects of therapy in inflammatory bowel diseases: antidiarrheal agents. J Clin Gastroenterol 10:57–63, 1988.

44. Kaplan MA, Korelitz BI: Narcotic dependence in inflammatory bowel disease. J Clin Gastroenterol 10:275–278, 1988.

45. Salomon P, Kornbluth AA, Janowitz: Treatment of ulcerative colitis with fish oil n-3-w-fatty, acid: an open trial. J Clin Gastroenterol 12:157–161, 1990.

46. Willoughby CP, Inflammatory bowel disease and pregnancy. In Allan RN, Keighley MRB, Alexander-Williams J, Hawkins C (eds): Inflammatory Bowel Diseases. New York, Churchill Livingstone, 1990, p 547.

47. Alstead EM, Ritchie JK, Lennard-Jones JE, et al.: Safety of azathiazoprine in pregnancy in inflammatory bowel disease. Gastroenterology 99:443–446, 1990.

48. Evans CM, Walker-Smith JA, Inflammatory bowel disease in childhood. In Allan RN, Keighley MRB, Alexander-Williams J, Hawkins C (eds): Inflammatory Bowel Diseases. New York, Churchill Livingstone, 1990, p 523.

49. Mason JB, Rosenberg IH, Nutritional therapy of inflammatory bowel disease. In Allan RN, Keighley MRB, Alexander-Williams J, Hawkins C (eds): Inflammatory Bowel Diseases. New York, Churchill Livingstone, 1990, p 411.

50. Sitzmann JV, Converse RL Jr, Bayless TM: Favorable response to parenteral nutrition and medical therapy in Crohn's colitis. Gastroenterology 99:1647–1652, 1990.

CHAPTER 23

NAUSEA AND VOMITING

BRUCE D. CLAYTON, Pharm.D. and RICHARD E. THOMAS, Ph.D.

Vomiting is the reflex expulsion of the stomach contents via the esophagus and mouth and is usually associated with nausea and retching. Nausea and retching can occur without expulsion, and occasionally expulsion occurs without prior nausea and retching. This is known as projectile vomiting.

Retching is the involuntary but ineffectual effort to vomit, which involves mainly the respiratory muscles of the abdomen and chest and is often accompanied by bradycardia. *Nausea* is the premonition of vomiting and is often preceded or accompanied by a variety of autonomic signs such as pallor, sweating, tachycardia, salivation, and increased respiratory rate.

The vomiting reflex probably evolved as a protective mechanism to limit the effects of ingested toxic materials. In humans, the tendency to vomit and experience nausea varies greatly. The causes of nausea and vomiting are listed in Table 23.1. The treatment of nausea and vomiting depends on the cause, which should be determined before beginning therapy (refer to Table 23.1).

PHYSIOLOGIC BASIS OF VOMITING

The principal anatomic elements involved in vomiting are shown in Figure 23.1. Integration of the vomiting reflex occurs in the vomiting center (VC) located in the medulla. Afferent fibers from sensory receptors in the stomach, intestines, and other viscera connect directly with the VC, and when stimulated, produce vomiting. The center also responds to stimuli originating in other tissues, such as the cerebral cortex, vestibular apparatus, and blood. These so-called central stimuli are believed to travel first to the chemoreceptor trigger zone (CTZ), which then activates the VC to induce vomiting. The CTZ is located in the medullary region known as the area postrema which is located on the caudal margin of the fourth ventricle. An important function of the CTZ is to sample blood and spinal fluid for potentially toxic substances and, when these are detected, to initiate vomiting. It is therefore appropriate that the CTZ is located in the area postrema—a region of the brain that is not protected by the blood-brain barrier. Both the VC and the CTZ occur bilaterally and are much smaller than shown in the figure (1).

The higher centers of the brain can be a source of stimuli for the vomiting center (Fig. 23.1). The reaction to unpleasant sights and smells is a common example of this. Vomiting can occur as a conditioned response (e.g.,

the pretreatment nausea that occurs in some patients about to receive a course of anticancer chemotherapy). The cerebrum can greatly modify the vomiting response to stimuli from other sources such as visceral or vestibular nerve pathways, leading to enhancement or repression of vomiting. The large placebo response seen in many trials of antiemetics can be explained in these terms, as can suppression of motion sickness by the patient's concentration on some mental activity. Psychologic factors can thus play an important role in nausea and vomiting, although they are usually outweighed by physical factors.

There is some confusion in the literature as to whether vestibular and hypermedullary stimuli travel directly to the VC or reach it, as shown in Figure 23.1 via the CTZ. These pathways have not been properly elucidated, but the scheme shown in the figure is supported by recent publications (1). Evidence indicates that in humans the CTZ

Table 23.1.
Causes of Vomiting

Ingestion of certain substances present in food and the environment

Ingestion of certain drugs, particularly opiates, general anesthetics, and antineoplastic drugs

Motion or other effects on the vestibular apparatus

Infection—part of the prodrome of many infections

Respiratory problems such as violent coughing

Cardiovascular disease such as infarction

Disorders of the gastrointestinal tract

   Gastrointestinal tract obstruction

   Mucosal lesions such as ulcers, inflammation, and atrophy

   Liver disease

   Pancreatic and small intestinal diseases

   Diseases of the components of the gut wall (collagen, smooth muscle, nerve)

   Peritonitis

Renal diseases such as renal failure, pyelonephritis, uremia, and uretic colic

Metabolic and endocrine disorders such as diabetic ketoacidosis, uremia, hyperparathyroidism, adrenal insufficiency, and pregnancy

Gynecologic disorders such as pelvic inflammation and complications of pregnancy

Normal pregnancy

Neurologic disorders such as increased cranial pressure, hemorrhage, epilepsy, meningitis, migraine, vertigo and Ménière's syndrome and brain metastases

Psychiatric disorders including bulimia, rumination, and anorexia nervosa

Drug withdrawal syndromes

Radiation therapy

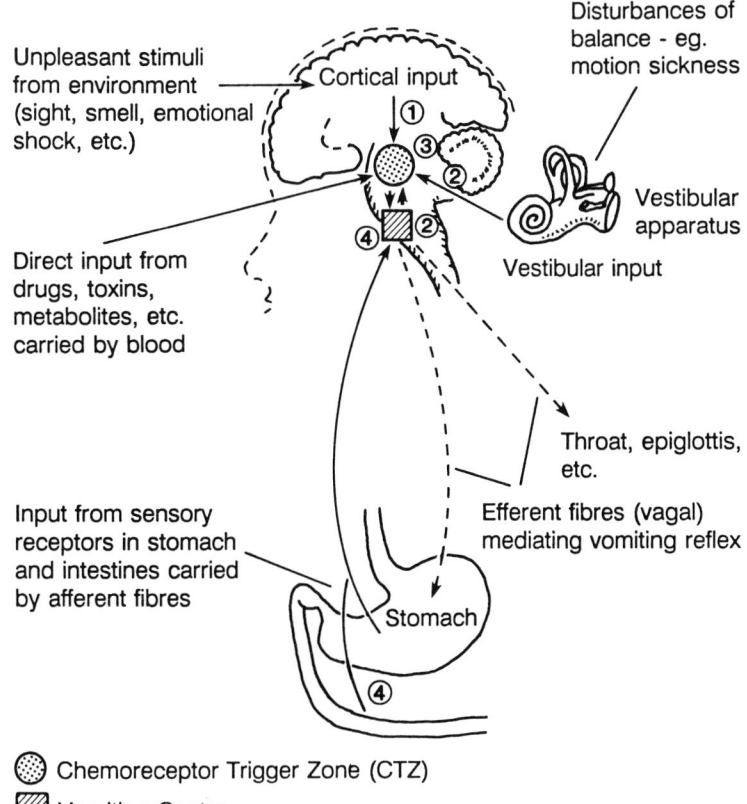

Unpleasant stimuli
from environment
(sight, smell, emotional
shock, etc.)

Cortical input

Disturbances of
balance - eg.
motion sickness

Vestibular
apparatus

Vestibular input

Direct input from
drugs, toxins,
metabolites, etc.
carried by blood

Throat, epiglottis,
etc.

Efferent fibres (vagal)
mediating vomiting reflex

Input from sensory
receptors in stomach
and intestines carried
by afferent fibres

Stomach

Chemoreceptor Trigger Zone (CTZ)

Vomiting Center

Figure 23.1. Anatomic structures involved in the vomiting reflex showing the site of action of common antiemetic drugs: 1, site of action of sedatives; 2, site of action of antihistamines and anticholinergics; 3, site of action of dopamine antagonists; and 4, proposed sites of action of serotonin antagonists. The vomiting reflex is mediated through the vomiting center. This center receives impulses from afferent fibers from the stomach and intestines and from fibers from the CTZ. It sends out impulses via efferent fibers to the muscles of the throat, epiglottis and stomach as shown in Figure 23.2.

may even influence the sensory input that the VC receives from the viscera. The variability in the literature is due to research on different species of experimental animals, which vary greatly in the anatomy and physiology of emesis.

Drugs that exert an emetic effect by acting on the CTZ include apomorphine, cardiac glycosides, morphine, the ergot alkaloids, anesthetics, and many antineoplastic agents. There is considerable species difference in the sensitivity of the CTZ to emetic drugs as well as great variation in the extent to which emesis is stimulated by other routes, such as stimulation of the sensory receptors of the viscera. Apomorphine is the only drug that produces vomiting solely by direct action on the CTZ in all species. The complexity of the pharmacology of emetic drugs is illustrated by morphine, which can act on the CTZ directly or indirectly via the vestibular afferent system. It can also antagonize the emetic action of other drugs by direct depression of the VC.

The neurochemical control of vomiting is not completely understood. Dopamine receptors are found in both the CTZ and the gastrointestinal tract. Dopamine agonists, such as apomorphine and l-dopa, produce emesis by acting on the CTZ and peripheral dopamine receptors that stimulate the CTZ, whereas dopamine antagonists, such as the phenothiazines, block emesis. Histamine (H_1 and

H_2) receptors are also found in the CTZ, but histamine receptor blockade results in antiemetic activity limited to vestibular causes. Recent studies indicate that 5-hydroxytryptamine$_3$ (5-HT$_3$) (serotonin) M-receptors appear to be principal mediators in the emetic reflex. About 90% of the 5-HT in the adult human body is located in the enterochromaffin cells of the gastrointestinal tract, while the remainder is present in platelets and the central nervous system. It is thought that these 5-HT$_3$ receptors are located on visceral afferent nerve terminals within the abdomen (2), sending sensory signals via the vagus and the greater splanchnic nerve to the central nervous system. High concentrations of 5-HT$_3$ receptors have also recently been identified in the area postrema-nucleus tractus solitarii region of the medulla (3). There may be other quite different receptors for drugs such as the cardiac glycosides. The vomiting of anaphylactic shock may involve the interaction of histamine receptors located in the CTZ, the viscera, and possibly elsewhere, and receptors for enkephalins may exist in the CTZ (1). Emesis is thus mediated through a variety of receptor types, and it is possible that more will be discovered.

The neurotransmitters involved in motion sickness are better understood. The sensory disorientation that occurs in motion sickness results in an imbalance in cholinergic and adrenergic activity in the region of the medulla near

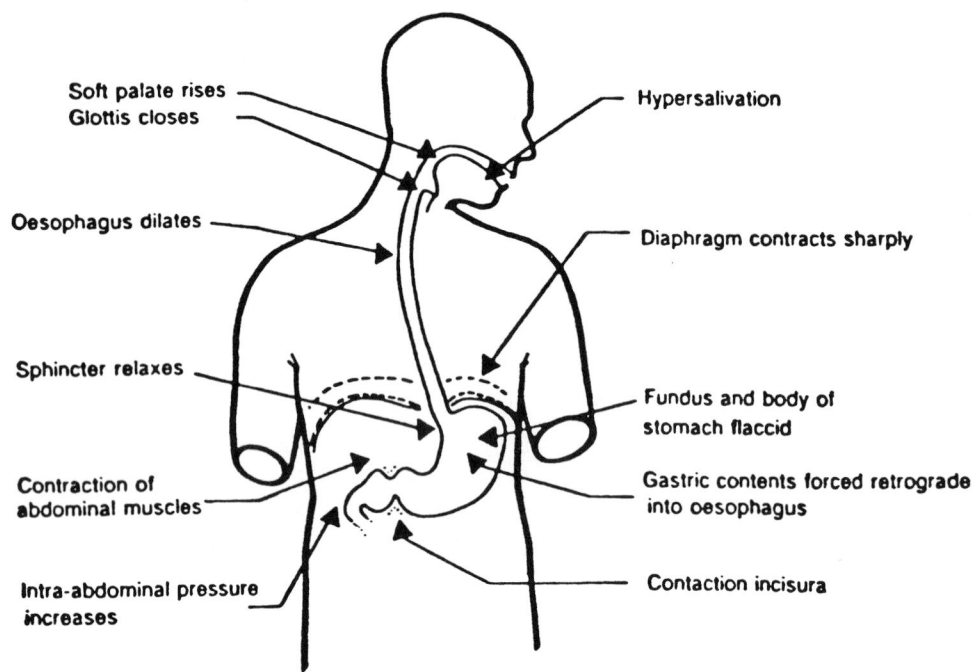

Figure 23.2.   The mechanism of the complex act of vomiting. (From Whelan G: Curr Therapeut 26(12):26, 1985, with permission.)

the VC and CTZ. The result is excess acetylcholine that affects the VC either directly, or more likely, through an effect on the CTZ (1).

Anatomically, the VC is well placed to coordinate the various efferent functions associated with vomiting (Fig. 23.2). The vomiting reflex begins with a sudden deep inspiration that increases abdominal pressure, which is further increased by contraction of the abdominal muscles. The soft palate rises and the epiglottis closes, thus preventing the aspiration of vomitus into the lungs. The pyloric sphincter contracts and the cardiac sphincter and esophagus relax. The flow of saliva increases to aid the expulsion of the stomach contents.

ANTIEMETIC DRUGS

Considerable effort has been spent in developing antinausea drugs. Initially the emphasis was on the treatment of motion sickness and nausea of pregnancy, but more recently it has focused on the treatment of nausea and vomiting caused by antineoplastic agents. Nausea and vomiting are common complications of chemotherapeutic regimens, often so severe as to cause the patient not to return for further treatment. Only recently have satisfactory antiemetic therapies begun to emerge.

When selecting drugs for the treatment of nausea and vomiting, it is important to appreciate that therapy must be individualized. Multiple pathways are available for a variety of stimuli to induce nausea and vomiting, and cor-

relations between serum levels and efficacy have not been established for most antiemetics. For these reasons, treatment regimens should be regarded only as guidelines.

Dopamine Antagonists

The dopamine antagonists include the phenothiazines, the butyrophenones and related compounds, and the substituted benzamides, which include metoclopramide. These compounds inhibit dopamine receptors and their antiemetic action is thought to be, at least in part, due to inhibition of dopamine receptors in the CTZ. Unfortunately, antiemetics that act as dopamine antagonists may also produce symptoms of dystonia, parkinsonism, akathisia, and tardive dyskinesia, since the extrapyramidal nigrostriatal system is highly innervated by dopaminergic fibers (4).

PHENOTHIAZINES

The phenothiazines have been the most widely used antiemetics since the 1950s. Two key modifications of the phenothiazine heterocyclic structure improve antiemetic activity. Halogenation (prochlorperazine, perphenazine) or thiethylation (thiethylperazine) of position 2 (R1), in combination with the attachment of a piperazine sidechain at the 10 position (R2), enhances antiemetic (as well as extrapyramidal) activity. The phenothiazines also have varying amounts of anticholinergic and antihistaminic activity that may inhibit the vestibular pathway and the vomiting center of the brain (4).

Adverse effects of the phenothiazines include orthostatic hypotension and excessive sedation, which may limit use in ambulatory patients. Extrapyramidal effects occur most frequently with perphenazine, but they are readily controlled with diphenhydramine or benztropine. Other adverse effects of the phenothiazines, such as cholestatic jaundice and blood dyscrasias, are potential complications, but they rarely occur because of the intermittent and short-term use of these agents as antiemetics. The phenothiazines can be given orally, parenterally, or rectally. The latter routes are useful when vomiting precludes the oral route.

Phenothrazines are primarily used as antiemetics for treatment of mild to moderate nausea and vomiting associated with anesthesia and surgery, radiation therapy, and anticancer chemotherapy. Prochlorperazine is the phenothiazine most widely used and studied as an antiemetic. Onset of action is 10 to 20 min for I.M. administration, 30 to 40 min for oral tablet administration, and 60 min for rectal suppository administration. The duration of action is 3 to 4 hr, irrespective of the route. Prochlorperazine has routinely been administered in a dose of 10 mg every 4 to 6 hours, orally or intramuscularly, to provide optimal antiemetic efficacy. In these dosages, comparative studies in cancer chemotherapy patients indicate that it is more effective than placebo, equivalent in potency to low-dose metoclopramide and droperidol, and less effective than tetrahydrocannabinol (THC), high-dose metoclopramide, and nabilone (4). Recent studies have demonstrated significantly improved antiemetic activity when doses of 30 to 40 mg of prochlorperazine are administered by slow IV infusion. No substantial increase in adverse effects occurs if diphenhydramine is administered prophylactically to prevent extrapyramidal reactions (5–7).

BUTYROPHENONES

The butyrophenones, like the phenothiazines, are dopamine antagonists and are effective antiemetic agents with similar uses and side effects. The main side effect is sedation, although extrapyramidal side effects do occur. The butyrophenones are less likely to produce hypotension than the phenothiazines. Haloperidol is the most widely used antiemetic of this class. It is usually given in doses of 1 to 3 mg orally or intramuscularly every 3 hours. Oral bioavailability is 60%. Peak plasma concentrations occur within 2 to 6 hr. Haloperidol appears to undergo first-pass metabolism and enterohepatic recirculation. Following i.m. administration, peak plasma concentrations occur within 10 to 20 min, with peak pharmacologic action in 30 to 45 min. Droperidol is also an effective antiemetic for use in cytotoxic therapy and in surgery, but is for parenteral administration only. The onset of pharmacologic action of droperidol occurs within 3 to 10 min, but peak pharmacologic effects may not be apparent until 30 min. Duration of action is 2 to 4 hr, but sedative and tranquilizing effects may persist for up to 12 hr after a single dose.

METOCLOPRAMIDE

Metoclopramide is an antagonist of both dopamine and 5-HT$_3$ receptors, protecting against the emetic effects of dopamine and serotonin agonists. The action of metoclopramide is more selective than that of the phenothiazines in that it shows neuroleptic activity only at very high doses. Through a peripheral action, possibly as a partial agonist of enteric postsynaptic neurones (8), metoclopramide also increases the motility of the stomach and small intestine and relaxes the pyloric sphincter, increasing the activity of the upper regions of the gastrointestinal (GI) tract. The antidopaminergic and antiserotonergic effects of metoclopramide on the gut complement the central antiemetic effect and are particularly useful in treating nausea and vomiting associated with GI cancer, gastritis, peptic ulcer, radiation sickness, and migraine. It must not be used in patients with intestinal obstructions who are at high risk for colonic rupture. It appears to be of little value in the treatment of motion sickness, although it has been widely used for this purpose in Europe.

Early clinical trials of metoclopramide at doses of 0.1 to 0.3 mg/kg showed only minimal antiemetic effect against a variety of antineoplastic agents. In 1981, after extensive animal testing, a phase 1 trial investigating the use of "high-dose" (1 to 3 mg/kg) metoclopramide gave very encouraging results (9).

There are no major differences in the pharmacokinetics of conventional- and high-dose metoclopramide (10). Oral doses are rapidly absorbed, but variable first-pass metabolism provides an oral bioavailability of 32 to 100% (11). Peak levels occur in about 1 hr. High lipophilicity results in a large volume of distribution (2.8 to 4.5 liter/kg). Approximately 85% of an orally administered dose appears in the urine within 72 hr. Of the 85% eliminated in the urine, about half is present as free or conjugated metoclopramide. The terminal half-life is 4.5 to 8.8 hr. One study indicates substantial pharmacokinetic variability between patients with various cancers. The authors attribute this variability primarily to differences in body weight and serum alkaline phosphatase levels (12). Although an early study indicated that serum levels >800 ng/ml were necessary to achieve maximum protection against cisplatin-induced emesis, more recent trials have failed to show that serum metoclopramide concentrations predict antiemetic response or adverse effects.

Several controlled and uncontrolled studies have investigated routes of administration for optimal antiemetic therapy, ease and expense of administration, and frequency of adverse effects. Although optimal doses and time schedules have not been completely delineated, the studies indicate that oral, continuous IV, and intermittent IV administration routes provide comparable antiemetic activity against a variety of chemotherapeutic agents. Oral therapy tends to be associated with a greater frequency of loose stools, and scheduled dosing may be difficult if vomiting occurs. Rectal administration shows significant variation in the bioavailability of extemporaneously compounded suppositories (30 to 86%), but is successful in reducing the frequency of emesis, as described in a case report of one patient (13). Other points such as legal aspects of compounding, formulation stability, and cost must also be considered (14).

Adverse effects associated with metoclopramide therapy include diarrhea, sedation, dizziness, and extrapyramidal symptoms. Diarrhea occurs in about 50% of patients receiving high-dose metoclopramide and cisplatin, but this may be related to cisplatin therapy. Mild sedation is observed in most patients who receive higher doses. The extrapyramidal symptoms include akathisia, restlessness, and dystonic reactions (including torticolis, oculogyric crisis, parkinson-like symptoms). The overall frequency is 3 to 5%, but as many as 30% of young men under the age of 30 years may suffer from extrapyramidal effects. Extrapyramidal symptoms are reversed within 5 min with intravenous diphenhydramine. Many cancer chemotherapy protocols now include both high-dose metoclopramide and routine doses of diphenhydramine when highly emetogenic cytotoxic agents are used. (See "Chemotherapy-induced Emesis").

Serotonin Antagonists

A relatively new group of compounds known as the serotonin (5-HT$_3$) receptor antagonists are currently under investigation as antiemetic agents. Cisplatin is known to induce an increase in 5-HT in the small intestine of the ferret, the standard animal model for cisplatin-induced emesis. The serotonin antagonist, ondansetron, has been shown to actively control nausea and vomiting associated with cisplatin and several other emetogenic chemotherapeutic agents in both animals and humans. Comparative studies between ondansetron and metoclopramide concluded that ondansetron is more effective than metoclopramide in the control of high-dose cisplatin-induced nausea and vomiting (15, 16). Side effects include mild-to-moderate diarrhea, headache, and sedation, lightheadedness, and dry mouth. A particular advantage to this group of compounds is that there is no dopaminergic blockade, and thus no extrapyramidal adverse effects have been reported (15).

Early pharmacokinetic studies of ondansetron in adult cancer patients report a mean elimination half-life of 4 hr. Pediatric cancer patients younger than 15 years exhibited a mean half-life of 2.4 hr. A reduction in clearance and an increase in elimination half-life was seen in patients over 75 years of age, but the number of patients was too small to allow a recommendation of dosage adjustment in the elderly. Ondansetron is extensively metabolized, with only 5% recovered in the urine as unchanged drug. The primary metabolic pathway is hydroxylation on the indole ring followed by glucuronide or sulfate conjugation. In vitro measurement of plasma protein binding of ondansetron is 70 to 76% (17).

Antimuscarinic Drugs

Antimuscarinic drugs include muscarinic antagonists such as scopolamine and antihistamines of the H$_1$-antagonist type. These drugs are used in the treatment of motion sickness, and in the case of the antihistamines, for treating nausea and vomiting associated with pregnancy. The antiemetic effects of the antihistamines are due to their anticholinergic activity and not to the blocking of histamine receptors (18). Motion sickness is believed to be mediated by an excess of acetylcholine in the medulla in the region of the VC and CTZ; The antimuscarinic antiemetics probably block acetylcholine in this central region and not peripherally.

In spite of the very extensive literature on anti-motion-sickness drug testing, there is a distinct lack of basic clinical pharmacology such as dose-response relationships and pharmacokinetic parameters. The most commonly used antimuscarinic antiemetic drugs include scopolamine (hyoscine) and the antihistamines promethazine, diphenhydramine, cyclizine, and meclizine. The choice of drug depends on the period for which antinausea protection is required and the side effects. Clinical studies indicate that scopolamine (0.2 to 0.6 mg) is the drug of choice for short periods of motion, and an antihistamine for longer periods (1). Of the antihistamines, promethazine (25 mg) is the drug of choice (18). Higher doses act longer, but usually sedation is a problem. Cyclizine (50 mg) has fewer side effects than promethazine but has a shorter duration of action and is less effective for severe conditions. Meclizine (50 mg) is similar to cyclizine, and both drugs are used when nausea is mild and protection is required for short periods. Diphenhydramine has a long duration, but excessive sedation is usually a problem. For very severe conditions, sympathomimetic drugs such as ephedrine are used in combination with scopolamine or antihistamines.

The transdermal delivery system for administering scopolamine ("scopolamine patch") has produced good results (19). The device, a 2-mm thick patch with a surface area of 2.5 cm^2, contains 1.5 mg of scopolamine. Part of the dose is contained in the hypoallergenic contact adhesive and is released immediately to saturate skin binding sites and to initiate absorption. The remainder of the dose is contained in a reservoir separated from the contact surface by a membrane that releases the drug at a constant rate of about 5 μg/hr for a period of approximately 66 hr. The patch is backed by a water-resistant layer. The manufacturers recommend that the patch be applied to the postauricular skin (the most permeable skin in the body) 4 to 6 hr before expecting motion.

About 40% of people using transdermal scopolamine complain of dryness of the mouth, although this is not a contraindication. Blurred vision is experienced by about 12% of users and is probably due in some cases to transfer of the drug to the eyes by the fingers. Potential users should be advised to try the patches before using them in a travel situation and to wash their hands after applying the patch. The patches should not be used in the young (certainly not in those under 10 years), in pregnancy, in patients with glaucoma or a family history of glaucoma, and in those with a psychosis.

Corticosteroids

A variety of studies have shown that dexamethasone, and to a lesser extent, methylprednisolone, can be effective antiemetics as single agents or in combination with other antiemetics. The mechanism of action by which the corticosteroids act as antiemetics is unknown, but it is suggested that the drugs act by inhibiting prostaglandin synthesis in the hypothalamus. Other actions of the corticosteroids such as mood elevation, increased appetite, and a sense of well-being may be responsible for patient acceptance and positive outcomes (20).

The antiemetic effects of dexamethasone are comparable to those of high-dose metoclopramide (1 to 2 mg/kg) in controlling nausea and vomiting associated with low-dose cisplatin (<60 mg/m^2) and standard doses of moderately emetogenic agents. However metoclopramide appears to be more effective than dexamethasone against high-dose cisplatin (120 mg/m^2) and other highly emetogenic cancer chemotherapy agents. Dexamethasone also appears to be more effective against emesis induced by moderately emetogenic agents than standard doses of oral prochlorperazine (10 mg) (20). More recent studies also indicate that the overall antiemetic activity can be improved when dexamethasone is added to metoclopramide and prochlorperazine therapy. A single dose of dexamethasone administered with metoclopramide shortly before administration of chemotherapy significantly reduces the frequency of emesis (21).

Although few studies have been completed, methylprednisolone may be useful as a single antiemetic agent during chemotherapy with mild-to-moderately emetogenic agents, but it is not recommended as a single-agent antiemetic with highly emetogenic agents such as cisplatin (20). Further trials are needed to establish the optimal regimens for use with the various antineoplastic agents and the advantages of combining corticosteroids with other antiemetics.

The other advantage of the steroids is their relative lack of side effects. Lethargy, weakness, euphoria, a sense of well-being, insomnia, increased appetite, and generalized swelling are more common side effects of corticosteroids used for short-course antiemetic therapy. Other (rare) effects include headache, metallic taste, abdominal discomfort, itchy throat, and a swollen feeling in the mouth (20). Adverse effects associated with the long-term use of corticosteroids are not applicable in this setting. Dexamethasone is also reported to decrease significantly the incidence of diarrhea and sedation associated with metoclopramide therapy (21).

Cannabinoids

Following numerous reports that smoking marijuana reduced nausea, the antiemetic properties of the active ingredients, Δ-8- and 9-tetrahydrocannabinol (THC), and synthetic analog such as nabilone and levonantradol have been studied extensively. Proposed mechanisms of action are that the cannabinoids act in the cerebral cortex to inhibit pathways to the vomiting center, exert an anticholinergic effect on cholinergic terminals in Auerbach's plexus, and possibly mediate the prostaglandin cyclic nucleotide system (22). Other studies indicate no dopaminergic antagonist activity (23).

Pharmacokinetic studies of THC show that absorption from the gastrointestinal tract is slow and erratic with bioavailability below 10%, although this may depend upon the formulation. THC is highly protein bound (97%). Peak plasma concentrations are attained in about 1 hr after oral administration, with serum levels in the 5 to 10 ng/ml range producing antiemetic activity. Higher serum levels are associated with greater antiemetic effect, but with substantially more adverse effects. The terminal half-life of THC is 20 to 30 hr, but other active metabolites require 1 to 2 days for elimination. Patients report a correlation with the peak serum concentrations and a "euphoric high." The "high" following oral administration usually begins 30 to 60 min after ingestion, peaks in 1 to 3 hr, and lasts for 4 to 6 hr. Smoking THC cigarettes raises bioavailability (about 20%), with onset of action in 6 to 12 min. Peak levels are attained in 30 to 120 min with a duration of 3 to 4 hr. Normal behavior is observed 24 hr after administration (22, 23).

THC has been shown to be more effective than placebo and equally as effective as prochlorperazine in patients receiving moderately emetogenic chemotherapy. It is less effective than metoclopramide and is associated with more side effects when used to prevent emesis secondary to cisplatin therapy. Most common adverse effects associated with THC therapy include dry mouth, sedation, orthostatic hypotension, dizziness, and confusion. Dysphoric effects such as depressed mood, dreaming or fantasizing, distortion of perception, and elated mood are more frequent with dosages >5 mg/m². Younger patients appear to tolerate these side effects better than older patients or patients who have not used marijuana (24).

Nabilone is rapidly and well absorbed orally (96%), with an elimination half-life of about 2 hr. Studies indicate that nabilone is more effective than placebo and prochlorperazine against moderately emetogenic chemotherapeutic agents. It is not as effective as metoclopramide with vomiting associated with cisplatin therapy. Nabilone has been reported to have fewer euphoric effects than THC (25).

Because of the mind-altering effects of the cannabinoids and the potential for abuse, these agents will probably serve as antiemetics only in patients receiving chemotherapy. The cannabinoids are of more use in those younger patients who are refractory to other antiemetic regimens and in whom combination therapy may be more effective.

Benzodiazepines

The benzodiazepines, diazepam, lorazepam, and midazolam, are quite effective in reducing not only the frequency of nausea and vomiting but also the anxiety often associated with chemotherapy (26, 27). This action is probably due to a combination of effects, including sedation, reduction in anxiety, possible depression of the VC, and an amnesic effect. Of these, the amnesic effect appears to be the most important as far as treating cancer patients is concerned, and in this respect, lorazepam and midazolam are superior to diazepam. The sedative and amnesic effects are dose-related, with higher doses (≥4 mg) of lorazepam inducing amnesic effects that persist longer and occur in a larger percentage of patients. Amnesia does not correlate well with sedation, since sedation may remain high, while the amnesic effects decline.

Following IV administration of either lorazepam or midazolam, the onset of sedative, anxiolytic, and amnesic action usually occurs within 1 to 5 min. The duration of action following IV administration of midazolam is usually less than 2 hr, however dose-dependent actions may persist for up to 6 hr in some patients. After i.m. administration, the onset of action of lorazepam is 15 to 30 min, and the duration of action is 12 to 24 hr. Following i.m. administration of midazolam, onset of action occurs within 5 to 15 min, but may not peak for 20 to 60 min; the duration of action is about 2 hr, although the range is 1 to 6 hr. The onset of action of orally administered lorazepam is about 30 min, with peak activity occurring within 2 hr. The duration of action is 4 to 6 hr. The elimination half-life of lorazepam is 10 to 20 hr, with no active metabolites, whereas that of midazolam is 1 to 12 hr, with active metabolites.

Clinically, midazolam and lorazepam are most useful in combination with other antiemetics such as metoclopramide and dexamethasone. The anxiolytic and amnesic effects result in marked subjective support by patients (28). The greatest benefit from benzodiazepine therapy is derived by patients without prior chemotherapy who have not developed negative conditioning from episodes of nausea and vomiting (see "Anticipatory Nausea and Vomiting). Side effects associated with benzodiazepine therapy are drowsiness and dizziness. Patients should not be left unattended in the sedated, amnesic state, since vomiting episodes may still occur. Because of its short half-life and short duration of action, midazolam may be an appropriate adjunctive antiemetic for outpatient use.

PATIENT ASSESSMENT AND MANAGEMENT

An accurate diagnosis is essential before beginning treatment for nausea and vomiting, because symptomatic therapy may be contraindicated (e.g. in gastrointestinal obstruction, acute appendicitis, or cerebral edema) or the underlying disease may be serious and require specific measures. The causes of vomiting should be kept in mind (Table 23-1) when deciding on the treatment plan.

The appearance, frequency, and timing of nausea and vomiting, together with associated specific and nonspecific symptoms such as jaundice, diarrhea, weight loss, pain, and fever are important in making a diagnosis. Blood in the vomitus, an important sign, can be fresh or altered, in which case it has the appearance of coffee grounds. Bile in the vomitus gives it a green or yellow color and suggests that the pyloric sphincter is open, allowing reflux of duodenal contents into the stomach.

The cause of vomiting is usually obvious (e.g., pregnancy, motion, or the use of certain drugs), but in some cases diagnosis can be difficult, especially if psychogenic factors are involved. With unexplained vomiting, the first step in assessment is elimination of the possibility of upper GI tract lesions or systemic conditions such as meningitis or uremia. The patient should also be assessed for the need to treat the sequelae of prolonged vomiting, such as fluid and electrolyte depletion.

Chronic vomiting, with or without weight loss, can be psychogenic. This is suggested when the vomiting has been occurring for some time (especially if the patient has delayed seeking help), when there is a family history of vomiting, or when the patient can suppress vomiting or vomits rarely in a public place.

The principles involved in treating vomiting are

1. Treat the cause if this can be identified.
2. Treat fluid and electrolyte loss. In most cases this involves giving adequate fluids orally, particularly those containing glucose. If fluid loss leads to metabolic disturbances, the patient should be hospitalized and given appropriate intravenous fluids.

3. Give appropriate symptomatic drug treatment, after considering contraindications and adverse drug reactions. The choice of drug and dose must be individualized.
4. For unexplained vomiting, continue diagnostic examinations (29).

The features of vomiting-induced metabolic disturbances include

1. Dehydration, suggested by oliguria, weight loss, mental confusion, and reduced tissue turgor;
2. Sodium depletion, suggested by thirst and hypotension;
3. Potassium depletion, suggested by muscle weakness;
4. Alkalosis, which can occur as a result of loss of hydrogen ions in the vomitus and the concentration of extracellular fluid secondary to fluid loss.

Sodium and potassium depletion occur mainly because of loss in vomitus but also as a consequence of other metabolic disturbances.

TREATMENT OF SELECTED CAUSES OF NAUSEA AND VOMITING
Chemotherapy-induced Emesis

Chemotherapy-induced emesis (CIE) is the most unpleasant adverse effect associated with the use of antineoplastic agents. Many patients regard it as the most stressful aspect of their disease, more so than the prospect of dying. Since the object of therapy in many cases is to prolong life for a relatively short period, the effect of CIE on the quality of life must be considered. Many patients whose prognosis is good find it difficult to comply and may request that therapy be discontinued because of CIE. In one multicenter survey, between 1 and 10% of patients refused to continue with chemotherapy because of nausea and vomiting (30).

Three types of emesis have been identified in patients receiving chemotherapy: (a) anticipatory nausea and vomiting; (b) acute chemotherapy-induced emesis; and (c) delayed emesis. Patients may have emesis for reasons other than chemotherapy, perhaps induced by medications such as analgesics or by tumor-related complications such as intestinal obstruction. Addressing these matters is usually more important than selection of antiemetic therapy (31). Apart from distressing the patient, severe vomiting complicates the patient's medical condition, causing dehydration, metabolic alkalosis, electrolyte deficiencies, nutritional impairment including cachexia, and physical injury including esophageal tears and bone fractures.

ANTICIPATORY NAUSEA AND VOMITING

The patient's fear of CIE may lead to anticipatory nausea and/or vomiting (ANV). Anticipatory nausea alone has been reported in up to 44% of patients and anticipatory vomiting in up to 38% (32). ANV correlates with the emetic potential of chemotherapy regimens and with the severity of nausea and vomiting after chemotherapy. Although considerable interpatient variability is observed, the onset of ANV usually occurs 2 to 4 hr before treatment and is most severe at the time of drug administration (33). Patients who experience ANV are more likely to be younger and to have received about twice as many courses of chemotherapy with more drugs for about three times as long as patients who do not experience ANV (32, 34). It is believed that ANV is a conditioned response triggered by the sight or smell of the clinic or hospital or by the knowledge that treatment is imminent. ANV tends to become more severe as treatments progress unless behavior therapy modifies the conditioned response (35). Such treatments include progressive muscle relaxation, mind diversion, hypnosis, self-hypnosis, and systematic desensitization. People with a negative attitude toward therapy, such as the belief that it will be of no benefit, are more likely to develop ANV than those with a positive attitude. Complications associated with ANV underscore the need for accompanying the initial course of emesis-producing chemotherapy with the most effective antiemetic regimen, and continuing vigorous therapy with each subsequent cycle of chemotherapy (31). Addition of lorazepam to antiemetic regimens induces an amnesic effect about chemotherapy and emesis in some patients (36) and has received more subjective support from patients (37). If delayed emesis is associated with any of the agents in the chemotherapeutic regimen, effective antiemetic therapy should be continued long enough to reduce the frequency of nausea and emesis, thus minimizing the risk of preconditioning the patient against further chemotherapy and ANV.

ACUTE CHEMOTHERAPY-INDUCED EMESIS

The choice of antiemetic therapy for patients receiving antineoplastic therapy should take into account both patient and drug factors.

Patient Factors. The incidence and severity of CIE are generally greater among people of advanced age, those in poor general health (especially if cachexic), and those with metabolic disturbances (i.e., dehydration, uremia, gastrointestinal tract obstruction, or infection). Age can influence the response to antiemetic drugs. For example, patients under the age of 30 are more sensitive to the extrapyramidal effects of dopaminergic blockade from phenothiazines or high-dose metoclopramide than are older patients. On the other hand, younger patients tolerate cannabinoids better than older people. Patients with a history of chronic heavy alcohol use (more than five mixed drinks per day) tolerate chemotherapy with fewer bouts of emesis than those without this history (31). Patients prone to motion sickness seem to be more sensitive to the emetic effects of cytotoxic agents. Since these two types of emesis have different mechanisms, this correlation probably reflects a psychogenic component. Finally, the patient's mental out-

Table 23.2.
Relative Emetic Activity of Chemotherapeutic Agents[a]

Agent	Emetic Time Course (hr)	
	Onset	Duration
Very high emetic incidence (90%)		
Cisplatin	1–6	24–120
Dacarbazine	1–3	1–12
Streptozocin	1–4	12–24
Mustine	½–2	8–24
High emetic incidence (60–90%)		
BCNU (carmustine)	2–4	4–24
Cyclophosphamide (prop. to dose)	4–12	4–10
Mithramycin	2–6	4–6
Procarbazine (prop. to dose)	24–27	variable
Moderate emetic incidence (30–60%)		
Daunorubicin	2–6	24
Adriamycin	4–6	—
5-Fluorouracil	3–6	—
Low emetic incidence (10–30%)		
Bleomycin	3–6	—
Cytarabine	6–12	3–5
Etoposide	3–8	—
Methotrexate	4–12	3–12
6-Mercaptopurine	4–8	—
Vinblastine (prop. to dose)	4–8	—
Tamoxifen	12–24	—
Very low emetic incidence (10%)		
Chlorambucil	48–72	—
Corticosteroids	4–8	—

[a] Adapted from Borison HL, McCarthy LE: Neuropharmacology of chemotherapy-induced emesis. Drugs 25(suppl 1):8–17, 1983.

look and attitude to therapy can influence the frequency and severity of emetic reactions considerably.

Drug Factors. The emetogenic potential of antineoplastic drugs varies greatly, ranging from a rate of 90% or more in the case of cisplatin to 10% or less with chlorambucil. Table 23.2 classifies chemotherapeutic agents in terms of emetogenicity, although emetogenicity is also influenced by the dose, duration, and frequency of administration. The effects of combinations of chemotherapeutic agents on vomiting are poorly understood.

The extensive literature on the testing of antiemetics for use with antineoplastic agents is often difficult to interpret. Comparisons between trials are difficult because of differences in protocol, cytoxic drugs, and patient characteristics (26, 39). Some studies rely entirely on objective data (i.e., the frequency of vomiting and the volume of vomitus) without investigating patient attitudes, performance capabilities, or quality-of-life issues. A patient who vomits only occasionally but experiences nausea continually may have a poorer quality of life than someone who vomits more frequently but with little intervening nausea.

However, it is clear that major progress has occurred in treating CIE (40), and some general recommendations

can be made. All patients being treated with chemotherapeutic agents of moderate to very high emetogenic potential (Table 23.2) should receive prophylactic antiemetic therapy before antineoplastic therapy is initiated. Combinations of high-dose metoclopramide, ondansetron, dexamethasone, lorazepam, and/or diphenhydramine are the drugs of choice in treating cisplatin-induced emesis (31, 41, 42). Haloperidol may be substituted for metoclopramide if it is not tolerated by the patient (31). Antiemetic therapy should be continued for 4 to 7 days to prevent delayed vomiting. Emesis induced by moderately emetogenic agents such as methotrexate and 5-fluorouracil may be treated prophylactically with metoclopramide and dexamethasone, and therapy should be continued for 24 hr (43). A phenothiazine (prochlorperazine) or dexamethasone alone is recommended if the chemotherapy is of low emetic potential. An alternative for this group is a cannabinoid plus a phenothiazine to ameliorate central nervous system side effects (43). The rationale for using combinations of antiemetic agents is based on the assumption that cytotoxic agents produce emesis by multiple mechanisms. Antiemetics also act by multiple mechanisms, and a combination could have a synergistic action. Side effects are also a factor in the choice of an antiemetic, and combinations of drugs acting by different mechanisms are less likely to produce adverse reactions than the highest dose of a single drug. In some cases a second antiemetic agent may reduce the side effects of the first drug (e.g., dexamethasone, diphenhydramine, or lorazepam added to high-dose metoclopramide). All antiemetics should be administered an adequate time before chemotherapy is initiated and should be continued through the characteristic time associated with vomiting for a particular chemotherapeutic agent (Table 23.2). Doses, efficacies, and adverse effects of some antiemetic drugs are given in Table 23.3. Therapy must be individualized, and the doses and treatment schedules given are meant as guidelines only. All antiemetics except antimuscarinics (anticholinergics and antihistamines) have been found useful in the treatment of CIE.

DELAYED EMESIS

Delayed emesis is a distinct syndrome that occurs 24 hr or more after the administration of chemotherapy. It has been reported in as many as 93% of patients receiving high-dose cisplatin. Symptoms may occur 24 to 120 hr after cisplatin administration, but they are most severe at 48 to 72 hr. Delayed nausea and vomiting is usually less severe than that which occurs acutely, but it can still be of importance in reducing activity, nutrition, and hydration. The causes of delayed nausea and vomiting are not known. Symptoms may be caused directly by the action of chemotherapeutic agents or their metabolites on the nervous system or gastrointestinal tract (44). Episodes of delayed

Table 23.3.
Efficacy, Dose, and Toxicity of Antiemetics Used in the Treatment of Cytotoxic-induced Emesis (CIE)

Drug	Antiemetic Activity[a]	Dosage Range (Doses Must Be Individualized)[b]	Adverse Effects[c]
Phenothiazines			
Prochlorperazine	+ +	5–10 mg q. 2–4 hr p.o.; 5–10 mg q. 3–6 hr i.m./IV[d]; 25 mg p.r. q. 6 hr	+/+ +
Chlorpromazine	+ +	25–50 mg q. 3–6 hr p.o. 25 mg q. 4–6 hr p.o./i.m./IV[d]/p.r.	+/+ +
Thiethylperazine	+ +	10 mg q. 8 hr p.o./i.m./p.r.	+/+ +
Butyrophenones			
Droperidol	+ +	1–3 mg q. 4–6 hr i.v. or 5 mg i.v. 30 min prior to chemotherapy then continuous infusion of 1–1.5 mg/hr for 9–12 hr	+/+ +
Haloperidol	+ +	1–3 mg q. 4–6 hr p.o./i.m./IV[d]	+/+ +
Metoclopramide			
High-dose	+ + +	1–3 mg/kg IVPB over 15 min 0.5 hr before and q. 2 hr × 3–4 doses after chemotherapy	+ +
Low-dose	0/+	0.1–0.3 mg/kg q. 4 hr p.o./i.m./IV	+
Corticosteroids			
Dexamethasone	+ + +	4–25 mg p.o./i.v. before chemotherapy and q. 4–6 hr × 1–2 days	0/+
Methylprednisolone	+ + +	125–500 mg p.o./i.v. 2 hr before chemotherapy and 2 hr after or as infusion	0/+
Benzodiazepines			
Lorazepam	+ +/+ + +	1–4 mg q. 4–6 hr p.o./IV; can commence when patient arrives for chemotherapy	+/+ +
Cannabinoids			
Δ-9-THC	+ +[e]	5–10 mg/m² q. 4 hr p.o.; commence night before chemotherapy	+ +/+ + +
Serotonin antagonist			
Ondansetron	+ + +	0.15 mg/kg IVPB q. 4 hr × 3 doses. Infuse first dose over 15 min beginning 30 min before start of emetogenic chemotherapy	+ +

[a] Antiemetic activity against cisplatin: 0, little or none, to + + +, high.
[b] Doses are examples only and represent the ranges given in the references cited in the text. Best results are usually obtained with a combination of antiemetics. Frequently dosing is begun before chemotherapy. IVPB = IV piggy-back, p.r. = per rectum.
[c] 0, little or none, to + + +, high incidence.
[d] Can be administered by slow (15–20 min) IV administration.
[e] May have marked efficacy in young patients.

vomiting are frequently associated with provocative events such as brushing teeth, using mouthwash, manipulating dentures, seeing food, and in the morning, standing up after getting out of bed. A combination of prochloperazine 10 mg, lorazepam 0.5 mg, and diphenhydramine 50 mg given orally 1 hr before breakfast, lunch, and dinner has been successful in controlling delayed emesis secondary to cisplatin therapy (45).

Motion Sickness

Motion sickness is a normal, healthy response to exposure to abnormal forms of motion, which occurs in animals as well as in humans. Susceptibility to motion sickness varies greatly, with approximately one-third of persons being very sensitive, one-third reacting to rough conditions only, and one-third reacting to extreme conditions only. While there is no question about the physical basis of motion sickness, psychological factors play an important part in both suppressing and enhancing the tendency to be sick.

Motion sickness usually begins with pallor, yawning, restlessness, and cold sweat, particularly on the brow and upper lip. The person then experiences nausea, which may lead to excessive salivation, vomiting, drowsiness, and depression. If not relieved, severe headache, prostration, and dehydration may develop. In very sensitive individuals these symptoms may progress rapidly; in less sensitive people, symptoms may wax and wane.

The stimuli that produce motion sickness arise in the labyrinth. They are carried by afferent fibers that synapse in the vestibular region of the medulla, where they are thought to stimulate the release of excessive amounts of acetylcholine that acts on the CTZ, which then stimulates the VC (1, 46). A proposed theory suggests that motion sickness arises when there is conflict between the sensory information being transmitted by the eyes, vestibular system, and nonvestibular proprioceptors, particularly as it relates to previous experience. As a result of this conflict, an imbalance of cholinergic and sympathetic transmitters occurs in the medulla, which can be corrected by giving anticholinergic drugs or sympathomimetics. The vestibular system plays the central role, since individuals with a nonfunctional vestibular system are immune to motion sickness.

The importance of conflicting sensory stimuli as a

Table 23.4.
Doses and Duration of Action of Anti-motion-sickness Drugs

Drug	Oral Dose[a]	Duration of Action (hr)	Condition
Scopolamine and dexamphetamine	0.2–0.6 mg scopolamine + 5–10 mg dexamphetamine[b]	6	Severe
Promethazine and ephedrine	25 mg promethazine + 25 mg t.d.s. ephedrine	12	Severe
Scopolamine	0.2–0.6 mg q.q.h.[c]	4	Severe
Promethazine	25 mg t.d.s.	12	Severe
Dimenhydrinate	50 mg 2–3 × daily	6	Moderate
Cyclizine	50 mg 2–3 × daily	4	Mild
Meclizine	50 mg 2–3 × daily	6	Mild

[a] Antimotion drugs are most effective if therapy is commenced before exposure to motion. Usually therapy should be commenced about 30 min before departure and repeated if necessary.

[b] Used only under special circumstances (e.g., by service personnel).

[c] Not more than four doses should be taken in 24 hr.

cause of motion sickness is illustrated in a practical way by the relief obtained when a person can establish a satisfactory visual earth reference. For example, looking out a car window (particularly from the front seat) can give marked relief, whereas reading in a car (particularly in the back seat, can provoke motion sickness.

Tolerance to motion sickness usually develops after a few days of continuous motion of a particular kind (getting one's "sea legs"), which emphasizes the fact that motion sickness is a response to unfamiliar motion. If exposure to an emetogenic stimulus is sufficiently prolonged, motion sickness may be experienced after cessation of the motion—"mal de debarquement." Many people experience motion sickness before commencing a journey.

Drug Therapy For Motion Sickness. In accordance with the theory of motion sickness, drugs used in the treatment of motion sickness include sympathomimetics and anticholinergics (Table 23.4) The choice of drug or drug combination depends on the expected duration and severity of the reaction. For very severe conditions, such as might be experienced by service personnel in a landing craft, combinations of scopolamine and dexamphetamine are the most effective therapy and have the advantage that the stimulatory effects of the dexamphetamine offset the drowsiness caused by the scopolamine. Unfortunately the tendency for dexamphetamine to be abused limits its use. However, combinations of ephedrine and promethazine are also very effective and have been ranked just below the dexamphetamine-scopolamine combination (18). Doses are given in Table 23.4.

Of the single drugs, scopolamine (0.2 to 0.6 mg) is the most effective for short periods of exposure (less than 6

hr). For longer periods or for moderate to mild conditions, antihistamines are the drugs of choice. Of these, promethazine 25 mg appears to be the most effective (18). Transdermal scopolamine can be used successfully for the treatment of motion sickness of several days duration. All anti-motion-sickness drugs are more effective if used prophylactically rather than after sickness has developed.

For persons with severe motion sickness, the oral route is unavailable, and therapy is given by the intramuscular route. Scopolamine (0.2 mg) or promethazine (50 mg) (adult doses) may be given. Promethazine is probably the preferred therapy for acute motion sickness.

In therapeutic doses, all drugs used for the treatment of motion sickness cause side effects. Antimuscarinic drugs produce dry mouth, sedation, and blurred vision, and the sympathomimetics produce tachycardia. In the case of scopolamine, the total dose should not exceed 1 mg in 24 hr because of effects on the central nervous system.

Psychogenic Vomiting

Psychogenic vomiting can be self-induced or occur involuntarily in response to situations that the person considers threatening or distasteful (e.g., eating food whose origin is considered repulsive).

When a person has chronic or recurrent vomiting, a diagnosis of psychogenic vomiting is made after elimination of all other possible causes (Table 23.1). The person with psychogenic vomiting usually does not lose weight and can control vomiting in certain situations (e.g., in public). The identification of the causes of psychogenic vomiting and successful resolution of the problem may not be possible. A short course of an antiemetic drug such as metoclopramide or antianxiety drugs may be prescribed, along with counseling to treat psychogenic vomiting.

CONCLUSION

Nausea and vomiting vary from minor inconveniences of a transient GI infection to severe and limiting adverse reactions to drug therapy. The consequences of vomiting can be severe. The cause of nausea and vomiting should be determined before treatment is begun, and specific therapy should be chosen for each of the causes. Drug regimens specifically designed for the patient and the cause of nausea and vomiting, based on good clinical studies, have a high success rate for the treatment of this disorder. However, care should be taken to minimize any side effects from the antiemetic drugs.

REFERENCES

1. Barnes JH: The physiology and pharmacology of emesis. Mol Aspects Med 7:397–508, 1984.
2. Bermudez J, Boyle EA, Miner WD, et al.: The antiemetic potential of the 5-hydroxytryptamine₃ receptor antagonist BRL 43694. Br J Cancer 58:644–650, 1988.

3. Cubeddu LX, Hoffmann IS, Fuenmayor NT, et al.: Efficacy of on-dansetron (GR38032F) and the role of serotonin in cisplatin-induced nausea and vomiting. N Engl J Med 322:810–816, 1990.

4. Wampler G: Pharmacology and clinical effectiveness of phenothia-zines and related drugs for managing chemotherapy-induced emesis. Drugs 25(S1):35–51, 1983.

5. Carr B, Doroshow J, Blayney D, et al: Toxicity and dose-response studies of prochlorperazine for cisplatin-induced emesis [abstr]. Proc Am Soc Clin Oncol 5:252, 1986.

6. Olver IN, Bishop JF, Hollcoat BL, et al.: A phase-I dose finding study for intravenous prochlorperazine as an antiemetic for chemo-therapy induced emesis [abstr]. Proc Am Soc Clin Oncol 7:287, 1988.

7. Carr BI, Somlo G, McDevitt J, et al.: Pharmacokinetic profiles of high and low dose prochlorperazine [abstr]. Proc Am Soc Clin Oncol 7:294, 1988.

8. Fozard JR: Neuronal 5-HT receptors in the periphery. Neurophar-macology 23:1473–1486, 1984.

9. Gralla RJ: Metoclopramide: a review of antiemetic trials. Drugs 25:63–73, 1983.

10. McGovern EM, Grevel J, Bryson SM: Pharmacokinetics of high-dose metoclopramide in cancer patients. Clin Pharmacokinet 11:415–424, 1986.

11. Bateman DN: Clinical pharmacokinetics of metoclopramide. Clin Pharmacokinet 8:523–529, 1983.

12. Grevel J, Whiting B, Kelman AW, et al: Population analysis of the pharmacokinetic variability of high-dose metoclopramide in cancer patients. Clin Pharmacokinet 14:52–63, 1983.

13. Parrish RH, Bonzo SM: Use of metoclopramide suppositories. Clin Pharm 2:395–396, 1983.

14. Tami JA, Waite WW: Metoclopramide suppository considerations. DICP 22:268–269, 1988.

15. Marty M, Pouillart P, Scholl S: Comparison of the 5-hydroxy-tryptamine₃ (serotonin) antagonist ondansetron (GR38032F) with high-dose metoclopramide in the control of cisplatin-induced emesis. N Engl J Med 322:816–821, 1990.

16. De Mulder PHM, Selynaeve C, Vermorken JB, et al.: Ondansetron compared with high-dose metoclopramide in prophylaxis of acute and delayed cisplatin-induced nausea and vomiting. Ann Intern Med 113:834–840, 1990.

17. Product Information "Zofran". Glaxo Pharmaceuticals, Research Tri-angle Park, NC, January, 1991.

18. Wood CD: Antimotion sickness and antiemetic drugs. Drugs 17:471–479, 1979.

19. Clissold SP, Heel RC: Transdermal hyoscine (scopolamine)—a pre-liminary review of its pharmacodynamic properties and therapeutic efficacy. Drugs 29:189–207, 1985.

20. Cersosimo RJ, Karp DD: Adrenal corticosteroids as antiemetics dur-ing cancer chemotherapy. Pharmacotherapy 6:118–127, 1986.

21. Kris MG, Gralla RJ, Tyson LB, et al.: Improved control of cisplatin-induced emesis with high-dose metoclopramide and with combi-nations of metoclopramide, dexamethasone and diphenhydramine. Cancer 55:527–534, 1985.

22. Vincent BJ, McQuiston DJ, Einhorn LH, et al.: Review of canna-binoids and their antiemetic effectiveness. Drugs 25(S1):52–62, 1983.

23. Anderson PO, McGuire GG: Delta-9-tetrahydrocannabinol as an an-tiemetic. AJHP 38:639–646, 1981.

24. Devine ML, Dow GJ, Greenberg BR, et al.: Adverse reactions to delta-9-tetrahydrocannabinol given as an antiemetic in a multicenter study. Clin Pharm 6:319–322, 1987.

25. Ward A, Holmes B: Nabilone: a preliminary review of its pharma-cological properties and therapeutic use. Drugs 30:127–144, 1985.

26. Kearsley JH, Tattersall MHN: Recent advances in the prevention and reduction of cytotoxic-induced emesis. Med J Aust 143:341–346, 1985.

27. Bishop JF, Olver IN, Wolf MM, et al.: Lorazepam: a randomized double-blind crossover study of a new antiemetic in patients receiving cytotoxic chemotherapy and prochlorperazine. J Clin Oncol 2:691–695, 1984.

28. Kris MG, Gralla RJ, Clark RA, et al.: Consecutive dose-finding trials adding lorazepam to the combination of metoclopramide plus dex-amethasone: improved subjective effectiveness over the combination of diphenhydramine plus metoclopramide plus dexamethasone. Cancer Treat Rep 69:1257–1262, 1985.

29. Malagelada JR, Camilleri M: Unexplained vomiting: a diagnostic challenge. Ann Intern Med 101:211–218, 1984.

30. Penta JS, Poster DS, Bruna S, et al.: Cancer chemotherapy induced nausea and vomiting in adult and pediatric patients. Am Soc Clin Oncol 4:396, 1981.

31. Gralla RJ, Tyson LB, Kris MG, et al.: The management of chemo-therapy-induced nausea and vomiting. Med Clin North Am 70:289–301, 1987.

32. Moher D, Arthur AZ, Pater JL: Anticipatory nausea and/or vomiting. Cancer Treat Rev 11:257–264, 1984.

33. Dolgin MJ, Katz ER, McGinty K, Siegel JSE: Anticipatory nausea and vomiting in pediatric cancer patients. Pediatrics 75:547–552, 1985.

34. Alba E, Roma B, de Andres L, et al.: Anticipatory nausea and vom-iting: prevalence and predictors in chemotherapy patients. Oncology 46:26–30, 1989.

35. Stoudemire A, Cotanch P, Laszlo J: Recent advances in the phar-macologic and behavioral management of chemotherapy-induced emesis. Arch Intern Med 144:1029–1033, 1984.

36. Laszlo J, Clark RA, Hanson DC, et al.: Lorazepam in cancer patients treated with cisplatin: a drug having antiemetic, amnesic and anx-iolytic effects. J Clin Oncol 3:864–869, 1985.

37. Kris MG, Gralla RJ, Clark RA, et al.: Consecutive dose-finding trials adding lorazepam to the combination of metoclopramide plus dex-amethasone: improved subjective effectiveness over the combination of diphenhydramine plus metoclopramide plus dexamethasone. Can-cer Treat Rep 69:1257–1262, 1985.

38. Borison HL, McCarthy LE: Neuropharmacology of chemotherapy-induced emesis. Drugs 25(suppl 1):8–17, 1983.

39. Pater JL, Willian AR: Methodologic issues in trials of antiemetics. J Clin Oncol 2:484–497, 1984.

40. O'Brien MER, Cullen MH: Are we making progress in the man-agement of cytotoxic drug-induced nausea and vomiting? J Clin Pharm Ther 13:19–31, 1988.

41. Smith DB, Newlands ES, Spruyt OW, et al.: Ondansetron (GR380032F) plus dexamethasone: effective antiemetic prophylaxis for patients receiving cytotoxic chemotherapy. Br J Cancer 61:323–324, 1990.

42. Cunningham D, Turner A, Hawthorn J, et al.: Ondansetron with and without dexamethasone to treat chemotherapy-induced emesis. Lan-cet (8650):1323, 1989.

43. Craig JB, Powell BL: Review: The management of nausea and vom-iting in clinical oncology. Am J Med Sci 293:34–44, 1987.

44. Kris MG, Gralla RJ, Clark RA, et al.: Incidence, course, and severity of delayed nausea and vomiting following the administration of high dose cisplatin. J Clin Oncol 3:1379–1384, 1985.

45. Sridhar KS, Donnelly E: Combination antiemetics for cisplatin chemotherapy. Cancer 61:1508–1517, 1988.

46. Reason JT, Brand JJ: Motion Sickness. New York: Academic Press, 1975.

CHAPTER 24

DIARRHEA AND CONSTIPATION

VALERIE W. HOGUE, Pharm.D.

Constipation and diarrhea are common disorders of the gastrointestinal system experienced by most of the population sometime in their lives. Generally, these symptoms are self-limiting and may not require any intervention. However, intervention may be considered necessary by patients because of their beliefs and attitude toward normal bowel function. Constipation and diarrhea can affect the ability to carry out work or school responsibilities and loss of productivity usually necessitates prompt and effective intervention.

Symptoms of diarrhea and constipation may result from various diseases, medications, dietary changes, food or water contamination, and even psychological distress. Many over-the-counter (OTC) products are available in the United States for resolving the symptoms. The pharmacist's consultation is important for proper use of these products for self-treatment. The pharmacist must ascertain the possible cause of these symptoms in an effort to prevent masking a serious medical problem and to deter laxative and antidiarrheal abuse.

The financial impact of constipation and diarrhea in the United States is significant. In 1989, $619 million dollars was spent on antacids and digestive aids, primarily antidiarrheals and laxatives. It is expected that by 1994 this figure will increase to $2 billion (1). One factor contributing to the increased use is the rise in patient self-treatment with OTC products. A recent survey of consumer OTC use trends revealed that of 1356 household respondents, 26% used products for constipation and 28% used products for diarrhea over a 6-month period (2). Women and persons over the age of 60 years used nonprescription laxatives more often. No correlation was observed with these two populations and the use of antidiarrheals.

The decision to self-medicate for constipation or diarrhea depends largely upon the individual's perception of "abnormal" bowel habits. In a survey of public perceptions of digestive health and disease, researchers found that 62% of American respondents believed that a bowel movement each day is necessary for good digestive health (3). This idea may have been influenced by the theory of "autointoxication," which stated that noxious substances in the colon increase cellular degeneration and promote the aging process (4). While this theory is obsolete, the belief appears to be common among the elderly, whose concern for regularity of bowel movements is shown by their frequent use and abuse of laxatives.

Normal bowel habits may range between 3 and 21 stools per week (5). This demonstrates a wide variation of bowel habits among healthy individuals. Recently, results were published from a national, population-based survey that evaluated the prevalence of self-reported constipation, diarrhea, and defecation frequency in the United States (6). Respondents ranged in age from 25 to 74 years. The majority of the respondents reported daily defecation (73.3% whites; 63.7% blacks). The frequency of defecation differed significantly with regard to race and gender, but not age. Regardless of gender or race, self-reported constipation was positively correlated with age. This difference may reflect a difference in the perception of constipation by older persons, since the frequency of defecation did not change as age progressed.

DEFINITION

The definitions of diarrhea and constipation have been debated for several years, primarily because of variations in the definition of normal bowel habits. Most clinicians will agree that a single definition does not describe either medical problem effectively.

Clinicians generally incorporate two primary aspects in the definition of constipation: (a) difficulty passing stools and (b) infrequent stools. However, patients may describe constipation as less frequent defecation than is normally observed, lower stool volume, difficulty passing stool, hard or firm stool, straining upon defecation, a sensation of incomplete evacuation of the bowel, or the lack of an urge to stool. A study of young adults not seeking healthcare asked 568 subjects to define constipation. They emphasized function (straining) and consistency (hard stools) rather than the number of stools in their definition (7). Therefore, determining the patient's definition before management is essential.

Diarrhea has been defined with more consistency than constipation. Generally, it is defined as three or more loose or unformed bowel movements per day accompanied by symptoms of fever, abdominal cramps, or vomiting. It has been further described as a condition of abnormal increases in stool weight and liquidity. An increase in stool water excretion above 150 to 200 ml every 24 hr is an objective parameter for acute diarrhea (8).

NORMAL INTESTINAL PHYSIOLOGY

Understanding the normal physiologic flow rate of fluid and electrolytes and a knowledge of the process of defecation provide the basis for discussing the development of constipation and diarrhea. Three major aspects of bowel function exist: colonic absorption, colonic motility, and defecation reflexes.

The daily volume of fluid transversing the duodenum is 9 liters for persons consuming three meals daily. Approximately 8 liters per day are absorbed by the small bowel, of which 1 to 1.5 liters are presented to the colon. The colon absorbs 0.9 to 1.4 liters per day, which is 90% of the fluid presented initially. The absorptive capacity of the colon exceeds that of the small intestine, which absorbs only 75% of the fluid presented initially. Daily fecal output is less than 200 ml, which contains approximately 5 mEq of sodium and 8 mEq of potassium.

Colonic motility involves three patterns of muscle contractions controlled by the autonomic nervous system: (a) nonpropulsive segmental contractions, which churn the contents of the lumen; (b) short segmental propulsive contractions, which move contents forward and backward, promoting absorption; and (c) long-segment propulsive contractions, which move contents forward over long distances. The urge to defecate occurs when gastric filling and increased physical activity trigger the gastroenteric reflex to produce massive peristalsis. The feces move from the sigmoid colon to the rectum, producing a sensation to defecate. This occurs most often after breakfast (4).

Defecation is initiated via the distension of the rectum by feces. Normally, the rectum can differentiate distension produced by fluids, flatus, and feces, through defecation reflexes. Evacuation occurs after relaxation of the internal and external anal sphincters in conjunction with the contraction of the rectosigmoid segment and increased intraabdominal pressure. Voluntary relaxation of the external anal sphincter allows evacuation of the bowel. Conversely, voluntary contraction of the sphincter inhibits defecation.

ETIOLOGY

Constipation may be secondary to underlying disorders or idiopathic (Table 24.1). Diseases producing constipation may be systemic or be localized to the gastrointestinal tract. Drugs may cause constipation, including the chronic use of laxatives (Table 24.2). In addition, psychological factors may cause changes in bowel habits leading to constipation (e.g., irritable bowel syndrome).

Diarrhea may be caused primarily by inhibition of ion absorption, stimulation of ion secretion, retention of fluid in the intestinal lumen, and disorders of intestinal motility. Retention of fluid in the bowel lumen may be precipitated by carbohydrate malabsorption, disaccharidase deficiencies, lactulose therapy, poorly absorbable salts (magnesium sulfate, sodium phosphate, sodium citrate, antacids), and ingestion of mannitol and sorbitol. Secretagogues from tumors, such as vasoactive intestinal polypeptide (VIP), serotonin, and calcitonin, may mediate secretory diarrhea.

Table 24.1.
Medical Problems Associated with Constipation

Endocrine/metabolic disorders
  Amyloidosis
  Diabetes mellitus
  Hyperparathyroidism
  Hypothyroidism
  Hypokalemia
  Hypercalcemia
  Porphyria
  Pseudohypoparathyroidism
  Uremia
Gastrointestinal disorders
  Anorectal disorders (anal fissures, hemorrhoids)
  Carcinoma of colon or rectum
  Colonic pseudoobstruction
  Cystocele, rectocele
  Diverticular disease
  Hirschsprung's disease
  Hypomotility disorders
  Inflammatory bowel disease
  Irritable bowel syndrome
  Ischemic bowel disease
  Rectal prolapse
Neurologic disorders
  Autonomic neuropathy
  Cerebrovascular accidents
  Cauda equina tumor
  Chagas' disease
  Multiple sclerosis
  Parkinson's disease
Psychiatric disorders
  Anxiety
  Depression
  Psychosis

Table 24.2.
Drug-induced Constipation

Antacids (e.g., calcium- and aluminum-containing)
Anticholinergics
Barium sulfate
Bismuth
Calcium-channel blockers (e.g., verapamil, diltiazem)
Central α-adrenergic agonists (e.g., clonidine, guanabenz, guanfacine)
Diuretics
Ganglionic blocking agents
Iron
Laxative (overuse)
MAO inhibitors
Opiates
Phenothiazines
Resins (e.g., cholestyramine, colestipol, polystyrene sulfonate)
Tricyclic antidepressants
Vincristine

Certain laxatives, such as docusates, phenolphthalein, and senna, may serve as mediators also. Disorders of motility may lead to symptoms of diarrhea in the irritable bowel syndrome, diabetic neuropathy, or thyrotoxicosis. Bacterial and viral infections cause diarrhea commonly (e.g., traveler's diarrhea). Food intolerance associated with disaccharidase (lactose) deficiency may result in diarrhea.

PATHOPHYSIOLOGY
Constipation

An intact nervous system is vital for normal defecation. Many patients develop constipation secondary to colonic motility disorders caused by congenital or acquired abnormalities of the nervous system. Outlet obstruction, a mechanism of constipation, may be secondary to a hyperactive rectosigmoid junction, increased rectal storage capacity, rectal spasticity, or hypertonicity of the anal canal (9).

Diarrhea

Four physiologic mechanisms may contribute to the development of diarrhea: (*a*) increased osmolality, (*b*) intestinal ion secretion, (*c*) impaired absorption, and (*d*) inflammatory and ulcerative processes. An understanding of these mechanisms of fluid loss aids in comprehending the mechanism of action of antidiarrheals.

INCREASED OSMOLALITY (OSMOTIC DIARRHEA)

Osmotic diarrhea is generally caused by the retention of fluid by nonabsorbable solutes in the bowel lumen. Peristalsis is stimulated by the increased fluid volume in the lumen, resulting in increased transit of the fecal matter by the colon. Since the colon is very efficient in the reabsorption of NaCl and water, increased transit through the colon promotes diarrhea.

Osmotic diarrhea also occurs when enzymes such as lactase are deficient. Lactase deficiency is common among certain racial groups, such as those of African and Asian descent. Lactase degrades lactase to glucose and galactose, which are then absorbed by the mucosa. In the absence of this enzyme, lactose retains fluid, thereby increasing the volume of water in the stool.

INTESTINAL ION SECRETION (SECRETORY DIARRHEA)

Two factors contribute to secretory diarrhea: (*a*) inhibition of ion absorption and (*b*) intestinal ion secretion. As a result, the stool contains an excess of monovalent ions and water. Enterotoxins produced by certain bacteria stimulate intestinal fluid secretion. Laxatives such as phenolphthalein, senna, and dioctyl sodium sulfosuccinate may also cause this type of diarrhea. Certain hormones such as serotonin, calcitonin, prostaglandin E1, and vasoactive in-

testinal peptide have been implicated as mediators of secretory diarrhea (8).

ALTERED INTESTINAL MOTILITY

Changes in intestinal motility may affect absorption of fluids and electrolytes within the gut lumen. Increased activity may reduce the surface area and limit the contact time for nutrient absorption.

INFLAMMATORY AND ULCERATIVE PROCESSES

Inflammation and ulceration of the intestinal mucosa often result in the release of mucus, serum proteins, and blood into the lumen. The absorption of water and electrolytes is impaired. This malabsorption of fluid and electrolytes is the presumed cause of diarrhea in patients with ulcerative colitis.

CONSEQUENCES OF DIARRHEA

Although diarrhea may be uncomplicated and self-limiting, persistent diarrhea may have serious consequences. Sodium and water deficits secondary to fluid loss are common in persistent diarrhea. Potassium losses of approximately 6 to 7 mEq/kg may be observed in untreated patients, which places the patient at risk of developing paralytic ileus and cardiac arrhythmias if potassium is not appropriately replaced. Fecal loss of bicarbonate and impaired renal excretion of acids may subsequently cause a metabolic acidosis.

DIAGNOSIS AND CLINICAL FINDINGS
Constipation

Diagnosis of constipation requires cooperation of the patient with the clinician to provide a complete history. During the interview the patient's definition of normal bowel function must be ascertained to determine the impact of the change in bowel habit. The onset and duration of constipation, a description of the stool, and the presence of other symptoms are necessary information. Medication use should be determined, especially that of OTC laxatives. The physical examination should include an abdominal examination, a digital examination of the rectum, and a proctosigmoidoscopy. A barium enema should be initiated in chronically constipated patients and those with a recent history of constipation, to determine whether obstruction is present.

Diarrhea

A careful history and physical examination are essential for the diagnosis of diarrhea. Ascertaining from the patient the duration of diarrhea, the description of the stool (consistency, color, odor, presence or absence of melanic stool), the frequency of bowel movements, associated symptoms, and any underlying disorders is essential to a thorough history. Distinguishing between large-stool and small-stool diarrhea helps determine whether the underlying disorder originates from the small bowel or proximal colon or the left colon and rectum, respectively.

Several signs and symptoms of diarrhea have been noted and suggest underlying disease states. Generally, the passage of blood may indicate inflammatory, infectious, or neoplastic disease. Inflammation or infection may be detected by pus or exudate in the stool. Infection caused by *Shigella* has a characteristic blood-tinged mucus without an odor. *Salmonella* infections and *Escherichia coli* infections of infants are usually characterized by green "soupy" stools. Passage of nonbloody mucus often suggests irritable bowel syndrome, particularly when it is associated with intermittent diarrhea and constipation. Fecal incontinence and nocturnal diarrhea are associated with rectal sphincter dysfunctions secondary to neurologic problems. Less specific signs of diarrhea associated with a patient's desire to lose weight may suggest laxative abuse.

TREATMENT OF CONSTIPATION

There are primary causes of constipation that may require nonpharmacological intervention for relief of symptoms. Deficient fluid and fiber intake is often a significant factor, since the American diet generally lacks sufficient fiber content. The average American consumes less than half the recommended daily amount (20 to 35 g) of fiber (10). Fiber is useful in preventing constipation. Fiber increases stool bulk, based on the ability of the polysaccharides to absorb and retain water and the extent of bacterial fermentation of these polysaccharides in the gut. A dietary bulk-forming agent such as bran is appropriate in constipation because it is only partially fermented by bacteria, resulting in increased stool bulk, accelerated transit time, and promotion of normal defecation (11).

Recommendations for increased fiber should be made cautiously. Rapid increases in dietary roughage may cause abdominal bloating and flatulence. Adequate fluid intake is necessary in order to prevent fecal impaction. Generally, 240 to 360 ml of fluid with each tablespoon of bran is sufficient.

Immobility, common among debilitated and elderly patients, may contribute to the development of constipation. Regular exercise such as walking or jogging may improve constipation associated with a sedentary lifestyle. Pharmacologic intervention may be necessary if modification in diet, increased fluid intake, and exercise are unsuccessful. The recommendation of certain laxatives would be appropriate.

The classification of laxative is controversial. They have been categorized primarily by their mechanisms of action, though the exact mechanisms are unclear. Most laxatives alter intestinal fluid and electrolyte transport mechanisms thereby causing defecation (12). The therapeutic options are many. Agents available for use are varied and include bulk-forming agents, hyperosmotic agents, stool softeners, lubricants, saline, and stimulant laxatives (Table 24.3).

Bulk-forming Agents

Bulk-forming agents include nonabsorbable polysaccharide and cellulose derivatives. These agents swell in water, forming an emollient gel, which increases bulk in the intestines. Peristalsis is stimulated by the increased fecal mass, which decreases the transit time. It is proposed that microflora metabolize polysaccharides to osmotically active metabolites that may alter intestinal motility and electrolyte transport.

Bulk-forming agents generally produce a laxative effect within 12 to 24 hr, but they may require 2 to 3 days to exert their full effect. They are generally safe products with minimal side effects. Flatulence may occur if doses are increased rapidly. Intestinal and esophageal obstruction may occur when insufficient liquid is administered with the dose. Therefore, patients should be cautioned to take each dose with at least one 2 240-ml glass of liquid. Bulk-forming laxatives should not be recommended for patients with intestinal stenosis, ulceration, or adhesions. Rare allergic reactions to karaya are characterized by urticaria, rhinitis, dermatitis, and bronchospasm (12).

Hyperosmotic Agents

Glycerine and lactulose are hyperosmotic laxatives. They increase the osmotic pressure within the intestinal lumen, which results in luminal retention of water, softening the stool. Lactulose is an unabsorbed disaccharide metabolized by colonic bacteria, primarily to lactic acid and formic and acetic acids. It has been proposed that these organic acids contribute to the osmotic effect.

Glycerin is only available for rectal administration (suppository or enema) for treatment of acute constipation. Its laxative effect occurs within 15 to 30 min. Lactulose may require 24 to 48 hr for its effect. Lactulose should also be reserved for acute constipation since it is as equally effective as other less costly medications.

Side effects of glycerin include rectal irritation and burning; hyperemia of the rectal mucosa may occur. Lactulose is associated with flatulence, abdominal cramps, and diarrhea. Caution should be exercised when administering this agent as it may also cause significant electrolyte imbalances and dehydration (13).

Stool Softeners

Stool softeners are also referred to as emollient laxatives. They include calcium, potassium, and sodium salts of dioctyl sulfosuccinate. Stool softeners are anionic surfactants that lower the fecal surface tension in vitro, allowing water and lipid penetration. It has been proposed that in vivo

Table 24.3.
Laxatives for the Management of Constipation

Laxative Catagory	Dose Per Day		Dosage Form[a]	Onset of Action	Patient Information
	Adult	Pediatric			
Bulk-forming					
Bran	>12 yr: up to 14 g	6–11 yr: up to 7 g 2–5 yr: up to 3.5 g	O	12–72 hr	Should be administered with 240 ml liquid/dose; additional fluid intake encouraged; recommended laxatives in pregnancy
Karaya	>12 yr: up to 14 g	——	O		
Malt soup extract	>12 yr: up to 64 g	6–11 yr: up to 32 g 2–5 yr: up to 16 g	O		
Methylcellulose and sodium carboxymethylcellulose	>12 yr: up to 6 g	6–11 yr: up to 3 g	O		
Polycarbophil	>12 yr: up to 6 g	6–11 yr: up to 3 g 3–5 yr: up to 1.5 g	O		
Psyllium hydrophilic muciloid	>12 yr: up to 30 g	6–11 yr: up to 15 g	O		
Stimulants					
Bisacodyl	>12 yr: 5–15 mg >12 yr: 10 mg	>3 yr: 0.3 mg/kg 2–11 yr: 5–10 mg <2 yr: 5 mg	O RS	6–12 hr 15 min–2 hr	May cause a pink or red discoloration of the urine; may cause rash; discontinue medication and contact pharmacist or physician; tablets should not be chewed
Casanthranol	>12 yr: 30–90 mg	2–12 yr: 15–45 mg <2 yr: 7.5–22.5 mg	O		
Dehydrocholic acid	>12 yr: 750–1500 mg		O		
Phenolphthalein	>12 yr: 30–270 mg	6–11 yr: 30–60 mg 2–5 yr: 15–30 mg	O		
Sennosides	>12 yr: 12–75 mg >12 yr: 30–60 mg	6–11 yr: 6–33 mg 2–6 yr: 3–12.5 mg	O RS		
Saline agents					
Magnesium citrate	>12 yr: 11–25 g	6–11 yr: 5.5–12.5 g 2–5 yr: 2.7–6.25 g	O	30 min–6 hr	
Magnesium hydroxide	>12 yr: 2.4–4.8 g	6–11 yr: 1.2–2.4 g 2–5 yr: 0.4–1.2 g	O		
Magnesium sulfate	>12 yr: 10–30 g	6–11 yr: 5–10 g 2–5 yr: 2.5–5 g	O		
Sodium phosphate, monobasic	>12 yr: 9.1–20.2 g >12 yr: 18.24–20.16 g	10–11 yr: 4.5–10.1 g 5–9 yr: 2.2–5.05 g 2–11 yr: 9.12–10.08 g	O RE	 2–15 min	
Sodium phosphate, dibasic	>12 yr: 3.42–7.5 g >12 yr: 6.84–7.56 g	10–11 yr: 1.71–3.78 g 5–9 yr: 0.86–1.89 g 2–11 yr: 3.42–3.78 g	O RE	 2–15 min	
Hyperosmotic agents					
Glycerin	> 12 yr: 3 g	 >6 yr: 2–3 g 5–15 ml <6 yr: 1–1.7 g 2–5 ml	RS RS RE RS RE	15–30 min	May cause rectal burning or irritation
Lactulose	>12 yr: 10–20 g, then up to 40 g	[b]<12 yr: 5 g	O, RE		May be mixed in fruit juice to increase palatability; may cause belching, flatulence, or abdominal cramps; pediatric dose should be given after breakfast

(continued)

Table 24.3. *(Continued)*

Laxative Catagory	Dose Per Day		Dosage Form[a]	Onset of Action	Patient Information
	Adult	Pediatric			
Lubricants					
Mineral oil	>12 yr: 15–45 ml	6–11 yr: 5–15 ml	O	6–8 hr	Should not be administered to children <6 yrs, pregnant women, or debilitated persons; bedtime doses should be avoided; may cause pruritis ani especially when administered rectally
	>12 yr: 120 ml	6–11 yr: 30–60 ml	R		
Surfactants					
Dioctyl sulfosuccinate (calcium, potassium, sodium)	(No official recommendation)		O, RE	12–72 hr	Oral solutions may be diluted with 120 ml milk, fruit juice, or infant formula; solutions may cause throat irritation

[a] O, oral; RE, rectal enema; RS, rectal suppository.
[b] Use is not currently included in the FDA-approved labeling.

these agents stimulate water and electrolyte secretion into the colon.

Softening of the feces generally occurs after 1 to 3 days. Some products (casanthrol and docusate sodium) contain a laxative in addition to the stool softener. Adverse effects are rare with docusates. Mild gastrointestinal cramping may occasionally develop. Throat irritation has occurred following the use of docusate sodium solution. Docusate has been associated with hepatotoxicity when used in combination with oxyphenisatin or dantrol (14).

Lubricants

The primary lubricant laxative is mineral oil. Its mechanism of action involves lubrication of the feces and hindrance of water reabsorption in the colon. Mineral oil is indigestible and its absorption is limited considerably in the nonemulsified formulation. Greater absorption from the emulsion formulation has been reported, but the clinical significance is unsubstantiated.

The onset of action of mineral oil orally is 6 to 8 hr. Although adverse effects occur rarely with mineral oil, potentially significant effects may occur. Chronic use of mineral oil has been reported to cause impaired absorption of fat-soluble vitamins (A, D, E, and K). Aspiration of the product may cause a lipoid pneumonia, therefore its oral use should be avoided in young children (<6 years), the elderly, and debilitated patients. Administration at bedtime should be avoided to prevent aspiration. Foreign-body reactions in the lymphoid tissue of the intestinal tract have resulted from its limited absorption. Seepage of the product from the rectum following high-dose oral or rectal administration may cause pruritus ani, increased infection, and decreased healing of anorectal lesions.

Saline Laxatives

Magnesium, sulfate, phosphate, and citrate salts are used when rapid bowel evacuation is required. The mechanism of action of these poorly absorbed ions is unclear, but it is believed that they produce an osmotic effect that increases intraluminal volume and stimulates peristalsis. Magnesium may cause cholecystokinin release from the duodenal mucosa, promoting increased fluid secretion and motility of the small intestine and colon (15).

The laxative effect of the orally administered magnesium and sodium phosphate salts occurs within 0.5 to 6 hr. Phosphate-containing rectal enemas evacuate the bowel within 2 to 15 min.

Saline laxatives are safe when administered for short-term management. They are useful in preparation for endoscopic examinations, elimination of parasites and toxic antihelmintics before and/or after therapy, removal of poisons, and fecal impaction. They may cause significant fluid and electrolyte imbalances when used for prolonged periods or in certain patients. Dehydration may occur from repeated administration without appropriate fluid replacement. The risk of hypermagnesemia in patients with renal dysfunction should be considered when initiating magnesium salts, because 10 to 20% of the dose may be absorbed systemically. Caution should be exercised when administering the sodium phosphate salts to patients with congestive heart failure when sodium restriction is necessary. These agents are not recommended for children under 2 years of age because of the potential for hypocalcemia in this population.

Stimulant Laxatives

Anthraquinone (casanthrol, cascara sagrada, danthron, sennosides, and aloe) and diphenylmethane (bisacodyl, phenolphthalein) derivatives, castor oil, and dehydrocholic acid are stimulant laxatives. They are termed "stimulants" because they stimulate peristalsis via mucosal irritation or intramural nerve plexus activity, which results in increased motility. While this has been long regarded as the mechanism of action for these agents, their activity may actually be related to their effect on the colonic mucosal cells. It is proposed that stimulant laxatives modify the permeability of these cells, which results in intraluminal fluid and electrolyte secretion.

Defecation occurs between 6 and 12 hours after oral administration. Therefore, a single bedtime dose promotes a morning bowel movement. The laxative effects of phenolphthalein may persist for several days because up to 15% of the oral dose is absorbed and undergoes enterohepatic recirculation. Unlike the other stimulant laxatives, dehydrocholic acid is administered at least three times daily. Rectal administration of bisacodyl and senna produces catharsis within 15 min to 2 hr.

Adverse effects of these medications include abdominal cramps, nausea, electrolyte disturbances (e.g., hypokalemia, hypocalcemia, metabolic acidosis, or alkalosis), and rectal burning and irritation with suppository use. Anthraquinone derivatives have been noted to cause melanosis coli (discoloring of colonic mucosa), which is harmless and reversible. Hypersensitivity reactions may occur (rarely) with phenolphthalein and dehydrocholic acid, causing dermatological manifestations (e.g., skin eruptions, rashes, pigmentation, pruritus). These agents may also cause a pink or red discoloration of the urine.

Chronic use of stimulant laxatives should be discouraged, and use beyond 1 week should be avoided. These agents may produce a "cathartic colon" if used for years (15 to 40). The colon develops abnormal motor function and on roentgenography resembles ulcerative colitis. Usually discontinuation of laxative use restores normal bowel function.

Danthron-containing laxatives were removed from the market in 1987 because of their potential for causing intestinal and hepatic tumors in humans. Chronic administration of danthron at high doses produced tumors in rats (16). While insignificant amounts are distributed into the milk of nursing mothers, stimulant laxatives should be avoided during lactation.

Other Agents

Recent data have suggested a role for other agents in the management of constipation. Cisapride (investigational) and naloxone have been used in the treatment of chronic idiopathic constipation.

Cisapride is a piperidinyl benzamide chemically related to metoclopramide. It is a prokinetic agent that enhances gastrointestinal motility throughout the entire length of the gastrointestinal tract. The mechanism by which cisapride facilitates gastrointestinal motility has not been clearly elucidated. However, a proposed mechanism involves its indirect effect on acetylcholine release in the myenteric plexus of the gut (17). Cisapride is devoid of antidopaminergic effects.

Cisapride in oral doses of 5 to 20 mg is absorbed rapidly, and its absorption is enhanced by food. The oral bioavailability is approximately 50%. Its tissue distribution in man is not known; however, it is metabolized extensively to metabolites with minimal pharmacological activity. Its elimination half-life after oral administration is approximately 7 to 10 hr. Some evidence suggests that the half-life of cisapride may increase in elderly patients and those with hepatic impairment (17).

Cisapride was investigated at a dose of 20 mg twice daily in patients with chronic idiopathic constipation or chronic laxative use. Cisapride increased stool frequency by 50%, and reduced mean laxative intake by half (18).

Reports have been published on the use of cisapride in other intestinal dysmotilities such as intestinal pseudoobstruction, constipation in paraplegics, and diabetic patients (19–21). Starting doses of 5 to 10 mg orally or 10 mg IV three times daily have been studied.

The side-effect profile of cisapride is moderate, based on current experience. Common side effects include abdominal cramping, borborygmi, and diarrhea. Central nervous system side effects include somnolence and fatigue.

Concomitant administration of cisapride with specific agents has caused drug interactions. Administration with digoxin slightly reduces digoxin C_{max} (peak plasma concentration) and AUC (area under the plasma concentration-time curve), however these decreases were not clinically significant (22). Cimetidine coadministration may cause a 45% increase in the bioavailability of cisapride (23). Cisapride enhances the absorption rates of diazepam and cimetidine; however the clinical significance of this appears to be minimal (23, 24).

It has been postulated that endogenous opiates regulate colonic propulsive activity (25). Consequently, the role of opiate receptor antagonists in the treatment of constipation has been investigated. Naloxone (an opiate receptor antagonist) has reversed chronic idiopathic constipation at intravenous and oral doses of 20 to 30 mg/day (26). In addition, naloxone causes acceleration of colonic transit, although it has not been shown to affect the number of bowel movements per 48 hr (27). Further studies are necessary to define the role of this agent in the management of chronic constipation.

PATIENT MEDICATION COUNSELING

Providing patient medication counseling for constipation requires determining the patient's perception of normal bowel habits. Only then can the pharmacist decide whether nonpharmacological or pharmacological treatment is appropriate. A discussion of bowel habits should emphasize that while constipation is often self-limiting, it may be a symptom of a more serious disease. Consequently, counseling should include questions about the onset and duration of constipation, as well as a history of medical illnesses. The patient's medication profile should be reviewed for possible drug-induced constipation and for a history of the patient's laxative use. Diet and lifestyle activities are ascertained because lack of exercise (e.g., walking and jogging) and fiber are associated with the development of constipation. Finally, educating patients (especially children) to respond to the urge to defecate is essential to prevent constipation.

If a recommendation of a laxative is appropriate, the pharmacist should consider the following guidelines:

1. Laxative use should not exceed 1 week of self-medication.
2. Laxatives are inappropriate in the presence of abdominal pain or cramping, nausea, vomiting, or bloating.
3. Daily administration of bulk-forming agents should be the first choice in uncomplicated chronic constipation.
4. Pharmacists may recommend one of the following for 1 week or less: a low-dose saline laxative, a stimulant laxative at bedtime, or a glycerin suppository.
5. Institutionalized or bedridden patients may require laxatives in addition to daily bulk-forming agents to prevent fecal impaction (e.g., weekly intermittent doses of stimulant laxatives, lactulose (30 ml/day), or milk of magnesia).
6. Mineral oil should be avoided in elderly or debilitated patients because of the risk of aspiration.
7. Patients with histories of myocardial infarction, anal fissures, hernias, and colorectal surgery are candidates for prophylactic laxative therapy to prevent straining. Acceptable agents include docusate, milk of magnesia, glycerin suppositories, or bulk-forming products.
8. Pregnant patients should use only bulk-forming agents and stool softeners if a laxative is required.

TREATMENT OF DIARRHEA

For most persons, diarrhea is a self-limiting complaint of short duration. This form of diarrhea is often referred to as acute, nonspecific diarrhea that is not caused by underlying diseases or etiological agents. However, the symptoms may often interfere with activities and contribute to loss of productivity. The management of acute, nonspecific diarrhea consists of adequate oral rehydration and relief of symptoms. Several nonprescription agents are effective in managing the associated symptoms of diarrhea (Table 24.4).

Rehydration

Fluid losses in acute, nonspecific diarrhea in adults are generally not severe and require only simple replacement of fluid and electrolytes lost in the stool. Patients should be advised to ingest 2 to 3 liters of clear liquids (e.g., ginger

Table 24.4.
FDA-Recommended OTC Antidiarrheals

Medication	Dose	Maximum Dose per Day
Attapulgite	>12 yr: 1.2 g at onset, then repeat after each loose stool	8.4 g
	6–11 yr: 0.6 g at onset, then repeat after each loose stool	4.2 g
	3–5 yr: 0.3 g at onset, then repeat after each loose stool	2.1 g
Polycarbophil and calcium polycarbophil	>12 yrs: 1–2 g t.i.d. to q.i.d.	4–6 g
	6–11 yrs: 0.5–1 g t.i.d.	3 g
	3–5 yrs: 0.33–0.5 g t.i.d.	1.5 g
Loperamide	>12 yrs: 4 mg at onset, then 2 mg after each loose stool	8 mg; 16 mg[a]
	9–11 yrs: 2 mg at onset, then 1 mg after each loose stool	6 mg
	6–8 yrs: same as above	4 mg
	[a]<6 yrs: 1 mg at onset, then 1 mg after each loose stool	3 mg

[a] Receive only under medical supervision.

Table 24.5.
WHO Oral Rehydration Salts Solution[a]

Ingredient	Ion Concentration mEq/liter (diluted)
Sodium	90
Potassium	20
Chloride	80
Citrate[b]	30
Glucose	20

[a] U.S. Department of Health and Human Services: Health Information for International Travel 1990. Atlanta: HHS Publication No. (CDC) 90–8280.
[b] May be replaced by 2.5 gm/liter of sodium bicarbonate

ale, decaffeinated cola, tea, broth, or gelatin) within the first 24 hr. The following 24-hr diet should consist of bland foods including rice, soup, bread, salted crackers, cooked cereals, baked potatoes, eggs, and applesauce (28). A regular diet may be resumed after 2 to 3 days.

Infants and young children are more susceptible to acute loss of fluid caused by diarrhea because the intestinal surface area of infants and children is greater, in relation to their body size. Consequently, oral rehydration salt (ORS) solutions are recommended for acute diarrhea. Infants and children with a 5 to 7.5% weight loss should receive ORS solution at doses of 40 to 50 ml/kg administered in the first 5 to 6 hr. Oral maintenance can be administered at a rate of 150 ml/kg/day after rehydration is achieved (29). The World Health Organization (WHO) provides the standard oral rehydration salt solution (Table 24.5). Several ORS solutions are available commercially.

Table 24.6.
CDC Formula for Home Rehydration Solution[a]

Glass 1:	
Orange, apple, or other fruit juices	240 ml (8 oz)
Honey or corn syrup	2.5 ml (¼ tsp)
Table salt	1 pinch
Glass 2:	
Water (carbonated or boiled)	240 ml (8 oz)
Baking soda	1.25 ml (¼ tsp)

[a] U.S. Department of Health and Human Services: Health Information for International Travel 1990. Atlanta: HHS Publication No. (CDC) 90–8280.

An alternative for rehydration has been recommended by the Centers for Disease Control (CDC) for the treatment of traveler's diarrhea (Table 24.6). This formula may be prepared extemporaneously but the solution must be prepared correctly to avoid electrolyte imbalances. The solution should be administered alternatively from each glass until the patient is no longer thirsty. Supplementation with carbonated beverages, water, or tea is appropriate. Nursing infants should receive water and breast milk as desired in addition to the solution (30).

Pharmacologic Agents

Various medications, both prescription and OTC are available for the symptomatic relief of diarrhea. Recently, the FDA has reevaluated the safety and efficacy of OTC products for diarrhea. The Advisory Review Panel on OTC Laxative, Antidiarrheal, Emetic, and Antiemetic Drug Products reviewed several products in 1975 for their safety and efficacy (31). The FDA evaluated the recommendations of the Panel and published tentative rulings on the products in 1986 (32). In 1990, the status of these agents was updated, and the OTC ingredients not recognized as safe and effective for diarrhea were listed (Table 24.7). The results on the FDA rulings for bismuth subsalicylate and kaolin and pectin are being deliberated. Currently, the only OTC products considered to be safe and effective treatments of diarrhea are attapulgite, polycarbophil, and loperamide.

Attapulgite is a naturally occurring hydrous magnesium aluminum silicate that adsorbs approximately eight times its weight in water because of its large surface area. This adsorbent property reduces the liquidity of the stool. Side effects are minimal with attapulgite, since it is not absorbed systemically. It is administered at the onset of symptoms, and followed by smaller doses after each loose stool (Table 24.4).

Polycarbophil has been used in the management of diarrhea and constipation. It is a hydrophilic polyacrylic resin that like attapulgite possesses adsorbent properties.

It is not absorbed systemically, making it devoid of systemic side effects. Epigastric pain and bloating are common sequelae. Administering smaller doses spaced more evenly throughout the day may provide relief from bloating. Minimal fluid intake is encouraged for patients in the treatment of diarrhea.

Loperamide, a synthetic congener of meperidine, decreases gastrointestinal motility through its effect on the circular and longitudinal muscles of the intestines. CNS penetration of the drug is small. It does not elicit the CNS side effects associated with opiate use and lacks potential for abuse.

Loperamide relieves symptoms of acute, nonspecific diarrhea and is effective in the treatment of nondysenteric traveler's diarrhea (33–35). It has been compared with attapulgite in treatment of acute diarrhea (34). The dose of loperamide was 4 mg initially, then 2 mg after every unformed stool, not exceeding 8 mg in 24 hr. Attapulgite was administered initially at 3 g, followed by up to 6 g after each unformed stool to a maximum dose of 9 g in 24 hr. The mean number of unformed stools was significantly lower in the loperamide group in the first and second 12-hr intervals. However, no significant difference was observed in duration of relief from diarrhea following the initial dose.

Although generally well tolerated, loperamide may cause abdominal pain, constipation, drowsiness, fatigue,

Table 24.7.
FDA Categorization of OTC Antidiarrheals[a]

Category I[b]
  Glycine
  Scopolamine hydrochloride
Category II[c]
  Aluminum hydroxide
  Atropine sulfate
  Calcium carbonate
  Carboxymethylcellulose
  Homatropine methylbromide
  Hyocyamine sulfate
  Lactobacillus acidophilus
  Lactobacillus bulgaricus
  Opium, powdered[d]
  Opium tincture[d]
  Paregoric
  Phenyl salicylate
  Zinc phenolsulfonate

[a] Anon: Antidiarrheal drug products for over-the-counter human use: tentative final monograph. Federal Register 51:16138–16149, 1986.
[b] Not generally recognized as safe and effective or misbranded.
[c] Insufficient data to classify as safe and effective; further investigation necessary.
[d] Opium products must be in combination with other antidiarrheals in order to be marketed as OTC.

dry mouth, nausea, and vomiting. Doses for adults should not exceed 8 mg/day for OTC use, however maximum daily doses of 16 mg are permitted under medical supervision. Children under 6 years of age should not receive loperamide unless medically supervised. The medication should be discontinued after 48 hr if clinical improvement is not evident.

Opiates (opium powder, tincture, and paregoric) have been used extensively in the treatment of acute, nonspecific diarrhea. Opiates contain morphine, which promotes increased smooth muscle tone of the gastrointestinal tract, inhibits gastrointestinal motility and propulsion, and reduces digestive secretions. Paregoric is commonly used at dosages of 5 to 10 ml one to four times daily for adults and 0.25 to 0.5 ml/kg one to four times daily for children (36). Opium tincture contains 25% more morphine than paregoric, therefore the dose is 0.3 ml to 1 ml q.i.d. with a maximum dose of 6 ml. While these agents are currently considered to be safe and effective antidiarrheals, they are not recommended in nonprescription combination products (37).

Other derivatives of morphine such as codeine and the meperidine congener, diphenoxylate, may be used for diarrhea. At doses of 15 to 30 mg orally every 6 hr, codeine reduces the frequency of loose stools. However, its use has been limited in favor of the various nonnarcotic alternatives for diarrhea currently available. Diphenoxylate,

with activity similar to that of morphine on intestinal smooth muscle, is used in combination with atropine sulfate at doses of 2.5 mg to 5 mg orally q.i.d. Unlike loperamide, diphenoxylate has potential for producing euphoria and suppressing opiate withdrawal symptoms at high doses. Consequently, abuse potential exists with diphenoxylate alone. Atropine sulfate has been added to discourage abuse.

The role of antiperistaltic agents in infectious diarrhea has been questioned. The body normally defends itself from invading bacteria by eliminating these organisms during diarrhea. Antiperistaltic agents such as diphenoxylate and loperamide inhibit this process by increasing gastrointestinal transit time. Therefore, these agents are not recommended for treatment of diarrhea induced by invasive organisms such as enterotoxigenic E. coli, Salmonella, or Shigella (38, 39). They should also be avoided in patients with fecal leukocytes, fever, or blood in the stools. The risk of toxic megacolon exists when administering these agents in patients with pseudomembranous colitis or ulcerative colitis (39).

Although infectious diarrhea may be treated with antimicrobial therapy, the use of these agents is controversial. Generally, acute diarrhea is self-limiting and only requires symptomatic relief and fluid replacement. Antimicrobial therapy is indicated in severe cases persisting for more than 48 hours, passing six or more loose stools in 24 hours,

Table 24.8.
Antiinfective Treatment for Common Causes of Infectious Diarrhea

Organism	Therapy of Choice	Alternative	Duration	Considerations
Salmonella				
Uncomplicated	None	None		
Hyperpyrexia and systemic toxicity	Ampicillin 150 mg/kg/day	TMP/SMX[a] Chloramphenicol	14 days	
Carrier state	Amoxicillin 6 g/day	Ampicillin	4–6 weeks	[b]Chloramphenicol acceptable but not preferred because of development of resistance
Shigella	TMP/SMX 160 mg/800 mg b.i.d.	—	3–5 days	
E. coli (ETEC)	TMP/SMX 160 mg/800 mg b.i.d.	Ampicillin	5 days	
Campylobacter jejuni	Erythromycin 500 mg q.i.d.	—	7 days	Treatment necessary in debilitated or patients with septicemia
Yersinia enterocolitica	Tetracycline 500 mg q.i.d.	—	7 days	Most cases remit spontaneously
Vibrio cholera	Tetracycline 500 mg q.i.d.	Doxycycline [c]Furazolidone	2–5 days	Ampicillin preferred in pregnant women
Clostridium difficile	Vancomycin 125–500 mg p.o. q.i.d.	Metronidazole	10 days	Relapse may occur requiring a repeat course of therapy
Giardia lamblia	Quinacrine 100 mg t.i.d.	Metronidazole Furazolidone	7 days	Furazolidone available in liquid form and may be administered to children
Entamoeba histolytica	[d]Metronidazole 750 mg t.i.d.		5–10 days	May treat in conjunction with iodoquinol or diloxanide furoate

[a] Trimethoprim/sulfamethoxazole.
[b] In patients with hyperpyrexia and systemic toxicity.
[c] Indicated for cases resistant to tetracycline.
[d] Acute intestinal disease.

and/or associated with fever, blood, or pus in the stools (40). Table 24.8 describes the common organisms and their therapy (41).

TRAVELER'S DIARRHEA

Each year 10% of the American population travels to international countries. Specifically, more than 8 million travel to developing countries (30, 42). Often their excursion is interrupted by a syndrome known as traveler's diarrhea (TD). TD is defined as an infectious disease of the gastrointestinal tract in persons traveling outside their country, which results in a twofold or greater increase in the frequency of unformed bowel movements with associated symptoms. The risk of TD depends on the destination of the traveler. Approximately 20 to 50% of travelers reportedly develop TD (30). The disease primarily affects individuals traveling from industrialized nations to developing countries. Persons traveling from the United States, Canada, or Northern Europe are at risk of developing TD when traveling to Latin America, Africa, the Middle East, or Asia.

The abrupt onset of diarrhea is generally self-limiting, with a median duration of 3 to 4 days. Although persistent diarrhea is uncommon in TD, 10% of cases may continue for more than 1 week. Travelers should be aware that TD may occur more than once during a trip, so appropriate precautions should be taken throughout the travel period. TD develops from food or water that is contaminated with fecal material containing bacteria, viruses, parasites, or combinations of microbes. The most common offending organism is enterotoxigenic *E. coli* (ETEC), which accounts for more than 40 to 50% of cases. *Salmonella* and *Shigella* spp. and *Campylobacter jejuni* also cause TD. Other potential bacterial pathogens include *Aeromonas hydrophila, Yersinia enterolytica, Plesiomonas shigelloides, Vibrio parahaemolyticus,* and other *Vibrio* spp. Viruses such as rotavirus and Norwalk virus often contaminate water, but they are not frequent causes of TD in adults. Parasitic enteric pathogens including *Giardia lamblia, Entamoeba histolytica,* and *Cryptosporidium* cause fewer cases of TD.

Prevention

Instructions to travelers about safe food and water precautions are the mainstay of TD prevention. Travelers should be advised to avoid drinking or brushing their teeth with tap water. Ice cubes should be avoided because they may have been made with contaminated water. Boiled water as (is found in hot tea or coffee), carbonated beverages, beer, and wine are generally safe to consume. Two reliable methods of purification are vigorous boiling of water and chemical disinfection with tincture of iodine. However, disinfection with iodine often leaves an unpleas-

ant taste. Foods that should be avoided are undercooked or raw food, salads, and unpasteurized milk and milk products. Foods safe for consumption include bread or crackers, peeled fruit or vegetables, and well-cooked foods.

Although there is consensus in the health community about food and water precautions for TD, chemoprophylaxis for the prevention of TD is controversial. Several studies have provided data that demonstrate efficacy for both antimicrobial and nonantimicrobial agents in decreasing the incidence of diarrhea. The nonantimicrobial agent bismuth subsalicylate has been shown to prevent diarrhea in up to 65% of subjects receiving two tablets (524 mg) four times daily for 21 days beginning on the first day of travel. Lower protection rates (40%) were observed in subjects receiving one tablet (262 mg) four times daily (43). In a previous trial of the liquid preparation, 60 ml four times daily for 3 weeks produced a 62% reduction in illness (44). Bismuth subsalicylate has side effects, including darkening of the tongue and stool and mild tinnitus. Patients taking aspirin concurrently for arthritis may be at increased risk for developing tinnitus secondary to the salicylate component in bismuth subsalicylate. There is concern about patients with renal insufficiency or allergies to aspirin who may consume large quantities of subsalicylate unsupervised. Concurrent use of anticoagulants is also contraindicated with this agent. Because of the modest benefit with the use of this drug at higher doses and the risk of side effects, it is not recommended by the CDC for widespread prophylaxis of TD.

Several antibiotics have been investigated for chemoprophylaxis of TD. One of the earliest agents studied was doxycycline. Doses of 100 mg/day for 21 days are effective in areas where enterotoxigenic *E. coli* (ETEC) were sensitive to the drug (45, 46). However, the protection rate decreased in geographical areas with resistant strains (45). In addition, side effects, including photosensitivity and diarrhea, and contraindications in pregnancy and lactation and in children (<8 years of age) increase its risk/benefit ratio for prophylactic use.

Trimethoprim/sulfamethoxazole (TMP/SMX) at doses of 160 mg/800 mg twice daily for 21 days and daily for 14 days has demonstrated efficacy in preventing TD (47, 48). Trimethoprim alone at doses of 20 mg daily for 14 days is effective for prevention of diarrhea (48). Although significant compared with placebo, the protection rate of TMP alone was less than that of the combination (95% vs. 52%). Side effects noted in the studies were primarily dermatologic, including rashes and skin eruptions. Since TMP/SMX can potentially cause serious skin eruptions such as Stevens-Johnson syndrome, the risk of taking these agents for prophylaxis of TD is of concern.

Quinolone carboxylic acid derivatives such as norfloxacin have also been investigated for prophylactic use. Norfloxacin 400 mg orally once daily for 14 days is effective

(49). Fewer patients developed diarrhea on norfloxacin than on placebo (7% vs. 61%). Norfloxacin provided an 88% protection rate from the development of TD. Resistance was not evident among aerobic Gram-negative bacilli. Adverse reactions were limited to one case of a generalized rash 11 days after therapy with norfloxacin, which resolved upon discontinuation.

While prophylactic management of TD with antimicrobial agents has demonstrated significant benefits, the risks of widespread use must be evaluated. These agents have the potential for side effects such as rashes, photosensitivity reactions, blood disorders, Stevens-Johnson syndrome, and staining of the teeth in children. Therefore, prophylactic antimicrobial agents are not recommended for widespread use by travelers.

Treatment

Approaches to the treatment of traveler's diarrhea include many of the remedies for treating acute nonspecific diarrhea: fluid replacement and symptomatic relief with adsorbents, antimotility agents, and short-term antimicrobial therapy. The self-limiting nature of traveler's diarrhea generally allows successful management with nonspecific agents. However, antimicrobial agents may be useful in persistent diarrhea.

Bismuth subsalicylate is effective for the relief of symptoms of mild to moderate TD. Doses of 30 ml every 30 min for 8 doses are generally effective in relief of abdominal pain and cramping and reduction of unformed stools (50, 51). Bismuth subsalicylate has not been shown to improve the nausea and vomiting of TD.

Antimotility agents such as loperamide are effective for the symptomatic relief of TD despite the concern of prolonging shigellosis in patients infected by this organism. Loperamide was compared with bismuth subsalicylate for the treatment of TD. Doses of loperamide were administered at 4 mg initially then 2 mg after each unformed stool, while bismuth subsalicylate was administered at recommended doses. Loperamide demonstrated significantly more relief (disappearance) of diarrhea and abdominal pains/cramps or decrease in severity than bismuth subsalicylate. There was no significant difference in the duration of diarrhea. Loperamide-treated patients with shigellosis did not experience prolongation of diarrhea (51). This is consistent with results from a study involving 43 patients with two reported cases of loperamide-treated patients with *Shigella* spp. without prolongation of diarrhea (52).

Although use of antimicrobial agents in the treatment of TD is controversial, they may be appropriate in patients who develop persistent diarrhea. Travelers with (a) diarrhea unresponsive to conventional therapy, (b) three or more loose stools in an 8-hr period, and (c) associated symptoms of nausea, vomiting, abdominal cramps, fever, or blood in the stools may benefit from a short course of therapy. The recommended duration of treatment is 3 days (30).

Trimethoprim/sulfamethoxazole (160 mg/800 mg) b.i.d. or trimethoprim 200 mg alone b.i.d. for 3 to 5 days is effective in reducing the number of unformed stools and decreasing symptoms, including abdominal cramps or pain and nausea (53). The efficacy of ciprofloxacin 500 mg b.i.d. and TMP/SMX (160 mg/800 mg) b.i.d. each for 5 days was compared with placebo (54). Both agents were equally effective. Ciprofloxacin may offer an alternative for patients with hypersensitivities to TMP/SMX.

Other agents that have been effective include furazolidone 100 mg q.i.d. It is a broad-spectrum antibiotic that includes coverage for *Giardia* and *Campylobacter* (55). However, its effectiveness is less than that of TMP/SMX or TMP alone. Recent data have suggested the use of combination therapy with antimotility agents (loperamide) and antibiotics (TMP/SMX) initially in patients with moderate to severe diarrhea (56). However, further study on the efficacy and safety is warranted.

IRRITABLE BOWEL SYNDROME

One of the most frequently encountered disorders of the gastrointestinal tract among young to middle-aged adults is the irritable bowel syndrome (IBS). Although this syndrome accounts for up to 70% of gastrointestinal consultations, little is known about the pathogenesis of IBS (57). It is believed that IBS results from disordered intestinal motility, with stress contributing to its recurrence and exacerbation.

The clinical manifestations of IBS may vary. Common symptoms in the absence of organic disease include abdominal pain (frequently associated with distension), flatus, and alternating constipation and diarrhea. Generally the abdominal pain is relieved by defecation and exacerbated by food. IBS is not usually associated with blood in the stools or weight loss.

Treatment

Treatment of IBS incorporates dietary interventions, bowel habit changes, and pharmacologic management based on the patient's symptoms. If patients have symptoms of constipation, then increased fluid intake, high-fiber diet, and exercise should be encouraged before the use of laxatives. If constipation persists, psyllium preparations are appropriate. Patients with symptoms of diarrhea should avoid foods that may precipitate diarrhea such as dairy products, coffee, alcoholic beverages, sorbitol-containing foods, and highly seasoned foods. Bulk-forming agents may be appropriate for resolving diarrhea after the dietary changes.

Several pharmacologic agents have been investigated

for management of IBS. Anticholinergics such as propantheline bromide 15 mg three times daily have been used, although no evidence supports its efficacy. Neuroleptics, antidepressants, and tranquilizers have been used in IBS patients with a history of psychiatric disorders. The benefit of these agents is questionable. Other agents used include phenytoin, verapamil, and cromolyn; however further study on the efficacy of these agents is warranted (58–60).

Recently, data have suggested the use of an opiate agonist, loperamide, in the management of diarrhea of IBS. Studies indicate that IBS patients taking loperamide experience improvement in diarrhea with decreases in stool frequency, passage of unformed stools, and incidence of urgency (61, 62). Caution must be exercised in IBS patients with constipation, as loperamide may worsen the symptoms (62). An appropriate dose for loperamide in IBS has not been determined. However, doses ranging from 2 mg twice daily to 4 mg three times daily have been used for relief of symptoms. Although loperamide appears to have a significant role in the management of diarrhea in IBS, it is presently only approved by the FDA for OTC use for the relief of symptoms in acute, nonspecific diarrhea.

CONCLUSION

Constipation and diarrhea are common among healthy persons. They are self-limiting, but may require intervention of short duration. Changes in diet and lifestyle may eliminate the need for laxatives in constipation. If laxatives are appropriate, an agent may be selected that is tailored to individual patient needs. A variety of agents are effective including, bulk-forming, stimulant, surfactant, hyperosmotic, lubricant, and saline laxatives.

Acute diarrhea may require intervention to prevent excessive fluid loss and dehydration. Rehydration and adsorbents or antiperistaltic agents are effective in most patients with acute nonspecific diarrhea. Persistent diarrhea secondary to bacterial organisms may require antiinfective agents in addition to conventional measures.

The pharmacist is essential in counseling patients on the self-management of constipation and diarrhea. As more products become available for OTC use, this role will become larger.

REFERENCES

1. Gannon K: The next five years: the hot and not so hot otc drugs. Drug Topics (May 7):28–32, 1990.
2. Gannon K: Who's buying what in otcs. Drug Topics (Jan. 8):32–48, 1990.
3. Ruben BD: Public perceptions of digestive health and disease. Pract Gastroenterol 10:35–40, 1986.
4. Haubrich WS, Constipation. In Berk JE: Bockus Gastroenterology, ed. 4. Philadelphia, WB Saunders, 1985. p 111.
5. Cohnell AM, Hilton C, Irvine G, et al.: Variation of bowel habit in two population samples. Br Med J [Clin Res] 2:1095–1102, 1965.
6. Everhart JE, Liang V, Johannes RS, et al.: A longitudinal survey of self-reported bowel habits in the United States. Dig Dis Sci 34:1153–1162, 1989.
7. Sandler RS, Drossman DA: Bowel habits in young adults not seeking health care. Dig Dis Sci 32:841–845, 1987.
8. Binder HJ: Pathophysiology of acute diarrhea. Am J Med 88 (suppl 6A):2S–4S, 1990.
9. Devroede G, Constipation. In Sleisinger MH, Fordtran JS: Gastrointestinal Disease: Pathophysiology, Diagnosis, and Management, ed. 4. Philadelphia, WB Saunders, 1989, p 331.
10. Cerrato PL: Is America really constipated? RN (May):81–86, 1989.
11. Edwards CA, Tomlin J, Read NW, et al.: Fibre and constipation. Br J Clin Pract 42:26–32, 1988.
12. Brunton LL, Laxatives. In Gilman AG, Goodman LS: Goodman and Gilman's The Pharmacological Basis of Therapeutics, ed. 7. New York, Macmillan, 1985, p 994.
13. Tedesco FJ, Dipiro JT: Laxative use in constipation. Am J Gastroenterol 80:303–309, 1985.
14. Anon: Safety of stool softeners. Med Lett 19:45–46, 1977.
15. Donowitz M: Current concepts of laxative action: mechanisms by which laxatives increase stool water. Clin Gastroenterol 1:77–84, 1979.
16. Anon: Laxatives. Replacing danthron. Drug Ther Bull 26:53–56, 1988.
17. McCallum RW, Prakash C, Campoli-Richards DM, et al.: Cisapride. A preliminary review of its pharmacodynamic and pharmacokinetic agent in gastrointestinal motility disorders. Drugs 36:652–681, 1988.
18. Muller-Lissner SA. Treatment of chronic constipation with cisapride and placebo. Gut 28:1033–1038, 1987.
19. Binnie NR, Creasy G, Edmond P, et al.: Action of cisapride on the chronic constipation of paraplegics. Gut 27:1241, 1986.
20. Camilleri M, Brown ML, Malogelada JR: Impaired transit of chyme in chronic intestinal pseudo-obstruction. Gastroenterology 91:619–626, 1986.
21. Cohen NP, Booth IW, Parashar K, et al.: Successful management of idiopathic intestinal pseudo-obstruction with cisapride. J Pediatr Surg 23:229–230, 1988.
22. Kirch W, Jamisch HD, Santos SR, et al.: Effect of cisapride and metoclopramide on digoxin bioavailability. Eur J Drug Metab Pharmacokinet 11:249–250, 1986.
23. Kirch W, Jamisch HD, Ohnhaus EE, et al.: Cisapride-cimetidine interaction: enhanced cisapride bioavailability and accelerated cimetidine absorption. Ther Drug Monit 11:411–414, 1989.
24. Bateman DN: The action of cisapride on gastric emptying and the pharmacodynamics and pharmacokinetics of oral diazepam. Eur J Clin Pharmacol 30:205–208, 1986.
25. Hedner T, Cassieto J: Opioids and opioid receptors in peripheral tissues. Scan J Gastroenterol Suppl 130:36–40, 1987.
26. Kreek MJ, Schaefer RA, Hahn EF, et al.: Naloxone, a specific opioid antagonist reverses chronic idiopathic constipation. Lancet 1:261–262, 1983.
27. Kaufman PN, Krevsky B, Malmud LS, et al.: Role of opiate receptors in the regulation of colonic transit. Gastroenterology 94:1351–1356, 1988.
28. Brownlee HJ: Family practitioner's guide to patient self-treatment of acute diarrhea. Am J Med 88(suppl 6A):27S–29S, 1990.
29. Anon: Oral fluids for dehydration. Med Lett 29:63–64, 1987.
30. U.S. Department of Health and Human Services: Health Information for International Travel 1990. Atlanta: HHS Publication No. (CDC) 90-8280.
31. Anon: Antidiarrheal drug products for over-the-counter human use: proposed monograph. Federal Register 40:12902–12944, 1975.

32. Anon: Antidiarrheal drug products for over-the-counter human use: tentative final monograph. Federal Register 51:16138–16149, 1986.

33. DuPont HL, Sanchez JF, Ericsson CD, et al.: Comparative efficacy of loperamide hydrochloride and bismuth subsalicylate in the management of acute diarrhea. Am J Med 88(suppl 6A):15S–19S, 1990.

34. DuPont HL, Ericsson CD, DuPont MW, et al.: A randomized open-label comparison of non-prescription loperamide and attapulgite in the symptomatic treatment of acute diarrhea. Am J Med 88(suppl 6A):20S–23S, 1990.

35. Johnson PC, Ericsson CD, DuPont HL, et al.: Comparison of loperamide with bismuth subsalicylate for the treatment of acute travelers' diarrhea. JAMA 255:757–760, 1986.

36. Anon: Opium Preparations. American Hospital Formulary Service Drug Information 1990: American Society of Hospital Pharmacists, Washington, D.C. Section 28:08:08, p 1084.

37. Anon: Status of certain over-the-counter drug category II and III ingredients. Federal Register 55:20434–20438, 1990.

38. DuPont HL, Hornick RB: Adverse effect of lomotil therapy in shigellosis. JAMA 226:1525–1528, 1973.

39. Brown JW: Toxic megacolon association with loperamide therapy. JAMA 241:501–502, 1979.

40. DuPont HL, Ericsson CD, Johnson P: Chemotherapy and chemoprophylaxis of traveler's diarrhea. Ann Intern Med 102:260–261, 1985.

41. Suarez J, Salamone FR: Management and prevention of bacterial diarrhea. Clin Pharm 7:746–759, 1988.

42. Salata RA, Olds GR, Infectious diseases in travelers and immigrants. In Warren KS, Mahmoud AF: Tropical and Geographical Medicine, ed. 2. New York, McGraw-Hill, 1990, p 228.

43. DuPont HL, Ericsson CD, Johnson PC: Prevention of traveler's diarrhea by the tablet formulation of bismuth subsalicylate. JAMA 257:1347–1350, 1987.

44. DuPont HL, Sullivan P, Evans DG, et al.: Prevention of traveler's diarrhea (emporiatic enteritis): prophylactic administration of bismuth subsalicylate. JAMA 243:237–241, 1980.

45. Sack DA, Kaminsky DC, Sack RB, et al.: Prophylactic doxycycline for traveler's diarrhea: results of a prospective double-blind study of peace corps volunteers in Kenya. N Engl J Med 298:758–763, 1978.

46. Sack RB, Frochlich JL, Zulich AW, et al.: Prophylactic doxycycline for traveler's diarrhea: results of a prospective double-blind study of Peace Corps volunteers in Morocco. Gastroenterology 76:1368–1373, 1979.

47. DuPont HL, Evans DG, Rios N, et al.: Prevention of traveler's diarrhea with trimethoprim-sulfamethoxazole. Rev Infect Dis 4:533–539, 1982.

48. DuPont HL, Galindo E, Evans DG, et al.: Prevention of traveler's diarrhea with trimethoprim-sulfamethoxazole and trimethoprim alone. Gastroenterology 84:75–80, 1983.

49. Johnson PC, Ericsson CD, Morgan DR, et al.: Lack of emergence of resistant fecal flora during successful prophylaxis of traveler's diarrhea with norfloxacin. Antimicrob Agents Chemother 30:671–674, 1986.

50. DuPont HL, Sullivan P, Pickering LK, et al.: Symptomatic treatment of diarrhea with bismuth subsalicylate among students attending a Mexican university. Gastroenterology 73:715–718, 1977.

51. Johnson PC, Ericsson CD, DuPont HL: Comparison of loperamide with bismuth subsalicylate for the treatment of acute traveler's diarrhea. JAMA 255:757–760, 1986.

52. Van Loon FP, Bennish ML, Butler C: Double-blind trial of loperamide for treating acute watery diarrhea in expatriates in Bangladesh. Gut 30:492–495, 1989.

53. DuPont HL, Reves RR, Galindo E, et al.: Treatment of traveler's diarrhea with trimethoprim/sulfamethoxazole and with trimethoprim alone. N Engl J Med 307:841–844, 1982.

54. Ericsson CD, Johnson PC, DuPont HL, et al.: Ciprofloxacin or trimethoprim-sulfamethoxazole as initial therapy for traveler's diarrhea. Ann Intern Med 106:216–220, 1987.

55. DuPont HL: Furazolidone versus ampicillin in the treatment of traveler's diarrhea. Antimicrob Agents Chemother 26:160, 1984.

56. Ericsson CD, DuPont HL, Mathewson JJ, et al.: Treatment of traveler's diarrhea with sulfamethoxazole and trimethoprim and loperamide. JAMA 263:257–261, 1990.

57. McGill B: Functional diarrhea. Evaluation and management. Pract Gastroenterol 4:16–20, 1980.

58. Dlatorre R, Navarro JL, Aldrete JA, et al.: Comparison between phenytoin and conventional treatment for irritable bowel syndrome. Curr Ther Res Clin Exp 38:661, 1985.

59. McLeod J: Verapamil effective in irritable bowel syndrome? [letter] Med J Aust 2:119, 1983.

60. Stefanni GF, Bazzocchi G, Prati E, et al.: Efficacy of oral disodium cromoglycate in patients with irritable bowel syndrome and positive skin prick tests to foods. Lancet 1:207–208, 1986.

61. Cann PA, Read NW, Holdsworth CD, et al.: Role of loperamide and placebo in the management of irritable bowel syndrome. Dig Dis Sci 29:239–247, 1984.

62. Hovdenak N: Loperamide treatment of the irritable bowel syndrome. Scand J Gastroenterol (suppl)130:81–84, 1987.

CHAPTER 25

HEPATITIS: VIRAL AND DRUG-INDUCED

ARCELIA M. JOHNSON-FANNIN, Pharm.D.

Hepatitis is an inflammation of the liver that may be caused by viral or bacterial infections, chemical toxicity (primarily drugs), or autoimmune hypersensitivity reactions.

VIRAL HEPATITIS

Virology and Etiology

Viral hepatitis is a major health concern worldwide. Reports from developing countries increase the number of viruses that can cause hepatitis. Viral agents currently implicated in hepatitis are hepatitis A virus (HAV), hepatitis B virus (HBV), hepatitis D virus (HDV), hepatitis C virus (HCV), hepatitis E virus (HEV), and (theoretically) hepatitis F (HFV). The symptoms of hepatitis may be mimicked by other viral infections such as cytomegalovirus, Epstein-Barr virus, and mononucleosis (1–4).

HEPATITIS A

Hepatitis A virus causes clinical hepatitis A. HAV is a 27-nm particle composed of four polypetides that form a tight protein shell (capsid) around the virion RNA. The virus belongs to the family Picornaviridae and replicates like the polioviruses. HAV differs significantly from the polioviruses in that HAV is more heat-stable and replication of HAV is not blocked by substances known to block poliovirus replication (2, 5, 6).

Hepatitis A (previously called infectious hepatitis) is spread primarily by the fecal-oral route. The incubation period is about 28 days, with a range of 15 to 50 days (2, 5). Fecal shedding of the virus is maximal late in the incubation period and immediately before and after the onset of symptoms. Propagation from person to person occurs during viral shedding. Antibodies to HAV (anti-HAV, or HA-Ab) can be detected in the serum after the onset of symptoms. The initial antibodies are primarily of the IgM class, with detectable levels of IgA in some patients. As the symptoms resolve, anti-HAV antibodies of the IgG class predominate, with levels remaining high indefinitely. With the appearance of high titers of anti-HAV, the patient is no longer infectious and is considered to be protected from further infection as long as IgG anti-HAV titers remain high (1–3, 5).

HEPATITIS B

Hepatitis B virus causes of hepatitis B infections. The intact virion is a 42-nm sphere called the "Dane particle." However, serum known to be HBV-positive contains the intact virion and other materials of varying size and shape. One of these is a 22-nm lipoprotein that probably represents excess external viral coating. This material is the hepatitis B surface antigen, HBsAg. It may exist in spherical or filamentous form. There are at least 10 major antigenic subtypes of HBsAg and several less important subtypes. The "parent" virion codes for its specific subtypes. However, the "a" specificity appears to be common to all HBsAg subtypes (2, 7). Disruption of the intact virion with mild detergent elutes two other important antigens: the 7-nm polypeptide coat of the nucleocapsid, called hepatitis B core antigen (HBcAg), and the 27-nm soluble protein internal substance of the nucleocapsid, called hepatitis Be antigen (HBeAg) (2, 8).

Hepatitis B (formerly called serum hepatitis) infections may be acquired by a number of mechanisms, including close personal contact. However, the primary mode of transmission is percutaneous contact with infected body fluids, i.e., blood, saliva, sputum, semen, or vaginal discharges. The incubation period ranges from 30 to 150 days (2). HBsAg is the first serologic marker to appear in the serum, detectable as early as 1 week, but usually evident by the fourth week after inoculation. HBsAg disappears from the serum within 2 months after onset of jaundice. HBeAg appears concurrently with or within days of HBsAg. This is the stage of intensive viral replication and maximal infectivity. HBeAg and HBsAg decline over the next 4 to 5 weeks, with HBeAG becoming undetectable before HBsAG. After HBeAg disappears, anti-HBe becomes detectable. HBcAg is not usually detectable in sera, but anti-HBc is usually found within 2 weeks of the appearance of HBsAg. The final serologic marker to appear is anti-HBsAg (Fig. 25.1). Increased sensitivity of test methods has closed the previously described "serologic window" (10). Anti-HBs can usually be detected before HBsAg completely disappears from the serum (2, 7, 9–11). The clinical implication of the pattern of serologic markers is discussed later in this chapter.

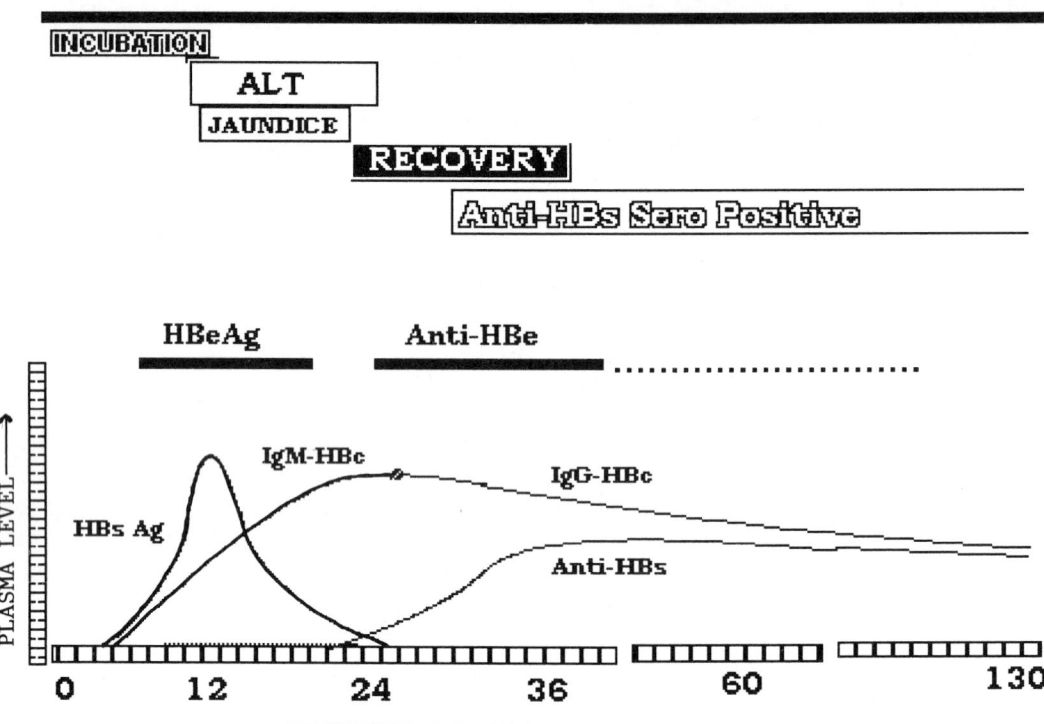

Figure 25.1.   Relative time course of hepatitis B clinical picture and serological markers.

HEPATITIS D (DELTA)

Hepatitis delta virus (HDV) is an incomplete or defective RNA virus that requires the hepatitis B virus to replicate. It is a 37-nm virus whose nucleocapsid core is thought to be encoated with HBsAg. Although hepatitis delta infections can only occur as coinfections with hepatitis B, simultaneously or as superinfection, HDV can replicate in cells where HBV is not present (2, 12). How this occurs has not been explained. Hepatitis delta antigen is only occasionally detectable in the serum. Anti-delta IgM is detectable during an acute infection. HDAg and anti-HDAg disappear from the serum when HBsAg is cleared. Delta infections cannot last longer than hepatitis B infections, but they can alter the severity, chronicity, and morbidity and mortality of hepatitis B infections (12).

HEPATITIS NON-A, NON-B

Hepatitis C virus (HCV) is thought to be the cause of blood-transmitted non-A, non-B hepatitis. The virus is known to belong to the flaviviridae family, however the exact structure and size of the virion remain unknown. Recent evidence suggests that more than one strain of the virus may exist and be able to cause hepatitis (3, 13). It is estimated that 5 to 15% of persons transfused with whole· blood develop hepatitis. Recent development of assay techniques to detect the HCV antibody should allow con-

firmation or rejection of HCV in transfusion-transmitted hepatitis (14, 15).

Hepatitis E virus is the waterborne pathogen of non-A, non-B hepatitis. It has been credited with causing epidemics in developing countries where sanitation is a problem. The virus can be recovered from the stool of infected persons 4 to 7 weeks after inoculation. The viral genome has been replicated, making the possibility of serologic testing and development of a vaccine more feasible (3, 16).

Hepatitis F, another distinct non-A, non-B hepatitis virus, is likely to exist. This is supported by the development of hepatitis in persons receiving coagulation factor concentrates from pooled blood who have already recovered from HCV infections. Such persons should be protected from subsequent HCV infections and should be HCV seropositive. A significant number of these persons are HCV seronegative. Little is known about the virus, suggesting the need for further research (1).

Epidemiology and Transmission

In 1985 almost 60,000 cases of hepatitis were reported to the CDC. In 1986 the number of reported cases was about 55,000. In 1988, the number was approximately 53,500. And through the 51st week of 1990 a total of 50,845 cases of hepatitis had been reported to the CDC, of which 28,500 were hepatitis A, 19,650 hepatitis B, and 2,695 non-A, non-B hepatitis (17–20). During the time period 1983 to 1988, the reported cases of hepatitis A increased from approximately 9/100,000 to almost 11/100,000 population. This apparent increased incidence of hepatitis A could be due to better detection and/or better reporting (18). The hepatitis B trend has not been as predictable. The incidence of reported cases rose from approximately 18,000 in 1984 to more than 25,000 in 1986, in spite of the availability of a hepatitis B vaccine since 1982. Final statistics for 1990 are expected to show about 21,000 cases reported. The recent development of assay techniques to detect the hepatitis C virus and alterations in guidelines for use of hepatitis B vaccine may alter the epidemiological pattern.

Hepatitis A is spread almost exclusively by virus shed in the feces and transmitted to the oral cavity. The vehicle for transmission may be contaminated water, food, shellfish, or even fresh produce (2, 21, 22). Transmission is enhanced by poor hand washing, poor personal hygiene, and crowded conditions. Outbreaks in North America are sporadic; however hepatitis A is endemic to certain areas where outbreaks are more common and last longer (23). Approximately 40 to 50% of urban Americans are seropositive for HAV. At particular risk for HAV are male homosexuals and child-care facility employees.

Hepatitis B is transmitted percutaneously. However, hepatitis from blood transfusions is not likely to be caused by HBV (3). HBsAg can be found in almost every body fluid of an infected person. The most noted transmission vehicle is contaminated needles, but transmission of hepatitis B through sexual contact (24, 25) and perinatal inoculation (11) is gaining in importance. For the American population at large, the risk of hepatitis B infection is estimated to be under 5%. For intravenous drug users, healthcare workers, residents and workers in mental health facilities and prisons, spouses/relatives of infected patient, the sexually promiscuous, the homosexual male, and persons with Down's syndrome, the risk ranges from an estimated 12 to 26% (20, 25–28). More than 200 million persons worldwide are estimated to carry HBsAg. It is estimated that HBV infects more than 200,000 persons in the United States each year, leading to more than 11,000 hospitalizations (20).

Hepatitis delta is endemic in hepatitis B patients in Mediterranean countries. In North America, HDV is seen primarily in hepatitis B patients who are drug users or hemophiliacs (12, 29).

Hepatitis C is transmitted primarily by blood transfusion, particularly when pooled blood is the source of the blood product. At increased risk are hemophiliacs, dialysis patients, and patients with bleeding disorders requiring blood products. Hepatitis E is thought to be endemic in developing countries (3, 4).

Clinical Presentation and Diagnosis

Hepatitis is a systemic disease. The preicteric symptoms are varied and unpredictable and include flu-like complaints such as loss of appetite, GI complaints, fatigue, headache, arthralgias, sore throat, and cough. Most persons infected with a hepatitis virus do not develop the clinical disease, show no alterations in liver function nor hepatocyte damage, and do not associate the flu-like symptoms with liver disease (nonapparent hepatitis). Others may show evidence of mild disease, with minor changes in the liver not progressing to icterus (anicteric symptomatic hepatitis) (2).

In patients with clinical disease (icteric symptomatic hepatitis), the flu-like symptoms (prodromal) precede jaundice by 1 to 2 weeks. In hepatitis A, a high fever may also be noted. One to 5 days before the onset of jaundice, the urine may become dark and the stools appear chalky. With the onset of jaundice, the prodromal symptoms subside. The patient may complain of right upper quadrant pain as the liver enlarges. Splenomegaly is observed in approximately 15% of patients. Some patients develop transient spider angiomas. In a small percentage of patients, biliary obstruction may give rise to a cholestatic presentation. The liver begins to return to normal usually within 2 weeks of the onset of jaundice. The duration of icterus is about 6 weeks, with complete resolution of hepatitis A in 1 to 2 months. In uncomplicated cases of hepatitis B and in hepatitis C, recovery takes 3 to 4 months after the onset of icterus. In the patient with jaundice, a diagnosis of hepatitis is a standard suspicion. Serum aspartate aminotransferase (AST) and alanine aminotransferase (ALT) levels (formerly called SGOT and SGPT, respectively) become elevated prior to the onset of jaundice, indicating hepatocyte necrosis (Fig. 25.1). Alkaline phosphatase levels do not rise unless a biliary obstruction leading to cholestasis is present. Bilirubin levels rise later than AST levels, but they are elevated at the onset of jaundice. There is no correlation between the degree of hepatic damage and enzyme or bilirubin levels. In the anicteric symptomatic patient, AST levels are also elevated. However, in the absence of jaundice, the diagnosis requires a high degree of suspicion. Albumin levels generally remain normal, while globulin levels are predictably elevated. In some patients, prothrombin time is prolonged. This is consistent with extensive hepatocyte necrosis and may signal a poorer prognosis (2, 11).

Serologic tests can determine the type of hepatitis virus responsible for the infection. The diagnosis of hepatitis A is made by confirming the presence of anti-HAV (IgM) in the serum of the patient. The diagnosis of hepatitis B depends on finding HBsAg in the serum of the patient. Recently, serologic tests have become available to detect anti-HCV. The tests are based on radioimmune assay and enzyme-linked immunosorbent assay for anti-C100-3 (13, 14).

Development of a DNA/polymerase chain reaction assay to detect HCV RNA has recently been approved (13).

Table 25.1.
Significance of Serologic Markers in Hepatitis B

Clinical State	Serologic Marker					
	HBsAg	HBeAg	Anti-HBc		Anti-HBe	Anti-HBs
			IgM	IgG		
Active disease	+	+	+	+[a]	−	−
Chronic disease						
Active	+	+	−	+	+	+[b]
Persistent	±		−	+	+	+
Carrier	+	+	−	−	+[b]	+[b]
Recovered	−	−	−	+[c]	±	+[c]

[a] Usually appears during recovery at about 24 weeks.
[b] Low titers of nonprotective antibody may be present in 10–20% of patients.
[c] Titers persist indefinitely in the recovered patient.

This assay should allow the confirmation of HCV in liver and plasma samples. Follow-up serology should be done to determine the outcome of the infection. The pattern of antigen/antibody expression can be used to delineate recovery, chronic states, and carriers (Table 25.1).

Pathogenesis

During acute viral hepatitis, the liver is described as enlarged, red and glistening, smooth-surfaced, and flabby. The morphologic lesions are consistent, regardless of which virus causes the hepatitis. The characteristic picture is a combination of hepatocyte necrosis and regeneration, a diffuse mononuclear cell infiltration, hyperplasia of Kupffer cells, and varying degrees of bile stasis. The mononuclear cells are primarily lymphocytes, with some eosinophils noted. Lobular disarray is apparent, probably due to the presence of ballooned hepatic plates that obliterate the sinusoids; smudging of hepatocyte cell membranes; and inflammatory cells. Large hepatocytes with a "ground-glass" cytoplasm because of HBsAg are characteristic in chronic hepatitis B but are not seen in acute hepatitis B. Although the liver cell plates may be disrupted, leading to focal disruption of the reticulin network, this framework is generally preserved because the necrosis tends to be limited to single or adjacent groups cells. In severe cases of hepatitis, this framework is destroyed, leading to the characteristic pattern of bridging necrosis and a poorer prognosis (30, 31).

Complications

In most cases of hepatitis, resolution of the biochemical changes and complete clinical recovery occur within 4 months. Mortality is quite low for hepatitis A infections, approximating 0.1%. For hepatitis B the mortality statistic varies. Five to 20% mortality in persons with HBV and HDV has been reported during some outbreaks. Current estimates place mortality for hepatitis B at about 1% for hospitalized patients and 10% for the population at large (17). Age (very young or old) and pregnancy are significant risks affecting mortality (11).

In 10 to 20% of patients with hepatitis B, the disease does not resolve but lingers over months to years. This chronic hepatitis may take on of two forms: chronic persistent hepatitis or chronic active hepatitis. Chronic persistent hepatitis is characterized by a mild focal lymphocyte infiltration. The lobular structure is retained, there is no fibrosis, and treatment is not usually required. The prognosis is good, with resolution to full recovery in almost all cases. In chronic active hepatitis (CAH) the liver biopsy shows greater lymphocyte infiltration, involving the portal and periportal areas, collapse with bridging necrosis, and often fibrosis. Continuation of the active inflammatory process in CAH is associated with a poor prognosis, and cirrhosis is likely (32, 33).

A major reservoir for hepatitis virus is the human carrier. Chronic carriers of the HBsAg harbor the virus without evidence of clinical infection but are a major source of infection for others. This group appears to be at greater risk for developing hepatocellular carcinoma. (See Chapter 78, "Liver Tumors"). Approximately 80% of hepatocellular carcinoma patients have a positive history of hepatitis B. A most interesting hypothesis to explain the differing responses to hepatitis B involves the type of cellular immune response mounted by the patient to virus. Theoretically, if the immune response is adequate, the disease follows its usual benign course. If the response is inadequate, the patient develops chronic hepatitis. If the response is absent or severely depressed, the patient becomes a carrier. This theory implies that much of the hepatocellular injury is autoimmune (31).

A small percentage (1 to 5%) of recovered hepatitis patients redevelop symptoms of acute hepatitis. In most instances the recurrence resolves without sequelae. In some cases the relapse progresses to massive hepatic necrosis. The liver shrinks rapidly, bilirubin levels rise rapidly, and the prothrombin time is markedly prolonged. This fulminant hepatic failure progresses to ascites, esophogeal bleeding, sepsis, encephalopathy, cardiovascular failure, coma, and death in less than 2 weeks in about 60 to 90% of patients. The only definitive treatment is liver transplantation (Table 25.2) (30).

Less common extrahepatic complications of hepatitis include rashes, cardiac changes, pleural effusions, altered thyroid function, gastritis, steatorrhea, pancreatitis, and aplastic anemia. Rare complications of hepatitis thought to be related to the immune system include focal glomerulitis, Raynaud's phenomena, acropapular dermatitis (Gianotti-Crosti disease) in children, arthralgias, and a serum-sickness-like syndrome associated with the prodromal symptoms in hepatitis B infections (2, 3, 11).

Table 25.2.
Prognosis of Acute Viral Hepatitis

Indicator	HAV All Ages (%)	Hepatitis B Age < 1 Year (%)	Hepatitis B Older Children Adults (%)	NANB All Ages (%)
Recovery	>98	90–95	85–90	50–90
Chronic disease	N/A[a]	<5	10–15	15–50
Carrier state	N/A[a]	90	10–20	10–20
Fulminant disease	<0.1	1–2	1–2	<5[b]
Cirrhosis	N/A[a]	Rare	Low	1–5
Hepatocellular carcinoma	N/A[a]	High[c]	Rare	Rare

[a] There is no known chronic or carrier state for hepatitis A. It is not implicated in progression to cirrhosis or hepatocellular carcinoma.

[b] Data are sketchy at best due to underreporting and lack of a serological testing method for HCV until recently.

[c] An estimated 80% of the cases of hepatocellular carcinoma show a positive history for hepatitis B.

Treatment

ACUTE VIRAL HEPATITIS

As with many viral infections, acute viral hepatitis is self-limiting. The goals of management in hepatitis, regardless of viral etiology, are (a) early, accurate diagnosis and virus classification, (b) support and monitoring during the acute illness, (c) recognition of the chronic disease state, and (d) prevention of disease transmission. The patient with uncomplicated disease does not require hospitalization. Hospitalization is indicated for patients who have become dehydrated, are suspected of having a more severe form of hepatitis, or are at particular risk of complications (e.g., pregnancy).

No specific treatment is available. Drugs are of little value and do not alter the severity or time course of the disease. In general, drugs should be avoided to prevent potentiating the liver problem. Drug therapies that must be continued (e.g., antihypertensives) can present therapeutic dosing problems, because predictions about liver metabolism are not reflected accurately by levels of liver enzymes. Generally speaking, the capacity of the liver to metabolize drugs is expansive and is not significantly depressed in uncomplicated hepatitis. However, drugs known to cause cholestasis should be specifically avoided.

Bed rest with exercise as tolerated, an appropriate diet, fluids and electrolytes, and education about hepatitis and its transmission are basic to patient management. In patients for whom nausea/vomiting/diarrhea is a problem, feeding the larger portion of the caloric allowance in the morning may be beneficial. Tube feeding may be required for patients who are too ill to eat. Antihistamines may be used to treat the pruritis. However, normal doses of a drug like diphenhydramine (25 to 30 mg q6h p.r.n.) may cause more drowsiness than usual, because of prolonged hepatic clearance in the acute phase of hepatitis. Mild analgesics may be prescribed for the patient complaining of pain. Acetaminophen, the agent most often prescribed in hospitals, has a wide margin of safety, but is implicated in drug-induced liver disease. Doses of 325 to 650 mg q6h should be adequate and appropriate. Aspirin should be avoided because of the potential for gastrointestinal bleeding, the antiplatelet effect, and suppression of the inflammatory response. Antiinflammatory agents (e.g., corticosteroids) should be avoided in acute viral hepatitis. If the prothrombin time is prolonged, 2 to 3 doses of vitamin K given as phytonadione 10 mg/day, p.o. or s.c., may be given. If biliary obstruction is present, the pruritis may be persistent and intense because of deposition of excess bile acids in the skin. Cholestyramine and colestipol HCl are anion-exchange resins capable of binding bile salts into a nonabsorbable, insoluble complex for excretion in the feces. The dose of cholestyramine is 4 g orally, 3 to 4 times a day before meals. The dose of colestipol is 15 to 30 g/day, divided in 2 to 4 doses. Therapy should continue for 14 to 21 days. Both of these agents are powders that must be mixed with 60 to 90 ml of liquid prior to administration. Because of the poor palatability of the drink, preparing the drug with an appropriate vehicle is important for compliance. Strong fruit juices, pulpy fruit, or cereal may mask the taste and texture sufficiently (2, 11).

The hospitalized patient should be discharged when the symptoms improve and AST levels, bilirubin levels, and prothrombin time return to acceptable values. Follow-up is essential to document biochemical recovery, to ensure clearance of HBsAg, and to recognize chronic or carrier states. The patient who develops fulminant hepatic disease should be treated as a patient with hepatic encephalopathy (see Chapter 26).

CHRONIC HEPATITIS

Chronic hepatitis represents a medical challenge. The goals of any treatment plan are to halt the progression to cirrhosis, liver failure, and death, and to reduce infectivity and transmission. Many treatment options have been proposed, with studies aimed primarily at chronic hepatitis B. Two classes of drugs have been investigated most extensively: immunomodulators and antiviral agents. The premise of these approaches is that suppression of viral replication and immune-mediated killing of virus-infected cells will lead to a decrease in both the infectivity and the severity of the disease (33).

Corticosteroids. The use of corticosteroids in the treatment of chronic hepatitis B grew out of their usefulness in the treatment of autoimmune chronic active hepatitis. These patients have high titers of antinuclear antibodies (ANA), indicating an ongoing immune mechanism. Several well-controlled, long-term studies have investigated prednisone and prednisolone in doses of 20 to 60 mg/day against nontreated patients. The conclusion was that long-term prednisone or prednisolone is of no benefit in the treatment of chronic active hepatitis B and may in fact be deleterious (3). Recent investigations have studied the use of pulse therapy (brief periods of steroids) in the treatment of chronic hepatitis B. Prednisone was given in a high dose, 60 mg/day, and tapered rapidly to 0 mg over a 4-week period. A significant reduction in AST levels was noted during drug therapy. However, rebound hepatitis occurred between 4 and 10 weeks after cessation of therapy. When compared with similar patients, the nontreated group faired better (34, 35). Less than 20% of patients with chronic active hepatitis achieve permanent remission with steroids. The question of whether to use steroids at all, initiate long-term steroid therapy, or use intermittent (pulse) therapy is not resolved. As long as there is a chance for improvement in the clinical picture, steroids will be used.

Antiviral Agents. Vidarabine (ARA-A) is a synthetic nucleoside that inhibits multiplication of DNA viruses. Studies conducted with similiar protocols have produced varying results. ARA-A has been tried in doses of 5 mg/kg/day for 4 weeks. Some patients showed a loss of HBeAg, others did not. All patients experienced the rather severe side effects of ARA-A, with painful persistant neuropathies the most frequently reported adverse effect. This agent is not considered to be clinically useful in chronic hepatitis (11, 36).

Acyclovir is an antiviral agent that inhibits the replication of varicella viruses. Its selective activity for viral cells over host cells is due to its higher affinity for viral thymidine kinase than for host cellular enzymes. Acyclovir has been given in doses of 45 mg/kg/day to patients with chronic hepatitis, with some evidence of inhibition of viral replication in HBsAg-positive patients. However, since the hepatitis B virus does not make its own thymidine kinase, the usefulness of this drug is questionable (11, 36).

α-Interferon has thus far demonstrated the most promise in the treatment of chronic hepatitis and was approved in 1991 for this indication. The interferons are a family of glycoproteins secreted by monocytes and lymphocytes in response to viral infections. The currently marketed agents are from recombinant technology. α-Interferon elicits an antiviral response in cells by binding to specific cell receptors and activating intracellular enzymes. This enzyme activation results in destruction of viral mRNA within the infected cell. α-Interferon has been used with some success in the treatment of chronic hepatitis B and chronic hepatitis C (37, 38). The drug is thought to be as effective in low doses (100,000 u/day) as in high doses. The current trend is to use doses ranging from 1,000,000 u/day to 3,000,000 u/day 3 times a week for 24 weeks. The recommended adult dose is 3,000,000

u/day 3 times a week for 16 weeks. For nonresponders, therapy may be continued for 24 weeks. The response rate is reported to be as high as 85%, with a range of 40 to 85% (38). The response is often transient, with as many as 60% of the patients relapsing within 6 to 12 months. Doses up to 5,000,000 u/day 3 times a week for 12 months have produced long-term remission in as many as 40% of treated patients (11, 35–39). Some population groups (e.g., patients of Mediterranean descent) show a lower response to interferon therapy. For those who do respond the relapse rate is high (36).

MISCELLANEOUS AGENTS

Other antiviral agents have been studied without much promise. Ribavirin has activity against a variety of RNA and DNA viruses, including other flaviviridae (11). Oral ribavirin has recently been tried in chronic hepatitis C infections. The response, similiar to α-interferon, is a rapid decrease in AST levels, breakthrough of disease in some patients (despite treatment), and rapid relapse when therapy is discontinued (40). A recent investigation into the use of prostaglandin E for fulminant hepatitis has suggested that it may be of remarkable benefit (41, 42), but controlled studies are needed to substantiate its usefulness. Ursodeoxycholic acid reduces bile acid levels in chronic hepatitis patients. It is given in a dose of 600 mg/day for 2 months and is reported to increase liver perfusion in patients with cholestatic disease (43).

Combination Therapy. The results of single-agent therapy for chronic hepatitis have been disappointing. Since it is likely that most agents studied for the treatment of viral hepatitis act at different stages of viral replication, combination therapy is logical. Azathioprine in combination with prednisone has been used with some success. Prednisone is started at a moderate dose and tapered to a low maintenance dose. The usual regimen of azathioprine 50 to 100 mg/day plus prednisone 30 to 40 mg/day for 1 week, 20 to 25 mg/day for 1 week, and 10 to 15 mg/day maintenance, appears to be well tolerated. The most promising combination therapy is corticosteroids plus α-interferon. Prednisone is given in a regimen of 30 to 60 mg/day for 6 weeks and is followed by 4 to 6 months of α-interferon in doses of 1,000,000 to 3,000,000 u 3 times a week. As many as 30% of patients treated with this regimen have become HBsAg-negative. The most often reported side effects of α-interferon, chills, fever, and neutropenia, are usually mild and well tolerated (11, 32, 33).

Prophylaxis and Prevention

As with all viral infections, prevention of hepatitis is the key to control. Unfortunately, vaccines capable of inducing active immunity to each of the hepatitis viruses are not available. The only vaccine currently marketed is for hepatitis B. Prophylaxis for other hepatitis infections involves the use of immune globulin, which can at best provide passive or "passive-active" immunity.

Passive immunity is accomplished when exogenous antibody (immune globulin) to a particular infectious agent is administered. These antibodies neutralize the infectious agent before extensive colonization can occur, thus preventing infection and clinical disease. Timing of the antibody administration is important. Active immunization is accomplished by the administration of a vaccine. The noninfectious viral material of the vaccine induces the host to produce antibodies to the specific agent. The vaccine should be administered before exposure so that upon exposure to the pathogen, an anamnestic response will occur, preventing infection and clinical disease. In nonimmunized persons, "passive-active" immunity may be accomplished by administering the vaccine and/or immune globulin. Replication of the infectious agent is not prevented, but the disease may be inapparent, with mild symptoms.

Agents used to confer immunity to hepatitis viruses include (a) immune globulin (IGIM), (b) hepatitis B immune globulin (HBIG), and (c) hepatitis B virus vaccine. Immune globulin is a sterile, nonpyrogenic solution containing many antibodies common in human serum. The intramuscular preparation is prepared from the pooled venous blood of at least 1000 persons. The donor blood has been tested for HBsAg and HIV. IGIM contains 15 to 18% protein, of which not less than 90% is IgG. The preparation also contains IgA and IgM. IGIM has a cold-storage life of 3 years from date of manufacture. Hepatitis B immune globulin (HBIG) is a sterile, nonpyrogenic solution containing 10 to 18% protein, of which not less than 80% is IgG. It is prepared from the serum of persons who have high titers of anti-HBs but who do not show evidence of HBsAg. The preparation is free of anti-HIV. HBIG should be refrigerated. There are two types of hepatitis B vaccine preparations, plasma-derived and recombinant DNA. The plasma-derived product is a noninfectious subunit viral vaccine containing HBsAg. It is a suspension prepared from plasma of individuals who are carriers of HBsAg. The manufacturing process inactivates hepatitis B virus and numerous other human viruses, including HIV. The vaccine contains HBsAg in a 20 μg/ml concentration and thimerosal as a preservative. The vaccine is marketed as Hepatavax by Merck Sharpe Dohme. The two recombinant products are sterile suspensions containing HBsAg produced by common bakers yeast, *Saccharomyces cerevisiae*. The yeast strain has been altered to contain the hepatitis B gene code for the HBsAg, subtype adw. Since the specificity is contained in all HBsAg subtypes, the vaccine promotes the production of endogenous antibodies which are effective against all HBsAg subtypes. The recombinant preparations are free of all human blood products but may contain yeast protein. Strict quality controls have assured products which are consistent from lot to lot. The plasma-derived product and the recombinant products are immunologically comparable in vivo (44). Recombivax HB, marketed by Merck Sharpe & Dohme, contains 10 μg/ml HBsAg or 5 μg/ml for pediatric dosing. Energix-B, marketed by SmithKline Beckman, contains 20 μg/ml HBsAg. Both preparations are adsorbed on aluminum hydroxide and contain thimerosal as a preservative.

HEPATITIS A

IGIM contains anti-HAV in titers high enough to provide protection in hepatitis A infections. If IGIM is given prior to exposure or within 2 weeks of exposure it is usually effective in conferring passive immunity and preventing clinically apparent hepatitis A. A dose of 0.02 ml/kg is recommended for persons who have had intimate contact with a hepatitis A patient. Prophylaxis is not recommended for casual contact. In day-care centers for children, identification of hepatitis A cases should be the stimulus for IGIM. For travelers to areas at high risk for hepatitis A, an IGIM dose of 0.06 ml/kg every 4 to 6 months is recommended if the stay is to exceed 3 months. If the visit is for 3 months or less, the standard prophylactic dose is given. There is currently in clinical trials a cell culture–derived hepatitis A vaccine. It is not expected to be available for general distribution for 2 to 3 years.

HEPATITIS B

For preexposure prophylaxis of hepatitis B infection in individuals who are at risk, hepatitis B vaccine should be given in three intramuscular injections into the deltoid muscle. The second injection is given 1 month after the first, and the third at 6 months after the first. For each injection using the plasma-derived vaccine, the adult dose is 20 μg for immunocompetent persons and 40 μg for immunocompromised persons. The dose for persons under age 10 years is 10 μg per vaccination. The adult dose for the recombinant vaccine is 10 μg/injection. For children under 10 years, the dose is 5 μg/injection. For exposure to a known HBsAg-positive person, the nonimmunized person should receive HBIG, 0.06 ml/kg within 24 hr of exposure, and the hepatitis B vaccine series beginning within 7 days of exposure. In neonates born to HBsAg-positive mothers, a 0.5 ml dose of HBIG immediately after birth, along with the hepatitis B vaccine series (5 μg/dose-recombinant) should confer "passive-active" immunity. The child is considered protected if at 1 month after the last vaccination, HBsAg is not detected and anti-HBs is found (Table 28.3) (44, 45).

Neither IGIM nor HBIG contain immunoglobulins specific for hepatitis C (non-A, non-B) in titers high enough to provide immunity. There is no hepatitis C virus vaccine available.

Table 25.3.
Hepatitis B Vaccination Recommendation (µg)

Vaccine	Neonate		Child < 10	Adult	
	(+)[a]	(−)[b]		Non-Ic[c]	Ic[d]
Plasma-derived (MSD)	10	10	10	20	40
Recombinant DNA (MSD)	5	2.5	5	10	20
Recombinant DNA (SmithKline Beechman)	5	2.5	5	10	20

[a] Neonate born to HBsAg/HBeAg-positive mother.
[b] Neonate born to HBsAg/HBeAg-negative mother.
[c] Nonimmunocompromised.
[d] Immunocompromised.

There is considerable controversy in the U.S. medical community about the status of vaccination in general. The question is of particular interest to the pediatric population, but with the availability of a cost-effective hepatitis B vaccine, the argument engulfs a larger segment of the population. Who should be vaccinated for hepatitis B (and hepatitis A when available) has been addressed by the Centers for Disease Control (CDC), the Immunization Practices Advisory Committee (ACIP), and the American Academy of Pediatrics (AAP). These groups agree that residents of mental retardation facilities and other institutions where carriers are likely, chronic recipients of blood products, dialysis patients, adoptees of countries where HBV is endemic, sexual partners of carriers, homosexual men, heterosexually active persons with multiple partners, intravenous drug users, international travelers, and U.S. populations with endemic hepatitis B should be vaccinated prior to exposure. They agree that postexposure vaccinations should be given to neonates born to HBsAg-positive mothers, those with accidental percutaneous exposures, sexual partners of HBV-active persons, and household contacts of HBV-active persons. There is still controversy about the routine vaccination of healthcare workers and the incorporation of hepatitis B vaccinations into the standard battery of pediatric vaccinations. It is suggested that hepatitis B could be eliminated with widespread immunization of infants and adolescents (44–48).

Conclusions

Acute viral hepatitis is a self-limiting disease with low morbidity and mortality. Treatment of the mild disease is supportive. Mortality from hepatitis B is greater than that from either of the other forms of viral hepatitis. Hepatitis B can progress to the chronic active disease or massive necrosis can develop, creating the potential for fulminant hepatic disease. Successful treatment of these more severe illnesses is difficult at best. Corticosteroids and antiviral

agents should be used appropriately. The best therapy is aimed at prevention. Proper sanitation, good hygiene, and avoiding high-risk situations (drug users, high-risk sexual situations) are of primary importance in controlling the spread of hepatitis. The most significant new therapeutic approach, recombinant hepatitis B vaccine, is still centered on prevention. Expanding the current vaccination protocol to include infants, adolescents, and high-risk persons could significantly reduce the incidence of hepatitis B. If the clinical trials of hepatitis A vaccine are successful, spread of the two most prevalent hepatitis viruses, A and B, could be controlled.

DRUG-INDUCED HEPATITIS
Etiology

By definition, any agent that induces a "hepatitis" causes necrosis and/or inflammation of hepatocytes. Injury caused by drugs may start out with a picture quite unlike that of hepatitis, but eventually creates necrotic lesions and inflammation. The list of drugs implicated in drug-induced liver disease is extensive. However it is estimated that fewer than 15 drugs account for more than 80% of the acute hepatic reactions (49). Acetaminophen heads this list. Halothane, methyldopa, isoniazide, oral contraceptives, rifampin, oxyphenisatin, and valproic acid are included. Drug-induced hepatic injury is thought to account for 2 to 5% of hospitalizations in the U.S. and as many as 10% in European countries. In the geriatric population, the incidence is much higher (50).

PATTERNS OF DRUG-INDUCED INJURY

Two major types of hepatotoxicity have been noted: (a) direct or toxic, also called predictable and (b) idiosyncratic, or nonpredictable. Idiosyncratic reactions are sometimes referred to as hypersensitivity reactions. The reaction caused by some drugs cannot be called direct or idiosyncratic even though necrosis and fatty changes may be evident. Oral contraceptives are an example. There are seven basic mechanisms for drug-induced hepatic injury. The characteristic morphological lesions seen in drug-induced injury can be related to these mechanisms (Tables 25.4 and 25.5) (51).

MORPHOLOGICAL CHANGES

Necrosis. The lesions occur in response to a dose-related, predictable injury. Necrosis is usually localized, but it may be massive and diffuse if the response is idiosyncratic rather than toxic. The extent of the necrosis is paralleled by equivalent rises in AST and ALT levels. Focal necrosis often occurs when a nontoxic parent drug is converted to a toxic metabolite. This process, called bioactivation, is often associated with drugs cleared through the cytochrome P-450 system (51–53). Acetaminophen conversion

Table 25.4.
Mechanisms of Drug-induced Hepatic Injury

No.	Description
[a]1	Disruption of metabolic processes
[a]2	Toxic destruction of essential cell structures
[a]3	Induction of immunological reaction
4	Carcinogenesis
5	Disruption of hepatocyte blood supply
6	Transmission of infections
7	Exacerbation underlying disease

[a] Implicated in drug-induced hepatitis.

Table 25.5.
Morphological Changes Induced by Frequently Encountered Drugs

Mechanism	Morphology	Drug Class	Sample Agents
2	Necrosis (toxic)	Mushrooms	*Amanita phalloides*
		Metals	Phosphorus
		Hydrocarbon	Carbon tetrachloride
		Analgesics	Acetaminophen
		Anesthetics	Halothane[a]
2	Hepatitis	Anesthetics	Halothane[a]
		Antituberculin	Isoniazid
		Antihypertensive	Methyldopa
		Chemotherapeutic	Nitrofurantoin
			Ketoconazole
1	Steatonecrosis	Sedative	Alcohol
		Chemotherapeutic	Methotrexate
			Tetracycline
		Anticonvulsant	Valproic acid
		Cardiovascular	Amiodarone
1	Cholestasis	Chemotherapeutic	Erythromycin
		Antipsychotic	Chlorpromazine
		Anabolic steroids	Testosterone
		Homones	Oral contraceptives
		Cardiovascular	Captopril
		Analgesic	Propoxyphene
3	Granulomas	Xanthine oxidase inhibitor	Allopurinol
		Chemotherapeutic	Sulfonamides
		Antiinflammatory	Phenylbutazone

[a] May be toxic or idiosyncratic reaction.

to a toxic metabolite is an important example. This toxic metabolite is detoxified by conjugation with glutathione. When large amounts of the metabolite are formed, glutathione is depleted. With the sulfhydryl group of glutathione unavailable, the metabolite then binds covalently to the hepatocyte, which is thought to cause the necrosis. A 10-g dose of actaminophen is likely to produce a toxic necrosis. Acetaminophen blood levels correlate well with liver damage. A blood level of at least 200 μg/ml 4 hours after ingestion or 100 μg/ml at 8 hr after ingestion is an indication for treatment. The goal of treatment is to supply sulfhydryl groups. *N*-acetylcysteine is given in a dose of 140 mg/kg for 1 dose, followed by 70 mg/kg q4h for a total of 17 doses (See Chapter 4, "Clinical Toxicology"). Damage already done cannot be corrected with treatment; however, survivors usually have adequate liver function (54, 55).

Halothane causes a focal necrosis in some persons and a idiosyncratic necrosis on subsequent exposure in others. Obese adults and women appear to be more susceptible. A genetic predisposition has been postulated. If the necrosis is massive, postmortem pathology shows changes indistinguishable from those of viral hepatitis (56).

Hepatitis. The hepatocyte damage is identical to the lesion seen in viral hepatitis. Methyldopa is thought to act as a hapten, creating a complex capable of inducing an autoimmune reaction in the hepatocyte. The resulting inflammatory response is responsible for the hepatitis. Isoniazid causes hepatocellular necrosis very similar to that in viral hepatitis in as many as 10% of persons taking the drug. A severe toxic hepatitis occurs in about 1%. Patients who are rapid acetylators are thought to be at greater risk for developing drug-induced hepatitis (57).

Fatty Liver (Steatonecrosis). Microvesicular (small droplets) fat accumulates in the hepatocyte. Inflammatory cells may be present, especially if necrosis coexists. AST and ALT levels may be normal or elevated, depending on severity. Alcohol is the most common cause of this type of lesion. Alcohol indirectly increases the synthesis of fatty acids, which are taken up by hepatocytes. If the hepatocyte becomes engorged and breaks open, an inflammatory response occurs, leading to necrosis. Valproic acid and tetracycline are thought to produce similiar hepatitis-like lesions (49, 95).

Cholestasis. Hepatic obstruction of biliary micelles by drugs leads to cholestatic hepatitis. The reaction may be hypersensitivity-induced as with chlorpromazine, erythromycin, and other antibiotics. The cholestasis may appear alone or with hepatocellular necrosis. Mortality is low, but recovery can sometimes take a long time (58).

Diagnosis

Establishing the diagnosis of drug-induced hepatitis is usually difficult because the evidence is circumstantial. The clinical illness and liver function tests may be so like those of viral hepatitis as to be indistinguishable. Complete serology should be done to rule out viral hepatitis. A thorough drug history, including all nonprescribed and over-the-counter agents is essential. Association of symptoms with the start of a new drug might provide initial evidence. If the drug reaction is idiosyncratic, eosinophilia should be evident. Examination of biopsy specimens is not indicated, as it defines only the lesion, not its cause. The decision to call the hepatitis drug-induced is to some extent based on what is not found (52, 57).

Treatment and Prognosis

The first line of therapy is to remove the offending agent. The patient may improve rapidly, often within 1 to 2 weeks. Cholestatic hepatitis caused by drugs like chlorpromazine does not show rapid improvement. Alcoholic hepatitis resolves rapidly; however hepatitis from amiodarone does not. While the liver is healing, other organs of the body which may have been affected by the drug must be supported. If the hepatitis is severe and fulminant hepatic failure seems possible, corticosteroids may be indicated. With the exception of acetaminophen overdose (discussed earlier), there is no definitive treatment for drug-induced hepatitis (48, 53, 59).

Conclusions

While drug-induced liver disease is not as predictable as other medical problems, understanding the potential for hepatocellular injury with certain drugs provides an edge. For patients who are at risk (e.g., age, underlying liver disease, renal disease), monitoring for hepatic damage should be routine. For patients who are not considered to be at risk, routine monitoring of liver function is of questionable value. The best treatment is prevention or early intervention. Appropriate patient education is probably the best method of providing that treatment.

REFERENCES

1. Anon: The A to F of viral hepatitis. Lancet 336:1158–1160, 1990.
2. Anon: Hepatitis knowledge base. Ann Intern Med 93:191–222, 1980.
3. Tabor E: The three viruses of non-A, non-B hepatitis. Lancet 1:743–745, 1985.
4. Bradley DW: Hepatitis non-A, non-B viruses become identified as hepatitis C and hepatitis E viruses. Prog Med Virol 37:101–135, 1990.
5. Lemon SM: Type A viral hepatitis-new developments in an old disease. N Engl J Med 313:1059–1067, 1985.
6. Koff RS: Viral hepatitis, ed. 1. New York: John Wiley & Sons, 1978, ch 1.
7. Holland PV, Hepatitis B surface antigen and antibody (HBsAg/anti-HBs). In Gerety RJ: Hepatitis B, ed. 1. Orlando, Academic Press, 1985, pp 5–25.
8. Koff RS: Viral hepatitis, ed. 1. New York: John Wiley & Sons, 1978, ch 2.
9. Gerety RJ, Hepatitis B core antigen and antibody (HBcAg-antiHBc). In Gerety RJ: Hepatitis B, ed. 1. Orlando, Acdemic Press, 1985, pp 27–43.
10. Ahtone J, Maynard JE: Laboratory diagnosis of hepatitis B. JAMA 249:2067–2069, 1983.
11. Balistreri WF: Viral hepatitis. Ped Clin North Am 35:637–669, 1988.
12. Nishioka NS, Dienstag JL: Delta hepatatis—a new scourge? N Engl J Med 312:1515–1516, 1985.
13. Weiner AJ, Kuo G, Bradley DW: Detection of hepatitis C viral sequences in non-A, non-B hepatitis. Lancet 335:1–3, 1990.
14. Kuo G, Choo Q-L, Alter HJ, et al.: An assay for circulating antibodies to a major etiologic virus of human non-A, non-B hepatitis. Science 244:362–364, 1989.
15. Choo Q-L, Kuo G, Weiner AJ, et al.: Isolation of a cDNA clone derived from a blood-borne non-A, non-B viral hepatitis genome. Science 247:359–361, 1990.
16. Reys GR, Kim JP, Luk KC, et al.: Isolation of a cDNA from the virus responsible for enterically transmitted non-A, non-B hepatitis. Science 247:1335–1339, 1990.
17. Anon: Summary—cases of specified notifiable diseases. MMWR Jan 4, vol 1, 1991.
18. Kane MA, Alter MJ, Hadler SC, et al.: Hepatitis B infection in the United States. Am J Med 87:11s–13s, 1989.
19. Alter MJ, Hadler SC, Margolis HS, et al.: The changing epidemiology of hepatitis B in the United States: need for alternative vaccination strategies. JAMA 263:1218–1222, 1990.
20. Francis DP, Hadler SC, Prendergast TJ, et al.: Occurrence of hepatitis A, B, and non-A/non-B in the United States. Am J Med 76:69–74, 1984.
21. Bloch AB, Stramer SL, Smith JD, et al.: Recovery of hepatitis A virus from a water supply responsible for a common source outbreak of hepatitis A. Am J Public Health 80:428–431, 1990.
22. Rosenblum LS, Mirkin IR, Allen DT, et al.: A multifocal outbreak of hepatitis A traced to commercially distributed lettuce. Am J Public Health 80:1075–1080, 1990.
23. Shaw FE, Shapiro CN, Welty TK, et al.: Hepatitis transmission among the Sioux Indians of South Dakota. Am J Public Health 80:1091–1094, 1990.
24. Alter MJ, Margolis HS: The emergence of hepatitis B as a sexually transmitted disease. Med Clin North Am 74:1529–1541, 1990.
25. Solomon RE, VanRader M, Kaslow RA, et al.: Association of hepatitis B surface antigen and core antibody with acquisition and manifestations of human immunodeficiency virus type 1 (HIV-1) infection. Am J Public Health 80:1475–1478, 1990.
26. Alter MJ, Coleman PJ, Alexander WJ: Importance of heterosexual activity in the transmission of hepatitis B and non-A, non-B hepatitis. JAMA 262:1201–1204, 1989.
27. Rosenblum LS, Hadler SC, Castro KG, et al.: Heterosexual transmission of hepatitis B virus in Belle Glade, Florida. J Infect Dis 161:407–411, 1990.
28. Evans MR, Henderson DK, Bennett JE: Potential for laboratory exposures to biohazardous agents found in blood. Am J Public Health 80:423–427, 1990.
29. Hershow RC, Chomel BB, Graham DR, et al.: Hepatitis D virus infection in Illinois state facilities for the developmentally disabled. Ann Intern Med 110:770–785, 1989.
30. Katelaris PH, Jones DB: Fulminant hepatic failure. Med Clin North Am 73:955–970, 1989.
31. Koff RS: Viral Hepatitis, ed. 1. New York: John Wiley & Sons, 1978, ch 11.
32. Bruckstein AH: Chronic hepatitis. Postgrad Med 85:67–74, 1989.
33. Garcia G, Gentry KR: Chronic viral hepatitis. Med Clin North Am 73:971–981, 1989.
34. Hoofnagle J, Davis GI, Pappas C, et al.: A short course of prednisolone in chronic type B hepatitis: report of a randomized, double-blind, placebo-controlled trial. Ann Intern Med 104:12–17, 1989.
35. Perrilo PR, Regenstein FG, Peters MG, et al.: Prednisone withdrawal followed by recombinant alpha interferon in the treatment of chronic type B hepatitis: a randomized controlled trial. Ann Intern Med 109:95–100, 1988.
36. Di Bisceglie AM, Hoofnagle JH: Antiviral therapy of chronic viral hepatitis. Am J Gastroenterol 85:650–654, 1990.
37. Di Bisceglie AM, Martin P, Kassianides C, et al.: Recombinant interferon alfa therapy for chronic hepatitis C. N Engl J Med 321:1506–1510, 1989.
38. Davis GL, Balart LA, Schiff ER, et al.: Treatment of chronic hepatitis C with recombinant interferon alfa. N Engl J Med 321:1501–1505, 1989.
39. Hoofnagle JH, Mullin KD, Jones DB, et al.: Treatment of chronic non-A, non-B hepatitis with recombinant human alpha interferon. N Engl J Med 315:1575–1578, 1986.

40. Jain S, Thomas H, Oxford J, et al.: Trial of ribavirin for the treatment of HBsAg positive chronic liver disease. J Antimicrob Chemother 4:367, 1978.

41. Sinclair SB, Greig PD, Blendis LM, et al.: Biochemical and clinical response of fulminant viral hepatitis to administration of prostaglandin E. A preliminary report. J Clin Invest 84:1063–1069, 1989.

42. Feldman M: Selected summaries: revolutionary lifesaving therapy for acute hepatic failure, or yet another false hope?. Gastroentrology 98:1088–1093, 1990.

43. Podda M, Ghezzi C, Battezzati M, et al.: Effects of ursodeoxycholic acid and taurine on serum liver enzymes and bile acids in chronic hepatitis. Gastroenterology 98:1044–1050, 1990.

44. West DJ, Calandra GB, Ellis RW: Vaccination of infants and children against hepatitis B. Pedatr Clin North Am 37:585–601, 1990.

45. Tong MJ: Hepatitis B vaccination of neonates and children. Am J Med 87:33s–35s, 1989.

46. Blumberg BS: Feasibility of controlling or eradicating the hepatitis B virus. Am J Med 87:2s–3s, 1989.

47. Pasko MT, Beam TR: Persistence of anti-HBs among health care personnel immunized with hepatitis B vaccine. Am J Public Health 80:590–593, 1990.

48. Hollinger FB: Factors influencing the immune response to hepatitis B vaccine, booster dose guidelines, and vaccine protocol recommendations. Am J Med 87:365–395, 1989.

49. Tredger JM, Neuberger JM, Williams R, Drugs in acute hepatic necrosis. In Testa B, Perrissoud D: Liver Drugs: From Experimental Pharmacology to Therapeutic Application, ed. 1. Florida, CRC Press, 1988, p 67.

50. Lewis JH, Zimmerman HJ: Drug-induced liver disease. Med Clin North Am 73:775–792, 1990.

51. Stricker BH, Spoelstra P: Drug-induced Hepatic Injury. Amsterdam: Elsevier, 1985, ch I–II.

52. Kaplowitz N: Drug-induced hepatotoxicity. Ann Intern Med. 104:826–839, 1986.

53. Lee MG, Hanchard B, Williams NP: Drug-induced acute liver disease. Postgrad Med J. 65:367–370, 1989.

54. Seeff LB, Cuccherini BA, Zimmerman HJ, et al.: Acetaminophen hepatotoxicity in alcoholics: a therapeutic misadventure. Ann Intern Med 104:399–404, 1986.

55. Maddrey WC, Drug-induced chronic active hepatitis. In Cohen S, Soloway RD: Chronic Active Liver Disease, vol 2. New York, Churchill Livingstone, 1986, p 131.

56. Dienstag JL: Halothane hepatitis, allergy or idiosyncracy. N Engl J Med 303:102–104, 1990.

57. Pohl LR: Drug induced allergic hepatitis. Hepatology 9:785–788, 1989.

58. Zimmerman JH, Lewis JH: Drug-induced cholestasis. Med Toxicol 2:112–160, 1987.

59. Colt HG, Shapiro AP: Drug induced illness as a cause for admission to a community hospital. J Am Geriatr Soc 37:323–326, 1989.

CHAPTER 26

CIRRHOSIS

WAYNE A. KRADJAN, Pharm.D.

Cirrhosis is characterized by a diffuse increase in the fibrous connective tissue of the liver, with areas of both necrosis and regeneration of parenchymal cells imparting a nodular or glandular texture. In later stages, cirrhosis leads to such deformity of the liver that it interferes with hepatobiliary function and the circulation of blood both to and from the liver. Currently, no specific medical therapy exists for cirrhosis, except prevention. However, drugs are used to treat the complications of this disorder.

ETIOLOGY

Several major types of cirrhosis have been described (Table 26.1), but cirrhosis associated with alcohol abuse of *Laënnec's cirrhosis* is by far the most commonly encountered form in the United States (1). Alcoholic liver disease usually begins with severe fatty changes in the liver. In the early stages this fatty infiltration is not associated with fibrosis and scarring. Later stages are marked by a prominent inflammation, an increase in fibrous tissue, and a progressive shrinkage and nodularity of the liver.

In experimental animals, dietary derangements can induce fatty changes in the liver, with subsequent development of cirrhosis. Thus, it is often claimed that dietary indiscretion in alcoholics may be an important underlying associated cause of cirrhosis. This concept is supported by the observation that when a chronic alcoholic is hospitalized and placed on an adequate diet, excess fat can be mobilized and the liver structure and function may return to normal. This reversibility is less clear if fibrosis has already occurred. Other evidence implicates alcohol as a direct hepatotoxin. One group of investigators were able to demonstrate development of cirrhosis in baboons maintained on a balanced diet, but given large daily doses of alcohol (2).

Biliary cirrhosis refers to cirrhosis following chronic obstruction of bile flow (cholestasis). Primary biliary cirrhosis follows long-standing cholestasis that is generally of unknown etiology, but it may have an underlying immunologic basis with elevated IgM, autoantibodies, and circulating complement-fixing immune complexes. Secondary biliary cirrhosis may be caused by stones or a tumor obstructing bile flow, leading to an inflammatory reaction and scarring.

Less common causes of cirrhosis are related to chronic viral hepatitis, immune-mediated chronic hepatitis, and various metabolic disorders (Table 26.1).

EPIDEMIOLOGY

It is difficult to cite an incidence of cirrhosis since patients often do not exhibit any signs or symptoms. Autopsies at various hospitals have shown a frequency ranging from 3 to 15%. Cirrhosis is a leading cause of death in the United States (3). Worldwide the annual death rate from cirrhosis of all causes is as high as 15 to 40 persons per 100,000 population (4). It also appears that cirrhosis has increased in frequency over the past 50 years. Various explanations for this increase have been proposed including (*a*) better medical care enabling patients to survive the initial acute liver disease, (*b*) increased incidence of alcoholism, and (*c*) a greater exposure to hepatotoxic drugs and chemicals that cause diffuse liver toxicity leading to cirrhosis. Table 26.1 lists the relative frequencies of the various types of cirrhosis encountered clinically. The largest percentage is Laënnec's cirrhosis, which occurs principally in patients between 40 and 60 years of age and is found most often in males. A history of chronic alcoholism can be obtained in 50 to 90% of these patients in the United States. In Third World countries, children are frequently affected following maternally acquired hepatitis (1, 3, 4).

CLINICAL FINDINGS AND DIAGNOSIS

Cirrhosis is insidious in its development and often produces no clinical manifestations. Up to 50% of all cases are discovered only at the time of postmortem examination. Many patients seek medical help complaining of vague, nonspecific symptoms such as weight loss, loss of appetite, nausea, vomiting, and ill-defined digestive disturbances. Others enter the hospital acutely ill with the full syndrome of acute *alcoholic hepatitis* (a precursor to cirrhosis). These patients have *jaundice* (bilirubin levels range from 34 μmol/liter (2 mg/dl) to more than 684 μmol/liter (40 mg/dl), mildly elevated serum aminotransferase (ALT and AST) and alkaline phosphatase levels, a low serum albumin level, evidence of impaired coagulation (prolonged prothrombin time) and right upper quadrant pain. In the later stages of cirrhosis, patients may have the complications of cirrhosis: ascites, gastrointestinal (GI) bleeding, and mental deterioration. Hepatocellular carcinoma develops in as many as 10% of subjects with long-standing cirrhosis.

COMPLICATIONS

The complications of cirrhosis generally relate to abnormalities in the portal venous system. The portal vein re-

Table 26.1.
Types of Cirrhosis: Incidence and Etiology

Type	Frequency (%)	Etiology
Alcohol-associated (Laënnec's)	60–70	Alcohol abuse and protein deficiency inducing fatty changes, inflammation, and scarring in liver
Biliary (primary and secondary)	10–15	Obstruction to bile flow, e.g., immune complexes, stones, and carcinoma; often secondary to long-standing bacterial infection
Postnecrotic	10–15	Scarring following massive hepatic necrosis such as that seen in chronic viral hepatitis, after exposure to hepatotoxic drugs, or immune-mediated hepatitis
Metabolic	5–10	Excessive iron (hemochromatosis) or copper (Wilson's disease) deposition, α-1-antitrypsin deficiency, other inborn errors of metabolism

ceives blood draining from the arterial and capillary system of the entire GI tract. This system is unique in that while it is a venous system, it has a second set of capillaries (or sinusoids) that run throughout the liver and then rejoin to empty into the hepatic veins and ventually the inferior vena cava. The main function of the portal venous network is to act as a pathway for detoxification and metabolism by the liver of substances absorbed from the GI tract. The portal venous system does not provide oxygenated blood to the liver (this is done by the hepatic artery). The anatomy of the portal system allows "first pass" (presystemic) metabolism of orally administered drugs such as propranolol, verapamil, and morphine. As scarring and nodularity increase in the liver during cirrhosis, the blood flow through the portal system becomes obstructed, leading to a dramatic rise in the pressure of the portal vein and its tributaries in the GI tract (i.e., *portal hypertension*). Blood may also be shunted around the liver to empty directly into the systemic circulation (inferior vena cava). The clinical problems arising secondary to portal hypertension include ascites, GI bleeding (varices), and encephalopathy.

Ascites

Ascites, characterized by the accumulation of protein-rich fluid in the peritoneal cavity, is one of the most striking features of cirrhosis. Complaints associated with ascites include a rapidly developing inability to fit into one's clothes, abdominal and back pain, gastroesophageal reflux, and shortness of breath secondary to impaired diaphragm movement. The amount of fluid in the abdomen can vary from a few liters to 20 or more liters, leading to a large protuberant abdomen and an umbilical hernia. Ascitic

fluid is a good culture medium for bacterial growth, and infections can occur spontaneously (spontaneous bacterial peritonitis). An unexplained high fever or elevated white blood cell count is an indication for obtaining a culture of an aspirate from the ascitic fluid or initiating appropriate antibiotic therapy.

Several postulates exist to explain the mechanism underlying the formation of ascites, none of which is fully accepted as the definitive answer (5–6). Most authors agree that one element of ascites formation is intrahepatic obstruction causing an elevated lymphatic pressure within hepatic sinusoids, which eventually causes excessive transudation (weeping) of protein-rich fluid from the surface of the liver into the peritoneal cavity. According to the "underfill" theory, both the lymphatic leakage and high prehepatic venous pressure (portal hypertension) cause a net flow of volume from the vascular spaces to the "third space" of the peritoneal cavity via hydrostatic forces. The high protein content of the ascitic fluid may also help to draw volume out of the vasculature. As a result "effective vascular volume" throughout the body is decreased, causing secondary sodium and water retention by the kidney. The renin-angiotensin system is a major mediator of the sodium and water retention, ultimately causing release of aldosterone by the adrenal gland. Release of antidiuretic hormone (ADH) may also be increased. Serum levels of aldosterone and ADH remain elevated because of impaired metabolism secondary to liver failure.

A major inconsistency with the underfill theory is that some patients have an increased, not decreased, total blood volume and not all patients have demonstrable hyperaldosteronism. According to another (the "overfill") theory, the primary defect in ascites formation is excessive renal reabsorption of sodium and water for unknown reasons. As plasma volume expands, ascites results due to "overflow" of fluid out of the splanchnic circulation and from increased pressure in the portal system.

Schrier (5) proposes an integration of these two theories, citing a possible systemic intravascular vasodilation that causes a relative decrease in effective plasma volume or pressure, followed by excessive renal retention of sodium and water. Rocco and Ware (6) believe that both intrahepatic hypertension and a primary renal defect are responsible for the early stages of ascites.

Hypoalbuminemia, secondary to decreased hepatic synthesis and lymphatic leakage into the peritoneum, may contribute to further accumulation of ascites. A low serum albumin concentration causes a reduced serum osmotic (oncotic) pressure that again favors flow of fluid from the vasculature into the extravascular third space. Not all patients with cirrhosis have hypoalbuminemia, but those that do may have both ascites and extensive peripheral edema with a relative systemic hypovolemia.

Fluid and Electrolyte Balance

Patients often have hyponatremia from retention of free water, induced by elevated antidiuretic hormone (ADH) levels. Hypokalemia develops secondary to hyperaldosteronism and excessive vomiting.

GI Bleeding (Varices)

GI hemorrhage occurs in about one-fourth to one-third of patients. In about one-third of these cases, the patient dies from the initial hemorrhage. Even nonfatal GI hemorrhages tend to be massive. The major cause of GI bleeding associated with cirrhosis is shunting of blood away from the high-pressure portal system to low-pressure systemic collaterals in the esophagus (esophageal varices), rectum (hemorrhoids), and other parts of the GI tract. Bleeding may be increased by an impaired clotting system caused by deficiencies in the vitamin K–dependent clotting factors. *Esophageal varices* account for about 50 to 60% of the GI bleeding observed in cirrhosis, and peptic ulcer disease accounts for another 25%.

Hepatic Encephalopathy

The ultimate result of advanced cirrhosis or severe hepatitis is liver failure and hepatic coma (hepatic encephalopathy). This is characterized by increasing drowsiness, personality changes, and mental confusion, with a characteristic flapping tremor of the fingers and hands when the wrists are hyperextended (liver flap or asterixis). Eventually, a deepening coma and death follow. Neurological complications include incoordination, tremor, nystagmus, and incontinence. As the disease progresses, a characteristic sweet, pungent odor (fetor hepaticus) may be present in the patient's breath. The cause of the odor is unclear but may be related to exhalation of mercaptans.

The diagnosis of hepatic encephalopathy may be complicated by other neurologic disorders including alcohol withdrawal-induced tremors, Wernicke's disease (mental disturbances, ataxia, and mystagmus from acute thiamin deficiency), Kursakorf syndrome (Psychosis and comfabulation from chronic thiamin deficiency), and cerebellar damage from chronic alcohol ingestion. The presence of asterixis is a motor differentiating factor.

The pathogenesis of hepatic encephalopathy is not well understood, but it is related to increased arterial and CNS ammonium levels. Although a direct cause-and-effect relationship has not been shown between encephalopathy and blood ammonium concentration, when factors that influence ammonium production are decreased, the patient's sensorium often clears. Dietary ingestion of food or bleeding into the gastrointestinal tract (e.g., esophageal bleeding) introduces a rich source of protein into the intestinal tract. Ammonia is produced in the lower gastrointestinal tract when these proteins and urea are metab-

olized by bacterial enzymatic action. The ammonia is then absorbed into the blood stream and converted to ammonium ion. Normally, the liver converts the ammonium into urea for excretion by the kidney, but when the liver is malfunctioning or the blood is being shunted away from it, as in advanced cirrhosis, serum ammonium levels increase and encephalopathy ensues. It is theorized that the cerebrotoxicity of ammonia is due to inhibition of oxidative metabolism by the citric acid cycle in the brain. α-Ketoglutarate combines with ammonia to produce high CNS levels of *glutamine* (a by-product of ammonium metabolism), while at the same time robbing the citric acid cycle of the α-ketoglutarate needed for production of high-energy adenosine triphosphate (ATP). Serum ammonium levels and cerebrospinal fluid (CSF) glutamine are sometimes measured to confirm hepatic encephalopathy.

An alternative explanation for the pathogenesis of hepatic encephalopathy concerns derangements in plasma and brain amino acid patterns (7–9). Characteristically, there is a relative elevation in methionine and *aromatic amino* acid levels (e.g., phenylalanine, tyrosine, and tryptophan) and a corresponding relative deficiency in *branched-chain* amino acids (e.g., valine, leucine, and isoleucine). These derangements lead to an imbalance of brain neurotransmitters, causing elevated levels of serotonin, octopamine, and phenylethanolamine and a decrease in dopamine and possibly norepinephrine. Serotonin is an end product of tryptophan metabolism, while phenylethanolamine and octopamine are by-products of phenylalanine and tyrosine metabolism.

While the exact reason for these derangements in plasma and brain amino acids is unknown, a number of observations have been made (7–9). The normal ratio of branched-chain amino acids (BCAAs) to aromatic amino acids (AAAs) is 4:1 to 6:1. In both sepsis and liver failure, catabolic states lead to a negative nitrogen balance and preferential use of BCAAs as a source of energy. As ammonia levels rise, glucagon secretion is stimulated, which in turn stimulates hepatic gluconeogenesis to convert amino acids into glucose for energy. In response to gluconeogenesis, insulin is secreted, which leads to increased uptake and metabolism of BCAAs by skeletal muscle. As liver failure progresses, the liver can no longer store or release glucose in adequate amounts, and thus greater quantities of BCAAs must be metabolized by skeletal muscle for energy.

Simultaneously, the plasma clearance of AAAs and methionine, which depends upon hepatic metabolism, is diminished. The net result is an alteration of the BCAA/AAA ratio. In acute liver failure the AAAs rise dramatically, while BCAAs remain normal. In chronic hepatic disease, the AAAs remain abnormally high, while BCAA concentrations drop to low levels, thus further lowering the BCAA/AAA ratio. In addition to alterations in amino acid metabolism, there appears to be a derangement of the blood brain barrier during chronic liver disease. In persons with hepatic encephalopathy, there is a selective increase in transport of AAAs across the blood brain barrier, possibly via an exchange of CSF glutamine (from ammonia metabolism) for AAAs in the plasma. The arterial concentration of ammonium and other amines may be accentuated by excessive dietary protein consumption, GI hemorrhage (source of protein), overdiuresis leading to dehydration, or other conditions that lead to severe electrolyte imbalance and metabolic alkalosis.

An entirely different avenue of research suggests that the γ-aminobutyric acid (GABA)–benzodiazepine receptor complex is involved in the pathogenesis of hepatic encephalopathy (10). GABA is the primary inhibitory neurotransmitter in the CNS. According to this theory, an increase in CNS GABA-ergic neurotransmission may partially account for the behavioral and electrophysiologic manifestations of encephalopathy. This hypothesis is based on the observation that an accentuation of CNS inhibitory neurotransmitter tone can cause ataxia, sedation, and coma. While GABA levels do not seem to be elevated in patients with encephalopathy, it is speculated that other endogenous or exogenous GABA-like ligands may be involved. Not surprisingly, these patients also demonstrate unusual sensitivity to benzodiazepine-like drugs that elicit GABA-ergic-like activity.

Other Associated Disorders

Anemia and other hematologic disorders commonly accompany cirrhosis. Chronic alcohol abusers tend to malabsorb *folic acid*, as well as iron. In addition, their diets may be deficient in both iron and folate. *Iron deficiency* may be further aggravated by a block of iron uptake into the bone marrow induced by chronic alcoholism and by slow GI bleeding due to gastritis. Thrombocytopenia and leukopenia may occur because of folic acid deficiency and hypersplenism secondary to portal hypertension.

Endocrine disorders are seen in advanced cirrhosis because of the inability of the liver to metabolize the steroid hormones of the adrenals and gonads. In the male, increased circulating estrogen levels cause gynecomastia, loss of body hair, impotence, spider angiomas, and palmar erythema.

Hepatorenal Syndrome. The concurrent impairment of renal function with hepatic failure is termed the hepatorenal syndrome. The exact cause for the progression to renal failure, if a cause and effect relationship exists, is unknown. Often no structural abnormalities can be found in the kidneys at postmortem examination, and some of the kidneys have performed well when used for renal transplant. It is possible that there is simply a functional change in the kidney, caused by fluid and electrolyte disturbances, diuretic-induced volume depletion, shock, or accumulation of unmetabolized toxic substances. The use of neomycin to treat encephalopathy has also been implicated as a cause of the change in renal status.

TREATMENT OF CIRRHOSIS

Management of cirrhosis is largely symptomatic (Table 26.2). In Laënnec's cirrhosis the primary treatment is to encourage the patient to abstain from alcohol. Fluid and electrolyte balance should be maintained either by parenteral administration or by oral therapy. If the patient is vomiting, antiemetics may be used. However, the phenothiazine-type antiemetics (e.g., prochlorperazine) have been associated with causing jaundice. Analgesics may be administered for abdominal pain, but aspirin-containing products or nonsteroidal antiinflammatory drugs may worsen gastritis or GI bleeding. Narcotics may lead to profound CNS and respiratory depression if the patient's liver status is severely compromised or if the patient is already obtunded. Sedatives and hypnotics should be avoided if there is any danger of the patient developing hepatic coma. If there are no signs of impending hepatic coma, the patient should be maintained on a 2000 to 3000 calorie diet with 1 g of protein per kg of body weight. If encephalopathy is present, dietary supplements rich in branched-chain amino acids and low in aromatic amino acids (e.g., Hepatic Aid) have been used in an attempt to prevent negative nitrogen balance. The value of these latter products is unproven, and their use is to be discouraged.

Vitamin replacement is essential in most cirrhotic patients, especially those with a recent alcoholic history. Replacement of thiamine at 50 to 100 mg per day along with a good diet may improve mentation as well as decrease peripheral neuritis and improve gait disorders. Continuation of thiamin therapy beyond 1 or 2 weeks is of questionable value, since it is a water-soluble vitamin whose stores are rapidly replaced. Up to 1 g per day may occasionally be required if the patient displays severe nystagmus, Wernicke's encephalopathy, or oculogyric crisis. Iron replacement or folic acid supplements are required if the patient is anemic. Iron deficiency is confirmed by measurement of serum iron, TIBC, and ferritin concentrations (see Chapter 12, "Iron Deficiency and Megaloblastic Anemias").

Vitamin K, 10 mg subcutaneously daily for 3 or more days, is given if the prothrombin time is elevated. If the prothrombin time is not reversed after 3 to 5 doses, further doses should be avoided, as an occasional patient will demonstrate a paradoxical lengthening of the prothrombin time from excessive vitamin K. This paradoxical effect is theorized to be a result of "consumptive processes" induced by overstimulation of the production of clotting factors, leading to an eventual depletion of the body stores. Vitamin K_1, or *phytonadione (Aquamephyton)*, gives a more rapid response when given parenterally than does

Table 26.2.
Drugs Used in Cirrhotic Patients

Thiamin
  Reason: reverse mental confusion secondary to thiamine deficiency
    (Wernicke's syndrome) and decrease peripheral neuropathies
  Dose: 100–200 mg/day, occasionally higher
  Monitoring parameters:
    Mental status
    Decrease in nystagmus, peripheral neuropathies; more than 10 days
      of therapy is unwarranted
Vitamin K (phytonadione) (AquaMethyton preferred)
  Reason: prevent bleeding secondary to decreased production of factors
    II, VII, IX, and X (vitamin K–dependent factors)
  Dose: 10–15 mg/day, not to exceed 3 doses
  Monitoring parameters:
    Hypersensitivity—fever, chills, anaphylaxis, flushing, sweating
    Prothrombin time
Spironolactone
  Reason: diuresis in ascites; specific for antagonism of preexisting hy-
    peraldosteronism
  Dose: 200–400 mg/day, occasionally higher; may be given as a single
    daily dose
  Monitoring parameters:
    Weight (avoid more than 1-kg weight loss per day)
    Mental status
    Serum K^+
    Urine Na^+ and K^+ (Na^+ should exceed K^+ at therapeutic doses)
    Abdominal girth
    BUN (increases in dehydration)
    Gynecomastia—prolonged use
    Blood pressure
Loop diuretics
  Reason: diuresis in ascites after failure of high-dose spironolactone
  Dose: start at 40mg, titrate to 1-kg weight loss per day; occasionally
    very high doses (200–600 mg/day) required
  Monitoring parameters:
    Same as spironolactone except urine electrolytes of no value
    Possible hearing loss with rapid IV bolus
Vasopressin
  Reason: vasoconstrictor for esophageal bleeding
  Dose: 0.2–0.4 u/min IV infusion
  Monitoring parameters:
    Rate of GI bleeding
    Signs of ischemia—chest pain, elevated blood pressure, bradycardia
    GI cramping
    Serum Na^+
Sodium tetradecyl sulfate or ethanolamine oleate
  Reason: sclerosing agent for esophageal bleeding
  Dose: 0.5–2 ml of 1 to 1.5% tetradecyl or 5% ethanolamine solution
    into each varix about 2 cm apart
  Monitoring parameters:
    Signs of GI bleeding
    Chest pain, fever, local ulceration

Propranolol
  Reason: prevent GI bleeding
  Dose: 40–320 mg/day
  Monitoring parameters:
    Signs of GI bleeding
    Mental changes
    Vital signs: pulse >60; BP >100/70
    Signs of congestive heart failure, bradycardia
    Signs of bronchospasm
    Renal function
Lactulose
  Reason: hepatic encephalopathy; converted to lactic acid to lower
    bowel pH and prevent absorption of NH_3
  Dose: 20–30 g q.i.d. or to 3–4 soft stools per day
  Monitoring parameters:
    Mental status, liver flap
    Diarrhea
Neomycin
  Reason: hepatic encephalopathy; sterilizes gut to prevent bacterial
    breakdown of protein and thus decreases serum NH_3 levels
  Dose: 2–6 g/day, orally or rectally
  Monitoring parameters:
    Mental status, liver flap
    Diarrhea, bacterial overgrowth
    Renal function
    Signs of ototoxicity
Hepatamine and Hepatic-Aid[a]
  Reason: hepatic encephalopathy; replace branched-chain amino acids
  Dose: Titrate to caloric and nitrogen needs
  Monitoring parameters:
    Mental status
    Serum ammonia, CSF glutamine
    Serum amino acid levels (BCAA:AAA ratio)
    Electrolyte balance
Dopamine[a]
  Reason: hepatorenal syndrome
  Dose: 1–4 µg/kg/min
  Monitoring parameters:
    Mental status, liver flap
    Urine output
    Blood pressure
Colchicine[a]
  Investigational use only; efficacy unclear
  Reason: antiinflammatory and antifibrotic effects
  Dose: 0.6 mg p.o. b.i.d. or 1 mg p.o. q.d. 5 days/week
  Monitoring parameters:
    Nausea, abdominal pain, diarrhea

[a] Not recommended for all patients.

either vitamin K₃ (mendadione) or vitamin K₄ (menadiol). When giving vitamin K parenterally, the subcutaneous or i.m. route is preferred, but it may also be given by very slow IV infusion in 50 ml of 5% dextrose in water (D₅W) over 15 to 20 min. I.M. injections are contraindicated if the patient has a prolonged prothrombin time or thrombocytopenia. Since phytonadione is a colloidal suspension, there is a small risk of development of fever, chills, and even anaphylactic reactions with rapid IV injection. If the patient is malabsorbing fats, menadiol is the vitamin K of choice for oral administration, since it is water-soluble and is absorbed independent of bile acids.

Ascites

The reversal of ascites is a time-consuming process requiring weeks and even months of conservative management including bed rest, salt restriction (500 mg to 2 g/day), and in some cases, fluid restriction. Approximately 5% of patients will have a spontaneous diuresis with bed rest alone, and another 10 to 25% will respond to salt restriction (6). Fluid restriction is warranted only in cases of hyponatremia, since excessive fluid restriction may lead to decreased renal blood flow and azotemia.

Diuresis is the cornerstone of drug therapy of ascites, but the diuresis must be slow. If urinary losses exceed the volume of fluid reabsorbed from ascites or peripheral edema, volume depletion with hypotension and renal insufficiency can ensue. In patients treated with sodium restriction alone, no more than 300 ml of ascites can be reabsorbed per day, and even with the use of a diuretic, the maximum rate of reabsorption is 750 to 1440 ml per 24 hours (11, 12). Diuresis should be limited to 0.2 to 0.3 kg weight loss per day in those without edema and 1 kg per day in patients with edema (6). Others allow a slightly more liberal diuresis of 0.75 to 2 kg weight loss per day (12). These recommendations assume that each liter of volume lost is equivalent to a 1-kg weight loss. In patients with concurrent peripheral edema, a greater diuresis may be acceptable for the first 1 to 2 days because peripheral edema equilibrates more readily with the vasculature than does ascitic fluid. Other monitoring parameters include volume of urine output, changes in abdominal girth, postural blood pressures, BUN (avoiding prerenal azotemia), and changes in mental status.

Although slow diuresis with any diuretic is acceptable for the treatment of ascites, the first diuretic given is usually *spironolactone (Aldactone)*. It is a gentle, slow-acting diuretic, specific for antagonizing the effects of the hyperaldosteronism that exists in many of these patients. In contrast to the small doses of spironolactone used as an adjunct in hypertension, the dose in ascites is begun at 50 to 100 mg per day. A several-day lag period exists for the onset and maximum response from spironolactone, so frequent dose adjustments should be avoided. Doses are ti-

trated upward in 50- to 100-mg intervals every 3 to 5 days with 400 mg per day being needed eventually in 75% of patients. Even greater doses, up to 1 g per day, have been used, but this is expensive and other diuretics are usually added before doses of this magnitude are tried. The delayed onset and long duration of spironolactone is due to the long half-life of its active metabolite, canrenone. For patients convenience, once-daily dosing should be recommended. Multiple daily doses are not necessary unless the patient cannot swallow the required number of tablets without gastric distress. Triamterene (Dyrenium) or amiloride (Midamor) may be slightly more rapid in onset, but they are not specific aldosterone inhibitors. Clinically, they are probably equal in effect to spironolactone, although the response of ascites to these drugs in comparison with spironolactone has not been studied.

Beside the general monitoring parameters cited above for diuretic therapy, serum and urine electrolyte levels, especially potassium, must be monitored. If hyperaldosteronism is present, it is not uncommon to see very small or nonexistent urinary sodium excretion and exceedingly large urinary potassium losses. One measure of having achieved the desired spironolactone dose is a reversal of the urine electrolyte pattern to normal (i.e., sodium loss greater than potassium loss). Patients with urine sodium-to-potassium ratios greater than 1 tend to respond to lower dosages of spironolactone (100 to 150 mg/day); those with ratios less than one (<1) often require larger doses, averaging 400 mg/day (6).

Hyperaldosteronism, if present may also cause a reduction in serum potassium concentration. While the use of spironolactone with potassium supplements is nearly always contraindicated in treatment of other diseases because of a high risk of inducing hyperkalemia, this combination may be necessary early in the treatment of ascites, especially if the patient has GI losses of potassium secondary to vomiting or diarrhea. Serum potassium must be monitored daily to avoid either hypo- or hyperkalemia. Long-term use of spironolactone can lead to gynecomastia, a problem that is frequently present in cirrhosis independent of diuretic use.

High spironolactone doses may fail to produce the desired diuresis in some patients or may cause hyperkalemia. In these situations, the addition of more potent diuretics such as thiazides and loop diuretics may be warranted. The dose should be started low, 50 mg per day of hydrochlorthiazide or 20 to 40 mg per day of furosemide, and gradually increased. Some patients are especially refractory, requiring several hundred milligrams per day of furosemide to obtain the desired 0.5 to 1 kg per day weight loss. One drawback to the use of thiazides and loop diuretics is that they cause a significant natriuresis, which negates the value of monitoring urine electrolytes.

Paracentesis (aspiration of peritoneal fluid with a

needle), except for removal of small volumes (250 to 1500 ml) to decrease pain and respiratory distress from abdominal stretching has traditionally been discouraged because of the risk of abdominal perforation and introduction of infection. Of greater concern is that if large volumes are removed, 15 to 100% (mean 58%) of the fluid reaccumulates over the next 24 to 48 hr, leading to transient hypovolemia and the possibility of shock, encephalopathy, or acute renal failure (11).

Recently, however, the combination of therapeutic paracentesis with intravenous albumin infusions (to hold volume in the vascular space) has become an accepted mode of therapy (13, 14). A typical regimen is removal of 4 to 6 liters per day via paracentesis, with replacement of 40 to 50 gm of albumin after each tap. Paracentesis with albumin replacement is superior to diuretic therapy; it decreases ascites faster and shortens hospital stay without significant worsening of hepatic, renal, or cardiovascular function. Single large-volume (5 liter) paracentesis without albumin replacement also appears to be safe in patients with painful, tense ascites (15); but repeated large volume paracentesis without albumin replacement may result in hyponatremia or renal impairment in some patients (14). One other possible concern over paracentesis is an increased risk of spontaneous bacterial peritonitis secondary to reduced ascitic fluid opsonic activity (16). Arguments about the high cost of albumin are counterbalanced by decreased hospitalization time. Albumin has also been used without paracentesis in an attempt to increase intravascular volume and to induce diuresis. The drawbacks to this treatment are a short duration of response, the risk of inducing variceal hemorrhage, and high cost. Generally, treatment with albumin without paracentesis is to be avoided unless all other therapies have failed. In Europe, ascites recirculation with removal, concentration, and reinfusion of peritional fluid has been found to be safe and effective (17).

A *peritoneovenous shunt* (*LeVeen shunt*) has been devised for use in refractory cases of ascites (18, 19). This consists of a surgically implanted one-way valve in the abdominal wall, an intraabdominal cannula, and an outflow tube tunneled subcutaneously from the valve to a vein that empties directly into the inferior vena cava. As the diaphragm descends, the pressure in the intrathoracic veins drops, and intraperitoneal pressure rises. This pressure differential pumps the ascitic fluid into the venous system. The results may be dramatic, with urine output as high as 15 liters occurring during the first 24 hours. Supplemental diuresis with furosemide may be required to prevent vascular overload. However, use of this procedure is limited by such complications as fever, shunt occlusions, hypokalemia, infection, shunt leaks, disseminated intravascular coagulopathy (DIC), and (less frequently) variceal hemorrhage, bowel obstruction, pulmonary edema, and pneu-

mothorax (18). A Veterans Administration Cooperative study involving 300 patients demonstrated no improved survival and significant morbidity in patients treated with peritoneovenous shunt compared with diuretic therapy (19). However, shunting alleviated disabling ascites more rapidly than medical management.

GI Bleeding

Bleeding from esophageal varices is a grave sign and may be difficult to stop. It often requires multiple transfusions. Even if the bleeding is stopped, the chances of the patient hemorrhaging again are high. Placement of a four-lumen balloon tube (Sengstaken-Blakemore tube) to slow the bleeding by compression is sometimes tried, with varied results. This procedure is complicated by vomiting and a high rate of aspiration or recurrence of bleeding as soon as the balloon is deflated.

Injecting sclerosing agents into esophageal varices is receiving increased interest (20–25). Although not a new technique, *sclerotherapy* remained impractical until the widespread availability of the flexible, fiberoptic esophagoscope in the 1970s. Percutaneous transhepatic sclerotherapy or embolization is a major operative procedure involving insertion of a catheter into the gastric and coronary veins via initial entry into the portal vein. Hypertonic glucose or Gel Foam is then injected into the vessels to obliterate them and prevent flow to the esophageal vessels. A less invasive procedure involves direct injection of bleeding varices with a sclerosing agent via an endoscope (esophagoscope). The most commonly used sclerosants in the United States are *sodium tetradecyl sulfate (Sotradecol)* and *ethanolamine oleate (Ethamolin)*. Sodium morrhuate has been used in Europe and investigationally in the U.S. Injection of these agents into a bleeding varix leads to intense inflammatory response, thrombus formation, and cessation of bleeding within 2 to 5 min. A more permanent fibrotic obliteration of the vessel will develop over several days.

Sclerotherapy controls acute variceal bleeding in 90 to 95% of patients, nearly twice the rate of benefit achieved with either balloon tamponade or vasopressin (20). A single treatment controls bleeding in 90% of subjects, with the remainder requiring one or more repeated treatments over several weeks. Success rates are lower in patients who are treated while actively bleeding, as opposed to controlling bleeding initially by more conservative methods. Compared with portacaval and splenorenal shunt procedures, sclerotherapy is almost equally effective in stopping bleeding, there is no difference in survival, and much lower morbidity (22, 23). Prophylactic sclerotherapy in patients with endoscopic evidence of varices, but with no history of past or current bleeding, is of no apparent clinical benefit (24, 25).

A 1% solution of tetradecyl for injection is prepared

by mixing 1 part saline, 1 part absolute alcohol and 1 part of commercially prepared 3% tetradecyl. Alternatively, a 1.5% solution can be prepared by combining 10 ml 50% dextrose plus 10 ml of 3% tetradecyl. Ethanolamine comes mixed in 5% 2-ml ampules. After passing the endoscope, approximately 0.5 to 2 ml of sclerosing solution is injected into each varix at points about 2 cm apart. If bleeding recurs, therapy can be repeated. While it appears that sclerotherapy is effective in stopping acute bleeding and in preventing rebleeding, compared with more conventional therapy, over 50% of patients rebleed and long-term mortality does not decrease. Side effects associated with sclerotherapy include pericarditis, cardiac tamponade, formation of esophagobronchial fistulae, fever, and local ulcerations.

Following sclerotherapy, prophylaxis with antacids, histamine 2 (H_2) antgonists and/or sucralfate may be initiated. Dosing of these drugs is the same as that recommended for treatment of peptic ulcer disease or reflux esophagitis (see Chapter 21 "Acid Peptic Disorders"). An unapproved method of administering sucralfate to prevent ulcers at the sclerosis site is as a suspension (26). Until a commercial suspension is marketed, the product must be prepared extemporaneously. Twelve 1-g tablets are ground by a pestle in a mortar and then suspended with 20 to 30 ml of 70% sorbitol. Sterile water is added to yield a total volume of 120 ml. Alternatively, the tablets can be placed directly in water and shaken until completely dissolved. Although easier to prepare, aqueous solutions may not be as occlusive as the sorbitol preparation. The products are stable for 2 weeks with refrigeration. One gram (10 ml) is sipped four times daily. Investigators using endoscopy have shown that the drug complex coats the varices and decreases ulcer formation (26).

The natural hormone vasopressin (also known as antidiuretic hormone or ADH) was frequently used to treat bleeding varices before the advent of sclerotherapy. Vasopressin significantly decreases portal blood flow and pressure by constricting portal and other splanchnic arterioles. This slows or stops bleeding long enough to allow thrombus formation at the site of bleeding. The use of this drug is declining and remains controversial as the benefits in morbidity and mortality have never been clearly proven (27). Sclerotherapy has been shown consistently to be more effective than vasopressin, but vasopression may be given first to slow bleeding and make visualization of bleeding varices by endoscope easier.

The major limitation to vasopressin therapy is side effects. The intense vasoconstrictor action decreases cardiac output and may cause coronary ischemia. This is especially a problem in patients with coronary artery disease or hypertension, but ECG changes have also been reported in patients with no prior evidence of heart disease (43). Bradycardia due to stimulation of the vagus nerve is the most widely observed side effect of vasopressing (27). It also may produce skin blanching, GI cramping, and even bowel necrosis due to stimulation of smooth muscle contraction. Women may experience uterine pain similar to menstrual cramps. Finally, vasopressin may lead to excess water retention and a dilutional hyponatremia (27).

In an attempt to reduce toxicity, continuous intravenous infusions starting at 0.2 to 0.4 unit per min or direct intraarterial infusion via a catheter into the superior mesenteric artery at 0.05 to 0.4 unit per min have been tried (27). The maximum recommended intravenous infusion rate is 0.9 units per min. Infusions may be continued for up to 72 hr with a slow tapering of the dose over time. The results have been varied, with some authors claiming up to 50 to 70% effectiveness (27). Others claim poor response and a high incidence of complications, including bleeding from the site of catheter insertion and septicemia (28).

A combination of vasopressin infusion and intravenous nitroglycerin (40 μg/min titrated according to blood pressure to a maximum of 400 μg/min) (29) or sublingual nitroglycerin (0.6 mg every 30 min for 6 hr) (30) may cause an additional decrease in portal pressure. In the study using intravenous nitroglycerin, there was less bleeding in the combination therapy group; while in the trial with sublingual nitroglycerin, the rate of bleeding cessation was equal to that with vasopression alone. In both studies, combination therapy led to a marked reduction in cardiac complications.

Bleeding from other GI sites, especially that due to gastritis and peptic ulcer, is usually treated with nasogastric suction, iced saline, H_2 antagonists and hourly antacids. Occasionally 20 units of vasopressin or 1 to 2 ampules of norepinephrine are used in a gastric lavage to cause localized vasoconstriction in an attempt to slow the bleeding. No evidence documents these latter maneuvers to be any more effective than antacids or H_2 antagonists alone.

It has been suggested that since propranolol and other β-adrenergic blockers decrease portal venous pressure, they may prevent gastrointestinal bleeding associated with portal hypertension (31–36). Primary therapy is defined as treatment of patients with known varices, but without a history of active bleeding. Secondary intervention is administration of the drug following resolution of an acute bleeding episode. Although data are still somewhat limited, overall analysis of the benefit of primary therapy is positive (31–33). For example, in the European Cooperative study group, a median dose of 160 mg per day (range 40 to 320 mg) led to a cumulative 74% of patients in the propranolol group who were free of bleeding after 2 years, compared with 39% in the placebo group. Two-year survival was 72% in the treated patients and 37% in the untreated subjects (33).

The results for secondary prophylaxis are also encouraging, but somewhat more complex. Lebrec (34) showed that oral propranolol in doses that reduced the heart rate by 25% significantly reduced the frequency of rebleeding, compared with placebo, during a 2-year study in chronic alcoholics with a history of prior esophageal bleeding. Only 21% of patients in the propranolol group had recurrence of bleeding, compared with 68% in the placebo group. Cumulative survival was 90% in the propranolol group and 57% in the placebo group. None of the patients showed deterioration of hepatic or renal function while taking propranolol, but because propranolol may decrease cardiac output and liver blood flow, patients should be monitored closely.

A similar study by Burroughs et al. (35) failed to confirm the findings of Lebrec. However, the patients in Burrough's study had more severe liver disease and included some with cirrhosis from causes other than chronic alcoholism. Selective β-blockade with atenolol or metoprolol is less effective than sclerotherapy in arresting acute variceal bleeding (31, 32).

A follow-up study by Poynard and Lebrec (36) confirms the benefits of propranolol, with 71% of subjects free of bleeding at 1 year and 57% in 2 years. In this study, five factors were identified that increased the risk of rebleeding: hepatocellular carcinoma, continued alcohol abuse, lack of suppression of pulse rate by propranolol, a previous history of rebleeding, and noncompliance with drug therapy. Of particular concern, 12 of 14 (86%) patients who discontinued β-blocker therapy abruptly rebled. The time of greatest risk for rebleeding is within the first 3 to 4 days of stopping therapy, but it may occur up to 150 days later (31, 32, 36–38). It is not possible to be certain that drug discontinuation is responsible for rebleeding in those cases where the occurrence is delayed.

Surgical treatment may be required for patients who have repeated GI bleeding (especially esophageal varices) or those who have bleeding that cannot be stopped by the more conservative measures already described (20). A *portacaval shunt* involves anastomosis of the portal vein directly to the inferior vena cava, thus bypassing the cirrhotic liver. This decreases portal hypertension and lowers backpressure on the abdominal venous system. Unfortunately, these patients have a poor prognosis since the only way to carry toxins to the liver for detoxification is now the hepatic artery. If they survive the initial surgery, patients may die of sepsis or develop hepatic failure and enephalopathy. The Warren shunt decompresses varices by shunting splenic blood flow to the renal vein (splenorenal shunt) and may decrease hepatic perfusion less.

Hepatic Encephalopathy

If the patient develops signs of an impending hepatic coma (e.g., confusion, drowsiness, asterixis), lactulose is indicated, and dietary protein should be decreased to 20 to 30 g per day. Use of CNS depressants should be minimized. Diuretics should be withheld at this stage, since hypovolemia, hypokalemia, and metabolic alkalosis tend to aggravate encephalopathy.

Lactulose is a synthetic disaccharide of galactose and fructose, which is neither absorbed nor hydrolyzed in the small bowel. It is degraded by colonic bacteria to lactic, acetic, and formic acids, thus decreasing the pH of the colonic contents to about 5.5. The effect of lactulose was originally attributed to replacement of proteolytic bacteria such as *Escherichia coli*, *Proteus* and *Bacteroides* with organisms like *Lactobacillus*, that thrive in a more acidic medium and lack urease and other enzymes used in the production of ammonia. However, most investigators cannot demonstrate a marked change in the colonic flora and attribute the effects of lactulose solely to the pH changes that occur. As the colon becomes more acidic, the ratio of ammonium ion to ammonia increases, and less absorption of the ammonia occurs. There may also be back-diffusion of ammonia from the blood to the intestinal lumen under acidic pH conditions. In any event, lactulose therapy results in a decrease in arterial ammonium levels (39).

Each 15 ml of lactulose contain 10 g of lactulose, and it is usually given in a dose of 30 to 45 ml, 3 to 4 times daily. Use of retention enemas (40) of 300 ml of 50% lactulose diluted to 700 to 1000 ml with tap water has also been reported. Onset of effect by either route is 12 to 48 hr. Once improved mental state has been achieved, the dose can be tapered slowly to identify the smallest effective dose. Patient tolerance may be improved by diluting the drug in fruit juice or carbonated beverages. In most patients, lactulose may be discontinued after several days to a few weeks if the patient's mental status improves. In a few patients, prolonged therapy for months or years may be required if discontinuation of the drug causes a recurrence of symptoms.

The most common complaints of patients treated with lactulose are nausea (because of the sweet taste of the drug), gaseous distension, bloating, belching, or diarrhea caused by osmotic effects in the bowel. Diarrhea may account for part of the therapeutic effects of lactulose (41), but compared with sorbitol, lactulose is more effective in overcoming the encephalopathy, indicating that other mechanisms are working. The dose is usually adjusted so that the patient has two to three soft, semiformed stools daily, but watery diarrhea is avoided. Of course, if the patient's mental state improves at a dose that produces fewer than 2 to 3 stools per day, it is not logical to give a larger dose.

The success rate with lactulose has been reported to be around 85%. Unfortunately, a few patients become resistant after prolonged therapy, and others die from complications of the disease, even though their encephalopathy has cleared. Fluid losses secondary to diarrhea should be considered when monitoring lactulose therapy. Serum sodium should be monitored to detect hyponatremia associated with loss of free water from osmotic diarrhea.

An alternative to lactulose is neomycin in doses of 1 to 2 g four times daily. Neomycin destroys colonic bacteria which slows the degradation of protein to ammonia. If the patient does not respond, the dose of the neomycin should be increased to 8 to 12 g per day and the protein restriction lowered to 0 to 20 g per day. For those unable to take medications orally, a retention enema of 2 to 4 g of neomycin in 200 ml of saline thickened with methylcellulose may be used morning and night. When the patient improves, the maintenance dose of neomycin may be lowered to 2 to 4 g per day.

The duration of therapy varies with both lactulose and neomycin and may last for less than 1 week in most cases or up to months and even years in poorly controlled patients. The importance of protein restriction cannot be overemphasized. Many patients who look well compensated can rapidly deteriorate after eating a single high-protein meal.

One well-controlled study (42) failed to show a clear superiority of either neomycin (83% effective) or lactulose (90% effective) in the treatment of acute encephalopathy. For long-term use lactulose has the potential advantage of less toxicity, but it is considerably more expensive. The possibility that sterilization of the gut by neomycin might decrease the effectiveness of lactulose appears to be of minimal consequence (43); in fact the two drugs have added effectiveness when used together (44).

Neomycin is considered a "nonabsorbable" antibiotic. However, from 1 to 3% of a dose is absorbed (45), and there are several reported cases of ototoxicity in patients on chronic oral neomycin therapy (46). Most of these patients had been taking neomycin for at least 8 months and had coexisting renal dysfunction. Annual auditory testing should be performed and the patient observed for subjective changes in hearing status if the drug is to be used for prolonged periods.

Neomycin has also been implicated in development of the hepatorenal syndrome. Although neomycin is renal toxic when given parenterally, it is difficult to determine if the renal changes with oral dosing are drug induced or a progression of the disease process itself. The consensus is that the latter mechanism prevails.

Another consequence of neomycin therapy is diarrhea from changes in the bowel flora. This may not be a serious problem, since patients are often given cathartics to cleanse the bowel and eliminate excess ammonia. However, cathartics alone are not effective in moderating encephalopathy, and they should always be accompanied by lactulose or neomycin and protein restriction. Since cathartics can cause fluid and electroyte imbalance, they may worsen encephalopathy. Adequate intravenous infusions of dextrose or saline with potassium supplements be maintained.

Branched-Chain Amino Acids

One of the goals of management of progressive liver disease is to provide adequate nutritional support, including protein and calories. Positive nitrogen balance must be established without exacerbating hepatic encephalopathy caused by giving inappropriate combinations of amino acids. In experimental animals and to a lesser extent in humans, administration of diets high in branched-chain amino acids and low in aromatic amino acids and methionine may help restore normal amino acid balance and reduce encephalopathy (7–9, 47). An 8% amino acid solution (Hepatamine) is marketed that contains more branched-chain amino acids than standard parenteral nutrition solutions. The ratio of BCAAs to AAAs in *Hepatamine* is 37:1, compared with 5:1 in conventional crystalline amino acid solutions. Mixing 500 ml of Hepatamine with 500 ml of 50% dextrose in water yields 40 g/liter of amino acids. Indications for use of this therapy and its efficacy are debated. The high cost and questionable efficacy of Hepatamine (compared with more conventional therapy) has led most institutions to limit the use of branched-chain amino acid solutions to patients with life-threatening encephalopathy refractory to conventional therapy and those with documented elevated serum ammonia and CSF glutamine levels. In most cases an amino acid screen is used to assess the ratio of BCAA:AAA in the patient. The cost of an amino acid screen is approximately equal to one day's therapy with Hepatamine.

For the alert patient without central venous access, enteral therapy has been proposed. One such dietary supplement is *Hepatic-aid*, a complex of carbohydrate, protein, and fat in a readily digestible form. One package of Hepatic-aid mixed in a blender with 250 ml of water yields 340 ml of suspension for oral or nasogastric administration, which contains 2.2 g of nitrogen (15 g protein), 98 g of carbohydrate, 12 g of fat, and 560 calories (500 nonprotein calories). One to four packages may be given per day, but the administration rate should be slow at first to prevent glucose overload. Use of oral branched-chain amino acids is discouraged because of questionable efficacy, high cost, and disagreeable taste.

Benzodiazepine Receptor Antagonists

As introduced in the section on clinical findings and diagnosis, some investigators believe that endogenous or exogenous GABA-ergic-like compounds that stimulate the GABA-benzodiazepine receptor complex in the brain may be responsible for symptoms of encephalopathy (10). Preliminary data suggest that the benzodiazepine antagonist, flumazenil, may be valuable in both short-term and long-term management of encephalopathy. In a series of 14 subjects, 71% of patients had short-term improvement in symptoms after intravenous administration of flumazenil (48). Arousal was greatest in patients with deeper coma (stage III to IV encephalopathy). Although response was rapid, the duration of effect was only 1 to 2 hr with parenteral therapy. The usual dose was 0.2 to 0.4 mg, with some subjects receiving up to ten doses. A single case report describes long-term use of oral therapy (49). A patient given 25 mg twice daily experienced complete reversal of symptoms for 14 months. Previously, this patient had experienced 12 attacks of coma over a 2-year period. Discontinuation of the drug led to a recurrence of symptoms within 48 hr. Benzodiazepine receptor antagonist therapy remains investigational, and flumazenil is not commercially available.

Dopamine

Dopamine and norepinephrine are important mediators of normal sympathetic activity in both the central nervous system and in the periphery, especially in the kidney. Some of the neurological manifestations of hepatic failure, as well as the hepatorenal syndrome, may be due to accumulation of other β-hydroxylated phenylethylamines such as octopamine and serotonin. These compounds may replace normal transmitters and act as false neurotransmitters in sympathetic nerve terminals and granules. Precursors of false neurotransmitters, such as phenylalanine and tyrosine (Fig. 26-1), are produced from protein in the gut by bacterial amino acid decarboxylases. Normally these precursors are metabolized rapidly in the liver by monoamine oxidase (MAO), allowing norepinephrine that is formed elsewhere in the body to predominate. When hepatic function is impaired or when blood is shunted away from the liver, these false neurotransmitters may replace normal transmitters. Systemically this may lead to lowered peripheral vascular resistance and shunting of blood away

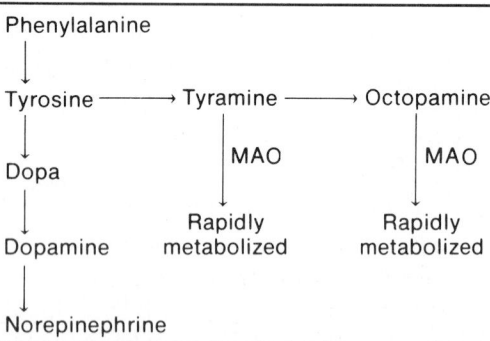

Figure 26.1. Synthetic pathway of neurotransmitters. Monoamine oxidase (MOA) action occurs mainly in the liver and is depressed in hepatic disease and shunting.

from the kidney. Similarly, asterixis and other signs of hepatic encephalopathy might result from displacement of transmitters such as dopamine and norepinephrine in the basal ganglia and other areas in the brain.

If the displacement of normal central and peripheral transmitters by less active amines can account for hepatic coma and its cardiovascular complications, then the restoration of normal transmitter stores might restore normal function. For hospitalized patients this is accomplished by administering low-dose infusions of dopamine (1 to 4 μg/kg/min). This may increase renal blood flow and help reverse the hepatorenal syndrome. Unfortunately, the mortality rate of persons with the hepatorenal syndrome approaches 100%, even in those who receive dopamine. Failure to improve urine output or increase blood pressure within the first 24 hours of dopamine treatment is a poor prognostic sign. Since dopamine does not cross the blood-brain barrier, encephalopathy may not be helped. However by referring to Figure 26.1, it can be seen that dopamine is also a precursor to norepinephrine, which may help to restore natural neurotransmitter balance in a second way.

Primary Biliary Cirrhosis: Colchicine and Other Drugs

Colchicine, a drug with both antiinflammatory and antifibrotic properties has been evaluated as a potential disease-modifying agent for several years. In one study, 57 patients with biopsy-proven primary biliary cirrhosis were treated with either 0.6 mg of colchicine twice daily or placebo (50). The colchicine-treated patients had significant improvement in biochemical parameters (serum bilirubin and transferase levels), but no difference (compared with placebo) in histological progression. A second group of investigators conducted a randomized, double-blind, placebo-controlled trial of colchicine, 1 mg per day, 5 days per week, in 100 patients with cirrhosis caused by alcohol abuse or a prior history of hepatitis (51). Median survival improved from 3.5 years in the placebo group to 11 years in the colchicine-treated patients, and deaths from liver failure were reduced from 24% in the placebo group to 15% in the treatment group. Side effects in both trials were mild, primarily consisting of nausea, abdominal pain, and diarrhea. Although these results are encouraging, flaws in the study design and the relatively small number of subjects treated prevent widespread endorsement of colchicine therapy at this time.

Numerous other drugs have been tried in the treatment of primary biliary cirrhosis including penicillamine, chlorombial, azathioprine, cyclosporin, corticosteroids, and methotrexate (52). Each of these therapies is based on the hope that antiinflammatory or immunmodulating effects may alter the disease process. In addition, sequestration of copper by penicillamine may have a therapeutic effect. Unfortunately, most of the trials with these drugs have either been limited by a small sample size without adequate controls or the improvement obtained has only been marginal. At this time, none of these drugs can be recommended.

PROGNOSIS

The outlook for patients with cirrhosis depends entirely upon the stage of the disease and the presence of complications. If the cause of the cirrhosis is alcoholism and the patient continues to drink, the prognosis is poor; conversely discontinuation of drinking increases survival. In one large series of 1155 patients with cirrhosis from a variety of causes, the overall 5-year survival was about 40% (53). The causes of death were liver failure in 49%, hepatocellular carcinoma in 22%, bleeding in 14%, hepatorenal syndrome in 8%, and other causes in the remainder. Patients who entered the study with compensated cirrhosis (mild or absent symptoms) became symptomatic at the rate of 10% per year. Survival was higher in this groups of patients, 54% at 6 years. Persons who entered the study with symptoms already present (ascites, history of bleeding, or encephalopathy) had a survival rate of only 21% at 6 years and a much higher incidence of hepatocellular carcinoma. In the United States, cirrhosis has become one of the 5 most frequent causes of death in persons over the age of 40 (3).

CONCLUSION

Despite extensive investigation of liver function and pathologies, there is no effective therapy for many liver diseases. At best only symptomatic management of the complications of chronic liver disease is possible. However, although the lesions of advanced cirrhosis are irreversible, it is estimated that 70% or more of liver tissue must be destroyed before the body is unable to eliminate drugs and toxins via the liver (54). Unfortunately it is difficult to tell which patients have reached this stage of involvement, so practitioners should always be aware of the potential inability of patients with advanced liver disease to excrete certain drugs and adjust doses accordingly.

REFERENCES

1. Cotran R, Kumar V, Robbins S: Pathological Basis of Disease, ed. 4. Philadelphia: WB Saunders, 1989, pp 941–957.
2. Rubin E, Lieber C: Fatty liver, alcoholic hepatitis, and cirrhosis produced by alcohol in primates. N Engl J Med 290:128, 1974.
3. Anon: Trends in mortality from cirrhosis and alcoholism—United States. MMWR 35:703–705, 1983.
4. World Health Statistics Annual. Geneva: World Health Organization, 1985.
5. Schrier R, Arroyo V, Bernardi M, et al.: Peripheral arterial vasodilation hypothesis: a proposal for the initiation of renal sodium and water retention in cirrhosis. Hepatology 8:1151–1157, 1988.
6. Rocco V, Ware A: Cirrhotic ascites; pathophysiology, diagnosis, and management. Ann Intern Med 105:573–585, 1986.
7. Fraser C, Arieff A: Hepatic encephalopathy. N Engl J Med 313:869–873, 1985.
8. Bode J, Shafer K: Pathophysiology of chronic hepatic encephalopathy. Hepatogastronenterology 32:259–255, 1985.
9. Sax H, Talamini M, Fischer J: Clinical use of branched-chain amino acids in liver disease, sepsis, trauma and burns. Arch Surg 121:358–366, 1986.
10. Basile A, Gammal S: Evidence for the involvement of benzodiazepine receptor complex in hepatic encephalopathy; Implications for treatment with benzodiazepine receptor anatgonists. Clin Neuropharmacol 11:401–422, 1988.
11. Shear L, Ching S, Gabuzda G: Compartmentalization of ascites and edema in patients with hepatic cirrhosis. N Engl J Med 282:1391–1396, 1970.
12. Pockros P, Reynolds T: Rapid diuresis in patients with ascites from chronic liver disease: the importance of peripheral edema. Gastroenterology 90:1827–1833, 1986.
13. Gines P, Arroyo V, Quintero E, et al.: Comparison of paracentesis and diuretics in the treatment of cirrhotics with tense ascites; results of a randomized study. Gastroenterology 93:234–241, 1987.
14. Gines P, Tito L, Arroyo V, et al.: Randomized comparative study of therapeutic paracentesis with and without intravenous albumin in cirrhosis. Gastroenterology 94:1493–1502, 1988.
15. Pinto P, Amerian J, Reynolds T: Large-volume paracentesis in nonedematous patients with tense ascites: its effect on intravascular volume. Hepatology 8:207–210, 1988.
16. Runyon B, Antillon M, Montano A: Effect of diuresis versus therapeutic paracentesis on ascitic fluid opsonic activity and serum complement. Gastroenterology 97:158–162, 1989.
17. Smart H, Triger D: A randomised prospective trial comparing daily paracentesis and intravenous albumin with recirculation in diuretic refratory ascites. J Hepatol 10:191–197, 1990.
18. Epstein M: Peritoneovenous shunt in the management of ascites and the hepatorenal syndrome. Gastroenterology 82:790–799, 1980.
19. Stanley M, Ochi S, Lee K, et al.: Peritoneovenous shunting as compared with medical treatment in patients with alcoholic cirrhosis and massive asictes. N Engl J Med 321:1632–1638, 1989.
20. Terblanche J, Burroughs A, Hobbs K: Controversies in the management of bleeding esophageal varices. N Engl J Med (part 1) 320:1393–1397, 1989; (part 2) 320:1469–1475, 1989.
21. Cello J, Crass R, Grendell J, et al.: Management of the patient with hemorrhaging esophageal varices. JAMA 256:1480–1484, 1986.
22. Rice T: Treatment of esophageal varices. Clin Pharm, 8:122–131, 1989.
23. Henderson J, Kutner M, Millikan W, et al.: Endoscopic variceal sclerosis compared with distal splenorenal shunt to prevent recurrent variceal bleeding in cirrhosis. Ann Intern Med 112:262–269, 1990.
24. Santangelo W, Dueno M, Estes B, et al.: Prophylactic sclerotherapy of large esophageal varices. N Engl J Med 318:814–816, 1988.
25. Sauerbruch T, Wotzka R, Kopcke W, et al.: Prophylactic sclerotherapy before the first episode of variceal hemorrhage in patients with cirrhosis. N Engl J Med 319:8–15, 1988.
26. Roark G: Treatment of postsclerotherapy esophageal ulcers with sucralfate. Gastrointest Endosc 30:9–10, 1984.
27. Stump D, Hardin T: The use of vasopressin in the treatment of upper gastrointestinal haemorrhage. Drugs 39:38–53, 1990.
28. Fogel M, Knaver C, Andres L, et al.: Continuous intravenous vasopressin in active upper gastrointestinal bleeding: a placebo controlled trial. Ann Intern Med 96:565–569, 1982.
29. Gimson A, Westaby D, Hegarty J, et al.: A randomized trial of vasopressin plus nitroglycerin in the control of acute variceal hemorrhage. Hepatol 6:410–413, 1986.

30. Tsai Y, Lay C, Lai K, et al.: Controlled trial of vasopressin plus nitroglycerin versus vasopression alone in bleeding esophageal varices. Hepatology 6:406–409, 1982.

31. Lewis J, Davis J, Allsopp D, et al.: Beta-blockers in protal hypertension; an overview. Drugs 37:62–69, 1989.

32. Hayes P, Davis J, Lewis J, et al.: Meta-analysis of value of propranolol in prevention of variceal hemorrhage. Lancet 336:153–156, 1990.

33. Pascal J, Cales P, et al.: Propranolol in the prevention of first upper gastrointestinal tract hemorrhage in patients with cirrhosis of the liver and esophageal varices. N Engl J Med 317:856–861, 1987.

34. Lebrec O, Poynard T, Bernuau J, et al.: A randomized controlled study of propranolol for prevention of recurrent gastrointestinal bleeding in patients with cirrhosis. Hepatology 4:355–384, 1984.

35. Burroughs A, Jenkins W, Sherlock S, et al.: Controlled trial of propranolol for the prevention of recurrent gastrointestinal bleeding in patients with cirrhosis. N Engl J Med 309:1539–1542, 1983.

36. Poynard T, Lebrec D, Hillon P, et al.: Propranolol for prevention of recurrent gastroinstestinal bleeding in patients with cirrhosis: a prospective study of factors associated with rebleeding. Hepatol 7:447–451, 1987.

37. Lebrec D, Bemuau J, Rueff B, Benhamou J: Gastrointestinal bleeding after abrupt cessation of propranolol administration in cirrhosis. N Engl J Med 307:560, 1982.

38. Alabaster S, Gogel H, McCarthy D: Propranolol withdrawal and variceal hemorrage. JAMA 250:3047, 1983.

39. Avery GS, Davies EF, Brogden RN: lactulose; a review. Drugs 4:7–48, 1972.

40. Kersh ES, Rifkin H: Lactulose enemas. Ann Intern Med 78:81–84, 1973.

41. Rodgers JB Jr, Kiley JE, Balint JA: Comparison of results of long term treatment of chronic hepatic encephalopathy with lactulose and sorbitol. Am J Gastroenterol 60:459–465, 1973.

42. Conn HO, Leevy CM, Vlahcevic J, et al.: Comparison of lactulose and neomycin in the treatment of chronic portal systemic encepahlopathy. Gastroenterology 72:573, 1977.

43. Conn HO: Interactions of lactulose and neomycin. Drugs 4:4–6, 1972.

44. Weber F, Fresard K, Lally B: Effects of lactulose and neomycin on urea metabolism in cirrhotic subjects. Gastroenterology 82:213–217, 1982.

45. Breen K, Bryant R, Levinson J, et al.: Neomycin absorption in man. Ann Intern Med 76:211–218, 1972.

46. Berk D, Chalmer T: Deafness complicating antibiotic therapy of hepatic encephalopathy. Ann Intern Med 73:393–396, 1970.

47. Horst D, Grace N, Conn H, et al.: Comparison of dietary protein with an oral, branched chain-enriched amino acid supplement in chronic portal-systemic encephalopathy: a randomized controlled trial. Hepatology 4:279–287, 1984.

48. Bansky G, Meier P, Riederer E, et al.: Effects of the benzodiazepine receptor antagonist flumazenil in hepatic encephalopathy in humans. Gastroenterology 97:744–750, 1989.

49. Ferenci P, Grimm G, Meryn S, et al.: Successful long-term treatment of portal-systemic encephalopathy by benzodiazepine antagonist flumazenil. Gastroenterology 96:240–243, 1989.

50. Bodenheimer H, Schaffner F, Pezzullo J: Evaluation of colchicine therapy in primary biliary cirrhosis. Gasteroenterology 95:124–129, 1988.

51. Kershenobich D, Vargas F, Barcia-Tsao G, et al.: Colchicine in the treatment of cirrhosis of the liver. N Engl J Med 318:1709–1713.

52. Stavinoha M, Soloway R. Current therapy of chronic liver disease. Drugs 39:814–840, 1990.

53. D'Amico G, Morabito A, Pagliaro L, Marubini E: Survival and prognostic indicators in compensated and decompensated cirrhosis. Dig Dis Sci 31:468–475, 1986.

54. Bass N, Williams R: Guide to drug dosage in hepatic disease. Clin Pharmacokinet 15:396–420, 1988.

CHAPTER 27

PANCREATITIS

GAIL W. McSWEENEY, Pharm.D.

The pancreas is a gland with complex endocrine and exocrine functions. The substances it manufactures and releases are responsible for transport of glucose across cell membranes, maintenance of serum glucose within the normal range, synthesis of glycogen, gluconeogenesis, and digestion of protein and fat. Pancreatitis is the term used to describe any inflammatory process within the gland. While usually mild and self-limiting, permanent injury or destruction of the gland and surrounding tissues can result if the disease becomes widespread or chronic. To understand the pathophysiology, treatment, and consequences of pancreatitis, it is necessary to understand the normal structure and function of the gland.

PANCREATIC FUNCTION

The pancreas is an elongated gland fixed in the retroperitoneal space by attachment to the duodenum at its head. It extends 20 to 25 cm across the midepigastrium and is subdivided anatomically into the head, neck, body, tail, and uncinate process. It is in close contact with the bile ducts, stomach, spleen, aorta, transverse colon, left adrenal gland and kidney, superior mesenteric artery, portal vein, hepatic artery, and omentum. The pancreas draws its blood supply from the superior mesenteric, gastroduodenal, splenic, and common hepatic arteries. Venous drainage is into the portal, splenic, and superior mesenteric veins. Lymphatic drainage, although not completely understood, appears to be into 12 regional nodal groups. Sympathetic innervation is through the greater, lesser, and lowest splanchnic nerves via the celiac ganglia and plexus; parasympathetic is via the celiac branch of the right vagus. During or following an attack of pancreatitis, any or all of these structures can become inflamed or damaged.

The endocrine function of the pancreas involves glucose metabolism and the synthesis and metabolism of glycogen. The best-understood hormones released by the gland are insulin, glucagon, and somatostatin. In pathologic and neoplastic conditions other substances (e.g., gastrin and parathyroid hormone) can be manufactured by the pancreas, but they are not included in this discussion. Insulin facilitates glucose transport across cell membranes and stimulates glycogen deposition in the liver. Glucagon directs the conversion of glycogen to glucose and the manufacture of "new" glucose (gluconeogenesis) from amino acids. Somatostatin inhibits secretion of insulin and glucagon, decreases GI motility, and reduces the volume of secretion from the pancreas, liver, and gastrointestinal tract (2).

The exocrine pancreas secretes a variety of substances and is second only to the breast during lactation in the amount and range of proteins it manufactures and releases. The secretory unit of the exocrine pancreas is the acinar cell. It contains zymogen granules, which enclose enzymes during the entire process of their synthesis, storage, and transport to the pancreatic duct. Lipase and amylase are released from the zymogen granules in active forms, but the proteolytic enzymes, trypsin, chymotrypsin, and the carboxypeptidases, are activated in the duodenum by enterokinase. Pancreatic enzyme output must fall below 10% of normal before maldigestion and malabsorption become important enough to cause malnutrition. In addition to responding to the gut hormones, enzymes are released in response to vagal stimulation (1). The pancreas secretes large quantities of water and electrolytes in response to the gut hormones secretin and cholecystokinin-pancreozymin. The cells that release water and electrolytes line the pancreatic ductal system extending from the acinar cell clusters to the duodenum. The volume of pancreatic output can be as high as 4 liters per day, with a protein content of 0.1 to 10% by weight. The fluid is isotonic with plasma, having a sodium concentration of 135 mmol/liter (mEq/liter), and the pH (although generally around 8) varies as the gland changes the bicarbonate-chloride ratio of the anions secreted.

ETIOLOGY

The specific cellular insult that leads to pancreatitis remains unknown, and etiologies of the disease are grouped by clinical association rather than by any uniform pancreatic histology. Lacking a unifying hypothesis, the etiologies have been divided arbitrarily into mechanical, metabolic, and infectious groups.

The mechanically based etiologies share the theory that activated enzymes reflux up the pancreatic duct and precipitate the inflammatory process. Duodenal obstruction, blunt abdominal trauma, biliary tract disease, and gallstones (cholelithiasis), alcoholism, and cystic fibrosis are situations in which an extraglandular process may cause pancreatitis. Clinically, 40% of cases of acute pancreatitis occur in patients with biliary tract disease, and 5% of patients with gallstones develop pancreatitis. Similarly, alcohol-induced pancreatitis has proteinaceous plugs obstructing the ductal system of the gland, which disappear when the patient stops drinking (3). Cystic fibrosis is a generalized process that results in pancreatic fibrosis as well as pulmonary insufficiency.

Metabolic processes that cause pancreatitis cover a broad range of seemingly unrelated conditions for which a unifying hypothesis does not exist. Alcoholic pancreatitis is the most common, accounting for 40% of all cases of acute and 90% of chronic pancreatitis. The cellular morphology of alcoholic pancreatitis is diffuse inflammation, periductal fibrosis, and calculi in addition to the protein plugs mentioned above. Alcoholism may cause the disease secondarily, as a result of the hyperlipidemia it often induces. Free pancreatic lipase acts on circulating triglycerides to raise the level of intraglandular free fatty acids, which may damage capillary membranes, with resultant enzyme release and inflammation. Other metabolic causes of pancreatitis include hypercalcemia, familial hyperlipidemia, and Reye's syndrome, but cause-and-effect relationships have not been determined and the number of case reports is low (1).

Few infectious diseases are thought to cause pancreatitis, and they are diverse. Patients with mumps, salmonellosis, hepatitis B, mononucleosis, coxsackie B, and hemolytic streptococcal infections have developed pancreatitis, but with only 1 or 2 case reports per disease, a causal relationship is difficult to establish (4).

More than 80% of all cases of pancreatitis appear to be caused by biliary tract disease and/or alcoholism.

Drug-induced Pancreatitis

The role of drugs in causing or exacerbating pancreatitis remains controversial. The literature often contains a few case reports per drug in which it is difficult to demonstrate an irrefutable causal relationship. Many patients had multiple coexisting diseases (some of which cause pancreatitis) and were receiving numerous medications prior to and during their illnesses.

Several drugs seem to be involved in development of pancreatic inflammation, as pancreatitis recurred when patients were rechallenged with the suspected agent. Corticosteroids are probably the agents most clinicians associate with drug-induced pancreatitis. More than 40 cases of steroid-induced pancreatitis have been reported, many of them in children. This is important because the disease occurs rarely in children, and in most instances, no other etiologic factor (such as cystic fibrosis) could be found. There is also autopsy evidence of incidental pancreatitis in 28 to 40% of patients who had received steroids as part of the therapy for their final illnesses. Many kidney transplant patients reported to have developed pancreatitis with azathioprine had also been receiving high-dose steroid therapy, which further complicates the issue. A patient treated with steroids for bullous pemphigoid died of acute

pancreatitis (5). Another case report describes a patient who redeveloped pancreatitis when rechallenged with steroids (6).

The evidence against steroids causing pancreatitis is that, in many cases, the patients had multiple diseases and treatments that could have caused the disease, but the preponderance of data supports the conclusion that steroids can cause pancreatitis (7, 8). In the National Cooperative Crohn's Disease Study, patients treated with azathioprine as sole therapy had a 6.2% occurrence rate of pancreatitis, which was statistically significant. Symptoms appeared 13 to 21 days after the initiation of therapy and subsided promptly when azathioprine was discontinued (9). Pancreatitis has also been reported frequently in patients taking azathioprine as part of an immunosuppressive regimen.

Sulfonamides and structurally similar agents, such as furosemide and chlorothiazide, appear to cause pancreatitis. Some patients rechallenged with these drugs redeveloped pancreatitis (10, 11). An interesting relationship appears to exist between estrogens, tetracycline, and pancreatic inflammation. Estrogen therapy, either as birth control pills or as postmenopausal replacement therapy, can cause hyperlipidemia, which may secondarily cause pancreatitis. Pancreatitis has not been reported in patients on estrogens who were not simultaneously hyperlipemic. Tetracycline is known to cause fatty necrosis of the liver leading to pancreatitis, but there are two reports of the disease in patients without preexisting liver damage (12).

Didanosine (ddI) is an antiviral agent currently undergoing clinical trials in patients infected with HIV. Doses above 12 mg/kd/day have caused unacceptable toxicity, including an incidence of pancreatitis that may have approached 2% (13). For other drugs, the evidence is less compelling and often confined to reports of a few cases (10, 11, 14). Medications implicated in the development of pancreatitis are listed in Table 27.1.

The clinical conditions and drugs discussed account for approximately 90% of the reported cases of pancreatitis. The remaining 10% are classified as idiopathic.

INCIDENCE

The incidence of pancreatitis varies widely depending on the population studied and the diagnostic criteria applied. The median age of individuals with acute pancreatitis is 53 years, and the disease is closely associated with alcoholism and biliary tract disease. It occurs more often in military personnel, patients in VA hospitals, and urban populations than in the population as a whole. The distribution is equal for men and women, because alcoholism is more common in men and gallbladder disease more common in women. The overall incidence is 3.5 to 36 per 100,000 per year. Death occurs in 10% of patients during an initial acute attack and 1% of the time in patients with

Table 27.1.
Drug-induced Pancreatitis

Definite
  Azathioprine
  Chlorothiazide
  Corticosteroids
  Didanosine (ddI)
  Estrogens
  Furosemide
  6-Mercaptopurine
  Methyldopa
  Sulfonamides
  Tetracycline
  Valproic acid
Possible
  L-Asparaginase
  Chlorthalidone
  cis-Platinum
  Cytosine arabinoside
  Ethacrynic acid
  H2 antagonists
  Metronidazole
  Pentamidine
  Sulindac

chronic, recurrent disease. Survival from pancreatitis has improved in recent years, probably because of more sophisticated supportive therapy (1).

PATHOPHYSIOLOGY

Pancreatitis runs a highly variable and unpredictable course. While usually mild, it can cause permanent functional injury to the gland, chronic pain, maldigestion, diabetes, and bowel obstruction as a result of the generalized retroperitoneal inflammation. Once the autodigestive process begins, it can be self-perpetuating and devastating.

Pancreatitis has two systems of nomenclature. One classifies the disease as acute or chronic. In acute pancreatitis the gland returns to normal after or between attacks; in chronic pancreatitis there is permanent and continuing damage.

Histology of the glandular lesion distinguishes edematous (interstitial) from necrotizing (hemorrhagic) pancreatitis. The edematous type is characterized by edema of the interstitial space, infiltration of tissue with polymorphonuclear leucocytes, congestion of capillaries, and lymphatic dilatation around areas of focal necrosis. The necrotizing type of pancreatitis further includes rupture of blood vessels, bleeding into the parenchymal space, and contiguous, widespread necrosis. Necrotizing pancreatitis has a higher morbidity and mortality rate; it can be quite virulent and is associated with more damage to surrounding structures. Edematous pancreatitis occurs more often than the necrotizing type, is usually of 10 to 14 days in duration, and has a low occurrence of late complications.

Fat necrosis with calcium soap formation can occur with either type. In both types of pancreatitis, intraglandular enzyme activation and acinar cell destruction is pathognomonic. The severity and duration of the inflammatory process and the degree to which surrounding tissues are compromised are the primary determinants of patient outcome (15).

DIAGNOSIS AND CLINICAL FINDINGS

There is no pathognomonic sign or symptom of pancreatitis. The gland is deep in the retroperitoneal space and direct physical examination is difficult. The physician must rely on a variety of clinical and laboratory parameters to make the diagnosis. Severe midepigastric pain, often exacerbated in food, which radiates to the back occurs in 50% of cases. Patients also report that assuming the knee-chest position while lying on the right side reduces pain. This is a classic sign of retroperitoneal inflammation, but it can be caused by conditions other than pancreatitis.

Laboratory findings can include elevated serum and urinary amylase levels, elevated bilirubin levels, hyperglycemia, hypertriglyceridemia, and hypocalcemia. Normal values from any or all of these tests do not rule out pancreatitis, and the only presenting symptom may be abdominal pain. An elevated serum amylase level is closely associated with this disease, but amylase is also present in the salivary glands, small intestine, fallopian tubes, prostate, liver, and lungs. Serum amylase activity may fall rapidly to normal during an attack as renal clearance of amylase is increased. Calculating a serum to urinary amylase activity ratio does not rule out hyperamylasemia from other organ sources and rarely adds useful information.

Elevated triglyceride levels may occur, but it is unclear how pancreatitis causes hypertriglyceridemia. Approximately 30% of patients with pancreatitis who did not have hypertriglyceridemia prior to their illness have elevations in serum triglyceride levels during an attack, but the importance of this in exacerbating or prolonging the disease is not known.

Hyperglycemia is seen in 50% of patients and probably indicates impaired insulin and glucagon release from injured tissue and the insulin receptor insensitivity seen under any severe metabolic stress. The blood glucose level returns to normal quickly as the disease subsides, and diabetes usually will not result unless 90% or more of the gland is destroyed. Hypocalcemia is seen in the most severe cases, secondary to the saponification of calcium with necrotic fat. The diagnosis of pancreatitis is based on an accumulation of information from physical findings, laboratory data, known or suspected concomitent diseases, and social history.

TREATMENT

There is no specific treatment for pancreatitis. The disease runs a course determined by unknown factors that appear to be unaffected by therapeutic interventions. The goals of therapy are to correct or remove any possible causes of the disease; to reduce enzyme release by the gland; to correct fluid, electrolyte, and acid-base disturbances; and to maintain cardiopulmonary function until the inflammatory process subsides.

Initial Treatment

Salts and water move from the vascular to the interstitial space whenever there is disruption of capillary integrity or permeability, an alteration in relative arteriole and venule hydrostatic pressures, and/or a low total body albumin concentration. The migration of fluid occurs at a rate and in an amount determined by the extent of injury; it can reach 6 to 10 liters per day in patients with massive peritoneal inflammation. The intravascular volume can become so low that perfusion of body tissues is impossible. Vigorous and rapid replacement of intravascular water and electrolytes is often required to prevent circulatory collapse. The kidneys and extremities are particularly susceptible to hypovolemia, and acute tubular necrosis, renal shutdown, and tissue necrosis can occur quickly.

The fluid used for resuscitation and its rate of administration are based on the amounts needed to maintain or reestablish adequate circulating volume and electrolyte values and a urine output of at least 0.5 ml/kg/hr. This level of urine output indicates adequate perfusion of the kidneys and other tissues. Normal saline or lactated Ringer's solutions are given most commonly, since they approximate the composition of the fluid being lost to the interstitial space. Colloid solutions (e.g., normal serum albumin, plasma protein fraction, and hetastarch) are not recommended for routine use because they will diffuse into the interstitial space, increase interstitial oncotic pressure, and cause further depletion of the intravascular volume. Blood pressure and cardiac support with vasopressors such as dopamine, dobutamine, and vasopressin may be required if fluid resuscitation alone cannot maintain perfusion.

Once homeostasis is achieved, therapies aimed at reducing stimulation of the gland are instituted. Although ordinary pancreatic stimulation and enzyme release through the pancreatic duct does not cause pancreatitis, it is thought that reducing glandular output may slow or stop the inflammatory, autodigestive process. Nasogastric suction reduces the volume of gastric fluid reaching the duodenum; acidic fluid stimulates secretin, which then causes release of enzymes and bicarbonate-buffers from the pancreas. This logical therapeutic intervention has not been shown to improve patient condition or change the course of the disease (16).

Many patients require placement of a nasogastric (NG)

tube to prevent vomiting, as ileus is a common feature in severe disease; but NG suction should not be considered a treatment for pancreatitis. Cimetidine has yielded equally disappointing results. Patients treated with cimetidine had more prolonged courses of hyperamylasemia than placebo-treated groups, and they derived no apparent benefit from the drug (17, 18). Glucagon and various anticholinergic drugs that might reduce neural and hormonal stimulation of the gland independent of the presence of acid in the duodenum have also been studied with no apparent benefit to patients (19–21). Octreotide, a synthetic analog of somatostatin, has been tested in a variety of gastrointestinal disorders. As a treatment for pancreatitis, one author reported dramatic improvements in abdominal pain and tenderness during a continuous infusion of somatostatin, but a randomized, double-blind, multicenter trial showed no significant differences in clinical and laboratory parameters or in patient outcomes (22–24).

Peritoneal lavage is used in severe cases to remove necrotic debris from the abdomen. A catheter is inserted into the peritoneum, and 1 to 6 liters of 1.5 or 4.5% aqueous dextrose solutions are introduced and removed from the cavity every day. This procedure has the risk of complications. The catheter can perforate abdominal structures and allow organisms to enter the peritoneum. The dialysate solution can also cause rapid changes in blood glucose levels and intravascular volume. While early mortality has been reduced with this intervention, the overall complication and death rate in patients undergoing peritoneal lavage remains unchanged (25).

The routine use of antibiotics to prevent infections is very questionable. While pancreatitis can result in perforation of an abdominal viscus and bacterial peritonitis, this complication occurs in only 3 to 6% of the most severe cases and should be managed with antibiotics when it occurs. Gram-negative aerobic and anaerobic organisms found in the gastrointestinal tract (e.g., *Escherichia coli*, microaerophilic *Streptococcus*, and *Bacteroides* species) are the most commonly cultured organisms. Empiric antibiotic therapy is directed at eradication of these organisms until more specific information is available from blood and peritoneal cultures (4).

The current consensus is that these interventions are useful in the management of pancreatitis and associated complications, but they are not treatments. A variety of therapies and medications may be required to minimize morbidity and mortality. Only those demonstrated to have caused pancreatitis must be avoided.

The pain associated with pancreatitis can be severe, and prolonged use of high-dose analgesics is often required. All narcotics can increase pressure in the biliary tree causing spasm of the sphincter of Oddi, which theoretically, can exacerbate pain. In equipotent doses, there appear to be no significant differences among the narcotic analgesics in their effect on the sphincter of Oddi, and therapy must be directed at providing adequate analgesia.

Ventilatory support may become necessary if abdominal distension, pleural effusions, or fluid sequestration in the lungs are severe enough to compromise breathing or oxygenation of the blood. In cases of hemorrhagic pancreatitis, replacement of red blood cell mass may become necessary, but serious blood loss is unusual and almost never a problem in edematous pancreatitis.

Nutrition Support

The role of nutritional support in pancreatitis raises several questions: (a) does bowel rest influence the course and severity of the disease? (b) can patients be fed enterally or parenterally so the pancreas is not stimulated? and (c) does improved nutritional status influence patient outcome? Elemental enteral or parenteral feeding has not been shown to improve survival or overall patient outcome in pancreatitis as a direct result of decreasing pancreatic stimulation (26). Studies done to evaluate the degree to which nutrients stimulate the exocrine pancreas have yielded conflicting results. Intravenous and oral administration of amino acids and fat have increased gastrin levels in dogs and humans (27, 28). It might be inferred from this that pancreatic secretion will increase in response to higher gastric acid production, but pancreatic secretion was not measured in the human study and the individuals evaluated were normal volunteers, not patients with pancreatitis. Several studies that evaluated pancreatic protein secretion in dogs given intravenous amino acids and fat showed no effect on gastrin, cholecystokinin, or pancreatic polypeptide release and either no effect or a decrease in pancreatic output (29, 30). Conflicting results were also obtained when the effect of intravenous fat on pancreatic secretion was studied; one author reported an increase in the volume of pancreatic output and two reported no change (31–33). From these data, it is not possible to assume that any form of nutritional support will put the pancreas completely at rest. Furthermore, no controlled prospective study demonstrates that nutrition support influences the course of the disease. Thus enteral and parenteral feeding appear to have no value in influencing the course or outcome of the disease.

The value and need for nutrition support in patients with pancreatitis should be determined using the same criteria applied in other diseases. The goal of the therapy is to stop the development of or to repair nutritional deficits, which may enable the patient to tolerate or recover more quickly from the underlying disease. In most instances, particularly in edematous pancreatitis, the course of the disease is short. Nutritional deficits important enough to increase morbidity and mortality will not develop if the patient was in good nutritional condition prior to the illness. No improvement in outcome as a result of nutrition support has been demonstrated in any previously well-nourished patient who is to not eat for a period of time less than 10 days. In individuals with mild to moderate nutritional deficits at the onset of their illness, no benefit that outweighs the risks of parenteral feeding has been demonstrated unless the feeding continued for at least 10 days. This leads to the conclusion that the patients with pancreatitis who will benefit from nutrition support are those who will be without feeding for at least 10 days, have some initial nutritional deficits, and may be at risk of developing important deficits before normal oral feeding can be resumed (34).

Selection of patients to be fed is based on the severity of the disease, the probable time course to resolution, current nutritional status, and the probability of complications from nutritional therapy itself. If the need for nutrition support outweighs its risk in an individual patient, it should be instituted as it would be in any other condition. The nutritional regimen should be made determined by the accepted criteria for calculating the energy and protein necessary to meet metabolic needs and repair any existing nutritional deficits.

Nutritional support regimens, whether oral, enteral, or parenteral, are composed of combinations of protein, carbohydrate, and fat. Because one of the classic symptoms of pancreatitis is abdominal pain exacerbated by food, much attention has been given to modifying the diet to provide adequate nutrition without exacerbating the disease or its symptoms. The macronutrient in food that appears to cause pain is fat. Amylase and lipase secreted by the pancreas break down the fats and long-chain triglycerides in food to absorbable molecules. Low-fat diets or those in which MCT (medium-chain triglyceride) oil has been substituted for vegetable oils are better tolerated by patients with pancreatitis. Medium-chain triglycerides do not require enzymatic digestion or micelle formation for absorption, so their presence in the gastrointestinal tract does not stimulate the pancreas to any appreciable degree. Usually patients are not fed by mouth until the acute pain of the attack has subsided, even if abdominal distension and ileus have resolved. Refeeding is usually begun with a fat-free clear diet. If the patient does not experience pain, nausea, or vomiting, the diet is advanced slowly with foods low in fat. When tube feeding is indicated or commercially available enteral products are preferred as a transitional diet, attention is given to fat content. A product low in the long-chain fatty acids found in vegetable oils (corn, safflower, soybean, and sunflower) or one composed of fats and proteins in a predigested form is usually well tolerated.

Parenteral nutrition is indicated only in patients who cannot tolerate being fed by the gastrointestinal tract; there is no therapeutic advantage to parenteral nutrition over oral or tube feeding. TPN (total parenteral nutrition) is appropriate for patients with ileus, fistulas, peritonitis, obstruction, and perforation of the GI tract.

The use and safety of intravenous fat emulsions in patients with pancreatitis is an area of controversy. Some clinicians are reluctant to give intravenous long-chain fatty acids, assuming the same sorts of problems seen with fat given by mouth will occur. Triglycerides are cleared from the blood after being converted to free fatty acids by lipoprotein lipase released from capillary endothelium, not by amylase and lipase released from the pancreas. The area of controversy is whether intravenous administration of long-chain fatty acids will cause or exacerbate pancreatitis. Patients with dyslipoproteinemias have exhibited elevated triglyceride levels when given intravenous fat. One patient developed a syndrome mimicking acute pancreatitis, but the problem appeared to result from the dyslipoproteinemia and be unrelated to the administration of intravenous long-chain fatty acids (35). All the available products are soybean or safflower oil emulsions composed entirely of long-chain fatty acids. Administration of these products to normal volunteers does not increase pancreatic enzyme output (36). Additionally, patients with pancreatic fistulas do not have an increase in fistula output when treated with intravenous fat. Eleven patients with acute pancreatitis and 25 patients with a history of pancreatitis have also been studied. In no instance was there an exacerbation of the disease (37, 38). The only report in the literature implicating fat emulsions in the development of pancreatitis involved two children with Crohn's disease who were simultaneously receiving steroids. As steroids can cause pancreatitis, it is difficult to implicate IV fat in these cases (39).

Patients with pancreatitis should be evaluated in the same manner as any patient requiring parenteral nutrition. A baseline triglyceride level is obtained. If it is within normal limits, fat emulsions can be given to meet requirements for essential fatty acids and calories. In the instances of hyperglycemia so often seen in these patients, a higher percentage of calories given as fat may enable the clinician to meet nutritional requirements without exacerbating preexisting difficulties with blood glucose management. A diagnosis of pancreatitis does not automatically preclude the use of intravenous fat emulsions as part of a complete nutrition support regimen.

COMPLICATIONS

Early complications of pancreatitis result from the autodigestive inflammatory process. Phlegmons are areas of inflamed necrotic tissue. They usually resolve with the disease, but they can cause bleeding, thrombosis of blood vessels, infarction of the colon and/or spleen or esophageal varices or progress to become pseudocysts. Fifty percent of patients with severe pancreatitis develop enzyme-and-

fluid-filled sacs (pseudocysts) within or near the gland. Fifty percent of the time, pseudocysts resolve spontaneously, but they may require surgical drainage if they expand, rupture, or become chronic. Pancreatic abscesses, enterocutaneous fistulas, and bacterial peritonitis can develop if the inflammatory process damages the gut and liberates enteric organisms and bowel contents. Bleeding can occur if there is erosion into any of the major blood vessels near the inflammation.

The late complications of pancreatitis are chronic pain, recurrent pseudocysts, and pancreatic insufficiency. Pain can result from continuing subclinical pancreatitis or from fibrotic tissue impinging on nerves. Treatment is with narcotic analgesics, but in the most severe, unremitting cases, destruction of the celiac ganglia by injection of alcohol may be necessary.

Pancreatic Insufficiency

Usually endocrine or exocrine pancreatic insufficiency develops only after 90% or more of the gland has been destroyed or removed. Endocrine insufficiency is managed as it is with diabetes mellitus, but one additional factor must be considered. In addition to low or absent insulin production, these patients also lack glucagon. Glucose control should not be too tight, because profound hypoglycemia can occur if oral hypoglycemia or insulin doses are too high. Patients must be educated carefully on the use of their medications and on the symptoms and management of hypoglycemic episodes.

Exocrine insufficiency results in maldigestion and malabsorption of fat and protein. Weight loss and life-threatening malnutrition can become serious problems. The most common symptom of exocrine pancreatic insufficiency is steatorrhea (fat in the stool), but there is often concomitent protein malabsorption (azotorrhea). Carbohydrate, vitamin, mineral, and electrolyte malabsorption are not features of the syndrome (1). The patient will complain of anorexia, postprandial bloating, and weight loss and report greasy, bulky, foul-smelling feces that float.

The goal of treatment is to provide enough pancreatic enzyme activity to allow normal digestion. The amount of pancreatic extract required varies as a function of the fat content of the patient's diet and the amount of enzyme that reaches the duodenum. Pancreatic enzymes are destroyed rapidly at a pH below 4, so much of an ingested supplement is inactivated in the stomach. Also, because pancreatic bicarbonate secretion is low or absent in pancreatic insufficiency and intraduodenal pH is often below 5, bile acids precipitate and fat solubilization and micelle formation are impaired. These factors make the treatment of malabsorption difficult for the patient and the clinician.

Often a large number of pancreatic extract capsules must be taken because the available products have much less activity than is usually provided by the gland. Assuming no inactivation in the stomach, 6 to 8 capsules of pancreatin or pancrelipase is equivalent to 5% of maximal pancreatic secretion in response to a meal. Eight to 20% of lipase and trypsin activity survives transit through the stomach. Fortunately, this is usually sufficient to reduce malabsorption by 60 to 70% (40, 41). In patients on high-dose replacement therapy with continuing steatorrhea, attempts have been made to raise the pH of the stomach and thereby improve enzyme delivery to the duodenum. Antacids and enteric-coated pancreatic enzyme preparations were given as adjunctive therapy, but only cimetidine was found to be useful and then only in patients with normal or high gastric acid production (42).

Patients with pancreatic insufficiency must understand the purpose and goals of therapy. They will be required to titrate their ingestion of pancreatic enzymes according to the changing composition of meals, on a schedule that will minimize steatorrhea. Enzyme ingestion is simultaneous with eating. Patients often taken the capsules in divided doses before, during, and shortly after each meal to achieve the best result. The end point of therapy is reduction or abolition of malabsorption and postprandial bloating, and improvement in nutritional status. The monitoring parameters for this therapy are relief from symptoms, normal-appearing feces, and weight gain. Available

Table 27.2.
Pancreatic Enzyme Supplements

	Lipase	Amylase	Protease
	(USP Units of Activity)		
Pancreatin			
Dizymes Tablets (Recsei)	6000	30000	20000
Hi-Vegi-Lip (Freeda)	12000	60000	60000
Pancreatin Enseals (EC Capsules, Lilly)	2000	25000	25000
Tablets (Lilly)	650	8125	8125
Pancrelipase			
Tablets			
Festal II (Hoescht-Roussel)	6000	30000	20000
Ilozyme (Adria)	11000	30000	30000
Viokase (Robins)	8000	30000	30000
Powder			
Viokase (Robins) (per 0.7 gm)	16800	70000	70000
Capsules			
Cotazym (Organon)	8000	30000	30000
Cotazym S EC (Organon)	5000	20000	20000
Creon (Reid-Rowell)	8000	30000	13000
Ku-Zyme HP (Kremens-Urban)	8000	30000	30000
Pancrease EC (McNeil)	4000	20000	25000
Pancrease MT4 EC (McNeil)	4000	12000	12000
Pancrease MT10 EC (McNeil)	10000	30000	30000
Pancrease MT16 EC (McNeil)	16000	48000	48000

Table 27.3.
Negative Prognostic Indicators in Pancreatitis

Admission
  Age greater than 55 years
  WBC > 16×10^6/liter (16×10^3/mm^3)
  Blood glucose > 11.1 mmol/liter (200 mg/dl)
  LDH > 5.8 μkat/liter (350 μ/liter)
  AST > 250 SFU/liter, 4.2 μkat/liter (250 μ/liter)
Within 48 hours
  Hematocrit drop > 10%
  BUN rise > 1.8 mmol/liter (5 mg/dl)
  Serum Ca < 2 mmol/liter (8 mg/dl)
  pO2 < 60 mm Hg
  Base deficit > 4
  Estimated fluid sequestration > 6 liters

pancreatic enzyme replacement products are listed in Table 27.2.

PROGNOSIS

The course of pancreatitis cannot be predicted or influenced to any appreciable degree. Patients who initially appear to be quite ill may recover completely within a matter of days. Others, whose symptoms were less impressive, may die just as quickly. Prognostic criteria can statistically predict mortality, but they are not useful in designing or modifying the treatment regimen for an individual patient. Ranson's prognostic criteria are most commonly used, and they are listed in Table 27.3. In his experience, mortality was less than 1% in patients with fewer than three indicators and 100% in those with seven or more signs within 48 hours of admission to the hospital (43). Most cases of acute pancreatitis resolve spontaneously and the patient recovers completely. Alcoholic patients who continue to drink and individuals with recurrent or chronic biliary tract disease are at greatest risk for recurrent acute attacks and development of chronic pancreatitis. Patients must understand the serious consequences of recurrent pancreatitis and know how to modify their behavior to avoid problems in the future.

CONCLUSION

Pancreatitis is easier to prevent than to treat. In 90% of acute cases, alcohol, biliary tract disease, or drugs were the precipitating agents. Alcoholism causes 90% of cases of chronic, recurrent pancreatitis. Abstinence from alcohol, cholecystectomy, or modification in drug therapy usually prevents reappearance of the disease. Patient management involves removing factors that may have caused the pancreatic inflammation, providing cardiopulmonary support, managing complications as they arise, and educating the patient in ways to prevent recurrence of the disease.

REFERENCES

1. Sleisenger MH, Fordtran JL: Gastrointestinal Diseases, ed. 4. Philadelphia: WB Saunders, 1989, pp 1765–1986.
2. Debas HT: Clinical significance of gastrointestinal hormones. Adv Surg 21:157–188, 1987.
3. Wilson JS, Korsten MA, Pirola RC: Alcohol-induced pancreatic injury (part 1). Unexplained features and ductular theories of pathogenesis. Int J Pancreatol 4(2):109–125, 1989.
4. Mandell GL, Douglas RG, Bennett JE: Principles and Practice of Infectious Diseases. New York: Churchill Livingston, 1990, pp 636–670.
5. Keefe M, Munro F: Acute pancreatitis: a fatal complication of treatment of bullous pemphigoid with systemic steroids. Dermatologica 179(2):73–75, 1988.
6. Levine RA, McGuire RF: Corticosteroid-induced pancreatitis: a case report demonstrating recurrence with rechallenge. Am J Gastroenterol 83(10):1181–1184, 1988.
7. Mallory A, Kern F: Drug-induced pancreatitis. Ballieres Clin Gastroenterology 2(2):293–307, 1988.
8. Scarpelli DG: Toxicology of the pancreas. Toxicol Appl Pharmacol 101(3):543–554, 1989.
9. Singleton JW, Law DH: National Cooperative Crohn's Disease Study: adverse reactions to study drugs. Gastroenterology 265:870–882, 1979.
10. Alberti-Flor JJ, Hernandez ME, Ferrar JP: Fulminant liver failure and pancreatitis associated with the use of sulfamethoxazole-trimethoprim. Am J Gastroenterol 84(2):1577–1579, 1989.
11. Stenveinkel P, Alvestrand A: Loop diuretic–induced pancreatitis with rechallenge in a patient with malignant hypertension and renal insufficiency. Acta Med Scand 224(1):89–91, 1988.
12. Torosis J, Vonder R: Tetracycline-induced pancreatitis. J Clin Gastroenterol 9(5):580–581, 1987.
13. Cooley TP, Kunches LM, Saunders CA: Treatment of AIDS and AIDS-related complex with 2,3-didooxyinosine given once daily. Rev Infect Dis 9(12):9552–9560, 1990.
14. Lott JA, Bond LW, Bobo RC: Valproic acid associated pancreatitis: report of three cases and a brief review. Clin Chem 38(2):395–397, 1990.
15. Geokas MC, Baltake HA: Acute pancreatitis. Ann Intern Med 103:86–100, 1985.
16. Field BE, Hepner GW: Nasogastric suction in alcoholic pancreatitis. Dig Dis Sci 24:339–344, 1979.
17. Regan PT, Malagelada JR: A prospective study of the antisecretory and therapeutic effects of cimetidine and glucagon in human acute pancreatitis. Mayo Clin Proc 56:499–503, 1981.
18. Meshkinpour H, Molinari MD: Cimetidine in the treatment of acute alcoholic pancreatitis: a randomized, double-blind study. Gastroenterology 77:687–690, 1979.
19. Durr HK, Maroske D: Glucagon therapy in acute pancreatitis. Gut 19:175–179, 1978.
20. Gilsanz V, Oteyza CP: Glucagon vs anticholinergics in the treatment of acute pancreatitis: a double-blind controlled study. Arch Intern Med 138:535–538, 1978.
21. Cameron JL, Mehigan D: Evaluation of atropine in acute pancreatitis. Surg Gynecol Obstet 148:206–208, 1979.
22. Mulvihill S, Pappas TN, Passaro E: The use of somatostatin and its analogs in the treatment of surgical disorders. Surgery 100:467–476, 1986.
23. Ellison CE, O'Dorisio TM, Sparks BS: Observations of the effect of a somatostatin analog in the Zollinger-Ellison syndrome: implications for the treatment of apudomas. Surgery 100:437–444, 1986.
24. Rosenberg JM: Octreotide: a synthetic analog of somatostatin. Drug Intell Clin Pharm 22:748–754, 1988.
25. Ranson JHC, Spencer FC: The role of peritoneal lavage in severe acute pancreatitis. Ann Surg 187:565–570, 1978.
26. Goodgame JT, Fischer JF: Parenteral nutrition in the treatment of acute pancreatitis: effect on complications and mortality. Ann Surg 186:651–658, 1977.
27. Konturek SJ, Tasler J: Intravenous amino acids and fat stimulate pancreatic secretion. Am J Physiol 236:E676–E684, 1979.
28. Isenberg JI, Maxwell J: Intravenous infusion of amino acids stimulates gastric acid secretion in man. N Engl J Med 298:27–29, 1978.
29. Stabile BE, Debas HT: Intravenous versus intraduodenal amino acids, fats, and glucose as stimulants of pancreatic secretion. Surg Forum 32:224–226, 1981.
30. Fried GM, Ogden WD: Pancreatic protein secretion and gastrointestinal hormone release in response to parenteral amino acids and lipids in dogs. Surgery 92:902–905, 1982.
31. Klein E, Shnebaum S: Effects of total parenteral nutrition on exocrine pancreatic secretion. Am J Gastroenterol 78:31–33, 1983.
32. Bivins BA, Bell RM: Pancreatic exocrine response to parenteral nutrition. JPEN 8:34–36, 1984.
33. Grundfest S, Steiger E: The effect of intravenous fat emulsions in patients with pancreatic fistula. JPEN 4:27–31, 1980.
34. Kirby DF, Craig RM: The value of intensive nutritional support in pancreatitis. JPEN 9:353–357, 1985.
35. Miller A, Lees RS: The natural history and surgical significance of hyperlipemic abdominal crisis. Ann Surg 190:401–408, 1979.
36. Edelman K, Valenzuela JE: Effect of intravenous lipids on human pancreatic secretion. Gastroenterology 85:1063–1066, 1983.
37. Silberman H, Dixon NP: The safety and efficacy of a lipid-based system of parenteral nutrition in acute pancreatitis. Am J Gastroenterol 77:494–497, 1982.
38. Buch A, Buch J: Hyperlipidemia and pancreatitis. World J Surg 4:307–314, 1980.
39. Noseworthy A, Kern F: Pancreatitis and intravenous fat: an association in patients with inflammatory bowel disease. J Pediatr Surg 18:269–272, 1983.
40. Heizler WD, Cleveland CR: Gastric inactivation of pancreatic supplements. Bull Johns Hopkins Hosp 116:261–265, 1965.
41. DiMagno EP, Malagelada JR: Fate of orally ingested enzymes in pancreatic insufficiency: comparison of two dosage schedules. N Engl J Med 296:1318–1322, 1977.
42. Regan PT, Malagelada JR: Comparative effects of antacids, cimetidine and enteric coating on the therapeutic response to oral enzymes in severe pancreatic insufficiency. N Engl J Med 297:854–858, 1977.
43. Ranson JHC, Rifkind KM: Prognostic signs and the role of operative management in acute pancreatitis. Surg Gynecol Obstet 139:69–81, 1974.

CHAPTER 28

RHEUMATOID ARTHRITIS AND ITS THERAPY

ERIC G. BOYCE, Pharm.D.

Rheumatoid arthritis is a highly variable, chronic inflammatory condition of unknown etiology affecting mostly the joints but often with periarticular and systemic involvement. The word *rheuma* was used by ancient Greek physicians to mean flowing, which fit well with their humoral theory of disease. Rheumatism was linked to joint ailments in the 1600s by a French physician who used it as an inexact label for a systemic condition. *Rheumatoid arthritis* was coined in 1858 as a label for cases reported earlier in the century. Although many refinements and developments in the understanding of rheumatoid arthritis have ensued, the pathogenesis of the disease is unknown, and current therapies are nonspecific and rarely curative. Patients with rheumatoid arthritis are extensive users of healthcare systems, incurring outpatient and hospital visits and costs at rates that are 2 to 3 times greater than those of the general population, when matched for age and gender (1). The goals of drug and nondrug therapy should be to provide safe, effective, and inexpensive treatment that will improve well being, diminish the progression of rheumatoid arthritis, and possibly diminish the need for healthcare and disability services.

ETIOLOGY

The etiology of rheumatoid arthritis is unknown, but theories implicate genetic, hormonal, viral, mycobacterial, autoimmune, atmospheric, environmental, and other factors. Rheumatoid arthritis is associated with HLA-DR4 and HLA-DR1, which are class II major histocompatibility complex antigenic products, and with the homozygous C-κ genotype, which codes for the κ constant portion of immunoglobulins (2, 3). These associations imply that genetics and the immune system play an important role in rheumatoid arthritis since the class II major histocompatibility complex antigens are involved in immune regulation and immunoglobulins are part of the immune response.

A hormonal link is supported by the female preponderance of this disease and the decreased risk of developing rheumatoid arthritis generally associated with a history of pregnancy or possibly oral contraceptive use (4, 5). Additionally, less severe rheumatoid arthritis is found in patients who used oral contraceptives prior to its onset (5). Infectious etiologies of rheumatoid arthritis are sup-

ported by a number of findings. Sera from rheumatoid arthritis patients demonstrates hyperreactivity to Epstein-Barr virus antigens, and RANA (rheumatoid arthritis nuclear antigen) is found in patients with rheumatoid arthritis and may be similar to Epstein-Barr nuclear antigens. White blood cells from patients with rheumatoid arthritis are hyperreactive to *Mycobacterium tuberculosis*. Also, rheumatoid arthritis has responded to antiinfectives. Although the etiology of rheumatoid arthritis is unknown, it appears to result in an altered immune response.

EPIDEMIOLOGY

Rheumatoid arthritis affects 0.3 to 1.5% of the population and is two to three times more common in women than in men. It can be seen in any culture or race. Rheumatoid arthritis occurs at any age, with the peak incidence in women occurring between 30 and 60 years of age. Genetic predisposition is suggested by the increased incidence of rheumatoid arthritis in certain families, monozygotic twins, and individuals with specific genetic markers for HLA-DR4, HLA-DR1, C-κ (2), or subtypes of HLA-DR4, HLA-DR1, or HLA-DQ (3). HLA-DR4, a product of the class II genes of the major histocompatibility complex, occurs in 36% of the population as a whole, 58 to 65% of those with rheumatoid arthritis, 60% of those with rheumatoid factor–negative (or seronegative) rheumatoid arthritis, 69 to 75% of those with rheumatoid factor–positive (or seropositive) rheumatoid arthritis, and more commonly in patients with more severe rheumatoid arthritis (2).

PATHOGENESIS

The pathophysiology of the joint changes seen in rheumatoid arthritis has been well described at the tissue level, but more recent studies on blood, tissue, and synovial fluid have begun to explore the pathogenesis of rheumatoid arthritis at cellular, biochemical, and molecular levels. The chronic inflammation, synovial proliferation, and bone and cartilage destruction seen in rheumatoid arthritis appear to be associated with abnormalities in immune, inflammatory, and repair responses that involve the direct actions, secretions, or regulation of macrophages, lymphocytes, neutrophils, fibroblasts (which may be specialized macrophages), and other cells.

A normal diarthrodial joint is a functional interface that supports and limits the relative movement of two or more bones over defined ranges. The joint capsule surrounds the joint space and connects to the bones. The synovium, or synovial tissue, is the internal structure of the joint capsule, which secretes synovial fluid and contains many immunologically active cells and blood vessels. Connective tissue surrounds the synovial tissue and provides stability to the joint capsule and the synovial lining membrane. Tendons, ligaments, and muscles also help stabilize the joint. Cartilage, which is composed of proteoglycan groups and 70% water, is bathed in synovial fluid and acts as a transition between the bones to cushion the forces between opposing bones during movement or compression. Synovial fluid provides nutrients and removes wastes from the cartilage, and also helps maintain the structure of the cartilage through hydration. In rheumatoid arthritis, the normal anatomy and physiology of joints are altered by immunologically mediated changes in bone, cartilage, supporting tissues, and synovial tissue and fluid. Portions of this immunologic dysfunction are becoming better understood, but many questions remain unanswered.

The event initiating immunologic abnormalities in rheumatoid arthritis is unknown, but it may involve an altered reaction to an exogenous or autoantigen. Potential antigens include the Fc (constant) portion of IgG, type II collagen found in cartilage, type III collagen found in synovium and blood vessels, chondrocyte membrane, and *Mycobacterium tuberculosis*. The overreactivity to antigens may be related to the major histocompatibility complex (MHC) class II products HLA-DR4 or HLA-DR1 (which occur more commonly in patients with rheumatoid arthritis) or to adhesion molecules on fibroblasts (6). MHC class II products are expressed on the surface of macrophages and other antigen-processing cells in association with processed antigen and appear to regulate the reaction of T lymphocytes.

Macrophages appear to be highly involved in rheumatoid arthritis through their release of interleukin-1 (IL-1) and tumor necrosis factor (TNF) in response to antigens, immune complexes, complement split products, γ-interferon (IFN-γ), and cartilage and synovial collagen (Table 28-1). (7) IL-1 stimulates the activation and proliferation of lymphocytes and secretion of a tissue growth factor. IL-1 and TNF are chemotactic and stimulate the release of immune, inflammatory, and enzymatic factors including IL-6, granulocyte-macrophage colony stimulating factor (GM-CSF), prostaglandin E_2 (PGE$_2$), collagenase, proteinase, and neuropeptide substance P. TNF-α is secreted with IL-1, but it appears to be less important than IL-1 in inflammation and enzyme release (7). IL-1, TNF-α, GM-CSF, and soluble IL-2 receptors increase in the blood, synovial fluid, and/or synovial tissue in patients with rheumatoid arthritis and may correlate with disease

Table 28.1.
Actions of Immunological Mediators in Rheumatoid Arthritis[a]

Substance	Source	Stimulates (Inhibits)
IL-1, TNF	Macrophages	MHC-I expression; chemotaxis; release of PGE$_2$, IL-6, GM-CSF, collagenase, proteinase, substance P
IL-1	Macrophages	Lymphocyte proliferation & activation; growth factor release
IL-6	Fibroblasts T lymphocytes	T cell & B cell function GM-CSF release
IFN-γ	T lymphocytes	MHC-I & MHC-II expression; (Inhibits collagenase & PGE$_2$ release)
GM-CSF	Macrophages	Bone marrow cell formation; IL-1 production
	Lymphocytes	PMN activation; monocyte attraction
PGE$_2$	Fibroblasts	Growth factor release; cartilage degradation; inflammation; pain
Collagenase	Fibroblasts	Cartilage degradation
Growth factors		Synovial tissue proliferation
Transforming growth factor		Synovial tissue proliferation; IL-1 production; monocyte chemotaxis; (Inhibits lymphokine and protease secretion; synoviocyte growth; HLA-DR expression)

[a] Abbreviations: GM-CSF, granulocyte macrophage colony stimulating factor; IFN, interferon; IL, interleukin; MHC, major histocompatibility complex; PG, prostaglandin; PMN, neutrophils; TNF, tumor necrosis factor.

activity (7, 8). Expression of MHC class I antigens, which are associated with cytotoxicity, and an adhesion molecule on the surface of rheumatoid synovial fibroblasts is enhanced by IL-1, TNF-α, and IFN-γ, but not by IL-6 or GM-CSF (6). IFN-γ increases the expression of MHC class II antigens (6). Inhibitors to IL-1 and TNF-α have also been identified (7).

T lymphocytes appear to play an important role in immune reactions. T lymphocytes from patients with rheumatoid arthritis demonstrate markers for activated (CD3+) and suppressor/cytotoxic (CD8+) T cells, activation by enhanced HLA-DR antigen expression, hyperreactivity to soluble antigen and chondrocyte membrane, and mature and hyperreactive memory T cells (9, 10). Patients with rheumatoid arthritis have gone into remission when infected with the human immunodeficiency virus (11), implicating a role of helper T lymphocytes in rheumatoid arthritis. However, patients with rheumatoid arthritis have T lymphocytes hyporesponsive to mitogenic stimuli, small numbers of activated inducer (CD4+) T cells, low levels of activated T lymphocyte products IL-2 and IFN-γ in synovial fluid, and a low degree of expression of activation receptors on the surface of synovial T cells

(9, 10). These effects may indicate a defect in inducer T lymphocytes in patients with rheumatoid arthritis, leaving the role of T lymphocytes in rheumatoid arthritis unclear.

IL-6, which is increased in inflammatory synovial fluid, increases production of GM-CSF, immunoglobulins, and liver acute-phase reactants following secretion from monocytes, T lymphocytes, and fibroblasts (Table 28.1) (7, 10). GM-CSF is secreted by synovial tissue, macrophages, fibroblasts, endothelial cells, and activated lymphocytes and acts to promote growth of certain bone marrow cell lines, increase MHC class II expression on synovial macrophages, stimulate IL-1 production, activate neutrophils, and attract monocytes (Table 28.1) (7, 10). IL-2, IL-4, and IFN-γ levels do not appear to be elevated in rheumatoid arthritis (10).

Antibodies, immune complexes, complement, and complement split products also increase in patients with rheumatoid arthritis. Rheumatoid factor is an antibody of IgM (or possibly IgG or IgA) type that is directed against Fc portion of IgG. It is found in 80% of patients with rheumatoid arthritis. Hyaluronic acid, a normal component of synovial fluid, may facilitate the formation of immune complexes of rheumatoid factor and IgG. Other autoantibodies may also be seen in rheumatoid arthritis.

Prostaglandin E_2 (PGE_2) and leukotriene B_4 (LTB_4) are inflammatory mediators that are increased in patients with rheumatoid arthritis. PGE and PGE_2 production by synovial fibroblasts is increased by IL-1 and TNF-α, but this effect is diminished by IFN-γ (Table 28.1) (7, 12). Neuropeptides may prove to be important in the pathogenesis of rheumatoid arthritis. Substance P, a neuropeptide, is increased in the synovial fluid of rheumatoid arthritis patients, possibly stimulated by IL-1 or TNF-α (13).

Synovial tissue proliferates and develops into an invasive tissue known as the pannus. Platelet-derived growth factor, epidermal growth factor, transforming growth factor, basic fibroblast growth factor and receptors for these growth factors have been found in synovial fluid and tissue (7). These growth factors cause uncontrolled proliferation in vitro and may lead to the tumor-like growth of synovial tissue in rheumatoid arthritis, possibly in an autocrine manner. Platelet-derived growth factor is regulated by IL-1 and PGE_2 in a complex interrelationship (Table 28.1) (7). Migrating circulatory macrophages may also help maintain the hyperplastic synovium. Additionally, transforming growth factor decreases lymphokine and protease secretion, synoviocyte growth, and HLA-DR expression, but enhances collagen and fibronectin gene transcription, protease inhibitor and IL-1 production, monocyte chemotaxis, and immunosuppression (7). Hypervascularity is also a feature of hypertrophic rheumatoid synovium.

The bone resorption and cartilage destruction of rheumatoid arthritis are due to cellular activities and secretions. Collagenase, PGE_2, plasminogen activator (a neutral proteinase of both tissue and urokinase types that is converted to plasmin), and stromelysin can degrade cartilage or collagen and are produced by synovial fibroblasts or chondrocytes after stimulation by IL-1 or TNF (7, 12, 14). The effect of IL-1 and TNF on collagenase and PGE_2 production is diminished by IFN-γ (Table 28.1) (12). Hyperreactivity of peripheral blood and synovial T lymphocytes to chondrocyte membrane may also explain the cartilage destruction. Phagocytes from rheumatoid synovial fluid have contained type II collagen, indicating active phagocytosis of cartilage. Plasma parathyroid hormone and calcitriol concentrations may also correlate with periarticular bone loss in rheumatoid arthritis patients (15). Plasmin inhibitor–plasmin complexes are slightly increased in patients with rheumatoid vasculitis and may correlate with prolongation of partial thromboplastin time possibly due to release of plasminogen activator from vessel walls (16). Activated macrophages may secrete a procoagulant that enhances the formation of fibrin or fibrinoid material over synovial lining or within a rheumatoid nodule.

The inflammation, synovial proliferation, and collagen destruction of rheumatoid arthritis lead to changes in synovial fluid, synovial tissue, cartilage, and bone. The pressure within the joint increases from vacuum or subatmospheric pressures in the normal joint to supraatmospheric pressures when inflamed. Rheumatoid synovial fluid is similar to that seen in other inflammatory joint diseases with respect to leukocytosis (particularly polymorphonuclear cells) and decreased viscosity. The synovial tissue becomes hypervascular, and blood flow increases as a result of vasodilation, but it may not increase enough to meet the metabolic demands resulting from the inflammation. Lactate levels are high in inflamed synovial fluid. Increased synovial fluid, synovial tissue proliferation, and cartilage destruction may lead to limitation of movement and discomfort. Cartilage and bone destruction further destabilize the joint.

DIAGNOSIS AND CLINICAL FINDINGS

The 1958 criteria for the classification of rheumatoid arthritis were revised in 1988 by the American College of Rheumatology using a "traditional" list (Table 28.2) and a "tree" format (Table 28.3) (17). The recent classification system also dropped the previous list of exclusions and the "possible," "probable," "definite," and "classic" classifications. These criteria are intended to serve as the standard for investigational purposes and to aid in the clinical setting, but they are not intended to impede making a diagnosis of rheumatoid arthritis based on clinical findings and impressions. These classification criteria emphasize the chronic, symmetrical, and small peripheral joint involvement in rheumatoid arthritis in conjunction with signs of the underlying pathophysiology of the disease.

Mild-to-moderate rheumatoid arthritis is character-

Table 28.2.
Classification of Rheumatoid Arthritis Based on the 1987 Revised "Traditional" Method[a]

The patient must meet 4 of the following 7 criteria to be classified as having rheumatoid arthritis:

1. Morning stiffness of or near joints, lasting 1 hour before maximum benefit[b]
2. Arthritis, demonstrated by soft tissue swelling or fluid, in three or more joint areas including right or left PIP, MCP, wrist, elbow, MTP, ankle, or knee joints[b,c,d]
3. Arthritis, demonstrated by soft tissue swelling or fluid, in the hand joints (PIP, MCP, or wrist)[b,c,d]
4. Symmetric arthritis in the areas noted in criterion 2; PIP, MCP, and MTP joint area symmetry does not need to be absolute in order to meet this criterion[b,c,d]
5. Rheumatoid nodules, as noted by subcutaneous nodules near bones or joints or on extensor surfaces[c]
6. Positive rheumatoid factor determined by a test positive in less than 5% of normal subjects
7. Radiologic changes of the hands or wrists including erosions or bone decalcification in or next to involved joints

[a] Adapted from Arnett FC, Edworthy SM, Bloch DA, et al.: The American Rheumatism Association 1987 revised criteria for the classification of rheumatoid arthritis. Arthritis Rheum 31:315–324, 1988.
[b] Present for at least 6 weeks.
[c] Must be observed by physician.
[d] PIP, proximal interphalangeal joint(s); MCP, metacarpophalangeal joint(s); MTP, metatarsophalangeal joint(s).

ized by mild-to-moderate tenderness on palpation or pain on movement of involved joints with or without reversible joint capsule swelling due to synovitis or increased synovial fluid. Patients with moderate-to-severe disease may exhibit signs similar to those with milder disease, but the signs will be more severe and the joint swelling may also be due to synovial proliferation. In patients with progressive disease, joint malformations may become evident within a few years of disease onset and may progress until joint instability and disabling deformities are seen. Restricted activity is noted in 70% of patients with rheumatoid arthritis and 89% of patients with rheumatoid arthritis and comorbid disorders (1). Functional classification allows monitoring of a patient's global ability to perform daily living activities. Functional class I indicates the ability to perform daily living activities without restriction, class II describes those who experience moderate restrictions but can still do normal activities, class II indicates major restriction in performing work or self-care activities, and class IV refers to patients unable to perform self-care or confined to bed or wheelchair.

Joints are the primary area of involvement in rheumatoid arthritis, ranging from quiescent or mild synovitis to severe synovitis, considerable synovial thickening or proliferation, detectable synovial fluid, and obvious bone malformations. Rheumatoid arthritis usually affects diarthrodial joints, including the joints of the hands and feet such as the proximal interphalangeal (PIP) joints, metacarpophalangeal (MCP) joints, metatarsophalangeal (MTP) joints, wrists, and/or ankles. Elbows, shoulders, sternoclavicular joints, temporomandibular joints, knees, and hips also may be commonly involved. Cervical spine involvement may lead to considerable pain and joint derangement.

Joint deformities in rheumatoid arthritis result from destruction of articular or periarticular bone by inflammatory mediators, enzymes, phagocytosis, and physical stress. Common deformities seen in rheumatoid arthritis include ulnar deviation, swan-neck deformities, boutonnière deformities, hammer- or cock-up toe formation, ankylosis, and a variety of other changes. Opposing or compensating forces appear to affect adjacent joints and lead to a zigzag pattern of deformity. In ulnar deviation of the fingers, for example, the fingers point toward the ulnar side of the hand but the metacarpal bones in the palm of the hand deviate or point to the radial side. In the very late stages of progressive disease, bony deformities may predominate and acute inflammation may be absent or minimal. Joints may become destabilized as a result of alterations in the functions or integrity of tendons, ligaments, and the joint capsule and by muscular weakness. Muscle weakness in patients with rheumatoid arthritis is related to decreased muscle mass, compared with normal subjects, which results from inactivity and the catabolic effects of inflammatory mediators.

Joint x-rays are helpful in working-up and following patients with rheumatoid arthritis. Early x-ray findings include some loss of joint space and soft tissue swelling. Periarticular bone loss may occur within 3 to 4 months of

Table 28.3.
Classification of Rheumatoid Arthritis (RA) Based on the 1987 Revised "Tree" or Step Format[a] **(See Table 28.2 for definition of criteria used to define each step.)**

Step	Question	If No	If Yes
1.	Arthritis of 3+ joints?[b,c]	Step 5	Step 2
2.	Radiologic changes or MCP swelling[b,c,d]	Step 3	RA
3.	Positive rheumatoid factor or wrist swelling[b,c]?	Step 4	RA
4.	MCP and wrist swelling?[b,c,d]	No RA	RA
5.	Positive rheumatoid factor or wrist swelling[b,c]?	No RA	Step 6
6.	Symmetric swelling?[b,c]	No RA	Step 7
7.	MCP or wrist swelling?[b,c,d]	No RA	RA

[a] Adapted from Arnett FC, Edworthy SM, Bloch DA, et al.: The American Rheumatism Association 1987 revised criteria for the classification of rheumatoid arthritis. Arthritis Rheum 31:315–324, 1988.
[b] Present for at least 6 weeks.
[c] Must be observed by physician.
[d] MCP, metacarpophalangeal joint(s).

onset of rheumatoid arthritis. Bone erosions, bone cysts, and deformities may become evident as the disease progresses. Radiography may serve as the "gold standard" for analysis of rheumatoid arthritis over time, but it must be evaluated appropriately. Radiographic classification may be useful in following patients over time. Joint scintigraphy may be useful in detecting soft tissue swelling in early rheumatoid arthritis.

Morning stiffness is a gel-like sensation experienced in the joints of patients with rheumatoid arthritis when they attempt to move after waking in the morning or after a period of inactivity. The degree of stiffness diminishes with movement. Plasma concentrations of keratan sulfate, a large cartilage-proteoglycan degradation product, are inversely proportional to the duration of morning stiffness.

Extraarticular involvement includes rheumatoid nodules, vasculitis, rheumatoid lung, renal disorder, Sjögren's syndrome, Felty's syndrome, anemia, depression, ocular inflammation, pericarditis, and general constitutional symptoms. Extraarticular involvement may be more common in rheumatoid factor–positive men than in rheumatoid factor–positive women, and in patients with circulating immune complexes than without. Extraarticular involvement may indicate more severe joint disease.

Subclinical renal dysfunction may be found, particularly in patients with chronic progressive rheumatoid arthritis. Rheumatoid lung disease occurs in up to 20% of rheumatoid arthritis patients, and is characterized by pulmonary effusions, pleuritis, and possibly fibrosis. It may also be associated with therapy for rheumatoid arthritis, rheumatoid nodules, and genetic or environmental factors. Sjögren's syndrome or keratoconjunctivitis sicca is an immunologic disorder that causes decreased function of tear and salivary glands. Interestingly, Sjögren's syndrome developed in a patient with rheumatoid arthritis who became infected with the human immunodeficiency virus (11). Felty's syndrome is a syndrome of neutropenia, splenomegaly, and lymphadenopathy that occurs in patients with rheumatoid arthritis and is associated with increased incidence of infection. Joint infections may occur more commonly in patients with rheumatoid arthritis, particularly in those with prosthetic joints. A mild anemia of chronic disease is seen in patients with rheumatoid arthritis. The anemia responds poorly to iron therapy, but will respond to improvements in the activity of rheumatoid arthritis and to erythropoietin administration (18). Anemia of chronic disease may occur in conjunction with iron deficiency. Hemolytic anemia is a rare feature of rheumatoid arthritis. Depression is seen commonly in patients with rheumatoid arthritis and may affect their perception of their arthritis, but the association between depression and disease activity is not clearly established. Keeping active may diminish signs of depression in rheumatoid arthritis patients. Anxiety and social problems also occur commonly in patients

with rheumatoid arthritis. Fatigue is seen in many patients with rheumatoid arthritis, particularly during active disease. It may be related to a variety of factors including abnormal sleep patterns, anemia, depression, muscle weakness, or neuropeptides. These features demonstrate the systemic nature of rheumatoid arthritis.

Rheumatoid nodules, which contain monocytes and macrophages surrounding a necrotic area, are a systemic feature of rheumatoid arthritis. Rheumatoid nodules are seen in 25% of patients with rheumatoid arthritis, almost all of whom are rheumatoid factor–positive, and are almost considered to be pathognomonic when seen in a patient with persistent arthritis. Rheumatoid nodules generally occur subcutaneously over bone in pressure point areas, but they may be found in other tissues and organs. The pathogenesis of rheumatoid nodules may parallel that of the synovial involvement in rheumatoid arthritis.

Rheumatoid factor is an antibody (usually IgM, but IgG and IgA are also found) that is directed against the Fc portion of IgG. Plasma titers of rheumatoid factor are positive in 80% of patients with rheumatoid arthritis and in up to 5% of the population at large. Rheumatoid factor is also detected in rheumatoid synovial fluid and in the plasma of patients with other inflammatory or infectious disorders. Plasma titers of rheumatoid factor above 1:160 are usually associated with more active rheumatoid arthritis. Plasma titers can be useful in following one patient's rheumatoid arthritis, but they cannot define the activity if no previous values are provided. Rheumatoid factor from patients with rheumatoid arthritis bind better to the Fc portions of IgG3 and IgG4 than to IgG1 and IgG2. False-positive hepatitis C antibody test results are found in many patients with rheumatoid arthritis and may be due to a rheumatoid factor directed against hepatitis C.

Other antibodies may be seen in patients with rheumatoid arthritis. Antinuclear antibodies (i.e., autoantibodies directed against nuclear proteins and commonly seen in patients with systemic lupus erythematosus and other disorders) are sometimes found in low titers in patients with rheumatoid arthritis. Other autoantibodies may also be associated with rheumatoid arthritis.

Erythrocyte sedimentation rate is a nonspecific indicator of inflammation that correlates with the number of joints with effusions in rheumatoid arthritis. Erythrocyte sedimentation rate is measured by placing whole blood in a small tube for 1 hr, allowing red blood cells to fall to the bottom of the tube, and measuring the number of millimeters that the red blood cells have vacated. Normal erythrocyte sedimentation rates range from 0 to 20 mm/hr for women and 0 to 10 mm/hr for men, but this may vary depending upon the method and the laboratory used. Particularly high erythrocyte sedimentation rates are associated with vasculitis. C-reactive protein levels, platelet counts, and orosomucoid levels, also known as α-1-acid glycoprotein, are acute phase reactant measurements and nonspecific indicators of inflammation which are elevated in patients with active rheumatoid arthritis. Plasma hyaluronic acid levels, which are also elevated in rheumatoid arthritis patients, correlate with the number of joints that are tender or have effusions.

TREATMENT

The goals of therapy in rheumatoid arthritis are to improve or maintain current function in the patient's daily living activities, diminish progression of the patient's joint and extraarticular disease, and minimize adverse drug effects using beneficial, safe, and cost-effective means. Therapy should be individualized based upon the course of rheumatoid arthritis, degree of articular and extraarticular disease, concurrent diseases and therapies, age, need for relief, and many other factors. Early in the course of disease it may be difficult to predict whether or not a patient's rheumatoid arthritis will follow a rapidly progressive, slowly progressive, unprogressive, or remitting course. This complicates some therapeutic decisions.

Nonspecific drug and nondrug therapies are used to control the acute inflammation and attempt to control the progression of the disease, but very few patients will achieve a cure. Specific measures such as surgery are useful in correcting deformities and enhancing the ability to perform certain tasks. Better understanding of the etiology and pathogenesis of rheumatoid arthritis may lead to a more specific and less toxic therapies.

Traditionally, the treatment of rheumatoid arthritis is described as a pyramid in which education, rest, exercise, and nonsteroidal antiinflammatory drugs serve as the base and are used in most if not all patients. The next levels of the pyramid involve the addition of one of a group of more toxic agents or experimental therapies to patients with progressive disease or sustained severe synovitis. Corticosteroids and orthopaedic surgery are used as adjunctive measures at any level of the pyramid. Many investigators have begun to promote approaches other than this traditional pyramid.

Nondrug therapies are widely used in all stages of rheumatoid arthritis. Patients should understand the nature and possible progression of their disease to promote self-awareness, self-determination, and self-reliance. They must know when to seek help from others. Family support is essential; negative attitudes toward the patient's disease lead to less coping, less adaptation, and more stress. Rest spares joints, decreases inflammation, and may lead to repair of damaged tissues. Patients with rheumatoid arthritis should not diminish activity completely because of fatigue, but they should be encouraged to rest on a routine basis each day. Prolonged immobility may lead to increased stiffness and diminished mobility of joints and strength. For

selected patients, hospitalization with rest and possibly minor revisions in drug therapy may have drastic results. Intensive hospitalization for 14 days resulted in a 3-fold improvement in rheumatoid arthritis at a 2.5-fold increase in cost over no hospitalization (19). An appropriate exercise program decreases joint inflammation, maintains range of motion, and increases overall well-being through range of motion, cardiovascular fitness, or strength building programs that do not overstress joints and muscles. Such exercise programs may also diminish the development of osteoporosis in those on corticosteroids or otherwise prone to develop it. Nutrition is important to help patients lose weight (if overweight) and to maintain protein and calcium intake. Fish oils or certain plant seed oils may be of some benefit in rheumatoid arthritis (see below). Specially designed eating utensils, grooming aids, working aids, and other self-help aids help maintain the patient's self-reliance. Splints may be useful in stabilizing a weak joint, resting an active joint, or possibly diminishing the rate of joint destruction. Walking aids or wheelchairs may improve a patient's mobility dramatically, and improve stability when mobile. Hot paraffin wax treatments may decrease inflammation and discomfort. Surgery can repair or replace damaged joints, fuse joints for stability, correct tendon or ligament instability, release carpal tunnel syndrome, or perform synovectomies. These nondrug therapies must be individualized to the patient's needs and current state.

Systemic and topical analgesics may benefit selected patients. Systemic analgesics, such as acetaminophen and opioid analgesics are generally considered to be of limited benefit because of the inflammatory nature of this disease, but they may help occasionally as adjuncts to antiinflammatory medications. Topical ointments, creams, and liniments may provide local relief, but systemic absorption is possible and may lead to toxicity or drug interactions (e.g., the increased effect of warfarin in patients using topical salicylates (20)).

NONSTEROIDAL ANTIINFLAMMATORY DRUGS

Nonsteroidal antiinflammatory drugs (NSAIDs) are used to treat acute synovitis in all stages of rheumatoid arthritis because of their inhibition of prostaglandin synthesis, membrane-related enzyme activities, membrane anion transport, arachidonate precursor uptake and insertion into monocyte membranes, collagenase release, and neutrophil function (21). Only the d-isomer of the propionate derivatives (Table 28.4) is active. Prostaglandin E concentrations in synovial fluid continue to be suppressed when synovial concentrations of these drugs drop to very low levels. Subtherapeutic concentrations of NSAIDs may enhance the secretion of prostaglandins in vitro (22). NSAIDs enhance cytotoxic and suppressor T lymphocyte activity, which may result in inhibition of B lymphocyte

Table 28.4.
Nonsteroidal Antiinflammatory Drugs Used in Rheumatoid Arthritis

Classes	Drug (Active Metabolite)	Half-life (hr) Normal	Half-Life (hr) in ESRD[a]	Daily Dose (mg/day)	Doses per Day
Fenamates	Meclofenamate	2–3		300–400	3–4
Indoles	Etodolac	7	NC[b]	800–1200	3–4
	Indomethacin	1–16	NC	100–200	3–4
	Indomethacin SR	1–16	NC	150	1–2
	Sulindac (Sulfide)	8	NC	300–400	2
		16–18			
	Tolmetin	0.5–3		1600–2000	3–4
Oxicams	Piroxicam	26–137	44	10–20	1
Phenylacetates	Diclofenac	1–2	1–2	150–200	3–4
Propionates	Fenoprofen	1.5–4		1600–3200	3–4
	Flurbiprofen	3–6		200–300	2–4
	Ibuprofen	1–2.5	2.5	1600–3200	3–4
	Ketoprofen	1–4	3.2	150–300	3–4
	Naproxen	9–17	15	500–1500	2–3
Salicylates	Aspirin (Salicylate)	0.2–0.3	NC	2400–6500	3–5
		2–30	NC		
	Diflunisal	5–20	15–138	500–1500	2–3
	Salsalate	2–30	NC	2000–3000	3–4
	Other salicylates	2–30	NC	2400–6500	3–5

[a] End-stage renal disease.
[b] No change in half-life.

activity. Most currently available NSAIDs do not alter or actually increase leukotrienes, but ketoprofen and possibly other investigational agents inhibit leukotriene synthesis and bradykinin activity (the consequences of which are unknown). Glycosaminoglycan synthesis in joint cartilage is inhibited by some NSAIDs, such as sodium salicylate (21), but others inhibit cartilage destruction. The balance of the antiinflammatory effects and the effects on the cartilage destruction in rheumatoid arthritis is not yet understood.

NSAIDs are generally well absorbed following oral administration and are highly bound to albumin. The half-lives and dosing of these agents vary considerably (Table 28.4). Following oral administration, synovial fluid concentrations of NSAIDs rise and fall more slowly than serum concentrations, with synovial fluid concentrations becoming greater than serum concentrations at times after administration that are proportional to approximately 2 to 3 times the half-life of the drug (23). Synovial fluid concentrations of NSAIDs with longer half-lives do not exceed serum concentrations during the dosing interval (23). Aspirin is rapidly deacetylated in plasma to salicylic acid, which displays nonlinear pharmacokinetics at antiinflammatory plasma concentrations of 150 to 250 mg/liter. Most NSAIDs undergo some hepatic metabolism, but appreciable amounts are excreted unchanged in urine. Sulindac is metabolized to an active product and to an inactive, renally excreted product. Naproxen is unusual; at high doses its excretion is increased, and serum concentrations are lower than those expected from the increase in dose. End-stage renal disease prolongs the half-life of diflunisal (Table 28.4) (24). Dosage adjustments may be needed in patients with end-stage renal or hepatic disease, depending upon the drug.

Adverse effects from NSAIDs involve many organ systems. Indomethacin, phenylbutazone, meclofenamate, and aspirin appear to be more frequently associated with severe adverse effects. Gastrointestinal effects are most common and include distress, nausea, vomiting, diarrhea, bleeding, and ulceration. Meclofenamate has a high incidence of diarrhea. Microbleeding from aspirin is greater than that from other NSAIDs. Gastric ulceration or bleeding occurs in up to 30% of individuals on chronic NSAIDs, depending upon the definition of the event (25). Misoprostol, a PGE_1 analog, protects against gastric ulceration associated with chronic NSAID use, particularly in high-risk groups such as the elderly, or those with a history of peptic ulcer disease or gastrointestinal bleeding from NSAIDs. Misoprostol may be cost-effective in patients with a history of gastrointestinal bleeding. Sucralfate is somewhat effective as preventative therapy. Histamine-2 receptor antagonists have little effect in preventing or treating NSAID-associated gastric ulceration or bleeding, but they may provide better protection than misoprostol against duodenal ulceration or bleeding in high-risk patients (26). Omeprazole may also prove to be protective against gastrointestinal damage. NSAIDs are also associated with cholestatic and cellular hepatotoxicity, particularly in patients with active rheumatoid arthritis.

NSAIDs cause interstitial nephritis, tubular necrosis, papillary necrosis, and decreased renal blood flow by prostaglandin inhibition. Patients with cardiovascular conditions or cirrhosis, those who are elderly, and patients on loop diuretics (if elderly), on high doses of NSAIDs, or renally insufficient appear to be at increased risk of effects on renal prostaglandins. Sulindac may have less effect on renal prostaglandins that other NSAIDs because of an inactive metabolite that is the major renal excretory product.

NSAIDs inhibit platelet aggregation in a concentration-dependent manner related to the inhibition of platelet thromboxane production. Production of vascular prostacyclin, an antithrombosis substance, may also be inhibited. Nonacetylated salicylates do not affect thromboxane or prostacyclin production. Aspirin causes irreversible inhibition of platelet aggregation, but the effect is reversible with other NSAIDs. Other hematologic abnormalities, such as agranulocytosis, are rarely associated with NSAIDs but occur more commonly when phenylbutazone is used in the elderly or for longer than 14 days.

Commonly occurring central nervous effects include dizziness, fussiness, and headache. Indomethacin use is limited by a high percentage of central nervous system effects including hallucinations, dizziness, headaches, confusion, and disorientation. Aseptic meningitis is a rare adverse reaction of NSAIDs, reported mostly in patients with systemic lupus erythematosus taking ibuprofen, but other NSAIDs have also been implicated.

Allergic reactions to NSAIDs include bronchoconstriction, nasal polyps, urticaria, rhinitis, angioedema, and anaphylaxis. These reactions may be due to the inhibition of prostaglandin synthesis, which is consistent with the cross-sensitivity of allergy among these drugs (27). Nonacetylated salicylates have been suggested as safe alternatives in allergic patients, but cross-sensitivity with nonacetylated salicylates has occurred (28). Photosensitivity may also be associated with NSAIDs.

Drug interactions associated with NSAIDs are generally mediated by pharmacodynamic or pharmacokinetic effects. These drugs may diminish the effectiveness of antihypertensives, but the effect may or may not be clinically important. Inhibition of renal function may alter the pharmacokinetics of renally excreted drugs. Salicylates inhibit the action of uricosurics. Aspirin and phenylbutazone interact with warfarin. High-dose methotrexate may be much more toxic when used with NSAIDs, but the low doses of methotrexate used to treat rheumatoid arthritis are usually administered safely with other NSAIDs. However, aspirin plus methotrexate was associated with increases in liver enzyme levels (29). NSAIDs interact with each other in pharmacokinetic, pharmacodynamic, and

toxic manners but combinations of these drugs are occasionally beneficial.

Efficacy of the various NSAIDs in rheumatoid arthritis do not differ overall. Onset of effect is within a few days to a week, possibly longer for agents with half-lives greater than 24 hr, with maximum effects seen in 1 to 4 weeks. NSAIDs decrease erythrocyte sedimentation rate, C-reactive protein levels, rheumatoid factor titers, and the number of circulating activated T lymphocytes in rheumatoid arthritis patients, but may not increase hemoglobin levels (30), possibly because of increased bleeding or limited effects on the underlying disease process. Patients more likely to respond to NSAIDs have more aggressive disease, based on clinical or nonspecific inflammatory measures such as C-reactive protein levels and erythrocyte sedimentation rate (30). Adverse effects, cost, and ease of administration should be major factors in choosing the initial and subsequent NSAIDs. If a patient does not tolerate or respond to antiinflammatory doses of one of them, subsequent selections can be made from a different or from the same chemical class.

SECOND-LINE ANTIRHEUMATIC DRUGS

Second-line agents, also known as disease-modifying or slow-acting antirheumatic drugs, include the antimalarials chloroquine and hydroxychloroquine, injectable gold salts, auranofin, methotrexate, sulfasalazine, penicillamine, azathioprine, and cyclosphamide. These drugs have varied effects on the immune system, but their mechanisms of action in rheumatoid arthritis remain unclear. Second-line agents should be used only in patients with potentially reversible or preventable severe disease because of the frequency of toxicity and inefficacy and the cost of therapy and monitoring. Beneficial effects of second-line agents are seen over 1 to 6 months and may lead to remission or decreased progression of the disease in a few patients (31, 32). Only injectable gold and cyclophosphamide have definitively slowed or reversed the radiographic progression of rheumatoid arthritis (31). Of those patients initiating therapy with a second-line drug, 50% or more will stop the drug within 5 years because of loss of effect or adverse drug reactions (33). The elderly do not differ from younger patients in the efficacy or toxicity of second-line agents (34).

Injectable gold salts have been used to treat rheumatoid arthritis since the 1920s as a result of their effects against tuberculosis and the possible association between rheumatoid arthritis and tuberculosis. The high doses used initially (100 to 200 mg per week) were associated with considerable toxicity, but the current maintenance doses of 25 and 50 mg per week are more tolerable. Generally, two test doses, one of 10 mg then one of 25 mg, are used for the first two weekly intramuscular injections of the injectable gold salt. If the patient responds to weekly maintenance doses, then the dosage interval may be widened to every 2 weeks, then every 3 weeks, and so on. An oral form of gold, auranofin, became available in the early 1980s and is effective at doses of 3 to 9 mg daily. Auranofin appears to be less effective but also less toxic than injectable gold (32).

Injectable gold salts and auranofin, which are 50 and 28% elemental gold, respectively, differ in many aspects of their pharmacokinetics. Two injectable gold-salt forms are available, aurothiomalate is the more water-soluble solution and aurothioglucose is a less water-soluble suspension. Injectable gold is very poorly absorbed orally, but auranofin is 20 to 25% absorbed. Gold is bound extensively to serum albumin and widely distributed to human tissues including the kidneys, liver, reticuloendothelial system, spleen, synovial membrane, skin, hair, and nails. Skin serves as a large storage site in some patients following injectable gold administration. A higher percentage of injectable gold is retained in body tissues than of auranofin. The half-lives of both forms of gold are at least 1 to 3 weeks. Most of the absorbed gold salt is excreted in urine, but 85% of auranofin is recovered in feces. Gold is removed by peritoneal dialysis (35), but not hemodialysis (24). Serum gold concentrations after aurothiomalate may not correlate with efficacy or toxicity, but lower whole blood concentrations are seen in those with a better response (36).

In pooled data from clinical studies, injectable gold was discontinued because of adverse effects more than other second-line agents (32). The reasons for withdrawal included rash (13%), proteinuria (3.7%), mucous membrane effects (1.8%), leukopenia (1.5%), thrombocytopenia (1.1%), gastrointestinal effects (1.3%), hepatic effects (0.9%), blood effects (0.9%), and less commonly, diarrhea, fever, alopecia, and renal, lung, and ocular effects (32). Nitritoid reactions, characterized by flushing and syncope, may occur up to 30 minutes following an injection of gold salts, particularly aurothiomalate. A trial with aurothioglucose may be considered or the patient may be asked to sit or lie down for 20 to 30 minutes following each injection if such reactions occur. Gold storage in skin can lead to chrysiasis, a bronze-like appearance. Injectable gold-induced proteinuria (but not hematologic or dermatologic toxicity) occurred much more commonly in HLA-DRw3+ and HLA-B8+ patients (37). Safe monitoring of injectable gold salts requires complete blood and platelet counts, urinalysis, and skin and mucous membrane inspections just prior to each injection. Auranofin adverse reaction withdrawals from pooled clinical studies were below those with other second-line agents and included diarrhea (3.9%), rash (3.2%), gastrointestinal (1.1%), proteinuria (0.9%) and less commonly, thrombocytopenia, leukopenia, anemia, alteration in taste, nausea, vomiting, and mucous membrane, hepatic, lung, and central nervous system effects (32). Auranofin monitoring includes a complete blood and platelet counts, urinalysis, and evaluations of skin, mucous membranes, and the gastrointestinal tract every 2 to 4 weeks. Other organ toxicity, such as lung and liver, also require monitoring for either type of gold. Severe diarrhea, bloody gastroenteritis, proteinuria, mucositis, rash, hematologic toxicity, or other serious abnormalities usually indicate a discontinuation of auranofin.

Methotrexate is effective in rheumatoid arthritis at doses ranging from 7.5 to 15 mg weekly administered orally or intramuscularly in one dose or in three equal doses every 12 hours. Subcutaneous injections may be an alternative to intramuscular injections of methotrexate (38). Methotraxate differs from other second-line agents in its rapid response at 6 weeks (39) and the arthritis flare seen soon after its withdrawal (40). Methotrexate was most effective in decreasing tender joint counts in a recent metaanalysis of second-line agents (32), but it may or may not alter the bony progression of the disease (39).

Methotrexate absorption is highly variable. Cholecystectomy may decrease the bioavailability of low-dose methotrexate from 85 to 39% (41). Methotrexate is metabolized to an active metabolite, 7-hydroxymethotrexate. Biliary excretion may account for 9 to 26% of methotrexate elimination and 2 to 5% of 7-hydroxy metabolite elimination after low doses of methotrexate (41). Methotrexate elimination may be decreased in patients with end-stage renal disease (24). Methotrexate is removed by hemodialysis, but not by peritoneal dialysis (24).

Patients are monitored every 2 to 6 weeks for adverse effects from methotrexate. Pooled clinical studies have revealed withdrawals for methotrexate due to hepatic effects (10.3%), mucous membrane effects (2.6%), nausea and/or vomiting (2.1%), gastrointestinal effects (2.1%), leukopenia (1%), blood effects (1.5%), and diarrhea (0.5%) (32). The majority of the liver effects were elevations of liver enzyme levels rather than abnormalities in liver biopsy specimens, which is the preferred method of detecting methotrexate-induced liver toxicity. Liver biopsies are not routinely recommended in patients with rheumatoid arthritis receiving methotrexate because of the low incidence of hepatotoxicity. Increased incidence of abnormalities in liver enzyme levels are noted in patients on methotrexate plus aspirin, but less commonly in patients also on hydroxychloroquine (29). Although usually irreversible, severe liver toxicity may be reversible. Sustained elevation of mean corpuscular volume in a patient treated with methotrexate may indicate folate deficiency and may serve as a predictor for methotrexate hematologic toxicity (42). Severe neutropenia may develop at low doses in rheumatoid arthritis in patients with end-stage renal disease. Concurrent folic acid administration may diminish the toxicity of methotrexate (43). Methotrexate also causes pneumonitis and rashes.

Drug interactions involving methotrexate may have serious consequences. As noted previously, NSAIDs cause clinically important increases in methotrexate toxicity when given with high (but not low) doses of methotrexate. Cholestryamine binds to methotrexate and enhances its excretion. Folinic acid may reverse the methotrexate-induced suppression of immunoglobulin production in a dose-related manner in vitro (44). Salicylate and probenecid inhibit methotrexate excretion.

Antimalarials have been used in rheumatoid arthritis since a 1951 report of a patient whose rheumatoid arthritis improved after an antimalarial, mepacrine, was used to treat the patient's discoid lupus (45). Chloroquine became widely used, but has been replaced by hydroxychloroquine in the treatment of rheumatoid arthritis. Although both are effective, chloroquine is possibly more effective (32). Hydroxychloroquine is used at doses of 2 to 4 mg/kg or 200 to 400 mg per day orally. Chloroquine oral doses are 200 to 300 mg daily of the base.

Hydroxychloroquine is absorbed readily following oral administration, with peak concentrations seen in 1 to 3 hr. Hydroxychloroquine is 45% bound to serum albumin and distributes into red blood cells and extensively into other tissues. Hydroxychloroquine pharmacokinetics are linear within usual therapeutic ranges and are best fit by a three-phase model with a terminal half-life of approximately 40 days. Dosage adjustment is not needed in renal dysfunction because only 22 to 34% of hydroxychloroquine is excreted unchanged in urine. Chloroquine pharmacokinetics are very similar, with a half-life of 6 to 50 days and lack appreciable removal by hemodialysis (24).

Pooled data from clinical studies involving second-line agents revealed that chloroquine and hydroxychloroquine adverse effects led to the fewest withdrawals, which included gastrointestinal tract (4.6%), rash (2.3%), ocular (0.7%), and less commonly, mucous membrane, leukopenia, and central nervous system effects (32). Corneal deposits occur in 20% plus and symptomatic retinopathy in 2 to 17% of those receiving chloroquine, with higher frequencies seen in those receiving higher doses and the elderly. Hydroxychloroquine appears to be discontinued rarely because of retinopathy at the dosage ranges listed above, but patients should see an ophthalmologist every 3 to 12 months for a full ophthalmic examination. Hydroxychloroquine may also exacerbate psoriasis, cause allergic reactions, or (rarely) cause bone marrow, neurologic, neuromuscular, or cardiac toxicity. Chloroquine has decreased the normal response to intradermal rabies vaccine in normal subjects (46).

Sulfasalazine was designed in the 1940s to treat rheumatoid arthritis but is being used more extensively following promising studies (32, 47). Compared with hydroxychloroquine, sulfasalazine may be associated with less progression of radiographic changes in rheumatoid ar-

thritis (47). The sulfapyridine component of sulfasalazine is responsible for its activity against rheumatoid arthritis.

Pooled data from studies involving second-line agents found that the adverse effect withdrawal rate from sulfasalazine was less than that for gold but similar to that of penicillamine (32). Sulfasalazine was withdrawn for nausea and/or vomiting (12.5%), rash (3.8%), liver effects (1.6), leukopenia (1.1%), mucous membranes (1.1%), fever (1.1%), anemia (0.5%), and lung effects (0.5%) (32). Monitoring for toxicity is based mostly upon the clinical presentation of the patient.

Azathioprine has demonstrated efficacy in treating rheumatoid arthritis at doses of 1.0 to 2.5 mg/kg or 50 to 200 mg per day. Azothioprine has a half-life of 0.2 to 1 hr, is removed by hemodialysis, and is converted to 6-mercaptopurine, its active form (24). Allopurinol inhibits the metabolism of azathioprine, requiring the dose of azathioprine to be decreased by 67 to 75%.

Adverse effects of azathioprine have been of concern, but postmarketing surveillance has revealed a relatively safe adverse effect profile in rheumatoid arthritis (48). Monitoring with complete blood counts, liver function tests, and examination of mucous membranes every 2 to 6 weeks is still necessary to evaluate azathioprine-induced gastrointestinal distress, leukopenia, mucous membrane effects, and liver toxicity.

Penicillamine is effective in the treatment of severe, progressive rheumatoid arthritis at doses from 250 to 1500 mg per day. Starting at low doses of 125 to 250 mg per day and increasing every 2 to 4 weeks to a maximum of 500 or 750 mg per day may decrease the incidence of adverse drug reactions and is currently preferred. Efficacy and toxicity do not correlate with serum concentration.

Peak plasma concentrations of penicillamine are seen 1 to 3 hr after administration, but only 30 to 70% is absorbed in fasting individuals and less in patients recently fed or given iron tablets or antacids containing aluminum or magnesium hydroxides (49). Penicillamine is 70 to 80% bound to serum albumin. In animals, penicillamine disappears rapidly from kidney and liver tissue, but more slowly from skin and bone. Approximately 2 to 8% of penicillamine is metabolized hepatically to its methyl metabolite, but the major route of elimination is urinary excretion (49). The half-life of penicillamine is 1.5 to 3 hr. In two patients with rheumatoid arthritis and end-stage renal disease, on hemodialysis 3 times a week, penicillamine doses of 250 mg three times weekly yielded serum concentrations of the drug and its metabolite that were similar to those seen after higher daily doses in patients with normal renal function (50). Penicillamine is removed by hemodialysis (50).

Use of penicillamine is limited by adverse effects that increase as the dose increases. The pooled metaanalysis data for second-line agents demonstrated withdrawals from penicillamine for rash (7.1%), proteinuria (5%), thrombocytopenia (2.5%), alterations in taste (2.5%), nausea or vomiting (2%), leukopenia (1%), and less commonly, gastrointestinal, fever, hepatic, diarrhea, renal, lung, breast, and mucous membrane effects (32). Patients with poor sulfoxidation capacity are 3.9 times more likely to experience toxicity to penicillamine at comparable doses than those with ample sulfoxidation capacity, but without a difference in efficacy (51). Penicillamine-induced proteinuria (but not dermatologic or hematologic toxicity) may occur more commonly in HLA-DRw3+ and HLA-B8+ patients (37). Penicillamine induces a variety of autoimmune disorders, including myasthenia gravis, systemic lupus erythematosis, Goodpasture's syndrome, polymyositis, hemolytic anemia, and pemphigus. Penicillamine-induced peripheral neuropathy may respond to pyridoxine. Since penicillamine is a metabolic byproduct of penicillin, caution should be used when administering penicillamine to penicillin-allergic patients, although it is generally considered safe. Fetal abnormalities may occur when penicillamine is given during pregnancy, including connective tissue defects such as lax skin syndrome. At the initiation of therapy, patients should be monitored every 2 to 4 weeks for adverse effects with urinalysis, complete blood count, and examination of skin and mucous membranes. Once stable, monitoring every 4 to 6 weeks may suffice. Penicillamine may chelate iron salts and lead to malabsorption of both agents from the gastrointestinal tract.

Cyclophosphamide is effective in rheumatoid arthritis at doses of 75 to 150 mg (0.68 to 3.4 mg/kg) per day, but causes considerable short- and long-term toxicity, even at lower doses. Doses are adjusted to keep the white blood cell count within the normal or low-normal range. Intravenous cyclophosphamide at high doses (500 mg/m^2) every 4 to 6 weeks for 6 cycles may be useful in treating rheumatoid vasculitis, but is poorly tolerated and minimally effective in patients with refractory rheumatoid arthritis (52).

Cyclophosphamide is inactive until converted in the liver to active metabolites, which are 56% plasma protein bound. Following the administration of radioactive cyclophosphamide, the half-life of radioactive material was 6.5 hr, and 68% was excreted in urine. The half-life of cyclophosphamide increases from 5 to 7 hr in normal renal function to 4 to 12 hr in end-stage renal disease (24). Renal dysfunction decreases the excretion of cyclophosphamide metabolites, leading to increased toxicity and requiring a decrease in dose. Cyclophosphamide is removed by hemodialysis (24).

Cyclophosphamide is associated with short- and long-term toxicity, even in the doses used to treat rheumatoid arthritis. Leukopenia, hemorrhagic cystitis, hair loss, gastrointestinal disturbance, infertility, inappropriate secretion of antidiuretic hormone, and immunosuppression are serious effects. Immunosuppression leads to an increased incidence of viral and bacterial infections. Cyclophosphamide causes pneumonitis and pulmonary fibrosis. The occurrence of malignancies is four times higher in a group of rheumatoid arthritis patients who received cyclophosphamide than in those who had not. Physical findings, complete blood counts and urinalyses are used to monitor cyclophosphamide therapy. Cyclophosphamide interacts with other agents that affect bone marrow function.

Choosing among second-line agents is difficult. A recent review (31) and metaanalyses (32) of published data concluded that gold sodium thiomalate and methotrexate were among the most efficacious, but methotrexate was among the least toxic and injectable gold salts among the most toxic second-line agent (5). Hydroxychloroquine and auranofin were ranked as least effective, with hydroxychloroquine among the least toxic and auranofin among the least (32) to intermediate (31) in toxicity. Sulfasalazine was ranked as both least (31) and most (32) effective, and intermediately toxic. Azathioprine was of intermediate efficacy and among the least toxic (31). Penicillamine was ranked as among agents with both intermediate (31) and most (32) efficacy, but also most toxic. Cyclophosphamide was not included in either analysis.

Currently, methotrexate is widely considered the initial second-line drug of choice in severe rheumatoid arthritis, but gold salts are still preferred by many practitioners. Antimalarials are used widely in certain clinics, but in less severe disease or as adjuncts to other second-line agents. If sulfasalazine proves to be as promising in practice as clinical studies have indicated, its use will increase because of its lack of serious adverse effects. Azathioprine and auranofin are used less often, and penicillamine and cyclophosphamide even less because of their lower benefit to toxicity ratio. Methotrexate, azathioprine, or cyclophosphamide may also be of benefit in extraarticular manifestations of rheumatoid arthritis such as steroid-resistant pulmonary disease or vasculitis.

Use of second-line agents is controversial in patients with recently diagnosed, early rheumatoid arthritis. Auranofin has been shown to retard disease progression in early rheumatoid arthritis (53), demonstrating that early rheumatoid arthritis may be more reversible or preventable. However, it is difficult to predict which patients will go on to progressive, erosive disease and if the toxicity and cost will be offset by the potential benefits.

Combined second-line agents have been considered since the early 1960s to increase efficacy without additive toxicity by initiating the agents at the same time or adding second or third agents when the first agent becomes less effective (54–65). Injectable gold plus either an antimalarial, sulfasalazine, or chlorambucil is more effective, but has increased toxicity over each drug alone (54, 55, 58). Auranofin plus methotrexate had more toxicity, and no improvement in efficacy over methotrexate or auranofin alone (65). Combinations of penicillamine with an antimalarial, azathioprine, gold, or sulfasalazine have been less predictable and more limited by adverse effects (56–59). Pulse cyclophosphamide provided little added benefit to gold plus pulse methylprednisolone (60). Three or more drug combinations using anticancer drugs with gold, penicillamine, or an antimalarial have also been evaluated. Full-dose hydroxychloroquine and methotrexate plus full- or low-dose azathioprine are efficacious with some toxicity (64), even following initial failure of methotrexate or azathioprine (63). Hydroxychloroquine, low-dose cyclophosphamide, and low-dose azathioprine or methotrexate were highly effective, with reversal of bony erosions (61, 62). Use of cyclophosphamide in combinations is limited by long-term toxicity, and it has been replaced by either azathioprine or methotrexate.

CORTICOSTEROIDS

Corticosteroids have been used to treat rheumatoid arthritis by oral low-doses daily, occasional intraarticular injections, and intravenous pulses of high doses. Corticosteroids inhibit T and B lymphocyte activity, leukocyte chemotaxis, number of mast cells in rheumatoid synovium, and release of collagenase and lysosomal enzymes. Low-dose oral corticosteroids, at prednisone-equivalent doses of 2.5 to 15 mg per day, can decrease the swelling and tenderness dramatically and improve the sense of well-being in patients treated with NSAIDs or just started on slow-acting antirheumatic drugs. However, risk of cumulative toxic effects on the skeleton, metabolism, and other organ systems limits the chronic use and dose of corticosteroids. Corticosteroids may increase the incidence of peptic ulcer and gastrointestinal hemorrhage, particularly in patients receiving NSAIDs. Hypothalamic-pituitary-adrenal suppression can be seen even with low-dose corticosteroids. An unconventional, experimental use of corticosteroids in selected patients includes an approach similar to patient-controlled analgesia, and may result in lower average daily doses (66). Corticosteroids are also useful in treating extraarticular features of rheumatoid arthritis, such as vasculitis and rheumatoid lung.

Intraarticular injections of corticosteroids use insoluble salt forms of active corticosteroids. Intraarticular injections of corticosteroids should be used only when indicated, including only one or two joints that are inflamed to the point of limiting the patient's ability to function or rehabilitate considerably and occur despite an adequate therapeutic regimen. A needle with attached syringe is inserted into a joint space under aseptic conditions prior to withdrawal and brief visual analysis of the synovial fluid. With the needle still in place, the syringe is changed and the corticosteroid is injected. A dose of 2.5 to 10 mg of prednisolone tebutate equivalents is used in a small joint

such as a PIP, MCP, or MTP joint of a hand or foot; 10 to 25 mg in a wrist, ankle, or elbow; and 20 to 50 mg in a shoulder, ankle, knee, or hip. These insoluble corticosteroid salts may also benefit tenosynovitis, bursitis, and carpal tunnel syndrome. Following injection of the joint or other structure, passive or small-load range of motion or activity can be used to enhance spread of the drug, followed by resting the joint for 24 to 48 hr. Earlier, strenuous activity may damage the joint. Intraarticular corticosteroids may cause a crystal synovitis because they are insoluble and may be safe in children, except in hip joint injections (67). Joint infections are rare, but multiple repeat injections to the same joint may result in breakdown of articular cartilage. The effects of this modality can be dramatic and may last for months to years. The joint fluid removed should be analyzed for white blood cells and differential, bacteria, crystals, and other features.

Pulse, high-dose methylprednisolone (1 g daily intravenously for one to three days) may produce short-term benefits in the treatment of refractory rheumatoid arthritis or prior to response from slow-acting agents, but it does not appear to have long-term effects or retard disease progression (68, 69). Pulse methylprednisolone can decrease synovial fluid polymorphonuclear cells, lymphocytes, immune complexes, and C-reactive protein (70). Severe adverse effects to high-dose, pulse corticosteroids include the rare occurrence of cardiac arrhythmias and sudden death.

EXPERIMENTAL THERAPIES

Numerous experimental therapies for patients with intractable disease attack various components of the immune and inflammatory systems. Total lymphoid irradiation, which kills lymphocytes in lymph nodes, may produce considerable benefit in patients with intractable rheumatoid arthritis, but long-term toxicity is of concern (71). Plasmapheresis, which attempts to remove immune complexes, improves laboratory markers but has only slight or temporary effect on the clinical measures of rheumatoid arthritis (72).

Fish oil, which contains the omega-3 fatty acids eicosapentanoic acid (EPA) and docosahexaenoic acid (DHA), has been of some benefit in treating rheumatoid arthritis in a slow-developing, dose-related manner, without changes in rheumatoid factor titer hemoglobin levels or erythrocyte sedimentation rate (73). EPA and DHA lead to formation of PGD_3 and PGE_3 over more inflammatory prostaglandins. Fish oil decreases LTB_4 and IL-1 production (73), chemotactic action of LTB_4, plasma arachidonic acid levels, and blood pressure in untreated mild hypertensives (74). However, fish oil inhibits proteoglycan synthesis and leads to osteoarthritic-type cartilage in rats (75).

Evening primrose oil and borage seed oil contain gamma linolenic acid (GLA) and may be of some benefit in rheumatoid arthritis with few adverse drug events (76).

GLA is a precursor of dihomogamma linolenic acid, which favors the formation of PGE_1 over an inflammatory prostaglandin PGE_2, cannot be converted to leukotrienes, and competes with arachidonic acid for oxidation enzymes. GLA administration for 12 weeks resulted in reduced PGE_2, LTB_4, and LTC_4 production in ex vivo stimulated monocytes (76). GLA has also inhibited the production and/or activity of IL-1, IL-2 and TNF. The formation of PGE_1 may also confer cytoprotective activity in the gastrointestinal tract. Corn oil, which contains linoleic acid, did not alter plasma arachidonic acid but lowered EPA and DHA levels in untreated mild hypertensives (74). Olive oil, which contains oleic acid, decreased the neutrophil production of LTB_4, monocyte stimulation, and macrophage production of IL-1 (p>.5), but was only marginally beneficial in treating rheumatoid arthritis (73). GLA-containing products seem to be the most promising.

Cyclosporine, which inhibits T lymphocyte function, has been of benefit in rheumatoid arthritis at initial doses of 2.5 to 10 mg/kg per day (77, 78). Nephrotoxicity, hypertension, hypertrichosis, fatigue, and gastrointestinal and neurologic complaints were frequent. Cyclosporine plus an oral corticosteroid was beneficial in rheumatoid lung (79). Use of cyclosporine in rheumatoid arthritis is currently limited by adverse effects, cost, monitoring, and unknown proper dosage or target blood concentrations.

Rheumatoid arthritis may also respond to other immunologically active compounds such as gamma globulin (80), antilymphocyte globulin (81), antithymocyte globulin (82), anti-CD4 antibody (83), IL-1 antagonists, interferon-γ (84), thymopoietin derivatives (85), levamisole (86), ciamexon (87), and others. Future advances in rheumatology, immunology, and molecular biology may prove useful in designing specific treatments for rheumatoid arthritis that may act specifically against possible defects in the HLA-DR4 antigen, macrophages, lymphocytes, mast cells or other components of the immune system.

Patients must be cautioned about use of quack therapies including copper bracelets, herbal remedies, megadose vitamins, bee venom, and snake venom. Such remedies may provide relief in anecdotal reports, but they do not stand up to the rigor of controlled clinical study.

PROGNOSIS

The prognosis in most patients with rheumatoid arthritis is expected to be good. Approximately 10 to 20% of patients with rheumatoid arthritis have a mild single cycle or the disease which remits spontaneously, 70 to 80% have multiple cycles of mild-to-moderate arthritis, and 10 to 20% have multiple cycles of progressive, severe disease. Patients with rheumatoid arthritis may experience temporary or permanent disability, considerable morbidity from medications or the systemic features of the disease, and some decrease in survival, particularly those with more severe disease. Quality of life, (which can be assessed by questionnaire) is affected in many patients at some time during the course of the disease. A very small number of patients become confined to a wheelchair or bed because of rheumatoid arthritis.

CONCLUSIONS

Rheumatoid arthritis is a chronic, autoimmune disease of unknown etiology which affects joints and other tissues and organs. Alterations in the immune, inflammatory, and related systems result in the tumor-like proliferation of synovial tissue and destruction of bone and cartilage in a minority of patients. The cyclic, variable course of rheumatoid arthritis may or may not be altered by the nonspecific drug and nondrug therapies used.

Nondrug therapies are used to help the patient cope and to maintain or correct the problems associated with rheumatoid arthritis. Nonsteroidal antiinflammatory drugs are used as one of the baseline measures to treat the acute inflammation, but may also have effects on the immune system and on cartilage formation and destruction. Chronic adverse effects may limit their use. In patients with progressive or probable progressive disease, a group of more toxic second-line agents are used, despite a poor therapeutic ratio, inability to sustain therapy with any one agent, questionable effects on the progression of the disease, and lack of consensus on which agent or agents to use and how early to initiate this type of therapy. Methotrexate, injectable gold salts, or antimalarials appear to be the current second-line drugs of choice, but sulfasalazine and azathioprine are still used frequently. Hopefully, research will lead to effective, more specific, and less toxic therapies.

REFERENCES

1. Yelin EH, Felts WR: A summary of the impact of musculoskeletal conditions in the United States. Arthritis Rheum 33:750–755, 1990.
2. Moxley G: Immunoglobulin kappa genotype confers risk of rheumatoid arthritis among HLA-DR4 negative individuals. Arthritis Rheum 32:1365–1370, 1989.
3. Gao X, Olsen NJ, Pincus T, Stastny P: HLA-DR alleles with naturally occurring amino acid substitutions and risk for development of rheumatoid arthritis. Arthritis Rheum 33:939–946, 1990.
4. Hazes JMW, Dijkmans BAC, Vandenbroucke JP, et al.: Pregnancy and the risk of developing rheumatoid arthritis. Arthritis Rheum 33:1770–1775, 1990.
5. van Zeben D, Hazes JMW, Vandenbroucke JP, et al.: Diminished incidence of severe rheumatoid arthritis associated with oral contraceptive use. Arthritis Rheum 33:1462–1465, 1990.
6. Chin JE, Winterrowd GE, Krzesicki RF, Sanders ME: Role of cytokines in inflammatory synovitis. The coordinate regulation of intercellular adhesion molecule 1 and HLA class I and class II antigens in rheumatoid synovial fibroblasts. Arthritis Rheum 33:1776–1786, 1990.
7. Arend WP, Dayer JM: Cytokines and cytokine inhibitors or antagonists in rheumatoid arthritis. Arthritis Rheum 33:305–315, 1990.

8. Rubin LA: The soluble interleukin-2 receptor in rheumatic disease. (Editorial) Arthritis Rheum 33:1145–1148, 1990.

9. Rème T, Portier M, Frayssinoux F, et al.: T cell receptor expression and activation of synovial lymphocyte subsets in patients with rheumatoid arthritis. Phenotyping of multiple synovial sites. Arthritis Rheum 33:485–492, 1990.

10. Firestein GS, Zvaifler NJ: How important are T cells in chronic rheumatoid synovitis? (Editorial) Arthritis Rheum 33:768–773, 1990.

11. Calabrese LH, Wilke WS, Perkins AD, Tubbs RR: Rheumatoid arthritis complicated by infection with the human immunodeficiency virus and the development of Sjögren's syndrome. Arthritis Rheum 32:1453–1457, 1989.

12. Meyer FA, Yaron I, Yaron M: Synergistic, additive, and antagonistic effects of interleukin-1β, tumor necrosis factor α, and γ-interferon on prostaglandin E, hyaluronic acid, and collagenase production by cultured synovial fibroblasts. Arthritis Rheum 33:1518–1525, 1990.

13. Marshall KW, Chiu B, Inman RD: Substance P and arthritis: analysis of plasma and synovial fluid levels. Arthritis Rheum 33:87–90, 1990.

14. Campbell IK, Piccoli DS, Roberts MJ, et al.: Effects of tumor necrosis factor α and β on resorption of human articular cartilage and production of plasminogen activator by human articular chondrocytes. Arthritis Rheum 33:542–552, 1990.

15. Sambrook PN, Shawe D, Hesp R, et al.: Rapid periarticular bone loss in rheumatoid arthritis. Possible promotion by normal circulating concentrations of parathyroid hormone or calcitriol (1,25-dihydroxyvitamin D_3). Arthritis Rheum 33:615–622, 1990.

16. Kawakami M, Kawagoe M, Harigai M, et al.: Elevated plasma levels of $α_2$-plasmin inhibitor-plasmin complex in patients with rheumatic diseases. Possible role of fibrinolytic mechanism in vasculitis. Arthritis Rheum 32:1427–1433, 1989.

17. Arnett FC, Edworthy SM, Bloch DA, et al.: The American Rheumatism Association 1987 revised criteria for the classification of rheumatoid arthritis. Arthritis Rheum 31:315–324, 1988.

18. Pincus T, Olsen NJ, Russel IJ, et al.: Multicenter study of recombinant human erythropoietin in correction of anemia in rheumatoid arthritis. Am J Med 89:161–168, 1990.

19. Helewa A, Bombardier C, Goldsmith CH, et al.: Cost-effectiveness of inpatient and intensive outpatient treatment of rheumatoid arthritis. A randomized, controlled trial. Arthritis Rheum 32:1505–1514, 1989.

20. Yip ASB, Chow WH, Tai YT, Cheung KL: Adverse effect of topical methylsalicylate ointment on warfarin anticoagulation: an unrecognized potential hazard. Postgrad Med J 66:367–369, 1990.

21. Abramson SB, Weissmann G: The mechanisms of action of nonsteroidal antiinflammatory drugs. Arthritis Rheum 32:1–9, 1989.

22. Lindsley HB, Smith DD: Enhanced prostaglandin E_2 secretion by cytokine-stimulated human synoviocytes in the presence of subtherapeutic concentrations of nonsteroidal antiinflammatory drugs. Arthritis Rheum 33:1162–1169, 1990.

23. Netter P, Bannwarth B, Royer-Morrot MJ: Recent findings on the pharmacokinetics of non-steroidal anti-inflammatory drugs in synovial fluid. Clin Pharmacokinet 17:145–162, 1989.

24. Bennett WM: Guide to drug dosage in renal failure. Clin Pharmacokinet 15:326–354, 1988.

25. Roth SH: NSAID and gastropathy: a rheumatologist's review. J Rheumatol 15:912–919, 1988.

26. Roth SH, Bennett RE, Mitchell CS, Hartman RJ: Cimetidine therapy in nonsteroidal anti-inflammatory drug gastropathy. Double-blind long-term evaluation. Arch Intern Med 147:1798–1801, 1987.

27. Szczeklik A, Gryglewski RJ, Czerniawska-Mysik G: Relationship of inhibition of prostaglandin biosynthesis by analgesics to asthma attacks in aspirin-sensitive patients. Br Med J 1:67–69, 1975.

28. Chudwin DS, Strub M, Golden HE, et al.: Sensitivity to non-acetylated salicylates in a patient with asthma, nasal polyps, and rheumatoid arthritis. Ann Allergy 57:133–134, 1986.

29. Fries JF, Singh G, Lenert L, Furst DE: Aspirin, hydroxychloroquine, and hepatic enzyme abnormalities with methotrexate in rheumatoid arthritis. Arthritis Rheum 33:1611–1619, 1990.

30. Cush JJ, Jasin HE, Johnson R, Lipsky PE: Relationship between clinical efficacy and laboratory correlates of inflammatory and immunologic activity in rheumatoid arthritis patients treated with nonsteroidal antiinflammatory drugs. Arthritis Rheum 33:623–633, 1990.

31. Furst DE: Rational use of disease-modifying antirheumatic drugs. Drugs 39:19–37, 1990.

32. Felson DT, Anderson JJ, Meenan RF: The comparative efficacy and toxicity of second-line drugs in rheumatoid arthritis. Results of two metaanalyses. Arthritis Rheum 33:1449–1461, 1990.

33. Alarcón GS, Tracy IC, Blackburn WD: Methotrexate in rheumatoid arthritis. Toxic effects as the major factor in limiting long-term treatment. Arthritis Rheum 32:671–676, 1989.

34. Dahl SL, Samuelson CO, Williams HJ, et al.: Second-line antirheumatic drugs in the elderly with rheumatoid arthritis: a post hoc analysis of three controlled trials. Pharmacotherapy 10:79–84, 1990.

35. Combs RJ, Dentino MM, Lehrman L, Szwed JJ: Gold toxicity and peritoneal dialysis. Arthritis Rheum 19:936–938, 1976.

36. Gottlieb NL, Smith PM, Smith EM: Pharmacodynamics of [197]Au and [195]Au labeled aurothiomalate in blood. Correlation with course of rheumatoid arthritis, gold toxicity and gold excretion. Arthritis Rheum 17:171–182, 1974.

37. Wooley PH, Griffin J, Panayi GS, et al.: HLA-DR antigens and toxic reaction to sodium aurothiomalate and D-penicillamine in patients with rheumatoid arthritis. N Engl J Med 303:300–302, 1980.

38. Brooks PJ, Spruill WJ, Parish RC, Birchmore DA: Pharmacokinetics of methotrexate administered by intramuscular and subcutaneous injections in patients with rheumatoid arthritis. Arthritis Rheum 33:91–94, 1990.

39. Nordstrom DM, West SG, Andersen PA, Sharp JT: Pulse methotrexate therapy in rheumatoid arthritis. A controlled prospective roentgenographic study. Ann Intern Med 107:797–801, 1987.

40. Kremer JM, Rynes RI, Bartholomew LE: Severe flare of rheumatoid arthritis after discontinuation of long-term methotrexate therapy: Double-blind study. Am J Med 82:781–786, 1987.

41. Nuernberg B, Koehnke R, Solsky M, et al.: Biliary elimination of low-dose methotrexate in humans. Arthritis Rheum 33:898–902, 1990.

42. Weinblatt ME, Fraser P: Elevated mean corpuscular volume as a predictor of hematologic toxicity due to methotrexate therapy. Arthritis Rheum 32:1592–1596, 1989.

43. Morgan SL, Baggott JE, Vaughn WH, et al.: The effect of folic acid supplementation on the toxicity of low-dose methotrexate in patients with rheumatoid arthritis. Arthritis Rheum 33:9–18, 1990.

44. Nesher G, Moore TL: The in vitro effects of methotrexate on peripheral blood mononuclear cells. Modulation by methyl donors and spermidine. Arthritis Rheum 33:954–959, 1990.

45. Page F: Treatment of lupus erythematosus with mepacrine. Lancet 261:755–758, 1951.

46. Pappaioanou M, Fishbein DB, Dreesen DW, et al.: Antibody response to preexposure human diploid-cell rabies vaccine given concurrently with chloroquine. N Engl J Med 314:280–284, 1986.

47. van der Heijde DM, van Riel PL, Nuver-Zwart IH, te al.: Effects of hydroxychloroquine and sulphasalazine on progression of joint damage in rheumatoid arthritis. Lancet 1:1036–1038, 1989.

48. Singh G, Fries JF, Spitz P, Williams CA: Toxic effects of azathioprine in rheumatoid arthritis. A national post-marketing perspective. Arthritis Rheum 32:837–843, 1989.

49. Netter P, Bannwarth B, Péré P, Nicolas A: Clinical pharmacokinetics of D-penicillamine. Clin Pharmacokinet 13:317–333, 1987.

50. Matthey F, Perrett D, Greenwood RN, Baker LRI: The use of D-

penicillamine in patients with rheumatoid arthritis undergoing hemodialysis. Clin Nephrol 25:268–271, 1986.

51. Madhok R, Zoma A, Torley; HI, et al.: The relationship of sulfoxidation status to efficacy and toxicity of penicillamine in the treatment of rheumatoid arthritis. Arthritis Rheum 33:574–577, 1990.

52. Arnold MH, Janssen B, Schrieber L, Brooks PM: Prospective pilot study of intravenous pulse cyclophosphamide therapy for refractory rheumatoid arthritis. (Letter) Arthritis Rheum 32:933–934, 1989.

53. Borg G, Allander E, Lund B, et al.: Auranofin improves outcome in early rheumatoid arthritis. Results from a 2-year, double blind, placebo controlled study. J Rheumatol 15:1747–1754, 1988.

54. Sievers K, Hurri L. Combined therapy of rheumatoid arthritis with gold and chloroquine: I. Evaluation of the therapeutic effect. Acta Rheum Scand 9:48–55, 1963.

55. Scott DL, Dawes PT, Tunn E, et al.: Combination therapy with gold and hydroxychloroquine in rheumatoid arthritis: a prospective, randomized, placebo-controlled study. Br J Rheumatol 28:128–133, 1989.

56. Bunch TW, O'Duffy JD, Tompkins RB, O'Fallon WM: Controlled trial of hydroxychloroquine and D-penicillamine singly and in combination in the treatment of rheumatoid arthritis. Arthritis Rheum 27:267–276, 1984.

57. Taggart AJ, Hill J, Astbury C, et al.: Sulphasalazine alone or in combination with D-penicillamine in rheumatoid arthritis. Br J Rheumatol 26:32–36, 1987.

58. Dawes PT, Sheeran TP, Fowler PD, Shadforth MF: Improving the response to gold or D-penicillamine by addition of sulphasalazine. A pilot study in 25 patients with rheumatoid arthritis. Clin Exper Rheumatol 5:151–153, 1987.

59. Berry H, Huskisson EC: Experience with penicillamine and azathioprine in rheumatoid arthritis. Postgrad Med J 50(suppl 2):61–62, 1974.

60. Walters MT, Cawley MID. Combined suppressive drug treatment in severe refractory rheumatoid disease: an analysis of the relative effects of parenteral methylprednisolone, cyclophosphamide, and sodium aurothiomalate. Ann Rheum Dis 47:924–929, 1988.

61. Csuka ME, Carrera GF, McCarty DJ: Treatment of intractable rheumatoid arthritis with combined cyclophosphamide, azathioprine, and hydroxychloroquine. A follow-up study. JAMA 255:2315–2319, 1986.

62. Tiliakos NA: Low-dose cytotoxic drug combination therapy in intractable rheumatoid arthritis: two years later. (Abstract) Arthritis Rheum 29(suppl):S79, 1986.

63. Biro JA, Segal AM, Mackenzie AH, et al.: The combination of methotrexate (MTX) and azathioprine (AZA) for resistant rheumatoid arthritis (RA). (Abstract) Arthritis Rheum 30(suppl):S18, 1987.

64. Langevitz P, Kaplinsky N, Ehrenfeld M, Pras M: Intractable RA-treatment with combined methotrexate, azathioprine and hydroxychloroquine. (Letter) Br J Rheumatol 28:271–272, 1989.

65. Williams HJ, Ward JR, Reading JC: Comparison of auranofin, methotrexate, and the combination of both in the treatment of rheumatoid arthritis. (Abstract) Arthritis Rheum 33(suppl):s10, 1990.

66. Wilder RL: Neuroendocrine control of inflammation: Update in Rheumatology, University of Pennsylvania School of Medicine, Philadelphia PA, September 25, 1990.

67. Sparling M, Malleson P, Wood B, Petty R: Radiographic followup of joints injected with triamcinolone hexacetonide for the management of childhood arthritis. Arthritis Rheum 33:821–826, 1990.

68. Neumann V, Hopkins R, Dixon J, et al: Combination therapy with pulsed methylprednisolone in rheumatoid arthritis. Ann Rheum Dis 44:747–751, 1985.

69. Liebling MR, Leib E, McLaughlin K, et al.: Pulse methylprednisolone in rheumatoid arthritis. A double-blind cross-over trial. Ann Intern Med 94:21–26, 1981.

70. Bertouch JV, Roberts-Thomson PJ, Smith MD, et al.: Methlyprednisolone infusion therapy in rheumatoid arthritis patients: The effect on synovial fluid lymphocyte subsets and inflammatory indices. Arthritis Rheum 29:32–38, 1986.

71. Tanay A, Field EH, Hoppe RT, Strober S: Long-term followup of rheumatoid arthritis patients treated with total lymphoid irradiation. Arthritis Rheum 30:1–10, 1987.

72. Dwosh IL, Giles AR, Ford PM, et al.: Plasmapheresis therapy in rheumatoid arthritis. A controlled, double-blind, crossover trial. N Engl J Med 308:1124–1129, 1983.

73. Kremer JM, Lawrence DA, Jubiz W, et al.: Dietary fish oil and olive oil supplementation in patients with rheumatoid arthritis. Clinical and immunologic effects. Arthritis Rheum 33:810–820, 1990.

74. Bønaa KH, Bjerve KS, Straume B, et al.: Effect of eicosapentaenoic and docosahexaenoic acids on blood pressure in hypertension: A population-based intervention trial from the Tromsø Study. N Engl J Med 322:795–801, 1990.

75. Lippiello L, Fienhold M, Grandjean C: Metobolic and ultrastructural changes in articular cartilage of rats fed dietary supplements of omega-3 fatty acids. Arthritis Rheum 33:1029–1036, 1990.

76. Pullman-Mooar S, Laposata M, Lem D, et al.: Alteration of the cellular fatty acid profile and the production of eicosanoids in human monocytes by gamma-linolenic acid. Arthritis Rheum 33:1526–1533, 1990.

77. Yocum DE, Klippel JH, Wilder RL, et al.: Cyclosporin A in severe, treatment-refractory rheumatoid arthritis. A randomized study. Ann Intern Med 109:863–869, 1988.

78. Tugwell P, Bombardier C, Gent M, et al.: Low-dose cyclosporin versus placebo in patients with rheumatoid arthritis. Lancet 335:1051–1055, 1990.

79. Alegre J, Teran J, Alvarex B, Viejo JL: Successful use of cyclosporine for the treatment of aggressive pulmonary fibrosis in a patient with rheumatoid arthritis. (Letter) Arthritis Rheum 33:1594–1596, 1990.

80. Silverman ED, Laxer RM, Greenwald M, et al.: Intravenous gamma globulin therapy in systemic juvenile rheumatoid arthritis. Arthritis Rheum 33:1015–1022, 1990.

81. Binder AI, So A, Ansell BM, Denman AM: Intensive immunosuppression in intractable rheumatoid arthritis. Br J Rheumatol 25:380–383, 1986.

82. Shmerling RH, Trentham DE: Prolonged improvement in refractory rheumatoid arthritis after antithymocyte globulin therapy of brief duration. (Letter) Arthritis Rheum 32:1495–1496, 1989.

83. Herzog C, Walker C, Pichler W, et al.: Monoclonal anti-CD4 in arthritis. (Letter) Lancet 2:1461–1462, 1987.

84. Lemmel EM, Brackhertz D, Franke M, et al.: Results of a multicentre placebo-controlled double-blind randomised phase III study of treatment of rheumatoid arthritis with recombinant human interferon gamma. Rheumatol Int 8:87–93, 1988.

85. Malaise MG, Hauwaert C, Franchimont P, et al.: Treatment of active rheumatoid arthritis with slow intravenous injections of thymopentin. A double-blind placebo-controlled randomised study. Lancet 1:832–836, 1985.

86. Runge LA, Pinals RS, Lourie SH, Tomar RH: Treatment of rheumatoid arthritis with levamisole. A controlled trial. Arthritis Rheum 20:1445–1448, 1977.

87. Baerwald C, Goebel KM, Krause A, Heymanns J: A randomized controlled trial of ciamexon versus placebo in the immunomodulatory treatment of rheumatoid arthritis. Arthritis Rheum 33:733–738, 1990.

CHAPTER 29

OSTEOARTHRITIS

JANELLE M. MAHONEY, Pharm.D., MICHAEL L. SCHMITZ, M.D., and STANLEY J. BIRGE, M.D.

Osteoarthritis (OA), also known as degenerative joint disease (DJD), is a common, progressive disorder initially affecting joint soft tissue with subsequent involvement of underlying bone and secondary inflammation of the contiguous synovium. OA commonly affects the spine, knees, hips, shoulders, and the interphalangeal joints of the hands and feet, and is characterized by pain, deformity, and limitation of joint function. In contrast to rheumatoid arthritis and other joint disorders, systemic abnormalities are not present in OA. The disease usually becomes symptomatic between the fourth and sixth decades of life (1).

EPIDEMIOLOGY

OA is the most common arthritis disorder in the United States, although precise prevalence is hard to determine because of diagnostic discrepancies and the low correlation between clinical symptoms and radiologic evidence of the disease. It is estimated that by age 30, approximately 35% of the population will demonstrate symptoms or radiologic changes consistent with OA (2). Disease prevalence appears to increase in direct proportion to the age of the patients, becoming almost universal in the geriatric population. Eighty-five percent of those over age 75 demonstrate signs and/or symptoms of OA (2). OA symptoms affect approximately 60 million Americans, resulting in more loss of time from work than any other chronic disease (1, 2).

OA does not show a predilection for a particular race, geographic area, climate, or socioeconomic class. Gender differences do exist, with male incidence greater before age 45 and female incidence greater after age 45 (3–5). Women are also more prone to knee and hand joint involvement than are men (6). Chronic excessive body weight has also been correlated with OA.

NORMAL JOINT FUNCTION

The diarthroidal joints are principally affected by OA, however, the fibrocartilaginous joints of the spine are also frequently involved. Diarthroidal joints consist of hyaline cartilage-covered bone ends that are juxtaposed and united by a fibrous capsule lined with synovial tissue. Typical examples are the knee and hip joints. Fibrocartilaginous joints, such as intervertebral disks, consist of bone united by fibrous tissue. The diarthroidal joints have a greater range of motion than fibrocartilagenous joints at the expense of joint stability.

Articular cartilage covers and protects bone from the forces encountered with normal joint activity. Cartilage is a matrix of hydrophilic proteoglycan complexes enclosed in a collagen fibril structure and is 80% water by weight (7). The proteoglycan molecules confer shock-absorbing and lubricative properties onto cartilage because of their capacity to retain and release great amounts of water. Analogous to a water-filled sponge, compressive forces cause an expulsion of water from the pressure region, resulting in matrix deformation (4).

This deformation increases the contact area under the compressive force and reduces stress on the cartilage and underlying bone. The highly polyanionic proteoglycans retard continued deformity by attracting water and inhibiting further outflow. When the pressure load is relieved, the matrix regains its original form through proteoglycan rehydration. The maintenance of a function joint depends upon the ability of the chondrocytes (cartilage cells) to synthesize and degrade the matrix components (proteoglycans, collagen) in equilibrium (7). A hallmark feature of OA is the disruption of this balance, with the degradative processes overwhelming the synthetic processes and causing a net loss of proteoglycan matrix.

The synovial tissue of the diarthroidal joints provides lubrication, nutrition, and elimination of waste products for articular hyaline cartilage. The synovial lubrication lowers the hyaline-hyaline coefficient of friction to approximately that of two pieces of wet ice sliding across each other. OA alters the hyaline-hyaline interface and surrounding tissues to increase drastically this coefficient of friction and ultimately reduce joint mobility.

ETIOLOGY

Although a number of investigators have proposed pathophysiologic mechanisms for OA, the etiology of OA appears to be multifactorial, and as of yet, incompletely elucidated. Advanced age is clearly a prominent influence, but OA is not limited to the elderly. Evidence suggests that genetic, hormonal, nutritional, and environmental factors influence the development and progression of the disease (8). Evidence suggesting that the development of OA is related to joint overuse remains equivocal (3, 8).

PATHOPHYSIOLOGY

OA is marked by concurrent anabolic and catabolic processes (4, 9–13). Articular cartilage and subchondral bone are the principal loci for the pathologic changes associated with OA. Unlike rheumatoid arthritis, the effects of OA are limited to the joints.

OA results from alterations in the biochemical composition of articular cartilage. Histologically, collagen content may remain stable, but the structure becomes disorganized and weakened. A resultant increase in cartilage hydration associated with proteoglycan swelling dilutes the proteoglycan component of cartilage (14–16). Proteolytic and lysosomal enzyme activity induced by interleukin-1 further degrades the proteoglycan structure (17). A reduction in osmotic pressure causes a loss of cartilage resiliency. Loss of the elastic properties of cartilage results in fibrillation, fissuring, and eventual ulceration of the surface, thus decreasing surface congruity and precipitating further injury.

Subchondral bone proliferates in an attempt to increase the surface area available for load bearing. As subchondral bone becomes more sclerotic, it is more susceptible to microfractures and further sclerosis. Osteophytes, a cardinal feature of OA, are osseous outgrowths that appear at the bony margins of the joint (18). These masses may enlarge the joint, compress spinal nerves, and severely limit joint mobility. Subchondral cysts surrounded by sclerotic bone begin to appear in advanced disease and are most evident in the hip joint. The subchondral bone loses elasticity and the ability to absorb shock from continued sclerosis, resulting in increased vascularity and intraosseous venous pressure (19). Continuous destruction of the cartilage may eventually result in the exposure of subchondral bone. Completely denuded bone grinds against the bone of the adjacent joint surface and becomes eburnated, shiny, and smooth. Points of maximum pressure show the most damage.

Proliferation of subchondral bone is accompanied by hypertrophy of all soft tissues (i.e., ligaments, tendons, muscles) in the joint, including the synovium (4). Hypertrophic changes are physiologic attempts to repair damage. However, the resultant tissue enlargement and synovial effusions are responsible for joint deformity, further limitation of motion, and pain (20).

Chronic synovitis (inflammation of the synovium) is thought to be caused by the presence of proteoglycan and collagen fragments following proteolytic attack. Neovascularization and focal hemorrhages may be marked in the synovial tissue. Crystals of calcium pyrophosphate dihydrate, calcium hydroxyapatite, or both may or may not be present and appear to be correlated with advanced radiographic disease and greater frequency of intraarticular corticosteroid injections (14).

CLINICAL PRESENTATION

Joint pain is the most common complaint of patients with OA. The pain is exacerbated by increased joint activity, especially weight-bearing activity, and relieved with rest in the early stages of the disease. Pain is generally characterized as dull and aching with episodes of lancinating pain usually related to certain movements. Pain is initially intermittent but eventually becomes constant and disabling.

Patients frequently complain of joint stiffness after rest, which is generally short in duration. Morning stiffness may be present but usually subsides within minutes, compared with the prolonged stiffness associated with rheumatoid arthritis. Affected joints may manifest restricted range of motion, tenderness, bony enlargement, effusion, and crepitus (a frequently audible crackling sensation) (21–23). Erythema and palpable warmth are rare but possible in OA.

Patients with OA of the fingers commonly have firm nodules located on the dorsolateral and dorsomedial aspects of the distal interphalangeal joints. The nodules, called Heberden's nodes, represent cartilage-covered bony spurs. Nodule formation is usually painless and may occur in the thumb as well as the feet (24). Women are 10 times more likely than men to develop Heberden's nodes (6).

Although OA affecting the hip may be the most incapacitating, due to mobility limitations, spinal OA can be the most painful. Nerve root compression from spinal involvement of facet joints may lead to local or referred pain, paresthesias, muscle spasms, and eventual muscle atrophy. OA of the knee is characterized by tenderness, synovitis, crepitus, palpable osteophytes, limited range of motion, and joint deformity (18, 21).

DIAGNOSIS

The diagnosis of OA is based primarily on clinical symptoms and exclusion of other disease processes. Radiographic findings typically include joint-space narrowing, sclerosis of subchondral bone, subchondral cysts, and osteophyte formation, in contrast to the juxtaarticular osteoporosis associated with rheumatoid arthritis. However, radiographic findings without symptomatic complaints are common and do not warrant treatment.

The increased volume of synovial fluid from affected joints shows decreased viscosity, increased protein concentration, and normal hyaluronate concentrations. The cartilage and fibrin fragments and crystal deposition suggest OA but do not constitute a definitive diagnosis. Probably important to the destructive process, increased concentrations of lysosomal enzymes, prostaglandins (PGs), and interleukin-1 are present in the synovial fluid of affected joints, although these findings are not exclusive to OA.

Results of hematologic studies are usually normal with the exception of a slightly elevated erythrocyte sedimentation rate (ESR) during episodes of inflammation. Rheu-

Table 29.1.
Osteoarthritis Classification Criteria[a]

Presence of osteophytes
Pain
Joint stiffness less than 30 min duration
Crepitus
Bony enlargement and tenderness with no palpable warmth
Age over 50 years

[a] Adapted from Schuomacher HR: Primer on Rheumatic Diseases Ninth Edition. Atlanta: National Arthritis Foundation, 1988, pp 172–177.

matoid factor and antinuclear antibody serology are generally negative.

Most investigators believe OA to result from several diverse causes. If the cause is unknown or thought to be genetic, the term primary OA is applicable. Secondary OA refers to all other situations in which a causative factor is known or presumed (e.g., trauma). Regardless of the cause, efforts to standardize reporting have generated several classification criteria including (a) the presence of osteophytes, (b) pain, (c) joint stiffness of less than 30 min duration, (d) crepitus, (e) bony enlargement and tenderness with no palpable warmth, and (f) age over 50 years (Table 29.1). These criteria are not intended to be diagnostic, but the presence of all six is a sensitive and specific indicator for OA (9).

TREATMENT

The treatment of OA is primarily directed toward alleviating pain, the chief reason for patients to seek medical attention (25). Preservation or improvement of joint function, minimization of disability, and maintenance of a good quality of life are also primary goals of therapy. OA treatment programs include nonpharmacologic therapy (psychosocial counseling, education, and physiotherapy), pharmacologic therapy, and surgical intervention. Treatment modalities may vary, depending upon the clinical severity of disease, and must be individualized for each patient.

NONPHARMACOLOGIC THERAPY

Nonpharmacologic modes of therapy are paramount to the management of OA and are usually effective for managing mild-to-moderate OA. The early stages of OA may respond to nonpharmacologic measures alone, and initial attempts to achieve acceptable therapeutic outcomes should reflect this. As in other pain syndromes, the symptoms of OA are magnified and possibly worsened by anxiety. Patients with OA should be assured that the disease is not the rapidly crippling illness that rheumatoid arthritis can be and that several effective treatment options exist (1).

Patient education is aimed at reducing irrational fears and providing accurate information on the course of the disease. Because of joint stiffness associated with rest, pa-

tients may fear erroneously that joints will "freeze" if not in constant motion. Patients should be taught the principles of joint protection and pain alleviation. Gentle range-of-motion exercises during periods of prolonged inactivity can prevent associated joint stiffness. Patients should be encouraged to comply with prescribed physiotherapeutic regimens and curtail weight-bearing, high-impact exercises to limit excessive joint stress.

Physiotherapy focuses on maintenance of a proper balance between exercise and rest. Short periods of isometric (not isotonic) exercises throughout the day should be encouraged to preserve or improve range of motion, relieve joint stiffness, minimize joint stress, and strengthen periarticular muscle groups. Characteristically, periarticular muscles are atrophied in patients with OA, because of inactivity due to pain (26). Increased pain, lasting for more than 1 hour after exercising, is an indication for reducing but not eliminating exercises. Alternating exercise with non-weight-bearing rest two to four times daily for an hour or more will allow cartilage rehydration and promote reparative processes. Excessive joint-loading activities (e.g., heavy lifting) should be avoided. The use of walking aids (i.e., canes, crutches, walkers), running shoes for walking, or specifically designed orthopaedic shoes may relieve some joint pressure and pain. Application of moderate heat for muscle relaxation or of ice packs for acute inflammation prior to exercising can reduce joint stiffness and increase exercise tolerance. Weight reduction is imperative in obese patients to reduce excessive joint stress. Patients should be instructed to continue nonpharmacologic therapy to minimize the need for drug therapy (24).

PHARMACOLOGIC THERAPY
Analgesics

Since there is no cure for OA, pharmacologic intervention is palliative and directed toward alleviation of pain and improving joint function. Therapy traditionally includes the use of analgesics and nonsteroidal antiinflammatory drugs (NSAIDs). Analgesics are usually employed early in the disease to minimize NSAID-associated renal and gastrointestinal adverse effects and decrease the potential for NSAID-induced inhibitory effects on cartilage proteoglycan synthesis. Acetaminophen in doses of 325 to 650 mg three to four times daily, not to exceed 2.6 g/day with prolonged use, is a useful and effective analgesic regimen. Scheduled dosing is more effective than "as needed" administration for the management of chronic pain. Propoxyphene alone provides no better analgesic effects than acetaminophen alone, but there may be additive effects when the two agents are combined. However, the use of centrally active medications (e.g., propoxyphene) increases the incidence of CNS adverse effects. These agents should not be used in patients particularly susceptible to adverse CNS effects (e.g., the elderly). Codeine and other narcotic analgesics are rarely appropriate and should be used only briefly if required.

NSAIDs

In the early stages of OA, there may be no evidence of inflammation. However, advanced disease is commonly associated with synovial inflammation, which is a likely source of pain. NSAIDs have both analgesic and antiinflammatory activity and are therefore a logical choice for the treatment of OA after failure with analgesics alone. Although the exact mechanism of action is unknown, NSAIDs are thought to inhibit peripheral prostaglandin synthesis through reversible cyclooxygenase inhibition (27). Inhibition of histamine and kinins and release of free oxygen radicals purportedly prevents pain receptor sensitization and inflammation (27, 28).

PHARMACOKINETICS

Following oral administration, all NSAIDs are rapidly absorbed. Food and various dosage formulations (e.g., enteric-coated, delayed release) may delay the rate of absorption, but the extent of absorption generally remains unaffected. Salicylate levels can be detected in the serum 5 to 30 min after oral administration, and peak concentrations are usually attained within 0.25 to 2.0 hr, depending on the dosage form and specific formulations. Maximum therapeutic effects may not be attained, however, for 2 to 3 weeks after starting therapy. All NSAIDs are highly protein bound ($\geq 90\%$), primarily to albumin. These agents are metabolized chiefly by hepatic biotransformation and excreted primarily through the kidneys. The half-life of NSAIDs varies from 1 to 8 hr following ingestion of a single oral dose with the exception of piroxicam ($t_{1/2} = 50$ hr). A half-life of sulindac is 7.8 hr and 16.4 hr for its active metabolite.

SPECIFIC AGENTS

The NSAIDs currently available include derivatives of salicylates, propionic acids, indoleacetic acids, pyrroleacetic acids, fenamates, pyrazoles, oxicams, and phenylacetic acids and are listed in Table 29.2. Selection of a particular agent should depend upon efficacy, side effect profile, patient preference, and cost.

Caution should be used when giving NSAIDs to patients with a history of hypersensitivity to NSAIDs, including aspirin, as cross-sensitivity may occur among different structural derivatives. NSAIDs are contraindicated in patients with a history of pulmonary or anaphylactoid manifestations of hypersensitivity associated with prior NSAID use.

EFFICACY

All currently approved NSAIDs are equipotent in providing symptomatic relief of OA if taken at the recommended doses. The potential for NSAIDs to alter disease progression remains controversial, and research is ongoing. Several NSAIDs have been implicated in the acceleration of joint destruction. Numerous in vitro investigations have shown NSAIDs to effectively reduce hyaluronic acid synthesis (the core of the proteoglycan molecule) and inhibit proteoglycan formation (29–31). Aspirin, indomethacin, sulindac, flurbiprofen, diclofenac, and ketoprofen have been identified as being deleterious to hip joints in human subjects (29). It has been proposed that osteoarthritic joints require adequate perfusion to maintain joint structure reparative processes (30). This perfusion is enhanced by inflammation. Inhibition of PG synthesis may interfere with joint blood flow and cause the already compromised joint to deteriorate more rapidly (30). This hypothesis was tested in 105 patients with OA of the hip who were randomly allocated to receive indomethacin (a *potent* PG inhibitor) 50 to 75 mg/day or azapropazone (a *weak* PG inhibitor) 600 to 900 mg/day (30). The time to reach arthroplasty, the end point in the OA process, was 50% longer and cartilage proteoglycan content was substantially higher in the group treated with azapropazone. Finally, overuse of a pain-free joint is another potential mechanism of enhanced joint destruction associated with NSAID use. Therefore, NSAIDs may not be indicated in the long-term treatment of OA.

Conversely, several investigators have demonstrated an NSAID-induced inhibition of proteinase activity, release of collagenase, and proteoglycan degradation in experimental models (31). These effects would seemingly protect joint structure integrity and/or enhance reparative processes. However, valid conclusions on either the deleterious or beneficial effects of NSAIDs on osteoarthritic joints cannot be drawn from comparisons of such diverse experimental systems (32).

Until further research provides definitive answers, simple analgesia is recommended for mild-to-moderate OA. Dosing with NSAIDs during periods of severe pain or inflammation in moderate-to-severe disease should be alternated with analgesics or low-potency NSAIDs during periods of quiescence (31).

ADVERSE EFFECTS

Although the use of NSAIDs is relatively safe, they are not without adverse effects, some of which may be severe in certain patient populations. All NSAIDs may produce adverse gastrointestinal (GI) effects including nausea, vomiting, dyspepsia, diarrhea, constipation, and gastritis. Severe effects include GI ulceration, perforation, and hemorrhage. Although the nonacetylated salicylates (i.e., salsalate, choline salicylate) have been associated with a lower incidence of gastric bleeding, no NSAID is completely free of the risk of causing gastric injury when taken on a chronic basis (33). The proposed mechanisms of GI

Table 29.2.
Nonsteroidal Antiinflammatory Agents

Drug	Usual Daily Dose	Maximum Daily Dose	Usual Dosing Interval	Trade Name	Relative Cost[a]
Salicylates					
Aspirin	3.9–5.1 g	5.1 g	4–6 times/day	Various	+
Sodium salicylate	3.9–5.1 g	5.1 g	4–6 times/day	Uracel 5	+
Choline salicylate	5.2–7.0 g	7.0 g	4–6 times/day	Arthropan	+ +
Magnesium salicylate	3.9–5.1 g	5.1 g	4–6 times/day	Doan's	+ +
Salsalate	3.0–4.0 g	4.0 g	b.i.d.–t.i.d.	Disalcid	+ + +
Diflunisal	0.5–1.5 g	1.5 g	b.i.d.–t.i.d.	Dolobid	+ + + +
Proprionic acids					
Fenoprofen	1200–3200 mg	3200 mg	t.i.d.–q.i.d.	Nalfon	+ + + +
Ibuprofen	1200–3200 mg	3200 mg	t.i.d.–q.i.d.	Motrin	+ +
Ketoprofen	150–300 mg	300 mg	t.i.d.–q.i.d.	Orudis	+ + + +
Naproxen	500–1000 mg	1200 mg	b.i.d.	Naprosyn	+ + +
Flurbiprofen	100–200 mg	300 mg	b.i.d.	Ansaid	+ + +
Indoleacetic acids					
Indomethacin	75–150 mg	200 mg	b.i.d.–t.i.d.	Indocin	+ +
Pyrroleacetic acids					
Sulindac	300–400 mg	400 mg	b.i.d.	Clinoril	+ + +
Tolmentin sodium	500–1000 mg	1250 mg	t.i.d.–q.i.d.	Tolectin	+ + +
Fenamates					
Mefenamic acid	750–1000 mg	1000 mg	t.i.d.–q.i.d.	Ponstel	+ + +
Meclofenamate sodium	200–400 mg	400 mg	t.i.d.–q.i.d.	Meclomen	+ + +
Pyrazoles					
Phenylbutazone	200–400 mg	400 mg	t.i.d.–q.i.d.	Butazolidin	+
Oxicams					
Piroxicam	20 mg	20 mg	q.d.	Feldene	+ +
Phenylacetic acids					
Diclofenac	100–150 mg	200 mg	b.i.d.–q.i.d.	Voltaren	+ + +

[a] Relative costs based on AWP cost of maximum daily dosage.

Table 29.3.
Factors Related to Increased Risk
of NSAID-induced GI Complications

History of peptic ulcer disease
History of GI bleeding
Advanced age
Short duration of exposure
Large NSAID doses
Cigarette smoking
Concurrent corticosteroid therapy
Concurrent anticoagulant therapy

injury include local irritation, inhibition of prostaglandin synthesis (prostaglandins inhibit gastric acid secretion), decreased availability of sulfhydryl donors (which are required for prostaglandin receptor activation), and inhibition of platelet aggregation (34, 35). Factors related to an increased risk of GI complications include (*a*) a history of peptic ulcer disease or gastrointestinal bleeding, (*b*) advanced age, (*c*) short duration of exposure, (*d*) cigarette smoking, (*e*) corticosteroid use, and (*f*) anticoagulant therapy (Table 29.3) (36,37). Since the appearance of GI adverse effects is a dose-related phenomenon, initiation with

low-dose NSAIDs is warranted in these high-risk patients (37). Instructing patients to take their medication with meals may also prevent or lessen most GI discomfort. Buffered aspirin is associated with the same GI toxicity as regular aspirin and should not be considered safe. However, because of its delayed release, enteric-coated aspirin is a reasonable alternative. The use of topical NSAIDs (e.g., trolamine salicylate, Aspercreme) or rectal suppositories may circumvent GI injury, but extensive studies have not yet demonstrated efficacy in OA. Further investigation of these formulations is warranted.

Until recently, no treatment has been proven to prevent NSAID-induced gastric ulcers and bleeding. The addition of H_2-antagonists or sucralfate has not been shown to reduce the severity or incidence of NSAID-induced ulcers or bleeding. Misoprostol, a synthetic prostaglandin analog with antisecretory and cytoprotective effects, has been shown to prevent and heal gastric ulcers associated with long-term NSAID therapy (38). Prophylactic misoprostol is indicated in (*a*) patients at high risk of developing gastric ulceration (such as those with a history of upper GI ulcers), and (*b*) patients at high risk of developing complications (i.e., bleeding, perforation, death) from NSAID-induced ulcers, including the elderly and patients with debilitating disease. The most common adverse effects are dose-related and include a self-limiting diarrhea in 5 to 40% of patients, abdominal pain, nausea, and flatulence. Halving the normal dose of 200 μg four times daily may decrease the incidence of adverse effects. Misoprostol is contraindicated in pregnant women and women of child-bearing potential unless adequate birth control is practiced, because of its ability to induce uterine contractions and cause expulsion of uterine contents.

The effects of NSAIDs on renal function may be problematic in some patients, particularly those with preexisting renal insufficiency, and are usually detected by increases in serum creatinine and BUN levels. Because normal renal function depends at least partially upon prostaglandin (PG) synthesis, the administration of agents that inhibit PG synthesis (i.e., NSAIDs) may induce renal injury. Vasodilatory PGs are released in response to the vasoconstriction produced by angiotensin II in patients with CHF, intravascular volume contraction, or on chronic diuretic therapy. When this compensatory mechanism is blocked, renal blood flow and glomerular filtration rate are reduced and secondary ischemia may occur. Decreased renal blood flow associated with aging puts the elderly population at increased risk for complications. NSAID-induced reduction in renal blood flow may also increase sodium reabsorption, resulting in edema and possible interference with antihypertensive therapy.

NSAIDs have been associated with hypoaldosteronemia and resultant hyperkalemia due to inhibition of aldosterone release secondary to PG inhibition (39). Papillary necrosis has also been reported, but definite drug causation has not been established (39). Interstitial nephritis has been observed and is generally considered to be an allergic manifestation consisting of eosinophilia, rash, arthralgias, fever, proteinuria, and nephrotic syndrome.

Renal function should be evaluated at baseline, 1 week after starting therapy and every 3 months during chronic therapy with NSAIDs in susceptible patients (i.e., the elderly, patients with preexisting renal disease). Sulindac appears to be the only renal-sparing NSAID and is a reasonable alternative in these patients (40).

All NSAIDs, except the nonacetylated salicylates, inhibit platelet aggregation. Therefore, these agents are relatively contraindicated in patients with coagulation defects, those with either active or a history of ulcers, and those currently receiving anticoagulant therapy. Leukopenia, thrombocytopenia, and agranulocytosis may occur rarely and are generally reversible. Periodic assessment of hematologic indices (i.e., hemoglobin, hematocrit, red blood cell count, white blood cell count, platelets) will afford early detection and possible prevention of these adverse events.

Some NSAIDs, especially indomethacin, have been as-

sociated with altered mental status. Dizziness, tinnitus, headache, vertigo, nervousness, excitation, somnolence, fatigue, confusion, depression, emotional lability, psychiatric disturbances, and syncope may result from NSAID use, particularly in the elderly. Dosage reduction is indicated to ameliorate these signs and symptoms. Confusion, agitation, and/or seizures may represent serious salicylate intoxication in the elderly. Since acid-base disturbances (i.e., respiratory alkalosis followed by metabolic acidosis) often accompany salicylate toxicity, a wide anion gap is generally diagnostic. However, serum salicylate levels should be determined to confirm the diagnosis. Elevated liver function test results have been reported rarely in association with NSAID use and are an indication for discontinuation of therapy (24).

The potential for fetal adverse effects is not clearly defined. The risks of prolonged maternal labor, perinatal mortality, and teratogenicity have not yet been established. Therefore, conservative approaches are recommended, and avoidance of these agents during pregnancy is ideal (41). While most NSAIDs are excreted in breast milk, toxicology data for nursing infants are not conclusive, and these agents are not recommended in lactating females.

DRUG INTERACTIONS

Although numerous drug interactions involving the NSAIDs have been reported, few are clinically important. Drug interactions of importance are those involving anticoagulants, sulfonylureas, corticosteroids, and uricosuric agents. Because NSAIDs are highly protein bound, other highly protein bound drugs, including warfarin, tolbutamide, and phenytoin, may be displaced. As a result, hypoprothrombinemia, hypoglycemia, and other toxicities may develop. GI toxicity may be compounded when combining NSAIDs with corticosteroid therapy because of additive cytotoxic effects. Finally, the uricosuric effects of NSAIDs, probenecid, and sulfinpyrazone are antagonistic when used concomitantly.

STEROIDS

Systemic corticosteroids are not indicated for the treatment of OA. Intraarticular administration of corticosteroids, however, appears to be beneficial for the temporary relief of pain and inflammation, while improving joint mobility. Like the NSAIDs, the mechanism of action of steroids is not clearly defined. It is thought that the inhibition of polymorphonuclear leukocyte (inflammatory cell) migration and extravasation along with reduction of vascular permeability results in diminished inflammatory response and secondary pain prevention (42).

Corticosteroids available for intraarticular administration include hydrocortisone, betamethasone, methylprednisolone, triamcinolone, and dexamethasone (Table 29.4).

Table 29.4.
Corticosteroids Available for Intraarticular Injection

Corticosteroid	Formulation	Dosage Range[a]
Betamethasone sodium phosphate/ acetate	Suspension	1.5–12 mg
Dexamethasone acetate	Suspension	4.0–16 mg
Dexamethasone sodium phosphate	Solution	1.0–4.0 mg
Hydrocortisone acetate	Suspension	10–50 mg
Methylprednisolone acetate	Suspension	4.0–80 mg
Prednisolone acetate	Suspension	2.0–30 mg
Prednisolone tebutate	Suspension	4.0–40 mg
Prednisolone sodium phosphate	Solution	2.0–30 mg
Triamcinolone acetonide	Suspension	2.5–40 mg
Triamcinolone hexacetonide	Suspension	2.0–20 mg

[a] Dosages may vary, depending on the size and location of the affected joint and the degree of inflammation.

Administration is performed with the use of a local anesthetic, usually 1 to 2% lidocaine. Aseptic technique is recommended. Dosages vary with the degree of inflammation and the size and location of the affected joint. Beneficial effects usually occur within 24 hr after an injection, reach a maximum in 1 week and last for 2 to 4 weeks, when using the suspension formulations. Activity should be limited for 48 hr following injection, to avoid exacerbating joint destruction from overuse of the pain-free joint (42).

Long-term use of intraarticular corticosteroids is still controversial because of the potential for serious adverse effects including arthropathy, infection, postinjection flare, and tendon rupture. Steroid arthropathy is a condition of accelerated degeneration of articular cartilage, subchondral bone, and surrounding ligaments, caused by repeated corticosteroid injections (43). Originally thought to result from overuse of an abnormal joint, steroid arthropathy has been shown to result from a specific effect of the steroids on the metabolism of articular cartilage (42, 43). Since the progression of destruction is proportional to the number of injections administered, conservative use is recommended, and administration should be no more frequent than every 4 to 6 weeks.

Joint infection secondary to intraarticular steroid therapy occurs rarely (<1%) and is usually caused by *Staphylococcus aureus*. Complications due to this infection can be devastating, so early diagnosis and treatment is critical. Immunocompromised individuals, including those taking systemic corticosteroids, are at an increased risk for joint infection and should be closely monitored. Joint aspiration should be performed to differentiate between infection and postinjection flare, a self-limited synovitis caused by deposition of steroid crystals in the joint cavity. Joint infection should be suspected if inflammation persists for 72 hr, even if cultures are negative.

Ruptured tendons may also occur with the use of in-

traarticular steroids, not only as a result of direct injury during administration, but as a consequence of overactivity. Several investigators have reported reduced tendon tensile strength and slowed repair processes after repeated intraarticular injections for prolonged periods. Overuse of a pain-free joint can intensify the strain on weakened tendons and result in ruptures.

CHONDROPROTECTIVE AGENTS

Because of the risk of severe adverse effects associated with the use of long-term NSAIDs and the deleterious effects of chronic steroid administration, the search for novel therapeutic approaches to OA has received much attention. Extensive research has produced two agents that appear to be "chondroprotective," that is, they retard further progression of cartilage breakdown. These agents, glycosaminoglycan-peptide complex (GP-C, Rumalon) and glycosaminoglycan polysuflate (GAGPS, Arteparon), not yet available in the United States, are isolated from bovine lung, tracheal cartilage, and bone marrow.

Long-term studies with GP-C and GAGPS in Europe have demonstrated significant improvement in OA symptoms, joint status, joint function, quality of life, and ability to work in afflicted patients (44). Surgical interventions and use of NSAIDs were significantly decreased in patients treated with GP-C and GAGPS, compared with controls (44). The percentage of stable radiographic findings indicating no further disease progression occurred seven (GAGPS) and nine (GP-C) times more than in control patients (44). Reports of heparin-related anticoagulant effects associated with GAGPS preclude the use of this agent in patients with coagulopathies, those with a history of gastrointestinal ulcers, or those receiving anticoagulant therapy. Caution is advised when using this agent in elderly patients. Otherwise, adverse effects and contraindications appear to be minimal with both GP-C and GAGPS. Both drugs are administered intramuscularly twice weekly at 2- to 6-month intervals.

Although the exact mechanism of action is unknown, most beneficial effects are believed to result from inhibition of the catabolic and lysosomal enzymes (collagenases, metalloproteinases) responsible for structural damage in OA (44, 45). The chondroprotective agents also purportedly stimulate reparative processes in injured articular cartilage (44, 45). Whatever the mechanism, numerous investigations have demonstrated GP-C and GAGPS to be effective in the treatment of OA. These agents may herald a major breakthrough in the therapy of OA. Delineation of the biochemical mechanisms of action and efficacy will be the primary focus of further research with these agents.

Intraarticular injections of orgotein (superoxide dismutase) are also being investigated for the treatment of OA. This novel antiinflammatory agent, isolated from bovine liver, purportedly eliminates the generation of superoxide free radicals and stabilizes the membranes of inflammatory cells (46). Oxygen free radicals are responsible for direct degradation of collagen and proteoglycans. Although orgotein has no central or peripheral analgesic properties, inhibition of inflammatory mediators may reduce or prevent the pain associated with OA. Dosing, dosage intervals, and place in therapy have not been established for this agent.

SURGERY

Surgical intervention may provide the most immediate improvement in patients with OA. Arthroscopic procedures focus on joint debridement to prevent further destruction of joint surfaces and stimulate repair by the remaining healthy tissue. Although osteotomies are rarely performed now, total or partial prosthetic joint replacement remains a treatment option for patients with advanced OA. However, surgery can be very costly and carries the risk of morbidity and mortality which may not be acceptable in some patients, especially the elderly. Risks and costs are unfortunately additive in patients with multiple joint disease, and surgery is not always curative. Surgical treatment of OA is generally reserved for patients with severe, debilitating disease for whom the potential benefits outweigh the potential risks.

CONCLUSION

Osteoarthritis is a painful, progressive condition that may cause significant disability and compromised quality of life. Recent therapeutic advances have resulted from progress in understanding the etiology and pathogenesis of OA. Pharmacologic therapy has been aimed primarily at relief of pain and inflammation associated with advanced disease; however, it is now being carefully scrutinized for efficacy and possible deleterious effects to osteoarthritic joints. New developments have revitalized interest in the reversibility of disease progression. Future research will be directed toward the identification of risk factors and specific markers of cartilage destruction in the hope of arresting progression before it is too late and assessing the role of inflammation in the disease process and clinical presentation. Eliciting mechanisms of interleukin-1 regulation, delineating the role of extraarticular structures in the disease process, and stimulating subchondral bone reparative processes are also primary areas of interest. Monoclonal antibody technology and cartilage growth and transformation factors will also play a prominent role in future investigations. If disease progression cannot be altered, the area of cartilage autotransplantation remains an option to be explored.

REFERENCES

1. Howell DS, Altman RD, Brown HE, Gorrlieb NL: A comprehensive regimen for osteoarthritis. Med Clin North Am 55(2):457–69, 1971.

2. Brown R, Lingg C: Musculoskeletal complaints in an industry, annual complaint rate and diagnosis, absenteeism and economic loss. Arthritis Rheum 4:283–302, 1961.

3. Lawrence JS: Generalized osteoarthritis in a population sample. Am J Epidemiol 90:381–389, 1969.

4. Bland JH, Cooper SM: Osteoarthritis: a review of the cell biology involved and evidence for reversibility. Management rationally related to known genesis and pathophysiology. Semin Arthritis Rehum 14(2):106–133, 1984.

5. Hartz AJ, Fischer ME, Bril G, Kelber S, Rupley D, Oken B, Rimm AA: The association of obesity with joint pain and osteoarthritis in the HANES data. J Chronic Dis 39:311–319, 1986.

6. Bjelle A: Epidemiological aspects of osteoarthritis. Scand J Rheumatol 43(Suppl):35–48, 1981.

7. Kuettner K, Thonar EJMA, Aydelotte MB: Modern aspects of articular cartilage biochemistry. Verh Dtsch Ges Inn Med 95:436–474, 1989.

8. Puranen J, Ala-Ketola L, Peltokallio J: Running and primary osteoarthrosis of the hip. Br Med J 2:242–245, 1975.

9. Schuomacher HR: Primer on Rheumatic Diseases Ninth Edition. Atlanta: National Arthritis Foundation, 1988, pp 171–177.

10. Ehrlich GE: Osteoarthritis beginning with inflammation. JAMA 232(2):157–159, 1975.

11. Johnson L: Kinetics of osteoarthritis. Lab Invest 8(6):1223–1241, 1959.

12. Altman RD, Kapila P, Dean DD, Howell DS: Future therapeutic trends in osteoarthritis. Scand J Rheumatol 77(suppl):37–42, 1989.

13. Mankin H: The response of articular cartilage to mechanical injury. J Bone Joint Surg 64A:460–466, 1982.

14. Schumacher R: The role of inflammation and crystals in the pain of osteoarthritis. Semin Arthritis Rheum 18(suppl 2):81–85, 1989.

15. Redler I, Zimny ML: Scanning electron microscopy of normal and abnormal articular cartilage and synovium. J Bone Joint Surg 52A:1395–1404, 1970.

16. McDevitt CA, Gilbertson EMM, Muir H: An experimental model of osteoarthrosis: Early morphological and biochemical changes. J Bone Joint Surg 59B:24–35, 1977.

17. Pujol JP, Loyau G: Interleukin-1 and osteoarthritis. Life Sci 41:1187–1198, 1987.

18. Bjelle A: The management of degenerative joint disease. Scand J Rheumatol 42(suppl):7–67, 1987.

19. Radin EL, Paul IL, Rose RM: Role of mechanical factors in the pathogenesis of primary osteoarthritis. Lancet 1:519–521, 1972.

20. Merritt JL: Soft tissue mechanisms of pain in osteoarthritis. Semin Arthritis Rheum 18(suppl 2):51–56, 1989.

21. Bienstock H, Fernando KR: Arthritis in the elderly—an overview. Med Clin North Am 60:1173–1189, 1976.

22. Blechman W: Managing the older arthritic. Geriatrics 39:131–132, 1984.

23. Gross M: Psychosocial aspects of osteoarthritis: helping patients cope. Aging 13:40–43, 1983.

24. Covington TR, Mallow LP, Hendersen RP, Stevenson JG: Degenerative joint disease. Consult Pharm 2:404–412, 1987.

25. Ehrlich GE: Future directions in therapy of pain in osteoarthritis. Semin Arthritis Rheum 18(suppl 2):100–104, 1989.

26. Sirca A, Susec-Michieli M: Selective type II fibre muscular atrophy in patients with osteoarthritis of the hip. J Neurol Sci 44:149–159, 1980.

27. Trang LE: Prostaglandins and inflammation. Semin Arthritis Rheum 9(3):153–190, 1980.

28. Hart FD, Huskisson EC: Nonsteroidal anti-inflammatory drugs—current status and rational therapeutic use. Drugs 27:232–255, 1984.

29. Newman NM, Ling RSM: Acetabular bone destruction related to non-steroidal anti-inflammatory drugs. Lancet 2:11–14, 1985.

30. Rashad S, Revell P, Hemingway A, Low F, Rainsford K, Walker F: Effect of nonsteroidal anti-inflammatory drugs on the course of osteoarthritis. Lancet 2:519–522, 1989.

31. Furst DE: Comments on possible long-term consequences of nonsteroidal anti-inflammatory use. J Clin Pharmacol 28:550–553, 1988.

32. Calin A: Clinical aspects of the effect of NSAID on cartilage. J Rheumatol 16(suppl 18):43–44, 1989.

33. Elliott DP: Preventing upper gastrointestinal bleeding in patients receiving nonsteroidal antiinflammatory drugs. DICP 24:954–8, 1990.

34. Seifert CF, Stanaszek WF: Arthritis in the elderly: Update 1990. J Geriatric Drug Ther 4(4):7–41, 1990.

35. Soll AH, Mechanisms by which nonsteroidal anti-inflammatory drugs damage the mucosa, pp 308–309. In Soll AH (moderator): Nonsteroidal anti-inflammatory drugs and peptic ulcer disease. Ann Intern Med 114:307–319, 1991.

36. Lanza FL: Endoscopic studies of gastric and duodenal injury after use of ibuprofen, aspirin and other nonsteroidal anti-inflammatory agents. Am J Med 77:19–24, 1984.

37. Griffin MR, Piper JM, Daugherty JR, Snowden M, Ray WA: Nonsteroidal anti-inflammatory drug use and increased risk for peptic ulcer disease in elderly persons. Ann Intern Med 114:257–263, 1991.

38. Graham DY, Agrawal NM, Roth SH: Prevention of NSAID-induced gastric ulcer with misoprostil: multicentre, double-blind, placebo-controlled trial. Lancet 12:1277–1280, 1988.

39. Clive DM, Stoff JS: Renal syndromes associated with nonsteroidal antiinflammatory drugs. N Engl J Med 310:563–572, 1984.

40. Bunnign RD, Barth WF: Sulindac: a potentially renal-sparing nonsteroidal anti-inflammatory drug. JAMA 248:2864–2867, 1982.

41. Martinez EM, Lopez JR: Use of analgesics during pregnancy. DICP 20:850–851, 1986.

42. Stefanich RJ: Intraarticular corticosteroids in treatment of osteoarthritis. Orthop Rev 15(2):27–33, 1986.

43. Chandler GN, Jones DT, Wright V, Hartford SJ: Charcot's arthropathy following intra-articular hydrocortisone. Br Med J 1:952, 1959.

44. Rejholec V: Long-term studies of antiosteoarthritic drugs: an assessment. Semin Arthritis Rheum 17(suppl 1):35–53, 1987.

45. Burkhardt D, Ghosh P: Laboratory evaluation of antiarthritic drugs as potential chondroprotective agents. Semin Arthritis Rheum 17(suppl 1):3–34, 1987.

46. McIlwain H, Silverfield JC, Cheatum DE, Poiley J, Taborn J, Ignaczak T, Multz CV: Intra-articular orgotein in osteoarthritis of the knee: a placebo-controlled efficacy, safety, and dosage comparison. Am J Med 87:295–300, 1989.

CHAPTER 30

GOUT AND HYPERURICEMIA

MARK S. SHAEFER, Pharm.D. and PIERRE A. MALOLEY, Pharm.D.

Gout is a chronic metabolic disease, most commonly afflicting males over 30 years of age. It was recognized as a human malady and treated before the ancient Greeks ruled the Mediterranean world. Gout was associated with wealthy intellectuals known to overindulge in food and drink. Despite this long history, it was not until the 19th century that a specific cause was identified. Sir Alfred Garrod identified uric acid as the cause of gout in 1848. One of the major therapeutic advances of the 19th century was the use of colchicine to treat the symptoms of the disease. Specific dietary recommendations were also made for patients with gout, as the role of purines in the disease process was discovered. Treatment improved in the 20th century with the development of new drugs. Acute attacks were treated with colchicine and later with indomethacin or phenylbutazone. The use of uricosuric agents closely followed these advances, and since 1965, allopurinol has also been used for the long-term management of gout.

Uric acid is an end product of protein catabolism. In humans, it is the final product from the breakdown of purines. DNA and RNA are degraded, yielding the nucleosides adenosine and guanosine. The enzyme xanthine oxidase (XO) converts guanosine directly to xanthine and converts adenosine first to hypoxanthine then to xanthine; finally, xanthine is converted into uric acid. At a physiologic pH of 7.4, the monovalent form of uric acid is the predominant form (1).

Total body content of uric acid ranges from 1.0 to 1.2 g in a normal man, with a daily turnover rate of 600 to 800 mg. These values are slightly lower for women. In a normal person, this turnover constitutes 50 to 60% of the urate pool each day. Almost 70% of the uric acid is excreted in the urine; the remainder is secreted into the gastrointestinal tract by a passive process and degraded by intestinal microorganisms to ammonia and carbon dioxide (2, 3).

A four-component hypothesis for urate handling by the kidney best explains the actions of drugs to increase or decrease uric acid levels. These four components are filtration, reabsorption, secretion, and postsecretory reabsorption, either in the later part of the proximal tubule, in the distal tubule, or in both. Approximately 95% of the serum uric acid is filtered freely across the glomerulus. The other 5% of plasma urate is protein bound. Ninety-eight to 100% of this filtered urate is reabsorbed in the early part of the proximal tubule. A variable percentage of the filtered load is secreted back into the tubular lumen in a more distal part of the proximal tubule. The fourth component may occur in the distal part of the proximal tubule, in the distal tubule, or in both (2).

Hyperuricemia is defined as a urate level greater than 480 μmol/liter (8.0 mg/dl) in men and 420 μmol/liter (7.0 mg/dl) in women. These values are more than two standard deviations above the mean population values. The lower value for females is because of an estrogen-dependent sex difference. This difference, which manifests at puberty and is related to greater urate clearance, diminishes or disappears after menopause (4).

Two laboratory methods are used to measure serum urate concentrations. This colorimetric method is used by most autoanalyzers. It is nonspecific, and false elevations can occur from amino acids in the test sample, uremia, high doses of vitamin C, and other xanthines such as caffeine, theobromine, and theophylline, as well as levodopa.

The uricase method is more specific and yields levels that are lower by 20 to 60 μmol/liter (0.4 to 1.0 mg/dl) than the colorimetric values. The clinician must know which method is used to analyze uric acid serum levels. The definitions of hyperuricemia given in the text above are based on colorimetric determinations (1).

ETIOLOGY

Hyperuricemia and gout are traditionally classified as either primary or secondary. Primary gout refers to cases in which the basic metabolic defect is unknown, or if known, the main manifestation is that of hyperuricemia and gout. Secondary gout refers to those cases in which hyperuricemia is part of some other acquired disorder, or in which the basic metabolic defect underlying the hyperuricemia is known but the main clinical characteristics are not those of gout. The distinctions may not always be clear (2).

Patients with primary hyperuricemia and gout have elevated serum uric acid levels caused by either an increased production of uric acid, an impaired clearance of uric acid, or a combination of both. Ten to 20% of patients with primary gout and hyperuricemia are overproducers of uric acid. Overexcreters of uric acid can be identified with a 24-hr urinary uric acid excretion test. Patients who overproduce uric acid generally have a miscible urate pool that is greater than two to three times normal. On a diet that is essentially free of purine-containing foods for greater than 5 days, normal men excrete from 975 to 3497 mmol (164 to 588 mg) of uric acid/day (5). Patients who excrete more than 3569 mmol (600 mg) of uric acid in 24 hr on a purine-restricted diet or more than 4758 to 5948 mmol (800 mg to 1 g) of uric acid on a normal diet can be classified as overexcreters (3). Another method for quantitative analysis of uric acid production involves the use of a spot urine specimen. This method expresses uric acid in terms of excretion per deciliter of glomerular filtrate. With this method, a value of 0.4 mg of urinary uric acid/dl (20 μmol/liter) of glomerular filtrate is considered normal. Patients who are overexcreters have values above 0.7 mg/dl (42 μmol/liter) (6).

Primary hyperuricemia and gout may also (rarely) result from one of two identified enzymatic defects. Patients who lack hypoxanthine guanine phosphoribosyltransferase (HGPRT) activity show one of two phenotypes. Complete HGPRT deficiencies present as the Lesch-Nyhan syndrome. This syndrome is associated with hyperuricemia, hyperuricaciduria, renal calculi, and a neurologic disorder characterized by self-mutilation, mental retardation, choreoathetosis, and spasticity. Patients with partial deficiency may have only gouty arthritis, hyperuricemia, hyperuricosuria, and renal calculi in a second or third decade of life. Patients with phosphoribosyl-1-pyrophosphate (PRPP) synthetase variants have increased de novo purine production. These patients may have gouty arthritis in the teens or early twenties (7).

Secondary hyperuricemia is associated with increased nucleic acid turnover, decreased renal function, increased purine production, or drug-induced decreased elimination of uric acid. A deficiency of glucose-6-phosphatase can also lead to hyperuricemia from infancy. This results from increased purine biosynthesis as well as decreased uric acid clearance from hyperlactacidemia (7).

Drug-induced hyperuricemia is the more common of the secondary hyperuricemias. Of the drugs responsible, diuretics are the most frequently implicated. The mechanism of diuretic-induced hyperuricemia is not clear, but it may relate to an increased reabsorption of uric acid in the proximal tubule. Another possible explanation is a decreased tubular secretion or an increased postsecretory reabsorption of uric acid. Spironolactone is the only diuretic that does not cause hyperuricemia.

Aspirin can cause increased serum urate concentrations when ingested in doses of less than 2 g/day. Doses of more than 2 g cause a uricosuric effect. Low doses preferentially inhibit tubular secretion, and high doses inhibit reabsorption of uric acid.

Pyrazinamide inhibits urate secretion. It markedly decreases urinary excretion of urate even when there are high levels of filtered urate. Another antitubercular drug, ethambutol, is also associated with decreased renal clearance of uric acid. Other drugs known to increase serum levels of uric acid are nicotinic acid, methoxyflurane, levodopa, and epinephrine (2, 8).

Hyperuricemia may be associated with any disorder that causes an increase in the rate of proliferation of cells. This leads to an increase in purine production and an elevation of the urate pool. Hyperuricemia occurs with lymphoid and myeloid proliferative disorders and may also occur with diseases such as psoriasis and dissemination of solid tumors.

Hyperuricemia occurs in up to half of the patients with chronic myelogenous leukemia. Patients with chronic lymphocytic leukemia rarely present with hyperuricemia. Hyperuricemia often occurs in myeloid metaplasia and polycythemia vera. Patients with sickle cell anemia, hemolytic anemia with secondary erythrocytosis, and thalassemia may have hyperuricemia, even though it is uncommon in primary red blood cell disorders (2).

Chronic lead ingestion leading to nephropathy is associated with gout and hyperuricemia. Lead presumably causes a defect in the tubular secretion of urate as well as inhibiting guanase, the enzyme that deaminates guanine to xanthine. In these cases of saturnine gout, uric acid clearance is reduced markedly, even though creatinine clearance may be only slightly decreased (2).

Patients who fast for 1 or 2 days have increased levels of serum urate. In most cases, these elevations in urate levels result from a decreased urinary output of uric acid because urate excretion is inhibited by elevated ketone levels. Doses of alcohol of 112 to 135 g given with food are associated with an important increase in blood lactate concentration, decreased urinary uric acid output, and hyperuricemia. The combination of fasting and ethyl alcohol may have an additive effect on uric acid retention (9).

Hyperuricemia may also result from other causes of increased ketoacids and lactic acid, such as exercise and uncontrolled diabetes. Additionally, hypothyroidism, hyperparathyroidism, and hypoparathyroidism have all been associated with hyperuricemia, presumably because of a reduction in the renal excretion of urate (3).

EPIDEMIOLOGY

Many studies have related gout to racial, geographic, dietary, and other socioecomonic factors. The one consistent marker is the relationship between elevated uric acid levels and gout. The epidemiology of gout was studied as a part of the Heart Disease Epidemiology Study at Framingham, Massachusetts. This study involved a total of 5127 subjects ages 30 through 59 on initial evaluation. Thirteen subjects had experienced a gouty attack prior to entry in the study, 0.2% of the total population. The mean age of the population at the beginning of the study was 44 years. Fourteen years later, when the mean age of the population was 58, 1.5% (76) of the population had experienced an attack of gout. Gout had occurred in 2.8% of the men and 0.4%

of the women. The prevalence of gouty arthritis was found to increase with increasing uric acid levels. In men with uric acid levels under 360 μmol/liter (6 mg/dl), the frequency of gout was 0.6%. The rate progressed to 1.9% with levels of 360 to 410 μmol/liter (6 to 6.9 mg/dl), and when levels exceeded 530 μmol/liter (9 mg/dl), 90% of the men had gout. The frequency of gout for all men with uric acid levels above 420 μmol/liter (7 mg/dl) was 20% (10).

PATHOGENESIS

A combination of factors is most likely responsible for the formation of urate crystals in patients with gout. The degree of hyperuricemia, location of the joint, abrupt changes (increases or decreases) in serum uric acid levels, physical state of the joint, resolution of joint effusions, the presence of certain protein polysaccharides, and the temperature of the joint are all involved in urate crystal formation.

Acute attacks of gout develop when monosodium urate crystals deposit in the synovium of joints involved. These crystals are derived from either preformed synovial deposits or de novo synthesis. Characteristically, acute attacks affect the peripheral joints; the most distal joints are more likely to be affected. A possible explanation for this involves the temperature of the joints, since monosodium urate solubility varies directly with temperature. The solubility of urate in physiologic saline is 400 μmol/liter (6.8 mg/dl) at 37°C, but only 270 μmol/liter (4.5 mg/dl) at 30°C. Joint temperatures decrease distally. The average temperature of the knee is 33°C, and that of the ankle is 29°C. However, this factor alone cannot explain why gout develops in some people and not in others with similar uric acid levels. Also involved may be the increased solubility of urate in proteoglycans, chondroitin sulfate, and hyaluronic acid, which are all abundant in the synovial fluid and cartilage. Urate solubility may be affected by genetic or environmental alterations in these substances that predispose to or even initiate attacks of gout (2).

Another explanation was proposed by Simkin, who was concerned with the predisposition of gout for the first metatarsophalangeal joint. Gout in this joint is referred to as "podagra," and more than 50% of first attacks of gout occur in this joint. Ultimately, most patients with gout experience podagra. The base of the big toe is subjected to extreme forces in the normal process of walking. Shoes compound the problem by forcing the joint to endure these forces in an unnatural position. The joint that has experienced degenerative changes or recent trauma, including trauma that may have been unnoticed, is likely to be the site of a synovial effusion. At night while the patient sleeps, the effusion resolves. Water leaves the joint faster than urate, which causes a transiently high intraarticular urate concentration that favors crystal formation. This explains the common nocturnal onset of gout in the big toe and may

help to explain the occasional attack of gout that develops in a person with a normal urate serum concentration (11).

Urate crystals in the synovial fluid or surrounding tissues and the reaction of the body's defense mechanisms to these crystals cause the typical gouty attack. This reaction begins within 4 to 8 hr of the presence of these crystals in the synovial fluid. Many factors are involved in this acute inflammatory response. Monosodium urate (MSU) crystals have sharp irregular crystal facets with multiple outward projections. These surface irregularities favor the absorption of immunoglobulin G (IgG) and other polypeptides. Adsorption of these polypeptides increases crystal phagocytosis by polymorphonuclear leukocytes (PMNs). In addition, MSU crystals are electronegative and therefore bind, denature, and cleave Hageman factor (clotting factor XII). This activates the clotting, kininogen, plasminogen, and complement cascades. Prostaglandins play a role in the inflammatory response of gout, causing vasodilation, increased vascular permeability, and release of chemotactic substances that attract PMNs. Although the extent of involvement of these other factors is unclear, the role of PMNs is well established (2).

Synovial fluid from patients with gout has an average leukocyte count of 19.5×10^9/liter (19,500 cells/mm^3), 90% or more of which are neutrophils. PMNs, monocytes, and synovial cells phagocytize MSU crystals that are coated with protein. This causes a fusion of lysosomes with a phagosome, producing a phagolysosome that contains enzymes. The protein coat on the crystal is digested by the enzymes, allowing hydrogen bond–mediated membranolysis to occur. Cellular autolysis results when the phagolysosome is lysed and hydrolytic enzymes are released into the cytoplasm. This also leads to increased permeability of the outer membrane of the cell and a subsequent release of enzymes into the extracellular medium. Urate crystals are digested by peroxidases in phagocytic cells, which can also adsorb leukocyte-derived proteins that may terminate the stimulus for further phagocytosis. This series of events causes the clinical findings that mark the beginning and the resolution of an acute attack of gout (12).

DIAGNOSIS AND CLINICAL FINDINGS

Acute attacks of gout are most often characterized by the sudden onset of unbearable pain in one joint of the lower extremities. The first attack is not associated with other symptoms and is usually monoarticular, although polyarticular involvement in a first attack occurs in about 10% of the general population. The attack lasts a variable but limited period of time and is followed by a completely asymptomatic period. Over time the periods between attacks become shorter, and the symptoms of the attack fail to resolve completely. This leads to chronic crippling arthritis. The peak age of onset of gout is between 30 and 50 years in men. When women develop gout, it is almost always after menopause. Gout in patients of either sex before the age of 30 should lead to an investigation for possible enzyme defects, purine overproduction, or renal disease. Gout rarely effects patients this young.

Other commonly affected joints, in order of frequency of involvement, are the instep, ankle, heel, knee, wrist, finger, and elbow. Although acute gout is predominantly a disease of the joints of the lower extremities, any joint may be involved. Rare sites of involvement are the shoulder, hip, spine, sacroiliac, sternoclavicular, and temporomandibular joints (11, 13).

Patients may report several trivial episodes of pain in the big toe or ankle prior to the first attack of gout. Most patients have their initial attack during periods of good health. Attacks commonly occur while the patient is sleeping; many patients are awakened by excruciating pain. Occasionally patients first detect the symptoms as their feet touch the cold floor when they get up in the morning. Three or 4 hr after the onset of an attack, the skin over the affected joint becomes red, hot, swollen, and exquisitely painful and tender. Inflammation is slight at first but progresses and can resemble a bacterial cellulitis. The systemic signs of the attack include fever, leukocytosis, and elevation of the erythrocyte sedimentation rate (4, 7). Systemic signs are more likely in patients with polyarticular involvement. Temperatures may reach values as high as 39.4°C. In one study, neither fever nor leukocytosis correlated with the number of joints involved (13). Untreated attacks of gout may last for hours to several weeks. As the patient recovers, the skin over the affected joint often desquamates. Even though an attack may have been severe, with marked swelling and incapacitation, recovery is generally complete with the first attack. Patients return to their preattack state of health, until the next attack (7).

The periods between attacks, called intercritical periods, vary in length. Some patients never experience a recurrence, and (rarely) some patients have an almost chronic involvement from the onset. Most patients experience a second attack within 6 months to 2 years. As the disease progresses, the intercritical periods become shorter and the attacks polyarticular, more severe, and longer lasting. Eventually patients enter a phase of chronic gout without pain-free intercritical periods.

Modern treatment of gout with allopurinol and uricosurics has all but eliminated the occurrence of chronic tophaceous gout. Before these agents become available, 50 to 70% of patients with gout had the chronic tophaceous form. It now affects approximately 3% of patients. Tophaceous gout is a consequence of consistently elevated levels of uric acid, and it correlates directly with the levels of urate. In one series, the mean serum urate concentration was 540 µmol/liter (9.1 mg/dl) (uricase method) in 722 nontophaceous patients, 590 to 650 µmol/liter (10 to 11 mg/dl) in 456 patients with minimal-to-moderate to-

phaceous deposits, and above 650 µmol/liter (11.0 mg/dl) in 111 patients with extensive tophaceous deposits. Tophi are usually firm and moveable with thin and reddened overlying skin. They are commonly found on the helix or antihelix of the ear, the finger, hand, knee, foot, or toe, the ulnar surface of the forearm, the olecranon bursa, or the Achilles tendon. The thin skin overlying the tophi may break down and extrude a milky white substance composed mainly of urate crystals. Infection by skin flora may develop in these areas and will heal slowly. Eventually these deposits lead to the destruction of the articular cartilage and portions of the subchondral bone (7, 14, 15).

Renal involvement in gout is the most serious, and second most common, clinical manifestation. Two forms of renal disease are possible, urate nephropathy or uric acid nephropathy. Urate nephropathy results from the deposition of MSU salt crystals in the renal interstitium and the accompanying inflammation. This progresses slowly but is not thought to decrease life expectancy. It is not known whether the urate deposits cause a deterioration in renal function. Uric acid nephropathy results from the deposition of uric acid crystals in the collecting tubules. Acute renal failure occurs in patients who overproduce and overexcrete uric acid as a result of aggressive chemotherapy, lymphoma, leukemia, or enzymatic defects. This renal failure does not correlate with the serum urate concentration but with the amount of uric acid excreted. Prior to the advent of hemodialysis, renal failure accounted for 17 to 25% of deaths in the gouty population. Kidney damage in gout usually occurs with either diabetes, hypertension, renal vascular disease, glomerulonephritis, pyelonephritis, renal calculi with urinary tract infection, congenital nephropathy, or some other cause of primary nephropathy not associated with gout. It is currently accepted that asymptomatic hyperuricemia does not result in renal destruction until uric acid levels exceed 650 µmol/liter (11 mg/dl) for prolonged periods (16–18).

Many criteria have been developed for establishing the diagnosis of gout. A diagnosis of gout must be firmly established before the institution of expensive and potentially toxic therapy. Gout should be considered in a patient with an acute onset of monoarticular or asymmetric polyarticular arthritis of the distal extremities. The diagnosis of acute gouty arthritis may be established by the demonstration of MSU crystals in white cells of synovial fluid or a tophus. The synovial fluid in gouty patients is cloudy and less viscous than normal. Leukocyte counts average 13.5×10^9/liter (13,500 cells/mm^3) (range 1.0 to 70.0 × 10^9/liter (1000 to 70,000 cells/mm^3)), with a predominance of PMNs. Total protein is normal, as is the glucose concentration. The Gram stain and culture of the aspirate should be negative. Needle-shaped crystals 2 to 10 µm long are present. When viewed with a polarized light microscope with a first-order red decompensator, the crystals

Table 30.1.
Criteria for Diagnosis of Acute Gout[a]

Definite
  Demonstration of sodium urate crystals in affected joints
Suggestive[b]
  1. More than one attack of arthritis
  2. Development of maximum inflammation within 1 day
  3. Oligoarthritis attack
  4. Redness over joint
  5. Painful or swollen first metatarsophalangeal joint
  6. Unilateral attack on first metatarsophalangeal joint
  7. Unilateral attack on tarsal joint
  8. Tophus
  9. Hyperuricemia
  10. Asymptomatic swelling within a joint

[a] Criteria established by the American Rheumatism Association.
[b] A minimum of six criteria should be present to be suggestive of gout.

are negatively birefringent. Urate crystals may not be found in patients with gout, because of the difficulty in aspiration of fluid from involved joints. Acutely inflamed joints have intracellular urate crystals in 85% of patients with gout. A probable diagnosis of gout may be established using criteria established by the American Rheumatism Association (Table 30.1). In addition to these criteria, complete resolution of synovitis with colchicine treatment may help establish a diagnosis. The clinical findings of pseudogout, acute sarcoidosis, psoriatic arthritis, and acute calcific tendonitis may mimic those of gout. Pseudogout and sarcoidosis may even respond to a trial of colchicine therapy, especially if given intravenously. If uric acid levels are normalized in a patient for a prolonged period without resolution of joint symptoms, another diagnosis should be sought (4, 7, 19).

Assessment of the gouty patient should begin with a detailed history and physical examination. A family history may demonstrate a predisposition for gout, and all medications should be checked for their potential to induce hyperuricemia. It is also important to classify the hyperuricemia as a problem with overproduction or underexcretion or possibly both. A 24-hr urine collection should be obtained to measure urine uric acid and creatinine. At the same time, samples for serum creatinine and blood urea nitrogen levels should be obtained, as a measure of kidney function. Uric acid excretion above 3569 mmol (600 mg) in 24 hr in a patient on a low-purine diet for 4 to 5 days should be considered abnormal. In the absence of a purine-free diet, excretion of more than 5948 mmol (1000 mg) per 24 hr is diagnostic of overproduction. Hyperuricemia with a normal 24-hr excretion indicates inadequate renal elimination (19).

TREATMENT

Treatment of gout and hyperuricemia has a two-step approach. The first step is to terminate the acute attack and resolve the pain. Once the acute attack is resolved, the goal is to gradually reduce the serum uric acid concentration. Antiinflammatory agents that are useful for acute attacks include colchicine, indomethacin, phenylbutazone, and the newer nonsteroidal antiinflammatory drugs (NSAIDs). Serum uric acid levels should not be reduced until the acute attack has been terminated. The process of lowering uric acid levels should proceed slowly and cautiously, because rapid lowering of uric acid levels may precipitate another acute attack. In some mild cases, patients may be able to control the hyperuricemia by diet modifications and weight reduction. Agents available to decrease uric acid levels include the xanthine oxidase inhibitor, allopurinol, and the uricosuric drugs, probenecid and sulfinpyrazone. Hypouricemic therapy is used to decrease the body stores of urate in an attempt to prevent or reverse the complications due to deposition of urate.

Acute Gouty Arthritis

The treatment of acute gout is directed at alleviating the pain rapidly and attempting to restore joint mobility. It is often beneficial to immobilize the affected joint and use analgesics in addition to antiinflammatory therapy. Antiinflammatory medications should be started as soon after the onset of pain as possible.

COLCHICINE

Extracts of colchicine have been used to treat acute episodes of gout for more than 1200 years. Colchicine, an alkaloid of colchicum, was isolated in 1820, and although one of the oldest treatments for gout, it still remains useful in certain cases. It is effective in alleviating acute attacks of gout as well as in prophylaxis of future attacks. Colchicine is also effective in the treatment of pseudogout, sarcoid arthritis, and calcific tendonitis. Colchicine may be used to establish a probable diagnosis of gout, since the antiinflammatory action is limited to these conditions (20). This action is particularly useful in cases where small joints are involved; aspiration of synovial fluid and isolation of uric acid crystals from these joints is often difficult. Response to colchicine is between 75 and 90%. Response rates depend on how quickly therapy is initiated after the onset of an attack. Colchicine is most effective when given within the first 12 to 36 hr of an attack. Signs and symptoms of inflammation abate within 12 to 24 hr; in 90% of patients the pain is gone within 24 to 48 hr. Most patients should be treated first with indomethacin, or another of the nonsteroidal antiinflammatory drugs that tend to be less toxic than colchicine (3, 7, 21–23).

Colchicine has antiinflammatory but no analgesic activity. It has no effect on serum levels of urinary excretion of uric acid. The mechanism of action of colchicine is not yet fully understood. Possible mechanisms include diminished PMN chemotaxis, metabolism, and lysosomal enzyme release. The mechanism of decreased chemotaxis is related to the ability of colchicine to impair chemotactic factor. Additionally, colchicine also interferes with sodium urate deposition by decreasing lactic acid production by PMNs (24).

After oral administration, colchicine is rapidly absorbed from the gastrointestinal (GI) tract and partially metabolized in the liver. Unchanged drug may be reabsorbed from the intestine after biliary secretion. Concentrations of colchicine and metabolites decrease after 1 to 2 hr and then increase as a result of reabsorption of unchanged drug. The acute GI toxicity related to colchicine is possibly related to this drug recycling. Colchicine is concentrated in leukocytes but also appears in other tissues, including the kidneys, liver, and intestinal tract. The plasma half-life after intravenous dosing is approximately 20 min. The half-life in leukocytes averages 60 hr. Colchicine and its metabolites are excreted primarily in the feces, with smaller amounts excreted in the urine. Patients with severe renal disease may have prolonged half-lives of colchicine as a result of large decreases in renal excretion, and measurable quantities of drug have been found in urine for up to 10 days after therapy has been discontinued in patients with normal renal function (22, 25).

Colchicine has a very narrow therapeutic index. Acute gout attacks are treated with an initial oral dose of 0.5 to 1.2 mg of colchicine. This is followed by a dose of 0.5 to 0.6 mg every hr or 1.0 to 1.2 mg every 2 hr. Therapy is continued until the patient improves, GI side effects develop, or a maximum of 8 to 10 mg is administered. The effective dose is usually between 4 and 8 mg (3, 7, 22). Death has occurred after administration of as little as 7 mg (26). As many as 80% of patients experience some GI side effects that require dosage modification. Patients with preexisting Crohn's disease, diverticulitis, peptic ulcer disease, or a history of GI bleeding should not be given oral colchicine. If treatment with colchicine is deemed necessary in these patients, the dose may be given intravenously. Colchicine for intravenous use should be mixed with 0.9% sodium chloride or sterile water for injection since dextrose 5% in water or bacteriostatic saline may cause precipitation. A dose of 1 to 2 mg should be mixed with 10 to 20 ml of the appropriate diluent and injected slowly over a period of 2 to 5 min or into the line of a flowing intravenous solution. Care should be taken to assure that the intravenous injection site is patent and not infiltrating. Colchicine causes severe local irritation to the skin and tissues and should never be given subcutaneously or intramuscularly. After an initial dose of 2 mg intravenously, 0.5 mg may be given every 6 hr until a response occurs. Alternate dosing methods include a one-time dose of 3 mg or 1 mg initially, followed by 0.5 mg once or twice

daily if needed. The total daily recommended intravenous dose is 4 mg. A total intravenous dose of more than 5 mg should not be given during any one treatment period. Additional courses of therapy should not be given for at least 3 days because of risk of GI toxicity (3, 25, 26).

Colchicine may cause bone marrow depression with agranulocytosis, thrombocytopenia, leukopenia, and aplastic anemia. These side effects are rare and usually only occur in patients who have received excessive doses or who have decreased renal or hepatic function. Other rare side effects that may occur with prolonged administration include loss of body and scalp hair, rashes, peripheral neuropathy, myopathy, vesicular dermatitis, anuria, renal damage, or hematuria. Increased serum concentrations of alkaline prosphatase may also occur with colchicine administration (27).

Colchicine may still be considered as primary therapy in patients who have used it successfully in the past. These patients generally know the total dose of colchicine that worked for them previously and should be given half the total dose at one time and the rest in 0.5 to 0.6 mg increments every hour until the total dose is given. Patients who have hypersensitivity reactions to aspirin and the NSAIDs may also be candidates for colchicine therapy. Some patients taking warfarin should not take NSAIDs and should use colchicine. Other patients with a relative contraindication to NSAIDs include those with renal failure, congestive heart failure, and hypertension. NSAIDs in these patients can cause decreased renal function and sodium and water retention. If colchicine cannot be tolerated in these patients, sulindac, which perhaps has a safer renal profile, should be tried cautiously (28).

Patients with alcoholic cirrhosis should also be treated with colchicine. Since these patients may have preexisting GI distress, renal insufficiency, and ascites, the intravenous dose of colchicine should be reduced by one-half (29).

Recurrent attacks of gout may be reduced by prophylactic treatment with colchicine. Patients who experience fewer than one attack per year may be given 0.5 to 0.6 mg of colchicine one to four times each week. If attacks are more frequent, the dose is usually 0.5 to 0.6 mg each day. Some patients may require as much as three times this dose each day to control the disease. Patients with a history of gout undergoing surgical procedures should receive 0.5 to 0.6 mg of colchicine three times daily for 3 days before and 3 days after surgery (30).

INDOMETHACIN

Indomethacin is a potent antiinflammatory drug that also has antipyretic and analgesic properties. It is considered by many to be the agent of choice for the treatment of acute gouty attacks. Indomethacin should be started as soon as possible after the onset of an acute gouty attack.

Unlike colchicine, it is usually effective even when treatment is delayed by several days. The probable mechanism of action of indomethacin is potent inhibition of prostaglandin synthesis. In addition, indomethacin may exert an inhibitory effect on the mobility of PMNs (3, 7, 21, 29).

Indomethacin given by the oral route is rapidly and completely absorbed. Peak plasma concentrations are attained within 30 to 120 min. Absorption of indomethacin administered with food is delayed, but the serum concentration-time profile is similar to that observed in fasting subjects. Indomethacin suppositories are available for patients unable to take oral doses. Peak concentrations from rectal administration are generally more rapid but lower than those achieved with similar oral doses. Bioavailability from suppositories is approximately 80%. The half-life of indomethacin ranges from 1 to 16 hr. Possibly, this large range results from extensive enterohepatic recycling and unpredictable biliary discharge. Indomethacin is metabolized primarily by the hepatic microsomal enzyme system and extramicrosomal deacylation. All metabolites are inactive (30).

An initial dose of 50 to 75 mg of indomethacin should be given, followed by 50 mg every 6 hr. This dose is continued for 24 to 48 hr, and then it is gradually tapered over the next several days. Common side effects include headache, dizziness, nausea, and vomiting. These side effects are generally better tolerated than those seen with colchicine. Additionally, sodium and water retention, hyperkalemia, and renal dysfunction may occur in some patients (2, 3, 29). Because it irritates the gastric mucosa,

indomethacin should be given with food, milk, or an antacid (29). Indomethacin should be used with caution in elderly patients, patients with congestive heart failure (21), and patients with a history of peptic ulcer disease.

When given concurrently with probenecid, indomethacin serum levels are increased. This is most likely due to decreased biliary secretion (30).

OTHER ANTIINFLAMMATORY AGENTS

There are many other NSAIDs, and most are useful in the treatment of gout. Agents such as sulindac, tolectin, ibuprofen, piroxicam, naproxen, and ketoprofen are just a few of the many drugs available. These compounds also inhibit the synthesis of prostaglandins. Many of the newer agents may have a lower overall rate of side effects than indomethacin. Doses of the drugs for the treatment of gout are usually the same as or higher than the doses used to treat rheumatoid arthritis (Table 30.2). These drugs should not be used in patients allergic to aspirin or in asthmatics with nasal polyps. The most common side effect with these agents is GI disturbance, and they should all be taken with food or milk to decrease this problem. These drugs should be used with caution in patients with a history of gastrointestinal bleeding. Gastrointestinal hemorrhage can be life threatening and has occurred with all of these drugs (31–34).

PHENYLBUTAZONE

Phenylbutazone has been used quite effectively in the past for the treatment of gout. Because of the risk of agranu-

Table 30.2.
Nonsteroidal Antiinflammatory Drugs for Gout

Drug (Trade Name)	Dose[a] (mg)	Dosing Interval	Dosage Form (mg)
Piroxicam (Feldene)	40	q.d.	Capsules (10, 20)
Sulindac (Clinoril)	200	b.i.d.	Tablets (150, 200)
Naproxen (Naprosyn) (Anaprox—Na⁺ salt)[b]	750 load then 250	t.i.d.	Tablets (250, 375, 500)
			Tablets (275, 550)
Ketoprofen (Orudis)	100	t.i.d.	Capsules (25, 50, 75)
Ibuprofen (Motrin, Rufen)[c]	800	t.i.d.	Tablets (200, 300, 400, 600, 800)
Indomethacin (Indocin)	50	t.i.d.–q.i.d.	Capsules (10, 25, 50, 75)
			Suspension (25/5 ml)
			Suppositories (50)
Tolmetin (Tolectin)	400	t.i.d.–q.i.d.	Tablets (200, 600)
			Capsules (400)
Fenoprofen (Nalfon)	800	q.i.d.	Capsules (200, 300, 600)
			Tablets (600)
Phenylbutazone (Butazolidin)	400 load then 100	q 4 h until relief	Tablets and capsules (100)
Flurbiprofen (Ansaid)	400 load then 50	100 q.i.d. q.i.d.	Tablets (50, 100)

[a] Recommended doses for the treatment of acute gouty attacks.
[b] 275 mg of naproxen sodium is equivalent to 250 mg of naproxen.
[c] Also available over the counter under various trade names.

locytosis and aplastic anemia, phenylbutazone is not recommended as initial therapy for any of its indications. It should be used only after all other nonsteroidal antiinflammatory drugs have been tried and found unsatisfactory.

Phenylbutazone is a potent antiinflammatory drug that works as well as or better than colchicine for acute attacks of gout. It is absorbed rapidly and completely from the GI tract. Peak plasma levels are achieved within 2 hr of ingestion. The half-life of phenylbutazone ranges from 48 to 72 hr. It is highly protein bound and is almost completely metabolized. In addition to its antiinflammatory and antipyretic activity, phenylbutazone has a paradoxical effect on urate excretion. At doses of 600 mg/24 hr or more it increases uric acid excretion; at lower doses it can decrease the rate of renal urate clearance (22).

If all other therapy fails and the decision is made to use phenylbutazone, a dose of 600 to 800 mg, divided in three to four doses, can be given initially; thereafter the dose should be reduced to a maximum of 400 mg/day divided into four doses. The dose should be tapered over the next few days and then discontinued (29). The rate of taper should be dictated by the clinical signs of the disease. Patients should not be given this drug for a period longer than 7 days because of the potential toxicity. Adverse effects are similar to those experienced with indomethacin. Gastrointestinal discomfort, reactivation of peptic ulcer disease, and fluid and salt retention are common and sometimes extreme. This drug should be used with extreme caution in patients with congestive heart failure or preexisting renal dysfunction. Hypersensitivity reactions such as rashes, and less commonly, hepatitis or nephritis may occur (2, 3, 21, 29).

Asymptomatic Hyperuricemia

Hyperuricemia exists when the serum concentration of urate exceeds the solubility limits. This level is generally considered to be 420 μmol/liter (7 mg/dl) with the uricase method or 480 μmol/liter (8 mg/dl) with the less specific colorimetric method (4). Once hyperuricemia is diagnosed, the decision to treat must be based on careful evaluation of the patient's clinical condition. If treatment is begun it requires lifelong therapy and therefore includes the risk of adverse reactions and a substantial cost to the patient. Controversy exists as to when asymptomatic hyperuricemia should be treated. It is impractical and perhaps imprudent to treat every person with mild hyperuricemia, since the risks of gout and its sequelae are small

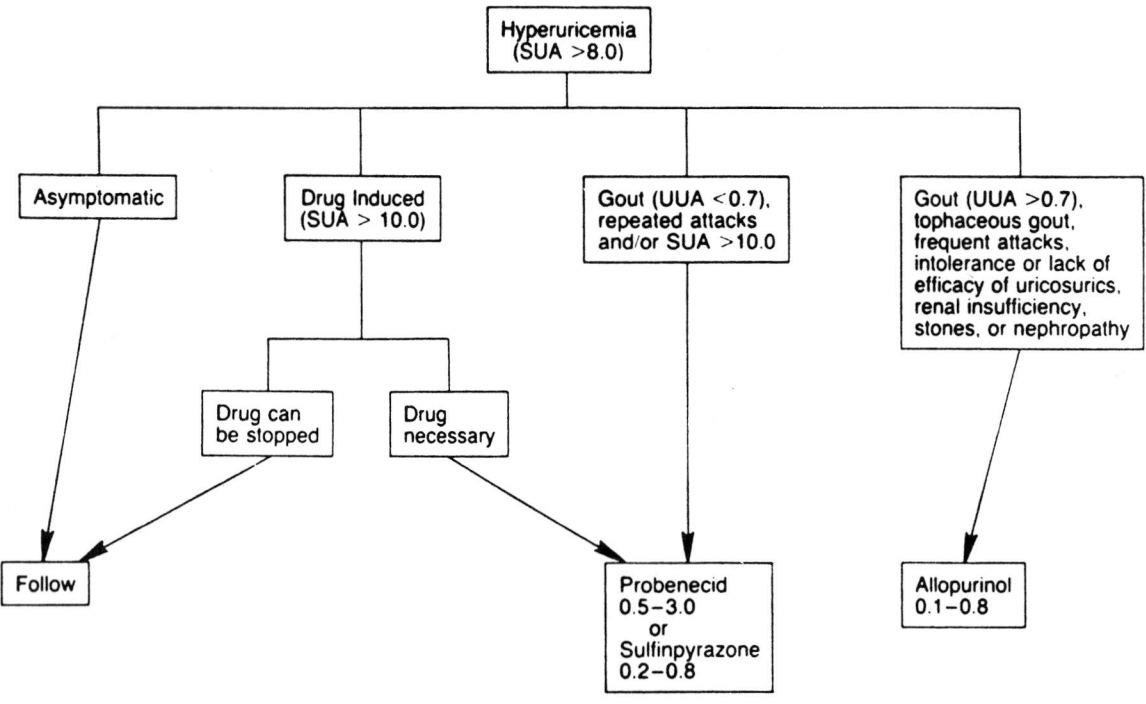

Figure 30.1. The management of hyperuricemia. Serum urate (SUA) is in milligrams per deciliter, measured by the colorimetric method. The excretion rate of urinary uric acid (UUA) is in milligrams per deciliter of glomerular filtrate. Doses of hypouricemic drugs (probenecid, sulfinpyrazone, and allopurinol) are in grams, with values indicating the starting dose on the left progressing toward a maximal dosage on the right. The hyperuricemia of most patients is well controlled by intermediate doses. (Adapted from Nashel DJ, Chandra M: Acute gouty arthritis, special management considerations in alcoholic patients. JAMA 247:58–59, 1982.)

Table 30.3.
Drugs For Acute and Chronic Gout and Hyperuricemia

Drug	Dosage Form (mg)	Initial Dose (Average Maintenance)	Comments
Probenecid (Benemid)	Tablets (500)	250 mg b.i.d. (500 mg b.i.d.)	Hydrate well; avoid salicylates; caution in PUD & renal impairment; take with meals
Sulfinpyrazone (Anturane)	Tablets (100) Capsules (200)	50 mg b.i.d. (100–200 mg b.i.d.)	Same as probenecid
Allopurinol (Zyloprim, Lopurin)	Tablets (100, 300)	100 mg q.d. (300 mg q.d.)	Hydrate well; adjust dose in renal impairment; report any rash; take with meals
Colchcine	Tablets (0.5, 0.6) Injection (½ ml)	p.o. 0.5–1.2 mg followed by 0.5–1.2 mg q 1–2 hours i.v. Refer to text	Caution in GI, renal, & hepatic disorders; bone marrow depression with long-term use
Probenecid/colchicine (ColBenemid)	Tablets (500/0.5)	1 tablet q.d. (1 tablet b.i.d.)	

(16, 35). Patients who have developed hyperuricemia as a result of other medications may require treatment. This may be especially true in patients on long-term diuretic therapy for hypertension, especially if the hyperuricemia is pronounced and alternative antihypertensive therapy cannot be used. When drugs cause serum urate levels to exceed 530 µmol/liter (9 mg/dl) from the uricase method of 590 µmol/liter (10 mg/dl) using the colorimetric method, a uricosuric agent should be added to overcome decreased tubular secretion of uric acid, because these concentrations are often associated with joint changes and renal complications (2, 16, 21). Hypouricemic agents should also be used in patients with recurrent episodes of gout. Patients who have developed tophi or other complications of gout should be candidates for treatment with urate-lowering drugs, even in the absence of clinical disease.

Once the decision to treat is made, there are two options available, xanthine oxidase (XO) inhibitors or uricosurics (Fig. 30.1). Two uricosuric agents, probenecid and sulfinpyrazone, are available to increase renal elimination of uric acid. Allopurinol is the XO inhibitor (Table 30.3). Therapy is generally based on the etiology of the hyperuricemia and overall physical condition of the patient. Uricosuric agents are considered the logical choice in patients who are underexcreters of uric acid. Overexcreters should be started on therapy with allopurinol. Allopurinol is also a rational choice in patients with tophi, renal stones, or moderate-to-severe renal dysfunction. All forms of hyperuricemia may be treated with allopurinol, but the toxicity profiles of the agents must be taken into consideration.

PROBENECID

Probenecid competitively inhibits the active reabsorption of uric acid at the proximal convoluted tubule. This tubular blocking action promotes the urinary excretion of uric acid, thereby decreasing serum urate concentrations (36). Absorption of probenecid is rapid and complete; peak levels are achieved in 1 to 5 hr. The peak action of the drug occurs at about 2 hr and lasts for about 8 hr. Probenecid is highly protein bound, primarily to albumin. The drug accumulates in the kidney but not in other organs. Probenecid is metabolized by oxidation of the alkyl side chains and glucuronide conjugation. These processes account for about 90% of the metabolism. The elimination half-life is dose dependent, approximately 2 to 6 hr with 0.5 to 1 g doses and 4 to 12 hr with a 2 g dose. Renal elimination is dose independent but does depend on the pH and rate of urine formation. Alkalinization of the urine results in an increased elimination of probenecid (37).

Doses of 1 to 2 g of probenecid can cause a four- to sixfold increase in the elimination of uric acid (21). Active metabolites of probenecid contribute little to the elimination of uric acid (37). Probenecid therapy should not be started during an acute attack of gout because it may exacerbate and prolong the inflammatory phase. Therapy should begin with 250 mg twice a day during the first week of therapy and then increase gradually in increments of 250 to 500 mg/week. A dose of 1 g/day will result in adequate urate lowering in approximately 60% of patients (3). Doses should be adjusted to maintain serum uric acid levels below 420 µmol/liter (7 mg/dl). The dose may also be increased if the 24-hr urine uric acid excretion is not above 4160 mmol (700 mg) (7). The drug may increase the frequency of acute attacks during the first year of therapy, even if urate concentrations are maintained at or below normal.

Patients should be advised to drink large quantities of fluid, at least 2 liters/day, while taking probenecid. This decreases the risk of formation of uric acid stones (3). Alkalinization of the urine to a pH > 6 greatly increases the solubility of uric acid; the resulting increased elimination of probenecid is not therapeutically important (37). Probenecid may not be effective and should not be used in patients with renal impairment who have a creatinine clearance of less than 0.83 ml/sec (50 ml/min) (22).

Probenecid is usually well tolerated; side effects most commonly associated with probenecid are GI in 8 to 18% of patients, hypersensitivity reactions in 5%, precipitation of uric acid stones in 10%, and precipitation of acute gouty attacks in 10%. Gastrointestinal complaints may be decreased by taking each dose with food (3, 36).

Probenecid should be used cautiously in patients with a history of peptic ulcer disease, and it should not be used in patients with a blood dyscrasia or uric acid kidney stones. The drug should never be used to treat hyperuricemia caused by cancer chemotherapy, myeloproliferative neoplastic diseases, or radiation because of greatly increased risks of uric acid nephropathy.

Because probenecid inhibits renal tubular secretion of many weak organic acids, it causes many interesting drug interactions. Probenecid inhibits the secretion of the penicillins, cephalosporins, nalidixic acid, rifampicin, and nitrofurantoin. This leads to higher levels of antibiotics for prolonged periods. This drug interaction has been used therapeutically to increase the duration and plasma concentrations of the penicillins and cephalosporins. The efficacy of nitrofurantoin is decreased by this interaction, and the toxicity is increased. The renal elimination of naproxen, indomethacin, and sulfinpyrazone is also decreased. The doses of naproxen and indomethacin must be decreased, but the concomitant use of probenecid and sulfinpyrazone does not cause increased adverse reactions. In contrast, the clearance of allopurinol is increased in the presence of probenecid, but the effects of the two drugs are additive, and the combination may be used to therapeutic advantage.

The diuresis produced by furosemide and the thiazides is increased because their renal elimination is decreased when they are given with probenecid. Concomitant administration with heparin has been reported to increase clotting time. Patients receiving chlorpropamide should have their blood sugar levels monitored closely at the start of probenecid therapy, since the half-life of chlorpropamide may be increased and result in hypoglycemia. Interactions with other sulfonylureas may occur but are controversial. Low-dose aspirin is an absolute contraindication with probenecid or sulfinpyrazone therapy, because the aspirin will block the excretion of uric acid and therefore block the therapeutic effect of these uricosuric agents.

SULFINPYRAZONE

Like probenecid, sulfinpyrazone competitively inhibits active reabsorption of uric acid at the proximal convoluted tubule, thereby promoting the urinary excretion of uric acid and reducing serum urate concentrations. Sulfinpyrazone is a potent uricosuric agent that is chemically related to phenylbutazone. In addition, it reduces platelet adhesiveness and can result in prolonged platelet survival (22).

Oral administration of sulfinpyrazone results in rapid and complete absorption. Peak plasma levels are usually obtained within 1 hr. The half-life is relatively short, ranging from 1 to 3 hr. Approximately 98% of plasma sulfinpyrazone is bound to proteins. Twenty to 45% of a dose is excreted unchanged in the urine, with most of the excretion occurring within 6 hr. The uricosuric action of the drug results from inhibition of the tubular reabsorption of uric acid in the nephron (36).

On a weight-for-weight basis sulfinpyrazone is three to six times as potent as probenecid as a uricosuric. Therapy should be started with a dose of 100 mg daily, given as 50 mg twice a day, for about the first week. The dose is then increased by 100-mg increments each week until an effective dose is reached. A typical regimen might be: 50 mg twice a day for 1 week, 100 mg twice a day for 1 week, 150 mg twice a day for 1 week and so on, until a maintenance dose of 200 to 400 mg daily is achieved. The drug may increase the frequency of acute attacks during the first year of therapy, even if urate concentrations are maintained at or below normal. There is some evidence that the administration of prophylactic doses of colchicine, 1 mg/day or less, during the first 6 months will decrease the frequency of subsequent attacks. Not all clinicians agree with the prophylactic use of colchicine in patients taking uricosuric drugs (7, 21, 22).

As with probenecid, this drug should not be used when creatinine clearance is less than 0.83 ml/sec (50 ml/min). Periodic blood counts should be performed during sulfinpyrazone therapy because of the rare occurrence of anemia, leukopenia, thrombocytopenia, and agranulocytosis. No uricosuric should be used in patients who are overproducers of uric acid.

When used in recommended doses, sulfinpyrazone is usually well tolerated, with a low rate of side effects. The most common side effects are those affecting the GI tract (nausea or peptic ulcer reactivation). These may occur in as many as 10 to 15% of patients. As with probenecid, there is the risk of inducing uric acid crystalluria, and therefore large quantities of fluid should be consumed by patients on this therapy (36). Bronchoconstriction may occur in some patients who are aspirin sensitive. In addition to these side effects, sulfinpyrazone has been noted to cause an immunoallergic acute interstitial nephritis. These changes are for the most part reversible.

Although sulfinpyrazone inhibits the renal tubular secretion of many weak organic acids, the elevation in plasma concentrations of penicillins and cephalosporins is not clinically useful. The antiinfective action of nitrofurantoin is decreased and the toxicity increased by sulfinpyrazone. Salicylates should not be used with sulfinpyrazone because they block the uricosuric action.

ALLOPURINOL

Allopurinol is the most commonly used agent for the long-term control of chronic gout. Allopurinol inhibits XO, the enzyme that catalyzes the conversion of xanthine to uric acid and hypoxanthine to xanthine. Allopurinol itself is metabolized by XO to oxypurinol, which also inhibits XO (Fig. 30.2). The inhibition of XO by allopurinol and oxypurinol decreases the concentrations of serum and urinary uric acid. The decrease in uric acid concentrations is accompanied by an increase in urinary concentrations of xanthine and hypoxanthine. The solubilities of uric acid, xanthine, and hypoxanthine are independent, thus greatly reducing the chances of crystalluria (38–40).

These actions are due not only to XO inhibition but also to a decrease in de novo purine biosynthesis. Allopurinol is converted to a ribonucleotide by HGPRT. The critical rate-limiting enzyme in purine biosynthesis, PRPP amidotransferase, is inhibited by the allopurinol ribonucleotide. Patients who are deficient in HGPRT activity, such as those with Lesch-Nyhan syndrome, do not demonstrate this decrease in purine biosynthesis (2, 41).

Allopurinol is well absorbed from the intestinal tract and has a short half-life of only 2 to 3 hr. The half-life of oxypurinol is much longer than that of allopurinol (18 to 30 hr). The long half-life of the active metabolite allows once-daily dosing in chronic therapy (25).

Allopurinol is the drug of choice for overproducers of uric acid, but it is also efficacious for patients who are underexcreters. Many clinicians prescribe allopurinol because of the decreased risk of nephrolithiases. However, because of uncommon but potentially dangerous side effects associated with allopurinol, it should be recommended only in the following cases: tophaceous gout, major uric acid overproduction (urinary excretion of > 5350 mmol (900 mg) of uric acid/24 hr on a diet with rigid purine restriction), frequent gouty attacks unresponsive to prophylactic colchicine, intolerance or lack of efficacy of uricosuric agents, recurrent uric acid calculi, renal insufficiency, recurrent calcium oxalate, renal calculi when associated with hyperuricosuria, and prevention of acute urate nephropathy in patients receiving cytotoxic therapy for malignancies. Asymptomatic hyperuricemia, uncom-

plicated gout, and acute gouty attacks are not considered proper indications for the use of allopurinol (42).

Allopurinol is effective in doses of 100 to 300 mg daily. The average adult dose for a patient with gout and normal renal function is 300 mg once a day. For cases of moderately severe tophaceous gout, doses of 400 to 600 mg daily in divided doses may be required. A single daily dose is possible in normal patients because of the prolonged half-life of the active allopurinol metabolite, oxypurinol. In patients with impaired renal function, allopurinol and oxypurinol may accumulate, and the dose should be reduced. The usual dose of 300 mg daily should be reduced to 200 mg when the creatinine clearance is (10 to 20 ml/min) 0.17 to 0.33 ml/sec, and to 100 mg when the creatinine clearance is less than (10 ml/min) 0.17 ml/sec. In patients with a creatinine clearance less than (3 ml/min) 0.05 ml/sec, a 300-mg dose twice a week should be adequate to reduce serum urate concentrations. To reduce the risk of an acute gouty attack when initiating therapy, the dose should begin at 100 mg per day and be increased by 100 mg weekly until serum urate levels fall below 360 μmol/liter (6 mg/dl) or the maximum recommended dose of 800 mg/day is reached. When begun after an acute gouty attack, prophylactic colchicine may be administered concurrently in doses of 0.5 to 1.2 mg/day to decrease the risk of another acute attack. If acute attacks occur after therapy has been started, doses should not be adjusted. Allopurinol therapy should be continued indefinitely; intermittent therapy is of little benefit and may place the patient at risk of an acute attack (7, 21, 22).

Allopurinol is also used to treat or prevent hyperuricemia associated with tissue breakdown resulting from cancer chemotherapy or radiation. It also reduces the chances of the patient developing secondary uric acid nephropathy from myeloproliferative neoplastic diseases.

Allopurinol is generally well tolerated. The overall rate of side effects is less than 1%. The most frequently occurring side effect is a pruritic maculopapular rash. Exfoliative, urticarial, erythematosus, hemorrhagic, and purpuric skin eruptions also occur. Stevens-Johnson syndrome has (rarely) been reported. Skin reactions may be delayed and have been reported as occurring as long as 2 years

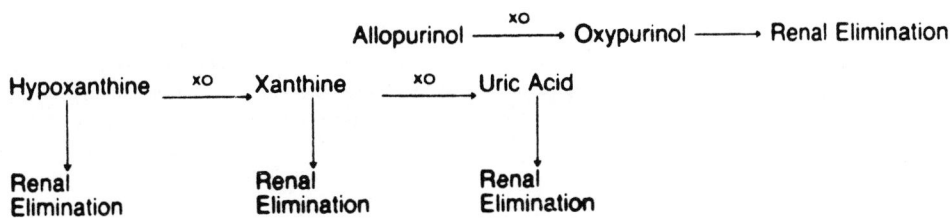

Figure 30.2. Inhibition of xanthine oxidase (*XO*) by allopurinol and oxypurinol. Note that both allopurinol and oxypurinol inhibit every XO-catalyzed reaction. Further note that the solubilities of each renally eliminated product are independent, increasing the ability of the body to eliminate products of purine metabolism.

after starting therapy. These are sometimes severe and associated with a hypersensitivity reaction that can be fatal. Symptoms include a variety of skin eruptions, fever, lymphadenopathy, eosinophilia, and generalized vasculitis. Renal and hepatic damage may occur if the reaction is severe and generalized. Other less common side effects include alopecia, exfoliative dermatitis, leukopenia and neutropenia, hepatitis as part of a generalized hypersensitivity reaction, and nephrolithiases (41–46).

Drug Interactions

Allopurinol and oxypurinol inhibit the metabolism of azathioprine and 6-mercaptopurine, increasing their potential toxicity. When administered concomitantly, the dose of these drugs should be reduced by 25 to 33%. Patients receiving allopurinol with either ampicillin or amoxicillin have an increased frequency of rash. In addition, patients receiving uricosuric therapy with allopurinol have an increased excretion of oxypurinol. This effect can reduce the inhibition of XO. Even though this occurs, the combination of allopurinol and a uricosuric is generally additive, and no dosage adjustments are necessary (21, 22).

PROGNOSIS AND CONCLUSIONS

Gout is characterized by hyperuricemia that results from an overproduction of an underexcretion of uric acid, or both. It is an acute inflammatory joint disease with deposition of uric acid crystals in the affected joints. Progression of the disease is variable and patient dependent. The risk of progression to a debilitating chronic disease is decreased today as a result of effective treatments. Treatment with hypouricemic agents for long-term control should be based on careful patient assessment. In patients where this therapy is deemed necessary, treatment is lifelong. Occasional gout or asymptomatic hyperuricemia may not require drug treatment. In these cases alterations in diet and lifestyle may be enough to keep a patient symptom free.

REFERENCES

1. Bell JE: Uric acid. Hosp Pharm 7:356–357, 1972.
2. Boss GR, Seegmiller JE: Hyperuricemia and gout—classification, complications and management. N Engl J Med 300:1459–1468, 1979.
3. Mangini RJ: Drug therapy reviews: pathogenesis and clinical management of hyperuricemia and gout. Am J Hosp Pharm 36:497–504, 1979.
4. Lo B: Hyperuricemia and gout [topics in primary care medicine]. West J Med 142:104–107, 1985.
5. Seegmiller JE, Grayzel AI, Laster L, et al.: Uric acid production in gout. J Clin Invest 40:1094–1098, 1962.
6. Simkin PA, Hoover PL, Paxson CS, et al.: Uric acid excretion: quantitative assessment from spot, midmorning serum and urine samples. Ann Intern Med 91:44–47, 1979.
7. German DC, Holmes EW: Hyperuricemia and gout. Med Clin North Am 70:419–436, 1986.
8. Demartine FE: Hyperuricemia induced by drugs. Arthritis Rheum 8:823–829, 1965.
9. Maclachlan MJ, Rodnan GP: Effects of food, fast and alcohol on serum uric acid and acute attacks of gout. Am J Med 42:38–57, 1967.
10. Hall AP, Barry PE, Dawber TR, et al.: Epidemiology of gout and hyperuricemia, a long term population study. N Engl J Med 42:27–37, 1967.
11. Simkin PA: The pathogenesis of podagra. Ann Intern Med 86:230–233, 1977.
12. McCarty DJ, Pathogenesis and treatment of crystal-induced inflammation. In McCarty DJ (ed): Arthritis and Allied Conditions, ed. 10. Philadelphia, Lea & Febiger, 1985, pp 1494–1514.
13. Hadler NM, Franck WA, Bress NM, et al.: Acute polyarticular gout. Am J Med 56:715–719, 1974.
14. Krane SM, Crystal-induced joint disease. In Rubenstein E, Federman DD (eds): Medicine. New York, Scientific American, 1982, vol 2 sect IX, pp 1–15.
15. Holmes EW, Clinical gout and the pathogenesis of hyperuricemia. In McCarty DJ (ed): Arthritis and Allied Conditions, ed. 10. Philadelphia, Lea & Febiger, 1985, pp 1445–1480.
16. Liang MH, Fries JF: Asymptomatic hyperuricemia: the case for conservative management. Ann Intern Med 88:666–670, 1978.
17. Yu TF, Berger L: Impaired renal function in gout, its association with hypertensive vascular disease and intrinsic renal disease. Am J Med 72:95–100, 1982.
18. Yu TF, Berger L: Renal function in gout. IV, An analysis of 524 gouty subjects including long-term follow-up studies. Am J Med 59:605–613, 1975.
19. Palella TD, Kelley WN: An approach to hyperuricemia and gout. Geriatrics 39:89–102, 1984.
20. Wallace SL, Bernstein D, Diamond H: Diagnostic value of the colchicine therapeutic trial. JAMA 199:525–528, 1967.
21. Bergman HD: Drug therapy in gout. US Pharm Jan, pp 58–64, 1977.
22. Emmerson BT: Drug control of gout and hyperuricemia. Drugs 16:158–166, 1978.
23. Lomen PL: Flurbiprofen in the treatment of acute gout. Am J Med 80(3A):134, 1986.
24. Spilberg I, Mandell B, Mehta J, et al.: Mechanism of action of colchicine in acute urate crystal-induced arthritis. J Clin Invest 64:775–780, 1979.
25. Flower RJ, Moncada S, Vane JR, Analgesic-antipyretics and anti-inflammatory agents; drugs employed in the treatment of gout. In Gilman GA, Goodman LS, Rall TW, Murad F: (eds): The Pharmacological Basis of Therapeutics, ed. 7. New York, Macmillan, 1985, pp 674–715.
26. Freeman DL: Frequent doses of intravenous colchicine can be lethal (letter). N Engl J Med 309:310, 1983.
27. Naidus RM, Rodvien R, Mielke CH: Colchicine toxicity, a multi-system disease. Arch Intern Med 137:394–396, 1977.
28. Ciabattoni G, Cinotti GA, Pierucci A, et al.: Effects of sulindac and ibuprofen in patients with chronic glomerular disease. N Engl J Med 310:279–283, 1984.
29. Nashel DJ, Chandra M: Acute gouty arthritis, special management considerations in alcoholic patients. JAMA 247:58–59, 1982.
30. Simkin PA: Management of gout. Ann Intern Med 90:812–816, 1979.
31. Helleberg L: Clinical pharmacokinetics of indomethacin. Clin Pharmacokinet 6:245–258, 1981.
32. Brogden RN, Heel RC, Speight TM, et al.: Piroxicam—a reappraisal of its pharmacology and therapeutic efficacy. Drugs 28:292–323, 1984.
33. Widmark PH: Piroxicam: its safety and efficacy in the treatment of acute gout. Am J Med 72(2A):63–65, 1982.
34. Schweitz MC, Nashel DJ, Alpea P: Ibuprofen in the treatment of acute gouty arthritis. JAMA 239:34–35, 1978.

35. Warnock DG: Treatment of hyperuricemia and gout (letter). N Engl J Med 301:1240, 1979.

36. Kantor T: Ketoprofen: a review of its pharmacologic and clinical properties. Pharmacotherapy 6(3):93–103, 1986.

37. Gutman AB: Uricosuric drugs, with special reference to probenecid and sulfinpyrazone. Adv Pharmacol 4:91–136, 1966.

38. Cunningham RF, Israili ZH, Dayton PG: Clinical pharmacokinetics of probenecid. Clin Pharmacokinet 6:135–151, 1981.

39. Yu TF: The effect of allopurinol in primary and secondary gout. Arthritis Rheum 8:905–906, 1965.

40. Houpt JB: The effect of allopurinol (HPP) in the treatment of gout. Arthritis Rheum 8:899–904, 1965.

41. Klineberg JR: The effectiveness of allopurinol in the treatment of gout. Arthritis Rheum 8:891–895, 1965.

42. Rundles RW: The development of allopurinol. Arch Intern Med 145:1492–1502, 1985.

43. Singer JZ, Wallace SL: The allopurinol hypersensitivity syndrome—unnecessary morbidity and mortality. Arthritis Rheum 29:82–87, 1986.

44. Vincent PC: Drug-induced aplastic anemia and agranulocytosis: incidence and mechanisms. Drugs 31:52–63, 1986.

45. Ohsawa T, Ohtsubo M: Hepatitis associated with allopurinol. Drug Intell Clin Pharm 19:431–433, 1985.

46. Worth CT, Hussein SM: Peripheral neuropathy due to long term ingestion of allopurinol. Br Med J 291:1688, 1985.

CHAPTER 31

SYSTEMIC LUPUS ERYTHEMATOSUS AND OTHER AUTOIMMUNE JOINT DISORDERS

Stephen H. Fuller, Pharm.D. and Thomas W. Wiser, Pharm.D.

Systemic lupus erythematosus (SLE) is a multisystem inflammatory disorder of unknown etiology characterized by autoantibody production. In recent years advances in immunology and immunopharmacology have led to increased recognition of the disease, insight into the pathogenesis, and improved therapeutic interventions. These events have allowed better application of scientific knowledge to the disease, which has resulted in a decrease in morbidity and mortality from SLE.

Lupus is the Latin word for *wolf* and has been used since at least 1230 AD to describe the cutaneous lesions that resemble the malar erythema of a wolf. Cazenave first used the term *lupus erythemateux* in 1851, and Kaposi first described systemic involvement of the disease in 1872. Kaposi subsequently correlated and described the resemblance of the rash to a butterfly, in 1875. Clinical recognition of the disease was greatly enhanced when Hargraves first discovered the lupus erythematous (LE) cell in 1948 and Friou developed the immunofluorescent antinuclear factor test in 1957 (1). Since the 1960s, advances have occurred through increased practitioner recognition of the disease (recent revision of diagnostic criteria), expanded diversity and refinement of diagnostic tests, and an enhanced understanding of the disease mechanisms. The increased use of immunosuppressant drug therapy has improved the prognosis of patients with major organ (central nervous system and renal) involvement (11, 15, 23).

Most of the symptoms of SLE relate to the key pathology, inflammation. Clinically distressing symptoms including heat, swelling, pain, tenderness, and local tissue destruction all relate to the inflammatory process. However, no single theory can completely explain the pathological process, so researchers suspect multifactorial causes and triggering mechanisms (e.g., one defect to trigger the immune response and another to permit a significant antibody reaction). Other etiological factors include genetic predisposition, drugs, viral infections, ultraviolet rays, hormones, environmental pollutants, and emotional stress. Hence, SLE may not be a single disease but rather a constellation of signs and symptoms from a number of causes.

There is no known cure for SLE, so therapy is primarily palliative. Newer therapies aim to relieve symptoms, prevent the inflammatory response and subsequent tissue destruction, and prolong survival.

EPIDEMIOLOGY

Systemic lupus erythematosus (SLE) is estimated to occur in 40 to 50.8 per 100,000 of the population with five new cases per 100,000 reported each year. SLE can occur in all races, but is observed two to three times more often in blacks, Hispanics, and Asians, compared with Caucasian patients. Sexual differences in SLE suggest an underlying hormonal role in the development of the disease, since it is primarily seen in women (8:1) versus men, with 65% of patients diagnosed during the childbearing years (ages 15 to 45 years). Sexual predominance fades in older patients, with the sex ration being 2:1 (female:male) in the 10% of SLE patients who are diagnosed after 65 years of age. A hereditary component also appears to be involved in the development of SLE. First-degree family members have SLE rates of 5 to 12%, with a rate of 14 to 57% in monozygotic twins. Although SLE occurs primarily in women in childbearing age, many etiological factors are still not understood concerning this disease (2–6).

PATHOPHYSIOLOGY

Systemic lupus erythematosus is thought to result primarily from a variety of defects in immune regulation leading to polyclonal activation of B cells and exaggerated production of autoantibodies that react with cellular (cell membrane) and subcellular (nuclear and cytoplasmic) antigens to form immune complexes. These complexes may be seen in the circulation or form on the cell or tissue surfaces, and they correlate with the clinical manifestations. It is also postulated that patients with SLE have a defect in removing these immune complexes.

During immune complex formation and deposition, the complement system is activated. Fixation occurs, resulting in low complement levels that give an indirect measure of immune complex formation. Chemotactic factors are released, attracting phagocytic cells, and phagocytosis is stimulated, which releases lysosomal enzymes and produces tissue destruction. The characteristic SLE pathologic changes include three histologic lesions: (*a*) hematoxylin bodies (bluish, globular masses suspected of being the inclusion bodies of LE cells), (*b*) onion-skin lesions (characteristic concentric perivascular fibrosis found in central and penicillary arteries of the spleen), and (*c*) Lib-man-Sacks verrucous endocarditis (characteristic lesions consisting of nonbacterial vegetations on heart valves (especially the mitral valve), chordae tendineae, and endocardium of the papillary muscle). Other pathologic involvement in most other organs relates to vasculitis or mononuclear cell infiltrates (1).

The immunoregulatory defect is considered to involve a combination of factors including genetic, viral, hormonal, or environmental; however, the exact mechanism is unknown. Many of these variables implicated in the development of the disease are discussed here.

Genetic factors play a significant role in the disease with immunologic abnormalities found more often in family members of SLE patients than in the general population (6). In addition, certain ethnic groups have a high prevalence of SLE, e.g., blacks develop the disease three times more often than the general population. Other relationships that implicate genetic causality include an increased prevalence in certain HLA phenotypes (A1, B8, DR3, and null C4 alleles), increased Gm markers of immunoglobulins, and decreased C3b receptors on erythrocytes (1).

Viruses and other transmissible infectious agents have received a lot of attention recently because of electron microscopic observations in SLE tissues that resemble tubuloreticular structures and the nucleoprotein core of paramyxoviruses. Serologic studies of antiviral antibodies in patients with SLE often show elevated titers. However, these antibodies are usually directed against several unrelated viruses, which suggests a nonspecific B lymphocyte activation rather than a unique antigenic exposure. Although direct viral isolation from tissue of SLE patients has been attempted, the current cultivation techniques have not been successful (7). Hence, although viral etiologies are suspected in SLE, it still remains to be determined if virus expression is the result or cause of SLE, so ultrasensitive research techniques and continued research in this area are needed.

The high incidence of SLE in women of reproductive age suggests that hormonal factors may play an important role in the development of the disorder. Selected mouse animal-model studies indicate that females have an earlier appearance of double-stranded DNA (dsDNA) antibodies, more severe complications (e.g., nephritis), and a shorter life span. Furthermore, administration of androgens appears to improve survival and reduce the nephritis complications in the female animals.

Environmental influences may also contribute to the development of SLE. Sunlight, thermal burns, and other physical stress (e.g., infection, pregnancy, or surgery) have been implicated in modifying the disease process. Drug-induced SLE, the presence of antibodies in laboratory workers exposed to SLE sera and household contacts of SLE patients, and dietary effects on clinical symptoms also support the involvement of environmental influences in SLE (1).

CLINICAL FEATURES

The most common complaints of SLE patients are fatigue, fever, and weight loss, which occur in 60 to 100% of patients (Table 31.1) (8). Fatigue, often a patient's initial complaint, responds to exercise or medication but will recur with acute exacerbations of the disease. Episodic fevers (>101°F) occur in 80% of patients with SLE; however, infectious disease processes must be ruled out. Weight loss (>5 pounds) experienced by SLE patients is thought to be related to the loss of appetite from SLE-induced gastrointestinal inflammation. This results in dyspepsia, difficulty swallowing, and gastroesophageal reflux disease. Gastrointestinal symptoms can also occur from medications for the treatment of SLE (NSAIDs, prednisone) (5).

Musculoskeletal manifestations are found in 95% of SLE patients and often precede the diagnosis by several months. Joint involvement is symmetrical and involves primarily the knees, ankles, wrists, and small joints of the hands. The arthritis of SLE is migratory, with symptoms moving between the affected joints over 24 to 48 hr (5). Morning stiffness, arthritic deformities (swan-neck, ulnar deviation), and tendon and ligament inflammation (tenosynovitis) are seen in 10 to 15% of patients but are less severe than deformities in rheumatoid arthritic patients. Overall, most patients with SLE arthritis have nonerosive, nondeforming joint involvement (9, 10). Patients receiving long-term steroid therapy (in high doses) for SLE may suffer from avascular necrosis (osteonecrosis) or steroid-induced osteopenia, which can result in demineralization of trabecular bone in the leg or in the vertebrae. The adverse effects of steroids on bone plus the water retention some patients experience while on steroids can complicate any joint pain and swelling. Seventy-percent of patients also experience muscle tenderness and pain, which may be caused by glucocorticoid therapy received by lupus patients (5, 9).

Skin lesions are present in 80% of SLE patients and occur with systemic flares of lupus or upon exposure to sunlight or other sources of ultraviolet light (fluorescent light). Fifty percent of patients experience the classic "butterfly" or malar rash that derives its name from the butterfly-shaped erythema covering the cheeks and the bridge of the nose (11). Other patients develop maculopapular rashes that are distributed in areas exposed to ultraviolet light (such patients are considered to be photosensitive). Subacute cutaneous lupus erythematosus (SCLE) and discoid lupus erythematosus (DLE) lesions develop in 10 to 25% of SLE patients, respectively. SCLE lesions are small, erythematous, papules located typically on the neck and upper torso areas. Discoid rashes are round, erythematous,

Table 31.1.
The 1982 Revised Criteria for Classification of Systemic Lupus Erythematosus[a,b]

Criterion	Definition
Malar rash	Fixed erythema, flat or raised, over the malar eminences, tending to spare the nasolabial folds
Discoid rash	Erythematous raised plaques with adherent keratotic scaling and follicular plugging; atrophic scarring may occur in older lesions
Photosensitivity	Rash as a result of unusual reaction to sunlight by patient history or physician observation
Oral ulcers	Oral or nasopharyngeal ulceration, usually painless, observed by a physician
Arthritis	Nonerosive arthritis involving two or more peripheral joints characterized by swelling, tenderness, or effusion
Serositis	Pleuritis—convincing history of pleuritic pain or rub heard by physician or evidence of pleural effusion OR pericarditis—documented by ECG, rub, or evidence of pericardial effusion
Renal disorder	Persistent proteinuria >0.5 g/day or $>3+$ if quantitation not performed OR cellular casts (red cell, hemoglobin, granular, mixed)
Neurologic disorder	Seizures OR psychosis—in the absence of offending drugs or known metabolic problems (uremia, ketoacidosis, or electrolyte imbalance)
Hematologic disorder	Hemolytic anemia—with reticulocytosis OR leukopenia—$<4 \times 10^6$/liter (<4000/mm^3) total on two or more occasions OR lymphopenia—$<1.5 \times 10^6$/liter (<1500/mm^3) on two or more occasions OR thrombocytopenia—$<100,000$/mm^3 in the absence of offending drugs
Immunologic disorder	Positive LE cell preparation OR anti-DNA antibodies OR anti-Sm antibodies OR false-positive serologic test for syphilis known to be positive for at least 6 months and confirmed by *Treponema pallidum* immobilization or fluorescent treponemal antibody absorption test
Antinuclear antibody	An abnormal titer of antinuclear antibody by immunofluorescence or an equivalent assay at any point in time and in the absence of drugs known to cause "drug-induced lupus" syndrome

[a] Adapted from Tan Em, Cohen AS, Fries JF, et al.: The 1982 revised criteria for the classification of systemic lupus erythematosus. Arthritis Rheum 25:1271–1277, 1982.
[b] The proposed classification is based upon 11 criteria. For the purpose of identifying patients in clinical studies, a person shall be said to have systemic lupus erythematosus if any 4 or more of the 11 criteria are present, serially or simultaneously, during any interval of observation.

gray-scaly plaques that occur primarily on the head and neck area. The severity of the rash often depends upon the intensity of the ultraviolet exposure, and rashes tend to last only hours to days if the aggravating source is removed. These rashes can be confused with psoriasis, so biopsies are often helpful for the appropriate diagnosis. The rashes usually heal without scarring; however, hyperpigmentation can occur. Vascular lesions (resulting from leukocyte infiltration) affect different vessel locations and can result in urticaria, purpura, and petechiae on the hands or feet (11).

Renal involvement occurs in 50 to 75% of SLE patients and has been associated with an increase in complications such as hypertension, nephrotic syndrome, and renal failure, if not treated adequately. The onset and progression of renal disease is variable among patients with clinical nephritis, and renal histological changes are usually observable within the first 5 years after onset of SLE. However, the clinical presentation does not always correlate well with the extent of renal cellular damage. The most common renal abnormalities seen are proteinuria (70% of patients), hematuria, pyuria, and casts in the urine of 30% of patients (5, 12). Glomerular damage induced by SLE may not result in clinical symptoms until later. The World Health Organization (WHO) classifications of the stages of lupus glomerulonephritis are often used to help determine the renal prognosis for an individual patient (Table 31.2) (12–15).

As indicated in Table 31.2, mesangial glomerulonephritis (type II) has a mild clinical presentation (minimal proteinuria, hematuria) with an excellent renal prognosis; however, up to 40% of these patients may progress to focal proliferative (mild-moderate, type III) or diffuse proliferative (severe, type IV) glomerulonephritis, which has a worse prognosis. It is difficult to determine which patients will progress to more severe stages of lupus nephritis. Therefore, an activity/chronicity index has been developed to determine the number of active and chronic renal lesions in patients with lupus nephritis (Table 31.3). Patients who have a higher chronicity score and more active lesions (upon renal biopsy specimens) have a poorer prognosis and are most likely to progress to more severe stages of lupus nephritis, placing them at a higher risk for renal failure. Therefore, a combination of clinical symptoms, renal histology (on biopsy material), and the activity/chronicity rating are used to determine the prognosis and therapeutic alternatives for different stages of lupus nephritis (12–15).

Pulmonary manifestations occur in approximately 50% of lupus patients, with pleurisy, coughing, and dyspnea as the most frequently reported complaints. Pleurisy, or chest wall pain, is often the only patient complaint and occurs on moving or changing position and frequently disturbs the patient's sleep. A pleural effusion occurs in about one-third of patients with pleuritic chest pain; therefore, patients with pleurisy usually undergo chest radiography to check for fluid accumulation.

Table 31.2.
Clinical, Laboratorty, and Pathologic Findings in Lupus Nephritis Patients[a]

Parameter	Class				
	Normal Glomeruli (I)	Mesangial GN (II)	Focal Proliferative GN (III)	diffuse Proliferative GN (IV)	Membranous GN (V)
Incidence	Rare	10–30%	10–25%	40–60%	10–20%
Hypertension	None	None	Occasional	Common	Late onset
Proteinuria g/day	None	<1	<2	1–20	3.6–20
Hematuria RBC/HPF	None	5–15	5–15	Many	None
Pyuria WBC/HPF	None	5–15	5–15	Many	None
Casts	None	Occasional	Many	Many	None
GFR ml/min	NL	NL	60–80	<60	NL
C3	NL	NL to decreased	Decreased	Largely decreased	NL
Anti-DNA	NL	NL to increased	Increased	Largely increased	NL
Immune complexes	NL	NL to increased	Increased	Largely increased	
Renal prognosis	Excellent	Excellent	Good	Severe, if not treated	Renal failure in 50%
Transformation	To class II or IV 15–20%	To class IV 20–40%	To class V 2–5%	To class III or V 5–10%	

[a] Adapted from Schur PH, Clinical features of SLE. In Kelley WN, Harris ED, Ruddy S, Sledge CB (eds): Textbook of Rheumatology, ed. 3. Philadelphia, WB Saunders, 1989, pp 1101–1129; and Ponticelli C: Current treatment recommendations for lupus nephritis. Drugs 40(1):19–30, 1990.

Table 31.3.
Renal Pathology Scoring System[a,b]

Activity Index	Chronicity Index
Glomerular changes	
Fibrinoid changes	Glomerular sclerosis
Cellular proliferative	Fibrous crescents
Cellular crescents	
Hyaline thrombi	
Leukocyte infiltration	
Tubulointerstitial changes	
Mononuclear cell infiltration	Interstitial fibrosis
Tubular atrophy	

[a] Adapted from Balow JE: Lupus as a renal disease. Hosp Pract 15:129–146, 1988.
[b] Each factor is scored from 0 to 3. Fibrinoid necrosis and cellular cresents are weighted by a factor of 2 because such lesions are more ominous than the other active lesions.

Atelectasis is seen in many SLE patients, causing basal infiltrates and diaphragmatic elevation leading to dyspnea. Acute lupus pneumonitis (ALP) occurs less frequently (5%) but has a short-term mortality rate of 50%. Patients experience high fevers, dyspnea, and tachycardia and can become cyanotic. This fatal pulmonary manifestation is thought to be caused by acute alveolar damage from immune complexes. Other pulmonary manifestations include chronic lupus pneumonitis, pulmonary hypertension, and pulmonary hemorrhage. Most pulmonary manifestations of SLE show restrictive lung disease patterns on pulmonary function tests, with reduction of carbon monoxide diffusion capacity and fibrosis of the lungs (16).

Almost every patient with SLE experiences some type of neurological manifestation. Central nervous system events are considered to be psychiatric or neurologic. The psychiatric manifestations include depression, anxiety, dementia, and psychoses. Depression or anxiety are diagnosed in most patients and are often seen soon after the diagnosis of SLE. Psychoses and dementia occur in approximately 25% of patients and often lead to impairment of intellectual ability and the ability to function in society. However, lupus nephritis (uremic encephalopathy), steroid therapy, NSAIDs, β-blockers, and other medications used by lupus patients can cause similar manifestations (17).

Neurologic disorders seen in lupus patients include headaches, seizures, and neuropathies. Headaches usually originate from muscle tension, and virtually all patients complain of headaches sometime during progression of their lupus. Seizures occur in 10 to 20% of patients and are generalized tonic-clonic seizures. Ten percent of patients experience either cranial or peripheral neuropathy. Cranial neuropathies occur as diplopia, nystagmus, visual field deficits, or hallucinations. Other neurologic manifestations seen less frequently include strokes, weakness of the lower extremities, and loss of rectal and bladder continence (17).

Up to 50% of SLE patients have cardiac manifestations, predominantly affecting the pericardium. Substernal chest pain and/or an audible pericardial rub are common in pericarditis. Myocarditis is suspected when patients have resting tachycardia and unexplained cardiomegaly, which can lead to CHF.

Patients with SLE have a high incidence of coronary artery disease and hypertension associated with chronic lupus nephritis. Frequently, SLE patients also have systolic murmurs that are secondary to anemia, cardiomegaly, and tachycardia (18).

Anemia occurs in approximately 50% of SLE patients and is thought to be caused by a combination of the chronic inflammatory process of lupus and the decrease of erythropoiesis from renal insufficiency. Therefore, most patients have a normochromic, normocytic anemia with a decrease in the number of reticulocytes. Hemolytic anemia is seen in over 10% of SLE patients. Up to 50% of lupus patients have leukopenia (WBC $< 4.5 \times 10^9$ (4500/mm^3)) and/or thrombocytopenia (less than 150×10^9 (150,000/mm^3)), which alone do not appear to expose lupus patients to infection or bleeding abnormalities. Some patients (25%) have antibodies to several clotting factors (lupus anticoagulant), which results in a prolonged partial thromboplastin time (PTT) with a normal prothrombin time (PT). This is usually not associated with bleeding unless thrombocytopenia coexists in the patients (19).

These clinical signs and symptoms (which are part of the 1982 ARA criteria) used in the diagnosis of SLE are combined with laboratory findings to diagnose a patient with SLE appropriately. Although the LE cell test is still used in some laboratories, this test lacks sensitivity and specificity and has been replaced by other diagnostic tests. The most commonly used laboratory test is the fluorescent antinuclear antibody (ANA) test. Although the ANA test is positive in up to 95% of patients with SLE, 5% of patients with clinical lupus will be ANA-negative. Although the ANA is a sensitive test, it is not completely specific, since up to 50% of patients with rheumatoid arthritis and scleroderma will have a positive ANA titer. Therefore, the pattern of the fluorescence of the ANA test is observed to increase the specificity of the diagnosis. Four ANA patterns are observed: diffuse (homogeneous), peripheral, speckled, and nucleolar, with the peripheral and speckled patterns being more specific for SLE. If further analysis is needed, laboratory tests can evaluate specific antibody levels. Each antibody test should be used discriminately, since many are not specifically diagnostic for SLE (Table 31.4). The presence of dsDNA (double-stranded DNA nuclear proteins), Sm (RNA nuclear proteins) antibodies, and decreasing levels of complement (C3, C4) is highly specific for SLE. Although ssDNA (single-stranded DNA) is detected in over 75% of patients with SLE, this test is not very useful because it lacks specificity and is positive in approximately 60% of patients with rheumatoid arthritis, chronic active hepatitis, and procainamide-induced lupus. Ro (RNA cytoplasmic proteins) antibodies can be found in approximately 60% of patients with SCLE or with signs, and symptoms of SLE who are ANA-negative. Histone antibodies (antibodies against drug-nuclear protein complexes) are found in 98% of patients experiencing drug-induced lupus (1, 5, 20).

Table 31.4.
Antinuclear Antibodies in Several Diseases[a]

Condition	ANA (% positive)	Antibodies[b]			
		dsDNA	Sm	ssDNA	Histone
Normal	<5	0	0	0	0
SLE	>95	75	25	>75	25
Rheumatoid arthritis	35–50	70	Rare	50–60	—
Scleroderma	40–55	0	Rare	—	—
Sjögren's syndrome	75	Rare	Rare	14	—
Drug-induced lupus	95	Rare	Rare	60	90

[a] Adapted from Alarcon-Segovia D, Systemic lupus erythematosus: pathology and pathogenesis. In Schumacher HR: Primer on Rheumatic Diseases, ed. 9. Atlanta, Arthritis Foundation, 1988, pp 96–100; Schur PH, Clinical Features of SLE; and Reichlin M, Antinuclear antibodies. In Kelley WN, Harris ED, Ruddy S, Sledge CB (eds): Textbook of Rheumatology, ed. 3. Philadelphia, WB Saunders, 1989.
[b] Percentage of patients haveing specific antibodies in each condition.

Table 31.5.
Drug-induced Lupus: Implicated Medications[a]

Definite	Possible	Unlikely
Hydralazine	Phenytoin	Griseofulvin
Procainamide	Quinidine	Phenylbutazone
Isoniazid	Sulfonamides	Oral contraceptive
Chlorpromazine	Propylthiouracil	Gold salts
Methyldopa	Lithium	Penicillin
	p-aminosalicylate	Hydrazine
	Nitrofurantoin	
	Atenolol	
	Trimethadione	
	Ethosuximide	
	Methimazole	
	Captopril	

[a] Adapted from Schur PH, Clinical features of SLE. In Kelley WN, Harris ED, Ruddy S, Sledge CB (eds): Textbook of Rheumatology, ed. 3. Philadelphia, WB Saunders, 1989, pp 1101–1129.

Drug-induced Lupus Syndrome

The first drug-induced lupus (DIL) syndromes were reported in the 1940s and 1950s and involved sulfonamides and penicillins. Since that time, more than 25 drugs have been implicated, with procainamide and hydralazine associated most clearly with DIL (Table 31.5).

Although several theories have been proposed to explain DIL, the etiology is unknown. Originally, drugs were thought to only exacerbate symptoms in patients with existing lupus conditions. A more popular hypothesis associates drug-induced lupus with HLA-DR4. These patients are genetically slow acetylators, which results in a slow rate of drug acetylation by N-acetyltransferase. Drug (procainamide or hydralazine) accumulates and forms a complex with nuclear proteins (DNA, histones). Antinuclear antibodies are then formed against the complexes, resulting in stimulation of T and B cells, formation of antibodies, and an inflammatory response. However, experts agree that DIL is probably multifactorial and that acetylator phenotype is only one predisposing factor (5, 21, 22).

Patients experiencing DIL differ vastly from patients with idiopathic SLE. Drug-induced lupus occurs most often in older patients (averaging 53 years for hydralazine and 62 years for procainamide), compared with the average age of onset of 29 years for idiopathic SLE. This probably reflects the older population of patients using procainamide and hydralazine. Women account for approximately 90% of patients with idiopathic SLE compared with 40 to 60% of patients with DIL. Caucasian patients account for 90 to 95% of DIL and approximately 65% of patients with idiopathic SLE. Although the populations that acquire DIL and SLE differ, many of the clinical presentations are similar (21, 22).

Patients with DIL typically have a milder clinical presentation with less organ involvement. Predominating clinical features include arthralgias, myalgias, weight loss, and malaise (Table 31.6). Joint involvement tends to be non-deforming, migratory, and similar to that of idiopathic SLE, involving the smaller joints of the hands, elbows, knees, shoulders, and feet. Other manifestations include cardiopulmonary lesions (dyspnea, hemoptysis, pleuritis, and pericarditis) in 30 to 50% of patients, and rashes (malar, photosensitive, purpura, urticaria) in 10 to 30%. Renal, central nervous system, and hematologic involvements are not common. Signs and symptoms of drug-induced lupus usually occur within 3 months to 2 years after initiating drug therapy; however, a few cases of DIL occur as early as 2 weeks and as late as 4 years after initiation of drug therapy. Drug-induced lupus is also different from idiopathic SLE because it is reversible and signs and symptoms fade within days to months after discontinuation of the medication (5, 22).

Laboratory tests commonly used to help diagnose drug-induced lupus in patients presenting with signs and symptoms consistent with lupus include ANA, dsDNA, and histone antibody tests. The commonly used ANA is positive in 95% of DIL and idiopathic SLE patients, so it may not differentiate between DIL and idiopathic SLE. However, if the ANA test is negative, DIL can be ruled out. Since many patients develop a positive ANA test result prior to having signs and symptoms of drug-induced lupus, the combination of a positive ANA result and clinical features is necessary for DIL to be considered. A positive dsDNA antibody test result indicates idiopathic SLE (but not DIL); whereas, a positive histone test result is very common (90%) with DIL and less common (25%) with idiopathic SLE (Table 31.4) (21, 22).

PROCAINAMIDE

Procainamide-induced SLE is the most common drug-induced lupus, with 50 to 100% of patients having positive ANA titers within 2 months of starting therapy. Approximately 5 to 30% of these patients will develop clinical signs of lupus within 3 months to 2 years (21, 22). There appears to be a total dose relationship to procainamide-induced lupus, with most patients having received 14 g or more (total dose) or a daily dose above 1600 mg. The most common signs and symptoms of procainamide-induced lupus are arthritis, pleuritis, and pleural effusions (21, 22).

HYDRALAZINE

The number of patients reported to have a positive ANA test result on hydralazine varies from 25 to 100%. The incidence of hydralazine-induced lupus is directly related to the dose, with no cases reported in patients receiving less than 50 mg per day. Incidence rates increase from 5.4 to 10.4% as patients receive 100 mg and 200 mg per day, respectively. Hydralazine-induced symptoms are characterized as early or late onset. Patients suffering from early onset hydralazine-induced lupus complain primarily of fever and malaise that occur usually within the first 30 days of hydralazine therapy. Patients complaining of late onset hydralazine-induced lupus have signs and symptoms that usually start 2 years after initiation of therapy and include arthritis, myalgias, and rash, and a few patients have been reported to have renal manifestations (21, 22).

Other medications that cause positive ANA test results include isoniazid, chlorpromazine, and methyldopa. Although 25% of patients receiving these medications develop positive ANA test results, few patients develop clinical feature (21, 22). Treatment of drug-induced lupus consists of discontinuing the medication and observing for resolution of signs and symptoms of lupus. Medical symp-

Table 31.6.
Clinical Manifestations of Drug-induced Lupus[a]

Problem	Hydralzaine[b]	Procainamide[b]
Arthalgias	92–93	77
Arthritis	57–76	18
Malaise	24–37	—
Fever	14–27	45
Rashes	24–34	5
Myalgias	2–34	48
Renal involvement	2–20	0–5
Pleuritis	14–25	52
Pericarditis	2	15
Seizures	0	0
Neuropathy	7	1
Hepatomegaly	3–45	20

[a] Adapted from Stratton MA: Drug-induced systemic lupus erythematosus. Clin Pharm 4:657–663, 1985.

[b] Percentage of patients with each manifestation.

toms usually resolve in days to months; however, patients may have a positive ANA result for months to years after discontinuation of the medication. Medications are often used to treat the signs and symptoms of drug-induced lupus, based upon the severity of the clinical features. Aspirin and other NSAIDs are used for patients complaining of arthralgias and myalgias. Patients suffering from more severe signs and symptoms may receive glucocorticoids (prednisone 0.5 to 1.0 mg/kg) for several weeks to resolve the drug-induced lupus more quickly (22).

Prognosis

The prognosis of SLE patients has improved over recent years, with 80% of patients with lupus nephritis surviving at least 10 years, compared with a survival of 1 to 2 years when such patients were diagnosed 20 years ago. Several factors have been related to a poor outcome in SLE patients, and many of these prognostic indicators are used along with clinical signs and symptoms to monitor progression of the disease. Patients who are diagnosed with SLE early in life (15 to 30 years of age) are considered to be at an increased risk for major organ involvement. This includes central nervous system or renal involvement and is considered to be a poor prognostic indicator. Patients discovered to have diffuse proliferative or membranous proliferative glomerulonephritis (types IV and V) upon renal biopsy are found to have a particularly poor prognosis. Patients diagnosed with mesangial or focal proliferative glomerulonephritis (types II, III) have a smaller chance of developing renal failure. Patients at risk for poor outcomes also include those with nonmajor organ symptoms (fevers, pleurisy, pericarditis) that are unresponsive to high-dose glucocorticoid therapy, and those frequently experiencing acute exacerbations upon tapering high-dose steroid therapy (5, 23). Laboratory values associated with a poor prognosis and active disease include azotemia, high levels of DNA antibodies, low levels of complement (C3, C4), prolonged and severe anemia, and a diffuse ANA pattern. A speckled ANA pattern is associated with less renal involvement and a better prognosis. Since many of these laboratory values change with acute and active disease, they are used along with clinical symptoms to monitor the progression of SLE. High levels of DNA antibodies and low levels of C3 are associated with active renal disease, and these laboratory values normalize as the disease is successfully treated (15, 23).

TREATMENT

General Principles

SLE is an inflammatory disease that results in acute and chronic complications; therefore, treatment is aimed at relieving acute symptoms and preventing chronic complications. Specific goals of therapy must be tailored to the clinical manifestations of each patient. These include minimization of the signs and symptoms of active disease and normalization of laboratory values used to monitor SLE disease activity. These goals are achieved through the use of treatment (nonpharmacologic and pharmacologic) and the discriminate use of laboratory tests (Table 31.7).

Nonpharmacologic therapy includes education of the patient and family; development of proper exercise, diet, and rest habits; and psychological and supportive therapies. Patients should learn about the irreversibility of SLE and its acute manifestations, the need for compliance with medications, and the adverse effects of the medications (5, 23). Patients should be instructed to minimize their exposure to direct sunlight, especially if they have a history of "photosensitivity" upon exposure to ultraviolet light. These patients should never sunbathe, should apply sunscreen to exposed body parts, and should wear long-sleeved shirts and broad-brimmed hats to minimize sun exposure when outdoors during the summer (23).

Pharmacologic treatment varies with the severity of the disease. Nonmajor organ involvement usually requires short-term symptomatic treatment, since clinical features are not life threatening. Major organ manifestations carry a poorer prognosis and usually require higher doses of medications for longer treatment periods. Nonmajor organ involvement includes arthritis/arthralgias, rashes, pleurisy, pericarditis, myositis, and constitutional symptoms such as fever, fatigue, and alopecia. Patients experiencing arthritis, arthralgias, pleurisy, and fevers can often be managed with nonsteroidal antiinflammatory drugs (NSAIDs), with a few patients requiring an antimalarial drug or low-dose glucocorticoids (15 to 30 mg/day of oral prednisone) to relieve symptoms. Rashes often do not require therapy, but when medication is necessary the lesions often respond to antimalarial therapy. A rash experienced during tapering of steroid therapy will usually resolve when the steroid dose is increased. Myositis usually resolves as systemic symptoms dissipate; however, glucocorticoids may help decrease muscle weakness and enzyme abnormalities. Although fever is often seen in lupus patients and does respond to NSAID therapy, infection must be considered in all lupus patients as a source of the fever (23).

Major organ involvement includes renal, central nervous system, pulmonary, and hematologic manifestations. Selection of the appropriate therapy for lupus nephritis varies with the prognosis for each classification of nephritis. Although the exact role of glucocorticoid and immunosuppressive therapy for the treatment of lupus nephritis is not completely clear, patients with mesangial (mild, type II) nephritis usually receive little treatment, whereas patients with type IV nephritis are treated aggressively (Table 31.2). Patients with mesangial nephritis are treated initially with prednisone (0.5 mg/kg/day), with renal and immune abnormalities reversing in 2 to 4 weeks.

Table 31.7.
Specific Goals of Therapy in Treating SLE

Minimize Signs/Symptoms	Treatment		Normalize Laboratory Values	Desired Goal
	Nonpharmacologic	Pharmacologic		
Fatigue	Rest, minimize exercise		Antibody levels (ANA, dsDNA, Sm, Histone)	Decrease levels
Arthralgias/myalgias	Rest	NSAIDs, steroids (if severe)		
Fever	Watch for infection	Acetaminophen, antibiotics	Complement levels (C4, CH_{50})	Increase levels
Rash	Avoid sun, use sunscreen	Antimalarials, steroids	Immunocomplexes	Decrease levels
Pulmonary signs	Avoid smoking	NSAIDs, steroids, antimalarials, antibiotics	GFR	Increase
			Proteinuria (g/day)	Decrease levels
Nephritis		Steroids, immunosuppressants	Hematuria RBC/hpf	Decrease
CNS signs	Psychotherapy	Antidepressants, antipsychotics		
Hematologic		Steroids, therapy for anemia type		

If a response is not seen after 4 weeks, steroid doses can be increased or another medication added (5, 23). Patients with moderate renal disease usually display high levels of proteinuria and hematuria, have a creatinine clearance under 0.83 ml/sec (50 ml/min), and have large increases and decreases of DNA antibodies and C3 levels, respectively. Treatment must be more aggressive, with oral prednisone 1 mg/kg/day for 4 weeks of pulse steroid therapy consisting of intravenous methylprednisolone (1 g or 15 mg/kg/day for 3 days). Cyclophosphamide or azathioprine may be added in patients with mild-to-moderate lupus nephritis not responding to prednisone alone (15, 23).

Patients with severe renal impairment should receive high-dose glucocorticoids (oral prednisone 1.5 mg/kg for 4 to 8 weeks or pulse doses of methylprednisolone for 3 days) and cyclophosphamide (0.5 to 1.0 g/M^2/month). Plasmapheresis (plasma exchange to reduce the concentration of circulating antibodies in the bloodstream) can be performed 2 to 4 times a week for 4 weeks along with immunosuppressive drugs to treat acute, severe glomerulonephritis. If all of these therapeutic modalities fail, the patients will progress to end-stage renal disease and require dialysis or renal transplantation (15, 23).

Diagnosis of lupus involvement in the central nervous system (CNS) is difficult, since the clinical presentation can be caused by other factors. There are no laboratory tests specific for CNS involvement in lupus patients and high DNA antibody level and low serum complement (C3) levels do not correlate with CNS manifestations. Therefore, CNS involvement in lupus is a diagnosis of exclusion, and therapy consists of medications to treat each manifestation. Antidepressants and antipsychotics are used to treat depression and psychoses, respectively. Patients with seizure disorders secondary to CNS lupus are treated with anticonvulsant therapy (17, 23).

Many of the pulmonary manifestations in lupus (such as pulmonary edema) may be secondary to other problems associated with lupus (renal failure CHF) and are treated by controlling the primary problems. Two serious pulmonary complications seen in SLE patients are diffuse pneumonitis and bacterial pneumonia. The problem may be diagnosed by clinical presentation and the occasional use of a lung biopsy. Antibiotics should be used to treat the pneumonia and steroid therapy for the pneumonitis (16, 23).

Patients with active SLE often develop severe anemia of chronic disease, which occasionally reverses with NSAID therapy but most frequently with low-dose steroid therapy. Some patients suffer from a mild and transient thrombocytopenia that does not usually require therapy. If platelet levels are below 100×10^9/liter (100,000/mm^3), patients will often respond to oral prednisone in doses of 30 to 50 mg/day. Patients should receive prednisone therapy until the platelet count rises within the normal limits (19, 23).

Nonsteroidal Antiinflammatory Drugs (NSAIDs)

The first line of therapy for mild manifestations of SLE includes aspirin (salicylates) or other nonsteroidal antiinflammatory drugs (NSAIDs) (Table 31.8). Salicylates and NSAIDs both have antipyretic, analgesic, and antiinflammatory effects, making them good for the signs and symptoms of lupus. These agents work primarily by inhibition of cyclooxygenase, which is responsible for converting arachidonic acid to prostaglandins that mediate inflammation. Since these agents are all equally effective, selection of an NSAID for SLE is empiric. Therefore, factors such as physician/patient preference, patient's tolerance to side effects, frequency of administration, and cost of therapy (all of which can affect compliance) are considered when selecting an NSAID (25).

Both salicylates and NSAIDs are absorbed rapidly and completely. Food may decrease the rate of absorption but usually does not affect the extent of absorption. NSAIDs are highly protein bound (>90%) to albumin binding sites and can displace other highly protein bound drugs (war-

Table 31.8.
Nonsteroidal Antiinflammatory Drugs (NSAIDs)

Drug	Trade Name	Half-life (hr)	Daily Dose	Dosing Schedule
Fenoprofen	Nalfon	2–3	1.2–3.2 g	t.i.d.–q.i.d.
Flurbiprofen	Ansaid	5–6	200–300 mg	b.i.d.–t.i.d.
Ibuprofen	Motrin, Rufen	1–3	1.2–3.2 g	t.i.d.–q.i.d.
Ketoprofen	Orudis	2–4	150–300 mg	t.i.d.–q.i.d.
Naproxen	Naprosyn, Anaprox	12–15	0.5–1.1 g	b.i.d.
Indomethacin	Indocin	3–4	50–200 mg	b.i.d.–q.i.d.
Sulindac	Clinoril	16–18	200–400 mg	b.i.d.
Tolmetin	Tolectin	1–2	0.6–2.0 g	q.i.d.
Meclofenamate	Meclomen	2–3	200–400 mg	q.i.d.
Piroxicam	Feldene	30–86	20 mg	q.d.
Diclofenac	Voltaren	2–3	100–200 mg	b.i.d.–q.i.d.

farin, oral hypoglycemics), resulting in their toxicity. This is usually not considered to be clinically significant unless a toxic dose of a salicylate or NSAID is administered (26, 27). Both salicylates and NSAIDs are metabolized extensively, with metabolites and small amounts of unchanged drug excreted by the kidneys. Salicylates display saturation kinetics, so the elimination half-life varies with the dose administered. Salicylates display first-order kinetics with an elimination half-life of 2 to 3 hr when using analgesic-antipyretic doses (325 mg q.i.d.). Serum concentrations corresponding to these doses will range between 2.2 and 7.2 mmol/liter (30 and 100 µg/ml). As doses are increased to achieve antiinflammatory effects (975 mg q.i.d.), enzymatic elimination pathways become saturated and zero-order kinetics result in a prolonged half-life of 15 to 30 hr. Serum concentrations corresponding to antiinflammatory effects range between 10.9 and 14.5 mmol/liter (150 and 200 µg/ml). Although many signs of salicylate toxicity are not well correlated with serum concentrations, most patients experience toxicity (tinnitus, respiratory stimulation, metabolic disturbances) with serum concentrations above 22.3 mmol/liter (300 µg/ml). Salicylate levels are generally not monitored unless toxicity is expected or patient compliance is being evaluated (23, 25, 26).

Although salicylates and NSAIDs are tolerated by most patients, common adverse effects seen in patients receiving NSAIDs involve the gastrointestinal tract, kidney, liver, and the hematopoietic and central nervous systems. Most adverse effects are dose-related and can be minimized by titrating doses upward slowly (25, 27).

Gastrointestinal symptoms range from mild gastric irritation because of direct irritation of the gastric mucosa) to peptic ulceration and gastrointestinal bleeding (from inhibition of prostaglandins). Suppression of prostaglandin production leads to an increase in gastric acid production and a decrease in the production of gastric mucus, which

provides a cytoprotective layer in the stomach (25–27). Mild gastric irritation can be minimized by administrating salicylates or NSAIDs with food or antacids or by using an enteric-coated product. However, if a patient has a history of severe gastrointestinal bleeding while using NSAIDs, then such therapy is considered to be contraindicated. Patients who have no history of gastrointestinal bleeding but are at increased risk of NSAID-induced ulcers/bleeding should use NSAIDs cautiously. These include patients who are elderly, have a history of NSAID-induced gastritis or gastric ulcers, consume ethanol regularly, or who are on chronic NSAID therapy. If chronic NSAID therapy is necessary, patients may benefit from receiving misoprostol (Cytotec, a synthetic prostaglandin) or an H-2 antagonist to prevent NSAID-induced gastropathy (28–30). However, this additional therapy can cause adverse effects and can be very expensive.

Although NSAIDs are primarily metabolized hepatically, NSAIDs and their metabolites inhibit renal prostaglandin synthesis, which can further reduce renal blood flow and the glomerular filtration rate, resulting in renal failure. Patients at risk for this usually have decreased renal perfusion (patients suffering from CHF, dehydration, or hypovolemia) or prior renal insufficiency (31). Hepatotoxicity consisting of transaminase level elevations and occasional increases in bilirubin level and prothrombin time are seen in some patients receiving salicylates and NSAIDs and usually return to baseline after discontinuation of the medication (25).

Aspirin and NSAIDs also affect platelet aggregation. Aspirin irreversibly decreases platelet aggregation, which lasts approximately 2 weeks after the aspirin is discontinued. Therefore, aspirin should be withheld 2 weeks prior to surgical procedures to allow complete excretion from the body. NSAIDs reversibly inhibit platelet aggregation, and this effect is lost with discontinuation of therapy. Toxic concentrations of salicylates can result in alteration of the hepatic synthesis of coagulation factors, increasing prothrombin times by 3 to 5 seconds. This usually occurs when patients receive doses above 6 g/day and have serum concentrations greater than 300 µg/ml. Hypersensitivity reactions have been noted in patients receiving salicylate therapy. Patients at risk for this reaction usually have a history of nasal polyps, asthma, and aspirin-induced rhinitis. This reaction, characterized by bronchospasm, occurs in 0.3% of the general population and 4% of patients with asthma. Since cross-sensitivity occurs with NSAIDs, these agents should not be used in patients with a history of bronchospasm due to aspirin. Aseptic meningitis can occur in SLE patients, but it has also been reported to be induced by NSAID therapy, primarily with ibuprofen. Patients suffering from aseptic meningitis have fever, headaches, facial edema, and meningism (25, 27, 32).

Table 31.9.
Corticosteroids and Immunosuppressive Agents

Drug	Trade Name	Dose/Schedule	Indications
Hydroxychloroquine	Plaquenil	200–600 mg p.o. divided b.i.d.	Mild disease
Chloroquine	Aralen	125–500 mg p.o. divided b.i.d.	Rashes, arthritis, serositis
Prednisone	Various	0.5–1.0 mg/kg p.o. daily	Moderate-severe disease
		1.0–2.0 mg/kg p.o. daily	Renal, CNS, refractory symptoms
Methylprednisolone	Various	1 g IV daily × 3 days	Severe disease
Azathioprine	Imuran	1–4 mg/kg p.o. daily	Severe disease
Cyclophosphamide	Cytoxan	2–4 mg/kg p.o. daily	Severe disease
		0.75–1.0 g/m^2 every 1–3 months	

Upon selection of NSAID therapy for treatment of lupus, patients should receive therapy for 2 to 4 weeks to evaluate the efficacy of the NSAID. If a particular NSAID is found to be ineffective or causes adverse effects, another NSAID should be selected and used for another 2- to 4-week trial period. More than one NSAID should not be used at a time, since no increase in efficacy has been demonstrated but increased side effects are possible (25, 32). If NSAID therapy fails, patients are often tried on immunosuppressive agents such as glucocorticoids or antimalarials, depending upon the lupus manifestation (Table 31.9).

Antimalarials

Patients presenting with lupus-induced rashes (from SLE or discoid lupus) are candidates for antimalarial treatment. The efficacy of antimalarial treatment for rashes is well documented, with most patients showing regression of skin manifestations within 1 to 2 weeks after initiating antimalarials (33). Although antimalarials are not considered to be effective for the major organ manifestations of SLE, antimalarials have been shown to have some beneficial effects for the treatment of mild or nonmajor organ involvement (arthritis, fever, fatigue, serositis). Antimalarial therapy has allowed a reduction in steroid doses in some patients, when treating these conditions (33, 34). Several mechanisms of action have been proposed for antimalarial medications including stabilization of lysosomal membranes, inhibiting lysosomal enzyme release; binding to DNA substrates, thus interfering with DNA antibody attacks; and inhibition of chemotaxis and phagocytosis by neutrophils (33).

The antimalarials most frequently used to treat SLE manifestations are chloroquine and hydroxychloroquine. Patients receive chloroquine (250 mg/day) or hydroxychloroquine (400 to 600 mg/day) for the first 1 to 2 weeks of therapy, with maintenance doses of chloroquine (125 to 250 mg/day) or hydroxychloroquine (200 mg/day) until the SLE manifestations have been completely resolved. The optimal duration of therapy is not well established, but attempts should be made to taper antimalarial therapy by administrating very low doses 2 to 3 times weekly before discontinuation of therapy. Unfortunately, in most patients (90%), symptoms will return within 3 years of stopping therapy (33).

The antimalarials are rapidly and almost completely absorbed from the gastrointestinal tract upon oral administration, with food enhancing absorption. These drugs are widely distributed, which explains adverse effects such as mild neurotoxicity, retinal deposits, and drug-induced rashes. Antimalarials are eliminated primarily by renal excretion (75%), with the remainder being metabolized. Little information exists on alteration of doses in hepatic or renal impairment (23, 33).

Antimalarial medications cause several adverse effects but are generally considered to be safe, and hydroxychloroquine is reported to have fewer adverse effects than chloroquine. The most common adverse effects are gastrointestinal (epigastric burning, abdominal bloating, nausea, vomiting), which usually begin shortly after initiation of therapy. These and other adverse effects appear to be dose-related and can be minimized by splitting the total daily dose (200 mg b.i.d. instead of 400 QAM, by administrating antimalarials with food, and by using small maintenance doses after the initial treatment period (33, 34).

Since antimalarial medications are well distributed to the skin, patients may experience cutaneous lesions or pigmentary changes. Rashes tend to be maculopapular or urticarial. Pigmentation changes include graying of the hair or blue-black discoloration of the skin. Neurologic side effects include headache, insomnia, and nervousness, are usually mild, and can be minimized by using lower doses. Muscle weakness in the proximal lower extremities has been reported after patients have received at least 1 year of antimalarial therapy, and it is often confused with glucocorticoid-induced muscle weakness (33). The most serious and publicized adverse effect of antimalarials is retinal toxicity. Early manifestations include changes in color vision caused by destruction of rods and cones because of deposition of these medications in the pigment layers of the retina. Retinal lesions also lead to visual field defects and decreases in visual field acuity (33, 35). The risk of retinal toxicity appears to be related to the total daily dose and not the duration of therapy or the cumulative dose. Patients at risk for retinal toxicity are usually above 65 years of age and have received daily doses above 6.5 mg/kg of hydroxychloroquine or 4 mg/kg of chloroquine. If patients are discovered to have retinal lesions (even if asymptomatic), therapy should be discontinued. If these doses are not exceeded, retinal toxicity is not common. Although many of the retinal lesions will reverse upon discontinuation of antimalarial therapy, patients should have ophthalmic examinations before initiation of therapy and every 6 months while receiving antimalarial therapy (33, 35).

The use of antimalarials in women desiring to become pregnant is controversial. Although doses used for prophylaxis of malaria do not seem to predispose the fetus to risk of teratogenic abnormalities, doses of antimalarials used for SLE have been associated with congenital abnormalities. Despite the possible risk of antimalarials, most experts agree that a patient with uncontrolled (active) lupus has a greater chance of experiencing spontaneous abortion or neonatal death. Therefore, if patients are on antimalarial medications when they become pregnant, they should remain on these medications throughout the pregnancy (36).

Corticosteroids

Corticosteroid therapy is considered a mainstay for SLE in reducing signs and symptoms during the first or acute episodes of the disease. The antiinflammatory and immunosuppressive actions of corticosteroids are responsible for their pharmacologic effect. However, their antiinflammatory actions are palliative, because the underlying cause of the disease remains, and their immunosuppressive actions are not completely understood (37).

Steroid therapy is not initiated automatically for mild SLE manifestations, and steroids should be reserved for conditions that are serious/life-threatening or in circumstances where the patient is not responsive to NSAIDs or antimalarial therapy and still has troublesome signs or symptoms. Specific indications for corticosteroid use include severe serositis (pleuritis or pericarditis), immune-mediated hematologic abnormalities (thrombocytopenia or hemolytic anemia), renal disease, severe CNS disease, or severe constitutional symptoms.

The goals of treatment with corticosteroids are to relieve the symptoms, sustain improvement in the clinical manifestations, and normalize laboratory abnormalities (Table 31.4). Prednisone is used more frequently than other corticosteroids (e.g., dexamethasone) because of its shorter biologic half-life and the subsequent ability to switch to alternate day therapy. Prednisone doses vary from 10 to 20 mg/day in mild SLE to 0.5 to 2 mg/kg/day in acute, severe SLE (37).

Once the therapeutic goals are achieved, treatment decisions are based upon controlling signs and symptoms and minimizing drug toxicity. After the disease has been controlled for at least 2 weeks, the steroid regimen should be changed to once daily dosing. After the patient has been asymptomatic for at least 2 weeks, the dose should be tapered, with the ultimate goal of alternate-day dosing. Special precautions are warranted when tapering prednisone doses of 20 mg/day or less and when transferring to alternate-day dosing, since adrenal insufficiency due to HPA (hypothalamic-pituitary-adrenal) suppression from steroid use can occur. An example of a tapering schedule is as follows: 20 mg/day for 2 weeks, 17.5 mg/day for 3 weeks, 15 mg/day for 4 weeks, then 15 mg/day alternating with 12.5 mg/day for 2 to 4 weeks, 15 mg/day alternating with 10 mg/day for 2 to 4 weeks, 15 mg/day alternating with 7.5 mg/day for 2 to 4 weeks, 15 mg/day alternating with 5 mg/day for 2 to 4 weeks, 15 mg/day alternating with 2.5 mg/day for 2 to 4 weeks, then 20 mg alternating with 0 mg every other day for 4 weeks, then 17.5 mg alternating with 0 mg every other day for 4 weeks, and so on until the patient is off the prednisone therapy. This schedule may take 6 months to a year or even longer if flares occur. A patient with nonmajor organ involvement may require a faster tapering schedule, and patients with severe disease may require slower tapering schedules. Flares without major organ involvement (e.g., fatigue, fever, arthralgias, or serositis) may respond to reverting to the previous dose until the symptoms resolve or to the addition of NSAIDs or hydroxychloroquine. Major organ involvement during a flare (e.g., nephritis) may not be controlled by reverting to the previous dose; therefore, it may be necessary to use very high doses to control signs and symptoms, which will require a new, slower tapering schedule.

In addition to the previously described HPA suppression with chronic steroid use, other complications that result from prolonged steroid therapy include fluid and electrolyte disturbances, hypertension, peptic ulceration, osteoporosis, myopathy, increased susceptibility to infections (including tuberculosis), cataracts, growth arrest, hyperglycemia, and Cushing's habitus.

Cyclophosphamide

A group of medications used more frequently for severe manifestations are the cytotoxic agents. These agents work by inhibiting DNA formation, resulting in death of cells that contribute to the inflammatory response (neutrophils, T and B lymphocytes). Suppression of B lymphocytes results in a direct suppression of antibody (IgG) formation, which aids in the inflammatory response. Unfortunately, if high doses of these medications are given, the death of these cells results in immunosuppression, placing patients at risk for neutropenia and infection (38). Cyclophosphamide is currently used for the treatment of serious lupus manifestations (kidney, CNS).

Cyclophosphamide is well absorbed, so it can be administered either orally or intravenously. Approximately 70% of cyclophosphamide is metabolized; metabolites and 30% of unchanged drug are excreted by the kidney. Despite the fact that cyclophosphamide is metabolized by the cytochrome oxidase pathways, medications known to affect microsomal enzymes (cimetidine and barbiturates) do not usually cause clinically important drug interactions.

Oral doses of cyclophosphamide range between 2 and 4 mg/kg/day or 750 to 1000/M^2 every 4 weeks for undetermined lengths of time (38, 39). Clinical effects are usually seen within 2 to 3 weeks of therapy, with white blood cell counts (primarily neutrophils) also reaching nadirs at this point. Immunosuppressive effects are thought to be worse with daily oral cyclophosphamide, compared with intermittent monthly IV boluses. Therefore, patients must have their granulocyte count monitored frequently to maintain cell counts at or above 1×10^6/liter (1000 to 1500/mm^3). If granulocyte levels fall below 1.5×10^6/liter (1500/mm^3), doses should be adjusted appropriately (38).

Hemorrhagic cystitis can occur in 20 to 30% of patients receiving chronic cyclophosphamide therapy. In most patients, the cystitis resolves after a dose reduction or discontinuation of cyclophosphamide; however, chronic administration can result in further hemorrhage and bladder carcinomas. This can be minimized by using IV bolus doses (rather than oral administration) and by increasing fluid intake to maintain adequate hydration of the bladder 24 hr before, during, and after administration of the drug. This enhances excretion of the cyclophosphamide and decreases contact with the bladder, which is the cause of the hemorrhagic cystitis (38). Other adverse effects of cyclophosphamide include dose-related nausea and vomiting (which is prevented with antiemetics) and alopecia (which is reversible). Adverse effects from chronic administration include gonadal suppression (temporary or permanent decreases in sperm or ova production) and pulmonary and cardiac inflammatory complications (38).

Cyclophosphamide has been shown to decrease proteinuria and DNA antibody and serum creatinine levels (slightly) and increase complement (C3) levels when the lupus nephritis is resolving. Addition of cyclophosphamide to the drug therapy of patients with lupus nephritis refractory to high-dose steroid therapy reduces the progression to end-stage renal disease and lowers the daily requirements for glucocorticoids (38–40). Studies must be conducted to evaluate the long-term efficacy and safety of intermittent boluses of cyclophosphamide in preventing lupus nephritis deterioration.

Azathioprine

Azathioprine used alone, like other cytotoxic agents (e.g., cyclophosphamide), is not as effective as corticosteroids in the treatment of symptomatic, multisystem systemic lupus erythematosus. However, azathioprine augments glucocorticoid therapy in SLE patients with renal disease and during acute, severe episodes of SLE not fully controlled with prednisone. Azathioprine is most effective in patients with resistant discoid lupus and in SLE patients with minimal renal involvement (38, 39). Austin and colleagues (41) demonstrated better outcomes in patients treated with either azathioprine or cyclophosphamide at low doses along with low-dose prednisone than in patients given prednisone alone. Azathioprine is generally considered to be less toxic than cyclophosphamide, but serious adverse effects may occur with its use including herpes zoster, sterility, cancer, hepatic toxicity, and hematological toxicity (leukopenia, thrombocytopenia) (39, 41, 42).

Azathioprine is given orally in doses starting at 0.5 mg/kg/day and titrated upward to doses of 2 mg/kg/day. Patients on azathioprine should be monitored for hematologic toxicity (anemia, leukopenia, thrombocytopenia) every 2 weeks during the first 3 months of therapy while doses are being adjusted, then monthly while patients are receiving therapy. Baseline liver function tests should be performed, and liver function should be monitored every 6 months during therapy (23, 38).

CONCLUSION

Systemic lupus erythematosus is a multisystem disease consisting primarily of abnormal autoantibody production. The disease course and prognosis is highly variable, but marked improvement is survival and quality of life provides hope to the patients. Today, healthcare providers have greater opportunities in disease identification, prognosis indicators, refined therapies, and improved guidelines for drug therapy use.

REFERENCES

1. Alarcon-Segovia D, Systemic lupus erythematosus: pathology and pathogenesis. In Schumacher HR: Primer on Rheumatic Diseases, ed. 9. Atlanta, Arthritis Foundation, 1988, pp 96–100.
2. Fessel WJ: Systemic lupus erythematosus in the community: incidence, prevalence, outcome and first symptoms; the high prevalence in black woman. Arch Intern Med 134:1027–1035, 1974.
3. Michet CJ Jr, McKenna CH, Elvaback LR: Epidemiology of systemic lupus erythematosus and other connective diseases in Rochester, Minnesota, 1950 through 1979. Mayo Clin Proc 60:105–113, 1985.
4. Hochberg MC: The incidence of systemic lupus erythematosus in Baltimore, Maryland, 1970–1977. Arthritis Rheum 28:80–86, 1985.
5. Schur PH, Clinical features of SLE. In Kelley WN, Harris ED, Ruddy S, Sledge CB (eds): Textbook of Rheumatology, ed. 3. Philadelphia, WB Saunders, 1989, pp 1101–1129.
6. Hochberg MC: The application of genetic epidemiology to systemic lupus erythematosus. J Rheumatol 14:867–869, 1987.

7. Woods VL, Zvaifler NJ, Pathogenesis of systemic lupus erythematosus. In Kelley WN, Harris ED, Ruddy S, Sledge CB (eds): Textbook of Rheumatology, ed. 3. Philadelphia, WB Saunders, 1989, pp. 1077–1100.

8. Tan EM, Cohen AS, Fries JF, et al.: The 1982 revised criteria for the classification of systemic lupus erythematosus. Arthritis Rheum 25:1271–1277, 1982.

9. Stevens MB, Musculoskeletal manifestations. In Schur PH: The Clinical Management of Systemic Lupus Erythematosus. Orlando, Grune & Stratton, 1983.

10. Buyon JP, Zuckerman JD, Articular manifestations of systemic lupus erythematosus. In Lahita RG: Systemic Lupus Erythematosus. New York, John Wiley & Sons, 1987, pp 791–820.

11. Gilliam JN, Systemic lupus erythematosus and the skin. In Lahita RG: Systemic Lupus Erythematosus. New York, John Wiley & Sons, 1987, pp 615–642.

12. Pollack VE, Kant KS, Systemic lupus erythematosus and the kidney. In Lahita RG (ed): Systemic Lupus Erythematosus. New York, John Wiley & Sons, 1987.

13. Appel GB, Cohen DJ, Pirani CL, et al.: Long-term follow of patients with lupus nephritis: a study based on the classification of the World Health Organization. Am J Med 83:877–885, 1987.

14. Balow JE: Lupus as a renal disease. Hosp Pract 15:129–146, 1988.

15. Ponticelli C: Current treatment recommendations for lupus nephritis. Drugs 40(1):19–30, 1990.

16. Segal AM, Calabrese LH, Ahmad M, et al.: The pulmonary manifestations of systemic lupus erythematosus. Semin Arthritis Rheum 14(3):202–224, 1985.

17. Perry SW, Psychiatric aspects of systemic lupus erythematosus. In Lahita RG (ed.): Systemic Lupus Erythematosus. New York, John Wiley & Sons, 1987, pp 821–846.

18. Stevens MB, Systemic lupus erythematosus and the cardiovascular system. In Lahita RG (ed): Systemic Lupus Erythematosus. New York, John Wiley & Sons, 1987, pp 673–690.

19. Schoenfeld Y, Schwartz RS, Hematologic manifestations. In Schur PH (ed): The Clinical Management of Systemic Lupus Erythematosus. Orlando, Grune & Stratton, 1983.

20. Reichlin M, Antinuclear antibodies. In Kelley WN, Harris ED, Ruddy S, Sledge CB: Textbook of Rheumatology, ed. 3. Philadelphia, WB Saunders, 1989, pp 1101–1130.

21. Hess EV, Drug related lupus: the same or different? In Lahita RG (ed): Systemic Lupus Erythematosus. New York, John Wiley & Sons, 1987, pp 869–880.

22. Stratton MA: Drug-induced systemic lupus erythematosus. Clin Pharm 4:657–663, 1985.

23. Steinberg AD, Management of systemic lupus erythematosus. In Kelley WN, Harris ED, Ruddy S, Sledge CB: Textbook of Rheumatology, ed. 3. Philadelphia, WB Saunders, 1989, pp 1130–1146.

24. Klippel JH, Systemic lupus erythematosus: treatment. In Schumacher HR: Primer on Rheumatic Diseases, ed. 9. Atlanta, Arthritis Foundation, 1988, pp 107–110.

25. Hart FD, Huskisson EC: Nonsteroidal antiinflammatory drugs: current status and rational therapeutic use. Drugs 27:232–255, 1984.

26. Brater DC: Drug-drug and drug-disease interactions and nonsteroidal anti-inflammatory drugs. Am J Med 80(suppl 1A):62–73, 1986.

27. Schlegel SI, Paulus HE: Nonsteroidal antiinflammatory drugs—use in rheumatic disease, side effects, and interactions. Bull Rheum Dis 36(6):1–8, 1986.

28. Griffen MR, Ray WA, Schaffner W: Nonsteroidal anti-inflammatory drugs use and death from peptic ulcer in elderly persons. Ann Intern Med 109:359–363, 1988.

29. Graham DY: Prevention of gastroduodenal injury induced by chronic nonsteroidal anti-inflammatory drug therapy. Gastroenterology 96:675–81, 1989.

30. Garris RE, Kirkwood CF: Drug Review: misoprostol: a prostaglandin E_1 analogue. Clin Pharm 8:627–644, 1989.

31. Clive DM, Stoff JS: Renal syndromes associated with nonsteroidal antiinflammatory drugs. N Engl J Med 310:563–572, 1984.

32. Miller DR: Combination use of nonsteroidal antiinflammatory drugs. Drug Intell Clin Pharm 15:3–7, 1981.

33. Rynes RI, Antimalarial drugs, In Kelley WN, Harris ED, Ruddy S, Sledge CB: Textbook of Rheumatology, ed. 3. Philadelphia, WB Saunders, 1989, pp 792–803.

34. Rothfield N: Efficacy of antimalarials in systemic lupus erythematosus. Am J Med 85(suppl 4A):53–56, 1988.

35. Bernstein HN: Ophthalmologic considerations and testing patients receiving long-term antimalarial therapy. Am J Med 75:25–34, 1983.

36. Parke A: Antimalarial drugs in pregnancy. Am J Med 85(suppl 4A):30–33, 1988.

37. Haynes RC, Adrenocorticotropic hormone; adrenocortical steroids and their synthetic analogs; inhibitors of the synthesis and actions of adrenocortical hormones. In Gilman AG, et al (eds): The Pharmacological Basis of Therapeutics, ed. 8. New York, Pergamon Press, 1990, pp 1431–1462.

38. Fauci AS, Young KR Jr, Immunoregulatory agents. In Kelley WN, Harris ED, Ruddy S, Sledge CB: Textbook of Rheumatology, ed. 3. Philadelphia, WB Saunders, 1989, pp 862–888.

39. Dinant HT, Decker JL, Klippel JH, et al.: Alternate modes of cyclophosphamide and azathioprine therapy in lupus nephritis. Ann Intern Med 96:728–736, 1982.

40. McCune WJ, Golbus J, Zeldes W, et al.: Clinical and immunologic effects of monthly administration of intravenous cyclophosphamide in severe systemic lupus erythematosus. N Engl J Med 318(22):1423–1431, 1988.

41. Austin HA, Klippel JH, Balow JE, et al.: Therapy of lupus nephritis. Controlled trial of prednisone and cytotoxic drugs. N Engl J Med 314:614–619, 1986.

42. Balow JE: Lupus nephritis: natural history, prognosis and treatment. Clin Immunol Allergy 6:353–366, 1986.

CHAPTER 32

OSTEOPOROSIS AND OSTEOMALACIA

JEAN DEVENPORT, Pharm.D. and DAVID J. HARPER, Pharm.D.

The two most common metabolic bone disorders are osteoporosis and osteomalacia, with the prevalence of osteoporosis far exceeding that of osteomalacia. These disorders usually occur as separate entities, but they can develop concurrently, particularly in debilitated patients with inadequate nutrition. Bone disorders can be insidious in their evolution. For example, bone pain or fractures may be the first indication of significant loss of bone mass that occurs with aging. As longevity of the U.S. population continues to increase, an escalation in hip fractures is occurring at a rate projected to double with each decade beyond 65 years. It is estimated that the annual cost of medical care for these fractures alone exceeds the research budget of the National Institutes of Health and surpasses by 100 times the dollars spent on osteoporosis research. However, widespread use of estrogens and calcium to avert postmenopausal osteoporosis may not be cost-effective when considering the potential risks of prolonged drug therapy. Further examination of these issues is likely to reveal the need for an individualized approach to evaluation, prevention, and treatment of osteoporosis and osteomalacia.

BONE REMODELING

The human skeleton grows until about age 14 years in females and age 16 years in males. After closure of the epiphyses, bone continues to restore itself through a process of turnover called bone remodeling. Bone remodeling occurs in discrete areas called bone remodeling units, or bone multicellular units, and follows a specific series of events (Fig. 32.1). Activation of remodeling is followed by an initial resorption phase when osteoclasts on the bone surface begin to mature. Within 1 to 3 weeks, these osteoclasts remove a layer of bone approximately 0.1 mm thick and are replaced by osteoblasts. The osteoblasts lay down a matrix of collagenous material known as osteoid. Approximately 10 days after this matrix is laid down, mineralization occurs. Since the extracellular fluid is supersaturated with calcium and phosphorus, a mechanism must be present to prevent metastatic calcification. This is accomplished by pyrophosphate. The enzyme alkaline phosphatase is responsible for cleaving the pyrophosphate and allowing normal calcification to occur. The new osteoid is initially composed of amorphous calcium phosphate and is later converted to hydroxyapatite. This second phase, or formation phase, takes about 3 months to complete. These processes of bone resorption and subsequent formation

are closely coupled. Since the resorption phase is much more rapid than the formation phase, there is a substantial period of time in which a weakened layer of bone is present. Therefore, it is easy to see the necessity of a tightly controlled coupling mechanism.

Homeostasis of bone remodeling is controlled normally by several endogenous hormones, including gonadal hormones, vitamin D and its metabolites, parathyroid hormone, and calcitonin. Vitamin D, obtained from the diet (as vitamin D_2) or endogenously synthesized in the skin (as vitamin D_3), is metabolized in the liver to 25-hydroxycholecalciferol ($25[OH]D_3$) and hydroxylated in the kidney to form the biologically active 1,25-dihydroxycholecalciferol ($1,25[OH]_2D_3$). This metabolite has many important effects on bone remodeling; it increases calcium and phosphate absorption from the gastrointestinal tract, it influences the maturation of osteoclasts, and it causes an increase in alkaline phosphatase synthesis.

Circulating parathyroid hormone (PTH) concentration is closely regulated by changes in serum calcium concentration. An increase in serum calcium concentration causes a decrease in the production and secretion of PTH. A decrease in serum calcium has the opposite effect. Like vitamin D, PTH also affects bone remodeling in different ways. It stimulates bone resorption by osteoclasts, increases reabsorption of calcium in the renal tubules, and increases hepatic hydroxylation of $25[OH]D_3$ to $1,25[OH]_2D_3$.

Calcitonin, a hormone produced by the thyroid gland, primarily inhibits the resorption of bone. It decreases serum concentrations of both calcium and phosphorus. Serum calcitonin is closely regulated by changes in serum calcium. An increase in serum calcium concentration leads to a corresponding increase in calcitonin production by the thyroid, whereas a decrease in serum calcium decreases calcitonin production.

The gonadal hormones (estrogens, progestins, testosterone) primarily stimulate bone formation. Their effects on skeletal growth subside with closure of the epiphyses. The absence of these hormones contributes dramatically to bone loss after menopause in women and after the seventh decade in men.

OSTEOPOROSIS
Etiology

Osteoporosis is defined as abnormally low bone tissue that can fracture during normal mechanical usage, and it is

Figure 32.1. Bone remodeling phase. Factors known to stimulate each phase. PTH, parathyroid hormone; PGE, prostaglandin E series; cytokines, γ-interferon, tissuenecrosis factor, colony-stimulating factor, interleukin-1.

PHASE	BONE	STIMULATORS*
ACTIVATION	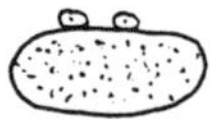	
RESORPTION	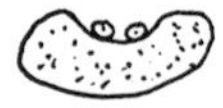 (3 weeks)	PTH, thyroxine, PGE, cytokines, vitamin D
FORMATION	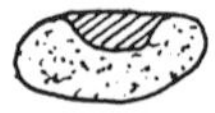 (3 months)	gonadal hormones, growth hormone, calcitonin, fluoride

Table 32.1.
Classification of Osteoporosis

I. Primary
  A. Involutional
    1. Type I (postmenopausal)
    2. Type II (age-related)
  B. Idiopathic osteoporosis
II. Secondary
  A. Endocrine
    1. Hypogonadism
    2. Hyperthyroidism
    3. Hypercortism
    4. Hyperparathyroidism
  B. Gastrointestinal
    1. Malabsorption syndromes
    2. Gastrectomy
  C. Immobilization
  D. Drugs
    1. Heparin
    2. Glucocorticoids
    3. Methotrexate

classified according to primary and secondary causes (Table 32.1). Primary osteoporosis describes two groups of individuals, those with involutional osteoporosis who demonstrate bone loss due to changes with age or menopause and those for whom a specific cause for bone loss is unidentifiable (idiopathic). Hormonal influences on aging bone include a decrease in gonadal hormone production and decreased circulation of active vitamin D. Nonhormonal factors in age-related osteoporosis include bone cell senescence resulting in dysfunctional bone remodeling; negative calcium balance caused by inadequate

intake; genetic predisposition, with Caucasians having lower maximum bone density than blacks; and physiologic stress or chronic illness. Secondary osteoporosis includes many disease entities, mechanical forces, and chemical substances. Normal bone metabolism requires a complex balance of physiologic factors, the interruption of which can result in localized or generalized bone loss.

Recently, an association was made between female endurance athletes and osteoporosis. Factors such as composition of diet, exercise-associated gonadal hormone changes, and physical and emotional stress were postulated as pathogenic mechanisms. However, a study of premenopausal women distance runners revealed twice the rate of trabecular bone loss (4% vs. 2% per year) in the group with ovulatory disturbance than that in the group with normal cycles (1). Thus, it appears that anovulatory cycles and cycles with a short luteal phase place women at risk for osteoporosis.

Young women experiencing anorexia may be at significant risk for early osteoporosis. Case reports of women with 2- to 14-year histories of anorexia reveal multiple vertebral compression fractures and a loss of 2 inches in height. While serum calcium and vitamin D levels are reported to be normal, these women were 35 to 50% of ideal body weight (2).

Incidence

Because bone loss occurs with normal aging, the incidence of osteoporosis could reflect the entire population over the age of 70 years. However, fractures secondary to osteoporosis are the critical element in assessing the morbidity and cost of this disease. It is generally agreed that 40% of women will experience a fracture by the age of 70 years. A lack of physical activity also produces bone loss. Healthy patients at bed rest for disk surgery lose bone mass in the lumbar vertebrae at a rate of almost 1% a week.

Drug-induced

Drug-induced osteoporosis is associated with glucocorticoids, heparin, and methotrexate. At least 50% of patients receiving exogenous glucocorticoids at high doses for prolonged periods experience fractures from nontraumatic events (3). Glucocorticoids directly stimulate osteoclasts and inhibit osteoblasts. There is more trabecular bone loss than cortical bone loss.

Heparin-induced osteoporosis is seen less frequently than the glucocorticoid-induced disorder. The effect of heparin appears to be a dose- and duration-related phenomenon. Patients receiving a course of heparin therapy for 14 days or less, regardless of dose, are unlikely to develop osteoporosis. Those receiving 20,000 units daily for 3 months will have clinically unimportant osseous changes. However, patients receiving more than 20,000 units daily for more than 6 months are at significant risk of developing osteoporosis. Co-morbid conditions in patients who developed osteoporosis from heparin therapy include pregnancy, menopause, and old age (4).

High-dose methotrexate use in children is associated with osteoporosis. The pathogenesis is unknown, but clinical findings suggest an increase in bone resorption.

Pathogenesis

The human skeleton is made up of two types of bone, cortical and trabecular. Cortical bone makes up ¾ of the total skeletal mass. It forms the outer wall of bones, predominantly the shafts of the long bones, or appendicular skeleton. Trabecular (or cancellous) bone represents the remaining skeletal mass. It is a network of plates and rods which contains the hematopoietic or fatty marrow, predominantly the vertebrae, pelvis, and ends of long bones, or the axial skeleton. Bone turnover occurs in both types of bone at differing rates and magnitudes of loss with aging.

Normal bone turnover requires a coupling between bone resorption (osteoclastic activity) and bone formation (osteoblastic activity). The pathogenesis of osteoporosis involves uncoupling of this turnover. Osteoclastic activity is thought to be stimulated directly or indirectly by PTH, prostaglandin E series, active vitamin D, growth factors, tumor necrosis factor, colony stimulating factor, γ-interferon, and interleukin-1 (5). Osteoblastic activity is stimulated by gonadal hormones, growth hormone, and calcitonin. Characteristic of osteoporotic mechanisms are increased resorption with inadequate replacement of normally mineralized bone, decreased resorption in aging bone, and increased resorption with defective bone formation. When sufficient bone is lost and the trabeculae become more widely spaced, bone becomes mechanically incompetent.

Two different rates of bone loss are described. An accelerated loss of bone, attributed to estrogen deficiency, is characterized by an increased number and depth of resorptive cavities. The trabeculae are fewer in number but relatively unchanged in thickness. A slower phase of bone loss demonstrates a slow thinning of the trabeculae with little further reduction in their number. This phase of senescent osteoblastic function represents later menopause and age-related osteoporosis.

An examination of differences between postmenopausal and age-related bone loss reveals a small subset (5 to 10%) of postmenopausal women, under 75 years of age, who demonstrate an excessive and disproportionate loss of trabecular bone (6). This finding supports the claim of an acceleration in bone loss in the first 3 to 5 years after menopause. Normal female subjects demonstrate a proportionate loss of both cortical and trabecular bone, with male subjects showing less bone loss, particularly of the proximal femur, than female subjects. These findings account, in part, for the difference in fracture rate between men and women, where hip fractures occurred at a 2:1 ratio (female:male) and vertebral fractures occurred at an 8:1 ratio.

An explanation for the accelerated and disproportionate trabecular bone loss may be found in a study of perimenopausal and postmenopausal women, suggesting that bone resorption increases gradually during the last perimenopausal years, but accelerates sharply within the first postmenopausal year (7). Bone formation increases until 2 years after the last menstrual cycle. Women with a long perimenopausal transition period, long intervals without menstruation, and low circulating estrogen levels appear to be at risk for greater bone resorption during the last perimenopausal years.

The mechanisms of drug-induced osteoporosis are similar to those described above. The pathogenesis of glucocorticoid-induced osteoporosis is understood better than that of heparin and methotrexate. Glucocorticoids cause osteoporosis by enhancing bone resorption, inhibiting bone formation, decreasing intestinal calcium absorption, increasing renal excretion of calcium, and inhibiting gonadotropin secretion (3). This state is characterized by greater trabecular bone loss. Glucocorticoids also can induce a proximal myopathy that may contribute to osteoporosis by decreasing normal forces on bone. The mechanisms by which heparin produces osteoporosis include potentiation of PTH effect, inhibition of osteoblasts, stimulation of osteoclastic activity due to heparin-related collagenase, and abnormalities of vitamin D metabolism (8).

Bone loss can begin as early as 24 hr after acute immobilization. Individuals with traumatic injury of the spinal cord demonstrate increased urinary calcium excretion 2 to 3 days after immobilization. Weight-bearing bones will lose abut 4% per month during the initial period of immobilization (9). Mechanical forces on the bone are necessary to maintain bone mass. While inactivity under gravitational forces can be accommodated to an extent, the weightlessness of prolonged space travel will demand unique measures to minimize bone loss (10).

Diagnosis and Clinical Findings

Suspicion of osteoporosis occurs when a patient has a fracture from a nontraumatic event, such as falling from a standing position, and has risk factors for osteoporosis, e.g., elderly, early menopause. Location of fracture sites is commonly the wrist (from attempting to brace the fall), vertebrae (where the majority of trabecular bone is lost), and hip (where bone loss of the femoral neck is significant). The patient may be asymptomatic or may complain of low back pain, frequently radiating to the abdomen, secondary to vertebral compression fractures. The vertebral regions most susceptible to fractures are midthoracic, thoracolumbar junction, and lower lumbar spine. Loss of height and kyphosis of the thoracic spine can cause the thoracic cage to rest on the pelvis, producing a "pot belly" appearance.

Laboratory tests are not diagnostic of osteoporosis. Although urine calcium and hydroxyproline levels may be elevated, serum concentrations of calcium, phosphate, and alkaline phosphatase are typically within normal limits. Increases in alkaline phosphatase usually reflect fractures. Parathyroid hormone levels may be normal or slightly increased. Conventional radiographs do not reflect changes until more than 30% of bone mass is lost. Quantitative assessment of bone density is accomplished through single- or dual-photon absorptiometry, CT scan, or bone biopsy. While quantitation is unnecessary for a clinical diagnosis, an estimation of baseline bone density in selected patients may be useful in following the progression of bone loss and assessing the efficacy of therapeutic interventions.

The type of bone to be studied determines the absorptiometry method. Single-photon absorptiometry is a sensitive measure of bones such as the wrist, which reflects cortical bone. It cannot accurately measure axial skeleton, where trabecular bone is predominant. Dual-photon absorptiometry is used to measure the density of the lumbar spine and hips. One limitation of the latter technique is that it measures bone mineral content of all mineral-containing areas, not just the vertebral body. Newer technology will offer greater precision in bone density measurement.

Bone biopsy after tetracycline labeling can be used in the differential diagnosis of osteoporosis, osteomalacia, osteitis fibrosa, and other rare bone disorders. While used primarily as a research tool, tetracycline labeling can help

to distinguish high and low bone turnover states, which in the future may assist in selection of treatment. For example, fluoride may be useful in a low turnover state to activate the bone remodeling surface.

Medical Treatment

Medical treatment of osteoporosis is extremely limited. Surgical removal of tissue causing excessive circulating thyroid hormone or cortisol may be indicated for secondary forms of osteoporosis. Weight-bearing exercise is important to bone development during growth. Since peak trabecular bone mass occurs at approximately 30 years of age and peak cortical bone mass occurs at 35 to 40 years, weight-bearing exercise as a preventative measure can minimize the effects of bone loss with aging. Studies suggest that weight-bearing exercise in postmenopausal and age-related osteoporosis can increase bone density over a 9 to 12 month period (11). While studies are needed to define the type, frequency, and duration of exercise, walking for 1 hour four times weekly is beneficial (9).

Pharmacologic Treatment

Current issues on the pharmacologic treatment of osteoporosis include single or combination drug therapy, risk-to-benefit estimate of long-term estrogen therapy, and continuous or sequential (coherence) therapy. Traditionally, treatment of postmenopausal osteoporosis has included minerals, hormones, vitamins, or biphosphonates. In 1987 a consensus development conference addressed several areas for prophylaxis and treatment of osteoporosis (Table 32.2) (12). The treatment of osteoporosis is un-

Table 32.2.
Consensus Conference Recommendations for Prophylaxis and Treatment of Osteoporosis[a]

Estrogen/ progestin	Estrogen is only prophylactic measure that reduces fractures; cycle with progestin to eliminate endometrial hyperplasia and reduce risk of endometrial carcinoma
Calcium	Negative calcium balance suggests need for calcium supplementation, but studies are needed to determine usefulness in adulthood
Vitamin D	Use only for coexisting vitamin D deficiency
Fluoride	Should be reserved for severe osteoporosis
Exercise	In moderation, at least to improve agility and reduce risk of fractures from falls
Anabolic steroids	Adverse effects limit use to selected subsets of patients
Calcitonin	May be useful in women for whom estrogen therapy is contraindicated
Cyclic and coherence therapy	More studies are needed to confirm efficacy and safety

[a] Adapted from Anon: Consensus development conference: prophylaxis and treatment of osteoporosis. Br Med J 295:914–915, 1987.

certain in spite of numerous clinical trials. A lack of consistency in study design with sometimes highly variable outcomes creates more questions than answers. Small sample size, differing outcome measures, inadequate length of study period, and unmatched subjects are a few of the design problems that create difficulty in interpreting study results. In spite of these inadequacies, there are sufficient patient-specific criteria that can be examined when selecting the appropriate drug regimen. Additionally, the adverse effects of each drug must be considered.

ESTROGEN

Estrogens decrease bone resorption, probably by a direct effect on bone. A decrease in urinary calcium and hydroxyproline levels indicate decreased resorption. Estrogen is the treatment of choice for osteoporosis secondary to estrogen deficiency, whether the cause is natural or surgical menopause, if there is no contraindication to estrogen therapy, such as breast cancer. The positive effects of estrogen replacement are seen immediately after menopause. It is unlikely that initiating estrogen therapy more than 15 years after menopause will be beneficial when weighed with the potential adverse effects. Changes in bone density and the ability to estimate fracture rate require at least 2 to 3 years of pharmacologic intervention and observation. However, the duration of treatment is not defined, but is considered to be at least 10 years (12). Equivalent daily doses of estrogen based on clinical response are conjugated equine estrogen 0.625 mg, estradiol 2 mg, and ethinyl estradiol 0.025 mg.

Transdermal estradiol is comparable to oral conjugated estrogen in physiologic effects (13). At two different doses of the two dosage systems, similarities are noted in increased circulating estrogen levels, decreased gonadotropin concentrations, and decreased urinary calcium excretion. Transdermal estradiol does not appear to decrease urinary hydroxyproline levels, while 1.25 mg of conjugated estrogen seems to produce a significant reduction. Oral estrogens can increase hepatic protein synthesis including renin substrate, which may be a link to the increased blood pressure associated with estrogen use. The transdermal preparation appears to produce none of these hepatic effects. While 1.25 mg of conjugated estrogen may increase HDL cholesterol, the effect of replacement doses of estrogen on lipoproteins remains unclear because of incomplete study methods.

The most serious potential complication of estrogen therapy is cancer, endometrial and breast. The risk of breast cancer from estrogen therapy is variably reported. However, women with a personal or family history of breast cancer should avoid estrogen therapy. Hyperproliferation of the endometrium from unopposed estrogen use can progress to atypical hyperplasia and adenocarcinoma. Cyclic administration of a progestin minimizes that risk by inducing a full secretory transformation of the endometrium. Preliminary studies suggest that the dose of progestin to achieve secretory transformation and to minimize dose-related adverse effects is determined by adjusting the progestin dose to achieve withdrawal bleeding on or after day 11 of each cycle (14). Clinical data indicate that the dosage range of norethindrone to achieve this effect is 0.35 to 1.05 mg or 5 to 10 mg of medroxyprogesterone acetate. The cyclic regimen is estrogen daily on days 1 through 21 and progestin daily on days 16 through 25 each month.

PROGESTIN

When estrogen therapy is contraindicated, progestins alone may be an alternative hormonal therapy to prevent bone loss. In middle-aged women (mean 48 years) who were within 3 years of natural or surgical menopause, norethisterone administration was associated with a 1.6% increase in bone mineral content (BMC) annually over 2 years, when compared with placebo (15). The placebo group demonstrated a 5% loss of BMC in the first year of the 2-year trial. The dose of norethisterone studied was 5 mg p.o. b.i.d. However, additional work is needed to better define the target population and to elucidate adverse effects of long-term usage, particularly on HDL cholesterol.

Progestins produce several unwanted effects including acne, depression, irritability, breast tenderness, and suppression of high-density-liproprotein cholesterol. A greater than normal annual bone loss (4%) is associated with short luteal phases and anovulatory menstrual cycles that are correlated with a low serum progesterone concentration. It appears that an adequate dose of progestin is necessary for beneficial effects on bone formation and prevention of endometrial abnormalities, while excessive doses may produce unacceptable adverse events.

ANDROGENS

Androgens are reported to inhibit bone resorption and stimulate osteoblastic activity. Controlled studies in postmenopausal osteoporosis using nandrolone decanoate 50 mg i.m. every 2 to 3 weeks over 12 to 24 months report an increase in trabecular bone density of the vertebrae, no significant increase in cortical bone density, a decrease in urinary hydroxyproline concentration, and a decrease in bone pain (15, 16). A relative increase in muscle mass with a decrease in fat mass is seen, which would be expected of androgens. Serum creatinine level increases of approximately 115% over 12 months reflect the increased muscle mass (17). Positive effects on bone metabolism can be seen for 2 years after withdrawing nandrolone decanoate treatment.

An examination of lipid metabolism in patients taking nandrolone decanoate reveals a slight decrease in high density lipoprotein (HDL) cholesterol without a significant effect on total cholesterol, low density lipoprotein (LDL) cholesterol, or triglycerides (18). The intramuscular route of administration, by avoiding the first-pass effect on the liver, may produce less risk for atherogenesis than oral androgenic preparations.

Androgens can produce significant adverse effects in the postmenopausal population. Nandrolone decanoate produces hoarseness of the voice in most study subjects. While hoarseness improves in most patients after discontinuation of the drug, there are complaints of persisting hoarseness 2 years after discontinuation of nandrolone. Increased facial hair and acne occur less frequently. Although serum aminotransferase values remain within the reference range, caution should be used because of the potential for hepatic lesions that have been reported with high-dose, long-term oral anabolic steroid use.

CALCITONIN

Calcitonin inhibits bone resorption, which results in a significant increase in total body calcium. Long-term synthetic salmon calcitonin use in patients with postmenopausal osteoporosis produces a significant increase in trabecular bone mass, with no effect on cortical bone mass (19). A plateau effect after 20 months is thought to reflect development of resistance through antibody formation. However, additional work is needed. Symptomatically, calcitonin reduces bone pain to the extent of decreasing the patient's need for narcotic analgesics (20). A threefold decrease in fracture rate is reported in the same study. Calcitonin appears to be an effective alternative for postmenopausal women who cannot take estrogen therapy.

Repeated injections of salmon calcitonin can cause local adverse reactions, which may be a limiting factor in prolonged therapy. An intranasal product, available in Europe, at a dose of 200 IU daily produces results similar to those reported with intramuscular or subcutaneous administration of salmon calcitonin at 50 to 100 IU daily (21).

Other adverse effects of salmon calcitonin include nausea, vomiting, facial flushing, and rash. Because of the potential for this foreign protein to cause an acute hypersensitivity reaction, a test dose of 0.1 ml of a solution containing 10 IU in 1.0 ml of normal saline is administered intracutaneously on the inner forearm and observed after 15 min for a reaction more severe than a wheal.

CALCIUM

Calcium, in the form of calcium carbonate or other salts, continues to be included in the management of osteoporosis. The calcium requirement in men and young women is calculated to be 800 mg daily. A decrease in consumption of dairy products among U.S. consumers, because of concern about elevated serum cholesterol, may contribute to a calcium deficiency in the U.S. diet. Although the absorption of calcium carbonate when taken preprandially is reported to be adequate, results of studies in postmenopausal osteoporosis suggest that calcium alone cannot effect a change in bone loss.

No relationship between dietary calcium intake and rates of change in bone density in the axial and appendicular skeleton is found in normal adult premenopausal and postmenopausal women with a calcium intake up to 1500 mg daily (22). Although the Consensus Development Conference recommends a calcium intake of 1500 mg daily, the dose may be determined best by the patient's dietary intake and concurrent drug use. Higher doses of calcium must be examined in the prevention of bone loss.

Calcium salts in large doses or taken with excessive doses of vitamin D can produce hypercalcemia. Clinical manifestations vary and depend to some extent on serum concentration, but can include nausea, vomiting, fatigue, and somnolence. In most cases, discontinuation of calcium supplementation and assuring adequate hydration will resolve the symptoms, unlike hypercalcemia of malignancy, which requires more aggressive therapy. A less severe but troublesome adverse effect from supplemental doses of calcium carbonate is constipation. Adequate fluid intake and dietary fiber usually correct this problem.

FLUORIDE

Fluoride enhances mineral uptake from the circulation into bone through stimulation of osteoblastic activity. This dose-related effect increases bone mass, but there appears to be a defect in mineralization associated with fluoride therapy that results in fractures. Forty to 80 mg daily of sodium fluoride is considered the effective dose range. A slow-release sodium fluoride preparation administered on an intermittent schedule of 25 mg twice daily for 3 of 5 months demonstrated a significant increase in vertebral mineral content, lower incidence of fractures, and lower incidence of gastrointestinal and rheumatic side effects (23). Supplementation of dietary calcium to a total intake of 1500 mg daily appears to be important in reducing the risk of the mineralization defect with fluoride.

Oral fluoride commonly causes nausea and gastritis at the doses used for osteoporosis, which frequently results in discontinuation of therapy. Sodium monofluorophosphate is reported to be more soluble than calcium fluoride and is associated with minimal gastrointestinal irritation. Pain and swelling in large joints is reported in up to 33% of patients receiving high doses of fluoride. Stress microfractures are found upon detailed examination and are thought to be the cause of bone pain in patients taking fluoride. The adverse effects related to inadequate mineralization are the primary reasons for disinterest in continuous fluoride therapy for osteoporosis.

VITAMIN D

Vitamin D is described as the major determinant of intestinal calcium absorption. It also stimulates bone resorption and inhibits collagen synthesis. In recent studies, patients with a relative deficiency of circulating $1,25[OH]_2D_3$ responded to calcitriol therapy with normalized intestinal absorption of calcium and improved calcium balance (24). Postmenopausal women with decreased estrogen production increase bone resorption, which decreases PTH, and 1,alpha-hydroxylase, resulting in decreased production of $1,25[OH]_2D_3$. This finding would suggest therapy with estrogen rather than vitamin D. Hyperphosphatemia also decreases 1α-hydroxylase activity. Depending on the cause of hyperphosphatemia, phosphate-binding agents may be more useful than vitamin D alone.

Hypercalcemia and hypervitaminosis D can result from combined calcium, vitamin D, and thiazide diuretic therapy. It is estimated that 17% of patients taking calcium and vitamin D at 50,000 units once or twice weekly will develop hypercalcemia (25). Elderly patients taking this triad of drugs who are volume-depleted may be at greater risk for hypercalcemia (26). Vitamin D doses should be limited to 400 to 800 units daily. Thiazide diuretics enhance distal tubular reabsorption of calcium and should be used cautiously, with frequent monitoring of serum calcium. Management of hypercalcemia includes discontinuation of calcium and vitamin D and following recommendations outlined previously. Depending on the accumulated body stores of vitamin D, symptoms may persist for weeks.

BIPHOSPHONATES

Etidronate disodium is an analog of pyrophosphate which binds strongly to hydroxyapatite crystals. It inhibits soft tissue calcification and can inhibit normal calcification in certain circumstances. Because of potent inhibition of bone resorption by a nonhormonal agent, etidronate has received much interest for use in postmenopausal women for whom estrogen is contraindicated. Divergent results with etidronate in osteoporosis come from limitations in study design. A 14-day course of etidronate 400 mg orally daily every 3 months for 8 cycles produced increases in trabecular bone density and decreased the rate of vertebral fractures by one-half (27). Oral phosphate therapy, given for 3 days prior to administration of etidronate, has no additional effect on bone. Etidronate is reported to cause dose-related gastrointestinal disturbance, but this is unlikely at the low doses used in osteoporosis.

Etidronate is absorbed poorly, with approximately 1% of a 5 mg/kg oral dose absorbed. It binds to di- and trivalent anions. Ingestion of etidronate should occur 2 hr before/after food, antacids, or other drugs containing calcium, aluminum, or magnesium. It is recommended to be taken only with water or fruit juice. Lack of strict adherence to these instructions may be a partial reason for reports of inefficacy.

Clodronate was studied in paraplegic patients shortly after spinal cord injury (28). Acute bone loss with immobilization was prevented, with no evidence of mineralization defects. Clodronate appears to be more effective in preventing osteoporosis due to immobilization than etidronate, which is the only available biphosphonate in the U.S.

COHERENCE AND INTERMITTENT THERAPY

Coherence therapy was proposed by Frost (29). This approach is based on principles of bone remodeling that entail activation of the remodeling cycle, 7 to 21 days for resorption to occur, and 90 days for bone formation and mineralization to be complete. Agents are selected for their positive effect on each interval to activate remodeling, while inhibiting resorption and stimulating bone formation. Applying the same principle, investigators have examined intermittent drugs use to minimize adverse effects and cost. Remodeling units do not function in unison, and each step of the remodeling cycle cannot be isolated completely. Drugs studied this way include etidronate, calcitonin, and phosphate. Preliminary results are promising, and further work will help identify populations who may benefit from this approach in addition to those for whom estrogen therapy is contraindicated.

Treatment Recommendations

The most effective approach to osteoporosis is prevention. Attention to proper nutritional intake, including calcium and vitamin D, reasonable exposure to sunlight, and a program of weight-bearing exercise will maximize peak bone mass in adulthood. While men achieve a 25 to 30% greater peak bone mass than women, longevity necessitates preventive measures by both groups. Where prevention is not possible, pharmacologic treatment of osteoporosis will vary with etiology, patient factors, and cost (Fig. 32.2 and Table 32.3).

In spite of the potential risks, estrogen is the drug of choice for most osteoporosis secondary to menopause. The choice of continuous estrogen therapy or cyclic therapy with a progestin depends on whether the uterus is intact. Hysterectomy allows continuous therapy, whereas cyclic therapy is more appropriate for the woman with an intact uterus who is at risk for hyperplastic endometrial changes. Estrogen is not recommended in women who are more than 15 years past menopause or who have a history of breast cancer.

Postmenopausal women unable to take estrogen may benefit from progestin-only therapy. While norethisterone is not currently available, continuous therapy with med-

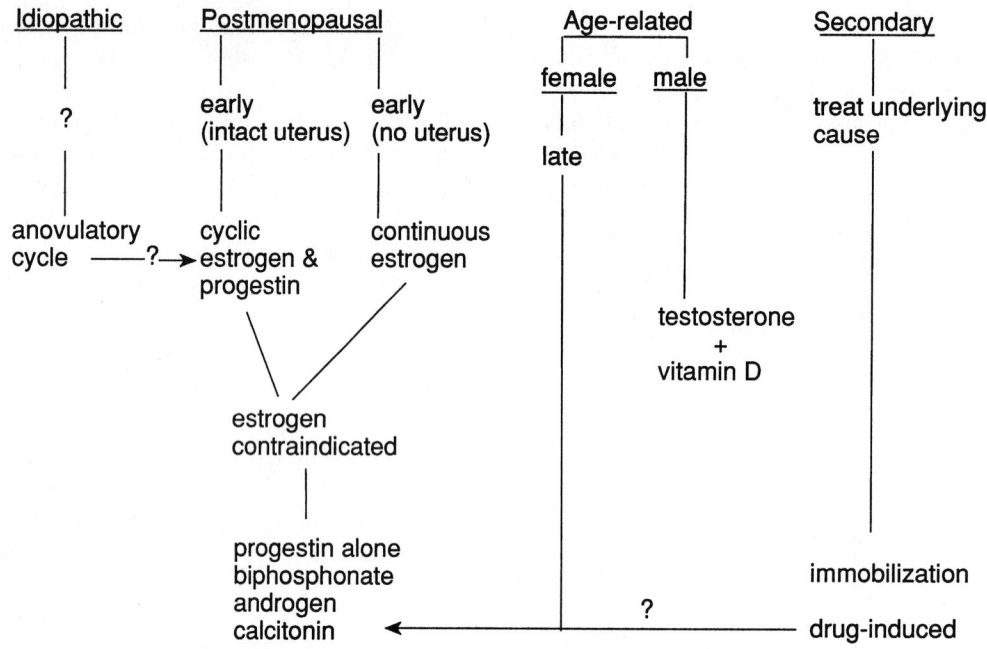

Figure 32.2.   Treatment choice of osteoporosis.

Table 32.3.
Annual Cost of Treatment for Osteoporosis

Drug	Unit	Dose & Frequency	Cost ($)[a]
Calcitonin (salmon)	200 IU/2 ml	100 IU daily	6480
Calcitriol	0.5 μg cap	0.5 μg daily	504
	0.25 μg cap	0.25 μg daily	315
Calcium	1250 mg tab	1250 mg daily	26
Estradiol	0.1 mg patch	0.1 mg twice weekly, continuous	204
		0.1 mg twice weekly, 21-day cycle	157
Estrogen (conjugated)	0.625 mg tab	0.625 mg daily, continuous	73
		0.625 mg, 21-day cycle	50
	1.25 mg tab	1.25 mg daily, continuous	91
		1.25 mg, 21-day cycle	63
Etidronate	400 mg tab	400 mg, 14 days q 3 month	157
Etinyl estradiol	0.05 mg tab	0.05 mg daily, continuous	122
		0.05 mg, 21-day cycle	84
Medroxyprogesterone	10 mg tab	10 mg daily, continuous	186
		10 mg, 10-day cycle	61
Nandrolone	50 mg/ml	50 mg q 2 weeks	104

[a] AWP 1991 Drug Topics Redbook, Medical Economics Data, Oradell, N.J. 1991.

roxyprogesterone acetate may reduce bone loss. Intermittent etidronate therapy is cost-effective, with less than 60 tablets used annually. The main limitation is adherence to a quarterly drug administration schedule that requires strict attention to dosage scheduling. Salmon calcitonin appears to be an effective and relatively safe alternative. However, the cost of daily treatment is prohibitive. Additional intermittent dosing regimens would help to reduce costs. Finally, androgens may be considered in the patient with severe, symptomatic osteoporosis where the potential benefits outweigh the risk of masculinization and hepatic and cardiovascular adverse effects.

Elderly male patients with osteoporosis should be evaluated for testosterone and vitamin D therapy. The hormone produces an increase in bone mass and the vitamin D corrects an associated malabsorption of calcium. An alternative is intermittent etidronate therapy.

Other populations at risk for osteoporosis include

young women with anovulatory cycles or short luteal phases. Early identification of that population with initiation of cyclic estrogen and progestin therapy should be considered. Women experiencing persistent anorexia who are at risk for osteoporosis may benefit from weight-bearing exercise initially. The alternative approaches previously described may be useful if weight-bearing is ineffective.

Glucocorticoid-induced osteoporosis may be minimized by using less than 8 mg daily of prednisone. While alternate-day dosing of glucocorticoids prevents adrenal suppression, this approach does not prevent bone loss. Short-acting glucocorticoids are recommended. An investigational agent, deflazacort, is reported to have less negative effect on calcium balance and bone loss than prednisone. Drugs that can interfere with the elimination of glucocorticoids should be avoided. Coadministration of ethinyl estradiol is reported to decrease the metabolism of prednisone and prednisolone. When preventive measures are inadequate, treatment of symptomatic glucocorticoid-induced osteoporosis can be instituted with salmon calcitonin, etidronate, fluoride, or anabolic steroids.

Vitamin D therapy is indicated in patients who have inadequate dietary intake or exposure to sunlight. Patients who have low serum concentrations of $1,25[OH]_2D_3$ or decreased intestinal calcium absorption may be appropriate candidates.

Prognosis

The natural course of postmenopausal osteoporosis suggests that accurate prediction of risk for fractures would minimize morbidity. Although there are a variety of risk factors associated with the development of osteoporosis, those risk factors are not predictive of fractures. However, long-term estrogen replacement therapy in postmenopausal patients is shown to prevent bone loss and decrease fracture risk by 50%. Untreated, the risk of fractures in the older postmenopausal population exceeds 60%. While the cost of estrogen therapy as prevention in all postmenopausal women is not warranted when compared with the cost of fracture treatment, the groups at risk for osteoporosis should be identified for early intervention.

OSTEOMALACIA

Osteomalacia and rickets both refer to disorders of bone mineralization. Osteomalacia describes a group of disorders characterized by a delay in the initiation of calcification of new bone matrix. Rickets refers to a similar disorder seen in children and adolescents, with the primary difference being a defect in the growth plate because of altered mineralization of epiphyseal cartilage.

Etiology

Osteomalacia may be caused by various underlying problems, each producing the disorder by a different mechanism. The etiology of osteomalacia can thus be divided into four general classifications: (a) vitamin D deficiency, (b) an alteration in vitamin D metabolism, (c) a deficiency of phosphate, or (d) a primary defect in mineralization (Table 32.4). The most common cause is a deficiency of vitamin D or its active metabolites, $25[OH]D_3$ and $1,25[OH]_2D_3$. It is important to determine the underlying cause of the osteomalacia and consider it when designing a therapeutic regimen for a specific patient.

Incidence

The incidence of osteomalacia has not been studied extensively in the United States. It is believed that osteomalacia is not a major issue because of adequate nutritional practices in the U.S. A problem encountered in attempting to determine incidence is that differing criteria are used in the diagnosis of osteomalacia. Investigators have used serum concentrations of vitamin D metabolites, radiologic determinations, serum alkaline phosphatase concentrations, and decreased serum calcium and phosphate levels. Thus, the incidence is reported from 1 to 4% to 75%, depending on the patient population and criteria by which osteomalacia is determined.

Table 32.4.
Etiology of Osteomalacia

Vitamin D deficiency
  Dietary deficiency
  Deficiency in endogenous synthesis (lack of sunlight exposure)
  Deficiency due to gastrointestinal malabsorption
    Gastrectomy
    Small intestinal diseases
    Hepatobiliary disease
    Chronic pancreatic insufficiency
Alteration of vitamin D metabolism
  Impaired hepatic 25-hydroxylation of vitamin D
    Primary biliary cirrhosis
    Biliary atresia or fistula
    Neonatal rickets
  Impaired renal 1-hydroxylation of 25-hydroxyvitamin D
    Hypoparathyroidism
    Chronic renal failure
    Tumor-induced
    Rickets
  Impaired target organ response
    Anticonvulsants
Phosphate deficiency
  Dietary deficiency
  Excessive aluminum intake (antacids)
  Impaired renal tubular reabsorption of phosphate
Primary defects in mineralization
  Chronic renal failure
  Generalized renal tubular disorders
  Hereditary: hypophosphatemia
  Drug-induced (etidronate, fluoride)
  Parenteral alimentation
  Aluminum intoxication

Drug-induced

Several drugs are associated with increased risk of osteomalacia. These include aluminum and aluminum-containing antacids, anticonvulsants, diphosphonates (disodium etidronate), fluoride, and parenteral alimentation. A variety of mechanisms are involved in the pathogenesis.

Osteomalacia is reported in groups of patients on chronic dialysis in isolated geographic locations (30, 31). A higher incidence of osteomalacia was seen in areas with high aluminum dialysate concentrations, and cases disappeared after purification processes were instituted. Increased bone aluminum content is seen in dialysis patients with osteomalacia. It appears that aluminum interferes with normal mineralization of bone.

Chronic use of aluminum-containing antacids may contribute to the development of osteomalacia through intestinal absorption in a patient predisposed to aluminum bone toxicity or by binding phosphates in the diet. This may cause hypophosphatemia and result in osteomalacia over time.

Anticonvulsants are perhaps the best-known causes of drug-induced osteomalacia, most commonly phenytoin, phenobarbital, and primidone (32). These agents apparently produce osteomalacia by induction of hepatic microsomal enzymes, which leads to increased metabolism of vitamin D and metabolites. These drugs also may inhibit intestinal transport of calcium. Multiple anticonvulsant therapy, larger daily doses, prolonged usage, dietary deficiency of vitamin D, or inadequate sun exposure are the key risk factors in this disorder (33).

Because of its potent inhibition of osteoblast action and its ability to crystallize calcium phosphate, etidronate prevents normal mineralization of the bone osteoid matrix. This is especially noteworthy because of recent interest in the use of etidronate in the treatment of osteoporosis. This agent may produce clinical osteomalacia at doses greater than 10 mg/kg/day.

Fluoride has been used to promote bone formation. Large doses of fluoride may cause accumulation of unmineralized bone matrix, resulting in osteomalacia. Generally this is seen only in patients not receiving concurrent calcium supplementation, and the mechanism is unknown.

Parenteral alimentation (TPN) is also associated with osteomalacia. The mechanism is not known, but decreased serum $1,25[OH]_2D_3$ occurs in patients on total parenteral nutrition for extended periods of time.

Pathogenesis

In patients with osteomalacia, osteoblasts lay down normal bone matrix, but normal mineralization does not occur. This weakened, nonmineralized bone may appear in both cortical and trabecular bone. Vitamin D deficiency appears to impair osteoblast function, leading to defective mineralization of the new matrix (1). The vitamin D deficiency may also interfere with osteoblastic activity to retain phosphate; therefore, a person may develop osteomalacia and without becoming hypophosphatemic.

Diagnosis and Clinical Findings

The most frequent finding in osteomalacia is bone pain. This can be a very severe, debilitating pain that commonly affects the ribs, spinal column, pelvis, and lower extremities. The pain is generally worsened by muscle strain, pressure, and weight-bearing, and many patients complain of increased pain during the night.

Skeletal deformities are often seen as a result of the weakened bone. It is common in moderate-to-advanced cases of osteomalacia to see bowing of the extremities, gibbus (hunch-backed), and pigeon chest. Spinal manifestations are common and include scoliosis, kyphosis, and spinal shortening. However, the substantial changes in height commonly associated with vertebral collapse are generally not seen in osteomalacia unless the patient also suffers from concurrent osteoporosis.

Muscle weakness is common in osteomalacia. This may often present as a waddling gait caused by proximal weakness in the lower extremities or as an unwillingness to tense muscles because of the pain caused by that action. Paresthesias, muscle cramps, and occasionally, tetany may be observed in patients with an underlying hypocalcemia.

Laboratory findings in osteomalacia are not diagnostic but relate to the underlying cause of the disorder. Serum calcium and phosphorus levels are often decreased, whereas alkaline phosphatase levels are commonly increased. Although a high false-positive rate (approaching 30%) may be seen, serum alkaline phosphatase measurements appear to be the best biochemical indicator of underlying osteomalacia. However, it is not uncommon to see normal laboratory results in patients with mild disease. Twenty-four hour urinary excretion of calcium is often diminished, at less than 100 mg. Serum $25(OH)D_3$ and $1,25[OH]_2D_3$ levels will vary, depending on the cause of the disorder.

Although uncommon, the most diagnostic radiologic finding in osteomalacia is the pseudofracture (also known as Milkman's fractures or Looser's zones). They are found primarily on the surfaces of bones affected by osteomalacia, including the femur, ribs, pubic rami, clavicles, and the scapulae. These pseudofractures form at right angles to the bone surface, at locations where major blood vessels cross the bone. They appear to be produced by inadequate healing of microfractures in these areas of high stress. They may progress to cause severe deformity or worsened fractures. The most prominent radiologic features include bowing of the long bones and subperiosteal resorption in the phalanges and metacarpals. However, radiologic determination of bone density is generally not useful in the diagnosis or prognosis of osteomalacia because density may be decreased in patients with vitamin D deficiency and increased in chronic renal failure patients.

Documentation of histological changes consistent with osteomalacia is the only accurate diagnostic method. Because the histological changes are distributed throughout the body in both cortical and trabecular bone, biopsy with tetracycline labeling is usually performed at the iliac crest for ease of acquisition.

Medical Treatment

The prognosis of osteomalacia is very good with appropriate treatment. Therapy is aimed at relieving symptoms and slowing the progression of the disease. Medical treatment includes treatment of the underlying cause, adequate nutrition, sun exposure, withdrawal of offending drugs such as anticonvulsants, and timely dialysis in patients with chronic renal failure.

Pharmacologic Treatment

Pharmacologic treatment of osteomalacia must be initiated aggressively to achieve a therapeutic response as rapidly as possible. Primary treatment is vitamin D or one of its active metabolites, with dose and duration of therapy varying with the etiology. The choice of agent should be based on underlying hepatic and renal function, cost, and success of implementing medical treatment (Fig. 32.3).

For the treatment of patients with osteomalacia secondary to nutritional deficiency ,vitamin D therapy may be initiated with cholecalciferol (vitamin D_3) at 2000 to 4000 IU daily for several months, followed by a maintenance dose of 200 to 400 IU per day (ergocalciferol, or vitamin D_2 may also be used). Response should be seen within a few months of initiation of therapy.

In patients with a vitamin D deficiency secondary to malabsorption, much larger doses are usually required to achieve a therapeutic response. Ergocalciferol with an initial dose of 25,000 to 100,000 IU daily should be given, with a corresponding decrease in dose once the desired response is achieved. Many patients may not respond to even these large doses. In those cases, administration of calcifediol (25[OH]D_3) may be more effective at maintenance doses of 50 to 100 µg/day. These patients should generally receive calcium supplementation of 1 to 2 g per day. Serum calcium should be monitored closely to avoid hypercalcemia.

Osteomalacia secondary to hypophosphatemia should be treated with a combination of phosphate replacement (1 to 3 g/day) and ergocalciferol (25,000 to 100,000 IU/day). Use of calcitriol (1,25[OH]$_2$D$_3$) at 0.25 to 1.0 µg/day may be substituted if underlying renal and/or hepatic dysfunction is present. The laxative effect of the phosphate replacement may prevent maximum doses from being reached.

In patients with primary defects of mineralization, it is important to control underlying factors. In cases of drug-induced osteomalacia, removal of the offending agent may be desirable, although not always feasible. The benefit of continued use of an anticonvulsant, for example, may outweigh the risk of worsened osteomalacia. If anticonvulsant therapy is continued and the patient has limited exposure to sunlight, prophylactic vitamin D therapy may be considered. If prophylaxis is desired, administration of cholecalciferol at a dose of 1000 to 2000 IU/day along with calcium supplementation (500 to 1000 mg of elemental calcium daily) may be recommended for patients on more than 6 months of therapy (34).

In patients with chronic renal failure, restriction of aluminum-containing antacids may be beneficial. Administration of calcitriol, 0.25 to 1.0 µg/day, along with calcium

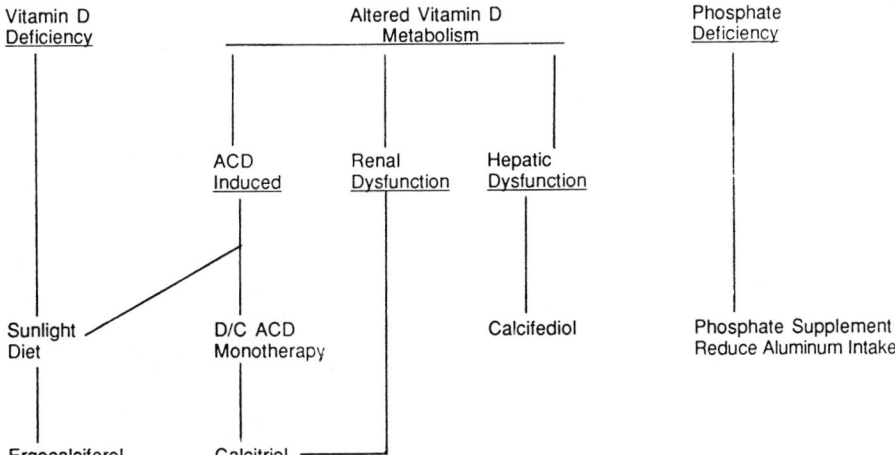

Figure 32.3. Treatment choice of osteomalacia. ACD, anticonvulsant drug; calcifediol, 25[OH]D_3; calcitriol, 1,25[OH]$_2$D$_3$.

Calcium intake should be assessed and supplemented with caution to avoid inducing hypercalcemia.

supplementation, 1 to 2 g/day, is recommended. Serum phosphate must be closely monitored. If a phosphate binder is necessary, calcium carbonate may be used both as calcium supplementation and for phosphate-binding. Cautious addition of aluminum-containing antacids may achieve the desired effect.

For chronic dialysis patients who also receive aluminum-based phosphate binders, periodic monitoring of serum aluminum concentrations is important. If patients demonstrate a serum aluminum concentration of >100 μg/ml or signs of encephalopathy or osteomalacia due to accumulation of aluminum, intravenous deferoxamine therapy should be considered in addition to discontinuation of aluminum products (35). Deferoxamine acts as a chelating agent, producing an initial increase in serum aluminum and promoting removal of aluminum from bone and the systemic circulation. Administration of deferoxamine, 4 to 6 g in 500 ml of dextrose 5%, infused IV over 2 hr once weekly before dialysis, will gradually correct the osteomalacia over a 6 to 12 month period. Signs of encephalopathy should improve earlier. Patients should be monitored for hypotension during administration of deferoxamine and cataracts and retinitis with chronic use.

For patients receiving large doses of fluoride for an extended period of time, calcium may be administered concurrently in a dose of 1 to 2 g/day to minimize their risk of developing osteomalacia.

Drug Interactions

Several interactions with vitamin D therapy are reported. Cholestyramine and mineral oil may both decrease the absorption of vitamin D in the intestine. Vitamin D in conjunction with magnesium-containing antacids may actually promote absorption of magnesium, leading to hypermagnesemia in some patients. Because of the potential for antagonism, the combination of vitamin D and calcium supplementation should be used with extreme caution in patients taking calcium-channel antagonists. Thiazide diuretics have been reported to cause both hypocalcemia and hypercalcemia in patients also receiving vitamin D.

CONCLUSION

Osteoporosis and osteomalacia represent common, but heterogeneous metabolic bone disorders. Both entities can be prevented if risk factors are identified and appropriate measures instituted early. Treatment of each bone disorder varies with etiology. The alert pharmacist can identify patients at risk for developing osteomalacia, including chronic dialysis patients, patients receiving chronic anticonvulsants, patients receiving chronic TPN therapy, and elderly patients. In most instances, osteomalacia carries a good prognosis if appropriate treatment is initiated and the regimen is followed carefully. While estrogen remains the only confirmed therapy for postmenopausal osteoporosis, future studies will elucidate treatment of subsets of the population, the place of intermittent drug therapy, the efficacy of new biphosphonates, and the long-term safety of progestins and androgens. However, it is clear that excessive vitamin D and calcium therapy can lead to significant adverse effects and may offer no benefit beyond adequate dietary intake in many patients.

REFERENCES

1. Prior JC, Vigna YM, Schechter MT, Burgess AE: Spinal bone loss and ovulatory disturbances. N Engl J Med 323:1221–1227, 1990.
2. Brotman AW, Stern TA: Osteoporosis and pathologic fractures in anorexia nervosa. Am J Psychiatry 142:495–496, 1985.
3. Lukert BP, Raisz LG: Glucocorticoid-induced osteoporosis: pathogenesis and management. Ann Intern Med 112:353–364, 1990.
4. Levine MN: Nonhemorrhagic complications of anticoagulant therapy. Semin Thromb Hemost 12:63–66, 1986.
5. Pacifici R, Rifas L, Teitelbaum S, Slatopolsky E, McCracken R, et al.: Spontaneous release of interleukin 1 from human blood monocytes reflects bone formation in idiopathic osteoporosis. Proc Natl Acad Sci 84:4616–4620, 1987.
6. Riggs BL, Wahner HW, Seeman E, Offord KP, Dunn WL, et al.: Changes in bone mineral density of the proximal femur and spine with aging. Differences between the postmenopausal and senile osteoporosis syndromes. J Clin Invest 70:716–723, 1982.
7. Nilas L, Christiansen C: The pathophysiology of peri- and postmenopausal bone loss. Br J Obstet Gynaecol 96:580–587, 1989.
8. Alvioli LV: Heparin-induced osteoporosis: an appraisal. Adv Exp Med Biol 52:375–387, 1975.
9. Sinaki M: Exercise and osteoporosis. Arch Phys Med Rehabil 70:220–229, 1989.
10. Nicogossian AE, Parker JF Jr: Space Physiology and Medicine. Washington, D.C.: U.S. Government Printing Office, 1982, ch 18.
11. Dalsky GP, Stocke KS, Ehsani AA, Slotpolsky E, Lee WC, Birge SJ: Weight bearing exercise training and lumbar spine bone mineral content in postmenopausal women. Ann Intern Med 108:824–828, 1988.
12. Anon: Consensus development conference: prophylaxis and treatment of osteoporosis. Br Med J 295:914–915, 1987.
13. Chetkowski RJ, Meldrum DR, Steingold KA, Randle D, Lu JK, et al.: Biologic effects of transdermal estradiol. N Engl J Med 314:1615–1620, 1986.
14. Padwick ML, Pryse-Davies J, Whitehead MI: A simple method for determining the optimal dosage of progestin in postmenopausal women receiving estrogens. N Engl J Med 315:930–934, 1986.
15. Abdalla HI, McKay Hart D, Lindsay R, Leggate I, Hooke A: Prevention of bone mineral loss in postmenopausal women by norethisterone. Obstet Gynecol 66:789–792, 1985.
16. Geusens P, Dequeker J, Verstraeten A, Nijs J, Van Holsbeeck M: Bone mineral content, cortical thickness and fracture rate in osteoporotic women after withdrawal of treatment with nandrolone decanoate, 1-α hydroxyvitamin D₃, or intermittent calcium infusions. Maturitas 8:281–289, 1986.
17. Need AG, Horowitz M, Bridges A, Morris HA, Nordin BEC: Effects of nandrolone decanoate and antiresorptive therapy on vertebral density in osteoporotic postmenopausal women. Arch Intern Med 149:57–60, 1989.
18. Hassager C, Podenphant J, Juel Riis B, Sidenius Johansen J, Jensen J, Christiansen C: Changes in soft tissue body composition and plasma lipid metabolism during nandrolone decanoate therapy in postmenopausal osteoporotic women. Metabolism 38:238–242, 1989.

19. Gruber HE, Ivey JL, Baylink DJ, Matthews M, Nelp WB, Sism K, Chesnut CH III: Long-term calcitonin therapy in postmenopausal osteoporosis. Metabolism 33:295–303, 1984.

20. Palmieri GMA, Pitcock JA, Brown P, Karas JG, Roen LJ: Effect of calcitonin and vitamin D in osteoporosis. Calcif Tissue Int 45:137–141, 1989.

21. Overgaard K, Hansen MA, Herss Nielsen VA, Juel Riis B, Christiansen C: Discontinuous calcitonin treatment of established osteoporosis—effects of withdrawal of treatment. Am J Med 89:1–6, 1990.

22. Riggs BL, Wahner HW, Melton LJ III, Richelson LS, Judd HL, O'Fallon WM: Dietary calcium intake and rates of bone loss in women. J Clin Invest 80:979–982, 1987.

23. Pak CYC, Sakhaee K, Zerwekh JE, Parcel C, Peterson R, et al.: Safe and effective treatment of osteoporosis with intermittent slow release sodium fluoride: augmentation of vertebral bone mass and inhibition of fractures. J Clin Endocrinol Metab 68:150–159, 1989.

24. Gallagher JC, Riggs BL, Recker RR, Goldgar D: The effect of calcitriol on patients with postmenopausal osteoporosis with special reference to fracture frequency. Proc Soc Exp Biol Med 191:287–292, 1989.

25. Schwartzman MS, Franck WA: Vitamin D toxicity complicating the treatment of senile, postmenopausal, and glucocorticoid-induced osteoporosis. Am J Med 82:224–230, 1987.

26. Drinka PJ, Nolten WD: Hazards of treating osteoporosis and hypertension concurrently with calcium, vitamin D, and distal diuretics. J Am Geriatr Soc 32:405–407, 1984.

27. Watts NB, Harris ST, Genant HK, Wasnich RD, Miller PD, et al.: Intermittent cyclical etidronate treatment of postmenopausal osteoporosis. N Engl J Med 323:73–79, 1990.

28. Minaire P, Depassio J, Berard E, Meunier PJ, Edouard C, et al.: Effects of clodronate on immobilization bone loss. Bone 8(suppl 1):S63–S68, 1987.

29. Frost HM. Coherence treatment of osteoporoses. Orthop Clin North Am 12:649–669, 1981.

30. Llach F, Felsenfeld AJ, Coleman MD, Keveney JJ, Pederson JA, Medlock TR: The natural course of dialysis osteomalacia. Kidney Int 29(suppl. 18): S74–S79, 1986.

31. Ihle BU, Becker GJ, Kincaid-Smith PS: Clinical and biochemical features of aluminum-related bone disease. Kidney Int 29(suppl. 18):S80–S86, 1986.

32. Hahn TJ: Bone complications of anticonvulsants. Drugs 12:201–211, 1976.

33. Bogliun G, Beghi E, Crespi V, Delodovici L, d'Amico P: Anticonvulsant drugs and bone metabolism. Acta Neurol Scand 74:284–288, 1986.

34. Christiansen C, Rodbro P, Lund M: Incidence of anticonvulsant osteomalacia and effect of vitamin D: controlled therapeutic trial. Br Med J 4:695–701, 1973.

35. Felsenfeld AJ, Rodriguez M, Coleman M, Ross D, Llach F: Desferrioxamine therapy in hemodialysis patients with aluminum-associated bone disease. Kidney Int 35:1371–1378, 1989.

CHAPTER 33

ASTHMA

R. PETER IAFRATE, Pharm.D. and KATHRYN BLAKE, Pharm.D.

The treatment of asthma has been extensively investigated in the past 10 years. After diagnosis, the management of this disease involves drug combinations that often include different routes of administration for the individual drugs.

The optimal treatment for asthma, which may be lifelong, is still evolving. However, considerable progress has been made, including better symptom control as well as few adverse effects, although the prevalence of asthma is increasing, as are the number of hospitalizations, morbidity, and perhaps mortality.

EPIDEMIOLOGY

The natural occurrence of asthma has been studied for many years. Despite this, the prevalence of asthma, the incidence of new cases, and etiologic factors of this disease remain unclear. Much of the confusion lies with the definition of the disease itself. In the past, an allergic component was required for the diagnosis; however, recently the focus has been on airway hyperreactivity to various stimuli and on inflammation of the airways.

The prevalence of active asthma in the United States is approximately 3% or 10 million people, while the cumulative prevalence is around 11%. From 1980 to 1987 the asthma prevalence rate has increased 29%, with a disproportionate increase in younger persons. The current incidence in children in the United States ranges from 4 to 9%.

In 1985, approximately 1% of all estimated ambulatory care visits reported asthma as the first listed diagnosis. Hospitalizations for asthma have increased 45% per year from 1979 to 1987 in children 17 years or younger, with the greatest increase occurring in black children under 4 years of age. Twenty percent of all hospitalizations in children under 15 years of age are for asthma. More discouraging, the mortality rate has increased 31% from 1980 to 1987. It is not known whether the increased morbidity is from an increase in asthma prevalence or from changes in the dynamics of the disease itself. However, socioeconomic status, clinical management, and changes in the external environment have been implicated.

In 1975 an epidemiologic study of Lebowitz et al. (1) tried to overcome some of the difficulties of previous studies. Nearly 4000 subjects in the Tucson area were entered into the study and followed longitudinally. This report found the prevalence of asthma in 5 to 14-year-olds to be virtually identical for girls and boys (8.74% versus 8.23%). During the late teens, the prevalence rate for females decreased while the rate for males remained high. In the age range from 30 to 49 years, female prevalence was nearly double the male rate; over 50, the male rate was generally higher. The overall prevalence was not different (5.6% for males, 5.9% for females).

Although the Tucson study was an advance in determining the epidemiology of asthma, until a clear, consistent definition of the disease is available for all age groups, the precise incidence and prevalence of asthma will remain unknown.

ETIOLOGY

The underlying abnormality of asthma appears to be hyperreactivity to certain stimuli. The hyperreactivity may or may not genetically transmitted. The stimuli may include atmospheric irritants, cold air, allergens, viral respiratory tract infections, exercise, and emotional stress.

Certain drugs and chemicals can also precipitate an asthmatic attack (2). The most notable of these is aspirin. The prevalence of aspirin sensitivity in patients with asthma varies between 3 and 19%. β-Adrenoreceptor blockers can also elicit an asthmatic attack in susceptible individuals. This effect is more common with the nonselective agents such as propranolol and nadolol than it is with the β_1-selective agents like atenolol and metoprolol. The β_1 selectivity of available agents is not absolute and may be lost at higher doses, resulting in the potential for increasing airway resistance and precipitating an asthmatic attack. Timolol eye drops, a β-blocker used for glaucoma, has resulted in deaths when given to asthmatic patients.

Sulfur dioxide and sulfites, commonly used as sanitizers and preservatives of foods and pharmaceuticals, may precipitate acute asthma in 5% or more of asthmatic patients. Other agents, including tartrazine (FDA Yellow No. 5), provoke asthmatic reactions; however, virtually none of the reports include blinded and placebo-controlled challenges. As of June, 1980 all pharmaceuticals that contain tartrazine must be so labeled. Sulfites were banned from food in 1986, but they may be found in alcoholic beverages such as wine. These products have warning labels.

Three theories for the cause of asthma have been widely accepted. Szentivanyi proposed in 1986 that asthma resulted from abnormal β-adrenergic receptor–adenylate cyclase function that decreased adrenergic responsiveness (3). Recently however, it was shown that the decreased number of β-receptors on leukocytes of asthmatic patients which had been used to support this theory may be due to the treatment of these patients with β-adrenergic drugs (4). Others have proposed that the fundamental defect is caused by increased cholinergic activity in the airways (5). This theory is supported by the seemingly lower threshold for irritant stimuli found in asthmatic patients. Although asthma seems to incorporate both concepts, neither theory can explain all the available data. Middleton (6) has proposed that the final common pathogenic pathway for asthma is an altered regulation of intracellular calcium, since mast cell release of mediators, smooth muscle contraction, mucus secretion, vagus nerve impulse initiation and conduction, and inflammatory cell infiltration are all calcium-dependent processes.

DEFINITION

The American Thoracic Society defines asthma as an obstructive disease of the airways that is due to spasm of airway smooth muscle, increased mucus secretion, and/or inflammation and is completely reversible either spontaneously or with treatment. Both large and small airways are affected to some degree with the hyperresponsiveness resulting from a variety of stimuli. This hyperresponsiveness is present at some time in all patients with the disease. However, the condition is intermittent, and hyperresponsiveness, smooth muscle tone, edema, and hypersecretion of the airways can vary greatly from one person to the other as well as within an affected individual.

Since asthma results from a variety of stimuli and presents in various ways even within the same patient, it is not useful from a pharmacologic viewpoint to place asthmatics in one of the traditional categories (i.e., extrinsic or intrinsic asthma). The National Heart, Lung and Blood Institute has developed a scheme for classification of asthma (mild, moderate, or severe) based in part upon the severity and frequency of symptoms, pulmonary function, and response to pharmacologic treatment. Classification by severity assists in determining the number and types of medications required for control. In addition, asthma can be intermittent, chronic, or seasonal. Patients with intermittent asthma are totally free of symptoms between episodes, and weeks, months, or years may pass between episodes. In such patients the as-needed use of an inhaled β2-selective agonist is most likely to provide rapid relief of symptoms without side effects, whereas a slow-release theophylline product, for example, would be totally inappropriate. On the other hand, the patient who has continuous symptoms of frequently recurring attacks is classified as a chronic asthmatic. In such a patient the goal of therapy is to suppress the symptoms by the use of a prophylactic drug regimen such as cromolyn or inhaled corticosteroids. In between these two classifications is the seasonal or indeterminate asthmatic who has continuous symptoms during a particular season and thus requires prophylactic medication during that time period. During the remainder of the year such a patient may have symptoms only intermittently and thus require only as-needed medication.

Because of the intrapatient variability of the disease, intermittent, chronic, and seasonal asthmatics may vary in their classification over time. The severity of asthmatic symptoms varies within both intermittent and chronic categories and thus determines the number and the types of medication required for control. For example, there are intermittent asthmatics whose symptoms become so severe that they require an emergency room visit or hospitalization, whereas in others, the episode may resolve spontaneously or with minimal treatment such as the as-needed use of an inhaled β-agonist. Similarly some chronic asthmatics may be completely controlled with a slow-release theophylline product administered on a continuous basis, whereas others may require treatment with additional drugs such as corticosteroids. The goal of therapy therefore is the adequate control of symptoms with the least pharmacologic intervention possible (Table 33.1).

Under certain circumstances an asthmatic may progress to a potentially life-threatening condition referred to as status asthmaticus. Status asthmaticus is defined as a prolonged severe episode of asthma that does not respond to usual treatment. The pathogenesis of this condition involves bronchoconstriction, mucus plugging, and inflammation causing a decrease in airway diameter. Status

Table 33.1.
Criteria for Adequate Control of Asthma[a]

Asthma Type	Criteria
Intermittent	No emergency physician visits
	Absence of symptoms not promptly relieved with the therapeutic measures
Chronic	No emergency physician visits
	Absence of symptoms not promptly relieved with as-needed therapy including: inhaled sympathomimetic ≤ twice/day and not after bedtime and corticosteroids ≤ 10-day course averaging < 5 days/month
	Nocturnal symptoms and interference with activities < once/week
	Postbronchodilator pulmonary function tests within normal limits[b]

[a] From Ekwo E, Weinberger MM: Evaluation of a program for the pharmacologic management of children with asthma. J Allergy Clin Immunol 61:240–247, 1978, with permission.
[b] Normal limits defined as forced expiratory flow rate from 25 to 75% of vital capacity of ≥75% of predicted, with forced vital capacity ≤80% of predicted.

asthmaticus develops over a period of hours to days. The symptoms worsen steadily, and the need for bronchodilator therapy increases. Both of these should be used as monitoring parameters by the patient and the clinician.

DIAGNOSIS

Since asthma presents in various ways and results from numerous stimuli, the diagnosis of asthma is generally made by a comprehensive history and confirmed by physical examination and laboratory tests. A thorough medical history includes a description of the current of symptoms (cough, wheeze, sputum production) and pattern of symptoms (yearly, daily, onset/duration) and precipitating factors. Pertinent past history includes age of onset and diagnosis, progression of the disease, previous therapy, and any family history. Determining the probability of successful treatment includes psychosocial issues relating to the impact of the disease on the patient's lifestyle and family dynamics. Objective physiologic data includes pulmonary function tests and response to bronchodilators and/or corticosteroids; x-rays; bronchoprovocation challenges with methacholine, histamine, or exercise; sputum or nasal smear examination; blood eosinophil count; and serum IgE antibodies to specific allergens (Table 33.2).

Since an allergic component to asthma may be present in 20 to 80% of patients, depending upon age and definition of atopy, a thorough history of allergic disease should be obtained. Skin testing may be used to evaluate the presence of an allergic stimulus. This procedure presents the patient's immune system with a small amount of allergen and allows a controlled and carefully monitored type I, immunoglobulin E (IgE)-mediated, reaction to take place. A positive reaction (a large wheal and flare) indicates IgE-reagenic antibody. However, an exacerbation of asthma must correlate with exposure to the antigen, since synthesis of IgE may occur in patients other than those with clinical allergy. Many patients with an allergic component to their asthma have positive skin tests to multiple antigens, implying the presence of IgE antibody, but have asthmatic symptoms that correlate with only a few antigens or none at all. Negative reactions provide strong evidence against an IgE-mediated immunologic reaction, but they can be misleading if the antigen causing the allergic response is not included in the panel of skin tests. The antigen is first applied with a needle prick. The results are read in 10 to 15 min by measuring the millimeters of wheal and flare. If negative, the antigen is then injected intradermally, because the prick test can give a false-negative result. In certain individuals who cannot undergo skin testing (e.g., dermatographic or severely eczematoid patients), a radioallergosorbent test (RAST) can be used (7). It is more expensive than skin testing, requires a delay for results, must be directed at specific antigens (i.e., not just grass, but bluegrass), and still must be correlated with the history.

Table 33.2.
Criteria for Diagnosis of Asthma[a]

Presenting Symptoms[b]	Supportive Data
Any one of the following: Wheezing Coughing Shortness of breath or labored respirations History of recurrent pneumonia of bronchitis	Demonstration of reversible airways obstruction by: Abnormal chest roentgenogram at some point in time with no abnormalities other than peribronchial thickening and Pulmonary function tests that demonstrate airway obstruction that is readily reversible either spontaneously or immediately following bronchodilator or subsequent to sustained therapy with bronchodilators and/or corticosteroids[c] or For younger children, history and clinical course that demonstrate reversibility of the symptoms of airway disease as a result of therapy with bronchodilators or bronchodilators plus corticosteroids.

[a] From Ekwo E, Weinberger MM: Evaluation of a program for the pharmacologic management of children with asthma. J Allergy Clin Immunol 61:240–247, 1978, with permission.
[b] The diagnosis is only finally accepted when the supportive data are obtained. The presenting symptoms only raise the question and do not themselves constitute final acceptance of the diagnosis.
[c] Defined as a 25% or greater increase in predicted force expiratory flow rate from 25 to 75%, with force vital capacity at least 80% of predicted.

Pulmonary function testing confirms the diagnosis and evaluates the severity of obstruction. Baseline pulmonary function studies may be abnormal, showing evidence of obstruction by means of a decrease in the FEV_1 (the volume of air that can be blown out in the first second of a forced expiratory maneuver) below that predicted for the patient's height, weight, and age. Inhalation of a bronchodilator medication may cause 15 to 20% improvement, leading to the diagnosis of reversible bronchospasm. When the diagnosis of asthma is suspected and the pulmonary function tests are abnormal but not reversible with an inhaled β-agonist, a short course of oral corticosteroids may be required to document reversibility of airway obstruction and thus confirm the diagnosis. In some patients, however, baseline pulmonary function values may be entirely within normal limits at the time the physician is seeing the patient. In these patients, graded inhalations of methacholine or histamine (8) are used to induce a 20% drop in FEV_1. If the provocative dose of methacholine or histamine required to decrease FEV_1 by 20% (PD_2O) is <16 mg/ml, the diagnosis of asthma can be confirmed. However, nonasthmatic patients may also have a positive methacholine or histamine test (e.g., patients with cystic fibrosis, chronic obstructive pulmonary disease (COPD), allergic rhinitis) so these results must be interpreted with regard to the patient's clinical history. Alternatively, the patient can be given a standardized exercise stress test on a treadmill. In asthmatics with a history of exercise intolerance, FEV1 will drop by 20% or more after exercise.

PHARMACOLOGIC MANAGEMENT OF ASTHMA

β-Adrenergic Receptor Agonists

The use of β-adrenergic receptor agonists can be traced back to the ancient Chinese; ephedrine was the major ingredient in the Chinese herb Ma-huang. It was not until the turn of this century, however, that β-adrenergic agents were used as bronchodilators by Western physicians.

There are three main categories of adrenergic receptor effects: α, β_1, and β_2. In asthma β_2 effects are desirable, whereas α and β_1 effects contribute greatly to the side effects of these agents. Although epinephrine and isoproterenol have been the mainstays in the treatment of acute asthma for many years, recent changes in the basic catechol ring resulted in more β_2 selective and longer-acting agents that are orally bioavailable. As a result, these agents are playing an increasingly greater role in the treatment of asthma and other obstructive airway diseases.

CHEMISTRY AND PHARMACOLOGY

All of the currently available sympathomimetic amines have the phenylethylamine structure as their nucleus (Fig. 33.1). Alterations of this structure, usually at the 3, 4, or 5 positions on the benzene ring, on the α carbon, or at the terminal nitrogen, produce variations in activity im-

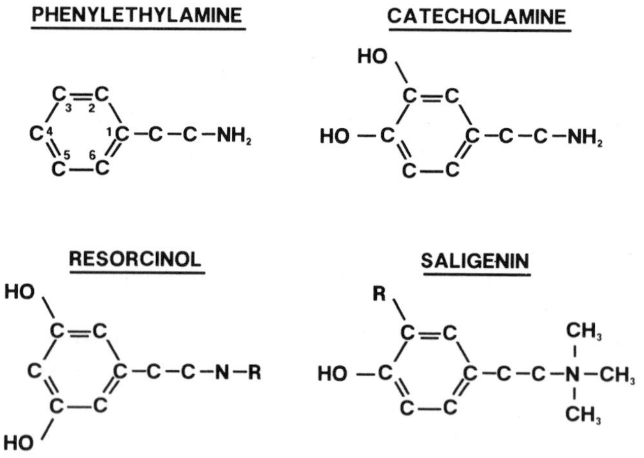

Figure 33.1. Basic structure of the sympathomimetic amines. The carbon atoms of the basic phenylethylamine structure are labeled in the conventional manner, with numbers used to identify the positions in the benzene ring. (R) represents various carbon moieties.

portant for the treatment of asthma. Epinephrine and other catecholamines contain adjacent hydroxyl groups on the 3 and 4 positions of the benzene ring. Catechol-O-methyltransferase (COMT) methylates the 3-hydroxy group, leading to biologic inactivation. Monoamine oxidase (MAO) degrades the natural adrenergic compounds by removing the amine portion of the phenylethylamine moiety. Thus the catecholamines are short acting and not orally bioavailable.

In an attempt to develop longer acting agents that were more β_2 selective, the catechol nucleus was replaced by a resorcinol or saligenin ring (Fig. 33.1). The resorcinols consist of metaproterenol, terbutaline, and fenoterol. These drugs differ from the catecholamines in a shift of the hydroxyl groups from the 3–4 position on the ring to a 3–5 configuration. The saligenins, albuterol and carbuterol, represent substitutions onto the 3-hydroxy position. Longer lipophilic N–side chains have resulted in two investigational β_2-receptor agonist, formeterol and salmeterol. These agents have shown a duration of activity of 8 to 12 hr. These structural modifications increase specificity, prevent metabolism by COMT, and provide resistance to the actions of sulfatases. In addition, the large amino group substitutions prevent the action of MAO, improve β_2 selectivity, and increase oral absorption (9). Thus the saligenins and resorcinols are effective by oral administration, have an increased duration of action, and improve selectivity for β-receptors.

Bitolterol mesylate represents a different approach. This β-agonist is a prodrug that requires hydrolysis by esterases to colterol, a catecholamine similar to terbutaline and albuterol in pharmacologic activity (10).

The stimulation of β-receptors by these agents results in an activation of the enzyme adenylcyclase, which results in an increase in production of cyclic AMP. This compound disinhibits protein kinase and stimulates the binding of calcium ions to the cell membrane and to the mycoplasmic reticulum. Thus, the mycoplasmic calcium concentration is reduced in both polarized and depolarized smooth muscle, and relaxation occurs (10). It is probable that these same mechanisms are involved in the regulation of the mast cell release of mediators. β-agonists in asthma also increase mucociliary transport; however, the clinical relevance of this effect has not been demonstrated.

Although there are both β_1 and β_2 receptors in the lung, β_1-receptors do not mediate any important bronchodilating effect. Selectively stimulating β_2-receptors therefore has the greatest effect on increasing airway caliber while minimizing the tachycardia and the potential for arrhythmias that can result from β_1 stimulation.

ABSORPTION/FATE/EXCRETION

A relatively close correlation between changes in serum concentration and pulmonary function has been demonstrated with systemically administered β₂-agonists. Little pharmacokinetic information is available on these products because of the difficulties with serum analyses. In general, they all have relatively short half-lives and a large first-pass metabolism. However, data from single-dose terbutaline studies indicate that the terminal half-life of terbutaline in healthy subjects is about 17 hr, compared with about 6 to 8 hr for albuterol.

TOXICITY

Side effects from β-receptor agonists result from the stimulation of adrenergic receptors other than those responsible for the therapeutic effect. Skeletal muscle tremor, tachycardia, palpitations, and a certain degree of nervousness result from administration of these drugs. Cardiac stimulation can be either direct, by β₁ activation, or reflex, through β₂-mediated peripheral vasodilation (11). The muscle tremor is principally a β₂-mediated effect. Both effects appear to be dose-related.

The frequency and severity of these side effects is directly related to the route of administration. After inhalation of normal doses of all β₂-selective agents, minor tremors and headaches may occur if any side effects occur at all. This is a result of the drug being delivered directly to the site of action, with only trivial amounts reaching the systemic circulation. Conversely, side effects are relatively common for orally or parenterally administered agents that produce higher concentrations of drug in many regions of the body.

An ongoing issue among researchers in asthma is whether the combined use of β-agonist and theophylline increases the potential for cardiac toxicity in patients. Although evidence in animals supports this contention, a lack of data in the clinical literature keeps this question unresolved. In those patients in whom concomitant administration is required, the aerosolized route of β-agonist is recommended to minimize this potential toxicity. Studies with continuous ambulatory electrocardiographic (ECG) monitors have not revealed any additive cardiac toxicity when inhaled β-agonists are combined with therapeutic serum concentrations of theophylline.

Although never conclusively established, there is circumstantial evidence of an increase in asthma mortality with one particular β₂-agonist, fenoterol. In the year that fenoterol was introduced into the New Zealand market, the incidence of asthma-related deaths increased. Possible explanations include (a) combined use of β₂-agonists with theophylline and (b) patients delaying seeing a physician in acute asthma attacks because of home nebulizers. Many patient variables including age, number of medications being taken, and severity of asthma confound any conclusions about the specific role of fenoterol in these deaths. Recent evidence suggests that the overreliance on any β₂ agonist increases the risk of death in asthmatics (11a).

TOLERANCE

The long-term use of β₂-agonists in the treatment of chronic asthma has raised the question of tolerance developing to these agents. Tolerance does develop to the nonbronchial β₂ responses in both animals and humans. These include reduced effects on tremor, heart rate, and lymphocyte and leukocyte cyclic AMP levels and a decrease in the number of β-adrenergic receptors on cell surfaces.

Numerous studies have attempted to determine if tachyphylaxis to the bronchodilating effects of β₂-agonists develops after long-term use. Although results have been conflicting, results of a recent study suggest that 6-month continuous, rather than "as-needed" use of β₂-agonists may lead to deterioration of asthma control (12).

CLINICAL USE

β-Agonists are the treatment of choice for acute exacerbations in either intermittent or chronic asthmatics, and for prevention of exercise-induced asthma.

Traditionally, acute exacerbations of asthma have been treated with subcutaneous epinephrine. As newer, longer-acting β₂-receptor agonists were developed, such as terbutaline and albuterol, their longer duration of action and their β₂ selectivity gave them the therapeutic advantage over epinephrine. Studies have clearly demonstrated that an inhaled β-adrenergic agent produces greater bronchodilation acutely than does the intravenous administration of sufficient theophylline to produce therapeutic blood concentrations (13).

A growing body of information indicates that the inhaled route has the greatest likelihood of relieving symptoms of acute asthma with minimal or no side effects. Inhalation via metered-dose inhalers or by nebulization delivers the drug to the target organ (Fig. 33.2). The theoretical advantage of injected β-agonists is improved bronchodilation of the smallest peripheral airways in patients with severe bronchoconstriction. However, studies in patients with acute asthma, in whom bronchial deposition of aerosols might be expected to be compromised, have failed to show any benefit of systemic therapy over aerosols, unless the patient is very short of breath (dyspneic) (11).

The intravenous use of β-agonists has been advocated for asthmatic children in impending respiratory failure, to eliminate the need for mechanical ventilation. Potentially life-threatening side effects limit the safety of this route of administration, and such treatment should be conducted only in an intensive care unit by an experienced physician.

PRODUCT SELECTION

Except in rare instances, β₂-receptor agonists should be administered by inhalation via metered-dose inhalers or

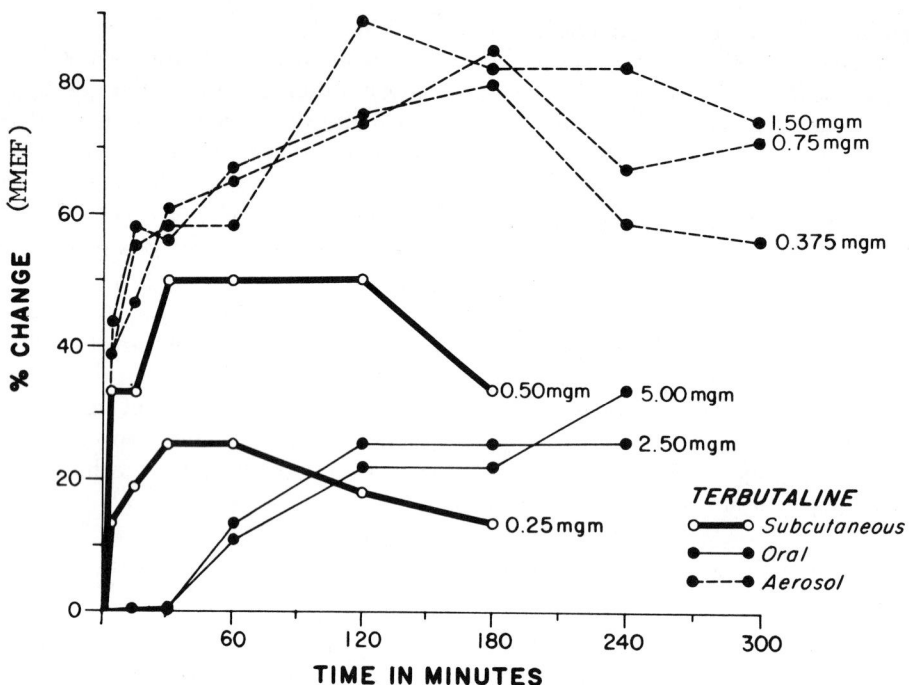

Figure 33.2. Changes in maximal mid-expiratory flow rate (MMEF), a measure of small airways obstruction, after three different routes of administration of terbutaline to adult asthmatics in no acute distress. Maximum increase was observed following the administration of terbutaline via inhalation. (From Dulfano MJ, Glass P: The bronchodilator effects of terbutaline: route of administration and patterns of response. Ann Allergy 37:357–366, 1976, with permission.)

by nebulization. In addition, albuterol may be given via a powdered capsule (Rotocaps, Allen & Hanburys) placed in a device called a Rotahaler. In patients who cannot master a metered-dose inhaler, the Rotahaler may be a viable alternative. In choosing between the available aerosol β-receptor agonists one should evaluate the β₂ selectivity, potency, and duration of action (Table 33.3). All other factors may be considered to be equal. However, the duration-of-action values reflect the ability of these products to reverse spontaneous bronchoconstriction in stable asthmatics, which may not truly reflect the length of activity. Bronchoprovocation tests result in a more uniform degree of bronchoconstriction and thus may provide a better means of demonstrating differences between β₂-agonists, although the clinical usefulness of this method of testing has not been clearly established (14).

Using in vitro data, differences in all the β₂-agonists can be demonstrated. From a practical clinical standpoint, albuterol, terbutaline, and fenoterol are probably as potent as isoproterenol in relieving acute bronchospasm, with metaproterenol and the catecholamines being considerably less potent (15). Contrary to some advertisements, the duration of action seems to be about the same for equipotent doses of metaproterenol, albuterol, and bitolterol (16). Terbutaline protects against histamine-induced broncho-

constriction for a longer period than the other agents, but this may not correlate with a longer duration of relief of symptoms.

For the treatment of acute asthmatic symptoms, there is probably little difference between the efficacy of inhaled β₂-agonists. In some patients, if a β₂-receptor agonist is used on a scheduled basis for protection against asthmatic symptoms, two puffs of terbutalie given four times a day is likely to provide greater efficacy than two puffs of albuterol four times a day. This is the recommended dose. However, the recommended dose of any β₂-agonist may not be the optimal dose for a given patient, and an every-4-hr dosing schedule may be required for short periods of time. Abuse of β-agonists has been reported, however. In addition to the side effects already mentioned, patients may experience euphoria or even hallucinations (17). These effects are probably the result of the fluorinated hydrocarbons used as a propellants rather than from the β-agonist. Formoterol, currently under investigation in Europe, has a duration of 8 to 12 hr.

Theophylline

Theophylline has become one of the most frequently reviewed agents in the drug literature. Since the early 1970s, the pharmacodynamics and pharmacokinetics of this drug

Table 33.3.
Adrenergic Stimulants Used in the Treatment of Obstructive Airways Disease[a]

Agent	Route of Administration[a]			Relative Potency	Duration (hr)	Receptor Stimulation		
	Injected	Inhaled	Oral	(Scale of 4)		β₂	β₁	α
Catecholamines								
Ephedrine	−	−	+	1	2–3	+	+	+
Epinephrine	+	+	−	3 (injected[d])	1–2	+	+	+
Isoproterenol	+	+	−	4	2–3	+	+	−
Isoetharine	+	+	−	2+	2–3	+ +	+	−
Rimiterol[b]	+	+	−	2+	2–3	+ +	+	−
Hexoprenaline[b]	+	+	+	2+	2–3	+ +	+	−
Bitolterol[c]	−	+	−	3+	4–6	+ + +	±	−
Resorcinols								
Metaproterenol	+	+	+	3	2–3	+ +	+	−
Terbutaline	+	+	+	4	4–6	+ + +	±	−
Fenoterol[b]	+	+	+	4	4–6	+ + +	±	−
Formeterol[b]	−	+	−	4	8–12	+ + +	±	−
Saligenins								
Albuterol	+	+	+	4	4–6	+ + +	±	−
Carbuterol[b]	+	+	+	3	4	+ + +	+	−
Salmeterol[b]	−	+	−	4	8–12	+ + +	±	−

[a] Not all dosage forms are marketed in the U.S.
[b] Drug not available in U.S.
[c] Active moiety is colterol.
[d] By the inhaled route, epinephrine is the least potent β-agonist, with the shortest duration of action. Available O.T.C. (Primatene-Mist, others).

have been more clearly defined, resulting in safer and more efficacious use. Although this drug has been used as a respiratory stimulant for Cheyne-Stokes respirations, in acute pulmonary edema, and in the treatment of apnea in premature newborns, its major use has been for the prophylactic treatment of chronic asthma. It is a weaker bronchodilator than β₂-receptor agonists and causes more side effects; therefore, it is of limited usefulness for the treatment of acute symptoms.

CHEMISTRY AND PHARMACOLOGY

Theophylline is a dimethylated xanthine that is similar in structure to caffeine and theobromine that are found in coffee, tea, cola beverages, and chocolate. At this time, theophylline is the only xanthine marketed in the United States that has been demonstrated to be effective in treating chronic asthma. Although diphylline, a 7-dihydroxypropyl derivative of theophylline, is available, several studies have shown it to be only 20% as potent as theophylline and thus not a viable alternative to theophylline. Diphylline has markedly different pharmacokinetics and requires a different assay for serum concentration measurements, the results of which have not been correlated with efficacy or toxicity.

Various substances have been added to theophylline to either increase its solubility (i.e., ethylenediamine in

intravenous aminophylline) or improve oral absorption. Since absorption of the methylxanthines relates more to the lipophilic characteristics than to water solubility, and plain theophylline is rapidly, completely, and consistently absorbed orally, there is no rationale for oral formulations that contain ethylenediamine, calcium salicylate, sodium glycinate, choline, or other bases aimed at improving water solubility and thus oral absorption.

The primary effect of theophylline in the treatment of asthma is the prevention of bronchospasm, mucosal edema, and excessive mucus secretion. Inhibition of phosphodiesterase resulting in an increase of 3′, 5′-cyclic AMP (cAMP) was proposed as a mechanism of action. However, this hypothesis is no longer tenable because toxic concentrations would be needed to inhibit phosphodiesterase and not all inhibitors of this enzyme cause bronchodilation (18). Other suggested mechanisms include prostaglandin antagonism, effects on intracellular calcium levels, and increased binding of cAMP to cAMP-binding protein. In addition to effects on the lung, other related pharmacologic actions of theophylline include an increase in right and left ventricular ejection fraction and a reduction in fatigue of the diaphragmatic muscles, which may in turn decrease the work of breathing. Although the clinical relevance of these effects has not been demonstrated, some investigators have proposed that they may offer benefit for patients with chronic obstructive pulmonary disease who do not show a hyperreactive airway component to their disease.

TOXICITY

The major drawback to theophylline therapy is the potential for severe toxicity when inappropriate doses are prescribed. However, when dosed properly, the frequency and severity of the adverse effects of theophylline can be greatly minimized. Upon initiation of therapy, theophylline can cause minor caffeine-like side effects, including some central nervous system stimulation and slight nausea. In an outpatient setting these effects can generally be avoided by starting with low doses and slowly titrating to full therapeutic doses.

More severe and persistent adverse effects are generally associated with serum concentrations above 110 μmol/liter (20 μg/ml) (Fig. 33.3), including hyperglycemia, hypotension, cardiac arrhythmias, seizures, permanent brain damage, and death (19). It must be noted that minor symptoms of toxicity such as nausea and vomiting may not

be a harbinger to more severe toxicity and cannot be relied upon as a dosing end point. In one report, seven of eight patients who developed theophylline-induced seizures had no evidence of any minor side effect of theophylline (20). Only serum theophylline concentration monitoring can reliably predict the potential for severe or life-threatening toxicity.

Acute overdoses from theophylline ingestion in a suicide gesture are generally life-threatening. As in chronic therapy, if seizures occur they are difficult to control and carry a mortality rate as high as 50% (20). Repeated doses of activated charcoal can greatly increase the clearance of theophylline, regardless of the route of administration (21). Charcoal hemoperfusion, which can reduce very high concentrations in a few hours, is recommended for theophylline concentrations above 333 to 388.5 μmol/liter (60 to 70 μg/ml) (19).

CLINICAL USE

Theophylline is considered by some experts to be the athrid-line agent for the prophylaxis of chronic asthma (Fig.

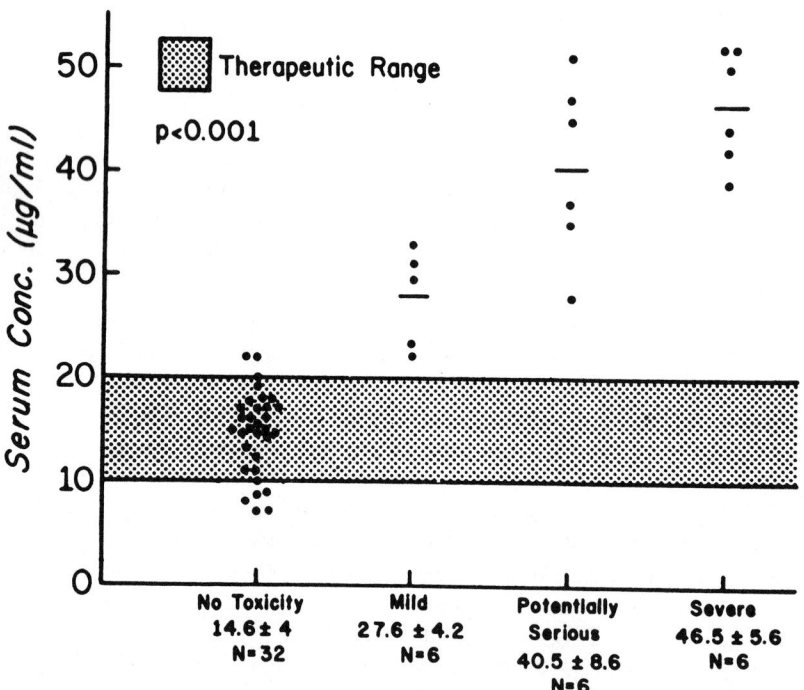

Figure 33.3. Relationship of serum concentration and symptoms of toxicity among 50 adults monitored consecutively in the Medical Intensive Car Unit of the University of Iowa during constant intravenous infusions of theophylline averaging 0.9 mg/kg/hr as aminophylline. Symptoms of toxicity were recorded by a pulmonary physician before the results of the serum concentration measurement became available. Mild toxicity included nausea, vomiting, headache, nervousness, and insomnia. Moderate toxicity consisted of mild symptoms in conjunction with sinus tachycardia and occasional premature ventricular contrac-

tions (PVCs). Patients in the severe category experienced serious arrhythmias such as multiple PVCs or ventricular tachycardia and/or grand mal seizures that occurred in two patients, one of whom died. Previous symptoms of nausea and vomiting or other minor symptoms of toxicity were absent in half of the patients in the moderate and severe categories. (From Hendeles L, Bighley L, Richardson RH, et al.: Frequent toxicity from I.V. aminophylline infusion in critically ill patients. Drug Intell Clin Pharm 11:12–18, 1977, with permission.)

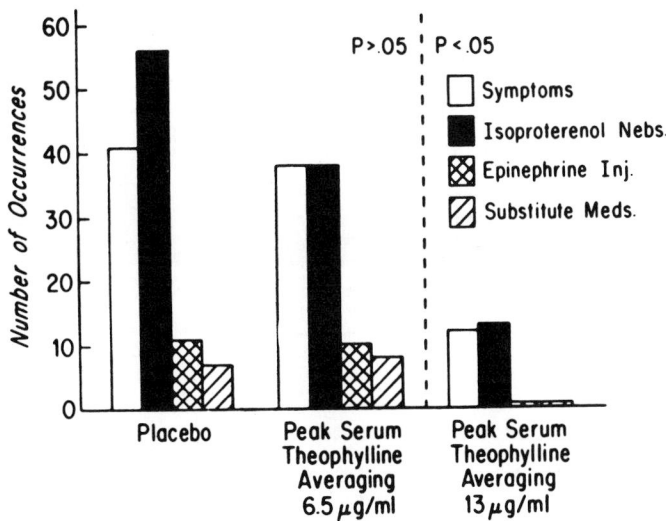

Figure 33.4. Frequency and severity of asthmatic symptoms among 12 children with chronic asthma at a residential treatment center. Each patient received, in a double-blind randomized sequence, 1 week's treatment with placebo, an ephedrine-theophylline combination in conventional doses that resulted in serum theophylline concentrations averaging 36 μmol/liter (6.5 μg/ml), and individualized theophylline doses that resulted in serum concentrations averaging 72 μmol/liter (13 μg/ml). Asthmatic symptoms during each 1-week period were promptly treated, when necessary, with inhaled isoproterenol; if symptoms were not rapidly relieved, subcutaneous epinephrine was administered. If the patient was unresponsive to these measures, known drugs were substituted for the double-blind medications. (Data from Weinberger MM, Bronsky EA: Evaluation of oral bronchodilator therapy in asthmatic children. J Pediatr 84:421–427, 1974.)

33.4). There is increasing evidence that (see "Corticosteroids") inhaled corticosteroids are preferred. In patients with intermittent asthma, prophylactic therapy with theophylline is not the most efficient, effective, or safe means of therapy, regardless of the severity of the symptoms. These patients are treated more effectively with an initial inhaled β-agonist and a short course of oral corticosteroids when symptoms become unresponsive to an inhaled β-agonist.

When used correctly, theophylline can provide a high degree of efficacy with relatively few side effects. However, the narrow therapeutic range and the great variability in rates of metabolism pose a therapeutic challenge.

Various studies have defined the therapeutic range for theophylline as 55 to 110 μmol/liter (10 to 20 μg/ml). In this range, efficacy is optimized, and the chance for toxic effects is minimized. This does not imply that antiasthmatic effects are not seen with serum concentrations below 55 μmol/liter (10 μg/ml). However, studies that argue for an extension of the therapeutic range to 28 to 110 μmol/liter (5 to 20 μg/ml) have not shown that the effect is maximized at lower concentrations nor that fewer side effects are seen (22). Further benefit from serum concentrations 100 μmol/liter (20 μg/ml) may occur but at the risk of toxicity.

Dosing requirements for theophylline vary inversely with the elimination rate. Although the rate of elimination (i.e., $t_{1/2}$) is relatively constant within an individual in a stable clinical setting, variability between patients is great. Consequently, doses must be individualized on the basis of serum concentration measurements.

The initial dose of theophylline is best predicted by using population averages, and subsequent doses by serum concentration monitoring and dose titration. For patients with chronic asthma where there is no urgent need to

attain a therapeutic serum concentration rapidly, the initial dose should be low (e.g., 400 mg/day for adults and 16 mg/kg/day for children over 1 year old) and titrated upward slowly over a 9- to 10-day period to the median dose for the age of the patient (Fig. 33.5). These median doses will result in concentrations below 55 μmol/liter (10 μg/ml) in 30% of patients and concentrations above 110 μmol/liter (20 μg/ml) in 20% of patients. The final dose adjustment must be based on a serum concentration measurement. This slow titration procedure can avoid caffeine-like side effects in more than 90% of patients.

When rapid attainment of therapeutic theophylline concentrations is desired (e.g., status asthmaticus) an intravenous loading dose is indicated (although an oral liquid can be used) under the following guidelines (19):

1. Give 5 mg/kg of theophylline intravenously over 20 to 30 min if the patient has not received theophylline in the past 24 hr.
2. Give 2.4 mg/kg of theophylline intravenously over 20 to 30 min if the patient has received theophylline within the past 24 hr and there is insufficient time to obtain an immediate serum concentration.
3. If the serum concentration is measured initially, then 1 mg/kg of theophylline can be given for every 11 μmol/liter (2 μg/ml) rise in serum concentration desired (this assumes an average volume of distribution of 0.5 liter/kg).

Following this, if a constant intravenous infusion of theophylline is required, dosing should be based on age and concurrent disease (Table 33.4). Therapy can be individualized quickly and accurately using the appropriate equations (23).

When determining the dose of theophylline, the factors that can influence how theophylline is handled in the body must be considered. Several drugs and diseases alter the clearance of theophylline (Table 33.5), and their pres-

Figure 33.5. Scheme for establishing optimal oral theophylline dosage in ambulatory patients. (Adapted from information appearing in *NEJM*. Weinberger MM, Hendeles L: Slow-release theophylline, rationale and basis for product selection. N Engl J Med 308:760–764, 1983, with permission.)

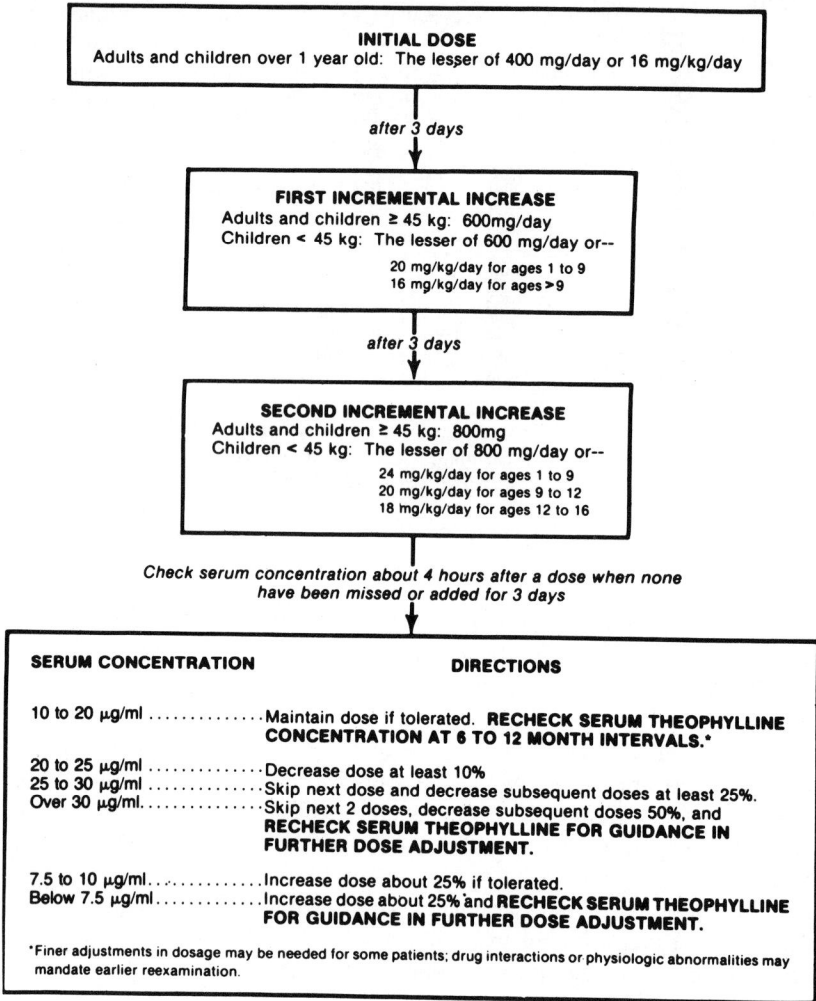

ence requires careful dose adjustment based upon serum concentration measurements.

PRODUCT SELECTION

Over 150 theophylline-containing products are currently available in the United States. Only single-entity theophylline products are recommended in the treatment of asthma. Ephedrine-containing combination products that previously dominated the market cause an increased frequency of adverse effects as a result of the synergistic toxicity of the combination, with no added therapeutic benefit.

Selection of a theophylline product is based on the specific clinical indication and the expected pharmacokinetics of the patient. The goal is to maintain serum concentrations within the therapeutic range for the entire dosing interval.

There are no clinically important differences between the rapid-release oral formulations available, and thus these can be used interchangeably. Plain, uncoated theophylline tablets or alcohol-free oral liquid is preferred.

These products are used most often in infants and children who are unable to swallow a sustained-release product or in some nonsmoking adults with slow elimination who have an acceptable peak-trough fluctuation on an every-8-hr interval.

Rectal solutions offer a convenient alternative in patients who tend to vomit medication for reasons other than theophylline toxicity during acute exacerbations of asthma or for patients fasting before surgery. Rectal administration should not exceed 24 to 36 hr to avoid local irritation from this very alkaline solution.

Slow-release theophylline products are designed to maintain serum concentrations within the therapeutic range around the clock, by minimizing peak-trough fluctuations in serum concentrations, while allowing dosing intervals that are compatible with normal lifestyles (i.e., no shorter than every 8 hr). Presently, 15 brands of slow-release theophylline formulations with varying absorption profiles are available, under 29 brand names (Table 33.6). They differ in the rate and sometimes in the extent of absorption and thus are not interchangeable. Of these

Table 33.4.
Initial Intravenous Theophylline Maintenance Dosages[a]

Patient Population	Age	Theophylline Infusion Rate (mg/kg/hr)[b,c]
Neonates	Postnatal age up to 24 days	1 mg/kg q 12 hr[d]
	Postnatal age beyond 24 days	1.5 mg/kg q 12 hr[d]
	6–52 weeks old	mg/kg/hr = (0.008) (age in weeks) + 0.21
Young children	1–9 years old	0.8
Older children	9–12 years old	0.7
Adolescents (cigarette or marijuana smokers)	12–16 years old	0.7
Adolescents (nonsmokers)	12–16 years old	0.5[e]
Adults (otherwise healthy cigarette or marijuana smokers)	16–50 years old	0.7[e]
Adults (otherwise healthy nonsmokers)	Beyond 16 years old (including the elderly)	0.4[e]
Adults with cardiac decompensation, cor pulmonale, or liver dysfunction (or a combination of these factors)	Beyond 16 years	0.2[f]

[a] Adapted from Hendeles L, Weinberger M: Theophylline, "a state of art" review. Pharmacotherapy 3:2–44, 1983.

[b] Assumes an appropriate loading dose has been given. To achieve a target concentration of 55 μmol/liter (10 μg/ml). Aminophylline = theophylline/0.8. Use lean body weight for obese patients. While these doses are generally safe, many patients will require higher infusion rates as determined by serial serum measurements. These dosages differ from the current FDA recommendations, which include a higher infusion rate for the first 12 hr.

[c] Further dosage reductions may be required for patients receiving other drugs (i.e., cimetidine) that decrease theophylline clearance.

[d] For a target concentration of 42 μmol/liter (7.5 μg/ml) (for neonatal apnea).

[e] Not to exceed 900 mg/day unless serum levels indicate the need for a larger dose.

[f] Not to exceed 400 mg/day unless serum levels indicate the need for a larger dose.

products only Theo-Dur and Slo-Bid are absorbed slowly enough to be dosed on an every-12-hr basis in nearly all individuals (24). Other products must be dosed at least every 8 hr (especially in patients who metabolize the drug rapidly) to ensure minimal peak-trough fluctuations (24). Factors such as circadian variation in absorption (25) and the administration of slow-release products with meals affect some formulations, while having little effect on others (Fig. 33.6).

Recently, three products were approved by the FDA for once-a-day dosing. Evidence suggests that unacceptable fluctuations in serum concentrations are likely if TheoDur (Key Pharmaceuticals) is given once a day in patients with average or rapid metabolism (27).

In contrast Theo-24 (Searle) is absorbed slowly enough when taken by a fasting patient to achieve acceptable fluctuations with once-a-day dosing in most subjects (23, 28). However, only 71 to 78% of the dose is absorbed under fasting conditions, thereby requiring higher doses (26). When Theo-24 is given with food, "dose dumping" occurs, which can result in potentially toxic theophylline concentrations (26).

Similarly, T-Phyl (Purdue Frederick) is only 55 to 65% absorbed when taken by a fasting subject; however, food increases the extent of absorption to about 80%, without affecting the rate of absorption. Thus serum levels increase slowly after multiple doses of T-Phyl taken with food.

In addition to the shortcomings of the individual products, there is insufficient evidence to support the contention that once-a-day dosing results in improved compliance over twice-a-day dosing. At this time once-a-day dosing seems to be more a marketing ploy than a breakthrough in pharmaceutical technology.

Cromolyn Sodium

Cromolyn, also known as cromolyn sodium or (di)sodium comoglycate, was synthesized in 1965 as part of an effort to improve upon the known bronchodilator potential of khellin, a naturally occurring chromone. This drug has gained wide acceptance in other countries, and although its acceptance in the United States has been slow, there has been a gradual increase in its use as a first-line drug for the prevention of chronic asthma (29).

CHEMISTRY AND PHARMACOLOGY

Cromolyn blocks the release of the chemical mediators of the type I(IgE-related) hypersensitivity reactions. It appears to do this through direct activity at the mast cell

Table 33.5.
Factors Reported to Affect Theophylline Elimination

Increase Elimination (Decrease $t_{1/2}$)	Decrease Elimination (Increase $t_{1/2}$)
Smoking (cigarettes or marijuana)	Hepatic cirrhosis
Phenobarbital	Cor pulmonale
High-protein/low-carbohydrate diet	Congestive heart failure
Charcoal-broiled beef	Fever
Phenytoin	Propranolol
Carbamazepine	Allopurinol (>600 mg/day)
Rifampin	Erythromycin
Isoproterenol	Cimetidine
	Troleandomycin
	Oral contraceptives
	Quinolone antibiotics
	Verapamil
	Thiabendazole

[a] Adapted from Hendeles L, Weinberger M: Theophylline, "a state of art" review. Pharmacotherapy 3:2–44, 1983.

Table 33.6.

Extent of Absorption and Predicted Fluctuations in Serum Concentrations during a 12-hour Dose Interval of Various Slow-Release Theophylline Products[a]

Manufacturer	Brand Name	Extent of Absorption (%)	Fluctuation[b] $t_{1/2} + 3.7$ hr	$t_{1/2} = 8$ hr
Plain tablets				
Rorer, Johnson & Johnson, Riker	Slo-Phyllin, Theophyl, Theolair	100	465	125
Bead-filled capsules				
Central Pharmacal	Physpan			
	Quibron-BID			
	Theoclear LA	95	240	73
	Theon-300			
	Theospan-SR			
Cord Laboratories	Bronkodyl S-R			
	Slo-Phyllin Gyrocaps	99	230	73
Graham Laboratories	Aerolate			
	Somophyllin-CRT	101	130	47
K-V Laboratories	Elixophyllin SR			
	Theobid	94	140	54
	Theovent-LA	94	167	60
Rorer	Slo-bid	101	43	18
Searle	Theo-24	71/100[c]	[d]	[d]
Schering	Theo-Dur Sprinkle	91/44 [c]	[d]	[d]
Slow-release tablets				
Cord Laboratories	Constant-T	76	155	57
Mead Johnson	Quibron T/SR	99	128	48
Mundipharma	Phyllocontin	95	165	58
Norwich-Eaton	LaBID	87	252	77
Parke-Davis	Choledyl SA	93	154	57
Purdue Frederick	T-Phyl	61/83 [c]	[e]	[e]
Riker	Theolair-SR, Respbid	99	[f]	[f]
Schering	Theo-Dur 200, 300	97	39	17
	Theo-Dur 100	103	88	35
	Uni-Dur	94	29	58[g]

[a] Adapted from Hendeles L, Weinberger M: J Allergy Clin Immunol 1985;76:285–291.

[b] Percentage fluctuation = (Peak − trough serum concentration)/Trough serum concentration × 100; actual fluctuations may somewhat exceed predictions because of circadian variation in absorption. The $t_{1/2}$ value is the median value for the average child (3.7 hours) or otherwise healthy nonsmoking adult (8 hr). Fluctuations >100% indicate that peak serum concentrations will be more than double the trough level and thus not compatible with maintaining serum concentrations within the therapeutic range even if peak levels as high as 110 μmol/liter (20 μg/ml) are attained; 8-hr intervals are then advisable, regardless of advertising claims for twice-daily or 12-hr dosing.

[c] Extent of absorption when taken fasting and with food, respectively.

[d] Because rate and completeness of absorption change with food, meaningful predictions of fluctuations cannot be made.

[e] Measured fluctuations at steady state with once-daily dosing in subjects with mean $t_{1/2} = 8.3$ hr were 232% fasting and 109% (range 22% to 240%) after food.

[f] pH-dependent dissolution may alter the rate of absorption depending on gastric pH and emptying. Therefore, meaningful predictions of fluctuations cannot be made.

[g] In one study of 18 adults (11 of whom smoked) with a mean $t_{1/2} = 6.4$ hr, fluctuations averaged 139% (44–415) with Uni-dur 600 mg q24h compared with 72% (range 39–127) with Theo-dur 300 mg q12h.

surface, only when the cell is exposed to cromolyn prior to antigen exposure. It does not interfere with the antigen-antibody interaction, nor does it oppose the action of the mediators once they are released. Instead, the mast cells simply do not degranulate and thus do not release the pharmacologically active substances that mediate allergen-induced asthma. The effect of cromolyn is nonspecific, and it blocks the nonimmunologic stimulation of mediator release from mast cells that results from exposure in vitro to such compounds as phospholipase A, dextran, and polymyxin B.

The mechanism by which cromolyn sodium inhibits mediator release at the cellular level is still unclear. A proposed mechanism is that it stabilizes the mast cell membrane during the antigen-dependent, calcium-dependent, activation stage of mediator release by affecting membrane or cytoplasmic control of "calcium gating" (29). The calcium transmembrane flux is regulated either by the binding affinity of cromolyn for the calcium cation at the surface or by binding to a basophilic membrane protein.

Other investigators have suggested that cromolyn acts on the irritant receptors in the airways, which could reduce

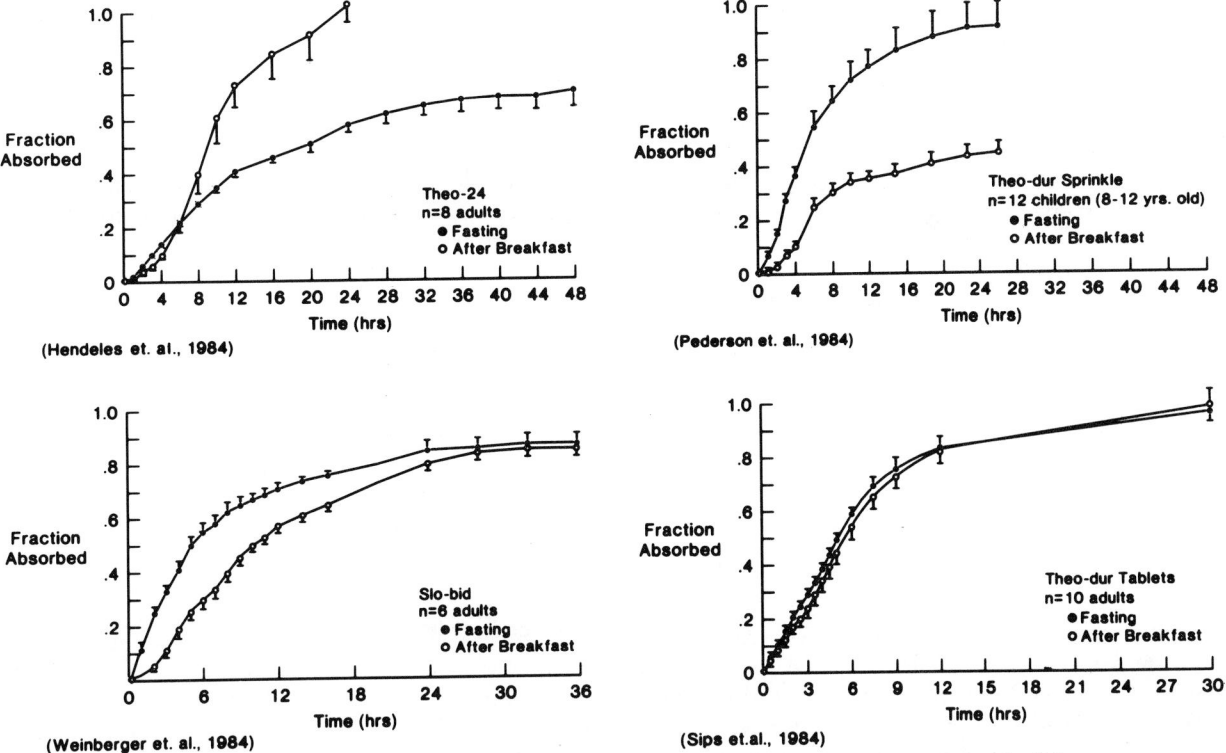

Figure 33.6. The effect of food on the bioavailability of four slow-release theophylline products. Theo-24 (*top left*), food increases both rate and extent of absorption (26). With Theo-Dur Sprinkle (*top right*), food decreases both rate and extent of absorption (57). Slo-Bid (*bottom left*), food decreases rate, while the extent of absorption remains the same (58). Theo-Dur tablets (*bottom right*) neither the rate nor extent of absorption are altered by food to a clinically important degree (59).

the vagal reflex pathways for bronchospasm (30, 31). This theory would explain the clinical efficacy of cromolyn in preventing asthmatic symptoms in nonallergic individuals.

ABSORPTION/FATE/EXCRETION

Less than 1% of a cromolyn dose is absorbed after oral administration. When administered by inhalation using a turboinhaler device (Spinhaler) for powder insufflation, only about 75% of the dose is delivered to the patient. Of that, only 10% reaches the peripheral airways, where it is rapidly eliminated by systemic absorption. The remainder is deposited in the mouth and pharynx, swallowed, and passed intact in the stool. The absorbed fraction is eliminated rapidly in bile and urine, with a biological half-life of 46 to 99 min. No biotransformation occurs.

TOXICITY

Cromolyn is the least toxic of all medications used for asthma. The 50% lethal dose (LD_5O) in rodents and primates is greater than 1000 mg/kg parenterally, as compared with the usual inhaled dose of 20 mg, of which less than 0.1 mg/kg is absorbed (32). No clinically important

adverse effects from cromolyn were detected in a large multicenter study of its long-term safety.

The most common adverse effects from cromolyn given as the powder are transient bronchospasm and cough, and dryness of the throat. The former may be avoided by concurrent administration of an inhaled β-agonist and the latter may be avoided by drinking water before and after inhalation or by switching to the metered dose inhaler or nebulized solution. Anaphylaxis, generalized or facial dermatitis, myositis, gastroenteritis, and immunologic reactions in the lung (granuloma) have been reported very rarely.

CLINICAL USE

Cromolyn is of value exclusively as a prophylactic medication for chronic asthma. It has no bronchodilating effect and is not appropriate for the treatment of acute asthmatic symptoms. The most important advantage of this drug is its safety. Unfortunately, there are no reliable means of identifying cromolyn "responders." Initial expectations of benefit only in "extrinsic" or allergic asthma have not been supported in controlled trials; patients with nonallergic asthma respond equally well.

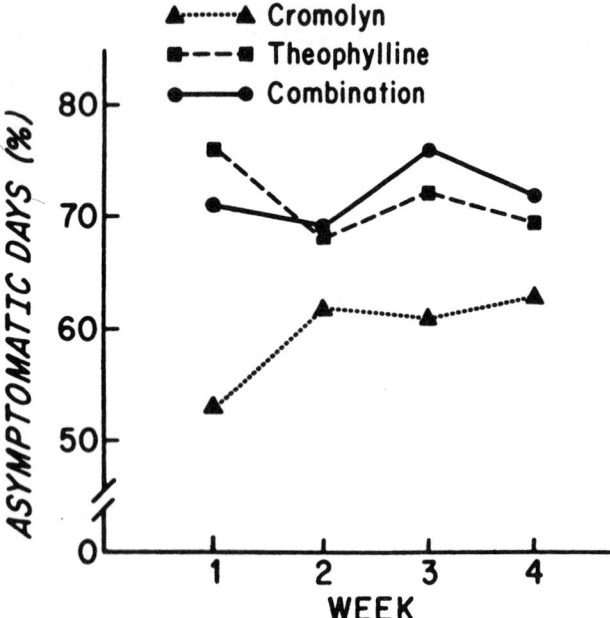

Figure 33.7. Frequency of asymptomatic days in 28 asthmatic children treated in a double-bind randomized manner for 4 weeks each with doses of theophylline that achieved a peak serum concentration in the 55 to 110 μmol/liter (10 to 20 μg/ml) therapeutic range, cromolyn 20 mg q.i.d. by spinhaler, and the combination. While significant differences between cromolyn and theophylline were observed (p < .025), differences between weeks during the same regimen were not significant for any of the three patients (33).

Most clinicians believe that cromolyn sodium is more effective in patients with mild-to-moderate asthma. In comparisons with slow-release theophylline preparation in these patients, results are mixed. Some studies have shown the theophylline group to have more symptom-free days (33) (Fig. 33.7), whereas in others no differences between the two treatments were found (34, 35). In most cases, cromolyn had fewer side effects, but the dose of theophylline in those studies was not titrated slowly as recommended. In comparison with regularly scheduled inhaled terbutaline, peak flow measurements, cough, and airway reactivity to methacholine have shown greater improvement with cromolyn alone or with the combination of cromolyn and terbutaline (36).

In some situations, such as patients with seizure disorders, active peptic ulcer disease, migraine headache, or intolerance to theophylline even at low serum concentrations, cromolyn may be preferred over theophylline.

The usual starting dose is one 20-mg capsule taken four times a day by inhalation with the turboinhaler or two puffs (2 mg) four times a day using the metered-dose inhaler. The frequency of dosing can be reduced to every 8 hr in some patients, whereas every-4-hr dosing may be required in others. A full trial on the drug should last at least 6 weeks, although improvement generally can be seen after 1 to 2 weeks. Proper inhalation technique is required to ensure delivery of the drug to the lungs.

PRODUCT SELECTION

In most individuals, the 20-mg cromolyn capsule given by inhalation via the turboinhaler is well accepted. Cromolyn is also available as a metered-dose inhaler in 8.1-g (112 metered sprays) and 14.2-g (200 metered sprays) sizes. This offers the patient the convenience of a metered-dose inhaler and may be of benefit in those experiencing a dry mouth or bronchospasm from the powdered capsule. Some evidence exists that 20 mg by the Spinhaler may provide greater protection against exercise-induced asthma than 2 puffs (2 mg) by the MD1 (37). For young children or others who cannot use these devices properly even when used with a spacing device, the nebulizer solution is a safe and effective alternative.

Corticosteroids

Soon after the beneficial effects of cortisone in rheumatoid arthritis were reported, corticosteroids were introduced for the treatment of asthma. As experience with these agents increased, corticosteroids were quickly recognized as a valuable adjunct in the management of this disease. Only after use of these agents increased did the large array of adverse effects (especially after prolonged administration) become evident.

Corticosteroids are uniquely effective for bronchodilator-unresponsive symptoms. Modification of the corticosteroid molecule and improved methods of administration have helped to minimize the adverse effects.

CHEMISTRY AND PHARMACOLOGY

The corticosteroids useful in the treatment of asthma have a heterocyclic carbon nucleus with potent glucocorticoid and antiinflammatory effects. In general, all corticosteroids act through the same cellular mechanisms. Circulating, unbound steroids (25%) can easily pass through cellular membranes and bind to specific cytoplasmic receptors. This combination moves to the nucleus, where new mRNA is synthesized. The result is new protein synthesis, which may alter cellular function.

Corticosteroids may affect β-adrenergic receptors, adenylate cyclase and cAMP, leukocyte distribution, inflammation, IgE synthesis, mast cells, basophils, and mediators. Hydrocortisone increases the number of β-adrenergic receptors both in vitro and in vivo (38). These effects are seen 4 hr after administration of corticosteroids, with maximal effects occurring within 24 hr. Corticosteroids increase cAMP levels, increase adenyl cyclase activity, and decrease the number of lymphocytes entering the blood stream and arriving at a site of inflammation. Numbers of monocytes, eosinophils, and basophils are also reduced, while the circulating neutrophil pool is increased.

The primary effect of corticosteroids in asthma is inhibition of the arachidonic acid cascade (Fig. 33.8). Corticosteroids stimulate the production of an intercellular protein, lipomodulin, which prevents all arachnoid formation. Therefore, the release of prostaglandins, hydroxyeicosatetraenoic acid (HETE), and the leukotrienes, all mediators in asthma, is inhibited. Finally, corticosteroids suppress mucus secretion by both spontaneous and secretogogue-stimulated release. The effects of corticosteroids on IgE production, mast cell degranulation, and reduction in histamine resynthesis are not likely to be important in the treatment of asthma. The antiinflammatory effects of glucocorticoids are associated with suppression of the redness, heat, pain, and swelling of the acute inflammatory reaction. They appear to do this by inhibiting neutrophil influx through reduced margination, reduced sticking of the neutrophils to endothelial walls, and inhibition of chemotaxis. Corticosteroids also seem to inhibit lysozymal enzyme release.

ABSORPTION/FATE/EXCRETION

Corticosteroids can be administered parenterally, orally, or topically. Phosphate and hemisuccinate conjugates suitable for both intravenous and intramuscular administration are absorbed rapidly and reach plasma concentrations similar to those following administration of the unconjugated steroids. Acetate derivatives frequently used as depot injections are absorbed over a long period of time and have no place in the treatment of asthma. Oral absorption of corticosteroids such as prednisone and prednisolone occurs quite rapidly, depending on the product. Absorption from topical administration varies widely with the steroid used. Betamethasone and dexamethasone appear to be absorbed efficiently from the lungs and capable of causing systemic effects. In contrast, triamcinolone acetonide, beclomethasone dipropionate, flunisolide, budesonide, and fluticasone (the latter two are under investigation in the U.S.) are active topically and either are poorly absorbed in the active form or, once absorbed systemically, are rapidly inactivated.

The onset and duration of action of corticosteroids depends on the effect being monitored and the dose used. Within 2 hr after an oral dose of prednisone or intravenous prednisolone there is a fall in numbers of circulating eosinophils and lymphocytes that may last for 12 to 72 hr (39). The onset of hypothalamic-pituitary-adrenal axis suppression occurs within minutes to hours after a single dose and may take up to 24 to 48 hr for restoration. Reversal of airway obstruction occurs roughly 4 to 12 hr after dosing, with the duration of effect increasing with the dose (40). The delay in the onset of effects from corticosteroids is consistent with the indirect mechanism of steroid action,

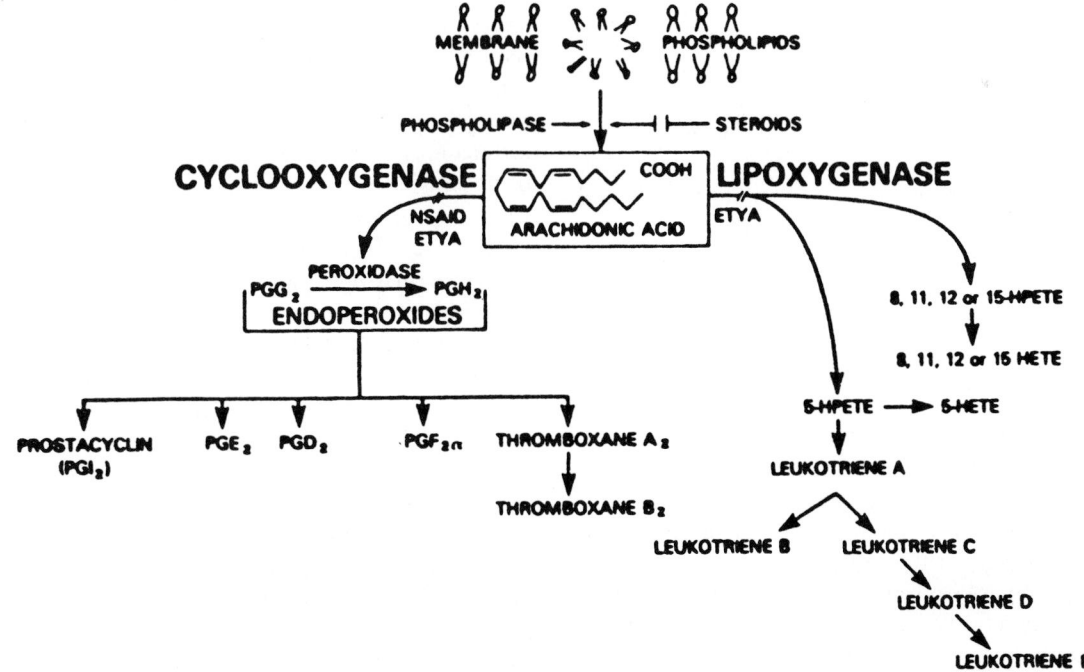

Figure 33.8. The arachidonic acid cascade. Arachidonic acid is the pivotal point for two important enzymatic pathways: cyclooxygenase and lipoxygenase. Various drugs affect this cascade. Corticosteroids inhibit the release of arachidonic acid from membrane phospholipids by stimulating the synthesis of a polypeptide, lipomodulin, that inhibits the enzyme phospholipase A_2. (From Kaliner M: Mechanisms of glucocorticosteroid action in bronchial asthma. J Allergy Clin Immunol 76:321–329, 1985.)

which involves the synthesis of new protein that inhibits formation of inflammatory mediators.

TOXICITY

Adverse effects from corticosteroids vary from severe to inconsequential. The frequency and severity of the adverse effects are influenced by the route, frequency, duration, total dose, albumin and transcortin concentrations, preexisting diseases, and specific properties of the agent being used. The duration of therapy seems to be the most important variable for serious adverse effects.

The side effects can be classified into systemic and local effects. There are virtually no risks of long-term toxicity with short-term (less than 2 weeks) use of daily oral or parenteral corticosteroids (41). However, psychosis, hyperglycemia, hypokalemia, and gastrointestinal bleeding may occur. The risks from long-term use of oral corticosteroids can be minimized by administering the shorter-acting agents (e.g., prednisone, prednisolone, or methylprednisolone) on an every-other-morning schedule. However, when used in large doses for long periods of time, alternate-day drug therapy can still result in all of the serious side effect noted. (See Chapter 15 "Adrenal Dysfunction and Clinical Use of Corticosteroids.")

Systemic side effects can be virtually eliminated by using inhaled corticosteroids. Doses up to 1.6 mg/day of beclomethasone or the equivalent are not associated with clinically important systemic side effects (42), although some suppression of the hypothalamic-pituitary-adrenal axis may occur. A budesonide dose of 1.0 mg/day (higher than doses currently being studied in the U.S.) produces the same systemic effect on serum cortisol as approximately 8 mg/day of prednisone (43). Local adverse effects from inhaled steroids include primarily thrush and dysphonia. These effects rarely lead to stopping therapy and can be minimized by rinsing the mouth after administration or by the use of extension devices for the inhalers.

CLINICAL USE

Corticosteroids are the only currently available antiasthmatic agents that can reverse the bronchodilator-unresponsive inflammatory component of asthmatic airway obstruction. They do not inhibit exercise-induced bronchospasm, nor do they inhibit experimental bronchospasm provoked by inhalation of methacholine or histamine. In patients with allergic asthma, continuous use of steroids during the pollen season can decrease airway reactivity.

The indication for the use of corticosteroids in asthma is the loss of response to bronchodilators. Although corticosteroids do not produce immediate benefit in the treatment of acute asthma, there is general agreement that their use hastens recovery and may diminish morbidity in these patients (39). In one study, acute asthmatics discharged

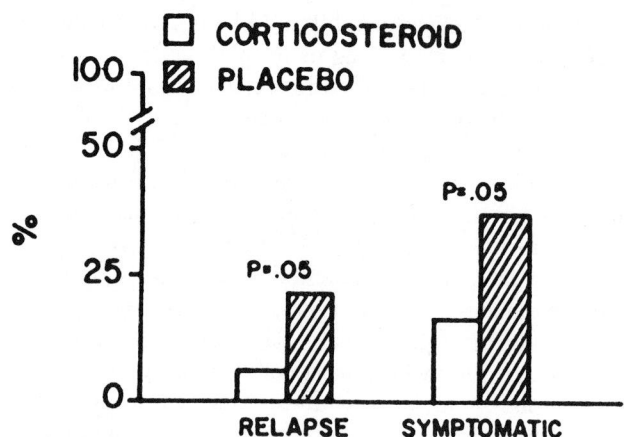

Figure 33.9. Comparison of outcomes for patients discharged on a controlled regimen of theophylline and randomly receiving either placebo or an intravenous bolus of methylprednisolone followed by an 8-day tapering dose of oral methylprednisolone, starting at 32 mg twice a day. The relapse rates (episodes followed by return to an emergency facility) and the number of episodes in which the patient was "symptomatic" at follow-up were significantly better in the corticosteroid treated group. (From Feil SB, Swartz MA, Glanz K, et al.: Efficacy of short-term corticosteroid therapy in outpatient treatment of acute bronchial asthma. Am J Med 75:259–262, 1983.)

on oral theophylline regimens received either oral steroids or placebo, randomly. Both the relapse rate and symptoms at follow-up were significantly decreased in the corticosteroid-treated group (Fig. 33.9). Recent evidence in pediatric patients suggests that prompt initiation of oral steroids at the first sign of a respiratory infection (which can precipitate severe asthma) can reduce the number of asthma episodes by 50% (44). In a second study, the use of an inhaled corticosteroid (budesonide) was compared with a β_2-agonist, terbutaline, in newly detected asthmatics (45). Results indicated that budesonide was more effective as first-line therapy in mild asthmatics than terbutaline.

Empirically determined doses of prednisone used for the treatment of acute symptoms are 10 mg for infants under 1 year, 20 mg for toddlers from 1 to 3 years old, 30 mg for children from 3 years to adolescence, and 40 to 60 mg for adolescents and adults. Once- or twice-daily oral administration of these doses is adequate for ambulatory patients. Hospitalized patients with more serious dyspnea may need more frequent administration of parenteral corticosteroids.

The recommended dose of parenteral corticosteroids for both adults and children is controversial. Doses equivalent to the oral prednisone dose above are used, but much larger doses are advocated by some clinicians, although the superiority of the higher doses is not documented. Parenteral steroids are given more frequently, usually every 6 hr, but every-4-hr dosing may be required, especially when there is concern of impending respiratory failure. Once the acute symptoms have been relieved, daily corticosteroids can usually be discontinued. Tapering over 2 weeks is advisable if steroid treatment was required for >14 days. With shorter courses of therapy, tapering only increases the risk of steroid toxicity by prolonging exposure to the drug. If there is concern that abrupt discontinuation of steroids would result in the exacerbation of asthmatic symptoms, the patient should be changed to alternate-day therapy with prednisone rather than tapering daily doses.

Patients with chronic asthma controlled inadequately by bronchodilators or cromolyn, who repeatedly develop symptoms that do not clear after an inhaled β_2-receptor agonist, and who require frequent emergency care for their asthma should be considered for chronic corticosteroid therapy. Once the airway obstruction is cleared by an oral regimen of steroids, the patient should be converted to alternate-day therapy or an inhaled agent. A patient is converted to alternate-day steroid by increments of no more than 5 mg prednisone/day. For example, a patient requiring 20 mg prednisone/day would follow the schedule outlined in Table 33.7. Once complete control is attained for more than a month, a cautious reduction in dose, such as 5 mg/dose for prednisone, at intervals no shorter than 1 to 2 weeks, is recommended to establish the minimal dose of corticosteroids necessary to keep the patient free of symptoms. If asthmatic symptoms increase, the dose should be increased to a previous dose that kept the patient relatively symptom-free, further tapering should be postponed, and a more gradual taper adopted. If patients are placed on an inhaled steroid, they are also maintained on the oral steroid for about 2 weeks. The inhaled steroid is begun at a dose proportional to the dose of oral steroid. After the 2 weeks of combined therapy, the oral prednisone may be tapered slowly. Most patients can discontinue systemic steroids. After the systemic steroids are discontinued, the inhaled steroid may be tapered slowly (e.g., at a rate of 50 mg of beclomethasone) at intervals of 1 to 2 weeks until the lowest effective dose that maintains control is determined.

For intermittent or seasonal asthmatics a short course of prednisone (up to 10 days) may be necessary to clear a bronchodilator-unresponsive event. Under these circumstances, the likelihood of adverse effects is minimal. However, when short courses become necessary more than once every other month, chronic administration as alternate-day or inhaled corticosteroid therapy will be required to provide benefit while minimizing toxicity.

Recent developments in the pathophysiology of asthma indicate that the chronicity of the disease is due to an inflammatory process. In Europe and Canada, inhaled corticosteroids are being investigated as second-line agents inpatients with mild chronic asthma. One-year treatment with budesonide (400 μg daily) significantly decreased airway reactivity asthma symptoms, and bronchodilator use in patients with mild asthma (46). In the U.S., inhaled steroids are recommended as second-line agents for patients with chronic moderate-to-severe asthma. Patients who are not controlled on PRN β_2-agonists should receive inhaled steroids (46a).

Currently, no corticosteroids are approved for administration by nebulization. Dexamethasone is active topically when given by nebulization, but enough is absorbed across the lung membranes to cause systemic effects. Methylprednisolone sodium succinate has little topical effect when given by nebulization and can cause systemic adverse effects. Administration of the intranasal corticosteroid solutions or suspensions via nebulization have been reported by some clinicians to clog the nebulizer.

PRODUCT SELECTION

In most patients with asthma who require oral corticosteroid therapy, a short-acting preparation such as prednisone, prednisolone, or methylprednisolone is preferred. These agents have a decreased potential for adverse effects, compared with those with longer half-lives. Since prednisone must be converted to prednisolone to become active, there would seem to be no reason to use prednisone. However, prednisone is equally effective clinically, and is much less expensive than either prednisolone or methylprednisolone. A liquid form of prednisone at a concentration of 1 mg/ml is also available for oral use, but it is not very palatable. Crushing a prednisone tablet and mixing it with jam is acceptable to children too small to swallow tablets whole.

When parenteral corticosteroids are indicated, methylprednisolone should be used (rather than hydrocortisone) because of its lower cost. It has fewer mineralocorticoid effects than hydrocortisone, but this is unlikely to be clinically significant. Parenteral steroids that contain

Table 33.7.
Example of How to Switch a Patient to Every-Other-Day Prednisone

Day	Dose (mg)
1	20
2	25
3	15
4	30
5	10
6	35
7	5
8	40
9	0
10	45

metabisulfites should not be used in asthmatics, since the sulfite can induce bronchospasm in the susceptible individual.

There are currently three aerosol corticosteroids available for use in the United States: beclomethasone dipropionate (BDP), triamcinolone acetonide (TAA), and flunisolide (FLN). Many studies have compared these agents with placebo or other asthma therapies or established their ability to decrease oral steroid use. Comparative studies of these agents are nonexistent. Several studies comparing beclomethasone and budesonide have found similar efficacies and adverse effects. There are certain pharmacologic differences between the aerosol corticosteroids. However, to date, none of these differences has translated into any clinically important advantage or disadvantage of one product over another. All are effective when given twice a day in mild-to-moderate asthmatics, however four doses per day are usually required in patients with more severe disease (47, 48). With the maximum recommended daily doses, beclomethasone (Beclovent, Vanceril) may be 50% more expensive than triamcinolone (Azmacort or flunisolide (Aerobid).

Other aerosol corticosteroid products include a recently released BDP metered-dose inhaler in the United Kingdom, with a higher dose per actuation (250 μg/actuation). Also available outside the United States is a powdered aerosol of BDP actuated by inspiration (rotohaler) and marketed to improve patient compliance with aerosol devices. Finally, an investigational 16α, 17α-acetal corticosteroid (budesonide) and a trifluorinated corticosteroid (fluticasone), both with 5 to 10 times higher antiinflammatory activity than BDP, are currently being evaluated. Budesonide metered-dose inhaler is available in several European countries and Canada, under the trade name Pulmicort.

Anticholinergic Agents

The treatment of asthma-like conditions by inhaling smoke from burning stramonium leaves was described as early as the 17th century. The use of stramonium or belladonna inhalation therapy spread throughout Europe and the United States until the introduction of the safer and more effective β-sympathomimetic agents in the middle of the 20th century. Considerable advances in the understanding of autonomic control of the airways coupled with the development of an aerosolized atropine derivative, ipratropium bromide, has renewed interest in anticholinergic therapy for pulmonary diseases.

CHEMISTRY AND PHARMACOLOGY

Anticholinergic bronchodilators are competitive antagonists of acetylcholine at the muscarinic receptor of the parasympathetic postganglionic effector-cell junctions. Atropine is the classic anticholinergic agent whose activity is believed to be highly specific for the muscarinic receptor. The parasympathetic (versus the sympathetic) nervous system is largely responsible for the control of baseline airway caliber. Stimulation of the distal end of cut vagal nerves in animals results in bronchoconstriction that can be prevented with atropine. The airway narrowing is due to smooth muscle contraction rather than to mucosal edema or mucus production and is believed to occur predominantly in the large central airways. In experiments of laboratory-induced bronchoconstriction, ipratropium bromide provides the greatest protection against methacholine, a parasympathomimetic, with variable or no protection against histamine-, allergen-, bradykinin-, or serotonin-induced bronchospasm. In addition, ipratropium bromide affords no clinically important protection against exercise-induced bronchoconstriction. Although less effective than β2-receptor-selective agonists, it does produce significant bronchodilation (49).

Anticholinergic agents available for respiratory use include the tertiary ammonium compound, atropine, and two quaternary ammonium compounds, ipratropium bromide (Atrovent) and glycopyrrolate (Robinul), although the latter is not approved for use in asthma (50).

ABSORPTION/FATE/EXCRETION

Atropine is absorbed rapidly from the respiratory and gastrointestinal mucosa, and peak concentrations are reached in approximately 1 hr. Its large volume of distribution indicates wide distribution throughout the body, including the central nervous system and breast milk. The elimination half-life is approximately 3 hr in adults but may be longer in children and the elderly. Elimination is primarily by the kidneys, occurring with 24 hr.

Ipratropium bromide is absorbed poorly (approximately 30%) from and reexcreted rapidly by the gastrointestinal tract. Absorption following inhalation is minimal as a result of the quaternary ammonium structure, with peak concentrations of 0.06 ng/ml following inhalation of 555 μg.

One to 6 hr after intravenous administration of radiolabeled drug in the rat, the greatest activity is found in the gastrointestinal tract, liver, and kidneys, with minimal concentrations in the brain, lung, and muscle. The volume of distribution in humans has not been elucidated.

Most of an inhaled dose is swallowed and excreted unchanged in the stool. Eighty-seven percent of the small amount that is systemically absorbed is metabolized to eight metabolites that possess either minimal anticholinergic activity or are inactive in vitro. The remainder is eliminated unchanged in the urine. The elimination half-life of ipratropium bromide is about 3 hr.

TOXICITY

The adverse effects from atropine are dose-related. At low dosages (0.5 mg absorbed dose), dry mouth occurs; at higher doses (5.0 mg), tachycardia, meiosis causing blurred vision, difficulty swallowing, and flushing occur; and at even higher doses, confusion develops. Patients with glaucoma or urinary retention can have a worsening of these conditions when given atropine. Unlike atropine, ipratropium bromide is remarkably free of unwanted side effects because of its minimal systemic absorption. Indeed, it is rare to see any side effects other than dryness of the mouth, scratching of the throat, or a bitter taste in the mouth.

CLINICAL USE

The following discussion on the clinical use is limited to ipratropium; however, the concepts apply equally to atropine.

In double-blind trails, ipratropium bromide 40 to 80 µg resulted in maximum improvement in airway function similar to that of isoproterenol 75 to 200 µg by inhalation, but the effect was much more prolonged. In placebo-controlled, double-blind trials with fenoterol and albuterol, the β-agonist produced an earlier and more prolonged maximum increase in FEV_1. While the peak effect with albuterol was consistently greater, this difference disappeared 3 to 4 hr after inhalation, and the two agents had a similar duration of action.

As a result of different mechanisms of action, combination of ipratropium with albuterol, fenoterol, metaproterenol, and theophylline has resulted in enhanced maximum effect and prolonged duration of action.

Studies with ipratropium bromide by inhalation show it to be somewhat inferior to the commonly used β-agonists in asthmatics. Although significant bronchodilation is seen rapidly following inhalation (50% of the eventual maximum in the first 3 to 5 min and 80% within 30 min), the maximum effect occurs relatively slowly (1.5 to 2 hr).

Ipratropium bromide appears to be indicated primarily as an alternative in patients who fail to respond adequately or experience troublesome side effects with β-agonists. When added to inhaled albuterol in the treatment of children with acute asthmatic symptoms, inhaled ipratropium provides important clinical benefit. There are no data on concomitant use of ipratropium with a β-agonist, theophylline, or cromolyn for long-term prophylaxis of chronic asthma. Since it does not block experimentally induced bronchospasm with histamine, antigen, or exercise and it provides less bronchodilation, ipratropium is unlikely to be beneficial for the prophylaxis of chronic asthma.

PRODUCT SELECTION

Ipratropium bromide is the anticholinergic agent of choice in the treatment of asthma because of the low incidence of adverse effects compared with atropine. Atropine is not available in the U.S. as a solution for inhalation, but the preservative-free parenteral formulations have been used via nebulization. Ipratropium is available only as a metered-dose inhaler in the U.S. A solution for nebulization is available in Europe and Canada and is expected to be available in the U.S. in 1994.

Miscellaneous Antiasthmatic Drugs

Several agents used in the treatment of asthma either are still under investigation or current data do not support their routine use. Calcium-channel blockers appear to have some potentially desirable effects on airway function and mediator release. The clinical usefulness of these drugs has, for the most part, not been encouraging, at least with the agents currently available. Potent H_1-receptor blockers such as astemizole antagonize histamine-induced bronchoconstriction and require further study in seasonal asthma. Ketotifen, an orally administered drug with antihistaminic and cromolyn-like activity, is being promoted in Europe for the long-term prophylaxis of bronchial asthma and other allergic disorders. In studies to date, however, it appears to be less effective than cromolyn. Also, ketotifen possesses marked antihistamine-like side effects (sedation and weight gain).

Troleandomycin (TAO) is a macrolide antibiotic with apparent steroid-enhancing effects in severe steroid-dependent asthmatics. This effect is specific for methylprednisolone and appears to be independent of any pharmacokinetic interaction.

Nedocromil the disodium salt of pyranoquinoline dicarboxylic acid, is similar in activity (as a mast cell stabilizer) to cromolyn sodium. Some studies have suggested that it has greater antiinflammatory effects than cromolyn. Nedocromil is available as a metered-dose inhaler under the brand name Tilade in Europe and Canada.

Recent research has shown that leukotrienes may be important medicators of asthma because of their potent bronchoconstrictor activity. Leukotrienes are released from cells in the airways which are involved in responses to stimuli such as inhaled allergens. Leukotriene-receptor antagonists are likely to result in a significant breakthrough in the next several years.

Mucolytic and expectorant agents have long been popular but have never been demonstrated to be effective. Iodides have sufficient toxicity to be contraindicated for use in children and in women of childbearing age. Controlled trials indicate that iodides neither increase volume nor decrease tenacity of sputum. Since even purulent-appearing sputum in the asthmatic patient usually is not infected with bacteria, infectious exacerbations of asthma are viral rather than bacterial in origin. Antibiotics have no specific indications in asthma unless there is evidence of a concurrent pyogenic infection such as acute otitis media. Moreover, controlled trials in patients with acute asthmatic symptoms have demonstrated no benefit from the addition of antibiotics.

The past decade of research into the pathophysiology of asthma has clarified the role of mediators from the cyclooxygenase and lipoxygenase pathways in producing airway inflammation. Leukotrienes, prostaglandins, thromboxanes, and platelet-activating factor are only a few of the mediators implicated. Clinical studies of leukotriene D4–receptor antagonists, platelet-activating-factor antagonists and lipoxygenase synthesis inhibitors in asthmatics have been encouraging. Preclinical trials of other mediator antagonists are underway.

Inhalation Devices

In most instances, administration of β_2-agonists and corticosteroids is best accomplished by the inhaled route. β_2-Agonists can be administered via a nebulizer, intermittent positive-pressure breathing (IPPB), or a metered-dose inhaler (MDI).

Several studies have been conducted comparing these three methods of aerosol administration, mostly with β-agonists. In a recent study conducted by the National Institutes of Health, bronchodilator drugs given by IPPB did not produce a significantly different effect than did the same drugs given by nebulization (51). Since IPPB can also result in a pneumothorax, it is not recommended. β-Agonists given by nebulization also require large, expensive equipment and at least 5 to 10 times the dose given by an MDI to produce the same bronchodilator effect. In addition, several of the commercially available bronchodilator solutions for nebulization (metaproterenol, isoetharine, isoproterenol) contain salts of bisulfite and metabisulfite as antioxidants. When nebulized, these solutions produce sufficient SO_2 to elicit bronchospasm in about 5 to 10% of asthmatics (52). Thus, sulfite-free products should be selected for nebulization in asthmatics.

MDIs have gained wide acceptance as a convenient dosage form that rapidly and selectively administers drugs to the site of action, the lung, while decreasing drug-induced side effects (53). Advantages of MDIs over IPPB and nebulizers include: lower required doses, convenience, portability, shorter administration time, maintenance of sterility and stability of the aerosol, and cost-effectiveness. However, administration technique with MDIs has come under close scrutiny. Between 14 and 72% of patients tested do not use their MDIs correctly, in some cases even after repeated instruction. When used correctly, only 10% of the drug reaches the lungs, with roughly 80% being deposited in the oropharynx, swallowed, or systemically absorbed.

Four main factors affect aerosol deposition in the lung. First, particle size is controlled mainly by the aerosol manufacturer. Most aerosol medications have a particle size between 2.8 and 4.3 μm. The propellants increase particle size, and they must evaporate partially to obtain optimal particle diameter. Most evaporation occurs within the first 10 cm from the canister, with only a marginal amount evaporating up to 25 cm from the canister. The second factor is inspiratory volume. It has recently been demonstrated that a 750-ml reservoir volume is optimal for particle deposition. The third factor, breath-holding, allows for sedimentation (gravitational deposition) of the aerosol particles into the lung. Studies have shown that a breath-hold of 10 sec is optimal for promoting aerosol deposition into the lung (53). This maneuver is difficult for certain patients to perform. Inspiratory flow rate is the fourth component necessary for optimal aerosol deposition. A greater and more uniform deposition pattern is found when an aerosol is inhaled at a slow flow rate of 0.2 to 0.3 liters/sec (54). Without a proper, slow inspiratory flow rate, the effects of breath-holding, inspiratory volume, and the particle size of aerosol deposition decrease, resulting in most of the drug being deposited in the oropharynx and upper airways (inertial impaction).

Several auxiliary aerosol delivery systems have been developed to facilitate the administration of MDIs (Table 33.8). These devices provide a way to assess the proper rate and depth of each inhalation while eliminating the need for "hand-lung" coordination. The devices provide significantly greater lung deposition of metered-dose aerosols, compared with a correctly used MDI, while reducing oropharyngeal deposition approximately ninefold.

The clinical relevance of auxiliary devices is still in question. There has been marginal enhancement of bronchodilator action with some devices but not with others. The dose-response curve of these agents is such that a small change in deposition may not alter the physiological effect from the drug. Improved deposition may be more important when bronchoprovocation tests are used in the evaluation. In young children or the elderly, in whom coordination of the MDI may not be ideal, an auxiliary device may improve response.

In contrast to bronchodilator aerosols, the effect from aerosolized corticosteroids is dose-dependent. Thus, the more delivered, the better the oral corticosteroid-sparing effect (53). Auxiliary devices reduce the rate of oral candidiasis and dysphonia significantly and double the therapeutic potency of an inhaled corticosteroid (56). Improved deposition, especially with larger doses, may have an effect on systemic side effects as a result of absorption from alveoli and distal airways.

Sequence for the Treatment of Asthma

Acute asthma is treated most effectively with inhaled β_2-agonists such as albuterol, metaproterenol, or terbutaline. If repeated administration of these aerosol bronchodilators

Table 33.8.
Comparison of Aerosol Delivery Systems[a]

Feature/Characteristics[b]	Metered-Dose Inhaler	Azmacort (William H. Rorer, Inc.) and Brethancer (Geigy Pharmaceuticals)	Aerochamber (Monaghan)	Inhal-Aid (Key Pharmaceuticals)	InspirEase (Key Pharmaceutical)
Simple construction	−	+	±	±	±
Compact and portable	+	+	+	±	+
Reduces aerosol impaction loss in oropharynx	−	+	+	+	+
Requires minimal training/ coordination	−	−	+	+	+
Promotes drug conservation	−	−	±	±	+
Allows even distribution of drug in inhaled air	−	−	−	±	+
Incorporates a means for awareness of flow rate and volume of air inhaled	−	−	+	±	+
Promotes reproducible dosing	−	−	−	±	+
More effective drug action than conventionally administered metered-dose inhaler used correctly	N/A	−	−	−	+

[a] Adapted with permission from Tobin MJ, Jenouri G, Danta I, et al.: Response to bronchodilator drug administration by a new reservoir aerosol delivery system and a review of other auxiliary delivery systems. Am Rev Respir Dis 126:670–675, 1982.
[b] Key: +, the characteristic is present; −, the characteritic is not present; ±, the presence of the characteristic is equivocal.

produces an inadequate effect, and administration technique is adequate, a bolus of systemic corticosteroids should be started. While waiting for the steroids to exert an effect, inhaled β-agonist therapy should be continued at frequent intervals up to every hour. Since theophylline is three to four times less effective in relieving airflow obstruction than repetitively administering β_2-agonists, a therapeutic theophylline concentration is not important in achieving immediate bronchodilation. Adequate hydration, correction of metabolic acidosis, and oxygen are essential supportive measures. Arterial blood gases should be followed closely. A rising pCO_2 indicates respiratory failure. If CO_2 levels are rising, an inhaled anticholinergic agent such as atropine or ipratropium can be tried to prevent respiratory failure. Intravenous use of isoproterenol may also prevent the need for intubation and ventilator support when other pharmacologic measures are unsuccessful. There are few data on the use of intravenous terbutaline in this situation (60), but it may be tried as an alternative to isoproterenol in the older patient who might be a greater risk of myocardial necrosis.

For treatment of intermittent asthma, use of an inhaled β_2-agonist (2 puffs repeated every 3 to 4 hours p.r.n.) is usually sufficient. Inhaled cromolyn may also be used before exposure to exercise, allergen, or other stimuli.

For treatment of chronic asthma, theophylline appears to be the most effective noncorticosteroid agent. Theophylline should be used in doses that attain therapeutic serum concentrations, and a product should be selected that maintains these therapeutic concentrations for the entire dosing interval. In selected individuals, cromolyn is an acceptable therapeutic alternative.

Recently, an expert panel of the National Asthma Education Program (NAEP) has recommended the use of inhaled corticosteroids early in the sequence of therapy. For patients who have an incomplete response to the repeated administration of β_2-agonists, the use of inhaled corticosteroids should be encouraged.

Additional sympathomimetic bronchodilator therapy should be used on an as-needed basis to treat breakthroughs in symptoms, and short courses of oral corticosteroids may be needed for symptoms that become unresponsive to bronchodilators. When cessation of corticosteroids for acute symptoms is followed consistently by a relapse of symptoms that respond poorly to bronchodilators, a continuous corticosteroid regimen or alternate-day prednisone must be considered. After control is achieved with a continuous corticosteroid regimen, the dose should be decreased slowly to the lowest dose that maintains adequate control.

Other therapeutic measures for the treatment of asthma include removing specific environmental factors such as household allergens (e.g., dog or cat) or cessation of cigarette smoking. Immunotherapy is indicated if rhinitis symptoms related to these specific inhalant allergens are present in addition to asthmatic symptoms and are not controlled by a reasonable number of pharmacologic measures alone.

CONCLUSION

Asthma continues to be a major cause of morbidity, particularly in children. Asthma has been classified as mild, moderate, and severe, based in part on the severity and frequency of symptoms. The pathophysiology of the disease is still not entirely known, however, most research has been focused recently on the inflammatory component of asthma. Although bronchodilator agents such as theophylline and β_2-agonists are still the mainstay of therapy, increasing evidence indicates that antiinflammatory drugs such as the corticosteroids (particularly by the inhaled route) are more effective in mild-to-moderate asthmatics. In addition, agents such as cromolyn are having an increased role as well, primarily because of their low side-effect potential.

REFERENCES

1. Lebowitz MD, Knudson RJ, Burrows B: Tucson epidemiologic study of obstructive lung disease: I. Methodology and prevalence of disease. Am J Epidemiol 102:137–152, 1975.
2. Mathison DA, Stevenson DD, Simon RA: Precipitating factors in asthma; aspirin, sulfites, and other drugs and chemicals. Chest 87:505–545, 1985.
3. Szentivanyi A: The β-adrenergic theory of the atopic abnormality in bronchial asthma. J Allergy 42:203–210, 1968.
4. Gallant SP, Duriseti L, Underwood S, et al.: Decreased β-adrenergic therapy. N Engl J Med 299:933–938, 1978.
5. Ellis EF: Asthma in childhood. J Allergy Clin Immunol 72(suppl):526–539, 1985.
6. Middleton E: Antiasthmatic drug therapy and calcium ions: review of pathogenesis and role of calcium. J Pharm Sci 69:243–251, 1980.
7. Cohen SH: Advances in the diagnosis and treatment of asthma. Chest 87(suppl):26S–30S, 1985.
8. Hargreave FE, Dolovich J, Boulet L: Inhalation provocation tests. Semin Respir Med 4:224–236, 1983.
9. McFadden ER Jr: β₂ receptor agonist: metabolism and pharmacology. J Allergy Clin Immunol 68:91, 1981.
10. Wallser SB, Kradjan WA, Bierman CW: Bitolterol mesylate: a β-adrenergic agent. Pharmacotherapy 5:127–137, 1985.
11. Nelson HS, β-Adrenergic therapy. In Middleton E, Reed CE, Ellis EF (eds): Allery: Principles and Practice, ed. 2. St. Louis, CV Mosby, 1983, pp 511–527.
11a.Spritzer WO, Suissa S, Ernst P, et al.: The use of β-agonist and their risk of death or near death from asthma. N Engl J Med 326:501–506, 1992.
12. Sears MR, Taylor DR, Print CG et al.: Regular inhaled β-agonist treatment in bronchial asthma. Lancet 336(8728):1391–1396, 1990.
13. Rossing TH, Fanta CH, Goldstein DH, et al.: Emergency therapy of asthma: comparison of the acute effects of parenteral and inhaled sympathomimetics and infused aminophylline. Am Rev Respir Dis 122:365–371, 1980.
14. Ahrens RC, Bonham AC, Maxwell GA, et al.: A method for comparing the peak intensity and duration of action of aerosolized bronchodilators using bronchoprovocation with methacholine. Am Rev Respir Dis 129:903–906, 1984.

15. McFadden ER: Clinical use of β-adrenergic agonist. J Allergy Clin Immunol 76:352–356, 1985.
16. Cockcroft DW, Berscheid BA, Dosman JA, et al.: Comparison of bitolerol mesylate and metaproterenol sulphate. Curr Ther Res 30:817–824, 1981.
17. Wickramasinghe H, Liebeschuetz HJ: Addiction to aerosol treatment. Br Med J 287:1877, 1983.
18. Bergstrand H: Phosphodiesterase inhibition and theophylline. Eur J Respir Dis 61(suppl 109):37–44, 1980.
19. Hendeles L, Weinberger M: Theophylline, "a state of art" review. Pharmacotherapy 3:2–44, 1983.
20. Zwillich CW, Sutton FD, Neff TA, et al.: Theophylline-induced seizures in adults: correlation with serum concentrations. Ann Intern Med 82:784–787, 1975.
21. Berlinger WG, Spector R, Gulberg MG, et al.: Enhancement of theophylline clearance by oral activated charcoal. Clin Pharmacol Ther 33:351–354, 1983.
22. Weinberger MM, Hendeles L: Theophylline use: an overview. J Allergy Clin Immunol 76:277–284, 1985.
23. Vozeh S, Kewitz G, Wenk M, et al.: Rapid prediction of steady-state serum concentration in patients treated with intravenous aminophylline. Eur J Clin Pharmacol 18:473–477, 1980.
24. Hendeles L, Iafrate RP, Weinberger M: A clinical and pharmacokinetic basis for the selection and use of slow-release theophylline products. Clin Pharmacokinet 9:95, 1984.
25. Scott PH, Tabachnik E, MacLeod S, et al.: Sustained release theophylline for childhood asthma: evidence for circadian variation of theophylline pharmacokinetics. J Pediatr 99:476–479, 1981.
26. Hendeles H, Weinberger M, Milavetz G, et al.: Food-induced dose dumping from a "once-a-day" theophylline product as a cause of theophylline toxicity. Chest 87:758, 1985.
27. Gonzalez MA, Golub AL, Meyer ML, et al.: Disposition kinetics of controlled-release theophylline dosed at 12 and 24 hour dosing intervals. Presented at the Thirty-sixth Annual Meeting of the American Pharmaceutical Association Academy of Pharmaceutical Sciences, Montreal. J Pharm Sci 14:108, 1984 (abstr).
28. Karim A, Burns T, Janky D, et al.: Food-induced changes in theophylline absorption for controlled-released formulations. Part II. Importance of meal composition and dosing time relative to meal intake in assessing changes in absorption. Clin Pharmacol Ther 38:642–647, 1985.
29. Bernstein IL: Cromolyn sodium in the treatment of asthma: coming of age in the United States. J Allergy Clin Immunol 76:381–388, 1985.
30. Gold WM, Kessler GH, Yu DYC: Role of vagus nerves in experimental asthma in allergic dogs. J Appl Physiol 33:719–725, 1972.
31. Mills JE, Sellick H, Widdicombe JG: Activity of lung irritant receptors in pulmonary microembolism, anaphylaxis and drug induced bronchoconstriction. J Physiol 203:337–357, 1969.
32. Shapiro GG, Konig P: Cromolyn sodium: a review. Pharmacotherapy 5:156–176, 1985.
33. Hambleton G, Weinberger MM, Taylor J, et al.: Comparison of cromoglycate (cromolyn) and theophylline in controlling symptoms of chronic asthma. Lancet 1:381–385, 1977.
34. Newth CJL, Newth CV, Turner JAP: Comparison of nebulized sodium cromoglycate and oral theophylline in controlling symptoms of chronic asthma in preschool children: a double-blind study; Aust NZ J Med 12:232–238, 1982.
35. Selcow JE, Mendelson L, Tosen JP: A comparison of cromolyn and bronchodilators in patients with mild to moderately severe asthma in an office practice. Ann Allergy 50:13–18, 1983.
36. Shapiro GG, Clifton TF, William E, et al.: Double-blind evaluation of nebulized cromolyn, etrburaline, and the combination for childhood asthma. J Allergy Clin Immunol 81:449–454, 1988.

37. Plit M, Amirav I, Dowdeswell R: Comparison of sodium cromoglycate spincapsule and aerosol in the prevention of exercise induced asthma (EIA) in adults. Am Rev Respir Dis 137:36(abstr), 1988.

38. Fraser CM, Venter JC: The synthesis of β-adrenergic receptors in cultured human lung cells: induction by glucocorticoids. Biochem Biphys Res Commun 94:390, 1980.

39. Siegel SC: Overview of corticosteroid therapy. J Allergy Clin Immunol 76:312–320, 1985.

40. Jusko WJ, Rose JQ: Monitoring prednisone and prednisolone. Ther Drug Monit 2:169, 1980.

41. Weinberger MM, Hendeles L, Ahrens R: Clinical pharmacology of drugs used for asthma. Pediatr Clin North Am 28:47–75, 1981.

42. Gaddie K, Reod IW, Skinner C, et al.: Aerosol beclomethasone dipropionate: a dose response study with chronic bronchial asthma. Lancet 2:280, 1973.

43. Toogood JH, Baskerville J, Jennings B, et al.: Bioequivalent doses of budesonide and prednisone in moderate and severe asthma. J Allergy Clin Immunol 84:688–700, 1989.

44. Brunette MG, Lands L, Thibodeau LP: Childhood asthma: prevention of attacks with short-term corticosteroid treatment of upper respiratory tract infection. Pediatrics 81:624–629, 1988.

45. Haahtela T, Jarvinen M, Kava T, et al.: Comparison of a β₂-agonist terbutaline, with an inhaled corticosteroid budesonide, in newly detected asthma. N Eng J Med 325:388–392, 1991.

46. Juniper EF, Kline PA, Vanzieleghem MA, et al.: Effect of long-term treatment with an inhaled corticosteroid (Budesonide) on aerway hyperresponsiveness and clinical asthma in nonsteroid-dependent asthmatics. Am Rev Respir Dis 142:832–836, 1990.

46a. Anon: Management of asthma. J Allergy Clin Immunol 88:(Part 2) 477–492, 1991.

47. Toogood JH: Concentrated aerosol formulations in asthma. Lancet 2:790–791, 1983.

48. Toogood JH, Lefcoe NM, Haines DSM, et al.: Minimum dose requirements of steroid-dependent asthmatic patients for aerosol beclomethasone and oral prednisone. J Allergy Clin Immunol 61:355–364, 1978.

49. Stemman EA, Kosche F: Comparison of the effect of SCH 1000 MDI, sodium cromoglycate and β-adrenergic drugs on exercise-induced asthma in children. Postgrad Med J 51(suppl 7):105–106, 1975.

50. Schroecksnstein DC, Bush RK, Chevinsky P, et al.: Twelve-hour bronchodilation in asthma with a single aerosol dose of the anticholinergic compound glycopyrrolate. J Allergy Clin Immunol 82:115–119, 1988.

51. Anon: Intermittent positive pressure breathing therapy of chronic obstructive pulmonary disease: a clinical trial. Ann Intern Med 99:612–620, 1983.

52. Koepke JW, Selner JC, Danhill AL: Presence of sulfur dioxide in commonly used bronchodilator solutions. J Allergy Clin Immunol 72:504–508, 1983.

53. Lee H: Comparison of oral and aerosol adrenergic bronchodilators in asthma. J Pediatr 99:805–807, 1981.

54. Newman SP, Bateman JRM, Pavia D, et al. The importance of breath-holding following the inhalation of pressurized aerosol bronchodilators. In Baron D (ed): Recent Advances in Aerosol Therapy. Brussels, UCB Pharmaceuticals. 1979, pp 117–122.

55. Newhouse MT, Ruffin RE: Deposition and fate of aerosolized drugs. Chest 73:936–943, 1978.

56. Toogood JH, Baskerville J, Jennings B, et al.: Use of spacers to facilitate inhaled corticosteroid treatment of asthma. Ann Rev Respir Dis 129:723–729, 1984.

57. Pedersen S, Moller-Pederson J: Erratic absorption of a slow-release theophylline sprinkle product caused by food. Pediatrics 74:534–538, 1984.

58. Hendeles L, Weinberger MM: Selection of slow-release theophylline products. J Allergy Clin Immunol 78:743–751, 1986.

59. Sips AP, Edelbroek BM, Dulstad S, et al.: Food does not affect bioavailability of theophylline from Theolin Retard. Eur J Clin Pharmacol 26:405–407, 1984.

60. O'Connell MB, Iber C: Continuous intravenous terbutaline infusions for adult patients with status asthmaticus. Ann Allergy 64:213–218, 1990.

CHAPTER 34

CHRONIC OBSTRUCTIVE PULMONARY DISEASE

TRACEY L. GOLDSMITH, Pharm.D.

The term *obstructive pulmonary disease* encompasses several separate and distinct sets of pathologic changes, including asthma, chronic bronchitis, and emphysema. Interference with ventilation from an obstruction to airflow is the common element, in contrast to restrictive lung disease where the defect is reduced capability for lung expansion. Asthma is discussed in detail in Chapter 33, but it can be summarized as a clinical syndrome characterized by narrowing of the airways as a result of bronchial hyperreactivity, excessive bronchial secretions, and inflammatory changes of the airways. The resulting obstruction to airflow is usually reversible. Chronic obstructive pulmonary disease (COPD), also known as chronic obstructive airways disease (COAD) or chronic obstructive lung disease (COLD), includes chronic bronchitis and emphysema. Airflow obstruction in these patients may respond to various therapeutic efforts, but these diseases are largely irreversible (1).

INCIDENCE

Chronic obstructive pulmonary disease is the fifth leading cause of mortality in the United States. In 1986, over 71,000 deaths were attributed to COPD. Current best estimates suggest that 82% of those deaths were attributable to smoking. COPD mortality currently is higher in males than females and is higher in whites than blacks. It is estimated that over 14 million persons in this country alone have COPD. Approximately 750,000 hospitalizations could be attributed to COPD during that same year (2).

PATHOPHYSIOLOGY

The normal function of the respiratory system is to exchange oxygen (O_2) and carbon dioxide (CO_2) so that oxygen is delivered to and carbon dioxide is removed from the blood. CO_2 is the major stimulus for the respiratory center, located in the medulla of the brain. When pCO_2 levels increase, ventilation is stimulated, resulting in increased removal of CO_2. Anatomically, the respiratory tract has three components that support this process: a conducting system, respiratory exchange units, and a vascular supply. The conducting system is composed of the nose, pharynx, larynx, trachea, and bronchi. Obstructions of the upper airway can result from foreign objects, tu-

mors, etc. The lower respiratory tract, or the respiratory exchange units, include the bronchioles, alveolar ducts, alveolar sacs, and alveoli. Normal airway integrity is maintained through the relationship of pressures in and around the airway and the elasticity of the airway. Exchange of O_2 and CO_2 occurs between the alveoli and the vascular supply (capillaries). With obstructive pulmonary disease, changes in these normal processes occur. If airway integrity is compromised through diseases such as chronic bronchitis or emphysema, obstruction of the lower airway results. Changes in pulmonary vasculature result from hypoxia. Pulmonary hypertension may result and is seen as elevated mean pulmonary artery pressures and pulmonary vascular resistance (3). Cor pulmonale, or hypertrophy of the right ventricle due to primary lung disease, may then result and progress to heart failure (3). These alterations in normal lung structure and function may occur in the course of chronic bronchitis and emphysema.

Chronic bronchitis is characterized by chronic or recurrent excessive mucus secretion and inflammation in the bronchi that interferes with normal mechanisms to maintain airway integrity. Excessive mucus production is the result of irritation of the airway by smoke or other irritants. With chronic irritation, the mucous glands increase in number and size, and their ducts dilate within the bronchial mucosa. Airway obstruction results from narrowing of the airway by thick, tenacious mucus and from bronchiolar inflammation and edema. Excess mucus secretion results in plugs or consolidations. Occlusion of the respiratory exchange units can occur from these plugs, reducing the functional air exchange area, and causing destruction of the alveoli. Importantly, airway obstruction is not necessarily always present in chronic bronchitis and may occur only during acute exacerbations. Chronic or recurrent bacterial infection is common in chronic bronchitis.

Emphysema is defined as a condition of the lung characterized by abnormal permanent enlargement of the airspaces distal to the terminal bronchiole, accompanied by destruction of their walls, and without obvious fibrosis (4). The result is loss of elastic recoil. Elastic recoil contributes to the force of expiration; if decreased, distal airways will collapse during expiration and trap air (5). Pathologically there are two types of emphysema. Centri-acinar (centri-lobular) emphysema is characterized by deposition of carbon pigment at the center of the pulmonary lobule, with distal alveoli left intact. This form is most common in emphysema caused by cigarette smoking. Panacinar (panlobular) emphysema is characterized by destruction of all areas of the pulmonary lobule and is more commonly associated with hereditary emphysema. This distinction is made at postmortem examination of lung tissue. Chronic bronchitis and emphysema are frequently indistinguishable on clinical examination, and many patients have components of both diseases.

ETIOLOGY

Chronic bronchitis is associated strongly with cigarette smoking but can occur in persons who have never smoked. Other factors such as pollution or occupational exposures have also been associated with bronchitis. Emphysema is also associated with smoking, although other environmental factors may be important. Cigarette smoking causes increased bronchial reactivity and inflammation. Ciliary function is depressed, resulting in decreased clearance of mucus and particles. Macrophage function is similarly inhibited. Release of lysosomal enzymes destroys the connective tissue in the lung.

A history of chronic bronchitis can often be elicited in patients with centri-acinar emphysema. Inborn errors resulting in enzyme deficiencies are rare causes of emphysema. If an imbalance occurs between elastase (enzyme that degrades elastin in the lung parenchyma) and elastase inhibitors, alveolar destruction results (6). A deficiency of α_1-antitrypsin (or α_1-proteinase inhibitor), an elastase inhibitor, has been demonstrated in some patients with panacinar emphysema, indicating a genetic basis for alveolar wall destruction (6).

CLINICAL PRESENTATION AND DIAGNOSIS

By the time they seek medical attention, patients are usually far advanced in their disease, with symptoms of airway obstruction. This delay in medical intervention occurs because the pathologic changes have been progressing for years, but overt clinical symptoms occur later. The usual presentation of COPD begins with cough and increased sputum production, reminiscent of chronic bronchitis. The patient may have noticed a decline in exercise tolerance. Weight loss (sometimes profound) may be reported by the patient with primary emphysema; however, the patient with chronic bronchitis is typically obese. Dyspnea, or breathlessness, is the sensation of labored or difficult breathing (7). It occurs later in the course of COPD and may be worsened by exposure to cold, dampness, pollution, and/or acute infection. Considerable individual variation exists in the subjective perception of dyspnea. There

is a close correlation between dyspnea and the degree of airway obstruction in patients with COPD (7).

Infections due to viruses, *Haemophilus influenzae*, *Mycoplasma pneumoniae*, or *Streptococcus pneumoniae* can trigger an acute deterioration in patient status, especially in the patient with chronic bronchitis (8–11). Patients with mucus hypersecretion are predisposed to repeated bacterial, viral, or mycoplasma infections. Decreased removal of bronchial secretions physically impairs the defenses of the lungs against infection (5), and the mucus provides a good growth medium for bacteria. Colonization of the airways by the above organisms has been clearly demonstrated. There is no conclusive evidence that colonization or recurrent infection contributes to the progression of COPD by contributing to further airway inflammation.

Certain characteristic signs of COPD may be noted on physical examination. A prolonged expiratory effort may be seen as a sign of airway obstruction in primary emphysema. These patients may also exhale through pursed lips in an attempt to control the rate of expiration. Grunting may be heard on inspiration. The patient may be using the accessory respiratory muscles to aid in breathing. An overall increase in respiratory rate is common. Wheezes may be heard during bouts of airway obstruction in both chronic bronchitis and emphysema. An increase in the anteroposterior diameter of the chest and the classic "barrel chest" may occur in both diseases. These signs and symptoms do not correlate well with severity of illness. The chest x-ray may be helpful if emphysematous bullae or marked vascular changes are present.

Pulmonary function tests provide good information on the degree of airway obstruction and also help assess the efficacy of drug therapy. Lung volumes and rates of flow can be measured by spirometry. Several important parameters should be reviewed. Vital capacity (VC) is a measure of the volume of air moved during a forced respiratory cycle (i.e., forced inspiration and expiration). The volume of air moved with a normal inspiration or expiration is termed tidal volume (TV). After a maximal expiration, the volume of air left in the lungs is called the residual volume (RV). The same volume of air remaining in the lungs after a normal expiration is then called functional residual capacity (FRC). VC plus RV equals the total lung capacity (TLC). In COPD, RV is increased because of obstruction to airflow, while TLC can be either normal or increased. Vital capacity is reduced in COPD.

Other parameters that should be understood are forced expiratory volume (FEV_1), forced vital capacity (FVC) and FEV_1/FVC ratio. FEV_1 is the volume of air exhaled during forced exhalation in the first second. This parameter is decreased in the patient with an obstruction to outflow, such as COPD. An FEV_1 above 2 liters is usually not associated with dyspnea with normal activity, while an FEV_1 under 1 liter is associated with dyspnea on mild exercise. FVC denotes the volume of gas expelled from the lungs during rapid and complete exhalation. The FEV_1/FVC ratio is normally 0.8. Therefore, a patient with chronic or acute airway obstruction would have an FEV_1/FVC ratio less than 0.8 because of a decrease in FEV_1. These tests are of limited value in distinguishing between chronic bronchitis and emphysema.

No specific laboratory information is useful in differentiating the various forms of COPD, with the exception of emphysema due to α_1-antitrypsin deficiency. This diagnosis is made by a serum protein electrophoretic study. Sputum and blood eosinophilia, usually associated with asthma, may be present if the COPD patient also has an asthma component. This information could be useful in determining the role of bronchodilator therapy.

Although chronic bronchitis and emphysema are closely related both in etiology and presentation, some attempt to characterize the predominant form of COPD is desirable. Most patients will have changes consistent with both diseases, but predominance of one is common. Many definitions have been proposed which suffer from the lack of easily obtainable objective criteria. The diagnosis of chronic bronchitis, as defined by the American Thoracic Society (12), is based on clinical symptoms. It is described as a chronic cough, producing more than 30 ml of sputum in a 24-hr period which must be present for at least 3 months/year for at least 2 consecutive years (12). Unfortunately, there is no simple definition to aid in diagnosing emphysema. Emphysema should be suspected in the patient with progressive dyspnea (unrelated to cardiac disease) and a history of heavy smoking.

As COPD progresses, other acute and chronic complications may develop. Patients in whom chronic bronchitis is the predominant feature of COPD may undergo repeated episodes of acute respiratory failure. These patients may develop cor pulmonale and right-sided congestive heart failure. The term "blue-bloater" has been associated with this type of COPD patient. Hypoxia and respiratory acidosis are common findings. In patients with predominant emphysema, acute respiratory failure is rare until the end stages of the disease. These patients are referred to as "pink-puffers" since alveolar ventilation is maintained until the terminal stages of the disease. Table 34.1 summarizes the pertinent clinical features distinguishing chronic bronchitis and emphysema.

GOALS OF THERAPY

The treatments for chronic bronchitis and emphysema are very similar. Therefore, the therapy of COPD will be discussed, with areas of particular benefit in primary chronic bronchitis or primary emphysema highlighted. Therapy of COPD should be aimed at halting or slowing the progression of the pathologic changes, improving the patient's quality of life, and preventing acute exacerbations of the disease. General recommendations can be summarized as follows:

Alter Environmental Influences. A normal decline in FEV_1 occurs with ageing; however, environmental influences can accelerate that decline. Since cigarette smoking is involved in most COPD cases, the patient must be persuaded to stop smoking. Patients should be encouraged to pursue a smoking cessation program as part of their overall therapeutic regimen. The patient should be counseled about formal smoking cessation programs, drug treatments such as nicotine-containing gum, and other alternatives. Many of the changes seen in COPD are reversible with cessation of smoking, although some damage will remain (13). Exposure to other pollutants such as environmental

Table 34.1.
Clinical Presentation of COPD

	Chronic Bronchitis ("Blue Bloater")	Emphysema ("Pink Puffer")
Symptoms	Chronic cough, heavy sputum production	Dyspnea, minimal cough, minimal sputum production
Weight	Obesity common	Marked weight loss
Smoking history	Common	Common
Blood gases	Low PaO_2	Normal or slightly low PaO_2
	Elevated $PaCO_2$	Normal or slightly high $PaCO_2$
	Respiratory acidosis	Normal pH or mild respiratory acidosis
Cor pulmonale	Early development	Late development
Respiratory failure	Repeated episodes	Rare until end stage
Pulmonary function tests	Decreased FEV_1	Decreased FEV_1
	Decreased FVC	Decreased FVC
	Increased residual volume	Greatly increased residual volume

or industrial pollutants should also be limited as much as possible. Humidification may help remove mucus.

Correct Air Flow Obstruction. Several therapeutic modalities have been studied, including bronchodilators, sympathomimetics, anticholinergics, corticosteroids, and mucolytics. Individual agents or combinations of agents have met with varying rates of success.

Improve Patient's Functional Status. Many attempts to demonstrate objective improvement in pulmonary function tests with drug therapy have resulted in slight but statistically significant improvement. Significant subjective improvement noted by the patient has varied between studies. However, if the patient's outlook improves, subjective improvement should not be taken lightly. A perception of increasing dyspnea and decreasing exercise tolerance can be detrimental to the treatment program. Both maximum exercise and exercise endurance are decreased with COPD. Effective programs aimed at improving overall conditioning and respiratory muscle performance can be very helpful in managing dyspnea and respiratory fatigue (7).

Prevent Acute Disease Exacerbations. Since acute respiratory decompensations are frequently associated with respiratory infections, vaccination against common sources of infection is warranted. The long-term use of prophylactic antibiotics is controversial and certainly not without risk of adverse effects. The patient should be protected from rapid environmental changes including cold, dampness, or heavy pollution, because these frequently trigger acute deterioration.

Optimize Drug Therapy Regimens. Although no specific drug or combination of drugs will reverse the damage already done to the respiratory tract, drug therapy is very important in controlling symptoms and managing progression of the disease. The patient may be exposed to any number of drugs with additive adverse effect profiles, and close monitoring is essential to ensure compliance and limit adverse effects. Concomitant drug therapy that could reduce ventilatory drive should be avoided whenever possible. Drugs that aggravate sequellae of COPD, such as arrhythmias, should also be used with caution.

Maintain Adequate Nutrition. COPD is often associated with significant weight loss. Many patients have a body weight less than 90% of ideal. The degree of weight loss affects time of survival—almost 50% of patients die within 5 years of the onset of substantial weight loss (14). There is some suggestion that COPD patients who develop acute respiratory failure may have a poorer nutritional status than those with stable COPD (15). Substantial weight loss has been noted in both hospitalized and nonhospitalized (16) COPD patients. Decreased caloric intake and increased energy expenditure due to the increased work of breathing are two possible explanations (14). Malnu-

Table 34.2.
Drug Therapy of COPD[a]

β₂-Agonists—Dose based upon product elected; begin with β₂-selective inhaler; instruct patient on use of MDIs; monitor for tremor and tachycardia

Anticholinergics—Ipratropium bromide inhaler, 2 inhalations 4 times a day; instruct patient on the use of MDI; counsel patient about dryness of mouth and throat and bitter taste

Theophylline—8 to 20 mg/kg/day orally; determine responsiveness of patient to theophylline with a therapeutic trial; if no objective or subjective improvement is noted, discontinue therapy; individualize dose based upon patient history and serum theophylline concentrations; monitor for GI side effects, nervousness, tremor, and tachycardia

Corticosteroids—Prednisone 30 mg p.o. q.d. × 1 to 2 weeks to ascertain response; if response is noted, continue with steroid therapy as inhaled steroids, if possible; if no response is noted, discontinue steroid therapy; patients unable to maintain similiar response with inhaled steroids as with initial oral therapy can be restarted on oral steroids or a combination of inhaled and oral steroids may be used; taper to the lowest possible dose or preferably switch to alternate-day therapy; if possible wean from steroids once the patient's condition stabilizes; monitor for oral candidiasis or systemic infection

[a] May include single agent or combination therapy as dictated by response of the patient.

trition can result in decreased respiratory muscle function and depressed immune function, which may predispose the patient to infection. Hypophosphatemia also contributes to poor respiratory muscle function, so nutritional supplementation should provide adequate phosphates to avoid this complication.

SPECIFIC DRUG THERAPY

A summary of the drug therapy of COPD can be found in Table 34.2.

Methylxanthines

Although the role of theophylline and other methylxanthines is established in asthma, the risk/benefit ratio for their use is less clearly defined in COPD. Chronic bronchitis and emphysema can have a bronchoconstrictive component, but bronchoconstriction is usually not a primary factor. However theophylline may be beneficial, especially if a bronchoconstrictive component can be identified. Patients may be given a trial of theophylline followed by pulmonary function testing to assess response to therapy. Small but significant improvement can be demonstrated through pulmonary function testing in some patients (17, 18).

The benefits of theophylline in COPD may occur through several proposed effects on the cardiac and respiratory systems. These include (*a*) bronchodilation, (*b*) improved respiratory muscle contractility, (*c*) stimulation of central ventilatory drive, (*d*) increased mucociliary clearance, (*e*) decreased mean pulmonary artery pressure and pulmonary vascular resistance, and, (*f*) improved biventricular cardiac performance (19, 20). Although demonstrated in several small trials, the significance of these effects has not been fully examined in COPD patients on a large scale. The ability to lower mean pulmonary artery pressure and decrease pulmonary vascular resistance has been demonstrated in both acute and long-term studies of theophylline, although study populations have been small (21). Infusion of intravenous aminophylline results in a significant decrease in these parameters as well as a direct inotropic action; both are advantageous in the patient who has progressed to cor pulmonale and heart failure. Ventricular afterload is reduced, and biventricular cardiac function is improved as a result.

Theophylline probably produces these effects through a number of actions including inhibition of phosphodiesterase, alteration in calcium movement, blockade of adenosine receptors, prostaglandin antagonism, and alteration of cyclic AMP binding to the binding protein (19, 20). Phosphodiesterase inhibition has traditionally been accepted as the mechanism of action of theophylline, but it is questionable whether this accounts for its effects at clinically used doses. The other effects have been noted at clinically useful levels and thus may be responsible for the efficacy of the drug (20, 22).

The clinician has several choices to make when initiating theophylline therapy. A multitude of dosage forms and salts of theophylline are available. The acuity of the situation dictates the choice of dosage form (e.g., the patient in acute respiratory failure is best managed by parenteral therapy). However, chronic therapy decisions must include an assessment of patient compliance, dosage form preference, factors that influence the clearance of theophylline, and cost. The reader should refer to Chapter 33, "Asthma" for a detailed discussion of theophylline, including dosage form comparisons, detailed pharmacokinetics, and drug interactions.

Recommendations for dosing of theophylline in COPD are similar to those for asthma. Continuous infusions for acute therapy are generally in the range of 0.2 to 1.0 mg/kg/hr (23), whereas oral doses range from 10 to 20 mg/kg/day. Although associated with optimal therapeutic effect in asthma, serum concentrations of 10 to 20 μg/ml do not correlate well with pulmonary function testing in the COPD patient (20). Symptomatic control may be reported by patients receiving theophylline, but it does not correlate well with measured serum concentrations or pulmonary function testing (20). When used in COPD, theophylline therapy should be monitored closely to assess the degree of benefit the patient is receiving. Careful monitoring is also warranted to prevent or limit adverse effects that may be more common in these patients (e.g., they may be particularly sensitive to the arrhythmogenic effects of theophylline) (24). Many COPD patients continue to smoke, thereby increasing theophylline clearance. The

Table 34.3.
Theophylline in COPD[a]

Patient	Total Body Clearance (ml/kg/min)	Intravenous Dose
Adult, nonsmoker	0.65 ± 0.19 to 0.86 ± 0.35	0.4 mg/kg/hr
Adult, cigarette or marijuana smoker	1.05 ± 0.32 to 1.5 ± 0.4	0.7 mg/kg/hr
Adult, cardiac decompensation or cor pulmonale	0.48 ± 0.2	0.2 mg/kg/hr

[a] Adapted from Hendeles L, Weinberger M: Theophylline—a state of the art review. Pharmacotherapy 3:2–44, 1983.

clearance of theophylline may be reduced in advanced stages of COPD or in the presence of cor pulmonale with or without heart failure (20). Table 34.3 contains a summary of pharmacokinetic parameters that must be considered when initiating and monitoring theophylline therapy in COPD (25).

Given the adverse effect profile of theophylline, evidence of significant benefit should be obtained before subjecting the patient to long-term therapy. Preferably, pre- and post-theophylline pulmonary function testing should be used. The clinician must be able to monitor the patient for side effects and toxicity such as nausea, vomiting, tremors, headaches, confusion, arrhythmias, and seizures. Further evidence of objective benefits on diaphragmatic contractility, stimulation of hypoxic drive, and improved cardiac performance may define the role of theophylline in COPD more clearly.

Sympathomimetics

Sympathomimetics, or β-agonists, are used in COPD to control dyspnea and improve exercise tolerance. These drugs work by activating adenyl cyclase and increasing levels of cAMP, resulting in airway smooth muscle relaxation. There is also some evidence that these drugs may increase diaphragmatic contractility (26) and improve cor pulmonale (27). β-Agonists were considered by many to be first-line therapy in COPD patients. This practice is currently controversial, since anticholinergic inhalers are also efficacious.

The earliest β-adrenergic agonists included drugs such as epinephrine, ephedrine, and isoproterenol. Epinephrine was particularly useful in acute reversal of bronchospasm, but its short duration of action, nonselectivity, development of refractoriness (28), and lack of an oral dosage form limited chronic use. Ephedrine was widely used because of its oral dosage form, but nonselectivity, short duration of action, and adverse effects limit its current utility. Newer agonists with β_2 selectivity have overcome many of the original drawbacks to β-agonist therapy.

The most commonly used β-agonists are administered

via inhalation, although oral and parenteral products are also used. Systemic therapy is associated with more frequent adverse effects. Rapid airway response is seen with inhaled β-agonists, whereas the onset of action with oral therapy in acute airway obstruction may be delayed. Therefore, most clinicians prefer to use inhaled β-agonists in patients capable of using the devices. Table 34.4 reviews the currently available β-agonists, dosage forms, and dosing recommendations (29, 30).

β-Agonists should be compared on the basis of selectivity for β2-receptors, available dosage forms, duration of action, and cost. Metaproterenol, terbutaline, albuterol, bitolterol, and pirbuterol are all relatively β2-specific agents. β2-Selectivity results in a decreased rate of systemic adverse effects, particularly adverse cardiovascular effects, compared with the nonselective agents. Because of this specificity, these drugs are frequently prescribed. Isoproterenol, isoetharine, metaproterenol, albuterol, bitolterol, and pirbuterol are all available for inhalation. They vary in duration of action, with bitolterol having the longest duration of action at 4 to 8 hr. The side effect profiles are similar but vary in frequency. Minimal cardiovascular adverse effects are seen with the β2-selective agonists. Tremor is common to all the agents. Combined therapy with inhaled and oral β2-agonists is likely to cause additive adverse effects.

Metered-dose inhalers (MDIs) are a convenient way to deliver β-agonists. However, many patients find it difficult to actuate the inhaler properly and to synchronize inhalation and exhalation for maximum drug deposition. It is estimated that up to 70% of adults are unable to correctly use MDIs (31). Aerosol deposition within the airways is decreased in these cases. Patients have also been known to exhale during actuation of the inhaler, preventing any airway deposition of drug. Pharmacologic activity occurs only when sufficient drug is deposited at bronchial receptors. Many authorities have made recommendations on the optimal use of MDIs. One group recommends inhalation of the aerosol during a slow, deep inhalation with breath-holding for 10 sec (32). Actuation of the MDI between tightly closed lips and actuation up to 2 inches in front of widely opened lips are both recommended, and study results disagree on the optimal technique. Add-on MDI auxiliary devices decrease deposition of drug in the upper airway and decrease particle size. These devices may protect against deposition of β-agonist in the oral mucosa and systemic absorption. These auxiliary systems may be useful in the patient with very poor MDI use technique. Other patients may benefit from thorough explanation of correct MDI use. Instructions to the patient for appropriate use of β-agonist MDIs should include:

1. Use the inhaler only at the frequency and dose prescribed. If symptoms worsen, seek medical attention before increasing the dose.
2. Shake the MDI canister thoroughly immediately before use.
3. Exhale normally and completely.
4. Inhale slowly and deeply while depressing the MDI canister.
5. Hold breath for 10 sec (or as long as possible if not able to do so for 10 sec).

Table 34.4.
β-Adrenergic Agonists[a]

Drug (Generic/Trade)	Receptor Activity	Routes of Administration	Usual Dose	Onset of Action	Duration of Action (hr)
Epinephrine	α, β1, β2	s.c.	Varies	5–10 min	1–4
		i.m.	with product		1–4
		Inhalation		1–5 min	1–3
Ephedrine	α, β1, β2	p.o.	25–50 mg q 3–4 hr	15–60 min	2–4
		s.c.	25–50 mg	1 hr	
		i.m.	25–50 mg	10–20 min	1
Isoproterenol	β1, β2	Inhalation	Varies with product	2–5 min	0.5–1
Isoetharine	Primarily β2	Inhalation	Varies with product	1–5 min	1–4
Metaproterenol/(Alupent, Metaprel)	Primarily β2	p.o.	20 mg t.q.i.d.	15 min	4
		Inhalation	2–3 inhalations q. 3–4 hr	1 min	3–4
Terbutaline/(Brethane, Brethine, Bricanyl)	Primarily β2	p.o.	2.5–5 mg t.i.d.	30 min	4–8
		s.c.	0.25 mg–0.5 mg q. 4 hr	6–15 min	1.5–4
		Inhalation	2 inhalations q. 4–6 hr	5–30 min	3–6
Albuterol/(Proventil, Ventolin)	Primarily β2	p.o.	2–4 mg t.q.i.d.	30 min	4–6
		Inhalation	2 inhalations q. 4–6 hr	5–15 min	3–4
Bitolterol/(Tornalate)	Primarily β2	Inhalation	2–3 inhalations q. 8 hr	3–5 min	4–8
Pirbuterol/(Maxair)	Primarily β2	Inhalation	1–2 inhalations q. 4–6 hr	within 5 min	5 hr

[a] Data from Olin BR (ed): Bronchodilators (Sympathomimetics). Facts and Comparisons. St. Louis: JB Lippincott, 1991, pp 173a–177a; and McEvoy GK (ed): Sympathomimetic Agents. AHFS Drug Information 90. Bethesda, MD: American Society of Hospital Pharmacists, 1990, pp 612–658.

6. Wait 5 to 10 min between multiple doses.
7. Clean MDI case and cap thoroughly with water at least once per day.

β-agonists may also be delivered via nebulization. Metered-dose inhalers are preferable to nebulizers because of their decreased cost, convenience, transportability, and efficacy in stable COPD patients. The relative doses of β-agonist required for nebulization are higher than those for MDI inhalation because of the reduced efficiency of nebulizers in delivering the drug. However, patients who are severely dyspneic may benefit from nebulizer therapy if the MDI has not proven effective. Part of this improved response may relate to delivery of the drug as a wet aerosol. Considerable debate still exists about the role of nebulizers in inhalational therapy.

Anticholinergics

In patients with a bronchospastic component to their COPD, anticholinergic therapy may be beneficial, especially during acute exacerbations. Cholinergic stimulation increases the activity of guanyl cyclase, the enzyme responsible for catalyzing the formation of cyclic GMP. Cyclic GMP stimulates bronchoconstriction; therefore, administration of an anticholinergic agent will prevent the formation of cyclic GMP. The result is inhibition of bronchoconstriction. The predominant effect appears to be in the large airways.

Anticholinergic therapy is gaining greater acceptance as a first-line alternative in stable COPD. Parentual atropine has been used for COPD, but nebulization is the preferred way to deliver the drug. This method may help decrease the incidence of systemic adverse effects. Some systemic absorption does occur, so the patient should be closely monitored for signs of systemic adverse effects, such as dry mouth, blurred vision, or tachycardia. Since atropine therapy is associated with tachycardia, care should be exercised when using combinations of atropine and β-agonists or theophylline. Atropine inhalation does not seem to cause clinically important worsening of airway obstruction. The dose of atropine by nebulization is 0.025 mg/kg three to four times a day, with a range of 1 to 2.5 mg.

Ipratropium bromide is an analog of atropine. It acts as a bronchodilator by the same mechanism as atropine; however, because it is a quaternary compound, little systemic absorption occurs. Studies comparing ipratropium to β-agonists in stable COPD patients show that ipratropium bromide produces equal or greater bonchodilation (33, 34). Ipratropium bromide produces a response within 15 min when inhaled, with effects seen for 4 to 6 hr (33, 35). Because of its slower onset, compared with β-agonists, patients may prefer β-agonists for acute bronchospasm. Some studies have shown that combination therapy with β-agonists produces greater increases in FEV_1 than either agent alone (35, 36).

Ipratropium bromide is administered as two inhalations four times a day, increasing to four inhalations if needed. The patient should be counseled on the proper technique for administration, as with any MDI. Adverse effects occur infrequently and consist of dryness of the mouth and throat, bitter taste, cough, and nausea.

Corticosteroids

The role of corticosteroids in chronic bronchitis and emphysema has been the subject of much debate. Asthmatic patients receive substantial benefit from steroid therapy, and many investigators believe that steroid responders in COPD are patients with some component of airway hyperreactivity. The lack of large-scale, well-controlled clinical trials designed to positively exclude the patient with an asthmatic component has contributed to the controversial role of corticosteroids in COPD.

Patients with severe airway obstruction secondary to COPD seem to respond better to steroids than do the more stable patients. In other words, the subset of patients with acute respiratory insufficiency or severe obstruction may benefit most from a trial of corticosteroids. Studies in more stable COPD patients have reported improvements in pulmonary function by up to 30%. In general, only a certain subset of patients have responded, many with eosinophilia or a demonstrated response to isoproterenol (36–39). Subjective improvements in exercise tolerance and dyspnea have been reported (40). Subjective improvement can occur without actual improvement in pulmonary function tests, exercise tolerance, or arterial oxygen saturation (41, 42). Since corticosteroids can result in euphoria, especially in higher doses, reports of subjective improvement may reflect a side effect of corticosteroid therapy. Overall, 15 to 25% of patients with severe COPD will show improvement in FEV_1 on corticosteroids (43).

Corticosteroids can be tried in patients uncontrolled on bronchodilators. Hudson et al. (44) recommend a trial of oral steroids for 1 to 2 weeks in patients with significant airflow obstruction. Methylprednisolone 32 mg daily or prednisone 30 to 60 mg daily may be initiated. Improvements in FEV_1 of 20% or more indicate a positive response, and therapy with oral or inhaled steroids should be continued. Subjective improvements in dyspnea and exercise tolerance should also be noted. If the patient responds, the dose of steroid should be tapered to the lowest effective dose. Therapy can be continued with oral steroid, but inhaled steroids should be tried. Less than 50% of COPD patients responding to oral steroids will maintain that response with inhaled steroids such as beclomethasone (37). Several inhaled corticosteroid products are available, although beclomethasone is commonly used. A beclomethasone dose of 2 puffs 3 to 4 times daily is recommended, although some clinicians prefer a regimen of 10 puffs twice daily. Inhaled dexamethasone 3 puffs 3 to 4 times daily, triamcinolone 2 puffs 3 to 4 times daily, or flunisolide 2 to 4 puffs twice daily are alternatives. Alternate-day steroid use in severe COPD appears to be an effective alternative. Studies comparing daily to alternate-day therapy in equivalent doses have shown a similar degree of improvement in pulmonary symptoms (43). Both inhaled and alternate-day oral steroids produce fewer systemic side effects than daily oral steroids. The use of inhaled steroids or alternate-day therapy can also significantly reduce dependence on oral steroids.

Patients who have not responded to corticosteroids during stable periods of their disease may benefit from steroids in acute exacerbations or respiratory insufficiency. High steroid doses are usually recommended, although the effects of lower doses have not been studied adequately. Methylprednisolone 0.5 mg/kg intravenously every 6 hr or hydrocortisone 100 to 250 mg intravenously every 6 hr for 72 hr can be used in acute respiratory insufficiency. Tapering over several days should be done to avoid precipitation of another episode of acute respiratory insufficiency. A small clinical trial of parenteral methylprednisolone versus placebo in patients with COPD undergoing abdominal surgery indicated that methylprednisolone hastened recovery of pulmonary function following surgery (45).

If inhaled steroids are to be used, the patient should receive adequate instructions on the use of the MDI. Instructions like those discussed under the β-agonist MDIs should be provided. Additional counseling to rinse the mouth thoroughly after use of the steroid inhaler is necessary, since this may decrease the risk of oral candidiasis associated with steroid deposition in the oral cavity. The patient should be instructed to seek medical attention at the first sign of oral candidiasis. Oral candidiasis is characterized by a sore throat, patchy white exudates, and an underlying erythematous mucosa. This usually responds to temporarily discontinuing the steroid inhaler and treating with local antifungal therapy. The patient should also be told to use the β-agonist inhaler first if combination inhaler therapy is prescribed, so that maximal deposition of steroid in the lower airway will occur.

Mucolytic Agents

The chronic bronchitis patient has increased sputum production, either episodic or continuous. Agents that reduce the viscosity of mucus will aid in its expectoration, although the absolute value of such treatments has not been clearly demonstrated in large-scale trials. Acetylcysteine may be used for this purpose, especially in the hospital setting. Acetylcysteine, with its free sulfhydryl group, works by interfering with disulfide linkages. With the disulfide bonds broken, mucus becomes less viscous and more amenable to removal. Although acetylcysteine may be effective in lowering mucus viscosity, the efficacy of chronic administration in reducing the frequency of exacerbation of airway obstruction has not been demonstrated (46).

Acetylcysteine may be administered via inhalation, nebulization, intratracheal instillation, or orally. Direct instillation of acetylcysteine has been shown to be effective, especially in the presence of mucous plugging. Oral acetylcysteine also improves mucus clearance. After administration, mucus liquefies, and the patient must cough or use other measures to remove it. Acetylcysteine can induce airway irritation and bronchospasm. In addition, the drug has a strong, foul odor that many patients find intolerable. It may also cause nausea.

Oral iodinated glycerol has been shown to be effective in improving symptoms in patients with stable, chronic bronchitis. Patients reported decreases in cough frequency and severity and chest discomfort with doses of 60 mg four times daily (47). Expectorants such as guaifenesin, terpin hydrate, and saturated potassium iodide solutions have also been used to improved mucus clearance. These agents do not have clearly demonstrated efficacy in COPD and can be associated with side effects. If a 4- to 6-week trial of the mucolytic/expectorant does not produce improvement, therapy should be discontinued. Adequate hydration and effective cough can do much to remove mucus from the airway and are preferable to the expectorants.

Respiratory Stimulants

Doxapram is a central nervous system stimulant that increases the rate and depth of respiration by stimulating central medullary respiratory centers. It has been used in short-term infusions in acute respiratory failure secondary to COPD in an attempt to prevent or reverse hypercapnia and respiratory depression. The benefit of this therapy is questionable, since arterial oxygenation is usually not improved due to the increased work of breathing induced by the drug. Carbon dioxide concentrations usually do not improve for the same reason. When used to prevent mechanical ventilation, doxapram therapy is usually unsuccessful.

Doxapram therapy is highly controversial in COPD because of its questionable efficacy and adverse effects. The drug is associated with hypertension, tachycardia, dyspnea, and muscle hyperreflexia. With its narrow margin of safety, overdosage may occur if therapy is not managed carefully. Seizures can result from severe overdosage.

If used in acute respiratory failure, a continuous infusion of doxapram at 1 to 2 mg/min to a maximum of 3 mg/min should be administered. The recommended duration of therapy is not to exceed 2 hr. Vital signs and arterial blood gas levels should be monitored in addition to observing the patient for signs of toxicity.

Other respiratory stimulants that have been tried in

COPD include medroxyprogesterone and acetazolamide. Medroxyprogesterone 20 mg orally 3 times daily has been shown in small clinical trials to improve carbon dioxide elimination and alveolar ventilation (48, 49). Acetazolamide, although potentially useful in acute respiratory failure to increase alveolar ventilation and correct metabolic alkalosis, does not appear to be beneficial in the chronic management of COPD. Further large-scale studies are required before routine use of these agents can be recommended.

α_1-Proteinase Inhibitors

A small percentage of emphysematous patients suffer from α-1-antitrypsin deficiency. This deficiency of α-1-proteinase inhibitor leads to progressive destruction of elastin tissues and alveolar destruction caused by unopposed elastase activity. α-1-Proteinase inhibitors were released in 1987 under the Orphan Drug Act as chronic replacement therapy for patients with this congenital disorder who have demonstrable panacinar emphysema. α_1-Proteinase inhibitor is not indicated for patients who have not developed signs and symptoms of emphysema or in those patients with other forms of emphysema. It is a purified human product prepared from pooled plasma of normal donors. Although it is found to be nonreactive for HIV antibody and hepatitis B surface antigen, hepatitis B immunization is still recommended with hepatitis B vaccine. Hepatitis B immune globulin may be given as an alternative to the vaccine if therapy with α-1-proteinase inhibitor therapy is indicated before the vaccination regimen can be administered. Treatment with α_1-proteinase inhibitor requires weekly therapy. A dose of 60 mg/kg/week appears to maintain the inhibitor at an appropriate level within the lungs.

Antibiotics and Vaccines

Certain organisms, particularly Streptococcus pneumoniae and Haemophilus influenzae, are often cultured from the respiratory tract of COPD patients. Frequently this represents colonization of the airway and is not associated with infection. Bacterial colonization or infection does not appear to alter the natural history of COPD. Although widely used in COPD, the role of antibiotics in the absence of signs of infection is clearly debatable. Studies evaluating the prophylactic use of antibiotics during high-risk months (i.e., winter) in chronic bronchitis patients have not shown a difference in the frequency of acute exacerbations. Antibiotic use at the onset of purulent sputum production, symptoms consistent with a head cold, increased cough, fever, or other subjective symptoms is a common practice that has not been associated with a decreased number of acute exacerbations. However, some evidence indicates that duration of illness may be decreased (50). The most commonly prescribed antibiotics include ampicillin, tetracycline, cotrimoxazole, and erythromycin. Duration of antibiotic therapy is usually 7 to 10 days. Exacerbations of COPD may be precipitated or complicated by infections. Antibiotic use during acute respiratory exacerbations is clearly beneficial in established infections such as pneumonia (51).

Vaccination with pneumococcal and influenzae virus vaccines has been recommended in high-risk patient groups. Pneumococcal vaccine is formulated to provide prophylaxis against the most common strains of Streptococcus pneumoniae. Clear evidence that COPD patients are at an increased risk of infection by Streptococcus pneumoniae and thus increased mortality has not been presented (52). Antibody titers to the organisms may be elevated in COPD, probably as a result of chronic upper airway colonization. When given the vaccine, these patients respond by further increasing their antibody titers. Therefore, many clinicians recommend giving the vaccine to individuals with COPD. The most current dosing recommendation for adults is 0.5 ml by subcutaneous or intramuscular injection. Although readministration after 5 years was initially recommended, experience has shown an increased frequency of adverse effects. Therefore, only one administration is recommended.

Influenza virus vaccine provides active immunity to the virus. As opposed to pneumococcal vaccine, influenza virus vaccine should be given annually. It is recommended in high-risk groups such as patients with COPD. The vaccine is reformulated periodically to cover the most common strains. The clinician must remember that transient increases in theophylline levels have occurred with use of the vaccine, so the patient should be monitored for signs of theophylline toxicity for 24 hr after vaccination. The usual adult dose is 0.5 ml intramuscularly. Amantadine 100 mg twice daily for 14 days may be given during outbreaks of influenza A to high-risk patients who have not been immunized.

Oxygen Therapy

Oxygen therapy is an option for patients with severe chronic hypoxemia, cor pulmonale, or nocturnal or exercise-induced hypoxemia. Oxygen can be administered by nasal cannulae, even in the home setting. It can be administered continuously, during exercise, or nocturnally. The number of hours per day the patient uses oxygen continuously seems to relate to the effectiveness of this therapy. Patients are usually reluctant to use continuous oxygen therapy, so nocturnal use may be more attractive. Oxygen use in combination with a structured exercise program may improve exercise tolerance. One to 4 liters of oxygen by nasal cannulae is usually required.

INVESTIGATIONAL TREATMENTS

Calcium-Channel Antagonists

Calcium plays in integral role in regulating bronchomotor tone. Calcium is involved in the release of immune-mediated substances such as histamine. Flux of calcium into the respiratory contractile cells is important in regulating bronchomotor tone. In vivo studies with both nifedipine and verapamil have been conducted, and no clear role has been established for the use of calcium-channel antagonists in COPD.

Nifedipine was effective in acutely reducing bronchospasm induced by histamine in the asthmatic patient (53). Verapamil, given by nebulization, was reported effective in preventing histamine- and acetylcholine-induced bronchoconstriction (54). Sublingual nifedipine and inhaled verapamil have been studied in exercise-induced asthma and appear to have some efficacy (55, 56). Effects on mucociliary transport are unclear. Further work must be done to assess the role of these effects in the chronically obstructed patient with an asthmatic component.

Some work has been done on the role of calcium-channel antagonists in COPD patients with vascular sequellae of hypoxia. Hypoxia induces several changes in the pulmonary vasculature, including pulmonary vasoconstriction and vascular smooth muscle hypertrophy. These changes theoretically contribute to pulmonary hypertension in COPD (57). In acute respiratory failure, nifedipine was shown to reduce pulmonary artery pressure and pulmonary vascular resistance (58). Similar results were seen in patients with COPD and hypoxemia (57). The combination of low-flow oxygen and a calcium-channel antagonist seemed to further improve pulmonary vascular resistance.

Leukotriene Inhibitors

The role of leukotrienes in airway obstruction is an area of current research (59). Leukotrienes directly induce bronchospasm in animals and humans. Certain leukotrienes increase the airway response to histamine. An increase in bronchial edema and increased mucus secretion have also been noted. Effects on pulmonary vascular smooth muscle have been observed. Several inhibitors or leukotriene receptor antagonists have been synthesized, but few are in clinical trials. These agents will likely be a source of great research interest over the next several years.

Lung Transplantation

A complete discussion of the indications, complications, and success of lung transplantation for cardiopulmonary diseases is beyond the scope of this chapter. However, experimental double-lung transplantations in a limited number of patients with advanced obstructive lung diseases are being undertaken (60). Early successes have been noted, and work in the surgical management of COPD is continuing.

COR PULMONALE

Cor pulmonale is hypertrophy of the right ventricle as a result of primary lung disease. Right ventricular or biventricular failure may result. Cor pulmonale develops in approximately 6% of COPD patients per year, which translates into approximately 50,000 patients with cor pulmonale due to COPD (3).

Since sustained hypoxemia is postulated to be the major stimulus behind increased pulmonary vascular resistance and pulmonary hypertension, oxygen therapy is one of the primary therapies used in cor pulmonale. Diuretics have been used to manage dyspnea and edema. Digoxin may be beneficial in the patient with biventricular failure resulting from cor pulmonale, but its usefulness in isolated right ventricular failure is limited. Vasodilators reduce right ventricular afterload and may be used in patients with resistant pulmonary hypertension or right ventricular failure. Calcium-channel antagonists are being investigated to determine their possible contribution to the management of cor pulmonale. Aggressive management of the underlying pulmonary disease, prevention of sustained hypoxemia, and patient education are the best means of reducing the incidence of this complication.

ACUTE RESPIRATORY FAILURE

Acute respiratory failure may be precipitated by infection, use of central nervous system depressant drugs, bronchospasm, mucus plugging, or changes in environmental pollutants. Other stresses (e.g., surgery) may precipitate acute respiratory failure. The patient may have signs of diaphragmatic fatigue noted as asynchronous breathing. The PaO_2 is usually below 50 mm Hg, the $PaCO_2$ above 45 mm Hg, and the pH acidotic. Oxygen therapy and possible mechanical ventilation will be required. Mechanical ventilation is reserved until absolutely necessary, because it is difficult and slow to wean the COPD patient from ventilatory support. Physiotherapy aimed at improving drainage of secretions and relieving obstruction is beneficial. Supportive drug therapy, including theophylline, β-agonists, corticosteroids, anticholinergics, and/or respiratory stimulants may be instituted based on clinical symptoms (Table 34.5). Antibiotic therapy should be initiated in the patient with signs of infection. Cardiac failure or arrhythmias should be treated by appropriate measures. Invasive cardiopulmonary monitoring should be instituted at this time. Nutritional support should be instituted early to prevent further loss of muscle mass. With treatment of

Table 34.5.
Drug Therapy of Acute Respiratory Failure[a]

Maintain adequate oxygenation and acid/base status

Ensure adequate fluid, electrolyte, and nutrition support

Assess likelihood of infection; institute antibiotics if necessary

Institute physiotherapy for removal of secretions; mucolytics such as *N*-acetylcysteine may be required

β_2-Agonist dose is based upon product selected; may require use of an inhaler, nebulizer, or parenteral administration; monitor for tremor and tachycardia, especially with parenteral administration

Anticholinergics—Ipratropium bromide inhaler, 2 inhalations four times a day; higher doses may be required

Theophylline (aminophylline equivalent)—5.6 mg/kg load (if not already receiving theophylline) followed by 0.2 to 1.0 mg/kg/hr continuous infusion; individualize dose based upon patient history and serum theophylline concentrations; monitor for nervousness, tremor, tachycardia, and gastrointestinal side effects

Corticosteroids—Hydrocortisone 100 to 250 mg IV q6h or methylprednisolone 0.5 mg/kg IV q6h × 72 hr; taper slowly to avoid relapse; monitor for signs of infection

Respiratory stimulants—(Use is controversial); doxapram 1 to 2 mg/min continuous infusion; do not use for periods exceeding 2 hr; monitor vital signs and blood gases

[a] Treatment generally involves a combination of therapies and should be individualized to the situation.

the underlying cause and adequate supportive care, the in-hospital mortality rate is currently under 7%.

PROGNOSIS

The best indicators of prognosis are degree of obstruction and age (61). Development of complications such as cor pulmonale and hypoxia are negative indicators for survival. FEV_1 obtained after bronchodilators is a good predictor of survival (61). Patients who maintain an FEV_1 above 2 liters generally do not experience dyspnea during ordinary activity. A decrease in FEV_1 to less than 1 liter is associated with dyspnea during ordinary physical activity such as level walking or climbing more than one flight of stairs. Once FEV_1 decreases below 0.75 liters, the severe airway obstruction is associated with increased 5-year mortality. When the patient has dyspnea, the rate of mortality increases; up to 50% of patients die within 5 years. Their course will likely be characterized by multiple exacerbations, hospitalizations, and multiple drug therapies to treat symptoms or prevent progression. Poor nutrition and exercise intolerance frequently develop, and patients undergo important alterations in lifestyle in severe disease.

CONCLUSIONS

Chronic obstructive pulmonary disease is a potentially preventable disease. Recognition that smoking contributes to the majority of COPD cases logically leads to the conclusion that cessation of smoking would dramatically decrease the incidence of COPD. Public education about the haz-

ards of smoking should continue. Once COPD develops, those with moderate-to-severe disease are faced with a multitude of drug therapies with clearly debatable efficacy. The progressive nature of the disease means the cost to the patient, both personally and financially, and the cost to society are high. It is hoped that results of current and future investigations will improve the outlook for those affected by COPD.

REFERENCES

1. Petty TL: Future trends in the management of asthma and chronic obstructive pulmonary disease. Am J Med 79(6Asuppl):38–42, 1985.
2. Anon: Chronic disease reports: chronic obstructive pulmonary disease mortality—United States, 1986. MMWR 38(32):549–552, 1989.
3. Murphy ML, Bone RC: Cor Pulmonale in Chronic Bronchitis and Emphysema. New York: Futura Publishing Company, 1984, ch 2, 4.
4. National Heart, Lung, and Blood Institute, Division of Lung Diseases Workshop Report. The definition of emphysema. Am Rev Respir Dis 32:182–185, 1985.
5. Snider GL: Distinguishing among asthma, chronic bronchitis, and emphysema. Chest 87(1suppl):35S–39S, 1985.
6. Maurell CB, Eriksson S: The electrophoretic α-1-globulin pattern of serum in α-1-antitrypsin deficiency. Scand J Clin Lab Invest 15:132–140, 1963.
7. Altose MD: Assessment and management of breathlessness. Chest 88(2suppl):77S–83S, 1985.
8. Alexander MR, Taylor JW, Dull WL, et al.: Therapy of chronic obstructive airways disease. Drug Intell Clin Pharm 18:279–291, 1984.
9. Leeder SR: Role of infection in the cause and course of chronic bronchitis. J Infect Dis 131:731–742, 1975.
10. Tager I, Speizer FE: Role of infection in chronic bronchitis. N Engl J Med 292:563–571, 1974.
11. Gump DW, Phillips CA, Forsyth BR, et al.: Role of infection in chronic bronchitis. Am Rev Respir Dis 113:465–474, 1976.
12. American Thoracic Society: Definitions and classification of chronic bronchitis, asthma, and pulmonary emphysema. Am Rev Respir Dis 85:762–769, 1962.
13. Surgeon General: Introduction, overview, and conclusions. In The Health Consequences of Smoking—Chronic Obstructive Lung Disease. A Report of the Surgeon General. Rockville, MD, U.S. Department of Health and Human Services, 1984, pp 5–15.
14. Wilson DO, Rogers RM, Hoffman RM: Nutrition and chronic lung disease. Am Rev Respir Dis 132:1347–1365, 1985.
15. Driver AG, McAlvey MT, Smith VL: Nutritional assessment of patients with COPD and acute respiratory failure. Chest 82:568–571, 1982.
16. Braun SR, Keim NL, Dixon RM, et al.: The prevalence and determinants of nutritional changes in chronic obstructive pulmonary disease. Chest 86(4):558–563, 1984.
17. Eaton ML, MacDonald FM, Church TR, Niewoehner DE: Effects of theophylline on breathlessness and exercise tolerance in patients with chronic airflow obstruction. Chest 82:538–542, 1982.
18. Alexander MR, Dull WL, Kasik JE: Treatment of chronic obstructive pulmonary disease with orally administered theophylline: a double-blind, controlled study. JAMA 244:2286–2290, 1980.
19. Aubier M, Roussos C: Effect of theophylline on respiratory muscle function. Chest 88(2suppl):91S–97S, 1985.
20. Hendeles L, Massanari M, Weinberger M: Update on the pharmacodynamics and pharmacokinetics of theophylline. Chest 88(2suppl):103S–111S, 1985.
21. Matthay RA: Effects of theophylline on cardiovascular performance in chronic obstructive pulmonary disease. Chest 88(2suppl):112S–117S, 1985.

22. Lakshminarayan S, Sahn SA, Weil JV: Effect of aminophylline on ventilatory responses in normal man. Am Rev Respir Dis 117:33–38, 1978.

23. Hendeles L, Massanari M, Weinberger M: Theophylline. In Evans WE, Schentag JJ, Jusko WJ: Applied Pharmacokinetics—Principles of Therapeutic Drug Monitoring, ed. 2. Spokane, Applied Therapeutics, 1986, ch 32.

24. Levine JH, Michael JR, Guarnieri T: Multifocal atrial tachycardia: a toxic effect of theophylline. Lancet pp 12–14, Jan, 1985.

25. Hendeles L, Weinberger M: Theophylline—a state of the art review. Pharmacotherapy 3:2–44, 1983.

26. Aubier M, Vires N, Murciano D, et al.: Effects and mechanism of action of terbutaline on diaphragmatic contractility and fatigue. J Appl Physiol 56:922–929, 1984.

27. Brent BN, Mahler D, Bueger HJ, et al.: Augmentation of right ventricular performance in chronic obstructive pulmonary disease by terbutaline: a combined radionuclide and hemodynamic study. Am J Cardiol 50:313–319, 1982.

28. Nelson HS, Black JW, Branch LB, et al.: Subsensitivity to epinephrine following the administration of epinephrine and ephedrine to normal individuals. J Allergy Clin Immunol 55:299–309, 1975.

29. Olin BR (ed): Bronchodilators (Sympathomimetics). Facts and Comparisons. St. Louis: JB Lippincott, 1991, pp 173a–177a.

30. McEvoy GK (ed): Sympathomimetic Agents. AHFS Drug Information 90. Bethesda, MD: American Society of Hospital Pharmacists, 1990, pp 612–658.

31. Gayrad P, Orehek J: Mauvaise utilisation des aerosol–doseurs par les asthmatiques. Respiration 40:47–52, 1980.

32. Newman SP, Clark SN: Inhalation technique with aerosol bronchodilators: does it matter? Pract Cardiol 9:157–164, 1983.

33. Tashkin DP, Ashutosh K, Bleecker ER et al.: Comparison of the anticholinergic bronchodilator ipratropium bromide with metaproterenol in chronic obstructive pulmonary disease. Am J Med 81(5A):81–90, 1986.

34. Ashutosh K, Lang H: Comparison between long-term treatment of chronic bronchitic airway obstruction with ipratropium bromide and metaproterenol. Ann Allergy 53(5):401–406, 1984.

35. Massey KL, Gotz VP: Ipratropium bromide. Drug Intell Clin Pharm 19(1):5–12, 1985.

36. Douglas NJ, Davidson I, Sudlow MF et al.: Bronchodilatation and the site of airway resistance in severe chronic bronchitis. Thorax 34:51–56, 1979.

37. Mendella LA, Manfreda J, Warren CPW, Anthonisen NR: Steroid response in stable chronic obstructive pulmonary disease. Ann Intern Med 96:17–21, 1982.

38. Shim C, Stover DE, Williams MH Jr: Response to corticosteroids in chronic bronchitis. J Allergy Clin Immunol 62:363–367, 1978.

39. Harding SM, Freedman S: A comparison of oral and inhaled steroids in patients with chronic airways obstruction: features determining response. Thorax 33:214–218, 1978.

40. Strain D, Kinazewitz GT, Franco DS, George RB: Effect of steroid therapy on exercise performance in patients with irreversible chronic obstructive pulmonary disease. Am Rev Respir Dis 129:A65, 1984.

41. Strain DS, Kinasewitz GT, Franco DS, George RB: Effect of steroid therapy on exercise performance in patients with irreversible chronic obstructive pulmonary disease. Chest 88(5):718–721, 1985.

42. Evans JA, Morrison IM, Saunders KB: A controlled trial of prednisone, in low dosage, in patients with chronic airflow obstruction. Thorax 29:401–406, 1974.

43. Blair GP, Light RW: Treatment of chronic obstructive pulmonary disease with corticosteroids—comparison of daily vs alternate-day therapy. Chest 86(4):524–528, 1984.

44. Hudson LD, Monti CM: Rationale and use of corticosteroids in chronic obstructive pulmonary disease. Med Clin North Am 74(3):661–690, 1990.

45. Fraser IM, Hyland RH, Hutcheon MA, et al.: Preliminary study of the effects of postoperative methylprednisolone therapy on lung function recovery in patients with chronic obstructive pulmonary disease. Clin Pharm 8:214–219, 1989.

46. British Thoracic Society Research Committee: Oral N-acetylcysteine and exacerbation rates in patients with chronic bronchitis and severe airways obstruction. Thorax 40:832–835, 1985.

47. Morgan EJ, Petty TL: Summary of the national mycolytic study. Chest 97(2):24S–27S, 1990.

48. Dolly ER, Block AJ: Medroxyprogesterone acetate and COPD: effect on breathing and oxygenation in sleeping and awake patients. Chest 84:394–398, 1983.

49. Skatrud JB, Dempsey JA: Determinants of chronic carbon dioxide retention and its correction in humans. J Clin Invest 65:813–821, 1980.

50. Anthonisen NR, Manfreda J, Warren CPW, et al.: Antibiotic therapy in exacerbations of chronic obstructive pulmonary disease. Ann Intern Med 106:196–204, 1987.

51. Bates JH: The role of infection during exacerbations of chronic bronchitis. Ann Intern Med 97:130–131, 1982.

52. Williams JH, Moser KM: Pneumococcal vaccine and patients with chronic lung disease. Ann Intern Med 104:106–109, 1986.

53. Williams DO, Barnes PJ, Vickers HP, Rudolf M: Effect of nifedipine on bronchomotor tone and histamine reactivity in asthma. Br Med J 283:348, 1981.

54. Popa VT, Somani P, Simon V: The effect of inhaled verapamil on resting bronchial tone and airway contractions induced by histamine and acetylcholine in normal and asthmatic subjects. Am Rev Respir Dis 130:1006–1013, 1984.

55. Barnes PJ, Wilson NM, Brown MJ: A calcium antagonist, nifedipine, modifies exercise-induced asthma. Thorax 36:726–730, 1981.

56. Patel KR: Calcium antagonists in exercise-induced asthma. Br Med J 282:932–933, 1981.

57. Michael JR, Selinger S, Parham W, et al.: Use of calcium channel blockers in hypoxic lung disease. Chest 88(4suppl):260S–263S, 1985.

58. Simmonneau G, Escourrou P, Duroux P, Lockhart A: Inhibition of hypoxic pulmonary vasoconstriction by nifedipine. N Engl J Med 304:1582–1585, 1981.

59. Lewis RA: A presumptive role for leukotrienes in obstructive airways disease. Chest 88(2suppl):98S–102S.

60. Cooper JD, Patterson GA, Grossman R, Maurer J and the Toronto Lung Transplant Group: Double-lung transplant for advanced chronic obstructive lung disease. Am Rev Respir Dis 139:303–307, 1989.

61. Anthonisen NR, Wright EC, Hodgkin JE, and the IPPB Trial Group: Prognosis in chronic obstructive pulmonary disease. Am Rev Respir Dis 133:14–20, 1986.

CHAPTER 35

HYPERTENSION

ROBERT T. WEIBERT, Pharm.D.

Hypertension is currently the most common reason for physician office visits in the United States. Important changes in the approach to treating hypertension have occurred during the past decade. Blood pressure (BP) control continues to be an important factor in reducing cardiovascular risk, but there is an increased emphasis on control of other risk factors, especially lowering cholesterol, and the importance of nonpharmacologic measures to reduce blood pressure has received renewed attention. Drug treatment has evolved to an individualized approach using a variety of drugs tailored to individual patients, based on considerations of age, race, other diseases, the effect of quality of life, drug costs, and compliance. Now evidence suggests an increase in mortality from excessive lowering of blood pressure. The adverse consequences of antihypertensive drugs must be considered carefully, and it now appears reasonable to "step-down" drug therapy following a sustained period of controlled blood pressure.

Most hypertensive patients require long-term antihypertensive drug treatment, and more pharmacologic agents are available for the treatment of hypertension than for any other condition. Pharmacists can provide information about the pharmacology, pharmacokinetics, drug interactions, and adverse effects of these agents. In addition, maintaining patients on long-term drug treatment is an opportunity for pharmacists to participate cooperatively in providing follow-up care. Although cardiovascular deaths have been reduced over the past 20 years, achieving long-term BP control in millions of patients with hypertension remains an important objective.

DEFINITION

Blood pressure varies from minute to minute and is influenced by measurement technique, time of day, emotion, pain, discomfort, hydration, temperature, exercise, posture, and drugs. The dividing line between normal blood pressure and hypertension is arbitrary. Early insurance actuarial data showed a continuum, where the higher the blood pressure the greater risk of developing complications. The 1988 Report of the Joint National Committee on Detection, Evaluation and Treatment of High Blood Pressure (JNC IV) set forth the following guidelines for establishing a diagnosis of hypertension:

After screening, the diagnosis of hypertension is confirmed when the average of two or more diastolic blood pressure measurements on at least two subsequent visits is 90 mm Hg or higher or the average of two or more systolic blood pressure measurements is consistently greater than 140 mm Hg. JNC IV classifies blood pressures as shown in Table 35.1. Single, casual measurements of blood pressure may inaccurately classify individuals as having hypertension and cause unnecessary emotional, social, and financial problems.

ETIOLOGY

More than 90% of patients with sustained elevation of arterial blood pressure have essential hypertension with no identifiable cause. This term evolved from the mistaken concept that high blood pressure was "essential" for adequate tissue perfusion. A small percentage of patients may have potentially curable hypertension caused by renal disease, adrenal disease, coarctation of the aorta, or other rare conditions (1). Renovascular hypertension, considered the most prevalent remediable type of hypertension, is estimated to occur in less than 0.5% of the hypertension population (2).

Drug-induced Hypertension

Hypertension may occur in up to 5% of patients taking oral contraceptives. However, most women show small, but measurable, increases (9/5 mm Hg) in blood pressure during the first 2 years on the "pill" (3). Factors that may increase the likelihood of oral contraceptive hypertension include age >35 years, smoking, obesity, and a family history of hypertension. Although the estrogen is the most important component, the amount and type of progestin may further influence the effect on blood pressure. Proposed mechanisms for contraceptive-induced hypertension include stimulation of the renin-angiotensin-aldosterone system and sodium and fluid retention. Oral contraceptive hypertension may develop gradually over 1 to 2 years and is usually reversible within 1 to 8 months after therapy is stopped. However, if blood pressure does not normalize within 3 months, further evaluation and therapy is appropriate. Oral contraceptive–induced hypertension is best prevented by checking blood pressure every 6 months and using the agent with the lowest effective estrogen dose (<30 μg) and a progestin content of

Table 35.1.
Classification of Blood Pressure

Classification	Diastolic Pressure (mm Hg)
Normal blood pressure	<85
High normal blood pressure	85–89
Mild hypertension	90–104
Moderate hypertension	105–114
Severe hypertension	>115

1 mg or less (3). Women who are at higher risk or who actually develop hypertension may need alternative forms of contraception (see Chapter 87, "Contraception and Infertility").

Other drugs may also increase blood pressure significantly. A double dose of the sympathomimetic diet drug phenylpropanolamine (PPA) increases blood pressure to a peak of 173/103 mm Hg (4). There are reports of intracranial hemorrhage following PPA use. Additional drugs that may increase blood pressure include corticosteroids, monoamine oxidase (MAO) inhibitors, cyclosporine, erythropoietin, and products containing large quantities of sodium such as effervescent solutions.

INCIDENCE

The JNC IV states that nearly 60 million Americans have blood pressure of ≥140/90 mm Hg or are taking antihypertensive medications (1). The majority have mild hypertension, with diastolic blood pressures ranging from 90 to 104 mm Hg. The incidence of hypertension increases with age and is higher among blacks than whites. In adults about 7% have high normal blood pressure, 15% have mild hypertension, 2% have moderate or severe diastolic hypertension, and 2% have isolated systolic hypertension (5). Men and women of the same race are affected approximately equally (6).

Massive public health efforts have increased the awareness of patient and the medical community of the need to identify and treat hypertension (7). Most patients are now aware that they have hypertension; the major challenge for healthcare providers is to maintain long-term treatment.

PATHOGENESIS

Blood pressure is maintained within a relatively constant range despite changes in posture and wide variations in the demand for blood supply. While much is known about the complex system that regulates blood pressure, the pathogenesis of essential hypertension remains mysterious. Early theories suggested that renal sodium retention expanded vascular volume, increasing cardiac output. The increased cardiac output was believed to lead to increased

vascular resistance (6). Further investigations suggest that natriuretic hormones may initiate sodium retention (6). Another theory suggests that inherited cellular defects cause increased intracellular sodium concentrations leading to increases in ionic calcium and increased vascular tone and reactivity (6, 8). A possible primary role of the sympathetic nervous system has also been suggested (6). It is likely that several interrelated mechanisms control blood pressure in essential hypertension, rather than a single causative defect. A relationship between hypertension and obesity, insulin resistance, hyperinsulinemia, glucose intolerance, and hypertriglyceridemia has been reported (see ref. 81, 87). This relationship has been termed the deadly quartet or syndrome (see ref. 81, 87, 88). This has led to the theory that hyperinsulinemia is a possible etiologic abnormality causing hypertension (see ref. 87, 88). However, even with continued insights into the regulation of blood pressure, essential hypertension remains a process that must be controlled, rather than a curable disorder.

DIAGNOSIS, SYMPTOMS, AND CLINICAL FINDINGS

Hypertension is usually an asymptomatic disease and is most often detected by screening. Because hypertension is easily detected and effective therapy is available, screening is recommended for all adults (9). Although headache, epistaxis, and tinnitus were once thought to be symptoms of high blood pressure, no relationship has been demonstrated between these symptoms and either systolic or diastolic blood pressure (10). It now appears that work-site screening programs produce minimal psychosocial consequences (11). Increased absenteeism following a diagnosis of hypertension is associated with higher baseline anxiety levels, and reassurance may be beneficial for these patients (11).

The initial evaluation of patients with possible hypertension is an important process with several objectives:

Establishing a Diagnosis of Hypertension (1, 12). The average of two or more measurements of blood pressure with the subject seated and the diastolic pressure reported as the disappearance of sound (phase V) on two subsequent visits after an elevated blood pressure at screening confirms the diagnosis of hypertension. JNC IV classifications are shown in Table 35.1.

Measurement. Correct techniques are crucial in determining if a casual screening or office blood pressure reflect a true increase in blood pressure (12). Accurate measurement of blood pressure requires correct cuff width (two-thirds of the length between the shoulder and elbow), correct arm position, a bared arm, and the lightest possible pressure on the stethoscope head. Patients should be comfortably seated, relaxed, with the arm held passively at the level of the heart. Ideally, both phase 4 (muffling) and phase 5 (disappearance) Korotkoff sounds should be recorded (12). Twenty-one percent of patients with untreated borderline hypertension were shown to have "white coat hypertension" based on ambulatory monitoring of blood pressure (13). This exaggerated pressor response is more pronounced when blood pressure is measured by a physician than by a technician, and it may be specific to the physician's office. White coat or office hypertension occurs more often in females, younger patients, and patients recently diagnosed as hypertensive (13).

Ambulatory blood pressure monitoring (ABPM) for 24 hr or longer is possible using newer monitoring devices (14). ABPM is not cost-effective for all patients, but it may have clinical utility in evaluation of patients with high normal blood pressure with target organ damage, resistant hypertension, episodic hypertension, transient hypotension, office hypertension, and myocardial ischemia (14). Damage to target organs appears to correlate best with data from ABPM (14).

Avoiding Early Dropout. The problem of early dropouts from hypertension treatment programs is well documented. Dropouts from care during the first year of treatment frequently approach 50% (15). The most important part of the initial visit is insuring that the patient will return for further follow-up.

Evaluation for the Presence of Cardiovascular Risk Factors and Quantitation of Hypertensive Vascular Disease. The medical history, physical examination, and laboratory testing are directed toward identifying risk factors, assessing the extent of any existing vascular damage, and detecting any concurrent diseases. The Joint National Committee has provided guidelines for evaluating patients (Table 35.2) (1).

Screening for Secondary Causes of Hypertension. Most patients with elevated blood pressure have essential hypertension. Any patient whose medical history or physical examination suggests a possible cause of secondary hypertension warrants additional diagnostic evaluation (Table 35.3) (1).

Explanation of Findings. To avoid early dropout and to work toward long-term control of hypertension, patients must become active participants in their own care. To do so requires that patients understand

- The potential benefits and risks of therapy;
- That their blood pressure exceeds normal limits;
- The possible consequences of uncontrolled hypertension;
- That hypertension is usually asymptomatic and symptoms do not reliably indicate the level of blood pressure;
- Prolonged follow-up and therapy are needed;
- Treatment will control but not cure high blood pressure;
- Their target blood pressure;
- The presence of any other cardiovascular risk factors and how these indicate their own probability of developing cardiovascular disease.

The initial evaluation documents the hypertension, begins

Table 35.2.
Evaluation Of Hypertensive Patients

Medical history
  Family history of hypertension and hypertensive complications
  History of cardiovascular, cerebrovascular, or renal disease or diabetes mellitus
  Duration and level of elevated blood pressure
  Effectiveness and side effects of previous drug treatment
  Medication history for drugs that elevate blood pressure
  Lifestyle and health habits:
    Smoking
    Ethanol excess
    Sodium intake
    Caffeine
    Exercise
    Emotional stress
Physical examination
  Two or more BP measurements with patient supine or seated and standing
  Verification of BP in the contralateral arm
  Height and weight
  Fundoscopic examination for arteriolar narrowing, A-V compression, hemorrhages, exudates, and papilledema
  Neck examination for carotid bruits, distended veins, and enlarged thyroid
  Cardiac examination for increased rate, size, precordial heave, murmurs, arrhythmias, and S3, S4 heart sounds
  Abdominal examination for bruits, enlarged kidneys, and aortic dilation
  Extremity examination for edema and decreased or absent pulses
  Neurologic assessment
Laboratory tests
  Hemoglobin and hematocrit
  Urinalysis
  Serum potassium
  Serum creatinine
  Fasting plasma glucose
  Total and HDL-cholesterol
  Serum uric acid

Table 35.3.
Clinical Findings Suggestive of Secondary Hypertension

Finding	Secondary Cause
Abdominal bruit	Renovascular disease
Abdominal or flank mass	Polycystic kidney disease
Hypokalemia	Hyperaldosteronism
Headache, palpitations, sweating, "spells"	Pheochromocytoma
Delayed or absent femoral pulse	Aortic coarctation
Truncal obesity	Cushing's syndrome

to establish long-term compliance, and establishes the extent of target organ damage and the existence of other risk factors. This provides a rational basis for treatment planning.

COMPLICATIONS

The major organs damaged by arterial hypertension are the brain, heart, and kidneys. The risk of complications

Table 35.4.
Effect of Combined Risk Factors on Total Deaths/1000 in MRFIT[a]

Risk Factor	Men Age 35–45 years Deaths/1000	Increase[a]	Men Age 46–57 years Deaths/1000	Increase
None	5.4		19.3	
DBP >90	8.4	1.6	25.8	1.3
Cholesterol >6.5 mmol/liter (250 mg/dl)	10.0	1.9	25.4	1.3
Smoker	12.8	2.4	38.8	2.0
DBP + cholesterol	15.8	2.9	37.9	2.0
DBP + smoker	23.2	4.3	56.4	2.9
DBP/cholesterol/smoker	33.2	6.1	70.7	3.7

[a] Data from Kannel WB, Neaton JD, Wentworth D, et al.: Overall and coronary heart disease mortality rates in relation to major risk factors in 325,348 men screened for MRFIT. Am Heart J 112:825–836, 1986.
[b] Increased risk = deaths for men with risk factor/deaths for men with no risks.

Table 35.5.
Risk Factors for Cardiovascular Disease

Correctable	Noncorrectable
Hypertension	Family history of hypertension, stroke, or heart disease
Cigarette smoking	
Elevated cholesterol	Diabetes mellitus
Reduced HDL-cholesterol	Male
Target organ damage	Older age
Obesity	

and premature death is related to the degree of elevation of blood pressure. Hypertension is additive with other risk factors in the development of coronary artery disease (CAD) and stroke. The Multiple Risk Factor Intervention Trial (MRFIT) study describes the combined effects of cardiovascular risk factors (16). In men <45 years a DBP>90 mm Hg increased deaths 1.6 times the rate for men without risks; two risk factors increased the rate 3 to 4 times, and all three major risk factors increased the death rate 6-fold (Table 35.4). The major correctable and noncorrectable risk factors are shown in Table 35.5.

Left ventricular hypertrophy (LVH) and left ventricular dysfunction are important complications related to hypertension (17–20). Echocardiography shows that left ventricular muscle mass is increased in 20 to 40% of patients with mild hypertension (18). Cardiovascular events occur more than twice as frequently in mildly hypertensive patients with LVH (26%) than in those without LVH (12%) (19). Patients with LVH have a 5 to 6 times higher risk of sudden death or other cardiovascular mortality than those without LVH (12, 17).

The major complications associated with hypertension are stroke and coronary artery disease. A meta-analysis of

nine prospective observational studies of 420,000 patients with a mean 10 years follow-up provided an assessment of these risks (21). The combined data demonstrated a positive, continuous increase in risk within the range of DBP 70 to 110 mm Hg. There was no evidence of a "threshold" DBP and lower blood pressures were always associated with less risk. Higher blood pressures (even within the range considered to be normotensive) are associated with increasing cardiovascular risks. A prolonged difference in DBP of 10 mm Hg was associated with 56% less stroke and 37% less coronary artery disease (21).

TREATMENT

Observational studies have clearly demonstrated that a lower DBP is associated with a lower risk of stroke and CAD. However, the effects of differences in blood pressure may develop over decades. Whether maintaining blood pressure reductions over a few years will decrease these cardiovascular risks has been examined in randomized trials. A detailed epidemiological analysis has recently summarized the findings from 14 unconfounded randomized trials of antihypertensive drugs, which were reported between 1965 and 1986 (22). There were a total of 37,000 patients, with 30,000 treated for mild hypertension (22). Most trials used a "stepped-care" approach, starting with a diuretic. Two trials started with a β-blocker. The usual goal of treatment was to reduce DBP to 90 mm Hg or less, and the mean follow-up time was 5 years. The average difference in blood pressure between the treatment and control groups was 6 mm Hg. This reduction in blood pressure produced a highly significant reduction in stroke, a decrease of 42%. This benefit of stroke reduction appears soon after the lowering of blood pressure. The effect of blood pressure reduction in CAD was much smaller (14%), and the reduction in fatal CAD (11%) was not significant. The reduction in the odds of stroke was 33 to 50% in the clinical trials, which corresponds to the 35 to 40% predicted from observational studies. The reduction in the odds of CAD was 4 to 22% in the clinical trials, which was less than the 20 to 25% predicted from epidemiology. The shortfall in CAD reduction could be due to chance, to the influence of chronic processes (e.g., atherosclerosis) that were not reversed by BP reduction, or to cardiotoxic adverse effects of the treatments that limited CAD reduction.

In summary, a 5 to 6 mm Hg reduction of DBP with diuretic-based regimens produced risk reductions of 42% for stroke and 14% for CAD. Improved compliance with antihypertensive therapy and an 8 to 10 mm Hg reduction in DBP should reduce stroke by 50% and CAD by 20%. Because CAD occurs more frequently, the absolute benefit of a 20% decrease in CAD could exceed the benefit of a 50% decrease in stroke. But, other therapies for CAD (cholesterol reduction, smoking cessation, aspirin, and β-blockers) have stronger evidence of cardiac benefit and should be emphasized for high-risk patients. A high risk of stroke is a clearer indication for antihypertensive therapy than is an increased risk of CAD. Elderly patients have a 2% annual incidence of stroke, and patients with a prior TIA have a 5% incidence.

Antihypertensive Therapy Trials

VETERANS ADMINISTRATION COOPERATIVE STUDY

The VA Cooperative Study clearly demonstrated that reducing blood pressure to normal or near normal levels decreases the occurrence of complications, and it provided the early evidence of the benefits of drug treatment (23–25). Complications developed 3 times as frequently in untreated patients. The treatment of moderate hypertension (DBP >104 mm Hg) abolished hypertensive complications (congestive heart failure, accelerated hypertension, renal failure) and reduced cerebrovascular accidents by 75%. However, treatment did not decrease the incidence of myocardial infarction. Finally, the VA study showed that even partial reduction of blood pressure (DBP <105>90 mm Hg) decreases cardiovascular complications (26).

HYPERTENSION DETECTION AND FOLLOW-UP PROGRAM COOPERATIVE STUDY

The Hypertension Detection and Follow-up Program (HDFP) randomized almost 11,000 patients to referred care or stepped-care groups (26–28). Seventy percent of the patients had "mild hypertension" (DBP 90 to 104 mm Hg). The treatment goal for HDFP patients was the lesser of a 10 mm Hg decrease from entry blood pressure or a DBP <90 mm Hg. The 5-year DBP averaged 84 mm Hg for the SC group and 89 mm Hg for the RC group, a difference of only 5 mm Hg. Strokes were reduced by 45%, and death from myocardial infarction was decreased 26%. The 5-year mortality was 16.9% lower for the SC group, compared with the RC group. Mortality was 20.3% lower for the SC subgroup with entry DBP of 90 to 104 mm Hg (5.9 vs. 7.4 per 100). The subgroup with DBP 90 to 140 mm Hg and no evidence of end-organ damage at entry had 28.6% fewer deaths at 5 years. The HDFP did not demonstrate a significant reduction in mortality for white women or for patients under age 50 years, as the death rate was low in both groups. A Postrial Surveillance Study (PTS) followed HDFP participants for an additional 2 years, providing 6.7-year mortality data. Mortality differences increased further to 95.1/1000 SC patients vs 116.3/1000 RC patients (29).

MULTIPLE RISK FACTOR INTERVENTION TRIAL (MRFIT)

The MRFIT trial followed 12,800 men over 7 years (30). A special intervention group (SI) that received stepped-care treatment for hypertension, counseling for cigarette smoking, and dietary advice to lower cholesterol was compared with usual-care (UC) group. Risk factors in the SI group decreased, compared with the usual are (UC) group. However, the SI group showed only a nonsignificant 7% lower rate of CAD mortality. The possibility that antihypertensive drug therapy had an adverse effect on some patients has been raised as a potential explanation for the similar mortality despite reduction of risk factors. Hypertensive men in the SI group with resting ECG abnormalities at the start of the study had 65% more deaths from CAD than the UC group with the same ECG abnormalities (30). In contrast, men with a normal resting ECG but an abnormal exercise ECG had a 57% lower rate of CAD mortality in the SI group than the UC group (31).

EUROPEAN WORKING PARTY ON HIGH BLOOD PRESSURE IN THE ELDERLY TRIAL (EWPHE)

The EWPHE trial assessed the effects of antihypertensive drug therapy in patients over 60 years of age (32). In this trial 840 patient with entry DBP of 90 to 119 mm Hg were randomized to treatment or placebo and followed over 12 years. Treatment reduced total mortality (9%) and cardiovascular mortality (27%). Therapy with combined hydrochlorothiazide/triamterene adversely affected glucose tolerance and serum uric acid and creatinine levels. Subanalysis shows little or no benefit from the treatment of patients over 80 years of age, most of whom were women (33).

SUMMARY OF TREATMENT STUDIES

Early studies clearly demonstrated the benefit of treating moderate and severe hypertension. The JNC recommends that patients with DBP of 90 to 94 mm Hg first attempt to lower blood pressure by nonpharmacologic methods for 3 to 6 months (1). If this fails, then drug treatment should be started in all patients over 50 years of age. Trials of antihypertensive drugs in mild hypertension have shown a reduction in stroke, LVH, CAD, and accelerated hypertension. Drug treatment for DBP ≥95 mm Hg is recommended if nondrug methods fail. The goal of therapy is a DBP <90 mm Hg.

NONPHARMACOLOGIC THERAPY

Nonpharmacologic methods of reducing blood pressure should be the initial approach for young patients with mild hypertension and no other cardiovascular risk factors, and they are also continued to augment drug therapy.

Sodium Restriction

While there is clear epidemiological evidence of a direct relationship between dietary sodium intake and blood pressure, severe dietary sodium restriction is usually not sustainable and is not needed. Moderate sodium reduction to an intake of 80 to 100 mmol sodium per day (5 to 6 g

NaCl) may lower blood pressure in some patients. Sodium restriction to 50 mmol daily (3 g salt) from a 200 mmol sodium diet reduced blood pressure 16/9 mm Hg (34). Modest dietary sodium restriction has also been shown to have adjunctive benefit with most antihypertensive drug therapy (35). This degree of sodium restriction can be achieved by refraining from adding salt at the table and avoiding highly salted processed foods.

Obesity

The prevalence of hypertension is 50% higher among overweight than normal-weight adults (36). Weight reduction can reduce arterial blood pressure independent of sodium restriction. The JNC recommends that all obese hypertensive patients participate in weight-reduction programs, with a goal body weight of within 15% of desirable weight (1). It is well recognized that weight reduction is difficult to achieve and sustain.

Exercise

Exercise training decreases blood pressure in hypertensive patients an average of 11/8 mm Hg (37). Exercise training also is beneficial for weight reduction, lowers plasma triglycerides, and improves insulin sensitivity (37). The addition of either diltiazem or propranolol did not produce additive benefit to exercise training (38). Exercise training lowered blood pressure and total and LDL cholesterol, while increasing HDL cholesterol. Propranolol limited the exercise-induced increase in HDL cholesterol (38). A regular exercise training program should be started gradually and may control blood pressure without drug therapy in mild hypertension.

Dynamic endurance exercises (walking, running, cycling, swimming) are recommended, while isometric exercises (rowing, competitive sports) are not suitable (39). Because hypertensive patients may show exaggerated blood pressures during exercise, intensive training should not be started until diastolic blood pressures are below 105 mm Hg (39). Drugs effective in treating superelevated blood pressures (SBP >200 mm Hg) during exercise include cardioselective β_1-blockers, verapamil, clonidine, and angiotensin converting-enzyme inhibitors (39).

Cigarettes

Smoking increases the risk of cancer and pulmonary disease, and more than doubles the risk of cardiovascular disease (1). Cigarette smoking raises blood pressure acutely from 3/5 mm Hg to 12/10 mm Hg (40). While office blood pressures do not differ for smokers, 24-hr ambulatory blood pressure monitoring has shown higher daytime blood pressures in smokers, particularly in Caucasians above the age of 50 years (40). Also, smoking interferes with the reduction of blood pressure by propran-

olol in black patients (41). Finally, the reduction of cardiovascular risk by antihypertensive treatment is not as great in smokers as in nonsmokers (1). The JNC recommends a smoking-cessation program as a key component of the treatment of hypertension.

Alcohol

Moderate-to-heavy alcohol intake increases the incidence of hypertension (1, 42). Alcohol also interferes with antihypertensive drug treatment, independently of noncompliance. A substitution of low-alcohol beer led to a 5/3 mm Hg reduction in the blood pressure of treated hypertensive men (43). The JNC recommends limiting alcohol consumption to 30 ml of ethanol daily (2 oz whiskey, 8 oz wine, or 24 oz beer) (1). Alcohol use should be evaluated in patients with resistant hypertension.

Caffeine

Caffeine increases blood pressure in people who do not regularly consume methylxanthines, while habitual consumption of caffeine is believed to be associated with the development of complete tolerance to its pressor effect (44). In infrequent caffeine users blood pressure increases an average of 5.3/3.6 mm Hg (44). Ambulatory monitoring of habitual coffee drinkers demonstrated a consistent 4/4 mm Hg work site increase in blood pressure and a 12/9 mm Hg increase during formal stress testing (45). Recent epidemiologic analysis did not show an increased risk of coronary artery disease or stroke from coffee or caffeine consumption (46). Because of the potential to increase blood pressure, hypertensive patients should be advised to avoid coffee or limit coffee to 2 cups daily and to avoid coffee consumption prior to blood pressure measurement.

Cation Supplementation and Stress Reduction

Both calcium and potassium supplementation have been used for possible modest blood pressure lowering effects (1). The role of these cations in treating hypertension is still under investigation. The use of relaxation and biofeedback therapy to reduce behavioral stress may reduce blood pressure modestly in some patients (1). Behavioral techniques should not be considered as alternatives to pharmacologic therapy, but rather as supplements to other therapy.

Summary of Nonpharmacologic Methods

The JNC has concluded that weight control, alcohol restriction, and sodium restriction independently reduce blood pressure and are additive with pharmacologic agents (1). These three approaches are recommended for all hypertensive patients. A nutritional program to lose weight and restrict sodium and alcohol achieved a 39% success in normalizing blood pressure without drug therapy (47).

Smoking cessation and exercise programs are recommended for all hypertensive patients. Nonpharmacologic therapy alone should be used for all patients with DBPs between 90 and 94 mm Hg. Patients who do not normalize blood pressure after 3 to 6 months of nonpharmacologic therapy should be considered for drug treatment.

DRUG THERAPY

Drug therapy is reserved for patients with DBPs $\geq$95 mm Hg or those who have DBPs of 90 to 94 mm Hg and at least one of the following additional risk factors: smoking, diabetes, or hypercholesterolemia (1). When initiating drug therapy it is important to remember that hypertension is a disease of decades. Unless hypertension is severe, it is preferable to start a simple drug regimen that minimizes side effects and encourages long-term compliance.

Understanding the site and mechanism of action of the various antihypertensive drugs is important in planning therapy. All current drugs impair normal homeostatic mechanisms and most reduce peripheral vascular resistance. The pharmacologic classification and dosage information are presented in Table 33.6. Common adverse effects and special precautions for antihypertensive drugs are in Table 33.7 and the hemodynamic and hormonal effects are in Table 33.8. Drug interactions are listed in Table 33.9.

Diuretics

Thiazide and related diuretics were the mainstay of therapy in most antihypertensive drug trials. Thiazide-type diuretics are effective in small doses, equivalent to 12.5 to 25 mg of hydrochlorothiazide, for most patients (48). Using lower doses may reduce the frequency and severity of some the metabolic abnormalities of hypokalemia, hyperglycemia, and hyperuricemia. Reducing hydrochlorothiazide from 50 mg daily to 25 mg daily resulted in a 5 mm Hg increase in SBP, with no change in DBP (85). This dose reduction led to a decrease in uric acid and an increase in serum potassium, but fasting and postprandial glucose, hemoglobin A_1C and serum lipid concentrations were unchanged. (see ref. 89) Serum lipid and hemoglobin A_1C concentrations decreased significantly after discontinuation of diuretics. Diuretics add to the effectiveness of most other antihypertensive drugs and can reverse the fluid retention that is associated with some antihypertensive drugs. Hydrochlorothiazide has proven efficacy, can be administered once daily, and is inexpensive.

The development of hypokalemia is dose-related, with moderate hypokalemia (<3.5 to >3.0 mmol/liter (mEq/liter) developing in only 2% of patients treated with HCTZ 25 mg daily, compared with 11% of patients treated with HCTZ 50 mg daily (49). Hypokalemia is exacerbated by high-sodium diets and can be minimized by sodium restriction (50). The risk of ventricular arrhythmias and sudden death may be increased by hypokalemia in patients with baseline ECG abnormalities (30). Follow-up studies suggested that mild-to-moderate hypokalemia from diuretic therapy was not a cause of cardiac arrhythmias (51). Nonetheless, hypokalemia should be minimized by using low-dose thiazide therapy, restricting sodium intake, using potassium supplements, and, if needed, adding potassium-sparing drugs. Particular caution is warranted in hypertensive patients with myocardial infarction, left ventricular hypertrophy, and/or electrocardiographic abnormalities (52).

Thiazide diuretics may produce other metabolic abnormalities, including an increase in total cholesterol, LDL-cholesterol, and triglyceride concentrations. A low-fat diet decreases the thiazide-induced change in cholesterol. Thiazide glucose intolerance is related to the degree of hypokalemia and is minimized by preventing potassium depletion. In the VA Cooperative studies the average increase in fasting glucose was 0.3 mmol/liter (6 mg/dl), with 3% of patients having a fasting glucose level above 7.8 mmol/liter (140 mg/dl) (50). Thiazides produce a mean increase in serum uric acid concentration of approximately 59.5 μmol/liter (1 mg/dl), which is not associated with adverse effects on renal function and does not require uric-acid-lowering drugs unless it is accompanied by symptomatic gout (53). Diuretics were associated with impotence at a frequency of 19.6 per 1000 patient-years in the MRC trial (52).

Thiazide diuretics are particularly effective in patients with low-renin hypertension, which is often seen in the elderly and in blacks (50, 52). Finally, thiazide diuretics may slow the rate of bone loss in the elderly and reduce the incidence of hip fractures (50, 54).

LOOP DIURETICS

The loop diuretics furosemide and bumetanide have a shorter duration of action than the thiazide diuretics and generally reduce blood pressure less (48). Loop diuretics should be reserved for patients with fluid retention unresponsive to thiazide diuretics or patients with decreased renal function. Thiazide diuretics are ineffective in patients with impaired renal function [creatinine clearance 0.83 ml/sec (<50 ml/min)]. These patients can be treated with loop diuretics, metazolone, or indapamide. Furosemide (40 mg daily) has been shown to produce less hypokalemia than hydrochlorothiazide (50 mg daily) in hypertensive patients (59).

THIAZIDE-LIKE DIURETICS

Chlorthalidone is a long-acting diuretic similar to thiazides, which produces greater hypokalemia. Metolazone is a thiazide-like diuretic that is effective in patients with renal impairment and produces a synergistic diuresis when com-

Table 35.6.
Antihypertensive Drugs

Drug	Class	Dosage Sizes (mg)	Dose Range (mg)
Diuretics			
Hydrocholrothiazide	Diuretic	25/50/100	12.5–50
Chlorthalidone	Diuretic	25/50/100	12.5–50
Indapamide	Diuretic	2.5	2.5–5.0
Metolazone	Diuretic	2.5/5/10	2.5–5.0
Bumetanide	Loop diuretic	0.5/1.0	0.5–10.0
Ethacrynic acid	Loop diuretic	25/50	25–400
Furosemide	Loop diuretic	20/40/80	20–600
Potassium-sparing diuretics			
Amiloride	Potassium-sparing diuretic	5	5–20
Spironolactone	Potassium-sparing diuretic	25/50/100	25–100
Triamterene	Potassium-sparing diuretic	50/100	50–300
β-Blockers			
Acebutolol	β-Blocker	200/400	200–1200
Atenolol	β-Blocker	50/100	50–100
Betaxolol	β-Blocker	10/20	10–40
Carteolol	β-Blocker	2.5/5	2.5–10
Metoprolol	β-Blocker	50/100	100–450
Nadolol	β-Blocker	20/40/80/120/160	40–320
Penbutolol	β-Blocker	20	20–80
Pindolol	β-Blocker	5/10	10–60
Propranalol	β-Blocker	10/20/40/60/80/90 SR: 80/120/160	40–320
Timolol	β-Blocker	5/10/20	10–40
α-β-Blocker			
Labetalol	α-β-Blocker	100/200/300	200–2400
Central adrenergic agnoists			
Clonidine	Central antiadrenergic	0.1/0.2/0.3	0.1–0.6
Clonidine TTS	Central antiadrenergic	TTS 1/2/3	0.1–0.3
Guanabenz	Central antiadrenergic	4/8	8–32
Guanfacine	Central antiadrenergic	1	1–3
Methyldopa	Central antiadrenergic	125/250/500	500–2000
Peripheral adrenergic blockers			
Guanadrel	Peripheral antiadrenergic	10/25	10–75
Guanethidine	Peripheral antiadrenergic	10/25	10–50
Reserpine	Peripheral antiadrenergic	0.1/0.25/0.5/1.0	0.1–0.25
α₁-Adrenergic blockers			
Prazosin	α₁-Blocker	1/2/5	1–20
Terazosin	α₁-Blocker	1/2/5/10	1–20
Doxazosin	α₁-Blocker	1/2/4/8	1–16
Vasodilators			
Hydralazine	Vasodilator	10/25/50/100	40–200
Minoxidil	Vasodilator	2.5/10	10–40
Angiotensin-converting-enzyme inhibitors			
Benazepril	CEI	5/10/20/40	20–80
Captopril	CEI	12.5/25/50/100	50–450
Enalapril maleate	CEI	2.5/5/10/20	2.5–40
Lisinopril	CEI	5/10/20	5–40
Ramipril	CEI	1.25/2.5/5/10	2.5–20
Fosinopril	CEI	5/10/20/40	10–80
Quinapril	CEI	5/10/20/40	10–80
Calcium-channel blockers			
Diltiazem	Calcium-entry blocker	30/60/90/120 SR: 60/90/120	120–240
Felodipine	Calcium-entry blocker	5/10	5–20
Nifedipine	Calcium-entry blocker	10/20 SR: 30/60/90	10–120
Nicardipine	Calcium-entry blocker	20/30	40–120
Isradipine	Calcium-entry blocker	2.5/5	5–20
Verapamil	Calcium-entry blocker	80/120/240 SR: 120/180/240	240–480

Table 35.7.
Adverse Antihypertensive Drug Effects

Drug	Adverse Effects	Special Precautions
Thiazide diuretics	Hypokalemia, hyperuricemia, glucose intolerance, increased serum cholesterol, trigylerides, sexual dysfunction, dehydration	LVH, CAD, diabetes mellitus/gout, renal failure, digitalis
Loop diuretics	Same as thiazide diuretics	Effective in renal failure
β-Blockers	Fatigue, insomnia, nightmares, depression, sexual dysfunction, bronchospasm, bradycardia, increased triglycerides, decreased HDL-cholesterol, dermatitis, GI upset, withdrawal rebound, psoriasis	Asthma, COPD, CHF, heart block, diabetes mellitus, hyperlipidemia, peripheral vascular disease
Central antiadrenergics	Sedation, dry mouth, fatigue, sexual dysfunction, postural hypotension, impaired concentration, withdrawal rebound hypertension, contact dermatitis from patch	Depression, caution when discontinuing to avoid rebound
Methyldopa	Hepatitis, Coombs-positive hemolytic anemia, colitis, lupus-like syndrome	
Peripheral antiadrenergics	Sexual dysfunction, nasal congestion, orthostatic hypotension, diarrhea, sodium/fluid retention	Caution in elderly, asthma, CHF
α₁-Blockers	First-dose syncope, orthostatic hypotension, headache, dizziness, drowsiness, tachycardia, sodium/fluid retention, priapism	Caution in elderly, caution with first dose
α-β-Blocker	Asthma, nausea, fatigue, dizziness, headache, orthostatic hypotension, fever, hepatotoxicity	Asthma, COPD, CHF, heart block, diabetes mellitus
Converting-enzyme inhibitors	Hyperkalemia, cough, hypotension, angioedema, rash, loss of taste, proteinuria, renal failure, neutropenia, cholestasis	Renal failure, pregnancy
Calcium-entry blockers	Headache, flushing, hypotension, dizziness, palpitations, nausea	Caution in CHF/heart block
Dihydropyridine CEB (Nifedipine)	Edema	
Verapamil	Constipation, conduction defects, CHF, bradycardia	Caution with digitalis
Vasodilators	Headache, tachycardia, dizziness, sodium/fluid retention	Angina pectoris, CHF
Hydralazine	Positive ANA, lupus-like syndrome, hepatitis, nasal congestion, GI disturbances	
Minoxidil	Hypertrichosis, facial coarsening, pleural/pericardial effusion	

Table 35.8.
Hemodynamic and Hormonal Effects of Antihypertensive Agents

Drug	PVR	CO	HR	PRA	GFR	PV
α₁-Blockers	−	0	0	−	0	+/0
α₂-Agonists	−	−/0	−	−	0	0/+
β-Blockers	0/−	−	−	−	0	0
Calcium-entry blockers	0/−	−/0	−/0/+	0/+	0	+/0
Converting-enzyme inhibitors	−	0/+	0	+	+/0	0/+
Labetalol	−	0	−	−	0/+	+
Loop diuretics	−	−	0	+	+	−
Preipheral adrenergic blockers	−	−/0	−	−	0/−	+
Thiazide diuretics	−	−	0	+	−	−
Vasodilators	−	+	+	+	+	+

a Symbols: +, increase; −, decrease; 0, no change.

Table 35.9.
Antihypertensive Drug Interactions

	α₁-Blockers	α₂-Agonists	β-Blockers	Calcium-Entry Blockers	Converting-Enzyme Inhibitors
Antacids			Decreased effect		Decreased effect (captopril)
Antiinflammatory drugs	Decreased effect	Decreased effect	Decreased effect		Decreased effect/ nephrotoxicity
Antipsychotics	Postural hypotension	Postural hypotension	Increased effect of both drugs	Postural hypotension	Postural hypotension
Barbiturates		Additive CNS depression	Decreased effect (hepatic β-blockers)	Decreased effect (verapamil)	
Barbiturates β-Blockers	First-dose syncope	Decreased guanfacine Rebound hypertension/ bradycardia		Additive cardiac depression	
Carbamazepine			Decreased effect (hepatic β-blockers)	Decreased effect (verapamil)	
Calcium blockers	First-dose syncope		Additive cardiac depression		
Cholestyramine/ colestipol Cimetidine			Increased effect (hepatic β-blockers)	Increased effect	
CNS depressants		Additive CNS depression			
Corticosteroids Cyclosporine				Increased cyclosporine	
Digitalis			Additive cardiac depression	Increased digitalis	
Diuretics	First-dose syncope	Additive effect	Additive effect	Additive effect	Postural hypotension/ additive effect
Epinephrine			Severe increase BP (nonselective) Vasoconstriction		
Ergot alkaloids Ethanol Indomethacin	Postural hypotension Decreased effect	Postural hypotension Decreased effect	Postural hypotension Decreased effect	Postural hypotension	Postural hypotension Decreased effect
Insulin			Hypoglycemia, masked symptoms, hypertension	Decreased insulin (diltiazem)	Possible hypoglycemia
Levodopa		Levodopa toxicity			
Lidocaine			Increased lidocaine		
Lithium		Lithium toxicity with methyldopa			Lithium toxicity
Monoamine oxidase inhibitors Phenothiazines		Markedly increased BP/CNS toxicity Increased BP with methydopa			
Phenytoin				Decreased effect	
Potassium/potassium-retaining drugs					Hyperkalemia
Probenecid Propafenone			Increased effect (hepatic β-blockers)		
Quinidine			Increased effect (hepatic β-blockers)	Hypotension, bradycardia (verapamil)	
Rifampin			Decreased effect (hepatic β-blockers)	Decreased effect	
Salicylates Sulfonylureas			Hypoglycemia/ hypertension		Decreased effect
Sympathomimetics	Decreased effect	Decreased effect	Decreased effect	Decreased effect	
Theophylline			Pharmacologic antagonism/increased theophylline		
Tricyclic antidepressants		Decreased effect	Increased depression		

Table 35.9. (Continued)

Loop Diuretics	Peripheral Adrenergic Blockers	Reserpine	Thiazide Diuretics	Triampterene	Vasodilators
Decreased effect	Decreased effect	Decreased effect	Decreased effect	Decreased effect	Decreased effect
Postural hypotension	Decreased effect	Decreased effect	Postural hypotension	Postural hypotension	Postural hypotension
Additive effect		Hypotension/ bradycardia	Additive effect		Additive effect
Additive effect			Additive effect		
			Decreased effect		
		Additive CNS depression			
Potassium loss			Potassium loss		
Digitalis toxicity		Arrhythmias	Digitalis toxicity		
	Additive effects	Additive effect		Decreased potassium loss	
Postural hypotension Decreased effect	Postural hypotension	Postural hypotension	Postural hypotension Decreased effect	Postural hypotension Decreased renal function	Postural hypotension
Hyperglycemia			Hyperglycemia		
	Postural hypotension	Decreased levodopa			
Lithium toxicity			Lithium toxicity		
	Decreased effect	CNS excitation			
				Hyperkalemia	
Decreased effect					
Decreased effect			Decreased effect		
Hyperglycemia Decreased effect	Decreased effect/ increased effect of direct SANS	Decreased effect/ increased effect of direct SANS	Hyperglycemia		
	Decreased effect	CNS excitation			

bined with furosemide. Indapamide is a sulfonamide diuretic with antihypertensive effects, which does not appear to elevate serum lipids.

POTASSIUM-SPARING DIURETICS

The potassium-sparing diuretics amiloride, spironolactone, and triamterene are used mainly to prevent or correct hypokalemia from other diuretics. Neither amiloride nor triamterene has a significant antihypertensive effect.

AMILORIDE

Amiloride is a potassium-sparing diuretic that acts in the distal tubule. Amiloride is excreted in the urine as unchanged drug and has natriuretic and antikaluretic effects for approximately 24 hr. The primary adverse effect is hyperkalemia. Diabetes mellitus, cirrhosis, renal insufficiency, concomitant angiotensin-converting enzyme inhibitor therapy, or potassium supplements increase the risk of hyperkalemia.

SPIRONOLACTONE

Spironolactone is a competitive aldosterone antagonist that is used in combination with thiazide diuretics to prevent or correct hypokalemia or as an alternative diuretic for patients with gout or diabetes. Food enhances the absorption of spironolactone, which is rapidly metabolized to pharmacologically active metabolites including canrenone (55). Spironolactone may be superior to potassium supplements in correcting diuretic-induced hypokalemia, and it also corrects coexisting magnesium deficiency. Hyperkalemia occurs in 3% of spironolactone-treated patients who have normal renal function and are not taking potassium supplements (55). In contrast, 25% of patients with renal insufficiency and taking potassium supplements can develop hyperkalemia. Gynecomastia is related to dosage and duration of treatment and has occurred in more than 50% of male patients (55). Impotence, hirsutism, menstrual irregularities, and gastrointestinal symptoms are adverse effects that can limit therapy. Limiting spironolactone dosage to ≤100 mg/day appears to reduce the incidence of adverse effects.

TRIAMTERENE

Triamterene is used principally in combination products to reduce the potassium loss with thiazide diuretics. Triamterene-hydrochlorothiazide combinations can produce hypokalemia or hyperkalemia. The risk of hyperkalemia is increased by other risks including renal impairment, potassium supplementation, converting-enzyme inhibitors, and diabetic mellitus. A triamterene urinary sediment (triamterene crystals) developed in over 50% of patients. This has caused nephrolithiasis and may be a risk factor for interstitial nephritis (56). Triamterene-hydrochloro-

thiazide decreases production of renal PGE_2, a renoprotective prostaglandin, while amiloride-hydrochlorothiazide increases renal PGE_2 production (57). Finally, the combination of indomethacin and triamterene may cause reversible acute renal failure (58).

Combination therapy with potassium-sparing diuretics may not be needed for most hypertensive patients treated with 25 mg of hydrochlorothiazide or less. In high-risk patients or when hypokalemia develops, potassium-sparing agents are effective in preventing or reversing hypokalemia.

β-Blockers

β-Blockers are effective antihypertensive agents, particularly in young white patients (hyperkinetic circulation), and have additive benefit for patients with coronary artery disease.

PHARMACOLOGY

β-blockers competitively inhibit catecholamine neurotransmitters throughout the body at both cardiac receptors ($β_1$) and noncardiac receptors ($β_2$) (59). Cardiac effects include a reduction in heart rate, venous return, cardiac output, and cardiac work. In addition, β-blockers reduce plasma renin activity, reduce norepinephrine release, and prevent the pressor response to exercise or stress catecholamine release.

EFFECTIVENESS

In the VA Cooperative Study Group, β-blockers were equivalent to hydrochlorothiazide in white patients, but hydrochlorothiazide was more effective in black and elderly patients (50, 59). Recent evidence suggests that β-blockers may provide primary protection from CAD, and β-blockers reduce the secondary risk following myocardial infarction (5, 50, 59). β-blockers are effective in producing LVH regression (59).

COMPARISON OF β-BLOCKERS

While the available β-blockers are similar in both efficacy and safety, there are two important differences in pharmacology (Table 35.10). Cardioselective ($β_1$-selective) agents produce less negative effects on the heart in patients with congestive heart failure or conduction system disease (5, 59). They are better tolerated by patients with chronic obstructive pulmonary disease, asthma, and peripheral vascular disease. Cardioselective ($β_1$-selective) blockers produce less impairment in response to hypoglycemia in diabetic patients. Unfortunately cardioselectivity is relative, and at higher doses these agents lose cardioselectivity. Drugs with β-agonist activity or intrinsic sympathomimetic activity (ISA) appear to avoid the decrease in cardiac output and heart rate (48, 59). ISA β-blockers

Table 35.10.
Pharmacologic Properties of β-Blockers

Drug	β₁-Selectivity	Intrinsic Sympathomimetic Activity	Lipid Solubility	Metabolism/Excretion
Acebutolol	+	+	Low	Hepatic/renal
Atenolol	+	−	Low	Renal
Betaxolol	+	−	Low	Hepatic
Carteolol	−	+ +	Low	Renal
Labetalol	−	−	Moderate	Hepatic/renal
Metoprolol	+	−	Low	Hepatic/renal
Nadolol	−	−	Low	Renal
Penbutolol	−	+	High	Hepatic
Pindolol	−	+ + +	Moderate	Hepatic/renal
Propranolol	−	−	High	Hepatic
Timolol	−	−	Low	Hepatic

are preferred for patients who experience bradycardia with other β-blockers. ISA β-blockers may also produce fewer problems for patients with peripheral vascular disease, lipid disorders, or diabetes mellitus. However, ISA β-blockers are not cardioprotective.

β-Blockers can be classified into two groups, based on their pharmacokinetic properties (59). The β-blockers eliminated by hepatic metabolism are highly lipophilic, absorbed in the small intestine, undergo extensive "first-pass" metabolism, have variable bioavailability, have relatively short plasma half-lives, and more readily penetrate the blood-brain barrier. The β-blockers eliminated unchanged by the kidney are water-soluble, are incompletely absorbed throughout the gut with longer plasma half-lives, and are less able to penetrate the CNS. Because the antihypertensive effect of β-blockers appears to outlast the presence of the drug in plasma, all agents can be used on a twice-daily schedule, and the longer-acting drugs can be given once daily. The bioavailability of propranolol and metroprolol is increased approximately 60% when they are taken with food. Propranolol, in particular, has a wide dose range, and plasma concentrations from a specific dose may vary 20-fold between patients. The hydrophilic agents (atenolol and nadolol) have relatively flat dose-response curves, but will accumulate in renal failure.

Several diseases contraindicate β-blockers or influence the selection of a β-blocker, and the choice of agents should be individualized for patients.

ADVERSE EFFECTS

Many adverse effects are related to β-adrenergic blockade in predisposed patients. Adverse effects from β₁-blockade include bradycardia, conduction abnormalities, and left ventricular failure (59). Adverse effect from β₂-blockade include bronchospasm, cold extremities, and worsening claudication. These adverse effects tend to occur early in therapy, even at low doses. CNS effects may be most common with propranolol, and frank depression or vivid visual hallucinations can occur. Some patients have a pressor response to propranolol with worsening hypertension. Dermatologic reactions include marked exacerbation of psoriasis. The addition of propranolol doubled the hydrochlorothiazide-induced increase in fasting glucose and glycosylated hemoglobin concentrations (60). β-blockers decrease HDL cholesterol concentrations, increase LDL cholesterol concentrations, and blunt the effectiveness of dietary modification to lower cholesterol (50). Lipid changes are not associated with ISA β-blockers.

The withdrawal of β-blockers may produce β-adrenergic supersensitivity. Both abrupt cessation and gradual withdrawal over 4 to 8 days has caused overshoot hypertension and cardiovascular complications within 48 to 72 hr after the last β-blocker dose (61). Symptoms of the withdrawal syndrome are nervousness, restlessness, anxiety, malaise, fatigue, headaches, insomnia, vivid dreams, tachycardia, palpitations, tremors, diaphoresis, excessive salivation, abdominal cramps and pain, anorexia, nausea, and vomiting (61). Cardiovascular morbidity has included encephalopathy, cerebrovascular accidents, unstable angina, myocardial infarction, and sudden death (61). β-Blocker withdrawal syndrome can be reversed by readministration of small doses of the β-blocker. To prevent β-adrenergic supersensitivity, the β-blocker dose should be reduced over 7 to 10 days to the equivalent of 30 mg of propranolol a day and then maintained at this low dose for 2 additional weeks (61). The risk of β-blocker withdrawal is not only in patients with known ischemic heart disease. The withdrawal of β-blockers in patients free of coronary artery disease resulted in a fourfold increase in new onset of coronary artery disease (62). Interestingly, ISA β-blockers do not cause a withdrawal syndrome and are not cardioprotective (62).

α-β-BLOCKER

Labetalol is a nonselective β-blocker and an α-blocker that reduces the β₂-blockade increase in PVR and sustains blood flow to the extremities and kidney. Labetalol does not reduce HDL-cholesterol concentrations, but may cause orthostatic hypotension and sexual dysfunction. Labetalol may be more effective than other β-blockers in elderly or black patients, and it has been used in patients with pulmonary disease.

Angiotensin-converting-Enzyme Inhibitors

Converting-enzyme inhibitors (CEI) block the generation of angiotensin II, which is a potent vasoconstrictor and stimulates aldosterone secretion. Angiotensin-converting-enzyme inhibitors have antihypertensive efficacy comparable to that of diuretics and β-blockers in monotherapy for hypertension. Converting-enzyme inhibitors are more effective in younger and white patients and less effective in black patients, unless higher doses are used or they are combined with diuretics (5, 63). The combination of low-dose diuretic therapy and converting-enzyme inhibitors may control up to 85% of patients (63, 64). Converting-enzyme inhibitors are also synergistic with calcium-entry blockers and additive with β-blockers. Converting-enzyme inhibitors prolong the survival of patients with severe congestive heart failure and produce regression of left ventricular hypertrophy (5). They are also used to treat renovascular hypertension (5). Another unique benefit of converting-enzyme inhibitors is the reduction of angiotensin II–mediated intraglomerular capillary pressure. This effect appears to retard the progression of diabetic renal disease, stabilize renal function, and decrease proteinuria (5, 63). Converting-enzyme inhibitors avoid many of the adverse effects common to earlier antihypertensive drugs. They do not alter plasma lipid, glucose, or uric acid concentrations or aggravate bronchospastic or peripheral vascular disease. Converting-enzyme inhibitors also do not cause CNS depression or sexual dysfunction. They may increase alertness and produce mood elevation, which may contribute to the positive effect on the quality of life seen with captopril (63).

CEI therapy has been suggested as initial antihypertensive therapy because it will control about 50% of patients and has few side effects (64). Initial CEI therapy is also an indirect means of classifying renin status. Patients with a poor decrease in blood pressure from CEI are likely to have low-renin hypertension (64).

COMPARISON OF CONVERTING-ENZYME INHIBITORS

The available converting-enzyme inhibitors differ in pharmacokinetics. Captopril binds to angiotensin-converting enzyme by a sulfhydryl and the other ACE inhibitors do not (63). Enalapril, ramapril, and fosinopril are administered as prodrugs, which delays their onset of action and prolongs the effect. Captopril should be taken without food and requires twice-daily dosing. All of the other agents are administered once daily. The primary route of elimination is the kidney, and doses should be reduced in renal insufficiency. Fosinopril is eliminated by both renal excretion and hepatic metabolism, and dose reductions are not needed for patients with renal dysfunction.

ADVERSE EFFECTS

Adverse effects common to all converting-enzyme inhibitors are hypotension, hyperkalemia, cough, angioedema, and renal insufficiency (63). Hypotension occurs when patients are sodium-depleted or have high renin and is more common with captopril because of its rapid onset of action (63, 64). To reduce this risk, diuretics should be discontinued for 3 days prior to the initial CEI dose. The risk of hyperkalemia is greater in patients with diabetes or renal insufficiency, if sodium intake is restricted, and if potassium-sparing diuretics, potassium supplements, or nonsteroidal antiinflammatory agents are given. An intractable, dry cough, requiring discontinuation of CEI therapy, may develop in more than 20% of patients (65). Cough develops more frequently with enalapril than with captopril, and it is believed to be caused by an effect of CEI on vagal C fibers (63, 65). Adverse effects of captopril also have included neutropenia, rash, proteinuria, and taste disturbances (63). Using lower doses of captopril has dramatically reduced the incidence of these complications.

Calcium-Entry Blockers

Calcium-entry blockers (CEB) are the fourth class of drugs considered to be effective monotherapy for the initial treatment of hypertension (1). Calcium-entry blockers impair the transport of calcium through the voltage-sensitive calcium channels in smooth muscle cells, which decreases contractile force, vascular smooth muscle tone, and peripheral resistance (66). The CEB may be particularly effective in patients with low-renin hypertension (i.e., elderly and black hypertensives) and have greater antihypertensive efficacy with higher pretreatment blood pressures (66). Verapamil is equally effective in black or white hypertensive patients (67). Calcium-entry blockers are also used to treat angina, variant angina, certain arrhythmias, and migraine headaches, making them attractive antihypertensive agents for patients with those conditions (5). The calcium-entry blockers also do not adversely affect asthma, gout, or peripheral vascular disease and appear to have minimal effect on diabetes mellitus.

COMPARISON OF CALCIUM-ENTRY BLOCKERS

The calcium-entry blockers, diltiazem, felodipine, isradipine, nicardapine, nifedipine, and verapamil used for hypertension have similar efficacies, but differ chemically and in their adverse-effect profiles. The CEB have limited oral bioavailability because of first-pass hepatic metabolism. Only diltiazem (35%) has important renal elimination. Because of short plasma half-lives, extended-release products are available for verapamil, diltiazem, and nifedipine, which allow once or twice daily administration. Extended-release products may also decrease dose-related adverse effects. In elderly patients verapamil produced a greater reduction in LVH than atenolol, or has reduced the progression of atherogenic lesions (50). Calcium-entry blockers have important antiarrhythmic effects and produced a 74% decrease in premature ventricular contractions and a decrease in LVH in hypertensive patients (68). Hydrochlorothiazide did not decrease LVH, and the prevalence of ventricular arrhythmias was unchanged. However, postinfarction trials of CEB have not demonstrated cardioprotection (66). Addition of a diuretic to a CEB usually has only minimal additive effect; this may be due in part to the natriuretic effect of the calcium-entry blockers (66, 70).

ADVERSE EFFECTS

The adverse effects of the calcium-entry blockers are primarily extensions of their pharmacologic actions: vasodilation, negative inotropic effects, conduction disturbances, gastrointestinal effects, and metabolic effects (69). Vasodilatory side effects include headaches, flushing, palpitations, hypotension, and peripheral edema. Vasodilation is more common with dihydropyridine CEB, nifedipine, nicardapine, and isradipine. Negative inotropic effects are least with the dihydropyridines, and verapamil has the greatest negative inotropic action. Diltiazem is intermediate in negative inotropic effect, but can produce new or worsen congestive heart failure in patients with preexisting left ventricular dysfunction. Conduction disturbances are also greatest with verapamil, intermediate with diltiazem, and infrequent with dihydropyridines. Verapamil often causes constipation, which may be relieved with stool softeners (5). Verapamil decreases digoxin elimination and can increase serum digoxin levels by 50 to 75%. Other calcium-entry blockers may also interact with digoxin, but usually to a lesser degree. If a CEB is used in combination with a β-blocker, a dihydropyridine agent is preferred, to reduce the additive cardioinhibitory and cardiodepressive effects (5, 69).

SYMPATHETIC INHIBITORS

Many antihypertensive drugs interfere with the sympathetic nervous system. These agents may act in the central nervous system, the peripheral nervous system, or both.

α₁-Adrenergic Blocking Agents

These drugs produce a selective postsynaptic α_1-adrenoceptor inhibition, causing decreased peripheral resistance and vasodilation without reducing cardiac output or inducing a reflex tachycardia. They produce a slightly greater decrease in standing blood pressure than in supine blood pressure. They have additive effects with β-blockers and diuretics. While α_1-adrenergic inhibitors are not currently recommended as initial therapy for hypertension by the JNC, their advantages include a favorable lipid profile effect, equal efficacy in all age and race groups, and a favorable effect on plasma glucose (71). Doxazosin, in contrast to enalapril, reduced total cholesterol and triglyceride levels and increased HDL cholesterol levels, while producing a similar reduction in blood pressure (72). This resulted in a greater reduction in calculated coronary artery disease risk than that found with enalapril (72). α_1-Adrenergic inhibitors may also reduce preload and afterload in severe chronic congestive heart failure. Patients with benign prostatic hypertrophy (BPH) may benefit from α_1-adrenergic inhibitors. α_1-Adrenergic inhibitors increase urine flow and decrease urinary frequency in patients with BPH by inhibition of norepinephrine-induced contraction of prostate smooth muscle (73).

COMPARISON OF α₁-ADRENERGIC BLOCKERS

The three α_1-adrenergic inhibitors appear to have similar antihypertensive effects and adverse effects. They undergo substantial hepatic first-pass metabolism. The newer agents, doxazosin and terazosin, have a longer duration of action than prazosin and can be dosed once daily (71).

ADVERSE EFFECTS

The most striking adverse effect with α_1-adrenergic inhibitors is the "first-dose syncope." Profound orthostatic hypotension with syncope can occur 1 to 3 hr after the first dose in patients with a low plasma volume from diuretic therapy and those who are taking other antihypertensive drugs that blunt their response to the acute decrease in blood pressure. To avoid this problem, the initial dose should be limited to the equivalent of 1 mg of prazosin and taken at bedtime or when the patient can be observed.

Central α₂-Agonists

Central α_2-adrenergic agonists stimulate α_2-adrenergic receptors in the lower brainstem, which decreases sympathetic outflow to the cardiovascular system. Some agents also block peripheral α_2-adrenergic receptors. The combined sympatholytic effects cause a decrease in peripheral vascular resistance (74). The central α_2-adrenergic agonists are equally effective in all age and race subgroups and can be used for patients with renal insufficiency, diabetes mellitus, bronchospastic disease, and ischemic heart disease. These drugs have similar efficacy to other antihypertensives when used as monotherapy for the initial treatment of hypertension. Unlike peripheral sympatholytics, the central α_2-adrenergic agonists do not cause significant sodium and fluid retention. They do not adversely effect glucose metabolism and have neutral or favorable effects on plasma lipid levels (74). These agents also produce a regression in left ventricular hypertrophy. Clonidine has increased the success of smoking cessation, particularly in women, decreasing craving as well as withdrawal symptoms (75).

COMPARISON OF α_2-ADRENERGIC AGONISTS

Newer formulations of the central α_2-adrenergic agonists provide sustained antihypertensive efficacy with less frequent dosing and have fewer symptomatic side effects. Clonidine can be given twice daily, and often a daily bedtime dose is effective and lessens sedation. A clonidine-suppression test has been used to assess the contribution of increased sympathetic outflow in patients with essential hypertension. Clonidine is also available as a transdermal therapeutic system (TTS) that is applied once weekly. Transdermal clonidine controls blood pressure in 60 to 80% of patients with mild hypertension (76). Severe withdrawal rebound hypertension is less likely to occur with transdermal therapy than with oral clonidine (76). The transdermal system is a convenient form of treatment with equal efficacy and fewer adverse effects than oral clonidine. The principle adverse effect is a contact dermatitis that develops in 10 to 15% of patients.

Guanfacine is a long-acting central α_2-adrenergic agonist that is metabolized by the liver (70%) and excreted unchanged by the kidneys (30%), with a prolonged elimination half-life of 16 to 23 hr (77). The long duration of action allows once-daily dosing and reduces adverse effects. Guanfacine also has a relatively flat dose-response curve, with little increase in antihypertensive effect from doses greater than 1 mg (74).

Guanabenz is a guanidine derivative that blocks central sympathetic vasomotor impulses and also produces a guanethidine-like postganglionic blockade. Guanabenz decreases cholesterol and triglyceride concentration without changing HDL cholesterol (75). It is used in a twice-daily dosing schedule.

Methyldopa, the first central α_2-adrenergic agonist, has been largely replaced by the newer agents. A methyldopa metabolite, α-methylnorepinephrine, is the active agonist that reduces CNS sympathetic outflow. Methyldopa has an greater orthostatic effect than clonidine, but both cardiac output and renal function are usually preserved. Because salt/water retention can produce a "pseudotolerance," methyldopa is normally combined with a diuretic. Methyldopa can be used with a twice-daily dosing schedule.

ADVERSE EFFECTS

Sedation and dry mouth are the most frequent adverse effects of central α_2-adrenergic agonists (78). These symptoms often disappear after the first few weeks. Saliva substitutes or sugarless gum or candy can provide relief from the dry mouth. Sedation is additive to that of other sedating drugs including alcohol, and patients should be cautioned about these combinations and driving. Serious hypersensitivity reactions have occurred with methyldopa, including drug fever, colitis, hepatotoxicity, a positive Coombs test, and hemolytic anemia. The risk of serious toxicity and impaired mental function make alternative antihypertensive drugs preferable to methyldopa.

Abrupt discontinuation of clonidine has caused an acute withdrawal syndrome (AWS) characterized by a rapid increase in blood pressure, headaches, palpitations, tremor, restlessness, diaphoresis, and nausea. AWS appears to be rare with transdermal clonidine and guanfacine (77, 78). The risk of AWS is higher in younger patients with severe hypertension who are treated with high doses and multiple antihypertensive agents. Combination with β-blockers increases the risk of a hypertensive episode on discontinuation of clonidine (79). This combination should be avoided, and if used, the β-blocker should be tapered and stopped before decreasing the clonidine. Avoiding excessive doses, encouraging patient compliance, and tapering clonidine slowly may help prevent an AWS. However, patients should be warned to seek immediate medical help if they develop signs and symptoms of AWS. Restarting the medications usually reverses an AWS, and labetalol has been effective for combined central agonist/β-blocker AWS (79).

Peripheral Sympatholytics

Guanethidine is actively transported into the peripheral adrenergic neuron, where it depletes norepinephrine and produces a postural hypotension. Guanethidine decreases venous return to the heart, decreases cardiac output, and interferes with the sympathetic reflexes that control the resistance (arteriolar) and capacitance (venous) vessels. Because guanethidine depletes myocardial catecholamines, it can worsen congestive heart failure. Guanethidine is absorbed slowly and variably, undergoing partial first-pass hepatic metabolism. With chronic administration the half-life of guanethidine is 5 days, with 50% of the drug excreted unchanged in the urine. Because of the long half-life, guanethidine can be taken once daily, and dosage adjustments should be made only after 2 to 3 weeks. Prolonged standing, exercise, and heat increase postural hypotension. The dose of guanethidine should be adjusted based on standing blood pressure, and blocks can be used to elevate the head of the bed to sustain a nighttime postural effect. Guanadrel is an adrenergic blocking agent that also depletes norepinephrine from peripheral neurons. Guanadrel has a more rapid onset and shorter duration of action than guanethidine. Because of the postural effect, standing blood pressure must always be measured. These agents are reserved for treating resistant hypertension.

ADVERSE EFFECTS

The major problem with both guanethidine and guanadrel is postural and exercise hypotension. Patients should be warned to rise slowly from supine or sitting positions, to flex their arms and legs before arising, and to avoid additive vasodilating factors such as prolonged standing, hot showers, and drinking alcohol. Postural effects are most pronounced in the morning on arising. Other dose-related problems include sexual dysfunction and diarrhea, which may require discontinuation of therapy. A "pseudotolerance" due to fluid retention may develop unless diuretic therapy is adequate. Because guanethidine diffuses poorly into the CNS, sedation and depression are infrequent problems. Several drugs can interfere with the uptake of peripheral sympatholytics into the adrenergic neuron and rapidly block the antihypertensive effects. Guanadrel may cause less sexual dysfunction and orthostasis than does guanethidine. However, patients should be given similar precautions to minimize the risks of postural hypotension. Diuretics are needed to reduce sodium/water retention and weight gain.

Reserpine

Reserpine acts in both the central and the peripheral sympathetic nervous systems, depleting norepinephrine and serotonin stores in the brain and peripheral adrenergic nerve endings. Reserpine also increases vagal tone, which contributes to the reduced heart rate and increased gastric acid secretions. The onset of action of reserpine may take several days, with maximal hypotensive effects taking weeks. Adverse effects are frequent and include nasal congestion from cholinergic stimulation. CNS changes include drowsiness, sedation, dizziness, sleep disturbances, difficulty in concentration, poor memory, and depression. Other antihypertensive agents are preferred because of greater efficacy and fewer adverse effects.

Vasodilators

Vasodilators directly relax arteriolar smooth muscle and decrease peripheral vascular resistance. They do not interfere with autonomic reflexes or produce postural hypotension. This stimulates carotid sinus baroreceptors producing reflex increases in heart rate, renin release, and sodium and water retention. These drugs have usually been used in combination with a diuretic and β-blocker or sympatholytic agent to prevent the reflex increases in cardiac output and fluid retention that blunt the effect of vasodilators when used alone. The elderly develop less reflex tachycardia.

COMPARISON OF VASODILATORS

Hydralazine is metabolized by hepatic acetylation with substantial first-pass elimination. Hydralazine is effective when taken twice daily, and food increases bioavailability. The acetylation rate is genetically determined, and slow acetylators experience greater hypotensive effects and should not receive more than 200 mg of hydralazine daily.

Minoxidil is a potent vasodilator that markedly reduces peripheral vascular resistance and is reserved for the treatment of severe hypertension. It can produce blood pressure reductions of 30 to 40 mm Hg when combined with diuretics and β-blockers. Minoxidil is well absorbed and undergoes hepatic metabolism. Despite a relatively short half-life, the antihypertensive effect persists 12 to 24 hr, and minoxidil is dosed twice daily. Minoxidil produces marked sodium/water retention, and large doses of loop diuretics are often needed to control the edema. Reflex tachycardia and increased cardiac output are prevented by adequate β-blocker therapy.

Diazoxide is a nondiuretic thiazide that dilates peripheral arterioles and is used to treat hypertensive emergencies. Intravenous injection produces a profound decrease in both systolic and diastolic blood pressure, which does not require continuous infusion and infrequently causes hypotension. Diazoxide is metabolized in the liver and excreted in the urine with a duration of action from 2 to 24 hr. Diazoxide is administered as a minibolus (1 to 3 mg/kg) every 10 min, with a maximum of 150 mg, or as a 15 mg/min infusion. Diazoxide produces sodium and water retention, and diuretic therapy is necessary to maintain blood pressure control. Hyperglycemia is a problem with prolonged use. Patients with renal failure or myocardial ischemia are predisposed to the adverse effects of diazoxide.

Nitroprusside is an instant-acting vasodilator that is useful in virtually all hypertensive emergencies. Nitroprusside relaxes both arteriolar and venous smooth muscles. It reacts with cysteine to form nitrocysteine, which activates guanylate cyclase, leading to increased cyclic GMP, which relaxes vascular smooth muscle. Controlled intravenous infusions of nitroprusside are highly effective in treating hypertensive emergencies. The onset and cessation of the hypotensive action is immediate. Nitroprusside is unstable and must be protected from light. The nitroprusside metabolite thiocyanate may accumulate rapidly with impaired renal function, and plasma thiocyanate concentrations above 1.7 mmol/liter (10 mg/dl) are toxic. Nitroprusside decreases peripheral resistance and can improve left ventricular function in patients with congestive heart failure or with impaired cardiac output after a myocardial infarction.

ADVERSE EFFECTS

Adverse effects from reflex sympathetic stimulation or direct vasodilation include headache, dizziness, postural hypotension, tachycardia, and palpitations (80). The reflex tachycardia can precipitate or aggravate angina pectoris. Hydralazine commonly causes throbbing headaches and also causes a pyridoxine-deficiency-induced peripheral neuropathy. A positive antinuclear antibody (ANA) develops in 15 to 20% of hydralazine-treated patients, which can lead to a lupus-like syndrome, particularly if doses above 200 mg/day are used. Symptoms can include arthralgia, arthritis, fever, malaise, rash, and weight loss. Symptoms can resolve rapidly and often disappear within 6 months; however, rheumatoid symptoms and a positive ANA can persist for years.

Minoxidil causes marked sodium and water retention leading to weight gain, peripheral edema, cardiac enlargement, pulmonary hypertension, and pericardial effusion (80). Minoxidil causes hypertrichosis in nearly all patients. This can be partly controlled with dipilatories, but it limits minoxidil use in women. Coarsening of facial features can also occur.

CLINICAL USE OF ANTIHYPERTENSIVE DRUGS

Drug treatment remains empiric because the etiology of essential hypertension is unknown (7). The JNC recommends an individualized stepped-care approach, with the initial antihypertensive drug selected for each patient from either a converting enzyme inhibitor, calcium-entry blocker, thiazide-type diuretic, or β-blocker (1). The central sympatholytics or α₁-blockers may also be appropriate initial therapy for some patients (81). If the response is not adequate, one approach is to gradually increase the dose of the initial drug to the recommended maximum. In many patients it may be appropriate to use sequential individualized monotherapy by discontinuing the initial drug and substituting an agent from a different class before combining two drugs. An alternative concept is to use synergistic combinations in very low doses as initial therapy (7). For hypertension not controlled by two drugs, the choices are to substitute for one of the drugs or to add a third drug from a different class. Additional drugs should be added or substituted in gradually increasing doses until blood pressure is controlled, side effects are intolerable, or maximal recommended doses are reached. Usually an interval of 1 to 2 months will allow maximal antihypertensive action before changes are made. In many instances using smaller doses of drugs with different sites of action is preferred to maximal doses of a single drug. This has the advantage of additive drug effects while minimizing side effects.

Refractory Hypertension

Blood pressure not controlled by multiple drugs or difficult to control may be caused by

- Patient noncompliance;
- Inadequate drug doses;
- Drug combinations that act at the same site;
- Volume overload:
    Excess sodium intake
    Inadequate diuretic therapy
    Renal insufficiency;
- Obesity;
- Renovascular hypertension;
- Excess alcohol intake;
- Drug-induced hypertension.

Step-Down Therapy

In patients who have maintained control of their blood pressure (DBP ≤85 mm Hg) for 6 months to 1 year, a stepwise reduction in antihypertensive medications may be attempted (1). Short-term studies described a relatively high success rate (40 to 50%) of discontinuation of drug treatment, but a long-term evaluation found that only 8% of previously treated patients remained normotensive off medications (82). Virtually all hypertensive patients off medication can be expected to relapse unless effective nonpharmacologic treatments are implemented. A reasonable approach is to stepdown to one medication after blood pressure control for 6 months to 1 year on multiple drugs. Cessation of drug therapy should be reserved for patients with no medical complications and mild hypertension, who have demonstrated weight loss, sodium reduction, and/or increased exercise. Patients off drugs should have blood pressure measurements every 3 to 6 months and should be informed that permanent remission is rare and that eventual reinstitution of drug treatment is likely.

Hypertensive Emergencies and Urgencies

Hypertensive crisis is a severe elevation of blood pressure, usually a diastolic blood pressure above 120 to 130 mm Hg (83). Severe blood pressure elevation with acute or progressive end-organ damage is a hypertensive emergency. If end-organ damage is absent, it is a hypertensive urgency. Hypertensive crisis is thought to involve an abrupt increase in vascular resistance, secondary to increased circulating vasoconstrictor substances leading to ischemia that triggers the further release of vasoconstrictors (83). Therapy should interrupt this cycle and decrease blood pressure, while avoiding an abrupt decrease to normotensive or hypotensive blood pressures that may cause ischemia or infarction. For a hypertensive emergency the target is usually to lower blood pressure by 25% to a DBP of 100 to 110 mm Hg. Sodium nitroprusside infusion is the current therapy of choice (83). Other treatment options include intravenous nicardipine or intravenous labetalol (83, 84). Hypertensive urgencies are encountered more commonly than emergencies and can be effectively managed with oral or sublingual therapy. Both oral nifedipine and oral clonidine are effective for urgent hypertension, but nifedipine acts more rapidly and controls 96% of patients within 2 hr (85). Sublingual or buccal nifedipine has an onset of action of 5 to 10 min. Oral therapy can be administered quickly, rarely causes hypotension, and facilitates the transition to long-term treatment.

Complicated Hypertension

Hypertensive complications or coexisting diseases can influence the selection of antihypertensive drugs.

Congestive Heart Failure and LVH

Left ventricular hypertrophy (LVH) is an independent risk factor for cardiac dysrhythmias and sudden death. Premature ventricular contractions are 40 to 50 times more prevalent in hypertensive patients, and the risk of sudden death is increased 5 to 6 times by their presence (17). Many antihypertensive drugs reduce LVH, including β-blockers, calcium-entry blockers, converting-enzyme inhibitors, and central adrenergic agonists (1). Diuretics are less effective in reversing LVH and may increase cardiac risk by causing electrolyte disturbances. Vasodilators increase left ventricular mass and should not be used as monotherapy. In patients with overt congestive heart failure, converting-enzyme inhibitors in combination with diuretics can reduce mortality.

Diabetes Mellitus

Hypertension is twice as frequent in diabetic patients than in nondiabetics (86). Eventually, 50% of diabetic patients become hypertensive. Insulin resistance and hyperinsulinemia may contribute to the pathogenesis of hypertension in these patients (86–88). Diabetic vascular disease and associated serum lipid abnormalities compound the cardiovascular risks. Nephropathy develops in up to 50% of patients with insulin-dependent diabetes mellitus (IDDM) and 40% of patients with non-insulin-dependent diabetes mellitus (NIDDM) (86).

Treatment of hypertension should lower blood pressure without worsening diabetic control, serum lipid concentrations, or diabetic complications. Thiazide diuretics worsen glucose control and increase cholesterol levels, and these effects may not reverse with dose reduction (50, 86, 89–91). Loop diuretics may produce less impairment of glucose control (90). The diuretic glucose elevation is likely caused hypokalemia, which suppresses insulin secretion (86). Patients with IDDM whose glycemic control is from exogenous insulin do not have this complication. β-Blockers adversely affect glucose by blocking insulin release and glycogenolysis (60, 86). β-Blockers also abolish catecholamine-mediated symptoms of hypoglycemia (86). These agents can worsen peripheral vascular disease, which is 30 times more common in diabetics. β-Blockers that are cardioselective and not lipophilic are preferred for patients with NIDDM (90). Converting-enzyme inhibitors do not adversely affect glycemic control or lipid metabolism and have the potential to decrease proteinuria and slow the progression of diabetic renal disease (63, 91–92). Information about the effect of calcium-entry blockers on glycemic control is conflicting. Nifedipine has increased serum glucose levels, while verapamil has improved glycemic control (83). Diltiazem can decrease massive proteinuria in diabetic patients as effectively as lisinopril can (93). Guanfacine may improve glycemic control, and α-blockers can blunt the deterioration in glucose tolerance caused by β-blockers (92). Autonomic neuropathy and orthostatic hypotension are 30 times more common in diabetic patients, and drugs that produce postural hypotension should be used cautiously. Finally, sexual dysfunction is a common problem in male diabetics, and drugs that cause sexual dysfunction are best used as secondary choices.

Renal Insufficiency

Treatment of hypertension can slow the progression of renal disease (1, 89). If the serum creatinine concentration is above 34 μmol/Liter (2 mg/dl), furosemide, bumetanide, or metolazone are needed, as thiazide diuretics are ineffective (1, 94). Sodium retention becomes a major factor in treating patients with renal insufficiency, and larger doses of loop diuretics may be added to most regimens. Other drugs that are effective in patients with renal disease and that do not adversely affect renal blood flow or glomerular filtration are converting-enzyme inhibitors, calcium-entry blockers, central antiadrenergics, and vasodilators (95, 96). Converting-enzyme inhibitors and calcium-entry blockers appear to have unique benefits for patients with renal disease. These agents increase renal blood flow and glomerular filtration rate, prevent tubular sodium reabsorption, and may limit the progression of renal disease (95, 96). Dosage reductions are needed for antihypertensive drugs excreted by the kidney, and patients with chronic renal failure may exhibit an increased sensitivity to some drugs, including α-blockers and converting-enzyme inhibitors (96).

Coronary Artery Disease

The benefits of antihypertensive treatment on the prevention of the complications of coronary artery disease are modest. To prevent the development of the complications of coronary artery disease, emphasis should be given to correcting other cardiovascular risk factors, especially smoking, hyperlipidemia, and diabetes mellitus (1). Calculating an individual coronary risk profile can aid in the management of patients (97). Patients with angina pectoris or a previous myocardial infarction can be treated with β-blockers or calcium blockers that reduce angina. β-Blockers also reduce mortality following myocardial infarction, at least in men. Because of the increased arrhythmias, caution must be exercised to avoid diuretic-induced hypokalemia and hypomagnesemia. Drugs that cause reflex tachycardia, like hydralazine, should be avoided.

Cerebrovascular Disease

Antihypertensive therapy can reduce the risk of recurrent stoke by 42% and is an important component of therapy in patients with cerebrovascular disease (22). It is important to avoid orthostatic hypotension. Even diuretic therapy should be started cautiously, as elderly patients with cerebrovascular disease are more likely to develop hypotension from these drugs.

Elderly

Nearly two-thirds of the 29 million people 65 years of age or older have some elevation of blood pressure (1). The HDFP and EWPHE trials have demonstrated benefit for elderly patients (up to age 80) treated for diastolic hypertension (DBP ≥90 mm Hg) (98). Isolated systolic hypertension (ISH), defined as an SBP >160 mm Hg and DBP <90 mm Hg, is more prevalent about age 60 (99). ISH is associated with an increased risk of stroke and cardiovascular disease, which is independent of other risk factors (99). The Systolic Hypertension in the Elderly Program (SHEP) trial demonstrated a 36% reduction in stroke from the treatment of ISH for 4.5 years in patients age 60 years and older (99). Drug treatment in SHEP was low-dose chlorthalidone (12.5 to 25 mg) and atenolol 25 mg, with potassium supplements if required (99).

Selection of drug therapy for the elderly may be complicated by the physiologic changes of aging. Elderly hypertensives usually have a reduced cardiac output, intravascular volume, and heart rate, and an increased peripheral vascular resistance (100). They often have LVH, which impairs coronary reserve and is associated with a possible increased risk of ventricular ectopy and sudden death (100). Diminished baroreflexes increase the risk of postural hypotension, and renal function may be reduced. Both thiazide diuretics and β-blockers have lowered cardiovascular mortality in controlled trials; however, these agents appear to be inappropriate for the physiologic changes seen in the elderly, and they are associated with significant adverse effects (100). α_1-Blockers, labetalol, guanethidine, and guanadrel can increase orthostatic hy-

potension, which limits their use in the elderly. Calcium-entry blockers are effective, physiologically appropriate, and do not adversely effect renal function. Their adverse effects in the elderly are similar to those seen in younger patients. Although plasma renin activity decreases with age, the converting-enzyme inhibitors are effective in the elderly. The converting-enzyme inhibitors do not have adverse metabolic effects and reduce the incidence of arrhythmias in cardiac failure (100). The elderly should be treated with an individualized approach to drug therapy, and treatment should be started with low doses of antihypertensive drugs.

Pregnancy

Hypertension complicates 10% of pregnancies and is more frequent in nulliparous women and multiple pregnancies (101). Hypertension during pregnancy can be caused by chronic hypertension, preeclampsia, preeclampsia plus chronic hypertension, or transient hypertension. Chronic hypertension is well tolerated during pregnancy if DBP remains <100 mm Hg. Preeclampsia can be life-threatening to both fetus and mother. Preeclampsia develops most often in nulliparous women, occulting near term, with a marked increase in peripheral resistance (101). Signs of preeclampsia include proteinuria, edema, hemoconcentration, hypoalbuminemia, increased urate, and hepatic or coagulation abnormalities (101). Life-threatening complications are hemolytic anemia and marked hepatic dysfunction. Progression to seizures is termed eclampsia, a major cause of maternal death. Methyldopa has a long history of safe use in pregnancy, with normal follow-up evaluations in children up to 10 years after treatment (101). β-Blockers, labetalol, thiazide diuretics, and hydralazine have also been used to treat hypertension during pregnancy with apparent success. Limited information is available for the use of calcium-entry blockers in pregnancy, and converting-enzyme inhibitors are avoided because they reduce uterine blood flow (101). Intravenous hydralazine is the current choice for treatment of severe hypertension during pregnancy (101). Diazoxide is used for refractory patients, and parenteral labetalol may become the second-choice agent. Calcium-entry blockers are also effective, but concurrent magnesium sulfate may potentiate their effect and cause a precipitous fall in blood pressure. Calcium-entry blockers also reduce uterine blood flow (101).

Racial Differences

The prevalence of hypertension among black African-Americans is substantially higher and hypertension-related morbidity and mortality is three- to fivefold higher in blacks than in caucasians (102–103). Hypertension is often poorly controlled in black patients. Environmental factors, particularly dietary excess, high sodium consumption, and low dietary potassium, calcium, and magnesium intake may contribute to these differences (103). The development of obesity and insulin resistance may be an important mechanism in black hypertensives. Approximately 50% of black hypertensives demonstrate salt sensitivity, and their hypertension is usually associated with low plasma renin and volume dependence (102). Thiazide diuretics continue to be effective and affordable therapy for black hypertensive patients. However, approximately 50% of black hypertensives require two or more drugs (103). Blacks have a lower response rate to β-blockers and converting-enzyme inhibitors than white hypertensives. This difference may be less if higher drug doses are used or if β-blockers and converting-enzyme inhibitors are use in combination with diuretics. A comparison of different antihypertensive drugs in black hypertensives demonstrated blood pressure control of 60% with atenolol, 57% with captopril, and 73% with verapamil (104).

The prevalence of hypertension in Hispanics appears to be lower than that in caucasians (103). Hispanic men also have a slightly lower mortality from hypertensive disease than caucasian men, but Hispanic women have a higher mortality rate than caucasian women.

Asians and Pacific-Islanders also have a lower incidence of hypertension than caucasians, but this appears to be modified by socioeconomic factors (103). Racial differences in drug response may be particularly important in the Asian population. Chinese men have a twofold greater sensitivity to the β-blocking effects of propranolol (105). Chinese men had a greater decrease in both heart rate and blood pressure, despite a significantly higher metabolic clearance of propranolol than the white subjects (105). Asian patients also have reduced nifedipine metabolism and frequently develop palpitations (106). Because of possible racial differences in drug response and metabolism, antihypertensive drugs should be started with reduced doses when treating Asian patients.

Adverse Drug Effects

Because of the long-term treatment of hypertension, drug therapy must have minimal adverse effects. Adverse drug effects are listed in Table 35.7.

Quality of Life and Cost of Care

Because hypertension is usually a lifelong condition, the cost of treatment and the effects of antihypertensive drugs on the quality of life are important concerns. Drug therapy may produce subtle changes in emotion, behavior, and physical and cognitive function (1). In an early study, physicians felt that all patients had improved, but only 48% of the patients agreed (50). However, 99% of relatives felt the patient had gotten worse since starting antihyperten-

sive treatment. Problems observed included decreased memory, irritability, depression, hypochondria, and decreased sexual interest (50). Captopril improved general well-being, caused fewer side effects, and had higher quality-of-life scores than methyldopa or propranolol (107). Addition of a diuretic worsened outcome for all drug-treatment groups. Black hypertensives showed no difference in quality of life with atenolol, captopril, or verapamil (108). However, verapamil produced a significantly greater decrease in blood pressure. The Trial of Antihypertensive Interventions and Management (TAIM) evaluated the effects of a low-sodium and high-potassium diet, a weight-loss diet, a placebo, chlorthalidone, or atenolol on sexual function and quality of life (109). Few drug-related side effects were found. Chlorthalidone produced erection problems in 28% of men on a usual diet, but a weight-loss diet removed this effect. The weight-loss diet reduced physical complaints and increased health satisfaction. The TAIM findings emphasize the importance of weight reduction in addition to drug regimens for overweight hypertensives (109).

The assessment of cost-benefit issues is needed to reduce medical costs while providing quality patient care. The costs of antihypertensive medications vary widely (110). Combination diuretic products are three times as expensive as hydrochlorothiazide, or more. β-Blockers and calcium-entry blockers also show wide cost variation (110). The converting-enzyme inhibitors and calcium-entry blockers are 4 to 20 times more expensive than generic diuretics or generic β-blockers (50). With the increasing cost of antihypertensive medications, some patients are not compliant because they cannot afford expensive drugs. Estimates of long-term cost-effectiveness projected the cost per year of life saved were $10,900 for propranolol; $16,400 for hydrochlorothiazide; $31,600 for nifedipine; $61,900 for prazosin; and $72,100 for captopril (111). Lowering DBP by 1 mm Hg was estimated to be equivalent to lowering cholesterol by 6% (111). However, these cost estimates have been severely criticized because of the multiple assumptions and wide differences in the patient populations between the many studies that were compared (112). The choice of antihypertensive agent should still be based on patient characteristics, concomitant diseases, and the cost of drug therapy.

Sexual Dysfunction

Antihypertensive drugs can cause impotence and ejaculation difficulties and decrease libido (113). Sexual dysfunction is reported by 4 to 7% of normotensive controls. The incidence of antihypertensive-induced sexual dysfunction is difficult to quantitate. Reports frequently range from 9 to 25% or higher, with increased frequency when multiple drug therapy is used and with advancing age (113). The MRC trial reported an increased frequency of impotence with both bendrofluazide and propranolol. Sexual-symptom-distress scores were worsened by methyldopa or propranolol, but not by captopril, either alone or combined with a diuretic (114). The risk of sexual dysfunction is greatest with peripheral adrenergic inhibitors, less with central α-agonists and diuretics. Lower incidences of sexual problems are also described with β-blockers (113). The drugs least likely to cause sexual problems are the converting-enzyme inhibitors, calcium-entry blockers, α₁-blockers, and direct vasodilators (113).

Depression

Depletion of biogenic amines may be pathogenic in depression. Antihypertensive medications that interfere with the sympathetic nervous system and neurotransmitter concentrations may induce depression (115). There is substantial evidence that reserpine and methyldopa can induce or worsen depression. β-blockers may produce CNS effects, and increased use of antidepressant drugs has been seen in β-blocker-related patients (115). Diuretics, calcium-entry blockers, and converting-enzyme inhibitors have the lowest association with depression and are the preferred agents for patients at risk for depression (115).

J Curve

There is growing evidence of a "J-shaped curve" relationship between treated DBP and cardiac mortality, where lowering blood pressure below a critical point leads to an increase in mortality. The J curve appeared to cause an increase in mortality in patients with preexisting ischemic heart disease whose DBP was lowered to less than 85 mm Hg (116). In the EWPHE trial, a U-shaped relation was described, where total mortality was increased in patients in the lowest third of treated SBP and DBP (117). A review of 13 studies with 48,000 combined patients found a consistent J-shaped relationship between cardiac events and treated blood diastolic blood pressure (118). There was no increase in stroke at lower treated blood pressures. Perhaps there is increased myocardial ischemia in hypertensive patients with left ventricular hypertrophy when the DBP is lowered below 85 mm Hg. A suggested compromise is to "be cautious in lowering blood pressure levels below 85 mm Hg in patients with known ischemia heart disease" (118).

Serum Lipids

The combination of elevated blood pressure and blood cholesterol creates a synergistic increase in the risk of cardiovascular disease (119). Nonpharmacologic interventions of diet, exercise, weight reduction, and smoking cessation are the foundation for the management of both hypertension and high blood cholesterol. The potential effects of antihypertensive drugs on serum lipid concentrations must be considered when treating patients who are hypertensive and dyslipidemic (119, 120). Thiazide-type diuretics produce a modest [1.3 to 2.6 mmol/liter (5 to 10 mg/dl)] increase in total cholesterol, LDL-cholesterol, and triglyceride levels. β-Blockers, except those with ISA or α-blocking properties, reduce HDL-cholesterol and increase serum triglycerides. Drugs with minimal effects on serum lipids include calcium-entry blockers, converting-enzyme inhibitors, ISA β-blockers, labetalol, hydralazine, minoxidil, and possibly indapamide. The α₁-adrenergic blockers and the central α₂-adrenergic agonists may decrease total and LDL-cholesterol levels slightly. In the Coronary Primary Prevention Trial, the thiazide diuretics reduced the effect of lipid-lowering drugs on LDL-cholesterol (119). However, not all patients on diuretics experience adverse lipid alterations, and a low-fat, low-cholesterol diet may minimize lipid changes. Some studies suggest that the hyperlipemic effects of diuretics may not persist more than 1 year (119, 120). Patients with coronary artery disease (CAD) and hypertension need aggressive cholesterol-lowering therapy and careful lowering of blood pressure.

β-Blockers may be needed in patients with CAD for antianginal effects and secondary prevention of myocardial infarction, despite their adverse effects on serum triglyceride and HDL-cholesterol levels. Antihyperlipidemic treatment may slow the progression of atherosclerosis and possibly induce plaque regression. The Primary Prevention Trial demonstrated that a reduction of both blood pressure and cholesterol is needed to reduce cardiovascular morbidity (121).

Drug Interactions

The effect of many antihypertensive drugs can be increased or decreased by the concurrent use of other drugs (122, 123). In addition, antihypertensive drugs can interact with other drugs. Often potentially interacting drugs can be successfully used in combination, if the possibility of the interaction is recognized, the effects are monitored, and drug doses are adjusted if needed. Common interactions are listed in Table 35.9.

Compliance

The single most important factor in the successful treatment of hypertension is patient compliance. Untreated and uncontrolled hypertension in aware hypertensive patients remains an important problem (124, 125). Public awareness programs have identified most people with hypertension, but the problems of patient dropouts and noncompliance with treatment still result in less 50% of hypertensive patients with controlled blood pressure. Continuous effort is needed to prevent patient dropout, encourage lifestyle changes, and improve medication compliance.

Noncompliance is a complex problem and prediction of compliance by clinicians is poor. A systematic procedure to screen for medication noncompliance can help to identify patients who require extra attention to achieve blood pressure control. A patient tracking system and missed-appointment follow-up program are needed to achieve long-term attendance and blood pressure control. Failure to achieve blood pressure control is twice as great in non-attenders (no appointment in 6 months) as in attenders (67% vs 30% (125).

Several important areas must be considered in attempting to overcome noncompliance, and combinations of techniques are usually needed.

- Education about the consequences of untreated hypertension and the role of drug and nondrug treatments serves as a foundation for compliance.
- The patient must understand and believe that hypertension is a serious condition that needs treatment.
- Simplification of the drug regimen can improve compliance.
  - Avoid side-effects by starting with low doses and individually selected drugs.
  - Schedule drugs once or twice daily.
- Label prescriptions with clear, explicit directions and indicate the purpose of the drug.
- Tailor medication times to coincide with existing daily habits.
- Provide written schedules or "pillbox" organizers for patients taking multiple drugs.
- Encourage the use of promoting cues like stickers or calendars to remind patients to take medications.
- Discuss potential problems such as drug costs, confusion with other drugs, or previous problems with drug therapy.
- Activate the patient by providing feedback of blood pressure response or self-monitoring of blood pressure.
- Encourage or reward patients for keeping appointments, taking medications, and reducing blood pressure.
- Screen for noncompliance by monitoring attendance, patient self-reports, blood pressure response, and changes in biochemical or physical parameters (e.g., pulse or serum potassium levels).
- Provide close professional supervision and establish a positive relationship with patients.

Pharmacists and Hypertension

The major opportunity for pharmacists is to assist cooperatively in achieving long-term control of blood pressure. Pharmacists can provide patient education, monitor prescription drug use for noncompliance, implement medication refill reminder systems, screen for drug interactions and adverse drug reactions, and monitor blood pressure response (126–128). In specialized settings clinical pharmacists have managed hypertensive patients with improved compliance and blood pressure control (129–132).

CONCLUSIONS

Hypertension continues to be a national health problem. However, it must be viewed as one of several major cardiovascular risk factors. Treatment in the 1990s must address all cardiovascular risks. The greatest patient benefit may be from controlling blood pressure by nonpharmacologic interventions. For patients unable to control blood pressure by these methods, long-term drug therapy can reduce risks effectively, if long-term control of hypertension is achieved.

REFERENCES

1. The 1988 Report of the Joint National Committee on Detection, Evaluation and Treatment of High Blood Pressure. Arch Intern Med 148:1023–1038, 1988.
2. Working Group on Renovascular Hypertension. Detection, evaluation and treatment of renovascular hypertension. Arch Intern Med 147:820–824, 1987.
3. Woods JW: Oral contraceptives and hypertension. Hypertension 11(suppl I):11–14, 1988.
4. Lake CR, Zaloga G, Bray J, et al.: Transient hypertension after two phenylpropanolamine diet aids and the effects of caffeine: a placebo-controlled follow-up study. Am J Med 86:427–432, 1989.
5. Sambhi MP, Chobanian AV, Julius S, Noth RH, Borhani NO, Perry HM Jr: University of California Davis, conference: mild hypertension. Am J Med 85:675–696, 1988.
6. Zachariah PK: Hypertension—an overview. Mayo Clin Proc 64:1403–1415, 1989.
7. Schwartz GL: Initial therapy for hypertension-individualizing care. Mayo Clin Proc 65:73–87, 1990.
8. Ives HE: Essential hypertension—where are we going? West J Med 153:415–420, 1990.
9. Littenberg B, Garber AM, Sox HC Jr: Screening for hypertension. Ann Intern Med 112:192–202, 1990.
10. Weiss NS: Relation of high blood pressure to headache, epistaxis and selected other symptoms. N Engl J Med 287:631–633, 1972.
11. Rudd P, Price MG, Graham LE, et al.: Consequences of worksite hypertension screening: differential changes in psychosocial function. Am J Med 80:853–860, 1986.
12. Williams Larson AW, Strong CG: Initial assessment of the patient with hypertension. Mayo Clin Proc 64:1533–1542, 1989.
13. Pickering TG, James GD, Boddie C, Harshfield GA, Blank S, Laragh JH: How common is white coat hypertension? JAMA 259:225–228, 1988.
14. National High Blood Pressure Education Program Coordinating Committee: National High Blood Pressure Education Program Working Group Report on Ambulatory Blood Pressure Monitoring. Arch Intern Med 150:2270–2280, 1990.
15. Klein LE: Compliance and blood pressure control. Hypertension 11(suppl II):61–64, 1988.
16. Kannel WB, Neaton JD, Wentworth D, et al.: Overall and coronary heart disease mortality rates in relation to major risk factors in 325,348 men screened for MRFIT. Am Heart J 112:825–836, 1986.
17. Messerlii FH, Schmieder R: Left ventricular hypertrophy: a cardiovascular risk factor in essential hypertension. Drugs 31(suppl 4):192–201, 1986.
18. Devereux RB: Does increased blood pressure cause left ventricular hypertrophy or vice versa? Ann Intern Med 112:157–159, 1990.
19. Shepherd RFJ, Zachariah PK, Shub H: Hypertension and left ventricular diastolic function. Mayo Clin Proc 64:1521–1532, 1989.
20. Koren MJ, Dveereux RB, Casale PN, et al.: Relation of left ventricular mass and geometry to morbidity and mortality in uncomplicated essential hypertension. Ann Intern Med 114:345–352, 1991.
21. MacMahon S, Peto R, Cutler J, et al.: Blood pressure, stroke, and

coronary heart disease. Part 1, prolonged differences in blood pressure prospective observational studies corrected for regression dilution bias. Lancet 335:765–774, 1990.

22. Collins R, Peto R, MacMahon S, et al.: Blood pressure, stroke, and coronary heart disease. Part 2, short-term reductions in blood pressure: overview of the randomised drug trials in their epidemiological context. Lancet 335:827–838, 1990.

23. Veterans Administration Cooperative Study Group on Antihypertensive Agents: Effects of treatment on morbidity in hypertension: results in patients with diastolic blood pressure averaging 115 through 129 mm Hg. JAMA 202:1028–1034, 1967.

24. Veterans Administration Cooperative Study Group on Antihypertensive Agents: Effects of treatment on morbidity in hypertension: results in patients with diastolic blood pressure averaging 90 through 104 mm Hg. JAMA 213:1143–1152, 1970.

25. Taguchi J, Freis ED: Partial reduction in blood pressure and prevention of complications in hypertension. N Engl J Med 291:329–331, 1974.

26. Hypertension Detection and Follow-up Program Cooperative Group: Five year findings of the hypertension detection and follow-up program. I. Reduction in mortality of persons with high blood pressure, including mild hypertension. JAMA 242:2562–2571, 1979.

27. Hypertension Detection and Follow-up Program Cooperative Group: Five year findings of the hypertension detection and follow-up program. II. Mortality by race, sex, and age. JAMA 242:2572–2577, 1979.

28. Hypertension Detection and Follow-up Program Cooperative Group: The effect of treatment on mortality in mild hypertension. N Engl J Med 307:976–980, 1982.

30. Multiple Risk Factor Intervention Trial Group: Risk factors changes and mortality results. JAMA 248:1465–1477, 1982.

31. Multiple Risk Factor Intervention Trial Group: Baseline rest electrocardiographic abnormalities, antihypertensive treatment, and mortality in the Multiple Risk Factor Intervention Trial. Am J Cardiol 55:1–14, 1985.

32. European Working Party on High Blood Pressure in the Elderly Trial (EWPHE): Mortality and morbidity results from the European Working Party on High Blood Pressure in the Elderly Trial. Lancet 1:1349–1354, 1985.

33. European Working Party on High Blood Pressure in the Elderly Trial (EWPHE): Efficacy of antihypertensive drug treatment according to age, sex, blood pressure, and previous cardiovascular disease in patients over the age of 60. Lancet 2:589–592, 1986.

34. MacGregor GA, Sagnella GA, Markandu ND, et al.: Double-blind study of three sodium intakes and long-term effects of sodium restriction in essential hypertension. Lancet 2:1244–1247, 1989.

35. Weinberger MH: Is salt restriction relevant and feasible as adjunctive treatment of hypertension? Drugs 39:809–813, 1990.

36. Schotte DE, Stunkard AJ: The effect of weight reduction on blood pressure in 301 obese patients. Arch Intern Med 150:1701–1704, 1990.

37. Hagberg JM, Seals DR: Exercise training and hypertension. Acta Med Scand Suppl 711:131–136, 1990.

38. Kelemen MH, Effron MB, Valenti SA, et al.: Exercise training combined with antihypertensive drug therapy: effects on lipids, blood pressure and left ventricular mass. JAMA 263:2766–2771, 1990.

39. Klaus D: Management of hypertension in actively exercising patients: implications of drug selection. Drugs 37:212–218, 1989.

40. Mann SJ, James GD, Wang RS, et al.: Elevation of ambulatory systolic blood pressure in hypertensive smokers: a case control study. JAMA 265:2226–2228, 1991.

41. Materson BJ, Reda D, Freis ED, et al.: Cigarette smoking interferes with treatment of hypertension. Arch Intern Med 148:2116–2119, 1988.

42. Beevers DG, Maheswaran R, Potter JF: Alcohol, blood pressure and antihypertensive drugs. J Clin Pharm Ther 15:395–397, 1990.

43. Puddy JB, Beilin LJ, Vandongen R: Regular alcohol use raises blood pressure in treated hypertensive subjects: a randomised controlled trial. Lancet 1:647–651, 1987.

44. Sharp DS, Bentowitz NL: Pharmacoepidemiology of the effect of caffeine on blood pressure. Clin Pharmacol Ther 47:57–60, 1990.

45. Jeong D-U, Dimsdale JE: The effects of caffeine on blood pressure in the work environment. Am J Hypertens 3:749–753, 1990.

46. Grobbee DE, Rimm EB, Giovannucci E, et al.: Coffee, caffeine, and cardiovascular disease in men. N Engl J Med 323:1026–1032, 1990.

47. Stamler R, Stamler J, Grimm R, et al.: Nutritional therapy for high blood pressure: final report of a four-year randomized controlled trial—the hypertension control program. JAMA 257:1484–1491, 1987.

48. Anon: Drugs for hypertension. Med Lett 33:33–38, 1991.

49. Licht JH, Haley RJ, Pugh B, Lewis SB: Diuretic regimens in essential hypertension: a comparison of hypokalemic effects, BP control, and cost. Arch Intern Med 143:1694–1699, 1983.

50. Perez-Stable EJ: Management of mild hypertension: selecting an antihypertensive regimen. West J Med 154:78–87, 1991.

51. Papademetriou V, Burris JF, Nootargiacomo A, et al.: Thiazide therapy is not a cause of arrhythmia in patients with systemic hypertension. Arch Intern Med 48:1272–1276, 1988.

52. Weinberger MH: Diuretics and their side effects: dilemma in the treatment of hypertension. Hypertension 11(suppl II):16–20, 1988.

53. Langford HG, Blaufox D, Borhani NO, et al.: Is thiazide-produced uric acid elevation harmful? Analysis of date from the Hypertension Detection and Follow-up Program. Arch Intern Med 147:645–649, 1987.

54. Wasnich R, Davis J, Ross P, Vogel J: Effect of thiazide on rates of bone mineral loss: a longitudinal study. Br Med J 301:303–305, 1990.

55. Skluth HA, Gums JC: Spironolactone: a re-examination. DICP, The Annals of Pharmacotherapy 24:52–59, 1990.

56. Spence JD, Wong DG, Lindsay RM: Effects of triamterene and amiloride on urinary sediment in hypertensive patients taking hydrochlorothiazide. Lancet 2:73–75, 1985.

57. Zawada ET: Antihypertensive therapy with triamterent-hydrochlorothiazide vs amiloride-hydrochlorothiazide: comparison of effects on urinary prostaglandin E2 excretion. Arch Intern Med 146:1312–1314, 1986.

58. Favre L, Glasson P, Valloton MB: Reversible acute renal failure from combined triamterene and indomethacin: a study in healthy subjects. Ann Intern Med 96:317–318, 1982.

59. Nadelmann J, Frishman WH: Clinical use of β-adrenoceptor blockade in systemic hypertension. Drugs 39:862–876, 1990.

60. Dornhorst A, Powell SH, Pensky J: Aggravation by propranolol of hyperglycaemic effect of hydrochlorothiazide in type II diabetics without alteration of insulin secretion. Lancet 1:123–126, 1985.

61. Houston MC, Hodge R: β-Adrenergic blocker withdrawal syndromes in hypertension and other cardiovascular diseases. Am Heart J 116:515–523, 1988.

62. Psaty BM, Koepsell TD, Wagner EH, et al.: The relative risk of incident coronary heart disease associated with recently stopping the use of β-blockers. JAMA 263:1653–1657, 1990.

63. Williams GH: Converting-enzyme inhibitors in the treatment of hypertension. N Engl J Med 319:1517–1525, 1988.

64. Townsend RR, Holland OB: Combination of converting-enzyme inhibitor with diuretic for the treatment of hypertension. Arch Intern Med 150:1175–1183, 1990.

65. Gibson GR: Enalapril-induced cough. Arch Intern Med 149:2701–2703, 1989.

66. Kaplan NM: Calcium entry blockers in the treatment of hypertension: current status and future prospects. JAMA 262:817–823, 1989.

67. Cubeddu LX, Aramda K, Somgj B, et al.: A comparison of verapamil and propranolol for the initial treatment of hypertension: racial differences in response. JAMA 256:2214–2221, 1986.

68. Messerli FH, Nunez BD, Nunez MM, et al.: Hypertension and sudden death: disparate effects of calcium entry blocker and diuretic therapy on cardiac dysrhythmias. Arch Intern Med 149:1263–1267, 1989.

69. Russell RP: Side effects of calcium channel blockers. Hypertension 11:(suppl II):II-42-4, 1988.

70. Nicholson JP, Resnick LM, Laragh JH: Hydrochlorothiazide is not additive to verapamil in treating essential hypertension. Arch Intern Med 149:125–128, 1989.

71. Young RA, Brogden RN: Doxazosin: a review of its pharmacodynamic and pharmacokinetic properties, and therapeutic efficacy in mild or moderate hypertension. Drugs 35:525–541, 1988.

72. Wessels F: Double-blind comparison of doxazosin and enalapril in patients with mild or moderate essential hypertension. Am Heart J 121:299–303, 1991.

73. Lepor H, Knapp-Maloney G, Wozniak-Petrofsky J: The safety and efficacy of terazosin for the treatment of benign prostatic hypertrophy. Int J Clin Pharmacol, Ther Toxicol 27:392–397, 1989.

74. Weber MA: Clinical pharmacology of centrally acting antihypertensive agents. J Clin Pharmacol 29:598–602, 1989.

75. Glassman AH, Stetner F, Walsh T, et al.: Heavy smokers, smoking cessation, and clonidine: results of a double-blind, randomized trial. JAMA 259:2863–2866, 1988.

76. Langley MS, Heel RC: Transdermal clonidine: a preliminary review of its pharmacodynamic properties and therapeutic efficacy. Drugs 35:123–142, 1988.

77. Cornish LA: Guanfacine hydrochloride: a centrally acting antihypertensive agent. Clin Pharm 7:187–197, 1988.

78. Engelman K: Side effects of sympatholytic antihypertensive drugs. Hypertension 11:(suppl II):II-30–33, 1988.

79. Mehta JL, Lopez LM: Rebound hypertension following abrupt cessation of clonidine and metoprolol: treatment with labetalol. Arch Intern Med 147:389–390, 1987.

80. Pettinger WA, Mitchell HC: Side effects of vasodilator therapy. Hypertension 11:(suppl II):II-34–36, 1988.

81. Schoenberger JA: Epidemiology and evaluation: steps toward hypertension treatment in the 1990s. Am J Med 90(suppl 4B):4S–7S, 1991.

82. Dannenberg AL, Kannel WB: Remission of hypertension: the 'natural' history of blood pressure treatment in the Framingham study. JAMA 257:1477–1483, 1987.

83. Calhoun DA, Oparil S: Treatment of hypertensive crisis. N Engl J Med 323:1177–1183, 1990.

84. Weber MA: Immediate treatment of severe hypertension: widening the options. Arch Intern Med 149:2635–2637, 1989.

85. Jaker M, Atkin S, Soto M, et al.: Oral nifedipine vs oral clonidine in the treatment of urgent hypertension. Arch Intern Med 149:260–265, 1991.

86. Christlieb AR: Treatment selection considerations for the hypertensive diabetic patient. Arch Intern Med 150:1167–1174, 1990.

87. Kaplan NM: The deadly quartet: upper-body obesity, glucose intolerance, hypertriglyceridemia, and hypertension. Arch Intern Med 149:1514–1519, 1989.

88. Reaven GM: Insulin resistance, hyperinsulinemia, and hypertriglyceridemia in the etiology and clinical course of hypertension. Am J Med 90:(Suppl 2A):7S–11S, 1991.

89. Kochar MS, Landry KM, Ristow SM: Effects of reduction in dose and discontinuation of hydrochlorothiazide in patients with controlled essential hypertension. Arch Intern Med 150:1009–1011, 1990.

90. O'Bryne S, Feely J: Effects of drugs on glucose tolerance in non-insulin dependent diabetics (part I): Drugs 40:6–18, 1990.

91. Pollare T, Lithell H, Berne C: A comparison of the effects of hydrochlorothiazide and captopril on glucose and lipid metabolism in patients with hypertension. N Engl J Med 321:868–873, 1989.

92. O'Bryne S, Feely J: Effects of drugs on glucose tolerance in non-insulin dependent diabetics (part II). Drugs 40:203–219, 1990.

93. Bakris G: Effects of diltiazem or lisinopril on massive proteinuria associated with diabetes mellitus. Ann Intern Med 112:707–708, 1990.

94. National High Blood Pressure Program Working Group Report on Hypertension and Chronic Renal Failure: National Heart, Lung, and Blood Institute. NIH Publication No. 90-3032, 1990, pp 1–20.

95. Schlueter WA, Batle DC: Renal effects of antihypertensive drugs. Drugs 37:900–925, 1989.

96. Heyka RJ, Vidt DG: Control of hypertension in patients with chronic renal failure. Cleveland Clin J Med 56:65–76, 1989.

97. Anderson KM, Wilson WF, Odell PM, Kannel WB: An updated coronary risk profile: a statement for health professionals. Circulation 83:356–361, 1991.

98. Applegate WB: Hypertension in elderly patients. Ann Intern Med 110:901–915, 1989.

99. SHEP Cooperative Research Group. Prevention of stroke by antihypertensive drug treatment in older persons with isolated systolic hypertension: final results of the systolic hypertension in the elderly program (SHEP). JAMA 265:3255–3264, 1991.

100. O'Malley K, Cox JP, O'Brien E: Choice of drug treatment of elderly hypertensive patients. Am J Med 90(suppl 3A):27S–33S, 1991.

101. National High Blood Pressure Education Program Working Group Report on High Blood Pressure in Pregnancy. Am J Obstet Gynecol 163:1691–1712, 1990.

102. Eisner GM: Hypertension: racial differences. Am J Kidney Dis XVI (suppl 1):35–40, 1990.

103. Cooper ES, Kuller LH, Saunders E, et al.: Cardiovascular diseases and stroke in African-Americans and other racial minorities in the United States: a statement for health professionals. Circulation 83:1462–1480, 1991.

104. Saunders E, Weir MR, Kong W, et al.: A comparison of the efficacy and safety of a β-blocker, a calcium channel blocker, and a converting enzyme inhibitor in hypertensive blacks. Arch Intern Med 150:1707–1713, 1990.

105. Zhou H-H, Koshakji RP, Silbertein DJ, et al.: Racial differences in drug response: altered sensitivity to and clearance of propranolol in men of Chinese descent as compared to American whites. N Engl J Med 320:565–570, 1989.

106. Ahsan CH, Macklin RB, Challenor VF, et al.: Ethnic differences in the pharmacokinetics of oral nifedipine. Br J Clin Pharm 31:399–403, 1991.

107. Croog SH, Levine S, Testa MA, et al.: The effects of antihypertensive therapy on the quality of life. N Engl J Med 314:1657–1664, 1986.

108. Croog SH, Kong W, Levine S, et al.: Hypertensive black men and women: quality of life and effects of antihypertensive medications. Arch Intern Med 150:1733–1741, 1990.

109. Wassertheil-Smoller S, Blaufox D, Oberman A, et al.: Effect of antihypertensives on sexual function and quality of life: the TAIM study. Ann Intern Med 114:613–620, 1991.

110. Friedman RB, Katt JA: Cost-benefit issues in the practice of internal medicine. Arch Intern Med 151:1165–1168, 1991.

111. Edelson JT, Weinstein MC, Tosteson ANA, et al.: Long-term cost-effectiveness of various initial monotherapies for mild to moderate hypertension. JAMA 263:407–413, 1990.

112. Kaplan NM: Cost-effectiveness of antihypertensive drugs: fact or fancy? Am J Hypertens 4:478–480, 1991.

113. Materson BJ: Sexual dysfunction during antihypertensive treatment. Prog Pharmacol 6:117–124, 1985.

114. Croog SH, Levine S, Sudilovsky A, et al.: Sexual symptoms in hypertensive patients. Arch Intern Med 148:788–794, 1988.

115. Beers MH, Passman LJ: Antihypertensive medications and depression. Drugs 40:792–799, 1990.

116. Cruickshank JM, Thorp JM, Zacharias FJ: Benefits and potential harm of lowering high blood pressure. Lancet 1:581–583, 1987.

117. Staessen J, Bulpitt C, Clement D, et al.: Relation between mortality and treated blood pressure in elderly patients with hypertension: report of the European Working Party on High Blood Pressure in the Elderly. Br Med J 298:1552–1556, 1989.

118. Farnett L, Mulrow CD, Linn WD, et al.: The J-curve phenomenon and the treatment of hypertension: is there a point beyond which pressure reduction is dangerous? JAMA 265:489–495, 1991.

119. Working Group on Management of Patients with Hypertension and High Blood Cholesterol. National education programs working group report on the management of patients with hypertension and high blood cholesterol. Ann Intern Med 114:224–237, 1991.

120. Lardinois CK, Neuman SL: The effects of antihypertensive agent on serum lipids and lipoproteins. Arch Intern Med 148:1280–1288, 1988.

121. Samuelsson O, Wilhelmsen L, Andersson OK, et al.: Cardiovascular morbidity in relation to change in blood pressure and serum cholesterol levels in treated hypertension: results from the Primary Prevention Trial in Goteborg, Sweden. JAMA 258:1768–1776, 1987.

122. Francis Lam YW, Shepherd MM: Drug interactions in hypertensive patients: pharmacokinetic, pharmacodynamic and genetic considerations. Clin Pharmacokinet 18:295–317, 1990.

123. Brown J, Dollery C, Valdes G: Interaction with nonsteroidal anti-inflammatory drugs with antihypertensive and diuretic agents: control of vascular reactivity by endogenous prostanoids. Am J Med 81(suppl 2B):43–57, 1986.

124. Winickoff RN, Murphy PK: The persistent problem of poor blood pressure control. Arch Intern Med 147:1393–1396, 1987.

125. McClellan WM, Hall W, Brogan D, et al.: Continuity of care in hypertension: an important correlate of blood pressure control among aware hypertensives. Arch Intern Med 148:525–528, 1988.

126. Lachman BE: Increasing patient compliance through tracking systems. Calif Pharmacist 34:54–58, 1987.

127. Oto-Kent DS: Controlling hypertension: pharmacists can make a difference. Calif Pharmacist 36:42–43, 1989.

128. McKenney JM, Slining JM, Henderson HR, et al.: The effect of clinical pharmacy services on patients with essential hypertension. Circulation 48:1104–1111, 1973.

129. Hawkins DW, Fiedler FP, Douglas HL, Eschbach RE: Evaluation of a clinical pharmacist in caring for hypertensive and diabetic patients. Am J Hosp Pharm 36:1321–1326, 1979.

CHAPTER 36

CONGESTIVE HEART FAILURE

CYNTHIA L. RAEHL, Pharm.D. and PAUL E. NOLAN, JR., Pharm.D.

Congestive heart failure (CHF) can be defined as a clinical syndrome that is characterized by congestion of both the pulmonary and systemic circulations. The congestion results from the body's excessive reflex activation of various physiologic processes that attempt to compensate for decreased perfusion pressure (1). Consequently the usual clinical findings of pulmonary congestion, peripheral edema, and diminished exercise tolerance often reflect inadequate systolic function of the heart. Until recently, the term *congestive* heart failure seemed appropriate as almost all patients exhibited the typical signs of pulmonary congestion such as dyspnea on exertion. It is now known that some patients may not have congestive symptoms. Aggressive diuretic therapy can alleviate the usual complaints of dyspnea. Also in some patients, the heart still contracts efficiently (systolic function preserved) but does not relax properly (diastolic dysfunction). Patients with primarily diastolic dysfunction may have dyspnea only with exertion. Therefore, the term *failing heart syndrome* may replace the older term *congestive heart failure*. The failing heart syndrome is characterized by cardiac systolic and/or diastolic dysfunction with reduced exercise tolerance. Cohn's definition of the failing heart syndrome helps clinicians understand treatment goals: "a syndrome in which cardiac dysfunction is associated with reduced exercise tolerance, a high incidence of ventricular arrhythmias, and shortened life expectancy" (2). The three overlapping components of heart failure (left ventricular dysfunction, arrhythmias, and reduced exercise tolerance) require individualization of drug therapy.

CHF is a clinical condition with a number of etiologies. The incidence of CHF appears to be increasing as the number of elderly individuals increases. Even though the pharmacological management of CHF is improving, the disease remains a lethal condition with a poor prognosis.

ETIOLOGY

In 1971 the Framingham Study demonstrated that hypertension (HTN) preceded CHF in 75% of all cases; coronary artery disease (CAD) was implicated in 39%, whereas 29% of all patients had CAD with accompanying HTN; rheumatic heart disease (RHD) was observed in 21%; and both RHD and HTN in 11% of all patients. Miscellaneous causes accounted for 5% of the cases and included congenital heart disease, thyrotoxicosis, atrial fibrillation, and dilated cardiomyopathy (3). More recent data

from the Henry Ford Hospital involving 100 consecutive patients discharged with CHF demonstrated that HTN was found in only 31%, CAD in 26%, diabetes mellitus in 25%, and valvular heart disease in 16% (2). Rheumatic heart disease was responsible for only 6 of the 16 cases of valvular heart disease. The only drugs that have been consistently implicated as causes of CHF are anticancer agents such as doxorubicin (adriamycin) (4). In summary, the principal causes of CHF include advanced age, HTN, diabetes mellitus, and overt heart disease including ischemic, valvular, rheumatic, idiopathic, and congenital heart disease.

INCIDENCE

Using data from the Framingham Study (3), the estimated incidence of CHF in the Untied States in 1983 was almost 400,000 persons. Of these new cases, 214,000 (54%) were male and 184,000 (46%) were female. Although CHF can occur at any age, there was a remarkable increase with advancing age as evidenced by a doubling of age-specific incidence rates for both men and women at each subsequent decade of life. When these estimates were applied to the 1981 census data, approximately 2.3 million persons had CHF. CHF accounts for 1.8 million physician's office visits and over 1.5 million hospital discharges yearly (5). Thus, CHF represents an enormous challenge to all healthcare practitioners.

PATHOGENESIS

Several generalized pathophysiological conditions can lead to the development of heart failure. These include pressure overload of the heart (e.g., HTN or aortic stenosis), volume overload (e.g., valvular regurgitation), loss of viable myocardium (e.g., chronic ischemic heart disease or myocardial infarction), or generalized decrease in myocardial contractility (e.g., several types of dilated cardiomyopathies) (6). Each of these conditions diminishes the functional ability of the heart to maintain effective cardiac output.

Understanding the cellular and biochemical abnormalities of progressive heart failure holds the promise of more effective therapeutic measures. It appears that two pathogenetic mechanisms contribute to the decline in myocardial performance (7). The first is chronic energy starvation in the heart, causing both impaired cellular function and ultimately cell death. Energy starvation may be the result of cellular hypertrophy representing an increase in the number of sarcomeres or a deficiency in high-energy phosphate compounds. Energy starvation could also result from diminished tissue nutrient supply caused by increased distances between the capillaries due to myocardial hypertrophy. The second proposed pathogenetic mechanism for myocardial deterioration is alteration in the composition of the hypertrophied muscle such as exaggerated formation of myocardial proteins. Whatever cellular changes occur in heart failure, the outcome is stimulation of a number of myocardial, circulatory, and neurohumoral compensatory mechanisms.

In response to the decreased myocardial performance, a number of cardiac and peripheral compensatory mechanisms become activated. The ventricular chamber may dilate to increase its preload and ultimately its output during systole (i.e., stroke volume). Preload can be considered as the end-diastolic pressure (or volume). As the ventricular chamber size increases during diastole, the end-diastolic pressure and volume increase. This allows the ventricle to increase its stroke volume, because it is receiving a greater volume during diastole. This response is often depicted by the Frank-Starling relationship between systolic performance and diastolic filling. Preload is determined in part by the extracellular fluid volume and venous return. There are, however, limitations to this adaptive response. As the preload continues to increase, the resultant increase in filling pressure is transmitted back to the pulmonary circulation. When this pressure exceeds the oncotic pressure within the pulmonary vasculature, there is a transudation of fluid into the pulmonary interstitial spaces, resulting in pulmonary congestion.

The heart may also increase its wall thickness, especially in response to pressure overload. This is analogous to a weightlifter's increase in muscle size in response to lifting heavier weights. The increased wall thickness would result in a reduction of wall stress (or afterload). Afterload refers to the hemodynamic load against which the ventricle must contract in order to deliver its stroke volume. A major component of afterload is the systemic arteriolar tone (or the systemic vascular resistance). Increases in afterload can result in decreased stroke volume, especially in CHF, where in the setting of decreased myocardial systolic function, the heart becomes increasingly afterload-dependent (8). Afterload corresponds to systolic wall stress. According to the LaPlace relationship, systolic wall stress equals the product of aortic pressure (P) times the internal radius of the ventricle (R) divided by the wall thickness of the ventricle (h) or $[(P \times R)/h]$. Preload in effect is a component of afterload in that it corresponds to the internal radius of the ventricular chamber.

In addition to the heart's adjustments, peripheral adaptations attempt to compensate for the reduced cardiac output and perfusion pressure to vital organs. Increases in arteriolar vasoconstriction, which decrease potential vascular space, and increases in the effective circulating blood volume via sodium and water retention are the major peripheral adjustments. Unfortunately, these compensatory changes ultimately lead to the development of many of the signs and symptoms of CHF.

These peripheral adaptations result from a complex interplay among a number of neurohumoral factors (9). Activation of the sympathetic nervous system (SNS) and the renin-angiotensin-aldosterone (RAA) system along with increased secretion of arginine vasopressin (AVP) are observed in many patients, especially in those with more advanced CHF. Elevated circulating levels of norepinephrine (NE) increase myocardial contractility and heart rate, principally via stimulation of cardiac β_1-adrenergic receptors. The enhanced SNS activity (via stimulation of renal β_2-adrenergic receptors) and decreased renal perfusion (secondary to vasoconstriction) result in increased circulating levels of renin. This eventually leads to increased formation of angiotensin II (A II). A II directly stimulates aldosterone release from the adrenal gland. Aldosterone stimulates sodium and water retention by the kidneys. The increased circulating levels of the antidiuretic hormone, AVP, also assist in increasing water reabsorption by the kidneys. These compensatory mechanisms interact to increase plasma volume and thus augment cardiac output via the Frank-Starling mechanism.

These extracardiac attempts to optimize preload and increase contractility result in a number of secondary, deleterious consequences. Norepinephrine, A II, and AVP are all potent vasoconstrictors. They increase afterload and subsequently cause a greater impairment of cardiac function. This in turn stimulates further compensatory attempts to maximize contractility and preload. A vicious cycle of events (Fig. 36.1) ultimately results in both pulmonary and systemic venous congestion. Increased circulating levels of NE also serve to convert principally the cardiac β_1-adrenergic receptors to forms with a lower affinity for β-agonists, as well as decrease the number of available β-receptors (i.e., receptor down-regulation) (10). These effects contribute ultimately to the diminished ventricular systolic function.

In addition to the neurohumoral factors noted previously, patients with CHF have impaired cardiac parasympathetic (PNS) control (11) and increased circulating levels of atrial natriuretic peptide (ANP) (12) and vasodilatory prostaglandins (11). There is evidence that suggests that impairment of inhibitory vagal afferent fibers (i.e., impaired parasympathetic control) might contribute to the increased sympathetic activity in CHF as evidenced by elevated resting heart rates (11). Although we do not completely understand why the baroreflex control mechanism is blunted in heart failure, several proposed pathophy-

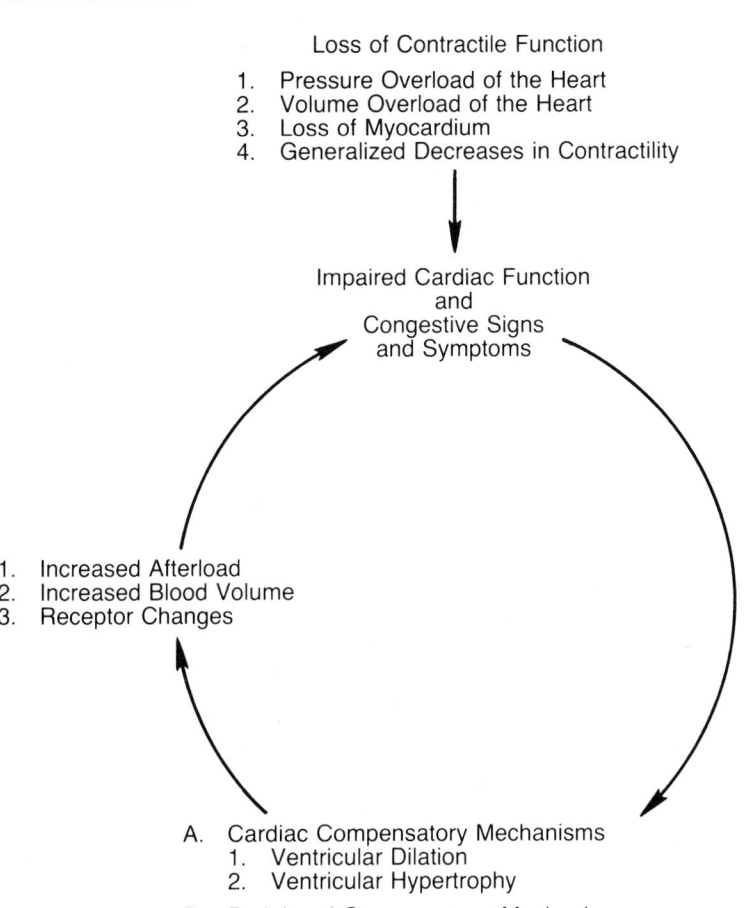

Loss of Contractile Function
1. Pressure Overload of the Heart
2. Volume Overload of the Heart
3. Loss of Myocardium
4. Generalized Decreases in Contractility

Impaired Cardiac Function
and
Congestive Signs
and Symptoms

1. Increased Afterload
2. Increased Blood Volume
3. Receptor Changes

A. Cardiac Compensatory Mechanisms
   1. Ventricular Dilation
   2. Ventricular Hypertrophy
B. Peripheral Compensatory Mechanisms
   1. Increased Sympathetic Activity
   2. Activation of the Renin-Angiotensin-Aldosterone
      System
   3. Increased Release of Arginine Vasopressin

Figure 36.1. Pathogenesis of congestive heart failure.

siologic mechanisms include circulatory congestion leading to increased vascular sodium content and ultimately changes in the mechanical properties of the atrial wall (13). These baroreflex control abnormalities appear to resolve as patients are treated with standard medical therapy such as bed rest, diuretics, and vasodilators (13).

ANP, an amino acid peptide in human atria, promotes natriuresis, decreases arterial pressure, and inhibits the RAA system; its concentration is elevated in patients with CHF (12). Vasodilatory prostaglandins I_2 and E_2 are also elevated in patients with CHF in an attempt to offset the systemic and regional vasoconstriction (14). Thus, complex interrelationships exist between ventricular dysfunction and subsequent abnormalities in sodium and water excretion.

SIGNS AND SYMPTOMS
Knowledge of CHF pathophysiology easily predicts the expected signs, symptoms, and associated laboratory findings (15). Weight gain, secondary to salt and water retention, is common in heart failure patients. Increases

in extracellular and plasma volume lead to congested pulmonary and systemic circulations. Pulmonary congestion is manifest by varying degrees of breathlessness: dyspnea on exertion (DOE); orthopnea (dyspnea that occurs in the recumbent position and requires elevation of the head with one or several pillows to prevent its recurrence); paroxysmal nocturnal dyspnea (PND, an exaggerated form of orthopnea, which occurs when the patient is awakened abruptly at night with a feeling of suffocation); dyspnea at rest; and pulmonary edema (fluid accumulation within the alveoli). Some patients complain of cough or asthma symptoms. Rales and dullness to percussion, usually over the bases of the lung, are common pulmonary physical findings.

Systemically, inadequate perfusion of the skeletal muscles often leads to easy fatiguability and weakness. Exercise tolerance is diminished, and patients adjust their lifestyle accordingly, such as no longer walking up a flight of steps. Nocturia (increased urine formation at night), which results from redistribution of blood flow to the kidney during recumbency, often occurs early in the course of CHF.

Oliguria may become manifest later as the patient's failure worsens. A host of cerebral symptoms may also be observed and can include impairment of memory, confusion, insomnia, and anxiety.

A number of cardiac and systemic physical findings are observed with varying frequencies. An early diastolic third heart sound, S_3 (Ken-tuc-ky), is believed to be related to impaired diastolic relaxation of the ventricle and suggests an elevated end-diastolic pressure. An S_3 is a hallmark finding of moderate-to-severe heart failure. A resting sinus tachycardia is often present. Objective cardiac findings often include an enlarged heart (palpable as a cardiac heave) and increased cardiothoracic ratio as determined by chest x-ray, a diminished ejection fraction as determined by radionuclide or other techniques, and an enlarged left ventricular chamber size as evidenced by echocardiography.

Systemic venous congestion may manifest as dependent peripheral edema, jugular venous distension (JVD), and congestive hepatomegaly. A minimal gain of approximately 10 pounds of extracellular fluid volume is necessary before peripheral edema is noted. This edema usually develops in the dependent areas of the body such as the ankles, feet, or above the shinbone (i.e., pretibial) in ambulatory patients and in the sacral area in bedridden individuals. Peripheral edema may be physically uncomfortable as well as cosmetically unattractive. Central venous pressure (CVP) is estimated by elevating the patient's head to a 45° angle and observing the peak of the maximal venous pulsation within the internal jugular vein. In this position, the CVP does not normally exceed 2 cm of vertical distance above the sternal angle. Because the sternal angle usually lies about 5 cm above the right atrium, the CVP can be estimated by noting the vertical distance and adding 5 cm to this value. The liver is also characteristically congested in CHF and is generally palpable several centimeters below the right costal margin. Hepatic edema may cause right upper quadrant pain. Generalized visceral edema may also occur and cause abdominal distention and anorexia.

Understanding the cardiovascular physical examination is essential to monitoring the efficacy of heart failure drug regimens. Along with medical history and chest x-ray, physicians have relied on the presence of an S3, pulmonary rales, an abnormal jugular venous pulse, and peripheral edema to monitor CHF. However, in chronic heart failure (systolic dysfunction), cardiocirculatory compensatory mechanisms make these physical signs less reliable. Patients can have very high left ventricular filling pressures but no detectable rales because the lymphatic drainage has increased proportionately (16). Third heart sounds are commonly present and therefore are nonspecific for changes in filling pressures. Signs of venous congestion are often absent, given the effect of diuretics

and vasodilators. The blood pressure measurement, however, can provide information that helps assess the adequacy of heart failure treatment. Neither systolic blood pressure (SBP) nor diastolic blood pressure (DBP) alone is an adequate measure. Rather, the proportional pulse pressure [(SBP-DBP)/SBP] is used because it represents the activation of compensatory mechanisms and cardiac output. The pulse pressure can identify patients with a low cardiac index. Because most patients with severe chronic heart failure have a SBP of 100 mm Hg or less, the pulse pressure as a proportion of total systolic pressure is useful. Stevenson et al. (16) found a proportional pulse pressure <25% in 91% of patients with a cardiac index of ≤2.2 liter/min/m².

Numerous laboratory abnormalities are observed in patients with CHF. Simple laboratory tests (body weight, serum electrolytes, chest x-ray, and serum digoxin levels) are used most frequently in monitoring ambulatory patients with congestive heart failure (17). Body weight is monitored at home by the patients every several days, while serum electrolytes are checked about every 2 months provided there are no changes in drug therapy. Hyponatremia is observed frequently despite the increase in total body sodium. The hyponatremia is dilutional, as there is a diminished ability to excrete free water. Hyponatremia may worsen with diuretic treatment. Patients with CHF generally have deficits of both total body and intracellular potassium and magnesium, which may or may not be reflected in the serum concentrations of these cations (18). Potentially lethal or lethal ventricular arrhythmias may occur as secondary consequences. Impaired hepatic function may be characterized by elevations in liver enzyme levels. Reductions in renal blood flow and glomerular filtration rate will be reflected by increases in both serum creatinine and blood urea nitrogen levels. The urine is usually concentrated, with a high urine specific gravity, and there may be associated proteinuria. More sophisticated measures of cardiac function are used less frequently and at longer intervals (usually every 12 to 24 months): echocardiography, radionuclide ventriculography, or exercise testing.

To evaluate both the severity of heart failure and the effects of treatment modalities, two classification systems have been developed: The New York Heart Association (NYHA) Functional Classification (15) and a classification based upon exercise tolerance (19) (Table 36.1). Unfortunately, these two classification systems do not correlate well. The NYHA classification, despite its reliance upon subjective findings during exertion, is very popular. Because patients often downgrade their expectations for exercise tolerance as their failure progresses, they may underestimate the impact of their disease. Most likely the NYHA classification will remain popular among practitioners because of its simplicity and convenience. The ex-

Table 36.1.
Classification Systems for Congestive Heart Failure

New York Heart Association functional classification

Class I: No limitation; ordinary physical activity does not cause symptoms

Class II: Slight limitation of physical activity; ordinary physical activity results in symptoms

Class III: Marked limitation of physical activity; less than ordinary activity leads to symptoms

Class IV: Inability to carry on any activity without symptoms; symptoms are present at rest

Classification of heart failure based upon exercise tolerance

Class A: No impairment; VO_{2max}[a] > 20 ml/min/kg

Class B: Mild to moderate impairment; VO_{2max} = 16–20 ml/min/kg

Class C: Moderate to severe impairment; VO_{2max} = 10–15 ml/min/kg

Class D: Severe impairment; VO_{2max} < 10 ml/min/kg

[a] VO_{2max}, maximal oxygen uptake. It is a function of the maximum cardiac output that the heart can generate and the maximal amount of oxygen (O_2) that the exercising tissues can extract.

ercise tolerance classification system uses an incremental treadmill exercise protocol and noninvasive monitoring of respiratory gas exchange, heart rate, and blood pressure to grade the severity of chronic CHF. Maximal oxygen uptake (VO_{2max}, expressed in ml/min/kg) is determined by maximal cardiac output and by maximal oxygen extraction by the exercising muscles. Despite its relative objectivity, it is a more complex, costly, and time-consuming method for evaluating levels of CHF and responses to therapy.

TREATMENT OF CHRONIC CHF

The two basic goals in the treatment of CHF are to relieve the symptoms that occur secondary to this syndrome and to prolong life. All therapies are directed to one or both of these goals, and new therapies should neither worsen symptoms nor shorten life. Difficulty in measuring these goals has resulted in several surrogate measures for symptomatology and mortality rates. Surrogates include cardiac ejection fraction and short-term and long-term hemodynamic responses to drug therapy. Symptoms, usually exercise intolerance, are not apparent until a patient is in NYHA functional class II. Salt restriction, reduction of the heart's workload with rest, and identification and treatment of precipitating causes are all general measures that relieve symptoms. Inotropic drugs (traditionally digoxin) by increasing contractility, diuretics by decreasing circulatory congestion, and vasodilatory drugs by diminishing cardiac workload, are also useful in relieving symptoms to varying degrees. Because improvement in exercise tolerance is a fundamental goal of heart failure treatment, new heart failure treatment drugs are tested using exercise criteria. Yet, these standardized tests using treadmills and bicycles often do not predict the exercise response in daily living activities. Symptomatic relief, such as a change from

NYHA class IV to class III, remains a lifelong goal for treatment of heart failure patients.

The second basic goal of heart failure treatment, prolongation of life, can only be measured in large-scale, controlled studies of mortality rates. CHF has an extremely high mortality rate. Patients in severe congestive heart failure, such as those with acute myocardial infarction and cadiogenic shock, have a short-term mortality rate as high as 90%. In the mid-1980s, the 5-year mortality rate of CHF was estimated to be about 50% (5). To date, the only drug therapies that have been proven to prolong life are vasodilator therapy using (*a*) a combination of hydralazine and isosorbide dinitrate (20) or (*b*) an ACE-inhibitor (21, 22). Left ventricular ejection fraction (LVEF) has been used as a surrogate study end point for mortality rates. However, improvement in LVEF and reduction in mortality are not always directly associated. Other physiologic parameters, often neurohumoral markers such as plasma NE, A II, or plasma ANP, are often evaluated in mortality studies. However, alteration of these markers toward normal levels is not necessarily associated with an improvement in mortality rates. Survival rates, despite the cost and difficulty of conducting mortality studies, remain the primary end point of heart failure treatment efficacy and safety studies.

Most of this chapter is devoted to treatment of systolic heart failure; diastolic heart failure is treated much differently and is therefore discussed in a separate section.

General Measures

Restricting physical activity to some degree is a therapeutic maneuver used in the management of virtually any patient with CHF (23). The restriction of physical activity should disturb the patient's lifestyle as little as possible. The degree of restriction will vary not just from patient to patient, but also from week to week (or month to month) for the same patient. The restriction of physical activity may range from discontinuing exhausting sports to confinement of the patient to a bed or chair.

Many heart failure patients will benefit from a prescribed cardiac rehabilitation program. General improvement in physical condition can be accompanied by hemodynamic benefits including reduction of the resting heart rate, reduction of exercise-associated peak systolic blood pressure, and an improvement in the tissue extraction of oxygen. Patients' capacity to exercise will vary widely, therefore each patient should receive individualized instruction. It is not possible to accurately predict exercise tolerance from either the LVEF or other clinical parameters. However, patients who cannot increase their cardiac output with exercise will probably do poorly. These patients often drop their systolic pressure when exercising—a finding that suggests no cardiac reserve remains. Such patients may not tolerate any exercise program. Similarly, patients who have recently experienced a myocardial infarction should begin exercising only under the direction of a healthcare practitioner. Heart failure patients should "begin low and go slow," thereby avoiding overexerting themselves. Many patients prefer walking programs.

Limiting a patient's salt intake helps counteract the exaggerated renal retention of sodium. Elimination of the saltshaker from the table and removal of high-sodium-containing foods (e.g., salted nuts, pretzels, salt-cured meats, potato chips, pickles, olives, processed meats, some canned vegetables, and soups) will decrease daily sodium intake to about 1.5 to 3.0 g (3.75 to 7.5 g of sodium chloride, as 1.0 g Na = 2.5 g of NaCl) (23). The typical American diet usually contains twice this amount of sodium. Exclusion of all salt from cooking will further reduce the patient's sodium intake to between 1.2 and 1.5 g. However, excessive sodium restriction may reduce the palatability of food and secondarily compromise adequate nutrition. The use of spices to flavor various foods may enhance patient compliance with a low-sodium diet. Over-the-counter medications may be a hidden source of sodium intake.

It is important to identify, promptly treat, and subsequently prevent aggravating factors of CHF. These factors include arrhythmias (particularly tachyarrhythmias such as uncontrolled atrial fibrillation), systemic infection, pulmonary embolism, hypocalcemia, anemia, prolonged myocardial ischemia, acute myocardial infarction, and endocrine disorders. Patient noncompliance with prescribed medical and pharmacological regimens often precipitates CHF worsening. In a study of patients admitted to a Chicago hospital for heart failure treatment, 64% were noncompliant with their medical regimen (24). Almost one-half of the patients in this study had uncontrolled hypertension as a precipitating factor for heart failure. Addition of negative inotropes, such as β-blockers or some of the antiarrhythmic agents, can worsen preexisting heart failure. Overexertion, cold exposure, and stress are three common environmental precipitants of heart failure. Stricter attention to these precipitating factors could decrease the number of hospitalizations significantly and ease the burden of congestive heart failure for both patients and society.

DIGOXIN

Digoxin and the other digitalis glycosides have been used as inotropic drugs for the treatment of CHF and other congestive states. However, considerable controversy still remains over the true benefit of cardiac glycosides in the management of CHF, particularly in the chronic treatment of patients with CHF in sinus rhythm. In the discussion that follows, digoxin is the only cardiac glycoside reviewed extensively, because of its predominant use in clinical medicine.

Mechanism of Action. The inotropic effects of digoxin are produced indirectly, through inhibition of the transport enzyme, sodium-potassium adenosine triphosphatase (Na^+-K^+ ATPase) (25). This enzyme complex catalyzes Na^+ afflux from the myocardial cell in exchange for K^+. When Na^+ afflux is inhibited, relatively high intracellular concentrations of Na^+ result. Sodium is subsequently exchanged for calcium (Ca^{+2}) via a Na^+-Ca^{+2} exchange carrier. The increased intracellular concentrations of Ca^{+2} ultimately enhance myocardial contractility through a complex series of intracellular Ca^{+2} movements. Digoxin also has effects on the autonomic nervous system, which at nontoxic doses result in a slowing both in heart rate and in atrioventricular conduction (26).

Pharmacokinetics. A vast amount of literature describes the absorption, distribution, metabolism, and elimination of digoxin (27–29). Digoxin is available as a parenteral product and as a tablet, elixir, and capsule. The systemic availabilities of the tablet, elixir, and capsule are 70 to 80%, 75 to 85%, and 90 to 100%, respectively. The upper portion of the small intestine is the major site of absorption. Digoxin undergoes very little first-pass effect. The extent of digoxin absorption appears to be independent of the dose administered.

Digoxin is distributed into a number of tissues. On a mg/g basis, the highest concentrations of digoxin are found in the kidneys, heart, liver, adrenal glands, diaphragm, and intestinal tract. However, approximately 50% of the apparent total body stores of digoxin are found in the skeletal muscles. As a result of this extensive distribution to lean tissue, digoxin should be dosed using an estimate of the patient's ideal body weight. The plasma protein binding of digoxin is independent of concentration and averages 20 to 30%. Albumin is the principal binding protein. In patients with normal renal function, the volume of distribution at steady-state (V_{SS}) averages 6 to 7 liters/kg, with a standard deviation of 1.4 liters/kg.

Digoxin undergoes metabolism primarily by two different pathways. One of these pathways involves sequential hydrolysis of digitoxose sugar moieties, and the other route results in the formation of reduced metabolites. The reduced (dihydro) metabolites are inactive. In contrast, the hydrolysis products, digoxigenin bis- and monodigitoxosides, have potencies that approach that of the parent compound. However, the contribution of these two metabolites to the overall activity of digoxin in humans is unknown at this time. In adults with normal renal and hepatic function, the systemic clearance (CL_S) of digoxin averages approximately 180 ml/min/1.73 m². Renal clearance (CL_R), which exceeds both creatinine and inulin clearances, generally accounts for about 70% of the CL_S. The nonrenal clearance (CL_{NR}) of digoxin includes metabolism, biliary excretion, and possibly intestinal secretion and resultant fecal elimination. CL_S of apparent digoxin is correlated linearly with creatinine clearance (CL_{CR}) in the presence of renal impairment. The apparent terminal elimination half-life ($t_{1/2}$) of digoxin in adults with normal renal and hepatic function averages 36 hr.

A number of clinical conditions and drugs (Table 36.2) can alter the pharmacokinetics of digoxin (27–29). The bioavailability of digoxin tablets can be reduced by abdominal radiation and by various malabsorption syndromes such as hypermotility, diarrhea, and subtotal villus atrophy. Cholesterol-binding resins (cholestyramine and colestipol), kaolin-pectin, large doses of antacids, oral metoclopramide, sulfasalazine, activated charcoal, and oral neomycin also decrease the absorption of digoxin tablets. In contrast, the absorption of digoxin may be enhanced by propantheline (and perhaps other anticholinergic drugs) and oral antibiotics such as tetracycline or erythromycin. These antibiotics decrease the number of colonic bacteria that metabolize digoxin to the inactive reduced metabolites. The V_{SS} of digoxin is reduced in chronic renal failure, whereas it is increased by physical activity. Chronic renal failure also increases the elimination $t_{1/2}$. Drugs that have reduced the CL_S of digoxin consistently include quinidine, verapamil, spironolactone, and amiodarone. Captopril, hypothyroidism, and advanced CHF also decrease the CL_S of digoxin. Hyperthyroidism and orally administered activated charcoal increase the CL_S of digoxin. In addition to the pharmacokinetic interactions between the above drugs and digoxin, the β-blocking agents, amiodarone, and the calcium-blocking drugs verapamil and diltiazem enhance the effects of digoxin on slowing atrioventricular (AV) nodal conduction and on decreasing sinoatrial (SA) nodal rate.

Serum Concentration-Response Relationship. Despite the abundant literature describing the pharmacokinetics of digoxin, a relationship between the intensity of the inotropic response, the development of toxicity, and the apparent serum concentration of digoxin is difficult to define (27–30). This lack of a definitive therapeutic range in part reflects both digoxin's rather modest inotropic effects and

Table 36.2.
Conditions of Altered Digoxin Pharmacokinetics or Pharmacodynamics

Condition	Clinical Management
A. *Reduced bioavailability*	
1. Abdominal radiation	1. Consider administering digoxin as elixir or capsule
2. Malabsorption syndromes	2. As in #1
a. Hypermotility	
b. Diarrhea	
c. Subtotal villus atrophy	
3. Drugs	3. Consider administering digoxin 1 to 2 hr before or 2 to 3 hr following a, b, c, e, f; consider administering digoxin as capsule or elixir for d
a. Cholesterol-binding resins	
b. Kalolin-pectin	
c. Large doses (e.g., 30 ml) of antacids	
d. Metoclopramide (oral)	
e. Sulfasalazine	
f. Neomycin (oral)	
B. *Enhanced bioavailability*	
1. Propantheline (and perhaps other anticholinergics)	1. Be alert for possible occurrence of digoxin toxicity
2. Oral antibiotics	2. Thought only to be a problem in 10% of population who extensively metabolize digoxin to inactive reduction products by colonic bacteria; avoid antibiotics if possible; if antibiotics must be administered, be alert for possible occurrence of digoxin toxicity
a. Erythromycin	
b. Tetracycline	
C. *Reduced systemic clearance*	
1. Renal failure	1. Adjust doses of digoxin to the reductions in creatinine clearance
2. Drugs	
a. Quinidine	a. Reduce digoxin dose by 50% upon start of quinidine; monitor serum digoxin levels (SDCs)
b. Verapamil	b. Consider reducing digoxin dose by about 50% upon initiation of verapamil; monitor serum digoxin levels and look for additive effects on SA and AV nodes
c. Spironolactone	c. Consider reducing digoxin dose by about 50%; monitor SDCs and be alert for signs and symptoms of toxicity
d. Amiodarone	d. Consider reducing digoxin dose by about 50%; monitor SDCs and look for additive effects on SA and AV nodes
e. Captopril	e. Routine reduction of digoxin appears unnecessary; monitor SDCs and be alert for signs and symptoms of toxicity
f. Propafenone	f.˙ Routine reduction of digoxin appears unnecessary; monitor SDCs and be alert for signs and symptoms of toxicity

the overlap that exists between therapeutic and toxic serum concentrations. In addition, many of the commercially available assays used to quantitate apparent serum digoxin concentrations (SDCs) are relatively nonspecific. Both active and inactive metabolites as well as endogenous digoxin-like substances can cross-react in many of these assays. A radioimmunoassay using a double antibody system and a newer monoclonal antibody assay appear to be the most specific laboratory tests (29). Nonetheless, many clinical laboratories and reference texts list the therapeutic range for digoxin as 0.5 or 0.8 to 2.0 ng/ml. In a review of about 50 studies that attempted to correlate the SDC to both nontoxic and toxic effects, a mean level of 1.4 ng/ml was observed in patients without toxicity, whereas patients with overt toxicity demonstrated serum levels 2 to 3 times greater (30). Even though statistical significance was achieved in most of these reports, the overlap between therapeutic and toxic concentrations in many of the studies was considerable. This overlap may be related to any one of the many factors that tend to predispose patients to the development of digoxin toxicity.

Dosing Guidelines. Several pharmacokinetic equations provide prospective dosing guidelines for digoxin (27–28). A study that compared several of these equations universally demonstrated a poor correlation between the predicted and measured SDC (31). Because the equations tend to overestimate the measured SDC, any one provides safe initial approximations of a patient's digoxin dose. The method of Koup et al. (32) using a CL_{NR} of 20 ml/min/1.73 m^2, provided the best correlation between the predicted and measured steady-state SDC.

To utilize the method developed by Koup and his colleagues (32), the patient's body weight must first be estimated:

$$LBW_{male} = 50 \text{ kg} + 2.3$$
$$\times \text{ (height in inches above 5 feet)}$$

$$LBW_{female} = 45 \text{ kg} + 2.3$$
$$\times \text{ (height in inches above 5 feet)}$$

If the patient's actual weight is less than the estimated LBW, use the actual weight. An estimate of the patient's body surface area (BSA) in square meters (m^2), using the patient's LBW is then needed:

$$BSA \text{ m}^2 = LBW \text{ (kg)}^{0.425}$$
$$\times \text{ Height (cm)}^{0.725} \times 0.007184$$

Thereafter, the patient's creatinine clearance (CL_{CR}) can be estimated: If the patient is female, multiply the above result by 0.85. Next the CL_S for digoxin must be estimated:

$$CL_S = (1.303 \times CL_{CR}) + 20 \text{ ml/min/1.73 m}^2$$

The initial estimate of the patient's daily digoxin dose can now be calculated using the steady-state equation and an intended SDC (i.e., 1.0 to 1.5 ng/ml):

where: D = dose (ng)

C_{SS} = steady-state digoxin level (1.0 ng/ml)

CL_S = systemic clearance (ml/min/1.73 m^2)

T = dosing interval (1440 minutes/day)

F = fraction absorbed (0.75 for tablets)

The above equation provides initial dosing guidelines for patients with CHF so that there is a low probability of achieving a potentially toxic SDC. A trough SDC can be obtained either after a few days, to verify that a serious underprediction of the measured SDC has not occurred, or at the attainment of steady-state (7 to 10 days for most adult patients). General indications for further determinations of SDCs in an individual patient are (a) to confirm the suspicion of the occurrence of digoxin toxicity; (b) to verify compliance; (c) to assess the effects of diseases or drugs on the pharmacokinetics of digoxin; and (d) to evaluate the lack of response to therapy. Again it must be remembered that SDCs do not predict efficacy or toxicity and should, therefore, only be used to supplement clinical judgment. Strict attention should be given to the timing of blood collection for serum digoxin assay and its relationship to the time of last dose. Collecting blood during the distribution phase (lasting up to 12 hr after an oral dose) will cause the SDC to be falsely elevated and useless in evaluating potential toxicity.

Digoxin Toxicity. Despite the objective means used to develop rational dosing guidelines for digoxin, digoxin toxicity remains a common clinical problem. Estimates of the frequency of digitalis toxicity in hospitalized patients taking digoxin range from 4 to 35%. The incidence in ambulatory patients is unknown. A retrospective review of medical records in a large urban teaching hospital provided contemporary insight into the pattern of digoxin intoxication (33). Between 1980 and 1988, 241 patients were discharged with a diagnosis of digoxin intoxication. Only 20% of these patients met the criteria for definite digoxin intoxication, while 60% were possibly intoxicated, and 20% had no evidence of digoxin intoxication. Eleven patients died, but 9 of the 11 deaths were due to multiple organ disease, suggesting a digoxin intoxication mortality rate of 1.1% (2 of 176). Only 9% of patients had life-threatening arrhythmias, and 5% required insertion of a temporary pacemaker. Digoxin toxicity can be acute or chronic, and it generally results from either excessive ingestion, a change in disposition, or an increased sensitivity to digoxin. Even though the mortality rate appears to be decreasing, diagnosis of digoxin toxicity remains a challenge.

Digoxin intoxication can manifest as a number of noncardiac and cardiac symptoms (Table 36.3) (30). Anorexia, nausea, and vomiting are the most common but nonspe-

Table 36.3.
Signs and Symptoms of Digoxin Intoxication

Noncardiac
    Gastrointestinal: anorexia, nausea, vomiting
    Neurologic: fatigue, malaise, delirium, acute psychosis, neuralgic pain
    Ocular: halo vision, green or yellow vision
    Miscellaneous: gynecomastia and sexual dysfunction (males)
Common cardiac arrhythmias[a]
    Ventricular premature depolarizations (VPDs): including multifocal
        VPDs and bi- or trigeminy
    First-degree AV block
    Mobitz type I AV block
    Nonparoxysmal junctional tachycardia
    Supraventricular tachycardia with block
    Ventricular tachycardia (including bidirectional ventricular
        tachycardia)

[a] Virtually every known cardiac arrhythmia has occurred secondary to digitalis intoxication.

cific symptoms of digoxin toxicity. Dizziness, fatigue, and malaise are common neurological findings, whereas headache, delirium, acute psychoses, and neuralgic pain (including trigeminal neuralgia) are uncommon ones. Seeing halos around lights or perceiving greens or yellows more prominently are classic visual disturbances associated with digitalis intoxication, but in reality are rarely reported by patients (33). Gynecomastia and sexual dysfunction have been reported occasionally in males and may be the result of digitalis-induced increases in estradiol levels. True digoxin allergy is reported rarely.

Virtually any cardiac arrhythmia or conduction disturbance can be associated with digoxin toxicity. Digoxin-induced arrhythmias can be generally classified as (*a*) decreases in impulse conduction; (*b*) enhancement of automaticity; or (*c*) combinations of *a* and *b*. In patients with definite digoxin toxicity, the most common arrhythmias were atrioventricular block and sinus bradycardia (66% and 26%, respectively) (33). Junctional rhythms are probably the next most common rhythm at time of presentation with digoxin toxicity, followed by sinus pauses. Ventricular premature depolarizations (VPDs or ventricular ectopy), especially multifocal or those that occur in a bigeminal pattern, are common. Atrial fibrillation with a ventricular response rate <50 may suggest digoxin toxicity. Ventricular tachycardia and ventricular fibrillation can occur and mandate consideration of digoxin-specific antibodies (Fab fragments, Digibind). However, ventricular rhythm disturbances are common in patients with left ventricular dysfunction. Finally, some patients may have paroxysmal atrial tachycardia, often with a 2:1 block. In short, rhythm disturbances are common outcomes of digoxin toxicity and may be the first sign of digoxin toxicity.

A number of factors predispose patients to digoxin toxicity (Table 36.4), with the most common being increased age with reduced renal function (27). Hypokalemia and

hypomagnesemia are associated with an increased incidence of digitalis-induced arrhythmias. Hypokalemia appears to increase myocardial uptake of digoxin. Magnesium (Mg^{+2}) serves as a cofactor for the enzyme, Na^+-K^+ ATPase, and thus hypomagnesemia may decrease intracellular potassium. Acid-base disturbances, particularly alkalosis, can alter the serum concentrations and total body stores of electrolytes and subsequently may increase the sensitivity to digitalis. Diuretic-induced alkalosis, even in the setting of normal serum potassium, increases the frequency of digitalis-associated arrhythmias. Elderly patients are at greater risk for developing digoxin toxicity either as a result of age-related decreases in renal function, or perhaps secondary to increased sensitivity of Na^+-K^+-ATPase to the inhibitory effects of digoxin. Renal dysfunction alone predisposes patients to digoxin toxicity because of decreases in both the volume of distribution and elimination of digoxin. Hypothyroidism and hypoxia, through unidentified mechanisms, increase a patient's sensitivity to digoxin. Lastly, the development of digoxin toxicity may be enhanced by drugs that either diminish the CL_S of digoxin or increase its absorption, or which share similar pharmacodynamic properties with digoxin.

Treatment of Digoxin Toxicity. The severity of digoxin toxicity should be considered before initiating a treatment plan (33). In general, blood should be obtained for determination of serum K^+, Mg^{+2}, and digoxin levels. Efforts should be made to identify and remove any factors that may predispose the patient to digoxin toxicity. Discontinuance of the digoxin and supportive treatment may be all that is necessary to manage noncardiac symptoms such as nausea, vomiting, and anorexia. Withdrawing digoxin may also suffice to treat asymptomatic cardiac manifestations such as first-degree AV block, or Mobitz type I second-degree AV block.

In the management of many of the digoxin-induced ectopic arrhythmias (e.g., nonparoxysmal AV junctional tachycardia, atrial tachycardia with block, VPDs, and ven-

Table 36.4.
Factors That May Predispose Patients to the Development of Digoxin Intoxication

Electrolyte abnormalities
    Hypokalemia
    Hypomagnesemia
    Hypercalcemia
Advanced age
Acid-base disturbances
    Alkalosis
Hypoxia
Renal dysfunction
Hypothyroidism
Drug interactions (see Table 36.2)

tricular tachycardia), potassium can be administered, unless serum K⁺ levels are elevated (e.g., 5.0 mEq/ml or greater), the patient is ingesting K⁺-sparing drugs, severe renal insufficiency is present, markedly delayed AV conduction (i.e., greater than first-degree AV block) is observed, or the patient has ingested a massive overdose of digoxin (30, 33). Potassium chloride is the salt used, as many digoxin patients may be hypochloremic secondary to concomitant diuretic therapy. If possible, K⁺ should be given orally at doses of up to 40 mEq every 1 to 4 hr. Alternatively, K⁺ can be administered intravenously at rates not exceeding 0.5 to 1.0 mEq/min. The concentration of the potassium solution should not exceed 80 Meq/liter. Normal saline may be a better choice than 5% dextrose solution for diluting the potassium, to avoid the occasional paradoxical worsening of the hypokalemia sometimes observed in the severely K⁺-depleted patient.

Magnesium can suppress digitalis-induced ectopic rhythms, especially those of ventricular origin (34). Ten milliliters of a 20% magnesium sulfate solution can be administered intravenously over 1 to 2 min followed by 0.5 to 1.0 mEq/kg intramuscularly every 4 hr for 5 doses. Daily magnesium replacement therapy may be required thereafter. Lymphocyte Mg^{+2} content may need to be monitored to guide repletion of this cation, because serum Mg^{+2} does not reflect total body magnesium stores. Magnesium supplementation should be avoided in patients with severe renal insufficiency, a greater than first-degree AV block, or hypermagnesemia.

The type IB antiarrhythmic drugs lidocaine and (rarely) phenytoin are frequently useful in treating digitalis-induced ventricular arrhythmias (30–33). Lidocaine is administered intravenously as a dose of 1 to 2 mg/kg at a rate of 50 mg per min. Within 20 to 30 min a second bolus dose, one-half of the initial dose, should be given. An infusion of 15 to 50 μg/kg/min should be started at the time of the first bolus dose. The most common adverse effects of lidocaine involve the central nervous system and can include drowsiness, paresthesias, feelings of dissociation, agitation, muscle twitching, or generalized convulsions. These adverse effects are likely dose- and serum level–dependent. Alternatively 15 to 20 mg/kg of intravenous phenytoin at a rate not greater than 25 to 50 mg per min can be given. Hypotension and myocardial depression, which can occur secondary to phenytoin administration, appear to be related to the rate of drug administration. Phenytoin can be diluted in normal saline at concentrations ranging from 1 to 10 mg/ml. Other antiarrhythmic drugs that have been used in treating digitalis-induced ectopic rhythms include β-blockers, bretylium, procainamide, quinidine, mexiletine, tocainide, and amiodarone. For reversing symptomatic digoxin-induced bradycardia or SA or AV conduction delays, atropine administered in IV doses of 0.5 to 2.0 mg may be useful. If the

bradycardia or conduction delays are hemodynamically important and refractory to atropine, temporary intravenous pacing is indicated.

In the setting of an accidental or suicidal ingestion of large amounts of digoxin, syrup of ipecac can decrease absorption if administered within an hour of ingestion (30). Gastric lavage can also be used. Orally administered activated charcoal, cholestyramine, or colestipol can also minimize absorption of digoxin.

If attempts to remove digoxin are unsuccessful and the patient is experiencing potentially life-threatening ventricular arrhythmias, refractory hyperkalemia, or conduction deficits resistant to conventional therapy, digoxin-specific antibodies (Fab fragments, Digibind) are indicated. The Fab antibodies bind to both intravascular and intersitital digoxin. An initial response consisting of an increase in total serum digoxin, a decrease in serum potassium, and a reversal of the adverse electrophysiological effects of digoxin is frequently observed within ½ to 1 hr after the Fab infusion. These digoxin-specific antibodies often completely reverse the toxic effects of digoxin (and digitoxin) within a few hours. A treatment response is expected in at least 90% of patients with definitive life-threatening digoxin toxicity (35).

A postmarketing surveillance study of Digibind administration to 717 adults provides excellent pharmacoepidemiologic data on life-threatening digoxin toxicity (36). Most patients were elderly (>70 years) and developed toxicity during maintenance digoxin therapy. About one-third of the patients had severely impaired renal function, and 43% had mild or moderate renal dysfunction. Signs of digoxin toxicity prompting Digibind therapy included ventricular ectopy in 29% of patients, third-degree atrioventricular block in 27%, supraventricular arrhythmia in 27%, hyperkalemia in 26%, ventricular tachycardia in 20%, second-degree heart block in 14%, ventricular fibrillation in 10%, and asystole in 9% of patients. Fifty percent of the patients appeared to have a complete response to Digibind administration, and 24% a partial response, with the remainder either not responding or having an uncertain response. Six patients had an allergic reaction to Digibind, while 20 patients developed recurrent digoxin toxicity after the first Digibind dose was administered. In summary, Digibind is a significant therapeutic advance in combating all too commonly observed life-threatening digoxin toxicity.

Digoxin Controversy. In the last decade several investigators have attempted to determine if digoxin has a clinically meaningful role in the management of patients with chronic CHF who are also in normal sinus rhythm (37). Many of these studies involved the withdrawal of digoxin from the therapeutic regimen of patients with CHF, most of whom were in normal sinus rhythm. Unfortunately, because of the variability both in study design and patient populations, it remains very difficult to provide strict guidelines for the use of digoxin in CHF. Some studies suggest that perhaps patients with more poorly compensated CHF (i.e., those patients with an S_3 gallop rhythm, with a greater left ventricular end-diastolic dimension, with a lower ejection fraction, or with previously unknown episodes of atrial fibrillation) may benefit from the chronic administration of digoxin. However, many patients who decompensated upon withdrawal of digoxin were neither maximally managed with diuretics nor being treated with vasodilators. Other studies suggest that the etiology of a patient's CHF may be important in predicting a beneficial response to digoxin therapy. For example, patients who develop CHF secondary to multiple myocardial infarctions or from a dilated idiopathic cardiomyopathy may demonstrate a continued response to digoxin, whereas patients with CHF secondary to hypertension or chronic ischemic heart disease may have no symptoms upon withdrawal of digoxin. Thus, even though clear-cut indications for digoxin are not evident at this time, it is not a therapy that should be employed universally in the management of each patient with CHF (38). This is especially true in light of its relatively low therapeutic-to-toxic ratio and its apparent inability to improve mortality. The etiology of a patient's clinical condition, the presence or absence of coexisting atrial fibrillation, and perhaps alternative treatments should be considered before committing a patient to long-term therapy with digoxin. In summary, digoxin, having never been shown to improve mortality rates, should be considered an agent to improve CHF symptoms in patients who have heart failure due to systolic dysfunction.

DIURETICS

Diuretics remain a cornerstone of the treatment of patients with chronic CHF, because these agents diminish the characteristic pulmonary and systemic circulatory congestion by removing sodium and water (39). Thus, even though diuretics as monotherapy have not been shown to prolong life, their effect in relieving symptoms justifies their widespread use. Most patients with clinically diagnosed CHF are maintained on some diuretic regimen. Diuretics may also indirectly provide favorable hemodynamic effects by decreasing intraventricular wall tension. This occurs principally through a reduction in preload. Preload reduction can sometimes improve systolic function slightly. Nevertheless, the major effect of chronically administered diuretics in the management of CHF remains the relief of congestive symptoms.

Principles of Diuretic Usage. Before initiation of a diuretic regimen for a patient with chronic CHF, a number of general principles of diuretic usage should be considered: (*a*) Therapy to rid patients of all traces of peripheral edema is often unnecessary and potentially harmful; (*b*) Begin therapy with the smallest effective dose and titrate upward to minimize a patient's weight loss to 0.5 to 1.0 kg/day, except in extreme cases of pulmonary edema; (*c*) The more proximally a diuretic acts within the nephron, the greater will be the loss of both fluid and electrolytes; (*d*) Diuretics that act proximal to the terminal portion within the distal tubule, where sodium is exchanged for both potassium and hydrogen, will likely produce both hypokalemia and metabolic alkalosis; (*e*) Diuretics that produce hypokalemia frequently also cause hypomagnesemia; (*f*) Diuretics should be administered as frequently (or infrequently) as necessary; (*g*) Combination diuretic therapy is often required as a patient's CHF worsens; and (*h*) Osmotic diuretics are not generally useful in the management of CHF.

CLASSIFICATION OF DIURETICS

Thiazides. The major site of diuretic action of the thiazides is the distal convoluted tubule, where they induce a maximal fractional excretion of sodium of approximately 3 to 6% (Table 36.5). Thus, these compounds are considered to be moderately potent diuretics. The individual thiazide agents are essentially interchangeable in terms of diuretic effectiveness; therefore, hydrochlorothiazide (HCTZ) is generally prescribed because of its relative low cost. HCTZ or another thiazide usually is the initial diuretic for CHF, unless the patient has either impaired renal function (creatinine clearance of less than 40 ml/min) or severe congestive symptoms. In each of these instances a loop diuretic would be a more logical initial choice. Adverse effects that may occur secondary to thiazide administration include hypokalemia, hyponatremia, hypomagnesemia, hyperuricemia, hyperlipoproteinemia (i.e., increases in total cholesterol, LDL-cholesterol, and triglyceride levels and decreases in HDL-cholesterol levels), and impaired carbohydrate tolerance. The latter adverse effect is probably of concern only in insulin-dependent diabetics. Mild heart failure usually responds to low thiazide doses, such as 12.5 or 25 mg of hydrochlorothiazide. Hydrochlorothiazide doses above 50 mg provide little symptom relief and are more likely to cause electrolyte imbalances.

Metolazone. Metolazone is a thiazide-type drug in that its principal site of action is the distal convoluted tubule of the nephron (Table 36.5). This drug has also been demonstrated to have proximal tubular effects to reduce sodium reabsorption. Major differences between metolazone and the thiazides are that metolazone retains its effectiveness even when renal function is markedly reduced and that metolazone has a duration of action much longer than most thiazides. Metolazone and the thiazides produce similar adverse effects. Metolazone can be used as a single diuretic in doses such as 2.5 mg daily. However, it is often used in combination with loop diuretics (se-

Table 36.5.
Diuretics Commonly Used in the Management of CHF

Class	Principal Site of Action within Nephron	Usual Oral Maintenance Dose Range	Adverse Effects
Thiazides	Distal convoluted tubule		Hypokalemia, hyponatremia, hypomagnesemia, azotemia, hyperlipoproteinemia, hyperglycemia
Hydrochlorothiazide		12.5–50 mg q 24 hr	
Many others			
Metolazone	Distal convoluted tubule	2.5–10 q 24 h	As for thiazides
Loop diuretics	Thick ascending limb of the loop of Henle		As for thiazides plus hypocalcemia and deafness
Furosemide		20–300 mg q 12–24 h	
Ethacrynic acid		25–200 mg q 12–24 h	
Bumetanide		0.5–10 mg q 12–24 h	
Potassium-sparing			
Spironolactone	Distal convoluted tubule; aldosterone-dependent Na+/K+ exchange site	25–50 mg q 12–24 h	Hyperkalemia, gynecomastia
Triamterene	Distal convoluted tubule; Na+/K+/H+ exchange site, not aldosterone-dependent	50–150 mg q 12–24 h	Hyperkalemia, azotemia, renal stores
Amiloride	Same as triamterene	2.5–5 mg q 12–24 h	Hyperkalemia, azotemia

quential diuresis) and therefore may be prescribed as 2.5 mg every 3 or 4 days.

Loop Diuretics. These drugs act principally at the thick ascending limb of the loop of Henle, where they may increase the fractional excretion of sodium up to 25% (Table 36.5). Loop diuretics also increase renal blood flow by enhancing production of the renal vasodilatory prostaglandin, PGE. This effect contributes to the natriuretic effects of the loop diuretics. Furosemide, ethacrynic acid, and bumetanide represent this most potent subgroup of diuretics available for the treatment of CHF. Furosemide is the most commonly prescribed agent within this subgroup. Adverse effects that occur secondary to the administration of loop diuretics are similar to those caused by the thiazide diuretics. In addition, the loop diuretics uniformly may produce adverse effects such as hypocalcemia and deafness, which are not shared with either the thiazide compounds or metolazone. Initial doses of furosemide (20 to 40 mg daily) and bumetanide (0.5 to 1.0 mg daily) can promote a prompt diuresis. However, as heart failure progresses, increasingly larger doses are needed. Although doses vary widely, patients suffering from endstage heart failure may require twice-daily furosemide, with daily doses ranging from 20 mg to 320 mg or more.

Potassium-sparing Diuretics. Spironolactone, triamterene, and amiloride exert their diuretic effects at the terminal portion of the distal convoluted tubule (Table 36.5). Spironolactone (which is primarily converted to the active metabolite, canrenone) acts at an aldosterone-sensitive site, whereas triamterene and amiloride act at a site that is not under the control of aldosterone. These compounds are considered weak diuretics, as they induce a fractional excretion of sodium of only 2 to 5%. Potassium-sparing diuretics are useful principally as adjuncts with thiazides, metolazone, and loop diuretics to counteract the hypokalemia and hypomagnesemia frequently induced or exacerbated by these other drugs. Hypokalemia and hypomagnesemia are directly arrhythmogenic, and they may potentiate arrhythmias secondary to either digoxin or circulating catecholamines. These combined electrolyte disturbances appear to be best prevented by the administration of potassium-sparing diuretics. However, therapy with potassium-sparing agents should be individualized.

In selecting a potassium-sparing diuretic it should be noted that spironolactone is only effective in relative hyperaldosteronemic states. Triamterene and amiloride are effective even when levels of aldosterone are not increased. Elevated levels of aldosterone are observed frequently in patients with CHF. The effects of spironolactone do not become maximal for several days, because it takes 3 to 4 days for canrenone to attain steady-state concentrations. Likewise, the effects of spironolactone persist for several days following cessation of therapy, because of the presence of the active metabolite. Both triamterene and amiloride attain steady-state effects in about 1 to 1.5 days. A potential consequence of prescribing any of the potassium-sparing diuretics is hyperkalemia. However, this is more likely to occur in patients with severe renal dysfunction or in patients receiving concomitant potassium supplements or angiotensin-converting-enzyme (ACE) inhibiting drugs. Spironolactone may cause gynecomastia, and triamterene-containing renal stones have occasionally been reported to result from its use. No heart failure patients should be advised to use a salt substitute (which contains potassium) without first seeking the advice of their physician or pharmacist (who is aware of recent serum potassium, serum BUN, and serum creatinine levels), especially if they are taking a potassium-sparing diuretic.

Diuretic Resistance. To optimize diuretic therapy in patients with CHF, a practitioner must be familiar with the physiological and pharmacological factors that mediate a diminished clinical response to diuretics (i.e., diuretic resistance) (40). Patient noncompliance with the prescribed diuretic regimen will minimize the effectiveness of the drug. Also an increase in sodium intake can offset the natriuretic effects of the diuretic. Therefore, a reduction in sodium consumption must usually accompany the institution of diuretic therapy.

Uremia may diminish the response to loop diuretics, which are organic acids. Therefore, to reach their site of action within the nephron, these drugs depend upon the organic acid secretory pump, which can be blocked by the increased circulating concentrations of endogenous organic acids seen in uremia. This example of diuretic resistance may be overcome either by using much higher doses of the loop diuretic or by combining the loop diuretic with a diuretic that has a different site of action within the nephron, such as a thiazide or metolazone.

Nonsteroidal antiinflammatory drugs (NSAIDs) lessen the natriuretic effects of loop diuretics. NSAIDs block the renal hemodynamic effects of these agents by inhibiting prostaglandin synthesis. This effect was initially reported with indomethacin and has subsequently been demonstrated with ibuprofen, sulindac, naproxen, and aspirin. NSAID-induced diuretic resistance can be counteracted by discontinuing the offending agent, if possible; by using larger or more frequently doses of the loop diuretic; or by combining the loop diuretic with a thiazide or metolazone.

CHF can also partially attenuate the response to loop diuretics by a number of mechanisms. The rate of gastrointestinal absorption and the corresponding peak serum concentrations of oral doses of loop diuretics are decreased in CHF, especially in patients in the decompensated state. These effects slow the rate of delivery of the drug to its site of action within the nephron, which results in a diminished maximal response. The administration of an IV dose of the loop diuretic or very large doses of the oral formulation (e.g., 500 mg or more of furosemide per day), or combination of the oral loop diuretic with a thiazide or metolazone may result in a more effective diuresis. Individual patients with CHF will even become resistant to IV doses of a loop diuretic because of an unexplained alteration in the patient's pharmacodynamic response to the drug. Larger single IV doses, more frequent and smaller IV doses, or a short-term IV infusion of the loop diuretic are useful initial strategies to overcome the diminished response. However, if a patient with relatively good renal function does not respond to approximately 400 to 500 mg

of IV furosemide (or the equivalent dose of another loop diuretic), then a second diuretic such as a thiazide or metolazone, or an afterload-reducing agent such as hydralazine or captopril should be added to produce a satisfactory diuretic response. Patients can often assume responsibility for making minor adjustments in their own diuretic regimen, based on weight, dyspnea, and peripheral edema. A simple but useful monitoring tool is a daily log of a patient's weight.

VASODILATORS

Vasodilator therapy has brought new promise to the treatment of congestive heart failure (41). Alteration of both the capacitance (preload) and resistance (afterload) compensatory mechanisms of the peripheral vasculature beds can profoundly improve cardiac function. Physiological performance of the diseased left ventricle is improved, dyspnea symptoms relieved, exercise tolerance improved, and (hopefully) life is prolonged. Since investigations of the early 1970s, vasodilator therapy has become an integral component in the treatment of patients with chronic CHF. In addition, recent evidence strongly suggests that vasodilator therapy is the only drug treatment modality that can favorably alter the grim prognosis of patients with CHF (41).

Classification of Vasodilators. Two classification schemes have been developed (Table 36.6) to guide the clinician in selecting the most appropriate vasodilator drug for the chronic management of a patient with CHF. However, each of these is limited in its long-term application (42). One system classifies vasodilators according to their peripheral site of action: either a venodilator (preload reducer) or arterial dilator (afterload reducer) or a combination venous and arterial dilator. This led early investigators to characterize an individual patient hemodynamically in the acute care setting and use these data to select the appropriate chronic oral vasodilator and starting dose. Unfortunately, the immediate hemodynamic response to a vasodilator does not appear to predict long-term clinical outcome. The other system categorizes vasodilators according to their mechanism of action: a drug may possess a direct effect on the peripheral vasculature or its circulatory effects may be secondary to selective neurohumoral inhibition. However, the concentration of such neurohumoral factors as circulating catecholamines or renin before the initiation of treatment does not predict either the acute or the long-term effects of vasodilator drugs. The selection of a vasodilator drug for chronic CHF management is therefore based on results of studies that have evaluated both the long-term beneficial and adverse effects of an agent. As the following sections describe in detail, most clinicians use either an ACE-inhibitor or (less

Table 36.6.
Vasodilator Drugs

Drug	Principal Site of Action	General Mechanism(s) of Action	Usual Oral Maintenance Dosing Range	Adverse Effects
Isosorbide dinitrate[a]	Venous vasodilator	Direct-acting vasodilator	20–80 mg t.i.d.-q.i.d.[b]	Headache, dizziness, flushing, postural hypotension
Hydralazine[c]	Arteriolar vasodilator	Direct-acting vasodilator	75–150 mg q6h	Headache, palpitations, postural hypotension, nausea, vomiting, systemic lupus erythematosus, increases in heart rate, myocardial ischemia, fluid retention
Angiotensin-converting-enzyme (ACE) inhibitors	Balanced vasodilators	Neurohumoral (see text)		Maculopapular rash, dysgeusia, leukopenia, proteinuria, hypotension, dizziness
Captopril			12.5–100 mg q 8–12 h	
Enalapril			2.5–20 mg q 12–24 h	

[a] Used alone for symptoms relief or with hydralazine to improve survival.

[b] Maintain 8–12 hr nitrate-free interval.

[c] Used in combination with oral isosorbide dinitrate to improve survival.

frequently) a combination of oral isosorbide dinitrate and hydralazine.

Nitrates. Nitrates were one of the first group of vasodilator drugs used in the management of CHF (43). These agents decrease preload predominantly through vasodilation of venous capacitance vessels. Nitrates may also improve cardiac function by decreasing afterload via dilation of the large arteries and arterioles, especially after acute administration and when using relatively high doses (e.g., in the management of patients with CHF). Generally, nitrates should be combined with other vasodilators with greater afterload-reducing effects, such as hydralazine. However, nitrates alone are often effective in relieving the pulmonary congestion symptoms of heart failure. Therefore, they are often added to other regimens, especially for patients on digoxin and diuretics.

Of the available nitrate formulations used in treating chronic CHF, oral isosorbide dinitrate (ISDN) is the most frequently prescribed. It is given at doses of 20 to 60 mg t.i.d.-q.i.d., often retaining an 8- to 12-hr nitrate-free interval. It no longer appears important to give the highest dose tolerated by an individual patient. Rather, it is more important to use a dosing regimen that causes fluctuating levels, to avoid the problem of nitrate tolerance induced by continuous nitrate serum levels.

Nitrate tolerance has been demonstrated consistently if the vascular endothelium is constantly exposed to nitroglycerin. If oral ISDN is given four times daily, with the last dose given at 10 PM, tolerance will develop. However, tolerance will not develop if oral ISDN is given three times daily such as 7 AM, 12 noon, and 5 PM. Similarly, if nitroglycerin patches are prescribed, they should be applied for 12 to 16 hr and then removed (44). Because most patients experience dyspnea on exertion during the waking hours, the nitrate-free interval is usually at night. These inter-

mittent dosage regimens do not preclude administration of short-acting sublingual or lingual spray nitroglycerin for either acute anginal episodes or acute dyspnea. Because nitrate tolerance is a critical issue in CHF management, both basic and clinical research is ongoing. Two mechanisms have been proposed for nitrate tolerance: depletion of intracellular sulfhydryl groups and activation of counter-regulatory hormones (45). Efforts to prevent nitrate tolerance by augmenting sulfhydryl availability have had mixed results. A small-scale study showed that methionine administration (a sulfhydryl donor) potentiated the venodilatory effects of both sublingual nitroglycerin and nitroglycerin patches (46). In a study of 14 patients with NYHA class IV heart failure receiving a continuous nitroglycerin infusion, nitrate tolerance was accompanied by an increase in intravascular fluid volume and increased plasma renin activity and plasma ANP (47). A concomitant infusion of *N*-acetylcysteine (another sulfhydryl donor) did not prevent nitrate tolerance. Efforts to prevent tolerance to high-dose intravenous nitroglycerin in CHF by coadministering captopril have failed (48). Even though captopril did not prevent nitrate tolerance in these patients with NYHA class IV failure, the combination nitrate-captopril regimen did exert synergistic hemodynamic benefits. Nitrates will most likely remain part of a vasodilator regimen that is based on the use of an ACE-inhibitor (41, 49).

The most frequently encountered adverse nitrate effect is headache, which often responds to mild analgesics such as acetaminophen. Headaches usually disappear after several days of nitrate administration. Some patients will always experience severe headaches with nitrates and therefore may not tolerate any nitrate administration. Dizziness, flushing, postural hypotension, weakness, and occasionally rash are also reported. In summary, nitrates are safe and effective vasodilators useful as adjunctive therapy to ACE-inhibitors in the treatment of heart failure.

Hydralazine. Hydralazine is a direct-acting arteriolar dilator that principally reduces afterload. Reductions in afterload by hydralazine may also result in moderate reductions in preload, because of the dependence of ventricular filling pressure on the resistance to ventricular emptying during systole (42). However, hydralazine may reduce left ventricular filling pressures markedly in patients with either mitral or aortic valve regurgitation. Clinically, hydralazine is commonly used with other vasodilators possessing greater preload-reducing properties, such as nitrates or angiotensin-converting-enzyme inhibitors.

Two investigations have evaluated the long-term clinical effects of hydralazine monotherapy in CHF (50–51). The first study was a double-blind, randomized trial comparing hydralazine, approximately 50 mg every 6 hr, to placebo for up to 26 weeks (50). There were no differences between the two groups in clinical status, maximal treadmill exercise duration, or mortality. The second trial was of similar design and compared hydralazine at an average dose of 50 mg every 8 hr to placebo for 1 year (51). The hydralazine group improved in both exercise duration and symptomatic status. However, almost one-half of the patients originally enrolled in the hydralazine group dropped out (40% in the placebo group), and the 1-year mortality rate was approximately 30% for both groups. Thus, when administered as a single vasodilator at maximal doses of up to 225 mg per day, hydralazine may possibly improve the quality of a patient's life, but it does not appear to improve the patient's chances of survival.

The first study to demonstrate that drug regimens can lower mortality rates in heart failure used combination oral ISDN and hydralazine. The Veterans Administration Cooperative Study on Vasodilatory Therapy of Heart Failure-I (V-HeFT-I) showed that the ISDN-hydralazine combination, when added to digoxin and diuretic therapy, decreased the 2-year CHF mortality by 34% (20). The average isosorbide dinitrate and hydralazine doses for patients receiving both drugs were 136 mg per day and 270 mg per day, respectively. Another vasodilator, prazosin at an average daily dose of 19 mg, did not improve mortality rates. Interestingly, even though the ISDN-hydralazine combination improved overall mortality, it did not improve exercise tolerance. Unfortunately, this combination therapy was often associated with adverse reactions. Side effects forcing discontinuation of therapy occurred for 19% of patients assigned to the ISDN-hydralazine combination.

Hydralazine doses for treating patients with chronic CHF are exceedingly variable, even though the placebo-controlled trials used relatively fixed dosage regimens (52). Baseline estimates of a patient's CVP (i.e., right atrial pressure), systolic blood pressure (SBP), resting heart rate (HR), and renal function should be determined before starting therapy. Single doses below 75 mg of oral hydralazine are often not effective in patients with CHF. Many patients respond favorably to 300 mg per day divided into equal doses administered every 6, 8, or 12 hr. Unfortunately, side effects increase with increasing daily doses. The dose should be titrated to responses in CVP, SBP (not less than 95 mm Hg), and HR (avoidance of a resting tachycardia); to improvements in pulmonary and systemic symptoms; and to the appearance of adverse effects. Patients with the highest elevations in CVP may require doses as large as 2400 mg per day, and those with creatinine clearances less than 35 ml/min/m^2 may exhibit the longest duration of action (at least 12 hr). The most common adverse effects, which are generally dose-related, include headache, palpitations, postural hypotension, nausea, vomiting, and systemic lupus erythematosus. Salt and water retention may occur during long-term therapy with hydralazine. Mild-to-moderate increases in resting heart rate and myocardial ischemic events in patients with CHF have also been reported after the administration of hydralazine.

Prazosin. Prazosin is a specific, competitive antagonist of postsynaptic α_1-receptors located in the walls of precapillary arteriolar resistance vessels and postcapillary venous capacitance vessels. Prazosin, therefore, is considered a balanced vasodilator, because it reduces both preload and afterload to approximately the same extent. Prazosin therapy was one of the treatment arms in the V-HeFT-I trial (20). However, prazosin therapy did not improve mortality rates, therefore little enthusiasm remains for using prazosin as a primary vasodilator in congestive heart failure.

Angiotensin-converting-Enzyme Inhibitors. The angiotensin-converting-enzyme (ACE) inhibitors, such as captopril, enalapril, and lisinopril, competitively block the conversion of angiotensin I (A I) to angiotensin II (A II). A II is a potent peripheral arteriolar vasoconstrictor. A II also stimulates the release of aldosterone and AVP and facilitates both central and peripheral activity of the sympathetic nervous system (9). In addition, the enzyme that converts A I to A II is identical to the enzyme that degrades a number of endogenous vasodilatory substances. Therefore, the vasorelaxant effects of these substances may be accentuated in the presence of ACE-inhibitors. Thus, the reductions in preload and afterload, seen after the administration of an ACE-inhibitor, may result from a number of different but interrelated mechanisms. Captopril binds directly to the converting enzyme. Enalapril is a prodrug that is hydrolyzed to the active ACE-inhibitor enalaprilat. The ACE-inhibitors are now the fundamental treatment for congestive heart failure (41), with only captopril and enalapril currently approved for this indication.

One of the landmark trials in the history of heart failure studies was the CONSENSUS trial (Cooperative North Scandinavian Enalapril Survival Study) (21). This study evaluated the effect of enalapril (compared with placebo) on mortality of severe congestive heart failure. All patients were treated optimally with digoxin and diuretics at the start of the trial; they could also receive other vasodilators (nitrates, hydralazine, prazosin). Enalapril and placebo treatments were assigned in a randomized, double-blind fashion. Enalapril therapy started with 5 mg twice daily, and was increased to 10 mg twice daily if no adverse effects were observed. The dose was titrated upward to a maximum of 20 mg twice daily. The overall mortality rate in the enalapril group was 26%, compared with 44% in the placebo group, a 40% reduction (P = .002). Mortality at 1 year was reduced by 31% in the enalapril group. A striking improvement in NYHA classification was also observed in the enalapril group and was accompanied by a decrease in the heart size and the number of required medications. The proportion of patients withdrawn from both the placebo and enalapril groups was the same, substantiating the excellent tolerance of enalapril.

Both captopril and enalapril have been evaluated prospectively in randomized, double-blind, placebo-controlled trials, each of 3 months duration (53, 54). Captopril, administered as an average dose of almost 75 mg three times daily (over 50% of the patients received 100 mg three times daily), improved clinical signs and symptoms, treadmill exercise duration, and NYHA functional class, compared with placebo (53). There were also fewer deaths and treatment failures in the captopril group. In patients with mild-to-moderate heart failure who were receiving diuretic maintenance therapy, captopril treatment was a suitable alternative to digoxin therapy (53). Exercise tolerance improved significantly, as did NYHA classification in the captopril-treated patients but not the digoxin-treated patients. At doses of 5 mg twice daily, enalapril improved NYHA functional class, treadmill exercise duration, patients' feelings of well-being, and hemodynamic findings, compared with placebo (54). There were fewer deaths in the enalapril group. ACE-inhibitors, therefore, appear to consistently improve the clinical status of patients with CHF and improve their longevity.

The doses of both captopril and enalapril are variable and should be titrated upward from relatively small doses. Clinical observations that can be used to guide the dosing of these agents include a decrease in systolic blood pressure (to levels not less than 85 to 90 mm Hg), the relief of signs and symptoms, improvements in physical activity, and the appearance of other adverse effects. The initial dose of captopril can range from 6.25 to 25 mg every 8 hr. A typical maintenance dose ranges from 12.5 to 50 mg every 8 hr. The initial dose of enalapril used frequently by many U.S. investigators is 2.5 to 5 mg every 12 hr. The maintenance dose usually ranges from 5 to 20 mg every 12 hr. Low starting doses for both of these agents should be used in patients who are hyponatremic or who are taking large diuretic doses. Daily maintenance doses can probably be reduced and the dosing interval extended (i.e., every 12 hr for captopril and every 24 hr for enalapril) for elderly patients and for patients with diminished renal function (i.e., creatinine clearance less than 40 ml/min/m^2).

The most common adverse effect of an ACE-inhibitor is hypotension. The peak hypotensive response to captopril generally occurs within 30 to 90 min postdose, whereas this effect frequently occurs within 2 to 4 hr following enalapril. One study showed that hypotension was often more severe and prolonged following enalapril than following captopril (55). However, this investigation used large fixed doses of both drugs, rather than optimizing the dose of each agent to either hemodynamic or clinical effects, as well as fixed doses of diuretics. It is best to administer the first ACE-inhibitor dose under the watchful eye of a clinician so that first-dose syncope or presyncope can be treated appropriately. Patients who are dehydrated or have low intravascular fluid volume or a low serum sodium level are particularly susceptible to ACE-inhibitor-induced orthostasis and syncope. Therefore, diuretic dosages are usually held the day of first-dose administration or perhaps for 24 hr before administering the first ACE-inhibitor test dose.

Increases in blood urea nitrogen and serum creatinine levels can occur after the administration of an ACE-inhibitor and may be related to the degree and duration of observed hypotension and secondary renal hypoperfusion. Serum potassium and magnesium levels tend to normalize with chronic administration of ACE-inhibitors, irrespective of changes in blood pressure or renal function. Consequently, oral potassium supplementation or the administration of potassium-sparing diuretics is generally unnecessary for patients with CHF who are taking ACE-inhibitors. All diuretic and electrolyte therapy should be assessed before beginning ACE-inhibitor therapy. Two weeks after beginning the ACE-inhibitor, the following laboratory tests should be repeated: serum BUN, serum lytes including both potassium and magnesium levels, and urinalysis. A maculopapular rash, cough, taste disturbances, leukopenia, and proteinuria have occurred secondary to the administration of ACE-inhibitors and perhaps with greater frequency with captopril. Therefore, it is prudent to check a baseline CBC with differential and repeat it 2 weeks and again every 6 months after beginning ACE-inhibitor therapy. Captopril has also been demonstrated to decrease the CL$_S$ of digoxin slightly.

Special attention is needed to detect patients who may have both CHF and bilateral renal artery stenosis (single renal artery stenosis in patients with only one kidney). Because many patients with CHF have severe coronary artery disease, atheroslcerosis of other arteries is expected. In a study of 89 patients referred to a heart failure unit, 6 (7%)

had renal artery stenosis (56). The suspicion of renal artery stenosis is usually raised after the serum creatinine level increases abruptly after beginning ACE-inhibitor vasodilator therapy. Another clue to renal artery stenosis is late-onset (>50 years) hypertension. Once renal artery stenosis is confirmed (usually with digital subtraction angiography), either angioplasty or surgery can correct the stenosis. The patient can then safely receive ACE-inhibitor therapy for CHF. If surgical or mechanical correction of the renal artery stenosis is not possible, the ACE-inhibitor must be discontinued.

Impact of Vasodilators on Mortality in CHF. The Multicenter Veterans Administration Cooperative Study (V-HeFT-I) (20) demonstrated a favorable effect of vasodilator therapy on the mortality of patients with moderately severe CHF. Specifically, the combination of hydralazine (75 mg four times per day) and ISDN (40 mg four times per day) was superior to both prazosin (5 mg four times per day) and placebo (four times per day) in reducing cumulative mortality up to a mean follow-up period of 2.3 years. The cumulative mortality in the hydralazine-ISDN group was 38.7%, in the prazosin group, 49.7%, and in the placebo group, 44%. This investigation was the first to demonstrate that a pharmacological intervention could improve survival of patients with CHF. The enalapril CONSENSUS (21) trial (discussed earlier in this chapter) later demonstrated the efficacy of an ACE-inhibitor in reducing heart failure mortality.

Ongoing Questions in Vasodilator Therapy. Although long-term vasodilator therapy has improved the survival of patients with chronic CHF, several questions remain. The first question is: when in the course of CHF should vasodilator therapy be introduced? Most patients in all of the previous vasodilator studies were at least NYHA functional class III and were already taking digoxin and diuretics. Should vasodilator therapy be introduced when signs and symptoms of CHF are mild (i.e., NYHA class II) as well as before initiating digoxin and/or diuretics? Hydralazine alone, the combination of hydralazine and ISDN, and captopril have all caused regression of myocardial hypertrophy in experimental models. However, it remains to be seen whether these experimental findings will result in an earlier implementation of vasodilator therapy and a consequent improvement in patient survival.

Researchers and clinicians are anxiously awaiting complete results of the Studies of Left Ventricular Dysfunction (SOLVD) currently in progress. SOLVD is a multicenter study with two trials. One ongoing trial will test the prevention hypothesis (i.e., will enalapril prevent the development of clinical heart failure and reduce mortality in patients with a decreased ejection fraction who do not yet require digoxin or diuretics for control of heart failure symptoms?) (57). The other study, a treatment trial, was recently completed (22). Enalapril reduced mortality in patients with an ejection fraction ≤35% and symptomatic failure requiring digoxin, diuretics, and/or converting-enzyme inhibitors, which confirmed the benefit of ACE-inhibitor therapy. In the SOLVD treatment trial, 90% of patients were NYHA class II and III and were already receiving digoxin, diuretics, and non-ACE-inhibitor vasodilators (22). Enalapril (2.5 to 20 mg daily) lowered mortality rates by 16%, compared with the placebo group. The major effect was observed within the first 6 months and was most evident in patients with more severely depressed ejection fractions. Enalapril appeared to reduce mortality by decreasing death attributable to progressive myocardial pump failure.

Another large-scale multicenter trial is in process to test the hypothesis that preventative treatment with captopril will prove beneficial to post-myocardial-infarction patients with asymptomatic left ventricular dysfunction. The SAVE study (Survival and Ventricular Enlargement) is ongoing in patients with an ejection fraction of ≤40%, who are randomized to either placebo or captopril. These ongoing trials (SAVE and SOLVD) will contribute immensely to our understanding of the pharmacologic treatment of heart failure.

A second question to answer is: which vasodilator regimen will offer the best chance for survival? The results of V-HeFT-I (20) suggested that the combination of hydralazine and ISDN might be the vasodilator regimen of choice. A related question is: what is the optimal dose for a vasodilator regimen? In V-HeFT-I (20), each vasodilator regimen was titrated to a predetermined ceiling dose in the absence of adverse effects. This multicenter trial did not address the issue of optimal dosages.

The second Vasodilator-Heart Failure Trial (V-HeFT-II) (58) was a logical extension of V-HeFT-I (20). V-HeFT-II (58) compared the isosorbide dinitrate–hydralazine combination with enalapril in patients with mild-to-moderate heart failure who were also receiving digoxin and diuretics. Enalapril proved superior to the nitrate-hydralazine combination, as it reduced the 2-year mortality by 28%. Interestingly, this reduction in mortality was due to a reduction in sudden cardiac deaths, which was more likely to occur in patients with less severe heart failure (NYHA class I or II). Thus, results of current studies suggest that ACE-inhibitor therapy and combination nitrate-hydralazine therapy can be used together in CHF patients, probably because of their different physiologic effects. The potential for second- and third-generation ACE-inhibitors to decrease mortality in CHF is currently under investigation. In summary, drug therapy for systolic dysfunction CHF will begin when the patient has NYHA class II failure. Therapy will be based on diuretics and ACE-inhibitors, and probably include digoxin and nitrates or perhaps the nitrate-hydralazine combination.

Table 36.7.
Causes of Diastolic Heart Dysfunction and Heart Failure[a]

Cardiac valve disorders
  Mitral stenosis
  Tricuspid stenosis
  Aortic regurgitation
  Mitral regurgitation
Constrictive pericarditis
Restrictive cardiomyopathy
Acute volume overload
Dilated cardiomyopathy
Myocardial ischemia (coronary artery disease)
Advanced cardiac hypertrophy due to chronic pressure overload of hypertension
Hypertrophic cardiomyopathy

[a] Adapted from Grossman W: Diastolic dysfunction and congestive heart failure. Circulation 81(suppl III):III-1–III-7, 1990.

DIASTOLIC HEART DYSFUNCTION

Traditional heart failure pathophysiology mechanisms and management methods have defined heart failure as an abnormality of systolic function. The heart's contractility and cardiac output are insufficient to adequately perfuse the tissues (1). In reality, the heart has two functions; both systolic (contraction phase) and diastolic (relaxation phase). Clinical heart failure can occur with either systolic or diastolic dysfunction.

For many years, the congestive heart failure syndrome was thought be the result of only systolic dysfunction. It is known that clinical manifestations of heart failure, such as dyspnea and orthopnea, can occur even when the left ventricle is contracting normally. These patients, with normal systolic function and clinical heart failure, exhibit abnormalities of diastolic function. Impaired diastolic function is caused by the heart's inability to relax. Because the heart muscle receives blood during diastole, relaxation dysfunction prevents the ventricles from receiving enough blood. Table 36.7 illustrates the common causes of diastolic heart dysfunction (59).

Sometimes even though the ventricles are pumping normally or even more than normal, an obstruction to filling prevents the ventricles from receiving enough blood. The resultant increased diastolic filling pressures cause the classic signs and symptoms of heart failure. Often the left ventricle pressures are normal at rest or with moderate exercise. However, with strenuous exercise, the left-sided heart pressures rise dramatically, and the patient complains of dyspnea on exertion (59, 60). A patient with a history of rheumatic fever and subsequent valvular disorders could exhibit this classical picture of impaired diastolic filling with normal systolic function.

Diastolic heart failure with a normal ejection fraction has different patient demographics, different hemodynamics, and a different prognosis than heart failure with a low ejection fraction. In the V-HeFT-I Study (20), 83 of 623 patients were identified with an ejection fraction of at least 0.45, but they still had clinical heart failure (61). When compared with the V-HeFT-I patients who had ejection fractions under 0.45, these patients had a higher incidence of hypertension and a lower incidence of coronary artery disease. Heart failure patients with preserved systolic function had a higher systolic blood pressure, a slower heart rate, and a smaller cardiothoracic ratio than patients with impaired systolic function. Yet, exercise tolerance capacity was only slightly better in patients with normal systolic function. The annual mortality rate in the normal ejection fraction heart failure group was 8%, compared with 19% for heart failure patients with a low ejection fraction. Both ventricular tachycardia observed on 24-hr ambulatory electrocardiographic monitoring and a severe decrease in exercise tolerance were signs of a poor prognosis for the failure patients with a normal ejection fraction.

Given the pathophysiologic differences between isolated diastolic dysfunction and systolic dysfunction, different therapeutic approaches are emerging. Drugs that lower cardiac filling pressures (diuretics, nitrates, nitroprusside) or relax the ventricles (verapamil) will likely relieve the dyspnea associated with diastolic dysfunction (60, 62). Drugs that increase contractility (digoxin) will be less useful. Converting-enzyme inhibitors (captopril, enalapril, lisinopril) can also decrease left ventricular filling pressures and improve exercise tolerance. Drugs that primarily reduce afterload should be used cautiously in lone diastolic dysfunction because they can cause severe hypotension. Abnormalities of diastolic dysfunction may occur in 30 to 40% of patients with clinical heart failure. Much more information is needed before general treatment recommendations for diastolic heart failure can be stated more emphatically.

Other Treatment Modalities

Newer Inotropic Drugs. A number of inotropic drugs are being investigated in the management of chronic CHF (63, 64). Each of these agents somehow increases calcium concentrations within myocardial cells, ultimately resulting in an increase in contractility. Some of these agents also possess peripheral vasodilatory effects. Thus far the major pharmacological categories investigated are (*a*) the orally active β-adrenergic receptor agonists such as xamoterol, pirbuterol, and prenalterol; (*b*) the dopaminergic receptor agonists such as levodopa and ibopamine; and (*c*) the phosphodiesterase inhibitors such as amrinone, milrinone, and enoximone. The β-agonists appear to be limited principally by the development of β-receptor down-regulation and increased mortality (10). Initial enthusiasm for β-adrenergic agonists has waned since most long-term studies failed to demonstrate improvement in symptoms or mortality. Xamoterol, a β-selective adrenergic partial agonist appeared to offer potential in patients with mild-to-moderate failure (65). However, it increased the mortality of patients with severe heart failure (66). The overall effect of xamoterol is that of a mild β_1-agonist while a patient is at rest or doing light exercise. However, with more strenuous exercise, xamoterol exerts greater β_1-receptor antagonism. The Xamoterol In Severe Heart Failure Study Group (66), treated 516 patients with NYHA class III and IV failure already receiving ACE-inhibitors and diuretics with placebo or xamoterol 200 mg daily. No differences between the xamoterol and placebo patients were observed in clinical symptoms or exercise duration. However, 100-day follow-up revealed 9.1% mortality in the xamoterol-treated patients, and 3.7% mortality in the placebo group.

Even though few long-term study results are available for accurate assessment of the clinical utility of the dopaminergic receptor agonists, ibopamine may offer some promise in treating heart failure. A prodrug, ibopamine exerts a positive inotropic effect through β_1-agonism and dopamine$_1$ agonism (67). In early studies, it appeared to improve exercise tolerance like digoxin. However, long-term studies are needed before its potential role in heart failure management can be considered.

Phosphodiesterase inhibitors appear to increase mortality rates in severe heart failure patients. Oral amrinone was the first phosphodiesterase inhibitor to undergo long-term, prospective, placebo-controlled trials. However, the frequent occurrence of a number of intolerable adverse effects resulted in the discontinuance of further investigations with this agent. Both milrinone and enoximone can increase mortality of heart failure patients (67, 69).

Cardiac Transplantation. Miscellaneous medical and surgical procedures have important roles in the management of chronic CHF (23). Ultrafiltration, a method of selectively removing body water, can be used to acutely relieve gross peripheral edema. During the last 20 to 25 years, cardiac transplantation has evolved from hopeful clinical experimentation to an accepted and vital therapeutic option for selected patients with CHF (70). At experienced centers, 1- and 5-year posttransplant survival approaches 90 and 70%, respectively. However, the limited availability of donor hearts restricts the number of active transplant candidates to fewer than 2000 per year.

Patients referred for cardiac transplantation undergo specific evaluation to prioritize those individuals most likely to benefit (70). Most patients referred for cardiac transplantation are adults between 20 and 65 years of age. Patients usually have a resting ejection fraction under 20 to 25%. The cause of the CHF is established for each patient, and potentially reversible and precipitating factors are corrected. Other systemic diseases (such as infection or cancer) that can diminish transplant survival should be identified. Patients referred for cardiac transplantation

undergo hemodynamic monitoring and receive medical therapy tailored to specific hemodynamic objectives. These diagnostic and therapeutic efforts are used to stratify potential heart recipients as critical, unstable, or stable with respect to the urgency for transplantation. Patients awaiting transplantation may require antiarrhythmic therapy for life-threatening or symptomatic ventricular tachyarrhythmias, hemodynamic support with inotropic agents such as dobutamine, or a ventricular assist device.

Proper selection and management of donor hearts and donor-recipient matching are essential to transplant success (70). Donors are usually considered up to 60 years of age. Cerebral blood flow imaging to certify brain death is useful in salvaging potential donor hearts, and echocardiography can identify cardiac dysfunction in the donor heart. ABO-identical blood type donors are generally preferred to ABO-compatible blood types. Recipients also undergo screening to detect selected IgG circulating antibodies that are likely to trigger hyperacute rejection during the immediate posttransplant period.

The improved survival following orthotopic cardiac allograft transplantation is largely due to advances in immunosuppression, such as cyclosporine therapy (70). Typically, cyclosporine is prescribed concomitantly with azathioprine and prednisone (i.e., triple-drug therapy) following transplantation. Cyclosporine therapy must be tailored for each patient, using cyclosporine whole blood concentrations as guidelines (71). Trough cyclosporine blood concentrations of 200 ng/ml are associated with a moderate incidence of rejection and minimal heptotoxicity and nephrotoxicity. In addition, clinicians must become familiar with the large number of other drugs that interfere with the metabolism of cyclosporine (72). Inhibition of cyclosporine metabolism results in increased blood concentrations and possible toxicity, whereas induction of cyclosporine metabolism could result in rejection. Interestingly, ketoconazole, an antifungal agent that inhibits cyclosporine metabolism, can be coadministered with low doses of cyclosporine with favorable clinical and financial results (73). Induction therapy with antilymphocyte antibodies (usually either antithymocyte globulin or OKT3) may facilitate earlier corticosteroid withdrawal and delay mean time to initial allograft rejection (70). These agents, alone or in combination with intravenous methylprednisolone, appear to be useful in the treatment of refractory allograft rejection. FK 506 is a novel anti-T-cell agent with a mechanism of action like that of cyclosporine (70). Ongoing and future investigations will help determine its usefulness in cardiac transplantation.

Posttransplant complications may include a variety of bacterial, viral, fungal, and protozoal infections. Posttransplant hypertension is another common complication. Accelerated graft atherosclerosis is the principal cause of death in long-term cardiac transplant survivors.

In summary, cardiac transplantation is an important and highly efficacious therapeutic option for small numbers of patients with CHF. Successful transplantation requires appropriate recipient and donor selection, effective immunosuppression, vigilant patient monitoring, and treatment of posttransplant complications. (See Chapter 92, "Transplantation.")

TREATMENT OF ACUTE HEART FAILURE

Acute heart failure is a common medical emergency generally occurring in one of two clinical settings. Patients with chronic failure may decompensate acutely. This condition is either a natural progression of heart failure or precipitated by factors such as infection, onset of arrhythmias, or medication noncompliance. Acute heart failure may also occur in association with acute myocardial infarction (Chapter 39). Although similar agents are used to treat acutely decompensated chronic heart failure and acute failure caused by myocardial infarction, selection of specific drugs depends on which compensatory mechanisms have been activated. The following discussion is limited to acute decompensation of chronic heart failure.

PATHOPHYSIOLOGY OVERVIEW

Acute decompensation of chronic severe heart failure is characterized by failure of compensatory mechanisms to maintain adequate perfusion to vital organs. Most patients exhibit some or all of the following: (a) increased afterload or impedance to left ventricular ejection, (b) increased preload or elevated left ventricular filling pressures, (c) myocardial hypertrophy, (d) sodium retention, (e) peripheral edema, (f) myocardial ischemia, (g) neurohumoral responses, including the sympathetic nervous system, the RAA system, and the vasopressin-antidiuretic hormone. Excessive activity of each of these mechanisms contributes to the vicious circle of congestive heart failure ultimately resulting in death. Therapy for patients with acutely depressed left ventricular function is aimed at augmenting cardiac output by parenteral vasodilator therapy or inotropic agents. Because clinical examination alone cannot identify and quantify the compensatory mechanisms, clinicians often rely on hemodynamic monitoring in making prognostic and therapeutic decisions.

Unlike the earlier stages of heart failure, which may require exercise testing for diagnosis, the patient with severe decompensation is easily recognized. Classically, hypotension occurs, but blood pressure may be maintained by peripheral vasoconstriction. Compensatory tachycardia is often observed and is especially ominous if it persists. The patient's skin may appear cool and pale due to vasoconstriction. However, diaphoresis may occasionally be observed. Skin mottling and cyanosis indicates shunting of blood from the periphery in an effort to maintain perfusion

to the heart and brain. Urine output decreases, and in severe failure, inadequate cerebral perfusion alters mental status. Dyspnea and tachypnea are often present. Systemic venous and pulmonary congestion may manifest as elevated central venous pressure, peripheral edema, and pulmonary rales.

Acute cardiogenic pulmonary edema is the most dramatic sign of left ventricular failure (15). The terrified patient is sitting bolt upright and expectorating pink frothy sputum. The patient has the sensation of drowning. Diaphoreses may be accompanied by cool and ashen skin. The respiratory rate is rapid, and accessory muscles are used for respiration. Pulmonary auscultation reveals rhonchi, wheezes, and rales. Heart sounds may be difficult to hear, although an S_3 is usually present. Overt signs of venous congestion are usually evident. Strategy for treating this emergency involves (a) immediate institution of nonspecific measures; (b) identification and removal of precipitating causes; (c) initiation of invasive hemodynamic monitoring; and (d) implementation of patient-specific drug treatment based upon clinical and hemodynamic findings.

HEMODYNAMIC MONITORING

The use of bedside hemodynamic monitoring with flow-directed pulmonary artery (i.e., Swan-Ganz) catheters and systemic arterial catheters has revolutionized critical care medicine. Although some experts contend that this procedure is overutilized, there is little disagreement over its

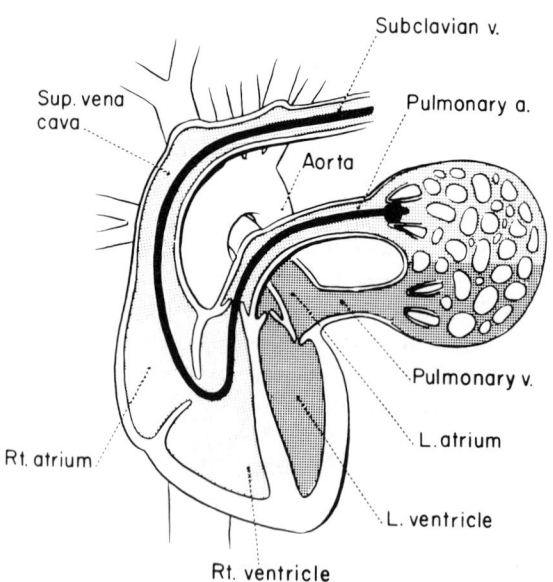

Figure 36.2. Final anatomic positioning of the Swan-Ganz catheter, depicting balloon inflation in the pulmonary artery. (From Bollish SJ, Foster TS: Swan-Ganz catheter: an important tool for monitoring drug therapy in the critically ill. Hosp Formul 15:99–113, 1980, with permission.)

value in managing patients with acutely decompensated chronic congestive heart failure.

Insertion of the pulmonary artery catheter is performed by a physician at the bedside, usually with the aid of fluoroscopy. A balloon is attached to the tip of the catheter, which when inflated allows the catheter to follow the blood flow (74). Right heart catheterization entails antegrade passage of the catheter into the superior vena cava, the right atrium, across the tricuspid valve, and into the right ventricle (Fig. 36.2). The catheter is advanced into the pulmonary artery until the inflated balloon is as large as the pulmonary artery. The catheter is then wedged, yielding the pulmonary capillary wedge pressure (PCWP). Potential complications of right heart catheterization (pulmonary infarction, arrhythmias, thromboembolism, perforation, balloon rupture, and catheter knotting) are usually minimized in the hands of an experienced physician.

HEMODYNAMIC DATA

The systemic arterial pressure (via arterial line) is monitored continuously, but in severe failure it will not provide a reliable indicator of tissue perfusion. The pulmonary capillary wedge pressure (Table 36.8, PCWP) is extremely important, as it accurately indicates pulmonary venous pressure and correlates with signs of pulmonary congestion. It also indirectly measures the filling pressure of the left ventricle or preload. The pulmonary artery diastolic pressure (PADP) is also a valuable index of left ventricular filling pressure. Systemic vascular resistance (SVR) is the most common measure of ventricular afterload. Even

though SVR does not accurately reflect the interaction of factors both internal and external to the myocardium, it remains the best indirect estimate of left ventricular afterload. Stroke volume (SV) is the volume of blood ejected with each heartbeat. Cardiac output (CO) is the amount of blood ejected by the heart per unit time and is usually expressed as liters per minute. Cardiac output varies with body size and is normalized by dividing by the patient's body surface area, yielding cardiac index. Estimates of cardiac output are generally obtained by thermodilution technique. A thermal indicator (usually cooled sterile D5W) is injected into the right atrium. A thermistor at the end of the catheter measures the change in blood temperature downstream. The cardiac output is then computer-calculated, using a modification of the Fick principle.

Even though it is not widely used, the ateriovenous oxygen difference is a better indicator of tissue perfusion than is cardiac index (cardiac output/body surface area) (75). It is fairly constant and independent of body surface area, metabolic rate, or oxygen uptake. The arteriovenous oxygen difference assesses the adequacy of CO in relation to the metabolic needs of the tissues. It requires withdrawal of blood samples from the pulmonary and radial arteries. If the patient is not hypoxemic, the mixed venous oxygen content (or saturation) is a good predictor of clinical outcome. A mixed venous oxygen saturation below 40% is associated with a very poor prognosis.

THERAPY OF DECOMPENSATED HEART FAILURE

Nonspecific measures designed to decrease pulmonary congestion and improve oxygenation are indicated in all patients with acute failure (23). Supplemental oxygen, perhaps facilitated by mechanical ventilation, improves oxygen delivery. The patient should be sitting, to minimize respiratory distress. Morphine sulfate administration is beneficial, owing to its potent venodilatory effect and anxiolytic action. Small doses (2 to 4 mg) are repeated as often as necessary until acute pulmonary congestion is relieved or alternative parenteral vasodilator therapy is begun. Respiratory depression and systemic hypotension may limit morphine use. Intravenous furosemide exerts an almost immediate venodilatory effect and should not be delayed because hemodynamic monitoring capability is not yet available (76, 77). Blood pressure support may be achieved safely with dopamine infusions prior to hemodynamic monitoring. Once the Swan-Ganz catheter and arterial line are inserted, patient-specific regimens may be tailored to the hemodynamic profile and the clinical signs and symptoms.

Diuretics. A mainstay of treatment for acute decompensation and pulmonary edema, intravenous furosemide causes venous dilation and reduces PCWP and pulmonary artery pressures (77). The venodilatory action of intravenous furosemide is observed within several minutes of ad-

Table 36.8.
Normal Hemodynamic Values[a]

Systemic arterial pressure (systolic/diastolic)	120/80 mm Hg
Mean arterial pressure	70–80 mm Hg
Pulmonary artery pressure (systolic/diastolic)	30/15 mm Hg
Pulmonary capillary wedge pressure	< 10–12 mm Hg
Left atrial pressure	5–12 mm Hg (mean)
Left-ventricular end-diastolic pressure	5–12 mm Hg (mean)
Pulmonary vascular resistance	150–250 dynes/sec/cm^{-5}
Systemic vascular resistance	900–1200 dynes/sec/cm^{-5}
Stroke volume	70–130 ml
Right ventricular stroke work	10–15 g•m
Left ventricular stroke work	60–80 g•m
Cardiac output	4–8 liters/min
Cardiac index	2.0–4.0 liters/min/m^2
Mixed venous oxygen content	13–16 ml/dl
Arterial oxygen content	18–20 ml/dl
Pulmonary capillary oxygen content	20 ml/dl
Arterial-mixed venous oxygen difference	4–5.5 ml/dl
Oxygen consumption	22 ± 40 ml/min

[a] Adapted from McGrath RB: Invasive bedside hemodynamic monitoring. Prog Cardiovasc Dis 29:129–144, 1986.

ministration and proceeds its naturetic effect (Fig. 36.3) (78). Intravenous furosemide (initial dose, 20 to 40 mg) may dramatically relieve the signs and symptoms of pulmonary congestion. Oral furosemide does not exert venodilatory activity. Until recently, investigators thought that diuretics had little effect on improving cardiac output. This concept has now been challenged, so that less concern prevails for furosemide-induced decreases in cardiac output secondary to overaggressive lowering of elevated filling pressures (76). Bumetanide is an alternative potent loop diuretic, although furosemide is usually given first. The initial intravenous bumetanide dose is 0.5 to 1.0 mg administered over 1 to 2 min. As with furosemide, the frequency of repeated doses is governed by hemodynamic data, urine output, and relief of pulmonary congestive symptoms.

Vasodilators. By blocking the vicious positive-feedback mechanisms of severe heart failure, parenteral vasodilators may abruptly improve cardiac output and relieve pulmonary congestion. The patient's hemodynamic profile guides selection of specific vasodilators, relative to effects on preload and afterload. Sodium nitroprusside is often the first vasodilator used, as it acts on both preload and afterload (23). It exhibits a fast onset and short duration of action,

so sodium nitroprusside is easily titrated. In many patients, it will lower pulmonary artery pressures, PCWP, and SVR, resulting in increased cardiac output. The initial infusion rate is 0.25 to 0.5 μg/kg/min, and it is titrated upward, based on clinical response and hemodynamics. Generally BP, pulmonary artery pressures, and urine output are monitored continuously. Cardiac output and SVR are determined every 2 to 6 hr to aid in dosage adjustment. The most common hazard of nitroprusside in treating severe heart failure is hypotension. Combination nitroprusside and dopamine therapy is common. Dopamine maintains blood pressure, and depending on the dose, it may improve renal and coronary blood flows.

Intravenous nitroglycerin is especially useful in acute decompensation, as it easily titrated. Because it predominantly increases venous capacitance (i.e., decreases preload), its effect is primarily to decrease PCWP and pulmonary artery pressures (79). Thus, it provides dramatic relief for patients with severe pulmonary congestion. It may also decrease SVR moderately and thus improve cardiac output. Intravenous nitroglycerin doses vary widely, however initial therapy may begin at 5 to 10 μg/min. Dangers of nitroglycerin represent extensions of its pharmacologic action and are usually limited to hypotension.

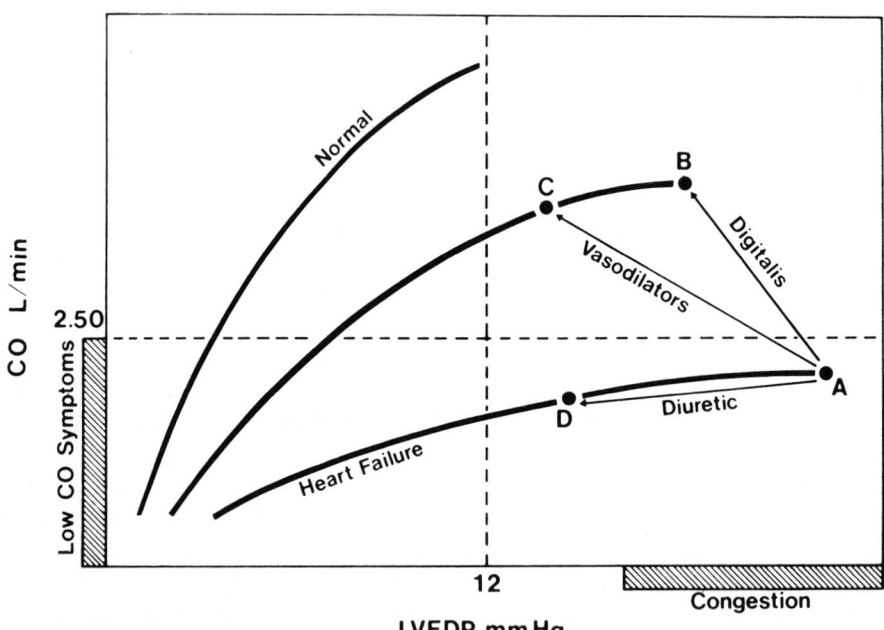

Figure 36.3. Illustration depicting Starling's law of the heart, where cardiac output (CO) normally depends on left ventricular end-diastolic pressure (LVEDP) as shown at the *top*. Through its inotropic activity, digitalis may shift the curve in failure (as shown at the *bottom*) toward normal (point *B*). Diuretics do not shift the curve but rather decrease LVEDP (point *D*), thereby relieving congestive symptoms such as shortness of breath. Va-

sodilators such as sodium nitroprusside may both reduce afterload, thereby increasing cardiac output, and decrease LVEDP and relieve pulmonary congestion (point *C*). (Reproduced from Grantham JJ, Chonko AM, The physiologic basis and clinical use of diuretics. In Brenner BM, Stein JH (eds): Sodium and Water Homeostasis. New York, Churchill Livingstone, 1978:178–211, with permission.)

Amrinone is a phosphodiesterase inhibitor possessing both positive inotropic actions and significant vasodilator activity. Although its pharmacology is not yet fully appreciated, its vasodilatory action is probably more prominent than its inotropic effect. Therefore, its indications are more similar to those for intravenous nitroglycerin or nitroprusside than for dopamine or dobutamine (80). In contrast to nitroglycerin and nitroprusside, amrinone has a relatively long terminal half-life (about 8 hr). It may also accumulate in renal failure. Dose- and duration-dependent thrombocytopenia is of special concern. Other side effects reflect vasodilation and an inotropic effect: hypotension and arrhythmias. Therapy is usually begun with a 0.75 mg/kg intravenous bolus given slowly over 2 to 3 min. Maintenance infusions vary between 5 and 10 μg/kg/min. Combination amrinone and dobutamine therapy may provide greater improvement in left ventricular performance than either agent used alone (81).

Sympathomimetic Amines. Because severe chronic congestive failure is complicated by overstimulation of the sympathetic nervous system, administration of exogenous catecholamines is generally reserved for acute decompensatory episodes.

Dopamine is especially useful in patients with mild-to-moderate hypotension. The initial dose is 0.5 μg/kg/min, and it is titrated upward according to filling pressures, cardiac output, and urine output. If hypotension is severe, dopamine doses in the range of 10 to 20 μg/kg/min will provide the α-stimulation necessary to maintain perfusion to the vital organs and improve cardiac output. Dopamine side effects include tachycardia, ventricular arrhythmias, and excessive vasoconstriction, especially at higher doses. Nevertheless, it remains a valuable agent, especially when used in combination with nitroprusside.

Dobutamine, a synthetic catecholamine, is a selective β_1-agonist (82). Its use is directed toward improving ventricular function, as evidenced by increased cardiac output. The improvement in cardiac output may then cause a reflex decrease in both filling pressures and SVR. Dobutamine infusions are begun at 1 to 2 μg/kg/min and titrated upward every 10 to 30 min. with optimal maintenance infusions generally between 5 and 15 μg/kg/min. Side effects are usually limited but may include tachycardia, arrhythmias, headaches, anxiety, and tremor. Recent uncontrolled clinical experiences have demonstrated the benefit of outpatient dobutamine infusions in patients with end-stage CHF awaiting cardiac transplantation (83). Important guidelines to follow include (*a*) limiting the dose of the dobutamine infusion to 5 μg/kg/min; (*b*) attempting to titrate the infusion to a minimum number of days per week; (*c*) careful monitoring of serum potassium and magnesium and treatment of electrolyte imbalances; and (*d*)

monitoring for ventricular arrhythmias and use of antiarrhythmic agents (including amiodarone) when indicated.

ARRHYTHMIA MANAGEMENT IN HEART FAILURE PATIENTS

Prevention of sudden cardiac death in heart failure patients remains an unmet therapeutic challenge. About 40% of the 400,000 patients who die of heart failure each year die of sudden cardiac death. Heart failure is an independent predictor of sudden death, and almost all heart failure patients exhibit asymptomatic ventricular arrhythmias on 24-hr electrocardiographic recordings. Despite our knowledge that sudden death is common among heart failure patients, no clear consensus on the treatment of asymptomatic ventricular arrhythmias in patients with heart failure has emerged (84). Many risks predispose heart failure patients to sudden death. Structural changes in the myocardium, such as enhanced protein deposition and stretching of tissues, may enhance arrhythmogenesis. Neurohumoral activation with elevated circulating catecholamines may stimulate arrhythmia development, as can hemodynamic derangements. Electrolyte disturbances, often induced by diuretic therapy, are common predisposing factors to arrhythmia development. Even the inotropes used to enhance myocardial contractility (such as digoxin and the experimental newer inotropes) are known to produce arrhythmias. Finally, antiarrhythmic drugs themselves are known to produce proarrhythmic results, most markedly in patients with depressed myocardial contractility.

Although not usually considered antiarrhythmic agents, antianginal drugs may decrease the risk of arrhythmias by reducing myocardial ischemia. Optimization of nitrate, calcium-channel blocker, ACE-inhibitor, and antiplatelet therapy is especially important for patients with heart failure. V-HeFT-II (58) showed that enalapril can decrease sudden cardiac death rates in patients with mild CHF.

The Cardiac Arrhythmia Suppression Trial (CAST) (85) demonstrated the danger of trying to suppress asymptomatic ventricular arrhythmias in postmyocardial infarction patients who had mild to moderate left ventricular dysfunction but no overt CHF. Two class Ic antiarrhythmic agents (encainide and flecainide) increased the mortality in all patients and particularly in patients with ejection fractions less than 30%. Recently the CAST 2 trial (i.e., that arm only comparing moricizine with placebo) was stopped, because of a trend in increasing mortality in the patient group receiving moricizine. Therefore, mere suppression of premature ventricular complexes in at least this patient population is not a desired therapeutic goal.

Treatment of life-threatening ventricular arrhythmias, such as sustained ventricular tachycardia or ventricular fibrillation, in heart failure patients should be guided by invasive electrophysiologic testing. If antiarrhythmic agents are selected, the patients should be carefully monitored for a drug-induced exacerbation of heart failure. Agents likely to cause worsening heart failure include quinidine, procainamide, disopyramide, and class Ic drugs. Patients who do not respond to or who do not tolerate antiarrhythmic medications may be candidates for surgical or device antiarrhythmic treatment. Much basic science and clinical study will be required before a definitive approach to managing ventricular arrhythmias in heart failure patients can be identified.

USE OF β-ADRENERGIC BLOCKERS IN CONGESTIVE HEART FAILURE

Despite the often assumed risk of using β-blocking agents in patients with heart failure, new evidence suggests that certain heart failure patients can benefit from carefully titrated β-blocker therapy. Many investigators have postulated that the benefit or β-blocker therapy in heart failure patients results from blunting the stimulated sympathetic nervous system. Another possible explanation for the therapeutic benefit of β-blockers may involve up-regulation of β-receptors (86). Most studies have demonstrated that chronic heart failure is associated with a reduction in myocardial β-receptors and decreased sensitivity to β-receptor stimulation. Perhaps a β-antagonist can restore β-receptor responsiveness by decreasing catecholamine stimulation. Clinical trials testing these hypotheses have generally enrolled patients with idiopathic cardiomyopathy (87).

Analysis of the Muticenter Diltiazem Post-Infarction Trial (which permitted β-blocker use) showed that β-blockers, if used cautiously in patients with decreased ventricular function, can benefit post-myocardial-infarction patients (88). However, in patients with severe myocardial depression, often heralded by presence of an S3 gallop, the risk of β-blocker therapy will probably outweigh any potential benefit (89). If a β-blocker is used in a heart failure patient, a low dose should be prescribed initially and the patient closely monitored. If heart failure symptoms do not increase, the β-blocker therapy could be gradually titrated upward.

USE OF CALCIUM-CHANNEL BLOCKERS IN HEART FAILURE

Concern that calcium-channel blockers could worsen preexisting heart failure has been widespread, given the usefulness of calcium blockers in treating ischemic syndromes and supraventricular arrhythmias. All calcium-channel blockers exert negative inotropic effects, but these effects may be counterbalanced by their vasodilatory effects. In the post hoc analysis of the Multicenter Diltiazem Post Infarction Trial (88), postinfarction patients with reduced ejection fractions were at increased risk for developing heart failure when treated with diltiazem. Furthermore, studies attempting to use dihydropyridine calcium-channel blockers as first-line vasodilator therapy for congestive heart failure have not shown any therapeutic benefit (90). Therefore, continuous caution should be exercised when calcium blockers are prescribed for patients with congestive heart failure (90). The dihydropyridines (such as nifedipine, nitrendipine, and nicardipine) are less likely to worsen heart failure than either verapamil or diltiazem.

PROGNOSIS

No information describes the natural history of heart failure in the absence of any treatment (5). Nonetheless, it is apparent from a number of epidemiological studies involving patients receiving active treatment that the prognosis of these individuals is grim. In the Framinghan Study the probability of death within 5 years of the diagnosis of CHF was 62% for men and 42% for women (3). A recent study, which included only men with CHF secondary to either CAD or idiopathic dilated cardiomyopathy, demonstrated that the mortality rate in the patients with CAD was 46% and 69% at 1 and 2 years, as compared with 23% and 48% at 1 and 2 years for those with idiopathic dilated cardiomyopathy (91). Approximately 45% of all deaths were sudden (i.e., secondary to presumed ventricular fibrillation), and the remainder were due to progressive CHF. The V-HeFT-I demonstrated that even in the hydralazine-ISDN group the cumulative mortality at 3 years was about 36% (20). In the V-HeFT-II (58) trial, the 2-year mortality of 18% in the enalapril group illustrates continued high mortality due to CHF. Thus, CHF remains a highly lethal clinical syndrome despite medical intervention.

CONCLUSIONS

Congestive heart failure remains a commonly occurring clinical syndrome whose prevalence is increasing as the general population ages. Many different treatment modalities are presently available for managing these increasing numbers of patients. A sound working knowledge of how to implement, monitor, and integrate these varying therapies is essential, to achieve the therapeutic goals of improving both the quality of life and the longevity of patients with CHF.

REFERENCES

1. Harris P: Congestive cardiac failure: central role of the arterial blood pressure. Br Heart J 58:190–203, 1987.
2. Cohn JN: Current therapy of the failing heart. Circulation 78:1099–1107, 1988.
3. Mckee PA, Castelli WP, McNamara PM, Kannel WB: The natural history of congestive heart failure: The Framingham Study. N Engl J Med 285:1441–1446, 1971.
4. Saltiel E, McGuire W: Doxorubicin (adriamycin) cardiomyopathy: a critical review. West J Med 139:332–341, 1983.

5. Smith WM: Epidemiology of congestive heart failure. Am J Cardiol 55:3A–8A, 1985.

6. Willerson JT: What is wrong with the failing heart? N Engl J Med 307:243–245, 1982.

7. Katz AM: Future perspectives in basic science understanding of congestive heart failure. Am J Cardiol 66:468–471, 1991.

8. Ross J: Afterload mismatch and preload reserve: a conceptual framework for the analysis of ventricular function. Prog Cardiovasc Dis 18:255–264, 1976.

9. Francis GS: Neurohumoral mechanisms involved in congestive heart failure. Am J Cardiol 55:15A–21A, 1985.

10. Fowler MB, Laser JA, Hopkins GL, Minobe W, et al.: Assessment of the β-adrenergic receptor pathway in the intact failing human heart: progressive receptor down-regulation and subsensitivity to agonist response. Circulation 74:1290–1302, 1986.

11. Mark AL: The Bezold-Jarisch reflex revisited: clinical implications of inhibitory reflexes originating in the heart. J Am Coll Cardiol 1:90–102, 1983.

12. Raine AEG, Erne P, Burgisser E, Muller FB, et al.: Atrial natriuretic peptide and atrial pressure in patients with congestive heart failure. N Engl J Med 315:533–537, 1986.

13. Marin-Neto JA, Pintya AO, Gallo L, Maciel BC: Abnormal baroreflex control of heart rate in decompensated congestive heart failure and reversal after compensation. Am J Cardiol 67:604–610, 1991.

14. Dzau VJ, Packer M, Lilly LS, Swartz SL, et al.: Prostaglandins in severe congestive heart failure: relation to activation of the renin-angiotensin system and hyponatremia. N Engl J Med 310:347–352, 1984.

15. Braunwald E, Clinical manifestations of heart failure. In Braunwald E: Heart Disease: A Textbook of Cardiovascular Medicine, ed. 2. Philadelphia, WB Saunders, 1984, pp 488–502.

16. Stevenson LW, Perloff JK: The limited reliability of physical signs for estimating hemodynamics in chronic heart failure. JAMA 261:884–888, 1989.

17. Fleg JL, Hinton PC, Lakatta EG, Marcus FI, et al.: Physician utilization of laboratory procedures to monitor outpatients with congestive heart failure. Arch Intern Med 149:393–396, 1989.

18. Packer M, Gottlieb SS, Kessler PD: Hormone-electrolyte interactions in the pathogenesis of lethal cardiac arrhythmias in patients with congestive heart failure. Am J Med 80(suppl 4A):23–29, 1986.

19. Weber KT, Janicki JS: Cardiopulmonary exercise testing for evaluation of chronic cardiac failure. Am J Cardiol 55:22A–31A, 1985.

20. Cohn JN, Archibald DG, Ziesche S, Franciosa JA, et al.: Effect of vasodilator therapy on mortality in chronic congestive heart failure. N Engl J Med 314:1547–1552, 1986.

21. CONSENSUS Trial Study Group: Effects of enalapril on vasodilatory therapy on mortality in severe congestive heart failure. N Engl J Med 316:1429–1435, 1987.

22. The SOLVD Investigators: Effect of enalapril on survival in patients with reduced left ventricular ejection fractions and congestive heart failure. N Engl J Med 325:293–302, 1991.

23. Smith TW, Braunwald E, The management of heart failure. In Braunwald E: Heart Disease: A Textbook of Cardiovascular Medicine, ed. 2. Philadelphia, WB Saunders, 1984, pp 503–559.

24. Ghali JK, Kadakia S, Cooper R, Ferlinz J: Precipitating factors leading to decompensation of heart failure: trait among urban blacks. Arch Intern Med 148:2013–2016, 1988.

25. Smith TW: Digitalis. Mechanisms of action and clinical use. N Engl J Med 318:358–365, 1988.

26. Watanabe AM: Digitalis and the autonomic nervous system. J Am Coll Cardiol 5:35A–42A, 1985.

27. Reuning RH, Geraets DR, Digoxin. In Evans WE, Schentag JJ, Jusko WJ: Applied Pharmacokinetics: Principles of Therapeutic Drug Monitoring, ed. 2. Spokane, Applied Therapeutics, 1986, pp 570–623.

28. Mooradian AD: Digitalis: an update of clinical pharmacokinetics, therapeutic monitoring techniques and treatment recommendations. Clin Pharmacokinet 15:165–179, 1988.

29. Mojaverian P, Green PJ, Jhangiania RK, Chase GD: Digoxin-like immunoreactive substance: monoclonal and polyclonal RIA and FPLA compared. J Pharm Biomed Anal 7:585–592, 1989.

30. Smith TW, Antman EM, Friedman PL, Blatt CM, et al.: Digitalis glycosides: mechanisms and manifestations of toxicity. Prog Cardiovasc Dis 26:413–458, 495–540; 27:21–56, 1984.

31. Jones WN, Perrier D, Trinca CE, Hager WD, et al.: Evaluation of various methods of digoxin dosing. J Clin Pharmacol 22:543–550, 1982.

32. Koup JR, Jusko WJ, Elwood CM, Kohli RK: Digoxin pharmacokinetics: role of renal failure in dosage regimen design. Clin Pharmacol Ther 18:9–21, 1975.

33. Mahdyoon H, Battilana G, Rosman H, Goldstein S, et al.: The evolving pattern of digoxin intoxication: observations at a large urban hospital from 1980 to 1988. Am Heart J 120:1189–1194, 1990.

34. Cohen L, Kitzes R: Magnesium sulfate and digitalis-toxic arrhythmias. JAMA 249:2808–2810, 1983.

35. Antman EM, Wenger TL, Butler VP, Haber E, et al.: Treatment of 150 cases of life-threatening digitalis intoxication with digoxin-specific Fab antibody fragments. Circulation 81:1744–1752, 1990.

36. Hickey AR, Wenger TL, Carpenter VP, Tilson HH, et al.: Digoxin immune Fab therapy in the management of digitalis intoxication: safety and efficacy results of an observational surveillance study. J Am Coll Cardiol 17:590–598, 1991.

37. Jaeschke R, Oxman AD, Guyatt GH: To what extent do congestive heart failure patients in sinus rhythm benefit from digoxin therapy? A systematic overview and meta-analysis. Am J Med 88:279–286, 1990.

38. Parmley WW: Should digoxin be the drug of first choice after diuretics in chronic congestive heart failure? I. Introduction. J Am Coll Cardiol 12:265–273, 1988.

39. Young JB, Roberts R, Heart failure. In Dirks JH, Sutton RAL: Diuretics: Physiology, Pharmacology and Clinical Use, ed. 1. Philadelphia, WB Saunders, 1986, p 151–167.

40. Ellison DT. The physiologic basis of diuretic synergism: its role in treating diuretic resistance. Ann Intern Med 114:886–894, 1991.

41. Braunwald E: ACE-inhibitors—a cornerstone of the treatment of heart failure. N Engl J Med 325:351–353, 1991.

42. Packer M: Conceptual dilemmas in the classification of vasodilator drugs for severe chronic heart failure. Am J Med 76(suppl 6A):3–13, 1984.

43. Cohn JN: Nitrates for congestive heart failure. Am J Cardiol 56:19A–23A, 1985.

44. Jordan RA, Seth L, Casebolt P, Hayes MJ, et al.: Rapidly developing tolerance to transdermal nitroglycerin in congestive heart failure. Ann Intern Med 104:295–298, 1986.

45. Katz RJ, Levy WS, Buff L, Wasserman AG: Prevention of nitrate tolerance with angiotension converting inhibitor. Circulation 83:1271–1277, 1991.

46. Levy WS, Katz RJ, Wasserman AG: Methionine restores the venodilative response to nitroglycerin after the development of tolerance. J Am Coll Cardiol 17:474–479, 1991.

47. Dupuis J, Lalonde G, Lemieux R, Rouleau JG: Tolerance to intravenous nitroglycerin in patients with congestive heart failure: role of increased intravascular volume, neurohumoral activation and lack of prevention with N-acetylcysteine. J Am Coll Cardiol 16:923–931, 1990.

48. Dakak N, Makhoul N, Flugelman MY, Merdler A, et al.: Failure of captopril to prevent nitrate tolerance in congestive heart failure secondary to coronary artery disease. Am J Cardiol 66:608–613, 1990.

49. Leier CV, Huss P, Magorien RD, Unverferth DV: Improved exercise

capacity and differing arterial and venous tolerance during chronic isosorbide dinitrate therapy for congestive heart failure. Circulation 67:817–822, 1983.

50. Franciosa JA, Weber KT, Levine TB, Kinasewitz GT, et al.: Hydralazine in the long-term treatment of chronic heart failure: lack of difference from placebo. Am Heart J 104:587–594, 1982.

51. Conradson T-B, Ryden L, Ahlmark G, Saetre H, et al.: Clinical efficacy of hydralazine in chronic heart failure: one-year double-blind placebo-controlled study. Am Heart J 108:1001–1006, 1984.

52. Packer M, Meller J, Medina N, Gorlin R, et al.: Hemodynamic evaluation of hydralazine dosage in refractory heart failure. Clin Pharmacol Ther 27:337–346, 1980.

53. The Captopril Multicenter Research Group: A placebo-controlled trial of captopril in refractory chronic congestive heart failure. J Am Coll Cardiol 2:755–763, 1983.

54. Sharpe DN, Murphy J, Coxon R, Hannan SF: Enalapril in patients with chronic heart failure: a placebo-controlled, randomized, double-blind study. Circulation 70:271–278, 1984.

55. Packer M, Lee WH, Yushak M, Medina N: Comparison of captopril and enalapril in patients with severe chronic heart failure. N Engl J Med 315:847–853, 1986.

56. Meissner MD, Wilson AR, Jessup M: Renal artery stenosis in heart failure. Am J Cardiol 62:1307–1308, 1988.

57. Francis GS: Heart failure management: the impact of drug therapy on survival. Am Heart J 115:699–701, 1988.

58. Cohn JN, Johnson G, Ziesche S, Cobb F, et al.: A comparison of enalapril with hydralazine-isosorbide dinitrate in the treatment of chronic congestive heart failure. N Engl J Med 325:303–310, 1991.

59. Grossman W: Diastolic dysfunction and congestive heart failure. Circulation 81(suppl III):III-1–III-7, 1990.

60. Packer M: Abnormalities of diastolic function as a potential cause of exercise tolerance in chronic heart failure. Circulation 81(suppl III):III-78–III-86, 1990.

61. Cohn JN, Johnson G, and the Veternas Administration Cooperative Study Group: Heart failure with normal ejection fraction: the V-HeFT study. Circulation 81(suppl III):III-48–III-53, 1990.

62. Setaro JF, Zaret BL, Schulman DS, Black HR, et al.: Usefulness of verapamil for congestive heart failure associated with abnormal left ventricular diastolic filling and normal left ventricular systolic performance. Am J Cardiol 66:981–986, 1990.

63. Colucci WS, Wright R, Braunwald E: New positive inotropic agents in the treatment of congestive heart failure. N Engl J Med 314:290–299; 349–358, 1986.

64. Packer M: Vasodilator and inotropic drugs for the treatment of chronic heart failure: distinguishing hype from hope. J Am Coll Cardiol 12:1299–1317, 1988.

65. The German and Austrian Xamoterol Study Group: Double-blind placebo-controlled comparison of digoxin and xamoterol in chronic heart failure. Lancet 1:489–493, 1988.

66. The Xamoterol in Severe Heart Failure Study Group: Xamoterol in severe heart failure. Lancet 336:1–6, 1990.

67. Alicandri C, Fariello R, Boni E, Zaninella, et al.: Ibopamine vs digoxin in chronic heart failure: a double-blind, crossover study. J Cardiovasc Pharmacol 14(suppl 8):S77–S82, 1989.

68. Uretsky BF, Jessup M, Konstam MA, Dec CW, et al.: Multicenter trial of oral enoximone in patients with moderate to moderately severe congestive heart failure. Circulation 82:774–780, 1990.

69. DiBainco R, Shabetai R, Kostuk W, Moran J, et al.: A comparison of oral milrinone, digoxin, and their combination in the treatment of patients with chronic heart failure. N Engl J Med 320:677–683, 1989.

70. Stevensen LW, Miller LW: Cardiac transplantation as therapy for heart failure. Curr Prob Cardiol 16:219–305, 1991.

71. Rodighiero V: Therapeutic drug monitoring of cyclosporine. Practical applications and limitations. Clin Pharmacokinet 16:27–37, 1989.

72. Yee GC, McGuire TR: Pharmacokinetic drug interactions with cyclosporine. Clin Pharmacokinet 19:319–332, 400–415, 1990.

73. Butman SM, Wild JC, Nolan PE, Fagan TC et al.: Prospective study of the safety and financial benefit of ketoconazole as adjunctive therapy to cyclosporine after heart transplantation. J Heart Lung Transplant 10:351–358, 1991.

74. Bollish SJ, Foster TJ: Swan-Ganz catheter: an important tool for monitoring drug therapy in the critically ill. Hosp Formul 16:99–113, 1980.

75. McGrath RB: Invasive bedside hemodynamic monitoring. Prog Cardiovasc Dis 29:129–144, 1986.

76. Stevenson LW, Tillisch JH: Maintenance of cardiac output with normal filling pressures in patients with dilated heart failure. Circulation 74:1303–1308, 1986.

77. Narins RG, Chusid P: Diuretic use in critical care. Am J Cardiol 57:26A–32A, 1986.

78. Grantham JJ, Chonko AM: The physiologic basis and clinical use of diuretics. In Brenner BM, Stein JH (eds): Sodium and Water Homeostasis. New York, Churchill Livingstone, 1978, pp 178–211.

79. Bayley S, Valentine H, Bennett ED: The hemodynamic responses to incremental doses of intravenous nitroglycerin in left ventricular failure. Intensive Care Med 10:139–145, 1984.

80. Konstam MA, Cohen SR, Weiland S, Martin TT, et al.: Relative contribution of inotropic and vasodilator effects to amrinone-induced hemodynamic improvement in congestive heart failure. Am J Cardiol 57:242–248, 1986.

81. Gage J, Rutman H, Lucido D, LeJemtel TH: Additive effects of dobutamine and amrinone on myocardial contractility and ventricular performance in patients with severe heart failure. Circulation 74:367–373, 1986.

82. Leier CV, Unverferth DV: Dobutamine. Ann Intern Med 99:490–496, 1983.

83. Miller LW: Outpatient dobutamine for refractory congestive heart failure: advantages, techniques, and results. J Heart Lung Transplant 10:482–487, 1991.

84. Podrid PJ, Wilson JS: Should asymptomatic ventricular arrhythmias in patients with congestive heart failure be treated? An antagonist's viewpoint. Am J Cardiol 66:451–457, 1990.

85. Cardiac Arrhythmia Suppression Trial (CAST) Investigators: Increased mortality due to encainide or flecainide in a randomized trial of arrhythmia suppression after myocardial infarction. N Engl J Med 321:406–412, 1989.

86. Lichstein E, Hager WD, Gregory JJ, et al.: Relation between β-adrenergic function and the chance of developing congestive heart failure. J Am Coll Cardiol 16:1327–1332, 1990.

87. Krukemyer JJ. Use of β-adrenergic blocking agents in congestive heart failure. Clin Pharm 9:853–863, 1990.

88. Goldstein RE, Boccuzzi SJ, Cruess D, et al.: Diltiazem increases late-onset congestive heart failure in postinfarction patients with early reduction in ejection fraction. Circulation 83:52–60, 1991.

89. Fisher ML, Plotnick GD, Peters RW, Carliner NH: Beta-blockers in congestive cardiomyopathy: conceptual advance or contraindication? Am J Med 80(suppl 2B):59–66, 1986.

90. Baughman KL: Calcium channel blocking agents in congestive heart failure. Am J Med 80(suppl 2B):46–50, 1986.

91. Franciosa JA, Wilen J, Ziesche S, Cohn JN: Survival in men with severe chronic left ventricular failure due to either coronary heart disease or idiopathic dilated cardiomyopathy. Am J Cardiol 51:831–836, 1983.

CHAPTER 37

CARDIAC ARRHYTHMIAS

JEAN K. NOGUCHI, Pharm.D. and MARK A. GILL, Pharm.D.

The appropriate selection of treatment for any arrhythmia is aided by an understanding of cardiac anatomy and electrophysiology. This chapter reviews the aspects of anatomy and electrophysiology that support an understanding of antiarrhythmic agents. The frequency of serious adverse reactions from antiarrhythmic drugs should be compared with the morbidity associated with the particular disturbance under consideration. This balance (when known) is presented under each type of arrhythmia. Once a drug is chosen, the principles of pharmacokinetics may be applied to tailor the regimen to each patient. This chapter provides examples of equations used to calculate drug dosage regimens.

ELECTROPHYSIOLOGY

The electrical system of the heart consists of intrinsic pacemakers and conduction tissues. It is convenient to conceptualize the progression of normal cardiac rhythm in terms of anatomical basis (Fig. 37.1). Figure 37.2 correlates the standard electrocardiogram with this normal electrical pathway.

The rate of electrical firing of the heart depends upon the most rapid pacemaker. Spontaneous electrical firing or automaticity can occur anywhere in the heart under certain conditions. Normally the sinoatrial node (SA node), which is located where the superior vena cava meets the right atrium, has the most rapid intrinsic rate (60 to 100 per min). Therefore, any electrical activity not initiated by a normal impulse generated by the SA node is considered an arrhythmia. Most arrhythmias are labeled by anatomical location and rate.

Firing of the SA node initiates contraction in the atria. The electrical impulse is conducted through the atria via internodal tracts to the atrioventricular (AV) node near the coronary sinus, between the two atria. The AV node has pacemaker properties but normally serves to coordinate atrial and ventricular contraction. The AV node normally limits excessively rapid atrial rates from activating the ventricles.

The conduction system in the ventricles is more elaborate than that in the atria since the muscle mass is larger. Rapid and effective excitation is critical because the ventricles contribute the most to cardiac output.

Fibers leaving the AV node are called the bundle of His. They separate into the bundle branches, which traverse the septum between the ventricles. Conduction between the AV node and the bundle of His is measured by the PR interval (Fig. 37.2). The final conducting components of the ventricles are the Purkinje fibers, which emanate from the bundle branches to stimulate the ventricular cardiac muscle to contract. The QRS complex measures depolarization of the ventricles. The QT interval reflects repolarization of the ventricles.

THE ACTION POTENTIAL

Conduction and electrical firing in myocardial cells may be analyzed by measuring the membrane potential of various tissues. The electrical potential of these membranes is established by the flow of ions. When electrodes are placed into these tissues, a characteristic repetitive pattern is seen, called an action potential (Fig. 37.3). This action potential may be divided into five phases. Phase 0 is the period of depolarization. It is mediated by two ionic currents. The initial event is the rapid transfer of sodium ions into the cardiac cell. As the sodium depolarizes the tissues, the threshold for the slow response is reached. The slow response depends on the transfer of calcium. Phase 1, the rapid repolarization of the tissue, may depend on inactivation of the sodium current and activation of chloride flow. Phase 2 is a plateau maintained primarily by calcium flow. Phase 3 is the repolarization of the cells initially begun by inhibition of calcium flow. Repolarization is accelerated by potassium flow outward. The rate of fall of phase 3 and its depth will determine the membrane responsiveness. Tissues may only depolarize after reaching a particular level of repolarization, at least -50 to -55 mV for normal Purkinje fibers. The tissue cannot be reactivated regardless of the stimulus until falling below the threshold potential (x in Fig. 37.3). This level of repolarization will therefore determine the end of the absolute refractory period (ARP). The ARP varies in length depending upon the action potential duration (APD). Phase 4 is the depolarization of the cells. In Purkinje fibers, it is brought on by stimulation from the sinus node. Phase 4 may develop spontaneously if the slope is increased. The action potential of pacemaker tissue, such as the sinus node, differs from that of Purkinje fibers. The depth of depolarization is less dramatic, and phase 4 has a steeper slope that determines the rate of sinus firing and its automaticity. The precise ionic currents responsible for pacemaker cells are not entirely known.

Figure 37.1. Anatomy of the electrical system of the heart. The impulse is generated by the sinoatrial (*S-A*) node and is conducted through the atria to the atrioventricular (*A-V*) node, which directs the current to the *bundle of His*, into the *bundle branches*, and finally to the *Purkinje fibers*.

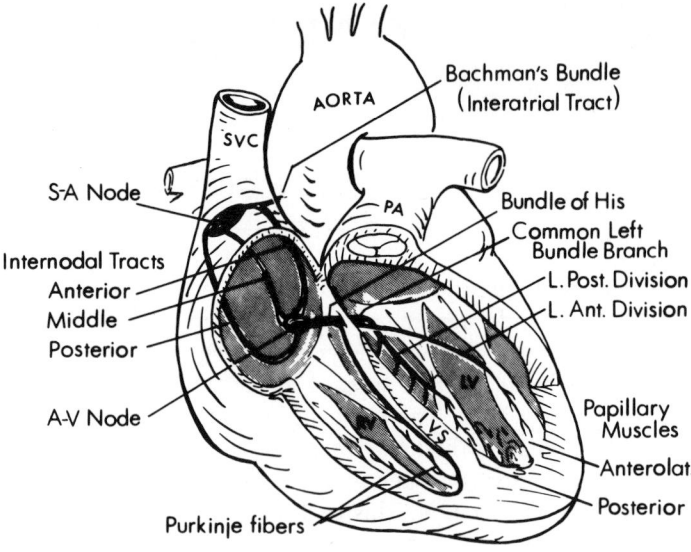

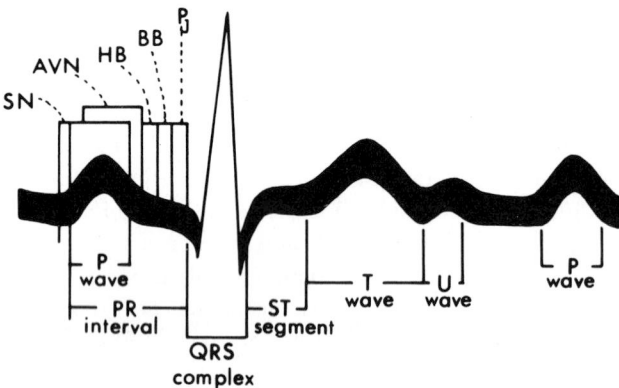

Figure 37.2. The normal electrocardiogram. The *P wave* is atrial depolarization. The *PR interval* (0.12 to 0.20 sec) is formed from the firing of the S-A node (*SN*) and conduction through the A-V node (*AVN*), bundle of His (*HB*), the bundle branches (*BB*) and Purkinje fibers (*P*). The *QRS complex* (0.05 to 0.10 sec) is ventricular depolarization. The *S-T segment* is the refractory period. The *T wave* is ventricular repolarization. The QT interval is 0.35 to 0.44 seconds in duration.

ARRHYTHMIA GENESIS

In general, arrhythmias may be described as abnormalities in electrical development, as ectopic tachyarrhythmias; in electrical conduction, as in reentry arrhythmias; or in a combination of both mechanisms.

Abnormalities in electrical development result from automaticity or triggered activity producing ectopic beats (1). Ectopic beats may develop as pacemaking cells emerge when anoxia, stretch, catecholamine excess, or edema increase the slope of phase 4. Abnormal automaticity may develop at any site in the heart. Generally the fastest firing tissue drives the heart. In the normal heart, atrial pacemakers have faster intrinsic rates than ventricular pace-

makers. When the sinus node rate falls below the intrinsic rate of another tissue, that tissue then drives the heart. Triggered activity is caused by early after depolarizations requiring a preceding action potential for their induction. After depolarizations can occur with oscillations in the plateau phase of the action potential leading to a second depolarization before the first is completed. Hypoxia, fiber stretch, catecholamines, high pCO_2, and an overdose of digitalis can lead to triggered activity.

Reentry arrhythmias depend upon different velocities along adjacent fibers and unidirectional block in electrical conduction (Fig. 37.4). This allows for continuing excitation in a repetitive manner. This circus rhythm may develop as areas of infarcted tissue block or delay conduction. A single circuit of fibers may induce a premature contraction, while continuous cycling of impulses might produce sustained tachycardia. This process may occur in both atrial and ventricular tissue.

Antiarrhythmics have varying effects on reentry mechanics. One effect might be to inhibit membrane responsiveness in fiber 2 such that block is produced in both directions (Fig. 37.5). Another effect might be to enhance conduction in the damaged portion of fiber 2 such that the impulse down fiber 1 finds depolarized fiber and cannot maintain the circuit (Fig. 37.6).

Conduction velocity may decrease by blocking the fast response and allowing emergence of the slow response as in infarction or digoxin toxicity. In addition, since ARP depends on the APD, if repolarization is accelerated, cardiac tissue may be more excitable. A measure of this is the maximum upstroke velocity of phase 0, referred to as $\dot{V}$max. Mechanisms (primarily drugs) that prolong the APD also lengthen the ARP and thereby reduce excitability. This prolongation of repolarization is associated with lengthening of the QT interval (called QTc when corrected

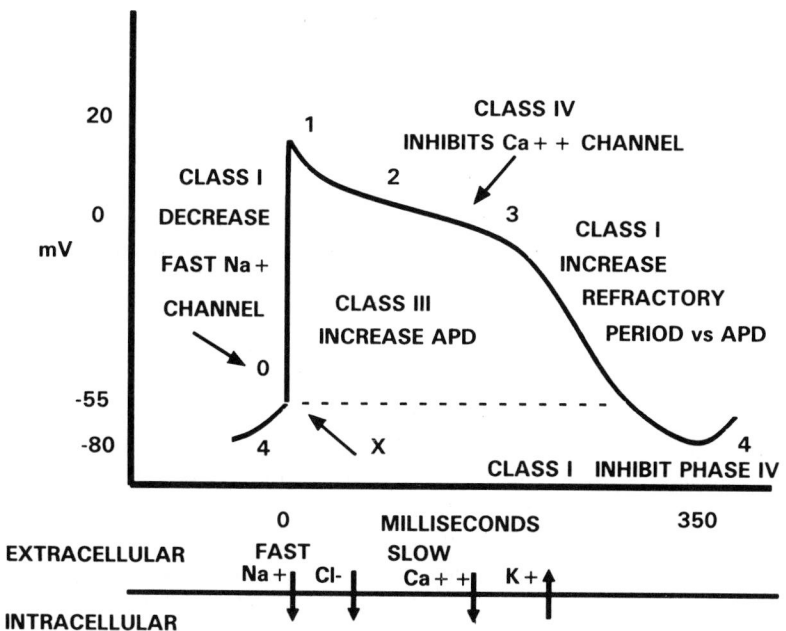

Figure 37.3. The action potential of a cardiac conduction cell correlated with electrolyte shifts. *X* is the threshold potential. The effects of the antiarrhythmic drug classes (see Table 37.1) are noted for the phases of the action potential.

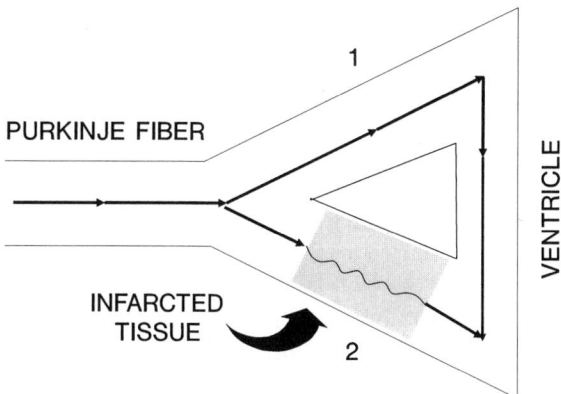

Figure 37.4. Reentry. A conduction fiber that bifurcates into fibers 1 and 2 to stimulate ventricular tissues. The normal pattern is for conduction through fibers 1 and 2 at similar rates. In this figure, fiber 2 was infarcted, which slows conduction until it is blocked by refractory cells. The impulse is impeded along fiber 1. Fiber 2 is activated by the impulse crossing the ventricular muscle tissue. The retrograde impulse finds fiber 2 repolarized and crosses, but at a slow rate. This circuit may be repeated or may terminate if fiber 1 is depolarized.

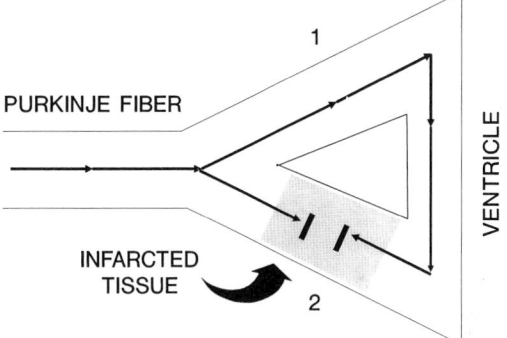

Figure 37.5. Antiarrhythmic drug effect on reentry. Antiarrhythmics may inhibit reentry by slowing conduction in both directions in fiber 2 so that the cells are still refractory when the impulses arrive.

for heart rate) (Fig. 37.2). Prolongation of depolarization also serves to lengthen the QRS duration.

DRUG ACTION

Antiarrhythmic drugs are classified according to their electrophysiologic properties (Table 37.1). Class I drugs depress myocardial membranes with varying ability to slow dV/dt of phase 0 through inhibition of sodium transport. This class is further separated into three groups based upon differing effects on repolarization and conduction. Class Ia drugs (quinidine, procainamide, and disopyramide) lengthen refractory periods and the duration of action potentials. Prolongation of the PR and QT intervals and widening of the QRS is expected. In contrast, Ib agents (lidocaine, tocainide, mexiletine, and phenytoin) shorten repolarization and the QT interval. Conduction and the QRS are altered minimally. Lastly, Ic antiarrhythmics are the most potent depressants of phase 0 in Class I. Class Ic (flecainide, propafenone, and encainide) is noted for slowing of conduction as seen by widening of PR and QRS intervals.

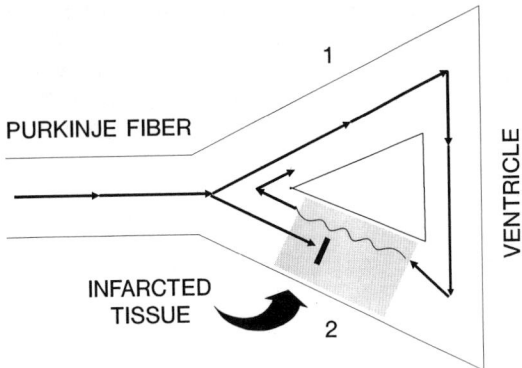

Figure 37.6. Antiarrhythmic drug effect. Another effect enhances conduction in the damaged portion of fiber 2 so that the impulse down fiber 1 finds depolarized fiber and cannot maintain the circuit.

Table 37.1.
Classification of Antiarrhythmic Agents

Class	PR Interval	QRS Duration	Q-Tc Duration	Agent
Ia	0, +[a]	+ + +	+ + +	Quinidine Procainamide Disopyramide Moricizine[b]
Ib	0	0	0, −	Lidocaine Tocainide Phenytoin Mexiletine
Ic	+	+ + +	+ + +	Flecainide Encainide Propafenone
II	+ + +	0	0, −	β-Blockers
III	+	+	+ + +	Bretylium Amiodarone NAPA
IV	+ + +	0	0	Calcium-channel blockers

[a] Symbols: 0, no activity; −, slight shortening; +, slight prolongation; + + +, significant prolongation.
[b] Moricizine has been placed in various categories, e.g. Ia, Ib and I without any subgroup.

Class II includes the β-blocking drugs. Many arrhythmias are produced or exacerbated by hyperactivity of the sympathetic nervous system. The clinical effects of class II agents depend on several variables, including the presence or absence of membrane stabilizing effects (i.e., propranolol, pindolol, and acebutolol act like class I with a decrease in dV/dt of phase 0), intrinsic sympathomimetic activity (pindolol or acebutolol) that in theory would counter the bradycardia and AV conduction depression of β-blockade. The effects of class II drugs depend upon the ambient sympathetic tone. In state of increased adrenergic

activity, such as myocardial infarction, class II will decrease the resting membrane potential, decrease dV/dt of phase 0, and slow conduction velocity, whereas in normal sympathetic tone these three parameters are unchanged.

Class III agents include bretylium, *N*-acetylprocainamide (NAPA) and amiodarone, drugs that prolong action potential duration from phase 2 lengthening and to a similar degree prolong the refractory period. Bretylium and amiodarone have other differing effects on electrophysiology. For example, bretylium initially increases sympathetic tone followed by a decrease, whereas amiodarone is sympatholytic. In addition some effects of amiodarone are felt to derive from a decrease in thyroid hormone activity. Class III agents include bretylium, amiodarone, and NAPA. NAPA does not alter QRS duration but does prolong Q-Tc intervals.

Class IV includes the calcium-channel blockers verapamil, diltiazem, nicardipine nifedipine, and isradipine. These agents block the calcium-mediated current passing through the slow channel. The predominant effect is to prolong the action potential duration. They also decrease phase 4 depolarization and increase the threshold potential. The result is a slowing in A-V conduction, except with nifedipine, which if it produces vasodilation, may increase A-V conduction through reflex sympathetic stimulation.

Some have questioned the utility of this classification system because arrhythmia suppression by an agent within a subclass (e.g., Ic) may not predict positive response from another Ic antiarrhythmic (2). There is evidence that this disparity exists for other classes, e.g., Ia and Ib (3, 4).

SINUS BRADYCARDIA

Sinus bradycardia is defined in adults as a heart rate below 60 per min, with each impulse originating in the SA node, followed by normal conduction through the AV node and His-Purkinje system. The normal range in children varies according to age. In most cases, sinus bradycardia is a normal physiologic variant. It usually reflects diminished SA node automaticity, though it may also be caused by improper impulse propagation out of the SA node.

SA node automaticity is regulated by underlying autonomic tone (sympathetic and vagal), and is lower during sleep and in trained athletes. Sinus rates as low as 30 per min as well as sinus pauses of up to 2.8 sec with first- and second-degree AV block have been observed in completely asymptomatic individuals (5). The slow heart rate results in a longer ventricular filling time and larger end-diastolic volume. Ventricular wall stretching produces an increased force of contraction by the Frank-Starling mechanism. The higher stroke volume results in an unchanged cardiac output despite the bradycardia. As long as the heart rate increases appropriately in response to elevations in sympathetic tone (e.g., exercise), many patients with resting sinus bradycardia remain asymptomatic. Asymptomatic sinus bradycardia is a benign condition that does not require treatment, aside from elimination of underlying factors that may worsen the bradycardia. These include drugs (e.g., β-blockers, digitalis, calcium-channel blockers, or cholinergic agents), hypothyroidism, increased intracranial pressure, and certain electrolyte abnormalities.

Sinus bradycardia is seen in 10 to 41% of patients with acute myocardial infarctions, especially the inferior type (6). It is most often caused by increased vagal tone associated with inferior ischemia or infarction. Ischemic sinus node dysfunction may also occur, but it is less common. Sinus bradycardia is usually seen in the early hours after infarction and is frequently asymptomatic. Uncomplicated asymptomatic sinus bradycardia does not require treatment aside from careful observation.

Therapy is indicated when hypotension, heart failure, or ventricular irritability is seen. Initial treatment should include leg elevation and infusion of volume expandus. Drugs that may further worsen hypotension (e.g., morphine, nitroglycerin) or bradycardia (e.g., β-blockers, calcium-channel blockers) should be titrated carefully. Severe bradycardia may increase ventricular irritability and result in arrhythmias such as premature ventricular contractions (PVCs). These often resolve after correction of the bradycardia and do not require conventional antiarrhythmics.

Atropine. The direct vagolytic action of atropine increases sinus node automaticity and accelerates conduction, usually producing a prompt increase in heart rate and blood pressure. The initial recommended dose is 0.4 to 0.6 mg IV, repeated as needed to a maximum of 2 mg. Lower doses should be avoided, since they may produce a vagal *stimulation* with worsened bradycardia or a biphasic response of slowing followed by acceleration in 2 to 3 min. Adverse cardiovascular effects include excessive tachycardia with increased myocardial oxygen consumption and a potential increase in infarct size, and an increase in ventricular irritability (7). This mandates cautious use in patients with acute myocardial infarction. Noncardiac effects include urinary retention, blurred vision, dry mouth, mydriasis, and toxic psychosis. Adverse reactions are minimized by using the lowest effective dose. Patients with sinus node disease may exhibit an inadequate response to atropine and require pacemakers.

Isoproterenol. Isoproterenol, a β-adrenergic agonist, is a second-line drug that should be used with extreme caution in an acute myocardial infarction because it increases heart rate, ventricular irritability, and myocardial oxygen consumption. Peripheral vasodilation may exacerbate hypotension, which further limits use.

Pacemakers. Patients not responding to atropine or those with persistent symptoms require pacemakers. Either the transvenous or transcutaneous route may be used. Transvenous pacing is the most reliable, with ventricular pacing the traditional mode. Atrial pacing gives the best hemodynamic response but requires intact and reliable AV conduction. Dual-chamber pacemakers that sequentially pace the atrium and ventricle may be preferred in patients with severe heart failure. In transcutaneous cardiac pacing, a low-density current is passed between two self-adhesive pads located anteriorly and posteriorly over the apex of the heart. This gives a hemodynamic response comparable to that of transvenous pacing and has the advantages of faster, easier, and less invasive implementation (8). Its primary limitation is a lower reliability, with successful pacing in 40 to 80% of patients.

Sinus bradycardia associated with an acute myocardial infarction is usually transient, therefore temporary pacemakers generally suffice. It is not associated with a higher incidence of complications or mortality. With proper management, this arrhythmia carries a good to excellent prognosis.

SICK SINUS SYNDROME

The sick sinus syndrome (SSS) encompasses a wide spectrum of impulse formation and/or conduction abnormalities in the SA node, perinodal tissues, atria, and AV node. It may be idiopathic or seen in patients with cardiac or other diseases such as amyloidosis, collagen vascular diseases, or endocrine imbalances. SSS is more common in the elderly and is thought to be caused by a degenerative process associated with an increase in conducting system fibrous tissue (9). Its many ECG and electrophysiologic manifestations include (*a*) sinus bradycardia with an inadequate chronotropic response to exercise, (*b*) sinus pauses or arrest, (*c*) SA node exit block, (*d*) paroxysmal supraventricular tachyarrhythmias (usually atrial fibrillation or flutter), alternating with sinus bradycardia, called the *tachycardia-bradycardia syndrome*, (*e*) prolonged suppression of SA node activity after conversion from supraventricular achycardia, or (*f*) carotid hypersensitivity, seen as abnormal sinus slowing or pauses after carotid sinus massage.

Some patients with ECG or electrophysiologic evidence of SSS are asymptomatic, have a good prognosis, and do not require treatment (10). Others develop a broad spectrum of central nervous system or hemodynamic symptoms, ranging from brief periods of fatigue, irritability, dizziness, and confusion, to syncope (Stokes-Adams attacks), seizures, and congestive heart failure. Angina and palpitations may also be seen in patients with the tachycardia-bradycardia syndrome.

Before initiating treatment, reversible or transient causes of sinus node dysfunction should be excluded or minimized. Drug-induced causes include digitalis, β-blockers, calcium-channel blockers (especially verapamil), class Ia and Ic antiarrhythmics, and certain antihypertensives. Treatment is justified in *symptomatic* patients with a documented correlation between inadequate sinus node activity and the symptoms. Pharmacologic attempts to increase SA node automaticity (e.g., chronic administration of atropine) are not effective. Antiarrhythmic drugs are likewise not useful, with the exception of the tachycardia-bradycardia syndrome, where they may be used in the management of the tachycardic component. Many tachycardia-bradycardia patients require concomitant pacemakers because of prolonged pauses when converting from the tachyarrhythmia to sinus rhythm, or an exacerbation of the bradycardic episodes caused by the antiarrhythmic. Those with intermittent atrial fibrillation may also benefit from anticoagulants (discussed under atrial fibrillation).

Pacemakers. Permanent pacemakers are the therapy of choice. SSS is the most common indication for permanent pacemakers, accounting for 40 to 50% of the pacemaker population. Several pacing options are available. Atrial, ventricular, or dual-demand pacemakers sense and pace the atria, ventricle, or both chambers, respectively. Rate-responsive pacemakers respond to various signals (motion sensors, respiratory rate, oxygen saturation, or lactate levels) with a faster pacing rate, thereby simulating a more physiologic response to exercise. Recent evidence has shown an association between traditional ventricular-demand pacemakers and adverse events, including chronic atrial fibrillation, congestive heart failure, and thromboembolism (11). Causes include a lack of AV synchrony and abnormal retrograde ventriculoatrial conduction. Atrial-demand pacemakers are therefore preferable; patients must first be carefully screened to exclude AV node and His-Purkinje system conduction defects, and drugs with negative AV chronotropic or dromotropic effects must be administered carefully.

Pacing relieves symptoms and is generally well tolerated. Previous studies in SSS patients did not demonstrate improved morbidity or mortality (50% at 5 years) (9), possibly because of underlying poor cardiac function. Recognition of the deleterious effects of ventricular-demand pacemakers now raises the question of whether they may have offset a trend toward higher survival. Recent studies have shown an improved short-term survival in elderly patients with atrial pacemakers (11). Long-term studies in large populations should also be performed.

ATRIOVENTRICULAR BLOCK

Abnormalities of atrioventricular conduction are classified into three types, based on the extent of impulse transmission across the AV node. The anatomic location of the conduction block determines the clinical significance, prognosis, and therapy.

First-Degree AV Block. First-degree AV block is defined as a prolongation of the PR interval to ≥0.20 seconds, with 1:1 atrioventricular conduction of all impulses. This is a relatively common ECG finding, with a prevalence of 0.5 to 10%. Conduction delay in the AV node is the most common cause. Both cardiac (AV nodal disease, acute myocardial infarction, myocarditis) and noncardiac (enhanced vagal tone) etiologies have been identified. Patients are rarely symptomatic, and treatment is not generally required (10). Digitalis, β-blockers, calcium-channel blockers, and potassium may cause or worsen this pattern. First-degree AV block is not an absolute contraindication to these drugs, but close observation is necessary because they may produce higher grade block.

Second-Degree AV Block. In second-degree AV block, there is intermittent failure of atrioventricular impulse conduction. The anatomic site of block may be the AV node, His bundle, or bundle branch system. This type of block is subdivided into Mobitz types I and II.

Mobitz type I, or Wenckebach block, is characterized by a gradual prolongation of atrioventricular conduction (PR interval on ECG) until a sinus impulse (P-wave) is not conducted to the ventricles. The cycle then begins anew with a short followed by progressively longer PR intervals and a nonconducted P-wave. Electrophysiologic studies usually implicate a conduction abnormality in the AV node proximal to the bundle of His. The presence and extent of Mobitz type I AV block is influenced by underlying autonomic tone. It may be seen in normal individuals (especially trained athletes), or may be caused by drugs (e.g. digitalis, β-blockers, or verapamil), electrolyte abnormalities or inflammation. This pattern is also seen in acute inferior myocardial infarctions. It usually appears within the first 72 hr after infarction, is transient, and infrequently progresses to higher grade block (6).

Many patients with Mobitz type I AV block are asymptomatic, in which case drugs or pacemakers are not required (10). Close observation of patients with acute myocardial infarction or digitalis toxicity is warranted. Treatment is indicated when the patient exhibits symptoms (central nervous system or hemodynamic), there is ventricular irritability, or the ventricular rate persists at <40 per min (8). Atropine facilitates AV nodal conduction by decreasing the effective and functional refractory periods of the AV node. It frequently restores 1:1 conduction in patients with Mobitz type I block and normal AV nodes (7) and may be useful in managing digitalis toxicity. However, this effect is unpredictable in patients with acute myocardial infarction, and temporary pacemakers are therefore indicated. β-blockers, verapamil, and digoxin should be dosed with caution in these patients.

Mobitz type II block is present when the PR interval of conducted beats remains constant, with unpredicted intermittent nonconduction of atrial impulse(s). It reflects a conduction abnormality distal to the bundle of His and is frequently associated with a wide QRS (bundle branch block) pattern on ECG. This type of block is seen in acute anterior or anteroseptal myocardial infarction, usually during the first 72 hr after infarction. It reflects extensive ischemia and necrosis of the septum, bundle branches, and Purkinje fibers. Almost all patients are symptomatic. Mobitz type II AV block with bundle branch block is an unstable rhythm with an ominous prognosis, often progressing abruptly to complete heart block, severe bradycardia, or asystole. Atropine is generally ineffective. Pacemakers are therefore mandatory and usually permanent (10).

Third-Degree AV Block. Third-degree AV block occurs when no P-waves are conducted to the ventricles. Also known as complete heart block, it reflects a total absence of atrioventricular conduction. This results in an escape rhythm with the AV junctional, His bundle, or Purkinje cells serving as the pacemaker. The site of block is related to the symptoms, prognosis, and therapy. When conduction is blocked within the AV node (proximal conducting system), the AV junctional or proximal His bundle cells function as the pacemaker. Normal-appearing QRS complexes are seen, reflecting normal ventricular impulse conduction. The physiologic escape rate for the AV junctional cells is 40 to 60 beats per min, which increases in response to elevated sympathetic tone. Complete heart block with AV junctional escape may be a congenital rhythm or be seen (usually transiently) in acute inferior myocardial infarction. This is a relatively stable rhythm. Normal ventricular conduction along with the ability to increase the rate with exercise allows some patients to remain asymptomatic. Infants and children with congenital proximal complete heart block may tolerate this rhythm well for long periods of time, requiring close observation but no intervention (5, 10). Treatment is indicated in patients with (*a*) symptoms (hypotension, syncope, persistent chest pain, heart failure), (*b*) inadequate chronotropic response to exercise, or (*c*) ventricular arrhythmias. Atropine may be used in the emergency situation, but it is of limited value and without long-term effectiveness. Permanent pacemakers are the therapy of choice. Pacemakers are reliable and well tolerated in infants and children with the congenital form of this rhythm. The role of pacemakers in myocardial infarction patients remains unclear.

Complete heart block in the distal His bundle or Purkinje system (distal conducting system) results in an idioventricular escape rhythm with wide QRS complexes occurring at a rate of 30 to 40 per min. This reflects abnormal impulse conduction through the ventricles and the slow intrinsic rate of ventricular pacemaker tissues. This pattern may be seen in acute myocardial infarction as well as other diseases such as myocarditis, cardiomyopathy, and sarcoidosis. The slow rate coupled with abnormal ventricular conduction usually causes hemodynamic or central nervous system symptoms. In patients with acute anterior or anteroseptal myocardial infarction, this is an unstable rhythm with abrupt progression to asystole or ventricular arrhythmias. Atropine is not effective (7). Patients with third-degree AV block and an idioventricular rhythm require permanent pacemakers (8, 10), regardless of symptoms. The abrupt occurrence of this type of block in the setting of an acute myocardial infarction carries an ominous prognosis and a high risk of sudden death.

SINUS TACHYCARDIA

Sinus tachycardia is characterized by a rate of over 100 and usually less than 180 beats per min, with impulses originating in the SA node and conducted normally to the AV node and His-Purkinje system. In most cases it reflects increased SA node automaticity. A gradual acceleration and deceleration may allow differentiation from other supraventricular tachycardias. The rate varies with sleep or changes in posture. Sinus tachycardia is a normal physiologic response to a myriad of conditions, including exercise, anxiety, pain, stress, fright, fever, hypoxia, anemia, hypovolemia, hypotension, early congestive heart failure, hyperthyroidism, and pheochromocytoma. It is seen in about one-third of patients with acute myocardial infarction and is attributed to sympathetic overactivity. Drugs with direct or indirect sympathomimetic or vagolytic activity may cause or contribute to sinus tachycardia. Common causes include sympathomimetics, catecholamines, β-agonists, methylxanthines, and anticholinergics.

Most individuals with sinus tachycardia are asymptomatic, except perhaps for palpitations. Patients with coronary artery disease may experience angina due to increased myocardial oxygen consumption. Those with poor cardiac reserve and sustained episodes of tachycardia may develop congestive heart failure.

The treatment of sinus tachycardia consists of management of the underlying condition. Treatment of the tachycardia itself is not necessary and may have deleterious effects, since decreasing the heart rate will decrease the cardiac output and oxygen delivery to the tissues. In the rare instance (e.g., hyperthyroidism) where sinus tachycardia is sustained and symptomatic, propranolol or another β-blocker may be given, provided the patient is not in congestive heart failure.

AV NODAL REENTRY

Paroxysmal supraventricular tachycardias are a group of common arrhythmias seen frequently in healthy individuals with otherwise normal cardiovascular systems. Reentry (sometimes called circus-movement tachycardia) is the mechanism for >90% of cases. Several variants may be seen. AV nodal reentry is sometimes known as paroxysmal supraventricular tachycardia (PSVT) and accounts for 50 to 60% of cases. Reentry using an accessory atrioventricular pathway (AV reentry, Wolff-Parkinson-White syndrome or concealed bypass tract conduction—discussed in a separate section) causes 30% of cases. Finally, reentry within the SA node (4%) or atria (4 to 8%) may also occur, primarily in patients with underlying heart disease. Typical features of reentry include (*a*) abrupt initiation and termination, (*b*) a regular rate of 150 to 250 beats per min (up to 325 in infants), (*c*) narrow QRS complexes of normal morphology, and (*d*) 1:1 AV conduction. Abrupt initiation and ventricular rate regularity are specific characteristics of AV nodal reentry, often used as clues in differentiating it from ectopic atrial tachycardia, atrial fibrillation, or atrial flutter.

An understanding of the electrophysiology of reentry is useful in the evaluation of therapeutic modalities. Under normal conditions, impulses begin in the SA node and terminate in the Purkinje fibers where the surrounding tissue is refractory. In reentry, the impulse is able to reactivate the conducting system by "hiding" in the heart long enough for the surrounding tissue to regain excitability. Slow conduction in the AV node makes this a likely site for reentry. In AV nodal reentry there are at least two functional pathways in the AV conducting system, sharing common proximal and distal limbs (Fig. 37.7). The α-pathway has slow conduction velocity and a short refractory period, while the β-pathway has fast conduction velocity and a long refractory period. During sinus rhythm, each impulse arrives at the AV junction, travels antegrade (toward the ventricles) down both pathways, reaches the His bundle via the fast β-pathway, and terminates in the His-Purkinje system. Conduction down the slow α-pathway ceases at the His-bundle, where the tissue is refractory (Fig. 37.7A). The relatively long cycle length in sinus rhythm allows both pathways to recover excitability before the next sinus impulse arrives at the AV junction.

In reentry (Fig. 37.7B), a premature impulse enters the AV node at a time when the slow α-path will conduct, but the fast β-path is refractory. The impulse travels through the AV junction via the α-pathway. The His-Purkinje system and ventricles are then activated in normal fashion. Additionally, retrograde transmission (toward the atria) occurs up the now recovered β-pathway, creating an atrial echo. Should the α-pathway be recovered, the impulse will travel antegrade (toward the ventricles), and a reentry circuit is created. The impulse travels antegrade down the slow α-pathway and retrograde up the fast β-pathway, with the atria and ventricles as "innocent bystanders" (1). In AV nodal reentry, the entire circuit is located in the AV junction. Clearly, to induce and sustain reentry the premature impulse must be critically timed, and a fine balance must exist between conductivity and refractoriness. The impulse must always find excitable tissue in the direction in which it is propagating. If refractory tissue is encountered, the circuit is broken and the rhythm terminates abruptly. On ECG, the premature atrial beat has a prolonged PR-interval. Subsequent P-waves are frequently buried in the QRS complex, reflecting simultaneous activation of the atria and ventricles. QRS morphology

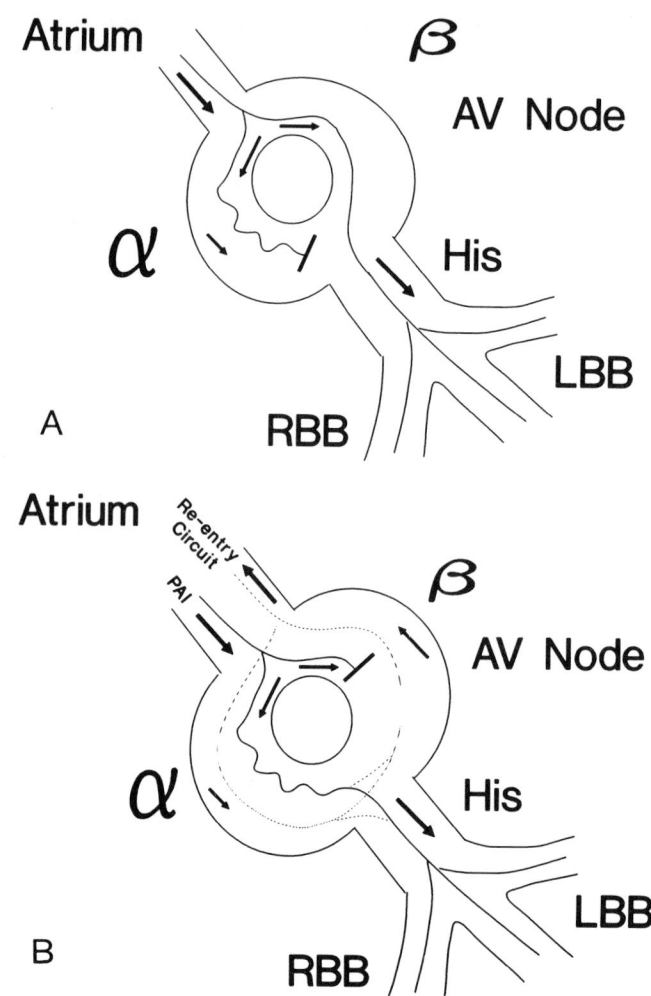

Figure 37.7. **A,** nodal reentry. Sinus rhythm. The impulse is blocked in the α-pathway and reaches the ventricles via the β-pathway. **B,** *PAI,* premature atrial impulse; *His,* bundle of His; *RBB,* right bundle branch; *LBB,* left bundle branches; *solid line,* PAI. The premature impulse is blocked in the β-pathway and reaches the ventricles via the α-pathway. If the β-pathway is recovered, AV nodal reentry may be initiated. *Dotted line,* reentry circuit.

is normal unless there is aberrant conduction or antegrade preexcitation down an anomalous AV connection (Wolff-Parkinson-White syndrome).

AV nodal reentry may be seen at any age from infancy to adulthood. It is a common arrhythmia in infants, children, and young adults. Approximately 50% of patients have no underlying heart disease. Brief runs are often detected on 24-hr ECG monitors of asymptomatic persons. Many cases are idiopathic. Noncardiac causes such as fever, infection, or drugs (sympathomimetics, catecholamines, β-agonists) may be seen in a minority of patients.

The clinical manifestations depend on the heart rate, the duration of the arrhythmia, and the presence of underlying heart disease. Reentrant rhythms are not usually life-threatening, except in patients with the Wolff-Parkinson-White syndrome. Most patients will notice the fast heart rate almost immediately, and may complain of dizziness, lightheadedness, weakness, or nonspecific chest discomfort. Less common symptoms include dyspnea, syncope, and angina. Congestive heart failure is uncommon, because ventricular (His-Purkinje) conduction remains normal in most patients. However, the shortened ventricular filling time lowers stroke volume and may induce congestive heart failure in patients with tenuous cardiovascular status. Infants often have nonspecific symptoms such as fussiness, lethargy, poor feeding, or rapid breathing, yet may present with severe congestive heart failure and shock.

Acute Treatment

The goal of treatment for AV nodal reentry is to interrupt the circuit by slowing conduction or prolonging refractoriness in either AV junctional pathway. When the impulse encounters refractory tissue, the tachycardia will terminate abruptly. Correctable contributing factors such as fever, infection, hypoxia, anemia, or hyperthyroidism should be treated. The arrhythmia may be terminated using pharmacologic, electrical, or other measures. The immediate treatment is dictated by the hemodynamic status of the patient.

DC Cardioversion. In patients with hemodynamic instability (severe hypotension or heart failure, pulmonary edema, myocardial ischemia, acute alteration in mental status), electrical cardioversion is the therapy of choice. Direct current (DC) cardioversion depolarizes a critical number of myocardial cells simultaneously, allowing the sinus node to reestablish dominance as the pacemaker. For conversion of supraventricular tachycardias, lower energies (10 to 50 joules, or 0.5 joules/kg) are often adequate. This is a uniformly effective, immediate method of termination with minimal adverse effects. The only major adverse effect is the induction of ventricular arrhythmias, which are avoided by synchronizing the electrical discharge to the QRS complex. Myocardial damage is rare with lower energies. Short-acting sedatives may be given before the procedure in older children and adults. Electroconversion is not advised in patients with stable cardiovascular status, because other measures are considered less invasive and safer. Moreover, DC cardioversion precludes a direct assessment of the efficacy of various maneuvers and drugs on the arrhythmia. This information is useful in managing recurrent episodes.

Vagal Maneuvers. In hemodynamically stable patients, interventions to increase vagal tone are performed first. These measures decrease conductivity and increase refractoriness in the AV node and decrease automaticity in the SA node. Used either alone or in conjunction with antiarrhythmic drugs, vagotonic maneuvers will terminate 50 to 80% of cases of AV nodal reentrant tachycardia.

The most common vagal measures are carotid sinus massage (or pressure) and the Valsalva maneuver. Carotid sinus massage stimulates the baroreceptors of the carotid artery, which slows the sinus rate, prolongs AV conduction, lowers cardiac output, decreases venous return, and decreases peripheral vascular resistance (12). Alteration in the critical balance between conduction and refractoriness disrupts the cycle and terminates the rhythm. The Valsalva maneuver (prolonged forced expiration against a closed glottis) may be induced by blowing into a blood pressure manometer tube to maintain a pressure of 30 to 60 mm Hg for 10 to 30 sec. Conversion to sinus rhythm occurs during the relaxation phase, when a parasympathetic surge induces antegrade AV nodal block. Other vagotonic procedures include deep breathing or gagging.

Carotid sinus massage and the Valsalva maneuver may not be successful in infants and young children. In these patients, the diving reflex may be initiated by immersing the face in a pan of ice water for 10 to 15 sec or by placing a washcloth soaked in ice water on the face. This causes an acute vagal surge that is more prominent and clinically effective in young patients. A slowing of the tachycardia rate is followed by abrupt conversion to sinus rhythm. The diving reflex may induce asystole and should be used only under monitored conditions.

Background increases in sympathetic tone may attenuate the effectiveness of vagal maneuvers (13). This may explain the lower efficacy when standing, as compared with the supine position. These measures are generally more effective in the young, probably relating to a reduction in overall autonomic tone associated with aging. Vagal maneuvers should be performed as early as possible after arrhythmia initiation, before elevated sympathetic tone reduces efficacy (13).

Vagotonic procedures of all types should not be used in patients with a history of sinus node dysfunction, since prolonged sinus node recovery time may cause sinus arrest after the reentry circuit is terminated. Carotid sinus massage or pressure may cause carotid artery ischemia in patients with preexisting atherosclerotic narrowing or (rarely) ventricular tachyarrhythmias (12). Both carotid arteries should be examined *before* the procedure, and it should not be attempted in patients with evidence of cerebrovascular insufficiency. Because of the prevalence of sinus node and cerebrovascular disease in the elderly, vagotonic stimuli should be avoided or used with great caution in this population.

Verapamil. If vagal maneuvers are unsuccessful, either verapamil or adenosine is the drug of choice for terminating AV nodal reentry. Verapamil inhibits channel-mediated entry of calcium into the cell. Effects are most evident in the SA node, AV node, and the cardiac and

Table 37.2.
Sites of Primary Drug Action in AV Nodal Reentry

AV node antegrade slow-conduction pathway
   Calcium-channel blockers (verapamil, diltiazem)
   Digoxin
   Adenosine
   β-Blockers
AV node retrograde fast-conduction pathway
   Class Ia drugs (quinidine, procainamide, disopyramide)
   Class Ic drugs (flecainide, encainide, propafenone)
Suppression of atrial ectopy
   Class Ia drugs (quinidine, procainamide, disopyramide)
   Class Ic drugs (flecainide, encainide, propafenone)
   β-Blockers

peripheral vascular smooth muscles, since these tissues depend calcium flux for action potential generation. In contrast, atrial and ventricular myocardium and the His-Purkinje system are normally fast-channel (sodium flux–dependent) tissues. This explains the lack of efficacy of verapamil in ventricular arrhythmias.

The net effect of verapamil results from an interplay between direct and indirect effects. Direct actions include a depression of automaticity in the SA and AV nodes (negative chronotropic effect), a reduction in conduction velocity in the AV node (negative dromotropic effect), a reduction in myocardial contractility (negative inotropic effect), and a dilation of coronary and peripheral arteries. These effects are modified by reflex sympathetic stimulation evoked by the peripheral arterial dilation. Increased cardiac automaticity and contractility largely offset the negative chronotropic and inotropic effects. The net cardiac effect is a negative dromotropic effect on antegrade conduction through the AV node (Table 37.2). Other effects become important only in diseased hearts (e.g., sinus node disease or congestive heart failure).

Amongst the calcium-channel blocking agents, verapamil has the lowest degree of peripheral arterial dilation relative to its effects on the heart. This characteristic is advantageous in treating arrhythmias, but the relatively prominent negative inotropic effect may be a limitation in some patients. In contrast, nifedipine is a much more potent vasodilator, causing marked hemodynamic alteration before conduction effects are seen; this drug is therefore not useful as an antiarrhythmic. Diltiazem has electrophysiologic and hemodynamic effects comparable to those of verapamil and has demonstrated efficacy and safety in clinical trials (14). Its potential advantage of a less marked negative inotropic effect than verapamil deserves further investigation.

Intravenous verapamil doses of 5 to 10 mg or 0.075 to 0.15 mg/kg over 2 min (3 min in elderly patients) will convert 60 to 90% of adult patients with AV nodal reentry to normal sinus rhythm within 5 to 10 min. If there is no response, a second dose of 0.15 mg/kg IV may be given 15 to 30 min later. Vagal maneuvers should be performed before the second dose.

After oral administration, ≥90% of the dose is absorbed, but extensive first-pass metabolism limits systemic availability to 20 to 35% (15, 16). Food prolongs the time to peak concentration but not the extent of absorption. Large inter- and intrapatient variability exists, with serum levels after administration of the same dose varying by as much as 10-fold. Verapamil is approximately 90% protein bound to albumin and α-1-acid glycoprotein (16). The volume of distribution of 4.5 to 7 liters/kg in healthy adults is increased in cirrhosis. It is converted rapidly and extensively in the liver to multiple metabolites that are largely inactive. The only active metabolite, norverapamil (the N-demethylated derivative), has approximately 20% of the potency of the parent drug. Verapamil undergoes bi- or triexponential decline with an elimination phase half-life of 3 to 5 hr after a single dose (15, 16). Long-term administration may result in nonlinear accumulation with a decreased clearance and prolonged half-life (16). Seventy percent of a p.o. or IV dose is recovered in the urine in 5 days, almost exclusively as metabolites, with 10 to 15% found in the feces (17).

Patients with cirrhosis demonstrate a significantly higher bioavailability (52.3% versus 22% for normals) due to a less marked first-pass effect, as well as a longer half-life and lower clearance (16, 18). Those with arrhythmias or congestive heart failure may have altered hepatic clearance related to hepatic blood flow.

After single IV doses, verapamil displays a good relationship between serum levels and electrophysiologic effects. Studies of oral administration have however yielded a poor correlation of serum levels with clinical efficacy. This is explained in part by stereoselective differences in its pharmacodynamics and pharmacokinetics. Commercially available preparations of verapamil are racemic mixtures of the d- and l-isomers. The l-isomer has more potent negative chronotropic, inotropic, and dromotropic effects (19). Stereoselective first-pass metabolism after oral dosing results in preferential extraction of the l-isomer. The bioavailability of the l-isomer (20%) is therefore lower than that of the d-isomer (50%) (18). The l-isomer has a distribution volume, clearance, and unbound fraction approximately twice that of the d-isomer (18). The relative ratios of l- and d-isomers after IV and p.o. administrations are therefore different, with IV dosing giving a larger fraction of total verapamil concentration as the more active l-isomer. Serum levels required for a given PR-interval prolongation after IV doses are 2 to 3 times lower than those after p.o. administration (16). This may explain the higher efficacy after acute IV versus chronic p.o. administration and wide inter- and intrapatient variability in response to a fixed serum level. Another explanation for the discrepancy in clinical effect of IV versus p.o. dosing is preferential myocardial uptake after IV administration (16). Alteration of response by underlying sympathetic tone further disrupts the relationship between serum level and drug effect. Conventional assays measuring total verapamil concentration are not useful in assessment of efficacy. Analytic methods to isolate the individual enantiomers are not widely available.

Adverse reactions occur in 10 to 14% (17) of patients receiving verapamil but require discontinuation in only 1 to 5%. Adverse effects after IV administration are an extension of the pharmacologic effect and include hypotension, disturbances in AV conduction, bradycardia or sinus arrest, and congestive heart failure. These reflect calcium-channel blockade in the vascular smooth muscle, AV node, SA node, and myocardium, respectively. Mild, transient hypotension is the most common adverse reaction. Most patients do not require treatment; in some, the reduction in afterload may even allow an *increase* in the cardiac output. In symptomatic patients, placement in Trendelenburg's position with IV fluid administration is usually adequate treatment. Patients with borderline blood pressures before verapamil (systolic pressure ≤90 to 100 mm Hg) may develop severe hypotension. These patients should receive adenosine. Alternatively, pretreatment with 1 g of IV calcium chloride or gluconate is thought to block the peripheral but not the cardiac receptors (20, 21). Calcium therefore blunts or abolishes the hypotensive effect while preserving AV nodal effect, when given either before or after verapamil. Sudden cardiovascular collapse with profound hypotension, bradycardia, apnea, and death has been reported after verapamil administration in neonates and infants (22). While verapamil is an excellent drug in older children, it should be avoided in children under 1 year of age (23).

Verapamil is not thought to have a significant proarrhythmic effect, but it requires cautious use in patients with preexisting conduction disorders. Premature atrial or ventricular impulses occasionally reactivate reentry. Atrial fibrillation and serious ventricular arrhythmias are uncommon. Bradycardia or heart block caused by excess AV nodal effect may require treatment with isoproterenol, atropine, calcium, or pacemakers. Verapamil is contraindicated in patients with preexisting SA nodal disease (sick sinus syndrome), because of the high risk for prolonged sinus arrest after termination of the arrhythmia. While verapamil is a first-line drug in most patients, it is contraindicated in sinus node disease, marked hypotension, heart failure, and neonates. Adenosine is preferred in these patients.

An important drug interaction occurs between verapamil and β-blockers. Concomitant administration of these drugs results in AV blocking and negative inotropic effects by independent mechanisms. This increases the risk of serious cardiovascular side effects such as congestive heart failure (24), high-degree AV block, or hypotension. Serum levels of digoxin may be increased by verapamil (25) via an increase in half-life and reduction in distribution volume and total clearance. Furthermore, verapamil should be used with caution in suspected digoxin toxicity, because of its additive effects on the AV node.

Monitoring parameters for intravenous verapamil in arrhythmias include cardiac rhythm and rate and blood pressure. Continuous ECG monitoring is strongly advised. Routine serum level assessment is not recommended.

Adenosine. Adenosine is an ubiquitous endogenous purine nucleoside. Its myriad biologic effects include regulation of coronary, cerebral, renal, and skeletal blood flow, modulation of neurotransmission and immune response, inhibition of platelet aggregation, stimulation of gastrin secretion, inhibition of lipolysis, and induction of bronchoconstriction. The actions of adenosine on cardiac tissues include a very transient powerful negative dromotropic effect on the AV node and a similar negative chronotropic effect in the sinus node, AV junction, and ventricles. In electrophysiologic studies, the primary effects are a lengthening of sinus cycle length and a prolongation of the AH-interval, followed by complete or partial AV nodal block (26). Adenosine has no effect on the His-Purkinje interval. Cardiac activity is thought to be related to alterations in calcium and potassium ion currents, but the precise mechanisms are unclear (27). Adenosine exerts minimal effect on vagal tone.

Adenosine is produced in many tissues and organs, but plasma concentrations are low because of rapid transport and metabolism. Local effects are mediated through interactions with intracellular and extracellular receptors, which may be up-regulated, down-regulated, supersensitized, and desensitized under different conditions. Analogs with agonist and antagonist activity and variable receptor affinity further modulate the effect. The effects of adenosine depend primarily on binding to the cell surface receptors; therefore the concentration in the extracellular space correlates directly with the magnitude of the effect. Extracellular fluid concentrations are linked to adenosine production and elimination via multiple pathways.

Adenosine is continuously produced and released by erythrocytes and cells in the liver, heart, skeletal muscle, and endothelium. At physiologic concentrations (0.1 to 1 μM), it is taken up avidly by erythrocytes and phosphorylated into adenosine monophosphate by adenosine kinase. At higher concentrations, it is deaminated by adenosine deaminase to inosine, which is further metabolized to hypoxanthine and uric acid. These metabolites have no antiarrhythmic effect. The balance between production and elimination is tightly regulated at the local level.

Adenosine is closely related to another endogenous compound, adenosine-5'-triphosphate (ATP). ATP and adenosine share similar biologic actions but have different potencies at the various receptors. Exogenous ATP is rapidly dephosphorylated to adenosine in vivo, and most of its cardiac effect is caused by adenosine formation. ATP also has vagal stimulant properties that contribute minimally to the antiarrhythmic effect (28). ATP has been used as an antiarrhythmic for many years in Europe, but is not available in the United States.

Adenosine restores sinus rhythm within 10 to 20 sec in 85 to 100% of adults and children with spontaneous or induced AV nodal reentrant tachycardias (27, 29–31). Antegrade pathway conduction block occurs in the majority of patients (Table 37.2) (27, 28, 31). In patients with sinus node or intraarial reentry, atrial fibrillation or flutter, or ectopic atrial tachycardia, adenosine induces a higher grade AV block (27)—the transiently (<20 sec) slower ventricular rate may allow visualization of P-waves and therefore aid in diagnosis, but atrial activity is unchanged, and these arrhythmias are rarely terminated.

In randomized (29) and nonrandomized (31, 32) comparative trials of adenosine and verapamil, conversion rates are comparable or favor adenosine for patients with AV nodal reentry or AV reentry involving an accessory pathway. Termination of the tachycardia is generally more rapid with adenosine than with verapamil, but the clinical importance of this is unclear. Repetitive administration results in consistent conversion at a similar dosage each time or repeated failures.

Adenosine is not absorbed by the oral route. After IV injection it is rapidly distributed into intracellular, extracellular, and interstitial spaces. It crosses the blood-brain barrier, and a vasodilatory effect on the cerebral vessels may account for the common occurrence of headache. In vitro studies have measured a half-life of <10 sec (33). Traditional pharmacokinetic studies are hampered by rapid clearance, with ongoing metabolism as specimens are collected. Parameters such as volume of distribution and clearance have therefore not been reported.

Noncardiac adverse effects occur in 15 to 81% of patients (26, 28, 29, 31). The most common are flushing, dyspnea or a feeling of suffocation, and headache. Chest pain or pressure may mimic angina. Cough, malaise, and nausea have also been observed. Inhaled adenosine has been reported to induce bronchoconstriction in asthmatics (26)—the effect of IV adenosine in patients with preexisting obstructive airway disease is not known, as most clinical trials have excluded asthmatics. Adenosine should therefore be used with caution in these patients. Adverse effects after IV adenosine abate within 1 to 2 min and are therefore limited in most patients.

Despite the action of adenosine to reduce systemic vascular resistance, IV boluses are well tolerated hemodynamically. Blood pressure remains unchanged or may even increase at the time of conversion to sinus rhythm. Masking of peripheral vasodilation in conscious subjects receiving bolus doses may be the result of autonomic reflexes. The lack of negative inotropic effect gives a theoretic advantage for adenosine in patients with severe heart failure, however trials in this population are lacking.

Postconversion arrhythmias or conduction disorders occur in up to 60% of patients receiving adenosine. Sinus bradycardia, sinus tachycardia, sinus arrest, and various degrees of AV block last less than 1 to 2 min and do not require intervention in most patients. However caution should be exercised in patients with sinus node disease, as sinus arrest for up to 4 sec has been observed (29). Premature atrial or ventricular impulses after conversion to sinus rhythm occur in 33 to 60% of patients (28, 29). This may reinitiate reentry, an effect that is more common after adenosine than after verapamil.

Drug interactions with adenosine may involve alterations in extra- and intracellular transport as well as receptor affinity. While many drugs have in vitro or theoretic mechanisms for interaction, systematic clinical trials are lacking. Interactions with dipyridamole and theophylline have the strongest documentation. Dipyridamole blocks the cellular uptake of adenosine, thereby inhibiting its metabolism (33). This may enhance the negative chronotropic and dromotropic effects of adenosine. Very limited evidence suggests a similar effect with diazepam. Aminophylline and theophylline bind to the extracellular adenosine receptor sites and therefore act as competitive antagonists (26). Patients receiving these drugs (and possibly caffeine) may exhibit a blunted response to adenosine. The possible role of calcium in the pharmacologic effect of adenosine suggests potential interactions with calcium-channel blockers and digoxin, however these have not been well studied. The clinical implications of these interactions have not been established. Adenosine's ultrashort duration of action should minimize long-term effects of any drug interactions observed.

The standard adult dose of adenosine is 6 mg given by rapid IV bolus over 1 to 2 sec, followed by a normal saline flush. If no response is observed in 2 min, 12 mg IV may be given. A second 12-mg dose may be given in 1 to 2 min if needed. Clinical trials in infants and children have used doses of 0.0375 to 0.25 mg/kg (30), but the drug is not FDA-approved for pediatric use. The ultra-short half-life of the drug mandates careful attention to the site and rate of administration. The pharmacologic effect depends on the amount of drug delivered to the heart. A slow administration rate or slow rate of blood flow (e.g., heart failure) may result in significant metabolism before the drug reaches the heart and therefore attenuate the effect of the drug. Conversely, administration into central veins (e.g., femoral vein during electrophysiologic studies) may result in a more marked response. Reflex tachycardia due to vasodilation has been reported after slow administration. Individual variation in underlying autonomic tone as well as the administration of other antiarrhythmics may enhance or attenuate the effect of adenosine.

The very high efficacy rate of adenosine is comparable to or perhaps even better than that of verapamil. It can restore sinus rhythm more rapidly than verapamil, although the clinical importance of this is unclear. The lack of negative inotropic and hypotensive effects makes it especially useful in patients with heart failure or hypotension. However DC cardioversion remains the treatment of choice in severe hemodynamic instability. The very short half-life allows rapid titration of individual doses, reduces concern for long-lasting or cumulative adverse effects and minimizes the importance of drug interactions. Adenosine is an ideal drug for studying arrhythmias in the electrophysiology laboratory. However, the short half-life may also be a limitation, because of the recurrence of reentry and lack of utility for long-term prophylaxis. Moreover the prevalence of adverse reactions is high compared with verapamil. Verapamil and adenosine share the need for cautious use in patients with sinus node dysfunction, conduction system disease, or Wolff-Parkinson-White syndrome. Adenosine is preferred in patients with hypotension or heart failure, while verapamil is favored in patients with obstructive airway disease or those taking dipyridamole or methylxanthines (and possibly benzodiazepines, β-blockers, and digoxin).

Monitoring parameters include heart rate and rhythm and blood pressure. Patient's subjective assessment of side effects can be a major limitation in treatment—some clinical trial participants have refused to complete studies because of adverse effects. The pharmacist should inform the patient of the likelihood and nature of noncardiac adverse effects, as well as their duration and lack of cardiac significance.

Pharmacologic Vagal Stimulation. If vagal maneuvers, verapamil, and adenosine are unsuccessful, pharmacologic vagal stimulation may be attempted. Edrophonium (5 to 10 mg IV) inhibits acetylcholinesterase, resulting in a direct vagal effect. Metaraminol (0.5 to 2 mg IV), phenylephrine (0.5 mg IV), or methoxamine (5 to 15 mg IV) will transiently raise blood pressure (to a goal of systolic 160 to 170 mm Hg), stimulate the carotid baroreceptors, and induce a reflex increase in vagal tone. These drugs should be preceded and followed by vagotonic maneuvers. They should be used with caution in patients with baseline sinus node dysfunction. Further caution is advised when using edrophonium in patients receiving digoxin, and with pressor agents in patients with severe congestive heart failure. Although their use in adults has been largely surpassed by verapamil and adenosine, these drugs maintain their usefulness in infants and children.

Other Drugs. Digoxin, propranolol, quinidine, and procainamide may also be used to terminate AV nodal or AV reentry. Digoxin has a lower response rate and a longer onset of action for conversion to sinus rhythm (several hours) than verapamil. It produces direct slowing of AV conduction by a different mechanism (vagal and antiadrenergic effects block AV nodal conduction) (Table 37.2). Patients who fail to respond to other drugs or maneuvers may respond to digoxin, especially children without accessory pathway conduction. Digoxin is also useful in patients with severe left ventricular dysfunction. Specific aspects of digoxin therapy are discussed under "Atrial Fibrillation."

Propranolol prolongs antegrade AV conduction and refractoriness and also depresses automaticity at the SA node, AV junction, and His-Purkinje fibers (Table 37.2). Propranolol is not a first-line drug because it is less efficacious than verapamil and adenosine and is contraindicated in patients who have received verapamil, because of the additive effects on cardiac conduction and contractility. It is primarily used in infants and children who have not received verapamil when digoxin is not desirable (e.g., accessory pathway conduction). Metoprolol and esmolol have the advantages of cardioselectivity and an ultra-short half-life, respectively.

Quinidine, procainamide, encainide, flecainide, and propafenone block conduction in the fast (usually retrograde) pathway (Table 37.2). They are not as effective in AV nodal or AV reentry and are reserved for refractory cases. They may be useful in cases where supraventricular and ventricular tachyarrhythmias cannot be distinguished.

Pacemakers. Patients who fail to respond to pharmacologic strategies should receive electrical therapy, which may include DC cardioversion (as above) or specialized pacing techniques. Pacing techniques include 1 to 2 critically timed extra stimuli or a rapid sequence of impulses (burst overdrive pacing) (34). As a rule, burst-pacing techniques are more effective. The goal of pacing is to create a strategically timed region of refractoriness. The paced impulse enters the circuit, collides with the advancing wavefront, blocks the succeeding wavefront, and stops the reentry circuit. Close proximity of the pacing site to the anatomic origin of the arrhythmia enhances the likelihood of success. Though highly effective, pacing is an invasive technique requiring transvenous or transesophageal catheter placement and electrophysiologic studies for application. Complications include tachycardia acceleration and fibrillation of the paced chamber(s).

Chronic Treatment

The need for prophylaxis is dictated by the frequency of episodes, the tachycardia rate, and its hemodynamic effects. In general, the presence and extent of symptoms are related to the rate and duration of the arrhythmia. The benefits of arrhythmia suppression must be balanced carefully against the risks and inconveniences of long-term antiarrhythmic therapy. In the absence of heart disease, most patients have infrequent attacks of short duration without cardiovascular compromise and do not require chronic suppression. Patients with underlying heart disease, frequent attacks, or debilitating symptoms (syncope, angina, hypotension, heart failure) may benefit from prophylaxis.

The goal of chronic prophylaxis is to prevent or minimize the frequency of attacks and their hemodynamic consequences. Complete abolition is not necessary and may be worse than no therapy because of proarrhythmic or other adverse drug effects. Precipitating factors such as sympathomimetics, β-agonists, caffeine, tobacco, or ethanol should be limited or discontinued. Patients with arrhythmias responsive to physical maneuvers such as carotid sinus pressure should be instructed in their proper application. This may obviate the need for pharmacologic prophylaxis.

Ideally, treatment should be guided by electrophysiologic studies (EPS). Percutaneously inserted catheters are positioned in the heart to permit repetitive initiation and termination of arrhythmias, to identify the site of origin and mechanism of the arrhythmia, as well as to evaluate the efficacy of drugs and other maneuvers. Suppression of induced arrhythmias in the laboratory is often a valuable predictor of efficacy for subsequent episodes. EPS therefore serve the following functions:

1. To rapidly achieve a therapeutic regimen in patients with hemodynamically serious consequences such as syncope, hypotension, or heart failure. EPS permit expeditious trials of multiple antiarrhythmic drugs or techniques. Identification of serum level–antiarrhythmic effect relationships may allow individualized targeting of drug doses.
2. To accurately characterize the electrophysiologic mechanism of the arrhythmia. This allows more rational drug or technique selection.
3. To identify the underlying mechanism prior to the institution of nonpharmacologic options such as pacemakers, surgery, or catheter ablation.
4. To identify symptomatic patients with Wolff-Parkinson-White syndrome who are at risk for developing life-threatening arrhythmias.

EPS are limited by poor predictability of response in as many as one-third of patients. This is sometimes explained by alterations in autonomic tone at the time of spontaneous arrhythmia recurrence—EPS are performed in the resting, supine state whereas arrhythmias recur in ambulatory patients. These differences in sympathetic tone alter the electrophysiologic characteristics and response to drugs. Furthermore, EPS are costly and uncomfortable. Some practitioners therefore prefer to treat patients with well-tolerated arrhythmias empirically, reserving EPS for patients who fail initial strategies.

Strategies for the pharmacologic prophylaxis of AV nodal reentry are not as well established as those for managing acute episodes. Many therapeutic options exist, some or all of which may give a satisfactory outcome. As a rule, patient response is not as predictable and efficacy rates are lower than for acute episodes, with no one drug emerging as the treatment of choice. Initial selections are based on specific patient considerations, dosing intervals, side-effect profile, cost of drugs and monitoring tests, and physician preference or experience. Treatment may be directed at either the antegrade or retrograde pathway. Calcium-channel blockers, digoxin, or β-blockers are common initial choices. Quinidine is also efficacious, but it requires hospitalization for the first few days of therapy, because of potential proarrhythmic events. Nondrug therapies include antitachycardia pacemakers and surgery to ablate or modify the AV node.

Verapamil. Despite its excellent IV efficacy for acute episodes of AV nodal reentry, oral verapamil has been less successful in the prophylaxis of recurrent arrhythmias. Efficacy varies between 40 and 90%. Successful termination with IV verapamil does not predict long-term efficacy with p.o. treatment. Serum levels required for specific AV node conduction effects are higher after p.o. (in comparison to IV) administration (15, 18). The lower potency of oral dosing may result from stereospecific presystemic metabolism of racemic verapamil, which causes preferential hepatic extraction of the more active l-isomer (18, 19). Since the l-isomer accounts for most of the AV nodal effect, this may explain both the more frequent therapeutic failures as well as the wide variability in serum level–response data (19). Alterations in autonomic tone at the time of arrhythmia recurrence further modulate the efficacy of verapamil.

Initial daily doses of 120 to 240 mg are titrated to average maintenance doses of 240 to 480 mg. The sustained-release preparations offer comparable bioavailability, slower absorption with less fluctuation, and more sustained serum levels, permitting once- or twice-daily dosing. Observations of significant nonlinear accumulation with a prolonged half-life after chronic oral dosing may permit a longer dosing interval for the conventional tablets as well (16).

Oral verapamil is very well tolerated in most patients. Smooth muscle relaxation in the gastrointestinal tract may cause constipation. Peripheral edema and headache may also be seen. Verapamil does not aggravate bronchospastic or vasospastic disorders and so is safer in patients unable to take β-blockers.

Monitoring parameters for oral verapamil therapy include cardiac rhythm and rate, constipation, and peripheral edema. Routine serum-level monitoring is not advised.

Digoxin. The suppressant effect of digoxin on AV nodal conduction occurs via a mechanism different from that of verapamil. It is particularly useful in infants and children, often as a single agent, after Wolff-Parkinson White syndrome with antegrade accessory pathway conduction has been excluded. Its positive inotropic effect is unique amongst the common antiarrhythmics and permits its use in patients with heart failure. The ideal digoxin dose is one that controls the ventricular rate during the tachyarrhythmia yet does not cause bradycardia while in sinus rhythm. Specific aspects of digoxin therapy are discussed under "Atrial Fibrillation."

Quinidine. Quinidine is a prototype class Ia drug that differs from digoxin and verapamil by its action on the fast (sodium) channel. Its net effect reflects a modification of its direct action by an indirect vagolytic effect. The direct action is a generalized slowing of both automaticity and conduction velocity in the SA node, AV node, and His-Purkinje systems. Vagolysis overrides many of these effects, resulting in a *net increase* in sinus rate and AV nodal conduction velocity. His-Purkinje conduction time remains delayed, reflecting minimal autonomic influence in these tissues. The effects of quinidine are minimal in healthy well-polarized tissues and most marked at rapid heart rates, in ectopic pacemakers, and in hypoxic or ischemic tissues. Peripheral α-adrenergic blockade and relaxation of vascular smooth muscle associated with IV administration may further influence cardiac action. Alteration of baseline susceptibility to the direct or indirect action of quinidine may explain interpatient variation in net effect.

The efficacy of quinidine in supraventricular tachycardias results from a decrease in atrial ectopy, thus suppressing the inciting premature impulses, as well as a slowing of conduction in the retrograde fast path (Table 37.2). It is not useful after reentry has begun and may even be deleterious because of an increase in AV nodal conduction velocity. Patients should therefore be "digitalized" before initiation of quinidine therapy for supraventricular tachyarrhythmias. Interestingly, controlled studies of quinidine in AV nodal reentry are lacking, despite widespread clinical use.

After oral administration, quinidine demonstrates variable absorption and first-pass effect, resulting in about 70% bioavailability (range 45 to 100%) (35). Peak serum concentrations are seen at 1 to 2 hr for the standard formulation of the sulfate salt and 3 to 5 hr with the sustained-release formulations of the sulfate and gluconate salts. The rate and extent of absorption is reduced in patients with heart failure (36). Quinidine is 80 to 89% protein-bound to albumin and α-1 acid glycoprotein. It demonstrates two-compartment kinetics, with average distribution and elimination phase half-lives of 7 min and 6 to 7 hr, respectively (35). The steady-state distribution volume in normals is 3 liters/kg (35). About 85% is metabolized to several active and inactive forms, including 3-hydroxyquinidine, 2-oxo-quinidinone, and quinidine-*N*-oxide. Ten to 20% is eliminated unchanged in the urine in 24 hr, primarily by glomerular filtration. Total clearance averaging 4.5 ml/min/

kg is widely variable and may be dose- and route of administration–dependent (35, 37).

Quinidine metabolites may contribute to both the antiarrhythmic and proarrhythmic effects (38). Total serum levels of 3-hydroxyquinidine are lower than those of the parent compound, but a higher unbound fraction results in free metabolite levels comparable to those of the parent drug (37). Both quinidine and 3-hydroxyquinidine may accumulate with multiple dosing, resulting in higher serum levels as well as an increase in QTc interval prolongation (37).

Patients with congestive heart failure have a decreased volume of distribution and total clearance, without an alteration in half-life (36). Increased levels of α-1 acid glycoprotein concentration commonly observed after acute myocardial infarction may result in diminished drug effect because of more extensive protein binding (39). Patients with cirrhosis demonstrate decreased protein binding, an increased half-life and volume of distribution, and no change in total clearance (35). A diminished volume of distribution and renal clearance without change in half-life are seen with renal failure.

Quinidine is available in several salts: quinidine sulfate (83% base), quinidine gluconate (62% base), and quinidine polygalacturonate (60% base). Since dosages are expressed as the salt rather than the base, it is important to account for the different potencies when switching forms. The usual daily dose is 200 to 400 mg of the sulfate salt or its equivalent 3 to 4 times daily for the conventional tablets. Dosage should be decreased in congestive heart failure and (possibly) cirrhosis. Children and young adults (<30 years) may require higher doses. Dosage adjustment in renal insufficiency is controversial.

IV administration has traditionally been discouraged because of dose- and rate-related hypotension caused by α-adrenergic blockade and a direct peripheral venodilation. Reports suggest that IV administration is safe when given no faster than 0.5 mg/kg/min to a total dosage of 10 mg/kg of quinidine gluconate, with careful blood pressure monitoring (40). Administration i.m. is not advised, as it gives erratic absorption, is painful, and may result in sterile abscess formation.

The utility of serum level monitoring is hindered by the nonspecificity of common analytic methods. The parent drug, its metabolites, and dihydroquinidine (a known impurity in commercial grade drug) may all be detected to varying degrees. The different pharmacokinetic and pharmacodynamic profiles of these compounds obscure the relationship between serum levels and therapeutic or adverse effects. Assays of total (bound and unbound) quinidine are further limited in diseases such as acute myocardial infarction, where the extent of protein binding can vary from day to day. High-performance liquid chromatography (HPLC) is considered the most specific and therefore the reference procedure, with a therapeutic range of 1 to 3 to 4 μg/ml (39). The double extraction photofluorometric and enzyme immunoassay (EMIT) assays have therapeutic ranges of 2 to 5 μg/ml. Individualized "target serum level" goals based on clinical or EPS response may be more useful than values based on population parameters. It is also important to recognize that "therapeutic range" estimates derived from trials of ventricular arrhythmias may not be applicable to supraventricular tachycardias. Serum level measurement is therefore useful in suspected noncompliance or toxicity but may not be necessary in well-controlled patients without clinical toxicity.

Adverse effects occur in as many as 30 to 50% of patients taking quinidine, with 14% of 652 patients in the Boston Collaborative Drug Surveillance Program (41) requiring drug discontinuation. Gastrointestinal reactions, primarily diarrhea with or without nausea, were particularly troublesome and the most common reason for discontinuing therapy, accounting for 7.8%. Fever was seen in 1.7%. Various dermatologic reactions, cinchonism (tinnitus, dizziness, hearing and visual disturbances) and hematologic reactions (thrombocytopenia, hemolytic anemia) each occurred in less than 1% of patients. As a rule, patients who do not have disabling gastrointestinal side effects have excellent long-term tolerance of quinidine.

The most serious cardiac reaction is exacerbation of arrhythmias. This may manifest as the induction of a new arrhythmia or conversion of an existing stable arrhythmia to an unstable one. Paroxysmal syncope or presyncope is correlated on ECG with intermittent pleomorphic ventricular tachycardia or fibrillation, often of the *torsade de pointes* pattern. It typically follows a pause or abrupt decrease in ventricular rate. The first tachycardic QRS complex occurs as a triggered response, emerging from a large postpause U-wave. The intervening sinus beats often demonstrate a markedly prolonged QTc interval. *Torsade de pointes* occurs in 2 to 3% of patients begun on quinidine (38). Patients with pretreatment QT prolongation, bradycardia, hypokalemia, hypomagnesemia, heart block, and heart failure (or possibly those taking digoxin) (25) are at increased risk. Proarrhythmic effects can appear at any time, generally within 3 to 5 days after initiation of therapy or dose increase. As many as 50% will have serum levels <2 μg/ml, reflecting the idiosyncratic rather than toxic nature of the reaction (38). In vitro testing suggests that quinidine metabolites or impurities may also contribute to the proarrhythmic effect (38). Proarrhythmic events are less common in patients with SVTs, compared with ventricular arrhythmias, possibly because SVT patients are more likely to have structurally normal hearts. Most episodes are self-limiting and usually abate 12 to 24 hr after discontinuing the drug. Some patients develop cardiovascular insufficiency or collapse. Treatment is limited to dis-

continuation of the drug, maintaining serum potassium levels at or above normal, DC cardioversion, or overdrive pacing; most antiarrhythmic drugs are ineffective.

Other cardiovascular reactions include bradyarrhythmias or an increased ventricular rate in patients with atrial fibrillation. Hypotension following IV administration of quinidine is minimized by slow infusion rates. Symptomatic hypotension is treated by administration of fluids and a reduction in the infusion rate.

The interaction of quinidine with digoxin is particularly important in the management of supraventricular tachycardias, as the concomitant use of digoxin is important to protect the AV node from the vagolytic effect of quinidine. Reduction of the digoxin dose is often necessary. Other drug interactions of quinidine include those with hepatic enzyme inducers (phenobarbital, phenytoin, rifampin) or inhibitors (cimetidine), and warfarin.

Monitoring guidelines for quinidine in AV nodal reentry prophylaxis include heart rate and rhythm, QRS and QTc intervals, and gastrointestinal symptoms. Patients with intolerable gastrointestinal reactions should be evaluated on a different salt or on a sustained-release preparation (at an equivalent dose) before switching to another drug. Administration with food may also lessen symptoms. Serum levels may be monitored, but the laboratory should be contacted to determine assay methodology, its limitations, and the recommended therapeutic range. To facilitate detection and treatment of proarrhythmic events, patients should be hospitalized for the first 3 to 5 days of therapy.

β-Blockers. Propanolol and the other β-blocking agents have many effects on cardiac conduction and contractility. Their efficacy in supraventricular tachycardias results from a slowing of automaticity in sinus and ectopic pacemakers, a decrease in conduction velocity through the AV node, and an increase in the refractory period of the AV node (Table 37.2). "Quinidine-like" membrane-stabilizing properties are seen only at very high doses and do not contribute to arrhythmia control. When successful during EPS evaluation, long-term efficacy is very good. Despite their numerous adverse effects and contraindications, these agents retain their usefulness in the prophylaxis of AV nodal reentry because their mechanism of action differs from that of the other commonly used drugs. They are especially useful in supraventricular tachycardias associated with excessive catecholamine release as in hyperthyroidism, pheochromocytoma, exercise, or emotional upset. A reduction in exercise tolerance may be bothersome in young patients. In theory, most of the currently available β-blocking drugs should be effective in supraventricular tachycardias; however large-scale studies are lacking. Dosage requirements for propranolol and the other β-blockers are difficult to predict, because of variation in the response of individual patients to fixed concentrations of drug. Underlying sympathetic tone and variations in pharmacokinetics further modify patient response. Other aspects of β-blockers are discussed under "Sudden Death."

Other Drugs. Procainamide, disopyramide, flecainide, encainide, and amiodarone all have good efficacy in controlling AV nodal reentry. Unfortunately, adverse effects relegate them to a secondary role. The proarrhythmic effects of flecainide and encainide are major limitations. These drugs should be used with careful observation, especially in patients with structural heart disease.

Nonpharmacologic Therapies. Nonpharmacologic therapies for AV nodal reentry include pacemakers, surgical interruption of the reentry circuit, and percutaneous catheter ablation or modification. They are indicated when medical therapy is ineffective or not tolerated. Since these modalities allow patients to remain drug-free, noncompliant patients, younger patients unwilling to comply with lifelong drug treatment, or females desiring pregnancy may also be candidates. Extensive EPS and cardiac-mapping studies are important in maximizing success.

Pacemakers. Permanent pacemakers have been used in the chronic management of AV nodal reentry for many years. They either minimize arrhythmia genesis or terminate tachycardias after they occur. Overdrive pacing at a rate slightly faster than the sinus rate, or programmed atrial and ventricular stimulation will alter refractoriness in the limbs of the reentrant circuit and therefore prevent the arrhythmia. Techniques for terminating tachycardia are the same as those discussed under "acute management" (34). The most sophisticated devices are activated automatically by a sensing function, may be programmed both before and after insertion, and have a memory function that remembers and delivers an algorithm of previously successful terminating sequences. Unfortunately, reliable termination of AV nodal reentry requires concomitant antiarrhythmic drug therapy in as many as 50% of patients receiving pacemakers (34). Adverse effects include precipitation of tachyarrhythmias, syncope, and sudden death, especially in patients with accessory pathways. Additionally, pacemakers require regular checks and reprogramming, may not eliminate symptoms, and are not curative. This last limitation has become more meaningful as surgical methods offering complete cure have evolved. Patients with sinus node disease are ideal candidates, as the pacemaker can manage both tachycardic and bradycardic episodes. They are also useful in those who are not candidates for surgery or who refuse surgery.

Surgery. Surgical techniques include (*a*) careful dissection of the perinodal tissue to alter intranodal or accessory pathway conduction, which is especially useful in the Wolff-Parkinson-White syndrome or (*b*) cryoablation of atrial fibers around the AV node to abolish extranodal retrograde pathways while preserving antegrade conduction (42). These procedures have been studied in both adults and children, primarily with AV nodal reentry or AV reentry using an accessory pathway. They are highly successful on short-term evaluation but incur the typical risks and limitations of open chest procedures.

Percutaneous Catheter Modification of the AV Node. Recent refinements in technique have allowed the sophisticated goal of selective modification of the AV node using percutaneously placed catheters. Antegrade conduction is preserved, but retrograde pathway conduction is abolished or impaired, by using various energy sources (direct current, radiofrequency, or laser) to modify the AV node and surrounding tissues. Complications include complete AV block or new atrial arrhythmias. The percutaneous approach has the advantage of avoiding an open chest procedure with cardiopulmonary bypass. However, present experience is limited, and large-scale trials with long-term follow-up are lacking.

Nonpharmacologic strategies for the management of AV nodal reentry and AV reentry associated with an accessory pathway are evolving rapidly. Their primary use at present is limited to patients who are resistant or intolerant to antiarrhythmic drug therapy. Their expeditious, cost-effective, and curative features are major attributes. As technologies are developed and refined, nonpharmacologic therapy is likely to be useful in a wide spectrum of populations.

ECTOPIC ATRIAL TACHYCARDIA

Enhanced automaticity (ability to generate spontaneous impulses) of an ectopic atrial focus may result in an arrhythmia known as ectopic atrial tachycardia. Like reentry, it is initiated by a premature atrial impulse. Unlike reentry, this arrhythmia is characterized by a "warm-up period" with gradual acceleration and termination via a gradual deceleration. The ventricular rate ranges from 100 to 280 beats per min. Periods of AV block are common. This arrhythmia is important because ectopic atrial tachycardia with block in a patient taking digitalis is highly suspicious for toxicity. Other acute causes include acute myocardial infarction, trauma, chronic lung disease, or certain metabolic abnormalities.

Multifocal atrial tachycardia (MAT) is a form of ectopic atrial tachycardia thought to be caused by either enhanced automaticity or triggered activity (43). On ECG, at least three different ectopic P-wave morphologies are seen, representing ≥3 ectopic foci, with irregular PR- and PP-intervals. The ventricular rate of 130 to 220 beats/min is variable ("irregularly irregular") during the tachycardic episodes. This allows differentiation from AV nodal or AV reentry but may result in confusion with atrial fibrillation. MAT is seen in 0.3 to 0.4% of hospitalized patients. It occurs typically in elderly patients with chronic lung or heart disease who are critically ill with acute pulmonary or cardiac failure or sepsis. It is associated with an elevation in circulating catecholamines and may be precipitated by hypoxia, electrolyte disturbances, acid-base disorders, or drugs such as methylxanthines or β-agonists.

Ectopic atrial tachycardia is often nonresponsive to standard antiarrhythmics or pacing. Vagal maneuvers, verapamil, adenosine, and digoxin commonly initiate or increase AV block, thereby slowing the ventricular rate. However, the atrial rate remains unchanged and the arrhythmia persists. Special care must be exercised in treatment with digoxin, as this drug may *induce* ectopic atrial tachycardia. In cases of suspected digitalis-induced arrhythmia, potassium is the agent of choice, as it will counteract the action of digitalis at the cellular level. Phenytoin, lidocaine, propranolol, or digoxin-immune Fab fragments may also be used. DC cardioversion is dangerous in digitalis toxicity, as it may precipitate intractable ventricular arrhythmias.

MAT is often difficult to manage. Pharmacologic attempts to block the AV node or decrease ectopic activity are rarely successful. Trials of digoxin, quinidine, procainamide, phenytoin, and lidocaine have been disappointing. Surgery to resect or ablate the ectopic foci, as well as electrical modalities (pacing or DC countershock), are also ineffective. Treatment of the underlying disease is the only reliable therapy. Correction of predisposing factors will terminate the arrhythmia in most patients, though recurrence is common. Verapamil (44) and metoprolol (45) have been reported to slow the ventricular rate, reduce atrial ectopy, and/or reduce abnormal atrial or AV junctional-triggered activity. In one trial, metoprolol was associated with a larger reduction in ventricular rate and higher rate of conversion to sinus rhythm (46) than verapamil. However, the hypotensive and adverse pulmonary effects of these drugs limit their utility. They should be reserved for patients with symptoms of hypoperfusion. The high mortality rate of patients with MAT (40 to 50%) is due to the underlying condition, not the arrhythmia. Antiarrhythmics have not been shown to reduce mortality.

ATRIAL FIBRILLATION

Atrial fibrillation (AF) is characterized by rapid, chaotic atrial firing at a rate of 350 to 600 beats/min ("auricular delirium"). The AV node blocks most impulses, resulting in random, irregular ventricular conduction averaging 100 to 180 impulses/min in untreated cases. Ventricular (His-Purkinje) conduction is usually normal. AF is thought to be caused by intraatrial reentry. Uneven refractoriness of adjacent atrial tissues allows the formation of multiple reentrant wavelets. These wavelets become wandering reentry circuits completely dissociated from one another. AF may be chronic, paroxysmal, or a single, isolated occurrence. Transition from paroxysmal to chronic AF depends on the underlying etiology and the duration of paroxysmal episodes. AF is the most common *sustained* arrhythmia, and the second most common overall.

The prevalence of AF is about 0.4% in individuals under 60 years old and 2 to 4% for those over 60 years (47). Paroxysmal or single isolated episodes of AF are seen with cardiac surgery, fever, infection, pulmonary embolism, ethanol intoxication, or drug toxicity (sympathomimetics, β-agonists, methylxanthines). AF is also seen in 10 to 15% of patients with acute myocardial infarction (6), usually lasting less than 24 hr. Chronic AF is associated with congestive heart failure, coronary artery disease, rheumatic heart disease, dilated or hypertrophic cardiomyopathy, hypertensive heart disease, hyperthyroidism, and certain congenital heart diseases. AF without associated cardiovascular disease ("lone AF") occurs in 0.5 to 30%, with the wide range reflecting different definitions and populations (48).

The principal hemodynamic effects of AF result from (*a*) a shortened diastolic filling time, leading to decreased left ventricular end-diastolic volume and stroke volume and (*b*) a loss of synchronized atrial contraction, resulting in increased mean left atrial pressure in addition to the above two effects. Loss of atrial systole causes a 20 to 30% reduction in stroke volume in normals, which is increased in patients with heart disease. When coupled with incomplete ventricular filling, the net effect is a decrease in cardiac reserve. Elevations in heart rate are initially associated with an increased cardiac output. Once a critical rate is exceeded, ventricular filling time becomes a limiting factor, and further increases in heart rate result in reduced cardiac output.

The nonhemodynamic consequence of AF is embolism resulting from turbulent blood flow through the atria with mural thrombus formation. Embolic risk is highest in the first 2 to 4 weeks after the onset of AF and at the time of transition from paroxysmal to chronic AF. In some patients the embolic event is the presenting manifestation of previously undetected AF. Embolism to arteries in the cerebral circulation is most common and accounts for about 7% of all strokes (49). Other locations include the extremity, mesenteric, coronary, and renal circulations. Framingham study patients with chronic AF due to rheumatic mitral valve disease were found to have a 17.6-fold increase in stroke risk, with a 5.6-fold increase for AF of other causes (50). Risk factors for embolism in chronic AF include a history of embolic stroke or an association with advanced age, congestive heart failure, and possibly left atrial enlargement (48). In patients with lone AF, stroke risk is low in young but probably higher in older patients and those with hypertension.

The clinical manifestations of AF include the signs and symptoms of congestive heart failure, most commonly in the pulmonary system, and are exacerbated with exercise. Some patients may develop angina or symptoms of cerebral insufficiency such as confusion, fatigue, or syncope. Palpitations may be especially troublesome in patients with paroxysmal AF. Elderly patients with diseased AV nodes may have slow ventricular rates at rest but will nonetheless have reduced cardiac reserve with exercise or stress. As many as 30% of patients with AF are asymptomatic at the time of diagnosis (51). Irregular apical and radial pulses result from random impulse transmission through the AV node and are the classic physical signs of AF. ECG findings include a lack of discrete atrial activity, variable R-R intervals, normal-appearing QRS complexes (unless aberrant conduction or bundle branch block are present), and an irregular baseline between QRS complexes.

ACUTE TREATMENT

The primary goal of the acute management of AF is to correct the hemodynamic manifestations by increasing cardiac output. This is usually accomplished by pharmacologic slowing of the ventricular rate, which lengthens diastolic filling time and increases stroke volume. Conversion to sinus rhythm in the acute phase is reserved for patients with hemodynamic instability. The optical ventricular rate for maximizing cardiac output is unknown. An arbitrary ventricular rate of less than 100 beats/min is often chosen as a therapeutic goal. However, the following therapeutic aspects must be emphasized: (a) Strict attention to ventricular rate should not be at the expense of objective and symptomatic relief or of drug intoxication; (b) Underlying factors favoring tachycardia should be considered, especially excess catecholamine release as in infection, hyperthyroidism, or sympathomimetic drug overdose. In these patients, a rate of 100 to 120 beats/min may be acceptable as long as the signs and symptoms are controlled. Strict adherence to a goal of a rate less than 100 beats/min may result in bradycardia when the underlying problem is corrected. Rate titration should consider the clinical appearance of the patient as well as the anticipated rapidity of catecholamine correction. (c) Aggressive treatment of coexisting conditions such as fever, infection, hypoxia, anemia, or hyperthyroidism is essential.

A review of the role of the AV node in AF is useful in understanding the pharmacologic management. The AV node is not involved in the initiation and perpetuation of AF per se, but plays a critical role as a "filter" of atrial impulses. The AV node is the primary determinant of ventricular rate n AF. In contrast, the SA node determines the rate in sinus rhythm. The intrinsic conductivity of AV nodal tissues as well as extracardiac factors that may alter conduction (autonomic tone, drugs) have a critical influence on ventricular rate. Vagal stimulation results in increased "filtering" and less conduction across the AV node. Increased sympathetic tone enhances AV nodal conduction, resulting in an inappropriate excessive increase in ventricular rate with exercise or stress. Control of ven-

tricular rate both at rest and during exercise is important in maintaining the function of the patient. However changes in AV nodal conductivity will not terminate the arrhythmia.

Digoxin. Digitalis is generally considered the drug of choice for the acute control of ventricular rate. Digitalis has positive inotropic and negative chronotropic and dromotropic properties. The last effect accounts for its efficacy in AF, is seen only at higher doses, and occurs via a variety of mechanisms. The predominant effect is indirect via vagal stimulation, with direct AV nodal action having a minor role. This vagotonic effect is largely attenuated by catecholamines, explaining the limited ability to control ventricular rates during exercise or stress (52–54). Digitalis does not suppress ectopy; most patients remain in AF. The effect of digitalis on accessory pathways differs from that on the AV node, and it should not be used in patients with AF and the Wolff-Parkinson-White syndrome (referred to in a separate section).

Optimally, individual digoxin-loading doses are determined based on the observed response to initial therapy. Doses of 0.5 mg IV are followed by 0.125 to 0.25 mg IV or p.o. every 4 to 8 hr until the desired response is seen. The dose and interval should take into account the time for tissue distribution of 6 to 8 hr. This regimen will usually result in rate control in 12 to 24 hr. Administration i.m. is not advised because of erratic absorption and excessive pain at the injection site. Infants, children, and patients with hyperthyroidism may require higher than estimated doses, while those with coronary artery disease or obstructive airway disease may be especially sensitive to digitalis. Oral maintenance doses for AF average 0.25 to 0.375 mg daily in adult patients with normal renal function. Calculated doses may be used as a guideline, but the clinical response of the patient is a better criterion of efficacy.

Monitoring parameters for digoxin in AF include ventricular rate (apical pulse) and the signs and symptoms of congestive heart failure. The radial (peripheral) pulse is NOT an appropriate monitoring criterion, as it may not reflect efficacy in patients with very high apical rates. In these patients, some ventricular contractions may not elicit detectable peripheral pulses, causing a "pulse deficit." Renal function and serum electrolytes (especially potassium and magnesium) should also be monitored, along with observation for signs and symptoms of toxicity. The use of serum levels as a guide to dosage requirements is not advised in the management of supraventricular tachycardias such as AV nodal reentry and AF. Correlation between therapeutic response (i.e., ventricular rate) and serum levels is poor (55, 56). This is probably because other factors (underlying autonomic tone, exogenous catecholamines, electrolyte concentrations) alter cardiac sensitivity to digitalis, independent of serum levels. Despite this limitation, serum levels may be useful in evaluating patient compliance, suspected toxicity, or drug interactions. Levels should be drawn at least 6 to 8 hr after dosage administration to allow for tissue distribution.

Two drug interactions with digoxin are relevant to the management of supraventricular tachyarrhythmias. An elevation of serum digoxin levels to 2 to 3 times baseline occurs in most patients taking digoxin and quinidine concomitantly. Digoxin levels increase within hours after quinidine administration, reaching a new steady state in several days. This interaction depends on the serum level of quinidine but not that of digoxin and is caused by a decrease in volume of distribution and renal and nonrenal clearance of digoxin by quinidine. Since there is no evidence for an alteration of digoxin receptor site activity or sensitivity, digoxin toxicity may ensue. Reducing the dose by 50% as well as careful serum level monitoring are advised (25). Serum digoxin levels may be increased by a similar mechanism in patients receiving verapamil, with new steady-state digoxin levels achieved in 7 to 14 days. The clinical importance of this reaction is not well established, although some have recommended a digoxin dosage reduction by 50% (25).

The subjective evaluation of patients for digoxin toxicity is difficult because of the nonspecific nature of the symptoms. Anorexia, nausea, vomiting, weakness, and lethargy are the most common symptoms. Vision changes, disorientation, and hallucinations are less common. Elevated serum levels may assist in the diagnosis, however there is overlap between toxic and therapeutic values. Moreover, electrolyte abnormalities (hypokalemia, metabolic alkalosis, hypomagnesemia, or hypercalcemia) or hypoxia may contribute to clinical toxicity even at "nontoxic" serum levels. Toxic cardiac effects result from enhanced automaticity, promotion of triggered activity, and/or a depression of AV nodal conduction. A useful monitoring tool for toxicity in AF patients is the ECG. The excessive effects of digoxin result in an exaggerated AV nodal block, seen initially as occasional long equal pauses (intermittent junctional escape). Eventually, the ventricular rate becomes *regular* at 35 to 30 beats/min, reflecting complete junctional escape. At higher levels, junctional pacemaker firing may accelerate, causing a junctional tachycardia. PVCs caused by enhanced firing of ectopic ventricular foci are also common. As toxicity progresses, essentially all arrhythmias may be seen. Toxicity is managed by discontinuation of the drug, potassium unless contraindicated, antiarrhythmics, and/or digoxin-immune Fab fragments. Refer to the section "Digitalis-induced PVCs" for management details.

Other aspects of digoxin therapy may be found in Chapter 36, "Congestive Heart Failure."

Verapamil. Verapamil exerts a direct effect on the AV node, which is not mediated by the autonomic nervous system. Thus, in contrast to digoxin, verapamil retains its usefulness during exercise or stress. Some patients may demonstrate regularization of ventricular rate while remaining in AF; however this does not augment hemodynamic function (57). A lack of suppressant effect on ectopic foci results in conversion to sinus rhythm in only 10 to 15%, probably through improved hemodynamic function. Verapamil is prompt, reliable, effective, and relatively safe. The dose for AF is the same as that for AV nodal reentry: 5 to 10 mg (0.075–0.15 mg/kg) IV over 2 to 3 min, repeated in 30 min if needed. It has an onset of action of 5 to 10 min and duration of about 30 min after a bolus injection. Constant infusions of 5 mg/hr initially, titrated to a ventricular rate <100 per min, a systolic blood pressure ≥90 mm Hg, and a maximum dose of about 10 mg/hr for up to 7 days have been reported (58), although this is not an FDA-labeled method of administration. Infusions should be preceded by bolus doses as above. Because of its rapid onset of action and more predictable effect in patients with high circulating catecholamine levels, some practitioners consider verapamil to be the drug of choice over digoxin in AF (59). The primary limitation of verapamil is its negative inotropic effect. Downward dosage adjustment should be considered in patients with heart or liver failure because of impaired drug elimination. It should be used cautiously in patients receiving digoxin (because of the previously discussed drug interaction) and patients with Wolff-Parkinson-White syndrome. Monitoring parameters include the ECG, ventricular rate, blood pressure, and the signs and symptoms of heart failure. Other aspects of verapamil are discussed in the section "AV Nodal Reentry."

Successful treatment of AF and atrial flutter with intravenous diltiazem has been reported (60). This drug may be advantageous in its relative lack of hypotensive effect compared with verapamil; however the intravenous dosage form is not currently available in the United State.

Esmolol. The β-blocker esmolol demonstrates the typical effects of a cardioselective β-blocker without intrinsic sympathomimetic activity or membrane-stabilizing effects and demonstrates the additional unique property of an ultra-short duration of action. This permits its use to slow AV nodal conduction directly, with minimal concern for long-lasting adverse effects. Esmolol is hydrolyzed rapidly by red cell esterases, with distribution and elimination half-lives of 2 and 9 min, respectively (61). The total clearance of 17 to 20 liters/kg/hr reflects the largely hepatic elimination to methanol and a metabolite with minimal β-blocking activity (61, 62). Esmolol is initiated with a loading dose of 500 μg/kg for 1 min, followed by maintenance infusions of 50 to 300 μg/kg/min. If control is not established, the loading dose is repeated and the infusion rate increased. Dosage adjustments may be made as often as every 5 to 15 min. Most patients respond at 100 μg/kg/min.

Clinical trials have shown esmolol to be comparable to propranolol in reducing the ventricular rate in supraventricular tachycardias, with an overall response rate of 64 to 72%, including 6 to 14% who converted to sinus rhythm (61–63). Comparative studies with verapamil have shown similar reductions in ventricular rate, with a higher number of patients converting to sinus rhythm after esmolol (64). The onset of action is less than 5 min, with a return to baseline heart rate 10 to 20 min after discontinuation. Esmolol therefore offers the flexibility to continually and rapidly titrate the dosage to the desired effect. Further, there is an added element of safety should adverse effects occur.

The primary adverse effect is hypotension, occurring in 33 to 44% of patients (61, 63). Hypotension is most common at doses ≥200 μg/kg/min, in postoperative or elderly patients over 65 years old, or in those with baseline hypotension (63). Most patients remain asymptomatic and are managed by a reduction in dosage. Severe hypotension may require discontinuation, with blood pressure returning to normal in 20 to 30 min. Local injection-site irritation is concentration- and duration-related and occurs in up to 8% of patients. This effect is minimized by diluting infusions to <10 mg/ml, which may hamper use in volume-restricted patients. Limited data support the safety of esmolol in patients with traditional contraindications to β-blockers, such as diabetes mellitus or obstructive airway disease (61, 63). In general, however, it should be avoided or used with caution in these patients.

β-Blockers are particularly useful in AF caused by high circulating catecholamine levels, including hyperthyroidism or sympathomimetic overdose, because they pharmacologically attenuate the underlying cause of the arrhythmia. Critically ill perioperative and cardiac patients should be managed with esmolol. β-Blockers may be necessary for only a short time in these patients, as correction of the precipitating cause may "restore" digoxin sensitivity or even allow conversion to sinus rhythm.

Pacing. At the present time, cardiac pacemakers or other devices are not considered first-line treatments in the acute management of AF.

CHRONIC TREATMENT

After initial control of ventricular rate, pharmacologic or electrical methods may be used for conversion to sinus rhythm. If successful, maintenance therapy (generally with the same antiarrhythmic used for conversion) is begun in an attempt to sustain sinus rhythm. Patients who remain in AF or who revert shortly after conversion are given drugs to slow the ventricular rate and maximize cardiac output. Chronic AF patients may also be candidates for long-term anticoagulation. Therapeutic goals in chronic AF include relief of symptom, reduction in embolic risk, and improvement in overall cardiac function and exercise tolerance.

Conversion to sinus rhythm is desirable since it will improve cardiac performance, relieve clinical symptoms, and decrease the risk of embolism markedly. Patients with AF of recent onset may convert spontaneously to sinus rhythm during initial drug treatment or after the inciting stress is eliminated. Unfortunately, not all patients will remain in sinus rhythm. Although conversion to sinus rhythm is crucial for some patients (e.g., those with hemodynamic instability), in others it may be neither practical nor useful. Ideally, an assessment of the likelihood of sustained sinus rhythm should be made before attempted conversion. Higher success rates are seen in patients with a corrected or controlled underlying cause and in those with recent arrhythmia onset. Patients likely to revert to AF include those with cardiomegaly (particularly left atrial enlargement), mitral valve disease, AF of more than 3 to 6 months duration, and moderate-to-severe heart failure (65). A curious finding has been a lack of atrial mechanical function (systole) for several days or weeks after cardioversion, despite a return of normal electrical activity (66). This may account for the lack of improvement in exercise tolerance and cardiac output, as well as the continued risk for embolism in the period immediately following conversion.

DC Countershock. Cardioversion may be accomplished either electrically or pharmacologically. Direct current (DC) countershock depolarizes a critical number of myocardial cells simultaneously, allowing the SA node to reestablish control as the pacemaker. The current should be synchronized with the QRS complex on ECG, to avoid delivery during the vulnerable period of ventricular recovery. Lower initial energies are often used, though as many as 300 to 400 joules may ultimately be required. An antiarrhythmic (usually quinidine) is initiated 1 to 2 days before cardioversion, to help maintain sinus rhythm. Short-acting sedatives or anesthetics are given immediately before the procedure. DC countershock is initially successful in 80 to 95% of patients (51, 65, 67). Data compiled from 824 patients demonstrated a 2.4% frequency of complications, including emboli in 1.3%, ventricular arrhythmias in 0.4% and miscellaneous complications in 0.6% (65). DC cardioversion should be performed with caution in patients with digitalis toxicity, because of the higher risk of ventricular arrhythmias. It is generally not necessary to withhold digoxin immediately before countershock in *nontoxic* patients (68). Patients with known or suspected sick sinus syndrome should be evaluated carefully for possible pacemaker insertion before attempted cardioversion, especially if they are receiving drugs that exacerbate bradycardia, such as calcium-channel or β-blockers. Short-term anticoagulation is appropriate, to decrease the embolic risk. See "Anticoagulants" below.

Drugs for Conversion to Sinus Rhythm. Pharmacologic conversion to sinus rhythm, although less invasive than DC countershock, is also less successful. Digitalis, verapamil, and diltiazem rarely convert patients with AF to sinus rhythm, probably because of their minimal effects on atrial automaticity.

Quinidine. Quinidine is the most commonly used agent for pharmacologic cardioversion and is also used to maintain sinus rhythm postconversion. Quinidine may have both beneficial and deleterious effects in AF. A decrease in atrial ectopy accounts for its efficacy, whereas its vagolytic effect at the AV node may *enhance* impulse transmission, resulting in a very rapid ventricular rate. Therefore patients with AF should be digitalized before administration of quinidine. Because of the possibility of quinidine-induced long QT syndrome or torsade de pointes, all patients should be hospitalized with cardiac monitoring for attempted conversion. A typical therapeutic strategy is to administer quinidine for several days, then proceed to DC countershock if conversion does not occur with quinidine alone. Common dosage regimens for conversion are 300 to 400 mg of the sulfate salt p.o. q6h. IV quinidine may also be given with close hemodynamic monitoring, as discussed under "AV Nodal Reentry." The reported success rate with quinidine conversion averages 71% (65).

After the first successful conversion, the risks and cost of prophylactic antiarrhythmics to sustain sinus rhythm must be weighed against the likelihood of reversion to AF. Patients thought to be at low risk for reversion to AF may be observed off antiarrhythmics, with the proviso that only about 30% (51, 67) of untreated patients will maintain sinus rhythm for 1 year. If AF recurs, prophylactic antiarrhythmic therapy is initiated. There is no superior drug for maintaining sinus rhythm. Strategies are often influenced by personal experience, local tradition, and theoretical considerations. Quinidine has the strongest literature evidence for efficacy, but adverse effects, including death from proarrhythmic events, are severe limitations. Maintenance doses of 200 to 400 mg of the sulfate salt (or its equivalent) p.o. q6h have yielded success rates of 40 to 50% after 1 year (51). Subtherapeutic serum concentrations, poor compliance, and inappropriate initial selection of patients for conversion contribute to the lower long-term success.

Other Drugs. Patients who do not convert or who fail to sustain sinus rhythm with quinidine may be given procainamide or disopyramide in standard doses. Flecainide is also effective, but reports of proarrhythmic effects in AF patients (69, 70) limit its use. Trials of amiodarone for induction and maintenance of sinus rhythm have demonstrated efficacy in maintaining sinus rhythm, as well as

controlling ventricular rate if AF recurs. However the high response rate must be balanced against its toxicity, which is common and may be severe. Flecainide and amiodarone therapy are discussed under "Ventricular Flutter/Fibrillation."

Drugs to Control Ventricular Rate. In some patients, conversion is not attempted because the likelihood of sustained sinus rhythm is thought to be low. Others convert initially but revert to AF shortly thereafter. Therapy in these patients is directed at regulation of the ventricular rate. The optimal rate for maximizing cardiac output has not been established. A reasonable goal is a ventricular rate of less than 80 to 90 beats/min at rest and 100 to 110/min with mild exercise. Most are given digoxin, with or without other agents. As reviewed earlier, sympathetic stimulation may override the effect of digoxin resulting in an unacceptably high rate. Trials comparing digoxin with either verapamil or diltiazem have yielded conflicting results. While all have noted better rate control with the calcium-channel blocker, some have shown an associated improvement in exercise capacity (54, 71), while others have observed no change (52, 53). Therefore better control of the ventricular rate may not improve cardiac output or exercise tolerance, thus negating any major advantage of calcium-channel blockers over digoxin. β-Blockers may be used in patients with excess catecholamine effect, but they can worsen heart failure and decrease exercise tolerance (24). Quinidine is not useful in patients with chronic AF and may even be detrimental because of its vagolytic effect.

Monitoring parameters for chronic AF patients include subjective symptoms such as dyspnea, fatigue, angina, and palpitations, as well as objective criteria such as ventricular (or apical) rate. Objective measurements of exercise tolerance and cardiac output may be performed, but they do not always correlate with a subjective sense of improvement.

Anticoagulants. Anticoagulants are used to reduce the embolic risk associated with AF. Imprecise data have resulted in treatment and preventative strategies that are controversial and empiric. The decision to anticoagulate must be made on an individual basis, taking into account both the potential benefit and risk. Cerebral embolism commonly results in large neurologic deficits with severe residual disability, occurs without warning symptoms, is recurrent in 30 to 75% of patients, and carries a mortality of up to 25% (49). On the other hand, the incidence of major bleeding with anticoagulants at conventional intensities has been estimated at 2 to 4% yearly, with 1% per year suffering brain hemorrhage (72). These values may be even higher in the elderly, who comprise the majority of patients with AF.

After the onset of AF, several days are required for thrombus formation. Anticoagulants are therefore not indicated for AF of less than 2-days duration. On the other hand, once thrombi are formed, several weeks of anticoagulants are necessary to allow fibrotic organization and adherence to the atrial wall. Moreover, atrial mechanical function (i.e., atrial systole) may be delayed for several weeks after ECG-documented conversion to sinus rhythm (66). The embolic risk in the Framingham study was 14% within the first year after onset, and 5% per year thereafter (50). Risk is similar after pharmacologic or electric cardioversion. The American College of Chest Physicians recommendations for anticoagulants at the time of cardioversion include (73) (a) for AF of >3 days duration, anticoagulate with warfarin to an international normalized ratio (INR) intensity of 2.0 to 3.0 for 3 weeks before and 2 to 4 weeks after cardioversion; (b) no anticoagulants for AF of <2-days duration, unless other risk factors for embolism are present; and (c) for patients requiring emergent cardioversion, anticoagulate with heparin on the day of cardioversion if AF is of several days duration, there is a high risk of recurrence, or other risk factors are present.

Assessment of embolic risk in chronic AF patients remains an enigmatic clinical problem. Stein et al. (49) have devised a simplified assessment of embolic risk with suggested management strategies (Table 37.3). Generalized consensus exists regarding the high embolic risk in patients with documented recent embolism, AF associated with older mechanical heart valve prostheses, and mitral valve disease. Patients with cardiomyopathies, heart failure, thyrotoxicosis, and modern mechanical valves are at a high but somewhat lower risk. The medium-to-low risk group comprises the largest number of patients, yet data regarding risk-benefit aspects of anticoagulants in this group are limited. Two recent large trials in patients with chronic nonvalvular AF (74, 75) have demonstrated efficacy of warfarin therapy to an INR of 2.0 to 4.2, compared with placebo. Aspirin was also found to be beneficial in one of the two trials (75). While these trials provide convincing evidence for the efficacy of warfarin, careful assessment of bleeding risk remains a critical element in the decision for or against anticoagulant use in individual patients. A literature review of comparative anticoagulant trials found a strong association between major bleeding and underlying risk factors such as ulcer disease, cancer, recent surgery, or hypertension (76). Patients unable to comply with medication regimens or laboratory follow-up, as well as those with dementia or alcohol abuse, may be poor candidates for anticoagulation, regardless of embolic risk. Bleeding risk is also reduced by maintaining anticoagulants in the less intense range (INR 2.0 to 3.0) whenever possible (76). Scrupulous monitoring is essential and can lower bleeding risk substantially. In the Stroke Prevention in Atrial Fibrillation trial the annual rate of major hemorrhage for patients anticoagulated with warfarin to an INR of 2.0 to 3.5 was limited to 1.7% by meticulous supervision (versus 0.9% for aspirin 325 mg p.o. daily and 1.2% for placebo) (75). Refer to chapter 40 for specific aspects of anticoagulant therapy.

Nonpharmacologic Therapy. Surgical procedures to eliminate or control AF have not been well studied. Surgical ablation of the AV node with pacemaker placement is considered only in patients resistant to other therapies. Innovative surgical techniques have been described but require further research.

Prognosis. The long-term prognosis in patients with chronic AF is poor, with a twofold increase in yearly cardiovascular mortality (10%) over age-matched controls (5%) (47). Mortality is related to age at onset as well as to the presence and extent of coexisting heart disease.

WOLFF-PARKINSON-WHITE SYNDROME

Wolff-Parkinson-White (WPW) syndrome is a congenital heart disease characterized by the presence of an anatomically distinct atrioventricular connection in addition to the

Table 37.3.
Stratification of Thromboembolic Risk in Atrial Fibrillation[a,b]

	Thromboembolic Risk (per Year)			
	High (> 6%)	Medium-High (4–6%)	Medium-Low (2–4%)	Low (< 2%)
Underlying heart disease	Prior embolism Old mechanical prostheses	Mitral stenosis Thyrotoxicosis Heart failure Modern mechanical prostheses	Mitral regurgitation Aortic valve disease Coronary disease Hypertensive disease Bioprostheses	Lone AF (age<60) Isolated mitral value prolapse
Long-term A/C therapy	A/C (INR = 3.0–4.5)[c]	A/C (INR = 2.0–3.0)[d]	A/C (INR = 2.0–3.0)[e]	No therapy

[a] Reprinted with permission from Stein B, Halperin JL, Fuster V: Should patients with atrial fibrillation be anticoagulated prior to and chronically following cardioversion? Cardiovasc Clin 21(1):231–247, 1990.
[b] Abbreviations: AF, Atrial fibrillation; A/C, anticoagulant; INR, international normalized ratio of prothrombin suppression.
[c] In high-risk patients with old mechanical prostheses, dipyridamole may be added to warfarin.
[d] In patients with mechanical prostheses, INR range should be 3.0–4.5.
[e] The decision for anticoagulation in this group should be individualized.

AV nodal tissue. This anomalous pathway, called the accessory AV pathway (or Kent bundle), can be located anywhere in the heart and consists of working myocardium that forms an "electrical bridge" connecting the atrium and the ventricle. Impulse conduction may occur both antegrade and retrograde. Patients with WPW typically have sinus rhythm at baseline, with paroxysmal episodes of supraventricular tachycardias (SVTs). While in sinus rhythm, antegrade conduction is over both the AV node and accessory pathway; ventricular activation is thus a fusion of the two impulses. Since the accessory pathway can activate the ventricular muscle directly (bypassing all or part of the AV node and His-Purkinje system), early or "preexcitation" of part of the ventricle occurs (Fig. 37.8A).

The accessory pathway and AV node may form reentry circuits that allow SVTs, most commonly AV reentry or AF (77). AV reentry is distinguished from AV nodal reentry by the use of the accessory pathway as part of the circuit. Accessory pathway conduction in the reentry circuit may be antegrade (called antidromic reentry) or retrograde (orthodromic reentry). Orthodromic reentry is 15 times more common than antidromic. In this form, impulses travel antegrade from the atrium to the ventricle via the AV node and retrograde from the ventricle to the atrium via the accessory pathway (Fig. 37.8B). Multiple accessory pathways are seen in 5 to 15% of patients, usually associated with antidromic reentry.

WPW syndrome is often seen in young otherwise healthy infants, children, and young adults. The clinical importance of the arrhythmias varies from relatively benign to life-threatening, depending on the electrophysiologic properties of the accessory pathway and the AV node. Arrhythmias seen in infancy may persist, disappear, or disappear then recur many years later (77). This is thought to reflect a change in the conduction properties of the accessory pathway over time. Orthodromic AV reentry is the most common SVT. The most feared arrhythmia in WPW is AF with antegrade conduction down an accessory pathway with a short refractory period. In this case, the protective effect of the AV node against very rapid ventricular rates is lost. Extremely rapid impulse transmission directly from the atrium to the ventricle may lead to ventricular flutter or fibrillation and sudden death.

The classic ECG in sinus rhythm includes a short PR-interval, with a delta wave preceding the QRS complex representing preexcitation. The QRS complex has abnormal morphology due to the fusion of normal conduction down the AV node–His bundle system and preexcitation of the left ventricular free wall. The initiating arrhythmic event is usually a critically timed premature atrial or ventricular impulse. Ventricular rates average 100 to 280/minute in AV reentry (higher in children) and 140 to 320/minute in AF. The direction of the reentry circuit (orthodromic or antidromic), variation in mode of ventricular

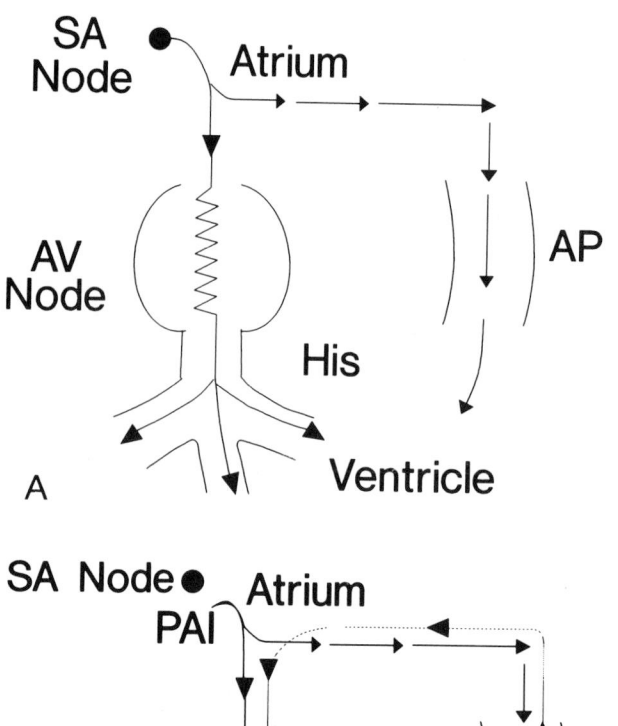

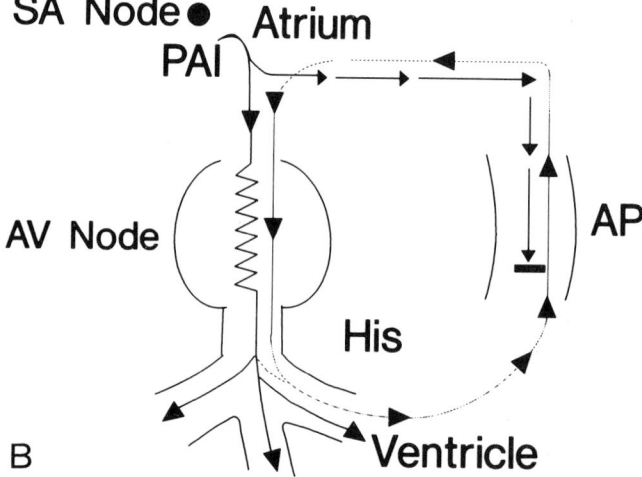

Figure 37.8. A, Wolff-Parkinson-White syndrome. Sinus rhythm. The impulse reaches the ventricles via the AV node–His-Purkinje system with simultaneous preexcitation via the accessory pathway. **B,** Orthodromic AV reentry. *PAI,* premature atrial impulse; *AP,* accessory pathway; *His,* bundle of His; *solid line,* PAI. The premature impulse is blocked in the AP and reaches the ventricles via the AV node–His-Purkinje system. If the AP is recovered, AV reentry may be initiated. *Dotted line* is a reentry circuit.

activation, and different accessory pathway anatomies all contribute to marked inter- and intrapatient ECG variation during SVTs. Detection of WPW syndrome and differentiation of its associated arrhythmias require an experienced ECG interpreter.

The clinical manifestations and hemodynamic consequences of AV reentry and AF are the same in patients with or without WPW syndrome, ranging from palpitations to syncope and sudden death. WPW patients may be difficult to manage because the effect of the drug on the accessory pathway is not predicted by effect on the AV node. Moreover, drug action on antegrade conduction may differ from that on retrograde. Underlying autonomic tone may alter conduction independent of drug effect. A drug may therefore be beneficial for one patient yet deleterious for another. Management should be individualized by electrophysiologic studies. These studies locate and characterize the accessory pathway, identify the mechanism of the arrhythmia, and evaluate the effects of the drug on each anatomic component. Other termination techniques such as atrial pacing may also be evaluated.

As a rule, *AV reentry* associated with WPW syndrome is readily terminated using traditional maneuvers and drugs, as discussed in the section "AV Nodal Reentry." In patients with *AF*, however, great care must be exercised to avoid enhanced atrioventricular conduction with subsequent acceleration of the ventricular rate and degeneration into ventricular fibrillation. This is a primary consideration in only a small minority (with a short antegrade accessory pathway refractory period). Unfortunately, it is not possible to identify susceptible patients on clinical grounds alone. Some may be entirely asymptomatic, yet have an electrophysiologic risk for sudden cardiac death. Moreover, the population at risk based on electrophysiologic studies is much larger than that which will ultimately have a fatal arrhythmia. Little is known about the natural history of asymptomatic WPW syndrome. Extensive testing and treatment to prevent sudden death in asymptomatic individuals remains controversial.

After conversion to sinus rhythm, patients with recurrent symptomatic attacks may receive prophylactic therapy to minimize further episodes of SVT. Regimens commonly include class Ia or Ic drugs, amiodarone, or β-blockers. Controlled comparative trials have not been performed, and no drug has demonstrated superiority. Drug treatment is often suboptimal due to limited efficacy and excessive toxicity. Preventative therapy is reserved for patients with recurrent disabling arrhythmias.

The effects of drugs on AV nodal and accessory pathway conduction is summarized in Table 37.4. The type Ia drugs quinidine, procainamide, and disopyramide slow or block antegrade accessory pathway conduction, with a lesser and more variable effect on retrograde conduction. These drugs also block retrograde AV nodal conduction and suppress atrial and ventricular ectopy. The effects of the drugs may vary with different accessory pathway refractory periods, emphasizing the importance of electrophysiologic studies.

Digitalis and verapamil maintain their AV nodal effects. Digitalis however may *shorten* the accessory pathway refractory period. Verapamil generally has minimal effects on the accessory pathway, but may also produce a refractory period shortening. These drugs are very effective first-line agents for terminating and preventing the recurrence of AV reentry. However, in AF or flutter, they may ac-

Table 37.4.
Sites of Primary Drug Action in Wolff-Parkinson-White Syndrome

AV node antegrade conduction
  Calcium-channel blockers (verapamil[a], diltiazem)
  Digoxin[a]
  Adenosine
  β-Blockers
AV node retrograde conduction, accessory pathway antegrade conduction
  Class Ia drugs (quinidine, procainamide, disopyramide)
AV node and accessory pathway, antegrade and retrograde conduction
  Class Ic drugs (flecainide, encainide, propafenone)
  Amiodarone
Suppression of atrial ectopy
  Class Ia drugs (quinidine, procainamide, disopyramide)
  Class Ic drugs (flecainide, encainide, propafenone)
  β-Blockers

[a] Digoxin and verapamil may *decrease* the accessory pathway antegrade refractory period, a dangerous effect in WPW with atrial fibrillation. See text for explanation.

centuate conduction and accelerate ventricular rate in those (unusual) patients with antegrade accessory pathway conduction. Potentially lethal ventricular tachycardia or fibrillation may ensue. Digitalis and verapamil should therefore not be used in AF with documented or suspected preexcitation, unless previous electrophysiologic studies have shown them to be safe.

Most trials of adenosine in AV reentry have shown its primary site of action to be the AV nodal loop of the reentrant circuit, with a lesser or no effect on accessory pathway conduction. Coupled with its lack of hypotensive properties, some investigators believe that adenosine is safer than verapamil or digitalis in documented or suspected WPW syndrome (78).

Propranolol and the other β-blockers alter AV nodal conduction but have minimal effect on accessory pathway conduction in either direction. They are not often used as single agents in WPW, but are sometimes combined with other drugs such as digoxin or quinidine.

Amiodarone, flecainide, encainide, and propafenone have additional unique antiarrhythmic mechanisms, as compared with the older agents. These drugs slow AV nodal *and* accessory pathway conduction *in both directions* and lengthen atrial and ventricular refractory periods. They can therefore be expected to terminate or control SVTs associated with WPW and also prevent their recurrence by suppressing ectopy. These drugs offer the best antiarrhythmic profile for SVTs associated with accessory pathways. Studies have demonstrated promising results. Unfortunately, the proarrhythmic effects of the class Ic drugs (69) and the toxicities of amiodarone limit use.

Because of the unpredictable and often inadequate response to drugs, nonpharmacologic therapy is an important component of the treatment of WPW syndrome. DC countershock retains its near-uniform reliability and efficacy and is the treatment of choice in patients with hemodynamic instability. Atrial pacing may be used in AV reentry, though it may induce transient AF with rapid ventricular rate in patients with rapid antegrade accessory pathway conduction. Permanent ventricular pacing may be necessary in patients requiring large doses of antiarrhythmics or those with sinus node disease (pacing will eliminate excessive bradycardia while the patient is in sinus rhythm).

Surgical interruption of the accessory pathway is an effective, usually curative treatment. Following detailed electrophysiologic and cardiac mapping studies, the accessory pathway is transected or ablated using either an endocardial or epicardial approach (77). AV nodal conduction is preserved. Surgical division of accessory pathways is 90 to 100% effective in experienced centers, with <1% mortality in uncomplicated cases and rare early or late recurrences (42). It may therefore be the treatment of choice in (a) patients unresponsive or intolerant to antiarrhythmics, (b) those with arrhythmias associated with marked adverse hemodynamic effects, (c) patients with AF with rapid antegrade accessory pathway conduction, (d) young patients who would otherwise require lifelong drug therapy, or (e) females desiring pregnancy. Percutaneous catheter ablation of the accessory pathway using DC countershock, radiofrequency energy, or lasers are less invasive experimental techniques.

PREMATURE VENTRICULAR CONTRACTIONS

Premature ventricular contractions (PVCs) are ectopic beats originating in the ventricular muscle. These beats are not initiated by the SA node but are stimulated by the spontaneous electrical firing of the local tissue. PVCs are the most common arrhythmia. Depending on the length of the observation, the frequency of PVCs in otherwise healthy subjects is variable. One-half of young males have PVCs with 24-hr monitoring (79). The frequency of PVCs increases with advancing age and the presence of cardiac disease. In most patients, this arrhythmia produces no symptoms whatsoever. However, it is also the most common arrhythmia (40 to 80%) seen with myocardial infarctions, where it may adversely affect survival.

Several classes of drugs may induce PVCs. These include the sympathomimetic amines (epinephrine, pseudoephedrine, phenylephrine, phenylpropanolamine, amphetamine); the methylxanthines (caffeine, theophylline); digitalis; cocaine; and certain general anesthetics (cyclopropane and halothane). Type Ia antiarrhythmics and flecainide may also induce PVCs and ventricular tachycardia. These drugs should be discontinued or their doses should be reduced.

Not all PVCs require treatment. This arrhythmia in otherwise healthy persons, when it is asymptomatic, does not require suppression. PVCs may compromise cardiac output and produce syncope, even in a patient without a history of cardiac disease. These PVCs should be treated. Yet, many patients complain merely of palpitations. If this is the only symptom, the benefit of PVC suppression must be balanced against the cost and toxicity of treatment. A variety of noncardiac events may induce PVCs, such as anemia, surgery, hypoxia, and stress. Elimination of the precipitating event should resolve the PVCs and obviate the need for an potential toxicity of antiarrhythmics.

PVCs may be separated into simple and complex arrhythmias. PVCs seen in asymptomatic, noncardiac disease subjects are usually simple, in that they are isolated beats, occurring singly, with a wave pattern on the ECG that repeats itself, indicating that the beat originates from the same site (unifocal). These appear to be well tolerated until their frequency compromises ventricular filling. Complex PVCs are uncommon in noncardiac disease subjects but are frequent in patients with coronary artery disease. They may be subclassified as multiform or multifocal, which means that the ECG wave form is different between ectopics, suggesting more than one site in the ventricles is showing automaticity. Another complex classification refers to paired PVCs or runs of PVCs. These are consecutive PVCs without intervening sinus beats. The final type of complex PVC is one that is termed early R-on-T, referring to the R wave of the PVC interrupting the T wave of the sinus beat. Complex PVCs are highly correlated with sudden death.

In the setting of coronary artery disease, a grading system has been proposed by Lown and Graboys (80) to separate patients according to risk of sudden death. This system gives a numerical grade from 0 to 5, with increasing risk of sudden death, according to the following descriptions:

0 = no PVCs;

1 = occasional simple, less than 30/hr;

2 = frequent simple, greater than 30/hr;

3 = multiform;

4 = runs of PVCs;

5 = early PVCs.

In an epidemiologic study over 7 months, the mortality rate varied from zero in class 0 to 30% in classes 3 to 5 (81).

Despite the fact that PVCs may predispose to sudden death, the cause of death is not known. It may be a random event precipitated by the unfortunate timing of PVCs. Procainamide, lidocaine, and quinidine reduce the frequency of, although they do not totally eliminate, PVCs. However, studies evaluating the response to these drugs do not demonstrate a significant decrease in mortality rate. On the other hand, death may be a result of acute ischemia, which is not altered by antiarrhythmic drugs. The agents shown to improve survival rate may act on ischemia not on the basis of their antiarrhythmic effects.

Lidocaine. Lidocaine is the drug of choice for the parenteral treatment of PVCs. The therapeutic serum concentration for lidocaine is 1.5 to 5.5 μg/ml. Lidocaine is usually initiated with an intravenous loading dose to produce rapid arrhythmia control. Any loading dose must account for the small central compartment, 0.5 liters/kg in normal subjects, reduced to 0.3 liters/kg with congestive heart failure, and increased to 0.6 liters/kg in liver disease (82). A minimum concentration in the central compartment must be reached, since the heart acts as if it belongs in this compartment, while limiting the maximum concentration since the brain is also present in this compartment. The loading dose (LD) may be calculated to produce a plasma concentration (Cp) of 3 μg/ml using the central volume (Vc) of 0.5 liters/kg as follows and administered over 1 to 2 min:

$$LD = Cp \times Vc$$
$$= 3 \ \mu g/ml \times 0.5 \ liters/kg$$
$$= 1.5 \ mg/kg$$

Since the loading dose will be rapidly distributed away from the heart and the central compartment with an alpha phase half-life of about 10 min, arrhythmias may recur after the initial dose. Additional boluses, using one-half the initial dose, may be given after 10 to 20 min or when ectopics recur. Unfortunately all bolus doses are effective only transiently because of the rapid distribution.

An alternative is to give the initial load, followed by a high-dose infusion of 120 μg/kg/min for 25 min, followed by an appropriate maintenance infusion. The high-dose infusion is intended to avoid the subtherapeutic levels produced on a constant infusion of lidocaine for suppression of PVCs. This constant infusion may be calculated based upon the therapeutic steady-state serum level of about 3 μg/ml (Cpss), and the clearance of lidocaine (Cl), which is 15.6 ml/min/kg in normal males, 20.2 ml/min/kg in normal females, 5.5 ml/min/kg in congestive heart failure, and 6.0 ml/min/kg for chronic liver disease (83), as follows:

$$R = Cpss \times Cl$$
$$= 3 \ \mu g/ml \times 6 \ ml/min/kg$$
$$= 18 \ \mu g/kg/min \ (with \ liver \ failure)$$

Other factors that may reduce lidocaine clearance include advanced age, propranolol, and cimetidine. Only 5% of lidocaine is eliminated unchanged in the urine, and renal failure does not decrease the clearance of lidocaine. Certain metabolites of lidocaine such as monoethylglycinexylide (MEGX) and glycinexylidide (GX) are active compounds. GX is cleared by the kidneys and may accumulate in renal impairment. MEGX and GX may contribute to the toxicity of lidocaine when it is administered for extended periods of time.

Lidocaine blood concentrations may be obtained at any point during the first 12 hr of therapy. There are advocates for early (1 to 2 hr after the start of the infusion) and late (2 to 4 hr) sampling followed by a delayed sample at 8, 12, or 24 hr (84). Levels of 1 to 2 μg/ml are only rarely effective. Many patients have control of their arrhythmia with concentrations of 3 to 5 μg/ml, and neurologic toxicity may limit any further dose increases. Paresthesias, dizziness, drowsiness, and euphoria may be seen. Resistant arrhythmias may require concentrations of 6 to 8 μg/ml at the risk of further confusion, nausea, vomiting, dysarthria, and psychoses. Pushing lidocaine beyond 9 μg/ml is rarely justified. Sweating, tremors, and muscle fasciculation may precede seizures, respiratory arrest, and coma. Lidocaine metabolites may contribute to the neurologic toxicity.

Prolonged infusions of lidocaine beyond 24 hr may require a downward adjustment in the dose. Steady-state concentrations should be expected by approximately four times the normal lidocaine half-life of 100 min. In patients with liver disease, steady state may be delayed because of the half-life of 300 min (83). Patients with uncomplicated myocardial infarction (AMI) receiving constant infusions of lidocaine have developed progressive accumulation after 30 hr. Such patients have prolonged elimination half-lives for lidocaine of 3 to 4 hr after lidocaine. A partial explanation for this phenomenon has derived from changing aspects of plasma protein binding of lidocaine. In normal subjects, lidocaine is 60 to 80% plasma protein–bound (30% to albumin and 70% to α_1-acid glycoprotein or AAG). The magnitude of the binding correlates closely with concentrations of AAG. As total lidocaine blood concentrations rise in these AMI patients, AAG accumulates. The drug redistributes out of red blood cells into AAG, decreasing free lidocaine concentrations. Free lidocaine clearance does not change with the AMI (85). It is probable that the free concentration of lidocaine is responsible for toxicity. A therapeutic range for the free lidocaine concentration has not been established. To avoid accumulation of lidocaine with prolonged administration, it has been suggested that the infusion rate be reduced by one-half after the first 24 hr of dosing (86).

Procainamide. Procainamide is an alternative when lidocaine toxicity or arrhythmias resistant to lidocaine develop. Procainamide is a versatile drug that can be administered orally and parenterally, but toxicity, not therapeutic inadequacy, has relegated procainamide to a secondary role.

After oral administration, procainamide averages 75% bioavailability, but certain patients may absorb as little as 10%. In addition, the rate of absorption and time to peak serum concentration varies considerably. First-pass hepatic metabolism may account for some of the reduced bioavailability. Food may delay the absorption. There are various manufacturers of both immediate-release and sustained-release procainamide. Switching between generic and proprietary immediate-release procainamide may result in arrhythmia recurrence (87). Similarly, interchange of the sustained-release procainamide may also result in arrhythmia relapse in certain patients, yet mean data suggest bioequivalence for at least two products (88). Sustained release of procainamide is accomplished by either a wax matrix or a nondisintegrating core. Generally the areas under the curve, maximum to minimum serum procainamide concentrations, and steady-state procainamide concentrations for the two types of products are similar; however the time to maximum serum concentration is delayed for the nondisintegrating matrix (89). Patients may complain of whole or partial tablets appearing in the stool, but this may not reflect incomplete absorption. Patients should be cautioned not to chew or crush the sustained-release tablets. Drug interactions and altered procainamide concentrations may be observed when procainamide is given along with trimethoprim, quinidine, cimetidine, and ranitidine.

Intravenous procainamide displays two-compartment kinetics similar to lidocaine. A rapid distribution phase with a half-life of 5 min occurs, with the drug binding extensively to tissues. There is evidence that procainamide does not penetrate well into fat. Thus total weight should not be used in calculating doses; ideal weight is preferred. Rapid arrhythmia control may require intravenous bolus doses. The negative inotropic and hypotensive effects of procainamide limit the rate at which the drug may be given. Even in emergency situations procainamide should not be given at a rate exceeding 50 mg/min. There is a trend suggesting even slower rates are preferred to avoid hypotension (i.e., 20 mg/min). The loading dose (LD) will be influenced by the therapeutic range for procainamide (Cp) of 4 to 8 µg/ml, the distribution volume (Vdss) of 2 liters/kg, and the procainamide content (S) of the hydrochloride salt, 0.82, as follows:

$$LD = CP \times Vdss/0.82$$
$$= 6 \ \mu g/ml \times 2 \ liters/kg/0.82$$
$$= 14.6 \ mg/kg$$

In renal impairment and congestive heart failure, the volume of distribution may be decreased by 25%. Loading doses have been given as small boluses of 50 to 100 mg every 5 min until arrhythmia control is seen or toxicity develops. An alternative is a loading infusion of 17 mg/kg over 1 hour, followed by the maintenance dose (see below). The generally accepted therapeutic range for procainamide is 4 to 8 µg/ml. However the indication for the drug may influence the therapeutic range. This range of

4 to 8 µg/ml may be appropriate for patients with acute or chronic coronary artery disease with the intent of suppressing PVCs. On the other hand, suppression of ventricular tachycardia may require higher doses, producing concentrations in the range of 10 to 20 µg/ml.

The selection of procainamide maintenance doses is intimately related to its metabolic fate. Procainamide may be excreted unchanged in the urine to the extent of 50%. The liver and other sites will transform 7 to 24% of procainamide to its major metabolite, N-acetylprocainamide (NAPA). The rate of acetylation varies between patients, who may be grouped as fast or slow. Fast acetylators convert a higher percentage of procainamide to NAPA than slow acetylators. About 85% of NAPA is excreted unchanged by the kidneys; thus NAPA accumulates more than procainamide as renal function deteriorates. It seems that procainamide and NAPA compete for renal tubular secretion. NAPA may thus prolong the procainamide half-life (90).

The typical patient receiving intravenous procainamide is placed on a dose of 2 to 4 mg/min. This may be tailored to the patient, using 2.8 mg/kg/hr as a standard, reduced in cardiac or renal impairment by one-third for moderate impairment and two-thirds for severe impairment (91). Calculations using population averages of kinetic variables for oral procainamide have not been particularly accurate. In general, patients may be started on 50 mg/kg/day and titrated to response or toxicity. The dose should be reduced in cardiac or renal impairment by one-third for moderate impairment and two-thirds for severe impairment. In renal impairment, the procainamide half-life may be increased from a normal of 2 to 4 hr to 5 to 10 hr, whereas the NAPA half-life is greatly increased from a normal of 6 hr to as much as 42 hr. Age, independent of renal function, may also affect procainamide clearance (Cl) as follows:

$$Cl \ (ml/min/kg) = 11.9 - (0.143 \times age)$$
$$+ (0.0321 \times ClCr) - (1.11 \times CHF)$$

where CHF is a constant of 1 if moderate heart failure is present (92).

Although the metabolite NAPA has some antiarrhythmic activity, the two drugs do not have the same electrophysiologic effects, and in patients they may be additive or antagonistic. Thus the use of ratios or sums of the two serum concentrations has met with mixed results. Some clinicians use a minimum sum of 10 µg/ml and maximum of 25 to 30 µg/ml (91, 93). There is probably more benefit to the use of NAPA concentrations in monitoring for toxicity than for predicting efficacy.

A limiting factor in the compliance with procainamide is the dosing interval for the immediate-release product. With normal renal function, the maintenance dose of 50 mg/kg/day must be given at 3- to 4-hr intervals. The sustained-release formulations allow a 6-hr dosing interval. There is evidence that an 8-hr interval may be appropriate in some cases, although the FDA indication is for 6 hr (94, 95). It is suggested that patients receive the immediate-release product first, for titration, then be converted to a sustained-release product if necessary. The total daily dose of the immediate-release product should be the initial daily dose of the sustained-release product. It has been suggested that sustained-release procainamide preparations should be avoided in patients with colostomies (96) or in other rapid gastrointestinal transit states.

Adverse effects commonly seen with procainamide include gastrointestinal distress, weakness, dizziness, nervousness, and blurred vision. These symptoms resolve if the dose is reduced, but many patients develop tolerance to these effects with continued procainamide use without a dose reduction. Cardiac toxicity seen with procainamide concentrations exceeding 12 µg/ml may include progressive lengthening of the Q-Tc interval and QRS complex duration, hypotension, and myocardial depression. However, procainamide may be less likely to produce an exacerbation of heart failure than other agents such as encainide or tocainide (97). A lupus-like syndrome may develop in more than 20% of patients taking procainamide. Procainamide lupus differs from systemic lupus erythematosus in that arthritic features are more prominent while dermatologic, hematologic, and renal changes are rare. Symptoms may develop as early as 2 weeks after initiating procainamide or as long as 2 years later. Risk factors include high doses, high serum concentrations, and slow acetylation status. Recently, a hepatic mixed-function oxidase metabolite, procainamide-hydroxylamine, has been implicated in causing the lupus (98). Common signs and symptoms for monitoring include fever, rash, myalgias, arthralgias, pericarditis, pleuritis, hepatosplenomegaly, and rarely pericardial tamponade. Many more patients will have positive serologic tests for lupus than will have symptoms. (See Chapter 31 "Systemic Lupus Erythematosus.") Originally the sustained-release product was reported to produce neutropenia more frequently than immediate-release procainamide (99). More recent data suggest that the rate of neutropenia is less than 1% and the risk is independent of formulation (100). All patients should be monitored for this hematologic complication with frequent white blood cell counts at the beginning of therapy. Patients should be followed for unexplained fevers because of the risk of infection related to the neutropenia.

Disopyramide. Disopyramide is currently available for oral use in the treatment of ventricular arrhythmias. It may also be as effective as quinidine in the management of atrial fibrillation. Parenteral disopyramide is as effective as lidocaine in the treatment of ventricular arrhythmias, but it is not yet available in the US (101).

Disopyramide is well absorbed (F = 0.83). With the immediate-release product, peak serum concentrations occur in 2 hr. Disopyramide is 50 to 65% protein-bound, with the majority bound to AAG and a small amount (5 to 10%) to albumin. The degree of binding is nonlinear, with higher disopyramide concentrations a greater amount of the drug is free (102). It is assumed that the free drug is active (103). The distribution volume in normal persons is 0.8 liters/kg. Variable amounts of disopyramide (36 to 71%) have been reported to be cleared by the kidney as unchanged drug. The remainder is an N-dealkylated metabolite with some antiarrhythmic activity. Healthy subjects have half-lives ranging from 4.4 to 8.2 hr. Renal impairment may prolong the half-life from 8.4 to 53 hr. The half-life may also be prolonged in patients with AMI. There appears to be an interaction with phenytoin and disopyramide, where phenytoin increases the metabolism of disopyramide (104).

The therapeutic range for disopyramide appears to be 3 to 6 µg/ml. This therapeutic range may not apply in certain diseases, using the conventional assay measuring total disopyramide. In cirrhosis, the AAG content decreases and the free disopyramide concentration increases in comparison with normal subjects (105). Postmyocardial infarction patients have the opposite problem, a rise in AAG with decrease in free disopyramide concentration (106). In some studies, atrial arrhythmias responded to lower concentrations than ventricular ectopics. Although steadily increasing, the plasma concentration of disopyramide progressively reduces the frequency of ectopics, responders and nonresponders have similar mean levels. Therefore patients should be titrated to response rather than selecting an arbitrary drug serum level.

Oral disopyramide may be initiated with a loading dose of 300 mg of the immediate-release product (200 mg for moderate renal impairment, moderate liver dysfunction, or decompensated heart failure). Maintenance doses of 100 to 150 mg may be given at 6-hr intervals; the lower dose is indicated for renal, liver, and cardiac insufficiency. The recommended maximum daily dose is 800 mg, yet up to 1600 mg has been used with close monitoring. For patients with severe renal impairment, the dosing interval may be prolonged to 12, 24, or 36 hr for creatinine clearances of 15 to 40, 5 to 15, or 1 to 5 ml/min, respectively.

A sustained-release preparation of disopyramide has been marketed. It has been studied in both normal volunteers and patients with arrhythmias (107). The dosing interval may be prolonged from 6 hr with the immediate-release to 12 hr with the sustained-release product. A proposed theoretical advantage of the sustained-release product is the avoidance of a transient high-peak serum disopyramide concentration. This, coupled with the potential for higher free drug concentration as a result of the nonlinear protein-binding characteristics of disopyramide, may lead to fewer side effects, yet this has not been proven.

Common adverse reactions observed with disopyramide have been anticholinergic symptoms of dry mouth, blurred vision, constipation, and urinary retention. Anticholinergic reactions may occur in as many as 45% of patients receiving disopyramide, and 25% may require cessation of therapy (108). Acetylcholinesterase inhibitors, such as pyridostigmine, may effectively prevent the anticholinergic side effects of disopyramide (109). Hypoglycemia has been associated with disopyramide with risk factors of advanced age, chronic renal impairment, and malnutrition. Death has resulted from persistent hypoglycemia (110). Like quinidine, disopyramide may prolong the Q-Tc interval and QRS complex duration. Initial reports on disopyramide were encouraging, indicating that quinidine produced more frequent adverse effects, yet the reports of acute heart failure developing during chronic disopyramide have dampened enthusiasm for this drug. Disopyramide has a negative inotropic effect. The risk of developing symptomatic heart failure may be as high as 16% (111). The drug has been used without complications in patients with heart failure, but such patients are at a much greater risk for decompensation. The onset of symptoms is variable, and there is no apparent correlation with the dose. Patients developing signs and symptoms of heart failure should have disopyramide discontinued. Symptoms usually resolve over a few days, but some patients may require diuretics or digitalis. As with other antiarrhythmics that prolong the Q-Tc interval, disopyramide may cause ventricular arrhythmias, at times with symptoms similar to those of quinidine syncope. Many patients revert after discontinuing the disopyramide; others may require suppression with lidocaine.

Encainide. Encainide is a class Ic antiarrhythmic agent that is structurally dissimilar to other currently available drugs. Electrophysiology studies must be interpreted with care, since the effects of encainide differ between single-dose and multiple-dose studies because of the presence of active metabolites [O-desmethylencainide (ODE), 3-methoxy-O-desmethylencainide (3-MODE), N-desmethylencainide (NDE), and N-O-didesmethylencainide (DDE)] that accumulate with multiple dosing. ODE is more potent than the parent compound. The effects observed are believed to be due to metabolites and include increases in effective atrial refractory period, ventricular refractoriness, and prolongation of the atrial, AV nodal, and His-Purkinje conduction, with little change in repolarization. Encainide is classed as Ic because it produces a decrease in the rate of rise of phase 0, with little effect on APD.

Absorption of encainide after oral dosing is rapid, with peak blood concentrations in 1.5 hr, but the extent of absorption varies from 7 to 82% (112). Encainide is oxidized extensively with a genetically determined rate, showing polymorphism. Most subjects are extensive metabolizers (EM), with ODE and MODE higher than encainide, and NDE absent in plasma. In slow or poor metabolizers (PM, 7 to 10% of population) ODE is lower and NDE is the major metabolite. In EM subjects, encainide undergoes a substantial first-pass effect with a short half-life of 1.5 hr, ODE has a half-life of 13 hr. In PM subjects, the bioavailability is greater, with concentrations of parent drug some 20 times higher than in EMs. The major metabolite present in PM is NDE, which has little activity; thus the antiarrhythmic effects are due to encainide. Renal impairment in EMs produces slower clearance of ODE and MODE metabolites (113). Cirrhosis in EMs produces higher oral availability and higher serum encainide concentrations but equivalent concentrations of ODE and MODE (113). Quinidine may interact with encainide, particularly in EM (114). Quinidine is a potent inhibitor of the enzyme responsible for encainide polymorphism, cytochrome P-450$_{dbl}$. Quinidine prolongs the half-life of encainide, decreases nonrenal encainide clearance, and reverses encainide EKG changes, but only in EM. In PM, quinidine has no effect on encainide pharmacokinetics. Diltiazem also interacts with encainide and with ODE and MODE in EM. Diltiazem is a hepatic enzyme inhibitor that decreases the first-pass metabolism of encainide, but electrophysiologic changes do not occur (115).

Encainide appears to be effective in suppressing PVCs and ventricular tachycardia (VT). It is superior to quinidine in the suppression of PVCs, with fewer side effects (116). The therapeutic range for encainide is not established, although in PMs concentrations of >265 ng/ml may be necessary. The daily dose of encainide has been 100 to 250 mg given in three to four doses. Higher doses may be proarrhythmic. QRS complex prolongation may predict arrhythmia suppression. With a baseline of <0.12 sec, a prolongation of 40 to 50% is suggested, whereas a QRS >0.12 sec should only be prolonged by 25 to 30%.

Minor toxicity may occur in as many as 60% of patients and includes dizziness, lightheadedness, visual disturbances, tremor, headache, gastrointestinal intolerance, or metallic taste. More serious are the proarrhythmic effects not seen in normal persons or in SVT but in VT or ventricular fibrillation (VF). Marked hypotension and progressive VF have occurred without associated QRS or Q-Tc prolongation as with other agents.

CARDIAC ARRHYTHMIA SUPPRESSION TRIAL

The National Heart, Lung and Blood Institute sponsored the Cardiac Arrhythmic Suppression Trial (CAST), a trial of encainide, flecainide, moricizine, or placebo in post-AMI with asymptomatic or mildly symptomatic ventricular arrhythmias (117). The trial was suspended for encainide and flecainide when excessive mortality was observed with these agents, in contrast to placebo. Subsequently the results were released to the public, and the manufacturers notified all physicians. Prior to CAST, encainide and flecainide had approved indications of non-life-threatening nonsustained VT or frequent symptomatic PVCs. After CAST, the FDA had the manufacturers suggest that these agents should be used only in patients with life-threatening ventricular arrhythmias. The mechanism for the higher mortality rate with encainide and flecainide is not known. Deaths occurred throughout the trial, thus proarrhythmia may not be a factor, because this adverse effect of antiarrhythmics usually is seen at the outset of therapy. It does appear though that elimination of PVCs may not improve mortality. These results should not be extrapolated to patients with ejection fractions <40% or to those with structural heart disease (factors associated with morbid events). **Propafenone.** Propafenone has recently been marketed in the U.S. after originating in West Germany in 1977, where it is the most frequently prescribed antiarrhythmic (118). Propafenone is a type Ic antiarrhythmic that blocks the fast inward sodium channel, producing a slowed rate of rise of phase 0 of the action potential. Propafenone also has weak β-blocking and calcium-channel blocking effects (119). There is a dose-related increase in PR interval and QRS duration.

Currently propafenone is marketed only in an oral dosage form in the U.S. Absorption is complete (>95%), with a time to maximal concentration of 1 to 3 hours. The drug is highly protein bound (77 to 95%) and undergoes saturable metabolism leading to variable bioavailability of 11 to 39%. Propafenone is almost completely cleared by the liver with polymorphic oxidative metabolism via cytochrome P-450$_{dbl}$ (120). Extensive metabolizers (EM) have a half life of 5.5 hr, while poor metabolizers (approximately 7% of the U.S. population) have a half life of 17.2 hr. The major metabolite of propafenone is 5-hydroxypropafenone, which is active and only detectable in EM.

Propafenone appears to be comparable to other antiarrhythmics such as quinidine, disopyramide, and flecainide in suppressing PVCs. In one trial, propafenone was inferior to lidocaine in suppressing arrhythmias shortly after an AMI (121).

The most common adverse reaction to propafenone is a metallic or bitter taste that may resolve without changing the dose. Propafenone may cause central nervous system effects such as dizziness, headache, paresthesias, and fatigue. Despite the β-blocking properties of propafenone, the risk of bronchospasm seems low. Patients that are poor metabolizers exhibit greater β-blocking effects, possibly due to higher blood concentrations of the parent compound, which tends to accumulate with chronic dosing.

DIGITALIS-INDUCED PVC
PVCs are the most common arrhythmia produced by digitalis. Generally this arrhythmia resolves when the digitalis is discontinued. For frequent or symptomatic PVCs, potassium replacement in hypo- or normokalemic patients may suppress the arrhythmia. For sustained PVCs induced by digitalis, lidocaine or phenytoin has been used successfully. Phenytoin is considered an ideal agent to treat digitalis-induced arrhythmias, since it improves AV conduction while it suppresses ventricular irritability. Unfortunately, phenytoin is not nearly as effective in PVCs of different etiology. For refractory arrhythmias that are life-threatening, especially when an overdose of digitalis has produced hyperkalemia, digoxin immune Fab (antigen-binding fragments from antibodies to digoxin in sheep) can be administered intravenously over 30 min or IVP if an arrest is imminent (122). The amount of antibody depends upon the quantity of digitalis to be bound, based upon the formula:

Dose Fab (in # of vials)

$$= \text{Digoxin stores (in mg)} \times 0.6 \text{ (mg/vial)}$$

Phenytoin. For the treatment of digitalis-induced PVCs, phenytoin would most likely be given parenterally, yet its hypotensive effects via this route are particularly troublesome. Phenytoin may lower blood pressure in 2 to 8% of patients given intravenous doses, through vasodilation and myocardial depression. Parahydroxylation by the liver accounts for 50 to 76% of an administered dose of phenytoin, while 5% is eliminated unchanged in the urine. Phenytoin is 93% protein-bound, primarily to albumin. The degree of binding may be reduced in renal or hepatic disease, where serum albumin concentrations may be reduced. In addition, in uremia and cirrhosis, the extent of binding to albumin is reduced. In such situations the free drug concentration may be adequate, while the total measured phenytoin concentration may not be within the therapeutic range, despite adequate arrhythmia suppression. Most arrhythmias are controlled by phenytoin plasma levels of 10 to 20 μg/ml.

In most situations phenytoin should be initiated with a loading dose. The diluent in the parenteral product may cause cardiovascular collapse and central nervous system depression. These complications may be reduced or avoided with rates of administration of 50 mg/min or less. Intramuscular injection may obviate this problem, but absorption is erratic and slow as a result of precipitation of phenytoin in the muscle. Phenytoin distributes into a volume (Vd) that approaches total body water (0.7 liters/kg), which may be used to estimate loading dose (LD), based upon the desired plasma concentration (Cp) of 15 μg/ml as follows:

$$LD = CP \times Vd$$
$$= 15 \text{ μg/ml} \times 0.7 \text{ liters/kg}$$
$$= 10.5 \text{ mg/kg}$$

The entire dose may be infused intravenously no faster than 50 mg/min or by intermittent bolus infusions of 100 mg over 2 min given every 5 min until arrhythmia suppression, a maximum dose of 1 g, or toxicity occurs. Digitalis-induced PVCs may be eliminated by the loading dose of phenytoin and not require a maintenance dose. Sustained PVCs require maintenance doses of phenytoin that are influenced by the capacity-limited metabolism of the drug. With therapeutic concentrations, the rate of metabolism is often near saturation. The Michaelis-Menton kinetics of phenytoin suggest that changes in dose lead to exponentially greater increased in serum concentration. Therefore, the typical patient should be given 300 to 400 mg/day as a single dose or divided into two doses. Subsequent adjustments should be made in 100 mg/day increments at approximately 2-week intervals. Additional bolus doses may be given to treat ectopic beats to avoid the delay to steady-state conditions. (For further information refer to Chapter 48, "Seizure Disorders.")

Parenteral therapy with phenytoin may produce bradycardia, hypotension, and a prolonged Q-Tc interval and QRS complex, related to rate of administration. Central nervous system toxicity may be related to blood concentrations. Nystagmus may be the initial sign of toxicity when levels exceed 20 μg/ml. Phenytoin levels above 30 μg/ml may produce ataxia. Mental changes are common with concentrations above 40 μg/ml. Toxic responses such as gingival hyperplasia, folate deficiency, peripheral neuropathy, hypertrichosis, and osteomalcia are seen with chronic therapy.

Other than for digitalis-induced arrhythmias, phenytoin has limited usefulness as an antiarrhythmic. Phenytoin does appear to be particularly effective in suppressing PVCs in pediatric patients, especially in those with an arrhythmia after surgery for congenital heart disease (124).

VENTRICULAR TACHYCARDIA

Ventricular tachycardia (VT) is a rapid (100 to 250 beats/min), regular, ectopic rhythm of three or more consecutive ventricular complexes. VT is more serious than PVCs, producing more marked hemodynamic deterioration as a result of decreased diastolic filling and loss of coordinated ventricular contraction with atrial kick. VT is also ominous since it often degenerates into ventricular fibrillation. VT may be seen in the prehospital phase of an AMI, as a result of enhanced automaticity. At this stage the rhythm is somewhat more stable. The third phase of VT seen in ischemic heart disease is noted after several days to weeks.

There are two general types of VT. Nonsustained VT is three or more coupled PVCs occurring at rates greater than 100 beats/min and terminating spontaneously in <30 sec. These may require only close observation if they are asymptomatic. VT beyond 30 sec is considered to be sustained VT. Sustained VT is often associated with hemodynamic instability. The drug therapy of sustained VT may be defined by laboratory-programmed electrical stimulation of the rhythm to determine the most efficacious drug, dose, and plasma concentration. This laboratory model is reported to reflect clinical VT and predict appropriate therapy. The successful drug concentration in the acute laboratory situation correlates well with the therapeutic level observed chronically for drugs such as quinidine and procainamide but not for propranolol, which depends upon prevailing sympathetic tone (125). Patients whose arrhythmia is not controlled during laboratory-programmed electrical stimulation usually have a relapse of their VT while on chronic suppression drug therapy.

In the patient with VT and hemodynamic instability, the therapy of choice is electrical cardioversion. In patients without a pulse, the rhythm should be treated as it is with ventricular fibrillation. VT with a pulse but in an unstable patient may be cardioverted with a synchronized shock of 50 joules. VT in the late hospital phase of an AMI is often asymptomatic, but it is a highly important risk, since patients with VT are five times more likely to die within 1 year than those without the arrhythmia (126). However, whether antiarrhythmics influence the mortality rate is not known. In drug-refractory VT, options include surgical ablative techniques and implantable cardioverter defibrillator (127).

Lidocaine is the preferred agent for rapid control of VT. Procainamide is also effective, yet many patients require plasma concentrations that are considered to be in the toxic range (>8 μg/ml).

TORSADE DE POINTES

Torsade de pointes is a proarrhythmia characterized by rapid series of ventricular tachycardia with varying axis on the ECG. Torsade de pointes may or may not be associated with the prolonged Q-T interval. Torsade de pointes may be a result of type Ia antiarrhythmics, metabolic derangements, or idiopathic mechanisms. Type Ia antiarrhythmics should be monitored closely for Q-Tc prolongation, to avoid episodes of torsade de pointes that may impair hemodynamics or lead to malignant ventricular arrhythmias. In the absence of the prolonged Q-T interval syndrome, torsade can be managed as VT. On the other hand, the prolonged Q-T interval syndrome is commonly caused by quinidine and in the past was termed "quinidine syncope." The syncope most frequently occurs within 1 to 3 days of initiation of quinidine, although occasionally patients may be receiving the drug for longer than a year when symptoms develop. However, this delayed syndrome is typically at or below the therapeutic range. When the syndrome develops in patients receiving quinidine for atrial fibrillation, the VT occurs typically after conversion to sinus rhythm. The frequency of the long QT syndrome is higher for quinidine than for the other class Ia agents disopyramide or procainamide (128). The most effective therapy for torsades is rapid pacing. An alternative therapy, effective even in normomagnesemia, is intravenous magnesium 2 g given over one min. Magnesium may cause hypotension and hypokalemia (129). Bretylium has also been used in quinidine-induced VT (130).

Flecainide. Flecainide is a fluorinated analog of procainamide currently available in oral form only. FDA indications before the CAST reports included sustained VT, symptomatic nonsustained VT, and frequent PVCs.

Absorption after oral dosing of flecainide is fairly rapid, with peak serum concentrations occurring in 3 to 4 hr. The bioavailability is nearly 100%. There is no apparent first-pass effect. Food does not affect the absorption of flecainide. Flecainide has a large volume of distribution, 8 to 10 liters/kg, reflecting substantial tissue distribution. The protein binding of flecainide is 37 to 58%. The free fraction of flecainide is proportional to serum albumin and AAG concentrations. The binding of flecainide is loose however, and in a situation such as immediately post-AMI where AAG levels rise, flecainide is displaced, producing higher free flecainide concentrations. About one-quarter of flecainide is excreted unchanged by the kidneys, and the remainder is primarily conjugated by the liver as inactive metabolites. The normal half-life of flecainide is about 14 hr and is prolonged by ventricular arrhythmias, heart failure, and renal impairment (131). Flecainide is marketed as a racemic mixture. The enantiomers of flecainide are metabolized with a genetically determined rate showing polymorphism. Patients are termed poor metabolizers (PM) and extensive metabolizers (EM) (132). Significantly longer half-lives may be expected in patients with liver cirrhosis (133). It is recommended that initial dosing should be low, 50 to 100 mg orally twice daily, and increased at 4-day intervals as needed and tolerated. The usual maintenance dose is 100 to 200 mg twice daily. The therapeutic range for flecainide is 318 ng/ml (with a reported 50% probability of efficacy) to 710 ng/ml (with <10% probability of cardiovascular toxicity) (134).

Interactions with flecainide have been observed with digoxin, cimetidine, and propranolol. Cimetidine may reduce the clearance of flecainide. Propranolol and flecainide may be additive in terms of negative inotropism. Flecainide may raise serum digoxin concentrations by an apparent decrease in distribution volume.

Unlike other class I drugs, flecainide does not produce frequent gastrointestinal toxicity. Dizziness and blurred vision may occur. A prolongation of the P-R interval and QRS complex duration should be expected and up to 30% is well tolerated. Flecainide may induce serious arrhythmias that may not be preceded by conduction changes. A history of sustained ventricular tachycardia, daily doses of flecainide over 400 mg, high flecainide concentrations (>1 μg/ml), and reduced ejection fractions may contribute to

drug-induced arrhythmias. This proarrhythmic effect of flecainide may occur in 6.6% of patients with sustained VT but only 0.9% with nonsustained VT (135). The mortality rate of the proarrhythmic events was also higher in sustained VT. Structural heart disease may also predict higher proarrhythmias from flecainide. The results of the CAST trial suggest that flecainide (and perhaps any class Ic agent) should not be used in anything but a life-threatening arrhythmia. Even in such a situation, flecainide may be considered after class Ia and class Ib drugs.

Moricizine. Moricizine is a class I agent that was developed in the Soviet Union and used there since 1971. Moricizine structurally resembles the phenothiazines, but the antiarrhythmic does not possess antidopaminergic effects. Moricizine cannot be assigned to a subgroup of class I because it has properties of all three. Moricizine prolongs QRS duration like class Ia agents, shortens APD like class Ib agents, and prolongs the PR interval like agents in class Ic. Moricizine has been described as a membrane-stabilizer with anticholinergic properties and the ability to suppress both normal and abnormal automaticity (136).

Moricizine is completely absorbed after oral administration, with peak blood levels occurring at 1 to 3 hr, but bioavailability is limited to 34 to 38% by pronounced first-pass metabolism. Food may lower peak moricizine levels, but the extent of absorption is not decreased (137). Moricizine has a large apparent distribution volume (300 liters) and is highly protein bound (~95%) to albumin and α_1-acid glycoprotein. Moricizine is metabolized by sulfooxidation, ring hydroxylation, N-dealkylation, and glucuronide and sulfate conjugation to at least 26 metabolites. The drug induces cytochrome P-450 activity, causing a decrease in its own elimination half-life with chronic dosing from 1.9 hr (single dose) to 1.4 hr. Drug blood levels do not predict response, and in fact the onset of antiarrhythmic action is substantially delayed (~16 hours) beyond the time to peak level of the drug (138).

Moricizine may be effective as quinidine or disopyramide with fewer side effects in treating patients with ventricular arrhythmias (137). In the CAPS trial (Cardiac Arrhythmia Pilot Study) moricizine was less effective than encainide and flecainide in suppressing PVC and nonsustained VT (139). However, in patients with depressed left ventricular function (ejection fraction <0.45) the agents were similar. In contrast, moricizine continued to be studied in the CAST trial, while encainide and flecainide were withdrawn because of excessive mortality compared with moricizine or placebo (140). Subsequently, moricizine was found to produce excess mortality relative to placebo and the trial was stopped. The current FDA-approved indication for moricizine is life-threatening, sustained VT.

Adverse effects from moricizine are infrequent and include dizziness, nausea, headache, and perioral paresthesia. Moricizine has proarrhythmic effects observed in

3.2 to 15% of patients (more common in potentially lethal as opposed to benign ventricular arrhythmias) (136). Cimetidine may reduce the clearance of moricizine, and moricizine may reduce the clearance of theophylline.

The starting dose of moricizine is 200 mg t.i.d. There is evidence that b.i.d. dosing is equivalent to t.i.d. dosing. The dose may be increased to 300 mg t.i.d. with small incremental adjustments at 3-day intervals.

Mexiletine. Mexiletine is classified as a class Ib agent with a structure and mechanism of action similar to those of lidocaine. At the present time mexiletine is available in an oral dosage form only, with FDA approval for symptomatic VT, couplets, and frequent PVCs.

Mexiletine is well absorbed orally, with a bioavailability of 80 to 90% in healthy volunteers and peak concentrations occurring at 2 to 4 hr. Absorption may be delayed and incomplete in patients with AMI. Antacids, cimetidine, and atropine delay the time to peak concentration but not the serum concentration–time profile for mexiletine. On the other hand, metoclopramide increases the rate of absorption with no effect on serum concentration–time profile. Mexiletine after intravenous administration is thought to exhibit three-compartment kinetics. It has a large volume of distribution, about 5 liters/kg, extensive tissue protein binding, and <1% of the drug remains in the blood (141). Mexiletine is primarily metabolized by the liver, with about 8% of the drug recovered unchanged in the urine in healthy volunteers. Urine excretion is pH-dependent, with a more rapid clearance as pH decreases (141). The elimination half-life of mexiletine is 9.4, 12.1, and 16.7 hr after oral dosing in healthy subjects, patients, and AMI patients, respectively. Cigarette smoking may induce the conjugation of mexiletine, reducing the half-life from 11.1 to 7.2 hr (142). Phenytoin enhances the metabolism of mexiletine, with a decrease in mexiletine half-life of about 50% (141). Renal function does not appear to affect the clearance of mexiletine, and the drug does not seem to be dialyzable (143).

The therapeutic range for mexiletine is 0.75 to 2.0 µg/ml. Because of the slow clearance of mexiletine, a loading dose may be required, but full loading doses are rarely tolerated. A compromise is to give a starting dose of 400 mg once, followed by 200 mg every 8 hr, or 10 to 15 mg/kg/day. There is evidence that a 12-hr regimen with the same total daily dose is as effective as the 8-hr regimen (144).

There is a high frequency of adverse reactions, in the induction phase of mexiletine, but with chronic use, it is considered to be comparable to quinidine or procainamide (145). Side effects frequently limit the dose of mexiletine and reduce the ability to suppress arrhythmias. When this occurs, it may be possible to add other drugs to a tolerated but ineffective dose of mexiletine. In fact, the combination of quinidine and mexiletine has been more effective than quinidine alone with fewer side effects (146). A side benefit is that mexiletine may block the increase in Q-Tc interval produced by quinidine (147). The additive antiarrhythmic effect is also demonstrated with mexiletine and disopyramide (148). Mexiletine effectively reduces the frequency of PVCs in most patients, even those who have failed to respond to other agents. Chronic, sustained recurrent VT does not respond well to mexiletine, but if electrophysiologic studies show mexiletine to control induced VT, it is usually effective chronically (149). The frequency of side effects may be as high as 54% of patients receiving chronic mexiletine, usually involving neurologic or gastrointestinal effects. Tremor, dizziness, vertigo, paresthesias, nystagmus, diplopia, ataxia, and confusion may occur. Nausea, vomiting, and dyspepsia are common. Cardiovascular effects include hypotension, sinus bradycardia, AV dissociation, and in overdosage, widened QRS complex. In usual doses, mexiletine does not reduce left ventricular function.

Tocainide. Tocainide, an amine analog of lidocaine, is indicated for the suppression of symptomatic ventricular arrhythmias, especially if the arrhythmias responded first to lidocaine. It currently is available only in an oral dosage form. It appears to be absorbed rapidly and completely, but food may decrease the peak plasma concentration without altering the extent of absorption. About one-half the tocainide is cleared unchanged by the kidneys; the rest is glucuronidated by the liver. The normal elimination half-life of 11 hr may be prolonged in patients with chronic arrhythmias, ventricular dysfunction, and renal impairment (150). The therapeutic range for tocainide concentrations is 3 to 9 µg/ml. Toxicity may occur with concentrations above 10 µg/ml. Rifampin may induce metabolism of tocainide leading to a shortened half-life (151). Cimetidine, on the other hand, decreases the bioavailability of tocainide (152).

Tocainide is indicated for the suppression of ventricular arrhythmias. It has very limited utility in atrial arrhythmias. Although tocainide may reduce the frequency of PVCs, it may not be as effective or as well tolerated as older drugs such as quinidine (153). Tocainide may be effective when class Ia drugs have failed.

The utility of tocainide chronically is limited by the high frequency of adverse reactions (up to 70%). Ataxia, tremor, dizziness, paresthesias, night sweats, nausea, and vomiting are common toxicities. As with lidocaine and procainamide, tocainide may produce confusion, psychoses, and seizures. Symptoms may resolve if the drug is administered with meals, by reducing the magnitude of the peak serum concentration without altering the extent of absorption. There are case reports of an association between the use of tocainide and the development of pulmonary fibrosis and interstitial pneumonitis. The pulmonary toxicity may resolve after discontinuing tocainide (154).

Agranulocytosis has been reported with tocainide. Although neutropenia is rare, it may be life-threatening. It is suggested that white blood cell counts be monitored frequently, particularly early in therapy. Rash and fever have also been reported. Cross-reactivity may occur in patients allergic to lidocaine or procainamide.

VENTRICULAR FLUTTER AND FIBRILLATION

Some consider ventricular flutter to be a separate entity from ventricular fibrillation (VF). Ventricular flutter is a rapid ectopic firing at one or more sites in the ventricles at a fairly regular rate of 150 to 300 beats/min. QRS complexes appear to run into each other, obliterating S-T segments and P waves, but the wave appears "saw-toothed." Classically, VF was a rapid (150 to 500 beats/min), disorganized ventricular rhythm. In VF, the ectopic beat does not develop from a single area. Instead the firing is random and changing. Individual fibers or groups of fibers contract independently. When observed, the heart shows areas of twitching. Consequently, there is no effective net contraction and no pumping of blood.

Almost 50% of patients who develop VF do not have warning arrhythmias (see "PVC"), especially during the early phase of AMI. Often the time period between warning arrhythmias and VF is very short (measured in seconds). In the setting of an AMI, 88% of patients with VF will develop it within the first 6 hr of the infarct. If resuscitated, such patients in general have a good prognosis. VF associated with or caused by heart failure may occur at any time after an infarct and is associated with a higher mortality rate because myocardial damage is more extensive.

Since the criteria for predicting VF are not very accurate, some centers use prophylactic antiarrhythmics to prevent fatal VF. This therapy is highly controversial. Some studies, using relatively low-dose infusions (2 mg/min), report that lidocaine does not prevent VF, particularly in the first few hours of the infarct (155). Higher doses of lidocaine (3 mg/min) have been shown to prevent VF at the expense of frequent toxicity (15%) in patients under 70 years old without heart failure or block (156). This regimen is recommended for the first 24 hr only. Recently, prophylactic lidocaine has come under intense criticism because of unacceptable toxicity (in 51% of patients) and questionable efficacy (157). Unfortunately, serum lidocaine concentrations provided little help in preventing these adverse reactions. This lack of efficacy was confirmed by meta-analysis of multiple trials suggesting that prehospital mortality was not decreased with lidocaine and the in-hospital mortality was actually increased by lidocaine (158).

Electrical Cardioversion. The primary treatment of VF is electrical cardioversion. The likelihood of successful conversion is increased if coronary artery perfusion is maintained. In 80% of patients, a single shock is adequate to convert to a more stable rhythm. Nonresponders should receive cardiopulmonary resuscitation with repeated shock therapy, epinephrine, and lidocaine. Lidocaine has been the preferred pharmacologic agent for VF. Bretylium is an effective alternative.

Bretylium. Bretylium is considered by some to be an alternative for patients resistant to lidocaine, although there are others who advocate bretylium before lidocaine in the management of DC conversion–resistant VF. Clearly a distinction should be drawn in indications for these agents. The prevention of VF is different from the suppression of active PVC. To complicate matters further, VF in sudden death syndrome may respond differently than VF in ischemia. Bretylium may have poor-to-adequate activity in PVC suppression, but it has excellent antifibrillatory activity. Bretylium is taken up by the amine pump in the adrenergic neuron. It displaces norepinephrine, then blocks subsequent release of catecholamines. The temporary period of sympathetic excess may produce hypertension and arrhythmias, particularly in patients with digitalis toxicity. The antiarrhythmic action of bretylium may be independent of its sympatholytic effects. The hypertension observed with bretylium, however, correlates well with changes in norepinephrine plasma concentration (159). The ability of bretylium to reduce the disparity in refractory periods between normal and infarcted tissues may indicate why it is effective in VF, which is felt to be sustained by reentry between these two tissues. Since bretylium does not depress automaticity, PVC frequency is largely unaffected.

Bretylium exhibits two-compartment kinetics. Elimination of bretylium is primarily 70 to 80% via the kidneys. In normal volunteers the half-life is 7.8 hr, compared with 33.4 hr in patients with impaired renal function. The relationship between total body clearance of bretylium (TBC) and creatinine clearance (CC) may be defined by the following: (160)

$$TBC = 0.362\ CC + 3.242 \qquad (r = 0.93)$$

This equation may be useful if infusions of bretylium are administered. The antiarrhythmic concentration is not well established; a range of 0.5 to 1.5 μg/ml has been suggested.

Bretylium may produce chemical defibrillation without electric shock when it is given undiluted by rapid injection of 5 mg/kg. Rapid administration should be reserved for emergency use, as in cardiopulmonary resuscitation. The average time to reversion after bretylium is 9 to 10 min. If after 15 to 30 min there is no response, another 10 mg/kg may be given, up to a maximum of 30 mg/kg. For less serious arrhythmias, bretylium can be given over 8 to 10 min, with 5 to 10 mg/kg as the loading dose. If the arrhythmia persists, the dose may be repeated at 1-hr intervals up to 30 mg/kg. For chronic suppression, bretylium may be given intramuscularly or by intermittent infusions (over 8 to 10 min), every 6 to 8 hr. Bretylium has also been given by constant infusion at 1 to 2 mg/min.

The common adverse effects of bretylium are related to its adrenergic-blocking actions producing transient hypertension followed by hypotension, worsened arrhythmias, and angina. Rapid intravenous injection often produces nausea and vomiting. Hyperthermia is an unusual reaction to bretylium. A reported temperature of 108.2°F was ascribed to bretylium infusion (161). The febrile illness resolved when the infusion was stopped.

Amiodarone. Amiodarone is a class III agent that is generally restricted to the treatment of drug-resistant arrhythmias because of its side effects. Amiodarone at this time has a restricted indication from the FDA for recurrent ventricular fibrillation or recurrent hemodynamically unstable ventricular tachycardia where other agents have failed through ineffectiveness or toxicity. Amiodarone resembles thyroxine structurally.

Amiodarone is currently available in an oral dosage form. Bioavailability is poor and erratic with 22 to 85% absorption (162). The time to peak absorption is about 6 hr. After absorption, the drug is widely distributed to fat, lung, liver, muscle, and spleen, with a very large volume of distribution, approximately 5000 liters. The elimination half-life varies from 26 to 107 days and appears biphasic. Amiodarone is metabolized with its major metabolite desethyamiodarone. The utility of monitoring serum concentrations of amiodarone is controversial. There is some evidence that arrhythmias may recur if concentrations fall below 1.0 μg/ml. Toxicity may occur if serum concentrations exceed 2.5 μg/ml. Variable correlations have been made with red cell concentrations of amiodarone. Various dosing schemes have been suggested to avoid the delay in reaching steady-state serum amiodarone concentrations. Up to 1600 mg daily for a week, then 800 mg daily for 2 to 4 weeks, and finally the dose is reduced to the minimally tolerable dose, usually 400 to 600 mg daily in two divided doses.

A wide range of side effects may be encountered with long-term use of amiodarone. Corneal deposits occur often. In one series, 79% of patients developed microdeposits but no change in visual acuity (163). Some cardiologists suggest observing only for visual symptoms such as photophobia or blurring, which develop less frequently than the microdeposits (164). Abnormal liver enzymes may be encountered in up to 55% of patients (163). The drug appears to concentrate in liver tissue. While enzyme levels may increase threefold, hepatic function may not change, and the drug may be continued with ultimate resolution of the problem. Dermatologic reactions to amiodarone may occur in up to 11.6% of patients (164) and have been described as sun sensitivity or a blue-grey skin discolora-

tion. Pulmonary abnormalities associated with amiodarone are considered to be a justification for discontinuing therapy. The pulmonary fibrosis is usually symptomatic, may be reversible upon discontinuation with or without administration of glucocorticoids, and may be fatal. Amiodarone interferes with the metabolism of thyrosine, resulting in increased serum concentrations. Patients typically are not symptomatic of hyperthyroidism, in fact TSH levels may be increased, which suggests insensitivity to the effects of thyroid hormone. There is controversy over the predictability of antiarrhythmic response and toxicity with the use of the serum reverse T3 concentrations (rT3). Very high rT3 levels (in excess of 130 ng/dl) have been associated with the development of pulmonary fibrosis, arrhythmogenicity, and sudden cardiac death (165). Cardiovascular side effects include sinus bradycardia that may reduce cardiac output.

Amiodarone may produce drug interactions with warfarin, digoxin, procainamide, and quinidine (166). It has been suggested that the dose of quinidine or procainamide be reduced by 30 to 50% when amiodarone is added and that QT and QRS intervals should be monitored for excessive prolongation. An interaction is observed with amiodarone and warfarin. It is suggested that the warfarin maintenance dose be decreased by one-half when amiodarone is added, and prothrombin times should be monitored carefully. When amiodarone is given to patients receiving digoxin, it is suggested that the digoxin maintenance dose be halved and adjusted according to serum digoxin concentrations.

SUDDEN DEATH

The predominant cause of sudden death is ventricular fibrillation. In approximately 25% of cases, sudden death (presumably via VF) is not preceded by a history of cardiac symptoms. Thus the prevention of VF with chronic antiarrhythmics becomes a question of patient selection. Sudden cardiac collapse via VF in ambulatory patients often (55%) is not associated with an AMI. After resuscitation these patients have a very high (three times greater than primary VF with an AMI) mortality rate. Chronic antiarrhythmics have produced mixed results in sudden death.

When considering the choices for chronic management of VF and prevention of sudden death, β-blockers deserve a prominent role. Unfortunately a variety of conditions may preclude patients from the potential benefit of β-blockage, such as uncontrolled heart failure, bradycardia, second- or third-degree heart block, sinoatrial block, insulin-dependent diabetes mellitus, peripheral vascular disease, and chronic obstructive pulmonary disease. The following discussion is limited to β-blockers, with substantial literature supporting their use in sudden death, AMI, or arrhythmias.

Propranolol has not met with exceptional results in ventricular ectopic suppression. It may not be effective in preventing ectopics after an AMI. In the treatment of VT, propranolol has been disappointing. However, it may be useful in exercise-induced arrhythmias, ventricular arrhythmias associated with mitral valve prolapse, digitalis-induced arrhythmias, and arrhythmias associated with a long QT interval.

Propranolol has been studied in post-AMI with mixed results in lowering the risk of sudden death. The report from the National Heart, Lung and Blood Institute revealed a 26% lower mortality rate for propranolol, compared with placebo (167). The site of the infarct, age, and sex had no influence on the response to propranolol. The initial dose of propranolol, 40 mg three times daily, was adjusted to 60 or 80 mg three times daily, depending upon the serum propranolol concentrations.

Propranolol is felt to have the highest membrane-stabilizing potency of the β-blockers. Called a "quinidine-like" action, it is manifest only in overdose situations. Propranolol is a nonselective antagonist to β_1 (cardiac) and β_2 (lungs and blood vessels) receptors. It is well absorbed (more than 90%), but first-pass hepatic extraction may reduce bioavailability to about 30%. Protein binding is of the order of 90%. Propranolol is cleared rapidly by hepatic metabolism, with a half-life of 3.5 to 6 hr.

Propranolol may be given intravenously under rare situations, 0.5 to 0.75 mg repeated every 2 min up to a maximum of 0.1 mg/kg. The effective dose may be repeated at 6- to 8-hr intervals. The oral propranolol dose is much higher, but variable. A typical starting dose is 10 mg every 6 hr. The dosing interval may not correlate with the short half-life; a twice-daily regimen has been effective.

The most common adverse reactions seen with propranolol involve the central nervous system and include fatigue, hallucinations, weakness, insomnia, and nightmares. These effects may not be related to β-blockade, and differences between the various β-blockers have not been demonstrated. Since it is nonselective, propranolol may exacerbate bronchospasm. Although propranolol may precipitate or worsen congestive heart failure, if the arrhythmia is felt to have induced symptoms, propranolol may relieve the symptoms because it suppresses the arrhythmia. β-Blockers with intrinsic sympathomimetic activity may produce less cardiac depression and may be indicated in patients prone to heart failure. Propranolol (by β-blockade) may allow α-vasoconstriction, producing cold or painful extremities. Gangrene, skin necrosis, and claudication have been observed. Nonselective agents should be avoided after such symptoms develop; cardioselective or high intrinsic sympathomimetic agents are preferred.

Timolol is a nonselective antagonist with good absorption (over 90%) and bioavailability (75%). Protein binding is low at 10%. Timolol is cleared primarily by the liver, with slight (20%) renal excretion. The half-life is short, 3 to 4 hr. Adverse effects are similar to those of propranolol.

Timolol has been compared with placebo in the chronic prophylaxis of post-AMI (168). Placebo patients had nearly three times as many arrhythmias requiring treatment as the timolol group. Besides a decrease in overall mortality rate with timolol, the incidence of sudden death and presumably fatal VF was reduced by approximately one-half. The study used a fixed-dose regimen (5 mg twice daily for 2 days then 10 mg twice daily), which was associated with a significant reduction in resting heart rate. Whether beneficial effects on mortality might be seen without bradycardia is not known.

Metoprolol, although currently limited to the treatment of hypertension, may be considered an alternative to propranolol for arrhythmias because it is somewhat selective for β_1-receptors, and it may be preferred over propranolol for patients with chronic or acute obstructive pulmonary disease. Metoprolol should be used with caution because in high doses it may also block β_2-receptors.

Metoprolol is well absorbed, over 95%, with greater bioavailability than propranolol, about 50%. Protein binding is slight, 12%. Metoprolol is cleared hepatically with a half-life of 3 to 4 hr. The typical patient is started at 20 mg four times daily. Metoprolol has adverse effects similar to those of propranolol, with less risk for patients with asthma or peripheral vascular disease.

Metoprolol has been compared with placebo in patients with AMI treated for 90 days (169). Metoprolol was initiated as 15 mg intravenously, followed by an oral dose of 100 mg twice daily. It reduced mortality by 36%, with beneficial effects in all age groups.

Alprenolol is a nonselective β-blocker with intrinsic sympathomimetic activity. It is cleared rapidly by the liver, with a half-life of 2 hr. The usual dose is 200 mg twice daily.

Alprenolol has produced a beneficial response in reducing sudden death, limited to patients under 65 years old (170).

As a class, β-blockers appear to be beneficial in the management of post-AMI patients. The efficacy seems to be independent of intrinsic sympathomimetic activity, β_2-receptor blockade, and membrane-stabilizing properties. However, these properties may aid individual drug selection in certain patients. The duration of therapy has not been established. The onset of therapy has varied between the studies, but immediate β-blockade (e.g., within 12 hr after the onset of pain) may limit the enzyme-estimated infarct size.

CONCLUSION

Cardiac arrhythmias are complex, have various etiologies and alterations in electrophysiology, differ in severity and prognosis, and require individualized treatment with potentially toxic drugs. A thorough understanding of the pharmacology, pharmacodynamics, pharmacokinetics, and adverse reactions for each antiarrhythmic drug is required for safe and effective treatment of patients with arrhythmias. No one drug is effective for any arrhythmia in all patients, although certain drugs are clearly first-line agents. Doses of many antiarrhythmics should be calculated, using known values for the pharmacokinetic variables. However, these doses are usually only estimates of the required dose for a patient, and adjustments may be required. Patients must be monitored carefully, which frequently involves drug-level monitoring. Many new antiarrhythmics have been marketed. The ultimate question remains unresolved for most arrhythmias—will these drugs improve mortality?

REFERENCES

1. Wit AL: Cellular electrophysiologic mechanisms of cardiac arrhythmias. Cardiol Clin 8:393–409, 1990.
2. Saini V, Podrid PJ, Slater W: Encainide and flecainide: are they interchangeable. Am Heart J 117:1253–1258, 1989.
3. Wyse DG, Mitchell LB, Duff HJ: Procainamide, disopyramide, and quinidine: discordant antiarrhythmic effects during crossover comparison in patients with inducible ventricular tachycardia. J Am Coll Cardiol 9:882–889, 1987.
4. Hession M, Blum R, Podrid PJ, Lampert S, Stein J, Lown B: Mexiletine and tocainide—does response to one predict response to the other? J Am Coll Cardiol 7:338–343, 1986.
5. Dreifus LS, Michelson EL, Kaplinsky E: Bradyarrhythmias: clinical significance and management. J Am Coll Cardiol 1:327–338, 1983.
6. Hindman MC, Wagner, GS: Arrhythmias during myocardial infarction: mechanisms, significance, and therapy. Cardiovasc Clin 11(1):81–102, 1980.
7. Schweitzer P, Mark H: The effect of atropine on cardiac arrhythmias and conduction (Parts 1 and 2). Am Heart J 100:119–127, 251–261, 1980.
8. Wood M, Ellenbogen KA: Bradyarrhythmias, emergency pacing, and implantable defibrillation devices. Crit Care Clin 5(3):551–568, 1989.
9. Rodriguez RD, Schocken DD: Update on sick sinus syndrome, a cardiac disorder of aging. Geriatrics 45(1):26–36, 1990.
10. Council on Scientific Affairs: The use of cardiac pacemakers in medical practice: Excerpts from the report of the advisory panel. JAMA 254(14):1952–1954, 1985.
11. Santini M, Alexidou G, Ansalone G, Cacciatore G, Cini R, Turitto G: Relation of prognosis in sick sinus syndrome to age, conduction defects and modes of permanent cardiac pacing. Am J Cardiol 65:729–735, 1990.
12. Schweitzer P, Teichholz LE: Carotid sinus massage: its diagnostic and therapeutic value in arrhythmias. Am J Med 78:645–654, 1985.
13. Mehta D, Ward DE, Wafa S, Camm AJ: Relative efficacy of various physical manoeuvres in the termination of junctional tachycardia. Lancet 1:1181–1185, 1988.
14. Huycke EC, Sung RJ, Dias VC, et al.: Intravenous diltiazem for termination of reentrant supraventricular tachycardia: a placebo-controlled, randomized, double-blind, multicenter study. J Am Coll Cardiol 13(3):538–544, 1989.
15. McAllister RG, Kirsten EB: The pharmacology of verapamil. IV.

Kinetic and dynamic effects after single intravenous and oral doses. Clin Pharmacol Ther 31(4):418–426, 1982.
16. Hamann SR, Blouin RA, McAllister RG: Clinical pharmacokinetics of verapamil. Clin Pharmacokinet 9:26–41, 1984.
17. McCall D, Walsh RA, Frohlich ED, O'Rourke RA: Calcium entry blocking drugs: mechanisms of action, experimental studies and clinical uses. Curr Probl Cardiol 10(8):2–80, 1985.
18. Hoon TJ, Bauman JL, Rodvold KA, Gallestegui J, Hariman RJ: The pharmacodynamic and pharmacokinetic differences of the d- and l-isomers of verapamil: Implications in the treatment of paroxysmal supraventricular tachycardia. Am Heart J 112(2):396–403, 1986.
19. Echizen H, Vogelgesang B, Eichelbaum M: Effects of d,l-verapamil on atrioventricular conduction in relation to its stereoselective first-pass metabolism. Clin Pharmacol Ther 38(1):71–76, 1985.
20. Weiss AT, Lewis BS, Halon DA, Hasin Y, Gotsman MS: The use of calcium with verapamil in the management of supraventricular tachyarrhythmias. Int J Cardiol 4:275–280, 1983.
21. Haft JI, Habbab MA: Treatment of atrial arrhythmias: effectiveness of verapamil when preceded by calcium infusion. Arch Intern Med 146:1085–1089, 1986.
22. Epstein ML, Kiel EA, Victorica BE: Cardiac decompensation following verapamil therapy in infants with supraventricular tachycardia. Pediatrics 75(4):737–740, 1985.
23. Garson A Jr: Medicolegal problems in the management of cardiac arrhythmias in children. Pediatrics 79(1):84–88, 1987.
24. Packer M, Meller J, Medina N, et al. Hemodynamic consequences of combined β-adrenergic and slow calcium channel blockade in man. Circulation 65(4):660–668, 1982.
25. Bussey HI: The influence of quinidine and other agents on digitalis glycosides. Am Heart J 104(2 Pt 1):289–302, 1982.
26. Parker RB, McCollam PL: Adenosine in the episodic treatment of paroxysmal supraventricular tachycardia. Clin Pharm 9(4):261–271, 1990.
27. DiMarco JP, Sellers TD, Lerman BB, Greenberg ML, Berne RM, Belardinelli L: Diagnostic and therapeutic use of adenosine in patients with supraventricular tachyarrhythmias. J Am Coll Cardiol 6(2):417–425, 1985.
28. Rankin AC, Oldroyd KG, Chong E, Dow JW, Rae AP, Cobbe SM: Adenosine or adenosine triphosphate for supraventricular tachycardias? Comparative double-blind randomized study in patients with spontaneous or inducible arrhythmias. Am Heart J 119(2Pt1):316–323, 1990.
29. DiMarco JP, Miles W, Akhtar M, et al.: Adenosine for paroxysmal supraventricular tachycardia: Dose ranging and comparison with verapamil. Ann Intern Med 113(2):104–110, 1990.
30. Till J, Shinebourne EA, Rigby ML, Clarke B, Ward DE, Rowland E: Efficacy and safety of adenosine in the treatment of supraventricular tachycardia in infants and children. Br Heart J 62:204–211, 1989.
31. Rankin AC, Rae AP, Oldroyd KG, Cobbe SM: Verapamil or adenosine for the immediate treatment of supraventricular tachycardia. Q J Med 74(274):203–208, 1990.
32. Garratt C, Linker N, Griffith M, Ward D, Camm AJ: Comparison of adenosine and verapamil for termination of paroxysmal junctional tachycardia. Am J Cardiol 64(19):1310–1316, 1989.
33. Klabunde RE: Dipyridamole inhibition of adenosine metabolism in human blood. Eur J Pharmacol 93:21–26, 1983.
34. De Belder MA, Malik M, Ward DE, Camm AJ: Pacing modalities for tachycardia termination. PACE 13:231–248, 1990.
35. Ueda C, Quinidine. In Evans WE, Schentag JJ, Jusko WJ: Applied Pharmacokinetics, ed. 2. Spokane, Applied Therapeutics, Inc, 1986, pp 712–734.
36. Woosley RL, Echt DS, Roden DM: Effects of congestive heart failure on the pharmacokinetics and pharmacodynamics of antiarrhythmic agents. Am J Cardiol 57:25B–33B, 1986.

37. Wooding-Scott RA, Smalley J, Visco J, Slaughter RL: The pharmacokinetics and pharmacodynamics of quinidine and 3-hydroxyquinidine. Br J Clin Pharmacol 26:415–421, 1988.

38. Roden DM, Thompson KA, Hoffman BF, Woosley RL: Clinical features and basic mechanisms of quinidine-induced arrhythmias. J Am Coll Cardiol 8(1):73A–78A, 1986.

39. Wooding-Scott RA, Darling IM, Slaughter RL: Comparison of assay procedures used to measure total and unbound concentrations of quinidine. Drug Intell Clin Pharm 23:999–1004, 1989.

40. Swerdlow CD, Yu JO, Jacobson E, et al.: Safety and efficacy of intravenous quinidine. Am J Med 75:36–42, 1983.

41. Cohen IS, Jick H, Cohen I: Adverse reactions to quinidine in hospitalized patients: findings based on data from the Boston Collaborative Drug Surveillance Program. Prog Cardiovasc Dis 20(2):151–163, 1977.

42. Ferguson B Jr, Cox JL: Surgical therapy for patients with supraventricular tachycardia. Cardiol Clin 8(3):535–555, 1990.

43. Scher DL, Arsura EL: Multifocal atrial tachycardia: mechanisms, clinical correlates, and treatment. Am Heart J 118(3):574–580, 1989.

44. Hazard PB, Burnett CR: Verapamil in multifocal atrial tachycardia: hemodynamic and respiratory changes. Chest 91(1):68–70, 1987.

45. Hazard PB, Burnett CR: Treatment of multifocal atrial tachycardia with metoprolol. Crit Care Med 15(1):20–25, 1987.

46. Arsura E, Lefkin AS, Scher DL, Solar M, Tessler S: A randomized, double-blind, placebo-controlled study of verapamil and metoprolol in treatment of multifocal atrial tachycardia. Am J Med 85:519–524, 1988.

47. Alpert JS, Petersen P, Godtfredsen JG: Atrial fibrillation: natural history, complications, and management. Annu Rev Med 39:41–52, 1988.

48. Petersen P: Thromboembolic complications in atrial fibrillation. Stroke 21(1):4–13, 1990.

49. Stein B, Halperin JL, Fuster V: Should patients with atrial fibrillation be anticoagulated prior to and chronically following cardioversion? Cardiovasc Clin 21(1):231–247, 1990.

50. Wolf PA, Kannel WB, McGee DL, Meeks SL, Bharucha NE, McNamara PM: Duration of atrial fibrillation and imminence of stroke: the Framingham study. Stroke 14(5):664–667, 1983.

51. Lundström T, Rydén L: Chronic atrial fibrillation: long-term results of direct current conversion. Acta Med Scand 223:53–59, 1988.

52. Lewis RV, Irvine N, McDevitt DG: Relationships between heart rate, exercise tolerance and cardiac output in atrial fibrillation: the effects of treatment with digoxin, verapamil and diltiazem. Eur Heart J 9:777–781, 1988.

53. Lewis RV, Laing E, Moreland TA, Service E, McDevitt DG: A comparison of digoxin, diltiazem and their combination in the treatment of atrial fibrillation. Eur Heart J 9:279–283, 1988.

54. Lang R, Klein HO, Di Segni E, et al.: Verapamil improves exercise capacity in chronic atrial fibrillation: double-blind crossover study. Am Heart J 105(5):820–825, 1983.

55. Beasley R, Smith DA, McHaffie DJ: Exercise heart rates at different serum digoxin concentrations in patients with atrial fibrillation. Br Med J 290:9–11, 1985.

56. Goldman S, Probst P, Selzer A, et al.: Inefficiency of "therapeutic" serum levels of digoxin in controlling the ventricular rate in atrial fibrillation. Am J Cardiol 35:651–655, 1975.

57. Klein GJ, Twum-Barima Y, Gulamhusein S, Carruthers SG, Donner AP: Verapamil in chronic atrial fibrillation: variable patterns of response in ventricular rate. Clin Cardiol 7(4):474–483, 1984.

58. Frisolone JA: Continuous verapamil infusion. DICP 23(12):1005–1006, 1989.

59. Klein HO, Kaplinsky E: Digitalis and verapamil in atrial fibrillation and flutter: Is verapamil now the preferred agent? Drugs 31:185–197, 1986.

60. Salerno DM, Dias VC, Kleiger RE, et al.: Efficacy and safety of intravenous diltiazem for treatment of atrial fibrillation and atrial flutter. Am J Cardiol 63:1046–1051, 1989.

61. The Esmolol Multicenter Study Research Group: Efficacy and safety of esmolol vs propranolol in the treatment of supraventricular tachyarrhythmias: a multicenter double-blind clinical trial. Am Heart J 110(5):913–922, 1985.

62. The Esmolol vs Placebo Multicenter Study Group: Comparison of the efficacy and safety of esmolol, a short-acting β-blocker, with placebo in the treatment of supraventricular tachyarrhythmias. Am Heart J 111:42, 1986.

63. Sung RJ, Blanski L, Kirshenbaum J, et al.: Clinical experience with esmolol a short-acting β-adrenergic blocker in cardiac arrhythmias and myocardial ischemia. J Clin Pharmacol 26(suppl A):A15–A26, 1986.

64. Platia EV, Michelson EL, Porterfield JK, Das G: Esmolol versus verapamil in the acute treatment of atrial fibrillation or atrial flutter. Am J Cardiol 63:925–929, 1989.

65. Morris DC, Hurst JW: Atrial fibrillation. Curr Probl Cardiol 5(1):1–50, 1980.

66. Lewis RV: Atrial fibrillation: the therapeutic options. Drugs 40(6):841–853, 1990.

67. Karlson BW, Herlitz J, Edvardsson N, Olsson SB: Prophylactic treatment after electroconversion of atrial fibrillation. Clin Cardiol 13(4):279–286, 1990.

68. Mann DL, Maisel AS, Atwood JE, et al.: Absence of cardioversion-induced ventricular arrhythmias in patients with therapeutic digoxin levels. J Am Coll Cardiol 5:882–888, 1985.

69. Feld GK, Chen P-S, Nicod P, Fleck RP, Meyer D: Possible atrial proarrhythmic effects of class 1C antiarrhythmic drugs. Am J Cardiol 66:378–383, 366–367, 1990.

70. Sihm I, Hansen FA, Rasmussen J, Pedersen AK, Thygesen K: Flecainide acetate in atrial flutter and fibrillation. Eur Heart J 11:145–148, 1990.

71. Roth A, Harrison E, Mitani G, Cohen J, Rahimtoola SH, Elkayam U: Efficacy and safety of medium- and high-dose diltiazem alone and in combination with dogixin for control of heart rate at rest and during exercise in patients with chronic atrial fibrillation. Circulation 73(2):316–324, 1986.

72. Cerebral Embolism Task Force: Cardiogenic brain embolism. Arch Neurol 43:71–84, 1986.

73. Dunn M, Alexander J, de Silva R, Hildner F: Antithrombotic therapy in atrial fibrillation. Chest 95(suppl 2):118S–127S, 1989.

74. Petersen P, Godtfredsen J, Boysen G, Andersen ED, Andersen B: Placebo-controlled, randomised trial of warfarin and aspirin for prevention of thromboembolic complications in chronic atrial fibrillation: The Copenhagen AFASAK study. Lancet 1(8631):175–179, 1989.

75. Anderson DC: Progress report of the Stroke Prevention in Atrial Fibrillation study. Stroke 21(11 suppl III):III-12–III-17, 1990.

76. Levine MN, Raskob G, Hirsch J: Hemorrhagic complications of long-term anticoagulant therapy. Chest 95(2 suppl):26S–36S, 1989.

77. Prystowsky EN: Diagnosis and management of the preexcitation syndromes. Curr Probl Cardiol 13(4):225–310, 1988.

78. Porter RS: Adenosine: Supplementary considerations about activity and use. Clin Pharm 9(4):271–274, 1990.

79. Brodsky M, Wu D, Denes P, Kanakis C, Rosen KM. Arrhythmias documented by 24 hour continuous electrocardiography in 50 male medical students without apparent heart disease. Am J Cardiol 39:390–395, 1977.

80. Lown B, Graboys TB: Management of patients with malignant ventricular arrhythmias. Am J Cardiol 39:910–924, 1977.

81. Schulze RA, Strauss HW, Pitt B: Sudden death in the year following myocardial infarction. Am J Med 62:192–199, 1977.

82. Pieper JA, Rodman JH, Lidocaine. In Evans WE, Schentag JJ, Jusko WJ (eds): Applied Pharmacokinetics, ed. 2. Spokane, WA, Applied Therapeutcs, 1986, p 642.

83. Pieper JA, Rodman JH, Lidocaine. In Evans WE, Schentag JJ, Jusko WJ (eds): Applied Pharmacokinetics, ed. 2. Spokane, WA, Applied Therapeutics, 1986, pp 648–649.

84. Vozeh S, Berger M, Wenk M, Ritz R, Follath F: Rapid prediction of individual dosage requirements of lidocaine. Clin Pharmacokinet 9:354–363, 1984.

85. Shand DG: α-1-Acid glycoprotein and plasma lidocaine binding. Clin Pharmacokinet 9:27–31, 1984.

86. LeLorier J, Grenon D, Latour Y, et al.: Pharmacokinetics of lidocaine after prolonged intravenous infusions in uncomplicated myocardial infarctions. Ann Intern Med 87:700–702, 1977.

87. Grubb BP: Recurrence of ventricular tachycardia after conversion from proprietary to generic procainamide. Am J Cardiol 63:1532–1533, 1989.

88. Hilleman DE, Patterson AJ, Mohiuddin SM, Ortmeier BG, Destache CJ: Comparative bioequivalence and efficacy of two sustained-release procainamide formulations in patients with cardiac arrhythmias. Drug Intell Clin Pharm 22:554–558, 1988.

89. Baker BA, Reynolds JR, Gleckel L, A'Zary E, Bodenheimer MM: Comparative bioavailability of two oral sustained-release procainamide products. Clin Pharm 7:135–138, 1988.

90. Funck-Brentano C, Light RT, Lineberry MD, Wright GM, Roden DM, Woosley RL: Pharmacokinetic and pharmacodynamic interaction of N-acetylprocainamide and procainamide in humans. J Cardiovasc Pharmacol 14:364–373, 1989.

91. Coyle JD, Lima JJ, Procainamide. In Evans WE, Schentag JJ, Jusko WJ (eds): Applied Pharmacokinetics, ed. 2. Spokane, WA, Applied Therapeutics, 1986, p 699.

92. Bauer LA, Black D, Gensler A, Sprinkle J: Influence of age, renal function and heart failure on procainamide clearance and n-acetylprocainamide serum concentrations. Int J Clin Pharmacol Ther Toxicol 27:213–216, 1989.

93. Lima JJ, Goldfarb AL, Conti DR, et al.: Safety and efficacy of procainamide infusions. Am J Cardiol 43:98–105, 1979.

94. Kuehl P, Arquin P, Fridahl J: Steady state bioavailability of a sustained release procainamide preparation. Drug Intell Clin Pharm 16:475–476, 1982.

95. Giardina EG, Fenster PE, Bigger JT Jr, Mayersohn M, Perrier D, Marcus FI: Efficacy, plasma concentrations and adverse effects of a new sustained release procainamide preparation. Am J Cardiol 46:855–862, 1980.

96. Flanagan AD: Pharmacokinetics of a sustained release procainamide preparation. Angiology 33:71–77, 1982.

97. Gottlieb SS, Kukin ML, Medina N, Yushak M, Packer M: Comparative hemodynamic effects of procainamide, tocainide, encainide in severe chronic heart failure. Circulation 81:860–864, 1990.

98. Rubin RL, Curnutte JT: Metabolism of procainamide to the cytotoxic hydroxylamine by neutrophils activated in vitro. J Clin Invest 83:1336–1343, 1989.

99. Ellrodt AG, Murata GH, Riedinger MS, Stewart ME, Mochizuki C, Gray R: Severe neutropenia associated with sustained release procainamide. Ann Intern Med 100:197–201, 1984.

100. Meyers DG, Gonzalez ER, Peters LL, Davis RB, Feagler JR, Egan JD, Nair CK: Severe neutropenia associated with procainamide: comparison of sustained release and conventional preparations. Am Heart J 109:1393–1395, 1985.

101. Sparboro JA, Rawling DA, Fozzard HA: Suppression of ventricular

arrhythmias with intravenous disopyramide and lidocaine: efficacy comparison in a randomized trial. Am J Cardiol 44:513–520, 1979.

102. Lima JJ, Boudoulas H, Blanford M: Concentration dependence of disopyramide binding to plasma protein and its influence on kinetics and dynamics. J Pharmacol Exp Ther 219:741–747, 1981.

103. Whiting B, Holford NHG, Sheiner LB: Quantitative analysis of the disopyramide concentration-effect relationship. Br J Clin Pharmacol 9:67–75, 1980.

104. Nightingale J, Nappi JM: Effect of phenytoin on serum disopyramide concentrations. Clin Pharm 6:46–50, 1987.

105. Pedersen LE, Bonde J, Graudal NA, Backer NV, Hansen JE, Kampmann JP: Quantitative and qualitative binding characteristics of disopyramide in serum from patients with decreased renal and hepatic function. Br J Clin Pharmacol 23:41–46, 1987.

106. Caplin JL, Johnston A, Hamer J, Camm AJ. The acute changes in serum binding of disopyramide and flecainide after myocardial infarction. Eur J Clin Pharmacol 28:253–255, 1985.

107. Capparelli EV, DiPersio DM, Zhao H, Kluger J, Chow MS: Clinical pharmacokinetics of controlled-release disopyramide in patients with cardiac arrhythmias. J Clin Pharmacol 28:306–311, 1988.

108. Zema MJ: Serum drug concentrations and adverse effects in cardiac patients after administration of a new controlled-release disopyramide preparation. Ther Drug Monit 6:192–198, 1984.

109. Teichman S: The anticholinergic side effects of disopyramide and controlled release disopyramide. Angiology 36:767–771, 1985.

110. Cacoub P, Deray G, Balou A, Grimaldi A, Soubrie C, Jacobs C: Disopyramide-induced hypoglycemia: case report and review of the literature. Fundam Clin Pharmacol 3(5):527–535, 1989.

111. Podrid PJ, Shoenberger A, Lown B: Congestive heart failure caused by oral disopyramide. N Engl J Med 302:614–617, 1980.

112. Wehmeyer AE, Thomas RL: Encainide: a new antiarrhythmic agent. Drug Intell Clin Pharm 20:9–13, 1986.

113. Bergstrand RH, Wang T, Roden DM, et al.: Encainide disposition in patients with renal failure. Clin Pharmacol Ther 40:148–154, 1986.

114. Funck-Brentano C, Turgeon J, Woosley RL, et al.: Effect of low dose quinidine on encainide pharmacokinetics and pharmacodynamics. Influence of genetic polymorphism. J Pharmacol Exp Ther 249:134–142, 1989.

115. Kazierad DJ, Lalonde RL, Hoon TJ, Mirvis DM, Bottorff MB: The effect of diltiazem on the disposition of encainide and its active metabolites. Clin Pharmacol Ther 46:668–673, 1989.

116. Morganroth J, Somberg JC, Pool PE, et al.: Comparative study of encainide and quinidine in the treatment of ventricular arrhythmias. J Am Coll Cardiol 7:9–16, 1986.

117. The Cardiac Arrhythmia Suppression Trial (CAST) Investigators: Preliminary report: effect of encainide and flecainide on mortality in a randomized trial of arrhythmia suppression after myocardial infarction. N Engl J Med 321:406–412, 1989.

118. Anon: Propafenone: an antiarrhythmic come in from the cold. Lancet 2:1490–1491, 1989.

119. Parker RB, McCollam PL, Bauman JL: Propafenone: a novel type Ic antiarrhythmic agent. Drug Intell Clin Pharm 23:196–203, 1989.

120. Lee JT, Kroemer HK, Silberstein DJ, et al.: The role of genetically determined polymorphic drug metabolism in the β-blockade produced by propafenone. N Engl J Med 322:1764–1768, 1990.

121. Touboul P, Moleur P, Mathieu MP, et al.: A comparative evaluation of the effects of propafenone and lidocaine on early ventricular arrhythmias after acute myocardial infarction. Eur Heart J 9:1188–1193, 1988.

122. Lee AJ: Digibind: emergency treatment for digitalis toxicity. J Emerg Nurs 15:266–268, 1989.

123. Boucher BA, Lalonde RL: Digoxin-specific antibody fragments for the treatment of digoxin intoxication. Clin Pharm 5:826–827, 1986.

124. Huang SK, Marcus FI: Antiarrhythmic drug therapy of ventricular arrhythmias. Curr Probl Cardiol 11:178–240, 1986.

125. Horowitz LN, Josephson ME, Farshidi A, Spielman SR, Michelson EL, Greenspan AM: Recurrent sustained ventricular tachycardia. Circulation 58:986–997, 1978.

126. Bigger JT, Weld FM: Rolnitzky LM: Prevalence, characteristics, and significance of ventricular tachycardia detected with ambulatory electrocardiographic recording in the late hospital phase of acute myocardial infarction. Am J Cardiol 48:815–823, 1981.

127. Manolis AS, Linzer M, Salem D, Estes NA III: Syncope: current diagnostic evaluation and management. Ann Intern Med 112:850–863, 1990.

128. Sasyniuk BI, Valois M, Toy W: Recent advances in understanding the mechanisms of drug-induced torsades de pointes arrhythmias. Am J Cardiol 64:29J–32J, 1989.

129. Iseri LT, Allen BJ, Brodsky MA: Magnesium therapy of cardiac arrhythmias in critical-care medicine. Magnesium 8:299–306, 1989.

130. Manolis AS, Linzer M, Salem D, et al.: Syncope: current diagnostic evaluation and management. Ann Intern Med 112:850–863, 1990.

131. Roden DM, Woosley RL: Drug therapy: flecainide. N Engl J Med 315:36–40, 1986.

132. Gross AS, Mikus G, Fischer C, Hertrampf R, Gundert-Remy U, Eichelbaum M: Stereoselective disposition of flecainide in relation to the sparteine/debrisoquine metaboliser phenotype. Br J Clin Pharmacol 28:555–566, 1989.

133. McQuinn RL, Pentikainen PJ, Chang SF, Conard GJ: Pharmacokinetics of flecainide in patients with cirrhosis of the liver. Clin Pharmacol Ther 44:566–572, 1988.

134. Salerno DM, Granrud G, Sharkey P, et al.: Pharmacodynamic and side effects of flecainide acetate. Clin Pharmacol Ther. 40:101–107, 1986.

135. Morganroth J, Anderson JL, Gentzkow GD: Classification by type of ventricular arrhythmia predicts frequency of adverse cardiac events from flecainide. J Am Coll Cardiol 8:607–615, 1986.

136. Fitton A, Buckley MMT: Moricizine: a review of its pharmacological properties, and therapeutic efficacy in cardiac arrhythmias. Drugs 40:138–167, 1990.

137. Mann HJ: Moricizine: a new class I antiarrhythmic. Clin Pharm 9:842–852, 1990.

138. Nestico PF, Morganroth J, Horowitz LN: New antiarrhythmic drug. Drugs 35:286–319, 1988.

139. CAPS Investigators: Effects of encainide, flecainide, imipramine, and moricizine on ventricular arrhythmias during the year after acute myocardial infarction. Am J Cardiol 61:501–509, 1988.

140. Bigger JT: The events surrounding the removal of encainide and flecainide from the CAST and why CAST is continuing with moricizine. J Am Coll Cardiol. 15:243–245, 1990.

141. Gillis AM, Kates RE: Clinical pharmacokinetics of the newer antiarrhythmic agents. Clin Pharmacokinet 9:375–403, 1984.

142. Grech-Belanger O, Gilbert M, Turgeon J, LeBlanc PP: Effect of cigarette smoking on mexiletine kinetics. Clin Pharmacol Ther 37:638–643, 1985.

143. Wang T, Wuellner D, Woosley RL, Stone WJ: Pharmacokinetics and nondialyzability of mexiletine in renal failure. Clin Pharmacol Ther 37:649–653, 1985.

144. Steen SN, Hughes EM, Sharon G, MacGregor TR: Efficacy of oral mexiletine therapy at a 12-h dosage interval. Chest 97:358–363, 1990.

145. Singh JB, Rasul AM, Shah A, Adams E, Flessas A, Kocot SL: Efficacy of mexiletine in chronic ventricular arrhythmias compared with quinidine: a single blind randomized trial. Am J Cardiol 53:84–87, 1984.

146. Giardina EG, Wechsler ME: Low dose quinidine-mexiletine combination therapy versus quinidine monotherapy for treatment of ventricular arrhythmias. J Am Coll Cardiol 15:1–45, 1990.

147. Duff HJ, Roden D, Primm RK, Oates JA, Woosley RL: Mexiletine in the treatment of resistant ventricular arrhythmias: enhancement of efficacy and reduction of dose-related side effects by combination with quinidine. Circulation 67:1124–1128, 1983.

148. Kim SG, Mercando AD, Tam S, Fisher JD: Combination of disopyramide and mexiletine for better tolerance and additive effects for treatment of ventricular arrhythmias. J Am Coll Cardiol 13:659–664, 1989.

149. DiMarco JP, Garan H, Ruskin JN: Mexiletine for refractory ventricular arrhythmias: results using serial electrophysiologic testing. Am J Cardiol 47:131–138, 1981.

150. Roden DM, Woosley RL: Drug therapy: tocainide. N Engl J Med 315:41–45, 1986.

151. Rice TL: Patterson JH, Celestin C, Foster JR, Powell JR: Influence of rifampin on tocainide pharmacokinetics in humans. Clin Pharm 8:200–205, 1989.

152. North DS, Mattern AL, Kapil RP, Lalonde RL: The effect of histamine-2 receptor antagonists on tocainide pharmacokinetics. J Clin Pharmacol 28:640–643, 1988.

153. Wassenmiller JE, Aronow WS: Effect of tocainide and quinidine on premature ventricular contractions. Clin Pharmacol Ther 28:431–435, 1980.

154. Feinberg L, Travis WD, Ferrans V, Sato N, Bernton HF: Pulmonary fibrosis associated with tocainide: report of a case with literature review. Am Rev Respir Dis 141:505–508, 1990.

155. Chopra MP, Thadani U, Portal RW, Aber CP: Lignocaine therapy for ventricular ectopic activity after acute myocardial infarction: a double-blind trial. Br Med J 3(776):668–670, 1971.

156. Lie KI, Wellens HJ, van Capelle FJ, Durrer D: Lidocaine in the prevention of primary ventricular fibrillation. A double-blind, randomized study of 212 consecutive patients. N Engl J Med 291(25):1324–1326, 1974.

157. Rademaker AW, Kellen J, Tam YK, Wyse DG: Character of adverse effects of prophylactic lidocaine in the coronary care unit. Clin Pharmacol Ther 40:73–80, 1986.

158. Hine LK, Laird N, Hewitt P, Chalmers TC: Meta-analytic evidence against prophylactic use of lidocaine in acute myocardial infarction. Arch Intern Med 149:2694–2698, 1989.

159. Duff HJ, Roden DM, Yacobi A, et al.: Bretylium: relations between plasma concentrations and pharmacologic actions in high-frequency ventricular arrhythmias. Am J Cardiol 55:395–401, 1985.

160. Adir J, Narang PK, Josselson J: Nomogram for bretylium dosing in renal impairment. Ther Drug Monit 7:265–268, 1985.

161. Perlman PE, Adams WG Jr, Ridgeway NA: Extreme pyrexia during bretylium administration. Postgrad Med 85:111–114, 1989.

162. Naccarelli GV, Rinkenberger RL, Dougherty AH, Giebel RA: Amiodarone: pharmacology and antiarrhythmic and adverse effects. Pharmacotherapy 5:298–313, 1985.

163. Heger JJ, Prytowsky EN, Jackman WM, et al.: Amiodarone, clinical efficacy and electrophysiology during long term therapy for recurrent ventricular tachycardia or ventricular fibrillation. N Engl J Med 305:539–545, 1981.

164. Peter T, Hamer A, Mandel WJ: Evaluation of amiodarone therapy in the treatment of drug resistant cardiac arrhythmias: long term follow up. Eur Heart J 6:151–162, 1985.

165. Kerin NZ, Blevins RD, Benaderet D, et al.: Relation of serum reverse T3 to amiodarone antiarrhythmic efficacy and toxicity. Am J Cardiol 57:128–130, 1986.

166. Saal KA, Werner JA, Greene HL, Sears GK, Graham El: Effect of amiodarone on serum quinidine and procainamide levels. Am J Cardiol 53:1264–1267, 1984.

167. National Heart, Lung, and Blood Institute: The β blocker heart attack trial. JAMA 246:2073–2074, 1981.

168. Norwegian Multicenter Study Group: Timolol induced reduction in mortality and reinfarction in patients surviving acute myocardial infarction. New Engl J Med 304:801–807, 1981.

169. Hjalmarson A, Elmfeldt D, Herlitz J, et al.: Effect on mortality of metoprolol in acute myocardial infarction. A double-blind randomised trial. Lancet 17;2(8251):823–827, 1981.

170. Anderson MP, Fredericksen J, Bechsgard P, Hansen DA, Jurgensen HJ, et al.: Effect of alprenolol on mortality among patients with definite or suspected acute myocardial infarction. Lancet 1979;2:865–868, 1979.

CHAPTER 38

ANGINA PECTORIS

BRADLEY G. WULF, Pharm.D., DAVID G. MEYERS, M.D., and KIMBERLY A. CANTRAL, Pharm.D.

Angina pectoris is a clinical syndrome of chest discomfort caused by myocardial ischemia, where ischemia refers to a lack of oxygen secondary to reduced perfusion. Myocardial ischemia is caused by an imbalance between oxygen supply and demand because of an inability to increase coronary blood flow in response to increased myocardial demands. This is nearly always related to atherosclerosis in the large epicardial coronary arteries, which causes a narrowing of the vessel lumen and thus a reduction of blood flow, modulated by the "tone" of the smaller resistance coronary arteries. It may also (rarely) be due to either focal or generalized vasospasm of the major coronary arteries.

RISK FACTORS

The cause of atherosclerotic-ischemic heart disease has not been clearly established, although it is likely to be a complex interaction of genetic, physical, biologic, and social factors. Risk factors associated epidemiologically with the development of ischemic heart disease include (1) family history of premature ischemic heart disease, elevated serum low-density lipoprotein cholesterol levels, decreased levels of high-density lipoprotein cholesterol, cigarette smoking, hypertension, obesity, sedentary lifestyle, diabetes mellitus, gout, type A personality, advanced age (>50 years), and being of the male sex. The more risk factors a patient has, the greater the risk of developing ischemic heart disease.

SIGNS AND SYMPTOMS

Angina pectoris is characterized by substernal discomfort that occurs with exertion or emotional stress and is relieved by rest or nitroglycerin. Actually, the word *angina* means a sense of strangling and not pain. Patients with angina may not use the word *pain* to describe their discomfort and instead may report squeezing, tightness, choking, pressure, burning, or heaviness. This discomfort may radiate to the neck, lower jaw, shoulder, and arms. Occasionally the discomfort may occur only in the arms or wrists. The anginal episode can last from 30 sec to 30 min. The typical anginal episode begins gradually, reaches peak intensity over minutes, then gradually dissipates after the precipitating activity has been halted. Precipitating factors include exertion such as walking up a flight of stairs, household chores, or manual labor. Other precipitating factors include the use of the arms above the head, exposure to cold temperatures, coitus, or emotional states such as anger or fright. The threshold for developing an anginal episode may also vary with the time of day, with most episodes occurring between 6 AM and 12 PM. A patient may have angina pectoris while shaving in the morning, yet later in the day he may be capable of performing moderate manual labor after he has "warmed up."

TYPES OF ANGINA

Angina may be classified as classical angina, unstable angina, or Prinzmetal's angina. Classical angina is precipitated by exertion or emotional stress, lasts only a few minutes, and is relieved by rest or nitroglycerin. It is commonly caused by a fixed atherosclerotic obstruction in a coronary artery.

Unstable angina, also referred to as crescendo angina or preinfarction angina, probably is caused by a combination of atherosclerotic stenosis, coronary thrombosis, and vasospasm. Unstable angina is most simply defined as any significant change in an individual patient's usual pattern of angina, i.e., any change in frequency, duration, intensity, or ease of onset of angina. Patients with unstable angina are more likely to suffer a myocardial infarction than patients with stable angina; thus the syndrome sometimes is called preinfarction angina.

Prinzmetal's angina or variant angina is a syndrome in which the patient develops anginal episodes while at rest which are associated with ST segment elevation on the electrocardiogram and are caused by focal coronary artery vasospasm. These episodes typically occur at the same times of the day, usually in the morning. Prinzmetal's angina does not require atherosclerotic coronary stenoses to produce an imbalance of oxygen supply and demand. Indeed, "spastic" arteries may appear normal.

CLINICAL FINDINGS
Physical Examination

Results of the physical examination of patients not experiencing an attack of angina pectoris are generally normal. However, changes in ventricular function may occur during an anginal episode and cause transient auscultatory changes, including third and fourth heart sounds, heart murmurs, or a precordial bulge. The physical examination may uncover factors that exacerbate angina such as thyrotoxicosis, anemia, hypoxemia, hypertension, and aortic stenosis.

Electrocardiography

A 12-lead electrocardiogram (ECG) is noninvasive, quick, and simple to perform. It supports the diagnosis of ischemic heart disease if specific changes are present. Lack of alterations does not rule out the diagnosis of ischemic heart disease, although the absence of ECG changes lessens the probability of angina as the explanation of chest pain. For instance, if the ECG is done in the absence of an anginal episode, it may appear normal, since approximately 25 to 50% of patients with ischemic heart disease have a normal ECG in the absence of chest discomfort. When the ECG is performed during an anginal episode, the most characteristic change is a transient displacement of the ST segment below baseline (ST segment depression). Inversion of the T wave may develop alone or with the ST segment depression. In contrast, patients who have Prinzmetal's angina show a dramatic elevation of the ST segment during an anginal episode, imitating acute myocardial infarction.

Exercise Tolerance Testing

Exercise tolerance testing (stress testing) can measure a patient's capability to increase coronary blood flow in response to increased myocardial oxygen demands. This test is done by walking on a motorized treadmill at increasing speed and grade or by pedaling a bicycle against increasing resistance until a target heart rate is achieved or until the patient's typical angina symptoms are reproduced. The Bruce protocol for treadmill stress testing is one common example (2) (Table 38.1). Patients are monitored with an ECG during and after the stress test. When ST segment depression of more than 1.0 mm is used to define a result indicating myocardial ischemia, the stress test has a sensitivity of 60 to 70% and a specificity of 90% (2). Digitalis glycosides, cardiac conduction abnormalities, and ventricular hypertrophy can cause ST segment depression, thus producing a false-positive result (2). β-Adrenergic blocking agents can blunt the heart rate response to exercise and thus affect the patients' ability to achieve their target heart rate (2).

Table 38.1.
Exercise Tolerance Testing: Bruce Protocol

Stage	Grade (%)	Speed (MPH)	Duration (Min)
1	10.0	1.7	3
2	12.0	2.5	3
3	14.0	3.4	3
4	16.0	4.2	3
5	18.0	5.0	3
6	20.0	5.5	3
7	22.0	6.0	3

Radionuclide Imaging

Exercise thallium-201 myocardial imaging involves exercising patients until peak exercise is attained. At that moment, thallium-201 is injected intravenously, and the patient is exercised for 1 more min. The patient's heart is scanned immediately after exercise and again in 3 to 4 hr (3). The uptake of thallium-201 depends on regional coronary blood flow and normal myocyte metabolism. Regions of the myocardium that develop poor perfusion and become ischemic with exercise will have little or no thallium-201 taken up by the cells and appear as "cold spots" (3). A "cold spot" will also appear in areas of infarction. The myocardial scan 3 to 4 hr after exercise will help differentiate between ischemia and infarction. If an area was ischemic, a redistribution of coronary blood flow and thallium uptake will occur, and the "cold spot" should disappear. Infarcted myocardium will remain as a "cold spot." This test has a higher sensitivity than a standard exercise tolerance test. The sensitivity has been reported to be 80%, 83%, and 96% for patients with one-, two-, and three-vessel disease, respectively (3). This test poses no higher risk than a standard exercise tolerance test, but it costs much more.

Coronary Arteriography

This procedure is done by inserting a catheter into either the femoral or brachial artery to gain access to both the left ventricle and the coronary arteries. Iodinated contrast medium is injected through the catheter into each coronary artery ostium at the base of the aorta. This allows the coronary arteries to be visualized on x-ray (cineangiography) and delineates stenotic lesions in the main branches of the coronary arteries. Complications secondary to this procedure, occurring in about 1% of patients, include bleeding, infection, embolism, arterial dissection, myocardial infarction, arrhythmias, and death. Renal toxicity may occur as a result of the iodinated contrast medium, as well as allergic reactions. The non-IgE-mediated "allergic reactions" are related to the iodine and are usually mild, typically appearing as hives and rarely as bronchospasm. An anaphylactic reaction is extremely rare. Patients with a mild contrast reaction may still receive the contrast medium if they are premedicated with an H_1-antihistamine, steroid, and an H_2-antagonist. An example for dosing is prednisone 30 to 60 mg on the evening before the procedure and diphenhydramine 25 to 50 mg, prednisone 30 to 60 mg, and ranitidine 300 mg the morning of the procedure.

If Prinzmetal's angina is suspected and no critical fixed stenoses are present, ergonovine, in increasing doses, may be injected though the catheter. The sections of the coronary arteries that are prone to vasospasm will be sensitive to the ergonovine stimulation and produce focal vasospasm. Intravenous nitroglycerin should be available to reverse the vasospasm if it does not subside spontaneously.

DIAGNOSIS

Classical angina pectoris may be diagnosed by history alone if the substernal discomfort is always precipitated by exertion and relieved by rest or nitroglycerin. However, esophageal spasm also presents as chest pain and is relieved by nitroglycerin. If the symptoms are somewhat atypical, then exercise tolerance testing, with or without thallium-201 scintigraphy, may be warranted. In rare cases, coronary arteriography becomes necessary for diagnosis of angina. This should not be confused with the very frequent use of exercise testing and coronary arteriography as aids in the selection of candidates for coronary artery bypass graft surgery (CABG) or percutaneous transluminal coronary angioplasty (PTCA) in patients with known angina pectoris.

Unstable angina also may be diagnosed by history alone. Because of the very real risk of myocardial infarction with this syndrome, no exercise tolerance testing is done. Almost all patients with unstable angina undergo coronary arteriography in contemplation of CABG surgery of PTCA.

Prinzmetal's angina requires either documented transient ST segment elevation by electrocardiography during chest discomfort or arteriographically visualized focal coronary artery spasm for diagnosis.

MANAGEMENT OF ANGINA PECTORIS

Symptoms of angina may be caused by disorders like thyrotoxicosis or anemia. If there is an identifiable underlying cause it should be treated. However, this is possible in only a small percentage of patients. Most patients will require symptomatic treatment of angina. The goal of therapy is to reduce the frequency and severity of the anginal episodes.

Avoidance of activities that can precipitate anginal attacks should be attempted, if feasible. Such activities include strenuous physical activity, exposure to cold weather, use of caffeine-containing beverages, cigarette smoking, eating heavy meals, and emotional stress. Preparations containing caffeine, thyroid hormones, or sympathomimetic agents (i.e., cold preparations and diet aids) should be avoided. Treatment of risk factors such as hypertension, diabetes mellitus, and hypercholesterolemia may be beneficial.

DRUG THERAPY

Medications, such as the nitrates, β-adrenergic blocking agents, and calcium-channel blockers, alone or in combination are very effective in preventing the onset of anginal episodes. The specific needs of the patient should be considered when deciding on the optimal antianginal treatment.

NITRATES

Organic nitrates are potent vasodilators of vascular smooth muscle. Nitrates are converted intracellularly in the presence of sulfhydryl groups, probably provided by cysteine, to inorganic nitrites. The inorganic nitrites are then cleaved to form nitric oxide, which reacts with sulfhydryl groups to produce S-nitrosothiols. The S-nitrosothiols, or nitric oxide itself, activates guanylate cyclase, which increases the production of cyclic guanosine monophosphate (cGMP) (4). It is suggested that cGMP causes a reduction in intracellular calcium levels by increasing calcium extrusion from the cell (5). A dephosphorylation of myosin light-chain kinase may also contribute to the mechanism of vasodilation (5). Nitrate-induced vasodilation is not mediated by endothelial cell prostacyclin production (6).

The mechanism of action by which nitrates relieve the symptoms of typical angina pectoris is generally believed to be a reduction in myocardial oxygen demand secondary to a reduction in preload and afterload. The organic nitrates exert their effect on both venous capacitance and arteriolar resistance vessels. At low doses, the primary effect is a vasodilation of the peripheral veins. This causes an increase in venous capacitance, which in turn decreases venous return to the heart. Left ventricular end-diastolic pressure and volume decrease, thus reducing myocardial work and oxygen consumption. At high doses, the nitrates also cause arterial dilation, which reduces systemic vascular resistance. These systemic vascular effects, coupled with diminished ventricular volume, reduce ventricular wall tension in accordance with Laplace's law, which results in a decrease in myocardial oxygen demand. Although nitrates also cause a reflex increase in both heart rate and myocardial contractility, which increase myocardial oxygen demands, the net effect is a decrease in myocardial oxygen demand.

Nitrates dilate the large coronary arteries selectively. This is probably the mechanism for relief of coronary artery spasm.

Nitrates do not increase total coronary blood flow in patients with angina pectoris due to atherosclerosis. Instead, they produce a redistribution of coronary blood flow in favor of the subendocardial regions of the heart that have undergone a disproportionate reduction in blood flow from atherosclerosis. It is believed that this effect is related to the ability of the nitrates to dilate the large epicardial vessels without altering the autoregulatory mechanism of the smaller resistance vessels (7). Administration of sublingual nitroglycerin dilates epicardial stenoses in humans and leads to a reduction in resistance to blood flow in these regions (8).

NITROGLYCERIN (Table 38.2)

Nitroglycerin has been used to treat patients with angina pectoris for over 100 years. It has been demonstrated to

Table 38.2.
Nitrate Preparations

Generic Name (Trade Name)	Dosage Form	Doses Available
Nitroglycerin		
Nitrostat	Sublingual tablet	0.15, 0.3, 0.4, 0.6 mg
Nitrolingual spray	Oral spray	200 metered-dose canister (400 μg/spray)
Nitro-Bid	2% Ointment	30 and 60 gm tubes
Nitrol	2% Ointment	30 and 60 gm tubes
Nitrol-TSAR kit	2% Ointment	30 and 60 gm tubes
Nitrong	2% Ointment	30 and 60 gm tubes
Nitrostat	2% Ointment	30 and 60 gm tubes
Nitrogard	Buccal tablet	1, 2, 3 mg
Isosorbide dinitrate		
Isordil, Sorbitrate	Sublingual tablet	2.5, 5 mg
Sorbitrate-chewable	Chewable tablet	5 mg
Isordil	Chewable tablet	10 mg
Isordil, Sorbitrate	Oral tablet	5, 10, 20 mg
Isordil Tembid	Sustained-release tablet/capsule	40 mg
Sorbitrate	Sustained-release tablet	40 mg

be highly effective in relieving anginal pain and improving exercise tolerance. Sublingual nitroglycerin has even been utilized as a diagnostic aid for determining if a patient's chest pain is due to myocardial ischemia. It has a very rapid onset of action and will relieve the chest pain in 3 to 5 min. The usual dose is 0.3 to 0.4 mg as needed for chest pain. When an anginal attack starts, patients are to immediately stop their current activity, sit down, and place 1 tablet under the tongue. Patients should not wait for the pain to worsen to its peak before taking the nitroglycerin. If the pain is not relieved within 5 min, they should administer another tablet. No more than 3 tablets should be used in 15 min. If the pain is not relieved after 3 doses, patients should call their physician or go immediately to the nearest emergency room to be evaluated.

Sublingual nitroglycerin can also be used as intermittent prophylactic therapy. Administration of sublingual nitroglycerin prior to exercise stress testing can improve exercise tolerance dramatically (9). A patient can take a sublingual nitroglycerin tablet just before any activity that is known to precipitate an anginal episode (i.e., walking to the bus stop) and prevent symptoms from developing for up to 30 min (10).

Patients prescribed sublingual nitroglycerin should be told to keep the tablets in the original glass container. The cotton filler in the bottle should be discarded after the bottle is first opened. After each use, the cap should be replaced immediately and screwed on tightly. The bottles should not be stored in hot, humid locations. These steps will help prevent any loss in drug potency. Patients should keep a bottle close by at all times. With normal use, nitroglycerin tablets (Nitrostat) have demonstrated potency until the expiration date printed on the bottle. The stinging or burning sensation one may get under the tongue after a dose is not an indication of potency.

There is an alternative to the sublingual tablets. A lingual nitroglycerin spray is available in a metered-dose canister that will deliver a 400-μg dose with each spray. Like the sublingual tablets, the onset of action is within a few minutes. The nitroglycerin spray is effective in the treatment of acute anginal episodes and has been found to improve exercise tolerance during exercise stress testing (11). This spray can also be used to prevent the occurrence of anginal symptoms for up to 30 min (11). Patients should not inhale the spray, rather they should hold the container upright, close to the mouth, and spray the inside of the mouth (preferably on the tongue) once. This procedure should be repeated if additional doses are required to alleviate the pain. No more than 3 doses are to be administered in 15 min, as with the sublingual tablets.

Buccal Nitroglycerin

Buccal nitroglycerin is a relatively new product in the United States. It contains nitroglycerin in an inert polymer matrix. The tablet is placed in the buccal cavity between the upper lip and gums. The tablet surface forms a gel-like coating that allows the tablet to adhere to the mucosal surface. The nitroglycerin will be absorbed as long as the tablet remains intact. The dissolution rate of the tablet varies between patients and is reported to be from 1 to 6 hr (12). This variation is related to saliva production, tongue manipulation of the tablet, displacement of the gel-like seal, and inadvertent chewing of the tablet. If the tablet is chewed, the patient could potentially receive an undesirable bolus of nitroglycerin via submucosal administration. Eating and drinking may disrupt the buccal tablet. This will most likely be only an occasional problem, and in only a few patients will it be a frequent problem. The onset of action is quite rapid (2 to 5 min), similar to sublingual nitroglycerin, but the effect can last for up to 5 hr (12). This product may be dosed 3 to 4 times daily and is available in 1, 2, and 3 mg tablets. Unfortunately, if larger doses are necessary for maximal efficacy (i.e., 5 mg) it is difficult to administer two tablets simultaneously. The advantage of the buccal nitroglycerin is that it can be used both to alleviate acute anginal episodes and as prophylactic therapy.

Nitroglycerin Ointment

Nitroglycerin ointment has been available for the last 30 years to control the symptoms of all types of angina. The onset of action is 30 min, similar to oral isosorbide dinitrate. Several studies have demonstrated effects lasting from 3 to 8 hr (13–15). The dose of the 2% nitroglycerin ointment ranges from ½ to 4 inches applied every 3 to 6 hr. Patients experiencing angina at night may be adequately controlled with a single application at bedtime. When changing from one route of administration to another (i.e., oral isosorbide dinitrate to nitroglycerin ointment), the dose cannot be converted directly—mg for mg. Instead, the dose must be initiated and titrated to achieve the optimal antianginal and hemodynamic response.

Before applying each dose, any remaining ointment should be wiped off the skin. The ointment should be carefully measured on and spread evenly over the applicator paper provided by the manufacturer, applied directly to the chest, abdomen, or thigh, and taped securely. Ideally, the ointment is applied over a 6-inch by 6-inch area and covered with an occlusive plastic wrap. The large surface area and occlusive wrap improve the absorption of nitroglycerin. The ointment should not be rubbed into the skin. The patients should wash their hands thoroughly after each application, to remove any ointment that might have gotten on the hands. Common patient complaints are that the ointment is messy and can stain clothes, especially when used without the occlusive plastic wrap.

Transdermal Nitroglycerin Patches

Transdermal nitroglycerin patches have a longer duration of action and a better aesthetic quality than nitroglycerin ointment. The patches are made with an impermeable backing and adhesive side, with the nitroglycerin incorporated in a polymer, a gel-matrix, or a drug reservoir and semipermeable membrane. These patches deliver a constant amount of nitroglycerin over a 24-hr period and sustain a constant plasma concentration (Table 38.3). Patients may apply the transdermal patches to any hair-free area

on the skin; usually the chest, thigh, abdomen, or upper arm is used. Areas with scar tissue, callouses, and skin irritation should be avoided, because absorption will be reduced. The site of administration should be rotated with each dose, to reduce the incidence of skin irritation. Again, patients should wash their hands after application, to remove any nitroglycerin that might have gotten on their hands from handling the patches.

These patches have become widely accepted by patients and physicians. However, rapid development of nitrate tolerance has become a problem with the use of these products. Several studies have demonstrated a reduction in antianginal efficacy (16–18). These studies raise doubts about the effectiveness of continuous therapy with transdermal patches.

Initial dosing should be 0.1 to 0.2 mg/hr patch, which can then be titrated up to 0.6 to 0.8 mg/hr, based on the frequency of angina, nitroglycerin consumption, blood pressure response, and exercise tolerance.

Intravenous Nitroglycerin

Intravenous nitroglycerin is used in the acute setting for patients with unstable angina. The onset of action is 1 to 2 min. The recommended initial dose is 5 μg/min, which can be titrated in 5 μg/min increments at 5 min intervals, based on control of chest discomfort and the patient's blood pressure and heart rate.

Intravenous nitroglycerin should be prepared in glass or non-PVC containers, because nitroglycerin binds to PVC. For the same reason, non-PVC intravenous tubing should be used when administering intravenous nitroglycerin.

ISOSORBIDE DINITRATE

Isosorbide dinitrate is available in sublingual, chewable, and oral tablets. The sublingual tablets may be used to treat acute episodes of chest pain just like the sublingual nitroglycerin tablets. Klaus and associates (10) showed that sublingual isosorbide dinitrate improved exercise tolerance for up to 45 min. Therefore, the sublingual isosorbide dinitrate is short-acting, but it can be administered before any exertion known to cause an anginal episode.

The chewable tablets are longer-acting than the sublingual tablets. The patient chews these tablets, then keeps the remaining particles in the mouth to be absorbed. Kattus and colleagues (19) demonstrated that the chewable tablets prevented exercise-induced angina for 2.5 to 3 hr.

The oral preparations of isosorbide dinitrate have a longer duration of action than the sublingual and chewable forms. The onset of action is reported to be 30 min. Several studies have shown that long-term administration of oral isosorbide dinitrate in doses ranging from 7.5 mg to 50 mg resulted in an increase in exercise tolerance for up to 8 hr (20–22).

Table 38.3.
Transdermal Nitroglycerin Patches

Name	Strengths Available (mg/hr)	Total Nitroglycerin Content
Transderm-Nitro	0.1	12.5 mg/5 cm²
	0.2	25 mg/10 cm²
	0.4	50 mg/20 cm²
	0.6	75 mg/30 cm²
Nitro-Dur	0.1	20 mg/5 cm²
	0.2	40 mg/10 cm²
	0.3	60 mg/15 cm²
	0.4	80 mg/20 cm²
	0.6	120 mg/30 cm²
Nitrodisc	0.2	16 mg/8 cm²
	0.4	32 mg/16 cm²
Deponit	0.2	16 mg/16 cm²
	0.4	32 mg/32 cm²

The goal of therapy is to eliminate all angina episodes, decrease nitroglycerin consumption, and increase exercise tolerance without causing hypotension, to improve the "quality of life" of the patient. The initial dosing regimen for oral isosorbide dinitrate is 10 mg three times daily. The dose can be increased in 10-mg increments up to 40 mg, although doses up to 100 mg have been used. Frishman suggests that titrating the dose until there are orthostatic changes, represented by an increase in resting heart rate of 10 beats/min and a decrease in systolic blood pressure of 10 mm Hg, should also result in adequate antianginal effects (23).

Parker and colleagues (24) demonstrated tolerance to hemodynamic and antianginal effects of isosorbide dinitrate when dosed four times daily. This study indicates that intermittent dosing that allows a substantial nitrate-free time period maintains the desired antianginal effect of isosorbide dinitrate.

Sustained-release tablets and capsules of isosorbide dinitrate are available, and the recommended dose is 20 to 40 mg every 12 hr. Tolerance has been demonstrated when the sustained-release products have been given twice daily, and it can be circumvented by dosing once daily or with an asymmetric twice-daily regimen (8:00 AM and 2:00 PM) (25). The sustained-release isosorbide dinitrate products do not appear to have any significant advantage over the other oral nitrate products.

NITRATE TOLERANCE

Over the past 10 years, considerable data have been published on the development of nitrate tolerance from continuous therapy of transdermal nitroglycerin patches, frequent dosing of oral nitrates, and use of sustained-release nitrates without an adequate nitrate-free period. Numerous studies have documented attenuation of the antianginal effects within 24 hr of intial use and little or no effect during long-term administration (16, 26–29). Some patients may not develop tolerance and be well controlled on continuous therapy. Many patients, however, will develop tolerance.

The mechanism of nitrate tolerance appears to be impaired intracellular conversion of organic nitrates to S-nitrosothiols and nitric oxide, probably because of depletion or reduced availability of intracellular sulfhydryl groups (cysteine).

Studies have shown that administering sulfhydryl groups as exogenous thiol donors (e.g., N-acetylcysteine) may prevent or reverse tolerance during continuous nitrate use (30, 31). However, this process is often impractical. Recently, it has been demonstrated that angiotensin-converting-enzyme inhibitors were ineffective in preventing nitrate tolerance (32). This study was based on a preliminary study suggesting that elevated norepinephrine levels and activation of the renin-angiotensin-aldosterone axis

correlated with a lack of response or tolerance to a single 20 mg/24 hr dose of a nitroglycerin patch (33).

The best option is a prolonged nitrate-free period. Several studies have demonstrated that a prolonged nitrate-free period can maintain the antianginal efficacy of nitrates (24, 25, 27–29). The specific length of a nitrate-free period is unknown and varies between patients. An 8 to 12 hr nitrate-free period will eliminate the development of tolerance. For transdermal nitroglycerin administration, this can easily be accomplished by having the patient remove the patch (or ointment) at bedtime and apply a new patch (or fresh ointment) in the morning. Dosing of oral nitrates 2 or 3 times daily, with the last dose in the early evening, results in little if any tolerance. Sustained-release isosorbide dinitrate dosed once daily or with an asymmetric twice-daily regimen (8:00 AM and 2:00 PM) prevents the development of tolerance.

A concern that arises with the use of this strategy is whether or not patients are being put at risk during the nitrate-free period. Patients with chronic stable angina have a low frequency of ST segment depression between midnight and 7:00 AM. These patients are at low risk during the nitrate-free period. However, if a patient has nocturnal angina, rest angina, or is at high risk of having a cardiovascular event, they should also be treated with a β-adrenegic blocker or calcium-channel blocker.

ADVERSE EFFECTS

The most common adverse effect occurring with nitrates is a headache. This may appear as a transient, throbbing sensation or as a feeling of fullness in the head lasting 20 to 30 min. It is generally relieved by acetaminophen or aspirin. The headache will usually disappear spontaneously within several days to weeks as treatment continues. Other adverse effects include orthostatic hypotension, flushing, lightheadedness, dizziness, and weakness. A reflex tachycardia and syncope may occur, but approximately 10% of the patients will develop hypotension and bradycardia.

β-ADRENERGIC BLOCKING AGENTS

The β-adrenergic blocking agents are effective in the treatment of stable and unstable angina pectoris, but they exacerbate coronary artery vasospasm. They are effective when used as monotherapy and in combination with nitrates or calcium-channel blockers. Normally, myocardial contractility and heart rate are increased in response to sympathetic stimulation during physical exercise and emotional stress. This produces an increase in myocardial oxygen demand, and consequently, angina in patients who have a slightly positive myocardial oxygen balance. The β-adrenergic blocking agents bind to the β-adrenergic receptor and competitively inhibit the binding of catecholamines (norepinephrine and epinephrine) to the receptor site, blunting the sympathetic effects on contractility, heart rate, and left ventricular wall tension, thereby preventing or at least reducing the increase in myocardial oxygen demand (34). This in turn allows a patient to endure more physical activity without angina.

To date, there are twelve β-adrenergic blocking agents available in the United States: acebutolol, atenolol, betaxolol, carteolol, esmolol, labetalol, metoprolol, nadolol, penbutolol, pindolol, propranolol, and timolol. These agents all possess competitive β-adrenergic blocking activity, but they differ in specific pharmacodynamic and pharmacokinetic characteristics (Table 38.4).

There are two distinct types of β-adrenergic receptors. β-Receptors are found primarily in the myocardium, and when stimulated by catecholamines, they cause an increase in heart rate, myocardial contractility, and cardiac output. When these receptors are occupied by β-adrenergic blocking agents, the opposite effects occur. The β$_2$-receptors are found in smooth muscle, such as the blood vessels and bronchioles. When these receptors are stimulated, dilation of the smooth muscle occurs. When a β-adrenergic blocking agent is bound to the β$_2$-receptors, the α-adrenergic effect is unopposed, resulting in an increase in smooth muscle tone causing vasoconstriction or bronchoconstriction.

The affinity with which the β-adrenergic blocking agents bind to the two receptor types varies. Some of these agents are more avidly bound to the β$_1$-receptors than the β$_2$-receptors. Since the β$_1$-receptors are located primarily in the heart, the selective binding to these receptors is referred to as "cardioselectivity." This is seen with acebutolol, atenolol, betaxolol, and metoprolol. These agents are less likely to cause vasoconstriction or bronchoconstriction. Unfortunately, they tend to lose their cardioselectivity as the dose is increased and behave like "nonselective" β-adrenergic blocking agents at high doses.

Acebutolol, carteolol, and pindolol possess intrinsic sympathomimetic activity (ISA). When bound to the β-receptor, they exhibit the usual β-adrenergic blocking activity, but they will cause some degree of receptor stimulation. These agents exhibit a smaller reduction in resting heart rate, less myocardial depression, and possibly less risk of bronchoconstriction. It is still unclear whether the ISA of these β-adrenergic blocking agents is advantageous in the clinical setting. However, there is evidence that ISA can cause an exacerbation of anginal symptoms in patients with rest angina.

Labetalol is unique in that it is both a nonselective β-adrenergic blocking agent and an α$_1$-adrenergic blocking agent. Unlike other β-adrenergic blockers, which typically

Table 38.4.
Dosages and Selected Pharmacologic Properties of Currently Available β-Blocking Agents

Drug: Generic Name (Trade Name)	Daily Dosage Range (mg)	No. of Daily Doses	Cardio-selective	ISA	Lipid solubility	Bioavailability (%)	Plasma Half-Life (hr)	Primary Route of Elimination
Acebutolol (Sectral)	400–1200	1–2	Yes	Yes	Low	20–60	3–4	Hepatic & renal
Atenolol (Tenormin)	50–200	1	Yes	No	Low	50–60	6–9	Hepatic & renal
Betaxolol (Kerlone)	10–20	1	Yes	No	Low	89	14–22	Hepatic & renal
Metoprolol (Lopressor)	50–200	2–3	Yes	No	Moderate	40–50	3–7	Hepatic
Carteolol (Cartrol)	2.5–5	1	No	Yes	Low	85	6	Hepatic & renal
Nadolol (Corgard)	40–320	1	No	No	Low	30–50	20–24	Renal
Penbutolol (Levatol)	10–20	1	No	No	High	100	5	Hepatic & renal
Pindolol (Visken)	10–40	2–3	No	Yes	Moderate	100	3–4	Hepatic & renal
Propranolol (Inderal)	40–480	2–4	No	No	High	30	3–5	Hepatic
(Inderal LA)	80–320	1	No	No	High	9–18	8–11	Hepatic
Timolol (Blocadren)	20–40	2	No	No	Low to moderate	75	4	Hepatic & renal
Labetalol[a] (Normodyne or Trandate)	200–1200	2–3	No	No	Moderate	30–40	5.5–8	Hepatic & renal

[a] Labetalol possesses combined β-blocking and α-blocking activity.

increase peripheral vascular resistance (PVR), labetalol decreases PVR, which results in a greater reduction in blood pressure and a smaller reduction in heart rate (35). Cardiac output and pulmonary capillary wedge pressure remain unchanged, and coronary vascular resistance is reduced, probably by the α-blocking effect (36). The importance of these effects in the treatment of angina remains unclear at this time.

The β-adrenergic blocking agents are effective in improving exercise tolerance and reducing the frequency of anginal episodes, along with a reduction of sublingual nitroglycerin consumption. β-Adrenergic blocking agents are used for prophylaxis of exercised-induced angina. They may be used as initial therapy or added to a nitrate regimen if anginal episodes are still occurring in spite of adequate nitrate therapy.

Since all of the β-adrenergic blocking agents appear to be effective in the treatment of angina, the choice of which agent to use depends on such factors as cardioselectivity, adverse effects, and duration of action. A cardioselective β-adrenergic blocking agent is preferred over a nonselective agent in patients with concomitant peripheral vascular disease or restrictive airway disease (a calcium-channel blocker would be the ideal choice). Acebutolol, atenolol, betaxolol, carteolol, nadolol, and penbutolol have the advantage of once-daily dosing, which may be helpful for patients whose compliance is a problem. The goals are to reduce the number of angina episodes and nitroglycerin consumption and improve exercise tolerance without development of major side effects.

ADVERSE EFFECTS

Adverse effects associated with β-adrenergic blocking agents include bradycardia (heart rate ≤50 beats/min), atrioventricular (AV) block, orthostatic hypotension, fatigue, lightheadedness, dizziness, peripheral edema, nausea, bizarre dreams, and mental depression. Some of these effects may be reduced by switching to a different β-adrenergic blocking agent. For example, if symptomatic bradycardia or AV block occur, a β-adrenergic blocking agent with ISA, such as acebutolol, carteolol, or pindolol, may be of benefit. It has been noted that β-blockers with ISA do not cause an increase in triglyceride levels or a decrease in HDL-cholesterol levels like that which occurs with non-ISA β-adrenergic blocking agents. When central nervous system effects like mental depression or bizarre, vivid dreams are a problem, switching to a more water-soluble agent such as atenolol, betaxolol, carteolol, or nadolol should decrease the incidence of these effects. β-Adrenergic blocking agents that are cardioselective, like acebutolol, atenolol, and metoprolol, have a lower incidence of fatigue reported with their use.

CAUTIONS

All of the β-adrenergic blocking agents exhibit a negative inotropic effect, and therefore they should be used cautiously, if at all, in patients with congestive heart failure. Patients with concomitant peripheral vascular disorders or restrictive airway disease should receive a cardioselective agent if β-adrenergic blockade is the desired therapeutic approach. Although the cardioselective agents pose less risk to these patients than the nonselective agents, the cardioselectivity is lost at higher doses, rendering these drugs dangerous to this subgroup of the population.

Although the occurrence of a "β-blocker withdrawal syndrome" is controversial, a hypersensitivity to catecholamines with exacerbation of angina and possible acute myocardial infarction can occur following the abrupt discontinuation of therapy. β-Adrenergic blocker doses should be tapered over 1 to 2 weeks for greatest safety.

DRUG INTERACTIONS
Calcium-Channel Blockers (37)

Since calcium-channel blockers and the β-adrenergic blockers cause reductions in blood pressure, the combined use of these agents may result in clinically significant hypotension. The use of verapamil and diltiazem in combination with any of the β-adrenergic blocking agents can cause enhanced slowing of conduction and an increased risk of developing bradycardia or AV block.

β-Adrenergic Agonists (38)

The use of a β-adrenergic blocking agent in a patient receiving a β-adrenergic agonist will result in antagonism of the desirable effects of both agents. This combination is not recommended.

Phenothiazines (39)

The phenothiazines can cause hypotension due to their α-adrenergic blocking activity. When combined with a β-adrenergic blocking agent, some patients may develop severe hypotension.

Oral Hypoglycemics/Insulin (40, 41)

The concomitant use of a β-adrenergic blocking agent and an oral hypoglycemic agent or insulin can place a patient at risk of developing severe hypoglycemia. β-Adrenergic blockers can delay the recovery from hypoglycemia by inhibiting epinephrine-induced hyperglycemia. This epinephrine release can lead to hypertension as a result of vasoconstriction in response to its action on the unopposed α-receptors. Also, β-adrenergic blocking agents can block the tachycardia and other symptoms that occur as a result of hypoglycemia. This may place the patient at an increased risk. The only symptom that is not blocked by a β-adrenergic blocker is sweating, which is mediated by the parasympathetic system. If a β-adrenergic blocker is needed, a cardioselective product is preferred, although it would not be entirely without risk.

CALCIUM-CHANNEL BLOCKERS

The calcium-channel blockers are a heterogenous group of compounds that have been widely accepted for the treatment of stable angina, unstable angina, and Prinzmetal's angina. Nifedipine, nicardipine, diltiazem, and verapamil are the agents currently available in the United States. Each of these drugs, with the exception of nicardipine, is available in an extended-release formulation.

There are two categories of calcium channels: receptor-operated channels and voltage-dependent channels. The voltage-dependent calcium channels are classified as L-, T-, or N-type, based on their electrophysiologic properties (42). The L-type voltage-dependent calcium channel is present in the brain and myocardial, skeletal, and smooth muscle. The L-type channel is also sensitive to the effects of the different types of calcium-channel blockers: dihydropyridines (nifedipine, nicardipine), phenylalkylamines (verapamil), and benzothiazepines (diltiazem). There are distinct binding sites for each type of calcium-channel blocker on the L-type channel (43). The binding sites are linked allosterically, so the binding of one type of calcium-channel blocker will affect the binding of a different type of calcium-channel blocker (e.g., binding of nifedipine to the dihydropyridine site reduces the ability of verapamil to bind to the phenylalkyamine site). These sites are also allosterically linked to the gating mechanism of the L-type channel.

The primary pharmacologic effect of these drugs is the inhibition of calcium influx through the slow calcium channels in the myocardial and vascular smooth muscle. These agents also interfere with the intracellular transport of calcium. This reduction in calcium influx leads to an inhibition of the excitation-contraction coupling mechanism in the myocardial muscle and vascular smooth muscle.

The calcium-channel blockers have four major physiologic effects (44):

1. They cause systemic arterial dilation leading to a decrease in systemic vascular resistance, which reduces myocardial oxygen demand. Therefore, they are useful for the management of chronic stable angina.
2. They dilate epicardial coronary arteries and reduce coronary vascular resistance. This improves coronary blood flow and myocardial oxygen supply. Thus, they are of benefit in the treatment of both unstable and Prinzmetal's angina.
3. They reduce myocardial contractility. This reduces myocardial oxygen consumption. Therefore, they are useful in the treatment of chronic stable angina.
4. Verapamil and diltiazem slow sinus node and AV node con-

Table 38.5.
Pharmacologic Effects of Calcium-Channel Blockers

Drug	Systemic Vasodilation	Coronary Vasodilation	Negative Inotropic Effect	Electrophysiologic Effects on SA/AV Nodes
Nifedipine	+ + +	+ +	+	0
Nicardipine	+ + +	+ + +	0, +	0
Diltiazem	+ +	+ +	+	+ +
Verapamil	+	+	+ +	+ + +

duction. This is not important for the treatment of angina pectoris, but is of benefit in the management of supraventricular tachyarrhythmias.

These agents differ in both the type and degree of systemic effects they produce (Table 38.5). Nifedipine and nicardipine produce more systemic vasodilation than diltiazem and verapamil (44, 45). Verapamil has the greatest negative inotropic effect (44), followed by nifedipine and diltiazem. Nicardipine can actually increase myocardial contractility, even in patients with severe congestive heart failure (45). Diltiazem and verapamil both reduce sinus node depolarization and AV nodal conduction, whereas nifedipine and nicardipine have no direct effects on cardiac conduction tissue when given in therapeutic doses (44, 45). All of these drugs can increase coronary blood flow, with nicardipine having the greatest effect (45). Secondary to their marked systemic vasodilatory effect, nifedipine and nicardipine produce a sympathetically mediated reflex tachycardia.

The efficacy of the calcium-channel blockers in the treatment of angina pectoris has been studied extensively. They all have been shown to reduce the frequency of anginal episodes, decrease nitroglycerin consumption, and improve exercise tolerance. These drugs can be added to existing nitrate and/or β-adrenergic blocking agent therapy or may be used as monotherapy. The pharmacokinetics of the calcium-channel blockers are outlined in Table 38.6.

The previously stated end-points of angina therapy must be monitored, as well as blood pressure and heart rate. All four agents can cause hypotension, so blood pressure must be monitored. Nifedipine and nicardipine can cause a reflex tachycardia, whereas diltiazem and verapamil can cause bradycardia. Therefore, heart rate must be followed, and if it drops below 50 beats/min or increases to more than 100 beats/min, then a drug from a different therapeutic class is recommended.

ADVERSE EFFECTS

Adverse effects of the calcium-channel blockers are generally associated with their pharmacologic effects. Nifedipine has the greatest frequency of adverse effects, and

Table 38.6.
Calcium-Channel Blockers Pharmacokinetic Parameters

Drug: Generic Name (Trade Name)	Total Daily Dose (mg)	No. of Doses per Day	Bioavailability (%)	Plasma Half-Life (hr)	Elimination
Diltiazem					
(Cardiazem)	180–360	3–4	40–67	3.5–6	60% via liver
(Cardiazem SR)	240–360	2	40–67	5–7	60% via kidney
Nicardipine					Extensively metabolized
(Cardene)	60–120	3	35	2–4	in the liver
Nifedipine					
(Procardia, Adalat)	30–120	3	45–70	2–5	Extensively metabolized
(Procardia XL)	30–90	1	86	2–5	in the liver
Verapamil					
(Calan, Isoptin)	240–360	3	20–35	3–7	Extensively metabolized
(Calan SR, Isoptin SR)	240–480	1–2	20–35	3–7	in the liver

diltiazem has the least. Adverse effects associated with nifedipine and nicardipine are related to their peripheral vasodilation and include headache, dizziness, lightheadedness, flushing, and hypotension. These effects also occur with diltiazem and verapamil, but are not as prevalent. Nifedipine, and to a lesser extent nicardipine, can also cause a noncardiac peripheral edema in the lower extremities, which can be reduced by administration of a diuretic. These two agents will cause a reflex tachycardia secondary to reduced systemic arterial pressure. Verapamil and diltiazem can produce bradycardia and AV block. Therefore, they should be used with caution when combined with a β-adrenergic blocking agent. Constipation can occur with all of these agents, but it is most common in patients receiving verapamil.

DRUG INTERACTIONS

Digoxin

Verapamil has been reported to raise the mean serum digoxin concentrations 60 to 80% (46, 47). Verapamil reduces the renal and nonrenal clearance of digoxin (48). There are conflicting data on the effects of nifedipine, nicardipine, and diltiazem on digoxin pharmacokinetics. However, it is advisable to monitor digoxin levels when a calcium-channel blocker is being coadministered.

Carbamazepine (49, 50)

Verapamil and diltiazem have been shown to decrease the metabolism of carbamazepine. As a result of this interaction, several patients have developed carbamazepine-induced neurotoxicity when verapamil or diltiazem was added to their regimen. If a calcium-channel blocker is desired in these patients, nifedipine or nicardipine is preferred. If verapamil or diltiazem is used, careful monitoring of serum carbamazepine levels is warranted.

Cyclosporine (51–53)

Serum cyclosporine concentrations are increased by concomitant administration of verapamil, diltiazem, or nicardipine. This reaction is caused by their ability to inhibit the cytochrome P-450 oxidative metabolic pathway. Close monitoring of serum cyclosporine concentrations is advisable when adding or discontinuing one of these agents from a medication regimen that also contains cyclosporine.

Quinidine (54–57)

It appears as though concomitant administration of nifedipine to a patient stabilized on quinidine can result in an increase in quinidine clearance. A specific mechanism has not been identified. On the other hand, verapamil inhibits the metabolism of quinidine, resulting in increases in serum quinidine concentration. Diltiazem has not been shown to have an effect on quinidine clearance.

Theophylline (57–59)

Verapamil appears to inhibit the metabolism of theophylline and increase its plasma concentration. In some patients, this interaction may result in theophylline toxicity. Diltiazem and nifedipine appear to have a similar effect.

CORONARY ARTERY BYPASS GRAFT SURGERY

Coronary artery bypass grafting is a surgical procedure in which a graft, usually a saphenous vein from the leg, is placed from the aorta to the distal segment of a stenosed coronary artery, or an internal mammary artery is inserted into the distal segment of a stenosed coronary artery. This should correct the imbalance between myocardial supply and demand by improving coronary blood flow to the ischemic region of the myocardium. Ideally, this procedure should prevent the recurrence of anginal attacks and allow patients to discontinue antianginal medications. Unfor-

Table 38.7.
Four-Year Survival (%) after Coronary Artery Bypass Grafting

	Extent of Cornary Artery Disease			
	1-vessel	2-vessel	3-vessel	LMCAD[a]
All patients	97%	95%	90%	95%
Normal LV function	98%	92%	94%	97%
Abnormal LV function	94%	97%	87%	94%

[a] LMCAD, left main coronary artery disease.

Table 38.8.
Five-Year Survival (%) of Medically Treated Patients with Angina Pectoris

	Extent of Cornary Artery Disease		
	1-vessel	2-vessel	3-vessel
All patients	89%	82%	68%
Normal LV function	94%	90%	79%
Abnormal LV function	62%	62%	33%

tunately, some patients still require medications (at lower doses) to control symptoms.

A problem with coronary artery bypass graft surgery is early and late occlusion of the graft. From early series, 5-year graft patency has been 80%, and 10-year patency has been 50%. Cigarette smoking markedly reduces graft patency. The incidence of graft occlusion can be reduced by administration of aspirin, 80 to 325 mg daily, with or without dipyridamole, 75 mg t.i.d. (60). Reduction of serum cholesterol levels may also improve graft survival, a concept that is evolving rapidly (61).

The survival rates of patients that have undergone coronary artery bypass graft surgery have increased over the last decade. In a study by Rahimtoola and co-workers (62), the overall survival rate was reported as 92.5%. The greater the obstruction of the coronary arteries and the greater the degree of left ventricular dysfunction, the worse the prognosis (Table 38.7). In comparison, the 5-year survival rate of patients receiving medical treatment is lower, as reported by Mock and colleagues (Table 38.8) (63). Coronary artery bypass graft surgery is recommended in patients with three-vessel disease, left main coronary artery disease, and persistent angina despite aggressive medical therapy (64). There are individuals who do not want to take medications, would not tolerate the symptoms of angina, and will accept the risks of surgery. The option of coronary artery bypass surgery should be offered to these patients.

PERCUTANEOUS TRANSLUMINAL CORONARY ANGIOPLASTY

Percutaneous transluminal coronary angioplasty (PTCA) is a remarkable alternative to coronary artery bypass grafting for the treatment of critical coronary artery disease. The technique, an extension of cardiac catheterization, involves threading a very small caliber catheter incorporating a 2 to 4 mm inflatable balloon down the involved coronary lumen. With the balloon straddling the coronary stenosis, it is inflated, often several times, with 2 to 10 atmospheres of CO_2 (Figs. 38.1 and 38.2). The desired result is fracture of the atherosclerotic plaque and stretching of the artery muscle layer (media). This technique can reduce severe arterial stenoses to nearly normal.

Since first developed by Gruentzig in 1977, many thousands of patients have undergone PTCA. With experience, operator skill and success have improved and indications for PTCA have expanded. With proper selection, the stenosis can be crossed and successfully dilated in over 90% of cases. Survival over 3 to 6 years is between 96 and 97%, with dramatic symptomatic improvement (65). Operative mortality is less than 1%. Abrupt occlusion during or immediately after balloon inflation occurs in about 3% of cases and requires emergency bypass surgery. PTCA is now performed safely in patients with multivessel disease, including complex, calcified, eccentric lesions. With these expanded indications, it is estimated that 39% of patients undergoing diagnostic coronary angiography are ultimately referred for PTCA, whereas only 28% are referred to bypass surgery (66). Much of the growth of PTCA has consisted of treating patients who are either too high a risk for bypass, or who have symptoms with medical therapy that are too mild to warrant surgery. While 60% of PTCAs are for stable angina, a substantial fraction of procedures are performed for unstable angina (27%) and for acute myocardial infarction (13%).

Over the 6 months after PTCA, restenosis occurs in 25 to 35% of patients (67). Further restenosis rarely occurs beyond that time. Restenosis is due to acceleration of atherosclerosis at the angioplasty site. It is more frequent with males; smokers; patients with hyperlipidemia, diabetes mellitus, unstable or variant angina or severe stenoses; those with calcified, eccentric, long or severe lesions, saphenous vein grafts, or lesions with significant residual stenosis or dissection after PTCA. Attempts to prevent restenosis have used antiplatelet agents, anticoagulants, calcium-channel blockers, corticosteroids, fish oils, prostaglandins, and platelet-derived growth-factor antagonists. All have failed to reduce the frequency of restenosis (67). Many physicians routinely prescribe antiplatelet agents (e.g., aspirin, dipyridamole) and calcium-channel blockers during and after PTCA. It is believed that these drugs reduce platelet-induced thrombosis and focal vasospasm,

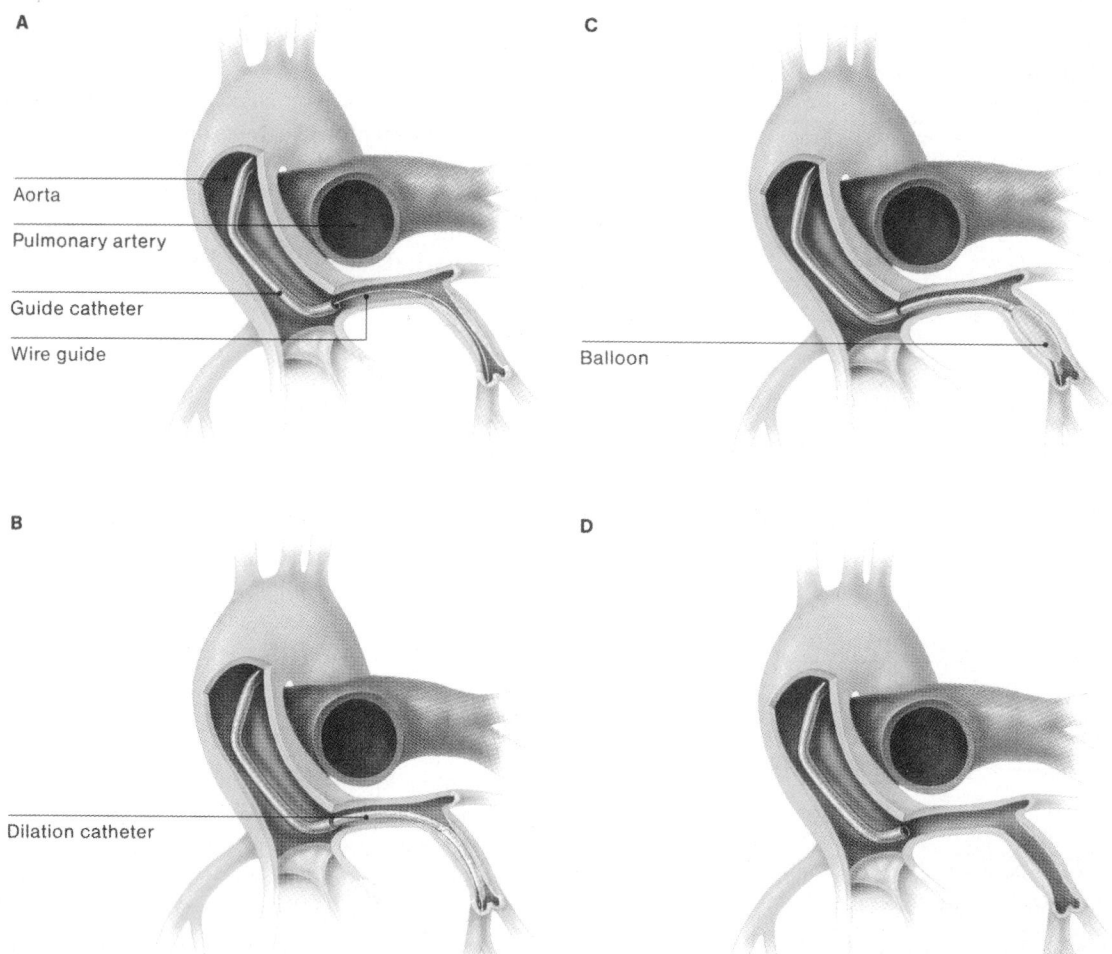

Figure 38.1. Schematic of percutaneous transluminal angio-plasty. **A,** The guide catheter is positioned at the coronary ostium, and the steerable wire guide is passed through the stenosis and into the distal coronary artery. **B,** The dilation catheter is passed over the wire guide and through the stenotic segment so that the dilation balloon lies within the area of stenosis. **C,** The balloon is inflated. **D,** The balloon is deflated and the dilation catheter is removed. Repeat angiography is performed to evaluate the size of the improved lumen. (From Block PC, Forrester JS: Intra-coronary interventions: balloon and laser angioplasty. Curr Con-cepts, p 7, 1986, with permission.)

which may precipitate early thrombotic occlusion without affecting restenosis.

TREATMENT OF ANGINA PECTORIS (Fig. 38.3)

Stable Angina

Patients who develop anginal attacks during exertion, once a week or less, can be initiated on sublingual nitroglycerin for treatment of the acute episodes. At this frequency of episodes, there is no need for prophylaxis. If some or all of these episodes occur from a specific activity, the patient can take a sublingual nitroglycerin just prior to the activity and will be protected for up to 30 min.

Once the frequency of anginal attacks exceeds 1 epi-sode a week, prophylaxis is recommended in addition to sublingual nitroglycerin. Nitrates, β-adrenergic blockers, and calcium-channel blockers are effective as monother-apy. In deciding which drug to use for a patient, the pa-tient's concurrent disease states and existing drug therapy must be considered. For example, a hypertensive patient on a diuretic will benefit from a β-adrenergic blocker or calcium-channel blocker.

Coronary artery bypass surgery and PTCA are also pos-sible options in patients with chronic stable angina pec-toris.

Unstable Angina

Plaque rupture with subsequent platelet activation and thrombus formation is believed to have a strong role in the pathophysiology of unstable angina. Unstable angina

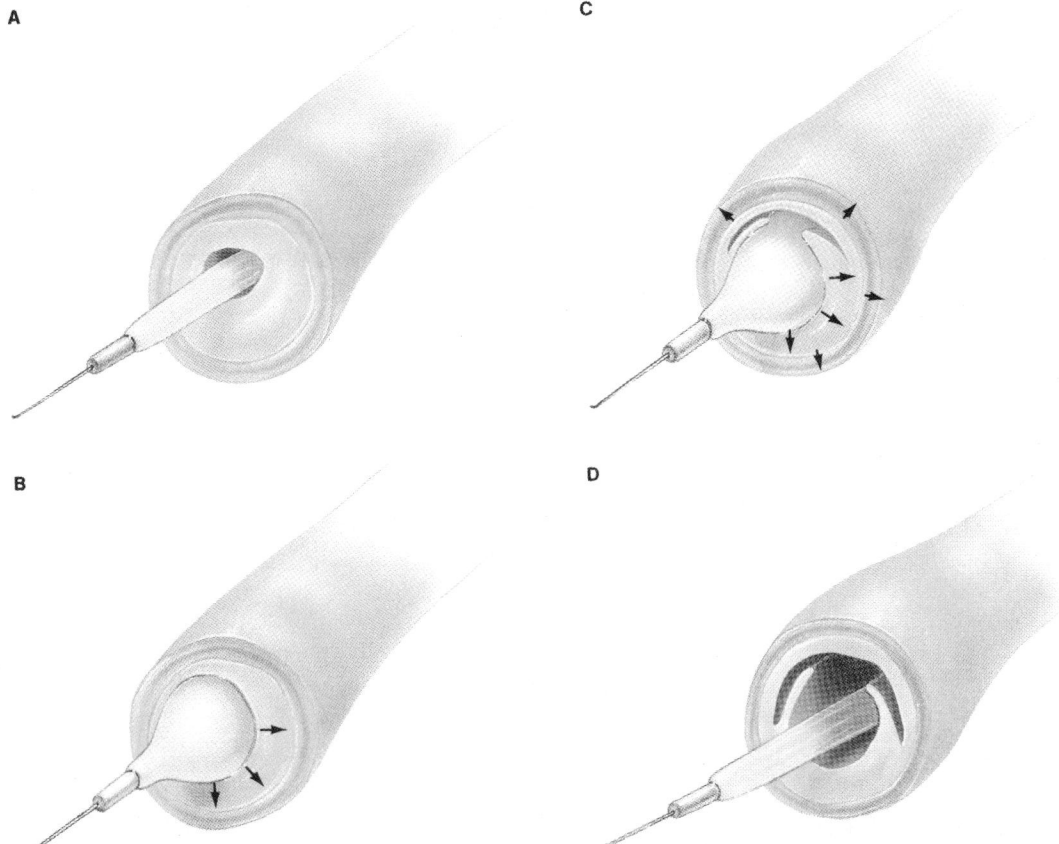

Figure 38.2. Schematic of the mechanism of transluminal angioplasty. **A,** the deflated dilation catheter lies within the coronary stenosis. **B,** As the balloon is inflated, the atherosclerotic plaque resists stretching. **C,** With additional inflation pressure, the atherosclerotic plaque splits at its weakest point. As the elastic outer media and adventitia are stretched, the lumen is enlarged. **D,** The balloon is deflated and withdrawn. This leaves a stretched, dilated vessel with an enlarged lumen. (From Block PC, Forrester JS: Intracoronary interventions: balloon and laser angioplasty. Curr Concepts, p 16, 1986, with permission.)

often proceeds to myocardial infarction. A patient presenting to the hospital with a changing pattern of chest pain occurring at rest (or with minimal exertion) or chest pain lasting more than 15 min should be admitted, and therapy should be initiated to control this process and prevent the development of acute myocardial infarction.

Heparin should be started as a continuous infusion (1000 units/hr), unless contraindications preclude its use. Heparin reduces the incidence of myocardial infarction in this patient population (68). After 2 days of heparin therapy, aspirin should be started. The optimal dose of aspirin is unknown at this time, but a dose of 325 mg daily is considered satisfactory. The use of aspirin in unstable angina does lead to a reduction in the incidence of myocardial infarction (68–70).

Intravenous nitroglycerin should be started immediately on these patients. β-Adrenergic blockers, calcium-channel blockers, or both may be added to the therapeutic regimen as needed to control the anginal symptoms.

Prinzmetal's Angina

As stated earlier, Prinzmetal's angina occurs predominately at rest and is caused by vasospasm of a coronary artery. The mechanism of the vasospasm is unknown. One hypothesis states that vasospasm may be caused by altered α-adrenergic activity (71). Coronary artery vasospasm can be documented by an ECG during an episode of chest pain. ST segment elevation occurs during the episode of pain and returns to baseline without Q wave formation upon relief of the pain. This can also be seen during 24-hr ambulatory continuous ECG (Holter) monitoring. The coronary arteriogram may show atherosclerotic lesions or appear normal. Intracoronary ergonovine may be administered as a provocative agent to induce vasospasm during arteriography. If vasospasm occurs secondary to the ergonovine, rapid administration of intracoronary nitroglycerin may be necessary to stop the vasospasm and avoid possible complications.

Treatment of Prinzmetal's angina involves relief of

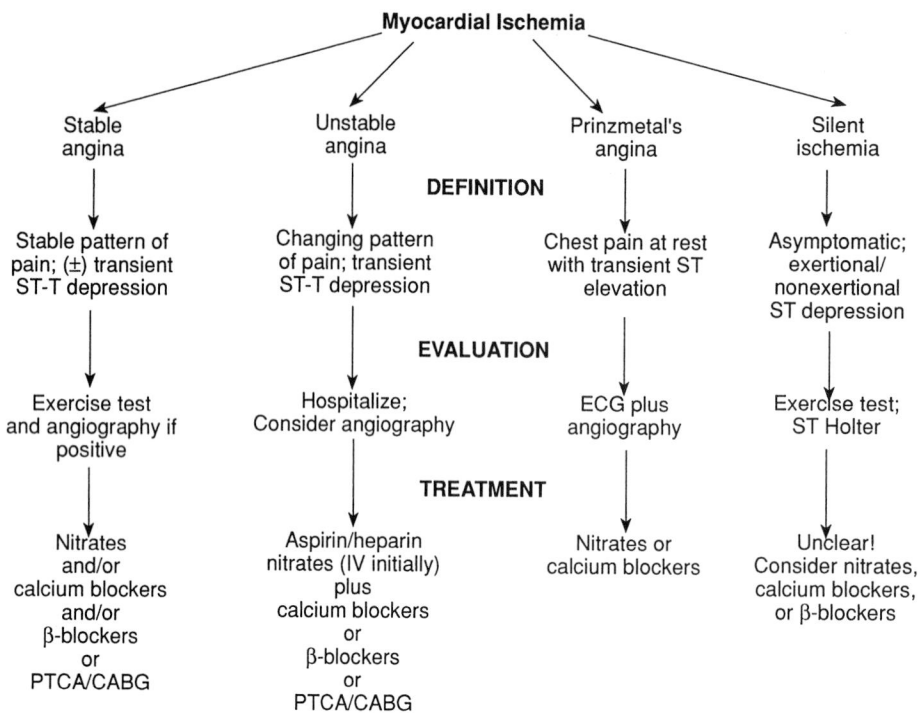

Figure 38.3.   Definition, evaluation, and treatment of myocardial ischemia.

acute episodes and prophylaxis for recurrent episodes. Sublingual nitroglycerin is used commonly for relief of acute vasospasm. Nitrates and calcium-channel blockers are used as prophylactic therapy; the calcium-channel blockers have become the more popular choice. Doses used for either class of drug are the same as those discussed earlier. All of the calcium-channel blockers have demonstrated efficacy in preventing Prinzmetal's angina. The β-adrenergic blocking agents are not of benefit in treating Prinzmetal's angina and have been shown to increase the frequency of vasospastic episodes (72).

SILENT ISCHEMIA

"Silent" myocardial ischemia is simply myocardial ischemia occurring in the absence of chest pain or anginal equivalents (73). Why ischemia is silent in some patients is unknown. Speculation has centered around three hypotheses: that silent ischemia represents less severe ischemia, not sufficient to meet pain thresholds; that there are important differences in pain perception thresholds or central transmission of painful stimuli among individuals; and that the pathophysiology may be varied, resulting in different patterns of disturbed myocardial blood flow during silent and symptomatic ischemia.

Silent ischemia has been detected by various methods, including metabolic studies such as positron emission tomography (PET scanning), thallium scintigraphy, and ST segment electrocardiography using either continuous am-

bulatory recording or exercise electrocardiography. Completely asymptomatic ischemia has occurred in 2.4% of healthy airmen (74). Silent ischemia has been produced during low-level exercise testing in about 30% of patients without recurrent angina several days after myocardial infarction (74). Silent ischemia occurs in most patients hospitalized with either stable or unstable angina (75). In these patients, up to 80% of the total ischemic episodes were silent and were unrelated to activity and heart rate, and nearly 50% occurred between 6:00 AM and 12:00 PM.

The fact that ischemia can occur spontaneously without a preceding increase in heart rate suggests that decreased blood supply, not increased myocardial oxygen demand, may be involved. The atherosclerotic plaque within a coronary artery is not fixed, but instead it can dilate and contract (76). Indeed paradoxical vasoconstriction can occur at a plaque, thus impairing blood flow. Other possible explanations for spontaneous ischemia include intermittent thrombus formation overlying the plaque and abnormal changes in distal coronary artery tone.

Silent ischemia suggests a relatively poor prognosis (74, 77). Patients with unstable angina have more untoward events (e.g., death and myocardial infarction) when frequent episodes of silent ischemia are present. The likelihood of death or infarction increases 4 to 6-fold when silent ischemia is identified after myocardial infarction.

Therapy is identical to symptomatic angina. Survival is improved in asymptomatic patients with left main coronary artery stenosis treated with bypass grafting. The number of both symptomatic and silent ischemia episodes can be diminished substantially with treatment using either nitrates, calcium-channel blockers, or β-adrenergic blocking agents. Aspirin appears to be ineffective. Except in left main stenosis, the impact of the treatment of silent ischemia on morbidity and mortality has not been identified.

CONCLUSION

Angina pectoris is a disease state that affects many people in the United States. Modification of risk factors and elimination of precipitating factors may help reduce the frequency of anginal attacks. Medications like nitrates, β-adrenergic blocking agents, and calcium-channel blockers have proven to be effective in controlling symptoms of ischemic heart disease and silent ischemia when used as monotherapy or in combination. Coronary artery bypass graft surgery is an acceptable alternative and is highly beneficial in patients with three-vessel disease, left main coronary artery disease, and persistent angina in spite of aggressive medical therapy. Also, percutaneous transluminal coronary angioplasty is an acceptable alternative to medication and/or surgery for patients who are intolerant to their medications and have limited activity as a result of their angina.

REFERENCES

1. Gotto AM, Farmer JA, Risk factors for coronary artery disease. In Braunwald E: Heart Disease: A Textbook of Cardiovascular Medicine, ed. 3. Philadelphia, WB Saunders, 1988, pp 1153–1190.
2. Sheffield LT, Exercise stress testing. In Braunwald E: Heart Disease: A Textbook of Cardiovascular Medicine, ed. 3. Philadelphia, WB Saunders, 1988, pp 223–241.
3. Gibson RS, Beller GA: Should exercise electrocardiographic testing be replaced by radioisotope methods? Cardiovasc Clin 13(1):1–31, 1983.
4. Ignarro LJ, Lippton H, Edwards JC, et al.: Mechanism of vascular smooth muscle relaxation by organic nitrates, nitrites, nitroprusside, and nitric oxide: evidence for the involvement of S-nitrosothiols as active intermediates. J Pharmacol Exp Ther 218:739–749, 1981.
5. Murad F: Cyclic guanosine monophosphate as a mediator of vasodilation. J Clin Invest 78:1–5, 1986.
6. Rehr RB, Jackson JA, Winniford MD, et al.: Mechanism of nitroglycerin-induced coronary dilation: lack of relaxation to intracoronary thromboxane concentrations. Am J Cardiol 54:971–974, 1984.
7. Cohen MV, Kirk ES: Differential response of large and small coronary arteries to nitroglycerin and angiotensin: autoregulation and tachyphylaxis. Circulation Res 336:445–453, 1973.
8. Feldman RL, Pepine CJ, Conti CR: Magnitude of dilation of large and small coronary arteries by nitroglycerin. Circulation 64:324–333, 1981.
9. Parker JO, West RO, DiGiorgi S: The effect of nitroglycerin on coronary blood flow and the hemodynamic response to exercise in coronary artery disease. Am J Cardiol 27:59–65, 1971.
10. Klaus AP, Zaret BL, Pitt BL, et al.: Comparative evaluation of sublingual long acting nitrates. Circulation 48:519–525, 1973.
11. Kimchi A, Lee G, Amsterdam E. et al.: Increased exercise tolerance

after nitroglycerin oral spray: a new and effective therapeutic modality in angina pectoris. Circulation 67:124–127, 1983.
12. Abrams J: New nitrate delivery systems: buccal nitroglycerin. Am Heart J 105:848–854, 1983.
13. Parker JO, Augustine RJ, Burton JR, et al.: Effect of nitroglycerin ointment on the clinical and hemodynamic response to exercise. Am J Cardiol 38:162–166, 1976.
14. Awan NA, Miller RR, Maxwell KS, et al.: Cardiocirculatory and antianginal actions of nitroglycerin ointment. Evaluation by cardiac catheterization, forearm plethysmography, and treadmill stress testing. Chest 73:14–18, 1978.
15. Abrams J: Transcutaneous nitroglycerin—ointment or disk? Am Heart J 105:1597–1600, 1984.
16. Parker JO, Fung HL: Transdermal nitroglycerin in angina pectoris. Am J Cardiol 54:471–476, 1984.
17. Thadani U, Hamilton SF, Olson E, et al.: Transdermal patches in angina pectoris. Ann Intern Med 105(4):485–492, 1986.
18. Sullivan M, Savvides M, Abouantoun S, et al.: Failure of transdermal nitroglycerin to improve exercise capacity in patients with angina pectoris. J Am Coll Cardiol 5:1220–1223, 1985.
19. Kattus AA, Alvaro AB, Zohman LR, et al.: Comparison of placebo, nitroglycerin, and isosorbide dinitrate for effectiveness of relief of angina and duration of action. Chest 75:17–23, 1979.
20. Danahy DT, Aronow WS: Hemodynamics and antianginal effects of high dose oral isosorbide dinitrate after chronic use. Circulation 56:205–212, 1977.
21. Lee G, Mason DT, DeMana AN, et al.: Effects of long-term oral administration of isosorbide dinitrate on the antianginal response to nitroglycerin: absence of nitrate cross-tolerance and self-tolerance shown by exercise testing. Am J Cardiol 41:82–87, 1978.
22. Thadani U, Fung HL, Darke AC, et al.: Oral isosorbide dinitrate in the treatment of angina pectoris: dose-response relationship and duration of action during acute therapy. Circulation 62:491–502, 1980.
23. Frishman WH: Pharmacology of the nitrates in angina pectoris. Am J Cardiol 56:8I–13I, 1985.
24. Parker JO, Farrell B, Lahey KA, et al.: Effect of intervals between doses on the development of tolerance to isosorbide dinitrate. N Engl J Med 316:1440–1444, 1987.
25. Silber S, Vogler AC, Krause KH, et al.: Induction and circumvention of nitrate tolerance applying different dosage intervals. Am J Med 83:860–870, 1987.
26. Reichek N, Priest C, Zimrin D, et al.: Antianginal effects of nitroglycerin patches. Am J Cardiol 54:1–7, 1984.
27. Cowan JC, Bourke JP, Ried DS, et al.: Prevention of tolerance to nitroglycerin patches by overnight removal. Am J Cardiol 60:271–275, 1987.
28. Demots H, Glasser SP: Intermittent transdermal nitroglycerin therapy in the treatment of chronic stable angina. J Am Coll Cardiol 13:786–795, 1989.
29. Schaer DH, Buff LA, Katz RJ: Sustained antianginal efficacy of transdermal nitroglycerin patches using an overnight 10-hour nitrate-free interval. Am J Cardiol 61:46–50, 1988.
30. May DC, Popma JJ, Black WH, et al.: In vivo induction of nitroglycerin tolerance in human coronary arteries. N Engl J Med 317:805–809, 1987.
31. Horowitz JD, Antman EM, Lorell BH, et al.: Potentiation of the cardiovascular effects of nitroglycerin by N-acetylcysteine. Circulation 68:1247–1253, 1983.
32. Dakak N, Makhoul N, Flugelman MY, et al.: Failure of captopril to prevent nitrate tolerance in congestive heart failure secondary to coronary artery disease. Am J Cardiol 66:608–613, 1990.
33. Muiesan ML, Agabiti-Rosei E, Beschi M, et al.: Transdermal nitroglycerin may activate adrenergic and renin-aldosterone systems. Effect on effort tolerance in angina pectoris. (abstr) J Am Coll Cardiol 11:184A, 1988.

34. Robinson BF: Mechanism of action of β-blocking drugs in angina pectoris: a review. Postgrad Med J 52:43–45, 1976.

35. Brittain RT, Levy GP: A review of animal pharmacology of labetalol, a combined α and β adrenoceptor-blocking drug. Br J Clin Pharmacol 3:681–684, 1976.

36. Gagnon RM, Morissette M, Présant S, et al.: Hemodynamic and coronary effects of intravenous labetalol in coronary artery disease. Am J Cardiol 49:1267–1269, 1982.

37. Packer M, Meller J, Medina N, et al.: Hemodynamic consequences of combined β-adrenergic and slow calcium channel blockade in man. Circulation 65:660–668, 1982.

38. Formgren H, Eriksson NE: Effects of practolol in combination with terbutaline in the treatment of hypertension and arrhythmias in asthmatic patients. Scand J Resp Dis 56:217–222, 1975.

39. Vestal RE, Kornhauser DM, Hollifield JW, et al.: Inhibition of propranolol metabolism by chlorpromazine. Clin Pharmacol Ther 25:19–24, 1979.

40. Mills GA, Horn JR: β-Blockers and glucose control. DICP: Ann Pharmacother 19:246–251, 1985.

41. Hansten PD: β-Blocking agents and antidiabetic drugs. DICP: Ann Pharmacother 14:46–50, 1980.

42. McCleskey EW, Fox AP, Feldman D, et al.: Different types of calcium channels. J Exp Biol 124:177–190, 1986.

43. Schwartz A: Calcium antagonists: review and perspective on mechanism of action. Am J Cardiol 64:3I–9I, 1989.

44. Conti CR, Pepine CJ, Feldman RL, et al.: Calcium antagonists. Cardiology 72:297–321, 1985.

45. Singh BN, Josephson MA: Clinical pharmacology, pharmacokinetics, and hemodynamic effect of nicardipine. Am Heart J 119:427–434, 1990.

46. Belz GG, Doering W, Munkes R, et al.: Interaction between digoxin and calcium antagonists and antiarrhythmic drugs. Clin Pharmacol Ther 33:410–507, 1983.

47. Klein HO, Lang R, DiSegni E, et al.: Verapamil-digoxin interaction. New Engl J Med 303:160, 1980.

48. De Vito JM, Friedman B: Evaluation of the pharmacodynamic and pharmacokinetic interaction between calcium antagonists and digoxin. Pharmacotherapy 6:73–82, 1986.

49. Macphee GJA, McInnes GT, Thompson GG, et al.: Verapamil potentiates carbamazepine neurotoxicity. Clinically important interaction. Lancet 1:700–703, 1986.

50. Eimer M, Carter BL: Elevated serum carbamazepine concentrations following diltiazem initiation. DICP: Ann Pharmacother 21:340–342, 1987.

51. Lindholm A, Henricsson S: Verapamil inhibits cyclosporin metabolism. Lancet 1:1262–1263, 1987.

52. Grino JM, Sabate I, Castelao AM, et al.: Influence of diltiazem on cyclosporin clearance. Lancet 1:1387, 1986.

53. Bourbiget B, Guiserix J, Airiau J, et al.: Nicardipine increases cyclosporin blood levels. Lancet 1:1447, 1986.

54. Edwards DJ, Lavoie R, Beckman H, et al.: The effect of coadministration of verapamil on the pharmacokinetics and metabolism of quinidine. Clin Pharmacol Ther 41:68–73, 1987.

55. Farringer JA, Green JA, O'Rourke RA, et al.: Nifedipine-induced alterations in serum quinidine concentrations. Am Heart J 108:1570–1572, 1984.

56. Matera MG, DeSantis D, Vacca F, et al.: Quinidine-diltiazem pharmacokinetic interaction in humans. Curr Ther Res 40:653–656, 1986.

57. Burnakis TG, Seldon M, Czaplicki AD, et al.: Increased serum theophylline concentrations secondary to oral verapamil. Clin Pharm 2:458–461, 1983.

58. Parrillo SJ, Venditto M: Elevated theophylline blood levels from institution of nifedipine therapy. Ann Emerg Med 13:216–217, 1984.

59. Sirmans S, Pieper JA, Lalonde RL, et al.: Effect of calcium channel antagonists on theophylline disposition. (abstr) DICP: Ann Pharmacother 21:16A, 1987.

60. Goldman S, Copeland J, Moritz T, et al.: Effect of dipyridamole and aspirin on late vein graft patency after coronary bypass surgery with antiplatelet therapy: results of the Veterans Administration cooperative study. Circulation 77:1324–1332, 1988.

61. Blankenhorn DH, Nessim SA, Johnson RL, et al.: Beneficial effects of combined colestipol-niacin therapy on coronary atherosclerosis and coronary venous bypass grafts. JAMA 257:3233–3240, 1987.

62. Rahimtoola SH, Grunkemeier G, Teply JF, et al.: Changes in coronary bypass surgery leading to improved survival. JAMA 46:1912–1916, 1981.

63. Mock MB, Ringqvist I, Fischer LD, et al.: The survival of non-operated patients with ischemic heart disease: the CASS experience. (abstr) Am J Cardiol 49:1007, 1982.

64. Loop FP: Current status of coronary bypass surgery. Contemp Int Med 6:56, 1989.

65. King SB III: Percutaneous transluminal coronary angioplasty: the second decade. Am J Cardiol 62:2K–6K, 1988.

66. Baim DS, Ignatius EJ: Use of percutaneous transluminal angioplasty: results of a second surgery. Am J Cardiol 61:3G–8G, 1988.

67. Fanelli C, Aronoff R: Restenosis following coronary angioplasty. Am Heart J 119:357–368, 1990.

68. Theroux P, Ouimet H, McCans J, et al.: Aspirin, heparin, or both to treat acute unstable angina. N Engl J Med 319:1105–1111, 1988.

69. Lewis Jr HD, Davis JW, Archibald DG, et al.: Protective effects of aspirin against acute myocardial infarction and death in men with unstable angina. N Engl J Med 309:396–403, 1983.

70. Cairns JA, Gent M, Singer J, et al.: Aspirin, sulfinpyrazone, or both in unstable angina. N Engl J Med 313:1369–1375, 1985.

71. Yasue H, Touyama M, Kato H, et al.: Prinzmetal's variant form of angina as a manifestation of α-adrenergic receptor-mediated coronary artery spasm: documentation by coronary arteriography. Am Heart J 91:148–155, 1976.

72. Kern MJ, Ganz P, Horowitz JO, et al.: Potentiation of coronary vasoconstriction by β-adrenergic blockade in patients with coronary artery disease. Circulation 67:1178–1185, 1983.

73. Rozanski A, Berman DS: Silent myocardial ischemia: I. Pathophysiology, frequency of occurrence, and approaches toward detection. Am Heart J 114:615–626, 1987.

74. Cohn PF: Detection and prognosis of the asymptomatic patient with silent ischemia. Am J Cardiol 61:4B–6B, 1988.

75. Selwyn AP, Shea M, Deanfield JE, et al.: Character of transient ischemia in angina pectoris. Am J Cardiol 58:21B–25B, 1986.

76. Singh BH, Nademanee K, Figueras J, et al.: Hemodynamic and electrophysiologic correlates of symptomatic and silent ischemia: pathophysiologic and therapeutic implications. Am J Cardiol 58:3B–10B, 1986.

77. Stern S, Gavish A, Zin D, et al.: Clinical outcome of silent myocardial ischemia. Am J Cardiol 61:16F–18F, 1988.

CHAPTER 39

ACUTE MYOCARDIAL INFARCTION

EDGAR R. GONZALEZ, Pharm.D.

Acute myocardial infarction (AMI) is a common manifestation of ischemic heart disease and a leading cause of admission to both community and university hospitals. In the United States, more than 500,000 people die each year from AMI (1). Approximately 50% of patients with AMI die within the first few hours as a result of ventricular fibrillation. Mortality among AMI victims ranges from 10 to 15% in the first year, and is 3 to 4% per year thereafter (2). Survival after myocardial infarction (MI) is determined by the extent of viable myocardium and by the occurrence of post-MI complications. Modern coronary care has decreased the mortality from fatal arrhythmias, but it has not significantly changed the number of deaths from other post-MI complications such as reinfarction or cardiogenic shock (3).

PATHOGENESIS

Infarcted myocardium is dead muscle, usually resulting from an occluded coronary artery. The involved area can be divided into three zones: the zone of infarction, the zone of injury, and the zone of ischemia (Fig. 39.1). The infarct may be confined to the interior of the myocardium (subendocardial) or may involve the full thickness of the myocardium (transmural).

The most common cause of myocardial infarction is atheroslcerosis of the coronary arteries, which narrows the coronary lumen and reduces myocardial blood supply. Below a certain critical level of blood flow, myocardial cells develop ischemic injury. Irreversible damage (i.e., myocardial infarction) results from prolonged ischemic injury to a region of cardiac muscle (4). Patients with significant disease (equal to greater than 70% luminal diameter narrowing) of one or more of the major coronary arteries (right, left main, left anterior descending, or left circumflex) are at greatest risk of ischemic insult (Fig. 39.2). The atherosclerotic plaque is usually not solely responsible for totally occluding a coronary artery (5). A thrombus is frequently superimposed on the plaque lesion in the coronary. The precipitants of thrombosis are not well understood, but they may relate to ulceration of the plaque or to regional changes in blood flow which trigger platelet aggregation (4). Less frequently, coronary vasospasm may precipitate clot formation and complete coronary occlusion (5). Rarely, myocardial infarction can occur in the absence of coronary narrowing if there is a marked disparity between myocardial oxygen supply and demand. Co-

caine abuse has been implicated as a possible cause of such a disparity. Myocardial infarction may occur in various locations on the left ventricle, or in the right ventricle, depending on which coronary artery is occluded.

SIGNS AND SYMPTOMS

The patient's chief complaint and history are invaluable in establishing a diagnosis of MI. Discomfort is the most common presenting complaint. The discomfort is described as oppressive, burning, a tightness, squeezing, choking, expanding, or indigestion-like. There may be a sense of "impending doom." The discomfort is typically substernal and may radiate to the neck, throat, jaws, shoulders, and arms. The discomfort is similar to angina pectoris in location and quality, but discomfort in angina is brief, whereas the discomfort of MI lasts for 30 min to several hours and is more severe. It usually begins while the patient is at rest, it does not subside, and it is only partially relieved by nitroglycerin. At least 15 to 20% of MI are not accompanied by any symptoms ("silent MI"). "Silent" infarction is seen most commonly in diabetes and elderly patients.

Most patients admit to prodromal symptoms: vague chest discomfort, weakness, fatigue, nausea, vomiting, and diaphoresis prior to the acute attack (1). Less commonly, an episode of light-headedness or syncope heralds the onset of MI.

Numerous factors associated with myocardial infarction include vasospasm, severe exertion, emotional stress, hemorrhage, trauma, respiratory dysfunction, hypoglycemia, administration of catecholamines and ergot alkaloids, and hypersensitivity reactions (1).

DIAGNOSIS AND CLINICAL FINDINGS

A detailed history may help to differentiate myocardial ischemic pain from noncardiac chest pain. Precipitating factors should be identified, and the patient's medication history and compliance should be assessed.

The patient is often anxious, restless, cool, sweaty, and pale. Heart rate varies widely; sinus tachycardia and mild fever are commonly observed. Sinus bradycardia is more common with inferior myocardial infarction. Blood pressure varies widely from patient to patient and temporally in a given patient; hypertension may accompany pain. Hypotension may result from the vasodilating effect of morphine, from left ventricular dysfunction, and/or from hy-

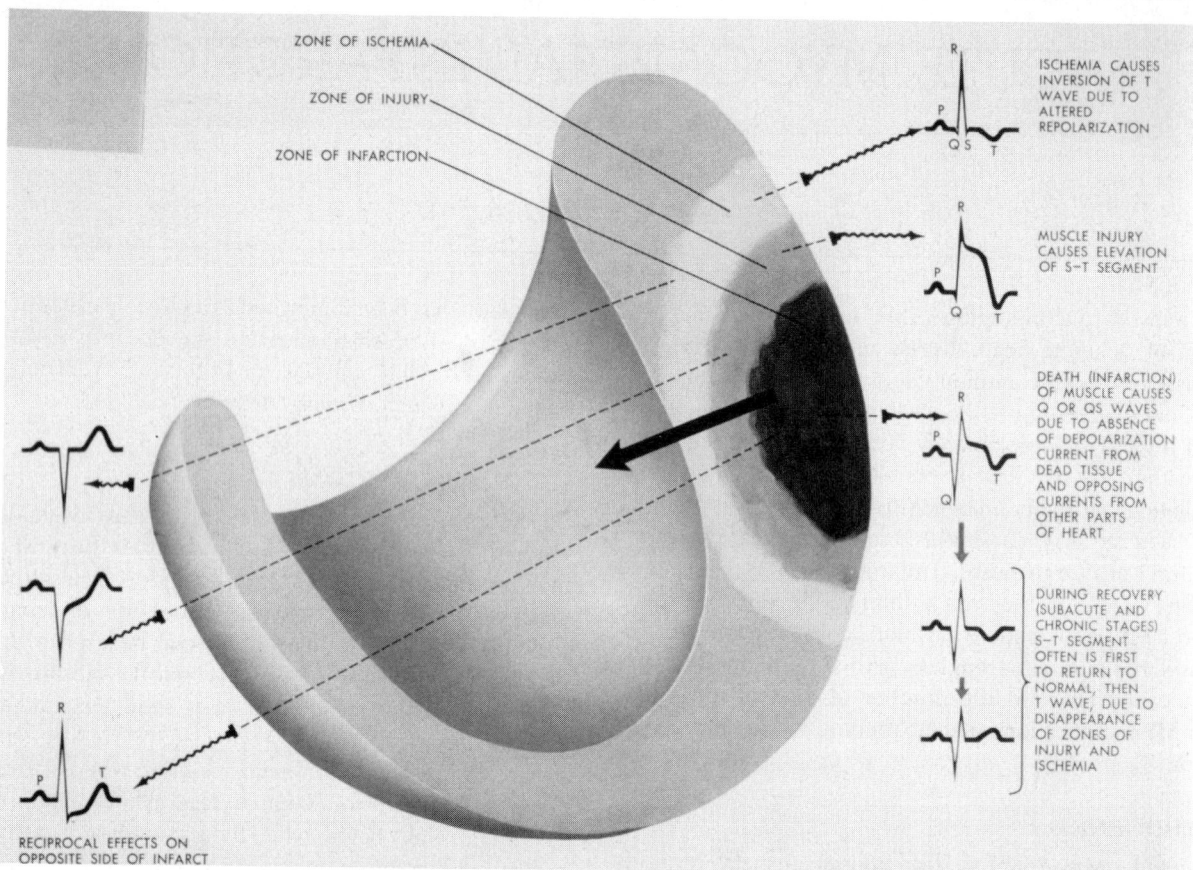

ZONE OF ISCHEMIA

ZONE OF INJURY

ZONE OF INFARCTION

ISCHEMIA CAUSES INVERSION OF T WAVE DUE TO ALTERED REPOLARIZATION

MUSCLE INJURY CAUSES ELEVATION OF S-T SEGMENT

DEATH (INFARCTION) OF MUSCLE CAUSES Q OR QS WAVES DUE TO ABSENCE OF DEPOLARIZATION CURRENT FROM DEAD TISSUE AND OPPOSING CURRENTS FROM OTHER PARTS OF HEART

DURING RECOVERY (SUBACUTE AND CHRONIC STAGES) S-T SEGMENT OFTEN IS FIRST TO RETURN TO NORMAL, THEN T WAVE, DUE TO DISAPPEARANCE OF ZONES OF INJURY AND ISCHEMIA

RECIPROCAL EFFECTS ON OPPOSITE SIDE OF INFARCT

Figure 39.1. Effects of cardiac infarction, injury, and ischemia. (With permission, from Yonkman FF (ed): The Ciba Collection of Medical Illustrations: *Heart*. New York, Ciba Pharmaceutical Company, 1969, p 62.)

povolemia. The respiratory rate is often rapid, and respiratory effort may be shallow. Heart sounds may be faint or normal. A fourth heart sound (atrial gallop) is common. Low-grade fever up to 38°C may be observed during the first week following AMI. Evidence of coronary risk factors may be present, such as retinopathy from hypertension and/or diabetes, and xanthomas or xanthelasmas due to hyperlipidemia.

ELECTROCARDIOGRAPHIC FINDINGS

The electrocardiogram (ECG) permits detection of the three pathophysiological events occurring during an AMI: ischemia (T wave inversion or elevation), injury (ST segment elevation), and infarction (pathologic Q waves) (Fig. 39.1). The diagnostic feature of MI is the deep, wide Q wave, or Q-S pattern, in the ECG leads corresponding to the injury. Transmural infarction (through and through; full thickness) is diagnosed if the ECG shows Q waves or loss of R waves. Nontransmural infarction (subendocardial or epicardial) is present if the ECG shows only ST-segment and T-wave changes. Nontransmural infarction may be less frequently associated with thrombosis. Although Q waves are seen more commonly in transmural than in nontrans-

mural infarction, both types of infarcts may occur with or without Q waves. Therefore, it is more appropriate to use the terms *Q-wave infarction* and *non-Q-wave infarction* (6).

SERUM ENZYME STUDIES

Enzymes are released into the systemic circulation from infarcted myocardium. The three enzymes most frequently assayed are creatine kinase (CK), lactate dehydrogenase (LDH), and aspartate aminotransferase (AST). Each enzyme has a particular time course for appearance in the systemic circulation following an AMI (Fig. 39.3). The temporal pattern of enzyme release is of diagnostic importance. Standard practice is to obtain serial cardiac enzyme determinations every 8 hr for the first 24 hr in patients with a suspected AMI. CK activity can be used to estimate infarct size. Blood CK concentrations peak (two to three times normal) within 24 hr and return to normal in 3 to 4 days. Serial CK measurements following infarction result in excellent clinical sensitivity. The major criticism of CK is its poor specificity. CK activity can be elevated following skeletal muscle trauma related to surgery, exercise, or intramuscular injections.

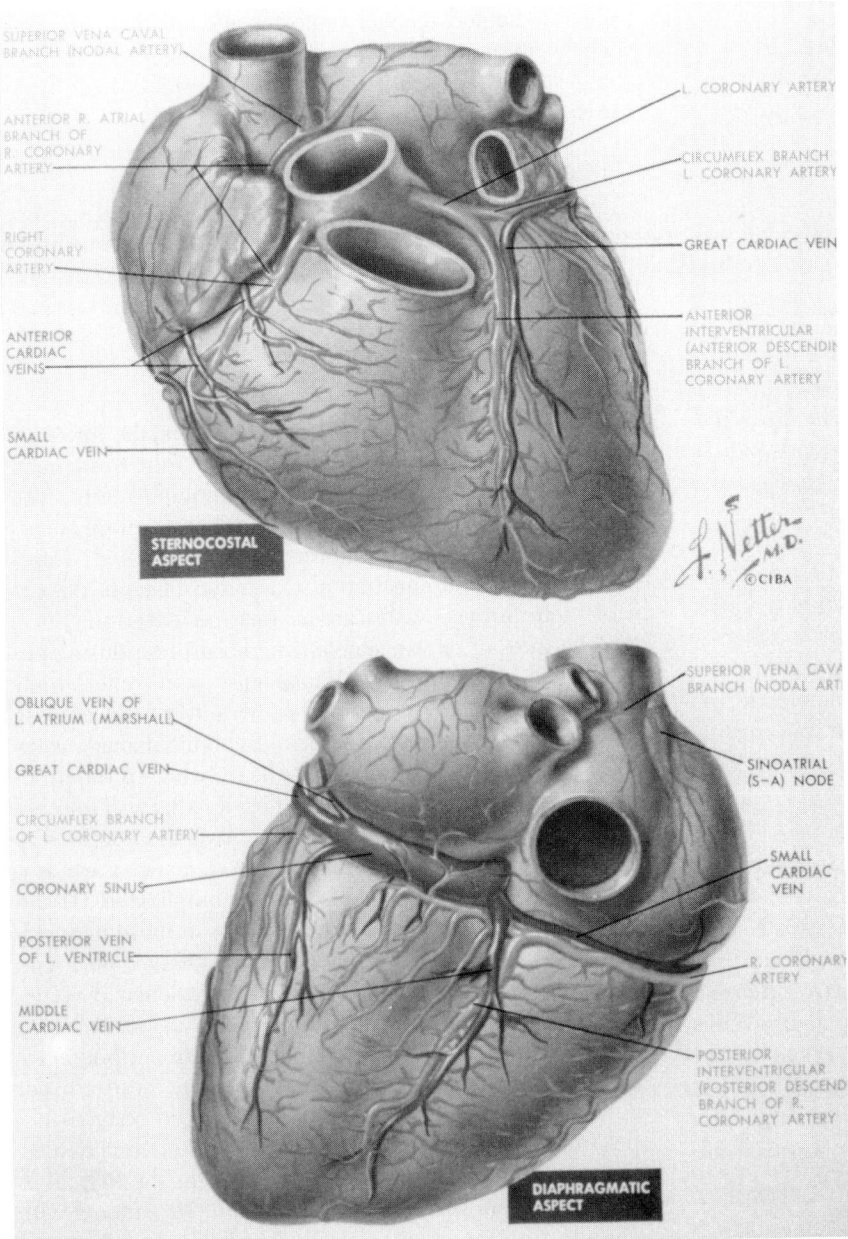

Figure 39.2. Coronary arteries and veins: blood supply of the heart. (With permission, from Yonkman FF (ed): The Ciba Collection of Medical Illustrations: *Heart.* New York, Ciba Pharmaceutical Company, 1969, p 16.)

LDH is the slowest rising enzyme activity following AMI. When assessed within the second and third days postinfarction, LDH has a relatively high specificity (94%) and good clinical sensitivity (85%) for AMI. The ubiquitous nature of AST makes it a relatively nonspecific indictor of myocardial cell damage. Therefore, AST activity is rarely used to diagnose AMI.

CK-MB and LDH-1 are the respective isoenzymes of CK and LDH with highest concentrations in the myocardium. The use of isoenzymes increases the specificity of the test for AMI. Within 48 hr after infarct, the sensitivity and specificity of CK-MB for myocardial injury approaches 100%. However, CK-MB is less specific for infarction be-

cause it can be elevated following traumatic injury to the heart due to cardiopulmonary resuscitation or electrical countershock. Since LDH_2 is normally the major LDH isoenzyme in blood, the usual serum pattern is $LDH_2 > LDH_1$. A change in this relationship is seen after MI, renal necrosis, and hemolysis. Within 48 hr post–acute episode, 80% of AMI patients have reversed their normal LDH isoenzyme pattern to $LDH_1 > LDH_2$.

RADIONUCLIDE IMAGING

Radionuclide imaging techniques are valuable in assessing myocardial ischemic injury. Acute infarct scintigraphy (hot-spot imaging) with infarct-avid ^{99m}Tc pyrophosphate

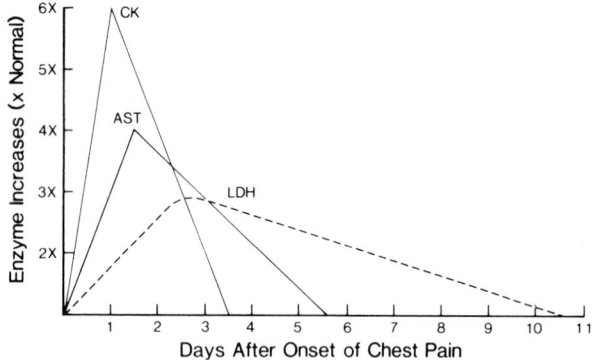

Figure 39.3. The time course of cardiac enzyme release during acute myocardial infarction. (With permission, from Zeller FP, Bauman JL: Current concepts in clinical therapeutics: acute myocardial infarction. Clin Pharm 5:556, 1986.)

aids in localizing and measuring the necrotic area. Scans are usually positive 2 to 5 days after infarction. Myocardial perfusion imaging with thallium-201, which is taken up and concentrated by viable myocardium, reveals a defect ("cold spot") within 6 hr after AMI. Radionuclide ventriculography frequently reveals wall motion abnormalities and reduced ventricular ejection in patients with AMI.

LABORATORY ABNORMALITIES

Nonspecific laboratory abnormalities associated with AMI include polymorphonuclear leukocytosis [12 to 15 $\times$ 10^6/liter (12,000 to 15,000 per mm^3)], which persists for 3 to 7 days, and an elevated erythrocyte sedimentation rate, which peaks during the first week. Electrolyte abnormalities, most notably hypokalemia and hypomagnesemia, should be sought and corrected. Hypokalemia and hypomagnesemia occur commonly in diuretic-treated patients with AMI. These electrocyte abnormalities can precipitate malignant ventricular arrhythmias in patients with ischemic, hypertrophied, or dilated hearts.

SUMMARY

In summary, AMI is diagnosed when any two of the three clinical features discussed are present: (*a*) ischemic chest pain, (*b*) new abnormal Q-waves or ST-segment changes, or (*c*) abnormally elevated cardiac enzymes.

COMPLICATIONS

Approximately 50% of hospitalized AMI patients will develop complications (7). Two general classes of complications have been defined: (*a*) electrical (arrhythmias) and (*b*) mechanical (pump failure). ECG monitoring and prompt recognition and treatment of electrical complications has reduced the in-hospital mortality from AMI. Unfortunately, a similarly favorable trend has not been observed with AMI-associated pump failure, despite ad-

vances in hemodynamic monitoring and inotropic support. Left ventricular failure with subsequent pulmonary congestion is the primary cause of in-hospital death from AMI.

TREATMENT

Reduction in mortality is the major goal of therapy in patients with AMI. The management of AMI is designed to relieve pain and anxiety, to recognize and control life-threatening arrhythmias, to limit infarct size, and to prevent complications.

General

Patients with suspected AMI are treated in the intensive or coronary care unit to permit close monitoring and prompt response to emergencies and complications. The ECG is monitored continuously. Peripheral venous access for intravenous drug administration is obtained. Intramuscular drug administration is avoided because of possible interference with cardiac enzyme determinations, and because of unpredictable drug absorption during episodes of hypoperfusion. Vital signs, pain relief, body weight, bowel habits, and diet are monitored closely.

Critical to limiting myocardial ischemic damage is reducing the oxygen demand of the heart, which is the product of heart rate, contractility, and myocardial wall tension. During the first 24 hr, patients with AMI are confined to bed rest to reduce myocardial oxygen demand. Early ambulation is feasible in patients with uncomplicated MI and may lessen the need for anticoagulation in these patients.

Hypoxemia usually results from ventilation perfusion abnormalities, commonly due to left ventricular dysfunction. Although oxygen therapy has been associated with theoretically deleterious effects (elevation of peripheral resistance and reduction of cardiac output), these are not clinically relevant. Administration of oxygen reduces hypoxemia and increases oxygen delivery to ischemic tissues. Oxygen is administered by nasal prongs for the first 24 to 48 hr at a flow rate of 3 to 4 liter/min. In patients with chronic obstructive lung disease, low flow rates of oxygen are appropriate, to avoid carbon dioxide retention. Endotracheal intubation and positive airway pressure mechanical ventilation should be used if adequate oxygenation (oxygen saturation $\geq$ 90%) cannot be maintained by mask. High-level, continuous positive airway pressure will improve tissue oxygenation and reduce the spontaneous respiratory effort without producing circulatory depression in AMI patients with left ventricular dysfunction (8). Arterial blood gas determinations should be avoided shortly after the administration of thrombolytics, to minimize the risk of arterial bleeding.

Analgesia

Pain relief is an initial therapeutic objective. Prompt pain relief attenuates the autonomic hyperactivity that increases myocardial oxygen demand and predisposes to tachyarrhythmias (9). Sublingual nitroglycerin is tried first unless the patient's systolic blood pressure is <90 mm Hg. In the presence of persistent ischemia and hypotension, a small amount of nitroglycerin paste may be applied and promptly removed if hypotension worsens. Nitroglycerin must be used with caution in patients with right ventricular infarction because precipitous hypotension may ensue. Intravenous access should be obtained for fluid resuscitation. Vasopressor agents should be avoided and are seldom required. If hypotension with bradycardia develops, intravenous atropine (0.5 to 1.0 mg) should be administered.

Numerous analgesic drugs (morphine, meperidine, pentazocine, and nalbuphine) have been used in AMI. Morphine is the agent of choice except in patients with well-documented morphine hypersensitivity. In addition to relieving pain and anxiety, the hemodynamic effects of morphine are invaluable in patients with pulmonary edema. Morphine is a potent vasodilator. It increases venous capacitance and decreases systemic vascular resistance (10). These effects are most pronounced in patients with heightened sympathetic tone. Four to 8 mg should be administered by slow intravenous injection, and doses of 2 to 8 mg repeated at 5 to 15 min intervals, until the pain is relieved or evident toxicity (i.e., hypotension, respiratory depression, or vomiting) precludes further administration. Morphine-induced hypotension can be minimized by maintaining the patient in a supine position. Concomitant administration of atropine, 0.5 to 1.0 mg intravenously, may help reverse the vagomimetic effects of morphine on blood pressure and heart rate. Meperidine, 25 to 75 mg by slow intravenous injection every 2 to 3 hr as needed for pain control, is a suitable alternative in morphine-intolerant patients. The anticholinergic effects of meperidine will counteract the heightened vagal tone in AMI patients with either bradycardia or nausea. Tachycardia is a potential adverse effect of meperidine administration. Patients should be monitored for the respiratory depressant effects of narcotic analgesics. Naloxone, 0.4 mg intravenously, may be administered at 5-min intervals as needed to reverse narcotic-induced respiratory depression. Nalbuphine is a useful agent in patients with AMI because it produces less respiratory depression, less hypotension, and less vagal stimulation than morphine.

The persistence of pain over several hours is a bad prognostic sign, usually indicating continued myocardial ischemia and necrosis. In this setting, nitroglycerin may effectively relieve refractory chest pain. Nitroglycerin decreases myocardial oxygen demand by reducing intramyocardial wall tension. Patients with signs and symptoms of pulmonary edema derive the most benefit from intravenous nitroglycerin administration. In addition, intravenous nitroglycerin may limit infarct size. This agent is discussed in greater detail later in this chapter.

Anticoagulation

Routine anticoagulation following AMI is controversial. Although anticoagulation has failed to unequivocally decrease mortality following AMI, it may prevent embolic complications: infarct extension, deep venous thrombosis, pulmonary emboli, and arterial emboli from cardiac mural thrombi (11). The incidence of anticoagulant-induced hemorrhagic complication in AMI patients ranges from 3 to 37%; the reported incidence of death due to hemorrhage is less than 1% with heparin and 2 to 4% with warfarin (11). The incidence of pulmonary embolism in AMI is between 1 and 2%; full-dose heparinization is not warranted in this setting. The incidence of cerebrovascular accident (CVA) after AMI is between 2 and 3%. Low-dose heparin (5000 units subcutaneously every 12 hr) safely and effectively reduces the risk of pulmonary embolization and CVA after AMI.

It is not justifiable to anticoagulate all patients after MI because the risk of anticoagulation exceeds the potential benefit. In patients at high risk of embolization (e.g., those with ventricular aneurysm, marked obesity, cardiogenic shock, present or past thrombophlebitis, or arterial or pulmonary embolism), full-dose anticoagulation for 5 to 7 days will reduce the risk of embolization and subsequent mortality. Thirty to 40% of patients with transmural anterior MI develop left ventricular thrombi (LVT); early anticoagulation with full-dose heparin may prevent LVT formation and subsequent CVA in these patients (11). To assess the risk of delayed embolization, a two-dimensional echocardiogram may be useful prior to hospital discharge. In the presence of LVT, oral anticoagulation for 3 to 6 months is warranted. In patients with normal wall motion and no LVT, anticoagulation can be safely discontinued prior to discharge from the hospital. Inferior wall MI is much less frequently complicated by LVT or CVA; routine anticoagulation is not justified except for certain high-risk patients (large MI, congestive heart failure, atrial arrhythmias, old anterior wall MI, and known apical akinesis or dyskinesis).

The use of full-dose anticoagulation in AMI patients must be based on the relative risk and potential benefit of treatment. In patients with absolute contraindication to anticoagulation (e.g., recent subarachnoid bleeding or active gastrointestinal tract bleeding), the potential benefits do not justify the risk. In patients with relative contraindications to anticoagulation (history of peptic ulcer disease, recent surgery), the risk of bleeding must be weighed against the risk of embolization.

TREATMENT AND PROPHYLAXIS OF ARRHYTHMIAS

The most common post-MI complication is disturbance of the cardiac rhythm. Pharmacologic manipulation of the cardiac conduction system and the autonomic nervous system and correction of electrolyte abnormalities reduce the morbidity and mortality associated with cardiac arrhythmia in AMI patients. An arrhythmia occurring in a patient with AMI requires vigorous treatment when it produces hemodynamic impairment, increases myocardial oxygen demands, or predisposes to malignant ventricular arrhythmias.

Ventricular fibrillation is the most common cause of death in the early hours post-MI, and it may occur without prior evidence of ventricular premature complexes (12). Ventricular fibrillation occurs in approximately 11% of patients with AMI, and carries a 46% mortality rate. Approximately 60% of episodes occur within 4 hr, and 80% within 12 hr of symptoms. Although there was no consensus regarding a reduction in morbidity and mortality, routine prophylactic antiarrhythmic therapy had been advocated during the initial 24 hr post-AMI (12). Today, the routine use of prophylactic antiarrhythmics in patients with AMI is disputed. Treatment with antiarrhythmics is commonly instituted in patients with warning arrhythmias (i.e., couplets, multifocal PVCs, runs of three or more consecutive PVCs). Lidocaine hydrochloride is the prophylactic antiarrhythmic agent of choice in AMI. This agent suppresses ventricular arrhythmogenicity by decreasing automaticity, blocking reentry pathways, and elevating the fibrillatory threshold. Prompt administration of lidocaine can reduce the incidence of malignant ventricular arrhythmias during the early phase of AMI. However, no data support a reduction in mortality with prophylactic lidocaine therapy in AMI, and lidocaine may produce asystole to aggravate myocardial dysfunction. Therefore, lidocaine is now reserved for AMI patients with warning arrhythmias, young patients presenting within 6 hr of symptoms, and patients treated with thrombolytic therapy.

Lidocaine, 1.0 mg/kg, is administered by intravenous injection over 1 min followed immediately by an intravenous infusion of 1 to 4 mg/min (20 to 50 μg/min). Because of the short distribution half-life (6 to 8 min) of lidocaine, an additional 0.5 mg/kg bolus should be given 10 min after the initial bolus to prevent the occurrence of subtherapeutic plasma lidocaine concentrations. If ventricular arrhythmias persist, 50 mg bolus injections can be repeated to a maximum of 250 mg of lidocaine over a 20-min period.

Lidocaine is metabolized by the liver, and has a half-life of approximately 90 min. The metabolism of lidocaine is impaired in the presence of AMI, circulatory shock, hepatic failure, cimetidine, and β-adrenergic blockers. Accumulation of the metabolites of lidocaine may occur in elderly patients, and in patients with hepatic and/or renal dysfunction. The dose of lidocaine should be reduced and individualized in such cases.

Excessive doses of lidocaine can produce central nervous system toxicity and possibly cardiovascular depres-sion. The toxicity of lidocaine is directly related to its concentration in blood. Plasma lidocaine concentrations should be maintained between 1.5 and 5 mg/ml. Patients with AMI may tolerate greater plasma concentrations (8 μg/ml). This may be related to increased binding of lidocaine to α-1-acid glycoprotein, which is released into the systemic circulation in large concentrations after AMI.

Procainamide and bretylium are alternatives to lidocaine in AMI patients with lidocaine hypersensitivity or refractory arrhythmia.

β-Adrenergic receptor blocking agents reverse the arrhythmogenic effect of circulating catecholamines and reduce electrical instability during ischemic insult to the myocardium (13). Both propranolol and metoprolol effectively reduce the incidence of ventricular fibrillation associated with AMI (14, 15). This effect is most noticeable in patients with hypertension or tachycardia on admission to the intensive care unit (15). The recommended dosage of propranolol for intravenous administration during AMI is 0.1 mg/kg in three divided doses given slowly at 5-min intervals, followed by a maintenance oral regimen of 180 to 320 mg/day (13). Intravenous metoprolol (15 mg) is administered in three equal doses at 5-min intervals, followed by a maintenance oral regimen of 200 mg/day. Patients should be monitored for signs and symptoms of excessive β-adrenergic blockade (bradycardia, atrioventricular conduction delay, hypotension). Circulatory collapse is a rare complication of β-adrenergic blockade in patients with AMI; patients with left ventricular impairment show only a modest fall in mean arterial pressure, heart rate, and cardiac output (13, 16, 17). These agents are contraindicated in patients with bradycardia, hypotension, bronchospastic airway disease, or overt congestive heart failure.

Sinus bradycardia is a common finding in patients with inferior wall MI. Transient episodes of bradycardia are often observed during the initial hours post-MI, and they may exert a protective function (18). If the bradycardia is associated with hypotension or a ventricular arrhythmia, atropine 0.5 to 1.0 mg should be administered by slow intravenous injection. Atropine may be repeated at 2- to 4-hr intervals as needed to maintain a heart rate above 60 beats per min. Asymptomatic bradycardia should not be treated, because the risk of increased myocardial oxygen demand outweighs any potential benefit from treatment. Atropine should not be administered in doses less than 0.5 mg because a paradoxical slowing of the heart rate may occur. Electrical pacing is used to manage atropine-refractory bradycardia. Intravenous isoproterenol (0.5 to 2.0 μg/min) should be used, if at all, only until a pacemaker can be inserted, because of the risks of tachyarrhythmias and hypotension or hypertension.

Sinus tachycardia occurs in 30% of AMI patients during the first few days postinfarction (19). Anxiety, pain, fever, and ventricular dysfunction commonly cause this arrhythmia. Young patients with their first anterior wall myocardial infarction may present in a hyperdynamic state with sinus tachycardia, hypertension, and ventricular ectopy. These patients may benefit from acute therapy with β-adrenergic blockers or ACE-inhibitors.

Atrial fibrillation/flutter occurs in up to 20% of AMI patients, often associated with left ventricular dysfunction (19). Because of this association, these rhythms are seen more often with anterior wall myocardial infarction and are associated with increased mortality. Therapy is indicated if the arrhythmia produces a rapid ventricular response and/or hemodynamic compromise. Restoration of normal sinus rhythm by electrical cardioversion is an immediate priority in acute hemodynamic instability. Patients may develop hemodynamic instability from supraventricular tachycardia. Verapamil, 5 mg over 2 min and repeated in 30 min to a total of 20 mg, may be used for conversion to normal sinus rhythm or for control of ventricular response rate. Verapamil should be used with caution, if at all, in patients with left ventricular dysfunction, hypotension, Wolf-Parkinsons-White syndrome, or wide complex tachycardias. Adenosine has the advantages of a shorter half-life and less propensity to produce hypotension than verapamil. The usual dose of adenosine is 6 mg, followed by 12 mg in 3 to 5 min if a response is not observed. Total doses above 18 mg increase the risk of atrioventricular block, flushing, chest pain, and bronchospasm.

CARDIOGENIC SHOCK
Pump Failure
Cardiogenic shock develops in 10 to 15% of hospitalized AMI patients (9). If untreated, cardiogenic shock follows a rapid downward spiral of progressive circulatory failure and impaired cellular metabolism leading to organ dysfunction and death (20). Despite aggressive pharmacologic and surgical intervention, 80 to 100% of cardiogenic shock victims do not survive to hospital discharge (21). This near-universal mortality reflects the self-perpetuating cycle of myocardial ischemia and power failure. Early therapeutic interventions aimed at increasing coronary perfusion pressure and decreasing myocardial oxygen demand should, at least theoretically, produce improved survival.

Clinical Assessment
The classic physical findings in cardiogenic shock are hypotension, tachycardia, diminished peripheral pulses, decreased urine output, clouded sensorium, and pulmonary edema. These indicate pump failure and circulatory insufficiency. Restlessness, agitation, and confusion are seen with mild-to-moderate impairment in cerebral blood flow, while lethargy and obtundation may indicate severe cerebral hypoperfusion. The clinical features of pulmonary edema include rales over the lower lung fields, bronchospasm, dyspnea, copious pulmonary secretions, and profound cyanosis with rapid shallow breathing. If cardiogenic shock occurs with relative hypovolemia, the lung fields may appear clear. Arterial blood gas determinations permit prompt assessment of the patient's respiratory function and acid-base status. Ventilatory adequacy can be determined by measuring the carbon dioxide tension in arterial blood ($PaCO_2$). A $PaCO_2$ above 50 torr in the presence of a low arterial pH suggests hypoventilation. The arterial oxygen tension (PaO_2) reflects the adequacy of oxygenation. Adequate arterial oxygenation ($PaO_2 \geq 70$ torr) in cardiogenic shock usually requires supplemental oxygen administration. While sinus tachycardia is generally present, sinus bradycardia, supraventricular tachycardia, ventricular tachycardia, or complete heart block may also occur in the cardiogenic shock victim. Diminished heart sound intensity may reflect reduced myocardial contractility. A systolic apical murmur may indicate mitral regurgitation due to papillary muscle dysfunction. With progressive loss of cardiac output, blood pressure will fall, despite compensatory sympathoadrenal reflexes. Weak, thready, or absent peripheral pulses result from both a reduction in arterial pressure and an increase in peripheral resistance with reduced peripheral blood flow. This leads to the cold, damp, mottled skin commonly seen in patients with cardiogenic shock. A urine output below 20 ml/hr with a spot urine sodium under 10 mg/liter suggests a reduced glomerular filtration rate and subsequent stimulation of the renin-angiotensin-aldosterone system.

Hemodynamics
Cardiogenic shock is best defined in hemodynamic terms: systolic arterial pressure <80 mm Hg, cardiac index < 1.8 liters/min/m², and pulmonary capillary wedge pressure > 18 mm Hg with urine output < 20 ml/hr. Because not only accurate diagnosis but also proper treatment requires hemodynamic guidance, it is almost always necessary to place a right heart (Swan-Ganz) catheter when signs of systemic hypoperfusion or severe pulmonary congestion are present. The Swan-Ganz catheter is designed to negotiate the right atrium, right ventricle, and pulmonary artery without radiographic guidance. This is performed by inflation of a small air-filled balloon that is carried by venous blood flow into proper position at a point where the balloon wedges into a pulmonary vein of similar diameter. A lumen beginning at the distal end of the catheter is connected to a transducer for continuous pressure monitoring. During insertion, central venous, right atrial, systolic right ventricular, and pulmonary arterial pressures may be recorded (Table 39.1). Additionally, this catheter provides a central infusion port for drugs.

The Swan-Ganz catheter has become an important tool for sorting out the differential diagnosis of peripheral hy-

Table 39.1.
Hemodynamic Parameters

	RAP[a]	RVP	PAP	PCWP
Normal range (mm Hg)	0–8	15–30	$\dfrac{15–30}{5–12}$	5–12
Increased in:	RVF, RVI, PE, COPD, PCT		Systolic: PE, COPD, VSD Diastolic: PE, COPD, LVI, MS	LVI, MS, PCT
Comments:	RAP = LVEDP in PE, COPD, MS	RVP not useful	PAD = PCWP (>5 mm Hg) in PE, COPD	PCWP ≤ 20–25 pulm. edema In AMI optimal PCWP: 14–18 mm Hg

[a] Abbreviations: RAP, right atrial pressure; RVP, right ventricular pressure; PAP, pulmonary artery pressure; PAD, pulmonary artery diastolic pressure; PCWP, pulmonary capillary wedge pressure; RVI, right ventricular infarction; PE, pulmonary embolus; COPD, chronic obstructive pulmonary disease; PCT, pericardial tamponade; LVI, left ventricular infarction; MS, mitral stenosis; AMI, acute myocardial infarction; RVF, right ventricular failure; LVEDP, left ventricular end-diastolic pressure.

Table 39.2.
Hemodynamic Classification and Relationship to Clinical Presentation and Percent Mortality based on Hemodynamic Signs[a]

>2.2	*Subset I* Normal hemodynamics Mortality = 3%	*Subset II* Pulmonary congestion Rales present Mortality = 9%
CI		
<2.2	*Subset III* Peripheral hypoperfusion Rales absent Mortality = 23%	*Subset IV* Pulmonary congestion Rales present Peripheral hypoperfusion Mortality = 51%
	<18	<18
	PCWP	

[a] With permission from Ornato JP (ed): Cardiovascular Emergencies. Churchill Livingston, New York, 1986, p. 123.
[b] Legend: CI, cardiac index (liters/min/m); PCWP, pulmonary capillary wedge pressure (mm Hg).

poperfusion and pulmonary congestion. In an AMI, the hemodynamic parameters define four subsets, based on the presence or absence of hypoperfusion and/or pulmonary congestion (Table 39.2). These subsets are useful diagnostically and therapeutically (22). Hemodynamic parameters are all normal in subset 1; the predicted mortality is 3%. Subset II clinically has pulmonary congestion without peripheral hypoperfusion and is defined hemodynamically by a cardiac index (CI) >2.2 liters/min/m^2 and a pulmonary capillary wedge pressure (PCWP) >18 mm Hg. The group mortality is 9%. Treatment generally includes diuretics and venodilators. Patients with peripheral hypoperfusion without pulmonary congestion constitute subset III, and their mortality rate is 23%. In this group, either relative volume depletion or slow heart rate cause a CI < 2.2 liters/min/m^2 with PCWP < 18 mm Hg. Lastly, cardiogenic shock from either myocardial failure or mechan-

ical lesions constitutes subset IV. Coexistent pulmonary congestion and peripheral hypoperfusion hemodynamically manifest as a CI < 1 liter/min/m^2 and a PCWP > 18 mm Hg. Systemic blood pressure cannot be maintained in spite of reflex vasoconstriction that elevates the systemic vascular resistance (SVR) > 1400 dyne-cm-sec^{-5}. Expected mortality in subset IV is 51%.

Medical Intervention

The goals of medical management of cardiogenic shock are to (a) optimize left ventricular filling pressure; (b) minimize the impedance to left ventricular ejection; and (c) maximize contractility without increasing myocardial oxygen demand excessively. Therapeutic agents used to remedy acute pump failure include diuretics, positive inotrope agents, and vasodilators.

Treatment of subset II is directed primarily at reducing PCWP. Diuretics are the cornerstone of therapy because they can be given by rapid intravenous administration with few adverse effects. In the cardiogenic shock patient, intravenous diuretics exert two distinctly important effects. The immediate effect is an increase in venous capacitance redistributing blood away from the lungs and decreasing pulmonary capillary pressures (23). The second effect is to increase sodium and water excretion by the kidneys. Loop diuretics produce renal vasodilation, which may increase their natriuretic effect (24). The resultant diuresis decreases both intravascular volume and left ventricular volume and filling pressure.

Overzealous diuresis should be avoided because excessive reductions in left ventricular filling pressure may worsen cardiac output. Diuretic-induced electrolyte abnormalities should be identified and corrected promptly. To minimize electrolyte abnormalities and to prevent the risk of suboptimal cardiac filling pressures, the smallest effective dose of the diuretic should be used. The patient's hemodynamic parameters and urine output should guide subsequent diuretic administration. If diuretics are inef-

Table 39.3.
Comparative Prices of Volume-expanding Agents[a]

Type	Amount (ml)	Average Cost ($)	Cost per 500 ml IV Expansion ($)
Albumin 5%	500	122.00	122.00
Albumin 25%	100	150.00	150.00
Hydroxyethyl starch (hetastarch)	500	24.79	25.00
Dextran 40	500	33.00	30.00
Dextran 70	500	21.00	20.00
Ringer's lactate	1000	1.50	4.00
Normal saline	1000	1.50	4.00

[a] Adapted from Chernow B (ed): The Pharmacologic Approach to the Critically Ill Patient. Baltimore: Williams & Wilkins, 1983, p 185.

fective and acute ischemia is present, topical or intravenous nitroglycerin might provide added preload reduction.

Isolated peripheral hypoperfusion (subset III) is of major prognostic importance because of the high mortality associated with it. These patients have hypovolemia and/or bradycardia. The goals of therapy are to improve the cardiac index and to reverse the hypoperfusion while minimizing myocardial oxygen expenditure.

Hypovolemia will abnormally reduce left ventricular filling pressure, which may contribute to hypotension and vascular collapse. Fluid loss may be due to chronic diuretic therapy, vomiting, diarrhea, diaphoresis, or internal hemorrhage. Hypovolemia should be identified and corrected before more aggressive circulatory support is initiated. Most of these patients demonstrate a reduction in stroke volume and a compensatory tachycardia. In general, cardiac output will increase with volume infusion until the PCWP reaches approximately 15 to 18 mm Hg, above which point further increases in cardiac output are minimal (25).

Initial volume therapy should consist of 5 to 100 ml of normal saline or 5% albumin administered intravenously over 5 to 10 min, with appropriate hemodynamic assessment and volume status monitoring. Table 39.3 lists the commercially available volume-expanding agents. No ideal agent for volume expansion has been identified. Crystalloids are less expensive but produce relatively short-lived volume expansion. Colloids increase plasma oncotic pressure and produce sustained volume expansion, but they are more expensive. There is no conclusive evidence that the type of fluid used in volume resuscitation influences the development of pulmonary complications.

A small group of patients in subset III have a normal stroke volume but a slow heart rate. Temporary transvenous pacing may restore cardiac output, but the increase in myocardial oxygen demand outweighs the marginal increase in cardiac output at rates beyond 90 to 100 beats per min (21). The most substantial rise in CI is observed in patients with resting heart rates of 50 to 70 beats per min (25).

Subset IV carries the highest mortality. The goal of therapy is simultaneous improvement in CI and PCWP (21). The choice of therapies lies between inotropic agents and peripheral vasodilators (25). Vasodilators are usually better because they impact more favorably on myocardial oxygen demand. However, when severe hypotension is present, a positive inotropic effect will prevent further circulatory collapse. The ideal inotropic agent must maintain or improve myocardial contractility while minimizing oxygen demand. Because no such agent exists, this is best accomplished by careful titration of combined therapy with inotropic and vasodilator drugs (Table 39.4).

Inotropic Agents

Inotropic agents increase the peak tension produced by the myocardium during systole and shorten the time spent in systole (26). All inotropes in clinical use have important effects on the peripheral arterial and venous vasculature as well as on myocardial oxygen demand. Sympathomimetic amines are the most commonly used inotropes. They stimulate both α- and β-adrenergic and dopaminergic receptors to varying degrees (26). α-Adrenergic stimulation mediates peripheral vasoconstriction. β_1-Adrenergic stimulation exerts positive chronotropic, dromotropic, and inotropic effects. β_2-Adrenergic stimulation produces vasodilation and bronchodilation. Stimulation of dopaminergic receptors mediates vasodilation of renal, adrenal, mesenteric, coronary, and cerebral vascular beds.

Norepinephrine. Norepinephrine increases myocardial contractility and causes vasoconstriction of arterial and venous vascular beds by stimulating β_1- and α-adrenergic receptors. In cardiogenic shock, it may increase cardiac output and redistribute blood flow to the heart and brain. The average adult dose is 2 to 12 μg/min, although higher doses may be needed to achieve what is believed to be an optimal mean arterial pressure of 75 mm Hg. Norepinephrine should be infused through a central line to minimize the risk of extravasation. If this should occur, 10 to 15 ml of sodium chloride solution containing 5 to 10 mg of phentolamine mesylate should be infiltrated liberally throughout the affected area, which is identified by a cold, hard, and pale appearance. Norepinephrine infusions require careful monitoring of arterial blood pressure. With increasing doses, the α-adrenergic effect becomes more pronounced, resulting in renal vasoconstriction, oliguria, and a marked increase in systemic vascular resistance. High doses will also increase the risk of tachyarrhythmia and myocardial ischemia. Anxiety, respiratory difficulty, angina, and headaches can also be observed.

Dopamine. Dopamine is a precursor of norepinephrine and it stimulates dopaminergic, β_1- and α-adrenergic receptors in a dose-dependent fashion (28). Dopamine also

Table 39.4.
Inotropes and Vasoactive Agents[a,b]

Drug Usual Dose	Receptor Specificity					Pharmacologic Effect				
	α	β₁	β₂	Dop	Sm Msc	VD	VC	INT	CHT	RBF
Norepinephrine (Levophed)										
IV 2–12 μg/min	+ + + +	+ +					+ + + +	+	+ +	↓
Dopamine (Inotropin)										
2–5 μg/kg/min		+		+ + + +		+		+ +	+	↕
6–10 μg/kg/min		+ + + +	+ +	+		+		+ + + +	+ +	
10–20 μg/kg/min	+ + +	+ + + +	+				+ + +	+ + +	+ + +	
Dobutamine (Dobutrex)			+ +			+ +	+	+ + + +	+ +	
2.0–15.0 μg/kg/min	+	+ + + +								↑
Amrinone (Inocor)		?				+ +		+ + +	+ + +	
0.75 mg/kg										
5–10 μg/kg/min										↑
Nitroprusside (Nipride)					+ + + + A = V					
0.5–10 μg/kg/min										↕
Nitroglycerin					+ + + + A < V					
5–300 μg/min										↕
Hydralazine (Apresoline)					A + + + +					
5–20 mg IV bolus										↑

[a] With permission, from Ornato JP (ed): Cardiovascular Emergencies. Churchill Livingston, New York, 1986, p 123.

[b] Key: α, α-adrenergic; β₁, β₁-adrenergic; β₂, β₂-adrenergic; DOP, dopaminergic; Sm Msc, smooth muscle; VD, vasodilation; VC, vasoconstriction; INT, inotropic; CHT, chronotropic; RBF, renal blood flow; MAP, mean arterial pressure; PCWP, pulmonary capillary wedge pressure; CO, cardiac output; SVR, systemic vascular resistance; UO, urine output; +, low; + + + +, high; A, arterial; V, venous; ↑, increase; ↓, decrease; →, no change.

releases endogenous norepinehprine. In low doses (2 to 5 μg/kg/min) dopamine produces vasodilation of renal, mesenteric, coronary, and cerebral arteries via direct dopaminergic stimulation. In the dosage range of 6 to 10 μg/kg/min, it increases cardiac output through β-adrenergic stimulation. At progressively higher infusion rates, (10 to 20 μg/kg/min), the α-adrenergic effects of dopamine become most prominent, producing peripheral vasoconstriction. Because there is a large interpatient variation in sensitivity to dopamine, infusions should be titrated slowly until the desired effect is seen (28). Dopamine infusions should not be discontinued abruptly; a gradual taper is recommended when the drug is no longer required. The ECG should be monitored for tachyarrhythmias. Dopamine may produce or exacerbate nausea, vomiting, and angina. The risk of extravasation is the same as that with norepinephrine and should be managed accordingly.

Comparative studies have shown that dopamine is more effective and less arrhythmogenic than isoproterenol in patients with cardiogenic shock (28). Dopamine appears to produce a greater increase in cardiac output and urine flow, compared with norepinephrine (28). Dopamine may not be a desirable agent in patients with elevated PCWP and SVR. However, it is invaluable when low SVR and

profound hypotension compromise coronary perfusion pressure (30).

Dobutamine. Dobutamine is a relatively selective positive inotrope. It was synthesized to minimize the arrhythmogenic side effects of isoproterenol (30). Dobutamine is a potent β₁-adrenergic agonist with mild β₂- and α-adrenergic activity. Experimental data suggest that dobutamine exerts a positive inotropic effect by stimulating α- and β-adrenergic receptors in the myocardium (31). Dobutamine produces a dose-related increase in cardiac output, which is accompanied by a significant reduction in left ventricular filling pressure (29). Dobutamine exerts little effect on SVR; the drug may often decrease this hemodynamic parameter (9). This effect and the lack of drug-mediated endogenous catecholamine release explains why dobutamine impacts more favorably than either norepinephrine or dopamine on myocardial oxygen demand (30).

Dobutamine is administered as a continuous intravenous infusion starting at 2 to 3 μg/kg/min and increased by 1 to 2 μg/kg/min every 10 to 30 min until optimal hemodynamic effects are achieved or side effects develop. The usual maintenance dose ranges from 7.5 to 20 μg/kg/min. Doses above 30 μg/kg/min frequently lead to side effects (30). Sinus tachycardia is the most frequent toxic

Table 39.4.
Continued

Hemodynamic Effect					Comments
MAP	PCWP	CO	SVR	UO	
↑	↑	↕	↑	↓	Decreased peripheral perfusion, painful extravasation, arrhythmias, angina
↑	↑	↕	↕	↕	Arrhythmias, headache, hypertension, decreased peripheral perfusion, painful extravasation
↕	↓	↑	→↓	↑	Headache, palpitation, hypotension
↕	↓	↑	↕	↑	Thrombocytopenia, nausea, flu-like syndrome, arrhythmias, hypotension
↓	↓	↕	↓	↕	Hypotension, nausea, abdominal pain, tremor, headache, confusion
↓	↓	↕	→↓	↕	Headache, tachycardia, hypotension, nausea
↓	→	↑	↓	↑	Hypotension, headache, reflex tachycardia, angina

effect of dobutamine, although it occurs less commonly than with dopamine or isoproterenol. Other side effects include nausea, headaches, anxiety, angina, tremors, hypotension, or hypertension.

Several studies have shown that the clinical and hemodynamic responses of dobutamine and dopamine are different and complementary (29, 32, 33). Dopamine exerts a greater increase in systemic blood pressure and an increase or no change in left ventricular filling pressure, when compared with equal doses of dobutamine. Dobutamine is indicated in clinical situations where pulmonary congestion and circulatory collapse are caused by loss of ventricular contractility with no significant loss of vascular tone (29). The combination of dobutamine plus dopamine may show more favorable results than either agent alone, especially in cardiogenic shock patients requiring mechanical ventilation (33).

The ability of dobutamine to increase cardiac output without increasing oxygen demand or reducing coronary blood flow through tachycardia, has led to its use in "pump failure" associated with an AMI. However, additional studies are needed to establish its role as the inotrope of choice in cardiogenic shock.

Amrinone. Amrinone, a nonglycosidic, noncatecholamine intravenous inotropic vasodilatory agent, is indicated for use in severe heart failure (34). Its positive inotropic effect develops within minutes and persists for 60 to 90 min following a single intravenous administration. This action is not impaired by β- or α-adrenoceptor blocking agents (26). Initial therapy with amrinone, 0.75 mg/kg by intravenous injection over 2 to 3 min followed by an infusion of 5 to 10 μg/kg/min, will increase cardiac contractility and decrease SVR. Improvements in CI, PCWP, and SVR average 50%, but greater benefits have been observed in some patients (35–37).

Amrinone is advertised as a "major advance" in inotropic therapy because of its sustained hemodynamic improvements and its reduction in myocardial oxygen demand (34). Few studies have compared amrinone with other inotropes in patients with severe refractory pump failure (38). Klein and coworkers reported that initial improvements in CI and SVR were greater with dobutamine than with amrinone. However, the hemodynamic effects of amrinone were maintained for 24 hr, whereas deterioration from initial response was noted to occur with dobutamine. These results are in conflict with those of other studies (34). Overall, amrinone does not appear to be superior to any other currently available inotropic agent and may actually be more prone to toxicity. Thrombocytopenia is reported to occur in up to 50% of patients treated with amrinone (39). The thrombocytopenia is rapidly reversible upon drug withdrawal. Short-term intravenous infusions may produce nausea, vomiting, liver function abnormalities, and influenza-like syndrome, dysrhythmias, and hypotension (34). Intravenous amrinone should be an agent of last resort.

Vasodilators

Generalized sympathetic vasoconstriction is a useful compensatory mechanism for maintaining systemic pressure and coronary perfusion in cardiogenic shock. However, excessive vasoconstriction decreases cardiac output and increases myocardial oxygen demand. By decreasing this reflex vasoconstriction, vasodilator drugs can reduce ventricular wall stress and produce an improvement in cardiac output similar to that observed with inotropic drugs. The primary effects of these agents appear to be related to their peripheral actions on arterial and venous beds. By dilating the arterial resistance bed, vasodilators reduce impedance, with a resultant increase in stroke volume. Vasodilating drugs that also reduce venous tone will decrease venous return to the heart, which will lower the filling pressure in both ventricles. These actions correct the combined hemodynamic abnormalities in cardiogenic shock and may improve the balance between myocardial oxygen supply and demand.

The use of vasodilators is limited by their potential to produce hypotension in patients with pump failure. These agents produce a triphasic response: (a) at low doses, cardiac output increases and PCWP decreases with little change in arterial pressure; (b) at moderate doses, cardiac output increases, PCWP decreases, and arterial pressures decrease or remain unchanged; and (c) at high doses, cardiac output, PCWP, and arterial pressure all decrease (40). Vasodilators should be avoided in patients without high filling pressures. Hemodynamic measurements should be followed closely in all patients receiving vasodilator therapy, particularly when concomitant diuretic therapy is employed.

Sodium Nitroprusside. Sodium nitroprusside is the most widely used vasodilator in the management of cardiogenic shock. Its rapid onset and short duration of action make it a suitable agent in hemodynamically unstable situations. Numerous studies have reported improvement in left ventricular function, tissue perfusion, coronary output, and clinical status in patients with low output and high SVR refractory to dopamine (41). However, nitroprusside should not be used routinely in patients who develop high left ventricular filling pressures within the first few hours after acute myocardial infarction, since it may produce a "coronary steal" phenomenon (42).

The recommended dosing range is 0.5 to 5 μg/kg/min, but higher doses (up to 10 μg/kg/min) may be needed. The major complication of nitroprusside is hypotension. Patients should be monitored for signs of cyanide or thiocyanate toxicity. Cyanide toxicity is detected by metabolic acidosis; thiocyanate toxicity is manifested by confusion, hyperreflexia, and convulsions. Thiocyanate levels above 2.1 mmol/liter (12 mg/dl) suggest thiocyanate toxicity (43). Low-dose infusions (under 3 μg/kg/min) for less than 72 hr rarely lead to toxicity.

Nitroglycerin. Nitroglycerin reduces intramyocardial wall tension, improves myocardial blood flow, and lowers systemic vascular resistance. Intravenous nitroglycerin is an effective adjunct in the management of pump failure associated with myocardial infarction. It is administered by continuous intravenous infusion at 10 to 20 μg/min and increased by 5 to 10 μg/min every 5 to 10 min until the desired hemodynamic or clinical response occurs. Low doses (30 to 40 μg/min) produce venodilation predominantly; high doses (250 μg/min), lead to arteriolar dilation as well (44).

In cardiogenic shock, the beneficial effects of nitroglycerin are due to systemic vasodilation, which increases cardiac output and lowers oxygen consumption, and to direct vasodilation of the coronary circulation, which increases blood supply to ischemic areas, compared with nitroprusside (45). The combination of nitroglycerin and an inotrope (dopamine or dobutamine), although not studied extensively, appears to produce marked hemodynamic improvements while reducing the risk of ischemia damage (46). Overall, patients with the most severe degree of left ventricular failure show the most beneficial hemodynamic effects.

Recent studies have suggested a difference between nitroglycerin and nitroprusside in their effects on myocardial blood flow (47). Nitroglycerin has a greater dilatory effect on collateral capacitance vessels. Nitroprusside has a greater dilatory effect on arteriolar resistance vessels. Therefore, nitroglycerin is less likely to produce coronary steal. Furthermore, nitroprusside has a greater propensity to lower coronary perfusion pressure, compared with nitroglycerin (48). The risk reduction in mortality in trials with nitroglycerin in AMI is 45%; this is greater than the 23% reduction in mortality observed with nitroprusside in AMI (49). These data suggest that intravenous nitroglycerin reduces mortality in AMI.

Potential complications of intravenous nitroglycerin include reversible hypotension and bradycardia, hypoxemia due to increased pulmonary ventilation-perfusion mismatch, methemoglobinemia, and headache. In general, the drug has been well tolerated.

Mechanical Circulatory Support

The near universal mortality among cardiogenic shock victims despite medical management has identified the need for other modalities to augment left ventricular function and reverse circulatory collapse. Mechanical circulatory support attempts to meet these needs while favorably affecting the balance between myocardial oxygen supply and demand. The decision to institute mechanical circulatory support is based on the presence of a low cardiac index (<1.8 liter/min) and an elevated PCWP (>20 mm Hg) despite maximum inotropic, vasodilator, and vasopressor support. The major uses of mechanical circulatory assist devices are in patients who are potential transplant recipients and in those with medically refractory unstable angina unamenable to invasive procedures.

The intraaortic balloon pump (IABP) was the first mechanical-assist device used for improving aortic and coronary blood flow and reducing left ventricular workload in cardiogenic shock (50). The IABP is a balloon-tipped arterial catheter that is placed just below the aortic arch via the femoral artery. Balloon inflation increases diastolic perfusion pressure and coronary blood flow; balloon deflation improves cardiac output by reducing afterload. The net effect of intraaortic balloon counterpulsation (IABC) is to improve the balance between myocardial oxygen supply and demand (5). Serious complications from IABC are common and include damage to or perforation of the aortic wall, limb ischemia, thrombocytopenia and hemolysis, systemic embolization, wound infection, and failure due to balloon rupture (51). Cardiac arrhythmias are relative contraindications to IABC and must be corrected for effective counterpulsation.

IABC can provide temporary hemodynamic improvement in cardiogenic shock patients (9, 50), but it impacts minimally on long-term survival. The failure to permanently reverse the shock syndrome following AMI is probably the result of preexisting irreversible tissue necrosis. Contraindications to IABC include aortic regurgitation, aortic dissection or aneurysm, near terminal or untreatable medical conditions, ventricular fibrillation, or asystole (4, 5, 11).

The IABP is not considered a true ventricular-assist device (VAD) because the term VAD is usually reserved for devices that are able to support the circulation totally (52). There are two types of VADs, nonpulsatile devices used for cardiopulmonary resuscitation and pulsatile devices used for long-term support. As the number of patients awaiting cardiac transplantation continues to increase, so will the need for VADs as a bridge to heart transplantation. The reader is referred to an excellent review on this topic by Miller (52).

Prognosis

Even under optimal conditions, the prognosis of the AMI patient with cardiogenic shock is grave. Of the 10 to 30% who do survive to hospital discharge, 50% will die within the following 24 months (2).

LIMITATION OF INFARCT SIZE

Irreversible myocardial ischemic injury in humans takes up to 6 hr to develop. If reperfusion of the ischemic zone is instituted within 3 to 4 hr the area of infarction may be reduced. Although direct measure of infarct size in human hearts can only be made at autopsy, infarct size can be assessed indirectly by trends in the ECG, by the pattern of myocardial enzyme release, or by radionuclide techniques. Because infarct size correlates with mortality, interventions capable of reducing MI size might be expected to reduce the rate of postinfarction death. Results obtained in animal models of AMI indicate that interventions designed to reduce myocardial oxygen demand, to enhance oxygen supply, or to reduce the acute inflammatory response can salvage ischemic myocardium (53). This section examines pharmacologic intervention that may limit infarct size by decreasing myocardial oxygen consumption or by improving myocardial oxygen demand.

β-Adrenergic Blocking Agents

β-Adrenergic blockade reduces myocardial oxygen consumption by reducing heart rate, contractility, and blood pressure. β-Adrenergic blockers can also reduce catecholamine levels in the ischemic heart and produce favorable redistribution of coronary blood flow (54–56).

Clinical trials with these agents can be divided into two groups: (a) those in which treatment was begun early and end points such as enzyme levels, ECG changes, and reinfarction rates are investigated, and (b) those in which treatment was begun later after resolution of the infarct, with mortality rate reduction as the end point. There is evidence that intravenous therapy followed by oral administration with atenolol, propranolol, metoprolol, sotalol, or timolol reduces serum enzyme levels. Reduction in ECG abnormalities post-AMI has been reported following acute intervention with propranolol, practolol, and metoprolol. Studies show that β-blockers limit infarct size, reduce the incidence of malignant ventricular arrhythmia, and reduce mortality following acute administration in patients with AMI (57). Intravenous β-blocker therapy reduces mortality and reinfarction rate when administered within 2 hr of the onset of symptoms in AMI patients receiving thrombolytic therapy (57). If intravenous β-blocker therapy is initiated within 4 hr of symptom onset, there is a reduction in nonfatal reinfarction and recurrent ischemia (57). β-Blockers may also reduce the risk of intracranial bleeding in AMI patients treated with thrombolytics.

Although β-adrenergic blockers are contraindicated in patients with serious myocardial dysfunction, cardiac conduction abnormalities, hypotension, peripheral hypoperfusion, or bronchospastic airway disease, it is reasonable to consider their use in AMI patients without contraindications, irrespective of concomitant thrombolytic therapy (57). β-Adrenergic blockers are also valuable in AMI patients with atrial tachyarrhythmias or rapid ventricular response rates in atrial fibrillation. Well-designed trials with large numbers of patients show that timolol, metoprolol, and propranolol significantly reduce long-term mortality of AMI. Because these agents were administered after resolution of the MI, the reduction in mortality is likely due to a decrease in the incidence of arrhythmias or reinfarction and not related to infarct size reduction.

Calcium-Channel Blockers

Experimental data in animals suggest that calcium-channel blockers may prevent the progression of ischemia and subsequent necrosis by decreasing myocardial oxygen demand without comprising cardiac output (1). Recent clinical trials indicate that these agents do not alter outcome in AMI patients. Verapamil may reduce infarct size, but it does not alter acute mortality (58). In the largest trial to date, verapamil (0.1/mg/kg intravenously, followed by 120 mg orally three times daily for 6 months) failed to alter acute mortality, long-term mortality, or reinfarction rate, when compared with placebo (59). Studies with nifedipine (20 mg orally every 4 hr for 14 days) failed to show a significant reduction in enzymatically assessed infarct size, compared with placebo (60). A slight trend for higher mortality was observed in the nifedipine group.

A placebo-controlled trial of diltiazem in AMI reported a reduction in early recurrent infarction (one-tailed, P = .03, two-tailed, P = .06) in patients with non–Q wave myocardial infarction (61). However, a small, nonsignificant, excess mortality and substantial side effects occurred in diltiazem-treated patients. Patients with Q-wave myocardial infarction and significant left ventricular dysfunction did not benefit from diltiazem therapy (62). Long-term diltiazem therapy in AMI patients failed to demonstrate any significant benefit and produced detrimental side effects in patients with left ventricular dysfunction.

Although there is laboratory evidence that calcium-channel blockers reduce infarct size, these results are not observed under clinical conditions. Currently, there is no reason to recommend general treatment with calcium-channel blockers to reduce infarct size. However, patients with documented or suspected vasospastic angina and AMI patients undergoing emergent angioplasty may benefit from the use of calcium-channel blockers as long as left ventricular function is relatively well preserved (57).

Nitrates

Organic nitrates, such as nitroglycerin and nitroprusside, reduce preload and afterload by their veno- and arteriolar-dilatory effects. Nitrates reduce myocardial oxygen demand and dilate the epicardial coronary circulation. Nitroglycerin infusion decreases both enzymatically assessed infarct size and hospital mortality in patients with left ventricular dysfunction (63). Intravenous nitroglycerin is preferred because it minimizes the risks of hypotension and tachycardia observed with oral nitrates and is less likely to produce "coronary steal," when compared with nitroprusside. Prompt initiation of intravenous nitroglycerin therapy can reduce infarct size and reduce the incidence of congestive heart failure in patients with AMI. Nitroglycerin is most useful in patients with ongoing ischemia, heart failure, or hypertension.

THROMBOLYTIC AGENTS

Thrombolytic therapy has assumed a central role in the management of patients with AMI. The interest in thrombolytic therapy stems from four clinical findings: (a) approximately 85% of transmural myocardial infarctions (evaluated within 4 hr of onset of symptoms) are caused by a coronary thrombus; (b) thrombolytic agents can lyse clots effectively; (c) myocardial salvage can occur if therapy is begun within 6 hr after the onset of symptoms; and (d) a reduction in mortality can be achieved in some patients who receive thrombolytic agents (57, 64–65).

Pharmacologic Thrombolysis

Thrombolytic agents activate both soluble plasminogen and surface-bound plasminogen to plasmin. Pharmacologic thrombolysis occurs when surface-bound plasminogen is converted to surface-bound plasmin. Plasmin, generated in close proximity to the fibrin clot, digests fibrin and dissolves the clot. Streptokinase, urokinase, and anisoylated plasminogen-streptokinase-activator complex (APSAC) are non-fibrin-selective thrombolytic agents. Recombinant tissue-type plasminogen activator and recombinant single-chain urokinase plasminogen activator (r-scu-PA) are fibrin-selective agents because they activate plasma plasminogen to a lesser extent than surface-bound plasminogen. However, fibrin-selectivity is relatively dose-dependent, and all agents will activate circulating plasminogen to different degrees (streptokinase > APSAC > urokinase > r-scu-PA > rtPA) (66). Table 39.5 lists the half-life, dose, advantages, and disadvantages for each of these agents (66).

The goals of thrombolytic therapy are (a) to lyse coronary thrombi during the early phase of AMI; (b) to limit infarct size by reperfusing jeopardized myocardium; and (c) to reduce morbidity and mortality. Thrombolytic agents can be infused by either the intracoronary or the intravenous route. Patients with recent onset of chest pain (usually less than 6 hr), with persistent ECG abnormalities indicating an evolving transmural AMI, are candidates for thrombolytic therapy (64). Patients with recent CVA, surgery, cardiopulmonary resuscitation, active bleeding, or bleeding diathesis should not receive thrombolytic therapy.

Intracoronary streptokinase is initiated with a 10,000 to 30,000 U bolus, followed by an infusion of 2000 to 4000

Table 39.5.
Comparison of Thrombolytic Agents[a,b]

Agent	Half-Life (min)	Dose	Advantages	Disadvantages
APSAC	105	30 U bolus	Long-acting bolus dose	Antigenicity, "lytic" effect
Streptokinase	90	1.5 million units over 1 hr	Proven value, inexpensive	Antigenicity, "lytic" effect
rtPA	36	100 mg over 3 hr	Proven value, clot-selective, nonantigenic	Expensive, inconvenient regimen
r-Pro-urokinase	7	70 mg over 1 hr	Clot-selective, nonantigenic	Short half-life, investigational
Urokinase	16	2 million unit bolus	Effective, nonantigenic	Expensive, "lytic" effect

[a] With permission, from Monk JP, Heel RC: Anisoylated plasminogen streptokinase activator complex (APSAC). A review of its mechanisms of action, clinical pharmacology and its therapeutic use in acute myocardial infarction. Drugs 34:25–49, 1987.
[b] Legend: anisoylated plasminogen-streptokinase activator complex (APSAC), recombinant tissue-type plasminogen activator (rtPA)

U/min. Clot lysis generally occurs within 30 min after initiation of the infusion and requires an average of 65,000 U of streptokinase. The infusion is continued for 30 to 60 min after successful reperfusion or until a predetermined maximal dose of streptokinase (150,000 to 500,000 U). Intravenous streptokinase is administered at a dose of 750,000 to 1.5 million U over 30 to 60 min. After streptokinase, patients receive full-dose, intravenous heparin for 24 to 72 hr. Early treatment reestablishes flow in the infarct-related coronary artery in 60 to 90% of patients treated with intracoronary and 35 to 62% of patients treated with intravenous streptokinase (65).

Urokinase may be used in patients with hypersensitivity to streptokinase or with high pneumococcal antibody titers. Patients who have received streptokinase within 1 to 2 months of a repeat course may require larger doses or treatment with urokinase, because streptokinase antibodies can be found in high concentrations for up to 3 months. Three units of urokinase are approximately equivalent to one unit of streptokinase. Urokinase is most commonly used by intracoronary administration to prevent acute closure in patients undergoing balloon dilatation of the right coronary artery or in patients requiring emergent coronary angioplasty after failed therapy with an intravenous thrombolytic.

Anisoylated human plasminogen-streptokinase-activator complex (APSAC) is a direct plasminogen-activator complex formed when streptokinase and human plasminogen are acylated with a p-anisoyl derivative. This renders the activator inactive, but the acylation of the catalytic site of the plasminogen molecule is reversible over time. The streptokinase-plasminogen complex of APSAC dissociates at a rate slower than the deacylation rate, ensuring that the fibrinolytic activity of the drug is controlled by the latter. The deacylation half-life is about 105 min in human plasma or whole blood in vitro, and the plasma clearance half-life of fibrinolytic activity has been reported at 90 to 112 min in patients with AMI. The extended half-life of APSAC allows it to be administered as a single intravenous injection over 4 to 5 min.

The main advantages of APSAC over alternative thrombolytic drugs is its ease of administration by the intravenous route in patients with AMI (57). At the recommended dose of 30 U injected intravenously over a period of 4 to 5 min in patients with AMI of less than 6-hr duration, reperfusion of occluded coronary arteries occurs in about 72% of patients at 90 min (range 53 to 91% in individual studies) (67–69). Subsequent reocclusion has been reported in 0 to 20% of patients in most studies, with an average reocclusion rate around 10% (67). Thrombolytic therapy with intravenous APSAC improves left ventricular function and survival in patients with AMI (57).

Unlike streptokinase, APSAC, and urokinase, tissue-type plasminogen activators (t-PA) have minimal affinity for free, circulating plasminogen. Tissue-type plasminogen activator produces clot-selective thrombolysis by activating fibrin-bound plasminogen; the activity of t-PAs is dose-dependent. Pharmacologic doses of t-PA activate circulating plasminogen, resulting in systemic fibrinogenolysis and a modest systemic lytic state (70–71). The short half-life of t-PA, approximately 5 min, does not assure prompt reversal of hemostatic abnormalities. This process depends upon the replenishment of fibrinogen and the elimination of fibrinogen breakdown products.

Successful reperfusion is indicated by the sudden relief of chest pain, resolution of ST segment elevation, or the onset of reperfusion tachyarrhythmias. These occur in 15% of patients but do not usually require treatment. Bleeding complications are the major concern with thrombolytic agents, as a result of their general interference with hemostatic mechanisms. Thrombolytics do not differentiate between pathologic clots and hemostatic plugs. Lysis of hemostatic plugs can lead to bleeding complications following pharmacologic thrombolysis. Clinical studies show a 5% risk of major bleeding complications from thrombolytic therapy (57, 65). Bleeding complications are minimized by avoiding drugs that affect hemostasis, and by avoiding excessive venipuncture.

Allergic reactions are more common with streptokinase and APSAC. Intravenous diphenhydramine may be required in some cases. Hypotension occurs in approximately 10% of patients treated with streptokinase or APSAC. Once the patient receives streptokinase, the patient is sensitized to the drug and should not receive it again for 6 months. Other side effects with thrombolytics include angina, flushing, dyspnea, mild febrile reactions, nausea/vomiting and occasionally rash, all of which may be symptoms of mild allergic reactions. Allergic reactions and hypotension are basically not an issue in patients treated with t-PA.

Successful thrombolytic therapy in AMI depends on more than just the ability to reperfuse the occluded coronary artery. Prevention of reocclusion and subsequent salvage of infarcted myocardium should reduce morbidity and mortality following thrombolytic therapy. Results of early studies that compared reperfusion rates achieved by t-PA and streptokinase suggested that t-PA was twice as effective as streptokinase in establishing reperfusion of acutely occluded coronary arteries (70–71). In recent trials, myocardial salvage, mortality reduction, or bleeding complications have not differed in AMI patients treated with t-PA versus streptokinase (72). Clinical experience provides little evidence for the superiority of t-PA over other thrombolytic agents in acute myocardial infarction. The largest trials measuring myocardial function after thrombolytic therapy failed to show that t-PA is more effective than streptokinase (73–74), urokinase (75), or APSAC (76). Additionally, t-PA is no safer than other thrombolytics (74, 77). The International Study of 20,749 AMI patients showed no difference in mortality rate between t-PA (8.9%) and streptokinase (8.5%) (78). There was also no difference in the incidence of ventricular fibrillation, reinfarction, or shock between treatment groups. The echocardiographically measured ejection fraction and the incidence of congestive heart failure also did not differ between treatment groups (74, 78). Available published data from direct comparative trials of large numbers of patients show that t-PA and streptokinase are equally safe and effective in salvaging myocardium during an evolving myocardial infarction and in assuring survival benefit after acute myocardial infarction (72).

POSTREPERFUSION MANAGEMENT

After successful thrombolysis, the stenotic vessel may reocclude. The rate of reocclusion varies but may be as high as 30% (64). The likelihood of reocclusion and recovery of regional ventricular function depends on the severity of residual stenosis. After successful thrombolysis, antico-

Table 39.6.

Proposed Indications for Percutaneous Transluminal Coronary Angioplasty in Patients with Acute Myocardial Infarction

Patients with inadequate response to pharmacologic thrombolysis
Patients with contraindications to pharmacologic thrombolysis
Patients requiring immediate reperfusion

agulation is advocated, although there is no consensus on the type, dosage, or duration of therapy. Most often, full-dose heparin is used for 24 to 72 hr. Aspirin (160 mg/day or 325 mg/day) is administered for 3 months or longer (64). There is no role for dipyridamole as an adjunctive antiplatelet agent after thrombolytic therapy.

Percutaneous transluminal coronary angioplasty (PTCA) provides a viable therapeutic alternative in some patients (Table 39.6). A major limitation of PTCA is that it requires a skilled team, a fully staffed catheterization laboratory, and a surgical team on stand-by. Potential complications of PTCA include catheter-induced occlusions caused by dissection, spasm, or subintimal hematoma and residual stenosis. Routine angioplasty performed within 24 hr of thrombolytic therapy offers no clinical benefit and is associated with an increased incidence of reocclusion and complications (57). Angioplasty is recommended in patients with ongoing ischemia or pump failure.

The safety and efficacy of coronary artery bypass-graft (CABG) surgery in AMI patients are well established (64). The systemic lytic state after thrombolysis may increase the morbidity of the surgical procedure if it is performed within 24 hr after infusion. Although the indications and timing for CABG surgery in AMI patients are still controversial, most clinicians agree that surgery can alter the natural history of AMI if reperfusion of the ischemic area can occur within 6 hr of symptoms (79). Emergency CABG surgery for AMI is successful in a few centers set up to perform cardiopulmonary bypass within 6 hr of symptoms, but this is not feasible in most hospitals.

Summary

The most important factor for successfully limiting infarct size is the prompt institution of therapy that salvages viable myocardium. The ability of any drug or intervention to reduce infarct size in humans is optimal when therapy can be started less than 4 hr after the onset of symptoms. Intravenous administration of a clot-specific thrombolytic agent may prove to be the initial therapy of choice. Because thrombolytic therapy dissolves only existing thrombi and does not affect the underlying causes of coronary artery occlusion, further study and therapy to reduce the risk of reinfarction and death should be initiated. Percutaneous transluminal coronary angioplasty may reduce the reocclusion rate after thrombolysis. β-Blockers and possibly nitroglycerin can provide valuable alternatives when thrombolysis is unavailable.

Prognosis

Considerable effort has been spent on the search for predictors of survival and factors determining the occurrence of reinfarction after AMI (80). Most patients who survive AMI initially have an uncomplicated event; the pain subsides and there is no evidence of heart failure or arrhythmias. Mortality after MI in unselected groups of patients ranges from 4 to 6% per year (80). Mortality is higher in patients with moderate impairment of left ventricular function and three-vessel coronary disease. These patients may benefit from elective CABG after AMI.

Survival after MI relates to the extent and location of the coronary obstructive lesion and to the adequacy of residual myocardial function. To prevent or retard the progression of atherosclerotic coronary heart disease, conventional coronary risk-factor reduction is necessary (81). Continued cigarette smoking after MI increases the likelihood of reinfarction and coronary death in men and women of all ages. Reduction of excess caloric and cholesterol intake is advisable. Control of systemic hypertension decreases both myocardial oxygen demand and the risk of stroke. Medical management with antianginal drugs reduces myocardial oxygen demand and decreases myocardial ischemia. Chronic therapy with β-adrenergic blockers decreases myocardial ischemia. Chronic therapy with β-adrenergic blockers reduces both the recurrence of MI and the incidence of sudden death for up to 2 years after AMI (82). Exercise training improves physical work capacity and favorably affects weight control and psychologic status.

In the absence of contraindications, one 325-mg tablet of aspirin should be taken after an AMI to prevent reinfarction (83). Aspirin in a daily dose of 325 mg reduces the rate of reinfarction by 21% (84) and mortality by 10% (85). The FDA approved aspirin for this indication in 1985. Higher doses of aspirin are no more effective, and lower doses have not been investigated. Neither dipyridamole nor sulfinpyrazone can be recommended for the prevention of recurrent myocardial infarction. The combination of aspirin and dipyridamole is no more effective than aspirin alone (85–86), and the efficacy of sulfinpyrazone has not been proven (87).

CONCLUSIONS

Myocardial infarction is one of the most common reasons for hospitalization in the Western World. The acute mortality rate is about 15%; approximately 10% of patients will die during the first year after their AMI. Short- and long-term survival depends on the extent and location of the coronary obstructive lesions and the prompt correction of post-MI complications. The presence or absence of mechanical, electrical, ischemic, and vascular abnormalities provides the necessary information to institute appropriate medical and/or surgical treatment.

REFERENCES

1. Zeller FP, Bauman JL: Current concepts in clinical therapeutics: acute myocardial infarction. Clin Pharm 5:553–572, 1986.
2. Alpert JS, Braunwald E, Acute myocardial infarction: pathological, pathophysiological, and clinical manifestations. In Braunwald E: Heart Disease, ed. 2. Philadelphia, WB Saunders, 1984, pp 1262–1270.
3. Sobel BE, Braunwald E, The management of acute myocardial infarction. In Braunwald E: Heart Disease, ed. 2. Philadelphia, WB Saunders, 1984, pp 1301–1321.
4. Epstein SE, Palmeri ST: Mechanisms contributing to precipitation of unstable angina and acute myocardial infarction: implications regarding therapy. Am J Cardiol 54:1245–1252, 1984.
5. Moseri A, L'Abbate A, Baroldi G, et al.: Coronary vasospasm as a possible cause of myocardial infarction. A conclusion derived from the study of "preinfarction" angina. N Engl J Med 299:1271–1277, 1978.
6. Zelma MJ: Q wave, S-T segment, and T wave myocardial infarction. Am J Med 78:391–398, 1985.
7. Rude RE: Acute myocardial infarction and its complications. Cardiol Clin 2:163–171, 1984.
8. Rasanen J, Vaisanen IT, Heikkila J, et al.: Acute myocardial infarction complicated by left ventricular dysfunction and respiratory failure: the effects of continuous positive airway pressure. Chest 87:278–360, 1985.
9. Dole WP, O'Rourke RA: Pathophysiology and management of cardiogenic shock. Circ Probl Cardiol 8:1, 1983.
10. Lee G, DeMaria AN, Amsterdam EA, et al.: Comparative effect of morphine, meperidine, and pentazocine on cardiopulmonary dynamics in patients with acute myocardial infarction. Am J Med 60:341–355, 1976.
11. Kaplan K: Prophylactic anticoagulation following acute myocardial infarction. Arch Intern Med 146:595–597, 1986.
12. Wyman MG, Gore S: Lidocaine prophylaxis in myocardial infarction: a concept whose time has come. Heart Lung 12:358–361, 1983.
13. Singh BN, Venkatesh N: Prevention of myocardial reinfarction and of sudden death in survivors of acute myocardial infarction: role of prophytactic β-adrenoceptor blockade. Am Heart J 108:450–455, 1984.
14. Norris RM, Brown MA, Clarke ED, et al.: Prevention of ventricular fibrillation during acute myocardial infarction by intravenous propranolol. Lancet 2:883–886, 1984.
15. Ryden L, Arniego R, Arnman K, et al.: A double-blind trial of metoprolol in acute myocardial infarction: effects on ventricular tachyarrhythmias. N Engl J Med 308:614–618, 1983.
16. Mueller H, Ayres SM, Religi A, et al.: Propranolol in the treatment of acute myocardial infarction. Circulation 49:1078–1081, 1974.
17. Chadda K, Goldstein S, Byington R, et al.: Effect of propranolol after acute myocardial infarction in patients with congestive heart failure. Circulation 73:503–510, 1986.
18. Wagner GS: Arrhythmias in acute myocardial infarction. Med Clin North Am 68:1061–1068, 1984.
19. Cristal N, Szwarcberg J, Gueron M: Supraventricular arrhythmias in acute myocardial infarction: prognostic importance of clinical setting; mechanisms of production. Ann Intern Med 82:35–39, 1975.
20. Swan HJ, Forrester JS, Danzig R, et al.: Power failure in acute myocardial infarction. Progr Cardiovasc Dis 12:508, 1970.

21. Berkley CE, Russell RO, Mantle JA, et al.: Cardiogenic shock. Recognition and management. Cardiovasc Clin 7:251, 1975.

22. Forrester JS, Diamond G, Chartterjee K, et al.: Medical therapy of acute myocardial infarction by application of hemodynamic subsets. N Engl J Med 295:1356, 1976.

23. Biddle TL, Paul NY: Effect of furosemide on hemodynamic and lung water in acute pulmonary edema secondary to myocardial infarction. Am J Cardiol 43:86, 1979.

24. Kilcoyne MM, Schmidt DH, Cannon PJ: Intrarenal blood flow in congestive heart failure. Postgrad Med J 51(suppl 6):54, 1975.

25. Gunnar RM, Leab HS, Scanlon PJ, et al.: Management of acute myocardial infarction and accelerating angina. Prog Cardiovasc Dis 22:1, 1979.

26. Scholz H: Inotropic drugs and their mechanisms of action. J Am Coll Cardiol 4:389, 1984.

27. Goldberg LI: Dopamine: clinical uses of an endogenous catecholamine. N Engl J Med 291:707, 1974.

28. Holzer J, Karliner JS, O'Rourke RA, et al.: Effectiveness of dopamine in patients with cardiogenic shock. Am J Cardiol 32:79, 1973.

29. Francis GS, Sharma B, Hodges M: Comparative hemodynamic effects of dopamine and dobutamine in patients with acute cardiogenic circulation collapse. Am Heart J 103:995, 1982.

30. Leier CV, Unverferth DV: Drugs five years later: dobutamine. Ann Intern Med 99:490, 1983.

31. Ruffolo RR: The mechanism of action of dobutamine. Ann Intern Med 100:313, 1984.

32. Maekawa K, Liang CS, Hood WB: Comparison of dobutamine and dopamine in acute myocardial infarction: effects of systemic hemodynamics, plasma catecholamines, blood flows, and infarct size. Circulation 67:750, 1983.

33. Richard C, Ricome JL, Rimailho A, et al.: Combined hemodynamic effects of dopamine and dobutamine in cardiogenic shock. Circulation 67:620, 1983.

34. Franciosa JA: Intravenous amrinone: an advance or wrong step? (editorial) Ann Intern Med 102:399, 1985.

35. LeJemtel TJ, Keung E, Ribner JS, et al.: Sustained beneficial effects of oral amrinone on cardiac and renal function in patients with severe congestive heart failure. Am J Cardiol 45:123, 1980.

36. Wynne J, Malacoff RF, Benotti JR, et al.: Oral amrinone in refractory congestive heart failure. Am J Cardiol 45:1245, 1980.

37. Naccarelli GV, Gray EL, Dougherty AH, et al.: Amrinone: acute electrophysiologic and hemodynamic effects in patients with congestive heart failure. Am J Cardiol 54:600, 1984.

38. Klein NA, Siskind SJ, Frishman WH, et al.: Hemodynamic comparison of intravenous amrinone and dobutamine in patients with chronic congestive heart failure. Am J Cardiol 48:170, 1981.

39. Chesebro JH, Foster V, Robertson JS, et al.: Shortened platelet survival in cardiac failure: predisposition to amrinone-induced platelet reduction. Circulation 66:II-382, 1982.

40. Forresters JS, Waters DD: Hospital treatment of congestive heart failure: management according to hemodynamic profile. Am J Med 65:173, 1978.

41. Parmley WW, Chatterjee K, Charuzi Y, et al.: Hemodynamic effects of noninvasive systolic unloading (nitroprusside) and diastolic augmentation (external counterpulsation) in patients with acute myocardial infarction. Am J Cardiol 33:810, 1974.

42. Cohn JN, Franciosa JA, Francis GS, et al.: Effect of short-term infusion of sodium nitroprusside on mortality rate in acute myocardial infarction complicated by left ventricular failure. N Engl J Med 306:1129, 1982.

43. Cohn JN, Burke LP: Drugs five years later: nitroprusside. Ann Intern Med 91:752, 1979.

44. Herling IM: Intravenous nitroglycerin: clinical pharmacology and therapeutic considerations. Am Heart J 108:141, 1984.

45. Roberts R: Intravenous nitroglycerin in acute myocardial infarction. Am J Med 74(6B):45, 1983.

46. Swan NA, Evenson MK, Needham KE, et al.: Effect of combined nitroglycerin and dobutamine infusion in left ventricular dysfunction. Am Heart J 106:35, 1983.

47. Chiarello M, Gold HK, Leinbach RC, et al.: Comparison between the effects of nitroprusside and nitroglycerin on ischemic injury during acute myocardial infarction. Circulation 54:766, 1976.

48. Flaherty JT: Comparison of intravenous nitroglycerin and sodium nitroprusside in acute myocardial infarction. Am J Med 74(6B):53, 1983.

49. Yusuf S, Wittes J, Friedman L: Overview of results of randomized clinical trials in heart disease. I. Treatments following myocardial infarction. JAMA 260:2088, 1988.

50. Weiss WR: Intra-aortic balloon pumping. Ann Thorac Surg 21:571, 1976.

51. Isner JM, Cohen SR, Virman R, et al.: Complications of the intra-aortic balloon counterpulsation device: clinical and morphologic observations in 45 necropsy patients. Am J Cardiol 45:260, 1980.

52. Miller LW: Mechanical assist devices in intensive care. Am Heart J 121:1887–1892, 1991.

53. Campbell CA, Przylenk K, Kloner RA: Infarct size reduction: a review of the clinical trials. J Clin Pharmacol 26:317–329, 1986.

54. May GS, Furbery CD, Eberlein KA, et al.: Secondary prevention after myocardial infarction. A review of short-term acute phase trials. Prog Cardiovasc Dis 25:335–359, 1985.

55. Mueller HS, Ayres SM: Propranolol decreases sympathetic necrosis activity reflected by plasma catecholamines during evolution of myocardial infarction in man. J Clin Invest 65:338–346, 1980.

56. Pitt B, Crown P: Effect of propranolol in regional myocardial blood flow in acute ischemia. Cardiovasc Res 4:176–179, 1970.

57. Gunnar RM, Bourdillon PD, Dixon DW, et al.: Guidelines for the early management of patients with acute myocardial infarction. J Am Coll Cardiol 16:249, 1990.

58. Bussman WD, Seher W, Gresengrus M: Reduction of creatinine kinase and creatinine kinase-MB indexes of infarct size by intravenous verapamil. Am J Cardiol 54:1224–1230, 1984.

59. Danish Multicenter Study Group: Verapamil in acute myocardial infarction. Eur Heart J 5:516–528, 1984.

60. Mueller JE, Morrison J, Stone PH, et al.: Nifedipine therapy for patients with threatened and acute myocardial infarction: A randomized double-blind, placebo-controlled comparison. Circulation 69:740–747, 1984.

61. Gibson RS, Boden WE, Theroux P, et al.: Diltiazem and reinfarction in patients with non Q wave MI. N Engl J Med 315:423, 1986.

62. The Multicenter Diltiazem Postinfarction Trial Research Group: The effect of diltiazem on mortality and reinfarction after myocardial infarction. N Engl J Med 319:385, 1988.

63. Mueller JE, Braunwald E: Can infarct size be limited in patients with acute myocardial infarction? Cardiovas Clin 13:147–161, 1983.

64. Gersh BJ: Role of thrombolytic therapy in evolving myocardial infarction. Mod Concepts Cardiovas Dis 54:13–17, 1985.

65. Schwartz DE, Yamaga CC: Thrombolysis for evolving myocardial infarction. Ann Intern Med 103:463–469, 1985.

66. Sherry S: Appraisal of various thrombolytic agents in the treatment of acute myocardial infarction. Am J Med 83(suppl 2A):31, 1987.

67. Monk JP, Heel RC: Anisoylated plasminogen streptokinase activator complex (APSAC). A review of its mechanisms of action, clinical pharmacology and its therapeutic use in acute myocardial infarction. Drugs 34:25, 1987.

68. Meinertz T, Kasper W, Schumacher M, et al.: The German multicenter trial of anisoylated plasminogen streptokinase activator complex versus heparin for acute myocardial infarction. Am J Cardiol 62:347, 1988.

69. AIMS Trial Study Group: Effect of intravenous APSAC on mortality after acute myocardial infarction: preliminary report of a placebo-controlled clinical trial. Lancet 1:545–549, 1988.

70. Crabbe SJ, Cloninger CC: Tissue plasminogen activator: A new thrombolytic agent. Clin Pharm 6:373–386, 1987.

71. Sherry S: Recombinant tissue plasminogen activator (r + -PA): is it the thrombolytic agent of choice for an evolving acute myocardial infarction. Am J Cardiol 59:984–989, 1987.

72. Sherry S, Marder VJ: Streptokinase and recombinant tissue plasminogen activator (rt-PA) are equally effective in treating acute myocardial infarction. Ann Intern Med 114:417–423, 1991.

73. White HD, Rivers JT, Maslowski AH, et al.: Effect of intravenous streptokinase as compared with that of tissue plasminogen activator on left ventricular function after first myocardial infarction. N Engl J Med 320:817–821, 1989.

74. Gruppo Italiano por lo Studio della Sopravivenza nell'Infarcto Miocardico.: GISSI-2: a factorial randomized trial of alteplase versus streptokinase and heparin versus no heparin among 12,490 patients with acute myocardial infarction. Lancet 336:65–71, 1990.

75. Neuhaus KL, Tebbe U, Gotwik M, et al.: Intravenous recombinant tissue plasminogen activator and urokinase in acute myocardial infarction: results of the German Activator Urokinase Study (GAUS). J Am Coll Cardiol 12:581–587, 1988.

76. Bassand JP, Cassagnes J, Machecourt T, et al.: A multicenter trial of intravenous APSAC versus rt-PA in acute myocardial infarction: assessment of efficacy and safety (Abstract). J Am Coll Cardiol 15(suppl A):214A, 1990.

77. Rao AK, Pratt C, Berke A, et al.: Thrombolysis in acute myocardial infarction (TIMI) Trial, Phase I: hemorrhagic manifestations and changes in plasma fibrinogen and the fibrinolytic system in patients treated with recombinant tissue plasminogen activator and streptokinase. J Am Coll Cardiol 11:1–11, 1988.

78. The International Study Group: In-hospital mortality and clinical course of 20,891 patients with suspected acute myocardial infarction randomised between alteplase and streptokinase with or without heparin. Lancet 336:71–75, 1990.

79. Robinson L, Surgical interventions for acute cardiothoric emergencies. In Ornato JP: Cardiovascular Emergencies, ed. 1. New York, Churchill Livingstone, 1986, p 43.

80. Sanz G, Castaner A, Betrice A, et al.: Determinants of prognosis in survivors of myocardial infarction. N Engl J Med 306:1065–1070, 1982.

81. Wenger NK: Uncomplicated acute myocardial infarction: long-term management. Am J Cardiol 52:658–660, 1983.

82. Turi ZG, Braumwald E: The use of beta blockers after myocardial infarction. JAMA 249:2512–2516, 1983.

83. Anon: Aspirin after myocardial infarction. Lancet 1:1172–1173, 1980.

84. Canner PL: Aspirin in coronary disease. Comparison of six clinical trials. Isr J Med Sci 19:413–423, 1983.

85. Klimt DR, Knatterud GL, Stamler J, Meier P: Persantine-aspirin reinfarction study. Part II. Secondary coronary prevention with persantine and aspirin. J Am Coll Cardiol 7:251–269, 1986.

86. Oates JA, Wood AJ: Dipyridamole. N Engl J Med 316:1247–1257, 1987.

87. Temple R, Pledger GW: The FDA's critique of the anturance reinfarction trial. N Engl J Med 303:1488–1492, 1980.

CHAPTER 40

THROMBOEMBOLIC DISEASE

STEVEN R. KAYSER, Pharm.D.

A prudent clinical approach to the management of thromboembolic disease depends upon a thorough understanding of and familiarity with the pharmacology of antithrombotic drugs. Recent national conferences on antithrombotic therapy sponsored by the American College of Chest Physicians have reevaluated many aspects of antithrombotic therapy and developed guidelines that may lead to more effective and safer use of antithrombotic drugs (1–3).

Presently however, arterial and venous thromboembolic disease still accounts for substantial morbidity and mortality and is costly in terms of healthcare dollars. Advances in the prevention of thrombotic diseases may be helpful in decreasing these.

ETIOLOGY

Many conditions contribute to the development of thromboembolic disease (Table 40.1). In general, any condition or combination of conditions leading to activation of blood coagulation, venous stasis, or damage to the vascular wall places a patient at risk for the development of a clot.

Immobilization and bed rest, with resultant stasis, frequently contribute to thrombosis, especially in elderly and obese persons. Prolonged partial occlusion of the veins in any person sitting for prolonged periods may also lead to stasis. A hypercoagulable state existing during the operative period may contribute to clotting. Trauma may initiate clotting and thus is a particular problem in patients suffering fractures of the hips and pelvis, who may also require prolonged bed rest. Congestive heart failure, ulcerative colitis, myocardial infarction, and other high-risk medical illnesses are associated with an increased risk of thrombosis. Carcinomas, particularly pancreatic, bronchogenic, gastric, and prostatic, may produce procoagulant substances that initiate clotting. The increased activity of many clotting factors during pregnancy contributes to an increased risk of thrombosis. Oral contraceptives have likewise been associated with an increased risk of clotting. Less frequently, some unusual blood diseases and hereditary causes have been associated with thrombosis (4, 5).

PATHOGENESIS

When injury occurs to the vascular endothelium, platelets adhere to exposed collagen as well as to other exposed subendothelial tissue. Following platelet adhesion, release of adenosine diphosphate (ADP) by the injured platelets leads to platelet aggregation (Fig. 40-1). Transformation of this temporary platelet plug to a permanent platelet fibrin clot is achieved through activation of the extrinsic or intrinsic blood clotting system (Fig. 40.2).

Throughout this process of platelet aggregation, a balance is maintained between certain prostaglandins that occur naturally and may be synthesized in vivo. Thromboxane A2 is found in platelets and is a potent stimulant for platelet aggregation, as well as a potent vasoconstrictor. Prostacyclin, in contrast, is found in vessel walls and is an inhibitor of platelet aggregation, as well as a vasodilator. Not only may the balance between prostacyclin and thromboxane be altered physiologically, but various drugs and even different doses of these drugs (e.g., aspirin) may alter this balance.

Each of the clotting factors circulates in the blood as an inactive protein. Before clotting can occur, each must be converted to an active or enzymatic form. Exposure of subendothelial collagen, in addition to interaction with platelets, initiates the intrinsic pathway by stimulating the activation of factor XII. Activated factor XII then stimulates the conversion of factor XI to the active form, which then stimulates activation of factor IX. Activated factor IX, in the presence of calcium, phospholipids (platelet factor 3), and factor VIII, stimulates the conversion of factor X to its active form. Activated factor X, in the presence of calcium, phospholipid (platelet factor 3), and factor V, stimulates the conversion of prothrombin to thrombin.

The extrinsic clotting pathway may also stimulate the

Table 40.1.
Conditions Associated with Venous Thromboembolism

Immobilization, especially in elderly and obese
Stasis
Surgery and the postoperative period
Trauma to lower limbs
High-risk medical illnesses
   Congestive heart failure
   Ulcerative colitis
   Myocardial infarction
Carcinoma of the pancreas, lung, stomach, and prostate
Pregnancy and contraceptives
Blood diseases
Heredity

conversion of prothrombin to thrombin. The release of material extrinsic to the blood, such as tissue extract or tissue thromboplastin, activates factor VII, which stimulates the activation of factor X. Factor X thus occupies a central position at the junction of the extrinsic and intrinsic systems.

Thrombin, which is generated by both pathways, stimulates the conversion of fibrinogen to fibrin in the presence ionized calcium. The initial soluble fibrin clot is further converted to an insoluble fibrin polymer when factor XIII is activated by thrombin. In addition to stimulating the conversion of fibrinogen to fibrin, thrombin stimulates platelet aggregation and potentiates the activity of factors V, VIIa, VII, and Xa.

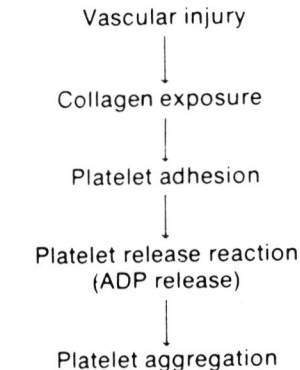

Figure 40.1. Formation of platelet plug.

Once thrombin is formed, it is partly removed by absorption into fibrin. This, plus other naturally occurring inhibitors of clotting factors, plays a role in localizing fibrin formation to the sites of injury and in maintaining the fluidity of circulating blood. Agents in normal blood inhibit the activated forms of factors II, X, XI, and XII. Deposition of fibrin also activates plasmin or fibrinolysin, a fibrinolytic enzyme that prevents excessive coagulation (Fig. 40.3).

Two types of thrombi are formed in response to appropriate stimuli. "White thrombi" or arterial thrombi are composed primarily of platelets, although they also contain fibrin and occasional leukocytes. They generally occur in areas of rapid blood flow and are formed in response to an injured or abnormal vessel wall. "Red thrombi" or venous thrombi are found primarily in areas of relative stasis, where dilution of activated clotting factors by blood flow prevented. They are almost completely composed of fibrin and erythrocytes, with a small number of platelets.

The choice of an antithrombotic drug is influenced by the type of thrombus. Heparin and the coumarins are used in the treatment of both "red" and "white" thrombi. Drugs affecting platelet behavior are still being studied for their effects in preventing and treating "white thrombi." Fibrinolytic agents dissolve both types of thrombi.

INDICATIONS FOR THERAPY

Thromboembolism may be associated with a large number of different conditions. Antithrombotic therapy has demonstrated a marked benefit for deep venous thrombosis,

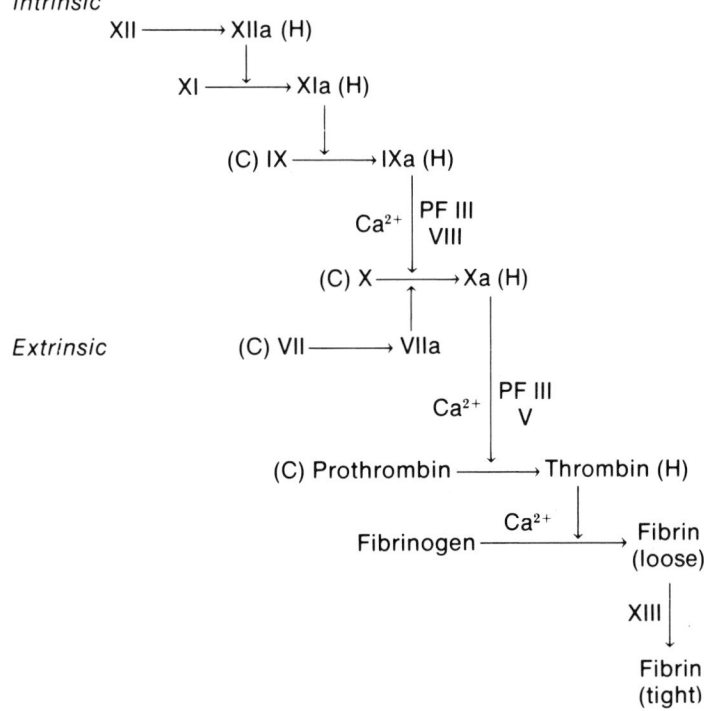

Figure 40.2. Soluble clotting cascade.

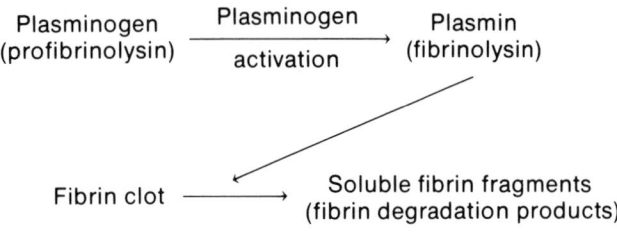

Figure 40.3.   Fibrinolysis.

Table 40.2.
Indications for Anticoagulant Therapy

Established benefit
  Deep venous thrombosis
  Pulmonary embolism
  Acute coronary syndromes, e.g., unstable angina, acute myocardial infarction
  Cerebral embolism associated with atrial fibrillation
  Atrial fibrillation
  Post-cardiac-valve replacement
  Acute peripheral arterial embolism
Other possible indications
  Congestive heart failure
  Transient ischemic attacks
  Disseminated intravascular coagulation (consumption coagulopathy)
  Prophylaxis of venous thromboembolism following hip surgery

pulmonary embolism, acute coronary syndromes (unstable angina, acute myocardial infarction), cerebral embolism associated with atrial fibrillation, atrial fibrillation, prophylaxis of thromboembolism following cardiac valve replacement, and peripheral arterial embolism. Other conditions where antithrombotic therapy may be useful include congestive heart failure, transient ischemic attacks, disseminated intravascular coagulation (consumption coagulopathy), and the prophylaxis of deep venous thrombosis following hip fractures. The selection of an antiplatelet, anticoagulant, or fibrinolytic agent depends upon the pathology of the disorder (Table 40.2).

Deep Venous Thrombosis and Pulmonary Embolism

The clinical diagnosis of deep venous thrombosis (DVT) is difficult and frequently misleading, with most venous clots occurring without prominent findings. Nevertheless, certain clinical signs are helpful. In 80% of cases of DVT reviewed, unilateral ankle edema was present, followed by calf tenderness in 50%, and a positive Homan's sign (pain upon dorsiflexion of the foot) in only 8%. Increased warmth and calf swelling are also consistent with DVT (6, 7).

Deep venous thrombi occur most frequently in the lower extremities, in association with one or more of the previously discussed risk factors. The progression of thrombosis in the calf veins to the iliofemoral system in the thigh is associated with a greater risk of pulmonary embolism. Early recognition and documentation of lower leg thrombosis is necessary to prevent pulmonary embolism.

The clinical manifestations of pulmonary embolism may include fever, pleuritic chest pain, hemoptysis, tachypnea, tachycardia, and shortness of breath. Electrocardiographic manifestations may include changes in the S-T segment and T waves. Chest x-rays are usually not very helpful. Arterial blood gases generally show a reduced pO_2 as well as a decreased pCO_2 caused by hyperventilation.

Objectively, the diagnosis of DVT may be confirmed by phlebography, impedance plethysmography (IPG), Doppler ultrasound, or radionuclide-labeled fibrinogen studies. Pulmonary embolism may be detected more specifically with the aid of pulmonary perfusion and ventilation scans and pulmonary angiography.

The effectiveness of anticoagulant therapy in proximal vein thrombosis is well established. The choice of heparin or fibrinolytic therapy depends upon the severity of symptoms and is discussed later in this chapter. Treatment of distal (calf) vein thrombosis is more controversial, and while most clinicians treat with heparin, this practice is not supported by all authors. The use of support stockings properly fitted for the patient, heat and elevation, and nonsteroidal antiinflammatory agents (NSAIDS) may be just as helpful for the treatment of calf-vein thrombosis. In either case if heparin is used, NSAIDS must be used cautiously, because they are potentially ulcerogenic and influence platelet function. Prompt treatment of pulmonary embolism is essential with heparin and or fibrinolytics because of the morbidity and mortality associated with it (8).

Cerebral Embolism

Acute vascular events leading to stroke may be embolic or hemorrhagic. Embolic etiologies account for 85% of strokes, and hemorrhagic events account for the remaining 15%. An accurate diagnosis must be made before therapy is initiated (9).

Anticoagulant therapy may be useful in preventing the recurrence of emboli responsible for strokes or in the treatment of evolving strokes or transient ischemic attacks. There is no place for anticoagulant therapy in the treatment of a completed stroke because of the risk of hemorrhage into the infarcted area, which could then lead to extension of neurologic damage.

Atrial Fibrillation

The prevention of stroke in patients with atrial fibrillation is important because the first stroke may be very debilitating. The primary source of cardioembolism is nonvalvular atrial fibrillation, which accounts for 45% of all cases. This is followed by ischemic heart disease which accounts for 15%, ventricular aneurysm 10%, rheumatic heart disease 10%, prosthetic heart valves 10%, and idiopathic sources 10%. The overall incidence of arterial thromboembolism varies, based upon several criteria, the most important being the presence of comorbid conditions. Patients at highest risk include those with anterior wall myocardial infarction, pedunculated thrombus located in the heart chamber, congestive heart failure, history of prior embolism, mitral stenosis, prosthetic heart valves, or bacterial endocarditis. Patients at lesser risk include those without a history of any of the above conditions, lone atrial fibrillation, mitral valve prolapse, or mild annular calcifications.

Anticoagulant treatment of patients at high risk is indicated. Treatment of patients with atrial fibrillation associated with nonvalvular heart disease has been more controversial. Recently, three studies have provided convincing evidence for the efficacy of anticoagulant therapy in these patients (10–12). The first trial to be published, the AFASAK trial (10) or Atrial Fibrillation, Aspirin, Anticoagulation study, investigated the role of aspirin, placebo, or high-dose warfarin therapy (international normalized ratio (INR) 2.8–4.2) in the prevention of stroke in patients with nonrheumatic valvular heart disease. The results strongly suggested that warfarin, but not aspirin (75 mg per day) or placebo, was effective in the prevention of stroke. The results were not statistically significant. The Stroke Prevention in Atrial Fibrillation (SPAF) study (11) and the Boston Area Anticoagulation Trial for Atrial Fibrillation (BAATAF) study (12) have provided statistically significant data that demonstrate the efficacy of warfarin in prevention of stroke in patients with nonvalvular heart disease. The SPAF study investigated the use of aspirin (325 mg q.d.) and warfarin (INR 1.7–4.6) individually, versus placebo. Patients followed up to a mean of 1.3 years demonstrated a 41% reduction in primary events (ischemic stroke and systemic embolism) with aspirin and a 67% reduction with warfarin. The trial is continuing to compare warfarin with aspirin, since too few events occurred to obtain definitive results. Aspirin did not appear to work in a subgroup of patients over 75 years of age. The incidence of bleeding requiring hospital admission and transfusion was greater in the warfarin group (1.7%, vs aspirin 0.9%, vs placebo 1.2%) and the incidence of cerebral bleeding was greater (0.4% vs 0.2% in both groups). The BAATAF study investigated the use of warfarin (adjusted to an INR 1.5–2.7) versus controls who were not given warfarin, but who could take aspirin. The results demonstrated an 86% reduction in the risk of stroke for patients taking warfarin over the average 2.2 years of follow-up. Patients receiving warfarin had a higher incidence of minor bleeding, but the incidence of major bleeding was the same in both groups.

Chronic anticoagulation with warfarin can be recommended for most patients with atrial fibrillation unless contraindicated. Evidence suggests that less intense therapy is effective and that anticoagulation to an INR (international normalized ratio) of 2.0–3.0 is adequate (see subsequent discussion of INR).

Myocardial Infarction

As early as 1948, the American Heart Association recommended anticoagulant therapy for patients who suffered a myocardial infarction. This has not been accepted universally as a treatment regimen. Inconsistent trial results, statistically significant but small clinical reductions in outcome, the availability of newer treatment regimens, the overall reduction in control group mortality, and the fear of bleeding may explain this reluctance.

The rationale for treatment with anticoagulants in acute myocardial infarction is to decrease mortality, decrease reinfarction, decrease systemic emboli, and decrease venous thromboembolism. The overall frequency of cerebral emboli in acute myocardial infarction is approximately 4%. The incidence of serious sequelae following these strokes may be very significant, with severe deficiency or death occurring in over half.

Several recent publications have provided stronger evidence favoring the use of anticoagulants in the treatment of acute myocardial infarction. Yusuf pooled the results from previous studies, subjected them to rigorous review, and concluded that there is on average a 22% reduction in mortality in patients receiving anticoagulant therapy (13). Smith randomized patients to warfarin (INR 2.8–4.8) or placebo within an average of 27 days following acute myocardial infarction regardless of site (anterior 47%, inferior 44%) and followed them for an average of 37 months. Overall there was a risk reduction of 24% for death, 34% for reinfarction, and 55% for cerebrovascular accident in the warfarin group, compared with placebo. The incidence of major bleeding was higher in the warfarin group and was often associated with underlying lesions (e.g., malignancy) or use of unauthorized antiplatelet drug therapy (14).

Antithrombotic agents are also useful in the management of unstable angina (see discussion in following sections) and in the acute stage of myocardial infarction. Aspirin and heparin decrease the incidence of subsequent infarction and death when used in unstable angina. Fibrinolytic therapy with streptokinase (SK), anisoylated plasminogen-streptokinse-activator complex (APSAC or anistreptlase), or recombinant tissue plasminogen activator (rt-PA or alteplase) in the acute phase of myocardial infarction reperfuses ischemic myocardium, decreases mortality, and preserves myocardial function. (See also further discussion in following sections.)

Heart Valve Prosthesis

Thromboembolism is one of the most frequent complications in survivors of prosthetic valve replacements. The greatest risk of embolism is to the brain. Patients with mechanical heart-valve prostheses should receive lifelong anticoagulation with oral agents such as warfarin. Bioprosthetic valves may offer some patients the option of not requiring long-term anticoagulation. For those receiving bioprosthetic valves in the aortic position, treatment with heparin for 7 to 10 days, followed by low-dose aspirin, may be adequate. Patients with bioprosthetic valves in the mitral position should receive oral anticoagulant for 3 months and then receive aspirin (15).

The addition of an antiplatelet agent to an oral anticoagulant regimen may protect against clotting in patients who develop systemic embolism despite therapeutic prothrombin times. Both aspirin and dipyridamole may be useful, but aspirin is associated with an increased incidence of bleeding.

Patients who receive anticoagulants should be followed closely to assure adequate intensity and control, since patients receiving anticoagulants who sustain an embolus are likely to have had inadequate anticoagulation.

TREATMENT OF THROMBOEMBOLIC DISEASE

Nonpharmacologic measures that contribute to the successful prevention or treatment of thromboembolic disease include proper education, use of support garments, and (infrequently) surgery.

Individualized patient education is important in an overall treatment plan. Prevention of stasis by avoiding prolonged sitting, leg crossing, or wearing constricting garments is extremely important. Properly fitted and prescribed support stockings are helpful. Embolectomy or surgical placement of an inferior vena cava umbrella is occasionally performed.

Heparin and the oral anticoagulants (primarily coumarins in the United States) are the major pharmacologic agents used in the treatment of clotting disorders.

Prevention of the interaction of platelets with the arterial wall and subsequent microthrombosis and microembolization from these sites with antiplatelet agents is useful. Drugs accelerating fibrinolysis increase the rate of resolution of emboli.

PHARMACOLOGIC TREATMENT OF THROMBOEMBOLIC DISEASE

Anticoagulant Therapy

LABORATORY ASSESSMENT

Laboratory assessment of anticoagulant therapy was thought by some early clinicians to be superfluous. Since response to a given dose of heparin or warfarin is highly variable, laboratory tests are now considered essential for monitoring for both hemorrhage or recurrent embolization.

Among the various tests available, the most commonly used ones are the prothrombin time (PT), the activated partial thromboplastin time (APTT), and the activated coagulation time (ACT), which is also called activated clotting time (Table 40.3). (*Note:* In most clinical laboratories the APTT has replaced the partial thromboplastin time (PTT). Only the APTT will be referred to subsequently.)

The prothrombin time of Quick is prolonged by deficiencies of factors V, VII, X, and II, by low levels of fibrinogen, and by high levels of heparin. The PT thus reflects alterations in the extrinsic and common pathways. A normal PT is approximately 11 sec. Prothrombin times are occasionally reported in percentage activity as determined by dilution of plasma. This should be avoided because of the risk of confusing a PT in seconds with percentage activity. They are not the same, and misinterpretation could lead to inappropriate changes in therapy. The PT is used to assess coumarin therapy.

Because of the variability in sensitivity of the thromboplastin reagent used in determining the prothrombin time, results from different laboratories usually differ. The ratio of the patient's prothrombin time to the laboratory control will subsequently differ among laboratories. To standardize interpretation of the intensity of anticoagulation, European investigators adopted the international normalized ratio (INR) in 1983. A World Health Organization primary international reference preparation of thromboplastin is used to standardize the commercial source of thromboplastin used by a given laboratory. The INR is calculated by raising the calculated PT ratio, PT of the patient/PT control from the laboratory, to the power of the international sensitivity index (ISI), which is assigned to each batch of thromboplastin. (INR = (PT patient/PT control) raised to the ISI.) For example, patient/ PT of 22 sec, control PT time of 11 sec, equals a ratio of 2 when raised to an ISI of 2, is equal to an INR of 4; i.e., 22/11 raised to the power of 2 = 4. Thromboplastin sources that are less sensitive have lower ISIs. This relationship has not only standardized interpretation of laboratory results but also has led to appreciation that less intense anticoagulation is often as effective as more intense treatment but is associated with a lower incidence of bleeding (16–19) (See Table 40.4 for recommendations for the intensity of anticoagulation).

The APTT is primarily a measure of the competency of the intrinsic and common clotting pathways. It is insensitive to factor VII and XIII. It is used in screening for deficiencies of the intrinsic clotting system in patients considered candidates for oral anticoagulation and in monitoring the response to heparin therapy. The APTT differs

Table 40.3.
Clotting Tests Used in the Management of Anticoagulant Therapy

Test	Factors Measured	Normal Value[a]	Drug Monitored
Prothrombin time (PT)	II, V, VII, X	11 sec	Warfarin
Activated partial thromboplastin time[b] (APTT)	All except VII	24–36 sec	Heparin (warfarin)
Activated coagulation time (ACT)[c]	All except VII	80–130 sec	Heparin

[a] University of California, San Francisco.
[b] May also be prolonged by warfarin.
[c] Also known as activated clotting time.

Table 40.4.
Relative Intensity of Anticoagulant Therapy[a]

Indication	International Normalized Ratio[b]
Prophylaxis of venous thrombosis	2.0–3.0
Treatment of venous thrombosis	2.0–3.0
Treatment of pulmonary embolism	2.0–3.0
Prevention of systemic embolism in patients with tissue valves	2.0–3.0
Acute myocardial infarction	2.0–3.0
Atrial fibrillation (valvular and nonvalvular)	2.0–3.0
Cerebral embolism	2.0–3.0
Congestive heart failure(?)	2.0–3.0
Mechanical heart valves	3.0–4.5
Recurrent systemic embolism	3.0–4.5

[a] Adapted from Hirsh J, Poller L, Deykin D, et al.: Optimal therapeutic range for oral anticoagulants. Chest 95(suppl 2):5S–11S, 1989.
[b] A prothrombin time ratio of 1.4–1.7 is approximately equivalent to an international normalized ratio of 2.0–3.0, where the thromboplastin has an international sensitivity index of 2. A ratio of 1.75–2.1 is equivalent to an INR of 3–4.5 for the same thromboplastin.

from the PTT only in being performed on activated plasma. It is generally a more sensitive test than the PTT. The APTT is performed with platelet-poor plasma and so does not reflect the activity of platelets. Normal values for the APTT are between 24 and 36 sec. Therapeutic heparinization is considered the dosage required to prolong the APTT to between 60 and 80 sec (see also Table 40.5).

The ACT of whole blood is sensitive to all clotting factors except factor VII, with undetermined sensitivity to factors V and II. The major advantage of this test is that it is a whole blood test; it does reflect the contribution of platelets in coagulation. The ACT is used to monitor heparin therapy, and normal values are 80 to 130 sec (18).

Disadvantages associated with the ACT include relatively limited experience with this test in monitoring anticoagulation by heparin therapy and lack of correlation with the APTT. The APTT thus remains the standard for the management of therapeutic doses of heparin.

DURATION

Little agreement exists regarding the optimal duration of anticoagulant therapy in the treatment of acute throm-

boembolic events such as deep venous thrombi or pulmonary embolism. The greatest risk for reembolization is immediately after an initial event. The risk decreases over the next 6 to 8 weeks, and it is during this period that adequate therapy is essential. After acute events, most clinicians continue anticoagulants for 6 weeks to 3 months (20). Most evidence supports treatment for 4 to 6 weeks for an initial event (21).

Treatment of recurrent embolic events or prophylaxis of emboli in patients with prosthetic heart valves continues longer and may be for life.

Heparin

MECHANISM OF ACTION

Heparin, a rapid-acting anticoagulant, exerts its antithrombotic effect by accelerating the action of a naturally occurring inhibitor of thrombin, an α_2-globulin, antithrombin III (AT III). Antithrombin III inhibits activated clotting factors that have a reactive serine residue at their enzymatically active center. Heparin, by binding at the lysine group of AT III (Fig. 40.4), induces a conformational change in AT III that allows more ready access of the arginine residue to the serine group on the activated clotting factors (22, 23).

Commercial heparin is obtained from hog mucosa or bovine lung. The anticoagulant activity of heparin from both sources appears to be equivalent. Differences may exist in the rate of thrombocytopenia, which appears to be greater with heparin of bovine lung origin. Because of this difference, the heparin source within an institution should be standardized (24).

Low-molecular-weight heparin, which has a longer half-life than standard heparin preparations, is presently under investigation and may be associated with a lower incidence of bleeding when administered in doses equivalent to the standard preparations (25).

PHARMACOKINETICS

Heparin is not absorbed orally and therefore must be administered parenterally. It is usually administered intravenously, with subcutaneous administration reserved for

Table 40.5.
General Guidelines for Heparin Administration

This information for therapeutic intravenous heparinization of adult patients is intended as a general guide only.
BEFORE BEGINNING HEPARIN THERAPY:
1. Order a STAT activated partial thromboplastin time (APTT); prothrombin time (PT), and platelet count.
2. Review current medications for:
   a. *i.m. injections:* Write an order that no i.m. injections be given while the patient is receiving anticoagulant therapy. If the patient is receiving a medication by the i.m. route, discontinue it, and if necessary, order the medication by another appropriate route or use an alternative.
   b. *Drugs inhibiting platelet function:* Avoid medications that may alter platelet function, especially aspirin, indomethacin, sulfinpyrazone, and dipyridamole. If a patient is receiving a medication known to alter platelet function, discontinue it, and if necessary, select an appropriate alternative. There are occasional therapeutic situations where a drug affecting platelet function may be indicated, in this event a statement should be included in the chart documenting this.
   c. *Known drugs that interact with heparin or warfarin.*
INITIATION OF HEPARIN THERAPY:
1. A typical bolus (loading) dose of heparin is 70–100 U/kg (dose to nearest 1000 U)
2. The initial bolus and infusion dose may require adjustment in the following conditions:

Increased	*Decreased*
Massive embolism	Recent bleeding history
	Age greater than 70
	Hematologic disorders resulting in
	bleeding tendencies
	Prior antithrombotic therapy
	Recent surgery (within 10 days)

3. Begin continuous infusion at that same time as the bolus administration. (See Maintenance Heparin Therapy No. 1 below for dosing information.)
MAINTENANCE HEPARIN THERAPY:
1. The usual beginning maintenance infusion rate is 10–15 U/kg/hr for DVT and 25 U kg/hr for pulmonary embolism. Order heparin as "Heparin Infusion ____ units per hour." Use a standardized heparin concentration of 15,000 U/250 ml D₅W. All heparin infusions must be delivered with an infusion device. Dosing sheets should be provided along with the solution.
2. Obtain a second APTT 4–6 hr after the bolus dose is given and the continuous infusion has begun.
3. Aim to achieve a therapeutic APTT of 60–80 sec.
4. Depending on the APTT value, a change in regimen may be necessary. Typical adjustments are as follows:
   a. <40 sec, re-bolus 100 U/kg and increase infusion by 200 U/hr
   b. 40–60 sec, re-bolus 50 U/kg and increase infusion by 100 U/hr
   c. 60–80 sec, maintain the current rate of infusion
   d. 80–100 sec, decrease infusion by 100 U/hr
   e. 100–135 sec, stop infusion for 1–2 hr and decrease infusion by 200 U/hr
   f. >135 sec stop infusion until APTT is within 60–80 sec, and decrease infusion by 300 U hr
   Note: If bleeding occurs at any time (regardless of APTT), discontinue heparin and treat appropriately
5. Obtain a repeat APTT approximately 6 hr after any dosage change.
6. Obtain an APTT daily when patient is stable.
GENERAL
1. Obtain CBC and platelets every other day, and a stool guiaic and urinalysis every third day.
2. Examine all sites (skin, nose, throat, urine, stool) for bleeding daily.
3. Begin oral anticoagulant therapy, usually within the first or second day of heparin therapy (*Note:* continuous infusion of heparin may cause a 1–3-sec prolongation of the PT.)

---

prophylactic, "low-dose" use. Heparin should not be given intramuscularly because of the risk of hematoma.

Once absorbed, heparin is bound to a number of plasma proteins. It is metabolized primarily in the liver and reticuloendothelial system and is partly eliminated by excretion into the urine.

The half-life of the anticoagulant effect of heparin in normal persons and in patients with venous thromboembolism, as measured by changes in APTT, is approximately 1.5 hr. The half-life, when plasma heparin activity is measured, depends upon the dose and increases with an in-creased dose. Limited studies show that patients with pulmonary embolism have a greater heparin clearance and shorter half-life than those with venous thrombosis. This may be due to the continuing thrombin formation on the surface of the embolus, leading to an increased rate of heparin clearance (26, 27).

DOSING AND ADMINISTRATION

Intravenous administration of a large bolus dose of heparin assures that therapeutic anticoagulation is achieved without delay. Initial doses of at least 50 to 100 U/kg of body

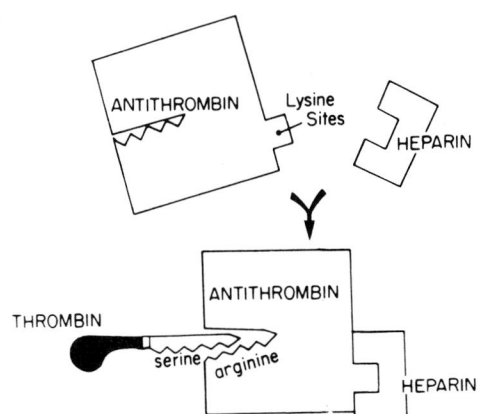

Figure 40.4. Model of heparin-induced conformation change in antithrombin, resulting in rapid inhibition of thrombin. (Reprinted, by permission of the New England Journal of Medicine from Rosenberg RD: Actions and interactions of antithrombin and heparin. N Engl J Med 292:146, 1975.)

weight are needed to overcome the initial resistance during early thromboembolic disease. Following an initial bolus dose, heparin is continued by intermittent or continuous intravenous administration.

General dosing guidelines can be applied to subsequent changes in the APTT (Table 40.5).

Prior to the initiation of heparin, baseline clotting studies must be performed and should include at least the prothrombin time (in anticipation of oral anticoagulant therapy) and the APTT or ACT.

Continuous infusion of heparin is the desired route of administration because it avoids the wide swings in heparin concentration and thus the periods of supratherapeutic and subtherapeutic anticoagulation seen with intermittent administration. In addition, with continuous infusion, less heparin is required, and laboratory tests for anticoagulation may be performed at any time. One disadvantage is that the rate must be controlled with an infusion pump. The usual dose needed to maintain the APTT from 1.5 to 2.5 times the control is 1000 U/hr. However, this must be adjusted, based upon individual response.

Intermittent infusion, although not requiring an infusion pump, has numerous disadvantages. Larger doses and frequent injections are required. Laboratory tests may be performed only at certain times for proper interpretation. In addition, intermittent infusion, with or without laboratory control, is associated with more bleeding than continuous infusion to an APTT of 1.5 to 2.5 times the control.

The initial resistance to heparin therapy returns to normal within several days; reductions in dose should be anticipated. Laboratory tests should be performed frequently in the beginning and at least daily thereafter.

Heparin therapy has generally been continued for 7 to 10 days following a thromboembolic event, since it is during this time that the incidence of recurrence is the greatest. Shorter-course therapy may be as efficacious in the treatment of proximal vein thrombosis. Treatment for 5 days versus 10 days was compared in patients with proximal vein thrombosis, and a similar incidence of recurrent venous thromboembolism was noted (7.1% vs 7.0%). Both therapies were followed with warfarin therapy for 12 weeks. Additional evidence is required before shorter-course therapy can be recommended for patients with thromboembolism at other sites.

Subcutaneous heparin administration is normally reserved for "low-dose" or "minidose" therapy. Small amounts of the initial coagulation enzymes (activated factors XII, XI, and IX) eventually lead to large amounts of thrombin. Heparin in relatively low concentrations can prevent this initiation of clotting, while much higher levels of heparin are required to inhibit fibrin formation after thrombin has been generated. Heparin in low subcutaneous doses especially augments the activity of an inhibitor of activated factor X. This inhibitor of factor Xa is probably AT III.

Most experience in the use of low-dose heparin has been accumulated in the prophylaxis of venous thromboembolism and pulmonary embolism during the surgical period and provides the strongest evidence for the efficacy of this route (29). The results show clinically significant benefits in the reduction of venous thrombosis and pulmonary embolism. Low-dose heparin is associated with a small risk of bleeding.

Heparin is most effective in elective gynecologic and abdominothoracic surgery. The efficacy in patients undergoing elective orthopaedic surgery has been less well established. A recent review of randomized trials of perioperative heparin and its impact on reduction of fatal pulmonary embolism and venous thromboembolism following general, orthopaedic and urologic surgery demonstrates a decrease in the incidence of deep venous thrombosis, pulmonary embolism, and death from pulmonary embolism (29).

Certain high-risk medical patients such as those with congestive heart failure, myocardial infarction, or malignancy may also benefit, with a decrease in pulmonary embolism and subsequent mortality (30).

Administration regimens generally include 5,000 to 10,000 U subcutaneously from 12 to 2 hr preoperatively, followed by 5,000 to 10,000 U every 8 to 12 hr postoperatively or until the patient is ambulatory. Although the APTT may be moderately elevated for several hours following administration, laboratory monitoring is not necessary following initial assessment of clotting status.

Low-dose warfarin has been investigated for its role in prevention of venous thrombosis after elective total hip or knee replacement. Doses of warfarin sufficient to prolong the prothrombin time by 1 to 3 sec were started 1 to 2 weeks preoperatively. This regimen was followed by doses increased to prolong the prothrombin time 1.5 times control immediately after surgery. A decrease in the incidence of venous thrombosis to 21% was observed. Further study with an appropriate control group is required to confirm this observation (31).

In a group of medical and surgical patients, more traditional low-dose heparin (5,000 to 10,000 units every 12 hr) without laboratory adjustment is as effective as warfarin in the prevention of recurrent calf vein thrombosis, but it is not as effective as warfarin in the prevention of recurrent proximal vein thrombosis (32).

Adjusted subcutaneous heparin therapy has recently been compared to warfarin therapy in the treatment of DVT and pulmonary embolus. Heparin in doses adequate to prolong the midinterval APTT to 1.5 times the control value was administered to one group of patients, while another group received warfarin in traditional doses. Both groups initially received high-dose intravenous heparin for 14 days. Recurrent proximal vein thromboembolism was prevented in both groups: the frequency of bleeding was greater in patients on warfarin (33).

ADVERSE REACTIONS

Hemorrhage is the most frequent adverse reaction to heparin and is generally, but not always, associated with clotting tests outside the recognized therapeutic range. Spontaneous bleeding is rare (34).

Minor hemorrhage occurs in approximately 4% of courses of anticoagulant therapy, usually into the skin or urine or from the nose. Major hemorrhagic events occur in approximately 2% of courses, usually in the gastrointestinal tract or the central nervous system.

Other adverse effects include thrombocytopenia (35), osteoporosis, hypoaldosteronism (36), and generalized hypersensitivity reactions. Thrombocytopenia secondary to heparin appears during the first 3 to 12 days of therapy, is unrelated to dose, and reverses within 3 to 5 days following discontinuation. It may occur in 5 to 10% of patients and can occur with therapeutic intravenous or prophylactic subcutaneous administration. The exact mechanism has not been established. Osteoporosis occurs with therapy of more than 10,000 U/day for 6 months or longer. Hypoaldosteronism with resultant hyperkalemia and sodium diuresis is uncommonly associated with heparin therapy.

DRUG INTERACTIONS

A direct interaction between heparin and nitroglycerin has been proposed as a mechanism for increased heparin requirements seen in some patients receiving both drugs concomitantly (37). This has not been a universal obser-vation however and a recent controlled trial provides evidence that there is no interference with nitroglycerin doses below 350 μg/min. At doses of nitroglycerin above 350 μg/min, a higher dose of heparin was required to achieve the same prolongation of the APTT. The proposed mechanism is a qualitative antithrombin III abnormality induced by nitroglycerin (38). Close patient monitoring is required, and any resistance can be overcome with appropriate dosage adjustments. Heparin is physically incompatible with many other drugs, and appropriate sources should be consulted before heparin is mixed with other solutions.

Drugs impairing platelet function should be avoided in patients receiving heparin since they further impair hemostasis (Table 40.5). However, there are certain situations where concomitant therapy is recommended.

TREATMENT OF OVERDOSE

Protamine sulfate, a strongly basic molecule, is a specific antidote that combines with and inactivates heparin. The appropriate dose of protamine depends upon the dose of heparin, the time since administration, and the route of administration. If administered immediately after intravenous heparin, 1 mg of protamine is given for every 100 U of heparin. If treatment is delayed, the dose of protamine must be decreased. Response can be assessed with the APTT or ACT.

Protamine has been reported to exert an anticoagulant effect if administered in excessive dosages. Clinically this is unlikely to be a problem. Of greater concern are the cardiovascular complications that may be associated with protamine. A decrease in blood pressure and systemic vascular resistance has been observed in humans. This appears to be associated most often with too rapid administration. Anaphylactoid reactions may occur in 2 to 5% of patients (39).

In the event of a major hemorrhage, whole blood or fresh frozen plasma should replace lost volume and clotting factors.

Oral Anticoagulants

Of the oral anticoagulants available in the United States, only warfarin and bishydroxycoumarin are used extensively.

Oral anticoagulants exert their pharmacologic effect by interfering with the synthesis of the vitamin K–dependent clotting factors in the liver. These factors and II, VII, IX, and X. Early investigators assumed a competitive antagonism to explain the relationship between warfarin and vitamin K. The has since been disproven. Presently it is believed that warfarin inhibits the effect of vitamin K at a postribosomal step in the hepatic synthesis of the vitamin K–dependent clotting factors. Vitamin K is required in the conversion of nonactive precursor proteins (precursors of active clotting factors), which lack calcium-binding capacity, to active precursor proteins (e.g., prothrombin) that have calcium-binding capacity. This calcium-binding capacity is needed to hold prothrombin onto phospholipid surfaces during its activation to thrombin. Vitamin K accomplishes this activation by carboxylation of glutamyl residues on the precursor protein to form γ-carboxyglutamic acid, which allows for calcium binding. Vitamin K probably carboxylates the glutamyl residues of factors VII, IX, and X. During the carboxylation of precursor proteins, vitamin K is converted to vitamin K epoxide. Vitamin K epoxide is then converted back to vitamin K. Warfarin prevents this reaction and thus produces a buildup of inactive precursor proteins. This effect of warfarin can be overcome by the administration of vitamin K (40).

The onset of anticoagulant effect of the coumarins depends not only on this interaction with vitamin K, but also on the metabolic clearance of clotting factors already present in the blood.

PHARMACOKINETICS

Warfarin is the most frequently administered oral anticoagulant in the United States. There are few exceptions where other agents should be used, since the pharmacokinetics of warfarin have been the most extensively studied. Warfarin is completely absorbed in the upper gastrointestinal tract, with peak blood levels occurring in 60 to 120 min. The volume of distribution (V_d) of warfarin is 12.5% of body weight. This small V_d is consistent with the extensive binding of warfarin to albumin, since it is equivalent to the V_d of albumin, 2.6 times the plasma volume.

The mean half-life of warfarin is independent of dose and is 42 hr (39). Warfarin is highly protein bound, on the order of 99.5%, to serum albumin. No apparent relationship exists between the extent of protein binding of warfarin and the concentration of albumin or total protein in the serum. Furthermore, there appears to be no correlation between the effect on prothrombin time and the dose of warfarin.

Warfarin is metabolized in the hepatic microsomes by mixed-function oxidase enzymes. It is administered as a racemate that contains equal parts of the R and S isomer. The S isomer is approximately five times more potent than the R isomer.

The reason why the R and S isomers differ in potency is unclear. The half-life of the R isomer is 45 hr, whereas the half-life of the S isomer is 33 hr, and they both have the same volume of distribution. It has been proposed that differences in permeability of affinity to the receptor site account for the differing potencies.

Knowledge of these two isomers is important because drugs interact with warfarin stereoselectively. Phenylbutazone and metronidazole inhibit the metabolism of the S isomer but have no effect on the R isomer (41).

DOSING

Oral anticoagulant therapy should be initiated without a loading dose. Many clinicians have traditionally started therapy with a large initial dose, followed by smaller doses over subsequent days. The belief was that therapeutic anticoagulation would be achieved more quickly.

The onset of the effect of warfarin depends not only upon the half-life of the parent drug but also upon the half-life of catabolism of the vitamin K–dependent clotting factors. These factors have half-lives of 5 hr for factor VII, 20 to 40 hr for factors IX and X, and up to 60 hr for factor II. Depression of any factor may predispose the patient to bleeding.

O'Reilly and Aggeler compared a loading dose of warfarin, 1.5 mg/kg, with two schedules (without a loading dose) of 10 mg and 15 mg daily. No significant difference was found in the rate of fall of factors II, IX, and X between the different schedules. However, there was a significantly faster decline in factor VII activity with the loading dose, versus the other two regimens. Because the PT is most sensitive to factor VII, a more rapid prolongation of the PT with the loading dose led many to consider this proof that loading doses achieved more rapid anticoagulation. Intrinsic coagulation depends most on factors IX and X and less on factor VII. In summary, depression of factor VII offers little, if any, protection against thromboembolism, and a rapid depression may lead to hemorrhage. Because of the many factors contributing to anticoagulant response, PTs should be obtained daily until therapy is stabilized (42).

To achieve a safe and rapid conversion from heparin to warfarin, it is recommended that both anticoagulants by administered concurrently, beginning from the first day. Since evidence exists that 5 days of therapeutic heparinization is as effective as 10 days for the treatment of proximal vein thrombosis, this technique may help decrease hospital stay. Heparin therapy must be sufficient to prolong the APTT into the therapeutic range. Once a stable therapeutic prothrombin time response to warfarin is achieved, heparin may be discontinued.

It has generally been recommended that the degree of oral anticoagulant–induced prolongation of the laboratory tests should be the same as with heparin, that is, prolongation of the PT to 1.5 to 2.5 times normal. The INR is the preferred standard for assessing the adequacy of anticoagulation with the coumarins. The ranges of therapeutic anticoagulation fall within two ranges, an INR of 2.0 to 3.0 and 3.0 to 4.5 (Table 40.4). More and more studies are demonstrating successful treatment and prophylaxis of proximal vein thrombosis and pulmonary embolism with less intense anticoagulation (INR 2.0 to 3.0). A lower incidence of bleeding has also been observed (43). Continued reevaluation of experience with less intense anticoagulation may reveal even broader applications.

TERMINATION OF THERAPY

When a therapeutic course is concluded, warfarin may be discontinued abruptly without a risk of "rebound" thromboembolism. Since the half-life of warfarin is prolonged, a tapering effect occurs.

DETERMINANTS OF RESPONSE

Many factors may alter response to warfarin (Table 40.6) (44–46).

Diet. Excessive intake of food rich in vitamin K may theoretically induce a relative resistance to warfarin. Clinically this is rarely a problem, and patients may still eat foods such as spinach, kale, cabbage, cauliflower, peas, cereals, and fish. Patients may occasionally be given supplements to improve their nutrition. Some of these (e.g., Ensure) contain vitamin K, which may cause resistance to warfarin, although reformulation of these products to decrease the amount of vitamin K minimizes this interference.

Conversely, poor nutrition may lead to an increased hypoprothrombinemic response. Fasting or malabsorption may lead to decreased vitamin K absorption and increased warfarin response. Any acute illness associated with diarrhea may quickly induce vitamin K deficiency and result in potentiation of warfarin response.

Drugs. Many drugs interfere with the effect of warfarin. The drugs that can cause important drug interactions with warfarin are listed in Table 40.7. Despite the small number of drugs that have been documented to interfere with warfarin, it is necessary to assume that all drugs have the potential for interaction unless proven otherwise.

Liver Function. Since the vitamin K–dependent clotting factors are synthesized in the liver, any disruption of normal liver function may lead to an increased PT, even without warfarin therapy. In the presence of warfarin, this prolongation will be exaggerated.

Hypermetabolic States. Fever of hyperthyroidism may result in increased sensitivity to warfarin because of the increased catabolism of the vitamin K–dependent clotting factors. This is the predominant effect, since the kinetics of warfarin appear unchanged. The response to warfarin in myxedema is conversely diminished.

Hereditary Resistance. A hereditary resistance has been

Table 40.6.
Determinants of Warfarin Response

Diet
Vitamin K
Drugs
Liver function
Hypermetabolic states
Hereditary resistance
Other

Table 40.7.
Significant Drug Interactions with Warfarin

Drugs enhancing anticoagulant effect
  Amiodarone
  Cimetidine
  Clofibrate (gemfibrozil?)
  Cotrimoxazole
  D-Thyroxine
  Disulfiram
  Glucagon
  Metronidazole
  Phenylbutazone
  Sulfinpyrazone
  Salicylcates (larger doses)
Drugs decreasing anticoagulant effect
  Barbiturates
  Carbamazepine
  Cholestyramine
  Griseofulvin
  Rifampin
  Vitamin K

Note: Many drugs have been reported to interact with oral anticoagulants. Many of these are based upon single or undocumented case reports. The drugs contained in this table have been reported to interfere more predictably. Whenever any drug is added to or discontinued from the regimen of a patient who is receiving warfarin, the patient must be followed carefully.

identified in animals and humans. Findings consistent with an altered affinity of the receptor for the oral anticoagulants or for vitamin K have been reported. This is apparently mediated by a single autosomal gene and is very rare.

Others. Many other, less well documented, determinants have been proposed, including climatic changes, smoking, race, age, plasma lipids, and renal function.

ADVERSE REACTIONS

Hemorrhage, the most important adverse effect of warfarin, is one of the most frequent reasons for admission to the hospital from adverse drug reactions. Patients should be told the most common sites of bleeding and should look routinely for any signs of bleeding.

Cutaneous. Warfarin may cause a hemorrhagic infarct, especially into soft, fatty tissues. This occurs 7 to 10 days after initiation of therapy, usually resolves with discontinuation of warfarin, but occasionally requires surgical intervention. Other skin lesions reported include urticaria, dermatitis, and the "purple toes" syndrome, a nonhemorrhage reaction occurring shortly after initiation of therapy.

Teratogenic. Warfarin crosses into the placental circulation and has been reported to cause chondromylasia punctata or stippling of the bones. Nasal bone deformities have been attributed to maternal consumption of warfarin during the first trimester.

Although heparin does not cross the placenta and may be safer during pregnancy, it is not without maternal risk, and it has also been associated with increased fetal risk.

It appears from the limited studies that warfarin does not cross into breast milk (47–50).

TREATMENT OF OVERDOSE

Excessive hypoprothrombinemia may be reversed by administration of vitamin K, or if associated with bleeding, with fresh frozen plasma or whole blood. Prolongation of the PT without evidence of hemorrhage may require no more than withholding further warfarin therapy until the PT returns to the therapeutic range. If there is evidence of minor bleeding or if the patient is at risk for bleeding, then administration of vitamin K is indicated. Vitamin K_1, or phytonadione, is the only vitamin K preparation that should be used because of its more rapid onset of action. It can be administered intravenously, subcutaneously, or orally, but intramuscular administration should be avoided because of the risk of hematoma formation. It should be administered slowly intravenously to prevent cardiorespiratory collapse. Administration of 5 to 10 mg results in a return of the PT to normal in 6 hr after intravenous and in 24 hr after oral administration (51, 52).

Patients who require continued anticoagulation may manifest resistance to subsequent warfarin administration for up to several weeks after vitamin K administration.

DRUG INTERACTIONS

Drugs may interact with warfarin by different mechanisms. Pharmacodynamically, drugs may interfere by antagonizing warfarin at the site of action (e.g., vitamin K) and by altering the synthesis of clotting factors (oral contraceptives), clotting factor catabolism (thyroxine), and the hemostatic process (by inhibiting platelet function).

Pharmacokinetically, drugs may interfere with warfarin by altering bioavailability, protein binding, metabolism, and excretion.

It has been proposed for many years that the administration of antibiotics, by suppressing intestinal synthesis of vitamin K by bacteria, would result in enhanced hypoprothrombinemia. It is most likely, however, that dietary sources of vitamin K are more important and that gut production is negligible. The interaction of broad-spectrum antibiotics and coumarins is clinically unimportant except in debilitated patients or those receiving prolonged parenteral nutrition. Cholestyramine decreases the absorption of warfarin as well as the absorption of vitamin K. High doses of salicylates may depress prothrombin synthesis by a direct effect on the liver.

Many drugs have been reported to interfere with coumarin absorption, protein binding, and biotransformation. Few drugs interact importantly via these mechanisms. Cholestyramine impairs the absorption of warfarin. Phenylbutazone, oxyphenbutazone, chloral hydrate, and perhaps some sulfonamides may potentiate the effect of warfarin by protein displacement. This effect should be transient if protein displacement is the mechanism, since the increased free level of drug will be metabolized and the levels will return quickly to the predisplacement level.

Phenylbutazone, metronidazole, disulfiram, cotrimoxazole, sulfinpyrazone, and perhaps cimetidine may stereoselectively inhibit the metabolism of warfarin, resulting in an enhanced anticoagulant effect.

Barbiturates, rifampin, and carbamazepine reduce the effect of warfarin by increasing its metabolism by induction of microsomal enzymes (53).

Drugs affecting prothrombin complex concentration may do so by depressing clotting factor synthesis or by increasing the rate of catabolism of clotting factors. Hepatotoxic drugs may potentiate coumarin-induced hypoprothrombinemia by destruction of the liver, resulting in decreased synthesis of the vitamin K–dependent clotting factors. Thyroid drugs may increase the response to warfarin secondary to a hypermetabolic state.

Any drug interfering with hemostasis may increase the risk of therapy with warfarin. Drugs interfering with platelet function by further impairing hemostasis potentiate the hemorrhagic risk of warfarin and should be avoided. Occasionally the combination of warfarin with an antiplatelet agent may be useful therapeutically. In these situations, close monitoring is essential.

The selection of a nonsteroidal antiinflammatory drug (NSAID) is a particularly difficult one because not only may these agents interfere with platelet function and cause gastric irritation, but some (like phenylbutazone) may interact pharmacokinetically with warfarin as well. Of the available NSAIDs, ibuprofen and naproxen appear to be the safest.

Antiplatelet Agents

The role of platelets in thrombogenesis was discussed in the section on the pathogenesis of thromboembolism. Drugs may affect platelet behavior by various mechanisms. They may reduce platelet adhesiveness, decrease or inhibit platelet aggregation, alter platelet membranes, prolong platelet survival, or interfere with platelet factor 3 availability.

The importance of drugs affecting platelet function in the clinical management of cardiovascular diseases has become more evident as a result of a number of recent trials. The primary benefit from antiplatelet drug therapy is in the maintenance of graft potency following coronary artery bypass graft (CABG) surgery, as an adjunct to oral anticoagulants in some patients with atrial fibrillation or mechanical heart valves who develop systemic embolization despite therapeutic anticoagulation, and in the management of patients with unstable angina. A trend toward benefit in preventing reinfarction after a myocardial infarction has been shown. Additionally some subsets of patients with a history of stroke may benefit from therapy with some antiplatelet agents (54). (See further discussion below).

ASPIRIN

Aspirin produces a detectable inhibitory effect on platelet aggregation that persists for 4 to 7 days following administration of a single dose. The inhibition of platelet aggregation occurs secondary to its interference with cyclooxygenase in the arachidonate pathway. The inhibitory effect of aspirin on cyclooxygenase is more pronounced on platelets and less so on the vessel wall (54). There has been considerable discussion about the optimal dose of aspirin in the prevention of thrombosis. No clear consensus exists. The inhibitory effect occurred in some studies with as little as 80 mg of aspirin/day, whereas benefit has been seen in other patients with doses much larger, up to 1 g/day or more. Other salicylates such as sodium salicylate or choline salicylate do not affect platelets. Aspirin has been proposed for the management of unstable angina and ischemia; several clinical trials support its use. The mechanisms for this benefit may be severalfold. Inhibition of platelet aggregation, which is frequently associated with arterial vasospasm (particularly in susceptible individuals), may help maintain adequate flow to the myocardium and prevent ischemia.

Aspirin treatment of unstable angina can decrease the incidence of subsequent infarction and is an accepted therapeutic approach. It is also used along with heparin and thrombolytic agents in the treatment of acute myocaridal infarction (55, 56).

Primary prevention of myocardial infarction with aspirin has been a topic of considerable interest and debate for years. The Physicians Health Study Research Group reports an overall 47% reduction in the risk of total (fatal and nonfatal) myocardial infarction in male physicians ages 40 to 84 years who were randomized to receive aspirin 325 mg every other day or placebo (57, 58). These results are not supported by a randomized trial of aspirin 500 mg per day that was undertaken in British male physicians (59). In this study, no difference in fatal and nonfatal myocardial infarctions was shown. In both the American and British studies there was an increased incidence of strokes in the active treatment groups. In the U.S. trial, the incidence of fatal and disabling hemorrhagic strokes was five times higher in the aspirin group (overall increase 0.02% per year), and in the U.K., trial disabling or fatal strokes were increased 75% (0.35% per year compared with 0.2% per year in controls). The overall risk of ulcer was 1.22 times greater in the U.S. trial for patients taking aspirin, and the relative risk for bleeding was 1.32 times. The incidence of adverse reactions is worrisome with aspirin. The decision to advise the use of aspirin in asymptomatic patients must be made on an individual basis, and consid-

erable attention must be made not only to the possible benefits and risks but to alternative risk factor reduction such as controlling hyperlipidemia hypertension, and obesity.

A number of studies have investigated aspirin for the prevention of a second myocardial infarction. None have detected a predictable benefit, although some have shown a favorable trend toward benefit. Results of the International Survival in Infarct Study II (ISIS-2), which randomized patients to streptokinase, aspirin, both, or placebo, did show a statistically decreased vascular morbidity in patients receiving either streptokinase, aspirin, or both, with the greatest benefit seen in patients receiving both. The 5-week difference was a 23% reduction with streptokinse, 21% reduction with aspirin, and a 40% reduction with the combination. Aspirin reduced the incidence of nonfatal reinfarction by 51%, and this effect persisted for 15 months (60). Further study is obviously needed, but the trend is to treat patients with aspirin postinfarction.

A Canadian Cooperative Study showed that aspirin in doses of 325 mg four times a day reduced the incidence of stroke and death in men with a previous history of transient ischemic attacks. Dipyridamole has not been shown to be effective (61, 62).

Aspirin prophylaxis of venous thromboembolism following total hip replacement was shown to be effective in men but not in women. Aspirin 600 mg twice daily resulted in a statistically significant prophylaxis in males assessed by radiographic phlebography (63, 64).

Aspirin is effective in maintenance of both early and late graft patency following coronary artery bypass grafting (CABG). Doses as low as 100 mg per day have been shown to be effective. Dipyridamole has not been shown to be effective individually, nor does it improve outcome when added to aspirin. Ideally, aspirin should be initiated preoperatively, but it is associated with increased incidence of chest tube drainage and reoperation for bleeding. A suggested alternative regimen is to treat with dipyridamole (300 to 400 mg per day) 24 to 48 hr preoperatively, start aspirin 6 hr postoperatively, discontinue the dipyridamole at 48 hr, and continue the aspirin indefinitely (65). Despite the lack of evidence for the role of dipyridamole, its use in this setting is to inhibit platelet deposition immediately without increasing the risk of bleeding, but then it should be discontinued, because it has not been shown to prevent reocclusion (65).

DIPYRIDAMOLE

Dipyridamole may exert an antiplatelet effect by one of several mechanisms. It increases the concentration of cyclic-AMP in platelets, thus potentiating prostacyclin-mediated platelet inhibition. It also increases uptake of adenosine and may stimulate the vascular endothelium to release eicosanoid. Dipyridamole is frequently administered in combination with aspirin; a potentiation of effect has been suggested but remains unproven. Clinically, dipyridamole has been investigated, almost always in combination with aspirin, for the prevention of a second myocardial infarction, prevention of transient cerebral ischemia and stroke, preservation of patency after CABG surgery, and prevention of venous thrombosis and the thromboembolic complications of cardiac valve disease. Very few studies used dipyridamole alone. In the studies where aspirin was used in combination with dipyridamole and compared with aspirin alone, there appeared to be no benefit from the addition of dipyridamole (58–60, 66–68).

The combination of dipyridamole and warfarin in the management of patients with mechanical prosthetic cardiac valves has recently been approved by the FDA. This combination should probably be reserved for patients who develop systemic emboli despite documented therapeutic anticoagulation. No evidence supports the use of dipyridamole alone for this indication.

In summary, there is little if any conclusive evidence to document the efficacy of dipyridamole as an antiplatelet agent, and its widespread use is not justified.

SULFINPYRAZONE

Sulfinpyrazone inhibits the platelet release reaction and prolongs platelet survival. The duration of action, unlike that of aspirin, is limited to the time when effective plasma concentrations of the drug are maintained.

The strongest evidence for the antithrombotic effect of sulfinpyrazone is in reducing the frequency of shunt thrombosis in patients with arteriovenous fistulas used in chronic hemodialysis. Doses of 200 mg four times daily were well tolerated and resulted in a decrease in clot formation.

The results of the Anturane Reinfarction Trial (ART) have been the subject of extensive controversy (69). Patients who received 800 mg (200 mg four times a day) of sulfinpyrazone within 25 to 35 days of a myocardial infarction demonstrated a reduction in sudden death from 6.3 to 2.7%, as well as a reduction in the annual death rate from 9.5 to 4.5%. These results have been questioned, however, because of problems in trial design and evaluation. Sulfinpyrazone is not presently approved for prevention of a second myocardial infarction. The efficacy of sulfinpyrazone in the prevention of venous thromboembolism and cerebrovascular disease remains to be established.

TICLOPIDINE

Ticlopidine is a new, nonsalicylate antiplatelet drug that is currently under investigation for the prevention of stroke recurrence in men and women. The effects of ticlopidine are dosage- and time-related, with an onset of action of 24 to 48 hr after oral administration. It has a half-life of 24 to 34 hr. Ticlopidine exerts its antiplatelet effect via inhibition of ADP-induced platelet aggregation (70).

The efficacy of ticlopidine in the treatment of stroke has been established by the results of two clinical trials performed in the late 1980s. The CATS study (Canadian American Ticlopidine Study) compared ticlopidine 250 mg b.i.d. with placebo and demonstrated after treatment and follow-up of 3 years an event rate for stroke, MI, or vascular death of 15.3% in the placebo group compared with 10.8% in the treatment group (71). The TASS study (Ticlopidine Aspirin Stroke Study) compared aspirin 1300 mg per day with ticlopidine 250 mg b.i.d. Follow-up ranged from 2 to 6 years. The overall event rate at 3 years was 10% in the ticlopidine group and 13% in the aspirin group. Side effects in both groups were similar and consisted mainly of diarrhea, rash, and neutropenia (72). Neutropenia secondary to ticlopidine must be monitored closely and the drug discontinued promptly if a reduction in white blood cell count is observed. It was observed in 0.9% of patients in the TASS study and resulted in one death. Ticlopidine appears to be slightly more effective than aspirin, although associated with a higher incidence of side effects. It is a promising alternative to aspirin, but it should be reserved for those intolerant of aspirin.

Fibrinolytic Agents

Fibrinolytic agents play an active role in the dissolution of clots, in contrast to heparin and warfarin, which only prevent the occurrence or propagation of them. There are four agents available for clinical use, streptokinase, anisoylated plasminogen-streptokinase-activator complex (APSAC or anistreplase), urokinase, and recombinant tissue-type plasminogen activator (rt-PA or alteplase).

These agents activate plasminogen (Fig. 40.3), urokinase by a direct mechanism, streptokinase by first complexing with plasminogen and then further activating plasminogen, and rt-PA by catalyzing the conversion of plasminogen to plasmin. APSAC is streptokinase-bound to plasminogen and protected from subsequent hydrolysis until it is in the blood stream. Once hydrolyzed, streptokinase is the active agent. The general properties of these agents are compared in Table 40.8.

Fibrinolysis induced by these drugs can induce widespread bleeding, because they will lyse not only thromboemboli but also hemostatic plugs. Careful patient selection is thus important. Fibrinolytic agents should be considered contraindicated in patients with a history of active internal bleeding, history of cerebrovascular accident or trauma within the last 2 months, known bleeding diathesis, severe uncontrolled hypertension, or other intracranial processes such as a neoplasm. Care should be taken and patients evaluated on an individual basis if there is a recent (within 10 days to 2 weeks) history of surgery,

Table 40.8.
Comparison of Fibrinolytic Agents

	SK[a]	APSAC	UK	rt-PA
Half-Life (min)	23	90–105	16	5
Dose (AMI) bolus/infusion	1.5 mU	30 U	2 mU	100 mg
	No/yes	Yes	No/yes	Yes/no
Fibrin specificity	+	+ +	+	+ + +
Antigenicity	Yes	Yes	No	No
Hypotension	+ + +	+ + +	+	+
Bleeding	+ + +	+ + +	+ + +	+ + +
Clotting defect (influence on tests)	+ + +	+ + +	+ + +	+ − + +
Rate of recanalization	+ − + +	+ +	+ − + +	+ + − + + +
Decrease in mortality	+ + +	+ + +	?	+ + +
Preservation of LV function	+ + +	+ + +	?	+ + +
Incidence of reocclusion	+	+	?	+ + +
Cost	+	+ +	+ +	+ + +

[a] Symbols and abbreviations: +, least; + + +, greatest; SK, streptokinase; APSAC, anistreplase; UK, urokinase; rt-PA, alteplase.

organ biopsy, bacterial endocarditis, puncture of noncompressible vessel, pregnancy, minor trauma (including CPR for greater than 5 min), acute pericarditis, or severe renal and/or hepatic disease. There are other conditions where they may be contraindicated and the patient must be evaluated to weigh the risk versus the benefits. Adverse reactions in addition to bleeding include hypotension, allergy, and fever.

The use of fibrinolytic agents in the treatment of pulmonary embolism is indicated for life-threatening symptoms associated with massive pulmonary embolism. This is usually the case where pulmonary embolectomy is being considered. Treatment with streptokinase is initiated with a loading dose of 250,000 units administered over 30 min, followed by an infusion of 100,000 units per hr for 24 to 72 hr. Urokinase is administered as a loading dose of 4400 units per kg over 10 min, followed by 4400 units per kg per hr for 12 to 24 hr. Tissue plasminogen activator is administered at a dosage of 100 mg over 2 hr. Heparin therapy is started following streptokinase and urokinase and given simultaneously with rt-PA.

The dose of streptokinase and urokinase for the treatment of deep venous thrombosis is the same as for pulmonary embolism. Treatment should be continued for 72 hr with both agents.

The hematologic status of the patient should be evaluated before administration of fibrinolytic agents. The thrombin time, prothrombin time, activated partial thromboplastin time, complete blood count and platelets should be measured. Once it is established that the patient's baseline coagulation profile is normal, clotting tests are performed to document that a "lytic" state has been achieved. If the thrombin time is prolonged two to five times the normal value, the dosage should not be increased.

The greatest impact of fibrinolytic therapy has been in the treatment of acute myocardial infarction. The three major goals of intervention with these agents in the treatment of acute myocardial infarction are to (a) recanalize the infarct-related artery, (b) preserve left ventricular function, and (c) decrease both short-term and long-term mortality. Many studies have been performed to establish the efficacy of fibrinolytic therapy and to define the differences between the agents (60, 73–88).

The percentage of successful recanalization of the infarct-related artery varies significantly from trial to trial. Tissue plasminogen activator achieves the highest patency rate (average approximately 75%), followed by APSAC and streptokinase (average 40 to 70%). Despite differences in recanalization rate, there is no difference between the agents and their ability to decrease mortality. Cumulative experience from the Italian Group for the Study of Streptokinase in Myocardial Infarction (GISSI-2) trial (86), which compared streptokinase and rt-PA, and the International Study of Infarct Survival III (ISIS-3) trial (87), which compared streptokinase, rt-PA (duteplase-rt-PA manufactured by Burroughs-Wellcome), and APSAC, demonstrated no difference in mortality.

The overall impact on mortality from comparative trials of thrombolytic agents is the same. The ISIS-3 trial showed a 5-week mortality of 10.5% for streptokinase, 10.3% for rt-PA, and 10.6% for APSAC. The reinfarction rate for the three drugs was 3.6%, 3.1%, and 3.8%, respectively, while the incidence of hemorrhagic stroke was 0.3%, 0.7%, and 0.6%, respectively. The results of the GISSI-2 trial are similar; there was no difference in mortality between the treatment groups (streptokinase and rt-PA).

Preservation of left ventricular function following fibrinolytic therapy has also been demonstrated with all of the available agents, with the greatest benefit shown when therapy is administered within 4 hr of symptoms.

Timing of administration of fibrinolytic therapy is important. Early (less than 3 hours from the onset of symptoms) administration results in the greatest decrease in mortality although benefit has been shown when therapy is given up to 24 hr.

Adjunctive therapy with aspirin is important in the treatment of myocardial infarction. The ISIS-2 trial (60) compared streptokinase, aspirin, and streptokinase and aspirin together. The greatest benefit on decreased mortality was seen with the combination. Heparin is another helpful adjunct, and the timing of administration and the intensity of treatment has become an area of controversy (87–89). Because the half-life of rt-PA is so short, heparin administration immediately following the conclusion of the rt-PA infusion is important. Heparin therapy is also used following streptokinase and APSAC but may need to be held if the APTT is greater than 100 sec, to allow minimal recovery of the hemostatic mechanism. It should be followed carefully however, and the APTT must not be allowed to fall below 60 to 80 sec. Other adjuncts such as β-blockers may further decrease mortality in selected patients. The ISIS-4 trial will be investigating the impact of angiotensin-converting-enzyme inhibitors, nitrates, and magnesium on mortality following myocardial infarction. The use of combination fibrinolytic agents (rt-PA and streptokinase) will be investigated in the GUSTO (Global Utilization of Streptokinase and TPA on Occluded Ateries) trial.

The most serious complication following fibrinolytic therapy is hemorrhage. Despite the reputed greater clot-selectivity of rt-PA, the incidence of bleeding following all of the agents is similar. The incidence of stroke was greater with rt-PA in the ISIS-3 trial than with streptokinase and APSAC.

Follow-up care of patients receiving fibrinolytic therapy is important, because these agents dissolve the clot but do not affect the underlying coronary lesion. Many patients will ultimately undergo percutaneous transluminal coronary angioplasty (PTCA) or CABG, but until that time they generally receive treatment with antiplatelet agents such as aspirin. Other agents such as calcium-channel blockers or nitrates may also be required.

In conclusion, fibrinolytic therapy is an important advance in the management of patients with acute myocardial infarction and in selected patients with deep venous thrombosis and pulmonary embolism. Based upon the published experience with them, efficacy, and cost, streptokinase should be the fibrinolytic agent of choice. In myocardial infarction there may be a slightly higher incidence of reinfarction with streptokinase, based upon the ISIS-3

results, but there is a higher incidence of hemorrhagic stroke and a higher incidence of reocclusion with rt-PA. The cost of rt-PA is approximately 12 to 20 times the cost of streptokinase, and APSAC is 8 to 10 times the cost of streptokinase. Upcoming trials may change our thinking over time, but now, streptokinase is the agent of choice.

CONCLUSION

The appropriate use of antithrombotic agents depends upon establishing well-defined therapeutic objectives. These objectives are determined to a large extent by the underlying pathophysiology of the thromboembolic event. For example, the patient with an acute myocardial infarction represents a different problem from the patient with a deep venous thrombosis or pulmonary embolism. In the patient with acute myocardial infarction there is a role for aggressive therapy with antithrombotic agents affecting acute fibrinolysis, platelet function, and fibrin deposition. This requires the use of a fibrinolytic agent such as streptokinase, and aspirin and heparin. It is thus important to be familiar with the pharmacology, dosing, and laboratory management of these agents to optimize the therapeutic outcome while minimizing the risk of adverse effects, particularly bleeding. Advances in antithrombotic therapy will most likely be in the area of developing even more specific antithrombotic agents or regimens of agents in the treatment of thromboembolic disease.

REFERENCES

1. Second American College of Chest Physicians Conference on Antithrombotic Therapy. Chest 95(suppl 2):1S–169S, 1989.
2. Stults BM, Dere WH, Caine TH: Long-term anticoagulation, indications and management. West J Med 151:414–429, 1989.
3. Stein B, Fuster V, Halperin JL, et al.: Antithrombotic therapy in cardiac disease. An emerging approach based on pathogenesis and risk. Circulation 80:1501–1513, 1989.
4. Goldhaber SZ, Savage DD, Garrison RJ, et al.: Risk factors for pulmonary embolism. The Framingham Study. Am J Med 74:1023, 1983.
5. Carter BL, Jones ME, Waickman LA: Pathophysiology and treatment of deep-vein thrombosis and pulmonary embolism. Clin Pharm 4:279–296, 1985.
6. Stein PD, Willis PW, DeMets DL: History and physical examination in acute pulmonary embolism in patients without preexisting cardiac or pulmonary disease. Am J Cardiol 42:218, 1981.
7. Hirsh J: Diagnosis of venous thrombosis and pulmonary embolism. Am J Cardiol 65:45C–49C, 1990.
8. Hyers TM, Hull RD, Weg JG: Antithrombotic therapy for venous thromboembolic disease. Chest 95(suppl 2):37S–51S, 1989.
9. Sherman DG: Cardiac embolism: the neurologists perspective. Am J Cardiol 65:32C–37C, 1990.
10. Wipf JE, Lipsky BA: Atrial fibrillation thromboembolic risk and indications for anticoagulation. Arch Intern Med 150:1598–1603, 1990.
11. Stroke Prevention in Atrial Fibrillation Study Group Investigators: Preliminary report of Stroke Prevention in Atrial Fibrillation Study. N Engl J Med 322:863–868, 1990.
12. Boston Area Anticoagulation Trial for Atrial Fibrillation Investiga-

tors: The effects of low-dose warfarin on the risk of stroke in patients with nonrheumatic atrial fibrillation. N Engl J Med 323:1505–1511, 1990.

13. Ysusf S, Wittes J, Friedman L: Overview of results of randomized clinical trials in heart disease. I. Treatment following myocardial infarction. JAMA 260:2088–2093, 1988.

14. Smith P, Arnesen H, Holme I: The effect of warfarin on mortality and reinfarction after myocardial infarction. N Engl J Med 323:147–152, 1990.

15. Chesebro JH, Adams PC, Fuster V: Antithrombotic therapy in patients with valvular heart disease and prosthetic heart valves. J Am Coll Cardiol 8:41B–56B, 1986.

16. Hirsh J, Deykin D, Poller L: Therapeutic range for oral anticoagulant therapy. Chest 89(suppl):11S–15S, 1986.

17. Poller L, Taberner DA: Dosage and control of oral anticoagulants: an international collaborative survey. Br J Haematol 51:479–485, 1982.

18. Hirsh J: Is the dose of warfarin prescribed by American physicians unnecessarily high? Arch Intern Med 147:769–771, 1987.

19. Hirsh J, Poller L, Deykin D, et al.: Optimal therapeutic range for oral anticoagulants. Chest 95(suppl 2):5S–11S, 1989.

20. Petitti DB, Strom B, Melmon K: Duration of warfarin anticoagulant therapy and the probabilities of recurrent thromboembolism and hemorrhage. Am J Med 81:255–258, 1986.

21. Holmgren K, Andersson G, Fagrell B, et al.: One-month versus six-month therapy with oral anticoagulants after symptomatic deep vein thrombosis. Acta Med Scand 218:279–284, 1985.

22. Rosenberg RD: Actions and interactions of antithrombin and heparin. N Engl J Med 292:146, 1975.

23. Wessler S, Gitel SN: Pharmacology of heparin and warfarin. J Am Coll Cardiol 8:10B–20B, 1986.

24. Coon WW: Heparin: a drug of varying composition and effectiveness. Clin Pharmacol Ther 23:139, 1978.

25. Hirsh J: Heparin. N Engl J Med 324:1565–1574, 1991

26. Estes JN: Clinical pharmacokinetics of heparin. Clin Pharmacokinet 5:204–220, 1980.

27. Hirsh J, Van A, Ken WG, et al.: Heparin kinetics in venous thrombosis and pulmonary embolism. Circulation 53:691, 1976.

28. Hull RD, Raskob GE, Rosenbloom D, et al.: Heparin for 5 days as compared with 10 days in the initial treatment of proximal vein thrombosis. N Engl J Med 322:1260–1264, 1990.

29. Collins R, Scrimgeour A, Yusuf S, et al.: Reduction in fatal pulmonary embolism and venous thrombosis by perioperative administration of subcutaneous heparin. Overview of results of randomized trials in general, orthopedic and urologic surgery. N Engl J Med 318:1162–1173, 1988.

30. Halkin H, Goldberg J, Modan M, et al.: Reduction in mortality in general medical in-patients by low-dose heparin prophylaxis. Ann Intern Med 96:561–565, 1982.

31. Francis CW, Marder VJ, Evarts CM, et al.: Two-step warfarin therapy: prevention of postoperative venous thrombosis without excessive bleeding. JAMA 249:374–378, 1983.

32. Hull R, Delmore T, Genton E, et al.; Warfarin sodium versus low-dose heparin in the long-term treatment of venous thrombosis. N Engl J Med 301:855–858, 1979.

33. Hull R, Delmore T, Carter C, et al.: Adjusted subcutaneous heparin vs. warfarin sodium in the long-term treatment of venous thrombosis. N Engl J Med 306:180, 1982.

34. Kelton JG, Hirsh J: Bleeding associated with antithrombotic therapy. Semin Hematol 17:259–291, 1980.

35. Bell WR, Tomasulo PA, Alving BM, et al.: Thrombocytopenia occurring during the administration of heparin: a prospective study in 52 patients. Ann Intern Med 85:155, 1976.

36. O'Kelly R, Magee F, McKenna J: Routine heparin therapy inhibits adrenal aldosterone production. J Clin Endocrinol Metab 56:108–112, 1983.

37. Habbab MA, Halt JL: Heparin resistance induced by nitroglycerin: a word of caution when both drugs are used concomitantly. Arch Intern Med 147:857–860, 1987.

38. Becker RC, Corrao JM, Bovill EG, et al.: Intravenous nitroglycerin-induced heparin resistance: a qualitative antithrombin III abnormality. Am Heart J 119:1254–1261, 1990.

39. Horrow JC: Protamine: a review of its toxicity. Anesth Analg 64:348–361, 1985.

40. Hirsh J: Oral anticoagulant drugs. N Engl J Med 324:1865–1875, 1991.

41. Holford NH: Clinical pharmacokinetics and pharmacodynamics of warfarin. Understanding the dose-effect relationship. Clin Pharmacokinet 11:483–504, 1986.

42. O'Reilly RA, Aggeler PM: Studies on coumarin anticoagulant drugs: initiation of therapy without a loading dose. Circulation 38:169, 1968.

43. Hull R, Hirsh J, Jay R, et al.: Different intensities of oral anticoagulant therapy in the treatment of proximal-vein thrombosis. N Engl J Med 307:1976, 1982.

44. O'Reilly RA, Aggeler PM: Determinants of the response to oral anticoagulant drugs in man. Pharmacol Rev 22:35, 1970.

45. Fenech A, Winter JH, Douglas S: Individualization of oral anticoagulant therapy. Drugs 18:48, 1979.

46. Breckenridge AM: Interindividual differences in the response to oral anticoagulants. Drugs 14:367, 1977.

47. Pettifor JM, Benson R: Congenital malformations associated with the administration of oral anticoagulants during pregnancy. J Pediatr 86:459, 1975.

48. Warkany J: A warfarin embryopathy. Am J Dis Child 129:287, 1975.

49. Hall JG, Pauli RM, Wilson KM, et al.: Maternal and fetal sequelae of anticoagulation during pregnancy. Am J Med 68:122, 1980.

50. Orme ML, Lewis PJ, de Swiet MS, et al.: May mothers given warfarin breast-feed their infants? Br Med J 1:1564, 1977.

51. Udall J: Don't use the wrong vitamin K. Calif Med 112:65, 1966.

52. Taberner DA, Thompson JM, Poller L, et al.: Comparison of prothrombin complex concentrate and vitamin K in oral anticoagulant reversal. Br Med J 1:83, 1976.

53. Serlin MJ, Breckenridge AM: Drug interactions with warfarin. Drugs 25:610–620, 1983.

54. Fuster J, Adams PC, Badimon JJ, et al.: Platelet-inhibitor drugs role in coronary artery disease. Prog Cardiovasc Dis 29:325–346, 1987.

55. Lewis HD, Davis JW, Archbald DG, et al.: Protective effects of aspirin against acute myocardial infarction and death in men with unstable angina. N Engl J Med 309:396–403, 1983.

56. Theroux TP, Quimet H, McCans J, et al.: Aspirin, heparin, or both to treat acute unstable angina. N Engl J Med 319:1105–1111, 1988.

57. Special Report: Preliminary report: findings from the aspirin component of the ongoing Physicians Health Study. N Engl J Med 318:262–264, 1988.

58. Steering Committee of the Physicians Health Research Group: Final report on the aspirin component of the Ongoing Physicians Health Study. N Engl J Med 321:129–135, 1989.

59. Peto R, Gray R, Collins R, et al.: Randomized trial of daily aspirin in British male doctors. Brit Med J 295:313–316, 1988.

60. ISIS-2 (Second International Study of Infarct Survival) Collagorative Group: Randomized trial of intravenous streptokinase, oral aspirin, both, or neither among 17,187 cases of suspected acute myocardial infarction. Lancet 2:349, 1988.

61. Canadian Cooperative Study Group: A randomized trial of aspirin and sulfinpyrazone in threatened stroke. N Engl J Med 299:53, 1978.

62. Mehta J: Platelets and prostaglandins in coronary artery disease. Ra-

tionale for the use of platelet-suppressive drugs. JAMA 249:2818, 1983.

63. Harris WH, Salzman EW, Athanasoulis CA, et al.: Aspirin prophylaxis of venous thromboembolism after total hip replacement. N Engl J Med 297:1246, 1977.

64. Powers PJ, Gent M, Jay RM, et al.: A randomized trial of less intense postoperative warfarin or aspirin therapy in the prevention of venous thromboembolism after surgery for fractured hip. Arch Intern Med 149:771, 1989.

65. Webster MWI, Chesebro JH, Fuster V: Platelet inhibitor therapy. Agents and clinical implications. Hematol Oncol Clin North Am 4:265–289, 1990.

66. Fitzgeral GA: Dipyridamole. N Engl J Med 316:1247–1257, 1987.

67. Bousser MG, Eschwege E, Haguenau M, et al.: "AICLA" Controlled trial of aspirin and dipyridamole in the secondary prevention of athero-thrombotic cerebral ischemica. Stroke 14:5–14, 1983.

68. American-Canadian Co-operative Study Group: Persantine aspirin trial in cerebral ischemia: Part II. End-point results. Stroke 16:606–615, 1985.

69. The Anturane Reinfarction Trial Research Group: Sulfinpyrazone in the prevention of cardiac death after myocardial infarction. The Anturane Reinfarction Trial. N Engl J Med 298:289, 1978.

70. Saltiel E, Ward A: Ticlopidine. A review of its pharmacodynamic and pharmacokinetic properties, and therapeutic efficacy in platelet-dependent disease states. Drugs 34:222–262, 1987.

71. Gent M, Easton JD, Hachinski VC, et al.: The Canadian American Ticlopidine Study (CATS) in Thromboembolic Stroke. Lancet 1:1215–1220, 1989.

72. Hass WK, Easton JD, Adams HP, et al.: A randomized trial comparing ticlopidine hydrochloride with aspirin for the prevention of stroke in high-risk patients. N Engl J Med 321:501–501, 1989.

73. The TIMI Study Group: The Thrombolysis in Myocardial Infarction (TIMI) trial: phase I findings. N Engl J Med 312:932, 1985.

74. Italian Group for the Study of Streptokinase in Myocardial Infarction (GISSI): Effectiveness of intravenous thrombolytic treatment in acute myocardial infarction. Lancet 1:397, 1986.

75. Chesebro JH, Knatterud G, Roberts R, et al.: Thrombolysis in Myocardial Infarction (TIMI) Trial, phase I: a comparison between intravenous tissue plasminogen activator and intravenous streptokinase. Clinical findings through hospital discharge. Circulation 76:142, 1987.

76. Van De Werf F, Arnold AER, and the European Cooperative Study Group for Recombinant Tissue-Type Plasminogen Activator: Effect of intravenous tissue plasminogen activator on infarct size, left ven-

tricular function and survival in patients with acute myocardial infarction. Br Med J 297:1374, 1988.

77. National Heart Foundation of Australia Coronary Thrombolysis Group: Coronary thrombolysis and myocardial salvage tissue plasminogen activator given up to four hours after onset of myocardial infarction. Lancet 1:203, 1988.

78. Wilcox RG, Olsson CG, Skene AM, Von Der Lippe G, et al.: Trial of tissue plasminogen activator for mortality reduction in acute myocardial infarction Anglo-Scandinavian Study of Early Thrombolysis (ASSET). Lancet 2:252, 1988.

79. AIMS Trial Study Group: Effect of intravenous APSAC on Mortality after acute myocardial infarction: preliminary report of a placebo-controlled clinical trial. Lancet 1:545, 1988.

80. O'Neill WW, Topel EJ, Pitt B: Reperfusion therapy of acute myocardial infarction. Prog Cardiovasc Dis 30:235–266, 1988.

81. White HD, Rivers JT, Maslowski AH, et al.: Effect of intravenous streptokinase as compared with that of tissue plasminogen activator on left ventricular function after first myocardial infarction. N Engl J Med 320:817, 1989.

82. Bleich SD, Nichols T, Schumacher R, et al.: The role of heparin following coronary thrombolysis with tissue plasminogen activator (t-PA) (abstract). Circulation 80(suppl II):13, 1989.

83. Magnani B: Plasminogen Activator Italian Multicenter Study (PAIMS): comparison of intravenous recombinant single-chain human tissue-type plasminogen activator (rt-PA) with intravenous streptokinase in acute myocardial infarction. J Am Coll Cardiol 13:19, 1989.

84. The TIMI Study Group: The Thrombolysis in Myocardial Infarction (TIMI) Phase II trial. N Engl J Med 320:618, 1989.

85. Tiefenbrunn AJ, Sobel BE: The impact of coronary thrombosis on myocardial infarction. Fibrinolysis 3:1, 1989.

86. Italian Group for the Study of Streptokinase in Myocardial Infarction (GISSI-2): A factorial randomized trial of alteplase versus streptokinase and heparin vs no heparin among 12,490 patients with acute myocardial infarction. Lancet 336:65, 1990.

87. The International Study Group: In-hospital mortality and clinical course of 20,891 patients with suspected acute myocardial infarction randomized between alteplase and streptokinase with or without heparin. Lancet 336:71, 1990.

88. Mahan EF III, Chandler JW, Rogers WJ: Heparin and infarct coronary artery patency after streptokinase in acute myocardial infarction. Am J Cardiol 65:967, 1990.

89. Sobel BE, Hirsh J: Principles and practice of coronary thrombolysis and conjunctive treatment. Am J Cardiol 68:382–388, 1991.

CHAPTER 41

ALLERGY AND DRUG-INDUCED SKIN DISEASE

ANN AMERSON, Pharm.D.

Allergic and drug-induced skin diseases encompass a wide variety of conditions, both acute and chronic, with varying morphology. The most commonly encountered allergic skin diseases are atopic dermatitis, contact dermatitis, and urticaria. In addition, ingestion of a number of drugs can produce varied dermatological reactions. A brief review of skin structure and function is provided as a basis for the discussion of the individual conditions. The etiology, pathogenesis, therapeutic interventions, and management of each condition are discussed. A glossary of common skin manifestations is included in Table 41.1.

SKIN STRUCTURE AND FUNCTION

The skin, the largest organ of the body, is divided into three (main) distinct layers, the epidermis, the dermis, and the hypodermis (subcutaneous tissue) as indicated in Figure 41.1 (1, 2). The nonvascular epidermis consists of stratified squamous epithelial cells that are of two distinct types, keratinocytes and dendritic cells (2). The dendritic cells are further classified into three types: (a) melanocytes, (b) Langerhans cells, and (c) indeterminate dendritic cells. The epidermis consists of five distinct layers from inside out:

1. Stratum germinativum (basal);
2. Stratum spinosum (prickle);
3. Stratum granulosum (granular);
4. Stratum lucidum (lucid);
5. Stratum corneum (horny).

The keratinocytes, located in the basal layer, are stem cells that differentiate into other cells in the upper layers of the epidermis. As the keratinocytes migrate toward the surface, they undergo gradual transformation from living cells to dead, thick-walled flat cells that contain keratin. The basal layer also contains melanocytes, which are the pigment-forming cells (1, 2).

The prickle layer also contains both kertinocytes and melanocytes. The cytoplasmic threads called prickles appearing prominently in this layer give it its name. The granular layer consists of several thicknesses of flattened cells with protein granules containing keratohyaline. These granules are changed to keratin, a fibrous substance in the outermost layers.

The lucid layer, which appears as a translucent line, is present only in thicker skin such as on the palms and soles. The outermost horny layer or the stratum corneum consists of flat, scaly dead tissue layers that are constantly shedding. The horny layer is the dead, end product while the other four layers are considered to be the living epidermis. A continual process occurs throughout the sublayers of the epidermis in which new cells from the lower layers push older cells toward the top, where they eventually fill with keratin and die. Under normal conditions the epidermis can replicate itself in 3 to 4 weeks.

The dermis or corium consists of connective tissue, cellular elements, and ground substance with a rich blood and nerve supply. The sebaceous glands and shorter hair follicles originate in the dermis, which can be divided into two distinct sublayers, the papillary and reticular units. The papillary layer is adjacent to the epidermis and has a rich supply of blood vessels. The reticular sublayer contains coarser tissue that connects the dermis and subcutaneous tissue (hypodermis).

The connective tissue of the dermis is comprised of collagen fibers, elastic fibers, and reticular fibers, which provide support and elasticity to the skin. The cellular elements consist of three types of mesodermal cell groups: (a) reticulohistocytes, (b) myeloid, and (c) lymphoid. The reticulohistocyte group consists of fibroblasts, histiocytes, and mast cells, with immature cells called reticulum cells. Intracytoplasmic granules containing heparin and histamine are present in mast cells. The number of cells, normally few, are increased in itching dermatoses, such as contact or atopic dermatitis. Normally, histiocytes are present in small numbers around blood vessels. In pathologic conditions, they migrate in the dermis as monocytes. They may phagocytize bacteria and particulate matter and then are known as macrophages. Fibroblasts form collagen fibers and may serve as precursors for the other connective tissue cells. Polymorphonuclear leukocytes and eosinophils, members of the myeloid group, are quite common in dermatoses, particularly when an allergic component is involved. Lymphocytes from the lymphoid group are common in inflammatory lesions of the skin (1, 2).

The hypodermis is composed of relatively loose connective tissue. This layer provides pliability to the skin, and its thickness varies. In most areas, it contains a unit for formation and storage of fat. The fat layer functions in thermal control, food reserve, and cushioning. The hypodermis supports the blood vessels and nerves that pass from tissues beneath to the dermis. Deeper hair follicles and sweat glands originate in the hypodermis (1, 2).

The skin confines underlying tissue and provides a barrier between the body and the environment. It prevents

Table 41.1.
Terms Associated with Allergic and Drug-induced Skin Diseases

Angioedema	An allergic skin disease characterized by patches of circumscribed swelling involving the skin and its subcutaneous layers, the mucous membranes, and sometimes the viscera; also called angioneurotic edema, giant urticaria
Bullae	Large vesicles or blisters
Dermographism	Pressure or friction on the skin gives rise to a transient, raised usually reddish mark, sometimes white, so that a word traced on the skin become visible
Desquamation	Peeling of skin in the form of scales
Eczema	An inflammatory condition of the skin characterized by redness; itching, and oozing vesicular lesions that become scaly, crusted, or hardened
Erythema	Abnormal redness of the skin caused by capillary congestion
Exanthem (exanthematous)	An eruptive disease (as measles) or its symptomatic eruption
Excoriation	A raw irritated lesion; the act of abrading or wearing off the skin
Exfoliation	Peeling of the horny layer of the (exfoliative) skin
Lichenoid	Resembling lichen, characterized by the eruption of flat papules
Macule	A patch of skin that is altered in color but usually not elevated
Maculopapular	Combining the characteristics of macules and papules
Morbilliform	Resembling the eruption of measles
Papule	A small, solid, usually conical, elevation of the skin caused by inflammation, accumulated secretion, or hypertrophy of tissue elements
Plaque	A localized abnormal patch on a body part or surface, especially on the skin
Pruritus	Localized or generalized itching due to irritation of sensory nerve endings from organic or psychogenic causes
Urticaria	An allergic disorder marked by raised edematous patches of skin or mucous membrane and usually intense itching; caused by contact with a specific precipitating factor, either externally or internally; also called hives
Vesicle	A small abnormal elevation of the outer layer of skin enclosing a watery liquid; blister

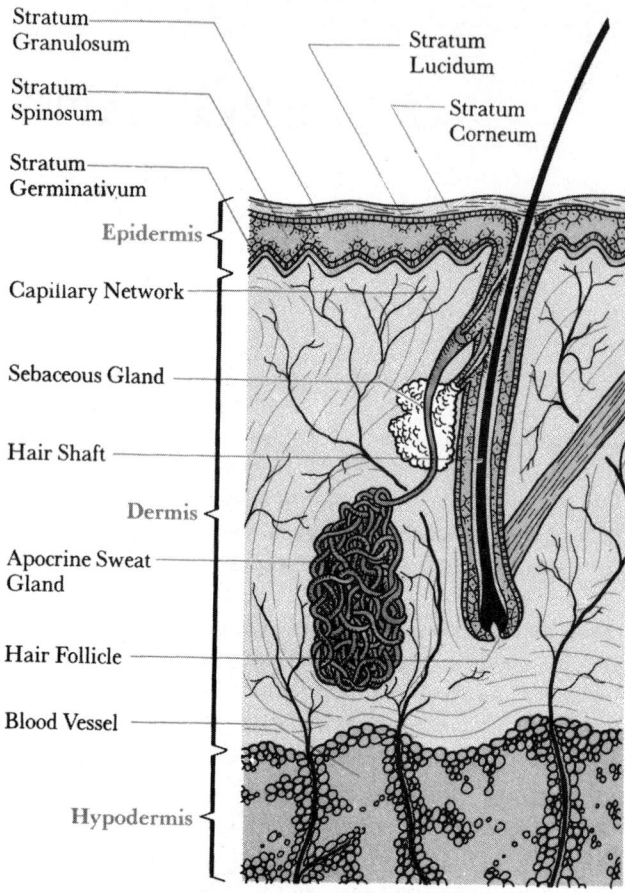

Figure 41.1. Cross-section of human skin. (Reprinted with permission from Handbook of Nonprescription Drugs. Washington, D.C., American Pharmaceutical Association, 1990.)

harm from external agents such as ultraviolet radiation, pathogenic organisms, and chemicals. Various factors can alter the effectiveness of the barrier including age, underlying diseases, use of medications (topical or systemic) and the integrity of the stratum corneum. Other skin functions involve sensation, temperature control, development of pigment, and synthesis of some vitamins. Moisture regulation is another important function (1).

Skin appendages are of two types, cornified and glandular (1, 2). Cornified appendages are hair and nails. Glandular appendages are the sebaceous glands and sweat glands, both eccrine and apocrine. Since these appendages are not usually involved in allergic and drug-induced disease, they will not be discussed further.

MECHANISMS

While many of the conditions discussed in this chapter are believed to result from allergy, nonimmunologic mechanisms are postulated or known to play a role (3, 4). For example, contact dermatitis may be caused by immunologic mechanisms or result from direct irritant properties. The clinical presentation is essentially identical (4).

The basic immunologic mechanisms of allergic reactions are of four types (5). Immediate or anaphylactic reactions (type I) result from the production of IgE antibodies that attach to the surface of basophils or mast cells. With reexposure, the offending substance binds to the antibodies on the cell surface, causing release of chemical mediators. These substances may include histamine, serotonin, peptides, leukotrienes, and prostaglandins (5, 6). The clinical effects are determined by the interaction of the mediators with the various target organs and may include pruritus, urticaria, bronchospasm, laryngeal edema, and hypotension.

Type II reactions result in antibody-dependent cytotoxicity. The offending substance interacts with surface components of a cell, thus making it appear foreign. Antibodies are produced that react with the cell-bound substance. The antigen-antibody reaction may trigger the complement system or permit attack by mononuclear killer cells, resulting in cell death (e.g., drug-induced hemolysis) (5).

Type III reactions involve immune complexes. The antigen-antibody complex forms in blood or tissue spaces. IgG and IgM antibodies are usually involved (6). Inflammation or complement activation may result if these complexes deposit on blood vessel walls or basement membranes. Serum sickness and allergic arteritis are examples of type III reactions (5).

Type IV reactions are termed cell-mediated, delayed, or tuberculin type reactions. The offending substance interacts with skin proteins, evoking a cell-mediated immune response. Sensitized T lymphocytes release lymphokines in response, which cause local edema and inflammation (5).

Type I and type IV reactions are most commonly involved in allergic skin manifestations. In some cases, skin manifestations may occur from circulating immune complexes (type III). Type II reactions are unlikely to produce cutaneous manifestations (5, 6). Some cases of drug-induced urticaria are an example of a type I reaction, and allergic contact dermatitis is an example of a type IV reaction.

Immunologic involvement is supported by certain clinical features described by Bigby (3). The reaction

1. Occurs in a small percentage of patients;
2. Is not dose-dependent;
3. Occurs (onset of rash) within 1 to 2 weeks after initiation of therapy;
4. Is accompanied by other signs and symptoms, e.g., fever, pruritus, eosinophilia;
5. Resolves upon withdrawal of agent and recurs if patient is rechallenged.

The immunologic mechanisms involved are discussed and the role of nonimmunologic mechanisms for each condition are identified.

ATOPIC DERMATITIS

Atopic dermatitis, frequently referred to as eczema, is a chronic pruritic skin disorder that occurs in individuals with a personal or family history of allergic diseases such as rhinitis, asthma, or conjunctivitis (7). It is estimated to be the eighth most common of all dermatoses in persons under 25 years of age (8). The disorder occurs in infants, children, and adults, with males more commonly affected in the infant/child group and females more commonly affected in the older child/adult group. Estimated cumulative incidence is 10 to 15% in children up to 14 years of age (9). Occurrence is more frequent in "well-developed" countries (8). Heredity plays a role, but the mechanism of inheritance is undefined (8).

Etiology

The exact cause of atopic dermatitis is unknown. Two theories are proposed: the immunologic hypothesis and the β-adrenergic-receptor blockade hypothesis (7, 8). Several factors support the immunologic hypothesis: (a) the frequent association of atopic dermatitis with other allergic disorders; (b) substantial elevations of serum IgE; (c) positive wheal-and-flare reactions to a wide variety of scratch tests; (d) increased susceptibility to viral and fungal infections; and (e) association with immunodeficiency disorders.

The β-adrenergic-receptor blockade theory suggests that a malfunction of β-receptors produces a pattern of hyperactivity that can be triggered by varied stimuli including psychic, immunologic, infectious, chemical, and physical factors (7).

Pathogenesis

The immunologic theory receives the most attention of the two theories, but the event that initiates the reaction is yet to be identified (7–10). Abnormalities of both humoral and cell-mediated immunity are present. Apparently IgE is stimulated by specific antigens; it attaches to mast cells and triggers release of mast cell inflammatory mediators (including histamine) that are released upon reexposure to the antigens (7). Other factors must play a role, because atopic dermatitis occurs in patients with a deficiency of immunoglobulins, e.g., agammaglobulinemia or Weskott-Aldrich syndrome.

Evidence for cell-mediated factors relates to susceptibility and recurrence of viral infections, including herpes simplex, molluscum contagiosum, and warts (7–9). Patients are frequently resistant to sensitization to poison ivy and dinitrochlorobenzene (DNCB) (8, 9). The demonstration of decreased numbers of T lymphocytes may indicate a lack of sufficient T cells to control B cell production of immunoglobulin, so that high levels of IgE are produced (7, 8). As well, phagocytic capacity is decreased, and chemotaxis of neutrophils and monocytes is impaired (7, 9).

Another factor supporting an immunologic basis is the demonstration of significant numbers of *Staphylococcus aureus* bacteria on both diseased and normal skin of atopic patients (8, 9). Skin infections secondary to *S. aureus* may exacerbate eczema (9).

The β-adrenergic theory is supported by a number of abnormal cutaneous responses. These include an exaggerated constrictor response by cutaneous vessels, white dermographism (white line is produced when skin is stroked), delayed blanch to cholinergic stimuli, and paradoxical response to application of nicotinic acid (9). A postulated defect in the enzyme adenyl cyclase, which results in decreased levels of cyclic AMP is supported by work showing abnormally low levels of cyclic AMP produced by leukocytes of atopic patients challenged with isoproterenol, prostaglandin E_1, and histamine (7, 9). Decreased cyclic AMP levels may enhance release of inflammatory mediators from mast cells and basophils (7). Evidence suggests that phosphodiesterase activity is increased, reducing cyclic-AMP levels and diminishing responsiveness of cyclic AMP when challenged with β-agonists. While this enzymatic abnormality might be a primary defect in patients with atopic dermatitis, subsequent studies have questioned earlier results (9). Further work is necessary to unravel the puzzle of atopic dermatitis.

Diagnosis and Clinical Findings

The diagnostic hallmark is pruritis, often accompanied by erythema and dry skin. The cutaneous features vary greatly, depending on age and chronicity of disease. Environmental factors, termed flare factors, which may induce or exacerbate atopic dermatitis are listed in Table 41.2.

Laboratory tests and histologic analysis of a skin biopsy do not provide confirmatory information. Measurement of IgE levels may be helpful (7, 8). Conditions that should

Table 41.2.
Flare Factors in Atopic Dermatitis

Dry skin (xerosis)	Heat
Sweating	Cold
Exercise	Temperature change
Infection	Allergic contact dermatitis
Anxiety	Allergies to foods or inhalants
Scratching	Coexisting diseases (e.g., scabies)
Light touch	Greasy ointments
Prickly clothes	

be considered in the differential diagnosis include seborrheic dermatitis, contact dermatitis, nummular dermatitis, scabies, and psoriasis (7).

Atopic dermatitis is divided into three stages, based on age: infantile, childhood, and adolescent/adult. In infants, atopic dermatitis is most likely to occur around 3 months of age. It frequently coincides with the introduction of foods, which have been blamed for its occurrence. However, a causal relationship is not well established (7, 10).

The eruption generally begins as erythematous patches on the cheeks and spreads to the extensor surfaces of the extremities. The diaper area is usually spared. Intense itching is evident, as the infant scratches constantly and rubs against garments and bedding. Many infantile cases clear over months to years. Some cases continue into the childhood stage or may recur years after resolution of the infantile form.

In the childhood stage, the flexor surfaces are usually involved, rather than extensor areas. The eruption is usually either lichenoid, consisting of small, discrete, brown or red-brown papules, or papular, consisting of larger papules with a central crust. Such lesions tend to be chronic, may disappear around the age of 10 to 12 years, or may continue into adolescence (7, 8).

In the adolescent/adult phase, papules tend to become confluent, forming large lichenified areas. Crusts result from scratching caused by intense itching. The lichenoid plaques are poorly marginated and vary in color from bright pink-red to brown or gray-brown. Areas commonly involved are the neck, eyelids, forehead/scalp, anterior chest, and wrists. Dorsal areas of the fingers, toes, and feet may be affected as well (7, 8).

The course of atopic dermatitis is quite variable and generally is marked by remissions and exacerbations (8, 9). Most cases begin in infancy, but onset may not occur until childhood or after puberty. Reported frequency of peristance varies widely, from 10 to 83% (9). Part of the variability can be explained by the imprecise diagnostic criteria available. Some factors that suggest an unfavorable prognosis are severe, widespread dermatitis in childhood, family history of atopic disease, presence of allergic rhinitis and/or asthma, female sex, and early age of onset (<1 year of age) (9).

Treatment

Strategies involve a variety of nondrug and drug treatment measures, depending on the acuteness or chronicity of the condition. The most common measures include environmental change, skin-maintenance care techniques, use of topical corticosteroids, systemic antihistamines, topical or systemic antibiotics, and selectively, systemic corticosteroids.

Where environmental factors are identified as contributory, avoidance is advised. This might include avoiding extremes of temperature and humidity, strenuous exercise, rough scratchy clothing, bathing with harsh soaps and hot water, irritant chemicals, and allergens (7, 8). These factors and others can precipitate or perpetuate the itch-scratch cycle. Stress, anger, or anxiety may contribute to exacerbations of atopic dermatitis in some patients.

Dry skin and itch are the two problems addressed in managing atopic dermatitis. The stratum corneum is inadequately hydrated, and attempts at rehydration can use either a "lubricating" method or a "dry" method. Many patients find relief from the application of greasy ointments such as petrolatum, while others find that such substances worsen their condition (7). Various types of topical therapy are described below.

TOPICAL THERAPY

Several forms of topical therapy are available. Patients with mild or localized atopic dermatitis may require treatment only with a topical corticosteroid ointment or cream. For patients with extensive disease, a combination of topical measures may be necessary.

Baths. Itching can be relieved, at least temporarily, by tepid baths containing oatmeal (Aveeno, plain or oilated), bath oils, or tar preparations. Bathing helps to rehydrate the skin, but it should not be frequent. Strong soaps should be avoided, although mild soaps can be used. A lubricating lotion (Cetaphil, Lubriderm, or Nutraderm) can be used instead of soap. Soaking in lukewarm water followed by application of a water-in-oil emulsion (e.g., Eucerin) while the skin is still wet will assist in rehydrating the keratin layers (8, 11).

Wet Dressings. When lesions are oozing, acute, and possibly infected, use of wet dressings such as Burow's solution 1:20 or tap water is appropriate. Compresses are applied generally for 20 to 60 min, three to six times a day. The dressings cool and dry by evaporation, thus stimulating vasoconstriction. In very acute situations, compresses can be applied continuously (7, 8).

Topical Corticosteroids. Topical corticosteroids are effective in treating many cases of atopic dermatitis. Nonfluorinated (hydrocortisone 1% or desonide 0.05%) or low-potency fluorinated preparations (triamcinolone 0.025%) are preferred for long-term use, although high-potency agents may be considered in the acute phase, switching to less potent preparations later (7, 8, 11). Use of fluorinated corticosteroids should be minimized by application only during acute flares, by applying only to the most problematic areas, or by once-daily or alternate-day application (7). Long-term use of fluorinated corticosteroids, particularly high-potency agents, causes thinning of the skin and can lead to atrophy and telangiectasia, particularly on the face and skin-fold areas (groin, armpits) (7).

Topical Antibacterial Agents. Secondary infection, fre-

quently due to *S. aureus,* can be treated with topical antibiotics (7, 8, 11). Preparations containing erythromycin or bacitracin are preferred, because of less sensitization than with agents such as neomycin (7, 8). Mupirocin is another agent to consider, but it is more costly.

Combined Topical Treatments. "Wet" and "dry" methods have been suggested (7). The "wet," or lubricating, method includes short baths or showers in tepid water (hot water stimulates pruritis). Mild soaps can be used, but sparingly. Following bathing, the skin is lubricated while still wet, to help hold water in the stratum corneum. Bath oil, petrolatum, hydrophilic ointment, or topical corticosteroids may be used (7, 8).

The "dry" method uses either short showers in tepid water or short baths with oilated oatmeal. Bathing with soap and water is not allowed, except for use of a moist cloth to cleanse the arms, groin, and axillae. A nonlipid cleanser is applied to the skin surface twice a day and gently wiped off. Oily or greasy lubricants are not used. Topical corticosteroids can be applied using products that are in a water/propylene glycol emollient base (Synalar solution) (7). Obviously, a great deal of patient effort and cooperation is necessary with either method.

SYSTEMIC THERAPY

Agents such as antihistamines, corticosteroids, and antibiotics may be useful under certain circumstances. Two possible benefits from oral administration of antihistamines include relief of pruritis and sedation. Histamine plays some role in atopic dermatitis but probably is not the only mediator involved in pruritis (1). The benefits of antihistamines in relieving pruritis are controversial (7, 8, 10–12). Studies have shown conflicting results and often suffer from insufficient numbers of patients (12). Use of antihistamines may relieve pruritis in some patients (7, 8, 12), at least initially (11), but sedation is seen as the primary benefit by some investigators (10, 11, 13). If sedation is the desired goal, then patients may benefit more from the traditional H_1-blockers rather than the newer, less sedating antihistamines (13).

Oral corticosteroids may be used for acute flares, to break the itch-scratch cycle (7, 8, 10, 11). Duration of use should be short-term, in the range of 5 to 7 days. Oral corticosteroid therapy generally is discouraged, except in the case of very refractory episodes (7, 8).

Systemic antibiotic therapy may be indicated to treat secondary bacterial infections (7, 8, 11). Therapy is directed toward Gram-positive cocci, particularly *S. aureus.* A 7-day course of erythromycin is often used (7).

CONTACT DERMATITIS

Allergic contact dermatitis is an inflammatory skin disease that represents a delayed hypersensitivity reaction to ex-

Table 41.3.
Common Causes of Contact Dermatitis[a]

Pharmaceutical agents	*Hobby materials*
Corticosteroids	Epoxy glues
Neomycin	Paints
"Caine" anesthetics	Solvents
Merbromin	*Occupational contactants*
Thimerosal	Chrome
Transdermal patches	Epoxy glues
Lubricants	Other glues
Lotions	Formaldehyde
Hand creams	Nickel
Face creams	Cobalt
Bath oils	Solvents
Cosmetics and fragrances	Resins
Deodorants	Dyes
Hair dyes	Oils and greases
Makeup	Solvents and waterless cleaners
Perfumes	*Metals*
Surfactants	Jewelry
Hand, bath, and shower soaps	*Plants*
Soaps used at work	Poison oak/ivy
Kitchen and laundry soaps	Algerian ivy
Waterless cleaners	Chrysanthemums
Rubber materials	House plants
Gloves	
Finger protectors	

[a] Adapted from Jacobs MR, Zanowiak P, Topical antiinfective products. In Feldman EG, Blockstein WL (eds): Handbook of Nonprescription Drugs, 9th ed. Washington, D.C., American Pharmaceutical Association, 1990, pp 771–773; Hanifin JM: The role of antihistamines in atopic dermatitis. J Allergy Clin Immunol 86:666–669, 1990; and Advenier C, Queille-Roussel C: Rational use of antihistamines in allergic dermatological conditions. Drugs 38:634–644, 1984.

ternal stimuli (4, 14). Not all contact dermatitis is allergic; it may be caused by the irritant properties of some substances that come in contact with the skin. The occurrence of contact dermatitis is widespread, partly because of the wide variety of substances that cause allergic contact dermatitis (Table 41.3). The prevalence within the general population is not well documented. Some studies have attempted to determine prevalence of allergy to specific substances in the normal population, and positive patch-test results have occurred in the following percentages: nickel (5.8%), neomycin (1.1%), ethylenediamine (0.43%), and benzocaine (0.17%) (15). Gender differences are observed regarding specific allergies. For example, nickel allergy is more frequent in women than in men, but this may reflect a higher rate of contact through jewelry and clothing (15). Irritant contact dermatitis is considered to be more common than allergic contact dermatitis, particularly in the industrial setting (15, 16).

Etiology

Causes of contact dermatitis are varied and commonly include plants, nickel compounds, rubber compounds, and ethylenediamine (14). Often the dermatitis is related to

occupational exposure (16). The origin, allergic or irritant, usually cannot be differentiated by the clinical presentation (4, 16, 17), and irritants may also be allergens (15).

Pathogenesis

In allergic contact dermatitis, certain physiologic events must occur (4) including

1. Penetration of the corneal barrier by the allergen;
2. Interaction with epidermal or dermal cells;
3. Interaction with the immune system;
4. The inflammatory response.

The development of contact hypersensitivity involves combination of the chemical (hapten) and skin protein to form an antigen. The antigen is carried to the regional lymph nodes by epidermal Langerhans cells and probably interacts at these sites to produce specifically sensitized T cells (14, 15). In addition, secretion of interleukin-1 by macrophages is required to initiate the response. Interleukin-1, which enhances many types of immunologic responses, is also produced by epidermal keratinocytes and Langerhans cells. Helper T cells then differentiate into effector cells that release lymphokines, producing local inflammation (14). A period of 8 to 10 days is generally required for presentation of the allergy once sensitization has begun (15).

The histopathologic features include perivascular infiltrates of lymphocytes and monocytes in the upper dermis. Edema is usually present and may involve intra- and intercellular edema in the epidermis, with a condition called spongiosis. Basophils and mast cells are present in the cellular infiltrate and may participate in the inflammatory reaction. Chronically, hyperkeratosis, acanthosis, and a cellular infiltrate in the superficial dermis containing basophils are present (14).

Patients may report no problem associated with the previous handling of a material, sometimes for prolonged periods (years). The latest exposure results in an eruption termed the elicitation dose (17). An earlier exposure resulted in the initial sensitization, and generally a latent period can be identified.

In the case of irritant contact dermatitis, direct cellular damage occurs with no latent period. Damage is proportional to the toxic properties of the irritant, but it may depend on repeated exposure for substances that are mild irritants. With irritant contact dermatitis, those exposed to the same dose under the same conditions for the same length of time would be expected to react. Reduction of the irritant dose (exposure) often means a good prognosis (17).

Diagnosis and Clinical Findings

Acute contact dermatitis frequently involves erythema, edema, and vesicle formation. More chronic forms involve scaling, excoriations, and plaque formation. Severe itching in the acute phase is prominent and may persist in the chronic phase. The history and physical examination can provide critical information to establish the diagnosis. An acute, patchy and streaky dermatitis of the extremities, coupled with a recent history of outdoor plant exposure, might lead to a diagnosis of poison ivy/oak dermatitis. A dermatitis occurring on a woman's eyelids or face might be associated with the use of cosmetics, perfumes, or hair sprays. A careful and thorough history regarding general activities, occupation, hobbies, known allergies or previous skin disorders, and family history, along with careful examination of the distribution and extent of the lesions may suggest possible causes. A listing of common causes of contact dermatitis is provided in Table 41.3, and the substances most likely involved with reactions in certain body areas are indicated in Table 41.4. In many patients, the diagnosis remains unclear and patch testing may be indicated, particularly in conditions that become chronic or

relatively resistant to treatment or those suspected to be occupationally related.

Patch testing may assist in diagnosis of delayed hypersensitivity contact dermatitis. Standardized methods and concentrations for testing for a variety of substances have been recommended (15). Even with standardized approaches, both false-positive and false-negative reactions may occur (16, 17). For example, an irritant reaction may be difficult to differentiate from a weak allergic reaction.

Treatment

Successful treatment requires the identification and/or removal of the allergen (irritant). This may be accomplished more easily with poison ivy dermatitis than with dermatitis caused by industrial exposure.

Specific drug therapy depends more on the stage of the dermatitis than on the cause (15). Severe, acute reactions characterized by blistering, swelling, and oozing may require systemic corticosteroids (15, 17). Daily doses of 60 mg of prednisone are commonly used for a period of 7 to 10 days. Doses of 100 mg/day are used in severe cases. Topical corticosteroids are of little benefit in acute edematous blistering dermatitis because of inadequate penetration. Topical steroid therapy once or twice a day can be instituted once the acute symptoms are controlled and continued after oral therapy is stopped. Ointments are usually preferred because cream preparations have a greater variety of ingredients, including fragrances and preservatives, to which the patients may be allergic (17). Oral antihistamines provide little if any benefit other than sedating properties, since they do not suppress contact allergy (14, 15). Soothing compresses or soaks with water, aluminum acetate, or dilute vinegar (2 tablespoons white vinegar per quart) may be beneficial (15).

For subacute (moderate) or chronic dermatitis, topical corticosteroid therapy is used, rather than systemic therapy. A high-potency agent may be applied twice daily in subacute conditions. Often the skin is dry, so ointment or cream preparations of corticosteroids are preferred over solutions. Compresses and soaks are usually not indicated, and other lotions (e.g., Calamine) should be avoided because of a drying effect. In chronic situations, low-, medium-, or high-potency corticosteroid preparations are selected, based on the degree of skin thickening (lichenification). Overnight occlusion with plastic enhances penetration of the steroid. Caution should be exercised with high-potency agents because of the potential problem mentioned previously (thinning atrophy of the skin, telangiectasia), particularly on the face and in skin-fold areas. Generally, lubrication is needed, with frequent application in a thin layer. White petrolatum is a good choice. If secondary infection is present, systemic antibiotic therapy is usually preferred (15).

Table 41.4.
Causes of Contact Dermatitis by Body Region[a]

Scalp	Hair dyes (paraphenylenediamine, a permanent dye), hair lotions, permanents (glyceryl thioglycolate), nickel in hair pins, wig attachments/adhesives
Face	Cosmetics, topical medicaments, plants; preshave and aftershave lotions, airborne allergens
Forehead	Hatbands, any hair products
Eyes	Eyelids affected by cosmetics, face creams, lubricants, hair spray, nail polish
Conjunctiva	Thimerosal
Lips and perioral areas	Lipstick, lip protectants, toothpastes, mouthwashes, mangoes
Ears	Nickel (earrings), perfume, earplugs, earphones, telephone receiver
Neck	Perfume, nickel (necklace), hair cosmetics, clothing; clothing labels, buttons, zippers
Armpits	Deodorants, depilatories, clothing, perfumes
Hands	Materials encountered at work and/or home, e.g., foods, chemicals, topical medicaments, hand lotions and lubricants, rubber gloves, rubber bands, jewelry, plants
Body (trunk, chest, waist)	Dyes, formaldehyde (fabric finisher), resin rubber in elastic of clothing, perfumes, scarves
Genitalia	Bubble bath, antiseptic cleansers, condoms, contraceptive creams or jellies, deodorant douches, scented menstrual pads or tampons
Feet	Shoes, shower sandals, fabrics, metal eye holes, sole inserts, adhesives, colorants, athelete's foot remedies

[a] Adapted from Jacobs MR, Zanowiak P, Topical antiinfective products. In Feldman EG, Blockstein WL (eds): Handbook of Nonprescription Drugs, 9th ed. Washington, D.C., American Pharmaceutical Association, 1990, pp 771–773; Hanifin JM: The role of antihistamines in atopic dermatitis. J Allergy Clin Immunol 86:666–669, 1990; and Advenier C, Queille-Roussel C: Rational use of antihistamimes in allergic dermatological conditions. Drugs 38:634–644, 1984.

URTICARIA

Urticaria and angioedema are vascular reactions of the skin (18). Another name for urticaria is hives. When edema extends into the dermis and hypodermis, it is termed angioedema. Urticaria is estimated to occur in about 15% of the population at some time in life. The prevalence in men and women is about equal. About one-third of the cases are acute, this form being more common in younger patients.

Etiology

The etiology of urticaria is varied and often obscure (10, 19). Urticaria may be associated with or caused by drugs, serums, foods, inhalants, insect bites/stings, contact substances, connective tissue diseases, neoplasms, and physical agents (10). The physical agents often include cold, heat, light, pressure, and dermographism (10, 19). The urticaria may be linked to cholinergic or adrenergic factors (19, 20). With adrenergic urticaria, stress was a factor in the development of attacks and elevated plasma concentrations of norepinephrine, epinephrine, and dopamine in a reported case (20). Hereditary angioedema constitutes about 1% of all cases of angioedema (19). In addition to childhood onset and family history, a specific test for Cl esterase inhibitor, a complement component, can be used to confirm the condition. A cause cannot be identified specifically in 70 to 80% of cases, and thus the urticaria is termed idiopathic (10, 18, 19).

Pathogenesis

Five pathophysiologic mechanisms have been proposed for urticaria and/or angioedema: IgE-mediated, complement-mediated, direct effects on mast cell membranes, alteration of arachidonic acid metabolism, and idiopathic (21). Skin biopsies of urticarial lesions show edema in the upper dermis, vascular dilation, and cellular infiltrates in the dermis around the small vessels, caused by leakage. The infiltrates consist mainly of mononuclear cells, with occasional eosinophils, neutrophils, and mast cells (10).

Histamine has been identified as a mediator in the urticarial response. The dermal mast cells produce and store histamine. When activated, the mast cells release histamine as well as other vasoactive substances including kinins, leucotrienes, and prostaglandins. Kinins are vasoactive peptides that may be important in the development of urticaria. They slow smooth muscle contraction, cause vasodilation, and increase vascular permeability. IgE antibodies can interact with antigens on the mast cell surface, producing histamine release. Complement-fixing antibodies can also react with antigens on the mast cell surface, producing histamine release. Direct histamine release may be caused by certain drugs and chemicals (18).

Diagnosis and Clinical Findings

A careful history, which describes the pattern of attacks, precipitating cause, duration of wheals, associated symptoms, and atopic background, should be taken. As a result, the presence or absence of the following can be established: relationship to any ingested, inhaled, or injected substance; a contact reaction; a systemic disease; a hormonal influence; an emotional cause; or infection. While the basic mechanism may still be unknown, the above factors can serve as triggers. For example, half of patients with idiopathic urticaria are made worse by aspirin or nonsteroidal antiinflammatory drugs. Thyroid disease, lymphoma, and systemic lupus erythematosus (SLE) have been linked to urticaria (18, 19).

The skin lesions are circumscribed, elevated, erythematous areas (wheals) that are pruritic (10, 21). The size of the wheal can vary from 1 to 2 mm to many centimeters. Individual lesions tend to resolve in 24 to 48 hr, but new lesions will appear (10). Some patients also develop angioedema that extends into the deeper tissue. If urticaria occurs continuously for longer than 6 weeks, it is termed chronic (10, 18).

Treatment

The best treatment is identification and removal of the cause. As indicated, in most cases this approach is unsuccessful, because either the cause cannot be identified or multiple factors are involved (10, 21). Treatment then is directed toward the effector cells and inflammatory mediators to block either release or effect. Therapy also may be directed toward receptor sites on target tissues, which involves the cutaneous microvasculature and cells (10).

Antihistamines, which are H_1-receptor antagonists, provide relief in about 65 to 70% of patients with urticaria or angioedema (13, 19). Other mediators are likely to be involved in patients not responding. The available H_1-antagonists are nearly equal in efficacy. Choice can be based on side effects (e.g., is sedation desirable or undesirable) or pharmacokinetic considerations (see section on antihistamines) (13, 21). If one agent is ineffective or not tolerated, a second agent from a different chemical group can be tried. On occasion, a combination of H_1-receptor antagonists can be used (13, 21). If treatment with H_1-receptor antagonists is successful, the agent should be tapered over several days to prevent flares, rather than discontinued abruptly (21).

H_2-receptor antagonists like cimetidine may be combined with H_1-receptor antagonists in treating urticaria (21, 22). Administered alone, the H_2-receptor blockers have little if any demonstrated benefit. Several studies have claimed greater benefit with the combination, but this is not a consistent observation. The H_2-receptor antagonists may be useful only in certain types of urticaria (e.g., cold, angioedema) (22). If a case is refractory, a trial of the combination may be appropriate (13). Doses of cimetidine have ranged from 400 to 1600 mg per day. Ranitidine has also been used in standard oral doses (22).

DRUG-INDUCED SKIN DISEASES

Cutaneous reactions to drugs result from immunologic or nonimmunologic mechanisms. Immunologic mechanisms require activation of host pathways, and their presence is supported by the clinical features identified by Bigby, which were noted earlier (3, 6). Cutaneous reactions caused by nonimmunologic mechanisms are more common than allergic reactions (6). Nonimmunologic mechanisms associated with cutaneous drug reactions include nonimmunologic activation of effector pathways, overdosage, cumulative toxicity, side effects, drug interactions, metabolic changes, and exacerbation of existing dermatologic conditions (6). The most relevant of these, the activation of effector pathways, is not antibody-dependent and actually involves at least three different mechanisms. The first involves direct release of mediators from mast cells, with presentation as urticaria or angioedema. Drugs implicated in this mechanism are opiates, polymyxin B, and radiographic contrast media. Radiographic contrast media also have activated complement in the absence of antibody, again resulting in urticaria. The third mechanism involves alteration of arachidonic acid metabolism, the most notable example being anaphylactic-like responses to aspirin and nonsteroidal antiinflammatory drugs. The other nonimmunologic mechanisms, for the most part, produce skin manifestations that are not the focus of this discussion (e.g., bruising with excess warfarin, color changes due to phenothiazines) (6). Drug-induced skin diseases have a variety of clinical manifestations (Table 41.5). Each of these will be reviewed briefly regarding clinical presentation, diagnostic considerations, and time course.

Drug Exanthem

Drug exanthem is the most common cutaneous reaction, comprising almost half of the skin reactions due to drugs

Table 41.5.
Dermatological Manifestations of Drug-induced Disease

Exanthematous rashes
Urticaria
Fixed drug eruption
Erythema multiforme
Exfoliative dermatitis
Photosensitivity
Toxic epidermal necrolysis
Vasculitis

(5). It is usually described as a morbilliform or maculopapular eruption, often generalized, but usually starting on the trunk or in areas where pressure and/or trauma occur. The rash is frequently symmetric and consists of erythematous macules and papules that may become confluent. Pruritus is commonly present (3, 6), and fever and eosinophilia may occur. A drug-induced exanthem must be differentiated from exanthems of viral origin, although this is difficult, since definitive diagnostic tests are lacking. The usual time course is occurrence within the first week of starting therapy with the offending agent, frequently within the first 3 days. Some antibiotics and allopurinol are considered exceptions. For penicillin, cephalosporins, and cotrimoxazole, exanthems may appear within the first 2 weeks, sometimes later, or even after therapy is stopped. With allopurinol, rashes can occur after 3 weeks or more. Most exanthems can be expected to disappear within 1 to 2 weeks after discontinuing the offending agent.

Some characteristics contribute to a higher risk of drug exanthem. Women have a 35 to 50% higher risk than men. Fifty to 80% of patients with infectious mononucleosis taking ampicillin (amoxicillin is also implicated) experience a rash. The combination of ampicillin and allopurinol produces a higher frequency of rashes than either agent alone. Patients with acquired immunodeficiency disease (AIDs) taking cotrimoxazole experience more drug exanthems (3).

Urticaria

Urticaria is responsible for about one-quarter of drug-induced skin reactions and is described as pruritic, red wheals or as firm, erythematous, round or oval plaques of varying sizes. The overlying epidermis appears normal, and no scaling is evident. A lesion generally is present for less than 24 hr, but it is replaced by new lesions at other sites. Edema of the reticular dermis is a prominent pathologic feature. The term angioedema is used to indicate swelling in deep dermal and subcutaneous tissues, often with mucous membrane involvement (3, 6).

If the reaction is IgE-dependent, onset can be within minutes but usually within 36 hr. Other systemic signs and symptoms of the immediate-type hypersensitivity may occur, including bronchospasm, diaphoresis, hypotension, and eosinophilia. Urticaria as a component of a serum sickness reaction will occur 4 to 12 days after challenge and will include systemic symptoms such as fever, arthralgias, hematuria, and possibly liver or neurologic symptoms. In some cases, the urticaria results from nonimmunologic mechanisms, but it is difficult to differentiate because the time course and presentation resemble the immediate hypersensitivity reaction (3, 6). This reaction is termed pseudoallergic (3).

Discontinuation of the offending agent results in prompt resolution, although some cases may persist for several weeks (3).

Fixed Drug Eruption

Fixed drug eruption is responsible for about 10% of drug-induced skin disorders. It involves the development of a lesion, often solitary, which appears as an erythematous macule and subsequently becomes an edematous plaque (3, 6, 23). Vesicles and bullae with desquamation may occur later (3, 23). After resolution of these acute phases, hyperpigmentation remains, with colors varying from brown to violet-brown or even black (28). Lesions most often occur on the face, lip, facial region, and genitalia. Pruritus and burning may accompany the reaction, and their severity reflects the intensity of the inflammatory response.

Also rare, systemic symptoms may range from malaise to severe prostration (23). As the name implies, lesions recur in the same place upon rechallenge by the offending substance. Symptoms recur usually between 30 min and 8 hr after reexposure. With repeated exposure, the number of lesions may gradually increase. Drugs most often implicated and phenolphthalein (used in over-the-counter laxatives), tetracycline, and oxyphenbutazone (23, 24).

Erythema Multiforme

Erythema multiforme is usually an acute, self-limited inflammatory disorder involving skin and mucous membranes, although the spectrum can vary widely (3, 6). A prodrome may occur consisting of malaise, sore throat, and possibly fever, with skin lesions developing over 2 to 7 days. Lesions have a distinctive iris or target appearance and are erythematous plaques with dusky centers, a surrounding ring of edema, and a darker erythematous outer border. The plaques are most perfuse peripherally and develop in groups over a period of a few days, fading after 1 to 2 weeks. Sites most commonly involved are the backs of the hands, palms, wrists, forearms, feet, elbows, and knees. Bullous or vesicular lesions accompanied by mucosal involvement and systemic symptoms is termed Stevens-Johnson syndrome. Usually, two or more mucosal surfaces are involved (3, 24).

Toxic Epidermal Necrolysis (TEN)

Toxic epidermal necrolysis, although uncommon, is a serious skin disorder with significant morbidity and mortality. It is somewhat similar to erythema multiforme but is more acute and catastrophic. A brief prodrome of sore throat, malaise, fever, and chills occurs with skin involvement within 24 hr. Lesions are small, dusky, necrotic macules with early and extensive involvement of periorificial areas and mucous membranes. The lesions enlarge progressively to produce large confluent areas of necrosis with extensive epidermal sloughing within 2 to 5 days. Patients are quite ill, with mortality ranging from 15 to 60% in reported series (3).

Staphylococcal scaled skin syndrome (SSSS), which usually occurs in children or immunocompromised patients, must be considered in the differential diagnosis. Some differentiating factors for (SSSS) are that epidermal separation is superficial (e.g., intraepidermal, usually the granular layer), periorificial and mucous membrane involvement is absent or mild, and skin pain is absent. Drug-induced TEN generally involves subepidermal separation (3, 24).

Drugs are the most common cause, particularly in adults. Nonsteroidal antiinflammatory drugs, particularly the butazolodins, sulindac and piroxicam, sulfonamides (cotrimoxazole), phenytoin, barbiturates and allopurinol are frequently implicated (6, 24).

Exfoliative Dermatitis

Exfoliative dermatitis involves redness of the entire skin, with widespread scaling due to exfoliation. Other than in cases of psoriasis, the condition is eczematous. Severe systemic symptoms that may accompany it include hypovolemia, heart failure, intestinal malabsorption, hypoprothrombinemia and hypothermia (24).

Photosensitivity

Photosensitivity is of two types, photoallergy and phototoxicity. Most reactions fall into the category of phototoxicity, with photoallergy being uncommon (6, 24). Phototoxic reactions can occur with the first exposure to a drug, even within a few hours, and are dose-related. The reaction resembles a sunburn and can in some cases progress to blister (6, 24). Removal of the offending agent usually brings resolution. Such reactions will occur in most patients given adequate amounts of drug and adequate exposure to ultraviolet (UV) light.

Photoallergy involves the combination of the drug, immune system, and light. A delayed hypersensitivity mechanism is suspected because the onset is usually delayed and recovery is slow. Such reactions occur in only a small percentage of exposed patients (3). The rash is usually eczematous but may involve lichenoid, urticarial, bullous, or purpuric lesions. The reaction typically occurs in sun-exposed areas but in severe cases may involve areas that are normally protected. Photoallergic reactions may persist for some time after the drug is withdrawn. Drugs commonly causing photoallergic reactions are tetracyclines, thiazides, diuretics, sulfonamides, phenothiazines, quinolones, and antihistamines (3, 6, 24).

Cutaneous Vasculitis

Cutaneous vasculitis commonly presents as palpable purpura and usually involves the lower extremities, although the reaction may be generalized. Other organs, such as the liver, kidney, joints, and gastrointestinal tract, may become involved. The cutaneous lesions at various times may be macules, papules, urticarial lesions, and in the most severe cases, hemorrhagic blisters. The origin of the reaction is thought to involve immune mechanisms, but the precise explanation is unknown (3, 6, 24).

ANTIHISTAMINES

The antihistamines (H_1-receptor antagonists) traditionally have been grouped according to chemical structure: ethanolamines, ethylenediamines, alkylamines, piperazines, piperadines, and phenothiazines (25, 26). However, this classification provides little information about the expected pharmacodynamic and pharmacokinetic properties. A more useful classification distinguishes first-generation (classic) and second-generation (nonsedating) H_1-receptor antagonists. This more clearly distinguishes differences in pharmacodynamic properties. Each group has

been examined for desirable pharmacokinetic properties (13, 25, 26). Table 41.6 summarizes many properties of the H_1-receptor antagonists, including some agents still under investigation.

H_1-receptor antagonists are reversible competitive inhibitors of the actions of histamine on H_1-receptors. The antihistamines block the bronchopulmonary and vasoactive effects of histamine, resulting in decreased vascular permeability, decreased pruritis, and relaxation of smooth muscle (25, 26). While differences in potency exist, the antihistaminic activity of the various agents is considered to be similar when equipotent doses are given (26). This effect is demonstrated by suppression of the wheal/flare reactions induced by histamine or allergens. The duration of effect varies among agents (Table 41.6) (25, 26). In addition, second-generation agents also prevent release of inflammatory mediators from IgE-sensitized mast cells and basophils (25, 26). An effect on calcium, either by

Table 41.6.
Antihistamine Activity and Pharmacokinetics

Generic Name (Trade Name)	Chemical Class	T max[27,31] (hr)	T$_{1/2}$[27,31] (hr)	Wheal/Flare[25,31] Suppression (hr)	Sedative[30] Activity[a]	Anticholinergic[30] Activity[a]
1st generation						
Azatadine (Optimine)	Poperidine	4	9–12	NF[b]	+ +	+ +
Brompheniramine (Dimetane)	Alkylamine	3.1 ± 1.1	24.9 ± 9.3	3–9	+	+ +
Chlorpheniramine (Chlortrimeton)	Alkylamine	2.5 – 3.4	24.4	24	+	+ +
Clemastine (Tavist)	Ethanolamine	3–5	4–6	12–24	+ +	+ + +
Cyproheptadine (Periactin)	Piperidine	6–9	[c]	NF	+	+ +
Diphenydramine (Benadryl)	Ethanolamine	2–3	3–5	NF	+ + +	+ + +
Hydroxyzine (Atavax, Vistaril)	Piperazine	2.0	20.0	2–36	+ +	+ +
Promethazine (Phenergan)	Phenothiazine	2.7	12.2	NF	+ + +	+ + +
Triprolidine (Actidil)	Alkylamine	2.0	2.1	NF	+	+ +
Tripelennamine (PBZ)	Ethylenediamine	2–3	[c]	NF	+ +	±
2nd generation						
Astemizole (Hismanal)	—	1–2	10 days	weeks	±	±
Loratadine[d] (Claritin)	—	1–2	11.0	24	±	±
Cetirizine[d] (Zyrtec)	Piperazine	0.5–1	7.4	24	±	±
Terfenadine (Seldane)	Butyrophenone	1–2	4.5	12–24	±	±

[a] Symbols: + + +, high; + +, moderate; +, low; ±, low to none.
[b] NF, Not found.
[c] Metabolic and excretory fate not fully elucidated.
[d] Not available in US.

inhibiting influx across the cell membrane or inhibiting intracellular release, is probably responsible. These agents may inhibit late-phase allergic reactions by effects on leukotrienes or prostaglandins (26).

Classic H_1-receptor antagonists possess anticholinergic activity. They also produce a number of central nervous system (CNS) effects that result from a CNS depression and are generally undesirable. These effects are clinically apparent at doses used therapeutically. In general, second-generation agents lack clinically apparent anticholinergic activity or CNS effects at therapeutic doses. These agents penetrate poorly into the CNS, and levels are insufficient to block central H_1 or cholinergic receptors. Binding is preferential for peripheral H_1-receptors (13, 25, 26).

Pharmacokinetics

All of the agents are generally well absorbed after oral administration, with peak serum levels reached at around 2 hr (21, 25, 27). Most agents undergo metabolism through the cytochrome P_{450} system in the liver, with clearance and elimination half-lives varying substantially. Active metabolites are formed for some agents like terfenadine and astemizole. The duration of wheal/flare suppression is related to both dose and the serum elimination half-life. Children usually exhibit shorter serum half-lives than adults, e.g., the half-life of chlorpheneramine has a mean of about 11 hr in children versus about 24 hr in adults, and the half-life of hydroxyzine is about 7 hr in children and 20 hr in adults. Serum half-lives are expected to be prolonged in elderly patients and those with liver disease (25).

The pharmacokinetic profile of astemizole differs considerably from that of other agents (25, 26). Astemizole and the primary active metabolite, desmethylastemizole, have a half-life of approximately 9 to 10 days after a single dose (26, 28). With once-daily administration of 10 mg, steady-state levels are achieved after 4 to 6 weeks of administration (26, 28). After continued administration, the half-life for astemizole and its metabolites is 18 to 20 days (26). Inhibition of the wheal/flare response may not be apparent until the second day of administration or later, so use of a loading dose (30 mg) is recommended to decrease the time to onset of effect (26). Suppression of the wheal/flare response may be seen for weeks to months, compared with a duration of 24 hr or less for most other agents (26, 28).

Adverse Effects/Drug Interactions

The adverse effects of first-generation agents include CNS and anticholinergic effects. The primary effects due to CNS depression include sedation, impaired cognitive function, diminished alertness, difficulty in concentrating,

confusion, dizziness, and tinnitus (25, 26). Sedation or drowsiness occurs in 10 to 25% of antihistamine users. These effects may result in impaired mental performance, as reviewed by Meltzer (29). Some first-generation agents such as diphenhydramine also cause dystonic reactions (25, 29). The common anticholinergic effects include dry mouth, blurred vision, and urinary retention. Some first-generation agents (e.g., tripelennamine) cause gastrointestinal symptoms including nausea, vomiting, epigastric distress, diarrhea, or constipation (25).

The second-generation agents generally lack sedative and anticholinergic effects. The prevalence of sedation is similar to that seen with placebo (25). In some of the skin diseases discussed, sedation may be a desired property and the only benefit from the use of an antihistamine.

Drug interactions are expected with the first-generation agents and other agents which have CNS depressant effects (alcohol, hypnotics, antianxiety agents, antipsychotics, analgesics) or anticholinergic activity (antispasmodics, tricyclic antidepressants, antipsychotics, antiparkinson drugs (13). These interactions do not occur with second-generation agents.

CONCLUSION

Allergic and drug-induced skin diseases encompass a varied group of diseases manifested through the skin. Although allergy is suspected in many cases, the specific allergen may be difficult to identify. Other mechanisms operate in some diseases, but the clinical presentation does not distinguish the etiology. Drug-induced conditions tend to be acute and resolve, particularly when the offending agent is removed. Atopic dermatitis, contact dermatitis, and idiopathic urticaria are more chronic, with exacerbations and remissions. Topical corticosteroids, occasional short-term systemic corticosteroids in severe conditions, and antihistamines are the mainstay of drug therapy, in addition to other nonspecific topical treatments.

REFERENCES

1. Jacobs MR, Zanowiak P, Topical antiinfective products. In Feldmann EG, Blockstein WL (eds): Handbook of Nonprescription Drugs, 9th ed. Washington, D.C., American Pharmaceutical Association, 1990, pp 771–773.
2. Sauer GC: Manual of Skin Diseases, 6th ed. Philadelphia: JB Lippincott, 1991, pp 1–8.
3. Bigby M, Stern RS, Arndt KA: Allergic cutaneous reactions to drugs. Prim Care 16:713–727, 1989.
4. Thestrup-Pedersen K, Larsen CG, Ronnevig J: The immunology of contact dermatitis. Contact Dermatitis 20:81–92, 1989.
5. Pratt WB, Drug allergy. In Pratt WB, Taylor P, (eds): Principles of Drug Action: The Basis of Pharmacology. New York, Churchhill Livingstone, 1990, pp 533–548.
6. Wintroub BU, Stern R: Cutaneous drug reactions: pathogenesis and clinical classification. J Am Acad Dermatol 13:167–179, 1985.
7. Oakes RC, Cox AD, Burgdorf WHC: Atopic dermatitis. A review of diagnosis, pathogenesis and management. Clin Pediatr 22:467–475, 1983.

8. Dahl MV, Lobitz WC, Dobson OL, Atopic dermatitis. In Demis DJ (ed): Clinical Dermatology, Vol 3. Philadelphia, JB Lippincott, 1985, unit 13–3:1–35.

9. Sampson HA: Pathogenesis of eczema. Clin Exp Allergy 20:459–467, 1990.

10. Dockhorn RJ: Atopic dermatitis, contact hypersensitivity, and urticaria. J Allergy Clin Immunol 84:1051–1054, 1989.

11. Rasmussen JE: Management of atopic dermatitis. Allergy 44(suppl 9):108–113, 1989.

12. Hanifin JM: The role of antihistamines in atopic dermatitis. J Allergy Clin Immunol 86:666–669, 1990.

13. Advenier C, Queille-Roussel C: Rational use of antihistamines in allergic dermatological conditions. Drugs 38:634–644, 1984.

14. Katz SI: Mechanisms involved in allergic contact dermatitis. J Allergy Clin Immunol 86:670–671, 1990.

15. Maibach H, Epstein E, Allergic contact dermatitis. In Demis DJ: Clinical Dermatology, Vol 3. Philadelphia, JB Lippincott, 1988, unit 13–1:1–46.

16. Nethercott JR, Holness DL: Occupational allergic contact dermatitis. Clin Rev Allergy 7:399–415, 1989.

17. Whittington C: Clinical aspects of contact dermatitis. Prim Care 16:729–738, 1989.

18. Maize JC: Urticaria and non-hereditary angioedema. In Demis DJ (ed): Clinical Dermatology, Vol 2. Philadelphia. JB Lippincott, 1985; unit 7–9:1–15.

19. Champion RH: A practical approach to the urticarial syndromes—a dermatologist's view. Clin Exp Allergy 20:221–224, 1990.

20. Haustein U: Adrenergic urticaria and adrenergic pruritis. Acta Derm Venereol 70:82–84, 1990.

21. Soter NA: Urticaria: current therapy. J Allergy Clin Immunol 86:1009–1014, 1990.

22. Theoharides TC: Histamine$_2$ (H$_2$)-receptor antagonists in the treatment of urticaria. Drugs 37:345–355, 1989.

23. Korkij W, Soltani K: Fixed drug eruption. A brief review. Arch Dermatol 120:520–524, 1984.

24. Felix RH, Smith AG, Stevenson CJ, Skin disorders. In Davies DM (ed): Textbook of Adverse Drug Reactions, 3rd ed. Oxford, Oxford University Press, 1985, pp 473–493.

25. Simons FER: H$_1$-receptor antagonists: clinical pharmacology and therapeutics. J Allergy Clin Immunol 84:845–861, 1989.

26. Woodward JK: Pharmacology of antihistamines. J Allergy Clin Immunol 86:606–612, 1990.

27. Paton DM, Webster DR: Clinical pharmacokinetics of H$_1$-receptor antagonists (the antihistamines). Clin Pharmacokinet 10:477–497, 1985.

28. Simons FER: Recent advances in H$_1$-receptor antagonist treatment. J Allergy Clin Immunol 86:995–999, 1990.

29. Meltzer EO: Performance effects of antihistamines. J Allergy Clin Immunol 86:613–619, 1990.

30. Olin BR (ed): Facts and Comparisons. St. Louis: JB Lippincott, 1991, pp 188–194.

31. Anon: Antihistamine Drugs. AHFS Drug Information 90. Washington, D.C.: American Society of Hospital Pharmacists, 1990, pp 1–31.

CHAPTER 42

COMMON SKIN DISORDERS: ACNE, PHOTODERMATOSES, WARTS, SEBORRHEIC DERMATITIS, AND PSORIASIS

LUELLA G. CHURCHWELL, M.D., PHI-VAN T. LE, M.D.,
MICHAEL A. SCHNEIDER, M.D., and KEN T. TAKEGAMI, M.D., M.P.H.

The skin is the largest organ of the body. It functions as a protective barrier from the external environment and maintains the homeostatic milieu of the internal environment. As such, the proper function and integrity of the skin is essential to life.

Many disease processes can attack this organ system alone. In addition, skin manifestations can give important clues to underlying systemic pathology, and many of these are discussed elsewhere. In this chapter we describe some common skin dermatoses that pose therapeutic challenges.

ACNE

Acne vulgaris is a chronic but usually self-limited disorder occurring within the pilosebaceous units of the face, neck, and upper trunk. It is the most common skin disorder and is estimated to occur to some degree in 85% of adolescents (1). The incidence of acne is the same in both sexes, with peak occurrence between the ages of 16 and 19 years. It resolves in the vast majority of patients by the age of 25. Females tend to develop the disorder at an earlier age, secondarily to the earlier onset of puberty (2). Acne persists more commonly into the third and fourth decade in females, in comparison to males (3). Males however tend to develop a more severe form of the disease. Genetic factors play a role, particularly in the more severe forms of acne. The high prevalence and the multifactorial origin of the disorder make genetic factors difficult to assess.

Clinical Features

Acne lesions occur within the specialized sebaceous hair follicular units found principally on the face, and to lesser degree the chest, shoulders, and back. The two basic lesions are noninflammatory and inflammatory. Noninflammatory lesions consist of open comedones (blackheads) and closed comedones (whiteheads). Comedones develop from an impaction of keratin and sebum within a dilated follicle and are considered the primary lesions in acne. Mild acne consists of only noninflammatory lesions, but unfortunately few cases fail to progress beyond this point.

Inflammatory lesions are derived from closed comedones. Papules and pustules represent superficial inflammatory lesions, and a preponderance of these lesions constitutes at least moderate acne. Deeper inflammatory lesions include nodules and cysts and are present in the more severe cases of acne. Patients with nodulocystic acne often have extensive involvement of the chest and back (Table 42.1).

Scarring can occur, particularly in the deeper inflammatory forms of acne. It is the most devastating clinical feature, prompting early aggressive therapy. The most common scar is the atrophic (ice-pick) form, which is permanent. Hypertrophic, keloid-like scars also occur and are more commonly seen on the trunk. These tend to flatten in time.

Often overlooked is the residual pigmentary alteration seen following resolution of inflammatory lesions. This is particularly noticeable in black patients, where hyperpigmentation predominates, and is often what prompts a physician visit. There is no effective treatment for the pigmentary alteration beyond preventing further inflammatory lesions from developing. Most pigmented lesions will fade, but it can take 6 months to a year.

Table 42.1.
Acne Lesions

Noninflammatory
Open comedones (blackheads)
Closed comedones (whiteheads)
precursor to inflammatory lesions
Inflammatory
Superficial
Papules
Pustules
Deep
Nodules
Cysts

Pathogenesis

The pathogenesis of acne is multifactorial, however active sebaceous glands are a prerequisite. The development of acne corresponds with the maturing of these glands under hormonal control at puberty. The only hormone known to stimulate the sebaceous gland directly is androgen (2). This is derived from the testes in males and the ovaries and adrenal glands in females. Circulating testosterone is converted at the tissue level by 5 α-reductase to dihydrotestosterone, a potent stimulator of sebum production. Sebum is composed of different lipids, including triglycerides and waxes that assist with hydration of the skin. On average, both male and female acne patients secrete more sebum than nonacne patients, and the level of secretion does correlate with the severity of acne. Acne-prone skin has shown an abnormally high 5 α-reductase activity in vitro. In addition, women with more severe acne frequently have biochemical androgen excess.

Excess sebum plays an important role, through a variety of mechanisms, in the development of an acne lesion. The earliest pathologic change in acne is a retention hyperkeratosis of the follicular epithelium. Sebum accumulates within this keratin and may cause the abnormal follicular keratinization (2). This mass of material plugs the follicle, causing it to dilate below the surface of the skin. If the follicular opening dilates enough to extrude this material, an open comedo results. The black color is attributed to the impacted keratinous material, not dirt, nor oxidized sebum or melanin as once thought (4). An open comedo is actually a mature lesion, not capable of becoming inflammatory. If the follicular opening does not dilate, a closed comedo results, which is the principal site for inflammatory lesion development.

Once the follicle has been occluded, an inflammatory lesion is initiated through an interaction between trapped bacteria, principally *Propionibacterium acnes*, and the retained contents. *P. acnes* is an anaerobe found in high levels in adolescents with acne but less so in nonacne patients. *P. acnes* secretes chemotactic factors for polymorphonuclear leukocytes, which can then invade the follicular wall leading to its disruption and eventual collapse. This results in spillage of its contents into the surrounding dermis, with a subsequent increased inflammatory response. In addition *P. acnes* produces lipases that hydrolyze the triglycerides of sebum into glycerol and free fatty acids. It utilizes the glycerol for growth, and the free fatty acids can further contribute to the inflammatory response. The depth and magnitude of the inflammatory response corresponds with the development of pustules, papules, nodules, and cysts (Fig. 42.1).

Immune response does play an associated role. Patients with acne have a much higher antibody titer against *P. acnes* than controls. Both the classical and alternative complement pathways are activated in acne lesions by *P. acnes*, which produce C5a neutrophilic chemotactic factor (5). Small numbers of *P. acnes* can produce profound in-

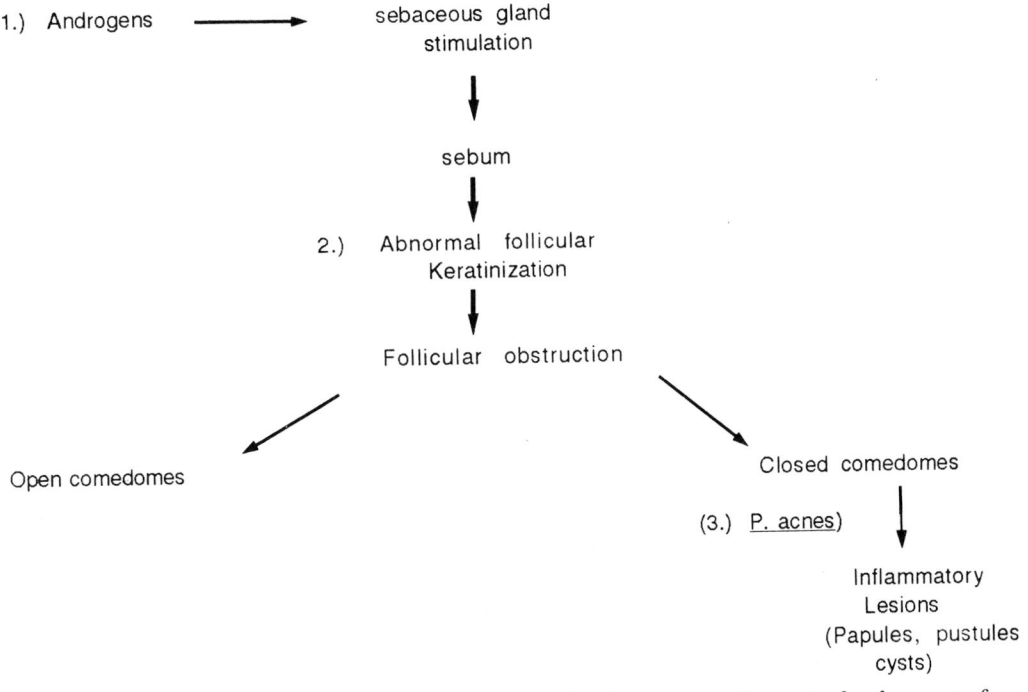

Figure 42.1. Treatment of acne is based on reversing the three primary factors in development of acne lesions, as numbered above.

Table 42.2.
Medications That Aggravate Acne

Hormonal
    Danazol
    High progesterone-containing OCP
    Anabolic steroids
    Gonadotropins
    Prednisone
Nonhormonal
    Azathioprine
    Bromides
    Cyanocobalamin
    Disulfuram
    Gold
    Hydantoin drugs
    Iodides
    Lithium
    Maprotiline
    Quinidine
    Quinine
    Rifampin
    Thiouracil

flammation in patients with high antibody titers against this organism. Finally, severe acne occurs rarely in females, perhaps because they have a better defense mechanism to *P. acnes* than males (6).

A number of exogenous factors can exacerbate acne. Oil-based makeup, pomades, and oily soaps and hair products can occlude the follicle, initiating a comedo. Physical pressure from a headband or hat can induce localized acne. Exposure to excessive heat and humidity can exacerbate acne, but the mechanism is not clear. The ingestion of certain drugs can aggravate acne. Danazol and birth control pills with a high progesterone component do this, presumably through increased androgenic activity. A list of other medications that aggravate acne is in Table 42.2. The mechanism for most of these is not understood. Diet and stress are frequently implicated, but controlled studies are lacking. Unless a patient implicitly believes a food is aggravating the condition, no food, including chocolate need be eliminated from the diet.

Treatment

The treatment of acne can often be difficult and disappointing. Acne is a chronic condition, at times requiring many months to years of individualized treatment in order to achieve control. Nevertheless, with the patient's commitment and compliance, it is certainly a treatable disease, and control should be expected. Compliance is enhanced if the patient understands both the nature of the disease and the rationale behind the therapy. Virtually all therapy is preventive, with little or no effect on the inflammatory lesions present at the outset. For that reason maximal efficacy is not reached for several months, even with the

most effective of treatments. Once control is achieved, the patient should understand that maintenance therapy will be required as long as the tendency to acne persists.

Important in the pathogenesis of acne are pilosebaceous obstruction by sebum and keratin, androgen-stimulated sebum production, and proliferation of *P. acnes*. Acne therapy is directed at correcting each of these factors. As in other diseases without a single best treatment, a multitude of therapies exist, each with merit in the individual patient. Many of the topical therapies are readily available over the counter, and while effective in some when used properly, are subject to misuse by the uninformed patient. Compliance with a single regimen, whether self-medicated or under a physician's care, should be stressed for optimal results. A summary of therapeutic agents in acne with their principal mode of activity is in Table 42.3.

General Skin Care

Cleansing the skin with soap and water can remove the oil so prominent on acne-prone skin and thereby improve the appearance. There is no evidence that excessive cleansing offers therapeutic benefit, and in fact it can be irritating. Surface sebum and bacteria are not felt to play a role in the development of lesions that begin deeper in the follicle. Patients should avoid soaps with a high oil content. These are usually reserved for dry, sensitive skin but can be counterproductive in acne. Expensive medicated soaps are usually not indicated as a supplement to other treatment plans. In noninflammatory acne, a mildly abrasive cleanser may be of some benefit by inducing a

Table 42.3.
Summary of Therapeutic Agents in Acne and Principal Mode of Activity

Topical Therapy	Oral Therapy
Antimicrobial (*P. acnes*)	Antimicrobial
Benzoyl peroxide	Antibiotics
Antibiotics	Tetracycline
Clindamycin	Minocycline
Erythromycin	Erythromycin
Meclocycline	Trimethoprim
Tetracycline	sulfamethoxazole
Azelaic acid	Isotretinoin
Sulfur—minor	Comedolytic
Salicylic acid—minor	Isotretinoin
Comedolytic	Decreased sebaceous gland
Tretinoin	activity
Azelaic acid	Isotretinoin (principal action)
Benzoyl peroxide—minor	Hormonal therapy
Salicylic acid—minor	Estrogen
Resorcin—minor	Cyproterone acetate
Decreased sebaceous gland activity	Spironolactone
None	

superficial exfoliation of the skin. In inflammatory acne, or in the patient with dry skin from previous acne therapy, a gentle soap is best.

Avoidance of all cosmetics is best. If they are to be used they should be water-based. Cosmetics should be removed by soap and water, not by cleansing creams.

Astringents are alcohol-based cleansers that are easy to use and leave the face feeling cool and refreshed. Unfortunately they are of limited value in the treatment of acne.

Topical Therapy

Topically applied medications remain the cornerstone of acne therapy. They are often effective alone in mild-to-moderate acne and are important adjuncts to oral antibiotics in more severe acne. The most widely used topical preparations are benzoyl peroxides and antibiotics, which inhibit the growth of *P. acnes*, and tretinoin, which reverses abnormal keratinization in the follicles.

BENZOYL PEROXIDE

Benzoyl peroxide was first formulated for dermatologic use in 1905, and the compound was recognized as useful for acne in 1934. The ointment vehicle was unsuitable for acne therapy though, and it was not until the mid 1960s that a stable preparation of benzoyl peroxide in a hydrous media was formulated. Since that time it has become the most frequently used topical medication in acne, because different preparations can be purchased over the counter and by prescription. When used properly it can be effective alone in mild acne, but it is used as an adjunct to other therapies in more severe disease.

The principal mode of action of benzoyl peroxide is thought to be its bactericidal activity against *P. acnes*. It is metabolized to benzoic acid in the skin, and its lipophilic properties allow it to penetrate better than other topical antimicrobials (7). Once it penetrates the follicle, the release of nascent oxygen from the peroxide exerts its effect on the bacteria. Studies have shown a twofold greater reduction of *P. acnes* counts with 5% benzoyl peroxide, compared with topical erythromycin or oral tetracycline at 4 weeks (8).

Benzoyl peroxide has also been thought to exert comedolytic and exfoliative properties, however reports are contradictory and this action is considered minor. Benzoyl peroxide has no effect on sebum production or concentration. By reducing the *P. acnes* counts, free fatty acids that contribute to the comedonal plug and inflammation are also reduced. Benzoyl peroxide can be irritating to the skin, leading to increased blood flow. Increased blood flow is felt to speed resolution of inflammatory lesions through a counterirritant mechanism (9).

Benzoyl peroxide is available over-the-counter as 2.5%, 5.0%, and 10.0% creams, lotions, washes, and soaps. It is available in the same concentrations by prescription, usually gel vehicles. Recently a 4% formulation in a hydrous medium with greater activity but a lower side-effect profile has been introduced. Selection of the appropriate vehicle is important. Gels are considered to be more effective for release of the active substance, however they can be more irritating. Although less effective, a wash or lotion may be all that is tolerated by a patient with more sensitive skin. During the winter months, when dry skin is a problem, switching from the gels to a cream or lotion may be necessary.

There is no difference among the three available concentrations in reducing *P. acnes* numbers in the skin (1). Therefore, when initiating therapy with benzoyl peroxide, it is reasonable to begin with a low concentration (2.5 to 5.0%) to decrease irritation. Initial therapy is once daily only. The patient should apply this sparingly, being careful to avoid the periorbital, perinasal, and perioral skin. Patients often experience mild erythema, burning, or stinging on initial application, and they should be instructed to expect this. By applying the medication at night, the erythema should be minimal by morning. If irritation persists, switching to every-other-night therapy is appropriate.

Tolerance to these side effects is usually achieved as therapy continues. Once tolerance is achieved, the patients should increase the frequency of application to twice a day. Switching to a more potent vehicle or a higher concentration should be done only after tolerance to the lower concentrations is achieved without significant improvement in the acne at 4 to 8 weeks. As a general rule, the side-effect profile increases more than the efficacy with increasing concentration of benzoyl peroxide.

The most frequent side effect of benzoyl peroxide is skin irritation, which may in part be responsible for its efficacy. It is known that 1 to 2% of people are allergic to this compound. Patients who continue to experience erythema and scaling at low concentrations applied on alternate days may have an allergic contact dermatitis. In these cases, stopping the medication is all that is required, and an alternative therapy will be necessary. Patients should be warned that benzoyl peroxide can bleach hair and clothes. Allowing the preparation to dry completely before contact with fabrics can minimize this problem.

The question of whether benzoyl peroxide is carcinogenic has been raised. Two earlier studies on rodents supported this, but case-controlled studies in humans have been negative. It is currently considered to be completely safe for use in humans (10).

TRETINOIN

Since being introduced for acne in 1969, this vitamin A derivative has probably become the single most effective agent for treatment of the disorder. Its mode of action was originally thought to relate to its ability to promote erythema and peeling of the skin. It is now known that its activity is directed at reducing the cohesiveness of keratinocytes within the sebaceous follicle, independent of clinical peeling (1). Inhibition of the retention hyperkeratoses prevents microcomedo formation. For that reason, tretinoin is superior to all other topical or oral therapies for comedonal acne. As inflammatory lesions are derived from comedones, tretinoin is an important adjunct to therapy in more severe acne.

The patient should understand that tretinoin can cause mild-to-severe irritation of the skin, which is more common at initiation of therapy. This is manifested by erythema, dryness, and peeling and is influenced by the formulation used. Tretinoin is now available in a 0.025, 0.05, and 0.1% cream, an 0.01 and 0.025% gel, and an 0.05% lotion. Therapy is usually initiated with the 0.025% cream, because the irritation can be much less while the efficacy is only slightly so (7). Tretinoin should not be applied more than once daily, initially. It should be applied to completely dry skin because moisture increases the permeability of tretinoin and therefore its irritant potential. The patient should avoid the periorbital, perinasal, and perioral skin. The erythema and dryness is not required for effectiveness, so if side effects continue to be a problem, using tretinoin every other, or every third night is recommended. As tolerance develops, the frequency can be increased.

Many patients offset the side effects of tretinoin with heavy emolliants, but this is counterproductive in the treatment of acne and should be discouraged. The use of other harsh skin-care products such as astringents can increase the irritant potential of tretinoin and should be eliminated if possible. A gentle soap should be used, and a mild lotion only if necessary.

Patients can experience a modest exacerbation of their acne on initiation of therapy. This is secondary to the ability of tretinoin to release the retained products of comedones to the skin surface. Patients should understand this so they will not become discouraged and possibly discontinue this therapy unnecessarily. This flare should resolve in 3 to 6 weeks.

Tretinoin decreases the thickness of the stratum corneum (9). The most superficial layer of the skin, it helps protect it from damage from the sun. Patients should avoid long exposure to UV radiation, but if it is necessary, should use a sunscreen with an SPF of at least 15. The thinned stratum corneum also allows better permeability of other topical agents, which is an advantage when tretinoin is used in conjunction with topical antibiotics. Systemic toxicity, as seen potentially with oral retinoids, is not a problem with topical tretinoin, even when applied in high concentrations. The small amount absorbed is metabolized rapidly by the liver. Although it is considered safe for use in pregnancy, it is not often used, for medicolegal reasons.

TOPICAL ANTIBIOTICS

Topical antibiotics are used in mild-to-moderate inflammatory acne and as an adjunct in more severe nodulocystic acne. They are not comedolytic, so are not useful alone in noninflammatory acne. The topical antibiotics most commonly used are clindamycin and erythromycin in a variety of vehicles. Meclocycline, a derivative of oxytetracycline, and topical tetracycline are also available. Studies have consistently shown that topical antibiotics are as efficacious as low-dose oral tetracycline in moderate inflammatory disease (11). Topical antibiotics are especially useful when tapering oral therapy.

The principal action of topical antibiotics is their antibacterial effect against P. acnes. Clindamycin is more lipophilic and appears to be more effective than erythromycin at reducing P. acnes counts (7). However, when comparing clinical efficacy of the different agents, similar results are obtained, so other factors play a role. Topical antibiotics may inhibit P. acnes metabolism without killing the organism. This would result in decreased lipase activity, FFAs, and chemotactic factors. Both oral and topical tetracycline have known antiinflammatory activities (12).

Topical antibiotics are usually applied twice a day to moist skin, after washing with soap and water. As with other topical products, the vehicle is important. Vehicles with a high alcohol content allow better absorption but can be more drying. A cream or ointment may be tolerated better initially in patients with more sensitive skin or during winter months.

A response to topical antibiotics is often evident before that of other topical therapies. Improvement is often noted within 2 weeks, but maximal efficacy cannot be determined for at least 12 weeks.

The most common side effect of topical antibiotics is mild erythema and stinging, secondary to the vehicle used. Organisms resistant to these antibiotics can develop, but this has not proven to be a clinical problem. Recolonization by susceptible strains of P. acnes occurs quickly on discontinuation of therapy (13). Oral clindamycin hydrochloride therapy is frequently complicated by pseudomembranous colitis (PMC). Commercially available topical clindamycin preparations are in the phosphate form and are less readily absorbed through the skin. However 10% of a daily application does reach the bloodstream, and cases of PMC have been described with topical use (14). This must be considered to be a rare but potential side effect, particularly when clindamycin is applied to large areas of skin. Topical meclocycline can impart a faint yellow tint to the skin, which will wash off. Topical tetracycline preparations will cause the skin to fluoresce under the black lights frequently used in discotheques.

COMBINED TOPICAL THERAPIES

Combining two topical therapies directed at different factors in the pathogenesis of acne makes sense from a practical standpoint. The most commonly used combination is that of tretinoin, with its comedolytic activity, with topical antibiotics or benzoyl peroxide. By thinning the stratum corneum tretinoin allows better absorption of the antimicrobials.

The combination of tretinoin and benzoyl peroxide appears to be less irritating than tretinoin alone, and it is more effective than either used individually. Therapy is initiated with low concentrations of each on an alternate-day basis. After tolerance to the irritant effect is acquired, they can each be used daily. The patient is usually instructed to use benzoyl peroxide in the morning and tretinoin at night. This should be strictly adhered to, because the irritant potential is additive when used concurrently. If the patient cannot tolerate benzoyl peroxide, one of the other topical antibiotics can be used.

A commercially available combination of benzoyl peroxide and erythromycin is now considered to be more effective than either alone. Erythromycin is more active than benzoyl peroxide against *P. acnes*, but it is not lipid soluble. It is thought that benzoyl peroxide somehow carries the more active erythromycin to the target tissue (7).

OTHER TOPICAL THERAPIES

Traditional therapies using salicylic acid (0.5 to 3.0%), sulfur (2 to 10%), or resorcin (2.0 to 6.0%) are not used frequently now. Their effectiveness correlated with their ability to induce erythema and desquamation. Salicylic acid is a keratolytic with some comedolytic activity, but tretinoin is more effective. Sulfur is not comedolytic, but it appears to hasten the resolution of inflammatory pustular lesions. The combination of sulfur and salicylic acid is synergistic, so they are frequently compounded together. Each also has weak antimicrobial activity. Resorcin, another keratolytic, has been shown to be less effective in acne in the most recent studies (15). If used extensively, systemic absorption can (rarely) cause methemaglobinemia, cyanosis, and convulsions. These treatments are best reserved for the patient with mild-to-moderate acne who is intolerant to other topical medications.

Some newer topical therapies have been promising in studies and may soon be available commercially. The combination of erythromycin 4.0% and zinc acetate 1.2% was more effective than clindamycin 1% and erythromycin 2% in controlled studies (16). The combination provided enhanced absorption of both products, and the zinc is thought to be antiinflammatory. Side effects include facial burning and redness in one patient. Azelaic acid, a naturally occurring dicarboxylic acid, has been effective for both noninflammatory and inflammatory acne. The dicarboxylic acids were initially found to have a beneficial effect on hyperpigmentary disorders such as melasma. When patients reported a coincidental improvement in their acne, studies were initiated to investigate this further. A 20%

azelaic acid cream was as effective as 0.5% tretinoin cream in reducing comedones, with less irritant side effects (17). The best results with azelaic acid cream were seen in papulo-pustular acne. Its efficacy is explained by both a strong comedolytic property and a bacteriostatic effect on *P. acnes*. No side effects beyond a low rate of local irritation were reported.

Systemic Therapy

ANTIBIOTICS

Oral antibodies are used at the outset of therapy for patients with moderate-to-severe inflammatory acne. They should be used in conjunction with topical benzoyl peroxide, tretinoin, or occasionally topical antibiotics. Tetracycline and its derivative minocycline are usually the drugs of choice. Erythromycin is a frequent alternative, and trimethoprim sulfamethoxazole is (rarely) prescribed as third-line therapy. They exert their effects principally by inhibiting *P. acnes*, resulting in decreased chemotactic factor and lipase production. They also exert a direct antiinflammatory response. This is more true of tetracycline than the other antibiotics.

Tetracycline in doses of 1 g/day in 2 to 4 divided doses is usually employed first. Occasionally doses up to 2 g are necessary in nodulocystic acne. It is best absorbed if not taken with food, dairy products, iron, or antacids. Patients should be instructed to take the medication 1 hr before or 2 hr after a meal. Tetracycline on an empty stomach can cause nausea in some patients, and in these instances it can be taken with a small amount of food.

Clinical improvement is usually noted within 2 to 4 weeks of therapy. The optimal time course for oral antibiotic therapy is not known. Frequently, maximal efficacy is not reached for 4 to 5 months so continuing therapy for this time period should be expected (12). If a good response is achieved, continued oral antibiotics for an additional 6 months offered no advantages over topical therapy alone (18). Once an adequate response is noted, tapering the dose by 250 mg/day over several weeks is recommended. The goal is to discontinue oral therapy and maintain control with topical therapy alone.

A common side effect of tetracycline is vaginal yeast infection, which can be controlled by oral and topical nystatin or other topical antiyeast preparations. Tetracycline can also cause a photosensitivity eruption, so patients should wear a sunscreen with a SPF of at least 15 if they plan to spend an extended period of time in the sun. A rare, but more serious side effect of tetracycline therapy is benign intracranial hypertension, manifested by headache and visual disturbances. Patients exhibiting these symptoms should discontinue the tetracycline and see their physician immediately. Tetracycline and its derivatives should never be administered in pregnancy because they may cause liver toxicity in the mother, and bone and teeth abnormalities in the fetus.

If cost were not a factor, minocycline would be the antibiotic of choice in acne. It is more lipophilic than tetracycline, allowing it to accumulate more readily in the sebaceous follicle, and its clinical efficacy is better than that of tetracycline (19). It is better absorbed with food and is less likely to cause nausea than tetracycline. It is also less likely to cause photosensitivity reactions. The usual initial dose is 50 mg twice a day, so patient compliance is improved.

Minocyline can more frequently cause esophagitis secondary to reflux, so it should not be taken just before retiring. A dose-dependent vestibular dysfunction can occur, leading to vertigo, ataxia, and nausea and vomiting. Lowering the dose can circumvent this, but often the medication must be discontinued. A blue-gray pigmentation of both skin and mucous membranes is reported with minocycline use. This is more prominent in sun-exposed areas and can take up to 7 months to resolve. Doxycycline, another derivative of tetracycline, has shown therapeutic equivalence to minocycline, but it is rarely used in the treatment of acne, because of a much higher incidence of photosensitivity reactions.

If a patient is unable to take tetracycline for any reason, erythromycin is an effective alternative. It is as effective as tetracycline, but a higher incidence of gastrointestinal problems and the more frequent development of resistant strains of P. acnes make it the second choice. Advantages of erythromycin include the lower rate of monilial overgrowth, the lack of photosensitivity, and the fact that it can be taken with food. It is considered safe in pregnancy, however consultation with the obstetrician is wise before initiating long-term therapy with any medication during pregnancy. The same dosing recommendations are made as for tetracycline. The safety of long-term antibiotics in the treatment of acne is well established. A concern over possible serious suprainfections has not been warranted clinically. There is also concern that broad spectrum antibiotics can decrease the effectiveness of oral contraceptives (OCP). A small study found two pregnancies in 163 woman-years, corresponding to a 6-fold increase in OCP failure (20). This remains controversial, but this possibility should be discussed with these patients and alternate forms of birth control suggested.

ISOTRETINOIN

Oral isotretinoin (13-*cis*-retinoic acid) is the most effective agent for the treatment of acne. This synthetic derivative of vitamin A, first introduced in 1982, is indicated for the treatment of the patient with resistant nodulocystic acne. It should be considered early in the therapy of patients who exhibit scarring. Dramatic improvement can be seen with isotretinoin, and in contrast to other acne therapies, prolonged remission can be expected. The teratogenicity and multiple potential side effects associated with isotretinoin preclude its use in less severe acne.

The mechanism of action of isotretinoin is multifactorial. It is the only known therapeutic agent that affects all the major factors in the pathogenesis of acne (21). Its most profound effect is on reduction of sebaceous gland size and sebum production. Sebaceous glands are reduced from 50 to 90% in size. This inhibition continues in most patients for more than a year after discontinuing therapy. Isotretinoin also normalizes the keratinization process within the follicle. It has no direct antibacterial properties, but isotretinoin reduces P. acnes counts indirectly by the reduction of sebum. Isotretinoin also has direct antiinflammatory properties by inhibiting chemotaxis of neutrophils and monocytes.

The usual starting dose of isotretinoin is 0.5 to 1.0 mg/kg/day. The lower dose is usually initiated and then gradually increased, based on clinical response and tolerance of side effects after 4 to 8 weeks. Therapy is continued for 16 to 20 weeks. Oral antibiotics and topical medications that can further dry the skin are discontinued before isotretinoin therapy. Improvement is usually noted within 2 months, and continued improvement can be seen for up to 6 months following therapy. Some patients have relapses after a course of isotretinoin, but they are usually much milder than the initial disease. This is seen more frequently in those treated with lower doses. If relapse occurs, a second course can be given but is not recommended until 6 months have elapsed, because of the delayed improvement that can occur.

Nearly all patients who receive isotretinoin experience mucocutaneous side effects, primarily dryness of the skin, eyes, nose, and mouth. Moisturizers can be used to combat the dry skin and chelitis. An antibiotic ointment is recommended for the nasal passages to prevent cracking, bleeding, and potential colonization by Staphylococcus aureus (9). Conjunctivitis is common, and corneal opacities can occur but usually resolve within 6 weeks after therapy. During this period, patients may be intolerant of contact lenses. Artificial tears can be used to offset this problem.

The most common laboratory abnormality in patients on isotretinoin is a dose-related elevation of serum triglyceride levels. Twenty-five percent of patients have a 10% or greater elevation (21). Less frequently seen are a decrease in high-density lipoprotein levels (15%) and an increase in cholesterol levels (8%). This is usually not a problem in the young patient treated for acne, but precautions should be taken. A baseline lipid profile should be determined, with repeat samples obtained after 1 week of therapy and every 2 weeks until levels stabilize. A low-fat diet and avoidance of alcohol is necessary in mild-to-moderate elevations. Close monitoring should be done in an obese or diabetic patient. This is reversible, with lipid levels returning to baseline within 8 weeks after therapy. Less frequently seen is an elevation of hepatic enzyme levels. These usually return to normal with continued therapy or a reduction in dose (21). Rarely, a decreased white blood cell count or hypercalcemia are seen. The need for laboratory monitoring of these parameters should be discussed with patients before therapy with isotretinoin.

Synthetic retinoid therapy has been associated with skeletal changes in a small percentage of patients. In acne patients treated for 20 weeks, significant abnormalities are rare. Most commonly seen are muscle and bone discomfort that respond to mild analgesic therapy. Skeletal hyperostosis, manifested by small spurs along the vertebral bodies, has been noted in 26% of acne patients in one study. However 23% of patients had these prior to therapy, and the significance of this finding on short-term therapy is not known (22).

Fewer than 10% of patients notice some hair loss during therapy, usually late in the course. Regrowth is to be expected. Photosensitivity can occur, and patients should use an SPF 15 sunscreen before prolonged exposure to the sun. Benign intracranial hypertension is a rare side effect of isotretinoin administration. This is manifested by headache, nausea, vomiting, and visual disturbances. If this occurs the patient should see the physician immediately.

The most serious side effect of isotretinoin is its teratogenicity. Miscarriage and stillbirth are common, and a 25-fold increase in major congenital anomalies is seen (2). These involve the cranium, face, heart, brain, and thymus during the period of organogenesis. The female patient must understand the teratogenic potential and the consequences of becoming pregnant while on this medication. A pregnancy test should be performed within 2 weeks of beginning therapy. Treatment should start on the second or third day of the next menstrual cycle. An effective method of birth control must be initiated at least 1 month before and continued until 1 month after cessation of therapy. Although teratogenic, isotretinoin is not mutagenic, and future pregnancies should not be affected (2). The drug has no known effect on spermatogenesis.

HORMONAL THERAPY

Estrogen therapy has long been noted to improve acne in women. This hormone counteracts the androgenic stimulation of the sebaceous gland, decreasing sebum production. Estrogen is usually given as the oral contraceptive pill. The most notable results were obtained using doses of 50 μg or more of ethinyl estradiol or mestranol daily. These have largely been withdrawn from the market now and OCP containing 30 μg of ethinyl estradiol or less are not as effective (2). However, estrogen therapy with or without antiandrogen therapy continues to be used with some success in female patients with other signs of hyperandrogenemia, (hirsurtism, obesity, and laboratory ele-

vations of testosterone). Androgen-dominant OCP containing norgestral can actually worsen acne and should be avoided; combinations containing norethisterone should be used instead (12).

Side effects of this therapy are common and include nausea, weight gain, spotting, breast tenderness, and amennorhea. Less commonly seen are a brown pigmentation of the skin (chloasma), telangiectasias, allergic reactions, and alopecia. Unfortunately, it can take several months to see noticeable improvement. Gynecomastia and decreased libido prevent its use in males.

Antiandrogens are a class of drugs that prevent androgen activity at the target sites by competing with dihydrotestosterone for the receptor. This therapy is used most commonly in women with hyperandrogenism secondary to polycystic ovarian disease and adrenal hyperactivity manifested by hirsutism and acne. Cyproterone acetate and spironolactone are two antiandrogens that have been used successfully in acne (23).

Excellent results are obtained in women using a combination of low-dose cyproterone acetate (2 mg/day) and ethinyl estradial (35 mg/day). This combination was twice as effective in reducing acne lesions as OCP alone. The seborrhea improves first, but by the end of 3 months, acne lesions also regress. Beneficial effects are maintained for many months after withdrawing therapy. A higher dose of cyproterone acetate (25 to 50 mg/day) may be needed in the resistant patient who also has hirsutism. Side effects of cyproterone are uncommon but include a low frequency of headache, dizziness, nausea, and menstrual irregularity. These tend to improve with continued therapy. Cyproterone acetate is not currently available in the United States.

Spironolactone is a weak potassium-sparing aldosterone-antagonist diuretic with antiandrogenic properties. It has been used alone in doses of 100 to 200 mg/day with excellent results achieved in acne regression at 4 to 6 months. Forty percent of cases relapse 6 to 12 months after therapy. It has been used in males at these doses without development of gynecomastia and decreased libido, but they have been seen in spironolactone therapy for other disorders. Potassium levels were not altered at this dose in subjects of one study, but spironolactone should be reserved for patients with normal renal function. Periodic evaluation of electrolytes should be done in any patient on long-term spironolactone therapy.

Conclusion

Frequently, optimal therapy of acne requires use of a combination of the topical and systemic medications discussed in this chapter. The patient may become confused about the proper use of the different therapeutic agents. When improperly used, the side-effect profile increases, and optimal results are not achieved. To insure compliance, evaluate the patient's understanding of the treatment program and address any questions.

PHOTODERMATOSES

Exposure to sunlight plays an essential part in many dermatologic diseases. Effects range from acute damage, including sunburn and photosensitive skin disorders, to chronic skin damage, including photoaging and carcinogenesis.

SOLAR RADIATION

The sun emits a broad spectrum of electromagnetic radiation, but at the earth's surface the solar spectrum consists of wavelengths between 290 and 3000 nm, divided into ultraviolet radiation (290 to 400 nm), visible radiation (400 to 760 nm), and near infrared radiation (wavelengths greater than 760 nm), as shown in Table 42.4. Ultraviolet radiation (UVR), the spectrum that most frequently affects the skin, is divided into three main categories, UVC (200 to 290 nm), UVB (290 to 320 nm), and UVA (320 to 400 nm) (24).

Ultraviolet C

Wavelengths between 200 and 290 nm are referred to as UVC or germicidal radiation, and they are lethal to microorganisms. UVC is attenuated during its passage through the atmosphere, where it is largely absorbed by the ozone layer, and thus it does not naturally reach the earth's surface. Mercury vapor lights and xenon lamps are artificial light sources that produce UVC for bacterial sterilization (24).

Ultraviolet B

UVB radiation, often referred to as the sunburn spectrum, includes wavelengths between 290 and 320 nm. This spec-

Table 42.4.
Parts of the Electromagnetic Spectrum

Radiation		Wavelength (nm)
X rays		0.01–10
Ultraviolet	UVC	200–290
	UVB	290–320
	UVA	320–400
Visible	Violet	
	Blue	
	Green	400–760
	Yellow	
	Red	
Infrared	Near	
	Middle	760–1,000,000
	Far	
Microwave, radiowave		> 1,000,000

trum reaches the earth's surface and is largely absorbed within the epidermis of the skin. UVB, a strong inducer of erythema or sunburn, can also produce delayed pigmentation or tanning. UVB contributes to chronic sun-damaged skin and skin carcinogenesis. A positive effect of UVB is its importance as a mediator of vitamin D_3 synthesis in the skin. UVB is produced by many artificial light sources for therapeutic purposes and can be blocked by window glass (25).

Ultraviolet A

Although the amount of UVA (320 to 400 nm) reaching the earth is about 10 times greater than that of UVB, it is 1000-fold less potent than UVB in producing erythema (26). In artificially high doses it can produce erythema and immediate pigment darkening of the skin. UVA may play some role in chronic skin damage (27). UVA is the solar spectrum that most frequently evokes drug photoallergy, phototoxicity, and other photosensitive disorders. It is emitted by many therapeutic appliances used to treat dermatologic diseases and is not blocked by window glass.

ACUTE EFFECTS OF ULTRAVIOLET RADIATION

The acute effects of UVR on the skin include sunburn, pigmentation, phototoxicity, and photoallergy.

Sunburn

SYMPTOMS

Erythema is the first visible sign of sunburn, which may be associated with soreness, swelling, and in severe cases blistering, nausea, and vomiting. Erythema produced by UVB occurs 12 to 24 hr after exposure, whereas UVA-induced erythema is more immediate, within the first 6 hr after exposure (26).

ETIOLOGY

UVB is the major cause of sunburn and is much more erythemagenic than UVA. Factors that may modify the effects of UVR on the skin include (*a*) time of day; (*b*) season; (*c*) geographic latitude; (*d*) clouds; (*e*) surface reflection; and (*f*) altitude. The skin type of the person is also important in the effects of UVR on the skin (28).

PATHOGENESIS

Damage to DNA and cell membranes with resulting elaboration of inflammatory mediators is thought to be involved in the skin's response to sun damage. Histamine has been detected in blisters, and prostaglandin levels have been elevated in the skin after UVB irradiation (26).

TREATMENT

Generally a sunburn patient must suffer through the course of the sunburn. Palliative therapy includes wet dressings, soothing zinc lotions, and spray formulations of topical steroids. Prostaglandin inhibitors, such as indomethacin or aspirin, have been found to block the earlier phases of erythema when prostaglandin levels are elevated, but they are of little use for the more delayed effects (29).

Tanning

There are two components of tanning, an immediate pigment-darkening produced by UVA, which occurs immediately after radiation, and delayed pigmentation, stimulated by UVB, which occurs 24 to 72 hr after exposure. Delayed pigmentation results in the formation of new melanin, which can be photoprotective (30).

PHOTOSENSITIVE DERMATOSES

Photosensitivity refers to an abnormal reaction in skin exposed to sun. This may be provoked by a number of substances that come in contact with the skin or are taken internally (Table 42.5). These reactions are divided into phototoxic, photoallergic, and miscellaneous disorders.

Phototoxic and photoallergic reactions require both a photosensitizer and ultraviolet radiation to the skin. Phototoxic reactions are nonimmunologic and occur 2 to 6 hr after sun exposure, causing a sunburn-type reaction. Photoallergic reactions occur only in people previously sensitized by a photoallergen and occur 24 to 48 hr after sun exposure, producing an eczematoid reaction confined to sun-exposed areas, usually the face, neck, and dorsum of hands. The porphyrias are a class of skin diseases thought to be a photoreaction to a porphyrin product of the host.

PHOTOAGGRAVATED DISEASES

Numerous diseases are adversely affected by sunlight, including lupus erythematosus and herpes simplex.

CHRONIC EFFECTS OF ULTRAVIOLET RADIATION

The chronic effects of UVR on the skin include photoaging and cancer.

Photoaging

Chronic sun exposure changes the appearance of the skin. Photoaged skin is deeply wrinkled, inelastic, coarse, and leathery with associated pigment changes, freckling, telangiectasias, easy bruising, and ultimately premalignant and malignant skin lesions. Actinic keratoses (solar keratoses) are common sun-induced lesions usually seen in elderly patients with fair complexions. They are most prominent in sun-exposed areas of the skin, especially the face and hands. They are small, rough, ill-defined erythematous lesions covered by adherent scales. When these lesions are present on the lip, they are called actinic cheilitis. Actinic keratoses and actinic cheilitis may go on to

Table 42.5.
Common Photosensitizers

Oral Photosensitizers	
Antidiabetics (sulfonylureas)	Antimicrobials
Chlorpropamide	Sulfanamides
Tolbutamide	Demeclocycline
Anthistamines	Doxycycline
Diphenhydramine	Tetracycline
Diuretics	Nalidixic acid
Chlorothiazide	Furocoumarins (drugs)
Hydrochlothiazide	Methoxpsoralen
Furosemide	Trimethylpsoralen
Phenothiazines	Antineoplastic
Chlorpromazine	Dacarbazine
Perchlorperazine	Vinblastine
Promethazine	Nonsteroidals
Trifluperazine	Feldene
Thioridazine	Benoxyprofen
Laxatives	Naproxen
Bisacodyl	Ibuprofen
Sweetener	Miscellaneous
Cyclamate	Amantadine
Antifungals	Quinidine
Griseofulvin	Quinine
	Amiodarone
Topical Photosensitizers	
Antiseptics, deodorants, soaps	Coal tar derivatives
Halogenated salicylanilides	
Hexachlorophene	Furocoumarins (plants)
Antifungals	Lime, figs, celery, dill, lemon,
Buclosamide	bergamot, rye, anise, mustard,
Fenticlor	parsnip, carrot, cow parsley,
Sunscreens	fennel, masterwort, angelica,
p-Aminobenzoic acid (PABA)	buttercup
Fragrances	
Musk ambrette	

form squamous cell carcinomas in a small percentage of patients, and for this reason some authors consider them to be precancerous lesions.

Photocarcinogenesis

Chronic sun exposure may lead to squamous cell and basal cell skin cancers. These are found more frequently in sun-exposed areas and are enhanced by the total exposure to UVR. Squamous cell cancers are commonly shallow ulcers with a raised border, but they may be red, raised, scaling lesions. Basal cell carcinomas are more often nodules on the skin, with a pearly, rolled border with prominent telangiectatic vessels on the surface, and they may ulcerate.

The risk of malignant melanoma appears to be increased by intermittent severe sunburn, especially during childhood (31). Malignant melanomas may have different clinical presentations, but any mole that appears to have a blue-black color or variegations in color, irregular borders, or a rapid change in size, should be evaluated by a dermatologist, because these skin cancers can have a grave prognosis if not treated adequately and promptly. The best treatment for skin cancers is usually surgical excision.

PHOTOPROTECTION

The goal of treatment for the photodermatoses is to block one or more steps in their pathogenesis. Although avoidance of sun is an obvious solution, this is not always feasible, and thus sunscreens are advocated to prevent sunburn and protect against acute and chronic photodamage.

SUNSCREENS

Sunscreens are topical preparations that block the effect of ultraviolet radiation on the skin by absorbing, reflecting, or scattering UVR. They are divided into physical sunscreens, which are usually opaque products that reflect and scatter UVR, and chemical sunscreens that contain agents that absorb UVR (Table 42.6).

Physical Sunscreens

Physical sunscreens are usually opaque and reflect or scatter UVR. They contain iron oxide, titanium dioxide, talc, zinc oxide, ferric chloride, or ichthammol. They absorb a broad spectrum of UVR, but many find them cosmetically unacceptable. The recent addition of coloring agents has made them more pleasing, but they can discolor clothes.

Table 42.6.
Sunscreen Chemicals Used in the United States

Chemical
  UVA Absorbers
    Benzophenones (UVA and UVB)
      Oxybenzone
      Dioxybenzone
      Sulisobenzone
    Avobenzone (Parsol 1789)
      Butylmethoxydibenzoylmethane
    Anthranilates
  UVB Absorbers
    PABA
      p-Aminobenzoic acid
    PABA esters
      Octyldimethyl PABA (Padimate-O)
      Glyceryl PABA
    Cinnamates
    Salicylates
  Physical (UVA and UVB)
    Red Petrolatum
    Titanium dioxide
    Magnesium oxide
    Zinc oxide
    Magnesium salicate
    Ferric chloride

They are not easily washed off, but they may melt with prolonged heat, requiring repeated application (32).

Chemical Sunscreens

The chemical sunscreens contain agents that absorb ultraviolet radiation. They may absorb UVA, UVB, or a combination of agents to give a broad spectrum of coverage.

UVB ABSORBERS

PABA Agents. One widely used chemical agent that absorbs UVB is *p*-aminobenzoic acid (PABA) and its esters. PABA penetrates the stratum corneum of the skin and attaches to proteins, so it is not easily washed off after swimming or bathing. It should be applied at least 1 hr before sun exposure, to allow adequate time for binding to the skin. A disadvantage of the PABAs is a yellow discoloration of clothing, but this is easily removed by washing. More significant are irritation and hypersensitivity reactions. The PABA esters have a lower potential for allergic or irritant reactions and staining. Currently the most frequently used ester is octyl-dimethyl-PABA, also known as padimate-O (33).

Cross-reactivity between PABA and sulfonylureas, sulfonamides, thiazides, and parapheneldiamine has been shown, and patients with sensitivity to these medications should avoid PABA-containing sunscreens (34).

Cinnamates. The cinnamates have been used increasingly in the United States for UVB absorption. They have a lower potential for hypersensitivity than the PABA agents and are nonstaining. However, they do not bind to the stratum corneum and are easily removed with water.

Salicylates. The salicylates are UVB absorbers and have been ingredients of sunscreens since the 1920s.

UVA ABSORBERS

The most widely used UVA absorbers are the benzophenone products such as oxybenzone and dioxybenzone. A new compound, butylmethoxydibenzoylmethane (Parsol 1789), has been found to be a more effective UVA sunscreen than oxybenzone (32).

SUN PROTECTION FACTOR

The concept of sun protection factor (SPF) was developed by Greiter of Austria (35) and was adopted by the FDA in 1978 (36). Currently, manufacturers specify the SPF on the labels of sunscreens. The SPF is a quantitative measure of the ability to absorb UVB only. By definition, the SPF is the ratio of the dose of UVB energy required to produce minimal erythema (MED) on sunscreen-protected skin to the dose of energy required to produce minimal erythema on skin without sunscreen protection (36).

$$SPF = \frac{MED \text{ of sunscreen-protected skin}}{MED \text{ of nonprotected skin}}$$

SPF ranges from 2 (minimal protection) to 15 or more for ultraprotection. Most of the sunscreens with SPFs above 30 contain at least three different sunscreen agents or greater concentrations of the agents to achieve increased photoprotection. This gives them an increased risk of allergic and irritant reactions (33).

There is controversy about whether superpotent sunscreens are needed. In a recent study by Kaidbey, sunscreens with SPF 30 prevented sunburn cell induction in the epidermis, compared with SPF 15, suggesting an advantage of SPF 30 in preventing photodamage (37). The SPF of sunscreens are determined indoors and may vary when used outdoors.

Currently there are no standardized guidelines for labeling products for their effectiveness in UVA protection. Two assays have been evaluated for testing the efficacy of UVA protection, a phototoxic protection factor (PPF) that requires psoralen-sensitized skin and a UVA protection factor, but which test would be more appropriate has not been determined (33).

SUBSTANTIVITY

The substantivity of a sunscreen is a measure of its ability to adhere to the skin and remain effective despite swimming, bathing, or sweating. A sunscreen is water-resistant if it maintains SPF after two 20-min immersions in a swimming pool, and it is waterproof if it withstands four such immersions (38).

Recommendations

There is strong evidence that sun exposure leads to photoaging and skin cancers, and sun protection should be stressed in the young, in people with fair skin, and in people prone to sun-sensitive disorders. Although the simplest and cheapest way to avoid sun exposure would be to avoid outdoor exposure during hours of intense sunlight (10:00 AM to 3:00 PM) and to wear protective clothing and hats, this is not always feasible, and sunscreens that provide maximal protection must be recommended (32).

Use of sunscreen by elderly people is more questionable, because sunscreens block ultraviolet-induced vitamin D synthesis in the skin and may make them more prone to vitamin D deficiency and thus bone fractures. When sunscreens are recommended to the elderly, Taylor et al. advised (a) three glasses of milk a day, (b) a vitamin D supplement, or (c) limited sun exposure without sunscreens (32). They should probably try to receive at least some sun exposure without sunscreen, especially during the winter months.

SYSTEMIC PHOTOPROTECTIVE AGENTS

There is currently no effective, safe systemic photoprotective agent that circumvents the shortcomings of topical sunscreens. Several agents have shown improvement in specific photosensitive diseases, but they are not effective as general photoprotecters.

Antimalarials

The aminoquinolines (chloroquine, hydroxychloroquine, quinacrine) are occasionally used to treat several light-sensitive diseases, including systemic lupus erythematosus, polymorphous light eruption, solar urticaria, and porphyria cutanea tarda.

Chloroquine has many diverse effects including enzyme inhibition; protein-, DNA-, and melanin-binding; and antihistaminic and antiinflammatory effects. It is also an effective absorber of UV light, but the exact mechanisms of action in photosensitive disorders is not known (39). Antimalarials have many toxicities and are not considered the first choice for treatment of photosensitive disorders. They should be used only after other therapies have failed and with close supervision.

Ocular toxicity is the greatest problem with the aminoquinolines. They can cause an irreversible retinopathy that is dose-related. To minimize the risk of ocular toxicity, the dose of chloroquine should not exceed 250 mg/day or hydroxychloroquine, 400 mg/day (in a patient weighing over 100 lbs). An ophthalmologic examination should be required before therapy and every 4 to 6 months during therapy. If any changes in vision occur, such as blurred vision or flashes of light, the drug should be stopped until the patient can be examined by an ophthalmologist (40).

Other reported side effects include headache, irritability, toxic psychosis, worsening of psoriasis, and leukopenia. They can cause a blue-black pigmentation of the skin, and quinacrine can give a yellow discoloration to the skin. The antimalarials, regarded as teratogenic, should be avoided during pregnancy (41).

Carotenoids

The carotenoids can exert a photoprotective effect in humans and chlorophyl-containing organisms. β-Carotene absorbs light in the visible spectrum (360 to 500 nm), however some think its photoprotective effect is due to its ability to quench singlet oxygen-derived photochemical reactions (39).

β-Carotene has been effective in the treatment of erythropoietic protoporphyria, a rare hereditary photosensitive disease caused by a defect in porphyrin metabolism, but its usefulness in other photosensitive diseases has been marginal. Oral ingestion should be regulated to keep a blood level between 600 and 800 μg/ml, which usually corresponds to an adult dose of 150 mg (39). The main side effect of β-carotene is a light orange discoloration of the skin, most notable on the palms and soles. Results are not expected until 1 to 2 months of therapy.

TREATMENT OF PHOTODAMAGE

Although sunscreens and sun avoidance are important to prevent photodamage, once chronic photodamage has occurred, treatment may be needed to obviate future need for surgical intervention. Recently, several products have been used to treat photodamaged skin.

Topical Tretinoin

Although topical tretinoin is currently not approved by the FDA to treat photodamaged skin, several studies have supported its beneficial effects. Weiss et al. (42) and Leyden et al. (43) have reported improvement in fine wrinkling, coarse wrinkling, and hyperpigmented lesions in patients treated with topical tretinoin.

For treatment of photodamaged skin or precancerous lesions, topical tretinoin is usually initiated at low strength (0.025% cream or 0.1% cream) and applied at bedtime, avoiding areas close to the eyes. The most significant side effect is irritation, which is readily treated by withholding treatment for 1 to 2 days and decreasing the dose or changing to alternate-day therapy. The patient should use sunscreens during the day (44). This treatment should be avoided in pregnancy, as it is considered nonessential.

Experience with topical tretinoids is limited, and their long-term effects are unknown. Whether their effects will persist past treatment is unanswered. They should be used only in motivated patients who are committed to future sun protection and sun avoidance.

α-Hydroxyacids

α-Hydroxyacids and α-ketoacids, including glycolic, pyruvic, and lactic acids, are powerful keratolytic agents that have been used to treat actinic keratosis and wrinkles with some success (45). Many different strengths and combinations of these acid produce varying degrees of epidermal damage, and they should be used only under dermatologic supervision.

Topical Fluorouracil

Topical 5-fluorouracil is an anticancer agent used to treat many precancerous lesions and dermatoses. It is most often used to treat severe actinic keratoses.

5-Fluorouracil (FU) is a structural analog of thiamine that blocks the synthesis of DNA. Rapidly growing cells, such as the cells in actinic keratoses, require more DNA and thus accumulate larger amounts of lethal FU and die (21). Normal skin is much less affected by fluorouracil (46).

Fluorouracil is available as a 1% cream or solution, a 2% solution, and a 5% cream or solution. It is usually applied twice daily for 2 to 4 weeks, depending on the response. The response includes an inflammatory phase followed by redness, burning, and oozing, then erosion or ulceration. This occurs over 1 to 3 weeks, depending on the site and strength used. Treatment is stopped when ulceration and crusting appear. The patient must be well informed of this expected response, or there will be many telephone calls. Oozing and erosion are expected, and patient information pamphlets with pictures, provided by pharmaceutical companies, should be given to the patient. If applied with the fingers, the hands should be washed immediately afterward, or gloves can be used during application. Fluorouracil should not be applied too close to the eyes.

Topical 5-fluorouracil is a very effective treatment of actinic keratoses, gives good cosmetic results, and may obviate the need for surgery. Side effects include an irritant dermatitis that is difficult to distinguish from the desired effect of 5-FU. If severe, the treatment may have to be interrupted and lubricants or topical steroids used. During therapy, the redness and oozing may be a cosmetic embarrassment, and patients should be forewarned of this. The most frequently encountered local reactions are pain, pruritus, hyperpigmentation, and burning at the site of application.

Other (rare) side effects include photosensitivity, concealing a cancer, nail changes, telangiectasias, and scarring (46). Actinic keratoses that do not respond to treatment should be biopsied.

Overall, when used with discretion and with consistent follow-up examinations, 5-fluorouracil is an effective and economic treatment for actinic keratoses and gives good cosmetic results.

In summary, a broad range of skin disorders are induced or aggravated by the sun, including sunburn, tanning, phototoxic reactions, photoallergic drug reactions, cutaneous changes in lupus erythematosus, photoaging, precancerous lesions, and skin cancers. These dermatoses usually occur on sun-exposed skin, which should aid in their recognition by the clinician, who can then determine the etiology and appropriate treatment.

WARTS
Clinical Features

Warts, also known as verrucae, are caused by human papillomaviruses (HPV). They are commonly classified by their clinical appearance and location as verruca vulgaris or common wart; myrmecia or deep palmoplantar wart; superficial, mosaic-type palmoplantar wart; verruca plana or flat wart; condyloma acuminata or anogenital wart; or epidermodysplasia verruciformis.

VERRUCA VULGARIS (COMMON WART)

Approximately 70% of warts are verruca vulgaris, or common warts, which are circumscribed, firm, rough, hyperkeratotic papules that may appear singly or grouped on any skin surface. They occur most commonly on the dorsum of hands and fingers and on knees of children. Warts can form at sites of trauma, a property known as the Koebner phenomenon. Although they are generally asymptomatic, periungual warts may become fissured, inflamed and tender and cause local dystrophic nails. Occasionally, warts consist of thread-like, thin, shrub-shaped projections. This variant called verruca filiformis, or filiform wart, occurs commonly on the face and scalp.

MYRMECIA WART (DEEP PALMOPLANTAR WART)

Myrmecia, meaning anthill, are deep, dome-shaped nodules often covered with a thick callus, which occur most commonly on the palms and soles. They are usually associated with inflammation and swelling, redness, and considerable tenderness. Although they can be multiple, they generally do not coalesce. Approximately 24% of warts occur on the plantar surfaces, including both deep and superficial plantar warts.

SUPERFICIAL, MOSAIC-TYPE PALMOPLANTAR WART

Superficial palmoplantar warts commonly form at points of pressure, especially the heel and the midmetatarsal area, causing pain with weight bearing. They have a rough, hyperkeratotic surface usually studded with punctate black dots ("seeds") representing thrombosed capillaries, and a firm, horny peripheral rim. Several lesions may coalesce to form a large plaque, known as a mosaic wart. Superficial palmoplantar warts may be difficult to distinguish from corns and calluses. Shaving off the keratotic surface may aid in differentiating the two entities; warts have a soft central core with black or bleeding points instead of a horny central core of corn.

VERRUCA PLANA (FLAT WART)

Flat warts, also known as juvenile warts, are smooth, slightly elevated, flat-topped papules that are usually less than 5 mm in diameter. They may be flesh-colored, gray, or brown and are usually multiple on the face, hands, and legs of children. Occasionally, men who shave their beards and women who shave their legs may develop numerous flat warts in the respective areas as a result of autoinoculation. Verruca plana make up approximately 35% of warts.

EPIDERMODYSPLASIA VERRUCIFORMIS

Epidermodysplasia verruciformis is a rare, lifelong, persistent disorder characterized by widespread flat warts with a tendency to coalesce into plaques. An autosomal recessive inheritance pattern has been suggested, and the disease usually begins in childhood. Lesions almost never regress spontaneously and approximately one-third of patients develop skin cancers in sun-exposed lesions (48). The lifelong HPV infection in these patients is thought to

be due to an altered immunity. A depressed cell-mediated immunity is found in 90% of these patients (49). This immune defect may be primary, perhaps leading to a predisposition to HPV infection and oncogenic transformation by these virtues, or it may be secondary to an overwhelming disseminated, chronic infection.

Extracutaneous, mucosal HPV infections are also recognized. Common warts and condyloma acuminata may occur on other mucosal surfaces such as the oral cavity and the larynx, which may lead to respiratory distress. Human papillomaviruses have been found in other entities such as focal oral hyperplasia in American Indian children and oral hairy leukoplakia.

Etiology

The papillomaviruses, which are members of the family Papovaviridae, contain double-stranded, circular, supercoiled DNA enclosed in an icosahedral capsid of 72 capsomers without an envelope. The viral particle has a molecular weight of approximately 5×10^6 and is 55 nm in diameter. DNA hybridization can classify the papillomaviruses into different types. If two isolates have less than 50% homology by DNA hybridization, they are considered to be two different types and are designated numerically. To date, 55 HPV types have been isolated, and each type tends to be associated with different clinical variants. Table 42.7 illustrates different HPV types correlated with common clinical lesions. Potential oncogenic transformation usually occurs in HPV types 5, 8, and 9 associated with epidermodysplasia verruciformis and HPV types 6, 11, 16, and 18 associated with anogenital and cervical condyloma. The incubation period of HPV varies from 1 to 20 months. Transmission of cutaneous warts is most likely by both direct contact and fomites. It is thought that HPV infection

Table 42.7.
HPV Types and Their Clinical Associations

HPV Types	Most Common Clinical Lesions	Less Common Lesions	Oncogenic Potential
1	Deep palmoplantar warts	Common warts	
2, 4	Common warts	Superficial, mosaic-type palmoplantar warts, anogenital warts	
3, 10	Flat warts		
5, 8, 9	Epidermodysplasia verruciformis		Yes
6, 11	Anogenital warts, cervical condyloma	Common warts	Yes
7	Common warts in butchers		
16, 18	Cervical condyloma	Anogenital warts	Yes

is acquired by inoculation of the epidermis via breaks in the skin. Thus trauma plays a role, which may explain the usual distribution of common warts on the hands, fingers, and knees of children. Autoinoculation of the virus may result in new lesions by direct contact. Anogenital warts are generally transmitted sexually with approximately a 60% chance of infectivity within 9 months of a single sexual contact (50). The immunologic state of the exposed individual is an important predisposing factor. More than 40% of kidney transplant patients with impaired cell-mediated immunity may develop warts (49).

Epidemiology

The prevalence of warts in the general population is unknown. They occur most frequently in children and young adults, in whom the incidence approaches 10% (48). In 1982, an estimated 4 million people saw physicians because of nonvenereal warts (49). The peak incidence of warts is between the ages of 12 and 16 years. Anogenital warts, on the other hand, are the most common sexually transmitted viral disease diagnosed in the United States. The annual incidence of these warts is 0.5 to 1.0% in young adults, with the age of onset ranging from late teens to early thirties (51). From 1966 to 1981, there has been a fivefold increase in the number of reported cases of anogenital warts in the United States (48). A study covering 1975 to 1978 estimated an annual incidence rate of 106.5 per 100,000 (48). HPV infection is also increased in patients with impaired cell-mediated immunity (as previously mentioned).

Histopathology

The histopathological features of warts generally consist of acanthosis (thickening of the stratum malpighii), papillomatosis (irregular undulation of the epidermis), hyperkeratosis (thickening of the horny layer), and parakeratosis (retention of nuclei in the horny layer). The distinguishing features of verruca vulgaris include large keratinocytes with a pyknotic nucleus surrounded by a perinuclear clear halo, called koilocytes, located in the upper stratum malpighii; vertical tiers of parakeratosis overlying the crests of papillomatous elevations; and foci of clumped keratohyaline granules in the intervening valleys. Anogenital warts have similar features but lack a granular layer because they occur on or near a mucosal surface. Although flat warts have diffuse koilocytes in the upper epidermis, they tend to lack papillomatosis and parakeratosis. Immunocytochemical studies have detected viral DNA, antigens, and mature virions in keratinocytes at and above the stratum granulosum.

Treatment

The approach to the treatment of warts depends on the patient's age, cooperation, immunologic status, previous

Table 42.8.
Treatment Modalities for Warts

Chemical destruction
  Acids
  Formalin
  Glutaraldehyde
  Cantharidin
Physical destruction
  Cryotherapy
  Electrosurgery
  Surgical excision
  CO_2 laser
Chemotherapeutic agents
  Podophyllin
  Podophyllotoxin
  5-Fluorouracil
  Bleomycin
  Interferons
  Retinoids
Immunotherapy
  Dinitrochlorobenzene (DNCB)
  Squaric acid dibutylester (SADBE)
  Diphenylcyclopropenone
  Inosine pranobex

treatments, and the location, number, size, duration, and type of the lesions. Studies have shown spontaneous regression of warts in two-thirds of children within 2 years, although new warts may continue to appear (49). All warts should be treated to prevent spreading to others and on the patients themselves.

Sexual partners of patients with anogenital warts should be examined and treated appropriately. During treatment, the patient should be instructed to avoid sexual contact or use condoms. Therapeutic options can be divided into broad categories: chemical destructive therapy including acids, formalin, glutaraldehyde, and cantharidin; physical destructive therapy including cryotherapy, electrosurgery, surgical excision, and CO_2 laser; chemotherapeutic agents including podophyllin, podophyllotoxin, 5-fluorouracil, bleomycin, interferons, and retinoids; and immunotherapy (Table 42.8). Most forms of wart treatment can be expected to have a 60 to 70% cure rate. Patients should be told that warts may need several treatments, often over a period of several weeks to months.

ACIDS

Salicylic acid in concentrations ranging from 10 to 60% can be used in paints, pastes, gels, or plasters. It is frequently used for common and palmoplantar warts, including periungual warts. Salicylic acid preparations can be used on all skin sites except the face and anogenital area. Other acids are frequently used in combination with salicylic acid. A popular preparation is equal parts of salicylic acid and lactic acid in 4 parts of flexible collodion.

Monochloroacetic acid crystals compounded with 60% salicylic acid have been found to be effective for plantar warts (52). Weekly applications of 50 to 85% trichloroacetic acid or less commonly bichloroacetic acid may be effective for anogenital warts when podophyllin is contraindicated; this acid does not have to be washed off as does podophyllin. Trichloroacetic acid may be compounded with salicylic acid for the treatment of common and palmoplantar warts.

In general, the acids act as keratolytic agents by physically destroying the keratin layer. Paints are most commonly used and are usually a collodion-based liquid. Treatment consists of soaking the wart in warm water for at least 5 min, then paring the wart as far as possible without causing bleeding. A pumice stone may be used if necessary. Next, a drop of the acid solution is applied to just cover the wart and allowed to dry to a white film. The wart is then kept covered for 24 hr, and the procedure is repeated daily until the wart is gone.

Salicylic acid plasters are especially suited for the treatment of multiple, mosaic plantar warts. After the lesion is pared and moistened with a drop of warm water, the plaster is cut to the size of the wart and applied for 24 to 48 hr, followed by repeated cycles until resolution of the wart. A 40% salicylic acid adhesive plaster is commonly used. Recently a topical transdermal 15% salicylic acid patch has been developed to provide continuous passive diffusion of the acid under occlusion (53). The acid is suspended in a karaya gum patch that acts as a self-adhesive and enhances absorption. Nightly application of this transdermal patch is repeated until the wart is gone.

Recently, the FDA has issued a monograph mandating that all salicylic acid–based wart therapy products be changed to nonprescription status, with a maximum of 17% concentration of salicylic acid (54). Lactic acid is no longer allowed as an active agent in over-the-counter products. However pharmacists may compound these acids using a higher concentration if necessary.

FORMALIN

Formalin preparations can be used for plantar or multiple warts. This chemical destroys the affected tissue. Three to 10% formalin in aqueous solution can be used to soak the pared wart for 10 to 30 min daily. The surrounding normal skin can be protected with petroleum jelly. Formalin 25% in hydrophilic petrolatum has also been used as a daily application. Development of allergic contact dermatitis is a potential complication of formalin treatment.

GLUTARALDEHYDE

Topical application of 10% glutaraldehyde may be less irritating for palmoplantar warts than formalin preparations.

CANTHARIDIN

Cantharidin, an extract of the green blister beetle, acts by destroying the epidermis and can dissociate oxidative phosphorylation. A solution containing 0.7% cantharidin in acetone or flexible collodion may be effective in treating common and plantar warts. The vehicle is applied to the pared wart, allowed to dry, and covered with adhesive tape for 24 hr, after which the process may be repeated weekly. It is not unusual for warts to recur in a doughnut-shaped ring around the original treated wart.

CRYOTHERAPY

Cryotherapy is considered to be more effective than topical medications, particularly for anogenital warts, with cure rates up to 90% (55). It is a popular treatment for many types of warts including common, palmoplantar, flat, anogenital warts, especially in pregnant women. Recently, the Centers for Disease Control stated that cryotherapy is first-line treatment for condyloma acuminata (56). Cure rates are similar to those of electrosurgery, but cryosurgery is preferred because it requires no local anesthesia. Liquid nitrogen is most commonly used, but solid carbon dioxide may also be effective. Cryotherapy causes cell injury by intracellular ice formation, cell shrinkage, and anoxia by intravascular thrombosis (57).

Before treatment, the wart should be pared down. A cotton-tipped applicator with liquid nitrogen is applied to the wart to create a white "ice ball" extending 1 to 2 mm beyond the visible wart. This process usually takes about 20 to 30 seconds, after which the lesion is allowed to thaw. The procedure is repeated a few times, depending on the size and site of the wart. The object is to produce epidermal necrosis, with the subsequent formation of a small blister. The lesion then dries and peels off with the wart. This regimen may require multiple treatments at 1- to 2-week intervals. A common method is a liquid nitrogen spray that delivers liquid nitrogen by spray canister rather than a cotton applicator. Carbon dioxide can be obtained from sparklet cylinders and mixed with acetone to form a slush. Freezing techniques with a cotton-tipped applicator are similar to those of liquid nitrogen.

ELECTROSURGERY

Electrosurgery is fairly common, but disadvantages include the need for local anesthesia, pain, and greater risk of scarring and infection. Cure rates are generally similar to those of cryotherapy (58). The treatment consists of low-current electrodesiccation followed by gentle curettage of the wart to minimize scarring. It should be used only on small warts.

SURGICAL EXCISION

In some series, simple surgical excision of anogenital warts has been reported to be more effective than podophyllin application (59). However, recurrence rates have been reported to be 20 to 30% in other series (57).

CO₂ LASER

Cure rates with the carbon dioxide laser reach 90%, but disadvantages include high expense, the possible necessity for general anesthesia, and HPV in the laser smoke (60). It is generally reserved for treating multiple, large, treatment-resistant anogenital, meatal, urethral, or vaginal condylomas.

PODOPHYLLIN

For many years, podophyllin or podophyllum resin has been used in the treatment of anogenital warts. It is a nonhomogeneous, unstable extract obtained from the plants *Podophyllum peltatum* (found in North America) and *Podophyllum emodi* (found in India, Tibet, and Afghanistan). The resin has four active agents, or lignans, including podophyllotoxin, 4-demethylpodophyllotoxin, α-peltatin, and β-peltatin. The maximal active content is about 40% in *P. emodi*, consisting predominantly of podophyllotoxin and trace amounts of 4-demethylpodophyllotoxin. *P. peltatum* has a maximal lignan content of approximately 20%, consisting of varying quantities of podophyllotoxin and the two peltatins. Podophyllin is most frequently used as a 20 to 25% solution in compound tincture of benzoin, although other vehicles have been used such as mineral oil or ethanol. The resin should be stored at room temperature and replaced at least every 2 years, or earlier if it contains precipitates.

Available studies include a cure rate ranging from 22 to 98% (56). Podophyllin provides the best results in patients with external, moist condylomas that are relatively new, small, and few in numbers. Before treatment, warts should be wiped dry. Podophyllin is then applied to the wart with a sterile cotton-tipped applicator, from which the excess solution is first wrung out. It is recommended that the area of treatment should not exceed 3 cm in diameter and the chemical be kept off the normal surrounding skin to avoid local and systemic side effects (47). Patients are instructed to wash off the podophyllin with rubbing alcohol or soap and water 4 hr after application. Treatment can be repeated at intervals of 1 to 2 weeks and should not exceed 1.0 ml per week (61).

Podophyllin acts as a strong irritant and arrests mitoses in metaphase by interfering with microtubule formation and causing subsequent epithelial cell death (62). After the application, an acute inflammatory reaction followed by necrosis usually develops over the treated area. Local irritation may range through erythema, burning, edema, pain, and ulceration. Uncircumcised men may occasionally develop balanitis and phimosis (62). Severe chemical burns, necrosis, scarring, and fistual formation have been reported with improper use of podophyllin. Thus podophyllin should not be used as a home remedy, but should be applied only by physicians, since both local and systemic side effects are potentially severe.

Systemic toxicity of podophyllin has been reported and usually occurs when the chemical has been applied in large volumes over an extensive area of the skin or has been in contact with the skin for a long period of time. Although podophyllin toxicity is multisystemic, neurologic manifestations are the hallmark features and may include mental status change, peripheral neuropathy, seizures, psychosis, and coma. Other manifestations include fever, nausea, vomiting, respiratory stimulation, tachycardia, renal failure, ileus, pancytopenia, leukocytosis, marrow suppression, and death (63).

Podophyllin is contraindicated in pregnancy. It is teratogenic in experimental animals, and intrauterine death has been reported following topical application of podophyllin in women (62). To minimize systemic absorption, podophyllin should not be used in the oral mucosa, vagina, cervix, rectum, urethra, or in infants. Alcoholic consumption should be avoided for several hours after treatment, since alcohol may facilitate absorption of podophyllin.

PODOPHYLLOTOXIN

Podophyllotoxin, a new treatment modality for anogenital warts, is the purified and most biologically active agent of podophyllin. Several clinical studies have reported the effectiveness of 0.5% podophyllotoxin on penile warts by self-application. Von Krogh reported a regimen of 0.5% podophyllotoxin applied by the patient twice daily for 3 consecutive days, resulting in a cure rate of 49% (64). In a subsequent study in which the same preparation was applied by the patient twice daily for 4 and 5 days, he found no significant improvement in efficacy, but an increase in local irritation (64). Edwards et al. compared 0.5% podophyllotoxin applied to penile warts by the patient for 3 consecutive days with a 4 day drug-free interval to 20% podophyllin treatment by a physician once a week (65). Each of these regimens was repeated for up to 6 weeks or cycles. He found an 88% cure rate in the self-treated patients and 63% in the podophyllin-treated patients. Beutner and von Krogh reported a placebo-controlled trial with 2 to 4 treatment cycles of 0.5% podophyllotoxin twice daily for 3 days; they noted an 82% clearance in the treated patients, versus 13% in the placebo group (64). In these trials, no systemic reactions were reported and local irritation was considerably less than that induced by podophyllin. Therefore, topical podophyllotoxin is a new, relatively safe, efficacious, cost-effective treatment for anogenital warts, which can be used as a home remedy.

5-FLUOROURACIL

5-Fluorouracil is a fluorinated pyrimidine antimetabolite that interferes with the synthesis of DNA and to a lesser degree inhibits the formation of RNA. When applied topically, it penetrates abnormal skin better than normal skin and has a direct immunostimulatory effect on the affected epidermis (66). It is used most frequently for the management of urethral and vaginal condylomas, but its effectiveness has also been reported in common, plantar, flat, and external genital warts. It has been used as a topical 1 to 5% cream. The patient can apply 5% 5-fluorouracil cream to the distal urethra with a cotton applicator after urination. Treatment of proximal urethral warts should be performed by a urologist. Applications four times a day for up to 2 weeks may be necessary (55). Intraurethral suppositories can be made by a pharmacist (60). Application of 5% 5-fluorouracil cream to penile warts for 8 weeks has resulted in an 84% response rate (66). Daily 5% 5-fluorouracil cream application at bedtime for 5 days may be effective for vaginal warts. Gynecologists use 5-fluorouracil cream prophylactically to minimize recurrences after laser surgery (67). A topical 1% solution of 5-fluorouracil in 70% alcohol applied twice daily for several weeks has also been used for condylomas (68). Because 5-fluorouracil can cause local inflammation, the vulva and urethra can be protected with zinc oxide or petrolatum.

For common, plantar, and flat warts, 1 to 5% 5-fluorouracil cream or ointment can be used as a single agent daily on a wart covered with a waterproof plaster or it may be compounded with other acids (69). Five percent 5-fluorouracil compounded with salicylic acid has been reported to be effective (47). α-Hydroxyacids, particularly pyruvic and glycolic acids, have been combined with 5-fluorouracil (45). 5-Fluorouracil powder dissolved in pyruvic acid to achieve a 1 to 2% solution can be applied to the pared wart with an artist camel-hair brush until the patient feels a burning sensation. Adhesive tape is then applied over the wart for a few hours, after which the chemical is washed off. The procedure may be repeated in 2 to 3 weeks if necessary. A 0.5% 5-fluorouracil in pyruvic acid:ethanol 1:1 preparation can be used as a home remedy. The patient applies the solution two to three times daily for 2 consecutive days, after which the cycle may be repeated in 1 week if needed.

BLEOMYCIN

Bleomycin is an antibiotic produced by *Streptomyces verticillus* with antiviral, antibacterial, and antitumor activity. It binds to DNA and prevents thymidine incorporation and single-stranded scission in DNA. Intralesional bleomycin has been reported to be effective as an alternative form of therapy, particularly for recalcitrant palmoplantar and periungual warts (70). A tuberculin syringe with a #30-gauge needle is used to inject 0.1 ml to 1.0 ml of 1 U/ml solution of bleomycin in saline, depending on the size of the wart. The object is to inject intralesionally so that the entire wart blanches. Local pain, erythema, and swelling may persist for 1 to 2 days after treatment. The wart usually blackens, thromboses, forms a eschar, and sloughs off several days after the injection. Cure rates of one or two treatments with a 2-week interval have been reported to exceed 80% (70). Complications, usually from infralesional or perilesional infiltration of bleomycin, may include extensive necrosis, permanent nail dystrophy, sclerodermoid changes, joint destruction, and subcutaneous abcesses (57).

Recently, intralesional bleomycin sulfate therapy using a bifurcated needle puncture technique resulted in a 90% cure rate with a single treatment (71). The procedure consists of soaking the wart for 10 min in warm water, after which the lesion is anesthetized with 2% lidocaine without epinephrine. Bleomycin sulfate solution (1 U/ml in normal saline) is placed onto the wart surface (0.02 ml/5 mm^2). A sterile, stainless steel, bifurcated needle, originally made for smallpox vaccination, is punctured rapidly through the base of the wart about 40 times per 5 mm^2 area of the lesion. The warts usually resolve in about 3 weeks. In reducing the amount of bleomycin introduced into the skin, this bifurcated needle carries only 0.001 of a unit and minimizes the bleomycin penetrating into the dermis. This type of treatment can be performed on many types of warts, except large condylomas, filiform warts, and warts on the loose skin of the penis and eyelid. It is especially suitable for paronychial warts.

INTERFERONS

Current studies show that interferons used alone or in combination with other conventional therapy are effective. All three types of interferons, α, β, and γ, have been shown to be effective intralesionally, subcutaneously, and intramuscularly. Topical treatment has been studied with disappointing results (72). Interferon has an antiviral property that theoretically can inhibit viral replication. Its antiproliferative activity may slow the rapidly dividing keratinocytes in warts, and its immunomodulatory effect may enhance the host's response to HPV infection (48). Most studies have indicated its effectiveness in condyloma acuminata. Intralesional injection of condyloma with 1×10^6 IU of recombinant α-2b interferon three times weekly for 3 weeks resulted in a 36% cure rate in one study (73) and 53% in another (74). A similar study achieved a response rate of 62% with intralesional injection of 1×10^6 IU of interferon-α weekly for up to 8 weeks (75). Systemic administration of interferon either subcutaneously or intramuscularly in the treatment of genital warts has also been shown to be effective. Dose comparison studies of systemic interferon have shown that intramuscular injection of 5×10^6 IU/mm^2 of interferon-α for 28 days followed by three times weekly for 2 weeks is highly effective, but the high incidence of systemic side effects make this dose unacceptable. Low-dose intramuscular injection of 1×10^6 IU/mm^2 for 14 days, followed by three times weekly for 1 month appears to be the best tolerated effective regimen (76).

Interferon-β 1×10^6 IU intralesional injections three times weekly for 4 weeks have been shown to have similar efficacy to recombinant α-2b and lymphoblastoid interferons (77). In a review of recombinant interferon-γ for the treatment of recalcitrant warts, the optimal dose of 50 to 100 μg/day subcutaneously resulted in an overall response rate of 50% (78).

Side effects of interferons are flu-like symptoms, including fatigue, malaise, fever, chills, nausea, vomiting, headaches, and transient leukopenia, even with intralesional injections. Relapse rates with interferon therapy are up to 25% (79). This and the high cost of treatment mean that interferon should be used only for very recalcitrant warts.

RETINOIDS

Retinoids are another mode of therapy for warts under recent investigation. Although the mechanism is unknown, vitamin A derivatives theoretically may block the production of viral particles, because these compounds affect cellular differentiation and keratinization, and HPV replication appears to be related to keratinocyte differentiation (48). Retinoids may prevent malignant transformation, which may be crucial in HPV-induced neoplasia. There are several anecdotal reports of topical and oral retinoids being effective in recalcitrant warts, particularly in immunosuppressive patients. Etretinate 1 mg/kg/day for 2 months improved a patient with epidermodysplasia verruciformis with widespread flat wart-like lesions and plaques (80). Other reports state its effectiveness in recalcitrant plantar warts, but relapses are common and results are not consistent (81). Topical retinoic acid has been used for flat warts, particularly on the face, to minimize scarring (82).

IMMUNOTHERAPY

Topical sensitizing agents such as dinitrochlorobenzene (DNCB), squaric acid dibutylester (SADBE), and diphenylcyclopropenone are also popular treatments for recalcitrant large nongenital warts. Immunotherapy usually involves initial sensitization of the patient to an agent, followed by applications of the same chemical to the wart to elicit a contact dermatitis at the base of the wart. The mechanism of contact immunotherapy may be related to induction of type IV hypersensitivity or cell-mediated immunity in the virus-infected tissue, resulting in wart destruction (83). It probably involves a nonwart-antigen-specific cell-mediated process. Also, the percentage of complement-binding wart antibodies in affected patients rose from 15% before treatment to 43% after therapy (84).

DNCB has been used frequently in the past. Two percent DNCB in acetone can be applied to an inconspicuous area on the body for 24 to 48 hr covered with a bandage, to sensitize the patient (85). The area usually becomes erythematous with blister formation. Two weeks after sensitivity develops, 0.1% DNCB in petrolatum is applied to the wart with a cotton-tipped applicator 2 to 3 times a week (86). This procedure may be repeated for an average of 3 to 6 weeks. DNCB therapy has about an 80% cure rate with low recurrence rates and low incidence of scarring. It is particularly effective for large, recurrent, recalcitrant, periungual, plantar, mosaic, and flat warts. Complications may include localized or severe generalized dermatitis and urticaria, pruritis, blistering, and (rarely) secondary infection. DNCB is no longer used in industry, but cross-reaction with other chemicals may occur. There are concerns about the mutagenicity of DNCB in the Ames test, although it has been used safely in the past for wart treatment.

SADBE and diphenylcyclopropenone may be used without concern about mutagenicity, although they are both unstable compounds. SADBE must be refrigerated because of its tendency to undergo hydrolysis, and diphenylcyclopropenone must be stored in dark glass and in a dark place to prevent photodecomposition (83). A 0.1% diphenylcyclopropenone solution in acetone may be used to sensitize the patient, followed by applications to the wart of a sequence of increasing strengths at weekly intervals. A 0.01% concentration is used initially followed by 0.025, 0.1, 0.5, and finally 1.0% (83).

Preliminary studies of systemic immunotherapy with inosine pranobex indicate a possible additive effect in treating genital warts when combined with conventional treatments such as podophyllin, trichloroacetic acid, and CO_2 laser. A 4-week course of 1 g three times a day of inosine pranobex as an adjunctive treatment resulted in a cure rate over 80% (87).

SEBORRHEIC DERMATITIS

Seborrheic dermatitis is a chronic inflammatory, erythematous, and scaling eruption recognized by its characteristic distribution on the body. These seborrheic areas include the scalp, eyebrows, glabella, eyelid margins (often with marginal blepharitis and conjunctivitis), cheeks, paranasal areas, nasolabial folds, beard area, presternal area, central back, retroaricular creases, and in and about the external ear canal. Other less commonly involved areas include the axillae, inframammary areas, umbilicus, groin, and intergluteal cleft. Seborrheic dermatitis in the intertriginous areas may exist alone or in conjunction with other seborrheic areas. Similarly, psoriasis may occasionally have an intertriginous distribution, called inverse psoriasis, along with scalp involvement. In this form, it has been designated as seborriasis.

The scales of seborrheic dermatitis vary from a dry to

thick powdery form with little to no erythema to an oily form with greasy or oily scales and crusts on an erythematous base. The former is usually located on the scalp and is referred to as simple dandruff. The greasier scales are found more commonly on the ears and central face such as the glabella, eyebrows, and nasaolabial folds.

Etiology and Pathogenesis

Seborrheic dermatitis is a common problem, and the onset is correlated with sebaceous gland activity. During infancy, it is commonly called cradle cap and spontaneous remission tends to occur by age 1 year, after which the disease is rare until puberty. In these infants, seborrheic dermatitis may become generalized to form an exfoliative erythroderma known as erythroderma desquamativum or Leiner's disease. Infants often have diarrhea, infection, and a failure to thrive. A small subset of infants with Leiner's disease have been reported with a dysfunction of the fifth component of complement, resulting in decreased opsonic activity. In adults, seborrheic dermatitis has a predilection for males and is more severe in the winter. The disorder is often asymptomatic, but pruritus is not uncommon and at times can be intense.

Seborrheic dermatitis is characterized by an increased epidermal cell turnover. The active ingredient of many antiseborrheic agents, such as coal tar, zinc pyrithione, and selenium sulfide, inhibits mitotic activity. It was once thought that this cytostatic effect was responsible for alleviating the scaling. Although no evidence establishes increased cell turnover as the primary defect, zinc pyrithione, selenium sulfide, and sulfur/salicylic acid preparations all kill yeast. Evidence now suggests that the hyperproliferative state may be secondary to the presence of a lipophilic, pleomorphic fungus, *Pityrosporum ovale* (88). When oral and topical ketoconazole, an imidazole derivative effective against *Pityrosporum*, is used in seborrheic dermatitis, the condition improves (89, 90). The primary mechanism of action is thought to be inhibition of ergosterol formation in the cell membrane of fungi. Improvement was correlated with a reduction in the number of yeast organisms. This was recently confirmed using a precipitated sulfur/salicylic acid (91). These observations fulfill all the requirements to implicate the organisms as the etiologic agent (Koch's postulates), but some investigators have demonstrated *P. ovale* on scalps of patients without the disease. This can be easily explained by the observation that patients with clinical disease inherit a heightened immune response to the alternate complement pathway, which overreacts to the cell walls of the *Pityrosporum* yeast (92). How can one explain the parallel occurrence of the disease with the onset of sebaceous gland activity? Recently, it was shown that when the sebum excretion rate was reduced by 70% with isotretinoin, the magnitude of rash improvement varied according to the body site. It was concluded that the residual pool of sebum was important for the growth of *P. ovale* and that, within the physiological range, sebum had a permissive effect on the growth of this yeast. This observation explains variations in disease activity at certain body sites and the greater prevalence in males, since androgens stimulate sebum production. Finally, the pathological increase in the residual pool of sebum due to immobility could explain the frequent occurrence of seborrheic dermatitis in patients with a variety of neurological disorders such as idiopathic and neuroleptic-induced Parkinson's disease (93).

Treatment

The mainstay of treatment of seborrheic dermatitis of the scalp is shampoos. As mentioned above, sulfur/salicylic acid, coal tar, and zinc pyrithione are available over the counter; but the most effective antifungal agents are 2.5% selenium sulfide and 2% ketoconazole, which can be obtained by prescription (94). The choice of shampoos depends on several factors including physician and patient preference, cost, and cosmetic appeal to the patient. Depending upon the severity of the disease, shampoos can be applied daily to twice weekly. Patients should be reminded that the scalp (not the hair) is being treated, so the shampoo should be left on to penetrate for at least 5 min before rinsing.

With the exception of accidental oral ingestion, systemic adverse reactions are minimal. Local adverse reactions include skin irritation (usually from the vehicle), occasionally reports of hair loss, and discoloration of hair, especially from selenium sulfide and coal tar. As with other shampoos, oiliness or dryness of the hair and scalp may occur. Topical corticosteroid lotions can be added if lesions are very inflammatory and pruritic. A 1% hydrocortisone lotion, applied one to three times daily, is usually safe and effective. Stronger preparations such as 0.025% triamcinolone lotion, 0.01% fluocinolone acetonide solution, 0.05% clobetasol solution or 0.1% betamethasone valerate lotion may be required for more severe instances, but they should be used only for very short periods to prevent hypothalamic-pituitary-adrenal (HPA) axis suppression or steroid rosacea. For thick, crusted, and scaly lesions, a mixture of liquid petrolatum, sodium chloride, and phenol can be applied overnight and rinsed off in the morning. Other preparations that use a similar application schedule include various concentrations of sulfur/salicylic acid in an ointment base.

Therapy for other seborrheic areas of the body including the scalp line, eyebrows, glabella, ears, and nasolabial can be successfully accomplished with 2% ketoconazole cream applied twice a day. Other alternatives include 1 to 2.5% hydrocortisone cream or 0.5% desonide applied two to three times a day.

If there is scaling in the auditory meatus, a polymyxin

B–hydrocortisone suspension, or 0.5% desonide and 2% acetic acid, 4 drops three to four times a day, is effective. The pruritus that sometimes accompanies the scaling is also relieved. Topical steroids should not be used for seborrheic blepharitis because of the potential to induce glaucoma and cataracts. Hot compresses and gentle debridement with a cotton-tipped applicator and baby shampoo one or more times daily are usually effective. If the lid margins are severely inflamed, 10% sodium sulfacetamide ointment may be added (95).

Special considerations must be made for infants with seborrheic dermatitis. Tar preparations should be avoided for fear they will rub it into their eyes. Topical corticosteroids should be limited to 0.5% to 1% hydrocortisone, to avoid HPA axis suppression. However, 2% ketoconazole cream should be the treatment of choice for infantile seborrheic dermatitis, because of its minimal percutaneous absorption and lack of accumulation in the plasma (96).

PSORIASIS

Psoriasis is an inflammatory disorder characterized by erythematous scaling plaques on virtually any area of the skin surface. The disease affects 1 to 2% of the general population in the U.S. It ranks third after acne and warts as the reason for the most office visits to a dermatologist. Psoriasis occurs with equal frequency in both sexes. It may be symptomatic throughout life and be progressive with age or wax and wane in severity. The condition can be present at birth, and an onset was reported at age 108 years. Most patients develop the initial lesions of psoriasis in the third decade of life. Symptoms appear in males at a mean age of 29, and in females at age 27 years. With earlier onset, there is a greater probability of a positive family history of psoriasis. Although psoriasis does not follow classic mendelian inheritance, studies of HLA phenotypes suggest a polygenic inheritance that requires environmental factors to induce the clinical expression of the disease. These include cutaneous or systemic microbial infection or colonization, trauma, drugs such as lithium, β-blockers, antimalarials, and nonsteroidal antiinflammatory agents, and corticosteroid withdrawal. Various HLA phenotypes have been reported to be associated with psoriasis, but the strongest association is with the HLA CW-6 antigen. Presence of this antigen increases the relative risk for development of psoriasis to 13 times that of the population without the antigen.

The morbidity associated with this disease is great. Psoriasis can cause functional impairment, skin disfigurement and emotional distress. Severe involvement of the hands, feet, and nails may make even routine activities, such as walking or dressing, difficult to perform, particularly in patients with severe psoriatic arthritis. As many as 30% of patients with psoriasis may have arthritis, and 5 to 10% of those patients may experience functional disability. There-

fore, psoriasis directly affects the quality of life and may cause difficulty in work performance, problems with social rejection, sexual dysfunction, and depression.

Psoriatic lesions are observed most commonly on the scalp, elbows, trunk, lower extremities, and nails. The primary lesion is an erythematous plaque covered with silvery scales. Scale removal may show punctate bleeding points, termed Auspitz sign, which help differentiate psoriasis from other chronic dermatoses. Several well-recognized clinical variants determine the treatment modality (see later discussion).

Plaque-type psoriasis is usually located on the extensor surfaces of elbows and knees, the lumbar region of the back, and the scalp. Guttate psoriasis, with small scaly teardrop shaped lesions, classically follows group A streptococcal pharyngitis. Psoriasis can also follow a seborrheic distribution called seborrhiasis. Inverse psoriasis is a form of psoriasis that often involves exclusively body folds such as the axillae, groin, inframammary folds, navel, intergluteal crease, and glans penis. Palmoplantar psoriasis differs from plaque-type in the variability of erythema, the loss of sharply marginated plaques, and replacement of the characteristic silvery scales by thickened fissured hyperkeratosis. Erythrodermic psoriasis is an acute inflammatory, erythematous, scaling disorder involving the entire skin surface. This is usually brought about by ingestion of concomitant medications, as mentioned above, or as a reaction to provoking factors (e.g., infections, chronic topical steroid use, or phototoxic erythema). These patients usually have difficulty in controlling body temperatures. Pustular psoriasis can be localized to the palms and soles or be generalized and may appear after withdrawal of corticosteroid therapy given inappropriately for plaque-type psoriasis. Erythrodermic and generalized pustular psoriasis may be life-threatening due to systemic infections, or cardiovascular or pulmonary complications. For example, in patients with preexisting cardiovascular disease, the erythroderma may precipitate high-output congestive heart failure or arrhthymia (97).

There is no agreement about the etiology of psoriasis, but increased epidermal cell proliferation and inflammation have been observed. In psoriatic lesions, all proliferation is 12 times the normal rate, with a 2-fold increase in proliferation in uninvolved skin. The increased rate found in uninvolved skin suggests a generalized skin abnormality in psoriasis. As a result of the hyperproliferative state, epidermal turnover and transit times are greatly reduced.

A key feature of newly formed psoriatic lesions is the attraction and migration of inflammatory cells, especially neutrophils. The neutrophils themselves are not abnormal; they are attracted to the epidermis by chemotactic mediators such as microbial products (peptides), complement components (C3a, C5), and the arachidonic acid products leukotriene B4 (LTB4) and hydroxyicosatetraenoic acids (HETEs).

Cytokines have also been implicated in the pathogenesis of psoriasis. These low-molecular-weight glycoproteins are regulatory molecules that mediate cell communication in both normal and pathologic conditions. When cytokines are released from inflammatory cells (T lymphocytes and monocytes) and keratinocytes they stimulate epidermal proliferation. Cytokine mediators that may be important in the pathogenesis of psoriasis include the interleukins, interferons, and growth factors, including epidermal growth factor. Although many of these cytokines are multifunctional, some have shown stimulation of epidermal proliferation (IL-6, and EGF) and attraction and mediation of neutrophils (IL-8) (98, 99).

The interrelationship between environmental influences, genetic predisposition, and the two pathologic features of psoriasis is best explained by the microbial association with psoriasis. Psoriatic lesions develop from microbial products that activate the alternate complement pathway to produce neutrophil migration and epidermal hyperplasia. The heightened responsiveness to the alternate complement pathway may be a phenotypic expression of a genetic predisposition to psoriasis (100).

The hyperproliferative and inflammatory bases of the disease offer two different therapeutic approaches. Most pharmacologic interventions act by modifying one or both of these processes. Therapeutic consideration must also be given to the type of psoriasis, the extent and location of involvement, and the psychological impact of the disease on the patient. Since psoriasis varies in its severity, its management can be similar to the stepped-care program used in the treatment of hypertension (Fig. 42.2). In the first step, side effects are minimal. If treatment resistance is encountered or if the disease is more severe, the second step includes the addition or a change to another form of therapy. Each step in the level of care carries an increased risk of side effects. Therefore, the risk to benefit ratio must be assessed before proceeding to the next program. When a patient reaches the highest step in the program, the therapy can be rotated for certain periods of time to minimize life-threatening side effects (Fig. 42.3).

Emollients and Keratolytics

Emollient agents hydrate the stratum corneum and prevent the increased transepidermal water loss observed in psoriasis patients. The hydrating effect softens the stratum corneum and assists in desquamation; the overall effect is moisturizing the skin. An occlusive oily film delivered to the skin surface seals the transepidermal water into the stratum corneum. With water retained in the skin, the stratum corneum becomes more pliable or softer, preventing fissuring and scaling in hyperkeratotic areas. Skin hydration also decreases the binding forces within the stratum corneum and facilitates desquamation.

Most emollient agents are mineral oils and paraffins

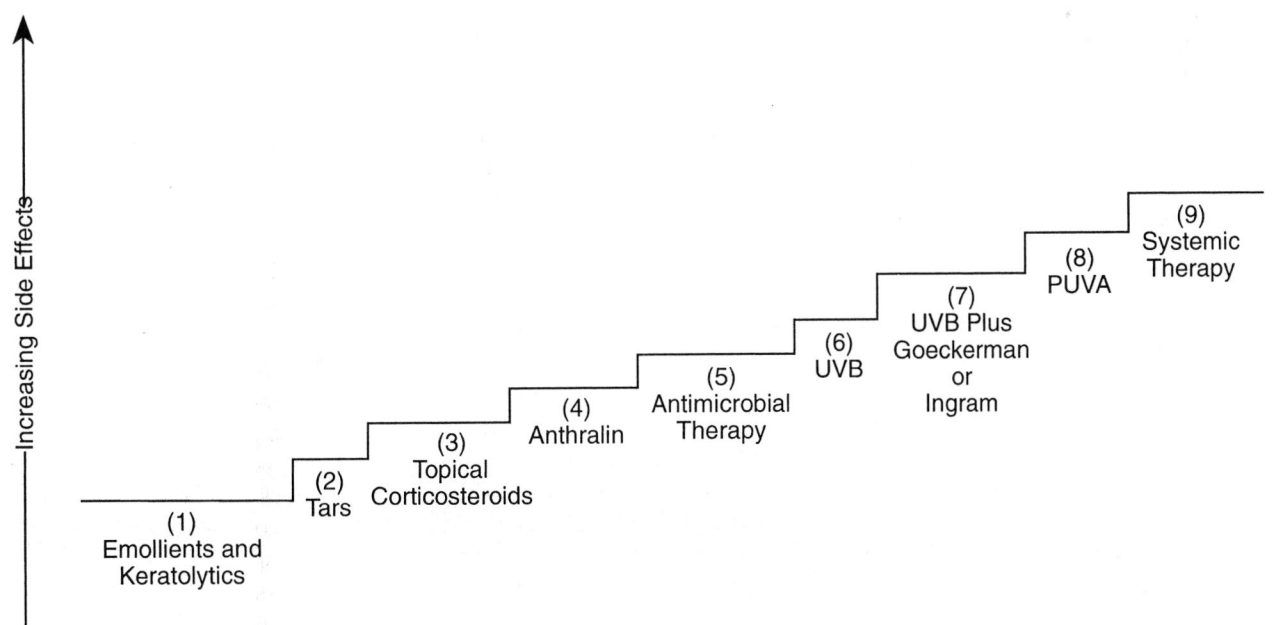

Figure 42.2. Stepped-care approach to psoriasis. Note that as one ascends each level of therapy there is an increased risk for more serious side effects.

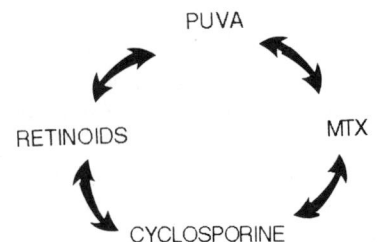

Figure 42.3. Rotation among higher levels of therapy to reduce the incidence of life-threatening side effects.

in an oil-in-water emulsion with emulsifiers, stabilizers, and antimicrobial preservatives. Humectants may be added to the emollient to enhance its water-retaining qualities. These include glycerin, urea, or pyrrolidone carboxylic acid, which hold water within the stratum corneum hygroscopically. Emollients in oil-in-water emulsion can be cosmetically acceptable, but the more "oily" or occlusive the preparation, the more effective the moisturizer. Some patients may find the oily feel to the skin unacceptable. Therefore, patients should be allowed input into the selection of emollients.

Patients should be instructed to apply the emollients three or more times a day. Side effects from frequent application may be acneiform folliculitis or an exacerbation of existing acne from occlusion of the follicular openings. Occlusion of the sweat ducts may produce miliaria, especially in hot and humid climates. The addition of urea or lactic acid may produce a stinging sensation unrelated to any toxic reaction to the skin, whose cause is not known. An occasional problem (as with any topical agent) is allergic contact dermatitis from the contents of the emulsifying agent or its antimicrobial preservatives.

Keratolytic agents promote desquamation of scales. Salicylic acid is the most frequently used keratolytic agent. Concentrations ranging from 2 to 20% are formulated in a variety of ways. For smaller, thinner scaling plaques or for healing patches, a 2% concentration in an ointment base is used. A lotion base, which is excellent for scalp applications, may have up to 6% salicylic acid. Higher concentrations are used for thicker and hyperkeratotic plaques, and concentrations above 6% show marked keratolytic activity. Lactic acid in concentrations of 5 to 12% can also be used to reduce scaling. A popular combination of keratolytics is 6% salicylic acid in 60% propylene glycol with 20% ethyl alcohol. The preparation is applied under occlusion at night to hydrate the skin to remove thick, adherent scales. During the day, topical steroids can be applied to enhance percutaneous penetration and healing. Salicylic acid at concentrations of 2 to 6% is used with tar in creams, ointments, and shampoos. The combination is very efficacious, but preparations are dark grey or brown,

may stain clothing, and have an unpleasant smell causing problems with patient compliance.

Side effects include allergic contact dermatitis to the vehicle and soreness of the treated area. The latter condition can be alleviated by discontinuing the treatment. Potential side effects of salicylic acid are tinnitus, nausea, and hyperventilation. These systemic side effects are more likely to occur when large areas of damaged skin are exposed to higher concentrations (101, 102).

Tars

The mechanism of action of coal tar is not known. It is currently believed to have antimitotic effects. The initial application of coal tars to normal skin transiently increases epidermal proliferation for the first 2 weeks of treatment. If the coal tar is continued for up to 40 days, a cytostatic effect eventually produces epidermal thinning. Coal tars in combination with ultraviolet-A (UVA) light produce photoadducts to inhibit DNA synthesis.

Coal tar is effective monotherapy, and although it takes longer to clear the psoriasis than other treatments, prolonged remission can be expected. Compliance is difficult because of odor, staining, and irritation. To reduce these problems, extracts or refined products of crude coal tar in a 10% concentration with alcohol may be used. This preparation, called liquor carbonis detergens (LCD), is incorporated into various cream-based vehicles and bath additives. Coal tar preparations can be applied once or twice a day, but patients should be warned of irritation to the groin, axillae, and around the eyes. Side effects include photosensitivity, acneiform eruptions, and folliculitis (103). There is a potential for an increased risk of skin cancer and internal malignancies with the chronic use of topical coal tars. Mutagenic substances in coal tars are absorbed percutaneously and excreted in urine (104). However, to date, no study has clearly shown that chronic use of coal tar alone increases the risk of carcinoma (105).

Topical Corticosteroids

Topical corticosteroids are the most frequently prescribed medication for psoriasis. They can be used alone or in combination with other agents. Several modes of action are probably important in explaining their antipsoriatic activity. The hyperproliferative response is altered by a reduction in DNA synthesis and epidermal mitoses. There is a reduction in phospholipase A activity, which decreases arachidonic acid production and ultimately affects the production of inflammatory mediators LTB4 and HETE.

Topical corticosteroids also cause vasoconstriction, and the vasoconstrictive properties correlate well with clinical efficacy and are used to rank preparations in order of anti-inflammatory potency (Table 42.9). The broad range of potency results, in part, from chemical modifications of

Table 42.9.
Potency Ranking of Topical Corticosteroids by Generic Names

Superpotent	Clobetasol propionate 0.05% cream and ointment
	Betamethasone diproprionate[a] 0.05% cream and ointment
	Diflorasone diacetate[a] 0.05% ointment
	Halobetasol propionate 0.5% cream and ointment
Potent	Amcinonide 0.1% cream and ointment
	Halcinonide 0.1% cream
	Fluocinonide 0.5% cream, ointment, and gel
	Desoximetasone 0.25–0.05% cream, ointment, and gel
	Triamcinolone acetonide 0.1% ointment
	Mometasone 0.1% lotion, cream, and ointment
	Betamethasone valerate 0.1% ointment
	Diflorasone diacetate 0.05% cream
Midstrength	Flurandrenolide 0.05% cream and ointment
	Triamcinolone acetonide 0.1% lotion and cream
	Fluocinolone acetonide 0.025% ointment and cream
	Desoximetasone 0.05% cream
	Hydrocortisone valerate 0.2% cream and ointment
	Hydrocortisone butyrate 0.1% cream and ointment
	Betamethasone dipropionate 0.02% lotion
	Betamethasone valerate 0.1% cream
	Fluticasone propionate 0.05% cream
Mild	Alclometasone dipropionate 0.05% cream and ointment
	Desonide 0.05% cream and ointment
	Fluocinolone acetonide 0.01% solution
	Betamethasone valerate 0.05% lotion
	Hydrocortisone, dexamethasone, flumethalone, prednisolone, methylprenisolone in all vehicles

[a] Some preparations have been placed in the potent category.

hydrocortisone. When the molecule is esterified with valerate, dipropionate, or acetonide groups, the potency increases dramatically from increased penetration to the skin. Penetration can also be increased between 10- and 100-fold by an occlusive dressing. However, HPA-axis suppression is more prevalent when a potent preparation is used. The potency of a corticosteroid preparation can be altered by its vehicle. Gels are generally more effective than ointments, and ointments have greater biological activity than the same corticosteroid in creams or lotions. Creams are generally more effective than lotions.

Ointments can be used on thick scaly plaques, but they should be avoided in the axilla and groin, where folliculitis may develop secondary to rubbing and maceration. In the intertriginous areas, creams are a better choice. For the scalp and other hairy areas, gels, lotions, or sprays are preferable to ointments and creams.

Topical corticosteroids are usually applied twice a day. Applications once or twice a day are as effective as multiple applications, and less frequent applications prevent the development of tachyphylaxis and other side effects.

The incidence of side effects is increased by use of high-potency preparations; application to areas of thin skin such as the face, scrotum, vulva, or intertriginous areas;

application to areas where the skin barrier is compromised; and the use of occlusive dressings. Children and patients with renal failure are more susceptible to side effects. To lessen both local and systemic side effects, a weaker potency should be used on the face or in intertriginous areas. On areas of the body requiring higher potency corticosteroids, the preparation should be reduced to a lower strength after clearing of the plaques begins. Local side effects include striae and atrophy, skin fragility producing bruising, poor wound healing, telangiectasia, acneiform eruptions, pigmentary abnormalities, and allergic contact dermatitis to the vehicle.

Topical steroids can mask clinically inapparent dermatophyte infections. Fluorinated corticosteroids and hydrocortisone butyrate and acetate used on the face commonly result in perioral dermatitis and acne rosacea–like eruptions. As in the systemic administration of corticosteroids, withdrawal of potent topical preparations can change a stable plaque-type psoriasis to a pustular form. On the other hand, chronic use can precipitate an erythrodermic flare, especially if topical steroids have been applied to extensive areas of the body surface.

Applications to large areas are more likely to produce systemic side effects, including HPA-axis suppression on doses as small as 2 g/day, glucose intolerance, and (rarely) Cushing's syndrome. HPA-axis suppression is reversible after short-term use of potent preparations. Topical corticosteroids should be used with caution around the eyes. Systemic absorption at this site can produce glaucoma, cataracts, or an exacerbation of an ocular infection (106).

Anthralin

Anthralin or dithranol is a topical treatment that has not achieved the popularity in the U.S. that it has in Britain and Europe. The compound, 1,8-trihydroxyanthracene, has several modes of action but inhibition of mitochondrial DNA synthesis and various cellular enzymes may be the main reasons for its clinical effectiveness. The overall effect is antiproliferative on the epidermis, which decreases mitoses to normalize the epidermal architecture (103).

Commercial preparations of anthralin ointment and creams are available in concentrations of 0.1 to 1%. Anthralin is oxidized easily by exposure to air. Salicylic acid in concentrations ranging from 0.2 to 0.4% is often added to a preparation called Lassar's paste to increase its shelf life. Lassar's paste consists of anthralin in concentrations ranging from 0.1 to 5% mixed into zinc oxide paste with paraffin as a hardener and salicylic acid. This stiff paste is used in the Ingram method of treating large, chronic, plaque-type psoriasis. The treatment program begins with a tar bath and UVB phototherapy, followed by Lassar's paste-anthralin application to the plaques. Talc or cornstarch is applied to the paste, which sets the paste and absorbs excess moisture, to prevent smearing. This is to prevent local irritation when anthralin comes in contact with normal skin. A soft loose garment such as pajamas or a sweatsuit can be worn over the paste. The paste is left on for 4 to 12 hours, and often can be left on overnight. It is removed with a cloth and light mineral oil or baby oil, and the excess is washed off in a shower or bath with soap. Lower concentrations of anthralin from 0.1 to 1% are used initially, but higher concentrations of up to 5% are needed as the psoriasis improves.

As the skin barrier is restored with clinical improvement, higher concentrations of anthralin are needed to provide adequate levels in the epidermis for continued therapeutic efficacy. This clinical observation and the fact that anthralin penetrates more rapidly through the altered stratum corneum of psoriasis led to short-contact therapy. Low concentrations of anthralin ointment (0.1 to 0.5%) are left on for 60 min or more, while higher concentrations (1%) may be left on for only 10 to 20 min. Anthralin is then removed with mineral oil, followed by a shower with soap and water. Short-contact anthralin therapy requires a well-motivated intelligent patient and can be used daily on an outpatient basis. Improvement is expected to occur in approximately 3 weeks. The advantages of short-contact therapy over the Ingram method are reductions in both irritation and staining of clothing, because earlier washings reduce penetration and irritation in nonlesional skin. Penetration of anthralin through the plaques is far greater and peaks much earlier than in normal skin, maintaining clinical efficacy (107). The inflammation and staining of clothing can be eliminated by the application of 10% triethanolamine in an aqueous cream. This is applied immediately after short-contact therapy, without interfering with the therapeutic effect (108).

Anthralin should not be used on the face, because of the potential for eye irritation. Intertriginous areas, especially the antecubital and popliteal fossae, axillae, retroaricular and inguinal folds, as well as the inner thighs should be avoided. Hair and nails may show discoloration, but low anthralin concentrations, short exposure time, and pretreatment with neutral henna to coat the hair prevent anthralin penetration into the hair shaft. Nail polish can prevent anthralin penetration of the nail plate. No systemic toxic effects are associated with topical anthralin use, and contact allergy is rare (102).

Antimicrobial Therapy

Antimicrobial therapy has recently been included in the American Academy of Dermatology revised guidelines for the care of psoriasis patients (109). Antimicrobial treatment of psoriasis includes oral and topical antifungals and antibacterials. This therapy is based on accumulating evidence suggesting that psoriasis is aggravated by cutaneous or systemic microbial infection or colonization and that the inflammatory and hyperproliferative response is a di-

rect result of microbial products activating the alternate complement pathway. Psoriasis patients are believed to inherit a heightened immune responsiveness to the alternate complement pathway to produce their disease (100). Over the years, the literature has cited frequent associations of psoriasis with streptococcal infections. The most common association is the guttate variant seen in children and young adults. Patients with either throat culture or serologic evidence of group A streptococcus have good-to-excellent clearing of their disease when treated with rifampin in combination with either penicillin or erythromycin orally (110).

Other indications for antimicrobial treatment include various topical imidazole and nystatin antifungal agents for *Candida albicans*–associated "napkin" (or diaper) psoriasis in infants; oral ketoconazole for scalp psoriasis, and topical 2% erythromycin ointment for inverse psoriasis, especially in the gluteal fold. Detailed accounts of the approach to antimicrobial treatment of psoriasis are outlined in another text (111).

Phototherapy

Phototherapy, either alone or in combination with other treatments, can be used for moderate-to-severe psoriasis. The ultraviolet spectrum is of interest in psoriasis. Within the ultraviolet spectrum, UVB defined between 290 and 320 nm, and in particular 313 nm, is beneficial in the healing of psoriasis. The UVA spectrum between 320 and 400 nm, by itself, is not effective, but used with psoralen (PUVA), either orally or topically, it is effective. This combination is referred to as photochemotherapy.

Some general comments can be made about its mode of action. In addition to its antiproliferative effect, ultraviolet radiation suppresses cell-mediated immunity, but the significance of the latter observation remains uncertain.

Phototherapy is indicated in patients who have failed to respond to topical therapy or when psoriasis is widespread. Patients should be selected carefully for phototherapy and excluded if they have psoriasis that is worsened by sunlight, a history of photosensitizing disorder, or are currently taking drugs that are known to photosensitize. Phototherapy can be used on an outpatient basis to produce comparatively long-lasting remission. UVB can also be used at home, but PUVA therapy should be supervised by a dermatologist familiar with photochemotherapy (112).

Ultraviolet B

If UVB is used as monotherapy, the best results are obtained when erythemogenic doses are used on nonlesional skin. In calculating the initial dose, the patient's skin type is considered. This is estimated on the individual's ability to sunburn and tan and is called the minimal erythema dose (MED), expressed in mJ/cm^2. A test grid is performed on the back using the initial dose, and the skin is examined 24 hr later. If the skin does not show a pink outline of the grid, the dose of light is increased by 15 to 20% of the initial dose. The dose that causes minimal erythema at 24 hr produces the optimal effect in clearing psoriasis. From the MED, time spent in the UVB cabinet can be calculated. In addition to time spent exposed to UVB, the dosage is determined by the intensity of radiation. Intensity varies as the inverse square of the distance from the radiation source, so the distance between the patient and the light source must be considered. Although this may not be a problem in UVB cabinets because of physical constraints, some patients use UVB fluorescent tubes at home where the light-source-to-patient distance will affect the therapeutic response. Various protocols have been developed, but the most common outpatient protocol is 3 times a week using variable exposure increments of MED with the application of emollients. Most patients will clear with 18 treatments using this protocol (112).

UVB combined with crude coal tar is more effective than either agent alone. This combination, known as the Goeckerman regimen, uses crude coal tar at concentrations of 1 to 5% applied during the evening. Since the tar layer prevents the ultraviolet light from reaching the skin, the tar is removed in the morning using mineral oil, before exposure to a suberythemogenic dose of UVB. It was once thought that the UVB would act on the tar to produce photoadducts, but (as previously stated) the photosensitizing wavelength of tar is in the UVA spectrum. Also, UVB does not enhance the tar-induced suppression of DNA synthesis by epidermal cells, so the reason for its synergy is not known.

A more popular treatment regimen used in the United Kingdom and in continental Europe is the Ingram method, where the tar bath and UVB radiation are followed by the application of anthralin in Lassar's paste directly onto the plaques. There are no advantages to adding anthralin to the UVB therapy, and with the potential for irritation and staining of clothing, this may be a reason why the Goeckerman regimen is used more frequently in the U.S.

A major side effect of UVB therapy is burning from excessive UVB. Sunscreen, zinc oxide, or cloth can be applied to the affected areas to prevent further burning. To prevent ultraviolet-induced conjunctival erosions, protective goggles are worn during treatment. Although premature aging of the skin is dose-dependent, tar and UVB used in the described manner seem to show no increase in skin cancers (113).

Photochemotherapy

Photochemotherapy consists of an oral administration of a photoactive drug (a psoralen), followed 2 hr later by exposure to UVA. The psoralens are thought to produce photoadducts from the absorption of UVA. The photochemically induced covalent binding of the psoralen to the pyrimidine bases in DNA inhibit its synthesis and cell replication. Psoralen belongs to the furocoumarin class of compounds. The two derivatives currently available in the U.S. are 8-methoxypsoralen (methoxsalen, 8-MOP) and 4,5′,8-trimethylpsoralen (trioxsalen, TMP). The third psoralen, 5-methoxypsoralen (bergapten, 5-MOP), is currently being investigated for clinical use in the U.S., but is available in Europe.

8-MOP, however, is more potent in causing suppression of DNA synthesis than the other compounds and is the main psoralen in dermatologic use at this time. 8-MOP is administered in a dose of 0.3 to 0.6 mg/kg. When 8-MOP is administered orally, the blood levels peak at 2 hr, producing maximum sensitivity to UVA. Blood levels can be increased by a low-fat meal. The highest tissue concentrations are found in the gastrointestinal tract, liver, blood, and skin. In the blood, 84% is bound to serum albumin, and tolbutamide can displace the drug from the binding sites to increase the free fraction of 8-MOP. As a result of the displacement, the free fraction of 8-MOP can produce a photosensitivity. 8-MOP is metabolized through the liver by several pathways, including hydroxylation, glucuronide formation, epoxidation, and hydrolysis.

Like PUVA therapy, the patient's skin type guides selection of the starting dose of UVA. Treatment is administered once every other day, because the erythema induced by PUVA may not be evident for up to 48 hr after exposure. In general, the dose of UVA is increased by 1.5 J/cm^2 for each consecutive treatment. Unlike UVB therapy, the time to produce clearing with UVA is longer, usually after 10 to 20 treatments over 4 to 8 weeks. Once clearing has been achieved, the dosage of UVA is held constant. Maintenance therapy must be used because PUVA is only a palliative treatment. The same dose of UVA that induced clearing is used, but the frequency of treatment is reduced gradually to twice a month (114).

Topical psoralens, known as bath-water PUVA, is a very popular method in Scandinavia. It can be effective for both extensive plaque-type psoriasis and selected parts of the body, such as the hands and feet. This method avoids the gastric side-effects of oral psoralens and is ideal for patients with hepatic impairment. The patient soaks in a bath containing a very low concentration of psoralen before exposure to UVA. TMP is usually used because it has less percutaneous absorption than 8-MOP; but this method carries a greater risk of photosensitivity. To reduce the amount of UVA exposure and the number of treatments, oral retinoid agents, such as etretinate, can be used along with PUVA (RE-PUVA). Although the mechanism of synergism is not known, it does not seem to involve the increased photosensitivity seen with the retinoid agents (114).

Aside from the erythema and blistering, other acute side effects include pruritis and nausea. Shielding with a drape or sunscreens during subsequent UVA exposure prevents further erythema, and the duration of UVA exposure can be reduced. Pruritis can be controlled with emollients or topical steroids. Dividing the psoralen into two doses given an hour apart, can reduce the incidence of nausea. A less desirable alternative, especially for severe refractory nausea, is to reduce the dosage and increase the UVA exposure. A potential chronic complication of PUVA therapy is the development of cataracts. The renal excretion of psoralens usually is completed within 8 hr, but the elimination of a psoralen from the lens of the eye takes about 24 hr. When UVA from natural sunlight reaches psoralens in the lens, there is a theoretical possibility of binding to the protein and DNA of the lens. Although the risk is small, this complication can be nearly eliminated by wearing UVA-blocking wraparound glasses for 12 to 24 hr after ingesting psoralen. Other more common chronic side effects include a dose-dependent increased incidence of squamous cell carcinoma and lentigines (114, 115).

Systemic Corticosteroid Therapy

Systemic corticosteroid therapy for psoriasis is included here to emphasize that it is not the treatment of choice because of the many side effects associated with prolonged administration and because of the potential severe rebound side effect. There is a potential for conversion of stable plaque-type psoriasis into a pustular flare after withdrawal of corticosteroid therapy (98).

Retinoids

Two synthetic analogs of vitamin A, etretinate and acetretin, have been used in the treatment of psoriasis. Etretinate, an aromatic retinoid, has been available for clinical use in the U.S. since 1986. Acitretin is an acid metabolite of etretinate with different pharmcokinetics than etretinate. Acitretin has a shorter half-life and is not stored in subcutaneous fat like etretinate. Although its efficacy is similar to that of its parent compound, etretinate, acitretin as of 1991 remains under investigation in the U.S. and Canada. The exact mechanism of action on psoriasis is not known, but its various effects on cellular differentiation may cause normalization of keratinization and proliferation. Retinoids also have an antiinflammatory effect by reducing the levels of leukotriene and HETE. Since adverse side effects are greater than those from topical therapies, UVB, and PUVA, retinoids should be reserved for psoriasis recalcitrant to these treatments. The usual starting dose is 0.75 to 1.0 mg/kg/day in divided doses. Maximum dosage of 1.5 mg/kg/day is recommended, and after

8 to 16 weeks of therapy, a maintenance dosage of 0.5 to 0.75 mg/kg/day is required (116).

Side effects are similar to those seen with hypervitaminosis A syndrome. Among the major side effects are the embryotoxic and teratogenic effects on animal models and humans. Women of childbearing years are required to use contraception, which should be continued for 2 years after completing treatment. Acitretin may be of more benefit than etretinate in these patients. Other side effects include elevation of triglyceride or cholesterol levels, mucocutaneous changes such as cheilitis, hepatoxicity, and musculoskeletal changes (117).

Methotrexate

Methotrexate (MTX) is a folic acid antagonist that inhibits dihydrofolate reductase, blocking key steps in DNA and RNA synthesis. The overall effect is inhibition of cell division and a subsequent decrease of epidermal hyperproliferation, a characteristic pathophysiologic feature of psoriasis. MTX also has some immunosuppressive activity. It probably inhibits DNA synthesis in immunologically competent cells. It affects both cell- and humoral-mediated immunity and decreases the levels of LTB4.

MTX taken orally is rapidly absorbed through the gastrointestinal tract, but peak levels occur more slowly than in intramuscular or intravenous routes. It is excreted through the kidneys almost unchanged, and the clearance of MTX correlates with endogenous creatinine clearance. A small amount, however, is excreted by active tubular secretion. MTX is 50 to 70% bound to albumin and may be displaced by acidic drugs such as phenylbutazone, sulfonamides, salicylates, tetracycline, chloramphenicol, and phenytoin. A potential for toxicity exists when these are used in combination with MTX, especially if renal excretion is impaired. Weak organic acids such as salicylates, probenecid, ketoprofen, and phenylbutazone can compete with MTX to prolong active tubular secretion of MTX. Also, direct renal toxicity occurs with the concomitant use of MTX and indomethacin. Therefore, both agents should be used cautiously in psoriatic arthritis patients who have poor renal function (118).

The Food and Drug Administration (FDA) has approved MTX for use in severe, recalcitrant psoriasis. However, patient selection for MTX should take into account not only the characteristics of the disease but also the socioeconomic impact to the patient and absolute and relative contraindications. The only absolute contraindications are pregnancy and lactation. Relative contraindications can be waived only when the probable benefits of therapy outweigh the potential risks.

One relative contraindication that needs further elaboration is alcohol abuse. With chronic administration of MTX, hepatotoxicity resulting in fibrosis and cirrhosis is a serious concern. Alcoholism significantly increases the risk of hepatotoxicity, and MTX should not be used in patients who abuse alcohol.

The usual oral dose of MTX is 10 to 20 mg in either a single weekly dose, or divided into 3 doses given 12 hr apart once weekly. A test dose of 5 to 10 mg is given, and a CBC and liver function test are done 7 days later. In general, 75 to 80% of psoriasis patients will respond within 4 weeks. If no response occurs, the dose is increased by 2.5 to 5.0 mg/week. Although the most common route of administration is oral, it may be given intramuscularly at doses of 10 to 25 mg/week. The total dose rarely exceeds 30 mg. Higher intramuscular doses are allowed because of the more rapid renal clearance. When the psoriasis is in control, MTX may be tapered by 2.5 mg/week until the lowest possible dose is found that provides disease control (119).

Common acute side effects of MTX are nausea and gastrointestinal upset related to dosing. MTX can also produce a phototoxic reaction similar to sunburn. If MTX is used with phototherapy, patients should omit their phototherapy treatments on the days MTX is administered. More serious long-term side effects include hepatotoxicity and bone marrow suppression. The hepatotoxicity seems to be related to the cumulative dose of MTX. Liver function tests are unreliable screening methods for MTX-induced hepatotoxicity, so liver biopsy is currently the only means of monitoring changes attributed to MTX. Guidelines for monitoring MTX toxicity have been published elsewhere (120). Folinic acid is the treatment of choice for accidental overdose. Leucovorin rescue, as this is called, bypasses the step in folic acid reduction that is blocked by MTX (118).

Hydroxyurea

Hydroxyurea is a hydroxylated molecule of urea that affects cell proliferation by inhibiting DNA synthesis. The exact mode of action is incompletely understood in psoriasis. Although not approved by the FDA for treatment of psoriasis, it has been reported to be effective. It is less effective than MTX; the response is slower (6 to 8 weeks), and the response is not as complete (i.e., the annular areas of psoriasis persist). A good and rapid response can be achieved with pustular psoriasis. Response to the drug ranges from a favorable response in 45 to 63% to an excellent response in 18 to 38%. This variation may reflect different doses, varying time intervals, and different criteria for evaluating disease activity. Although this medication is not a first-line agent, it may benefit patients with high alcohol intake because of the low prevalence of hepatotoxicity. A major disadvantage is the frequent occurrence of bone marrow suppression (121).

Evolving Treatments

The following discussion focuses on systemic therapies that have been designated as evolving treatments by the American Academy of Dermatology guidelines of care for psoriasis (109).

CYCLOSPORINE

Cyclosporine is a 11–amino acid cyclic peptide frequently used to facilitate organ transplantation. Although the precise mechanism of action is not known, the inhibition of lymphokine secretion by activated T cells may play a central role. Because of the cost and toxicity associated with the drug, it is currently recommended only in patients with severe psoriasis that is unresponsive to more conventional therapies. Cyclosporine appears to be as effective as PUVA, UVB, MTX, or retinoid therapy in the treatment of chronic severe plaque psoriasis, but less effective in pustular psoriasis. Relapse is common after therapy is withdrawn. A rebound phenomenon such as those seen in systemic corticosteroid withdrawal is usually not seen. Dosages required for transplantation (15 mg/kg/day) are not appropriate, but lower doses (2.5 to 5 mg/kg/day) lead to a good response within 4 to 8 weeks. Therapeutic response is faster and more complete with higher doses, but there is a dose-dependent increased incidence of nephrotoxicity and hypertension. These side effects are reported to be reversed after lowering the dose. Other side effects include hepatotoxicity, neurologic abnormalities, and an increased incidence of lymphoma. Because of the many potentially life-threatening side effects, it has been recommended that patients with hypertension, evidence of compromised renal function, concurrent immunosuppression, past history of malignancy, pregnancy, and infection be excluded from taking this medication. To date, little is known about the safety and efficacy of long-term maintenance therapy. One study showed hypertension and renal dysfunction to be a problem, but this was corrected with dose reduction, therapeutic intervention, or both. To reduce the daily dose, combination with UVB, PUVA, or etretinate has been suggested. Phototherapy may not be a desirable combination in view of cyclosporine's immunosuppression and the potential for carcinogenic effects with phototherapy. High-dose etretinate showed only a modest reduction in cyclosporine dose (122, 123).

In conclusion, although systemic cyclosporine is efficacious in clearing psoriasis, several life-threatening side effects limit its use. Because of the toxicity of systemically administered cyclosporine, current investigations are focusing on topical preparations and intralesional cyclosporine.

SULFASALAZINE

Sulfasalazine contains a sulfapyridine moeity attached to 5-aminosalicylate. This drug has been used commonly in the treatment of ulcerative colitis and Crohn's disease. About one-third of a given dose of sulfasalazine is absorbed from the small intestine. The remaining two-thirds pass to the colon where the compound is split, possibly by intestinal bacteria, into its two components. Most of the sulfapyridine is absorbed in the colon, but only one-third of the 5-aminosalicylate is absorbed. The remainder of the two components are excreted into the feces. There are several proposed mechanisms of action since the drug may act as a whole or in parts. Sulfasalazine has been reported to inhibit folic acid, and the salicylate moiety affects the arachidonic acid pathway by inhibiting 5-lipoxygenase. It also has antimicrobial effects on the gut microflora.

A double-blind trial has recently found it to be effective in moderate-to-severe, stable, plaque-type psoriasis. Marked improvement was found in 41% of these patients. Common side effects are related to the gastrointestinal tract, such as nausea and diarrhea. With the low incidence of severe side effects, it may be used in patients whose disease severity may not justify the use of PUVA, etretinate or MTX. Further studies are needed to clarify its use with other forms of therapy (124–126).

VITAMIN D₃, FISH OIL, AND FUMARIC ACID

Calcitriol (1,25-dihydroxycholecalciferol) is the active form of vitamin D_3. The skin has receptors for circulating calcitriol, and when bound keratinocyte proliferation is inhibited and basal cells are induced to differentiate to squamous cells. In vitro, cultured cells from psoriatic skin exhibit a partial resistance to these effects of calcitriol, which is overcome by large increases in calcitriol concentrations. Clinical studies have confirmed the effectiveness of both topical and systemic calcitriol. Unfortunately, the limiting factor is hypercalcemia from systemic administration. Topical therapy, however, has been well tolerated with little or no side effects in the treatment of localized psoriasis.

A synthetic analog of calcitriol, calcipotriol, is an effective topical therapy for psoriasis, without changes in serum levels of ionized calcium. Like calcitriol, calcipotriol shows receptor binding and effects on cell differentiation, but calcipotriol is 100 times less potent in its effect on calcium metabolism. With up to 100-µg/g concentrations of calcipotriol, marked improvement was seen in 88% of psoriasis patients. Calcipotriol can be used over a larger body surface area than calcitriol, without significant hypercalcemia. Within the near future, there will no doubt be synthetic analogs of vitamin D, such as calcipotriol, that can be effective orally with less effect on calcium metabolism (127, 128).

Deep-sea fish oil contains significant quantities of the fatty acids eicosapentaenoic acid and docosahexaenoic acid. These fatty acids have a variety of effects on arachidonic acid metabolism. Eicosapentaenoic acid competes with arachidonic acid as substrates for cyclooxygenase and lipoxygenase to form biologically less potent prostaglandins and leukotrienes, respectively. Docosahexaenoic acid inhibits prostaglandin production and weakly inhibits leukotriene production. Since elevated levels of leukotrienes are found in the lesions of psoriasis, modifying the levels may influence the course. However, fish oils give orally slightly reduced the redness, scaling, and itching. Although it may not be used as monotherapy, it may be useful as an adjuvant treatment (129).

Fumaric acid therapy for psoriasis has recently been investigated in placebo-controlled studies by Dutch investigators. It consists of an oral treatment with monoethyl and dimethyl esters of fumaric acids. Its mechanism of action against psoriasis is currently not known. Although the results are preliminary, considerable improvement was found in 50% of the patients. The drawback of this medication has been its significant side effects such as flushing, nausea, diarrhea, and fatigue. This may limit future use in psoriasis patients (130, 131).

Clinical Variants and Specific Treatment Modalities

As mentioned previously, several clinical variants of psoriasis have been recognized that will determine the type of treatment modality. The following discussion summarizes specific treatment modalities for these clinical variants. Children and adults with guttate psoriasis are usually given systemic antimicrobial treatment, based on either cultures or antibody titers showing group A streptococcal infection. For both erythrodermic and generalized pustular psoriasis, MTX and etretinate have been successful monotherapies in controlling these eruptions. Localized psoriasis of the palms and soles responds well to PUVA treatments concentrated in these areas, and the addition of etretinate to PUVA (RE-PUVA) is reported to be more effective than PUVA alone. Sebopsoriasis distributed over the scalp, central face, central chest, and groin may respond to oral ketoconazole. Localized psoriasis of the scalp can be treated with 2% ketoconazole shampoo or other antiseborrheic preparations. Inverse psoriasis of the body folds with associated group B streptococcus colonization has been reported to respond to 2% erythromycin ointment. Finally, the choice of treatment for plaque-type psoriasis depends on the extent of body surface involvement. For more localized disease, topical corticosteroids or anthralin may be used. If more than 50% of the body surface is involved, then phototherapy, photochemotherapy, or systemic therapy should be considered. The two most commonly used forms of systemic monotherapies for plaque-type psoriasis are MTX and retinoids, but the latter is less effective and is usually used in combination with other treatments (98, 132).

In summary, seborrheic dermatitis and psoriasis are cutaneous eruptions in which disease expression is based on genetic and environmental factors. The pathophysiology of both diseases involves epidermal cell proliferation and inflammation. Therapies for seborrheic dermatitis and psoriasis are directed at these two pathologic features. Seborrheic dermatitis can be treated with shampoos or with topical antifungals and corticosteroids in areas not involving the scalp. The treatment of psoriasis, however, not only depends on the location but also its clinical presentation. Since a wide range of therapies is available for psoriasis, consideration must be given to side effects. Ideally, the choice is a regimen that provides adequate therapeutic efficacy without compromising the patient's quality of life.

REFERENCES

1. Leyden JJ, Shalita AR: Rational therapy for acne vulgaris: an update on topical treatment. J Am Acad Dermatol 15:907–914, 1986.

2. Pochi PE: The pathogenesis and treatment of acne. Annu Rev Med 41:187–198, 1990.

3. Ebling FJG, Culiffe WJ, The sebaceous glands. In Rook A, Wilkinson DS, Ebling FJG, Champion RH, Burton JL; Textbook of Dermatology, ed. 4. Oxford, England, Blackwell Scientific Publications, 1986 p 1914.

4. Puissegur-Lupo ML: Acne vulgaris: treatments and their rationale. Postgrad Med 78:76–84, 1985.

5. Webster GF, Leyden JJ, Norman ME, et al.: Complement activation in acne vulgaris: in vitro studies with Propionibacterium acnes and Propionibacterium granulosum. Infect Immun 22:523, 1978.

6. Holland DB, Gowland G, Cunliffe WJ, et al.: Lymphocyte subpopulations in patients with acne vulgaris. Br J Dermatol 109:199–203, 1983.

7. Shalita AR, Leyden JJ: New insights into pathogenesis of acne. 15 Symp Digest 3(4):25–32, 1991.

8. Cunliffe WJ: Evolution of a strategy for the treatment of acne. J Am Acad Dermatol 16:591–599, 1987.

9. Wilson BB: Acne vulgaris. Prim Care 16(3):695–712, 1989.

10. Liden S, Lindelof B: Is benzoyl peroxide carcinogenic? Br J Dermatol 123:129–130, 1990.

11. Katsambas A, Towarky AA, Stratigos J: Topical clindamycin phosphate compared with oral tetraycyline in the treatment of acne vulgaris. Br J Dermatol 116:387–391, 1987.

12. Lever L, Marks R: Current views on the aetiology, pathogenesis and treatment of acne vulgaris. Drugs 39(5):681–692, 1990.

13. Hirschmann JV: Topical antibiotics in dermatology. Arch Dermatol 124:1691–1700, 1989.

14. Parry MF, Chan-Kook R: Pseudomembranous colitis caused by topical clindamycin phosphate. Arch Dermatol 122:583–584, 1986.

15. Mills OH, Kligman AM: Drugs that are ineffective in the treatment of acne vulgaris. Br J Dermatol 108:371–374, 1983.

16. Schachner L, Pestana A, Kittles C: A clinical trial comparing the safety and efficacy of topical erythromycin zinc formulation with a topical clindamycin formulation. J Am Acad Dermatol 22:489–495, 1990.

17. Katsambas A, Graups K, Stratigos J: Clinical studies of 20% azelaic acid cream in the treatment of acne vulgaris. Acta Dermatol Venerol (Stockh) 143(suppl):35–39, 1989.

18. Hughes BR, Murphy CE, Barnett J, Cunliffe WJ: Strategy of acne therapy with long-term antibiotics. Br J Dermatol 121:623–628, 1989.

19. Eady EA, et al.: Superior antibacterial action and reduced incidence of bacterial resistance in minocycline compared to tetracycline treated acne patients. Br J Dermatol 122:233–244, 1990.

20. Hugh BR, Cunliffe WJ: Interactions between the oral contraceptive pill and antibiotics. Br J Dermatol 122:717, 1990.

21. Shalita AR, Armstrong RB, Leyden JJ, et al.: Isotretinoin revisited. Cutis 42:1–19, 1988.

22. Killoyne RF: Effects of retinoids in bone. J Am Acad Dermatol 19(suppl):212–216, 1988.

23. Sciarra F, et al.: Antiandrogens: clinical applications. J Steroid Biochem Molec Biol 37(3):349–362, 1990.

24. Pathak MA, Fitzpatrick TB, Greiter F, Kraus EW, Preventive treatment of sunburn, dermatoheliosis, and skin cancer with sunprotective agents. In Fitzpatrick TB, Eisen AZ, Wolff K, Freedberg IM, Austen KF: Dermatology in General Medicine, ed. 3. New York, McGraw-Hill, 1987, pp 1507–1522.

25. Braun-Falco O, Plewig G, Wolff HH, Winkelmann RK: Dermatology. Berlin, Heidelberg: Spinger-Verlag, 1991, ed 3, ch 13.

26. Soter NA, Acute effects of ultraviolet radiation on the skin. In Maibach HI: Seminars in Dermatology. Philadelphia, WB Saunders, 1990, vol 9, no 1, pp 11–15.

27. Young AR, Cumulative effects of ultraviolet radiation on the skin. Cancer and photoaging. In Maibach HI: Seminars in Dermatology. Philadelphia, WB Saunders, 1990, vol 9, no 1, pp 25–31.

28. Diffey BL, Human exposure to ultraviolet radiation. In Maibach HI: Seminars in Dermatology. Philadelphia, WB Saunders, 1990, vol 9, no 1 pp 2–10.

29. Morrison WL, et al.: The effects of indomethacin on ultraviolet-induced delayed erythema. J Invest Dermatol 68:130, 1977.

30. Arnold HL, Odom RB, James WD: Diseases of the Skin: Clinical Dermatology, ed. 8. Philadelphia, WB Saunders, 1990, ch 3.

31. Green A: Sun exposure and the risk of melanoma. Australas J Dermatol 25:99–102, 1984.

32. Taylor CR, Stern RS, Leyden JJ, Gilchrest BA: Photoaging/photodamage and photoprotection. J Am Acad Dermatol 22:1–15, 1990.

33. Lowe NJ: Sunscreens and the prevention of skin aging. J Dermatol Surg Oncol 16:936–938, 1990.

34. Boger J, Araugo OE, Flowers F: Sunscreen efficacy, use, and misuse. South Med J 77:1421–1427, 1984.

35. Pathak MA: Sunscreens: topical and systemic approaches for protection for human skin against harmful effects of solar radiation. J Am Acad Dermatol 7:285–312, 1982.

36. Federal Register: Sunscreen drug products for over-the-counter human drugs: proposed safety, effective, and labeling conditions. Washington, D.C., Dept of Health, Education and Welfare, Food and Drug Administration: Aug 25, 1978; 43(166):28206–28269.

37. Kaidbey RH: The photoprotective potential of the new superpotent sunscreens. J Am Acad Dermatol 22:449–452, 1990.

38. Lowe NJ, Photoprotection. In Maibach HI: Seminars in Dermatology. Philadelphia, WB Saunders, 1990, vol 9, no 1, pp 78–83.

39. Black HS: Systemic photoprotective agents. Photodermatology 4:187–195, 1987.

40. Dubois EL: Antimalarials in the management of discoid and systemic lupus erythematosus. Semin Arthritis Rheum 8:33–51, 1978.

41. Swanbeck G, Aminoquinolones. In Fitzpatrick TB, Eisen AZ, Wolff K, Freedberg IM, Austen KF: Dermatology in General Medicine, ed. 3. New York, McGraw-Hill, 1987, pp 2574–2582.

42. Weiss JS, Ellis CN, Headington JT, et al.: Topical tretinoin improves photoaged skin: a double blind, vehicle-controlled study. JAMA 259:527–532, 1988.

43. Leyden JJ, Grove GL, Grove MJ, et al.: Treatment of photodamage skin with topical tretinoin. J Am Acad Dermatol 21:638–644, 1989.

44. Gardner SS, Weiss JS: Clinical features of photodamage and treatment with topical tretinoin. J Dermatol Surg Oncol 16:925–931, 1990.

45. Van Scott EJ, Yu RJ: Alpha hydroxyacids. Can J Dermatol 1:108–112, 1989.

46. Goette DR: Topical chemotherapy with 5-fluorouracil. J Am Acad Dermatol 4:663–649, 1981.

47. Arnold HL, Odom RB, James WD: Warts. In Andrews' Diseases of the Skin, ed. 8. Philadelphia: WB Saunders, 1990, pp 468–475.

48. Cobb MW: Human papillomaviruses infection. J Am Acad Dermatol 22:547–566, 1990.

49. Lowy DR, Androphy EJ: Warts. In Fitzpatrich TB, Eisen AZ, Wolff K, et al. (eds): Dermatology in General Medicine, ed. 3. New York, McGraw-Hill 1987, pp 2355–2372.

50. Highet AS: Viral warts. Semin Dermatol 7(1):53–57, 1988.

51. Beutner KR: Human papillomavirus infection. J Am Acad Dermatol 20(1):114–123, 1989.

52. Steele KS, O'Hare P, Merrett JD, et al.: Monochloroacetic acid and 60% salicylic acid as a treatment for simple plantar warts: effectiveness and mode of action. Br J Dermatol 118:537–544, 1988.

53. Bart BJ, Biglow J, Vance JC, et al.: Salicylic acid in karaya gum patch as a treatment for verruca vulgaris. J Am Acad Dermatol 20(1):74–76, 1989.

54. Food and Drug Administration Health and Human Services: Wart removal drug products for over the counter human use: final monograph. 21 CFR, part 358, 1991.

55. Silva PD, Micha JP, Silva DG: Management of condyloma acuminatum. J Am Acad Dermatol 13:457–463, 1985.

56. Marcus J, Camisa C: Podophyllin therapy for condyloma acuminatum. Int J Dermatol 29(10):693–698, 1990.

57. Mroczkowski TF, McEwen C: Warts and other human papillomavirus infections. Postgrad Med 78(7):91–98, 1985.

58. Stone KM, Becker TM, Hadgu A, et al.: Treatment of external genital warts: a randomized clinical trial comparing podophyllin, cryotherapy, and electrodessication. Genitourin Med 66:16–19, 1990.

59. Jensen SL: Comparison of podophyllin application with simple surgical excision in clearance and recurrence of perianal condyloma acuminata. Lancet 2:1146–1148, 1985.

60. Rapini RP: Venereal warts. Prim Care 17(1):127–144, 1990.

61. Campbell BJ: The treatment of warts. Prim Care 13(3):465–476, 1986.

62. Miller RA: Podophyllin. Int J Dermatol 24:491–498, 1985.

63. Cassidy DE, Drewry J, Fanning J: Podophyllum toxicity: a report of a fatal case and a review of the literature. J Toxicol Clin Toxicol 19(1):35–44, 1982.

64. Beutner KR, von Krogh G: Current status of podophyllin for the treatment of genital warts. Semin Dermatol 9(2):148–151, 1990.

65. Edwards A, Atma-Ram A, Thin RN: Podophyllotoxin 0.5% vs podophyllin 20% to treat penile warts. Genitourin Med 64:263–265, 1988.

66. Rosemberg SK: Sexually transmitted papillomaviral infections: v. prophylactic use of topical 5-fluorouracil in refractory infection in the male. Urology 34(2):86–88, 1989.

67. Ferenczy A: Comparison of 5-fluorouracil and CO_2 laser for treatment of vaginal condyloma. Obstet Gynecol 64:773–778, 1984.

68. Boyd S: Condyloma acuminata in the pediatric population. Am J Dis Child 144:817–824, 1990.

69. Hursthouse MW: A controlled trial on the use of topical 5-fluorouracil on viral warts. Br J Dermatol 92:93–99, 1975.

70. Shumer SM, O'Keefe EJ: Bleomycin in the treatment of recalcitrant warts. J Am Acad Dermatol 9:91–96, 1983.

71. Shelley WB, Shelley ED: Intralesional bleomycin sulfate therapy for warts. Arch Dermatol 127:234–236, 1991.

72. Keay S, Teng N, Eisenberg M, et al.: Topical interferon for treating condyloma acuminata in women. J Infect Dis 158(5):934–939, 1988.

73. Eron LJ, Judson F, Tucker S, et al.: Interferon therapy for condyloma acuminata. N Engl J Med 315(17):1059–1063, 1986.

74. Vance JC, Bart BJ, Hansen RC, et al.: Intralesional recombinant α-2 interferon for the treatment of patients with condyloma acuminatum or verruca plantaris. Arch Dermatol 122:272–276, 1986.

75. Friedman-Kien AE, Eron LJ, Conant M, et al.: Natural interferon α for treatment of condyloma acuminata. JAMA 259(4):533–538, 1988.

76. Weck PK, Buddin DA, Whisnant JK, et al.: Interferons in the treatment of genital human papillomavirus infections. Am J Med 85(suppl 2A):159–164, 1988.

77. Reichman RC: Treatment of condyloma acuminatum with three interferons administered intralesionally. Ann Int Med 108:675–679, 1988.

78. Mahrle G, Schulze HJ: Recombinant interferon-γ in dermatology. J Invest Dermatol 95(6 suppl):132s–137s, 1990.

79. Kirby P: Interferon and genital warts: much potential, modest progress. JAMA 259(4):570–572, 1988.

80. Lutzner MA: Oral retinoid treatment of human papillomavirus type 5-induced epidermodysplasia verruciformis. N Engl J Med 302(19):1091, 1980.

81. Gross G, Pfister H, Hagedorn M, et al.: Effect of oral aromatic retinoid (Ro 10-9359) on human papillomavirus-2 induced common warts. Dermatologica 166:48–53, 1983.

82. Bolton RA: Nongenital warts: classification and treatment options. Am Fam Physician 43(6):2049–2056, 1991.

83. Naylor MF, Neldner KH, Yarbrough GK, et al.: Contact immunotherapy of resistant warts. J Am Acad Dermatol 19:679–683, 1988.

84. Eriksen K: Treatment of the common wart by induced allergic inflammation. Dermatologica 160:161–166, 1980.

85. Sanders BB, Smith KW: Dinitrochlorobenzene immunotherapy of human warts. Cutis 27:389–392, 1981.

86. Davidson-Parker J, Dinsmore W, Khan MH, et al.: Immunotherapy of genital warts with inosine pranobex and conventional treatment: double blind placebo controlled study. Genitourin Med 64:383–386, 1988.

87. Taylor MB: Successful treatment of warts. Postgrad Med 84(8):126–136, 1988.

88. Shuster S: The aetiology of dandruff and the mode of action of therapeutic agents. Br J Dermatol 1:235–242, 1984.

89. Skinner RB Jr, Noah PW, Taylor RM, et al.: Double-blind treatment of seborrheic dermatitis with 2% ketoconazole cream. J Am Acad Dermatol 12:852–856, 1985.

90. Ford GP, Farr PM, Ive FA, et al.: The response of seborrhoeic dermatitis to ketoconazole. Br J Dermatol 111:603–607, 1984.

91. Heng MC, Henderson BA, Barker BA, et al.: Correlation of *Pityosporum ovale* density with clinical severity of seborrheic dermatitis as assessed by a simplified technique. J Am Acad Dermatol 23:82–86, 1990.

92. Belew PW, Rosenberg EW, Jennings BR: Activation of the alternative pathway of complement by *Malassezia ovalis (Pityrosporum ovale)*. Mycopathologia 70:187–191, 1980.

93. Cowley NC, Farr PM, Shuster S: The permissive effect of sebum in seborroeic dermatitis: an explanation of the rash in neurological disorders. Br J Dermatol 122:71–76, 1990.

94. Brown M, Evans TW, Tooley PJH: The role of ketoconazole 2% shampoo in the treatment and prophylactic management of dandruff. J Dermatol Treat 1:177–179, 1990.

95. White JW, Localized eczematous disease. In Sams WM, Lynch PJ: Principles and Practice of Dermatology. New York, Churchill Livingstone, 1990, p 403.

96. Taieb A, Legrain V, Palmier C, et al.: Topical ketoconazole for infantile seborrhoeic dermatitis. Dermatologica 181:26–32, 1990.

97. Christophers E, Krueger GG, Psoriasis. In Fitzpatrick TB, Eisen AZ, Wolff K, et al.: Dermatology in General Medicine, ed. 3. Philadelphia, WB Saunders, 1987, p 461.

98. Zanolli MD, Psoriasis and Reiter's disease. In Sams WM, Lynch

PJ: Principles and Practice of Dermatology. New York, Churchill Livingstone, 1990, p 307.

99. Karasek MA: New developments in our understanding of the biology of psoriasis. Cutis 46:307–310, 1990.

100. Rosenberg EW, Belew PW: Microbial factors in psoriasis. Arch Dermatol 118:143–144, 1982.

101. Felscher Z, Rothman S: The insensible perspiration of the skin in hyperkeratotic conditions. J Invest Dermatol 6:271–278, 1945.

102. Marks R: Topical therapy for psoriasis: general principles. Dermatol Clin 2:383–388, 1984.

103. Lowe NJ, Ashton R: Anthralin and coal tar therapy for psoriasis. Dermatol Clin 2:389–396, 1984.

104. Wheeler L, Lowe NJ: Mutagenicity of urines from patients undergoing coal tar therapy for psoriasis. J Int Dermatol 77:181–185, 1981.

105. Jones SK, Mackie RM, Hole DJ, et al.: Further evidence of safety of tar in the management of psoriasis. Br J Dermatol 113:97–101, 1985.

106. Trozak DJ: Topical corticosteroid therapy in psoriasis vulgaris. Cutis 46:341–349, 1990.

107. Fiore M: Practical aspects of anthralin therapy. Cutis 46:351–354, 1990.

108. Ramsay B, Lawrence CM, Bruce JM, et al.: The effect of triethanolamine application on anthralin-induced inflammation and therapeutic effect on psoriasis. J Am Acad Dermatol 23:73–76, 1990.

109. Guidelines of care for psoriasis. AAD Bulletin 9:10–15, 1991.

110. Rosenberg EW, Noah PW, Zanolli MD, et al.: Use of rifampin with penicillin and erythromycin in the treatment of psoriasis. J Am Acad Dermatol 14:761–764, 1986.

111. Rosenberg EW, Skinner RB Jr, Noah PW, Antimicrobial treatment of psoriasis. In Roenigk H, Maibach HA: Psoriasis, ed. 2. New York, Marcel Dekker, 1990 p 815.

112. Paul BS, Diette KM, Parrish JA, Therapeutic photomedicine. In Fitzpatrick TB, Eisen AZ, Wolff K, et al: Dermatology in General Medicine, ed. 3. Philadelphia, WB Saunders, 1987, p 1522.

113. Stern RS, Thibodeau LA, Kleinerman RA, et al.: Psoriasis and susceptibility of nonmelanoma skin cancer. J Am Acad Dermatol 12:67–73, 1985.

114. Skinner RB Jr: Psoralens. In Wolverton SE, Wilkins JK: Systemic drugs for skin diseases. Philadelphia, WB Saunders, 1991, p 219.

115. Wolff K: Side-effects of psoralen photochemotherapy (PUVA). Br J Dermatol 122(suppl 36):117–125, 1990.

116. Wolverton SE: Retinoids. In Wolverton SE, Wilkins JK: Systemic Drug for Skin Diseases. Philadelphia, WB Saunders, 1991, p 187.

117. Ellis CN, Voorhees JJ: Etretinate therapy. J Am Acad Dermatol 16:267–291, 1987.

118. Olsen EA: The pharmacology of methotrexate. J Am Acad Dermatol 25:306–318, 1991.

119. Tung JP, Maibach HI: The practical use of methotrexate in psoriasis. Drugs 40:697–712, 1990.

120. Roenigk HH, Auerbach R, Maibach HI, et al.: Methotrexate in psoriasis: revised guidelines. J Am Acad Dermatol 19:145–156, 1988.

121. Boyd AS, Neldner KH: Hydroxyurea therapy. J Am Acad Dermatol 25:518–524, 1991.

122. Griffiths CE: Systemic and local administration of cyclosporine in the treatment of psoriasis. J Am Acad Dermatol 23:1242–1246, 1990.

123. Guenther L, Cyclosporine. In Wolverton SE, Wilkins JK: Systemic Drugs for Skin Diseases. Philadelphia, WB Saunders, 1991, p 167.

124. Gupta AK, et al.: Sulfasalazine improves psoriasis. A double-blind analysis. Arch Dermatol 126:487–493, 1990.

125. Halasz CI: Sulfasalazine as folic acid inhibitor in psoriasis. Arch Dermatol 126:1516–1517, 1990.

126. Neumann VC, Shinebaum R, Cooke EM, et al.: Effects of sulphasalazine on faecal flora in patients with rheumatoid arthritis: a comparison with penicillamine. Br J Rheumatol 26:334–337, 1987.

127. Smrtnik-Davis L, New uses of old drugs. In Wolverton SE, Wilkins JK: Systemic drugs for skin diseases. Philadelphia, WB Saunders, 1991, p 364.

128. Kragballe K: Treatment of psoriasis by the topical application of the novel cholecalciferol analogue calcipotriol (MC 903). Arch Dermatol 125:1647–1652, 1989.

129. Bittiner SB, Tucker WF, Cartwright I, et al.: A double-blind, randomized, placebo-controlled trial of fish oil in psoriasis. Lancet 1:378–380, 1988.

130. Nugteren-Huying WM, van der Schroeff JG, Hermans J, et al.: Fumaric acid therapy for psoriasis: a randomized, double-blind, placebo-controlled study. J Am Acad Dermatol 22:311–312, 1990.

131. Nieboer C, de Hoop D, Langendijk PN, et al.: Fumaric acid therapy in psoriasis: a double-blind comparison between fumaric acid compound therapy and monotherapy with dimethylfumaric acid ester. Dermatologica 181:33–37, 1990.

132. Matsunami E, Takashima A, Mizumo N, et al.: Topical PUVA, etretinate, and combined PUVA and etretinate for plamoplantar pustulosis: comparison of therapeutic efficacy and the influences of tonsillar and dental focal infections. J Dermatol 17:92–96, 1990.

CHAPTER 43

BURNS

TED L. RICE, B.S., M.S.

Skin, the largest organ of the body, performs five major functions. It provides protection from the environment, sensory perception, vitamin production, excretion of water and some wastes, and regulation of body temperature. When the skin is damaged, bacteria are no longer prevented from invading, pain is produced (unless superficial sensory nerves are destroyed), and both fluid and heat are lost through the damaged area.

Extensive skin loss or damage requiring hospitalization can occur by many different mechanisms that produce similar effects: thermal injury from hot liquids (scalds), flames, or extreme cold (frostbite) and injury from chemicals, radiation (sunburn), electricity, or trauma (abrasion). In addition, patients with extensive exfoliative dermatoses (e.g., the Stevens-Johnson syndrome or toxic epidermal necrolysis) are treated in burn centers.

Fire victims can suffer severe injury or death without significant body surface burns. A classic demonstration of this is the 1942 Coconut Grove Nightclub fire in which 75 of the 114 deaths were due to smoke inhalation. Carbon monoxide (CO) poisoning is a frequent cause of death. CO binds preferentially to hemoglobin, displacing oxygen and shifting the oxyhemoglobin dissociation curve to the left, resulting in tissue hypoxia. Although a function of the material burning, smoke contains toxins other than CO, such as cyanide, acrolein, benzene, and phosgene (1, 2).

Outcome following thermal injury is determined by a combination of patient and burn factors. The very young, very old, and previously ill have a poorer prognosis than healthy, young adults following a similar injury. Burn factors determining outcome include depth, extent, and body surface location (3). A list of burn severity criteria is provided in Table 43.1. The important distinction in depth of burn is that partial-thickness injuries heal by cell regeneration; full-thickness injuries, unless very small, require skin-grafting. Small full-thickness burns heal by contraction and reepithelialization from progenitor cells at the edges of the wound.

WOUND ASSESSMENT

Traditionally the depth of burns is described in degrees of injury as listed in Figure 43.1. As the depth of injury increases, the number for degree of injury increases. A first-degree burn is very shallow and involves only the epidermis. A second-degree burn involves complete destruction of the epidermis and variable portions of the under-lying dermis. When destruction to the dermis is limited to the upper third or less, it is called a superficial second-degree burn. Conversely, a deep second-degree burn has tissue destruction below the top one-third, but not completely through the dermis. A third-degree, or full-thickness, burn has destruction of the entire epidermis and dermis. The terms fourth-degree and fifth-degree burn have been used to describe tissue destruction through subcutaneous fat and through muscle, respectively (4).

The typical first-degree burn is easily identified. It is painful, erythematous, and blanches to pressure. A superficial second-degree burn is painful, forms blisters, and blanches to pressure. A third-degree burn is usually not painful because superficial nerve endings are destroyed, can appear white, leather-like, or black (charred), and contains thrombosed blood vessels. This dead tissue is called eschar (es'kar). Unfortunately, sometimes even the most experienced clinician cannot differentiate a partial-thickness from a full-thickness injury. In addition, flame injuries are typically mixtures of full and partial-thickness injuries. This classic presentation as depicted in Figure 43.2 was described as a target or bull's-eye where the deepest injury is in the center, followed by increasingly superficial injury at increasing distance from the center. Early attempts to improve the accurate assessment of injury depth included histologic staining, injection of radioactive compounds or dyes such as bromphenol blue, and fiberoptic perfusion fluorometry. These methods suffered from being invasive, cumbersome, labor-intensive, and inaccurate. Although

Table 43.1.
Burn Injury Severity Classification[a]

Depth of Burn	Percentage of Body Surface Affected (TBSA)[b]					
	Minor Injury		Moderate Injury		Major Injury	
	Adult	Child	Adult	Child	Adult	Child
Partial-thickness						
First-degree	<50	<10	50–75	10–20	>75	>20
Second-degree	<15	<10	15–25	10–20	>25	>20
Full-thickness						
Third-degree	<2	<2	2–10	2–10	>10	>10

[a] Irrespective of burn extent, injuries are classified as major when they involve areas of special importance such as the eyes, ears, hands, feet, or genitals. Injuries are major when burns occur in conjunction with other major trauma (e.g., fractures) or are associated with inhalation injury.
[b] TBSA, total body surface area.

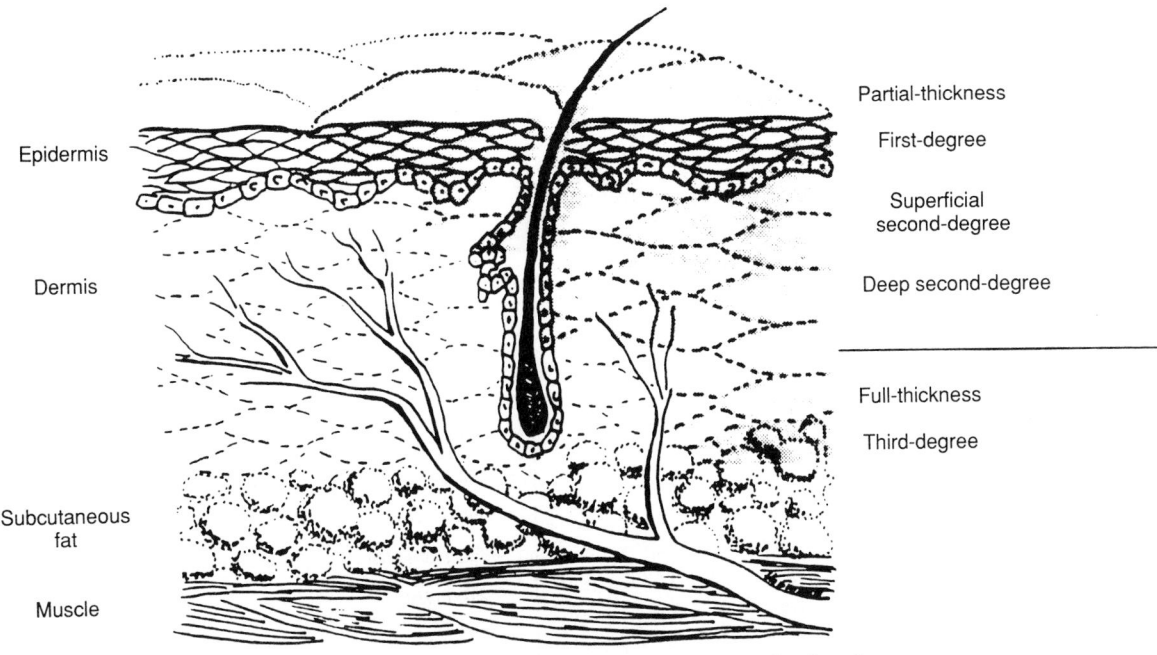

Figure 43.1. Diagram of burn depth in gross skin histology.

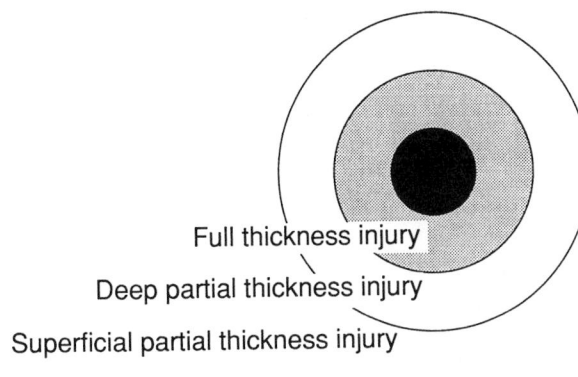

Figure 43.2. Typical pattern of injury following flame burn.

sensitive to variations in positioning and temperature, the recently developed laser doppler has better than 90% accuracy of correlation compared with histologic analysis of burn wound depth. The laser doppler documents a reduction in blood cell velocity in a burn wound, establishing the necessity for surgical removal and grafting. Clinicians must remain cognizant of the need for confirmation of initial assessments of burn depth. Reassessment is necessary because of the changing nature of deep partial-thickness injuries, which may become full-thickness because of inadequate resuscitation or infection (5).

A number of systems are used to calculate the relative percentage of total body surface area (TBSA) burned. The rule of nines is a simple system that can be used to estimate the extent of burn in adults. It represents regions of the body surface as 9% or multiples of 9%, e.g., the head and arms each represent approximately 9% TBSA, the torso 36%, each leg 18%, and 1% for the perineum. For burns with an uneven distribution, the patient's hand is a useful measuring tool. One side of the patient's hand is about 1% TBSA. Because the head of infants and children represents a larger TBSA than that of adults, the rule of nines does not hold. A more accurate assessment of TBSA can be made using the Lund-Browder chart. The chart used at the University of Michigan Burn Center is reproduced in Figure 43.3.

WOUND CLOSURE

When a large portion of the skin sustains full-thickness damage or destruction, the current surgical approach is staged eschar excision (debridement) and placement of autologous skin grafts. Split-thickness skin grafts (STSG) approximately 0.06 mm thick are harvested (using a dermatome), expanded by a ratio of 1.5:1 (using a meshing device), and applied to the wound after removal of devitalized tissue and achievement of hemostasis. Once adherent and vascularized, this STSG from the patient's own noninjured skin (autograft or isograft) permanently closes the wound (6).

Unfortunately, the amount of noninjured skin available for STSGs often cannot completely cover the open wound. A number of skin substitutes can be used to cover the open wound temporarily while waiting for donor site healing and reharvesting of autograft. Commonly used biologic

UNIVERSITY OF MICHIGAN HOSPITALS

BURN CENTER

ESTIMATION OF SIZE OF BURN BY PERCENT

LOCATION   DATE   SERVICE

Reg. No.   Class

Name

Address

① COLOR IN THE BURN

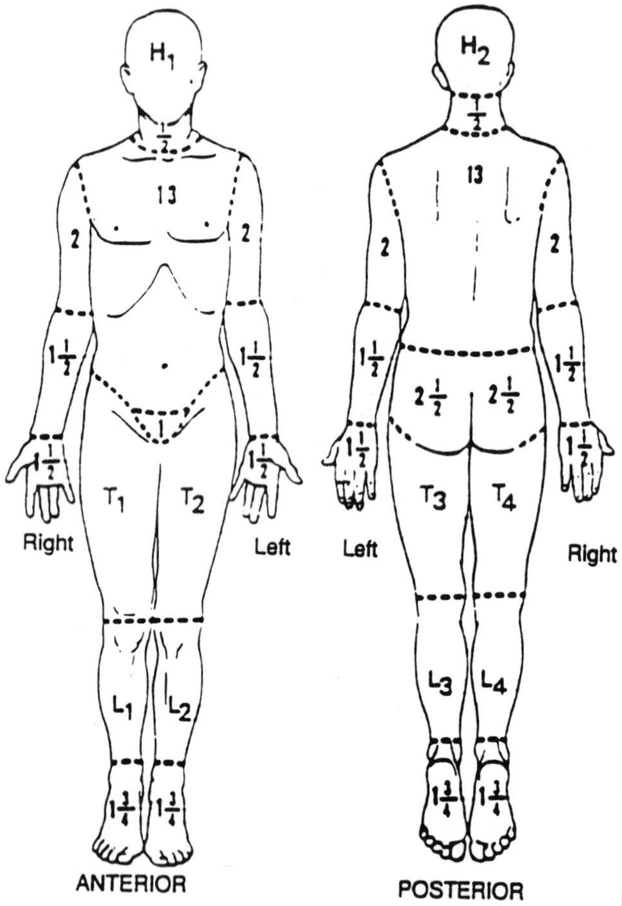

H₁   H₂

13   13

2   2   2   2

1½   1½   1½   1½

2½   2½

1½   1½   1½   1½

T₁   T₂   T₃   T₄

Right   Left   Left   Right

L₁   L₂   L₃   L₄

1¾   1¾   1¾   1¾

ANTERIOR   POSTERIOR

③ CALCULATE EXTENT BURN

	ANTERIOR	POSTERIOR
Head	H₁ _____	H₂ _____
Neck	_____	_____
Rt. Arm	_____	_____
Rt. Forearm	_____	_____
Rt. Hand	_____	_____
Lt. Arm	_____	_____
Lt. Forearm	_____	_____
Lt. Hand	_____	_____
Trunk	_____	_____
Buttock	_____	_____
Perineum	_____	_____
Rt. Thigh	T₁ _____	T₄ _____
Rt. Leg	L₁ _____	L₄ _____
Rt. Foot	_____	_____
Lt. Thigh	T₂ _____	T₃ _____
Lt. Leg	L₂ _____	L₃ _____
Lt. Foot	_____	_____
SUB TOTAL	_____	_____

▨   %   PARTIAL THICKNESS   _____ %

■   &   FULL THICKNESS   _____ %

%   TOTAL AREA BURNED   _____ %

② CIRCLE AGE FACTOR   PERCENT OF AREAS AFFECTED BY GROWTH

	AGE					
	0	1	5	10	15	ADULT
H (1 or 2) = 1/2 of the head	9 1/2	8 1/2	6 1/2	5 1/2	4 1/2	3 1/2
T (1,2,3, or 4) = 1/2 of a thigh	2 3/4	3 1/4	4	4 1/4	4 1/2	4 3/4
L (1,2,3, or 4) = 1/2 of a leg	2 1/2	2 1/2	2 3/4	3	3 1/4	3 1/2

H-2053949-DS   Rev. 3/89   **MEDICAL RECORD**   MED University of Michigan Medical Center   ESTIMATION OF SIZE OF BURN BY PERCENT

Figure 43.3. University of Michigan Hospitals Burn Center estimation of size of burn by percentage.

skin substitutes include cadaver skin (allograft or homograft) and animal skin (xenograft or heterograft). Less frequently used biologic skin substitutes are amniotic membranes and tissue-derived collagen. Synthetic skin substitutes include polyurethane films (e.g., OpSite) and petrolatum-impregnated fine mesh gauze (e.g., scarlet red and Xeroform). Biosynthetic skin substitutes have been developed which are combinations of biologic and synthetic materials, such as Biobrane, which combines collagen with a synthetic membrane (7).

Skin substitutes adhere to the wound, minimize pain, decrease protein, water and electrolyte loss, and simulate many important skin functions such as providing a barrier to bacteria. Although these skin substitutes provide important functions, they must eventually be replaced by autologous skin. An alternative to reharvesting STSG donor sites is the in vitro production of new skin by culture of autologous epidermis. Since the first successful transplantation of cultured autologous epidermis in 1981, keratinocyte growth techniques have been so improved that current methods allow a several thousandfold expansion of skin specimens within 3 to 4 weeks (8).

FLUID RESUSCITATION

Damaged skin loses the ability to serve as a barrier to percutaneous water loss. Evaporative water loss can be substantial (9). In contrast to the normal vapor pressure of approximately 3 mm Hg, the vapor pressure of full-thickness burns is about 30 mm Hg. The amount of water loss in ml/hr can be estimated using the following formula:

$$\text{Evaporative loss (ml/hr)} = (25 + \text{TBSA}) \times \text{BSA}$$

where *BSA* is body surface area in square meters. In addition, injury to capillaries in the burn wound causes them to leak a protein-rich fluid into the interstitial space, producing edema and blisters. Blood vessels are generally thought of as solid-walled tubes like plumbing, when in fact they are made of individual cells. When injured or under the influence of cytokines or inflammatory mediators these cells swell apart and produce small "holes" in the vessel wall. The problem resolves within 24 hr, but until then large macromolecules (molecular weights up to 80,000) can leak out of the intravascular space. When the TBSA burned exceeds 25%, a generalized "capillary leak" is produced throughout the body, and fluid exudes from unburned vessels into tissue and organs. The exact pathophysiology of this phenomenon is not clear, but the effects of leukotrienes, prostaglandins, arachidonic acid, and oxygen-derived free radicals have been implicated.

FLUID REQUIREMENTS

The treatment of resuscitation of the burned patient in shock has been the subject of much interest, research, and controversy. Focused interest was generated in the 1940s because hypovolemic shock was the leading cause of death in burned patients who survived their initial injury. The goal of initial fluid resuscitation is to restore and maintain tissue perfusion while minimizing edema formation (10, 11). The success of fluid administration is judged primarily by urine production at a rate of 0.5 to 1.0 ml/kg/hr. In addition, clinical observation of the adequately resuscitated patient should reveal a pulse rate less than 120 (adults) and a clear sensorium (12). Use of a physiologic salt solution (crystalloid) such as lactated Ringer's is recommended.

The major controversy regarding fluid resuscitation of the burn victim is the necessity of colloid infusion (13–17). Colloid is a general descriptive term for nondiffusible, large-molecular-weight molecules that affect osmotic pressure. Available colloid suspensions include fresh frozen plasma, plasma protein fraction, albumin, dextrans, hetastarch, and pentastarch. Clinicians who routinely use colloids suggest that they are more physiologic and can reduce nonburned tissue edema. Crystalloid proponents caution that administered colloids can escape from the intravascular space until the capillary leak is sealed. Although no definitive answer is available, it seems reasonable to exclude colloid infusion from resuscitation fluids for the first 12 hr. Representative resuscitation guidelines are listed in Table 43.2. Fluid requirements after the first 24-hr postburn period are determined in the usual fashion, with consideration of fluids lost through the burn wound and nasogastric suction. (See Chapter 8, "Fluid and Electrolyte Therapy and Acid-Base Balance.")

The main benefit of published guidelines is to alert the clinician unfamiliar with burn care that unusually large volumes of fluids and rates of administration are required for severely injured patients. Almost every author has acknowledged that patient variability prohibits development of a strictly calculated volume of resuscitative fluid and rate of administration.

In severe injuries, release of free hemoglobin from destroyed red cells and myoglobin from damaged muscle (especially following electrical injury) leads to destruction of renal tubules and acute renal failure. Binding of the free pigments to the renal tubules can be prevented by establishing a brisk urine flow (using mannitol if necessary) and alkalinizing the urine (pH $\geq$ 6.5) with parenteral sodium bicarbonate.

PHARMACOKINETIC CONSIDERATIONS IN BURN PATIENTS

The characteristic biphasic metabolic response to injury of an initial short ebb or shock phase (hypometabolic) followed by a flow phase (hypermetabolic) was described by Cuthbertson in 1930. A burn injury that exceeds 10 to 15% TBSA causes pathophysiologic alterations in the cardio-

Table 43.2.
Resuscitation Formulas for Postburn Fluid Requirements during the First 24 Hours Postburn[a]

Formula	Crystalloid	Colloid	Free Water
Adults			
Parkland	Lactated Ringer's 4 ml/kg/TBSA (%)	None	None
	½ in first 8 hr		
	¼ in next 8 hr		
	¼ in last 8 hr		
Evans	Lactated Ringer's 1 ml/kg/TBSA	1 ml/kg/TBSA	2000 ml/m^2
Brooke	Lactated Ringer's 1.5 ml/kg/TBSA	0.5 ml/kg/TBSA	2000 ml/m^2
Modified Brooke	Lactated Ringer's 2 ml/kg/TBSA	None	None
Children			
Graves	Lactated Ringer's 3 ml/kg/TBSA	None	Maintenance

[a] TBSA, total body surface area. Maintenance fluid requirements are 100 ml/kg/day for the first 10 kg body weight, 50 ml/kg/day for the second 10 kg body weight, and 20 ml/kg/day for weight in excess of 20 kg.

vascular, gastrointestinal, renal, and hepatic systems. The plasma proteins responsible for drug binding either increase or decrease in concentration, resulting in decreased or increased unbound drug concentrations, respectively. Finally, the movement of drugs into and out of the circulation is increased through the burn wound. The pharmacokinetics and pharmacodynamics of many drugs are changed after thermal trauma.

CARDIOVASCULAR CHANGES

Cardiac output has been demonstrated to decrease as much as 50% within 6 hr of severe thermal injury. This reduction in output has been attributed to hypovolemia, increased blood viscosity, increased peripheral vascular resistance, and the presence of a cardiotoxic protein termed "myocardial depressant factor" (18). Theoretically, intravenous drugs have a slower rate of distribution and elimination during this initial 48-hr period.

Following resuscitation, the hyperdynamic or recovery phase of injury is associated with increases of cardiac output to one and one-half to three times normal. This may not occur in the patient with preexisting myocardial disease. This increase in tissue perfusion is associated with an increased rate of drug distribution and elimination following intravenous administration (19).

GASTROINTESTINAL CONSIDERATIONS

Acute stress-related mucosal damage (SRMD) of the stomach and duodenum following severe burns is extremely common and is presumably related to increased acid secretion (20). The first case of acute gastroduodenal ulcer associated with thermal injury was reported by Swan in 1823. Following the 1842 report on a series of 12 patients by Curling, the syndrome was established and named Curling's ulcer. Prophylaxis and treatment of SRMD includes enteral feeding and administration of sucralfate, antacids, or H$_2$-receptor antagonists (H$_2$RAs). Cimetidine appears to be unique among the H$_2$RAs in that following burns, it reduces resuscitative fluid requirements and has increased clearance. A study in burned children demonstrated a reduced cimetidine pharmacodynamic response, in addition to an altered pharmacokinetic profile. The absorption of orally administered drugs may be either increased or decreased, depending upon the drug pKa and whether intragastric pH has been modified by antacids or H$_2$RAs. (See Chapter 21, "Acid Peptic Disorders.")

RENAL FUNCTION

The initial renal insults following a severe burn injury are general hypoxia and reduced perfusion. Following severe injury, liberation of free hemoglobin or myoglobin may result in acute renal failure. These problems can be reversed rapidly with resuscitative efforts and establishment of adequate urine flow. During the postburn hypermetabolic phase, renal blood flow and glomerular filtration rate (GFR) are increased, although tubular secretion may be impaired. This suggests that the elimination of freely filterable drugs such as the aminoglycosides and vancomycin will increase after burn injury. This effect was demonstrated in a study of 20 burn patients, which reported abnormal increases for both GFR and tobramycin elimination in 13 of 20 patients (21). The need for increased dosage of gentamicin in burn patients has been demonstrated in numerous studies of both adults and children (22–25). There are conflicting results about increased renal elimination of vancomycin following burn injury, but a need for increased dosing is commonly observed (26, 27).

HEPATIC FUNCTION

The hepatocyte is the most important site for drug metabolism, and in general it produces a metabolite that is more water soluble (facilitates urinary excretion) and of greater molecular weight (facilitates biliary secretion). The chemical reactions are classified into phase I and phase II biotransformations, which may occur in series. Phase I reactions include addition of a polar group (hydroxylation) or deletion of a nonpolar group (N-demethylation). Phase II conjugation with endogenous compounds such as glucuronic acid may follow phase I reactions. The most important enzymes catalyzing these reactions make up the microsomal enzyme oxidation system and include cytochrome P-450 and cytochrome P-450 reductase.

Although the mechanism is not completely clear, burn injury is associated with a marked depression of phase I reactions, while phase II reactions are unaffected. There is some evidence that decreased enzyme activity is due to oxygen-derived free radical damage to the hepatocyte. This discrepancy is evident in the postburn metabolism of diazepam and lorazepam (18). The phase I metabolism of diazepam is impaired, while the phase II metabolism of lorazepam (glucuronidation) does not differ from normal (28).

PLASMA PROTEIN BINDING

Although problems associated with changes in unbound drug concentration associated with inverse changes in plasma protein concentrations are theoretically possible, clinically important examples are few. The two proteins that account for most drug serum protein binding are albumin and α-1-acid glycoprotein (AAG) (29).

Albumin is a large molecule (approximately 69,000 daltons) capable of binding acidic, neutral, and basic drugs. Despite its large molecular weight, albumin is not confined to the intravascular space; 30% of total exchangeable albumin is in extravascular fluid. Postburn serum albumin concentration is commonly reduced by 50%, and often reaches critical levels of 10 g/l (1 g/dl) (normal: 3.5 to 4.9 g/dl in adults). The free fractions of diazepam, phenytoin, and salicylic acid increase following burn injury, which has been attributed to a decreased serum albumin concentration.

AAG is an acute-phase reactant that has a high affinity but low capacity for basic drugs and may be saturated at therapeutic concentrations (e.g., lidocaine). The concentration of AAG may increase to as much as 300% of normal during the first postburn week and not return to normal for 4 to 6 weeks. The free fractions of imipramine, lidocaine, meperidine, and propranolol decrease after the first postburn week, presumably in response to an increased AAG concentration.

The critically important breakpoint for drug serum protein binding is approximately 90%. When binding is less than 90%, the pharmacokinetic parameters change little following pathophysiologic changes in binding. Oral administration of drugs with a high hepatic extraction ratio

(such as propranolol) would be affected little by changes in plasma protein binding, because of the first-pass effect. Although the potential for problems is low, the clinician monitoring a patient receiving agents that have low therapeutic indices or steep dose-response curves should consider the effect of altered protein binding when evaluating drug toxicity or suboptimal response.

The efficacies of the nondepolarizing neuromuscular blocking agents tubocurarine chloride, metocurine iodide, pancuronium bromide, and atracurium besylate are reduced after the first postburn week, which implies that increased plasma protein binding to AAG is responsible (30, 31). Although increased binding does occur, the relatively small increase cannot explain the sometimes dramatic decrease in response. Investigations of the mechanism for this resistance have ruled out changes in drug clearance or volume of distribution. The decreased potency of these agents may be due to an unidentified substance in the plasma of burn patients.

DRUG MOVEMENT THROUGH BURN WOUNDS

Destruction of the normal barriers to percutaneous absorption occurs with burn injury. The diffusion resistance to water movement through injured skin can be less than one-tenth that of normal skin. Gentamicin is absorbed readily following topical application of a 0.1% cream and absorbed to a smaller extent with a 0.1% ointment (32). Eschar penetration has also been demonstrated in vitro for mafenide acetate, nitrofurazone, povidone-iodine, silver nitrate, and silver sulfadiazine (33).

Drug penetration of the burn wound is not unidirectional. Historically, it has been assumed that eschar penetration by systemically administered drugs was prevented by the avascular nature of the wound. However, systemically administered gentamicin and tobramycin both penetrate burn eschar (34). Drug loss through the burn wound may add substantially to total drug clearance.

INFECTION AND ANTIMICROBIALS

Despite therapeutic advances, infection in the burned patient remains the most important cause of death in those who survive initial resuscitation (35–37). Administration of tetanus immune globulin and/or tetanus toxoid when the patient's tetanus immunization history is not known should be based on the American College of Surgeons guidelines. Colonization of the burn wound has been demonstrated even when the patient is cared for in a laminar-flow room. Explanations for this phenomenon are that endogenous bacteria translocate from the gastrointestinal tract, that bacteria are iatrogenically transmitted, and that normal skin flora proliferate (38).

BURN WOUND INFECTION

Although the importance of bacteria in the burn wound has been recognized, the terminology describing the association between wound bacteria and systemic manifestations of infection is confusing. Moncrief and Teplitz suggested that "burn wound sepsis" be used to describe the events associated with bacterial proliferation to 100,000 colony forming units (cfu) per gram of burn wound tissue and subsequent invasion of adjacent nonburned tissue (39). Unfortunately, this number of bacteria per gram of tissue is not diagnostic of an invasive burn wound infection, and a complex classification scheme ranging from surface contamination to microvascular invasion (I, II, III, IV, V, VIa, VIb, VIc) has been suggested by Pruitt (40).

Whether or not the bacteria are localized to the burn or are disseminated, a rational method for selecting from the available topical antimicrobials is necessary. Similar to the Kirby-Bauer method of determining bacterial susceptibility to systemic agents, Nathan et al. first reported on the agar-well diffusion method for determining susceptibilities to topical antimicrobials (41). Support for this method was supplied by Heggers et al. who demonstrated that the agar-well diffusion test was more reliable than minimum inhibitory concentration determination for predicting bacterial susceptibility (42).

TOPICAL ANTIMICROBIALS

Silver Nitrate. The "modern" use of silver nitrate began in the late 1800s with the prevention of opthalmia neonatorum. Substantial improvement in the treatment of large burns by the use of continuously applied 0.5% silver nitrate solution was reported in 1965 (43). The characteristics that make 0.5% silver nitrate a useful topical antibacterial agent are its safety, water solubility, prolonged antibacterial action, lack of toxicity to viable skin, lack of antigenicity, and ease of preparation. Problems associated with its use include hypochloremia from formation of silver chloride salts, water intoxication because of the hypotonicity of the solution, and hyponatremia or hypokalemia from diffusion into the wet dressings. Other problems are a requirement for bulky dressings that restrict joint motion and ambulation, and black staining of everything that comes into contact with the solution.

Silver Sulfadiazine. The use of silver sulfadiazine (SSD) in burns was first reported in both a murine burn model and 16 patients (44). SSD is unique among the usual topical antibacterial agents in effectively inhibiting *Candida albicans*. The exact antimicrobial mechanism of action of SSD has not been clearly elucidated, but it is attributed to silver inhibition of DNA replication or cell membrane modification. Two studies imply that the sulfadiazine component is not necessary for in vitro bacterial sensitivity. In addition, clinical efficacy may be associated with a reversal of injury-induced suppression of lymphocyte natural killer cell cytotoxicity rather than strict antibacterial effects.

SSD is the topical agent of choice worldwide because of its safety and efficacy (45–47). Toxicity associated with

SSD application is infrequent and associated predominantly with the propylene glycol component of the cream base. The potential for allergic hypersensitivity is shown by circulating sulfadiazine antibodies (predominantly IgG) in the serum of treated patients. Although SSD-associated leukopenia has been reported, it is probably an artifact of the physiologic response to burn injury of WBC margination and/or diapedesis (movement through vessels) from the intravascular space (48). Clinicians continue to apply SSD to patients who develop leukopenia.

Because of its demonstrated efficacy, SSD has been incorporated into a number of biologic and synthetic dressings or skin substitutes, to take advantage of its benefits and eliminate the inconvenience of dressing changes with reapplication of cream. Another method used to improve upon SSD is the addition of other agents such as nitrofurazone, gentamicin, fluoroquinolones, and cerium nitrate. The most successful combination is with chlorhexidine; Silvazine (Smith & Nephew, Clayton, Australia), a commercially available combination has been used in Australia for over 10 years.

Mafenide Acetate and Nitrofurazone. Although causing pain upon application, mafenide acetate is a useful topical antimicrobial for the treatment of subeschar burn wound infections because of its ability to penetrate the burn wound. Mafenide is often used on burned ears to prevent chondritis. Although closely related chemically, mafenide is not a sulfonamide. The primary metabolite (*p*-carboxybenzene sulfonamide) is a sulfonamide, and it may cause allergic reactions in patients with sulfonamide hypersensitivity. When applied to large TBSA burns, mafenide can produce systemic metabolic acidosis secondary to carbonic anhydrase inhibition (49). Another disadvantage of mafenide is its high cost, approximately four times that of SSD. The antimicrobial usefulness of nitrofurazone has been demonstrated since the mid-1940s (50). Its primary use has been in prophylaxis of infection following skin grafting.

SYSTEMIC ANTIMICROBIALS

The use of prophylactic penicillin during the first postburn week was common during the 1950s and 1960s because of a justified concern of infection by *Streptococcus pyogenes*. This organism produced rapid conversion of partial-thickness to full-thickness wounds and fatalities. However, current laboratory methods for monitoring the burn wound and close clinical monitoring of patient allow the rapid recognition of infection. Recent prospective clinical trials have demonstrated no benefit for prophylactic penicillin. Indeed, subsequent wound cultures in penicillin-treated patients have a greater incidence of resistant organisms.

The choice of antibiotics for systemic infections in burn patients should be the same as for other patients (51).

However, because the pathophysiologic changes following burn trauma are dynamic, the dosing of systemic antimicrobials must be individualized when possible (52). Increased requirements for aminoglycosides and vancomycin have been demonstrated in burn patients (as discussed in the pharmacokinetics section).

NUTRITION SUPPORT

(See also Chapter 11, "Parenteral and Enteral Nutrition.")

METABOLIC RESPONSE TO TRAUMA

The hypermetabolism following trauma was initially explained as a physiologic response to increased heat loss. The rationale was that burned skin allows increased water loss that lowers the skin/wound temperature when it evaporates. However, the precise relationship between evaporative water loss and postburn hypermetabolism is unclear, since conflicting results have been reported from similar investigations.

Similarly, it has been assumed that increased thermogenesis was necessary to compensate for heat loss in a cold environment, since damaged skin cannot respond with decreased perspiration and cutaneous vasoconstriction. However, postburn hypermetabolism is not attenuated, even when the environmental temperature is increased above thermal neutrality. A resetting of the hypothalamic thermal regulatory setpoint is suggested by a study comparing burned patients to normal controls, in which the burn patients selected a significantly higher environmental temperature when placed in a metabolic chamber.

Metabolic rate may be reduced following relief of pain, although the degree of reduction is not well defined (53). Historically, pain management of hospitalized patients with opioids has been suboptimal because of unnecessary fears of addiction. Morphine requirements of burn patients can be substantial, exceeding 60 mg/hr before development of tolerance (54).

Other contributors to postburn hypermetabolism are prostaglandins, interleukins, components of the complement cascade, and the catabolic neurohumoral milieu of elevated serum cortisol, growth hormone, catecholamines, and glucagon levels. Initial insulin secretion inhibition is usually followed by normal or supranormal plasma insulin levels. Despite this insulin recovery, hyperglycemia persists, secondary to insulin resistance at the tissue insulin receptor.

The fuel stores that are mobilized to sustain postburn hypermetabolism include hepatic and muscle glycogen; visceral, plasma, and muscle protein; and fat. Because the major metabolic source of ATP provided to the burn wound is anaerobic glycolysis, the obligatory glucose requirement is increased. Production of glucose from glycogenolysis is relatively short-lived, because stores only approximate 100 to 200 g and endogenous glucose production can exceed 400 g per day. Significant endogenous glucose is provided by efficient recycling of pyruvate and lactate via the Cori cycle and the glucose-alanine cycle. Catabolism of muscle protein and direct oxidation of amino acids provide approximately 15 to 20% of the total caloric expenditure in the fasting injured patient. The body adapts to using fat as its main energy source and can mobilize abundant energy from the typical fat stores of approximately 160,000 kcals.

The specific cause of postburn hypermetabolism is not clear but appears to be multifactorial. Completely arresting postburn hypermetabolism is not currently possible. A reasonable approach is to provide the patient with a warm environment, adequate pain relief, early enteral nutrition, and aggressive wound coverage. In addition, an attempt should be made to minimize endogenous protein catabolism by providing exogenous protein and nonprotein calories.

METHOD OF NUTRIENT ADMINISTRATION

Patients with less than 20% TBSA burns can usually be maintained on a normal diet, unless there is an associated condition such as severe preburn malnutrition or an injury that prevents mastication. Patients with larger burns are often unwilling or unable to consume enough high-protein and caloric-dense food to fulfill requirements. For these patients, nutritional requirements can be met by insertion of a small-bore nasoenteric feeding tube and administration of commercially available enteral feeding formulations such as Osmolite-HN, TwoCal-HN, Traumacal, and Replete. Enteral nutrition is preferred to parenteral nutrition because it is more physiologic, less costly, and avoids complications associated with parenteral nutrition such as catheter-related sepsis.

In contrast to historical recommendations that focused on parenteral nutrition, current guidelines call for early enteral feeding (55). Even in severely burned patients with absent bowel sounds, feeding into the small intestine through a nasoenteric tube is still possible, because postburn ileus is confined primarily to the stomach (56). In these severely injured patients, a nasogastric tube is inserted and connected to suction for 2 to 3 days until gastric function returns. Experimental evidence favoring early enteral feeding demonstrated a reduction in catabolism and the hypermetabolic response in a guinea pig burn model. Another beneficial effect of early enteral feeding is the maintenance of gut mucosal mass. Improved gut wall homeostasis may prevent the increased intestinal permeability that allows translocation of enteric bacteria.

Macronutrient Needs

The metabolic demands associated with severe burns exceed those of any other hospitalized patient. The postburn

Table 43.3.
Various Formulas Used to Estimate Energy Requirements in Burn Patients[a]

Adults
(1) Harris-Benedict equation (estimates basal energy expenditure (BEE))

Male: BEE (kcal) $= 66 + (13.7 \times W) + (5 \times H) - (6.8 \times A)$

Female: BEE (kcal) $= 665 + (9.6 \times W) + (1.7 \times H) - (4.7 \times A)$

(2) Burke and Wolfe

Kcal per day $= 2 \times BEE$

(3) Curreri

Kcal per day $= 25 \times W + (40 \times TBSA)$

(4) Davies and Liljedahl

Kcal per day $= 20 \times W + (70 \times TBSA)$

Children
(1) Wolfe

Kcal per day $= 2 \times BEE$

(2) Curreri Junior

Kcal per day $=$ (0–1 years) $BEE + (15 \times TBSA)$

(1–3 years) $BEE + (25 \times TBSA)$

(3–15 years) $BEE + (40 \times TBSA)$

[a] W, weight in kg; H, height in cm; A, age in years; and TBSA, total body surface area burned (%).

energy expenditure increases with increasing burn size. However, there is an upper limit to required calories. This upper limit is approximately twice the calculated basal energy expenditure (BEE) using the Harris-Benedict equation. Numerous methods are available to calculate the burn patient's daily energy requirement, and representative formulas are listed in Table 43.3.

Although mathematical calculation to predict energy requirements is convenient, determination of the patient's specific calorie needs is desirable (57). A complex metabolic chamber is necessary to specifically measure energy expenditure, but a reasonably accurate estimation can be performed at the bedside using indirect calorimetry (58). Metabolic carts measure the respiratory gas exchange of oxygen (VO_2) and carbon dioxide (VCO_2) to indirectly measure energy expenditure (via the reverse Fick equation).

CARBOHYDRATE REQUIREMENTS

Energy liberated by oxidation of enterally administered carbohydrate is approximately 4 kcal/g. The carbohydrate commonly administered parenterally is hydrous dextrose, which liberates 3.4 kcal/g when completely oxidized. The optimal amount of administered carbohydrate will minimize gluconeogenesis without exceeding energy requirements and being stored as triglycerides.

The utilization of glucose for energy by burned patients has limits. When glucose is oxidized to liberate energy, equimolar concentrations of oxygen are consumed

and carbon dioxide produced (respiratory quotient (RQ) = 1). The normal, fed RQ is approximately 0.84, and it rises when the rate of administered glucose exceeds the maximum rate of utilization. When glucose is converted into fat, more than eight times as much carbon dioxide is released for each mole of oxygen (RQ > 1). Excretion of this extra carbon dioxide could be difficult for a burned patient with an associated inhalation injury. An additional negative aspect of lipogenesis is that it is an energy-consuming process. An elegant study of intravenous glucose, using isotopic tracers, demonstrated that the maximum rate of oxidation is approximately 5 mg/kg/min. At faster rates of glucose administration, the RQ rapidly increased above 1.0, suggesting lipogenesis. For a 70-kg patient, this maximum rate of glucose utilization translates into 2 liters of 25% dextrose-containing total parenteral nutrition solution (500 g) per day (59).

FAT REQUIREMENTS

Fat is an efficient provider of energy at 9 kcal/g, but it is vital only for supplying essential fatty acids to prevent essential fatty acid deficiency syndrome. The amount of fat necessary in burned patients is not known, but fat should provide a minimum 2% of total calories. Fat is an essential component of cell membranes, functions as a carrier for the fat-soluble vitamins, and is important for wound healing.

Patients with severe thermal injury may have reduced lipolytic capacity, especially following parenteral administration of fat emulsion. It appears that parenteral administration of long-chain triglycerides is associated with hepatomegaly, impaired clotting, and decreased resistance to infection. Preliminary evidence indicates that lipids high in linoleic acid (e.g., safflower or soybean oil) are associated with immunosuppression, presumably because linoleic acid is the precursor of arachidonic acid, which is the principal substrate for prostaglandins (PGE1 and PGE2) and certain leukotrienes. Another advantage of enteral administration is that medium-chain triglycerides are absorbed without the need for bile, and at the cellular level, they are transported into mitochondria without the need for carnitine.

Because of the constraint on the rate of carbohydrate administration, fat must usually be provided in substantial quantities as an energy source. Although not often important clinically, fat has a specific advantage over glucose in patients with pulmonary dysfunction, when a reduced carbon dioxide production for an equivalent amount of oxygen consumed is useful. The optimal fatty acid chain length and exact dietary fat requirements for burn patients remain to be determined.

PROTEIN REQUIREMENTS

Protein loss across burn wounds is considerable and is greatest in the first 3 postburn days. Although early protein loss across full-thickness burns is greater than that in partial-thickness burns, the rates become approximately the same after postburn day 3. The rate of protein loss is reduced by application of either antimicrobial creams or skin substitutes. Using the average protein loss during the first postburn week (0.5 mg/cm^2/hr) a formula that estimates the daily protein loss (g) across the burn wound can be devised: 1.2 × body surface area (m^2) × total body surface area burn (%). Protein loss across the burn wound during the second postburn week occurs at approximately half this rate.

The recommended daily allowance of protein for healthy adults is 0.8 g/kg. The optimal amount of protein required by burned patients to prevent catabolism of protein stores and promote wound healing is not well defined. The importance of protein-sparing by providing energy must be considered, but some clinicians advocate a high-protein diet aimed at achieving a 100:1 nonprotein calorie to nitrogen ratio in contrast to the standard 150:1 ratio.

In clinical practice, approximately 1.5 to 2 g/kg/day (using lean body weight) of protein is provided initially. Nitrogen-balance studies then determine the adequacy of this regimen. Although the nitrogen balance calculation appears simple:

$$\text{Nitrogen balance} = N(in) - N(out)$$

there is potential error in assessment of both $N(in)$ and $N(out)$. $N(in)$ is the number of grams of nitrogen ingested or infused, and it is common practice to multiply the number of grams of protein or amino acid by 0.16 to estimate grams of nitrogen. This calculation assumes that the protein is made up of 16% nitrogen, but the percentage nitrogen in available parenteral amino acid products varies from 11.1% to 16.9% (60). The $N(out)$ is calculated by adding the urinary urea nitrogen (UUN) from a 24-hr urine collection to an estimate of nitrogen excretion other than that measured as urine urea. This estimate is comprised of nonurea urinary nitrogen (ammonia, uric acid, creatinine) and nonurinary nitrogen loss (fecal and skin). A commonly used estimate for non-UUN losses is 4 g. As described above, significant quantities of protein (nitrogen) are lost through open burn wounds and must be included in this estimate.

The branched-chain amino acids (BCAAs) leucine, isoleucine, and valine are unique in that skeletal muscle can oxidize them directly for energy. In contrast, the other amino acids are metabolized almost wholly by the liver. Under ordinary circumstances, only 6 to 7% of the daily energy expenditure is provided through BCAA oxidation by skeletal muscle. The administration of supplemental BCAAs, especially leucine, to burn patients should (theoretically) reduce protein catabolism in skeletal muscle and increase protein synthesis. However, conclusive evidence of beneficial effects for BCAA-enriched solutions in burn patients has not been demonstrated, and further studies are needed (61).

Measurement of serum proteins such as albumin, prealbumin, transferrin, and retinol-binding protein is often regarded as a reliable index of nutritional status. However, because of surgical excision and grafting of wounds, associated blood loss and transfusions, and administration of exogenous albumin, changes in serum protein concentrations as an indication of nutrition regimen adequacy must be viewed with caution. Nitrogen-balance studies are probably the best assessment of protein status, despite the limitations described previously.

Micronutrient Needs

In contrast to the extensive information about macronutrient requirements, little information is available about the micronutrient needs of burn patients. There is evidence that micronutrient needs are increased following burns, although the exact amounts have not been defined (62, 63).

VITAMINS

At a minimum, burn patients should receive vitamin supplements based on the Recommended Dietary Allowance (RDA) for enteral or the American Medical Association Nutrition Advisory Group (AMA) for parenteral administration. In the absence of preexisting deficiency, there is little indication to administer increased amounts of fat-soluble vitamins. Vitamin C is often supplemented to 5 × RDA because it has little inherent toxic potential and has an important role in collagen deposition and wound healing. Because of their role as cofactors in metabolism and potential increased losses through the wound and urine, the B vitamin group is supplemented to 2 × RDA.

TRACE ELEMENTS

In the acute-phase reaction to trauma, plasma concentrations of zinc, iron, and copper are markedly diminished (64). Like vitamin C, zinc is thought to promote wound healing, and it is supplemented to 2 × RDA. Aggressive iron supplementation must be undertaken with some caution because of the potential for increased bacterial growth due to plasma unbound iron. Deficiency syndromes of copper, selenium, chromium, iodine, manganese, and molybdenum occur in patients on long-term total parenteral nutrition, but no cases of deficiency appear to have been reported as a direct result of burn trauma. These trace elements are administered according to RDA or AMA guidelines.

CONCLUSION

The complex clinical management and rehabilitation of a severely burned patient requires a multidisciplinary team including surgeons, nurses, a pharmacist, dietitian, physical therapist, occupational therapist, respiratory therapist, and social worker. A large TBSA full-thickness burn requires surgical excision and split-thickness skin grafting. Fluid requirements during the initial post-burn period are surprisingly large, and guidelines for fluid resuscitation have been devised by experienced clinicians. The pharmacist must be aware that the postburn hyperdynamic and hypermetabolic phase produces multiple pharmacokinetic and pharmacodynamic changes.

The nutritional requirements of burn patients can be substantial, with energy needs often approaching twice those of other hospitalized patients. A number of methods are available for estimating energy requirements by mathematical calculation, but determination of the patient's specific caloric needs by indirect calorimetry is desirable. The amount of dietary protein required by burn patients to promote wound healing, replace losses, and prevent catabolism of protein stores is not well defined. Usually, intravenous amino acids or enteral protein at 1.5 to 2 g/kg/day is provided, and nitrogen-balance studies are performed. Current guidelines call for the preferential use of enteral (rather than parenteral) nutrition.

Prevention and treatment of infection in the burned patient is of paramount importance, since it is the most common cause of death in patients who survive initial resuscitation. Treatment of systemic infection in burned patients is similar to methods used for other patients, with dose individualization by antimicrobial serum-concentration monitoring when possible. Microbial growth in the burn wound can be substantial following colonization by endogenous or exogenous organisms. The availability of topical antimicrobial agents has dramatically improved the control of burn wound infections.

REFERENCES

1. Arturson MG: The pathophysiology of severe thermal injury. J Burn Care Rehabil 6:129–146, 1985.
2. Silverman SH, Purdue GF, Hunt JL, et al.: Cyanide toxicity in burned patients. J Trauma 28:171–176, 1988.
3. Punch JD, Smith DJ, Robson MC: Hospital care of major burns. Postgrad Med 85:205–215, 1989.
4. Wachtel TL: Major burns. Postgrad Med 85:178–196, 1989.
5. Robson MC, Smith DJ, Heggers JP: Innovations in burn wound management. Adv Plast Reconstr Surg 4:149–176, 1987.
6. Demling RH: Burns. N Engl J Med 313:1389–1398, 1985.
7. Nowicki CR, Springer CK: Temporary skin substitutes for burn patients: a nursing perspective. J Burn Care Rehabil 9:209–215, 1988.
8. Teepe RGC, Kreis RW, Koebrugge EJ, et al.: The use of cultured autologous epidermis in the treatment of extensive burn wounds. J Trauma 30:269–275, 1990.
9. Rubin WD, Mani MM, Hiebert JM: Fluid resuscitation of the thermally injured patient. Current concepts with definition of clinical subsets and their specialized treatment. Clin Plast Surg 13:9–20, 1986.
10. Demling RH: Fluid replacement in burned patients. Surg Clin North Am 67:15–30, 1987.
11. Graves TA, Cioffi WG, McManus WF, et al.: Fluid resuscitation of infants and children with massive thermal injury. J Trauma 28:1656–1659, 1988.
12. Aikawa N, Ishibiki K, Naito C, et al.: Individualized fluid resuscitation based on haemodynamic monitoring in the management of extensive burns. Burns 8:249–255, 1982.
13. Horton JW, White DJ, Baxter CR: Hypertonic saline dextran resuscitation of thermal injury. Ann Surg 211:301–311, 1990.
14. Gunn ML, Hansbrough JF, Davis JW, et al.: Prospective, randomized trial of hypertonic sodium lactate versus lactated Ringer's solution for burn shock resuscitation. J Trauma 29:1261–1267, 1989.
15. Ross AD, Angaran DM: Colloids vs. crystalloids—a continuing controversy. DICP Ann Pharmacother 18:202–212, 1984.
16. Waters LM, Christensen MA, Sato RM: Hetastarch: an alternative colloid in burn shock management. J Burn Care Rehabil 10:11–16, 1989.
17. Bowser BH, Caldwell FT: The effects of resuscitation with hypertonic vs. hypotonic vs. colloid on wound and urine fluid and electrolyte losses in severely burned children. J Trauma 23:916–923, 1983.
18. Martyn J: Clinical pharmacology and drug therapy in the burned patient. Anesthesiology 65:67–75, 1986.
19. Bonate PL: Pathophysiology and pharmacokinetics following burn injury. Clin Pharmacokinet 18:118–130, 1990.
20. Czaja AJ, McAlhany JC, Pruitt BA: Acute duodenitis and duodenal ulceration after burns. Clinical and pathological characteristics. JAMA 232:621–624, 1975.
21. Loirat P, Rohan J, Baillet A, et al.: Increased glomerular filtration rate in patients with major burns and its effect on the pharmacokinetics of tobramycin. N Engl J Med 299:915–919, 1978.
22. Zaske DE, Sawchuck RJ, Gerding DN, et al.: Increased dosage requirements of gentamicin in burn patients. J Trauma 16:824–828, 1976.
23. Glew RH, Moellering RC, Burke JF: Gentamicin dosage in children with extensive burns. J Trauma 16:819–823, 1976.
24. Zaske DE, Bootman JL, Solem LB, et al.: Increased burn patient survival with individualized dosages of gentamicin. Surgery 91:142–149, 1982.
25. Zaske DE, Chin T, Kohls PR, et al.: Initial dosage regimens of gentamicin in patients with burns. J Burn Care Rehabil 12:46–50, 1991.
26. Garrelts JC, Peterie JD: Altered vancomycin dose vs. serum concentration relationship in burn patients. Clin Pharmacol Ther 44:9–13, 1988.
27. Brater DC, Bawdon RE, Anderson SA, et al.: Vancomycin elimination in patients with burn injury. Clin Pharmacol Ther 39:631–634, 1986.
28. Martyn J, Greenblatt DJ: Lorazepam conjugation is unimpaired in burn trauma. Clin Pharmacol Ther 43:250–255, 1987.
29. Bloedow DC, Hansbrough JF, Hardin T, et al.: Postburn serum drug binding and serum protein concentrations. J Clin Pharmacol 26:147–151, 1986.
30. Thompson DF: Neuromuscular blocking agents in burn patients. DICP, Ann Pharmacother 23:1006–1008, 1989.
31. Dwersteg JF, Pavlin EG, Heimbach DM: Patients with burns are resistant to atracurium. Anesthesiology 65:517–520, 1986.
32. Stone HH, Kolb LD, Pettit J, et al.: The systemic absorption of an antibiotic from the burn wound surface. Am Surg 34:639–643, 1968.
33. Stefanides MM, Copeland CE, Kominos SD, et al.: In vitro penetration of topical antiseptics through eschar of burn patients. Ann Surg 183:358–364, 1976.
34. Polk RE, Mayhall CG, Smith J, et al.: Gentamicin and tobramycin penetration into burn eschar. Arch Surg 118:295–302, 1983.

35. McManus WF: Patterns of infection over the past ten years: Historical patterns. J Burn Care Rehabil 8:32–35, 1987.

36. Gelfand JA: Infections in burn patients: a paradigm for cutaneous infection in the patient at risk. Am J Med 76(suppl 5A):158–165, 1984.

37. Luterman A, Dacso CC, Curreri PW: Infections in burn patients. Am J Med 81(suppl 1A):45–52, 1986.

38. Ziegler TR, Smith RJ, O'Dwyer RT, et al.: Increased intestinal permeability associated with infection in burn patients. Arch Surg 123:1313–1319, 1988.

39. Moncrief JA, Teplitz C: Changing concepts in burn sepsis. J Trauma 4:233–245, 1964.

40. Pruitt BA: The diagnosis and treatment of infection in the burn patient. Burns Incl Therm Inj 11:79–91, 1984.

41. Nathan P, Law EJ, Murphy DF, et al.: A laboratory method for selection of topical antimicrobial agents to treat infected burn wounds. Burns Incl Therm Inj 4:177–187, 1978.

42. Heggers JP, Velanovich V, Robson MC, et al.: Control of burn wound sepsis: a comparison of in vitro topical antimicrobial assays. J Trauma 27:176–179, 1987.

43. Moyer CA, Brentano L, Gravens DL, et al.: Treatment of large human burns with 0.5% silver nitrate solution. Arch Surg 90:812–867, 1965.

44. Fox CL: Silver sulfadiazine—a new topical therapy for *Pseudomonas* in burns. Arch Surg 96:184–188, 1968.

45. Monafo WW, West MA: Current treatment recommendations for topical burn therapy. Drugs 40:364–373, 1990.

46. Rice TL: Topical antibacterials. The Michigan Drug Letter 10, 1991.

47. Sawhney CP, Sharma RK, Rao KR, et al.: Long-term experience with 1 per cent topical silver sulphadiazine cream in the management of burn wounds. Burns Incl Therm Inj 15:403–406, 1989.

48. Thomson PD, Moore NP, Rice TL, et al.: Leukopenia in acute thermal injury: Evidence against silver sulfadiazine as the causative agent. J Burn Care Rehab 10:418–420, 1989.

49. Liebman PR, Kennelly MM, Hirsch EF: Hypercarbia and acidosis associated with carbonic anhydrase inhibition: a hazard of topical mafenide acetate use in renal failure. Burns 8:395–398, 1982.

50. Hooper G, Covarrubias J: Clinical use and efficacy of furacin: a historical perspective. J Int Med Res 11:289–293, 1983.

51. Dacso CC, Luterman A, Curreri PW: Systemic antibiotic treatment in burned patients. Surg Clin North Am 67:57–68, 1987.

52. Mason AD, McManus AT, Pruitt BA: Association of burn mortality and bacteremia. A 25-year review. Arch Surg 121:1027–1031, 1986.

53. Mackersie RC, Karagianes TG: Pain management following trauma and burns. Anesthesiol Clin North Am 7:211–227, 1989.

54. Wermeling DP, Record KE, Foster TS: Patient-controlled high-dose morphine therapy in a patient with electrical burns. Clin Pharm 5:832–835, 1986.

55. Enzi G, Casadei A, Sergi G, et al.: Metabolic and hormonal effects of early nutritional supplementation after surgery in burn patients. Crit Care Med 18:719–721, 1990.

56. Garrel DR, Davignon I, Lopez D: Length of care in patients with severe burns with or without early enteral nutritional support. A retrospective study. J Burn Care Rehabil 12:85–90, 1991.

57. Cunningham JJ, Hegarty MT, Meara PA, et al.: Measured and predicted calorie requirements of adults during recovery from severe burn trauma. Am J Clin Nutr 49:404–408, 1989.

58. Saffle JR, Medina E, Raymond J, et al.: Use of indirect calorimetry in the nutritional management of burned patients. J Trauma 25:32–39, 1985.

59. Bell SJ, Blackburn GL, Nutritional support of the burn patient. In Martyn JAJ (ed): Acute Management of the Burned Patient. Philadelphia, WB Saunders, 1990, pp 138–158.

60. Miller SJ: The nitrogen balance revisited. Hosp Pharm 25:61–65, 1990.

61. Oki JC, Cuddy PG: Branched-chain amino acid support of stressed patients. DICP, Ann Pharmacother 23:399–408, 1989.

62. Pasulka PS, Wachtel TL: Nutritional considerations for the burned patient. Surg Clin North Am 67:109–131, 1987.

63. O'Neil CE, Hutsler D, Hildreth MA: Basic nutritional guidelines for pediatric burn patients. J Burn Care Rehabil 10:278–284, 1989.

64. Shewmake KB, Talbert GE, Bowser-Wallace BH, et al.: Alterations in plasma copper, zinc, and ceruloplasmin levels in patients with thermal trauma. J Burn Care Rehabil 9:13–17, 1988.

CHAPTER 44

COMMON EYE DISORDERS

ANTON C. DREYER, D.Sc., ANDRIES G. GOUS, Pharm.D., and HERMIEN GOUS, Pharm.D.

A variety of disorders commonly affect the eye. These vary in severity from mild but annoying allergic conjunctivitis or dry eyes to sight-threatening infections. Some of these disorders may be treated with over-the-counter preparations, but the more serious disorders require aggressive therapy, frequently with multiple drugs and often by more than one route of administration. This chapter discusses the common ocular disorders and their treatment as well as general principles of ophthalmic medications. Fig. 44.1 depicts the various structures that may be affected by commonly occurring disorders.

OPHTHALMIC MEDICINES USED IN COMMON EYE DISORDERS

There are numerous ophthalmic preparations for topical application to the eye. For an enhanced effect, a systemic form of the same medications may be added to the therapeutic regimen. In such cases and in susceptible patients who are treated with topical medications, systemic side effects may occur. The following summarizes the ophthalmic products used and provides some general considerations to therapy. The tables provide a partial list of available ophthalmic products.

Antimicrobial Preparations

Most eye infections are caused by bacteria; viral and fungal infections are much less common. Superficial infections such as conjunctivitis and blepharitis are generally treated adequately with agents applied topically. More serious infections may require subconjunctival injections and/or other routes of administration. The precautions applying to systemic antibiotic use also apply to topical use. Indiscriminate use may lead to the emergence of resistance or hypersensitivity. This holds true especially for the use of the aminoglycosides for trivial conditions (1, 2).

For infections of a serious nature or those extending beyond the conjunctiva, cornea, and eyelids, culture and sensitivity tests are essential. In the absence of such, broad antiinfective coverage may be obtained (for serious infections) from combination of an aminoglycoside and a cephalosporin injected subconjunctivally plus appropriate topical therapy (3). Table 44.1 provides a partial list of ophthalmic antimicrobial agents.

Antivirals (3)
The topical antivirals are listed in Table 44.2.

Glucocorticosteroid-containing Preparations
The topical glucocorticosteroid-containing preparations are included in Table 44.3. Steroids are available in drop and ointment form and are used for a variety of inflammatory eye conditions. Applied topically, they are ineffective against inflammation of the optic nerve, choroid, and retina. In these cases, systemic steroids are required (2, 4, 5).

The inflammatory process may cause permanent tissue damage. Correctly applied steroid therapy, by suppressing inflammation, may save eye structures and preserve sight. Certain infections are absolute contraindications to the use of steroids, e.g., herpes simplex viral infections. The main dangers associated with the use of ocular steroids are given in Table 44.4.

Decongestants (Vasoconstrictors)
Commonly used sympathomimetics are listed in Table 44.5. These agents stimulate α_1-adrenergic receptors on small blood vessels, causing them to constrict. This reduces blood flow in the affected area of the eye, clearing red eyes and shrinking (decongesting) the engorged tissue. Sympathomimetics also cause the radial muscle of the pupil to contract, leading to mydriasis. This effect is less pronounced than the mydriasis that is produced by the application of parasympatholytics (anticholinergics) such as atropine. These sympathomimetics are nevertheless used for their mydriatic effect. The dose required for clinically significant mydriasis is much higher than that needed for decongestion. In some patients, a combination of an α-sympathomimetic and an anticholinergic provides optimal mydriasis, e.g., in patients with diabetic retinopathy (6, 7).

Mydriasis (whether produced by topical application or systemic use of anticholinergics or sympathomimetics) generally leads to obstruction of the trabecular meshwork—canal of Schlemm drainage system for aqueous humor, leading to an increased intraocular pressure (IOP) in angle-closure glaucoma. The side effects and precautions associated with the use of α-sympathomimetic eye drops are listed in Table 44.6.

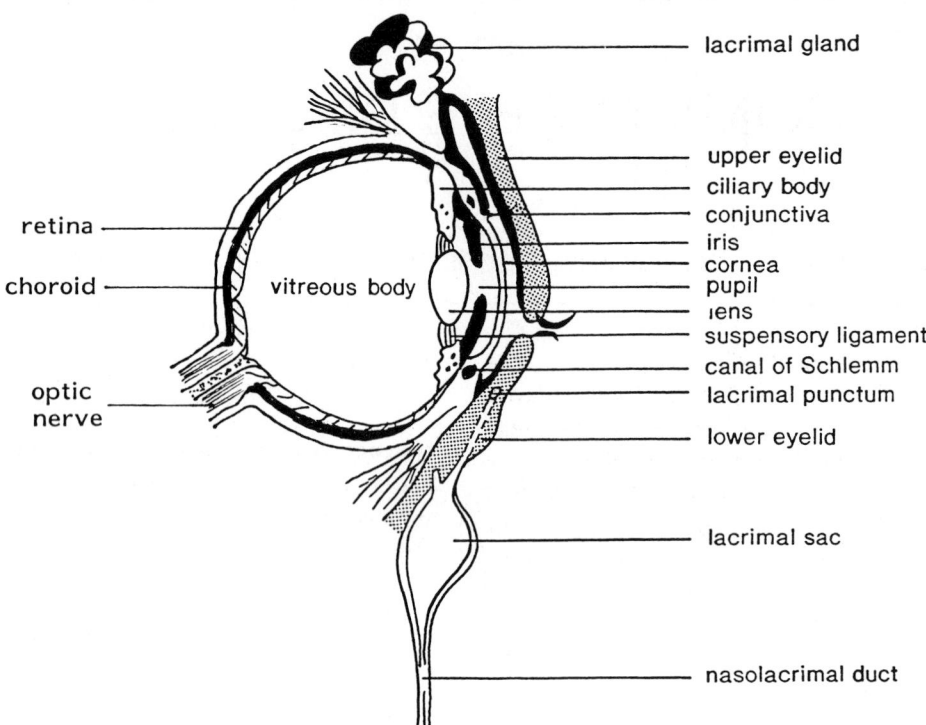

Figure 44.1. Cross-section of the eyeball and lacrimal passages.

Table 44.1.
Ophthalmic Antimicrobials

Drug	Dosage Form/Strength
Bacitracin	Ointment (500 units/g)
Chloramphenicol	Ointment (1%); soln. (0.05%, 0.16%, 0.5%, 1.0%)
Ciprofloxacin	Solution (0.3%)
Erythromycin	Ointment (0.5%)
Gentamicin	Ointment or solution (0.3%)
Norfloxacin	Solution (0.3%)
Sulfacetamide	Soln. (10.0%, 15.0%, 30.0%); ointment (10.0%)
Sulfisoxazole	Solution (4.0%); ointment (4.0%)
Tetracycline	Ointment (1.0%)
Chlortetracycline	Ointment (1.0%)
Tobramycin	Solution (0.3%); ointment (0.3%)
Combination products	

Neomycin 0.35%; polymyxin B 10,000 units/g, bacitracin 500 units/g in ointment
Polymyxin B 10,000 units/g; bacitracin 500 units/g in ointment
Polymyxin B 10,000 units/g or ml; neomycin 0.35% in ointment or solution
Oxytetracycline 0.5% and polymyxin B 10,000 units/g in ointment
Trimethoprim 0.1% and polymyxin B 10,000 units/g in ointment

Table 44.2.
Ophthalmic Antiviral and Antifungal Agents

Drug	Dosage Form/Strength	Usual Dose
Antiviral		
Idoxuridine	Soln. (0.1%); oint. (0.5%)	Soln-q.h. during the day, q2h at night for 10–21 days
		Oint-5 × day for 10–21 days
Vidarabine	Ointment (3.0%)	5 × day for 14–21 days
Trifluorothymidine	Solution (1.0%)	9 × day for 14 days
Antifungal		
Natamycin	Suspension (5%)	q. 1–2 hr for 3–4 days, then 8 times per day for 14–21 days

tions of action, with atropine being the most potent and having the longest duration of activity (mydriasis lasting 2 to 3 weeks in some patients and cycloplegia for up to 6 days). Tropicamide and cyclopentolate are used where a short-duration effect is required (3).

The mydriatics are used primarily:

1. To dilate the pupil, for easier examination of the fundus, tropicamide is the anticholinergic of choice for this purpose;
2. To produce cycloplegia for refraction, cyclopentolate or homatropine is used (atropine may be more suitable in children under 6 years);

Mydriatics (Cycloplegics)

Mydriatic agents are listed in Table 44.7. These anticholinergics produce a dilation of the pupil (mydriasis) and paralysis of accommodation (cycloplegia) when applied topically. They vary in their relative potencies and dura-

Table 44.3.
Opthalmic Corticosteroids

Drug	Dosage Form/Strength
Prednisolone	Acetate suspension (0.12% or 1.0%)
	Sodium phosphate solution (0.12%, 0.5%, or 1.0%)
Dexamethasone	Phosphate solution (0.1%)
	Suspension (0.1%)
	Phosphate ointment (0.05%)
Medrysone	Solution (1.0%)
Fluorometholone	Suspension (0.1% and 1.0%)

Combination products
Prednisolone acetate 0.25% and atropine sulfate 1.0%—solution
Hydrocortisone 0.5% and chloromycetin 2.5%—solution
Hydrocortisone 0.5%, Chloramphenicol 0.1%, and polymyxin B 10,000 units/g—ointment
Hydrocortisone 0.5% and neomycin 0.35%—solution
Hydrocortisone 1.0%; polymyxin 10,000 units/gm; bacitracin 400 units/g and neomycin 0.35%—ointment and suspension
Prednisolone 0.2% and sulfacetamide 10%—solution and ointment
Prednisolone 0.5% and sulfacetamide 10%—solution and ointment
Prednisolone 0.5%, neomycin 0.35%, and polymyxin B 10,000 units/ml—suspension
Prednisolone 1% and gentamicin 0.3%—suspension
Dexamethasone 0.1% and neomycin 0.35%—suspension or ointment
Dexamethasone 0.1%, neomycin 0.35%, and polymyxin 10,000 units/ml—suspension or ointment
Dexamethasone 0.1% and tobramycin 0.3%—suspension

Table 44.4.
Dangers Associated with the Use of Ocular Steroids[a]

- Aggravation of unrecognized herpes simplex corneal ulceration, which may lead to corneal perforation
- Steroid glaucoma may be produced after a week or more of treatment in patients predisposed to chronic simple glaucoma
- Aggravation of fungal or bacterial infection, by decreasing the immune response
- The production of cataracts (one drop of tropical steroid three times a day for 1 year is potentially cataractogenic)
- Masking of serious hypersensitivity reactions, as well as the signs and symptoms of infections
- Occasionally amounts sufficient to cause systemic effect (such as growth retardation in children) may be absorbed

[a] Adapted from Lavin MJ, Rose GE: Use of steroid eye drops in general practice. Br Med J 292:1448–1450, 1986; Jones BR, Coster DJ, Falcon MG: Prospects of prevention of recurrent herpetic eye disease. Trans Ophthalmol Soc UK 97:350–355, 1977; and Conradie EA, Straughan JL (eds): South African Medicines Formulary. Cape Town: Med Assoc S Afr 1988, p 223.

3. To produce cycloplegia and mydriasis prior to, during, and after intraocular surgery;
4. To treat inflammation of the anterior segment of the eye. Paralysis of the ciliary muscle relieves the pain and congestion associated with this condition. A longer-acting anticholinergic (atropine or homatropine) is more suitable.

Mydriasis causes the pupil to crowd and block the canal of Schlemm. This may impair drainage of the aqueous humor, precipitating an attack of acute angle-closure glaucoma in susceptible patients (see Chapter 46).

Local Anesthetics

The ophthalmic anesthetics are listed in Table 44.8. The opththalmic use of local anesthetics is reserved for eye surgery and for minor procedures such as the removal of a foreign body; *they should never be given for the relief of symptoms* (6, 8).

Side effects of local anesthetics are usually the consequence of overdose or protracted use. These include:

1. Systemic effects such as CNS stimulation followed by CNS depression, hypertension, and tachydrysrhythmias. Systemic side effects are also more likely to occur if the eye is red (increased blood flow will lead to increased absorption) or the patient has impaired kidney or liver function.
2. Minor local allergic reactions may occur, especially in patients who are prone to allergic reactions.
3. Mild, reversible corneal damage may occur. Severe damage and loss of vision have occurred in some cases. Because of possible corneal damage and retarded healing, local anesthetics should not be applied repeatedly to the eye as ongoing therapy in painful conditions.

Cocaine is not used to any great extent as a local anesthetic in ophthalmology because it causes severe damage to the cornea. Systemic side effects and addiction liability further justify not using it.

Artificial Tears

A listing of the artificial tear products is provided in Table 44.9. Artificial tears are specially formulated to replace the deficient or incomplete normal tear, so it completely "wets" the eye and resists breaking up into dry spots. The resulting ophthalmic preparations generally possess a greater viscosity than tears (which are much like water). Excessive viscosity leads to poor lid lubrication, corneal injury, crusting on the lid margins, and blockage of tear drainage. Vehicles used for artifical tear preparations today are less viscous. They are applied to improve the survival time of the natural tear film as well as providing an artifical layer. Artifical tear solutions should not contain chemicals that disrupt this basic film (6, 7).

Lubricating ointments (containing an oily substance such as lanolin or mineral oil) are usually used at night to provide lubrication during sleep. The drops should be used during the daytime, and depending on the severity of the deficiency, may be used hourly or even more frequently if required.

Pharmaceutics and Kinetics of Ophthalmic Medicines (7, 9)

The kinetic properties (rates and extents of absorption, distribution, metabolism, and excretion) of a medicine in-

Table 44.5.
Opthalmic Decongestant Product Table[a]

Product (MFGR.)	Viscosity Agent	Vasoconstrictor	Preservative
Absorbonac (Alcon)	Povidone		EDTA, 0.1%; thimerosal 0.004%
AK-Nefrin (Akorn)	Hydroxyethylcellulose 0.5%	Phenylephrine HCl 0.12%	Benzalkonium Cl 0.01%; EDTA
Allerest eye drops (Pharmacraft)		Naphazolone HCl 0.012%	
Clear Eyes (Ross)		Naphazoline HCl 0.012%	Benzalkonium Cl, EDTA
Collyrium w/tetrahydrozoline (Wyeth-Ayerst)		Tetrahydrozoline HCl 0.05%	Benzalkonium Cl 0.01%; EDTA 0.1%
Comfort eye drops (Sola/Barnes-Hind)	Hydroxyethylcellulose; polyvinyl alcohol	Naphazoline HCl 0.03%	Benzalkonium Cl 0.005%; EDTA 0.02%
Degest 2 (Sola/Barnes-Hind)	Hydroxyethylcellulose	Naphazoline HCl 0.012%	Benzalkonium Cl 0.0067%; EDTA 0.02%
Eye-Zine (Ocumed)		Tetrahydrozoline HCl 0.05%	
Isopto-Frin (Alcon)	Hydroxypropylmethylcellulose 0.5%	Phenylephrine HCl 0.12%	Benzalkonium Cl 0.01%
Mallazine (Hauck)		Tetrahydrozoline HCl 0.05%	Benzalkonium Cl 0.01%
Murine Plus		Tetrahydrozoline HCl 0.05%	Benzalkonium Cl 0.01%; EDTA 0.1%
Naphcon		Naphazoline HCl 0.012%	Benzalkonium Cl 0.01%
OcuClear (Schering)		Oxymetazoline HCl 0.025%	Benzalkonium Cl 0.01%; EDTA
Ocu-Phrin (Ocumed)		Phenylephrine HCl 0.12%	
Optigene III (Pfeiffer)	Povidone	Tetrahydrozoline HCl 0.05%	Benzalkonium Cl 0.004%; EDTA 0.1%
Optised (Various Mfgr)		Phenylephrine HCl 0.12%	
Phenylzin (Cooper Vision)	Hydroxypropylmethylcellulose	Phenylephrine HCl 0.12%	Benzalkonium Cl 0.01%; EDTA 0.01%
Prefrin Liquifilm (Allergan)	Polyvinyl alcohol 1.4%	Phenylephrine HCl 0.12%	Benzalkonium Cl 0.005%
Relief (Allergan)	Polyvinyl alcohol 1.4%	Phenylephrine HCl 0.12%	
Soothe (Alcon)	Povidone	Tetrahydrozoline HCl 0.05%	Benzalkonium Cl 0.004%; EDTA 0.1%
Tetrahydrozoline hydrochloride (various mfgr.)		Tetrahydrozoline HCl 0.05%	
20/20 Eye drops (S.S.S.)		Naphazoline HCl 0.12%	Thimerosal 0.005%
VasoClear (Iolab)	Polyvinyl alcohol	Naphazoline HCl 0.02%	Benzalkonium Cl 0.01%; EDTA
VasoClear A (Iolab)	Polyvinyl alcohol 0.25%	Naphazoline HCl 0.02%	Benzalkonium Cl 0.005%; EDTA
Visine (Leeming)		Tetrahydrozoline HCl 0.05%	Benzalkonium Cl 0.01%; EDTA 0.1%
Visine A. C.[b] (Leeming)		Tetrahydrozoline HCl 0.05%	Benzalkonium Cl 0.1%; EDTA 0.1%
Visine Extra[c] (Leeming)		Tetrahydrozoline HCl 0.05%	Benzalkonium Cl 0.013%; EDTA 0.1%
Zincfrin (Alcon)		Phenylephrine HCl 0.12%	Benzalkonium Cl 0.01%

[a] Adapted from Gourley, DR: Ophthalmic products. In Handbook of Nonprescription Drugs, ed 9. Washington: Am Pharm Assoc, 1990, pp 598–599.
[b] Includes zinc sulfate 0.25%.
[c] Includes PEG-400 1%.

fluence its local effects on the eye and its possible systemic effects.

Drug molecules generally move from one eye structure to another (or into the bloodstream and thus into the system) by means of passive diffusion. The ease of movement from one area of the eye to another or into the bloodstream, is determined by, among other things:

1. The condition of the eye tissue. Damage to tissue permits the passage of drug molecules that would not normally penetrate healthy tissue. Inflammation, for example, generally promotes drug penetration into the affected areas.
2. The increased perfusion that occurs when eyes are red leads to increased systemic absorption of ophthalmic preparations, and a greater likelihood of systemic side effects.
3. Age affects tear production. Decreased tear production, sagging lacrimal sacs, etc., in old age are believed to affect drug

absorption and distribution. The very young and very old tend to absorb topically applied ophthalmic drugs more readily and may consequently manifest systemic side effects.

The ophthalmic structures that lie anterior to (in front of) the lens (i.e., the conjunctiva, sclera, cornea, iris, and aqueous humor, Fig. 44.1) are readily penetrated by topically applied drugs. These drugs, however, rarely pass through anterior structures sufficiently to reach posterior structures (vitreous humor and retina) in therapeutic quantities.

Systemically administered medicines reach the eye via the bloodstream. The choroid and retina, being the most vascular structures, receive the greatest supply. Systemic drugs may, however, reach other areas of the eye by diffusing from other periocular vessels.

The formulation of the ophthalmic preparations largely

Table 44.6.
Side Effects and Precautions Associated with
α-Sympathomimetic Eye Drops[a]

- These eye drops should not be used in greater quantities or more often than prescribed, nor should they be used unnecessarily, because rebound vasodilation may lead to chronic congestion and red eyes. The chronic vasoconstriction that results from the excessive use of decongestant eye drops leads to the formation of new blood vessels as a means of compensation by the eye. The "neovascularization" adds to the chronic congestion and red eye.

Patients should be cautioned against the habitual use of OTC decongestant eye-drops.

- These eyedrops should not be used on young children, as absorption may cause marked CNS stimulation and serious hypertension.
- These agents should not be used by patients who may suffer attacks of angle-closure glaucoma. The pharmacist should note that many OTC preparations contain sympathomimetic decongestants.

Susceptible adults may absorb sufficient quantities to suffer cardiac tachyarrhythmias and hypertension. Patients who are known to have vascular problems, are elderly, debilitated, or are taking MAO inhibitors or tricyclics should use these eye drops only under supervision. Ophthalmic solutions that contain high concentrations of sympathomimetics should be avoided by these patients.

[a] Adapted from Plus Continuing Pharmacy Education Programme: Eye conditions and the pharmacists. (5:141) 1988. Published by Pharmaceutical Society of South Africa, compiled by TPS Drug Information Center Johannesburg; and Gourley DR: Ophthalmic products. In Handbook of Nonprescription Drugs, ed. 9. Washington, D.C.: Am Pharm Assoc, 1990, ch 20.

Table 44.7.
Mydriatic-Cycloplegic Agents

Drug	Dosage Form/Strength
Atropine sulfate	Ointment (0.5%, 1.0%) & solution (0.5%, 1%, 2%, 3%)
Cyclopentolate	Solution (0.5%, 1%, 2%)
Homatropine	Solution (2%, 5%)
Phenylephrine	Solution (2.5%, 10%)
Scopolamine	Solution (0.25%)
Tropicamide	Solution (0.5% or 1%)

Table 44.8.
Ophthalmic Topical Anesthetics

Drug	Dosage Form	Strength
Cocaine	Solution	1.0 to 4.0%
Benoxinate with fluorescein	Solution	0.4%
Proparacaine HCl with fluorescein	Solution	0.5%
Tetracaine HCl	Solution	0.5%

Note: 1–2 drops used for temporary anesthesia (lasts for 15–20 min) during examinations and procedures

determines their durations of action. Active ingredients in eye drops are more readily absorbed when in *solution* rather than *suspension*. Eye ointments have the most prolonged action. The drug particles that are found in aqueous or oily suspensions are released gradually as they dissolve in the tears.

INJURIES

Foreign Bodies in the Eye

Foreign bodies are a common occurrence, with symptoms ranging from little or no discomfort to severe pain. Failure to remove the foreign material may result in physical damage to the eye, development of a secondary infection, or eventual blindness. Objects such as dust particles or small insects can usually be removed by flushing the eye with sterile normal saline, any natural tears product, or if nothing else is available, tap water. If the objects are not removed by flushing the eye, the patient should be referred to an emergency room or an ophthalmologist.

Foreign bodies visibly lodged in the conjunctival area may be gently lifted out with a moist sterile cotton applicator. Removal of corneal foreign bodies requires proper instrumentation and should be referred to a physician. Foreign bodies not readily seen with the naked eye may be made visible by fluorescein staining. If the foreign body is deeply embedded or has penetrated the eye, it will probably require surgical removal. If wood splinters or metal shavings may have become lodged in the eye, patients should be referred to a physician immediately.

Topical anesthetic eye drops *should not* be used to relieve the painful irritation caused by a foreign body but only to facilitate its removal. The local analgesia produced may mask the presence of residual foreign material, which in turn may lead to severe corneal abrasions. Furthermore, chronic ophthalmic use of topical anesthesia can permanently damage the corneal epithelium (8).

After removal of the foreign body, a broad-spectrum antibiotic ophthalmic ointment such as tobramycin or gentamicin (Table 44.1) and a short-acting cycloplegic agent (e.g., 1 drop of cyclopentolate 1%) should be instilled in the lower cul-de-sac and a moderate pressure patch placed over the closed lids for 24 to 48 hr (10). The cyclopentolate should be instilled before the antibiotic. If there was a penetrating injury to the eye, antibiotic ointment should not be used because the injury may allow access to the anterior chamber of the eye (10). Ophthalmic corticosteroid preparations are contraindicated in eye injuries as they may delay healing and promote the development and spread of infection (4, 5) (Table 44.4).

Contusion Injuries of the Anterior Segment ("Black Eye")

A direct blow to the eye by an object such as a fist, racket ball, tennis ball, etc., can produce a combination of in-

Table 44.9.
Artificial Tear Products[a]

Product	Viscosity Agent	Preservative
Absorbotear	Hydroxyethylcellulose; povidone 1.67%	Edetate disodium 0.1%; thimerosal 0.004%
Akwa Tears	Polyvinyl alcohol	Benzalkonium Cl 0.01%; edetate disodium
Artificial Tears solution	Polyvinyl alcohol 1.4%	Edetate disodium, chlorobutanol
Celluvisc	Carboxymethylcellulose sodium 1%	
Comfort Tears	Hydroxyethylcellulose; polyvinyl alcohol	Edetate disodium 0.005%; benzalkonium Cl 0.02%
Hypotears	Polyvinyl alcohol 1%	Benzalkonium Cl 0.01%
Isopto Alkaline	Hydroxypropyl methylcellulose 1%	Benzalkonium Cl 0.01%
Isopto Plain	Hydroxypropyl methylcellulose 0.05%	Benzalkonium Cl 0.01%
Just Tears	Hydroxypropyl methylcellulose	Benzalkonium Cl 0.01%; edetate disodium 0.025%
Lacril	Hydroxypropyl methylcellulose 0.5%; gelatin A 0.01%	Chlorobutanol 0.5%
Liquifilm Forte	Polyvinyl alcohol 3%	Edetate disodium; thimerosal 0.002%
Liquifilm Tears	Polyvinyl alcohol 1.4%	Chlorobutanol 0.5%
Moisture Drops	Hydroxypropyl methylcellulose 0.5%; dextran 40, 0.1%	Edetate disodium; benzalkonium Cl 0.01%
Murine	Polyvinyl alcohol 1.4%; povidone 0.6%	Benzalkonium Cl; edetate disodium
Muro Tears	Hydroxypropyl methylcellulose; dextran 40	Benzalkonium Cl 0.01%; edetate disodium
Murocel	Methylcellulose 1%	
Refresh	Polyvinyl alcohol 1.4% povidone 0.6%	
TearGard	Hydroxyethylcellulose	Edetate disodium 0.1%
Tearisol	Hydroxypropyl methylcellulose 0.5%	Benzalkonium Cl 0.01%
Tears Naturale	Hydroxypropyl methylcellulose; dextran 70	Benzalkonium Cl 0.01%; edetate disodium 0.05%
Tears Naturale II	Hydroxypropyl methylcellulose 0.3%; dextran 70, 0.1%	Edetate disodium
Tears Plus	Polyvinyl alcohol 1.4%; povidone 0.6%	Chlorobutanol 0.5%
Tears Renewed	Hydroxypropyl methylcellulose; dextran 70	Benzalkonium Cl 0.01; edetate disodium 0.05%
Ultra Tears	Hydroxypropyl methylcellulose 1%	Benzalkonium Cl 0.01%

[a] Adapted from Gourley DR: Ophthalmic products. In Handbook of Nonprescription Drugs, ed. 9. Washington: Am Pharm Assoc, 1990, pp 596–597.

juries, including a dislocation of the crystalline lens, iridodialysis, traumatic iritis, and hyphema (blood in the anterior chamber). The patient should be checked in the emergency room (E.R.) and to make sure that no serious damage has occurred. A black eye is usually self-limiting. A "black eye" caused by trauma should be treated with cold compresses during the first 24 hr to inhibit swelling. The second day, hot compresses may aid absorption of the hematoma (10).

Chemical Burns

Chemical burns of the cornea and the conjunctiva must be treated immediately by extensive irrigation with sterile water or saline for 5 to 30 min to dilute and remove the offending agent. If sterile water is not available, any source of water should be used (e.g., shower, faucet, drinking fountain, hose). The eyelids should be held apart and water irrigated continuously for at least 5 min. The patient should be referred immediately to an ophthalmologist or the E.R. enroute, the eye should be kept irrigated. A wet towel will help maintain the irrigation. Once in the E.R., irrigation with at least 2000 ml of normal saline 0.9% for a minimum of 1 hr is necessary. Instillation of topical anesthetics every 20 min to relieve the pain is recommended. Irrigation should be continued until pH paper reveals that the conjunctival pH has returned to normal (pH between 7.3 and

7.7). Once a normal pH has been attained, a second reading should be done in 5 to 10 min to insure that the pH has not shifted to a more alkaline or acid range (10).

After the irrigation, topical antibiotics (e.g., gentamicin, tobramycin, or erythromycin) should be started to prevent a secondary infection. If there is an increase in the intraocular pressure due to the trauma, then a carbonic anhydrase inhibitor should be given. To prevent iris adhesions to the lens (posterior synechiae), a mydriatic-cyclopegic agent should be used (1 drop of cyclopentolate 1% or 1 drop of phenylephrine 2.5%). After the emergency is controlled, the eye should be patched and the antibiotic continued for 2 to 3 days.

Flash Burns ("Arc-Eye" and Snow-Blindness)

"Arc-eye" results from direct exposure of the eye to ultraviolet irradiation, e.g., from an arc-flame used for welding, reflection, or sunrays in the snow. Symptoms usually start a few hours after exposure and cause severe pain, lacrimation, and photophobia.

Although the pain associated with "arc-eye" may be quite severe, symptoms normally resolve within 24 hr. Emergency treatment should include application of cold compresses to the eye and administration of oral analgesics to relieve pain (ASA with codeine). Severe cases of "arc-eye" may require a topical anesthetic such as proparacaine

HCl 0.5% and a decongestant such as epinephrine 0.5–1.0% to reduce congestion. Patients should not be given topical anesthetic for routine use since it may mask the symptoms of other problems (e.g., welding burn that also has a foreign body present which if not detected could lead to further damage). A topical antibiotic ointment such as gentamicin, tobramycin, or neomycin may be needed to prevent infection. Chloramphenicol should be avoided because safer alternatives are available.

DISORDERS OF THE EYELIDS (11, 12)

Lid Edema

This condition manifests as swelling and itching of one or both eyelids in atopic individuals in response to certain allergens. Various ophthalmic medications, cosmetics, insect stings or bites on the eyelid, or plant allergens may act as contact allergens. Systemic allergens include certain foods (e.g., seafood, nuts, egg, milk products), inhalants (e.g., pollens, hair sprays, deodorant sprays), and drugs (e.g., penicillin, sulfonamides, salicylates).

Signs and symptoms include urticaria of the eyelids in a circumscribed area of subepidermal and epidermal edema with an erythematous margin and blanched center, which may disappear after a few hours.

Treatment includes identification and removal of the offending allergen. This may be the only treatment required. Cold compresses over the closed lids may speed resolution, but desensitization, cromolyn sodium, or oral antihistamine therapy is indicated where the responsible allergen(s) cannot be identified or avoided. Topical corticosteroid creams (e.g., triamcinolone 0.1%) may be required if swelling persists for longer than 24 hr.

Blepharitis

Blepharitis is a condition characterized by chronic redness of the lid margins, thickening, and often formation of scales sticking to the base of the eyelashes, presenting either as squamous or ulcerative blepharitis, depending on the etiology.

Nonulcerative (squamous or seborrheic) blepharitis may be associated with seborrheic dermatitis of the scalp or eyebrows or may be an allergic response to an ophthalmic medication (the medication, the vehicle, or the preservatives and/or buffers). Ulcerative blepharitis is caused by bacterial infection (usually *Staphylococcus*) of the lash follicles and meibomian glands.

Signs and symptoms of squamous blepharitis include redness of the lid margins, lid edema, loss of lashes, and a foreign-body sensation. Excessive itching may indicate an allergic component in the etiology. In ulcerative blepharitis, small pustules develop in the lash follicles and eventually break down to form shallow ulcers. A purulent discharge produces unsightly crusting on the lid margin.

The standard treatment of blepharitis consists of meticulous lid hygiene, with cleansing and debridement of the crusts on the eyelids. Use diluted baby shampoo on cotton swabs to cleanse the eyelids. Moist warm compresses will help to reduce the symptoms and increase blood flow (13).

Regular use of a dandruff shampoo may be helpful as well. *Pityrosporum* yeasts have been implicated in seborrheic dermatitis, and these organisms have been identified on the lid margin in patients with blepharitis. The antifungal agent ketoconazole may have some advantages over conventional antidandruff preparations in the treatment of blepharitis (14). Bacterial blepharitis requires antimicrobial therapy such as gentamicin, tobramycin, or erythromycin applied as an ointment 3 to 4 times a day for 3 days. Short-term topical steroids have been used concurrently in persistent cases (e.g., prednisolone acetate suspension 0.12%, 1 drop, 3 times a day). The nonprescription preparation, 1% mercuric oxide (yellow) ophthalmic ointment has been reported to offer a safe and effective alternative to topical antibiotics (9).

Hordeolum (Stye) and Chalazion

An external hordeolum or stye is a small abscess at the root of an eyelash in the glands of Zeis or Moll and is very painful, but not serious. An internal hordeolum is an infection of a meibomian gland on the conjunctival side of the lid. It may be more serious and painful than an external stye. A chalazion is a chronic enlargement of a meibomian gland from occlusion of its duct. It is painless and may disappear after a few months.

Infection of these glands is usually caused by *Staphylococcus*. Styes may sometimes develop secondary to blepharitis. An external hordeolum (stye) begins with redness and painful swelling of the lid margin, followed by a small, round area of induration. The patient suffers from a foreign-body sensation, photophobia, and lacrimation. A small spot, indicative of suppuration, forms in the center of the induration ("pointing"), and this little abscess ruptures spontaneously with relief of pain.

An internal hordeolum (stye) is more severe and the area of inflammation is away from the lid margin on the conjunctival side of the lid. A small yellow area can be seen at the site of the affected gland, but it seldom points through the skin and does not rupture spontaneously. A chalazion starts like a stye with lid edema, swelling, and irritation. After a few days it resolves, leaving a painless, slowly enlarging round mass in the lid. It can be seen subconjunctivally as a red or grey mass, and it may disappear after a few months.

Suppuration may be terminated in the early stages by antimicrobials (e.g., erythromycin, bacitracin, or sulfacetamide ophthalmic ointment used every 2 hr). Pointing of a stye may be enhanced by using hot compresses and then draining the stye by pulling the lash or incising with a fine-tipped blade to be able to express the contents of the abscess. If styes must be excised, patients should be advised to seek medical assistance and not to try it themselves. Pus should be removed carefully, and antimicrobial solutions or ointments used to prevent spreading of the infection (3 times a day for 3 days). Internal meibomian abscesses and chalazions should be referred to a physician for incision and curettage under local anesthesia.

Entropion

Entropion is a common condition occurring mainly in the elderly (over 65 years of age). The lower eyelids turn inward causing the eyelashes to abrade the cornea and conjunctiva. This causes a painful, red, watery eye. Surgical repair is the only permanent cure for this condition. Micropore tape is useful as a temporary measure in keeping the lid everted (15).

DISORDERS OF THE CONJUNCTIVA

The conjunctiva lines the back of the eyelid and extends into the space between the lid and the globe as well as over the sclera to the cornea. Dilation of the blood vessels in the conjunctiva and sclera results in a so-called red eye, which may be caused by various stimuli. Identifying the cause of a red eye has often proven difficult. One condition may be easily mistaken for another. Table 44.10 compares conditions that cause red eyes.

Conjunctivitis (16–19)

Conjunctivitis is a common eye disease that may be acute or chronic. The etiology includes various conditions that all have inflammation of the conjunctiva as a common symptom. It is usually bilateral, the eyes are uncomfortable rather than painful, and vision is not affected. Acute conjunctivitis is usually caused by bacteria, viruses, or allergy and sometimes chemical or mechanical irritants. Chronic conjunctivitis, characterized by exacerbations and remissions over long periods, even years, is also caused by bacteria, viruses, or allergens as well as disorders such as blepharitis and chronic dacryocystitis. Because the conjunctiva contains many small blood vessels, spontaneous subconjunctival hemorrhage sometimes occurs on sneezing or straining on defecation. The condition is painless, does not effect vision and is localized to one area of the conjunctiva. The situation should resolve spontaneously within 10 to 14 days without treatment. Recurrence warrants exclusion of hypertension and bleeding disorders. Most cases of conjunctivitis are treated based upon clinical diagnosis, without the aid of culture and sensitivity tests. For infections that do not respond to therapy in 2 to 3 days or those extending beyond the conjunctiva, cornea, and eyelids, a culture and sensitivity test is essential. In the absence of such tests, broad-spectrum antibiotic coverage may be obtained from the combination of an aminoglycoside and a cephalosporin injected subconjunctivally plus appropriate topical therapy (16–19).

BACTERIAL CONJUNCTIVITIS (1, 12, 16)

Infection by various bacteria causes inflammation of the conjunctiva with dilatation of its blood vessels. The goblet cells (mucus-secreting cells) and tiny lacrimal glands of the conjunctiva become overactive, which results in watering and a discharge containing many inflammatory white cells. *Staphylococcus aureus* (most common causative agent), *Staphylococcus epidermidis*, *Streptococus pneumoniae* (pneumococcus), *Streptococcus pyogenes*, and *Haemophilus influenzae* are common causative organisms. Newborn babies sometimes suffer from acute purulent conjunctivitis (Ophthalmia neonatorum) caused by *Neisseria gonorrhoeae* or *Chlamydia trachomatis*. The eyes are red and itch, and the purulent discharge tends to accumulate on the lashes, causing them to stick together. The lids may be moderately swollen.

Although the condition can be self-limiting, it often requires treatment with a topical broad-spectrum antibiotic in solution or ointment form. If the diagnosis is based on clinical diagnosis alone (no culture), then erythromycin or bacitracin ointment or sodium sulfacetamide 10 to 15% solution are usually effective. These agents cover the most common Gram-positive microorganisms that normally cause bacterial conjunctivitis. However, since about 50% of staphylococci are resistant to the sulfonamides, a product such as neomycin-polymyxin-bacitracin is effective. Approximately 6 to 8% of patients treated with this combination have a sensitivity reaction to the neomycin. If the affending microorganism is *Haemophilus* or *Moraxella*, chloramphenicol is very effective. Other broad-spectrum antibiotics include polymyxin B–bacitracin ointment, polymyxin B–trimethoprim, and gentamicin, or tobramycin drops or ointment are used as well. Tobramycin and gentamicin are usually used for conjunctivitis caused by Gram-negative microorganisms (16).

A poor clinical response after 2 or 3 days indicates resistant bacteria or a misdiagnosis. Culture and sensitivity tests should be done to determine the causative agent. Proper eye hygiene should be maintained to avoid transmitting the infection. Warm wet compresses improve the circulation and help cleanse the discharge. If the eyelids become crusted, the use of a dilute baby shampoo solution applied with a cotton swab is effective. Corticosteroids, either separately or with antibiotics, should not be used until a viral etiology has been positively excluded.

The World Health Organization (WHO) recommends use of a 1% silver nitrate solution in the eyes of newborns to prevent *Neisseriae gonorrhoeae* infection. The use of tetracycline or erythromycin ophthalmic ointment is pre-

Table 44.10.

Comparison of a Number of Conditions Causing Red Eyes[a]

Condition	Appearance of the Eye(s)	Lids and Lashes	Discharge	Other Features	Basic Treatment
Blepharitis	Eyes are moderately red	Lid margins inflamed, swollen, scaly, loss of lashes, pustules in lash follicles	Purulent discharge from pustules on lashes	Seborrheic dermatitis of scalp or eyebrows in nonulcerative type; vision unaffected	Antidandruff shampoo, topical antibiotic and steroid therapy where indicated
Conjunctivitis					
Bacterial	Conjunctiva red	Lids moderately swollen, lashes sticky and matted on wakening	Mucopurulent	Vision not affected	Topical antibiotic
Viral	Conjunctiva red	Lymphoid follicles inside upper lid	Profuse, clear, watery	Occasionally associated with sore throat and fever; preauricular adenopathy; vision unaffected	None
Allergic	Conjunctiva red	Lids inflamed, upper inner lid lumpy	Stringy, clear mucoid	Intense itching; usually part of larger allergic syndrome; vision unaffected	Cromolyn Na, antihistamine
Chlamydial (trachoma)	Conjunctiva red	Lids very swollen, upper inner lid lumpy	Watery	Corneal damage can occur; vision loss may ensue	Topical and oral tetracycline
Dry eyes	Eyes are moderately red and lusterless		Stringy, deficient	Corneal damage may occur, photophobia may exist, and impaired vision may ensure	Tear solution, treat underlying cause
Entropion	Eyes red	Lashes turned inwards, chafing cornea and conjunctiva	Watery		Surgery
Keratitis					
Bacterial	Red rim around cornea, ulcer, and pus visible in cornea		Mucopurulent	Very painful; occasionally visual disturbance	Topical/oral antibiotic; mydriatic to relieve painful iris spasm
Viral (herpes simplex)	Red rim around cornea, dentritic ulcer on cornea		Watery	Usually only one eye affected; painful, eye damage and loss of vision may occur	Topical antiviral; mydriatic to relieve painful iris spasm
Uveitis (iritis)	Red eyes, especially around corneal rim, (circumciliary injection of vessels)		No discharge or excessive tearing	Pain, photophobia, loss of visual acuity, miosis in affected eye	Topical steroids; mydriatic to relieve painful iris spasm and to prevent iris from adhering to lens

[a] Adapted from Plus Continuing Pharmacy Education Programme: Eye conditions and the pharmacists. (5:141) 1988. Published by Pharmaceutical Society of South Africa, compiled by TPS Drug Information Center Johannesburg.

ferred, as it will prevent both chlamydial and *N. gonorrhoeae* conjunctivitis.

VIRAL CONJUNCTIVITIS (11, 20)

The pathophysiology of viral conjunctivitis is the same as that of bacterial conjunctivitis. The most common virus is the adenovirus type 3 and 8 in populations with satisfactory hygiene. The herpes simplex virus may cause serious sight-threatening eye infections. It is often associated with other viral infections such as colds, sore throats, or influenzae.

The patient may feel generally ill and complain of red, watery, and gritty eyes. Lymphoid follicles are usually present on the upper lid conjunctiva, and swollen lymph nodes can often be detected in front of the ear (preauricular node). The discharge is profuse and watery with minimal lid edema.

Viral infections are usually self-limiting, and as antiviral agents currently available are effective only against the herpes viruses, treatment is often unsatisfactory. The antiviral agents that are effective against DNA herpesvirus are useful in the treatment of herpes simplex eye infections. A 14- to 21-day treatment regimen of either ophthalmic vidarabine 3% or idoxuridine 0.5% ointment administered 5 times a day or trifluridine 1% solution, 1 drop in the affected eye 9 times a day stops viral replication until the infected cells slough from the eye (16). Antibacterial ophthalmic preparations may prevent secondary bacterial infections and may be used in conjunction with the antiviral agents. Corticosteroids should be avoided in viral infections (16).

ALLERGIC CONJUNCTIVITIS (19, 20)

Allergic conjunctivitis, either acute or chronic, is usually part of a larger allergic syndrome such as hay fever. Patients with atopic diseases have an inherited predisposition to develop hypersensitivity to specific inhaled and ingested allergens, which is characterized by development of specific antibodies of the IgE immunoglobulin class. Symptoms of allergic conjunctivitis can be evoked by direct contact with airborne allergens like pollen, fungal spores, dust, and animal danders, or systemic allergens such as certain foods can stimulate an attack. The eye irritation due to indoor pollutants, as experienced by sufferers of the so-called sick-building syndrome, is also a form of allergic conjunctivitis (21).

The most commonly occuring types of allergic conjunctivitis are seasonal allergies and the acute allergic response. The seasonal type is characterized by transient attacks of severe itching, watery or mucoid discharge, and a pink eye. The patient may also suffer from asthma or other atopic disease. On examination, the lids and conjunctiva are swollen, and papillae can be seen lining the lid conjunctiva particularly on the upper lids. Symptoms of acute allergic conjunctivitis are similar to the seasonal type but more severe, often involving only one eye. Neither condition causes visual disturbance.

In allergic conjunctivitis, cold compresses are extremely useful in relieving the symptoms and reducing the swelling. The most effective treatment is removal of the allergen. The use of topical ophthalmic decongestants, antihistamines, or both will provide symptomatic relief. The treatment of allergic conjunctivitis resembles that of lid edema (Table 44.10). Cromolyn sodium 4% administered 4 to 6 times a day is a safe and effective agent in the treatment of allergic conjunctivitis in patients with a history of atopy, hay fever, eczema, or other systemic allergies and especially in children. Note that patients suffering from chronic allergic conjunctivitis should be warned against habitual use of OTC sympathomimetic decongestant eyedrops because of possible rebound vasodilatation.

Precipitation of an attack of angle-closure glaucoma is a danger with the use of sympathomimetic-containing eye drops.

VERNAL CONJUNCTIVITIS (16)

Vernal conjunctivitis is a seasonally recurrent, bilateral inflammation of the conjunctiva. It produces itching, watery eyes, photophobia, and a foreign body sensation in the eye. Positive diagnosis requires the scraping of the conjunctiva to show prominent eosinophils. The seasonal characteristic is usually in the spring and early summer and may include the fall. A thick, ropy, mucous discharge is a prominent characteristic of vernal conjunctivitis.

The primary treatment is topical steriods, but since this requires prolonged therapy in most cases, the sequele of cataract formation from the topical steriod or elevation of intraocular pressure (IOP) are major complications. When used, prednisolone 1/8% to 1% administered b.i.d. to q.i.d. is effective. Cromolyn sodium solution 4% administered 4 to 6 times a day may control the symptoms.

CHLAMYDIAL KERATOCONJUNCTIVITIS (TRACHOMA) (18, 21)

A chronic form of conjunctivitis is caused by *Chlamydia trachomatis*, which is characterized by subconjunctival hyperplasia and vascularization of the cornea. It occurs mainly in hot, dry, underdeveloped countries. It is also common among American Indians and in mountainous areas of the southern U.S.

It is a most contagious condition in its early stages and is transmitted by direct contact or possibly, by handling contaminated articles. Flies are well-known vectors. Another strain of *Chlamydia* is sexually transmitted and is a fairly common cause of neonatal conjunctivitis.

After an incubation period of about a week, swelling of the eyelids, photophobia, and lacrimation occur. Small follicles (appearing as bumps) appear on the inner surface of the upper lid. Exacerbations and remissions are a feature of this disease. Pannus formation with invasion of the cornea develops over time, and corneal scarring and blindness may ensue.

WHO recommendations for the prophylaxis and therapy for trachoma are

1. Improved hygiene and prevention of spread;
2. Mass prophylactic treatment with tetracycline hydrochloride ointment to both eyes, twice daily for 5 days;
3. Treatment of active trachoma in the individual: tetracycline ointment three times daily for 6 weeks, combined with oral sulfonamides in adults and erythromycin in children for 2 weeks.

Other authorities suggest that chloramphenicol be used topically instead of tetracycline, accompanied by trimethoprin/sulfamethoxazole by mouth (adults and children), a tetracycline derivative (adults only), or erythromycin (adults and children).

KERATOCONJUNCTIVITIS SICCA (DRY EYE) (12, 16)

Dry eye is a condition characterized by chronic dryness of the conjunctiva and cornea, which may lead to desiccation of the ocular surface. Most people who complain of "dry eyes" are seen, on examination, to have a perfectly normal supply of tears. The normal tear film consists of three distinct layers. The inner layer, which overlies the corneal and conjunctival epithelial cells and is produced by the goblet cells, is composed of mucin. This layer acts as a surfactant so that the cornea becomes hydrophilic. The middle layer is the saline layer produced by the accessory lacrimal glands in the conjunctiva, and the outer, oily layer comes from the meibomian glands. The main purpose of this outer layer is to retard evaporation of the saline.

Tear film deficiency can be due to shortage of any of these three constituents. A number of pathological or environmental conditions can cause such an imbalance. Diseases associated with the dry eye syndrome include rheumatoid arthritis, Sjögren's syndrome, Stevens-Johnson syndrome, the menopause, mumps and vitamin A deficiency. The use of certain medications, e.g., anticholinergics, diuretics and oral contraceptives, has been reported to contribute to dryness of the eyes.

Chronic eye discomfort and conjunctival redness accompanied by photophobia are common symptoms of the dry eye syndrome. In advanced cases, corneal damage and various degrees of impaired vision can occur. Frequent use of artifical tears containing methylcellulose or polyvinyl alcoholol as the vehicle may produce better results than hypotonic solutions because of their increased viscosity. The number of different natural tears products on the market indicates a great deal of variability in patient response from product to product. If tear replacement is not successful, other therapeutic measures such as ocular inserts, or a lubricant eye ointment may be effective. A topical antibiotic is required if secondary bacterial infections occur. Sometimes the unrecognized dry eye syndrome is treated with vasoconstrictors and local antihistamines. Treatment with these medications, however, is ineffective and may only worsen the condition (Table 44.6).

DISORDERS OF THE LACRIMAL SYSTEM (THE WATERING EYE) (13, 22)

The watering eye may be a result of either excess tear production (lacrimation) or deficient tear drainage (epiphora). Causes of lacrimation include corneal irritation by a foreign body or trauma. Causes of poor drainage include the following.

1. Stricture of the nasolacrimal duct (dacryostenosis) is often seen in newborn babies as a result of blockage by debris in the duct. In adults, dacryostenosis may result from inflammatory obstruction of the duct due to chronic nasal infection or from severe or chronic conjunctivitis.
2. Infection of the lacrimal sac (dacryocystitis) is usually secondary to obstruction of the nasolacrimal duct.
3. In senile ectropion, the lower lid of the eye sags away from the globe as a result of weakening of the muscles surrounding the eye. The opening (puncti) to the lacrimal drain is thus displaced resulting in epiphora.

A chronic overflow of tears and moderate edema of the lacrimal sac as well as redness are seen in dacryocystitis. Watery eyes are present in the dry eye syndrome when the tear composition lacks sufficient mucin.

Congenital obstruction resolves spontaneously, although fingertip massage of the lacrimal sac may speed resolution. Surgery may be necessary to correct epiphora due to ectropion. Antibiotic ointments (erythromycin or tobramycin q.i.d.) may be required in cases of secondary infection.

DISORDERS OF THE CORNEA (KERATITIS) (3, 16)

Keratitis is a condition characterized by inflammation of the cornea. As the cornea does not contain blood vessels, inflammation takes the form of edema, infiltration by white blood cells, and redness around the rim of the cornea. The abundant nerve endings in the cornea make the condition painful. Keratitis most commonly results from infection (by bacteria, viruses, or fungi) or is due to noninfectious causes like corneal oxygen deprivation brought about by excessive wearing of hard contact lenses, exposure to UV light, or an inability of the lids to close over the eye. The two more commonly occurring types of keratitis are bacterial and viral keratitis.

BACTERIAL KERATITIS (1, 16, 19)

Bacterial keratitis occurs when organisms like *Staphylococcus aureus*, *Streptococcus pneumoniae*, *Pseudomonas*, and enterobacterial species invade a small erosion on the corneal surface. The patient with a bacterial corneal ulcer complains of discomfort and a foreign body sensation, photophobia, and a mucopurulent discharge. The condition is painful, with redness around the rim of the cornea, and a white corneal ulcer visible upon examination. Visual disturbance occurs if the ulcer is in the center of the cornea.

Topical and/or oral antibiotic treatment is indicated. Initial therapy should be aggressive and be based upon the results of corneal scraping (culture and sensitivity reports). Therapy should not be started until these results are in hand. The scraping requires the use of a topical anesthetic such as proparacaine 0.5%. The eye should not be covered with a patch because this might encourage further bacterial growth. All corneal ulcers should be referred directly to an ophthalmologist.

VIRAL KERATITIS (11, 20)

Viral keratitis is caused by herpes simplex or herpes zoster. The herpes simplex virus is the most common cause of viral keratitis. The eye is red, gritty, photophobic, and painful. Usually only one eye is involved. Staining with fluorescein may reveal a branching corneal ulcer that may heal without damage but may result in serious corneal scarring.

The herpes zoster virus may attack neuronal tissue causing a painful condition known as shingles. The ophthalmic neurons may also become involved, in which case an extremely painful condition involving the cornea, tip of the nose, and forehead develops. Corneal scarring may occur, and secondary glaucoma may develop.

Topical antivirals such as acyclovir, idoxuridine, trifluridine, and vidarabine are indicated to treat herpes simplex keratitis (see treatment of viral conjunctivitis). If the 0.1% solution of idoxuridine is used, the regimen is 1 drop in affected eye hourly during the day and every 2 hr at night (unless the ointment is used at night) (16). Steroid-containing preparations are contraindicated as they may accelerate corneal damage (4, 5, 15) (Table 44.4). The oral and intravenous antivirals are not as effective as topical agents in viral keratitis.

Unlike herpes simplex, herpes zoster is an indication for the use of topical steroids. This prevents prolonged inflammation and nerve pain. Steroids should be used only after herpes simplex has been excluded. A 0.1% dexamethasone solution, instilled every 2 hours may be used concomitantly with a mydriatic such as 1% atropine or 0.5% to 1% cyclopentolate solution, one drop three times a day. Intraocular pressure (IOP) must be monitored in these patients, because the infection may cause an increase in IOP. Systemic corticosteroids, and recently, cimetidine have been used to prevent postherpetic neuralgia (21). Cimetidine (300 mg p.o. q.i.d.) is used for 2 to 3 weeks, and with therapy begun 48 to 72 hr after onset of the disease, it has been shown to reduce pain and pruritus in acute herpes zoster (11, 21). Oral acyclovir (200 to 800 mg 5 times a day with a maximum dosage of 4000 mg/day) for 10 days in the immunosuppressed patient has been effective, especially if therapy is started within 72 hr of onset of the disease.

DISORDERS OF THE UVEAL TRACT (1, 23)

The uveal tract consists of the iris, ciliary body, and choroid. Uveitis is the generic term for inflammatory conditions of the uveal tract. One or all three parts of the uveal tract may be affected simultaneously. Anterior uveitis is the term used for an inflammation of the iris (iritis) and/or the ciliary body (iridocyclitis), and posterior uveitis is the term used to describe inflammation of the choroid (choroiditis) and/or the retina (retinitis).

The etiology of uveitis is as yet unknown. It has, however, been associated with other inflammatory conditions such as arthritis, Crohn's disease, ankylosing spondylitis, and sarcoidosis. Chronic infection, trauma, and anatomical abnormalities such as cataracts have also been implicated. Patients are usually 20 to 50 years of age, and there is a decrease in patients over 70 (23).

A patient suffering from uveitis can be easily misdiagnosed as having conjunctivitis. Initially the patient will complain of a red, tender eye that feels bruised to the touch. There may be some photophobia while there is no discharge or excessive tearing, and initially the visual acuity is not affected. Uveitis may be unilateral or bilateral and there may be isolated attacks or repeated episodes (23). Gradually the eye becomes redder, more painful, and vision becomes disturbed. Careful examination of the eye will show that the pupil on the affected side is smaller than the other and possibly irregular.

No specific therapy is available for uveitis since the etiology is not known. Nonspecific measures include mydriatics, corticosteroids, nonsteroidal antiinflammatory agents, immunosuppressive drugs, and photocoagulation (11, 23). Treatment should be instituted immediately upon positive diagnosis to prevent the iris from adhering to the front surface of the lens. The pupil should be dilated using mydriatic drops to prevent adhesions and scarring between the pupillary border and the anterior lens capsule and to provide relief from photophobia. The mydriatic-cycloplegics used include moderately severe to severe uveitis—atropine (1 to 4%, 1 drop, 1 to 4 times a day); mild-to-moderate uveitis—homatropine (5%, 1 drop q.d. to b.i.d.). Cyclopentolate is not used in uveitis since it may further aggravate iritis (23).

Corticosteroids reduce the inflammation and are very effective. Table 44.4 lists the topical steroids and their relative potencies. Drops or ointments are effective in patients with anterior uveitis but are not effective in posterior uveitis. The dosage and frequency of the corticosteroids depends upon the severity of the disease and can vary from 1 drop every 2 to 4 hr to 1 drop every other day (23). If the patient does not respond to the topical agents, then systemic corticosteroids may be used. (Note: For further information on treatment regimens for uveitis, please refer to reference 23.)

CATARACTS

A cataract is a developmental or degenerative opacity of the crystalline lens. Developmental or congenital cataracts are present at birth, while the degenerative type develops slowly with age, leading to a gradual, painless loss of vision. Congenital cataracts are probably caused by chromosomal abnormalities. The degenerative type may be the result of senile degeneration, x-rays, systemic disease (e.g., diabetes), uveitis or certain drugs (e.g., corticosteroids). The patient experiences a progressive loss of vision, the degree of which depends on the location and extent of the opacity.

No medications currently available reduce the effect of a cataract once it is formed. The treatment of cataracts involves the surgical removal of the opacity (17).

OPTIC NEURITIS (PAPILLITIS) (18)

Inflammation of the part of the optic nerve that is ophthalmoscopically visible is optic neuritis (papillitis). The precise etiology remains obscure. Optic neuritis has been found to develop after viral illnesses, multiple sclerosis, certain chemicals (e.g., lead, methanol), bee stings, meningitis and syphilis. In patients over 60, an important cause may be temporal arteritis. Vision loss, which may develop within days, is the only symptom.

Removal of the cause in the early stages may restore vision, otherwise postneuritic optic atrophy develops with varying degrees of vision loss. Corticosteroids systemically (e.g., prednisone 60 mg/day orally) or retrobulbarly administered (e.g., methylprednisolone acetate 20 mg) may help. Nonsteroidal antiinflammatory agents have been used orally with some effectiveness as well (18).

CONCLUSION

The treatment of ocular disorders is dictated by the structure of the eye that is involved, the etiology, and the severity. Ophthalmic administration of drugs requires special patient education as well as precautions, and patients who overuse corticosteroid or decongestant ophthalmic preparations may develop adverse effects. Thus, the appropriate drug and dosage form must be selected, and it must be administered correctly for the successful treatment of common eye disorders.

REFERENCES

1. Riley GJ, Baker AS, Eye infections. In Reese RE, Gordon DR Jr: A Practical Approach to Infection Diseases, ed. 2. Boston, Little, Brown, 1986, p 156.
2. Vale J, Cox B: Drugs and the Eye. Durban: Butterworths (South Africa), 1978, p 17.
3. Youngson RM: Common eye disorders: Lid problems. SA Retail Pharmacist 38:25–29, 1989.
4. Lavin MJ, Rose GE: Use of steroid eye drops in general practice. Br Med J 292:1448–1450, 1986.
5. Jones BR, Coster DJ, Falcon MG: Prospects of prevention of recurrent herpetic eye disease. Trans Ophthalmol Soc UK 97:350–355, 1977.
6. Plus Continuing Pharmacy Education Programme: Eye conditions and the pharmacists. (5:141) 1988. Published by Pharmaceutical Society of South Africa, compiled by TPS Drug Information Center Johannesburg.
7. Gourley DR: Ophthalmic products. In Handbook of Nonprescription Drugs, ed. 9. Washington: Am Pharm Assoc, 1990, ch 20.
8. Burns RP, Gipson I: Toxic effects of local anesthetics. JAMA 240:347, 1978.
9. Hyndiuk RA, Burd EM, Hartz A: Efficacy and safety of mercuric oxide in the treatment of bacterial blepharitis. Antimicrob Agents Chemother 34:610–613, 1990.
10. Pavan-Langston D, Burns and trauma. In Pavan-Langston D (ed): Manual of Ocular Diagnosis and Therapy, ed. 3. Boston, Little, Brown, 1991, pp 31–46.
11. Fedukowixz HG: External Infections of the Eye. New York: Appleton-Century-Cofts, 1978, p 117.
12. Galloway NR: Common Eye Diseases and Their Management. Berlin: Springer-Verlag, 1985, p 44.
13. Grove AS Jr, Eyelids and lacrimal system. In Pavan-Langston D (ed): Manual of Ocular Diagnosis and Therapy, ed. 3. Boston: Little, Brown, 1991, pp 47–56.
14. Nelson ME, Midgley G, Blatchford NR: Ketoconazole in the treatment of blepharitis. Eye 4:151–159, 1990.
15. Mars S, Keightley S: The aging eye. Practitioner 233:1560–1564, 1989.
16. Pavan-Langston D, Foulks GN, Cornea and external disease. In Pavan-Langston D (ed): Manual of Ocular Diagnosis and Therapy, ed. 3. Boston: Little, Brown, 1991, pp 67–124.
17. Bankes JLK: Clinical Ophthalmology. Edinburgh: Churchill Livingstone, 1982, p 33.
18. Berkow R, Fletcher AJ (eds): The Merck Manual of Diagnosis and Therapy, ed. 15. Rahway: Merck & Co, 1987, ch 18.
19. Fox J: Conjunctivitis, keratitis and iritis. Nursing 3(45):20–23, 1989.
20. Allansmith MR: The Eye and Immunology. St. Louis: CV Mosby, 1982, p 113.
21. Conradie EA, Straughan JL (eds): South African Medicines Formulary. Cape Town: Med Assoc S Afr, 1988, p 223.
22. Klopfer J: Effects of environmental air pollution on the eye. J Am Optometric Assoc 60(10):773–778, 1989.
23. Pavan-Langston D, Uveal tract: iris, ciliary body, and choroid. In Pavan-Langston D (ed): Manual of Ocular Diagnosis and Therapy, ed. 3. Boston: Little, Brown, 1991, pp 173–218.
24. Miller A, Harel D, Laor A, Lahat N: Cimetidine as an immunomodulator in the treatment of herpes zoster. J Neuroimmunol 22(1):69–76, 1989.

COMMON EAR DISEASES

MICHAEL A. OSZKO, Pharm.D. and RICHARD D. LEFF, Pharm.D., F.C.C.P.

The ear is a complex structure consisting of bone and cartilage, sensory and nervous tissue, and fluid. In addition to facilitating the sense of hearing, the structures of the ear are intimately involved in the maintenance of balance and equilibrium.

Because of its anatomical complexity, there are a wide range of conditions that can alter normal ear function. This chapter describes three of the most common otological disease states that are likely to be encountered by the pharmacist in clinical practice: (*a*) otitis media; (*b*) otitis externa; and (*c*) vertigo.

ANATOMY OF THE EAR

The ear can be divided conveniently into three anatomical sections: the outer (or external), middle, and inner (or internal) ear (Fig. 45.1). The external ear consists of two structures, the *auricle* and the *external auditory canal*. The purpose of these structures is to collect and transmit sound waves to the middle ear.

The middle ear consists of the *tympanic membrane* (eardrum) and an air-filled *tympanic cavity* that houses three tiny bones known collectively as *ossicles* (Fig. 45.1). Incoming sound waves cause the tympanic membrane to vibrate. The first of the ossicles, the *malleus*, is attached at one end to the tympanic membrane and at the other to the second bone in the series, the *incus*. The incus, in turn, is attached to the third bone, the *stapes*, which sits against a membrane-covered aperture known as the *oval window*. The ossicles are designed so that the vibrations received from the tympanic membrane are amplified and transmitted to the sensory receptors located in the inner ear.

The middle ear is a relatively closed system, with a pressure approximately equal to atmospheric pressure. Pressure in the middle ear is maintained by the *eustachian tube*, which connects the tympanic cavity with the nasopharynx.

The inner ear consists of a complex series of canals containing two fluids known as *endolymph* and *perilymph*. These canals include the *cochlea*, which is involved with hearing, and the *labyrinth*, which is involved with maintaining equilibrium (Fig. 45.1). The movement of endolymph in the cochlea, which is caused by vibrations received from the middle ear, results in displacement of tiny hairs projecting out from specialized sensory cells. Such displacement transmits impulses to the cochlear (auditory) branch of the vestibulocochlear nerve (also known as the eighth cranial nerve).

Another series of fluid-filled canals in the inner ear (the labyrinth) functions to maintain balance. Movement of the head results in the movement of endolymph in these canals. Like the movement of endolymph in the cochlea, movement of tiny hairs projecting from specialized vestibular sensory cells transmits impulses to the vestibular branch of the vestibulocochlear nerve.

COMMON EAR DISORDERS
Otitis Media

Inflammation of the middle ear, *otitis media,* is one of the most frequent infectious diseases seen in pediatric patients. As many as 70% of children have had at least one episode by the time they are 3 years old (1). In the United States, otitis media is responsible for one in eight visits to office-based pediatricians (2) and accounts for 25 to 30 million prescriptions for oral antibiotics and more than two billion dollars in pharmacologic and surgical treatment annually (2, 3).

While the term otitis media commonly denotes an inflammation of the middle ear, the disease can be more accurately described as (*a*) either suppurative or nonsuppurative and (*b*) either acute, subacute, or chronic (4, 5). *Acute suppurative* otitis media refers to a clinically identifiable infection of the middle ear in which the symptoms appear suddenly (over several hours) and resolve completely within 3 weeks. If the inflammatory process persists for more than 3 weeks but less than 3 months, it is termed *subacute.* A middle ear discharge that persists for more than 3 months is termed *chronic* otitis media. If middle ear inflammation occurs in the absence of an identifiable infectious etiology, it is considered to be *nonsuppurative.*

Otitis media is frequently associated with an *effusion* in the tympanic cavity. *Secretory* otitis media is the term used if the effusion is located behind an intact tympanic membrane. The effusion may be further characterized as *serous* (i.e., serum-like, thin), *mucoid* (i.e., mucus-like, thick) or *purulent* (i.e., pus-like). A patient with secretory otitis media may be either symptomatic or asymptomatic.

PATHOGENESIS

The pathogenesis of otitis media is not completely understood, but is thought to be the result of two primary factors

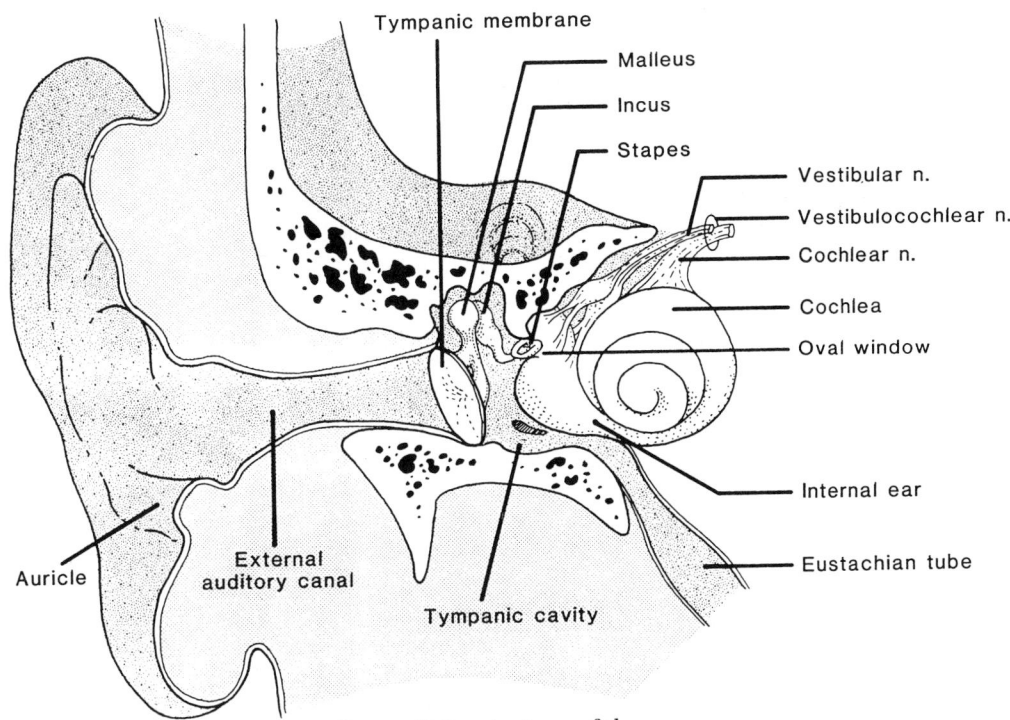

Figure 45.1. Anatomy of the ear.

(5, 6): (*a*) eustachian tube dysfunction and (*b*) introduction of infectious material (i.e., viruses and/or bacteria) into the middle ear.

The eustachian tube equalizes the pressure between the tympanic cavity and the atmosphere. Cilia located in the eustachian tube continuously sweep mucus and debris toward the nasopharynx and away from the middle ear. Obstruction of the eustachian tube may result from either mucous membrane edema (secondary to allergy or an upper respiratory infection) or blockage by a foreign body, tumor, or lymphatic (e.g., adenoid) tissue. In addition, developmental differences between children and adults with respect to anatomical positioning of the eustachian tube may predispose children to eustachian tube dysfunction.

Once an obstruction occurs, a negative pressure (relative to the atmosphere) develops in the tympanic cavity. This negative pressure is caused by the absorption of gases through the epithelial lining of the eustachian tube and tympanic cavity. If this obstruction is suddenly relieved, nasopharyngeal mucus and bacteria may be insufflated into the tympanic cavity. Alternatively, a strong positive pressure originating in the nasopharynx (e.g., nose-blowing) may also force nasopharyngeal contents into the middle ear.

Other etiologic factors of otitis media include anatomical and/or functional irregularities of the eustachian tube and/or its surrounding structures; viruses (e.g., influenza,

respiratory syncytial virus); trauma; and immunoglobulin deficiencies (particularly secretory IgA and IgG$_2$) (5, 6).

MICROBIOLOGY

Although viruses may play a concomitant role in the development of otitis media, the major etiologic pathogens are bacteria. In acute otitis media, the organisms most commonly isolated from middle ear fluid are *Streptococcus pneumoniae, Haemophilus influenzae,* and *Moraxella catarrhalis* (formerly *Branhamella catarrhalis*) (7). These organisms commonly colonize the nasopharynx of young children, but are less frequently found in older children (8). In infants less than 6 weeks old, *Escherichia coli* and group B streptococci are common pathogens. Other, less common organisms include staphylococci (both coagulase + and −), *Streptococcus pyogenes,* group A streptococci, other Gram-negative rods, *Chlamydia trachomatis,* and anaerobes. In chronic suppurative otitis media, the predominant organisms are staphylococci and *Pseudomonas* (5).

Up to 30% of *H. influenzae* and 80% of *M. catarrhalis* strains produce β-lactamases (3). The prevalence of β-lactamase-producing strains is highly variable and appears to depend on geographic location (9).

SIGNS AND SYMPTOMS

The classical presentation of acute suppurative otitis media is that of an acute (within hours) onset of unilateral otalgia (ear pain), fever, and nasal discharge (2). Neonates and small children display signs of otitis media, including excessive fussiness, irritability, and/or tugging at the affected ear. Older children may complain of a sore throat and/or a sensation of "fullness" or "pressure" in the ear. These symptoms may be associated with a decrease in hearing acuity. Seventy to 80% of patients with otitis media have a recent history of an upper respiratory tract infection, and approximately 50% have had a previous episode of otitis media (2). Less frequent symptoms include dizziness, lethargy, headache, anorexia (or reduced feeding in neonates), nausea, vomiting, diarrhea, and otorrhea (2, 5, 6).

DIAGNOSIS

The clinical diagnosis of otitis media is based largely on the patient's signs and symptoms. Otoscopic examination of the ear may reveal an erythematous tympanic membrane that is opaque or dull in appearance. The membrane is frequently bulging, and infrequently, the tympanic membrane may be perforated and draining pus. Tympanometric testing of the eardrum usually reveals reduced compliance.

Isolation of the causative organism may be accomplished by aspirating fluid from the middle ear (tympanocentesis). Unfortunately, cultures may be negative in one-third of patients with acute otitis media and two-thirds of patients with recurrent or secretory otitis media (7, 10). Cultures of the nasopharynx are more easily obtained, but are a poor predictor of the causative organism (11).

TREATMENT

Antibiotic Therapy. Despite the consensus that acute otitis media is primarily of bacterial etiology, there is disagreement on three issues: whether or not this condition should be treated with oral antibiotics; duration of antibiotic therapy; and the end point by which antibiotic efficacy should be assessed (12–14). In most patients, the symptoms of acute otitis media resolve spontaneously without treatment within 24 to 72 hr with resolution of the effusion within 2 weeks. Thus, it has been suggested that antibiotic therapy should be reserved for those who do not improve within this time (13). Unfortunately, it is impossible to identify a priori patients who will not improve spontaneously, and antimicrobial therapy is generally recommended to reduce the risk of suppurative complications (12, 15).

Since, in most cases, the causative organism is not isolated prior to initiating treatment, the choice of antibiotic is based on its efficacy against the most common pathogens. Table 45.1 lists antibiotics that are commonly used to treat acute otitis media.

Figure 45.2 presents a systematic approach to treating acute otitis media. For most patients, oral amoxicillin is an appropriate first choice. It is effective against the most likely causative organisms, relatively free of serious side effects (rash and diarrhea are most common), and is least expensive. If the patient is allergic to penicillins, either trimethoprim-sulfamethoxazole or erythromycin-sulfisoxazole are effective alternatives. Both of these contain a sulfonamide, but the prevalence of side effects (rash and gastrointestinal upset) is low (<5%), and hematologic toxicity is rare (16).

Although cross-sensitivity between penicillins and cephalosporins is infrequent, use of a cephalosporin in a patient who is allergic to penicillin is not recommended because of the risk of an anaphylactic reaction (17).

Because both *H. influenzae* and *M. catarrhalis* are capable of producing β-lactamases, an antibiotic that is stable against these enzymes should be considered if therapy with amoxicillin appears to be ineffective or if the prevalence of these organisms in a particular geographic area is high. Amoxicillin combined with potassium clavulanate (a β-lactamase inhibitor), erythromycin-sulfisoxazole, trimethoprim-sulfamethoxazole, cefaclor, cefixime, and cefuroxime axetil are equally effective. However, therapeutic failures

Table 45.1.
Oral Antibiotics Used In the Treatment of Acute Otitis Media[a]

Antibiotic	Pediatric Dose	Comments
Amoxicillin	20–40 mg/kg/day in 3 divided doses (q8h)	
Amoxicillin-potassium clavulanate (Augmentin)	20–40 mg/kg/day in 3 divided doses (q8h)	Dose based on amoxicillin content
Cefaclor (Ceclor)	40 mg/kg/day in 3 divided doses (q8h)	Maximum dose: 2 g/24 hr; ?stability vs β-lactamase-producing *M. catarrhalis*
Cefixime (Suprax)	8 mg/kg/day in 1 or 2 doses	?efficacy vs. *S. pneumoniae*
Cefuroxime axetil (Ceftin)	125–250 mg b.i.d.	Currently not available as a suspension
Erythromycin-sulfisoxizole (Pediazole)	200 mg/kg/day in 4 divided doses (q6h)	Dose based on erythromycin content
Trimethoprim-sulfamethoxazole (Bactrim, Septra)	8–10 mg/kg/day in 2 divided doses (q12h)	Dose based on trimethoprim content

[a] Adapted from: Greene MG (ed): The Harriet Lane Handbook, ed. 12. St. Louis: Mosby Yearbook 1991, pp 150–244.

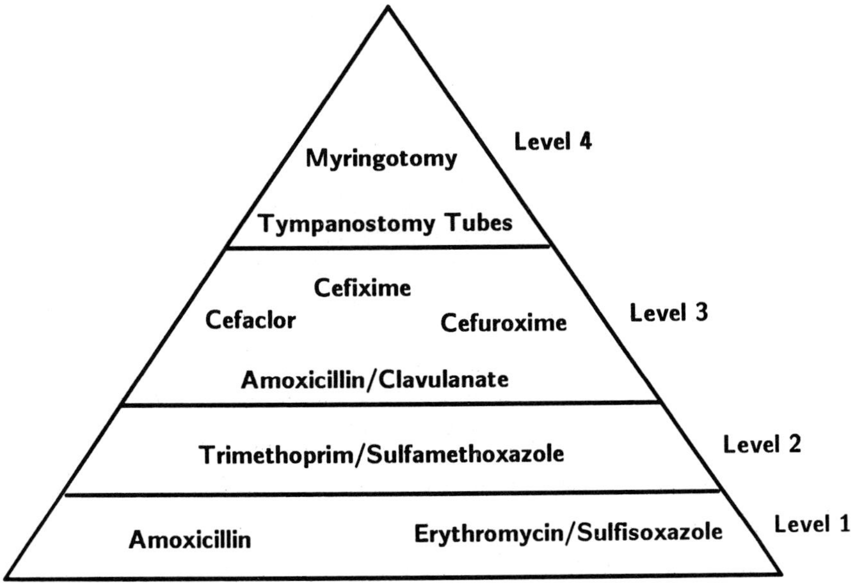

Figure 45.2. Systematic approach to the treatment of acute otitis media.

with cefaclor have been reported with certain β-lactamase-producing strains of *M. catarrhalis* (9). Although it is currently not approved for use in otitis media caused by *S. pneumoniae*, cefixime provides adequate coverage against *S. pneumoniae*, despite the fact that it is less active than other agents against this organism.

The usual length of antibiotic therapy in acute otitis media is 10 days. If the child's clinical response is unsatisfactory, a 10-day course of therapy with another antibiotic may be tried. This is unnecessary in most patients. However, middle ear effusion will persist for days to several months in a small number of patients. Recently, antibiotic treatment regimens of 2 to 7 days have been reported to be as effective as the 10-day regimen, but this finding awaits confirmation from well-designed clinical trials (6).

Many children experience several episodes of otitis media during their childhood. *Recurrent otitis media* is defined as three episodes within a 6-month period or four episodes within a 12-month period. Because of the discomfort and the risk of suppurative complications that are associated with each episode, low-dose, prophylactic antibiotic therapy has been advocated. Amoxicillin 20 mg/kg or sulfisoxazole 50 mg/kg in a single dose at bedtime for 3 to 6 months has been recommended (3). Recurrent episodes of otitis media despite prophylactic therapy may necessitate surgical intervention (discussed below).

Adjunctive Therapy. In addition to antibiotics, decongestants, antihistamines, corticosteroids, mucolytics, surfactants, immune globulins, and bacterial vaccines have been used to treat otitis media (5, 18, 19). None of these agents have been shown to improve the outcome of otitis media.

If antibiotic therapy fails and otitis media becomes chronic, it may be necessary to perform a myringotomy to place tympanostomy tubes. This allows the effusion to drain and the middle ear to be ventilated. This procedure is invasive (often requiring general anesthesia) and is associated with a number of complications (5).

PROGNOSIS

For most children, otitis media is a self-limiting condition that does not recur once adolescence is reached. In a small number of patients, however, otitis media becomes chronic. Intracranial (e.g., meningitis) or extracranial sequelae (e.g., labyrinthitis and permanent hearing loss) are rare but potentially serious complications of otitis media (6).

Otitis Externa

Otitis externa is an infectious condition of the external ear canal. While it may be associated with chronic otitis media, it is more frequently an independent condition that affects patients of all ages. It is characterized by pain, swelling, maceration and breakdown of the skin and subcutaneous tissues of the external ear canal. Two conditions produce an environment that is favorable for the development of otitis externa: (*a*) the introduction of a sharp object (e.g., toothpick, hairpin) into the external auditory canal, which disrupts the integrity of the lining of the canal and allows bacterial or fungal growth and (*b*) introduction and accumulation of moisture in the canal. Moisture not only softens the lining of the canal but also provides a medium for the growth of bacteria or fungi. Otitis externa commonly occurs when the ear is frequently exposed to water (e.g., swimming) and for this reason is sometimes referred to as "swimmer's ear."

The two most common organisms that are isolated in

otitis externa are *Pseudomonas aeruginosa* and *Staphylococcus aureus*. Together, these bacteria account for three-fourths of the organisms that are isolated (20). Fungi, primarily *Candida* and *Aspergillus* are found in about 10% of cases. Normally, the focus of infection is limited to the external ear. However, it may spread to the surrounding soft tissue and bone.

TREATMENT

The goal of treatment of otitis externa is to produce an environment in the external ear canal that promotes healing of the inflamed, infected tissue. This includes treating the infection and drying the external ear canal. Table 45.2 lists those substances commonly found in otic preparations used to treat otitis externa.

Antibiotics. Although antibiotics are found in many otic preparations, they may cause contact dermatitis, permit the overgrowth of resistant organisms, result in local (e.g., neomycin) or systemic (e.g., chloramphenicol) toxicities, and are generally not recommended (21). A 2% acetic acid solution is both antibacterial and antifungal, but does not cause any of the problems associated with antibiotics. Rarely, an otologist may instill antibiotic powders (e.g., amphotericin B, chloramphenicol, sulfanilamide) into the ear canal (22). Oral antibiotics are indicated only if the infection has spread to the surrounding soft tissue. In *malignant otitis externa* (described below), parenteral antibiotics may be necessary.

Other Agents. Corticosteroids possess antiinflammatory, antipruritic, and vasoconstrictive activity and may be useful topically in reducing swelling and inflammation in the external ear canal. A few drops of isopropyl alcohol 70% can serve as an excellent drying agent. It should be used sparingly to prevent excessive drying of the tissues and subsequent pruritis.

The direct instillation of local anesthetics or analgesics is not recommended. For severe pain, oral analgesics are preferred.

Administration of Otic Drops. In treating otitis externa, 3 to 4 drops of the desired solution should be instilled into the ear canal four times daily. To prevent the solution from escaping from the ear canal, the otic drops may be placed on a cotton or gauze wick, which is then inserted into the ear canal and left in place. In addition to keeping the solution in contact with the affected tissues, the wick also prevents occlusion of the ear canal due to swelling.

With proper attention to aural hygiene, most cases of otitis externa will resolve in 5 to 7 days. In a small number of cases, this condition becomes chronic and is characterized by dry, scaly, sometimes weeping skin covering the auricle and external ear canal. Again, meticulous aural hygiene, combined with the topical application of a steroid cream (e.g., hydrocortisone) 3 to 4 times daily, will manage the patient's symptoms.

Rarely, the superficial infection will spread to the underlying soft tissues and bone. *Malignant otitis externa* is a potentially life-threatening infection caused by *Pseudomonas aeruginosa*, predominantly in patients with underlying diseases (e.g., diabetes mellitus) (23). Patients with this condition are usually hospitalized and treated with parenteral antipseudomonal penicillins (e.g., mezlocillin, piperacillin, ticarcillin) or cephalopsorins (e.g., ceftazidime) (23, 24). Preliminary data suggest that ciprofloxacin, a 6-fluoroquinolone antibiotic with antipseudomonal activity, may also be effective in treating malignant otitis externa (25).

Vertigo

Most people have experienced dizziness at some point in their lives. Four classes of conditions are associated with dizziness (26): (*a*) vertigo; (*b*) syncope; (*c*) gait disturbances; and (*d*) miscellaneous head sensations. Vertigo is the most common of these and is discussed below.

Vertigo is the sensation of head motion when, in fact, there is none. This is an important point, since other conditions in which the head is moving (e.g., motion sickness) can produce sensations that are similar to vertigo. In most cases, vertigo is the result of vestibular dysfunction (*pe-*

Table 45.2.
Selectic Otic Preparations for Treatment of Otitis Externa

Drug Product	Antibiotic	Antibacterial/ Antifungal	Corticosteroid	Analgesic	Local Anesthetic
Auralgan Otic				Antipyrine 5.4%	Benzocaine 1.4%
Chloromycetin Otic	Chloramphenicol 0.5%				
Coly-Mycin S Otic	Neomycin SO$_4$ 3.3 mg/ml Colistin SO$_4$ 3 mg/ml		Hydrocortisone 1%		
Cortisporin Otic	Neomycin SO$_4$ 5 mg/ml Polymyxin B SO$_4$ 10,000 U/ml		Hydrocortisone 1%		
Otobiotic Otic	Polymyxin B SO$_4$ 10,000 U/ml		Hydrocortisone 0.5%		
Otic Tridesilon		Acetic acid 2%	Desonide 0.05%		
Vosol HC Otic		Acetic acid 2%	Hydrocortisone 1%		

ripheral vertigo), though it may also be due to disease of the central nervous system (*central vertigo*). The type of spinning sensation experienced by the patient may be also be used to classify vertigo. In *objective vertigo,* the environment appears to be turning about the patient, whereas in *subjective vertigo,* the patient himself appears to be turning in place. Vertigo can also be associated with cochlear dysfunction (e.g., Ménière's disease).

Diagnosis. The subjective nature of dizziness makes diagnosing vertigo difficult. Vertigo is often diagnosed without a clear etiology due to the inaccessibility of the inner ear structures. Thus, a careful history is essential to rule out unrelated conditions (e.g., orthostatic hypotension, gait disturbances).

The most objective sign of vertigo obtained upon physical examination is *nystagmus.* Whether nystagmus is spontaneous or positional can provide important clues to the etiology of vertigo (27).

Caloric stimulation is used to test vestibular function. In this procedure, irrigation of the ear canal with cold or warm water will induce vertigo and nystagmus in patients with normal vestibular function. An abnormal response (i.e., the inability to induce vertigo) to caloric stimulation can be helpful in establishing an etiology. Other tests include audiometry, electronystagmography, and radiologic visualization of the affected structures (26–28).

TREATMENT

The treatment of vertigo involves both pharmacologic and nonpharmacologic modalities. Unfortunately, no drugs are specific for treating vertigo. A number of drug classes, by virtue of their effects on the nervous system, are sometimes effective in alleviating the symptoms of vertigo. Table 45.3 lists those drugs that are commonly used. More recently, methylprednisolone (29) and flunarizine (30), an investigational calcium-channel antagonist, have been reported to be beneficial in the management of the symptoms of vertigo.

Long-term, nonpharmacologic therapies are often preferred. These include; (*a*) balancing exercises, designed to enhance the body's ability to adapt to vestibular, visual, or sensory mismatches; (*b*) surgery, to remove pathologic lesions or correct anatomic abnormalities; and (*c*) psychotherapy, particularly when an organic etiology cannot be found.

CONCLUSION

Three common ear disorders are encountered by the pharmacist: otitis media, otitis externa, and vertigo. As with other diseases, pharmacotherapy in otologic diseases must not be undertaken without a thorough understanding of the pathophysiology of the disease state.

REFERENCES

1. Teele GW, Klein JO, Rosner BA: Epidemiology of otitis media in children. Ann Otol Rhinol Laryngol 89(suppl 68):5–6, 1980.
2. Froom J, Culpepper L, Grob P, et al.: Diagnosis and antibiotic treatment of acute otitis media: report from International Primary Care Network. Br Med J 300:582–586, 1990.
3. Bluestone CD: Management of otitis media in infants and children: current role of old and new antimicrobial agents. Pediatr Infect Dis J 7:S129–S136, 1988.
4. Klein JO, Tos M, Hussl B, et al.: Recent advances in otitis media: definition and classification. Ann Otol Rhinol Laryngol 139(suppl):10, 1989.
5. Kemp ED: Otitis media. Prim Care 17:267–287, 1990.
6. Lisby-Sutch SM, Nemec-Dwyer MA, Deeter RG, Gaur SM: Therapy of otitis media. Clin Pharm 9:15–34, 1990.
7. Qvarnberg Y, Kantola O, Valtonen H, et al.: Bacterial findings in middle ear effusion in children. Otolaryngol Head Neck Surg 102:118–121, 1990.
8. Stenfors L-E, Räisänen S. Occurrence of middle ear pathogens in the nasopharynx of young individuals: a quantitative study in four age groups. Acta Otolaryngol 109:142–148, 1990.
9. Marchant CD: Spectrum of disease due to *Branhamella catarrhalis* in children with particular reference to acute otitis media. Am J Med 88(suppl 5A):15S–19S, 1990.
10. Karma P: Secretory otitis media—infectious background and its implications for treatment. Acta Otolaryngol Suppl 449:47–48, 1988.
11. Groothuis JR, Thompson J, Wright PF: Correlation of nasopharyngeal and conjunctival cultures with middle ear fluid cultures in otitis media. Clin Pediatr 25:85–88, 1986.
12. Bluestone CD: Otitis media in children: to treat or not to treat? N Engl J Med 306:1399–1404, 1982.
13. Browning GG: Childhood otalgia: acute otitis media—antibiotics not necessary in most cases. Br Med J 300:1005–1006, 1990.
14. Bain J: Childhood otalgia: acute otitis media—Justification for antibiotic use in general practice. Br Med J 300:1006–1007, 1990.
15. McCracken GH: Selection of antimicrobial agents for treatment of acute otitis media with effusion. Pediatr Inf Dis J 6:985–988, 1987.
16. Cunningham MJ: Chemoprophylaxis with oral trimethoprim-sulfamethoxazole in otitis media. Clin Pediatr 29:273–277, 1990.
17. Klein JO: Otitis externa, otitis media, mastoiditis. In: Mandell GL, Douglas RG, Bennett JE (eds): Principles and Practice of Infectious Diseases. ed. 3. New York, Churchill Livingstone, 1990, pp 505–510.

Table 45.3.
Drugs Used to Treat Vertigo

Drug Class	Drug	Adult Dose[a]
Antimuscarinic	Scopolamine	Topical: 1 patch (0.5 mg) q72h
H$_1$ Antagonists	Cyclizine (Marezine)	50 mg q4–6h
	Meclizine (Antivert)	12.5–25 mg 3–4 ×/day
	Dimenhydrinate (Dramamine)	50–100 mg q4–6h
Phenothiazines	Promethazine (Phenergan)	25 mg q8–12h
Antiemetics	Trimethobenzamide (Tigan)	Oral: 250 mg 3–4 ×/day Rectal: 200 mg 3–4 ×/day

[a] Oral route of administration unless otherwise specified.

18. Mandel EM, Rockette HE, Bluestone CD, et al.: Efficacy of amoxicillin with and without decongestant-antihistamine for otitis media in children. N Engl J Med 316:432–437, 1987.

19. Jørgensen F, Andersson B, Hanson LÅ, Nylén O, Edén: Gamma globulin treatment of recurrent acute otitis media in children. Pediatr Inf Dis J 9:389–394, 1990.

20. Farmer HS: A guide for the treatment of external otitis. Am Fam Physician 21(6):96–101, 1980.

21. Rutks J, Alberti PW: Toxic and drug-induced disorders in otolaryngology. Ololaryngol Clin North Am 17:761–774, 1984.

22. Amundson LH: Disorders of the external ear. Prim Care 17:213–231, 1990.

23. Rubin J, Yu VL: Malignant external otitis: insights into pathogenesis, clinical manifestations, diagnosis, and therapy. Am J Med 85:391–398, 1988.

24. Johnson MP, Ramphal R: Malignant external otitis: report on therapy with ceftazidime and review of therapy and prognosis. Rev Infect Dis 12:173–180, 1990.

25. Legett JM, Prendergast K: Malignant external otitis: the use of ciprogloxacin. J Laryngol Otol 102:53–54, 1988.

26. Daroff RB. Dizziness and vertigo. In: Braunwald E, Isselbacher KJ, Petersdorf RG, et al., (eds): Harrison's Principles of Internal Medicine. ed. 11. New York, McGraw-Hill, 1987, pp 76–79.

27. Barker LR, Moses H, Rothman W: Dizziness, vertigo, motion sickness, near syncope, symcope, and disequilibrium. In: Barker LR, Burton JR, Zieve PD (eds): Principles of Ambulatory Medicine. ed. 2. Baltimore, Williams & Wilkins, 1986, pp 1153–1163.

28. Paparella MM, Alleva M, Bequer NG: Dizziness. Prim Care 17:299–308, 1990.

29. Ariyasu L, Byl FM, Sprague MS, Adour KK: The beneficial effect of methylprednisolone in acute vestibular vertigo. Arch Otolaryngol Head Neck Surg 116:700–703, 1990.

30. Olesen J: Calcium entry blockers in the treatment of vertigo. Ann NY Acad Sci 522:690–697, 1988.

CHAPTER 46

GLAUCOMA

DICK R. GOURLEY, Pharm.D. and CONSTANCE A. McKENZIE, Pharm.D.

Glaucoma is a disease of the eye that is characterized by an increase in intraocular pressure (IOP). More than 2 million Americans have glaucoma (one-half of whom are undiagnosed) and approximately 80,000 of them have varying degrees of blindness caused by damage to the optic disk and visual field loss (1). Glaucoma is the leading cause of legal blindness in the United States. Glaucoma usually manifests itself after age 35, but can occur in younger people as well. One to 2% of the population over 40 years of age and 5 to 9% over 65 years of age suffer from glaucoma. The older the patient, the greater the need for evaluation for glaucoma.

Glaucoma is insidious in onset and often produces only minor symptoms of discomfort, such as headache or "tired eyes." Many patients do not seek medical attention until the disorder is well established because of this lack of symptoms. Some patients have a very high IOP, but still have no symptoms. Fortunately, optic nerve and retinal damage are late findings of end-stage disease. Symptoms such as persistent headache and eye pain usually cause patients to seek medical assistance before these serious consequences develop (2).

PATHOGENESIS

IOP is physiologically determined by the relative production and elimination of aqueous humor. Increased IOP can result from either increased production of aqueous humor, decreased elimination, or both. The major cause of increased IOP is decreased elimination.

There are more than 40 different types of glaucoma (Table 46.1), but the two major types of glaucoma are angle-closure and open-angle. The more acute type is angle-closure glaucoma. It occurs in only 5 to 10% of all cases, compared to 90% for open angle. Both types can be further classified into primary and secondary glaucoma. A third type is congenital glaucoma, which results from developmental ocular abnormalities and occurs in less than 2% of cases.

The familial relationship of glaucoma has been well established; whether the hereditary pattern is one consistent with a dominant or recessive autosomal trait remains equivocal. Patients with a familial history of glaucoma should have routine yearly eye examinations because of this increased risk. Although there are more males with primary open-angle glaucoma, sex predilections for the disease are not clinically apparent. Primary open-angle

glaucoma is relatively more common in Caucasians and blacks than in American Indians and Asians. Although many patients may have unilateral involvement initially, it can be anticipated that the other eye will become involved within 5 years. Myopia may be a high-risk factor for glaucoma. Although it is more common to find open-angle glaucoma in patients with myopia, especially in the younger age group, the evidence for association between the two factors remains equivocal (3). A summary of risk factors associated with an increase in probability of primary glaucoma screening in any given patient is listed in Table 46.2.

PATHOPHYSIOLOGY

Anatomic factors associated with acute angle-closure glaucoma include: (a) small hyperopic (farsighted) eyes, (b) tautness of the iris and large pupils, (c) anterior lens dislocations, (d) swollen hypermature lens, and (e) posterior or anterior synechiae (fibrous scars).

Farsighted individuals are particularly at risk for angle closure since the tissues of their eyeballs are relatively compacted and the lens is shifted anteriorly. In individuals with a lack of tautness of the iris diaphragm (usually in large pupils), a bulging iris (bombe) may occur because of increased iridotrabecular contact.

Two conditions that lead to anterior lens dislocation are ocular trauma or a severe blow to the eye, both of which may lead to pupillary blockage or direct obstruction of the angle. Similarly, a swollen lens, as in inflammatory conditions (uveitis), produces pupillary blockage.

Posterior synechiae can form in the eyes of patients with uveitis and, if present in sufficient numbers, occlude the pupil. An increase in IOP may then result. Anterior synechiae can form after long-standing iritis and produce adhesion of the anterior portion of the iris to the trabecular meshwork. The outflow of aqueous humor is further obstructed, increasing IOP.

The damage from either type of glaucoma is primarily due to the inhibition of aqueous humor outflow. Aqueous humor formation occurs at a rapid rate (approximately 1 ml/min) and depends on several interacting mechanisms within the ciliary processes. Aqueous humor is secreted by the ciliary processes into the posterior chamber (Fig. 46.1), where it flows to the trabecular meshwork and finally out through the canal of Schlemm. Since a decrease in the outflow facility of aqueous humor is the primary mechanism for producing an increase in IOP, the anatomic changes in open-angle and angle-closure glaucoma are important (3).

In open-angle glaucoma a physical blockage occurs within the trabecular meshwork that retards elimination

Table 46.1.
Classification of Glaucomas[a]

Primary glaucoma
    Primary open-angle glaucoma; synonyms: chronic open-angle glaucoma, chronic simple glaucoma, glaucoma simplex
    Low tension glaucoma
    Primary closed-angle glaucoma; synonyms: primary angle-closure glaucoma, narrow-angle glaucoma, iris-block glaucoma, acute congestive glaucoma
        Acute angle-closure glaucoma
        Chronic angle-closure glaucoma (may also be secondary to other ocular diseases)
        Intermittent angle-closure glaucoma
        Superimposed on chronic open-angle glaucoma (combined mechanism)
Variants of primary glaucoma
    Pigmentary glaucoma
    Exfoliation glaucoma; synonyms: pseudoexfoliation of the lens capsule, glaucoma capsulare
Developmental glaucoma
    Primary congenital glaucoma
    Infantile glaucoma with associated defects such as Axenfeld's and Reiger's anomalies
    Glaucoma associated with hereditary or familial diseases such as aniridia, encephalotrigeminal hemangiomatosis (Sturge-Weber syndrome), neurofibromatosis, oculocerebrorenal (Lowe's) syndrome
Secondary glaucoma
    Inflammatory glaucoma
        Uveitis of all types
        Fuchs' heterochromic iridocyclitis
    Phacogenic galucoma
        Angle-closure glaucoma with mature cataract
        Phacoanaphylactic glaucoma secondary to rupture of lens capsule
        Phacolytic glaucoma caused by phacotoxic meshwork blockage
        Subluxation of lens
    Glaucoma secondary to intraocular hemorrhage
        Hyphema
        Hemolytic glaucoma (erthroclastic glaucoma)
    Traumatic glaucoma
        Traumatic recession of chamber angle
        Postsurgical glaucomas
            Aphakic pupillary block
            Ciliary block (malignant) glaucoma
    Neovascular glaucoma (especially in diabetic patients)
    Drug-induced glaucoma
        Corticosteroid-induced glaucoma
        Postoperative ocular hypertension from use of α-chymotrypsin
    Glaucomas of miscellaneous origin
        Associated with intraocular tumors
        Associated with retinal detachments (rare)
        Secondary to severe chemical burns of the eye
        Associated with essential iris atrophy
Absolute glaucoma

[a] Reprinted with permission from Paton D, Craig JA: Glaucomas: diagnosis and management. Clin Symp 28:20, 1976.

Table 46.2.
Risk Factors Associated with Glaucoma

Age
Familial history
Race
Sex
Concurrent diseases
Ametropia

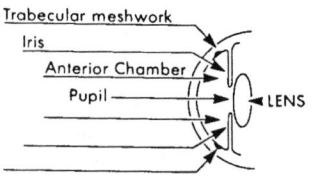

Figure 46.1.   Normal eye anatomy.

of aqueous humor. The obstruction is presumed to be between the trabecular sheet and the episcleral veins, into which the aqueous humor ultimately flows.

The impairment of aqueous drainage elevates the IOP to between 25 and 35 mm Hg (normal is 10 to 20 mm Hg), indicating that the obstruction is usually partial. This increase in IOP is sufficient to cause progressive cupping of the optic disk and eventually visual field defects. As the trabecular spaces become more involved, detachment of the cornea and formation of bullae may develop. Since visual acuity remains largely unaffected until late in the disease, scotomata must be regarded as a major indication for medical therapy.

In angle-closure glaucoma increased IOP is caused by pupillary blockage of aqueous humor outflow and is more severe. The basic requirements leading to an acute attack of angle closure are (a) a pupillary block, (b) a narrowed anterior chamber angle, and (c) a convex iris (iris bombe). The sequence of events leading to increased IOP is depicted in Figure 46.2. When a patient has a narrow anterior chamber (Fig. 46.2A) or a pupil that dilates to a degree where the iris comes in greater contact with the lens (Fig. 46.2B), there is interference with the flow of aqueous humor from the posterior to the anterior chamber. Since aqueous humor is continually secreted, pressure from within the posterior chamber forces the iris to bulge forward (Fig. 46.2C). This may progress to complete blockage (Fig. 46.2D).

The pathologic complications of angle-closure and open-angle glaucoma include the formation of cataracts, peripheral anterior synechiae, atrophy of the optic nerve and retina, and absolute glaucoma (complete blockage of aqueous outflow). The development of cataracts can increase existing pupillary block and the degree of angle closure.

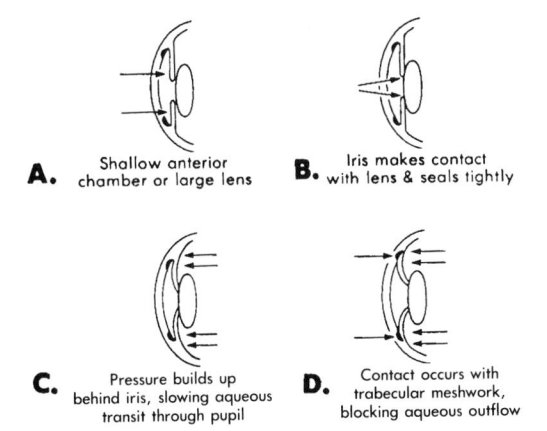

A. Shallow anterior chamber or large lens

B. Iris makes contact with lens & seals tightly

C. Pressure builds up behind iris, slowing aqueous transit through pupil

D. Contact occurs with trabecular meshwork, blocking aqueous outflow

Figure 46.2. Abnormal eye with development of pupillary block.

Table 46.3.
Factors Implicated in Potential Drug-induction of Angle-closure Glaucoma

Age—usually over 30
History—familial, genetic basis
Race—usually Caucasian
Sex—usually female
Anterior chamber angle—shallow and narrow
Vision—hyperopia, hypermetropia
Convexity of the iris—flattened
Dose and duration of the offending drug used
Duration of effect on eye—longer duration
Route of administration—topical more than systemic

ETIOLOGY

Drugs that have autonomic effects produce several types of ocular changes. Of great importance is the effect of anticholinergic agents on angle-closure glaucoma. Several factors appear to be associated with drug-induced glaucoma (Table 46.3).

In addition to drugs, glaucoma can occur as a secondary manifestation of systemic disorders or trauma. A list of systemic diseases associated with increased IOP is given in Table 46.4.

Congenital glaucoma is a rare disorder in which the IOP is increased as a result of developmental abnormalities of the ocular structures in the newborn. It may occur in association with other congenital abnormalities and anomalies such as homocystinuria and Marfan's syndrome. Congenital glaucoma should be considered in newborns who have sensitivity to light, excessive tearing, or spasm of the eyelids.

DIAGNOSIS AND CLINICAL FINDINGS
Open-Angle Glaucoma

The common signs of open-angle glaucoma may be minimal and do not appear immediately. As time progresses, the signs become more marked until they finally restrict vision. In some cases, there may be a total absence of signs. The common signs are (*a*) increased IOP, (*b*) visual field loss, (*c*) optic disk changes, (*d*) decreased outflow facility, (*e*) gonioscipically open angles, and (*f*) positive provocative tests (3).

An increased IOP can have several interpretations. Most normal individuals have pressures of 21 mm Hg or less. However, a small group of patients may sustain glaucomatous damage even with pressures under 20 mm Hg, "low tension glaucoma" (4, 5). In general, pressure readings in the high 20s are suspicious, and those above 30 are cause for serious concern. Patients between the ages of 50 and 75 with pressures above 30 mm Hg as the only sign of glaucoma should be treated medically, because decreased vascular perfusion in older people can endanger the optic nerve. The younger patient with similar readings may only require assessment for changes in the optic disk or visual fields at frequent intervals (2).

In the early stage of chronic open-angle glaucoma, symptoms of pain or visual field loss are usually not present (Table 46.5).

Angle-Closure Glaucoma

Acute angle-closure glaucoma usually presents with signs and symptoms of blurred vision (often with colored halos around light), severe ocular pain, and nausea with occasional vomiting (4). The eye appears red, the cornea is cloudy, the pupil is middilated and the anterior chamber is narrow, and the IOP is frequently above 50 mm Hg. Visual acuity is reduced by corneal changes or edema. Bullae may be present on the cornea if the acute attack is prolonged. Colored halos result from diffraction of light by the edematous cornea.

Ocular pain may vary from moderate to severe. The oculovagal reflex is thought to produce the nausea, vom-

Table 46.4.
Systemic Conditions Associated with Glaucoma (Secondary)[a]

Congenital rubella
Diabetes mellitus
Down's syndrome
Hallermann-Streiff syndrome
Homocystinuria
Idiopathic infantile hypoglycemia
Lowe's syndrome
Marfan's syndrome
Melanoma (intraocular tumors)
Neurofibromatosis (von Recklinghausen's)
Turner's syndrome
Uveitis (secondary)

[a] Modified from Scheie HG, Edwards DL, Yanoff MC: Clinical and experimental observations using alpha chymotrypsin. Am J Ophthalmol 59:469, 1965.

Table 46.5.
Clinical Findings and Symptoms of Primary Glaucoma

Glaucoma	Onset	Early Findings and Symptoms	Late Findings and Symptoms
Open-angle	Insidious	Asymptomatic slight rise in IOP: decreaased rate of aqueous humor outflow, optic disk changes (symptoms may be marginal or even at times absent)	Gradual loss of peripheral vision (over months to years); persistent elevation of IOP; optic nerve degenerations; retinal nerve atrophy; edema of the cornea; cataracts; trabecular meshwork degeneration
Angle-closure	Sudden	Blurred vision; severe ocular pain and congestion; conjunctival redness; cloudy cornea; moderately dilated pupil; poor pupil response to light; IOP markedly elevated; nausea and vomiting	Complete blindness in 2–5 days if not treated

iting, bradycardia, and sweating that may accompany an acute attack. With very high IOPs, the pupil may become fixed in middilation and eventually damaged. In severe cases, the pupil changes from a round to an oval shape and may resist constriction by topical parasympathomimetic agents.

Chronic angle-closure is a less severe form of glaucoma than acute angle-closure; the symptoms may range from none to intermittent and severe ocular pain along with halo formation and ocular congestion. Synechiae do not form without ocular congestion, which may be evident only with a moderately high pressure reading.

Diagnostic Procedures

With both major types of glaucoma, several diagnostic procedures (Table 46.6) are available to evaluate visual field loss, optic disk changes, outflow facility, angle measurements, and provocative tests.

DRUGS CONTRAINDICATED IN GLAUCOMA

Specific classes of drugs, such as anticholinergic, adrenergic, and corticosteroid, have been implicated in inducing glaucoma. Any drug with atropine-like side effects can produce pupillary dilation and paralysis of accommodation for near vision. Concern for this iatrogenic complication has prompted Food and Drug Administration (FDA) requirements for warnings on the systemic use of anticholinergics in the presence of glaucoma.

One must distinguish between open-angle and angle-closure glaucoma in arriving at a therapeutic decision about this warning because drug effects differ in the two cases. Drugs that dilate the pupil, for instance, may precipitate an acute attack of angle-closure glaucoma but usually do not produce harmful effects in open-angle cases. Dilation of the pupil in angle-closure glaucoma may cause the peripheral iris to bulge forward, blocking the trabecular meshwork. The aqueous humor is prevented from reaching the outflow channels, which results in an increased IOP. Since excessive resistance to outflow in open-

angle glaucoma is caused primarily by changes within the trabecular outflow channels, dilation of the pupil usually will not exacerbate the IOP.

Topical administration of some drugs (Table 46.7) is known to elevate IOP in various patients with glaucoma, and it has been assumed that systemic administration of such medications will have a similar effect. In patients with mild or controlled open-angle glaucoma it is unwarranted to prohibit the use of systemic sympathomimetic, anticholinergic, and other atropine-like drugs because the evidence that they exacerbate the condition is not well documented (6).

Anticholinergics

In patients with normal eyes, topically instilled anticholinergics such as atropine, scopolamine, and cyclopentolate produce no significant elevation in IOP. However, in patients over 30 years of age who have abnormally shallow anterior chambers, there is a risk of precipitating acute attacks of angle-closure glaucoma. The incidence has been estimated to be nearly 1 in 4000 (7). Atropine and scopolamine have a profound effect on the eye because of their longer durations of action than other agents with anticholinergic effects (i.e., phenothiazine, tricyclic antidepressants, and antihistamines). These locally instilled agents cause mydriasis and cycloplegia that may persist for as long as 2 weeks. In some open-angle patients, they produce a slight rise of IOP (less than 6 mm Hg) when instilled into the eyes (8). Other mydriatics, however, do not appear to have this effect.

Conventional doses of atropine systemically administered for preanesthesia have little ocular effect; in contrast, equivalent therapeutic doses of scopolamine can cause definite pupillary dilation (9). Prolonged use of anticholinergics can exacerbate open-angle glaucoma to some extent, but studies have shown that oral atropine at a dose of 0.6 mg every 4 hours for 1 week produces only slight elevations of IOP (10). In another study, the administration of proprietary cold remedies containing 0.2 mg of belladonna alkaloids (given twice daily for 4 days) caused

Table 46.6.
Diagnostic Studies for Glaucoma

Procedures	Comments
Tonometry	Measures intraocular tension; routinely used for mass screening studies; diurnal variations of intraocular tension in open-angle glaucoma should be considered; repeated readings should be done before definite diagnosis; between acute attacks of angle-closure glaucoma, the intraocular tension may be normal; applanation tonometry measures the force applied per unit area whereas indentation tonometry uses a plunger to produce a pit in the cornea, which serves as a measure of intraocular pressure
Gonioscopy	Differentiates the type of glaucoma; gonioscopic appearance of narrowed anterior chamber angle is usually diagnostic of angle-closure glaucoma
Tonography	May reveal impaired facility of aqueous humor outflow; early open-angle glaucoma can be detected by this technique; tonometer is applied to the eye and the resultant reduction in the intraocular tension is measured as an indicator of outflow facility
Water-drinking test	Rise in intraocular tension after rapid ingestion of a quart of water is significant indication of glaucoma; positive result occurs in 30% of open-angle glaucoma cases; negative result does not rule out glaucoma; tonography and water-drinking test will reveal open-angle glaucoma with 90% reliability
Ophthalmoscopy	Glaucomatous excavation or cupping of the optic disk is found in chronic primary open-angle and congenital glaucomas; glaucomatous changes of optic disk and/or occlusion of the central retinal vein in absence of elevated intraocular tension should arouse suspicion of glaucoma in early stage
Visual field examination	Isolated areas of impaired vision surrounded by normal areas in a visual field is indicative of open-angle glaucoma; visual field changes are irreversible; parallel optic disk changes
Corticosteroid instillation	Striking differences in ocular tension between primary open-angle glaucoma patients and normal subjects are produced by topically instilled corticosteroids; steroid provocative rest is used to evaluate genetic predisposition of glaucoma; response of primary angle-closure glaucoma to corticosteroid instillation is much more similar to normal subjects
Dark room test	Intraocular tension is assessed in patient before and after being placed in a dark room; in chronic angle-closure glaucoma, a considerable rise in the intraocular tension is observed after being in the dark

no changes in IOP in 27 normal volunteers and 37 patients with glaucoma (including 18 patients with chronic angle closure) (11).

Propantheline, a commonly used anticholinergic, produces no significant elevation in IOP in either normal or angle-closure patients. Anticholinergics, in fact, can deepen the anterior chamber by inhibiting the contraction of the ciliary body and produce cycloplegia, which widens rather than narrows the anterior chamber angle, making angle closure less likely to occur. No recent reports of exacerbations of glaucoma with diazepam or amitriptyline have appeared in the literature, although the manufacturers of these drugs contraindicate their use in patients with this disorder. Very high doses of phenothiazines given for schizophrenia have produced slight elevations of IOP (2). Treatment with miotics easily overcame the effect.

In summary, withholding systemic anticholinergics for fear of inducing open-angle glaucoma is not justified. This is true especially with parenteral atropine or scopolamine given preoperatively prior to general anesthesia. Sensitivity of the eye to systemic drugs is relatively low (1). Although these agents can induce angle-closure in rare instances, the concomitant use of parasympathomimetic miotics will prevent any of the IOP effects. However, ocularly instilled potent anticholinergics, such as atropine, scopolamine, cyclopentolate, and homatropine, should not be used in patients diagnosed with or predisposed to angle-closure glaucoma.

Sympathomimetics

Adrenergic agents commonly found in appetite suppressants, bronchodilators, central nervous stimulants, and vasoconstrictors produce slight pupillary dilation. No adverse effects on open-angle glaucoma have been reported. After systemic administration of these agents the frequency of deleterious effects on angle-closure glaucoma has been extremely small (13). Adrenergic agents such as epinephrine and phenylephrine have been used ocularly to treat open-angle-glaucoma. These agents *will* elevate the IOP by narrowing the anterior chamber angle when instilled into the eyes of angle-closure patients (6).

General anesthetics producing parasympathetic and sympathetic imbalance may cause pupillary block. Topical pilocarpine 1% may be instilled into the eye prior to inducing anesthesia to prevent this complication (6, 12).

Cardiovascular Drugs

There is no convincing evidence that vasodilators significantly aggravate glaucoma, despite the fact that subconjunctival injection of strong vasodilators such as isoxsuprine and tolazolline can induce transient elevations in IOP, particularly in chronic open-angle glaucoma (5). Nitrates, nitrites, aminophylline, nylidirin, and cyclandelate can be used safely in glaucoma (6, 7). Antihypertensives will decrease intraocular blood flow, which can lead to loss of small visual fields in patients with a high IOP. Therefore, it is best to decrease blood pressure gradually in angle-

Table 46.7.
Ability of Drugs to Induce Glaucoma

Drug	Route	Glaucoma Type	
		Open-Angle	Angle-Closure
Anticholinergics			
Atropine	Topical	Rare	Frequent
Scopolamine	Topical	Rare	Frequent
Belladonna	Topical	Rare	Frequent
Propantheline	Systemic	Rare	Rare
Adrenergics			
Phenylephrine 10%	Topical	Never	Occasional
Epinephrine	Systemic	Never	Rare
Miotics			
Pilocarpine 4–8%	Topical	Never	Occasional
Echothiophate	Topical	Never	Occasional
Isoflurophate	Topical	Never	Occasional
Carbonic anhydrase inhibitors			
Acetazolamide	Systemic	Never	Rare
Antihypertensives	Systemic	Never	Never
β-Chymotrypsin	Topical	Rare	Occasional
Prochlorperazine	Systemic	Never	Never
Promethazine (high doses)	Systemic	Never	Rare
Ganglionic blocking agents	Systemic	Rare	Occasional
Amphetamines	Systemic	Rare	Occasional
Tricyclic antidepressants	Systemic	Rare	Occasional
Corticosteroids (at equipotent doses)			
Betamethasone	Topical	Frequent	Never
Dexamethasone	Topical	Frequent	Never
Hydrocortisone	Topical	Occasional	Never
Prednisolone	Topical	Occasional	Never
Triamcinolone	Topical	Occasional	Never
Dexamethasone	Systemic	Occasional	Never
Hydrocortisone	Systemic	Occasional	Never
Prednisolone	Systemic	Occasional	Never

closure patients. If it is necessary to decrease blood pressure rapidly, one should either increase the patient's miotic medication or simultaneously lower the IOP rapidly with an agent such as acetazolamide.

Miscellaneous Agents

Amphetamines, tricyclic antidepressants, monamine oxidase inhibitors, indomethacin, and cocaine produce slight degrees of mydriasis, but the likelihood of inducing angle closure with these drugs is very low (6, 14). Strong miotics such as pilocarpine 4 to 8% and the indirect-acting nonreversible clolinesterase inhibitors may lead to pupillary block and inhibition of aqueous humor outflow and increase vascular congestion of the peripheral part of the iris so that the swollen iris block the canal of Schlemm and prevents the outflow of aqueous humor (6, 12, 14).

Polarizing neuromuscular blocking agents, such as succinylcholine, used as adjuvants to general anesthesia can cause a marked rise in IOP if the patient is not adequately anesthetized. They should not be used in glaucomatous

patients. A nondepolarizing neuromuscular blocking agent such as atracurium is effective in preventing the rise in IOP.

An acute transient myopia has occurred following vaginal absorption of AVC cream, which contains sulfanilamide, complicated by retinal edema, shallowing anterior chambers, and acute angle closure (16). Similar reactions have occurred with carbonic anhydrase inhibitors (17), tetracycline (18), prochloperazine, and promethazine (19). A few of these may be responsible for ocular hypertension, but more commonly they increase retinal fluid production. These reactions can be classified as idiosyncratic phenomena.

Patients who have received chymotrypsin B while undergoing cataract extraction characteristically show an increase in IOP 2 to 5 days after surgery, that lasts for a week or more (20). Deep anterior chambers and open angles are seen, differentiating chymotrypsin B from pupillary block-induced glaucoma. The induced ocular hypertension appears to be dose-related and self-limiting (21).

Corticosteroid-induced Glaucoma

Corticosteroid-induced glaucoma is well documented (6, 12, 13, 22–28). This form of glaucoma is usually without pain, physical findings in the eye, or visual field defects. The lesion probably occurs in the trabecular meshwork and severely decreases the outflow facility. Systematically or topically administered corticosteroids produce decreased outflow facility accompanied by a corresponding increase of IOP. After topical therapy, the glaucomatous change occurs in the eye instilled with the drug. This ocular hypertensive effect is usually fully reversible within 1 month after the discontinuation of the steroid.

The increase in IOP is approximately 10 mm Hg for patients with preglaucomatous anterior chambers and 5 mm Hg in normal persons. In some cases, irreversible eye damage occurs if ocular tension persists for 1 to 2 months or even longer. In addition, cupping of the optic disk and defects of the visual field may develop a few months after topical administration of corticosteroids is begun. Patients on chronic topical steroid therapy should therefore have tonometric examinations every 2 months.

The degree of rise in pressure appears to be associated with the antiinflammatory potency of the agents involved and is most marked with dexamethasone (23) and betamethasone. Equivalent doses of ophthalmic prednisolone and triamcinolone used four times daily gave elevations of IOP similar to those of betamethasone instilled only once daily. The duration of corticosteroid treatment and the age of the patient influenced the degree of ocular hypertension experienced. In some instances, topical epinephrine or systemic carbonic anhydrase inhibitors can maintain the ocular tension within normal limits. On other occasions, it may be necessary to reduce the frequency of administration or substitute a less potent steroid. Withdrawal of the drug may be necessary to return ocular tension to normal levels.

Steroids administered systemically can make preexisting open-angle glaucoma more difficult to control, but their effect on IOP is much smaller than that of topically applied steroids (25). Ocular hypertension may occur during prolonged systemic corticosteroid therapy, usually over a period of 1 year or more, in patients with such conditions as rheumatoid arthritis or systemic lupus erythematosus. However, this complication should not deter one from using systemic corticosteroid in situations where they are appropriate.

The ocular hypertension effect induced by topical steroids can be categorized for three groups of patients in the general population who do not have diagnosed glaucoma. Two-thirds of the general population (group 1) respond with an average rise in pressure of 1.6 mm Hg after 4 weeks of 0.1% dexamethasone 3 times daily (29). A second group (29%) responds with an average rise of 10 mm Hg. Finally, a third group (5%) responds with a rise greater than 16 mm Hg. For each group, the rate of IOP increase differs significantly. The clinical implication is that patients who are receiving corticosteroid for at least 1 month and who have tonometric pressures below 21 mm Hg are unlikely to have glaucomatous complications. In addition, since approximately one-third of the general population will have a group 2 or group 3 response to topical steroids, tonometric monitoring should be performed on a monthly basis.

Summary of Drug-induced Glaucoma

Table 46.7 lists drugs that can induce glaucoma. The following factors must be considered in assessing the problem of drug-induced glaucoma. Topically administered drugs induce glaucoma more frequency than those given systemically. Conditions under which any drugs are contraindicated are specific as to type of glaucoma and method of treatment for it. Seldom, if ever, does the warning against the use of a particular agent in glaucoma specify the type of glaucoma. Acute angle-closure glaucoma is an emergency, and any agent that might precipitate an attack must be used cautiously. Unfortunately, patients who are predisposed to angle-closure glaucoma are not accurately identified without a gonioscopic examination of the anterior angle. Patients with diagnosed angle-closure glaucoma will have had a corrective surgical procedure or be receiving medical therapy; these patients are not at risk for another episode of angle-closure glaucoma (30, 31). Patients with chronic open-angle glaucoma that is adequately controlled by therapy are not at risk when treated with either systemic anticholinergics or sympathomimetics. In general, remarkably few drugs, except ophthalmic preparations, worsen existing or potential glaucoma (6, 12).

Therapy

The goal of glaucoma therapy is the immediate and sustained reduction of IOP to prevent deterioration of the optic nerve and loss of vision. Drugs used in the treatment of glaucoma may be divided conveniently into those that increase the elimination of aqueous humor and those that decrease its formation. Parasympathomimetic miotic agents remove the obstruction to the outflow channels, thereby facilitating the elimination of aqueous humor. Sympathomimetic mydriatic agents lower elevated IOP by decreasing the rate of aqueous humor formation (14). β-Blockers such as timolol decrease the rate of aqueous secretion and also increase outflow, but the mechanism of action is not clearly understood (32–47). Secretion and inflow of aqueous humor are decreased most effectively by the carbonic anhydrase inhibitors (48). Hyperosmotic agents reduce IOP by increasing the osmolarity of the plasma relative to the aqueous and vitreous humor. Ocularly instilled parasympathomimetic miotics, sympathomimetic mydriatics, and orally administered carbonic anhydrase inhibitors find their greatest clinical application in primary open-angle glaucoma (Fig. 46.3 schematically shows the medical management of open-angle glaucoma) (49). Management of acute angle-closure glaucoma and congenital glaucoma is essentially surgical. Medical treatment is limited to preparing the patient for surgery (Fig. 46.4 contains a flowchart of the management of acute angle-closure glaucoma) (49). Treatment of secondary glaucoma should be directed at correcting the underlying cause as will as the elevation of IOP. Table 46.8 summarizes the basis of medical treatment of glaucoma.

Miotics

Miotics are cholinergic agents that facilitate the outflow of aqueous humor from the anterior chamber of the eye (Table 46.9). This is accomplished primarily by their action

Table 46.8
Basis of Medical Treatment for Glaucomas[a]

Because elevated intraocular pressure is responsible for glaucomatous damage in the majority of patients, therapeutic measures are directed at:

1. Increasing the rate of outflow of aqueous humor via the drainage system
   Drugs: Parasympathomimetics
         Sympathomimetics
         β-Blockers
2. Decreasing formation of aqueous humor by the ciliary processes
   Drugs: Sympathomimetics
         Carbonic anhydrase inhibitors
3. Reducing volume of aqueous humor in anterior chamber
   Drugs: Hyperosmotics

[a] From Leopold IH: Glaucoma Drug Therapy. Monograph IV-New Developments in Clinical Practice. Laguna Beach, CA: Allergan Pharmaceuticals, 1981.

Figure 46.3. Flowchart for the medical managment of primary open-angle glaucoma. Argon laser trabeculoplasty is used as an adjunct to drug therapy. (Adapted from Eskridge JB, Bartlett JD, The glaucomas. In Bartlett JD, Jaanus SD (eds): Clinical Ocular Pharmacology. Boston, Butterworths, 1988, p 766.)

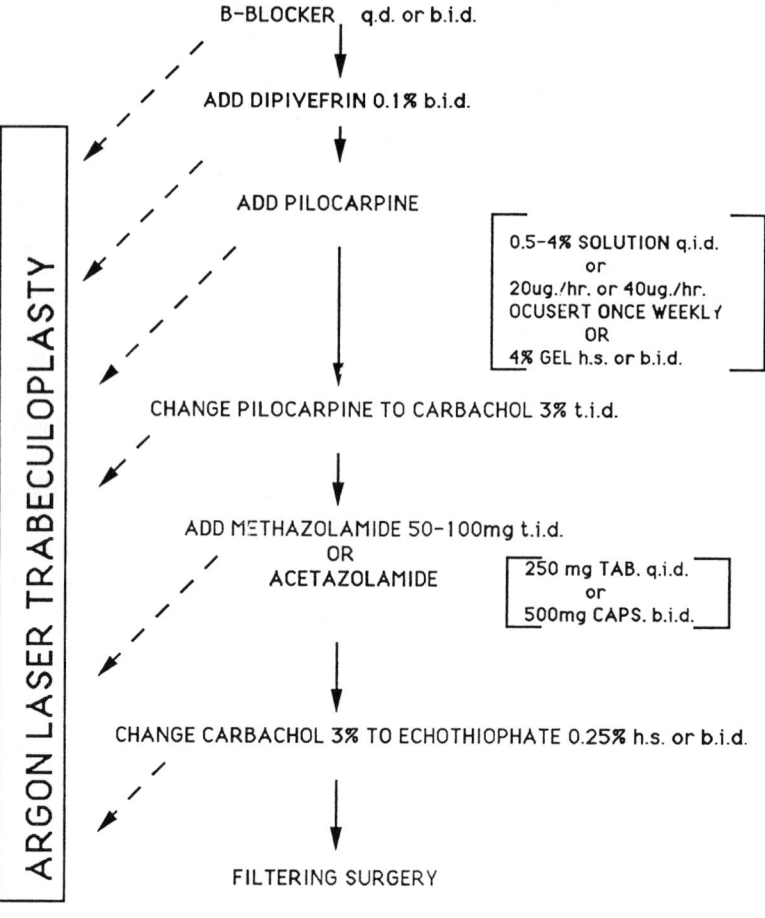

on the musculature of the iris and the ciliary body. The exact mechanism of improved fluid drainage remains poorly understood. The contraction of the ciliary muscle appears to be a primary mechanism by which the IOP is reduced. The trabecular meshwork and veins peripheral to the canal of Schlemm also may be dilated, thereby facilitating the outflow of aqueous humor. This action is independent of the pupillary constriction or miosis produced by the cholinergic miotic, since outflow is unaffected in the absence of miosis. Miotics can lower IOP directly by stimulating the postfunctional effector cells innervated by the cholinergic fibers. Structurally these agents are similar to acetylcholine. Cholinergic miotics are therapeutically beneficial for treatment of open-angle glaucoma and for preoperative preparation for surgery in angle-closure glaucoma. Their disadvantage is their short duration of action, requiring frequent administration.

PARASYMPATHOMIMETICS

Acetylcholine is not used in glaucoma therapy because of its poor corneal penetration upon ocular instillation and rapid inactivation by cholinesterase. Intraocular acetylcholine is used in ophthalmic surgery. Pilocarpine is the most common miotic used for initial and maintenance therapy of chronic primary open-angle glaucoma (2–4, 32). Pilocarpine penetrates the cornea after ocular instillation, with miosis and decreases in IOP reaching their maximum levels in 30 to 40 min (4, 31, 50–52). It is used in strengths varying from 0.5 to 10%, although there appears to be little if any therapeutic advantage in the use of concentrations above 4%. The duration of IOP lowering is 4 to 8 hr. The usual frequency of instillation is two or three times daily, but pilocarpine may be given as often as every 2 hr. The Ocusert system is an innovative method of pilocarpine administration. Slightly larger than a contact lens and containing pilocarpine solution in its core, it is worn in the conjunctival sac of the eye where the drug diffuses out at a constant rate. It is available as Pilo-20 or Pilo-40 and releases 20 and 40 μg of pilocarpine/hr, respectively. Patients previously using 0.5 or 1% drops are controlled with Pilo-20; those using 2 to 4% drops require Pilo-40. The Ocusert is replaced every 7 days. Advantages of the Ocusert include a constant rate of drug released and improved compliance. Disadvantages of the Ocusert include expense and irritation (foreign body sensation), which occasionally results in the patient having to return to pilocarpine drops (52, 53).

A pilocarpine HCL gel presoaked system is also avail-

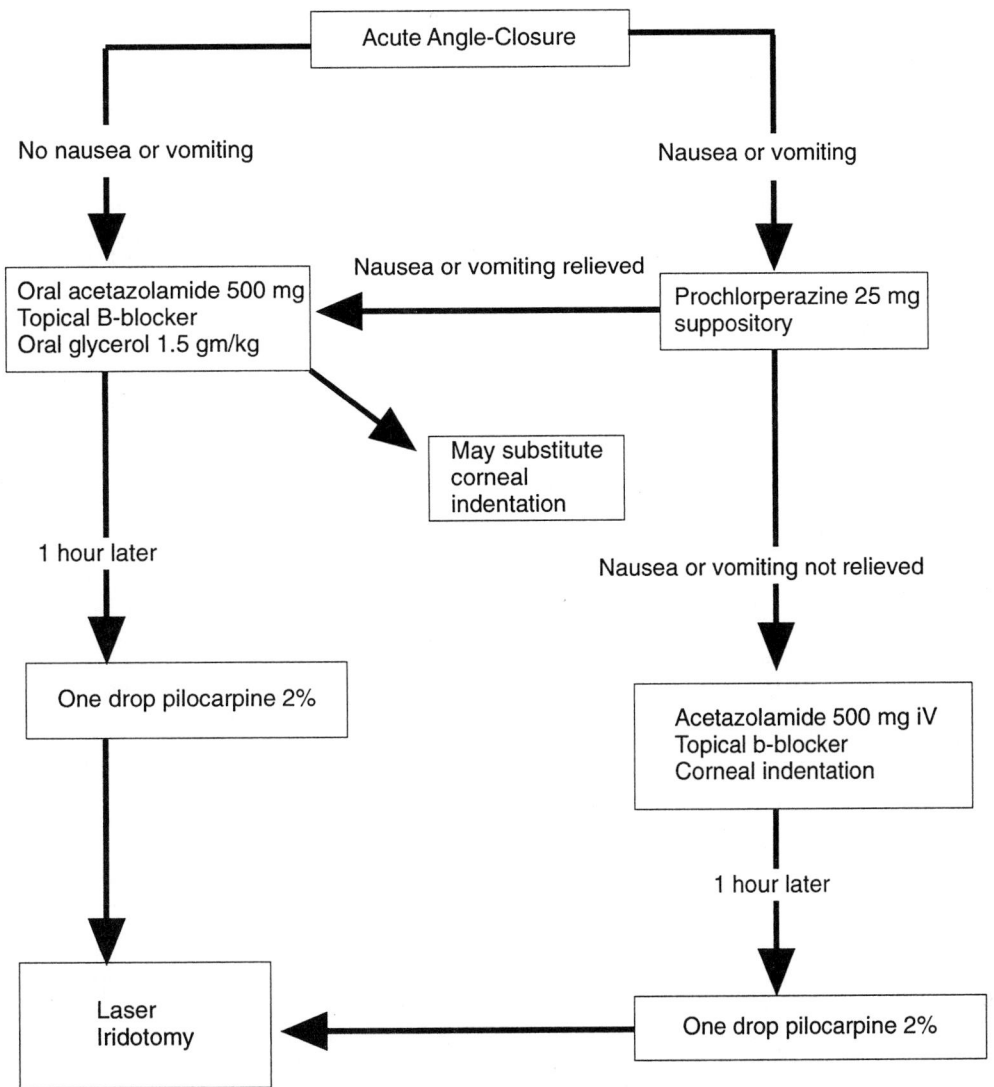

Figure 46.4. Flowchart for the managment of acute angle-closure glaucoma. (Reprinted with permission from Eskridge JB, Bartlett JD, The glaucomas. In Bartlett JD, Jaanus SD (eds): Clinical Ocular Pharmacology. Boston, Butterworths, 1988, p 743.)

able. Goldberg et al. compared 4% pilocarpine gel with 4% pilocarpine drops in 15 patients. The gel was applied only once a day in one eye and the drops were used four times a day in the other eye. IOP and pupil diameters were similar with both forms of pilocarpine except in the evening, when the eye treated with the gel showed no significant difference, compared to pretreatment values (54).

Carbachol is an unsubstituted carbamylester with a direct action like that of pilocarpine on parasympathetic receptors. It is totally resistent to hydrolysis by cholinesterase or acetylcholinesterase and therefore has a longer duration of action than pilocarpine in comparable strengths for IOP control. Solutions are available in strengths of 0.75 to 3%. In the treatment of open-angle glaucoma one drop is in-

stilled, usually two or three times daily. Response varies with the dose, and the weaker strength solutions require more frequent administration than usually suggested. When pilocarpine and other miotics cannot be used owing to either allergy or intolerable side effects, carbachol may be a suitable alternative. However, if the glaucoma is uncontrollable with pilocarpine, it is doubtful that carbachol would yield much, if any, therapeutic improvement.

Diurnal fluctuations of IOP are diminished more effectively by carbachol than by pilocarpine. The major disadvantage of carbachol is its poor corneal penetration. In addition, it must be prepared in a vehicle such as methylcellulose to ensure prolonged contact with cornea, or with a wetting agent such as benzalkonium chloride to enhance corneal penetration. In the treatment of none-

Table 46.9.
Miotic Drugs Used in the Management of Glaucoma

Drug	Dosage[a]	Comments
Parasympathomimetics		
Pilocarpine hydrochloride	0.25–10% instilled 1 or 2 drops in affected eye from q. 6–8 hr to as often as q. 4 hr	Onset of IOP lowering effect is rapid with a 4–6 hr duration; although strengths above 4% are available, there is little advantage to using any strength above 4%
Pilocarpine nitrate		
Pilocarpine gel	4% gel applied to affected eye h.s.	The gel dosage form is used as an adjunct to daytime medications
Ocuserts P-20 and P-40	Placed into the affected eye once a week.	Ocusert P-20 is generally used in patients controlled by a 2% solution or less; those requiring a greater strength use P-40
Carbachol	0.75–3% instilled 1 or 2 drops in affected eye from q. 8–10 hr to as often as q. 4 hr	Response varied with dose; may require frequent administration for weaker solutions than usually suggested; a suitable alternative when other miotics cannot be used because of allergy or side effects; poor corneal penetration; contraindicated in presence of corneal injury; longer acting than pilocarpine
Short-acting anticholinesterases		
Physostigmine salicylate	0.25–0.5% instilled 1 or 2 drops in affected eye q. 6–12 hr; 0.25% ointment applied at bedtime	Onset of IOP-lowering effect similar to pilocarpine; considered to be stronger miotic than pilocarpine; aqueous solutions unstable; decomposition on exposure to light
Physostigmine sulfate		
Neostigmine bromide	3–5% instilled 1 or 2 drops in affected eye q. 4–6 hr	More stable and less irritating than physostigmine; less effective because of poor corneal permeability
Long-acting anticholinesterases		
Echothiophate iodide	0.03–0.25% instilled 1 drop in affected eye no more frequently than q. 12 hr	Potent, long-acting; maximum effects in 10–20 hr and may persist for several days; unstable in solution; should be used when shorter-acting miotics are inadequate; contraindicated prior to filtering surgery; not used prior to cataract extraction
Demecarium bromide	0.125–0.25% instilled 1 or 2 drops in affected eye q. 12 hr	Potent, long-acting; should be used only when shorter acting miotics do not give desired result; duration of miosis is prolonged
Isoflurophate	0.025% instilled 1 or 2 drops in affected eye q. 12–24 hr. or longer weekly	Potent, long-acting; should be used when shorter-acting miotics are inadequate; unstable; ointment supposedly most stable and less irritating; blurring of vision common complaint with ointment

[a] For open-angle glaucoma.

dematous glaucoma, an ointment of carbachol applied locally twice daily causes blurring of vision, a disadvantage of any ophthalmic ointment.

Methacholine bromide is very similar pharmacologically to acetylcholine, except that it is hydrolyzed more slowly by acetylcholinesterase and is almost totally resistant to cholinesterase. However, poor corneal penetration and instability in solution make it an unsuitable miotic for clinical use in glaucoma.

ANTICHOLINESTERASE

The anticholinesterase miotics act by inhibiting the cholinesterase enzyme, thereby permitting the accumulation of acetylcholine and prolonging the parasympathetic activity on the effector end organs of the eye. Physostigmine and neostigmine are reversible agents with short durations of effect. Organophosphate compounds, such as demecarium, echothiophate, and isoflurophate, have long durations of action and are irreversible anticholinesterases. The essential pharmacologic difference between these compounds is the relative irreversibility or permanency of their parasympathomimetic activity. Although the direct- and indirect-acting parasympathomimetic miotics act pharmacologically on different sites, their clinical effects on lowering elevated IOP in glaucoma are quite similar (50, 55).

Anticholinesterase miotics are therapeutically beneficial for the treatment of primary open-angle glaucoma; they are not indicated for the treatment of angle-closure glaucoma or congenital glaucoma. Since these agents act indirectly by inhibiting cholinesterase activity and prolonging the effects of endogenous acetylcholine, parasympathetic fibers to the pupil must be functional. The anticholinesterases are not effective if given after retrobulbar injections of anesthesia such as during cataract extration, since liberation of acetylcholine is impaired.

Physostigmine lowers IOP by facilitating the outflow of aqueous humor. It has a longer duration of action and is considered to be a stronger miotic than pilocarpine. Physostigmine can be given in strengths of 0.25 to 1.0% every 4 to 6 hr. The onset of reduction in IOP usually occurs within 10 to 30 min, reaching its maximal effect within 1 to 2 hr and lasting 4 hr or more after instillation. The miotic effects may persist much longer. Aqueous solutions of physostigmine are unstable. Decomposition occurring with pH changes and upon exposure to light is detected by progressive darkening of the solution. Decomposition products of physostigmine are unstable, quite irritating, and therapeutically ineffective. Physostigmine ointment should be reserved for bedtime use because, the intense miosis produced soon after application is less discomforting for the patient while asleep. The prolonged duration of increased aqueous humor outflow facilitation is ideal and convenient because the patient need not be interrupted from sleeping to administer miotics (48, 54).

Neostigmine is more stable but less effective than physostigmine because of poorer corneal penetration. It is less irritating and has fewer unpleasant side effects than physostigmine. Ocular instillation of 3 to 5% aqueous solutions of neostigmine can be given every 4 to 6 hr alone or with pilocarpine on an alternating schedule. Demecarium is chemically similar to neostigmine, with miotic and IOP-lowering activity comparable to that of echothiophate and isoflurophate. In contrast to the organophosphates, the inhibition of cholinesterase activity by demecarium 0.06 to 0.25% instilled every 12 to 48 hr gives beneficial effects on IOP lasting from 12 hr to several days. In open-angle glaucoma, maximal reduction of IOP with demecarium is seen in 24 to 36 hr. The rapidity of the onset and duration of miosis is directly related to the concentrations used. Tolerance and refractoriness to demecarium occur earlier than with echothiophate and isflurophate.

Echothiophate has a slow onset but is a long-acting cholinesterase inhibitor (56). Aqueous solutions of 0.06 to 0.25% instilled 1 drop every 12 to 24 hr for open-angle glaucoma can produce miosis within 10 to 15 min, although maximal effect on lowering IOP is not seen until 10 to 20 hr later and may persist as long as 96 hr. Instillation of the 0.25% solution more often than twice daily does not appear to enhance the reduction if IOP (57).

The advantage of echothiophate is its long duration of action, requiring fewer installations and better control of the IOP on a diurnal basis. The intense miosis can produce a pupillary block and resultant shallowing of the anterior chamber of the eye. Therefore, in the presence of subacute narrow angles or angle-closure glaucoma, echothiophate should not be used. Aqueous solutions of echothiophate are unstable and must be prepared just before dispensing. Storage under refrigeration for no more than 6 months should be recommended to the patient.

Isoflurophate possesses the longest duration of action and is more potent than other anticholinestenases or parasympathomimetic miotics. A drop of 0.01 to 0.1% concentration once or twice daily produces effects on IOP similar to those of echothiophate in open-angle glaucoma. Miosis is maximal within 15 to 20 min. IOP is maximally reduced within 24 hr after instillation. Instillation of 0.1% solution more than twice daily yields very minimal additional therapeutic benefit.

ADVERSE SIDE EFFECTS

A direct and short-acting miotic such as pilocarpine can produce local conjunctival irritation as a result of frequent instillations. Allergic sensitivity or refractoriness to pilocarpine develops after prolonged use. Frequent instillation of the short-acting miotics can exacerbate chronic allergic conjunctivitis or blepharitis. Miosis itself can produce decreased night vision (58).

Discontinuation of the offending agent will most often eliminate the symptoms, or another miotic can be tried. Miotics may stimulate progressive deterioration of the visual field defect associated with glaucoma. Poor vision in dim light and blurring of vision from pupillary constriction and accommodative myopia are particularly troublesome for some patients. It is likely that the elderly patient already has diminished visual acuity and therefore should be made aware of the effect of the drug. This problem can be further complicated in aged patients who have cataracts in addition to impairment of vision.

Miotics can produce annoying side effects such as transient headaches, ocular and periorbital pain, twitching of the eyelids, ciliary congestion, and spasms. The direct long-acting anticholinesterase miotics produce the most severe symptoms, including discomfort associated with bright lights and close-up work. The affected eye is extremely myopic. This is particularly intense in younger patients who have active accommodation and are initially myopic. Patients should be reassured that these difficulties will usually diminish within a week or so. Severe fibrinous iritis can be induced by miotics and is most likely to occur with the long- and indirect-acting cholinesterase inhibitors. After intense and prolonged administration of the stronger miotics, pupillary cysts occur (59). These are seen more commonly in children, but the reason is not known.

Anticholinesterase miotics may also produce vitreous hemorrhaging, contact dermatitis, and allergic conjunctivitis. Retinal detachment and cataracts have been associated with the use of anticholinesterase miotics; however, their role is probably as a contributing factor secondary to underlying retinal pathology.

Glaucoma secondary to ocular inflammation may be exacerbated by these agents as a result of further vascular disruption. Lens opacities have been reported in patients treated with anticholinesterase miotics (60–64). Cataractogenic lens changes appear to be related to the drug, the concentration the patient is receiving, and the duration of treatment. Cataract formation does not appear to be directly associated with glaucomatous eyes; patients treated with miotics other than the anticholinesterase miotics are less likely to develop lens opacity. The lens changes may be partly reversible when the drug is discontinued. Progressive worsening of the cataract may occur, however, necessitating surgical extraction.

Systemic absorption of antiglaucoma drugs following ocular instillation may result in undesirable stimulating effects (65, 66). These are seen more commonly after administration of the indirect- and longer-acting anticholinesterase agents. Gastrointestinal disturbances (i.e., nausea, diarrhea, abdominal pain, muscle spasm and weakness, sweating, lacrimation, salivation, hypotension, bradycardia, bronchial constriction, and respiratory failure) have been experienced (67). Most systemic effects reverse rapidly after discontinuation of the drug. In severe cholinergic toxicity, atropine sulfate 2 mg or pralidoxine chloride 25 mg/kg intravenously or subcutaneously can be given without affecting the control of the glaucoma.

Any potent long-acting miotic agent should be used with caution when a patient has bronchial asthma, parkinsonism, peptic ulcer, or other gastrointestinal disease, since anticholinesterase systemic effects can exacerbate their clinical course. There is evidence that echothiophate and other organophosphates can traverse the placenta; therefore the potential risks and benefits must be considered during pregnancy (68).

When known sensitivities to these agents exist, they should not be used. Considerable inhibition of plasma cholinesterase can be produced by prolonged topical anticholinesterase therapy (69). A patient receiving these agents must be monitored closely for prolongation of apnea when given succinylcholine chloride during surgery (70).

Patients who may be exposed to organophosphate pesticides should be made aware of the potential problems and risks associated with prolonged topical anticholinesterase exposure. There is an additive and cumulative effect on the parasympathetic nervous system. Systemically administered cholinergic agents such as ambenomium, neostigmine, or physostigmine used in disorders such as myasthenia gravis can potentiate the action of the anticholinesterase miotics.

The long-acting, irreversible anticholinesterase miotics should be reserved for use in chronic primary noncongestive glaucoma and secondary glaucoma when the shorter-acting miotics or β-blockers have not successfully reduced the IOP. Undesirable side effects from these agents can also be minimized by instillation of their lowest effective concentrations at reasonable intervals.

Table 46.10.
β-Blockers Used in the Management of Glaucoma

Drug	Dosage[a]	Comment
Timolol	0.25% and 0.50% drops, intill 1 drop in affected eye q.d. or q. 12 hr	β-Blockers may be used in combination with other miotic agents or carbonic anhydrase inhibitors; may also be used with epinephrine, best results are obtained by administering the epinephrine about 4 hr after the timolol as the latter is releasing the receptors to which the epinephrine must bind
Levobunolol	0.50% drops, instill 1 drop q.d. or q. 12 hr	A nonselective β_1- and β_2-agent, it may in a number of patients be administered once a day
Betaxolol	0.50% drops, instill 1 drop q.d. or q. 12 hr	A cardioselective β-blocking agent, therefore it is advantageous over timolol in patients with respiratory diseases

[a] For open-angle glaucoma.

β-Blockers

The use of β-blockers in the treatment of glaucoma has been investigated for several years, and they are now the most widely prescribed drugs for the treatment of glaucoma (58). The reason for the initial clinical trials with these agents was the reduction of β-adrenergic activity, which seems to be beneficial in the reduction of IOP. These agents reduce or abolish β-adrenoreceptor stimulation caused by either catecholamine release from sympathetic nerve endings or the adrenal medulla or by injected sympathomimetic agents (32–47). Several β-blockers have been and are being used in the treatment of open-angle glaucoma, including timolol maleate (32–47), propranolol (71), pindolol (72), atenolol (73), levobunolol HCl, and betaxolol HCl. Only timolol, levobunolol, and betazolol are currently available (Table 46.10).

Timolol is a potent, short-acting, nonselective β-blocker. The ocular hypotensive effect is probably due to suppression of aqueous humor formation by the ciliary body (74, 75). An exact mechanism is not known at this time. Timolol is available as 0.25 and 0.5% solutions. The usual starting dose is one drop of 0.25% in the affected eye(s) twice a day. If this does not control the glaucoma, the dose may be increased to 0.5% solution, 1 drop twice a day (34). Timolol may be used alone or in combination with agents such as epinephrine, pilocarpine, carbachol, or acetazolamide (32, 76). The addition of timolol to the therapy of patients on these agents significantly reduced IOP (76). Conflicting reports about the reduction of IOP when timolol and epinephrine are combined have been clarified (77). The recommendation is that epinephrine be administered 3 hours after timolol.

Studies suggest that the effects of acetazolamide and timolol are similar in reducing IOP (78). However, the combination of these two agents may be more effective than either drug alone.

When adding timolol to a patient's therapy, the other agent should be continued as well. The other agents may be discontinued on the following day or doses adjusted, depending on the therapeutic response of the patient. Stabilization of timolol therapy may take several weeks. A reevaluation should take place 2 and 4 weeks after therapy is begun. If the IOP is maintained, the schedule may be decreased to one drop once a day because of the diurnal variations in IOP. Tonometer readings should be done at different times of the day (34–37, 39–42). If 1 drop of timolol (0.5% solution) twice a day is not effective (34), concomitant therapy with other agents is warranted.

Contraindications of timolol include use in patients with bronchospasm (including bronchial asthma or severe chronic obstructive pulmonary disease) and in those with congestive cardiac failure (79). β-Blockers should not be used alone in patients with angle-closure glaucoma (use with pilocarpine) (53, 55).

The newest β-blockers approved for treatment of ocular hypertension and chronic open-angle glaucoma are levobunolol and betaxolol. Levobunolol, a nonselective β_1 and β_2-blocking agent, successfully decreases IOP. It is available as a 0.5% solution and is recommended to be instilled once or twice a day. Wandel et al. (80) compared once-a-day dosing of levobunolol 0.5% or 1.0% and timolol 0.5% in 92 patients. Both levobunolol 0.5% and 1.0% were found to have an overall greater effect on IOP than timolol. This once-daily dosing of levobunolol improves patient compliance. If IOP is not controlled with a single dose of levobunolol, then the frequency of administration should be increased to twice a day; thus levobunolol offers no real advantage over timolol (80–83).

Betaxolol, a β_1-adrenergic blocking agent, is available as a 0.25% solution that is instilled into the eye every 12 hr. In a double-blind randomized study, betaxolol (0.5%) was compared with timolol (0.5%). The most frequently reported side effects were mild discomfort and tearing upon administration, but side effects were not sufficient to cause discontinuation of therapy. Both drugs had similar efficacy in reducing IOP (84). Betaxolol, unlike timolol, offers the advantage of little or no effect on pulmonary disease, but it should still be used with caution. In concentrations ranging from 0.125% to 1%, betaxolol has reduced IOP by as much as 10.1% (85). Because of its selective β-adrenergic activity, betaxolol produces a greater additive effect than timolol when administered concomi-

tantly with epinephrine. However, betaxolol, like other β-blockers, should not be administered to patients with heart failure (86–88).

Side effects of timolol and other β-blockers include burning or pain after instillation (most common), blurring of vision, and dilated pupils with epinephrine combination. Systemic side effects include cardiovascular problems (bradycardia, palpitations, hypertension, congestive heart failure), central nervous system disturbances (headaches, dizziness, drowsiness, anxiety, and depression), and pulmonary system side effects, including deaths due to precipitation or exacerbation of existing brochospasm (34–37, 39–42). Patients with diabetes should also use timolol with caution.

Sympathomimetics

Reduction of IOP in open-angle glaucoma may be accomplished successfully by ocular instillation of sympathomimetics. Their mechanism of action is not fully understood but the main effects appear to be decreasing the rate of aqueous humor production due to vasoconstriction and increasing its outflow.

Epinephrine, 1 to 2% solution instilled every 8 to 24 hr, can reduce IOP in open-angle glaucoma. The rate of aqueous secretion is initially decreased, probably by adrenergic stimulation at receptor sites in the ciliary epithelium. Improved facility of outflow is not immediate but may be seen after several months of epinephrine therapy. The probable mechanism suggested is α-adrenergic response to epinephrine at the trabecular meshwork. The pressure lowering by epinephrine of 3 to 15 mm Hg occurs in 6 to 8 hr and lasts from several hours to days. Patient response appears to be highly variable. Epinephrine is seldom used alone for open-angle glaucoma but is usually used with miotics (89–91). Epinephrine does not disturb accommodation and is especially beneficial in overcoming the disabling miosis induced by the parasympathomimetic. When used in combination, it should be given 5 to 10 min after the miotic has been instilled. Comparative effects of epinephrine bitartrate 2% and epinephrine borate 1% have been studied, and no statistical difference in ability to reduce IOP in glaucomatous eyes can be found between individual preparations (89). The commercial borate salt is buffered to enhance corneal penetration and is perhaps better tolerated than the others.

Dipivalyl HCl, a prodrug for epinephrine, is produced by the addition of two pivalyl side chains to epinephrine. Dipivalyl has better lipid solubility than epinephrine, and thus corneal penetration is better (approximately 17 times better). Studies have shown no significant difference in 0.1% dipivalyl (when compared with 2% epinephrine) in lowering IOP. Kass et al. (92) and Kohn et al. (93) compared 0.1% dipivalyl with 2% epinephrine in terms of their effect on lowering IOP, increasing pupil size, and the frequency of side effects. Both investigators found that these agents lowered IOP significantly. While dipivalyl was less effective in lowering IOP than epinephrine, fewer side effects were reported in patients receiving dipivalyl (33, 78, 92–94).

Phenylephrine has not proved to be any more effective than epinephrine in lowering IOP. A 10% solution of phenylephrine is used primarily in assisting with ophthalmoscopic examination, because it has disturbing cycloplegic effects. Propranolol is an α-adrenergic blocker used in the management of angina and cardiac arrhythmias. It has been demonstrated that 20 mg given orally is able to reduce IOP in open-angle glaucoma quite effectively. However, in many cases, the dose had to be increased with time, to maintain effective reduction of IOP. The fall in systemic blood pressure and the potential for cardiac difficulties associated with propranolol argue against its widespread use for the treatment of glaucoma.

Isoproterenol in a 5% solution produces comparable effects to those of epinephrine, with maximal reduction of IOP in 6 hr and persisting decreases for 12 to 60 hr. Widespread use of isoproterenol for ocular instillation is prevented by the common occurrence of systemic side effects such as tachycardia and palpitations (95).

Appreciable local and systemic side effects are experienced by patients who use ocular sympathomimetics for long periods of time (96). Local side effects include melanin deposits on the conjunctiva and cornea, hyperemia and corneal edema, and allergic blepharoconjunctivitis (96). Headache, periorbital pain, and lacrimation with intermittent visual blurring and distortion are common complaints. Although the frequency is relatively low, cardiac irregularities and elevations of blood pressure after ocular administration of epinephrine have been reported (97). Side effects, both local and systemic, are promptly relieved after the epinephrine is discontinued. Closer supervision and caution should be exercised for patients who are receiving anesthetics in preparation for surgery, because the reported rate of systemic side effects of the ocular sympathomimetic is higher in such cases. Sympathomimetics are contraindicated in angle-closure glaucoma prior to peripheral iridectomy. Gonioscopic examinations are advised before the ocular instillation of a sympathomimetic mydriatic, to rule out asymptomatic or subacute angle-closure glaucoma. After the iridectomy is performed, ocular epinephrine can be useful, especially if aqueous humor outflow is impaired. It should not be used if IOP can be adequately managed by miotics alone.

Carbonic Anhydrase Inhibitors

The lowering of IOP can be achieved by systemic administration of carbonic anhydrase inhibitors (Table 46.11) (48, 77, 99). These agents are of particular value where

control of glaucoma is unobtainable with parasympathomimethic miotics. Carbonic anhydrase, a widely distributed enzyme in the body, catalyzes the reversible reaction of water and carbon dioxide to form carbonic acid and subsequently the bicarbonate ion. In the eye, large concentrations of carbonic anhydrase are found in the ciliary process and retina. The mechanism of action of the carbonic anhydrase inhibitor on IOP is not clearly understood. Acetazolamide increases the outflow of aqueous fluid in some glaucoma patients, whereas a decrease in outflow occurs in normal eyes and in eyes with very early glaucoma. The lowering of the intraocular volume does not depend upon the diuretic effect of carbonic anhydrase inhibitors and cannot be explained simply as a depletion of the bicarbonate ion content. The buffer system necessary for maintaining secretory functions in the ciliary epithelium is probably impaired or inhibited, thus reducing aqueous humor formation. Only slight changes in IOP are experienced in normotensive eyes when carbonic anhydrase inhibitors are administered. There is no effect on the IOP when carbonic anhydrase inhibitors are instilled locally. These drugs are used concomitantly with cholinergic miotics and hyperosmotic agents for the emergency treatment of primary angle-closure glaucoma. Prompt and vigorous reduction of IOP to normal levels before peripheral iridectomy gives a better postoperative prognosis (100).

A single dose of oral or intravenous acetazolamide can reduce IOP for 4 to 6 hr. The maximum effect is seen about 2 hr after oral administration. Following intravenous administration, the maximum effect is attained within 20 min. Hypersecretion glaucoma that is infrequent can respond to treatment with carbonic anhydrase inhibitors alone. In chronic primary glaucoma where control has been difficult to obtain with miotics or during acute exacerbations, addition of a carbonic anhydrase inhibitor to cholinergic and sympathomimetic agents may produce satisfactory ocular tension control. Carbonic anhydrase inhibitors are useful in the short-term management of glaucoma secondary to trauma or uveitis and in the preoperative management of congenital glaucoma. Their use in chronic angle-closure glaucoma should be discouraged because symptoms of progressive angle narrowing can easily be obscured.

Long-term use of carbonic anhydrase inhibitors is frequently unsuccessful because of their side effects. Patients differ in their ability to tolerate the various carbonic anhydrase inhibitors, and some may be better tolerated.

The drug of choice is usually acetazolamide tablets. However, more than 50% of patients are unable to tolerate this therapy. Acetazolamide sustained-release capsules are somewhat better tolerated, but approximately 40% of patients cannot tolerate acetazolamide in this dosage form. Between 25 and 50% of patients who are intolerant of acetazolamide will be able to take methazolamide. There-

Table 46.11.
Carbonic Anhydrase Inhibitors Used to Manage Glaucoma[a]

Drug and Dosage Form	Dose	Onset	Duration	Comment
Acetazolamide tablets 125 & 250 mg	125–250 mg q.i.d.	½–1 hr	4–6 hr	Used in short-term therapy for primary and secondary glaucoma especially if refractory or uncontrollable by miotics; used with miotics and hyperosmotics in emergency treatment of primary angle-closure glaucoma; fair success with long-term use in open-angle glaucoma; failures frequently due to side effects; carbonic anhydrase inhibitor of choice in management of glaucoma
Acetazolamide sequels 500 mg	500 mg b.i.d.	1–2 hr	10–18 hr	
Acetazolamide IV 500 mg vials	500 mg IV	1 min	4 hr	
Methazolamide tablets 25 and 50 mg	25–100 mg b.i.d. or t.i.d.	1 hr	10–14 hr	50 mg is equivalent to 250 mg of acetazolamide; few significant differences from acetazolamide with exception of side effects and slower onset of action; drowsiness, fatigue, malaise with minimal gastrointestinal disturbance are common; main indication for chronic glaucoma insufficiently controlled by miotics or acetazolamide
Dichlorphenamide tablets 50 mg	25–50 mg b.i.d., t.i.d., or q.d.	½ hr	6–12 hr	Metabolic acidosis occurs less frequently with dichlorphenamide than with other carbonic anhydrase inhibitors; used with patient intolerant or refractory to acetazolamide; anorexia, nausea, paresthesias, dizziness, or ataxia and tremor should alert one of the possibility of toxicity

[a] Adapted from Flach AJ: Topical acetazolamide and other carbonic anhydrase inhibitors in the current medical therapy of the glaucomas. Glaucoma 8:20–27, 1986.

fore, patients suffering considerable adverse effects of acetazolamide can be tried on the sustained-release capsules or switched to methazolamide. A reduction in dose also may decrease the side effects. Other ways of minimizing the side effects of carbonic anhydrase inhibitors have not been substantiated. Dicholorphenamide and ethoxozolamide have a greater propensity to cause side effects leading to discontinuation of therapy and are rarely used. Older patients appear to be more intolerant to the carbonic anhydrase inhibitors than younger patients (101–103).

The gastrointestinal effects are a common cause of discomfort for the patient and often become so severe that the drug is discontinued. Nausea, vomiting, intestinal colic, diarrhea, anorexia, and paresthesia of the face and extremities are common side effects. Transient myopia is an unusual and rare occurrence. Long-term treatment with a carbonic anhydrase inhibitor does not appear to deplete intracellular potassium. Since there may be marked depletion of electrolytes, including potassium (104), when treatment with the agent is begun, serum potassium levels and clinical manifestations of cellular potassium depletion should be monitored (105). However, the routine supplementation of potassium for glaucoma patients receiving carbonic anhydrase inhibitors is not encouraged and is of doubtful value in the absence of depletion.

Acetazolamide produces hyperglycemia in prediabetics and diabetics receiving oral hypoglycemic agents. Hyperuricemia has occurred following treatment with carbonic anhydrase inhibitors. Prolonged use of these drugs can lead to urinary and renal colic secondary to formation of calcium calculi (105, 106). Alkalinization of the urine by acetazolamide results in an enhanced renal tubular reabsorption of drugs such as quinidine, amphetamine, and the tricyclic antidepressants. Alkalinization of the urine can also decrease the acid-dependent antibacterial activity of methenamine. Exfoliative dermatitis secondary to these agents is similar to dermatologic reactions encountered with the sulfonamides. Rare occurrences of idiosyncratic reactions such as cholestatic jaundice, drug fever, and blood dyscrasias including thrombocytopenia, agranulocytosis, and aplastic anemia have been reported. Carbonic anhydrase inhibitors are not recommended in patients with hemorrhagic glaucoma, hepatic or renal dysfunction, and renocortical hypofunction, or a history of prior sensitivities to the drug.

Hyperosmotic Agents
Hyperosmotic agents lower the IOP by creating an osmotic gradient between the plasma and aqueous humor from the anterior chamber of the eye (Table 46.12) (107). Given systemically, these agents draw fluids from the anterior chamber of the eye into the plasma. Hyperosmotic agents are most useful in the preoperative management of primary acute angle-closure glaucoma. The degree of IOP lowering depends upon the tension elevation and the osmotic gradient induced. The greatest effect of rapid changes in plasma osmolarity is on the eye, with very profound pressure elevations. The most commonly used hyperosmotics are mannitol, urea, and glycerol (108).

Mannitol can effectively reduce acutely elevated IOPs when given slowly by the intravenous route as a 20% solution to adults and a 10% solution to children (109, 110).

Table 46.12.
Hyperosmotic Agents Used in the Management of Glaucomas

Drug	Dosage (g/kg body wt)	Route	Comments
Ascorbic Acid	0.4–1.0	IV or oral	Gastric distress and diarrhea oral administration; seldom used since more effective agents are available
Glycerin (50% soln)	1.0–1.5	Oral	Nausea, vomiting, hyperglycemia can occur; caution in diabetic patients; as effective as intravenous hyperosmotic agents; less diuresis produced
Isosorbide	1–2	Oral	Can be given to diabetic; effects on intraocular tension comparable to those of intravenous hyperosmotics; diarrhea, nausea, and vomiting less frequently experienced
Mannitol (20% soln)	1.0–2.0	IV	Requires larger volumes than other hyperosmotics; rapid diuresis produced; not metabolized; can be used in diabetics; less irritating and free of tissue necrosis when solution extravasates; not contraindicated in patents with renal disease; monitor for cellular dehydration, hypokalemia, cardiac irregularities, urinary output, and chest pain; more effective for glaucoma with inflammation than urea or glycerol; avoid excessive hydration if therapeutic effect diminishes
Urea (30% soln)	1.0–1.5	IV	Given intravenously over 30 min; unstable; side effects are sloughing, phlebitis, acute psychosis, severe headaches, nausea, vomiting hemolysis "rebound diuresis"; contraindicated in nephrotic patients; caution in hepatic impairment; use freshly made solution only; maximal effect 1 hr

The ocular hypotensive effect is produced in 30 to 60 min and lasts from 4 to 6 hr. The effectiveness of the hyperosmotic agents depends upon the rate of administration. Mannitol is preferred in the management of secondary glaucoma accompanied by hyperemia or uveitis, because it penetrates the eye less readily, which is an advantage when inflammatory processes are active. Agents that enter the eye rapidly produce a lower osmotic gradient and a shorter duration of action than those that do so slowly or not at all. Inflammation greatly increases the ocular permeability of agents such as urea. Therefore, it is less desirable under those circumstances. There is relatively less local tissue irritation, thrombophlebitis, and necrosis occurring with mannitol than with urea when given intravenously. Renal disease does not contraindicate the use of mannitol.

Excessive thirst is a common sensation experienced by patients following infusion of hyperosmotic agents. However, these patients should not be given fluids during the period of osmotic dehydration. Secondary rises in IOP occur after administration of fluids, diminishing the therapeutic effects of the hyperosmotics. Headache is also a common complaint but can be minimized simply by bed rest. Symptoms of cellular dehydration, hypokalemia, and cardiac irregularities secondary to mannitol therapy should be monitored. On rare occasions, disorientation and severe agitation may be observed. Pulmonary edema and congestive heart failure may be precipitated in the elderly, especially with mannitol infusions. Potassium deficiency can accompany diuresis following hyperosmotic infusion, and cardiac patients and patients with hepatic or renal disorders should be cautiously monitored. Since mannitol is not absorbed orally, it is not effective when given by that route.

Urea given by the intravenous route as a 30% solution will reduce elevated IOP within 30 to 40 min (111). Miotics and carbonic anhydrase inhibitors are used concomitantly with urea in the management of acute glaucoma prior to surgery. Nausea, vomiting, confusion, disorientation, and anxiety are seen. Severe headache, a common complaint, can begin soon after the initiation and continue for the duration of the intravenous infusion. The patient's head should not be elevated during this time.

Although urea produces less cellular dehydration because of its ease of penetrability into the cell, a "rebound phenomenon" can occur as the plasma level of the hyperosmotic agent drops below that of the vitreous fluid. As the urea is cleared from the circulation rapidly with diuresis, the osmolality of the blood will decline. The hyperosmotic vitreous in turn draws fluid into the eye, resulting in an increased IOP or pressure "rebound" effect.

Ascorbic acid successfully reduces IOP in rabbits with glaucoma (112). In cases of refractoriness to acetazolamide and miotics, ascorbic acid given intravenously can lower the ocular hypertension. A 20% solution of sodium ascorbate at a pH of 7.2 to 7.4 can produce normal ocular tension in 60 to 90 min.

Oral hyperosmotic agents effectively reduce elevated IOP and are useful where the rapid-action infused preparations are not required. Glycerol is a convenient hyperosmotic agent when given as a 50 or 75% solution (114). The ocular penetration of glycerol is poor; therefore a substantial osmotic gradient can be produced between the plasma and aqueous humor. IOP reduction is as effective as with hyperosmotic agents given by intravenous infusion. IOPs normally return to pretreatment levels within 5 to 6 hours. Hyperglycemia and glycosuria can occur following glycerol and should be used with particular caution in labile diabetics (113, 114). Acute diabetic ketoacidosis has been reported following treatment with glycerol (113). Nausea, diarrhea, and headache are also common complaints following oral glycerol. (113).

The reduction of IOP with isosorbide is comparable

to that of intravenous mannitol, urea, or oral glycerol. Given as a 50% solution orally, its absorption is rapid, and it is primarily unchanged upon excretion in the urine. Effective reduction in IOP occurs within 30 min after ingestion and remains for 1 to 2 hr or more, depending on the dose. Side effects include transient headaches and diarrhea. Other gastrointestinal disturbances such as nausea are usually less of a problem with isosorbide than glycerol (115).

MEDICAL MANAGEMENT

Conservative medical treatment can successfully control most cases of chronic open-angle glaucoma. The stage or severity of the disease as evidenced by the condition of the optic disk and the quality of the visual field should be the major factors in choosing the treatment. Mild elevations of IOP (less than 30 mm Hg) in the presence of a normal optic disk and visual field is not an absolute indication for therapy. These patients should have routine periodic examinations to detect any optic changes, because such changes can be detected long before permanent visual field impairment. There is no absolute level of IOP that must be maintained to assure therapeutic success. The IOP should be maintained at a level that prevents further deterioration of the optic disk and impairment of visual field. If the disk is normal on gonioscopic examination, an IOP in the high 20s is not as important clinically as one with concurrent disk involvement or abnormal visual field. The former situation may warrant only close periodic follow-up, whereas in the latter appropriate medical treatment should be started. If there is the slightest indication of disk pathology, the IOP should be maintained at 20 mm Hg or even lower by medical management. In cases of considerable disk degeneration and visual field loss, vigorous treatment should be undertaken to obtain a level of 15 mm Hg or lower.

In situations where advanced cupping of the optic disk and visual loss is not apparent in the presence of high IOP (greater than 30 mm Hg), medical therapy should be initiated. The aim of therapy is to lower the IOP enough to interrupt the course of the disease. Problems common to antiglaucoma therapy must be considered before reducing IOP with drugs. The expense and inconvenience of the medications should be considered as well as whether the side effects and toxicities of the drugs constitute a greater risk to the patient than the increased level of IOP.

For primary open-angle glaucoma, a miotic agent should be given at its lowest effective concentration and at intervals no more frequent than necessary to maintain a satisfactory level of IOP. The IOP should be measured before beginning therapy. The effects of therapy on the IOP can be determined within a week or more. If the reduction of IOP is not satisfactory, the concentration of the miotic agent should be increased, keeping in mind,

however, that there is little advantage to using concentrations of pilocarpine solutions greater than 4% or its equivalent.

Refractoriness often occurs following prolonged use of cholinergic miotics. Rather than increase the frequency of instillation or strength used, an alternative agent should be selected. Responsiveness to the cholinergic miotics often is restored after their replacement for a brief period by an anticholinesterase miotic. Various combinations of glaucoma medications are often given together to potentiate their therapeutic effects. However, not all combinations produce an additive pharmacologic response.

Epinephrine or phenylephrine may be added to miotic therapy if IOP control is inadequate, provided that gonioscopic examination has failed to demonstrate excessive narrowing of the anterior chamber angle (116). There is evidence suggesting that greater activity is produced when pilocarpine and epinephrine are applied separately rather than in combination (117, 118). Combinations of anticholinesterase miotics can reduce rather than potentiate the effectiveness of each other. Prior installations of physostigmine or demecarium will reduce the activity of subsequently instilled echothiophate or isoflurophate by competitive inhibition of the acetylcholinesterase. Pretreatment with either echothiophate or isoflurophate will enhance only slightly the activity of physostigmine or demecarium. However, the actions of physostigmine on demecarium are additive rather than competitive, regardless of their order of instillation. Differences in the duration of action and type of cholinesterase-inhibiting activity inherent with each miotic given in combination contribute to these predictable responses. Concomitant instillation of miotics, particularly those that act indirectly, offers very few advantages and should not be used in attempts to treat difficult-to-control open-angle glaucoma.

β-Blocker therapy has recently become the most widely prescribed drug therapy for the treatment of glaucoma (timolol is the most widely used drug) (58, 120). Combination of β-blocker with pilocarpine, epinephrine, or acetazolamide have also been used effectively. Other agents may be used when glaucoma is refractory to the cholinergic miotics; however, a β-blocker should be selected first because it has fewer side effects and is more effective.

Addition of an agent from another class of antiglaucoma drugs is preferred to substitution or addition of an agent from the same group. Deterioration of the glaucoma should always be ruled out. The storage condition of the medication, expiration date, and method of administration should be assessed when a patient experiences diminished effects from the eye drops.

SURGICAL MANAGEMENT

Surgical management of open-angle glaucoma should be reserved for situations in which maximal efforts utilizing

Table 46.13.
Basis of Surgical Treatment for Glaucomas

- Reestablish circulation between posterior and anterior chamber
  Procedure—Peripheral iridectomy
- Create new outflow channels
  Procedures—Iridencleisis

          Trephine with iridectomy
          Sclerectomy
          Cyclodialysis
          Cyclodiathermy
          Cyclocryosurgery
          Goniotomy

miotics, sympathomimetics, β-blockers, and carbonic anhydrase inhibitors have been unsuccessful in maintaining an acceptable level of IOP and preventing progressive changes of the optic disk or the visual field. The surgical procedure involves creating a collateral drainage from the anterior chamber. An acute-closure glaucoma attack must receive prompt and intensive attention to avoid irreparable damage to the eye. Pilocarpine 1 to 4% or an equivalent cholinergic miotic is instilled into the affected eye at frequent intervals (every 15 min for 1 hr, then every hour for 4 to 6 hr) until the IOP is reduced to levels at which surgery can be performed. The surgical procedure is a peripheral iridectomy, which allows the anterior chamber to communicate with the posterior chamber.

Table 46.13 summarizes the basis of surgical treatment of glaucoma. Cholinesterase-inhibiting miotics should be avoided. Intravenous or oral carbonic anhydrase inhibitors or hyperosmotic agents may be required in a patient with an acutely dilated pupil not responsive to the miotic agent.

Control of an attack should be established within 1 to 2 hr following the initiation of this intensive treatment. The subsequent involvement in the unaffected eye is greatly reduced when pilocarpine is given as a prophylactic measure. Instillation of pilocarpine at normal intervals into the unaffected eye following an episode of acute angle-closure glaucoma is considered appropriate. Treatment of secondary glaucoma should be directed by the underlying and contributory factors. Medical treatment of congenital glaucoma may lower IOP levels, but this disorder can be successfully corrected only by surgery.

LASER THERAPY

Laser trabeculoplasty, an alternative to surgery, is now the most often used nonpharmacologic means of treating chronic open-angle glaucoma. Laser iridotomy, in most cases, is recommended over traditional surgery in angle-closure glaucoma. Remis et al. reported that laser surgery can reduce the IOP by 7 to 13 mm Hg in over 80% of patients (33).

ARGON LASER TRABECULOPLASTY (ALT)

At least 1 hr before laser trabeculoplasty, apraclonidine hydrochloride 1% is instilled into the operated eye for control of IOP. Apraclonidine hydrochloride is an α-adrenergic agonist that is used in a sterile isotonic solution. Ophthalmic apraclonidine when instilled into the eye has minimal cardiovascular effects and reduces IOP (123, 124). It does not have any significant local anesthetic activity and has minimal effect on cardiovascular parameters when instilled into the eye (123 124). It is used in conjunction with trabeculoplasty to prevent an acute elevation in IOP, which can occur after ALT. An elevated IOP is a risk factor in the pathogenesis of visual field loss. The mechanism of action of apraclonidine HCl has not been established, but it is postulated that its action may be related to a reduction in aqueous formation. Its onset of action is seen within 1 hr of instillation, and maximal effect is seen within 3 to 5 hr. It is used 1 hr prior to ALT, and a second drop is instilled immediately after completion of the laser surgical procedure (123–124). Apraclonidine hydrochloride has replaced pilocarpine as the agent of choice prior to ALT. A topical anesthetic is instilled prior to the procedure, and then the patient is seated at the slit lamp laser photocoagulator.

Using the argon laser coupled to a high-magnification biomicroscope, the surgeon places approximately 50 to 100 lesions in an evenly spaced sequence on the inner surface of the trabecular meshwork. Histopathologic studies have shown by scanning electron microscopy that laser light energy produces fibrosis at the treatment site. It is theorized that these laser "burns" cause localized shrinkage, which in turn produces tension on the adjacent, untreated trabecular beams. The previously collapsed spaces between the beams are then pulled open, allowing aqueous humor to pass more easily and resulting in a reduction in IOP (119, 121).

LASER IRIDOTOMY

Laser iridotomy is the treatment of choice for pupillary block or angle-closure glaucoma. In most cases, laser surgery is recommended over traditional surgery. It is performed on an outpatient basis. One hour prior to laser iridotomy surgery, topical apraclonidine hydrochloride 1% (Iopidine) is instilled in the eye, along with pilocarpine drops. The pilocarpine causes pupillary constriction, which thins the iris, making laser puncture much easier. At the time of laser surgery, a topical anesthetic is instilled. Using either the Nd:YAG laser or the Argon laser, an opening measuring approximately 50 to 100 microns in diameter is created in the peripheral iris. This iridotomy releases the pupillary block component of angle-closure glaucoma, thus breaking the attack of glaucoma or serving as prophylaxis against subsequent attacks (125).

Complications of laser treatment of glaucoma include

intraocular inflammation in the form of uveitis, intraocular bleeding, elevated IOP, diplopia, pigment dissemination, and lens injury (34, 85, 119–121).

CONCLUSION

The successful outcome of glaucoma treatment depends greatly upon the patient's proper use of medications. An asymptomatic patient who does not understand why expensive and inconvenient eyedrops are required will be less inclined to use them according to prescribed instructions. The blurring of vision and occasional discomfort associated with the use of these medications further enhance noncompliance. As a consequence, visual function is often irreversibly impaired, and drugs no longer influence the clinical course of the disease. The patient with glaucoma should understand the nature of the disorder and appropriate expectations for the drugs being used against it. Optimal therapeutic results can occur only in an environment of mutual cooperation and understanding between patients and the healthcare providers responsible for their care.

REFERENCES

1. Sommer A: Glaucoma screening: too little, too late? J Gen Intern Med 5:533, 1990.
2. Newell FW, The glaucomas. In: Ophthalmology: Principles and Concepts. St. Louis, CV Mosby, 1986, Ch 20.
3. Paton D, Craig JA: Glaucomas: diagnosis and management. Clin Symp 28:20, 1976.
4. Vaughan D, Glaucoma. In Vaughn D, Asbury T, and Tabbaka KF (eds): General Ophthalmology, ed. 12 Los Altos, CA, Lange Medical Publications, 1989, pp 190–205.
5. Margolis KL, Rich EC: Open-angle glaucoma. Prim Care 16:197, 1989.
6. Fraunfelder FT: Drug-Induced Ocular Side Effects and Drug Interactions, ed. 2. Philadelphia: Lea & Febiger, 1982.
7. Grant WM: Ocular complications of drugs-glaucoma. JAMA 207:2089, 1969.
8. Harris LS: Cycloplegic-induced intraocular pressure elevations. Arch Ophthalmol 79:242, 1968.
9. Mehra KS, Chandra P, Khare BB: Ocular manifestations of parenteral administration of scopolamine (hyoscine). Br J Ophthalmol 49:557, 1965.
10. Lazenby GW, Reed JW, Grant WM: Anticholinergic medications in open-angle glaucoma. Arch Ophthalmol 84:719, 1970.
11. Mulberger RD: Effect of a common cold product containing belladonna on intraocular pressure. Eye Ear Nose Throat Mouth 47:61–64, 1968.
12. Spaeth GL: General medications, glaucoma and disturbances of intraocular pressure. Med Clin North Am 53:1109, 1969.
13. Grant WM, Systemic drugs and adverse influence on ocular pressure. In Leopold IH (ed): Symposium on Ocular Therapy. St. Louis, CV Mosby, 1968, vol 3, p 57.
14. Willets GS: Ocular side effects of drugs. Br J Ophthalmol 53:252, 1969.
15. Drance SM: The effects of phospholine iodide on the lens and anterior chamber depth. In Liopold IH (ed): Symposium on Ocular Therapy. St. Louis, CV Mosby, 1969, vol 4, p 25.
16. Maddalena MA: Transient myopia associated with acute glaucoma

and retinal edema following vaginal administration of sulfanilamide. Arch Ophthalmol 80:186, 1986.
17. Galin MA, Baras I, Zweifach P: Diamox-induced myopia. Am J Ophthalmol 54:237, 1962.
18. Edwards TS: Transient myopia due to tetracycline, JAMA 186:69, 1963.
19. Bard LA: Transient myopia associated with promethazine therapy. Am J Ophthalmol 58:682, 1964.
20. Jocson VL: Tonograph and gonioscopy—before and after cataract extraction with alpha chymotrypsin. Am J Ophthalmol 60:318, 1965.
21. Havener WF, Alpha-chymotrypsin. In Havener WF (ed): Ocular Pharmacology, part I, ed. 4. St. Louis, CV Mosby, 1978, p 46.
22. Armaly MF: Inheritance of dexamethasone hypertension and glaucoma. Arch Ophthalmol 77:747, 1967.
23. Armaly MF: Effect of corticosteroids on intraocular pressure and fluid dynamics. II. The effect of dexamethasone in the glaucomatous eye. Arch Ophthalmol 70:492, 1963.
24. Becker B, Hahn KA: Topical corticosteroids and heredity in primary open-angle glaucoma. Am J Ophthalmol 57:543, 1964.
25. Bernstein HN, Schwartz B: Effects of long-term systemic steroids on ocular pressure and tonographic values. Arch Ophthalmol 68:742, 1962.
26. Burde RM, Becker B: Steroid-induced glaucoma and cataracts in contact lens wearers. JAMA 213:2075, 1970.
27. Kolker AE, Becker B, Mills DW: Topical corticosteroids in secondary glaucoma. Arch Ophthalmol. 72:772, 1964.
28. Smith CL: Corticosteroid glaucoma—a summary and review of the literature. AM J Med Sci 252:239, 1966.
29. Havener WF, Corticosteroid therapy. In Havener WF (ed): Ocular Pharmacology, part 1, ed. 4, St. Louis, CV Mosby, 1978, p 347.
30. Hiatt RL, Fuller JB, Smith L, et al.: Systemically administered anticholinergic drugs and introcular pressure. Arch Ophthalmol 84:735–740, 1970.
31. Durkee DP, Bryant BG: Drug therapy of glaucoma. Am J Hosp Pharm 35:682–690, 1978.
32. Leopold IH: Glaucoma Drug Therapy, Monograph IV-New Developments in Clinical Practice. Laguna Beach, CA: Allergan Pharmaceuticals, 1981.
33. Remis LL, Epstein DL: Treatment of glaucoma, Annu Rev Med 35:195, 1984.
34. Anon: Timoptic in the Management of Chronic Open-Angle Glaucoma, vol. II, West Point, PA: Merck Sharp and Dohme Publishers, 1979.
35. Wilcockson J, Wilcockson T: Long-term use of timolol in open-angle glaucoma. Curr Ther Res 27:545, 1980.
36. Anon: Beta blockers for glaucoma. Lancet 1:1064, 1979.
37. Boger WP III, Steinert RF, Puliafito CA, et al.: Clinical trial comparing timolol ophthalmic solution to pilocarpine in open-angle glaucoma. Am J Ophthalmol 86(1):8–18, 1978.
38. Korey MS, Hodapp E, Kass MA, et al.: Timolol and epinephrine, Long-term evaluation of concurrent administration. Arch Ophthalmol 100:742, 1982.
39. Phillips CI, et al.: Penetration of timolol eye drops into human aqueous humor. Br J Ophthalmol 65:593, 1981.
40. LeBlanc RP, Krip G: Timolol. Canadian multicenter study. Ophthalmology 88:244, 1981.
41. Lin Ll, Galin MA, Obstbaum SA, et al.: Long-term therapy. Surv Ophthalmol 23(6):377–380, 1979.
42. Thomas JV, Epstein DL: Timolol and epinephrine in primary open-angle glaucoma. Transient additive effect. Arch Ophthalmol 99:91, 1981.
43. Kass MA: Efficacy of combining timolol with other antiglaucoma medications. Surv Ophthalmol 28(suppl):274, 1983.
44. Keates EU, Stone RA: Safety and effectiveness of concomitant ad-

ministration of dipivefrin and timolol maleate. Am J Ophthalmol 91:243, 1981.

45. Levy NS, Boone L, Ellis E: A controlled comparison of betaxolol and timolol with long-term evaluation of safety and efficacy. Glaucoma 7(2):54, 1985.

46. Berry DP, Van Buskirk EM, Shields MB: Betaxolol and timolol. A comparison of efficacy and side effects. Arch Ophthalmol 102:42, 1984.

47. Stewart RH, Kimbrough RL, Ward RL: Betaxolol vs timolol. A six-month double-blind comparison. Arch Ophthalmol 104:46, 1986.

48. Ellis PP, Carbonic anhydrase inhibitors: pharmacologic effects and problems of long-term therapy. In Leopold IH (ed): Symposium on Ocular Therapy. St. Louis, CV Mosby, 1969, vol 4, p 32.

49. Eskridge JB, Bartlett JD: The glaucomas. In Bartlett JD, Jaanus SD (eds): Clinical Ocular Pharmacology. Boston, Butterworths, 1989, pp 733–798.

50. Drance SM: Comparison of action of cholinergic and anticholinesterase agents in glaucoma. Invest Ophthalmol 5:130, 1966.

51. Durkee DP, Bryant BG: Drug therapy review: drug therapy glaucoma. Am J Hosp Pharm 35:682, 1978.

52. Sugrue MF: The pharmacology of antiglaucoma drugs. Pharmacol Ther 43:91, 1989.

53. Pearson D: Complications with the use of Ocusert (letter). Arch Ophthalmol 94:168, 1976.

54. Goldberg I, Ashburn FB, Kass MA, Becker B: Efficacy and patient acceptance of pilocarpine gel. Am J Ophthalmol 88:843, 1979.

55. Leopold IH: Ocular cholinesterase and cholinesterase inhibitors: The Friedenwald Memorial Lecture. Am J Ophthalmol 51:885, 1961.

56. Kellerman L, King AC: Echothiophate iodide in glaucoma. Am J Ophthalmol 62:278, 1966.

57. Harris LS: Dose response analysis of echothiophate iodide. Arch Ophthalmol 86:502, 1971.

58. Everitt DE, Avorn J: Systemic effects of medications used to treat glaucoma. 112:120, 1990.

59. Chin NB, Gold AA, Breinin GM: Iris cysts and miotics. Arch Ophthalmol 71:611, 1964.

60. Axelsson J, Holmberg A: The frequency of cataracts after miotic therapy, Acta Ophthalmol 44:421, 1966.

61. DeRoetth A Jr: Lens opacities in glaucoma patients on phospholine iodide therapy. Am J Ophthalmol 62:619, 1966.

62. Drance SM, The effects of phospholine iodide on the lens and anterior chamber depth. In Liopold IH (ed): Symposium on Ocular Therapy. St. Louis, CV Mosby, 1969, vol 4, p 25.

63. Levene RZ, Echothiophate iodide and lens changes. In Leopold IH (ed): Symposium on Ocular Therapy, St. Louis, CV Mosby. 1969, vol 4, p 45.

64. Shaffer RN, Hetherington J: Anticholinesterase and cataracts. Am J Ophthalmol 62:613, 1966.

65. Ellis PP: Systemic effects of locally applied anticholinesterase agents. Invest Ophthalmol 5:146, 1966.

66. Leopold IH: Cholinesterases and the effects and side effects of drugs affecting cholinergic systemic. Am J Ophthalmol 60:425, 1965.

67. Hiscox PEA, McCulloch C: Cardiac arrest occurring in a patient on echothiophate iodide therapy. Am J Ophthalmol 60:425, 1965.

68. Birks DA, Prior VJ, Silk E: Echothiophate iodide treatment of glaucoma in pregnancy. Arch Ophthalmol 79:283, 1968.

69. Eilderton TE, Farmati O, Zsigmond EK: Reduction in plasma cholinesterase levels after prolonged administration of echothiophate iodide eyedrops. Can Anaesth Soc J 15:291, 1968.

70. Gesztes T: Prolonged apnea after suxamethonium injection associated with eyedrops containing an anticholinesterase agent. Br J Anesth 38:408, 1966.

71. Ohrstrom A, Pandolfi M: Long-term treatment of glaucoma with systemic propranolol. Am J Ophthalmol 86:340, 1978.

72. Smith SE, Smith SA, Reynolds F, Whitmarsh VB: Ocular and cardiovascular effects of local and systemic pindolol. Br J Ophthalmol 63:63, 1979.

73. Elliot MJ, Cullen PM, Phillips CI: Ocular hypertensive effect of atenolol (Tenormin, I.C.I.). Br J Ophthalmol 59:296, 1975.

74. Coakes RL, Brubaker R: The mechanism of timolol in lowering introcular pressure. Arch Ophthalmol 96:2045, 1978.

75. Lesar TS: Comparison of ophthalmic beta-blocking agents. Clin Pharm 6:451–463, 1987.

76. Keates EJ: Evaluation of timolol malcate combination therapy in chronic open-angle glaucoma. Am J Ophthalmol 88:565, 1979.

77. Cyrlin MN, Thomas JV, Epstein DL: Additive effect of epinephrine to timolol therapy in primary open-angle glaucoma. Arch Ophthalmol 100:414, 1982.

78. Daily RA, Brubaker RF, Bourne WM: The effects of timolol maleate and acetazolamide on the rate of aqueous formation in normal human subjects. Am J Ophthalmol 93:232, 1982.

79. Anon: Additions to timoptic contraindictions. FDD Drug Bull 11:1, 1981.

80. Wandel T, Charap AD, Lewis RA, et al.: Glaucoma treatment with once-daily levobunolol. Am J Ophthalmol 101:298, 1986.

81. Soll DB, Saxon AM: Drugs and glaucoma. Am Fam Physician 34:181, 1986.

82. Bersinger RE, Keates EJ, Gotman JD, Novack GD, Duzman E: Levbunolol. A three-month efficacy study in the treatment of glaucoma and ocular hypertension. Arch Ophthalmol 103:375, 1985.

83. Berson FG, Howard BC, Foerster RJ, Lass JH, Novack GD, Duzman E: Levobunolol compared with timolol for the long-term control of elevated introcular pressure. Arch Ophthalmol 103:379, 1985.

84. Stewart RH, Kimbrough RL, Ward RL: Betaxolol vs timolol. Arch Ophthalmol 104:46, 1986.

85. Goldberg I: Betaxolol. Aust NZ J Ophthalmol 17:9, 1989.

86. Richards RD: Glaucoma. Am Fam Physician 35:212, 1987.

87. Allen RC, Hertzmark E, Walker AM, Epstein DL: A double-masked comparison of betazolol vs timolol in the treatment of open-angle glaucoma. Am J Ophthalmol 101:535, 1986.

88. Berrospi AR, Leibowitz HM: A new β-adrenergic blocking agent for treatment of glaucoma, Arch Ophthalmol 100:943, 1982.

89. Becker B, Petitt TH, Gay AJ: Topical epinephrine therapy in open-angle glaucoma. Arch Ophthalmol 66:219, 1961.

90. Briswick VG, Drance SM: Epinephrine salts and introcular pressure. Arch Ophthalmol 75:768, 1966.

91. Vaughan G, Shaffer R, Riegelman S: A new stabilized form of epinephrine for treatment of open-angle glaucoma. Arch Ophthalmol 66:232, 1961.

92. Kass MA, Mandell AL, Goldberg I, Paine JM, Becker B: Dipivefrin and epinephrine treatment of elevated introcular pressure. Arch Ophthalmol 97:1865, 1979.

93. Kohn AN, Moss AP, Hargett NA, Ritch R, Smith H, Rodos SM: Clinical comparisons of divalyl epinephrine and epinephrine in the treatment of glaucoma. Am J Ophthalmol 87:196, 1979.

94. Carlstedt BC, Stanaszek WF: Glaucoma. US Pharmacist 12(4):7690, 1987.

95. Ross RA, Drance SM: Effects of topically applied isoproterenol on aqueous dynamics in man. Arch Ophthalmol 83:39, 1970.

96. Ballin N, Becker B, Goldman ML: Sustemic effects of epinephrine applied topically to the eye. Invest Ophthalmol 5:125, 1966.

97. Mooney D: Pigmentation after long-term usage of adrenaline compounds. Br J Ophthalmol 54:923, 1970.

98. Lansche RK: Reaction to epinephrine and phenylephrine. Am J Ophthalmol 61:95, 1966.

99. Gallin MA, Harris LS: Acetazolamide and outflow facility. Arch Ophthalmol 76:493, 1966.

100. Maren TH: Carbonic anhydrase: chemistry, physiology and inhibition. Physiol Rev 47:595, 1967.

101. Shrader CE, Thomas JV, Simmons RJ: Relationship of patient age and tolerance to carbonic anhydrase inhibitors. Am J Ophthalmol 96:730, 1983.

102. Lichter PR, Newman LP, Wheeler NC, Beall OV: Patient tolerance to carbonic anhydrase inhibitors. Am J Ophthalmol 85:495–502, 1978.

103. Lichter PR: Reducing side effects of carbonic anhydrase inhibitors. Ophthalmology 88:266, 1981.

104. Draeger J, Gtuttner R, Theilmann W: Avoidance of side-reactions and loss of drug efficacy during long-term administration of carbonic anhydrase inhibitors by concomitant supplement electrolyte administration. Br J Ophthalmol 47:467, 1961.

105. Parfitt AM: Acetazolamide and sodium bicarbonate induced nephrocalcinosis and nephrolithiasis. Arch Intern Med 124:736, 1969.

106. Peyes MB: Acetazolamide and renal stone formation. Lancet 1:837, 1970.

107. Becker B, Kolker AR, Kupin T, Hyperosmotic agents. In Leopold IH (ed): Symposium on Ocular Therapy. St. Louis, CV Mosby, 1968, vol 3, p 42.

108. Kronfeld PC: The efficacy of combinations of ocular hypotensive drugs. Arch Ophthalmol 78:140, 1967.

109. Adams RE, Kirschner RJ, Leopold IH: Ocular hypotensive effect of intravenously administered mannitol. Arch Ophthalmol 69:55, 1963.

110. Weiss DI, Shaffer RN, Harrington DD: Treatment of malignant glaucoma with intravenous mannitol infusion. Arch Ophthalmol 69:154, 1963.

111. Davis M, Duehr P, Javid M: The clinical use of urea for reduction of introcular pressure. Arch Ophthalmol 65:526, 1961.

112. Suzuki Y: Studies on the effect of ascorbic acid on the introcular pressure of rabbits. Acta Ophthalmol 75:201, 1966.

113. D'Alena P, Ferguson W. Adverse effects after glycerol orally and mannital parenterally. Arch Ophthalmol 75:210, 1966.

114. McCurdy DK, Schneider B, Scheic HG: Oral glycerol: the mechanism of introcular hypotension. Am J Ophthalmol 61:373, 1970.

115. Krupin T, Kolker AE, Becker B: A comparison of isosorbide and glycerol for cataract surgery. Am J Ophthalmol 69:373, 1970.

116. Becker B, Morton RW: Topical epinephrine in glaucoma suspects. Am J Ophthalmol 62:272, 1966.

117. Becker B, Round table discussion. In Armaly MF (ed): Fifteenth Annual Session of the New Orleans Academy of Ophthalmology. St. Louis, CV Mosby, 1967, vol 1, p 239.

118. Swan KC: Problems in the use of combinations of drugs in ophthalmology. In Leopold IH (ed): Ocular Therapy— Complications and Management. St. Louis, CV Mosby, 1967, vol 2, p 29.

119. Epstein DL, Laser methods in glaucoma. In Grant WM, Chandler PA (eds): Glaucoma. Philadelphia, Lea & Febiger, 1986, p 104.

120. Heuer DK: Glaucoma update. Ophthalmology 95:282, 1988.

121. Wise JB: Ten year results of laser trabeculoplasty. Does the laser avoid glaucoma surgery or merely defer it? Eye 45:1(part 1):4550, 1987.

122. Scheie HG, Edwards DL, Yanoff MC: Clinical and experimental observations using alpha chymotrypsin. Am J Ophthalmol 59:469, 1965.

123. Package insert, Iodipine (apraclonidine hydrochloride 1%). Fort worth: Alcon Surgical, 1991.

124. Pollack IP, Brown RH, Crandall AS, Steward RH, White GL: Prevention of the rise in intraocular pressure following neodymium-YAG posterior capsulotomy using topical 1% apraclonidine. Arch Ophthalmol 106:754–757, 1988.

125. Reid FR: Personal communication. Sept 17, 1991.

CHAPTER 47

HEADACHE

MARK D. WATANABE, Pharm.D., Ph.D.

Headache is the most frequently reported painful state in the clinical setting. In the United States, fully 75 to 90% of the population experiences isolated episodes of headache pain during any given year, and up to 50 million people may suffer from recurring pain (1). The potential social costs in terms of decreased function and productivity make headache a major public health problem. Headaches are consistently listed as among the 10 most common reasons for visits to outpatient clinics (2). This has prompted the development of designated headache clinics where specialists can focus their attention on diagnosis and therapy. Yet, a thorough understanding of this affliction remains elusive.

The general principles of pain management are applicable in the treatment of headache syndromes. The most common type of pain results from activation of peripheral nociceptors (pain receptors) in a normally functioning nervous system. Another type results from direct injury to the central or peripheral nervous system, which does not necessarily require the activation of specific receptors. Either mechanism may initiate head pain. Headache may be considered an ultimate consequence of the dysfunction, injury, or displacement of pain-sensitive cranial structures, which are primarily vascular in nature (e.g., the cerebral arteries, the large veins, and the venous sinuses). The blood vessels are innervated by branches of the trigeminal, glossopharyngeal, and vagal nerves, as well as the upper cervical roots of the spinal cord; this sensory innervation facilitates transmission of pain impulses. For years, the brain itself was deemed a pain-insensitive structure; however, recent studies suggest that this organ can indeed generate cephalic pain by its own headache-generating processes (3).

Headache can be particularly perplexing to the clinician, because the nature and severity of this symptom does not necessarily reflect the seriousness of the underlying pathology. Causative events such as vasodilatation, skeletal muscle tension, or changes in intracranial pressure are often associated with a variety of precipitating factors, e.g., depression, hypertension, stress, or organic disease. Therefore, extensive medical, neurologic, and when appropriate, psychiatric evaluations are essential for patients with severe or chronic headache symptoms, to eliminate such disorders as causal factors.

Neurologic testing in patients with primary headache disorder seldom reveals abnormalities beyond those detected by an extensive history and physical examination. The expense and limited accessibility of the more technologically sophisticated diagnostic imaging procedures usually limits them to patients refractory to conventional treatment. If organic etiologies have been ruled out, a thorough history is critical to characterize the headache subtype and to design appropriate therapeutic interventions. As with any painful state, determination of the quality, severity, location, duration, and frequency of headache symptoms is necessary, as is identification of any conditions that induce, exacerbate, or relieve them. The presence or absence of associated somatic (e.g., neurologic, visual, or gastrointestinal) symptoms, alterations in sleep patterns, or positive family history of headaches, anxiety, or depression may provide important diagnostic clues. It is also useful to obtain details regarding the age and circumstances when headaches first became a problem and any history of head trauma or seizure disorder. Because pain is a subjective experience, patients suffering from chronic headaches may lapse into states of anxiety and helplessness that aggravate the physical component of the pain.

An assessment of psychosocial and health factors affecting a patient's life may lend insight into the extent that emotional, personality, and physiological considerations contribute to the etiology of headache. Many situational conditions with significant psychological impact can induce head pain; stress, anxiety, depression, and emotional discord are common precipitants. Physical stress from hunger, poor nutrition, exertion, head trauma, and exposure to environmental extremes is also associated with headache attacks. Ingestion of certain foods, especially those containing vasoactive substances (e.g., tyramine, nitrites, monosodium glutamate), cigarette smoking, and hormonal changes can be a problem for patients with certain variants of headache. Careful probing for potential precipitating factors in headache patients is an important process.

A clinician's ability to obtain a thorough medication history is critical. In particular, details of previous use of both nonprescription and prescription analgesics should be elicited from the patient. Knowledge of the amounts taken, duration of treatment, therapeutic efficacy, and noted adverse effects is important information. All concomitant medications taken by the patient must be reviewed to probe for possible iatrogenic causes of headache. Examples of drugs that have been implicated in the development of headache either by their administration or withdrawal are listed in Table 47.1 (4). Patient attitudes about medication use or alternative nondrug treatments such as relaxation therapy or biofeedback may also assist in predicting overall therapeutic success. Once a comprehensive headache profile has been established, a diagnosis is made, and options for treatment are planned.

The simplest classification scheme considers four general types of headaches. *Vascular headaches*, which include migraine and cluster headaches, are those caused by an abnormal reaction of the cerebral arteries, usually vasodilatation. *Muscle contraction or tension headaches*, the most common type seen in clinical practice, may result from muscular overcontraction of the head, neck, and face area in conjunction with emotional stress, fatigue, or noise exposure. *Traction and inflammatory headaches* include all headaches caused by diagnosed organic disease of the skull and its components, e.g., cerebrovascular disease, brain tumor, infections, or inflammatory disease, which may involve compression of cranial and cervical nerves or displacement of large intracranial veins. *Idiopathic cranial neuralgias* describe head pain for which clear pathologic changes are not identified. The Ad Hoc Committee on Classification of Headache, in recognizing the distinction between primary and secondary headaches, outlined the classification scheme in Table 47.2 (5).

Often patients have a mixture of symptoms that cross diagnostic categories. Fortunately, headaches secondary to a significant underlying organic disorder are rare, with estimates of less than 1% of cases encountered by a general practitioner (2). Therefore, this chapter focuses on the clinical presentation, pathogenesis, and pharmacotherapy of the more common primary headache, i.e., tension or muscle contraction, migraine, and cluster headaches.

Table 47.1.
Representative Medications Implicated in Headache Etiology

Alcohol	Dopamine
Amphetamine	Ergotamine withdrawal
Atenolol	Estrogens
Barbiturates	Fenfluramine
Caffeine	Hydralazine
Caffeine withdrawal	Indomethacin
Cannabis	Isosorbide dinitrate
Captopril	Nifedipine
Cimetidine	Nitroglycerin
Corticosteroid	Oral contraceptives
Corticosteroid withdrawal	Reserpine
Digitalis	Theophylline

Table 47.2.
Classification of Headache[a]

Vascular headache of migraine type
  "Classic" migraine
  "Common" migraine
  "Cluster" headache
  "Hemiplegic" and "ophthalmoplegic" migraine
  "Lower-half" headache
Muscle-contraction (tension) headache
Combined headache: vascular and muscle-contraction type
Headache of nasal vasomotor reaction
Headache of delusional, conversion, or hypochondriacal states
Nonmigrainous vascular headaches
Traction headache
Headache due to overt cranial inflammation
Headache due to disease of ocular structures
Headache due to disease of aural structures
Headache due to disease of nasal structures and sinuses
Headache due to disease of dental structures
Headache due to disease of other cranial or neck structures
Cranial neuritides
Cranial neuralgias

[a] Adapted from Ad Hoc Committee on Classification of Headache: Classification of headache. JAMA 179:717–718, 1962.

CLINICAL PRESENTATION AND PATHOGENESIS
Tension Headache

Tension, or muscle contraction, headaches are the most commonly reported subtype. The estimated prevalence in the general population varies between 10 and 80%, with at least 80% of the adult population affected sometime during their lifetimes (6). There appears to be a 3:1 predominance in women (7), but men are less likely to report symptoms and seek treatment. The clinical features of tension headache include a characteristic dull, persistent, and steady pain; some patients may describe a sensation of tightness or pressure, as if a band were placed around the head. A throbbing sensation, associated more with vascular headaches, is not a typical component of tension headache (8), although it may evolve as the pain increases in severity. In such cases, there may be a mixed tension-vascular syndrome. The pain of tension headache is usually bifrontal, but it can also be occipital or in the neck and shoulders. Its onset is gradual, and its duration may range from only a few hours to episodes recurring over the course of weeks, months, or years at the same intensity. Tension headaches can occur at any age but are relatively infrequent in children (9). Sometimes the pain is diminished with positional changes or when the head is supported.

Although persistent muscle contraction with eventual compression of pain-sensitive cranial structures and localized ischemia is often thought to be the source of tension headaches, the precise etiology remains ambiguous. Despite the term, *muscle contraction* and *tension*, no direct evidence confirms a clear causal relationship between the degree of muscle contraction and the severity of tension headache (10). Contraction of neck and scalp muscles can certainly contribute to the generation of head pain, but this is probably secondary to a more central headache-generating mechanism. Vascular hyperactivity and serotonergic dysregulation models have been proposed as pathogenic factors (11, 12). Episodic tension headache can be associated with heightened emotions, fatigue, and psychological and environmental stress. Chronic tension headache can be a symptom of depression or anticipatory anxiety, a psychosomatic defense reaction against exacerbation of head pain by excess head movement, or (as previously mentioned) a manifestation of a concurrent vascular headache disorder. The effectiveness of biofeedback and relaxation techniques (13) is consistent with the assumption that tension headache has a significant psychosomatic component. Counseling or psychotherapy are useful adjunctive interventions for headaches known to be reactions to life stressors.

Migraine Headache

Migraine headaches are considerably more debilitating than tension headaches and are characterized by a different clinical profile. As a general category, it afflicts about 20 to 25% of the population (14) The usual age of initial onset is any time between the ages of 5 and 30 years, but first migraine attacks are commonly experienced during puberty (9). While male and female children are affected in equal numbers, a 3:2 predominance in women evolves by 40 years of age (15). The finding that a positive family history of migraine is present in 65 to 90% of migraine patients (16) suggests that there is a hereditary component affecting susceptibility to the disorder. Only anecdotal support exists for the idea of predisposing "migraine personality" traits, i.e., the tendency to be perfectionist, obsessive-compulsive, ambitious, and easily frustrated.

A typical migraine attack is described as pulsatile head pain of varying intensity, usually associated with uncomfortable somatic symptoms. Nausea, vomiting, diarrhea, perspiration, photophobia, visual disturbances, lightheadedness, and vertigo have all been reported, as have concurrent neurologic and mood disturbances (17). Although pain is unilateral in most cases, it may be unilateral or bilateral and may be frontal, temporal, or generalized (18). Unilateral pain does not necessarily recur on the same side. It may actually switch sides or become bilateral during the course of a migraine attack. Beginning as a dull ache, migraine pain intensifies in quality over a period of minutes to hours to an often incapacitating throbbing headache. The pulsating nature of the pain is an essential feature of a migraine headache. Physical stimuli such as movement, noise, and light exacerbate the pain. For this reason, migraine sufferers often want to lie down in a quiet, darkened room to sleep, a maneuver that successfully alleviates the

pain. Otherwise, an untreated attack may last from several hours to 1 to 3 days in the most severe cases. Migraine attacks are episodic, with considerable interpatient variability in the frequency of occurrence. Most patients do not experience them more than once every few weeks, but for others the incidence of suffering will vary from only a handful of attacks over the course of a lifetime to several times per week on a chronic basis.

Traditional classification of migraine headaches divided the malady into three diagnostic categories: classical migraine, common migraine, and complicated migraine. A recent revision by the Headache Classification Committee of the International Headache Society (19) proposes that "classical" and "complicated" migraine be redesignated "migraine with aura," while "common" migraine be reclassified as "migraine without aura." As the terminology, diagnostic criteria, and validity of this nosology may be unfamiliar to the practicing clinician, provisional reference to the traditional nomenclature will continue in this chapter.

Classical migraine attacks progress through three stages, of which the aura is the first (18). However, the aura may be preceded by an extended period of prodromal symptoms that occur 24 to 48 hr before an active attack. The prodrome may manifest itself as mental status changes (increased irritability, anxiety, depression, decreased concentration, somnolence) or autonomic disturbances (increased hunger, increased thirst, gastrointestinal fullness, chills). The aura consists of focal neurological symptoms that can precede the headache by 15 to 60 min or be experienced concurrently with pulsatile pain. The most common element is some form of visual disturbance. Frequently reported phenomena are scintillating scotomata (blind spots with luminous borders), photopsia (unformed flashes of light), and fortification spectra (slowly enlarging scotomata with surrounding "zig-zag" patterns). Other aura symptoms may include transient aphasia, vertigo, pallor, and paresthesia. The active headache phase has the previously described symptoms. The third, postheadache phase may find the patient exhausted and confused, with episodes of diuresis. Because the affected scalp area on the side of the attack remains tender, any physical exertion or head movement may result in reemergence of throbbing head pain.

Common migraine, which occurs in 85% of migraine patients, is distinguished from its classical counterpart in that the initial phase of the headache does not have an associated aura of focal neurologic deficits. The duration of pain tends to be longer per attack, sometimes lasting for days. It is not uncommon for patients with the classic migraine syndrome to experience intervening episodes of common migraine. Complicated migraine is best described as an unusual variant of classical migraine in which the neurologic disturbances persist after the headache has dissipated. Examples of the complicated subtype are ophthalmoplegic and hemiplegic migraines. In ophthalmoplegic migraine, paralysis of the third cranial nerve causes extraocular paresis, ocular muscle weakness, ptosis, and diplopia. These symptoms occur on the same side as the actual headache. Hemiplegic migraine, often familial in nature, can result in sudden hemiparesis or hemiplegia, as well as aphasia and confusion. The onset of these neurologic reactions may either precede or accompany an ipsilateral or contralateral headache. While their usual duration may be less than an hour, in some patients the paralysis may endure. A comprehensive neurologic examination is warranted for patients with unremitting complicated migraine (20).

Historically, two major theories have been advocated for the etiology of migraine: the humoral-vascular theory and the neurogenic theory (21, 22). The former postulates that circulating vasoactive substances, by constricting the cortical microcirculation and reducing cerebral blood flow, cause the neurologic symptoms associated with the aura. This is followed by a period of predominantly extracranial vasodilatation and the release of pain-mediating autacoids (e.g., histamine, serotonin, vasoactive peptides, kinins, prostaglandins), a phenomenon thought to be the source of head pain. An implicit assumption is that the vessel wall has been sensitized by both the adsorption of serotonin released from abnormally activated platelets and the local accumulation of histamine and bradykinin. As part of a vascular theory variation known as the "platelet theory," the hyperaggregation of platelets, induced by various stimuli (e.g., release of catecholamines, an imbalance of regulatory agents thromboxane A_2 and prostacyclin, the presence of excess adenosine diphosphate) forms microemboli that can lodge in the extracerebral microvasculature. The subsequent release of serotonin results in local changes in vasomotor tone and transient peripheral ischemia; a concomitant inflammatory tissue response involving the accumulation of pain-potentiating substances such as bradykinin and substance P (both potent vasodilators) may also contribute to the active headache phase. As the process of adsorption reduces the initial vasoconstricting effects of serotonin in the microcirculation, painful dilatation of the larger arteries may be another, synergistic mechanism for head pain.

While elegant in its simplicity, the humoral-vascular theory falters in view of recent studies that show inconsistent or no changes in cerebral blood flow in common migraine (migraine without aura). In classic migraine, reduction of regional cerebral blood flow has been demonstrated during the prodromal aura, and the pattern of hemodynamic changes is remarkably uniform in starting at the occipital region of the affected hemisphere and progressing anteriorly (23). This finding runs counter to the observation of asymmetry in migraine, as seen in the al-

ternating localization of head pain, i.e., the headache may appear as often as not on the side opposite that giving rise to the prodromal symptoms. It is apparent that the correlation between migraine attacks and regional cerebral blood flow changes caused by vascular mechanisms is incomplete. In addition, purely localized vascular involvement does not explain the following phenomena: prompt precipitation of attacks in some patients by an external stimulus such as a bright, flashing light, the lack of emesis and photophobia in patients who have temporal arteritis, and the presence of facial pallor secondary to vasoconstriction in many migraine patients. As the inadequacies of the vascular theory revealed themselves, some investigators invoked neural involvement as a complementary mechanism to the pathogenesis of migraine.

The neurogenic theory states that migraine is mediated primarily by activity in the cerebral cortex, with only secondary extracerebral vascular manifestations (24). Prodromal symptoms, such as altered behavior, mood changes, carbohydrate craving, yawning, altered bowel frequency, and feeling unduly tired or cold, cannot be explained by changes in vasomotor tone alone. These may represent autonomic disturbances that are centrally mediated by the hypothalamus and sent, as sensory inputs, to the cerebral cortex for processing. Other external factors such as stress, fatigue, ingestion of vasoactive substances (e.g., alcohol, some medications, certain foods), and hormonal changes may also provide afferent input to the cerebral cortex. In patients predisposed to migraine, the result is thought to be a gradually spreading cortical depression accompanied by a diffuse ischemia (25). This process presumably accounts for the focal neurologic symptoms associated with the classical migraine aura. The ensuing extracranial vasodilatation during the headache phase is probably a reflex response triggered by the ischemic prodrome. A schematic diagram that summarizes the fundamentals of a combined neurogenic-vascular etiology of migraine is shown in Figure 47.1. The roles that nucleotides, neuropeptides, and hormones play in this expanded theory are not known.

Cluster Headache

The precise incidence of cluster headache is not known; many investigators estimate that less than 1% of the general population is afflicted. However, unlike tension or migraine headache, there is a considerable predominance of the disorder in males to females, in a ratio approximating 5:1. Cluster periods, when attacks occur, generally last between 6 to 12 weeks. These are followed by remission periods averaging 12 months in duration, with considerable variation in length. The attacks can occur one to three times a day, are of short duration, and present with pain described as excruciating, boring, and nonthrobbing in character. It is always unilateral and occulotemporal or occulofrontal, with common associated symptoms of uni-

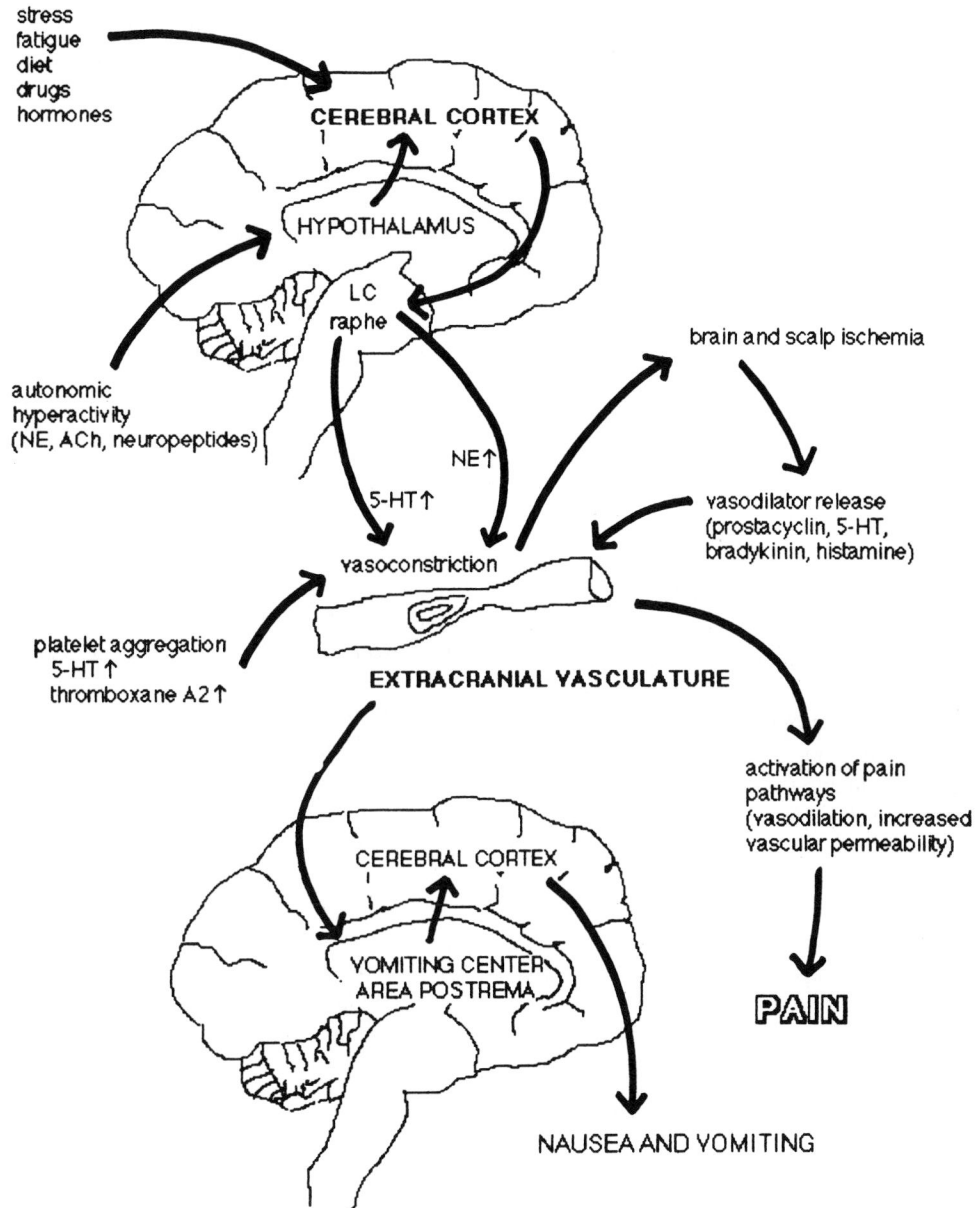

Figure 47.1. Schematic of the sequence of events proposed under the vascular-neurogenic theory of migraine. *NE*, norepi- nephrine; *ACh*, acetylcholine; *5-HT*, 5-hydroxytryptamine (se- rotonin); *LC*, locus coeruleus.

lateral lacrimation, rhinorrhea, or nasal stuffiness. Con- comitant neurologic symptoms are rare, which clearly dis- tinguishes this subtype of headache from migraine. Cluster headaches have been induced reportedly by the use of vasodilator medications such as nitroglycerin and alcohol ingestion. One clinic has reported a specific behavior pat- tern of pacing, walking, sitting, and rocking during an at- tack as being pathognomonic for cluster headache (26).

The etiology and pathogenesis of cluster headache is also not well characterized. Most of the clinical symptoms have been attributed to external carotid artery dilatation

(i.e., enlarged temporal artery, relief of pain with compres- sion, ipsilateral flushing or pallor, and increases in skin temperature by 1° to 2°C), but many exceptions to this association have been found in individual patients. A hor- monal contribution is suggested by the gender predomi- nance and a vascular contribution is likewise inferred from the precipitation of cluster headaches by vasodilators, but substantial supportive evidence is lacking. As with mi- graine headaches, there may be some association with al- tered blood serotonin concentrations, but the nature of the relationship is not clear. In contrast to migraines, there is no evidence that platelet dysfunction plays a role in the pathogenesis of the disorder. Other biochemical changes reported in patients during the cluster period include increased urinary excretion and blood concentrations of histamine, decreased testosterone and leutinizing hormone, decreased platelet monoamine oxidase B, and decreased erythrocyte choline levels. Substance P and bradykinin may also mediate cluster symptoms (27). To date, no comprehensive model for the pathogenesis of cluster headache has been proposed that adequately integrates each of the clinical findings.

TREATMENT
General Therapeutic Considerations

The approach to the treatment of headache should be multifaceted, taking into consideration the subjective needs of the patient as well as the specific clinical characteristics of the physical symptoms. Because of the significant psychological component to the perception of pain, the clinician must develop a solid empathic rapport with the headache patient. This forms the basis of a therapeutic relationship that facilitates the process of monitoring pain relief by patient report. Sincere and supportive reassurances provide much needed encouragement to a patient who is often anxious, frustrated, and unable to cope well with a potentially debilitating condition. Some patients may require the use of psychotherapy or biofeedback relaxation techniques as adjunctive measures. All patients should be educated continually about their headaches, so that precipitating factors can be avoided, realistic expectations can be set, and a sense of full participation in their own therapy is developed.

A comprehensive history and physical examination is of paramount importance. Once organic trauma or medical disease is eliminated as a primary cause of headache, the search for identifiable precipitants should follow. Known situational stressors should be minimized, if at all possible. Any medication prescribed for a concomitant medical problem should be assessed as a potential iatrogenic cause of headache. The remaining primary symptoms that persist are to be characterized carefully. Often, patients experience symptoms that overlap two or more defined headache subtype syndromes, e.g., the appearance of both tension and migraine headache profiles over the course of time. In such cases, the clinician must assign priorities based on the severity of the dominant symptoms. Pharmacotherapy can be useful in treating headache in two ways: as abortive intervention during an acute attack and as a prophylactic measure against future attacks. The clinician should be aware that the headache drug therapy literature is often riddled with study design inconsistencies that make it difficult to evaluate true therapeutic efficacy. Until a consensus is reached on standardized measurements of headache pain and medication effects, the choice of drug is generally based on previous clinical experience and studies and reports in the literature.

PHARMACOTHERAPY (Table 47.3)
Tension Headache Pharmacotherapy
SYMPTOMATIC TREATMENT

The choice of therapy for tension headache depends on the severity and chronicity of the pain. Most patients do not seek out treatment assistance for mild, infrequent episodes that often respond to self-medication or self-imposed behavior modification. Relaxation methods, such as massage, meditation, or local heat application, help alleviate the attendant stress and anxiety of tension headaches. For an acute attack of limited frequency, mild-to-moderate analgesics such as acetaminophen and nonsteroidal anti-inflammatory agents (commonly aspirin and ibuprofen) are effective if taken early in the course of the headache. One placebo-controlled study demonstrated that 1000 mg acetaminophen and 650 mg aspirin were equipotent in treating moderately severe tension headache pain (28). Ibuprofen, in doses of 400 to 600 mg, has been used successfully as well (29). Some patients find that a combination of acetaminophen, butalbital, and caffeine (Fiorinal) provides symptomatic relief when a milder analgesic is ineffective (30). Adjunctive usage of anxiolytics (e.g., diazepam and meprobamate) and skeletal muscle relaxants (e.g., orphenadrine) with analgesics has been shown to be useful (31–33). While support exists for the use of mild tranquilizers (barbiturates, benzodiazepines, and meprobamate) as effective monotherapy of acute attacks (34), these agents should be used judiciously in view of their potential to exacerbate chronic tension headache (16). Potentially addicting medications should be avoided in patients with chronic and frequent tension headaches. This particular patient population tends to exhibit passive and dependent personality traits that can complicate chances of symptomatic relief with even mild analgesics.

PROPHYLACTIC TREATMENT

In general, tricyclic antidepressants that inhibit the reuptake of serotonin released by presynaptic neuronal endplates are most effective in the prophylaxis of tension headache. The drug of choice is amitriptyline, by virtue of its long-standing status as a particularly effective agent (35). Interestingly, the effective daily dose required to achieve analgesia for most patients (50 to 100 mg) is significantly lower than the doses used to alleviate depressive symptoms (150 to 300 mg) (30). Likewise, the time frame expected for a therapeutic response from amitriptyline differs in patients suffering from tension headache (2 to 10 days) and patients with depressive symptoms (3 to 4 weeks). This suggests that the mechanisms of action in headache is different and that the analgesic response is not absolutely

Table 47.3.
Pharmacotherapy of Symptomatic Headache Attacks and Prophylaxis

Drug	Usual Adult Dose	Maximum Daily Dose	Route of Administration	Indication[a]
Vasoactive agents				
Dihydroergotamine	1 mg stat; repeat q 1 hr prn	3 mg	par	C, M
Ergonovine	0.2–0.4 mg stat	2 mg	par	M
Ergotamine	1–2 mg stat; repeat q 30 min prn	6 mg	po, sl, pr	C, M
	0.25–0.5 mg stat; repeat in 1 hr prn	3 mg	par	
	0.36 mg stat; repeat q 5 min prn	2.16 mg (6 doses)	inh	
Midrin	2 caps stat; repeat 1 cap q 1 hr prn	6 caps (10/week)	po	M
Sumatriptan	6 mg stat; repeat in 1 hr prn	12 mg	po	M
Antiemetics				
Chlorpromazine	25–50 mg stat; repeat q 4 hr prn	400 mg	po, pr, par	A, C
Metoclopramide	10 mg stat; repeat q 4 hr prn	40 mg	po, par	A
Prochlorperazine	5–10 mg stat; repeat q 4 hr prn	60 mg	po, pr, par	A
Thiethylperazine	10 mg stat; repeat q 4 hr prn	40 mg	po, pr, par	A
Trimethobenzamide	200–250 mg stat; repeat q 4 hr prn	1000 mg	par, po, pr	A
Analgesics/nonsteroidal antiinflammatory drugs				
Acetaminophen	325–650 mg stat; repeat q 4 hr prn	2600 mg	po, pr	M, T
Aspirin	325–650 mg stat; repeat q 4 hr prn	2600 mg	po, pr	M, T
Codeine	30–60 mg stat; repeat q 4 hr prn	240 mg	po, par	M
Ibuprofen	400–600 mg stat; repeat q 6 hr prn	2400 mg	po	M, T
Indomethacin	50–75 mg stat; repeat q 8 hr prn	300 mg	po, pr	C
Meperidine	25–100 mg stat	400 mg	po, par	M
Morphine	5–10 mg stat	60 mg	par	M
Naproxen	250–500 mg stat; repeat q 8 hr prn	1500 mg	po	M
Naproxen sodium	275–550 mg stat; repeat q 8 hr prn	1650 mg	po	M
Sedative/hypnotics				
Diazepam	5–10 mg stat; repeat q 6–8 hr prn	40 mg	po, par	T
Lorazepam	0.5–2 mg stat; repeat q 8 hr prn	8 mg	po, par	T
Triazolam	0.25–0.5 mg stat; repeat ×1 prn	1.0 mg	po	T
Steroids				
Prednisone	40–60 mg; taper dose over 21 days	80 mg	po	C, M
PROPHYLAXIS				
Amitriptyline	75–100 mg qd	200 mg	po	C, T
Aspirin	325 mg bid-tid	1300 mg	po	M
Chlorpromazine	25 mg bid-qid	400 mg	po	C, M
Cyproheptadine	4 mg tid	24 mg	po	C, M
Ergonovine	0.2 mg tid	2 mg	po	C, M
Ergotamine	1 mg bid	10 mg/wk	po	M
Ibuprofen	400 mg bid-qid	2400 mg	po	C
Lithium carbonate	300 mg tid-qid	1800 mg	po	C, M
Methysergide	2 mg tid	8 mg	po	M
Naproxen	250–500 mg bid	1500 mg	po	C, M
Nifedipine	10 mg tid	60 mg	po	C, M
Nimodipine	60 mg qd-bid	120 mg	po	C, M
Prednisone	20 mg bid-tid	80 mg	po	M
Propranolol	20 mg qid	320 mg	po	

[a] Abbreviations: C, cluster headache; M, migraine headache; T, tension headache; A, adjunctive antiemetic therapy.

dependent on the coexistence of the depressive symptoms found in about one-third of tension headache patients. Plasma concentrations of amitriptyline do not correlate well with the clinical effects. Addition of propranolol and biofeedback techniques to amitriptyline has been found to be more effective than monotherapy, without significantly increasing the incidence of adverse reactions (36). However, a clear disadvantage of amitriptyline is its ability to cause prominent sedative and anticholinergic effects. If therapeutic benefit from a given drug is achieved, treatment may continue for approximately 6 months, after which the dose should be tapered over the course of 3 to 4 weeks. If the headache recurs with an increase in frequency or severity, the effective medication can be readministered to initiate another 6-month drug trial. Other antidepressants, such as imipramine, doxepin, and mianserin, are reportedly effective in the treatment of migraine, but a rigorous comparison with amitriptyline has not been made.

Migraine Headache Pharmacotherapy

SYMPTOMATIC TREATMENT

As a general rule, the earlier the acute migraine attack is treated, the greater the chances that it can be aborted. One of the first patient responses to an attack is lying down in a quiet, darkened room with a cold pack applied to the forehead or temples and attempting to sleep. This rapid reduction in sensory input can be quite effective. If pharmacotherapy is indicated, it should be directed at relieving the migraine headache pain and its associated symptoms. In particular, nausea hinders the use of oral medication because of the possibility of vomiting. Decreases in gastric motility and emptying may delay the absorption of some drugs, such as salicylates. Ironically, the antiemetic phenothiazines commonly used can also potentially decrease gastrointestinal motility, prolong gastric emptying, and exacerbate gastric stasis. While some phenothiazines (e.g., chlorpromazine) can inherently produce analgesia in migraine, these should not be the first choice of antiemetic drugs to be used during an acute attack. That distinction belongs to metoclopramide, a selective D_2-receptor antagonist that accelerates gastrointestinal motility and gastric emptying in humans. Oral or intramuscular administration of 10 to 20 mg of metoclopramide is usually effective; greater doses will enhance the dopamine receptor blockade and increase the probability of abnormal involuntary movements (37, 38). Metoclopramide as monotherapy is not an effective analgesic in the treatment of migraine. Hydroxyzine, trimethobenzamide, and cyclizine can be used as alternative antiemetic agents, with varying degrees of success. Many medications are available in rectal suppositories that can be given when frequent vomiting and impaired gastrointestinal absorption precludes the use of oral medications.

Often the immediate ingestion of a simple analgesic, such as 1000 mg aspirin or acetaminophen is sufficient to provide pain relief (39, 40). Other nonsteroidal antiinflammatory drugs that have been shown to be effective include 400 mg of ibuprofen and 825 mg naproxen sodium (41, 42). The key to treatment success in the use of simple analgesics is that they be taken when the earliest symptoms appear. Any delay in treatment may coincide with the development of migraine-induced decreases in gastrointestinal motility, thereby diminishing the overall effectiveness of oral medications. If metoclopramide is given prior to aspirin, the absorption of the latter is enhanced, secondary

to the increase in gastric emptying. Other combinations of medications may help the patient by reducing the number of undesirable side effects while improving efficacy. One approach is the use of a mild analgesic with a sedative at the onset of an attack (e.g., administration of acetaminophen in tandem with a benzodiazepine). Another combination is the concomitant use of antacids with large doses of aspirin or nonsteroidal antiinflammatory agents to reduce the discomfort of gastrointestinal irritation.

The most reproducibly effective medication available for the abortion of migraine attacks is ergotamine. One report (43) found that 47% of patients under study promptly became headache-free, with an additional 34% noting that some of their attacks were aborted or the severity of headaches generally decreased. Its mechanism of action is probably related to its ability to cause vasoconstriction of the extracranial arterial blood vessels. This reduces the amplitude of pulsations seen in dilated scalp arteries, which tends to correlate, albeit imperfectly, with a decrease in the intensity of headache. Ergotamine exhibits selective vasoconstriction of the cranial arteriovenous anastomoses supplied by the external carotid artery and decreases the tendency for platelets to aggregate in migraine (44). Both actions result in a net blunting of the vascular responses to localized inflammation. Because ergot alkaloids inherently possess both α-receptor agonist and antagonist activity, the effect of ergotamine on arterial tone depends on the preexisting tonic state of the vascular bed. When the vascular resistance is low, ergotamine acts as a vasoconstrictor; in instances of increased resistance, it may induce vasodilatation. The effects of ergotamine may also be mediated by central serotonin activity. A growing body of evidence suggests that disturbances of serotonin (5-hydroxytryptamine; 5-HT) are crucial for the development of migraine (45). In some patients, platelet serotonin concentrations fall rapidly at the onset of a migraine attack, with increased excretion of the main metabolite of serotonin, 5-hydroxyindoleacetic acid (5-HIAA). Migraine attacks can be precipitated in predisposed patients by serotonin-enhancing agents such as reserpine and fenfluramine. The firing rate of serotonergic neurons in the brain stem raphe is diminished by several ergot alkaloid congeners (46). When a completely integrated vascular-neurogenic theory for migraine is developed, an understanding of the mechanism of action of ergotamine may lead to the development of more effective agents.

Ideally, ergotamine should be given during the prodrome phase of classical migraine; a delay in its administration often requires higher doses for an equivalent response. There is significant interpatient variability in both the oral and rectal absorption of ergotamine. Bioavailability approximates 1 to 2% for the oral and 5% for the rectal route of administration. Absorption is apparently enhanced by caffeine, which accounts for its inclusion in available ergot preparations. Peak plasma concentrations are detected from 1 to 2 hr following oral or rectal dosing. However, the pharmacological effects of ergotamine are not well correlated to the plasma concentrations of the parent drug. In fact, the therapeutic effects of ergotamine are prolonged beyond what would be expected from observed plasma levels, given its relatively short elimination half-life of 2 to 3 hr. One plausible explanation is that the actual biological activity is due to the formation of a long-acting active metabolite with a half-life that corresponds to the duration of peripheral vasoconstriction. The poor absorption associated with the sublingual route of administration often renders it less effective, resulting in poor clinical response. After parenteral administration, plasma concentrations decay bioexponentially. Ergotamine is metabolized extensively in the liver and excreted in the bile, but the details of drug biotransformation in humans are now known. Reports of ergotamine in cerebrospinal fluid after an oral dose are conflicting (47).

The most commonly used dosage forms are oral tablets and rectal suppositories. Proprietary preparations contain ergotamine tartrate alone or in combination with caffeine, belladonna alkaloids, or barbiturates. The appropriate dosing is 1 to 2 mg ergotamine tartrate at the onset of the prodrome, with additional 1-mg doses every 30 min as necessary for relief of pain. The maximum allowable dosage of ergotamine, which reduces the risk of complications secondary to arterial insufficiency, is 6 mg per attack or 10 mg per week. For patients who cannot tolerate oral medication, rectal suppositories containing 2 mg ergotamine per suppository may be substituted. An initial dose of one-half to one suppository inserted rectally may be repeated every hour up to 2 suppositories per episode or 5 suppositories per week. The onset of pain relief may average about 1 hr after oral or rectal administration. Ergotamine tartrate can also be given by aerosol inhalation. Pressurized, metered-dose inhalers are available that, properly used, dispense 0.36 mg ergotamine per inhalation. Patient education in the use of an inhaler is critical for maximal benefit. The mouthpiece of the inhaler should be held close to the open mouth as the patient exhales completely. Depression of the canister takes place as the patient inhales deeply. The inhalation should be held as long as possible before slow exhalation through pursed lips is allowed. Starting with an initial dose of one to two inhalations, the patient may repeat with a subsequent inhalation after 5 min if necessary. No more than 6 inhalations over a 24-hr period or 15 inhalations per week should be given. The relatively rapid onset of action, about 15 to 30 min, may make this the administration route of choice for patients with severe headaches without prodromes or those of short duration (48).

Most patients tolerate ergotamine well, especially when the dosage and frequency of dose are carefully monitored. The most common side effects of ergotamine include abdominal and muscle cramps, nausea, vomiting, vertigo, fatigue, diarrhea, numbness, and transient paresthesias of the extremities. Episodes of syncope, tremor, and dyspnea appear less frequently. The occurrence of angina pectoris, limb claudication pain, or persistent paresthesias may require discontinuation of the drug, as these symptoms often reflect the onset of serious arterial insufficiency. The potential for cumulative side effects precludes the use of ergotamine for prophylaxis of migraine. Among the most severe of the long-term side effects of ergotamine is gangrene of the limbs, a toxic sequela of a condition referred to as "ergotism." For this reason, ergot alkaloids are contraindicated in patients with severe peripheral vascular disease, coronary artery disease, and sepsis. Hypertension is a relative contraindication (49). Because of evidence of deleterious effects on animal fetuses, including increased postnatal mortality and abortion, ergotamine should not be given to pregnant women. Chronic dosing of ergotamine may lead to tolerance and physical dependence, often resulting in withdrawal headaches; this problem can also be minimized by compliance with maximum dosage recommendations.

For patients who either fail to respond to ergotamine or cannot tolerate its side effects, alternatives must be considered. The use of mild analgesics has been discussed previously. Isometheptene, an indirect sympathomimetic amine, is available in combination with the sedative dichloralphenazone and acetaminophen (Midrin). The efficacy of this combination, providing relief in about 50% of patients, is superior to that of each of the agents alone. The most frequently reported side effects are nausea, vomiting, insomnia, and transient numbness. The usual dosage is two capsules taken immediately at the onset of head pain, followed by one capsule every hour until the pain is relieved, with a maximum of five capsules within a 12-hr period (50). Intractable migraine may necessitate the use of parenteral ergot preparations. In such cases, the intramuscular administration of 1 mg dihydroergotamine in combination with an antiemetic (e.g., 10 mg metoclopramide) given every 8 hr has been found to be effective in 90% of afflicted patients within 48 hr (51). The maximum dose is 3 mg per headache or 6 mg per week, and the onset of pain relief varies from 15 min to 2 hr. Because of their addictive potential, potent narcotic analgesics should be reserved for patients refractory to parenteral dihydroergotamine. Corticosteroid antiinflammatory agents (e.g., 40 to 60 mg/day of prednisone) have also been used as alternatives in the treatment of intractable migraine.

PROPHYLACTIC TREATMENT

The frequency, duration, and severity of migraine attacks, as well as the extent of relief from abortive therapy, will determine the need for prophylactic pharmacotherapy. Usually, if attacks occur at a rate exceeding two or three per month, a trial of preventive medication may be warranted. Patients who have predictable patterns of headaches and who must avoid head pain in order to function are also candidates for migraine prophylaxis. In particular, women who experience incapacitating headaches during menses may benefit from short-term prophylactic therapy during this period. Certainly, any exogenous precipitating factors must be eliminated or minimized. If the frequency of attacks has recently increased, an assessment for pharmacological tolerance should also be made. One of the problems in the treatment of headache is the risk of medication overusage and generation of a dependency cycle. Prophylactic pharmacotherapy, by decreasing the frequency, duration, and severity of future attacks, may decrease the urgency that compels patients to seek relief by using more potent and possibly habituating drugs. Interestingly, a significant placebo effect has been observed during prophylactic treatment regimens for about one-third of migraine patients. The best placebo response was found in patients with more intense migraine symptoms, and within the first 4 weeks of therapy (52).

β-*Adrenergic Receptor Antagonists.* A serendipitous observation led to the identification of propranolol as an effective prophylactic agent in the treatment of migraine for up to 80% of patients (53). This nonspecific β-adrenergic receptor antagonist permits unopposed α-adrenergic activity, thereby preventing vasodilatation of a major site associated with migraine pain, the external carotid artery. Blockade of the uptake of serotonin by platelets, diminution of the platelet-aggregating properties of epinephrine, and inhibition of thromboxane synthesis have been proposed as possible mechanisms of action of propranolol (54). Nonselective β-receptor blockade, lack of intrinsic sympathomimetic activity, and significant distribution into brain tissue are the common features of beneficial antimigraine β-receptor antagonists. Recently, the optical isomers of propranolol, which are inequivalent in their β-blocking activity, were found to be equivalent in reducing migraine pain. This suggests that direct correlation between β-receptor antagonism and migraine headache relief is unlikely (55). An adequate explanation of the effects of β-adrenergic antagonists in migraine treatment remains elusive. The optimal dosage range of propranolol is quite variable. Initial doses are relatively low, 40 to 80 mg per day in two or three divided doses, followed by 20 mg incremental increases on a weekly basis to a maximum of 320 mg daily as needed for therapeutic effect. Dose-limiting side effects include fatigue, dizziness, bradycardia, hypotension, and depression. Risk-benefit considerations regarding the use of propranolol should be made for patients with diabetes and asthma; the drug is contraindicated for patients with congestive heart failure. A slow tapering schedule can be instituted after a patient has been headache-free for several months, a practice that avoids a potential β-blocker withdrawal syndrome. Isolated reports of severe peripheral vasoconstriction with the concomitant use of propranolol and ergotamine (56) may warrant caution in using these medications together.

Serotonin (5-HT) Receptor Antagonists. Methysergide maleate, a lysergic acid derivative, is a potent competitive antagonist of peripheral serotonin (5-HT) receptors, particularly the $5-HC_{1C}$ and $5-HT_2$ subtypes. Although its exact mechanism of action is unclear, it has been used for over four decades for migraine prophylaxis. Because methysergide has weak intrinsic vasoconstricting properties, it is not used for the treatment of acute migraine attacks. Prophylactic administration of methysergide has resulted in 60 to 70% of patients reporting a decrease in migraine pain (57). It is absorbed quickly, reaching peak plasma concentrations within 1 hr (58). As has been hypothesized for ergotamine and dihydroergotamine, the effects of methysergide may be mediated by active metabolites instead of by the parent drug. The contraindications for its use are also similar to those for the ergot alkaloids. In contrast to ergotamine, however, the primary elimination pathway of methysergide is through renal excretion.

The initial dosing of methysergide maleate starts at 2 mg daily, which can be gradually increased as tolerated to up to 8 mg in three or four divided daily doses. Unfortunately, 30 to 50% of patients experience at least one of the common side effects (57): nausea, vomiting, muscle cramps, drowsiness, dizziness, paresthesias, mood alterations, and edema. For about 10% of patients, some potentially reversible effects, such as coldness, numbness, intermittent claudication, and even mild angina, cause such persistent discomfort that the drug must be discontinued. Because gastrointestinal distress occurs frequently during methysergide therapy, it should be given with food, milk, or antacids. Some therapeutic effects may become evident after 7 to 10 days, but a 3- to 4-week course of medication is necessary for an adequate trial. If a therapeutic effect is not achieved after this time, continuation of treatment is not expected to provide any benefit. If improvement is sustained, the daily dose can be gradually decreased to determine the minimum amount of methysergide that can be given to suppress the recurrence of migraine. Among the most serious long-term adverse reactions associated with methysergide is the development of fibrotic disorders. Retroperitoneal, pleuropulmonary, and endocardial fibrosis has been reported in patients receiving daily doses above 8 mg or after continuous, uninterrupted use of the drug for 7 to 79 months (59). Therefore, scheduled prophylactic methysergide therapy should not be extended beyond 6 months without an intervening 3- to 4-week drug-free holiday. The fibrotic changes almost always remit when the drug is stopped and may recur upon rechallenge. Medication counseling should direct the patient to report any flank pain, angina, or dysuria to a physician. An annual intravenous pyelogram and chest x-ray to look for fibrosis is part of a thorough monitoring program. When methysergide is to be discontinued, it should be tapered over 2 to 3 weeks to minimize the potential for rebound headache.

Cyproheptadine is an antihistamine that is independently a potent serotonin receptor antagonist. It is effective in 40 to 50% of patients suffering from migraine (59), yet it does not antagonize the vasoconstrictor effects of serotonin to the same extent as methysergide. The usual dosage for migraine prophylaxis is 12 to 24 mg daily, given in divided doses as tolerated. Sedation and weight gain are the two most common side effects. Occasionally, patients may experience dry mouth, vertigo, nausea, pedal edema, or diarrhea.

Ergonovine maleate, an oxytocic drug, has been used as an alternative to methysergide and ergotamine to prevent migraine headaches (60). Ergonovine exerts a stronger peripheral serotonin-blocking effect than ergotamine (61). A clinical advantage to ergonovine is that it has a much lower frequency of nausea and vomiting than is seen with ergotamine therapy. Effective oral dosages range from 0.4 to 2 mg/day as needed or tolerated. Although the drug is generally well tolerated, ergonovine and ergotamine share the same precautions, warnings, and contraindications with respect to their clinical use.

Serotonin (5-HT) Agonists. Sumatriptan (Imitrex), a more specific 5-HT1D agonist, may be particularly useful in causing selective vasoconstriction in the cranial blood vessels, which this serotonin receptor subtype mediates. It is a new agent that is scheduled to be released in the United States sometime in 1992. Studies involving both oral and subcutaneous administration have been performed. Subcutaneous sumatriptan resulted in rapid relief of migraine pain after doses of 6 to 12 mg, with some patients reporting analgesia within 10 min. There was also improvement with respect to resolution of nausea and photophobia. Oral doses of 100 mg also elicit a favorable response. Sumatriptan appears to be generally well tolerated, with adverse reactions that are mild and transient. A tight feeling or tingling sensation in the head was the most commonly reported; others noted vertigo, malaise, fatigue, and local irritation at injection sites. No significant changes in heart rate, blood pressure, or electrocardiogram have been associated with sumatriptan. At present, no rigorous studies directly compare the efficacy of sumatriptan to more commonly used agents such as ergotamine.

Antidepressants. The use of tricyclic antidepressants in the treatment of headache was based on another fortuitous clinical observation. This class of antidepressants is characterized by shared pharmacological properties that may contribute to the mediation of pain: inhibition of presynaptic reuptake of norepinephrine and serotonin and interference with serotonin release from platelets. Amitriptyline is particularly efficacious in the prophylaxis of tension and mixed headaches. Patients without a mood disorder can experience head pain relief from selected antidepressants. In a report describing migraine patients receiving prophylactic amitriptyline, 72% of the subjects received more than 50% improvement (64). The usual required dosage range for migraine prophylaxis is 50 to 200 mg daily, with most patients receiving maximal benefit between 75 and 100 mg/day. Therapy should be initiated at lower, divided daily doses to allow for patient tolerance to the excessive sedation commonly experienced. Other potential side effects include dry mouth, weight gain, constipation, and orthostatic hypotension. About two-thirds of those patients who respond to amitriptyline will improve within 7 days. Amitriptyline can be discontinued after a patient has been essentially headache-free for 1 to 2 months.

The justification for use of a monoamine oxidase inhibitor in migraine prophylaxis rests on the critical role assigned to serotonin in the humoral-vascular theory of migraine. The hypothesis is that as a monoamine oxidase inhibitor blocks the metabolic degradation of serotonin, its plasma and tissue concentrations will increase, and uncontrolled localized vasodilatation will be prevented. The only uncontrolled clinical study that specifically examined this issue used phenelzine in patients who had previously failed on methysergide, cyproheptadine, and ergotamine (65). Fully 80% of the patients who participated experienced at least a 50% improvement on a daily regimen of 45 mg/day phenelzine for a period ranging from 5 to 24 months. The usual precautions about tyramine-free diet restrictions apply to all patients given phenelzine for migraine prophylaxis.

Calcium-Channel Antagonists. Intracellular calcium is known to regulate many physiological functions such as muscle contraction and the secretion of hormones and neurotransmitters. Since each of these functions may impact on the pathogenesis of migraine, the interference of calcium entry into cells by the calcium-channel antagonists could, in principle, alter the outcome of the syndrome. Specifically, since an increase in intracellular calcium is the penultimate stimulus for localized vasoconstriction, theoretically these agents block the reactive vasodilatation associated with headache. Calcium influx is also essential for initiation of the arachidonic acid cascade by activation of phospholipase A_2, marking the calcium-channel antagonists as inhibitors of the local inflammatory response as well. From a clinical standpoint, these agents reduce only the number of migraine attacks, not the severity or duration (66). There is also a delay of about 2 to 8 weeks before the onset of prophylactic efficacy. Agents currently available in the United States (and the associated daily dosage ranges reported to ameliorate migraine symptoms) are verapamil (240 to 480 mg), nifedipine (30 to 90 mg), diltiazem (90 to 270 mg), and nimodipine (60 to 120 mg). Side effects such as sedation and weight gain are common, but are mild in intensity. Therapeutic tolerance has developed in some patients after several months of calcium-channel antagonist treatment. Although the prospects for the use of this class of drugs in migraine prophylaxis are encouraging, their place in the pharmacotherapeutic armamentarium is yet to be validated by carefully designed studies and extensive clinical experience.

Nonsteroidal Antiinflammatory Drugs. Nonsteroidal antiinflammatory drugs are effective in the preventive treatment of migraine (67). In studies that compared the prophylactic activity of nonsteroidal antiinflammatory drugs with placebo or reference drugs, daily doses of 1300 mg aspirin, 600 mg fenoprofen, 400 mg ibuprofen, and 500 mg naproxen were found to be as effective as the reference drug and superior to placebo. These studies lasted from 8 to 12 weeks. Gastrointestinal irritation is associated with this drug class; nonsteroidal antiinflammatory drugs are better tolerated when taken with food or milk. Monitoring for symptoms of impaired renal function induced by nonsteroidal antiinflammatory drugs may be appropriate for certain high-risk patients.

Cluster Headache Pharmacotherapy

SYMPTOMATIC TREATMENT

Because of the relatively brief duration of acute cluster headache attacks, slowly absorbed drugs are essentially ineffective unless the attack is prolonged. Aerosol or parenteral ergotamine preparations, because of their rapid onset of action, have shown some benefit in cluster headache patients. Ergotamine dosages are similar to those useful in the treatment of migraine. Inhalation of 100% oxygen at a flow rate of 8 to 10 liters/min for 10 to 15 min results in dramatic relief, especially in nocturnal attacks. Oxygen inhalations can be repeated up to five times a day; each administration results in substantial vasoconstriction of the scalp and cerebral blood vessels and stimulated synthesis of serotonin in the central nervous system (68). Prednisone is effective as abortive therapy in patients suffering from either an episodic or chronic cluster headache. When given in divided doses of at least 40 mg/day, followed by tapering and discontinuation over 3 to 4 weeks, prednisone provides satisfactory pain relief in approximately 40 to 75% of patients. Paroxysmal pain sensations usually subside within hours of the first dose; otherwise, if there is no response after 48 hr, an alternative agent should be considered. Although considered standard therapy for prophylactic management, lithium carbonate can be effective in some episodic patients, especially those over the age of 45, when given in doses of 300 mg 2 to 4 times daily (69). As in the treatment of migraine, care should be taken to avoid overdosages of ergotamine in patients with frequent cluster headache attacks.

PROPHYLACTIC TREATMENT

Prophylactic management of cluster headache is often warranted for patients who experience attacks with some regularity. Prednisone has demonstrated some use in decreasing the duration, severity, and frequency of cluster attacks in 50 to 75% of patients (70, 71) in doses of 20 mg/day. If the cluster headaches recur in a predictable manner, 2 mg ergotamine tartrate taken orally 2 hr before an expected attack can be effective, especially for nocturnal attacks. Another prophylactic regimen of ergotamine is 1 to 2 mg used 2 to 3 times daily to a maximum weekly dose of 10 mg for up to 2 weeks. After 1 week, the drug should be stopped for 2 days to avoid ergot accumulation; after the second week, ergotamine can be discontinued easily with a tapering schedule. Methysergide is effective prophylaxis in about 70% of patients with episodic cluster headache; it is only 20% effective in preventing chronic cluster (70). The dosage range varies from 4 to 10 mg/day. Because this drug is used only for cluster periods of up to 3 months in duration, the long-term risks of fibrotic disorders resulting from chronic methysergide use are minimized. Response occurs within the first few days of therapy, but sometimes improvement is delayed for about 10 to 14 days.

Lithium carbonate (72) has been found to be effective in up to 85% of chronic cluster headache patients and is considered the drug of choice for prevention of this subtype. Episodic cluster attacks are relieved by lithium therapy, but not to as great an extent. The actual mechanism of action is not known, but lithium may stabilize central serotonergic neurotransmission. The starting dosage in patients with normal renal function is 300 mg orally three times a day. Therapeutic benefit occurs within 1 to 2 weeks after lithium therapy has been initiated, and this response can be maintained with continued administration. To reduce the risk of lithium toxicity or disruptions of renal or thyroid states after long-term use, the dosages should be adjusted so that the plasma concentration of lithium does not exceed 1.2 mmol/liter (1.2 mEq/liter). Plasma levels should be determined 12 hr after the last dose and monitored weekly during the initial titration period. After levels have stabilized and the patient appears free of side effects, plasma levels can be monitored at least quarterly (every 3 months). The most common side effects include tremor, polyuria, nausea, diarrhea, acne-like lesions, and muscle weakness; others, which include slurred speech, confusion, lethargy, dizziness, and hyperreflexia, are dose-related and can signal imminent toxicity. Because lithium is known to suppress thyroid function, flatten or invert electrocardiogram T-waves, induce renal concentrating defects, and cause leukocytosis with chronic use, a routine lithium baseline workup should include: urinalysis, electrolyte levels, electrocardiogram, serum creatinine and blood urea nitrogen levels, thyroid function tests, and a complete blood count with differential, hemoglobin, and hematocrit. In addition, a pregnancy test should be performed on all females not known to be sterile because of the well-documented teratogenic effects of lithium. Contraindications for the use of lithium include renal disease, thyroid disease, pregnancy, dehydration, congestive heart failure, and concomitant thiazide diuretic use. The clinician should be aware of many potentially adverse lithium interactions with other medications, which predispose the patient to central nervous system toxicity (cf. "Mood Disorders," Chapter 52).

Other agents have been used successfully in the prophylaxis of cluster headache (68). Cyproheptadine in doses of 4 to 16 mg/day demonstrates some utility, but the associated weight gain and sedation may be undesirable. Chlorpromazine (75 to 100 mg/day) and the calcium-channel antagonists (nimodipine at doses up to 240 mg/day; nifedipine at doses between 40 to 120 mg/day) reduce the frequency of chronic cluster headache attacks effectively. Combinations of drugs have been required for some relatively refractory patients, e.g., lithium and ergotamine, prednisone and methysergide, triamcinolone and ergotamine. A rare subgroup of cluster headache is chronic paroxysmal hemicrania, which is characterized by 15 or more focal attacks of head pain per day, each of about 15-min duration. This syndrome is particularly responsive to indomethacin during the cluster period at doses of 150 mg/day. Patients with persistent headache attacks who are completely resistant to medication may have to undergo more invasive procedures, such as injections of glycerol or corticosteroids into nerve tissue, as a last resort. Agents known to be ineffective as cluster headache pharmacotherapy include antihistamines, β-blockers, carbamazepine, nonprescription analgesics, and tricyclic antidepressants.

CONCLUSIONS

The seemingly ubiquitous and complex nature of headaches challenges the clinician to develop a rational therapeutic plan. Obtaining a careful history to define a headache profile and establishing a supportive relationship between clinician and patient are the critical first steps in individualizing a treatment strategy. If it has been determined that the headache is secondary to specific environmental, iatrogenic, or organic causes, the primary etiology must be addressed as part of the overall goal of pain resolution. Otherwise, the treatment approach to primary headache disorders can only be focused on relief or prevention of symptoms, not an ultimate cure for the syndrome. Recognition of differences in the clinical presentation of headache subtypes may guide the clinician when considerations of pharmacological or psychological interventions come to the fore. With respect to pharmacotherapy, symptomatic relief is most likely to be achieved when medication is taken early in the course of the attack. At best, prophylaxis results in prevention of future headaches, but for most patients the therapeutic end point is only a reduction in the severity, duration, and frequency of attacks. The medications used in the treatment of headache are not innocuous and often require careful patient monitoring and education. As research in the area continues, an evolving understanding of the underlying pathophysiologic basis of headache should allow further optimization of its management.

REFERENCES

1. Waters WE: Inheritance and epidemiology of headache. In Dalessio DJ: Wolff's Headache and Other Head Pain, ed. 5. New York, Oxford University Press, 1987, pp 51–57.
2. Diehr P, Wood RW, Barr V, et al.: Acute headaches: presenting symptoms and diagnostic rules to identify patients with tension and migraine headache. J Chron Dis 34:147–158, 1981.
3. Raskin NH: Headache, ed. 2. New York: Churchill Livingstone, 1988, ch 1, pp 1–33.
4. Askmark H, Lundberg PO, Olsson S: Drug-related headache. Headache 29:441–444, 1989.
5. Ad Hoc Committee on Classification of Headache: Classification of headache. JAMA 179:717–718, 1962.
6. Philips C: Headache in general practice. Headache 16:322–329, 1977.
7. Ziegler DK: Tension headache. Med Clin North Am 62:495–505, 1978.
8. Diamond S: Muscle-contraction headache. In Dalessio DJ: Wolff's Headache and Other Head Pain, ed. 5. New York, Oxford University Press, 1987, pp 172–189.
9. Diamond S, Medina JL: Headaches. Clin Symp 41:1–32, 1989.
10. Anderson CA, Franks RD: Migraine and tension headache: is there a physiological difference? Headache 21:63–71, 1981.
11. Martin PR, Mathews AM: Tension headaches: psychophysiological investigation and treatment. J Psychosom Res 22:389–399, 1978.
12. Rolf LH, Wiele G, Brune GG: 5-Hydroxytryptamine in platelets of patient with muscle contraction headache. Headache 21:10–11, 1981.
13. Nuechterlein KH, Holroyd JC: Biofeedback in the treatment of tension headache: current status. Arch Gen Psychiatry 37:866–873, 1980.
14. Waters WE: The prevalence of migraine. Headache 18:53–54, 1978.
15. Markush RE, Harp HR, Heyman A, et al.: Epidemiologic study of migraine symptoms in young women. Neurology 25:430–435, 1975.
16. Appenzeller O, Feldman RG, Friedman AP: Migraine, headache, and related conditions—Panel 7. Arch Neurol 36:784–805, 1979.
17. Ziegler DK, Hassanein RS, Couch JR: Headache syndromes suggested by statistical analysis of headache symptoms. Cephalagia 2:125–134, 1982.
18. Adams RD, Victor M: Principles of Neurology, ed. 4. New York: McGraw-Hill, 1989, ch 9, pp 134–154.
19. Headache Classification Committee of the International Headache Society: Classification and diagnostic criteria for headache disorders, cranial neuralgias, and facial pain. Cephalagia 8(suppl 7):1–96, 1988.
20. Adams HE, Feinstein M, Fowler JL: Migraine headache: review of parameters, etiology, and intervention. Psychol Bull 87:217–237, 1980.

21. Glover V, Sandler M: Can the vascular and neurogenic theories of migraine finally be reconciled? Trends Pharmacol Sci 10:1–3, 1989.

22. Lance JW: The pathophysiology of migraine. In Dalessio DJ: Wolff's Headache and Other Head Pain, ed. 5. New York, Oxford University Pres, 1987, pp 58–86.

23. Raskin NH: Headache, ed. 2. New York: Churchill Livingstone, 1988, ch 3, pp 99–133.

24. Lance JW, Lambert GA, Goadsby PJ, et al.: Brain stem influences on the cephalic circulation: experimental data from cat and monkey of relevance to the mechanism of migraine. Headache 23:258–265, 1983.

25. Leão AAP: Spreading depression of activity in cerebral cortex. J Neurophysiol 7:359–390, 1944.

26. Kudrow L: Cluster headache: diagnosis and management. Headache 19:142–150, 1979.

27. Sjaastead O: Cluster headache. In Rose FC: Handbook of Clinical Neurology, v. 4. New York, Elsevier, 1986, pp 217–246.

28. Peters BH, Fraim CJ, Masel BE: Comparison of 650 mg aspirin and 1000 mg acetaminophen with each other, and with placebo in moderately severe headache. Am J Med 74(suppl 6A):36–42, 1983.

29. Ryan RE: Motrin—a new agent for the symptomatic treatment of muscle contraction headache. Headache 16:280–283, 1977.

30. Raskin NH, Appenzeller O: Headache. Major Problems in Internal Medicine. XIX. Philadelphia: WB Saunders, 1980, ch 5, pp 172–184.

31. Weber MB: The treatment of muscle contraction headaches with diazepam. Curr Ther Res 15:210–216, 1973.

32. Friedman AP: The treatment of chronic headache with meprobamate. Ann N Y Acad Sci 67:822–827, 1957.

33. Elenbaas JK: Centrally acting oral skeletal muscle relaxants. Am J Hosp Pharm 37:1313–1323, 1980.

34. Lance JW: Headache. Ann Neurol 10:1–10, 1981.

35. Diamond S, Baltes BJ: Chronic tension headache treated with amitriptyline: a double-blind study. Headache 21:105–109, 1981.

36. Mathew NT: Prophylaxis of migraine and mixed headache: a randomized controlled study. Headache 21:105–109, 1981.

37. Hakkarainen H, Allonen H: Ergotamine vs. metoclopramide vs. their combination in acute migraine attacks. Headache 22:10–12, 1982.

38. Tfelt-Hansen P, Olesen J: Effervescent metoclopramide and aspirin (Migravess) versus effervescent aspirin or placebo for migraine attacks: a double-blind study. Cephalagia 4:107–111, 1984.

39. Ross-Lee L, Eadie MJ, Tyrer JH: Aspirin treatment of migraine attacks: clinical observations. Cephalagia 2:71–76, 1982.

40. Peatfield RC, Petty RG, Rose FC: Double-blind comparison of mefenamic acid and acetaminophen (paracetamol) in migraine. Cephalagia 3:129–134, 1983.

41. Pearce I, Frank GJ, Pearce JMS: Ibuprofen compared with paracetamol in migraine. Practitioner 227:465–467, 1983.

42. Johnson ES, Ratcliffe DM, Wilkinson M: Naproxen sodium in the treatment of migraine. Cephalagia 5:5–10, 1985.

43. Selby G, Lance JW: Observations on 500 cases of migraine and allied vascular headache. J Neurol Neurosurg Psychiatry 23:23–32, 1960.

44. Hilton BP, Zilkh KJ: Effects of ergotamine and methysergide in blood platelet aggregation responses of migrainous subjects. J Neurol Neurosurg Psychiatry 37:593–597, 1974.

45. Peatfield R: Drugs and the treatment of migraine. Trends Pharmacol Sci 9:141–145, 1988.

46. Aghajanian GK, Wang RY: Physiology and pharmacology of central serotonergic neurons. In Lipton MA, DiMascio A, Killam KF: Psychopharmacology: A Generation of Progress. New York, Raven Press, 1978, pp 171–183.

47. Perrin VL: Clinical pharmacokinetics of ergotamine in migraine and cluster headache. Clin Pharmacokin 10:334–352.

48. Raskin NH, Appenzeller O: Headache. Major Problems in Internal Medicine. XIX. Philadelphia: WB Saunders, 1980, ch 4, pp 111–171.

49. Tfelt-Hansen P, Paalzow L: Intramuscular ergotamine: plasma levels and dynamic activity. Clin Pharmacol Ther 37:29–35, 1985.

50. Diamond S: Treatment of migraine with isometheptene, acetaminophen, and dichlorphenazone combination: a double-blind, crossover trial. Headache 15:282–287, 1976.

51. Lance JW: The pharmacotherapy of migraine. Med J Aust 144:85–88, 1986.

52. Couch JR, Bearss CM, Verhulst S: The long-term effect of placebo on migraine. Neurology 37(suppl 1):238, 1987. Abstract.

53. Turner P: Beta-blocking agents in migraine. Postgrad Med J 60(suppl 2):51–55, 1987.

54. Campbell WB, Callahan KS, Johnson AR, et al.: Anti-platelet activity of beta-adrenergic antagonists: inhibition of thromboxane synthesis and platelet aggregation in patients. Lancet 2:1382–1384, 1981.

55. Tfelt-Hansen P: Efficacy of β-blockers in migraine. Cephalagia 6(suppl 5):15–24, 1986.

56. Venter CP, Joubert PH: Severe peripheral ischaemia during concomitant use of beta blockers and ergot alkaloids. Br Med J 289:288–289, 1984.

57. Graham JR: Methysergide for prevention of headache: experience in five hundred patients over three years. N Engl J Med 270:67–72, 1964.

58. Bredberg U, Eyjolfsdottir GS, Paalzow L, et al.: Pharmacokinetics of methysergide and its metabolite methylergometrine in man. Eur J Clin Pharmacol 30:75–77, 1986.

59. Lance JW, Anthony M, Somerville B: Comparative trial of serotonin antagonists in the management of migraine. Br Med J 2:327–330, 1970.

60. Raskin NH, Schwartz RK: Interval therapy of migraine: long-term results. Headache 20:336–340, 1980.

61. Cerletti A, Doepfner W: Comparative study on the serotonin antagonism of amide derivatives of lysergic acid and of ergot alkaloids. J Pharmacol Exp Ther 122:124–136, 1958.

62. Cady RK, Wendt JK, Kirchner JR, et al.: Treatment of acute migraine with subcutaneous sumatriptan. JAMA 265:2831–2835, 1991.

63. Groadsby PJ, Zagami AS, Donnan GA, et al.: Oral sumatriptan in acute migraine. Lancet 338:782–783, 1991.

64. Couch JR, Hassanein RS: Amitriptyline in migraine prophylaxis. Arch Neurol 36:695–699, 1979.

65. Anthony M, Lance JW: Monoamine oxidase inhibition in the treatment of migraine. Arch Neurol 21:263–268, 1986.

66. Greenberg DA: Calcium channel antagonists and the treatment of migraine. Clin Neuropharmacol 9:311–328, 1986.

67. Pradalier A, Clapin A, Dry J: Treatment review: non-steroidal anti-inflammatory drugs in the treatment and long-term prevention of migraine attacks. Headache 28:550–557, 1988.

68. Costa E, Meek JL: Regulation of the biosynthesis of catecholamines and serotonin in the CNS. Annu Rev Pharmacol 14:491–511, 1974.

69. Kudrow L: Cluster headache: diagnosis and management. Headache 19:142–150, 1979.

70. Kudrow L: Comparative results of prednisone, methysergide, and lithium therapy in cluster headache. In Green R: Current Concepts in Migraine Research. New York, Raven Press, 1978, pp 159–163.

71. Jannes JL: The treatment of cluster headaches with prednisone. Dis Nerve Syst 36:375–376, 1975.

72. Manzoni GC, Bono G, Lanfranchi M, et al.: Lithium carbonate in cluster headache: assessment of its short- and long-term therapeutic efficacy. Cephalagia 3:109–114, 1983.

CHAPTER 48

SEIZURE DISORDERS

BRIAN K. ALLDREDGE, Pharm.D.

Epilepsy affects approximately 1% of the worldwide population and is the second most common neurologic disorder after stroke. The incidence is highest in the first 10 years of life and declines thereafter through the age of 50 until the elderly years, when again the incidence increases. Epilepsy begins before the age of 18 years in over 75% of patients (1). The word *epilepsy* originates from the Greek, meaning "to seize," and is used to characterize a *self-sustained, spontaneously recurring seizure disorder*. This definition specifically excludes isolated seizures that have an identifiable cause, such as drug toxicity or metabolic abnormalities.

A *seizure* is defined as the clinical manifestation of excessive or hypersynchronous activity of neurons within the cerebral cortex (2). Though the term often refers to an event characterized by an abrupt loss of consciousness, with generalized muscle contraction and jerking (i.e., a *generalized tonic-clonic* or *grand mal* seizure) the clinical manifestations of various seizure types are quite heterogeneous. The specific signs and symptoms that accompany the event depend upon the functional area of the brain involved and may include various degrees of motor, sensory, or cognitive dysfunction. It is estimated that one of every 11 persons in the United States will experience a seizure at some time during life (3).

ETIOLOGY

Seizures may result from primary or acquired disturbances of central nervous system (CNS) function, from metabolic derangements, or from a variety of systemic diseases. Some of the common causes of new-onset seizures are listed in Table 48.1. Identification of the cause of seizures is of primary importance in the determination of subsequent management. If precipitating factors are identified that are amenable to therapeutic intervention (e.g., metabolic disorders, hypertensive encephalopathy, or drug overdose), then specific treatment should be instituted to correct the underlying cause. Rarely is there a need for chronic antiepileptic drug (AED) therapy. Conversely, when no cause of seizures can be identified by history, physical examination, or laboratory investigation, the seizure disorder is termed *idiopathic* and, if seizures recur, long-term AED therapy is warranted.

Drugs are a particularly common cause of new-onset seizures. In most instances, seizures are dose-related and more likely to occur in patients with a history of seizures or impaired drug elimination capacity (4). Table 48.2 lists drugs that have been implicated as causing seizures.

CLASSIFICATION AND CLINICAL MANIFESTATIONS

Whereas an etiologic diagnosis of seizures is needed to establish whether chronic AED therapy is necessary, the classification of epileptic seizures by their clinical and electrophysiologic manifestations is necessary to determine which AED is most likely to be effective. In most circumstances, the seizure can be classified after a complete patient history in which the patient describes the events that occurred during the attack. This should include questions about any symptoms that warn the patient of an impending seizure (i.e., the *aura*), the specific ictal manifestations, and any postictal abnormalities. Throughout this process, the patient should be discouraged from labeling the attacks, but rather guided to relate the events as they were experienced or described by observers. The current scheme used for the classification of epileptic seizures and syndromes was established by the International League Against Epilepsy (5, 6). A modified version of this classification is presented in Table 48.3.

Seizures are classified as either *generalized* or *partial*, based on their clinical and electroencephalographic features. *Generalized seizures* are those that appear to begin in both hemispheres of the brain. Previously, these seizures were subdivided into *convulsive* and *nonconvulsive* generalized seizures according to the severity of associated motor disturbances. Nonconvulsive generalized seizures included absence (*petite mal*), myoclonic, and atonic seizures. Clonic and tonic-clonic were previously referred to as *grand mal* seizures.

Generalized tonic-clonic seizures are characteristic of maximal involvement of neurons of both hemispheres of the brain. Typically, these seizures begin with tonic (rigid) flexion of the extremities, followed by extension. During this phase, air is forced from the larynx to produce an audible cry. The tonic phase of the seizure usually lasts 15 to 20 sec and is quickly followed by the clonic (jerking) phase, during which there are spasms of the trunk and extremities and often biting of the tongue. The clonic phase usually lasts 20 to 30 sec and is followed by a postictal state, during which the patient may sleep or awaken confused and disoriented. There is then a gradual return of consciousness and orientation over a period of 15 to 30

Table 48.1.
Common Causes of New-Onset Seizures[a]

Cause	Comment
Primary CNS disorders	
Benign febrile convulsions of childhood	Do not occur after age 5; always consider other causes first
Idiopathic epilepsy	Onset less common after age 25
Head trauma	Especially when associated with depressed skull fracture or intracerebral or subdural hematoma
Stroke	Embolic, or hemorrhage; thrombotic
CNS mass lesion	Primary or metastatic tumor; brain abscess; arteriovenous malformation
Metabolic or systemic disorders	
Cerebral hypoperfusion or hypoxia	Cardiopulmonary arrest; cardiac dysrhythmia; severe hypotension
Meningitis, encephalitis	Acute or chronic; bacterial, viral, fungal, tuberculous or parasitic
Hyponatremia	Usually with serum sodium level of 104–118 mmol/liter (104–118 mEq/liter), but rapid fall better correlated with seizures than actual level
Hypoglycemia	Usually with serum glucose level of 1.1–1.65 mmol/liter (20–30 mg/dl), but little correlation between hypoglycemic symptoms and glucose levels
Hypernatremia or hyperosmolar nonketotic hyperglycemia	Serum osmolality usually above 330 mOsm/liter
Hypocalcemia	Convulsant range 1.07 to 2.3 mmol/liter (4.3–9.2 mg/dl); common presentation of hypoparathyroidism and pseudohypoparathyroidism; tetany need not be present
Hypertensive encephalopathy	Blood pressure usually greater than 250/150 mm Hg or, when acutely elevated from normal BP, above 160/100
Uremic encephalopathy	Rapid development of uremia is more closely associated with seizures than is absolute serum urea nitrogen
Hepatic encephalopathy	Respiratory alkalosis nearly always present
Eclampsia	Phenytoin treatment is preferable to MgSO$_4$
Porphyria	Most anticonvulsants can exacerbate porphyric symptoms; anticonvulsant of choice is triple bromides
Drug overdose	See Table 9.2
Drug withdrawal	Anticonvulsants, ethanol, or sedative-hypnotic drugs (with habituation to daily doses of 600–800 mg secobarbital or its equivalent)
Hyperthermia	Temperature usually above 42°C (107°F); immediate reduction of body temperature to 39°C (102°F) mandatory

[a] Reprinted with permission from Simon RP, Aminoff MJ, Greenberg DA: Clinical Neurology. Norwalk: Appleton & Lange, 1989, ch 9.

min after which the patient has no recall of the event. Increases in blood pressure and heart rate, incontinence of urine or feces, as well as brief interruption of normal breathing with cyanosis commonly accompany this seizure type. Generalized tonic-clonic seizures often result from the progression of some other fundamental seizure type (e.g., simple partial or complex partial seizures) in which case they are termed *secondarily generalized tonic-clonic seizures. Primary generalized* seizures have no evidence of progression from another seizure type.

Absence (petit mal) seizures occur primarily during childhood and are characterized by an abrupt interruption of consciousness followed by a fixed stare and automatisms (e.g., lip smacking, chewing, grimacing) or mild clonic movements. During the seizure there is no loss of postural tone. The seizure usually last less than 45 sec and ends as abruptly as it begins, with the patient immediately regaining full alertness. Absence seizures may occur hundreds of times in a day and are often perceived initially by family or teachers as daydreaming. This seizure type is characterized by a classic pattern on the electroencephalogram

of bilateral 3 Hz spike-waves discharges. Absence seizures usually have their onset between the ages of 4 and 12 years. Rarely does this seizure type persist beyond the age of 20 years. *Atypical absence* seizures differ from traditional absence seizures by a longer duration, focal motor manifestations, and a greater association with developmental delay.

Atonic seizures are characterized by a sudden loss of muscle tone. Since the patient may fall abruptly, injuries are common, and it is often necessary to protect the patient's head by prescribing the use of a helmet during the daytime. *Myoclonic* seizures are characterized by jerking movements of a single or multiple muscle groups. *Tonic* seizures are similar to generalized tonic-clonic seizures except that they lack the usual clonic phase.

Partial seizures begin in an area of the brain limited to one hemisphere and often indicate some underlying focal brain lesion (e.g., perinatal injury, trauma, stroke, or CNS tumor). Partial seizures are differentiated according to whether or not consciousness is impaired during the event. *Complex partial seizures* are associated with im-

Table 48.2.
Drugs That Can Cause Seizures[a]

Antimicrobials	Anesthetic and antiarrhythmic agents
β-Lactam and related compounds	Class 1B
Cephalosporins	Lidocaine
Imipenem/cilastatin	Tocainide
Penicillin and its derivatives	β-Adrenergic blockers
Quinolones	Esmolol
Ciprofloxacin	Metoprolol
Enoxacin	Propranolol
Nalidixic acid	Local anesthetics
Norfloxacin	Bupivicaine
Isoniazid	Chlorprocaine
Psychotropic agents	Lidocaine
Antidepressants	Procaine
Amitriptyline	*Radiographic contrast agents*
Bupropion	Diatrizoate meglumine
Desipramine	Iohexol
Doxepin	Iopamidol
Fluoxetine	Ioxaglate sodium
Imipramine	Meglumine metrizoate
Maprotiline	Sodium iothalamate
Nortriptyline	*Drugs of abuse*
Protriptyline	Amphethamine
Antipsychotics	Cocaine
Chlorpromazine	Phencyclidine
Haloperidol	Methylphenidate
Perphenazine	*Sedative-hypnotic drug withdrawal*
Promazine	Alcohol
Thioridazine	Barbiturates
Trifluoperazine	Benzodiazepines
Lithium	Ethchlorvynol
Theophylline	Glutethimide
	Meprobamate
	Methaqualone
	Methyprylon

[a] Adapted from Alldredge BK, Simon RP, Drugs that can precipitate seizures. In Resor SR, Kutt H (eds): Medical Management of Seizures. New York, Marcel Dekker (in press).

pairment of consciousness whereas *simple partial* seizures are not.

Simple partial seizures are characterized by either motor manifestations (e.g., clonic jerking of one arm) or sensory symptoms (e.g., a foul odor or visual distortions). In some patients with motor symptoms, the seizure may spread to contiguous areas of the cortex resulting in the recruitment of additional muscle groups ("jacksonian march"). Autonomic symptoms such as piloerection or pupillary dilatation, or psychic symptoms such as feelings of deja vu or fear may also accompany simple partial seizures; however, they are less common. In all cases, patients can respond to the environment throughout the attack.

Complex partial seizures (*psychomotor* or *temporal lobe* seizures) are characterized by impaired consciousness and a heterogeneous group of abnormal symptoms. Although the variety of symptoms associated with complex partial seizures is wide, each individual usually reports ste-

reotypical attacks. Auras precede complex partial seizures in many patients. Unusual epigastric sensations are most common, although various motor, sensory, or psychic symptoms (as described for simple partial seizures) may occur. Consciousness is then impaired for an average duration of about 2 min. During this time patients may exhibit coordinated involuntary movements (automatisms) such as lip smacking, buttoning or unbuttoning of clothing, or wandering behavior. Less often, the behavioral abnormalities include violent outbursts, crying, or sexual actions. In some patients, there is diagnostic confusion between the symp-

Table 48.3.
International Classification of Epileptic Seizures and Syndromes[a]

Partial seizures (focal, local)
Simple partial seizures (consciousness preserved)
  With motor signs (jacksonian)
  With somatosensory or special sensory symptoms
  With autonomic symptoms or signs
  With psychic symptoms
Complex partial seizures (consciousness impaired)
  Simple partial onset followed by impaired consciousness
  Impaired consciousness at onset
Secondarily generalized seizures
  Simple partial seizures evolving to generalized tonic-clonic seizures
  Complex partial seizures evolving to generalized tonic-clonic seizures
  Simple partial seizures evolving to complex partial seizures evolving to generalized tonic-clonic seizures
Generalized-onset seizures (convulsive or nonconvulsive)
Tonic-clonic seizures
Absence seizures
  Typical absence seizures
  Atypical absence seizures
Myoclonic seizures
Tonic seizures
Atonic seizures
Localization-related (focal) epilepsies
Idiopathic
  Benign epilepsy of childhood
Symptomatic
  Temporal lobe epilepsy
  Extratemporal epilepsy
Generalized epilepsy
Idiopathic
  Benign neonatal convulsions
  Childhood absence epilepsy
  Juvenile myoclonic epilepsy
  Other
Idiopathic and/or symptomatic
  Infantile spasms (West syndrome)
  Lennox-Gastaut syndrome
  Myoclonic epilepsies
Special syndromes
Febrile seizures

[a] Adapted from Commission on Classification and Terminology of the International League Against Epilepsy: Proposal for revised clinical and electroencephalographic classification of epileptic seizures. Epilepsia 22:489–501, 1981; and Proposal for classification of epilepsies and epileptic syndromes. Epilepsia 26:268–278, 1985.

toms of absence and complex partial seizures. Table 48.4 compares usual clinical features of these two seizure types. Either simple or partial complex seizures may spread to involve both hemispheres of the brain (usually as a generalized tonic-clonic seizure). These events are termed *partial seizures with secondary generalization.*

In some cases, the seizure classification, etiologic diagnosis, patient age, and coexistent medical conditions can be used to define a specific *epileptic syndrome.* An epileptic syndrome is a constellation of signs and symptoms that tends to occur together. Identification of epileptic syndromes may provide useful information not necessarily implied by either the etiologic diagnosis or seizure classification, such as the anticipated duration of AED therapy and patient prognosis. Not all patients with epilepsy can be classified into an epileptic syndrome.

Febrile Seizures

Febrile seizures are defined as generalized tonic-clonic seizures associated with temperatures above 38°C that occur in the absence of other identifiable causes. Febrile seizures are the most common form of epilepsy in children, occurring in 2 to 5% of the population. Affected children are usually between the ages of 3 months and 5 years, and are otherwise neurologically and developmentally normal. Febrile seizures are classified as either *simple* or *complex. Complex febrile seizures* are prolonged (>15 min), occur in series (2 or more seizures in 24 h), or have associated focal features. The remainder are classified as simple febrile seizures. *Simple febrile seizures* are usually benign, self-limited, and associated with only a 3% risk of recurrent, nonfebrile seizures in later life (7). The risk of epilepsy is increased to 4 to 11% in children affected by complex febrile seizures.

Because most febrile seizures are self-limited and not associated with acute or long-term neurologic sequelae, aggressive treatment is not required. Most febrile seizures occur within 24 hr of a febrile episode and can be prevented by promptly instituting antipyretic measures as soon as the fever is evident. Parents should be told to sponge the child with tepid water for 10 to 15 min and administer acetaminophen every 4 hr for a temperature above 38°C. Acute treatment with AEDs is usually not necessary unless the seizure continues for longer than 10 or 15 min. In this case, either phenobarbital or diazepam are effective. Chronic administration of AEDs to children with a history of simple febrile seizures is not indicated.

Children with complex febrile seizures, preexisting neurologic abnormalities, or a family history of nonfebrile epilepsy are at greater risk for the development of epilepsy in later life. Drug therapy for the prevention of febrile seizures should be considered for these patients, although there is no evidence that the risk of nonfebrile epilepsy is reduced. Phenobarbital is effective for the treatment of febrile seizures, however, it must be administered continuously to ensure adequate drug levels at the onset of a febrile episode. Initiating oral phenobarbital at the onset of febrile illness is not appropriate. Rectal administration of diazepam (using the parenteral solution) results in rapid absorption and provides immediate protection from febrile seizures (7). This treatment is preferred by many clinicians since it does not require continuous administration.

DIAGNOSIS

Table 48.5 outlines a comprehensive evaluation for patients with new-onset seizures. The diagnosis of epilepsy and proper classification of epileptic seizures is based primarily upon the patient's history and observer's accounts of the events. Although a complete evaluation usually includes other laboratory and diagnostic studies, a diagnosis of epilepsy can only be clearly established when an accurate and unambiguous history is obtained. Most patients and witnesses can give a clear account of generalized tonic-clonic seizures, however more careful questioning is often necessary to elicit the subtle manifestations that accompany partial, absence, and other less dramatic seizure types.

Once it is apparent that a seizure has occurred, subsequent efforts should be directed toward establishing the cause. A thorough evaluation including medical history and physical and laboratory examinations should be directed toward the variety of primary, metabolic and systemic fac-

Table 48.4.
Comparison of the Clinical Features of Absence and Complex Partial Seizures

Feature	Absence Seizures	Complex Partial Seizures
Patients affected	Children	Children and adults
Preictal symptoms	No aura; abrupt interruption of consciousness	Aura common
Ictal phenomena	Automatisms common Average duration 10 sec	Automatisms common though more complex than in absence; average duration 2 min
Postictal symptoms	None; abrupt return of consciousness	Fatigue, confusion, drowsiness; gradual return of consciousness
Prognosis	Complete seizure control common	Less favorable response to drug therapy

tors that may cause new-onset seizures (Table 48.1). Seizures due to an acute metabolic or systemic disorder must be differentiated from those related to a primary CNS disorder. Even with extensive work-up, the etiology of epilepsy remains unidentified in 60 to 70% of patients. A genetic cause is suggested when the age at seizure onset is less than 25 years and there is a family history of epilepsy (8).

The electroencephalogram (EEG) is a useful tool for both the diagnosis and classification of seizures. Spike and wave discharges on the EEG in conjunction with a clinical history of spontaneously recurring seizures usually can establish the diagnosis of epilepsy. While epileptiform abnormalities on the EEG are almost always seen during a seizure, most EEG recordings are made between seizures (interictal EEG). Absence of EEG abnormalities on an interictal recording rarely can rule out the diagnosis of epilepsy. Epileptiform abnormalities are found in only about 50% of epileptic patients after a single interictal recording. Although the yield can be improved with repeated recordings, in 15% of epileptic patients no EEG abnormalities are ever found (8). Just as the diagnosis of epilepsy is rarely excluded on the basis of a normal interictal EEG, the presence of EEG abnormalities alone is not diagnostic for epilepsy. EEG abnormalities are seen in 10 to 15% of the nonepileptic population and do not indicate epilepsy unless strong evidence from the patient history supports the diagnosis (8).

Computer-assisted tomography (CT) and magnetic resonance imaging (MRI) scans are particularly useful when the history or neurological examination suggests a structural lesion of the brain (e.g., focal neurologic abnormalities or a history suggestive of partial seizures), although they are often used in the initial evaluation of pa-

Table 48.5.
Workup for the Patient with New-Onset Seizures

Patient history
  Seizure description
    Preictal phenomena (aura)
    Ictal manifestations
    Postictal state
    Provocative factors
  Perinatal and developmental history
  History of febrile seizures
  History of head trauma
  History of CNS infection
  Family history of epilepsy
Physical examination
Laboratory evaluation
  CBC, electrolytes, glucose, cerebrospinal fluid, BUN, osmolality
Electroencephalogram
Computed tomographic scanning
Magnetic resonance imaging

Table 48.6.
Disorders That May Mimic Epilepsy[a]

Gastroesophageal reflux
Breath-holding spells
Migraine
  Confusional
  Basilar
  With recurrent abdominal pain and cyclic vomiting
Sleep disorders (especially parainsomnias)
Cardiovascular events
  Pallid infantile syncope
  Vasovagal attacks
  Vasomotor syncope
  Cardiac arrhythmias
Movement disorders
  Shuddering attacks
  Paroxysmal choreoathetosis
  Nonepileptic myoclonus
  Tics and habit spasms
Psychological disorders
  Panic disorder
  Hyperventilation attacks
  Pseudoseizures
  Rage attacks

[a] Reprinted with permission from Schever ML, Pedley TA: The evaluation and treatment of seizures. N Engl J Med 323:1468–1474, 1990.

tients with new-onset seizures, regardless of the seizure type. MRI is more likely to detect lesions associated with partial epilepsy and is preferred over CT (1). Positron emission tomography (PET), an advanced imaging technique that allows more precise localization of areas of abnormal blood flow or metabolism, is useful for evaluation of patients in whom surgical intervention is considered, however, its availability is limited by high equipment costs.

Finally, in some patients, seizure-like activity may be a manifestation of some other nonepileptic condition (Table 48.6). The misdiagnosis of these events as seizures can result in unnecessary and potentially harmful therapy. Accordingly, the diagnosis of epilepsy should be reevaluated whenever the "seizure-like" events fail to respond to the usual treatments.

TREATMENT OVERVIEW
Lifestyle Adjustment and Social Issues

Although lifestyle adjustments may be required for patients with epilepsy, most patients respond well to medical therapy and can lead a life that is not severely restricted by their disorder. Nonetheless, some alteration of the patient's usual activities may be required, depending upon the timing and clinical manifestation of seizures. For example, patients affected by seizures associated with loss of consciousness or normal muscle control should restrict activities that place them or others at risk of injury. This may include partial or complete restriction of driving privileges and avoidance of activities such as swimming unattended, working at heights, or operating potentially dangerous machinery. Common sense should be the ultimate guide in the determination of specific lifestyle limitations necessitated by the patient's epileptic condition.

Certain changes in daily activities may reduce the occurrence of seizures by avoiding patient-specific risk factors. Conditions that are occasionally identified by patients as seizure precipitants include stress, exercise, alcohol or caffeine consumption, altered sleep schedules, and missed meals. When these or other precipitating conditions are identified, the patient and health provider should work cooperatively to establish guidelines that minimize these risks, yet do not unnecessarily encumber the patient's daily routine.

In addition to lifestyle limitations, many persons with epilepsy also deal with problems of self-image and the social stigma attached to this disorder. Many patient concerns can be dealt with effectively by proper education. The clinician should explain the disorder and its implications and establish an atmosphere in which the patient can voice questions and concerns. The Epilepsy Foundation of American and its local affiliates have a wide range of client services and brochures to help patients (and their families) deal with the condition and its psychosocial implications.

Drug Therapy

AED therapy is the mainstay of epilepsy treatment. The goals are to reduce the frequency of recurrent seizures and minimize the adverse effects associated with AED therapy. Specific therapeutic end points must be individualized for each patient. The choice of AED should be based on the seizure classification, the age and sex of the patient, concurrent medical conditions, potential adverse effects, and the pharmacokinetic features of the individual drugs. When these factors are considered and the guiding principles of AED therapy (discussed below) are followed, good-to-excellent seizures control can be attained in most patients. Nonetheless, some patients may continue to suffer from frequent seizures despite appropriate drug treatment.

PRINCIPLES OF ANTIEPILEPTIC DRUG SELECTION AND USAGE
Monotherapy with Nonsedating Agents is Preferred

Monotherapy is preferred to polytherapy with AEDs because of the lower cost associated with the medication and blood level monitoring, reduced potential for adverse reactions and undesirable drug interactions, and improved medication compliance with a simplified drug administration schedule. Furthermore, a growing body of evidence indicates that polytherapy offers no advantage over monotherapy for about 90% of patients with epilepsy (9). For patients in whom single drug therapy does not provide sufficient seizure control, polytherapy may be necessary to achieve the goals of treatment.

In addition to selecting the minimum effective number of AEDs, it is important to choose agents based on their adverse-effect profile. The specific adverse effects of each drug are discussed below; however, sedating AEDs should be minimized or avoided. Phenobarbital and benzodiazepine antiepileptic drugs are sedating; phenytoin, carbamazepine, valproate, and ethosuximide are not. Sedation and decreased mentation are particularly common upon initiation of barbiturate and benzodiazepine agents. Over time an adaptive process occurs during which these effects become less noticeable. Despite the development of tolerance to the overt sedative effect of these drugs, evidence suggests that subtle effects on intelligence, memory, complex motor skills, and behavior often persist during treatment. In some cases, these changes are noted by patients or their families only after the drug is discontinued (10). In this regard, therapy with nonsedating agents is preferred when possible, and the relative place of sedating AEDs has been reconsidered. For example, phenobarbital is as effective as phenytoin and carbamazepine for the treatment of generalized tonic-clonic seizures, but the latter agents are preferred because of their relative lack of CNS-depressant effects.

When possible, therapy should begin with one of the nonsedating AEDs such as phenytoin, carbamazepine, valproate, or ethosuximide. Except in some of the less common epilepsies (e.g., myoclonic epilepsy), phenobarbital and benzodiazepine should be reserved until nonsedating alternatives have filed. Nitrazepam and clobazam are benzodiazepine agents that may have advantages over clonazepam in terms of sedation-related adverse effects, but they are not available for use in the United States. In summary, sedating AEDs should be avoided when possible, and in many cases, substitution with nonsedating alternatives can result in noticeable improvement in cognitive, motor, and behavioral changes.

Drug Selection

After diagnosis of epilepsy, the choice of AED therapy is guided by the relative efficacy and toxicity of each agent. Proper classification of the patient's seizure type is the most important step in choosing the appropriate agent. Table 48.7 lists the preferred AEDs for the treatment of different seizure types.

PARTIAL SEIZURES

Carbamazepine, phenytoin, phenobarbital, and primidone are equally effective for the treatment of partial seizures, including those that secondarily generalize (11). However,

Table 48.7.
Antiepileptic Drugs of Choice Based on Seizure Classification[a]

	Partial Seizures[b]	Generalized Tonic-Clonic Seizures	Absence Seizures	Myoclonic Seizures
Drugs of choice	Carbamazepine Phenytoin	Valproate[c] Carbamazepine Phenytoin	Ethosuximide Valproate	Valproate
Alternatives Primary	Phenobarbital Valproate Primidone	Phenobarbital Primidone	Clonazepam	Clonazepam
Secondary	Clorazepate		Acetazolamide	

[a] Information from References (1, 3, 8, 11, 14)
[b] Includes simple partial seizures, complex partial seizures, and partial seizures that secondarily generalize.
[c] Probably the drug of choice for primary (generalized-onset) tonic-clonic seizures.

carbamazepine and phenytoin are usually tolerated better. Phenytoin has a long half-life that allows once-daily dosing, so this agent is preferred for patients unlikely to comply with a chronic regimen requiring multiple daily doses. Alternately, phenytoin is associated with cosmetic changes that make it less desirable for the treatment of epilepsy in children, adolescents, and women. Valproate is also useful for the treatment of partial seizures, but it has been studied less extensively, and its efficacy relative to other agents is yet to be determined (12). Overall, partial seizures do not respond to treatment as well as seizures that are generalized from their onset. Indeed, the prognosis for complete control of complex partial seizures in adults is often poor.

GENERALIZED TONIC-CLONIC SEIZURES

Carbamazepine, phenytoin, and valproate are the drugs of choice for the treatment of generalized tonic-clonic seizures. Evidence from some studies suggests that valproate is the drug of choice for the treatment of primary generalized tonic-clonic seizures. Approximately 75 to 85% of patients achieve complete seizure control with monotherapy with this agent (3). Carbamazepine or phenytoin is preferred for the treatment of children under the age of 2 years because of the higher risk of valproate-associated hepatotoxicity in these patients. Phenobarbital and primidone are also effective against generalized tonic-clonic seizures, but because of their adverse effects, they are usually reserved for use as second-line agents.

ABSENCE SEIZURES

Ethosuximide and valproate are equally effective for the treatment of absence seizures. Ethosuximide is preferred over valproate when only absence seizures are involved because it is associated with fewer serious adverse effects. Valproate is the preferred if generalized tonic-clonic seizures also occur (1). The response to these agents is dramatic. In controlled trials, 70 to 90% of patients treated with ethosuximide or valproate experience cessation or a dramatic reduction in absence seizures (13, 14). The combination of ethosuximide and valproate is often effective when monotherapy fails. Clonazepam is also effective against absence seizures, but because of frequent dose-related adverse effects and the development of tolerance to its antiepileptic effect, it should be reserved for patients in whom ethosuximide and valproate fail. Carbamazepine is ineffective for the treatment of absence seizures and may even exacerbate these and other seizure types when used in children with mixed seizures disorders (15).

MYOCLONIC SEIZURES

Valproate controls myoclonic seizures effectively in 75 to 90% of patients with generalized idiopathic and juvenile myoclonic epilepsy (14). Myoclonic seizures after anoxic encephalopathy are more resistant to treatment. Clonazepam is also effective as monotherapy or in combination with valproate when either drug alone does not provide adequate seizure control.

Initiating Antiepileptic Drug Therapy

Phenytoin and phenobarbital are usually tolerated well when initiated at maintenance doses (e.g., 300 mg and 90 mg daily, respectively, in adults). Carbamazepine, valproate, ethosuximide, primidone, and benzodiazepine agents are frequently associated with acute adverse effects, so therapy should begin with low doses and be titrated gradually according to the clinical status of the patient. Patients who experience uncomfortable adverse effects at the initiation of therapy may be unwilling to continue treatment with that agent despite a reduction in dosage. Patients should be told to report adverse effects immediately so an adjustment in therapy can be made as soon as possible. Patients should also know the goal of treatment and the time course over which seizure control is anticipated. The importance of strict compliance with the prescribed regimen should also be emphasized.

Adjusting and Monitoring Antiepileptic Drug Therapy

There is great interpatient variability in the dose-response relationship for all of the AEDs in common use. Therefore, after therapy is initiated, the optimal drug dose for each patient should be determined. This necessitates the titration of therapy until the desired clinical response is achieved or the patient experiences unacceptable dose-related adverse effects.

The determination of acceptable seizure control requires input from both patient and clinician. Though complete control of seizures is always desirable, patients may choose to continue therapy that allows minimal interruption of their lifestyle even though seizures occasionally recur. The clinician must assess the temporary disability and potential for harm (both to the patient and others) that may accompany a seizure and use this information, with input from the patient, to determine whether dosage adjustments should be made.

If the first agent does not achieve the desired therapeutic goal, then an alternate AED, appropriate for the patient's seizure type, should be substituted gradually rather than added. Tapering of the first drug should begin after a therapeutic effect (or blood level) of the new agent is attained. The rate of drug tapering is empiric. In this instance, most practitioners prefer to discontinue therapy gradually over several days to weeks (see "Withdrawal of Antiepileptic Drug Therapy"). Only after monotherapy has failed, should multiple AED treatment be tried.

AED therapy fails for many reasons. Although various drugs may demonstrate equal efficacy in large populations of patients, an individual may respond better to one agent than to others. Additional factors that should be considered include poor medication compliance, erroneous diagnosis or classification, progressive neurologic disease, or lifestyle factors that compromise the efficacy of treatment (e.g., recreational drug or alcohol abuse). Noncompliance with treatment is probably the most common cause of AED therapy failure and this possibility should be carefully investigated. Patients who report a change in the character of their seizures (e.g., seizures are now preceded by an aura whereas previously there was no warning) or frequent seizures after a long period of complete control should be referred for a thorough medical evaluation to rule out other neurologic disease (e.g., brain tumor).

Blood Levels

The widespread availability of blood-level monitoring of AED therapy has had a dramatic effect on the use of these agents. For example, patients were frequently begun on combination AED regimens (e.g., phenytoin and phenobarbital) before clinicians could individualize the doses for either agent. On the basis of past experience in which a single drug was occasionally ineffective and above average doses sometimes led to toxicity, it was assumed that most patients would benefit if multiple drugs were used. Blood-level monitoring, in addition to the pharmacokinetic properties of AEDs, is now used to maximize efficacy and minimize adverse effects.

The therapeutic range of plasma concentrations is a useful guide for titrating therapy. Within this range, many patients achieve seizure control without unacceptable side effects. However, it is also common to observe an adequate therapeutic response at concentrations below the usual therapeutic range, and some patients tolerate and indeed require blood levels above the upper limit of the therapeutic range to maintain seizure control. Thus, although these limits are useful guides to therapy, the clinician should strive to determine the optimum AED plasma concentration for each individual patient (16).

Plasma-concentration monitoring of AEDs is most useful under the following conditions: (*a*) to document therapeutic failures; (*b*) to evaluate noncompliance or drug malabsorption; (*c*) to guide subsequent dosage adjustments required on a clinical basis; and (*d*) to evaluate possible drug-related adverse effects. The timing of blood sampling for drug-level determination is important, particularly during therapy with AEDs that have a short half-life (e.g., carbamazepine and valproate). For these agents, blood levels can fluctuate greatly over the course of the dosing interval. Comparisons between drug levels may be inaccurate unless the blood is sampled at a consistent time relative to the dose. For most patients, it is recommended that blood samples be taken in the morning, before the first daily dose of medication. An exception is patients with repeated, transient symptoms that suggest dose-related drug toxicity. For these patients, blood sampling should coincide with the adverse experience so that the contribution of the drug level can be assessed.

Plasma-level monitoring of AEDs is often both overused and misused (9). It is common (and appropriate) to document drug levels occasionally in patients with well-controlled epileptic conditions (e.g., every 6 to 12 months), but other drug-level determinations should not be done unless there is clinical indication of their necessity. Likewise, there is often a tendency to adjust AED therapy on the basis of the level without considering the clinical status of the patient. For example, it may be tempting to decrease the drug dose when the reported blood level is above the usual therapeutic range. However, some patients require higher concentrations than usual to achieve the desired therapeutic effect. Likewise, patients whose seizures are controlled with levels below the therapeutic range neither need a dose increase nor should be assumed to no longer require AED treatment. In his editorial on the use of AED blood-level monitoring, W. Edwin Dodson wrote that "[c]hanging an antiepileptic drug dose based only on the drug level is like driving a car looking only at the speedometer and not out the window. Wrecks are inevitable and frequent" (16).

ANTIEPILEPTIC DRUGS

Clinical pharmacokinetic features of the common antiepileptic drugs are summarized in Table 48.8.

Carbamazepine

Carbamazepine is a highly lipophilic iminostilbene compound structurally related to the tricyclic antidepressant agent, imipramine. Carbamazepine is very effective for the treatment of generalized tonic-clonic and partial seizures, but it is not effective against myoclonic or absence seizures. The antiepileptic effect of carbamazepine may be related to its effects on sodium channels to limit sustained, repetitive firing and alter synaptic transmission.

Carbamazepine (Tegretol and generic) is available as oral (200 mg) and chewable (100 mg) tablets and as a suspension (100 mg/5 ml). No parenteral formulation of the drug is available. Therapy with carbamazepine is usually initiated at a dose of 100 to 200 mg twice daily with gradual dose titration, in 200 mg increments, every 3 to 7 days. Although the manufacturer recommends that daily

doses of carbamazepine not exceed 1200 mg, daily doses of 2000 mg and above are occasionally required for optimal therapy. Because of frequent gastric disturbances, loading doses of carbamazepine are not recommended for usual outpatient therapy. However, single carbamazepine doses of 8 to 10 mg/kg by the nasogastric route are useful for critically ill patients in whom attainment of a therapeutic level is desired (17).

Absorption of carbamazepine from the gastrointestinal tract is slow and erratic and often does not follow first-order kinetics. The time to peak plasma levels after oral administration may vary from an average of 4 to 8 hr to as long as 24 hr. Although prolonged absorption of the drug may be due to slow dissolution of the drug from tablet form, the suspension is also absorbed erratically. Food has no consistent effect on the bioavailability of carbamazepine.

Carbamazepine is cleared almost exclusively by hepatic metabolism. Oxidation of the parent drug to carbamazepine 10,11-epoxide (CBZ-E) is the major metabolic pathway for elimination. The remainder is glucuronidated, sulfur-conjugated, or oxidatively metabolized by other routes. Only 2% of the dose is recovered unchanged in the urine. The half-life of the drug after a single dose may range from 24 to 45 hr. With chronic administration, the half-life of carbamazepine is reduced, and interindividual dif-

Table 48.8.
Clinical Pharmacokinetics of Antiepileptic Drugs[a]

	Carbamazepine	Phenytoin	Valproate	Ethosuximide	Phenobarbital	Primidone	Clonazepam	Clorazepate
Adult daily dose (mg/kg)	5–20	4–6	10–20	15–40[b]	1–3	10–15	0.1–0.3	0.3–1.3
Initial dose	100–200 mg b.i.d.	300 mg q.d.	125–250 mg b.i.d.-t.i.d.	500 mg q.d.	90 mg q.d.	125–250 mg b.i.d.	0.5–1 mg q.d.	7.5 mg t.i.d.
Dosage schedule	b.i.d.-q.i.d.	q.d.-b.i.d.	t.i.d.-q.i.d.	q.d.-b.i.d.	q.d.-b.i.d.	b.i.d.-t.i.d.	q.d.-t.i.d.	q.d.-t.i.d.
Bioavailability (%)	75–85	85–95	100	90–95	95–100	90–100	80–90	—
Time to peak absorption (hr)	4–8	4–8	2–8	1–7	1–4	1–3	1–4	0.5–2[c]
Volume of distribution (liter/kg)	0.8–1.6	0.5–0.7	0.09–0.17	0.6–0.9	0.51–0.57	0.4–0.8	2.1–4.3	1–1.8[d]
Protein binding (%)	75–78	90–93	88–92	0	48–54	20–30	80–90	95–98[c]
Plasma half-life (hr)	24–45 (single dose) 8–24 (chronic therapy)	9–40	6–16	20–60	72–144	5–18	30–40	55–100[c]
Therapeutic plasma levels								
(μg/ml)	4–12	10–20	50–100	40–100	10–40	5–15	5–70 ng/ml	
(μmol/liter)	16–48	40–80	200–400	283–708	43–172	23–69	16–220 nmol/ml	

[a] Adapted from Brodie MJ: Established anticonvulsants and treatment of refractory epilepsy. Lancet 336:350–354, 1990; and Levy RH, Dreifuss FE, Mattson RH, Meldrum BS, Penry JK (eds): Antiepileptic Drugs, ed. 3. New York, Raven Press, 1989.
[b] The daily dose in children is 20–40 mg/kg.
[c] Pharmacokinetic values for DMD, the active metabolite of clorazepate.

ferences in clearance are enhanced. Increased clearance of carbamazepine occurs during the first few weeks of therapy because of autoinduction of cytochrome P-450 activity, leading to an increase in oxidation to CBZ-E. This metabolic conversion is also enhanced by other enzyme-inducing drugs, such as phenytoin, phenobarbital, and primidone. Thus, the metabolic clearance and half-life may vary significantly, depending upon the duration of treatment and concomitant drug therapy. It is not uncommon to observe a reduction in the half-life of carbamazepine from 30 hr after a single dose to 12 hr with chronic therapy, and a further reduction to 8 hr during polytherapy with other AEDs. Larger daily doses (>1200 mg) and more frequent administration (t.i.d.-q.i.d.) of carbamazepine is often necessary to minimize plasma level flutucations and the attendant risk of breakthrough seizures or transient adverse effects.

Because of the large interindividual variability in carbamazepine absorption and clearance, the time-dependent alterations in metabolism, and the potential for large fluctuations in drug concentrations over a dosage interval, careful plasma-level monitoring is often needed to determine optimal therapy. Steady-state concentrations of carbamazepine are reached several days after therapy is initiated, although levels may drop by as much as 50% during the first month of therapy, because of autoinduction of metabolism. After 1 month, autoinduction is complete, and plasma levels vary predictably with changes in dosage.

ADVERSE EFFECTS

Initial, dose-related adverse effects of carbamazepine are common and include dizziness, drowsiness, anorexia, and nausea. Although tolerance develops to these effects within the first few weeks of therapy, their occurrence can be minimized or avoided by gradual dose titration. Persistent gastrointestinal upset may be relieved by giving the drug with meals. Reversible, dose-related symptoms of carbamazepine toxicity include diplopia (most commonly the initial manifestation of toxicity), nausea, headache, dizziness, and ataxia. Because of large fluctuations in the blood level of carbamazepine over the course of a usual dosing interval, dose-related toxicities may occur transiently at times of peak drug-plasma concentrations.

Other dose-related neuropsychiatric adverse effects of carbamazepine include depression, irritability, mental sluggishness, and impairment of concentration and short-term memory. However, these adverse effects are less common than with phenobarbital and primidone. Furthermore, in several clinical epilepsy trials, patients with personality and behavioral disorders treated with carbamazepine had significant improvement during therapy (18). When dose-related adverse effects persist throughout the day, the total daily dose of carbamazepine should be decreased; when they are transient and occur 2 to 4 hr

after a dose, an adjustment in the dosing schedule may suffice. Unusual movement disorders and carbamazepine-induced seizures can occur acutely following an overdose.

Rash occurs in approximately 5% of patients treated with carbamazepine, usually between the first and second week of therapy. Benign, maculopapular, urticarial, and morbilliform reactions are most common, but exfoliative dermatitis and Stevens-Johnson syndrome may also occur. In some cases, rash may be accompanied by fever, generalized lymphadenopathy, hepatomegaly, splenomegaly, and less commonly, nephritis and vasculitis. Symptoms are reversible upon drug discontinuation, and corticosteroids may hasten recovery. Cross-reactivity between carbamazepine and other aromatic antiepileptic drugs (e.g., phenytoin, phenobarbital) may complicate the subsequent management of these patients. In such cases, valproate is usually well tolerated (19). Other idiosyncratic adverse reactions include hepatitis and systemic lupus erythematosus (SLE). Hepatitis usually occurs within the first few weeks of therapy and may coincide with eosinophilia and other symptoms of drug hypersensitivity. Carbamazepine may also cause a mild elevation of liver enzyme levels in less than 10% of patients, which appears to have no adverse clinical consequence. Carbamazepine-induced SLE is delayed, usually occurring after 6-12 months of therapy.

Among the most worrisome of idiosyncratic adverse reactions associated with carbamazepine is aplastic anemia. Although rare, this condition is fatal in about one-half of patients and is probably responsible for the low use of this agent. However, with additional postmarketing surveillance, the risk of serious hematologic toxicity is now more clearly known. The incidence of carbamazepine-associated aplastic anemia is estimated to be 0.5 per 100,000 treatment-years (20). Neither patient age, nor daily or total dosage significantly affect this risk. Carbamazepine is also associated with a dose-independent transient leukopenia, which occurs in about 10% of patients. In most cases, the leukopenia is mild and resolves, despite continuation of treatment. However, in about 2% of patients, leukopenia persists until the drug is discontinued (20). Carbamazepine-induced leukopenia does not appear to be a risk factor for aplastic anemia. While aplastic anemia can develop at any time during the first year of carbamazepine treatment, leukopenia is most common within the first month. The risk of serious hematologic reactions to carbamazepine can be minimized by patient education and laboratory monitoring. When therapy is initiated, patients should be counseled to seek immediate medical attention for abrupt onset of high fever, infection, petechiae, or unusual fatigue. If the diagnosis of aplastic anemia is confirmed, carbamazepine should be discontinued immediately, and the patient should not be rechallenged. Laboratory monitoring should include complete blood counts before initiation of treatment, and every 2 weeks for the first 2 months of therapy. If no abnormalities are detected, hematologic monitoring should continue either at intervals of 3 months or when the patient develops signs or symptoms of myelosuppression. If mild leukopenia develops, complete blood counts should be evaluated at 2-week intervals until they return to baseline values. Therapy should be discontinued if the absolute neutrophil count drops below 1500/mm^3 or if infection occurs.

Carbamazepine may also cause hyponatremia and water retention, probably by increasing antidiuretic hormone secretion. This effect appears to be dose-related as it is most often associated with blood levels of carbamazepine above the therapeutic range and often responds to a reduction in dose. At low serum-sodium concentrations (<120 mEq/liter), patients may report headache, confusion, dizziness, or loss of seizure control. Treatment consists of water restriction and/or reduction or discontinuation of carbamazepine therapy. Treatment with demeclocycline may be effective for patients who require continued carbamazepine therapy. Carbamazepine can cause cardiac conduction disturbances, primarily in older patients. Cardiotoxicity may be more common with higher doses and in patients with an underlying cardiac abnormality. A thorough history and baseline electrocardiogram should precede the initiation of carbamazepine in elderly patients.

DRUG INTERACTIONS

Carbamazepine, a potent inducer of drug metabolism, has been shown to increase the clearance of theophylline, doxycycline, haloperidol, warfarin, corticosteroids, valproate, clonazepam, ethosuximide, and various hormones. Thus, the potential for reduced effectiveness of these agents should be considered when carbamazepine therapy is begun. Because the failure rate of oral contraceptives is increased during coadministration with carbamazepine and other enzyme-inducing AEDs (e.g., phenytoin, phenobarbital), an alternate form of birth control should be recommended. The effect of carbamazepine on plasma levels of phenytoin, phenobarbital, and primidone is inconsistent and probably reflects various degrees of enzyme induction and inhibition. Routine monitoring of blood levels is recommended when carbamazepine is added to the regimen of any patient receiving AED therapy.

Drug interactions that affect the blood level and response to carbamazepine are common. Danazol, dextropropoxyphene, erythromycin, isoniazid, verapamil, and diltiazem can inhibit carbamazepine metabolism and induce clinical symptoms of toxicity. Cimetidine may inhibit the metabolism of carbamazepine, but ranitidine has no effect. Carbamazepine levels can also be affected by concomitant therapy with other AEDs. Phenytoin, phenobarbital, and primidone may increase the metabolism of carbamazepine and lead to a reduction in the steady-state plasma concentration. Carbamazepine blood levels may increase, decrease, or remain the same when valproate is added. This may reflect the variable effects of valproate displacement of carbamazepine from protein binding sites and valproate-mediated inhibition of carbamazepine metabolism.

Valproate

Valproate is a unique AED because of its chemical structure and its broad activity against both partial and generalized seizures. Unlike other AEDs, which have a substituted heterocyclic ring structure, valproate is a short, branched-chain fatty acid. Valproate is considered by many to be the drug of choice for the treatment of generalized idiopathic epilepsies including primary generalized tonic-clonic seizures (14). Ethosuximide and valproate are equally effective against absence seizures. Although there is less experience with valproate in the treatment of partial seizures, its efficacy is probably comparable to that of phenytoin and carbamazepine, especially for partial seizures that generalize secondarily. Valproate is the only available agent that can be used as monotherapy for treating patients with a combination of generalized tonic-clonic and absence or myoclonic seizures. The mechanism of action of valproate is not completely characterized but probably involves potentiation of γ-aminobutyric acid (GABA), an inhibitory neurotransmitter within the CNS.

Valproate is available as valproic acid (Depakene) in soft gelatin capsules (250 mg) and syrup (250 mg/5 ml) and as divalproex sodium (Depakote) in enteric-coated tablets (125 mg, 250 mg, and 500 mg) and sprinkle capsules (125 mg) that may emptied onto food. Divalproex sodium dissociates into valproate in the gastrointestinal tract. An intravenous dosage form is currently under investigation. In adults, valproate should be initiated at a dose of 125 to 250 mg b.i.d. to t.i.d. with gradual dose titration in 250-mg increments every 3 to 7 days. The usual effective dose of valproate is 750 to 1500 mg divided into three or four daily doses.

The bioavailability of valproate is close to 100% for all oral dosage forms, but the rate of absorption may vary. Peak levels occur within 2 hr after administration of valproate syrup and capsules. Enteric-coated tablets were developed to minimize the gastric distress associated with the plain capsule by prolonging the rate of drug dissolution. Consequently, the time to peak levels is delayed and may vary from 3 to 8 hr (21). Although food has no significant effect on the absorption of the soft gelatin capsules, the rate of valproate absorption from enteric-coated tablets is delayed.

Valproate is highly bound to plasma proteins, so the volume of distribution is small. The extent of protein binding varies and depends highly upon the dose and plasma level of the drug. At concentrations below 75 μg/ml, valproate is approximately 90% bound to plasma proteins, primarily albumin. As the total concentration of valproate increases above 100 μg/ml, albumin binding sites become saturated, and the free fraction of the drug may increase by up to 50% (21). The distribution and protein binding of valproate can be affected by a variety of other factors including albumin and free fatty acid concentrations, pregnancy, age, and the presence of displacing drugs.

The relationship between the dose and steady-state plasma levels of valproate is curvilinear. Thus, with increasing dosage, a less-than-proportional change in the plasma concentration occurs. Since only the unbound fraction of drug is available for metabolic transformation, this curvilinear relationship may be explained by the increase in valproate clearance that would be expected when free valproate concentrations rise as a consequence of saturable protein binding. Valproate is eliminated almost exclusively by hepatic metabolism, with a half-life of 12 to 16 hr in healthy volunteers. The half-life may be reduced during concomitant therapy with other AEDs. Oxidation of valproate at the β and ω positions, and glucuronide conjugation of the parent and metabolites are the primary routes of metabolism. The major metabolites of valproate are eliminated slowly and may also be active. This may explain the fact that maximal response to valproate can be delayed by several weeks beyond the time required to achieve steady-state plasma levels of the parent drug. Also, the anticonvulsant effect during valproate therapy outlasts its presence in plasma, further supporting the hypothesis that metabolites contribute to the antiepileptic effect of the drug.

ADVERSE EFFECTS

Valproate is generally well tolerated, and for this reason it is often preferred over other AEDs. Gastrointestinal adverse effects are most common during valproate therapy. As many as 35% of patients treated with either the capsule or syrup report nausea, vomiting, anorexia, or other symptoms of gastrointestinal discomfort. Patient tolerance can be improved by using the enteric-coated products (tablets or sprinkles), and most patients prefer them.

Although the dose-related neurologic adverse effects are like those seen with other AEDs, the incidence of adverse effects to valproate within the therapeutic range is lower. Fine tremor, a reversible, dose-related adverse effect, occurs frequently. When tremor occurs transiently during the day, adjustment of the drug regimen to minimize plasma-level fluctuations may alleviate the problem. Otherwise, a reduction in the total daily dose of valproate or concomitant treatment with a β-adrenergic blocking agent (e.g., propranolol) may be necessary. Behavioral and cognitive adverse effects are less common with valproate than with phenytoin, phenobarbital, and primidone (22).

Other dose-related adverse effects include weight gain,

loss or thinning of hair and increases in hepatic enzyme levels. Weight gain occurs in up to 50% of patients and may be related to an increase in appetite (22). Hair thinning or alopecia is transient and usually occurs upon initiation of therapy. Reduction of valproate dosage may help. Approximately 40% of patients experience a dose-related increase in hepatic enzymes during valproate therapy. This abnormality is usually asymptomatic and responds rapidly to a reduction in dose or discontinuation of the drug. Practitioners should discontinue valproate in the following instances: (a) an elevation in hepatic enzymes three times above baseline; (b) abnormalities in laboratory tests of hepatic synthesis or metabolism (e.g., elevated bilirubin or prothrombin time or decreased serum albumin concentration); or (c) the patient develops clinical signs or symptoms of hepatitis. Baseline laboratory values, including liver enzymes and hepatic function tests, should be determined prior to initiating valproate.

Valproate has also been associated with fulminant hepatotoxicity leading to coma and death. Although the overall incidence of hepatic fatalities is very low (1 in 49,000 treated patients), certain patients are particularly at risk. Specific risk factors include age less than 2 years, AED polytherapy, and developmental delay (23). The risk of fatal hepatotoxicity is exceedingly low in patients over the age of 10 years on monotherapy. When it occurs, fulminant hepatotoxicity is usually seen during the first 6 months of therapy. Gastrointestinal distress, anorexia, or sudden loss of seizure control may precede the development of fulminant hepatic failure, so patients should be counseled at the start of therapy to report these or other clinical signs or symptoms of hepatitis as soon as they develop. The prognosis may be improved if therapy is discontinued quickly.

Dreifuss et al. suggest the following guidelines for minimizing the risk of fatal valproate hepatotoxicity:

(a) avoid administering valproate as part of anticonvulsant polytherapy in children under age 3 years, unless monotherapy has failed or the potential benefits of polypharmacy outweigh the risks; (b) avoid administering valproate to patients with preexisting liver disease or a family history of childhood hepatic disease; (c) administer valproate in the lowest possible dose that is consistent with seizure control; (d) avoid concomitant administration of valproate and salicylates, and avoid fasting in children with intercurrent illnesses; (e) monitor clinically for such symptoms as nausea, vomiting, headache, lethargy, edema, jaundice, or seizure breakthrough, especially after febrile illness (23).

Greater recognition of patients at risk for valproate hepatotoxicity is probably responsible for the significant decrease in the number of hepatic fatalities despite the overall increased use of the drug (1).

ADVERSE EFFECTS

Metabolic interactions between valproate and other AEDs are common. Unlike phenytoin, carbamazepine, phenobarbital, and primidone, valproate is not an enzyme-inducing drug. Conversely, valproate may inhibit hepatic drug metabolism. This enzyme-inhibition has been implicated in valproate interactions with phenobarbital, phenytoin, and carbamazepine. Valproate inhibits the oxidative metabolism of phenobarbital, leading to an average increase of phenobarbital levels of 80% (24). However, because of variability in this increase (0 to 200%), routine adjustment of the dose of phenobarbital is not recommended. Rather, blood levels of phenobarbital should be monitored, with appropriate adjustment of the dose if necessary. The interaction between phenytoin and valproate is complex and probably involves both enzyme inhibition and protein binding displacement. Phenytoin levels commonly fall after initiation of valproate, probably due to displacement of phenytoin from protein binding sites and an attendant increase in phenytoin clearance and volume of distribution. The free fraction of phenytoin may increase further with subsequent increases in valproate dosage. During continued therapy with valproate, phenytoin levels may remain low or rise to the preadministration level or above. Regardless of the subsequent change in phenytoin levels, the free fraction of phenytoin likely remains elevated during polytherapy and may increase further with increasing doses of valproate. Thus, total plasma levels of phenytoin should be interpreted cautiously. Valproate has been reported to induce clinical symptoms of carbamazepine toxicity, but this is not well characterized.

The metabolism of valproate is susceptible to induction by other AEDs including phenobarbital, carbamazepine, phenytoin, and primidone. Serum levels of valproate decrease by an average of 30 to 40% (24), and the half-life is reduced to 6 to 9 hr. Because of the difficulty in maintaining consistent, therapeutic concentrations of valproate in patients taking other AEDs, monotherapy with valproate is highly recommended.

Antipyretic doses of aspirin may displace valproate from protein binding sites and competitively inhibit β-oxidation. Unlike other AEDs, valproate does not increase the failure rate of oral contraceptives (24). However, because of the potential teratogenic effects, this agent should be used cautiously in women of childbearing age.

Phenytoin

Phenytoin, a diphenyl-substituted hydantoin derivative, was introduced for the treatment of epilepsy in 1938. It soon became one of the most widely prescribed antiepileptic drugs because it possessed anticonvulsant activity at nonsedative doses. Phenytoin is effective for the treatment of partial and generalized tonic-clonic seizures, but it has no activity against absence and febrile seizures. Other hydantoin derivatives, including ethotoin and mephenytoin, also have anticonvulsant activity, but their clinical use is limited. Phenytoin blocks neuronal sodium and calcium conductance, as well as calcium-mediated excitatory neurotransmission, which probably is involved in its ability to regulate neuronal excitability under abnormal conditions. The specific mechanism of the anticonvulsant effect of phenytoin is unknown.

Phenytoin (Dilantin and generic) is available as the free acid in suspension (30 mg/5 ml and 125 mg/5 ml) and 50-mg chewable tablets. The sodium salt of phenytoin is contained in phenytoin capsules (30 and 100 mg) and phenytoin injectable (50 mg/ml); for these dosage forms, phenytoin content is expressed in milligrams of sodium phenytoin. Because of the difference in molecular weight between the acid and salt forms of the drug, the capsule and parenteral dosage forms contain 8% fewer phenytoin acid equivalents than the suspension and chewable tablets. This difference in drug content should be accounted for when changing products.

In adults, phenytoin can be initiated at a dose of 300 mg daily. The usual effective maintenance dose is 300 to 400 mg daily. Only Dilantin Kapseals, extended-release phenytoin capsules, is approved for once-daily maintenance dosing. The suspension and parenteral dosage forms should be given in divided daily doses. Loading doses of phenytoin help patients who require rapid attainment of a therapeutic level. The usual loading dose of phenytoin is 15 mg/kg. Oral loading doses of phenytoin should be given in individual increments of 200 to 400 mg, each separated by at least 2 hr. This reduces the gastrointestinal distress occasionally associated with large doses, and the rate of drug absorption is enhanced (25). Even when given in small increments, phenytoin is absorbed slowly after oral administration, and the resultant peak plasma concentration is approximately half that achieved after an equivalent intravenous loading dose (25). When given by the intravenous route, phenytoin should be administered at a maximal rate of 50 mg/min to reduce the risk of hypotension and cardiac arrhythmias. These adverse effects are likely related to the 40% propylene glycol diluent used in the parenteral formulation of the drug. Blood pressure and heart rate should be measured periodically when large doses of phenytoin are administered intravenously.

Phenytoin is poorly water-soluble at acidic pH. Very little drug exists in solution in the stomach, and phenytoin absorption takes place primarily in the proximal part of the small intestine. Because the rate of drug dissolution in intestinal fluid is dose-dependent, the time to peak drug concentration after an oral loading dose of phenytoin may be delayed (74). The bioavailability of phenytoin approaches 100% for most well-formulated products, but it is prudent to avoid changing dosage forms and products, because small changes in bioavailability can result in large changes in seizure control. Additional complications of the low water solubility of phenytoin are evident after intramuscular administration. Phenytoin crystallizes when injected into muscle resulting in a depot of drug that is both potentially damaging to local tissue, and is slowly and erratically absorbed from the injection site. Phenytoin should not be given by the intramuscular route. When oral administration is not feasible, the nasogastric or intravenous routes are preferred.

Under normal conditions, phenytoin is approximately 90% bound to plasma proteins, primarily albumin. Conditions that can alter protein binding include renal failure, a lowered plasma albumin concentration, and the presence of displacing drugs. In each case, these factors result in a decrease in phenytoin binding and an increase in the free fraction and volume of distribution. However, despite alterations in the free fraction, the free concentration of phenytoin is not changed significantly. Since the free drug exerts the therapeutic and toxic effects at receptor sites, the clinical response to a given dose of phenytoin is unchanged by altered protein binding. However, careful interpretation of the total (bound and unbound) phenytoin concentration is warranted. Equation 48.1 approximates the concentration of phenytoin that would be observed if the albumin concentration were normal (C_{normal}) from the total (bound and unbound) concentration ($C_{observed}$) and the patient's albumin concentration in gm/dl (Alb) (25).

$$C_{normal} = \frac{C_{observed}}{0.2 \cdot Alb + 0.1} \qquad (48.1)$$

In patients with end-stage renal disease (CrCl < 10ml/min), the affinity of albumin for phenytoin is reduced by approximately 50% and equation 48.2 should be used (25).

$$C_{normal} = \frac{C_{observed}}{0.1 \cdot Alb + 0.1} \qquad (48.2)$$

Free(unbound) concentration values are also available from many clinical laboratories.

Phenytoin is eliminated primarily by hepatic metabolism. The major metabolic route involves *para*-hydroxylation of the parent compound to yield (5-(p-hydroxyphenyl)-5-phenylhydantoin (p-HPPH). This metabolite is then glucuronidated and excreted primarily in the urine. Other hydroxylated metabolites are also generated during phenytoin metabolism, and all metabolites are inactive. Less than 5% of the drug is eliminated unchanged in the urine.

Unlike many drugs that are cleared from the body by a first-order elimination process, the clearance of phenytoin varies over the range of plasma levels that are clinically useful for the treatment of seizures. At very low plasma levels, phenytoin clearance is first-order, and small dosage changes result in a proportional change in the level. However, as the phenytoin concentration approaches the therapeutic range, the maximal capacity for phenytoin metabolism is approached, and a change in dosage can result in a disproportionately large change in the steady-state level.

Thus, phenytoin dosage adjustments must be made cautiously. The Michaelis-Menten model of saturable enzyme kinetics has been used to characterize the relationship between phenytoin dose and plasma level at steady state. Using equation 48.3, the rate of phenytoin administration (mg/day) can be calculated from the desired steady-state plasma level. Population estimates of V_{max} (maximal rate of phenytoin metabolism = 7 mg/kg/day in adults) and K_m (phenytoin concentration at which V_{max} is half-maximum = 4 mg/liter in adults) can be used if patient-specific data are not available (25).

$$R_i = \frac{V_{max} \cdot Cp_{ss}}{K_m + Cp_{ss}} \qquad (48.3)$$

ADVERSE EFFECTS

Acute, dose-related adverse effects of phenytoin include ataxia, diplopia, dizziness, drowsiness, encephalopathy, and involuntary movements. These symptoms usually occur at phenytoin levels above 30 μg/ml and are reversible when phenytoin is discontinued or the dose is reduced. Involuntary movements during phenytoin intoxication may include dyskinesias of the limbs, trunk, or face and are similar to those encountered with long-term antipsychotic drug therapy. Phenytoin has also been reported to exacerbate seizures at toxic levels, but this is rare. Nystagmus is a dose-related effect that may occur at plasma levels within the therapeutic range and does not necessitate a reduction in dosage.

Adverse effects associated with long-term therapy include gingival hyperplasia, facial coarsening, peripheral neuropathy, and vitamin deficiencies. Gingival hyperplasia is a dose-related effect that occurs in over 40% of adult patients taking phenytoin. It usually begins within the first 3 months and may progress during the first year of phenytoin therapy. Patients at risk for gingival hyperplasia include children and those with poor oral hygiene. Patients taking phenytoin should be counseled to brush and floss their teeth regularly and have regular dental check-ups. Mild gingival hyperplasia may respond to improved dental and periodontal care or a reduction in phenytoin dosage. In advanced cases, gum resection surgery may be required. Alternate AED therapy should be considered for these patients. Chronic phenytoin therapy is also associated with dysmorphic changes in the lips, nose, brow, and other facial structures as well as other cosmetic changes including hirsuitism and acne. These adverse effects are a major limitation to the use of phenytoin in children, adolescents, and young women.

Peripheral neuropathy with decreased deep tendon reflexes and sensory deficits may also occur during long-term phenytoin therapy. These symptoms are probably most common during polytherapy with phenytoin and pheno-barbital, and are not reversible. Phenytoin-induced meg-aloblastic anemia with folic acid deficiency occurs in less than 1% of patients and responds to folic acid supple-mentation. Prophylactic folic acid supplementation is un-necessary and may alter phenytoin metabolism. Alterations of bone density, mass, and mineral content have been as-sociated with phenytoin, usually when given in combina-tion with other enzyme-inducing AEDs. Although most patients with AED-related bone disease are asymptomatic, clinically apparent osteomalacia and osteoporosis may also occur and requires appropriate treatment. Whether pa-tients without clinical evidence of bone disease should re-ceive prophylactic vitamin D and calcium supplementation is not known. Certainly, patients with known risk factors for metabolic bone disease (e.g., inadequate diet, sunlight, or exercise) should be monitored closely. AED-induced metabolism of vitamin D to less active products and im-paired absorption of calcium may cause this complication of chronic therapy.

Idiosyncratic adverse reactions usually occur within the first 8 weeks of phenytoin therapy, including rash, hep-atitis, lymphadenopathy, and hematologic alterations. Rashes, which occur in less than 10% of patients, usually manifest within the first 14 days of phenytoin therapy and may be accompanied by hepatitis, lymphadenopathy, and fever. The rash is usually morbilliform but may progress to Stevens-Johnson syndrome, erythema multiforme, or toxic epidermal necrolysis. Thus, phenytoin therapy must be discontinued with even mild hypersensitivity reactions. Hepatitis usually occurs with fever, rash, and lymphade-nopathy during the first 3 weeks of therapy and necessi-tates the immediate discontinuation of phenytoin. Al-though drug discontinuation optimizes the chance of recovery, some patients continue to deteriorate and (rarely) phenytoin-induced hepatic injury leads to en-cephalopathy, coma, and death. Hematologic adverse re-actions during phenytoin therapy include a modest, tran-sient depression in leukocytes, and (very rarely) aplastic anemia or agranulocytosis. Patients with severe idiosyn-cratic reactions to phenytoin should not be rechallenged. Also, the potential for cross-reactivity with other aromatic AEDs should be considered (see Carbamazepine-Adverse Effects).

DRUG INTERACTIONS

Phenytoin, a potent inducer of hepatic microsomal en-zymes, can enhance the metabolism of other drugs eliminated by similar enzyme systems, including oral contraceptives, warfarin, corticosteroid, cyclosporine, theophylline, and other AEDs. Phenytoin increases the metabolism of carbamazepine, valproate, and clonazepam, resulting in decreased plasma concentrations and concom-itant reduction in the clinical anticonvulsant effect. Phen-ytoin also may increase the ratio of primidone to pheno-barbital when administered to patients stabilized on primidone. Although phenytoin may enhance warfarin me-tabolism, the effect is unpredictable and may even be man-ifested by a transient increase in the anticoagulant effect of warfarin. Thus, warfarin therapy should be monitored closely during phenytoin coadministration.

Drug interactions affecting phenytoin may involve al-terations in phenytoin absorption, metabolism, or protein binding. Antacids and nutritional formulas have been shown to reduce plasma levels of phenytoin, but in neither case is the interaction predictable. Steady-state phenytoin levels may fall during coadministration with aluminum- and magnesium-containing antacids, but the magnitude of the effect is variable. Given the potential for an interaction, it is reasonable to space antacid and phenytoin doses by 2 to 3 hr. Phenytoin levels drop after institution of naso-gastric feedings, but the mechanism of this interaction is unclear. With flushing of the nasogastric tube, phenytoin adsorption to the apparatus is probably minimal. Concur-rent administration with Isocal and Osmolite, but not En-sure, may reduce phenytoin levels (26). Patients should have their phenytoin levels monitored closely when enteral feedings are initiated or stopped, and if the formula is changed. Heparin, phenylbutazone, tolbutamide, and val-proate displace phenytoin from plasma protein binding sites. Many drugs alter the metabolism of phenytoin. It is important to be aware of drugs that can alter phenytoin metabolism, because small changes in phenytoin clearance can have a large effect on the steady-state plasma level. Folic acid, alcohol, and rifampin can increase the metab-olism of phenytoin. Drugs that can reduce the metabolism of phenytoin include valproate, isoniazid, amiodarone, ci-metidine, omeprazole, phenylbutazone, disulfiram, sul-fonamides, and chloramphenicol.

Ethosuximide

Ethosuximide is a member of the succinimide class of an-tiepileptic agents that includes phensuximide and meth-osuximide. The latter share similar antiepileptic effects with ethosuximide, but they are rarely used in the treat-ment of seizures because they are less effective and their use is associated with more serious adverse effects. Etho-suximide is as effective as valproate for the treatment of absence seizures, but ethosuximide is often preferred for use in young children because of the potential for val-proate-associated hepatotoxicity. Ethosuximide has no ac-tivity against partial and generalized tonic-clonic seizures. Although the mechanism of ethosuximide's antiepileptic effect is unknown, the drug may suppress seizures by al-teration of calcium flux in the thalamus or by the depletion of excitatory neurotransmitter stores within the CNS.

Ethosuximide (Zarontin) is available as capsules (250 mg) and syrup (250 mg/5 ml) for oral use. The initial dose of ethosuximide is 250 mg daily for children 3 to 6 years of age, and 500 mg for children 6 years and older. The dose should be increased weekly in 250-mg increments as necessary. Infants require larger doses on a weight basis than adolescents and adults. Despite the long half-life of ethosuximide, the drug is often given in divided doses to minimize gastrointestinal distress.

Ethosuximide is metabolized hepatically to inactive hydroxylated products that are then excreted. Approximately 20% of a given dose is excreted in the urine unchanged. Serum-level monitoring helps to guide therapy, but the upper end of the therapeutic range is loosely defined. Many patients tolerate levels above 100 µg/ml, and plasma concentrations of 150 µg/ml or greater are required occasionally for optimal treatment.

ADVERSE EFFECTS

Sedation, nausea, anorexia, and headache are the most common adverse effects reported upon initiation of ethosuximide. Tolerance to these symptoms usually develops within the first weeks of treatment, and they can be minimized by reducing the dose or by introducing the drug gradually as outlined above. Behavioral disturbances, including irritability, depression, and frank psychosis, occur independent of the drug dose. These symptoms are rare and usually occur in children or adolescents with a history of behavioral or psychiatric problems. Discontinuation of the drug is usually required. In most patients, ethosuximide has no detrimental effect on intellectual function. Idiosyncratic reactions during ethosuximide therapy include mild, transient leukopenia, rare pancytopenia, rash, and SLE. Periodic complete blood counts should be performed during the first 6 to 12 months of therapy, and the patient should be observed for development of clinical symptoms suggesting serious bone marrow suppression.

DRUG INTERACTIONS

Ethosuximide is not an enzyme inducer or inhibitor and has no important effect on the disposition of most other AEDs. Ethosuximide levels may be reduced by carbamazepine and increased by valproate, presumably by enzyme induction and inhibition, respectively. Phenytoin, phenobarbital, and primidone have no clinical effect on ethosuximide levels.

Phenobarbital

All barbiturates have anticonvulsant activity, but only phenobarbital and primidone are used commonly for the chronic treatment of epilepsy, because they are effective at subhypnotic doses. Phenobarbital was first used for the treatment of seizures in 1912, and it continues to be one of the most widely prescribed AEDs. However, because of adverse effects on the CNS, this agent is now used primarily as an alternative when monotherapy with first-line agents has failed. Phenobarbital is most useful for the treatment of partial and generalized tonic-clonic seizures. Phenobarbital elevates the seizure threshold and prevents the spread of electrical seizure activity. Although the precise mechanism of action is unknown, these effects may be related to the ability of phenobarbital to modulate the inhibitory action of GABA or attenuate the postsynaptic effects of excitatory neurotransmitters such as glutamate.

Phenobarbital is available as the sodium salt in a variety of dosage forms including oral capsules and tablets (various strengths), elixir (20 mg/5 ml), and injectable preparations (various concentrations). The usual maintenance dose of phenobarbital for adults is 1 to 3 mg/kg daily. In neonates and children, the usual daily dose is 3 to 4 mg/kg. Phenobarbital is usually given as a single daily dose at bedtime, to avoid peak sedative effects during the day. Although food may delay absorption, the absolute bioavailability of phenobarbital is unchanged. The long half-life of phenobarbital (approximately 4 days) may cause a delay of 2 to 3 weeks until steady-state levels are achieved. Therefore, a loading dose should be administered when a prompt therapeutic effect is needed. The usual loading dose of phenobarbital is 15 mg/kg. Given intravenously, the rate of administration should not exceed 100 mg/min. Oral loading doses may also be used. The oral loading doses of phenobarbital should be divided into 3 equal increments and separated by 24 hr. Patients should be monitored for the attendant sedation and incoordination that may occur.

Phenobarbital is nearly completely absorbed after oral and intramuscular administration, with peak concentrations occurring in less than 4 hr. Phenobarbital is not highly bound to plasma proteins, and for this reason, clinically important protein binding interactions are rare. Phenobarbital is eliminated by a first-order process. Thirty to 50% of phenobarbital is metabolized by the liver to inactive products that are glucuronidated or sulfated and excreted in the urine. Approximately 25% of the dose is excreted in the urine unchanged. Excretion of phenobarbital is enhanced significantly in alkaline urine and during forced diuresis.

ADVERSE EFFECTS

CNS adverse effects during phenobarbital therapy are generally dose-related and include sedation, nystagmus, dizziness, and ataxia. Mild drowsiness is common upon initiation of therapy, but tolerance to this effect usually develops within the first several weeks. Occasionally, sedation persists during chronic treatment, and in these patients, the dose should be reduced. Of greater concern are the subtle effects of phenobarbital on behavior, mood, and cognition. Reversible hyperactivity and insomnia occur in up to 40% of children treated with phenobarbital, and paradoxical excitation has been reported in the elderly as well. These behavioral changes usually occur within the first few months of therapy and are more prevalent in patients with organic brain disease. A noticeable improvement in behavior may be seen upon replacement of phenobarbital with valproate or carbamazepine therapy (27). Phenobarbital may also cause mild depression and lack of interest or ambition, only recognized by others or appreciated after discontinuation of the drug. Although the cognitive effects of phenobarbital are not well-characterized, several investigations have found a dose-related impairment of memory, intelligence and vigilance tests, work performance, and complex verbal and nonverbal tasks. These changes likely persist despite the development of tolerance to the sedative effects of the drug.

Serious adverse effects of phenobarbital are uncommon, and in general, it is associated with fewer idiosyncratic adverse effects than phenytoin or carbamazepine (11). Morbilliform rash is the most common idiosyncratic reaction, occurring in 1 to 3% of patients. Rarely, the rash may progress to Stevens-Johnson syndrome or exfoliative dermatitis or may occur in conjunction with symptoms of hepatitis or bone marrow suppression. Megaloblastic anemia with folic acid deficiency occurs in less than 1% of phenobarbital-treated patients and responds to folic acid supplementation. Like phenytoin, phenobarbital is also associated with bone disorders (e.g., osteomalacia) during chronic therapy.

DRUG INTERACTIONS

Most drug interactions with phenobarbital are characterized by alterations of metabolism. By increasing the synthesis and retarding the degradation of hepatic enzymes, phenobarbital accelerates the metabolism of many agents that are metabolized by the mixed-function oxidase system, including theophylline, warfarin, cyclosporine, chloramphenicol, valproate, chlorpromazine, haloperidol, and tricyclic antidepressants. The degree of enzyme induction and alteration of drug metabolism varies greatly among patients and is to some extent under genetic control. Enzyme induction may last for days to weeks after phenobarbital is discontinued. Carbamazepine levels may remain unchanged or decline during phenobarbital coadministration. Phenobarbital can also inhibit the metabolism of some drugs, presumably by competition for similar metabolic pathways. The effect of phenobarbital on plasma levels of phenytoin is unpredictable; levels may modestly rise, decline, or (as in most cases) show no change. Valproate often causes a clinically important reduction in the metabolism of phenobarbital, with resultant symptoms of phenobarbital toxicity (see Valproate—Drug Interactions). The effect of phenytoin on phenobarbital plasma levels is unpredictable, and in most cases, clinically important alterations are not seen.

Primidone

Primidone is structurally related to the barbiturates, and like phenobarbital, it is effective for the treatment of partial and generalized tonic-clonic seizures. Primidone is an active anticonvulsant agent, as are its two major metabolites, phenobarbital and phenylethylmalonamide (PEMA). Although the clinical use of primidone is similar to that of phenobarbital, adverse effects are more commonly a limiting factor during long-term primidone therapy. Some patients may respond to primidone therapy despite the failure of phenobarbital to control seizures.

Primidone (Mysoline and generic) is available as oral tablets (50 and 250 mg) and as an oral suspension (250 mg/5 ml). Primidone should be initiated slowly, to allow the development of tolerance to the acute gastrointestinal and sedative effects of the parent drug. In adults, therapy can be started at a dose of 125 to 250 mg b.i.d. with gradual dosage increases every 4 to 7 days in 125- to 250-mg increments until the effective dose is reached.

Metabolic transformation of primidone to phenobarbital and PEMA occurs by oxidative metabolism and pyrimidine ring cleavage, respectively. Primidone and its metabolites are also excreted by the kidney to a significant extent. Because the half-life of primidone is relatively short, the drug is usually given in divided doses, to maintain more consistent plasma levels of the parent drug and reduce the likelihood of transient side effects at times of peak primidone levels. Pharmacokinetic monitoring of primidone therapy includes routine assessment of both primidone and phenobarbital levels. Samples should be drawn at a consistent time relative to the dose. Whereas primidone reaches steady-state concentrations quickly, there is usually a delay of 2 to 3 weeks before plateau concentrations of phenobarbital are attained. During chronic treatment, plasma concentrations of phenobarbital are approximately 1 to 3 times higher than those of primidone. This fact is sometimes useful in monitoring compliance.

ADVERSE EFFECTS

The adverse effects of primidone are similar to those of phenobarbital. Thus, the potential for primidone-related neurotoxicity is also of concern during long-term therapy. In addition, primidone is frequently associated with initial dose-related adverse effects including sedation, dizziness, and nausea. Decreased libido and impotence appear to be more common during primidone therapy than with other AEDs. Serious adverse effects during primidone therapy are rare.

DRUG INTERACTIONS

The metabolism of primidone or its metabolites can be affected by other AEDs, including phenytoin and valproate. Phenytoin increases phenobarbital levels during coadministration with primidone. The result is an approximate doubling of the phenobarbital:primidone concentration ratio. Primidone levels do not appear to be affected significantly during phenytoin therapy. Valproate can reduce the metabolic clearance of metabolically derived phenobarbital and produce signs of barbiturate intoxication during primidone therapy. Valproate has a negligible effect on the plasma concentrations of primidone. Carbamazepine may increase the metabolism of primidone, although in many patients, this interaction is not clinically important.

Benzodiazepines

Diazepam, clonazepam, and clorazepate are the only benzodiazepine agents that are FDA-approved for the treatment of seizures. Diazepam and lorazepam have little utility in the chronic treatment of epilepsy, but they are frequently used intravenously for the termination of status epilepticus. In general, benzodiazepines are more effective in suppressing generalized epileptiform activity than focal discharges, and these agents limit the spread of epileptic discharges without suppressing the primary seizure focus. Nonetheless, clinical use of clonazepam and clorazepate for the chronic treatment of epilepsy includes both generalized and partial seizure types. Although the precise mechanism of the anticonvulsant effect of these agents is unknown, the benzodiazepines are thought to facilitate inhibitory neurotransmission in the CNS by enhancing the postsynaptic effects of GABA.

Clonazepam

Clonazepam is useful, alone or as an adjunct to other agents, for the treatment of Lennox-Gastaut syndrome and akinetic and myoclonic seizures. The drug is also useful for the treatment of absence seizures that fail to respond to valproate or ethosuximide. Clonazepam is not approved for the treatment of partial or generalized tonic-clonic seizures, and experience in the treatment of these seizure types is limited.

Clonazepam (Klonopin) is available as oral tablets in strengths of 0.5, 1, and 2 mg. An intravenous preparation is available for use in Europe, but it is not available in the United States. Clonazepam should be initiated at low doses (0.5 mg t.i.d. in adults; 0.01 to 0.03 mg/kg/day divided b.i.d. to t.i.d. in infants and children) and gradually titrated upward at 3- to 7-day intervals. The maximum recommended daily dose is 20 mg in adults and 0.1 to 0.2 mg/kg in infants and children. Although the half-life of clonazepam is long enough to allow once-daily dosing in many patients, the drug is often administered in divided doses. This is particularly important for patients who are intolerant of the transient sedative effects that occur after peak absorption

and for infants and children in whom the drug's half-life may be shortened.

Clonazepam is eliminated primarily by reduction of the nitro group to form 7-amino clonazepam, an inactive metabolite. Although loss of efficacy may occur during chronic therapy (see "Adverse Effects"), clonazepam does not induce its own metabolism. There is wide variation in the relationship between the dose and plasma levels of clonazepam. There is also significant overlap between the plasma levels associated with the antiepileptic effect of the drug and those associated with dose-related adverse effects. For these reasons, the therapeutic range of clonazepam levels is imprecisely defined, and therapeutic monitoring of clonazepam concentrations is not routinely done.

ADVERSE EFFECTS

Adverse effects are common during clonazepam treatment and necessitate drug discontinuation in up to one-third of patients (28). Dose-related adverse effects are particularly common and include drowsiness and ataxia. Although tolerance to the overt sedative effects of clonazepam and other benzodiazepines usually develops during the first few weeks of therapy, mild impairment of cognitive and motor skills may persist throughout treatment. In other patients, dose-related adverse effects are not tolerable, and clonazepam therapy must be discontinued. Clonazepam can also cause behavioral disturbances including hyperactivity, irritability, restlessness, and aggressive or violent behavior. Children are affected more frequently than adults. Dosage reduction may be attempted, but it does not always alleviate behavioral changes. Other noteworthy adverse effects include excessive salivation, bronchial hypersecretion, weight gain, and rarely, exacerbation of seizures. Abrupt discontinuation of clonazepam may precipitate seizures or status epilepticus. Thus, clonazepam should be withdrawn gradually when treatment is to be terminated.

The long-term clinical utility of clonazepam is limited by the development of tolerance to the antiepileptic effect. Approximately one-third of patients who benefit initially from clonazepam therapy experience some loss of efficacy, usually within the first 6 months of treatment (28). Although the antiepileptic effect may be restored by increasing the dose, as many as 30% of patients who develop tolerance do not regain adequate seizure control (28).

DRUG INTERACTIONS

Clinically important drug interactions with clonazepam are uncommon. Clonazepam has no significant effect on the pharmacokinetic disposition of phenytoin, carbamazepine, or primidone. However, phenytoin, carbamazepine, and phenobarbital can reduce the steady-state concentrations of clonazepam, presumably by induction of hepatic metabolism. The combined use of clonazepam and valproate has been reported to exacerbate absence seizures. Although the simultaneous use of these agents is not a strict contraindication, caution should be observed.

Clorazepate

Clorazepate dipotassium is approved for use as an adjunct to other agents for the treatment of partial seizures. Clorazepate is a prodrug that is rapidly decarboxylated in the acidic medium of the stomach to yield N-desmethyldiazepam (DMD), the primary active metabolite. This metabolite is responsible for the antiepileptic effect of the parent compound.

Clorazepate (Tranxene) is available as a prompt-release oral tablet (3.75, 7.5, and 15 mg) and as an extended-release oral tablet (11.5 and 22.5 mg) for once-daily dosing. Therapy with clorazepate should be initiated with the prompt-release form at a dose of 7.5 mg t.i.d in adults and 7.5 mg b.i.d. in children (ages 9 to 12 years). The dose should be increased at 7-day intervals, in increments of 7.5 mg or less, to a maximum daily dose of 90 mg in adults and 60 mg in children. Transient dose-related adverse effects may be minimized and compliance improved by switching patients stabilized on clorazepate to the extended-release dosage form.

DMD and its hydroxylated metabolites (including oxazepam) are conjugated and excreted in the urine. Plasma-level monitoring is of little use in the management of patients taking clorazepate.

ADVERSE EFFECTS

Adverse effects of clorazepate are similar to those of clonazepam and include sedation, dizziness, hypersalivation, and behavioral changes. Tolerance to the antiepileptic effect of clorazepate has been reported, but it does not seem to be as common, or develop as quickly, as with clonazepam.

DRUG INTERACTIONS

Concurrent antacid administration may significantly slow the rate of conversion from clorazepate to DMD, as can other diseases characterized by an increase in gastric pH. However, during prolonged administration, steady-state DMD levels are not significantly reduced. Smoking and concurrent AED therapy with enzyme-inducing agents can accelerate the metabolism of clorazepate. Clorazepate has no known effect on the disposition of other AEDs.

TREATING THE PREGNANT WOMAN WITH EPILEPSY

There is much controversy about the treatment of pregnant women with epilepsy. Central issues are the risk of fetal malformations attributable to individual seizures and to the epileptic diathesis, the degree of additional risk attributable to AED therapy, and the antiepileptic agent of choice for minimizing the risk of fetal malformations. Although a detailed discussion of these topics is beyond the scope of this chapter, several important principles should be considered. The reader is referred to other reviews for additional discussion in this topic (29, 30) and Chapter 88, "Drugs in Pregnancy and Lactation."

Therapeutic considerations that are unique during pregnancy include: (a) changes in maternal seizure control, (b) the choice of antiepileptic agents, (c) alteration of AED pharmacokinetics, and (d) the potential for AED-associated coagulopathy in the newborn. Approximately 50% of women with epilepsy will have no change in seizure frequency during pregnancy (1). Among the remaining patients, worsening of seizures occurs in approximately 40%, and only 10% experience a reduction in seizures (29). This may be attributable to several factors including reduced medication compliance caused by maternal fears that the medication may injure the developing fetus, pharmacokinetic changes in AED disposition, and sleep deprivation.

Overall, the incidence of fetal abnormalities in children of epileptic mothers is approximately 6%, roughly twice that found in the general population. Although there is considerable controversy about which AED has the lowest teratogenic risk, there is a clear association between some AEDs and fetal malformations. Trimethadione is clearly associated with a syndrome of anomalies, and this drug should be avoided during pregnancy. Affected infants may have craniofacial abnormalities including microcephaly and ocular defects, cardiac abnormalities, intrauterine growth retardation, short stature, and developmental delay. Valproate should also be avoided, if possible, because it is associated with a 1 to 2% incidence of neural tube defects in humans, and cleft palate and renal defects in animals (29, 30). A specific syndrome of fetal abnormalities has been associated with phenytoin (*fetal hydantoin syndrome*), which includes craniofacial anomalies, retardation or deficiencies in growth and mental or motor performance, and limb defects. Similar abnormalities have been associated with other AEDs. It is hypothesized that the arene oxide intermediates generated during the metabolism of aromatic AEDs may be responsible for these teratogenic effects (30). There is no conclusive evidence on which to base a preference for the use of phenytoin, phenobarbital, or carbamazepine during pregnancy. There also appears to be no good reason to switch therapy between these agents during pregnancy, particularly if the first trimester has passed (30). On the basis of published and personal experience, several authors recommended carbamazepine for the treatment of partial and generalized tonic-clonic seizures during pregnancy (1, 31). However, a recent report emphasized similarity between the fetal hydantoin syndrome and fetal abnormalities associated with carbamazepine therapy (32).

Pregnancy is associated with significant changes in the pharmacokinetic properties of AEDs. These changes include acceleration of hepatic drug metabolism, increased apparent volume of distribution, and alterations in plasma protein binding. The result is a decline in plasma AED concentrations, and in some patients, loss of seizure control. Consequently, AED plasma levels and the clinical status of the patient should be monitored at least monthly during pregnancy. Monitoring of unbound plasma concentrations of phenytoin and valproate is recommended for patients whose clinical response does not appear to correlate with the total plasma concentration. After delivery, AED plasma concentrations should be determined weekly and appropriate dosage adjustments made.

Approximately 50% of the infants born to mothers taking phenytoin, phenobarbital, and primidone during pregnancy are deficient in vitamin K–dependent clotting factors at birth. Although neonatal hemorrhage is uncommon, infants should be treated with vitamin K 1 mg intramuscularly immediately after birth. Clotting should then be monitored every 2 to 4 hr and repeat doses of vitamin K administered as needed. Alternately, coagulopathy can be prevented by treating the mother with vitamin K 20 mg orally each day for 2 weeks before delivery, or 10 mg intramuscularly 4 hr before delivery. The effect of maternal carbamazepine and valproate therapy on neonatal hemostasis is unknown.

All AEDs are excreted in breast milk to some degree. The ratio of breast milk to serum concentration is 80% for ethosuximide, 40 to 60% for phenobarbital, 40% for carbamazepine, 15% for phenytoin, and 3% for valproic acid (30). Although most epileptic mothers may safely breastfeed their infants, the potential effect of drug transfer to the baby should be considered, especially if the infant appears lethargic or feeds poorly.

Despite the concern of parents and clinicians about the risks of epilepsy and AED therapy during pregnancy, over 90% of epileptic women have normal children. However, epileptic women of childbearing age must understanding the value of prepregnancy planning and, once pregnant, be made aware of the risks for fetal abnormalities, the potential consequences of medication noncompliance, and the need for close therapeutic monitoring during and for several weeks following pregnancy.

WITHDRAWAL OF ANTIEPILEPTIC DRUG THERAPY

Several community-based studies have shown that, among patients with epilepsy who are followed for more than 10 years, over half will attain a 2- to 5-year remission from seizures during drug therapy. Remission rates tend to be

Table 48.9.
Factors That Affect the Risk of Seizure Recurrence after Antiepileptic Drug Withdrawal

Favorable Prognosis	Unfavorable Prognosis
Childhood-onset epilepsy	Adult-onset epilepsy
Longer seizure-free interval before drug withdrawal	Frequent, severe seizures before remission
Absence seizures	Partial seizures (with and without secondary generalization)
Primary generalized tonic-clonic seizures	EEG abnormalities at time of drug withdrawal
Normal or improved EEG at time of drug withdrawal	Abrupt withdrawal of benzodiazepine or barbiturate antiepileptic drugs
	Atypical febrile seizures

highest for patients with primary generalized seizures and range from 60% for those with tonic-clonic seizures to 80% for children with typical absence attacks.

In general, patients that remain free of seizures for 2 years or more may be considered candidates for AED withdrawal. The potential benefits of drug withdrawal include avoidance of the cognitive and behavioral adverse effects of AED therapy, reduction in the risk of adverse drug reactions and drug interactions, as well as a return by the patient to a lifestyle unencumbered by the need for chronic medication. However, the decision to withdraw AED therapy is complex, both medically and socially, and requires a clear explanation to the patient of both the risks and benefits.

Medical factors that appear to affect the risk of seizure recurrence after AED drug withdrawal are summarized in Table 48.9. In particular, it is important to consider the age of onset of epilepsy, seizure type, EEG abnormalities, and rate of drug withdrawal when assessing the risk of seizure recurrence. Relapse rates after AED withdrawal in patients free of seizures for 2 years or more are approximately 20% for childhood-onset epilepsy and 40% for adult-onset epilepsy (8, 33). Thus, 60 to 80% of patients will remain free of seizures when AED therapy is withdrawn after a 2-year remission. The risk of seizure recurrence is highest during the period of AED reduction and within the first year after drug withdrawal.

The rate of drug withdrawal may also affect seizure recurrence. Most authors agree that a gradual taper (usually over a period of 2 to 6 months) is preferred. Abrupt withdrawal is a risk factor for status epilepticus. Furthermore, rapid removal of AED therapy itself may precipitate seizures due to drug withdrawal (in distinction to a recurrence of seizures due to the underlying epileptic condition). Seizures during withdrawal are most common with benzodiazepine or barbiturate AEDs. Since there are no means to determine reliably whether recurrent seizures are truly epileptic in origin, the need for continued drug therapy is unclear unless the rate of taper is long enough to rule out a drug-withdrawal phenomenon.

Any decision to withdraw AED therapy based on a favorable medical prognosis must also include a careful assessment of the patient's work and social environments. Not only should patients clearly understand the risks and benefits of drug withdrawal, they must also be encouraged to participate actively in the decision. Patients who have been seizure-free for long intervals often have valid concerns about the possible recurrence of seizures at home, at work, or while driving. During AED withdrawal, it is often recommended that the patient not drive for a period of several months. Furthermore, in some areas, a recurrent seizure during this period may result in the suspension of driving privileges until AED therapy is restarted and adequate control is demonstrated. These, and other patient-

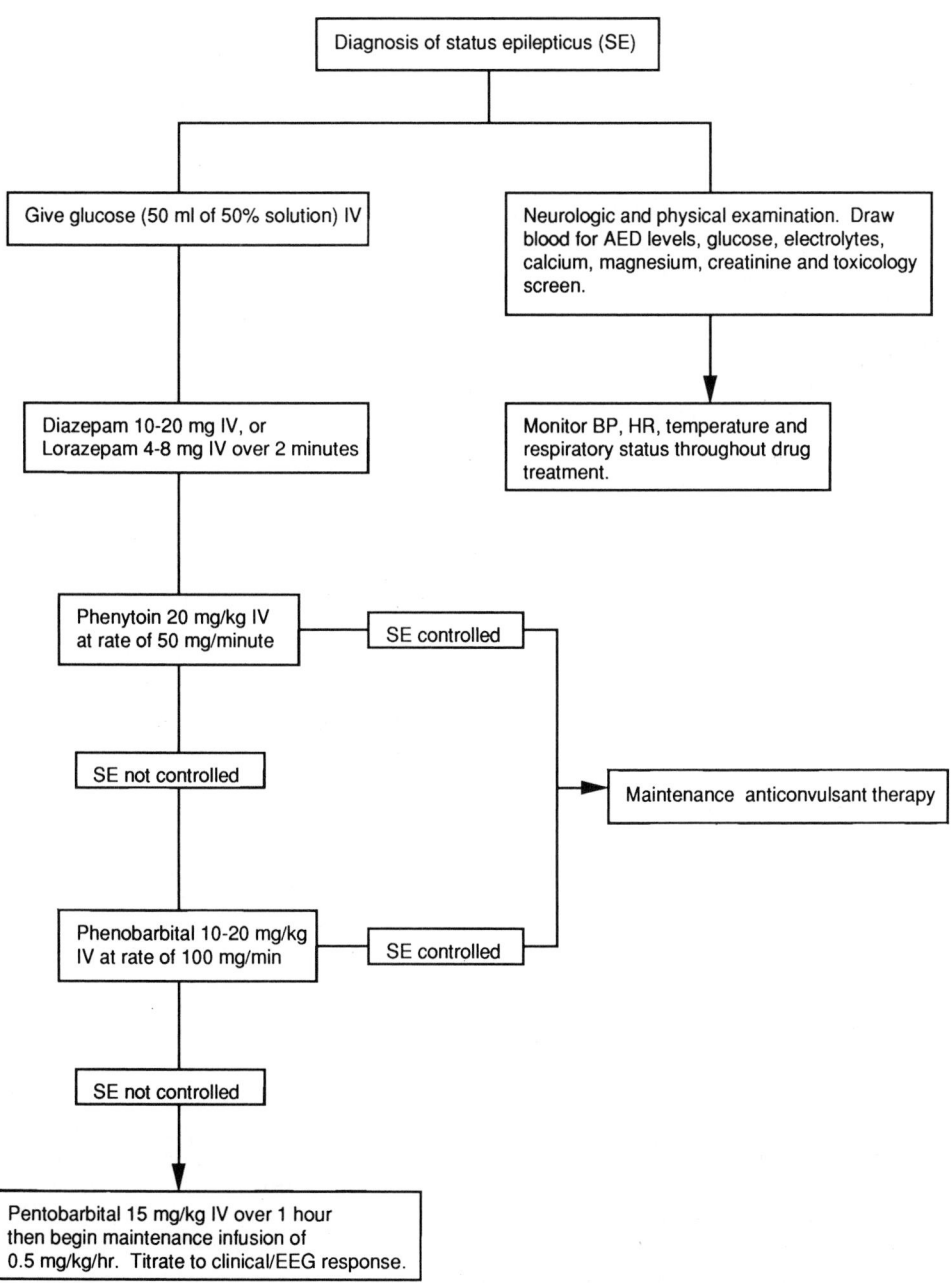

Figure 48.1. Treatment algorithm for status epilepticus in adults.

specific social factors, should be discussed with each individual for whom AED withdrawal is considered.

NONDRUG THERAPIES
Surgical Treatment

Approximately 300,000 patients in the United States have uncontrolled seizures despite medical therapy (1). For approximately 15% of these patients, surgical intervention may be a viable option. Patients most likely to benefit from surgery are those with partial seizures whose symptoms remain intractable despite optimal medical therapy. The degree to which seizures and drug toxicity impair the functional abilities of the patient must also be considered. Presurgical evaluation includes intensive medical and neurological testing to localize the lesion. CT and PET scans, as well as simultaneous EEG and video telemetry monitoring are very useful in this regard. Resection of a seizure focus from the anterior temporal lobe is the most common surgery performed. After temporal lobectomy, approximately one-half of patients are rendered free of seizures and one-third experience a significant reduction.

Behavioral Therapies

Psychological techniques for control of epileptic seizures are often successful for patients with seizures triggered by flashing lights or visual patterns, reading, or listening to music (referred to as *reflex epilepsies*). In these cases, behavioral conditioning has been used with success. The role of behavioral therapies in other types of epilepsy remains limited.

STATUS EPILEPTICUS

Status epilepticus (SE) is a medical emergency that requires prompt, effective treatment to minimize permanent neurologic damage and death. SE is defined as repetitive clinical convulsions without recovery of consciousness between attacks or repeated electrographic seizure activity in a comatose patient, usually lasting 30 min or more. Morbidity and mortality after SE are caused primarily by CNS injury due to the condition precipitating the episode and neuronal injury from continuous electrical and convulsive seizure activity. Even with aggressive medical therapy, SE is fatal in 10 to 12% of patients.

The most common cause of SE in patients with a history of epilepsy is noncompliance with AED therapy. Additionally, the factors listed in Table 48.1 which can cause seizures are also potential causes of SE. The initial work-up for patients should include a thorough evaluation to identify potentially treatable causes of SE.

Figure 48.1 is an algorithm that outlines the treatment of SE in adults. The goals of treatment are to (*a*) terminate the seizures as quickly as possible, but within at least 90 to 120 min after onset; (*b*) identify and treat any potentially

reversible causes; and (*c*) medically manage systemic complications that arise from prolonged convulsive seizures (e.g., hyperpyrexia, or hypoxia).

Benzodiazepines (diazepam or lorazepam) are the agents of choice for the initial treatment of SE. Diazepam and lorazepam terminate SE in 90% of patients, usually within 2 to 3 min after intravenous administration. The utility of diazepam is limited by its short duration of anticonvulsant effect (15 min to 2 hr). This drug is highly lipophilic and quickly redistributes out of the brain to other fat stores in the body. Lorazepam has a longer duration of action and is often preferred over diazepam for this reason. Phenytoin and phenobarbital are usually administered after benzodiazepines because they have a longer anticonvulsant effect. Barbiturate anesthesia (preferably with pentobarbital) offers definitive therapy of SE when other treatments are ineffective or when the duration of continuous seizure activity threatens to cause permanent neurologic damage.

CONCLUSION

The effective treatment of epilepsy requires the mutual participation of patient and clinician. The goal of epilepsy treatment is to reduce the frequency of recurrent seizures while avoiding adverse effects of drug therapy. The specific means by which this goal is attained must be individualized and take into account the seizure classification, age, sex, and concurrent medical problems of the patients. Monotherapy with nonsedating AEDs is both effective and well tolerated in most patients. Patients and their families also require education and support regarding their condition and its effect, if any, on daily activities.

REFERENCES

1. Porter RJ: Epilepsy. 100 Elementary Principles, ed. 2. London: WB Saunders, 1989.
2. Engel J: Seizure and Epilepsy. Philadelphia, FA Davis, 1989.
3. Scheuer ML, Pedley TA: The evaluation and treatment of seizures. N Engl J Med 323:1468–1474, 1990.
4. Alldredge BK, Simon RP, Drugs that can precipitate seizures. In Resor SR, Kutt H (eds): The Medical Treatment of Epilepsy. New York, Marcel Dekker, 1992, pp 497–523.
5. Commission on Classification and Terminology of the International League-Against Epilepsy: Proposal for revised clinical and electroencephalographic classification of epileptic seizures. Epilepsia 22:489–501, 1981.
6. Commission on Classification and Terminology of the International League Against Epilepsy: Proposal for classification of epilepsies and epileptic syndromes. Epilepsia 26:268–278, 1985.
7. Knudsen FU: Optimum management of febrile seizures in childhood. Drugs 36:111–120, 1988.
8. Chadwick D: Diagnosis of epilepsy. Lancet 336:291–295, 1990.
9. Brodie MJ: Established anticonvulsants and treatment of refractory epilepsy. Lancet 336:350–354, 1990.
10. Theodore WH, Porter RJ: Removal of sedative-hypnotic antiepileptic drugs from the regimens of patients with intractable epilepsy. Ann Neurol 13:320–324, 1983.

11. Mattson RH, Cramer JA, Collins JF, et al.: Comparison of carbamazepine, phenobarbital, phenytoin, and primidone in partial and secondarily generalized tonic-clonic seizures. N Engl J Med 313:145–151, 1985.

12. Dean JC, Penry JK: Valproate monotherapy in 30 patients with partial seizures. Epilepsia 29:140–144, 1988.

13. Sato S, White BG, Penry JK, et al.: Valproic acid versus ethosuximide in the treatment of absence seizures. Neurology 32:157–163, 1982.

14. Mattson RH, General principles: selection of antiepileptic drug therapy. In Levy RH, Dreifuss FE, Mattson RH, Meldrum BS, Penry JK (eds): Antiepileptic Drugs, ed. 3. New York, Raven Press, 1989, pp 103–115.

15. Snead OC, Hosey LC: Exacerbation of seizures in children by carbamazepine. N Engl J Med 313:916–921, 1985.

16. Dodson WE: Level off. Neurology 39:1009–1010, 1989.

17. Miles MV, Lawless ST, Tennison MB, Zaritsky AL, Greenwood RS: Rapid loading of critically ill patients with carbamazepine suspension. Pediatric 86:263–266, 1990.

18. Dalby MA, Behavioral effects of carbamazepine. In Penry JK, Dalby DD (eds): Advances in Neurology, vol 11. New York, Raven Press, 1975, pp 331–343.

19. Ferriero D, Alldredge BK, Knutsen AP: Anticonvulsant hypersensitivity syndrome: in vitro and clinical observations (Abstract). Neurology 41(suppl 1):385, 1991.

20. Hart RG, Easton JD: Carbamazepine and hematological monitoring. Ann Neurol 11:309–312, 1982.

21. Zaccara B, Messori A, Moroni F: Clinical pharmacokinetics of valproic acid—1988. Clin Pharmacokinet 15:367–389, 1988.

22. Dreifuss FE, Langer DH: Side effects of valproate. Am J Med 84(suppl 1A):34–41, 1988.

23. Dreifuss FE, Langer DH, Moline KA, Maxwell JE: Valproic acid hepatic fatalities. II. US experience since 1984. Neurology 39:201–207, 1989.

24. Bourgeois BFD: Pharmacologic interactions between valproate and other drugs. Am J Med 84(suppl 1A):29–33, 1988.

25. Winter ME, Tozer TN, Phenytoin. In Evans WE, Schentag JJ, Jusko WJ (eds): Applied Pharmacokinetics: Principles of Therapeutic Drug Monitoring, ed. 2. Spokane, Applied Therapeutics, 1986, pp 493–539.

26. Nation RL, Evans AM, Milne RW: Pharmacokinetic drug interactions with phenytoin (Part II). Clin Pharmacokinet 18:131–150, 1990.

27. Mattson RH, Kramer JA, Phenobarbital: toxicity. In Levy RH, Dreifuss FE, Mattson RH, Meldrum BS, Penry JK (eds): Antiepileptic Drugs, ed. 3. New York, Raven Press, 1989, pp 341–355.

28. Browne TR, Benzodiazepines. In Browne TR, Feldman RG (eds): Epilepsy: Diagnosis and Management. Boston, Little, Brown and Co, 1983, pp 235–245.

29. Dalessio DJ: Seizure disorders and pregnancy. N Engl J Med 312:559–563, 1985.

30. Donaldson JO, Epilepsy. In Donaldson JO: Neurology of Pregnancy. London, WB Saunders, 1989, p 229.

31. Saunders M: Epilepsy in women of childbearing age: if anticonvulsants cannot be avoided use carbamazepine. Br Med J 299:581, 1989.

32. Jones KL, Lacro RV, Johnson KA, Adams J: Pattern of malformations in the children of women treated with carbamazepine during pregnancy. N Engl J Med 320:1661–1666, 1989.

33. Chadwick D, The discontinuation of antiepileptic therapy. In Pedley TA, Meldrum BS (eds): Recent Advances in Epilepsy, 2. New York, Churchill Livingstone, 1985, pp 111–124.

34. Simon RP, Aminoff MJ, Greenberg DA: Clinical Neurology. Norwalk: Appleton & Lange, 1989, ch. 9.

35. Levy RH, Dreifuss FE, Mattson RH, Meldrum BS, Penry JK (eds): Antiepileptic Drugs, ed. 3. New York, Raven Press, 1989.

CHAPTER 49

PARKINSONISM

SAM K. SHIMOMURA, Pharm.D. and LEE HEADLEY, Pharm.D.

In 1817, a general practitioner in London, Dr. James Parkinson, first described a disease he called the "shaking palsy" or "paralysis agitans." It has since become known as Parkinson's disease, parkinsonism, or Parkinson's syndrome. Even today very little can be added to his description of the signs and symptoms of this disease. A brief excerpt from "An Essay on the Shaking Palsy" characterizes this disease as follows:

Involuntary tremulous motion, with lessened muscular power, in parts not in action and even when supported; with a propensity to bend the trunk forward and to pass from a walking to a running pace; the senses and the intellects being uninjured. . . (1)

Historically, anticholinergics have been the mainstay of treatment for Parkinson's disease. Traditional surgical treatment has benefited a few patients, but it has not been proven to ameliorate the signs and symptoms of the vast majority of patients. The introduction of levodopa has been hailed in an editorial in the *New England Journal of Medicine* as "the most important contribution to medical therapy of a neurological disease in the past 50 years because of its usefulness in one of the prevalent and disabling neurologic illnesses of man."

BIOCHEMICAL BASIS OF PARKINSONISM

In recent years, much has been elucidated about the biochemical basis of parkinsonism, but not all the information is in. A cholinergic component appears to be involved, since anticholinergics have been useful in the treatment of Parkinson's disease for over 100 years. This cholinergic overactivity has been confirmed by studies that show that centrally acting cholinesterase inhibitors, such as physostigmine, aggravate parkinsonian tremor, while centrally acting anticholinergics, such as benztropine, will reverse the effects.

Acetylcholine has predominantly excitatory effects on the central nervous system and is responsible for the positive signs of parkinsonism such as tremor. However, the primary defect in Parkinson's disease appears to be dopamine deficiency. It is estimated that symptoms of the disease do not appear until there is approximately 80% cell loss. Normally the effects of excitatory acetylcholine balance the inhibitory effects of dopamine. Although the concentration of acetylcholine seems to be unchanged in parkinsonism, the deficiency of dopamine disturbs the balance, and the cholinergic activity predominates. Other neurotransmitters, such as serotonin, norepinephrine, γ-aminobutyric acid, substance P, cholecystokinin, glycine, and somatostatin may also be involved in parkinsonism. Parkinsonism may be caused by any degenerative, toxic, infective, traumatic, or neoplastic pathology altering the balance between acetylcholine and dopamine in favor of cholinergic overactivity. Based on this hypothesis, anticholinergics are given to decrease central cholinergic activity, and dopamine, as its precursor levodopa, is given to increase dopaminergic activity (2).

EPIDEMIOLOGY

Approximately 500,000 patients in the United States are estimated to suffer from parkinsonism. Each year there are another 20 new cases per 100,000 population. The risk of developing parkinsonism sometime during one's lifetime is 2 to 3%. At least 66% of all those afflicted have onset of signs and symptoms between 50 and 69 years of age. The age of onset and incidence is the same for men and women (3).

ETIOLOGY

The signs and symptoms of parkinsonism are produced by many different causes (4). Before a diagnosis of primary parkinsonism is established, secondary causes must be ruled out. Unlike idiopathic parkinsonism, many of the secondary forms of parkinsonism can be cured.

Idiopathic Parkinsonism

The term *idiopathic* denotes a disease of unknown cause. Many theories have been proposed, and each in succession has been refuted or abandoned because of lack of supporting evidence. This chapter focuses on idiopathic parkinsonism, since secondary causes make up only a small percentage of cases.

Trauma-induced Parkinsonism

Severe injuries to the head very rarely produce tremor and extrapyramidal rigidity similar to that seen in primary parkinsonism. Usually this occurs soon after injury, and recovery is the general rule.

Chemical-induced Parkinsonism

Many chemicals produce parkinsonism-like symptoms upon acute ingestion of large amounts or occasionally upon chronic exposure. Acute carbon monoxide poisoning can be a cause of secondary parkinsonism. It is not a common sequela of carbon monoxide intoxication, but when it does occur, recovery may be slow. Chronic exposure to heavy metals, such as lead, manganese, and mercury, may cause symptoms of parkinsonism. Other chemicals that have been reported to produce some or all of the signs of parkinsonism are carbon disulfide, cyanide, methylchloride, and some photographic dyes. In most cases of chemical-induced parkinsonism, recovery is complete if the patient survives the acute exposure to the chemical.

Drug-induced Parkinsonism

Phenothiazines commonly produce extrapyramidal side effects that ultimately may manifest as a parkinsonism-like syndrome (Table 49.1). Early in the treatment with phenothiazine derivatives, a dystonic syndrome may develop. This side effect consists of torsional movements involving most of the muscles of the body, especially those of the tongue and face. Stiff neck (torticollis), facial grimacing, and retrocollis are common. Dystonic reactions occur twice as frequently in males, most often between 5 and 45 years of age. The parenteral administration of diphenhydramine 50 mg or benztropine 2 mg produces a dramatic response within 10 to 30 min. Akathisia may occur after a few weeks of phenothiazine therapy. Patients with akathisia appear jittery and very anxious. They may pace the floor, tap their fingers, and generally give the impression of restlessness. This occurs twice as often in females as in males and usually in patients between 12 and 65 years of age. The true parkinsonism-like syndrome usually becomes apparent 2 to 3 months after initiation of drug therapy. It consists of the usual symptoms associated with idiopathic parkinsonism, namely rigidity, tremor, bradykinesia, drooling, slurred speech, mask-like face, festinating gait, and seborrhea; and it occurs most frequently in patients over 50 years of age.

Even phenothiazines that are thought to have fewer extrapyramidal side effects, such as thioridazine, may cause

Table 49.1.
Examples of Phenothiazines That Produce Extrapyramidal Effects

Drug	Relative Degree
Trifluoroperazine	High
Perphenazine	High
Fluphenazine	High
Prochlorperazine	High
Promazine	Moderate
Chlorpromazine	Moderate
Thioridazine	Low

Table 49.2.
Drugs That May Produce a Parkinson-like Syndrome

Amitriptyline and other tricyclic antidepressants
Carbamazepine
Chlorpromazine and other phenothiazines
Chlorprothixene and thiothixene
Haloperidol and other butyrophenones
Metoclopramide
MPTP
Reserpine

or unmask parkinsonism-like signs and symptoms in low doses. Parkinsonism caused by phenothiazines may persist for a considerable time after discontinuation of the drug (up to 2 years in some cases). Therefore, all newly diagnosed parkinsonism patients should be questioned carefully about their prior use of neuroleptic agents. If there is any suspicion that the patient may have taken a phenothiazine in the past, a "drug holiday" every 6 months would reveal if the condition was entirely or partly drug-induced (5).

Other drugs besides the phenothiazines have the potential for producing a parkinsonism-like syndrome (Table 49.2). Haloperidol and other butyrophenones produce similar pharmacological effects, and the same precautions should be observed. Reserpine depletes the brain of dopamine and in high doses can produce a parkinsonism-like syndrome. Methyldopa is a decarboxylase inhibitor that can also produce parkinsonism-like symptoms when given in large doses. Metoclopramide has been shown to worsen Parkinson symptoms despite Sinemet treatment. Metoclopramide-induced parkinsonism is rare and usually associated with renal failure. Other drugs that have been reported to produce extrapyramidal symptoms are carbamazepine, thiothixine, and chloroprothixene.

In 1983, parkinsonism was reported in several young drug users after the intravenous administration of a meperidine analog, 1-methyl-4-phenyl-1,2,3,6-tetrahydropyridine (MPTP) (6). MPTP itself eventually turned out to be nontoxic, but its oxidation product, 1-methyl-4-phenylpyridinium ion (MPP$^+$) was determined to be highly toxic to melanin-containing neurons in the substantia nigra. MPP$^+$ is formed by the oxidation of MPTP by monoamine oxidase type B (MAO B). In studies involving monkeys, pretreatment with selegiline (a MAO B inhibitor) prevented the oxidation of MPTP to its toxic metabolite and prevented the signs and symptoms of parkinsonism. Selegiline has also been found to slow or perhaps even reverse the progression of idiopathic parkinsonism in humans. This fascinating research has caused many to speculate that some environmental contaminant resembling MPTP may be the cause of parkinsonism. The other side benefit of research with MPTP has been the development of an animal model for parkinsonism. Monkeys treated with MPTP appear to develop the same clinical, pathological, and chemical changes found in human parkinsonism (7).

Postencephalic Parkinsonism (Encephalitis Lethargica)

Between 1917 and 1925, there was an epidemic of encephalitis lethargica (van Economo's disease). A sequela of this viral infection was an onset of a syndrome similar to parkinsonism, which included seborrhea of the face, sialorrhea, occulogyric crisis, and a respiratory tic. Although new cases are rare, it is currently one of the major causes of secondary parkinsonism. Because of its viral origin, investigators have been trying to establish a viral basis for primary parkinsonism. At present, there is no evidence to support this hypothesis.

Infection-induced Parkinsonism

Besides the viral etiology of postencephalic parkinsonism, a number of other infectious diseases mimic parkinsonism as an occasional complication. A few examples are syphilis, poliomyelitis, malaria, typhoid, herpes zoster, coxsackie virus, measles, Western Equine encephalitis, and Japanese encephalitis.

Tumor-induced Parkinsonism

Another rare cause of a syndrome resembling parkinsonism is intracranial tumor. The signs are usually unilateral and very rarely produce a mask-like facies.

DIAGNOSIS AND CLINICAL FINDINGS

The signs of advanced parkinsonism are so striking and unique that it hardly ever poses a diagnostic challenge. The patient has rigidity, bradykinesia, seborrhea, festinating gait, flexed posture, drooling, and a characteristic "pill rolling" tremor. With further observation, the clinician notices a "reptilian stare" consisting of frozen, mask-like facies, infrequent blinking of the eyes, and the tendency to sit for long periods of time in a stationary position. The voice may be initially hoarse and harsh, and with time, decrease in volume and resonance into a low monotone.

Most of the clinical features of parkinsonism fall into three general categories: bradykinesia, rigidity, and tremor. Bradykinesia and akinesia are a slowing down of voluntary actions with apparent difficulty in initiating movement, respectively. This is often severe enough to cause the patient to "freeze" into immobility. This can be tested for by assessing the ability of the patient to perform rapid, alternating movements. Rigidity is the tendency to move en bloc. There is an increased hypertonicity with resistance to passive and active movements of muscles.

Table 49.3.
Staging Parkinson's Disease

Stage I	Unilateral involvement only
	Functional impairment usually minimal or absent
Stage II	Bilateral or midline involvement
	No impairment of balance
Stage III	Bilateral involvement
	First sign of impaired righting reflexes
Stage IV	Fully developed, severely disabling disease
	Unassisted standing and walking but markedly incapacitated
Stage V	Confined to bed or chair unless aided

Muscle control and normal associated movements are hampered. Cogwheel rigidity is seen upon applying force to bend the limbs; the muscles yield jerkily, giving the impression of cogwheels moving one upon another. It has a higher frequency and may not be related to the resting tremor. The tremor of parkinsonism is generally coarser, slower, and of wider amplitude than that associated with alcoholism, hyperthyroidism, or nervousness. A relaxed patient shows a slow, rhythmical resting tremor.

Although moderately advanced to advanced parkinsonism is easily diagnosed, early features and findings of the disease frequently can be confused with many other diseases. Hoehn and Yahr have described a staging of Parkinson's disease (see Table 49.3) (8).

The masking of facial expression is often an early feature of parkinsonism, appearing long before more overt signs such as the festinating gait. A friendly, outgoing, and smiling individual may slowly appear to become more restrained, emotionless, and depressed. There is a subtle restraint of smile, a drawing down of the lips and lower face into an unchanging and worried expression. A slight bulging of the eyes and the barely noticeable tremulousness of early parkinsonism can easily mislead the physician into a diagnosis of anxiety, nervousness, or depression. Not only can this diagnosis destroy the confidence and self-esteem of the patient, but it sets in motion a self-fulfilling prophecy wherein the patient actually becomes depressed, anxious, and nervous. The patient may be referred for psychiatric therapy where treatment with a phenothiazine may exacerbate the extrapyramidal signs of the disease.

Another patient may show weakness and stiffness of one hand. There may be no tremor or other signs of parkinsonism. The patient may also complain of stiff joints, difficulty in turning over in bed or getting up out of a chair, and the inability to perform activities of daily living such as buttoning a shirt or putting on cuff links. These presenting signs can often be misdiagnosed as arthritis, or when unilateral involvement is apparent, the possibility of a stroke may be raised.

Early features of parkinsonism frequently involve only

one of the three cardinal signs of rigidity, bradykinesia, and tremor. The signs are often unilateral and almost imperceptible at first, and they slowly progress in severity and spread from one area of involvement such as one finger, hand, or shoulder to the whole body. The upper part of the body is usually affected first, with involvement of the lower part of the body (e.g., shuffling gait) a later finding.

Dementia and impairment of intellectual function are encountered in a significantly higher percentage of parkinsonism patients than in age-matched controls (9). However, there is continuing debate over whether the dementia is a part of the disease process or due to concurrent drug therapy, Alzheimer's disease, or other factors (10).

TREATMENT

Treatment is aimed primarily at providing maximal relief of symptoms and maintaining the independence and movement of the patient. At present, there is no cure for this disease, but the use of levodopa has greatly improved the prognosis of parkinsonism. Successful treatment involves a total program of drug therapy, physical therapy, psychological support, and occasionally surgery.

Drug Treatment
ANTICHOLINERGICS

Although drugs with anticholinergic properties had been the mainstay of therapy for parkinsonism for over a century, many neurologists are now avoiding the use of anticholinergic agents even in mild-to-moderate cases of parkinsonism, because the modest benefits of the drugs are outweighed by their many side effects. The mechanism of action involves the suppression of cholinergic overactivity in the brain. Anticholinergics that do not cross the blood-brain barrier (e.g., quaternary ammonium compounds such as propantheline) are ineffective in parkinsonism. Centrally acting anticholinergics produce moderate improvement in tremor, rigidity, and akinesia in one-third to one-half of patients.

All of the anticholinergics share these common side effects; blurred vision, dry mouth, drowsiness, mental confusion, constipation, and urinary retention. In toxic doses, they may produce hallucinations, agitation, and elevation of body temperature. The older population in which parkinsonism usually occurs is particularly susceptible to these anticholinergic side effects.

The belladonna alkaloids such as atropine and scopolamine have been replaced in therapy by the synthetic anticholinergics. Although the synthetic agents are not more effective, they produce somewhat fewer side effects.

Of the synthetic anticholinergics, trihexyphenidyl is currently the most popular. A number of congeners such as procyclidine, cycrimine, and biperiden are also available. There is no clinically apparent difference among these agents. Any one of this group is suitable for initial therapy. One should begin with low doses and gradually increase the dose, weighing satisfactory response against undesirable side effects.

Benztropine is used widely because of its long duration of action. One to 2 mg at bedtime will allow most patients mobility upon arising during the night or getting up out of bed in the morning.

Diphenhydramine provides mild anticholinergic and antiparkinson effects. Diphenhydramine is also useful as a hypnotic in parkinsonism patients who have difficulty going to sleep or staying asleep.

The phenothiazine derivative ethopropazine has also been used for its anticholinergic properties in the treatment of parkinsonism. The recommended initial dosage is 50 mg once or twice a day, with gradual increases until optimal therapeutic effect or onset of toxic effects. Doses of up to 600 mg per day have been used.

AMANTADINE

Amantadine is an antiviral agent that produces moderate improvement in parkinsonism. Currently the mechanism of action is unknown, although it is postulated that amantadine may (a) inhibit the reuptake of dopamine and other catecholamines from neuronal storage sites, (b) release dopamine from intact dopaminergic terminals, or (c) have prominent anticholinergic effects. Side effects include slurred speech, ataxia, depression, hyperexcitability, insomnia, dizziness, livedo reticularis, and in extremely large doses, convulsions and hallucinations. In general, the side effects are mild, transient, and reversible. The usual dose is 100 mg per day with breakfast for the first week and then 100 mg with breakfast and lunch. The dose may be increased to a maximum of 400 mg per day. Approximately 90% of amantadine is excreted unchanged in the urine, and therefore, the dose must be reduced in patients with renal impairment (11). Early studies demonstrated that tachyphylaxis occurs after 4 to 8 weeks in about one-half of patients. A few patients may receive benefits for much longer. Therefore, it is often used for short-term, intermittent therapeutic assistance, since its effect is enhanced by concurrent use of levodopa. It has a rapid onset of action with effects seen within a few days. Amantadine is not a first-line drug, but it may be useful as an adjunct to therapy with anticholinergics and levodopa.

LEVODOPA

Cotzias (12) first demonstrated the efficacy of levodopa in parkinsonism in 1967. Although small doses of dopa were tried as early as 1961 in parkinsonism, most investigators reported transient or no improvement. By switching to the levo isomer of dopa and gradually increasing the dose of the drug, Cotzias and associates could push the dose high enough to achieve therapeutic results, while keeping the gastrointestinal side effects at a tolerable level.

The next major breakthrough in the use of levodopa was the addition of carbidopa, a decarboxylase inhibitor, to levodopa therapy. High doses of levodopa, 4 to 8 g per day, are generally needed, because much of the levodopa is wasted through extracerebral metabolism. Decarboxylase inhibitors that do not cross the blood-brain barrier are useful in preventing the conversion of levodopa to dopamine outside the brain. This enables the dose of levodopa to be reduced to one-fourth of the original dose, with concomitant decrease in nausea, vomiting, and cardiac arrhythmias (13).

Akinesia is generally the first symptom to improve, followed by improvements in rigidity and tremors. Overall, therapy with levodopa can be expected to produce 50% or greater improvement in about two-thirds of patients. Levodopa is approximately 3½ times more effective in treating parkinsonism than anticholinergic therapy.

The rationale for the use of levodopa is that parkinsonism may be caused by the depletion of dopamine in the basal ganglia. Dopamine seems to act as a specific transmitter at certain dopaminergic synapses. Dopamine itself was tried in the treatment of parkinsonism, but it does not cross the blood-brain barrier to any appreciable extent. However, the immediate precursor of dopamine, levodopa, does so easily, and it is therefore effective in restoring dopamine levels in the brain.

Dosage and Administration

The careful titration of dosage for each individual patient is of the utmost importance to achieving successful levodopa therapy. The usual effective dose of levodopa is 2 to 8 g per day in divided doses given with meals or food. With the introduction of the levodopa/carbidopa combination (Sinemet and Sinemet CR), it is no longer necessary to use such high doses. When the levodopa/carbidopa combination (Sinemet) is used, the dose of levodopa can be reduced by 75%. The patient may be started on 1 tablet of 100 mg levodopa and 25 mg carbidopa (Sinemet 25/100) 3 times a day. About 75 to 100 mg per day of carbidopa is needed to reach its optimal saturation point. The dose may be increased rapidly to effective levels, since the necessity to develop tolerance to the peripheral effects of dopamine is minimized. As the dose is increased, the patient may be switched to tablets containing 250 mg levodopa and 25 mg carbidopa (Sinemet 25/250). The maximum recommended dose of levodopa in such a combination is 2 g per day. When switching a patient from levodopa to the combination, wait at least 8 hr after the last dose of levodopa, to prevent toxic effects.

A controlled-release formulation of Sinemet called Sinemet CR contains levodopa 200 mg and carbidopa 50 mg and decreases fluctuations in response seen after prolonged use of levodopa. Sinemet CR is less bioavailable than Sinemet. When converting a patient to the sustained-release formulation, an additional 10 to 30% more levodopa may be required to achieve the same therapeutic effect. The dosing interval for Sinemet CR should be 4 to 8 hr during waking hours. A guideline for converting a patient from Sinemet to Sinemet CR is included in Table 49.4.

Sinemet and Sinemet CR offer several advantages over levodopa alone. In addition to being able to reduce the dose by 75%, there are generally fewer peripheral side effects, a more rapid onset, and greater improvement, because larger doses can be given before limited by toxic effects. Pyridoxine can be given with this combination without counteracting the effects of levodopa. On the other hand, central nervous system toxicities may be increased in onset and severity, since more levodopa is available to the brain.

Initiating Therapy with Levodopa

There has been significant controversy among clinicians about when to initiate levodopa therapy. There is no question that its effectiveness diminishes over time. If levodopa is effective only for a limited period of time, advocates of late initiation argue that it is most reasonable to save levodopa until there is significant disability. The proponents of early initiation argue that it is the progression of the disease that makes levodopa less effective over time, and so it should be used early, to obtain the maximum benefits of the drug.

Studies by Markham and Diamond (14, 15) provide persuasive data to show that the loss of effectiveness of levodopa is due to the progression of the disease not the time on levodopa. When groups who had equal durations of symptoms, (e.g., 8 years) but had different durations of levodopa therapy (3 years versus 6 years) were compared, their disability scores were similar. On the other hand, patients who had equal durations of levodopa therapy but different durations of symptoms had significantly different disability scores. These data support the proponents of early initiation of levodopa who implicate duration of disease rather than duration of levodopa therapy as the cause of the loss of effectiveness.

There is also convincing evidence that long-term levodopa therapy can alter the responsiveness of dopamine receptors. Only after prolonged levodopa therapy do we see a significant number of patients with the "on-off" effect and the "end-of-dose" or "wearing-off effect." This may be due to decreased sensitivity of dopamine receptors with prolonged therapy or to a decrease in dopamine receptors caused by levodopa therapy.

Most neurologists initiate levodopa therapy as soon as the disease interferes with the occupational or social func-

Table 49.4.
Antiparkinsonism Drugs

Drug	Dose
Anticholinergics	
Trihexyphenidyl (Artane)	1–5 mg t.i.d., start with low doses; doses over 20 mg/day are rarely tolerated
2 and 5 mg tablets; 5 mg time-released capsules	
Benztropine (Cogentin)	Initially 0.5–1 mg daily, with slow increase to 1–2 mg daily; maximum dose 6 mg in divided doses
0.5, 1, 2 mg tablets	
Diphenhydramine (Benadryl)	Usual dose is 75–150 mg per day in divided doses with a maximum of 300 mg
25 and 50 mg capsules; 12.5 mg/5 mg elixir	
Biperiden (Akineton)	2 mg 3–4 times a day
2 mg tablets	
Cycrimine (Pagitane)	1.25 mg 2–3 times a day; usual range 3.75–15 mg daily in divided doses
1.25 and 2.5 mg tablets	
Procyclidine (Kemadrin)	2.5 mg 2–3 times a day; usual dosage range 10–20 mg daily in 3–4 doses
5 mg tablets	
Ethopropazine (Parsidol)	Initially 50 mg once or twice daily; may increase to 600 mg/day
10 and 50 mg tablets	
Dopaminergic drugs	
Levodopa (Larodopa, Dopar, Levopa)	Initially 300–500 mg/day with slow increase to 2–8 g/day in divided doses
100, 250, and 500 mg capsules	
Carbidopa (Lodosyn)	75–100 mg daily
25 mg tablets	
Levodopa/carbidopa (Sinemet)	300/75 to 1500/150 mg/day in 3–4 divided doses; maximum dose 2000/200 mg per day
100 mg/10 mg, 100 mg/25 mg, and 250 mg/25 mg	
Levodopa/carbidopa sustained-release (Sinemet CR)	1 tablet b.i.d. = 300–400 mg Sinemet; 1½ tablet b.i.d. or 1 tablet t.i.d. = 500–600 mg Sinemet; 4 tablets in 3 or more divided doses = 700–800 mg Sinemet; 5 tablets in 3 or more divided doses = 900–1000 mg Sinemet
200 mg/50 mg	
Amantidine (Symmetrel)	100 mg with breakfast for 5–7 days, then 100 mg with breakfast and lunch
100 mg capsules, 50 mg/5 ml syrup	
Bromocriptine (Parlodel)	Start with 1.25 mg twice a day with meals; if necessary, dosage may be increased every 14–28 days by 2.5 mg with meals; maximum dose 100 mg/day
2.5 mg tablet and 5 mg capsule	
Pergolide (Permax)	Initiate with 0.05 mg for first 2 days; gradually increase the dosage by 0.1–0.15 mg/day every third day over the next 12 days of therapy; dosage may then be increased by 0.25 mg/day every third day until an optimal therapeutic dose is achieved; average dose is 3 mg per day, maximum dose is 5 mg/day
0.05, 0.25, and 1 mg tablets	
Selegiline (Eldepryl)	5 mg at breakfast and 5 mg at lunch
5 mg tablets	

tioning of the patient. This may be much earlier for a painter or surgeon than for someone not dependent on fine motor skills. The optimal time to initiate levodopa therapy, therefore, depends heavily on the wishes and needs of the individual patient.

Absorption, Metabolism, and Excretion

Approximately 80% of orally administered levodopa is absorbed, primarily in the small intestine. Peak levels occur ½ to 2 hr after an oral dose is given in a fasting state. Although food delays absorption, generally it is given with meals to decrease nausea and vomiting. Even before absorption begins, some levodopa is metabolized in the gut. Once it reaches the general circulation, metabolism is fairly rapid, with detectable levels present for only 4 to 6 hr. When used alone, only 1% of a levodopa dose crosses the blood-brain barrier. This is increased to about 3% by com-

bination with carbidopa. Levodopa is converted to dopamine in the stomach, liver, and kidneys, as well as the brain. The metabolic transformation is shown in Figure 49.1. It is initially decarboxylated to dopamine, and then it is further metabolized to norepinephrine, epinephrine, and a host of other metabolites. Most of these metabolites are excreted in the urine within 6 h, with very little excreted unchanged.

Side Effects

Gastrointestinal. Nausea and vomiting are seen at some time in almost all patients taking levodopa. Anorexia may occur in conjunction with the nausea and vomiting or occasionally may occur alone. The nausea and vomiting are probably a result of both the local and central effects of levodopa. To prevent the GI side effects, levodopa should be initiated with low doses and slowly increased as tol-

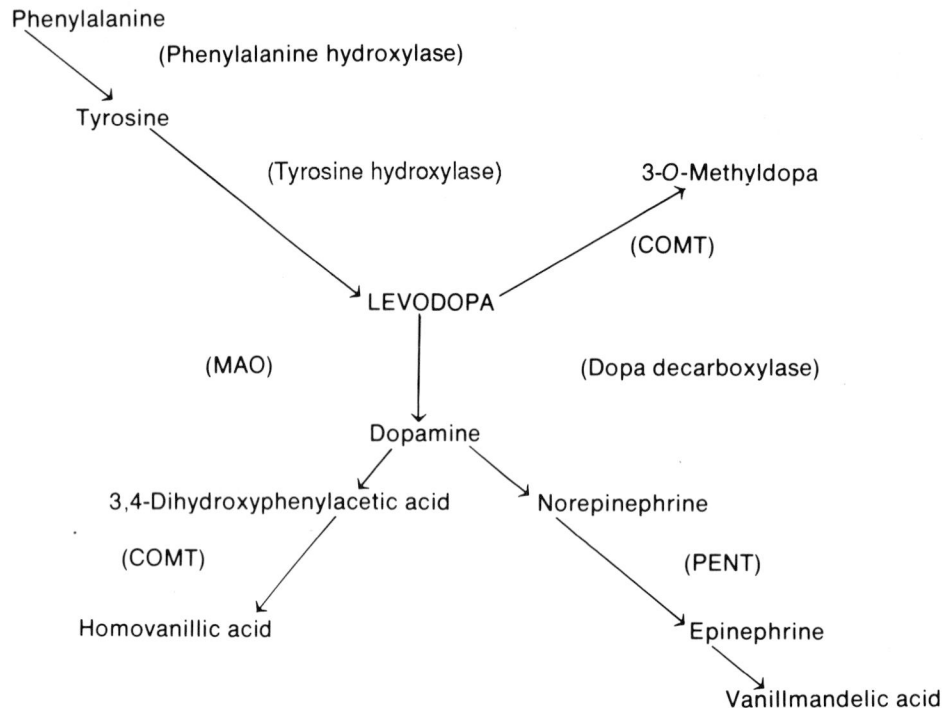

Figure 49.1.   Synthesis and metabolism of levodopa. *COMT*, catechol-*O*-methyltransferase; *MAO*, mono-amine oxidase; *PENT*, phenylethanolamine-*N*-methyltransferase.

erated by the patient. Administering the drug with food or antacid decreases the nausea. If nausea and vomiting become severe enough to limit the dosage despite slow increases in dose and administration with food, symptomatic treatment may be required. Phenothiazine derivatives, such as prochlorperazine (Compazine), should be avoided because they may counteract the therapeutic effects of levodopa.

Nausea and vomiting are decreased significantly when carbidopa is used in conjunction with levodopa. Other GI side effects include abdominal pain, diarrhea, constipation, peptic ulcer, and gastrointestinal bleeding.

Cardiovascular.   Cardiac arrhythmias, most commonly sinus tachycardia, and premature ventricular contractions occur in a small number of patients. This side effect can be attributed to the stimulation of β-adrenergic receptors in the heart by dopamine and its metabolites, such as norepinephrine. Treatment consists of discontinuing the levodopa and starting an antiarrhythmic agent. Propranolol is the logical agent because of its β-blocking actions. Decarboxylase inhibitors such as carbidopa may decrease the prevalence of cardiac arrhythmias.

The orthostatic hypotension frequently found in patients with parkinsonism can be aggravated by levodopa. Several different mechanisms have been proposed including direct β-effects of dopamine on blood vessels producing vasodilation, α-blockade of the peripheral vascular sys-

tem, and depletion of norepinephrine from adrengergic nerve endings by dopamine. Whatever the mechanism, it occurs in more than 25 to 35% of patients early in treatment, but, fortunately, the blood pressure usually returns to normal within 2 to 3 months after initiation of therapy. If symptoms are severe, treatment with elastic stockings, an increased salt intake, or sympathomimetic drugs such as ephedrine, is indicated.

Central Nervous System.   Levodopa causes behavioral changes manifested as hallucinations, depression, paranoia, agitation, delusions, and loss of judgment. The magnitude of these changes is difficult to determine, since parkinsonism occurs primarily in older patients who may develop impairment of memory, dementia, and other personality changes independent of levodopa therapy.

Abnormal involuntary movements are related to high doses and prolonged therapy with levodopa. After 6 months or more of therapy, over half the patients show symptoms of grimacing, chewing, active tongue movement, bobbing of the head and neck, and rocking movements of the trunk. When the carbidopa/levodopa combination is used, the onset of abnormal involuntary movements and other central nervous system reactions may be shortened to a few weeks, since more levodopa is available to enter the brain.

The "on-off" effect is a complication of levodopa therapy that often occurs after 2 to 3 years of treatment. There is an abrupt fluctuation in the patient's response to levodopa from being symptom-free "on" to experiencing full-blown parkinsonism signs and symptoms "off." It may occur at any time and persist in either phase for minutes to hours. In about half of the cases of the "on-off" effect, the "off" phase occurs 3 to 4 hr after the last dose of levodopa and is called "end-of-dose deterioration." Improvement "on" begins about an hour after the next dose. The exact mechanism for the "on-off" effect is unknown, but it may be due to factors that cause fluctuation in the blood level of levodopa or alter the sensitivity of dopamine receptors. The treatment of the "on-off" effect includes more frequent administration of levodopa, use of the levodopa/carbidopa sustained-release combination, substitution of a direct-acting dopamine agonist such as bromocriptine, or addition of selegiline.

Drug Interactions

A number of drugs can interact with levodopa. The clinical significance of these interactions is largely unknown, because most reports of interactions are either theoretical or anecdotal.

Pyridoxine (Vitamin B$_6$). Even small amounts of pyridoxine can antagonize the effects of levodopa by enhancement of its peripheral metabolism. A pyridoxine-dependent enzyme catalyzes the conversion of levodopa to dopamine. For this reason, pyridoxine was initially administered to potentiate the effect of levodopa, but instead it completely reversed it. By catalyzing the conversion of levodopa to dopamine in the gut, liver, and kidneys, pyridoxine decreases the amount of levodopa available to cross the blood-brain barrier. Although even 5 to 10 mg may antagonize the therapeutic effects of levodopa, in some patients such doses may be given to overcome the torsion dystonia produced by levodopa. However, reducing the dose slowly usually produces the same result and is the preferred method for treating this side effect. Small doses of pyridoxine may be given to overcome pyridoxine deficiency resulting from the large amount utilized in levodopa metabolism or to prevent the peripheral neuropathy associated with isoniazid or hydralazine therapy. Since most parkinsonism patients now receive carbidopa (a decarboxylase inhibitor) with their levodopa, even large doses of pyridoxine will not counteract the effects of levodopa. Therefore, pyridoxine restriction is unnecessary in patients receiving Sinemet.

Phenothiazines and Butyrophenones. Phenothiazines in large doses cause extrapyramidal side effects, apparently by their ability to block dopamine receptors in the brain. Although low doses of phenothiazines for short periods of time do not significantly reverse levodopa effects, it is best to avoid this combination if possible. An additive hypotensive effect may also complicate therapy with this combination. Clinicians unaware of this interaction may try to treat the nausea produced by levodopa with prochlorperazine (Compazine) or one of the other phenothiazine antiemetics. Haloperidol, a butyrophenone, has actions similar to those of the phenothiazines and also produces considerable extrapyramidal effect.

Reserpine. Reserpine antagonizes the "dopa effect." In fact the discovery that reserpine depletes the brain of dopamine and produces a parkinsonism-like syndrome was an important clue in determining the biochemical defect in parkinsonism. Reserpine should be avoided in parkinsonism patients whether or not they are on levodopa.

Food. High protein intake has been implicated in decreasing the beneficial effects of levodopa. Since levodopa is absorbed and transported like other amino acids, it has been suggested that high-protein diets may interfere with the absorption of levodopa or other common pathways. In summary, food does not interfere significantly with the action of levodopa.

Monoamine Oxidase Inhibitors. Levodopa may interact with monoamine oxidase type A inhibitors to produce a hypertensive reaction due to a buildup of dopa metabolites, such as norepinephrine, which have vasopressor activity. This combination is potentially dangerous and should be avoided. On the other hand, monoamine oxidase type B inhibitors such as selegiline have a beneficial interaction with levodopa, allowing a 30% reduction of the levodopa dose without causing a hypertensive reaction when given in its usual dose (16).

Phenytoin. Therapeutic doses of phenytoin (300 to 500 mg per day) have been reported to produce a return of hypokinesia, rigidity, and postural instability in five patients previously well controlled on levodopa or levodopa/carbidopa. When the phenytoin was discontinued, the patients returned slowly to their previous level of control over a 2-week period. While the mechanism for this interaction is unknown, it has been postulated that phenytoin may interfere with either the binding of dopamine or the reactivity of the brain to the dopamine.

Laboratory Test Interference

Very few laboratory abnormalities have been noted thus far with levodopa therapy. There is no significant interference with hematological, renal, endocrine, or liver tests. There have been reports of slight, transient elevations of AST and ALT levels and interference with determination of serum uric acid by the colorimetric method, but not by the more specific uricase test. Levodopa also produces an excess excretion of catecholamine metabolites in the urine. Certain metabolites of levodopa cause false-positive reactions for ketoacidosis by the dipstick method. Urine, saliva, and sweat may turn reddish and then black because of levodopa metabolites. Positive Coombs' test without frank hemolysis may also be noted. Phenistix, used to test for phenylketonuria, is relatively sensitive to levodopa. In fact, it can be used as a screening test for consumption of levodopa in patients who may not respond to levodopa therapy as expected.

Drug Holidays

The term *drug holiday* refers to the complete withdrawal of levodopa after chronic high-dose therapy. It is used when either reducing the dose or altering the frequency of dosage fails to relieve the adverse effects of long-term therapy or when the patient has become increasingly refractory to the therapeutic effects of levodopa. If the patient can tolerate a drug holiday from 1 to 2 days to 2 weeks, the dose may be reduced by 50% when levodopa is reinstated. During the drug holiday, the signs and symptoms may become very severe, and the patient must be hospitalized and kept under close supervision. Thrombophlebitis, pulmonary embolus, depression, and other complications have been reported during the drug holiday. Improvement is not immediate but comes gradually over a period of a few months and rarely lasts more than a year. Most neurologists feel that it is too dangerous and that the benefits do not outweigh the risks to the patient (17).

BROMOCRIPTINE

Although levodopa has helped most patients with Parkinson's disease, an increasing number of patients fail to maintain this beneficial response as their disease progresses. For levodopa to be active in the brain, it must be converted to dopamine by pigmented neurons in the substantia nigra. As parkinsonism progresses, the brain loses its ability to convert levodopa to dopamine, and the patient becomes more and more refractory to the beneficial effects of the agent. A drug that stimulates intact postsynaptic receptors directly would solve this problem. There are two distinct dopamine receptors known as D1 and D2; the main receptor of importance in Parkinson's disease is the D2 receptor.

Bromocriptine (Parlodel) is a direct-acting D2 dopamine agonist originally approved by the FDA for endocrine disorders such as amenorrhea/galactorrhea associated with hyperprolactinemia (18). Since late 1981, it has been approved for the treatment of parkinsonism. Bromocriptine acts directly in the brain to stimulate intact postsynaptic receptors. Bromocriptine appears to be about as effective as levodopa and is reserved predominantly for severely disabled Parkinson patients who no longer respond adequately to levodopa alone. It has a longer half-life (6 to 8 hr versus about 3 hr for levodopa), greater efficacy against tremors, and a reduction of the on-off effect caused by levodopa. Adverse reactions to bromocriptine are qualitatively similar to those of levodopa. Orthostatic hypotension and mental changes are more frequent with bromocriptine, and involuntary abnormal movements and the on-off effect are decreased, as compared with levodopa (19).

While most studies indicate that the optimum dose for parkinsonism patients not taking levodopa is 30 to 90 mg in three divided doses, one study gives hope that low-dose therapy (average dose 15 mg per day) may be just as effective. In this study (20), the patients were started on 1 mg of bromocriptine daily and slowly increased by not more than 1 mg daily at intervals of 1 week or more. At four dose-stage points (4, 7.5, 10, and 12.5 mg per day), the dose was not increased for 2 weeks to determine the status of the patients. In their study of 25 patients (14 levodopa-treated patients and 11 not on levodopa), there was a significant improvement (39%) in the combined scores of tremor, rigidity, and bradykinesia in those on bromocriptine therapy. More recent studies corroborate the efficacy of low-dose bromocriptine therapy (21). Because optimum response to low-dose bromocriptine is delayed for several weeks, rapid increases in drug doses may place the patient on a larger dose than necessary. The dosage recommendation in Table 49.4 is the FDA-approved dose from the package insert. Bromocriptine is very expensive and should be used in the lowest possible dose. Currently, most neurologists use bromocriptine only in parkinsonism patients who no longer respond to levodopa or who experience severe on-off phenomena or other intolerable adverse effects from levodopa.

PERGOLIDE

Pergolide (Permax) is a long-acting dopamine agonist that has recently been approved as an adjunct to levodopa/carbidopa treatment in parkinsonism. Pergolide stimulates both D1 and D2 receptors. When pergolide is combined with levodopa, the dosage of levodopa may be reduced by 5 to 30%. Both "on" time and motor function are increased, and the total disability score improves.

However, after 6 months, the degree of improvement has been shown to decline. The reason for this loss of efficacy with time is unknown. Pergolide has a longer duration of activity than the other direct-acting agonists, 4 to 8 hr, and appears to have fewer psychiatric side effects. Side effects are similar to those seen with bromocriptine and include nausea, somnolence, and dyskinesias. The manufacturer recommends taking a single 0.05-mg tablet daily for 2 days and then increasing the dosage over the next 12 days by 0.1 mg or 0.15 mg every third day. Further increases are made in 0.25-mg increments at 3-day intervals until the patient has a satisfactory response or experiences an adverse reaction. The doses should be divided into 3 daily doses, with a maximum of 5 mg per day. The average daily dose is 3 mg per day combined with an average of 650 mg of levodopa in the form of Sinemet (22, 23).

SELEGILINE

Selegiline (Eldepryl) is an MAO B inhibitor used primarily as an adjunct to levodopa/carbidopa therapy. Two isoenzymes oxidize monamines, MAO A and MAO B. Both are present in the periphery, while MAO B predominates in certain areas of the central nervous system having dopamine as one of its major substrates. Selegiline (1-deprenyl) is a specific MAO B inhibitor that allows a patient to eat tyramine-rich foods or take levodopa simultaneously without suffering side effects. When combined with Sinemet, it allows a reduction in the dose of levodopa by preventing its conversion in the brain by MAO B. It is effective in the treatment of the on-off and the dystonias and dyskinesias occurring in the transition between on and off. It appears to be most useful in those in early stages of disease or where the effectiveness of levodopa is greatly diminished and wide oscillations in motor performance are evident. About 10 to 20% do not respond at all to the addition of selegiline, and it appears to be of little use in advanced stages of the disease.

There is growing excitement that selegiline may slow the progression of parkinsonism and increase life expectancy for these patients. Birkmayer et al. (24) reported that their patients who received selegiline in addition to levodopa survived 12% longer than those who received levodopa alone. In another study (25) of 54 patients with early Parkinson's disease not receiving levodopa, those who received selegiline could function without requiring levodopa for 549 days, versus 312 days for those who received placebo. The largest study of this issue to date involved 800 patients with early untreated parkinsonism who were given selegiline alone, tocopherol alone, selegiline and tocopherol, or double placebo for 12 months. Of the 399 patients who received selegiline, 302 were able to function without levodopa compared with only 225 of 401 patients who did not receive selegiline (26). Results of the effects of tocopherol have not been reported because sufficient data have not yet been accumulated.

Side effects of selegiline include nausea, dizziness, abdominal pain, confusion, hallucinations, dry mouth, vivid dreams, headache, and dyskinesias. Selegiline is metabolized to amphetamine and methamphetamine, so insomnia may occur if evening doses are administered. The usual dose is 10 mg per day given 5 mg with breakfast and 5 mg with lunch. At higher doses selegiline loses its MAO B selectivity and has the potential to interact with products containing tyramine or other sympathomimetic amines. At the recommended dose, selegiline has very few side effects (27).

General Comfort Medications

Many of the minor signs and symptoms of parkinsonism can be corrected easily with simple over-the-counter medications. For example, constipation is common in parkinsonism. It is frequently aggravated by the anticholinergic drugs and levodopa. A stool softener such as docusate sodium or a mild laxative like milk of magnesia is usually effective, but a high-fiber diet and plenty of water will reduce the need for laxatives. Another common complaint in these patients is blurred vision, especially while watching television or movies. This can be attributed to the infrequent blinking of the eyes in parkinsonism. The lubricating action of artificial tears eye drops often gives relief. Blurred vision may result from therapy with anticholinergic drugs, and dosage reduction may be necessary in this case. Parkinsonism patients often have difficulty falling asleep and staying asleep. The drug of choice in this situation is diphenhydramine, because it is an effective hypnotic that possesses significant antiparkinson effects as well.

Diet

No particular diet has been found to be beneficial in parkinsonian patients. The best diet is one that is well-balanced and high in fiber, since many of these patients have constipation. Some parkinsonism patients have difficulty swallowing and cutting up their food and may require a soft mechanical diet.

Psychotherapy

The signs and symptoms of parkinsonism are frequently aggravated by psychologic factors. The patient usually has suffered much humiliation from the readily obvious signs of the disease and often becomes defensive, uncommunicative, and introverted. Since the patient's outlook and motivation can seriously influence the disease, members of the healthcare team must provide reassurance, empathy, and encouragement. To add to the problem, many of the drugs used to treat parkinsonism produce hallucinations, paranoid delusions, and changes in mood and behavior. Since the neuroleptics usually used to treat these symptoms may aggravate parkinsonism, the best course of action is to start by reducing the doses of the antiparkinson agents.

Physical Therapy

The purely neurologic signs, such as tremor and rigidity, do not respond to physical therapy. However, certain secondary disabling manifestations, such as bradykinesia, festinating gait and freezing of motion, can be lessened, although sometimes only temporarily. The goal is to turn a normally unconscious, automatic movement such as walking into a conscious, voluntary movement, where the patient attempts to place undivided attention on the performance of a series of small sequential acts. Activities such as getting up from a chair and walking are broken down into prearranged units so the patient can practice performing these acts in a flowing, coordinated motion.

Heat and massage help alleviate painful muscle cramps, while frequent walking and stretching exercises are very valuable in maintaining muscle tone and control. As a patient becomes more bedridden, a water or foam mattress helps prevent pressure sores. A program of physical therapy may slow the progression of the disabling features of parkinsonism and allow these patients added years of independence.

Speech Therapy

Often with the advance of the disease, the patient's voice becomes very soft, making it very difficult for them to be heard or understood. Voice exercises and socialization aid in relieving this problem.

PROGNOSIS

Parkinsonism is a slow, progressive disease. Transplantation of fetal or adrenal tissue has decreased the akinesia and rigidity in some cases, but these experimental surgical procedures are still unproven and controversial (28, 29). Drugs may relieve many of the signs and symptoms of parkinsonism, but they do not cure the disease.

Before the introduction of levodopa, a study found that parkinsonism significantly shortened life, with mortality being 2.9 times that of the general population of the same age, sex, and race. The average patient died about 9.4 years after onset of the disease, but some have survived for 30 years or more. The most common causes of death were cardiovascular complications, bronchopneumonia, and cancer.

Several studies indicate that introduction of levodopa may have decreased the mortality rate of parkinsonism almost to that of the general population. A multicenter study of 1625 parkinsonism patients followed for 4358 patient-years found a mortality rate of 1.03. When their data were adjusted for the mortality rate of the dropouts, the adjusted mortality rate was 1.33 (30). Another group (31) investigated 349 patients treated with either levodopa or levodopa combined with a decarboxylase inhibitor from 1969 to 1975, inclusive, and found a ratio of actual to expected deaths of 1.85. The excess mortality was accounted for by patients with severe disease at entry in the study.

CONCLUSION

The parkinsonism patient must be monitored closely to achieve maximum benefit from drug therapy. The complex combination of drugs often used in these patients must be adjusted frequently because there is a high potential for adverse reactions, drug-drug interactions, and laboratory test interference. With proper therapy, the signs and symptoms of parkinsonism may be controlled for many years, and the life-span of these patients may approach that of the general population.

REFERENCES

1. Parkinson J: An essay of the shaking palsy (1817). Reprinted in Critchley M (ed): James Parkinson. London: Macmillan, 1955.
2. Hoehn MM: Recent advances in the treatment of parkinsonism. Drug Ther Hosp 7:81–85, 1982.
3. Rajput AH: Epidemiology of Parkinson's disease. Can J Neurol Sci 11:156–159, 1984.
4. Calne DB, Duvoisin RC, McGeer E: Speculations on the etiology of Parkinson's disease. Adv Neurol 40:353–360, 1984.
5. Murdoch PS, Williamson J: A danger in making the diagnosis of Parkinson's Disease. Lancet 1:1212–1213, 1982.
6. Langston JW, Ballard P, Tetrud JW, et al.: Chronic parkinsonism in humans due to a product of meperidine-analog synthesis. Science 219:979–980, 1983.
7. Snyder SH, D'Amato RJ: MPTP: a neurotoxin relevant to the pathophysiology of Parkinson's disease. Neurology 36:250–258, 1986.
8. Hoehn MM, Yahr MD: Parkinsonism: onset, progression, and mortality. Neurology 17:427–442, 1967.
9. El-Awar M, Becker JT, Hammond KM, et al.: Learning deficit in Parkinson's disease. Arch Neurol 44:180–184, 1987.
10. Korczyn AD, Inzelberg R, Treves T, et al.: Dementia in Parkinson's disease. Adv Neurol 45:399–403, 1987.
11. Horadam VW, Sharp JG, Smilack JD, et al.: Pharmacokinetics of amantadine hydrochloride in subjects with normal and impaired renal function. Ann Intern Med 94:450–454, 1981.
12. Cotzias GC, Van Woert MH, Schiffer LM: Aromatic amino acid and modification of parkinsonism. N Engl J Med 276:374–378, 1967.
13. Boshes B: Sinemet and the treatment of parkinsonism. Ann Intern Med 94:364–370, 1981.
14. Markham CH, Diamond SG: Evidence to support early levodopa in Parkinson's disease. Neurol 31:125–131, 1981.
15. Markham CH, Diamond SG: Long-term follow-up of early dopa treatment in Parkinson's disease. Ann Neurol 19:365–372, 1986.
16. Robertson DRC, George CF: Drug therapy for Parkinson's disease in the elderly. Br Med Bull 46:124–146, 1990.
17. Mayeux R, Stern Y, Mulvey K, Cote L: Reappraisal of temporary levodopa withdrawal ("drug holiday") in Parkinson's disease. New Engl J Med 313:724–728, 1985.
18. Vance ML, Evan WS, Thorner MO: Bromocriptine. Ann Intern Med 100:78–91, 1984.
19. Parkes JD: Bromocriptine in the treatment of parkinsonism. Drugs 17:365–382, 1979.
20. Teychenne PF, Bergsrud D, Raly A, et al.: Bromocriptine: low-dose therapy in Parkinson's disease. Neurology 32:577–583, 1982.
21. Staal-Schreinemachers AL, Wesseling H, Kamphuis DJ, et al.: Low-dose bromocriptine therapy in Parkinson's disease: double-blind, placebo-controlled study. Neurolorgy 36:291–293, 1986.
22. Jankovic J: Long-term study of pergolide in Parkinson's disease. Neurology 35:296–299, 1985.
23. Langtry HD, Clissold SP, et al.: Pergolide. Drugs 39:491–506, 1990.
24. Birkmayer W, Knoll J, Reiderer P, et al.: Increased life expectancy resulting from addition of l-deprenyl to Madopar treatment in Parkinson's disease: a longterm study. J Neural Trans 64:113–127, 1985.
25. Tetrud JW, Langston JW: The effect of deprenyl (selegiline) on the natural history of Parkinson's disease. Science 245:519–522, 1989.
26. Parkinson Study Group: Effect of deprenyl on the progression of disability in early Parkinson's disease. N Engl J Med 321:1364–1371, 1989.
27. Golbe LI, Langston JW, Shoulson I: Selegiline and Parkinson's disease. Drugs 39(5):646–651, 1990.
28. Freed CR, Breeze RE, Rosenberg NL, et al.: Transplantation of human fetal dopamine cells for Parkinson's diseae. Arch Neurol 47:505–512, 1990.
29. Takeuchi J, Takebe Y, Sakakura T, et al.: Adrenal meducalla transplantation into the putamen in Parkinson's disease. Neurosurgery 26:499–503, 1990.
30. Joseph C, Chassan JB, Koch ML: Levodopa in Parkinson's disease: a long-term appraisal of mortality. Ann Neurol 3:116–118, 1978.
31. Martilla RJ, Rinne UK, Siirtola et al.: Mortality of patients with Parkinson's disease treated with levodopa. J Neurol 216:147–153, 1977.

CHAPTER 50

PAIN MANAGEMENT

LORI A. REISNER-KELLER, Pharm.D.

Divinum est opus sedare dolorem (Divine is the effort to subdue pain).

—Hippocrates

HISTORY OF PAIN RESEARCH

The mystery of pain has plagued mankind since its earliest days, and throughout time various remedies—some with scientific merit—have attempted to relieve this curse. Documentation of suffering from pain is found in Babylonian tablets and Egyptian papyrus writings. Throughout time, man has sought to understand and control pain, a noble venture since pain is linked with consciousness. Earliest treatments included massage, exposure to cold water, exposure to solar heat and later the heat of fire, and pressure over certain regions. The Egyptians, Greeks, and Romans used shocks from electric fish to treat painful disorders. Primitive peoples relied on witches, sorcerers, and medicine men.

In the early nineteenth century, the study of pain emerged as part of experimental science (1). Important advances were made in pain therapy as well, most notably the isolation of morphine from crude opium in 1806 and of codeine in 1832 (2). By the mid-1800s, acetylsalicylic acid was introduced, followed by development of ether as an anesthetic. Hypnosis, neurosurgery, electrotherapy, mechanotherapy, hydrotherapy, thermotherapy, and radiation therapy then joined pharmacologic treatments for both surgical and nonsurgical pain (3). Two theories of pain were formulated and expanded during this period. The first was the specificity theory, proposed in 1894 (4). It was based on works by ancient Romans, Arabians, and Europeans, and proposed that pain was a specific sensation with its own peripheral and central mechanisms, independent of the other five senses (3). Specific receptors (free nerve endings) were thought to cause pain when stimulated. Support for this theory came from experiments conducted from the late 1800s through the mid-twentieth century: a specific unique experience originated from the skin when an appropriate stimulus was applied (3).

The second theory of pain to evolve was known as the intensive, pattern, or summation theory. Pain was believed to result from excessive stimulation of the sense of touch. Pain signals were thought to originate as nerve impulses from a peripheral site and to be coded at that distant location instead of within the central nervous system. The theory also suggested that body damage would cause a reverberating circuit between the injured peripheral site and the spinal cord, and the reverberations would summate, or intensify in their effects. Observations that repeated pinpricks could cause intense pain showed that the stimulus-to-response relationship was not proportional, i.e., each successive pinprick overlapped the effect of the previous one, rather than being transmitted as a distinct and separate impulse (6). Furthermore, skin receptors were shown to have unique physiological properties by which they could transmit different degrees of stimulation in the form of impulse patterns (1).

Debate and controversy surrounded each theory, so a third postulate was introduced. In this theory, pain was regarded as an original physiologic sensation *and* the psychic reaction produced by that sensation. This marked the first time that an individual's *response* to pain-eliciting phenomena became an issue in pain research. In the 1940s, consolidation of these three theories led to a proposal that pain could be separated into two components: perception and reaction to pain (2).

Finally, in the 1960s, Melzack and Wall proposed the "gate-control" theory of pain, in which it was thought that a painful stimulus acted upon pain-sensitive receptors and caused a nerve impulse to travel to the brain, which then initiated the physical and psychologic responses to pain. Though certain key details of the gate-control theory have since been questioned, it is still widely accepted to explain the way pain signals are collected, transmitted, and interpreted within the central nervous system, as it allows for specific pain receptors as well as the role of the nervous system in pain medication. Essentially, the gate-control mechanism occurs as follows: afferent C fibers and A-delta (A-δ) nerve fibers transmit pain signals to an area known as the substantia gelatinosa, located in the dorsal horn of the spinal cord (Fig. 50.1). Cells within the dorsal horn collect and interpret these signals, and send them to transmission cells with terminals projecting to distant sites outside the dorsal horn. Some C fibers and A-δ fibers terminate in the dorsal root horn, whereas others form a complex known as the lateral spinothalamic tract. Pain impulses travel along this tract to the thalamus, and from there to the cerebral cortex of the brain (8). Other controls descend from the brain to inhibit firing of responsive neurons in the dorsal horn, and therefore blunt or stop pain signals.

Some researchers believe that humans can be divided

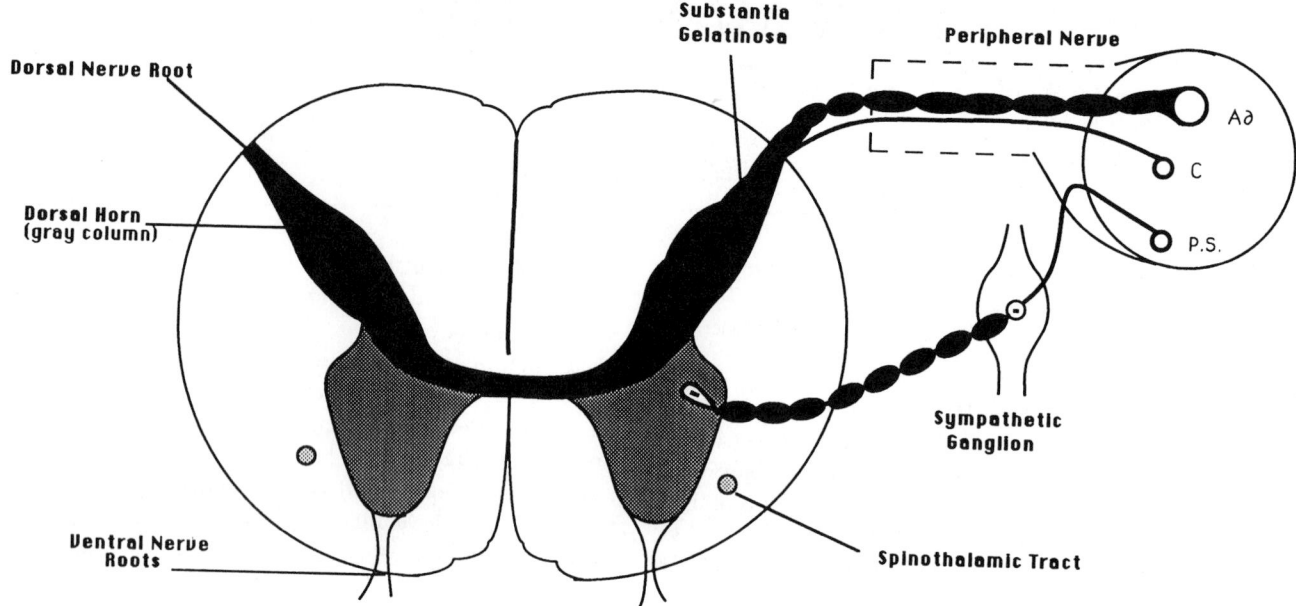

Figure 50.1. Transverse section of the spinal cord with peripheral nerve section illustrating two different types of axons: A- and C-fibers with cell bodies in the *dorsal root* and sympathetic fibers with cell bodies in the *sympathetic ganglion*. A- and sympathetic preganglionic fibers are myelinated, while both C- and postganglionic sympathetic (*P.S.*) fibers are unmyelinated.

The myelinated fibers carry impulses at a faster rate. Sympathetic fibers are thought to mediate some of the body's response to pain signals traveling along the peripheral nerve to the spinal cord. (Adapted from Fields HL: Pain. New York: McGraw-Hill, 1987, p 14; and Clement CD: Gray's Anatomy, (ed. 30.). Philadelphia: Lea & Febiger, 1985.)

into two categories: pain-sensitive (PS) or pain-tolerant (PT) subjects, who differ in aspects of pain behavior. PS subjects experience pain with qualitative differences, and the experience depends more on psychologic variables than with PT subjects. These experiences can be measured by electroencephalography (EEG) devices. Because of the role that stress plays in pain responeness and the higher stress level observed in PS subjects, PS subjects have a lower pain threshold (9). Further research will determine additional criteria for classifying pain response and whether these two categories can be generalized to include a broad range of painful stimuli.

Modern concepts of pain have been derived from these theories, and current therapy is directed at both the emotional and the sensory components of pain. Specific treatments are aimed at both the physiologic and psychologic aspects, using such interventions as medications, physical therapy, or surgical procedures for the former, and counseling, biofeedback, and stress-management training for the latter.

PHYSIOLOGY OF PAIN
PERIPHERAL PAIN SENSORY SYSTEM

When a painful (noxious) stimulus is applied to a sensitive area such as the skin, a series of events follows that are ultimately identified as a painful sensation. Sensitive tissues are those which contain pain receptors, also called

nociceptors. Nociceptors are primary afferent nerves with terminals outside the spinal cord that respond to noxious stimuli. Two phenomena occur via the nociceptors (10). The first is receptor activation, in which chemical, thermal, or mechanical energy is translated to an electrochemical nerve impulse in the primary afferent nerve. The second event is transmission of the impulse as coded information to structures in the central nervous system that interpret the signal as pain. Transmission occurs initially in the spinal cord, where neurons relay messages from the nociceptors to the brain. The messages elicit many responses, such as a withdrawal reflex or a subjective perceptual event ("Ouch!"). Most nociceptors conduct their signals in two velocity ranges. Larger diameter, myelinated A-δ, or rapid-firing fibers include muscle receptors, among other primary afferents, and constitute most of the known myelinated nociceptors. The A-δ fibers are most sensitive to stimulation by heat and by sharp, pointed instruments, hence they are known as mechanothermal or mechanical nociceptors. A third type of A-δ fiber may exist which is sensitive to irritant chemicals. A-δ fibers have the property of *sensitization* (i.e., repeated application of a noxious stimulus produces increased sensitivity of these receptors (11)).

The unmyelinated axons are known as C, or slow-firing, fibers and make up about 75% of the primary afferents in peripheral nerve. They have a smaller diameter than their fast-conducting counterparts, and are sensitive to noxious thermal, mechanical, and chemical stimuli. As with the A-δ fibers, C fibers also sensitize with repeated application of painful stimuli, although they may be less sensitive immediately after a stimulus (10).

Evidence of the role of both A-δ and C fibers in pain perception is found in observations that brief, intense, stimuli applied to a limb produce two distinct sensations: an early sharp, localized "pricking" pain of brief duration followed by a dull, diffuse, and prolonged unpleasant sensation (12). By using compression to selectively block A-δ fibers, the initial sharp pain is abolished. Likewise, blockade of the C fibers by local anesthetics like lidocaine leads to abolition of dull prolonged pain (13, 14).

How a pain sensation is perceived depends upon the size of the area stimulated, the frequency of stimulus application, and duration and location of the stimulus (15). Although pain is a definite, singular experience based upon activity in specific receptors, any single nociceptor's activity is influenced by simultaneous activity at nearby nociceptors. Thus the pain experience is a compound of concurrent inputs at multiple receptors (10).

When tissue injury occurs, the nociceptors undergo depolarization, leading to generation (transduction) of a nerve impulse. Depolarization is followed by pain and hypersensitivity lasting from minutes to days. Persistent pain can result from ongoing tissue damage or lingering chemical irritants released by cells during the initial insult. Other possibilities include a lasting change in the integrity of the receptor itself or even in the central nervous system. A combination of these factors is possible (10).

Stimuli above a nociceptor's pain threshold result in visible signs of tissue damage. More extensive injuries lead to local increased sensitivity to mild stimuli, or hyperesthesia. Hyperesthesia causes injured tissues to develop tenderness, so that normally innocuous stimuli produce pain. This hyperalgesia is paralleled by changes in the activity of the nociceptors, including sensitization. After superficial injury to the skin, an intense vasodilation occurs at the injury site (Fig. 50.2). This is rapidly followed by edema (a wheal) and secondary vasodilation that produces reddening (a flare), which spreads into adjacent, uninjured skin. The hypersensitive region enlarges progressively with time, and depends mainly on the activity of the C fibers, as both the flare and remote sensitization are blocked by local anesthetics. Thus, activity in C fibers causes vasodilation and sensitizes adjacent C fibers. The long-lasting changes that occur *after* application of the injurious stimuli may play a major role in determining both the intensity and the quality of clinically important pain (10).

CENTRAL PAIN TRANSMISSION

The cell bodies of the nociceptors are located in the dorsal root ganglion, and most of their axons terminate in the dorsal horn of the spinal cord. Some afferents project to the spinal cord through a ventral root as well, and both roots are thought to be important for pain transmission.

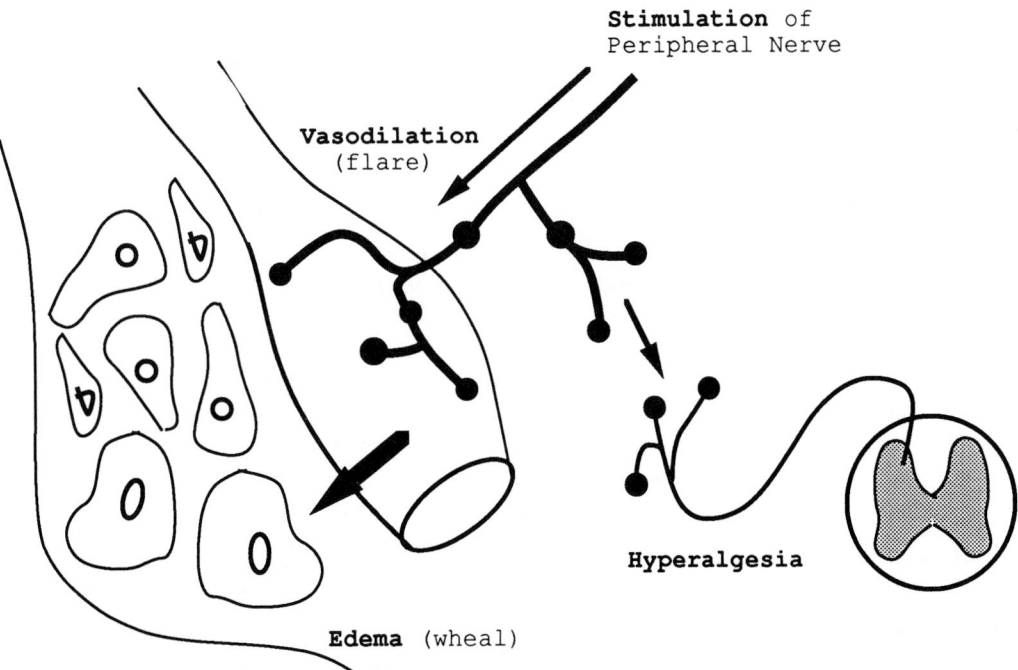

Figure 50.2. Events occurring after an insult to a peripheral nerve. Stimulation of the nerve ending produces a stimulus to vessel walls at the site of injury or trauma. Histamine, bradykinin, and other chemical mediators lead to vasodilation, then edema. Electrochemical signals across nociceptive synapses transmit the pain sensation to pathways in the spinal cord and ultimately to the brain (thalamus). (Taken with permission from Fields HL: Pain. New York: McGraw-Hill, 1987.)

There may exist different pain-transmitting pathways, including the spinothalamic, spinoreticular, spinocervical, and dorsal column tracts. Animal models of pain transmission have failed to precisely define the human pain pathways because of species differences, but it is understood that the various nociceptive pathways of the human, primate, cat, and rat reach their destination in the thalamus of the brain (16).

The lateral spinothalamic tract is thought to be the dominant spinal cord pathway for signaling pain in humans, as lesions of this tract result in the absence of pain below the lesion. In addition, stimulation of this tract induces pain in humans (17). The termination zone of the spinothalamic tract and that of some dorsal column nuclei appear to overlap in the thalamus, and low-threshold stimulation of the dorsal column either electrically or chemically can interrupt pain-signal transmission. This provides the basis for the use of transcutaneous electrical nerve stimulation (TENS) and dorsal column electrical stimulators in the treatment of chronic pain (18).

Central nervous system opioid receptors have been identified in high concentration in the dorsal horn. They have also been localized in the cerebrum (including the limbic system), the brainstem, medulla, pons, and amygdala. In man, administration of morphine into the brain's ventricles produces potent pain relief in terminal cancer patients (19). The mechanism of opiate analgesia is detailed later in this chapter.

PAIN-PRODUCING SUBSTANCES

Several chemical compounds accumulate near nociceptors after tissue injury. They may arise from cell leakage, from synthesis by local substrate released via enzymes induced by damage, or from release by the nociceptor itself (10) (Table 50.1).

Histamine from mast cells and potassium are among the substances released by tissue damage, both of which excite nociceptors and produce pain upon injection into human skin. Adenosine triphosphate (ATP) may also have this action. These compounds act either alone or in combination to sensitize nociceptors (20).

One substance known to produce pain is bradykinin, a polypeptide produced by cleavage of plasma proteins following tissue injury. Actions of bradykinin include both low-concentration indirect production of hyperalgesia, and high-concentration direct stimulation of nociceptors (21).

Other compounds synthesized in the area of tissue damage are the by-products of arachidonic acid metabolism, including prostaglandins and leukotrienes. These chemicals are present in high concentrations in inflammatory fluids, are potent mediators of inflammation, and elicit pain. Prostaglandins are formed from arachidonic acid via the enzyme cyclooxygenase; of these, prostaglandin E_2 (PGE_2) is the most potent. Prostacyclin (PGI_2) is also a potent inducer of pain and hyperalgesia. PGE_2 is thought to produce hyperalgesia by direct action on the nociceptors, but prostaglandins may also sensitize nociceptors via coupling to a cyclic AMP system (22). Other prostaglandins contribute to nociceptor activation by their interaction with additional chemical mediators. For example, prostaglandin E_1 produces pain only when injected with either bradykinin or histamine. Similarly, norepinephrine may produce peripheral hyperalgesia via enhanced production of prostacyclin. Aspirin and other nonsteroidal antiinflammatory drugs (NSAIDs) have analgesic activity because of their inhibition by cyclooxygenase (23). Bradykinin-induced hyperalgesia can be blocked by the NSAIDs and may occur by stimulation of specific PGE_2 production (24).

Leukotrienes are produced from arachidonic acid by lipooxygenase. Like prostaglandins, these agents produce hyperalgesia. However, leukotrienes are not notably blocked by cyclooxygenase inhibitors but by depletion of polymorphonuclear leukocytes (PMNs). Both prostaglandins and leukotrienes may exert their hyperalgesic effects by medication of other pain-eliciting compounds (25).

In contrast to substrates released in the region of injury, nociceptors themselves liberate pain-enhancing sub-

Table 50.1.
Chemicals Active in Nociceptive Transduction[a]

Substance	Source	Enzyme Mediator	Potency in Producing Pain
Nociceptor Activators			
Histamine	Release from mast cells	None known	+
Potassium	Release from damaged cells	None known	+ +
Bradykinin	Plasma proteins	Kallikrein	+ + +
Nociceptor Sensitizers			
Prostaglandins	Arachidonic acid released by damaged cells	Cyclooxygenase	+ / −
Leukotrienes	Arachidonic acid released by damaged cells	Lipooxygenase	+ / −
Substance P	Primary afferent	None known	+ / −

[a] Adapted from Fields HL: Pain. New York: McGraw-Hill, 1987, p 32.

stances. Substance P, a polypeptide, is released from some C-fibers and excites pain transmission pathways in the dorsal horn. In experimental arthritis, intramuscular gold sodium thiomalate, a neurotoxin, causes substance P depletion by decreasing the number of C-fibers in peripheral nerve. Substance P is a potent vasodilator and leads to release of histamine from mast cells, explaining its role in immunomodulation as well as the pain of arthritis. Histamine itself also activates nociceptors and produces vasodilation (26).

Modulation and Interruption of Central Pain Processing

OPIOID RECEPTORS

Opioids, also called narcotics, administered into the spinal fluid reduce nearly all manifestations of clinical pain in humans. Subpopulations of these receptors are characterized by their sensitivity to selective opioid agonists (27). Specific receptors in the central nervous system and peripheral tissues are responsible for modulating the effects of opiates, and they are subdivided into four types: the mu (μ), delta (δ), kappa (κ), and sigma (σ) receptors. The μ and κ receptors both produce analgesia, while the μ-receptor is responsible for the habituating and withdrawal effects of the opiates. μ-Receptors, located primarily in pain-modulating areas of the CNS, induce central analgesia and respiratory depression (28). κ-Receptors are responsible for analgesia at the levels of the spinal cord and the brain, and are found in greatest concentration in the cerebral cortex and in the substantia gelatinosa of the dorsal horn. Because they are thought to produce analgesia without inducing opiate habituation, there is a great deal of interest in the development of κ-specific receptor agonists. Though experimental κ-agonists such as spiradoline have shown low dependence and abuse liability, they are not ideal analgesics due to their psychotomimetic (hallucinogenic) and dysphoric effects. δ-Receptors are located in the limbic area of the brain and in the spinal cord and may play a role in the euphoria that selected opiates produce. Evidence also implicates them in analgesia at the spinal cord level. Some researchers consider δ-receptors to be a subpopulation of the μ-receptors or mediators of μ-receptors. σ-Receptors are believed to produce the psychotomimetic and dysphoric effects of some opiate agonists and partial agonists (29).

Endogenous opioids known as endorphins, enkephalins, and dynorphins are found in varying concentrations in the central nervous system (30). Their roles have not been fully elucidated, but dynorphins and enkephalins appear to be responsible for intrinsic regulation of pain perception within the medulla, while endorphins and enkephalins probably serve this function within the substantia gelatinosa. Each subclass of endogenous opioids has greater preference for a particular receptor type: β-endorphin and enkaphalins are potent at μ and δ-receptors, while the κ-receptor is the target for the dynorphins (31).

The site of action of opiates depends upon the method of administration. Systemically injected or ingested opiates produce high brain opiate concentrations with relatively low spinal concentrations. The reverse occurs with spinal administration of the drug, i.e., intrathecal (into the subarachnoid space) or epidural injection. At the spinal level, opiates are thought to inhibit pain signals carried by the A-δ and C fibers at their synapses in the substantia gelatinosa.

Opiates exert at least part of their analgesic action by inhibiting substance P release in the central and peripheral nervous systems. They also interfere with the actions of prostaglandins at peripheral sites, particularly μ-receptor-specific opioids that inhibit PGE_2 hyperalgesia in a dose-dependent fashion (32). It is speculated that opiates produce analgesia by causing adenosine release, since methylxanthines such as caffeine antagonize the effects of morphine (33, 34).

Opiates may exert their inhibitory actions via hyperpolarization of neurons through altered conductance of potassium or calcium. However, they also cause in vitro excitatory actions at the nerve terminals. This bimodal action is dose-dependent and helps explain the mechanisms of opiate tolerance and dependence (35).

Tolerance and tachyphylaxis probably result from repeated exposure of receptors to high doses of opiate analgesics (28). Continuously administered low-dose opiates can slow the development of tolerance. Patient-controlled analgesia (PCA), in which a controlled amount of drug is infused continuously, with bolus or "rescue" doses for breakthrough pain, produces less tolerance than intermittent high doses of an opiate. A second potential approach to delay tolerance is use of agents that are analgesic at a specific receptor; thus far, however, κ- or δ-specific agents are investigational only. Due to varying degrees of affinity for different receptors, narcotics do not produce complete cross-tolerance to each other. In general, cross-tolerance exists among opioids with high affinity to the same receptor, but little or no cross-tolerance is seen between opiates acting at different receptors. Since most available opioids have some affinity for each receptor type, the extent of cross-tolerance is variable and unpredictable (36). When changing from one opiate agonist to another, half the calculated equianalgesic dose may be used initially and then the dose is titrated upward as needed (37).

Besides their analgesic effects, opiates produce drowsiness, sedation, mood changes, and mental clouding manifested by disorientation and memory impairment. Respiratory depression occurs by a direct action on the medullary respiratory and ventilation centers to reduce their responsiveness to carbon dioxide tension (PCO_2), and by depression of brain centers responsible for the rate and rhythm of respirations. Studies comparing morphine with other opioids have shown that equianalgesic doses of these agents do not differ significantly in their abilities to depress respiration. Nausea and vomiting occur by opioid stimulation of dopamine release in the chemoreceptor trigger zone of the medulla, and opiate-induced emesis is treated with phenothiazines that exert dopamine-blocking action, e.g., chlorpromazine or prochlorperazine. Dopaminergic actions are also involved in the euphoria experienced with opioids (38). Miosis occurs through a stimulatory effect on the oculomotor nerve, and pinpoint pupils are pathognomonic for opiate toxicity. Central stimulation by opioids can also induce convulsions, which may not be suppressed by anticonvulsant agents (39).

Opiate receptors have been localized outside the nervous system. In the gastrointestinal tract, opiates increase smooth muscle tone in portions of the stomach, duodenum, ileum, and large intestine, leading to decreased motility and spasm. Morphine reduces secretion of hydrochloric acid and pancreatic enzymes and inhibits mucosal transfer of fluids and electrolytes across the intestinal epithelium. Digestion and propulsion of food is delayed, and absorption of oral drugs may be slowed. These properties have led to the development of the piperidine opioid congeners diphenoxylate, diphenoxylic acid, and loperamide to treat hypersecretory diarrhea.

Therapeutic doses of meperidine, morphine, codeine, or their analogs can lead to increased pressure in the common bile duct with elevations of serum lipase or amylase levels. Spasm and constriction of the sphincter of Oddi are probably responsible for this effect. Methadone, fentanyl, or narcotic agonist-antagonist combinations do not raise biliary pressure to the same degree as other opiates and can be used to treat pain from biliary colic or pancreatitis (39).

In the cardiovascular system, opiates produce orthostatic hypotension by peripheral arteriolar and venous dilation. This is either a direct effect or the result of opioid-stimulated histamine release. Vasodilation can be reversed partially by histamine-receptor (H_1) blocking agents and completely by opiate antagonists such as naloxone. Patients with coronary artery disease or evolving myocardial infarction may experience reduced myocardial oxygen consumption, but effects on the normal heart are insignificant. Opiate-induced respiratory depression can result in cerebrovascular dilation and increased cerebrospinal fluid pressure, effects that are hazardous in patients with cor pumonale or in persons with cerebrovascular compromise who may suffer further damage from increased CSF pressure. A second factor that discourages use of opiates is depression of cognitive function and masking of cerebral damage secondary to pathophysiologies such as stroke.

In the smooth muscle of the bladder and ureter, opioids increase tone of the ureter and the vesical sphincter, leading to urinary hesitancy or retention. In the uterus, morphine reverses oxytocin-stimulated hyperactivity, leading to prolonged labor. Opiates also depress respiration in the infant, as all narcotics cross the placenta. Epidurally administered opiates are often used during parturition. Preferred intravenous agents in obstetrics are the opiate agonist-antagonists butorphanol and nalbuphine, due to their "ceiling effect" on respiration, i.e., higher doses do not increase the degree of neonatal respiratory depression (40).

Cutaneous blood vessels dilate with opiates, making the skin flushed and warm. Histamine release is partly responsible for these effects and for the pruritis and sweating that often follow narcotic administration. Urticaria is particularly problematic following spinal administration of opiates (39).

OTHER RECEPTORS (Table 50.2)
Adrenergic agonists norepinephrine and clonidine, an α-2 agonist, produce significant analgesia in man when administered into the spinal fluid, highlighting the role of adrenergic modulation of pain. Although it can produce peripheral hyperalgesia by enhancing prostacyclin production, norepinephrine acts centrally on dorsal horn synapses via pain-inhibiting descending impulses from the brain. The antinociceptive actions of both clonidine and norepinephrine can be reversed in a dose-dependent manner with adrenergic antagonists such as yohimbine (41, 42).

Serotonin receptors are found along the spinothalamic tract. Serotonin appears to reduce pain centrally by modulating descending impulses from the brain, and this effect may be enhanced by selective serotonin-reuptake inhibitors such as fluoxetine. This forms the basis of treatment of neuropathic pain syndromes with antidepressants that block presynaptic reuptake of serotonin (43).

Cholinergic binding sites have been discovered in the dorsal horn. Application of the muscarinic agonist acetylcholine produces analgesia that can be reversed by atropine. Such antinociceptive effects are not reduced by opiate antagonists (44).

GABAergic receptors are divided into two types: $GABA_A$ receptors are sensitive to muscimol and $GABA_B$ receptors to baclofen. Of known GABAergic compounds, only baclofen has been shown to produce analgesia. $GABA_B$ agonists inhibit firing of the nociceptors, particularly the C fibers. Unlike opiates, baclofen does not inhibit substance P release in the spinal column. Baclofen is used in central pain syndromes resulting from injury to the spinal cord, especially if consequent muscle spasms are involved (45, 46).

ACUTE VERSUS CHRONIC PAIN

Pain is defined as "an unpleasant sensory and emotional experience associated with actual or potential tissue dam-

Table 50.2.
Receptors Involved in Modulation of Pain Pathways

Receptor	Subtypes	Agonist	Action	Location	Antagonist
Opioid	μ,∂,κ	Morphine	Analgesia	Brain and spinal cord	Naloxone
Adrenergic	alpha-1		Reduction in sympathetic	Dorsal column	Prazosin
	alpha-2	Clonidine	nervous system output	Dorsal column	Yohimbine
	alpha & beta	Norepinephrine		Dorsal column	Yohimbine
Serotonergic		Tricyclic antidepressants	Modulation	Spinothalamic tract	
Cholinergic		Acetylcholine	Antinociception	Dorsal horn	Atropine
GABAergic	A, B	Baclofen	Inhibits firing of	Peripheral	
			nociceptors	Dorsal horn	

age, or described in terms of such damage" (47). Pain is always subjective, and no specific tests can quantitatively or qualitatively measure pain. Tests such as a visual analog scale can be used by the clinician in an attempt to measure pain objectively, as can observations of grimacing, limping, and tachycardia, but these are crude methods at best, and can only be used to support a patient's report of pain.

Acute pain is that arising from an injury, trauma, spasm, or disease to the skin, muscles, somatic structures, or viscera of the body. It is perceived and communicated via the peripheral mechanisms identified as classic pain pathways, i.e., the A-δ and C fibers. The intensity of pain is usually proportional to the degree of damage. Acute pain may be accompanied by signs of autonomic nervous system activity—tachycardia, hypertension, diaphoresis, mydriasis, and pallor—that mimic those of anxiety, which often coexists with acute pain. It is characterized by limited duration, and diagnosis is not difficult. Acute pain decreases in intensity as the damaged area heals and tissue repair takes place (48).

Superficial pain is that derived from the skin or underlying subcutaneous and mucous tissue. It is characterized by local throbbing, burning, or pricking. It may be associated with tenderness, allodynia (pain from a stimulus that normally does not provoke pain), or hyperalgesia. Visceral pain is diffuse, dull, aching pain that is poorly localized and is noticed at the onset or early stages of disease. It may be associated with nausea and other autonomic symptoms. Deep somatic pain is dull and aching and can be localized, though there may be radiating components. Injury or disease of deep somatic structures produces the same response as injury to the skin or viscera (1).

Treatment of acute pain is based upon whether the pain is superficial or deep in origin, and it is directed toward the underlying etiology. Acute pain management involves the use of agents aimed at short-term symptomatic treatment, and the goal is to provide relief during the period of tissue healing. Opiates such as morphine, meperidine, and hydromorphone are used acutely in postsurgical

pain treatment, but other important agents are the nonsteroidal antiinflammatory agents that can limit the inflammatory response at the site of trauma, thereby reducing pain, swelling, and erythema.

Chronic pain is that which has lasted 6 months or longer and is separated into cancer pain and nonmalignant or "benign" pain. The term benign is a misnomer, however, as persons with noncancer pain often suffer a great deal of physical and psychologic damage. Chronic pain persists beyond the expected healing time of the precipitating insult and is rarely accompanied by autonomic symptoms. Persons who report chronic pain often fail to show evidence of any underlying pathophysiology upon physical or radiologic examination, although patients who have undergone multiple surgeries can develop fibrotic (scar) tissue, which may be apparent in imaging studies. Chronic pain is further characterized by its location: it may arise from visceral locations, from myofascial (muscle and connective) tissue, or from neurologic causes such as herpes zoster infection or diabetic neuropathy. Treatment is directed not only toward symptoms but also to the suffering and disability produced. Symptoms of depression (e.g., hopelessness, helplessness, loss of weight, and sleep disturbance) may accompany chronic pain and must be treated concomitantly (48). Cancer or malignant pain exhibit characteristics of both acute and chronic pain. It may be constant or intermittent. A definable cause is usually present and is related to tumor recurrence and treatment. As with chronic nonmalignant pain, therapy is composed of psychologic and disability interventions, with analgesics in effective and tolerable doses.

In the treatment of chronic pain, narcotic and nonopiate analgesics should be dosed on an around-the-clock basis, as there is no evidence that such pain will abate abruptly, and pain perceived as "minor" can proceed to intolerable pain within a few hours. Once this phenomenon occurs, a larger dose of analgesic is required to overcome pain-associated anxiety and bring the pain below the threshold of patient tolerance. For malignant pain, habituation is not a concern, as pain modulates the body's response to opiates, and tolerance is slow to develop.

FACTORS INFLUENCING PAIN PERCEPTION

Pain intensity varies with each individual, and pain perception is determined by a person's psychologic background in addition to physiologic factors. Since pain is multifactorial, it can be classified on emotional, social, spiritual, and physical spheres (Fig. 50.3). Emotional pain consists of isolation, depression, and fear; factors that can reinforce each other. Social pain is comprised of strained or broken relationships as well as financial problems resulting from disability. Spiritual pain includes feelings of guilt, regret, or worthlessness, and physical pain encompasses disease and debilitation. Chronic pain can dull the normal sympathetic responses to stress (hypertension, sweating, etc.). Signs of depression may emerge, most often sleep disturbance and irritability. Delayed sleep onset and frequent waking may occur, and patients report exhaustion from lack of sleep and from inability to tolerate the stresses

imposed by continuous pain. Chronic pain often leads to anxiety and depression, which in turn exacerbate the pain. This cycle ultimately leads to adoption of a "pain lifestyle" in which polypharmacy and polysurgery become overrepresented in a patient's medical history. If secondary gain such as increased attention from family members or financial reward becomes an issue, there is less incentive to recover from a pain syndrome. Pain may also mask underlying psychologic or physical abuse and can present itself as a symptom of emotional need (49).

A distinction can usually be made between the "pain patient" and the patient in pain. The patient in pain exhibits findings seen more often with acute pain such as pacing, grimacing, or alterations in heart rate and blood pressure. These persons will likely fully recover psychologically from the painful episode once adequate pain control is achieved. Even in many such patients with chronic pain, reliance on medications is stable at a minimal level, and the patient demonstrates a high degree of self-dependence in overcoming disability due to pain. Interaction

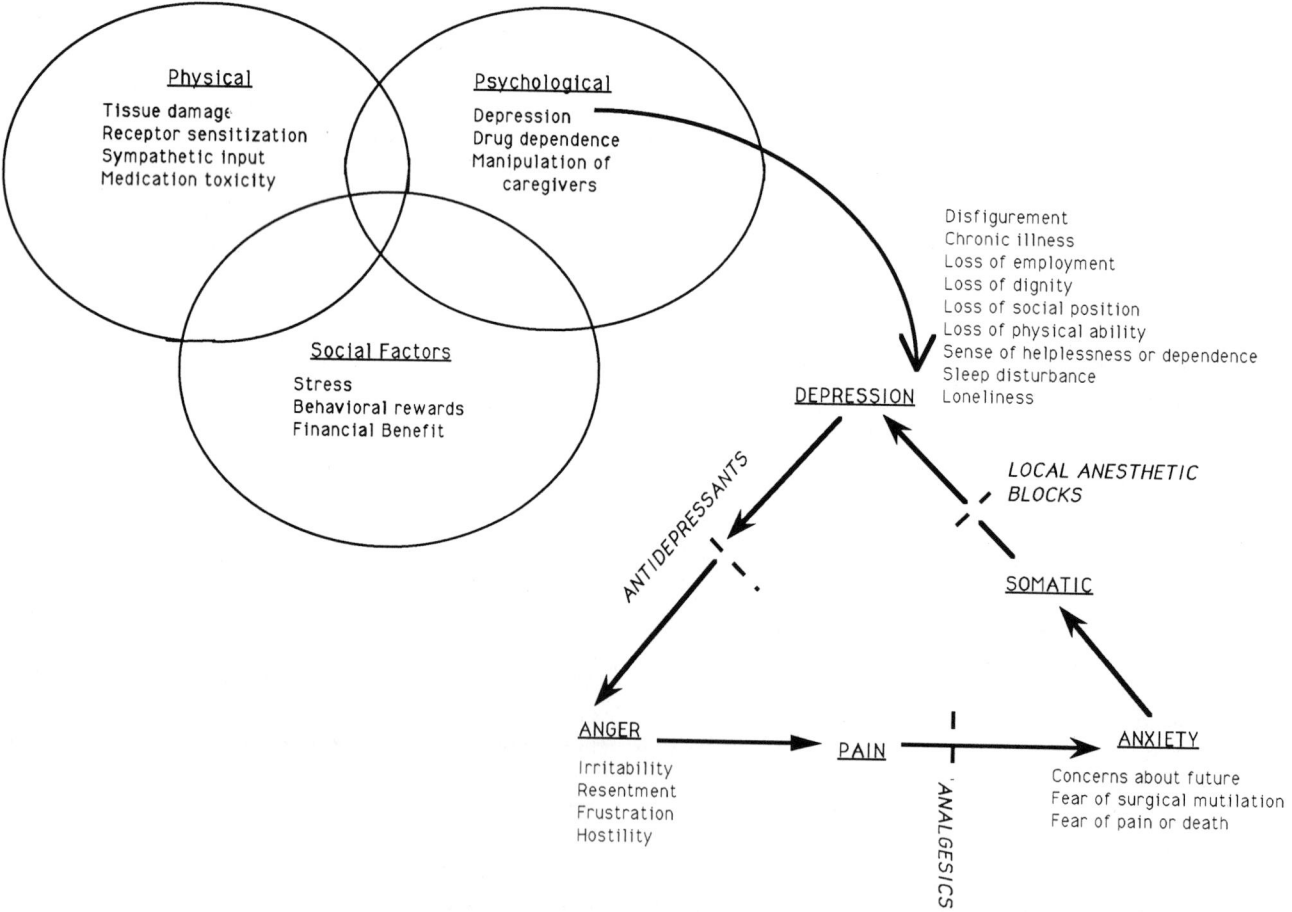

Figure 50.3. Determinants and modifiers of pain response and behavior. Portions of the pain triangle interrupted by pharmacologic interventions are shown.

with healthcare providers is not extensive, and the patient exhibits self-motivation in returning to a premorbid life style.

The "pain patient," on the other hand, is an individual who has suffered pain long enough to produce notable changes in lifestyle, such as a discharge from employment and heavy reliance on family members or the healthcare system to offer relief. These patients may be tearful and anxious and may also exhibit symptoms of acute pain, which abate when the patient is distracted during conversation. Patients with extreme pain behaviors visit and/or call their healthcare providers often and may manipulate their medication regimens without the advice of a physician or pharmacist. Patients who use their medications more often than directed may be required to "contract" with their providers, a system in which they are dispensed a specific quantity of medicines for a predetermined period of time. Pain patients may have difficulty establishing realistic goals for their therapy and request a "cure" for their pain syndrome, though no such cure exists.

EVALUATION OF PAIN

A simple "PQRST" mnemonic can aid the practitioner in evaluating pain. P represents the *palliative* or *precipitating* factors associated with the pain, such as diet, stress, or physical exertion. Q represents the *quality* of the pain, i.e., whether it is sharp dull, constant, aching, shooting, etc. R stands for *"region"* or *"radiation"* and is used to locate the pain. S is the *subjective* description by the patient of the pain's *severity* and its effects on daily habits and lifestyle. For example, does pain cause waking or appetite loss? Finally, T represents the *temporal*, or time-related nature of the pain. It is useful to ask the patient whether the pain is worse in the evening or the morning, whether it is related to any habitual daily activity, or other questions designed to detect diurnal, weekly, or monthly patterns. Women may experience differences in pain at various points in their menstrual cycles, as estrogen induces hyperalgesia (50).

In addition to knowing how, where, and when the pain began and what leads to its continuation, other pertinent facts about a patient's lifestyle are relative to accurate pain assessment. A pain questionnaire will aid in the evaluation and treatment of the chronic pain patient in the ambulatory care setting (51). Such questionnaires should evaluate personal information such as marital status, education, and employment, as these are germane to the pain experience. The practitioner should ask: have these factors changed since the pain began? If so, was it due to the adoption of a pain lifestyle?

Detailed information about the pain should be gathered to supplement the more general PQRST scale. It is necessary to determine what help the patients request and

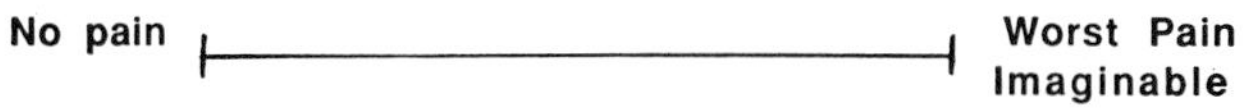

No pain ├─────────────────────────────┤ Worst Pain Imaginable

Figure 50.4. VAS Pain Scale. The subject is asked to draw a hash mark at a point on the line corresponding to his or her pain. A ruler is used to measure placement of the mark, and a number value (in cm) is assigned to the measurement.

whether their goals are consistent with the treatment offered. Chronic pain patients cannot expect to be pain-free, as underlying altered or degenerative pathophysiology are often permanent. Changes in lifestyle such as exercise and exertion, employment, and emotional approaches to living with chronic pain may reduce pain's dominance in one's life, however.

The pain is located with anatomic drawings on which the patient shades areas where it is worse. For pain intensity, a visual analog scale (VAS) is a reproducible method to objectively measure and quantify pain. The VAS is a 10-cm line without subdivision marks. On the left extreme of the line "zero" or "no pain" is written. On the right extreme of the line, "10" or "worst pain I've ever had" is written. (Fig. 50.4) A subject is asked to draw a hash mark on the line at the point best corresponding to the pain. Successive VAS scales are compared over time to evaluate response to therapy.

An important portion of the questionnaire for the pharmacist is a section concerned with past medication history as well as current pain medication and other treatments. From this portion of the evaluation, proper selection of analgesics, analgesic adjuncts, and patient compliance can be assessed. Patients who are compulsive in their consumption of pain medications and those on subtherapeutic doses of appropriate medication are identified.

Finally, a checklist of problems related to major organ systems should be included. Patients who complain of multiple somatic symptoms along with pain may be experiencing depression or another affective disorder. Correction of the underlying depression may lead to remission of pain and somatic complaints.

Assessing pediatric pain is more difficult, as young children are often unable to adequately describe pain intensity and quality. Children can use a modified visual scale, the Faces Pain Scale (Fig. 50.5) (52).

CLINICAL PAIN SYNDROMES

An algorithm for medication selection in various pain syndromes is illustrated in Figure 50.6.

Cancer pain arises at the primary site as a result of tumor expansion, nerve compression or infiltration by the tumor, malignant obstruction, or infections in malignant ulcers. It may also occur at distant metastatic sites. Furthermore, treatment for tumors (such as radiation therapy)

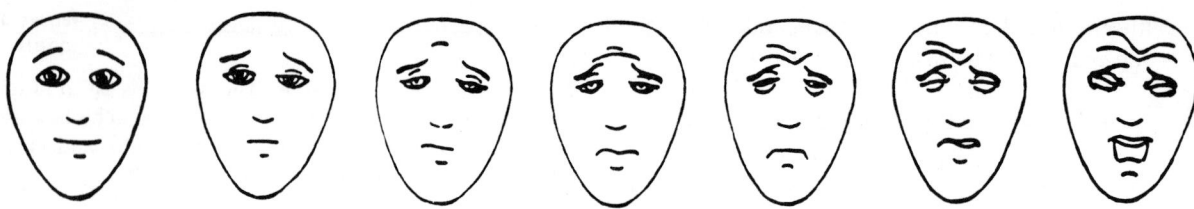

Figure 50.5.   The Faces Pain Scale for assessment of pain in pediatric patients. Children are asked to point to the face that best describes their pain.

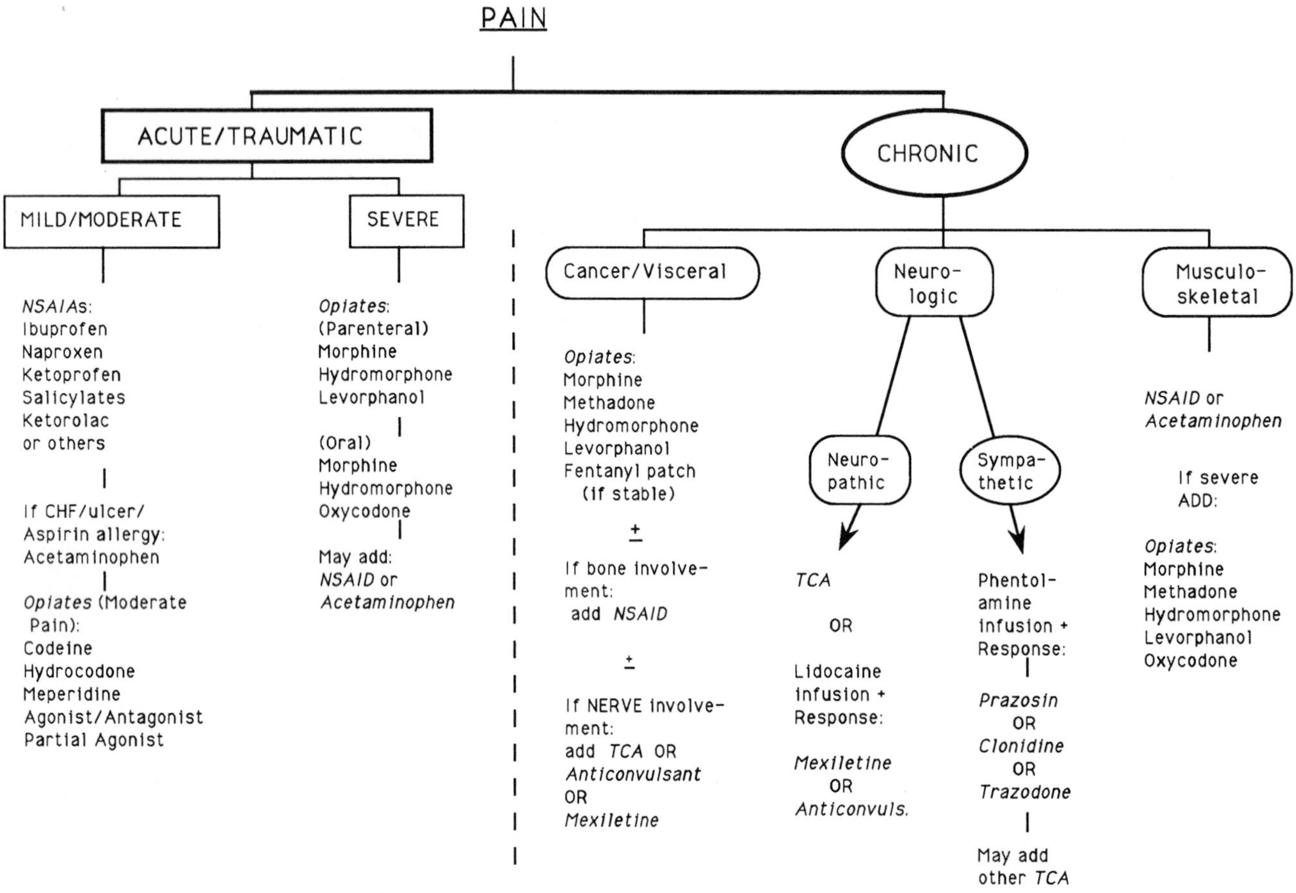

PAIN

ACUTE/TRAUMATIC

MILD/MODERATE

NSAIAs:
Ibuprofen
Naproxen
Ketoprofen
Salicylates
Ketorolac
or others

If CHF/ulcer/
Aspirin allergy:
Acetaminophen

Opiates (Moderate
Pain):
Codeine
Hydrocodone
Meperidine
Agonist/Antagonist
Partial Agonist

SEVERE

Opiates:
(Parenteral)
Morphine
Hydromorphone
Levorphanol

(Oral)
Morphine
Hydromorphone
Oxycodone

May add:
NSAID or
Acetaminophen

CHRONIC

Cancer/Visceral

Opiates:
Morphine
Methadone
Hydromorphone
Levorphanol
Fentanyl patch
(if stable)

±

If bone involve-
ment:
add *NSAID*

±

If NERVE involve-
ment:
add *TCA* OR
Anticonvulsant
OR
Mexiletine

Neuro-
logic

Neuro-
pathic

TCA

OR

Lidocaine
infusion +
Response:

Mexiletine
OR
Anticonvuls.

Sympa-
thetic

Phentol-
amine
infusion +
Response:

Prazosin
OR
Clonidine
OR
Trazodone

May add
other *TCA*

Musculo-
skeletal

NSAID or
Acetaminophen

If severe
ADD:

Opiates:
Morphine
Methadone
Hydromorphone
Levorphanol
Oxycodone

Figure 50.6.   Medication selection in the treatment of pain.

may lead to mucositis and subsequent pain. Some of the more commonly encountered symptoms of cancer pain occur in the musculoskeletal tissue and in the nervous system. Although most bony metastases do not produce pain, infiltration of bone is the most common cause of cancer pain. A constant, unpleasant, burning sensation often indicates compression of somatic nerves by tumor. This pain can also be accompanied by an intermittent lancinating pain (53).

For cancer pain, analgesics should be given at regular intervals and in adequate doses (Table 50.3). Medication should never be prescribed on a "p.r.n." basis, as the objective is to maintain maximum possible patient comfort at all times through maintenance of therapeutic tissue levels. Oral medication is preferred, especially long-acting drugs, unless factors prohibit such administration. These include malignant bowel obstruction or severe nausea from emetogenic chemotherapeutic agents. Sublingual narcotic administration has also been studied, with more lipophilic agents providing better analgesia than the less lipophilic morphine, presumably due to absorption characteristics related to lipophilicity. Rectal suppositories may suffice,

Table 50.3.
Principles of Analgesia for Cancer Pain

Choose appropriate analgesic(s)
Determine the dose by individual requirement
Time doses to regular schedule (not p.r.n.)
Anticipate pain; do not "chase" it
Minimize sedation or untoward effects
Use oral route whenever feasible
Tolerance and dependence are not problems
Treat nausea and constipation early
Use adjuvant medications whenever necessary

although this method is less reliable because of variable absorption of drugs from the rectal mucosa. Subcutaneous infusion is a reliable method of analgesic delivery that can be used in the home as well as the hospital with portable, programmable infusion pumps. Many such pumps are now available with syringe drivers that require infrequent changes of the syringe. Medication can thus be prepared by a home-health agency and supplied to the patient on a regular basis (54, 55).

Treatment of mild-to-moderate cancer pain should begin with nonnarcotic analgesics; when these drugs alone are ineffective, they are combined with intermediate opiate agonists such as codeine. Nonsteroidal antiinflammatory agents are effective in relieving many symptoms of bone-associated cancer pain, as are corticosteroids. However, the extensive side-effect profile of the steroids makes the nonsteroidal agents preferable. Bony metastases release prostaglandin E_2, which sensitizes peripheral nociceptors, and NSAIDs act by inhibiting elaboration of PGE_2. In addition to relieving pain, the nonsteroidals reduce stiffness, swelling, and tenderness (56). Finally, potent opiate agonists such as morphine or methadone should be used in the pain management regimen (57). A common agent for treatment of advanced cancer pain is morphine, because of its flexibility in dosing and potency. It is generally well tolerated by patients with a terminal illness. Alternatives include hydromorphone, methadone, and levorphanol. Diacetylmorphine (heroin) is not available in the United States for the treatment of pain and has not been shown to possess any advantage, since it is metabolized hepatically to morphine, its active analgesic component, in vivo. Heroin has a slightly faster onset of action but a shorter duration of analgesia than morphine. It is more soluble than morphine, allowing its use via the intramuscular route; however, methadone is as appropriate a selection (58).

Analgesic adjuvants, such as tricyclic antidepressants may be added to the drug regimen for cancer pain, particularly if neural involvement occurs. The benefits of analgesia may be enhanced by the psychotropic effects of the drugs upon depression. Other adjuncts include anti-

histamines, phenothiazines, anticonvulsants, and amphetamines (56, 59).

Neuropathic pain can arise from either discrete or generalized sites of nerve injury, or it may be idiopathic in nature. Two common neuropathic pain syndromes are postherpetic neuralgia ("shingles") and peripheral neuropathies arising from various causes such as diabetes mellitus or acquired immune deficiency syndrome. Less common are neuropathies induced by agents such as dideoxycytosine (ddC), used to treat AIDS. Neuropathic pains are most often sharp, lancinating, burning, hot, electrical, shocking, or searing. They can be intermittent and/or constant, and may involve paresthesias manifested by tingling or numbness of a limb. Neuropathic pain is relatively unresponsive to opioids, but this may reflect inadequate dosing and underlying patient variables rather than the pharmacology of the opiates (60).

Postherpetic neuralgia is a persistent, often lifelong pain syndrome resulting from infection with varicella-zoster virus (herpes zoster). The infection is initially manifested by fever, headache, lymphadenopathy, and malaise. It is followed by increasing pain or itching over a local area known as a dermatome, which is innervated by a specific nerve branch. Treatments for acute herpes zoster infection include systemic corticosteroids, antiviral agents, interferon, adenine arabinoside, and cimetidine. More invasive procedures, including somatic and sympathetic nerve blocks with local anesthetics and/or corticosteroids have proven efficacious (61). Rarely, herpes zoster can leave an elderly or immunocompromised patient with permanent nerve damage, resulting in persistent pain characterized by lancinating, burning, or itching. Regions commonly affected by postherpetic neuralgia are the thoracic, cranial/trigeminal, lumbar, and cervical. Herpes zoster is a reactivation of a latent virus originally acquired through acute varicella (chickenpox) infection. The afferent nerve pathways undergo degeneration and interruption, causing deafferentation followed by nerve reorganization (62). The cornerstone of treatment of PHN is the use of tricyclic antidepressants. In addition to their pain-remitting effects, tricyclic antidepressants treat the vegetative signs of depression such as sleep disturbance or anorexia (63). Anticonvulsants are also used. Carbamazepine and valproic acid have been used in doses of 600 to 1200 mg per day or 500 to 1500 mg per day, respectively. These drugs reduce complaints of lancinating pain. They are gradually adjusted upward from low starting doses, particularly in elderly patients (64). Topical local anesthetics also help reduce pain of the affected dermatome. A cream containing capsaicin, a purified derivative of red chili found in tabasco sauce, can be applied directly to the area of itching and inflammation. A few studies comparing this agent with placebo show favorable response, but its use is accompanied by 1 to 2 days of intense burning, since it acts as a nerve-ending counterirritant by stimulating and then desensitizing afferent C fibers (65). Intravenous administration of lidocaine (5 mg/kg) has also been beneficial in PHN, as have its oral congeners mexiletine and tocainide. Other cardiovascular agents such as clonidine may prove beneficial as well. Baclofen is also useful for refractory PHN pain of the trigeminal distribution (66, 67).

Diabetic neuropathy is usually reported as distal sensorimotor loss, and is a long-term complication of diabetes mellitus. Like PHN, diabetic neuropathies respond well to the tricyclic antidepressants. Intravenous lidocaine has been administered with encouraging results, and mexiletine may also prove useful for this condition. Aldose reductase inhibitors, which counteract hyperglycemia-induced metabolic changes at peripheral nerve sites, show promise for reversing early changes associated with functional nerve loss (68, 69).

Phantom-limb pain has been described variously as burning, tingling, throbbing, shooting, and stabbing. Neurosurgical procedures are not permanently successful in reducing pain. Biofeedback has a role in increasing temperature and blood perfusion and in reducing discomfort at the amputation site. Anticonvulsants help reduce paroxysms of pain, as do tricyclic antidepressants (70).

A syndrome known as reflex sympathetic dystrophy (RSD), causalgia, posttraumatic spreading neuralgia, or more recently, sympathetically maintained pain, predominates in areas of the extremities innervated by thoracolumbar branches of the nervous system. It may coexist with other forms of neuropathic pain. Causalgia is marked by burning pain, allodynia, and hyperpathia, and occurs in a hand or foot following nerve injury. RSD is continuous pain in a portion of an extremity following injury and is associated with sympathetic hyperactivity (47). Causes include multiple fractures or surgery in a localized area without involvement of a major nerve. Manifestations of RSD, in addition to burning pain stimulated by activity of the extremity, include vascular phenomena of coldness, numbness, or pain with changes in skin color. Trophic changes such as shiny, hairless skin or loss of bone mass may occur later. Sympathetic dystrophy may be lifelong, and treatment involves vasoactive agents such as prazosin as well as analgesic medications. Initial episodes usually respond to local glucocorticoid injections; more refractory cases respond to regional sympathetic blockade with local anesthetics or instillation of a sympatholytic agent such as guanethidine. Topical application of clonidine or capsaicin to the affected area is promising (71, 72).

Musculoskeletal pain arises from the muscles (myalgias), bones, joints (arthralgias), or connective tissue. Like neuropathies, it can be idiopathic, iatrogenic, or injurious in origin. Muscle pain arising from exertion or strain is treated easily with the nonsteroidal antiinflammatory agents, as is bone pain following dental or orthopaedic

procedures. Idiopathic musculoskeletal pain includes myofascial disorders and fasciitis, which are treated with local injections of anesthetics. Inflammatory diseases of muscle include polymyositis, dermatomyositis, and polymyalgia rheumatica. These may respond to low-dose intermittent steroids, e.g., prednisone 10 to 60 mg/day tapered over a 2-week period (73).

Examples of iatrogenic, or drug-induced musculoskeletal pains include those arising from the use of zidovudine (AZT), an agent used in treatment of acquired immune deficiency syndrome, and amphetamine or phancyclidine overdose leading to rhabdomyolysis and myoglobinuria (74). In October 1989, an illness associated with consumption of L-tryptophan for insomnia was reported that included myalgia, weakness, fever, arthralgia, dyspnea, rash, extremity edema, and pneumonia. Congestive heart failure, cardiac arrhythmias, hypoxemia, liver enzyme abnormalities, muscle creatinine phosphokinase elevations, and perivascular inflammatory infiltrates were also noted. A striking component in all cases was marked eosinophilia. By May 1990, approximately 1500 cases of eosinophilia-myalgia syndrome (EMS) were recorded, and of these approximately 20 patients have died thus far. The acute phase is notable for severe myalgia followed by proximal muscular weakness. Sensory and motor neuropathy are late complications that mimic rheumatic diseases such as systemic sclerosis, polymyalgia rheumatica, or fibrositis. A contaminant of L-tryptophan that causes a dramatic increase of eosinophils and subsequent release by these cells of toxic granule-related proteins is suspected. Degranulation of mast cells is also thought to occur, with activation of fibroblasts and subsequent development of fibrotic disease. Alternatively, the syndrome may be related to lymphokine secretion abnormalities leading to uncontrolled collagen synthesis. Though treatment is experimental, patients have not responded adequately to NSAIDs, hydroxychloroquine sulfate, or penicillamine. High-dose corticosteroids produce a modicum of success, though these drugs are often discontinued because of severe muscle cramping. Muscular injections of local anesthetic/steroid combinations (e.g., lidocaine/triamcinolone or bupivacaine/hydrocortisone) produce short-term reduction of myalgia pain. In extreme cases, pain may be opiate-responsive (75, 76).

Sickle cell disease results in acute infarctions and necrosis of organs secondary to vaso-occlusive episodes ("crises"). Chronic pain is experienced when arthritis develops secondary to bleeding into the joints. Painful episodes are attributed to tissue injury from obstruction of blood flow by the deformed erythrocytes; however, a small population of persons affected with sickle cell disease reports constant pain that persists between such episodes. NSAIDs and acetaminophen are the mainstay of therapy for mild-to-moderate pain. Opiate analgesics such as meperidine, morphine, or methadone are reserved for severe acute episodes and are dosed according to duration of action and relative potency. Consideration of hepatic or renal dysfunction caused by veno-occlusion of these organs is required. When a crisis begins to abate, narcotic tapering is instituted, with pharmacologic emphasis placed on the nonopiate drugs (77).

PRINCIPLES OF PAIN MANAGEMENT

Pain therapy is begun with nonnarcotic analgesics where possible, followed by the step-wise addition of opiates and analgesic adjuncts (Figure 50.7).

OPIOID ANALGESICS (Table 50.4)

Opioids include natural and synthetic agents. They reduce moderate-to-severe pain and are unique in their ability to do this without producing loss of consciousness. All opiates have the potential for habituation and addiction. There are three classes of opiates: the phenanthrene (morphine-like) derivatives, which include morphine, codeine, opium, hydrocodone, hydromorphone, levorphanol, oxycodone, oxymorphone, and dihydrocodeine; the phenylpiperidine derivatives, which include meperidine (pethidine), fentanyl, sufentanil, and alfentanil; and the diphenylheptane derivatives, which include methadone and propoxyphene. Methadone was synthesized in Germany during the 1940s to treat war casualties when morphine supplies were exhausted.

Several agonist/antagonist combinations and partial opiate agonists are available which are weaker than their pure agonist counterparts and are purported to be less habituating.

POTENT OPIATES

Morphine and other potent opioids are used to treat severe acute, chronic, or terminal malignant pain. They can be given orally, rectally, as a continuous subcutaneous or intravenous infusion, intramuscularly, or directly into the CNS via epidural or intrathecal administration. The CNS route allows minute doses without sensory, motor, or sympathetic dysfunction. Meperidine is used in moderate traumatic or postoperative pain, and like morphine is given for pain from myocardial infarction or for sedation in patients with pulmonary edema. However, caution is advised with atrial flutter or supraventricular tachycardia, as meperidine can increase systemic vascular resistance and heart rate. Some preparations contain metabisulfite preservatives that produce anaphylaxis or hypersensitivity reactions, especially in asthmatic patients. Parenteral meperidine reduces rigors associated with amphotericin B administration and is used as a premedication for patients receiving this antifungal agent. Methadone was initially approved for narcotic detoxification, and in the 1980s approval was extended to analgesia. It is popular for treatment of terminal painful conditions, as a longer duration of action allows less frequent dosing. Levorphanol is a potent, semisynthetic opiate agonist for moderate-to-severe pain, including intractable pain in terminally ill patients. It produces more sedation and smooth muscle stimulation than does morphine in equianalgesic doses and has the same potential for habituation or addiction as naturally occurring opi-

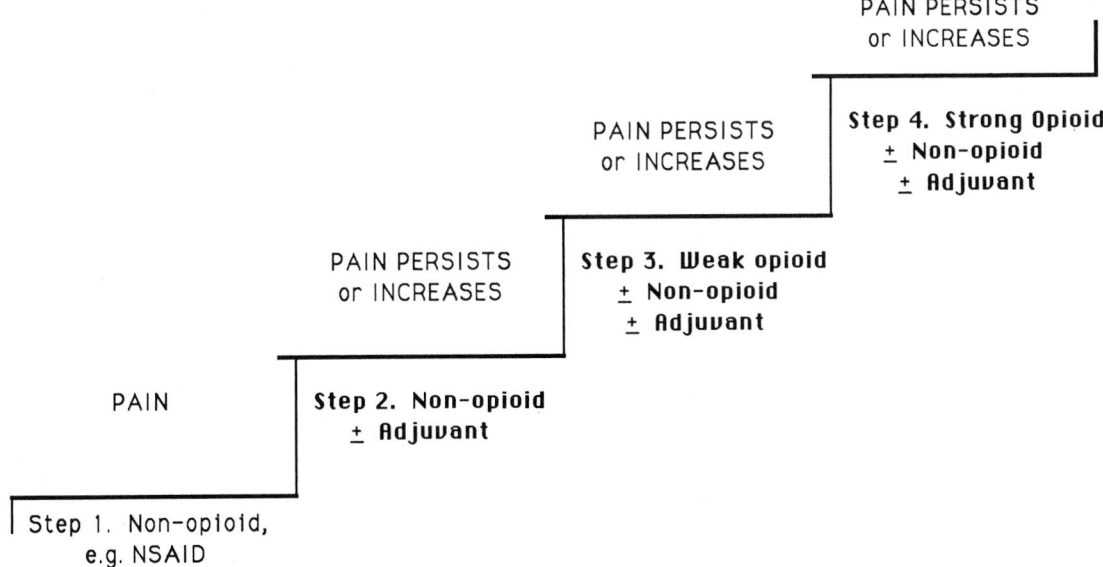

Figure 50.7. Analgesic stepladder for chronic pain management. (Adapted from World Health Organization: Cancer Pain Relief. Geneva: World Health Organization, 1986.)

Table 50.4.
Centrally Acting Analgesic Characteristics

	IM Dose (mg)[a]	Oral Equiv.[a]	Routes	Time to Onset (min)	Duration Plasma (hr)	$t_{1/2}$ (hr)
Opioid agonists for severe pain						
Morphine	10	60	PO, SC, IV, IM, PR	IV = 5; PO = 60+	3–6	2–3
Hydromorphone	1.5	3	PO, SC, IV, IM, PR	See morphine	4–5	2–4
Levorphanol	2	4	PO, SC, IM	30–90	4–6	10–12
Methadone	10	20	PO, SC, IM	SC, IM = 60	6–8	21–25
Oxymorphone	1	6	PO, SC, IV, IM	10 to 90	3–6	3–4
Fentanyl	0.1	N/A	IV, Intraspinal	10	1–2	3–4
Opioids for mild-to-moderate pain						
Codeine	120	200	PO, SC, IV, IM	See morphine	4–6	
Hydrocodone	N/A		PO		4–6	
Oxycodone	15	30	PO		4–6	
Dihydrocodone	N/A		PO		4–6	
Meperidine	100	400	PO, SC, IV, IM	15–60	2–4	3–4
Propoxyphene	N/A	65–130	PO	60–90	4–6	6–12
Partial agonists/antagonists						
Nalorphine	0.4	N/A	SC, IV, IM	15	3–6	2–3
Buprenorphine	2	N/A	SC, IV, IM	15	4–6	2–3
Pentazocine	30–60	150	SC, IV, IM	10	3–4	2–4
Nalbuphine	10	N/A	SC, IV, IM	15	2–3	2–3
Dezocine	10–15	N/A	SC, IV, IM	15	3–6	4–6
Opioid antagonists						
Naloxone	0.4–0.8					1–1.5
Naltrexone						

[a] Based on single doses.

ates. Like methadone, it has a long half-life and a longer duration of action than morphine, hydromorphone, or meperidine. It is often used as a substitute when large requirements lead to the need for frequent morphine dosing.

Morphine and hydromorphone exert major pharmacodynamic effects on μ- and κ-receptors. Large doses of morphine can reduce systemic vascular resistance, producing a transient fall in blood pressure. Hydromorphone has less potential to produce nausea, vomiting, constipation, sedation, or euphoria than morphine and can be used as a substitute when these adverse effects warrant a therapeutic alternative. Concentrated parenteral preparations are useful for opiate-tolerant cancer patients whose high narcotic requirements have posed a problem because of volume required for administration. All narcotics can lead to muscular rigidity, presumably by accumulation in the striatum and nucleus accumbens (78).

Oral morphine is absorbed variably, with bioavailability of approximately 20%. It is also absorbed rectally. Peak analgesia occurs about 20 to 60 min after a dose and lasts longer in opiate-naive individuals. The major metabolite of morphine is morphine-3-glucuronide, which is inactive. Minor active metabolites include morphine-6-glucuronide and normorphine, with a small amount biotransformed to codeine. Approximately 90% of morphine is excreted unchanged by the kidneys, with most of the remaining 10%

excreted via biliary elimination (79). Hydromorphone, a semisynthetic opiate, has a more rapid onset and shorter duration of action than morphine. Hydromorphone is converted mainly to a glucuronide metabolite, with urinary excretion (80). Levorphanol is well absorbed and like morphine, undergoes hepatic metabolism to a glucuronide conjugate excreted by the kidneys. Peak analgesia occurs approximately 20 to 90 min after intravenous or subcutaneous injection, respectively. Duration of analgesia may be shorter in opiate-tolerant individuals (81). Meperidine is poorly absorbed, and oral doses are 25% as effective as parenteral. It is metabolized to meperidinic acid, which is excreted by the kidneys as a glucuronide metabolite. Of greater importance is normeperidine, which can accumulate with renal impairment to induce central nervous stimulation and tonic-clonic seizures. Approximately one-third of meperidine is converted to this N-demethyl metabolite, which has twice the convulsant activity and half of the analgesic potency of meperidine and a half-life of 12 to 16 hr. Meperidine is shorter-acting than morphine and produces the same degree, but a shorter duration of, respiratory depression. It is preferred for analgesia during labor, because of less extensive placental penetration with less respiratory and CNS depression than morphine in the newborn infant (82).

Methadone has unique pharmacokinetic properties.

Oral absorption is nearly complete and the half-life of the drug is 13 to 47 hr, with an average of 25 hr. Analgesic duration increases from 4 to 6 hr for a single dose to 6 to 8 hr after repeated administration. However, CNS depression persists up to 36 hr following overdosage, an important factor in reversing the effects with the opiate antagonist naloxone. The half-life of naloxone is about 60 to 90 min, and a patient requires naloxone by continuous infusion until the critical period has ended (83).

Doses of opiates vary according to a patient's prior exposure, severity of pain, hepatic or renal function, and route of administration. The oral:parenteral morphine ratio is approximately 5:1, owing to a large first-pass effect. Oral preparations include short-acting tablets and elixers as well as extended-release tablets. Conversion from short-acting to longer duration formulations requires consideration to active drug and metabolite accumulation. One approach is to reduce the total daily dose by 25%, and divide this amount by three or four and administer the resulting amount every 8 or 6 hr, respectively. When increasing the dose, an extra tablet is initially added at night to eliminate daytime somnolence, followed by the addition of subsequent tablets until effective analgesia is seen.

Parenteral hydromorphone and levorphanol are about five times as potent as morphine, with oral to parenteral ratios of 2:1 and 3:1, respectively. Both are available as tablets and as parenteral formulations for intravenous, intramuscular, or subcutaneous use. Hydromorphone can also be administered intraspinally or rectally as a suppository (83).

Parenteral meperidine has one-tenth the potency of morphine, and the oral to parenteral ratio is approximately 4:1. Meperidine is available as tablets, a solution, and an injectable preparation. Oral combinations with promethazine or acetaminophen and parenteral combinations with promethazine or atropine also exist, though there is little rationale in using fixed-dose combinations of analgesics, because patient-specific dosing is required. Combination products are more expensive than individual constituents and can produce additive side effects without providing added benefit.

Methadone is equivalent to morphine on a single-dose basis, but with repeated administration accumulation in CNS and lipid tissues occurs, so the morphine to methadone conversion is 4:1. Once initiated, methadone can be decreased 10% per day until a stable analgesic regimen is obtained. In detoxifying opiate-dependent patients with chronic pain, a "blind taper" can be used, in which methadone oral solution is mixed with acetaminophen elixir or cherry syrup. The methadone dose is thus decreased gradually, while the same total volume is administered to the patient. Methadone is available as tablets, an oral solution, and parenterally for intramuscular use.

NARCOTIC ANALGESICS FOR MILD-TO-MODERATE PAIN

Codeine (methylmorphine) is a natural opiate derivative produced in the liver by morphine metabolism. It is a less potent analgesic, as are its derivatives hydrocodone and dihydrocodeine. Oxycodone, a third codeine derivative, exhibits intermediate potency. All of these drugs are effective for mild-to-moderate pain, and dihydrocodeine enjoys popularity as an analgesic following dental procedures.

AGONIST/ANTAGONISTS

Agonists and antagonists have varying effects at different opiate receptors, and their affinity for any particular receptor is dose-related. A characteristic of agonist/antagonist combinations is a "ceiling" effect with regard to analgesia and respiratory depression (28). This means that higher doses (i.e., those above the ceiling) do not increase the degree of analgesia or the potential for respiratory failure. Butorphanol, a nonscheduled opiate agent, is only available parenterally. Pentazocine, a benzomorphan derivative, does not decrease propulsive activity of the intestines in therapeutic doses (39). It is contraindicated in myocardial infarction and has been combined with naloxone in oral preparations to discourage abuse. Nalbuphine, also nonscheduled, may have fewer psychotomimetic effects than either butorphanol or pentazocine (84).

Picenadol, an experimental mixed agonist-antagonist, has moderate analgesic activity, comparable to codeine or meperidine. It is a μ-receptor agonist, with weak activity at the κ-receptor. Picenadol, a phenylpiperidine derivative, can be reversed by naloxone. Side effects include drowsiness, dizziness, and lightheadedness (85).

PARTIAL AGONISTS

Buprenorphine and dezocine have less reported abuse liability than morphine, but either drug can precipitate withdrawal in narcotic-addicted patients. Dezocine is a nonscheduled opiate analgesic approved for parenteral administration. Both agents are indicated for postoperative or posttraumatic acute pain. Like other opioids, they are metabolized by glucuronidation, and dezocine also appears to have a sulfate metabolite. Side effects of these agents include constipation or diarrhea, hyper- or hypotension, nausea, vomiting, anxiety, and sedation. Dezocine reportedly has high μ-receptor affinty, moderate δ- and κ-affinity, and low σ-affinity. The threshold dose for respiratory depression is 30 mg (86).

NARCOTIC ANTAGONISTS

Naloxone is a short-acting, specific opiate receptor antagonist used to reverse untoward side effects of the narcotics such as pruritis and respiratory depression. It is a competitive saturable inhibitor of the opiate receptor, usually administered in doses of 0.2 to 0.4 mg as needed. Care should be taken not to administer an excessive amount, as large doses reverse opioid analgesia (83).

NONOPIOID ANALGESICS

NONSTEROIDAL ANTIINFLAMMATORY DRUGS (NSAIDs)

Aspirin and other nonsteroidal antiinflammatory drugs are useful for the treatment of pain from injury, surgery, trauma, arthritis, or cancer. The NSAIDs are especially effective in the management of bone pain secondary to tumor metastases. Acetaminophen, though not possessing antiinflammatory properties, is the most commonly used nonprescription pain reliever. NSAIDs differ from opiate analgesics in several ways: an analgesic ceiling exists for these agents, they do not induce tolerance or physical or psychological dependence, and they are also antipyretics. In addition, their actions (with the exception of acetaminophen) occur through inhibition of cyclooxygenase, a catalyst in the formation of prostaglandins that sensitize nociceptors to the effects of pain-eliciting substances such as bradykinin. Because of predominant action in the peripheral nervous system, the NSAIDs and acetaminophen work synergistically with the centrally acting opiates. NSAIDs also have central effects that contribute to their analgesic activity, as they are thought to reduce C-fiber activity in the thalamus (87, 88).

The NSAIDs are approximately equipotent. Only ibuprofen and ketoprofen are superior analgesics at equivalent doses. Patient response varies considerably, so a patient who does not obtain therapeutic efficacy with one drug at a maximum dose should be given an alternative agent (48).

Absorption of the NSAIDs occurs in the stomach and duodenum. The rate of absorption increases with slower gastric emptying or decreases when food or antacids are present in the stomach, although the total amount of drug absorbed is unchanged. Extent of absorption can be affected by the salt formulation. NSAIDs are eliminated primarily through biotransformation in the liver, with metabolites excreted by the kidney. Some may undergo enterohepatic recirculation (89).

The propionic acid class of agents includes ibuprofen, naproxen, fenoprofen, flurbiprofen, and ketoprofen. Ketoprofen is unique in that it also inhibits lipooxygenase at normal doses, decreasing leukotriene production. Whether this has clinical relevance is unknown, as other NSAIDs inhibit lipooxygenase at high doses. Ketoprofen is as effective in treating cancer pain as an acetaminophen and codeine combination in single-dose comparisons (90).

Ketorolac, a pyrrolacetic acid structurally related to zomepirac and tolmetin, possesses potent analgesic and moderate antiinflammatory activity. In postoperative pain ketorolac is as effective as morphine, meperidine, or pen-

tazocine, although its onset of action is slightly longer. Like other NSAIDs, it inhibits platelet aggregation and can prolong bleeding time, induce gastric ulceration, or decrease renal function. The most common side effects are somnolence and other central effects such as nausea and dizziness. Available for intramuscular administration, it is well absorbed with a time to maximum effect of approximately 45 min. The major metabolite is a glucuronide and elimination is mostly renal, with approximately 90% excreted in the urine. Usual initial loading doses are 30 to 60 mg, followed by 15 to 30 mg every 6 hr as needed. The role of ketorolac in pain therapy is for acute (24 to 72 hr) postoperative analgesia when opiates are undesirable, as it is nonhabituating and does not appear to decrease respiratory drive. There is little rationale to support the use of ketorolac in a patient tolerating oral medications or in one for whom intramuscular narcotics are appropriate, and conversion to ibuprofen, naproxen, or a similar agent is indicated. Oral ketorolac is planned for future release in the United States (91).

Anthranilic acids are also called fenamates, and although mefenamic acid is reported to have greater prostaglandin inhibition at the myometrium, it does not provide greater analgesia than other NSAIDs. Frequently reported adverse effects, such as diarrhea and central nervous system impairment have limited its use (92).

Piroxicam has an extended plasma half-life and is dosed once daily (93). This makes it unsuitable for treatment of chronic pain, as plasma levels drop below analgesic threshold before the next dose is due.

New agents include etodolac, a pyranocarboxylic acid used for acute pain and osteoarthritis. Usual doses are 200 to 400 mg every 6 to 8 hr for analgesia, not to exceed 1200 mg per day.

ANALGESIC ADJUNCTS

ANTIDEPRESSANTS (Table 50.5)

Human response to pain includes the "fight-or-flight" reaction mounted against physical or emotional stresses. Two simultaneous phenomena occur: corticoadrenal and sympathetic responses. The first results in production of endogenous glucocorticoid steroids to mobilize energy sources and inhibit prostaglandins. The sympathetic response induces an outpouring of norepinephrine, a catecholamine, and serotonin, an indoleamine, within neuronal synaptic junctions. Tricyclic antidepressants that inhibit the reuptake and storage of these neurogenic amines have analgesic properties related to their ability to increase pain tolerance (94, 95). This effect occurs in the absence of depression, and the onset of analgesia is often more rapid than the antidepressant effect (96). In addition, vegetative symptoms associated with chronic pain such as sleep disturbance and depression are reduced by central serotonin enhancement. Serotonergic processes are an integral part

Table 50.5.
Antidepressants Used as Analgesic Adjuvants

Medication	Daily Dose	Conc. (ng/ml)	Receptor Blockade			
			Cholinergic	Histaminergic	Adrenergic	
					α_1	α_2
Tertiary amines						
Amitriptyline	75–300 mg	110–250[a]	Very high	Very high	High–v. high	Moderate
Doxepin	30–300 mg	30–150[b]	Moderate	Very high	High–v. high	Moderate
Imipramine	75–300 mg	100–350[a]	Moderate-high	Moderate	High	Insignificant
Secondary amines						
Amoxapine	100–300 mg	Not established	None-slight	Slight	Slight-mod.	Slight
Desipramine	75–300 mg	125–250	Slight	Slight	Moderate	None-slight
Nortriptyline	50–150 mg	50–150	Moderate	Moderate	Slight-mod.	Insignificant
Protriptyline	15–60 mg	100–200	Mod.-high	Slight	Moderate	Insignificant
Bicyclic						
Fluoxetine	20–60 mg	160–700[a]	None-slight	None-slight	None-slight	None-slight
Triazolopyridine						
Trazodone	150–600 mg	800–2100	None-slight	Moderate	Very high	Moderate

[a] Parent compound + active metabolite.
[b] Parent compound alone.

of endogenous pain inhibitory mechanisms, so tricyclic antidepressants have proven useful as adjuncts in chronic pain management (97). Patients should be told that 1 to 3 weeks are typically required before such analgesia occurs.

The antidepressants include several classes of agents, which can be organized into three categories: the tricyclic antidepressants (TCAs), the monoamine oxidase inhibitors (MAOIs), and newer heterocyclic compounds. Clinical effects include improvement in mood and sleep, anxiolysis, and a decreased perception of pain. The tricyclic agents are commonly used in the management of neuropathic pains and related conditions. The monoamine oxidase inhibitors have not been used as frequently for treatment of painful conditions and are reserved for patients refractory to the TCAs. MAOIs are more difficult to use, and their benefits in treating pain have not been well-documented. Newer agents include fluoxetine and buproprion, an aminoketone that like MAOIs is reserved for persons with refractory depression. Neither of these have been thoroughly studied for their effects on chronic pain.

The most commonly used antidepressant for painful conditions is amitriptyline in doses of 50 to 300 mg per day. Persons with chronic pain usually have poor sleep habits, making this drug useful in overcoming insomnia or nighttime waking. An agent with less anticholinergic effects such as nortriptyline may be substituted for amitriptyline. Desipramine, an active metabolite of imipramine, is also less sedating and has fewer anticholinergic effects than its parent compound.

Antidepressants scheduled for release include analogs of fluoxetine with shorter half-lives to prevent their ac-

cumulation in slow metabolizers such as the elderly. Paroxetine is an investigational selective serotonin reuptake inhibitor modeled after the prototype agent zimelidine, and it significantly decreases symptoms of painful diabetic neuropathy without withdrawal effects or changes in nerve function measurements. Paroxetine at 40 mg/day is also devoid of autonomic side effects that limit the use of TCAs (98).

NEUROLEPTICS

Of the neuroleptics, fluphenazine potentiates the effects of amitriptyline in patient with diabetic neuropathies. It also aids sleep onset and is typically given in doses of 1 mg at bedtime, up to a maximum of 3 mg per day in divided doses or all at bedtime (99). Methotrimeprazine is available as a treatment for mild-to-moderate pain. Its duration of action is equal to that of morphine, and it possesses analgesic efficacy equivalent to morphine or meperidine, without similar habituating and addictive potentials or likelihood of respiratory depression. It has been underutilized in chronic pain management because of sedative and anticholinergic effects that decrease patient tolerance. The use of other neuroleptics is controversial, and phenothiazine analgesia is unproven, with the exception of these agents (100).

ANTICONVULSANTS

The mechanism of action of carbamazepine and valproate is suppression of spontaneous neuronal firing. Lancinating, burning pains are best treated by these drugs, which are typically long-acting but can induce their own metabolism.

Carbamazepine and valproate are prescribed for tic douloureux (trigeminal neuropathy), cranial nerve disorders, neural invasion by cancerous tumor, radiation fibrosis, surgical scarring, deafferentation syndromes, and other neuralgic conditions. Doses of carbamazepine and valproate are the same as those used for treatment of convulsive disorders. Plasma levels should be monitored, as side effects can be serious and include hematologic changes associated with bone marrow suppression, ataxia, diplopia, nausea, lymphadenopathy, and hepatic dysfunction. Periodic liver function tests, blood counts, and serum drug levels should be obtained for patients on chronic therapy (101).

OTHER AGENTS

Lidocaine is also given for neuropathic syndromes, and like all local anesthetics, it enters the central nervous system after intravenous administration. Mexiletine has been used in lidocaine-responsive patients requiring a longer-acting substitute, as the effects of lidocaine are short-lived. Both agents reduce neuronal firing through stabilization of sodium-conducting channels in nerve cell membranes. When administered systemically, they diffuse into the peripheral nerves. Analgesic doses of mexiletine are the same as those needed for antiarrhythmic effects (i.e., approximately 10 mg/kg per day to produce plasma levels of 0.75 to 2.0 μg/ml). The use of tocainide, an oral lidocaine analog, is not widespread because of a higher incidence of serious adverse effects such as aplastic anemia. Side effects of both lidocaine and mexiletine include dizziness, light-headedness, ataxia, nausea, and vomiting. High doses of these agents can lead to tremor and convulsions. Gastrointestinal effects of mexiletine can be reduced by taking the medication with food (102).

Two centrally acting α_2-agonists, clonidine and guanethidine, are under investigation for pain management. They block sympathetic outflow from the central nervous system by presynaptic inhibition of norepinephrine release. Clonidine may interact with opiate receptors by inducing the release of the endogenous peptide dynorphin, and it has been used with some success in suppressing the symptoms of opiate withdrawal attributed to a hypernoradrenergic state, including agitation, diarrhea, and sweating. This drug may also be used during surgery to reduce inhalation and opiate anesthetic requirements, as it potentiates morphine analgesia. Unlike morphine, however, clonidine is not reversed by naloxone, though its actions can be blocked by κ-specific antagonists. Clonidine may also prove useful in patients with spinal cord injury, and neuropathic and sympathetically mediated pain syndromes. It is available as an oral tablet or as a patch that provides consistent blood levels of the drug for a period of 5 to 7 days, increasing compliance. Clonidine may produce orthostatic hypotension, so a candidate for therapy

should first receive a baseline evaluation of blood pressure (103, 104). Guanethidine, with a mechanism of action similar to that of clonidine, is also used in patients with sympathetic pain. Guanethidine produces significant vasodilation, counteracting the vasoconstriction noted with sympathetic activity, with resultant warming of an affected extremity and a reduction in pain. Guanethidine holds promise in the treatment of pain associated with rheumatoid arthritis, as patient response to regional guanethidine blockade has been favorable (105).

Prazosin is used for the relief of sympathetically mediated pains such as reflex sympathetic dystrophy. It has high specificity and affinity for the α_1-adrenergic receptor. Like clonidine, it produces vasodilation with significant orthostasis. Prazosin should be dosed initially at bedtime to reduce the risk of falling because of a precipitous drop in blood pressure. Doses can be increased gradually according to patient response and tolerance of side effects. Other agents used to relieve sympathetically mediated pain include intravenous phentolamine and oral phenoxybenzamine. However, these agents are nonselective for the α_1-receptor and also produce α_2-adrenergic effects. A test infusion of phentolamine can be used to predict guanethidine or prazosin response (106). Use of clonidine, guanethidine, or prazosin should include frequent monitoring of patients, since these agents may worsen depression observed to coexist with chronic pain.

Benzodiazepines such as diazepam and clonazepam are used for skeletal muscle relaxation in the treatment of chronic spasm and neuropathic pain. Side effects include sedation, cognitive impairment, and depression, all of which decrease activity of the pain patient, and some researchers believe benzodiazepines may even exacerbate pain. In addition, they produce habituation and serious withdrawal reactions, including seizure. The elderly are more susceptible to these effects. Therefore, tricyclic antidepressants are more rational choices for relieving the insomnia and anxiety that accompany chronic pain (107).

Antihistamines such as hydroxyzine and promethazine have been used to augment the sedative effects of opiates. They may have some analgesic activity, although their use is controversial.

Dextroamphetamine 5 to 10 mg per day can be used in patients with cancer pain to overcome the sedation of opiates. It also relieves some vegetative effects of depression that often accompany a terminal diagnosis (108).

ADVANCES IN PAIN THERAPY

NEW METHODS OF DRUG ADMINISTRATION—
PATIENT-CONTROLLED ANALGESIA (PCA)

Patient-controlled devices take advantage of intravenous bolus injections to produce rapid analgesia along with slower infusion to produce steady-state opiate concentrations for sustained pain control. Since opioid kinetics vary greatly between patients, the rates of infusion must be tailored. Many computerized PCA devices rely on the principle of a baseline infusion plus optional rescue doses. Boluses are self-administered and can be controlled by a predetermined lockout period. PCA is useful for patients with chronic malignant pain, allowing a greater degree of ambulation and independence. Many PCA devices are compact enough to be worn on a belt or carried in a pocket (109).

INTRASPINAL

Opiates administered into the spinal fluid give important information about nociceptive pharmacology at their active sites, in addition to being clinically useful for pain relief. They are justified for patients with malignant pain, those in whom neurolytic techniques have failed, those with acquired tolerance to systemic opiates, and those whose pain undergoes a sudden exacerbation such as postsurgical amputees. Morphine was the first opiate used in this manner. Unfortunately, spinal opiates may produce more urinary retention, biphasic respiratory depression, urticaria, pruritus, nausea, and vomiting than opiates administered parenterally or orally. Agents that undergo significant migration up the spinal column toward the head are most often associated with these side effects, and drug polarity influences such migration. Morphine is more polar than meperidine and undergoes more migration, leading to delayed respiratory depression. This agent reaches the respiratory center approximately 3 hr after administration. Because of this, efforts have been made to reduce the severe side effects through combinations of opiates and local anesthetics such as bupivacaine. By taking advantage of analgesic synergism via different mechanisms of action, smaller doses of each drug may be administered. Several other analgesic opioid and nonopioid drugs have been studied since the initiation of intraspinal morphine. Spinally infused opiates have the potential for precipitating abstinence syndrome when withdrawn, but it is not clear if intraspinal opioids produce differences in the development of narcotic tolerance when compared with oral administration. Changes in opioid receptor number and/or drug-receptor affinity because of chronic occupation of the opioid receptors are believed to account for the tolerance phenomenon, but removal of opiate for 7 to 14 days can result in recovery of drug efficacy. Long-term spinal infusion of opiates does not cause permanent sensory or motor functional loss or histophysiologic changes, though it may lead to mild dorsal column degeneration. Disadvantages include risk of infection or puncture of the dura mater and catheter displacement (110, 111).

The entire volume of CSF turns over approximately every 5 hr. Any drug placed into the CSF is distributed rapidly and eliminated into the systemic circulation. Bulk flow of CSF upward (toward the head) will cause a lumbar

injection of an opiate to reach the brainstem, leading to effects such as drowsiness and vomiting, within 2 to 4 hr. A bolus will cause concentrated drug to reach the brainstem, whereas a continuous infusion pump will establish a steady-state after 5 drug half-lives. Distribution across the dura from epidural administration occurs within 10 to 40 min. More lipid-soluble agents, such as methadone, distribute along the spinal cord in a very limited manner because of rapid crossing of the dura and consequent migration out of the CSF (112).

The action of morphine in the spinal cord makes it ideal for powerful and relatively selective inhibition of pain information processing. Repeated bolus administration and continuous infusion of narcotics into the epidural space for terminal cancer pain have both demonstrated utility and efficacy. An implantable pump allows continuous infusion of opiates or other agents into the spinal space without requiring an external port. In addition, the lack of repeated bolus injections theoretically limits the development of narcotic tolerance. Spinal morphine has the advantage of providing adequate pain relief when other forms of the drug are not tolerated. Cancer patients receiving highly emetic antineoplastic drugs, for example, may lose significant amounts of oral drug by vomiting. A third advantage of this method of drug delivery is facilitation of ambulation, allowing a patient to leave the hospital. Epidural administration of narcotics or other analgesic agents has also found use in the postoperative and obstetrical settings for short-term pain relief (i.e., 2 to 5 days) following surgical procedures (113, 114).

Intrathecal opiate administration has also received widespread attention. For morphine, normorphine, methadone, meperidine, fentanyl, buprenorphine, and the experimental agent etorphine, in vitro and in vivo data suggest a strong inverse relationship between intrathecal potency and lipophilicity. This can be explained by the rapid migration of highly lipophilic agents out of the cerebrospinal fluid. Etorphine has greater analgesic properties than would be predicted by lipophilicity alone, and its high affinity for the δ-receptor is believed to compensate for the effects of lipophilicity on its spinal potency. Therefore, generalizations about relative intravenous or intramuscular narcotic efficacy do not correlate with intrathecal or epidural potency, and specific δ-receptor agonists may prove useful for spinal infusion with minimal μ-receptor cross-tolerance. Similarly, clonidine via intrathecal administration shows promise for producing analgesia without morphine cross-tolerance. Hormones as diverse as somatostatin and calcitonin have been administered intraspinally for analgesia, and intrathecal baclofen is under investigation for treatment of intractable pain and spasm caused by spinal cord injury. Like clonidine, baclofen can potentiate morphine analgesia or produce analgesic effects alone. Intrathecal methadone 5, 10, and 20 mg has been used for patients following orthopaedic surgery. However because of its higher side-effect profile and lower efficacy when compared with morphine, it is not widely used via the intraspinal routes (115–119).

TRANSDERMAL AND INNOVATIVE METHODS OF DRUG DELIVERY

Fentanyl is a synthetic opioid derivative of the 4-anilinophenyl-piperidine class, and it is approximately 80 times as potent as morphine. It is used clinically as an analgesic, administered either intraspinally or intraveneously, and as a preoperative anesthetic agent because of its potency, rapid onset, and short duration of action. Fentanyl is a highly lipophilic agent, leading to rapid uptake and fast elimination, and orally the drug undergoes extensive first-pass metabolism. Parenteral administration has therefore been the typical route, but the large initial doses required to sustain analgesia lead to a risk of overdose. Stable levels can be achieved through continuous intravenous administration when the infusion rate matches the plasma elimination rate. Transdermal administration has widened the clinical use of this agent because it also supplies the drug at a stable rate. Transdermal fantanyl is available in four strengths, with patches releasing 25, 50, 75, or 100 μg per hour of fentanyl. These patches are most applicable in treatment of stable terminal cancer pain, as each patch lasts approximately 72 hr but requires several days to reach steady-state concentrations. Similarly, the drug is not rapidly eliminated if the patch must be removed because of untoward effects. Transdermal patches are noninvasive and offer an advantage in facilitating patient mobility. Conversion to an oral opiate can be done easily if such conversion becomes feasible. Sufentanil, another synthetic phenylpiperidine derivative, which is approximately 10 times more potent than fentanyl and more lipophilic, may also find future use with this novel route of administration (39). Unlike previous permeability studies with other drugs, percutaneous penetration of these weak bases depends on pH but not upon the anatomical location of the patch (120).

Morphine can be administered directly into the brain's cerebral ventricles for treatment of cancer pain. Morphine administered in this fashion is effective and naloxone-reversible. The disadvantages of this technique are risk of meningitis, nausea, vomiting, and pruritis (121).

Intrapleural administration of bupivacaine has been performed in patients with rib fractures and in patients with abdominal and thoracic pain following surgery, which exemplifies one of the many newer modalities available to the practitioner (122).

AGENTS UNDER INVESTIGATION

Cholecystokinin antagonists have gained recent attention for their role in analgesia based on observations that mor-

phine-induced analgesia can be antagonized in vivo by cholecystokinin. Administration of proglumide, an investigational agent, potentiates morphine-induced analgesia in both animals and humans. Calcium-channel blockers may also potentiate morphine analgesia by modulation of calcium availability to the cell. These drugs, like proglumide, are devoid of any analgesic activity when given alone. Endogenous opioid peptides (endorphine, dynorphin, and enkephalins) have not proven superior to exogenous opioids in the management of pain. Their analgesic effects are short-lived, and they produce the same side effects as drugs like morphine. Other (nonopioid) endogenous peptides have been suggested for their role in pain modulation. Calcitonin has been studied rigorously, but it produces severe respiratory depression. Specific δ-receptor agonists have risen to the forefront of opioid research, as recent evidence suggests that they may produce analgesia without inducing habituation. Opioid peptides also show promise as therapeutic agents, since they differ from opiates in several ways. Peptide analogs of enkephalins are expected to undergo degradation by placental enzymes, inhibiting or preventing their transfer across placental membranes. This would make them ideal agents for obstetrics, placing the fetus at less risk. Moreover, no δ-receptors have been demonstrated in fetal brain tissue, increasing the safety margin of future δ-specific peptides. A third advantage the peptides may have over their opiate counterparts is degradation to constituent amino acids instead of to active and possibly toxic metabolites. There is less potential for renal or hepatic damage with such peptides. Third, peptide δ-agonists, as mentioned, are likely to have less dependence and abuse liability than μ- and κ-agonists. Patients who have become tolerant to μ-agonists such as morphine may benefit from little or no analgesic cross-tolerance with the δ-opioid peptides (123).

NONPHARMACOLOGIC MODALITIES

SURGICAL

Cordotomy is a method of severing the sympathetic chains that emanate from the spinal cord. Indications for such intervention are short life expectancy and specific unilateral or focal pain. In percutaneous cordotomy, a lesion is produced in the spinothalamic tract, most often at the level of the first or second cervical vertebra. This method has virtually replaced open cordotomy, in which a quadrant of the spinal cord is almost completely severed at the cervical or thoracic level. Pain relief by either technique is transient, rarely lasting more than 2 years. The advantage of cordotomy includes analgesia without significant loss of motor function or touch sensation (124).

NEUROABLATIVE BLOCKS/CHEMONEUROLYSIS

Chemical destruction of nerves (neurolysis) at spinal nerve roots is a relatively simple and painless procedure that can be done with minimal equipment. It is shorter-acting than cordotomy, but unlike this procedure, can be done in the elderly and those with poor general health. Agents used include absolute alcohol and phenol.

NERVOUS SYSTEM STIMULATORS

Various types of central and peripheral nervous system stimulators are used for neurogenic, neuropathic, and ischemic pain syndromes. Dorsal column stimulators (DCS) operate on a principle similar to that of transcutaneous electrical nerve stimulators (TENS), as both produce analgesia by inducing partial depolarization of neurons. DCS consists of an electrode placed in the epidural space and attached to a programmable continuous-pulse pacemaker implanted into a subcutaneous pocket in the abdomen. A sensory thalamic stimulator (STS) consists of an electrode placed into the thalamus of the brain. DCS and STS are used in cases of intractable neurogenic pain unresponsive to medications or other therapies. Peripheral nerve stimulators (PNS) are implantable devices that are most successful in pain syndromes caused by injury to a peripheral nerve. Newer stimulators are taking the form of thermal, vibrotactile, and magnetic stimulators, though these methods have not evolved sufficiently for widespread use in pain management (125).

SPECIAL CONSIDERATIONS IN ANALGESIC PHARMACOTHERAPY

Narcotics exert anticholinergic effects that can be compounded by concomitant use of anticholinergic agents such as diphenhydramine, hydroxyzine, tertiary tricyclic antidepressants, or atropine. The most serious consequence of combined use of these drugs is precipitation of an anticholinergic crisis, manifested by psychosis, tachycardia, cardiac conduction abnormalities with possible first-, second-, or third-degree heart block, coma, and death by cardiorespiratory failure.

Alcohol is often used by patients with chronic pain to decrease suffering. They may drink themselves into a stupor to achieve pain relief through decreased consciousness. Combining analgesics and ethanol produces additive CNS depression with mood changes, depression of respiratory drive, and the danger of lethal overdose. Alcohol in combination with NSAIDs can lead to increased CNS side effects of the NSAIDS, such as disorientation and dizziness, as well as increased gastric irritation and ulceration.

As with alcohol and antihistamines, narcotics can potentiate effects of barbiturates, meprobamate, etchlorvinol, or benzodiazepines, including transient delirium and respiratory failure. Of particular concern is the interaction between fentanyl and midazolam, an ultra-short-acting benzodiazepine used in preoperative anesthetic "cocktails." This combination produced a few deaths from cardiorespiratory failure until lower doses of midazolam with more judicious perioperative monitoring of the patient were used (126).

Patients with obstructive respiratory diseases such as asthma and emphysema or structural abnormalities like kyphoscoliosis are at greater risk of respiratory-drive depression with opiates. Half of the usual starting dose should be prescribed, titrating upward with careful attention to respiratory rate and oxygen saturation. Narcotic suppression of the cerebellar chemoreceptor response to carbon dioxide can have catastrophic consequences in patients whose response to carbon dioxide is already blunted from chronic respiratory disease.

Patients with hepatic failure are at potential risk for drug-induced sequellae when given opiate or NSAIDS, because the liver cannot glucuronidate these agents for renal excretion. In addition, the NSAIDs have been shown to induce hepatocellular necrosis. Acetaminophen is commonly combined with centrally acting opioids. In patients with hepatic dysfunction secondary to alcoholic cirrhosis or hepatitis, chronic doses can precipitate hepatic failure. Cirrhosis also affects the disposition of opiates, as meperidine, pentazocine, and propoxyphene all exhibit increased bioavailability and decreased clearance (127, 128).

Most of the opioids are conjugated and demethylated in the liver to form normetabolites as well as glucuronide metabolites, both of which are excreted by the kidneys. In renal impairment or dysfunction, these metabolites accumulate and produce side effects that last longer than the biological half-lives of the parent compounds. This is particularly true of morphine, dihydrocodeine, propoxyphene, and meperidine. Methadone appears to be safe to use in renal dysfunction when administered at 12- or 24-hr intervals (129, 130).

INTERDISCIPLINARY PAIN MANAGEMENT

Multidisciplinary methods of pain management are emerging as an effective treatment option for complex chronic pain syndromes. The goal of centers using these methods is not to "cure" pain, as this is often unachievable, but to ease the suffering of chronic pain patients and to reduce their reliance on opiate analgesics. These centers strive to improve pain control and improve both psychological and physical functioning and conditioning by involving specialists in the fields of anesthesia, neurology/neurosurgery, internal medicine, physical therapy, pharmacy, psychology, and nursing.

CONCLUSION

Pain management has progressed a great deal scientifically throughout the last century, due in large part to the introduction of more effective pharmacologic agents and a better understanding of their use. Though ancient civilizations did not understand the reason behind applying electric fish to an area affected by neuropathic pain or of using acupuncture to induce analgesia, they did learn through trial and error the methods available to them which gave a therapeutic response. There is still a great deal for practitioners to learn about the mechanisms and treatments for pain.

The pharmacist has a unique role in helping other practitioners develop useful medicinal tools to ease suffering brought on by acute or chronic pain. Through rational drug prescribing and education of both patients and care-givers, effective regimens can be designed to increase pain control while decreasing untoward drug side effects. The pharmacist can help implement such regimens to reduce drug dependence and overall drug use while increasing patient activity. A nationwide movement toward pharmacist involvement with pain-management teams is gaining momentum, as government and third-party issuers seek ways to reduce the financial burden of chronic pain in terms of dollars spent and work days lost.

The pharmacist's role in researching nontraditional medicines for pain relief is integral. Studies involving the use of lidocaine and antidepressants for relief of chronic pain have had pharmacists serving as coinvestigators. Even in the areas of traditional pain management, pharmacists can serve as monitors of medication compliance and efficacy. In the multidisciplinary setting, the pharmacist can provide counseling and guidance to patients who are adjusting their intake of antidepressants, anticonvulsants, or other nonopiate medications, while providing direction in decreasing opiate use. A lucid understanding of pharmacology and pharmacokinetics is invaluable, since opiate habituation and symptoms of withdrawal are highly undesirable and counterproductive. Many such settings allow the pharmacist to see patients on a regular basis, documenting pain relief scores, monitoring side effects, determining when and by how much medication doses should be increased or decreased, selecting alternatives to nontolerated medications, and obtaining pharmacokinetic data or other laboratory parameters. The pharmacist's knowledge of real or potential drug interactions can help providers predict which regimens will be most useful in treating patients, especially those with chronic and debilitating pain syndromes.

REFERENCES

1. Melzack R, Wall PD: On the nature of cutaneous sensory mechanisms. Brain 85:331–356, 1962.
2. Hardy JD, Wolff HG, Goodell H: Pain Sensations and Reactions. Baltimore: Williams & Wilkins, 1952.
3. Bonica JJ: The Management of Pain, ed. 2. Philadelphia: Lea & Febiger, 1990, ch 1.
4. Melzack R, Wall PD: Pain mechanisms: a new theory. Science 150:971–979, 1965.
5. Bonica JJ: The Management of Pain: Philadelphia: Lea & Febiger, 1953.
6. Livingston, WK: Pain Mechanisms. New York: The Macmillan Co., 1943.
7. Wall PD: Presynaptic control of impulses at the first central synapse in the cutaneous pathway. In Physiology of Spinal Neurons. Progress in Brain Research 12. Amsterdam: Elsevier, 1964, pp 92–118.
8. Ganong WF: Review of Medical Physiology. Los Altos, California: Lange Medical Publications, 1985, pp 105.
9. Peters ML, Schmidt AJM: Human pain responsivity. Pain 41:117–119, 1990.
10. Fields HL: Pain. New York: McGraw-Hill, 1987, pp 13–28.
11. Adriaensen H, Gybels J, Handwerker HO, Van Hees J: Response properties of thin myelinated (A-α) fibers in human skin nerves. J Neurophysiol 49:111–122.
12. Price DD, Hu JW, Dubner R, Gracely RH: Peripheral suppression of first pain and central stimulation of second pain evoked by noxious heat pulses. Pain 3:57–68, 1977.
13. Torebjork HE: Afferent C units responding to mechanical, thermal and chemical stimuli in human non-glabrous skin. Acta Physiol Scand 92:374–390, 1974.
14. Torebjork HE, Hallin RG: Perceptual changes accompanying controlled preferential blocking of A and C fibre responses in intact human skin nerves. Exp Brain Res 16:321–332, 1973.
15. Wall PD, McMahon SB: Microneuronography and its relation to perceived sensation: A critical review. Pain 21:209–229, 1985.
16. Willis WD: The origin and destination of pathways involved in pain transmission. In Wall PD, Melzack R: Textbook of Pain, ed. 2. New York: Churchill Livingstone, 1989, pp 112–123.
17. Vierck CJ, Luck MM: Loss and recovery of reactivity to noxious stimuli in monkeys with primary spinothalamic cordotomies, followed by secondary and tertiary lesions of other cord sectors. Brain 102:233–238, 1979.
18. Wall PD, Sweet WH: Temporary abolition of pain in man. Science 155:108–109, 1967.
19. Yaksh TL, Aimone LD: The central pharmacology of pain transmission. In Wall PD, Melzack R: Textbook of Pain, ed. 2. New York: Churchill Livingstone, 1989, p 190.
20. Perl ER: Sensitization of nociceptors and its relation to sensation. In Bonica JJ, Albe-Fessard D: Advances in Pain Research and Therapy, Vol I. New York: Raven Press, 1976, pp 17–28.
21. Beck PW, Handwerker HO: Bradykinin and serotonin effects on various types of cutaneous nerve fibres. Pflugers Arch 347:209–222, 1974.
22. Taiwo YO, Bjerknes LK, Goetzl EJ, Levine JD: Mediation of primary afferent peripheral hyperalgesia by the cAMP second messenger system. Neurosci 32:577–580, 1989.
23. Ferreira SH: Prostaglandins, aspirin-like drugs, and analgesia. Nature 240:200–203, 1972.
24. Taiwo YO, Levine JD: Characterization of the arachidonic acid metabolites mediating bradykinin and noradrenaline hyperalgesia. Brain Res 458:402–406, 1988.
25. Levine JD, Lau W, Kwiat G, Goetzl EJ: Leukotriene B$_4$ produces hyperalgesia that is dependent on polymorphonuclear leukocytes. Science 225:743–745, 1984.
26. Levine JD, Moskowitz MA, Basbaum AI: The effect of gold, an anti-rheumatic therapy, on substance P levels in rat peripheral nerve. Neurosci Lett 87:200–202, 1988.
27. Yaksh TL: Multiple opioid receptor systems in brain and spinal cord: parts 1 and 2. Eur J Anaesth 1:171–243, 1984.
28. DiFazio CA: Pharmacology of narcotic analgesics. Clin J Pain 5(suppl 1):S5–S7, 1989.
29. Millan MJ: κ-Opioid receptors and analgesia. Trends Pharmacol Sci 11:70–76, 1990.

30. Carmody JJ: Opiate receptors: an introduction. Anaesth Intens Care 15:27–37, 1987.

31. Goldstein A, James IF: Multiple opiate receptors: criteria for identification and classification. Trends Pharmacol Sci 5:503–505, 1984.

32. Ferreira SH, Nakamura M: II. Prostaglandin hyperalgesia: the peripheral analgesic activity of morphine, enkephalins, and opioid antagonists. Prostaglandins 18:191–200, 1979.

33. Levine JD, Taiwo YO: Involvement of the mu-opiate receptor in peripheral analgesia. Neuroscience 32:571–575, 1989.

34. DeLander GE, Hopkins CJ: Spinal adenosine modulates descending antinociceptive pathways stimulated by morphine. J Pharmacol Exp Ther 239:88–93, 1986.

35. Duggan AW, North RA: Electrophysiology of opioids. Pharmacol Rev 35:219–282, 1983.

36. Martin WR: A homeostatic and redundancy theory of tolerance to and dependence on narcotic analgesics. Proc Assoc Res Nerv Ment Dis 46:206–225, 1968.

37. Foley KM: Treatment of cancer pain. N Engl J Med 313:84–95, 1985.

38. Bozarth MA, Wise RA: Anatomically distinct opiate receptor fields mediate reward and physical dependence. Science 224:516–517, 1984.

39. Jaffe JH, Martin WR: Opioid analgesics and antagonists. In Gilman AG, Goodman LS, Rall TW, Murad F: The Pharmacological Basis of Therapeutics, ed. 7. New York: Macmillan, 1985, pp 491–531.

40. Romagnoli A, Keats AS: Ceiling effect for respiratory depression by nalbuphine. Clin Pharmacol Ther 27:478–485, 1980.

41. Tamsen A, Gordh T: Epidural clonidine produces analgesia. Lancet i:231–232, 1984.

42. Howe JR, Wang J-Y, Taksh TL: Selective antagonism of the antinociceptive effect of intrathecally applied alpha-adrenergic agonists by intrathecal prazosin and intrathecal yohimbine. J Pharmacol Exp Ther 224:552–558, 1983.

43. Schmauss C, Hammond DL, Ochi JW, Yaksh TL: Pharmacological antagonism of the antinociceptive effects of serotonin in the rat spinal cord. Eur J Pharmacol 90:349–357, 1983.

44. Post C, Gordh T Jr, Jansson I, Hartvig P, Gillberg P-G: Interactions between spinal noradrenergic and cholinergic mechanism of antinociception. Pain (suppl 4):S408, 1987.

45. Panerai AE, Sacerdote P, Bianchi M, Ripamonte C, Manfredi L, Tiengo M, Mantegazza P: Neuropharmacological approach to nociception. In Lipton S, Tunks E, Zoppi M: Advances in Pain Research and Therapy, Vol 13. The Pain Clinic. New York: Raven Press, 1990, pp 41–44.

46. Dickinson AH, Brewer CM, Hayes NA: Effects of topical baclofen on C-fibre evoked neuronal activity in the rat dorsal horn. Neuroscience 14:557–562, 1985.

47. Merskey H (ed): IASP Committee on Taxonomy, Classification of chronic pain: descriptions of chronic pain syndromes and definitions of pain terms. Pain (Suppl 3):S28–S217, 1986.

48. American Pain Society: Principles of analgesic use in the treatment of acute pain and chronic cancer pain, ed. 2. Clin Pharm 9:601–611, 1990.

49. Sternbach RA: Clinical aspects of pain. In Sternbach RA: The Psychology of Pain, ed. 2. New York: Raven Press, 1986, pp 223–239.

50. Levine JD, Taiwo YO: β-Estradiol induced catecholamine-sensitive hyperalgesia: a contribution to pain in Raynaud's phenomenon. Brain Res 487:143–147, 1989.

51. Fields HL: The Medical Center at the University of California, San Francisco Pain Questionnaire, copyright 1988.

52. Bieri D, Reeve RA, Champion GD, Addicoat L, Ziegler JB: The Faces Pain Scale for the self-assessment of the severity of pain experienced by children: development, initial validation, and preliminary investigation for ratio scale properties. Pain 41:139–150, 1990.

53. Foley KM: Cancer pain syndromes. J Pain Symp Manag 2:T3–T7, 1987.

54. Ferrer-Brechner T: Rational management of cancer pain. In Raj PP: Practical Management of Pain. Chicago: Year Book Medical Publishers, 1986, pp 312–328.

55. Inturrisi CE: Newer methods of opioid drug delivery. In IASP Refresher Course on Pain Management: Book of Abstracts. Hamburg, Germany: International Association for the Study of Pain, 1987; 1:27–39.

56. Bennett A: The role of biochemical mediators in peripheral nociception and bone pain. Cancer Surv 7:55–67, 1988.

57. World Health Organization: Cancer Pain Relief. Geneva: World Health Organization, 1986.

58. Inturrisi CE, Max MB, Foley KM, et al.: The pharmacokinetics of heroin in patients with chronic pain. N Engl J Med 210:1213–1217, 1984.

59. Halpern LM: Psychotropics and ataractics and related drugs. Adv Pain Res Ther 2:275–283, 19799.

60. Portenoy RK, Foley KM, Inturrisi CE: The nature of opioid responsiveness and its implications for neuropathic pain: new hypotheses derived from studies of opioid infusions. Pain 43:273–286, 1990.

61. Satterthwaite JR: Acute herpes zoster: diagnosis and treatment. Pain Management 3:17–28, 1990.

62. Loeser JD: Prostherpetic neuralgia: A review of pathophysiology and treatment. Presented at the Annual Meeting of the American Pain Society, Washington, D.C., Nov 8, 1986.

63. Portenoy RK, Duma C, Foley KM: Acute herpetic and postherpetic neuralgia: clinical review and current management. Ann Neurol 20:651–664, 1986.

64. Davis EH: Clinical trials of tegretol in trigeminal neuralgia. Headache 9:77–82, 1969.

65. Bernstein JE, Korman NJ, Bickers DR, Dahl MV, Lawrence LE: Topical capsaicin treatment of chronic postherpetic neuralgia. J Am Acad Dermatol 21:265–270, 1989.

66. Chabal C, Russell LC, Burchiel KJ: The effect of intravenous lidocaine, tocainide and mexiletine on spontaneously active fibers originating in rat sciatic neuromas. Pain 38:333–338, 1989.

67. Max MB, Schafer SC, Culnane M, Dubner R, Gracely RH: Association of pain relief with drug side effects in postherpetic neuralgia: a single-dose study of clonidine, codeine, ibuprofen, and placebo. Clin Pharmacol Ther 43:363–371, 1988.

68. Bach FW, Jensen TS, Kastrup J, Stigsby B, Dejgård A: The effect of intravenous lidocaine on nociceptive processing in diabetic neuropathy. Pain 40:29–34, 1990.

69. Masson EA, Boulton AJM: Aldose reductase inhibitors in the treatment of diabetic neuropathy. A review of the rationale and clinical evidence. Drugs 39:190–202, 1990.

70. Sherman R, Sherman C, Gall N: A survey of current phantom-limb pain treatment in the United States. Pain 8:85–99, 1980.

71. Fine PG: The pharmacologic management of sympathetically maintained pain. Hosp Formul 23:796–808, 1988.

72. Davis KD, Campbell JN, Raja SN, et al.: Topical application of an α-2 agonist relieves hyperalgesia in sympathetically-maintained pain (Abstr.). Pain (suppl):S421, 1990.

73. Currie S: Inflammatory myopathies. Polymyositis and related disorders. In Walton JN: Disorders of Voluntary Muscle, ed. 4. Edinburgh: Churchill Livingstone, 1981, pp 525–568.

74. Lane RJM, Mastaglia FL: Drug-induced myopathies in man. Lancet ii:562–566, 1978.

75. Criswell LA, Sack KE: Tryptophan-induced eosinophilia myalgia syndrome. West J Med 153:269–274, 1990.

76. Jimenez SA, Varga J: The eosinophilia-myalgia syndrome (editorial). West J Med 153:322–323, 1990.

77. Shapiro BS: The management of pain in sickle cell disease. Pediatr Clin North Am 36:1029–1055, 1989.

78. Melzacka M, Neßelhut T, Havemann U, Vetulani J, Kuschinsky K: Pharmacokinetics of morphine in striatum and nucleus accumbens: relationship to pharmacological actions. Pharmacol Biochem Behav 23:295–301, 1985.

79. Hoskin PJ, Hanks GW, Aherne GW, et al.: The bioavailability and pharmacokinetics of morphine after intravenous, oral and buccal administration in healthy volunteers. Br J Clin Pharmacol 27:499–505, 1989.

80. Reidenberg MM, Goodman H, Erle H, et al.: Hydromorphone levels and pain control in patients with severe chronic pain. Clin Pharmacol Ther 44:376–382, 1988.

81. Foley KM: Controversies in cancer pain: Medical perspectives. Cancer 63:2257–2265, 1989.

82. Kaiko RF, Foley KM, Grabinsky PY, et al.: Central nervous system excitatory effects of meperidine in cancer patients. Ann Neurol 13:180–185, 1983.

83. AHFS Drug Information. Bethesda, MD: American Society of Hospital Pharmacists, 1990, pp 1025–1060.

84. Meyers FJ, Meyers FH: Management of chronic pain. Am Fam Practitioner 36:139–146, 1987.

85. Weintraub M, Standish R: Picenadol: a mixed agonist-antagonist narcotic analgesic. Hosp Form 24:71–77, 1989.

86. O'Brien JJ, Benfield P: Dezocine: a preliminary review of its pharmacokinetic properties, and therapeutic efficacy. Drugs 38:226–248, 1989.

87. Stambaugh JE: The use of nonsteroidal anti-inflammatory drugs in chronic bone pain. Orthop Rev 18:54–60, 1989.

88. Jurna I, Brune K: Central effect of the non-steroid anti-inflammatory agents, indometacin, ibuprofen, and diclofenac, determined in C fibre-evoked activity in single neurones of the rat thalamus. Pain 41:71–80, 1990.

89. Harris RH, Vavra I, Ketoprofen: In Rainsford KD: Anti-inflammatory and anti-rheumatic drugs, vol II. Newer anti-inflammatory drugs. Boca Raton, Florida: CRC Press, 1985, pp 151–170.

90. Sunshine A, Olson NZ: Analgesic efficacy of ketoprofen in postpartum, general surgery, and chronic cancer pain. J Clin Pharmacol 28:S47–S54, 1988.

91. Buckley MMT, Brogden RN: Ketorolac: a review of its pharmacodynamic and pharmacokinetic properties, and therapeutic potential. Drugs 39:86–109, 1990.

92. Stambaugh J, Drew J: A double-blind parallel evaluation of the efficacy and safety of a single dose of ketoprofen in cancer pain. J Clin Pharmacol 28:S34–S39, 1988.

93. Wiseman EH: Pharmacologic studies with a new class of nonsteroidal anti-inflammatory agents—the oxicams—with special reference to piroxicam (Feldene). Am J Med 72:2–8, 1982.

94. Krishnan KRR, France RD: Antidepressants in chronic pain syndromes. Am Fam Pract 4:233–237, 1989.

95. Lee R, Spencer PSJ: Antidepressants and pain: a review of the pharmacological data supporting the use of certain tricyclics in chronic pain. J Int Med Res 5(supp 1):146–156, 1977.

96. Feinmann C: Pain relief by antidepressants: Possible modes of actino. Pain 23:1–8, 1985.

97. Messing RB, Lytle LD: Serotonin-containing neurons: their possible role in pain and analgesia. Pain 4:1–21, 1977.

98. Sindrup SH, Gram LF, Brøsen K, Eshøj O, Mogenson EF: The selective serotonin reuptake inhibitor paroxetine is effective in the treatment of diabetic neuropathy syndromes. Pain 42:135–145, 1990.

99. Davis JL, Lewis SB, Gerich JE, et al.: Peripheral diabetic neuropathy treated with amitriptyline and fluphenazine. JAMA 238:2291–2292, 1977.

100. McGee JL, Alexander MR: Phenothiazine analgesia: fact or fantasy. Am J Hosp Pharm 36:633–650, 1979.

101. Hatangdi VS, Boas RA, Edwards EG: Postherpetic neuralgia: management with antiepileptic and tricyclic drugs. Adv Pain Res Ther 1:583–587, 1976.

102. Chabal C, Russell LC, Burchiel KJ: The effects of intravenous lidocaine, tocainide and mexiletine on spontaneously active fibers originating in rat sciatic neuromas. Pain 38:333–338, 1989.

103. Crawley JN, Laverty R, Roth RH: Clonidine reversal of increased norepinephrine metabolite levels during morphine withdrawal. Eur J Pharmacol 57:247–250, 1979.

104. Maze M, Segal IS, Bloor BC: Clonidine and other alpha$_2$ adrenergic agonists: strategies for the rational use of these novel anesthetic agents. J Clin Anesth 1:146–157, 1988.

105. Levine JD, Fye K, Heller P, Basbaum AI, Whiting-O'Keefe Q: Clinical response to regional intravenous guanethidine in patients with rheumatoid arthritis. J Rheumatol 13:1040–1043, 1986.

106. Exton JH: Mechanisms involved in α-adrenergic phenomena. Am J Physiol 248 (Endocrinol Metab 211):E633–E647, 1985.

107. King SA, Strain JJ: Benzodiazepines and chronic pain. Pain 40:3–4, 1990.

108. Forrest WH, Brown BW, Brown CR, et al.: Dextroamphetamine with morphine for the treatment of postoperative pain. N Engl J Med 296:712–715, 1977.

109. Barkas G, Duafala ME: Advances in cancer pain management: A review. Patient-controlled analgesia. J Pain Symp Manag 3:150–160, 1988.

110. Magora F: The spinal route. In Lipton S, Tunks E, Zoppi M: Advances in Pain Research and Therapy, vol 13. The Pain Clinic. New York: Raven Press, 1990, pp 309–314.

111. Max MB, Inturrisi CE, Kaiko RF, et al.: Epidural and intrathecal opiates: cerebrospinal fluid and plasma profiles in patients with chronic cancer pain. Clin Pharmacol Ther 38:631–641, 1985.

112. Gourlay GK, Cherry DA, Plummer JL, Armstrong PJ, Cousins MJ: The influence of drug polarity on the absorption of opioid drugs into CSF and subsequent cephalad migration following lumbar epidural administration: application to morphine and pethidine. Pain 31:297–305, 1987.

113. Arner S, Rawal N, Gustaffson LL: Clinical Experience of long term treatment with extradural and intradural opioids—a nation wide follow-up survey. Br J Anaesth 59:791–799, 1987.

114. Onofrio BM, Yaksh TL: Long-term pain relief produced by intrathecal morphine infusion in 53 patients. J Neurosurg 72:200–209, 1990.

115. Dickinson AH, Sullivan AF, McQuay HJ: Intrathecal etorphine, fentanyl and buprenorphine on spinal nociceptive neurones in the rat. Pain 42:227–234, 1990.

116. Coombs DW, Saunders RL, Fratkin JD, et al.: Continuous intrathecal hydromorphone and clonidine for intractable cancer pain. J Neurosurg 64:890–894, 1986.

117. Mollenholt P, Post C, Paulsson I, Rawal N: Intrathecal and epidural somatostatin in rats: can antinociception, motor effect and neurotoxicity be separated? Pain 43:363–370, 1990.

118. Yaksh TL, Reddy SVR: Studies in the primate on the analgetic effects associated with intrathecal actions of opiate, α-adrenergic agonists and baclofen. Anesthesiology 54:451–467, 1981.

119. Jacobson L, Chabal C, Brody MC, Ward RJ, Wasse L: Intrathecal methadone: a dose-response study and comparison with intrathecal morphine 0.5 mg. Pain 43:141–148, 1990.

120. Roy SD, Flynn GL: Transdermal delivery of narcotic analgesics: pH, anatomical, and subject influences on cutaneous permeability of fantanyl and sufentanil. Pharmaceut Res 7:842–847, 1990.

121. Yaksh TL, Stevens CW: Properties of the modulation of spinal no-

ciceptive transmission by receptor-selective agents. In Dubner R, Gebhart GF, Bond MR: Proceedings of the Fifth World Congress on Pain. Amsterdam: Elsevier, 1988, pp 417–435.

122. Rocco A, Reiestad F, Gudman J, MacKay W: Intrapleural administration of local anesthetics for pain relief in patients with multiple rib fractures. Reg Anesth 12:10–14, 1987.

123. Rapaka RS, Porreca F: Development of delta opioid peptides as nonaddicting analgesics. Pharmaceut Res 8:1–8, 1991.

124. Siegfried J: Neurosurgical treatment of neurogenic pain. In Lipton S, Tunks E, Zoppi M: Advances in Pain Research and Therapy, vol 13. The Pain Clinic. New York: Raven Press, 1990, pp 207–215.

125. McGlone FP, Marsh D: Stimulators for treatment of pain. In Lipton S, Tunks E, Zoppi M: Advances in Pain Research and Therapy, vol 13. The Pain Clinic, New York: Raven Press, 1990, pp 79–82.

126. Forster A, Morel D, Bachmann M, Gemperle M: Respiratory depressant effects of different doses of midazolam and lack of reversal with naloxone—a double-blind randomized study. Anesth Analg 62:920–924, 1983.

127. Seeff LB, Cuccherini BA, Zimmerman HJ, et al.: Acetaminophen hepatotoxicity in alcoholics. Ann Intern Med 104:399–404, 1986.

128. Neal EA, Meffin PJ, Gregory PB, Blaschke TF: Enhanced bioavailability and decreased clearance of analgesics in patients with cirrhosis. Gastroenterology 77:96–102, 1979.

129. Wolfert AI, Sica DA: Narcotic usage in renal failure (editorial). Int J Artif Organs 11:411–415, 1988.

130. Kreek MJ, Schecter AJ, Gutjahr CL, et al.: Methadone use in patients with chronic renal disease. Drug Alc Depend 5:197–205, 1980.

CHAPTER 51

ANXIETY DISORDERS

BARBARA G. WELLS, Pharm.D.

Anxiety is an unpleasant feeling of apprehension or nervousness. It may be a normal, reasonable, and expected response to a stressful situation or perceived danger, or it may be an excessive, irrational feeling state that signifies a mental disorder. The distinction between the two may be difficult to make. Generally in the former, anxiety serves adaptive purposes, while in the latter, it is clearly maladaptive.

ETIOLOGY

Various psychodynamic, psychoanalytic, behavioral, cognitive, and biologic theories have been proposed to explain the pathophysiology of anxiety disorders. Biologic theories of greatest interest include the noradrenergic and benzodiazepine receptor models.

According to the noradrenergic model, the autonomic nervous system of patients with anxiety disorders becomes overreactive to various stimuli. This model may have particular relevance for panic disorder. It is clear that patients with anxiety disorders exhibit symptoms of peripheral autonomic hyperactivity including tremulousness, palpitations, and hyperventilation (1). The locus ceruleus (LC) is a brain stem nucleus that contain 70% of the noradrenergic neurons in the brain. It has extensive projections to the limbic system, cerebral cortex, and cerebellar cortex. In general, drugs with anxiolytic or antipanic efficacy (e.g., tricyclic antidepressants and benzodiazepines) decrease neuronal firing in the LC (2). A notable exception to this is buspirone, which increases LC firing (3). Drugs that stimulate LC activity (e.g., caffeine and yohimbine) are usually anxiogenic, and patients with anxiety disorders are often more susceptible to the anxiogenic effects of these drugs (4).

γ-Aminobutyric acid (GABA) is the major inhibitory neurotransmitter. Two types of GABA receptors have been described, $GABA_A$ receptors that are coupled to chloride channels and $GABA_B$ receptors that are coupled to calcium and possibly cAMP. When GABA interacts with the $GABA_A$ receptor, this facilitates opening of the chloride channel linked to the receptor. The result is augmentation of chloride ion influx intraneuronally (hyperpolarization), making depolarization less likely (5).

Benzodiazepine binding sites have been identified on human neurons. Although an endogenous benzodiazepine receptor agonist has not been identified, an endogenous inverse agonist called diazepam-binding inhibitor (DBI) has been identified. DBI decreases GABA receptor affinity and is anxiogenic (6). The level of anxiety in an individual may be explained by the balance between the action of such inverse agonists, unidentified benzodiazepine agonists and other neurotransmitters whose activity is modulated by GABA receptors (5).

There is some evidence that central serotonin (5HT) activity is involved in controlling anxiety and arousal (7). This area of investigation is in its embryonic stages, but it is likely that 5HT has a complex role in the chain of biologic events that leads to anxiety.

EPIDEMIOLOGY

The National Institute of Mental Health (NIMH) Epidemiologic Catchment Area Study (ECA) provides the most comprehensive information on the epidemiology of anxiety disorders (8). The annual prevalence rate for anxiety disorders overall is 4 to 8:100. Sixteen percent of the population will experience an anxiety disorder during their lifetime. Generally, these disorders begin early in life (before the age of 30 years) and may have a genetic basis, especially panic disorders, phobic disorders, and obsessive compulsive disorder (OCD).

DIAGNOSIS AND CLINICAL FINDINGS

Evaluation of the anxious patient requires a thorough physical examination, psychiatric examination (including the mental status examination), appropriate laboratory workup, and an understanding of the patient's history, including a drug history. It is important to determine whether the symptoms of anxiety represent situational anxiety or an anxiety disorder. Situational anxiety is a normal response to a stressful situation and usually lasts only 2 to 3 weeks. Short-term treatment with an antianxiety agent may be helpful, but more prolonged therapy is unnecessary.

Symptoms of anxiety may be associated with numerous medical illnesses including the cardiovascular (e.g., arrhythmias, angina, myocardial infarction, hypertension, mitral valve prolapse), pulmonary (e.g., chronic obstructive pulmonary disease, pulmonary embolism), digestive (e.g., ulcerative colitis, peptic ulcer disease, irritable bowel syndrome), and endocrine (thyrotoxicosis, pheochromocytoma, hypoglycemia) systems. Symptoms of anxiety may be part of the presentation of these medical illnesses. Furthermore, knowledge that one has a chronic and perhaps disabling medical illness can precipitate anxiety that may in turn complicate treatment and rehabilitation (9).

Anxiety may also be a symptom of an underlying primary psychiatric disorder. Almost all major psychiatric illnesses may be associated with symptoms of anxiety. These include schizophrenia, major depression, dysthymia, mania, delirium, dementia, and substance-use disorders (10).

When symptoms of anxiety are secondary to an underlying medical or psychiatric illness, treatment of the primary illness is the treatment of choice. Use of an antianxiety agent may also be necessary, preferably short-term. Several pharmacologic agents are known to produce anxious symptoms, most notably central nervous system (CNS) stimulants and depressants. CNS stimulants most commonly incriminated include albuterol, amphetamines and other appetite suppressants, cocaine, fenfluramine, isoproterenol, and methylphenidate. Nonprescription drugs well known to cause anxiety include caffeine, nicotine, and decongestants (e.g., ephedrine, pseudoephedrine, oxymetazoline, phenylephrine, phenylpropanolamine, and naphazoline) (11). The elderly and patients with panic disorder may be especially sensitive to the anxiety-producing effects of these agents. CNS depressants (e.g., alcohol, narcotic analgesics, barbiturates, meprobamate, benzodiazepines) may cause anxiety and agitation as a paradoxical reaction, but far more commonly anxiety associated with the use of these agents is a part of the physiologic withdrawal phenomenon following abrupt discontinuation of chronic administration of these agents (10).

The official classification of anxiety disorders according to the American Psychiatric Association is detailed in the Diagnostic and Statistical Manual, 3rd edition, revised (DSM-III-R) (Table 51.1) (1). This manual also specifies

Table 51.1.
DSM-III-R Classification of Anxiety Disorders

Generalized anxiety disorder
Panic disorder
   Panic disorder with agoraphobia
   Panic disorder without agoraphobia
Agoraphobia without history of panic disorder
Social phobia
Simple phobia
Obsessive compulsive disorder
Post-traumatic stress disorder
Anxiety disorder not otherwise specified

Table 51.2.
DSM-III-R Diagnostic Criteria for Generalized Anxiety Disorder[a]

A. Unrealistic or excessive anxiety and worry about two or more life circumstances for a period of 6 months or longer
B. At least 6 of the following 18 symptoms are often present when anxious (do not include symptoms present only during panic attacks)
  Motor tension
    1. Trembling, twitching, or feeling shaky
    2. Muscle tension, aches, or soreness
    3. Restlessness
    4. Easy fatigability
  Autonomic hyperactivity
    5. Shortness of breath or smothering sensation
    6. Palpitations or tachycardia
    7. Sweating or cold clammy hands
    8. Dry mouth
    9. Dizziness or lightheadedness
    10. Nausea, diarrhea, or other abdominal distress
    11. Hot flashes or chills
    12. Frequent urination
    13. Trouble swallowing or "lump in throat"
  Vigilance and scanning
    14. Feeling keyed up or on edge
    15. Exaggerated startle response
    16. Difficulty concentrating or "mind going blank" because of anxiety
    17. Trouble falling or staying asleep
    18. Irritability
C. It cannot be established that an organic factor initiated and maintained the disturbance (e.g., hyperthyroidism, caffeine intoxication)

[a] Adapted from American Psychiatric Association: Diagnostic and Statistical Manual of Mental Disorders, ed. 3, revised (DSM-III-R). Washington, D.C., American Psychiatric Association, 1987, pp 252–253.

the diagnostic criteria and differential diagnosis for each disorder.

Generalized Anxiety Disorder

The diagnostic criteria for generalized anxiety disorder (GAD) (1) are shown in Table 51.2. The age of onset of this disorder is most commonly in the 20s and 30s. It is equally common in males and females, and genetic factors are considered less relevant to the etiology of GAD than panic disorder (10). The essential feature of GAD is excessive and unrealistic worry about two or more life circumstances for 6 months or longer. At least 6 of the 18 specified symptoms are required and are characteristic of motor tension, autonomic hyperactivity, and vigilance. Mild depressive symptoms are common, and social or occupational impairment is rarely more than mild (1).

Panic Disorder

This disorder has an average age of onset in the late 20s. Panic disorder without agoraphobia (phobic avoidance behaviors) is about equally common in males and females; panic disorder with agoraphobia is about twice as common in females as males. It is often a chronic relapsing illness that may require lifetime treatment. Genetic factors play an important role, with approximately 15 to 20% of patients having at least one first-degree relative (mother, father, sister, or brother) with a similar condition, compared with only 2% among relatives of healthy controls (10). Disturbances in LC (12) and parahippocampal (13) structures are implicated in the pathophysiology. Gorman and colleagues (14) hypothesize that the neuroanatomic loci for the acute panic attack, anticipatory anxiety, and phobic avoidance are the brainstem, limbic system, and prefrontal cortex, respectively.

An infusion of lactate or inhalation of 5% carbon dioxide will precipitate panic attacks in patients with panic disorder, but the precise metabolic mechanism underlying this phenomenon has not been delineated (15). Interestingly, one-fourth of panic disorder patients have mitral valve prolapse (MVP), a generally benign valvular lesion, compared to one in 20 in the general population (16).

Essential features of this disorder are recurrent panic attacks with at least four symptoms as described in Table 51.3. Panic attacks are episodes of intense, unprovoked fear or discomfort that usually last minutes, or more rarely, hours. These attacks do not occur just prior to or on exposure to a situation that almost always causes anxiety as

Table 51.3.
DSM-III-R Diagnostic Criteria for Panic Disorder[a]

A. One or more panic attacks have occurred that were unexpected (unrelated to exposure to an anxiety provoking situation) and not triggered by the patient being the focus of attention
B. At least four attacks have occurred within a 4-week period or at least one attack has been followed by a period of at least 1 month of persistent fear of having another attack.
C. At least four of the following symptoms developed during at least one of the attacks:
   1. Shortness of breath (dyspnea) or smothering sensations
   2. Dizziness, unsteadiness, or faintness
   3. Palpitations or tachycardia
   4. Trembling
   5. Sweating
   6. Choking
   7. Nausea or abdominal distress
   8. Depersonalization or derealization
   9. Numbness or tingling (paresthesias)
   10. Hot flashes or chills
   11. Chest pain or discomfort
   12. Fear of dying
   13. Fear of going crazy or of losing control
D. During at least some of the attacks, at least four of the above symptoms developed suddenly and increased in intensity within ten minutes of the beginning of the first symptoms noticed.
E. Not caused by an organic factor, e.g., amphetamine or caffeine intoxication, hyperthyroidism.

[a] Adapted from American Psychiatric Association: Diagnostic and Statistical Manual of Mental Disorders, ed. 3, revised (DSM-III-R). Washington, D.C., American Psychiatric Association, 1987, pp 252–253.

is the case in simple phobia. Additionally, these attacks are not triggered by situations in which the person is the focus of others' attention as is the case in social phobia. Initially the panic attacks are unexpected, but later in the course of the illness certain situations (e.g., being in a crowded place or driving a car) may become associated with having an attack. Entering these situations may then increase the likelihood of an attack occurring, although not immediately upon entering the situation. Panic attacks usually begin with the sudden onset of intense apprehension and fear. There may be feelings of impending doom. Symptoms experienced may include dyspnea, dizziness, palpitations, trembling, sweating, numbness, and chest pain (1).

Most patients who seek treatment have also developed some symptoms of agoraphobia, a fear of being in places or situation where help may be unavailable or where escape might be difficult or embarrassing. As result of this, patients often come to avoid these situations, placing travel restrictions on themselves or only venturing out in the presence of a companion. Common agoraphobic situations include being away from home alone, being in a crowd, standing in line, being on a bridge, and traveling in a bus, train, or car (1).

Most panic disorder patients have recurrent panic attacks several times a week or even daily, and typically this pattern lasts for years, with periods of partial or full remission and exacerbation. Although panic disorder without agoraphobia may cause limited or no social or occupational impairment, panic disorder with agoraphobia is associated with constriction in lifestyle. In severe cases patients may be unable to leave the house alone. Complications of this disorder include psychoactive substance use, particularly alcohol and antianxiety agents, social and occupational impairment, and suicide (1).

Agoraphobia without History of Panic Disorder
Agoraphobia may also occur in the absence of a history of panic disorder. In clinical samples this disorder is rare, but impairment is usually severe. It is diagnosed far more commonly in females than in males and typically persists for many years. In agoraphobia without history of panic disorder, the common agoraphobic situations are the same as described above. Typically, the person is afraid of having a limited symptom attack, that is, developing one to three symptoms of panic attack (not enough for diagnosis of panic disorder) or loss of bladder or bowel control, vomiting, or having cardiac distress. In some cases, patients have experienced such symptoms in the past; in others they have not, but fear developing them. Some of these patients subsequently develop panic disorder (1).

Social Phobia
Social phobia with symptoms of fear of eating in public places, writing in public, or using public restrooms is con-

sidered rare. However, social phobia involving fear of public speaking and fear of many social situations is common. In clinical samples this disorder is more common in males than in females, but this may not be the case in unselected samples. This disorder often begins in late childhood or early adolescence (1).

Social phobia is characterized by a fear of one or more social situations when the person is exposed to scrutiny by others and fears doing something humiliating. The fear may be circumscribed, as in fears of having a hand tremor when writing in the presence of others or fears of choking when eating in front of others. In other cases, the fears may involve most social situations. The feared situations are usually avoided, but less commonly they may be endured with intense anxiety. The diagnosis is made only if the avoidant behavior interferes with social or occupational functioning. This disorder is rarely incapacitating, but it usually causes some interference with social or occupational functioning. Fear of public speaking may in some cases interfere with occupational advancement. Complications of social phobia include depression and abuse of alcohol and anxiolytics (1).

Simple Phobia

Simple phobias are common but rarely cause marked impairment. This disorder is more common in females than in males. Animal phobias usually begin in childhood, blood-injury phobias in adolescence or early adulthood. Phobias of heights, driving, closed spaces, and air travel most commonly begin in the fourth decade of life. The most common simple phobias involve animals, especially dogs, snakes, insects, and mice. Other simple phobias involve closed spaces (claustrophobia), heights (acrophobia), air travel, and witnessing blood or tissue injury (blood-injury phobia). During some phase of the disturbance, exposure to the phobic stimulus predictably provokes an immediate anxiety response, such as panicky feelings, sweating, and tachycardia. These situations are therefore usually avoided, but they may be endured with intense anxiety. As in the case of social phobia, these persons invariably recognize that the fear is excessive and unreasonable. Impairment is usually minimal, as the phobic object or situation is merely avoided. However, impairment may be considerable if the phobic object is common and cannot be avoided (1).

Obsessive Compulsive Disorder

Obsessive compulsive disorder (OCD) usually begins in adolescence or early adulthood. The course is usually chronic, but with some waxing and waning of symptoms. Until recently the disorder was thought to be relatively rare. The prevalence rate is now considered to be approximately 2% (17). The essential feature of OCD is re-current obsessions or compulsions that cause marked distress, are time-consuming, or interfere significantly with normal occupational functioning, social activities, or relationships.

Obsessions are persistent ideas, thoughts, impulses, or images that are experienced as intrusive and senseless. Examples include recurrent thoughts of harming a loved one, recurrent blasphemous thoughts, or recurrent thoughts of contamination. Compulsions are repetitive, intentional, purposeful behaviors performed in response to an obsession in a certain stereotyped fashion. However, the activity is not realistically connected with the obsession it is designed to neutralize, or it is clearly excessive. Usually the person recognizes that the behavior is excessive or unreasonable. Although the behavior provides some decrease in anxiety, these persons do not derive pleasure from carrying out the activity. Examples of common compulsions are repetitive hand-washing, counting, checking (door locks, light switches, burners on the stove, etc.), and touching. When these patients resist a compulsion or are prevented from performing the compulsive behavior, there is a sense of mounting anxiety. Patients with OCD are often moderately to severely impaired, and in some cases acting on compulsions may become the major life activity. Complications of OCD include major depression and abuse of alcohol or antianxiety agents.

Post-traumatic Stress Disorder

Post-traumatic stress disorder (PTSD) can occur at any age. The lifetime prevalence is reported to be 1% (18). Patients with this disorder develop symptoms following a severely stressful event that is outside the realm of usual human experience and is usually experienced with fear, terror, and helplessness. Characteristic symptoms of PTSD involve avoidance of stimuli associated with the event, numbing of general responsiveness, increased arousal and reexperiencing the event through intrusive thoughts, flashbacks, or nightmares. Usually the traumatic events involve a serious threat to the life or physical integrity of the individual (or a close friend or loved one). The traumatic events often have violent themes, such as injury, physical violence, and torture, and many involve natural disasters (e.g., earthquakes), accidents (e.g., airplane crashes, fires), and deliberately caused disasters (e.g., bombing, concentration camps, torture). The disorder is more likely to occur and more likely to be severe after a traumatic event of human design (1).

The traumatic event can be reexperienced through recurrent and intrusive recollections, recurrent distressing dreams, or dissociative states lasting a few seconds to a few days. Patients with PTSD commonly attempt to avoid thoughts of feelings about the event and situations that rekindle memories of the event. There may be amnesia for selected aspects of the event. These individuals may manifest a "psychic numbing," which is a diminished responsiveness to the external world, and this symptom usually begins soon after the traumatic event. The person may feel estranged from others and unable to feel emotions of any type, especially intimacy and sexuality.

Symptoms of increased arousal may include sleep disturbance, hypervigilance, and exaggerated startle response. Patients may complain of poor concentration and irritability, and in severe cases may exhibit unpredictable explosions of aggressive behavior (1).

Impairment may be mild to severe. In severe cases, symptoms may affect nearly every aspect of life including ability to hold employment and interpersonal relationships. Emotional lability, depression, and guilt may lead to suicidality. Psychoactive substance use disorders are also common complications (1).

TREATMENT
Nonpharmacologic Approaches

Several nonpharmacologic interventions are available for treating primary anxiety disorders, and when combined with drug therapy, can yield greater improvement than is achieved with either approach alone (19). Supportive therapy usually consists of listening to the patient's problems and offering encouragement and support. A few sessions of supportive therapy may significantly mitigate anxiety complaints and may even obviate the need for pharmacotherapy, especially in the case of GAD. Education on the anxiety disorders and the role of the autonomic nervous system in mediating signs and symptoms may allay fears in GAD, mild cases of panic disorder, and PTSD.

Behavior therapy involving some form of exposure to the phobic situation is the treatment of choice for most phobias and for the phobic avoidance behavior in panic disorder and OCD (20). Exposure therapy involves gradual exposure to and increasingly prolonged contact with the phobic situation. Cognitive therapy is most often used to treat GAD, but it may also have applications in treatment of phobias (21). In this treatment approach it is assumed that anxious symptoms are caused by cognitions (thoughts or images) and schemata (silent assumptions). Cognitive therapy is directed at reducing anxious symptoms that are derived from these cognitions. The patient is assisted in developing new cognitions that do not produce anxious symptoms. Treatment is also directed toward modifying the schemata.

Relaxation techniques that depend on systematically tensing and relaxing muscle groups are used with variable success in the treatment of panic disorder, GAD, and situational anxiety. The underlying premise of this treatment approach is that anxiety and relaxation cannot coexist. Electromyographic biofeedback is sometimes used to facilitate learning muscle relaxation techniques (22).

Nonpharmacologic interventions alone are insufficient in many patients with anxiety disorders, especially when they are severe. Many OCD patients are either resistant to behavioral approaches or are unresponsive. In panic disorder, behavioral approaches are known to be effective for reducing phobic avoidance, but pharmacotherapy is usually necessary to eliminate panic attacks (23).

Pharmacologic Approaches

As a general rule, if anxiety is associated with a medical disorder, then the first line of treatment should be directed at the underlying medical condition. In addition, a brief trial of a benzodiazepine may be a reasonable adjunct. Similarly, if the anxiety is associated with an underlying major psychiatric disorder, treatment should be directed toward the underlying psychiatric disorder (e.g., antipsychotics for schizophrenia). If anxiety is situational, in most cases antianxiety agents are unnecessary, as situational anxiety is short-term and self-limiting. However, some cases may merit short-term intervention with a benzodiazepine.

Psychotherapy is generally the preferred treatment approach for GAD, especially if symptoms are mild. However, for patients whose symptoms cause significant discomfort or impairment, short-term antianxiety agents may be indicated. The benzodiazepines, buspirone, and to a lesser extent the β-adrenergic blocking agents are the most appropriate pharmacologic alternatives. Because of high abuse potential and narrow therapeutic index, meprobamate and the barbiturates are largely of historical interest. Diphenhydramine, hydroxyzine, and other antihistamines are sometimes prescribed, especially for elderly patients. Their primary advantage is lack of potential for physiologic dependence, however, their efficacy is not well established, and anticholinergic side effects can be troublesome (24).

The pharmacotherapeutic armamentarium for treatment of panic disorders continues to grow. Most clinicians combine antipanic medications and behavioral therapy, with moderate-to-marked improvement in approximately 85% of patients (23). The monoamine oxidase inhibitor (MAOI) phenelzine is an effective treatment for panic disorder (25). Several double-blind studies have demonstrated the efficacy of imipramine in this disorder as well (23, 26, 27). More recently, two additional tricyclic antidepressants (TCAs), desipramine (28) and clomipramine (29) have shown possible efficacy, and preliminary evidence supports the efficacy of fluoxetine, a 5HT-reuptake inhibitor (30, 31). Alprazolam is more effective than placebo, (32) and is the only drug that is FDA-approved for use in this disorder. Imipramine and alprazolam are probably equally effective, but more patients discontinue imipramine therapy, especially early in treatment, because of side effects (33). Further, alprazolam may not be unique among benzodiazepines in its antipanic effects, as diazepam, clonazepam (34), and lorazepam (35) have been shown to have similar therapeutic effects.

In treatment of social phobias, both the β-adrenergic blockers (36, 37) and the MAOI phenelzine (37) are effective. The β-blockers (propranolol or atenolol) are more useful in treating the specific form of social phobia (anxiety in one situation, e.g., public speaking), whereas phenelzine appears more useful for the generalized form of the disorder (characterized by anxiety in several social situations) (38).

Although most investigators consider simple phobias to be unresponsive to drug therapy, it is usually responsive to behavioral treatments.

Double-blind trials support the efficacy of clomipramine in treating OCD (39). It is the only FDA-approved drug for treating OCD. Evidence from open trials supports efficacy for fluoxetine (40), and double-blind data show effectiveness of fluvoxamine (41), which is still in premarketing trials. Behavior therapy (exposure therapy with response prevention) combined with pharmacotherapy is preferred for most patients, provided compulsions are present. Behavior therapy would be expected to offer little if obsessions but no compulsive rituals are present (42).

Pharmacotherapy alone is rarely sufficient to provide complete remission of PTSD, but it can facilitate participation in individual or group psychotherapy. The literature is replete with case reports and open trials of drug therapy in treating this condition, but there is a paucity of double-blind investigation. Preliminary reports suggest that phenelzine and imipramine may be effective (43). In addition, amitriptyline was superior to placebo in a double-blind trial in 46 patients (18). Uncontrolled reports, usually in small samples, have touted the potential usefulness of

doxepin, desipramine, carbamazepine, clonidine, and propranolol. Clearly, these reports require corroboration by rigorous investigation (18).

Benzodiazepines

INDICATIONS

Anxiety disorders where benzodiazepines are useful include GAD and panic disorder. All benzodiazepines are effective in treatment of GAD, and they are considered by most clinicians to be the class of first choice in treating of this disorder. Benzodiazepine antianxiety agents are shown in Table 51.4. They are the most widely prescribed agents for GAD and account for approximately 5% of prescriptions dispensed by community pharmacies (44). Predictors of response to benzodiazepines in patients with GAD include acuteness of symptoms, presence of a precipitating stress, high level of psychic and somatic anxiety, low level of depression and interpersonal problems, lack of previous treatment or good response to previous treatment, expectation of recovery, desire for medications, awareness that symptoms are psychologic, and improvement during the first week of treatment (5).

Nearly 500 patients have participated in 12 published controlled trials establishing the efficacy of alprazolam as an antipanic agent (45). Nine studies were placebo-controlled. Alprazolam is an effective antipanic and antiphobic agent that is superior to placebo and probably has efficacy equal to that of imipramine and phenelzine. Furthermore, alprazolam is better tolerated and has a more rapid onset of antipanic effects than the antidepressants. There is evidence to support the efficacy of clonazepam (45), diazepam (46), and lorazepam (35).

There is no drug of choice in treating panic disorder.

Table 51.4.
Benzodiazepines Used in Treatment of Anxiety Disorders

Generic Name	Brand Name/Manufacturer	Approximate Equivalent Dose (mg/day)	Usual Dosage Range (mg/day)[a]
Alprazolam	Xanax/Upjohn	0.5	0.75–4 (anxiety)
Chlordiazepoxide	Librium/Roche, Generics	10	1.5–10 (panic)[b] 15–75 (anxiety)
Clonazepam	Klonopin/Roche	0.25	1–6 (panic)
Clorazepate	Tranxene/Abbott Generics	7.5	15–60 (anxiety)
Diazepam	Valium/Roche, Generics	5	5–40 (anxiety) 30–40 (panic)
Halazepam	Paxipam/Schering	20	60–160 (anxiety)
Lorazepam	Ativan/Wyeth, Generics	1	2–6 (anxiety) 2–10 (panic)
Oxazepam	Serax/Wyeth, Generics	15	30–120 (anxiety)
Prazepam	Centrax/Parke-Davis Generics	10	20–60 (anxiety)

[a] Elderly patients usually require approximately one-half the doses required for younger adults. Dosage in the elderly must be carefully individualized.
[b] FDA-approved for treating panic disorder.

TCAs are sometimes used as first-line treatment because they lack abuse and physiologic dependence potential. Benzodiazepines frequently cause physiologic dependence with chronic dosing, however in general, panic disorder patients without a history of alcohol or substance abuse do not seek to increase or prolong dosing unnecessarily. A relatively rapid onset of action and benign side-effect profile make the benzodiazepines an appealing choice. Of the benzodiazepines, some clinicians prefer clonazepam over alprazolam because of its longer half-life of elimination, sustained therapeutic effect, and lack of euphoriant properties. Clearly, in patients with a history of prior alcohol or other substance abuse, an antidepressant is the preferred therapeutic option (45). Benzodiazepines should be used with caution in patients whose panic disorder is complicated by depression. Antidepressants should be chosen first for panic patients who are clinically depressed or have a family history of depression (47).

MECHANISM OF ACTION

Benzodiazepines may exert antianxiety effects through the potentiation of the inhibitory neurotransmitter, GABA. Benzodiazepine-binding sites have been identified in cortical and limbic forebrain areas in the CNS. These receptors are linked to GABA receptors. When benzodiazepines interact at the benzodiazepine receptor, the affinity of the GABA receptor for GABA is increased. This causes an amplification of the GABA-mediated chloride ion influx intracellularly, with resultant hyperpolarization (5). Benzodiazepines inhibit firing in the LC (10).

PHARMACOKINETICS

The pharmacokinetics of the benzodiazepine antianxiety agents are summarized in Table 51.5. Subtle differences in the pharmacokinetic profiles may aid clinicians in selecting the most appropriate agent. When immediate effects are desired, as in treatment of acute anxiety or in as-needed (p.r.n.) treatment of anxiety, it is important to select an agent with rapid onset. In treating anxiety of a more chronic nature with more prolonged dosing, this becomes less important. Similarly, if panic attacks occur between doses of alprazolam, it may be helpful to switch the patient to clonazepam, as the longer half-life of elimination seems to be associated with a more sustained duration of action (45).

The highly lipophilic benzodiazepines, diazepam and clorazepate, are rapidly absorbed and distributed into the CNS. As a result, an anxiolytic effect can be anticipated within 1 hr of dosing with these agents. This rapid entry into the CNS may be associated with a "rush" in some patients that may contribute to the likelihood of abuse. Similarly, the highly lipophilic agents are rapidly distributed peripherally to inactive storage sites (adipose tissue).

This accounts for the short duration of action seen with single dosing of clorazepate and diazepam (48). Lorazepam and oxazepam are less lipophilic. This results in a slower onset of antianxiety effect but a more prolonged effect than might be expected based on half-life, because extensive tissue distribution does not occur (44).

Clorazepate and prazepam are prodrugs and do not have antianxiety activity until they are converted to the metabolite, N-desmethyldiazepam (N-DMDZ). Clorazepate is converted rapidly in the acidic gastric environment to N-DMDZ by a pH-dependent process. Administration of antacids may elevate the pH of the stomach and significantly decrease the rate of N-DMDZ formation. Conversion of prazepam to N-DMDZ is a much slower process, as transformation occurs in the liver. Consequently, several hours are required to achieve peak plasma concentrations of N-DMDZ after administration of prazepam. Prazepam would not be an appropriate drug to choose when acute (rapid) antianxiety effects are desired.

In the unusual circumstance that an intramuscular preparation is to be used, lorazepam provides the most predictable absorption. Diazepam and chlordiazepoxide intramuscular injections can be painful and are absorbed erratically (48).

With chronic dosing, the rate and extent of accumulation depend upon clearance and half-life of elimination of parent compound and active metabolites. The benzodiazepines are biotransformed by two primary metabolic processes, hepatic microsomal oxidation (N-dealkylation and aliphatic hydroxylation) and glucuronide conjugation. Oxidation may be impaired by aging, liver disease, and concurrent administration of drugs that inhibit oxidative processes. In this situation greater plasma concentrations and total body stores at steady state would be expected (48). Conjugation is not affected by these factors.

As shown in Table 51.5, several benzodiazepines are converted by N-dealkylation to N-DMDZ, which is an active metabolite with a half-life of elimination of 36 to 200 hr. Further oxidation converts N-DMDA to oxazepam, which is then conjugated and excreted. Extensive accumulation of N-DMDZ at steady-state provides a long duration of antianxiety effects, allowing once or twice daily dosing if desired. In the presence of impaired oxidation, prolonged half-life and increased accumulation may be associated with excessive sedation and ataxia in some patients (48).

Alprazolam, oxazepam, and lorazepam have short-to-intermediate half-lives of elimination, so a shorter time is required to achieve steady-state accumulation and plasma concentrations. Alprazolam is oxidized to α-hydroxyalprazolam, which is present in small amounts and probably does not contribute substantially to clinical efficacy. Oxazepam and lorazepam do not undergo oxidation; they are simply glucuronidated and excreted (48). For this reason,

Table 51.5.
Pharmacokinetic Profile of the Benzodiazepine Antianxiety Agents[a]

Generic Name	Time to Peak Plasma Concentration (hr)	Half-Life of Elimination[b]	Protein Binding (%)	Biotransformation Pathway	Clinically Important Metabolites
Alprazolam	1–2	12–15	80	Oxidation	None
Chlordiazepoxide	1–4	5–30	96	N-Dealkylation	Desmethchlordiazepoxide
					Demoxepam
					N-DMDZ[c]
					Oxazepam
Clonazepam		20–80			
Clorazepate	1–2	Prodrug	97	Oxidation	N-DMDZ[c]
					Oxazepam
Diazepam	0.5–2	20–80	98	Oxidation	N-DMDZ[c]
					Oxazepam
Halazepam	1–3	7–14	97	Oxidation	3-Hydroxyhalazepam
					N-DMDZ[c]
					Oxazepam
Lorazepam	2–4	10–20	85	Conjugation	None
Oxazepam	2–4	5–20	87	Conjugation	None
Prazepam	6	Prodrug	97	Oxidation	3-Hydroxyprazepam
					N-DMDZ[c]
					Oxazepam

[a] Modified from Dommisse CS, Hayes PE: Current concepts in clinical therapeutics: anxiety disorders, Part 2. Clin Pharm 6:196–215, 1987.
[b] Parent compound.
[c] N-Desmethyldiazepam half-life 36–200 hours.

oxazepam and lorazepam are considered good choices for the patient suspected of having impaired oxidative processes.

Patients with hypoalbuminemia may have a significantly greater free (pharmacologically active) fraction of benzodiazepines that are highly protein bound. For these patients lorazepam or oxazepam would be a rational choice because of its lower percentage of protein binding.

DOSING

Usual doses of benzodiazepines in treatment of anxiety and panic are shown in Table 51.4. Benzodiazepines with long half-lives of elimination may be dosed once daily at bedtime if desired, thereby providing hypnotic effects as well as daytime antianxiety effects. Agents with shorter half-lives (oxazepam, lorazepam, and alprazolam) are usually administered in divided daily doses. Patients should be started on low doses and titrated upward to the lowest effective dose. Treatment duration should be as brief as possible.

In treating panic, alprazolam is usually begun at 0.5 mg three times daily. The average maintenance dose is approximately 3 to 4 mg/day, although some patients require up to 10 mg/day or more. Some patients require five or six doses daily to prevent interdose increases in anxiety or panic attacks. These patients may do better if switched to clonazepam, because it can be administered twice daily.

Clonazepam is started at a dose of 0.5 mg or less once daily. Panic attacks are often controlled at a dose of 1 to 2 mg/day in two divided doses; however, many patients require more (3 to 6 mg/day). When a benzodiazepine is to be given for panic disorder, some clinicians select clonazepam initially over alprazolam because of the more continuous control of anxiety afforded some patients with less frequent dosing (45). Diazepam in doses of 10 to 60 mg/day (mean dose of 30 to 40 mg/day and lorazepam in doses of up to 16 mg/day (mean dose of 6 mg/day) may be effective in treating panic disorder (45).

ADVERSE DRUG REACTIONS

The most common adverse effect associated with benzodiazepine therapy is CNS depression manifested as sedation, psychomotor impairment, and ataxia, Many patients experience mild drowsiness during the first few days of treatment, but tolerance usually begins to develop during the first week. Anterograde amnesia (loss of memory for events occurring after drug ingestion) is reported with benzodiazepine use. This often goes unnoticed, but any complaints of forgetfulness by patients on benzodiazepines should be explored further for possible drug-induced amnesia. In addition, a paradoxical excitement, aggressiveness, confusion, and disorientation may occur, especially in the elderly (44). Depression may be aggravated by benzodiazepines in some patients (5). The risk of being involved in a serious accident is fivefold greater in drivers taking benzodiazepines, and the risk is even greater if the driver concurrently uses alcohol (5).

Benzodiazepines are surprising well tolerated, even at the higher end of the dosage range, in patients with panic disorder. In patients taking alprazolam, the dropout rate due to side effects is less than 5%. Depression and nausea are side effects reported with clonazepam treatment of panic attacks (44).

DRUG INTERACTIONS

Drug-drug interactions involving benzodiazepines are summarized in Table 51.6. Concurrent use of alcohol and a benzodiazepine increases sedation and has an additive or synergistic deleterious effect on psychomotor performance. This combination is potentially lethal. Several drugs may impair the oxidative metabolism of benzodiazepines. These include propranolol, metoprolol, cimetidine, disulfiram, isoniazid, omeprazole, oral contraceptives, and valproic acid. If an interaction is suspected with one of these drugs, the clinician should consider decreasing the dose of the oxidatively metabolized benzodiazepine. In some cases it may be prudent to select lorazepam or oxazepam instead of a benzodiazepine metabolized by oxidative processes. Conversely, rifampin stimulates oxidative metabolic pathways. Antacids decrease the rate of absorption of diazepam and chlordiazepoxide and decrease both the rate and extent of absorption of N-DMDZ from clorazepate. It is therefore recommended that the administration times for benzodiazepines and antacids be staggered. Ranitidine may cause decreased gastrointestinal absorption of diazepam. Concurrent administration of procarbazine with the benzodiazepines may cause increased sedation, and co-administration of theophylline may antagonize diazepam-induced sedation and impairment of psychomotor performance. Elevated serum digoxin concentrations with signs and symptoms of toxicity may occur with the addition of diazepam or alprazolam to the regimen. Both increased and decreased serum concentrations of phenytoin have been reported with addition of diazepam or chlordiazepoxide. In addition, increased oxazepam elimination has been reported in patients taking phenytoin alone or in combination with phenobarbital. In parkinsonian patients, addition of benzodiazepines may impair the therapeutic effects of levodopa by an unknown mechanism. There is a single case report of hypothermia occurring on three occasions in one patient when diazepam was given with lithium. The mechanism underlying this interaction is unknown. Another poorly understood interaction is the reported enhancement of and resistance to the neuromuscular blocking effect of nondepolarizing muscle relaxants (49). Lastly, a particularly troubling interaction between temazepam and diphenhydramine has been reported, resulting in the stillbirth of an infant (50).

Cigarette smokers may have a decreased response to diazepam, and the stimulating effects of caffeine (via coffee consumption or other modes of ingestion) may counteract the antianxiety effects of the benzodiazepines.

PATIENT EDUCATION

Patients should be told (in terminology they can understand) about the expected benefits, expected length of therapy, common side effects, and precautions to be observed with any medications they are taking. Detailed patient-education information can be found in the USP-DI published by the United States Pharmacopeial Convention, Inc. (51). Patients should be told that although they will likely experience some antianxiety and/or antipanic effects during the first weeks, they should maintain regular contact with the prescriber as long as they are on this medication. The prescriber should regularly assess side effects and make a decision on the need to continue drug therapy. If depression emerges or becomes more pronounced, the prescriber should be notified (51).

Patients should understand that with continued dosing, their medication can cause a physical dependence and that stopping the medication abruptly may result in withdrawal side effects. They should, therefore, not discontinue medication abruptly without first checking with the prescriber, who may elect to gradually taper the dose downward before discontinuing it (51).

Female patients of child-bearing potential should understand that taking benzodiazepines during pregnancy may be associated with risks including birth defects (if taken during the first trimester), physiologic dependence in the baby, and other selected problems in the newborn, such as drowsiness, slow heart beat, and difficulty breathing (51).

DEPENDENCE, WITHDRAWAL, TOLERANCE, AND ABUSE

Physiologic dependence is defined by the emergence of withdrawal symptoms upon discontinuation of therapy. Benzodiazepine dependence is well documented, and a mild withdrawal syndrome occurs in up to 44% of patients receiving therapeutic doses of benzodiazepines for 4 to 6 weeks (52). Mild withdrawal symptoms include anxiety, insomnia, irritability, anorexia, diaphoresis, irritability, and sensitivity to light and sound. In more severe cases, withdrawal may include confusion, depersonalization, myoclonus, nausea, delirium, and psychosis. The onset of withdrawal usually occurs 1 to 2 days after discontinuing (or reducing the dose of) short-to-intermediate half-life benzodiazepines and 5 to 10 days after discontinuing (or reducing the dose of) the long half-life entities. Although prominent withdrawal symptoms generally subside within 1 to 3 weeks, mild symptoms may persist for several

Table 51.6.

Drug-Drug Interactions with the Benzodiazepine Antianxiety Agents[a]

Drug	Effect	Management
Antacids	Decreased rate of diazepam and chlordiazepoxide absorption; decreased rate and extent of DMDZ absorption from clorazepate	Stagger administration times
β-Adrenergic blockers	Propranolol and metroprolol cause a small reduction in oxidative metabolism of diazepam and DMDZ	If interaction suspected, consider lowering dose of benzodiazepine
Cimetidine	Decreased oxidative metabolism of diazepam, chlordiazepoxide, desalkylmetabolites, alprazolam, and triazolam	Of limited clinical significance in healthy adults; consider diazepam dosage reduction, selection of lorazepam or oxazepam, or selection of H_2 antagonist that does not affect oxidative metabolism of benzodiazepines (famotidine or nazatidine)
Digoxin	Elevated digoxin serum concentrations with sign/symptoms of toxicity reported with addition of alprazolam or diazepam	If interaction suspected, consider decreasing the dose of digoxin during concurrent benzodiazepine administration; monitor digoxin serum levels
Diphenhydramine	Stillbirth reported following coadministration of temazepam and diphenhydramine	Avoid this combination
Disulfiram	Decreased oxidative metabolism of diazepam, chlordiazepoxide, and desalkylmetabolites	Consider lowering dose of oxidatively metabolized benzodiazepines during concurrent disulfiram administration
Ethanol	Decreased volume of distribution and impaired elimination of diazepam and other benzodiazepines; increased sedation and additive or synergistic deleterious effects on psychomotor performance	Avoid ethanol ingestion during concurrent benzodiazepine administration
Fluoxetine	Decreased oxidative metabolism of diazepam	Probably not of clinical relevance; if interaction suspected, lower dose of diazepam or other oxidatively metabolized benzodiazepine
Hydantoins	Increased and decreased phenytoin serum concentrations reported with addition of diazepam or chlordiazepoxide; increased oxazepam elimination in patients taking phenytoin alone or in combination with phenobarbital	If interaction suspected, monitor hydantoin serum concentrations and adjust dose accordingly
Isoniazid	Decreased oxidative metabolism of diazepam and triazolam	If interaction suspected, consider lowering dose of diazepam and other oxidatively metabolized benzodizepines
Levodopa	Worsening of rigidity, bradykinesia, and tremor	If interaction suspected, consider increasing dose of levodopa
Lithium	Hypothermia reported with lithium and diazepam combination (1 case report)	If hypothermia occurs, discontinue this drug combination
Nondepolarizing muscle relaxants	Both enhancement of and resistance to the neuromuscular blocking effects of nondepolarizing muscle relaxants have been reported	
Omeprazole	Decreased oxidative metabolism of diazepam	If interaction is suspected, lower dose of diazepam or other oxidatively metabolized benzodiazepine
Oral contraceptives	Oral contraceptives decrease clearance of diazepam, chlordiazepoxide, and triazolam, and perhaps alprazolam; metabolism of oxazepam, lorazepam, and temazepam may be increased	Lower dose of diazepam and other oxidatively metabolized benzodiazepines may be required during concurrent administration of oral contraceptives
Procarbazine	Increased sedation can occur when CNS depressants are used with procarbazine	Adjust benzodiazepine dose to minimize sedation, or avoid combination; questionable clinical significance
Rantidine	Decreased gastrointestinal absorption of diazepam; increased oral bioavailability and hypnotic action of midazolam	Undetermined clinical significance
Rifampin	Increased oxidative metabolism of diazepam and N-DMDZ	If interaction suspected, consider increased dose of oxidatively metabolized benzodiazepine
Theophyllines	Theophyllines may antagonize diazepam-induced impairment of psychomotor performance and sedation	If interaction is suspected, consider increasing dose of diazepam
Valproic acid	Decreased oxidative metabolism of diazepam; protein binding of diazepam may also be altered	Undetermined clinical significance; if interaction suspected, consider decreasing dose of oxidatively metabolized benzodiazepines

[a] Modified from Drug Therapy Screening System.

months (5). Withdrawal is more likely to occur and to be severe if the duration of therapy has been long and if high doses have been used. Withdrawal may also be more severe following the use of the short-to-intermediate half-life drugs lorazepam, oxazepam, and alprazolam (44).

Withdrawal symptoms after discontinuation or gradual downward tapering of benzodiazepines in panic patients may be particularly difficult, as high doses are often used for prolonged periods. A lack of cross-tolerance with diazepam has been reported (44).

Two other discontinuation syndromes are described and may be confused with withdrawal. Relapse is simply a return of the original symptoms of anxiety, which may occur weeks to months after drug discontinuation. Rebound refers to a return of the original symptoms, but with greater intensity. This may occur hours to days after drug discontinuation, and it is followed by recovery to pretreatment status (5).

Benzodiazepines should be discontinued gradually, by one-eighth to one-fourth of the total dose every few weeks to allow careful monitoring and to reduce the risk of withdrawal or rebound. Substituting a long half-life benzodiazepine for a short-to-intermediate half-life drug before downward tapering may reduce the severity of withdrawal symptoms (5). In some cases, patients taking alprazolam will require more gradual downward tapering (0.25 to 0.5 mg/week) than that recommended by the package insert (0.5 mg/3 days) (44).

In treating GAD, the lowest effective dose for the shortest possible period should be used. Periodic attempts at drug discontinuation should be made. For patients who relapse, intermittent treatment coinciding with the fluctuating nature of the illness is often effective. Many clinicians believe that some patients need to continue the medication long-term. This may include those who relapse frequently, face persistent stresses, are unable to resolve conflict, or may suffer physical harm from chronic anxiety. Major risks associated with long-term use (e.g., physical dependence and impaired psychomotor performance) must be weighed against the benefits of benzodiazepine therapy (5, 53).

Recommendations about appropriate duration of benzodiazepine treatment in panic disorder are more difficult to make. There is a relatively high rate of relapse after discontinuation of all pharmacotherapy (benzodiazepines and antidepressants). Side effects of antidepressant therapy are a significant cause of morbidity and noncompliance. Antidepressant therapy poses an important risk for overdose in these patients, as well. The high-potency benzodiazepines, which are safe, well-tolerated, and apparently without therapeutic tolerance in most patients, are a reasonable option for maintenance therapy in these patients. Clonazepam may offer important advantages over alprazolam and lorazepam in long-term treatment because

of the less frequent occurrence of interdose panic attacks, and patients may experience less discomfort and difficulty during discontinuation (54).

It is crucial to recognize that abuse is a separate issue from dependence. Abuse is persistent or sporadic excessive drug use inconsistent with or unrelated to acceptable medical practice. Individuals with a history of alcohol or other drug abuse are at greatest risk of becoming benzodiazepine abusers. In individuals without this history, benzodiazepine abuse is rare (55). Diazepam, followed by alprazolam and lorazepam, has been judged to have the greatest liability for abuse among the benzodiazepines (5).

Although tolerance develops to the sedative, muscle relaxant, and anticonvulsant properties of the benzodiazepines, tolerance does not appear to develop to the antianxiety or antipanic effects in most patients (54, 56). Consequently, most patients are unlikely to attempt to escalate the dose. It is notable, however, that there is a paucity of data from clinical trials addressing the issue of long-term efficacy. Nevertheless, it is clear, based on extensive worldwide clinical experience, that many patients continue to obtain antianxiety effects with chronic administration of these agents.

CLINICAL APPLICATION

All benzodiazepines are considered to be equally effective as antianxiety agents, and selection of one agent over another is usually based on pharmacokinetic properties and the patient's clinical situation, medical status, and past history of response and tolerability. All patients taking benzodiazepines should see their clinician regularly to permit monitoring for response of target symptoms, adverse effects, drug interactions, and physical dependence and to be assessed for the necessity to continue therapy.

Clorazepate and diazepam are preferred choices where a rapid onset of antianxiety effect is desired. For elderly patients, patients with hepatic disease, and those receiving concurrent pharmacotherapy that may impair oxidative metabolism, lorazepam or oxazepam are preferred. The long half-life drugs can be used in this situation, but excessive drug and metabolite accumulation may occur with resultant side effects unless the dosage and/or frequency of administration is reduced accordingly. Elderly patients taking benzodiazepines require more careful monitoring than younger adult patients, as they are more likely to experience side effects, such as sedation, agitation, aggression, falling, and memory impairment.

In treatment of panic disorder, imipramine, phenelzine, alprazolam, and clonazepam are probably equally effective, but comparative trials are sorely needed. Selection of one drug over another is usually made by consideration of desired onset of antipanic effect, anticipated problems with drug discontinuation, anticipated patient tolerance of side effects or dietary restrictions, presence of depression, patient's age, history of prior response and tolerability, and costs of drug therapy.

Benzodiazepine therapy of panic disorder is generally well tolerated, and except for sedation, side effects are unusual. Benzodiazepine-treated patients should be monitored carefully for emergence of depression, which occurs in 33% of alprazolam-treated patients. It is unclear in this situation whether depression is secondary to the illness or to benzodiazepine treatment. Antidepressants are a better choice than benzodiazepines for panic disorder patients with depression or those who have a family history of depression. Regardless of choice of pharmacotherapeutic agent, most patients continue to improve for 6 to 10 months. There is a relatively high rate of relapse associated with pharmacotherapy discontinuation, but many patients can be successfully tapered off medication during the second year of therapy (48).

Buspirone

INDICATIONS

Buspirone is a member of a unique chemical class called the azapirones. It is as yet the sole member of this class to be marketed. It is structurally dissimilar to previously marketed agents and exhibits no cross-tolerance with the benzodiazepines. It is approved for the management of anxiety and for the short-term relief of symptoms of anxiety. However, it lacks anticonvulsant, muscle relaxant and hypnotic properties. Several double-blind studies have demonstrated that buspirone has antianxiety activity superior to placebo and equal to that of clorazepate, lorazepam, oxazepam, clobazam, bromazepam, and alprazolam (57, 58). An additional two studies found buspirone unsatisfactory compared to lorazepam and diazepam, especially in patients with severe anxiety (44). Preliminary work suggests that buspirone may be effective in treatment of depressive symptoms secondary to anxiety and in outpatients with major depression. Additional investigation is needed to substantiate these findings (57).

MECHANISM OF ACTION

The mechanism of action of buspirone in exerting antianxiety effects is poorly understood, but it clearly does not interact with benzodiazepine receptors and may increase rather than decrease brain noradrenergic and dopaminergic activity. Buspirone is a $5HT_{1A}$ partial agonist and reportedly inhibits spontaneous firing in the dorsal raphe. 5HT has a complex role in anxiety and interacts in multiple ways with other neurotransmitters. The effect of buspirone in treating anxiety may involve multiple systems in the midbrain; hence the term "midbrain modulator" (5).

PHARMACOKINETICS

Buspirone is absorbed rapidly and undergoes extensive first-pass metabolism. After oral administration, plasma concentrations of unchanged buspirone are low. Peak plasma concentrations of 1 to 6 ng/ml occur 40 to 90 min after a single oral dose of 20 mg. Food may decrease the presystemic clearance of buspirone, resulting in an increased area under the plasma-concentration-time curve and an increased peak-plasma concentration. Buspirone demonstrates nonlinear pharmacokinetics. Therefore, a dosage increase may result in a greater increase in steady-state plasma concentrations than would have been predicted. Buspirone is approximately 95% protein bound. Buspirone is metabolized primarily by oxidative mechanisms producing several hydroxylated metabolites, one of which is active, 1-pyrimidinylpiperazine (1-PP). 1-PP has about one-fourth the antianxiety activity of buspirone but probably contributes little or nothing to antianxiety effects, as it is present in small amounts in humans. The mean half-life of elimination of unchanged buspirone after single doses of 10 to 40 mg is 2 to 3 hr (manufacturers information). Although not studied extensively, clearance appears to be unaffected by age, but it decreases markedly in patients with cirrhosis and to a lesser extent in patients with renal impairment (59).

DOSING AND ONSET OF ACTION

The recommended initial dose if 5 mg three times daily. Dosage may be increased by 5 mg per day at 2- to 3-day intervals as needed. Maximum daily dose should not exceed 60 mg daily. In most clinical trials that allowed flexible dosing, 20 to 30 mg/day were the commonly employed doses (60).

The onset of antianxiety effects is not immediate. At least 1 week is required before onset of antianxiety activity, and maximal antianxiety effects may required 4 to 6 weeks (44). Rickels observed that clorazepate produced significantly more improvement than did buspirone early in treatment, but the two drugs produced equal degrees of improvement after 4 weeks of treatment. Further, he observed that the somatic (not psychic) symptoms of anxiety accounted for the perceived slower onset of clinical improvement (57).

ADVERSE DRUG REACTIONS

The more commonly observed side effects associated with buspirone treatment (not reported in an equivalent incidence in placebo-treated patients) are dizziness (12%), nausea (8%), headache (6%), nervousness (5%), lightheadedness (3%), and excitement (2%). These data are taken from pooled data from 17 controlled trials of 4-weeks duration. Ten percent of patients participating in premarketing efficacy trials lasting 3 to 4 weeks discontinued treatment because of an adverse event (60).

Comparative studies generally report a greater incidence of sedation in benzodiazepine-treated patients than in buspirone-treated patients. However, although the incidence of sedation appears to be less with buspirone than with equipotent doses of benzodiazepines, buspirone can cause drowsiness, especially when doses exceed 20 mg/day. Dysphoria has been reported, especially with single doses of 20 to 40 mg. Symptoms suggestive of postsynaptic dopamine receptor blockade (e.g., extrapyramidal symptoms, galactorrhea, gynecomastia) occurred in less than 0.57% of patients in clinical trials (44). Tollefson and colleagues failed to find an increase in prolactin or growth hormone levels at mean doses of 25 mg/day after 28 days of treatment (61).

DRUG INTERACTIONS

The concurrent administration of trazodone and buspirone has been reported to cause a 3- to 6-fold elevation in ALT (formerly SGPT) levels in a few patients; however, a similar study failed to replicate an effect on hepatic transaminases. A study in normal volunteers found that concomitant administration of single doses of buspirone (45 mg) and haloperidol resulted in increased serum haloperidol concentrations. There is a single report of a prolonged prothrombin time when buspirone was added to warfarin.

In vitro buspirone may displace digoxin from its protein binding site, but not phenytoin, propranolol, or warfarin. Four occurrences of elevated blood pressure were reported in patients taking concurrent MAOIs with buspirone. This combination should, therefore, be avoided. Buspirone 20 mg/day in divided doses and 30 mg of flurazepam at bedtime resulted in slight impairment of daytime psychomotor performance, compared with that produced by either drug alone. Unlike the benzodiazepines, buspirone lacks a pharmacokinetic interaction with alcohol and does not potentiate the impairment in psychomotor performance caused by alcohol (44). Levels of buspirone metabolites may be increased by cimetidine (5).

PATIENT EDUCATION

As with most medications, patients taking buspirone should inform the clinician if they are pregnant, plan to become pregnant, or are breast-feeding. Although buspirone is known to cause less sedation than equipotent doses of benzodiazepines, patients are well advised to not drive or engage in other potentially hazardous activities until they know how the medication affects them.

Patients prescribed buspirone should be well educated on the relatively low sedative profile (relative to benzodiazepines) and on the delayed onset of therapeutic effects. Specifically, they should understand that they will probably not have the immediate sedative effects they may have experienced with prior benzodiazepine therapy. Further, they should understand that onset of antianxiety effects may not occur for 1 week or more, and optimal effects

may be delayed for approximately 6 weeks. In addition, if they are educated on the lack of potential for causing physiologic dependence, they are more likely to willingly sacrifice immediate antianxiety effects and comply with treatment.

DEPENDENCE, WITHDRAWAL, AND ABUSE

Early studies in animals and humans failed to demonstrate physical dependence (62). A more recent study provides evidence that may allow a more in-depth understanding of this issue. This was a double-blind study in 51 outpatients with GAD who were treated with either diazepam or buspirone for 6 or 12 weeks, after which they were withdrawn abruptly and continued on placebo to week 14. Forty patients completed the study. Not surprisingly, diazepam was rapidly effective, and buspirone did not achieve antianxiety efficacy similar to diazepam until week 6. The data taken as a whole showed buspirone to cause few or no withdrawal symptoms; however, similar numbers in each group experienced a temporary increase in symptoms occurring within 2 weeks of discontinuation. Interestingly, 5% of buspirone-treated patients, compared with 30% of diazepam-treated patients, experienced emergence of 2 or more new symptoms after discontinuation which were not present before or during treatment. The temporary increase in symptoms in 3 of 10 patients treated with buspirone for 6 weeks suggests that buspirone should not be regarded as entirely free from dependence potential (63). Another study reported no observed adverse effects after abrupt discontinuation of buspirone treatment for 6 months (64). In view of these two reports, it is reasonable to conclude that buspirone has significantly less potential for dependence than the benzodiazepines. Human trials suggest that buspirone has a low potential for abuse, and postmarketing experience is consistent with this conclusion.

CLINICAL APPLICATION

Because buspirone is associated with minimal sedative effects and a lagtime of 1 to 2 weeks before onset of antianxiety activity, it is not an appropriate choice for patients requiring immediate relief of anxiety or for patients who require antianxiety treatment on an as-needed basis. It is, however, a good choice for patients unable to tolerate sedation or psychomotor impairment. For these reasons it may be a good choice in the elderly, although data from controlled double-blind trials in this population are sparse. Buspirone is also a good choice for anxious patients with a prior history of drug abuse and patients likely to need long-term treatment, because of its low potential for dependence and abuse. It is not recommended for routine treatment of panic disorder.

As buspirone is not cross-tolerant with the benzodiazepines, it will not block withdrawal signs and symptoms that may ensue with discontinuation of benzodiazepine therapy (65). Early recommendations for switching a patient from a benzodiazepine to buspirone involved slowly tapering downward and discontinuing the benzodiazepine before initiating buspirone. A recent placebo-controlled double-blind study demonstrates that buspirone and alprazolam may be used together safely, and buspirone may be started early in the alprazolam-tapering process (65). Rickels (57) recommends that patients receive buspirone at least 4 weeks before the benzodiazepine taper begins.

Schweiger and colleagues (66) reported that prior benzodiazepine use may predict a less favorable therapeutic outcome with buspirone, perhaps because patients with prior experience with benzodiazepines expect immediate response and sedation. As buspirone fails to meet these expectation, patient acceptance and compliance may be compromised. A more recent trial found no clear association between previous benzodiazepine use and clinical improvement; however, the sample size was small (n = 13 in previous experience group; n = 7 in no previous experience group) (63).

Antihistamines

The antihistamines diphenhydramine and hydroxyzine have limited application in treating anxiety. Although they do have sedative effects in many patients, their efficacy as antianxiety agents has not been well established, when compared with placebo. They are considered to be less effective than the benzodiazepines, and their primary advantage is that they have essentially no liability for physical dependence. Diphenhydramine is used in usual doses of 10 to 25 mg four times daily, and hydroxyzine in doses 10 to 50 mg one to four times daily for mild anxiety (67).

The antihistamines have anticholinergic side effects that are particularly problematic in elderly patients. At least additive CNS depression should be expected when antihistamines are taken concurrently with alcohol or other CNS-depressant drugs, such as narcotic analgesics and tricyclic antidepressants (44).

β-Adrenergic Blockers

Many studies of propranolol in treatment of GAD are marked by flawed design. Propranolol has no sedative properties and is considered to be a less effective antianxiety agent than diazepam (68). Although somewhat controversial, propranolol may be considered useful in selected patients with prominent cardiovascular symptoms of anxiety, such as tachycardia, palpitations, and tremulousness (69).

Single-dose β-blocker treatment is likely to be effective for specific social phobias (fear of specific social situations, such as public speaking or taking examinations)

(38). Preliminary results from a double-blind trial suggest that atenolol may be useful in treating the specific form of social phobia, as well (37).

One study suggests that propranolol may be of benefit to patients with PTSD. Propranolol-treated patients were reported to have fewer intrusive thoughts and nightmares and to experience less explosiveness and autonomic instability (70). Propranolol is considered to be unsatisfactory in treating panic disorder.

Propranolol therapy is generally well tolerated if patients are well selected. Propranolol is contraindicated in patients with sinus bradycardia, greater than first-degree block, bronchial asthma, and congestive heart failure. It may worsen Raynaud's syndrome. Side effects reported in propranolol-treated anxious patients are similar to those seen in patients treated for hypertension. These include lightheadedness, fatigue, insomnia, nausea, bradycardia, and hypotension.

Propranolol doses used in treatment of most anxiety symptoms are 40 to 360 mg/day. It should be dosed at least twice daily. Initial doses are 10 mg twice daily, titrated to individual needs. In PTSD, propranolol can be initiated at a dose of 20 mg three times daily and increased by 60 mg every 3 days to a maximum of 640 mg/day if needed and if tolerated. When the drug is to be discontinued, it is generally gradually tapered downward to avoid adverse cardiovascular effects and rebound anxiety (69). In treatment of specific social phobias, 20 to 40 mg of propranolol 1 hr before the performance is usually adequate.

Cyclic Antidepressants

INDICATIONS

TCAs are not traditionally considered to be treatments for GAD, however two studies have shown doxepin to be more effective than placebo in treating GAD. Amitriptyline, imipramine, and desipramine may also be effective in treating this disorder (5), and up to 8 weeks may be required for efficacy.

Imipramine is the most widely studied TCA in treating panic disorder (23, 26, 27) and is well-documented to be effective. Other TCAs may also be effective, including amitriptyline, desipramine, doxepin, and nortriptyline (71). Mild depressive symptoms that are common in these patients also frequently respond to TCA treatment. More recently, clomipramine has been demonstrated to be an effective alternative (29, 72), and fluoxetine treatment produced complete remission of panic attacks for 4 successive weeks in 7 of 16 patients in an open trial (30). In an additional study, 19 of 25 patients showed a moderate-to-marked improvement on fluoxetine (31).

Clomipramine is well-documented in several double-blind trials to be effective in treatment of OCD (39). It is the only drug with FDA approval for this indication. Multiple open trials demonstrate fluoxetine to also be useful in this disorder (40). Double-blind data also support the effectiveness of fluvoxamine (not yet unavailable in the U.S.). (41). After response to medication, most patients still meet the diagnostic criteria for OCD. Even patients who are markedly improved usually remain sufficiently symptomatic to justify the continued diagnosis of OCD.

Rigorous trials are sparse in the PTSD literature. A preliminary report from a controlled trial suggests efficacy of imipramine (43), and amitriptyline has been shown to be superior to placebo in a double-blind trial in 46 patients. Although depression was improved at 4 weeks, 8 weeks of treatment was required to detect overall clinical improvement. At the end of the study, almost two-thirds of patients who received amitriptyline still met the diagnostic criteria for PTSD (18). The effect of desipramine was studied in 18 veterans with PTSD in a double-blind placebo-controlled crossover-study design. They found no response for the PTSD symptoms. However, short duration of treatment (4 weeks) and subtherapeutic dosages of desipramine (maximum, 200 mg/day) may have decreased the likelihood of detecting response (73). Uncontrolled reports in small samples suggest usefulness of doxepin, desipramine, carbamazepine, clonidine, and propranolol. However, conclusions on the efficacy of these agents must await more rigorous study. When TCA therapy is effective, it reduces traumatic recollections and nightmares, represses flashbacks, and dampens hyperarousal. It is important to note that pharmacotherapy alone rarely provides complete remission of symptoms (74).

DOSING

Although a few patients respond to dose of imipramine as low as 25 mg/day, many patients require doses in excess of 150 mg/day for treating panic disorder. Indeed, doses up to 200 to 300 mg/day can be used, if necessary. Ordinarily, doses are initiated at 10 to 25 mg/day and increased gradually (25 mg every 3 days) to maximize compliance and minimize side effects, especially a hyperstimulatory reaction. The key to response for many patients is to push to an adequate dose and treat for an adequate period of time. Panic attacks respond to fluoxetine in doses of 10 to 80 mg/day. It is recommended that dosing be initiated at 2.5 to 5 mg/day and increased gradually, based on individual needs and tolerability. This can be accomplished using the liquid formulation that provides 20 mg/5 ml.

For treating OCD, 150 to 250 mg/day of clomipramine is usually required, although in many cases the dose can be reduced by approximately one-third after a favorable response is achieved. Although fluoxetine-treated patients may respond to 20 to 80 mg/day, most patients required 60 to 80 mg/day. In treating PTSD, typical antidepressant doses of the TCAs (50 to 300 mg/day) are required.

ADVERSE DRUG REACTIONS

Twenty percent of panic disorder patients taking imipramine (and other TCAs) experience a hyperstimulatory reaction characterized by intensification of anxiety symptoms, agitation, tachycardia, and insomnia. Medication compliance suffers in many patients who manifest this side effect (75). Initiating dosage at 10 to 25 mg/day with gradual escalation often helps to minimize this side effect. Other side effects commonly seen are sedation, tremor, dry mouth, blurred vision, constipation, delayed micturition, and orthostatic hypotension.

A hyperstimulatory reaction occurred in 43% of panic disorder patients taking fluoxetine. For this reason it is also often started at a very low dose and increased gradually (30). Although fluoxetine is free from anticholinergic, orthostatic, and sedative effects, it may be associated with nausea, nervousness, insomnia, diarrhea, and dizziness.

Clomipramine treatment of OCD has been associated with lethargy, constipation, anorgasmia, weight gain, and lowering the seizure threshold. Interestingly, in spite of several side effects, OCD patients usually tolerate clomipramine with minimal complaints.

CLINICAL APPLICATION

In addition to the hyperstimulatory reaction, another problem associated with imipramine in treatment of panic disorder is a lag time of 3 to 5 weeks before antipanic response and up to 12 weeks before antiphobic effect is maximal. Patients unable to tolerate the anticholinergic effects of imipramine may be switched to desipramine (44). Imipramine is available as an inexpensive generic.

A diagnosis of MVP does not preclude the use of TCAs in patients with panic disorder, and evidence suggests these patients respond as well to imipramine as patients without MVP (76).

The lag time before antipanic response to fluoxetine is similar in length to the one for imipramine. As previously noted, the side-effect profile of fluoxetine offers some advantages over imipramine, and it is also less toxic on overdose. The half-life of fluoxetine and its metabolite, norfluoxetine, are 1 to 3 days and 7 to 15 days, respectively. Theoretically, substantial drug could be accumulated in the elderly or patients with hepatic disease, but this has not been reported to be a problem to date. Fluoxetine may increase serum concentrations of concurrently administered TCAs and carbamazepine, which can lead to toxicity. A "serotonergic syndrome" was reported when the MAOI tanylcypromine was initiated only 2 days after discontinuing fluoxetine. This syndrome was characterized by shivering, nausea, anxiety, and confusion. Fluoxetine should be discontinued 5 weeks before starting MAOIs (77).

In clomipramine treatment of OCD, a lag time of 4 to 6 weeks is required before onset of effects. Obsessive-compulsive symptoms are reduced by about 45 to 55%, and improvement occurs in 65 to 80% of patients. No tolerance to antiobsessive-compulsive effects occurs. Although definitive trials comparing clomipramine with fluoxetine have not been published, a meta-analysis of previous studies suggests a larger antiobsessive-compulsive effect for clomipramine than for fluoxetine (78). Although the evidence in support of the efficacy of fluoxetine is fairly compelling, controlled investigations are needed to confirm the findings of preliminary open trials.

Monoamine Oxidase Inhibitors (MAOIs)

INDICATIONS

Most early studies assessing the efficacy of MAOIs in panic disorder were methodologically flawed. The best-designed trial compared phenelzine, 45 mg/day, with imipramine, 150 mg/day, and placebo. Both active treatments were effective and superior to placebo in reducing phobic anxiety, fears, general anxiety, avoidance behaviors, and disability. Phenelzine treatment was slightly, but not significantly, superior to imipramine on several scales (25).

The most extensive study on the use of phenelzine in social phobia is still in progress. Preliminary data analysis reveals 64% of patients much improved on phenelzine, 36% on atenolol, and 31% on placebo. Phenelzine appeared to be particularly effective for the generalized (rather than the specific) form of social phobia. The mean dose of atenolol was 95 mg/day, and for phenelzine, 72 mg/day.

Several open studies suggest possible effectiveness of phenelzine in treating PTSD (79). The efficacy of phenelzine was confirmed in an 8-week, double-blind, randomized trial in 34 veterans comparing imipramine (mean dose, 240 mg/day), phenelzine (mean dose, 71 mg/day), and placebo. Patients in both active treatment groups improved. Symptoms most improved were nightmares, flashbacks, and intrusive recollections. Avoidance symptoms were resistant to treatment (43).

DOSING

The average therapeutic dose of phenelzine in treatment of panic disorder is 60 mg/day (range 45 to 90 mg/day). The initial dose is 15 mg/day, and increases can be made every 3 to 4 days until 60 mg/day is reached. If there is no improvement after 8 to 12 weeks, the dose can be increased further. However, 90 mg/day is considered the dosage ceiling (44).

Phenelzine dosing is similar in treating social phobia. The mean phenelzine dose used in the study by Liebowitz et al. (37) was 72 mg/day. Studies of phenelzine treatment of PTSD used doses ranging from 45 to 90 mg/day (79). In treatment of social phobia and PTSD, a dosage escalation schedule similar to the one for panic disorder can be used. If a patient has been taking a TCA, a 7- to 10-day waiting period must be observed before initiating an MAOI.

ADVERSE DRUG REACTIONS

Adverse effects associated with phenelzine therapy include insomnia, irritability, hypomania, disinhibition, orthostatic hypotension, anorgasmia, edema, and weight gain. Anticholinergic side effects are less severe than with the TCAs, but postural hypotension and insomnia are more of a problem. Hyperstimulatory reactions at the beginning of treatment of panic disorder patients may also occur, but they are less likely to occur with phenelzine than with imipramine (80).

CLINICAL APPLICATION

In panic disorder, response to phenelzine occurs after approximately 3 to 6 weeks at therapeutic doses. Maximal response may not be achieved for 6 to 10 weeks. The most feared event associated with MAOI therapy is a hypertensive crisis following ingestion of tyramine-containing foods or concurrent administration of selected drugs. Eight percent of patients taking MAOIs are reported to experience such reactions. This reaction is characterized by elevated blood pressure, severe headache, diaphoresis, neck stiffness, and neuromuscular excitation. Intracerebral hemorrhage may occur (81). Patients should be carefully counseled about dietary and drug restrictions, side effects, and lagtime before response is expected.

Imipramine, phenelzine, and alprazolam are probably equally effective in treatment of panic disorder, but controlled trials comparing them are sorely needed. A clear disadvantage of phenelzine is patient acceptance. Patients are often apprehensive about the dietary and drug restrictions necessary to avoid precipitating a hypertensive crisis. Patient acceptance of alprazolam is not usually a problem. Many physicians initiate therapy of panic disorder with either imipramine or alprazolam. Alprazolam offers rapid antipanic effects, few side effects, but more problems than imipramine with discontinuation. Imipramine is often the first choice, based on its long history of safety and proven efficacy. However, some patients do not respond to imipramine or cannot tolerate its side effects. An alternative is to start with imipramine and alprazolam simultaneously, to take advantage of the rapid onset of antipanic efficacy of alprazolam, but to withdraw alprazolam after antipanic effects are achieved and when therapeutic levels of imipramine are presumed to have been attained (82).

The appropriate duration of treatment for panic disorder is not well studied. Many clinicians continue treatment for 6 to 12 months, then discontinue medication gradually over 2 to 3 months. If relapse occurs, treatment is continued for another 12 to 14 months, when discontinuation can again be attempted. Some patients may need to continue medications indefinitely (82).

In the treatment of social phobias, both phenelzine and β-blockers have demonstrated efficacy. The β-blockers may be more useful in treating the specific form of social phobia, whereas phenelzine may be more beneficial for the generalized form of the disorder. Psychotherapy can play an important role in reducing negative cognitions and avoidance behavior.

Pharmacotherapeutic studies have demonstrated that the positive symptoms of PTSD (e.g., increased arousal and reexperiencing the event) often respond to medication. Negative symptoms, including avoidance and withdrawal, usually respond poorly. Comorbid psychiatric conditions must definitely be identified so that they may be addressed in the therapeutic plan. Concomitant psychiatric diagnoses may include major depression, panic disorder, generalized anxiety disorder, or alcohol and substance abuse (79).

In most situations when there is no comorbid condition, a TCA is the first-choice treatment of PTSD. Treatment should last at least 6 to 8 weeks before assessing response. Phenelzine is just as effective as TCAs, but it is usually reserved for patients with refractory depression. For persistent symptoms of hyperarousal, (e.g., hypervigilance, startle response), propranolol can be initiated. Residual aggression and irritability may be managed with antiaggressive medications such as propranolol, carbamazepine, or lithium (79).

PROGNOSIS

It is difficult to predict with confidence the course of the anxiety disorders over a lifetime. However, the symptoms and disability associated with most of these disorders can be impacted positively by well-selected and carefully monitored pharmacotherapy. Benzodiazepine treatment and buspirone treatment of GAD generally produces a moderate-to-marked improvement in approximately 70% of patients (57). In treatment of panic disorder, 70 to 90% of patients treated with TCAs, phenelzine, or alprazolam experience a reduction or elimination of panic attacks (82). Sixty-four percent of patients with social phobia were much improved on phenelzine (37). Clomipramine treatment of OCD resulted in 58% of patients rating themselves as much improved or very much improved (39). It is clear, however, that most patients receiving clomipramine for OCD or TCAs for PTSD still meet the diagnostic criteria for OCD or PTSD, respectively, after successful treatment. Progress continues to be made in improving outcome of pharmacotherapeutic interventions in anxiety disorders, but nonpharmacologic interventions remain a key part of the treatment plan.

CONCLUSIONS

Our understanding of the anxiety disorders, their pathophysiology, epidemiology, and treatment, continues to advance. Not all patients with anxiety disorders should receive pharmacotherapy, and many of those who are appropriate candidates for antianxiety medications, should also have the benefit of nonpharmacologic interventions. Accurate diagnosis is crucial to the selection of the most rational pharmacotherapy. It is now recognized that many patients with anxiety disorders have important morbidity and that some patients are, in fact, profoundly disabled by their illness. These patients deserve the same meticulous assessment and concern as that afforded patients with chest pain. It is the responsibility of the prescriber, dispenser, clinical pharmacist, and nurse to take an active role in educating patients about their therapy, monitoring for therapeutic benefit and real and potential drug-related problems, and intervening whenever possible to maximize positive clinical outcomes.

REFERENCES

1. American Psychiatric Association: Diagnostic and Statistical Manual of Mental Disorders, ed. 3, revised. Washington, D.C.: American Psychiatric Association, 1987, pp 235–253.
2. Charney DS, Heninger GR: Noradrenergic function and the mechanism of action of antianxiety treatment. I. The effect of long-term alprazolam treatment. Arch Gen Psychiatry 42:458–467, 1985.
3. Sanghera MK, McMillan BA, German CD: Buspirone, a nonbenzodiazepine anxiolytic, increases locus coeruleus noradrenergic neuronal activity. Eur J Pharmacol 48:107–110, 1983.
4. Charney DS, Heninger GR, Breier A: Noradrenergic function in panic anxiety. Arch Gen Psychiatry 41:751–763, 1984.
5. Dubovsky SL: Generalized anxiety disorder: new concepts and pharmacologic therapies. J Clin Psychiatry 51(suppl):3–10, 1990.
6. Costa GA, Neuropeptides as cotransmitters: modulatory effects at GABAergic synapses. In Meltzer HY (ed): Psychopharmacology: The Third Generation of Progress. New York, Raven Press, 1987, pp 425–437.
7. Eison AS, Eison MS, Stanley M, et al.: Serotonergic mechanisms in the behavioral effects of buspirone and gepirone. Pharmacol Biochem Behav 24:701–707, 1986.
8. Weissman MM, Merikangas KR: The epidemiology of anxiety and panic disorders: an update. J Clin Psychiatry 47:11S–17S, 1986.
9. Schuckit MA: Anxiety related to medical disease. J Clin Psychiatry 44:31–36, 1983.
10. Hayes PE, Dommisse CS: Current concepts in clinical therapeutics: anxiety disorders, part I. Clin Pharm 6:140–147, 1987.
11. Cameron OG: The differential diagnosis of anxiety: psychiatric and medical disorders. Psychiatr Clin North Am 8:3–23, 1985.
12. Redmond DE, Huang UH: Current concepts II. New evidence for a locus coeruleus-norepinephrine connection with anxiety. Life Sci 25:149–153, 1979.
13. Reiman EM, Raichle ME, Robins E, et al.: The application of positron emission tomography to the study of panic disorder. Am J Psychiatry 143:469–477, 1986.
14. Gorman JM, Liebowitz MR, Fyer AJ, et al.: A neuroanatomical hypothesis for panic disorder. Am J Psychiatry 146:148–161, 1989.
15. Pitts FNJ, McClure JNJ: Lactate metabolism in anxiety neurosis. N Engl J Med 277:1329–1336, 1977.
16. Savage PD, Garrison RJ, Deveraux RB, et al.: Mitral valve prolapse in the general population. I. Epidemiological features: the Framingham Study. Am Heart J 106:571–576, 1983.
17. Robins LN, Helzer JE, Weissman M, et al.: Lifetime prevalence of

specific psychiatric disorders in three sites. Arch Gen Psychiatry 41:949–958, 1984.

18. Davidson J, Kudler H, Smith R, et al.: Treatment of posttraumatic stress disorder with amitriptyline and placebo. Arch Gen Psychiatry 47:259–266, 1990.

19. Shader RI, Greenblatt DJ: Some current treatment options for symptoms of anxiety. J Clin Psychiatry 44:21S–29S, 1983.

20. Marks I: Behavioral psychotherapy for the anxiety disorders. Psychiatr Clin North Am 8:25–35, 1985.

21. Ursano RJ, Hales RE: A review of individual psychotherapies. Am J Psychiatry 143:1507–1517, 1986.

22. Silver BV, Blanchard EB: Biofeedback and relaxation training in the treatment of psychophysiologic disorders: or are the machines really working? J Behav Med 1:217–239, 1978.

23. Zitrin CM, Klein DF, Woemer MG: Treatment of agoraphobia with group exposure in vivo and imipramine. Arch Gen Psychiatry 37:63–72, 1980.

24. Ballenger JC: Psychopharmacology of the anxiety disorders. Psychiatr Clin North Am 7:757–771, 1984.

25. Sheehan DV, Ballenger JC, Jacobsen G: Treatment of endogenous anxiety with phobic, hysterical and hypochondriacal symptoms. Arch Gen Psychiatry 37:51–59, 1980.

26. Klein DF, Zitrin CM, Woemer MG, et al. Treatment of phobias: II. behavior therapy and supportive therapy: are there any specific ingredients. Arch Gen Psychiatry 40:139–145, 1983.

27. Mavissakalian M, Perel JM: Imipramine in the treatment of agoraphobia: dose-response relationships. Am J Psychiatry 142:1032–1036, 1985.

28. Lydiard BR: Desipramine in agoraphobia with panic attacks: an open fixed-dose study. J Clin Psychopharmacol 7:258–260, 1987.

29. Johnson DG, Troyer IE, Whitsett SF: Clomipramine treatment of agoraphobic women. Arch Gen Psychiatry 45:453–459, 1988.

30. Gorman JM, Liebowitz MR, Fryer AJ, et al.: An open trial of fluxoetine in the treatment of panic attacks. J Clin Psychopharmacol 7:329–332, 1987.

31. Schneier FR, Liebowitz MR, Davies SO, et al.: Fluoxetine in panic disorder. J Clin Psychopharmacol 10:119–121, 1990.

32. Ballenger JC, Burrows GD, DuPont RL, et al.: Alprazolam in panic disorder and agoraphobia: results from a multicenter trial. I. Efficacy in short-term treatment. Arch Gen Psychiatry 45:413–422, 1988.

33. Noyes R, DuPont RL, Pecknold JC, et al.: Alprazolam in panic disorder and agoraphobia: results from a multicenter trial. III. Patient acceptance, side effects and safety. Arch Gen Psychiatry 45:423–428, 1988.

34. Tesar GE, Rosenbaum JF: Successful use of clonazepam in patients with treatment resistant panic disorder. J Nerv Ment Dis 174:477–482, 1986.

35. Charney DS, Woods SW: Benzodiazepine treatment of panic disorder: A comparison of alprazolam and lorazepam. J Clin Psychiatry 50:418–423, 1989.

36. Liebowitz MR, Gorman JM, Fyer AJ, et al.: Social phobia: review of a neglected anxiety disorder. Arch Gen Psychiatry 42:729–736, 1985.

37. Liebowitz MR, Gorman JM, Fyer AJ, et al.: Pharmacotherapy of social phobia: an interim report of a placebo-controlled comparison of phenelzine and atenolol. J Clin Psychiatry 49:252–257, 1988.

38. Agras WS: Treatment of social phobias. J Clin Psychiatry 51(suppl 10):52S–55S, 1990.

39. DeVeaugh-Geiss J, Katz RJ, Landau P, et al.: Preliminary results from a multicenter trial of clomipramine in obsessive-compulsive disorder. Psychopharmacol Bull 25:36–40, 1989.

40. Jenike MA, Buttol PHL, Baer L, et al.: Fluoxetine in obsessive-compulsive disorder: a positive open trial. Am J Psychiatry 46:909–911, 1989.

41. Goodman WK, Price LH, Rasmussen SA, et al.: Efficacy of fluvoxamine in obsessive-compulsive disorder: a double-blind comparison with placebo. Arch Gen Psychiatry 46:36–44, 1989.

42. Greist JH: Treating anxiety: therapeutic options in obsessive compulsive disorder. J Clin Psychiatry 51(suppl 1):29S–34S, 1990.

43. Frank JB, Kosten TR, Giller EL, et al.: A randomized clinical trial of phenelzine and imipramine for posttraumatic stress disorder. Am J Psychiatry 145:1289–1291, 1988.

44. Dommisse CS, Hayes PE: Current concepts in clinical therapeutics: anxiety disorders, Part II. Clin Pharm 6:196–215, 1987.

45. Tesar GE: High-potency benzodiazepines for short-term management of panic disorder: the U.S. experience. J Clin Psychiatry 51(9 suppl):4S–10S, 1990.

46. Noyes R, Anderson DJ, Claney J, et al.: Diazepam and propranolol in panic disorder and agoraphobia. Arch Gen Psychiatry 41:287–292, 1984.

47. Ballenger JC: Pharmacotherapy of the panic disorders. J Clin Psychiatry 47:27S–32S, 1986.

48. Greenblatt DJ, Shader RI, Abernethy DR: Current status of benzodiazepines, part I. New Engl J Med 309:354–358, 1983.

49. Medi-Span Drug Therapy Screening System (DTSS), Medi-Span Development Corporation, 1990.

50. Kargas GA, Kargas SA, Bruyere HJ, et al.: Perinatal mortality due to interaction of diphenhydramine and temazepam. N Engl J Med 313:1417–1418, 1985.

51. United States Pharmacopeial Convention: USP-DI, ed. 3. Rockville, MD, United States Pharmacopeial Convention, 1990, pp 595–615.

52. Power KG, Jerrom DWA, Simpson RJ, et al.: Controlled study of withdrawal and rebound anxiety after six week course of diazepam for generalized anxiety. Br Med J 290:1246–1248, 1985.

53. Gorman JM, Papp LA: Chronic anxiety: deciding the length of treatment. J Clin Psychiatry 51(suppl 1):11S–15S, 1990.

54. Pollack MH: Long-term management of panic disorder. J Clin Psychiatry 51(suppl 5):11S–13S, 1990.

55. Busto U, Seller EM, Naranjo CA, et al.: Patterns of benzoidazepine abuse and dependence. Br J Addict 81:87–94, 1986.

56. Roth M: Anxiety disorders and the use and abuse of drugs. J Clin Psychiatry 50(11suppl):30–35, 1989.

57. Rickels K: Buspirone in clinical practice. J Clin Psychiatry 51(9 suppl):51S–54S, 1990.

58. Strand M, Hetta J, Rosen A, et al.: A double-blind controlled trial in primary care patients with generalized anxiety: a comparison between buspirone and oxazepam. J Clin Psychiatry 51(9 suppl):40–45, 1990.

59. Gammans RE, Mayol RF, Labudde JA: Metabolism and disposition of buspirone. Am J Med 80:41S–51S, 1986.

60. Mead Johnson Pharmaceutical Division/Bristol Myers. Buspar package insert. Evansville, IN, 1990.

61. Tollefson GD, Godes M, Montague-Clouse J, et al.: Buspirone: effects on prolactin and growth hormone as a function of drug level in generalized anxiety. J Clin Psychopharmacol 9:132–136, 1989.

62. Tyrer P, Murphy S, Owen RT: The risk of pharmacological dependence with buspirone. Br J Clin Pract 39:91–93, 1985.

63. Murphy SM, Owen R, Tyrer P: Comparative assessment of efficacy and withdrawal symptoms after 6 and 12 weeks' treatment with diazepam or buspirone. Br J Psychiatry 154:529–534, 1989.

64. Rickels K, Schweizer E, Csanalosi I, et al.: Long-term treatment of anxiety and risk of withdrawal: prospective comparison of clorazepate and buspirone. Arch Gen Psychiatry 45:444–450, 1988.

65. Udelman HD, Udelman DL: Concurrent use of buspirone in anxious patients during withdrawal from alprazolam therapy. J Clin Psychiatry 51(suppl 9):46–50, 1990.

66. Schweizer E, Rickels K, Lucki I: Resistance to the antianxiety effects of buspirone in patients with a history of benzodiazepine use. N Engl J Med 314:719–720, 1986.

67. Bernstein JG: Handbook of Drug Therapy in Psychiatry. Boston: John Wright, PSG, Inc., 1983, p 33.

68. Cole JO: The drug treatment of anxiety and depression. Med Clin North Am 72:815–830, 1988.

69. Noyes R: Beta-adrenergic blocking drugs in anxiety and stress. Psychiatr Clin North Am 8:119–132, 1985.

70. Kolb LC, Burris BC, Griffiths S, Propranolol and clonidine in the treatment of post traumatic stress disorder of war. In van der Kolk BA (ed): Post Traumatic Stress Disorders Psychological and Biological Sequelae. Washington, D.C., American Psychiatric Press, 1984, pp 29–42.

71. Lydiard RB, Ballenger JC: Antidepressants in panic disorder and agoraphobia. J Affective Disord 13:153–168, 1987.

72. Gloger S, Grunhaus L, Gladic D, et al.: Panic attacks and agoraphobia: low dose clomipramine treatment. J Clin Psychopharmacol 9:28–32, 1989.

73. Reist C, Kauffmann CD, Haier RJ, et al.: A controlled trial of desipramine in 18 men with posttraumatic stress disorder. Am J Psychiatry 146:513–516, 1989.

74. Freidman MJ: Toward rational pharmacotherapy for posttraumatic stress disorder: an interim report. Am J Psychiatry 145:281–285, 1988.

75. Noyes R, Garvey MJ, Cook BL, et al.: Problems with tricyclic antidepressant use in patients with panic disorder or agoraphobia: results of a naturalistic follow-up study. J Clin Psychiatry 50:163–169, 1989.

76. Crowe RR: Mitral valve prolapse and panic disorder. Psychiatr Clin North Am 8:63–71, 1985.

77. Ciraulo DA, Shader RI: Fluoxetine drug-drug interactions: I. antidepressants and antipsychotics. J Clin Psychopharmacol 10:48–50, 1990.

78. Jenike MA, Baer L, Greist JH: Clomipramine versus fluoxetine in obsessive-compulsive disorder: a retrospective comparison of side effects and efficacy. J Clin Psychopharmacol 10:122–124, 1990.

79. Silver JM, Sandberg DP, Hales RE: New approaches in the pharmacotherapy of posttraumatic stress disorder. J Clin Psychiatry 51(suppl 10):33–38, 1990.

80. Rabkin J, Quitkin FM, Harrison W, et al.: Adverse reactions to monamine oxidase inhibitors. Part I. a comparative study. J Clin Psychopharmacol 4:270–278, 1984.

81. Brown CS, Bryant SG: Monoamine oxidase inhibitors: safety and efficacy issues. Drug Intell Clin Pharm 22:232–235, 1988.

82. Sargent M: NIMH report: panic disorder. Hosp Comm Psychiatry 41:621–623, 1990.

CHAPTER 52

MOOD DISORDERS

GLEN L. STIMMEL, Pharm.D.

Disturbances of mood include both full and partial manic or depressive syndromes. Mood disorders involve prolonged disturbances of the expression of emotion that go beyond brief emotional upset from negative life experiences. At least one in ten people in the United States will experience a diagnosable mood disorder in their lifetime. Such a high prevalence in the general population suggests that pharmacists in all treatment settings will encounter patients with mood disorders and must be familiar with their recognition and treatment.

ETIOLOGY

While the exact etiology of mood disorders is not known, much is known about neurotransmitter and neuroendocrine systems and their relationship to mood disorders. The most clearly established biologic fact regarding mood disorders is the existence of a genetic substrate, with genetic loading greatest in bipolar illness. Sixty to 65% of bipolar patients have a positive family history of mood disorder. Since recurrence is fundamental to most mood disorders, hypotheses that incorporate sleep and circadian rhythm as well as kindling and sensitization are being investigated. Much more is known about the mechanisms of action of antidepressants, which provides only indirect evidence about an etiology for mood disorders. There is a long list of drugs that can produce depression, but establishing a direct causative relationship is very difficult. With a lifetime prevalence of major depression at 7 to 13% in the United States, there are no drugs that cause depression with such frequency. Of greatest concern is use of drugs reported to cause depression in patients with a history of depressive illness. These drugs include many antihypertensives (reserpine, propranolol, methyldopa, clonidine), hormones (estrogen, progesterone), corticosteroids, and several antiparkinson agents (levodopa, amantadine) (1).

PREVALENCE AND COURSE OF ILLNESS

The 6-month prevalence of all mood disorders is about 8% in women and 4% in men. In any 6-month period, 4% of women and 2% of men could be diagnosed as having major depression, with a similar number being diagnosed as having dysthymia. Lifetime prevalence for major depression is 5 to 9% in women and 2 to 4% in men, while bipolar disorder is 0.6 to 0.9% in women and men. The lifetime prevalence for cyclothymia is from 0.4 to 3.5%.

For major depression, 40% will recover fully and not experience another depressive episode in their lifetime, while another 40% will have an episodic course with recurring depressive episodes. The remaining 20% of patients with major depression will have a chronic course with persistent residual symptoms and social impairment. The ultimate risk of completed suicide in patients with primary mood disorders is 15%, which is 30 times the risk for the general population. About 60 to 80% of bipolar patients begin with a manic episode. Without treatment, episodes last 6 months to 1 year for depression and 4 months for mania. Bipolar patients are more likely than major depression patients to have multiple subsequent episodes (1).

DIAGNOSTIC CLASSIFICATION

There are four major categories of mood disorders (Table 52.1)(1, 2). Bipolar disorder is typically characterized by distinct episodes of mania and depression separated by intervals without mood disturbance. There is no category of manic disorder, since one manic episode is sufficient to be classified as bipolar. Most bipolar patients with one or more manic episodes will eventually have a depressive episode. At any one time, a bipolar patient may be a manic, depressed, or between episodes. Frequently a manic or depressive episode is followed by a short episode of the other without an interval between. Two or more complete cycles of mania and depression within 1 year is termed rapid cycling. Another common but unofficial classification of bipolar illness is bipolar I versus bipolar II. Bipolar I is the more classic picture of manic and depressive episodes, while bipolar II is characterized by hypomanic and depressive episodes. Hypomania is a predominantly elevated, expansive, or irritable mood but much less severe than a manic episode.

Major depression includes patients who experience only one episode of depression and those who have recurrent depressive episodes. Patients with major depression are commonly referred to as unipolar. The frequency of episodes is quite variable, with some patients having episodes separated by many years of normal functioning, while others have clusters of episodes. Up to 80% of patients return to their premorbid level of function after a major depression.

Cyclothymia is a chronic mood disturbance of longer than 2 years involving numerous periods of depression and

924

Table 52.1.
Classification of Mood Disorders

Bipolar disorder
    Manic
    Depressed
Major depression
    Single episode
    Recurrent
Cyclothymia
Dysthymia
Seasonal affective disorder
"Unofficial" subtypes of depression
    Double depression
    Psychotic depression
    Atypical depression

hypomania (mild mania). Symptoms are of shorter duration and of less severity than those of bipolar disorder. Intervals of normal mood last no more than 2 months between episodes of depression and hypomania. Cyclothymic patients do not develop psychotic symptoms, rarely require hospitalization, only occasionally require drug treatment, but often become substance abusers in an attempt to self-treat their mood fluctuations. Cyclothymia is frequently found in relatives of bipolar patients and is thought to represent a mild form of bipolar disorder.

Dysthymia, previously termed depressive neurosis, is a chronic mood disturbance of longer than 2 years in which the severity of depressed mood is insufficient to meet criteria for major depression. Periods of normal mood last only a few days to a few weeks, but never more than 2 months at a time. Symptoms include either prominent depressed mood or marked loss of interest in or pleasure in most usual activities and pastimes. Dysthymic patients do not have psychotic symptoms, rarely require hospitalization, and are most often seen by primary care physicians.

A fifth category of mood disorder more recently recognized is seasonal affective disorder. These patients are predominantly women with bipolar II illness whose episodes of hypomania or depression begin in a particular 60-day period of the year (winter, e.g., October-November), and full remission occurs within a 60-day period of the year (spring, e.g., mid-February to mid-April). This syndrome is most commonly seen in northern latitudes where sunlight is limited in the winter, and it responds well to phototherapy (light therapy) (2, 3).

CLINICAL FEATURES
Manic Episode

The essential feature of a manic episode is a distinct period of elevated, expansive, or irritable mood accompanied by at least three of the symptoms listed in Table 52.2. Common examples of excessive involvement in pleasurable ac-

tivities that may cause great harm to the patient and/or family include unrestrained buying sprees, sexual indiscretions, or foolish business investments. While most manic episodes have a predominance of euphoria and grandiosity, others may show a more dysphoric and paranoid pattern. The onset of mania is usually sudden and dramatic. Frequently, manic patients do not recognize that they are ill and resist treatment. Lability of mood is also common, in which there are rapid shifts in mood. The manic patient has considerable impairment in social and occupational functioning, though many bipolar patients have a good work history between episodes. The acute course of a manic episode has been described in three stages. The first stage corresponds to hypomania, in which euphoria predominates. These patients are perceived as happy, hyperactive, somewhat tangential in thinking, impulsive, distractable, hyperverbal, but not psychotic nor markedly impaired in occupational or social functioning. Stage II, usually called acute mania, finds the euphoria replaced by irritability and anger. The racing thoughts of the first stage lead to definite flight of ideas, with rapid skipping from one thought to another. The grandiose or paranoid ideas of stage I become more intense and often become fixed false beliefs (delusions). With treatment, few patients progress to stage III, which can be indistinguishable from any florid psychosis, including schizophrenia or an organic psychosis. The rate of progress through these stages can be very rapid, but the sequence of symptom progression is usually consistent and predictable. Use of longitudinal sequential analysis of changing symptom patterns rather than merely depending upon the acute presenting symptoms results in improved diagnosis for bipolar disorder (1, 4).

Major Depressive Episode

Depression is characterized by a persistent dysphoric mood accompanied by a variety of other symptoms (Table 52.3) (1). Major depression is diagnosed when at least five

Table 52.2.
Clinical Features of Mania

- Distinct period of persistently elevated, expansive, or irritable mood characterized by:
    Inflated self-esteem or grandiosity
    Decreased need for sleep
    More talkative than usual; pressure to keep talking
    Flight of ideas; subjective experience that thoughts are racing
    Distractibility
    Increase in goal-directed activity; psychomotor agitation
    Excessive involvement in pleasurable activities that have a high potential for painful consequences
- Marked impairment in occupational functioning; or necessity to hospitalize to prevent harm to self or others

Table 52.3.
Clinical Features for Depression

Physiologic
  Sleep disturbance, typically decreased
  Change in appetite and weight, typically decreased
  Loss of energy, fatigue
  Psychomotor agitation or retardation
  Decreased libido
  Menstrual irregularities
  Palpitations, constipation, headache
  Other nonspecific bodily complaints
Psychologic
  Dysphoric mood (sad, despondent, discouraged)
  Excessive guilt
  Pessimism, hopelessness, self-pity
  Loss of interest in usual activities
  Social withdrawal
Thinking
  Decreased concentration and attention span
  Confusion, poor memory
  Slowed thought processes
  Persecutory, somatic, or religious delusions
  Suicidal ideation

of the following nine symptoms are present nearly every day for at least 2 weeks: depressed mood, markedly decreased interest or pleasure in most activities, significant change in appetite and weight, change in sleep, psychomotor agitation or retardation, fatigue or loss of energy, feelings of worthlessness or guilt, diminished ability to think or concentrate, and recurrent thoughts of death or suicide ideation/attempt. Most depressed patients describe their mood as sad, hopeless, or blue. Others deny depressed mood, but describe loss of interest and caring or an inability to experience pleasure in normal activities. Sleep and appetite are typically decreased, but occasionally both may be increased. Change in weight must exceed 5% of body weight in a month. Psychomotor agitation is manifest as pacing, wringing of the hands, pulling or rubbing hair, skin, clothing, and outbursts of shouting. Psychomotor retardation is manifest as slowed speech, increased pauses in speech, slowed body movements, and sometimes, muteness (1, 2).

TREATMENT OF DEPRESSION

Treatment options for depression include various psychotherapies, electroconvulsive therapy (ECT), monoamine oxidase inhibitors (MAOIs), tricyclic antidepressant drugs (TCAs) and the newer nontricyclic antidepressant drugs. Selection of a treatment option depends primarily on the type and subtype of depression. Treatment of a depressive episode in a bipolar patient usually requires both lithium and an antidepressant drug. While the remainder of this chapter focuses on treatment of major depression and bi-

polar disorder, depressive subtypes whose treatment is different are considered first.

Dysthymia

Patients with dysthymia have chronic mild depression that is often unresponsive to antidepressant drug treatment. Efficacy of antidepressant drug therapy correlates directly with presence of symptoms that support the diagnosis of major depression, which means dysthymic patients usually do not have the symptoms to justify drug treatment. A study of mild-to-moderate depression in outpatients found desipramine to be significantly more effective than placebo in patients meeting criteria for major depression, while patients with dysthymia did no better on desipramine than on placebo (5). Patients with dysthymia probably represent the largest group who receive inappropriate antidepressant drug therapy. Dysthymic patients have a mood of depression that is mild but persistent, and they too often receive long-term small-dose antidepressant drug treatment that provides no therapeutic benefit beyond the value of regular interactions with the treating clinician. The most effective treatment for dysthymia is a nondrug, psychotherapeutic approach.

Double Depression

Dysthymic patients can have a superimposed major depressive episode. Up to 20% of patients hospitalized with a major depressive episode have underlying dysthymia. Antidepressant drugs are effective in treating the major depressive episode, but patients return to their baseline, which is dysthymia. The chronic mild depression remains, and the unsuspecting clinician will incorrectly view the patient as a partial responder and continue to increase antidepressant dosage or change drugs. Thus an adequate history is necessary on all patients being treated for major depression to establish a realistic therapeutic end point (6).

Delusional Depression

Patients with major depressive disorder may have psychotic symptoms, delusions being most common. The presence of delusions means that antidepressant drug therapy alone will be much less effective. Electroconvulsive therapy (ECT) is the most effective treatment for psychotic depression. When drugs are used, higher doses and longer durations of treatment are necessary, and most patients will benefit from use of an adjunctive antipsychotic drug. Antidepressant drug treatment alone for delusional depression has been shown to be effective only in 41% of patients, while a combination of an antidepressant and an antipsychotic drug has a response rate of 78%. These differences in efficacy are not due to the antipsychotic drug increasing the plasma level of the antidepressant (7, 8).

Fixed combination products (e.g., Triavil) are not recommended, since use of the antipsychotic is needed for only a few weeks whereas the antidepressant will be used for at least 6 months.

Atypical Depression

A final unofficial subtype of major depression is atypical depression, defined as a reversal of many symptoms that are typically seen in major depression. While most patients with major depression have decreased sleep, decreased appetite with weight loss, and a worse mood in the morning (compared with the evening), patients with atypical depression have the opposite of these symptoms, showing hypersomnolence, increased appetite and weight gain, and worse mood in the evening. Others have suggested that a reactive mood is a necessary feature and have added lethargy and rejection-sensitivity (rejection-precipitated depressive episodes) as features of atypical depression. For these atypical major depressions, MAOIs have been shown to be at least as effective if not more effective than TCAs (9, 10).

Treatment Options for Major Depression and Bipolar Depression

Psychotherapy. Once-weekly interpersonal psychotherapy has been shown to be equal in efficacy to antidepressant drug therapy for ambulatory depressed patients, and the combination of both is superior to either treatment alone. Maintenance drug therapy is effective in reducing relapse rates and preventing symptom return, while psychotherapy improves psychosocial function, interpersonal relationships, and day-to-day coping. Pharmacotherapy and psychotherapy should be viewed as complementary and necessary components of an effective total treatment plan (11, 12).

Electroconvulsive Therapy. ECT remains the most effective treatment for major depression. ECT is more effective, more rapid in onset of effect, and safer in patients with cardiovascular disease than TCAs. Disadvantages of ECT (compared with TCAs) include frequent relapse after treatment termination, temporary memory loss, a significant social stigma concerning its use, and in many states, legal barriers to its use. Following a successful course of ECT, there is a 50% risk to relapse during the next 12 months unless maintenance antidepressant drugs are given. Although ECT has a history of gross misuse and overuse, drug modification of ECT by anesthetic and neuromuscular blocking drugs, and unilateral rather than bilateral ECT now make it a safe, effective, and humane treatment option (13, 14). Atropine 0.4 mg is usually administered i.m. 30 min before the treatment or IV immediately before the anesthetic, to reduce oral secretions and postictal bradycardia. Glycopyrrolate 0.2 mg has been

suggested as an alternative treatment that is less likely than atropine to cause tachycardia. Methohexital 0.75 to 1.0 mg/kg is given as a bolus, followed immediately by succinylcholine 0.75 to 1.0 mg/kg to induce unconsciousness and muscle paralysis. The dose of methohexital must usually be adjusted up or down in subsequent treatments, based upon response during the first ECT treatment (14–17). In addition to being a valuable treatment option for major depression, ECT is especially effective and indicated for treatment of delusional depression and drug-treatment-resistant depression. While a highly charged political and emotional issue, ECT should be viewed as a treatment option that can be a life-saving treatment for patients who otherwise would not recover from their depressive illnesses.

Stimulants. Controversy continues among clinicians about the role of psychostimulants in the treatment of depression. A review of English-language literature found 16 reports on the efficacy of dextroamphetamine and methylphenidate in patients with primary depression (18). Of the 10 placebo-controlled studies, only one found clear support for the effectiveness of stimulants in a group of outpatients with mild-to-moderate depression with prominent apathy and fatigue. Stimulants clearly have no place in the treatment of major depression. The best evidence for efficacy is brief, low-dose therapy in apathetic "senile" institutionalized geriatric patients, with the expectation that depressed mood will only partially improve. Methylphenidate 20 to 30 mg/day for 2 to 4 weeks is usually tolerated better than tricyclic antidepressants, with exacerbation of preexisting anxiety the only consistent adverse effect.

Monoamine Oxidase Inhibitors. After nearly 20 years of being viewed as less effective and more toxic than TCAs, MAOIs have become recognized as effective agents for selected patients. Table 52.4 lists currently available MAOI antidepressants. MAOIs are most effective in atypical depression, panic disorder, and some phobic disorders, and they are an alternative treatment for patients with major depression who fail to respond to other antidepressant drugs (19, 20).

Phenelzine and tranylcypromine, the more commonly used MAOIs, are equal in efficacy and very similar in adverse effects. MAOIs should be given in divided doses, with the last dose administered no later than 6 PM to prevent drug-induced insomnia. The initial dose should be low (e.g., phenelzine 15 mg twice daily) to allow assessment of adverse effects before titration up to a therapeutic dose (Table 52.5). MAOIs have a delay in onset of clinical efficacy of several weeks, similar to TCAs. Inhibition of MAO enzyme and subsequent increased synaptic neurotransmitter levels requires 2 to 4 weeks for peak effect. About 60% of the clinical improvement of symptoms of depression occurs in 2 weeks, and maximum improvement

Table 52.4.
Available Antidepressant Drugs

Monoamine oxidase inhibitors
  Phenelzine (Nardil)
  Tranylcypromine (Parnate)
  Isocarboxazid (Marplan)
Tricyclics
  Amitriptyline (Elavil, Endep)
  Nortriptyline (Pamelor)
  Protriptyline (Vivactil)
  Imipramine (Tofranil, Janimine)
  Trimipramine (Surmontil)
  Desipramine (Norpramin, Pertofrane)
  Doxepin (Sinequan, Adapin)
Tetracyclics
  Maprotiline (Ludiomil)
Dibenzoxazepine
  Amoxapine (Asendin)
Triazolopyridine
  Trazodone (Desyrel)
Bicyclic
  Fluoxetine (Prozac)
Monocyclic aminoketone
  Bupropion (Wellbutrin)

Table 52.5.
Effective Antidepressant Dosage Ranges (Acute)

Drug	Dose mg/day
Amitriptyline	150–300
Nortriptyline	50–150
Protriptyline	30–60
Imipramine	150–300
Desipramine	150–250
Trimipramine	150–300
Doxepin	150–300
Maprotiline	150–225[a]
Amoxapine	200–600
Trazodone	200–600
Fluoxetine	20–40
Bupropion	300–450[a]
Phenelzine	45–90
Tranylcypromine	20–60
Isocarboxazid	20–30

[a] Maximum daily dose due to risk of seizures.

from a given dose is attained by the end of the fourth week.

Common adverse effects with MAOIs include orthostatic hypotension, delayed ejaculation and anorgasmia, weight gain, and edema. Orthostatic hypotension may often limit the rate of dosage titration. MAOIs also lower supine blood pressure, which does not occur with TCAs. In contrast to TCAs, MAOIs do not prolong cardiac conduction and have little effect on heart rate. For these rea-

sons, MAOIs may offer some advantages to patients with angina and conduction defects, while TCAs may be preferred for patients with preexisting dysrhythmias (21). Phenelzine is the MAOI most likely to cause weight gain; tranylcypromine does not (22). Generalized edema is more common with phenelzine and usually subsides within a week. The anticholinergic effects are the same as seen with TCAs but are much less frequent and severe. Restlessness, agitation, and insomnia can occur, and MAOIs can switch bipolar patients into mania. Unlike TCAs, MAOIs do not lower seizure threshold (23).

Severe hypertensive reactions following ingestion of food containing high amounts of tyramine is rare, but the risk can and should be minimized by careful patient education. MAO inhibition prevents the metabolism of tyramine in the GI tract and liver, causing release of norepinephrine. The clinical result is a sudden onset, painful, throbbing occipital headache, which if severe may progress to severe hypertension, profuse sweating, pallor, palpitation, and occasionally death. The severity of the reaction depends upon many factors. Six mg of tyramine produces mild elevation of blood pressure, 10 mg has a marked pressor effect, and 25 mg of tyramine can result in a severe hypertensive crisis. There are only a few foods that must be absolutely restricted: all aged cheeses, concentrated yeast extracts, pickled fish (herring), sauerkraut, and broad bean pods (fava beans) (20, 24). Although foods have received the most attention in hypertensive reactions, several drugs are more dangerous than these foods when combined with MAOI drugs. These drugs include sympathomimetics (ephedrine, phenylpropanolamine), stimulants (amphetamine, methylphenidate), levodopa, and meperidine (25).

Changing a patient from an MAOI to a TCA or from a TCA to an MAOI is done safely with a 2-week washout period between the two drug treatments. However there is rarely such luxury of time when dealing with a severely depressed patient. Fortunately, the more common clinical situation involves switching a patient from a TCA to an MAOI when the TCA has failed. This switch can be done without a washout period because there is no immediate double effect on neurotransmitters. Changing from an MAOI to a TCA, however, can not be done quickly, because there is an immediate doubling effect of neurotransmitter levels. TCAs block presynaptic reuptake of neurotransmitters and do so immediately, while MAOIs slowly increase levels of neurotransmitters released into the synapse over several weeks (26).

Antidepressant Drugs. There are currently seven tricyclic and five newer nontricyclic antidepressant drugs available for use in the United States (Table 52.6). Most of these drugs are potent inhibitors of the uptake of norepinephrine, serotonin, or both, into the presynaptic nerve ending. A common belief is that tertiary amine TCAs are

Table 52.6.
Antidepressant Adverse-Effect Profiles[a]

Drug	Sedation	Anticholinergic Effect	Orthostatic Hypotension
Amitriptyline	4	4	4
Trimipramine	4	3	4
Doxepin	4	3	4
Maprotiline	3	2	3
Trazodone	3	0	3
Amoxapine	2	2	3
Imipramine	2	2	3
Protriptyline	1	4	2
Nortriptyline	2	2	2
Desipramine	1	2	3
Fluoxetine	−1	0	0
Bupropion	−1	1	0
MAOIs	−1	1	4

[a] 1 is low, 4 is high.

serotonin (5-HT) reuptake blockers, while the secondary amine TCAs are norepinephrine (NE) reuptake blockers. This gave rise to the idea that there may be 5-HT-deficient depressions and NE-deficient depressions, and one had only to pick the drug that would specifically treat the deficiency. More recent work has challenged this concept, showing that trazodone and fluoxetine have greater potency for reuptake blockade for 5-HT, trimipramine has equal potency for blockade of both neurotransmitters, and the other drugs have a higher potency for blockade of NE reuptake (27). The exception is bupropion, which has virtually no effect on NE or 5-HT.

Antidepressants also are potent antagonists of several other neurotransmitter receptors. TCAs are histamine H_1-receptor blockers, with doxepine, trimipramine, and amitriptyline several hundred times more potent than diphenhydramine. Least potent H_1-blockers include protriptyline, trazodone, and desipramine. With the exception of trazodone, these potencies correlate well with the sedative properties of these drugs. Early reports claimed that some antidepressants were more potent than cimetidine as H_2-blockers. Improved assays have now shown that antidepressants are not potent H_2-blockers.

All antidepressants block muscarinic receptors, which leads clinically to peripheral and central anticholinergic effects. Amitriptyline and protriptyline are most potent; trazodone, fluoxetine, and bupropion are virtually devoid of this effect.

α_1-Adrenergic blockade helps explain the postural hypotension and reflex tachycardia seen with some antidepressants. Doxepine, trimipramine, and amitriptyline are most potent, while protriptyline and desipramine are least potent as α_1-adrenergic blockers. Blockade of 5-HT reuptake in the brainstem vasomotor center also contributes to orthostatic hypotension. Imipramine and nortriptyline, for example, have about equal activity at α_1-adrenergic re-

ceptors, yet imipramine causes significantly more orthostatic hypotension than nortriptyline. The difference between these two drugs is that imipramine is a much more potent 5-HT-reuptake blocker, and nortripyline is more potent as a 5-HT-receptor blocker. Antidepressants are very weak antagonists of dopamine (D-2) receptors, while β-adrenergic, GABA, opiate, and benzodiazepine receptors are not antagonized by antidepressants (27).

Mechanism of Action

While it has long been known that antidepressant drugs increase neurotransmitter levels by reuptake blockade, their proposed mechanism of antidepressant action has moved past this simplistic notion, and depression is no longer thought to be caused by a deficiency of these neurotransmitters. Studies with chronic administration of antidepressants have revealed different effects on neurotransmitters and receptors than is seen with acute administration. With chronic administration, sensitivities of several neurotransmitter receptors are altered in response to the acute effects of increased neurotransmitter levels from reuptake blockade. These changes in receptor sensitivity develop over 2 to 4 weeks, which coincides with the time necessary to see clinical antidepressant response. The major functional consequence of chronic TCA treatment is a gradual facilitation of postsynaptic α_1-adrenergic receptor function, as well as increased physiologic sensitivity to 5-HT in the brain. There is also a down-regulation (fewer receptor sites) and decreased sensitivity of α_2-adrenergic autoreceptors and β-adrenergic receptor function (28). While much is known about the acute and chronic effects of TCA treatment on neurotransmitter systems and their relative sensitivities, the exact mechanism of action of antidepressants is not yet precisely defined.

There have also been attempts to correlate neuroendocrine findings in depression to drug responsiveness and drug effect. The finding of corticotropin dysregulation in depressive disorders led to the use of several endocrinologic tests to aid in the diagnosis and treatment of depressive disorders. The most studied is a modified dexamethasone-suppression test (DST), with claims that it is useful in differential diagnosis of depressive disorders, prediction of antidepressant drug responsiveness, and prediction of when to discontinue antidepressant drug therapy. These claims have been greatly overstated, the DST is no longer used clinically, but it remains an interesting research tool in the search for simple biologic tests to help validate the diagnosis of depressive disorders and aid in predicting treatment response and long-term prognosis (29).

Drug of Choice

Two factors are important in selecting an antidepressant drug for a patient: past history of response and differences in adverse-effect profile. There are no differences among antidepressant drugs in relative overall efficacy, no differences in efficacy for certain types of symptoms except for atypical depression and delusional depression previously discussed, and no differences in onset of effect. While it is not possible to predict which drug will be effective, individual patients do sometimes show a better response to particular drugs. It is for this reason that a past history of response should be a major factor in drug selection. The drug history should include a determination of which antidepressant drugs have been used in the past, which one was most effective, what type of adverse effects were experienced, and which drugs are viewed positively or negatively by the patient. For many patients, this information will be a more important drug selection factor than differences in adverse-effect profile among antidepressant drugs. Patient attitude, while of no pharmacological value, is crucial to future patient compliance with drug therapy.

All TCAs cause the same type of adverse effects, but there are significant differences in the relative frequency of sedation, anticholinergic, and orthostatic hypotensive effects. The nontricyclic antidepressants have a much different adverse-effect profile than TCAs (Table 52.5). Sedation is often a desirable effect since most depressed patients have insomnia, and some patients have psychomotor agitation. Use of a more sedating antidepressant also eliminates the need for a hypnotic drug. Patients with important psychomotor retardation, even if there is insomnia, usually do best with a less sedating antidepressant. The relative frequency of anticholinergic effects varies greatly among antidepressant drugs. In comparison with antipsychotic drugs, thioridazine is about equal to desipramine, meaning antidepressant drugs as a class are much more likely to cause anticholinergic effects. Dry mouth, blurred near vision, and constipation are usually only bothersome effects for most patients and can be minimized by once-daily bedtime dosing. For some patients, however, anticholinergic effects can become intolerable. Drugs with higher anticholinergic effect should be avoided in patients with preexisting prostatic hypertrophy, to prevent worsened urinary hesitancy or retention. Dementia, glaucoma, and constipation can also be aggravated by anticholinergic effects. The elderly are of particular concern, since they are most likely to have these intercurrent illnesses. Orthostatic hypotension is not an important problem for most patients properly educated about its cause and how to prevent dizziness and syncope. For the elderly with decreased cerebral perfusion or for patients taking other drugs with hypotensive effects, nortriptyline, fluoxetine, or bupropion may offer an advantage. No drug has an ideal adverse-effect profile. Information from a patient's medical history, past drug history, and current symptoms must be considered in selecting the most appropriate antidepressant drug.

TCA Pharmacokinetics

TCAs are tertiary and secondary amines with pKa's in the range of 8 to 10 and a high degree of lipid solubility. These basic drugs are rapidly and well absorbed following oral administration, and most undergo significant first-pass metabolism. Peak plasma levels occur within 2 to 6 hr for all TCAs except protriptyline, which peaks in 6 to 12 hr. Systemic availability is markedly reduced by pronounced hepatic first-pass metabolism. Peak plasma levels occur within 2 to 6 hr for all TCAs except protriptyline, which peaks in 6 to 12 hr. Systemic availability is markedly reduced by pronounced hepatic first-pass metabolism. Doxepin has the highest first-pass metabolism (75%), while protriptyline is the least metabolized on first pass (15%). All other TCAs are 50 to 60% metabolized on first pass. TCAs are widely distributed, more than 90% protein-bound, and have high volumes of distribution of 10 to 40 liters/kg. Secondary amine TCAs tend to have slightly longer elimination half-lives averaging 12 to 44 hr while the tertiary amine TCAs range from 10 to 25 hr. Protriptyline is the exception, with an elimination half-life of 67 to 89 hr. Tertiary amine TCAs are demthylated to their respective secondary amine compounds, which are then hydroxylated, glucuronidated, and excreted. The hydroxy metbolites were once considered to be inactive, but recently have been shown to contribute to antidepressant efficacy and adverse effects. The rate of hydroxylation can vary greatly among individuals, resulting in variation of steady-state plasma levels as high as 30-fold in individuals given the same oral dose (23, 30, 31).

TCA Plasma Levels

Three antidepressant drugs have a well-established correlation of plasma level range with antidepressant response—nortriptyline, desipramine, and imipramine. Other TCAs have proposed therapeutic levels, but they should not be viewed as well-established (Table 52.7) (23, 32–34). Studies with nortriptyline have impressively consistent results, indicating that the minimum effective concentration of nortriptyline is 50 ng/ml, with an upper limit of 150 ng/ml above which therapeutic response declines. Nortriptyline is the only TCA to consistently demonstrate this curvilinear response, or so-called therapeutic window. Imipramine response has been shown to correlate with plasma levels of imipramine plus its metabolite desipramine at concentrations above 200 ng/ml. No decline in response is found at higher levels, with beginning toxicity seen above 500 ng/ml, and seven toxicity becoming apparent when levels reach 1000 ng/ml. Desipramine is less adequately studied, but a linear relationship seems to exist

Table 52.7.
Therapeutic Antidepressant Plasma Levels

	ng/ml
Well established	
Nortriptyline	50–150
Imipramine (plus desipramine)	>200
Desipramine	100–160
Tentative	
Amitriptyline (plus nortriptyline)	100–250
Doxepin (plus desmethyldoxepin)	150–250
Protriptyline	>70
Maprotiline	200–600
Amoxapine (plus 8-OH amoxapine)	200–600
Trazodone	800–1600

between plasma level and therapeutic effect. All other antidepressants lack sufficient data to allow any correlation between plasma level and response. Blood samples for TCA concentration determination should be drawn 10 to 12 hr after the last dose. Indications for TCA plasma level determinations include lack of response at usual therapeutic doses, intolerable adverse effects at relatively low doses, suspected noncompliance, concurrent use with other drugs known to affect TCA metabolism, stopping or starting cigarette smoking, and use of TCAs in the very young or elderly. Patients given nortriptyline are definite candidates for plasma-level monitoring, since the maximum therapeutic plasma level of 150 ng/ml can be unknowingly exceeded and full response never achieved as the dosage is increased beyond the therapeutic window. Patients given imipramine or desipramine should have one steady-state measurement if compliance is not an issue. Repeat determinations are indicated in situations listed above that can alter TCA elimination or when noncompliance is suspected. For all other antidepressants, plasma-level monitoring should not be considered routine because the cost is high and correlation with clinical response is uncertain.

Nontricyclic Antidepressants

After nearly a 10-year gap without introduction of new antidepressants during the 1970s, a number of nontricyclic antidepressant drugs were marketed in the United States in the 1980s. Clinicians had high expectations of these newer antidepressant drugs, since the TCAs have several important disadvantages. TCAs have a slow onset of effect of several weeks, are not effective in more than 20% of patients with major depression, have troublesome anticholinergic effects, have serious cardiovascular effects, and are extremely toxic in overdose. Thus far, no antidepressant offers a faster onset of effect, and all are equally effective to TCAs but not more effective. The nontricyclic antidepressants do offer some advantages in terms of ad-

verse effects and safety in overdose, though most have their own unique disadvantages, compared with TCAs.

Maprotiline has been shown to be an equally effective antidepressant when compared with TCAs. Structurally it is a tetracyclic, but it behaves no differently than other TCAs. Postmarketing experience has revealed that seizures are about three times more likely with maprotiline than with TCAs. Seizures have occurred in patients without a seizure history when doses were given at the top end of the initially recommended range of 150 to 300 mg daily. Because of its high seizure potential, the maximum recommended daily dose has been decreased to 225 mg. It is unknown if maprotiline is equal in efficacy to TCAs with its lowered maximum daily dose. In 13 cases of fatal overdose with maprotiline alone, the ingested dose ranged from 1.75 to 6 g, making it as toxic in overdose as TCAs. Compared with TCAs, maprotiline overdose involves more seizures, more delirium, and fewer cardiac arrhythmias (35, 36). Maprotiline offers no advantages but an increased likelihood of seizures over TCAs.

Amoxapine is as effective an antidepressant as the TCAs. In the early 1980s amoxapine seemed to be another effective antidepressant with a relatively modest adverse-effect profile. Subsequent reports of extrapyramidal effects and tardive dyskinesia have now significantly reduced its consideration for use. One of the hydroxy metabolites of amoxapine has dopamine-blocking activity, giving this drug some antipsychotic activity as well as antidepressant activity. While amoxapine could be considered as an option for delusional depression, the amount of neuroleptic activity is not predictable, and as a "fixed-combination" product, there is not the needed flexibility of dosage titration of each drug nor the ability to discontinue the antipsychotic and continue treatment with the antidepressant. For nonpscyhotic depressions, amoxapine is not an appropriate choice since it is the only antidepressant capable of causing extrapyramidal effects, tardive dyskinesia, and neuroleptic malignant syndrome. Amoxapine is less potent than most TCAs, so the daily dose must be higher (Table 52.5). Because most clinicians prescribe antidepressants in doses of 150 to 300 mg daily, patients given amoxapine in these doses will not receive an adequate therapeutic trial. Of 8 documented fatalities with amoxapine alone, the lethal dose ranged from 2.6 to 6 g, which provides no additional safety in overdose over TCAs. Amoxapine toxicity includes fewer cardiac effects but carries an increased risk of renal failure, seizures, and irreversible neurological damage (36–38).

Trazodone was the first of the newer antidepressant drugs to offer several important advantages to TCAs. Efficacy studies completed before marketing showed trazodone to be equal to TCAs. Postmarketing experience has led many clinicians to question whether trazodone is as effective as the TCAs. The differences between earlier studies and clinical use is a matter of dose. Trazodone is one-half as potent as TCAs such as amitriptyline and imipramine, meaning trazodone must be given in daily doses of 200 to 600 mg. Many clinicians abandon trazodone at doses of 300 to 400 mg, claiming it to be ineffective (39). Others find that some patients can not tolerate the sedation at daily doses of 500 to 600 mg. Trazodone, in doses of 100 to 400 mg daily, can be given in a single daily bedtime dose with no loss of efficacy and less daytime sedation (40). Trazodone commonly causes orthostatic hypotension, but administration of doses after meals eliminates this effect. Trazodone has no anticholinergic effects, making it a useful consideration for patients who must avoid anticholinergic effects. Trazodone has a much greater margin of safety in overdose than TCAs. Of 43 cases of trazodone overdose, the greatest 9.2 g, there was uneventful recovery. Trazodone has no effect on cardiac conduction in contrast to TCAs, which slow cardiac conduction defects. This lack of effect on cardiac conduction means that trazodone has no antiarrhythmic effect, and there are case reports of some ventricular arrhythmias being aggravated by trazodone (36, 41).

Since 1982, 207 cases of abnormal penile erectile activity have been reported with trazodone. These cases include increased nocturnal tumescence, return of erectile activity in previously impotent males, and true priapism. Priapism is defined as often painful sustained penile erection unaccompanied by sexual desire. Fifty-two of these cases required surgical intervention, with about half leading to permanent impotence. Priapism has been reported with many drugs, most commonly with phenothiazine antipsychotics, antihypertensives (mostly prazosin), and trazodone (42). Other common causes include sickle cell disease, solid tumors, leukemia, and trauma. Drug-induced priapism is caused by the inhibition of sympathetically controlled detumescence through direct α-blockade. Most cases with trazodone occur at daily doses of 150 mg or less, and most occur within the first 28 days of treatment. The incidence of priapism with trazodone is estimated to be between 1 in 1,000 and 1 in 10,000. Male patients given trazodone should be advised to report prolonged erections, and information should be given concerning the need for early reporting and intervention. Once priapism occurs, it should be considered a urologic emergency. Any erection lasting longer than 4 hr must be treated quickly before local hypoxia occurs. After 72 hr untreated priapism may lead to fibrosis of the corpora cavernosa and gangrene. Early recognition allows pharmacological treatment rather than surgical treatment, with no risk of permanent impotence. Deoxygenated blood can be removed, through angiocatheters, and irrigation with saline and an α-agonist (norepinephrine or metaraminol) often successfully promotes detumescence (43). Only one case of a priapism equivalent in females has been reported, although there are case reports of clitoral enlargement and increased libido in women receiving trazodone (42, 44, 45).

Fluoxetine, a bicyclic antidepressant, is a specific and potent inhibitor of presynaptic 5-HT reuptake. Fluoxetine has no significant binding to α- or β-adrenergic, muscarinic, serotonin, dopamine, or histamine receptors (46, 47). The elimination half-life of fluoxetine after long-term use is 4 days, while its active metabolite, norfluoxetine, averages 7 days. An effective antidepressant dose for most patients is 20 mg administered in the morning. Although the manufacturer recommends a daily dosage range of 20 to 80 mg, increased response is seldom seen in doses above 20 mg, and some patients respond to daily doses of only 5 to 10 mg (48). Because of an extremely long half-life, fluoxetine can be given in a dosing schedule of every other day. Fluoxetine has antidepressant effects equal to those of TCAs, but it differs greatly in its profile of adverse effects (Table 52.5). It lacks sedative, anticholinergic, and cardiovascular effects, which represents an advantage over TCAs for some patients. The common adverse effects of fluoxetine include nausea, anxiety, insomnia, anorexia, diarrhea, nervousness, and headache. Thus the psychomotor activity, sleep, and appetite of the patient may suggest whether fluoxetine would be a good choice or should be avoided. Akathisia, or severe motor restlessness, reported with fluoxetine is clinically indistinguishable from antipsychotic-induced akathisia (49). Anorgasmia or delayed orgasm that persists with continued treatment has been reported in 5 to 8% of patients treated with fluoxetine (50).

Anorexia and weight loss can be considered to be a positive or negative effect of fluoxetine for a depressed patient. Most fluoxetine studies for depression that mention weight change indicate weight loss of 1 to 2 kg over 5 to 6 weeks. Case reports and a few controlled studies for obesity suggest weight loss of up to 5 kg over 8 weeks. There is no information about whether the weight loss is maintained after the initial loss (51). Though many questions remain about weight loss with fluoxetine, the lack of weight gain gives it a definite advantage over TCAs for some patients. The emergence of intense suicidal preoccupation during fluoxetine treatment is not yet a clearly determined effect of the drug. The initial six case reports of intense suicidal preoccupation after treatment with fluoxetine, and subsequent completed suicides during fluoxetine treatment have raised clinical and legal concerns (52). Emergence of suicidal ideation during treatment with antidepressants is not unique to fluoxetine; it is a component of necessary clinical monitoring of any severely depressed patient (53). The primary clinical concern with fluoxetine is its many drug-drug interactions. Fluoxetine impairs oxidative metabolism, resulting in increased plasma levels and adverse effects of many drugs. Addition of fluoxetine to TCAs can increase TCA plasma levels by

100%, and adverse effects of antipsychotics can be aggravated by the addition of fluoxetine (54). The combination of fluoxetine and MAOIs can lead to a serotonin syndrome consisting of confusion, hypomania, myoclonus, hypertension, tremor, and diarrhea. One death has resulted from initiation of MAOI therapy shortly after discontinuation of fluoxetine (55). These interactions may occur up to 5 weeks after discontinuation of fluoxetine (54, 55). Fluoxetine is safer in overdose than TCAs, with ingestions of up to 1400 mg producing few adverse effects (56).

Bupropion is a monocyclic antidepressant, unique as a dopamine-uptake inhibitor with no direct effect on norepinephrine, serotonin, or monoamine oxidase, and essentially devoid of anticholinergic, antihistaminic, and adrenergic effects. Elimination $t_{1/2}$ is 10 to 20 hr but an active hydroxy metabolite has a $t_{1/2}$ of more than 24 hr. Bupropion produces no clinically important effect on cardiac conduction or orthostatic hypotension, has minimal anticholinergic effect, and causes little or no weight gain. Frequent adverse effects include insomnia, agitation, headache, and nausea (57). Its lack of sedation and its activating effect may be advantageous for patients with decreased psychomotor activity and lethargy. Disadvantages of bupropion include seizures and the inability to dose once daily. With daily doses of 450 mg or less, seizures are observed in 0.4% of patients, with a 1-year cumulative incidence of 0.5% (58). Bupropion is contraindicated in patients with psychotic disorders, as its dopamine-agonist effect causes increased psychotic symptoms. Although still too early to assess, bupropion seems to offer additional safety in overdose over the tricyclic antidepressants. The original efficacy studies were done at daily doses of 300 to 750 mg, but seizures at the higher doses caused the maximum recommended daily dose to be decreased to 450 mg. Subsequent studies have demonstrated that the lower daily doses of 300 to 450 mg is more effective than placebo (59). Bupropion must be dosed three times daily, with a maximum single dose of 150 mg. The initial dose is 100 mg twice daily, increasing to 100 mg three times daily no sooner than 3 days after the start of therapy. After several weeks, the dose may be increased to a maximum of 450 mg/day in divided doses in those not responding to 300 mg/day.

INITIATION OF TREATMENT

Antidepressant drug therapy should begin with small divided doses to assess tolerance to side effects, sedation and orthostatic hypotension in particular. For a healthy hospitalized young adult, 25 mg three times daily for imipramine is reasonable. If that dose is tolerated well, the dose can be quickly titrated upward to 50 mg three times daily within the first 3 or 4 days. Dosage increments should be done more slowly in outpatients whose appointments are usually weekly. Once the lower end of the therapeutic dosage range is reached (Table 52.7), doses can be increased weekly. The physiologic manifestations of depression are expected to show improvement within the first week, and the psychological symptoms should improve after 2 to 4 weeks of an effective dose (Table 52.3). If the patient given imipramine 150 mg daily for 1 week shows improvement in sleep, appetite, and energy level, then the dose should remain at 150 mg with the expectation that the pessimism and dysphoric mood will respond after another week or two. If no change is noted in physiologic symptoms after 1 week at 150 mg daily, the dose should be increased in 50-mg increments weekly until response in physiological symptoms is seen. When an effective dose is achieved, most patients benefit from once-daily bedtime dosing. Adverse effects may slow the rate of upward dosage titration, while patients given a more sedating antidepressant drug may initially benefit from having most or all of the dose administered at bedtime. The elderly require more conservative initial dosing and subsequent dosage titration. The elderly are more sensitive to both the therapeutic and the toxic effects of antidepressants because of reductions in neurotransmitters, increased receptor-site sensitivity, and age-related alterations in the pharmacokinetics of antidepressants (60). Initial daily doses in geriatric patients should be 10 mg for all drugs except trazodone and amoxapine, which should begin at 25 mg daily. Dosage titration should be slower in the elderly, but dose increases should be continued until clinical response or adverse effects prevent undertreatment (61, 62).

Patients must have reasonable expectations for a drug response with antidepressant drugs. Adverse effects may start the first day, while the patient will notice no improvement in mood for several weeks. Add to this the pessimistic nature of the depressed patient, and noncompliance within the first several weeks of treatment becomes a reasonable option to the patient. Patients should be counseled on expected adverse effects and what to do if they occur, and understand that there is a lag time in onset of effect. Patients should consider the improved sleep and energy seen in the first week of treatment to be a good predictor that the drug is working and expect a beneficial effect on mood.

Treatment-resistant Depression

Approximately 30% of patients with major depression do not respond to a trial of antidepressant therapy, which suggests that clinicians must often decide upon a second and sometimes third treatment option. The first approach to nonresponse is to reassess diagnosis, and ensure the adequacy of dose, duration, and plasma levels with the first drug treatment. Many studies of so-called treatment-resistant depression show that less than one-half of these patients received at least 200 mg of imipramine or its equivalent for at least 4 weeks (63). A 4-week trial of 250 to 300 mg daily of amitriptyline or imipramine is adequate, and if symptoms remain unresponsive, an alternative drug should be considered. Plasma levels should be determined for nonresponders if possible. There are no clear guidelines for choosing an alternative antidepressant. It should have a favorable adverse-effect profile for the patient and should be of a different chemical subclass. Because all TCAs primarily affect norepinephrine and have similar effects on receptor sensitivities (27), the serotonin-specific drugs (trazodone and fluoxetine) represent commonly used alternatives for a TCA-resistant patient. Trials of two different antidepressants at the top end of their dosage range for at least 4 weeks each, along with plasma-level monitoring represents a logical initial approach to the treatment-resistant patient. Despite this common clinical practice, studies that evaluate differential efficacy suggest that serotonin and noradrenergic-selective drugs are not effective alternatives for nonresponders to other cyclic antidepressants, and that nonresponders to noradrenergic antidepressants do not appear to have much chance of responding to serotonin antidepressants and vice versa (64). The differences in adverse effects determine how quickly one can switch from an ineffective drug to an alternative drug (Table 52.6). Differences in sedation and orthostatic hypotension are of most concern, while switching from a drug high in anticholinergic activity to one without can cause a cholinergic rebound.

Two antidepressant failures suggest the use of augmentation therapy. Lithium, triiodothyronine (T₃), and MAOIs are the most effective antidepressant adjunctive treatment options. T₃ has the advantage of an onset of effect within 1 week, while lithium and MAOIs must be used for 4 weeks to determine their efficacy as adjunctive therapy (64, 65). The potential benefit of augmentation drugs must be weighed against the increasing illness morbidity and the likelihood of increased adverse effects of the combination therapy. The risks of combination therapy are more often greater than the potential benefit in the elderly, particularly when lithium is added to antidepressants (66).

MAINTENANCE THERAPY

Once a depressive episode has successfully responded to drug treatment, the clinician must decide how long to continue drug therapy. Because both bipolar depression and major depression are episodic, with periods of normal or near normal mood between episodes, maintenance treatment is divided into continuation therapy and prophylaxis. Continuation therapy is defined by the time period that the underlying pathophysiology of the depressive episode continues to run its course. Since the natural duration of an untreated major depressive episode is approximately 6 months, continuation therapy is usually that used 6 months after onset of the depressive episode. Prophylactic therapy

is given when the patent would normally be between episodes of depression, and the drug is being used to prevent future episodes. Virtually all depressed patients should receive continuation antidepressant therapy. When antidepressant drugs are discontinued immediately after drug response, relapse is almost certain. At a minimum, a patient should remain free of depressive symptoms for 16 to 20 weeks before treatment is discontinued. The first 8 weeks following discontinuation of drug therapy is the period of highest risk for relapse. Even mild symptoms in patients with a previous baseline of better functioning between episodes suggest that the depressive episode has not run its course, and drug therapy should not be discontinued (67). It is common clinical practice to decrease the maintenance antidepressant dose by 30 to 50% of the dose necessary to treat the acute depressive episode, even though the efficacy of higher versus lower maintenance doses has not been directly evaluated (68). Prophylactic use of TCAs is for patients with an established history of frequent relapse of their major depressive disorder, and for patients who have infrequent but severe depression with serious suicide attempts. Lithium is also effective in prevention of recurrent major depression. For bipolar patients, lithium is equal in prophylactic efficacy to a combination of lithium and a TCA for prevention of depressive episodes and manic episodes in bipolar patients (69, 70).

Antidepressant Withdrawal

Antidepressant drugs must be discontinued by gradual tapering of the dose, rather than by abrupt discontinuation. A variety of withdrawal effects can occur with abrupt discontinuation, including excessive anxiety, restlessness, insomnia, and autonomic symptoms such as diaphoresis, diarrhea, hot and cold flashes, and piloerection. The mechanism of these withdrawal symptoms is related to rebound cholinergic effects as well as noradrenergic hyperactivity (71). Estimates of the frequency of withdrawal effects with abrupt discontinuation of TCAs ranges from 20 to 55%. Patients who experience these effects often fear that they are becoming depressed again. Prevention of withdrawal effects is best achieved by decreasing the antidepressant dose by no more than 25% every 1 to 2 weeks. Discontinuation of an antidepressant drug must be done with careful monitoring, because early signs of relapse are a major concern in addition to possible withdrawal effects. Patients should be told about the possibility of withdrawal effects and urged not to abruptly discontinue drug therapy on their own. Withdrawal effects are not a concern when switching from one antidepressant to another with a similar profile of adverse effects.

Adverse Effects and Toxicity

Common adverse effects of antidepressants include sedation, and anticholinergic and cardiovascular effects (72)

(Table 52.6). Sedation can be selected or avoided, based upon drug choice, and excessive sedation can usually be managed by switching to a once-daily bedtime dosing schedule. For patients with daytime psychomotor agitation, a divided schedule of a more sedating antidepressant may be most appropriate. Common anticholinergic effects include dry mouth, blurred near vision, and constipation. These effects can also be minimized by a once-daily bedtime dosing schedule. Many more patients taking antidepressants experience these effects than patients receiving antipsychotic drugs. There is no treatment of proven value for dry mouth and blurred near vision except changing the dosing schedule or decreasing the dose. The severity of these effects often decreases after 2 weeks of treatment. Constipation requires more careful attention, because untreated, it can progress to fecal impaction and ileus. Because constipation is caused by decreased GI motility, resulting in hard, dry stools, the best treatment is use of a stool softener and increased fluid intake. Docusate 100 to 500 mg daily, with increased fluid intake, is usually effective. Treatment need not be continuous, but it is given for treatment periods of 4 to 7 days. Less common, but of more concern, are urinary retention and central anticholinergic intoxication effects. Men with prostatic hypertrophy are at risk for urinary retention, as are patients with any preexisting difficulty in initiating urination. Central anticholinergic intoxication manifests as confusion, delirium, and sometimes, psychotic symptoms. Urinary retention may require acute treatment with catheterization and bethanechol, but both urinary retention and central intoxication indicate a significant reduction in antidepressant dose or a switch to an alternative drug with very low anticholinergic effect.

Cardiovascular Effects

Cardiovascular effects of concern with antidepressants include orthostatic hypotension, tachycardia, and decreased cardiac conduction. Orthostatic hypotension is a common effect of TCAs, with the exception of nortriptyline (Table 52.5). About 20% of patients given imipramine will be seriously affected by orthostatic hypotension, with 10% requiring a dose reduction and/or discontinuation. Subjective complaints of dizziness and lightheadedness often decrease with time, but no tolerance develops to the objective drop in blood pressure. The risk of TCA-induced orthostatic hypotension increases greatly in patients with impaired cardiac conduction or congestive heart failure and in patients taking antihypertensive drugs. MAOIs cause orthostatic hypotension more frequently than TCAs, and also cause a fall in supine blood pressure (73, 74). Fluoxetine and bupropion cause no orthostatic hypotensive effect.

Sinus tachycardia resulting from the anticholinergic effect of vagal inhibition of the SA node is of clinical concern only in patients with ischemic heart disease and marginally compensated congestive heart failure. In these cases, the patient should be given an antidepressant low in anticholinergic effect. Tricyclic antidepressants have properties similar to class I antiarrhythmic drugs like quinidine and lidocaine. Clinically, imipramine has an antiarrhythmic effect, suppressing ventricular premature contractions. TCAs have little effect on A-V nodal conduction, but do prolong conduction below the A-V node. These effects are of no clinical significance in patients with no evidence of preexisting conduction defects. Of concern, however, are patients whose pretreatment ECGs show prolonged PR interval, higher degrees of A-V block, bundle-branch or fascicular block, or intraventricular conduction delay. For these patients, trazodone, fluoxetine, bupropion, and MAOIs represent safer treatment options (73, 74).

Other Adverse Effects

Several types of sexual dysfunction are commonly caused by TCAs and MAOIs. Erectile impotence is the more common of the sexual dysfunctions associated with TCAs, while MAOIs are more likely to impair ejaculation and cause anorgasmia. Sexual dysfunction is common in both males and females, though men have a higher incidence (72). Drug-induced sexual dysfunction is often difficult to identify in depressed patients who often have decreased libido as a symptom of depression. When most symptoms of depression have improved but sexual dysfunction continues or worsens, drug-induced dysfunction should be suspected.

Weight gain is common with TCAs and MAOIs. Patients can gain 2 pounds per week for many weeks on TCAs. MAOIs can also cause edema of the legs and ankles, which contributes to weight gain. When compliance is threatened by weight gain, fluoxetine or bupropion offers an alternative that does not contribute to continued weight gain and may cause slight weight loss.

Virtually all antidepressants, TCAs, MAOIs, nontricyclic antidepressants, and ECT switch some bipolar patients from depression to hypomania or mania. When a patient is switched to mania or hypomania, the antidepressant should be discontinued and lithium initiated. TCAs have been reported to be capable of exacerbating psychotic symptoms in schizophrenic patients, though the evidence is scarce. Of special concern, however, is bupropion, which can definitely exacerbate psychotic symptoms, because of its unique dopamine agonist activity.

Antidepressant toxicity in overdose is manifest as CNS effects (toxic psychosis, seizures, coma with respiratory depression), cardiovascular effects (sinus and supraventricular tachycardias, impaired conduction leading to A-V block, intraventricular block, ventricular arrhythmias or fibrillation, and asystole), and peripheral anticholinergic effects (urinary retention, decreased bowel sounds, ileus). Treatment consists of first preventing absorption and interfering with enterohepatic recirculation by gastric lavage and activated charcoal. Physostigmine is not an antidepressant antidote, and should be reserved for treating supraventricular tachycardias causing significant problems. Fluids require careful monitoring, since too vigorous hydration may lead to pulmonary edema. Intensive cardiac monitoring can be discontinued when plasma levels fall below 500 ng/ml for drugs like amitriptyline or imipramine or when the ECG has been normal for more than 2 days (75). An ingestion of a 1-week supply of any TCA, amoxapine, and maprotiline represents a serious medical emergency. Clinicians must exercise care in selecting the amount of medication given to depressed patients and not give 1-month supplies routinely to all patients.

TREATMENT OF BIPOLAR PATIENTS
Acute Mania
Lithium is the treatment of choice for acute manic episodes. It remains the most effective and most specific treatment, compared with antipsychotic and anticonvulsant drugs. Because lithium has a lag time in onset of effect of 7 to 10 days, an antipsychotic drug often must be given with lithium for the first 1 to 2 weeks. High-potency antipsychotics like haloperidol or fluphenazine are preferred over low-potency antipsychotics like chlorpromazine because of their virtual lack of sedative and cardiovascular effects (76, 77). Once lithium plasma levels are within therapeutic range, the antipsychotic drug should be tapered and discontinued to allow assessment of the efficacy of lithium when used alone. Use of high-potency benzodiazepines has recently become a preferred adjunctive treatment to lithium instead of antipsychotic drugs. Lorazepam intramuscularly and clonazepam orally are equally effective in managing manic symptoms while waiting for onset of lithium effect, and cause fewer adverse effects than antipsychotic drugs (78, 79). A reasonable expectation of the efficacy of lithium for an acute manic episode is remission or remarkable improvement of manic symptoms in 70 to 80% of patients after 2 weeks (76). Indicators of favorable lithium response include a definitive diagnosis of bipolar disorder, occurrence of fewer than 4 episodes of mania or depression in 1 year, psychotic features, presence of the more typical euphoric-grandiose symptoms, family history of bipolar illness, and response of family members to lithium. Patients with a history of psychomotor-retarded depressions, severe anxiety, and thought disorder are less likely to be responsive to lithium. These positive and negative factors cannot be separated individually, but together become reliable indicators of lithium responsiveness (80, 81). There is some suggestion that lithium nonresponse may be episode-specific. The 20 to 30% of patients who do not respond to lithium for an acute

manic episode are not necessarily unresponsive to lithium for future episodes (82). This is contrary to the common clinical practice of labeling a patient a lithium nonresponder and seeking alternative drugs for prophylaxis and future manic episodes.

Prophylaxis
Lithium is the most effective treatment for preventing future manic and depressive episodes in bipolar patients (83). Lithium is somewhat more effective in preventing manic episodes than depressive episodes. Relapse rate studies of manic and depressive episodes show 34% relapse in 1 year for lithium-treated patients, compared with 79% relapse with placebo (84). Lithium prophylaxis is effective in recurrent major depressive episodes, but not as effective as antidepressant prophylaxis. Lithium should not be considered an antidepressant, but it is effective in treating a very small percentage of depressed bipolar patients and is reserved as an alternative treatment option for bipolar patients unresponsive to antidepressant drugs (85). Bipolar patients who receive antidepressant drugs should be given lithium to prevent the antidepressant drug from switching the patient into a hypomanic or manic state (86). In spite of its efficacy, lithium prophylaxis is not indicated for every bipolar patient. The decision to initiate lithium prophylaxis depends upon the past history of episode frequency and the impact of another episode on the patient, and his or her job and family. Bipolar patients with good insight into their illness, who can recognize early signs of relapse, who have a good family support system, who do not have significant residual symptoms between episodes, and whose episodes are less frequent than every 2 years often do not need lithium prophylaxis.

Lithium prophylaxis is the preferred treatment for cyclothymic patients who require drug therapy. While no published studies compare various treatment alternatives for cyclothymia, clinical experience suggests that lithium can decrease the frequency of cycling and/or the severity of the hypomanic or depressive episodes. There is some concern that antidepressant drugs alone may in fact increase the frequency of cycling in both bipolar and cyclothymic patients (87).

LITHIUM PHARMACOKINETICS
Lithium carbonate is almost completely absorbed from the gastrointestinal tract within 8 hr of oral administration, with peak blood levels achieved in 2 to 4 hr for rapid-release and 4-12 hr for slow-release preparations. The peak concentration achieved from a single 600 mg dose is 0.45 to 0.85 mEq/liter. The initial volume of distribution corresponds to the extracellular fluid space, with a final volume of distribution of 0.8 to 1.2 liter/kg. Tissue uptake is not uniform, with levels in the brain, thyroid, and saliva

exceeding plasma levels. Lithium is not bound to proteins or metabolized but is excreted unchanged in the urine. Lithium is freely filtered through the glomerulus, about 80% being reabsorbed in the proximal tubule, competing with sodium. The average plasma elimination half-life is 18 to 24 hr (88, 89). Compared with younger patients, elderly patients eliminate lithium more slowly from a smaller volume of distribution. The elimination half-life of lithium in the elderly is about 25% longer than that in younger patients, typically ranging up to 36 hr. The elderly require one-third to one-half less lithium than do younger patients (90).

Blood Levels

There is very good correlation between clinical response and adverse effects to lithium levels. The traditional recommendation for acute manic episodes is a plasma level for 0.8 to 1.5 mEq/liter, while a level of 0.6 to 1.2 mEq/liter is effective for prophylaxis. More recently, the recommended plasma levels have been adjusted downward to maximize therapeutic benefits while minimizing adverse effects. For acute mania, levels of 0.9 to 1.2 mEq/liter are often adequate, and maintenance levels of 0.6 to 0.8 mEq/liter are effective for most patients (91, 92). Levels above 1.5 mEq/liter are regularly associated with signs of toxicity, and levels above 2.0 mEq/liter result in serious toxicity. The narrow range between therapeutic and toxic levels makes plasma-level monitoring mandatory for all patients receiving lithium. A 12-hr interval between the last dose and drawing the blood sample in a patient receiving the same divided daily dose for at least 1 week will yield a standardized lithium level that is reproducible.

Use of erythrocyte lithium concentrations and saliva lithium concentrations have not been adopted clinically and remain of only research interest. The RBC lithium level was thought to more reflect CNS lithium levels more accurately than plasma lithium levels (i.e., there should be a better correlation with clinical response and toxicity). The only potential clinical use of the RBC lithium to plasma lithium ratio is in assessing lithium compliance. The noncompliant patient who takes lithium only a few days before the clinic appointment will have an apparent therapeutic plasma level, but the ratio will be very low. Similarly, the patient with relatively stable plasma levels but significant swings in the ratio over repeated visits is probably not compliant (93). While saliva lithium levels have been studied for over a decade, there is little clinical use of this information. Some clinicians question the predictive value of saliva levels, while others suggest that it is valuable only in clinically stabilized patients (94).

LITHIUM DOSING

For acute manic episodes, a daily dose of 1500 to 2400 mg is usually necessary to achieve a plasma level near 1.0

Table 52.8.
Lithium Steady-State Prediction[a]

Day	Lithium Received	Plasma Level (mEq/liter)
1	900	—
2	900	—
3	900	0.51

Blood drawn on morning of day 3 prior to lithium administration, so 0.51 represents 2 days of 900 mg. Assume 24-hr half-life, 0.51 represents 75% of steady-state (ss) level at 900 mg/day.

Estimated ss level at 900 mg/day = 100/75 × 0.51 = 0.68 mEq/liter.

For each 300 mg/day added, the new ss level will increase 0.15–0.35 mEq/liter. Thus, to reach desired level of 1.0, you should increase dose by 300 mg:

Estimated ss level at 1200 mg/day = (0.68 + 0.15) to (0.68 + 0.35)
= 0.83 to 1.03 mEq/liter

[a] Adapted from Gutierrez MA, Walker NR, Kramer BA: Evaluation of a new steady-state lithium prediction method. Lithium 2: in press, 1991.

mEq/liter. The initial dose, however, should be small and divided, to assess tolerance of initial adverse effects. A typical starting dose of 300 mg three times daily is conservative and can be increased by 300-mg increments every 2 or 3 days, if necessary. More aggressive therapy may be necessary for inpatients whose manic symptoms are severe or whose past history of response indicates the need for higher doses. A plasma-level determination from a sample drawn 2 or 3 days after initiation of therapy can be used to calculate the steady-state level at that dose, with subsequent 300-mg dosage increments yielding a plasma level increase of 0.15 to 0.35 mEq/liter (Table 52.8) (95). Its relatively simple pharmacokinetics allows consideration of lithium-loading doses and prediction of dosage based upon a single test dose. A loading dose of 30 mg/kg of slow-release lithium administered in 3 divided doses over a 6-hr period has been shown to accurately predict a 12-hr plasma level of 1.0 mEq/liter without adverse effects (96). A number of studies have attempted to predict lithium doses based upon a single test dose and plasma-level determination, as well as a priori predictive dosing methods with relatively positive results (97, 98). Once the desired lithium level is reached and reproduced on the same daily dose, monthly plasma-level determinations suffice. Initiation of lithium for prophylaxis should be done very conservatively because the patient is not symptomatic and no adverse effects are desired. A starting dose might be 300 mg twice daily with weekly dosage increments of 300 mg following steady-state plasma-level determinations. An oral daily dose of 900 mg to 1200 mg will usually yield lithium plasma levels within the maintenance range of 0.6 to 0.8 mEq/liter.

Before lithium is begun, a physical examination and history should focus on detection of cardiovascular, endocrine, and renal disease. Baseline tests should include serum creatinine and blood urea nitrogen levels, complete blood count, urinalysis, thyroid function tests, electrolytes, serum calcium concentration, and an ECG if the patient is over 40 or has cardiovascular disease.

Concern about adverse renal effects of lithium has led to investigation of once-daily or every-other-day dosing regimens. Most evidence suggests that trough plasma lithium concentrations are more important than peak concentrations in causing nephrotoxicity. A disadvantage of daily or every-other-day dosing schedules is the possibility of increased adverse effects, especially gastrointestinal and neurologic, which can be minimized by using slow-release lithium preparations. Whether the total daily dose is divided into two, three, or four doses does not appear to alter the 12-hr/steady-state serum lithium concentration. Once-daily dosing at bedtime, however, will increase the 12-hr concentration by 12 to 33%. Because the kinetics of single daily doses of lithium influence the standardized 12-hr serum level, patients should be stabilized on a twice-daily dosing schedule, with a switch to once-daily dosing if renal dysfunction occurs (91).

LITHIUM ADVERSE EFFECTS

Adverse effects and their relationship to therapeutic or toxic lithium levels, as well as non-dose-related adverse effects are listed in Table 52.9. While the list is long and adverse effects dramatically worsen when plasma lithium levels exceed 1.5 mEq/liter, most patients with a therapeutic lithium level experience few if any important adverse effects. The most common adverse effects are polyuria, polydipsia, and weight gain. The most bothersome adverse effects that lead to noncompliance, however, are weight gain, confusion, and mental slowness (99).

Dose-related Adverse Effects

Adverse effects seen with therapeutic lithium levels are worse in the first week or two of therapy, and for most patients are bothersome but not severe. When plasma levels are maintained near 0.7 mEq/liter, the frequency and severity of these effects are well below those previously reported with mean levels of 0.85 mEq/liter. At the lower levels, diarrhea occurs in 6% of patients, polydipsia 60%, and tremor 15% (100).

Gastrointestinal effects are most apparent during the first week of lithium therapy and usually result from the peak plasma level being too high. If further dividing the daily dosage does not treat the nausea, then a slow-release lithium preparation will further reduce the steepness of the rise of the peak plasma level, which usually eliminates GI complaints. Almost 25% of patients continue to experience polyuria and secondary polydipsia after 1 to 2 years of lithium therapy. For most patients it is of little concern and does not interfere with continued treatment. Cognitive impairment is usually manifest as confusion, mental slowness, poor concentration, and memory problems. While it is difficult to distinguish lithium-induced cognitive effects from those caused by depressed mood, patients attribute these symptoms to lithium and frequently become noncompliant. Muscle weakness is present in about 30% of patients initially but disappears quickly. Fine hand tremor is noticeable in over 50% of patients initially, and it may persist. Lithium tremor is a fine hand tremor that is seen at rest, worsens with voluntary movement, is not an extrapyramidal symptom, and is not responsive to anticholinergic drugs. Most patients are unaware of the tremor, which becomes noticeable only when delicate movements are attempted such as drinking coffee or eating soup. Management of the tremor includes reduction of the lithium dose if clinically possible, reduction in caffeine intake, and as a last resort, addition of a β-adrenergic blocking agent. Propranolol 40 to 80 mg daily or metoprolol 50 to 100 mg daily are effective treatments (101). About 50% of patients given lithium in the therapeutic range demonstrate T-wave flattening, and cases of reversible sinus node abnormalities and other conduction disturbances have been reported rarely.

Lithium Toxicity

Lithium toxicity is usually seen when the plasma level exceeds 1.5 mEq/liter, though many cases of lithium toxicity have been reported with therapeutic levels, particularly in the elderly. Many of the effects seen at therapeutic levels

Table 52.9.
Lithium Adverse Effects

Dose-related	
(Therapeutic levels)	Nausea, diarrhea
	Polyuria, polydipsia
	Cognitive impairment
	Fine hand tremor
	Muscle weakness
	ECG T-wave alteration
(Signs of toxicity)	Coarse hand tremor
	Persistent nausea, diarrhea
	Slurred speech, confusion
	Seizures
	Increased deep-tendon reflexes
	Irregular pulse, hypotension
	Coma
Non-dose-related	
	Nephrogenic diabetes insipidus
	Goiter, hypothyroidism
	Hypercalcemia
	Weight gain
	Macropapular or acneiform reactions
	Leukocytosis

worsen, and central effects of slurred speech, increased confusion, or seizures predominate in lithium toxicity. Patients and family members should be familiar with these effects and should be instructed to temporarily discontinue lithium and immediately contact their physician if they are seen. Lithium intoxication represents a serious medical emergency. Mild intoxication can quickly become serious when the nausea and diarrhea cause the patient to stop eating. Several days of fasting and diarrhea dramatically decrease sodium intake and increase sodium loss, causing significant lithium reabsorption and higher lithium levels. Hemodialysis is indicated when the lithium plasma level exceeds 4.0 mEq/liter, the patient has renal failure, or if electrolyte and fluid balance can not be maintained. For levels between 2.0 and 4.0 mEq/liter, most patients can be treated with supportive care. Use of diuresis to hasten lithium elimination is no longer recommended, and diuretics that act in the distal renal tubule may actually increase lithium retention. Lithium levels should be measured every 3 hr to follow the decline and aid in initial decision making. Fatalities are uncommon and are usually caused by renal failure or cardiovascular collapse; persistent neurologic and renal sequelae are more common (102, 103).

Non-Dose-related Adverse Effects

A variety of non-dose-related effects are possible with lithium, many of which develop only with long-term lithium therapy. The polyuria and polydipsia seen in many patients may progress in a few patients to a nephrogenic diabetes insipidus, manifest as 3 or more liters of urine output per day and a urine specific gravity as low as 1.002 to 1.005 following a 12-hr water-deprivation test. This nephrogenic diabetes insipidus is unresponsive to vasopressin and is usually fully reversible upon discontinuation of lithium therapy. Lithium blocks the effect of antidiuretic hormone on adenylate cyclase, which reduces water reabsorption in the distal tubules and collecting ducts, leading to polyuria. Because many patients must continue lithium therapy in spite of this adverse effect, attention has focused on treatment rather than discontinuation of lithium therapy. Hydrochlorthiazide has been used to reduce extracellular volume and thus decrease urine output, but increased lithium reabsorption with resultant increased lithium levels and hypokalemia are important clinical concerns. Amiloride is equally effective, causes volume contraction similar to that seen with thiazide diuretics, but also blocks reuptake of lithium into the cells of the distal tubules and collecting ducts. Amiloride has a very weak natriuretic effect, predisposing less to lithium toxicity, and no hypokalemia. Treatment of lithium-induced diabetes insipidus should begin with amiloride 5 to 10 mg twice daily, and if no response is seen, a thiazide diuretic can be added (100, 104). Renal-function monitoring (urine specific gravity,

serum creatinine, and BUN) should be done in all lithium patients every 6 to 12 months.

The potential for actual functional renal damage with long-term lithium therapy and its possible relationship to the persistence of nephrogenic diabetes insipidus is much less clear. Large prospective studies of renal function in patients receiving long-term lithium therapy have found no evidence of progressive deterioration of renal function, only an impaired renal concentrating ability (100, 105). Lithium may also cause several endocrine and metabolic adverse effects. In about 5% of patients, lithium will induce a diffuse nontender goiter, and an equal number of patients may become hypothyroid. Lithium inhibits the synthesis and release of thyroid hormone from the thyroid gland as well as inhibiting the action of thyroid-stimulating hormone (TSH). The most consistent laboratory finding is an elevated TSH seen in the first several months of therapy in about 30% of patients. An elevated TSH level persisting for more than 3 months implies impaired thyroid reserve, and replacement with L-thyroxine is required. An adequate dose will produce a normal TSH assay result in 6 weeks. To prevent the development of these complications, thyroid function should be monitored every 6 to 12 months. Evaluation of thyroid function should include inspection of the patient's neck for signs of goiter and eyes for exophthalmos, and TSH, T_3 uptake, and free T_4. Hypercalcemia is occasionally seen in lithium-treated patients, although its importance is not clearly understood. Complications of hyperparathyroidism and hypercalcemia have not been observed in lithium-treated patients, but baseline and yearly serum calcium levels should be part of routine lithium monitoring.

Weight gain is a common and important adverse effect of lithium. In the first year of therapy, patients gain an average of 4 kg, with 20% of patients gaining more than 10 kg. Intake of high caloric fluids is common because of the polyuria and polydipsia, which contribute greatly to this weight gain. Weight measurement must be a routine part of lithium monitoring, since this effect is a common cause for noncompliance (99). Lithium may aggravate psoriasis and acne, and may cause maculopapular eruptions, exfoliative dermatitis, and hair loss. Unfortunately, aggravated acne or psoriasis is often not responsive to common treatments, and discontinuation of lithium may be necessary. Hair loss, although rare, can be severe and a cause for discontinuation of therapy. Thyroid function must be evaluated in cases of hair loss to determine whether hypothyroidism is the cause (106). Leukocytosis during lithium therapy is secondary to neutrophilia accompanied by lymphocytopenia. The mean increase is 3000 to 4000/mm^3, without the shift to the left seen in an infectious process. Although a benign effect, it is useful to obtain a baseline complete blood count before lithium therapy.

LITHIUM AND PREGNANCY

Any woman of child-bearing age should be using a contraceptive method while taking lithium; lithium should be discontinued before a planned pregnancy; and lithium should be discontinued as soon as an unplanned pregnancy has been discovered. The teratogenicity of lithium is well established, with demonstrated malformations of the heart and large vessels. Because the cardiovascular system is formed during the third to ninth week after conception, lithium is contraindicated in the first trimester of pregnancy. Lithium may be used if necessary in the second and third trimesters, but lithium should be discontinued or the dose decreased by 50% several weeks prior to the delivery date. The dehydration associated with labor and fluid shifts during delivery may lead to lithium toxicity in the mother. Maternal lithium levels of 1.0 mEq/liter at term have been associated with neonatal toxicity manifest by cyanosis, bradycardia, impaired respiratory function, "floppy baby syndrome," and nephrogenic diabetes insipidus. Lithium therapy should be resumed a few days after delivery, with a reduced dose to counteract the increased risk of postpartum mania and depression. Lithium does pass from the mother's blood to milk. Infants breast-fed by mothers taking lithium have serum lithium concentrations 10 to 50% of the mother's serum lithium concentrations, causing most clinicians to recommend that women taking lithium abstain from nursing their children (107, 108).

DRUG INTERACTIONS WITH LITHIUM

There are relatively few drug interactions of concern with lithium, but several can quickly lead to lithium toxicity if not recognized and prevented. Thiazide diuretics reduce lithium clearance within several days, causing lithium levels to rise as much as 50%. When a thiazide diuretic must be used in a patient receiving lithium, the lithium dose must be decreased and lithium levels monitored more closely. Nonsteroidal antiinflammatory drugs, particularly indomethacin, declofenac, naproxen, and ibuprofen decrease the renal clearance of lithium, thus increasing serum lithium levels by 20 to 60% after 3 to 7 days of concurrent use. Sulindac and aspirin do not significantly affect lithium levels (109). Electroconvulsive therapy (ECT) should be used cautiously in a patient receiving lithium since memory loss and confusion are increased, and lithium can potentiate and prolong the effect of neuromuscular blocking agents (110).

ALTERNATIVES TO LITHIUM

Increasing attention has been devoted to alternative drugs to lithium for the treatment of acute manic episodes as well as for prophylaxis in bipolar patients. Such drugs are needed because there are patients who are unresponsive to lithium and others who discontinue lithium because of adverse effects. Carbamazepine has clearly demonstrated its efficacy both for acute manic episodes and for prophylaxis of bipolar disorder, and valproate has also shown some efficacy. Efficacy of these agents has been demonstrated both alone and in combination with lithium. Carbamazepine demonstrates an overall response rate of 70% in acute mania, with a more rapid onset of effect than lithium. Carbamazepine has been shown to be effective in patients with severe mania, or with rapid cycling that has not been responsive to lithium. For prophylaxis, carbamazepine has an overall efficacy of 65%, though most of these studies added carbamazepine to lithium. The efficacy of carbamazepine alone to prevent future manic and depressive episodes is not as well established (111, 112). Valproate is an alternative drug for bipolar disorder that has shown efficacy for rapid-cycling patients as well as an adjunct to lithium (113). Clonazepam has not been shown to be a useful alternative treatment for bipolar disorder. It is useful as an alternative to antipsychotic drugs for insomnia in mania, but there is no evidence of clonazepam having a specific antimanic effect. Lorazepam has been shown to be superior to clonazepam in acute mania (112, 114).

CONCLUSION

Mood disorders are very common, and effective treatments are available for most patients. Because of the slow onset of clinical effect and many possible adverse effects, patient education about antidepressant drugs is critical. Advances in antidepressant therapy include increased use of therapeutic plasma-level monitoring and introduction of newer antidepressant drugs with unique differences compared with tricyclic antidepressants. Lithium remains the standard for treatment of bipolar illness. Careful patient monitoring can significantly minimize the likelihood of adverse effects and drug interactions. The high prevalence of mood disorders requires all pharmacists to be familiar with their appropriate treatment.

REFERENCES

1. Hirschfeld RMA, Goodwin FK, Mood disorders. in Talbott JA, Hales RE, Yudofsky SC: Textbook of Psychiatry. Washington D.C., American Psychiatric Press, 1988, pp 403–441.
2. American Psychiatric Association: Diagnostic and Statistical Manual of Mental Disorders, ed. 3—revised. Washington, D.C.: American Psychiatric Press, 1987, pp 213–233.
3. Rosenthal NE, Light therapy. In Treatment of Psychiatric Disorders, vol 3. Washington D.C.: American Psychiatric Association, 1989, pp 1890–1896.
4. Garvey MJ, Tuason VB: Mania misdiagnosed as schizophrenia. J Clin Psychiatry 41:75–78, 1980.
5. Stewart JW, McGrath PJ, Liebowitz MR, et al.: Treatment outcome validation of DSM-III depressive subtypes. Arch Gen Psychiatry 42:1148–1153, 1985.

6. Keller MB, Lavori PW, Endicott J, et al.: "Double depression": two year followup. Am J Psychiatry 140:689–694, 1983.

7. Spiker DG, Weiss JC, Dealy RS, et al.: The pharmacological treatment of delusional depression: part I. Am J Psychiatry 142:430–436, 1985.

8. Spiker DG, Perel JM, Hanin I, et al.: The pharmacological treatment of delusional depression: part II. J Clin Psychopharmacol 6:339–342, 1986.

9. Quitkin FM, Harrison W, Liebowitz M, et al.: Defining the boundaries of atypical depression. J Clin Psychiatry 45(7, sec 2):19–21, 1984.

10. Quitkin FM, McGrath PJ, Stewart JW, et al.: Atypical depression, panic attacks, and response to imipramine and phenelzine. Arch Gen Psychiatry 47:935–941, 1990.

11. Frank E, Kupfer KJ, Perel JM, et al: Three year outcomes for maintenance therapies in recurrent depression. Arch Gen Psychiatry 47:1100–1105, 1990.

12. Weissman MM, Psychotherapy in the treatment of depression: new technologies and efficacy. In Treatment of Psychiatric Disorders, vol 3. Washington, D.C., American Psychiatric Association, 1989, pp 1814–1823.

13. Fink M: Myths of shock therapy. Am J Psychiatry 134:991–996, 1977.

14. Welch CA, Electroconvulsive therapy. In Treatment of Psychiatric Disorders, vol 3, Washington, D.C., American Psychiatric Association, 1989, pp 1803–1813.

15. Kramer BA, Allen RE, Friedman B: Atropine and glycopyrrolate as ECT preanesthesia. J Clin Psychiatry 47:199–200, 1986.

16. Allen RE, Pitts FN, Summers WK: Drug modification of ECT: methohexital and diazepam. Biol Psychiatry 15:257–264, 1980.

17. Marco LA, Randals RM: Succinylcholine drug interactions during electroconvulsive therapy. Biol Psychiatry 14:433–445, 1979.

18. Satel SL, Nelson JC: Stimulants in the treatment of depression: a critical overview. J Clin Psychiatry 50:241–249, 1989.

19. Nies A: Differential response patterns to MAO inhibitors and tricyclics. J Clin Psychiatry 45(7,sec.2):70–77, 1984.

20. Brown CS, Bryant SG: Monoamine oxidase inhibitors: safety and efficacy issues. Drug Intell Clin Pharm 22:232–235, 1988.

21. Goldman LS, Alexander RC, Luchins DJ: Monoamine oxidase inhibitors and tricyclic antidepressants: comparison of their cardiovascular effects. J Clin Psychiatry 47:225–229, 1986.

22. Cantu TG, Korek JS: Monoamine oxidase inhibitors and weight gain. Drug Intell Clin Pharm 22:755–759, 1988.

23. Bryant SG, Brown CS: Major affective disorders, parts I and II. Clin Pharm 5:304–318, 385–395, 1986.

24. Shulman KI, Walker SE, MacKenzie S, et al.: Dietary restriction, tyramine, and the use of monoamine oxidase inhibitors. J Clin Psychopharmacol 9:397–402, 1989.

25. Walker JI, Davison J, Zung WWK: Patient compliance with MAO inhibitor therapy. J Clin Psychiatry 45(7, sec 2):78–80, 1984.

26. Kahn D, Silver JM, Opler LA: The safety of switching rapidly from tricyclic antidepressants to monoamine oxidase inhibitors. J Clin Psychopharmacol 9:198–202, 1989.

27. Richelson E: Pharmacology of antidepressants in use in the United States. J Clin Psychiatry 43(11, sec 2):4–11, 1982.

28. Baldessarini RJ: Current status of antidepressants: clinical pharmacology and therapy. J Clin Psychiatry 50:117–126, 1989.

29. Arana GW, Baldessarini RJ, Ornsteen M: The dexamethasone suppression test for diagnosis and prognosis in psychiatry. Arch Gen Psychiatry 42:1193–1204, 1985.

30. Potter WZ, Calil HM, Stutfin TA, et al.: Active metabolites of imipramine and desipramine in man. Clin Pharmacol Ther 31:393–401, 1982.

31. Amsterdam J, Brunswick D, Mendels J: The clinical application of tricyclic antidepressant pharmacokinetics and plasma levels. Am J Psychiatry 137:653–662, 1980.

32. Orsulak PJ: Therapeutic monitoring of antidepressant drugs: current methodology and applications. J Clin Psychiatry 47(10, suppl):39–50, 1986.

33. Preskorn SH: Tricyclic antidepressants: the whys and hows of therapeutic drug monitoring. J Clin Psychiatry 50(7,suppl):34–42, 1989.

34. Glassman AH, Schildkraut JJ, Orsulak PJ, et al.: Tricyclic antidepressants—blood level measurements and clinical outcome: An APA Task Force Report. Am J Psychiatry 142:155–162, 1985.

35. Stimmel GL: Maprotiline. Drug Intell Clin Pharm 14:585–590, 1980.

36. Coccaro EF, Siever LJ: Second generation antidepressants: a comparative review. J Clin Pharmacol 25:241–260, 1985.

37. Lydiard RB, Gelenberg AJ: Amoxapine—an antidepressant with some neuroleptic properties? Pharmacotherapy 1:163–178, 1981.

38. Madakasira S: Amoxapine-induced neuroleptic malignant syndrome. Drug Intell Clin Pharm 23:50–51, 1989.

39. Bryant SG, Hokanson JA, Brown CS: A drug utilization review of prescribing patterns for trazodone versus amitriptyline. J Clin Psychiatry 51(9,suppl):27–29, 1990.

40. Fabre LF: Trazodone dosing regimen: experience with single daily administration. J Clin Psychiatry 51(9,suppl):23–36, 1990.

41. Georgotas A, Forsell TL, Mann JJ, et al.: Trazodone hydrochloride. Pharmacotherapy 2:253–265, 1982.

42. Thompson JW, Ware MR, Blashfield RK: Psychotropic medication and priapism: a comprehensive review. J Clin Psychiatry 51:430–433, 1990.

43. Branger B, Ramperez P, Oules R: Metaraminol for haemodialysis-associated priapism. Lancet 1:641, 1985.

44. Lorzano GB, Cataneda PF: Priapism of the clitoris. Br J Urol 53:390, 1981.

45. Gartrell N: Increased libido in women receiving trazodone. Am J Psychiatry 143:781–782, 1986.

46. Sommi RW, Crismon ML, Bowden CL: Fluoxetine: a serotonin-specific second-generation antidepressant. Pharmacotherapy 7:1–15, 1987.

47. Fuller RW: Pharmacologic properties of serotonergic agents and antidepressant drugs. J Clin Psychiatry 48(3,suppl):5–11, 1987.

48. Schweizer E, Rickels K, Amsterdam JD, et al.: What constitutes an adequate antidepressant trial for fluoxetine? J Clin Psychiatry 51:8–11, 1990.

49. Lipinski JF, Mallya G, Zimmerman P, et al.: Fluoxetine-induced akathisia: clinical and theoretical implications. J Clin Psychiatry 50:339–342, 1989.

50. Herman JB, Brotman AW, Pollack MH, et al.: Fluoxetine-induced sexual dysfunction. J Clin Psychiatry 51:25–27, 1990.

51. Kinney-Parker JL, Smith D, Ingle SF: Fluoxetine and weight: something lost and something gained? Clin Pharm 8:727–733, 1989.

52. Teicher MH, Glod C, Cole JO: Emergency of intense suicidal preoccupation during fluoxetine treatment. Am J Psychiatry 147:207–210, 1990.

53. Damluji NF, Ferguson JM: Paradoxical worsening of depressive symptomatology caused by antidepressants. J Clin Psychopharmacol 8:347–349, 1988.

54. Ciraulo DA, Shader RI: Fluoxetine drug-drug interactions: antidepressants and antipsychotics. J Clin Psychopharmacol 10:48–50, 1990.

55. Feighner JP, Boyer WF, Tyler DL, et al.: Adverse consequences of fluoxetine-MAOI combination therapy. J Clin Psychiatry 51:222–225, 1990.

56. Finnegan KT, Gabiola JM: Fluoxetine overdose (letter). Am J Psychiatry 145:1604, 1988.

57. Preskorn SH, Othmer SC: Evaluation of bupropion hydorochloride,

the first of a new class of atypical antidepressants. Pharmacotherapy 4:20–34, 1984.

58. Davidson J: Seizures and bupropion: a review. J Clin Psychiatry 50:256–261, 1989.

59. Lineberry CG, Johnston JA, Raymond RN, et al.: A fixed-dose (300 mg) efficacy study of bupropion and placebo in depressed outpatients. J Clin Psychiatry 51:194–199, 1990.

60. Salzman C: Practical considerations in the pharmacologic treatment of depression and anxiety in the elderly. J Clin Psychiatry 51(1,suppl):40–43, 1990.

61. Small GW: Tricyclic antidepressants for medically ill geriatric patients. J Clin Psychiatry 50(7,suppl):27–31, 1989.

62. Blazer D: Depression in the elderly. N Engl J Med 320:164–166, 1989.

63. Post RM, Treatment of refractory mood disorders. In Review of Psychiatry, vol 9, Washington, D.C., American Psychiatric Press, 1990, pp 7–202.

64. Nolen WA, vandePutte JJ, Dijken WA, et al.: Treatment strategies in depression. Part I and II. Acta Psychiatr Scand 78:668–675, 676–683, 1988.

65. Nierenberg AA, Amsterdam JD: Treatment-resistant depression: definition and treatment approaches. J Clin Psychiatry 51(6,suppl):39–47, 1990.

66. Austin LS, Arana GW, Melvin JA: Toxicity resulting from lithium augmentation of antidepressant treatment in elderly patients. J Clin Psychiatry 51:344–345, 1990.

67. Prien RF, Kupfer DJ: Continuation drug therapy for major depressive episodes: how long should it be maintained? Am J Psychiatry 143:18–23, 1986.

68. Kupfer DJ, Perel JM, Frank E: Adequate treatment with imipramine in continuation treatment. J Clin Psychiatry 50:250–255, 1989.

69. Prien RF, Kupfer DJ, Mansky PA, et al.: Drug therapy in the prevention of recurrences in unipolar and bipolar effective disorders—a comparison of lithium, imipramine, and a lithium combination. Arch Gen Psychiatry 41:1096–1104, 1984.

70. Consensus Development Panel: NIMH/NIH Consensus Development Conference Statement. Mood disorders: pharmacologic prevention of recurrences. Am J Psychiatry 142:469–476, 1985.

71. Charney DS, Heninger GR, Sternberg DE, et al.: Abrupt discontinuation of tricyclic antidepressant drugs: evidence of noradrenergic hyperactivity. Br J Psychiatry 141:377–386, 1982.

72. Cole JO, Bodkin JA: Antidepressant drug side effects. J Clin Psychiatry 51(1,suppl):21–26, 1990.

73. Jefferson JW: Cardiovascular effects and toxicity of anxiolytics and antidepressants. J Clin Psychiatry 50:368–378, 1989.

74. Roose SP, Glassman AH: Cardiovascular effects of tricyclic antidepressants in depressed patients with and without heart disease. J Clin Psychiatry Monograph 7(2):1–18, 1989.

75. Preskorn SH, Irwin HA: Toxicity of tricyclic antidepressants—kinetics, mechanism, intervention: a review. J Clin Psychiatry 43:151–156, 1982.

76. Goodwin FK, Zis AP: Lithium in the treatment of mania. Arch Gen Psychiatry 36:840–844, 1979.

77. Shopsin B, Gershon S, Thompson H, et al.: Psychoactive drugs in mania: a controlled comparison of lithium, chlorpromazine, and haloperidol. Arch Gen Psychiatry 32:34–42, 1975.

78. Busch FN, Miller FT, Weiden PJ: A comparison of two adjunctive treatment strategies in acute mania. J Clin Psychiatry 50:453–455, 1989.

79. Bodkin JA: Emerging uses for high-potency benzodiazepines in psychotic disorders. J Clin Psychiatry 51(5,suppl):41–46, 1990.

80. Taylor MA, Abrams R: Prediction of treatment response in mania. Arch Gen Psychiatry 38:800–803, 1981.

81. Ananth J, Engelsmann F, Kiriakos R, et al.: Prediction of lithium response. Acta Psychiatr Scand 60:279–286, 1979.

82. Carroll BJ: Prediction of treatment outcome with lithium. Arch Gen Psychiatry 36:870–878, 1979.

83. Prien RF, Kupfer DJ, Mansky PA, et al.: Drug therapy in the prevention of recurrences in unipolar and bipolar affective disorders. Arch Gen Psychiatry 41:1096–1104, 1984.

84. Klerman GL, Long term treatment of affective disorders. In Lipton MA, DiMascio A, Killam KF: Psychopharmacology: A Generation of Progress. New York, Raven Press, 1978. pp 1303–1311.

85. Donnelly EF, Goodwin FK, Walkman IN, et al.: Prediction of antidepressant responses to lithium. Am J Psychiatry 135:856–859, 1978.

86. Nasrallah HA, Lyskowski J, Schroeder D: TCA-induced mania: difference between switchers and nonswitchers. Biol Psychiatry 17:271–275, 1982.

87. Wehr TA, Goodwin FK: Rapid cycling in manic-depressives induced by tricyclic antidepressants. Arch Gen Psychiatry 36:555–559, 1979.

88. Amdisen A: Serum level monitoring and clinical pharmacokinetics of lithium. Clin Pharmacokinet 2:73–92, 1977.

89. DeVane CL: Fundamentals of Monitoring Psychoactive Drug Therapy. Baltimore: Williams & Wilkins, 1990, pp 82–138.

90. Hardy BG, Shulman KI, Mackenzie SE, et al.: Pharmacokinetics of lithium in the elderly. J Clin Psychopharmacol 7:153–158, 1987.

91. Jefferson JW: Lithium: a therapeutic magic wand. J Clin Psychiatry 50:81–86, 1989.

92. Gelenberg AJ, Kane JM, Keller MB, et al.: Comparison of standard and low serum levels of lithium for maintenance treatment of bipolar disorder. N Engl J Med 321:1489–1493, 1989.

93. Frazer A, Mendels J, Brunswick D, et al: Erythorcyte concentrations of the lithium ion: clinical correlates and mechanisms of action. Am J Psychiatry 135:1065–1069, 1978.

94. Rosman AW, Sczupak CA, Pakes GE: Correlation between saliva and serum lithium levels in manic-depressive patients. Am J Hosp Pharm 37:514–518, 1980.

95. Gutierrez MA, Walker NR, Kramer BA: Evaluation of a new steady-state lithium prediction method. Lithium 2:57–59, 1991.

96. Kook KA, Stimmel GL, Wilkins JN, et al.: Accuracy and safety of a priori lithium loading. J Clin Psychiatry 46:49–51, 1985.

97. Lobeck F: A review of lithium dosing methods. Pharmacotherapy 8:248–255, 1988.

98. Browne JL, Huffman CS, Golden RN: A comparison of pharmacokinetic versus empirical lithium dosing techniques. Ther Drug Monitoring 11:149–154, 1989.

99. Gitlin MJ, Cochran SD, Jamison KR: Maintenance lithium treatment: side effects and compliance. J Clin Psychiatry 50:127–131, 1989.

100. Jefferson JW: Lithium: the present and the future. J Clin Psychiatry 51(suppl,8):4–8, 1990.

101. Zubenko GS, Cohen BM: Comparison of metoprolol and propranolol in the treatment of lithium tremor. Psychiatr Res 11:163–164, 1984.

102. Hansen HE, Amdisen A: Lithium intoxication. Quart J Med 47:123–144, 1978.

103. Rose SR, Klein-Schwartz, Oderda GM, et al.: Lithium intoxication with acute renal failure and death. Drug Intell Clin Pharm 22:691–694, 1988.

104. Battle DC, von Riotte AB, Gaviria M, et al.: Amelioration of polyuria by amiloride in patients receiving longterm lithium therapy. N Engl J Med 312:408–414, 1985.

105. Johnson GFS, Hunt GE, Duggin GC, et al.: Renal function and lithium treatment: initial and followup tests in manic-depressive patients. J Affective Disord 6:249–263, 1984.

106. Deandrea D, Walker NR, Mehlmauer M, et al: Dermatological reactions to lithium: a critical review of the literature. J Clin Psychopharmacol 2:199–204, 1982.

107. Schou M: Lithium treatment during pregnancy, delivery, and lactation: an update. J Clin Psychiatry 51:410–413, 1990.

108. Cohen LS, Heller VL, Rosenbaum JF: Treatment guidelines for psychotropic drug use in pregnancy. Psychosomatics 30:25–33, 1989.

109. Ragheb M: The clinical significance of lithium-nonsteroidal anti-inflammatory drug interactions. J Clin Psychopharmacol 10:350–354, 1990.

110. Small JG, Milstein V: Lithium interactions: lithium and electroconvulsive therapy. J Clin Psychopharmacol 10:346–350, 1990.

111. Sachs GS: Adjuncts and alternatives to lithium therapy for bipolar affective disorder. J Clin Psychiatry 50(suppl 12):31–39, 1989.

112. Post RM: Non-lithium treatment for bipolar disorder. J Clin Psychiatry 51(suppl 8):9–16, 1990.

113. McElroy SL, Keck PE, Pope HG, et al: Valproate in psychiatric disorders: literature review and clinical guidelines. J Clin Psychiatry 50(suppl 3):23–29, 1989.

114. Bradwejn J, Shriqui C, Koszycki D, et al.: Double-blind comparison of the effects of clonazepam and lorazepam in acute mania. J Clin Psychopharmacol 10:403–408, 1990.

CHAPTER 53

SCHIZOPHRENIA

GLEN L. STIMMEL, Pharm.D.

The emphasis on community treatment and the closing of many state mental hospitals has ensured that virtually all healthcare settings treat schizophrenic patients. Community hospitals and health maintenance organizations now provide care to many psychiatric patients, and community pharmacy practitioners increasingly serve residential care facilities and board-and-care facilities. Thus schizophrenia and other major psychiatric disorders whose treatment is largely pharmacologic is part of all pharmacists' practice.

Schizophrenia is one of the more misunderstood psychiatric disorders. Schizophrenia is not a split personality. Portrayal of schizophrenia as a Dr. Jekyll–Mr. Hyde syndrome or as multiple personalities is inaccurate. Multiple personality disorder exists, but is classified as a personality disorder, not a psychotic disorder. Schizophrenia is also not associated with mental retardation. Television and movie productions tend to portray schizophrenic patients as intellectually impaired, but schizophrenia is not a cause or result of mental retardation. While schizophrenic patients may at times be floridly psychotic and bizarre, between these psychotic episodes they often remain in total control of their behavior, feelings, and thoughts.

ETIOLOGY

There is no clear etiologic explanation for schizophrenia. Hypotheses about the etiology and pathophysiology fall into several different categories, including genetic, developmental, environmental, sociocultural, and neurobiologic causes. Schizophrenia is best viewed as set of syndromes with a large continuum of pathophysiologic disruptions. The simple hypothesis of overactive dopaminergic pathways can no longer explain schizophrenia. Schizophrenics have diminished dopaminergic autoregulatory functions, abnormal patterns of response to stressors, and disturbed homoeostatic function within the dopaminergic system and between other systems. These findings suggest that a dysregulation hypothesis may best account for the diversity of neurochemical, neuroanatomic, and clinical findings in schizophrenia (1).

Schizophrenia is not synonomous with pyschosis. Psychosis has many causes and is merely a clinical descriptor defined as being out of touch with reality. Psychosis can be caused by many drugs (e.g., amphetamines, hallucinogens, anticholinergics, alcohol, phencyclidine, as well as sedative-hypnotic withdrawal), and psychotic symptoms may accompany dementias and delirium from many causes (infectious, metabolic, and endocrine). Psychotic symptoms are also very common in mood disorders, including mania and some major depressive disorders. The diagnostic criterion of a minimum 6-month duration of symptoms for schizophrenia ensures that schizophrenia can usually be distinguished from the more brief drug-induced psychoses.

PREVALENCE

In the United States the total lifetime prevalence for schizophrenia ranges from 1.0 to 1.9%, with an average prevalence of 1.1% for men and 1.9% for women. The prevalence rates for schizophrenia appear to be very similar in different countries and cultures. In 1980, there were 1.6 million admissions for patients with schizophrenia to inpatient facilities in the United States. Surveys find that up to 50% of schizophrenics at the time of the survey are not receiving any type of mental health care, even though all were deemed to be in need of care. Over 10% of schizophrenic patients ultimately commit suicide. A survey in Baltimore found that 14% of schizophrenics had never received treatment for their disorder (2).

DIAGNOSIS AND CLINICAL FINDINGS

Schizophrenia is best understood as a thought disorder. Diagnostic criteria for all psychiatric disorders are set by the American Psychiatric Association and published in the Association's Diagnostic and Statistical Manual (3). The essential features of schizophrenia include characteristic psychotic symptoms during the active phase of the illness, deterioration from a previous level of social and occupational functioning, and continuous signs of the disturbance for at least 6 months. If an illness otherwise meets the criteria but has a duration under 6 months, it is termed schizophreniform disorder (2, 3). Characteristic symptoms involve disturbances in content and form of thought, perception, affect, sense of self, volition, relationship to the external world, and psychomotor behavior.

Content of Thought. The major disturbance in content of thought involves delusion, defined as a fixed false belief. Delusions can vary in theme and content (e.g., somatic, religious, or persecutory). Common delusions in schizophrenia include a belief of thought insertion, thought broadcasting, thought withdrawal, or being controlled by an outside force. Paranoid delusions and delusions of reference are also common. False beliefs or concerns that are not yet firmly held are termed ideation (e.g., paranoid ideation, ideas of reference).

Form of Thought. A formal thought disorder is regarded as the symptom most diagnostic for schizophrenia. Form of thought disturbances are manifest as "loose associations" in which the patient may shift from one thought to another without any awareness that the topics are unrelated, illogical, or overinclusive thinking. Other common descriptors include tangentiality, circumstantiality, or in the most severe cases, derailment of thought processes. The tangential patient is one whose thinking goes off on a tangent, never to return to the original thought; the circumstantial patient talks in general terms around an idea but never addresses the topic directly. Derailment involves a patient jumping from one idea to another without any connection between the two ideas. "Concrete thinking" is the loss of an ability to think in abstract terms.

Changes in Perception. Perception disturbance primarily involves hallucinations, in which there is a sensory awareness without a sensory stimulus. While perceptual disturbance is possible in any of the five senses, auditory hallucinations are most common in schizophrenia. Voices or noises are perceived as coming from outside the head, not from within the mind as in the imagination. Visual and tactile hallucinations are possible in schizophrenia, but they are more characteristic of a drug-induced psychosis.

Affect. Disturbances of affect involve blunting, flattening, or inappropriateness of the expression of the mood. This is manifest as an unchanging facial expression, decreased spontaneous movements, poverty of gestures, poor eye contact, lack of vocal inflection, and slowed speech. These symptoms may be interpreted by others as apathy or indifference and must be differentiated from antipsychotic drug-induced pseudoparkinsonism as well as depression.

Other Symptoms. Most schizophrenics have some disturbance in self-initiated goal-directed activity, which interferes with work and other role functioning. Most schizophrenics do not comfortably relate to the world around them and have great difficulty in interpersonal relationships. This is manifest as social withdrawal and isolation, emotional detachment, and lack of friends. Schizophrenics may neglect themselves, become unkempt, and wear dirty or bizarre clothing. Psychomotor activity may be increased or decreased, sometimes so severely that the patient becomes stuporous and immobile or exhibits uncontrolled and aimless motor activity. Stereotypical behavior (non-goal-directed repetitive movements) and odd mannerisms are common in chronic schizophrenic patients.

Positive and Negative Symptoms. A more recent classification of symptoms of schizophrenia, which correlates well with responsiveness to drug therapy, is the separation of symptoms into positive and negative symptoms (2, 4).

Positive symptoms include delusions, hallucinations, marked thought disorder, and bizarre behavior, which correspond to an acute stage and reflect increased dopamine function. Negative symptoms include flat affect, social withdrawal, volitional impairment, poverty of speech, difficulty in interpersonal relationships, and attentional impairment, which correspond to a chronic state and possibly organic pathology involving hypoactive prefrontal dopaminergic pathways. Antipsychotic drugs are generally very effective in treating the positive symptoms of schizophrenia, but they are much less effective in treating the negative symptoms. The atypical antipsychotic drug clozapine is a more effective drug for negative symptoms, suggesting a different mechanism of action and hope that other atypical drugs will improve the ability to treat these symptoms (1, 4).

Course and Outcome. The natural course and outcome of schizophrenia is very poor (2, 5). It is a chronic disorder that either recurs repeatedly with incomplete recovery and subsequent persistent dysfunction or follows a progressive deteriorating course. There are three stages of a schizophrenic illness. The prodromal phase consists of the gradual development of social withdrawal, peculiar behavior, and strange ideation, with resultant work impairment, inappropriate affect, and lack of motivation. The prodromal phase varies in length, but commonly lasts about 1 year before the first acute psychotic episode. The active phase is when psychotic symptoms predominate and usually requires medical intervention. The residual phase follows and is similar to the prodromal phase except that role impairment and flattening of affect may be worse. Active-phase exacerbations often intrude repeatedly during the residual phase. Over time, the symptoms of the illness may change, with a tendency for persistence of negative symptoms. There is some evidence that antipsychotic drugs can alter the natural course of the illness; effectively treating an acute psychotic episode does provide for a better outcome for at least several years. Several 15- to 35-year follow-up studies of schizophrenics show that 60% were completely incapacitated economically and two-thirds of the patients were functioning marginally or worse at follow-up. Only 6 to 20% of patients at follow-up were completely free of psychiatric symptoms and judged to be recovered (2).

SCHIZOAFFECTIVE DISORDER

Distinguishing an acutely manic bipolar patient from an acutely psychotic schizophrenic patient is often very difficult because so many symptoms are common to both disorders. Likewise, the patient with a major depression with psychotic features may be very difficult to distinguish from the schizophrenic with a secondary depression. The diagnostic criteria for schizoaffective disorder require a manic or major depressive disorder concurrent with symptoms that meet criteria for schizophrenia. During an episode, delusions or hallucinations must be present for at least 2 weeks without any prominent mood symptoms (3). Schizoaffective disorder is too convenient a diagnosis, and it is often used in place of an adequate diagnostic assessment. Most patients given this diagnosis are found on follow-up to be either schizophrenic or to have bipolar disorder. Although primarily a diagnostic issue, there must be some concern about the validity of a diagnosis of schizoaffective disorder since these patients often receive unnecessary polypharmacy.

TREATMENT

Antipsychotic drug therapy is by no means the only component of effective therapy for schizophrenic disorders. Drug treatment can eliminate or reduce symptoms of schizophrenia, but psychologic, vocational, and social therapies are most effective in facilitating day-to-day coping and improving long-term outcome of schizophrenia (5).

Pharmacology of Antipsychotic Drugs

There are 15 antipsychotic drugs available for use in the United States, although only about 6 are commonly used in the treatment of schizophrenia (Table 53.1). The aliphatic and piperidine phenothiazines are commonly referred to as low-potency drugs, while the piperazine phenothiazines, thiothixene, and haloperidol are commonly called high-potency drugs. This terminology of low and high potency

Table 53.1.
Available Antipsychotic Drugs

Phenothiazines
  Aliphatic
    Chlorpromazine (Thorazine)
    Trifluopromazine (Vesprin)
  Piperidine
    Thioridazine (Mellaril)
    Mesoridazine (Serentil)
  Piperazine
    Trifluoperazine (Stelazine)
    Fluphenazine (Prolixin, Permitil)
    Perphenazine (Trilafon)
    Acetophenazine (Tindal)
    Prochlorperazine (Compazine)
Thioxanthenes
  Thiothixene (Navane)
  Chlorprothixene (Taractan)
Butyrophenones
  Haloperidol (Haldol)
Dibenzoxazepines
  Loxapine (Loxitane)
Dibenzazepines
  Clozapine (Clozaril)
Dihydroindolones
  Molindone (Moban)

refers only to the milligram doses used for these drugs and does not suggest any difference in effectiveness.

All antipsychotic drugs have in common an ability to antagonize dopaminergic, muscarinic, histaminic, and α-adrenergic neurotransmitter receptors, although the relative affinity for each receptor varies greatly among the drugs. Both the therapeutic and many of the adverse effects of antipsychotic drugs can be explained by their antagonism of neurotransmitter receptors (6).

Antagonism of dopamine receptors explains the therapeutic and some adverse effects. Specifically, the antipsychotic activity of these drugs is related to their antagonism of D-2 receptors in the meso-limbic area. Antagonism of the D-2 receptors in other areas of the brain explains the occurrence of extrapyramidal effects and endocrinologic effects. Antagonism of muscarinic (acetylcholine) receptors explains the occurrence of anticholinergic effects. Antipsychotic drugs antagonize histamine receptors, with a much greater affinity for H_1 receptors than for H_2 receptors. This antagonism explains sedation, drowsiness and appetite stimulation and contributes to their hypotensive effects. Molindone's virtual lack of H_1-blockade explains its lack of weight gain and reported weight loss effect, compared with other antipsychotic drugs. Finally, these drugs antagonize both α_1- and α_2-receptors. α_1-Blockade explains the occurrence of postural hypotension and reflex tachycardia, while α_2-blockade explains the mechanism of blocking the antihypertensive effect of drugs like clonidine and methyldopa. The most potent α_1-blockers are mesoridazine, chlorpromazine, and thioridazine, while molindone has virtually no effect on α_1-receptors. Most antipsychotic drugs do not have sufficient α_1-blockade effect to be of clinical significance, but when it is advisable to avoid this effect, haloperidol is least potent.

Drug of Choice

An examination of factors important in the drug selection process provides a useful way to present the clinically significant differences among antipsychotic drugs. The drug of choice for a patient should ideally be the most effective and have the fewest side effects for that patient, and the patient should have a positive past history of response to the drug. For compliance reasons, the patient should have a positive attitude or at least a neutral attitude toward the drug selected. No single drug can be predicted to be more effective than any other prior to its use. This does not suggest that all patients respond equally well to all antipsychotic drugs. While it is not possible to predict the most effective drug, individual patients do sometimes show a better response to particular drugs. This is why a history of response should be a major factor in drug selection. Important questions to ask in the drug history include: "Which drug helped you in the past?" and "Which side effects gave you the most difficulty?" Most schizophrenic patients have been treated with several or many different drugs, and they often have definite opinions about individual drugs. If a negative attitude is elicited about a particular drug, it makes no sense to choose that drug, since compliance will likely be very poor. Some chronic patients have very negative attitudes about most of the antipsychotic drugs, and will refuse to take them if prescribed. In this case, drug selection becomes a matter of reviewing the record to find a drug untried by the patient. Other patients are firmly committed to taking one drug and will refuse to try anything else in spite of other considerations such as side effects. These two types of patients make a strong case for the need for a very liberal formulary of antipsychotic drugs. Based upon efficacy, there is no need for more than one drug. Based upon side effects, maybe four or five drugs could be justified. But based upon patient attitudes and past history, virtually all antipsychotic drugs should be available for use in the treatment of schizophrenic disorders. A patient's early subjective response to an antipsychotic drug can be used as a predictor of symptomatic outcome (7). Response to questions such as: "How does the medication agree with you?," "Did it make you feel calmer?," "Did it affect your thinking?," and "Do you think this would be the right medicine for you?" were rated, based upon euphoric or dysphoric responses after a test dose of chlorpromazine. Patients with an early euphoric response improved more than patients with an early dysphoric response during the subsequent hospital stay. The early dysphoric response persists, since 88% of the dysphoric responders eventually refused to continue taking chlorpromazine because of persisting dysphoria, against only 23% of the early euphoric responders. Thus, in addition to seeking a patient's past history of response and attitude, it is worth assessing a patient's early subjective response to an antipsychotic drug.

The final important factor in drug selection is the clinically important differences in frequency of adverse effects. Relative frequencies of four of the more common adverse effects are listed in Table 53.2. Unfortunately, no drug is least likely to cause all adverse effects. Rather, drug selection requires tailoring the drug to the individual patient. Sedation may be an undesirable effect in some patients, but for those with significant agitation or insomnia, sedation may be advantageous. A history of extrapyramidal symptoms (EPS) or noncompliance due to EPS might suggest the use of thioridazine, as opposed to haloperidol or fluphenazine. For the patient with dementia, glaucoma, prostatic hypertrophy, or chronic constipation, a drug low in anticholinergic effects is most desirable. For the patient already taking another drug with orthostatic hypotensive effects or for elderly patients in whom hypotension can decrease cerebral blood flow and worsen confusion, a drug low in orthostatic hypotensive effects would be most de-

Table 53.2.
Adverse-Effect Profiles[a]

Drug	Sedation	Extrapyramidal	Anticholinergic	Postural Hypotension
Haloperidol	1	4	1	1
Fluphenazine	1	4	2	1
Thiothixene	2	3	2	1
Trifluoperazine	2	3	2	1
Perphenazine	2	3	2	1
Molindone	1	2	1	1
Loxapine	2	2	2	2
Chlorpromazine	4	2	3	4
Thioridazine	4	1	4	4
Clozapine	4	<1	4	4

[a] 1 is low, 4 is high.

Table 53.3.
Oral Dosage and Potency

Drug	Acute Dosage (mg/day)	Maintenance Dosage (mg/day)	Potency[a]
Haloperidol	10–60	3–20	2
Fluphenazine	10–60	3–20	2
Thiothixene	20–80	5–30	4
Trifluoperazine	20–80	5–30	5
Loxapine	40–160	20–80	9
Molindone	50–200	20–100	12
Clozapine	300–600	150–400	50
Thioridazine	400–800	100–300	100
Chlorpromazine	400–1000	100–300	100

[a] Chlorpromazine, 100 mg, has equal antipsychotic activity to haloperidol, 2 mg.

sirable. Information from a patient's medical and drug histories and current symptoms must be used in selecting the most appropriate drug.

Treatment of Acute Psychosis

Once a particular drug has been selected for a patient, the lower end of the daily dosage range is given in divided doses initially (Table 53.3) (8, 9), for example, haloperidol 5 mg b.i.d. or thiothixene 5 mg q.i.d. An initial divided dose allows evaluation of tolerance of adverse effects and a patient's subjective response to the medication. The dose can then be titrated upward by 25 to 33% increments of the initial dose, weekly. No change in target symptoms after 1 week suggests that an increased dose is necessary, while partial reduction of some psychotic symptoms after 1 week suggests that the dosage should be left at its current level. This titration schedule must be slowed in the elderly or patients experiencing adverse effects and can be accelerated in patients whose psychotic symptoms and agitation are severe.

Full therapeutic effect from a given dosage is seen at 6 to 8 weeks, but at least some response should be seen within 1 week to justify maintaining the current dose. Psychomotor agitation and insomnia are likely to resolve first, while auditory hallucinations, delusions, and thought disorder typically require several weeks of treatment for significant improvement. If no improvement is seen at the top end of the dosage range, the diagnosis should be reevaluated, drug compliance should be questioned, and an alternative drug considered. If partial response is seen at the top end of the dosage range, the dose can be increased further. The one exception is thioridazine, whose pigmentary retinopathy at high doses restricts its maximum daily dosage to 800 mg. Some acutely psychotic patients will require very high doses for response, such as haloperidol 100 mg or more daily. However these patients should constitute a minority in a treatment facility. The best candidate for high-dose therapy is the patient whose psychosis is acute, past history of episodes brief, and physical examination and medical history unremarkable. Nonresponse to one antipsychotic drug suggests a trial of different classes of antipsychotic drugs used for at least 4 weeks in doses in excess of 500 mg/day chlorpromazine equivalents. Failure of three antipsychotic drugs justifies consideration of clozapine or adjunctive drugs (9).

Rapid High-Dose Strategies

Attempts have been made to hasten the response of acute psychotic episodes by rapidly administering intramuscular doses of the high-potency drugs. Fluphenazine hydrochloride or haloperidol are given intramuscularly, 5 to 10 mg every hour until resolution of symptoms, excessive sedation, or intolerable adverse effects occur. Often patients may receive 40 to 100 mg within the first 24 hr of therapy. While an appealing concept, indications for such rapid titration are very few. Rapid dosing is most effective for quick control of psychotic agitation and bizarre acting-out of psychotic ideation. This technique does not shorten the time these drugs require to exert their therapeutic benefit for the core psychotic symptoms of thought disorder, delusions, and hallucinations, when compared with traditional dosing regimens. Doses of oral haloperidol or fluphenazine 5 to 20 mg daily are equally effective and are better tolerated than high-dose therapy (9). Equally effective for acute psychotic agitation is use of a benzodiazepine as an adjunct to the antipsychotic drug, which allows elimination of p.r.n. antipsychotic orders, fewer adverse effects, and up to a 50% reduction of antipsychotic drug dose. Lorazepam is the preferred drug, as it is quickly and reliably absorbed parenterally and has been most studied (10, 11).

Dosage Schedule

After an effective dosage is found, all antipsychotic drugs can be shifted to once-daily bedtime dosing. Once-daily dosing is equally effective, enhances compliance, reduces anticholinergic effects, often eliminates the need for a hypnotic drug, and decreases cost. Occasionally, a patient may require or prefer the daytime sedative effect provided by a divided-dosing schedule.

Maintenance Therapy

After an acute psychotic episode has resolved and the patient is free of overt psychotic symptoms, a decision must be made about maintenance drug therapy. A comparison of controlled studies of continuing antipsychotic drugs versus placebo treatment for 6 weeks to 2 years found overall relapse rates of 58% in placebo-treated patients and 16% in drug-treated patients (12). For the schizophrenic patient stabilized on drug therapy and virtually asymptomatic for several years, it is not clear whether low-dose maintenance therapy or an attempt to taper and discontinue drug treatment is preferred. Although 60 to 80% of patients will relapse within 1 year when placebo-treated, 20 to 40% of patients may manage for a year or longer without drug treatment (9). There continue to be attempts to characterize schizophrenic patients who can benefit from drug discontinuation without significant risk of relapse. Discontinuing antipsychotic therapy requires that warning signals of relapse be detected quickly and that drug treatment be instituted immediately. The prodromal of early signs of relapse typically include dysphoric affect, sleep disturbance, suspiciousness, and increase in preexisting psychotic symptoms such as hallucinations or paranoid delusions. Such clinical changes usually occur several days to several weeks before full relapse, allowing time for intervention. Patients selected for drug withdrawal should be those whose exacerbations have been drug-responsive, whose episodes are infrequent, who are noncompliant with maintenance therapy, or whose risks outweigh benefits of maintenance medication (e.g., early tardive dyskinesia). This approach also requires close monitoring of patients by a therapist, patient and family education about early signs of relapse, and the availability at all times of a crisis intervention team. A comparison of this targeted, intermittent treatment approach to continuous drug treatment found that the targeted approach substantially reduced the use of medication, which has a presumptive bearing on the development of tardive dyskinesia. The continuous drug-treatment approach, was superior in preventing relapse and hospitalization and in the extent of employment (13).

An alternative strategy is very low dose maintenance therapy, which has been evaluated using fluphenazine decanoate. An average maintenance dose is 25 mg intramuscularly every 2 weeks, but low-dose studies have found that 5 mg i.m. every 2 weeks is the minimal effective dose. Risk of relapse was higher with 5 mg than with 25 mg after 2 years, but raising the dose to 10 mg i.m. every 2 weeks was sufficient to treat and prevent psychotic exacerbations (14). Results of these low-dose studies suggest that all stable chronic schizophrenic patients should be tapered down to a very low maintenance dose with careful monitoring. A reasonable goal for maintenance therapy is to reduce the antipsychotic dosage to one-half the discharge dose by the end of 1 year (15). It must be remembered, however, that 10 to 15% of chronic patients will continue to require high-dose maintenance therapy of greater than 15 mg/day of haloperidol equivalents (16).

Depot Formulations

The use of fluphenazine decanoate or haloperidol decanoate represents a unique option for maintenance drug therapy. The advantage of these preparations is that a patient can receive an intramuscular injection every 2 to 4 weeks instead of ingesting capsules or tablets daily. Depot drugs are indicated for patients who respond well to antipsychotic drugs but are consistently noncompliant or refuse to take oral medication. Depot therapy is not an appropriate treatment for an acute psychotic episode because of the variable onset and duration of depot drugs. Treatment of acute psychotic symptoms requires the flexibility of dosage titration offered by oral or nondepot intramuscular preparations. The contribution of depot drugs to maintenance drug therapy is substantial, considering the magnitude of noncompliance with antipsychotic drugs. Several danger areas must be avoided when using these preparations. The convenience and success of depot therapy can result in routine doses and schedules that lack individualization. Continuous monitoring is needed to ensure that the convenience of staff remains secondary to the patient needs. Drug-usage evaluation for depot drugs in a group of patients should reveal varying doses and different frequencies of injections. Use of depot therapy for outpatients contradicts the basic philosophy of community treatment, which is to allow patients to assume as much responsibility as possible for their own care. Giving a patient a depot preparation should not be viewed as a life sentence to depot therapy. After a patient demonstrates capability for assuming responsibility for other activities, a switch from depot to oral medication should be considered.

Fluphenazine decanoate (FD) is best initiated after acute psychotic symptoms have resolved from oral treatment. There are many techniques for conversion from oral to depot, but most are based upon clinical experience rather than validated by clinical trial. If it is known early that the patient will be converted to FD for maintenance, it is easiest to give the patient oral fluphenazine for the acute phase of the psychosis. If the patient happens to be taking another antipsychotic orally, it is not necessary to convert to oral fluphenazine before instituting FD. The average initial dose of FD following successful treatment of an acute psychotic episode is 12.5 to 75 mg i.m. every 2 weeks. A practical approach to conversion, developed by this author, is to convert based upon the relationship of oral and FD usual dosage ranges. The oral dose of fluphenazine for treatment of an acute episode is 10 to 60 mg daily, while the usual FD dose initially is 12.5 to 75 mg every 2 weeks. To maintain this relationship, take the daily oral fluphenazine dose or its equivalent, increase it to the nearest 0.5 ml amount of FD (25 mg/ml), and give that amount every 2 weeks (for example, 10 mg p.o. equals 12.5 mg (0.5 ml), 25 mg p.o. equals 25 mg (1.0 ml). It is not practical or necessary for FD to be administered in amounts more precise than 0.5-ml increments. Because of the delayed onset of effect with FD, conversion from oral to FD is not a simple matter of stopping one and starting the other. Although the peak plasma concentration of fluphenazine occurs within 2 days after a single FD injection, it is often necessary to reduce but continue oral treatment until the second injection. With continuous dosing, FD requires at least 6 weeks to reach steady state (17). For maintenance therapy, FD dosage can be gradually reduced, with most patients requiring 12.5 to 25 mg every 2 to 3 weeks.

Haloperidol decanoate (HD) is the newer depot preparation, offering an alternative to FD. While the two depot drugs are virtually identical in efficacies and adverse effect profiles, doses and frequencies of administration differ. The initial dose of HD is 10 to 15 times the oral dose of haloperidol or its equivalent, up to a maximum initial dose of 100 mg. The target monthly maintenance dose should be approximately 20 times the oral daily dose. In geriatric or hepatically impaired patients, a 15-fold conversion should be used. Experience with doses over 500 mg is limited, and administration of more than 5 ml should be divided into two equal injections given in two sites. Peak haloperidol concentrations occur between 3 and 9 days, with an apparent half-life of 3 weeks, and steady-state levels with multiple dosing are reached after 12 to 16 weeks. Adverse effects, notably extrapyramidal effects, occur with the same frequency as with oral haloperidol, although the severity of extrapyramidal effects tends to be worse with depot than with oral therapy (18). HD is available at 50 to 100 mg/ml, whereas FD is available at 25 mg/ml. While HD doses seem low relative to their oral equivalents, efficacy at these low doses reinforces recent efforts to significantly lower the maintenance doses used for most schizophrenic patients.

Plasma Levels

Monitoring plasma levels would be very useful since there is no clear dose-response relationship for antipsychotic drugs, and achieving the lowest therapeutic dosage could minimize adverse effects. Unfortunately, therapeutic plasma concentrations are not well established. Haloperidol has been most studied, since it has only one active metabolite. A review of 16 fixed-dose studies with haloperidol suggests that acutely psychotic patients respond best when plasma levels range from 3 to 40 ng/ml, with most the studies suggesting a range of 5 to 18 ng/ml. There is some suggestion of a therapeutic window, with clinical response decreasing when levels are either above or below the therapeutic range. Chlorpromazine has been suggested to require plasma concentrations above 30 ng/ml for clinical efficacy, with some claiming a ceiling of 300 ng/ml above which clinical response is reduced. All studies suffer from serious methodologic flaws including variable dose, different stages of illness, and different diagnoses and most have a very small sample size. Even less evidence exists for the other antipsychotic drugs (9, 19). Plasma levels are not yet useful routinely in the clinical management of schizophrenic patients.

Clozapine

Clozapine is the first marketed atypical antipsychotic drug that has unique pharmacological effects and indications as well as significant adverse effects. While typical antipsychotic drugs exert their effects primarily via blockade of type 2 dopamine receptors, clozapine has effects on both types 1 and 2 dopamine receptors. Peak plasma levels do not correlate with onsets of therapeutic effect. Clozapine is almost completely absorbed after oral administration, with about 50% oral bioavailability because of extensive first-pass metabolism. Clozapine is more effective than typical antipsychotic drugs for refractory schizophrenia and more effective for the negative symptoms of schizophrenia (20). Frequent adverse effects include sedation, orthostatic hypotension, anticholinergic effects, fever (13 to 21%), and excessive salivation (32%). Seizures are dose-related, with a frequency up to 5% with therapeutic doses and a 1-year cumulative incidence of 10%. Agranulocytosis is the other major adverse effect of concern, occurring in 1.6% of patients after 6 weeks, with a 1-year cumulative incidence of 2%. Weekly WBC monitoring is mandatory. Substantial weight gain has been reported in most patients receiving clozapine (21). Extrapyramidal effects are rare with clozapine, a unique advantage among typical antipsychotic drugs.

ADVERSE EFFECTS (Table 53.4)

Extrapyramidal Effects. Extrapyramidal symptoms (EPS) are the most significant adverse effect in terms of frequency and reason for patients' noncompliance with antipsychotic drug therapy. There are three categories of EPS: dystonic reactions, pseudoparkinsonism, and akathisia. A fourth, tardive dyskinesia, while technically an extrapyramidal effect, is treated separately since its cause, mechanism, and treatment in many respects are the op-

Table 53.4.
Adverse Effects

Extrapyramidal	*Cardiovascular*
Dystonic reaction	Orthostatic hypotension
Pseudoparkinsonism	ECG changes
Akathisia	*Endocrine*
Tardive dyskinesia	Amenorrhea
Autonomic	Galactorrhea
Dry mouth	Gynecomastia
Constipation, ileus	Weight change
Blurred near vision	*Pigmentation*
Urinary retention	Corneal, lenticular
Delayed ejaculation	Retinopathy
Central	Skin
Sedation	*Allergic*
Toxic psychosis	Skin
Seizures	Hepatic
Neuroleptic malignant syndrome	Hematologic

Table 53.5.
Extrapyramidal Effects

Dystonic reactions
Oculogyric crisis: fixed upward gaze
Torticollis: neck twisting
Opisthotonus: arching of back
Trismus: clenched jaw
Others: spasm of muscle group resulting in facial grimaces, exaggerated posturing of head or jaw, difficulty in speech, swallowing, breathing (laryngospasm)

Pseudoparkinsonism
Akinesia: rigidity and immobility; stiffness and slowness of voluntary movement; mask-like facial expression; drooling (sialorrhea); stooped posture; shuffling, festinating gait; slow, montonous speech
Tremor: regular rhythmic oscillations of extremities, especially hands and fingers; pill-rolling movement of fingers

Akathisia
Inability to sit still, constant pacing, continuous agitation and restless movements, rocking and shifting of weight while standing, shifting of legs, tapping of feet while sitting

Tardive dyskinesia
Mouth: rhythmical involuntary movements of tongue, lips, or jaw; protrusion of tongue, puckering of mouth, chewing movements (bucco-lingo-masticatory triad)
Choreiform: irregular purposeless involuntary quick movements of the extremities; flailing movements
Athetoid: continuous worm-like slow movements of the extremities
Axial hyperkinesia: to-and-fro clonic movement of spine

posite of the first three. Table 53.5 provides a description of EPS (22, 23).

Dystonic reactions involve an acute spasm of a muscle group, which is frightening and often painful for the patient. About 90% of all dystonic reactions occur in the first 72 hr of therapy, and they can occur after a single dose. Dystonic reactions are most frequent in younger patients and in males (24). The high-potency drugs are more likely to cause dystonic reactions than are low-potency drugs. Haloperidol caused dystonia in 65% of acute psychotic patients (25). Dystonic reactions are generally brief, and are most responsive of all EPS to treatment. Laryngospasm is the only potentially life-threatening EPS, because it can interfere with respiration.

Pseudoparkinsonism manifests like Parkinson's disease. Early signs or milder forms consist of a reduction of facial expression and arm movements. Of special concern is akinesia, which can sometimes be misdiagnosed as depression, demoralization, and/or negative symptoms of schizophrenia. Pseudoparkinson symptoms typically begin after several weeks of antipsychotic drug therapy and may occur up to 3 months after initiation of treatment. Pseudoparkinsonism is more commonly seen in the elderly and is usually very responsive to treatment.

Akathisia is the most common and troublesome EPS. It is often difficult to distinguish akathisia from psychotic agitation, which can result in the antipsychotic dose being increased, thus worsening the akathisia. Akathisia has no preference for any age group and has its onset days to weeks after drug therapy begins. Akathisia is the least likely EPS to respond to treatment and is the primary cause for antipsychotic drug noncompliance. Akathisia is caused more often by the high-potency drugs (23).

The approximate frequency of EPS caused by treatment with thioridazine is 10 to 15%, chlorpromazine 20 to 25%, and fluphenazine and haloperidol, 40 to 50%. The depot preparations of fluphenazine and haloperidol have the same EPS frequency as oral dosage forms, but the severity of akathisia in particular is greater with depot drugs. It is not uncommon to be forced to discontinue depot drugs because of intolerable and untreatable akathisia and switch to another drug with less likelihood of causing EPS.

The pathophysiology of EPS is now understood to be much more complex than a simple model of cholinergic-dopaminergic balance in the striatum. Blockade or dysregulation of dopamine-2 receptors appears to be responsible for most EPS. Additionally, GABA, adrenergic, and cholinergic influences on nigrostriatal dopaminergic activity can directly affect whether EPS will be manifest, and drugs affecting each of these systems can be used as treatments for EPS. Dystonias are the result of rapid shifts in dopaminergic transmission, whereas pseudoparkinsonism results from postsynaptic dopaminergic blockade. Akathisia is thought to result from dopaminergic dysregulation in limbic or cortical pathways, explaining why it is the EPS most resistant to treatment (1).

Drug Treatment of EPS

The commonly used drugs and doses to treat EPS are listed in Table 53.6. The two most commonly used drugs are trihexyphenidyl and benztropine. They are equal in

Table 53.6.
Drugs for Extrapyramidal Effects

Drug	Daily p.o. Dose (mg)	Daily Dosing Frequency	i.m./i.v. Dose (mg)
Benztropine (Cogentin)	2–6	1–2	2
Trihexyphenidyl (Artane, Tremin)	4–15	3–4	—
Procyclidine (Kemadrin)	5–15	3–4	—
Biperidin (Akineton)	4–12	3–4	—
Diphenhydramine (Benadryl)	100–300	3–4	50
Amantadine (Symmetrel)	200–400	2–3	—

efficacy and adverse effects, but three differences should be noted. Both are available as 2-mg tablets, but benztropine is twice as potent as trihexyphenidyl. This potency difference has led to the incorrect clinical impression that benztropine causes more adverse effects. The duration of effect of benztropine is longer than that of trihexyphenidyl, allowing benztropine to be dosed once daily or at most twice daily. Trihexyphenidyl must be dosed at least three times daily. When benztropine is given once daily, it should be given in the morning. Bedtime dosing is of no value because the extrapyramidal tracts shut down during sleep and EPS is not present during the night. Also benztropine does not have a reputation for abuse or street value. Trihexyphenidyl is a common drug of abuse among patients, because some euphoria is possible along with other possible CNS intoxication symptoms including confusion, delirium, and psychosis. Clinicians should become suspicious when a patient claims that trihexyphenidyl is the only drug that works for EPS. Procyclidine and biperiden are used rarely, but they can be viewed as virtually identical to trihexyphenidyl. Diphenhydramine is a less effective oral treatment for EPS and is best considered an effective drug parenterally for dystonic reactions and an adjunct to the other anticholinergic drugs orally. Acute dystonic reactions are best treated with parenteral diphenhydramine 50 mg or benztropine 2 mg. Nonresponse within 1 min (IV) or 15 to 20 min (i.m.) justifies administration of a second dose. For pseudoparkinsonism, oral benztropine 1 to 2 mg twice daily or trihexyphenidyl 2 mg three or four times daily are usual starting doses, within maximum doses usually 6 mg and 15 mg, respectively. While pseudoparkinsonism is usually responsive to anticholinergic agents, akathisia only responds to anticholinergic drugs when accompanied by pseudoparkinsonism (23). The two classes of drugs commonly used to treat akathisia include benzodiazepines and β-adrenergic antagonists. Diazepam 15 to 30 mg daily, lorazepam 2 to 5 mg daily, and propranolol 20 to 80 mg daily are most commonly used to treat akathisia. Case reports suggest that other benzodiazepines (clonazepam) and β-blockers (nadolol, pindolol) are also effective in the treatment of akathisia. The variety of treatment approaches to akathisia suggests that there is no optimal treatment approach and that many patients will not be treated effectively. The best treatment for akathisia remains antipsychotic dose reduction (if clinically possible), trials of drug treatments, and as a last choice, switching to an antipsychotic drug less likely to cause EPS.

Amantadine is considered to be an alternative drug for EPS when anticholinergic drugs fail or cause intolerable adverse effects. Amantadine causes no anticholinergic effects, thus offering a useful alternative for the elderly and for patients whose medical status could be worsened by these effects. Amantadine also has no significant effect on memory or time perception, whereas anticholinergic drugs impair storage of new information and perception of time (26). A daily dose of amantadine 200 mg has the efficacy of 8 mg of trihexyphenidyl. There is yet no explanation why amantadine is effective in overcoming the antipsychotic postsynaptic dopaminergic blockade to treat EPS while levodopa is not effective in treating neuroleptic-induced EPS. A formidable literature in the 1970s recommended against the automatic prescribing of an anticholinergic agent when antipsychotic drugs are initiated. This literature fails to consider that more recent prescribing trends favor use of the high-potency antipsychotics in higher doses than those used in the 1970s, thus creating a much greater potential for EPS, and in particular, dystonic reactions. Use of benztropine 2 mg twice daily for the first week of high-potency antipsychotic therapy has been shown to significantly reduce dystonic reactions, while placebo-treated patients given high-potency drugs experienced a 47% incidence of dystonic reactions (27). Most studies suggest that prophylaxis reduces the rate of dystonia twofold in all patients, and 5- to 8-fold in patients given high-potency antipsychotic drugs (28). Anticholinergic prophylaxis is justified when at least two risk factors for developing EPS are present: a patient with a past history of EPS, a young male, and administration of high-potency antipsychotic drug. In these cases, prophylaxis is a high-benefit, low-risk adjunctive treatment to antipsychotic drug therapy.

The appropriate duration of anticholinergic drug treatment is not well established. Again, studies in the 1970s suggest that only 20% of patients who remain on antipsychotic drugs require anticholinergic drugs after 3 months. With the increased use of high-potency drugs, this generalization may or may not still be true. After 3 months, the anticholinergic drug dose should be reduced gradually, and if no EPS recur, the drug should be discontinued. Withdrawal of unnecessary anticholinergic agents is desirable to minimize adverse effects of memory impairment and anticholinergic effects (29).

Tardive Dyskinesia (TD). TD is a late-appearing effect that looks like an EPS but whose etiology and treatment are very different. The clinical features of TD are the bucco-linguo-masticatory triad (Table 53.5). These mouth movements are usually mild, and many patients are unaware of them until told by others. TD often looks like the patient is chewing gum or has ill-fitting dentures. The more severe cases may include movements of fingers, toes, arms, and legs. Although rare, severe axial movements may interfere with walking, respiratory dyskinesia may make breathing labored, and intense facial grimacing can produce marked discomfort as well as social and physical disability (30). The jerky choreiform movements are often made to look like purposeful movements, so that a patient is constantly readjusting glasses, hair, or clothing. Observation of fingers and toes at rest may reveal constant involuntary dyskinetic movement. In elderly patients, dyskinesias can develop spontaneously, independent of antipsychotic drug therapy. One study in a retirement home found a prevalence of spontaneous dyskinesia of 18% in patients who had never received antipsychotic drug therapy, while 42% of those who had received antipsychotic drugs had dyskinesia (31).

The clinical manifestations of TD are similar to those of EPS, but there are some significant differences between EPS and TD. TD typically appears upon antipsychotic dose reduction or discontinuation, improves when the antipsychotic dose is increased, worsens with administration of anticholinergic drugs, and may persist for months or years after antipsychotic drugs are discontinued. All antipsychotic drugs are capable of causing TD, including drugs such as prochlorperazine, which are not typically considered to be antipsychotic drugs but do cause postsynaptic dopaminergic blockade. Clozapine, the one exception, is much less likely to cause TD. Prevalence of TD cannot be precisely stated because so many variables are involved with a long-term adverse effect. The incidence of TD based on a prospective study of young adults was 19% after 4 years of cumulative antipsychotic drug exposure, with an incidence of about 4% per year for the first 5 to 6 years. Higher incidence rates have been found consistently in older populations (32). Increasing age remains the most consistent factor associated with increased risk of TD. Other risk factors include female sex in older populations and diagnosis of affective disorder. The risk of more severe TD is higher in males under 40 and in females over 71 years old. Patients with moderate TD have more drug-free periods in their drug histories than than do patients with mild TD (33). Follow-up of patients for up to 3 years suggests that the severity of TD does not increase over time but remains constant or decreases, despite continued antipsychotic drug treatment (9).

Withdrawal dyskinesia must be distinguished from TD. Withdrawal dyskinesias have virtually identical symptoms, usually appear within 1 to 2 weeks of discontinuation of antipsychotic drug therapy, are self-limited, and slowly decrease and disappear within 12 weeks (34). Withdrawal dyskinesia is thought to be caused by a temporary hyperdopaminergic state in the basal ganglia following discontinuation of the dopamine-blocking neuroleptic drug. Emergence of TD after drug withdrawal is differentiated from withdrawal dyskinesia by the persistence of symptoms beyond 12 weeks.

The pathophysiology of TD can be deduced from clinical observation of changes induced by various drugs. Improvement of symptoms with an increase in dose of antipsychotic drug and worsening with an anticholinergic drug or decrease in dose of an antipsychotic drug suggests a relative striatal hyperdopaminergic activity. TD is thought to result from long-term blockade of striatal dopaminergic receptors with resultant hypersensitivity of those receptors. TD may remain reversible if only hypersensitivity develops but become irreversible if dopaminergic receptors undergo structural changes and/or an increased number of dopaminergic receptors develop (34, 35). Early in the use of a neuroleptic drug, there is up-regulation of dopamine-2 receptors with later denervation supersensitivity, which causes a further proliferation of dopamine-2 receptors in those parts of the striatum controlling mouth-lips-tongue motion. Upon dose reduction or discontinuation of treatment, younger patients are more able to down-regulate their dopamine-2 receptors and have their TD reverse. Older patients are less able to down-regulate dopamine-2 receptors, accounting for a more persistent form of dyskinesia (36).

Treatment approaches to TD are based on an understanding of its pathophysiology. Symptoms should improve upon administration of GABAergic agonists, noradrenergic antagonists, dopaminergic antagonists, or cholinergic agonists (37). Studies of all treatment attempts can be summarized as being moderately effective at best for up to several months, but not effective in the long-term management of irreversible TD. Although there is no consistently effective treatment of TD, there are several necessary steps in the management of the patient with TD. First, the patient should have any anticholinergic drug discontinued and the antipsychotic drug dose lowered as far as clinically possible. Clozapine has been suggested as the antipsychotic drug least likely to contribute to a worsening of TD and may become the drug of choice for patients with severe TD. Because treatment of tardive dyskinesia is so disappointing, prevention becomes most important. While TD is an acceptable risk for patients with schizophrenia with its possibility of severe disruptive psychotic episodes, antipsychotic drugs should not be used casually for nonpsychotic indications. Anxiety disorders, insomnia, personality disorders, gastrointestinal disorders, and bipolar patients are more effectively treated with other drug classes. Patients who receive maintenance antipsychotic drug therapy should be assessed for early signs of TD at least semiannually and preferably quarterly. Early signs include worm-like muscular movements on the surface of the tongue, facial tics such as frequent blinking, and choreoathetoid finger or toe movements. Early detection is crucial in identifying TD while it is still reversible.

Anticholinergic Effects. Peripheral anticholinergic effects may commonly accompany thioridazine and chlorpromazine therapy (Table 53.2). Additionally, patients on the high-potency drugs often require anticholinergic agents for EPS, so they too are often bothered by dry mouth, blurred near vision, and constipation. These effects are directly dose-related and additive. Usually, anticholinergic effects are bothersome but not significant unless there is preexisting prostatic hypertrophy, glaucoma, or constipation. Anticholinergic effects can often be minimized by switching to once-daily bedtime dosing or by decreasing antipsychotic or anticholinergic drug doses. The dry mouth and blurred vision are worse in the beginning of therapy and some tolerance develops. Patients should be told that these effects should decrease after the first 2 weeks of therapy. There is no treatment of proven value except alteration of dose or dosing schedule. Constipation, the more serious concern, should be part of routine monitoring. Reduction in GI motility and secretions typically results in constipation characterized by hard dry stools. Use of stool softeners is the most appropriate treatment, such as docusate 100 to 500 mg daily accompanied by increased fluid intake. Treatment need not be continuous, but on an interrupted basis for 4 to 7 days at a time. Often patients also require information about normal physiology and the role of exercise and diet. Untreated constipation can become a significant medical concern and emergency. Fecal impaction, ileus, megacolon requiring surgery, and fatalities have resulted from untreated chronic constipation caused by antipsychotic drugs. Rarely, more severe anticholinergic effects can occur such as urinary retention and a central anticholinergic intoxication characterized by confusion, delirium, and psychotic symptoms. Urinary retention is a particular problem in older men with benign prostatic hypertrophy. Treatment may require catheterization and bethanechol, accompanied by significant reduction of the dose of the causative drug or change to another drug with much less anticholinergic activity (Table 53.2). Central anticholinergic effects are of most concern in the elderly and patients with dementia. A patient's entire drug regimen must be reviewed to detect all drugs capable of contributing to the anticholinergic effect, including antihistamines and tricyclic antidepressants.

Cardiovascular Effects. The most frequent cardiovascular effect caused by antipsychotic drugs is orthostatic hypotension. It is much more common with the aliphatic and piperidine phenothiazines and unusual with the high-potency drugs, except when they are given parenterally (22). Orthostatic hypotension is most common in the first hours or days of treatment, and most patients develop a compensatory tolerance to the subjective effect of dizziness during the first week of therapy. This effect must be part of initial patient education since it is easy to prevent. When aliphatic or piperidine phenothiazine therapy is started or when the dose is increased, patients should be warned to rise slowly from a sitting or reclining position. Elderly patients and those taking other drugs with hypotensive effects are at much greater risk of significant hypotensive effects. Treatment of orthostatic hypotension usually requires only elevating the feet of the patient in a prone position. Nonresponse, which is unusual, will then require administration of fluids, and in rare cases, pressor agents. Pure α-adrenergic agents are preferred over a drug like epinephrine to overcome the antipsychotic drug's α-adrenergic blockade. Thioridazine, and to a lesser extent chlorpromazine, may induce ECG changes, T-wave abnormalities in particular. Doses above 300 mg daily are necessary to elicit this effect in most patients. This change is thought to represent a benign disturbance of myocardial repolarization, and it does not represent a significant clinical concern.

Neuroleptic Malignant Syndrome (NMS).
NMS is an uncommon but serious adverse effect that occurs in 1.4% of patients treated with antipsychotic drugs. NMS is characterized by fever; severe EPS such as lead-pipe rigidity, trismus, choreiform movements, and opisthotonus; signs of autonomic instability such as tachycardia, labile hypertension, diaphoresis, and incontinence; and fluctuating levels of consciousness. Some cases have been followed by permanent neurological sequelae, including dementia and signs of parkinsonism. Through 1980, there was a mortality rate of 22% in reported cases, which has now dropped to a 4% mortality rate in the last 50 cases reported, because of improved early recognition and treatment (38). Fatalities have been associated with rhabdomyolysis and myoglobinuria with acute renal failure, cardiovascular collapse, intravascular thrombosis with pulmonary embolism, and respiratory arrest. NMS occurs typically after 3 to 9 days of treatment with antipsychotic drugs and is not related to dose or previous antipsychotic drug exposure. Once NMS begins, symptoms progress rapidly over 24 to 72 hr. Symptoms usually last 5 to 10 days after discontinuing oral antipsychotic drugs and 13 to 30 days with depot drugs. NMS occurs more often in patients under 40 years of age and is almost twice as common in males; 40% of cases occurred in patients with affective disorder rather than schizophrenia. Early diagnosis of NMS is crucial to successful treatment. The antipsychotic drug should be discontinued quickly, and supportive measures provided, particularly hydration. Though controlled trials are not likely to be possible, dantrolene and dopaminergic agonists such as bromocriptine and levodopa have been effective in treating many cases of NMS. Because many patients who experience NMS will require resumption of an antipsychotic drug, rechallenge is often necessary. Successful rechallenge seems to depend primarily upon waiting a minimum of 5 days and preferably 2 weeks after complete resolution of the NMS (39, 40).

Endocrine Effects.
Common endocrine effects of antipsychotic drugs include galactorrhea and menstrual irregularities in females, with a prevalence of 30% (41). Galactorrhea results from suppression of prolactin inhibitory factor in the median eminence of the hypothalamus by antipsychotic drugs, allowing secretion of prolactin from the anterior pituitary. No specific treatment is necessary, and lowering the dose may lessen or eliminate this effect. The patient should be assured that it is a reversible effect. There is no information about a differential incidence of galactorrhea among antipsychotic drugs—all drugs should be capable of causing this effect since it is caused by dopaminergic blockade in the hypothalamus. Amenorrhea and irregular menses are common findings in the psychiatric patients. A 1942 study (pre–drug era) of schizophrenic women of child-bearing age showed an 18% incidence of amenorrhea, and 31% had delayed or prolonged menstrual cycles (42). With the introduction of antipsychotic drugs, the incidence seems not to have increased, although there is recognition that antipsychotic drugs can interfere pharmacologically with the menstrual cycle. All women of child-bearing age should have a menstrual history taken to use as a baseline before drug therapy is initiated. Women experiencing amenorrhea should be cautioned that the antipsychotic drug is not a reliable contraceptive.

Phenothiazines, thiothixene, and haloperidol have been reported to cause weight gain, while loxapine and molindone have no effect on weight or may in fact cause slight weight loss (43). This difference may influence drug selection for some patients. The mechanism of weight change is unknown but may involve a combination of effects on several neurotransmitters. A high affinity for blockade of histamine-1 receptors and dopamine-2 receptors correlates with weight gain, and serotonin-agonist effects contribute to weight loss. Molindone may have a central anorexigenic effect via serotonin-agonist activity, coupled with its low affinity for histamine-1 and dopamine-2 receptors. Loxapine's lack of weight gain is not as well understood but may involve its serotonin agonist effect.

Temperature Regulation.
Antipsychotic drugs interfere with normal temperature regulation centrally. The most common effect is relative poikilothermia, in which the environmental temperature can produce either hypothermia or hyperthermia. Hyperthermia is more frequently reported in patients taking antipsychotic drugs in hot humid climates. Hyperthermia not only results from central effects on temperature regulation but also is aggravated by an increased peripheral vasodilation and diminished heat

loss due to decreased sweating from anticholinergic effects.

Sexual Dysfunction. The most frequent adverse effect is a disorder of ejaculation. Most common is absence of ejaculation on masturbation or sexual intercourse, with some patients reporting suprapubic pain on orgasm. In addition to the effect on α-adrenergic receptors in the pelvic plexus to interfere with the ejaculatory mechanism, antipsychotic drugs with high anticholinergic effects can also relax the internal sphincter muscle of the bladder, resulting in retrograde ejaculation by reflux of semen into the bladder. Patients should be reassured that these effects are reversible, and if necessary, a drug with less anticholinergic activity should be substituted. Impotence or ejaculation complaints should not be routinely assumed to be drug-induced because sexual dysfunction is common in psychiatric disorders.

Pigmentary Effects. Pigmentary effects in the skin and eye occur with high-dose long-term use of low-potency phenothiazine drugs. Piperazine phenothiazines and thioxanthenes can also contribute to pigmentation, but the risk is low because they are given in tens of milligrams instead of hundreds of milligrams daily. Haloperidol, loxapine, and molindone do not cause these pigmentary effects, and should be substituted if a patient develops skin or eye pigmentation. Ocular pigmentation is described as a light dusty pigment on the lens capsule, which eventually may take the form of a stellate cataract. Skin pigmentation may range from a slate gray to a metallic purple color and is confined to skin exposed to sunlight. The color changes are so gradual that the patient may not notice. Any patient with skin pigmentation should be referred for ophthalmologic examination because there is close correlation of skin and eye changes. Patients who have received a total of 600 g or 200 g of chlorpromazine in 1 year have a 30% likelihood of eye pigmentation (44). Most evidence suggests that these pigmentary changes are slowly reversible over a period of months after the patient is switched to an antipsychotic incapable of causing pigmentation. Thioridazine is unique in its ability to cause pigmentary retinopathy when given in doses over 1200 mg daily for several months. Because retinal pigmentation can interfere directly with visual acuity, thioridazine has a dosage limit of 800 mg daily to prevent this effect.

Allergic Reactions. Skin eruptions take a variety of forms, but the most common antipsychotic drug reaction is a rash on the face, neck, upper chest, and extremities, which occurs between 14 and 60 days after starting the neuroleptic drug. Often allergic skin reactions are mild and transitory and can be treated with antihistamines without discontinuing the antipsychotic drug. Allergic skin manifestations must be differentiated from photosensitivity reactions, which are characterized by erythematous lesions in sun-exposed areas of the body.

Other Adverse Effects. Hepatic toxicity is now rare with antipsychotic drugs. Cholestatic jaundice with chlorpromazine typically occurs within the first 4 weeks of therapy, and most cases have classic prodromal symptoms that precede the jaundice by about 1 week. Laboratory findings are consistent with those seen in other types of obstructive jaundice. Onset of prodromal symptoms is usually abrupt. Chlorpromazine-induced hepatitis is usually short-lived and self-limiting. With the exception of clozapine, hematologic effects of antipsychotic drugs are varied but extremely rare. Agranulocytosis, the most significant hematologic effect, has an abrupt onset in which the leukocyte count drops rapidly, reaching its low point in 2 to 5 days. Ninety percent of cases occur within the first 8 weeks of phenothiazine drug therapy, whereas clozapine-induced agranulocytosis has a delayed onset of 6 to 8 weeks and will usually occur within the first 6 months of treatment. Agranulocytosis begins with symptoms of localized infection, usually in the pharynx, and includes fever, pharyngeal erythema, and adenopathy (20, 45).

Seizures occur in approximately 1% of patients given antipsychotic drugs. A history of seizures is not an absolute contraindication to use of an antipsychotic drug. Among typical antipsychotic drugs, thioridazine, molindone, thiothixene, fluphenazine, and haloperidol are least associated with seizure production, while seizures have been reported most with chlorpromazine and to a moderate extent with trifluoperazine and perphenazine. Clozapine, by far the most likely psychotropic drug to cause seizures, has a 1-year prevalence of approximately 10%. Of additional significant importance are drug factors that increase the likelihood of seizures: rapid dosage titration, abruptly switching from one antipsychotic drug to another, use of two antipsychotics simultaneously, and discontinuation of concurrently used benzodiazepines (46).

CONCLUSION

Schizophrenia is best characterized as a chronic thought disorder manifested by various psychotic symptoms and (usually) a gradual decline in functioning. Drug treatment is most effective in treating the acute psychotic symptoms and preventing relapse with maintenance therapy. Antipsychotic drug selection must be individualized to each patient. The drug of choice should be determined by an evaluation of the patient's history of drug response and adverse effects, the patient's attitude toward individual drugs (which may affect compliance), and clinically significant differences in the antipsychotic drugs' adverse-effect profiles. Most schizophrenics will require lifelong drug treatment to prevent psychotic exacerbations of their illness. Although antipsychotic drugs cause many adverse effects, most can be ameliorated by patient education, manipulation of doses and schedule, and sometimes adjunctive drug treatments. Thus patients being treated with antipsychotic drugs require careful monitoring to maximize response and minimize adverse effects. The philosophy of community mental health care means that most pharmacists, regardless of practice setting, will care for schizophrenic patients and must have some expertise and experience in this area of therapeutics.

REFERENCES

1. Ereshefsky L, Tran-Johnson TK, Watanabe MD: Pathophysiologic basis for schizophrenia and the efficacy of antipsychotics. Clin Pharm 9:682–707, 1990.
2. Black DW, Yates WR, Andreasen NC, Schizophrenia, schizophreniform disorder, and delusional disorders. In Talbott JA, Hales RE, Yudofsky SC: Textbook of Psychiatry. Washington, D.C., American Psychiatric Press, 1988, pp 357–402.
3. American Psychiatric Association: Diagnostic and Statistical Manual of Mental Disorders, ed. 3—revised. Washington, D.C., American Psychiatric Association, 1987, pp 187–211.
4. Andreasen NC: Positive vs. negative schizophrenia: a critical evaluation. Schizophr Bull 11:380–389, 1985.
5. Davis JM, Andriukaitis S: The natural course of schizophrenia and effective maintenance drug treatment. J Clin Psychopharmacol 6(1:suppl):2S-10S, 1986.
6. Richelson E: Pharmacology of neuroleptics in use in the United States. J Clin Psychiatry 46(8:Sec 2):8–14, 1985.
7. Van Putten T, May PRA: Subjective responses as a predictor of outcome in pharmacotherapy. Arch Gen Psychiatry 35:477–480, 1978.
8. Ortiz A, Gershon S: The future of neuroleptic psychopharmacology. J Clin Psychiatry 47(5, Suppl):3–11, 1986.
9. Kane JM: The current status of neuroleptic therapy. J Clin Psychiatry 50:322–328, 1989.
10. Bodkin JA: Emerging uses for high-potency benzodiazepines in psychotic disorders. J Clin Psychiatry 51(5 suppl):41–46, 1990.
11. Garza-Trevino ES, Hollister LE, Overall JE, et al.: Efficacy of combinations of intramuscular antipsychotics and sedative-hypnotics for control of psychotic agitation. Am J Psychiatry 146:1598–1601, 1989.
12. Davis JM, Andriukaitis S: The natural course of schizophrenia and effective maintenance drug treatment. J Clni Psychopharmacol 6:2S-10S, 1986.
13. Carpenter WT Jr, Hanlon TE, Heinrichs DW, et al.: Continuous versus targeted medication in schizophrenic outpatients: outcome results. Am J Psychiatry 147:1138–1148, 1990.
14. Marder SR, Van Putten T, Mintz J, et al.: Low and conventional dose maintenance therapy with fluphenazine decanoate. Arch Gen Psychiatry 44:518–521, 1987.
15. Johnson DAW: Antipsychotic medication: clinical guidelines for maintenance therapy. J Cln Psychiatry 46(5 sec 2):6–15, 1985.
16. Brotman AW, McCormick S: A role for high-dose antipsychotics. J Clin Psychiatry 51:164–166, 1990.
17. Jann M, Ereshefsky L, Saklad SR: Clinical pharmacokinetics of the depot antipsychotics. Clin Pharmacokinet 10:315–333, 1985.
18. Hemstrom CA, Evans RL, Lobeck FG: Haloperidol decanoate: a depot antipsychotic. Drug Intell Clin Pharm 22:290–295, 1988.
19. Sramek JJ, Potkin SG, Hahn R: Neuroleptic plasma concentrations and clinical response: in search of a thearpeutic window. Drug Intell Clin Pharm 22:373–380, 1988.
20. Ereshefsky L, Watanabe MD, Tran-Johnson TK: Clozapine: an atypical antipsychotic agent. Clin Pharm 8:691–709, 1989.
21. Cohen S, Chiles J, MacNaughton A: Weight gain with clozapine. Am J Psychiatry 147:503–504, 1990.
22. Simpson GM, Pi EH, Sramek JJ Jr: Adverse effects of antipsychotic agents. Drugs 21:138–151, 1981.
23. Fleischhacker WW, Roth SD, Kane JM: The pharmacologic treatment of neuroleptic-induced akathisia. J Clin Psychopharmacol 10:12–21, 1990.
24. Keepers GA, Casey DE: Prediction of neuroleptic-induced dystonia. J Clin Psychopharmacol 7:342–345, 1987.
25. Remington GJ, Voineskos G, Pollock B, et al.: Prevalence of neuroleptic-induced dystonia in mania and schizophrenia. Am J Psychiatry 147:1231–1233, 1990.
26. Gelenberg AJ, VanPutten T, Lavori PW, et al.: Anticholinergic effects on memory: benztropine versus amantadine. J Clin Psychopharmacol 9:180–185, 1989.
27. Winslow RS, Stillner V, Coons DJ, et al.: Prevention of acute dystonic reactions in patients beginning high-potency neuroleptics. Am J Psychiatry 143:706–710, 1986.
28. Arana GW, Goff DC, Baldessarini RJ, et al.: Efficacy of anticholinergic prophylaxis for neuroleptic-induced acute dystonia. Am J Psychiatry 145:993–996, 1988.
29. Baker LA, Cheng LY, Amara IB: The withdrawal of benztropine mesylate in chronic schizophrenic patients. Br J Psychiatry 143:584–590, 1983.
30. Singh H, Simpson GM, Tardive dyskinesia. In Wolf ME, Mosnaim AD: Tardive Dyskinesia, Washington, D.C., American Psychiatric Press, 1988, pp 69–84.
31. Bourgeois M, Bouilh P, Tignol J, et al.: Spontaneous dyskinesia vs. neuroleptic induced dyskinesia in 270 elderly subjects. J Nerv Ment Dis 168:177–178, 1980.
32. Kane JM, Woerner M, Lieberman J: Tardive dyskinesia: prevalence, incidence, and risk factors. J Clin Psychopharmacol 8:52S–56S, 1988.
33. Yassa R, Nair NPV, Iskandar H, et al.: Factors in the development of severe forms of tardive dyskinesia. Am J Psychiatry 147:1156–1163, 1990.
34. Baldessarini RJ: Clinical and epidemiologic aspects of tardive dyskinesia. J Clin Psychiatry 46(4,Sec 2):8–13, 1985.
35. Klawans HL, Carvey P, Tanner CM, et al.: The pathophysiology of tardive dyskinesia. J Clin Psychiatry 46 (4, sec.2):38–41, 1985.
36. Seeman P: Tardive dyskinesia, dopamine receptors, and neuroleptic damage to cell membranes. J Clin Psychopharmacol 8:3S–9S, 1988.
37. Jeste DV, Lohr JB, Clark K, et al.: Pharmacologic treatments of tardive dyskinesia in the 1980s. J Clin Psychopharmacol 8:38S–48S, 1988.
38. Pearlman CA: Neuroleptic malignant syndrome: a review of the literature. J Clin Psychopharmacol 6:257–273, 1986.
39. Wells AJ, Sommi RW, Crismon ML: Neuroleptic rechallenge after neuroleptic malignant syndrome: case report and literature review. Drug Intell Clin Pharm 22:475–480, 1988.
40. Rosebush PI, Stewart TD, Gelenberg AJ: Twenty neuroleptic rechallenges after neuroleptic malignant syndrome in 15 patients. J Clin Psychiatry 50:295–298, 1989.
41. Zito JM, Sofair JB, Jaeger J: Self-reported neuroendocrine effects of antipsychotics in women: a pilot study. DICP Ann Pharmacother 24:176–180, 1990.
42. Ripley HS, Papanicolaou GN: The menstrual cycle with vaginal smear studies in schizophrenia, depression and elation. Am J Psychiatry 98:567–573, 1942.
43. Doss FW: The effect of antipsychotic drugs on body weight: a retrospective review. J Clin Psychiatry 40:528–530, 1979.
44. Wheeler RH, Bhalerao UR, Gilkes MJ: Ocular pigmentation, extrapyramidal symptoms and phenothiazine dosage. Br J Psychiatry 115:687–690, 1968.
45. Swett C: Outpatient phenothiazine use and bone marrow depression. Arch Gen Psychiatry 32:1416–1418, 1975.
46. Cold JA, Wells BG, Froemming JH: Seizure activity associated with antipsychotic therapy. DICP Ann Pharmacother 24:601–606, 1990.

CHAPTER 54

SLEEP DISORDERS

MICHAEL Z. WINCOR, Pharm.D.

On average, we spend one-third of our lives sleeping, yet many of us take this psychophysiologic phenomenon for granted. Only when it becomes disturbed, do we pay some attention to it; even then, we probably heed the warnings of daytime fatigue less than we should. We do not know why, but we definitely need to sleep, and the exact sleep need varies a great deal among individuals. It has been found in various national surveys that during the course of a year 25 to 35% of the adult population have some complaint concerning sleep (1). Up to 17% of the population experience the problem as serious. The serious insomniacs tend to be older women with high levels of psychic distress and somatic anxiety as well as multiple health problems. Between 2 and 4% of those surveyed use hypnotics or other psychotherapeutic agents to promote sleep. The vast majority of hypnotic users take these drugs for short periods (1 day to 2 weeks); only 11% (0.3% of all adults) report using the drugs regularly for a year or more (2). An additional 3 to 4% use nonprescription sleep aids. However, a small survey of community pharmacists indicated little involvement in counseling patients about over-the-counter sleep aids (3). Although insomnia and daytime sleepiness are two of the most common human complaints, most serious insomniacs (85%) are untreated by either prescription or nonprescription hypnotics. It is becoming increasingly clear that poor sleep and resultant daytime sleepiness play a major role in work-related accidents, traffic accidents, and lost productivity. With a reasonable familiarity with sleep disorders, the pharmacist can make an important contribution in assessing the appropriateness of a sleep aid, stimulant, or referral.

SLEEP PHYSIOLOGY

Sleep has been studied in various ways. Behaviorally, one can observe changes in body position, responsiveness to external stimuli, and eyelid closure. Anatomically, sleep-regulating centers in the brainstem have been identified. Neurochemically, various neurotransmitters are involved in sleep mechanisms. Not long ago, we simply pointed to norepinephrine as being involved in wakefulness and dreaming sleep and serotonin as involved in nondreaming sleep. Then it became clear that there is an interaction between the cholinergic systems and noradrenergic systems. In the future, contributions of other neurotransmitters and various endogenous peptides will likely be elucidated (4).

Electrophysiology and Sleep Stages

Currently, the standard method for observing and measuring sleep is electrophysiologic (5). In the laboratory, sleep is recorded polygraphically, with electroencephalograms (EEGs), electro-oculograms (EOGs) from each of the two eyes, and electromyograms (EMGs) generally of the mentalis and submentalis muscles. Two EOGs, one EEG, and one EMG are the minimal recordings used for scoring sleep stages. A number of other physiologic variables may be needed to identify specific sleep disorders, as will be discussed. The entire recording process is often referred to as polysomnography. Currently, by means of portable devices, such recordings are possible in the patient's home.

By means of these recordings, sleep can be divided into nonrapid eye movement (NREM) sleep that is further subdivided into stages 1 through 4 and rapid eye movement (REM) sleep. Wakefulness is characterized by a low-voltage, fast EEG, high muscle tone, and various types of eye movements including blinks. Stage 1 sleep is characterized by a low-voltage, mixed-frequency EEG, slightly decreased muscle tone, and slow, rolling eye movements; the subjective experience of this transition stage varies widely among individuals, some experiencing it as wakefulness, others as drowsiness, and yet others as sleep. Stage 2 is characterized by sleep spindles and K-complexes on EEG and is recognized as unequivocal sleep. Stages 3 and 4 are characterized by high-amplitude, slow activity in the EEG known as delta waves; hence, these two stages together are often referred to as delta sleep. Delta sleep appears to be the deep, restorative sleep that most people (especially insomniacs) think of when they visualize sleep.

REM sleep is characterized by a low-voltage, mixed-frequency EEG, in many ways quite similar to that seen in stage 1, but with very low muscle tone and bursts of bilaterally conjugate rapid eye movements. It appears as though the sleeper is watching a movie or actively observing some activity. Classical dreaming occurs in REM sleep; dream reports can be obtained 80 to 90% of the times that subjects are awakened during or at the end of REM periods. Brain and autonomic activity may be greater and more variable than during relaxed wakefulness.

Sleep Cycle

The architecture of sleep in the normal young adult is cyclic. The sleeper quickly passes from wakefulness through stages 1 and 2, spending a moderate block of time in delta sleep. Some 90 min after sleep onset, the sleeper enters the first REM period of the night, which may last only 5 to 7 min. The cycle is repeated four to five times each night. As the night progresses, less time is spent in delta sleep, with most delta sleep occurring in the first half of the night. REM periods become longer and more intense, both physiologically and psychologically, as the night goes on. The final REM period of the night may last as long as 30 to 60 min. Most individuals who recall a dream in the morning are waking from this REM period and remembering the dream's content. In general, one spends approximately 75% of the night in NREM sleep and the remaining 25% of the night in REM sleep.

In the elderly, however, the typical sleep architecture described above may be quite different, with a considerable decrease in delta sleep, an increase in light sleep, an increase in awakenings during the night, and a generally more disrupted night of sleep. There may be a slight decrease in total sleep time during the night, compared with young adults, but how much daytime napping and specific sleep pathology (e.g., sleep apnea and periodic limb movements) contribute to this apparent decrease is unclear. Even in randomly selected, noncomplaining, elderly individuals, the combined incidence of sleep apnea and periodic limb movements is as high as 58% (6–8).

The parameters that can be measured objectively in the sleep laboratory which are of particular interest with respect to insomnia and drug effects on sleep are listed in Table 54.1. Latency to sleep onset (or sleep latency) is defined as the length of time taken to fall asleep after getting into bed. The number of awakenings and number of stage shifts during the night are indications of how disrupted sleep has been. REM intensity, or the frequency of bursts of rapid eye movements, may at times be a more subtle indicator of changes in REM sleep than simply the total number of minutes spent in REM sleep during the night. Finally, other physiologic measurements may include electrocardiogram, respiration, oxygen saturation, and activity of the anterior tibialis muscles.

Table 54.1.
Sleep Parameters

Latency to sleep onset
Total sleep time
Sleep stage durations
Sleep stage percentages of total sleep time
Number of awakenings during the night
Number of stage shifts during the night
REM intensity
Other physiologic measurements

Table 54.2.
International Classification of Sleep Disorders (ICSD)[a]

1. Dyssomnias
    A. Intrinsic sleep disorders
    B. Extrinsic sleep disorders
    C. Circadian rhythm sleep disorders
2. Parasomnias
    A. Arousal disorders
    B. Sleep-wake transition disorders
    C. Parasomnias usually associated with REM sleep
    D. Other parasomnias
3. Medical/psychiatric sleep disorders
    A. Associated with mental disorders
    B. Associated with neurologic disorders
    C. Associated with other medical disorders
4. Proposed sleep disorders

[a] Adapted from Diagnostic Classification Steering Committee of the American Sleep Disorders Association (Thorpy MJ, Chair): International Classification of Sleep Disorders—Diagnostic and Coding Manual. Rochester, MN: American Sleep Disorders Association, 1990.

DIAGNOSIS AND CLINICAL FINDINGS

In the 1970s, a group of clinically oriented sleep researchers developed an organization, the Association of Sleep Disorders Centers, as well as a scheme for classifying sleep disorders (9). Simply stated, disorders of initiating and maintaining sleep (DIMS) were equivalent to insomnia, the disorders of excessive somnolence (DOES) were equivalent of excessive daytime sleepiness, the disorders of the sleep-wake schedule involved disturbances of biologic rhythms, and the parasomnias included a number of miscellaneous disorders associated with sleep, sleep stages, or partial arousals. There was a considerable amount of overlap in possible etiologies among the major categories of disorders, with the exception of the parasomnias. In fact, the determining factor in applying a label to the patient was often the nature of the subjective complaint (e.g., "Doctor, I'm not sleeping well at night" versus "Doctor, I'm always sleepy").

As sleep-disorder clinicians worked with this classification scheme over the years, an international effort for revision and modification began. The result was *The International Classification of Sleep Disorders* (ICSD) (10) a very extensive listing and description of the sleep disorders (as outlined in Table 54.2). It was published by what is now called the American Sleep Disorders Association, in cooperation with the European Sleep Research Society, the Japanese Society of Sleep Research, and the Latin American Sleep Society. A bit earlier, however, a committee of the American Psychiatric Association was revising its official *Diagnostic and Statistical Manual of Mental Disorders* (DSM-III-R). The result was a somewhat abbreviated nomenclature for the sleep disorders most likely to be encountered in a psychiatric practice (11). It is out-

Table 54.3.
DSM-III-R Classification of Sleep Disorders[a]

Dyssomnias
 Insomnia disorders
  307.42 Insomnia related to another mental disorder (nonorganic)
  780.50 Insomnia related to a known organic factor
  307.42 Primary insomnia
 Hypersomnia disorders
  307.44 Hypersomnia related to another mental disorder (nonorganic)
  780.50 Hypersomnia related to a known organic factor
  780.54 Primary hypersomnia
 Sleep-wake schedule disorder
  307.45 Sleep-wake schedule disorder
 Other dyssomnias
  307.40 Dyssomnias not otherwise specified
Parasomnias
  307.47 Dream anxiety disorder (nightmare disorder)
  307.46 Sleep terror disorder
  307.46 Sleepwalking disorder
  307.40 Parasomnia not otherwise specified

[a] Adapted from American Psychiatric Association: Diagnostic and Statistical Manual of Mental Disorders, ed. 3, revised. Washington, D.C.: American Psychiatric Association, 1987, pp 297–313.

lined in Table 54.3 for the sake of completeness; however, since the ICSD is the more exhaustive, international classification, it will serve as the basis of this discussion. Eighty-four specific sleep disorders are described in the ICSD. It is beyond the scope of this chapter to cover each of them in detail; however, each of the major categories is expanded in Tables 54.4 through 54.7 to provide the reader with an idea of the progress made in the past 15 years in identifying and classifying sleep disorders.

The entire field of sleep-disorders medicine is in its infancy, at most approaching adolescence. For many of the sleep disorders, both etiology and prevalence are as yet unclear (in instances where these are established or even postulated such information will be mentioned). The remaining discussion is focused on the disorders that have been best studied, are seen most frequently, or are most likely to have a pharmacotherapeutic component to treatment. Particular emphasis is placed on insomnia and the use of hypnotics.

PARASOMNIAS

The parasomnias, as indicated in Table 54.5, include 23 distinct disorders. Only sleepwalking (somnambulism), sleep terrors (pavor nocturnus), and nightmares are discussed in detail here.

Somnambulism

Sleepwalking, or somnambulism, is a phenomenon occurring in delta sleep. At least one episode of sleepwalking

in seen in about 15% of children, as compared with 2 to 5% of adults. Peak prevalence occurs between ages 4 and 8 years. Typically, the sleeper sits up, gets out of bed, walks around, and returns to bed. The individual appears to be navigating well, but critical skills and reactivity are impaired (e.g., if you were to rearrange the furniture in the house, the sleepwalker would probably stumble over it). Fortunately, the disorder is usually "outgrown." Treatment consists primarily of protecting the individual from harm. This may include locking doors and windows at night and giving the sleepwalker a first-floor bedroom. Medications that may exacerbate or induce sleepwalking (e.g., thioridazine, chloral hydrate, lithium, fluphenazine, perphenazine, and desipramine) should be discontinued if possible. Theoretically, sleepwalking could be reduced by suppressing delta sleep. Most benzodiazepines suppress delta sleep, and in an adult with frequent episodes, especially with a history of injury to self or others, a benzodiazepine may be a very appropriate and efficacious intervention. However, in the case of childhood sleepwalking, the benefit of treatment over simply protecting the individual from injury is questionable in light of the unknown risks of long-term exposure of the child's developing central nervous system to benzodiazepines (12).

Sleep Terrors

Sleep terrors (pavor nocturnus or night terrors), also a delta sleep phenomenon, is seen in approximately 3% of children and less than 1% of adults. It is characterized by extreme vocalizations, motility, and autonomic variability. Recall of frightening content is minimal or absent. Hence, the phenomenon may be more disturbing to others in the house than to the child experiencing it. The parents of the child may hear a "blood-curdling" scream, run into the sleeper's bedroom, and find the child wet from perspiration, breathing forcefully, and experiencing tachycardia. Fortunately, the absence of frightening content results in nothing psychologic with which to associate the event. Generally, there is amnesia for the event. Again, treatment consists primarily of waiting for the disorder to be "outgrown," since sleep terrors are typically observed in children between the ages of 4 and 12 years and resolve spontaneously during adolescence. The same reservations about use of delta sleep suppressants discussed in regard to somnambulism apply for this disorder (12).

Nightmares

Unlike sleep terrors, nightmares ("bad dreams") occur in REM sleep (in about 5% of the general population) and are associated with elaborate and frightening content. There is less motility and autonomic variability than in sleep terrors. It is estimated that 10 to 50% of children

Table 54.4.
ICSD Classification of Dyssomnias[a]

Disorders that are characterized by difficulty in initiating or maintaining sleep or by excessive sleepiness

Intrinsic sleep disorders

Developing within the body or from causes within the body

307.42-0 Psychophysiological insomnia

Somatized tension and learned sleep-preventing associations resulting in a complaint of insomnia and associated decreased functioning during wakefulness

307.49-1 Sleep state misperception

A complaint of insomnia or excessive sleepiness without objective evidence of sleep disturbance

780.52-7 Idiopathic insomnia

A lifelong inability to obtain adequate sleep that is presumably due to an abnormality of the neurologic control of the sleep-wake system

347 Narcolepsy

Characterized by excessive sleepiness typically associated with cataplexy and other REM sleep phenomena such as sleep paralysis and hypnagogic hallucinations

780.54-2 Recurrent hypersomnia

Characterized by recurrent episodes of excessive sleepiness that typically occur weeks or months apart

780.54-7 Idiopathic hypersomnia

Characterized by a normal or prolonged major sleep episode and excessive sleepiness consisting of prolonged (1–2 hours) sleep episodes of NREM sleep, presumably due to a central nervous system abnormality

780.54-8 Posttraumatic hypersomnia

Excessive sleepiness as a result of a trauma to the central nervous system

780.53-0 Obstructive sleep apnea syndrome

Characterized by repetitive episodes of upper airway obstruction that occur during sleep, usually associated with a reduction in blood oxygen saturation

780.51-0 Central sleep apnea syndrome

Characterized by a cessation or decrease of ventilatory effort during sleep, usually with associated oxygen desaturation

780.51-1 Central alveolar hypoventilation syndrome

Characterized by ventilatory impairment, resulting in arterial oxygen desaturation that is worsened by sleep, which occurs in patients with normal mechanical properties of the lung

780.51-1 Periodic limb movement disorder

Characterized by periodic episodes of repetitive and highly stereotyped limb movements that occur during sleep

780.52-5 Restless legs syndrome

Characterized by disagreeable leg sensations, usually prior to sleep onset, that cause an almost irresistible urge to move the legs

780.52-9 Intrinsic sleep disorder NOS

An intrinsic dyssomnia not otherwise specified (i.e., none of the above)

Extrinsic sleep disorders

Developing from causes outside of the body

307.41-1 Inadequate sleep hygiene

Due to the performance of daily living activities that are inconsistent with the maintenance of good quality sleep and full daytime alertness

780.52-6 Environmental sleep disorder

Due to a disturbing environmental factor that causes a complaint of either insomnia or excessive sleepiness

289.0 Altitude insomnia

An acute insomnia, usually accompanied by headaches, loss of appetite, and fatigue, that occurs following ascent to high altitudes

307.41-0 Adjustment sleep disorder

Temporally related to acute stress, conflict, or environmental change causing emotional arousal

307.49-4 Insufficient sleep syndrome

Occurs in an individual who persistently fails to obtain sufficient nocturnal sleep required to support normally alert wakefulness

307.42-4 Limit-setting sleep disorder

Primarily a childhood disorder that is characterized by the inadequate enforcement of bedtimes by a caretaker, with resultant stalling or refusal to go to bed at an appropriate time

307.42-5 Sleep-onset association disorder

Characterized by impaired sleep onset due to the absence of a certain object or set of cirumstances

780.52-2 Food allergy insomnia

Disorder of initiating and maintaining sleep due to an allergic response to food allergens

780.52-8 Nocturnal eating (drinking) syndrome

Characterized by recurrent awakenings, with the inability to return to sleep without eating or drinking

780.52-0 Hypnotic-dependent sleep disorder

Characterized by insomnia or excessive sleepiness that is associated with tolerance to or withdrawal from hypnotic medications

780.52-1 Stimulant-dependent sleep disorder

Characterized by a reduction of sleepiness or suppression of sleep by central stimulants, and resultant alterations in wakefulness following drug abstinence

780.52-3 Alcohol-dependent sleep disorder

Characterized by the assisted initiation of sleep onset by the sustained ingestion of ethanol that is used for its hypnotic effect

780.54-6 Toxin-induced sleep disorder

Characterized by either insomnia or excessive sleepiness produced by poisoning with heavy metals or organic toxins

780.52-9 Extrinsic sleep disorder NOS

An extrinsic dyssomnia not otherwise specified (i.e., none of the above)

Circadian rhythm sleep disorders

Related to the timing of sleep in the 24-hour day

307.45-0 Time zone change (jet lag) syndrome

Characterized by varying degrees of difficulty in initiating or maintaining sleep, excessive sleepiness, decrements in subjective daytime alertness and performance, and somatic symptoms (largely gastrointestinal) following rapid travel across multiple time zones

307.45-1 Shift work sleep disorder

Insomnia or excessive sleepiness that occurs as transient phenomena in relation to work schedules

307.45-3 Irregular sleep-wake pattern

Temporally disorganized and variable episodes of sleep and waking behavior

780.55-0 Delayed sleep phase syndrome

Characterized by the major sleep episode being delayed relative to the desired sleep time, resulting in sleep-onset insomnia or difficulty in awakening at the desired time

780.55-1 Advanced sleep phase syndrome

Characterized by the major sleep episode being advanced relative to the desired sleep time, resulting in symptoms of compelling evening sleepiness, an early sleep onset, and an awakening that is earlier than desired

780.55-2 Non-24-hour sleep-wake disorder

Characterized by chronic steady patterns composed of 1- to 2-hour daily delays in sleep onset and wake times

780.55-9 Circadian rhythm sleep disorder NOS

A circadian rhythm dyssomnia not otherwise specified (i.e., none of the above)

---

[a]Adapted from Diagnostic Classification Steering Committee of the American Sleep Disorders Association (Thorpy MJ, Chair): International Classification of Sleep Disorders—Diagnostic and Coding Manual. Rochester, MN: American Sleep Disorders Association, 1990.

Table 54.5.
ICSD Classification of Parasomnias[a]

Undesirable physical phenomena occurring predominantly during sleep, including disorders of arousal, partial arousal, and sleep stage transition

Arousal disorders

Disorders of impaired arousal from slow wave (delta) sleep

307.46-2 Confusional arousals

Characterized by confusion during and following arousals from sleep, most typically from deep sleep in the first part of the night

307.46-0 Sleepwalking

Characterized by a series of complex behaviors that are initiated during slow wave (delta) sleep, resulting in walking during sleep

307.46-1 Sleep terrors

Characterized by a sudden arousal from slow wave (delta) sleep with a piercing scream or cry, accompanied by autonomic and behavioral manifestations of intense fear

Sleep-wake transition disorders

Occurring in the transition from wakefulness to sleep, from sleep to wakefulness, or, more rarely, from one stage of sleep to another; regarded as altered physiology rather than pathophysiology

307.3 Rhythmic movement disorder

Characterized by stereotyped, repetitive movements involving large muscles, usually of the head and neck, which typically occur immediately prior to sleep onset and are sustained into light sleep

307.47-2 Sleep starts

Characterized by sudden, brief contractions of the legs, sometimes also involving the arms and head, which occur at sleep onset

307.47-3 Sleep talking

The utterance of speech or sounds during sleep without simultaneous subjective detailed awareness of the event

729.82 Nocturnal leg cramps

Characterized by painful sensations of muscular tightness or tension, usually in the calf, but occasionally in the foot, that occur during the sleep episode

Parasomnias usually associated with REM sleep

307.47-0 Nightmares

Frightening dreams that usually awaken the sleeper from REM sleep

780.56-2 Sleep paralysis

Characterized by an inability to perform voluntary movements either at sleep onset (hypnagogic or predormital form) or upon awakening (hypnopompic or postdormital form) either during the night or in the morning

780.56-3 Impaired sleep-related penile erections

Inability to sustain a penile erection during sleep that would be sufficiently large or rigid to engage in sexual intercourse

780.56-4 Sleep-related painful erections

Characterized by penile pain that occurs during erections, typically during REM sleep

780.56-8 REM sleep-related sinus arrest

A cardiac rhythm disorder that is characterized by sinus arrest during REM sleep in otherwise healthy individuals

780.59-0 REM sleep behavior disorder

Characterized by the intermittent loss of REM sleep electromyographic (EMG) atonia and by the appearance of elaborate motor activity associated with dream mentation

Other parasomnias

306.8 Sleep bruxism

A stereotyped movement disorder characterized by grinding or clenching of the teeth during sleep

780.56-0 Sleep enuresis

Characterized by recurrent involuntary micturition that occurs during sleep

780.56-6 Sleep-related abnormal swallowing syndrome

Characterized by inadequate swallowing of saliva, resulting in aspiration, with coughing, choking, and arousals or awakenings from sleep

780.59-1 Nocturnal paroxysmal dystonia (NPD)

Characterized by repeated, stereotyped dystonia or dyskinetic (ballistic, choreoathetoid) episodes that occur during NREM sleep

780.59-3 Sudden unexplained nocturnal death syndrome (SUND)

Characterized by sudden death during sleep in apparently healthy young adults, particularly of Southeast Asian descent

780.53-1 Primary snoring

Characterized by loud upper airway breathing sounds in sleep, without episodes of apnea or hypoventilation

770.80 Infant sleep apnea

Characterized by central or obstructive apneas that occur during sleep

770.81 Congenital central hypoventilation syndrome

Characterized by hypoventilation, which is worse during sleep than wakefulness, and unexplained by primary pulmonary disease or ventilatory muscle weakness

798.0 Sudden infant death syndrome

Unexpected sudden death in which a thorough postmortem investigation fails to demonstrate an adequate cause for death

780.59-5 Benign neonatal sleep myoclonus

Characterized by asynchronous jerking of the limbs and trunk that occurs during quiet sleep in neonates

780.59-9 Other parasomnia NOS

A parasomnia not otherwise specified (i.e., none of the above)

---

[a] Adapted from Diagnostic Classification Steering Committee of the American Sleep Disorders Association (Thorpy MJ, Chair): International Classification of Sleep Disorders—Diagnostic and Coding Manual. Rochester, MN: American Sleep Disorders Association, 1990.

Table 54.6.
ICSD Classification of Sleep Disorders Associated with Medical/Psychiatric Disorders[a]

Associated with mental disorders
292-299 Psychoses
    Insomnia or excessive sleepiness commonly associated with psychiatric disorders characterized by the presence of delusions, hallucinations, incoherence, catatonic behavior, or inappropriate affect that causes impaired social or work functioning
296-301 Mood disorders
    Insomnia typically and, rarely, excessive sleepiness associated with psychiatric disorders characterized by either one or more episodes of depression, or partial or full manic or hypomanic episodes
300 Anxiety disorders
    A sleep-onset or maintenance insomnia due to excessive anxiety and apprehensive expectation about one or more life circumstances associated with psychiatric disorders characterized by symptoms of anxiety and avoidance behavior
300 Panic disorder
    Sudden awakenings from sleep associated with panic episodes which are characterized by discrete periods of intense fear or discomfort, with several somatic symptoms that occur unexpectedly and without organic precipitation
303 Alcoholism
    Insomnia or excessive sleepiness associated with excessive alcohol intake, both abuse and dependence
Associated with neurological disorders
330-337 Cerebral degenerative disorders
    Insomnia, excessive sleepiness, abnormal movement activity, or circadian rhythm disturbances associated with slowly progressive conditions characterized by abnormal behavior or involuntary movements, often with evidence of other motor system degeneration
331 Dementia
    Delirium, agitation, combativeness, wandering, and vocalization without ostensible purpose occurring during the early evening or nighttime hours associated with the loss of memory and other intellectual functions due to a chronic, progressive degenerative disease of the brain
332-333 Parkinsonism
    Insomnia associated with the group of neurological disorders characterized by hypokinesia, tremor, and muscular rigidity
337.9 Fatal familial insomnia
    A progressive disorder that begins with a difficulty in initiating sleep and leads within a few months to total lack of sleep and later to spontaneous lapses from quiet wakefulness into a sleep state with enacted dreams (oneiric stupor)

345 Sleep-related epilepsy
    Facilitatory effects of sleep on epileptic activity in disorders characterized by an intermittent, sudden discharge of cerebral neuronal activity
345.8 Electrical status epilepticus of sleep
    Characterized by continuous and diffuse spike-and-slow-wave complexes persisting through NREM sleep
346 Sleep-related headaches
    Severe, mainly unilateral headaches that often have their onset during sleep
Associated with other medical disorders
086 Sleeping sickness
    A protozoan-caused illness characterized by an acute febrile lymphadenopathy followed, after a period of latency usually of 4 to 6 months, by an excessive sleepiness associated with a chronic meningoencephalomyelitis
411-414 Nocturnal cardiac ischemia
    Characterized by myocardial ischemia that occurs during the major sleep episode
490-494 Chronic obstructive pulmonary disease
    Altered cardiorespiratory physiology during sleep or a complaint of insomnia associated with a disorder characterized by a chronic impairment of airflow through the respiratory tract between the atmosphere and gas exchange portion of the lung
493 Sleep-related asthma
    Asthma attacks that occur during sleep
530.1 Sleep-related gastroesophageal reflux
    Characterized by regurgitation of stomach contents into the esophagus during sleep
531-534 Peptic ulcer disease
    Awakenings from sleep with pain or discomfort in the abdomen, resulting in a complaint of insomnia, associated with a disorder characterized by gastric or duodenal ulceration by acid and pepsin
729.1 Fibrositis syndrome
    Unrefreshing, light sleep and chronic fatigue associated with a disorder characterized by diffuse musculoskeletal pain, and increased tenderness in specific localized anatomic regions, but without laboratory evidence of contributing articular, nonarticular or metabolic disease

[a] Adapted from Diagnostic Classification Steering Committee of the American Sleep Disorders Association (Thorpy MJ, Chair): International Classification of Sleep Disorders—Diagnostic and Coding Manual. Rochester, MN: American Sleep Disorders Association, 1990.

between ages 3 and 6 years suffer from enough nightmares to disturb the parents. Approximately 50% of the adult population admit to having at least an occasional nightmare, and perhaps 1% experience frequent nightmares (one or more per week). After REM suppressant drug withdrawal is ruled out as the cause, psychological intervention is the usual treatment. This may be as simple as a parent providing comfort and reassurance to a child with an occasional nightmare or as complex as intensive psychotherapy for an adult with frequent, highly disturbing nightmares (12).

SLEEP APNEA
Definition and Overview

Sleep apnea, a sleep-induced respiratory impairment, is a condition characterized by episodes of cessation of breathing (13). Each apneic episode, often lasting 20 to 30 sec, is terminated by a brief arousal from sleep during which

Table 54.7.
ICSD Classification of Proposed Sleep Disorders[a]

Disorders for which insufficient or inadequate information is available to substantiate their unequivocal existence

307.49-0 Short sleeper

An individual who habitually sleeps substantially less during a 24-hour period than is expected for his or her age group

307.49-2 Long sleeper

An individual who consistently sleeps substantially more (although with basically normal sleep architecture and physiology) in 24 hours than the conventional amount of sleep for his or her age group

307.47-1 Subwakefulness syndrome

An inability to sustain daytime alertness without polysomnographic evidence of nocturnal sleep disruption or severe excessive sleepiness

780.59-7 Fragmentary myoclonus

Characterized by jerks that consist of brief involuntary "twitchlike" local contractions involving various areas of both sides of the body in an asynchronous and asymmetrical manner during sleep

780.8 Sleep hyperhidrosis

Characterized by profuse sweating that occurs during sleep

780.54.3 Menstrual-associated sleep disorder

Characterized by a complaint of either insomnia or excessive sleepiness that is temporally related to the menses or menopause

780.59-6 Pregnancy-associated sleep disorder

Characterized by either insomnia or excessive sleepiness that develops in the course of pregnancy

307.47-4 Terrifying hypnagogic hallucinations

Terrifying dream experiences that occur at sleep onset which are similar to, or at times indistinguishable from, those taking place within sleep

780.53-2 Sleep-related neurogenic tachypnea

Characterized by a sustained increase in respiratory rate during sleep, which occurs at sleep onset, is maintained throughout sleep, and reverses immediately upon return to wakefulness

780.49-4 Sleep-related laryngospasm

Characterized by episodes of abrupt awakenings from sleep with an intense sensation of inability to breathe, and stridor

307.42-1 Sleep choking syndrome

Characterized by frequent episodes of awakening with a choking sensation

[a] Adapted from Diagnostic Classification Steering Committee of the American Sleep Disorders Association (Thorpy MJ, Chair): International Classification of Sleep Disorders—Diagnostic and Coding Manual. Rochester, MN: American Sleep Disorders Association, 1990.

breathing resumes. There may be as many as several hundred of these "mini-arousals" during a single night, but the patient may not be aware of their occurrence. The patient may instead complain of morning headache, irritability, and general difficulty with daytime functioning. Often, the bed partner is the best source of information, reporting that the patient snores very loudly or has periods in which breathing stops followed by gasps for air. Often there is a recent history of weight gain associated with onset of symptoms. Sleep apnea generally has an onset in adulthood, usually over the age of 30, probably with a prevalence of 1 to 2% of the population, and, in the case of obstructive sleep apnea, is at least eight times more prevalent in men than in women. Although the incidence is high in the elderly, many are asymptomatic (i.e., they have no complaints that would have brought this condition to the attention of a physician or sleep-disorders specialist). Common complications of sleep apnea include arrhythmias, systolic or diastolic hypertension, and signs of pulmonary arterial hypertension and right-sided heart failure.

Sleep apnea is often described as obstructive, central, or mixed. Obstructive sleep apnea is caused by something obstructing the airway. The problem may be the tongue falling back across the airway, enlarged tonsils, or some other craniofacial abnormality. Respiratory effort continues as is demonstrated by strain gauge recordings around the thorax and abdomen in the absence of nasal/oral airflow (measured by a device attached to the face below the nostrils). In central sleep apnea, respiratory effort ceases, indicating a problem in the respiratory centers of the brain, with resultant absence of nasal/oral airflow. In mixed sleep apnea, there seems to be a cessation of central respiratory effort, followed by an obstructive event, and then even when respiratory effort resumes, there is no airflow. In any of these cases, as oxygen saturation falls (which can be measured with an earlobe oximeter), the brain automatically produces a "mini-arousal" resulting in resumption of breathing. Whether the patient complains of insomnia or excessive daytime sleepiness is subjective, but obstructive sleep apnea seems to be more highly associated with complaints of excessive daytime sleepiness, while central sleep apnea appears to be more closely associated with complaints of insomnia (14).

Treatment

Treatment varies with the type of sleep apnea under consideration. For obstructive sleep apnea, sometimes simple weight loss or removal of enlarged tonsils may solve the problem. Sometimes preventing the patient from sleeping on his back, by sewing a tennis ball to the back of the night shirt, can lead to a significant decrease in apneic episodes. When life-threatening complications of repeated episodes of hypoxemia (e.g., arrhythmias, pulmonary hypertension, right ventricular failure) are present, a tracheostomy can dramatically change how the patient feels. The opening can be plugged during the day, with the plug removed during sleep. A more elegant plastic surgical procedure, performed in some patients, is the uvulopalatopharyngoplasty (UPPP). It involves major reconstruction of the pharyngeal airspace. Unfortunately, in many cases, long-term follow-up has been lacking. A most promising, recent approach is continuous positive airway pressure (nasal CPAP) (15). This involves the use of a small device that sits beside the bed, connected by a tube to a facial mask worn by the patient throughout the night. The device, initially calibrated during one or two nights in a sleep-disorders center, provides a continuous flow of air that keeps the airway open. The community pharmacist might consider including the apparatus in the pharmacy's inventory of durable medical equipment. For the many patients who are appropriately counseled and learn to tolerate the noise, mucosal drying, and minor discomfort of the facial mask, the technique can have a major impact on the quality of sleep and resultant daytime functioning. Finally, various dental appliances designed to pull the tongue forward and maintain an open airway are being tested.

The single most important pharmacologic intervention in the treatment of any type of sleep apnea is the careful avoidance of all drugs that have central nervous system (CNS) depressant activity. These include anxiolytics, hypnotics, narcotics, and alcohol. Any agent that can interfere with the ability of the brain to produce an apnea-terminating "mini-arousal" is potentially lethal. Even CNS depressants that appear to have little or no effect on respiration during wakefulness must be avoided, since some evidence indicates differential effects during sleep. Preliminary data indicate that a subset of patients with central sleep apnea may be an exception to this rule of avoiding CNS depressants. In fact, triazolam improved sleep quality, increased total sleep time, and decreased apneic episodes (16). However, until these findings are confirmed in further studies, it remains safest to avoid CNS depressants in all patients with sleep apnea. Active pharmacologic intervention in treating sleep apnea has met with mixed, fairly unimpressive results. Tricyclic antidepressants, particularly protriptyline, have been used in both obstructive and central sleep apnea. Protriptyline may act by decreasing REM sleep or by increasing oropharyngeal muscle tone (17). Respiratory stimulants, such as medroxyprogesterone (18) and acetazolamide (19) show only limited efficacy with no studies demonstrating long-term effectiveness.

NARCOLEPSY

Definition and Overview

Narcolepsy, along with obstructive sleep apnea, is a major cause of excessive daytime sleepiness and is found in approximately 0.1% of the population. Its onset is often during adolescence. Patients suffering with narcolepsy are extremely sleepy throughout the day and find themselves falling asleep at inopportune moments. There are four classic features: excessive daytime sleepiness, cataplexy, sleep paralysis, and hypnagogic hallucinations. Cataplexy is described as brief (lasting only seconds to minutes) episodes of muscle weakness that may result in the patient collapsing. They are often precipitated by emotionally charged stimuli (e.g., laughter, anger, excitement). Sleep paralysis and hypnagogic hallucinations occur during the

transition between wakefulness and sleep. Sleep paralysis involves inhibition of the musculature before the individual is unconscious. This is particularly frightening because the patient is aware of the paralysis. Hypnagogic hallucinations are brief dreamlike events but perhaps more fragmented and bizarre than a typical dream (14, 20).

Sleep-laboratory findings strongly suggest that narcolepsy involves a dysregulation of REM sleep. In addition to cataplexy and sleep paralysis (which represent the loss of muscle tone in REM sleep), narcoleptics have sleep-onset REM periods (i.e., instead of the normal latency of 90 min following sleep onset to the first REM period, they can make a transition from wakefulness immediately to REM sleep). The genetic basis of the disorder is supported by an extremely strong association between the human leucocyte antigen-DR2 phenotype (HLA-DR2) and narcolepsy (21).

Treatment

Treatment consists of both pharmacologic and nonpharmacologic interventions. The patient and family members must be educated about the disorder to dispel the misconception that the patient is simply a lazy, amotivated, nonproductive individual. There are local and national support groups. In addition, careful scheduling of daytime naps can be particularly helpful. The patient may feel fairly refreshed for up to several hours after a 15- or 20-min nap.

Pharmacologic treatment is directed toward the excessive daytime sleepiness on the one hand and the cataplexy on the other (22). CNS stimulants are used for the sleepiness. Hesitation in prescribing amphetamines (due to concerns over abuse, tolerance, and dependence) has led to the more common use of methylphenidate starting at 2.5 mg twice daily. Occasionally, pemoline is started at a dose of 18.75 mg/day. For the cataplexy, imipramine (in the past) and now, more commonly, the less sedating protriptyline (at an initial dose of 5 mg titrated up to 60 mg daily) have been used.

General principles of pharmacologic management include using the lowest effective dose possible, with gradual titration and careful monitoring for therapeutic and adverse effects (particularly the anticholinergic and hypotensive effects of the tricyclic antidepressant), and temporarily withdrawing the stimulant when tolerance has developed. It is ideal if the temporary withdrawal can be scheduled at a time when a return of daytime sleepiness will have the least impact on the general functioning of the patient (e.g., during a vacation break from work or school). Cataplexy, in some patients, can be treated on a PRN basis. A patient who recognizes specific situations with which the cataplexy is associated can use the protriptyline for a day or two before and during the time of expected occurrence.

INSOMNIA

Definition and Dimensions

Insomnia is a problem that 95% of all adults have experienced at least once in their lives. It must be defined in terms of both amount of sleep and its perceived quality. No absolute number of hours of sleep per se constitutes insomnia, since sleep need among individuals is highly variable. The individual who sleeps 5 hr per night, only needs 5 hr per night, and functions in his daily activities at peak performance does not have insomnia. However, the individual who needs 8 hr per night, sleeps only 7 with a perception of fragmented sleep, and complains of daytime impairment may indeed by suffering from insomnia. Hence, insomnia must be seen as a perceived relative decrease in the quantity and/or quality of sleep along with some perceived consequences in waking life. These perceptions take the form of a subjective complaint on the part of the patient. In many respects, insomniacs' sleep is not that dramatically different from that of good sleepers, but they perceive it as poor sleep. Unfortunately, at present, there is no definitive way to measure the quality of sleep in the sleep laboratory; however, it appears likely that fragmentation of sleep (as indicated by arousals, stage shifts, and perhaps subtle findings in EEG frequencies) is most closely associated with perceived quality (12, 23).

Insomnia can be viewed from various perspectives. The severity (i.e., from mild to severe) will clearly have implications with respect to treatment decisions. Whether the insomnia is transient or chronic is important in both diagnosis and treatment. Finally, the pattern of a typical night may be characterized by difficulty falling asleep, difficulty staying asleep (numerous awakenings during the night), early morning awakening (3 to 4 hr earlier than expected, with an inability to return to sleep), or some combination of these problems.

Etiology

The actual neurochemical or pathophysiologic bases for the various types of insomnia are, in general, unknown. There are numerous "causes" for insomnia; some of the more common ones are listed in Table 54.8. They can be divided into medical, psychologic/psychiatric, and miscellaneous causes. Medical causes include pain of various types (e.g., arthritis, pruritus, duodenal ulcer). Pain not only interferes with the ability to fall asleep but also may lead to increased nocturnal arousals and a generally "lighter" sleep. Nocturia may be part of a medical disorder or a result of too late a dose of a diuretic; the result in either case is fragmentation of sleep. Psychologic or psychiatric causes of insomnia can be as common as worry or excitement (e.g., over an important examination or job interview). Almost everyone is familiar with an occasional bout of insomnia associated with emotional arousal. In addition, it is almost certain that some type of sleep disturbance will accompany an acute episode of any of the major psychiatric disorders (e.g., schizophrenia, major depression, mania), and often the sleep disturbance is one of the diagnostic criteria. The ICSD has 19 specific mental, neurologic, and medical disorders with which sleep disturbances are associated. Additional causes may include disruption of circadian rhythms (e.g., jet lag or work shift change), change of environment (e.g., sleeping for the first night or two in a hotel room in a strange city), sleep apnea, periodic limb movements, stimulant drugs, drug dependence, and drug withdrawal.

Table 54.8.
Causes of Insomnia

Medical	*Psychologic/psychiatric*
Pain	Worry
Pruritus	Excitement
Nocturia	Anxiety
Inflammatory bowel disease	Stressful life event
Cardiovascular disorders	Serious illness
Neoplasms	Schizophrenia
Infections	Depression
Endocrinologic and metabolic disorders	Mania
	Panic Disorder
Fever	Alcoholism
Chronic obstructive pulmonary disease	

Others	
Disruption of circadian rhythms (jet lag, shift work)	Sleep apnea
	Periodic limb movements
New sleeping environment	Drug dependence/withdrawal
Drugs—Alcohol and other CNS depressants, antihypertensives, caffeine and other CNS stimulants, monoamine oxidase inhibitors, nicotine, steroids, theophylline, and thyroid preparations	

Classification by Duration

Often it is useful to classify insomnia as transient, short-term, or persistent (also called long-term or chronic). This distinction is valuable for both diagnosis and treatment decisions. Transient insomnia occurs in an otherwise normal sleeper, has a duration of only several days, and is often associated with an acute stress or disruption of the biological clock. Short-term insomnia is very similar to transient insomnia except that its duration is 1 to 3 or 4 weeks. It too is often associated with some situational stress (e.g., loss of a loved one, family conflict, work conflict) or serious medical illness.

Persistent insomnia has a duration longer than 3 or 4 weeks and is often associated with psychiatric or medical conditions. Sleep apnea syndrome and the association of insomnia with psychiatric disorders have already been discussed. Periodic limb movement disorder (also called periodic leg movements, nocturnal myoclonus, or PMS for periodic movements during sleep) is characterized by periodic (every 20 to 40 sec), stereotypic, myoclonic movements of the anterior tibialis or other limb muscles during sleep, resulting in arousals. Like the arousals of sleep apnea, the patient may experience several hundred per night and yet not be aware of them the following day. Often, as with sleep apnea, the bed partner will voice the complaint, in this case about the sleeper's "kicking" throughout the night. The condition is age-related, showing a marked increase in incidence in individuals over the age of 40 years. It can be exacerbated by tricyclic antidepressants and levodopa. A related condition that can affect the ability to fall asleep, is restless legs syndrome. This is characterized by uncomfortable sensations in the legs at rest which can be relieved by movement; hence, the patient feels the need to get out of bed and move around.

A number of biological rhythm disorders can be associated with a complaint of persistent insomnia, for example, delayed sleep phase syndrome (24). The patient wants to fall asleep at 11:00 PM and awaken at 7:00 AM. He gets into bed at 11:00 PM and finds that he cannot fall asleep for 4 or 5 hr. When he wakes up (usually with the help of an alarm or two) at 7:00 AM to meet his and society's daily demands, he feels unrefreshed and tired. This pattern is repeated night after night. If he is asked how late he would sleep if he did not have to get out of bed at 7:00 AM, he would probably say 11:00 AM or noon; hence, he could indeed sleep 8 hr. The patient's ability to sleep simply does not coincide with the time period set aside for sleep; his body (i.e., his internal biological clock) is not sleepy at the time that he wants to be sleeping.

Drugs and alcohol can be associated with insomnia in numerous ways. Any drug with stimulant properties can disrupt sleep, especially if taken late in the day. The use of CNS depressants, including alcohol, can lead to dependence; then, upon withdrawal, it is common to see more disturbed, restless sleep. Even within a single night, alcohol can disrupt sleep. Although it may make the individual feel more relaxed and able to fall asleep, the short duration of action may allow a mild withdrawal in the middle of the night, associated with more disrupted sleep and increased dreaming due to a REM rebound (i.e., early in the night, the alcohol suppresses REM sleep, and as the effect of the alcohol wears off, there is a tendency to make up the lost REM sleep later in the night).

Psychophysiological insomnia may be transient, short-term, or persistent. It is a conditioned or learned insomnia that the sleeper has associated with the bed, bedroom, or sleep process. The harder the patient tries, the more difficult it becomes to sleep. The patient becomes more and more focused on the inability to sleep and the resultant daytime impairment. Interestingly, such individuals sleep remarkably well in the laboratory or in a strange hotel room, away from the conditions with which insomnia is associated, or at times when they are not thinking about trying to fall asleep (e.g., while watching TV or reading).

Finally, sleep-related gastroesophageal reflux, characterized by regurgitation of gastric contents or fluid into the esophagus during sleep, can awaken the patient from sleep, with heartburn or a sour taste in the mouth.

Epidemiology

As stated earlier, 35% of all adults will be afflicted with insomnia in a given year. Other surveys estimate that this is the percentage of people who have a sleep problem at any given time (1). The results of a prevalence study of randomly selected elderly (age 65 and older) individuals indicate that sleep apnea can be found in 24% and periodic limb movements during sleep can be found in 45%, with 10% showing both (6, 7).

The largest analysis of patients studied objectively in sleep-disorders centers found that the most prevalent diagnosis for a complaint of insomnia was insomnia associated with psychiatric disorders (35%). Approximately half had a major affective disorder and half had personality disorders; less than 5% had major psychoses. Psychophysiological insomnia (15%) was the second most frequent diagnosis, followed by drug and alcohol dependence (12.4%). Nearly 9% of people with complaints of insomnia had no significant sleep pathology. Sleep apnea syndromes accounted for 6.2% of insomnia. Only 2.9% of the patients were diagnosed with circadian rhythm disorders; however, this category may be underrepresented because of a lesser awareness at that time (25).

The results, unfortunately, may not be representative of the population at large since they represent findings in sleep-disorders centers. Most individuals with a sleep problem probably do not seek medical attention. No adequate, large-scale epidemiologic study has yet been done in the general population (i.e., individuals seen in a primary care practice or in a community pharmacy). The most common sleep disorders may be adjustment sleep disorder (i.e., transient situational insomnia), insomnia associated with anxiety disorders, psychophysiological insomnia, inadequate sleep hygiene, insomnia associated with mood disorders, obstructive sleep apnea syndrome, delayed or advanced sleep phase syndromes, shift work sleep disorders, alcohol/hypnotic/stimulant-dependent sleep disorders, and periodic limb movement disorder.

Treatment

Treatment of insomnia depends highly upon the type. Again, an extremely important distinction exists between persistent or chronic versus transient or short-term insomnia. Hypnotics are reserved primarily for transient or short-term insomnia. The persistent insomnias often have other specific interventions of choice. For instance, delayed sleep phase syndrome is treated by chronotherapy (24). Since the patient with delayed sleep phase syndrome can sleep but is sleepy at the wrong time of the 24-hr day, chronotherapy is a means of adjusting the internal clock in 2- to 3-hr blocks each day until sleep occurs at the desired time. The persistent insomnias associated with major psychiatric disorders are most appropriately treated with the specific class of agents targeted for the particular disorder. For example, the patient with a major depressive disorder should be receiving an antidepressant as the primary drug treatment. The sleep disturbance, one symptom of the depressive episode, will be one of the first target symptoms to respond to the treatment. For the psychotic patient, selection and titration of an antipsychotic would be the most appropriate treatment. If the insomnia is associated with drug dependence or drug withdrawal, gradual tapering of the offending agent or the equivalent amount of a cross-tolerant long-acting agent is the primary treatment. If the insomnia is associated with a stimulant, in many cases the agent should simply be discontinued abruptly.

In the case of insomnia associated with medical disorders, adjunctive, short-term use of a benzodiazepine to promote sleep may be reasonable, while a specific treatment is directed to the primary problem. Also, there are times when a patient is best served by education. The elderly individual whose sleep has become more fragmented or the "short sleeper" whose sleep need is small and who shows no daytime impairment may both simply need assurance that they are sleeping normally.

Periodic limb movements of sleep, a persistent insomnia, is an exception to the general rule of not using hypnotics for chronic insomnias because it is occasionally treated with these agents. Originally treated with clonazepam (Klonopin), it appears that an equivalent response can be obtained with any benzodiazepine (26). The benzodiazepines do not significantly reduce the number of movements, but patients report an improved quality of sleep and feeling more refreshed in the morning. For restless legs syndrome, codeine and related compounds (e.g., oxycodone) or carbamazepine (Tegretol), typically one Percodan tablet or 200 mg of carbamazepine given at bedtime, have helped some patients (27).

Some general rules of sleep hygiene can be recommended for both persistent and transient insomnias (Table 54.9). In addition, other nonpharmacologic approaches are available. These include desensitization, meditation, biofeedback, stimulus control, and others (28, 29). There are, however, times when hypnotics should be and are appropriately used.

Table 54.9.
Sleep Hygiene—Suggestions for Improved Sleep

1. Set a regular time to go to bed and a regular time to wake up.

    Regularity is a key component to improving sleep. The patient must set these times and adhere to them as diligently as possible. A patient who cannot fall asleep within a reasonable period of time should get out of bed, leave the bedroom, and do something nonstimulating; for some this would be watching a late night talk show on television and for others it might be reading one's professional journals. After 30 to 60 min, another attempt should be made to fall asleep. The idea is to not spend too much time in bed awake; an association between the bed and an inability to fall sleep can simply compound the problem. At least as important is the establishment of a regular wake-up time. No matter how long it took to fall asleep, no matter how little sleep the patient has had, and no matter how flexible the morning schedule is, there should be no "sleeping in." This would only further confuse and disorganize the internal biological clock (i.e., the circadian pacemaker).

2. Make the sleep environment as comfortable and secure as possible.

    The patient should attempt to see that the bedroom is dark and quiet, and is neither too hot nor too cold. Although minor fluctuations in room temperature and firmness of the mattress probably have little impact on sleep, extremes can be disturbing. A sense of security can be important especially to the elderly, who may feel more vulnerable to intruders or who may be increasingly concerned as old neighborhoods change.

3. Omit alcohol and cafferine in the late afternoon and evening.

    Each individual must discover how late such ingestion can be tolerated. However, for the very sensitive, caffeine intake may need to be discontinued each day by noon. Although alcohol is often used as a self-treatment for relaxation and sleep induction, the patient must be told about the rapid elimination of the substance during the first half of the night, resulting in some degree of withdrawal, characterized by increased dreaming and nightmares as well as a general disruption of sleep, during the latter half.

4. Develop a sleep habit or ritual and use the bedroom primarily as a place to sleep.

    Although many of us, while in bed, use the bedroom for watching television, preparing work for the following day, eating snacks, and paying bills, the individual with a sleep problem needs to set the bedroom aside for sleep only. (Sexual activity may be an exception.) Just as warm milk and cookies become a ritual for some children prior to bedtime, some adults must develop a similar relaxing ritual that can be a part of the stimulus for a sleep response.

5. Carefully time meals and exercise.

    A heavy meal late in the evening can severely disrupt sleep in the patient with gastroesophageal reflux. Heavy exercise too late in the evening can also lead to a worsening of sleep in all but the best-conditioned athlete; therefore, for most of us, heavy exercise should be scheduled earlier in the day.

6. Relaxation techniques or hypnosis may be useful.

    Some people simply need to be able to relax sufficiently to allow sleep to occur. Perhaps on the counter displaying all of the nonprescription sleep aids, there should be available relaxation tapes as well.

7. Consider psychotherapy.

    Since at least 35% of all patients seen in sleep-disorders centers for a complaint of insomnia have an identifiable psychiatric or psychologic cause, some form of psychotherapy or psychiatric treatment should be considered.

HYPNOTICS

The Ideal Hypnotic

It is helpful to describe the ideal hypnotic. Although it does not exist, keeping the ideal characteristics in mind helps to place the existing agents into perspective. Ideally, the drug should induce sleep rapidly after ingestion. It should maintain sleep for the entire duration expected, without lasting so long that it produces a "morning hangover" and impaired daytime performance. It should not induce development of tolerance or dependence when used over a number of consecutive nights, and abrupt withdrawal should not result in a drug-withdrawal or rebound insomnia. It should have a wide margin of safety, and it should make abnormal sleep normal, while not making the sleep of a normal sleeper abnormal. Finally, it should have no potential for drug-drug interactions.

Classification and Pharmacology of Selected Agents

Many of the more commonly used hypnotic agents are presented in Table 54.10. Note that for the elderly, dosing should begin at or below the low end of the dosage ranges shown. The old-time barbiturates lost popularity as a result of their narrow margin of safety, moderately high abuse potential, potential drug-drug interactions as a result of liver enzyme induction, suppression of delta and REM sleep, with a REM rebound following abrupt discontinuation, and loss of efficacy in inducing and maintaining sleep within 14 consecutive nights of use at a consistent dose (30).

The nonbarbiturate nonbenzodiazepines were thought

to be superior to the barbiturates because of their lack of the barbiturate structure. However, with the exception of chloral hydrate, they share many of the disadvantages of the barbiturates, and they have additional ones as well. For instance, methaqualone, which is no longer available, was found to have an even higher abuse potential than the barbiturates. Glutethimide, in an overdose situation, presents the emergency room staff not only with a CNS depressant overdose but also with anticholinergic toxicity. In several European countries agents such as ethchlorvynol, glutethimide, and methyprylon are not available. Although there has been controversy over their ability in the United States for the past 15 years, they remain on the market. Chloral hydrate, an exception, lacks some of these disadvantages, but it does displace other protein-bound drugs (e.g., warfarin), it causes gastrointestinal irritation in some individuals, and in the higher doses (1 to 2 g) needed for some patients, it may lose its effectiveness in inducing and maintaining sleep at least as rapidly as the barbiturates (31).

The antihistamines, primarily diphenhydramine and doxylamine, are used by taking advantage of their sedative side effects. Some would argue that this drug class is a good choice for patients with a high potential for abusing the benzodiazepines (i.e., those with a history or current problem of substance abuse). Unfortunately, little research into the hypnotic efficacy of these drugs has been done in the sleep laboratory. By subjective report, patients assess the soporific effect of diphenhydramine 50 mg to be equivalent to 60 mg of pentobarbital (32). Increasing the dose of diphenhydramine does not produce a linear increase in hypnotic effect, but it does produce greater anticholinergic side effects, which can be particularly troublesome in the elderly. Not only are they bothered by constipation, urinary retention, dry mouth, and blurred near vision, but they are particularly sensitive to the central anticholinergic effects of confusion, disorientation, impaired short-term memory, and, at times, visual and tactile hallucinations. Hence, the patient should be monitored for and counseled about these side effects as well as drug interactions with other CNS depressants.

One amino acid, L-tryptophan, became popular as a natural hypnotic since it is a precursor to serotonin, a neurotransmitter that seems to be significantly involved in NREM sleep. L-Tryptophan has never been approved by the FDA as a hypnotic; it has been sold as a food supplement. The overall efficacy of this agent is unclear. Positive response is unpredictable as the predictors of response have not been identified (33). Some 1500 cases (including 24 fatalities) of an eosinophilia-myalgia syndrome associated with the use of L-tryptophan have been reported to the U.S. Centers for Disease Control (CDC) in Atlanta (34). The CDC defines this L-tryptophan-associated eosinophilia-myalgia syndrome as (a) an increase of eosin-

Table 54.10.
Hypnotics—Classification and Dosages

Generic Name	Trade Name	Dosage Range
Barbiturates		
Pentobarbital	Nembutal	100–200 mg
Secobarbital	Seconal	100–200 mg
Amobarbital	Amytal	100–200 mg
Nonbarbiturate nonbenzodiazepines		
Ethchlorvynol	Placidyl	0.5–1.0 g
Glutethimide	Doriden	0.5–1.0 g
Methyprylon	Noludar	200–400 mg
Chloral hydrate	Noctec	0.5–2.0 g
Antihistamines		
Diphenhydramine	Benadryl, Sominex-2	25–100 mg
Doxylamine	Unisom	25–100 mg
Benzodiazepines		
Flurazepam	Dalmane	15–30 mg
Temazepam	Restoril	15–30 mg
Triazolam	Halcion	0.125–0.5 mg
Quazepam	Doral	7.5–15 mg
Estazolam	ProSom	1.0–2.0 mg
Amino acids		
L-Tryptophan	Trofan	1.0–4.0 g

ophils to counts above 1000/mm³; (*b*) myalgia that interferes with daily activities; and (*c*) the absence of some other identifiable cause (e.g., parasites, leukemia). Although the nature of this association is unclear (for instance, there has been strong speculation that some contaminant was accidentally introduced through use of a new strain of bacillus in the production process into the bulk supplies shipped from overseas), as of this writing, the FDA and CDC have recommended that people stop using the agent and that physicians stop prescribing it. If it should come back into use, it should be noted that it is not a totally innocuous substance. Most commonly, people are bothered by its gastrointestinal irritation, which previously pregnant women have compared with morning sickness. In addition, chronic use has been associated with both niacin and pyridoxine deficiencies. The combination of L-tryptophan and a monoamine oxidase inhibitor (e.g, phenelzine or tranylcypromine) or fluoxetine can produce a "serotonin syndrome," characterized by disorientation, agitation, hyperthermia, hyperreflexia, diaphoresis, ocular oscillations, and myoclonic jerking. Finally, low doses have been associated with changes in liver ultrastructure in normal rats and have been lethal in rats with adrenal insufficiency.

The benzodiazepines come closest to the ideal hypnotic. Indeed, this was one of several major conclusions of the Consensus Development Conference on Drugs and Insomnia at the National Institute of Mental Health in November, 1983 (35). Three conclusions of significance to this discussion were that (*a*) hypnotics should be used primarily in the treatment of transient or short-term insomnia (e.g., situational, jet lag, and work shift change); (*b*) when pharmacotherapy is indicated, a benzodiazepine is generally the drug of choice; and (*c*) selection of the specific agent should be based on its pharmacokinetic/pharmacodynamic characteristics in relation to the individual patient and situation.

Flurazepam was the first of the benzodiazepines marketed as a hypnotic. Its favorable profile, as compared with the barbiturates and the nonbarbiturate nonbenzodiazepines, includes a wider margin of safety, lower abuse potential, and fewer drug-drug interactions. In addition, it produces little or no REM suppression at lower doses (15 mg), and even at higher doses (30 mg) REM suppression is not followed by a REM rebound upon abrupt discontinuation of the drug, probably because of the slow elimination of its long-acting active metabolite, *N*-desalkylflurazepam. Whether it demonstrates no withdrawal phenomena has yet to be clarified; one may need to look at sleep patterns several weeks beyond discontinuation of the drug. It has the additional advantage of remaining effective at a consistent dose for at least 28 consecutive nights of use. It does suppress delta sleep, and the long-acting metabolite (with an elimination half-life of 47 to 200 hr) accumulates over time. This can cause impaired daytime functioning, especially in the elderly, leading to falls resulting in injuries (36). Peak plasma levels are achieved within 30 to 60 min.

Temazepam has the advantage of a short-to-intermediate elimination half-life of 9 to 15 hr. However, it can be as long 20 to 30 hr in the elderly, so one must watch for possible accumulation and morning hangover with repeated use. It shares many of the properties of flurazepam with respect to effects on sleep. In doses of 15 to 30 mg, it increases total sleep time and decreases the frequency and duration of nocturnal awakenings in insomniac patients. It suppresses delta sleep, and, although there is a decrease in REM sleep during the first half of the night, there is a corresponding increase in the second half. However, there is an ongoing question about its ability to shorten sleep latency significantly in the patient who has difficulty falling asleep because it can take 1 to 2 hr to work. Initial studies of the drug included two dosage forms, a hard gelatin capsule with a powder inside (available in the United States) and a soft gelatin capsule containing a solution of the drug in polyethylene glycol. With the soft gelatin capsule, the drug appears to be absorbed more quickly. This formulation issue has yet to be adequately addressed by the manufacturer.

Triazolam is unique in being ultrashort to short acting, with an elimination half-life of 2 to 3 hr (5.5 at the most). Peak plasma levels are achieved within 30 to 80 min. Triazolam appears to be absorbed about as quickly as flurazepam, but eliminated much more rapidly. Although it suppresses REM sleep in the first half of the night, there appears to be compensation for this in the second half (probably as drug levels are decreasing). It seems to have little effect on delta sleep, which distinguishes it from flurazepam, temazepam, and other benzodiazepines. It is least likely of the benzodiazepines to produce morning hangover. Indeed, at the 0.25-mg dose, the effect is equal to that with placebo. Like flurazepam and temazepam, it increases the general quality of sleep, decreases nocturnal awakenings, and increases total sleep time (37–41).

There has been some concern among clinicians and the public that triazolam is more likely to produce psychomotor impairment, psychologic adverse effects, and anterograde amnesia than other benzodiazepines. However, this may be a function of the dose and pattern of use, potency, combination with other CNS depressants, and the mechanism of adverse drug reaction reporting, rather than a unique risk of triazolam (42). In a meeting of the FDA's Psychopharmacological Drugs Advisory Committee (September 22, 1989), the consensus was that the issue of amnesia should receive greater attention in the product labeling (i.e., the package insert) and that patient information should be developed about the use and risks of the entire class of benzodiazepine hypnotics. Some of the concern over triazolam has been associated with "traveler's amnesia." This is the situation in which an individual flying across a number of time zones decides to force sleep during the flight with a short-acting hypnotic, perhaps having ingested some ethanol on the plane as well. Later the traveler has little or no recall for a number of hours following ingestion of the drug (e.g., arrival at the airport and subsequent activities). Until we fully understand this form of anterograde amnesia, it may simply be safer to readjust the internal biological clock after arriving at our destination. Whatever the actual incidence (as yet still unclear) of psychomotor impairment, psychological adverse affects, and anterograde amnesia, especially at the lower doses currently being recommended and used, it is prudent to carefully monitor and counsel patients using triazolam.

Most recently, quazepam and estazolam have been marketed in the United States. Although quazepam has an intriguing specificity for the BZ_1 benzodiazepine receptor subtype, the clinical importance of this property is unclear. Indeed, although the parent compound has a 39-hr half-life of elimination, one of its metabolites, N-desalkyl-2-oxoquazepam, is identical to N-desalkylflurazepam, which is the long-acting active metabolite of flurazepam. Peak plasma levels are achieved in 1 to 2 hr (43). With greater use, it may be discovered to offer few, if any, advantages over flurazepam.

Estazolam, the second triazolobenzodiazepine hypnotic, at the time of this writing is so new that its place in our benzodiazepine hypnotic armamentarium is yet to be established. It appears to decrease sleep latency and nocturnal awakenings, while increasing total sleep time and improving depth of sleep and sleep quality (44). Peak plasma levels are achieved within 0.5 to 4 hr, although with the doses generally employed, onset of action appears to be similar to that seen with flurazepam and triazolam. The half-life of elimination is 8 to 28 hr. Based on its onset of action and elimination half-life, it appears to be a "faster-acting temazepam." This would make it an agent that can significantly decrease sleep latency (a distinct advantage over temazepam) and provide a duration of action intermediate between flurazepam and triazolam. However, results of objective, sleep laboratory studies are mixed with respect to estazolam's ability to significantly decrease latency to sleep onset.

Drug-Withdrawal Insomnia and Rebound Insomnia

When barbiturates were used more commonly for the treatment of insomnia, drug-withdrawal insomnia was described as a phenomenon associated with the abrupt discontinuation of the hypnotic after long-term use (45). After chronic REM suppression, discontinuation led to a REM rebound, accounting for as much as 40% of total sleep time. This REM rebound was accompanied by very intense and frightening dreams as well as a generally disrupted night of sleep. The patient, not understanding the nature of the phenomenon, was likely to immediately return to chronic, high-dose use. With gradual tapering of the drug or an equivalent amount of a longer-acting agent and patient education about the possibility of temporarily increased dreaming and decreased quality of sleep, patients are better able to tolerate discontinuation of their hypnotics.

More recently, rebound insomnia has been described as a phenomenon associated with the abrupt discontinuation of the shorter-acting benzodiazepines (e.g., temazepam and triazolam) (46). It involves a worsening of sleep, even beyond what it was like before the patient was started on the drug. The exact incidence of the phenomenon is unclear, but it is prudent to warn the patient about a possible transient worsening of sleep immediately after stopping the drug. Gradual tapering of the drug, rather than abrupt discontinuation, may lessen the severity of these withdrawal symptoms (47). As an example, a patient taking 0.25 mg of triazolam every night for several weeks could reduce the dose by half (to 0.125 mg) for 3 nights, by half again (to one half of a 0.125-mg tablet) for the next 3 nights, and then finally discontinue the medication.

Problems/Controversies

Two important issues with insomnia and hypnotics are that no one drug is ideal for every insomniac and that not all insomniacs should be treated with hypnotics. As previously stated, hypnotics are to be used almost exclusively for the treatment of transient or short-term insomnia. The implication is that a thorough assessment will be made of every patient with a complaint of insomnia. Although hypnotic-induced sleep may be unnatural in some respects, an ultimate measure of efficacy must be seen as optimal daytime performance (48, 49).

Some prescribers and patients believe that all hypnotics should be avoided because of the possible development of dependence. If they are used appropriately—for brief periods and at low doses—the risk is low. Also, drug-dependence insomnia, in which sleep worsens with long-term use of hypnotics even while the patient continues to take the drug (44), should not be a problem. In many respects, our society has been responsible for many of the transient insomnias (e.g., jet lag, work shift change, and situational) and must take responsibility, either pharmacologically or nonpharmacologically, for dealing with the problem.

General Clinical Guidelines

A careful diagnostic assessment is necessary before treating any insomnia. The pharmacist can play a major role in assessing sleep and arousal disorders (Table 54.11).

Once a decision is made to treat insomnia pharma-

Table 54.11.
Pharmacist's Guide to Assessment of Sleep and Arousal Disorders

1. Don't allow your own experiences to interfere with your assessment.
   Unfortunately, because most of us have had at least an occasional bout of insomnia, we may too easily assume that everyone else's problem is similar to our own.
2. Clarify the complaint.
   Every time a patient is seen standing in the nonprescription products area looking at sleep aids or stimulants, the pharmacist can be of major service. How likely is it that the patient has thoroughly assessed his problem?
3. Do a drug history.
   Assess the possibility that the problem is drug-induced. Look for stimulating drugs such as sympathomimetic decongestants or caffeine. Look for CNS depressant withdrawal such as moderate-to-heavy ethanol intake at dinner time. Assess the contribution of street drugs. In addition, look for sedating drugs as causes of excessive daytime sleepiness. Finally, find out what, if anything, has worked for the same problem in the past.
4. Ask if the problem is one of insomnia or excessive daytime sleepiness.
   Patients who are looking at the nonprescription stimulants may be excessively sleepy secondary to obstructive sleep apnea or narcolepsy. If it's a case of self-induced sleep deprivation (e.g., studying for examinations), caffeine tablets may be appropriate short-term, but evaluate possible drug-disease interactions (e.g., hypertension) and tell the patient about sleep hygiene.
5. If the complaint is insomnia, determine if it is transient or chronic.
   If transient, a nonprescription sleep aid containing doxylamine or diphenhydramine may be worth a try for a few nights; but tell the patient about anticholinergic effects and suggest visiting a physician if the antihistamine is either ineffective or intolerable.
6. If the insomnia is chronic, encourage the patient to see a physician.
   There are many reasons for chronic insomnia, and a number of them are treatable. The patient with chronic insomnia deserves as meticulous an evaluation as the patient who comes in with a complaint of chronic stomach pain or unremitting, chronic headache
7. Be prepared for appreciation and praise.
   You may refer only one patient a year for assessment. But if that patient has a treatable and responsive chronic insomnia, the change in quality of life will make that patient forever grateful.

cologically, pharmacokinetic differences play a major role in selecting a benzodiazepine. Drug selection must take into account onset of action and duration with respect to single versus multiple dosing and past history of response. If possible daytime impairment associated with accumulation of long-acting active metabolites (especially in the elderly) is a concern, avoid flurazepam and quazepam; choose one of the shorter-acting agents. Also, recall that accumulation becomes a much greater concern with continuous use over several nights than with infrequent p.r.n. use (in which drug action is terminated as quickly as it can be redistributed out of brain tissue). If the possible delayed onset of action of temazepam is a concern, choose the more rapidly acting flurazepam, triazolam, or perhaps estazolam. If possible anterograde amnesia with triazolam is a concern, use very low doses, caution the patient, and

consider avoiding its use in situations in which the drug effect may not have worn off by the time the individual needs to be awake, alert, and fully functioning. The choices do not always have to be limited to the five agents specifically marketed as hypnotics. For instance, diazepam is superior to flurazepam in onset of action and yet shares the property of accumulation of a long-acting active metabolite under multiple-dosing conditions. In general, the choice of drug depends upon pharmacokinetic profile and benefits sought.

The hypnotics should be avoided in patients with sleep apnea, patients who use alcohol or other CNS depressants heavily, pregnant patients, and individuals in whom alert nighttime performance is mandatory (e.g., firemen, pilots). Although the benzodiazepines are relatively safe, one must be cautious in giving them to patients with a high suicidal risk. Patients who overdose often use combinations of agents, frequently washing down everything with alcohol. Combination of benzodiazepines with alcohol can be fatal.

The benefit that the patient is seeking must be determined. Ideally, the patient is looking for both improved sleep and improved daytime functioning. Simply increasing the number of hours of sleep is generally not a sufficient reason for prescribing hypnotics. Once the hypnotic is chosen, the lowest effective dose to achieve a clear-cut benefit is used. This requires following the patient regularly, quantifying the results, and educating the patient about the need to begin with a low dose and give it an adequate trial. For flurazepam, this is 15 mg; with triazolam in an elderly patient, the dose is 0.125 mg, or perhaps even half a 0.125-mg tablet. The importance of starting with a low dose cannot be overstated. For instance, with flurazepam the optimal effect may not be experienced for 2 to 3 days; this may be due to the slow accumulation of N-desalkylflurazepam. In addition, especially in the elderly, daytime sequelae must be monitored. These are important educational and monitoring roles for the pharmacist. Drug-drug and drug-disease interactions should be identified and avoided. Examples of drug-drug interactions include additive CNS depression when the hypnotics are combined with other CNS depressants; and accumulation of flurazepam, quazepam, and their long-acting metabolite N-desalkylflurazepam in the presence of cimetidine (which interferes with oxidative metabolic processes). A primary drug-disease interaction is the use of an agent requiring oxidative metabolic transformation (e.g., flurazepam and quazepam) in the presence of liver disease or old age. If a nonbenzodiazepine is being prescribed, the effect of liver enzyme induction must be kept in mind in addition to additive effects with other CNS depressants.

The issue of hypnotic use in chronic insomnia is complex. Few data are available regarding the efficacy and safety of hypnotics when taken for more than 1 to 2 months. In addition, there is no evidence to indicate that chronic hypnotic use will produce lasting, objective improvement in sleep and daytime function in the persistent insomnias. Indeed, for many chronic insomniacs the underlying problem is a psychiatric condition, drug or alcohol dependence, sleep apnea, or delayed sleep phase syndrome. Treatments specific to the disorder and nonpharmacologic approaches should be tried first. If psychiatric and medical disorders have been ruled out and nonpharmacologic approaches have failed, referral to a sleep-disorders center would be appropriate. In the rare instances in which a thorough sleep evaluation has been done and a hypnotic is used in treating a chronic insomnia (e.g., periodic limb movement disorder), the patient should be evaluated frequently for improvement in both sleep and daytime functioning, as well as the persistence of the therapeutic effect at a constant dose. The reason for this is that longer-term use carries an increased risk of dependence, tolerance with resulting escalation of dose, and difficult withdrawal.

Patient education should include emphasis on short-term use, discussion of possible daytime sedation and impairment with the longer-acting agents, the importance of avoiding other CNS depressants, and the risks of tolerance and dependence if used for too long and/or at excessively high doses. Where hypnotics are to be used for extended periods of time, it may be useful to suggest skipping a night or two once in a while. This allows the patient to see if the drug is still really needed, and perhaps it can reduce the development of tolerance. When the drug is discontinued, ideally in a gradual, tapered style, the patient must be told about possible temporary withdrawal phenomena.

PROGNOSIS

Insomnia and the other sleep disorders can be crippling for many people. As life becomes more complex, it would not be surprising to see an increase in the incidence of transient insomnia. However, with appropriate assessment and treatment, the transient insomnias can be managed, to improve both nighttime sleep and daytime performance. Although there may be no cures for many persistent insomnias such as sleep apnea, increased understanding of these disorders is leading to prevention of harm to patients by inadequate assessment or inappropriate use of hypnotics. Also, with better assessment and increased referral by pharmacists, many patients with some of the persistent insomnias (e.g., psychiatric disorders and delayed sleep phase syndrome) can be helped significantly.

CONCLUSION

Sleep is a fascinating psychophysiologic phenomenon that is cyclic and can be measured electrophysiologically. Much

is now known about sleep and its disorders, but sleep-disorders medicine is still in its infancy. Millions of our patients are afflicted by a variety of sleep disorders. They are a heterogeneous group of disorders capable of producing major social/occupational disability; disturbed sleep can be crippling for many people. Sleep complaints deserve the same meticulous assessment and concern as that afforded a complaint of chest pain, flank pain, or coughing up blood. Disorders of excessive daytime sleepiness (obstructive sleep apnea and narcolepsy), insomnia (transient as well as persistent types), and unusual behaviors and mental activity during sleep (sleepwalking, sleep terrors, and nightmares) have been described. Not all sleep complaints should be treated with hypnotics; indeed, some of the sleep disorders may be worsened by hypnotics or other drugs.

Hypnotic use is generally most appropriately reserved for the treatment of transient or short-term insomnias. Although a number of hypnotics are available, the benzodiazepines are currently accepted as the drugs of choice; selection within the group is based primarily on differences in pharmacokinetic profiles. The practicing pharmacist has the opportunity to play an important role in assessing, recommending treatment, or recommending further evaluation for the many patients with complaints of insomnia or excessive daytime sleepiness. In addition, the pharmacist can play a major role in educating the patient about therapy and monitoring for therapeutic and adverse effects. With careful diagnosis and treatment tailored to the individual and the particular problem, more people will be sleeping better and also performing considerably better in their daily activities.

REFERENCES

1. Bixler EO, Kales A, Soldatos CR, et al.: Prevalence of sleep disorders in the Los Angeles metropolitan area. Am J Psychiatry 136:1257–1262, 1979.
2. Mellinger GD, Balter MB, Uhlenhuth EH: Insomnia and its treatments. Arch Gen Psychiatry 42:225–232, 1985.
3. Wincor MZ, Johnson KA: Non-prescription hypnotics: purchase and pharmacist-patient interaction in the community pharmacy. Presented to the 14th European Symposium on Clinical Pharmacy. Stockholm, October, 1985.
4. Hobson JA, Lydic R, Baghdoyan HA: Evolving concepts of sleep cycle generation: from brain centers to neuronal populations. Behav Brain Sci 9:371–448, 1986.
5. Rechtschaffen A, Kales A (eds): A Manual of Standardized Terminology, Techniques and Scoring System for Sleep Stages of Human Subjects. (Publication 204, Public Health Service Publications.) Washington, D.C.: U.S. Government Printing Office, 1968.
6. Ancoli-Israel S, Kripke DF, Klauber MR, et al.: Sleep-disordered breathing in community-dwelling elderly. Sleep 14:486–495, 1991.
7. Ancoli-Israel S, Kripke DF, Klauber MR, et al.: Periodic limb movements in sleep in community-dwelling elderly. Sleep 14:496–500, 1991.
8. Prinz PN, Vitiello MV, Raskind MA, et al.: Geriatrics: sleep disorders and aging. N Engl J Med 323:520–526, 1990.

9. Sleep Disorders Classification Committee, Association of Sleep Disorders Centers: Diagnostic classification of sleep and arousal disorders. Sleep 2:1–137, 1979.

10. Diagnostic Classification Steering Committee of the American Sleep Disorders Association (Thorpy MJ, Chair): International Classification of Sleep Disorders—Diagnostic and Coding Manual. Rochester, MN: American Sleep Disorders Association, 1990, 396 pp.

11. American Psychiatric Association: Diagnostic and Statistical Manual of Mental Disorders, ed. 3, revised. Washington, D.C.: American Psychiatric Association, 1987, pp 297–313.

12. Kales A, Soldatos CR, Kales JD: Sleep disorders: insomnia, sleepwalking, night terrors, nightmares, and enuresis. Ann Intern Med 106:582–592, 1987.

13. Guilleminault C: Obstructive sleep apnea syndrome: a review. Psychiatr Clin North Am 10:607–621, 1987.

14. Kales A, Vela-Bueno A, Kales JD: Sleep disorders: sleep apnea and narcolepsy. Ann Intern Med 106:434–443, 1987.

15. Handelsman H, Carter E: Continuous Positive Airway Pressure for the Treatment of Obstructive Sleep Apnea in Adults. (Health Technology Assessment Reports 1986, no 3.) Rockville, MD: National Center for Health Services Research and Health Care Technology Assessment, 1986.

16. Bonnet MH, Dexter JR, Arand DL: The effect of triazolam on arousal and respiration in central sleep apnea patients. Sleep 13:31–41, 1990.

17. Whyte KF, Gould GA, Airlie MA: Role of protriptyline and acetazolamide in the sleep apnea/hypopnea syndrome. Sleep 11:463–472, 1988.

18. Strohl KP, Hensley MJ, Saunders NA, et al.: Progesterone administration and progressive sleep apneas. JAMA 245:1230–1232, 1981.

19. Tojima H, Kunitomo F, Kimura H, et al.: Effects of acetazolamide in patients with the sleep apnea syndrome. Thorax 43:113–118, 1988.

20. Dement WC, Carskadon MA, Guilleminault C, et al.: Narcolepsy: diagnosis and treatment. Prim Care 3:609–623, 1976.

21. Inoko H, Ando A, Tseuji K, et al.: HLA-DQ chain DNA restriction fragments can differentiate between healthy and narcoleptic individuals with HLA-DR2. Immunogenetics 23:126–128, 1986.

22. Campbell RK: The treatment of narcolepsy and cataplexy. Drug Intell Clin Pharm 15:257–262, 1981.

23. Carskadon MA, Dement WC, Mitler MM, et al.: Self reports versus sleep laboratory findings in 122 drug-free subjects with complaints of chronic insomnia. Am J Psychiatry 133:1382–1388, 1976.

24. Weitzman ED, Czeisler CA, Coleman RM, et al.: Delayed sleep phase syndrome. Arch Gen Psychiatry 38:737–746, 1981.

25. Coleman R, Roffwarg H, Kennedy S, et al.: Sleep-wake disorders based on a polysomnographic diagnosis: a national cooperative study. JAMA 247:997–1003, 1982.

26. Mitler MM, Browman CP, Menn SJ, et al.: Nocturnal myoclonus: treatment efficacy of clonazepam and temazepam. Sleep 9:385–392, 1986.

27. Telstad W, Sorenson O, Larsen S, et al.: Treatment of restless legs syndrome with carbamazepine: a double blind study. Br Med J 288:444, 1984.

28. Killen J, Coates T, The complaint of insomnia: what is it and how do we treat it? In Franks CM: New Developments in Behavior Therapy: From Research to Clinical Application. New York, Haworth Press, 1984, pp 377–408.

29. McClusky HY, Milby JB, Switzer PK, et al.: Efficacy of behavioral versus triazolam treatment in persistent sleep-onset insomnia. Am J Psychiatry 148:121–126, 1991.

30. Kales AK, Bixler EO, Kales JD, et al.: Comparative effectiveness of nine hypnotic drugs: sleep laboratory studies. J Clin Pharmacol 17:207–213, 1977.

31. Kales A, Allen C, Scharf MB, et al.: Hypnotic drugs and their effectiveness: all night EEG studies of insomniac subjects. Arch Gen Psychiatry 23:226–232, 1970.

32. Teutach G, Mahler DL, Brown CR, et al.: Hypnotic efficacy of diphenhydramine, methapyrilene, and pentobarbital for nighttime sedation. Clin Pharmacol Ther 17:195–201, 1975.

33. Schneider-Helmert D, Spinweber CL: Evaluation of L-tryptophan for treatment of insomnia: a review. Psychopharmacology 89:1–7, 1986.

34. Raphals P: Disease puzzle nears solution. Science 249:619, 1990.

35. National Institute of Mental Health, Consensus Development Conference: Drugs and insomnia: the use of medications to promote sleep. JAMA 251:2410–2414, 1984.

36. Ray WA, Griffin MR, Downey W: Benzodiazepines of short and long elimination half-life and the risk of hip fracture. JAMA 262:3303–3307, 1989.

37. Dement WC: Rational basis for the use of sleeping pills. Pharmacology 27(suppl 2):3–38, 1983.

38. Wincor MZ: Insomnia and the new benzodiazepines. Clin Pharm 1:425–432, 1982.

39. Kales A, Kales JD: Sleep laboratory studies of hypnotic drugs: efficacy and withdrawal effects. J Clin Psychopharmacol 3:140–150, 1983.

40. Rickels K: Clinical trials of hypnotics. J Clin Psychopharmacol 3:133, 1983.

41. Greenblatt DJ, Harmatz JS, Englehardt N, et al.: Pharmacokinetic determinants of dynamic differences among three benzodiazepine hypnotics. Arch Gen Psychiatry 46:326–332, 1989.

42. Griffiths RR, Lamb RJ, Ator NA, et al.: Relative abuse liability of triazolam: experimental assessment in animals and humans. Neurosci Biobehav Res 9:133–151, 1985.

43. Kales A: Quazepam: hypnotic efficacy and side effects. Pharmacotherapy 10:1–12, 1990.

44. Pierce MW, Shu VS: Efficacy of estazolam: the United States clinical experience. Am J Med 88(suppl 3A):6–11, 1990.

45. Kales A, Bixler E, Tan T, et al.: Chronic hypnotic-drug use: ineffectiveness, drug-withdrawal insomnia, and dependence. JAMA 227:513–517, 1974.

46. Kales A, Scharf M, Kales J: Rebound insomnia: a new clinical syndrome. Science 201:1039–1041, 1978.

47. Schweizer E, Rickels K, Case G, et al.: Long-term therapeutic use of benzodiazepines—II. Effects of gradual taper. Arch Gen Psychiatry 47:908–915, 1990.

48. Gillin JC, Byerley WF: The diagnosis and management of insomnia. N Engl J Med 322:239–247, 1990.

49. Everett DE, Avorn J, Baker MW: Clinical decision-making in the evaluation and treatment of insomnia. Am J Med 89:357–362, 1990.

CHAPTER 55

ATTENTION-DEFICIT HYPERACTIVITY DISORDER

ROBERT W. PIEPHO, Ph.D., F.C.P. and JOHN W. HILL, Ph.D.

The term "attention-deficit hyperactivity disorder" (ADHD) is a contemporary term used to describe a behavioral disorder of childhood. Historically, behavioral and cognitive disorders were linked together and characterized as the notion of minimal brain dysfunction (MBD). Included were a broad array of characteristics such as hyperactivity, distractibility, impulsivity, learning disabilities, and emotional instability (1). The term ADHD is used throughout this chapter as it reflects the separation of this syndrome from learning disabilities, except as a related disorder. This term also implies no specific etiology, no pathognomonic signs, and no particular similarity in course of the disorder, or treatment duration. Evolution of operational definitions can be traced through three revisions of the Diagnostic and Statistical Manual of Mental Disorders (DSM) published by the American Psychiatric Association. In the second edition, DSM II published in 1968, the phrase "hyperkinetic reaction of childhood" was used (2). DSM III (1982) presented two subtypes of a more broad-based concept, attention-deficit disorder with and without hyperactivity (3). The most recent revision, DSM III-R, (1987) combines the subtypes into one disorder to reflect the prominent and often disturbing role that hyperactivity plays in the disorder.

Table 55.1, shows the behaviors that a child with ADHD may exhibit with corresponding treatment goals and multimodal treatment plans for increasing the availability of the child to learning. Current practice suggests a patient-oriented healthcare team, including a primary care physician, clinical pharmacist, special educator, psychologist, and parent, and interactive pharmacologic and behavioral management that occurs within the child's primary environments. The primary concern is for children who are producing chronic ADHD behaviors at home, at school, and in their communities because they present the greatest challenges, and with multimodal treatment, they may experience recovered potential rather than failure and despair (5).

ADHD is more common in boys than girls. The exact cause is unknown, although it is presumed to be neurologic. The affected children are not "available" for learning whether it is academic, social, or emotional skills that are involved.

A major and obvious symptom of ADHD is excessive motor activity. Movement, however, is also a primary form of normal expression in young children. During the first 6 years of their lives, children learn by touching, tasting, feeling, holding, and manipulating. Furthermore, children tend to translate their anxiety into excessive motor behavior; this often helps them communicate their unhappiness to adults in the absence of language. These normal developmental conditions often complicate diagnosis, particularly for for 4- and 5-year-old children enrolled in inappropriately structured and overly demanding academic preschool programs, where they must sit still to "learn" before they are ready to do so.

Therefore, ADHD could be described as purposeless, chronic, pervasive, driven behavior that interferes with a child's availability to social, emotional and academic learning. The definition is assessed by an examination of the three characteristics—hyperactivity, impulsivity, and distractibility.

The term hyperactivity brings to mind the stereotypical wound-up child, unable to slow down for anything short of a brick wall. However, to label a child hyperactive simply on the basis of miles traveled per hour is to disregard some of the hallmarks of ADHD. Any child who is producing behavior that is purposeful, even at high energy, need not be considered hyperactive. To illustrate purposeless behavior in the extreme, consider a sandbox situation where four or five 6-year-old children are making roads in the sand and playing with toy trucks. The child with ADHD might use the truck to knock down another child's sand house or throw the truck while moving rapidly from one part of the play area to the next, but this child will not typically be observed playing together or in common with the other children or "driving" the toy truck on the roads while making contextually appropriate "truck" sounds.

The impulsive ADHD child is likely to be viewed as disruptive and perhaps mean or "bad" by his peers and by adults. Very often with the impulsive ADHD child there is a one-to-one correspondence between feelings a child might have and the expression of these feelings—no matter how inappropriate—through verbal behavior or physical action. Therefore, a feeling of anger will be expressed without reflectivity or any recognition as to what impact

Table 55.1.

Behavior of Child with Attention Deficit–Hyperactivity Disorder, Treatment Goal, and Multimodal Treatment Plan for Increasing Availability to Learning

ADHD Behavior (Child may exhibit one or more)	Treatment Goal	Multimodal Treatment Plan
Hyperactivity	Decrease motor activity	Drug intervention with behavioral management at home and school
Distractibility	Increase attention span and response to appropriate stimuli	Drug intervention with behavioral management at home and school and educational modification
Impulsivity	Increase reflectivity before acting	Drug intervention with behavioral management at home and school and family therapy

the words "I hate you" or "I want to smash you" for example, might have on the recipient. Even a hug, impulsively given at the wrong time and wrong place, can result in embarrassment and surprise for the unwilling recipient and corresponding rejection and hurt feelings for the ADHD teen. Adults and children often react negatively, which sets up a vicious cycle with the child producing even more impulsive behavior.

The distractible ADHD child has a short attention span and seems to be more interested in what is going on in the next room than in the activity at hand. However, distractible children often are more on-task than they might appear and respond well to behavioral modification techniques and educational modifications.

While the young ADHD child may be observed producing purposeless motor behavior, the ADHD adolescent may be sophisticated enough to control the external behavior, even though his mind is racing a mile a minute. Distracted by anything and everything, he is preoccupied with his own thoughts.

Although often described as a disease of childhood, some symptoms of ADHD, such as impulsivity and distractibility may persist into adult life (6, 7).

PATHOGENESIS

Studies of causative factors have focused on the relationship between scholastic underachievement and central nervous system (CNS) disorder. Table 55.2 lists abnormalities and lesions that have been postulated to be responsible for the symptoms of ADHD, which is presumed

to be a neurological disorder (8). The most promising of the contemporary postulates on CNS-related causative factors is assumed neurotransmitter deficiency or breakdown. It is thought that psychostimulants increase the production of norepinephrine so that the child can function as normally as possible (9). However, the actual etiology of ADHD remains elusive.

DIAGNOSTIC AND CLINICAL FINDINGS

Diagnosing ADHD begins the process of change, but making that diagnosis is complex. The typical ADHD child has good health, but the history reveals that, from the earliest days, the child has been different and his purposeless behavior has been chronic. Whereas ADHD was once thought of as a global syndrome, it is now differentiated into two general types: the chronic or neurologically based and the situational or anxiety-based (10).

The two types have striking similarities in that the child may be producing hyperactive behavior. The chronic or neurologically based hyperactivity however, is recognized very early in life. Some mothers report that even in utero, the child was very active. Often the medical history will indicate a child who was very colicky and had very disruptive sleeping and eating patterns. From early on, the child was fearless and charged headlong into situations that were dangerous or even life-threatening, such as running out into the street, whereas normally developing preschoolers are more likely to be put off by loud noises made by cars and, therefore, tend to avoid the street. Approximately 1% of the school-aged population would be considered ADHD if only those children who fit the "chronic rule" were considered.

In contrast, situational or anxiety-based hyperactivity has no chronic history of problems with attention deficits. For example, the child may be 10 years old, with a good disposition and perfect school attendance record. Then, suddenly, the child no longer pays attention in class, and is fidgety, nervous, and upset. His behavior is suddenly and acutely purposeless, and not directed toward goal completion. In most cases, these are young people experiencing anxiety over an unpleasant situation in their lives,

Table 55.2.

Postulated Causative Factors in Attention Deficit–Hyperactivity Disorder

Prenatal or perinatal insult
Neurotransmitter (norepinephrine) deficiency or breakdown
Neurochemical lesions
Congenital anomalies
Low CNS arousal level
Genetic disorders
Exposure to environmental toxins

such as a parent's impending divorce or loss or change of jobs, the death of a pet, problems with a bully who wants to fight or a visit by relatives. The anxiety is then translated into motor behavior. Children sometimes become symptom-bearers for family issues, particularly when family routine, predictability, and structure are altered or lost. These children are not thought to be good candidates for drug treatment, and individual counseling and family therapy are indicated. While controversial, it might be best to not consider these children as ADHD patients.

Although there is not a critical diagnostic test for ADHD, it is important to attempt to rule out other syndromes, such as borderline schizophrenia. The schizophrenic child will usually appear more fearful, will have pronounced phobic symptoms, and will avoid social contact while exhibiting undue preoccupation with violent or sexual matters.

Learning disabilities and ADHD are now no longer thought of as a common syndrome with differing clinical manifestations. Rather they are conceptualized as distinct conditions (11). Table 55.3 highlights the similarities and differences noted for both syndromes. Similarities include: (a) presumed neurological cause and (b) school failure. Differences include (a) impact of presumed neurological involvement; (b) reason for school failure; and (c) entitlement to special education classes by law. On this last point, federal lawmakers have recently agreed to drop a proposal explicitly entitling ADHD children to special education classes under the federal special education law. How this will turn out is of serious concern to education, mental health, and civil rights groups who believe that a disproportionate number of minority children could be mislabeled and consequently placed in special education classes. Furthermore, services for deserving special education children might be diluted (12). For children with learning disabilities, ADHD should be thought of as a separate but

Table 55.3.
Comparison of Attention Deficit–Hyperactivity Disorder and Learning Disabilities Syndromes

Attention Deficit–Hyperactivity Disorder	Learning Disabilities
Presumed to be neurological resulting in impaired control of motor activity levels	Presumed to be neurological resulting in impaired basic psychological learning processes
School failure due to not being available to learning	School failure due to imperfect ability to listen, read, write, etc.
Not entitled to special education classes	Entitled to special education classes[a]

[a] *Note:* 15–20% of children with learning disabilities have ADHD as a "related" disorder (13).

"related" disorder when these children also demonstrate hyperactivity, distractibility, and/or impulsivity.

GENERAL MEASURE OF TREATMENT

The major nonmedical treatment approaches for children with ADHD are behavior therapy and individual and family psychotherapy. Behavior therapy techniques include (a) establishing baseline data; (b) recognizing and reinforcing desirable behaviors; and (c) modifying instructional sequences at home and school. Because desirable and undesirable behaviors cannot occur at the same time, it is often advantageous to use a behavior therapy approach referred to as incompatible alternatives, where the ADHD child's desirable behaviors, which occur spontaneously and fleetingly, are recognized and reinforced by the teacher and/or parents (14). According to Bax, "manipulation of the external environment of the hyperactive child, rather than changing the internal environment pharmacologically, is in the long run the most likely to be helpful" (15).

Individual psychotherapy is indicated so the child can learn to cope with family and friends during the recuperative phase. The child is often acclimated to censure from teachers and parents along with abuse from peers, resulting in the formation of many psychological scars. These problems must be ameliorated with adequate psychotherapy because most of the medications currently used can only relieve the immediate symptoms of ADHD. They will not aid coping with the indirect consequences of the child's former behavior on the other individuals.

Family psychotherapy is indicated when family relationships and interactions become dysfunctional. Child-focused and problem-oriented parenting, which may serve to keep a child dependent, confused, and defensive are a concern when special needs are present (16, 17). In many families the behavior of the parent mirrors that of the child. For example, if the child with ADHD is angry, a parent is angry. If a child starts crying, a parent starts crying, and if the ADHD child is happy, a parent is happy. If parents are that emotionally enmeshed with their child, they only heighten the child's anxiety. A family with this structure needs to work on becoming less emotional and more cognitive through family therapy, which also focuses on building predictability, limits, consequences, and routines for all members of the family, not just the child with ADHD.

Most parents seek help for their hyperactive, distractible, and/or impulsive child because the purposeless behavior has caused problems for the whole family. When family members are willing to look at their part in this relational-systemic process (understanding that if one member of a relational system has a problem then every member of that system also has a problem), the use of available technology results in a very positive prognosis. Unfortunately, there are cases where families hope that the problem will just go away. That may be encouraged, unfortunately, by well-meaning professionals, who say "your child is just immature" or "boys will be boys."

In families with other achieving children, the sibling with ADHD may be subjected to unfavorable comparisons or simply be written off as the only one with the problem. In those cases, there may be enough positive relational activity going on that the family is not hurting to the point where they are motivated to seek needed family therapy.

PHARMACOTHERAPY

Many pharmacotherapeutic approaches have been taken in the treatment of ADHD. The use of medications in these children is most likely to be effective when it is an aspect of a multimodal treatment plan along with instructional modification, behavioral intervention, and family therapy. The use of selected drugs, such as dextroamphetamine or methylphenidate, is considered an acceptable therapy for managing specific inappropriate motor activity behaviors of children with ADHD, particularly where the hyperactivity is neurologically and not anxiety-based (10). Medications do not cure ADHD, but they may help make the child more available to the learning experience. The likelihood that medications will be effective is enhanced when there is an interdisciplinary diagnostic approach and when there is complete cooperation and communication between the physician and the child's home and school, where the ADHD child is most likely to be at odds with his parents and school authorities because of hyperactivity, impulsivity, and distractibility. Perhaps the greatest difficulty with drug use is that children are often put on medications before any specific baseline behaviors have been identified and documented. Without this information from home and school, positive changes in behavior become difficult to evaluate. Furthermore, with pinpointed behaviors, other forms of behavior management, such as positive reinforcement and modified curriculum, can be instituted once the child becomes available to learning, with the ultimate goal being the gradual withdrawal of the drugs.

Centrally Acting Sympathomimetics

The primary agents used in the treatment of ADHD are the centrally acting sympathomimetics, such as methylphenidate, dextroamphetamine, and magnesium pemoline (18). Dextroamphetamine was used initially in 1937 and continued to be the agent of choice until the late 1960s, when the use of methylphenidate increased in association with reports of a lower rate of side effects with the latter drugs. It would appear that these reports of greater safety with methylphenidate are of questionable clinical importance (19). There are also studies attesting to the greater clinical efficacy of methylphenidate (20) over dextroamphetamine by some authorities who prefer the former

Table 55.4.

Dosage Parameters for CNS Stimulants in Children with Attention–Deficit Disorder

Drug (Reference)	Daily Dosage (mg/kg)	Dosing Interval (hr)	Elimination Half-Life (hr)
Dextroamphetamine (26)	0.3–1.5	4–6	6.6
Methylphenidate (27)	0.3–2.5	4–6	2.5
Pemoline (28)	2.0–6.7	8–12	7.2

drug; proponents of dextroamphetamine indicate that, in their hands, it has comparable clinical efficacy at a lower cost (21). Some clinicians recommend that a trial of both dextroamphetamine and methylphenidate be given to each child. This allows identification of the most useful agent, i.e., whichever one gives the greatest improvement and lowest incidence of adverse effects (22). With the availability of sustained-release preparations, many clinicians now prefer to use these formulations. They provide sustained therapeutic levels with a single daily dose: methylphenidate, 20 mg SR; pemoline, 56.25 mg; or dextroamphetamine Spansule, 10 mg. The duration of effect was noted to be from 1 to 9 hr after ingestion, and all were equieffective; however, pemoline was associated with a greater frequency of difficulty in falling asleep (23).

Many studies have demonstrated that the centrally acting sympathomimetics are effective in 70 to 80% of affected children. The drugs are most effective in improving attentiveness and decreasing hyperactivity, but they may also be of use in ameliorating deficits in fine motor coordination, particularly handwriting. Although the action of these drugs on cognition is questionable, the improvement in attention span may help create a more positive atmosphere for learning (24). Identification of target symptoms is of particular importance, since some researchers have reported that low doses of stimulants improve cognitive performance, while higher doses are recommended for controlling undesirable behavior (25). A summary of the dose characteristics of CNS stimulants is provided in Table 55.4.

Use of the psychostimulant medications also carries inherent risk, as these agents are known to cause a number of adverse effects (29). The most commonly reported side effects include anorexia, weight loss, GI pain, and insomnia. These tend to decrease with time in many patients, but they must be carefully monitored. The sympathetic activation of these agents, particularly methylphenidate or dextroamphetamine can cause palpitations, tachycardia, and increased blood pressure. Routine monitoring *must* include measurement of blood pressure and pulse, as there is a risk of myocardial hypertrophy from the chronic use of agents of this type (30). If significant increases in either

BP or HR are noted, the drug dosage should be reduced or an alternative agent (usually pemoline) should be used.

The actual decision to initiate drug therapy with CNS stimulants must be based on the characteristics of each case; however, two factors considered to be critical are proper class placement and use of target symptoms (24). Proper class placement appears to be most critical, so it is imperative that the school system properly evaluate the academic level of the child. Otherwise, medication will be of little use because of the problems of inappropriate coursework and negative peer interaction. Identification of target symptoms, i.e., hyperactivity, impulsivity, cognitive skills, or social interactions is also imperative for proper selection and dosage adjustment.

Methylphenidate

Methylphenidate is the most commonly used agent for pharmacotherapy of ADHD (31). In contrast to therapeutic agents used in other childhood disorders, the dosing of methylphenidate and other agents used in ADHD is somewhat empirical because of the lack of sensitive analytical methods prior to the 1980s. Recent studies indicate that oral methylphenidate has a lag phase of 0.5 to 1.0 hr and reaches a peak 2.5 hr after administration (24), with a positive correlation between plasma levels and response in ADHD (32). The drug is given orally in doses of 5 to 10 mg/twice daily (in the morning and at noon, to avoid the potential iatrogenic insomnia that can ensue from the drug) or in a single 20-mg sustained-release form (Ritalin-SR) in the morning. Therapy should be initiated with a dose of 0.3 mg/kg either in the morning or twice daily. If a satisfactory response is not noted after 2 weeks, the dose is increased by 0.1 mg/kg every 2 weeks until the maximal dose is reached. If there is still no response at this point, switching to another medication is considered.

Most patients respond well at 10 to 20 mg twice a day, and the daily dose should be limited to 80 to 120 mg maximum. A single-dose study of methylphenidate revealed that a morning dose of 20 mg had clinical efficacy similar to a sustained-release form of dextroamphetamine. However, 15% of the children did not retain a therapeutic response for the entire school day (33). In addition, children will often experience decreased blood levels in the hours after school and social conflicts may develop, so the SR preparation is particularly useful in these cases.

Methylphenidate has a 72 to 85% response rate and appears to reduce hyperactivity and restlessness, prevent distraction, and increase the attention span. These factors all aid in making the child more available for the learning environment, so that a secondary, but important effect of the drug is to increase learning ability. Motor ability and coordination are also enhanced by the drug (34).

Methylphenidate has also been used for treatment of ADHD, residual type, which is noted in adult patients.

Doses of 10 to 80 mg/day were significantly more effective than placebo in the amelioration of attention difficulty, affective lability, motor overactivity, and impulsivity (35).

In children with ADHD, methylphenidate can cause certain undesirable side effects. Suppression of growth has been reported, with both decreased weight and height being noted (36); however, when medication was discontinued over vacations, a spurt in growth returned the treated children to control levels (37, 38). A subsequent study in 100 patients has revealed no stunting of growth in children treated with methylphenidate, dextroamphetamine, or imipramine/desipramine on a long-term basis (39). It appears that a temporary decrease in the rate of growth in weight or height occurs during the first few years of therapy at conventional doses, dependent upon both dose and use of drug holidays. Any weight or height decrement should be compensated for during the drug-free period, and there does not appear to be any effect on adult height or weight (40). The current treatment approach allows the child to remain drug free, if pragmatically possible, over weekends and vacations, to both prevent any transient growth retardation and allow for continual reevaluation of the need for pharmacotherapy (41). If a child's hyperactive behavior is pronounced at home as well as in school, drug-free holidays may be difficult to institute in the absence of behavioral and counseling therapies. The child whose hyperactive behavior was primarily a school problem is a better candidate for intermittent drug therapy.

Cardiovascular side effects, usually either increased diastolic blood pressure or tachycardia, have been reported. It is important to monitor both blood pressure and pulse rate to evaluate excessive systemic sympathetic response (see above). Insomnia and anorexia resulting in weight loss have also been reported, but they occur less commonly than with other amphetamine derivatives. Cases of Gilles de la Tourette's syndrome have also been precipitated or exacerbated by this drug (42). Methylphenidate has been reported to inhibit hepatic drug metabolism, and the half-lives of several substances, such as desipramine and phenytoin, may be prolonged, resulting in potential toxicity. It is particularly important to consider the potential interactions with the anticonvulsant drugs, because these are often used concurrently in the child with ADHD, and there have been several reports of ataxia in patients on phenytoin and methylphenidate (34).

The use of methylphenidate (or other CNS sympathomimetic agent) is contraindicated in patients with symptomatic cardiovascular disease, hypertension, hyperthyroidism, or glaucoma, and in patients that are using or have taken monoamine oxidase inhibitors within the previous 14 days due to the drug interaction between indirect sympathomimetic agents and the MAOI drugs (29).

Dextroamphetamine

Dextroamphetamine is used similarly to methylphenidate in the treatment of ADHD, and although some studies indicate similar clinical efficacy (21), most of the clinical literature indicates an approximately 10 to 15% higher symptom improvement rate with methylphenidate (20, 36). The use of dextroamphetamine in ADHD rather than levoamphetamine or racemic amphetamine mixtures is based on the established superiority of the former agent in various clinical trials (43). The usual dosing schedule for dextroamphetamine is 2.5 to 20 mg twice daily, morning and at noon, or the sustained-release dosage forms that are available can be used in a single morning dose. The use of 5-mg tablets allows greater latitude in dose adjustment and better evaluation of clinical response over time (41). Dextroamphetamine in the ADHD child has a peak effect at 1 to 2 hr after dosing and a duration of action of 4 to 6 hr. The dose is generally titrated from an initial dose of 5 mg twice a day up to an effective level by increasing the dose by 5 mg/day every 2 to 3 days until either the symptoms subside or side effects occur.

Side effects reported with dextroamphetamine are similar to those of methylphenidate and usually tend to decrease a few weeks after initiation of therapy. Persistent insomnia may be treated with a mild hypnotic agent such as diphenhydramine (25 mg) or can occasionally be alleviated by taking the child off dextroamphetamine and initiating therapy with methylphenidate. When this type of change in stimulant therapy is attempted, a 24-hr period should elapse prior to initiation of therapy with the new stimulant drug (21).

The question of potential abuse of psychostimulant drugs by children previously treated with these agents has been one of concern to many health professionals. However, at present, studies indicate that abuse of drugs in later life is not a sequel to amphetamine therapy in childhood (19, 44, 45).

Magnesium Pemoline

Magnesium pemoline has also been used in children with ADHD. This drug is a CNS stimulant with psychostimulant actions, similar to dextroamphetamine. It possesses similar beneficial actions to those of dextroamphetamine as well as similar side effects, with insomnia and anorexia being most prevalent. However, a more serious problem is hypersensitivity reactions that usually involve the liver; these are noted in 1 to 2% of patients, and liver function tests should be performed periodically in treated children (24, 29). Pemoline has a slower onset of action than the other CNS stimulants (2 to 4 hr), but a longer duration of action (8 to 12 hr). It may be given as a single morning dose or in two divided doses (morning/after school), depending upon patient response. The initial dose should be 37.5 to 75 mg/day, with incremental increases of 18.75 mg/day at weekly intervals until maximal therapeutic response or a maximum recommended dose of 112.5 mg/day is attained. Magnesium pemoline does not give as rapid a clinical response as dextroamphetamine, but after 8 weeks of treatment with either drug, a similar clinical response can be anticipated. This drug may be considered as an alternate agent for those patients that cannot tolerate either of the stimulants previously discussed.

Tricyclic Antidepressants

A variety of other agents have been used in attempts to treat cases of ADHD that are nonresponsive to or inappropriate for psychostimulant therapy. Many reports have indicated that tricyclic antidepressants, usually imipramine or desipramine, may benefit these patients, even though the only childhood use approved by the FDA is in the treatment of enuresis. However, although most studies have indicated their superiority over placebo, they are still not as effective as the psychostimulants. When a response is noted, it is usually seen within 3 to 4 days, as contrasted to the 2 to 4 weeks necessary for the antidepressant action. Effective doses range from 1 to 2 mg/kg/day in the majority of patients (29). Prior to starting therapy, patients should have a baseline EKG, CBC, platelet count, and liver and renal function tests. Drawbacks to the use of tricyclics include the development of tolerance in some children and the numerous side effects of these agents (46). Side effects may be somewhat limited by the maximum daily dose approved by the FDA (5 mg/kg/day), but autonomic effects, weight loss, gastrointestinal irritation, fine tremors, hyperirritability, and mood alterations must be evaluated continually. The incidence of anticholinergic side effects with desipramine is generally less than with other first-generation tricyclic antidepressants, so it may be preferred in some patients. In addition, the more severe effects on the CNS (e.g., seizures) and the cardiovascular system (e.g., increased pulse and diastolic blood pressure) must be monitored. Sudden death has also been reported in three prepubertal boys that received desipramine for ADHD (47). Since abrupt withdrawal of these drugs can cause rebound cholinergic symptoms, it is important to taper the dose during drug discontinuation. This cholinergic syndrome is marked by anxiety, nausea, diarrhea, and flu-like symptoms (48). Thus, although the tricyclic antidepressants are useful in the child with ADHD, their use at this point is limited primarily to nonresponders to CNS stimulants, and precautions must be taken if they are used (19, 49).

Antipsychotic Agents

Several antipsychotic drugs have been used in ADHD, including chlorpromazine, thioridazine, haloperidol, and reserpine. Chlorpromazine has been reported to be significantly more effective in treatment of hyperactivity than placebo, and in some studies it has equivalent efficacy to that of dextroamphetamine, which is generally effective in approximately 55 to 70% of cases. However, the psychostimulants have a broader spectrum of action in ADHD, because chlorpromazine was found to control hyperactivity, but failed to result in significant attention improvement (50). Studies with thioridazine have provided results essentially similar to those described for chlorpromazine (50). A report of the effect of haloperidol on cognitive behavior in children with hyperactivity indicated that methylphenidate and low-dose haloperidol (0.025 mg/kg) both facilitated cognitive performance, while high-dose haloperidol (0.05 mg/kg) appeared to cause a slight deterioration of performance (51). Therefore, low doses of the antipsychotic agents should be used to obtain an optimal response. Use of these drugs in combination with psychostimulants is inappropriate, since haloperidol has been shown to block the positive effects of methylphenidate (52). Reserpine has been shown to produce improvement in 34% of the children with ADHD, and this limited success rate negates its use in this disorder (20). Thus, the antipsychotic agents may be useful occasionally in therapy of ADHD, but they are capable of depressing the higher CNS functions of attention, and more importantly, cognition. These latter concerns coupled with the multiple autonomic and extrapyramidal side effects associated with the antipsychotic agents, including the potentially irreversible syndrome of tardive dyskinesia, preclude their use as primary agents. They can be viewed as an alternate choice of therapy only in patients who are poor candidates for psychostimulant therapy.

Other Therapeutic Approaches

Many other therapeutic approaches have been used in an attempt to find the ideal drug for treatment of ADHD. The *monoamine oxidase inhibitors* clorgyline and tranylcypromine have been shown to be equieffective to dextroamphetamine in ADHD, but they must be carefully monitored and strict dietary compliance is mandatory (29). These drugs have an "immediate" clinical effect, in contrast to the time lag to their antidepressant response. *Clonidine*, an α_2-receptor agonist in the CNS, has also been reported to produce improvements in both behavior and attentional difficulties, with minimal side effects (53). In one clinical trial, clonidine, 0.05 to 0.6 mg/kg/day was found to have equal activity to methylphenidate in ADHD. The availability of a transdermal administration system for this drug, its low abuse potential, and the relative lack of adverse effects (as contrasted to the oral preparations of this agent) make it an agent worthy of further investigation. *Antianxiety agents* have been evaluated on a limited basis and appear to be of little use. The benzodiazepines are of no value in therapy (54), and phenobarbital is similarly not

useful and has been reported to worsen the child's behavior (19, 55). Therefore, use of these agents should be avoided in the child with ADHD. Similarly, anticonvulsant drugs (19, 55), caffeine (56), antihistamines (57), lithium salts (58), and fenfluramine (59) are either unacceptable for therapy or inadequately evaluated.

There is evidence that chronic low-level lead exposure can result in subtle CNS damage and hyperactivity. In one reported study, 13 hyperkinetic children with blood and urinary lead levels that were elevated, but in a nontoxic range, were treated with the lead-chelating agents penicillamine or calcium disodium acetate. Six of the children had a positive medical history of perinatal or developmental CNS insult and did not respond, while the other seven ADHD children that had unremarkable histories and a possible lead-induced hyperactivity showed marked improvement. The authors concluded that lead may play an important role in the etiology of ADHD, and measurements of blood and urinary lead levels may become a part of the standard work-up in cases of ADHD with no previous history of CNS insult (60).

There have also been isolated reports on the use of megavitamin therapy in ADHD (61). This approach is to be discouraged because of the potential toxic effects of vitamins A and D (62, 63); however, it is important to ensure adequate nutrition in the child with ADHD via monitoring of diet.

In 1973 an allergist postulated that hyperactivity was caused by food additives (64). Subsequent studies have failed to demonstrate any benefit of dietary regulation deleting food additives in the treatment of children with ADHD (65, 66). As mentioned previously, the causes of ADHD are not definable and may be multiple; therefore, the success of the Feingold diet should be viewed with some pessimism. Although there are individual testimonials to the positive outcome of dietary treatment of hyperactivity, studies carried out by numerous investigators over a 5-year period provide "sufficient evidence to refute the claim that artificial food colorings, artificial flavorings, and natural salicylates produce hyperactivity" (66).

THE ADULT ADHD PATIENT

Children with ADHD do not always "outgrow" this disorder. Longitudinal studies indicate that 31% of these patients will continue with full symptoms (attention deficit, hyperactivity, impulsivity), with another 9% showing two of the three symptoms. Twenty percent of these patients had an antisocial disorder of some type, while another 12% had a substance abuse disorder. In another study, 66% of ADHD patients were found to have residual symptoms after 15 years (67).

The psychostimulants (methylphenidate, pemoline) have demonstrated efficacy in both adolescent and adult ADHD patients (67). However, the distribution of these scheduled substances in the adult population may result in diversion. The antidepressant drug bupropion or the monoamine oxidase inhibitors pargyline and deprenyl may offer therapeutic alternatives. Pargyline (68) and deprenyl (69) provide moderate-to-marked improvement of symptoms in approximately 60% of adults with ADHD. Bupropion was found to benefit 14 of 19 patients in an open trial. However, tolerance to the therapeutic action was noted, and dosage had to be increased to an average of 359 mg/day. Ten of the 19 patients elected to remain on the drug rather than return to their former medication (70). Further studies are needed on this agent and on other therapeutic alternatives to psychostimulant therapy for the adult ADHD patient.

THERAPEUTIC CONSIDERATIONS

Methylphenidate or dextroamphetamine are the drugs of choice in this disorder. When these drugs are not effective, magnesium pemoline is the second agent to consider. If none of these agents are successful, the use of tricyclic antidepressants, antipsychotic agents, or clonidine might be attempted in hope of a response. Appropriate doses for commonly used agents are given in Table 55.5

The child and family will need supportive counseling to promote compliance with the medication regimen as well as to ensure therapeutic success. As mentioned previously, behavior therapy, remedial education, and individual and family psychotherapy may all be indicated in addition to pharmacotherapy.

The duration of therapy is somewhat empirical, based on the response of the child during drug-free periods such as weekends and vacations. A number of children with ADHD continue to show characteristics of the disorder into adult life, and therapy of some type may be needed for the remainder of the patient's life. Some clinicians have treated patients into the fourth decade of life, and interestingly, these patients do not appear to become tolerant to the effects of the psychostimulant drugs, and they do

not become dependent upon the psychological attraction of their euphoric actions (45, 46). However, there may be concern for patients who view drugs as responsible for the control of their behavior without a corresponding increase in the development of personality skills, such as assertiveness and open, direct communication.

PROGNOSIS

The prognosis of the ADHD child is questionable. It is generally assumed that ADHD is outgrown by puberty or in early adolescence. However, ADHD has been causally linked to a variety of persistent disorders into adult life. Adjustment to continued schooling, jobs, and intimate personal relationships may continue to be a source of extreme reaction for the ADHD adult. Academic underachievement due to unavailability to learning during younger years, impulsive character disorder, sociopathy, and other recognized psychiatric disorders may then become the diagnosis. It is difficult with the present medical evidence to give an adequate prognosis on recovery per se, in light of limited follow-up data.

CONCLUSIONS

ADHD is a common disorder of primary grade school children which can persist into adult life. The cardinal features involve hyperactivity, impulsivity, and distractibility in the presence of normal intelligence. Treatment with psychostimulants is effective in approximately 75 to 80% of affected children when used as part of a multimodal treatment plan including behavior management, both at home and school, and educational modification. However, lingering affective aspects of the disorder are rarely totally alleviated by drug therapy, and other nonpharmacologic individual and family psychotherapy measures must be used concomitantly with these agents. When all of these approaches are used effectively, there is no reason for the quality of life of these patients to be any different from that of the rest of the populace.

Table 55.5.
Daily Dosage Ranges of Drugs Useful in Therapy of Attention-Deficit Disorder

Drug	Dosage Range (mg/day)
Psychostimulants	
Methylphenidate	5–120
Dextroamphetamine	2.5–60
Pemoline	56.25–112.5
Phenothiazines	
Chlorpromazine	10–1000
Thioridazine	20–600
Tricyclic antidepressants	
Imipramine	10–175
Desipramine	10–175

REFERENCES

1. Clements SD: Minimal brain dysfunction in children. Terminology and identification. Public Health Service Publication No. 1415. Washington, D.C., U.S. Department of Health, Education, and Welfare, 1966.
2. American Psychiatric Association: Diagnostic and Statistical Manual of Mental Disorders, ed. 2. Washington, D.C., American Psychiatric Association, 1968.
3. American Psychiatric Association: Diagnostic and Statistical Manual of Mental Disorders, ed. 3. Washington, D.C., American Psychiatric Association, 1982.
4. American Psychiatric Association: Diagnostic and Statistical Manual of Mental Disorders, ed. 3, revised. Washington, D.C., American Psychiatric Association, 1987.
5. Herskowitz J, Rosman NP: Hyperactivity and attentional problems. In Pediatrics, Neurology and Psychiatry—Common Ground. Be-

havioral, Cognitive, Affective and Physical Disorders of Childhood and Adolescence. New York, Macmillan, 1982, p. 403.

6. Weiss G, Hectman L, Perlman T, et al.: Hyperactives as young adults. Arch Gen Psychiatry 36:675–681, 1979.

7. Wender PH, Reimkerr FW, Wood DR: Attention deficit disorder (minimal brain dysfunction) in adults. Arch Gen Psychiatry 38:449–456, 1981.

8. Shaywitz SE, Shaywitz BE: Attention deficit disorder: current practice. In Learning Disabilities: Proceedings of the National Conference. Parkton, MD, York Press, pp. 369–523, 1988

9. Mercer CD: Students With Learning Disabilities. Columbus: Merrill, 1987, pp 67–69.

10. Silver LB: The Misunderstood Child. A Guide for Parents of Learning Disabled Children. New York: McGraw-Hill, 1984, pp 135–142.

11. Silver LB: Attention deficit-hyperactivity disorder: Is it a learning disability or a related disorder? J Learn Disabil 23:394–397, 1990.

12. Viadero D: Lawmakers tentatively agree to drop proposal on attention-deficit disorder. Educ Week 10(4):21, 1990.

13. Silver LB: The relationship between learning disabilities, hyperactivity, distractibility, and behavioral problems. J Am Acad Child Psychiatry 20:385–397, 1981.

14. Madsen LJ Jr, Madsen CK: Teaching Discipline: A Positive Approach for Educational Development. Boston: Allyn & Bacon, 1974.

15. Bax M: Who is hyperactive? Dev Med Child Neurol 20:277–278, 1978.

16. Hill JW, Parker T, Leimbeck J: Family self-esteem at the crisis apex before one family member's special education evaluation and the family's therapy assessment. Fam Ther 15:175–184, 1988.

17. Parker T, Hill JW, Goodnow J: The impact of special-needs children on their parents perceptions of family structural interaction patterns. Fam Ther 16:259–270, 1989.

18. Sprague RL, Sleator EK: Effects of psychopharmacologic agents on learning disorders. Pediatr Clin North Am 20:719–735, 1973.

19. Werry JS: Medication for hyperkinetic children. Drugs 11:81–89, 1976.

20. Millichap JG: Drugs in management of hyperkinetic and perceptually handicapped children. JAMA 206:1527, 1968.

21. Winsberg BG, Yepes LE, Bialer I: Pharmacologic management of children with hyperactive/aggressive/inattentive behavior disorders. Clin Pediatr 15:471–477, 1976.

22. Elia J, Borcherding WZ, Potter IN, et al.: Dextroamphetamine and methylphenidate treatment of hyperactivity: differing effects on monoamines, and on clinical response. Poster presented at 28th Annual Meeting of the American College of Neuropsychopharmacology. Maui, HI: 1989.

23. Pelham WE, Grenslade KE, Vodde-Hamilton M, et al.: Relative efficacy of long-acting stimulants on children with a attention-deficit-hyperactivity disorder: a comparison of standard methylphenidate, sustained-release methylphenidate, sustained-release dextroamphetamine, and pemoline. Pediatrics 86:226–237, 1990.

24. Shaywitz SE, Shaywitz BA: Diagnosis and management of attention deficit disorder: a pediatric perspective. Pediatr Clin North Am 31:429–457, 1984.

25. Sprague RL, Sleator EK: Methylphenidate in hyperkinetic children: differences in dose effects on learning and social behavior. Science 198:1274–1276, 1977.

26. Brown GL, Ebert MH, Mikkelson EJ, et al.: Behavior and motor activity response in hyperactive children and plasma amphetamine levels following a sustained release preparation. J Am Acad Child Psychiatry 19:225, 1980.

27. Chan Y, Soldin S, Swanson T, et al.: Gas chromatographic/mass spectrometric analysis of methylphenidate (Ritalin) in serum. Clin Biochem 13:266–272, 1980.

28. Tomkins C, Soldin S, MadLead S, et al.: Analysis of pemoline in serum by high performance liquid chromatography: clinical application to optimize treatment of hyperactive children. In Therapeutic Drug Monitoring. New York, Raven Press, 1980, vol 2, pp 255–260.

29. Calis KA, Grothe DR, Elia J: Attention-deficit hyperactivity disorder. Clin Pharm 9:632–642, 1990.

30. Fischer VW, Barner H: Cardiomyopathic findings associated with methylphenidate. JAMA 238:1497, 1977.

31. Wolraich ML, Lindgren S, Stromquist, A, et al.: Stimulant medication use by primary care physicians in the treatment of attention deficit hyperactivity disorder. Pediatrics 86:95–101, 1990.

32. Shaywitz SE, Sebrects MM, Vatlow P, et al.: Plasma methylphenidate levels predict attention and activity: results in a double-blind placebo study. Pediatr Res 16:93A, 1982.

33. Safer DJ, Allen RP: Single daily dose methylphenidate in hyperactive children. Dis Nerve Syst 34:325–328, 1973.

34. Fischer KC, Wilson WP: Methylphenidate and hyperkinetic state. Dis Nerv Syst 32:695–698, 1971.

35. Wender PH, Reimherr FW, Wood D, et al.: A controlled study of methylphenidate in the treatment of attention deficit disorder, residual type, in adults. Am J Psychiatry 142:547–552, 1985.

36. Safer DJ, Allen RP: Factors influencing the suppressant effect of two stimulant drugs on the growth of hyperactive children. Pediatrics 51:660, 1973.

37. Safer DJ, Allen RP, Barr E: Growth rebound after termination of stimulant drugs. J Pediatr 86:113, 1975.

38. Satterfield JH, Cartwell DP, Schnell A, et al.: Growth of hyperactive children treated with methylphenidate. Arch Gen Psychiatry 36:212–217, 1979.

39. Gross MD: Growth of hyperkinetic children taking methylphenidate, dextroamphetamine, or imipramine/desipramine. Pediatrics 58:423–431, 1976.

40. Roache AF, Lipman RS, Overall JE, et al.: The effects of stimulant medication on the growth of hyperkinetic children. Pediatrics 63:847–850, 1979.

41. Piepho RW, Gourley DR, Hill JW: Current therapeutic concepts: minimal brain dysfunction. J Am Pharm Assoc 17 (NS):500–504 1977.

42. Lowe TI, Cohen DJ, Detlor J, et al.: Stimulant medications precipitate Tourette's syndrome. JAMA 247:1168, 1982.

43. Arnold LE, Huestis RD, Smeltzer DJ, et al.: Levoamphetamine vs. dextroamphetamine in minimal brain dysfunction. Arch Gen Psychiatry 33:292–301, 1976.

44. Laufer MW: Long-term management and some follow-up findings on the use of drugs with minimal cerebral syndromes. J Learn Disabil 4:55, 1971.

45. Charles L, Schain RJ, Guthrie D: Long-term use and discontinuation of methylphenidate with hyperactive children. Dev Med Child Neurol 21:758–764, 1979.

46. Wender PH: The minimal brain dysfunction syndrome. Annu Rev Med 26:45–62, 1975.

47. Anon: Sudden death in children treated with a tricyclic antidepressant. Med Lett Drugs Ther 32(819):53, 1990.

48. Dilsaver SC, Feinberg M, Greden JF: Antidepressant withdrawal symptoms treated with anticholinergic agents. Am J Psychiatry 140:249–251, 1983.

49. Werry JS, Aman MG, Diamond E: Imipramine and methylphenidate in hyperactive children. J Child Psychol Psychiatry 21:27–35, 1980.

50. Klein-Gittelman R, Klein DF, Katz S, Saraf K, Pollack E: Comparative effects of methylphenidate and thioridazine in hyperkinetic children. Arch Gen Psychiatry 23:1217–1231, 1976.

51. Werry JS, Aman MG: Methylphenidate and haloperidol in children. Arch Gen Psychiatry 32:790–805, 1975.

52. Levy F, Hobbes G: The action of stimulant medication in attention deficit disorder with hyperactivity: Dopaminergic, noradrenergic, or both? J Am Acad Child Adolesc Psychiatry 27:802–805, 1988.

53. Hunt RD, Minderaa RB, Cohen DJ: Clonidine benefits children with attention-deficit disorder and hyperactivity: report of a double-blind placebo crossover therapeutic trial. J Am Acad Child Psychiatry 5:617–629, 1985.

54. Greenblatt D, Shader R: Benzodiazepines in Clinical Practice. New York: Raven Press, 1974.

55. Erenberg G: Drug therapy in minimal brain dysfunction: a commentary. J Pediatr 81:359–365, 1972.

56. Gittelman-Klein R: Pharmacotherapy of childhood hyperactivity: an update. In Meltzer HY (ed): Psychopharmacology: The Third Generation of Progress. New York, Raven, pp 1215–1224, 1987.

57. Connors C: Pharmacotherapy. In Quay HC, Werry JS (eds): Psychopathological Disorders of Childhood. New York, John Wiley & Sons, pp 316–347, 1972.

58. Greenhill LL, Reider RO, Wender PH, Buchsbaum M, Zahn TP: Lithium carbonate in the treatment of hyperactive children. Arch Gen Psychiatry 28:636–640, 1973.

59. Donnelly M, Rapoport JL, Potter WZ, et al.: Fenfluramine and dextroamphetamine treatment of childhood hyperactivity: clinical and biochemical findings. Arch Gen Psychiatry 46:205–212, 1989.

60. David OJ, Hoffman SP, Sverd J, Clark J, Voeller K: Lead and hyperactivity: behavioral response to chelation: a pilot study. Am J Psychiatry 133:1155–1158, 1976.

61. Shaywitz BA, Siegel NJ, Pearson HA: Megavitamins for minimal brain dysfunction. JAMA 238:1749, 1977.

62. White PL: The lid is off (editorial). JAMA 138:1761, 1977.

63. Vaisrub S: Vitamin abuse (editorial). JAMA 238:1762, 1977.

64. Feingold BF: Hyperkinesis and learning disabilities linked to artificial food flavors and colors. Am J Nurs 75:797–803, 1975.

65. Wender PH: Food additives and hyperkinesis. Am J Dis Child 131:1204–1206, 1977.

66. Final report to the Nutritional Foundation, October 1980. National Advisory Committee on Hyperkinesis and Food Additives: New York: Nutrition Foundation, 1980.

67. Laird LK, Saklad JJ: Attention-deficit hyperactivity disorder. J Pharm Pract 3:241–251, 1990.

68. Wender PH, Wood DR, Reimherr FW, et al.: An open trial of pargyline in the treatment of attention deficit disorder, residual type. Psychiatry Res 9:329–336, 1983.

69. Wood DR, Reimherr FW, Wender PH: The use of L-deprenyl in the treatment of attention deficit disorder, residual type (ADD, RT). Psychopharmacol Bull 19:627–629, 1983.

70. Wender PH, Reimherr FW: Bupropion treatment of attention deficit hyperactivity disorder in adults. Am J Psychiatr 147:1018–1020, 1990.

CHAPTER 56

OBESITY AND EATING DISORDERS

MARTIN J. JINKS, Pharm.D. and MARK W. GARRISON, Pharm.D.

OBESITY

Leave gourmandizing, know that the grave doth gape for thee thrice wider than for other men.
—William Shakespeare, 16th Century

Despite these perceptive words, Shakespeare and his contemporaries admired an ample form. Suppleness denoted a person graced by God, and was the hallmark of the opulent and idly rich. Rubens would certainly have scoffed at the idea of Twiggy as a model of beauty. It took the industrial revolution to give obesity a bad reputation. Mechanization caused voluntary or forced reduction in average activity without a decrease in calorie intake, and obesity became the single most prevalent metabolic disorder in the United States.

Obesity can be defined as a condition occurring from the sum total of environmental, emotional, and familial factors that have as the lowest common denominator an abnormal energy balance, usually resulting from excessive caloric intake and inadequate caloric loss. In simplest terms, obesity exists when there is excess energy stored as body fat. In man, moderate obesity is present when fat accounts for more than 25% of ideal weight. The upper limit in females is 30%. Massive obesity is defined by adiposity in excess of 100% of ideal weight (1).

Prevalence

Currently it is estimated that close to 50% of men and women in the United States have some degree of obesity. Over age 50, 34% of men and 49% of women are moderately obese, and the overall incidence of adults seriously overweight ranges from 5 to 7% (1, 2).

The incidence of obesity appears to be increasing over time. Evaluation of military records reveals a consistent pattern of weight increase in service men over the years 1918, 1943, and 1950 (3). The degree of body fat is influenced by age, gender, race, and extent of physical activity.

At the start of life, adipose tissue accounts for approximately 12% of body weight, and it rapidly increases to an average of 25% at 6 months of age. During early adulthood, the percentage of body fat in males is 15 to 18% and in females, 20 to 25%. A gradual increase in body fat occurs with age, approaching an average of 30 to 40% in adult men and women (3).

Differences in racial background and socioeconomic status appear to influence body fat, but it is often difficult to accurately distinguish the individual effects that each of the factors have. Reports indicate a greater prevalence of obesity in black versus white women; however, the reverse is true with males—obesity is more likely to occur in white rather than black men (4). Furthermore, individuals in lower socioeconomic classes tend to have a higher rate of obesity than their middle- and upper-class counterparts. This relationship holds true particularly in females, and does not appear to be as pronounced in males (3).

As one might expect, an inverse relationship exists between level of physical activity and development of obesity. Individuals with sedentary lifestyles or a physical handicap that restricts activity are prone to obesity. Increasing the degree of physical exercise is associated with a reduction in body fat as lean body mass increases; however, this relationship is rapidly reversed upon discontinuation of the energy expenditure.

Pathogenesis

In a small percentage of patients, obesity has an identifiable organic cause (5). Weight gain in excess of 1 kg/day invariably implies fluid retention and is frequently a signal of cardiovascular, renal, or hepatic disorders (6). Medications can produce weight gain by inducing fluid retention in susceptible individuals, through either direct (steroids and related drugs) or indirect mechanisms (medicinals high in sodium). Only rarely is obesity a symptom of a specific endocrinopathy, such as insulinoma or Cushing's disease. These uncommon disorders are easily differentiated by their peculiar fat distribution, attendant symptoms, and a history of sudden appetite changes.

Idiopathic obesity is a complex interplay of physiologic, hereditary, psychologic, and metabolic influences that have as their ultimate manifestation, chronic dietary indiscretion.

PHYSIOLOGIC FACTORS

Since the discovery nearly 70 years ago that obesity can be induced surgically in animals, a great deal of interest has developed in the relationship between abnormal appetite and possible aberrations within the hypothalamus. Lesions in the ventromedial nucleus of the hypothalamus (satiety center) result in hyperphagia, whereas lesions in the lateral hypothalamic areas (feeding center) result in cessation of eating (7, 8). Factors controlling these centers are unknown, but have been associated with endocrine and metabolic determinants.

Obese individuals exhibit behavior that might indicate a derangement in the satiety center. When obese and nonobese individuals are allowed to ingest freely, the nonobese regulate food intake based on internal cues, such as hunger sensations and caloric density of the food, while obese individuals regulate food intake by external cues such as time and environment, regardless of the caloric density of the food (9).

In the first year of life, the number of existing fat cells is relatively fixed. Storage of excess energy is accommodated by increasing the size of adipose cells (hypertrophic). Prior to adolescence, the number of adipose cells multiply as young children grow. In obese children, this rate of multiplication is greater than in nonobese children, resulting in a larger number of adipose cells (hypercellular) throughout life. In contrast, adult-onset obesity is primarily the result of hypertrophic obesity (10).

Weight loss is more rapid and prolonged in persons with hypertrophic obesity, compared with hypercellular obesity. Attempts to reduce weight to norms in hypercellular individuals are very difficult and can result in extreme hunger symptoms similar to those seen with starvation and also psychological and physical disability (11).

Since evidence favors the increased likelihood of chubby infants becoming obese adults (12), preventative measures are important. These measures include avoiding overfeeding of infants, encouraging the use of unsugared foods, keeping junk foods and snacks out of the house, and encouraging activity.

GENETIC FACTORS

The role of heredity in obesity is a matter of great speculation and research. Often environmental factors pertaining to food intake greatly confound this issue, making it difficult to determine the true impact of genetics on obesity. Studies involving adopted children and twins have been performed in an attempt to overcome these environmental influences. Results reflect little correlation of relative body weight between adopted children and their adoptive parents; however, definite trends do exist when the weights of the children are compared with those of their biological parents (13). Furthermore, the body weights of twin siblings appear to correlate well; identical twins showing greater correlation than fraternal twins (14). These observations lend to support to a genetic component of obesity.

Statistically, when both parents are of normal weight, the incidence of having an obese child is approximately 9%. If one or both parents are obese, there is a 50% and 80% incidence of obese offspring, respectively (13).

PSYCHOLOGIC FACTORS

Familial and cultural eating habits are implanted in individuals at an early age. As a society, we place great emphasis on food—to most, one of life's enduring pleasures is a rich, hearty meal. The obese patient carries this gratification to an extreme level.

These obese individuals often exhibit an immense appetite for psychological reasons. Overeating may be a manifestation of anxiety or depression, where the pleasures of food serve as a substitute for the satisfactions missed from other sources. As a result, the obese characteristically dine until the food is completely gone or until they are overtly uncomfortable, while the nonobese usually stop eating when their hunger is gone.

Because obesity is often associated with neurotic traits, overeating is commonly considered to be a behavioral defect. In the pathologically obese, where no distinct underlying problem exists, psychological factors undoubtedly play a major role. Obviously, obesity is a complicated mix of psychological, genetic, and metabolic influences that manifest as abnormal appetite and resultant overweight.

METABOLIC ABNORMALITIES

Insulin refractoriness is the most significant metabolic deviation in obesity, since insulin regulates the major pathways for fat accumulation and storage. Insulin-induced lipogenesis is an attractive hypothesis to explain the cause of obesity, but current evidence suggests that insulin refractoriness is a result, rather than cause, of obesity.

Adrenal overactivity is a common finding in massively obese patients. This is reflected by elevated urinary corticosteroids, mild hirsutism, borderline hypertension, and glucose intolerance (15). Again, these abnormalities are most likely the result of obesity rather than its cause, since they develop in nonobese subjects following gorging and disappear as weight returns to normal.

Metabolic enzyme deficiency may also result in abnormalities in thermogenic dissipation of calories in obese patients. Cellular enzyme systems account for much of thermogenic calorie loss, and there is evidence that the obese may have inefficient catalytic rates (16). Impaired hormonal control by catecholamines and insulin may be involved, but this hypothesis is controversial (17).

Diagnosis

Individuals with massive obesity, peculiar fat distribution, or sudden, rapid weight gain require extensive evaluation. However, common idiopathic obesity does not usually demand elaborate evaluation techniques.

Quantifying obesity is not difficult. The patient who is 136 kg (300 lb) overweight is readily recognized as obese. Moderately obese patients are easily diagnosed using standard height-weight charts. These charts have a 90% cor-

Table 56.1.
Disorders Associated with Obesity

Hypertension
Congestive heart failure
Diabetes
Cerebrovascular disease
Gall bladder disease
Hyperlipidemia
Respiratory distress syndrome (Pickwickian)
Obstetric complications
Osteoarthritis
Varicose veins
Flat feet
Hiatus hernia
Intertriginous dermatitis

relation with much more elaborate densiometry and radioisotope dilution techniques (1). However, height-weight charts are not without deficiencies, and the easiest and most accurate method of quantifying body fat involves measuring triceps, subscapular, or suprailiac skinfold thickness with constant-pressure calipers. Skinfold-thickness measurements coupled with height-weight data give a convenient and accurate evaluation of the degree of obesity.

Complications

Many serious disorders are associated with severe obesity (Table 56.1). Significant excess weight is clearly detrimental to longevity, and a definite statistical link exists between obesity and hypertension, diabetes, cardiovascular disease, and gastrointestinal disorders (Figs. 56.1 and 56.2). This link pertains primarily to moderate and severe obesity, since the marginally or slightly obese individual compares favorably in longevity with nonobese persons. In addition, significantly underweight persons are also at risk for digestive and pulmonary disease.

Massive obesity during pregnancy is associated with a 7-fold increase in toxemia, a 10-fold increase in diabetes, and a 2-fold risk of maternal mortality (18). Substantial excess weight is also associated with altered pharmacokinetics of certain drugs (19).

Despite evidence of the detrimental effects of obesity on health, the prevalent factor motivating most individuals to lose weight is not health but cosmetic ideals.

Treatment

Successful approaches to the management of obesity are often difficult and pose a significant challenge to individuals interested in reducing their weight. There is no "standard treatment" that is effective in most or even a large fraction of obese patients, and weight-reduction programs must be designed to fit the personality, lifestyle, and health status of each patient. Success depends on the individual's motivation and behavioral modification and the establishment of reasonable goals and expectations. Crash programs and demands for extreme alterations from established lifestyles are uniformly unsuccessful in the long run and potentially dangerous.

A comprehensive weight-reduction program incorporates components of diet restriction, exercise, counseling, and possibly pharmacologic and invasive approaches. The critical factors are that caloric expenditures exceed caloric demands and that permanent change in caloric intake must be achieved to maintain the desired weight.

REGULATION OF CALORIC INTAKE

Modest reduction of caloric intake through dieting and setting realistic goals and expectations is the most palatable and available method of treatment. A good diet prevents the patient from becoming too hungry and noncompliant. The importance of learning good eating habits and familiarity with the caloric content of various foods should be strongly emphasized.

The primary goal of any diet is to reduce the caloric intake below expenditure so excess energy stored in the form of fat can be utilized. Weight loss should not exceed 1 kg (2 lb) per week unless close medical supervision is involved (20). Any program resulting in weight loss of more than 0.3 kg (0.7 lb) per day usually involves more fluid than tissue loss. Obligatory water loss accounts for the accelerated weight loss frequently observed during the initial weeks of dieting. Although use of diuretics for weight reduction exploits this phenomenon, this practice is both illusory and hazardous (21).

In obese subjects, approximately a 3500-calorie deficit is required to lose 0.5 kg (1 lb) of tissue. To achieve this deficit, a bewildering array of diets have been advocated, each differing in ratios of carbohydrate, fat, and protein, and each claiming superiority over all the others. Easy weight-loss diets tend to exploit the obese individual who is not ready for a permanent level of change and discipline. Items like dietary drinks offer easy, short-term solutions, but their simplicity and convenience merely put off the essential need to learn about food and food values. Diet books appear with great regularity, and despite their guarantees and initial effectiveness, few effectively induce the permanent solutions of discipline and lifestyle changes.

"Crash diets" are dangerous in susceptible individuals when applied to extremes. Diets involving limited foods, such as the "Beverly Hills Diet," promote nutritional misinformation and can result in severe health problems (22, 23). "Very low calorie diets" (VLCDs) consisting of 200 to 500 kcal/day are designed to cause a calorie deficit while preserving lean body mass. One such diet, the "Last Chance Diet," resulted in dozens of cardiovascular fatalities due to negative nitrogen balance and consequence

Mortality Associated with Obesity

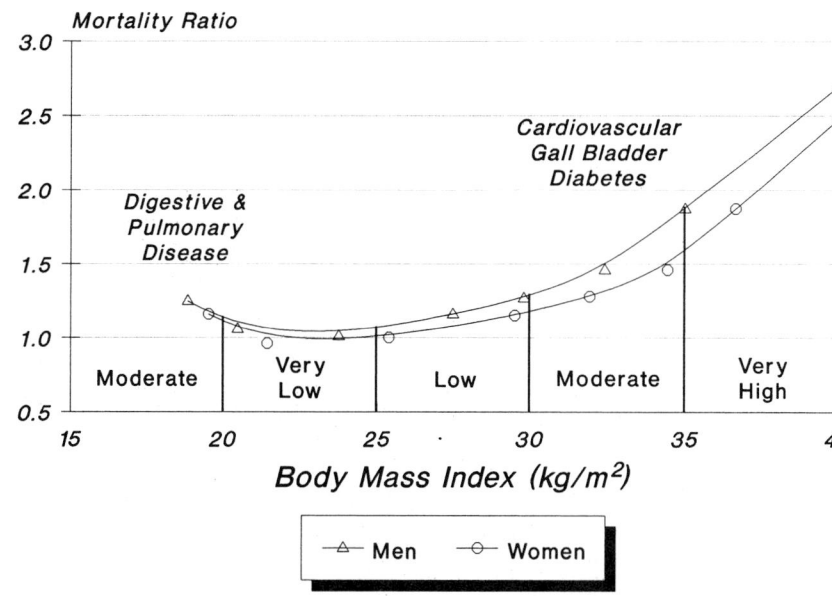

Figure 56.1. Overall mortality risk at various levels of body mass index. (Reprinted with permission from Bray GA, Gray DS: Obesity. Part I-Pathogenesis. West J Med 149:429, 1988.)

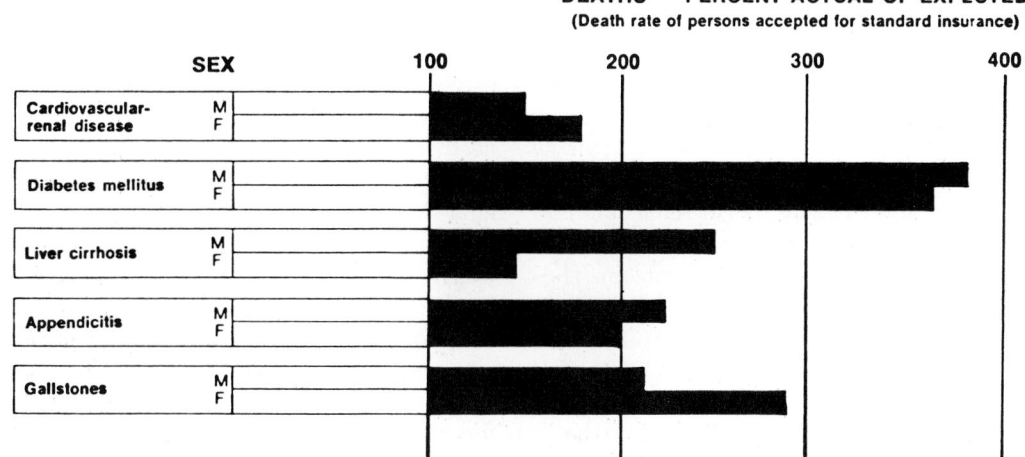

Figure 56.2. Relationship between obesity and serious medical disorders. (Reprinted with permission from the Metropolitan Life Insurance Company.)

protein tissue loss (24). Newer VLCDs, such as the Cambridge diet, appear improved by higher quality protein sources (egg albumin, casein, or soy) and adequate nutritional content, but concern persists that such diets are inherently dangerous when used as sole nutritional sources (25, 26). The use of VLCDs should be restricted to patients with moderate-to-severe obesity who are under close medical supervision, with special attention to cardiovascular monitoring (26).

With all VLCD diets, fluid and electrolyte abnormalities, arrhythmias, dehydration, ketoacidosis, hyperuri-

cemia, alopecia, and teratogenesis are potential complications. These diets are contraindicated in patients with diabetes, cardiovascular disorders, kidney and liver disease, and pregnancy.

Diets based on starvation represent an extreme form of caloric restriction with intake under 200 kcal/day. Starvation diets are associated with very rapid and significant reductions in body weight; however, their use is limited by potential side effects, the need for extremely close medical supervision, and the high percentage of weight regain that occurs following discontinuation of the diet.

EXERCISE

Inclusion of physical exercise in a weight-reduction program can be a valuable supplement to dieting. Regular exercise increases the degree of energy expenditure, favoring adipose reduction and prolonged maintenance of weight loss. Due to reductions in caloric intake associated with dieting, individuals may experience a compensatory decrease in their basal metabolic rate (BMR) of up to 40% in 6 months (27). Regular exercise generates an increase in BMR, which counteracts this adaptive response to dieting.

For exercise to be useful, it must be regular and of high quality. A regimen of thrice-weekly exercise that expends in excess of 300 kcal over at least 30 min is recommended (28). The selection of an activity of moderate intensity and longer duration is preferred because the longer time-frame favors use of fat stores. In mild-to-moderate obesity, exercise results in a significant reduction in adipose tissue; however, in some instances overall body weight may not change significantly because of increases in lean body mass.

Unfortunately, quality exercise is not acceptable to many obese patients. They often turn to "effortless" weight-reduction devices, such as mechanical vibrators, inflatable weight-reducing clothing or "spot reducers." As one author noted, these devices are little better than doing nothing, and the primary reduction often occurs in the exerciser's wallet (28).

BEHAVIORAL MODIFICATION

Behavior therapy can also facilitate weight reduction, especially in the massively obese patient who requires assistance in accepting the seriousness of the problem. The primary goal of behavioral treatment is to modify behaviors that are associated with or promote eating (29). Therapy can be divided into three separate components. First, self-monitoring forces obese individuals to record on a daily basis, the type of food items eaten and when and where they are eaten. Daily record keeping increases the individual's awareness and identifies specific eating patterns or behaviors. Once these patterns are identified, the second phase of behavioral therapy focuses on breaking the relationship between repetitive patterns or events (external cues) and actual ingestion of the meal. Often this is done through limiting specific times and places in which meals can be eaten, chewing food a specific number of times, or taking sips of water between each bite. Finally, behavioral modification incorporates a system of positive self-feedback to reinforce and maintain an optimal attitude toward weight reduction. Most studies evaluating the effectiveness of behavioral therapy on weight reduction indicate a greater duration of maintenance of weight loss, compared with programs that lack a behavioral modification component (30).

A number of self-help programs such as Weight Watchers, NutriSystems, Overeaters Anonymous, and Take Off Pounds Sensibly (TOPS), provide obese individuals with important psychological support and motivation to bring about permanent weight control measures. Membership levels are high in these programs; Weight Watchers alone claims several million active members.

APPETITE SUPPRESSANTS

Obese patients who are adequately instructed on dietary management and are treated with appetite suppressants tend to lose more weight on average than patients on diet alone. In a review of over 200 studies of appetite suppressants involving 10,000 patients, pooled data demonstrate an average loss of 0.25 kg (0.56 lb) per week more than with placebo (31). However, since these drugs are typically labeled for durations of 2 to 4 weeks only, the average patient will lose only one additional kilogram when they are used as recommended. When appetite suppressants are used, it becomes critical for the patient to realize that improved dietary compliance is the goal of therapy and that diet, not the drug, is responsible for weight loss. Drug use is only temporary, and restoration of drug-free dieting through behavior changes is the desired outcome.

Unfortunately, the routine use of appetite suppressants in the initial phases of a weight-reduction program may detract from the importance of dietary/behavioral measures and provide a psychological escape from the need to change lifelong eating habits. A comparison of patients treated with either pharmacotherapy or behavioral therapy indicates that while pharmacotherapy produces more weight loss, the benefits are short-lived, and weight is rapidly regained when the drug is discontinued. At the end of a 1-year follow-up, patients treated with behavioral therapy alone weighed significantly less than patients treated with drugs alone. Also, combined pharmacotherapy and behavioral therapy produce results inferior to behavioral therapy alone (32).

Appetite suppressants should be reserved for use in situations where (a) a reducing diet has been established and an unsatisfactory response observed; (b) a plateau is reached after initial success with dieting alone; or (c) a relapse is encountered after a prolonged period of progress. Unfortunately, many physicians prescribe appetite suppressants early in therapy because they cannot resist the pressures placed on them by patients who have invariably experienced failure with do-it-yourself dieting and present to the physician expecting more. Better long-term results could be realized if physicians would lend their esteem and credibility to dietary/behavioral approaches, including vigorous monitoring for compliance, rather than undermining the importance of self-motivated dieting by prescribing appetite suppressants in the initial stages.

Pharmacology. Appetite suppressants are thought to exert their effect directly on the hypothalamic satiety center, which is under adrenergic control. Most suppressants augment brain catecholamine action, with the exception of fenfluramine, which acts specifically on serotonin. Fenfluramine and mazindol also affect peripheral energy metabolism, such as triglyceride and glucose uptake and utilization, but the relationship of these effects to appetite suppression is unclear (33). Many authorities feel that the drugs act by inducing euphoria and suppressing appetite as a manifestation of a psychological defect.

Conventional wisdom holds that tolerance develops rapidly to the anorectic effects of these agents, as evidenced by the decelerating weight loss curves with continued use. This belief has led to recommendations that appetite suppressants be limited to short-term use. However, appetite suppressants appear to maintain weight loss for the duration of administration, and discontinuation following long-term use results in a rapid rebound of increased appetite and weight regain (34). Therefore, tolerance to the appetite suppressant effects may not be significant at doses usually employed, and long-term treatment may be plausible for selected patients (35). In addition, a recent study demonstrated that phentermine, diethylpropion, and mazindol were as effective, cheaper, and less prone to drug abuse when administered intermittently (i.e., 4 weeks every second month) for an extended period of time (36).

The antidepressant agents fluoxetine and femoxetine are selective inhibitors of serotonin reuptake that are currently being evaluated for the management of obesity. Study results suggest similar rates of effectiveness and fewer side effects than with currently available anorectic agents (37). Fluoxetine has recently been approved by the FDA for the treatment of depression; however, use of this drug in obesity has not yet been approved.

Abuse Potential. Because several of these agents are reinforcing (i.e., euphorigenic) central nervous system stimulants, their misuse potential is high. However, misuse of these agents is not associated with anorectic use in motivated, obese patients. Misuse is more a result of indiscriminate prescribing with subsequent diversion for nonmedial, "recreational" use. Among the anorectic drugs, amphetamines account for most of the abuse episodes, and estimates are that over 10% of the legitimately manufactured amphetamines wind up in the hands of abusers (35).

In December 1978, the Advisory Review Panel on OTC Miscellaneous Internal Drug Products found the nonprescription ingredient, phenylpropanolamine (PPA) to be safe and effective for weight control. The widespread promotion of PPA as the "ultimate diet pill" and its close association with prescription ingredients (e.g., Dexatrim, Dex-A-Diet) have led to special problems of misuse. PPA

Table 56.2.
Appetite Suppressants Used to Treat Obesity

Drug (Common Trade Name)	Usual Doses (mg)	Frequency of Administration[a]
Schedule II[b]		
Amphetamine (Biphetamine)	5, 10	t.i.d. (before meals)
Dextroamphetamine (Dexedrine)	5, 10	t.i.d. (before meals)
	10, 15	q.d. (before breakfast)
Methamphetamine (Desoxyn)	2½, 5	b.i.d.-t.i.d. (before meals)
	10, 15	q.d. (before breakfast)
Phenmetrazine (Preludin)	75	q.d. (midmorning)
Schedule III[b]		
Benzphetamine (Didrex)	25, 50	q.d. (midmorning)
Phendimetrazine (Plegine, Phenazine)	35	b.i.d.-t.i.d. (before meals)
	105	q.d. (before breakfast)
Schedule IV[b]		
Diethylpropion (Tenuate)	25	t.i.d. (before meals)
	75	q.d. (midmorning)
Fenfluramine (Pondimin)	20	t.i.d. (before meals)
Mazindol (Mazanor, Sanorex)	1	t.i.d. (before meals)
	2	q.d. (before lunch)
Phentermine (Ionamin, Fastin)	8	t.i.d. (before meals)
	15, 30	q.d. (before breakfast)
Fluoxetine[c]		
Femoxetine[c]		
Over-the-counter		
Phenylpropanolamine (Dexatrim, Acutrim)	25, 37.5	b.i.d.-t.i.d. (before meals)
	50, 75	q.d. (midmorning)

[a] t.i.d., three times daily; b.i.d., twice daily; q.d., once daily.
[b] Drug Enforcement Agency (DEA) controlled-substance schedule.
[c] Investigational agents not yet approved by the Food and Drug Administration (FDA)

is the most common ingredient in "look-alike" counterfeit drugs that are packaged in tablets and capsules to look virtually identical to amphetamines and are sold as "legal stimulants."

Drug Selection. No superiority has been shown for the appetite-suppressant effects of any of these agents. Thus, product selection is determined primarily by trial and error, using the entire spectrum of available agents (Table 56.2). Patients often tolerate an agent from one chemical class better than one from another. Restlessness, insomnia, tremors, tachycardia, nausea, diarrhea, constipation, dry mouth, and mydriasis are commonly reported side effects. In susceptible patients, elevated blood pressure and cardiac arrhythmias may occur. Agents acting on serotonin (fenfluramine, fluoxetine and femoxetine) are an exception, producing sedation and hypotension, especially in combination with other sedating or hypotensive agents (36). Pulmonary hypertension has been reported in two patients receiving 120 mg and 160 mg of fenfluramine continuously for 8 months (38).

The duration of action can also help determine the

best anorectic agent for a given patient. If overeating occurs in the evening, little benefit is derived from morning doses. Likewise, long-acting agents are irrational when dietary indiscretion is limited to a particular time of day. In both instances, short-acting agents are preferred. Patients who overindulge in the evening, but suffer from drug-induced insomnia, may benefit from fenfluramine, which exhibits unique sedating properties (36, 39). Combinations of anorectic agents with other ingredients, such as barbiturates or phenothiazines, probably possess no greater efficacy and exhibit an expanded array of side effects.

Persons receiving appetite suppressants should be advised about stimulant side effects, dry mouth and possible insomnia. Dry mouth is minimized by sucking on sugarless hard candy. Insomnia from long-acting agents can be minimized by taking the dose early in the day. Patients receiving fenfluramine should be warned about possible drowsiness and additive depressant effects with ethanol or other sedatives. Drug interactions can occur with all of these agents, and the pharmacist should be alert to their concomitant use with monoamine oxidase inhibitors, antihypertensives, tricyclic antidepressants, and caffeine. Lithium toxicity has been reported to be precipitated by mazindol (40).

Appetite suppressants are dispensed with caution to pregnant patients. In studies involving amphetamines and morpholines, an increased incidence in oral clefts was noted when the drug was taken during the first 56 days of pregnancy (41).

BULK-FORMING AGENTS

Bulk formers are indigestible hydrophilic colloids that swell when hydrated to give a sense of fullness. Clinical studies have been contradictory, and bulk can be easily obtained by eating high-fiber fruits and vegetables. These are less expensive and more palatable, and they should become a part of the patient's lifelong diet.

In addition, various inhibitors of carbohydrate and lipid absorption as well as lipid synthesis inhibitors are being evaluated as potential weight-reducing agents (37). Gastrointestinal side effects appear to limit the effectiveness of these agents, and further studies are needed to characterize their potential role in the management of obesity.

THYROID HORMONES

Thyroid has been advocated for the treatment of obesity. Its early use was based on the incorrect observation that obesity was accompanied by an abnormally low BMR. This observation was later shown to be an artifact of the poor correlation between body surface area and BMR in grossly obese patients (6). Currently, advocates claim thyroid hormone may prevent the compensatory drop in BMR caused by caloric restriction. Critics argue that very substantial doses of thyroid are required (6 to 14 grains) to increase BMR even slightly, and these pharmacological doses can have deleterious cardiovascular effects in obese patients already predisposed to heart problems. In view of the risks, use of thyroid hormone in obese individuals should be avoided unless there is clear evidence of thyroid deficiency.

Additional drugs that appear to enhance thermogenesis include ephedrine, caffeine, nicotine, and investigational β-agonists (30, 37). A limited number of studies have evaluated these agents and, despite an apparent effect on increased energy expenditure, associated side effects tend to limit the usefulness of these agents.

Invasive Treatment Approaches

At the extreme end of the treatment continuum, more invasive approaches to obesity are available including mandibular fixation, vagotomy, surgical manipulation of the gastrointestinal tract, and liposuction. These methods should be restricted for use in morbidly obese individuals refractory to the previously mentioned approaches.

Limited data suggest that fixation of the mandible (jaw wiring) can effectively reduce weight by restricting solid food intake. Although this particular procedure is associated with significant weight reduction, rapid weight regain is encountered in roughly 70% following removal of the wires (30). Truncal vagotomy is another approach involving surgical interruption of the vagal nerve in an attempt to reduce the stimuli responsible for triggering eating. Unfortunately, the additional side effects associated with such a procedure limit its usefulness (30).

Jejunoileal and gastric surgery involves bypassing a significant portion of the small intestine and stomach, respectively. Weight loss with either proceeds more slowly than with fasting, and unfortunately, may stop quite short of ideal weight. Jejunoileal bypass works by inducing a malabsorptive state and is associated with significant digestive discomfort, nutrient malabsorption, polyarthritis, fatty liver degeneration, oxalate nephrolithiasis, and tuberculosis (2, 42). Gastric bypass surgery produces a decreased gastric reservoir, which results in epigastric distress or vomiting when the capacity is exceeded. Gastric bypass may have fewer long-term complications, but it is technically more difficult and associated with a higher incidence of early postoperative complications. Nevertheless, despite these many complications, surgery remains the only viable solution in selected patients to avoid permanent disability or death.

Liposuction should be viewed as more of a cosmetic method for body contouring than a means of weight reduction. A frequently misconstrued notion is that significant amounts of adipose can be eliminated via liposuction. Often, if excessive tissue is extracted, serious complications such as blood loss, nerve damage, infection, and disfiguration of the skin contour may occur. Furthermore, successful operations tend to involve younger individuals in whom the elasticity of the skin structure is intact (30). Therefore, the number of obese individuals potentially able to benefit from the procedure is limited. For the above-mentioned reasons, liposuction should not be advocated for managing obesity.

Conclusion

In virtually all cases, obesity is preventable. When it occurs, the cure is simple and noninvasive. Despite this, a significant fraction of the population is suffering from what can be depicted as a "human energy crisis." This is caused largely by the insensitivity of our society to the unfavorable health outcomes associated with sustained obesity and the unwillingness of obese individuals to undertake lifetime treatment (i.e., good dietary habits). Our acceptance of obesity as a benign condition leads to poor motivation and poor patient compliance.

Pharmacists can play an important role in the management of obesity. As has been emphasized, the use of drugs, though temporarily beneficial, can detract from the attainment of permanent solutions. The pharmacist is in a position to put the many components of treatment into perspective, and with educational and reinforcing techniques, assist the obese patient to achieve lasting results.

EATING DISORDERS

The two common eating disorders (EDs) are anorexia nervosa (AN) and bulimia. AN is a syndrome characterized by self-starvation, extreme weight loss, body image disturbance, and an intense fear of becoming obese (43). Bulimia was described as a clinical entity only a decade ago (44) and is characterized by binge eating usually followed by some form of purging, such as self-induced vomiting, laxative abuse, or associated behaviors such as diuretic use, diet pill use, or compulsive exercising (45). Almost half of anorectics have bulimic symptoms, and one-third of bulimics have a history of anorexia or a major depressive order (46). Thus, most eating-disordered patients fall on a spectrum between the purely food-restrictive anorectic and the binging and purging bulimic (47).

Etiology and Incidence

An intense preoccupation with food is common to both anorectics and bulimics. Bulimia is characterized by mild or marked weight fluctuations, while severe weight loss is found in AN. The bulimic's weight typically does not fluctuate to the dangerously low levels seen in AN. The most common type of ED is normal-weight bulimia, i.e., patients who are within 10% of ideal weight despite purging (48). A normal weight, coupled with characteristic secre-

tiveness regarding binging/purging behavior, makes these patients very difficult to detect.

This preoccupation with food stems in part from the cultural value Western society places on thinness and the belief that fat is disgusting and that weight gain means one is bad or out of control. Susceptible individuals have an unfettered drive to achieve society's ideal figure. AN usually begins between the ages of 12 years and the mid-30s, but most commonly first afflicts females in their early teens. Commonly, the teenager perceives a real or imagined weight problem and progresses from a modest effort to lose weight to a compulsive preoccupation with food restriction. "Anorexia" is a misnomer, because most patients do not lose their appetites.

Bulimia has a similar pattern of onset. It begins later in adolescence, usually after a period of being overweight. Unsuccessful attempts at dieting, coupled with self-imposed or family pressure to lose weight, lead the individual, either accidently or through a friend, to the discovery that self-induced vomiting or laxative use may control weight. This ultimately escalates into the binge-and-purge bulimic behavior.

Ninety percent of anorectic and bulimic patients are young females, often from middle- or upper-class backgrounds (43, 48). Five to 10% of adolescent girls and young women are affected to some degree, and it is estimated that the incidence of AN and bulimia has doubled over the past two decades (49, 50). Up to 2% of teenaged girls from upper socioeconomic backgrounds develop AN, and 3 to 5% of college women suffer from bulimia. Twenty percent of patients with EDs have a history of alcohol or other drug abuse (48).

Diagnosis

EDs are classified as psychiatric illnesses. Diagnostic criteria from the third edition of the American Psychiatric Association's *Diagnostic and Statistical Manual (DSM-III-R)* (51) are presented in Table 56.3.

Complications

The complications of AN are mainly those of starvation. The most consistent medical findings, aside from cachexia, are amenorrhea and estrogen deficiency (52). In extreme cases, every physiological system may be disturbed, including the endocrine, cardiovascular, renal, gastrointestinal, and hematological systems (53). Bradycardia is reported in up to 87% (47), and cardiac arrhythmias, a common cause of death, may be precipitated by a diminished heart muscle mass and hypokalemia and other severe electrolyte imbalances (43). Mortality associated with AN (excluding suicide) may be as high as 9%, and suicide may account for an additional 2 to 5% of deaths (54).

The complications of bulimia tend to be less severe

Table 56.3.
DSM III-R Criteria for Anorexia Nervosa and Bulimia

Anorexia nervosa

A. Refusal to maintain body weight over a minimal normal weight for age and height, e.g., weight loss leading to maintenance of body weight 15% below that expected; or failure to make expected weight gain during period of growth, leading to body weight 15% below that expected

B. Intense fear of gaining weight of becoming fat, even though underweight

C. Disturbance in the way in which one's body weight, size, or shape is experienced, e.g., the person claims to "feel fat" even when emaciated, believes that one area of the body is "too fat" even when obviously underweight

D. In females, absence of at least three consecutive menstrual cycles when otherwise expected to occur (primary or secondary amenorrhea); (a woman is considered to have amenorrhea if her periods occur only following hormone, e.g., estrogen, administration)

Bulimia nervosa

A. Recurrent episodes of binge eating (rapid consumption of a large amount of food in a discrete period of time)

B. A feeling of lack of control over eating behavior during eating binges

C. The person regularly engages in either self-induced vomiting, use of laxatives or diuretics, strict dieting or fasting, or vigorous exercise in order to prevent weight gain

D. A minimum average of two binge eating episodes a week for at least 3 months

E. Persistent overconcern with body shape and weight

---

and are the consequences of chronic binging and purging. Unlike the anorectic, whose emaciation attracts attention, the bulimic may be near ideal weight and easily hide the problem. If weight loss is substantial, menstrual irregularities are common (43). Subtle changes in serum electrolytes may be seen in chronic vomiters, and laxative and diuretic abuse further contribute to hypokalemia with muscle weakness and fasciculations. Parotid gland swelling and infections, complaints of frequent sore throats, poor dentition, and scarring on the fingers and nails may be observed in chronic vomiters. Vomiting following use of central nervous system depressants, such as alcohol, predisposes the bulimic to aspiration pneumonia. A particularly dangerous practice is the repeated induction of vomiting with syrup of ipecac. Chronic absorption of ipecac can lead to a potentially fatal cardiotoxicity (55).

A comprehensive list of complications of AN and bulimia are compared and reviewed in Table 56.4.

Treatment

The treatments of AN and bulimia are among the most unsatisfactory in clinical medicine. Anorectic patients and their families tend to deny the existence and severity of the illness and fail to obtain adequate medical and psychiatric care (43). Bulimia patients are more likely to seek treatment, but have a low tolerance for extended compliance and a high relapse rate (56).

Psychotherapy is the mainstay of treatment of EDs, producing a full or partial recovery in 75% (57). Psychotherapy includes individual, group, family, and behavioral therapy, with the objective of helping patients to overcome denial of the problem and to reconstruct self-identity and self-confidence.

In addition to psychotherapy, pharmacologic interventions may benefit ED patients. Recent studies have suggested a possible link between EDs and major depressive illness, including a blunted dexamethasone-suppression test (53) and lowered urinary metabolites of norepinephrine (58). More than 20% of bulimic patients satisfy DSM-III-R criteria for major depressive illness (59). Other evidence disputes a definitive connection between EDs and depression. One of the best studies demonstrating the effectiveness of the tricyclic antidepressant desipramine in bulimia carefully excluded subjects with major depressive disorder (63), suggesting that these agents may have a direct antibulimic effect. In addition, AN and bulimia are associated with changes in the noradrenergic, serotonergic, and opioid systems, which are thought to perpetuate pathological eating behavior (60). Thus, drugs modifying activity of these neurotransmitters may prove useful in the treatment of EDs.

In double-blind controlled studies, imipramine, desipramine, and phenelzine produced a striking reduction in binging behavior in bulimics (61–63). Antidepressants are preferred to monoamine oxidase inhibitors because they preclude dietary restriction problems in patients with diet-indiscreet illness. Also, the phenelzine study group exhibited a high dropout rate, indicating poor patient acceptability of this drug. In another study, amitriptyline produced disappointing results, compared with controls, but suboptimal amitriptyline doses (150 mg/day) and mixed therapy, including psychotherapy for both study and control groups, may have confounded the results (64).

Based on current evidence, desipramine and imipramine are the preferred agents for the drug treatment of bulimia (65). Doses for the tricyclic antidepressants are essentially the same as those used for major depressive disorders and are administered for at least 6 to 8 weeks. In the successful treatment of bulimia with antidepressants alone, most patients relapsed after the drug was stopped, emphasizing that drugs are only a part of a multifocal strategy. Bulimic patients have been maintained successfully on antidepressants for 2 years or more (66).

Several second-generation antidepressants have been studied in open trials in the treatment of bulimia. Fluoxetine, a serotonin reuptake inhibitor, produced complete or partial response in 30 female bulimic patients (67). In addition to its role in depression, serotonin selectively suppresses carbohydrate intake (60). Because binge-eating often involves massive carbohydrate intake, fluoxetine may have a direct antibulimic action. In contrast to fluoxetine, open studies of trazodone, another serotonergic antide-

Table 56.4.
Complications of Anorexia Nervosa and Bulimia[a]

Manifestation	Anorexia nervosa	Bulimia
Endocrine/metabolic	Amenorrhea Osteoporosis Euthyroid sick syndrome Decreased norepinephrine secretion Decreased somatomedin C Elevated growth hormone Decreased or erratic vasopressin secretion Abnormal temperature regulation Hypercarotenemia	Menstrual irregularities
Cardiovascular	Bradycardia Hypotension Arrhythmias	Ipecac poisoning
Renal	Increased blood urea nitrogen Decreased glomerular filtration rate Renal calculi Edema	Hypokalemia (diuretic-induced)
Gastrointestinal	Decreased gastric emptying Elevated hepatic enzymes	Acute gastric dilatation, rupture Constipation Parotid enlargement Dental-enamel erosion Esophagitis Mallory-Weiss tears, esophageal rupture Hypokalemia (laxative-induced)
Hematologic	Anemia Leukopenia Thrombocytopenia	
Pulmonary		Aspiration pneumonia

[a] Reprinted with permission from Herzog DB, Copeland PM: Eating disorders. N Engl J Med 313:295–303, 1985.

pressant, produced mixed results and even worsening of bulimic behavior (68, 69). In 1986, a trial of bupropion in a bulimic population resulted in a relatively high incidence of seizures, which forced the temporary withdrawal of bupropion from the market (70). Clearly, further controlled studies of these newer agents in a large number of bulimics are required to establish their safety and specific role in the treatment of EDs.

A number of other drug modalities have been employed in EDs. In a double-blind study of 72 patients with AN, cyproheptadine in high doses (32 mg/day) produced modest weight gain, compared with amitriptyline and placebo (71). The anticonvulsants phenytoin, carbamazepine, and valproic acid have all been studied in the treatment of bulimic patients (72–74). Results have been generally disappointing, but there have been isolated cases of symptomatic improvement. There may be a subgroup of binge eaters whose behavior is secondary to a neurological disorder analogous to epilepsy, and some bulimic patients may respond to an anticonvulsant agent (75).

The Pharmacist's Role in Recognizing Eating Disorders

As the most approachable and accessible health professional, pharmacists can play an important role in recog-

Table 56.5.
Recognizing Patients with Eating Disorders

- Typical ED patient is a female in early to late teens who (a) exhibits weight loss or no significant weight gain during development (AN), or (b) exhibits frequent significant weight fluctuations (bulimia)
- Young women fitting ED stereotype who repeatedly purchase laxatives, enemas, appetite suppressants, syrup of ipecac or diuretics
- Complaints of irregular menstrual cycles or amenorrhea
- History of depression or alcohol/other drug abuse
- Other nonspecific complaints, e.g., swollen parotid glands, poor dentition, frequent sore throats from vomiting; abdominal complaints from laxative abuse

nizing and counseling patients with EDs. ED patients exhibit typical symptoms and behaviors, which are listed in Table 56.5. Based on these symptoms and behaviors, pharmacists may have to make rapid judgments about whether a patient is suffering from one of these serious, potentially life-threatening disorders. Since many of the drugs misused by bulimics are purchased in pharmacies without a prescription, pharmacists can monitor and restrict repeated sales to young women of stimulant laxatives, enemas, appetite suppressants, and syrup of ipecac. Suspicious use of prescription diuretic agents, such as furosemide or thiazides, in apparently healthy young women should be questioned (76). In one study of 275 bulimic patients, 34% admitted to using a prescription diuretic for weight control (44). Finally, pharmacists must be knowledgeable about community services available to help ED victims once they are identified. Information about regional and local support groups can be obtained from:

Anorexia Nervosa and Associated Disorders (ANAD)
P.O. Box 271
Highland Park, IL 60035
312/831-3438

Conclusion

Current evidence suggests a relationship between depression or other neurotransmitter abnormalities and EDs, particularly bulimia. Antidepressants probably are effective in treating depression in ED patients, and moreover, they appear to provide symptomatic relief in patients who are not clinically depressed. At the present time, a trial of antidepressants is considered appropriate in patients with EDs.

Pharmacists must remember that these patients are often noncompliant and tend to misuse and overuse drugs. They may not comply with a prescribed diet regimen when treated with monoamine oxidase inhibitors, and they require education and monitoring. Relapses are heralded by excessive purchases of laxatives (especially of the phenolphthalein, bisacodyl, and anthraquinone stimulant type), syrup of ipecac and over-the-counter weight control products and by surreptitious diuretic use.

Through vigilance of patient compliance in psychotherapy and pharmacotherapy strategies, and observing for evidence of relapses, the pharmacist can play an important role in the interdisciplinary management of patients with EDs.

REFERENCES

1. Gray DS: Diagnosis and prevalence of obesity. Med Clin North Am 73:1, 1989.
2. Van Itallie TB, Kral JG: The dilemma of morbid obesity. JAMA 246:999, 1981.
3. Bray GA, Gray DS: Obesity. Part I-Pathogenesis. West J Med 149:429, 1988.
4. Pi-Sunyer FX, Obesity. In Shils ME, Young VR: Modern Nutrition in Health and Disease, ed. 7. Philadelphia, Lea & Febiger, p 795, 1988.
5. Tan T, Handford HA, Soldatos CR: Current therapy of eating disorders II: Obesity. Ration Drug Ther 18:1, 1984.
6. Thorn GW, Cahill GF, Gain in weight; obesity. In Wintrobe MM, Thorn GW, Adams RD, et al.: Harrison's Principles of Internal Medicine, ed. 7. New York, McGraw-Hill, p 232, 1974.
7. Anand BK: Nervous regulation of food intake. Physiol Rev 41:667, 1961.
8. Celesia GG, Archer CR, Chung HD: Hyperphagia and obesity, relationship to medial hypothalamic lesions. JAMA 246:151, 1981.
9. Schacter S: Obesity and eating: internal and external values differ-

entially affect the eating behavior of obese and normal subjects. Science 161:751, 1968.
10. Knittle JL, Timmers K, Ginsberg-Fellner F, et al.: The growth of adipose tissue in children and adolescents. J Clin Invest 63:239, 1979.
11. Stunkard A, Rush J: Dieting and depression reexamined—a critical review of reports of untoward responses during weight reduction for obesity. Ann Intern Med 81:526, 1975.
12. Charney E, Goodman HC, McBride M, et al.: Childhood antecedents of adult obesity. N Engl J Med 295:6, 1976.
13. Price RA, Cadoret RJ, Stunkard AJ, et al.: Genetic contributions to human fatness: an adoption study. Am J Psychiatry 144:1003, 1987.
14. Stunkard AJ, Foch TT, Hrubec Z: A twin study of human obesity. JAMA 256:51, 1986.
15. Danowski TS: The management of obesity. Hosp Pract 11:39–46, 1976.
16. Bondy PK: Metabolic obesity? N Engl J Med 303:1057, 1980.
17. Newsholme EA: A possible metabolic basis for the control of body weight. N Engl J Med 303:400, 1980.
18. Edwards LE, Dickes WF, Alton IR, et al.: Pregnancy in the massively obese: course, outcome, and obesity prognosis of the infant. Am J Obstet Gynecol 131:479, 1978.
19. Sketris I, Lesar T, Zaske DE, et al.: Effect of obesity on gentamicin pharmacokinetics. Clin Pharmacol 21:288, 1981.
20. Stunkard AJ, Sorensen TIA, Hanis C, et al.: Adoption study of human obesity. N Engl J Med 314:193, 1986.
21. Van Itallie TB, Yang M: Diet and weight loss. N Engl J Med 297:1158, 1977.
22. Mazel J: The Beverly Hills Diet. New York: Macmillan, 1981.
23. Mirkin GB, Shore RN: The Beverly Hills diet: dangers of the newest weight loss fad. JAMA 246:2235, 1981.
24. Anon: Protein diets. FDA Drug Bull 8:2, 1978.
25. Wadden TA, Stunkard AJ, Brownell KD, Van Itallie TB: The Cambridge diet—more mayhem? JAMA 250:2833, 1983.
26. Felig P: Very-low-calorie-diets. N Engl J Med 310:589, 1984.
27. Straw WE, Sonne AC: The obese patient. J Fam Pract 9:317, 1979.
28. Franklin BA, Rubenfire M: Losing weight through exercise. JAMA 244:377, 1980.
29. Brownell KD, Kramer FM: Behavioral management of obesity. Med Clin North Am 73:185, 1989.
30. Bray GA, Gray DS: Obesity. Part II-Treatment. West J Med 149:555, 1988.
31. Scoville BA: Review of amphetamine-like drugs by the Food and Drug Administration: clinical data and value judgments. In Bray GA: Obesity in Perspective. Washington, D.C.: U.S. Government Printing Office, 1976, p 441.
32. Craighead LW, Stunkard AJ, O'Brien RM: Behavior therapy and pharmacotherapy for obesity. Arch Gen Psychiatry 38:763, 1981.
33. Sullivan AC, Comai K: Pharmacologic treatment of obesity. Int J Obes 2:167, 1978.
34. Stunkard AJ, Anorectic agents: a theory of action and lack of tolerance in a clinical trial. In Garattini S: Anorectic Agents: Mechanisms of Action and of Tolerance. New York: Raven Press, 1981.
35. Anon: The Green Sheet Dec. 5, 1977.
36. Galloway SML, Munro JF, Farquhar DL: The current status of anti-obesity drugs. Postgrad Med J 60:19, 1984.
37. Wilson MA: Treatment of obesity. Am J Med Sci 299:62, 1990.
38. Douglas JG, Munro JF, Kitchin AH, et al.: Pulmonary hypertension and fenfluramine. Br Med J 283:881, 1981.
39. Duhault J, Beregi L, deBoistesselin R: General and comparative pharmacology of fenfluramine. Curr Med Res Opin 6:3(suppl 1), 1979.
40. Hendy MS, Dove AF, Arblaster PG: Mazindol-induced lithium toxicity. Br Med J 280:684, 1980.
41. Milkovich R, van den Berg BJ: Effects of antenatal exposure to anorectic drugs. Am J Obstet Gynecol 129:637, 1977.

42. Bruce RM, Wise L: Tuberculosis after jejunoileal bypass for obesity. Ann Intern Med 87:574, 1977.

43. Herzog DB, Copeland PM: Eating disorders. N Engl J Med 313:295, 1985.

44. Russell G: Bulimia nervosa: an ominous variant of anorexia nervosa. Psychol Med 9:429, 1979.

45. Mitchell JE, Hatsukami D, Pyle RL, Eckert ED: The bulimia syndrome: course of the illness and associated problems. Comprehens Psychiatry 27:165, 1986.

46. Newman MM, Halmi KA: The endocrinology of anorexia nervosa and bulimia nervosa. Neurol Clin 6:195, 1988.

47. Brotman AW, Rigotti N, Herzog DB: Medical complications of eating disorders: outpatient evaluation and management. Comprehens Psychiatry 26:258, 1985.

48. Mickley D: Evaluating common eating disorders—ten questions to ask your patient. Female Patient 13:33, 1988.

49. Pope HG, Hudson JI, Yurgelun-Todd D, Hudson MS: Prevalence of anorexia nervosa and bulimia in three student populations. Int J Eat Disord 3:45, 1984.

50. Pope HG, Hudson JI, Yurgelun-Todd D: Anorexia nervosa and bulimia among 300 women shoppers. Am J Psychiatry 141:292, 1984.

51. American Psychiatric Association: Diagnostic and Statistical Manual of Mental Disorders, ed. 3, revised. Washington, D.C.: American Psychiatric Association, 1987.

52. Warren MP, Vande Weile RL: Clinical and metabolic features of anorexia nervosa. Am J Obstet Gynecol 117:435, 1975.

53. Weiner H: The physiology of eating disorders. Int J Eat Disord 4:347, 1985.

54. Seidensticker JF, Tzagournis M: Anorexia nervosa—clinical features and long term follow-up. J Chronic Dis 21:361, 1968.

55. Adler AG, Walinsky P, Krall RA, Cho SY: Death resulting from ipecac syrup poisoning. JAMA 243:1927, 1980.

56. Mitchell JE, Davis L, Goff G: The process of relapse in patients with bulimia. Int J Eat Disord 4:457, 1985.

57. Adams C, Koop L, Toce P: Current ideologies of eating disorders: an overview. Am Pharm NS28:41, 1988.

58. Biederman J, Herzog DB, Rivinus T, et al.: Urinary MHPG in anorexia nervosa patients with and without a major depressive disorder. J Psychiatr Res 18:149, 1984.

59. Bond WS, Crabbe S, Sanders MC: Pharmacotherapy of eating disorders: a critical review. Drug Intell Clin Pharm 20:659, 1986.

60. Fava M, Copeland PM, Schweiger U, Herzog DB: Neurochemical abnormalities of anorexia nervosa and bulimia nervosa. Am J Psychiatry 146:963, 1989.

61. Pope HG Jr, Hudson JI, Jonas JM, Yurgelun-Todd D: Bulimia treated with imipramine: a placebo-controlled, double-blind study. Am J Psychiatry 140:554, 1983.

62. Walsh BT, Stewart JW, Roose SP, et al.: Treatment of bulimia with phenelzine; a double-blind, placebo-controlled study. Arch Gen Psychiatry 41:1105, 1984.

63. Hughes PL, Wells LA, Cunningham CJ, Ilstrup DM: Treating bulimia with desipramine: a double-blind, placebo-controlled study. Arch Gen Psychiatry 43:182, 1986.

64. Mitchell JE, Groat R: A placebo-controlled, double-blind trial of amitriptyline in bulimia. J Clin Psychopharmacol 4:186, 1984.

65. Kim LE, Middleton RK: Antidepressants used in bulimia. DICP, Ann Pharmacother 23:882, 1989.

66. Mitchell PB: The pharmacological management of bulimia nervosa: a critical review. Int J Eat Disord 7:29, 1988.

67. Wilcox JA: Fluoxetine and bulimia. J Psychoactive Drugs 22:81, 1990.

68. Wold P: Trazodone in the treatment of bulimia. J Clin Psychiatry 44:275, 1983.

69. Pope HG, Hudson JI, Jonas JM: Antidepressant treatment of bulimia: preliminary experience and practical recommendations. J Clin Psychopharmacol 3:274, 1983.

70. Carson SW: Bupropion, is it here to stay? DICP Ann Pharmacother 23:704, 1989.

71. Halmi KA, Eckert E, LaDu TJ, et al.: Anorexia nervosa: treatment efficacy of cyproheptadine and amitriptyline. Arch Gen Psychiatry 43:177, 1986.

72. Wermuth BM, Davis KL, Hollister LE, et al.: Phenytoin treatment of the binge-eating syndrome. Am J Psychiatry 134:1249, 1977.

73. Kaplan AS, Garfinkle PE, Darby PL, et al.: Carbamazepine in the treatment of bulimia. Am J Psychiatry 140:1225, 1983.

74. Herridge PL, Pope HG Jr: Treatment of bulimia and rapid cycling bipolar disorder with sodium valproate: a case report. J Clin Psychopharmacol 5:229, 1985.

75. Moore SL, Rakes SM: Binge eating—therapeutic response to diphenylhydantoin: case report. J Clin Psychiatry 43:385, 1982.

76. Pomeroy C, Mitchell JE, Seim HC, Seppala M: Prescription diuretic abuse in patients with bulimia nervosa. J Fam Pract 27:493, 1988.

CHAPTER 57

ALCOHOLISM

THEODORE G. TONG, Pharm.D. and JEFFREY N. BALDWIN, Pharm.D.

Alcohol is the most misused drug in the United States today. Alcohol abuse and alcoholism are estimated to have cost the United States $136.3 billion in 1990, mostly from lost productivity and employment (1). According to knowledgeable estimates, the incidence of alcoholism in the United States ranges from 9 to 14 million, about 10% of the total number of adult Americans who use alcohol (2). This rate increases to 30 to 50% when close relatives are alcoholic (3). It is a condition far more common than generally perceived, with only 3 to 5% of the country's alcoholic population classified as the "skid row" of public inebriate type. Alcoholics come from all levels of our society; most are found in the working and homemaking population.

The largest percentage of American alcoholics are between the ages of 35 and 50 years. Professionals and business people have high rates of alcohol consumption and alcoholism. The proportion of alcohol use in the younger school-age population and "problem drinking" among women have increased alarmingly and appear to be continuing trends (4, 5). While the prevalence of alcohol misuse among the elderly is lower, detection of the problem is difficult and it is frequently unrecognized. Vulnerability of the older alcoholic to the harmful effects of alcohol is much greater (2). Alcoholism is among America's major health concerns along with cancer and heart disease, and problems related to alcohol abuse and alcoholism are increasing.

Alcoholism is an illness that can shorten one's life-span considerably. About 25% of hospitalized individuals are estimated to have an alcohol-related problem, and 20% of the total national health expenditure for hospital care is spent on alcohol-related illness (2, 6). Alcohol is involved in half of all fatalities from fire and highway traffic accidents, 67% of homicides and 33% of suicides (2). Death rates from alcohol abuse in the major risk age groups are more than twice those for the general population. Alcoholism is a treatable illness when diagnosed in its early stages. Unfortunately, there is a serious deficit of accessible and high quality alcoholism treatment services. Moreover, most the services available are designed to deal with only the late stages of alcoholism.

Alcoholism, like other diseases such as hypertension and diabetes mellitus, can be considered a biological disease with genetic predisposition that is activated by environmental factors (6, 7). Thus, a "biopsychosocial" ap-

proach is usually used in the identification, treatment, and ongoing recovery support systems for alcoholics. Difficulty in differentiating between alcohol abuse and alcoholism (alcohol dependence) may be cited by some as a reason for questioning the disease concept. However, other diseases such as hypertension may be equally difficult to define when borderline. A recent survey found that about 89% of the surveyed population considered alcoholics to be ill, yet 47% also felt that the alcoholic was morally weak (8). This reveals a fairly strong public sentiment that alcoholism represents "willful misconduct," which is an important societal impediment in the identification and treatment of the disease.

Alcohol abuse involves persistent patterns of heavy alcohol consumption with associated health or social consequences. Alcoholism is differentiated from abuse by the craving, tolerance, and physical dependence that result in behavioral changes and loss of control over drinking. Persons who are alcoholic experience both psychologic and physical dependency and tolerance. Psychologic dependency, perhaps the single most important factor, involves the compulsive use of and craving for a drug. Physical dependency is characterized by a series of physiologic events that occur when the drug is discontinued, including the withdrawal or abstinence syndrome. Tolerance develops when continued use of a drug is required, and increasing doses are needed to produce the same effect.

While the most important feature of addictive disorders is the psychologic dependency, it is the least understood. A person may be made physically dependent on alcohol, but abuse may not be recognized or diagnosed as such until behavioral effects secondary to psychologic dependence occur. Many persons consume alcoholic beverages, but relatively few develop physical and psychologic dependency on the drug. A commonly held belief is that someone who does not drink daily or who only drinks alcoholic beverages with relatively low alcohol content, such as wine or beer, cannot be alcoholic. The quantity, type, and frequency of alcohol consumption are relatively unimportant; loss of control over consumption once initiated and continued use despite clear evidence of adverse consequences (social, physical, legal) are more important in the diagnosis of alcoholism.

PHARMACOLOGY

Alcohol is a psychoactive agent that can be characterized pharmacologically as a sedative-hypnotic drug. At low doses, the action of alcohol is an excitatory and stimulatory effect caused by its depression of inhibitory centers in the brain. In a dose-response relationship, at sufficient doses, alcohol produces a depressant action. Although alcohol provides relief of anxiety and sedation at one dose level, it produces sleep and depression of the central nervous and respiratory systems at higher levels.

Alcohol is present in a variety of popular beverages: beer and ale are products of the fermentation of cereal grains and contain 3 to 6% alcohol; wine results from the fermentation of yeast on sugars present in fruits and contains 11 to 20% alcohol; brandy is produced from the distillation of wine products and usually contains 40% alcohol; hard liquors, the distillates of fermented products such as grain, are available as gin, rye, bourbon, scotch, and vodka and contain approximately 40 to 50% alcohol. Hard liquors are commonly labeled with a proof number that is twice the alcohol concentration by volume. Nonalcoholic ("N.A.") beers and wines rarely contain no alcohol; they often contain less than 1% alcohol, but this may be enough to cause a relapse in a recovering alcoholic. Such individuals should generally be advised to avoid products containing any alcohol.

METABOLISM

Alcohol is efficiently and rapidly absorbed by the stomach and small intestine in 30 to 120 min after ingestion. Absorption is direct and complete by simple (passive) diffusion. Alcohol distributes freely in body tissues and fluids. Its volume of distribution ranges from 0.58 to 0.70 liter/kg of body weight. The concentration of alcohol in the brain rapidly approaches that in the blood.

Factors that modify alcohol absorption are volume, dilution, rate of ingestion, and presence of food in the stomach. Protein and water both slow while carbonation facilitates the absorption of alcohol. Gastric alcohol dehydrogenase (ADH), which is involved in gastric metabolism of alcohol, is about 80% higher in nonalcoholic males than females, while chronic alcoholism results in a decrease of about 40% in men and 15% in women. This may help to explain why alcohol blood levels in females, corrected for size, are relatively higher than those in males and may partially explain the early onset of liver and brain damage in female alcoholics (9). Alcohol crosses the placenta and may be found in the milk of lactating mothers.

The liver is the main site of the first step in the oxidation of ethyl alcohol. Ethanol is oxidized by alcohol dehydrogenase to acetaldehyde, which is subsequently oxidized by acetaldehyde dehydrogenase (ALDH) to acetate or acetyl coenzyme A. This enters the Kreb's cycle to form carbon dioxide and water and also participates in protein and fat synthesis. Both oxidizing enzymes are responsible for converting nicotinamide adenine dinucleotide (NAD) to its reduced form, NADH, which contributes to the many metabolic abnormalities (e.g., hyperlipidemia, ketoacidosis, hyperlactacidemia, hyperuricemia) associated with chronic alcohol ingestion. Genetic predisposition may be explained in part by an inactive form of ALDH2 isoenzyme in many alcoholics, which impairs acetaldehyde metabolism. Acetaldehyde accumulation may lead to an increase in aldehyde condensation products, such as tetrahydropapaveroline and salsolinol, collectively known as tetrahydroisoquinolines (THIQs), and β-carbolinese. Infusion of these substances in rats and monkeys causes them to drink large quantities of alcohol. They probably have a relationship to the development of tolerance and habituation. Inactive ALDH2 isoenzyme may therefore be implicated in the pathogenesis of alcohol-induced tissue toxicity and dependence (7, 10, 11). A distinct microsomal ethanol-oxidizing system (MEOS) has also been characterized, which may be involved in increasing the clearance of alcohol and other drugs from the blood (12, 13).

Although most drugs are known to be metabolized or cleared from the body in a fixed percentage (first-order) of the dose taken, alcohol is unique in that nonlinear or saturation-elimination kinetics is followed, and therefore, it is removed from the blood in a fixed amount (zero-order) over time. Most of the ingested dose of alcohol is eliminated by liver metabolism. In a 70-kg (approximately 150-lb) person, the rate of alcohol metabolism approximates 7 g/hr. At this rate of metabolism, the blood alcohol level will decline at a rate of nearly 15 mg/100 ml/hr. An average shot of distilled spirit, 86 proof, contains about 15 g of ethyl alcohol. Because body water approximates 65% of body weight in a 70-kg person, the blood ethyl alcohol content after one shot will be 15 g/50 liters, or 30 mg/dl, with 50 liters being the approximate volume of total body water calculated from the percentage of weight. If taken in one swallow, it will take approximately 2 hr for the blood ethyl alcohol level to return to zero. Within 1 hr after drinking any of the following: five 12-ounce cans of beer, four 4-ounce glasses of table wine, five 1-ounce glasses of liqueur, five 1-ounce shots of distilled spirits, or three 3-ounce martinis, a 70-kg person would have a blood ethanol concentration of 100 mg/dl (the amount legally defined as intoxication in many states; some now use 50 mg/dl).

Ethanol elimination by the kidneys, lungs, and through sweat is minimal, with approximately 2 to 10% cleared by these routes, depending on the amount of alcohol ingested. Exercise or administration of thyroid hormone, oxygen, glucose, or multivitamins does not increase the rate of alcohol oxidation. Whether or not there are ethnic differences for developing tolerance to alcohol is unclear (12, 14).

BLOOD ALCOHOL CONCENTRATIONS AND INTOXICATION

The relationship between blood ethyl alcohol concentration and clinical signs and symptoms of intoxication is vari-

Table 57.1.
Blood Ethanol Concentrations and Clinical Effects in the Nontolerant Adult Drinker

Blood Ethanol Level (mg/100 ml)	Clinical Effects
20–99	Slight changes in mood and feelings progressing to muscular incoordination, impaired sensory function, personality and behavioral changes (talkative, noisy, morose)
100–199	Marked mental impairment, incoordination, clumsiness and unsteadiness in standing or walking, ataxia, prolonged reaction time, gross intoxication
200–299	Nausea, vomiting, diplopia, marked ataxia
300–399	Hypothermia, severe dysarthria, amnesia, stage 1 anesthesia
400–700	Coma, respiratory failure, and death

able and depends on the rate of ingestion, amount consumed, alterations in absorption, metabolism, excretion, and chronicity of exposure (Table 57.1). The correlation of the blood alcohol concentration to behavioral effects has obvious important medical and legal importance. As a consequence of tolerance, higher blood alcohol concentrations may be required to produce clinical effects in alcoholics than in occasional drinkers. There are drinkers who exhibit such extreme degrees of tolerance to alcohol that they will appear sober even with blood alcohol concentrations two to three times higher than the limit permitted by law for driving an automobile. The lethal blood alcohol level is variable, but in the range of 400 to 700 mg/dl. The lethal level may be substantially lowered when opiates, neuroleptics, or other sedative-hypnotics are taken with an excessive amount of alcohol.

DIAGNOSIS OF ALCOHOLISM

The diagnosis of alcoholism is difficult because of societal stigmatization of the disease, denial, and imprecise diagnostic criteria. The clinical signs and subtleties of the condition are varied, elusive, and without reliable parameters. Objective laboratory verification of the diagnosis is frequently unavailable or incomplete. Although a specific genetic marker for alcoholism has been recently suggested (15), this is not universally accepted and likely represents only one of a number of factors (e.g., multiple gene loci, environment, gender, ethnicity) that affect predisposition. Reliable biochemical or genetic markers for diagnosing alcoholism are not available. Much depends on the experience and motivation of the observer in deciding whether a patient is suffering from alcoholism or not. Unfortunately, many physicians and other health professionals are poorly informed about the diagnosis of alcoholism,

and therefore underdiagnose and mismanage alcohol-related problems. The first recognition of alcoholism often occurs during a hospitalization when an advanced manifestation of alcoholism, such as ascites or cirrhosis, is being treated. Many patients with unrecognized alcoholism probably experience minor withdrawal symptoms, such as agitation and insomnia, during the course of hospital stays or when admitted to nursing homes. Although not absolute, the DSM-III-R criteria established by the American Psychiatric Association can serve as a convenient starting point for the diagnosis of alcohol dependence (16).

Early identification of an existing alcohol problem is important because the prognosis from treatment is much more promising when the difficulty is recognized early in its course. Clues that provide early recognition are to be found in the demographic, social, familial, and cultural characteristics of alcohol consumers (17). Frequent episodes of drinking to the point of intoxication, an inability to control the intake of alcohol, alcoholic "blackout" periods (loss of memory while intoxicated, not passing out), drinking despite strong social contraindications such as job loss, legal problems such as drunk driving arrests, or family or marital discord resulting from pathologic drinking are signs of this condition. Common early physical signs and symptoms of alcoholism include hypertension, gastritis, diarrhea or irritable colon, burns, bruises, red face, puffy face and eyes, enlarged nose with prominent veins, reddened conjunctiva, obesity, insomnia, or impotence. Several identification or screening tests in common clinical use (Michigan Alcoholism Screening Test (MAST), the abbreviated MAST, and CAGE (Cutting down, Drinking, Annoyed by criticism of drinking, Guilty about drinking, and Eye-openers) were recently studied. Cyr and Wartman (18) found that, in addition to one of these tests, the specific questions "Have you ever had a drinking problem?" and "When was your last drink?" were helpful in establishing a diagnosis of alcoholism.

Equally important in obtaining assistance for alcoholics is getting them to agree to be evaluated for the problem. Denial is a common characteristic of chemical dependency, including alcoholism. Although some patients may respond to a personal expression of concern from a friend, employers, or physician, many patients require a formal intervention to get help. Normally a formal intervention is a carefully planned confrontation of the individual during which those who have observed alcohol-related behaviors report them in objective terms and define an ultimatum that the individual get help or suffer consequences such as loss of job, family, friends, or other significant support. Interventions are normally coordinated by an individual such as counselor. In some specific professions, such as pharmacy, interventions may also be done by trained teams of intervenors from within the profession. Normally, the individual is encouraged to obtain the formal evaluation or enter formal treatment as soon as possible, preferably that day. This helps to assure compliance and reduces the risk of suicide at a time when this is a major risk.

MAJOR ADVERSE EFFECTS FROM ALCOHOL

Alcohol affects almost every organ system in the body. The more important and known medical complications and pathologic consequences from excessive alcohol consumption are summarized in Table 57-2 (19).

Alcoholic Liver Disease

There are three distinct histologic patterns of alcohol-induced liver disease. All three may coexist simultaneously and do not represent a single progression. Cirrhosis may occur in the absence of prior hepatitis (35). The risk of developing alcoholic liver disease is related to the quantity and duration of alcohol consumption. Factors such as genetics, nutritional state, and environment also predispose to the development of alcoholic liver disease (22). Alcoholic "fatty liver" disease is the most common alcohol-induced hepatic abnormality, occurring in 90 to 100% of chronic alcoholics.

The postulated mechanism for fatty accumulation in the liver is that an increase in the NADH:NAD ratio during ethanol oxidation is responsible for accumulation of hepatic triglycerides. Uncomplicated fatty liver is usually asymptomatic or presents as nausea, vomiting, and right upper quadrant abdominal pain, rarely presenting with the usual signs of liver disease such as ascites, jaundice, or splenomegaly. Mild, usually reversible, elevation of liver enzyme levels is the most frequent laboratory finding. Not as relatively benign as once believed, fatty liver can progress to liver failure and occasionally death.

Alcoholic hepatitis is a much more serious disorder; 10 to 30% of alcoholics develop this complication, usually after years of excessive drinking or after an abrupt increase in alcohol intake. Liver injury results from the degenerative effects of alcohol on subcellular structures. The clinical course of alcoholic hepatitis ranges through acute or chronic asymptomatic, mild, severe, and fulminant forms. It is often an incidental diagnosis when hepatomegaly and mild elevations in liver function study results are detected during a physical examination. Some patients who develop the fulminant course progress rapidly to liver failure. The death rate in cases of severe alcoholic hepatitis is substantial. Approximately half of the survivors subsequently progress to development of cirrhosis of the liver.

The pathogenesis of alcoholic cirrhosis has not been determined completely. The liver is characterized as being finely nodular or grossly deformed, which may be smaller or larger than normal. Laboratory findings include hyperbilirubinemia, hypoalbuminemia, and prolonged pro-

thrombin time. Complications from cirrhosis include encephalopathy, portal hypertension with bleeding at the esophageal varices, portal vein thrombosis, and hepatorenal syndrome. As many as 30,000 deaths occur each year from alcohol-induced cirrhosis.

Alcohol and the Heart

Cardiac dysfunction may account for up to 50% of the difference between normal death rates and those in alcohol-abusing or -dependent individuals. Alcohol can cause cardiomyopathy and cardiac arrhythmias, is associated with a significant increase in hypertension when used chronically, and may cause ischemic heart disease and stroke (36).

Recognition of alcoholic cardiomyopathy has been made difficult by its similarity to two other types of alcohol-related cardiomyopathies (24, 25). Nutritional deficiency in thiamine can lead to an unusual type of cardiac disorder ("wet beriberi heart disease"), which is characterized by a state of high output failure, fluid retention, and cardiac dilatation. Another cause of cardiomyopathy has been associated with excessive consumption of beer containing cobalt, an added foaming agent. There are patients with a history of alcoholism who have heart disease that is unrelated to either of these possible causes. Recent evidence suggests that alcohol is metabolized in the heart to fatty acid ethyl esters that interfere with mitochondrial function, causing cardiomyopathy. With abstinence, alcohol-induced cardiomyopathy may be reversible in about 30% of patients (37, 38).

As many as 24% of cases of hypertension may have alcohol as a primary cause. Blood pressure elevation occurs with acute intoxication and often parallels the severity of alcoholism with chronic use. Regression of hypertension often occurs with abstention (37, 38).

Alcohol and the Hematopoietic System

The association of anemia, macrocytosis, and alcoholism was long held to be attributable to nutritional deficiencies. Studies have shown a direct role of alcohol on suppression of folate metabolism, depletion of folate from body stores, and malabsorption of folate. The direct toxicity of alcohol on erythropoiesis is demonstrated by vacuolation of erythroid and myeloid precursors (28, 29). A sideroblastic or "iron-loading" anemia can result from the impairment by alcohol of iron incorporation and metabolism in the red blood cell. Alcohol affects iron absorption by increasing jejunal absorption of iron, as reflected in hemochromatosis and a rise in serum iron levels. Iron deficiency anemia due to gastritis and to gastrointestinal bleeding can also occur. Alcoholic thrombocytopenia occurs in 25 to 30% of acutely ill alcoholics; platelets often have shorter than normal life spans, and thrombopoiesis is ineffective because of marrow suppression and folate deficiency.

Table 57.2.
Complications of Alcoholism

Complication	Usual Onset	Comments
Increased morbidity and mortality	Chronic	Most common causes are cirrhosis, cancers of respiratory and gastrointestinal tracts, accidents, suicide, and ischemic heart disease (19).
Fluid and electrolyte abnormalities	Acute	Alcohol has diuretic action as blood alcohol concentration increases. Stable or decreasing blood alcohol concentrations result in antidiuresis. Hyperosmolarity, hypokalemia, hypophosphatemia, and hypomagnesemia are common. Mild lactic acidemia may contribute to asymptomatic elevation of uric acid due to interference with renal secretion of uric acid (19).
Hypoglycemia	Acute or chronic	Alcohol depletes liver glycogen stores and decreases gluconeogenesis; blood sugar may drop precipitously. Stupor and coma, apart from the direct effects of alcohol on the nervous system, are experienced. A dramatic but relatively uncommon complication (20).
Hyperglycemia	Acute	During early phases of alcohol withdrawal, blood sugar may be elevated because of increased release of catecholamines. Alcoholic pancreatitis and decreased peripheral glucose utilization are contributing factors.
Hyperketonemia	Acute	Alcoholic patients frequently develop hyperketonemia and metabolic acidosis in the absence of hyperglycemia. Often the patient is hypoglycemic and without glycosuria. This is presumably due to alcohol-induced starvation ketosis. Insulin is not administered.
Hypothermia	Acute	Occurs frequently as a result of prolonged exposure to cold (not uncommon in unconscious or stuporous state); pancreatitis and meningitis may also contribute.
Liver disease		Best known sequela of chronic alcoholism and a leading cause of morbidity. Three common liver diseases are often associated with alcoholism: acute fatty liver, alcoholic hepatitis, and alcoholic cirrhosis. Individual sensitivity is variable and the degree of liver dysfunction does not appear to be related only to the amount of alcohol ingested. Nutritional status, genetic composition, and immunologic factors appear to interact in the development of alcoholic liver disease (21).
Acute fatty liver	Acute	Develops in nearly all who ingest alcohol excessively (defined by some as an intake of at least 70 g ethyl alcohol daily) even for only a few days. Treatment: to stop drinking and give a diet with adequate vitamin and protein replacement (21).
Alcoholic hepatitis	Acute or chronic	Apparently a toxic inflammatory response of the liver in 10–30% of chronic or acute alcoholics. A high percentage who continue to drink with alcoholic hepatitis develop cirrhosis within 5–10 years. Most patients require 8–12 weeks to show improvement from the acute stage. Treatment is supportive, an adequate diet, vitamin supplements, bed rest, and stopping drinking. In severe cases, liver failure (hepatic coma), variceal bleeding, and hepatorenal syndrome often are present. Clinical features are similar to those of other forms of toxic or viral liver injury. Hepatomegaly, jaundice, splenomegaly, fever and ascites are common. Corticosteroids may be of benefit in fulminant cases, but their exact role in treatment of this disorder is still being investigated. Some studies have failed to show any benefit from their use (21).
Alcoholic or Laennec's cirrhosis	Chronic	Symptoms are frequently nonspecific in character, e.g., fatigue, weight loss, lethargy. Other physical signs include slight hepatomegaly, splenomegaly, ascites, gynecomastia, spider angiomas, and palmar erythema. About 10–30% of alcoholics develop alcoholic cirrhosis, usually after drinking heavily for 10–15 years. The three most common causes of death in alcoholic cirrhosis are: bleeding esophageal varices, liver failure (encephalopathy and coma), and infection. The only treatment is to stop drinking (21).
Portal hypertension	Acute or chronic	A sequela of hepatitis. Return of blood from abdominal viscera to the heart is impaired as pressure rises and collateral blood vessels enlarge. All abdominal organs become congested; splenomegaly and ascites (result (21).
Ascites	Acute or chronic	Seen often in patients with portal hypertension and may be worsened by alcoholic liver disease and a low serum albumin. A low sodium diet, spironolactone, and sometimes diuretics are helpful. As liver disease improves, ascites will often resolve. Careful monitoring of electrolytes must be done when diuretics and aldosterone antagonists are used (21).
Esophageal varices	Acute	These thin-walled, collateral blood vessels of the portal system are prone to hemorrhaging. Hemorrhage usually occurs when the portal pressure rises because of expanded plasma volume, worsening liver involvement, or increased intraabdominal pressure. Thin walls and accompanying esophagitis are also contributing causes.
Encephalopathy	Acute	The central nervous system is depressed by toxins, e.g., ammonia that reaches it through shunted blood that has bypassed liver. The patient is usually lethargic, has "flapping tremor," deterioration of fine movement, and is unable to perform any purposeful activity before lapsing into coma. The central nervous system is more sensitive than usual to anoxia, sedative-hypnotics, opiates, or tranquilizers. Coma is frequently precipitated by gastrointestinal hemorrhage, hypokalemia, infection or large amounts of nitrogen from dietary sources such as proteins (22).
Gastrointestinal problems; e.g., pancreatitis, gastritis, peptic ulcer	Acute or chronic	Acute pancreatitis occurs more commonly in alcoholics and is most often seen in persons who have been drinking heavily for 8–10 years or more. Often no characteristic clinical picture except for abdominal pain is present. Nausea and vomiting are common. It is one of the more frequent causes for hospitalization of alcoholics following a drinking bout. Other manifestations of this condition include shock, hypocalcemia, hyperglycemia, marked fluid loss, or dehydration. Acute gastritis, often hemorrhagic, is common in alcoholics and is worsened by the chronic use of aspirin. The incidence of peptic ulcer is probably higher in alcoholics than nonalcoholics. Tearing of the gastroesophageal mucosa (Mallory-Weiss syndrome) with severe bleeding may occur as consequence of vomiting; this should be considered a medical and surgical emergency.

Table 57.2. (*Continued*)

Complication	Usual Onset	Comments
Malabsorption	Chronic	Changes in gastrointestinal morphology and decreased enzyme activity in the intestinal tract have been observed in chronic alcoholic patients, even with an adequate diet. Thiamine, vitamin B_{12}, folate, xylose, iron, and fat malabsorption occur. Alcohol consumption and poor diet are major contributors to malabsorption.
Hyperlipidemia	Acute or chronic	Alcohol ingestion induces an elevation of serum triglycerides in persons with type IV hyperlipoproteinemia. Because alcoholic liver disease begins with fatty infiltrates, hypertriglyceridemia may be an early contributory factor to the hepatic and cardiac disorders from alcohol.
Cardiomyopathies	Acute or chronic	Alcohol presumably affects the heart by depressing ventricular activity, reducing myocardial uptake of free fatty acids, enhancing uptake of triglycerides, and causing myocardial cell injury. Direct toxic effects of alcohol on the myocardium, multiple vitamin deficiencies, inadequate protein intake, and electrolyte disturbances are all contributory (23, 24).
Myopathy	Acute or chronic	Generalized and occasionally focal muscle weakness develops during or following heavy drinking bout. Muscle edema, pain, and cramps are common and may by accompanied by tenderness and edema. Elevated muscle enzymes (creatine phosphokinase and aldolase) may be present. In severe cases, myoglobulinuria can occur. Mortality is high (50%) when alcoholic myopathy occurs concomitantly with hyperkalemia and renal failure (25).
Infection	Acute or chronic	Acute and chronic alcohol ingestion decreases resistance to bacterial infection, especially in the respiratory tract. Most pulmonary infections in alcoholics are due to *Pneumococcus*. Susceptibility to *Klebsiella* and *Haemophilis* organisms is also greater. Because they are debilitated, alcoholics are at a higher risk of reactivated tuberculosis; it has been claimed that 20% of patients with active tuberculosis are alcoholics. Aspiration pneumonia is also a major complication. Absence of elevation of white blood cell counts or temperature should not preclude the possibility of infections in an alcoholic (26).
Hematologic disorders; e.g., anemia, leukopenia, thrombocytopenia	Chronic	Four major factors contribute to hematologic disorders: poor diet, blood loss, liver disease, and alcohol itself. Folate deficiency is probably the most important hematologic abnormality in alcoholics. Good diet alone cannot protect against the bone marrow toxicity of alcohol if a major portion of calories are ingested as ethanol. Stopping of alcohol, a nutritious diet including folic acid and multivitamins, and treatment of other medical complications nearly always reverse hematologic abnormalities (27, 28).
Neurologic disorders, polyneuropathy	Chronic	A degenerative process of nerve and brain tissues secondary to nutritional deficiency is common with a long history of alcoholism. Clinical and pathologic features of polyneuropathy are almost identical with beriberi. Subjective sensory disturbances and loss of reflexes and motor activity occur. Recovery is slow and often incomplete, even with complete alcohol abstinence (22, 29).
Wernicke's disease	Acute or chronic	The clinical presentation includes ocular disturbances (e.g., nystagmus), muscle weakness or paralysis, diplopia, ataxia, disorientation, and confusion frequently accompanying signs of thiamine deficiency. It can be treated by giving thiamine (22, 29).
Korsakoff's psychosis	Acute or chronic	More-apparent disturbances in this disorder are cognitive defect and personality changes. Memory may be affected to exclusion of other components of mental function. Recent memory is affected the most. Other clinical features often are confusion and confabulation. Recovery is slow and usually incomplete, despite treatment with thiamine and other vitamins and cessation of drinking (22, 29).
Amblyopia	Chronic	A disorder of the optic nerve occurring alone or in conjunction with other neuropathies; manifested by blurred vision (22).
Skin disorders	Chronic	Skin disorders are common (30–50%) in alcoholic patients and can result from vitamin deficiency diseases such as scurvy or pellagra. Neglected skin disorders often result in secondary infections; seborrhea, lacerations, abrasions, acne, scabies, and pediculosis are also frequent. When common skin conditions (e.g., psoriasis, eczema) are not responding to the usual treatment measures, alcoholism may play a role (30).
Teratogenesis	Chronic	Multiple congenital defects, prenatal growth retardation, and delay in development are fetal abnormalities that result from heavy alcohol abuse during pregnancy (31).
Neonatal intoxication and withdrawal	Chronic	Ethanol crosses the placental barrier freely. The clearance rate of alcohol is reduced in premature infants. Substantial impairment of motor activity, alertness, and respiration are reported in neonates after ethanol infusion just before delivery (32).
Sexual impotence, loss of libido	Chronic	Experienced frequently by male alcoholics. Endocrine effects of alcohol, characteristics of hypogonadism (i.e., gynecomastia), loss of facial hair, spider angiomata, and testicular atrophy, and testostrone deficiency are seen.
Cancer	Chronic	Excessive use of alcohol combined with tobacco has been implicated in greater risks for cancers, particularly of the head, neck, mouth, pharynx, larynx, esophagus, and liver. Alcohol may be a cocarcinogen promoting the activity of true carcinogens (33).

ACUTE ALCOHOL INTOXICATION

Intoxication from alcohol, like that of other sedative-hypnotics, is characterized by depressed deep tendon reflexes, slurred speech, staggering gait, stupor, and coma through a generalized depression of the central nervous system. Nystagmus and ataxia may also be present.

The lethal dose of alcohol varies in adults: it ranges from 5 to 8 g/kg of body weight. This is lower in children, approximately 3 to 4 g/kg of body weight is considered at risk. The therapeutic index of alcohol is about 1:5, which is low in comparison with other sedative-hypnotic drugs. Diazepam and chlordiazepoxide, for example, have a therapeutic index of approximately 1:7000. Occasionally, alcohol substitutes such as methanol or isopropyl alcohol are ingested. Differences in the clinical manifestations following ingestion of these agents distinguish each (Table 57.3).

Diagnosis

The severity of acute intoxication depends on the blood alcohol level and individual tolerance. Levels below 50 mg/dl, or 0.05%, rarely produce significant effects in adults. In children, signs of alcohol intoxication are often prominent at this level. The presence or absence of the odor of alcohol on a patient's breath cannot be used to establish a diagnosis of alcohol intoxication. Unique odors should still be noted since they may offer a diagnostic clue as to the overall clinical condition of a toxic patient. The plasma osmolality can be a useful indicator, since the relationship of osmolality with plasma alcohol is linear. A rise of approximately 25 to 30 milliosmoles/kg H_2O reflects a 100 mg/dl, or 0.1%, increase in plasma alcohol. Concomitant conditions such as trauma, blood loss, infection, multiple drug use, and hypoglycemia often complicate the recognition and assessment of an intoxicated patient. Therefore, the measurement or estimate of the blood alcohol level or comparable analysis of urine, saliva, and expired air is valuable for confirming alcohol intoxication and establishing an appropriate treatment plan (39).

Other toxicologic tests, particularly for barbiturates and other sedative drugs and also salicylates, may be indicated to detect suspected commonly occurring polydrug toxicity. In addition, specific laboratory studies for liver function, renal function, serum electrolytes (with particular attention to the potassium, magnesium, and phosphate levels and the anion gap), arterial blood gases, blood ketones, and glucose levels should be performed routinely. The urine should be examined for the appearance of any crystal-like material or myoglobin. Following a prolonged

Table 57.3.
Toxicities of Alcohol Substitutes

Substances	Sources	Signs and Symptoms	Management
Methanol (methyl alcohol, "denatured alcohol")	Found in solvents, denaturant, antifreeze; toxic amounts attained through inhalation and ingestion	Intractable metabolic acidosis and optic nerve injury can result 12–24 hr after ingestion; toxic metabolites are formic acid and formaldehyde; find both metabolites in urine	Approximate lethal dose: 1–4 ml/kg in adult; treat by administering intravenous ethanol to block the generation of toxic metabolites by alcohol dehydrogenase; administer sodium bicarbonate; peritoneal dialysis and hemodialysis can be useful
Isopropanol (isopropyl alcohol)	Found in rubbing alcohol, solvents; toxic amounts attained through inhalation and ingestion	Severe hypoglycemia, acidosis, and coma; hypothermia and convulsions also occur; infants and children at risk of hypoglycemia; gastrointestinal irritant; acetone on breath, in urine, and serum in absence of hyperglycemia or glycosuria	Approximate lethal dose: 250 g for adult; alkalinization to correct metabolic acidosis may be helpful; manage primarily with support
Ethylene glycol	Found in antifreeze	Clinical abnormalities of the central nervous and cardiopulmonary systems; oxidation of ethylene glycol by alcohol dehydrogenase to oxalic acid and calcium oxalate, which precipitate in kidney; oliguria and acute renal failure can occur	Approximate lethal dose: 100 mg for adult; in children, much lower doses are associated with renal, cardiac, and central nervous system toxicity; treatment by administration of intravenous ethanol; alkalinization to correct metabolic acidosis and to solubilize calcium oxalate useful; hemodialysis has been successful in removing ethylene glycol

drinking binge, myoglobinuria, hyperkalemia, and increased serum creatine kinase levels secondary to alcohol myopathy may occur. An electrocardiogram should be taken and changes characteristic of abnormal calcium, magnesium, and potassium levels or presence of hypoxia or hypothermia should be recognized. An abdominal x-ray examination (KUB) may offer useful clues to the identity of materials ingested in any possible multiple overdose involving an acutely alcohol-intoxicated patient. Some common drugs often taken in suicide attempts such as phenothiazines, tricyclic antidepressants, heavy metals including iron, arsenic and halides, iodides and bromides, chloral hydrate and enteric-coated tablets are radiopaque. X-rays of the skull and chest are also advisable at the time of initial examination.

Management

The basic treatment for acute alcohol intoxication is to maintain and support vital functions (i.e., maintain a patent airway and adequate blood pressure, avoid aspiration) until no longer needed during the detoxification process, which takes from 7 to 10 days (33, 40). In the comatose patient, particularly if this involves accidental ingestion of alcohol by a child, acute alcoholic hypoglycemia and other possible causes of coma such as subdural hematoma should be ruled out. Central nervous system stimulants should not be used. The major problems encountered in the management of acute alcohol intoxication are (a) pneumonia, a leading cause of morbidity; (b) overhydration; and (c) complications from unnecessary therapeutic maneuvers.

The possible presence of alcohol should not be overlooked when evaluating a suspected acute case of drug intoxication. One study revealed that almost one of every five acute drug-overdosed patients in whom the presence of alcohol was unsuspected or thought to be irrelevant were found to have high blood levels of alcohol. The notion that acute alcohol intoxication is benign should be dispelled. Diagnosis of any drug intoxication should include a blood ethanol determination in addition to other laboratory tests.

Alcoholic coma is a life-threatening situation that usually responds well to supportive treatment. Establishment of a clear airway and assisted ventilation are essential in this condition. Oxygenation and volume replacement with intravenous fluids generally improves the hypotension. Patients who are experiencing protracted vomiting may have substantial fluid deficits. If alcoholic hypoglycemia is suspected or if the blood glucose is at 70 mg/dl or lower, 50 to 100 ml of 50% glucose should be given intravenously. Thiamine 100 mg given to prevent the possible exacerbation of the Wernicke-Korsakoff syndrome should be administered before or along with the glucose. In circumstances where the recent ingestion of drugs is suspected, gastric lavage can be performed carefully in the unconscious patient with appropriate guarding of the airway to avoid the risk of aspiration. Emetics, such as syrup of ipecac, given to prevent the further absorption of drugs taken in an overdose should be used with great caution in any acutely intoxicated conscious alcoholic patient since tearing of the gastroesophageal mucosa may occur as a life-threatening consequence of ipecac-induced protracted vomiting.

The use of 10 and 40% solutions of fructose given either orally or intravenously in attempts to accelerate the metabolism of ethanol is not suggested. The minimal benefits from such an effort are outweighed by the disadvantages. Adverse effects from fructose include nausea, vomiting, hyperuricemia, worsening of metabolic acidosis, and volume depletion. Increasing the rate of clearance of alcohol from the body also leads to more rapid development of the alcohol withdrawal symptoms (44). Recent reports claim that administration of naloxone will reverse alcohol-induced coma and have some antagonistic effects in acute alcohol intoxication. In cases described, the responses were quite variable; in some, improvement was only slight. Difficulties encountered when trying to exclude concomitant opiate use in those patients reported to have responded and failed attempts to reproduce these findings in the laboratory have left the issue of naloxone use as an antagonist to alcohol-induced coma to be resolved (42, 43).

Treatment of hepatic encephalopathy precipitated by alcohol is to reverse the precipitating factors and lower serum ammonia levels. The immediate approach to bleeding esophageal varices is blood replacement, possible administration of vasopressin, and use of a Sengstaken-Blakemore tube if necessary. Injection of sclerosant solutions can be given for bleeding varices of the esophagus. Sodium morrhuate and sodium tetradecyl sulfate are available variceal sclerosing agents. Reduction of increased blood flow in the portal collateral system and increased intrahepatic resistance with vasoconstrictors such as vasopressin and somatostain, or with β-adrenergic blockers are beneficial in lowering variceal pressures. Surgery may be required to further decompress the varices by shunting the flow of the hepatic portal circulation after the patient has stabilized. This condition is further characterized by sodium retention, progressively worsening oliguria, and eventually, azotemia.

A toxic psychosis associated with acute alcohol intoxication occasionally presents as an emergency situation. It is characterized by a markedly impaired sensorium with confusion, amnesia, and disorientation. There is frequently a sudden onset of aggressive and hostile behavior with associated psychotic symptoms including hallucinations and delusions. The treatment of this agitated phase can be accomplished with sedation to produce a calm, but still arousable, condition. Benzodiazepines and haloperidol can be used judiciously in these circumstances.

A number of considerations should be kept in mind when treating and caring for the patient acutely intoxicated or overdosed with alcohol. Both symptoms of acute alcohol intoxication and response to treatment vary among patients. Factors such as age, weight, tolerance, and concomitant ingestion of other drugs must be considered. Polydrug abuse in the adult with alcohol intoxication should be suspected and withdrawal from barbiturates or opiates may be a further complication. In children, the toxicological effects of ingredients contained in alcoholic solutions that are used for cough and colds, pain, allergic symptoms, or sleep should be considered. Medical and surgical illnesses may contribute to the toxicologic problems of acute alcohol poisoning. The basis of treatment should be to maintain and support vital functions and to individualize all aspects of care and treatment (39).

CLINICAL FEATURES OF ACUTE ALCOHOL ABSTINENCE (WITHDRAWAL) SYNDROME

An acute abstinence, or withdrawal, syndrome is a common problem experienced by the alcoholic when alcohol is discontinued abruptly. Delirium tremens (DTs) is the most severe form. The severity of the withdrawal syndrome cannot always be predicted on the basis of the quantity or duration of alcohol ingestion. Although most patients experience only minor and moderate symptoms, described often as a "hangover," it is difficult to rule out the possibility that progressively more severe and even life-threatening withdrawal reactions may occur. There is a wide variability in the severity and duration of this syndrome; 5 to 6% of those undergoing this experience will progress to the most severe stage, delirium tremens.

The early physiologic and behavioral effects of acute alcohol abstinence experienced (8 to 36 hr after cessation of drinking) include anorexia; tremors ("shakes"); flushing; increased blood pressure, pulse, respiration rate, and temperature; intermittent hallucinations; seizures ("rum fits"); sleep disturbance; and sweating. Mild-to-moderate withdrawal may stimulate the alcoholic to resume drinking in order to reverse the symptoms. A common finding in the later progression of alcoholism is the use of morning drinks ("eye openers") to reduce these effects from drinking the previous night. Late effects, experienced 2 to 6 days after cessation of drinking, may include severe tremors, marked agitation, profound disorientation, excitation, persistent visual and auditory hallucinations, marked sleep disturbances, fever, tachycardia, and other life-threatening complications. Patients experiencing major alcohol withdrawal symptoms or delirium tremens, estimated to occur in 5% of hospitalized withdrawing alcoholics, are seriously ill. Although the mortality rate for this condition has decreased during the past 50 years, deaths from the DTs still occur (variously estimated at 5 to 20%), particularly in patients with underlying alcohol-associated diseases such as pan-

creatitis, cirrhosis, gastrointestinal bleeding, pneumonia, or sepsis.

It should not be taken for granted that the intoxicated or bizarre behavior in alcoholics is an effect of alcohol; hypoxia, hypersmolarity, hypomagnesemia, or hypoglycemia may be contributing (39).

The exact pathophysiologic mechanism for the acute alcohol withdrawal syndrome is uncertain. With hyperventilation and respiratory alkalosis, a corresponding rise in arterial pH and fall in serum magnesium takes place. Central nervous system excitability, altered sleep patterns, and other signs of withdrawal are experienced, probably as a result of decreased cerebral blood flow and oxygen delivery to the brain and electrolyte imbalance.

Management

The object of detoxification is to remove alcohol from the body with as few withdrawal symptoms as possible. This process involves the substitution and slow withdrawing of a long-acting sedative-hypnotic drug for the shorter-acting one, alcohol. Some patients in case of mild withdrawal may not require drugs for relief. In the past 25 years, over 100 different drugs and drug combinations have been described in the medical literature for the treatment of acute alcohol withdrawal (33, 44–53).

A review of studies that investigated the effectiveness of drugs in treating the withdrawal syndrome suggests that many are poorly controlled and lack objective comparisons of effects. In carefully conducted studies, some drugs have not been shown to be necessarily or universally much more effective than placebos. The major benefit of the antianxiety agents may be, in many instances, for the nursing and medical staff as the patient is made more manageable.

Drug Therapy

Benzodiazepines (diazepam, chlordiazepoxide, clorazepate, oxazepam, lorazepam). The sedative-hypnotic drugs of this group when compared with others in this class of agents are longer-acting, safer, do not produce gastritis, and have antiseizure activity. They are used also because of the convenient dosage forms available. Diazepam and chlordiazepoxide can be administered by oral and intravenous routes. Lorazepam is available in oral and parenteral dosage forms. Clorazepate and oxazepam are available in the oral form. The usual therapeutic end point in the management of acute alcohol withdrawal symptoms is to produce a calmed but awake patient, using whatever doses are required (33, 55).

The pharmacokinetics of these drugs in patients undergoing alcohol withdrawal or in patients with mild liver impairment have aroused a great deal of clinical and research interest. The elimination half-lives of oxazepam, lorazepam, chlordiazepoxide, clorazepate, and diazepam are 8, 16, 16, 24, and 32 hr respectively, with wide individual variations existing. In patients with alcohol cirrhosis, the elimination of diazepam from the body is presumably decreased because of decreased clearance by the liver and increased tissue distribution. Because the major metabolites of benzodiazepines, with the exception of oxazepam and lorazepam, are also psychoactive, accumulation of effects during chronic administration of these drugs should be evaluated carefully in patients with cirrhosis. No evidence suggests that any one of the benzodiazepines is better than another for use in acute alcohol detoxification. Most studies on the use of benzodiazepines in this situation have been conducted with chlordiazepoxide. Oxazepam and lorazepam might be considered the drugs of choice, particularly in patients with liver disease who are likely to have impaired metabolism of these drugs.

Dose requirements of these drugs for detoxification are quite variable. The usual range for diazepam is 30 to 200 mg during the first 24 hr, but a few cases may require 1000 mg or more. Withdrawing alcoholics may require more sedative-hypnotic drug than other agitated patients, probably because of tolerance and decreased sensitivity (54). Some alcoholic patients are calmed only by doses that would be severely depressive in nonalcoholic patients. Because dose requirements are variable, no fixed dose schedule can be predicted for a given patient. In a patient undergoing a mild-to-moderate withdrawal syndrome, an initial oral dose of 20 mg diazepam can be administered orally, followed by 10 to 20 mg every 2 to 3 hr. However, elderly patients should receive only 10 mg initially, followed by doses every 4 to 6 hr if needed. If chlordiazepoxide is the preferred drug, 25 to 100 mg can be given every 2 to 6 hr, depending on symptoms. A total dose of 400 to 600 mg may be needed by extremely tolerant individuals with severe symptoms. In the elderly patient, 50 mg two to four times a day should be sufficient for symptom relief.

Every patient should be reevaluated and drug requirements reassessed every few hr until initial sedation is achieved and then at least daily during the maintenance phase. Standing orders for repetitive doses are not advisable. In cases of severe withdrawal, intravenous diazepam should be administered cautiously in a dose of 10 to 30 mg every 30 min or more until the patient is calm. Once calmed, a maintenance regimen of 10 to 20 mg can be given intravenously or orally as needed during the day and in the evening to enable sleep. Because of the risks of hypotension and respiratory depression, the patient should be assessed before and periodically after every intravenous dose of a sedative-hypnotic drug. Intramuscular administration of the benzodiazepines should be avoided because of its slow and erratic absorption. With the shorter-acting benzodiazepines, loading doses are not required; however, to maintain blood levels sufficient to sustain relief from

withdrawal symptoms, doses of oxazepam and lorazepam at 15 to 30 mg and 1 to 4 mg, respectively, need to be given at 6- to 8-hr intervals. During the detoxification process these drugs should be withdrawn by lowering their dose rather than by lengthening their administration interval beyond 8 hr.

Phenothiazines. The major neuroleptics have not been shown to be any more effective than the sedative-hypnotic drugs and should not be used. They can result in increased seizures, impaired thermoregulation, extrapyramidal effects, and postural hypotension. The syncope and arrhythmias that can result from these drugs can produce serious consequences in the acutely withdrawing alcoholic.

Butyrophenones. Haloperidol in oral doses of 5 to 10 mg or 5 mg intramuscularly has been advocated for use in treating hallucinations and acute agitation associated with alcohol. Producing less sedation, hypotension, and hypothermia than the phenothiazines, haloperidol, like other dopamine antagonists, may cause extrapyramidal and centrally mediated anticholinergic reactions. Extreme caution should be exercised with the use of this drug because the central nervous system depression from the concomitant alcohol may be additive or potentiated.

Lithium. Lithium carbonate may also be an effective medication for the treatment of the acute alcohol withdrawal syndrome. Subjective symptoms of alcohol withdrawal appear to ameliorate when lithium is administered before discontinuation of the alcohol (50). The mechanism is unknown because catecholamine release, heart rate, blood pressure, and dopamine β-hydroxylase are not affected.

Clonidine. Clonidine, a centrally acting inhibitor of adrenergic vasomotor centers used in the treatment of hypertension, has been compared with benzodiazepines in the management of acute alcohol withdrawal. Used successfully to treat opiate withdrawal, clonidine can also relieve the tremors, tachycardia, systolic hypertension, and diaphoresis secondary to alcohol withdrawal and appears to be as effective as chlordiazepoxide. Since the ability of clonidine to protect against withdrawal seizures is uncertain, the drug should be given only in situations where the risks of seizures and serious medical or psychiatric complications are minimal (55).

Phenytoin. Phenytoin has been advocated for routine use in acute alcohol withdrawal to prevent seizures, but there is no evidence that the drug actually prevents seizures associated with alcohol abstinence. Prospective studies have examined the benefits of phenytoin in preventing additional seizures in alcohol withdrawal once the initial seizure has been experienced. Whether prophylaxis with phenytoin during alcohol withdrawal reduces the risk for seizures is unclear. The study most often cited as showing that the risk is reduced compared chlordiazepoxide alone and in combination with phenytoin 100 mg given orally three times a day for 5 days. While the combination was concluded to be more effective, the phenytoin blood levels were considerably lower than those usually required for seizure control (56).

The seizures associated with acute alcohol withdrawal ("rum fits") are usually self-limiting and frequently do not require anticonvulsant medication. The episode is brief, consisting usually of a single grand mal–like seizure and only occasionally appears as repeated seizures. This usually occurs in patients with a history of traumatic epilepsy or seizure onset in childhood or adolescence. In the postictal period following alcohol withdrawal seizures, very few will show electroencephalographic abnormalities. In the acute situation during status epilepticus, small doses (2 to 4 mg) of intravenous diazepam can be administered. Patients who have or are suspected to have alcohol-withdrawal seizures require careful observation and need thorough evaluation for traumatic, infectious, or metabolic causes. Withholding anticonvulsant medications over a 6 to 12 hr period may provide an opportunity to characterize any subsequent seizure that might occur (57).

Long-term antiepileptic drug therapy is unproven and not indicated for alcohol-withdrawal seizures. Focal seizures suggest a central nervous system lesion and are not alcohol-related. Patients with status epilepticus or focal seizures may experience greater risks for seizures during alcohol withdrawal. Prophylactic use of phenytoin during the detoxification process might offer some reduction of seizure risk in these circumstances.

Propranolol. Theoretically, a β-adrenergic blocking drug such as propranolol should be beneficial in preventing the adrenergic overactivity that occurs during alcohol withdrawal. The alcohol withdrawal syndrome is likely to be mediated in part by the autonomic system (58). Few clinical studies on the use of β-blockers in alcohol withdrawal have been published. A trial comparing atenolol, a β-blocker, with placebo in a large group of hospitalized alcohol-withdrawing patients, showed that the drug had an ameliorating effect on the symptoms experienced. Because β-blockers lack anticonvulsant activity, both groups also received oxazepam 15 or 30 mg q.i.d. The results showed a shorter hospital stay, a reduced need for benzodiazepines during hospitalization, and a more rapid return of vital signs to normal in the atenolol-treated patients (59). Propranolol has been shown to be effective in reducing tremor, blood pressure, heart rate, and urinary and total catecholamine levels in alcohol-withdrawing patients.

Potential hazards include the precipitation of congestive heart failure, asthmatic attacks, and peripheral vascular insufficiency, and the masking of symptoms of hypoglycemia. Benefits from the use of propranolol should, nevertheless, be weighed carefully in each case against its risks before it can be considered as a therapeutic agent for acute alcohol withdrawal syndrome.

Paraldehyde. The difficulty in administering this drug, the variability in dose response, and the currently recommended use of safer drugs (e.g., benzodiazepines) have reduced the use of paraldehyde in treating alcoholic withdrawal (44). This traditional and once popular drug was used widely in the treatment of alcohol withdrawal. A major complication of this drug is the ability to produce an acidosis from its acetaldehyde and acetic acid metabolites, which further complicate an already altered acid-base status. Paraldehyde is primarily metabolized in the liver, and its potential for hepatotoxicity should be recognized, particularly when administered to a patient where severe hepatic impairment may exist. Oral or rectal administration is impractical in an acutely agitated alcoholic and causes local irritation of mucous membranes.

Ethanol. The use of alcohol in the management of acute alcohol withdrawal symptoms is hazardous because of its short duration of action and the risk of continuing the metabolic, endocrine, and neurologic disturbances and pathologies.

Antihistamines-Hydroxyzine. These drugs have been recommended by some and are sometimes used, although clinical investigations suggest only equivocal therapeutic benefits. They are less effective in seizure control and their antianxiety effects have not been well established. Toxic doses of antihistamines may produce anticholinergic symptoms such as delirium and tachycardia that may be confused with acute alcohol withdrawal.

Thiamine (Vitamin B₁). The most serious consequences of thiamine deficiency experienced by chronic alcoholics are neuromuscular effects. Wernicke's syndrome and Korsakoff's syndrome, characterized by ophthalmoplegia, ataxia, peripheral neuropathy, and progressive confusion, are manifestations of the deficiency (23, 60). Thiamine is routinely administered intravenously (100 to 200 mg) to withdrawing alcoholics as a preventative measure. Because glucose solutions are invariably administered to such patients, deficient stores of thiamine may be further depleted as a result.

Vitamin K. Vitamin K is used particularly in patients with alcoholic hepatitis or cirrhosis because prothrombin production is frequently impaired.

Folic Acid. The moderate-to-severe anemia seen in alcoholics is usually of the megaloblastic type caused by folic acid deficiency. A combined megaloblastic anemia and microcytic anemia indicating iron deficiency usually results from blood loss in addition to nutritional deficits (24).

Fluids, Glucose, and Electrolytes. It is important to correct fluid and electrolytes imbalances, particularly sodium, potassium, and magnesium, accompanying acute withdrawal (61, 62). In some patients, water is retained and renal resorption of sodium, potassium, and chloride is increased, contrary to the notion that all acutely withdrawing alcoholics are dehydrated from the diuresis produced by alcohol (20). An observation common in patients with severe alcohol withdrawal is hypomagnesemia, with serum levels ranging from 0.7 to 1.4 mEq/liter. Since symptoms of withdrawal such as tremor, hyperreflexia, and seizures are similar to those associated with this condition, the administration of magnesium is thought to aid in reducing the severity and even preventing some of these symptoms.

Summary

The following considerations should be kept in mind when treating and caring for the alcoholic patient in the acute withdrawal phase. The acute alcohol-withdrawal syndrome and response to treatment will vary among alcoholic patients. Polydrug abuse occurs in the chronic alcoholic, and withdrawal from barbiturates or opiates would further complicate therapy. An opiate-dependent person who is also dependent on alcohol is generally detoxified from the alcohol while being maintained on methadone. Benzodiazepines are the drugs of choice for treating the acute alcohol-withdrawal syndrome because they are distinctly safer than other medications. Patient variables may influence the pharmacokinetics of benzodiazepines, the dose, and the route of administration. The doses of the medication used to treat withdrawal symptoms should be tapered to avoid delayed withdrawal symptoms. Complete eradication of withdrawal symptoms may indicate overmedication. Medical and surgical illness may worsen the acute withdrawal syndrome. Nondrug factors such as staff attitude and ward environment can be effective in helping with the anxiety, insomnia, depression, and other problems that often occur during acute detoxification. There is no evidence that drug therapy during acute alcohol detoxification modifies the outcome of long-term treatment of alcoholism. Detoxification is the first, not the final, step in therapy for alcoholism. The most important factors in successful treatment of and recovery from alcoholism are the motivation of the patient to stop drinking and ongoing participation in recovery support programs, such as Alcoholics Anonymous.

ACUTE INTOXICATION FROM ALCOHOL SUBSTITUTES

Occasionally, alcohol substitutes such as methanol, ethylene glycol, isopropyl alcohol or paraldehyde are ingested. Often the availability and low cost of products containing alcohol substitutes by comparison to alcoholic beverages, make it convenient for persons intent on drinking alcohol to seek out these products. Many of these products are readily found around the home; they are sweet smelling and pleasant tasting, often colorless, and appear innocuous enough to young children who might be attracted to them. Many of these products are packaged in an attractive man-

ner and not in child-resistant containers, thus contributing to risks of accidental ingestion. Differences in the clinical manifestations following ingestion of these agents distinguish each of them (Table 57.3).

Methanol

Following ingestion, methanol is rapidly absorbed and distributed throughout the total body water, like ethanol. The toxic dose is extremely variable; as little as 4 ml has been reported to cause blindness, while no permanent impairment was demonstrated after an alleged 500 ml had been consumed. Methanol is metabolized by alcohol dehydrogenase enzymes in the liver to formaldehyde and formic acid. The rate of this process is independent of the dose and blood concentration and is approximately one-seventh the rate for ethanol metabolism. Formic acid accumulation is associated with the clinical symptoms experienced.

Methanol produces slight central nervous system depression; unlike ethanol, inebriation is not often observed. Optic nerve and retinal injury from the toxic metabolites develop within 12 to 24 hr following acute exposure. An asymptomatic period of up to a day may follow an acute methanol poisoning before the onset of headache, nausea, and vomiting. Severe abdominal pain, occasionally presumed mistakenly to be the result of ethanol-induced pancreatitis, is experienced. Central nervous system depression, coma, and respiratory failure take place late in the course. The breath odor of alcohol or methanol is frequently not present. In the later stages of the intoxication, the breath odor of formalin and Kussmaul respiration may be noticed. Visual disturbances will occur. They range in severity from mild diminished vision to total blindness, very often accompanied by photophobia, pain, and conjunctival changes. Eye examination will show dilated, nonreactive pupils with optic disk hyperemia and retinal edema. The early recognition of the clinical presentation of acute methanol intoxication is commonly hampered by the effects of concomitant excessive ethanol ingestion.

Laboratory findings in acute methanol intoxication usually include metabolic acidosis, with a large anion gap and moderate ketonemia. Serum amylase activity is often markedly elevated. A significant leukocytosis is also part of this poisoning. Urine analysis will yield albuminuria with slight to moderate acetonuria. Differential diagnostic considerations would necessarily include diabetic ketoacidosis, lactic acidosis, uremic acidosis, and acute intoxication from ethylene glycol, paraldehyde, isoniazid, or salicylates. Detection of methanol and formic acid in the urine would confirm methanol poisoning.

Early diagnosis and vigorous treatment of methanol poisoning can be sight- and life-saving. A methanol blood level can be obtained. It is estimated that for each 40 mg/dl of methanol in blood, there is an accompanying rise in plasma osmolality of 15 mOsm/kg H_2O. Sodium bicarbonate to reverse the metabolic acidosis and ethanol, either intravenously or orally, should be administered. Ethanol with its greater affinity for alcohol dehydrogenase can competitively inhibit generation of the toxic metabolites of methanol. Blood ethanol levels of 100 mg/dl or higher are required to saturate the liver enzyme alcohol dehydrogenase. A loading dose of ethanol of 0.6 g/kg body weight, or about 40 g for a 70-kg person, is needed to achieve this desired concentration in the blood. This dose can be given conveniently by mouth with four 1-ounce shots of 80-proof whiskey or intravenously as 500 ml of a 10% ethanol solution. Maintenance doses of ethanol should average 7 to 10 g/hr or 109 mg/kg/hr. Hemodialysis is an effective method of treating methanol poisoning and should be initiated promptly when the blood methanol level exceeds 50 mg/dl. Rapid blood methanol level reduction appears to be critical for a favorable outcome. Doses of ethanol required to maintain a blood level of 100 mg/dl should be increased to 237 mg/kg/hr. Therefore, a total of 17 g of ethanol must be given hourly during dialysis for a 70-kg person to satisfactorily maintain the desired ethanol blood level. Blood levels of ethanol should be monitored frequently until the methanol has been cleared from the blood (63).

If an acute ingestion of methanol has taken place within several minutes to a few hours from the time of ingestion to initiation of treatment, further gastrointestinal absorption should be decreased with activated charcoal and removal by emesis or lavage. Respiratory and circulatory support should be established and maintained. Forced diuresis does not enhance elimination of either methanol or its metabolites.

Ethylene Glycol

The initial symptoms of acute ethylene glycol poisoning are similar to those for acute ethanol intoxication except for differences in their onset and duration. The earliest sign of ethylene glycol intoxication is inebriation. A breath odor of alcohol is conspicuously absent in persons who have ingested only ethylene glycol. Central nervous system depression and gastrointestinal distress are experienced early in the course. During the first 12 hr, hypertension and leukocytosis are frequently seen. Symptoms may progressively worsen until pulmonary edema, convulsions, respiratory failure, and coma occur (30). Ethylene glycol itself is relatively nontoxic, but its metabolic products are responsible for considerable toxicity. Severe metabolic acidosis, similar to that experienced with acute methanol poisoning, is seen. Glyoxylic acid, oxalic acid, and hippurate are the acid breakdown products of ethylene glycol which cause this profound acidosis. The overproduction and accumulation of lactate and other organic acids also contribute to the acidosis. Acute oliguric renal failure can occur. This is usually severe and believed to be irreversible,

although survival from this condition has occurred. There is marked renal pathology, including focal hemorrhagic necrosis, oxalate crystals in the convoluted renal tubules, and epithelial cell destruction. Calcium oxalate crystals, considered an important diagnostic marker for ethylene glycol poisoning, are frequently but not always seen on urinalysis. Urinalysis normally shows albumin, red blood cells, and casts.

Myopathy is another common feature of ethylene glycol poisoning. Searching for signs of ethylene glycol is not often helpful for establishing an early diagnosis. Blood ethylene glycol, if the test is rapidly available, is more useful. Serum osmolality can be used to provide an estimation of the toxic ethylene glycol concentration. For every 50 mg/dl of ethylene glycol, the plasma osmolality is increased by 10 mOsm/kg H_2O. A high anion and osmolal gap with metabolic acidosis is quite characteristic of this poisoning. Treatment of acute ethylene glycol poisoning is focused on preventing metabolism to the toxic metabolites and enhancing its elimination from the body. Ethanol inhibits the metabolism of ethylene glycol by competitively competing for alcohol dehydrogenase. The monitoring and pharmacokinetic considerations of ethanol administration, which have been described for methanol, are applicable for ethylene glycol. The necessity for rapid treatment in ethylene glycol cannot be overstated. Since the half-life of ethylene glycol is approximately 3 hr, ethanol administration should be initiated promptly. Alkalinization should be attempted, with consideration for risks of volume overload and exacerbation of existing electrolyte imbalance.

Hemodialysis readily eliminates ethylene glycol and its metabolites from the body. Blood ethylene glycol levels should be closely monitored because redistribution of the alcohol from tissue to the body water often occurs after dialysis. Repeated dialysis may be necessary to completely clear the ethylene glycol. Support of vital functions such as ventilation, perfusion, and volume are important as in all acute overdoses involving the alcohols.

Isopropyl Alcohol

Isopropyl alcohol is rapidly absorbed following ingestion. Peak plasma levels with distribution throughout body fluids and tissues may be reached within an hour. Inhalation of isopropyl alcohol vapors can produce considerable systemic absorption. With the exception of children, skin absorption is minimal. Coma has been experienced by children who were bathed with excessive amounts of rubbing alcohol. Isopropyl alcohol is metabolized in the liver by alcohol dehydrogenase enzymes to form acetone. Only 15% of this alcohol, when consumed, is eliminated as acetone via the saliva, lungs, and kidneys. The remainder is further converted to acetate, formate, and carbon dioxide. The rate of isopropyl alcohol metabolism to acetone is slower than that of ethanol. Both isopropyl alcohol and acetone are central nervous system depressants. Tolerance to the toxic levels of both is experienced similarly to the ethanol tolerance seen in chronic alcoholics. Toxic symptoms can occur with an ingestion of as little as 20 ml. Deaths from ingestion of 4 to 8 ounces of 70% isopropyl alcohol have been reported. The symptoms of acute isopropyl alcohol intoxication are similar to those of acute ethanol intoxication except for the absence of any early stimulatory phase. Dizziness, headache, confusion, flushing sensation, ataxia, stupor, hypothermia, and hypotension may be felt. Nausea, vomiting, diarrhea, and severe gastritis occasionally accompanied by bleeding are frequent. Children are often hypoglycemic. Respiratory failure and death can occur within a few hours following a sufficient ingestion of isopropyl alcohol. Marked hypotension and renal and hepatic dysfunction are ominous predictors of outcome on such occasions.

Volume for volume, the toxicity of isopropyl alcohol is considered twice that of ethanol. Toxic symptoms are noticed when blood isopropyl alcohol levels reach 50 mg/dl. In children, symptoms are likely to occur at even lower levels. Coma is associated with levels above 120 mg/dl. The range of blood isopropyl alcohol between fatal and severe nonfatal intoxication is narrow. Acetonuria and acetonemia in the absence of glucosuria, hyperglycemia, or acidemia in an acutely intoxicated patient should arouse suspicion of acute isopropyl alcohol poisoning. Unlike ethanol, there is no fixed relationship between the concentration of isopropyl alcohol in the blood and urine, therefore, blood level determination in such circumstances is necessary.

There is no specific treatment for an acute isopropyl alcohol overdose. Usual methods for preventing further and continuous absorption, giving symptomatic and supportive treatment to maintain vital function, should be used. Forced diuresis is of little value. Hemodialysis has been shown to be life-saving in severe and unresponsive isopropyl alcohol poisoning. Repeated gastric lavage to prevent continued reabsorption of isopropyl alcohol has been reported to successfully reverse severe acute toxic symptoms. Use of serial activated charcoal may be effective in removing this alcohol. Many manufacturers of rubbing alcohol have begun to substitute ethanol for isopropyl alcohol, presumably because it is less toxic. Whenever dealing with a history of acute rubbing alcohol ingestion, determine which of these alcohols is the product prior to treatment.

MANAGEMENT OF CHRONIC ALCOHOLISM

Although the period of detoxification is relatively short, it may take months for the physiologic processes to return to normal. Treatment of the chronic alcoholic is enhanced by maintaining a prolonged alcohol-free period after detoxification.

It is commonly thought that alcoholism is primarily a manifestation of underlying psychiatric problems, and most methods of treatment and dealing with those problems will not succeed while the patient continues to drink. A variety of pharmacotherapeutic approaches are available for management of chronic alcoholism, including use of medications either alone or in combination with behavior modification techniques. While some recovering alcoholics feel that recovery requires total abstinence from any medication, successful recovery maintenance for some depends upon pharmacotherapy under the direction of a physician experienced in addiction medicine.

Disulfiram

Disulfiram is considered best used in the context of a close physician-patient or therapist-patient relationship with attempts at behavioral modification (64). Although disulfiram has been available and used for more than 30 years, a consensus on its therapeutic utility has still not been developed because of methodologic problems inherent in studies without accurate definitions for the stages of the disorder or a method to assess compliance.

Mechanism of Action. When administered alone, disulfiram is relatively nontoxic, but in the presence of alcohol, it alters alcohol metabolism. Disulfiram causes an increase in the blood acetaldehyde levels by interfering with acetaldehyde dehydrogenase action, producing an acetaldehyde syndrome. It also inhibits dopamine β-hydroxylase, leading to the release and depletion of norepinephrine stores. The patient becomes flushed and develops a scarlet appearance, and as the vasodilation continues, palpitations, chest pain, hyperventilation, headache, tachycardia, weakness, hypotension, and syncope occur. Respiratory difficulty, nausea, vomiting, blurred vision, and vertigo may also occur. The reaction may be produced by as little as a few milliliters of alcohol and can last from 30 min to several hours. The action of disulfiram may last up to 10 days after the patient's last dose. At higher blood alcohol levels, more marked symptoms are experienced, including cardiac arrhythmias, heart failure, and death.

Treatment of the Disulfiram-Alcohol Reaction. The intensity and duration of symptoms are related to the disulfiram dosage, the amount of alcohol consumed, and individual sensitivity. Blood alcohol levels as low as 5 to 10 mg/dl can cause a mild reaction. Although the disulfiram-alcohol reaction is usually short-lived and without major sequelae, death can occur. In many fatal cases, the disulfiram dose was excessive, but others had no apparent explanation. In these inexplicable cases, the causes of death were intracranial hemorrhage, acute myocardial infarction, pulmonary edema, and cerebral edema (65).

There are reports of antidotal treatment of the disulfiram-alcohol reaction with ascorbic acid, iron salts, or antihistamines, but the results are not definitive. Intravenous administration of ascorbic acid (0.5 to 2.0 g) is based on experimental evidence that ascorbic acid appears to reverse the disulfiram inhibition of cellular oxidation. However, nonspecific supportive measures such as placing the patient in Trendelenburg posture, administration of oxygen, infusion of fluids and solutes, and (if needed) vasopressor agents are more beneficial than the unproved use of these questionable antidotes. Table 57.4 summarizes the special factors to be considered in the use of disulfiram.

Pharmacokinetics. Disulfiram is rapidly absorbed from the gastrointestinal tract and achieves full pharmacologic action in approximately 12 hr. Disulfiram is eliminated slowly; approximately 20% still remains in the body after a week.

Adverse Effects. Although disulfiram is relatively safe in most cases, it can cause acneform eruptions, fatigue, tremor, restlessness, impotence, and a garlicky or metallic taste in the mouth. With large doses, psychologic depression occurs, probably as a result of interference in dopamine β-hydroxylase activity in the brain. Disulfiram also retards the metabolism of oral anticoagulants, isoniazid, and other drugs (Table 57.5). Any patient receiving disulfiram should be warned to avoid medications that contain alcohol, particularly over-the-counter preparations such as some cough and cold medications, tonics, antihistamines, body and after-shave lotions, colognes, mouthwashes, and alcohol sponges (66).

Dosage. The usual initial dosage of disulfiram is 250 to 500 mg/day for 5 to 7 days. The dosage may then be reduced to 125 to 250 mg/day.

Sedative-Hypnotic Drugs

Anxiety, depression, and insomnia are common in chronic alcoholics. Under most circumstances, these symptoms can be treated supportively, without psychotropic medications. The indiscriminate prescribing of antianxiety agents is all too frequent, and they have a high abuse potential in the alcoholic population. There is no evidence to support outpatient use of psychotropic drugs in the long-term treatment of alcoholism. The use of placebos for relief of anxiety may be worthwhile when basic behavioral problems are dealt with concomitantly.

Tricyclic Antidepressants

Tricyclic antidepressants for patients in need of therapy for chronic and severe depression should be considered only after careful evaluation of the patient. Tricyclic antidepressant drugs are too frequently a convenient means of suicide in the depressed alcoholic patient. When antidepressants are prescribed for an alcoholic patient, the patient should be warned that the concomitant use of alcohol or other central nervous depressing agents with these drugs will produce severe impairment of motor and sensory function.

Lithium

Some studies suggest that lithium, which is indicated for manic depressive disorders, may prevent the progress of primary alcoholism; however, results of these investigations indicate that a comprehensive evaluation of lithium

Table 57.4.
Considerations in Use of Disulfiram

Assessment	Management	Evaluation
Assess for informed consent motivation, social stability	Adequate blood level may take up to 4 days, although effect begins within 12 hr; the effect may last up to a week after discontinuation of disulfiram	Check for side effects (usually transient, lasting 2 weeks), drowsiness, fatigue, impotence, acneform eruption, metallic taste
Persons with moderate to severe hypertension, psychiatric problems, suicidal ideation should not receive this drug	Metallic taste may cause anorexia; good oral hygiene may decrease taste	Nausea and vomiting, dizziness, hypotension, headache, syncope, and flushed face in disulfiram-alcohol reaction
Interview patient	Tell patient to avoid alcohol; give list of OTC drugs and foods containing alcohol	Check for other medications being taken; i.e., phenytoin, barbiturates, isoniazid, metronidazole, or warfarin; disulfiram can potentiate their therapeutic or toxic effects
	Paraldehyde may cause reaction and should not be given	
	Give with caution concurrently with central nervous system depressants; may potentiate their effects	
	Patient should carry appropriate medical alert identification with this drug	

Table 57.5.
Nutritional Problems Associated with Alcoholism

Source	Signs and Symptoms	Comments
Protein	Fatty liver and hypoalbuminema may be result of deterioration of liver function or low protein intake; others: hypocholesterolemia, edema, normocytic anemia	Association of alcohol with liver disease complicates the interpretation of many clinical signs of protein deficiency. Alcoholic liver disease is not prevented by eating well or by limiting alcohol consumption only to certain types of beverages. Administration of protein to patients with severe active alcoholic cirrhosis can precipitate hepatic coma. When protein is poorly tolerated or the patient becomes progressively disoriented, showing asterixis or flapping tremors, administration of protein should be discontinued.
Water-soluble vitamins, vitamin B complexes, thiamine	The signs and symptoms are variable depending on severity of the deficiency: opthalmoplegia, sixth-nerve palsy, nystagmus, weakness, ataxia, peripheral neuropathies, confusion, amnesia, coma, heart failure, Wernicke's syndrome, "beriberi" heart disease, sudden death	Most common deficiency in alcoholics. Polyneuropathy is the mildest and most common form of thiamine deficiency. Depressed tendon reflexes, muscle cramps, weakness, paresthesia and pain develop. The lower extremities are most often affected. Prognosis grave and must be recognized early. Treatment is to give thiamine. Administration of glucose without thiamine may further deplete stores of thiamine. Thiamine deficiency–induced heart failure does not respond well to digitalis or diuretics. Animal studies suggest that thiamine deficiency reduces myocardial oxygen consumption due to deficiency of the coenzyme thiamine pyrophosphate. Average requirement for is 1.5–2 mg/day thiamine for adults. Alcoholics often will require more; 100–200 mg results in dramatic reversal of signs and symptoms.
Niacin	Weakness, photosensitive dermatitis, stomatitis, gastritis, diarrhea, peripheral neuropathy, dementia, encephalopathy	Alcoholic pellagra is the result of the lack of dietary nicotinic acid or its precursor, tryptophan. Niacin contributes to formation of specific coenzyme nucleotides (NAD) which participate in intracellular metabolism and cell respiration. Replacement dose is 200 mg niacinamide three times a day.
Riboflavin	Weakness, photosensitive dermatitis, stomatitis, gastritis, diarrhea, peripheral neuropathy, dementia, encephalopathy	Riboflavin deficiency usually accompanies alcoholic pellagra. Riboflavin is an essential constituent of coenzymes responsible for oxidative and electron transport processes. Replacement dose is 10 mg per day.
Pyridoxine	Irritability, anemia, insominia, peripheral neuropathy, ataxia, skin lesions	Pyridoxine is responsible for a variety of enzymatic activities particularly related to nitrogen metabolism.
Ascorbic acid	Anorexia, petechial ecchymoses, gingivitis and bleeding gums, dry mouth, loss of hair, perifollicular hemorrhages, purpuric lesions, ecchymoses, itchy dry skin, weakness, lethargy	Ascorbic acid is a coenzyme involved in the metabolism of amino acids. Usual amount recommended is 10 mg/day.
Folic acid	Macrocytic anemia, reticulocytosis	Deficiency of folic acid is the primary cause of macrocytic anemia in chronic alcoholics. Alcohol directly affects the hemotopoietic activity and interferes with utilization of folic acid. Must discontinue alcohol. Usual amount recommended for replacement is 1.0 mg daily.
Magnesium	Lethargy, muscle weakness, coarse athetoid movements, gross tremors of hands and tongue, mental changes, convusions, stupor, coma	Alcohol promotes the renal excretion of magnesium. Renal effect and inadequate diet cause significant depletion. Symptoms of acute alcohol withdrawal are often complicated by coexisting magnesium depletion. The total body magnesium deficits are not reflected by serum magnesium levels.
Potassium	Weakness, lethargy	Poor dietary intake of potassium and loss by diuresis, vomiting, and diarrhea contribute to hypokalemia.

for further evidence of its efficacy is needed (67). The dual diagnosis of other psychiatric illnesses accompanying alcoholism has been increasing, with manic-depressive illness a not infrequent diagnosis. In such cases, lithium therapy may support recovery and might affect the course of alcoholism.

Diet

Malnutrition is commonplace among alcoholics (31). Chronic alcohol consumption results in impaired digestion and absorption of essential nutrients. Nearly all alcoholics have diminished food intake while drinking, because alcohol presumably suppresses appetite. Alcohol represents "empty calories" lacking in nutritive value. In excess, alcohol also prevents adequate gastrointestinal absorption of nutrients and contributes to debilitated and malnourished conditions. Nutritional problems that alcoholics are most susceptible to are deficiencies of protein, water-soluble vitamins, and minerals (Table 57.6).

Accumulation of fluids with resultant ascites is a frequent complication of alcoholic cirrhosis. It is secondary to nutritional, endocrine, and metabolic disorders resulting from alcoholism. The basis of management is to supply a normal or fortified diet with restricted sodium intake to replace only daily losses. "Hidden sources" of sodium such as intravenously administered fluids including plasma and drugs may be responsible for unexpected reaccumulation of fluids in these patients. Careful monitoring for problems of nutritional balance in the hospitalized alcoholic patient is essential for successful management and care.

Nondrug Treatment Methods

Often alcoholics enter treatment under threat from family, employer, or the courts; they may not initially want the help. Treatment initially attempts to break through the denial systems and help the alcoholic to realize that alcoholism is a disease that can be treated. Recovery from alcoholism is a life-long process. Relapse is only one drink away for alcoholics; they usually consider themselves "recovering" rather than "recovered" alcoholics.

Several techniques for behavioral modification are used with the chronic alcoholic. Individual psychotherapy is useful in patients who are intelligent, well-motivated, and financially secure. Group psychotherapy allows interaction among alcoholics to deal with difficulties they have in common. An estimated success rate of 80 to 90% of health professionals and 70% of employed people who participate in a full-recovery program for at least 2 years can be contrasted with a 4-year sobriety rate of less than 5% for "skid row" alcoholics. In managing the chronic alcoholic, the goal is to achieve and maintain sobriety or prolong the periods of sobriety to give the patient time to learn to identify and avoid factors that may promote drinking or so-called slips.

The preferred full-recovery program includes (a) education about the disease of alcoholism; (b) abstinence from alcohol and other psychoactive substances (not forever, but "one day at a time," as is recommended by Alcoholics Anonymous, or AA); (c) group therapy (regular attendance at Alcoholics Anonymous meetings or the equivalent; formal, interactive group therapy, preferably for at least 2 years; and family therapy, including participation of family members in Al-Anon or similar support group meetings). Initially, treatment may involve formal participation in an inpatient (residential) treatment program, usually for several weeks, followed by intensive outpatient therapy for a number of weeks, then regular aftercare meetings, usually

through the treatment provider. Difficult cases may require more prolonged inpatient therapy, while relatively uncomplicated, low-risk cases may be managed totally on an outpatient basis.

Employee assistance programs are available through most major employers; these programs often require employees to sign a recovery agreement. Such agreements assure understanding of the terms of continued employment, encourage ongoing sobriety, and provide employers with assurance of compliance. Random drug screening at employee expense is often a stated condition of the agreement.

For individuals who have inadequate support systems in place at home to assure sobriety during outpatient therapy or early in the recovery process following such therapy, halfway houses may be utilized. These provide a community living environment with fairly rigid rules, ongoing group therapy, and requirements, such as maintaining employment, that encourage responsibility and social adaptation during sobriety. Halfway houses are most often used by individuals recovering from drug addictions other than alcohol and by individuals with multiple addictions.

The group support approach of AA takes a more structured and evangelistic attitude in dealing with alcoholics; it has returned many alcoholics to sobriety and helped to maintain ongoing recovery. Basic tenants of AA's 12 steps are acceptance of the disease nature of alcoholism, acceptance of an internal locus of control in life, "cleaning house" (guilt reduction through the process of confession and maintenance of ongoing honesty), and helping other alcoholics. AA is a private organization whose members offer mutual support to each other to remain free of alcohol. Meetings occur regularly in most communities, and globally, in most countries. Individuals in early recovery are often encouraged to attend 90 AA meetings in 90 days; this encourages the alcoholic to maintain frequent contact with a support system and forces them to attend a number of different meetings. Since AA meetings vary in format and character, recovering alcoholics can eventually identify meetings that meet their specific needs and schedules. Other similar groups such as the Salvation Army and Volunteers of America also have help groups for assisting in the recovery of alcoholics. Alcoholism resources listed in the yellow pages of telephone books can identify these and other treatment and support resources in the community. Many support groups exist for specific populations, such as lawyers, physicians, pharmacists, and nurses. These exist to provide support for problems unique to recovery for each group and are not intended to replace participation in other support groups, such as AA.

ALCOHOL-DRUG INTERACTIONS

Because approximately 70 to 80% of adults consume alcoholic beverages, it is almost inevitable that medications

Table 57.6.
Summary of Selected Alcohol-Drug Interactions

Drugs Interacting with Alcohol	Mechanism	Effect	Significance
Anticoagulants (oral): warfarin	Metabolism enhanced with chronic alcohol abuse	Diminished anticoagulant effect	Moderate
	Metabolism reduced with acute alcohol intoxication	Increased anticoagulant effect	Moderate
Antihistamines	Additive	Increased central nervous system (CNS) depression	Moderate
Aspirin (and other salicylates)	Additive	Increased occult blood loss and damage to gastric mucosa	Moderate
Acetaminophen	Metabolism enhanced in chronic alcohol abuse	Increase risk for hepatotoxicity	Moderate
	Metabolism reduced in acute alcohol intoxication	Reduce risk for hepatotoxicity	Moderate
Anticonvulsants: phenytoin (Dilantin) and others	Metabolism enhanced with chronic alcohol abuse	Diminished anticonvulsant effect	Moderate
	Metabolism reduced with acute alcohol intoxication	Increased anticonvulsant effect	Moderate
Antimicrobials:			
isoniazid	Metabolism enhanced in chronic alcohol abuse	Diminished isoniazid effect	Moderate
		Increased incidence of isoniazid hepatitis	Not established
metronidazole, chloramphenicol, griseofulvin	Metabolism of alcohol reduced	Disulfiram-like reaction	Minor
Antidiabetic agents: sulfonylureas, tolbutamide (Orinase) chloropropamide (Diabinese)	Additive	Hypoglycemia effect increased	Moderate
	Metabolism enhanced in chronic alcohol abuse	Decreased effect	Moderate in chronic alcoholic
acetohexamide (Dymelor)	Accumulation of acetaldehyde	Disulfiram-like reaction	Moderate
phenformin (DBI)	Alteration of biochemical pathway	Lactic acidosis	Major
insulin	Interferes with hepatic gluconeogenesis	Increased hypoglycemic effects	Moderate but major if liver is damaged
Antihypertensives: methyldopa (Aldomet),	Additive	Sedation	Minor to moderate
reserpine, methyldopa (Aldomet), guanethidine (Ismelin), hydralazine (Apresoline)	Additive	Postural hypotensive effect increased	Minor to moderate
Disulfiram (Antabuse)	Inhibits intermediate metabolism of alcohol	Abdominal cramps, flushing, vomiting, confusion, hypotension	Major
Monoamine oxidase inhibitors: pargyline, tranylcypromine, procarbazine	Alteration of tryamine metabolism additive	Increased CNS depression, hypertensive crisis	Moderate to major
Narcotic analgesics: meperidine (Demerol), morphine, methadone	Additive	Increased CNS depression	Major
Nonbarbiturates: (ethchlorvynol, glutethimide, meprobamate), chloral hydrate	Tolerance with chronic alcohol use	Diminished CNS effect	Minor to moderate
	Additive with acute alcohol intoxication and competition for metabolic pathway	Increased CNS depression	Moderate
Nonsteroidal antiinflammatory drugs: indomethacin	Additive	Possible additive, gastric mucosal damage	Minor
Sedative-hypnotics: barbiturates (phenobarbital, pentobarbital, secobarbital)	Additive or metabolism enhanced with acute alcohol intoxication	Increased CNS depression	Major
Tranquilizers: phenothiazines (Thorazine, etc.)	Additive	Impaired coordination and judgment, also increased CNS depression	Moderate

(Continued)

Table 57.6. (*Continued*)

Drugs Interacting with Alcohol	Mechanism	Effect	Significance
Chlordiazepoxide (Librium), diazepam (Valium), flurazepam (Dalmane)	Additive	Increased CNS depression	Major
	Additive with acute alcohol intoxication	Increased CNS depression	Major
Tricyclic antidepressants: amitriptyline (Elavil, Triavil), imipramine (Tofranil), nortriptyline	Additive with acute alcohol intoxication	Possible increase in sedation, also additive to anticholinergic effects of tricyclics	Moderate
Vasodilators: nitroglycerin	Additive	Hypotension potentiated may cause cardiovascular collapse	Major
H-2 antagonist: cimetidine, ranitidine, nizatidine	Additive	Decrease gastric alcohol dehydrogenase activity resulting in increased alcohol absorption and effects	Major

either prescribed by a physician or bought over-the-counter will be taken concomitantly with alcohol or while alcohol is still in the body. Often these preparations are sources of the alcohol that interacts with prescribed medications to produce untoward effects in the unsuspecting patient (68).

Cimetidine, ranitidine, and nizatidine, but not famotidine, have been shown to decrease gastric alcohol dehydrogenase activity, resulting in increased alcohol absorption and effects (68, 69).

Alcohol administration in high concentrations results in increased metabolism by MEOS, with concurrent inhibition of metabolism of drugs that undergo microsomal degradation. Repeated administration of alcohol causes nonspecific hepatic microsomal enzyme induction, resulting in increased clearance of both alcohol and microsomally metabolized drugs, such as barbiturates (70–72). Following withdrawal of alcohol, enhanced hepatic metabolism of drugs may persist for some time, requiring higher doses of affected drugs. Metabolic pathways such as N-desmethylation of the longer-acting benzodiazepines and oxidation and glucuronidation are inhibited by acute alcohol intake. With chronic use, however, metabolism increases. This partially explains the "tolerance" to the action of sedatives observed in some chronic alcoholics. Warfarin, phenytoin, tolbutamide, procainamide, and isoniazid are nonpsychoactive drugs subject to hepatic microsomal enzyme activity. The plasma half-lives of these drugs are markedly decreased in some chronic and heavy users of alcohol as a result of their increased rate of clearance. Clinical reports of problems from such interactions, however, are few. Variable and unpredictable response to drugs in the alcoholic should suggest the possibility of some metabolic alteration of drug kinetics. It has become increasingly evident that toxicity to certain drugs and chemicals is enhanced in chronic alcoholics by this mechanism. The hepatotoxic risk with acetaminophen usage or with carbon tetrachloride ingestion is increased in chronic alcoholics because of increased formation of toxic metabolites of these chemicals caused by MEOS induction.

Alcohol is primarily a central nervous system depressant. When combined with other drugs with similar depressing action on the central nervous system, an additive or synergistic effect occurs. This is the most important type of interaction between alcohol and other drugs.

Alcoholics taking tolbutamide and other antidiabetic drugs, chloramphenicol, griseofulvin, quinacrine, or metronidazole have reported a mild disulfiram-like reaction (Table 57-6). Alcohol consumption during moxalactam, cefamandole, and cefoperazone therapy may precipitate a disulfiram-like reaction. Some alcoholic beverages such as chianti wines contain appreciable amounts of tyramine that cause an acute hypertensive episode when taken by patients using monoamine oxidase–inhibiting (MAOIs) drugs (i.e., procarbazine, pargyline). Interference with tyramine metabolism by the MAOIs results in the release of norepinephrine from the sympathetic nerve terminal.

Alcohol as a Therapeutic Agent

There is a prevailing notion that alcohol may have some usefulness in the treatment of a variety of disorders and conditions. Clinical evidence, however, is not encouraging about the role of alcohol in therapy, and it may actually worsen many conditions for which its use has been suggested (Table 57.7).

Intravenous administration of 10% volume/volume alcohol has been used with some success to delay premature labor and prolong gestation. The efficacy of this method has been compared with ritodrine to delay premature labor by inhibiting uterine contractions. Ritodrine, a synthetic sympathomimetic amine, was considered more effective. Blood alcohol levels of 100 to 150 mg/dl are required to inhibit uterine contractions. Studies of placenta and cord blood alcohol levels following delivery showed they were

Table 57.7.
"Therapeutic" Use of Alcohol

Proposed Use	Actual Effect
Relief of anxiety	Anxiety often worsens when blood alcohol level falls, as in withdrawal
Bedtime sedation	Sleeplessness is less common as blood alcohol level declines
Improvement of nutrition	Blood sugar levels become more labile; although each gram of alcohol = 7.1 calories on oxidation, "empty" calories are gained; overall nutrition not improved with alcohol because vitamins, minerals, or other essential dietary materials are absent in alcoholic beverages
Diuresis of edema	Diuretic response to alcohol occurs when blood alcohol level is on the rise; antidiuresis, hypersomality, and fluid retention occur as blood alcohol concentration falls
Anemia	Iron metabolism and bone marrow function are affected, and folate antagonism contributes to anemia in spite of frequent presence of iron in wines
Lowering of blood sugar in diabetics	Lowering of blood sugar is negligible; in fact, alcohol produces more labile blood sugar levels
Heart disease	The alcohol metabolite acetaldehyde is toxic to myocardium and not effective as a coronary vasodilator; alcohol is a myocardial depressant; although alcohol enhances coronary blood flow, myocardial oxygen consumption simultaneously increases
Antiinfective	Chronic alcoholism predisposes to systemic infections

slightly less than that of the mother. In fact, neonatal depression of respiratory and circulatory activity after administration of alcohol before delivery have been reported.

CONCLUSION

Much confusion has arisen in the midst of a widely publicized 1976 report by the Rand Corporation on alcoholism, which seems to imply that some alcoholics can return to social drinking (73). The goal of alcohol abstinence by the alcoholic has been long advocated. For instance, Alcoholics Anonymous considers abstinence as the only goal for anyone with an alcohol problem. Careful evaluation of data from this report does not support the notion that alcoholics can safely return to drinking. What it did point out was that after an 18-month period, relatively few alcoholics were practicing long-term abstinence despite an impressive improvement rate (70%). Most had intermittent periods of abstinence interspersed with "controlled" drinking. Relapse to uncontrolled drinking by those who continued to drink in a "controlled" manner and those who continued abstinence were found to be no different. Major methodological problems are suggested by the large number (more than 80%) of subjects lost to follow-up at the end of the 18-month study period. The same investigators in a 1980 follow-up report sharply modified their original claims; however, this has accomplished little to discourage the many and vocal advocates of "controlled drinking" for alcoholics (74).

Abstinence from alcohol should not be a goal for treatment but rather a means to an end. The treatment of alcoholism is best accomplished if conducted in a relationship of understanding and trust with others. This can be a concerned and interested friend or spouse; a professional person such as a pharmacist, therapist, or physician; or members of a therapeutic or rehabilitation group. The pharmacist is often asked by the recovering alcoholic or drug addict if a particular OTC or prescription medication is addicting. Pharmacists should maintain a notation of the patient's recovery status in patient profiles. Whenever possible, such individuals should avoid any psychoactive substance, including not only traditionally identified controlled substances but also alcohol in elixirs and sympathomimetics and antihistamines contained in OTC products. Relapses are documented that were caused by exposure to OTC decongestants that promote feelings similar to those experienced with the addiction. In general, a physician experienced in addiction medicine should manage therapy with any psychoactive medication. This does not mean that a recovering alcoholic or addict cannot receive controlled substances for specific, short-term uses, such as severe pain; the physician must limit the amount prescribed to no more than the amount required by most patients. The experienced physician must recognize the possibility that the recovering individual may lose control of use fairly rapidly and may attempt to obtain additional medication beyond the normal period of use.

Dependence on alcohol does not differ significantly from dependency on other addictive drugs such as opiates and barbiturates. Although there are differences in social attitudes toward drinking and drug abuse, many features of alcohol and hard drugs are remarkably similar. The similarities and differences should be appreciated and understood by those who are involved in the treatment, care, and rehabilitation of alcohol-dependent patients.

REFERENCES

1. Harwood HJ, Kristiansen P, Rachal JV: Social and economic costs of alcohol abuse and alcoholism. Issue Report No. 2. Research Triangle Park, NC: Research Triangle Institute, 1985.
2. West LJ, Maxwell DS, Noble EP, et al: Alcoholism. Ann Intern Med 100:405–416, 1984.
3. Cotton NS: The familial incidence of alcoholism. J Stud Alcohol 40:89–116, 1979.
4. Committee on Adolescence, American Academy of Pediatrics: Al-

cohol use and abuse: a pediatric concern. Pediatrics 79:450–453, 1987.

5. Blume SB: Women and alcohol. JAMA 256:1467–1470, 1986.

6. Seventh Special Report to the U.S. Congress on Alcohol and Health. Rockville, MD: National Institute on Alcohol Abuse and Alcoholism, 1990, pp 1–41.

7. Wallace J: The new disease model of alcoholism. West J Med 152:502–505, 1990.

8. Blum TC, Roman PM, Bennett N: Public images of alcoholism: data from a Georgia survey. J Stud Alcohol 50:5–14, 1989.

9. Frezza M, di Padora C, Pozzata G, et al.: High blood alcohol levels in women. N Engl J Med 322:95–99, 1990.

10. Morgan MY, Sherlock S: Sex-related differences among 100 patients with alcoholic liver diseases. Br Med J 1:939–941, 1977.

11. Ehrig T, Bosron WF, Ting-Kai L: Alcohol and aldehyde dehydrogenase. Alcohol Alcohol 25:105–116, 1990.

12. Mendelson JH: Biologic concomitants of alcoholism: Parts I and II. N Engl J Med 283:24, 71–81, 1970.

13. Lieber CS: Metabolism and metabolic effects of alcohol. Med Clin North Am 68:3–31, 1984.

14. Vessell ES, Page PG, Passananti GT: Gastric and environmental factors affecting ethanol metabolism in man. Clin Pharmacol Ther 12:192–201, 1971.

15. Blum K, Noble EP, Sheridan PJ, et al.: Allelic association of human dopamine D_2 receptor gene in alcoholism. JAMA 263:2055–2060, 1990.

16. American Psychiatric Association: Diagnostic and Statistical Manual of Mental Disorders, 3ed. rev. Washington, D.C.: American Psychiatric Association, 1987.

17. Ewing JA: Detecting alcoholism: the CAGE questionnaire. JAMA 252:1905–1907, 1984.

18. Cyr MG, Wartman SA: The effectiveness of routine screening questions in the detection of alcoholism. JAMA 259:51–54, 1988.

19. Eckardt MJ, Harford TC, Kaelbar CT, et al.: Health hazards associated with alcohol consumption. JAMA 246:648–666, 1981.

20. Kaysen G, Noth RH: The effects of alcohol on blood pressure and electrolytes. Med Clin North Am 68:221–246, 1984.

21. Williams HE: Alcoholic hypoglycemia and ketoacidosis. Med Clin North Am 68:33–38, 1984.

22. Pimstone NR, French SW: Alcoholic liver disease. Med Clin North Am 68:39–56, 1984.

23. Nakada T, Knight RT: Alcohol and the central nervous system. Med Clin North Am 68:121–131, 1984.

24. Segel LD, Klausner SC, Harney-Gnadt JJ, et al: Alcohol and the heart. Med Clin North Am 68:147–161, 1984.

25. Demakis JG, Proskey A, Rahimtoola SH: The natural course of alcohol cardiomyopathy. Ann Intern Med 80:293, 1974.

26. Haller RG, Knochel JP: Skeletal muscle disease in alcoholism. Med Clin North Am 68:91–103, 1984.

27. Adams HG, Jordan C: Infections in the alcoholic. Med Clin North Am 68:179–201, 1984.

28. Eichner ER: The hematologic disorder of alcoholism. Am J Med 54:621, 1973.

29. Larkin EC, Watson-Williams EJ: Alcohol and blood. Med Clin North Am 68:105–120, 1984.

30. Scully RE, Galdabini JJ, McNeely BU: Case records of the Massachusetts General Hospital: Case 38-1979: ethylene glycol poisoning. N Engl J Med 301:650–657, 1979.

31. Leevy C, Baker H: Vitamins and alcoholism. Am J Clin Nutr 21:1325, 1968.

32. Clarren SK, Smith DW: The fetal alcohol syndrome. N Engl J Med 298:1063, 1978.

33. Sellers EM, Kalant H: Alcohol intoxication and withdrawal. N Engl J Med 294:757–762, 1976.

34. Breeden JH: Alcohol, alcoholism and cancer. Med Clin North Am 68:163–177, 1984.

35. Lieber CS: Alcohol and the liver: 1984 update. Hepatology 4:1243–1260, 1984.

36. Altura BM: Introduction to the symposium and overview. Alcoholism (NY) 10:557–559, 1986.

37. Lange LG, Kinnunen PM: Cardiovascular effects of alcohol. Adv Alcohol Subst Abuse 6:47–52, 1987.

38. Klatsky AL: The cardiovascular effects of alcohol. Alcohol Alchohol 22(suppl 1):117–124, 1987.

39. Purdie FR, Honigman B, Rosen P: Acute organic brain syndrome: a review of 100 cases. Ann Emerg Med 10:455–461, 1981.

40. Khantzian EJ, McKenna GJ: Acute toxic withdrawal reactions associated with drug use and abuse. Ann Intern Med 90:361, 1979.

41. Coarse JF, Cardoni AA: Use of fructose in the treatment of acute alcoholic intoxication. Am J Hosp Pharm 32:518, 1975.

42. Lyon LJ, Antony J: Reversal of alcoholic coma by naloxone. Ann Intern Med 96:464–465, 1982.

43. Mattila MJ, Nuotto E, Seppala T: Naloxone is not an effective antagonist of ethanol. Lancet 1:775–776, 1981.

44. Thompson WL, Johnson AD, Maddrey WC: Diazepam and paraldehyde for treatment of severe delirium tremens. Ann Intern Med 82:175–180, 1975.

45. Golbert TM, Sanz CJ, Rose HD, et al.: Comparative evaluation of treatments of alcohol withdrawal syndrome. JAMA 201:99, 1967.

46. Kaim SC, Klett CJ, Rothefeld B: Treatment of the acute alcohol withdrawal state: a comparison of four drugs. Am J Psychiatry 125:1640–1641, 1968.

47. Kaim SC, Klett J: Treatment of delirium tremens. Q J Stud Alcohol 33:1065, 1072, 1972.

48. Sellers EM, Naranjo CA, Harrison M, et al.: Diazepam loading: simplified treatment of alcohol withdrawal. Clin Pharmacol Ther 34:822–826, 1983.

49. Zilm DH, Sellers EM: Effect of propranolol on tremor of alcohol withdrawal (letter). N Engl J Med 294:785, 1976.

50. Sellers EM, Cooper SD, Zilm DH, et al.: Lithium treatment of alcohol withdrawal. Clin Pharmacol Ther 20:199, 1976.

51. Miller WC Jr, McCurdy L: A double-blind comparison of the efficacy and safety of lorazepam and diazepam in the treatment of the acute alcohol withdrawal syndrome. Clin Therap 6:364–368, 1984.

52. Greenblatt DJ, Greenblatt M: Which drug for alcohol withdrawal? J Clin Pharmacol 12:429–431, 1972.

53. Viamontes JA: Review of drug effectiveness in the treatment of alcoholism. Am J Psychiatry 128:120, 1972.

54. Kloz UA, Avant GR, Hoyumpia A, et al: The effects of age and liver disease on the disposition and elimination of diazepam in adult man. J Clin Invest 55:347, 1975.

55. Baumgartner GR, Rowen RC: Clonidine versus chlordiazepoxide in the management of acute alcohol withdrawal syndrome. Arch Intern Med 147:1223, 1987.

56. Sampliner R, Iber FL: Diphenylhydantoin control of alcohol withdrawal seizures. JAMA 230:1430–1432, 1974.

57. Brown CG: The alcohol-withdrawal syndrome. West J Med 138:579–581, 1983.

58. Mendelson JH: Propranolol and behavior of alcoholic addicts after acute alcohol ingestion. Clin Pharmacol Ther 15:571, 1974.

59. Kraus ML, Gottlieb LD, Horwitz RI, et al.: Randomized clinical trial of atenolol in patients with alcohol withdrawal. N Engl J Med 313:905–909, 1985.

60. Victor M, Adams RD: On the etiology of the alcoholic neurologic diseases with special reference in the role of nutrition. Am J Clin Nutr 9:379, 1961.

61. Vetter WR, Cohn LH, Reichgott M: Hypokalemia and electrocardiographic abnormalities during acute alcohol withdrawal. Arch Intern Med 120:536, 1967.

62. Beard JD, Knott DH: Fluid and electrolyte balance during acute withdrawal in chronic alcoholic patients. JAMA 204:135, 1968.

63. McCoy HG, Cipolle RJ, Ehlers SM, et al.: Severe methanol poison-

ing: application of a pharmacokinetic model for ethanol therapy and hemodialysis. Am J Med 67:804–807, 1979.

64. Fuller RK, Branchey L, Brightwell DR, et al.: Disulfiram treatment of alcoholism: a Veterans Administration Cooperative study. JAMA 256:1449–1455, 1986.

65. Elenbaas RM, Ryan JL, Robinson WA, et al.: On the disulfiram-like activity of moxalactam. Clin Pharmacol Ther 32:347–355, 1982.

66. Tong TG, Bernstein LR, Alcoholism. In Herfindal E: Clinical Pharmacy and Therapeutics, ed. 3. Baltimore, Williams & Wilkins, 1983, pp 146–155.

67. Dorus W, Ostrow DG, Anton R, et al.: Lithium treatment of depressed and nondepressed alcoholics. JAMA 262:1646–1652, 1989.

68. Caballeria J, Baraona E, Rodamilans M, et al.: Effects of cimetidine on gastric alcohol dehydrogenase activity and blood ethanol levels. Gastroenterology 96:388–392, 1989.

69. Caballeria J, Baraona E, Rodamilans M, et al.: Cimetidine and alcohol absorption. Gastroenterology 97:1067–1068, 1989.

70. Lane EA, Guthrie S, Linnoila M: Effects of ethanol on drug and metabolite pharmacokinetics. Clin Pharmacokinet 10:228–247, 1985.

71. Hoyumpa AM, Schenker S: Ethanol-drug interaction. Annu Rev Med 33:113–149, 1982.

72. Lieber CS: Interaction of ethanol with drugs, hepatotoxic agents, carcinogens and vitamins. Alcohol Alcohol 25:157–176, 1990.

73. Armour DJ, Polich JM, Stambul HB: Alcoholism and Treatment. The Rand Corporation. R-1739-NIAAA, New York, John Wiley & Sons, 1978.

74. Polich JM, Armour DJ, Braiker HV: The Course of Alcoholism Four Years After Treatment. The Rand Corporation, R-2433-NIAAA, 1980.

CHAPTER 58

DRUG ABUSE

JAMES C. EOFF III, Pharm.D. and RITA G. BATES, Pharm.D.

Drug abuse in the United States reached epidemic proportions during the 1980s. Combined efforts at the local, state, and federal levels to attempt to curtail this problem have been implemented. The president has declared national "war on drugs" and many states have "drug free programs." Recent statistics indicate that drug use among junior and senior high school students has dropped slightly in the past year. While these statistics are encouraging, the war on drugs is far from being won, and the cost of drug abuse to our society continues to be great. There is a great cost to society in increased crime and violence, with 65% of all crime being drug-related. Drug abuse contributes to the rising medical costs through expensive rehabilitation and treatment programs and the spread of infectious diseases such as AIDS. Drug abuse is responsible for thousands of deaths by accidental overdosage and suicide and for half of the 45,000 traffic fatalities in the United States. Drug abuse also causes higher taxes to pay for the prevention, treatment, and rehabilitation programs, not to mention the burden to the criminal justice system, including the courts, prisons, and law enforcement agencies. Drug abuse disrupts families and schools; drug abuse lowers productivity and causes loss of creative potential. All health professionals need to be involved in education and prevention programs to help control and eliminate this problem to society.

Drug abuse is the self-administration of a drug that deviates from the approved medical or society patterns within a given society. People misuse drugs for a number of reasons. The primary factors in young people are peer pressure and the fear of being different, the desire to "fit in." Other well-known reasons for drug abuse are curiosity, boredom, escape, pleasure seeking, insecurity, and rebellion involving a desire to prove independence. Different classifications of drug abusers range from the experimental user who tries drugs only 1 or 2 times for curiosity, to the recreational users who occasionally use drugs, to the heavy users administering the drug on a daily basis. Compulsive drug users or drug dependents have a compelling desire to continue self-administration of a drug, either to experience its effects or to avoid the discomfort of its absence. This terminology is used in most reports of drug abuse and has generally replaced the term "drug addition." *Physical dependence* refers to an altered physiologic state resulting from the chronic administration of a drug, which requires the continued administration of the drug to prevent a characteristic set of withdrawal symptoms for that particular drug. *Psychologic dependence* refers to a pattern of behavior directed to the procurement and use of a drug, based on an attitude that the effects produced by this drug are essential to maintain an optimal state of well being. *Tolerance* is the condition in which the body is accustomed to the drug so that the larger doses of the drug must be taken to obtain the same effects produced by the smaller dose when the drug is first taken. Some authorities hold that genetically inherited traits may result in progression of addictive diseases when individuals are exposed to certain drugs. Though we do not know as much as we would like to about the biochemical basis for the addictive process, which may be the same for all drugs, the pharmacologic and psychosocial aspects have been described and vary considerably from drug to drug. The most common substances used for alteration of consciousness are the narcotics, the CNS sedatives, the CNS simulants, the hallucinogens, and a few inhalants.

NARCOTICS–OPIATES

Narcotics can be divided into three groups on the basis of their origin (Table 58.1). Morphine and codeine are naturally occurring constituents of the crude plant preparation opium. The semisynthetic agents are chemical derivatives of morphine and codeine. Lastly, the synthetic drugs produce the same pharmacological effects as the natural agents. Opium is the dried crude exudate of the incised unripe poppy pod. Opium contains about 10% morphine, 1% codeine, and 18 other alkaloids. Heroin is the most widely abused semisynthetic narcotic drug and was quickly marketed as a "cure" for morphine addiction shortly after its discovery in 1874. Several new synthetic drugs have a potency 600 times that of heroin (1).

The potential for physiologic and psychologic dependence on narcotics is high. Although these agents are used extensively in medical practice, long-term dependence produced by medical use is rare. The most common abusers of narcotics fall into the following categories: street addicts, drug-dependent health professionals, infants of addicted mothers, and methadone maintenance patients. Heroin, the most potent semisynthetic narcotic, is converted to morphine in the body. The rapid onset of action and marked euphoric properties of heroin produce a greater potential for dependence than with other semisynthetic or naturally occurring agents. However, addicts

Table 58.1.
Narcotics and Related Compounds

Naturally occurring and derivatives
   Opium
   Morphine
   Codeine
   Tincture of opium
   Camphorated tincture of opium (paregoric)
Semisynthetic derivatives
   Heroin (diacetylmorphine)
   Oxycodone (Percodan, Percocet, Tylox)
   Hydrocodone (various)
   Oxymorphone (Numorphan)
   Hydromorphone (Dilaudid)
Synthetic agents
   Meperidine (Demerol)
   Loperamide (Imodium)
   Diphenoxylate (Lomotil)
   Anileridine (Leritine)
   Fentanyl (Innovos, Sublimaze)
   Methadone (Dolophine)
   L-Acetylomethandol (LAAM)
   Propoxyphene (Darvon)
   Pentazcine (Talwin)
   Butorphanol (Stadol)
   Nalbuphine (Nubain)

have difficulty differentiating between heroin, morphine, and synthetic narcotics given in equivalent doses. Tolerance develops rapidly to most of the effects of heroin, with the exception of pupilary constriction and constipation. Tolerance for narcotics disappears after complete withdrawal and may result in unintentional overdosage following weeks or months of abstinence if the previous doses are taken.

Acute Intoxication—Overdose

A large percent of chronic heroin users have experienced an overdose on at least one occasion. A number of factors can contribute to accidental overdoses of narcotics. A major factor is considerable confusion about the precise quantity of heroin taken because of variation in the concentration of street heroin, which may range from 1 to 90%. The amount of powder that looks like a user's customary dose may contain a dose of heroin many times greater. On some occasions an overdose occurs soon after the addict has completed a jail sentence, during which tolerance to heroin is lost. Some of the "designer drugs," (e.g., α-methylfentanyl, referred to as "China White") are much more potent than the compounds they are derived from and are sometimes inadequately mixed with inactive powdered ingredients, causing a very high concentration of active drugs in one dose (2). "Mexican tar" is another example of a product with a particularly high concentration of heroin. It was available on the streets in a higher concentration than had previously been available and was re-

sponsible for a number of narcotic overdoses. Multiple-drug use may produce an overdose when the additive effects of agents such as CNS depressants are combined with narcotics.

Patients may have been treated through one of several "street methods" for resuscitation, such as the intravenous administration of salt, vinegar, or milk solutions. Salt and vinegar IV injections are extremely painful and may produce sclerosing of the veins, abscesses, infections, and hypernatremia. Intravenous milk may also cause lipoidal pneumonia and microscopic pulmonary emboli. External pain such as slapping the face, ice baths, and pinching the nipples or testicles are commonly used to attempt to revive the unconscious patient. Neither stimulation nor painful injections have any positive effect on an important narcotic overdose, and they may simply produce additional trauma and complicate the medical condition further.

Another street treatment known as "speed reversal" is the use of CNS stimulants (e.g. cocaine or methamphetamine) intravenously. These agents do not reverse the respiratory depressant effects of narcotics and may produce serious additional adverse effects (e.g., convulsions, hypertension, arrhythmias) producing further complications requiring treatment of stimulant overdosage in addition to the narcotic overdosage.

To escape apprehension by authorities, bags or balloons of heroin are sometimes swallowed to hide evidence. If these rupture or are released in the intestinal tract, they can produce an overdose.

Narcotic overdose produces a profound coma, depressed respiration (as low as 2 to 4 per min), and cyanosis. The pupils are symetric and pinpoint, characteristic of the narcotic effect. However, if hypoxia or asphyxia has occurred, mydriasis may develop at this state. As the respiratory rate becomes slower, the blood pressure drops, and bradycardia, hypothermia, and pulmonary edema are commonly seen.

Management of Narcotic Intoxication

Naloxone (Narcan) is the narcotic anatagonist of choice (3). It is a specific pure opioid antagonist with no agonist properties of its own. It lacks the adverse effects associated with nalorphine (Nalline) and levallorphan (Lorfan), which have both antagonist and agonist activity and are likely to worsen the respiratory depressant effects, especially in cases of overdoses of a mixture of nonnarcotic depressant drugs. Nalorphine and levallorphan may also produce CNS stimulant effects leading to hallucinations and acute psychosis.

Naloxone should be administered in an initial dose of 0.4 mg intravenously followed by a second dose within 10 to 20 min if the first dose does not revive the patient. The peak effect of naloxone occurs within 1 to 2 min, but the agent is very short acting, lasting only 30 to 60 min. The patient must be monitored carefully, as the toxic effects of the narcotics may last for 6 to 8 hr requiring multidose administration of the naloxone. Propoxyphene (Darvon), codeine, pentazocine and fentanyl derivatives may require much larger doses of naloxone, and their durations of action are longer than those of other narcotics, so the acutely intoxicated patient must be monitored from 12 to 24 hr. In these cases, it is more convenient to infuse naloxone in a dose sufficient to produce antagonistic effects, usually 0.8 to 1.2 mg/hr. Naloxone has a very high therapeutic index, with patients tolerating 80 to 100 mg of the drug intravenously with few side effects (4). As the dose of narcotic antagonist is increased, a narcotic-withdrawal syndrome may be precipitated. A serious attempt should be made to determine if any street therapies have been tried. In addition to narcotic antagonist therapy, there should be close monitoring as well as mechanical support of respiration and blood pressure.

Narcotic-Withdrawal Syndrome

Withdrawal can be precipitated by the administration of a narcotic antagonist (5). If compulsive narcotic users do not receive their drugs, a predictable sequence of symptoms occurs, depending upon the degree of tolerance, dose of the drug, and duration of use (Table 58.2). Initial signs of anxiety, hyperactivity, lacrimation, rhinorrhea, and yawning appear 8 to 12 hr after the last dose. This is followed by a restless sleep that may last only a few hours as the withdrawal progresses. Initial symptoms of narcotic withdrawal are followed by marked chills, excessive sweating, and pilomotor activity producing waves of "gooseflesh" of the skin (i.e., resembling that of a plucked turkey). This symptom is the basis of the term "cold turkey" used to describe abrupt withdrawal without treatment. Abdominal cramps, anorexia, nausea, vomiting, and diarrhea follow. Musculoskeletal pains of the back along with muscle spasms and kicking movements have been referred to as "kicking the habit." As the syndrome approaches peak intensity, the patient exhibits increasing irritability, insomnia, anorexia, lacrimation, and increases in heart rate and

Table 58.2.
Narcotic Withdrawal/Abstinence Symptoms

Dilated pupils	Vomiting
Elevation of pulse rate	Diarrhea
Elevation of blood pressure	Dehydration
Elevation of temperature	Weakness
Elevation of respiratory rate	Chills
Muscle aches	Rhinorrhea
Irritability	Lacrimation
Twitching	Gooseflesh
Tremulousness	Yawning
Nausea	Restlessness

blood pressure. Leukocytosis is common, and white cell counts are often above 14,000/mm³. Weight loss, dehydration, ketosis, and acid-base imbalance follow the vomiting, sweating, diarrhea, and failure to take foods and fluids. Although cardiovascular collapse has been reported during the peak of the withdrawal, this is a rare phenomenon. In fact, death due to narcotic withdrawal is very rare. Without treatment, the withdrawal syndrome subsides, with most of the observable symptoms disappearing in 7 to 10 days. Total restoration of the physiological equilibrium can take much longer and varies with the patient, the length of the dependence, and the total daily dose of the drug. Administration of any narcotic opiate completely suppresses the symptoms of withdrawal at any point (6,7).

All narcotic-opiate drugs produce the same withdrawal signs and symptoms. However, depending on the particular agents and their length of action, symptoms may vary in duration and severity. For example, methadone withdrawal is less intense, develops more slowly, and is more prolonged because of the longer duration of action of methadone. Symptoms are rare within the first 24 to 48 hr after the last dose. A similar picture of withdrawal as that with heroin or morphine is observed, with peak effects occurring in 5 to 6 days and subsiding within 2 or 3 weeks. Meperidine, a much shorter-acting synthetic narcotic, may produce withdrawal effects within 3 hr of the last dose, which reach their greatest intensity within 8 to 12 hr and subside rapidly within 3 to 5 days. The pupils may not be widely dilated, and there are fewer autonomic signs and symptoms with meperidine withdrawal. Nausea, vomiting, and diarrhea are not as common as the nervousness, restlessness, and muscle twitching characteristic of meperidine abstinence.

Infant Dependence

Since narcotics cross the placenta, babies born to narcotic-dependent mothers will be physically dependent. With heroin dependence, signs of withdrawal appear within 24 hr of birth and include irritability, excessive crying, tremors, hyperactivity, increased respiratory rate, frantic sucking of fists, sneezing, vomiting, and fever. These same symptoms will occur in 2 or 3 days in babies born to methadone-dependent mothers (8). Withdrawal symptoms in babies born to mothers maintained on methadone are generally more intense; however, infant mortality is reduced in mothers maintained on methadone because of the greater likelihood of appropriate prenatal care (9). Teratogenic effects have not been linked to methadone. Withdrawal of the narcotic can be fatal to the fetus, so dependent mothers should remain on low doses of methadone until after birth. Other agents used to treat infant narcotic withdrawal, in addition to paregoric, are tincture of opium, phenobarbital, diazepam, chlorpromazine, and clonidine (10). Mild symptoms may not require replacement therapy. If symptoms persist and become more severe, then paregoric (0.2 ml), orally every 3 to 4 hr and increased as needed until symptoms are controlled, provides effective relief.

Patients who have received 2 weeks of recommended doses of morphine 3 or 4 times daily may experience minor withdrawal symptoms when therapy is abruptly discontinued or a narcotic antagonist is administered. Treatment of pain with narcotics should be limited when possible, and patients should be withdrawn gradually to minimize the withdrawal symptoms. Patients on narcotics less than 2 weeks seldom experience more than mild anxiety, irritability, insomnia, and restlessness. However, only a small percentage of patients who receive narcotics for medical treatment of pain desire or seek continued use of narcotics when the pain subsides. This points to the insignificant role of physical dependence in the development of the compulsive narcotic addict.

Management of Detoxification with Methadone

Hospitalized patients who are narcotic-dependent are usually not withdrawn until their acute medical or surgical problems are treated. These patients are generally placed on methadone for short-term replacement therapy to avoid complication of their medical problems. Methadone is usually not administered until physiologic symptoms of the withdrawal syndrome are present. Doses of 5 to 10 mg are initiated and titrated to prevent further withdrawal symptoms. Total daily doses of 10 to 20 mg may be sufficient. The dose is titrated as low as possible without allowing withdrawal symptoms to continue (11). After the medical or surgical illness is treated, the patient should choose between detoxification or enrolling in a methadone-maintenance program (12). Some patients refuse therapy and are simply discharged. Long waiting lists and program prerequisites may make methadone maintenance less attractive. The most convenient alternatives are detoxification with methadone or Naltrexone-clonidine combination (13–15). The goal of detoxification is to transform the narcotic addict into a "recovering," psychologically and emotionally stable, responsible, and productive member of society. Unfortunately, failure rates remain high in most programs.

Methadone is a synthetic narcotic with a duration of action up to 24 hr. It possesses pharmacologic effects identical to those of morphine and carries a full dependence potential. The slow onset of action of methadone produces a less intense "rush" effect. However, methadone continues to be a desired street substitute for heroin among addicts, even though they consider the high it provides inferior to other narcotics.

The major method of management of narcotic dependence is detoxification, which is the initial substitution of heroin with methadone to minimize withdrawal symptoms,

followed by progressively decreasing doses until the patient is drug-free. Detoxification can be carried out by a daily or every other day reduction of up to 20% of the total methadone dose, while keeping the withdrawal symptoms minimal (16). Most programs can complete this process within 14 to 21 days, depending on the dose and severity (length of time) of dependence. Since street products vary in percentage of heroin, it is difficult to determine an exact dosage for replacement. If you are convinced that the daily narcotic dosage is known, then the conversion used is 1 mg methadone substituted for 2 mg heroin, 4 mg morphine, and 20 mg meperidine (17). If there is no evidence of how much narcotic is being ingested on a daily basis, a daily dose of 10 to 20 mg is initiated and increased until withdrawal symptoms stop. Since 20% reduction in dose is well tolerated with minimum withdrawal symptoms, the dose is reduced accordingly. Many clinicians question the benefits of large doses of methadone and recommend a maximum daily dose of 50 mg to avoid possible euphoric effects that reinforce drug dependence. A quick method of methadone detoxification used in some programs involves a 5-day regimen with the initial dose of methadone at 100 mg followed by 50 mg, 25 mg, 12.5 mg, and 6 mg on the last day; followed by nonnarcotic symptomatic therapy.

During detoxification, the patient is not informed of the dose of methadone, since addicts always exaggerate their need and tend to become argumentative over adjusted doses. For this reason, patients most often receive their methadone dose in liquid form that must be taken at the clinic in the presence of staff. Methadone may produce sedation and drowsiness, excessive sweating, constipation, and decreased libido. Methadone should be used only after narcotic addiction is clearly established because fatalities have resulted from overdoses of methadone in nontolerant persons (18).

Methadone Maintenance

The treatment of heroin addiction varies from program to program and ranges from an aggressive narcotic abstinence of the "cold turkey" approach with abrupt cessation and no supportive therapy to maintenance with a substitute narcotic agent (e.g., long-acting methadone). Methadone maintenance involves placing the addict on a large enough dose of methadone to prevent withdrawal symptoms without producing euphoria. Initial doses of 10 to 20 mg per day are titrated up to 60 to 80 mg per day. A single daily oral dose is given to maintain contact with the patient and prevent the patient hoarding or selling the drug on the street. Since methadone is less likely than other narcotics to produce euphoria and tolerance develops rapidly, the craving for narcotics disappears at approximately 40 mg per day. Higher doses appear to block the euphoric effects of additional use of other narcotics. Longer-acting narcotics (L-acetyl methadone) (LAAM) have been tested in clinical trials since they can be given every 3 days instead of daily (19). Other methadone analogs are D-acetyl-methadol and 1-methadyl acetate.

Methadone maintenance allows addicts a chance to escape from the illegal drug scene and refocus their goals and lifestyles. Controversy continues to surround long-term methadone-maintenance programs, and many practitioners see the replacement of illegal heroin with legally sanctioned methadone as incomplete and nonsuccessful therapy. Proponents think that time away from the illegal street scene will foster the attitudes and values necessary to conquer the dependency at a later time (18).

Supportive Treatment

A nonnarcotic technique for withdrawal involves management of the symptoms with a variety of nonnarcotic medications. Anxiety, irritability, and apprehension are usually treated with long-acting minor tranquilizers such as chlordiazepoxide (Librium), since the shorter-acting agents produce euphoric effects of their own that may reinforce or substitute a dependence. Phenobarbital is also effective in the treatment of anxiety. Insomnia has been treated with flurazepam (Dalmane), triazolam (Halcion), chloral hydrate, or diphenhydramine. Gastrointestinal symptoms of cramps, diarrhea, and nausea may be managed with the belladonna alkaloids, dicyclomine (Bentyl), or prochlorperazine (Compazine) if vomiting is present. Analgesic therapy is usually limited to nonsteroidal antiinflammatory agents (e.g., ibuprofen) to avoid mood-altering effects of mild analgesics such as propoxyphene. Nonsteroidal antiinflammatory drugs are also effective for musculoskeletal pain.

Clonidine, a centrally acting α_2-agonist, can suppress some components of the opiate withdrawal syndrome. Orthostatic hypotension and sedation have limited the outpatient use of oral clonidine therapy, but use of the drug in the hospital has been very effective. Clonidine side effects have been reduced by use of the sustained-release patches. After 2 days of oral clonidine therapy of 0.4 to 1.2 mg in daily divided doses, two Catapres-TTS-2 patches are applied. The patches should be replaced in 1 week, for a total therapy of 2 weeks (20, 21). Combination therapy of clonidine with nonsteroidal antiinflammatory agents for pain and sleep medications has been very successful.

The narcotic antagonists have been used to produce a block of the euphoric efforts of opioids. If a drug is needed to break the conditioning of a drug-seeking behavior, narcotic antagonist may be used. Naloxone and naltrexone can block the euphoria of narcotics and prevent development of physical dependence as well as protect the individuals from narcotic overdosage. Naltrexone (Trexan) is an orally effective narcotic antagonist and relatively free of side ef-

Table 58.3.
Medical Complications of Intravenous Drug Abuse

Skin	Abscesses, cellulitis, edema, emboli, excoriation, jaundice, macules, nodules, purpura, "tracks," ulcers
Lymph nodes	"Addict's lymphadenopathy," lymphatic hyperplasia
Eyes	Emboli from talc and cornstarch, quinine amblyopia, scleral icterus
Mouth	Poor dental hygiene
Pulmonary	Infections secondary to aspiration, bronchiectasis, atelectasis, septic emboli, tuberculosis, pulmonary hypertension, decreased vital capacity, asthma, noncardiogenic pulmonary edema
Cardiovascular	Arrhythmias, endocarditis complicated by systemic and pulmonary emboli, vasculities, gangrene
Hematologic	Anemia, hemolysis, malaria, neutropenia
Neurologic	Subarachnoid hemorrhage, neuropathies, meningitis, central and peripheral emboli, nerve damage
Gastrointestinal	Hepatomegaly, hepatitis, splenic abscess, portal hypertension, constipation, bowel obstruction, hemorrhoids
Genitourinary	Heroin nephropathy, vasculitis, glomerulonephritis secondary to hepatitis or infection, myoglobinuria from muscle destruction, acute tubular necrosis, acute renal failure
Extremities	Phlebitis, edema, arthritis, rhabdomyolysis, tetanus
Immunologic	False-positive VDRL, rheumatoid factor, hypergammaglobinemia, serologic abnormalities, increased risk for acquired immunodeficiency syndrome (AIDS)
"Cotton fever"	Pyrogenic reaction, shaking chills, headache, vomiting, gastrointestinal pain, leukocytosis shortly after intravenous administration subsiding in an hour or two

fects (22–24). Doses of 50 to 150 mg block narcotic effects for 2 to 3 days making a Monday, Wednesday, Friday schedule possible. Unlike methadone, naltrexone is non-addictive and without reenforcing properties. Poor compliance has limited this agent's use. However, some individuals who are motivated to abstain by their support groups have found additional help and long-term success with this drug (25, 26).

Medical Complications of Narcotic Dependence

Most medical complications of narcotic abuse are indirect and depend more on the method of use than on the direct effects of the drugs (e.g., toxic and withdrawal reactions) (Table 58.3). The repeated use of unsterile needles and syringes has led to acute hepatitis of the serum or viral type, bacterial endocarditis, aseptic abscesses, embolism, thrombophlebitis, and cellulitis. *Staphylococcus aureus* is the most common infecting organism, followed by streptococci, Gram-negative bacilli (*Pseudomonas* and *Serra-*

tia), and fungi (*Candida*). One study reported a 60% incidence of AIDS (Acquired Immunodeficiency syndrome) among addicts who commonly share needles and syringes (27). Some of the other infectious disease transmitted in this fashion are tetanus, viral hepatitis, tuberculosis, and syphilis (28).

A common practice of self-administration of heroin is the use of cotton to filter out adulterants. Allergic reactions caused by the tiny cotton fibers may cause shaking, chills, fever, tachycardia, and a low-grade fever mimicking sepsis within 30 min of injection. These symptoms commonly subside within 2 to 4 hr. Pulmonary complications may be secondary to injection of these and other foreign body emboli (e.g., starch, talc, or cotton fibers). Many patients with significant embolic complications have been previous users of methylphenidate or pentazocine. Subcutaneous use of heroin (skin popping) frequently produces infection at the site, with *Staphylococcus aureus* being the most frequent organism. Tetanus is also a possible serious infection (29).

CNS DEPRESSANTS

The most common sedative-hypnotic drug used and abused is alcohol. Most authorities still consider alcohol the major drug problem in the United States. Chapter 57 goes into detail on alcohol abuse and its management.

Barbiturates and other sedative hypnotic drugs produce their effects through generalized depression of the central nervous system and are all capable of producing physical dependence when used chronically and above the recommended maximum dosages. Short-acting barbiturates such as pentobarbital (Nembutal), secobarbital (Seconal), and amobarbital (Amytal) were the major sedative-hypnotics used and abused prior to the 1970s. Physician awareness of their dependence liability and toxicities coupled with stringent DEA controls has dramatically decreased both their use and abuse. However, a host of non-barbiturate sedative-hypnotics appeared on the market, with meprobamate (Milltown, Equanil) introduced in the 1950s as the first of many "minor tranquilizers" to be released. Several other nonbarbiturate agents were also used (glutethimide, methyprylon, ethinamate, ethchlorvynol, and methaqualone) but have been primarily replaced by the increasing use of benzodiazepines. However, there are marked similarities of all agents that depress the central nervous system in producing the same type dependence and withdrawal syndrome (30, 31).

Acute intoxication from combined use of alcohol with the barbiturates and benzodiazepines is a frequent problem. In addition, the number of attempted suicides with sedative-hypnotics is the largest of any class of prescription drugs. Some patients have accidently overdosed on the barbiturates, because although there is considerable tolerance to the sedative and intoxicating effects, the lethal dose is not much greater in addicts than in normal individuals. Consequently, acute barbiturate poisoning may be accidently superimposed on chronic intoxication at any time. Benzodiazepines appear to be safer than barbiturates and related sedatives, since an acute overdosage is much less likely to produce fatal respiratory depression. However, the combination of alcohol and benzodiazepines is a serious problem that can be life-threatening.

The signs and symptoms of barbiturate poisoning relate to their CNS depressant effects. Initial signs of minor intoxication resemble those of alcohol inebriation and progress in severe intoxication to slurred speech, ataxia, and coma. Lowered blood pressure and depressed respiration and tendon reflexes are common. Cerebral hypoxia and respiratory acidosis may lead to hypotension and arrhythmias. The patient develops shock, a weak but rapid pulse, cold and sweaty skin, increased hematocrit, and renal ischemia. Pulmonary complications and renal failure are the most common causes of death from severe barbiturate poisoning (32).

The basic treatment of barbiturate intoxication is general supportive care and maintenance of vital functions, which may include mechanical respiration, dialysis, and intensive-care continuous monitoring. Initial treatment should also prevent further intestinal absorption of the drug. Gastric lavage should be considered within the first 2 to 4 hr after the overdose, followed by repeated doses of activated charcoal given orally to decrease absorption of drug remaining in the intestinal tract. However, forced diuresis, urinary alkalization, and giving repeated doses of charcoal have not been shown to be more successful than general supportive care (33, 34). Use of CNS stimulants increases mortality and has no place in the treatment of sedative-hypnotic overdose. Special attention must be given to maintenance of the patient's airway and the prevention of pneumonia. Oxygen should be administered, and mechanical ventilation used when indicated. Patients with severe hypotension or shock must be rehydrated. Hypovolemia must be corrected with caution; overhydration may contribute to pulmonary edema. Should renal failure occur, the most effective method of eliminating barbiturate is hemodialysis.

Unlike the narcotics, the original contact with sedative-hypnosis is most commonly through a physician's prescription. Development of dependence may be gradual, beginning with prolonged use of these agents for anxiety or insomnia, progressing through increased doses at night for insomnia, to multidoses in the daytime for sedation, until drug use becomes a major part of the user's life. In such situations, a fine line separates psychologic and physical dependency. Neither the prescriber nor the patient may recognize the existence of a dependence until the patient attempts to withdraw from the drug.

Withdrawal Syndrome

There are marked similarities between the withdrawal syndromes of the barbiturates and the nonbarbiturate minor tranquilizers. The term *general depressant-withdrawal syndrome* refers to the manifestation and withdrawal from any of these agents. Initial withdrawal symptoms include restlessness, anxiety, sleep disturbances, tremulousness, and gastric distress. Withdrawal symptoms of shorter-acting sedatives appear within 24 hr and reach a peak in 2 to 3 days, including agitation, delirium, psychoses, postural hypotension, hyperthermia, cardiovascular collapse, tonic-clonic seizures, and even death. Presence of these later symptoms should be considered signs and symptoms of major withdrawal, and they require hospitalization. Abstinence from the longer-acting sedatives does not produce withdrawal symptoms until the 2nd or 3rd day, and they reach their peak much more slowly. Seizures may not occur until the 7th to 10th day.

Major signs of physiologic dependence and withdrawal have been observed after 30 to 60 days of use of depressants at minimum or threshold doses two to three times maximum recommended therapeutic doses. Daily doses of secobarbital and pentobarbital of 600 to 800 mg per day for 30 to 60 days have been reported as the minimum threshold dose to produce physical dependence. Thirty percent of patients taking 400 mg per day experience significant symptoms. The withdrawal or abstinence syndrome has been described for almost every sedative hypnotic drug, but the doses and times to produce withdrawal are not as well defined as with the barbiturates. Abrupt discontinuation of doses as low as 30 mg diazepam per day for 3 months has resulted in seizures. Obviously, the longer the therapy and the higher the daily dose, the more likely that serious withdrawal symptoms will occur upon discontinuing the drug. In addition, it takes 5 to 7 days for the longer-acting benzodiazepines to produce significant symptoms of abstinence after discontinuing the drug, resulting in a withdrawal that might last 2 to 3 weeks (35–41). In addition to the classic withdrawal symptoms, patients who are taking lower than threshold doses required to produce physical dependency may exhibit a *rebound phenomenon* with the abrupt discontinuation of the drug. Patients abruptly discontinuing commonly prescribed doses of benzodiazepines have experienced insomnia, anorexia, REM rebound, irritability, and anxiety, which could be mistaken for the symptoms that the drug was originally prescribed for (42, 43). All patients taking benzodiazopines should gradually taper their dose over a period of 2 to 4 weeks to avoid this effect.

Sedative Detoxification

Because of the severity of general depressant withdrawal, successful management must involve tapering the patient off the sedative agents slowly. Phenobarbital is considered the agent of choice for substitution withdrawal because of its long duration of action, its anticonvulsant effects, and its wide margin of saftey. Phenobarbial does not produce euphoric effects commonly seen with the short-acting barbiturates and benzodiazepines (44, 45). Most treatment centers will not allow the use of the agent the patient is dependent on to detoxify the patient. Because of the strong association with the patient's drug of choice and the psychologic dependency, use of the agent the patient is dependent on to detoxify the patient is not recommended. All sedatives and hypnotics can be withdrawn by phenobarbital. The dose of phenobarbital is 30 mg for each 100 mg of phenobarbital, pentobarbital, or secobarbital or for each 5 mg of diazepam, 25 mg of chlordiazepoxide, or 50 mg of butalbital. The total daily dose may be as high as 600 or 700 mg of phenobarbital and is administered in 3 or 4 divided doses. Some clinics orally administer 120-mg doses of phenobarbital hourly until sedative effects and/or horizontal nystagmus appear, and this total dose is then given in divided daily doses (46). A stabilization period of 1 to 2 days for short-acting drugs and 3 to 4 days for long-acting drugs is used. The patient is monitored for slurred speech, nystagmus, or ataxia during this stabilization period. An oral or intramuscular 200-mg dose of phenobarbital usually controls minor symptoms of withdrawal. Total daily dose is then adjusted, based on incidence and severity of symptoms. After the patient is stabilized, the total daily dose of phenobarbital is decreased 30 mg per day (47). The withdrawal schedule should be adjusted gradually, based on the signs of intoxication or withdrawal symptoms. The most successful withdrawal programs take place in supervised inpatient settings. If patients requiring detoxification have mixed addictions of the narcotic-sedative type, they are maintained on sufficient amounts of methadone until detoxification from the sedative hypnotic is completed (48).

Benzodiazepine Detoxification

Benzodiazepines (Table 58.4) have cross-tolerance with each other, alcohol, and other sedative/hypnotic drugs. Any benzodiazepine can be substituted for another ben-

Table 58.4.
Short and Long-Acting Benzodiazepines

Short-Acting Agents	Long-Acting Agents
Triazolam (Halcion)	Chlordiazepoxide (Librium)
Oxazepam (Serax)	Diazepam (Valium)
Temazepam (Restoril)	Halazepam (Paxipam)
Lorazepam (Ativan)	Clorazepate (Tranxene)
Alprazolam (Xanax)	Prazepam (Centrax)
	Clorazepam (Klonopin)
	Flurazepam (Dalmane)

Table 58.5.
Signs and Symptoms of Benzodiazepine Withdrawal

Neuropsychiatric symptoms	*Symptoms of hyperexcitability*
Ataxia	Agitation
Depresonalization	Anxiety
Depression	Hyperactivity
Fasciculations	Insomnia
Formications	*Gastrointestinal symptoms*
Headache	Abdominal pain
Hyperventilation	Constipation
Malaise	Diarrhea
Myalgia	Nausea
Paranoid delusions	Vomiting
Paresthesias	*Cardiovascular symptoms*
Pruritus	Chest pain
Tinnitus	Flushing
Tremors	Palpitations
Visual halluncinations	*Genitourinary symptoms*
	Incontinence
	Loss of libido
	Urinary urgency, frequency

zodiazepine or barbiturate, so conversion for equivalent doses can be calculated. The long-acting benzodiazepines are more effective than short-acting agents in suppressing withdrawal symptoms (Table 58.5) (35). Long-acting agents produce a gradual, smooth transition to the abstinent state, which improves patient compliance and reduces morbidity (49, 50). Benzodiazepines with lower euphoric properties are more effective during detoxification. For example, chlordiazepoxide is preferred to diazepam.

Medications should be prescribed on a regular schedule. Addicts need the structure of a drug schedule; they do not do well with as-needed (p.r.n.) prescriptions because their basic problem is loss of control over drugs. Unlike alcohol withdrawal, benzodiazepine withdrawal is not usually marked by hypertension and tachycardia, so p.r.n. doses are not necessary. Drug-seeking behavior must be differentiated from withdrawal-related anxiety and from anxiety caused by another disorder. Only anxiety secondary to benzodiazepine withdrawal should be treated with increasing doses of benzodiazepines. Alternative treatment is indicated for anxiety associated with another disorder (e.g., panic disorder) (35).

CENTRAL NERVOUS SYSTEM STIMULANTS

Caffeine is the most universal, socially accepted stimulant in the world, in the form of coffee, tea, and soft drinks, and has a wide margin of safety and rare toxicity. Use of central nervous system stimulants was recorded in ancient Asian and African writings. Amphetamines are the prototype prescription CNS stimulant, and they were heavily prescribed for weight control until the 1970s when the DEA moved most of them to schedule II controlled substances and limited their production.

The over-the-counter diet pills contain phenylpropanolamine, caffeine, or a combination. Phenylpropanolamine has a limited effect on suppressing appetite, but it is not defined as habit-forming because it is not self-administered by animals and does not produce the increase of energy, alertness, and euphoria of the amphetamines. Serious adverse effects of excessive use of these over-the-counter diet aids (including sudden death) have rarely been reported (51–53). "Look-alikes" are nonprescription tablets and capsules manufactured in colors, shapes, and sizes to resemble the prescription stimulants and marketed as diet aids. These agents most commonly contain phenylpropanolamine, pseudoephedrine, ephedrine, caffeine, and/or a combination of the above. They are commonly advertised as appetite suppressants but sold illicitly for methamphetamine, dextroamphetamine, or cocaine. Illicit production of methamphetamine (speed, crystal meth, crank) has attempted to meet the street demand for these agents.

Amphetamines were first used for treatment of depression and fatigue, increasing alertness, and as an anorexiant to suppress appetite. Because of a rapid tolerance that develops within a few weeks, these drugs have no medical place in the previously mentioned conditions. The only accepted medical uses for the amphetamine agents today are hyperkinesia, attention-deficit disorder, and narcolepsy. Amphetamines are sympathomimetic agents that produce systemic stimulation of the central nervous system. In addition to increasing alertness, amphetamines produce an elevation of mood, a sense of increased energy, and decreased appetite. Amphetamines initially increase productivity slightly, alleviate fatigue, and produce a euphoric sense of well-being, which can produce a quick, psychological habituation to the drug. Coupled with a rapid development of tolerance requiring increased doses on a weekly basis, dependence is common. Tolerance to the recommended 15 mg per day dosage leads to use of 80 to 100 times the initial dosages. Some users have been reported to inject up to 1 g of the drug several times daily without apparent toxicity.

Chronic users have not only used intravenous injections of amphetamines, but have also started freebasing methamphetamine (ice) and smoking it, similar to cocaine. Chronic amphetamine users, known as "speed freaks," tend to be hostile, impulsive, aggressive, mentally unstable, and subject to wide swings in behavior, including violence (Table 58.6) (35). An amphetamine binge or "speed run" is the continuous round-the-clock use of amphetamines for several days without sleep. The patient is referred to as "strung out" and may become hostile, overactive, and impulsive. Prolonged periods of paranoia and delusions can result. An acute psychotic episode induced by amphetamines does not generally respond to "talk-down" therapy. Mild nonviolent patients are treated with

Table 58.6.
Common Signs and Symptoms of Acute Amphetamine Intoxication

Restlessness	Parania
Anxiety	Delusional thoughts
Tremor	Visual hallucinations
Muscle tension	Auditory hallucinations
Repetitious body movement	Physical malnutrition
Facial grimacing	Needle tracks and abscesses
Dystonia	Hypertensive crisis
Temporary amnesia	Cardiac arrhythmias

oral benzodiazepines, and more seriously agitated patients should receive parenteral haloperidol (Haldol). If the patient is combative and hostile, physical restraints are indicated until the drug therapy controls the patient. After several days of a "speed run," the patient usually "crashes" from exhaustion. Psychological changes, including delusions, paranoia, and hallucinations, are problems with chronic amphetamine use. The fully developed toxic syndrome is characterized by vivid visual, auditory, and sometimes tactile hallucinations. In chronic users, a tolerance builds up to most of the sympathomimetic effects, and the blood pressure may be normal. It is very difficult to differentiate the toxic syndrome from a schizophrenic reaction. Chronic use of high-dose amphetamine has also been reported to produce microvascular neurologic damage and depletion of dopamine in the caudate nucleus (54). Other complications of chronic use are malnutrition due to appetite suppression and perception of "crank bugs" (i.e., imagining bugs crawling under the skin). The intravenous use of these agents carries with it all of the medical complications of other agents abused in this fashion (e.g., infectious diseases, microemboli, abcesses, hepatitis, AIDS, "cotton fever"). Intravenous injections of methamphetamines may produce a systemic necrotizing angitis and generalized spasm of the cerebral blood vessels. Cardiac arrhythmias and cerebral hemorrhages have been reported. Severe abdominal pain mimicking acute appendicitis is also seen.

Amphetamine overdosage-toxicity may result if an individual has lost tolerance and self-administers the previous dosage. Toxicity developing if the amphetamine dose has been increased too rapidly before tolerance develops is referred to as "overamped," with patients characterized by consciousness without the ability to move or speak. Physiologic signs and symptoms include high blood pressure and an extremely rapid pulse, intense pain, increased temperature, severe agitation, and insomnia. Higher doses produce cardiac arrhythmias, seizures, hallucinations, cardiomyopathy, and myocardial infarction. Dehydration associated with malnutrition, vomiting, and diarrhea is also possible. Death from overdosage is usually caused by cardiovascular collapse.

Abrupt cessation following chronic or high-dose amphetamine use will produce an abstinence syndrome that may last up to 1 week. Symptoms include fatigue, muscle aches, depression, headache, gastrointestinal disturbances, and craving for the drug. Withdrawal from amphetamines is not life-threatening and does not require gradual reduction of dose. Underlying psychiatric conditions, depression, and sleep disturbances may persist for months and require psychiatric management. Treatment of acute amphetamine withdrawal is supportive in nature: benzodiazepines are appropriate for mild-to-moderate symptoms, and haloperidol can be given if sedation is required. Chlorpromazine and other phenothiazines should not be given to treat mental or physiological disturbances caused by amphetamine reactions. There is a great risk of impulsive self-destructive behavior in the chronic amphetamine abuser. Treatment of the chronic amphetamine abuser is difficult with a high frequency of relapse. The number of chronic amphetamine users has been dramatically reduced in the past 2 decades, with a corresponding increase in cocaine abuse.

COCAINE

Cocaine is a local anesthetic drug with significant CNS-stimulant effects. Widespread abuse of cocaine began in the late 1800s, shortly after its isolation from the *Erythroxylon coca* plant. The use of cocaine goes back many centuries in Peru, Bolivia, Equador, and Columbia. Local natives in the upper Andes regularly chewed or sucked plugs of moistened coca leaves, smeared with a pinch of lime (ashes or limestone) to extract the cocaine from the leaves. Chewing coca leaves satisfies hunger, eliminates fatigue, and imparts great physical strength to its users working in the high altitudes (55). Cocaine is still obtained primarily from the natural plant source. As an alkaloid, it is extracted from the plant with organic solvents, precipitated into a paste, and then usually converted to the hydrochloride salt, producing the white powder seen on the street. The purity of street cocaine varies considerably. Pure cocaine is most commonly diluted with adulterants ("cut" or "stepped on") to help dealers support their own habits and/or increase their profit margin. Cheaper local anesthetics, mannitol, lactose, glucose, corn starch, flour, and talc are some of the agents used to cut the pure form. Samples of street cocaine may vary from 25 to 75%. Because of the high demand and popularity of the drug and the large profits, suppliers have increased the availability of higher quality product on the street. It is estimated that there are over 5 million regular users in the United States alone, with 30 million who have experimented with the drug. The Drug Enforcement Agency estimates range as high as 200 tons of cocaine sold on the street annually, representing a multibillion dollar business.

In addition to the crystalline powder form of cocaine

found on the street, "freebase" and "crack" became increasingly popular in the 1980s. Freebase is prepared by mixing cocaine hydrochloride with an alkali solution such as sodium bicarbonate, then extracting with a solvent, usually ethyl ether. This not only separates the cocaine from the adulterants but also cleaves the hydrochloride salt, leaving the free alkaloidal cocaine base as a colorless, transparent, crystalline substance, insoluble in water. Crack is a base form of cocaine prepared by dissolving the hydrochloride salt in water and alkali (bleach or sodium bicarbonate) (56). The free alkaloidal base precipitates out, leaving a brittle, milky-colored solid that crackles when it burns, hence the nickname crack. After the product is dried, it is broken into small pieces or chips known as "rocks" and usually sold in small glass vials or metal tubes.

Cocaine can be administered in a number of different ways (57). The oldest known method of using cocaine is orally, chewing the moistened leaves placed between the cheek and gum like a plug of chewing tobacco. The drug is also effective when ingested orally, although gastrointestinal absorption is slower and incomplete. However, these routes of administration do not produce as fast or as intense a high, or rush, and are rarely seen in the United States. The most common method of self-administration of cocaine is smoking crack, either by itself in a pipe or sprinkled in marijuana cigarettes called "primo joints" (58). Because of its purity, crack produces the quickest and most intense cocaine high, taking effect within 8 to 10 sec with a very short duration of 10 to 20 min. Many addictionologists believe that almost all crack users become addicts, unable to control their use of the drug.

Another common route of administration of cocaine is inhalation through the nose, "snorting." There is a ritual of using the drug by this method which involves placing the powder on a hard surface (counter top, book, or mirror), separating and chopping the powder into a small particle size, dividing the powder into a small narrow "line" or "hit," then sniffing the powder into the nostril with a rolled-up dollar bill or a short straw. A small spoon, "coke spoon," is a device to measure out single doses of the drug sufficient for one sniff. One "line" of street cocaine would usually contain 5 to 10 mg of cocaine, while one "coke spoon" may only contain half this amount. Most recreational cocaine users (those using the drug once a month or less and only in social settings) snort the powder.

Another method of use is freebasing. Using a modified water pipe with several layers of stainless steel screens fitted in the bowl, the freebase is placed on the top screen, melted to an oil, and heated slowly to vaporize the drug for inhalation. Absorption of cocaine through the lungs is very rapid, and users experience a more intensive, euphoric (rush) effect. Many users report binges lasting up to 3 or 4 days of uncontrolled craving and repeated drug use via freebasing. Freebase smokers and the intravenous cocaine users seldom return intranasal use (59).

Other patterns of cocaine drug use are smoking the crude paste with marijuana or tobacco and intravenous injection. Most users claim the euphoric rush of IV use to be of lower intensity than that with free-basing or crack smoking. For this reason a very small percentage of cocaine users administer the drug intravenously. A preparation called "speed ball" is a combination of heroin and cocaine administered together intravenously.

Pharmacologic Effects

The local anesthetic activity of cocaine is due to a direct effect on the nerve cell membrane to prevent the generation and conduction of nerve inpulses. Cocaine affects the sympathetic nervous system by blocking the reuptake of catecholamines at adrenergic nerve endings, thus potentiating both inhibitory and excitory responses of sympathetically intervated structures to endogenous and exogenous serotonin, norepinephrine, and epinephrine. Although cocaine blocks the reuptake of dopamine in the brain initally, it appears that chronic use actually depletes dopamine stores (60). The mechanism of reinforcing action and effects associated with cocaine may be related to this increase of synaptic concentration of dopamine. However, the cocaine high may be caused by altered serotonin and acetylcholine activity in the brain.

Cocaine is generally considered to have a rapid onset and short duration of action, depending somewhat on the method of administration (61). The onset is 2 to 3 min when the drug is snorted, less than 1 min when it is injected, and 8 to 10 sec when it is smoked. The elimination half-life of cocaine is 60 to 75 min, with peak plasma concentration occurring between 30 and 60 min, depending on the route of administration (intravenous vs. snorting). The physiologic effect of cocaine outlasts the euphoria and tends to correlate with the blood levels of the drug. However, most users want to repeat the use of the drug within 20 to 30 min after the first dose. This may indicate that the rate of rise of cocaine concentration in the brain is the major factor responsible for the subjective euphoric effects and the "rush," rather than the serum concentrations (62).

Cocaine produces many classic sympathomimetic manifestations (Table 58.7). Cocaine has powerful CNS-stimulant effects producing euphoria, restlessness, talkativeness, and gregariousness. Other physiologic effects include dry mouth, sweating, mydriasis, hyperthermia, tachycardia, increased blood pressure, vasoconstriction, increased muscle activity, tics, chills, and increased respiratory rate intially, followed by Cheyne-Stokes respiration with continued drug use. The euphoric rush, often referred to by users as being "better than orgasm," reinforces

Table 58.7.
Signs and Symptoms of Cocaine Toxicity

Phase	CNS	Circulatory	Respiratory
I (Early stimulation)	Euphoria/elation Mydriasis Talkativeness Excited/flighty Restless/irritable Nausea/vomiting Vertigo Sudden headache Cold sweats Tremor/twitching (especially face, fingers) Generalized tics Preconvulsive movements Pseudohallucinations Verbalization of impending doom	Initial decrease pulse rate, then increased Increase blood pressure Skin pallor (vasoconstriction) PVCs	Increased respiratory rate Dypsnea
II (Advanced stimulation)	Decreased responsiveness to stimuli Generalized hyperflexia Increased DTRs, incontinence Convulsions, status epilepticus Malignant encephalopathy possible	Increase pulse rate Increase blood pressure initially followed by decrease blood pressure due to decrease cardiac output with ventricular arrhythmias Rapid pulse, weak and irregular Peripheral then central cyanosis	Gasping, rapid or irregular respiratory rate Cheyne-Stokes progressive hypoxia
III (Depressive)	Flacid paralysis of muscle coma Pupils fixed and dilated Loss of reflexes Loss of vital support functions Paralysis of medullary brain center Death	Ventricular fibrillation Circulatory failure Ashen gray cyanosis No palpable pulse Cardiac arrest Paralysis of medullary brain center Death	Agonal gasps Respiratory failure Gross pulmonary edema Paralysis of medullary brain center Death

and contributes to repeated self-administration. Abusers claim they can not control their dose and may go on a "binge" or "run" of cocaine for several days. Continuous use after a few hours will begin the progression from the euphoric stage through dysphoria and hallucinosis to psychosis.

Medical Complications of Cocaine (Table 58.8)

The cardiovascular effects of cocaine are due to the increased central sympathetic stimulation. The initial effects of tachycardia, palpitations, angina, and hypertension will return to normal within several hours, depending on the dosage and whether the drug is being used repeatedly. However, increasing numbers of patients are developing life-threatening arrhythmias and infarctions (63). Ventricular tachycardia, fibrillation, and premature ventricular contractions have been reported (64, 65). These users frequently complain of chest pain from alveolar hemorrhage (crack lung) and may experience pulmonary edema, pneumonia, or respiratory depression. Other serious cardiovascular effects seen with cocaine use are myocardial

infarction, life-threatening ventricular arrhythmias, hypertensive crisis, endocarditis, thrombosis, and rupture of the ascending aorta (66–68). Many patients who have experienced the cardiovascular toxicities had no underlying heart disease previously. These effects have been reported following all routes of administration and with both large and small doses (69–72).

Pulmonary complications have increased dramatically with freebasing and the smoking of crack, and alveolar hemorrhage (crack lung), pulmonary edema, pneumomediastinum, pneumothorax, pneumopericardium, pneumonia, and respiratory arrest are commonly seen in regular users of cocaine in these manners (73–75). Stroke and subarachnoid and intracranial hemorrhage are some of the life-threatening CNS effects reported with cocaine use (76–78). High doses of cocaine have been associated with tonic-clonic convulsions (79). Intravenous use of cocaine has been associated with a variety of infectious diseases such as hepatitis, AIDS, bacterial endocarditis, and other complications (80). Excessive doses of cocaine may lead to cardiac arrhythmias, severe hypotension, hypothermia,

Table 58.8.
Medical Complications of Cocaine Use

System or Condition	Complication Examples
Cardiovascular	Myocardial infarction, premature ventricular contraction, ventricular tachycardia, ventricular fibrillation, congestive heart failure, chest pain, endocarditis, hypertension, pneumopericardium, rupture of ascending aorta, thrombosis, thrombophlebitis
CNS	Stroke, subarachnoid hemorrage, intercranial hemorrage, cerebral vasculitis, hyperpyrexia, dysphagia, dysarthria
Respiratory	Alveolar hemorrhage (crack lung), pneumonia, pneumomediastinum, pulmonary edema, pneumothorax, respiratory arrest
Opthalmic	Retinopathy, central retinal artery occulsion
Pregnancy	Abrupt placenta fetal hypoxemia, fetal death in utero, spontaneous abortion, preterm labor, convulsions in breast-feeding baby, feeding disorder, teratogenicity
Psychiatric	Panic disorder, psychosis, and violence
Miscellaneous	Renal artery thrombosis, midline granuloma, subcutaneous emphysema, nasal problems, rhadomyolipsis, sexual dysfunction, various infectious diseases and other complications with IV drug use (Table 58.3)

seizures, and renal and respiratory failure (81). Myocardial infarction and cardiac failure within 2 to 3 hr following cocaine use in young adults without prior heart disease have been reported (82–85). Toxic effects of acute cocaine exposure may be precipitated by physical exertion. Cases of sudden death following freebase use are probably caused by arrhythmias. Cocaine overdose has also been frequently reported in individuals smuggling cocaine. "Body packing" involves swallowing plastic bags filled with cocaine in order to pass through immigrations, with a plan to retrieve the containers from bowel movements. Occasionally, these bags will rupture in the gut, and in other cases the plastic may be semipermeable, allowing absorption of cocaine (86–88, 43).

Treatment of Overdosage

Treatment of acute cocaine intoxication includes general supportive care, fluid and electrolyte replacement, maintenance of vital functions (blood pressure, airway) and monitoring for suspected hyperadrenergic crisis (e.g., hypertension, arrhythmias) (89). Mild-to-moderate cocaine intoxication is self-limiting and lasts no longer than 2 to 3 hr without treatment. If symptoms progress in severity or persist longer than an hour, the patient should be monitored for arrhythmias with an ECG, since cardiac arrhythmias are the major cause of death due to cocaine toxicity. Respiratory arrest, seizures, myocardial infarction, or cardiovascular collapse are all possible, and preparations

should be made to manage any of these conditions should they arise. Ventricular arrhythmias are treated with lidocaine or phenytoin and may require cardioversion. Supraventricular arrhythmias have been managed effectively with the nonselective β-blocker propranolol (Inderal) in mild-to-moderate cocaine toxicity. There is a danger of unexpected hypertension because of unopposed alphadrenergic activity, so propronolol should be avoided in major toxicity (90–92). Several reports have indicated that labetalol may be more effective in managing cocaine toxicity (93). Intravenous nitroprusside sodium may be used to control hypertensive emergencies. Naloxone may be given to comatose patients suspected of cocaine intoxication, since a large percentage of patients use narcotics with cocaine. Seizures may be treated by diazepam, phenytoin, or phenobarbital (94). Anxiety and restlessness may be treated with benzodiazepines, and acute psychotic reactions with haloperidol (95). Caution is advised because haloperidol may lower the seizure threshold and increase the risk of convulsions.

Cocaine Withdrawal

There is no doubt that cocaine produces severe psychologic dependence or habituation. Many addictionologists claim that cocaine dependence is the most difficult drug dependence to treat. There has been debate about labeling cocaine as physically addicting, although there is no question that animals given cocaine will self-administer the drug. Furthermore, abrupt discontinuation of cocaine following chronic use results in depression, fatigue, craving for the drug, social withdrawal, eating and sleep disturbances, REM rebound, and electroencephalographic changes. These effects generally last less than a week, with the exception of the abnormal sleep patterns, which may last several weeks (96). These signs and symptoms are significant enough to meet the criteria for withdrawal syndrome as evidence of physical dependence (97, 98). The 3 phases of cocaine withdrawal are outlined in Table 58.9 (99).

Abrupt discontinuation of cocaine use is not life-threatening and does not cause the major physiological withdrawal symptoms associated with narcotics and sedatives. Pharmacologic treatment of chronic cocaine dependence is limited, unless efforts are made to include support and behavioral modification modeled after the Alcoholics Anonymous treatment program. The treatment modalities that are under investigation include the use of tricyclic antidepressants, which produce an alteration of dopamine receptors (100); bromocryptine (Parlodel), which restores dopamine depletion (101); lithium carbonate, which decreases the euphoria of cocaine through unknown mechanisms; and methylphenidate. The benefits of these agents are still under evaluation (102–104).

Table 58.9.
Phases of Cocaine Abstinence[a]

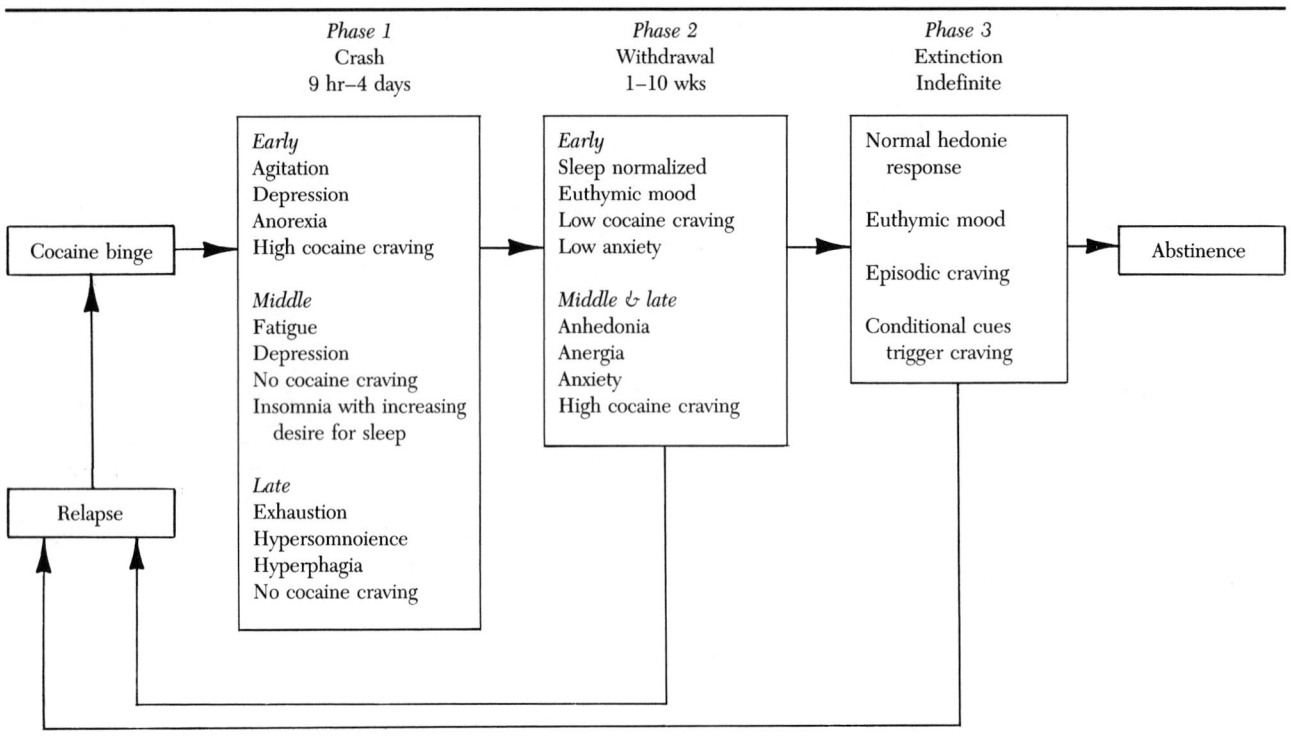

	Phase 1 Crash 9 hr–4 days	*Phase 2* Withdrawal 1–10 wks	*Phase 3* Extinction Indefinite	
Cocaine binge →	*Early* Agitation Depression Anorexia High cocaine craving *Middle* Fatigue Depression No cocaine craving Insomnia with increasing desire for sleep *Late* Exhaustion Hypersomnoience Hyperphagia No cocaine craving	*Early* Sleep normalized Euthymic mood Low cocaine craving Low anxiety *Middle & late* Anhedonia Anergia Anxiety High cocaine craving	Normal hedonie response Euthymic mood Episodic craving Conditional cues trigger craving	→ Abstinence

Relapse

[a] Modified from Hall WC, Talbert RL, Ereshefsky L: Cocaine abuse and its treatment. Pharmacotherapy 10:47–65, 1990.

PSYCHEDELICS

A wide variety of natural alkaloids and synthetic chemicals have been taken for their mind-altering and psychedelic effects. Other names used for this class of compounds are hallucinogens, psychotomimetics, and entactogens. In addition to their psychedelic effect, each of these drugs also has a wide range of physiologic and psychologic effects. A classic physical dependence has not been observed with the prototype hallucinoginic agents. Tolerance is seen with chronic use, and psychologic dependence is possible but rare. The normal drug-use cycle is an occasional self-administration for curiosity and to "explore the inner self." Adverse effects vary from agent to agent and depend not only on dose and duration of use but also on the user's personality and underlying psychiatric conditions.

The classic hallucinogenic agent is LSD (acid, white lightning, cubes, window panes, dots, blotteracid), first synthesized by Albert Hoffman at Sandoz laboratories in 1938. Five years later he accidentally discovered the intense visual hallucinations associated with this drug. Self-experimentation and illicit use of LSD peaked in the early 1970s, and it dropped steadily through that decade into the 1980s because of public attention to the serious adverse effects of this compound. However, the mid-1980s saw a resurgence in LSD use, particularly in high-school students, be-

cause of its low cost and increased availability and a renewed interest in self-exploration of the inner self.

LSD is a very potent agent active at doses averaging from 50 to 150 μg. LSD is usually taken orally, with an onset of 30 to 40 min. The first symptoms are mild to moderate sympathomimetic effects (pupillary dilation, tachycardia, sweating, blurred vision, etc.) followed by the sensory, psychologic, and cognitive effects of profound visual hallucinosis and the sensation of disordered integration of sensory input (Table 58.10) (105). For example, users may visualize sounds or music, feel odors, and hear color, and inanimate objects can assume life-like qualities. The peak intensity of effects is variable, depending upon the dose, and occurs within the first 2 or 3 hr and then wears off over the next 5 to 10 hr. Most users return to a normal psychologic state within 10 to 12 hr after ingestion. The user's personality and experience with LSD along with environmental factors play an important part in the sensory and psychologic effects seen with the drug.

The most common adverse effect is a temporary episode of panic and fear referred to as a "bad trip" (106). Although this is most common with first-time users, it is also possible with repeat users with increased dosages. Some users can control themselves by relaxation techniques involving breathing exercises and removing any ex-

Table 58.10.
Signs and Symptoms of Hallucinogenic Reactions

Sensory	Psychologic	Cognitive	Physiologic
Altered perception of color, objects, size, and shape	Anxiety	Impaired memory, recall, attention	Dilated pupils
Distortion of time, direction, and distance	Panic	Reduced mental performance	Tremor
Synethesias (e.g., "seeing sounds," "hearing colors")	Depression	Difficulty with problem solving	Piloerection ("gooseflesh")
	Mood alterations		Sweating
	Paranoid ideation		Dizziness
	Hallucinations (when sufficiently large doses are taken)		Weakness
			Paresthesias
			Ataxia
			Blurred vision
			Hyperreflexia
			Elevated blood pressure
			Hyperactivity
			Coma
			Elevated temperature
			Nausea
			Vomiting
			Hunger
			Tachycardia
			Bleeding (in massive LSD overdoses; thought to be evidence of platelet dysfunction)
			Clonic movements
			Blood pressure decline (in severe overdose)

ternal stimuli that might be producing acute stress. If the patient can not control the "bad trip," treatment is generally supportive and involves "talking down" the anxiety and fear. This is also referred to as reality therapy and involves the reassurance that these adverse effects are drug-related and will soon wear off. Placing the user in a quiet relaxed setting and removal of stress-producing stimuli is also helpful. If this method is not effective, oral benzodiazepines are useful in calming the patient and relieving the panic. However, since benzodiazepines do not reverse the LSD effects, talk-down reassurance should be continued. Even though phenothiazines antagonize the LSD effects, they are usually not needed and have produced orthostatic hypotension and anticholinergic toxicities. Sedative doses of a benzodiazepine like flurazepam 30 to 60 mg (Dalmane) should be used if panic reactions continue after initial therapy, which will allow the patient to sleep through the remainder of the drug effects (107).

Flashbacks are an acute but transient recurrence of past or all of the LSD experiences following a period of normal consciousness. The duration is usually a matter of hours. These events are more common in frequent users of LSD and may occur several years after the last LSD exposure. The incidence of flashbacks has been reported to range from 10 to 80%. However, most people who experimented only a few times with the drug have never had a flashback. Treatment of flashbacks is the same as for an acute anxiety-panic attack.

A small number of cases are reported of what appears to be permanent changes in patterns of thought and behavior developing after repeated use of large doses of LSD. These individuals have been referred to as acid burnouts or acid casualties, and they exhibit a condition indistinguishable from chronic undifferentiated schizophrenia (108). Whether such conditions would have resulted without the drug is unclear. It is possible that the drug simply exacerbated or unmasked an existing schizophrenia (109). Evidence linking these effects to direct neurologic toxicity (brain damage) is inconclusive at this time.

A number of mothers using LSD during pregnancy gave birth to children with birth defects. All of these cases involved multidrug use during pregnancy, preventing clear evidence that LSD is teratogenic when taken by either parent before or during pregnancy. However, all drugs used in pregnancy have a potential for producing teratogenic or fetotoxic effects, and they should be avoided, especially during the first trimester.

Mescaline (3,4,5-trimethoxyphenethylamine) is chemically similar to norepinephrine and its precursor, dopamine. Mescaline and its derivatives, have been referred to as the "hallucinogenic amphetamines." Mescaline occurs naturally in peyote, a plant preparation obtained from the mescal cactus. The dome-shaped head of this plant is made up of one or more discs (buttons) that have the potential for flowering and contain the principle peyote hallucinogen, mescaline. The peyote or mescal buttons are brown and hard and only rarely available in a powdered form. The buttons are usually softened by the user's saliva before being swallowed and contain, in addition to mescaline, numerous other β-phenylethylamine and isoquinoline alkaloids. This accounts for the common differences and effects of peyote and mescaline.

Mescaline and peyote have a slow onset, and initial effects are often unpleasant. Nausea, profuse perspiration, and static tremors are common for the first 1 to 2 hr followed by an hallucinogenic experience similar to that with LSD (110). The psychomimetic effects, lasting 8 to 12 hr, include alterations of sight, smell, touch, and hearing, but less mental reorganization than with LSD. Although some illicit users claim to prefer mescaline to LSD, most street samples of mescaline are in fact LSD, PCP, or combinations of LSD and PCP and contain no mescaline.

Other phenethylamine derivatives of mescaline include TMA (3,4,5-trimethoxyphenylisopropylamine) and DOM (STP) 2,5-dimethoxy-4-methyl phenylisopropanolomine. The original STP (serenity, tranquility, and peace) was in fact a variety of drug mixtures and not all of them contained DOM; today STP is a common synonym for DOM. These related conjurors produce a sense of euphoria and talkativeness; however, unlike amphetamines, they impair rather than improve concentration and rarely cause anorexia. They provide a mild psychedelic experience in lower doses and effects similar to mescaline and LSD in larger doses.

Another related chemical entity, MDA (3,4, methylenedioxyamphetamine) was synthesized in 1910, but its psychedelic effects were not discovered until the 1960s. MDA possesses both psychedelic and amphetamine-like effects. Initial effects with doses of 50 to 150 mg are described as euphoric and a sense of detachment or out-of-body experience. The drug has been used experimentally for introspection and to facilitate psychotherapy. Larger doses have produced hallucinations similar to the LSD experience (111). The N-methylation of MDA produces MDMA (methylenedioxymethamphetamine) (111). Street names for this drug are ecstasy, ice, XTC, M & M's, Adam and Eve. This drug appears to increase talkativeness and has a reputation as an aphrodisiac. Initial sympathomimetic activity includes a mild rise in blood pressure, tachycardia, increased motor activity (brusixm), and mild anxiety lasting 30 min to 1 hr. This state is followed by the relaxed introspection and euphoria seen with MDA. Users claim the psychedelic effects are easier to manage, increasing its popularity among college students as a "recreational drug" (113–118). This drug has a low therapeutic index with the possibility of chronic and possibly permanent neurologic toxicity at 2 to 4 times the hallucinogenic dose. There appears to be a selective destruction of tryptaminergic nerves in the cerebral cortex and hypothalamus in animals. Long-term recovery may occur but is generally incomplete (119).

Chronic users experience a withdrawal syndrome marked by severe depression (known as crash) and bruxism (120–122).

Compounds related to LSD and resembling serotonin are DMT (dimethyltryptamine), psilocybin, psilocin, harmine, and bufotenine. Psilocybin is a naturally occurring psychedelic found in mushrooms and used by the Mexican indians. Psilocybin is commonly taken by mouth and is one of the most rapidly acting psychedelics used orally. Initial effects are seen within 15 min after ingestion of doses 4 to 8 mg, reaching a peak effect in 1 to 2 hr. Total duration is 5 to 6 hr unless the dosage is increased above 8 mg. Physiologic effects include an increased pulse rate, respiratory rate, and body temperature, pupils are dilated, and systolic blood pressure increased, followed by a LSD-type hallucinogenic experience. As with the other exotic psychedelics (mescaline and DOM) most street sales of this compound contain LSD, PCP, amphetamines, or a combination of these or other drugs.

DMT (dimethyltryptamine) is one of the derivatives that has been isolated from the "hallucinogenic snuffs" used by the South American Indians. In its pure form, DMT is a very short acting agent with effects lasting less than 1 hr. Because of its short-acting effects, DMT is sometimes referred as the "businessman's psychedelic" or "businessman's trip."

Other agents that have been used recently to produce hallucinogenic effects are the anticholinergic preparations used in the treatment of extrapyramidal effects, trihexiphenidyl (Artane) and benzotropine (Cogentin). These agents may produce effects ranging from mild central nervous stimulation to a toxic delirium. High doses of these agents produce euphoria, confusion, hallucinations, and paranoia and may result in a state resembling toxic psychosis.

PHENCYCLIDINE

Phencyclidine was developed in the 1950s as a general anesthetic for veterinary and human use under the trade name of Sernyl. Although it was approved and marketed for human use for a short period of time, the postoperative delirium and unpleasant side effects resulted in withdrawal of the drug from the market in 1965. Phencyclidine was then marketed for veterinary use only in 1967 as Sernylan, until 1978 when it was classified as a schedule I controlled substance and removed from the market. Parke Davis continues to market a similar arylcycloalkylamine compound, ketamine (Ketalar), which causes similar adverse effects to PCP in a few patients and has also appeared with increasing frequency on the street scene as "monkey morphine." PCP appeared on the street scene in the late 1960s under the street names of "hog, PeaCe Pill, crystal, flakes, and angel dust." Its popularity increased in the mid-1970s, frequently as a substitute for less-available drugs such as

THC, peyote, mescaline, psilocyline, and LSD. Publicity about serious adverse effects led to a decline in PCP use in the late 1980s (123). PCP can be used orally, injected, or snorted, but it is most commonly smoked to allow users to monitor the dosage more carefully. PCP can be applied to tobacco, parsley, or marijuana (laced or dusted joint, or killerweed). It is also sold in combination with a variety of other drugs and many times substituted for street drugs that are difficult to obtain, such as THC, peyote, psylocyline, mescaline, or LSD.

In small doses PCP produces intoxication, with staggering gait, ataxia, slurred speech, numbness of the extremities, and a dissociative feeling. Horizontal and/or vertical nystagmus is often present and diagnostic. Muscular rigidity, sweating, apathy, and a blank stare may develop. Users report feelings of depersonalization and disordered thoughts. The effects of PCP generally last 4 to 6 hr depending upon the dosage. With doses in excess of 5 mg, a more pronounced analgesic effect is noticed. Hostile or unusual behavior is possible as doses are increased (124). The patient may show agitation, combativeness, and psychosis. Users perceive a superhuman strength, invulnerability, and body image distortions. Blood pressure is likely to be increased along with heart rate. Increased salivation, fever, repetitive movements, and muscular rigidity have also been reported. With increasing doses, analgesia is increased. Users do not perceive pain. Anesthesia, stupor, or coma and convulsions may occur, although the eyes may remain open. With higher doses, prolonged coma, muscle rigidity, opisthotonic posturing, and convulsions may occur. Nystagmus may or may not be present at toxic doses. Respiratory depression, seizures, acidosis, and rhabdomyolysis are also possible (125). Hypoglycemia, increased CPK, AST, ALT, and uric acid levels are also present. Isolation of patients from external stimuli to the degree compatible with support of vital functions and control of self destructive or violent behavior is recommended. Recovery is usually rapid, although some reports of overdosage include symptoms that last for several weeks. Mental status may take several days to weeks to return to normal. A psychotic phase has been reported for several weeks in some patients after a single dose of PCP.

Treatment of bad trips or an overdose of PCP often requires emergency care, because the patient is often violent and combative in behavior. Benzodiazapines are used to calm the patient. Attempts to talk-down the patient are generally ineffective and may often trigger violent behavior. Hostile and combative patients may require haloperidol (Haldol) to protect the patient and others from violent behavior. Chlorpromazine (Thorazine) is not recommended due to possible hypotensive effects and augmenting the anticholinergic actions of PCP (126). Treatment of overdosage is otherwise symptomatic and aimed at supporting vital functions (127). Hypersalivation may require suction, respiratory depression may require artificial ventilation, convulsions have been successfully treated with diazepam, and hypertension has been treated with hydralazine (Apresoline), sublingual nifedipine (Procardia), nitroprusside (Nipride), or phentolamine (Regitine). Anticonvulsants should be used to prevent seizures and excessive muscle contractions, since these along with hyperthemia may aggravate rhabdomyolysis.

There is considerable gastric recirculation of PCP when it reaches the alkaline environment of the duodenum. Continuous gastric suction can be of value in the treatment of an overdose. Other clinicians prefer to use repeated doses of activated charcoal to enhance elimination of the drug from the intestine. Urinary secretion of PCP is increased when urinary pH is acidic. However, since only a small percentage of the drug is excreted renally, urinary acidification may not play an important role in the elimination of the compound.

Serious neurologic and psychologic disorders have been reported with chronic PCP use, ranging from personality changes, confusional states, to psychotic states that may be long lasting. Patients with schizophrenia may be especially vulnerable to the psychotogenic effects of PCP. Other disorders that have been commonly reported with chronic PCP use are anxiety, nervousness, paranoia, delusions, memory disturbances, speech problems, anxiety, and mood swings ranging from social withdrawal and isolation to highly aggressive violent behavior that may last up to 1 year after cessation of drug use. Psychotic states have been reported to last several weeks after a single dose of PCP. Flashbacks have been reported to recur over a period of up to 2 months after discontinuing PCP use.

Chronic use of PCP can lead to both psychologic and physical dependence. Monkeys with implanted cathers will not administer LSD to themselves but they do self-administer PCP (128). Chronic users have reported continuous difficulty with memory, speech, and visual disturbances lasting up to one year after discontinuing the drug. Severe depression, nervousness, and personality changes are often resistant to treatment. The recovery phase of users discontinuing PCP is often marked with severe depression, stimulating recurrent drug abuse.

MARIJUANA

Marijuana is the flowering tops and leaves of the hemp plant known as *Cannabis sativa* (grass, pot, weed, Mary Jane). The dried leaves are most commonly smoked as cigarettes (joint, reefer, doobie, number) or in a pipe. The drug may be ingested orally in a prepared food (brownies) or beverage, but onset is slow (45 to 60 min) and absorption incomplete. While all parts of the male and female plant contain psychoactive substances, the highest concentrations are found in the flowering tops. The dried resinous exudate of the tops is called hashish. Over 60 cannabinoids have been isolated from marijuana. The euphoric and psychoactive effects may be due to a combination of several of them. However, Δ9-tetrahydrocannabinol (THC) is the agent believed to produce most of the characteristic effects. Hundreds of other compounds are produced by pyrolysis when marijuana is smoked and may be important in the long-term toxic effects of chronic use.

Another form of the drug, "hashoil," is extracted from the plant with organic solvents and may contain a concentration of up to 50 to 60% THC. However, much of the "pure THC" or hashoil that is found on the street is often PCP. The major effects of marijuana are seen in the central nervous system (CNS) and range from a mild relaxation and sedation to euphoria. Intoxication with marijuana is known as being "stoned or high." Users commonly describe a increased sense of well-being, giddiness, alteration of time and space perception, and subjective enhancement in senses of touch, taste, smell, and sound. Users experience unusual hunger and craving for food referred to as the "munchies." Some users claim that the drug increases their creativity and awareness of their surroundings. Many of the subjective effects appear to depend upon the expectations of the user and the circumstances under which the drug is used. Other physiologic effects are a mild increase in heart rate, dry mouth and throat, dryness of the eyelids, and conjunctival redding. Performance of simple motor tasks and reaction times are unimpaired in small doses but are significantly affected by doses equivalent to 1 or 2 cigarettes. Driving performance is clearly impaired for 4 to 8 hr, well beyond the time that the user thinks the subjective effects of the drug have worn off. Impairment produced by marijuana is additive to that of alcohol if the two are used concurrently. The effects of smoking marijuana occur rapidly within 5 to 10 min, may last 2 to 3 hr, depending on the dose, and are occasionally followed by a period of drowsiness (129).

Relative to narcotics, cocaine, depressants, and hallucinogens, emergency treatment of marijuana intoxication is rare (130, 131). Occasionally, a first-time user may experience a syndrome known as a "panic attack," consisting of anxiety, disorientation, and paranoid feelings. Users of the milder forms of the drugs may also experience this reaction if exposed to more potent forms of cannabis or THC. Treatment for this reaction is primarily reassurance and talking-down the fear and panic exhibited. Placing the patient in quiet surroundings and avoiding stimulants are also beneficial. Panic attacks seldom last more than 2 to 3 hr and may be relieved by small doses of benzodiazepines, if talk-down therapy is not fully effective. Patients with combative or aggressive behavior may have been using a product known as "super weed" that has been "laced" with phencyclidine (PCP).

Tolerance to the effects of marijuana clearly exists, even though chronic users have described a "reversed tolerance" and claim that smaller doses of the drug are necessary to produce the desired effects (132, 133). This effect is probably related to the manner of use and the expectations of the user. Chronic, high-dose cannabis users may experience an abstinance or withdrawal syndrome upon abrupt discontinuation of use. Signs and symptoms include irritability, restlessness, nervousness, anorexia, weight loss, insomnia, and REM rebound. Onset of this syndrome is several hours after the last dose, and it lasts 4 to 5 days. Since withdrawal is not life-threatening, treatment involves little more than supportive therapy with short-term, low doses of benzodiazopines.

In addition to the slowed psychomotor response while under the influence of the drug, there is a decrease in short-term memory that is reversible on discontinuing the drug (134–136). Several reported physiologic effects produce concern. The respiratory effects of long-term marijuana use produce chronic cough, laryngitis, bronchitis, and pathologic changes like those in chronic tobacco smokers (137–141). Chronic smoking of one marijuana cigarette daily will decrease vital lung capacity equal to that seen after chronic smoking of 1 pack of tobacco cigarettes daily (142–144). In addition, the smoke from a marijuana cigarette contains high concentrations of several key carcinogenic agents found in tobacco smoke (145). Another concern is the possibility of pulmonary fibrosis from smoking marijuana that has been sprayed with paraquat, other herbicides, or other insecticides. However, the latest reports indicate that smoking destroys paraquat by pyrolysis (146).

Other effects of marijuana are decreased testosterone concentrations and a reversible decreased spermatogenesis in males. Females experience decreased FSH and LH concentrations in the normal ovulatory cycle. Although THC crosses the placenta, there are no reports in humans of teratogenic effects directly attributable to marijuana alone (147–149). However, avoiding any unnecessary drug during pregnancy is advisable. Children born to mothers who were chronic marijuana smokers during pregnancy may be at increased risk for learning disabilities such as attention-deficit disorders (150, 151). *Salmonella* and *Aspergillus* contaminants have been reported to produce infections (152, 153).

Chronic use of marijuana has been implicated in producing psychologic changes and production of what has been called an "amotivational syndrome" characterized by diminished drive, lessened ambition, decreased motivation, loss of effectiveness, impairment of judgement, concentration, memory, and communication skills, and inability to set goals or manage stress. Cessation may lead to gradual improvement over several weeks, but may require months. It is difficult to determine whether these effects were present prior to and not caused by marijuana use, but they are observed very commonly. Several studies have implicated marijuana with structural brain damage, but much controversy exists about these (154, 155). Seizures have occurred in some epileptics.

There has been much recent information on the dangers of passive tobacco smoke. Concern could also be expressed over potential problems of passive marijuana smoke, although, intoxication is rarely reported from passive inhalation of marijuana. However, there are numerous reports of cannabis metabolites detected in the urine of the passive inhaler (156–158). THC metabolites may be present in the urine up to 3 months after heavy chronic use.

Marijuana is considered, along with alcohol and tobacco products, as one of the major "gateway" drugs. While this does not imply that users of marijuana will all progress to more dangerous drugs (e.g., cocaine), use of one or more of these commonly available agents is part of the history of most drug dependencies.

VOLATILE SUBSTANCES—INHALENTS

Many volatile liquids produce an intoxicated state when inhaled. Young children and adolescents most commonly experiment with this method of producing distorted consciousness. A wide variety of industrial solvents, anesthetics, and other chemicals may produce intoxication and coma (Table 58.11). They can be divided into 3 groups: (a) commercial solvents: toluene, xylene, benzene, naphtha, hexane, acetone, trichloroethylene, carbon tetrachloride, and many other volatile solvents found in model airplane glue, plastic cements, paint thinner, gasoline, cleaning fluids, nail polish remover, and lighter fluid; (b) aerosols: propellants in many household and commercial aerosols sprays, gases containing chlorinated or fluorinated

Table 58.11.
Commonly Abused Solvent Products

Glue	Toluene, xylene, acetone, benzene, n-hexane
Cleaning fluids	Trichloroethylene, toluene, carbon tetrachloride, tetrachlorethylene, 1,1,1-trichloroethane
Petrochemicals (gasoline)	Hydrocarbons, lead
Aerosols	Fluorocarbons
Lighter fluid	Butane
Acrylic paint	Toluene
Paints, varnishes, thinning lacquers	Trichloroethane, methylene chloride, toluene, alcohols, ketones
Cements	Acetone, toluene, hydrocarbons, trichlorethylene, hexane
Dyes	Acetone, methylene chloride
Nail polish remover	Acetone, amyl acetate, alcohol

Table 58.12.
General Effects of Inhaled Volatile Solvents

Common Acute Effects	Rare Dangers
Euphoria	"Sudden sniffing death"
Drowsiness	Suffocation
Headache	
Nausea	
Partial amnesia	
Visual disturbance	
Hallucination	
Ataxia	
Impaired judgment	
Reduced muscle and reflex control	
Tolerance	
Metabolic acidosis	
High anion gap	
Hypokalemia	

hydrocarbons including insecticides, deodorants, hairsprays and nonstick coating substances; and (c) anesthetics: nitrous oxide (laughing gas), and less frequently, chloroform and ether. Nitrous oxide is available commercially as a whipped-cream propellant, as a tracer gas to detect pipe leaks, and to reduce preignition in racing cars. Anesthetics have been abused since their discovery in the early 1800s. Glue sniffing became widespread in the late 1950s, and experimentation with many other inhalants proliferated during the 1960s. These compounds are commonly sniffed for their intoxicating effects. Solvents can be "bagged," or sprayed into a plastic bag prior to inhalation, or "huffed," sprayed into a cloth and held to the mouth.

Although there is a wide range of chemical entities, nearly all the abused volatile substances produce central nervous system depression. Decreased inhibition may produce an apparent stimulant effect and initial sense of euphoria preceding the classic sedative effects of ataxia, dizziness, impaired judgement, slurred speech, and somnolence. At larger doses, hallucinations and delusions including a sense of omnipotence or unusual strength may lead to impulsive behavior. The initial euphoric effects may last only a few minutes, with the depressant effects gradually wearing off in 1 to 2 h. At very high doses, loss of consciousness may occur, and recovery can take several hours.

All the inhalants share the hazard of inducing an intoxicated state in which judgment and motor function are impaired (Table 58.12). Accidents have occurred including fatalities where suffocation is the major cause of death. Most commonly, this occurs when the user becomes unconscious with the apparatus used covering the nose and mouth. High concentrations of any aromatic hydrocarbon can cause coma and death (159, 160). In addition to asphyxiation and trauma, reports of death due to sudden cardiac ventricular arrhythmias are most commonly preceded by physical exercise (161). Other adverse effects are direct organ toxicities associated with specific compounds (161). Chronic long-term inhalation of benzene may cause bone marrow aplasia, neurosis, and fatty degeneration of the liver and heart (163). Gasoline not only contains benzene, but some types contain enough lead to produce systemic lead poisoning (164–166). Toluene may produce permanent, neurologic dysfunction of the cerebral cortical, cerebellar, auditory, pyramidal track, brain stem, and peripheral nervous system (167–171). Hepatic and renal damage (renal tubular acidosis) have also been reported with chronic use (172).

Nitrous oxide has been recreationally abused since its discovery in 1844. However, it is a safe and valuable anesthetic when used appropriately, as is seen commonly in "painless" dental practice today. Misuse can cause hypoxia and asphyxia leading to permanent nerve damage and/or death when oxygen is not inhaled in appropriate concentrations with the gas. End-organ toxicity is rare with occasional use of nitrous oxide. However, chronic use of this gas has been reported to produce a number of transient neurotoxicities such as progressive paresthesia or neuropathy similar to vitamin B-12 deficiency (173). Contaminants of some consumer kits for production of nitrous oxide may produce respiratory distress (174). Intoxication with nitrous oxide clearly impairs muscle coordination and delays reaction time, decreasing the ability to drive.

A growing number of users of organic nitrites include abuse of amyl nitrite and its nonprescription analogs, butyl and isobuyl nitrite, which are sold as liquid incense or room deodorizers under such trade names as (Rush, Lockerroom, Sweat, Bolt, Quicksilver, Jock, Hardware, Aroma of Men, and Heart On.) Commonly known as "poppers," "snappers," or "disco drugs," these products have been popularized as aphrodisiacs among male homosexuals (175). The major pharmacological effects of the nitrites is a significant vasodilation due to their smooth muscle relaxant effect (Table 58.13). Peak effects following inhalation occur within seconds, last less than a minute, and may be followed by flushing, headaches, and dizziness. Hypotensive reflex tachycardia is common and may lead to syncope. Methemoglobinemia and death have been rarely reported following chronic use of these compounds and are more likely to occur if they are ingested (176, 177).

SUMMARY

Drug abuse is a complex multifaceted problem. There have been no simple or universally successful solutions. Increased public awareness programs, coordinated educational programs in elementary and junior high schools, increased law enforcement efforts to decrease the availability of illicit drugs, and more severe punishment from the judicial system have been the mainstays of coordinated efforts at both the local and national levels to decrease most forms of drug abuse among young people. However, at the same time alcohol abuse is at an all-time high in teenagers and is occurring at younger ages. There is a continued need for health professional involvement in drug abuse prevention programs. Pharmacists have the unique responsibility of drug use control in society as well as being the most knowledgeable health professionals in therapeutics and adverse drug effects. Therefore, all pharmacists should be proactive in drug abuse education and prevention programs.

Table 58.13.
Organic Nitrite Effects

Physiologic Effects	Adverse Effects
Vasodilation	Giddiness
Venous pooling	Headache
Hypotension	Nausea
Reflex tachycardia	Vomiting
Reduced cerebral blood flow	Flushing
Tissue hypoxia	Dermatitis
Sphincter relaxation	Methemoglobinemia
Tolerance	Weakness
	Dizziness
	Syncope
	Shortness of breath
	Chest pain
	Tracheobronchitis
	Increased intraocular pressure

REFERENCES

1. Ziporyn T: A growing industry and menace: makeshift laboratory's designer drugs. JAMA 256(22):3061, 1986.
2. LaBarbera M, Wolfe T: Characteristics, attitudes and implications of fentanyl use based upon reports from self-identified fentanyl users. J Psychoactive Drugs 15(4):293, 1983.
3. Moore RA, Rumack BH, Conner CS, et al.: Nalozone underdosage after narcotic poisoning. Am J Dis Child 134:156, 1980.
4. Jasinski DR, Martin WR, Haertzen CA: The human pharmacology and abuse potential of N-allylnoroxymorphone (Naloxone). J Pharmacol Exp Ther 157:420, 1967.
5. Heishman SJ, Stitzer ML, Bigelow GE, Liebson IA: Acute opioid physical dependence in postaddict humans: naloxone dose effects after brief morphine exposure. J Pharmacol Exp Ther 248:127–134, 1989.
6. Freitas PM: Narcotic withdrawal in the emergency department. Am J Emerg Med 3:456–460, 1985.
7. Hodding GC, Jann M, Ackerman IP: Drug withdrawal syndromes: a literature review. West J Med 133:383–391, 1980.
8. Ostrea EM, Chavez JS, Strauss ME: A study of factors that influence the severity of neonatal narcotic withdrawal. J Pediatr 88:642, 1976.
9. Bashore RA, Ketchum JS, Staisch KJ: Heroin addiction and pregnancy. West J Med 134:506, 1981.
10. Rosen TS: Infants of addicted mothers. In Farnoff AA, Martin RJ (eds): Neonatal-Perinatal Medicine St. Louis, CV Mosby, 1114, 1987.
11. Futz JM Jr, Senay EC: Guidelines for the management of hospitalized narcotic addicts. Ann Inter Med 82:815–818, 1975.
12. Gossop M, Johns A, Green L: Opiate withdrawal: inpatient versus outpatient programmes and preferred versus random assignment to treatment. Br Med J 293:103–104, 1986.
13. Vining E, Kosten TR, Kleber HD: Clinical utility of rapid clonibine-

naltrexone detoxification for opioid abusers. Br J Addiction 83:567–574, 1988.

14. Brewer C, Rezae H, Bailey C: Opioid withdrawal and naltrexone induction in 48–72 hours with minimal drop-out, using a modification of the naltrexone-clonidine technique. Br J Psychiatry 153:340–343, 1988.

15. Charney DS, Heninger GR, Kelber HD: The combined use of clonidine and naltrezone as a rapid, safe, and effective treatment of abrupt withdrawal from methadone. Am J Psychiatry 143:831–837, 1986.

16. Fultz JM, Senay EC: Guidelines to the management of hospitalized narcotic addicts. Ann Intern Med, 82:815–818, 1975.

17. Jaffe JH, Drug addiction and drug abuse. In Gilman AG, Rall TW, Nies AS, et al. (eds): The Pharmacological Basis of Therapeutics, ed. 8. New York, Macmillan, 1990.

18. Newman RG: Methadone treatment: defining and evaluating success. N Engl J Med 317:447, 1987.

19. Judson BA, Goldstein A, Inturrisi CE: Methadylacetate (LAAM) in the treatment of heroin addicts. Arch Gen Psychiatry 40:834–840, 1983.

20. Gossop M: Clonidine and the treatment of the opiate withdrawal syndrome. Drug Alcohol Depend 21:253–259, 1988.

21. Gold MS, Pottash AC, Sweeney DR: Opiate withdrawal using clonidine. JAMA, 243:343, 1980.

22. Crabtree B: Review of naltrexane, a long-acting opiate antagonist. Clin Pharm 3:273–280, 1984.

23. Kleber HD: Naltrexone. J Subst Abuse Treat 2:117, 1985.

24. Gonzales JP, Brogden RN: Naltrexone: a review. Drugs 35:192–213, 1988.

25. Gram DH, Marmo J, Holden R: Naltrexone treatment—the problem of patient acceptance. J Subst Abuse Treat 6:119–122, 1989.

26. Preston KL, Bigelow GE: Pharmacological advances in addiction treatment. Int J Addict, 20(6 & 7):185, 1985.

27. Chaisson RE, Moss AR, Onishi R: Human immunodeficiency virus infection in heterosexual intravenous drug users in San Francisco. Am J Public Health, 77(2):169, 1987.

28. Louria D, Hensle T, Rose J: Major medical complications of heroioin addiction. Ann Intern Med 67:1, 1967.

29. Becker CE: Medical complications of drug abuse. Adv Intern Med 24:183–202, 1979.

30. Khantzian EJ, McKenna GJ: Acute toxic and withdrawal reactions associated with drug use and abuse. Ann Intern Med 90:361, 1979.

31. Woods JH, Katz JL, Winger G: Abuse liability of benzodiazepines, Pharmacol Rev 39:251–419, 1987.

32. Arieff AJ, Friedmann EA: Coma following non-narcotic drug overdose: management of 200 adult patients. Am J Med Sci 266:405, 1973.

33. Hadden J, Johnson K, Smith S: Acute barbiturate intoxication concepts of management. JAMA 209:893, 1969.

34. Pond SM, Olson KR, Osterloh JD: Randomized study of the treatment of phenobarbital overdose with repeated doses of activated charcoal. JAMA 251:3104–3108, 1984.

35. Miller NS, Gold MS: Identification and treatment of benzodiazepine abuse. Am Fam Physician 40:175–183, 1989.

36. Owen RT, Tyrer P. Benzodiazepine dependence: a review of the evidence. Drugs 25:385, 1983.

37. Rifkin A, Quitkin F, Klein DF: Withdrawal reaction to diazepam. JAMA 236:2171, 1976.

38. Smith DS, Wesson DR: Benzodiazepine dependency syndromes. J Psychoactive Drugs, 15:85, 1983.

39. Rosenberg HC, Chiu TH: Time course for development of benzodiazepine tolerance and physical dependence. Neurosci Biobehav Rev 9:123–131, 1985.

40. Busto U, Sellers EM, Naranjo CA: Withdrawal reaction after long-term therapeutic use of benzodiazepines. N Engl J Med 313:854–859, 1986.

41. Sanchez-Craig M, Cappell H, Busto U, Kay G: Cognitive-behavioural treatment for benzodiazepine dependence: a comparison of gradual versus abrupt cessation of drug intake. Br J Addict 82:1317–1327, 1987.

42. Woods JH, Katz JL, Winger G: Use and abuse of benzodiazepines: issues relevant to prescribing. JAMA 260:3476–3480, 1988.

43. Kales A, Scharf MB, Kales JD: Rebound insomnia: a potential hazard following withdrawal of certain benzodiazepines. JAMA 241:1692, 1979.

44. Robinson GM, Sellers EM, Janecek E: Barbiturate and hypnosedative withdrawal by a multiple oral phenobarbital loading dose technique. Clin Pharmacol Ther, 30(1):71, 1981.

45. Smith DE, Wesson DR: Phenobarbital technique for treatment of barbiturate dependence. Arch Gen Psychiatry 24:56–60, 1971.

46. Robinson GM, Sellers EM, Janecek E: Barbiturate and hypnosedative withdrawal by a multiple oral phenobarbital loading dose technique. Clin Pharmacol Ther 30:71–76, 1981.

47. Martin PR, Kapur BM, Whiteside EA: Intravenous phenobarbital therapy in barbiturate and hyposedative withdrawal reactions: a kinetic approach. Clin Pharmacol Ther 26:856–864, 1979.

48. Wesson DR, Smith DE: Treatment techniques for narcotic withdrawal and special reference to mixed narcotic-sedative addiction. J Psychedelic Drugs 4:118, 1971.

49. Perry PJ, Alexander B: Sedative/hypnotic dependence: patient stabilization, tolerance testing, and withdrawal. Drug Intell Clin Pharm 20:532–537, 1986.

50. Harrison M, Busto U, Naranjo CA: Diazepan tapering in detoxification for high-dose benzodiazepine abuse. Clin Pharmacol Ther 36:527–533, 1984.

51. Mueller SM: Neurologic complications of phenylpropanolamine use. Neurology 33:650, 1983.

52. Dietz AJ: Amphetamine-like reactions to phenylpropanolamine. JAMA 245(6):601, 1981.

53. Ellinwood EH: Assault and homocide associated with amphetamine abuse. Am J Psych 127:1170, 1971.

54. Schmidt CJ, Gibb JW: Role of dopamine in the neurotoxic effects of methamphetamine. J Pharmacol Exp Ther 233:539, 1985.

55. Kleber HD: Cocaine abuse: historical, epidemiological, and psychological perspectives. J Clin Psychiatry 49:2(suppl), 3–6, 1988.

56. Washton AM, Gold MS, Pottash AC: Crack: early report on a new drug epidemic. Postgrad Med, 80(5):52, 1986.

57. Gawin FH, Ellinwood EH, Jr: Cocaine and other stimulants: actions, abuse, and treatment. N Engl J Med 318:1173–1182, 1988.

58. Siegel RK: Cocaine smoking. J Psychoactive Drugs 14(4):313, 1982.

59. Perez-Reyes M, DiGuiseppi S, Ondrusek G: Free-base cocaine smoking. Clin Pharmacol Ther 32(4):459, 1982.

60. Dakis CA, Gold MS: New concepts in cocaine addiction: the dopamine depletion hypothesis. Neurosci Biobehav Rev 9:469, 1985.

61. Jeffcoat AR, Perez-Reyes M, Hill JM: Cocaine disposition in humans after intravenous injection, nasal insufflation (snorting), or smoking. Drug Metab Dispos 17:153–159, 1989.

62. Chow MJ, Ambre JJ, Ruo TI; Kinetics of cocaine distribution, elimination, and chronotropic effects. Clin Pharmacol Ther 38:318, 1985.

63. Isner JM, Estes NAM III, Thompson PD: Acute cardiac events temporally related to cocaine abuse. N Engl J Med 315:1438–1443, 1986.

64. Itkonen J, Schnoll S, Glassroth J: Pulmonary dysfunction in "free-base" cocaine users. Arch Intern Med 144:2195, 1984.

65. Shesser R, Davis C, Edelstein S: Pneumomediastinum and pneumothorax after inhaling alkaloidal cocaine. Ann Emerg Med 10(4):213, 1981.

66. Karch SB, Billingham ME: The pathology and etiology of cocaine-induced heart disease. Arch Pathol Lab Med 112:225–230, 1988.

67. Cregler LL: Adverse consequences of cocaine abuse. J Natl Med Assoc 81:27–38, 1989.

68. Isner JM, Estes NAM III, Thompson PD: Acute cardiac events temporally related to cocaine abuse. N Engl J Med 315:1438–1443, 1986.

69. Lang RA, Cigarroa RG, Yancy CW: Cocaine-induced coronary-artery vasoconstriction. N Engl J Med 321:1557–1562, 1989.

70. Cregler LL, Mark H: Special report: medical complications of cocaine abuse. N Engl J Med 315(23):1495, 1986.

71. Coleman DL, Ross TF, Naughton JL: Myocardial ischemia and infarction related to recreational cocaine use. West J Med 136:444, 1982.

72. Wetli CV, Wright RK: Death caused by recreational cocaine use. JAMA 241(23):2519, 1979.

73. Ettinger NA, Albin RJ: A review of the respiratory effects of smoking cocaine. Am J Med 87:664–668, 1989.

74. Itkonen J, Schnoll S, Glassroth J: Pulmonary dysfunction in "free-base" cocaine users. Arch Intern Med 144:2195, 1984.

75. Shesser R, Davis C, Edelstein S: Pneumomediastinum and pneumothorax after inhaling alkaloidal cocaine. Ann Emerg Med 10(4):213, 1981.

76. Golbe LI, Merkin MD: Cerebral infarction in a user of freebase cocaine (crack). Neurology 36:1602, 1986.

77. Lichtenfeld PJ, Rubin DB, Feldman RS: Subarachnoid hemorrhage precipitated by cocaine snorting. Arch Neurol 41:223, 1984.

78. Mody CK, Miller BL, McIntyre HB, Cobb SK, Goldberg MA: Neurologic complications of cocaine abuse, Neurology 38:1189–1193, 1988.

79. Lathers CM, Tyau LSY, Spino MM, Agarwal I: Cocaine-induced seizures, arrhythmias and sudden death. J Clin Pharmacol 28:584–593, 1988.

80. Cregler LL, Mark H: Medical complications of cocaine abuse. N Engl J Med 315:1495–1500, 1986.

81. Sharff JA: Renal infarction associated with intravenous cocaine use. Ann Emerg Med 13:1145, 1984.

82. Isner JM, Chorkshi SK: Cocaine and vasospasm. N Engl J Med 321:1604–1606, 1989.

83. Nademanee K, Gorelick DA, Josephson MA: Myocardial ischemia during cocaine withdrawal. Ann Intern Med 111:876–880, 1989.

84. Pasternack PF, Colvin SB, Baumann FG: Cocaine induced angina pectoris and acute infarction in patients younger than 40 years. Am J Cardiol 55:847, 1985.

85. Howard RE, Hueter DC, Davis GJ: Acute myocardial infarction following cocaine abuse in a young woman with normal coronary arteries. JAMA 245(1):95, 1985.

86. Vandette JM, Cornish LA: Medical Complications of illicit cocaine use. Clin Pharm 8:401–411, 1989.

87. Caruana DS, Weinbach B, Goery D: Cocaine packet ingestion: diagnosis, management, and natural history. Ann Intern Med 100:73, 1984.

88. Roberts JR, Price D, Goldfrank L: The bodystuffer syndrome: a clandestine form of drug overdose. Am J Emerg Med 4:24, 1986.

89. Gay GR: Clinical management of acute and chronic cocaine poisoning. Ann Emerg Med 11:562, 1982.

90. Deriet RW: Cocaine intoxication. Postgrad Med 86:245–253, 1989.

91. Ramoska E, Sacchetti AD: Propranolol induced hypertension in treatment of cocaine intoxication. Ann Emerg Med 14:1112–1113, 1985.

92. Ramoska E, Sacchetti AD: Propranolol-induced hypertension in treatment of cocaine intoxication. Ann Emerg Med 14:1112, 1985.

93. Dusenberry SJ, Hicks MJ, Mariani PJ: Labetalol treatment of cocaine toxicity. Ann Emerg Med 16(2):235, 1987.

94. Jonsson S, O'Meara M, Young JB: Acute cocaine poisoning: importance of treating seizures and acidosis. Am J Med 75:106, 1983.

95. Louie AK, Lannon RA, Keller IA: Treatment of cocaine-induced panic disorder. Am J Psychiatry 146:40–44, 1989.

96. Fischman MW: Behavioral pharmacology of cocaine. J Clin Psychiatry 318:1173–1182, 1988.

97. Kalivas PW, Duffy P, DuMars LA, Skinner C: Behavioral and neurochemical effects of acute and daily cocaine administration in rats. J Pharmacol Exp Ther 245:485–492, 1988.

98. O'Brien CP, Childress AR, Arndt IO, McLellan T, Woody GE, Maany I: Pharmacological and behavioral treatment of cocaine dependence: controlled studies. J Clin Psychiatry, 49:17–22, 1988.

99. Hall WC, Talbert RL, Ereshefsky L: Cocaine abuse and its treatment. Pharmacotherapy 10:47–65, 1990.

100. O'Brien CP, Childress AR, Arndt IO: Pharmacological and behavioral treatments of cocaine dependence: controlled studies. J Clin Psychiatry 49:2(suppl):3–6, 1988.

101. Dackis CA, Gold MS: Bromocriptine as a treatment for cocaine abuse. Lancet, 1(8438):1151, 1985.

102. Gawin R, Kleber H: Pharmacologic treatment of cocaine abuse. Psychiatr Clin North Am 9(3):573, 1986.

103. Resnick RB, Resnick EB: Cocaine abuse and its treatment. Psychiatr Clin North Am 7(4):713, 1984.

104. Gawin FH, Kleber HD, Byck R, Rounsaville BJ, Kosten TR, Jatlow PI, Morgan C: Desipramine facilitation of initial cocaine abstinence. Arch Gen Psychiatry 46:117–121, 1989.

105. Sanders-Bush E, Burris KD, Knoth K: Lysergic acid diethylamide and 2,5-dimethozy-4 methylamphetamine are partial agonists at serotonin receptors linked to phosphoinositide hydrolysis. J Pharmacol Exp Ther 246:924–928, 1988.

106. McGlothlin WH, Arnold DO: LSD revised: 10 year follow up of medical LSD users. Arch Gen Psychiatry 24:35, 1971.

107. Hollister LE: Drug-induced psychiatric disorders and their management. Med Toxicol 1:428, 1986.

108. McWilliams S, Tuttle R: Long term psychological effects of LSD. Psychol Bull 79:341, 1973.

109. Vardy MM, and Kay SR: LSD psychosis or LSK-induced schizophrenia? Arch Gen Psychiatry 40:877–883, 1983.

110. Schuckit MA: The hallucinogens and related drugs. In Woods SM (ed) Drug and Alcohol Abuse: A Clinical Guide to Diagnosis and Treatment. New York, Plenum Press, pp 137–151, 1984.

111. Glass G. Psychedelic drugs, stress, and the ego. J Nerv Ment Dis 156:232, 1973.

112. Shulgin AT: The background and chemistry of MDMA. J Psychedelic Drugs 18(4):291, 1986.

113. Hayner GN, McKinney H: MDMA—the dark side of ecstasy. J Psychedelic Drugs 18(4):341, 1986.

114. Dowling GP, McDonough ET, Bost RO: Eve and ecstasy—a report of five deaths associated with the use of MDEA and MDMA. JAMA 257(12):1615, 1987.

115. Ricaurte G, Bryan G, Strauss L: Hallucinogenic amphetamine selectively destroys brain serotonin nerve terminals. Science 229:986, 1985.

116. Schmidt CJ, Wu L, Lovenberg W: Methylenedioxymethamphetamine: a potential neurotoxic amphetamine analog. Eur J Pharmacol 124:175, 1986.

117. Gehlert DR, Schmidt CJ, Wu L: Evidence for specific methylenedioxymethamphetamine (ecstasy) binding sites in the rat brain. Eur J Pharmacol 119:135, 1985.

118. Stone DM, Stahl DC, Hanson GR: The effects of 3,4-methylenedioxyamphetamine (MDA) and 3,4-methylenedioxymethamphetamine (MDMA) on monoaminergic systems in the rat brain. Eur J Pharmacol 128:41, 1986.

119. Battaglia G, Yeh SY, O'Hearn E, Molliver ME, Kuhar MJ, De Souza EB: 3,4-Methylenedioxymethamphetamine and 3,4-methylenedioxyamphetamine destroy serotonin terminals in rat brain: quantification of neurodegeneration by measurement of [^{3}H]paroxetine-labeled serotonin uptake sites. J Pharmacol Exp Ther 242:911–916, 1987.

120. Verebey K, Alrazi J, Jaffe JH: Complications of "ecstasy" (MDMA). JAMA 259:1649–1650, 1988.

121. Lamb RJ, Griffitys RR: Self-injection of d, 1-3, 4-methylenediox-

ymethamphetamine (MDMA) in the baboon. Psychopharmacology (Berlin) 91:268–272, 1987.

122. Peroutka SJ, Newman H, Harris H: Subjective effects of 3,4-methylenedioxymethamphetamine in recreational users. Neuropsychopharmacology 1:273–278, 1988.

123. Davis BL: The PCP epidemic: a critical review. Int J Addict 17:1137, 1982.

124. McCarron MM, Schulze BW, Thompson GA: Acute phencyclidine intoxication: incidence of clinical findings in 1000 cases. Ann Emerg Med 10:237, 1981.

125. Patel R, Connor G: A review of thirty cases of rhabdomyolysis associated renal failure among phencyclidine users. Clin Toxicol 23:547, 1986.

126. Giannini AJ, Eighan MS, Loiselle RH: Comparison of haloperidol and chlorpromazine in the treatment of phencyclidine psychosis. J Clin Pharmacol 24:202, 1984.

127. Aronow R, Miceli JN, Done AK: A therapeutic approach to the acutely overdosed PCP patient. J Psychedelic Drugs 12:259, 1980.

128. Nabeshima T, Fukaya H, Yamaguchi K, Ishikawa K, Furukawa H, Kameyama T: Development of tolerance and supersensitivity to phencyclidine in rats after repeated administration of phencyclidine. Eur J Pharmacol 135:23–33, 1987.

129. Dewey WL: Cannabinoid pharmacology. Pharmacol Rev 38:151–178, 1986.

130. Weil AT: Adverse reactions to marijuana. N Engl J Med 282(18):997, 1970.

131. Weil AT, Zinberg NE, Nelson JM: Clinical and psychological effects of marijuana in man. Science 162:1243, 1968.

132. Jones RT, Benowitz N: Clinical studies of cannabis tolerance and dependence. Ann NY Acad Sci 282:221, 1976.

133. Nowlan R, Cohen S: Tolerance to marijuana: heart rate and subjective "high." Clin Pharmacol Ther 22(5):550, 1977.

134. Vachon L, Sulkowski A, Rich E: Marijuana effects of learning, attention and time estimation. Psychopharmacologia 39–41, 1974.

135. Abel E: Marijuana and memory: acquisition and retrieval. Science 128:194, 1971.

136. Dornbush RL, Fink M, Freedman AM: Marijuana, memory and perception. Am J Psychiatry 128:194, 1971.

137. Huber GL, Simmons GA, McCarthy CR: Depressant effect of marijuana smoke on antibacterial activity of pulmonary alveolar macrophages. Chest 68:769, 1975.

138. Henderson RL, Tennant FS, Guerry R: Respiratory manifestations of hashish smoking. Arch Otolaryngol 95:248, 1972.

139. Abramson HA: Respiratory disorders and marijuana use. J Asthma Res 11:97, 1974.

140. Waldman MM: Marijuana bronchitis. JAMA 211:501, 1970.

141. Wu TC, Tashkin DP, Djahed GB, Rose JE: Pulmonary hazards of smoking marijuana as compared with tobacco. N Engl J Med 318:347–351, 1988.

142. Tashkin DP, Shapiro BJ, Lee YE: Subacute effects of heavy marijuana smoking on pulmonary function in healthy men. N Engl J Med 294(3):125, 1976.

143. Tashkin DP, Calvarese BM, Simmons MS: Respiratory status of seventy-four habitual marijuana smokers. Chest 78:699, 1980.

144. Gong H Jr, Taskin DP, Simmons MS: Acute and subacute bronchial effects of oral cannabinoids. Clin Pharmacol Ther 35:26, 1984.

145. Hoffman D: On the carcinogenicity of marijuana smoke. Res Adv Phytochem 9:63, 1975.

146. Landrigan PJ, Powell KE, James LM: Paraquat and marijuana: epidemiological risk assessment. Am J Public Health 73:784, 1983.

147. Fried PA, Buckingham M, VonKulmiz P: Marijuana use during pregnancy and perinatal risk factors. Am J Obstet Gynecol 146:992, 1983.

148. Linn S, Schoenbaum SC, Monson RR: The association of marijuana use with outcome of pregnancy. Am J Public Health 73:1161, 1983.

149. Greenland S, Staisch KJ, Brown N: The effects of marijuana use during pregnancy. Am J Obstet Gynecol June:408, 1982.

150. Hollister LE: Cannabis—1988. Acta Psychiatr Scand (Suppl. 345) 78:108–118, 1988.

151. Hollister LE. Health aspects of cannabis. Pharmacol Rev 38:1–20, 1986.

152. Taylor DN, Wachsmuth IK, Shangknan YH: Salmonellosis associated with marijuana: a multistate outbreak traced by plasmid fingerprinting. N Engl J Med 306(21):1249, 1982.

153. Kagen SL: *Aspergillus*: an inhalable contaminant of marijuana. N Engl J Med 304(8):483, 1981.

154. Hannerz J, Hindmarsh T: Neurological and neuroradiological examination of chronic cannabis smokers. Ann Neurol 13:207, 1983.

155. Co BT, Goodwin DW, Gado M: Absence of cerebral atrophy in chronic cannabis users. JAMA 237(12):1229, 1977.

156. Morland J, Bugge A, Skuterud B: Cannabinoids in blood and urine after passive inhalation of cannabis smoke. J Forensic Sci 30(4):997, 1985.

157. Cone EJ, Johnson RE: Contact highs and urinary cannabinoid excretion after passive exposure to marijuana smoke. Clin Pharmacol Ther 40(3):247, 1986.

158. Perez-Reyes M, DiGuiseppi S, Mason AP: Passive inhalation of marijuana smoke and urinary excretion of cannabinoids. Clin Pharmacol Ther 34(1):36, 1983.

159. Anderson HR, Macnair RS, Ramsey JD: Deaths from abuse of volatile substances: a national epidemiological study. Br Med J 290:304, 1985.

160. King GS, Smialek JE, Troutman WG: Sudden death in adolescents resulting from the inhalation of typewriter correction fluid. JAMA 253:1604, 1985.

161. Boon NA: Solvent abuse and the heart. Br Med J 21:722, 1987.

162. Engstrand DA, England DM, Huntington RW: Pathology of paint sniffer's lung. Am J Forensic Med Pathol 7(3):232, 1986.

163. Vigliani E, Forni A: Benzene and leukemia. Environ Res 11:122, 1976.

164. Coulehan JL, Hirsch W, Brillman J: Gasoline sniffing and lead toxicity in Navajo adolescents. Pediatrics 71(1):113, 1983.

165. Hansen KS, Sharp FR: Gasoline sniffing, lead poisoning, and myoclonus. JAMA 240(13):1375, 1978.

166. Robinson RO: Tetraethyl lead poisoning from gasoline sniffing. JAMA 240(13):1373, 1978.

167. Bass M: Death from sniffing gasoline. N Engl J Med 299(4):203, 1978.

168. Lazar RB, Ho SU, Melen O: Multifocal central nervous system damage caused by toluene abuse. Neurology 33:1337, 1983.

169. Streicher HZ, Gabow PA, Moss AN: Syndromes of toluene sniffing in adults. Ann Intern Med 94:758, 1981.

170. Fischman CM, Oster JR: Toxic effects of toluene: a new cause of high anion gap metabolic acidosis. JAMA 241(16):1713, 1979.

171. Rosenberg NL, Kleinschmidt-KeMasters BK, Davis KA: Toluene abuse causes diffuse central nervous system white matter changes. Ann Neurol 1988.

172. Moss AH, Gabow PA, Kaehny WD: Fanconi's syndrome and distal tubular acidosis after glue sniffing. Ann Intern Med 92(1):69, 1980.

173. Heyer EJ, Simpson DM, Bodis-Wollner I: Nitrous oxide: clinical and electrophysiologic investigation of neurologic complications. Neurology 36:1618, 1986.

174. Messina FV, Wynne JW: Homemade nitrous oxide: no laughing matter. Ann Intern Med 96(3):333, 1982.

175. Everett G: Effects of amyl nitrite ("poppers") on sexual experience. Med Aspects Human Sexuality 6:146, 1972.

176. Cohen S: The volatile nitrites. JAMA 241(19):2077, 1979.

177. Sharp CW, Stillman RC: Blush not with nitrites. Ann Intern Med 92(5):700, 1980.

CHAPTER 59

IMMUNIZATIONS

EMILY B. COCHRAN, Pharm.D., STEPHANIE J. PHELPS, Pharm.D., MICHAEL L. CHRISTENSEN, Pharm.D., and
KELLY J. BURCH, Pharm.D.

Active and passive immunization can effectively protect an individual from infectious disease and even eliminate certain infectious diseases. In 1972 the World Health Organization declared that smallpox had been eradicated by a successful worldwide vaccination program. While the protective effects of immunization are undisputed, recent studies suggest that fewer children and adults are receiving the immunizations currently recommended by the American Academy of Pediatrics (AAP) and the Immunization Practices Advisory Committee (ACIP) of the Centers for Disease Control (CDC) (1, 2).

Active immunization is the process of administering a microorganism or its products to stimulate the host's immunologic response to that antigen. Immunization with either vaccine or toxoid results in long-term but not necessarily lifelong protection against a specific disease. Vaccines are composed of live or inactivated microorganisms (e.g., bacteria, viruses) and are usually administered by subcutaneous (s.q.), intramuscular (i.m.), or intradermal (i.d.) injection. Live vaccines stimulate an immunologic response similar to natural infection (e.g., including S-IgA as with polio vaccination) and usually result in lifelong immunity. The response induced by killed vaccines is sufficient to confer long-lasting immunity; however, it may not be lifelong, and revaccination may be required. Unlike vaccines, toxoids are modified nontoxic exotoxins that retain the ability to stimulate an immunologic response. Revaccination is required at scheduled intervals to insure continued immunity. Split, subvirion, or purified surface antigen vaccines have been chemically treated to decrease pyrogen content, and thereby, decrease the risk for febrile reaction. Vaccines manufactured by recombinant DNA technology have no risk for transmission of infectious diseases such as human immunodeficiency virus (HIV) or hepatitis. The immunologic agents discussed in the text are listed in Table 59.1.

The antibody response usually begins soon after active immunization, but adequate antibody concentrations to provide immunity may not be achieved for weeks. Therefore, individuals should not be considered immune from disease immediately after immunization. While studies are limited, available data suggest that immunization against several diseases with killed or inactivated vaccines can be accomplished at the same time (3, 4). Injections should be administered at different sites unless efficacy with a combination product has been demonstrated.

Passive immunity results from direct administration of nonspecific (e.g., immunoglobulin) or specific antibodies (e.g., antitoxin) and is a prophylactic measure. The immunity resulting from immunoglobulin or antitoxin is short-lived, as the half-life is about 21 days, but it provides protection at or around the time of disease exposure. Individuals given specific or nonspecific immunoglobulins may not achieve the desired antibody response to simultaneous immunization with a vaccine or toxoid. In some cases vaccination immediately following immunoglobulin administration may be warranted, as in the case of neonatal hepatitis B exposure. However, failure to elicit an appropriate antibody response by 3 months may necessitate revaccination.

Specific groups of individuals require special thought when vaccination is being considered. Immunization of pregnant women, immunocompromised individuals, or dialysis patients may require modification of an immunization schedule, vaccine dose, or special consideration of the type of immunization (e.g., live vs. killed vaccine). Individuals traveling to countries where specific infectious diseases are endemic may require immunization or prophylactic therapies to prevent such diseases as yellow fever, rabies, or hepatitis A. Patients with hypersensitivity reactions to vaccine components (e.g., egg protein, stabilizers, preservatives) may require desensitization prior to immunization.

Proper storage and reconstitution of vaccines and immunoglobulin products are necessary to insure potency and concentration. Products ready for injection usually require refrigeration and protection from freezing. Lyophilized vaccines may require storage under refrigeration and protection from heat and freezing. The package insert should be consulted for proper storage conditions and reconstitution instructions.

New or improved products to provide immunity and more effective immunization schedules are continuously being evaluated. The AAP Committee on Infectious Dis-

Table 59.1.
Immunologic Agents

Vaccine	Type
BCG	Live bacteria
Cholera	Inactivated bacteria
Diphtheria	Toxoid
Hepatitis B	Inactived viral antigen
Haemophilus influenzae	
PRP	Bacterial polysaccharide
PRP-D	Bacterial polysaccharide conjugated to diphtheria toxoid
HbOC	Bacterial polysaccharide conjugated to diphtheria CRM$_{197}$
PRP-OMP	Bacterial polysaccharide conjugated to meningococcal outer-membrane protein
PRP-T	Bacterial polysaccharide conjugated to tetanus toxoid
Influenza	Inactivated virus
IPV	Inactivated virus
Measles	Live virus
Meningococcal	Bacterial polysaccharides (4 serotypes)
Mumps	Live virus
OPV	Live, attenuated virus
Pertussis	Inactivated bacteria
Pneumococcal	Bacterial polysaccharides (23 serotypes)
Rabies	Inactivated virus
Rubella	Live virus
Tetanus	Toxoid
Typhoid	Inactivated bacteria
Yellow fever	Live virus

eases publishes current recommendations for immunizations in the *Red Book*, which is updated every 3 to 5 years (4). As new information becomes available, revised recommendations are published in *Pediatrics* and the *Morbidity and Mortality Weekly Review* (*MMWR*).

ACTIVE IMMUNIZATIONS
Pediatric Immunizations

ONTOGENIC EVENTS

The immune system begins to develop early in fetal life. At 7-weeks gestation, small lymphocytes appear in the circulation, and at 9 weeks, B cells primarily involved in humoral immune response are seen in fetal liver. At birth, all of the components of the immune system are present and functional, but immunoglobulin concentrations are low. In early life, there is no immunologic memory, complement concentrations are reduced, opsonin activity is poor, and neutrophil chemotaxis and phagocytosis are reduced. While neonates can produce all classes of immunoglobulins, they cannot produce specific antibodies against all antigens. By 1 year of age, delayed hypersensitivity to *Candida* antigen is present, and complement concentrations have reached adult values. By 2 years of

age, memory function to polysaccharide antigen is present, and immune complex diseases begin to appear. Secretory IgA reaches maximal concentration by 2 to 4 years; however, the capacity for production of specific antibodies of the IgA class matures slowly, and adult values are not reached until 10 to 12 years. The IgG subclasses attain adult values at different times, requiring 8 to 12 years to achieve maximum concentrations.

The age at which a specific immunization is given is determined by the disappearance of transplacentally acquired antibodies and the capability of the immune system to respond to specific antigens. For example, maternally derived antibodies to measles, mumps, or rubella may be present in sufficient concentration to prevent the desired antibody response until 15 months of age; therefore, immunization for these viruses is delayed until that time. Likewise, infants respond poorly to immunization with polysaccharide capsular antigens from organisms such as *Streptococcus pneumoniae* and *Haemophilis influenzae* type b (Hib). Effective immunization to Hib capsular polysaccharide results if a particular type of protein is conjugated to the polysaccharide. For other polysaccharides such as that of *S. pneumoniae*, vaccination is delayed until the age when the desired response can be elicited.

In general, pediatric immunizations begin when an infant is 6 weeks to 2 months of age. Immunizations in preterm infants should begin at 2 months postnatal age and not 11 months postconceptional age. The AAP recommends using the standard vaccine dose, since use of half-dose vaccination in preterm infants may result in inadequate protection against disease (4, 5). To avoid confusion of a potentially serious adverse reaction to an immunization with disease occurrence, infants who experience an acute febrile illness or those with a developing neurologic illness should not be immunized at the time of the illness. Any systemic viral syndrome should be considered a contraindication to administration of a live viral vaccine, since elevated interferon concentrations resulting from the viral syndrome may result in loss of vaccine efficacy. On the other hand, a mild upper respiratory tract infection is not a contraindication to immunization.

DIPHTHERIA, PERTUSSIS, AND TETANUS VACCINE

Diphtheria. *Corynebacterium diphtheriae* is the causative agent for diphtheria, a highly contagious disease transmitted by aerosolized droplets. The mucous membranes of the upper respiratory tract are usually the site of local infection, but ocular and genital mucous membranes and even the skin can be infected. The toxin causes local tissue inflammation and necrosis that may form an exudate and further progress to a gray to black membrane. Local lesions may be sufficiently deep to allow hematogenous spread. Mild infection resembles the common cold, while severe disease resulting from the delayed action of the diphtheria toxin may result in cardiomyopathy, neuropathy, or liver necrosis. A single intravenous dose of diphtheria antitoxin is the specific treatment for the complications of diphtheria, but the appropriate antibiotics are required to kill the organism. Active infection does not necessarily confer immunity, and individuals who have had diphtheria should be immunized according to current recommendations.

Tetanus. The spores of *Clostridium tetani* are commonly found in soil and dust, and once introduced into a wound, they can be converted to the vegetative form that elaborates a neurotoxic exotoxin responsible for tetanus, commonly called "lockjaw." Local infection results in pain, muscle rigidity, and muscle spasm in adjacent areas. More commonly, the disease is generalized to involve virtually every muscle, including those involved with respiration. While the individual with tetanus can be neurologically alert, there may be intense pain or airway obstruction, cyanosis, and asphyxia associated with the muscle spasms. Treatment includes supportive care, administration of tetanus immune globulin, tetanus toxoid, and, in some cases, tetanus antitoxin. Active infection does not necessarily provide immunity, and therefore, patients with tetanus should be immunized during convalescence. As immunity to tetanus wanes with time, all individuals should receive tetanus toxoid every 8 to 10 years.

Pertussis. Humans are the only known reservoir for pertussis or "whooping cough," an acute respiratory infection that usually results from *Bordetella pertussis*. A milder form of "whooping cough" may be caused by *Bordetella parapertussis*. For the initial 1 to 2 weeks of infection, pertussis resembles an upper respiratory tract infection. During the following 2 to 4 weeks, the paroxysmal cough worsens and may be severe enough to result in asphyxia and cerebral anoxia leading to seizures, coma, and permanent neurologic damage. Exhaustion from coughing, dehydration, and weight loss are frequent findings. During the weeks to months of recovery, the number and severity of coughing episodes gradually decreases. In adults, pertussis may go unrecognized because the symptoms are often atypical, and a severe cough may be the only overt symptom of infection. Active infection with pertussis appears to provide lifelong immunity.

After the pertussis vaccine was introduced, the incidence of the disease decreased from over 250,000 cases in 1934 to only 1,010 in 1976. Since 1976, the number of cases has increased in some areas, despite attainment of greater than 90% vaccination rates in those areas. This increased incidence of pertussis may be due to vaccine failures (6) or to a gradual decrease in immunity after vaccination (7).

Immunizations. In most infants, immunization with diphtheria and tetanus toxoids and pertussis vaccine (DTP) begins at 6 weeks to 2 months of age (3, 4). Three primary immunizations are given at least 1 month apart, followed

Table 59.2.
Schedule for Routine Pediatric Immunizations

Age	Immunization
2 months	OPV, DTP, HbOC[a] or PRP-OMP[a]
4 months	OPV, DTP, HbOC[a] or PRP-OMP[a]
6 months	DTP, OPV[b], HbOC[a]
12 months	PRP-OMP[a]
15 months	MMR, HiB conjugate vaccine (HbOC[a], PRP-OMP[c], or PRP-D), TB skin test
18 months	OPV, DTP
6 years	OPV, DTP, MMR[c], TB skin test
12 years	MMR[c]
every 10 years	Td

[a] Immunization series should be completed with the same vaccine.
[b] Given during polio epidemic or for travel to an endemic area.
[c] Given at either at 6 years (recommended by ACIP) or at 12 years (recommended by AAP).

by booster doses at 18 months and prior to school enrollment. For increased compliance and convenience, the DTP immunization is usually scheduled every 6 weeks to 2 months to coincide with administration of the live, oral polio vaccine (OPV) (Table 59.2). Children with certain neurological disorders (e.g., a neurologic complication temporally associated with DTP administration, progressive neurological disorder, a personal history of seizures or a neurologic disorder that predisposes to seizures or neurologic deterioration) should not receive the pertussis vaccine (4). For these children <7 years old, diphtheria and tetanus toxoids adsorbed (DT) is available and should be administered according to the same schedule as the DTP.

Most older individuals have had pertussis and have permanent immunity for pertussis. In addition, pertussis immunization in individuals ≥7 years of age results in more significant adverse effects. Thus pertussis immunization is not recommended in those ≥7 years of age. Because diphtheria and tetanus immunity decreases with time, these immunizations should be repeated every 8 to 10 years (2). Adverse effects to diphtheria immunization increase with age, thus, individuals ≥7 years of age should not receive the larger dose of diphtheria toxoid in the pediatric DTP and DT products. Individuals ≥7 years old should receive the diphtheria immunization with a product formulated for adults that contains no pertussis vaccine and a lower dose of diphtheria toxoid (Td) every 8 to 10 years (2, 4).

The diphtheria and tetanus toxoids adsorbed are prepared from *Corynebacterium diphtheria* and *Clostridium tetani* exotoxins. Both are treated with formaldehyde and adsorbed onto a carrier (in this case aluminum hydroxide) that delays absorption and increases antigenicity. Unfortunately, carriers are responsible for increased tissue irritation at the injection site. The antitoxin content of diphtheria and tetanus toxoids is described in flocculating units (Lf). The pertussis vaccine currently in use in the United States is a whole-cell inactivated vaccine adsorbed onto aluminum. Potency is described in protective units.

The usual 0.5 ml dose of DTP contains 12.5 Lf units of diphtheria toxoid adsorbed, 5 Lf units of tetanus toxoid adsorbed, and 4 protective units of pertussis vaccine adsorbed for i.m. administration. DT for pediatric use contains 6.6 to 15 Lf units of diphtheria toxoid and 5 to 10 Lf units of tetanus toxoid adsorbed. For individuals >7 years old, Td is available with 5 to 10 Lf units of tetanus toxoid and the lower diphtheria toxoid dose of 1.5 to 2 Lf units. All diphtheria and tetanus toxoid-containing products contain thimerosal as a preservative.

Despite limited indications for single immunization, each is available individually. Diphtheria toxoid adsorbed is available in 15 Lf doses for pediatric use. Tetanus toxoid is marketed in doses of 4 or 5 Lf units or adsorbed in doses of 5 or 10 Lf units. Rarely, individuals ≥7 years of age who are increased risk for pertussis infection may require immunization with the pertussis vaccine adsorbed as a single immunization that is available through the Michigan State Department of Public Health.

The adverse effects seen with DTP immunization are usually mild and self-limiting but are more frequent and severe than with the DT (8). Local reactions, including redness, swelling, or pain at the injection site, occur in about 50% of patients immunized with DTP but in only 8 to 10% of patients immunized with DT. Similar findings were noted with systemic effects (e.g., fever (46% vs. 9%), drowsiness (31% vs. 15%), anorexia (21% vs. 7%), vomiting (6% vs. 3%), and persistent crying (3% vs. 1%)). DTP immunization may result in an increased risk for seizure that is probably related to a preexisting seizure disorder or associated with the development of fever, which is a relatively common adverse effect reported after DTP (9, 10). Currently the AAP recommends that those with a progressive neurological disorder, a personal history of seizures, or a neurologic disorder that predisposes to seizures or neurologic deterioration not be immunized with DTP. A family history of seizures does not warrant withholding the immunization (4). While uncommon, a sterile abscess may develop following DTP immunization and is probably related to the aluminum phosphate carrier (4). While a causal relationship between DTP immunization and sudden infant death syndrome (SIDS) has been suggested, it has not been proven in controlled studies (11).

Serious neurologic side effects have been temporally associated with the DTP immunization, and retrospective studies suggest that the pertussis component is responsible. Unfortunately, the age of onset of serious neurological disease coincides with the age of routine pediatric immunizations. This coincidental relationship coupled with the desire to establish a causal agent for serious neuro-logical diseases has probably influenced the linkage of pertussis immunization to serious neurologic sequelae (12, 13). Currently the AAP recommends that patients who experience one of the following events after DTP should not receive subsequent DTP or pertussis vaccine: (a) seizure within 3 days of immunization; (b) encephalopathy within 7 days; (c) persistant, unconsolable crying or screaming for ≥3 hr or an unusual high-pitched cry within 4 hr; (d) hypotonic or hyporesponsive episode within 48 hr; (e) fever of 40.5°C within 48 hr; or (f) severe or anaphylactic reaction immediately after vaccine administration (4). Any one of the aforementioned adverse effects following immunization must be reported to the CDC.

An acellular pertussis vaccine may replace the whole-cell pertussis vaccine in the DTP vaccine. Advantages of the acellular vaccine include a decrease in reactivity and increased immunogenicity. The efficacy of this vaccine has not been established in children <17 months of age (14).

POLIO VACCINE

Humans are the only known reservoir for the enteroviruses responsible for poliomyelitis. Infection with either type 1, type 2, or type 3 may result in progressive disease. Symptoms with the first stage or abortive poliomyelitis include fever, malaise, headache, and nausea. About 20% progress to the nonparalytic aseptic meningitis stage and have a stiff neck and spine. The nonparalytic stage may progress further to either spinal or bulbar paralytic polio. The spinal type involves the upper or lower extremities, abdomen, back, or thorax, while bulbar polio involves the cranial nerves and affects eyelids, tongue, facial muscles, and pharyngeal muscles. Rarely, the spinal and bulbar forms occur together.

The first poliovirus vaccine, developed by Jonas Salk in 1954, was an inactivated polio vaccine (IPV) that contained antigens for types 1, 2, and 3 polioviruses. Unfortunately, IPV did not confer long-term protection against polio. Recently, an enhanced potency IPV (Poliovirus Vaccine Inactivated, Connaught) that stimulates an enhanced antibody response was licensed, and it will likely replace the Salk IPV as the IPV of choice (4).

Currently, IPV is used primarily in adults and immunosuppressed individuals (including children with HIV infection). A total of 3 s.q. doses given 2 months apart is required to complete the immunization series. For immunocompromised infants who are to receive IPV, the immunization series should begin at 2 months of age. The initial immunization should be followed by repeat doses at 4 and 15 months of age and a booster prior to school enrollment (4). Booster doses of the Salk IPV must be given every 5 years to insure adequate immunity.

IPV is a trivalent vaccine containing at least $10^{6.5}$ infectivity titers of poliovirus types 1, 2, and 3, inactivated with formaldehyde. In addition to the virus titers, the vaccine contains human serum albumin, phenoxyethanol, streptomycin, and neomycin. Adverse effects described with IPV include erythema and tenderness at the injection site, fever, and urticarial rash.

In 1961 Albert Sabin developed a live, attenuated oral polio vaccine (OPV) that provided protection against poliovirus types 1, 2, and 3, induced gastrointestinal immunity, presumably S-IgA, and had a longer duration of immunity. In addition, OPV was less expensive, more immunogenic, and easier to administer than IPV. Use of OPV for immunization has virtually eradicated naturally occurring polio from the United States. While this polio vaccine has distinct advantages, there is an extremely low risk that a wild-type mutant may emerge from the attenuated virus pool. Infection with the wild-type virus may progress to paralytic polio (15, 16). Both the ACIP and AAP recommend OPV for primary pediatric polio immunization, but the debate over the preferred vaccine continues (17).

The current OPV is a trivalent vaccine containing the 3 types (1, 2, 3) of live, attenuated polio virus. The first OPV is given at 6 weeks to 2 months of age and is followed by a second dose in 6 weeks to 2 months (Table 59.2). For children residing in endemic areas or during polio outbreaks, a third dose of OPV may be given 6 weeks to 2 months after the second. Boosters are given at 18 months of age and prior to school enrollment. Because OPV is a live virus vaccine, the virus replicates in the gastrointestinal tract and is shed via stool and other body secretions for up to 6 weeks following immunization. Because of intestinal replication and carriage of the live virus, repeat immunization would not be effective if given more frequently than every 6 weeks.

During the weeks following OPV immunization, immunocompromised individuals, those receiving immunosuppressants (e.g., steroids, chemotherapy) (16, 17) and unimmunized adults (>18 years) who come in contact with infants shedding the live virus are at risk of contracting the rarely excreted mutant wild-type virus and developing polio. Most cases of paralytic polio in the United States are in immunocompromised individuals who come in direct contact with an infant who has been immunized with the OPV. For this reason, unimmunized adults should receive the IPV vaccination series prior to the administration of the OPV vaccine to an infant with whom they come in frequent contact. The infant can begin OPV immunizations when the adult receives the third IPV immunization.

Each dose of OPV contains infectivity titers of approximately 10^5 for each of the three virus types and the antibiotics streptomycin and neomycin. Two dosage forms are available, one in a 0.5 ml volume and the other a 2-drop dose. Both contain the same infectivity titers, but the 2-drop dose contains ≤5 μg of the antibiotics while the 0.5 ml dose contains ≤25 μg of the antibiotics. Individuals

immunized with OPV have an extremely low risk (1 case per 2.6 million doses) for the development of paralytic polio (15, 16). Although the actual number of polio cases is very small, 85 to 90 cases of paralytic polio that occurred in the United States from 1980 to 1986 were related to exposure of an unimmunized adult or immunocompromised individual to attenuated OPV and the subsequent emergence of a mutant wild-type virus.

MEASLES, MUMPS, RUBELLA VACCINE

Measles. Rubeola, or measles, is a highly contagious disease caused by the RNA virus *Morbillivirus*. Following 10 days of incubation, a prodrome characterized by Koplik spots on the buccal and pharyngeal mucosa, fever, conjunctivitis, photophobia, cough, and coryza occurs. During this time measles may be transmitted via aerosolized droplets. Following the prodrome, a high fever develops, and a maculopapular rash starts on the neck and face and progresses down the body. Although rare, encephalitis with potential permanent neurologic sequelae is a serious complication.

Immunization with the currently available live, attenuated vaccine has resulted in a highly significant decrease in the incidence of measles. Unfortunately, several measles outbreaks have occurred in appropriately immunized individuals (18, 19). Several factors, including past use of less immunogenic vaccines, primarily vaccine failures, immunization with a vaccine that was improperly stored, vaccination at an age when the appropriate immunologic response could not be achieved, and waning immunity with time, have been cited as potential reasons for these apparent vaccine failures (19).

When the vaccine was first available in the 1960s, children as young as 10 months of age were vaccinated. Because of an inadequate response in younger patients (20), the age for measles immunization was increased to 12 months and later to 15 months, when vaccine efficacy is estimated to be about 95% (19). However, vaccine failure rates up to 10% continue to be reported (19). Because disease outbreaks continue to occur in immunized individuals who have not had measles, it is recommended that a second dose of measles vaccine be administered to all individuals >15 months of age who are born after 1957 (3, 4, 18). Almost all individuals born before 1957 contracted measles and have natural immunity.

Mumps. Also known as epidemic parotitis, mumps is a highly contagious acute viral disease that is transmitted by aerosolized droplets. The 3-week incubation period is characterized by fever and complaints of neck muscle pain, headache, and malaise. This is followed in a matter of hours by unilateral or bilateral parotid gland swelling. Age-related complications associated with mumps are not uncommon and include meningoencephalomyelitis, orchitis, or epididymitis in up to 45% of postpubertal males, oophoritis in 7% of postpubertal females, pancreatitis and rarely, glomerulonephritis. A small number of males with orchitis may become sterile as a result of testicular infection. Mumps immunization has decreased the incidence by 98%, but mumps outbreaks continue to occur (21).

Rubella. German or three-day measles is a contagious disease caused by an RNA virus whose only known host is man. Following a 2 to 3 week incubation period, rubella is characterized by mild catarrhal symptoms culminating with a generalized morbilliform rash and enlarged, tender cervical lymph nodes lasting up to 7 days. Complications are relatively uncommon but include arthritis and neuritis, usually in adolescent and older females.

The most significant problem with rubella is the potential for fetal infection. Congenital rubella syndrome is most likely to occur when the mother is infected during the first trimester of pregnancy. From 50 to 80% of infants are affected if infection occurs during the first trimester. This decreases to 10 to 20% if infection occurs during the second trimester and is rare if infection occurs during the third trimester. Relatively common manifestations of congenital rubella syndrome noted at birth include low birth weight, hepatomegaly, splenomegaly, congenital heart disease, or cataracts. While newborns may be asymptomatic, up to 70% are eventually diagnosed with hearing loss, congenital heart disease, mental retardation, and cataracts.

Immunizations. Measles, mumps, and rubella vaccines (MMR) are administered as 2 immunizations, the first at 15 months of age and the second given either prior to school entry or any time thereafter (19) (Table 59.2). The ACIP and AAP suggest giving the second dose prior to school entry (6 years) or prior to middle-school enrollment (12 years) to standardize the time for immunization and increase compliance (3, 4). For children in a county with a measles outbreak, the monovalent measles vaccine (or MMR if the monovalent vaccine is not available) should be administered to infants >6 months of age. If the initial immunization is given prior to 12 months of age, MMR should be administered according to the AAP and ACIP recommendations at 15 months and >6 years of age. Individuals born prior to 1957 likely had measles infection and do not require immunization. However, for those born after 1957 who have only had one immunization and no documentation of measles immunity, a second immunization is indicated to insure immunity (19). In addition, most colleges and medical institutions require that incoming students or employees document that they have received two measles immunizations or provide evidence of immunity (19). Although individuals immunized with MMR can shed virus, there is no risk for transmission of disease.

Adverse effects associated with MMR have been reported in between 0.5 and 4% of vaccinees (22). Infants may experience irritability, fever, drowsiness, conjuncti-

vitis, generalized rash, and a willingness to stay in bed. Local reactions include redness and soreness at the injection site. Specific adverse effects attributed to the individual components of the MMR are discussed with the appropriate individual vaccine.

Measles vaccine is a preparation of live, attenuated measles virus (more attenuated Ender's line) grown in chick embryo cell cultures. The potency of the measles vaccine is described using tissue culture infective dose 50% ($TCID_{50}$). A 0.5 ml dose is administered s.q. and contains 1000 $TCID_{50}$ and 25 μg of neomycin. In addition to MMR that is most commonly used, measles vaccine is available as a single immunization or in combination with the rubella vaccine. The measles vaccine has been associated with burning at the time of injection, which is probably due to the low pH of the vaccine. Local reactions include induration, erythema, vesiculation, and edema at the injection site. From 6 to 11 days after immunization, a transient rash and fever up to 39.4°C representing a mild case of measles may occur. Although rare, seizures have been reported during the febrile episode. Very infrequent side effects include mild measles symptoms of headache, cough, sore throat, eye pain, and malaise.

Mumps vaccine is a preparation of live, attenuated mumps virus of the Jeryl Lynn (B level) strain grown in chick embryo cell culture. This s.q. immunization is usually given at 15 months of age as MMR. A 0.5 ml dose contains 5000 $TCID_{50}$ and neomycin. In addition to the MMR, mumps vaccine is available as a single immunization and in combination with rubella. As with measles, local reactions to mumps vaccine are likely caused by the low pH of the vaccine and include burning and stinging at the time of injection. Systemic reactions are rare, but mild fever has been reported.

Rubella vaccine is a live, attenuated virus vaccine of the Wistar Institute RA 27/3 strain that is given s.q. at 15 months of age, usually as MMR. A 0.5 ml dose contains 1000 $TCID_{50}$ and neomycin. Rubella vaccine is also available as a single immunization or in combination with the mumps or measles vaccines. Local reactions to rubella vaccine include stinging and burning sensation upon injection, probably related to the low pH of the product. While systemic effects are relatively rare, they resemble those seen with rubella infection and appear to be age-related. A transient arthralgia occurring 2 to 6 weeks after immunization has been reported in 1 to 3% of children and in up to 40% of adult females.

Several factors related to each component vaccine of the MMR must be considered before vaccine administration. MMR and the individual vaccines are live virus vaccines and should not be administered to immunosuppressed individuals (with the exception of young children with HIV infection), including those receiving immunosuppressive doses of steroids. Because each vaccine in the

Table 59.3.
Management of Immunizations in Individuals with Egg Allergy

1. *Scratch, prick, puncture test.* 1:10 dilution (in physiologic saline) applied to a scratch, prick, or puncture on forearm. Positive test result is denoted by a wheal ≥ 3 mm greater than that produced by the control (physiologic saline applied to scratch, prick, or puncture at another site).
2. *Intradermal test.* 0.02 ml of 1:100 dilution (in physiologic saline) is injected intradermally. Wheal > 5 mm greater than that produced by the control (physiologic saline injected intradermally at another site).
3. *Desensitization.* The following should be administered subcutaneously at 15- to 20-min intervals.
   - 0.05 ml of 1:100 dilution in physiologic saline
   - 0.05 ml of 1:10 dilution in physiologic saline
   - 0.05 ml of full-strength vaccine
   - 0.1 ml of full-strength vaccine
   - 0.15 ml of full-strength vaccine
   - 0.2 ml of full-strength vaccine

This procedure should be supervised by a physician experienced in the management of anaphylactic reactions, and the appropriate resuscitative medications and equipment should be available.

MMR is grown in chick embryo cultures, individuals with anaphylactic egg allergies may require desensitization prior to vaccine administration (23, 24) (Table 59.3). Finally, women who are pregnant or who intend to become pregnant within 3 months should not be immunized with the rubella vaccine because of the potential risk for congenital rubella syndrome.

NATIONAL CHILDHOOD VACCINE INJURY COMPENSATION ACT

All vaccines and toxoids can produce adverse effects that are predominantly mild and self-limiting. While extremely rare, certain side effects temporally associated with vaccines may result in severe permanent injury or death. Serious side effects temporally related to immunization (4) should be reported to the U.S. Department of Health and Human Services through the Vaccine Adverse Event Reporting System (VAERS) (4).

Historically, compensation for injury related to immunization was through litigation between the injured party and vaccine manufactures or healthcare professionals who prescribed or administered vaccines. A few law suits of sufficient magnitude forced several manufactures to suspend production of vaccines and toxoids and threatened the viability of the national immunization program. Because of the importance of the immunization program, the federal government passed the National Childhood Vaccine Injury Compensation Act. This legislation was designed to provide financial assistance to children who experienced serious adverse reactions that were temporally related to vaccination and to decrease the financial burden previously assumed by vaccine manufacturers. To finance

this program, the government appropriated monies through the general tax fund through 1992 and placed a tax on each vaccine, with the amount of tax directly related to the possibility of severe adverse reaction. For example the tax on DTP was $4.56, OPV $0.29, MMR $4.44, and TD $0.06 (25). On October 1, 1988, the National Childhood Vaccine Injury Act became effective and is applicable to children immunized with DTP; pertussis vaccine; MMR; MR; measles, mumps, or rubella single-antigen vaccines; DT; Td; OPV; and IPV. This route of compensation for proven vaccine related injuries allows more rapid settlement of claims and does not require expensive litigation. Funds are available to provide treatment and rehabilitation costs not covered by private insurance, with damages awarded for pain and suffering not exceeding $250,000. If parents of children who experienced vaccine-related severe adverse effects accept compensation via this route, they give up the right to institute legal proceeding against the manufacturer or individuals who prescribed or administered the vaccine (25, 26).

Haemophilus influenzae

Haemophilus influenzae type b (Hib) is an important cause of morbidity and mortality in children <5 years of age with up to 75% of Hib infections occurring in children <18 months of age. Hib is the most common cause of bacterial meningitis in children <4 years of age and is frequently responsible for epiglottitis, pneumonia, septic arthritis, osteomyelitis, cellulitis, and pericarditis. Neurologic morbidity including mild-to-moderate hearing loss and other neurologic sequelae occurs in 21%, and mortality occurs in 3 to 10% of patients with Hib meningitis (27). Hib is carried in the nasopharynx in <5% of people and may be transmitted by asymptomatic carriers via aerosolized droplets. Risk factors for acquiring Hib disease include age, attendance in a day-care center, anatomic or functional asplenia, and Hodgkin's disease (4). In addition, native Americans and Alaska natives are at increased risk for Hib infection (4, 28).

In 1985, the first Hib capsular polysaccharide vaccine (PRP) was licensed in the United States. Children ≥24 months of age achieved adequate seroconversion to confer protection against Hib disease (28). However, younger children who were most likely to acquire the infection failed to respond adequately to PRP vaccine. In addition, geographic differences in the response to immunization were noted in children >23 months of age (28, 29). Certain populations (e.g., native Americans, Alaska natives) did not have the desired immunologic responses to immunization that was thought to be related to socioeconomic factors, genetics, or differences in infecting strains of Hib (28).

To increase immunogenicity, the Hib polysaccharide was conjugated to various proteins. As of January 1992, three different conjugated vaccines had been licensed in the United States: diphtheria toxoid conjugate (PRP-D), diphtheria CRM_{197} protein conjugate (HbOC), and meningococcal outer-membrane protein conjugate (PRP-OMP). It is expected that a fourth, Hib-conjugate (tetanus toxoid conjugate) vaccine (PRP-T) will be licensed soon. After the conjugated vaccines were introduced, studies showed that younger children could respond sufficiently to the vaccine to warrant lowering the age for immunization with a conjugated vaccine (30) (Table 59.2). Children who are to be immunized with HbOC, can begin a primary immunization series at 2 months of age with 3 subsequent immunizations at 4, 6, and 15 months of age (31). PRP-OMP may be given to infants at 2, 4, and 12 months of age (31). Alternatively, any of the Hib-conjugated vaccines can be given as a single immunization at 15 months of age (30). Unimmunized children 18 months to 5 years of age should receive Hib immunization. Children >5 years old who are at increased risk for Hib disease (functional or anatomic asplenia, Hodgkin's disease) should be immunized. If necessary to insure compliance, the conjugated vaccines can be administered at the same time as IPV or OPV, MMR, or DTP (30, 32). Immunization with a conjugated-Hib vaccine does not provide immunity against diphtheria, tetanus, or meningococcal disease, therefore, routine immunization against these diseases should follow AAP and ACIP recommendations.

Children who have invasive Hib disease prior to 2 years of age may not develop adequate immunity following disease and should be immunized 2 months after the illness with the appropriate vaccine according to the usual immunization schedule. Active disease after the age of 2 years probably renders the child immune from further infection, and immunization is not recommended.

The PRP-D vaccine contains 25 μg of purified Hib capsular polysaccharide and 18 μg of diphtheria toxoid protein. HbOC contains 10 μg is purified Hib saccharide and 25 μg of CRM_{197} protein. PRP-OMP contains 15 μg of purified Hib polysaccharide and 251 μg of group B meningococcal OMP (outer-membrane protein). The full immunizing dose is contained in 0.5 ml for i.m. injection. Thimerosal is added to some products as a preservative.

The PRP causes few local (e.g., induration tenderness in <5%) or systemic (e.g., fever in about 2%) side effects (29). Likewise, immunization with the Hib-conjugated vaccines is associated with few local or systemic side effects.

RIFAMPIN PROPHYLAXIS (Haemophilus influenzae)
The Hib bacteria continue to colonize the nasopharynx even after the infection has been treated with systemic antibiotics. Rifampin therapy is used to eliminate nasopharyngeal colonization of Hib in the index case (patient with systemic disease) and in asymptomatic carriers,

thereby decreasing the occurrence of secondary Hib infections. Rifampin should be administered to the index case along with systemic antibiotics. Although nasopharyngeal colonization with encapsulated or pathogenic Hib occurs in 2 to 5% of all children, 60 to 70% of index case siblings, 9 to 20% of parents, 20% of patients in institutions, and up to 58% of children in day-care centers are colonized (34). Even though the risk for developing secondary systemic Hib is low, the attack rate for all household contacts is approximately 600 times higher than the endemic risk for the general population (33).

Regardless of immunization history, all patient with systemic Hib should be treated with rifampin (34). The indications for institution of rifampin prophylaxis against secondary infection are controversial. Generally, all pediatric and adult household contacts (e.g., individuals living with the index case or nonresidents who spent >4 hr/day with the index case for 5 to 7 days prior to hospitalization) in homes where at least one child is <48 months of age should receive prophylaxis. Children and personnel in day-care centers that house children <2 years of age for longer than 25 hr/week may require rifampin prophylaxis. The efficacy of large-scale prophylaxis of day-care-center children has not been well established (35). The ACIP recommends that prophylaxis be given to children <2 years of age in a day-care center where only one case of systemic Hib has occurred (33), while the AAP recommends that at least two cases occur before initiating rifampin therapy (35). Because recommendations vary from state to state and even within a state, the local health department should be contacted for information concerning prophylaxis criteria.

Prophylaxis should be initiated as soon as possible after identification of the index case, because 54% of all secondary cases of Hib occur within 1 week after hospitalization of the index case (35). Furthermore, those individuals identified as requiring prophylaxis should be treated during the same time period to prevent nasopharyngeal recolonization within a group. A 20 mg/kg dose (maximum 600 mg/day) of rifampin administered once a day for 4 days is 95% effective (4, 36). The dose of rifampin for infants <1 month of age has not been established; however, some experts recommend reducing the dose to 10 mg/kg per dose (4). Rifampin is not marketed in a dosage form suitable for pediatric use; however, a rifampin suspension extemporaneously compounded from the powder from rifampin capsule and simple syrup provides an acceptable method of delivering the prescribed dose (37). Rifampin is a potent inducer of hepatic microsomal enzymes, so potential drug interactions must be considered. In addition to usual cautions about adverse effects, patients taking rifampin should be counseled on the orange discoloration of various body secretions and potential permanent discoloration of soft contact lenses.

Delayed or Missed Immunizations

Should a child <7 years of age fail to receive all recommended immunizations on time, it is not necessary to repeat immunizations that have already been given. Rather, the immunizations that have not been given should be administered at the recommended intervals. Unimmunized children who are 15 months to 5 years can be given DTP, OPV, MMR, and any one of the Hib-conjugate vaccines at the same time but at different injection sites (3, 32). Those >5 years old should be given all the named immunizations except the Hib-conjugate vaccine, which they no longer require. To appropriately immunize children between 2 months and 15 months of age against Hib, either HbOC is given every 2 months for 3 doses with a booster at 15 months or PRP-OMP is administered every 2 months for 2 doses with a booster at 12 months of age. The second DTP and OPV should be given 2 months after the initial immunization, and the third DTP 2 months after the second. Six to 12 months after the third DTP, a second dose of MMR and booster doses of DTP and OPV are given.

Unimmunized children ≥7 years but <18 years of age should be immunized with Td, OPV, and MMR. Td and OPV are then repeated in 2 months. A third immunization with both Td and OPV is given after 6 to 12 months to complete the primary series. All individuals should receive Td every 8 to 10 years.

Other Vaccines

PNEUMOCOCCAL

Streptococcus pneumoniae, the leading pathogen in community-acquired pneumonia, is the second most common cause of meningitis in the United States and is the cause for otitis media in over a million pediatric patients each year. Although there are over 80 pneumococcal capsular polysaccharide serotypes worldwide, most pneumococcal disease is caused by 10 serotypes. The current pneumococcal vaccine contains 23 capsular polysaccharides, representing 85 to 98% of disease isolates worldwide (38). Approximately 88% of serotypes causing adult bacteremia and meningitis, 85% causing acute otitis media, and nearly 100% of the serotypes causing pediatric bacteremia and meningitis are contained in the current vaccine (39).

The polyvalent pneumococcal vaccine is indicated in individuals >2 years of age who are at high risk for acquiring serious pneumococcal infection (38, 40). Groups at high risk include those with anatomic or functional asplenia (e.g., sickle cell anemia), nephrotic syndrome, Hodgkin's disease, and immunosuppression, including

children with HIV infection (38, 40). The vaccine is also indicated in healthy patients >65 years of age (38). Patients undergoing elective splenectomy or those treated with immunosuppressive medications should be vaccinated at least 10 to 14 days before the procedure or initiation of therapy (4, 40). Influenza and pneumococcal vaccines can be administered concomitantly at different sites, thereby increasing compliance.

A 0.5 ml dose contains 25 μg of each of the 23 polysaccharide antigens and is given at an i.m. or s.q. injection. Phenol or thimerosal is added as a preservative.

Revaccination may be considered for very high risk patients who received the 14-strain pneumococcal vaccine or for patients who received the 23-serotype vaccine >6 years ago (38). However, individuals who are revaccinated may experience serious adverse reactions (4, 38).

Few serious adverse effects are associated with initial immunization with the pneumococcal vaccine. Discomfort, induration, and erythema at the injection site occur in 40 to 90% of patients. Systemic effects occur less frequently, but include fever, weakness, muscle aches, chills, headache, nausea, and photophobia. Patients with immune thrombocytopenia have experienced exacerbations of disease following pneumococcal immunization.

MENINGOCOCCAL

Neisseria meningitidis is a Gram-negative diplococcus that causes meningococcemia with or without meningitis. Onset of fever, chills, malaise, and a characteristic rash is abrupt. Fulminant disease can progress to disseminated intravascular coagulation, shock, coma, and death within hours of the initial symptoms. Individuals with asymptomatic colonization of the upper respiratory tract frequently transmit the disease via infected droplets. Meningococcal infections occur most frequently in children <5 years of age, with most disease occurring in those 6 to 12 months of age. Disease transmission requires close personal contact (e.g., family members, day-care attendance, military). About 3% of households will experience more than one secondary case of meningococcal disease. While 9 serotypes have been identified; groups B, C, Y, and W-135 are the most common in the United States.

The current quadrivalent vaccine provides protection against serotypes A, C, Y, and W-135 but does not provide protection against serotype B, the major cause of disease in children. Similarly, the immunologic response to types C, Y, and W-135 is poor in infants. However, the quadrivalent vaccine is very effective in preventing disease secondary to serotype A in children >3 months of age (41). By 2 years of age, children have an adequate immune response to serotype C (42).

Routine immunization with meningococcal vaccine is not recommended. However, individuals >2 years old who have functional or anatomic asplenia or complement deficiency should receive the vaccine. All military personnel are vaccinated.

The vaccine contains 50 μg of each of the purified bacterial capsular polysaccharides for types A, C, Y, and W-135. Individuals >2 years of age should be given a single 0.5 ml dose of the vaccine as a s.q. injection. Immunization of a child 3 to 18 months of age during an epidemic should include two 0.5-ml doses that are administered 3 months apart. The duration of protection in children <4 years of age is probably <3 years for serotype A (4).

Adverse effects seen with meningococcal vaccine include mild local and systemic effects. Fever is more common in younger children but is rarely >38.5°C (42).

RIFAMPIN PROPHYLAXIS (Neisseria meningitidis)

As with Hib infection, *Neisseria meningitidis* colonizes the naropharynx and is easily spread through direct contact. Secondary cases may not develop symptoms for several weeks after disease exposure (4). Because of the disease severity, all household contacts and children in day-care centers should receive prophylactic antibiotics within 24 hr of diagnosis of the index case. Antibiotics are also indicated for individuals who have come in contact with oral secretions (e.g., kissing, sharing beverages, or food) from the index case. Hospital personnel who care for a child with meningococcal disease have a very low risk for acquiring the disease; thus prophylaxis is not recommended unless biologic fluid exposure (e.g., mouth-to-mouth, intubation, or suctioning) occurs prior to beginning antibiotics. Neither the vaccine nor chemoprophylaxis prevents 33% of cases that occur within 72 hr of the disease onset in the index case; therefore, follow-up surveillance after exposure and chemoprophylaxis is essential. Rifampin 10 mg/kg up to 600 mg is given every 12 hr for 4 doses. The dose is decreased to 5 mg/kg in infants <1 month. An extemporaneously compounded rifampin suspension is stable for 30 days under refrigeration and allows reliable delivery to the prescribed dose (37). While rifampin is preferred, sulfisoxazole can be given every 12 hr for 4 doses. The dose for infants <1 year is 250 mg, children 1 to 12 years is 500 mg, and those >12 years is 1000 mg.

INFLUENZA

Influenza is a viral illness that is spread by direct contact and characterized by the abrupt onset of fever, headache, malaise, muscle aches, and cough. Later, respiratory symptoms become more prominent, and nausea and vomiting may occur.

Although the influenza vaccine is recommended for the general population, the CDC has defined high-risk target groups that may receive the greatest benefit from vaccination. These include individuals with chronic cardiovascular, metabolic (diabetes), renal, hemoglobinopa-thies (sickle cell disease), or pulmonary disorders (cystic fibrosis, bronchiectasis, obstructive pulmonary disease, asthma, and class 3 tuberculosis). Individuals >65 years of age, individuals in chronic-care facilities, and healthcare personnel who may spread nosocomial infections should be vaccinated. Likewise, patients who are pharmacologically or functionally immunosuppressed should be immunized (43). Children who are not in a high-risk group do not need to be immunized.

Generally, the vaccine is given in the fall 1 month before the expected influenza season begins. From 2 weeks to 6 months after vaccination, antibody concentrations should be protective. From September through March, hospitalized patients in any high-risk group should receive influenza vaccination as part of routine discharge procedures.

In March and April of each year, the vaccine is prospectively formulated, based on circulating influenza strains that are expected to be prevalent in the upcoming year. At least 6 months are required for production, quality control, and distribution. The vaccine is made from three virus strains of types A and B influenza that are grown in chick embryos.

An inactivated, whole-virus vaccine and a split (subvirion) vaccine are available for i.m. administration. Children 6 months to 13 years old who are in a high-risk group should receive the split, subvirion, or purified-surface-antigen virus vaccine because these are associated with fewer side effects (4, 43). The vaccine dose for children 6 to 35 months of age is 0.25 ml, while children 3 to 12 years of age should be given 0.5 ml. Individuals ≥9 years are given a single 0.5-ml dose of whole or split virus (43). The initial immunization should be followed in 4 weeks by a second immunization. For subsequent influenza immunizations, only one dose is required.

In general, few adverse effects are associated with the influenza vaccine. The whole virus is a better antigen, but adverse effects are greater than those seen with split (subvirion) vaccines that contain only the antigenic portions of the virus. The most common adverse effects include pain, induration, and erythema at the injection site. Common flu-like symptoms of fever, chills, myalgia, and malaise may begin within 12 hr and are more common in children given the whole-virus vaccine. Febrile seizures have been reported. Because chick embryo cultures are used to manufacture this vaccine, individuals with egg allergies may require a graded protocol for vaccine administration or desensitization prior to influenza immunization (23, 24) (Table 59.3).

Influenza and pneumococcal vaccines can be administered simultaneously at different sites, thereby increasing compliance. Conversely, the influenza vaccine should not be given within 3 days of the pertussis immunization.

HEPATITIS B VACCINE

The hepatitis B virus (HBV), a 42-nm, DNA virus of the class hepadnaviridae is a major cause of acute and chronic hepatitis, cirrhosis, and hepatocellular carcinoma. Hepatitis B infection has a variable clinical course characterized by (a) a subclinical infection followed by recovery, (b) an acute illness with jaundice followed by recovery, (c) a subclinical illness that progresses to chronic active hepatitis, (d) an acute illness that progresses to chronic active hepatitis, and (e) a fulminant fatal disease. Worldwide, more than 250 million chronic carriers provide a reservoir for viral transmission. The incubation period ranges from 6 weeks to 6 months.

The likelihood of becoming chronically infected with HBV varies inversely with the age at which infection occurs. Infants born to mothers who are hepatitis B surface antigen (HBsAg) positive have an 80 to 90% chance of contracting the virus. Only a very small percentage will contract the virus in utero, the remainder becoming infected during the perinatal or postnatal period. Thus, identification of HBsAg-positive mothers is important, since the carrier state can be prevented in about 90% of infants who are appropriately treated with the vaccine and hepatitis B immune globulin.

Healthcare workers, hospital staff, clients or staff of institutions for the mentally retarded, recipients of clotting factors, contacts of HBV carriers, hemodialysis patients, homosexually active males, and intravenous drug abusers are at increased risk for HBV infection and require preexposure hepatitis B vaccine. Persons requiring postexposure hepatitis B vaccine include infants born to carrier mothers, those with accidental percutaneous or permucosal exposure to HBsAg-positive blood, sexual partners of persons with acute HBV infection, and household contacts of persons with acute HBV infection. Primary vaccination consists of 3 i.m. doses of vaccine, with the second and third doses given 1 and 6 months after the first (4, 44).

Production of the plasma-derived hepatitis B vaccine was discontinued in December 1989. The two current hepatitis B vaccines, RECOMBIVAX HB (Merck, Sharp, and Dohme) and Engerix-B (SmithKline Beckman) are produced using recombinant DNA technology by inserting the plasmid containing the gene for HBsAg into common baker's yeast, *Saccharomyces cerevisiae*. The purified HBsAg is treated with formalin and adsorbed with aluminum. The vaccine contains >95% HBsAg protein, ≤5% yeast protein, and a preservative. HBsAg concentration is 10 (RECOMBIVAX HB) or 20 (Engerix-B) μg per ml. The recombinant HBV vaccines have no real or theoretical potential for contamination with the human immunodeficiency virus (HIV).

Newborns whose mothers are HBV carriers should receive 0.5 ml (5 μg) of RECOMBIVAX HB or Engerix-B (10 μg) as the primary vaccination. The dose for children ≤10 years is 0.25 ml (2.5 μg) of RECOMBIVAX HB or 0.5 ml (10 μg) of Engerix-B, 11 to 19 years should receive 0.5 ml (5 μg) of RECOMBIVAX HB or 1 ml of Engerix-B (20 μg), and those ≥20 years should receive 1 ml (10 μg) of RECOMBIVAX HB or 1 ml of Engerix-B (20 μg). Although protection continues for at least 5 years, it is not known whether a booster dose is needed to insure continued protection (44).

Patients undergoing hemodialysis or who are immunosuppressed require larger doses to induce antibody concentrations that are considered protective. Two 1-ml doses (40 μg) of Engerix-B can be given at different sites, or alternatively, RECOMBIVAX HB dialysis formulation (40 μg/ml) can be given as a 1-ml dose. Current Food and Drug Administration (FDA) recommendations are that the amount of aluminum adjuvant not exceed 1.25 mg. Use of RECOMBIVAX HB 10 μg/ml in patients requiring the larger vaccine dose would deliver 2 mg aluminum. While the amount of aluminum delivered with this product is probably not clinically important, it is recommended that the RECOMBIVAX HB dialysis formulation (40 μg/ml) be used in patients requiring increased doses of HBV vaccine.

The most common side effect of these vaccines is soreness at the site of injection. Occasionally a fever (usually <39°C), malaise, headache, chills, and gastrointestinal symptoms occur and may persist for a few days. Immediate hypersensitivity reactions have been reported rarely.

For a thorough discussion of hepatitis B, see Chapter 25.

VARICELLA VACCINE

Varicella-zoster virus, a herpesvirus, is responsible for both varicella (chickenpox) and herpes zoster (shingles, zoster). Varicella is spread by aerosolized droplets and is the primary varicella-zoster infection in children <10 years old. Herpes zoster results from reactivation of the latent virus and is more common in those >10 years old. Varicella is highly contagious, with >90% secondary infection rates for household contacts with an incubation period ranging from 10 to 20 days after exposure. Prodromal symptoms consist of malaise, fever, and anorexia. The constantly pruritic rash has an abrupt onset about 24 hr later and consists of small red papules that progress to fluid-filled vesicles. Individuals are contagious from 1 to 2 days before onset of the characteristic rash until the lesions have dried and crusted 5 to 6 days later. Because the disease is highly contagious, most children between 5 and 10 years of age have chickenpox with an uncomfortable but uncomplicated course and no serious sequelae. However, children who are immunocompromised have a more complicated course, a prolonged recovery, and potentially serious sequelae.

A varicella vaccine has been developed, clinically

tested, and may be licensed soon. The vaccine was developed by removing fluid from a vesicle and isolating and attenuating the virus by serial passages through various cell cultures. The protective effects of this vaccine were demonstrated by a decrease in the rate of postexposure infection and a milder course in immunized children who developed disease. Questions surrounding the usefulness of the varicella vaccine include persistence of immunity, value in immunosuppressed patients, and the incidence of zoster infection (45). Most importantly, the long-term consequences of injecting healthy individuals with an attenuated virus that may become latent in the body for years are unknown.

The reconstituted varicella vaccine contains 1000 to 2000 plaque-forming units (pfu) per 0.5 ml. Additional constituents include sucrose, buffering salts, and neomycin sulfate. The dose used in clinical trials has ranged from 200 to 8700 pfu given s.q. Vaccination by inhalation gives a satisfactory immune response; however, controlling the dose is difficult. Vaccination should be avoided for at least 3 months following administration of immunoglobulin.

About 17% of normal, healthy individuals experience rash and fever after immunization. The rate of adverse effects is increased to 47% in immunocompromised patients.

TUBERCULOSIS SKIN TESTING/BACILLUS CALMETTE-GUERIN (BCG) VACCINE

Tuberculosis (TB) is a necrotizing bacterial infection caused by *Mycobacterium tuberculosis*. The disease affects the lungs most commonly, but lesions can occur in the kidney, bones, lymph nodes, or meninges. Clinical disease may occur early after innoculation or after months to years of dormancy. After many years of decline, the incidence of TB in the United States has recently increased because patients with AIDS develop TB secondarily. The AAP suggests that children receive a TB skin test at the time of the first MMR immunization (about 15 months of age), before school entry (about 6 years of age), and during adolescence (14 to 16 years of age). Children in high-risk groups should receive annual TB skin tests (4).

BCG vaccine is a preparation of a live, attenuated Calmette-Guerin strain of *Mycobacterium bovis*. Two different preparations are available for percutaneous or i.d. injection. The Danish substrain product is preservative-free for percutaneous administration. The concentration of the bacteria is 1 to 8 × 10^8 cfu per 2 ml. Between 0.2 and 0.3 ml of the reconstituted vaccine is dropped on cleansed skin and a multiple puncture disc is applied to instill the dose percutaneously. Infants <1 month should be given half the dose. A Tice substrain product in concentrations of 8 to 26 million cfu per ml is available for i.d. injection. The usual dose is 0.1 ml; however, infants <3 months should receive 0.05 ml. Between 10 and 14 days after im-

munization, a lesion develops at the immunization site. Maximal effects are noted by 4 to 6 weeks, and by 6 months the lesion usually has completely healed and faded. In some patients, there may be a residual scar. A tuberculin skin test should be applied 2 to 3 months after immunization. If the skin test is negative, a second dose of the vaccine should be administered. Because a positive tuberculin skin test is an endpoint of BCG vaccination, this test is not useful for identifying TB after BCG vaccination.

Routine vaccination against TB using the Bacillus Camette-Guerin (BCG) vaccine is not recommended because its efficacy has not been well established. In addition, the duration of protection is not known, but sensitivity to tuberculin skin testing has persisted for 7 to 10 years following vaccination. In spite of lack of agreement on the efficacy of BCG, vaccination should be considered in individuals in close contact with infected patients who are untreated, ineffectively treated, or resistant to treatment; healthcare workers where other control measures do not prevent an annual new infection rate greater than 1%; and other groups with an excessive new infection rate in whom surveillance and treatment programs fail or are not feasible. The vaccine is contraindicated in immunosuppressed patients, individuals with a positive tuberculin skin test, or burn patients (4).

Adverse effects include skin ulceration at the injection site, regional adenitis, osteomyelitis, and occasionally, lupoid reactions.

For a more complete discussion of tuberculosis, see Chapter 62.

RABIES

Rabies is an acute viral disease of the central nervous system caused by a RNA virus of the rhabdovirus group. Known natural reservoirs for rabies include skunks, foxes, raccoons, and bats, but all mammals can be affected. Transmission is primarily by infected secretions, usually saliva. The incubation period for rabies is between 20 and 60 days but may be >6 months. Following the initial innoculation, the virus remains close to the wound; however, migration along a neuronal pathway to the central nervous system ultimately occurs. The clinical manifestations of rabies can be divided into 3 stages; a nonspecific prodrome, an acute encephalitis, and a profound dysfunction of brainstem centers. Recovery without intervention is rare and occurs slowly.

The original vaccine developed by Pasteur was a suspension of fragments of rabies virus–infected spinal cords. Because of adverse effects, the vaccine was modified several times. Work in the early 1960s led to development of the human diploid-cell rabies vaccine that is more immunogenic and has fewer side effects than previous vaccines. A second rabies vaccine has been prepared by growing virus on cell culture and adsorbing the product on aluminum phosphate (46). Both the human diploid-cell rabies vaccine and the rabies vaccine adsorbed contain not less than 2.5 IU/ml.

Individuals who have a high risk for exposure to rabies, such as veterinarians or dog catchers, should be immunized against rabies. The preexposure immunization schedule is 1 ml i.m. or 0.1 ml i.d. injection given on days 0, 7, and 21 or 28 (3 doses). Individuals who are repeatedly exposed to rabies should have antibody concentrations measured every 6 months and be revaccinated when serum concentrations are below the protective concentration (0.5 IU). Preexposure immunization does not eliminate the need for postexposure vaccination with two booster doses given 3 days apart. Rabies immune globulin should not be given to individuals who are immunized preexposure.

Those who have not been immunized previously but who are acutely exposed to rabies should be immunized with 1 ml of either vaccine given i.m. on days 0, 3, 7, 14, and 28 (45). Additionally, rabies immune globulin 20 IU/kg should be given, with half the dose instilled at the site of the bite and the remainder administered i.m.

Rabies vaccine should be administered i.m. for preexposure rabies prophylaxis in individuals receiving chloroquine for malaria prophylaxis. In this situation, i.d. injection of rabies vaccine may interfere with the antibody response to the rabies vaccine.

Vaccination causes local discomfort, swelling, erythema, and induration in up to 90% of individuals, which usually subsides in 1 to 3 days. Up to 10% of patients have systemic reactions that include nausea, vomiting, abdominal pain, headache, malaise, and low-grade fever. An immune complex–like reaction has been reported in up to 7% of individuals receiving booster vaccination and is characterized by urticaria with or without arthralgia, arthritis, or angioedema (47). Anaphylactic reactions have been reported rarely. Once initiated, rabies prophylaxis should not be discontinued because of local or mild systemic reactions to the vaccine.

VACCINATIONS FOR TRAVEL

Travel to developing countries may include exposure to diseases that are rarely encountered in the United States. Immunization or prophylactic measures will help decrease the likelihood of developing specific diseases that are endemic in certain areas of the world. Prior to travel outside the United States, the CDC should be contacted regarding information about immunizations or prophylactic medications and other measures that are advised or required for entrance into individual countries. This should be done as early as possible before anticipated travel, because immunizations for various diseases can not be administered at the same time, and others require a series of injections to induce adequate immunity (48, 49).

Cholera

Cholera results from colonization of the small intestine by *Vibrio cholerae*, a curved, aerobic, Gram-negative bacillus. In 1849, cholera was shown to be contracted by ingestion of contaminated water. Spread of the disease depends on the transfer of infected intestinal contents from one person to another (fecal-oral transmission), with food and water being the most common vehicle. The incubation period of 6 to 48 hr is followed by the abrupt onset of watery diarrhea. Infection results in lifelong immunity. Cholera is endemic in Africa, South America, and Asia but presents a small risk to travelers who eat and drink only safe food and beverages.

The vaccine is used primarily in travelers who will be visiting countries requiring an International Certificate of Vaccination against cholera. Because the vaccine approved for use in the United States only provides 40 to 60% protection against the disease and the duration of protection is only 3 to 6 months, the vaccine is considered to be of limited value. Inactivated oral vaccines used in other countries are safe and effective but protection decreases significantly 3 years after immunization. An attenuated live oral cholera vaccine is under development and will likely be more effective.

Primary immunization with the product approved for use in the United States consists of two doses administered s.q. or i.m. given 1 week to 1 month apart. The s.q. or i.m. dose for infants and children from 6 months to 4 years old is 0.2 ml, for those 5 to 10 years of age is 0.3 ml, and for individuals >10 years of age is 0.5 ml. Alternatively, 0.2 ml can be given i.d. to all ages. Because the duration of immunity is short-lived, booster doses of the same volume as the primary immunization series may be required at 6-month intervals by some countries. The cholera vaccine is not recommended for infants <6 months of age (48–50).

The current cholera vaccine is a sterile suspension of phenol-killed whole cell *Vibrio cholera* from two bacterial strains. Eight unit (4 billion organisms) of both strains are contained in each ml, with phenol added as a preservative.

Cholera vaccination frequently results in local discomfort, redness, and swelling that may persist for several days. Local reactions can be severe. Systemic manifestations occur in <1% of vaccinees and include fever, malaise, headache, and generalized aches and pains.

A 3-week interval between cholera and yellow fever immunizations is recommended because of reported decreased antibody response to both vaccines when given concomitantly. In spite of the decreased antibody response, there is no evidence that protection against these two diseases is decreased. While it is recommended that there be 3 weeks between immunization with these two vaccines, they can be administered concomitantly at different sites if time constraints do not permit the interval (49, 51).

Typhoid

Typhoid fever is an acute systemic infection caused by the bacillus *Salmonella typhi*. The disease is spread by ingestion of water or food contaminated by respiratory secretions, urine, or stool from typhoid carriers who may be asymptomatic. Oysters and shellfish grown in polluted water can be a source for infection. The 10- to 20-day incubation period is followed by symptoms of high fever, malaise, and abdominal discomfort. Within a week, the fever increases, abdominal pain and diarrhea increase in severity, the spleen enlarges, a maculopapular rash develops, and the patient may become lethargic. Major complications include intestinal hemorrhage and perforation.

Typhoid vaccination is recommended for individuals who travel to rural areas of tropical countries or to areas where there are unsanitary conditions and an increased risk for disease exposure. Although immunization results in antibody production in 50 to 90% of individuals, the degree of immunity is not great and can be readily overcome with a large inoculum. Immunity continues for 2 years after primary immunization. A booster dose is recommended at least every 3 years if continued or reexposure to typhoid is anticipated (4, 48, 49).

Several typhoid vaccines are in use currently. A phenol- and heat-inactivated vaccine of *Salmonella typhi* given by s.q. or i.d. injection is commercially available. This vaccine contains ≤1 billion organisms per ml, with phenol as a preservative. The phenol-inactivated typhoid vaccine is administered s.q. or i.d. in 2 doses given 4 weeks apart. The s.q. dose for children <10 years old is 0.25 ml and for individuals ≥10 years is 0.5 ml. The i.d. dose for all ages is 0.1 ml. An acetone-inactivated typhoid vaccine is provided by the U.S. government for military use.

Immunization with the vaccine, which contains significant quantities of organisms containing endotoxin, often results in 1 to 2 days of discomfort at the injection site, fever, malaise, and headache. Serious systemic adverse reactions of acute renal failure, thrombocytopenic purpura, and anaphylaxis are rare. I.D. injection may be associated with fewer adverse reactions than s.q. administration.

Vivotif Berna is a recently introduced typhoid vaccine for oral administration. Each enteric-coated capsule contains 2 to 6 × 10⁹ colony forming units (cfu) of live and 5 to 50 × 10⁹ cfu of nonviable *S. typhi* Ty21a. Individuals ≥6 years old take 1 capsule every other day for 4 doses. The oral vaccine is contraindicated in children <6 years old, those with an acute febrile illness or an acute gastrointestinal illness, and in individuals receiving sulfa drugs or antibiotics. Adverse effects with the oral vaccine are fewer than with the parenteral products and include nausea, vomiting, abdominal cramps, and urticarial rash.

Yellow Fever

Yellow fever is an acute viral disease caused by a group B arbovirus and transmitted by the *Aedes aegypti* mosquito. Symptoms occur 3 to 10 days after exposure and in mild to moderate cases include headache, fever, nausea, vomiting, conjunctival injection, albuminuria, and bone and joint pain. Recovery occurs in a few days. Severe disease or classic yellow fever consists of three distinct clinical periods. The active infection period is characterized by a sudden onset of high fever lasting 3 to 4 days. Symptoms abate during the remission period that lasts a few hours to several days. During the yellow period, the fever returns and is accompanied by jaundice, albuminuria, hematuria, epistaxis, and melena. Infection with yellow fever affords lifelong immunity.

The vaccine is recommended for persons who will be traveling to rural endemic areas or laboratory workers who may be exposed to the virus (49, 51). Yellow fever vaccine available in the United States is a live, attenuated virus prepared from the 17D strain of virus grown in chick embryo. Immunity is induced by a single s.q. injection of 0.5 ml of reconstituted vaccine and persists for >10 years. Infants <4 months of age should not be vaccinated because of the increased risk of encephalitis. Infants from 4 to 9 months of age should be immunized after consultation with the CDC (48, 50).

Reactions to the yellow fever vaccine are generally mild. Up to 10% of individuals vaccinated have mild headaches, myalgia, or low-grade fever from 5 to 10 days after immunization. Immediate hypersensitivity reactions are rare. Yellow fever vaccine should not be given to those who are immunocompromised or experience anaphylactic reactions to eggs. An immunization waiver from a physician or official immunization center stating the contraindication may be sufficient to gain entrance into certain countries. Should there be a high risk for yellow fever and immunization a requirement, skin testing may be performed to determine the allergic potential of the vaccine. If necessary a desensitization protocol can be followed to achieve full immunization (Table 61.3).

Cholera and yellow fever vaccines should be given at least 3 weeks apart because of reported decreases in antibody response to both vaccines with concomitant administration. However, if time constraints do not permit, the ACIP recommends they be administered at the same time but at different sites (51).

Malaria

Malaria is a protozoal disease caused by *Plasmodium* organisms (*P. falciparum, P. vivax, P. ovale,* and *P. malariae*) that are transmitted to humans by the *Anopheles* mosquito. The disease is characterized by rigors, fever, headache, splenomegaly, and anemia. Clinical symptoms of malaria may not be present until months after exposure. Forms of *P. vivax* and *P. ovale* can be harbored in the liver for up to 4 years after chemoprophylaxis, and once reactivated, symptoms of malaria will reappear. *P. falciparum* is often resistant to therapy and may cause renal failure, coma, and death. The CDC can provide information regarding specific organisms prevalent in a given area and advice as to the appropriate prophylactic measures that should be undertaken.

Since no vaccine is available currently, chemoprophylaxis remains the primary method for malaria prevention. The choice of therapy depends on the organism endemic to the area being visited. Usually therapy is with chloroquine 300 mg (base) given once per week, started 1 week prior to travel and continued for 4 to 6 weeks after exposure (48, 49, 52). The pediatric dose is 5 mg/kg up to 300 mg of the base drug. For those who use chloroquine, a dose of pyrimethamine (75 mg)-sulfadoxine (1500 mg) (3 tablets of Fansidar) should be available to take in the event that a febrile illness occurs when professional medical care is not available. However, those with a history of hypersensitivity to sulfonamides should not receive pyrimethamine-sulfadoxine. An alternative agent for nonpregnant individuals >8 years old is doxycycline, which can be started 1 to 2 days prior to travel in a dose of 2 mg/kg up to 100 mg per day and continues for 4 to 6 weeks after exposure.

Those traveling to areas known to have chloroquine-resistant malaria should receive one 250-mg dose of mefloquine salt (228 mg base) 1 week prior to arrival in the malarious area, and prophylaxis should continue with weekly doses until 4 weeks after exposure (53). The pediatric dose is ¼ tablet for 15 to 19 kg, ½ tablet for 20 to 30 kg, ¾ tablet for 31 to 45 kg, and one 250-mg tablet for >45 kg. Children <15 kg should not receive mefloquine. Individuals receiving β-blockers, calcium-channel blockers, chloroquine, quinidine or quinine, or valproic acid should not receive mefloquine because of the risk of drug interactions. An alternative to mefloquine is doxycycline in the previously described doses.

Travelers to areas endemic for *P. vivax* or *P. ovale* should be aware of the risk for relapse after infection with these organisms. To prevent relapse in individuals who have prolonged exposure to malaria, 15 mg primaquine (base) is taken daily for 14 days beginning the last 2 weeks of chloroquine prophylaxis after the traveler has left the malarious area. The pediatric dose of primaquine base is 0.3 mg/kg/day up to 15 mg. The CDC may be consulted for the appropriateness of therapy and an acceptable method to deliver primaquine in small doses.

Adverse effects associated with chloroquine therapy include dizziness, headache, gastrointestinal problems, and pruritis. Doxycycline causes photosensitivity and may

be upsetting to the gastrointestinal tract. With mefloquine, gastrointestinal disturbances and dizziness are reported. Occasionally, hallucinations and seizures have been reported; however, these are more frequent with higher doses than those used for malaria prophylaxis. Pyrimethamine-sulfadoxine has been associated with a risk for Stevens-Johnson syndrome, and fatalities have been reported. Therapy should be discontinued immediately upon appearance of a rash. Primaquine may cause hemolysis in individuals with G6PD deficiency.

A previously discussed, concomitant chloroquine prophylaxis during preexposure i.d. rabies vaccination may interfere with the antibody response to the rabies vaccine. The ACIP recommends that under these conditions, the rabies vaccine be given i.m. (47).

PASSIVE IMMUNITY

Passive immunity results from intravenous infusion of immune globulin or antitoxin that contains antibodies to disease. Certain precautions should be undertaken when administering these products. Individuals with a specific IgA deficiency may have anti-IgA antibodies, resulting in a risk of serious adverse effects. Because immune globulin infusion may interfere with the desired antibody response to live-virus vaccines, immune globulin should not be infused for 2 weeks after immunization. Further, should immune globulin be infused in a patient, immunization with a live-virus vaccine should be delayed for 3 months, except in the case of neonatal hepatitis B exposure, when the vaccine and immunoglobulin should be administered at the same time but at different sites. When concomitant administration of immune globulin and a live-virus vaccine occurs, the immunization should be repeated in 3 months unless seroconversion is documented. Immune globulin does not interfere with the antibody response to the OPV or yellow fever live-virus vaccine.

Immune Globulin

Immune globulin i.m. (IGIM) is used to provide passive immunity to individuals who may be or have been exposed within the past 2 weeks to certain infectious diseases including hepatitis A, hepatitis B, non-A non-B hepatitis, measles, rubella, and varicella zoster. Preexposure hepatitis A prophylaxis is primarily used for those traveling to developing countries. Persons who have close personal contact with an infected individual should receive IGIM within 2 weeks of exposure (44).

IGIM is prepared from >1000 donors to insure a broad spectrum of antibody content. Because of concern over potential transmission of viral diseases such as hepatitis and HIV, all donor units are tested prior to fractionation. Additionally, newer fractionation techniques have been effective in removing or inactivating HIV in donor units spiked with the virus. The risk for transmission of these viruses via IGIM remains theoretical, and no cases of HIV infection have been directly attributed to infusion of IGIM.

The protein content of IGIM is about 165 mg/ml, and the stabilizer glycine and preservative thimerosal are also included. Doses of 0.02 ml/kg given prior to or within 2 weeks of exposure to hepatitis A is 80 to 90% successful in preventing infection (4, 44). IGIM in a dose of 0.25 ml/kg up to 15 ml can be given within 6 days of exposure to measles to decrease morbidity or prevent the disease. Because of the relatively large volume required, the dose may need to be divided and administered at different sites. Adverse effects associated with IGIM are primarily pain at the injection site, and less commonly, flushing, headache, chills, and nausea (4). IGIM should not be infused intravenously because of the risk for serious side effects.

Immune globulin for intravenous infusion (IGIV) is a purified immune globulin product, and because it can be infused intravenously, it allows administration of a larger dose of immune globulin than can be achieved with IGIM. Primary immunodeficiency resulting from an immune globulin deficiency or from impaired function is the major indication for IGIV. In addition to immunodeficiency, IGIV has also been used to improve immunity and decrease infection in patients with thermal injuries, chronic lymphocytic leukemia, multiple myeloma, cytomegalovirus, idiopathic thrombocytopenic purpura, and neonatal sepsis (54). IGIV given within 7 days of the onset of Kawasaki disease is highly effective at decreasing the incidence of coronary vasculitis (54).

IGIV infusion is efficacious in preventing or reducing the number of infectious episodes in patients with immunodeficiency. Serum IgG concentrations <200 mg/dl are associated with an increased risk for sudden, overwhelming bacterial infection. Because concentrations >400 mg/dl are generally felt to be adequate, the goal of therapy is to increase serum concentrations to >400 mg/dl (54). Although the minimal effective dose is considered to be 150 mg/kg, an IGIV dose of 200 to 400 mg/kg per month is used in most patients (54). IGIV use in patients with IgG subclass deficiency is reserved for those who have recurrent infections. For sepsis prophylaxis in high-risk neonates, IGIV should be infused to attain an IgG serum concentration of 700 mg/dl (54).

As with IGIM, IGIV is prepared from >1000 donors to insure a broad spectrum of antibody content. Because of concern over potential transmission of viral diseases such as hepatitis and HIV, all donor units are tested prior to fractionation. Additionally, newer fractionation techniques have been effective in removing or inactivating HIV in donor units spiked with the virus. The risk for transmission of these viruses via IGIV remains theoretical, and

no cases of HIV infection have been directly attributed to infusion of IGIV. IGIV is produced by a variety of manufacturers and varies in immune globulin concentrations, manufacturing techniques, additives, product form, and FDA-approved indications.

Up to 10% of patients who receive IGIV experience adverse reactions including nausea, vomiting, chills, fever, malaise, fatigue, dizziness, headache, urticaria, tightness in the chest, flushing, dyspnea, and pain in the chest, hip, or back. These effects are usually related to the rate of infusion and are managed by stopping the infusion until the symptoms subside and restarting the infusion at a lower rate. Pretreatment with acetominophen, diphenohydramine and/or glucocorticoids has also been used to decrease side effects. Patients with IgA deficiency are at risk for the development of anaphylaxis due to anti-IgA antibody formation and should receive immune globulin products with as low a concentration of IgA as possible.

Hyperimmune Globulins

Passive immunity against specific diseases can be provided by infusion of immune globulin products with high concentrations of specific antibodies. These products are made from the serum of individuals with increased concentrations of the specific antibody. All plasma used to prepare hyperimmune globulin products is negative for HBsAg. Products contain glycine as a stabilizer and most contain thimerosal as a preservative. These products are administered i.m. because of the potential for serious reaction if infused intravenously. Currently available products include hepatitis, tetanus immune globulin, rabies, Rh$_o$(D), and varicella zoster; and many others are being developed.

In December of 1991, cytomegalovirus (CMV) immune globulin for intravenous infusion was released. CMVIG is approved for use in CMV-negative renal transplant patients who receive a graft from a CMV-positive individual.

Hepatitis B Immune Globulin

Hepatitis B immune globulin (HBIG) provides passive immunity against hepatitis B infection in individuals exposed to hepatitis B virus or HBsAg-positive individuals. ACIP currently recommends postexposure prophylaxis in individuals following percutaneous exposure (e.g. needlestick, bite), direct mucous membrane contact or ingestion, and in neonates born to an HBsAg-positive mother. Postexposure prophylaxis is also recommended following sexual or intimate contact (44).

For perinatal exposure of infants born to HBsAg-positive mothers, the newborn should be given 0.5 ml of HBIG i.m. within 12 hr of birth in addition to the HBV vaccine. The usual adult dose of HBIG is 0.06 ml/kg up to 5 ml i.m. within 24 hr of percutaneous exposure or within 14 days after sexual contact. HBIG should be administered concurrently with the first dose of hepatitis B virus vaccine. To avoid neutralization, the vaccine and HBIG should not be given in the same syringe nor administered near the same site.

Local pain and tenderness may occur at the site of injection. Urticaria, rash, pruritis, and body aches may also occur.

Rabies Immune Globulin

Rabies immune globulin is used to provide postexposure passive immunity to individuals exposed to rabies. When given in recommended doses at the time the first dose of rabies vaccine is given, rabies immune globulin does not interfere with formation of vaccine-induced antibodies. It is recommended that rabies immune globulin not be administered beyond 8 days after initiation of the vaccination schedule or in individuals previously immunized against rabies because of interference with the anamnestic response (46). Rabies immune globulin is a sterile, concentrated solution containing 150 IU/ml of rabies-neutralizing antibodies. The dose of rabies immune globulin is 20 IU/kg. If possible, half of the dose is infiltrated around the wound site, and the remainder is given i.m. at a site distant to the wound.

Efficacy with the combined use of rabies vaccine and rabies immune globulin has been well documented. Although mortality rates of 50 to 60% have been noted following postexposure immunization with the vaccine alone, mortality using the vaccine and rabies immune globulin is uncommon.

Side effects are rare and include local soreness at the site of injection and mild fever that may persist for 3 days. Sensitization to repeated injection has occurred in immunoglobulin-deficient patients. Angioneurotic edema, rash, nephrotic syndrome, and anaphylactic shock have been reported rarely.

$Rh_o(D)$ Immune Globulin

$Rh_o(D)$-negative women who are exposed to $Rh_o(D)$-positive blood during delivery or pregnancy termination are at risk for development of anti-$Rh_o(D)$ formation. If a subsequent pregnancy occurs, the infant may develop erythroblastosis fetalis (hemolytic disease of the newborn) (4). Infusion of $Rh_o(D)$ immune globulin suppresses the antibody response and anti-$Rh_o(D)$ formation and prevents this from occurring.

$Rh_o(D)$ is given as an i.m. injection to the mother within 72 hr of delivery. The dosage is usually 1 vial, which contains enough anti $Rh_o(D)$ to suppress 15 ml of $Rh_o(D)$-positive packed red blood cells. The dose may need to be increased in the event of a large fetal-maternal hemorrhage.

Adverse effects are usually mild and consist of tenderness at the injection site and low-grade fever.

Tetanus Immune Globulin

Tetanus immune globulin (TIG) is derived from human plasma obtained from adults hyperimmunized with tetanus toxoid. TIG is used to treat active tetanus infection by direct provision of antitoxin antibodies that neutralize the *Clostridium tetani* exotoxin. Tetanus-prone wounds are those contaminated by dirt, soil, feces, or saliva; puncture wounds; avulsions; and wounds resulting from missiles, crush injury, burns, or frostbite. The postexposure dose of prophylactically given human-derived TIG is 250 to 500 units given i.m. For treatment of active tetanus infection, the dose ranges from 3000 to 6000 units given as an i.m. injection. Some clinicians infiltrate part of the dose around the wound(s). Use of TIG does not obviate the need for administration of tetanus toxoid, and all individuals who have not completed the immunization series should do so. If the immunization status is unknown, the patient should receive the complete immunization series.

Varicella-Zoster Immunoglobulin

Varicella-zoster immune globulin (VZIG), derived from patients convalescent from zoster, provides passive immunity for postexposure prophylaxis of individuals at high risk for developing a complicated varicella infection. While attack rates of 80 to 90% were decreased to 20 to 65% with the use of VZIG, it is primarily used to decrease the severity of illness and, thereby, decrease morbidity and mortality. The incubation period may be prolonged after VZIG, but most cases occur within 28 days of exposure.

The indications for VZIG are based on a variety of factors. In general, patients <15 years of age who have not had varicella, who are immunocompromised (e.g., leukemia, lymphoma, immunosuppressive doses of steroids) and who are exposed to varicella (e.g., household contact; playmate, hospital, or school contact) should receive VZIG. In addition, newborns whose mother developed varicella 5 days before or 2 days after delivery, premature newborn ⩾28 weeks gestation whose mother has not had varicella infection, and premature newborns <28 weeks gestation regardless of maternal history should receive VZIG. Criteria for VZIG administration in immunocompromised individuals ⩾15 years of age is less clear because of difficulties determining susceptibility status. For maximum effectiveness, VZIG should be administered as soon as possible but within 96 hr of exposure (55).

Distribution of VZIG is through the American Red Cross Blood Services Northeast Region on a 24 hr a day basis. VZIG is administered i.m. in doses of 125 units/10 kg (maximum dose of 625 units or 5 vials). Duration of protection is unknown but is estimated to be at least one-half-life of the immunoglobulin or about 3 weeks.

Side effects include local discomfort at the injection site in 1% of individuals. Gastrointestinal symptoms, malaise, headache, rash, and respiratory symptoms have been reported in 0.2%. Severe reactions, angioedema, and anaphylactic shock have been reported rarely.

Antitoxin

Antitoxins differ from hyperimmune globulins in being derived from equine serum. Products derived from animal sera may result in severe allergic reactions, and therefore, require special precautions prior to their administration. First, a careful history of past allergic responses (especially to horses or animals) should be elicited, since these individuals may be extremely sensitive to antitoxin. Additionally, a scratch test or "eye test" should be performed to determine an individual's sensitivity. If this test is negative, an intradermal test using a small amount of very dilute antitoxin is performed. The scratch test or eye test should always be performed first, and an appropriately trained individual should be available in case of an acute anaphylactic response (4). Antitoxins are available through the CDC for the treatment of diphtheria, tetanus, and botulism. Because of the increased potential for serious adverse effects, indications for the use of antitoxin are very limited, and these products should be used under close supervision by an individual experienced in their use.

If the sensitivity tests are negative, the specified dose can be given i.m. In some cases, intravenous administration may be indicated; however, the risk for a systemic reaction with intravenous infusion is increased. Intravenous doses should be dilute, infused very slowly, and the patient observed for adverse effects.

IMMUNOCOMPROMISED HOST

Immunocompromised patients may respond poorly to immunization. The response to live-virus vaccines may result in enhanced or prolonged viral replication and potentially result in systemic disease. The immune response to inactivated vaccines, although lower than in normal individuals, is usually adequate in the immunocompromised patient.

Patients who are immunosuppressed due to disease (e.g., malignancy, immune deficiency syndromes) or those receiving immunosuppressants (e.g., high-dose steroids, chemotherapy, irradiation) should not be given live-virus vaccines (OPV, MMR, influenza, and yellow fever) with the exception of influenza and measles vaccines (MMR) for infants or children with HIV infection. In addition, immunocompromised individuals are at risk for the development of polio should they come in contact with an infant immunized with OPV who is shedding live virus via stool. Disseminated disease may occur in immunocompromised patients who receive BCG; thus, its use is contraindicated in those individuals (4).

A quantitatively normal immunologic response usually develops by 3 to 12 months after discontinuing immunosuppressive therapy. Corticosteroids given as replacement therapy (e.g., Addison's disease); short courses of high-dose steroids (<2 weeks); topical steroid therapy; long-term alternate-day therapy with low-to-moderate doses of short-acting steroid; or single-dose intra-articular, bursal, or tendon injection are not usually immunosuppressive and live-virus vaccine administration is not contraindicated in these patients (3).

Cancer patients may be immunosuppressed due to the malignancy, nutritional status, or anticancer therapy (e.g., irradiation, chemotherapy). Patients with active malignant disease should not be given live vaccines. While killed vaccines and toxoids may be given, the immune response to the immunization depends on the chemotherapeutic agent being used and may be inadequate to confer immunity. Whenever possible, vaccination should occur before radiation or chemotherapy. Patients >2 years old with Hodgkin's lymphoma should be immunized with pneumococcal and Hib vaccines 10 to 14 days before therapy is started. Patients who have not received chemotherapy for 3 to 4 weeks may have an adequate antibody response to influenza vaccine (1). Live virus vaccines can be given to patients who are in remission from leukemia when 3 months have lapsed since the last chemotherapy was administered.

Individuals with asymptomatic HIV infection may be safely immunized with inactivated vaccines. Both the AAP and ACIP recommend that children with HIV receive routine pediatric immunizations with the appropriate vaccines (DPT, IPV, MMR, *Haemophilus influenzae* type b protein-conjugate vaccine) regardless of symptoms (56). While MMR is a live-virus vaccine, no adverse effects were reported in 42 children with HIV who received MMR either during or following measles infection, and the current recommendation is that children with HIV receive MMR. In addition, the AAP and ACIP recommend vaccinating children with symptomatic HIV infection against pneumococcal and influenza infections (3, 4, 56).

Functional (e.g., sickle cell disease) or anatomic asplenia results in an increased risk of infection from encapsulated microorganisms that appears to be greater in children. Although other encapsulated organisms (e.g., meningococcus, *Haemophilus influenzae*) are common, pneumococcus is the most common pathogen in splenectomized individuals. Immunization with the polyvalent pneumococcal vaccine, quadrivalent meningococcal-polysaccharide vaccine, and *Haemophilus influenzae* type b protein-conjugate vaccines are recommended for all asplenic individuals >2 years old. Because the response to pneumococcal vaccine is poor, prophylactic penicillin is recommended for sickle cell patients <5 years of age. It is not clear at what age penicillin prophylaxis can be stopped.

PREGNANCY AND LACTATION

In determining the need for active immunization during pregnancy or lactation, the potential benefits and risks must be considered. The consequences of natural infection and the likelihood of exposure must be balanced against the risk of immunization for both the mother and fetus. In most cases, the decision to immunize must be made with limited or no data available regarding the risk for congenital anomalies or other adverse outcomes. Should it be decided that immunization is needed during pregnancy, vaccination should occur during the third trimester whenever possible. The ACIP and AAP publish guidelines that assist in managing complex or unusual situations.

In general, passive immunization with immune globulin is considered safe for pregnant women (3, 4). Active immunization with toxoids is relatively safe when performed in the third trimester. In fact, it is desirable to immunize previously unimmunized pregnant women against diphtheria and tetanus, preferably during the third trimester of pregnancy (3, 4). Furthermore, immunized women who have not received a Td booster within the last 10 years should receive Td prior to delivery.

Inactivated viral and bacterial vaccines present less risk than live vaccines because these organisms will not replicate. Pregnant women in high-risk groups should be immunized for influenza at the appropriate time of year (43). The risks of pneumococcal immunization to the fetus are unknown; therefore, the risk of infection in a high-risk mother must be weighed against the potential harm to the fetus (4).

Immunization with the MMR live, attenuated virus vaccine is contraindicated in pregnancy. Because of the potential risk of fetal infection, women who are of childbearing age who are vaccinated with these agents should be counseled to avoid conception for 3 months following immunization. While immunization with MMR should be avoided immediately prior to and during pregnancy, recently published findings of women who inadvertently received the rubella vaccine within 3 months of conception reported no evidence that the vaccination was responsible for congenital rubella syndrome (3).

If unimmunized and pregnant, a woman anticipating travel outside the United States and exposure to wild polio virus should be immunized with OPV, or alternatively, IPV (4). If travel to an area with a high risk for contracting yellow fever cannot be postponed, the yellow fever vaccine should be given (4, 51). Malaria prophylaxis with chloroquine or hydroxychloroquine is not contraindicated in pregnancy. However, travel to areas with *P. falciparum* that is resistant to chloroquine or hydroxychloroquine should be avoided, since both mefloquine and doxycycline are contraindicated in pregnancy (52).

The postpartum period is thought to be a good time to review immunization status and update any necessary immunizations. While there may be transfer of antibody to the infant who is fed with human milk, lactation is not a contraindication to immunization with any agent (3).

PHARMACEUTICAL CONSIDERATIONS

Understanding vaccine manufacturing techniques and the various excipients added to products to stabilize and preserve the final product is essential to minimize adverse reactions to vaccines. The package insert provides information about manufacturing procedures and provides a list of all excipients for vaccines and immunobiologics.

Should an allergic reaction occur, it is generally related to (*a*) viral vaccines grown in embryonic egg culture, (*b*) antibiotics or preservations, (*c*) stabilizers, or (*d*) antitoxin or antisera of animal origin. Individuals who experience anaphylactic reactions to eggs or egg products may experience a similar reaction to a viral vaccine grown in egg culture. MMR and influenza vaccines are grown in egg culture; however, they are highly purified and can generally be safely given to patients with a nonanaphylactic-type egg allergy. Desensitization or a graded protocol can be used successfully for vaccines grown in egg cell cultures to immunize individuals with egg allergies (23, 24) (Table 59.3). Trace amounts of antibiotics or preservatives (e.g., neomycin, thimerosal) added to immunobiologics may be responsible for hypersensitivity reactions. However, a causal relationship between the trace amounts of antibiotics in vaccines and adverse effects has not been established. Delayed minor reactions attributed to neomycin or streptomycin have been reported between 48 and 96 hr after immunization with MMR and IPV. Anyone with a history of anaphylactic reaction to neomycin or streptomycin should not receive vaccines that contain these antibiotics. No vaccine contains penicillin. Mercury may accumulate in individuals who receive repeated courses of IGIM. Those who are sensitive to mercury may experience a reaction; however, no specific causal relationship has been reported.

Antisera or antitoxins of animal origin are the most likely agents to cause allergic reactions. Horse serum is used to produce diphtheria, tetanus, and botulism antitoxins; equine antirabies serum; and antivenins. Biologicals of equine origin are inherently immunogenic; thus, all patients should undergo a scratch test or eye test using a dilution of the product to be administered prior to treatment. Positive reactions indicate the need to use a desensitization protocol before the therapeutic dose is given. However, failure to elicit a positive response does not preclude the occurrence of a systemic reaction. Patients who have received horse serum–containing products or who experience asthma or allergic symptoms when near horses should be desensitized prior to administration of antisera or antitoxins.

Safe handling and storage of vaccines and immunobiologics is essential to insure vaccine potency and prevent vaccine failure (57). Pharmacists should be familiar with the usual appearance of immunobiologics to help validate that product integrity was maintained during transport and to assure that product degradation did not occur during storage. The shelf life should be validated and expiration dates noted, and the appropriate storage conditions should be maintained. Care must be taken to insure timely reconstitution prior to immunization to maintain potency and prevent vaccine failure. The package insert should be consulted for specific information about the appropriate handling and storage of each vaccine.

FUTURE

Vaccine development is directed toward improving safety, increasing supplies, and producing new vaccines for diseases that currently are not preventable. Cytomegalovirus, hepatitis A, herpes simplex, and HIV vaccines are currently being investigated (45). Work continues in the development of avirulent polio vaccines to eliminate the small risk for polio infection that exists with the current OPV. While vaccines of today are usually composed of attenuated or inactivated microorganisms, vaccines of the future may be derived from a component of an organism that stimulates the immunologic response or an "empty" viral particle or be manufactured using recombinant DNA technology. In addition, different techniques of administration are being explored, including nasal sprays and time-release capsules. The further development of safer, more effective vaccines will have a positive impact on decreasing infectious disease provided immunizations are administered to the appropriate target population. As a highly visible and easily accessible healthcare professional, the pharmacist can facilitate the prevention of infectious diseases by providing accurate and timely information about immunizations. Further, the pharmacist has a professional obligation to promote wellness by educating the public about the essentiality of immunization programs.

REFERENCES

1. Breese C: Influenza: a shot or not? Pediatrics 79:564–566, 1987.
2. Williams WW, Hickson MA, Kane MA, et al.: Immunization policies and vaccine coverage among adults: the risk for missed opportunities. Ann Intern Med 108:616–625, 1988.
3. Immunizations Practices Advisory Committee (ACIP): General recommendations on immunizations. MMWR 38:205–214, 219–227, 1989.
4. American Academy of Pediatrics. Report of the Committee on Infectious Diseases (Redbook), ed. 21. 1988.
5. Bernbaum J, Draft A, Samuelson J, et al.: Half-dose immunization for diphtheria, tetanus, pertussis: response of preterm infants. Pediatrics 83:471–476, 1989.
6. Halperin SA, Bortolussi R, MacLean D, et al.: Persistence of pertussis in an immunized population: results of the Nova Scotia enhanced pertussis surveillance program. J Pediatr 115:686–693, 1989.
7. Bass JW, Stephenson SR: The return of pertussis. Pediatr Infect Dis J 6:141–144, 1987.
8. Cody CL, Baraff LJ, Cherry JD, et al.: Nature and rates of adverse reactions associated with DPT and DT immunizations in infants and children. Pediatrics 68:650–660, 1981.
9. Stetler HC, Orenstein WA, Bart KJ, et al.: History of convulsions and use of petussis vaccine. J Pediatr 107:175–179, 1985.
10. Walker AM, Jick H, Perera DR, et al.: Neurologic events following diphtheria-tetanus-pertussis immunization. Pediatrics 81:345–349, 1988.
11. Hoffman HJ, Hunter JC, Damus K, et al.: Diphtheria-tetanus-pertussis immunization and sudden infant death: results of the National Institute of Child Health and Human Development Cooperative Epidemiology Study of Sudden Infant Death Syndrome risk factors. Pediatrics 79:598–611, 1987.
12. Fulginiti VA: A pertussis vaccine myth dies. Am J Dis Child 144;860–861, 1990.
13. Golden GS: Pertussis vaccine and injury to the brain. J Pediatr 116:854–861, 1990.
14. Blumberg DA, Mink CM, Cherry JD, et al.: Comparison of an acellular pertussis-component diphtheria-tetanus-pertussis (DTP) vaccine with a whole-cell pertussis-component DTP vaccine in 17- to 24-month-old children, with measurement of 69–kilodalton outer membrane protein antibody. J Pediatr 117:46–51, 1990.
15. Gaebler JWW, Kleiman MB, French MLV, et al.: Neurologic complications in oral polio vaccine recipients. J Pediatr 108:878–881, 1986.
16. Rasch DK, Wells O, Fowlkes J: Fatal disseminated infection due to poliovirus type 2 vaccine. Am J Dis Child 140:1211–1212, 1984.
17. McBean AM, Modlin JF: Rationale for the sequential use of inactivated poliovirus vaccine and live attenuated poliovirus vaccine for routine poliomyelitis immunization in the United States. Pediatr Infect Dis 6:881–887, 1987.
18. American Academy of Pediatrics. Committee on Infectious Diseases: Measles: reassessment of the current immunization policy. Pediatrics 84:1110–1113, 1989.
19. Immunizations Practices Advisory Committee (ACIP). Measles prevention. MMWR 38(S-9):1–17, 1989.
20. Stetler HC, Orenstein WA, Bernier RH, et al.: Impact of revaccinating children who initially received measles vaccine before 10 months of age. Pediatrics 77:471–476, 1986.
21. Bakshi SS, Cooper LZ: Rubella and mumps vaccines. Pediatr Clin North Am 37:651–668, 1990.
22. Peltola H, Heinonen OP: Frequency of true adverse reactions to measles-mumps-rubella vaccine: a double blind placebo-controlled trial in twins. Lancet 1:939–942, 1986.
23. Herman JJ, Radom R, Schneider R: Allergic reactions to measles (rubeola) vaccine in patients hypersensitive to egg protein. J Pediatr 102:196–199, 1983.
24. Miller JR, Orgel HA, Meltzer EO: The safety of egg-containing vaccines for egg-allergic patients. J Allergy Clin Immunol 71:568–573, 1983.
25. Bartell LA, Charney SA: National vaccine injury compensation act: a viable alternative to litigation? J Pharm Pract 2:36–44, 1989.
26. Clayton EW, Hickson GB: Compensation under the National Childhood Vaccine Injury Act. J Pediatr 116:508–513, 1990.
27. Taylor HG, Michaels RH, Mazur PM, et al.: Intellectual, neuropsychological, and achievement outcomes in children six to eight years after recovery from Haemophilus influenzae menengitis. Pediatrics 74:198–205, 1984.
28. Ward JI, Brenneman G, Letson GW, et al.: Limited efficacy of a Haemophilus influenzae type b conjugate vaccine in Alaska native infants. N Engl J Med 323:1393–1401, 1990.
29. Peltola H, Kayhty H, Sivonen A, et al.: Haemophilus influenzae type

b capsular polysaccharide vaccine in children: a double-blind field study of 100,000 vaccinees 3 months to 5 years of age in Finland. Pediatrics 60:730–737, 1977.

30. American Academy of Pediatrics. Committee on Infectious Diseases. *Haemophilus influenzae* type b conjugate vaccines: immunization of children at 15 months of age. Pediatrics 86:794–796, 1990.

31. Anon. *H. influenzae* vaccine for infants. The Medical Letter 33:5–7, 1991.

32. Dahsefsky B, Wald E, Guerra N, et al.: Safety, tolerability, and immunogenicity of concurrent administration of *Haemophilus influenzae* type b conjugate vaccine (meningococcal protein conjugate) with either measles-mumps-rubella vaccine or diphtheria-tetanus-pertussis and oral poliovirus vaccines in 14- to 23-month-old infants. Pediatrics 85:682–689, 1990.

33. Immunizations Practices Advisory Committee (ACIP). Update: Prevention of *Haemophilus influenzae* type b disease. MMWR 35:170–180, 1986.

34. Phelps SJ, Hogue SL, Saluk S, et al.: Rifampin prophylaxis for *Hemophilus influenzae* infections. Hosp Pharm 25:861–864, 1990.

35. American Academy of Pediatrics. Committee on Infectious Diseases. Revision of recommendation for use of rifampin prophylaxis of contacts of patients with *Haemophilus influenzae* infection. Pediatrics 74:301–302, 1984.

36. Shapiro ED, Wald ER: Efficacy of rifampin in eliminating pharyngeal carriage of *Haemophilus influenzae* type b. Pediatrics 66:5–8, 1980.

37. Committee on Extemporaneous Formulations. Handbook on Extemporaneous Formulations. Bethesda, MD: American Society of Hospital Pharmacists Special Projects Division, ASHP, 1987, p. 43.

38. Immunizations Practices Advisory Committee (ACIP). Pneumococcal polysaccharide vaccine. MMWR 38:64–76, 1989.

39. Klein JO: The epidemiology of pneumococcal disease in infants and children. Rev Infect Dis 3:S246–S253, 1981.

40. American Academy of Pediatrics. Committee on Infectious Diseases. Recommendations for using pneumococcal vaccine in children. Pediatrics 75:1153–1158, 1985.

41. Greenwood BM, Hassan-King M, Whittle HC: Prevention of secondary cases of meningococcal disease in household contacts by vaccination. Br Med J 1:1317–1319, 1978.

42. Peltola H, Safary A, Kayhty H, et al.: Evaluation of two tetravalent

(ACYW$_{135}$) meningococcal vaccines in infants and small children: a clinical study comparing immunogenicity of O-acetyl-negative and O-acetyl positive group C polysaccharides. Pediatrics 76:91–96, 1985.

43. Immunizations Practices Advisory Committee (ACIP). Prevention and control influenza. MMWR 39(RR-7):1–15, 1990.

44. Immunizations Practices Advisory Committee (ACIP). Protection against viral hepatitis. MMWR 39(S-2):1–25, 1990.

45. Gershon AA: Viral vaccines of the future. Pediatr Clin North Am 37:689–707, 1990.

46. Centers for Disease Control. Rabies vaccine, adsorbed: a new rabies vaccine for use in humans. MMWR 37:217–223, 1988.

47. Immunizations Practices Advisory Committee (ACIP). Systemic allergic reactions following immunization with human diploid cell rabies vaccine. MMWR 33:185–187, 1984.

48. Hill DR, Pearson RD: Health advice for international travel. Ann Intern Med 108:839–852, 1988.

49. Wolfe MS: Vaccines for foreign travel. Pediatr Clin North Am 37:757–769, 1990.

50. Immunizations Practices Advisory Committee (ACIP): Cholera. MMWR 37:617–624, 1988.

51. Immunizations Practices Advisory Committee (ACIP). Yellow fever MMWR 39(RR-6):1–6, 1990.

52. Immunizations Practices Advisory Committee (ACIP). Recommendations for the prevention of malaria among travelers. MMWR 39(RR-3):1–10, 1990.

53. Centers for Disease Control. Revised dosing regimen for malaria prophylaxis with mefloquine. MMWR 39(36):630, 1990.

54. Phelps SJ, Reynolds MA, Tami JA, et al.: ASHP therapeutic guidelines for intravenous immune globulin. ASHP Commission on Therapeutics. Clin Pharm 11:117–136, 1991.

55. Immunizations Practices Advisory Committee (ACIP). Recommendations on varicella-zoster immune globulin for the prevention of chickenpox. MMWR 33:84–100, 1984.

56. Onorato IM, Markowitz LE, Oxtoby MJ: Childhood immunization, vaccine-preventable diseases, and infection with human immunodeficiency virus. Pediatr Infect Dis J 7:588–595, 1988.

57. Casto DT, Brunell PA: Safe handling of vaccines. Pediatrics 87:108–112, 1991.

CHAPTER 60

UPPER RESPIRATORY TRACT INFECTIONS

CHRISTINE E. HULS, Pharm.D., TIMOTHY A. MULLENIX, Pharm.D., M.S., and RANDALL A. PRINCE, Pharm.D.

Although coryza, laryngitis, pharyngitis, and other syndromes designated "upper respiratory tract infections" are usually discussed as separate entities, they actually represent a continuum of illness severity and a blend of symptoms and signs (1). The nose, paranasal sinuses, pharynx, larynx, trachea, and bronchi make up the upper respiratory system.

THE COMMON COLD

Acute coryza, better known as the common cold, is actually a group of diseases caused by various viral families, which result in a mild, self-limited, inflammatory syndrome. In the United States, adults average 2 to 4 colds per year and children have 6 to 8 such episodes (2, 3). An estimated 50 million days were lost from work or school in 1985 (4). Cold sufferers spend more than $2 billion yearly in the United States for the more than 800 cold remedies available (5).

Pathogenesis

Viral invasion of the upper respiratory tract is the triggering event in the pathogenesis of the common cold. Pathogenic agents thought to cause this disease include rhinoviruses, parainfluenza viruses, respiratory syncytial viruses, enteroviruses, coxsackie viruses, and coronaviruses. Of these, rhinoviruses are the cause of approximately 30% of all cases of colds. This virus alone has an estimated 100 antigenically different serotypes. This multiplicity of viruses and serotypes precludes the possibility of a simple cure to the common cold. The etiology of as many as 35% of colds in adults, however, is unknown (7). These would potentially represent presumed undiscovered viruses.

Several factors, such as age, season, weather, and smoking, are associated with the development of a cold. Cigarette smoking increases the severity, but not the incidence, of colds (8). The cold season in the United States begins in late August to mid-September. Incidence rates climb over the following weeks and remain elevated until March or May, when the attack rate declines (10). While some viral groups demonstrate a seasonal variation, exposure to cold or wet environments has not been shown to predispose one to the development of upper respiratory tract infections (11). Explanations for the seasonal fluctuations in the frequency of colds remain obscure, although factors such as bringing children together during the school year and increased crowding during winter months probably play important roles in the pathogenesis of this disease.

The principle mode of transmission of respiratory viruses remains controversial (12, 13). Suggested mechanisms include contamination by aerosolization or direct contact with respiratory secretions. Coughing allows small-particle aerosolization of respiratory secretions, whereas large-particle aerosolization may result from either coughing or sneezing. Direct contact with infectious secretions may involve handshaking or use of a contaminated telephone.

Once a patient is inoculated, the incubation period of the common cold is approximately 48 to 72 hr. As a response to viral insult, the body's defense mechanisms are activated, producing an inflammatory reaction at the sites of infection. One complication of viral presence is the effect on the resident bacterial flora, which may influence the development of a secondary bacterial infection. In children, a cold caused by parainfluenza virus and respiratory syncytial virus infection may progress to viral pneumonia, croup, or bronchiolitis. There is also a positive correlation between colds and the incitement of asthma, chronic bronchitis, and emphysema (14).

Clinical Characteristics and Diagnosis

The common cold produces a variety of complaints, which usually resolve after 1 week in adults and 2 weeks in children (2). Cardinal symptoms include rhinorrhea, nasal congestion, sneezing, sore throat, and nonproductive cough. Nasal discharge may progress from clear and watery to more tenacious and purulent. Maceration of the skin around the nares may result from frequent nose blowing. Some sufferers experience a loss in the sense of taste and smell and/or a feeling of fullness in the ears or paranasal sinuses. Nasal congestion may also impart a nasal quality to the voice. Fever, if present, is usually low grade. Other symptoms include headache, a feeling of general malaise, chills, and conjunctivitis.

Due to the ubiquitous nature and easy recognition of the syndrome, nearly everyone can diagnose the common cold. There is no definitive diagnostic test. While findings on physical examination are few, nasal discharge and reddened nose are common. Mucous membranes in the nose may appear glassy. Pharyngeal, nasal, or tympanic erythema may or may not be remarkable. Auscultation of the chest may reveal crackles. Because of the time and expense currently required in isolating viruses, the nonavailability of virus-specific therapy, and the benign, self-limiting nature of most colds, specific virologic diagnosis is impractical for clinical use.

Of the patients with cold symptoms, 0.5% will have secondary bacterial infections and 2% will have otitis media. A complete examination of the pharynx, nasal cavity, ears, and sinuses can help distinguish the small percentage of patients with these complications. Further testing, such as rapid antigen detection, cultures for β-hemolytic streptococci, or sinus radiography, may be used.

Treatment

Treatment for the common cold remains symptomatic. Besides symptom relief, other goals of therapy include minimizing communicability and decreasing complications. Antibiotic administration is not indicated. Simple measures, including bed rest, petroleum jelly to the nares, or saline gargles for sore throat, may provide relief. While antihistamines and decongestants are commonly used to ameliorate cold symptoms, scientific evidence to support the use of many of these agents is lacking. Many cold products are combination products, in which some of the active ingredients may not be in therapeutic doses. Some combinations may antagonize each other. Also, when using a combination product, patients may be exposing themselves to unneeded, possibly detrimental, agents. Rational symptomatic treatment dictates using one or more single product(s) at appropriate doses. Fixed-combination products may be appropriate in occasional, selected cases. The Food and Drug Administration (FDA) has devised a classification scheme for over-the-counter (OTC) products in an effort to communicate their safety and efficacy (15). Category I agents are drugs that the FDA has recognized as being safe and effective for the claimed therapeutic indication. Category II drugs are those that are neither safe nor effective. Category III agents are those about which there is insufficient data to permit a final classification. See Table 60.1 for a listing of FDA category I antihistamines, decongestants, and antitussives.

Antihistamines

Unlike allergic rhinitis, the role of histamine released by mast cells in the pathogenesis of colds has not been established. In allergic rhinitis, antihistamines block the binding of histamine to the H1 receptor, preventing increased capillary permeability and resultant rhinorrhea. Since histamine concentrations do not change in the nasal secretions during the course of rhinovirus colds, the role of this mechanism for coryza-associated rhinorrhea is questionable (16, 17).

Any therapeutic benefit of antihistamines may depend

Table 60.1.
F.D.A. Category I Over-the-Counter Cold Remedies[a]

Antihistamine (by Chemical Class)	Decongestants	Antitussives
Ethanolamines	*Topical*	Codeine
Diphenhydramine	Ephedrine 0.1%	Dextromethorphan
Doxylamine	Naphazoline 0.05%	Diphenhydramine
Ethylenediamines	Oxymetazoline 0.05%	
Pyrilamine	Phenylephrine 0.25%	
Thonzylamine	Xylometazoline 0.05%	
Alkylamines	*Oral*	
Pheniramine	Phenylephrine	
Brompheniramine	Phenylpropanolamine	
Chlorpheniramine	Pseudoephedrine	
Miscellaneous		
Phenindamine		

[a] Adapted from Handbook of Nonprescription Drugs, ed. 8. Washington, D.C.: American Pharmaceutical Association and the National Professional Society of Pharmacists, 1986.

on the ability of these drugs to block cholinergic receptors. Anticholinergic effects may dry up nasal and pharyngeal secretions, as well as worsen nasal blockage and sinus congestion. Antihistamine-associated sedation may contribute to the patient's perception of cold relief. Modest benefits of alkylamine-type antihistamines (e.g., chlorpheniramine and triprolidine) have been demonstrated in controlled trials. In one study, chlorpheniramine demonstrated up to a 15% reduction in nasal discharge, sneezing, and nose blowing, as well as excess sedation (20). The chlorpheniramine group also experienced excess drowsiness. Antihistamines do not prevent the development of complications, such as otitis media (21, 22). Terfenadine and loratadine, selective H1 antihistamines that have lower potential for sedation and lack anticholinergic effect, have not demonstrated efficacy against common cold symptoms (23, 24). Terfenadine and loratadine are available on prescription.

Choosing an antihistamine becomes a matter of trial and error. A product should be selected on the basis of individual efficacy, side effects, and cost. Expected side effects are those of an anticholinergic nature: sedation, tachycardia, mucosal drying, decreased gastrointestinal motility, and urinary retention. Sedation, the most common side effect, may interfere with the patient's daytime activities. The patient should be warned to avoid the concurrent use of other sedating agents such as tranquilizers or alcohol.

Sympathomimetics

Topical and systemic sympathomimetic agents are among the most commonly used decongestants for relief of nasal congestion due to colds. α-Adrenergic agonists vasoconstrict the microvasculature of the engorged nasal mucosa, reducing blood flow and shrinking venous capacitance. This results in inhibition of vascular leakage, drainage of sinuses, and clearing of airways. Most nasal decongestants are from the phenylethamine class, which includes pseudoephedrine, ephedrine, phenylephrine, and phenylpropanolamine (25). Phenylpropanolamine and phenylephrine are selective α-adrenergic agonists, whereas pseudoephedrine and ephedrine stimulate both α- and β-receptors. All but phenylephrine increase norepinephrine in the synapse.

Topical application of nasal sympathomimetics in the form of nasal sprays or drops provides immediate and effective relief from nasal congestion in the short term (26). The use of topical decongestants is limited by the rapid development of tolerance and the potential for rebound nasal congestion. Rebound congestion, which is severe nasal reengorgement upon drug withdrawal, occurs after 3 to 4 days of use and may be associated with vasoconstrictive ischemia and membrane irritation. Tachyphylaxis has also been reported. Systemic side effects, such as vasoconstriction in other vascular beds leading in an increase of blood pressure, are less with nasal sprays and drops than with oral sympathomimetics. The patient who desires to use these products should be counseled to not exceed the labeled regimen and to limit their use to a few days and to limit the frequency of use to every 4 to 8 hours.

Nasal spray should be administered with the patient in an upright position. After squeezing the flexible plastic container to administer one spray in each nostril, the nose should be blown a few minutes later to eliminate nasal mucus. If congestion is still present, an additional spray can be administered into each nostril. Sprays provide better coverage of the nasal mucosal surface and are preferred for adults and older children. Children younger than 6 years of age should receive nose drops because of their smaller nares. For optimal administration, the child should recline with the head tilted back during the administration and for an additional few minutes.

In the past, trials evaluating oral sympathomimetics have been hampered by nonquantifiable outcome measures. Studies quantifying nasal resistance and nasal mucus weights have documented a beneficial effect of pseudoephedrine and phenylpropanolamine (27–29). Reduction of sneezing and congestion was also noted (27–30).

Systemic side effects include restlessness, tachycardia, hypertension, and occasionally nausea, vomiting, or anorexia. Patients seeking relief from nasal congestion can substitute saline nasal sprays to irrigate nasal passages without fear of aggravating their underlying blood pressure abnormalities. Drinking hot liquids is an effective alternative to induce nasal mucus clearance (31). The risk of high blood pressure appears to be greater with phenylpropanolamine than with pseudoephedrine and with immediate-release forms than with slow-release forms (32).

Phenylpropanolamine, the most commonly used decongestant, has been infrequently associated with serious toxicities, including myocardial damage, when used in the recommended doses. If an overdose is taken, it can cause serious adverse effects, including stroke and death. However, the relatively low incidence of reports of serious toxicities associated with these frequently used agents implies a relatively low risk in otherwise healthy individuals (33).

Anticholinergics

While the role of parasympathetic-cholinergic mechanisms in the development of the nasal symptoms associated with colds is not clear, intranasal ipratropium nasal spray has been under scrutiny. In a recent study, intranasal ipratropium (80 μg three times daily × 5 days) produced a 40% reduction of mucus weights (34). Reported side effects included dry mouth, dry nasal passages, and epistaxis. There was no change in pulse or blood pressure in a second clinical trial (35). The clinical value of topical anticholinergic agents appears promising, but requires further study. The use of systemic anticholinergic agents has not been evaluated.

Analgesics

Aspirin and acetaminophen exert equipotent effects as analgesics and antipyretics. The usual adult dose for either agent is 650 mg every 4 hr as needed. Other nonsteroidal antiinflammatory analgesics, e.g., ibuprofen 200 mg every 4 hr as needed, may be used as well. Studies investigating the relationship of viral shedding to aspirin administration have yielded conflicting results (36, 37). Ibuprofen was shown to decrease the number of days of viral shedding by 44% (30). There is some evidence that aspirin may reduce lung and tracheal mucociliary clearance, thereby interfering with normal defense mechanisms (38). Since aspirin administration has been associated with Reyes syndrome in pediatric patients, acetaminophen 10 mg/kg every 4 hr is the recommended analgesic and antipyretic in this population.

Caffeine is in many over-the-counter analgesics and cold medications. While it does augment pain relief, it also disturbs sleep patterns, alters mood, and increases blood pressure and gastric acid secretion (39). It may also provoke cardiac arrhythmias (40).

Antitussives

Coughs due to colds tend to be nonproductive and are easily suppressed by available antitussives. Narcotic agents (codeine, hydrocodone, and noscapine), dextromethorphan, and diphenhydramine depress the cough reflex mediated in the medulla. Benzonatate depresses coughs by a local anesthetic action in the respiratory tree. The most common indication for antitussives is when coughing interferes with sleep. In this case, either a narcotic agent or diphenhydramine provides the added benefit of sedation. Some coughs may become self-perpetuating and cause injury to the nasopharynx, larynx, and/or other respiratory structures. Dextromethorphan is the safest antitussive for daytime cough relief and in the pediatric population. If the cough should become productive, antitussive administration should strive for suppression of excessive coughing, without elimination of this important mechanism for the clearance of bronchial secretions.

Side effects of these drugs are few. When used at the recommended dosages, narcotic antitussives may cause sedation and/or constipation. Diphenhydramine is likely to cause sedation, while dextromethorphan may occasionally produce gastrointestinal distress.

Topical anesthetics are weak cough suppressants, but may prove soothing. Products include gargles, sprays, and lozenges. These agents anesthetize the irritant and pain receptors in the oral pharynx. If used excessively, oral topical anesthetics may abolish the gag reflex, thereby increasing the risk of pulmonary aspiration.

Expectorants

Expectorants have long been promoted for decreasing sputum viscosity, thus facilitating the expectoration of bronchial secretions, and for an antitussive effect. Some of the more common expectorants include guaifenesin, terpin hydrate, syrup of ipecac, ammonium chloride, potassium guaiacol sulfonate, and potassium iodide. Despite their widespread use, there is no convincing evidence that expectorants are effective for their claimed indications (41). Likewise, it has never been proven that oral hydration will thin respiratory secretions; however, dehydration surely will not benefit the clearance of bronchial secretions and should be avoided. Steam or cool mist humidification does help to liquefy secretions.

Antivirals

α-Interferons have been comprehensively tested for both cold prophylaxis and treatment. Intranasal administration of recombinant interferon alpha-2 has demonstrated efficacy for prevention of experimentally induced rhinoviral and coronaviral infections (42, 43). There was a 40% incidence of nasal intolerance, primarily epistaxis. In an effort to minimize nasal side effects, short-term prophylaxis and reduced dosages have been studied. Two placebo-controlled trials of short-term intranasal interferon have confirmed that a shorter duration of treatment may be effective in decreasing the number of cold episodes and nasal side effects (44, 45). Therapeutic administration of intranasal interferon has yielded results ranging from modest benefit to worsened course of illness (46–48). Issues to be clarified include the role of other interferons as possible cold prophylaxis or therapy, combination therapy, or alternate routes of administration.

In the mid-1970s, zinc chloride was discovered to inhibit the in vitro replication of rhinovirus via inhibition of viral polypeptide cleavage (49). The zinc lozenges are large, unpalatable, and require every-2-hr administration while awake. Clinical studies have been hampered by the availability of an equally bad-tasting placebo and volunteers who will be compliant with the bitter lozenges. Although earlier trials demonstrated efficacy, subsequent studies with a suitable placebo failed to demonstrate reduced viral shedding or reduction of symptoms or nasal mucus production despite elevated serum zinc levels (50–52). Furthermore, the lozenges caused mouth soreness in 50% of the patients, as well as unpleasant aftertaste (75%) and nausea (30%).

Capsid-binding agents prevent uncoating of the viral capsid, a process that is required in viral replication. Capsid-binding agents, including flavans and flavones, such as dichloroflavan, chalcone, RMI 15731 and R61837, should theoretically be able to reduce viral shedding, and therefore, reinfection and communicability. With the exception of R61837, oral and intranasal administration of capsid-binding agents has yielded disappointing results (53–56).

Enviroxime, a benzimidazole derivative, inhibits in vitro rhinovirus replication. Significant therapeutic benefit has not been seen with oral or intranasal administration (57–59). One placebo-controlled study examining the combined use of oral and nasal administration tended to reduce symptoms and nasal mucus production (60). Oral administration of enviroxime is associated with a high incidence of nausea and vomiting. Enviradene, also a benzimidazole, is currently under investigation by both liposomal topical delivery and oral administration routes (61).

Vitamin C

Ascorbic acid (vitamin C) has received considerable attention in the lay literature and news media for its purported prophylactic benefits for colds. Nobel laureate Linus Pauling suggested that 1 to 5 g/day of ascorbic acid could prevent colds and 15 g/day could be curative (62). Pauling has received much acclaim as well as criticism for his research methods. Since Pauling's original investigations, large placebo-controlled trials have not been able to demonstrate any difference between the placebo group and the vitamin C group, when evaluating prophylaxis or cure of the common cold (63, 64). There is no long-term study that demonstrates the safety of vitamin C. Potential adverse effects of ascorbic acid taken regularly in large doses include diarrhea, precipitation of oxalate or urate renal stones, mobilization of calcium from bones, and hyperglycemia, as well as adverse effects on fertility and the fetus. Vitamin C may interact with many common drugs, e.g., vitamin C may inhibit the anticoagulant effect of warfarin (64).

Prevention

Vaccination would be a welcome method of cold prophylaxis, but it is a formidable task in view of the antigenic diversity and possible mutation of the many serotypes of the etiologic viruses. Cold vaccines for specific viruses have been effective in inducing local antibody and conferring protection (65). Unless some methods for combining viral antigens or using antigenic cross-relationships are discovered, prospects for the development of a practical vaccine are not good.

Intranasal monoclonal antibodies have reduced infection in a preliminary report. All the rhinovirus serotypes bind to one of two different receptors on the host cell. Monoclonal antibodies competitively inhibit attachment of the rhinovirus to the host cell by binding to those two sites (66). This area of cold prevention is still in its infancy.

SINUSITIS

Sinusitis is an inflammation of one or more of the four paired structures that make up the paranasal sinuses, including the maxillary, ethmoidal, sphenoidal and frontal sinuses. The primary functions of the paranasal sinuses are to warm and humidify inhaled air, remove airborne debris, increase olfactory sensitivity, and impart resonance to the voice. Sinusitis has been classified as acute, subacute, or chronic, based on the duration of illness, inflammatory response, and histopathology (67). Acute sinusitis consists of congestion, submucosal edema, and epithelial cellular debris lasting 2 to 4 weeks. Subacute sinusitis may last anywhere from 2 weeks to 3 months and is of lesser severity than acute sinusitis. Finally, chronic sinusitis, which is the consequence of recurrent and uncured acute sinusitis lasting more than 3 months, results in a change in the epithelium. The replacement of normal, ciliated columnar epithelium with stratified squamous epithelium compromises self-cleansing. While the exact incidence of sinusitis is unknown, it appears to parallel the incidence of acute infections of the upper respiratory tract, which are most prevalent during the fall, winter, and spring months. Adults are more likely to be afflicted than children (68, 69).

Pathogenesis

Acute sinusitis is most commonly precipitated by the effects of the common cold (70). Damage secondary to viral invasion provides an environment conducive to development of a secondary bacterial infection (71, 72). The inflammation and edema of viral respiratory infection, which cause obstruction of sinus drainage, allow the collection of a rich medium for bacteria. Viral infection interferes with ciliary clearance of mucus and bacteria, which encourages bacterial access to this growth medium. Other predisposing conditions include allergic rhinitis, nasal polyposis, tumors, foreign bodies, congenital malformations, nasal packing, and indwelling nasal tubes (73, 74). Due to close proximity, dental infections may spread to neighboring maxillary sinuses.

The microbial etiology of acute sinusitis has been well described in studies using direct puncture (75–77). *Streptococcus pneumoniae* and unencapsulated *Haemophilus influenzae* account for approximately half of all cases of adult and pediatric community-acquired, acute sinusitis. *Moraxella catarrhalis* is responsible for 20% of pediatric acute sinusitis. The incidence of β-lactamase-producing organisms, currently increasing in frequency, is estimated to be 25 to 40%. While a 6% incidence of *Staphylococcus aureus* has been reported in the past, it is likely that *S. aureus* was a contaminant harvested due to improper culturing. While *Bacteroides* spp. are the primary anaerobic organisms found in acute sinusitis in adults, anaerobic organisms are rarely found in children. A viral cause of sinusitis has been documented in 15 to 30% of cases studied, most commonly rhinovirus, influenza, and parainfluenza (72, 78). This may actually be an underestimation of the true incidence of viral sinusitis because of technical problems of viral culturing.

Chronic sinusitis studies have yielded a wider variety of Gram-positive and Gram-negative bacteria (79). Ongoing bacterial growth, especially anaerobic bacteria, *S. aureus*, and *Streptococcus viridans*, is secondary to the irreversible changes in the mucosal lining of the sinus. Anaerobic organisms, primarily *Bacteroides* spp., *Peptostreptococcus*, and *Fusobacterium* spp., are found in up to 88% of reported cases. Patients with chronic sinusitis can experience exacerbations of acute sinusitis with its own particular microbial milieu.

Other special patient groups have other prevalent organisms. Gram-negative enteric organisms predominate in hospital-acquired, acute sinusitis, which is often polymicrobial (74, 80). The most frequent isolate in sinus aspirates from cystic fibrosis patients was *Pseudomonas aeruginosa* (81). Immunocompromised patients and poorly controlled diabetics develop fungal sinusitis, commonly with *Aspergillus niger* (82). *Rhizopus* spp. (*Mucor*), most often occurring in uncontrolled diabetics, is rare but rapidly devastating.

Complications of the pathological process of sinusitis result from direct extension of the suppurative process of adjacent areas, such as the soft tissue (cellulitis), the orbit, the frontal bone (osteomyelitis), and the intracranial space (meningitis). When complications occur, hospitalization, intravenous antibiotics, prolonged therapy, and/or surgical intervention may be required (83).

Clinical Characteristics and Diagnosis

Facial pain, headache, purulent nasal discharge or nasal obstruction, and recent history of upper respiratory infection are the most typical presenting signs and symptoms in acute and chronic sinusitis. Concomitant symptoms include disorders of sense of smell, nasal quality to the voice, and tenderness to palpation over the involved sinus. While cough was the most frequent symptom in children, fetid breath was also frequently reported (77). Fever was reported in approximately one-half of cases of adult and pediatric, acute, maxillary sinusitis.

The differential diagnosis for the patient with signs and symptoms of sinusitis also includes allergic rhinitis, prolonged cold, headaches, and neoplasms. Besides assessing the patient's complaints and recent history, a complete examination must be done of the ears, nose, throat, teeth, and sinuses. Transillumination of the sinuses may provide valuable information in acute sinusitis (84). If the diagnosis of sinusitis is difficult or if serious complications are already present, a radiologic examination should be done. If the standard views, including Waters view, reveal an air-fluid level or mucosal thickening, this is strong evidence for an active sinus infection (84, 85). Whenever treatment is initiated without the benefit of x-rays and the symptoms persist or worsen, radiologic studies should be obtained. Transillumination and radiologic diagnosis are limited in patients with chronic sinusitis, because of persistent abnormalities. Sinus radiography is of limited utility in children under 1 year of age (85). Computed tomography (CT) and magnetic resonance imaging (MRI), very sensitive and costly evaluative techniques, are especially helpful for visualization of the ethmoid sinus, of sphenoid sinus, or for orbital extension of ethmoid sinusitis.

Cultures of nasal exudates are contaminated by the nasal passages. Cultures obtained by direct sinus puncture, using aseptic technique, can yield reliable information about the infecting organism. This invasive procedure is indicated in unusually severe sinusitis, suspected or documented intracranial extension, empiric antimicrobial failure, severe immunosuppression, or nosocomial sinusitis.

Treatment

In the absence of a definitive organism, empiric antimicrobial therapy effective for *S. pneumoniae* and *H. influenzae* should be initiated (70, 86). Acute sinusitis requires a 10-day course of therapy, while longer courses of therapy are required in cases of recurrent, subacute, and chronic sinusitis. In the absence of a penicillin allergy, amoxicillin and ampicillin are considered the drugs of choice. Erythromycin, co-trimoxazole, or tetracycline are viable alternatives for penicillin-allergic patients. Tetracycline should not be administered to children or pregnant females because of possible staining of teeth. Failure to respond to therapy within 72 hr is suspicious for β-lac-

tamase production. Co-trimoxazole, erythromycin/sulfisoxazole, cefaclor or amoxicillin/clavulanate potassium should be initiated, whenever there is a high suspicion of β-lactamase production. The choice of antibiotics is directed by the clinician's knowledge of likely infecting organisms, susceptibility patterns, patient tolerance, and drug cost (see Table 60.2 for dosage guidelines). Supportive therapy may consist of decongestants, humidification, nasal lavage, and analgesics. Systemic topical decongestants may be helpful in reopening blocked sinuses to promote drainage of purulent material and provide symptomatic relief, but their efficacy has not been rigorously established (86). The effectiveness of topical decongestants may be enhanced by positioning the head in a dependent position during administration. While oxymetazoline, xylometazoline, and phenylephrine are effective topical decongestants, oxymetazoline and xylometazoline impart the convenience of longer half-lives. Rebound phenomenon can be avoided by limiting decongestant usage to 3 or 4 days. Inhalation of hot water vapor liquefies and mobilizes tenacious nasal mucus. Nasal lavage with saline nasal drops can also help clear exudates. Antihistamines thicken purulent discharge, and antihistamine use should be discouraged, unless allergic rhinitis is the underlying cause of the sinusitis. If the relief of nasal congestion does not relieve the pain, the patient may need to use an analgesic, such as acetaminophen. If severe pain persists, the patient may require a short course of codeine or other mild narcotic. Intranasal steroids such as beconase reduce edema associated with allergic rhinitis, vasomotor rhinitis, rebound, or polyp degeneration. They should be avoided in acute sinusitis to eliminate their interference with the patient's immune response to bacterial invasion.

Identification of any underlying cause must be pursued in chronic disease. This may include culture via direct sinus puncture. Chronic sinusitis may require a 3- to 4-week course of broadened antibiotic coverage (73; 86). Addition of clindamycin to the regimen provides better coverage of *Bacteroides* spp., although it also adds the risk of pseudomembranous colitis. Surgical removal of diseased mucosa and/or obstruction may also be required.

Prevention

Methods of acute sinusitis prevention are intuitive, not proven. Since sinusitis is frequently initiated by colds, inroads to cold prevention and treatment should yield the benefit of reduced incidence of sinusitis. Therapies reducing obstruction promote normal sinus drainage and lessen the risk of sinus infection. Prompt attention to dental hygiene and infection would logically reduce the risk of maxillary sinusitis. The incidence of chronic sinusitis may be minimized by the effective antimicrobial treatment of acute sinusitis.

Table 60.2.
Commonly Used Antibiotics in Upper Respiratory Diseases[a]

Drug/Route	Pediatric Regimen[a]	Adult Regimen
Penicillins		
Ampicillin p.o.	50–100 mg/kg/day q6h	250–500 mg q6h
Amoxicillin p.o.	20–40 mg/kg/day q8h	250–500 mg q8h
Amoxicillin/clavulanate p.o.	20–40 mg/kg/day q8h (based on amoxicillin)	250–500 mg q8h
Dicloxacillin p.o.	12–25 mg/kg/day q6h	125–500 mg q6h
Nafcillin i.v.	150–200 mg/kg/day q4–6h (max. 10 g/24h)	0.5–3 g q4–6h (max. 12 g/24h)
Penicillin G i.v., i.m.	100,000–200,000 U/day q6h	5–24 million U/day q4h
Penicillin V p.o.	25–50 mg/kg/day q6h	250–500 mg q6h
Cephalosporins		
Cefaclor p.o.	40 mg/kg/day q8h	250–500 mg q8h
Cefuroxime p.o., i.v.	50–100 mg/kg/day q8h	0.76–3 g q8h
Cefotaxime i.v., i.m.	50–200 mg/kg/day q6–8h	1 g q8–12h
Ceftazidime i.v., i.m.	90–150 mg/kg/day q8–12h	1–2 g q8–12h
Miscellaneous		
Clindamycin HCl p.o.	15–40 mg/kg/day q6h	150–450 mg q6h
Cotrimazole p.o.	8 mg/kg/day q12h (based on trimethoprim)	160 mg q12h
Erythromycin p.o.	40–50 mg/kg/day q6h	250–500 mg q6h
Erythromycin/sulfisoxazole p.o.	50 mg/kg/day q8h (based on erythromycin)	250–500 mg q6h
Tetracycline p.o.	Not indicated	250–500 mg q6h

[a] Adapted from Benitz WE, Tatro DS: The Pediatric Drug Handbook, ed. 2. Chicago: Year Book Medical Publishers, 1988.
[b] Pediatric implies infant and children.

OTITIS MEDIA

Otitis media, inflammation of the middle ear, is the most common diagnosis in family practice and the second most common infectious diagnosis in pediatric patients (88). A study of the literature is complicated by the confusion of terms classifying otitis media. Although otitis media is usually described depending upon the presence and duration of middle ear effusion, other descriptive labels include quality of the effusion, presence of drainage, and recurrence of pathology. The effusion may be serous, mucoid, or purulent. Acute otitis media lasts less than 3 weeks, subacute otitis media lasts less than 3 months, and chronic otitis media lasts longer than 3 months. While emphasis is placed on acute otitis media with effusion, some consideration is given to chronic and recurrent otitis media.

Pathogenesis

Acute otitis media is primarily a disease of children, with only occasional episodes in adolescents or adults (89). The highest incidence occurs from the age of 6 to 24 months. Two-thirds of 3-year-old children have had at least one episode of acute otitis media. The earlier the first episode of otitis media, the more likely it is that the child will experience recurrent otitis media. While the incidence of acute otitis media declines with increasing age, a reversal of this trend occurs when these individuals enter day-care or begin school. Group situations expose children to colonization with *S. pneumoniae* and *H. influenzae*, as well as exposure to the common cold. Other factors positively correlated with increased incidence of otitis media include

male gender, bottle feeding, poverty, American Indian or Eskimo race, a sibling with recurrent otitis media, and cigarette smoking within the home.

The interplay of eustachian tube dysfunction and upper respiratory infection is the most important factor in the development of otitis media (90). Underlying allergies, congenital malformations, or immunodeficiency syndromes, when present, contribute to the development of otitis media. Critical functions of the eustachian tube are drainage of middle ear secretions into the nasopharynx, protection from nasopharyngeal secretions, aeration of the middle ear, and equilibration of air pressure. Dysfunction may be caused structurally, mechanically via obstruction, or functionally via immature neural control. While the angle and length of the eustachian tube in children is less conducive to effective drainage of secretions, the delayed innervation plays the more important etiologic role (91). Bacterial or viral upper respiratory infections not only colonize the nasopharynx with pathogenic organisms, the secretions associated with the upper respiratory infection overwhelm the eustachian tube's ability to function adequately. Therefore, seasonal variation of otitis media is a consequence of the increased incidence of upper respiratory infections in the winter months.

The pathogens responsible for otitis media in varied clinical situations are well documented (89). *S. pneumoniae* and nontypeable *H. influenzae* account for approximately 50% of cases in children and adults, while the importance of *M. catarrhalis* is increasing in many communities. Depending on geographical location, about

40% of *H. influenzae* and 75% of *M. catarrhalis* are β-lactamase-producing strains. Other common pathogens include β-hemolytic streptococci and Staphylococcus spp. One-third of cultures are sterile, but 3 to 4% of these may reflect anaerobic infections. One-fourth of cultures are positive for viral presence, not surprisingly respiratory syncytial virus, influenza virus, enteroviruses, and rhinoviruses. Diphtheroids may grow out of the middle ear effusion, but they are frequently considered to be normal flora. Since *Chlamydia trachomatis* is associated with respiratory infections in infants less than 6 months old, it is a frequent cause of otitis media in this age group and may in fact, be more common in other age groups than is presently appreciated. Neonates under 6 weeks most frequently experience otitis media due to *Escherichia coli* or *Klebsiella* spp. In addition to the acute otitis pathogens, *S. aureus* and *P. aeruginosa* are important pathogens in chronic otitis media.

While complications occur more commonly in recurrent and chronic otitis media, the overall incidence of serious complications is low. The tympanic membrane may tear because of the pressure of effusion against the membrane. Although surgical repair is occasionally required, the tear is usually small and heals spontaneously. Since the tear allows for drainage of infected material, this complication is frequently advantageous. Hematogenous or contiguous spread of the infective process may result in meningitis, abscesses, mastoiditis, labyrinthitis, facial paralysis, cholesteatoma, and hearing loss (88, 92, 93). Hearing loss is the most common complication. The relationship of hearing loss due to otitis media and cognitive, linguistic, and emotional development in children is controversial because of confounding variables in published studies (94). Chronic otitis media may influence a pathophysiologic change in the tympanic membrane.

Clinical Characteristics and Diagnosis

Symptoms of acute otitis media develop over minutes to hours and may occur as new symptoms in association with an ongoing upper respiratory infection. Mild-to-severe ear pain, hearing loss, and fever are common. Infants may display irritability and ear pulling. The tympanic membrane can spontaneously tear and allow drainage of purulent material and/or blood. Less frequent manifestations include lethargy, vomiting, dizziness, and nystagmus.

The diagnosis of otitis media can be made in the presence of middle ear inflammation with effusion and acute illness. The combination of history or recent upper respiratory infection, presence of symptoms, and physical examination constitute the required assessment. The physical examination consists of visualization of the tympanic membrane for erythema, drainage, and mobility of tympanic membrane. Loss of mobility of the tympanic membrane, which can be assessed by pneumatic otoscopy or tympanometry, implies middle ear effusion. Hearing loss can be assessed by a tuning fork. Published microbiological studies of middle ear effusions are usually sufficient for institution of empiric therapy. When bacteriological studies are justified, aspiration and culture of the middle ear effusion is the gold standard. Cultures of swabs of ear drainage do not predict the infecting organism. Pathogen confirmation is justified if the patient is toxic, has a focal infection, remains toxic after 48 to 72 hr of therapy, is critically ill at the onset, has an immunological defect, or is a newborn (89).

Treatment

Antimicrobial therapy is the standard of care for acute otitis media. Although 70 to 80% of episodes of otitis media resolve spontaneously within 72 hr, it is not possible to predict which cases will progress and develop complications (95). Not only does antibiotic therapy diminish the incidence and sequelae of complications but also antimicrobials are superior to placebo in improving symptoms and healing of the tympanic membrane (96).

The superior agent and regimen for the treatment of otitis media has not been established, partially because of the lack of consistent outcome measures in therapeutic studies. While bacteriologic clearance has been suggested as a sensitive measure, other clinical outcome measures suggested are duration of symptoms, recovery period, suppurative complications, recurrence, and chronicity (97, 98). Traditionally the duration of therapy has been 10 to 14 days, however, shorter courses (3 to 7 days) have demonstrated effectiveness in patients with intact tympanic membranes (99–101). Rapid institution of therapy may play a beneficial role (102). In selecting the antimicrobial agent, the prevalent pathogens and local patterns of resistance are high-priority considerations. Empiric therapy should be effective against *S. pneumoniae* and *H. influenzae* (89). In communities with a high incidence of β-lactamase-producing *H. influenzae* or *M. catarrhalis*, therapy should consist of agents effective in the presence of β-lactamase. Refinement of therapy further requires the consideration of allergy history, adverse-effect profile, cost, patient acceptance (compliance), and previous response to therapy. Cost, a prominent point of comparison, is a complicated issue that requires incorporation of extra expenses associated with failure of the first-line therapy. The most frequent cause of therapeutic failure is noncompliance, so patient acceptability issues, such as affordability, flavor, and dosage schedule, play a critical role. Thorough counseling by the pharmacist, with the inclusion of a calibrated measuring device, increases compliance from 5 to 51% (103).

Amoxicillin and ampicillin continue to be the first-line agents for the treatment of acute otitis media, because they are active against the likely organisms and are inexpensive

(89, 104) (see Table 60.2 for dosage guidelines). Amoxicillin is preferred over ampicillin because of its every-8-hr regimen and lower incidence of diarrhea and rash. If the patient has a penicillin allergy, erythromycin ethylsuccinate–sulfisoxazole is an appropriate substitute. Erythromycin, besides having variable penetration into middle ear effusion, is not reliably efficacious against *H. influenzae* (98, 105).

In the presence of proven or suspected β-lactamase-producing organisms, the choice between amoxicillin-clavulanate, erythromycin ethylsuccinate–sulfisoxazole (EES-SXZ), cotrimoxazole (TMP-SMX), cefaclor, cefixime, or cefuroxime axetil should be based on their specific advantages and disadvantages. Amoxicillin-clavulanate, which is expensive in comparison with TMP-SMX and EES-SXZ, has the same incidence of rash as amoxicillin, but a much higher incidence of gastrointestinal adverse effects. Serious adverse effects are rare. Amoxicillin-clavulanate offers the benefit of three dosage times per day, but has an unpopular flavor and smell.

TMP-SMX, which requires only two doses daily, is the least expensive of the alternatives. Thirty percent of *S. pneumoniae* strains are resistant to TMP-SMX (106). TMP-SMX may cause rash (5% incidence) and diarrhea. While TMP-SMX-associated rash develops into a fatal case of Stevens-Johnson syndrome in 1 in 100,000 cases and is even more rare in the short courses of therapy used to treat otitis media, the development of a rash on TMP-SMX is an indication to stop the therapy (107). Clinically significant bone marrow depression rarely occurs, however monitoring for blood dyscrasias, especially in longer courses of therapy, is warranted. Patients with glucose-6-phosphate dehydrogenase deficiency are at risk for hemolysis (98).

EES-SXZ offers the advantage of adequate coverage of both β-lactamase-producing organisms and *S. pneumoniae* at a moderate cost. The sulfonamide component of EES-SXZ insures the same adverse effect profile as TMP-SMX, while the erythromycin component may induce hepatotoxicity. Rare case reports of erythromycin-associated hepatotoxicity involved adults receiving erythromycin administration for longer than 14 days (108).

Cefaclor has enjoyed popularity as a second-line agent for otitis media, while experience with cefuroxime axetil and cefixime is limited. All of these agents are expensive. Although the incidence of cross-sensitivity is low, these agents are contraindicated if there is a history of anaphylaxis to penicillin. Adverse effects are similar to those with amoxicillin, primarily gastrointestinal upset and rash. Cefaclor is one of the most palatable agents used for otitis media. Disadvantages of cefaclor include a 2% incidence of serum sickness syndrome and unreliable efficacy against *M. catarrhalis* (109, 110). Cefuroxime axetil provides excellent efficacy against common organisms. The only oral preparation is a bitter tablet. Nausea and vomiting are reported side effects, which are aggravated by the formulation. Cefixime, which is also available only as a bitter tablet, seems to have a much higher incidence (up to 30%) of diarrhea and loose stools than alternative agents (111). Because the response rate of *S. pneumoniae* to cefixime is 10% less than to control agents, cefixime is only indicated for otitis media caused by *H. influenzae* or *M. catarrhalis* (112). This precludes the use of cefixime as an empiric agent.

In the case of recurrent otitis media, tympanostomy tube placement or antibiotic prophylaxis are viable options to reduce the incidence of acute otitis media. The definition of "recurrent" is controversial, but it may be defined as 3 or more episodes of otitis media in 6 months or 4 episodes in 12 months. Chemoprophylaxis, a reasonable initial intervention, reduces the recurrence of acute otitis media 40 to 90%, although failures are also documented (113). As with therapeutic regimens, noncompliance is the most frequent cause of failure. On the first episode of acute otitis media while on chemoprophylaxis, the patient should receive a complete therapeutic course of an effective antibiotic and then return to the prophylactic regimen. Insertion of tympanostomy tubes should be considered on repeated failures of chemoprophylaxis. While long-term antibiotic administration may contribute to resistance and adverse effects, the risk of damage associated with recurrent or chronic otitis media or tympanostomy tube placement is also of consideration.

Determination of the optimal chemoprophylaxis, the agent, the dosage, and the duration, awaits further trials. Amoxicillin (10 to 20 mg/kg/24 hr in one or two doses) and sulfisoxazole (50 mg/kg/24 hr in one or two doses) have emerged as the prevalent recommendations, although TMP-SMX, sulfamethoxazole, ampicillin, and cefaclor are potential therapies (90, 113, 114).

Since the microbiology of chronic otitis media is varied, middle ear fluid should be obtained for culture and sensitivity. Empiric therapy should include agents efficacious against *P. aeruginosa* and *Staphylococcus* species. The suggested regimen of 7 days of an intravenous antipseudomonal β-lactum, such as ticarcillin or ceftazidime, with daily aural hygiene is 89% effective (115). Ciprofloxacin, an oral antipseudomonal fluoroquinolone, may be effective for chronic otitis media, but is not approved by the Food and Drug Administration for use in children because ciprofloxacin administration to dogs resulted in cartilage degeneration. In a microbiological study (*n* = 48) of chronic otitis media, 46% of the infections were aerobic, 44% were mixed aerobic and anaerobic, and 69% were due to β-lactamase-producing organisms (116). The role of anaerobic coverage in empiric therapy of chronic otitis media is undefined. Following successful therapy, the patient requires prophylactic therapy, i.e., antibiotics or surgery.

Frequent adjunctive therapies include antihistamine and decongestant combination products, decongestant sprays, and otologic preparations. Numerous studies of antihistamines and decongestants, systemically and topically, failed to prove benefit for either treatment or prophylaxis of otitis media (117, 118). Patients on these agents have demonstrated a higher incidence of adverse effects. Irritability or lethargy were especially prominent. Antihistamines may play a role, presently unestablished, if allergy is the underlying cause. For now, there is no support for administration of either of these agents. Frequently prescribed ear drops, including antibiotic and acetic acid agents, have demonstrated ototoxic properties in recognized animal models (119). The causative component, whether active ingredient or vehicle, has not been identified. The relationship of the ototoxic results to sensorineural hearing loss associated with otitis media is unknown. Academic work cannot at this time support the use of ototopical agents, based on safety.

Because arachidonic acid metabolites are important inflammatory mediators in the pathogenesis of otitis media, both steroids and nonsteroidal antiinflammatory agents are theoretical therapies (120). Nonsteroidals, which actually increase effusion, have been eliminated as beneficial (120, 121). The role of steroids remains debatable, due to conflicting results (122–124). There may be a place for steroids in the treatment of persistent middle ear effusion in children over 4 years of age, who are without hypertrophic adenoids (125).

Prevention

Preventative measures have thus far yielded modest benefits. Antibiotic prophylaxis and surgical interventions, as described above, address otitis media after it has become a problem. The elimination of smoking in the household and regular handwashing to minimize the spread of upper respiratory infections are reasonable avoidance techniques of factors associated with increased incidence of otitis media. Screening programs may identify those who would benefit from early intervention (90). Although surfactants have been hypothesized to play a role in the pathogenesis of middle ear disease, clinical application of surface-tension-lowering agents as prevention or therapy is premature (126, 127).

Since *S. pneumoniae* and *H. influenzae* are the most prevalent organisms in acute otitis media, the availability of vaccines against these organisms stimulated a lot of interest. The vast majority of *H. influenzae* otitis media is nontypable, which is not prevented by *H. influenza* type-b vaccine. Pneumococcal polysaccharide vaccine does contain the prevalent serotypes of *S. pneumoniae* pathogenic for otitis media. While some parameters demonstrated statistically significant differences between pneumococcal vaccine groups and control groups, the overall clinical outcome between groups was the same (128). Exploration of vaccines with improved immunogenicity for the young are underway (129).

PHARYNGITIS

Eleven percent of school-aged children visit their physician annually with the complaint of pharyngitis or "sore throat" (130). Pharyngitis, an acute, inflammatory process involving the pharynx, may result from environmental causes or viral or bacterial infection. The incidence of pharyngitis due to environmental causes varies with exposure to the causative agent, including cigarette smoke, air pollution, and lack of humidity. Pharyngitis due to viral or bacterial invasion is more common in the winter months.

Pathogenesis

In older children and adults, pharyngitis may occur as an isolated event. In younger children and infants, pharyngitis frequently is part of a much larger picture that may include otitis media, sinusitis, or other upper respiratory infections. Viruses, including rhinovirus (20%) and coronavirus (5%), are the most common causes of relatively benign and self-limiting pharyngitis (131). Herpes simplex virus pharyngitis (4%) and adenovirus pharyngitis (5%) are usually more severe. *Mycoplasma pneumoniae* (<1%) has not been an important cause of sore throat. The role of Chlamydia species is under scrutiny. *Streptococcus pyogenes* (15 to 30%), a group A β-hemolytic streptococcus (GABHS), remains the primary bacterial cause of pharyngitis. Group C streptococci are becoming of increasing concern, with some areas of the U.S. reporting up to a 20% prevalence. *Neisseria gonorrhoeae* (<1%) should not be overlooked as a possible causative organism in those practicing oral sex. The microbiologic agent of as many as 40% of cases is unknown. Fungal and severe viral pharyngitis occur frequently in the immunocompromised host.

Pharyngitis is associated with few complications, with GABHS pharyngitis being the noted exception. GABHS pharyngitis is associated with rheumatic fever, glomerulonephritis, and suppurative complications, including otitis media, sinusitis, bacteremia, mastoiditis, lateral sinus thrombosis, and pneumonia. While treatment decreases rheumatic fever and suppurative complications, it has no proven effect on glomerulonephritis. Recent reports of outbreaks of rheumatic fever underscores the continued importance of accurate diagnosis and treatment of GABHS pharyngitis (132). Rare causes of pharyngitis, including *Yersinia enterocolitica* and *Corynebacterium diphtheriae*, may be fatal. Diphtheria has been essentially eliminated by the widespread availability of effective immunization.

Clinical Characteristics and Diagnosis

Pharyngitis has a wide range of symptoms. The patient may complain of mild-to-moderate soreness, hoarseness, and irritation of the pharynx. Pharyngeal erythema, edema, and hyperemia may be accompanied by exudates, abscesses, and/or palatal petechiae. Cervical adenopathy and tenderness may also be present. Abdominal pain is, surprisingly, a frequent complaint of children.

The diagnostic goal is to differentiate between benign viral pharyngitis (which requires palliative care), and GABHS pharyngitis (which requires antibiotic therapy), and rarer viral or bacterial causes. History of recent infection, community epidemiology, infected contacts, or immunosuppression provides invaluable aid in diagnosis. GABHS pharyngitis occurs primarily in children 3 to 18 years of age, during the winter and spring months. Due to the varied and nonspecific clinical presentation of "strep throat," diagnosis requires bacteriologic confirmation. Although the gold standard for diagnosis of GABHS pharyngitis ("strep throat") has been blood agar culture, rapid antigen detection is now readily available for use in the physician's office (133). Current recommendations are to treat the positive rapid antigen result in a sick patient and plate a sample from the negative result on agar for confirmation (134). Other possible causative agents should be considered, and appropriate culture media used. While culturing requires 2 days, late institution of therapy for a positive *S. pyogenes* culture does not adversely affect prevention of rheumatic fever. Nonetheless, the patient's clinical improvement is slowed and communicability prolonged. Up to 50% of children with positive *S. pyogenes* cultures may be merely carriers and not infected. When the physician wants to treat pharyngitis of suspected viral etiology, empiric therapy must be instituted based on clinical presentation, since results of viral testing requires several days.

Treatment

Penicillin is the treatment of choice for GABHS pharyngitis. A course of therapy consists of one intramuscular injection of benzathine or benzathine plus procaine penicillin or 10 days of oral penicillin (131). While the effectiveness of the 10-day course of therapy to decrease rheumatic fever is well substantiated, the frequency of dosing is controversial. Many authorities recommend oral penicillin three or four times daily, but several studies suggest that a twice-daily regimen is equally effective (133). Erythromycin is a suitable substitute, when the patient is allergic to penicillin (Table 60.3).

Circumstances in which eradication of the GABHS-carrier state should be considered include families with inordinate anxiety about "strep throat" or "ping-pong" spread of GABHS pharyngitis, families with a history of rheumatic fever, outbreaks of GABHS pharyngitis in closed or semiclosed communities, or when tonsillectomy is being considered to eradicate chronic carriage of *S. pyogenes*. Addition of a short course of rifampin to the pen-

Table 60.3.
Treatment of Acute Streptococcal Pharyngitis[a]

Drug	Regimen
Penicillin V K	50 mg/kg/day q.i.d. × 10 days (Maximum 250 mg q.i.d.)
Benzathine penicillin	600,000 U i.m. (<9 years old) 900,000 U i.m. (9–12 years old) 1.2 million U i.m. (>12 years old)
Erythromycin	40 mg/kg/day b.i.d. or q.i.d. (Maximum 1 g/day)
Elimination of carrier state:	
Rifampin	20 mg/kg/day q.d. × 4 days (Maximum 600 mg/day)

[a] Adapted from Littler JE, Momany T: The Family Practice Handbook. Chicago: Year Book Medical Publishers, 1990, pp 516–517.

icillin regimen has been successful in eradicating GABHS carriage (134, 136, 137).

Influenza A pharyngitis is treated effectively with amantadine (131). Herpetic infection should be treated with acyclovir in immunosuppressed patients only.

Palliative care for pharyngitis of all types include rest, analgesics, topical anesthetics/antiseptics, demulcents, and liquids. While liberal use of over-the-counter analgesics may be required, aspirin should be avoided in children, due to the association with Reye's syndrome. Controversy surrounds the efficacy of anesthetic/antiseptic topical sprays and gargles. Common nonprescription anesthetics include benzocaine (5 to 20%), phenol or phenol-containing salts (0.5 to 1.5%), and benzyl alcohol (10%). Warm saline (1 teaspoonful salt/8 ounces warm tap water) gargles may be soothing. No antiseptic mouthwash has been recognized as beneficial by the American Dental Association's Council on Dental Therapeutics (138). Demulcents, agents that soothe irritated tissues, are available in liquids in lozenges. The active ingredients of demulcent products include compound tincture of benzoin, elm bark, or linseed oil. Sugarless candies may also be comforting, without increasing dental caries. Product selection depends on patient preference.

Prevention

Immunization has minimized diphtheria as a practical concern (131). Vaccine against *S. pyogenes* are still in the developmental stage. While yearly influenza A and B immunization can minimize further the few cases of pharyngitis caused by these viruses, amantadine can be taken prophylactically in the case of local epidemics of influenza A. Rimantadine, when released for use, can be used as prophylaxis against both influenza A and B. Tonsillectomy is no longer recommended routinely to pharyngitis-prone children. Strict isolation within the home, combined with good handwashing and hygiene of food utensils, may prevent spread within families.

LARYNGITIS

Laryngitis, an acute inflammatory process of the larynx, is commonly associated with viral syndromes. Incidence varies in relation to upper respiratory infections, which peak in midwinter. Characteristic presentation consists of hoarseness or aphonia (loss of voice), either painless or mildly painful. Eight-seven percent of patients report recent upper respiratory infection, and 13% admit voice abuse (139). In addition to a significant history, diagnosis can be confirmed by visual examination of an edematous and hyperemic larynx. Laryngitis lingering longer than 10 days requires laryngoscopic examination.

Out of the 90% of cases of viral origin, influenza virus (22 to 37%), rhinovirus (10 to 25%), and adenovirus (6 to 25%) are the most often implicated pathogens (139). *S. pyogenes* (10%) is the prominent bacterial cause of laryngitis, but a recent study demonstrated the presence of *M. catarrhalis* in 55% of 40 patients with hoarseness (141, 142). There are rare reports of tubercular, herpetic, syphilitic, or fungal causes of laryngitis.

Treatment for this benign, self-limiting complaint consists primarily of voice rest and inhalation of moist air. Antibiotics are recommended only for laryngitis of bacterial etiology.

SUPRAGLOTTITIS

Supraglottitis, previously known as epiglottitis, is an infection of the epiglottis, aryepiglottic folds, and arytenoids. Although the incidence of this infrequent malady is unknown, when it does occur, it is a medical emergency. Acute and rapidly progressive cellulitis of these structures results in partial to complete airway obstruction.

Pathogenesis

While supraglottitis can occur from infancy to adulthood, the peak incidence occurs in children from 2 to 7 years old, more often in males. There is no relation between frequency and season. *H. influenzae* type b (HITB) is cultured from the epiglottis in the overwhelming majority of pediatric patients and in 26% of adults (143). Mode of spread appears to be person-to-person (144). Concurrent HITB bacteremia is reported in up to 100% of children with supraglottitis (145). Other implicated organisms include *Streptococcus* species, *Staphylococcus* species, and *Haemophilus paraphrophilus*. The role of viral invasion in supraglottis has not been elucidated, but it may explain the large number of negative cultures.

Rare serious complications are primarily limited to noncardiogenic pulmonary congestion and effusion, although increased pulmonary vascular resistance may result in right-sided heart failure (146, 147). While metastatic spread of HITB is unusual, the potential for meningitis, septic arthritis, pericarditis, and endocarditis should not be overlooked. Cervical lymphadenopathy is common.

Clinical Characteristics and Diagnosis

Supraglottitis is an acute and rapidly progressive process. The child seeking medical care usually has a 6- to 12-hour history of fever and dysphagia. Symptoms process more slowly in adults. The classical presentation includes a drooling, very sick child sitting erect, flexed at the waist, chin forward and tongue protruding (148). Children will often prop themselves in this position with their two hands, completing a "tripod" configuration. This posture allows the greatest possible relief from the airway obstruction caused by the swollen epiglottis. Drooling results from the refusal to swallow because of the severe sore throat. Soft, muffled, hissing sounds may accompany tachypnea. Tachycardia and retractions may also be present. Inspiratory stridor and hoarseness are common, but aphonia and barking cough are rare.

Any child with febrile dysphagia should be considered to have supraglottitis until proven otherwise. Until supraglottitis is ruled out, caregivers must be prepared to provide an endotracheal airway and resuscitation at all times. While diagnosis is confirmed by direct visualization of the cherry red, swollen epiglottis, forced examination can quickly lead to complete obstruction of the airway. Unless the child can be induced to "show" the throat, further inspection should take place in the operating room with the necessary personnel to provide an artificial airway. A lateral neck radiograph can be useful to rule out supraglottis in a child who probably does not have the disease. The child must remain upright throughout. However, if the clinical presentation suggests supraglottitis, the child should be taken to the surgical suite immediately for inspection under anesthesia and subsequent prophylactic placement of an airway. Positive blood and epiglottis cultures, leukocytosis with a "left shift," and evidence of pneumonia on chest x-ray occur in 25% of cases of supraglottitis.

Treatment

Prophylactic endotracheal intubation is the emergent therapy of choice. Intubation reduces to nearly zero the morbidity and mortality (6 to 25%) associated with supraglottitis. Only after the airway is secured, should cultures of the epiglottitis and blood be obtained. Empiric intravenous antibiotic therapy aimed at β-lactamase-producing HITB should be initiated, while awaiting the results of the microbiological studies. Intravenous ampicillin 200 mg/kg/day plus chloramphenicol 75 to 100 mg/kg/day, divided into every 6 hr, has been the conventional therapy. Recently, intravenous cefotaxime 100 to 150 mg/kg/day in four doses or cefuroxime 100 to 200 mg/kg/day in three doses have been used for initial therapy (148). Once the microbiological results are obtained, therapy can be streamlined accordingly. Within 48 to 72 hr after the initiation of antibiotics, the patient is usually afebrile, alert, and ready for extubation. Antibiotics should be continued for 7 to 10 days, but may be changed to an oral dosage form. While fluids should be adequate to maintain hydration, there are no data to support overhydration. Vigorous hydration may, in fact, induce pulmonary edema, a potential complication of supraglottitis (149). Although the use of nebulized bronchodilators has not been studied in supraglottitis, they are not of any theoretic value and may delay efficacious therapy. Corticosteroids have no role in the treatment of supraglottitis, and if used, may prolong and complicate the infectious process (150). If the patient has any household or day-care contacts under 6 years old, the patient and each contact, including adults, should receive rifampin 20 mg/kg/day (maximum dose 600 mg) × 4 days (147). The prophylactic regimen should be completed prior to release from the hospital and may be given concurrently with the therapeutic regimen.

Prevention

Early vaccination with recently available HITB polysaccharide vaccine should provide protection against supraglottitis. Contacts can be further protected by elimination of *H. influenzae* colonization via rifampin prophylaxis. An episode of HITB supraglottitis appears to provide adequate immunity against a recurrence, as second episodes are rare.

ACUTE LARYNGOTRACHEOBRONCHITIS

Acute laryngotracheobronchitis (croup) is a viral process of the upper and lower respiratory tract, resulting in inflammation in the subglottic area. Subglottic swelling produces dyspnea and a characteristic, inspiratory cough. Croup is usually benign and self-limiting.

Pathogenesis

Croup occurs most commonly in male children between the ages of 3 months and 3 years, with the peak incidence of 15% during the second year of life (151). Older children and adults, if affected with disorder, have the clinical picture associated with laryngitis. Seasonal variations reflect the prevalence of the different causative viruses. At all ages, parainfluenza viruses are the major causative agents. Parainfluenza type 1 (6 to 39%), the most common cause, tends to cause outbreaks of croup every other year in the fall. Parainfluenza type 3 (2 to 14%), the second most frequently associated agent, peaks in late spring and sum-

mer, while parainfluenza type 2 (2 to 7%) produces small outbreaks in the fall and early winter. Although influenza A croup (1 to 10%) occurs less frequently than parainfluenza-induced croup, it may produce a more severe illness in a broader age range of patients (152, 153). Influenza A and respiratory syncytial virus (1 to 11.4%) appear in the winter to spring months. Rhinoviruses, adenoviruses, enteroviruses and *Mycoplasma pneumoniae* contribute to a sporadic number of cases throughout the year. Secondary bacterial infection may occur as a result of virus-induced croup.

Complications are rare. Only 3% of patients with croup will require intubation (154). If a patient with mild disease develops an abrupt onset of high fever and toxicity, secondary bacterial tracheitis with *S. aureus* is the probable cause and will require antibiotic therapy (135).

Clinical Characteristics and Diagnosis

Croup often appears one to several days after an acute upper respiratory tract infection. During the prodrome, the child may experience rhinorrhea, sore throat, mild cough, and fever. The child exhibits increasing anxiety and hoarseness with a deepening, nonproductive cough (151). The characteristic inspiratory stridor, which has been described as "high-pitched," "seal's bark," and "musical," results from inflammatory obstruction and collapse of the airway. Stridor may be accompanied by suprasternal and supraclavicular retractions. Severely affected children may reveal crackles, wheezing, and expiratory stridor on auscultation, as well as cyanosis on physical examination. Hypoxemia occurs in 80% of all cases. Tachypnea ensues to compensate for inadequate tidal volumes. A distinguishing characteristic of croup is its fluctuating course. Children often improve in the morning, only to worsen later at night. This is sometimes termed "spasmodic croup," and may be aggravated by allergic or hyperactive airways (154). The usual duration of illness is 3 to 4 days, although the cough may persist longer. Rarely will croup be severe enough to cause an exhausted child to decline into respiratory failure.

Diagnosis of croup can be made correctly in 98% of cases, based on the clinical presentation alone (155). An anterior-posterior neck radiograph may demonstrate the nonspecific "hourglass" or "steeple" sign. The reliability and usefulness of the roentgenographic picture in the acute situation is controversial. Laboratory analysis is unremarkable. Leukocytosis, with neutrophils or lymphocytes predominating, may or may not be present. Blood gas analysis reveals hypoxemia and hypocarbia, changing to hypoxemia and normocarbia or hypercarbia with progression of respiratory failure. The differential diagnosis includes supraglottitis, foreign body aspiration, and retropharyngeal abscesses. Diphtheria has been virtually eliminated by vaccination programs.

Treatment

Antibiotic therapy is not indicated, since croup has a viral etiology. Otherwise, treatment varies with the severity of the disease. Due to the fluctuating course, it is difficult to decide when to hospitalize for observation and when to treat in the ambulatory setting. In croup's mildest forms, treatment can be delivered by a parent in the ambulatory setting. A time-honored treatment consists of the child sitting on the parent's lap, while steaming up the bathroom. Since crying and lack of rest aggravate croup, clinical improvement may result from the comfort and reassurance provided by this experience (156). The parent may elect to use a cool mist or steam humidifier. The risk of burning is eliminated with the cool mist humidifier, making it the preferred delivery system. The delivery of moist air and the hum of the machine may be soothing to the child. No drugs nor petroleum products should be added. The machine should be cleaned and fresh water added daily.

The child with stridor at rest or respiratory distress should be hospitalized. Once hospitalized, care should consist of support and observation for deterioration. Humidified air, often provided by a mist tent, is considered routine therapy. While no data show any effect of humid air on subglottic edema, humidified air moistens secretions, facilitating expectoration, and soothes inflamed laryngeal mucosa, increasing comfort (157, 158). If it is distressing to the child to be separated from parents and put into the mist tent, the mist tent should be eliminated from therapy (156). There are no controlled data on which to decide about the use of oxygen. Since the maximum attainable oxygen in a mist tent is approximately 40%, it is unlikely to be detrimental and may be of some theoretical advantage to a hypoxemic child.

Nebulized racemic epinephrine decreases airway obstruction from 10 to 30 min after administration. This effect declines to zero by 2 hr and may result in rebound constriction in some cases (155). Intermittent positive-pressure breathing, as compared with nebulization, did not provide any advantages, but is did provide more risks of therapy. The result of racemic epinephrine therapy included an improvement in stridor and retractions, but no change in arterial pO_2 (151). Therefore, while transient amelioration of clinical signs may deter fatigue, continued observation is necessary, and the degree of hypoxemia is unchanged.

Corticosteroid therapy remains controversial, in part because of studies that were flawed either in diagnostic criteria, steroid dosage, and/or outcome measures. Four of six studies using more than 0.3 mg/kg of dexamethasone phosphate or its equivalent, given in one intramuscular injection, showed a significant decrease in the length and severity of respiratory symptoms, and three studies demonstrated shorter hospital stays (159–164). The consequence of repeated doses of corticosteroids has not been examined. Since the risk of an adverse effect with a short course of corticosteroids is small and no study of corticosteroid use in croup has reported any adverse effects, it seems reasonable to recommend dexamethasone phosphate 0.6 mg/kg intramuscular injection on admission to the hospital with viral croup. This is consistent with a meta-analysis of randomized trials assessing corticosteroid use in viral croup (164).

Prevention

Prevention of croup is limited to avoidance of persons infected with the associated viruses. Conscientious hygienic practices, including handwashing, not drinking from the same cup, and washing shared toys, may decrease transmission. During influenza A outbreaks, amantadine administration may be considered.

CONCLUSION

Treatment of upper respiratory tract infections is a common, yet therapeutically demanding task. The interplay between the indigenous flora and the host's normal defense mechanisms must be appreciated to achieve successful patient outcomes. The large numbers of new antimicrobial and antiviral agents, coupled with changing bacterial susceptibility patterns, have created a difficult environment for clinician seeking to promote rational drug use. The pharmacotherapist involved in the management of patients with upper respiratory tract infections must stay informed about bacterial issues (e.g., resistance, flora) and therapeutic management issues (e.g., pharmacokinetics/dynamics, toxicities, cost effectiveness) to be of benefit to the patient and healthcare team.

REFERENCES

1. Anderson LJ, Patriarca PA, Hierholzer JC, et al.: Viral respiratory illnesses. Med Clin North Am 67:1009–1030, 1983.
2. Parrott RH, Rhinoviral infections. In Behrman RE, Vaughen VC (eds): Nelson Textbook of Pediatrics, ed. 12. Philadelphia, WB Saunders, 1983, pp 783–784.
3. Longini IM, Monto AS, Koopman JS: Statistical procedures for estimating the community probability of illnesses in family studies: rhinovirus and influenza. Int J Epidemiol 13:99–106, 1984.
4. National Center for Health Statistics: Current estimates from the National Health Interview Survey, United States, 1985. Vital and Health Statistics, 1986, Series 10, no. 160. Washington, D.C.: Public Health Service.
5. Anonymous: Cough remedies: Which ones work best? Consumer Reports Feb:58–61, 1983.
6. Huebner RJ, Rowe WP, Ward TG, et al.: Adenoidal-pharyngeal-conjunctive agents: a newly recognized group of common viruses of the respiratory system. N Engl J Med 251:1077–1086, 1954.
7. Gwaltney JM: Virology and immunology of the common cold. Rhinology 23:265–271, 1985.

8. Aronson MD, Weiss ST, Ben RL, et al.: Association between cigarette smoking and acute respiratory tract illness in young adults. JAMA 248:181–183, 1982.

9. Fox JP, Cooney MK, Hall CE: The Seattle virus watch: V. epidemiologic observations of rhinovirus infections, 1965–1969 in familes with young children. Am J Epidemiol 101:122–143, 1975.

10. Gwaltney JM Jr, Hendley JO, Simon G, et al.: Rhinovirus infections in an industrial population. I. The occurrence of illness. N Engl J Med 275:1261, 1966.

11. Douglas RG, Lindgren KM, Couch RB: Exposure to cold environment and rhinovirus common cold: failure to demonstrate effect. N Engl J Med 279:742–747, 1968.

12. Jennings LC, Dick EC: Transmission and control of rhinovirus colds. Eur J Epidemiol 3(4):327–335, 1987.

13. Gwaltney JM, Hendley JO: Rhinovirus transmission: one if by air, two if by hand. Am J Epidemiol 107:357–361, 1978.

14. Gwaltney JM Jr, The common cold. In Mandell GL, Douglas RG, Bennet JE (eds): Principles and Practices of Infectious Diseases. New York, John Wiley & Sons, 1990, pp 489–493.

15. Anonymous. Handbook of Nonprescription Drugs, ed. 8. Washington, D.C.: American Pharmaceutical Association and the National Professional Society of Pharmacists, 1986, ch. 1, 9, 23.

16. Eggleston PA, Hendley JO, Gwaltney JM Jr: Mediators of immediate hypersensitivity in nasal secretions during natural colds and rhinovirus infection. Acta Otolaryngol 413(suppl):25–35, 1984.

17. Naclerio RM, Proud D, Lichtenstein LM, et al.: Kinins are generated during experimental rhinovirus colds. J Infect Dis 157:133–142, 1988.

18. Smith TF, Remigio LK: Histamine in nasal secretions and serum may be elevated during viral respiratory tract infections. Int Arch Allergy Appl Immunol 67:380–383, 1982.

19. Welliver RC, Wong DT, Middleton E Jr., et al.: Role of parainfluenza virus–specific IgE in pathogenesis of croup and wheezing subsequent to infection. Pediatrics 101:889–896, 1982.

20. Howard JC Jr., Kantner TR, Lilienfield LS, et al.: Effectiveness of antihistamines in symptomatic management of the common cold. JAMA 242:2414–2417, 1979.

21. Randall JE, Hendley JO: A decongestant-antihistamine mixture in the prevention of otitis media in children with colds. Pediatrics 63:483–485, 1979.

22. Kjellman NIM, Harder H, Lindwall L, et al.: Longterm treatment with brompheniramine and phenylpropanolamine in recurrent otitis media—a double-blind study. J Otolaryngol 7:257–261, 1978.

23. McTavish D, Goa KL, Ferrill M: Terfenadine. An updated review of its pharmacological properties and therapeutic efficacy. Drugs 39(4):552–574, 1990.

24. Clissold SP, Sorkin EM, Goa KL: Loratadine. A preliminary review of its pharmacodynamic properties and therapeutic efficacy. Drugs 37(1):42–57, 1989.

25. Empey DW, Medder KT: Nasal decongestants. Drugs 21:438–443, 1981.

26. Lea P: A double-blind controlled evaluation of the nasal decongestant effect of Day Nurse in the common cold. J Int Med Res 12:124–127, 1984.

27. Dressler WE, Myers T, Rankell AS, et al.: A system of rhinomanometry and in the clinical evaluation of nasal decongestants. Ann Otol Rhinol Laryngol 86:310–317, 1977.

28. Roth RP, Cantekin EI, Welch RM, et al.: Nasal decongestant activity of pseudoephedrine. Ann Otol Rhinol Laryngol 86:235–241, 1977.

29. Sperber SJ, Swaltney JM Jr., Sorrentino JV, Hayden FG: Pseudoephedrine alone or combined with ibuprofen as treatment for experimental rhinovirus colds. Program and Abstracts of the Twenty-Seventh Interscience Conference on Antimicrobial Agents and Chemotherapy (ICAAC) 27:184, 1987. Abstract #501.

30. Bue CE, Cooper J, Empey DW, et al.: Effects of pseudoephedrine and triprolidine, alone and in combination, on symptoms of the common cold. Br Med J 281:189–190, 1980.

31. Sakethoo K, Januszkiewicz A, Sackner MA: Effects of drinking hot water and chicken soup on nasal mucus velocity and nasal airflow resistance. Chest 74:408, 1978.

32. Pentel P: Toxicity of over-the-counter stimulants. JAMA 252:1898–1903, 1984.

33. Anonymous: Phenylpropanolamine over-the-counter. Lancet (editorial) 1:839, 1982.

34. Gaffey MJ, Haden FG, Boyd JC, et al.: Ipratropium bromide treatment of experimental rhinovirus infection. Antimicrob Agents Chemother 32(11):1644–1647, 1988.

35. Dolovich J, Kennedy L, Vickerson F, et al.: Control of the hypersecretion of vasomotor rhinitis by topical ipratropium bromide. J Allergy Clin Immunol 3(1):274–278, 1987.

36. Stanley ED, Jackson GG, Panusarn C, et al.: Increased virus shedding with aspirin treatment of rhinovirus infections. Int Arch Allergy Appl Immunol 67:380–383, 1982.

37. Mogabgab WJ, Pollock B: Re: increased virus shedding with aspirin treatment of rhinovirus infection. JAMA 235:801, 1976.

38. Gerrity TR, Cotromanes E, Garrard CS, et al.: The effect of aspirin on lung mucociliary clearance. N Engl J Med 308:139–141, 1983.

39. Curatolo PW, Robertson D. The health consequences of caffeine. Ann Intern Med 98(1):641–653, 1983.

40. Dobmeyer DJ, Stine RA, Leier CV, et al.: The arrhythmogenic effects of caffeine in human beings. N Engl J Med 308:814–816, 1983.

41. Anonymous: AMA Drug Evaluations, ed. 6. Philadelphia: American Medical Association and WB Saunders, 1986, Ch 21, 58.

42. Scott GM, Phillpotts RJ, Wallace J, et al.: Prevention of rhinovirus colds by human interferon α-2 from Escherichia coli. Lancet 2:186–189, 1982.

43. Hayden FG, Gwaltney JM: Intranasal interferon α-2 for prevention of rhinovirus infection and illness. J Infect Dis 148:543–550, 1983.

44. Douglas RM, Moore BW, Miles HB, et al.: Prophylactic efficacy of intranasal α-interferon against rhinovirus infections in the family setting. N Engl J Med 314:65–70, 1986.

45. Hayden FG, Albrecht JK, Kaiser DL, et al.: Prevention of natural colds by contact prophylaxis with intranasal α-interferon. N Engl J Med 314:71–75, 1986.

46. Hayden FG, Gwaltney JM Jr: Intranasal interferon α-2 treatment of experimental rhinovirus colds. J Infect Dis 150:174–180, 1984.

47. Hayden FG, Kaiser DL, Albrecht JK: Intranasal recombinant α-2b interferon treatment of naturally occurring common colds. Antimicrob Agents Chemother 32:224–230, 1988.

48. Phillpotts RJ, Tyrrell DAJ: Rhinovirus colds. Br Med Bull 41:386–390, 1985.

49. Korant BD, Kauer JC, Butterworth BE: Zinc ions inhibit replication of rhinoviruses. Nature (London) 248:588–590, 1974.

50. Farr BM, Conner EM, Betts RF, et al.: Two randomized controlled trials of zinc gluconate lozenge therapy of experimentally induced rhinovirus colds. Antimicrob Agents Chemother 31:1183–1187, 1987.

51. Douglas RM, Miles HB, Moore BW: Failure of effervescent zinc acetate lozenges to alter the course of upper respiratory tract infections in Australian adults. Antimicrob Agents Chemother 31:1263–1265, 1987.

52. Farr BM, Gwaltney JM Jr: The problems of taste in placebo matching: an evaluation of zinc gluconate for the common cold. J Chronic Dis 40:875–879, 1987.

53. Al-Nakib W, Higgins PG, Barrow I, et al.: Intranasal chalcone Ro 09-0410, as prophylaxis against rhinovirus infection in human volunteers. J Antimicrob Chemother 20:887–892, 1987.

54. Phillpotts RJ, Wallace J, Tyrrell DAJ, et al.: Failure of oral 4',6-dichlorofavan to protect against rhinovirus infection in man. Arch Virol 75:115–121, 1983.

55. Al-Nakib W, Tyrrell DAJ: A "new" generation of more potent synthetic antirhinovirus compounds: comparison of their MICs and their synergistic interactions. Antiviral Res 8:179–188, 1987.

56. Al-Nakib W, Higgins PG, Tyrrell DAJ, et al.: Intranasal R61837 decrease of nasal symptoms and mucus weights in experimental rhinovirus infection. Abstracts of the 7th International Congress of Virology, 1987. Abstract no. 32.3.

57. Hayden FG, Gwaltney JM Jr: Prophylactic activity of intranasal enviroxime against experimentally induced rhinovirus type 39 infection. Antimicrob Agents Chemother 21:892–897, 1982.

58. Levandowski RA, Pachucki CT, Rubenis M, et al.: Topical enviroxime against rhinovirus infection. Antimicrob Agents Chemother 22:1004–1007, 1982.

59. Miller FD, Monto AS, DeLong DC, et al.: Controlled trial of enviroxime against natural rhinovirus infections in a community. Antimicrob Agents Chemother 27:102–106, 1985.

60. Phillpotts RJ, DeLong DC, Wallace J, et al.: The activity of enviroxime against rhinovirus infection in man. Lancet i:1342–1344, 1982.

61. Swallow DL, Kampfner GL: The laboratory selection of antiviral agents. Br Med Bull 42:322–332, 1985.

62. Pauling L: Vitamin C, the Common Cold and the Flu. San Francisco: WH Freeman, 1976, ch 14.

63. Pitt HA, Costrini AM: Vitamin C prophylaxis in marine recruits. JAMA 241:908–911, 1979.

64. Dykes MH, Meier P: Ascorbic acid and the common cold: evaluation of its efficacy and toxicity. JAMA 231:1073–1079, 1975.

65. Bittle JL, Houghten RA, Alexander H, et al.: Protection against foot-in-mouth disease by immunization with a chemically synthesized peptide predicted from the viral nucleotide sequence. Nature(London) 298:30–33, 1981.

66. Tomassini JE, Colonno RJ: Isolation of a receptor protein involved in attachment of human rhinoviruses. J Virol 58:290–295, 1986.

67. Bluestone DC: Preface. Pediatr Intect Dis S49:4, 1985.

68. Pennington JE: Respiratory Infections: Diagnosis and Management. New York: Raven Press, 1983, pp 79–111.

69. Gwaltney JM Jr, Sinusitis. In Mandell GL, Douglas RG, Bennett JE (eds): Principles and Practice of Infectious Diseases. New York, John Wiley & Sons, 1990, pp 510–514.

70. Anonymous: Acute sinusitis and its management. Drug Ther Bull 26(13):49–50, 1988.

71. Cuyler JP, Monaghan AL: Cystic fibrosis and sinusitis. J Otolaryngol 18(4):173–175, 1989.

72. Daley CL, Sande M: The runny nose, infection of the paranasal sinuses. Infect Dis Clin North Am 2(1):131–147, 1988.

73. Kern EB: Suppurative (bacterial) sinusitis. Postgrad Med 81(4):194–210, 1987.

74. Caplan ES, Hoyt NJ: Nosocomial sinusitis. JAMA 247:639, 1982.

75. Hamory BH, Sande MA, Sydnor A Jr, et al.: Etiology and antimicrobial therapy of acute maxillary sinusitis. J Infect Dis 139:197, 1979.

76. Axelsson A, Broson JE: The correlation and maxillary sinus in acute maxillary sinusitis. Laryngoscope 83:2003, 1973.

77. Wald ER, Milmoe GJ, Bowen AD, et al.: Acute maxillary sinusitis in children. N Engl J Med 304:749, 1981.

78. Sogg A: Long term results of ethmoid surgery. Ann Otol Rhinol Laryngol 98:699–701, 1989.

79. Simon H, Infections of the upper respiratory tract. In Rubenstein E, Federmann DD, (eds): Sci Am. New York, 1985, vol 7(19), pp 1–4.

80. Humphrey MA, Simpson GP, Grindlinger GA: Clinical characteristics of nosocomial sinusitis. Ann Otol Rhinol Laryngol 96:687–690, 1987.

81. Shapiro ED, Milmoe GJ, Wald ER, et al.: Bacteriology of the maxillary sinuses in patients with cystic fibrosis. J Infect Dis 146:589, 1982.

82. Parnes LS, Brown DH, Garcia B: Mycotic sinusitis: a management protocol. J Otolaryngol 18(4):176–180, 1989.

83. Gray WC, Blanchard CL: Sinusitis and its complications. Practical Therapeutics 35(3):232–243, 1987.

84. Evans FO, Sydnor JB, Moore WEC, et al.: Sinusitis of maxillary antrum. N Engl J Med 293:735, 1975.

85. Kovatch AL, Wald ER, Ledesma-Medina J, et al.: Maxillary sinus radiographs in children with non-respiratory complaints. Pediatrics 73:306, 1984.

86. Malow JB, Creticos CM: Nonsurgical treatment of sinusitis. Otol Clin North Am 22(4):809–819, 1989.

87. Benitz WE, Tatro DS: The Pediatric Handbook, ed. 2. Chicago: Year Book Medical Publishers, 1988, pp 503–608.

88. Blueston CD, Klein JO: Otitis Media in Infants and Children. Philadelphia: WB Saunders, 1988, pp 121–247.

89. Klein JO, Otitis externa, otitis media, mastoiditis. In Mandell GL, Douglas RG, Bennett JE (eds): Principles and Practice of Infectious Diseases. New York, John Wiley & Sons, 1990, pp 505–509.

90. Kemp ED: Otitis media. Disorders of the ears, nose, and throat. Prim Care 17(2):267–287, 1990.

91. Eichenwald H: Developments in diagnosing and treating otitis media. Am Fam Physician 31(3):155–164, 1985.

92. Giebink G, Canafax D: Controversies in the management of acute otitis media. Adv Pediatr Infect Dis 3:47–64, 1988.

93. Kamitsuka M, Feklman D, Richardson M: Facial paralysis associated with otitis media. Pediatr Infect Dis 4:682–684, 1985.

94. Paradise JL: Otitis media during early life: how hazardous to development? A critical review of the evidence. Pediatrics 68:869–873, 1981.

95. Wright PF: Indication and duration of antimicrobial agents for acute otitis media. Pediatr Ann 13:377–379, 1984.

96. Lorentzen P, Haugsten P: Treatment of acute suppurative otitis media. J Laryngol Otol 91:331–340, 1977.

97. Carlin SA, Marchant CD, Shurin PA, et al.: Host factors and early therapeutic response in acute otitis media. J Pediatr 118:178–183, 1991.

98. McCracken GH: Selection of antimicrobial agents for treatment of acute otitis media with effusion. Pediatr Infect Dis J 6:985–988, 1987.

99. Hendrickse WA, Kusmiesz H, Shelton S, et al.: Five vs ten days of therapy for acute otitis media. Pediatr Infect Dis J 7:14–23, 1988.

100. Chaput de Saintonge DM, Levine DF, Templae-Savage I, et al.: Trial of three-day and ten-day courses of amoxycillin in otitis media. Br Med J 284:1078–1081, 1982.

101. Meistrup-Larsen KI, Sorensen H, Johnson HJ, et al.: Two versus 7 days penicillin treatment for acute otitis media. Acta Otolaryngol 96:99–104, 1983.

102. Harder H, Ohman L, Strand E: Early or late start of treatment in acute otitis media, a comparative study. Acta Otolaryngol 449(Suppl):41–42, 1988.

103. Matter ME, Markello J, Yaffe SH: Pharmaceutic factors affecting pediatric compliance. Pediatrics 55:101–108, 1975.

104. Klein JO, Bluestone CD: Acute Otitis Media. Pediatr Infect Dis 1(1):66–73, 1982.

105. McLinn SE, Nelson JD, Haltalin KC: Antimicrobial susceptibility of Haemophilus influenzae. Pediatrics 45:827, 1970.

106. Henderson FW, Gilligan PH, Wait K, et al.: Nasopharyngeal carriage of antibiotic-resistant pneumococci by children in group day care. J Infect Dis 157:256–263, 1988.

107. Giebink G, Canafax D: Controversies in the management of acute otitis media. Adv Pediatr Infect Dis 3:47–64, 1988.

108. Eichwald HF: Adverse reactions to erythromycin. Pediatr Infect Dis 5:147–150, 1986.

109. Levine LR: Quantitative comparison of adverse reactions to cefaclor vs. amoxicillin in surveillance study. Pediatr Infect Dis 4:358–361, 1985.

110. Van Hare GF, Shurin PA: The increasing importance of *Branhamella catarrhalis* in respiratory infections. Pediatr Infect Dis J 6:92–94, 1987.

111. Tally FP, Desjardins RE, McCarthy EF, et al.: Safety profile of cefixime. Pediatr Infect Dis J 6:976–980, 1987.

112. Lederle Laboratories. Suprax package insert. Pearl River, NY. Apr. 1989.

113. Marchant CD, Collison LM: Serous and recurrent otitis media. Pharmacological or surgical management? Drugs 34:695–701, 1987.

114. McCracken GH: Management of acute otitis media with effusion. Pediatr Infect Dis J 7(6):442–445, 1988.

115. Nelson JD: Chronic suppurative otitis media. Pediatr Infect Dis J 7:446–448, 1988.

116. Brook I: Prevalence of β-lactamase-producing bacteria in chronic suppurative otitis media. Am J Dis Child 139:280–283, 1985.

117. Mandell EM, Rockette HE, Bluestone CD, et al.: Efficacy of amoxicillin with and without decongestant-antihistamine for otitis media with effusion in children. N Engl J Med 316:432–437, 1987.

118. Jenson JH, Niels L, Bonding P: Topical application of decongestant in dysfunction of the eustachian tube: a randomized, double-blind, placebo-controlled trial. Clin Otolaryngol 15:197–201, 1990.

119. Morizono T: Toxicity of ototopical drugs: animal modeling. Ann Otol Rhinol Laryngol 99:42–45, 1990.

120. Jung TT: Prostaglandins, leukotrienes, and other arachidonic acid metabolites in the pathogenesis of otitis media. Laryngoscope 98:980–993, 1988.

121. Abramovich S, O'Grady J, Fuller A, et al.: Naproxen in otitis media with effusion. J Laryngol Otol 100:263–266, 1986.

122. Macknin M, Jones PK: Oral dexamethasone for treatment of persistent middle ear effusion. Pediatrics 75(2):329–335, 1985.

123. Lambert PR: Oral steroid therapy for chronic middle ear perfusion: a double-blind crossover study. Otolaryngol Head Neck Surg 95:193–199, 1986.

124. Lildholdt T, Kortholm B: Beclomethasone nasal spray in the treatment of middle-ear effusion—a double-blind study. Int J Pediatr Otorhinolaryngol 4:133–137, 1982.

125. Podoshin L, Fradis M, Ben-David Y, Faraggi D: The efficacy of oral steroids in the treatment of persistent otitis media with effusion. Arch Otolaryngol Head Neck Surg 116:1404–1406, 1990.

126. Passali D, Zavattini G: Multicenter study on the treatment of secretory otitis media with ambroxol. Importance of a surface-tension-lowering substance. Respiration 51(suppl 1):52–59, 1987.

127. Grace A, Kwok P, Hawke M: Surfactant in middle ear effusions. Otolaryngol Head Neck Surg 96:336–340, 1987.

128. Makela PH, Leinonen M, Pukander J, Karma P: A study of the pneumococcal vaccine in prevention of clinically acute attacks of recurrent otitis media. Rev Infect Dis 3(suppl):S124–S132, 1981.

129. Anderson P, Betts R: Human adult immunogenicity of protein-coupled pneumococcal capsular antigens of serotypes prevalent in otitis media. Pediatr Infect Dis J 8:550–553, 1989.

130. National Center for Health Statistics: The National Ambulatory Health Care Survey, U.S. 1979 Summary. Viral and Health Statistics. U.S. Government Printing Office. 13(66), 1982.

131. Gwaltney JM, Pharyngitis. In Mandell GL, Douglas RG, Bennett JE (eds): Principles and Practice of Infectious Diseases. New York, John Wiley & Sons, 1990, pp 493–498.

132. Bisno AL, Schulna ST, Dajani AS: The rise and fall (and rise?) of rheumatic fever. JAMA 259:728–729, 1988.

133. Gerber MA, Markowitz M: Management of streptococcal pharyngitis reconsidered. Pediatr Infect Dis J 4(5):518–526, 1985.

134. Littler JE, Momany T: The Family Practice Handbook. Chicago: Year Book Medical Publishers, 1990, pp 516–517.

135. Loos GD: Pharyngitis, croup, and epiglottitis. Prim Care 17(2):335–345, 1990.

136. Chaudhary S, Bilinsky SA, Hennessy JL: Penicillin V and rifampin for the treatment of group A streptococcal pharyngitis. A randomized trial of 10 days penicillin vs. 10 days penicillin with rifampin during the final 4 days of therapy. J Pediatr 106:481–486, 1985.

137. Tanz RR, Shulman ST, Barthel MJ, et al.: Penicillin plus rifampin eradicates pharyngeal carriage of group A streptococci. J Pediatr 106:876–880, 1985.

138. Anon: Accepted Dental Therapeutics, ed. 40. Chicago: American Dental Association, 1984, sect II.

139. Schalen L, Christensen P, Eliasson I, et al.: Inefficacy of penicillin V in acute laryngitis in adults. Evaluation from results of double-blind study. Ann Otol Laryngol 94:14, 1985.

140. Gwaltney JM Jr, Acute laryngitis. In Mandell GL, Douglas RG, Bennett JE (eds): Principles and Practice of Infectious Diseases. New York, John Wiley & Sons, 1990, pp 499.

141. Gwaltney JM Jr: Rhinoviruses. In Evans AS (ed): Viral Infections of Humans: Epidemiology and Control. New York, Plenum, 1982, pp 507.

142. Schalen L, Christensen P, Kamme C, et al.: High isolation rate of *Branhamella catarrhalis* from the nasopharynx in adults with acute laryngitis. Scand J Infect Dis 12:277–280, 1980.

143. Mustoe T, Strome M: Adult epiglottitis. Am J Otolaryngol 4:393–399, 1983.

144. Ginsburg C: Epiglottitis, meningitis, and arthritis due to *Haemophilus influenza* type b presenting almost simultaneously in sibling. J Pediatr 87:492, 1975.

145. Sendi K, Crysdale WS: Acute epiglottitis: Decade of change—a 10-year experience with 242 children. J Otolaryngol 16:196–202, 1987.

146. Rivera M, Hadlock FP, O'Meara ME: Pulmonary edema secondary to acute epiglottitis. Am J Roentgenol 132:991, 1979.

147. Buda AJ, Pinsky MR, Ingels NB, et al.: Effects of intrathoracic pressure on left ventricular performance. N Engl J Med 301:453, 1979.

148. Burns JE, Hendley JO: Epiglottitis. In Mandell GL, Douglas RG, Bennett JE (eds): Principles and Practice of Infectious Diseases. New York, John Wiley & Sons, 1990, pp 514–516, 1990.

149. Galvis AG, Stool SE, Bluestone CD: Pulmonary edema following relief of acute upper airway obstruction. Ann Otol Rhinol Laryngol 89:124–128, 1980.

150. Deeb ZE: Approach to supraglottitis. Emerg Med Clin North Am 5(2):353–358, 1987.

151. Hall CB: Acute laryngotracheobronchitis (croup). In Mandell GL, Douglas RG, Bennett JE (eds): Principles and Practices of Infectious Diseases. New York, John Wiley & Sons, 1990, pp 499–505.

152. Kim HW, Brandt CD, Chanock RM, et al.: Influenza A and B virus infection in infants and young children during the years 1957–1976. Am J Epidemiol 109:464–479, 1979.

153. Denny FW, Murphy TF, Clyde WA Jr, et al.: Croup: An 11 year study in a pediatric practice. Pediatrics 71:871–876, 1983.

154. Clark WD, Bailey BS, Clegg TS: Epiglottitis and laryngotracheobronchitis. Am Fam Physician 28:189–194, 1983.

155. Skolnik NS: Treatment of Croup. A critical review. Am J Dis Child 143:1045–1049, 1989.

156. Henry R: Moist air in the treatment of laryngotracheitis. Arch Dis Child 58:577, 1983.

157. Lenney W, Milner AD: Treatment of acute viral croup. Arch Dis Child 53:704–706, 1978.

158. Bourchier D, Fergusson DM: Humidification in viral croup: a controlled trial. Aust Paediatr J 20:289–291, 1984.

159. James JA: Dexamethasone in croup. Am J Dis Child 117:511–516, 1969.

160. Kuusela AL, Vesidari T: A randomized double-blind, placebo-controlled trial of dexamethasone and racemic epinephrine in the treatment of croup. Acta Pediatr Scand 77:99–104, 1988.

161. Koren G, Frand M, Barzilay Z, MacLeod SM: Corticosteroid treatment of laryngotracheitis vs. spasmodic croup in children. Am J Dis Child 137:941–944, 1983.

162. Leipzig B, Oski FA, Cummings CW, et al.: A perspective randomized study to determine the efficacy of steroids in treatment of croup. J Pediatr 94:194–196, 1979.

163. Skowron PN, Turner JAP, NcNaughton GA: The use of corticosteroid (dexamethasone) in the treatment of acute laryngotracheitis. Can Med Assoc J 94:528–531, 1966.

164. Muhlendahl KE, Kahn D, Spohr HL, et al.: Steroid treatment of pseudo-croup. Helv Paediatr Acta 37:431–436, 1982.

165. Kairys SW, Olmstead BA, O'Connor GT: Steroid treatment of laryngotracheitis: a meta-analysis of the evidence from randomized trials. Pediatrics 83:683–693, 1989.

CHAPTER 61

LOWER RESPIRATORY TRACT INFECTIONS

TIMOTHY A. MULLENIX, Pharm.D., M.S. and RANDALL A. PRINCE, Pharm.D.

Despite improvements in diagnostic methods and the development of new antimicrobial agents, pneumonia remains the most common cause of life-threatening infectious disease and is the sixth most common cause of death in the United States (1). Pneumonia is defined as inflammation of the lungs caused primarily by bacteria, viruses, and chemical irritants. The term pneumonia usually refers to acute bacterial infection of the lungs.

Although almost any bacteria can cause pneumonia, certain organisms, depending upon the clinical situation, are more likely to cause it than others. It is not the diagnosis of pneumonia that is difficult; it is the identification of the causative agent that represents the greatest challenge. In most cases, the precise cause of infection is undetermined unless invasive methods are used. Thus, management is based upon an understanding of the pathogenesis of the disease and the determination of the most likely etiologic cause using the patient history, physical examination, and the microbiology laboratory.

PATHOGENESIS

The normal respiratory tract has elaborate and remarkably efficient defense mechanisms that maintain an essentially sterile airway distal to the larynx. The development of clinical infection in the lung is a rarity in healthy individuals and usually indicates a defect in host defenses, exposure to a particularly virulent organism, or an overwhelming infectious inoculum. Organisms reach the lower lungs via one of three possible routes. The first route is inhalation of aerosolized particles, which is associated with *Legionella* pneumonia and tuberculosis. The second route is metastatic spread of bacteria from an extrapulmonary source via the blood. Aspiration of oropharyngeal bacteria represents the third and most common cause of bacterial respiratory infections. Aspiration of oropharyngeal flora occurs most in patients with impaired consciousness, but it has been found to occur in over 50% of normal, sleeping subjects, as well (2).

Even though the inhalation of microorganisms and the aspiration of oropharyngeal contents occurs commonly in healthy individuals, the development of pneumonia is relatively rare because of several protective mechanisms present in the lungs. The normal defense mechanisms of the respiratory tract include mechanical, secretory, and phagocytic systems (Fig. 61.1) (3). In the upper airways, bacteria in inspired air are removed by filtration and humidification. In addition, the frequent branching of the pulmonary tree creates a physical barrier that also filters the inspired air. These defenses are augmented by airway reflexes. The epiglottis, under autonomic control, closes reflexly and prevents aspiration of material into the lower respiratory tract. Material that does reach the trachea and large bronchi stimulates the cough reflex, which expels the material.

Another integral part of the pulmonary defense mechanism is the mucociliary transport system. From the nasopharynx to the terminal bronchioles, mucus-secreting, ciliated epithelium helps trap and propel material from smaller airways to the large airways, where it can induce the cough reflex and be expectorated or swallowed.

Particles in the 0.2 to 3-micron range may escape the mechanical defense mechanisms and reach the terminal alveoli. The cell surface of the terminal air sacs consists of a single layer of epithelium that lacks mucus-secreting and ciliated cells. At this level, the clearance of organisms depends entirely upon cellular and humoral components of the immune system. Immunoglobulins and complement coat or opsonize the organism and prepare it for ingestion by alveolar macrophages. The alveolar macrophages are the first line of cellular defense in the lower respiratory tract. The macrophages may be able to kill or contain the organism and resolve the infection. Polymorphonuclear neutrophils found near the alveolar spaces can be stimulated by chemotactic factors released by the microorganism or macrophages following phagocytosis. This is the inflammatory response that occurs in pneumonia and often results in a pulmonary infiltrate and pathologic pneumonitis. Cellular immunity, specifically the T lymphocyte, may be required to further activate the phagocytic activity of the macrophage and enhance its killing ability.

Many factors may interfere with these normal host defenses and predispose patients to develop lower respiratory infections. Altered consciousness from alcoholism, cranial trauma, seizures, anesthesia, drug overdose, cerebrovascular disease, and old age can depress the cough reflex and compromise epiglottic closure, resulting in the aspiration of oropharyngeal contents into the lower lungs (4). An endotracheal tube eliminates glottic closure and impedes an effective cough. Also, severe obstructive lung disease, malnutrition, and neuromuscular disease can hinder coughing.

Mucociliary transport is impaired by alcohol, cigarette

smoke, and viral respiratory infections resulting in a reduced ability to clear secretions from the lungs (5, 6). Endobronchial obstruction from a foreign body or lung tumor, as well as cystic fibrosis, may impair this clearance mechanism.

Alveolar macrophage function may be inhibited by cigarette smoke, hypoxia, malnutrition, and pulmonary edema (7). Also, deficiencies in cellular and humoral immunity can predispose to the acquisition of pneumonia, particularly in acquired immune deficiency syndrome (AIDS) and congenital or acquired granulocyte abnormalities (8).

Most pneumonias develop as a result of aspiration of oropharyngeal contents. Thus, the microbiologic make-up of the oropharyngeal flora is important in the determination of the etiologic cause of pneumonia. Normally, a complex assortment of aerobic and anaerobic bacteria is present in the upper respiratory tract. Anaerobic organisms outnumber aerobes several fold in the oropharyngeal flora. Fortunately, the anaerobes are generally weak pathogens individually, and they usually cause pneumonia only when large numbers are aspirated or cause pneumonia in the presence of other pathogens (polymicrobial

Table 61.1.
Normal Flora of the Upper Respiratory Tract

Viridans group streptococci	*Moraxella* spp.
Streptococcus pyogenes	*Haemophilus influenzae*
Streptococcus pneumoniae	Lactobacillaceae
Staphylococci, including *S. aureus*	Corynebacteria
Neisseria spp.	Various obligate anaerobes

infection). Bacteria that colonize the normal upper respiratory tract are listed in Table 61.1. Each of these organisms is a potential pathogen that may cause pneumonia when aspirated into the alveoli.

Gram-negative organisms such as *Escherichia coli*, *Klebsiella* spp., *Proteus* spp., and *Pseudomonas* spp. are uncommon in the oropharynx of healthy individuals. These organisms are generally more pathogenic and are associated with a higher rate of morbidity and mortality. Many factors favor their growth and resulting colonization of the oropharynx (9), including hospitalization, serious underlying disease, confinement in an intensive care unit, use of endotracheal tube and ventilator support, contaminated respiratory equipment, and the use of broad-spectrum antimicrobial therapy therapy. Also, certain chronic illnesses result in colonization with Gram-negative bacteria, e.g., alcoholism, diabetes, chronic obstructive lung disease, and chronic granulocytic leukemia. The development of pneumonia depends upon which organisms are present in the flora, the quantity of material aspirated, and the underlying condition of the host.

DIAGNOSIS

The diagnosis of lower respiratory tract infections entails physical and laboratory examinations, chest roentgenograms, and isolation of the infecting pathogen(s). The presentation of nonbacterial pneumonias is significantly different from bacterial pneumonias and is summarized in Table 61.2.

The primary symptoms of bacterial pneumonia include cough, fever, chest pain, and the production of sputum that is often purulent. In certain patients, such as the elderly, alcoholic, or neutropenic patient, typical signs and symptoms may be absent or mild. In addition, the extrapulmonary symptoms, such as mental status changes, disorientation, and reduced appetite may predominate.

Common physical findings include fever, usually above 101°F, tachycardia, tachypnea, and decreased breath sounds over the affected area. Hypoxia and cyanosis are common and are the result of continued perfusion of nonventilated areas of the lung.

Radiologic examination is very useful in diagnosing pneumonias. The *classic* radiographic features of an advanced, typical bacterial pneumonia include dense con-

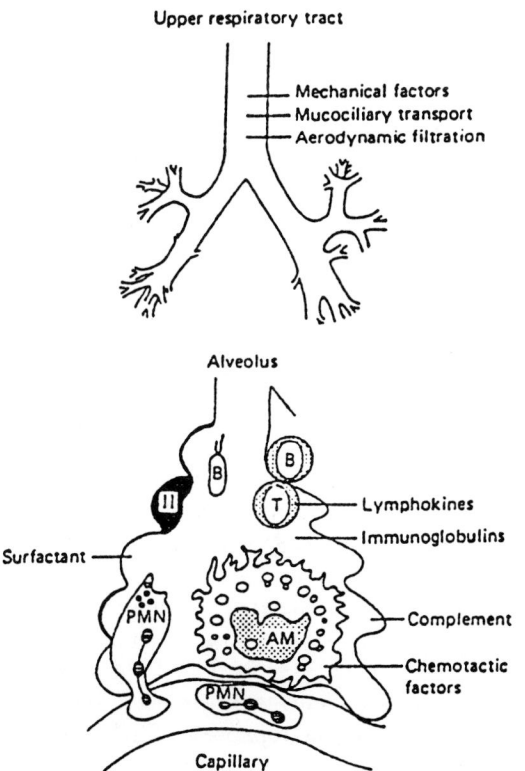

Figure 61.1. Defense mechanisms of the lung. (Reprinted with permission from Reynolds HY: Host defense impairments that may lead to respiratory infections. Clin Chest Med 8(3):344, 1987.)

Table 61.2.
Differential Diagnosis of Bacterial versus Nonbacterial Pneumonia

Feature	Bacterial	Nonbacterial
Onset	Sudden	Insidious
Fever	>39°C	<39°C
Rigors	May or may not be present	Usually absent
Cough	Productive	Nonproductive
Sputum	Purulent	Mucoid
General appearance	"Toxic"	General malaise, constitutional symptoms
Respiratory status	Cyanosis, tachypnea, tachycardia, pleuritic chest pain, splinting	Essentially unremarkable
Gram stain	Bacteria, white blood cells	Mixed oral flora, mononuclear cells
White blood cell count	Elevated	Normal
Chest x-ray	Defined infiltrate	Patchy infiltrate

solidation involving one or more lobes of the lung, either unilaterally or bilaterally. Often, the x-ray findings in acute pneumonia are those of a bronchopneumonia. Other features that may be seen with bacterial pneumonias include cavitation and large pleural effusions. Although certain findings on chest roentgenogram may suggest specific pathogens, such findings are neither sensitive nor specific enough to ascertain the etiology of the pneumonia. The radiographic diagnosis may be unreliable in pneumonias of acute onset and in patients who are dehydrated as well. In these settings, radiographic signs may be undetectable, despite prominent clinical symptoms.

A critical but difficult step in the diagnosis of pneumonia is the isolation of the infecting pathogen(s). The mainstay of laboratory evaluation of pneumonia is the microscopic examination and microbiologic culture of respiratory tract secretions or tissue. The most useful laboratory procedure in evaluating pneumonia is the procurement and microscopic examination of a Gram-stained sputum specimen. This noninvasive technique can provide valuable information in establishing the diagnosis of pneumonia by following specific guideline precautions. The most important guideline is to obtain a properly collected specimen that represents secretions from the lower respiratory tract and not simply saliva or oropharyngeal secretions that represent upper respiratory tract flora. The secretions are most appropriately obtained by inducing a deep cough and examining the most purulent areas of the stained sputum. To assure minimal oropharyngeal contamination of the specimen, the number of neutrophils and epithelial cells should be determined microscopically. Specimens with >25 neutrophils and <10 epithelial cells per low-power field (LPF) are usually properly collected specimens; specimens with >10 epithelial cells and few neutrophils per LPF should be discarded and considered improper (10).

Using the sputum specimen, the number and morphology of the bacteria should be noted by Gram stain. Although the exact identification of bacteria by Gram stain

is not possible, the appearance of the organisms can allow reasonable inference of their identity. Gram-positive lancet-shaped diplococci should suggest pneumococcal pneumonia, while staphylococci appear as Gram-positive cocci in tetrads and grape-like clusters. Small Gram-negative coccobacillary organisms are typical for *Haemophilus influenzae*.

If sputum cannot be obtained or its analysis is equivocal, more invasive diagnostic techniques may be used. One such method is transtracheal aspiration, which obtains specimens directly from the lower respiratory tract which are generally considered to be free from contamination by the upper airways. This technique is particularly useful in the diagnosis of anaerobic infections, but is not without potential serious complications. Subcutaneous emphysema, bleeding, and infection are potential adverse effects of this procedure. Additional methods of obtaining specimens for the diagnosis of pneumonia include fiberoptic bronchoscopy, transbronchial biopsy, and open lung biopsy. Lung biopsy may be necessary, and it remains the definitive procedure for the accurate diagnosis and treatment of pneumonias in patients who are immunocompromised or fail to respond to conventional therapy (11).

Other tests that aid in the diagnosis of pneumonia include blood and pleural fluid cultures and counterimmunoelectrophoresis of sputum or lung fluid. The incidence of pleural effusions associated with pneumonia depends upon the etiologic agent. Pleural fluid cultures, when positive, are highly specific. Approximately 20 to 30% of patients with bacterial pneumonia have positive blood cultures that provide positive identification of the organism involved (12). Thus, blood cultures should be obtained from all patients with suspected pneumonia.

Counterimmunoelectrophoresis (CIE) has been used to detect bacterial antigens in various body fluids including urine, serum, sputum, and pleural fluid. No available test is definitive for the diagnosis of pneumonia. CIE is most useful in patients with bacteremic pneumococcal pneumonia, where it is positive in 75 to 100% of sputum samples (13). Although a positive CIE can detect pneumococcal antigen in sputum, it cannot distinguish colonization from true infection.

Serologic testing has been used to diagnose a variety of agents causing pneumonia, which are difficult to isolate, e.g., *Legionella pneumophila*, *Mycoplasma pneumoniae*, *Chlamydia* spp., and *Cryptococcus* spp. (14). Acute and convalescent serum samples should be obtained when these agents are suspected. Unfortunately, seroconversion may not occur for a number of weeks and their usefulness in rapidly diagnosing pneumonia is limited. They are generally more helpful in confirming the clinical diagnosis after treatment has begun.

The clinical history is very important in the presumptive diagnosis of pneumonia because underlying conditions are known to predispose to specific etiologic causes of pneumonia (Table 61.3). Up to 50% of patients with pneumococcal pneumonia report a history of upper respiratory infection prior to the development of pneumonia (15). Anaerobic infections should be considered in patients with a history of alcoholism, seizures, sedative overdose, recent dental procedures, or loss of consciousness followed by aspiration of oral contents (16). Staphylococcal pneumonia has been found to occur commonly during outbreaks of influenza. Patients with a history of chronic obstructive lung disease have an increased risk of pneumococcal and *H. influenzae* pneumonia because they are frequently colonized with these agents. Cystic fibrosis patients frequently develop *Pseudomonas* and staphylococcal pneumonias (17). Pneumonias in patients who are frequently hospitalized or have chronic underlying disorders, such as congestive heart failure, COPD, diabetes, and alcoholism, are more commonly caused by Gram-negative bacteria

such as *Proteus* spp., *E. coli*, *Klebsiella* spp., and *Enterobacter* spp. The elderly are prone to pneumonia, especially those who reside in nursing homes or extended-care facilities. In addition, AIDS increases the risk for the development of *Pneumocystis carinii*, cytomegalovirus, *Mycobacterium tuberculosis*, and atypical tuberculosis, as well as other common bacterial causes of pneumonia (8).

ETIOLOGY

With a presumptive diagnosis of pneumonia, knowing the relative frequencies of the various etiologies helps in determining an initial antimicrobial therapy. Pneumonias can be categorized by the clinical setting in which they occur, community-acquired or hospital-acquired. Only a few organisms are commonly implicated in community-acquired pneumonia. *Streptococcus pneumoniae* is responsible for 30 to 60% of the cases of acute community-acquired pneumonia (18). *H. influenzae* is the most common causative Gram-negative pathogen, accounting for 2 to 20% of cases (19). Other, less common causes include *Staphylococcus aureus*, mixed infection by aerobic and anaerobic bacteria, and non-*Haemophilus* Gram-negative bacilli. *Legionella* spp. are an important cause of community-acquired pneumonia, but the relative frequency appears to relate to geographic location. *Moraxella catarrhalis* has been recently identified as a cause of community-acquired pneumonia. Nonbacterial causes of community-acquired pneumonia include *Mycoplasma pneumoniae*, *Chlamydia pneumoniae*, *Chlamydia psittaci* and various viruses.

In the hospital-acquired pneumonias (nosocomial), the predominate organisms isolated are aerobic Gram-negative rods. These organisms account for 60% of hospital-acquired pneumonias, with most belonging to the Enter-

Table 61.3.
Suspected Pathogens and Empiric Treatment of Pneumonia in Adults

Clinical Setting	Usual Pathogens	Presumptive Therapy
Previously healthy, community acquired	Pneumococcus, *Mycoplasma pneumoniae*	Erythromycin, penicillin
Nosocomial (hospital acquired)	*K. pneumoniae*, *P. aeruginosa*, *E. coli*, *S. aureus*	2nd/3rd-generation ceph,[a] extended-spectrum penicillin,[b] aztreonam, imipenem plus an aminoglycoside
Nursing home	Pneumococcus, *H. influenzae*, *K. pneumoniae*, *S. aureus*, *E. coli*	2nd/3rd-generation ceph, ampicillin/sulbactam, ticarcillin/clavulanate, extended-spectrum penicillin
COPD	Pneumococcus, *H. influenzae*, *M. catarrhalis*	Ampicillin, ampicillin/sulbactam, 2nd/3rd-generation ceph, TMP/SMX
Recent influenza	Pneumococcus, *S. aureus*, *H. influenzae*	Ampicillin/sulbactam, ticarcillin/clavulanate, extended-spectrum penicillin
Alcoholism	Pneumococcus, *H. influenzae*, *K. pneumoniae*, *S. aureus*	As above
Aspiration		
Community	Anaerobes	Penicillin, clindamycin
Hospital	Mixed: Gram-negative enterics, anaerobes, *S. aureus*	Ampicillin/sulbactam, ticarcillin/clavulanate, clindamycin plus aminoglycoside, imipenem

[a] If *Pseudomonas aeruginosa* is suspected, ceftazidime or cefoperazone.
[b] Pipercillin, mezlocillin, azlocillin.

obacteriaceae family (*Klebsiella pneumoniae*, *E. coli*, *Enterobacter* spp., *Proteus* spp.) and *Pseudomonas* spp. *S. pneumoniae* causes only 8% of hospital-acquired pneumonias and *S. aureus* approximately 13% (20). The high incidence of Gram-negative infections in the hospital setting is related to three closely linked events: colonization of the oropharyngeal flora with these organisms, aspiration, and the inability of the host lung defenses to clear or kill the aspirated challenges.

Other pathogens such as viruses, fungi, *Legionella* spp. and *P. carinii* may be responsible for nosocomial infections, especially in immunocompromised patients.

COMMUNITY-ACQUIRED PNEUMONIA

An estimated 2 to 2.5 million cases of pneumonia occur annually in the United States, with most being community-acquired pneumonia. The typical presentation is a patient in the mid-50s who becomes ill in mid to late winter or early spring. Most patients have one or more underlying chronic diseases, such as chronic obstructive lung disease, cardiovascular disease, alcoholism, or diabetes. The onset of symptoms is usually acute and marked by a sudden chill, sustained fever, chest pain, and a productive cough. Frequently, community-acquired pneumonia follows an upper respiratory tract infection or an influenza outbreak.

Laboratory evaluation reveals an elevated white blood cell count [15 to 35 × 10^9/liter (15,000 to 35,000/mm^3)] with an increased number of immature forms (bands) on the differential cell count. Leukopenia is a poor prognostic indicator, especially in the elderly. Microscopic examination of lower respiratory specimens reveals a polymorphonuclear exudate and usually a predominance of a single type of organism.

Pneumococcal Pneumonia

Streptococcus pneumoniae is the most common cause of acute bacterial pneumonia. It occurs more frequently in the winter and early spring, in middle-aged and elderly patients, as well as in infants and children under 5 years of age (21). Significant risk factors for the development of pneumococcal pneumonia include advanced age, cigarette smoking, dementia, chronic institutionalization, seizures, and splenectomy. Other groups at particular risk include those with underlying chronic diseases, such as cardiovascular disease, pulmonary disease, diabetes mellitus, and chronic alcoholism.

The onset is classically associated with an abrupt shaking chill or rigor, which is followed by a sustained high fever, dyspnea, and pleuritic chest pain. This typical presentation occurs in up to 70% of cases. Cough with production of rust-colored, purulent sputum is frequent, along with nausea, vomiting, malaise, and weakness (22). Most patients will be tachypneic, tachycardiac, and cyanotic. In the elderly or debilitated patient, confusion and stupor are often the principle findings, with the typical symptoms frequently absent. Herpes labialis occurs in as many as 30% of patients.

Chest x-rays typically show a lobar consolidation with occasional patchy infiltrates. Pleural effusions occur in 25% of cases, while cavitation occurs rarely and suggests another etiology. The white blood cell count usually reveals a leukocytosis of [15 × 10^9/liter (15,000 cells/mm^3)] or greater with a neutrophilia and an increased percentage of immature granulocytes i.e., a shift to the left. It should be noted that leukopenia may be seen in patients with fulminant disease. Gram staining of the sputum is one of the most important presumptive diagnostic procedures available. A preponderance of lancet-shaped diplococci with a large number of granulocytes is highly suggestive for pneumococcal pneumonia. Sputum culture is positive in less than 50% of patients with pneumococcal pneumonia (23). The 20% case fatality rate of bacteremic pneumococcal pneumonia underscores the importance of obtaining blood cultures in all patients (24).

The drug of choice for pneumococcal pneumonia is penicillin G. Most strains have a minimum inhibitory concentration of less than 0.02 μg/ml. Although penicillin-sensitive pneumococci are also sensitive to other penicillin derivatives, none are more active than penicillin and some are considerably less active. Uncomplicated pneumococcal pneumonia responds well to 600,000 units of procaine penicillin G i.m. every 12 hr for 7 to 10 days. In the outpatient setting, 1 g of oral penicillin V daily for 10 days is also effective. Some clinicians begin an outpatient regimen with a single 600,000 unit i.m. injection of procaine penicillin G, followed by oral therapy. In complicated pneumococcal pneumonia, aqueous penicillin G should be administered intravenously in a dose of 5 to 10 million units daily. In patients with meningitis, endocarditis, or arthritis, 20 million units/day of IV aqueous penicillin G would be appropriate.

In the penicillin-allergic patient, erythromycin 1 to 2 g daily is an effective alternative. Cephalosporins are also effective; but there is a 5 to 15% rate of cross-sensitivity in penicillin-allergic patients, and cephalosporins should be avoided in patients with a history of immediate hypersensitivity to penicillins.

The tetracyclines and aminoglycosides should be avoided because of resistance. Ciprofloxacin should also be used very cautiously in the treatment of pneumococcal pneumonia because of its moderate activity against the pneumococcus and reports of possible treatment failures (25, 26).

With appropriate therapy and in the absence of complications, response is often dramatic, with rapid defervescence and clearing of symptoms within 48 hr. Complete resolution of radiographic infiltrates may require longer than 6 weeks, even in uncomplicated cases. After the patient has responded to therapy and been afebrile for at least 48 hr, consideration should be given to continuing therapy with an oral agent.

Despite its commonplace occurrence and rapid response to therapy, complications of pneumococcal pneumonia can be fatal. Bacteremic patients have an increased mortality, as do patients with splenic dysfunction, multiple myeloma, chronic lymphocytic leukemia, chronic renal, hepatic, or cardiac failure, and diabetes mellitus. Also, pneumococcal meningitis is associated with a high mortality rate.

Because of the mortality rate associated with pneumococcal pneumonia in certain populations, prophylaxis against pneumococcal infections by active immunization is recommended. The currently available vaccine is a polyvalent pneumococcal vaccine composed of 23 types of purified, capsular polysaccharide antigens of *S. pneumoniae*, which represents 87% of bacterial types responsible for bacteremia in the United States. Although there is some controversy about the effectiveness of the vaccine, it is clearly effective in healthy adults and immunocompetent elderly patients in reducing the incidence of pneumococcal pneumonia (27). The efficacy appears to be directly related to the immune responsiveness of the population. Current recommendations for vaccination include adults with splenic dysfunction; chronic diseases such as Hodgkin's disease, cardiovascular disease, and pulmonary disease; immunosuppressive conditions including multiple myeloma, alcoholism, cirrhosis, renal failure, and cerebrospinal fluid leaks; healthy adults over 65 years of age; and persons over 2 years of age with human immunodeficiency virus. It is contraindicated in patients under 2 years of age, pregnant women, and those with a febrile illness (28).

About 50% of patients experience local reactions with soreness, pain, and erythema at the site of injection. Less than 1% of patients develop fever, myalgias, and severe local reaction. Severe anaphylactoid reactions are rare (5 reactions per one million doses). (See Chapter 59; "Immunization.")

Hemophilus influenzae Pneumonia

Haemophilus influenzae has become an increasingly common cause of bacterial pneumonia in adults. Its incidence is not known because of difficulties in identifying and isolating the organism from the sputum and distinguishing true infection from contamination. *H. influenzae* is an aerobic, Gram-negative rod that is frequently present in the normal flora of the upper respiratory tract. Respiratory infections are the result of aspiration of oropharyngeal contents, and less commonly, inhalation. The incidence of *H. influenzae* pneumonia is higher in the very young, in patients over the age of 50, and during the winter months.

The major predisposing factors include chronic obstructive lung disease and alcoholism. The clinical signs and symptoms of *H. influenzae* pneumonia include fever, chills, cough, purulent sputum production, dyspnea, sore throat, nausea, and vomiting. Hemoptysis and pleuritic chest pain may also be present. The radiographic pattern of *H. influenzae* pneumonia is indistinguishable from that of other types of bacterial pneumonias. As with other infectious processes, a leukocytosis with an increase in granulocytes and circulating immature granulocytes is present.

The diagnosis of *H. influenzae* pneumonia is based upon Gram staining of sputum and culture of transtracheal aspirates or pleural fluid and blood. Sputum examination usually reveals numerous granulocytes and a predominance of small, Gram-negative rods. Although most strains of *H. influenzae* are sensitive to ampicillin or amoxicillin, isolation of ampicillin-resistant strains has increased steadily in the community setting. The resistance is due to the plasmid-mediated production of β-lactamase and has been reported in as many as 31% of strains in the United States (29). Thus, it is imperative that *H. influenzae* isolates be tested for β-lactamase production or that standard sensitivity tests be performed.

In the β-lactamase-negative strains, ampicillin remains the drug of choice in a dose of 1 to 2 g every 4 to 6 hr intravenously. For ampicillin-resistant strains, several agents are effective: trimethoprim/sulfamethoxazole, the second-generation cephalosporins (cefuroxime, cefoxitin, cefotetan, and cefamandole), and the third-generation cephalosporins (ceftazidime, cefotaxime, ceftriaxone, cefoperazone, and ceftizoxime). Other agents that have good activity against *H. influenzae* include those that contain a β-lactamase inhibitor (clavulanic acid, sulbactam) in combination with ampicillin, amoxicillin, or ticarcillin. Chloramphenicol is also highly effective, but less toxic and equally effective alternative agents are available for use in most clinical situations. Ambulatory patients may receive any one of a number of effective agents including amoxicillin, amoxicillin-clavulanic acid, trimethoprim-sulfamethoxazole, cefuroxime axetil, cefixime, or ciprofloxacin. A vaccine for *H. influenzae* is available. (See Chapter 59, "Immunizations.")

Legionnaires' Disease

Legionella pneumophila is a Gram-negative bacillus found ubiquitously in aquatic environments, including rivers and lakes. However, it grows and proliferates in man-made habitats such as hot-water tanks, cooling towers, and whirlpools. *Legionella* pneumonia usually occurs sporadically, but localized outbreaks have occurred in institutions. Legionnaires disease occurs more frequently during the summer months and primarily affects older male smokers with chronic lung disease. The only documented route of transmission is via airborne inhalation (30). Legionnaires' pneumonia is an acute bacterial bronchopneumonia with an incubation period of 2 to 10 days. Onset is usually manifested by high fever, malaise, myalgias, chills, a nonproductive cough, headache, nausea, and vomiting. Diarrhea (25 to 50% of cases), a relative bradycardia, and changes in mental status are common findings (31). These characteristics are of limited value in differentiating Legionnaires' disease from other pneumonias. Leukocytosis and elevations in serum lactic acid dehydrogenase, aspartate aminotransferase, and alkaline phosphatase levels may be present.

The diagnosis is usually made by either culture or immunofluorescent-antibody testing of an expectorated sputum or pleural fluid specimen.

Erythromycin is the drug of choice in the treatment of *Legionella* infections. In retrospective reviews, erythromycin has had the lowest mortality rate associated with its use (32). A dose of 4 g per day should be given intravenously until clinical improvement is observed. Oral therapy may then be instituted at 2 g/day for a total of 14 to 21 days of therapy. If the patient is unable to tolerate erythromycin, tetracycline is an alternative. Other agents that have been used successfully (from anecdotal reports) include trimethoprim-sulfamethoxazole, imipenem/cilastatin, and ciprofloxacin. Penicillins, cephalosporins, and aminoglycosides are not effective in the treatment of Legionnaires' disease.

Atypical Pneumonia

Atypical pneumonia syndromes contrast with typical community-acquired pneumonias (33). They occur more commonly in older children, adolescents, and young adults, but can occur at all ages. Atypical pneumonias are insidious illnesses with low fever, nonproductive cough, and prominent constitutional symptoms including headache, malaise, and myalgias. Temperature, peripheral white blood count, pulse, and respiratory rate are not as markedly elevated as in typical bacterial pneumonia. Sputum is usually not produced or is nonpurulent.

Atypical pneumonia syndromes are caused by *Mycoplasma pneumoniae*, viruses, *Chlamydia* spp., *Rickettsia* spp., and fungi. The most common pathogen is *M. pneumoniae*. Influenza virus is also a common cause, and amantadine has been found to be effective for the early treatment and prophylaxis of influenza A (34).

Mycoplasma Pneumonia

Mycoplasma pneumoniae is primarily a human pathogen that produces upper respiratory infection as well as pneumonia. *Mycoplasma* pneumonia is common, occurring predominantly in school-age children and young adults between the ages of 5 and 35. It is an uncommon cause of pneumonia in the very young and old; however, people of

any age may become infected. *Mycoplasma* are transmitted by inhalation of aerosolized organisms, requiring close contact. High occurrence rates are found in enclosed populations such as college students, military recruits, and prisoners (35). *Mycoplasma* pneumonia has a wide spectrum of syndromes that range from benign and self-limited to life-threatening. Only 3 to 10% of patients infected with *M. pneumoniae* have clinically apparent pneumonia. Symptomatic involvement of the upper respiratory tract is the most commonly seen syndrome, with the vast majority developing pharyngitis or bronchitis. The onset of pneumonia is slow and follows an incubation period of 2 to 3 weeks. Fever, chills, cough, headache, and malaise are common symptoms in patients with pneumonia. Cough is most often nonproductive and reveals no predominate organism on Gram stain. One-third of patients with pneumonia also have upper respiratory tract symptoms, including sore throat, rhinorrhea, and earache. Chest x-ray usually shows a lobar bronchopneumonia that is not diagnostic.

The diagnosis of *M. pneumoniae* pneumonia may be made by the isolation of the organism from the sputum or other lung-washing samples or by a rise in the specific antibody titer. The results of these methods require several weeks to become positive, therefore, the diagnosis must initially be made upon clinical findings.

Most *M. pneumoniae* infections are self-limited and rarely require hospitalization. Treatment with tetracycline or erythromycin shortens the duration of clinical manifestations and pulmonary infiltrates, if present (36). These agents, in a dose of 500 mg every 6 hr, are the agents of choice. Because the diagnosis of *Mycoplasma* pneumonia is usually made on clinical grounds, erythromycin is chosen most often, due to its additional activity against *Legionella pneumophila* and *Streptococcus pneumoniae*. Therapy should be continued for 14 days to prevent relapse. Less severe or symptomatic infections confined to the upper respiratory tract usually do not require treatment. Agents that inhibit cell wall synthesis in bacteria (e.g., penicillins and cephalosporins) are not effective against *M. pneumoniae*.

HOSPITAL-ACQUIRED PNEUMONIA

It is estimated that 3.5 to 5% of all patients hospitalized in the United States develop a nosocomial infection. Lower respiratory tract infections account for about 15% of nosocomial infections and rank only behind urinary tract infections and wound infections in frequency (37). The reported mortality of nosocomial pneumonia is between 20 and 50%, which accounts for the greatest number of deaths from hospital-acquired infections.

Although pneumonias acquired during hospitalization may occur as a result of metastatic spread secondary to bacteremia, most pulmonary infections result from aspiration of organisms from the oropharynx. The critical first step in the pathogenesis of nosocomial bacterial pneumonia is colonization of the upper respiratory tract with enteric Gram-negative organisms. Pharyngeal cultures from normal, nonhospitalized individuals rarely reveal Gram-negative rods. In contrast, 75% of hospitalized patients become colonized by enteric gram-negative bacteria after only a few days of hospitalization (38). To develop pneumonia, a patient must have impaired host-defense mechanisms that prevent normal clearance from the lower respiratory tract. Factors that promote colonization of the oropharynx with Gram-negative bacteria include serious underlying disease, pulmonary disease, use of broad-spectrum antibiotics, use of respiratory equipment, and exposure to bacteria indigenous to the hospital and instrumentation (39). Recently, the use of antacids and histamine-type-2 blockers that raise the pH of the stomach has been found to promote colonization of the stomach with Gram-negative bacteria and increase the risk of aspiration pneumonia in the hospital setting (40).

The clinical features of hospital-acquired pneumonia are similar to those of community-acquired pneumonia and include fever, tachycardia, tachypnea, chest pain, leukocytosis, cough, purulent sputum production, and chest x-ray abnormalities. However, in the presence of serious underlying disease, these signs and symptoms may be overshadowed. Because culture material is frequently either nondiagnostic, pending examination, or unobtainable, antibiotic therapy must often be chosen empirically. Empiric therapy must be directed against the most likely infecting organisms, based upon Gram stain, culture results, and hospital surveillance data.

Staphylococcal Pneumonia

Staphylococcus aureus is an unusual cause of pneumonia and accounts for approximately 5 to 10% of all pneumonias. However, despite effective antimicrobial therapy, mortality from staphylococcal pneumonia is disturbingly high (30 to 50% in some series). Primary staphylococcal pneumonia most frequently develops from the upper respiratory tract and occurs as a complication of viral infection. Viral infections appear to predispose patients to secondary infections by destroying the ciliated surface epithelium. In addition, secondary staphylococcal pneumonia may develop from hematogenous spread to the lungs.

The clinical presentation of staphylococcal pneumonia is highly variable. Onset of infection may be acute or insidious. In severe cases, high fever, multiple shaking chills, confusion, vascular collapse, chest pain, hypoxia, and cyanosis may occur rapidly. Often the presentation is less dramatic, with only mental confusion present and no other signs of pulmonary infection, especially in the elderly. Additional signs and symptoms include fever, leukocytosis,

and cough, with sputum of a dirty, salmon-pink color. Staphylococcal skin lesions, including pustule formation, subcutaneous abscesses, and scarlatiniform rash, may be found and provide clues to the diagnosis. Chest x-ray results often demonstrate patchy, scattered infiltrates with empyema and abscess formation occurring in 10% and 25% of patients, respectively. Lobar consolidation, as in pneumococcal pneumonia, is uncommon.

The diagnosis of staphylococcal pneumonia is based on the recovery of *S. aureus* from pulmonary secretions. Gram-stain of sputum shows numerous polymorphonuclear leukocytes and Gram-positive cocci in clusters. If pleural fluid is present, smears and cultures of the fluid can confirm the diagnosis. In addition, 20 to 30% of patients have bacteremia, and blood cultures are very helpful in the diagnosis.

Most isolates of *S. aureus* produce penicillinase and are resistant to penicillin. Thus, the antibiotics of choice are semisynthetic penicillins that are β-lactamase resistant. These agents include methicillin, nafcillin, oxacillin, cloxacillin, and dicloxacillin. Nafcillin and oxacillin in a dose of 2 g every 4 hr parenterally are the preferred regimens. Nafcillin may be preferred in patients with renal impairment because it is primarily eliminated via the liver. A first-generation cephalosporin (e.g., cefazolin) may also be used, especially in a penicillin-allergic patient. Second- and third-generation cephalosporins are less active against *S. aureus* and are not generally recommended. If the patient has a history of an immediate-type penicillin allergy, cephalosporins should be avoided. In these patients, intravenous vancomycin is the drug of choice.

In addition to producing penicillinase, an increasing number of staphylococcal strains are also methicillin-resistant. These strains are resistant to all penicillins and cephalosporins in vitro and frequently to other antibiotics, as well. Infections due to this strain occur most frequently in hospitals. Vancomycin is the only reliable agent and is the drug of choice for these infections (41).

The response of staphylococcal pneumonia to adequate treatment is slow and usually requires 2 to 3 weeks of intravenous therapy, or longer if complications (abscess or empyema) are present. Treatment of bacteremic staphylococcal infections usually require 4 to 6 weeks.

Aerobic Gram-negative Bacillary Pneumonia

Aerobic Gram-negative bacilli (AGNB) account for 40 to 60% of hospital acquired pneumonias and only a small percentage of community-acquired pneumonias. This type of infection most commonly occurs in patients with chronic obstructive lung disease, alcoholism, and diabetes mellitus. AGNB pneumonias are associated with a high mortality rate and account for 60 to 70% of deaths from pneumonia. As with other pneumonias, Gram-negative pneumonias are typically the result of colonization of the upper airways with aspiration of oropharyngeal contents into the lower lungs. These pneumonias can also result from the aerosolization of bacterial particles with inhalation, especially with the use of respiratory equipment.

The most common Gram-negative organisms associated with the development of pneumonia include *Klebsiella pneumoniae, Enterobacter* spp., *Escherichia coli, Serratia marcescens, Proteus* spp., *Acinetobacter* spp., and *Pseudomonas aeruginosa* (42).

The clinical manifestations of AGNB pneumonia are similar to those of other bacterial pneumonias. High fever, chills, productive cough, pleuritic chest pain, and dyspnea are frequently present. The symptoms do not correlate with a specific etiology. In the hospitalized patient, the development of a new infiltrate on x-ray with fever, leukocytosis, and purulent sputum production suggests a nosocomial, Gram-negative pneumonia.

The treatment of Gram-negative pneumonia is difficult, prolonged, and often associated with a high mortality rate. The prognosis varies with the infecting organism and the underlying condition of the patient. The initial treatment regimen must often be empiric and should be selected based upon the underlying condition of the patient, past medical history, and the institution's epidemiologic data on causative organisms and antimicrobial sensitivities. Generally, an aminoglycoside plus an antipseudomonal penicillin or cephalosporin has been considered the treatment regime of choice. Such a combination regimen is required because of the poor penetration of the aminoglycosides into bronchial secretions. In addition, an aminoglycoside and a β-lactam antibiotic work synergistically and more rapidly than either agent alone because of their different mechanisms of action (43). In less severely ill patients or those who cannot receive an aminoglycoside, single-agent therapy with an extended-spectrum cephalosporin (third-generation) or aztreonam may be considered. The agent chosen depends upon the institution's susceptibility pattern and whether *Pseudomonas* is suspected. After 48 hr, the initial antibiotic regimen should be reevaluated, depending upon the patient response and the results of sputum and blood cultures. Once the etiologic organism is isolated, therapy should be tailored to provide adequate coverage with the least possible toxicity.

Enterobacteriaceae Pneumonia

Pulmonary pathogens among the Enterobacteriaceae include *Klebsiella pneumoniae, Escherichia coli, Enterobacter* spp., *Proteus* spp., and *Serratia marcescens*. The most common etiologic agent in this group is *Klebsiella pneumoniae*. *K. pneumoniae* infection is seem most frequently in middle-aged and elderly men and in patients with coexisting alcoholism, chronic obstructive lung disease, or diabetes mellitus. It occurs commonly in nursing home populations and in immunocompromised hosts, particularly those with granulocytopenia. Signs and symptoms of *Klebsiella* pneumonia are not diagnostic of *Klebsiella* pneumonia. The characteristic sputum is tenacious and brick-red, consisting of a mixture of blood and pus in up to 50% of patients.

K. pneumoniae is typically sensitive to a wide variety of agents including cephalosporins, extended-spectrum penicillins, aminoglycosides, aztreonam, imipenem, and ciprofloxacin. Initial treatment should consist of a third-generation cephalosporin or an extended-spectrum penicillin (pipercillin, mezlocillin) alone or in combination with an aminoglycoside, depending upon the clinical condition of the patient. This regimen should be modified once microbiological sensitivity data are available.

The other Enterobacteriaceae can all cause pneumonia, most commonly in the hospital setting. The clinical settings and clinical conditions in which these agents are found are similar to those seen with *K. pneumoniae*. The clinical signs and symptoms of pneumonia are also similar. *E. coli* is the second most common pathogen in this class. Unlike, *K. pneumoniae*, however, it is more commonly associated with bacteremic spread from the urinary and gastrointestinal tracts. Treatment of pneumonia caused by these Enterobacteriaceae depends upon the hospital susceptibility pattern. Many of these bacteria are susceptible to ampicillin or ampicillin plus a β-lactamase inhibitor and first- or second-generation cephalosporins. There are trends in areas of the country for increased resistance among these organisms, especially *E. coli* and *Serratia* spp. In these circumstances, the use of an extended-spectrum penicillin or third-generation cephalosporin would be appropriate. Addition of an aminoglycoside is warranted in severe infections, particularly bacteremic patients.

Pseudomonas Pneumonia

Pseudomonas aeruginosa pneumonia is a dreaded infection with a high mortality rate. Community-acquired *Pseudomonas* pneumonia is relatively rare, while *P. aeruginosa* causes 15% of nosocomial infections. Most of these pneumonias occur in intensive care units and in patients with granulocytopenia. Other predisposing factors include chronic lung disease, heart disease, cystic fibrosis, burns, nebulization, mechanical ventilation, and other immunosuppressive diseases. *P. aeruginosa* infections usually begin with aspiration of oropharyngeal contents. Colonization of the oropharyngeal flora usually occurs as a result of spread by hospital personnel from patient to patient, especially in intensive care units.

Clinical features include a very toxic and apprehensive appearance with confusion, chills, fever, and a productive cough with yellow-green sputum. *Pseudomonas* pneumonia typically produces microabscesses, which are seen as multiple, small, thin-walled radiolucencies, often involving both lungs or multiple lobes of a single lung.

P. aeruginosa is resistant to many antimicrobial agents. It is susceptible to aminoglycosides, with tobramycin having the greatest activity, antipseudomonal penicillins (carbenicillin, ticarcillin, pipercillin, mezlocillin, and azlocillin), and antipseudomonal third-generation cephalosporins (ceftazidime, cefoperazone). Amikacin is effective against many strains resistant to gentamicin and tobramycin. Newer agents active against *P. aeruginosa* include ciprofloxacin, aztreonam, and imipenem. Treatment of pneumonia should consist of a combination of an aminoglycoside and an antipseudomonal β-lactam. Single-agent therapy may be used, but the high mortality and severity of the infection, as well as the potential development of resistance during therapy, supports the use of combination therapies.

ASPIRATION PNEUMONIA AND LUNG ABSCESS

Aspiration pneumonia describes pneumonia in a patient who aspirates large quantities of microorganisms into the lower airways. This event may be termed macroaspiration as opposed to the microaspiration that is considered to be the underlying cause of most pneumonias. The pathogenesis of aspiration pneumonia involves the aspiration of material into the lower lungs, which results in an inflammatory reaction or pneumonitis. Aspiration does not always develop into an infection, especially if gastric contents have been aspirated. A necrotizing pneumonia may develop with multiple excavations and eventually evolve into a lung abscess and empyema. Development of aspiration pneumonia and lung abscess represents a continuum of changes involving the same process. The most common site of aspiration pneumonia is the posterior segment of the right upper lobe. However, other locations (depending on the position of the patient at the time of aspiration) are also frequently seen (44).

The bacteriologic cause of aspiration-related infections depends upon whether the infection is community-acquired or hospital-acquired. In community-acquired infections, anaerobic bacteria are the predominant pathogens in most aspiration pneumonias and lung abscesses (45). The anaerobes most commonly involved are those present in the oral cavity, e.g., *Bacteroides melaninogenicus*, *Fusobacterium nucleatum*, peptostreptococci, and peptococci. *Bacteroides fragilis* and other β-lactamase-producing *Bacteroides* spp. are found in 15% of cases. Thirty to 40% of community-acquired aspiration pneumonia also involve aerobic bacteria, primarily *Staphylococcus* spp. and Gram-negative bacilli.

Aspiration pneumonia occurring in the hospital is most often polymicrobial (46). Most of these pneumonias involve aerobic Gram-negative bacilli including *P. aeruginosa*, *S. aureus*, *S. pyogenes*, and Gram-positive and Gram-negative anaerobes. The development of lung abscess depends upon the organisms' ability to cause necrosis of lung tissue. This process occurs with anaerobic bacteria, *K. pneumoniae*, other enteric Gram-negative bacilli, and *S. aureus*.

Patients at the greatest risk of aspiration pneumonia are those with altered consciousness and those with disruption of the normal gag and swallowing reflexes.

Bacterial infection following aspiration is generally insidious in onset. After 1 to 2 weeks, abscess and empyema form. Patients have symptoms of malaise, weight loss, low-grade fever, and cough that gradually worsen over days to weeks. Following cavitation, putrid sputum is noted in over 50% of patients and is definitive evidence of anaerobic involvement. Additional symptoms include night sweats, pleuritic chest pain, and dyspnea. Other findings that are often noted are diseased gums, presence of an endotracheal tube, absence of gag reflex, history of alcoholism, or recent seizures. Chest x-ray is diagnostic of pneumonia and particularly of lung abscess. Because the normal flora of the oropharynx represent the leading causes of aspiration pneumonia and lung abscess, cultures of expectorated sputum are of little value. Cultures obtained by transtracheal aspiration are effective in determining the etiologic cause of infection. Because of the potential risks associated with this procedure, empiric therapy is most often chosen, based upon the suspected microbiology of the infection.

Treatment of aspiration pneumonia is based upon appropriate use of antibiotics and the drainage of infected material, i.e., abscess, empyema. Community-acquired aspiration pneumonia and lung abscess without serious underlying disease can generally be presumed to be caused by anaerobic organisms (Table 61.4). Penicillin has been considered the drug of choice in the treatment of anaerobic pleuropulmonary infections (47). Penicillin is cost-effective, has a low incidence of side effects, and is active against most anaerobic organisms found in the oropharyngeal flora. There has been some concern about the efficacy of penicillin because of the occurrence of penicillin-resistant *Bacteroides fragilis* in 15% of anaerobic infections, as well as increasing reports of other *Bacteroides* spp. that are penicillin-resistant. Clindamycin also has good anaerobic activity and is associated with fewer therapeutic failures in the treatment of anaerobic abscess (48). For this reason, many clinicians feel that clindamycin is the drug of choice for community-acquired aspiration pneumonia and lung abscess. Metronidazole has bactericidal activity against a wide range of anaerobic organisms and is highly effective in anaerobic infections of the abdomen and pelvis. However, metronidazole used alone is poorly effective in the treatment of pulmonary infections, probably because of its lack of activity against aerobic bacteria (49).

In the treatment of hospital-acquired aspiration pneumonias, combination therapy is often necessary because of the incidence of Gram-negative bacilli and the poly-

Table 61.4.
In vitro Sensitivities of Important Anaerobic Pathogens

Antibiotic	B. fragilis	B. melaninogenicus	Fusobacterium	Clostridium	Peptostreptococcus	Actinomyces
β-Lactam plus β-lactamase inhibitor	+ + +[a]	+ + +	+ + +	+ + +	+ + +	+ + +
Cefoxitin	+ +	+ + +	+ + +	+ +	+ + +	+ + +
Chloramphenicol	+ + +	+ + +	+ + +	+ + +	+ + +	+ + +
Clindamycin	+ + to + + +	+ + +	+ + +	+ +	+ + +	+ + +
Erythromycin[b]	+ to + +	+ + to + + +	+	+ + +	+ + to + + +	+ + +
Imipenem-cilastatin	+ + +	+ + +	+ +	+ + +	+ + +	+ + +
Metronidazole	+ + +	+ + +	+ + +	+ + +	+ + to + + +	–
Penicillin G	+	+ + to + + +	+ +	+ + +	+ + +	+ + +
Ureido/carboxy penicillins	+ + to + + +	+ + +	+ + +	+ + +	+ + +	+ + +
Vancomycin[b]	+	+	+	+ + +	+ + +	+ + +

[a] Key: – = no activity; + = poor or inconsistent activity; + + = moderate activity; + + + = good activity.
[b] Not approved by FDA for anaerobic infections.

microbial nature of these infections. Therapy should be directed against *S. aureus*, aerobic Gram-negative bacilli, and anaerobes. Treatment with an aminoglycoside and penicillin, clindamycin, or metronidazole have been used successfully. Newer agents that have broad spectrums of activity and excellent anaerobic coverage include ampicillin plus sulbactam, ticarcillin plus clavulanic acid, pipercillin, mezlocillin, azlocillin, and imipenem. Agents that lack significant activity against anaerobic bacteria include the aminoglycosides, aztreonam, and ciprofloxacin.

Resolution of aspiration pneumonia depends upon its severity and whether lung abscess or empyema are present. Necrotizing pneumonia usually requires 2 to 3 weeks of antimicrobial therapy. Lung abscesses respond slowly to therapy and often require weeks to months of treatment. In addition to antibiotics, drainage of empyema, if present, is required for adequate resolution. The overall mortality rate for lung abscess is 5 to 10% (50).

CONCLUSIONS

The clinician must take a systematic approach to the diagnosis and treatment of respiratory tract infections. With the use of empiric antimicrobial therapy as the rule, the clinician must be guided by the knowledge of the most likely infecting pathogens in various clinical settings. An understanding of host-defense mechanisms and predisposing conditions to certain pathogens is critical. Equally important is familiarity with the local institutional microbiologic sensitivity and resistance patterns, to tailor therapy as necessary. The use of so-called broad-spectrum antimicrobials should not replace the clinician's diagnostic acumen and clinical expertise in the management of respiratory tract infections. Once a causative pathogen has been identified, therapy should be directed by sensitivity data, underlying condition of the host, patient tolerance, severity of the disease, and cost of therapy. Without an organized approach to the diagnosis and choice of treatment of respiratory tract infections, antimicrobials will be overused and misused to the detriment of all.

REFERENCES

1. Anon: Premature mortality in the United States: public health issues in the use of years of potential life lost. MMWR 35(suppl):1S–11S, 1986.
2. Huxley EJ, Viroslav J, Gray WR: Pharyngeal aspiration in normal adults and patients with depressed consciousness. Am J Med 64:564–568, 1978.
3. Reynolds HY: Normal and defective respiratory host defenses. In Pennington JE, Respiratory Infections: Diagnosis and Management, ed. 2. New York, Raven Press, 1988, p 1–33.
4. Bartlett JG, Finegold AM: Anaerobic infections of the lung and pleural space. Am Rev Respir Dis 110:56–77, 1974.
5. Green GM, Carolin D: The depressant effect of cigarette smoke in the in vitro antibacterial activity of alveolar macrophages. N Engl J Med 226:421–427, 1967.
6. Afzelius BA: Immotile-cilia syndrome and ciliary abnormalities induced by infection and injury. Am Rev Respir Dis 124:107–109, 1981.
7. Green GM, Kass EH: The role of the alveolar macrophage in the clearance of bacteria from the lung. J Exp Med 119:167–176, 1964.
8. Murray JF, Mills J: Pulmonary infectious complications of human immunodeficiency virus infection. Am Rev Respir Dis 141:1356–1372, 1990.
9. Palmer LB: Bacterial colonization: pathogenesis and clinical significance. Clin Chest Med 8:455–466, 1987.
10. Murray PR, Washington JA: Microscopic and bacteriologic analysis of expectorated sputum. Mayo Clin Proc 50:339–344, 1975.
11. Tobin MJ: Diagnosis of pneumonia: techniques and problems. Clin Chest Med 8:513–527, 1987.
12. Seidenfeld JJ, Pohl DF, Bell RD, et al.: Incidence, site and outcome of infections in patients with the adult respiratory distress syndrome. Am Rev Respir Dis 134:12–16, 1986.
13. Sands RL, Green ID: The diagnosis of pneumococcal chest infection by counter-current immunoelectrophoresis. J Appl Bacteriol 49:471–478, 1980.
14. Campbell JF, Spika JS: The serodiagnosis of nonpneumococcal bacterial pneumonia. Semin Respir Infect 3:123–130, 1988.
15. Fekety FR, Caldwell J, Grump D, et al.: Bacteria, viruses, and mycoplasmas in acute pneumonia in adults. Am Rev Respir Dis 104:499–507, 1971.

16. Bartlett J, Corbach S, Finegold S: The bacteriology of aspiration pneumonia. Am J Med 56:202–207, 1974.

17. Hoiby N: Epidemiological investigations of the respiratory tract bacteriology in patients with cystic fibrosis. Acta Pathol Microbiol Scand B 82:541–550, 1974.

18. MacFarlane JT, Finch RG, Ward MJ, et al.: Hospital study of adult community acquired pneumonia. Lancet 2:255–258, 1982.

19. Wallace RJ, Musher D, Martin R: *Hemophilus influenzae* pneumonia in adults. Am J Med 64:87–93, 1978.

20. Gross PA: Epidemiology of hospital-acquired pneumonia. Semin Respir Infect 2:2–7, 1987.

21. Klein JO: The epidemiology of pneumococcal disease in infants and children. Rev Infect Dis 3:246–253, 1981.

22. Helms CM, Viner JP, Sturm RH, et al.: Comparative features of pneumococcal, mycoplasmal, Legionnaire's disease pneumonias. Ann Intern Med 90:543–547, 1979.

23. Barrett-Conner E: The non-value of sputum culture in the diagnosis of pneumococcal pneumonia. Am Rev Respir Dis 103:845–848, 1971.

24. Austrian R, Gold J: Pneumococcal bacteremia with special reference to bacteremic pneumococcal pneumonia. Ann Intern Med 60:759–776, 1964.

25. Davies BI, Maesen FPV: Quinolones in chest infections. J Antimicrob Chemother 18:296–299, 1986.

26. Anon: Ciprofloxacin. Med Lett 30:11–13, 1988.

27. Sims RV, Steinmann WC, McConville JH, et al.: The clinical effectiveness of pneumococcal vaccine in the elderly. Ann Intern Med 108:653–657, 1988.

28. Anon: Pneumococcal polysaccharide vaccine. MMWR 38:64–68, 73–76, 1989.

29. Doern GV, Jergensen JH, Thornsberry C, et al.: National collaborative study of the prevalence of antimicrobial resistance among clinical isolates of *Haemophilus influenzae*. Antimicrob Agents Chemother 32:180–185, 1988.

30. Edelstein PH, Meyer RD, *Legionella* pneumonias. In Pennington JE: Respiratory Infections: Diagnosis and Management, ed. 2. New York, Raven Press, 1988, pp 381–402.

31. Woodhead MA, MacFarlane JT: Legionnaire's disease: a review of 79 community acquired cases in Nottingham. Thorax 41:635–640, 1986.

32. Kirby BD, Snyder KM, Meyer RD, et al.: Legionnaires' disease: report of sixty-five nosocomially acquired cases and review of the literature. Medicine 59:188–205, 1980.

33. Tuazon CU, Murray HW, Atypical pneumonias. In Pennington JE: Respiratory Infections: Diagnosis and Management, ed. 2. New York, Raven Press, 1988, pp 341–363.

34. Oates JA, Wood AJJ: Prophylaxis and treatment of influenza. New Engl J Med 322:443–450, 1990.

35. Levine DP, Lerner AM: The clinical spectrum of *Mycoplasma* pneumonia infections. Med Clin North Am 62:961–978, 1978.

36. Shames JM, George RB, Holliday WB, et al.: Comparison of antibiotics in the treatment of mycoplasmal pneumonia. Arch Intern Med 125:680–684, 1970.

37. Haley RW, Culver DH, White JW, et al.: The nationwide nosocomial infection rate: a new need for vital statistics. Am J Epidemiol 121:159–167, 1985.

38. Johansen WG, Pierce AK, Sanford JP, et al.: Nosocomial respiratory infections with gram-negative bacilli: the significance of colonization of the respiratory tract. Ann Intern Med 77:701–706, 1972.

39. Toews GB, Nosocomial pneumonia. Clin Chest Med 8:467–479, 1987.

40. Driks MR, Craven DE, Celli BR, et al.: Nosocomial pneumonia in intubated patients given sucralfate as compared with antacids or histamine type-2 blockers. The role of gastric colonization. N Engl J Med 317:1376–1382, 1987.

41. Brumfitt W, Hamilton-Miller J: Methicillin-resistant *Staphylococcus aureus*. New Engl J Med 320:1188–1196, 1989.

42. Anon: Centers for Disease Control: National Nosocomial Infections Study report, annual summary 1984. MMWR 35:17S–29S, 1986.

43. Eliopoulos GM, Moellering RC: Antibiotic synergism and antimicrobial combinations in clinical infections. Rev Infect Dis 4:282–293, 1982.

44. Bartlett JG, Finegold SM: Anaerobic infections of the lung and pleural space. Am Rev Respir Dis 110:56–77, 1974.

45. Bartlett JG, Gorbach SL, Finegold SM: The bacteriology of aspiration pneumonia. Am J Med 56:202–207, 1974.

46. Lober B, Swenson RM: Bacteriology of aspiration pneumonia. A prospective study of community and hospital-acquired cases. Ann Intern Med 81:329–331, 1974.

47. Kirsch CM, Sanders A: Aspiration pneumonia. Medical management. Otol Clin North Am 21:677–689, 1988.

48. Levison ME, Mangura CT, Lorber B, et al.: Clindamycin compared with penicillin for the treatment of anaerobic lung abscess. Ann Intern Med 98:466–471, 1983.

49. Sanders CV, Hanna BJ, Lewis AC: Metronidazole in the treatment of anaerobic infections. Am Rev Respir Dis 120:337–343, 1979.

50. Bartlett JG, Corbach SL, Tally FP, Finegold SM: Bacteriology and treatment of primary lung abscess. Am Rev Respir Dis 109:510–518, 1974.

CHAPTER 62

TUBERCULOSIS

K. DALE HOOKER, Pharm.D. and PAUL M. JOST, M.D.

Tuberculosis is an infection caused by the bacterium *Mycobacterium tuberculosis*. It is usually chronic and may be almost lifelong in duration. While infection may affect almost any organ, it most commonly involves the lungs. Despite major strides in the therapy of this disease, tuberculosis continues to be an important health problem in the United States and worldwide. Drug therapy is key in both the treatment and prevention of tuberculosis.

ETIOLOGY

The genus *Mycobacterium* contains many species of bacteria, some of which can be pathogenic in humans. The type of disease caused by a species from the genus *Mycobacterium* varies widely, depending upon the specific species involved. The most important strict pathogens for this genus are *Mycobacterium leprae*, which is the causative organism of leprosy, and the tubercle bacilli *M. tuberculosis* and *M. bovis*. *M. avium* complex, an opportunistic pathogen, is being seen more frequently as a cause of disease, mostly in patients with the acquired immunodeficiency syndrome (AIDS), but more rarely, it can cause pulmonary disease in the nonimmunocompromised host, most notably the patient with chronic obstructive pulmonary disease. Infection with this organism frequently shows up late in the course of AIDS. *Mycobacterium bovis* is closely related to *M. tuberculosis* and it causes a symptom complex similar to that caused by *M. tuberculosis*. Infection due to this organism has become rare because of measures such as pasteurization of milk and skin testing of cattle.

In the laboratory, these organisms are difficult to stain so that they can be seen with the microscope, but once stained, they are resistant to decolorization with acid alcohol. Because of this property, they are frequently referred to as acid-fast bacilli. Many grow slowly on artificial media, and cultures often require 4 to 6 weeks of incubation before colonies appear. Identification and susceptibility testing may take several additional weeks. Methods are becoming available to shorten the processes of determining whether mycobacteria are present in a specimen, identifying the mycobacterial organism, and determining its sensitivity pattern. Culturing *M. tuberculosis* from a patient nearly always represents acute infection; other mycobacteria may be evidence of a disease process or simply indicate colonization.

INCIDENCE

A continual decline in the number of cases of tuberculosis was seen in the United States from 1953 through 1985. Since 1986, an increased number of cases has been reported (1). In 1989, there were 23,495 cases reported to the Centers for Disease Control from throughout the United States (2).

Males are twice as likely to have clinical tuberculosis as females. Age-specific risk is lowest in the 5- to 14-year-old group, with a steady increase with age after that. Among non-Hispanic whites, the largest number of cases is seen among the elderly. The largest number of cases among minorities occurs in younger adults. The annual risk of tuberculosis in nonwhites was 5.3 times the risk in whites in 1987. The increased risk for nonwhites (compared with whites) has been slowly increasing during the past three decades (2).

There are several reasons for the increasing incidence of tuberculosis. The current epidemic of infection with human immunodeficiency virus (HIV) is part of the reason. Tuberculosis is frequently the first infection seen in patients infected with HIV. A strong correlation has been noted between the recent rise in tuberculosis cases and the increasing incidence of HIV infection. The incidence of tuberculosis among AIDS patients in the U.S. varies widely, from 2 to 30%, but nationwide it is probably about 4.6%. This is 500 times the national incidence in the general population (3).

Immigrants to the United States constitute a large proportion of cases of tuberculosis. In 1987, 22.6% of persons with tuberculosis were foreign-born. Thirty-six percent of these persons were from Asia and 23.3% from Mexico. Poverty and homelessness may also be contributing to the increase in cases (1). An increasing incidence is seen in the elderly as well. The proportion of patients with tuberculosis over the age of 65 went from 18.9% to 29.7% from 1960 to 1982, while the proportion of the general population over age 65 went from 9.2% to 11.3% (4).

In 1989 the United States Department of Health and Human Services put forth a plan to eliminate tuberculosis in the U.S. by the year 2010. The actual goal is to reduce the case rate of tuberculosis in the U.S. to less than one case per one million population. For comparison, the case rate in the U.S. in 1987 was 9.3 cases per 100,000 population (5). A three-part plan was developed to achieve this goal. The first part is to make more effective use of current prevention and control methods. This is possible, in part, because the demographics of persons with tuberculosis are becoming better defined. The second part of the plan is to develop and evaluate new technologies for prevention, as well as diagnosis and treatment, of tuberculosis. The third portion of the plan involves rapid assessment and transfer of new technologies into clinical practice (5).

PATHOGENESIS

Mycobacterium tuberculosis can infect a number of mammals, but the only reservoir for the organism is humans. Almost all infections now seen in the U.S. are due to inhalation of droplet nuclei, which are tiny infectious particles produced by talking, coughing, or sneezing. These particles may remain suspended in the air for prolonged periods and are small enough to be inhaled into terminal air passages, resulting in infection. Prolonged exposure to an infectious environment is usually needed for infection. The risk of disease transmission depends on both the infectiousness of the patient and the amount of close contact (6). A patient with pulmonary tuberculosis and acid-fast bacilli on a sputum stain is considered to be infectious and should be placed in respiratory isolation. If three separate sputum smears are negative, the patient is not considered to be infectious, even though *M. tuberculosis* may subsequently be cultured from the sputum. The risk to hospital personnel probably depends mostly on the incidence in the local community. While an infected patient can infect healthcare workers, this is probably not a major occupational risk (7).

When tubercle bacilli are inhaled in particles small enough to reach the alveoli, they are ingested by alveolar macrophages (Fig. 62.1). If the individual has had no prior exposure to tuberculosis, the bacilli will multiply within the macrophage. These cells then die and release the bacilli, which are ingested by other alveolar macrophages and macrophages from the blood pool of monocytes. These infected cells may spread to nearby lymph nodes and from there to other parts of the body. As a result, if the infection is not subsequently contained, disseminated disease may occur (8).

Within 2 to 4 weeks, cell-mediated immunity develops. At this point a tubercle forms, with a caseous necrotic center surrounded by granulation tissue. Whether this lesion is contained or continues to spread depends on the balance between the virulence of the organism and the microbicidal capacity of the macrophages. Minute caseous foci can be eliminated, while larger foci undergo fibrous encapsulation, isolating the contained organisms. If the host resistance is lowered at some later time, these foci may reactivate (8).

Liquefaction of the caseous center results in material that is an excellent culture medium for the tubercle bacilli. Walls of nearby bronchi may necrose and rupture, forming a cavity and spreading the infection to other parts of the lung (8, 9).

In about 5% of patients infected with *M. tuberculosis*, the immune system is unable to control the infection and disease occurs within the first year. In another 5%, disease occurs later in life. For the remaining 90%, active disease never develops, although they may retain viable organisms for many years (9).

Tuberculous infection has traditionally been thought of as either primary (childhood) infection or reinfection (adult) pulmonary tuberculosis. Adult disease is generally thought to be a reactivation of infection acquired at an earlier age. This is probably true in most instances of disease occurring in the United States as the level of contagion is low, but a previously infected person with a high level of exposure to someone with active disease may acquire exogenous infection (6).

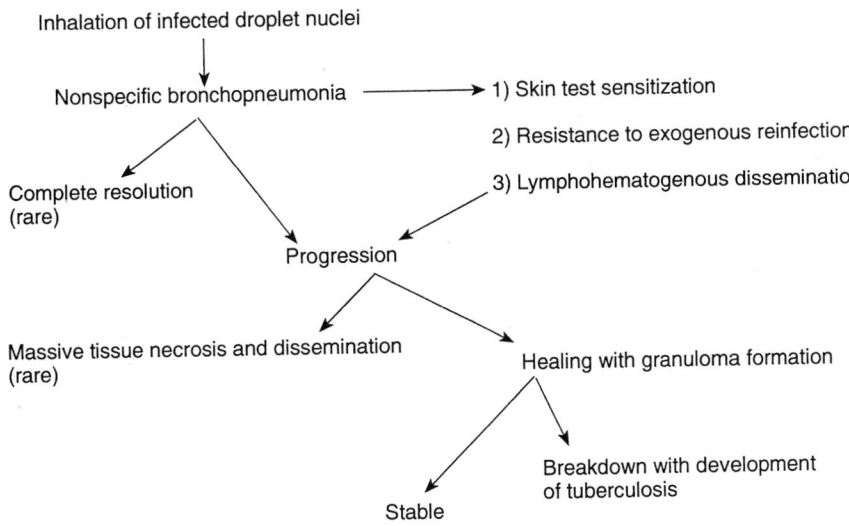

Figure 62.1. Results of infection with *M. tuberculosis*. (From Glassroth J, Robins A, Snider DE Jr: Tuberculosis in the 1980's. Reprinted, by permission of the New England Journal of Medicine, 302:1442, 1980).

A study of tuberculosis in patients in nursing homes demonstrated that while many of these persons were probably infected as children, their infections waned to the point that they were no longer skin-test positive. With subsequent exposure, these persons developed disease like the primary infection usually seen in childhood. Tuberculosis testing in the 1930s found that 80% of persons were infected by the age of 30. In contrast, in this study only 10.9% of persons were positive when tested within 1 month of admission to the nursing home (4). The annual rate of conversion in nursing homes with an infectious case of tuberculosis within the preceding 3 years was about 5%, while the rate in homes without a case was about 3.5% (4).

SIGN AND SYMPTOMS

If infection with *M. tuberculosis* has been controlled by the immune system, the patient is asymptomatic, and the only evidence of tuberculosis may be a positive skin test or possibly changes on chest roentgenogram. Signs and symptoms of active disease depend, in part, on the location of infection. Symptoms tend to be late in onset. Nonspecific constitutional symptoms may include anorexia, weight loss, fatigue, fever, and night sweats. Some patients may have an influenza-like illness, with acute onset of fever, chills, and malaise. Occasionally patients may have active disease and yet be totally asymptomatic.

With pulmonary infection, cough and sputum production usually occur. The cough is generally insidious in onset, progressing over weeks to months. The patient may have production of mucopurulent sputum. A patient who already has a chronic productive cough may have little or no change in pulmonary symptoms, making the diagnosis more difficult. Hemoptysis may occur in advanced disease, but blood is usually only present in small amounts. Dull chest pain or tightness may occur. If inflammation involves the pleura, acute or recurrent pleuritic pain may occur. Shortness of breath is unusual unless the patient has very extensive lung disease or a large pleural effusion (7).

Tuberculosis occurs occasionally at sites other than the lungs. The patient may have associated pulmonary infection or have evidence of disease only at an extrapulmonary site, even though the organisms usually enter the body through the lungs. Tuberculous meningitis may present as only a mild headache or slight change in mentation; it can also present as fulminant meningitis. Patients usually have a low-grade fever but can be afebrile. The peripheral white blood count is usually normal. As many as 25% of patients with tuberculous meningitis have no evidence of tuberculosis at any location outside the central nervous system (6).

Tuberculosis involving the skeleton is usually a combination of arthritis and osteomyelitis. Since there is generally no evidence of infection elsewhere, a high degree of suspicion is required to make the diagnosis. About half of such cases occur in the spine, termed Pott's disease. Paralysis of the lower extremities can occur as the result of extrinsic compression on the spinal cord from granulation tissue or from abscess formation (6).

Urinary tract infection due to *M. tuberculosis* is asymptomatic approximately 20% of the time. Even when symptoms are present, they generally do not include the constitutional symptoms associated with most forms of tuberculosis. Symptoms include gross hematuria, dysuria, frequency, and in late cases, flank pain. Patients may be found to have pyuria with a negative routine urine culture—so-called "sterile pyuria." An intravenous pyelogram is almost always abnormal. Tuberculosis may occur in any other part of the body, with signs and symptoms dependent upon the location (6).

Miliary tuberculosis involves infection throughout the body. The term "miliary" is used because the granulomas seen on chest roentgenogram resemble millet seeds. Symptoms in these patients are nonspecific constitutional symptoms that may be suggestive of the diagnosis but are not pathognomonic, making the diagnosis difficult. One recently reported series of 38 patients with miliary tuberculosis found that 89% of these patients had fever, three-fourths of them had anorexia and sweats, and two-thirds had weight loss. Approximately one-half of the patients had pulmonary symptoms such as cough and dyspnea. Very few patients had other symptoms that pointed to other specific sites of involvement. Most such patients are either PPD skin-test negative or anergic. While cultures of sputum and/or gastric aspirates were positive 80% of the time, sputum smears were positive for acid-fast bacilli only 36% of the time. Extensive cultures and biopsies may be necessary to confirm this diagnosis, which still carries a high mortality rate. In the series mentioned, 21% of such patients died (10).

Tuberculosis is a frequent problem in patients with HIV infection. This infection should not be confused with infection with *M. Avium-intracellulare* (MAI), which is also one of the most common complications of AIDS. For a discussion on MAI and its treatment, refer to the chapter on AIDS. Of patients with both HIV infection and tuberculosis, 85% will have tuberculosis diagnosed before or within 1 month of their diagnosis of AIDS (3). Symptoms in these patients are frequently nonspecific and may be indistinguishable from other symptoms of HIV disease and opportunistic infections, making the diagnosis difficult. Tuberculosis at both pulmonary and extrapulmonary sites is quite common in AIDS. Disseminated tuberculosis or miliary tuberculosis is the most common form of the disease seen in these patients, although any other presentation of tuberculosis may be seen as well. Extrapulmonary tuberculosis in AIDS patients with tuberculosis occurs in one-third to three-fourths of patients (3). Chest roentgenograms may be atypical, and rarely, may be entirely normal. The diagnosis is important both in terms of the public health problem of potential disease spread from an infected patient and because of the favorable response to treatment for tuberculosis in AIDS patients unless it is due to MAI, unlike many of the other infections these patients acquire.

DIAGNOSIS AND CLINICAL FINDINGS

Making a definitive diagnosis of tuberculosis requires isolation of *M. tuberculosis* in the laboratory. In the appropriate clinical setting, a strong presumptive diagnosis can be made on the basis of an appropriate chest roentgenogram, although other diseases (e.g., histoplasmosis) can cause the same clinical picture, including chest roentgenogram changes. A positive sputum smear for acid-fast bacilli is almost definitive. The best sample for analysis by staining and culturing is an early-morning sputum specimen. Generally three such samples are sufficient to make a diagnosis. Occasionally an induced sputum or a specimen obtained by fiberoptic bronchoscopy is needed. An alternative method is to obtain early-morning gastric aspirates and washings to acquire sputum that has been swallowed during the night, although this can be misleading.

Diagnostic measures for disease at sites outside the lung depend on the location of disease. Culture of appropriate fluids or biopsy specimens is necessary. If tuberculosis involving the urinary tract is suspected, three morning urine specimens should be examined. Finding caseating granulomas in a biopsy specimen is evidence for a presumptive diagnosis. Finding acid-fast bacilli in the biopsy specimen increases the likelihood of the disease being tuberculosis.

In patients infected with HIV, it is important to maintain a high index of suspicion for tuberculosis, since the clinical, laboratory and x-ray presentations are often atypical. Any time such patients have new or changing pulmonary symptoms, evaluation for tuberculosis should be included. Likewise, with evidence of an infectious process elsewhere, studies should always include an evaluation for tuberculosis. For example, failure to find evidence of granulomas on biopsies of potentially infected tissue should not preclude doing stains and cultures for acid-fast bacilli. If the diagnosis is considered, it is usually not difficult to make, because sputum cultures are usually positive with pulmonary tuberculosis. Blood cultures are an important aid in making a diagnosis in the AIDS population, as they are positive about 40% of the time (11).

Tuberculin skin testing helps make a diagnosis of tuberculosis. Purified protein derivative (PPD) is the reagent used, and the standard dose is 5 tuberculin units (TU) (also referred to as an intermediate-strength test). A first-strength test is 1 TU; a second-strength test is 250 TU. In the intracutaneous (Mantoux) test, the material is injected intradermally in the skin of the forearm. A small wheal should be produced, indicating the material has been injected into the proper site. The results are read between 48 and 72 hr after application. The amount of induration (not erythema) is then measured. Interpretation of the first- and second-strength tests has not been standardized, and these tests have limited usefulness in the diagnosis of tuberculosis (9).

Interpretation of the intermediate-strength test has recently been revised. The cutoff point for determination of a positive test result depends on the risk status of the patient and the ability of the immune system to react to the test. An area of induration ≥5 mm is considered a positive result in persons with HIV infection, those with risk factors for HIV infection who have an unknown HIV status, persons who have had close recent contact with infectious tuberculosis cases, or persons who have chest radiographs consistent with old, healed tuberculosis. Induration ≥10 mm is considered a positive test result in foreign-born persons from high-prevalence countries in Asia, Africa, and Latin America, intravenous drug users, medically underserved low-income populations (including high-risk racial or ethnic minority populations), residents of long-term care facilities, and persons with medical conditions that have been reported to increase the risk of tuberculosis. Such conditions include silicosis, gastrectomy, jejunoileal bypass, weight of 10% or more below ideal body weight, chronic renal failure, diabetes mellitus, immunosuppressive therapy (including but not limited to prolonged high-dose corticosteroid therapy), and malignancies including solid tumors, leukemias, and lymphomas. A reaction ≥15 mm is considered a positive result in all other individuals (9).

Multiple-puncture testes are available for use in screening large groups, but they should not be used for diagnostic purposes. With such a test, the results are based on the presence or absence of induration. If no induration is present, the test result is considered to be negative. If the individual develops vesiculation at the site of the test, it may be considered a positive result. If there is induration present, a Mantoux test should be performed and interpreted as indicated above (9).

If an individual was exposed to tuberculosis many years previously, the reaction may have weakened, and a negative result may occur. If there is strong suspicion, a repeat test should be given at least 1 week later. This may be positive as a result of a booster effect from the first test. A skin test alone will not induce immunity that would result in the development of a positive test result. A positive result in the repeated test does not indicate recent conversion requiring chemoprophylaxis.

Factors that may result in a positive skin-test result include infection with *M. tuberculosis*, a cross-reaction due to infection with a nontuberculous mycobacterium, vac-

Table 62.1.
Factors Causing Decreased Ability to Respond to Tuberculin[a]

Factors related to patient
  Infections
    Viral (measles, mumps, chickenpox)
    Bacterial (typhoid fever, brucellosis, typhus, overwhelming tuberculosis, etc.)
    Fungal (coccidiomycosis, blastomycosis)
  Live virus vaccine (mumps, measles, polio)
  Malnutrition
  Metabolic disorders (chronic renal failure)
  Extremes of age (newborns, elderly)
  Recent or overwhelming infection with *M. tuberculosis*
  Stress (surgery, burns, etc.)
  Drug therapy (corticosteroids, immunosuppressive or cytotoxic drugs)
  Lymphoid disorders (sarcoidosis, Hodgkin's disease, lymphoma, etc.)
Factors related to tuberculin
  Denaturation from light, heat, or contamination
  Improper dilution or diluent
  Adsorption (not Tween-stabilized)
  Contamination (bacterial)
Factors related to administration method
  Inadequate dosage (too little antigen)
  Delayed administration after drawing into syringe
  Injection too close or too deep
Factors related to reading of test
  Reader bias or inexperience
  Recording error
  Delay in interpretation

[a] Adapted from American Thoracic Society: Diagnostic standards and classification of tuberculosis. Am Rev Respir Dis 142:725–735, 1990.

cination for tuberculosis with BCG, and improper reading or interpretation of the test. False-negative results occasionally occur in otherwise healthy individuals infected with tuberculosis. This is more likely to occur in persons with depression of the immune system, for a variety of reasons. Improper handling or administration of PPD or problems in reading the test may also cause a false-negative results (Table 62.1) (6, 9).

It is important to remember that a true-positive skin test result simply indicates prior exposure to *M. tuberculosis*; it does not mean that the patient has active disease or necessarily needs drug therapy. Further clinical evaluation and testing is needed to make such a determination. Likewise, a negative test result does not rule out disease.

TREATMENT STRATEGIES

Chemotherapeutic regimens for tuberculosis have changed dramatically over the last 25 years. Significant reductions in mortality among patients with pulmonary tuberculosis were demonstrated in the 1940s after the discovery of streptomycin. The late 1950s and 1960s saw the introduction of other, more potent chemotherapeutic agents such as isoniazid, and *p*-aminosalicylic acid. Sani-

toria (tuberculosis hospitals) were closing by the early 1970s with evidence that spending long periods of time in these facilities was unnecessary, since patients treated with effective oral drug combinations promptly (approximately 2 weeks) became noninfectious. Recent reports suggest that most patients can be successfully treated with shorter regimens than previously required. In addition, today's combination regimens are generally well-tolerated, with a low rate of serious toxicities.

Selection of an effective chemotherapeutic regimen is the backbone of successful therapy of tuberculosis. Several principles have been used in the selection process. The first is that effective therapy requires the use of at least two active drugs. Most importantly, the use of drug combinations is desirable to prevent the emergence of drug-resistant organisms. The use of multiple active agents lowers the chance that resistance will occur, since the likelihood of an organism being spontaneously resistant to two drugs is extremely small. When drug resistance occurs, recommendations are that drugs should be changed in combination, rather than singly. Individuals harboring drug-resistant organisms are very likely to select out organisms resistant to the new, singly administered chemotherapeutic agent. The last principle is that curing tuberculosis requires extensive therapy, even after improvement of clinical disease. Inadequate treatment leads to an increased possibility of relapse months to years afterward. Single daily administration is preferred, because of the slow-growing nature of the tubercle bacillus. Single daily doses are also preferred because of greater patient compliance and acceptance. Patients should be monitored extensively for efficacy, drug toxicities, and compliance.

Three histological and functional populations of the tubercle bacilli can potentially coexist during an infection (6). The location of these organisms is contingent upon the physiologic environment. Appropriate antituberculous therapy should be directed against all three sites of mycobacterial growth in the body (Table 62.2). The first of

Table 62.2.
Principal Activity and Site of Action of the Major Antituberculous Agents

Agent	Activity	Site of Action
Isoniazid (INH)	Bactericidal	Intracellular bacilli Extracellular bacilli Bacilli in caseous lesions
Rifampin (RMP)	Bactericidal	Intracellular bacilli Extracellular bacilli Bacilli in caseous lesions
Pyrazinamide (PZA)	Bactericidal	Intracellular bacilli
Streptomycin (STM)	Bactericidal	Extracellular bacilli
Ethambutol (EMB)	Bacteriostatic	Intracellular bacilli Extracellular bacilli

these populations, comprising the most organisms, consists of the rapidly multiplying extracellular bacteria that thrive best at neutral pH (e.g., in a pulmonary cavity). These organisms are best treated with isoniazid, streptomycin, and to a lesser extent rifampin.

The second population is the slowly metabolizing organisms that seek out the acidic environment of solid caseous material. Therapy directed against these organisms should include rifampin, which is unique in its ability to kill these organisms. Isoniazid also has marginal activity against this subpopulation.

The remaining population of organisms is present within the activated macrophages (intracellular). These organisms appear low in number and seldom divide within cells. Because of the acidity within the macrophages, the activity of most chemotherapeutic agents is inhibited. Pyrazinamide (PZA) has demonstrated the greatest activity against this third population, followed to a lesser degree by rifampin and isoniazid.

Drug resistance in tuberculosis can be minimized by administration of combinations of drugs. An essential step in determining the antituberculous regimen is obtaining complete, detailed information from the patient of any prior tuberculosis history. Potentially one of two types of resistance can develop: genetic or acquired resistance and secondary resistance (12). Resistance is chromosomally rather than plasmid-mediated. Genetic or primary (before therapy) resistance occurs as a result of a mutation within the population of tubercle bacilli. The organisms have never been exposed to drugs, but chemotherapy gives a selective advantage to the drug-resistant mutants. Secondary resistance (after therapy) occurs when drug-resistant organisms in one individual infect a new host, a previously untreated patient. Several factors are known to contribute to emergence of genetic resistance (13). The first is the size of the bacterial population. The larger the bacterial load, the more likely there are to be resistant mutants. Resistance would be most common in a pulmonary cavity where the bacillary population approximates 10^9 to 10^{11} organisms. By comparison, low levels or resistance would be expected with lesions such as tuberculomata, bone, joint and renal tuberculosis, and tuberculous meningitis, which have populations estimated at 100 to 1000 bacilli (13).

The second factor contributing to emergence of resistance is the number of drugs used. Naturally occurring resistance to two drugs is very uncommon. The incidence of an organism developing resistance is the product of the rate of spontaneous mutation to resistance for each individual drug. Rates of mutation have been calculated for four of the major antituberculosis agents (12): isoniazid, 1 in 10^6; rifampin, 1 in 10^8; ethambutol, 1 in 10^6; and streptomycin, 1 in 10^5. For example, the probability of resistance when isoniazid and rifampin are given concur-

rently would be 1 in 10^{14} bacteria, a number that far exceeds the bacterial population seen in pulmonary disease.

The third factor, discussed later, is the activity of the individual antituberculous drugs. As will be seen, the effectiveness of a single antituberculous drug or a combination regimen depends upon the subpopulation of bacilli present.

Apparent resistance before therapy is the last factor contributing to the emergence of resistance (secondary resistance). This type of resistance usually develops in treated patients as a result of improper chemotherapy. Secondary resistance is relatively uncommon in native-born Americans, but in developing countries, resistance is quite high for some drugs. In a recently conducted study from Southern California, the country of origin and a history of previous treatment were the two most important predictors of drug resistance (14). For instance, in a recent study conducted in central Haiti, resistance to one or more drugs was found in 22% of the *Mycobacterium tuberculosis* isolates. In patients not known to have received antituberculous drugs in the past, resistance to isoniazid was significantly high at 19% (15). Other developing countries have reported rates of resistance to isoniazid and/or streptomycin as high as 50%. This has significance because patients with isoniazid-resistant tuberculosis receiving INH and rifampin alone are likely to develop resistance to rifampin within several weeks of initiation of therapy, which suggests the need to start all patients with tuberculosis on a three- or four-drug regimen. Certainly, immigrants from other countries, e.g., Asians and Hispanics should always be treated with at least three drugs (16).

PHARMACOLOGY OF ANTITUBERCULOUS DRUGS

Isoniazid. Since its introduction in 1952, isoniazid, or isonicotinicyl hydrazine (INH), has dominated as the single most vital drug in antituberculous chemotherapy. It is bactericidal for *Mycobacterium tuberculosis*, being especially effective against the rapidly dividing extracellular population of organisms. Its mechanism of action probably involves impairment of synthesis of certain long-chain fatty acids that are important components of the cell walls of mycobacteria. Isoniazid is very effective, with most strains of *M. tuberculosis* inhibited by concentration of approximately 0.05 µg/ml. The drug is generally administered as a single dose of 300 mg for adults and 10 mg/kg (up to 300 mg) for children (Table 62.3). Rapid, complete absorption occurs after oral administration, achieving peak concentrations approaching 5 µg/ml after a 3 to 5 mg per kg dose (17). Of equal importance is that the drug is widely distributed throughout the body, including pleural, ascitic, and cerebrospinal fluids. Protein binding of INH appears to be very low, only about 10 to 15%. Food and antacids

Table 62.3.
Drugs for the Treatment of Tuberculosis in Children and Adults

Drug	Daily Dose		Twice Weekly		Common Adverse Effects
	Children	Adults	Children	Adults	
First-line agents					
Isoniazid	10–20 mg/kg, p.o. or i.m., max 300 mg	5–10 mg/kg p.o. or i.m., max 300 mg	20–40 mg/kg, max 900 mg	20–40 mg/kg, max 900 mg	Hepatitis, peripheral neuropathy, hypersensitivity acne, CNS effects
Rifampin	10–20 mg/kg, p.o., max 600 mg	10–20 mg/kg, max 600 mg	10–20 mg/kg, p.o.	10 mg/kg, p.o.	Hepatitis, nausea, vomiting, febrile reaction, orange discoloration of secretions, purpura (rare)
Pyrazinamide	15–30 mg/kg, p.o., max 2 g	15–30 mg/kg, p.o., max 2 g	50–70 mg/kg	50–70 mg/kg	Hepatotoxicity, hyperuricemia arthralgias, rash
Streptomycin	20–40 mg/kg, i.m., max 1 g	15–20 mg/kg, i.m., max 1 g	25–30 mg/kg	25–30 mg/kg	Ototoxicity, nephrotoxicity
Ethambutol	15–25 mg/kg, p.o., max 2.5 g	15–25 mg/kg, p.o., max 2.5 g	50 mg/kg	50 mg/kg	Retrobulbar neuritis, rash
Second-line agents					
p-Aminosalicylic acid	150 mg/kg, p.o., max 12 g	150 mg/kg, p.o., max 12 g	—	—	Gastrointestinal upset, sodium load, hypersensitivity, hepatotoxicity
Ethionamide	15–20 mg/kg, p.o., max 1 g	15–20 mg/kg, p.o., max 1 g	—	—	Gastrointestinal upset, hepatotoxicity, hypersensitivity
Cycloserine	10–20 mg/kg, p.o., max 1 g	10–20 mg/kg, p.o., max 1 g	—	—	Personality changes, psychosis, depression, convulsions, rash
Capreomycin, kanamycin	15–30 mg/kg, i.m., max 1 g	15–30 mg/kg, max 1 g	25–30 mg/kg	25–30 mg/kg	Ototoxicity, nephrotoxicity

may decrease absorption, thus decreasing serum and tissue concentrations of the drug (18).

Metabolism by both acetylation and oxidation via the hepatic P-450 mixed oxidase drug-detoxifying system accounts for 70 to 90% of the elimination of INH. The major route is hepatic acetylation to inactive metabolites that are excreted by the kidneys. The rate of acetylation is a genetically determined trait. Individuals are categorized as being fast or slow acetylators. Slow acetylators have a relative lack of hepatic N-acetyltransferase. Half-lives of INH average approximately 0.5 to 2 hr in fast acetylators and 2 to 5 hr in slow acetylators (19). The slow acetylators may be more prone to toxic side effects related to higher serum concentrations, particularly peripheral neuropathy. Hepatitis, also common following INH administration, has been suggested to be more common in the rapid acetylators because of the metabolite acetylhydrazine (20). However, there is considerable disagreement on this point, and the most recent data suggest that rapid acetylators are not at increased risk and that the rate at which patients acetylate the drug does not appear to be of therapeutic significance. The mechanism of the hepatitis is not conclusively known, but attention has centered around these differences in metabolism. Recently, several studies have refuted these findings.

Because only a small amount of INH is eliminated unchanged by the kidneys, dosage adjustment in patients with renal impairment is necessary only in individuals who are slow acetylators with a creatinine clearance <10 ml/min. To prevent accumulation and reduce potential drug toxicities, these individuals as well as those with severe hepatic disease should receive 50% of the recommended daily dose. For the dialysis patient, significant amounts of INH are removed from the blood by both hemo- and peritoneal dialysis (21, 22).

Peripheral neuropathy and hepatotoxicity are the most frequently observed adverse effects of INH. Peripheral neuropathy is due to INH-induced depletion of pyridoxine stores by mechanisms that are not completely understood. Peripheral neuropathy appears to be dose-dependent but uncommon with INH doses under 5 mg/kg (23). Underlying pyridoxine deficiency seen in some alcoholics, uremics, malnourished persons, children, cancer patients, and pregnant women predisposes these individuals to an increased risk of peripheral neuropathy. As previously mentioned, this problem is more common in slow acetylators.

In some this condition is irreversible. However, the risk of developing this condition can be reduced from 20% to less than 1% by coadministration of supplementary pyridoxine hydrochloride (15 to 50 mg/day) (24). Routine administration of pyridoxine in otherwise healthy individuals is not necessary.

Hepatotoxicity is the other frequent adverse effect, with an incidence of approximately 1 to 2%. Hepatotoxicity is associated with either a clinical hepatitis or asymptomatic elevations in liver enzymes. The problem appears to be both dose-dependent and age-related. The incidence is extremely low in individuals under the age of 20, 0.3% between 20 and 34, 1.2% between 35 and 49, and 2.3% over the age of 50 (25). Recent studies have demonstrated that the incidence in those over 65 may be as high as 4% (26). Up to 15 to 20% of INH-treated patients experience transient elevations of transaminase values (sometimes up to three times normal). It is generally recommended that unless these values exceed five times normal or clinical signs or symptoms suggestive of hepatic damage (i.e., liver enlargement with tenderness, jaundice, dark urine, tiredness, fever, chills, nausea, vomiting, or loss of appetite) are present, discontinuation of the drug is not necessary. Prompt discontinuation of the drug almost always prevents progression. Hepatitis is the most serious side-effect of INH. As previously mentioned, the mechanism of the hepatitis is not known, but it is probably associated with hepatic metabolites. Advanced age and excessive or chronic alcohol use are risk factors associated with a higher incidence of INH-associated hepatitis. The risk of death from hepatitis has ranged from 6 to 12% (25, 27, 28, 30). In a U.S. Public Health Service Surveillance Study (25) that evaluated the toxicity of INH in 13,838 patients, the overall rate of hepatitis was 10.4 cases per 1000 patients treated. In this study there were 8 deaths among the 174 cases of hepatitis. Severe and fatal hepatitis associated with INH administration usually develops in the first 3 months of therapy but may occur after several months of treatment. As a result, patients should be carefully monitored and interviewed regularly during the first few months of INH therapy. Baseline measurement of liver enzyme levels should be completed on all patients treated for tuberculosis with INH-containing regimens.

Because of the high risk associated with INH-induced hepatotoxicity and peripheral neuropathy, patients should be instructed to report immediately any of the clinical signs or symptoms of hepatitis (i.e., malaise, anorexia, nausea, jaundice) or neurotoxicity (tingling, numbness, seizures, mental status changes, paresthesias).

Although peripheral neuropathy and hepatotoxicity are the two major adverse effects reported with INH administration, others have been reported. These include other CNS toxicities (i.e., hallucinations, convulsions) and dermatologic (i.e., acne, allergic rashes), hematologic (i.e., aplastic anemia), and gastrointestinal effects.

Several drug interactions are worth noting. Isoniazid has been shown to increase the serum concentration of phenytoin, disulfiram, carbamazepine, warfarin, benzodiazepines, and vitamin D by inhibiting the metabolism of these drugs. Concomitant administration of INH and theophylline has resulted in significant increases in theophylline serum concentrations (30). To avoid these or other potential drug interactions, patients should be monitored closely, with dosage adjustments made when appropriate.

Rifampin. Discovered in 1966, rifampin (RMP) is the newest of the major antituberculous drugs. While both the oral and parenteral forms of RMP have been available in other countries, the parenteral form of this drug has only recently become available in the U.S. Both forms of RMP are relatively expensive. A semisynthetic derivative of rifamycin B, rifampin has a wide spectrum of antibacterial activity. Its spectrum includes activity against *Neisseria*, *Staphylococcus*, *Haemophilus*, most streptococci, and several species of Enterobacteriaceae. It is best known for its activity against mycobacteria, having activity equal to that of INH. It acts by the inhibition of DNA-dependent RNA polymerase, preventing chain initiation. Most mycobacteria are inhibited by concentrations of 0.5 μg/ml. Rifampin is more active than INH against the slow- or intermittently growing organisms present in macrophages. It also seems to be the most active agent in killing the organisms in semisolid caseous material (24). The synergy obtained when INH and RMP are used together has enabled the duration of treatment for tuberculosis to be shortened from 18 to 24 months to 6 to 9 months (31). If used alone, resistance develops rapidly to RMP.

The usual adult dose is 600 mg, given as a single dose. The pediatric dose ranges from 10 to 20 mg/kg/day up to a maximum of 600 mg. Following oral administration, the drug is well absorbed from the gastrointestinal tract. Peak serum concentrations 1 to 4 hr after a 600-mg oral dose in adults or 10 mg/kg in children are approximately 7 μg/ml (range, 4 to 32) (32–35). Food interferes with absorption, lowering and delaying peak blood levels. Rifampin is 60 to 90% protein bound, is highly lipid soluble and penetrates well into the tissues, including the CNS, lungs, liver, and bone (24). Patients should be cautioned to expect orange discoloration of urine, sweat, tears, and saliva. Although these findings present no serious threat to the patient, soft contact lenses may be permanently discolored.

Approximately 60 to 80% of RMP undergoes metabolism by enterohepatic circulation. Nearly all RMP excreted into the bile is deacetylated to desacetylrifampin, a metabolite that is only slightly less active against mycobacteria than the parent compound (24). The metabolite has also been shown to undergo enterohepatic circulation in competition with bile (36). A small portion of the drug is found in the urine as formylrifampin. The serum half-life of RMP is dose-dependent, initially ranging from 1.5 to 5 hr. Because RMP is a potent inducer of the hepatic microsomal P-450 mixed oxidase drug-detoxifying system of enzymes, it induces its own metabolism as well as that of other drugs. With this increase in metabolism, the half-life of RMP drops to 2 to 3 hr (37). Dosage adjustments may be necessary in the presence of hepatic dysfunction, but they are not necessary in patients with renal impairment. Because RMP is a potent inducer of hepatic microsomal enzymes, clinically important interactions have occurred with cortisone, methadone, warfarin, oral contraceptive agents, ketoconazole, phenytoin, and cyclosporine. These interactions can result in such clinical effects as transplant rejection, adrenal insufficiency, seizures, and unplanned pregnancy (38). Rifampin also increases the clearance of thyroxine, and in patients receiving thyroid replacement therapy, it may result in hypothyroidism (39).

Adverse effects to RMP occur infrequently, usually in less than 4% of patients taking usual doses. The most common adverse effects are rash (0.8%), fever (0.5%), and gastrointestinal upset (i.e., nausea and vomiting; 1.5%). Other potential toxicities include hepatitis and thrombocytopenia. Hepatitis secondary to RMP administered alone or in combination with INH has been reported frequently (40–42). When RMP is administered alone, hepatitis with elevations in AST levels occurs in approximately 10% of patients. Though it remains controversial whether the concomitant use of RMP and INH increases the incidence of hepatotoxicity, in a study by Bassetti and associates (43), hepatotoxicity with hypertransaminasemia was evident in 4.4% and 9.6% of patients treated with INH alone or the combination of INH and RMP, respectively. Hepatitis rarely occurs in patients with normal liver function; however, as seen with INH administration, chronic liver disease, alcoholism, and old age appear to increase the risk of hepatotoxicity with RMP (24).

Intermittent administration of higher doses of RMP has been associated with the development of an immunologically mediated reaction, typically classified as a "flu-like" syndrome. This syndrome is rarely observed with daily administration, and classically occurs in individuals receiving more than 15 to 20 mg/kg/dose at twice-weekly intervals. The clinical picture consists of fever, chills, malaise, arthralgias, headache, and rarely, purpura with thrombocytopenia, hemolytic anemia, respiratory distress, and acute renal failure. Typically, the patient also describes flushing and/or pruritus with or without a rash, nausea, vomiting, and abdominal pain. Rifampin has also been demonstrated to have immunosuppressive effects in both human and animals, but the clinical importance of this remains unclear.

Although 600 mg/day is the usual adult dosage, 600 mg twice weekly has been well tolerated (44). Severe toxicities have been seen with higher dosages (900 to 1200 mg). Patients should be monitored for gastrointestinal symptoms, liver enzyme elevation, renal function, and complete blood counts. Patients should be instructed to adhere to the prescribed dosing schedule, since inconsistency in dosing may increase the incidence of toxicity.

Ethambutol. Introduced in the U.S. in 1967, ethambutol (EMB), or *d*-ethylenediimino-di-1-butanol dihydrochloride, is a synthetic antimycobacterial agent that is less active than INH or RMP. It is tuberculostatic and should be used primarily to supplement INH or RMP. Ethambutol has been shown to require about 24 hr before inhibition of the mycobacteria organism is seen. Its exact mechanism is unknown, although it appears to suppress multiplication by interfering with RNA synthesis. The drug appears to have in vivo activity against actively dividing mycobacteria. Most mycobacteria are inhibited by 1 to 4 μg/ml. The peak plasma concentration 2 to 4 hr after a 25 mg/kg oral dose is approximately 2 to 5 μg/ml (24).

Approximately 80% of EMB is absorbed from the gastrointestinal tract. Therapy is usually initiated with 15 to 25 mg/kg as a single dose for the first 6 to 8 weeks, then decreased to 15 mg/kg/day for the remainder of therapy. Food does not interfere with absorption. The maximum recommended dose is 2.5 g per day. As an alternative to the single daily dose, 50 mg/kg twice weekly has been used. Ethambutol penetrates well into most tissues and fluids. However, even in the face of inflamed meninges, the concentration in the CSF remains low. Approximately 80% of an oral dose is excreted in the urine; at least 50% is excreted unchanged through glomerular filtration and tubular secretion, the remaining amount as an inactive metabolite. Hepatic metabolism occurs through oxidation to the aldehyde or carboxylic acid form. Another 20% is eliminated unchanged through fecal excretion. The serum half-life for EMB is 3 to 4 hr in patients with normal renal function and increases up to 8 hr with renal impairment (24). Dosage adjustment is required in patients with impaired renal function; 50% reduction in the normal dose in individuals with creatinine clearances between 10 and 50 ml/min and 65% reduction in dose in individuals with clearances under 10 ml/min (45). Significant amounts of EMB are removed from the blood following hemodialysis and peritoneal dialysis. No dosage adjustment is necessary with hepatic dysfunction.

Ethambutol is relatively free of toxicities. The most serious adverse effect noted with EMB is retrobulbar neuritis, characterized by decreasing visual acuity and loss of red-green color vision. The frequency appears to be dose-related and is more common at doses above 50 mg/kg/day (46). The occurrence rate is reported to be 5% in patients receiving daily doses of 25 mg/kg and is less than 1% in patients treated with 15 mg/kg/day (24). Baseline examination of visual acuity should be done prior to prescribing EMB, followed by monthly eye examinations. The drug accumulates with renal dysfunction, contributing to an increased frequency of ocular toxicity. Patients should be warned to immediately discontinue the drug if they experience a decrease in visual acuity. Dosage adjustment, as outlined above, is mandatory. Other toxicities of EMB include hypersensitivity reactions (i.e., fever, rash), neuritis, gastrointestinal intolerance, headache, and hyperuricemia; the latter having the potential to cause clinical gout (47).

Pyrazinamide. Introduced in 1952, pyrazinamide (PZA) is a synthetic pyrazine analog of nicotinamide, with bactericidal activity against mycobacteria. In the past, PZA has been considered to be a second-line agent; however, the drug has recently been used as a first-time drug in short-course regimens with INH and RMP. Although its exact mechanism is unknown, the drug is unique in that it is rapidly bacteriostatic and slowly bactericidal against the slow-growing bacilli within the acidic pH of the macrophages (48). It is thus able to penetrate and kill tubercle bacilli that other antituberculous agents do not. Because of this unique intracellular ability, several clinical studies have suggested that PZA is most useful in the initial phase of therapy. These organisms are most responsible for relapse. The minimum inhibitory concentration (in an acidic environment) is 20 µg/ml against *Mycobacterium tuberculosis*. Within the monocytes themselves, the tubercle bacilli are killed by concentrations of 12.5 µg/ml. Pyrazinamide is also well absorbed from the gastrointestinal tract, achieving peak serum concentrations of 33 µg/ml 2 hr after a 1.5-g dose. The recommended dosage ranges from 15 to 30 mg/kg daily, up to a maximum of 2 g. The elimination half-life is 9 to 10 hr in normal individuals. It is widely distributed to most fluids and tissues, including the liver, lungs, and CSF. Pyrazinamide undergoes both renal and hepatic elimination. The drug is primarily (approximately 70%) excreted by glomerular filtration. PZA also undergoes extensive hepatic biotransformation. It is first hydroxylated to pyrazinoic acid, which is subsequently hydroxylated to 5-hydroxypyrazinoic acid, the major excretory product. Minor dosage adjustments may be required with kidney disease (24).

The major adverse effect of PZA is dose-dependent hepatotoxicity. Early studies using high doses of approximately 3 g daily reported a 15% incidence of hepatotoxicity (24). Also seen in these early studies were transient, asymptomatic elevation of serum transaminase levels. The incidence of hepatitis appears to be much lower in regimens where 2 g/day or less are used. Other untoward effects that have been observed with of PZA are arthralgias, hypersensitivity reactions, photosensitivity, anorexia, nausea and vomiting, dysuria, malaise, and fever. Pyrazin-

amide may cause elevations in the prothrombin time (by decreasing prothrombin concentration or activity), serum bilirubin levels, and serum uric acid levels (by inhibiting renal tubular secretion of uric acid). Precipitation of an acute gouty attack may be a problem in individuals with a history of gout and may warrant discontinuation of the drug (49).

Streptomycin. Released in 1947, streptomycin (STM) was the first clinically effective drug to become available for the treatment of tuberculosis. An aminoglycoside, its use has been limited by its significant ototoxicity and need for intramuscular administration. Streptomycin is bactericidal in the neutral pH of the extracellular environment and acts by inhibiting protein synthesis. Streptomycin diffuses poorly into granulomas and macrophages and lacks activity in the intracellular environment. Strains of *M. tuberculosis* are inhibited by serum concentrations as low as 0.4 µg/ml, but the majority are sensitive to 10.0 µg/ml (24).

The normal dose is 1 g daily for the first 2 to 8 weeks, followed by 1 g twice weekly. Peak serum levels averaging approximately 40 µg/ml are achieved 1 hr after a 15 mg/kg intramuscular dose. The drug is approximately 90% excreted unchanged in the urine. Its serum half-life is 2 to 5 hr in normal individuals. In the presence of renal impairment, STM half-life may be prolonged to 27 to 111 hr (50). Because the drug is excreted primarily via the kidney, the dose should be reduced in patients with impaired renal function. This can be accomplished easily by increasing the dosing interval. Bennett and associates (51) recommend a dosing interval of every 24 to 72 and 72 to 96 hr in patients with a GFR between 10 and 50 ml/min and less than 10 ml/min, respectively. Hemodialysis has been noted to reduce serum concentrations by 66% during a 12-hour dialysis (52). STM has moderate tissue distribution. However, it penetrates the CSF very poorly.

Major toxicities include eighth cranial nerve toxicity, usually causing vertigo and ataxia. Deafness may also occur. This has been more of a problem in older individuals or those with compromised renal function. Other toxicities include hypersensitivity, fever, and less commonly nephrotoxicity. Many drug interactions are known to occur with concomitant administration with STM. Perhaps the best known of these is the interaction of STM with neuromuscular blocking agents (e.g., pancuronium, tubocurarine), which results in prolonged respiratory depression (53). All patients should have baseline hearing and renal function tests. Patients receiving STM should then be monitored periodically for changes. Monitoring serum concentrations may be useful, particularly in those with renal impairment.

p-Aminosalicylate. *p*-Aminosalicylate (PAS) is a highly specific, tuberculostatic agent that is rarely used in today's antituberculous regimens. Once first-line, this now second-line agent has a mechanism of action that is believed to be similar to that of the sulfonamides, competitive antagonism of PABA. It inhibits most *M. tuberculosis* at concentrations of 1 μg/ml (24). The usual adult dose is 10 to 12 g/day in 2 or 3 divided doses and 200–300 mg/kg/24 hr in divided doses every 6 hr in children. The drug is readily absorbed from the gastrointestinal tract and distributes evenly to most tissues and fluids. Plasma concentrations reach between 75 and 100 μg/ml within 1 to 2 hr after a single 4-g oral dose (24). High doses are necessary because of an elimination half-life of about 1 hr. Protein binding is high (60 to 70%), and CSF concentrations are low. Approximately 50% of a dose of PAS is metabolized to the active, acetylated compound that is then eliminated in the urine (24). The dose should be reduced in patients with severe renal impairment but not necessarily in patients with hepatic disease.

The frequency of untoward effects associated with the use of PAS is approximately 10 to 30% (24). Gastrointestinal upset (nausea, vomiting, anorexia, diarrhea, and epigastric pain) is most frequently seen, and contributes to patient noncompliance. Other adverse effects include hypersensitivity reactions, acidosis, thrombocytopenia, and rarely hepatitis. *p*-Aminosalicylic acid interacts with both INH and RMP. Concomitant PAS and INH results in increases in INH serum levels through competition for hepatic metabolism. Administration of PAS and RMP impairs the GI absorption of RMP, decreasing serum concentrations (54). Patients should receive instruction on compliance with the medication and be advised to take PAS with meals, to minimize gastric irritation. Patients should have routine monitoring of a complete blood count.

Ethionamide. Ethionamide, or α-ethylthioisonicotinamide, is another second-line oral agent, structurally similar to INH, but with less activity. It is indicated in combination with other antituberculous agents following failure with the primary regimens. Its mechanism of action is unknown, but it appears to act by inhibiting protein synthesis. Most strains of *M. tuberculosis* are inhibited by concentrations of 0.6 to 2.5 μg/ml. This agent may be either tuberculostatic or tuberculocidal, depending upon the susceptibility of the organism and on drug concentration at the site of infection. Resistance develops rapidly in vitro; cross-resistance occurs between ethionamide and INH (24). The usual daily adult dose is 15 to 20 mg/kg, up to a maximum of 1 g. Rapid absorption from the gastrointestinal tract follows oral administration, yielding peak concentrations of about 20 μg/ml in 3 hr. The serum half-life is 3 hr. Ethionamide is rapidly and widely distributed; the concentrations in blood and various organs are approximately equal. Elimination occurs through hepatic metabolism (24). Anorexia, nausea, and vomiting are the most common untoward effects of ethionamide. In addition, increased salivation and a metallic taste in the mouth may occur.

Other adverse effects that occur include arthralgias, impotence, photosensitivity dermatitis, gynecomastia, hypotension, and hepatitis. Convulsions and peripheral neuropathy are rare. Patients should have periodic liver enzyme determinations, with the drug being discontinued if the hepatic enzymes reach five times normal levels. Gastrointestinal disturbances can be minimized by dividing the dose into 3 or 4 equal-sized doses and administering after meals.

Cycloserine. The use of cycloserine as an antituberculous agent, like ethionamide, is limited to certain situations. An analog of the amino acid D-alanine, cycloserine inhibits the processes that incorporate D-alanine in cell wall synthesis. Because of inhibitory concentrations of 5 to 20 μg/ml, the drug is normally considered to be bacteriostatic. Cycloserine is rapidly absorbed from the gastrointestinal tract following the usual dose of 15 to 20 mg/kg/day. It is well distributed throughout most body fluids and tissues, including the CSF. Cycloserine is used infrequently because of its high incidence of adverse effects. It frequently causes central nervous system disturbances such as mood changes, headaches, tremor, vertigo, confusion, visual disturbances, nystagmus, lethargy, and seizures. Use of this agent is contraindicated in those with a history of epilepsy, depression, or severe anxiety. Concurrent use with ethionamide, INH, and alcohol may increase the risk of CNS toxicities or seizures (24).

Capreomycin and Kanamycin. These agents are aminoglycoside antibiotics that require intramuscular administration in combination with other effective antituberculous agents. Concurrent use of more than one aminoglycoside should absolutely be avoided. Pharmacologically, they are similar to STM but somewhat less effective. Capreomycin and kanamycin are both bacteriostatic and act by inhibiting protein synthesis. Frequent adverse reactions that occur following administration are hearing loss, tinnitus, pain on injection, eosinophilia, and nephrotoxicity. Since these agents are eliminated via the kidneys, dose reduction is essential in renal impairment. Audiometry performed at baseline and then monthly intervals is recommended. Routine monitoring of serum creatinine levels as well as serum concentrations may prevent renal toxicity.

New Agents. The search for new antimycobacterial agents has been rejuvenated by the need to treat opportunistic infections associated with HIV infection. Until recently, research in this area had been hampered by the lack of economic incentives and the limited potential market for these drugs. It had been several years since new compounds with suitable antimycobacterial potential were developed. The last was RMP, introduced in 1971. Newer agents have now been studied in vitro, but the availability of in vivo data is limited. The quinolone class of antimicrobial agents has demonstrated bactericidal activity that would suggest that these agents will be useful as alternatives in the treatment of tuberculosis. The quinolones most active against *M. tuberculosis* appear to be ciprofloxacin and ofloxacin, with inhibitory concentrations ranging from 0.25 to 2.0 μg/ml (55, 56). They have suitable pharmacokinetic properties and penetrate into mammalian cells. Certainly, it should be borne in mind that the emergence of resistance is common within the quinolone class. Toxicities associated with the quinolones have been minimal.

Several new rifamycin derivatives have been studied. Rifapentine (MDL473) is a cyclopentyl derivative of RMP. In comparison with RMP, it has several pharmacokinetic advantages including higher peak serum levels, better tissue penetration, longer half-life, and less-effective induction of hepatic desacetylation. In vitro, it appears to be less active than RMP, however, human studies have not been reported. Rifabutine (ansamycin, LM 427), a semisynthetic derivative of rifamycin S, is reported to have broader antimycobacterial properties than RMP, even against some RMP-resistant strains. Rifabutin is often used in combination with other effective antimycobacterial agents for the treatment of MAI infections in AIDS patients. The drug is available from the CDC Drug Service for compassionate use. CGP 7040 is also a rifamycin derivative with activity comparable to RMP and a half-life of more than 30 hr (55).

Clofazimine, an oral phenazine dye, has been approved for use in the treatment of leprosy. It has also demonstrated in vitro and in vivo activity against *M. tuberculosis* and nontuberculous mycobacteria. While the drug appears to have good in vitro activity, with minimum inhibitory concentrations ranging from 0.1 to 3.3 μg/ml, the efficacy against tuberculous infections has not been established (55).

Gangamicin or CQQ, a dual vitamin K–coenzyme Q analog, has been found to have activity against both *M. tuberculosis* and *M. avium* complex. In one study, most *M. tuberculosis* isolates were inhibited by a CQQ concentration of 1 μg/ml. However, 24-hr drug exposure was required before inhibition of growth was seen (55). Other agents having activity against tuberculosis isolates include dihydromycoplanecin A, a cyclic peptide antibiotic, and fusidic acid. Little is known about these agents at this time. Immunomodulators (e.g., interferon-γ, interleukin-2, tumor necrosis factor) and novel drug delivery systems (i.e., liposome-encapsulation) are presently under study. Finally, several β-lactams, other aminoglycosides, sulfonamides, macrolides, and the folate antagonists are all presently under study.

TREATMENT REGIMENS

A positive sputum for acid-fast bacilli is sufficient evidence to begin therapy in patients with an appropriate clinical picture (57). Optimally, selection of appropriate antimicrobial agents should be based on culture and sensitivity testing; however, waiting for culture results (which may take up to 6 weeks) is undesirable and impractical. A decision to initiate early therapy must be based upon clinical and radiographic findings on chest roentgenograms (58). Hilar lymphadenopathy alone is sufficient evidence to initiate early therapy in children, even in the absence of a pulmonary infiltrate (59).

Currently available antituberculous drug regimens are highly effective, well-tolerated, and relatively easily administered. However, for nearly 30 years, treatment of active tuberculosis involved the use of two to three drugs for 18 to 24 months. Isoniazid, PAS, and STM were the major components of those chemotherapeutic regimens. Although these regimens were quite effective, compliance was poor because of lengthy treatments, relatively high cost of some of the drugs, and drug toxicities. As a result, relapse rates were high. Since the introduction of RMP, it has been possible to shorten the duration of treatment. Rifampin, in combination with INH and STM has shown a cure rate of almost 100% during a 9-month treatment period, i.e., half the time required with the three drug regimen of INH + STM + PAS (60, 61). Numerous investigators have studied the effectiveness of short-course chemotherapy.

Short-course antituberculous therapy (defined as treatment for 9 months or less) is divided into an initial bactericidal phase and a subsequent sterilizing phase (62). The initial bactericidal phase or "induction" phase of chemotherapy constitutes the first 2 to 3 months of therapy. The goal of this phase is to rapidly eliminate the extracellular organisms from the sputum and decrease the infectivity of the patient using agents such as INH, STM, RMP, and PZA. The second phase, also referred to as the "consolidation" or "continuation" phase, usually extends for at least 4 months. The objective is to destroy the slowly dividing intracellular organisms or "persisters," best accomplished with RMP and INH. Antimycobacterial agents that are actively bactericidal may not be the most active sterilizing agent; the opposite is also true. Not only was it important that the regimen of STM and INH used in the 1950s be administered for 18 to 24 months, but this regimen was effective only against extracellular organisms. For complete eradication it was essential that remaining populations of organisms (persisters) migrate from the extracellular site where these organisms would be more prone to destruction by the host's immune system (63).

Short-course chemotherapy represents an important advance in the treatment of tuberculosis. The combination of INH (300 mg) plus RMP (600 mg) administered once daily for 9 months is now an established regimen, effective against both pulmonary and extrapulmonary tuberculosis (60, 64). Six-month trial of INH plus RMP proved unacceptable, because of relapse rates between 7 and 9% (65, 66). Triple-drug regimens, (INH-RMP plus either STM or EMB), are often used during the early stages of treatment while awaiting drug sensitivity results in individuals where primary drug resistance is difficult to rule out. A number of studies have demonstrated that a 6-month regimen of INH-RMP-PZA plus either STM or EMB for 2 months followed by 4 months of INH-RMP-PZA treatment produces excellent results with low relapse rates (67). Still, additional studies with this regimen have demonstrated that the addition of PZA to RMP and INH during the first 2 months of treatment is the critical agent, and EMB and STM probably contribute very little (23, 31, 68, 69). A recently published study conducted by the United States Public Health Service (Study 21) clearly demonstrated that a 6-month regimen of INH-RMP-PZA had similar effectiveness, toxicities, and acceptability when compared with the 9-month regimen of INH-RMP (70). Another study has shown that addition of EMB to 6-month regimens of INH-RMP appears to be no more effective than the INH-RMP combination and results in relapse rates around 8 to 18% after completing therapy (71). An acceptable alternative for both 6- and 9-month regimens is intermittent administration of appropriate antituberculous agents following an initial daily phase. When a 9-month regimen is used, INH and RMP are administered daily as described above for 2 months, and then twice weekly with the same dose of RMP but with a larger (900 mg) dose of INH. Similarly, for a 6-month regimen, INH and RMP may be given either daily or twice weekly for the last 4 months. Twice-weekly dosing is less expensive and may be useful to achieve greater patient compliance.

In summary, short-course chemotherapy in most situations is the ideal treatment for new cases of tuberculosis unless drug resistance is suspected. In general, these regimens offer many advantages: reduction of total cost of the treatment, decreased cost of medications, and less toxicity than observed with the prolonged use of standard medications. Compliance and patient acceptance are also better. Two short-course treatment regimens have been routinely used in the United States. A 9-month regimen of INH in combination with RMP with or without STM or EMB (administered daily for 2 months) followed by 7 months of INH and RMP administered daily or twice weekly has been highly effective. A 6-month regimen consisting of 2 months of INH, RMP plus PZA followed by 4 months of INH-RMP therapy, daily or twice weekly, has also been successful.

Isoniazid and rifampin have similar activities and when possible all regimens should contain these agents. However, when INH or RMP cannot be used (i.e., resistance, adverse effects, allergy), EMB may replace either drug. In either case, this change results in a less effective regimen and treatment duration should be extended. The regimen

of INH and EMB requires 18 to 24 months of treatment, while the combination of RMP and EMB requires only 12 to 18 months for sufficient treatment (72). The addition of PZA for the first 2 months to the combination of RMP and EMB improves the efficacy and permits shortening of therapy to 9 months (73), however the effect of PZA on INH-EMB has not been assessed.

SPECIAL TREATMENT CIRCUMSTANCES

Children. Treatment of tuberculosis in children is essentially identical to that in adults. A 9-month course of INH and RMP, with 1 initial month of daily administration followed by 8 months of twice-weekly administration has had a high rate of success (74). A 6-month regimen with INH, RMP, and PZA has the same success in children as in adults. Doses of these agents should be based on mg/kg body weight. Because the major toxicity of EMB is retrobulbar neuritis and because ocular toxicity is difficult to monitor in young children, this agent is of limited usefulness in pediatric populations. Experience with PZA in children is also limited, but to date has been found to be safe and effective, particularly in the treatment of tuberculous meningitis (75).

Pregnancy. Treatment of tuberculosis during pregnancy should be initiated promptly with effective chemotherapeutic agents. The risk to the pregnant woman and her fetus is greater if the tuberculosis is left untreated than if treatment is initiated. Of the first-line drugs, INH, RMP, and EMB can be administered safely. The regimen of INH and RMP with or without EMB for 9 months is the treatment of choice (76). Pyridoxine should always be given with INH during pregnancy because of the increased requirement for this vitamin in pregnant women (77). Streptomycin is contraindicated in pregnancy because of the potential of ototoxicity in the fetus (23). Little to no data are available on the teratogenicity of PZA, however it should be avoided unless absolutely necessary. Although INH, RMP, and EMB cross the placental barrier, they have not been shown to have teratogenic effects. Ethionamide should also be avoided whenever possible, as it may cause serious gastrointestinal upset in the fetus. Little is known about the teratogenicity of the other second-line agents (78). Since the pregnant female often continues treatment after delivery, the question of whether it is safe for the mother to breast-feed her infant often arises. Snider and Powell (79) have shown that only small amounts of the antituberculous agents are excreted in the breast milk. However, should the infant also be receiving antituberculous therapy, then breast-feeding probably should be discontinued because of the increased risk for toxicities.

Renal Failure. Certain drugs used to treat tuberculosis may accumulate in the body in the situation of renal impairment. Agent-specific, this accumulation can often lead to serious adverse effects. Appropriate dosage adjustments can often prevent or minimize this problem. Of the first-line agents, INH, RMP, and PZA may be given at the usual dose in mild-to-moderate renal failure. With severe dysfunction, both INH and PZA should be given at two-thirds of the normal daily dose (80, 81). Recommendations concerning STM and EMB are that these agents should also be reduced in renal failure, since toxic serum levels may occur with the usual dose. Streptomycin, kanamycin, and capreomycin should all be used with caution because of the potential for nephrotoxicity. Pyridoxine supplementation should always be used in the uremic patient.

AIDS/HIV Infection. Treatment guidelines for the treatment of tuberculosis in patients with AIDS or HIV infection have been published by the American Thoracic Society and the Centers for Disease Control (23, 82). In general, tuberculosis can be treated effectively with standard drugs in patients with HIV infection. These patients should be given INH and RMP with the addition of 2 months of PZA or EMB if PZA can not be used. Ethambutol should be added as a fourth agent to the INH-RMP-PZA regimen if INH resistance is suspected. Optimal duration of therapy is not known. The CDC recommends that treatment should extend for a minimum of 9 months and for a least 6 months after documented culture conversion, as evidenced by three negative cultures. Others prescribe INH-RMP therapy for 12 to 18 months and a minimum of 9 months after culture conversion. Experience in treating AIDS-related tuberculosis using these regimens has shown a response comparable to non-HIV-infected tuberculosis patients. Isoniazid resistance is no more common in these individuals, however, adverse reactions are more common in patients with advanced HIV disease (82).

NONDRUG THERAPY

In general, tuberculosis can be treated on an outpatient basis unless the patient has a life-threatening infection or confounding factors requiring hospitalization. It must be recognized that patients receiving appropriate drug therapy remain infectious for a short period of time. According to the CDC, persons should be considered infectious if "cough is present, if cough-inducing procedures are performed, or if sputum smears are known to contain acid-fast bacilli (AFB), and if these patients are not on chemotherapy, have just started chemotherapy, or have a poor clinical or bacteriologic response to chemotherapy." Any infectious patient with pulmonary tuberculosis, hospitalized or in any other inpatient facility, should be placed in respiratory isolation until the patient becomes noninfectious. CDC defines this as "a person with tuberculosis who has been on adequate chemotherapy for at least 2 to 3 weeks and has had a definite clinical and bacteriologic response to therapy (reduction in cough, resolution of fever, and progressively decreasing quantity of bacilli on

smear)." Persons entering a room in which AFB isolation precautions are in effect should be instructed to wear properly fitted mask (e.g., PRs, which are valveless particulate respirators). Patients should receive instruction on such simple precautions as remaining in the room with the door closed, covering their nose and mouth when coughing, and wearing a properly fitted surgical mask when required to leave the room (83).

In past years there were two indications for surgery in the treatment of tuberculosis. The first was for the resection of cavitary lesions; the other for performing collapse procedures that created an unfavorable environment for organisms to grow. Now, because of effective antituberculous chemotherapy, surgery has been relegated to a minor role (84).

MONITORING RESPONSE TO TREATMENT

Noncompliance continues to be a significant problem in the treatment of tuberculosis, which reinforces the need for close monitoring of patients throughout therapy. Relapse is also a major concern in patients having received treatment for tuberculosis. Relapse can be defined as a subsequent recurrence of a positive sputum in a patient who has had a negative sputum upon completing a course of chemotherapy. Relapses usually occur within the first 12 months following chemotherapy. Because of this, patients should undergo routine bacteriologic evaluation during and for the first 6 to 12 months after completion of therapy. Serial chest radiographs are not a sensitive or efficient method of monitoring therapeutic response.

CHEMOPROPHYLAXIS

According to the American Thoracic Society and Centers for Disease Control (23) preventive therapy should consist of INH (10 to 15 mg/kg daily up to a maximum of 300 mg). An alternative is twice-weekly dosing of 15 mg/kg (up to 900 mg) if noncompliance is a problem and direct observation is needed. The recommended duration is controversial and has varied from 6 to 12 months of daily administration. Individuals with HIV infection and those with stable abnormal chest radiographs consistent with tuberculosis should definitely receive 12 months of therapy. Because of recent recommendation changes, it is unclear who should receive preventive therapy. It should be emphasized that the administration of INH is preventive therapy instead of prophylaxis. The purpose of INH therapy is to prevent latent (asymptomatic) infection from progressing to clinical disease or the recurrence of past, untreated disease. Individuals receiving preventive therapy have already been exposed to the tubercle bacilli. Despite its proven effectiveness, the CDC reports that less than 60% of persons at risk of contacting tuberculosis are being started on preventive therapy (CDC, unpublished data).

A reason may be the dilemma clinicians face in initiating INH therapy in individuals >35 years of age because of the untoward effects. To assist in who should receive chemoprophylaxis, the Advisory Committee for Elimination of Tuberculosis (ACET) has recommended that priority for preventive therapy be given to the following groups regardless of age (85):

1. Persons with HIV infection with a tuberculin reaction ≥5 mm and persons with risk factors for HIV infection whose HIV infection status is unknown but who are suspected of having HIV infection.
2. Close contacts of persons with newly diagnosed infectious tuberculosis and a tuberculin reaction ≥5 mm. In addition, tuberculin-negative (<5 mm) children and adolescents who have been close contacts of infectious persons within the past 3 months are candidates for preventive therapy until a repeat tuberculin skin test is done 12 weeks after contact with the infectious source.
3. Recent converters, as indicated by a tuberculin skin test. Recent conversion being: ≥10 mm increase within a 2-year period for those <35 years old or ≥15 mm increase for those ≥35 years of age.
4. Persons with abnormal chest radiographs that show fibrotic lesions likely to represent old healed tuberculosis and a tuberculin reaction of ≥5 mm.
5. Intravenous drug users known to be HIV-seronegative but having a tuberculin reaction of ≥10 mm.
6. Persons with medical conditions that have been reported to increase the risk of tuberculosis (e.g., diabetics, immunocompromised, postgastrectomy) and having a tuberculin reaction of ≥10 mm.

In the absence of any of the above factors, persons <35 years of age with a tuberculin skin test ≥10 mm who fall into one of the following high risk groups should also receive preventive therapy:

1. Foreign-born persons from high-prevalence countries;
2. Medically underserved low-income populations, including high-risk racial or ethnic minority populations, especially blacks, Hispanics, and Native Americans;
3. Residents long-term facilities (e.g., correctional institutions, nursing homes, and mental institutions).

Before giving INH preventive therapy, active tuberculosis must be ruled out. For this reason, a chest radiograph is recommended whenever a tuberculin test is reactive. When in doubt, it is better to initiate therapy with two or more agents until proven otherwise, to avoid the possibility of INH resistance. Preventive therapy is contraindicated in individuals allergic to or with documented adverse reactions to INH and those with active disease. Because of the potential for adverse reactions, particularly hepatotoxicity, patients should have liver enzyme levels monitored closely on a monthly basis (85).

USE OF VACCINES (BCG)

The only available vaccine for the prevention of tuberculosis is the bacillus Calmette-Guérin (BCG). BCG is a live attenuated strain of *M. bovis*, which is used as a vaccine against tuberculosis. It was first used against human tuberculosis in 1921, in France, and works by inducing tuberculin hypersensitivity. Despite its use today in more than 70% of the world's children, there is conflicting evidence of its safety and effectiveness in preventing disease (86). The controversy surrounds the results of the eight major controlled trials using BCG. The efficacy in these trials varied greatly, ranging from 0 to 80%. Why these disparate results occurred are unclear, but they are best explained by unequal potency and other differences in the vaccine strains, study methodology, and nutritional status of the patients. Several studies have suggested that the vaccine provides protection against childhood forms of the disease, such as pulmonary and disseminated forms of tuberculosis. The vaccine has limited use in prevention of tuberculosis in adults. BCG is most effective in areas with a high incidence of new infection; thus it is not recommended for routine use in the United States. It is recommended for infants and children who cannot receive INH chemoprophylaxis but who are at high risk because of close, prolonged contacts with infectious individuals (86, 87). Vaccination with BCG makes interpretation of the tuberculin skin test difficult, since vaccination converts most tuberculin-negative reactors to positive reactors. There can also be a booster effect of the tuberculin reaction to tuberculin after receiving BCG vaccination. It is impossible to clinically distinguish a reaction due to previous BCG vaccination from one due to *M. tuberculosis*. However, the BCG reactions are often less than 10 mm in induration, and tend to diminish over time (88). Vaccinated patients who have large reactions to a tuberculin skin test must be evaluated for clinical tuberculosis and treated accordingly.

The BCG vaccine is usually given as an intracutaneous inoculation, most commonly in the deltoid region. A wheal of about 8 mm in diameter normally results. A postvaccinal scar is common evidence of having received the vaccine. Though the current BCG vaccine is cheap, safe, and normally requires a single inoculation, it is less than ideal because of the unpredictable immunity for different populations. Serious complications following BCG administration are rare. Local ulceration and regional suppurative lymphadenitis are most common, occurring in 0.5% of the cases. The vaccination is contraindicated in pregnancy, with any other active infection, or in immunocompromised patients, including those with HIV infection (85, 86).

CONCLUSION

Tuberculosis is an infectious disease with major public health significance. Chemotherapy of tuberculosis is the cornerstone of effective treatment, and is usually initiated upon evidence of a positive sputum smear. The major determinant of the outcome of tuberculosis treatment is compliance. If a patient is to be noncompliant, it is likely to be during the first 6 to 8 weeks of a 6- to 9-month treatment period. Twenty to 50% of tuberculosis patients in a recent literature review failed to complete therapy within a 24-month period. The consequences were treatment failures, relapses, additional treatment, additional expense, increases in drug resistance, and death. After starting therapy, management of patients requires monitoring for adverse effects, ensuring patient compliance, and evaluating for bacteria eradication.

REFERENCES

1. Reider HL, Cauthen GM, Kelly GD, et al.: Tuberculosis in the United States. JAMA 262:385–389, 1989.
2. Centers for Disease Control: Summary of notifiable diseases, United States, 1989. MMWR 38:3, 1990.
3. Fertel D, Pitchenik AE: Tuberculosis in acquired immunodeficiency syndrome. Semin Respir Infect 4:198–205, 1989.
4. Stead WW, Lofgren JP, Warren E, et al.: Tuberculosis as an endemic and nosocomial infection among the elderly in nursing homes. N Engl J Med 312:1483–1487, 1985.
5. Centers for Disease Control: A strategic plan for the elimination of tuberculosis in the United States. MMWR 38(suppl S-3):1, 1989.
6. Des Prez RM, Heim CR, *Mycobacterium tuberculosis*. In Mandell GL, Douglas RG, Bennett JE: Principles and Practice of Infectious Diseases, ed. 3. New York, Churchill Livingstone, 1990, pp 1877–1906.
7. Price LE, Rutala WA, Samsa GP: Tuberculosis in hospital personnel. Infect Control 8:97–101, 1987.
8. Dannenbury AM: Immune mechanisms in the pathogenesis of pulmonary tuberculosis. Rev Infect Dis 11:S369–378, 1989.
9. American Thoracic Society: Diagnostic standards and classification of tuberculosis. Am Rev Respir Dis 142:725–735, 1990.
10. Kim JH, Langston AA, Gallis HA: Miliary tuberculosis: epidemiology, clinical manifestations, diagnosis and outcomes. Rev Infect Dis 12:583–590, 1990.
11. Modilevsky T, Sattler FR, Barnes PF: Mycobacterial disease in patients with human immunodeficiency virus infection. Arch Intern Med 149:2201–2205, 1989.
12. Iseman MD, Madsen LA: Drug-resistant tuberculosis. Clin Chest Med 10(3):341–353, 1989.
13. Al-Orainey IOM: Drug resistance in tuberculosis. J Chemother 2(3):147–151, 1990.
14. Barnes PF: The influence of epidemiologic factors on drug resistance rates in tuberculosis. Am Rev Respir Dis 136:325–328, 1987.
15. Scalcini M, Carré G, Jean-Baptiste M, et al.: Antituberculous drug resistance in central Haiti. Am Rev Respir Dis 142:508–511, 1990.
16. Mitchison DA, Nunn AJ: Influence of initial drug resistance on the response to short-course chemotherapy of pulmonary tuberculosis. Am Rev Respir Dis 131:423–430, 1986.
17. Dickinson JM, Aber VR, Mitchison DA: Bactericidal activity of streptomycin, isoniazid, rifampin, ethambutol, and pyrazinamide alone and in combination against *Mycobacterium tuberculosis*. Am Rev Respir Dis 116:625–635, 1977.
18. Hurwitz A, Schlozman DL: Effects of antacids on gastrointestinal absorption of isoniazid in rat and man. Am Rev Respir Dis 109:41–47, 1974.
19. Holdiness MR: Cerebrospinal pharmacokinetics of the antituberculosis drugs. Clin Pharmacokinet 10:532–534, 1985.
20. Palmer PE: Pulmonary tuberculosis-usual and unusual radiographic presentation. Semin Roentgenol 14:204–243, 1979.
21. Anderson RJ, Gambertoglio JG, Schrier RW: Clinical use of drugs in renal failure. Springfield, Illinois: Charles C Thomas, 1976.
22. Bennett WM, Aronoff GR, Morrison G, et al.: Drug prescribing in renal failure: dosing guidelines for adults. Am J Kidney Dis 3:155–193, 1983.
23. American Thoracic Society/Centers for Disease Control: Treatment of tuberculosis and tuberculosis infection in adults and children. Am Rev Respir Dis 134:355–363, 1986.
24. Mandell GL, Sande MA, Drugs used in the chemotherapy of tuberculosis and leprosy. In Gilman AG, Goodman LS, Gilman A: The Pharmacological Basis of Therapeutics, ed. 7. New York, Macmillan, 1985, pp 1205–1206.
25. Kopanoff DE, Snider DE Jr, Caras GJ: Isoniazid-related hepatitis. A U.S. Public Health Service cooperative surveillance study. Am Rev Respir Dis 117:991–1001, 1978.
26. Stead WW, To T: The significance of the tuberculin skin test in elderly persons. Ann Intern Med 107:837–842, 1987.
27. Taylor WC, Aronson MD, Delbanco TL: Should young adults with a positive tuberculin test take isoniazid? Ann Intern Med 94:808–813, 1981.
28. Black M, Mitchell JR, Zimmerman HJ, et al.: Isoniazid-associated hepatitis in 114 patients. Gastroenterology 69:289–302, 1975.
29. Dash LA, Comstock GW, Flynn PG: Isoniazid preventive therapy: retrospect and prospect. Am Rev Respir Dis 121:1039–1044, 1980.
30. Hoglund P, Nilsson LG, Paulsen O: Interaction between isoniazid and theophylline. Eur J Respir Dis 70:110–116, 1987.
31. Fox W: Whither short-course chemotherapy? Br J Dis Chest 75:331–357, 1981.
32. Kucer A, Bennett N: The use of antibiotics: a comprehensive review with clinical emphasis, ed. 3. Philadelphia: Lippincott, 1979.
33. Koup JR, Williams-Warren J, Viswanathan CT, et al.: Pharmacokinetics of rifampin in children II. Oral bioavailability. Ther Drug Monit 8:17–22, 1986.
34. McCracken GH, Ginsburg CM, Zweighaft TC, et al.: Pharmacokinetics of rifampin in infants and children: relevance to prophylaxis against *Haemophilus influenzae* type b disease. Pediatrics 66:17–21, 1980.
35. Council on Drugs, American Medical Association: Evaluation of a new antituberculous agent. JAMA 220:414–415, 1972.
36. Maggi N, Furesz S, Pallanza R, et al.: Rifampicin desacetylation in the human organism. Arzneim Forsch 19:651–654, 1969.
37. Acocella G: Clinical pharmacokinetics of rifampicin. Clin Pharmacokinet 3:108–127, 1978.
38. Baciewicz AM, Self TH, Bekemeyer WB: Update of rifampin drug interactions. Arch Intern Med 147:565–568, 1987.
39. Isley WL: Effect of rifampin therapy on thyroid function tests in a hypothyroid patient on replacement L-thyroxine. Ann Intern Med 107:517–518, 1987.
40. Most JA, Markel GB: A nearly fatal hepatotoxic reaction to rifampin after halothane anesthesia. Am J Surg 127:593–595, 1974.
41. Scheuer PJ, Lal S, Summerfield JA, et al.: Rifampicin hepatitis. A clinical and histological study. Lancet 1:421–425, 1974.
42. Pessayre D, Bentata M, Degott C, et al.: Isoniazid-rifampin fulminant hepatitis. A possible consequence of the enhancement of isoniazid hepatotoxicity by enzyme induction. Gastroenterology 72:284–289, 1977.
43. Bassetti D, Ciravegna B, Viscoli C: Rifampicin's tolerance in pediatrics. Drugs Exp Clin Res 8:255–257, 1982.
44. Dutt AK, Jones L, Stead WW: Short-course chemotherapy for tuberculosis with largely twice-weekly isoniazid-rifampin. Chest 75:441–447, 1979.
45. Holdiness MR: Clinical pharmacokinetics of the antituberculosis drugs. Clin Pharmacokin 9:511–544, 1984.
46. Leibold JE: The ocular toxicity of ethambutol and its relation to dose. Ann NY Acad Sci 135:904–909, 1966.

47. Postlethwaite AE, Bartel AG, Kelly WN: Hyperuricemia due to ethambutol. N Engl J Med 286:761–762, 1972.

48. Mackandess GB: The intracellular activation of pyrazinamide and nicotinamide. Am Rev Tuberc 74:718–728, 1956.

49. Cullen JH, Early LJA, Fiore JM: The occurrence of hyperuricemia during pyrazinamide-isoniazid therapy. Am Rev Tuberc Pulm Dis 74:289–292, 1956.

50. Kunin CM, Finland M: Persistance of antibiotics in blood of patients with acute renal failure. III. penicillin, streptomycin, erythromycin, and kanamycin. J Clin Invest 38:1509, 1959.

51. Bennett WM, Aronoff GR, Morrison G, et al.: Drug prescribing in renal failure: dosing guidelines for adults. Am J Kidney Dis 3:155–193, 1983.

52. Edwards KDG, Whyte HM: Streptomycin poisoning in renal failure. Br Med J 1:752, 1959.

53. Hansten PD, Horn JR: Drug interactions, ed. 6. Philadelphia: Lea & Febiger, 1989.

54. Hansten PD: Drug Interactions: clinical significance of drug-drug interactions and drug effect on clinical laboratory results, ed. 4. Philadelphia: Lea & Febiger, 1979.

55. Cynamon MH, Klemens SP: New antimycobacterial agents. Clin Chest Med 10:355–364, 1989.

56. Leysen DC, Haemers A, Pattyn SR: Mycobacteria and the new quinolones. Antimicrob Agents Chemother 33:1–5, 1989.

57. Penn RL, George RB, Respiratory infections. In George RB, Light RW, Matthay RA: Chest Medicine. New York, Churchill Livingstone, 1983, pp 403–480.

58. Bates JH: Diagnosis of tuberculosis. Chest 76(suppl):757–763, 1979.

59. Jacobs RF, Abernathy RS: The treatment of tuberculosis in children. Pediatr Infect Dis 4:513–517, 1985.

60. British Thoracic and Tuberculosis Association: Short-course chemotherapy in pulmonary tuberculosis: a controlled trial. Lancet 2:1102–1104, 1976.

61. General report: Overall methods and results. Trial 6,9,12. Rev Fr Mal Respir 5(suppl 1):3–63, 1977.

62. O'Brien RJ: Present chemotherapy of tuberculosis. Semin Respir Infect 4:216–224, 1989.

63. Alford RH, Manian FA, Current antimicrobial management of tuberculosis. In Remington JS, Schwatz MN: Current Clinical Topics in Infectious Diseases. New York, McGraw-Hill, 1987, pp 204–226.

64. Dutt AK, Moers D, Stead WW: Short-course chemotherapy for tuberculosis with mainly twice-weekly isoniazid and rifampin. Am J Med 77:233–242, 1984.

65. Snider DE Jr, Long MW, Cross FS, et al.: Six-months isoniazid-rifampin therapy for pulmonary tuberculosis. Report of a United States Public Health Service cooperative trial. Am Rev Respir Dis 129:573–579, 1984.

66. East Africa/British Medical Research Council: Controlled clinical trial of four 6-month regimens of chemotherapy for pulmonary tuberculosis. Second report. Second East African/British Medical Research Council Study. Am Rev Respir Dis 114:471–475, 1976.

67. Zierski M, Bek E: Side-effects of drug regimens used in short-course chemotherapy for pulmonary tuberculosis. A controlled clinical study. Tubercle 61:41–49, 1980.

68. Committee on Chemotherapy of Tuberculosis—National Consensus Conference on Tuberculosis: Standard therapy for tuberculosis, 1985. Chest 87:117S–124S, 1985.

69. Iseman MD: Short-course chemotherapy for tuberculosis: the harsh realities. Semin Respir Infect 1:213–219, 1986.

70. Combs DL, O'Brien RJ, Geiter LJ: USPHS tuberculosis short-course chemotherapy trial 21: effectiveness, toxicity, and acceptability. Ann Intern Med 112:397–406, 1990.

71. Zierski M, Bek E, Long MW, et al.: Short-course (6-month) cooperative tuberculosis study in Poland: results 30 months after completion of treatment. Am Rev Respir Dis 124:249–251, 1981.

72. Zierski M: Prospects of retreatment of chronic resistant pulmonary tuberculosis patient. A critical review. Lung 154:91–102, 1977.

73. Swai OB, Aluoch JA, Githui WA, et al.: Controlled clinical trial of a regimen of two durations for the treatment of isoniazid resistant pulmonary tuberculosis. Tubercle 69:5–14, 1988.

74. Abernathy RS: Tuberculosis in children and its management. Semin Respir Infect 4(3):232–242, 1989.

75. Holdiness MR: Management of tuberculosis meningitis. Drugs 39:224–233, 1990.

76. Jacobs RF, Abernathy RS: Management of tuberculosis in pregnancy and the newborn. Clin Perinatol 15(2):305–319, 1988.

77. Snider DE Jr: Pyridoxine supplementation during isoniazid therapy. Tubercle 61:191–196, 1980.

78. Holdiness MR: Teratology of the antituberculous drugs. Early Hum Dev 15:61–74, 1987.

79. Snider DE Jr, Powell KE: Should women taking antituberculous drugs breastfeed? Arch Intern Med 144:589–590, 1984.

80. Bowersox DW, Winterbauer RH, Stewart GL, et al.: Isoniazid dosage in patients with renal failure. N Engl J Med 289:84–87, 1973.

81. Stamatakis G, Montes C, Trouvin JH, et al.: Pyrazinamide and pyrazinoic acid pharmacokinetics in patients with chronic renal failure. Clin Nephrol 30:203–234, 1988.

82. American Thoracic Society/Centers for Disease Control: Mycobacterioses and the acquired immunodeficiency syndrome. Am Rev Respir Dis 136:492–496, 1987.

83. Centers for Disease Control: Guidelines for preventing the transmission of tuberculosis in healthcare settings, with special focus on HIV-related issues. MMWR 39:1–29, 1990.

84. Boyars MC: The microbiology, chemotherapy, and surgical treatment of tuberculosis. J Thorac Imag 5(2):1–7, 1990.

85. Centers for Disease Control: Screening for tuberculosis and tuberculous infection in high-risk populations and the use of preventive therapy for tuberculous infection in the United States: recommendations of the advisory committee for elimination of tuberculosis. MMWR 39:1–12, 1990.

86. Fine PM, Rodrigues LC: Mycobacterial diseases. Lancet 335:1016–1020, 1990.

87. Fine PEM: The BCG story: lessons from the past and implications for the future. Rev Infect Dis 11(suppl 2):S353–S359, 1989.

88. Hanson CA, Reichman LB: Tuberculosis skin testing and preventive therapy. Semin Respir Infect 4(3):182–188, 1989.

89. Cuneo WD, Snider DE Jr: Enhancing patient compliance with tuberculosis therapy. Clin Chest Med 10:375–380, 1989.

CHAPTER 63

URINARY TRACT INFECTIONS

DIANE R. ROMAC, Pharm.D.

Urinary tract infections continue to be one of the most common infectious diseases for which medical treatment is sought. These infections are responsible for approximately 6 million office visits in the United States annually, ranking second only to respiratory tract infections. Research continues in an attempt to resolve the controversial issues that remain and to seek new and better approaches to treatment.

DEFINITIONS

The urinary tract consists of the urethra, prostate gland (in males), urinary bladder, ureters, and kidneys. The term *urinary tract infection* (UTI) describes a variety of conditions relating to the parts of the tract in which microorganisms are present in significant quantities.

UTI may be seen solely as the presence of bacteria in the urine (bacteriuria)/or signs and symptoms of bacterial invasion of one or more components of the tract. However localized the infection is initially, once any part of the tract is invaded the entire tract is at risk of infection.

UTIs can be designated as asymptomatic or symptomatic, complicated or uncomplicated, and acute, chronic, or recurrent. The terms asymptomatic, symptomatic, chronic, and acute are self-explanatory. An uncomplicated UTI is defined as an infection in which there is no structural or neurologic abnormality of the urinary tract that interferes with the normal flow of urine in the voiding mechanism of an otherwise healthy patient. A complicated UTI is the result of a congenital abnormality or distortion of the tract, a stone, an indwelling catheter, an enlarged prostate gland, a neurologic deficit, or an infection of a normal tract in a patient with an underlying disease, or one that is hospital-acquired.

The term *recurrent* refers to the recurrence of UTI in a given patient. The recurrent infection is further categorized into relapse or reinfection. If a UTI is a relapse, it is the result of invasion by the same specific serotype of microorganism, usually within 7 to 10 days of completion of antibacterial therapy for the preceding UTI. Relapse accounts for approximately 20% of recurrent attacks. The remaining 80% of recurrent infections can be termed reinfection, occurring weeks to months after successful treatment, and are the result of a completely different microorganism or the same microorganism with a different serotype.

EPIDEMIOLOGY

In general, UTIs are predominantly found in females. It is only during the first year and after the fifth decade of life that the incidence of UTIs in males is high or begins to increase. These latter findings are attributable to the higher incidence of congenital abnormalities in male infants and the development of prostatic hypertrophy and interference with urinary flow in aging males. A recent review quantified the incidence of UTIs, pooling data from 17 studies and is presented in Table 63.1 (1).

Approximately 10 to 20% of all females will have at least one UTI in their lifetime. During the childbearing years, women appear to have a particular predisposition to UTIs. This is seen in the syndromes of "honeymoon" cystitis and pyelonephritis of pregnancy. Sexual intercourse produces a transient bacteriuria in most women, and several studies have associated sexual activity with an increased risk of UTI (2, 3). Recently the use of diaphragms has been implicated as another behavioral factor that may predispose young women to UTIs (2, 4).

Bacteriuria occurs in 4 to 7% of pregnant females, an incidence similar to that of nonpregnant women. However, if left untreated, bacteriuria can develop into symptomatic pyelonephritis in approximately 20% of pregnant women (5). An increased incidence of bacteriuria may be seen in patients with diabetes mellitus, renal transplants, advanced age, and other immunocompromising conditions. In the diabetic population, women appear to have a 2- to 3-fold higher incidence of bacteriuria, while men and children do not appear to be further predisposed to UTIs (6). In addition, these factors and conditions such as analgesic abuse may cause interstitial nephritis and papillary necrosis, leading to upper tract involvement and kidney damage. Urologic manipulation such as catheterization, and cystoscopy accounts for over 500,000 UTIs annually. UTIs account for 40% of all nosocomial infections, with more than 60% of these associated with the use of catheters (7).

PATHOGENESIS

Microorganisms invade the urinary tract by two routes, through the urethra and by hematogenous spread. The hematogenous route where the kidney is seeded from a primary site of infection such as a carbuncle, osteomyelitis, endocarditis, or empyema is much less common. (8). The UTI thus becomes a secondary infection.

The most common route of invasion of microorganisms

Table 63.1.
Prevalence of Bacteriuria in Various Populations[a]

Population	Prevalence (%)	
	Male	Female
Community-based		
Infants	2	0.5
Young children	0.1	1.5
College students	<0.01	5
Adults (30 to 65 years old)	0.1	10
Elderly persons		
65 to 85 years old	5	15
>85 years old	15	25
Patient-based		
Adults (medical clinic)	4	6
Adults (urology clinic)	8	—
Adult inpatient		
<70 years old	7.5	30
>70 years old	25	30
Institutionalized elderly persons	>30	>30
Patients after instrumentation		
Urethral catheterization	5	5
Transurethral procedures	20	40

[a] Percentages are approximations derived from a wide range of values from many studies in diverse settings; in these studies, specimens were obtained by various methods, and different definitions of bacteriuria were used. Table adapted from Lipsky BA: Urinary tract infections in men. Ann Intern Med 110(2):138–150, 1989.

into the urinary tract is via the urethra. The source of these organisms is the fecal reservoir of enteric bacteria; there is a 75 to 80% correlation between the etiologic microorganisms in bacteriuria and those cultured from a rectal swab. Bacteria progressively colonize the perineum, vagina, urethra, and bladder. Bacteria that adhere to the bladder mucosa remain behind after voiding, colonize, and produce infection. These bacteria may ascend into the kidneys, causing upper tract infection (8). Urologic manipulation can introduce bacteria into the bladder by contamination at the time of instrument insertion, by bacterial migration, and by breaks in the sterility of the catheter system. Normally bacteria inhabit the distal third of the urethra. Thus, the introduction of an instrument through the urethra can contaminate the bladder. With an indwelling urinary catheter, microorganisms can migrate from the periurethral area into the bladder via the fluid that separates the urethral mucosa and the catheter (7). Loss of sterility of the catheter system can contribute to catheter-associated UTIs. This can occur if the closed collecting system is broken or disconnected at any time, if retrograde urine flow occurs from bag to bladder, or if cross-contamination of patients in close proximity occurs as a result of improper hand cleansing by hospital personnel caring for the patients (9). Other factors that increase the rate of catheter-associated UTIs include age, sex, duration of the catheterization, catheter care techniques, training of the healthcare personnel inserting the

catheter, and clustering of catheterized patients. Elderly, debilitated men appear to be at highest risk for developing this form of infection.

A major intrinsic defense mechanism against UTI is the washing out of bacteria that occurs with each urinary void (8). This defense mechanism is compromised if urinary flow is slowed or obstructed or if a postvoid residual urine occurs. Since urine is a good culture medium, urinary stasis provides an ideal situation for bacterial growth. Obstructed or decreased urine flow can occur with urologic tumors, strictures, stones, or prostatic hypertrophy. Postvoid residual urine can occur with neurologic lesions affecting the bladder or sphincter muscles including bladder spasticity or flaccidity; with drugs, including anticholinergic and anesthetic medications; or with poor micturition habits.

Vesicoureteral reflux provides a mechanism for bacteria to ascend from the bladder to the kidney. This reflux occurs when the anatomic valve at the vesicoureteral junction is incompetent. This lesion may result from a congenital abnormality or a distortion of the bladder, such as occurs during pregnancy.

ETIOLOGIC AGENTS

The enteric bacteria—*Escherichia coli*, *Proteus*, *Klebsiella*, *Enterobacter*, *Enterococcus*, and *Pseudomonas*—are responsible for the vast majority of UTIs (Table 63.2). The predominant infecting agent is *E. coli*, accounting for over 80% of initial infections and approximately 50% of recurrent infections. When the UTI is hospital-acquired or if the urinary tract is complicated by obstruction, stone, catheter, or other urologic manipulation, it is difficult to predict the causative microorganism. The use of repeated

Table 63.2.
Etiologic Organisms of Urinary Tract Infections (UTIs)[a]

Organism	% of Total UTIs	% of Inpatient UTIs	% of Outpatient UTIs
Gram-negative			
Escherichia coli	52.2	31.9	72.5
Proteus mirabilis	6.4	7.5	5.3
Klebsiella aerogenes	6.5	8.7	4.3
Pseudomonas aeruginosa	5.8	11.7	0.0
Other coliforms	9.9	16.4	3.3
Gram-positive			
Enterococci	7.6	13.6	1.6
Staphylococci	9.3	5.6	13.0
Others	2.3	4.6	
	100.0	100.0	100.0

[a] Data from Hughes JM, Culver DH, White JW, et al.: Nosocomial infection surveillance, 1980–1982. MMWR Surveillance Summaries 32(Suppl 4ss):1ss, 1983; and Gruneberg RN: Antibiotic sensitivities of urinary pathogens, 1971–1982. J Antimicrob Chemother 14:17, 1984.

courses of antiinfectives and the presence of these complicating factors tend to select organisms other than *E. coli* and also result in an increased frequency of mixed infections. In this situation there is also an increased prevalence of *Staphylococcus saprophyticus* UTIs. Once thought to be a urinary contaminant, the subspecies is now recognized as a common cause of UTI in young women (11).

CLINICAL PRESENTATION

The clinical presentation of UTIs can be divided into findings associated with lower tract and and upper tract infections. Classically the signs and symptoms of lower tract infection have an abrupt onset and include dysuria, frequency, urgency, and a vague lower abdominal discomfort. Grossly, the urine is turbid, dark, and foul-smelling. Urinalysis reveals pyuria (more than 5 to 10 white blood cells (WBCs) per high-power field), bacteria, and hematuria in approximately 50% of patients. Leukocytosis is absent in a peripheral blood smear unless the upper tract or prostate is involved.

The presentation of prostatitis is primarily that of a lower UTI; however, fever, perineal pain, and urethral discharge may also be present. A rectal examination reveals an enlarged, tender, firm prostate gland. In the acute prostatic infection, leukocytosis is present. In chronic infection, the patient also typically complains of a lumbosacral backache.

The classical presentation of an upper UTI includes nonspecific complaints of headache, malaise, and nausea and vomiting. In association with these nonspecific findings, the patient may complain of suprapubic pain, costovertebral angle (CVA) tenderness, fever (to 39°C), and chills. Urinalysis will reveal bacteria, pyuria, and WBC casts in most patients. Hematuria and proteinuria will be detected in approximately 10 to 15% of patients, especially in the first few days of infection. Examination of the blood reveals a leukocytosis with a predominance of polymorphonucleocytes and band forms on the differential count. Blood cultures are positive for the infecting organism in approximately 20% of patients. In addition to these upper tract findings, lower tract symptoms can also be present.

Unfortunately not all UTIs have classical findings. For example, both upper and lower tract UTIs can be asymptomatic. Asymptomatic UTIs can occur in young children, with an incidence of approximately 1 to 2% in infants. Up to 30% of pregnant women with bacteriuria may be asymptomatic, while 25% of pregnant women with symptoms have sterile urine (5). Although pyuria can be a good predictor of a UTI, not all women with UTIs have pyuria on urinalysis. Conversely, pyuria can occur without bacteriuria. In this latter instance, vaginal contamination of the specimen, tuberculous infection, tumor, a foreign body, or medications can cause inflammation of the tract. Similarly, dysuria in the absence of a UTI can be caused by

irritation of the bladder or urethra by medications, including methenamine and cyclophosphamide, or by other genitourinary conditions in up to 50% of patients with dysuria (13).

DIAGNOSIS

The diagnosis of a UTI should be based on the demonstration of a significant quantity of bacteria in the urine. In addition, although other factors may not definitively diagnose a UTI, together they may be good predictive factors. A study involving three different groups of women (approximately 250/group) defined five common clinical findings as having high predictive value for positive urinary culture results: (*a*) history of UTI, (*b*) back pain, (*c*) urinalysis with >15 WBC/high-power field (HPF), (*d*) urinalysis with >5 red blood cells (RBCs)/HPF, and (*e*) urinalysis with more than a "few" bacteria. Patients without any findings had negative urine cultures, whereas 73% of women with two or more findings and 86% of women with four or five findings had positive urinary cultures (14).

Several studies have shown that pyuria accompanied by lower UTI symptoms is a good predictor of true infection (13). Gram-stain examination of the urine may provide information as to whether the microorganism is Gram-positive or Gram-negative, but does not specifically identify the organism nor does it provide quantitative information. Gram-staining can be also misleading, as is evidenced by a 20% error rate.

Consequently, the most reliable method of diagnosing the UTI is the properly performed urine culture and sensitivity test.

Collection of the Specimen

Collection of urine for culture and sensitivity testing is performed by one of three different methods: the suprapubic needle aspirate, single catheterization, and the midstream void collection (6). Each method has a different accuracy potential and a different level of bacteriuria indicative of the presence or absence of UTI.

Suprapubic aspiration is performed by inserting a needle in the midline, 2 cm above symphysis pubis, and aspirating the urine. The sample is then cultured. A colony count of 5×10^3/ml or above of the same organism is diagnostic of a UTI. A single culture using this technique is 99% accurate in detecting infection. Although not routinely done, this method may be necessary to obtain a specimen from infants and young children, as well as patients with spinal cord injury.

The single or in-and-out catheterization method can alleviate the problem of contamination of the specimen in the debilitated patient or may be useful in the patient who cannot void or follow instructions. However, the procedure itself can introduce bacteria into the bladder. The patient's periurethral area is cleansed and a catheter is aseptically inserted, the urine is drained, the catheter removed, and an aliquot of urine is cultured. A bacterial colony count of $1 \times 10^5/ml$ or above of the same microorganism is diagnostic of a UTI. This method is 95% accurate in detecting UTIs.

The most common technique for obtaining urine for culture is the midstream void method. The patient's periurethral area is cleansed with soap. The female patient is asked to separate her labia to avoid contamination. During the midpoint of the void, an aliquot of urine is collected, and this specimen is cultured. If the patient is asymptomatic, midstream samples from two separate voids should be obtained; if symptomatic, a single specimen is sufficient. A bacterial colony count of $1 \times 10^5/ml$ or above of the same microorganism is diagnostic of UTI. This method is 95% accurate in detection UTIs. Over recent years, the traditional colony count of $1 \times 10^5/ml$ as diagnostic of UTI has been disputed. Several studies have shown that women with bacterial counts as low as 1×10^2 who are symptomatic have been culture-positive and have benefited from treatment. One study found that one-third of all acute dysuric episodes in ambulatory women who had positive culture results were characterized by 10^2 to 10^4 organisms/ml of midstream urine (13).

The urine specimen from a patient with an indwelling catheter can be collected with relative ease. The catheter is clamped closed a short distance from the meatus for 1 hr. After this interval, the clamp is released and a few milliliters of urine are allowed to drain before the clamp is reapplied. An alcohol swab is used to clean the area on the catheter between the meatus and clamp. Finally, a needle and syringe are used to aspirate the urine from the catheter just distal to the meatus. The sample is then cultured.

Culture and Sensitivity Testing

The standard method of identifying, quantitating, and determining the sensitivity and resistance pattern to antiinfectives of the invading microorganism is the culture and sensitivity test. The most popular tests are the Kirby-Bauer method and microdilution testing.

After 24 hr of incubation, the organism can be delineated. After 48 hr, the sensitivities of the microorganism can usually be defined.

The concentration required to determine susceptibility varies with the agent and may reflect the concentration achievable in either the urine or serum. The concentration used by a laboratory should be investigated by the practitioner to gain the proper perspective of the sensitivity and resistance pattern of the microorganism. Many antiinfectives are excreted and concentrated in their active form in the urine. Therefore, sensitivities that used the antiinfective concentration achievable in the serum do not reflect the true resistance/sensitivity pattern of the microorganism infecting the urine, and may underestimate the ability of the drug to eradicate the infection. In addition, when treating an upper tract infection, the organism must also be susceptible in serum.

Methods other than the standard culture and sensitivity test for urinary infections are available. These methods are designed primarily to circumvent the cost and time factors required by the culture and sensitivity test. These alternative methods are most useful for diagnosis in uncomplicated UTIs or for posttherapy follow-up of complicated or upper tract infections. Since these tests do not provide information on organism identification or sensitivity testing, they are not useful in patients requiring an exact diagnosis for proper treatment. These patients include those with (a) recurrent or relapsing infection, (b) upper tract infection, (c) nosocomial infection, (d) infection associated with a catheter or instrumentation, and (e) kidney stones or other complicating factors.

Localization Studies

A positive culture and sensitivity test only confirms that bacteria are present in the bladder. It provides no information about infection in the kidney. Various tests, including renal concentrating ability and antibody titers, have been devised to detect pyelonephritis. Since in pyelonephritis the kidney often loses its ability to concentrate urine, a test of this function has been devised. This test unfortunately requires ureteral catheterization and can be influenced by other noninfectious renal conditions (e.g., analgesic nephropathy), but it still remains the most reliable diagnostic test.

The use of serum antibody titers to the infecting microorganism is based on the fact that patients who have classic upper UTIs have higher titers than patients with classic cystitis. However, since there is considerable overlap, the test is not definitive.

Another test for differentiating upper from lower tract UTIs is the presence or absence of antibody-coated bacteria (ACB) in urinary sediment. Theoretically, upper tract infections should evoke an immune response and the bacteria would be coated with antibody (ACB-positive). UTIs confined to the lower tract should not produce antibody (ACB-negative). Several factors, including poor standards for test results, have prevented widespread use of the test (6).

The intravenous pyelogram (IVP) is another study that can provide evidence of pyelonephritis. Classically, in the early states, localized scarring and calyceal distortion are present. In advanced cases of pyelonephritis, the above findings plus cortical scarring are found.

The indications for using localization studies in males revolve around the infrequent occurrence of UTIs. The presence of an infection, especially in boys and men under

50 years of age, usually indicates a structural deformity within the tract, which can possibly be corrected with surgery. Consequently, localization studies should be done with the first infection. Since the incidence of UTIs in women is quite high as a result of their anatomic predisposition, localization studies are usually not performed on a routine basis. Studies have shown that only a small percentage of women have abnormalities of the urinary tract. In addition, the outcome of these studies rarely influences clinical management. Therefore, these studies are usually reserved for women with relapsing infections after long-term antimicrobial therapy.

THERAPY

The therapeutic approaches available for the patient with urinary tract infection can be broadly classified as eradicative, prophylactic, suppressive, and preventive.

The approach used depends on the extent of the current illness; the patient's past history of UTIs; the patient's urologic status (complicated or uncomplicated); and the presence or absence of other diseases that predispose or affect the severity of the current and future UTIs.

Eradicative Therapy

The goal of eradicative therapy is sterilization of the urinary tract. The approach is used when there is bacterial colonization occurring in any part of the tract. It is indicated prior to the institution of prophylactic or suppressive therapy and prior to insertion of an indwelling catheter or other urologic manipulation, should an infection be present.

The efficacy of eradicative therapy is usually more dependent on the host environment than on the choice of drug. In the patient with a complicated infection, the structural abnormality, whether it be a stone, renal disease, prostatic hypertrophy, or vesicoureteral or ureterovesical reflux, can negatively affect the outcome of therapy by preventing adequate antimicrobial-organism contact. Similarly, should the patient have a disease such as diabetes mellitus, which predisposes or otherwise modifies the patient's response to infection, the outcome of therapy can be adversely affected. Control or correction of the underlying predisposing factors is essential to effective eradicative therapy.

The ideal antimicrobial agents for the treatment of UTI should meet the following criteria: a low rate of allergic/untoward reactions, once-daily dosing, complete upper gastrointestinal absorption so as not to change bowel flora, high urinary levels with glomerular filtration and secretion, minimal change in vaginal flora, excellent Gram-negative coverage, low cost, and finally, minimal development of resistance (15). To date, many agents are available for the treatment of UTI, but none satisfies all the requirements for the ideal agent.

The drug that is selected should reflect variables encountered in the individual patient. In this regard, the patient's immunologic status, age, allergy history, renal and hepatic function, previous history of UTIs, and sex can influence the choice of antimicrobial. In pregnant women, the selection of an agent should consider potential teratogenic or neonatal toxicity; for example, tetracyclines and tooth discoloration, sulfonamides and kernicterus.

Aside from these patient variables, the sensitivity of the organism to the available agents must be considered. Finally, the relative differences of the agents themselves, including kinetics, cost, dosage-form availability, and toxicity, are practical considerations that influence the choice of agents.

The agents available for the treatment of UTIs can be divided into two groups: (a) agents available for the treatment of acute, uncomplicated UTIs in the outpatient setting (Table 63.3) and (b) agents used in the treatment of serious, and/or complicated UTIs (Table 63.4). These agents will be discussed in the following section.

Acute, Uncomplicated UTI

The vast majority of women with urinary tract symptoms have simple, uncomplicated UTIs. Despite the overwhelming prevalence of these infections, controversy still exists concerning optimal therapy, especially in regards to the duration of treatment. Traditional treatment regimens consisted of 7- to 10-day antibiotic courses. In the past decade, numerous studies have been undertaken to demonstrate therapeutic efficacy of short-term antibiotic therapy including single-dose, 3-day, and 5-day regimens (16–19). Although many of these studies have shown single-dose therapy to be as effective as 7- to 10-day treatment, they have often involved small numbers of highly selected patients. Opponents point out that these studies do not parallel true patient populations so the results cannot be extrapolated to the general population (17, 18). Due to these factors, many physicians hesitate to adopt single-dose therapy as routine clinical practice, especially until definitive data are collected from large-scale double-blind trials. Single-dose therapy does offer several advantages, including a lower rate of adverse drug reactions, cost-effectiveness, better patient compliance, minimal change in bacterial flora, and a lower frequency of developing bacterial antibiotic resistance. Studies have shown that most women with lower tract infections are cured by single-dose treatment when the organisms are sensitive, whereas less than half of the women with upper tract involvement respond. Indications for patient inclusion are: females, acute uncomplicated UTI, no systemic symptoms, duration of local symptoms 48 hr or less, infrequent recurrence, and good follow-up available.

Single-dose studies have been carried out using several drugs including trimethoprim-sulfamethoxazole (TMP/

Table 63.3.
Eradicative Agents for Acute, Uncomplicated UTI

Class	Medication	Adult Dose	Half-Life (hr)		Common Toxicity	Comments
			Normal	Anuric		
Cephalosporins	Cefaclor	250–500 mg p.o., q. 8 hr	0.5–1	3	Gastrointestinal, hypersensitivity; moniliasis	Approximately 5–16% cross-sensitivity with penicillins; although categorized as second generation, may not offer greater Gram-negative coverage
	Cefadroxil	500–1000 mg, p.o. q. 12 hr	1.1	20–25	As above	Positive Coombs' anemia test, false-positive urine glucose (not with enzyme-based tests)
	Cephalexin	250–500 mg p.o. q. 6 hr	0.5–1.2	10–20	As above	As above
	Cephradine	250–500 mg p.o. q. 6 hr	0.7–2	8–15	As above	As above
Penicillins	Amoxicillin	250–500 mg p.o., q. 8 hr	0.7–1.4	7.4–21	Hypersensitivity; rash; gastrointestinal	Better gastrointestinal absorption than ampicillin; lower frequency of diarrhea, rash
	Amoxicillin-clavulanate	250–500 mg p.o., q. 8 hr; each tablet contains 125 clavulanic acid	As above	As above	As above	As above + clavulanic acid helps prevent inactivation of amoxicillin through β-lactamase inhibition; positive Coombs' anemia test
	Ampicillin	250–500 mg p.o., q. 6 hr	As above	As above	As above	Lower absorption with food; higher rate of diarrhea, rash
	Bacampicillin	400 mg p.o., q. 12 hr	As above	As above	As above	Prodrug of ampicillin; good gastrointestinal absorption; lower rate of diarrhea, rash
	Cyclacillin	250–500 mg p.o., q. 6 hr	0.5	3.5–10	As above	Good gastrointestinal absorption; lower rate of diarrhea, rash
Sulfonamides	Sulfacytine	250 mg p.o. q. 6 hr	4–8	?	Hypersensitivity; gastrointestinal; blood dyscrasias; crystalluria	Caution in patients with liver dysfunction or asthma; maintain adequate fluid intake; contraindicated in term pregnancy
	Sulfamethizole	500–1000 mg p.o., q. 6–8 hr	4–8	?	As above	As above
	Sulfamethoxazole	1 g p.o., q. 8–12 hr	7–17	30	As above	Greater risk of crystalluria over sulfisoxazole because of slower absorption and excretion; alkalinazation of urine usually unnecessary
	Sulfisoxazole	1 g p.o., q. 6 hr	4–8	10	As above	Relatively high solubility even in acid urine; risk of crystalluria low; alkalinization of urine usually unnecessary

(continued)

Table 63.3. (*Continued*)

Class	Medication	Adult Dose	Half-Life (hr)		Common Toxicity	Comments
			Normal	Anuric		
Tetracyclines	Tetracycline	250–500 mg p.o., q. 6 hr	6–12	57–120	Gastrointestinal, rash; suprainfection; dental staining	Contraindicated in last half of pregnancy and in children <8 years; avoid antacids, dairy products
	Doxycycline	50–100 mg p.o., q. 12 hr	14–25	20–30	As above	As above + administration with food or milk OK; high lipid solubility affords good prostatic penetration
	Minocycline	100 mg p.o., q. 12 hr	11–26	12–30	As above + vestibular disturbances	As above
Miscellaneous	Cinoxacin	500 mg p.o., q. 12 hr	1–1.5	16	Gastrointestinal; headache; dizziness; hypersensitivity	Chemically related to nalidixic acid—cross-resistance may occur
	Nalidixic acid	1 g p.o., q. 6 hr	1–2.5	21	Gastrointestinal, headache; visual disturbances; drowsiness; glucose 6-phosphate dehydrogenase hemolysis	Development of resistance may occur within 48 hr
	Nitrofurantoin	50–100 mg p.o., q. 6 hr	0.5	?	Gastrointestinal; eosinophilic pulmonary infiltrate; glucose 6-phosphate dehydrogenase hemolysis; peripheral neuropathy; hepatotoxicity	Contraindicated with creatinine clearance of <0.7 ml/sec (40 ml/min)
	Trimethoprim	100 mg p.o., q. 12 hr	8–11	26	Rash; gastrointestinal; blood dyscrasias	Contraindicated in pregnancy; use with caution in patients with folate deficiency because of megaloblastic anemia; penetrates prostatic tissue and fluid
	Trimethoprim/ Sulfamethoxazole	160 mg/800 mg (double-strength tablet) p.o. q. 12 hr	As above	As above	As above + see sulfonamides	As above + see sulfonamides

SMZ), amoxicillin, cefaclor, kanamycin, and tetracycline (19). Cure rates range from 70 to 100% with all of the agents except the cephalosporins, which have a success rate of 50% (6). TMP/SMZ (320 mg/1600 mg) appears to yield the most favorable outcome with single-dose therapy when compared with longer treatment regimens. This may be due to the longer plasma half-life of the drug with maintenance of therapeutic levels in the urine for up to 48 hr (17, 18).

In a recent review of 28 trials comparing treatment duration, the author pooled data on eradication rates (18).

TMP/SMZ, in studies of single-dose, 3-day, and 5-day courses, initially cured 89%, 94.6%, and 95.5% of UTIs, respectively, with follow-up cure rates of 81.8%, 84.8%, and 90.0%. Even though eradication rates were high, significant differences were noted between the groups. Amoxicillin therapy cured 71.4%, 80.8%, and 90% initially, with follow-up rates of 77% in all groups. The initial cure rates showed more highly significant differences, suggesting the need for longer therapy with this agent. The conclusions of the review indicated that the optimal duration of therapy may depend on the individual agents, but the

Table 63.4.
Commonly Used Eradicative Agents in Complicated UTI

Drug Class/Medications	Spectrum	Dose	Adjust Dose in Renal Impairment	Toxicity	Comments
Aminoglycosides (Gentamicin, Tobramycin, Amikacin)	Gram-negative, including *Pseudomonas aeruginosa*	(3–5 mg/kg/day IV q. 8 hr) (15 mg/kg/day IV q. 8 hr)	Yes	Nephrotoxicity; ototoxicity; neuromuscular blockade	Monitor serum levels: G T A Peak 4–8 15–30 Trough <2 5–10 Gentamicin least expensive; reserve amikacin for resistant organisms
Antifungals Amphotericin B	*Candida*	50 mg/liter sterile H$_2$O continuous irrigation	No	Minimal because of local effect—minimal systemic absorption	Continual irrigation for 5 days; efficacy is controversial and may depend on host factors
Flucytosine	*Candida, Cryptococcus*	50–150 mg/kg/day p.o., q. 6 hr	Yes	Gastrointestinal; hematologic disorders; rash; elevation of hepatic enzymes	Nausea/vomiting may be reduced by spacing capsules over 15 min
Fluconazole	*Candida, Cryptococcus*	50–100 mg q.d.	Yes	Minimal toxicity	High urinary concentrations
Cephalosporins	Gram-negative (3rd gen. > 2nd gen. > 1st gen.)			Hypersensitivity; gastrointestinal; blood dyscrasias, phlebitis; suprainfection; positive Coombs' anemia test	
Cefazolin	As above	1 g IV, q. 8 hr	Yes	As above	1st generation; organisms may be resistant
Cefixime	As above	200 mg p.o. q. 12 hr	Yes	As above	3rd generation; oral form
Cefotaxime	As above	1–2 g IV, q. 6–8 hr	Only if creatinine clearance <0.35 ml/sec (<20 ml/min)	As above	Enhanced Gram-negative coverage; 3rd generation
Ceftazidime	As above + *Pseudomonas*	0.5–1 g IV, q. 8–12 hr	Yes	As above	3rd generation; most active vs. *Pseudomonas*
Ceftizoxime	As above	0.5–1 g IV, q. 8–12 hr	Yes	As above	As above with slightly lower activity vs. *Pseudomonas*
Penicillins				Hypersensitivity; gastrointestinal; blood dyscrasias; neurotoxicity; thrombophlebitis; suprainfection	
Ampicillin	*E. coli, Proteus*	0.5–1 g IV, q. 6 hr	Only if creatinine clearance <0.5 ml/sec (<30 ml/min)	As above	Organisms may be resistant
Carbenicillin-indanyl sodium	Gram-negative, *Pseudomonas*	382–764 mg p.o., q. 6 hr	Contraindicated in creatinine clearance <0.2 ml/sec (<10 ml/min)	As above	Good prostatic penetration
Mezlocillin	As above	2–3 g IV, q. 6 hr	Only if creatinine clearance <0.5 ml/sec (<30 ml/min)	As above, possibly lower	
Piperacillin	As above	2–3 g IV, q. 6 hr	Only if creatinine clearance <0.7 ml/sec (<40 ml/min)	As above + bleeding abnormalities; electrolyte imbalances	Positive Coombs' anemia test; greatest in vitro activity vs. *Pseudomonas*; prostatic penetration

(continued)

Table 63.4. (*Continued*)

Drug Class/Medications	Spectrum	Dose	Adjust Dose in Renal Impairment	Toxicity	Comments
Ticarcillin–clavulanate potassium	As above	3.1 g IV, q. 6 hr	Yes	As for class	As above + greater activity vs. Gram-negative organisms because of addition of clavulanate to prevent inactivation of ticarcillin through β-lactamase inhibition
Miscellaneous Amdinocillin	Gram-negative	10 mg/kg IV, q. 4–6 hr	Only if creatinine clearance <0.5 ml/sec (<30 ml/min)	Hypersensitivity; gastrointestinal; blood dyscrasias	Synergistic activity vs. Gram-negative organisms when used in combination with other β-lactam antibiotics
Aztreonam	Gram-negative including *Pseudomonas*	500 mg–1 g IV, q. 8–12 hr	Only if creatinine clearance <0.5 ml/sec (<30 ml/min)	Gastrointestinal; phlebitis; rash; hypersensitivity; suprainfection	Monobactam; reserve for resistant organisms, patients with renal failure
Imipenem-Cilastatin	Gram-negative, *Pseudomonas*	250–500 mg IV, q. 6 hr	Yes	Gastrointestinal; blood dyscrasias; hypersensitivity; neurotoxicity; phlebitis	Reserve for serious infections resistant to other available agents; use with aminoglycoside in pseudomonal infection
Quinolones Norfloxacin	Gram-negative, *Pseudomonas*, Gram-positive	400 mg p.o., q. 12 hr	Only if creatinine clearance ≤0.5 ml/sec (≤30 ml/min)	Gastrointestinal; headache; dizziness; fatigue; rash; somnolence	Newer oral agent with good Gram-negative coverage; reserve for use against multiply resistant strains; contraindicated in pregnant women and children; avoid concurrent antacid administration
Ciprofloxacin	As above	250–500 mg p.o., q. 12 hr, or 200–400 IV, q. 12 hr	As above	As above	As above; greatest in vitro antimicrobial activity of the quinolones; good prostatic penetration; higher serum levels
Ofloxacin	As above	200 mg p.o., q. 12 hr	Only if creatinine clearance ≤0.2 ml/sec (≤10 ml/min)	As above	
Enoxacin[a]	As above	400 mg p.o., q. 12 hr[b]	N/A	As above	

[a] N/A, information unavailable at time of publication.
[b] Based on initial clinical trial data.

authors generally advocated therapy of not less than 3 days for short-term therapy.

Fihn et al. compared single-dose versus 10-day course of TMP/SMZ in acute, uncomplicated UTI in 255 women (20). Although no significant differences were found in resolution of symptoms in the two groups, they did find a significant difference in the recurrence rate at 13 days (24% single-dose versus 5% 10-day) and at 6 weeks (32% versus 21%). In analyzing the data, the authors found that that predictors for single-dose treatment failure included patients with colony counts ≥10^5 organisms and history of UTI within the preceding 6 weeks. Eliminating these two factors from the data, there was no longer a significant difference in failure rate at 6 weeks. A two-fold increase in the incidence of adverse effects was noted in the 10-day treatment group. The study demonstrated the importance of patient selection in determining appropriate candidates for single-dose therapy. The authors also concluded that 3-day regimens may prove to be more effective as a short-term course, while still retaining some of the major advantages of single-dose therapy. Single-dose therapy has not been shown to be effective in the treatment of upper urinary tract infections and is inappropriate for use in the patient with known renal involvement. In addition, short-term therapy is not indicated in the treatment of UTIs in pregnant women, children, elderly women, diabetics, women with recurrent infections, and in men (19). Therefore, standard 7- to 10-day regimens are recommended for these patient populations. Although treatment of uncomplicated UTI without complicating factors is often done empirically, without culture and sensitivity testing, infections in these patients must be guided by culture and sensitivity data. These patients may not have typical infecting organisms or sensitivities to antimicrobials, and therefore success of eradicative therapy will depend on appropriate selection of an antimicrobial agent. Many agents have been shown to be effective in the treatment of UTI with standard 7- to 10-day courses. The preferred agents include nitrofurantoin and TMP/SMZ (12, 15).

Most community-acquired pathogens remain sensitive to commonly prescribed antimicrobials. The in vitro susceptibilities of 295 isolates from adult female outpatients are presented in Table 63.5 (6). The breakpoint criterion for sensitivity was based on serum levels in all drugs but nitrofurantoin and nalidixic acid, and therefore it underestimates the ability of these agents to eradicate the UTI. This is because most antibiotics concentrate in the urine and achieve much higher levels there than in the serum.

Comparative clinical trials with newer agents such as the quinolones have not shown superiority over established regimens for the treatment of uncomplicated infections. In patients with UTIs due to organisms resistant to the preferred agents, alternate 10-day drug regimes include first-generation cephalosporins, amoxicillin-clavulanate, quinolones, and cefixime (12).

Pyelonephritis

In the treatment of mild pyelonephritis where the patient is not acutely ill and is able to tolerate oral antibiotic therapy, most patients can be treated as outpatients. Again there is some controversy about treatment duration, but most studies advocate treatment for 10 to 14 days (19). Culture and sensitivity testing is important to ensure appropriate antibiotic coverage. Commonly used regimens include TMP/SMZ, amoxicillin, and first-generation cephalosporins (12). Sensitivity data may warrant the use of newer, more expensive agents including amoxicillin plus clavulanate, norfloxacin, ciprofloxacin, ofloxacin, or oral third-generation cephalosporins such as cefixime (12, 21). The availability of these oral antibiotics has been a significant advantage in the treatment of mild cases of pyelonephritis. Prior to their development, many patients required hospitalization to receive parenteral antibiotic therapy to ensure adequate coverage of the infecting organisms. Because of their extended spectrum and enhanced susceptibilities, these agents can effectively eradicate these infections and substantially reduce costs when compared with hospitalization and parenteral antibiotic therapy. Adequate follow-up and posttherapy cultures are essential to document bacterial eradication.

The acutely ill patient with pyelonephritis is hospitalized and immediately started on empiric parenteral antimicrobial therapy until results of urine culture and sensitivity tests are known. Empiric therapy usually consists of a combination of ampicillin and an aminoglycoside or monotherapy with an extended-spectrum penicillin or a third-generation cephalosporin (12). When susceptibility is known, appropriate therapy is continued with the least expensive agent providing adequate coverage of the infecting organism. Therapy is converted to an oral regimen when the patient has been afebrile for 48 hr, and it is continued for a minimum of 2 weeks (19).

Complicated Infections

Complicated infections usually present a greater therapeutic challenge because they are often (a) caused by mul-

Table 63.5.

In Vitro Antimicrobial Susceptibilities of Isolates from Ambulatory Bacteriuric Women as Determined by Kirby-Bauer Assay: Experience in One Clinic[a]

Organism	Number of Isolates	AMP[b]	CEPH	NA	NITRO	SULFA	TCN	TMP-SMX	One or More	All
Escherichia coli	223	69	96	98	98	73	76	96	100	48
Proteus spp.	22	91	95	95	32	68	5	91	100	0
Klebsiella spp.	17	6	88	100	82	75	76	88	100	6
Pseudomonas spp.	10	0	0	0	0	0	0	0	0	0
Enterococcus	10	90	40	20	90	20	30	50	100	0
Other	13	15	31	100	54	77	69	92	100	8

[a] Adapted from Fowler JE: Urinary Tract Infection and Inflammation. Chicago: Year Book Medical Publishers, 1989.

[b] AMP, ampicillin; CEPH, cephalothin; NA, nalidixic acid; NITRO, nitrofurantoin; SULFA, sulfonamides; TCN, tetracycline; TMP/SMX, trimethoprim-sulfamethoxazole.

tiply-resistant organisms, (b) difficult to eradicate, and (c) precursors to chronic conditions and renal damage. It is important to attempt to correct the underlying problem (catheter, stone, enlarged prostate, etc.) if possible, as eradicative therapy is not usually successful or long-term if the condition remains.

In bacterial prostatitis, the efficacy of eradicative therapy depends on the ability of the medication to penetrate into the prostate gland as well as activity against the usual urinary tract pathogens. In acute bacterial prostatitis, penetration of the drug into the prostatic tissue and fluid is higher as a result of inflammation (1). The patient is usually hospitalized and treated with parenteral antibiotics. After the patient has been afebrile for 48 hr, the medication is changed to an oral agent. Trimethoprim, doxycycline, carbenicillin, and ciprofloxacin achieve high prostatic concentrations (1, 21). Doxycycline may not always offer Gram-negative coverage, and both carbenicillin and ciprofloxacin are usually reserved for resistant organisms. Therefore, trimethoprim, with good Gram-negative coverage, is the drug of choice in prostatic infections. It is usually given in combination with sulfamethoxazole, which does not penetrate the prostate gland well, in a dose of one double-strength tablet twice daily. These patients require long-term treatment of 4 to 6 weeks, followed by long-term suppression, treatment of relapses, or surgical correction (1).

Nosocomial infections contribute significantly to morbidity and mortality in the hospitalized patient. The urinary tract is the most common site of nosocomial infection and is associated with catheter placement in 60 to 70% of infections (7). *E. coli* accounts for only 30% of nosocomial UTIs with *Pseudomonas, Proteus, Klebsiella, Enterobacter, Serratia, Enterococcus, Staphylococcus,* and *Candida* being other likely pathogens (22). Many of these hospital-acquired strains are often resistant to the more frequently used antibiotics. In the patient who develops asymptomatic bacteriuria while catheterized, antibiotic therapy is not indicated and may, in fact, lead to the development of resistant organisms. In many cases, the urine clears spontaneously after catheter removal (11). In the symptomatic patient, every attempt should be made to remove the catheter before initiating therapy. In patients in whom urosepsis is likely, empiric therapy is initiated after urine and blood cultures have been obtained. The usual drugs of choice for nosocomial UTI are a combination regimen of an aminoglycoside (gentamicin) and ampicillin (23). Alternate regimens include third-generation cephalosporins and extended-spectrum penicillins. If the Gram stain reveals a Gram-negative organism, monotherapy with gentamicin is adequate treatment. Antibiotic therapy can be adjusted after culture and sensitivity data are obtained. New antimicrobials are constantly introduced and add to the armamentarium of agents available for the treatment of serious UTIs. These drugs, such as aztreonam, imipenem, and parenteral quinolones, should be reserved for use in patients with infections due to multiply-resistant organisms or in patients who cannot tolerate first-line agents because of allergy or toxicity. The restriction of these antibiotics is important for cost-containment measures and to help prevent widespread bacterial resistance.

The quinolone agents may also play an important role in the treatment of nosocomial infections. A recent study evaluated the use of norfloxacin, 400 mg orally twice a day, versus the physician's preferred parenteral regimen in a group of 94 patients with moderate-to-severe nosocomial UTI (24). Of the 46 patients in the norfloxacin group, 76% were cured, while of the 48 patients receiving parenteral therapy, 67% were cured. Outcome was similar in the norfloxacin versus parenteral regimen groups, with failures occurring in 0 and 4%, suprainfections in 2 and 8%, and reinfection in 2 and 0%, respectively. While the efficacy rates were similar, the cost differences were striking. As patients improved clinically, they could be discharged to home to continue norfloxacin treatment an average of 4.5 days earlier than the other group. The authors stated that 40% of the patients in the parenteral therapy group remained in the hospital for the additional 4.5 days solely to receive their intravenous antibiotics. The mean cost of drugs alone was $43.30 in the norfloxacin group versus $244.71 in the parenteral group. These figures do not include the additional hospitalization costs in the parenteral group. Another advantage of oral therapy was a lower incidence of adverse drug reactions likely to be caused by drug treatment, 9.8% versus 24.5%. Norfloxacin appeared to provide safe and effective therapy of nosocomial UTI, with the added benefit of substantial cost savings. More studies are needed to assess the efficacy of the quinolones in this setting, but their use in complicated UTIs seems promising.

Follow-up cultures after eradicative therapy of complicated UTIs are necessary to detect and treat bacterial persistence or suprainfection if it occurs.

Prophylaxis

Prophylactic therapy is used to prevent infection in patients who have uncomplicated urinary tracts and a history of closely spaced, recurrent UTIs. Since recurrent, uncomplicated UTIs are primarily a problem of women and are usually reinfections, a prophylactic agent should continue to be effective in low doses to minimize side effects (Table 63.6).

Women who have had three or more UTIs per year generally benefit from prophylaxis. At this rate, it is also cost-effective to use prophylaxis, when compared with treatment costs—office visits, urinalysis, medication, and time (25).

Table 63.6.
Prophylactic and Suppressive Agents for UTIs

Drug	Dose	Comments
Methenamine mandelate	1.0 g q.i.d.	Requires urine pH of <5.5; contraindicated in renal insufficiency, dehydration; can cause dysuria, gastrointestinal irritation; avoid concurrent use with sulfonamides
Methenamine hippurate	1.0 g b.i.d.	As above
Nitrofurantoin	50–100 mg q.h.s.	See Table 63.3
Trimethoprim-sulfamethoxazole	½–1 tab q.h.s.	See Table 63.3

Prophylactic therapy should not be instituted until an existing infection is cleared by eradicative therapy.

Several antiinfectives appear to be effective as prophylactic agents: TMP/SMZ, nitrofurantoin, methenamine, and others. Since uncomplicated reinfections result from periurethral contamination by colonic flora, the prophylactic agent should not alter the sensitivity-resistance pattern of these bacteria. Neither methenamine nor nitrofurantoin affect the sensitivity of these organisms, and thus they remain effective with continued use (26). The effectiveness of trimethoprim is based on the ability to achieve bactericidal concentrations in vaginal fluid and thus inhibit periurethral colonization of enteric flora (26).

The dose and regimens for nitrofurantoin or trimethoprim-sulfamethoxazole as prophylactic agents are much lower than those required for eradicative therapy. Nitrofurantoin in a dose of 50 to 100 mg at bedtime or one-half tablet of trimethoprim-sulfamethoxazole (80 to 400 mg/tablet) at bedtime is an effective prophylactic measure (26, 27). Recent reports have shown doses of trimethoprim-sulfamethoxazole as low as 1/2 tablet three times weekly to be as effective as daily dosing, with infection rates <0.2/patient year. A long-term prophylaxis study of 11 women demonstrated excellent results with this dosage regimen (28). Although the study was small, infection rates dropped from an average of 3 to 5 UTIs per year to 0.14 per patient year. In addition, these women were predisposed to UTI by underlying conditions: diabetes, 3 patients; renal transplant, 1; cancer patient on chemotherapy, 1; and one patient with systemic lupus erythematosus. Five of the seven UTIs were caused by resistant organisms (*E. coli*, *Staphylococcus epidermidis*, *Streptococcus faecalis*) that were sensitive to nitrofurantoin and ampicillin. In the 5-year study, no significant adverse reactions occurred. TMP/SMZ appeared to be a safe and effective

agent for long-term prophylaxis in the patient predisposed to UTI. Infections that do occur are caused by resistant organisms. This appears to be the only potential problem, and it needs to be further assessed with larger research trials.

A recent randomized, double-blind study of 132 renal transplant patients evaluated prophylaxis with TMP/SMZ versus placebo for an average of 8.5 months following transplantation (29). The authors found no benefit of prophylaxis in the immediate postoperative period when the patient was catheterized (27% placebo group versus 21% TMP/SMZ group). Additionally, they noted that infections during this period were likely to be caused by a resistant organism. Following catheter removal, the incidence of UTIs in the hospital dropped from 17% placebo versus 5% TMP/SMZ, with 2 of the 3 infections in the TMP/SMZ group caused by a resistant organism. TMP/SMZ also was highly effective in reducing the incidence of UTI following discharge from the hospital: 38% placebo versus 5% TMP/SMZ, with resistance rates of 24% versus 86%, respectively. Optimal results were achieved with doses of 160/800 mg twice daily during hospitalization and once daily following hospital discharge. The authors concluded that TMP/SMZ prophylaxis, following catheter removal, was highly effective, well-tolerated, and cost-effective.

Nitrofurantoin has also been shown to be effective in the prophylaxis of recurrent UTIs (27). The drug is well absorbed in the gastrointestinal tract and only achieves therapeutic concentrations in the urinary tract. Therefore, it does not alter normal bacterial flora. Another advantage is the lack of development of resistance among sensitive organisms, despite use of the drug for almost 40 years. The disadvantage of the drug is the potential for serious adverse drug reactions, including pulmonary fibrosis and liver toxicity, with long-term use. Although the incidence of these side effects is low, patients receiving nitrofurantoin therapy should receive careful monitoring for adverse effects.

Methenamine mandelate has been tried in a single bedtime dose of 1.0 g; however, this is less effective than the other agents. Consequently, full doses of 0.5 to 1.0 g four times a day of methenamine in addition to urinary acidification to a pH of 5.5 or lower are required if this agent is used for prophylaxis (Table 63.7) (6).

Methenamine hippurate, a different salt of the drug, was evaluated in a double-blind crossover study in a dose of 1 g twice daily (30). Patients received 6 months of drug or placebo and then were crossed over to the other agent. Prophylaxis continued for 2 years. A significant difference was noted between the two groups, with an infection rate of 2.1 per patient year in the placebo group versus 0.8 per patient year in the methenamine group. The drug provided effective prophylaxis and was well tolerated. This salt may be more efficacious because patient compliance is better with the simplified regimen. Methenamine does not alter

Table 63.7.
Urinary Acidifying Agents

Acidifying Agent	Dose	Comments
Ascorbic acid	6 g/day in divided doses	Titrate dose and urine pH; caution with patients who are receiving other medications, whose clearance will be affected by acidic pH
Ammonium chloride	2–3 g p.o., q. 6 hr	As above; caution in patients with decreased hepatic or renal function; effectiveness limited by renal compensation; can cause systemic acidosis

normal flora, and resistance does not develop since the agent is only an antiseptic.

In comparison with the other prophylactic regimens, methenamine does have a higher infection rate and may not be as effective in patients with high recurrence rates.

Currently, most patients are placed on prophylactic therapy for 6 months, and then the agent is discontinued. If the infection recurs, the patient again goes through the eradication treatment and is placed back on prophylactic therapy. Prophylaxis has not been shown to alter the natural course of UTIs, as demonstrated by rapid reinfection after the agent is discontinued in most studies, and therefore it may need to be continued indefinitely in the patient who suffers from unrelentless recurrences (6).

Because of the association of sexual intercourse with UTIs and concern over long-term continuous prophylaxis, more studies are now being done to assess the effectiveness of postcoital prophylaxis. Excellent results have been achieved with several agents, including TMP/SMZ, nitrofurantoin, cephalexin, nalidixic acid and cinoxacin (31). In a study of 31 women with recurrent UTIs (127 UTIs in 6 months), patients were instructed to take one 250-mg cephalexin tablet postcoitally (32). In the 12 months of the trial, only one UTI occurred. The infection rate dropped from 4 per patient year to 0.03 per patient year. Another interesting aspect of this trial was the inclusion of 16 pregnant women. This type of prophylaxis may prove to be particularly beneficial in this group of women who are predisposed to pyelonephritis. Potential benefits of this type of prophylaxis include lower cost, better tolerance, and increased patient compliance. The disadvantages of this prophylactic regimen as well as continuous prophylaxis, are emergence of resistant organisms and the possibility of drug-induced toxicity. Therefore, all patients on any prophylactic regimen who acquire an acute UTI require a urine culture with sensitivity testing to ensure effective eradicative therapy.

Another approach, although not truly prophylactic, is

self-treatment. The patient is instructed to initiated single-dose or short-course therapy with the selected antimicrobial at the first sign of an impending UTI. A recent trial proved the regimen to be effective, to be less costly than prophylaxis or standard treatment procedures, and to have a decreased rate of adverse drug reactions when compared with long-term prophylaxis (33). Patient selection is crucial for this regimen to be effective.

Suppressive Therapy

Long-term suppressive therapy is used primarily to reduce the frequency of recurrence and acute exacerbations of chronic infections. This form of therapy is indicated in patients who have a persistent focus of infection from which the microorganism cannot be eradicated. Examples of this type of infection include men with chronic bacterial prostatitis, patients with urinary calculi or other structural defects in the urinary tract, or those with a chronic indwelling catheter.

In patients in whom a stone is the nidus of infection, the goals of suppressive therapy are the maintenance of sterile urine and an asymptomatic patient. The antimicrobials used for suppressive therapy are similar to those used for prophylactic regimens. TMP/SMZ 80/4000 mg, nitrofurantoin 50 to 100 mg, or trimethoprim, all dosed once daily, have been shown to be effective. Methenamine may also be useful for long-term use, due to lack of resistance or toxicity. The hippurate salt can be dosed 1 g twice daily, with urinary acidification to maintain pH at 5.5 or less. Prior to instituting suppressive therapy, an attempt should be made to clear the urine of active infection (1).

Preventive Therapy

Preventive measures attempt to minimize the chance of developing a UTI. These measures are directed toward patient populations that are at particular risk of infection. Included in this group are patients who are or are about to be catheterized or have some other form of urologic manipulation, diabetics, and debilitated or otherwise compromised patients.

Since urologic manipulation is such a well-known risk factor for UTIs, the need for performing the procedure should be weighed against the potential risks. Should the necessity be compelling, proper preparation of both the patient and the practitioner should be made to minimize the risk of infection, and the procedure should be performed using aseptic techniques.

The urinary catheter poses a special predisposing problem and has been studied extensively. The frequently of catheter-associated UTIs is related to a variety of factors, including the method and duration of catheterization, the healthcare personnel inserting the catheter, the catheter system, and catheter care. The Centers for Disease Control

(CDC) have developed recommendations for the use of an indwelling catheter. Although the complete recommendations are too extensive for discussion in this text, a summary is presented (34):

1. Indwelling catheters should be used only when indicated and for as short a time as is possible.
2. Insertion should be done by adequately trained personnel using aspetic technique.
3. A sterile closed-drainage system should always be used.
4. At no time should the collecting bag be above the level of the patient's bladder. The urine flow should be "downhill" and unobstructed, but should be suspended off the floor to prevent bacterial contamination.
5. Any closed collecting system that is contaminated by inappropriate technique, accidental disconnection, or the like should be replaced.
6. If a patient is catheterized for 2 weeks or less, a routine catheter change is not required except when obstruction, contamination, or other malfunction of the system occurs.
7. In patients who are chronically catheterized, replacement is not necessary until a malfunction or obstruction occurs.
8. Patients who are catheterized should be in separate rooms and not in adjacent beds, to avoid cross-contamination.
9. Bacteriologic monitoring of the urine of catheterized patients may be useful; however, the cost-effectiveness requires evaluation.
10. Urine samples should be obtained from the aspiration port using aseptic technique.
11. The urethral meatus should be cleansed daily, with water used to reduce encrustations.
12. The use of systemic antibiotics may delay the development of bacteriuria but does not prevent it. In light of cost, adverse reactions, and development of resistance, prophylactic antimicrobial therapy is not recommended as routine practice. However, its use may be warranted in patients who require short-term catheterization and who are at high risk of complications from UTI.

The routine use of antibiotic irrigations, antiseptic instillation into the drainage bag, or meatal care with antimicrobial ointments has not been shown to be effective in preventing or reducing the incidence of UTIs (11, 35, 36).

Recently, the U.S. Preventive Task Force adopted new guidelines for screening of asymptomatic bacteriuria by dipstick urinalysis (37). They concluded that routine dipstick analysis is not recommended for asymptomatic persons. They did, however, recommend routine screening of all pregnant women, since early detection and treatment can prevent symptomatic infections that can cause serious morbidity in this patient population. They favored the routine use of urine culture over dipstick urinalysis in pregnant women, to prevent the occurrence of false-negative results.

They also recommend that dipstick urinalysis may be appropriate for women who are over age 60 or diabetic. At this time there are no definitive data to suggest that treatment of asymptomatic bacteriuria in these women af-

fects morbidity or mortality. Conflicting reports exist about the effect of bacteriuria on survival in the elderly. One trial demonstrated maintenance of sterile urine for 6 months of 63.6% of women given short-course antimicrobial therapy versus 34.5% in the untreated women (36). While a bacteria-free urine may be achievable in the elderly, the importance of this remains to be elucidated.

Maintenance of the patient in a well-hydrated state is a simple and worthwhile preventive measure that inhibits or minimizes the risk of developing pyelonephritis. The value of maintaining hydration is based on its effect on the activity of phagocytes in the renal medulla. Dehydration and resultant hypertonicity of the urine in the renal medulla inhibits leukocyte mobilization and phagocytic activity (36).

Follow-up

One of the most important yet most frequently omitted components in the total treatment of UTIs is adequate follow-up. A culture is indicated after the first 48 to 72 hr of therapy to check for antiinfective effectiveness. Since pyuria can persist during this initial phase of treatment, a urinalysis is a poor screening test for ineffective therapy.

While many clinicians do not insist on follow-up cultures after treatment for acute, uncomplicated UTIs, they should be performed routinely after therapy for complicated infections, those involving the upper tract, and in pregnant women. After achievement of sterile urine, cultures are only repeated for symptomatic episodes of bacteriuria.

PROGNOSIS

The prognosis for UTIs is highly variable, even with adequate therapy. Urologic structural abnormalities, presence of an indwelling catheter, and prostatitis favor the potential for recurrent infections. Concurrent predisposing conditions such as immunosuppression, pregnancy, diabetes, sex, advanced age, debility, and urologic manipulation favor the spread of infection beyond the urinary tract.

There is a high recurrence rate with children: 26% in neonates, 30 to 40% in girls, and 10 to 18% in boys. The prognosis is poor if these infections are not diagnosed early and treated adequately. In fact, 5 to 25% of these cases will progress to end-stage renal disease (39). Following an episode of bacteriuria during pregnancy, the possibility of recurrence is markedly enhanced, when compared with patients who did not have bacteriuria during pregnancy (30 versus 5%). Of note is the increased incidence, approximately 20%, of urologic abnormalities on radiographs on follow-up examination in the patients who had bacteriuria during pregnancy (5). Elderly men, especially those with prostatitis, also are prone to recurrent infections.

Eradication rates average 50%, even with long-term therapy.

Metastatic infections secondary to UTIs can occur. Men appear to be more prone to developing metastases from lower UTIs and women more prone to developing metastases from upper tract infections. In general, predisposing factors to developing these ectopic infections include an abnormal urinary tract, urologic manipulation, and impaired host defenses as seen in diabetes, malignancy, cirrhosis, uremia, malnutrition, anemia, and collagen vascular diseases. The sites of reported metastases include skeletal (59%), endocarditis (29%), chest (4%), eye (2%), and miscellaneous (3%). Of note is that within the skeletal metastatic lesions, 83% were to the vertebrae (40).

The uncomplicated UTI has the most favorable prognosis. In women with this type of infection up to 94% of uncomplicated infections can be eradicated.

CONCLUSION

UTIs are one of the most common infectious diseases and therefore are encountered in virtually all types of practices. A thorough knowledge of the pathogenesis, clinical course, and therapeutic choices is essential to the rational management of this disease. The pharmacist can be a key member of the healthcare team by understanding the controversies, the therapeutic options, and the rationale for drug selection in the management of UTI. The pharmacist can then provide recommendations for the optimal therapy of these infections.

REFERENCES

1. Lipsky BA: Urinary tract infections in men. Ann Intern Med 110(2):138–150, 1989.
2. Stamm WE, Hooton TM, Johnson JR, et al.: Urinary tract infections: from pathogenesis to treatment. J Infect Dis 159(3):400–406, 1989.
3. Leibovici L, Alpert G, Laor A, et al.: Urinary tract infections and sexual activity in young women. Arch Intern Med 147:345–347, 1987.
4. Fihn SD: Behavioral aspects of urinary tract infection. Suppl Urol 32(3):16–18, 1988.
5. Krieger JN: Complications and treatment of urinary tract infections during pregnancy. Urol Clin North Am 13:658–693, 1986.
6. Fowler JE: Urinary Tract Infection and Inflammation. Chicago: Year Book Medical Publishers, 1989.
7. Roberts JA, Fussell EN, Kaack MB: Bacterial adherence to urethral catheters. J Urol 144:264–269, 1990.
8. Sobel JD: Pathogenesis of urinary tract infections. Infect Dis Clin North Am 1(4):751–772, 1987.
9. Hughes JM, Culver DH, White JW, et al.: Nosocomial infection surveillance, 1980–1982. MMWR CDC Surveillance Summaries 32(suppl 4ss):1ss, 1983.
10. Gruneberg RN: Antibiotic sensitivities of urinary pathogens, 1971–1982. J Antimicrob Chemother 14:17, 1984.
11. Schaeffer AJ: Catheter-associated bacteriuria. Urol Clin North Am 13:735–747, 1986.
12. Johnson JR, Stamm WE: Urinary tract infections in women: diagnosis and treatment. Ann Intern Med 111:906–917, 1989.
13. Stamm WE: Protocol for diagnosis of urinary tract infection: reconsidering the criterion for significant bacteriuria. Suppl Urol 32:6–12, 1988.
14. Wigton RS, Hoellerich VL, Ornato JP, et al.: Use of clinical findings in the diagnosis of urinary tract infection in women. Arch Intern Med 145:2222, 1985.
15. Parsons CL: Protocol for treatment of typical urinary tract infection: criteria for antimicrobial selection. Suppl Urol 32:22–27, 1988.
16. Trienekens TAM, Stobberigh EE, Winkens RAG, et al.: Different lengths of treatment with co-trimoxazole for acute uncomplicated urinary tract infections in women. Br Med J 299:1319–1322, 1989.
17. Philbrick JT, Bracikowski JP: Single-dose antibiotic treatment for uncomplicated urinary tract infections. Arch Intern Med 145:1672–1678, 1985.
18. Norrby SR: Short-term treatment of uncomplicated lower urinary tract infections in women. Rev Infect Dis 12:458–467, 1990.
19. Gleckman RA: Treatment duration for urinary tract infections in adults. Antimicrob Agents Chemother 31:1–5, 1987.
20. Fihn SD, Johnson C, Roberts PL, et al.: Trimethoprim-sulfamethoxazole for acute dysuria in women: a single-dose or 10-day course. Ann Intern Med 108:350–357, 1988.
21. Wolfson JS, Hooper DC: Treatment of genitourinary tract infections with fluoroquinolones: activity in vitro, pharmacokinetics, and clinical efficacy in urinary tract infections and prostatitis. Antimicrob Agents Chemother 33:1655–1661, 1989.
22. Brettman LR: Nosocomial infection: risks associated with short-term and long-term inpatient care. Suppl Urol 32:21–23, 1988.
23. Cunha BA: Aminoglycosides in urology. Urology 36:1–14, 1990.
24. Scheife RT, Cox CE, McCabe RE, et al.: Norfloxacin vs best parenteral therapy in treatment of moderate to serious, multiply-resistant, nosocomial urinary tract infections: a pharmacoeconomic analysis. Suppl Urol 32:24–30, 1988.
25. Nicolle LE, Ronald AR: Recurrent urinary tract infections in adult women: diagnosis and treatment. Infect Dis Clin North Am 1(4):793–806, 1987.
26. Mulholland SG: Controversies in management of urinary tract infections. Urology (suppl) 26(2):3, 1986.
27. Cunha BA: Nitrofurantoin—current concepts. Urology 32(1):67–71, 1988.
28. Nicolle LE, Harding GK, Thompson M, et al.: Efficacy of five years of continuous, low-dose trimethoprim-sulfamethoxazole prophylaxis for urinary tract infection. J Infect Dis 157(6):1239–1242, 1988.
29. Fox BC, Sollinger HW, Belzer FO, et al.: A prospective, randomized, double-blind study of trimethoprim-sulfamethoxazole for prophylaxis of infection in renal transplantation: clinical efficacy, absorption of trimethoprim-sulfamethoxazole, effects on the microflora, and the cost-benefit of prophylaxis. Am J Med 89:255–274, 1990.
30. Cronberg S, Welin CO, Henriksson L, et al.: Prevention of recurrent acute cystitis by methenamine hippurate: double blind controlled crossover long term study. Br Med J 294:1507–1508, 1987.
31. Stapleton A, Latham RH, Johnson C, et al.: Postcoital antimicrobial prophylaxis for recurrent urinary tract infection. JAMA 264(6):703–706, 1990.
32. Pfau A, Sacks TG: Effective prophylaxis of recurrent urinary tract infections in premenopausal women by postcoital administration of cephalexin. J Urol 142:1276–1278, 1989.
33. Wong ES, McKevitt M, Running K, et al.: Management of recurrent urinary tract infections with patient-administered single-dose therapy. Ann Intern Med 102:302, 1985.
34. Stamm WE: Guidelines for prevention of catheter-associated urinary tract infections. Ann Intern Med 82:386–390, 1975.

35. DeGroot-Kosolcharoen J, Guse R, Jones J: Evaluation of a urinary catheter with a preconnected closed drainage bag. Infect Control Hosp Epidemiol 9(2):72–76, 1988.

36. Seiler WO, Stahelin HB: Practical management of catheter-associated UTIs. Geriatrics 43(8):43–45, 1988.

37. Pels RJ, Bor DH, Woolhandler S, et al.: Dipstick urinalysis screening of asymptomatic adults for urinary tract disorders. JAMA 262(9):1220–1224, 1989.

38. Boscia JA, Kobasa WD, Knight RA, et al.: Therapy vs no therapy for bacteriuria in elderly ambulatory nonhospitalized women. JAMA 257(8):1067–1071, 1987.

39. Spencer JR, Schaeffer AJ: Pediatric urinary tract infection. Urol Clin North Am 13(4):661–672, 1986.

40. Siroky MB, Moylan RA, Austin G Jr, et al.: Metastatic infection secondary to genitourinary tract sepsis. Am J Med 61:351, 1976.

Chapter 64

ABDOMINAL INFECTIONS

JOAN E. KAPUSNIK-UNER, Pharm.D.

Intra-abdominal infections present serious clinical problems because they are difficult to diagnose and treat successfully. Such infections generally occur after leakage of bacteria from the gastrointestinal (GI) tract into the sterile environment of the peritoneal cavity. The resulting infection may be a diffuse peritonitis and/or localized abscesses. These infections may seem to occur spontaneously, and so are named spontaneous bacterial peritonitis (SBP) (1), or they may be secondary to abdominal trauma, surgery, or intrinsic GI disease. Many cases of secondary peritonitis, especially when caused by anaerobic organisms, occur after hematogenous or lymphogenous bacterial spread.

The concept of mixed bacterial infection is especially relevant to these abdominal processes. Normal intestinal flora is comprised of both anaerobic and aerobic microorganisms. Thus, when infection occurs after GI content spillage, multiple organisms may be responsible. However, it may be difficult to determine which of the many microbes requires antimicrobial treatment. The mere presence of an organism on culture from a site of infection does not guarantee its pathogenicity. Therefore, knowledge of the flora encountered at the various levels of the GI tract in a given patient population provides the microbiologic basis for diagnosis and empiric antimicrobial therapy.

Even after identification of the pathogens from cultures, clinical outcome may be influenced by other factors including the bacterial load at the site of infection (i.e., the inoculum size); immunologic variables relating to local host defenses, as well as the general systemic immune response; progression or severity of the underlying intrinsic GI disease; and whether the antimicrobial agents administered penetrate to the site of the infection and are pharmacologically active in that environment. These factors should be considered prior to selection of therapy as well as when assessing clinical response.

Patients who receive dialysis via continuous ambulatory peritoneal dialysis (CAPD) are a particular challenge (2) with regards to treatment of intra-abdominal infections. These patients have a high incidence of primary peritonitis arising from contamination caused by the technical aspects of CAPD (3). The advantages of CAPD compared to hemodialysis have been tempered by this constant risk of peritonitis. Therefore, successful treatment of intra-abdominal infections in these patients holds a separate importance.

ETIOLOGY—INTESTINAL MICROFLORA

The great majority of intra-abdominal infections are caused by aerobic organisms (i.e., Enterobacteriaceae and streptococci), with the minority involving anaerobes from the GI tract. In general, the normal GI tract bacterial flora is of low virulence. The number of bacterial species and the colony counts increase as one moves from the mouth down along the GI tract. This flora is stable early in childhood, and for the most part does not differ with geographic location, race, diet, or age. In a human stomach there are usually fewer than 10^4 colony forming units/ml (cfu/ml) of aerobic and anaerobic microflora. Acidity and normal GI motility inhibit bacterial growth in this region (4). Trauma or diseases of the stomach and duodenal region may compromise these protective factors. Thus, medical conditions such as a gastric ulceration, achlorhydria or chronic H_2-antagonist use, obstructing duodenal ulcer, carcinoma, upper GI bleeding, or other drug therapies may result in the abnormal proliferation of the local flora (i.e., viridans streptococci, lactobacilli, and yeast).

The microflora of the proximal small bowel is similar to that observed in the stomach, though increased numbers of Enterobacteriaceae and *Bacteroides* spp. may be found. Peristalsis is most rapid in the jejunum and upper ileum, which explains in part the low bacterial counts relative to the distal ileum. Injury or disease of this upper portion of the GI tract results in a relatively low bacterial inoculum being introduced into the peritoneal cavity. Thus, the number and severity of clinical infections related to such injuries are less than with injuries of the large bowel. Between the proximal and terminal ileum is a bacterial transition zone. The composition of the normal flora changes toward greater numbers of aerobic and anaerobic Gram-negative bacilli. Finally, in the terminal ileum equal numbers of anaerobic and aerobic bacteria are found at counts up to 10^8 cfu/ml.

The highest concentration of microorganisms observed in the GI tract is in the colon. As many as 10^{11} cfu/g of anaerobes and 10^8 cfu/g of aerobic coliforms are present (5). Most organisms at this level of the gut are anaerobes. Under the usual conditions within the lumen of the GI tract, anaerobic organisms behave as harmless commensals, but when introduced into the surrounding host tissues they become pathogenic. Certain underlying clinical conditions, such as compromised vascular supply or tissue necrosis predispose a patient to anaerobic infections. Such clinical situations are associated with confined tissue spaces with a low oxidation-reduction potential and hypoxia, which provides an environment for uncontrolled anaerobic proliferation. Granulocytic killing of anaerobes (e.g., *Clostridium perfringens*) is impaired under anaerobic conditions as well. Although more than 400 species of anaerobes reside in the colon and 200 in the oral cavity, only a few produce most clinical anaerobic infections. *Bacteroides fragilis* accounts for only about 5% of the colonic microflora, yet *B. fragilis* causes many more clinical infections than any other *Bacteroides* species. The capsular polysaccharide of *B. fragilis* is probably an important virulence factor.

Intra-abdominal infections usually involve mixed microflora, both aerobic and anaerobic bacteria, with the potential for synergism. Coliforms have a lower oxygen tension or redox potential within the peritoneal cavity, thus promoting the growth of obligate anaerobes. Conversely, there is some evidence that low-virulence anaerobic organisms enhance the pathogenicity of aerobic Gram-negative bacilli such as *Escherichia coli*, *Klebsiella* spp., and *Proteus mirabilis*. One mechanism by which *B. fragilis* does this, is by secreting β-lactamases extracellularly (into the site of infection), thus creating a protected environment in which β-lactam drugs are rendered ineffective. Also, a variety of obligate anaerobes interfere with intracellular bacterial killing by polymorphonuclear leukocytes (PMNs), as well as PMN chemotaxis and phagocytosis (6).

Results from an animal model of intra-abdominal sepsis reveal a biphasic disease process. After intra-abdominal inoculation of intestinal flora, animals initially developed acute peritonitis, predominantly from aerobic Gram-negative bacilli and less frequently *Enterococcus* spp. This phase was associated with a 40% mortality rate. Surviving animals later developed intra-abdominal abscesses that were culture-positive most often for obligate anaerobes. However, in this model when a large inoculum of a single strain of bacteria was used (5×10^7 cfu/ml), no strain (either aerobic or anaerobic) was able to induce abscesses when used above. This evidence reaffirms the importance of synergism for abscess formation (7).

The microbiology of peritonitis in CAPD patients shows that most cases are caused by aerobic organisms from normal skin flora. Most episodes are caused by Gram-positive cocci (*Staphylococcus aureus* and *Staphylococcus epidermidis*). Aerobic Gram-negative bacteria and fungi less frequently cause infection. Anaerobic organisms rarely cause infection in this group of patients. A partial explanation may be the high oxygen tension of the CAPD dialysate.

PATHOGENESIS OF PERITONITIS

A general understanding of anatomic relationships within the peritoneal cavity is important for determining the pos-

sible sources of intra-abdominal infection and for anticipating the extent and routes of spread of infection. The peritoneal cavity in males is a completely closed space, whereas in females it is perforated by the free ends of the fallopian tubes. This distinction is important because pelvic peritonitis often accompanies pelvic inflammatory disease (PID), especially if infection of the fallopian tubes is severe. Organs found within the peritoneal cavity include the stomach, jejunum, ileum, transverse and sigmoid colon, cecum, liver, gallbladder, pancreas, spleen and appendix. The peritoneal cavity has various pouches and recesses where bacteria or infected exudate may potentially collect and become loculated. The peritoneal cavity is lined by a serous membrane consisting of a mesothelial cell monolayer below and lymphatics, blood vessels, and nerve endings. The peritoneal space usually contains sufficient fluid to maintain surface moistness, which facilitates movement of the viscera. This moist, peritoneal membrane is also highly permeable, so solutes and water are quickly transported bidirectionally.

Host defense mechanisms generally combat bacterial invasion of the peritoneal cavity (8). Humoral and cellular immune defense mechanisms form the immediate response to bacterial contamination, and the regional lymphatic circulation absorbs bacteria. Bacteria are rapidly cleared from the peritoneal cavity through stomata in the mesothelial cell layer. Stomata are openings that connect lacunae, which are larger lymphatic drainage structures.

The abdominal tissue may confine an inflammatory process by sequestration, which restricts infectious foci by the formation of adhesions between visceral surfaces and loops of bowel. This occurs after a fibrinogen-rich inflammatory exudate containing plasma opsonins appears and fibrin is laid down. Sequestration is important because otherwise the normal peristaltic movements of the viscera and the recumbent position would disperse infected exudate throughout the peritoneal cavity. Sequestration may also protect by trapping bacteria and preventing rapid lymphatic absorption, which could result in death from bacterial endotoxic shock.

Intra-abdominal infections result if the first-line host defense mechanisms become overwhelmed, e.g., (*a*) when the infecting inoculum is very large; (*b*) when the bacterial contamination is due to mixed flora that acts synergistically to evade the first-line defenses; and (*c*) when a foreign body (e.g., CAPD catheter) renders host defenses inefficient (9).

The peritoneal membrane responds next by exuding a fluid containing opsonins, antibodies, complement, PMNs, and macrophages into the peritoneal cavity. This inflammatory response is facilitated by local vasodilitation and increased vascular permeability. Inflammation increases the permeability of the membrane so that the transport of large molecules and protein is enhanced. This may additionally improve the penetration of an antimicrobial agent into the peritoneal cavity during peritonitis (10).

The natural host defenses are unfortunately not without problems under these circumstances, thus making the appropriate antimicrobial selection even more critical. Lymphatic drainage of bacteria from the peritoneal cavity may facilitate bacteremia and endotoxemia, resulting in increased morbidity and mortality. The fibrin/bacterial matrix that is formed on visceral structures may actually isolate the bacteria away from PMNs and macrophages to the extent that phagocytosis is ineffective. These highly protected organisms initiate abscess formation. They exist in this environment at a slowed metabolic rate. Not only are these organisms protected from host defenses, but when antimicrobials do penetrate to the site of infection they may not work optimally because their mechanisms of action may require rapidly multiplying organisms. Another well-known example of this bacterial isolation, is in bacterial infective endocarditis (IE).

INCIDENCE AND PROGNOSTIC FACTORS

Primary peritonitis (SBP) in adults with cirrhosis and ascites may occur in as many as 10% of patients (11), with the presence of hepatorenal syndrome and hepatic coma significantly increasing the mortality rate (12). The overall mortality in these severely ill patients may be as high as 95%. Because SBP often accompanies severe hepatic failure, discerning the mortality rate specific to the infection, is difficult.

The incidence and prognosis of secondary peritonitis are closely associated with the etiology GI tract disruption. Each surgical procedure has its own morbidity and mortality (13). Complication rates relate to the patient's age, duration/stage of illness, the adequacy of surgical procedures, and the presence of other chronic underlying illnesses.

CLINICAL FEATURES AND DIAGNOSIS
Systemic Effects

General malaise, prostration, nausea, vomiting, fever, dehydration, leukocytosis with a left shift, and electrolyte imbalance are systemic symptoms that are seen in patients with intra-abdominal infections. Intra-abdominal abscesses often "smolder" for long periods of time with no or inconsistent symptoms.

Aerobic and anaerobic Gram-negative bacteria may release endotoxin, a lipopolysaccharide from the bacterial cell wall, into the blood stream, which is responsible for some of the serious clinical symptoms observed: septic shock, adult respiratory distress syndrome (ARDS), and disseminated intravascular coagulation (DIC). None of these clinical findings are specific for intra-abdominal infections, and they may occur to a varying degree or not at all.

Hypotension may also be caused by reduced intravascular volume secondary to the massive influx of fluid from the vascular space into the peritoneum during peritonitis.

Abdominal Signs

Abdominal pain and tenderness may be localized or general. Specific abdominal pain on respiration or coughing, rebound tenderness (pain after release of mild pressure on abdomen), and tenderness with gentle percussion of the abdomen are signs of acute peritonitis. The musculature overlying the area of inflamed peritoneum may become spastic. Involuntary muscle rigidity of the entire abdominal wall ("guarding") may develop with diffuse peritonitis. This muscle rigidity is frequently absent or difficult to elicit in the latter stages of peritonitis, in obese patients, or in patients with significant third-spacing of fluid (e.g., ascites).

Specific Objective Findings

The normal serous fluid in the peritoneal cavity is clear yellow with a low specific gravity (less than 1.016) and a low protein concentration (usually less than 3 g/ml), with albumin being the predominant protein. Fibrinogen is not normally present. Solute concentrations are similar to those observed in plasma. A few leukocytes ($<300/mm^3$) and desquamated serosal cells may also be found (14).

Infected peritoneal fluid is visibly cloudy. Measurements used for immediate diagnosis include a pH ≤ 7.34 and a PMN count $>500/mm^3$ (15). Other predictive measures, which are less sensitive however, include a peritoneal fluid lactate concentration >25 mg/dl and glucose concentration <60 mg/dl. Diagnostic sensitivity improves when multiple parameters are used to establish the diagnosis (16).

Specimens from the infected tissue or fluid should be obtained during surgery or by needle aspirate and directly cultured for both anaerobic and aerobic bacteria. Gram-staining of the specimen sediment may help identify pathogens more quickly, so that empiric antimicrobial therapy can be tailored to the patient. The Gram-staining procedure is especially important in situations where the patient has been on antibiotics prior to obtaining the specimen, as cultures may never be positive.

The diagnosis of intra-abdominal abscesses has been improved, particularly with use of computerized tomography scans (CT scans), gallium scans, and ultrasonography (17).

TREATMENT
Surgical Management

Management of intra-abdominal infections is initially based upon any necessary operative procedures to repair GI perforations. Also important are debridement procedures for removal of any infectious foci. This includes drainage of abscesses and debridement of infected, necrotic tissue or bowel. The goal of surgical procedures is to debulk the infection and revitalize tissue with sufficient blood supply, which then allows antibiotics and host defenses to have an impact. Even death may result as a complication from undrained intra-abdominal abscesses (18). Radiologists have become adept at draining most abscesses by percutaneous catheters. Catheters are placed under ultrasound or CT-scan guidance (19).

The indication for Tenckhoff catheter removal in CAPD patients with peritonitis has not been established. Some experts think that continuing regular CAPD in patients with peritonitis improves outcome because infectious exudate can be physically removed with continued dialysis. Others feel that it is important to remove the catheter (thus losing dialysis access), because curing an infection that involves a foreign body (e.g., the catheter) is extremely difficult. Hemodialysis access is assessed in these patients. As a conservative recommendation, if a patient has not responded to appropriate parenteral antimicrobial therapy alone within 5 days, removal of the Tenckhoff catheter should be considered. Experience with fungal peritonitis in CAPD suggests that early catheter removal is probably indicated (3).

General Measures

Support of intravascular volume with fluid therapy is essential to maintain adequate blood pressure and renal perfusion. The so-called volume expanders, such as albumin and hetastarch, are not essential in this setting, and they are expensive. Electrolyte imbalances and metabolic acidosis should be corrected quickly with intravenous therapy.

Oral intake of foods should be discontinued temporarily and nasogastric (NG) suction started as soon as peritonitis is suspected, to prevent GI distension. Suction is continued until peristaltic activity returns and the patient begins to pass flatus. NG suctioning may contribute to the patient's overall fluid loss, dehydration, and acid/base and electrolyte disturbances. This must be taken into consideration when recommending a patient-specific fluid-replacement regimen.

Administration of oral medications should be discontinued in patients receiving NG suctioning. The GI absorption of oral medications in these clinical circumstances may be erratic because of changes in pH and motility. The drug may also be inadvertently removed from the GI tract by the suctioning procedure.

Antimicrobial Therapy

The choice of empiric antimicrobial therapy for intra-abdominal infections is controversial and has been reviewed in an excellent article by DiPiro et al. (20). Antibiotics were directed against only aerobic organisms before technical improvements in anaerobic culturing methods revealed the true incidence of anaerobic infection. Now, parenteral therapy for both anaerobic and aerobic organisms of the GI flora is most often administered. The rationale for such therapy is based upon observations in animal models of intra-abdominal sepsis and from clinical experience (Table 64.1). Therapy that includes antistaphylococcal and antipseudomonal activity is not empirically necessary, unless there are predisposing factors.

There are many acceptable antibiotic regimens, both monotherapy or combination regimens, for the treatment of intra-abdominal infections. Each regimen may have subtle or major advantages or disadvantages in a specific patient. Table 64.2 provides a listing of antimicrobial agents that may be used. The following descriptions of antibiotic therapies do not give exact recommendations for therapy, but they do provide a necessary framework and some important details for the formulation of patient-specific regimens.

Selection of empiric antimicrobial therapy should follow careful consideration of the suspected site(s) and source of infection and the most likely pathogens. Empiric therapy should be chosen to cover, as narrowly as possible, only the suspected organisms. Using antibiotic(s) with the narrowest spectrum reduces the rate of secondary drug-resistance, superinfections, and confusion when assessing clinical response.

The unique pharmacologic properties of each potential antimicrobial must next be considered with regards to the following properties: (a) ability to penetrate the site of infection; (b) "inoculum effect" (stability toward β-lactamases produced by large bacterial inocula); and (c) activity in an environment of potentially low metabolic activity (as in abscesses), or low pH or pO_2, as in necrotic tissue disease. Lastly, antimicrobial selection is based upon considerations of potential adverse reactions, drug-disease interactions, ease of dosing, and overall therapy costs.

Penicillin or ampicillin provide antibacterial coverage for aerobic and anaerobic Gram-positive cocci from the oropharyngeal region. Cephalosporins also are active against these organisms, but they have a broader antibacterial activity, including many aerobic/anaerobic Gram-negative bacilli. This broadened bacterial coverage may not be needed empirically.

Aminoglycosides are often used to provide specific antimicrobial activity against aerobic Gram-negative bacilli (e.g., Enterobacteriaceae) that are found further down the GI tract. These agents have a narrow therapeutic-toxic serum concentration range that makes dosage adjustments and monitoring more complicated. Aminoglycosides are highly active in vitro against most strains of facultative aerobes, which are important in producing bacteremia and

Table 64.1.
Positive Cultures from Intra-Abdominal Infections[a]

Aerobes	Positive Cultures (%)				
	Study 1 (*n* = 161)	Study 2 (*n* = 144)	Study 3 (*n* = 48)	Study 4 (*n* = 37)	Total[b] (*n* = 390)
Enterococci	19	17	6	49	19
Other streptococci	14	33	6	14	20
Staphylococci	7	24	8	32	16
E. coli	99	67	40	51	75
Proteus spp.	9	10	8	3	9
Enterobacter spp.	5	0	2	11	3
Klebsiella spp.	30	13	0	22	19
Pseudomonas spp.	15	10	2	14	12
Candida spp.	0	4	4	0	2
Misc. aerobes	22	14	2	14	16
Anaerobes	Study 1	Study 2	Study 3	Study 4	Total
Streptococci	0	1	13	0	2
Peptococcus	0	4	19	5	4
Peptostreptococcus	8	6	17	0	8
Fusobacterium	35	3	4	0	16
Clostridium spp.	29	36	31	0	29
B. fragilis	100	66	52	3	91
Other *Bacteroides*	19	36	58	14	29
Misc. anaerobes	0	25	8	0	6

[a] Data are from blood and peritoneal cultures; reported in Lau WY, et al. (21), Harding et al. (22), Jones et al. (23), and Smith et al. (24).
[b] Percentages do not add up to 100 because each culture may have been positive for more than one organism.

early mortality in intra-abdominal infections (i.e., endo-toxin-induced septic shock). This efficacy was illustrated in an animal model of intra-abdominal sepsis (25, 26), and they have become a component of the standard therapy. Aztreonam, a new monobactam antibiotic, has a similar narrow spectrum of activity and has the low adverse reaction profile of β-lactams. It deserves clinical study for these infections.

Various extended-spectrum penicillins and second- and third-generation cephalosporins have been more recently recommended over aminoglycosides, because their activity against most aerobic Gram-negative bacilli is comparable. The combination of a penicillin and an aminoglycoside compares with cefoxitin, with regards to susceptibility of aerobic Gram-negative bacilli and anaerobic/aerobic Gram-positive streptococci. Also, the penicillin/aminoglycoside combination provides bactericidal activity against *Enterococcus* spp. The toxicity of aminoglycosides remains the limiting factor. The prevalence of aminoglycoside-induced nephrotoxicity in patients being treated for intra-abdominal infections has been recently reviewed (27). Therapeutic failures from *Pseudomonas* and *Enterobacter* infections in patients receiving nonaminoglycoside regimens may justify their empiric use under certain circumstances. Also, aminoglycoside-containing regimens are thought by many experts to be specifically indicated in more severely ill patients manifesting symptoms of septic shock (i.e., hypotension, renal failure, unexplained acidosis). The aminoglycosides are generally not necessary for prophylaxis of infection (28, 29). After culture results are available, therapy may be switched to antimicrobials with less potential for toxicity. Future use of single-daily dose aminoglycoside regimens will maximize efficacy, minimize toxicity, and may further increase the use of aminoglycosides (30).

Studies have shown a loss of activity of some antibiotics in dialysis fluid because of the low pH and high osmolarity of the dialysate solution. Aminoglycosides, specifically, have reduced bactericidal activity when the pH of the test media is lowered to 5.5, which simulates infected dialysate (31). This may be a consideration when CAPD patients treated with aminoglycosides are not clinically responding as expected.

No cephalosporin has antimicrobial activity against the enterococcus. Penicillins such as penicillin, ampicillin, mezlocillin, azlocillin, and piperacillin, or vancomycin when given alone, are bacteriostatic against this organism. Imipenem has some activity against some strains of *Enterococcus*. The combination of one of these agents plus gentamicin is bactericidal against enterococci. This improved activity against the enterococcus is often another rationale for using aminoglycoside/penicillin combinations when

Table 64.2.
Usefulness of Antimicrobials for Empiric Therapy of Intra-Abdominal Infections: Activity against Suspected Pathogens

Generic Name (Trade Name)	Dose	Effective against		
		B. fragilis	Enterobacteriaceae	*Enterococcus* spp.
Metronidazole (Flagyl)	500 mg, q8h	Yes	No	No
Clindamycin (Cleocin)	900 mg, q8h	Yes	No	No
Chloramphenicol (Chloromycetin)	50 mg/kg/day, q6h	Yes	No	No
Cefuroxime (Zinacef, Kefurox)	750 mg–1.5 g, q8h	No	Yes	No
Cefotetan (Cefotan)	1–2 g, q12h	Yes	Yes	No
Cefoxitin (Mefoxin)	1–2 g, q6–8h	Yes	Yes	No
Cefmetazole (Zefazone)	1–2 g, q6–8h	Yes	Yes	No
Cefotaxime (Claforan)	1–2 g, q6–8h	Some	Yes	No
Ceftizoxime (Ceftizox)	1–2 g, q6–8h	Yes	Yes	No
Ceftazidime (Fortaz, Taxicef, Tazidime)	1–2 g, q8h	No	Yes	No
Cefoperazone (Cefobid)	1–2 g, q6–8h	Yes	Yes	No
Ceftriaxone (Rocephin)	1g, q12–24h	No	Yes	No
Ticarcillin/clavulanic acid (Timentin)	3.1 g, q4h	Yes	Yes	No
Ampicillin/sulbactam (Unasyn)	1.5–3 g, q6h	Yes	Some	Yes
Imipenem/cilastatin (Primaxin)	500 mg q6–8h	Yes	Yes	No
Gentamicin/tobramycin	5–10 µg/ml "peak"	No	Yes	No
Vancomycin (Vancocin)	1 g, q12h	No	No	Yes
Penicillin (various)	1–2 mU q4–6h	No	No	Yes
Ampicillin (various)	1–2 g, q4–6h	No	No	Yes
Mezlocillin (Mezlin)	4–5 g, q6–8h	Some	Yes	Yes
Piperacillin (Pipracil)	3–4 g, q4–6h	Some	Yes	Yes
Ticarcillin (Ticar)	3g, q4h	No	Yes	Yes
Aztreonam (Aztactam)	1 g, q6–8h	No	Yes	No

treating intra-abdominal sepsis. If enterococci are cultured from the blood of patients with intra-abdominal infections, therapy with enterococcal coverage should definitely be initiated.

Antimicrobial agents with good activity against obligate anaerobes, such as *B. fragilis* reduce the frequency of abscesses, a later complication of intra-abdominal infections. This coverage is needed in addition to, not instead of, therapy for aerobes. Chloramphenicol has a broad spectrum of activity against anaerobes, but few studies have evaluated its efficacy (22). In addition the potential for serious toxicity (e.g., aplastic anemia and bone marrow suppression) has minimized its usefulness as a first-line drug.

Clindamycin has been used successfully for treatment (32) and prophylaxis (23) of abdominal abscesses. It has the advantage of broad anaerobic Gram-positive and Gram-negative activity, and in addition has good antistaphylococcal activity, which may be needed in specific patients. The value of clindamycin has been reduced by concerns about drug-induced diarrhea and pseudomembranous colitis, though the latter toxicity may result from the use of any antimicrobial therapy. Clindamycin may also be higher in cost and regional sensitivity patterns have revealed significant resistance. Metronidazole has been directly compared to clindamycin for the

treatment of serious intra-abdominal infections caused by anaerobic organisms and has demonstrated equal efficacy and probably better safety (24, 33). Metronidazole is bactericidal, with a narrow spectrum of antianaerobic bacterial activity, mostly against the Gram-negative anaerobes. Bacterial resistance has not been an issue with metronidazole. The parenteral formulation is well tolerated by most patients, except for those with ethanol "on board" at admission and patients that may receive an alcohol-containing medication (i.e., elixirs) during therapy. The disulfiram-like reaction caused by metronidazole may be serious, with significant hypotension. There is also concern about metronidazole causing mutagenicity and carcinogenicity in animals (34). No studies have monitored the incidence of cancer in humans after prolonged administration of metronidazole, as might be encountered in the treatment of intra-abdominal processes. The uncontrolled observation of carcinomas in three young Crohn's disease patients who received 275 to 720 g of metronidazole is worrisome (35). Long-term controlled studies are warranted. During pregnancy and lactation metronidazole should be avoided (36).

Cefoxitin was the first of the β-lactams to show in vitro activity against *B. fragilis*. It is safe and effective for the treatment of mixed flora intra-abdominal infections, whether given alone or with an aminoglycoside (37). Not all of the second- and third-generation cephalosporins are appropriate for single-drug therapy. Each has its own problems. Cefamandole and cefoperazone have unacceptable failure rates; cefotetan, ceftizoxime, and cefmetazole lack widespread acceptance, though they should be as effective as cefoxitin in most circumstances; cefotaxime has less activity against *B. fragilis* group species, compared with metronidazole; and lastly, moxalactam has the potential for causing hypoprothrombinemia with clinical bleeding and also is associated with a significant rate of enterococcal superinfections. Imipenem, a new carbapenem antibiotic has excellent activity against all suspected organisms. However drug accumulation may occur in renal failure, which puts patients at risk for drug-induced seizures. The broad spectrum of activity of imipenem (including activity against *Pseudomonas* spp. and *Enterobacter* spp.) is unnecessary in an empiric drug for these infections, though it may be useful when bacterial resistance against traditional agents becomes a problem for particular patients or institutions. Penicillin plus β-lactamase-inhibitor drugs (i.e., ticarcillin plus clavulanic acid or ampicillin plus sulbactam) are broad-spectrum agents with excellent activity against β-lactamase-producing Gram-negative organisms including *B. fragilis*. In fact they have comparable activity to metronidazole against these pathogens (38). These agents may however be lacking in their coverage of important Enterobacteriaceae (e.g., *Klebsiella, Acinetobacter,* or *Citrobacter* spp.).

COMPLICATIONS
Paralytic Ileus

Adynamic or paralytic ileus occurs to some extent with any peritoneal injury or surgery. Early in the course of peritoneal irritation, the intestine may have a transient period of hyperperistalsis, followed by a decrease in motility or an absence to the point of obstruction. Severity and duration depend upon the type of insult but usually lasts from 2 to 3 days, even in an uncomplicated surgical case. Studies indicate that the pathogenesis of this condition involves neurogenic, hormonal, and local factors. The adrenergic response to intra-abdominal inflammation results in the slowing of peristalsis. The accumulation of gas and fluids within the bowel lumen distends the intestinal wall to the point that intraluminal pressure exceeds capillary perfusion pressure, causing bowel ischemia.

Symptoms of paralytic ileus include progressive abdominal distension and vomiting of pooled gastric contents and biliary secretions. Localized pain and profuse vomiting only occur if there is complete bowel obstruction and strangulation. Therapy consists of GI tract rest, NG suction, and treatment of the underlying GI disease.

Abdominal Adhesions

As a normal host defense, the body attempts to isolate infections of the abdomen into localized pockets. The peritoneum exudes large quantities of fibrin into the peritoneal fluid, while at the same time fibrinolytic activity is reduced. The result is the formation of a network of fibrinous strands between the loops of bowel and the adjacent visceral surfaces. If the fibrin is not reabsorbed, the strands are invaded by fibroblasts and develop a blood supply. Fibrin strands transform into firm adhesive bands. The absence of peristalsis allows these adhesions to form more easily. Surgical treatment may be necessary to free these attachments.

CONCLUSIONS

In the patient with intra-abdominal sepsis, the crucial therapy is prompt, adequate surgical intervention. Parenteral antibiotics are also used to decrease the rate of bacteremia and abscess formation. By necessity the empiric antimicrobial regimen is selected based upon patient-specific considerations. Thus, every clinician must be aware of the differences in the microflora at various levels of the GI tract, along with their usual antimicrobial susceptibilities. These data are then used to formulate empiric therapy regimens. Therapy usually includes antimicrobial coverage for the aerobic Gram-negative bacilli that cause early-infection morbidity, as well as coverage for *B. fragilis*, which causes late-infection morbidity. Antimicrobial selection is further refined by considering patient-specific issues such as concurrent medical problems and concommitant drug therapies. Next, the practical issues surrounding drug administration and overall therapy costs are considered. Lastly, future therapy regimens for intra-abdominal infection are likely to include new agents such as antiendotoxin (HA1A Centoxin). Recommendations for the appropriate use of these agents will be a multidisciplinary decision. Patient-selection criteria must be formulated and monitored, as these new biotechnology drugs will prove to be useful, but will be very expensive.

REFERENCES

1. Conn HO, Fessel JM: Spontaneous bacterial peritonitis. Medicine 50:161–197, 1971.
2. Popovich RP, Moncrief JW, Nolph KD, Ghods AJ, Twardowski ZJ, Pyle WK: Continuous ambulatory peritoneal dialysis. Ann Intern Med 88:449–456, 1978.
3. Rubin J, Rogers WA, Taylor HM, Everett ED, Prowant BF, Fruto LV, Nolph KD: Peritonitis during continuous ambulatory peritoneal dialysis. Ann Intern Med 92:7–13, 1980.
4. Nichols RL: Intraabdominal sepsis: characterization and treatment. J Infect Dis 135:S54–S57, 1977.
5. Gorbach SL: Treatment of intraabdominal infection. Am J Med 76:107–110, 1984.
6. Ingham HR, Tharagonnet D, Sisson PR, Selkin JB, Codd AA: Inhibition of phagocytosis in vitro by obligate anaerobes. Lancet 2:1252–1254, 1977.
7. Onderdonk AB, Shapiro ME, Finberg RW, Zaleznik DF, Kasper DL: Use of a model of intraabdominal sepsis for studies of the pathogenicity of *Bacteroides fragilis*. Rev Infect Dis 6:S91–S95, 1984.

8. Dunn DL, Simmons RL: The role of anaerobic bacteria in intraabdominal infections. Rev Infect Dis 6:S139–S146, 1984.

9. Buggy BP, Schaberg DR, Swartz RD: Intraleukocytic sequestration as a cause of persistent *Staphylococcus aureus* peritonitis in continuous ambulatory peritoneal dialysis. Am J Med 76:1035–1039, 1984.

10. Gerding DN, Wendell HH, Schierl EA: Antibiotic concentrations in ascitic fluid of patients with ascites and bacterial peritonitis. Ann Intern Med 86:708–713, 1977.

11. Kline MM, McCallum RW, Guth PH: The clinical value of ascitic fluid culture and leukocyte count studies in alcoholic cirrhosis. Gastroenterology 70:408–412, 1976.

12. Weinstein MP, Iannin PB, Stratton CW, Eickhoff TC: Spontaneous bacterial peritonitis. Am J Med 64:592–598, 1978.

13. Welch CE, Malt RA: Surgery of the stomach, duodenum, gallbladder, and bile ducts. N Engl J Med 316:999–1008, 1987.

14. Levison ME, Bush LM, Peritonitis and other intra-abdominal infections. In Mandall GL, Douglas RG Jr, Bennett JE: Principles and Practice of Infectious Diseases, ed. 3. New York, Churchill Livingstone, 1990, p 636.

15. Stassen WN, McCullough AJ, Bacon BR, Gutnik SH, Wadiwala IM, McLaren C, Kalhan SC, Tavill AS: Immediate diagnostic criteria for bacterial infection of ascitic fluid. Gastroenterology 90:1247–1254, 1986.

16. Garcia-Tsao G, Conn HO, Lerner E: The diagnosis of bacterial peritonitis: comparison of pH, lactate concentration and leukocyte count. Hepatology 5:91–96, 1985.

17. Moir C, Robins RE: Role of ultrasonography, gallium scanning, and computed tomography in the diagnosis of intraabdominal abscess. Am J Surg 143:582–585, 1982.

18. Fry DE, Garrison RN, Heitsch RC, Calhoun K, Polk HC: Determinants of death in patients with intraabdominal abscess. Surgery 88:517–522, 1980.

19. Gerzoh SG, Robbins AH, Johnson WC, Birkett DH, Nabseth DC: Percutaneous catheter drainage of abdominal abscesses. N Engl J Med 305:653–657, 1981.

20. DiPiro JT, Mansberger JA, Davis JB Jr: Current concepts in clinical therapeutics: Intra-abdominal infections. Clin Pharm 5:334–350, 1986.

21. Lau WY, Teoh-Chan CH, Fan ST, Yam WC, Lau KF, Wong SH: The bacteriology and septic complication of patients with appendicitis. Ann Surg 200:576–581, 1984.

22. Harding GKM, Buckwold FJ, Ronald AR, Marrie TJ, Brunton S, Koss JC, Gurwith MJ, Albritton WL: Prospective, randomized comparative study of clindamycin, chloramphenicol, and ticarcillin, each in combination with gentamicin in therapy for intraabdominal and female genital tract sepsis. J Infect Dis 142:384–393, 1980.

23. Jones RC, Thal ER, Johnson NA, Golihar LN: Evaluation of antibiotic therapy following penetrating abdominal trauma. Ann Surg 201:576–585, 1985.

24. Smith JA, Skidmore AG, Forward AD, et al.: Prospective, randomized, double-blind comparison of metronidazole and tobramycin with clindamycin and tubramycin in the treatment of intra-abdominal sepsis. Ann Surg 192:213–220, 1980.

25. Nichols RL, Smith JW, Fossedal EN, Condon RE: Efficacy of parenteral antibiotics in the treatment of experimentally induced intraabdominal sepsis. Rev Infect Dis 1:302–312, 1979.

26. Bartlett JG, Louie TJ, Gorbach SL, Onderdonk AB: Therapeutic efficacy of 29 antimicrobial regimens in experimental intraabdominal sepsis. Rev Infect Dis 3:535–542, 1981.

27. Ho JL, Barza M: Role of aminoglycoside antibiotics in the treatment of intra-abdominal infection. Antimicrob Agents Chemother 31:485–491, 1987.

28. Gentry LO, Feliciano DV, Lea AS, Short HD, Mattox KL, Jordan GL: Perioperative antibiotic therapy for penetrating injuries of the abdomen. Ann Surg 200:561–566, 1984.

29. Nichols RL, Smith JW, Klein DB, Trunkey DD, Cooper RH, Adinolfi MF: Risk of infection after penetrating abdominal trauma. N Engl J Med 311:1065–1070, 1984.

30. Kapusnik JE, Hackbarth CJ, Chambers HF, Carpenter T, Sande MA: Single-large daily dose versus conventional intermittent dosing of tobramycin for the treatment of guinea pigs with *Pseudomonas* pneumonia. J Infect Dis 158:7–12, 1988.

31. McCormick EM, Echols RM: Effect of peritoneal dialysis fluid and pH on bactericidal activity of ciprofloxacin. Antimicrob Agents Chemother 31:657–659, 1987.

32. Leigh DA, Simmons K, Williams S: The treatment of abdominal and gynecological infections with parenteral clindamycin phosphate. J Antimicrob Chemother 3:493–500, 1977.

33. Van der Auwera, Collier J, Goris RJA, Saario I, Willis AT: A comparison of metronidazole and clindamycin for the treatment of intra-abdominal anaerobic infection: a multicentre trial. J Antimicrob Chemother 10:57–66, 1982.

34. Finegold SM: Metronidazole. Ann Intern Med 93:585–587, 1980.

35. Krause JR, Ayuyang HQ, Ellis LD: Occurrence of three cases of carcinoma in individuals with Crohn's disease treated with metronidazole. Am J Gastroenterol 80:978–982, 1985.

36. Robbie MO, Sweet RL: Metronidazole use in obstetrics and gynecology: a review. Am J Obstet Gynecol 145:865–881, 1983.

37. Tally FP, Kellum JM, Ho JL, O'Donnell TF, Barza M, Gorbach SL: Randomized prospective study comparing moxalactam and cefoxitin with or without tobramycin for the treatment of serious surgical infections. Antimicrob Agents Chemother 29:244–249, 1986.

38. Cuchural GJ Jr., Tally FP, Jacobus NV: Susceptibilities of *Bacteroides fragilis* group in the United States: analysis by site of isolation. Antimicrob Agents Chemother 32:717–722, 1988.

CHAPTER 65

GASTROINTESTINAL INFECTIONS

VICTOR LAMPASONA, Pharm.D.

Gastroenteritis (GE) is a major cause of mortality in developing countries, where it is second to the common cold as a source of morbidity during the colder months (1). Some authors estimate that 25 million enteric infections with 10,000 deaths occur each year in the U.S. alone (2). The most common symptom of acute infectious GE is diarrhea, which may be severe enough in elderly, debilitated patients and infants to cause fluid and electrolyte depletion that may require hospitalization. However, many cases are self-limiting, requiring only supportive care and oral fluid and electrolyte replacement. Occasionally, patients may self-medicate with over-the-counter (OTC) antidiarrheal drugs.

ETIOLOGY AND EPIDEMIOLOGY

Viruses are the most common cause of infectious diarrhea in the United States; most cases are caused by rotavirus or Norwalk virus (3). Bacterial GE is less frequent and is caused by *Salmonella, Shigella, Campylobacter, Yersinia, Vibrio* and *Escherichia coli.* Certain parasites, such as *Giardia lamblia, Entamoeba histolytica* and *Cryptosporidium,* are also associated with diarrheal illness; these are discussed with other intestinal parasites in Chapter 64.

This discussion is limited to organisms that are common, are of increasing epidemiologic importance, or that merit special treatment considerations. Information about other viral infections, overgrowth of normal flora, antibiotic-induced *Clostridium difficile* colitis, and agents that cause diarrhea mainly through food poisoning may be found in other references (4, 5).

Viruses

Viral GE occurs in two major clinical forms. The first type is more often associated with epidemics and is typically responsible for family and community outbreaks among school-age children and adults. The second type is more sporadic and occurs in infants and young children. Both types of GE are thought to be associated predominantly with two viruses, Norwalk virus and rotavirus.

Rotavirus GE occurs during the winter months and primarily affects children under 3 years of age (3, 4). It is the cause of large outbreaks of diarrhea in infants, usually in day-care environments. The illness may be severe and is commonly accompanied by fever and vomiting. Transmission is usually by the fecal-oral route. The incubation period is 1 to 3 days, with the duration of illness ranging from 5 to 8 days (1). The virus is excreted in the feces throughout the illness.

Norwalk virus outbreaks occur in recreational camps, on cruise ships, in elementary schools and colleges, in nursing homes and after ingestion of contaminated water or inadequately cooked shellfish. GE from this organism may be epidemic in nature and affects adults and school-age children, whereas infants and young children are typically spared (3). The incubation period is usually shorter than with rotavirus, typically from 4 to 48 hr, with the duration of the illness from 1 to 2 days (1, 3). The virus can be detected in the feces for up to 72 hr after the onset of the illness. The infection is usually acquired by fecal-oral contamination, although some airborne transmission may occur. Clinical manifestation of Norwalk virus GE is usually abrupt, with patients experiencing vomiting or diarrhea, or both. Illness caused by this virus has been called "winter vomiting disease," indicating the association with vomiting and seasonal incidence, although outbreaks may occur in all seasons.

Enteric adenoviruses, calcivirus, and astrovirus have also been observed in the stools of individuals with diarrheal illnesses, although the role these agents play in the entire spectrum of GE illnesses is thought to be minimal (3, 6–9).

Bacteria

Salmonella are Gram-negative bacilli of the Enterobacteriaceae family and are represented by three primary serotypes—*S. choleraesuis, S. typhi* (the causative agent of typhoid fever), and *S. enteritidis.* They have been isolated from many animal species, including chickens, turkeys, ducks, cows, pigs, domestic pets, doves, pigeons, sheep, and donkeys. Although there are > 2000 serotypes of *Salmonella,* most cases of Salmonella-induced GE are caused by *S. enteritidis, S. newport,* or *S. anatum* and result from the ingestion of contaminated food or water, as demonstrated in home, community, or institutional outbreaks. Contaminated eggs or products made from eggs are major sources of infection. Person-to-person spread is via the fecal-oral route. Modern methods of food production and distribution increase the potential for *Salmonella* epidemic outbreaks. A good example of this was a six-state outbreak in the Chicago area affecting 16,000 individuals. This outbreak was eventually linked to a milk-processing plant where a malfunctioning valve resulted in the contamination of pasteurized milk with *Salmonella*-infected raw milk (11, 12). Forty-seven thousand cases of salmonellosis (excluding typhoid fever) were reported in the United States in 1989 (13). It appears that the states of the Northeast have higher reported rates of *S. enteritidis* compared with other parts of the country (14).

Symptoms occur from 6 to 48 hr after the ingestion of contaminated food or water. The major symptom, diarrhea, usually abates within 3 to 7 days.

Campylobacter are spiral-shaped Gram-negative rods known to cause systemic as well as gastrointestinal illnesses. The human pathogenic species are *C. jejuni*, *C. fetus*, and *C. coli*. These organisms are commonly found in the gastrointestinal tracts of wild or domesticated cattle, sheep, swine, fowl, cats, and dogs. Most human infections occur from ingestion of contaminated water or food. Unpasteurized milk, untreated surface water, undercooked meat, and raw clams have been associated with GE infections. Domestic pets such as young dogs or cats with diarrhea have been implicated as vectors (14). Person-to-person spread via the fecal-oral route has also been described and may be the major cause of intrafamilial infection. Evidence suggests that *Campylobacter* gastrointestinal infections may occur with greater frequency than *Salmonella* or *Shigella* infections, since it is more commonly isolated from fecal specimens (15). *Campylobacter* has also been implicated as a cause of traveler's diarrhea (16). The incubation period for *Campylobacter* GE is variable, from 24 hr to 10 days. Although the duration of illness is typically 1 week, it is not uncommon for symptoms to last up to 2 weeks.

Escherichia coli is a Gram-negative rod that is a common inhabitant in the human gastrointestinal tract. GE can be caused by five different types of the organism, each with different virulence properties. These five types of organisms are thought to cause diarrhea by up to seven possible mechanisms (17). Three of these mechanisms involve heat-labile (LTEC) and two types of heat-stable enterotoxin (ST_a and ST_b), found in enterotoxigenic *E. coli* (ETEC). Others involve enteropathogenic *E. coli* (EPEC), which cause diarrhea by enteroadherent organisms; enteroinvasive *E. coli* (EIEC), which cause inflammatory colitis; enterohemorrhagic *E. coli* (EHEC), which cause hemorrhagic diarrhea by producing a verocytotoxin; and *E. coli* that produce diarrhea by colonization. ETEC is the major cause of infant diarrhea and dehydration in less-developed countries. EPEC has been associated with outbreaks of diarrhea in hospitalized infants less than 3 months old in urban areas. Hemolytic uremic syndrome, a syndrome of unknown etiology that leads to acute renal failure in infants and small children worldwide, has been associated with GE caused by EHEC (18). Most cases of *E. coli* GE are associated with the ingestion of contaminated food or water. ETEC strains are a major cause of

traveler's diarrhea. The incubation period for ETEC infections appears to be about 1 to 2 days, with a duration of illness of about 3 days (7). The excretion of organisms in the stool ceases within 5 days in most patients.

Yersinia enterocolitica is another Gram-negative organism that causes GE in both children and adults (20). The organism can be isolated from a variety of animals, including swine, cattle, horses, sheep, cats, and dogs. Although the organism is widely found in water, most outbreaks of GE infection have been attributed to contaminated food or unpasteurized milk. The GE caused by this organism may last 1 to 3 weeks, with *Yersinia* being excreted in feces for weeks after symptoms subside.

Shigellae are Gram-negative rods that are known to cause a type of GE in humans that is also referred to as bacillary dysentery. Four types of *Shigella* have been implicated: *S. sonnei* (currently most prevalent in industrialized countries), *S. flexneri* (most important between the 1920s and 1930s, *S. boydii* rarely implicated), and *S. dysenteriae* (the most virulent and not commonly seen in developed countries since early this century). *Shigella* are notorious for the small inoculum of organisms needed to produce clinical illness. This fact explains the rapid spread seen in day-care centers and other closed populations. Transmission is usually by the fecal-oral route, with humans as the sole reservoir. Twenty-five thousand cases of shigellosis were reported in the United States in 1989 (13). The incubation period is from 2 to 20 days (7).

Several other Gram-negative organisms have been reported to cause clinical gastrointestinal illnesses in certain patient groups. *Pseudomonas*, *Aeromonas*, and *Plesiomonas* species can cause a GE that is most important in young infants or immunocompromised patients (7, 21, 22). The source of the infection can usually be credited to the colonization of the gastrointestinal tract of these patients during hospitalization (*Pseudomonas*) or the ingestion of contaminated water (*Aeromonas* and *Plesiomonas*) (23). *Vibrio* is a cause of GE in the United States and around the world. Major enteric pathogens are *V. cholerae* (the causative agent of cholera), *V. parahemolyticus*, and *V. mimicus* (24). *V. vulnificus*, a marine *Vibrio* associated with extraintestinal infections, has also been identified as a cause of GE (25). *Vibrio* GE is usually linked with the ingestion of raw or undercooked seafood, typically shellfish, and with travel to Mexico.

A summary of the epidemiology of GE is listed on Table 65.1.

PATHOGENESIS
Host Defenses
Among the host factors that act against pathogenic organisms, four have been well established as defense mechanisms: gastric acidity, peristalsis, immune response, and resident microflora. Most enteric pathogens are sensitive

Table 65.1.
Epidemiologic Characteristics of Gastroenteritis

Infecting Organism	Common Source of Isolation	Common Age Characteristics	Transmission	Other Characteristics
Campylobacter	Animals, water	All ages	Person-to-person, waterborne	Summer–fall
Salmonella	Poultry, pigs	Very young, very old	Foods of animal origin	Summer–fall
Shigella	Infected persons	1–4 years old	Person-to-person	Summer–fall
Escherichia coli	Water	All ages	Person-to-person, foodborne	Traveler's diarrhea
Vibrio	Shellfish	All ages	Foodborne, waterborne	Summer
Yersinia	Pigs, milk, water, domestic animals	<5 years old	Person-to-person, foodborne	May involve multiple organ systems, summer peak—USA? fall–winter peak—Europe
Aeromonas	Fresh water	All ages	Waterborne	Immunocompromised persons

to gastric acidity. The peristaltic action of the small intestine aided by mucus secretion also minimizes colonization and assists in eliminating pathogenic organisms. Enteric immunity consists of intraluminal phagocytic cells, cell-mediated immune processes, and secretory IgA production. Finally, resident microflora provide competition for pathogenic colonization by attaching to intestinal epithelium and acting synergistically with enteric immune-response mechanisms. Interference with these factors may increase host susceptibility to infection.

Patients with achlorhydria or gastric resection are more susceptible to enteric infection. Anatacids or H_2-antagonists reduce the inoculum required to produce clinically important GE from certain organisms. Slowing of intestinal motility caused by antiperistaltic compounds such as diphenoxylate or loperamide encourage colonization as a result of increased contact time of the organisms with the gastric mucosa. Immature or compromised immune status predisposes patients to infection. Antibiotics (especially broad-spectrum compounds) decrease normal flora of the intestinal tract and allow inappropriate overgrowth of pathogenic organisms or colonizing nosocomial organisms known to cause GE.

A recent report of an investigation into an outbreak of nosocomial *Salmonella enteritidis* infections affecting 28% of the patients in a 1045-bed hospital indicates that diabetics who require insulin or oral hypoglycemics are at an increased risk for infection, when compared with matched control patients. The increased risk may be due to decreased gastric acid production and disturbances in gastric and bowel motility commonly recognized as complications of diabetes mellitus (26). This report illustrates the need to consider underlying diseases when considering a patient's risk for gastrointestinal infections.

Viral and Bacterial Virulence
Norwalk and rotavirus both cause lesions of the mucosa cells of the small intestine, whereas colonic mucosa remains normal. The exact mechanism of diarrhea produc-

tion is uncertain, although the clinical features most closely resemble enterotoxin-mediated diarrhea. Alterations of duodenal mucosal function usually accompany these infections, as indicated by decreased xylose absorption and reduced fat absorption (27).

Among the many bacterial properties that promote infection, three of the most important are (*a*) the ability to produce enterotoxin, (*b*) the ability to adhere to mucosa and cause inflammation, and (*c*) the ability to invade intact intestinal mucosa. Organisms that cause disease mainly by enterotoxin production primarily colonize the upper small intestine and produce secretory diarrhea (isotonic fluid loss of more than 10 ml/kg/24 hr). *Salmonella*, *Shigella*, ETEC, and *Y. enterocolitica* produce enterotoxins that are also called exotoxins (28). These proteins are secreted by the organisms and bind to receptors located in the brush border of the villus epithelial cell. The bound exotoxin then stimulates adenyl cyclase or guanyl cyclase to dramatically increase intestinal secretion of water and electrolytes. When the volume of fluid overwhelms the reabsorptive capacity of the colon, diarrhea results. The importance of enterotoxin in the pathogenesis of ETEC is well documented, but it is much less well described for *Salmonella*, *Shigella*, and *Yersinia* GE (18, 29–31).

Cytotoxin, a type of exotoxin that alters mucosal cell histology, causes diarrhea by an unknown mechanism. It may assist in the inflammatory invasion of mucosa. *Salmonella dysenteriae*, EHEC, and possibly *C. jejuni* produce cytotoxins (31).

An important part of the pathogenesis of GE for *Salmonella*, *Shigella*, and *E. coli* is bacterial adherence to intestinal muscosa. These organisms possess structures called fimbriae, fine protein filaments protruding from their surfaces. They attach to specific receptor sites on the intestinal cell. The presence or absence of specific receptor sites is inherited, thus susceptibility or resistance to infection is partly genetic (32). *S. enteritidis*, *Shigella*, *C. jejuni*, and EIEC are present and multiplying in the colonic mucosa where they cause inflammation. The inflam-

Table 65.2.
Types of Enteric Infections

	I	II	III
Mechanism	Noninflammatory (enterotoxin)	Inflammatory (cytoxin invasion?)	Penetrating (intact mucosa)
Location	Proximal small bowel	Colon	Distal small bowel
Organisms	*Vibrio*	*Vibrio*	*S. typhi*
	ETEC	*Shigella*	*Yersinia*
	? *Salmonella*	ETEC	? *Campylobacter*
	Rotavirus	*Salmonella*	
	Norwalk virus	? *Campylobacter*	

[a] Adapted from Guerrant RL: Principles and syndromes of enteric infection. In Mandell GL, Douglas RG, Bennett JE (eds): Principles and Practice of Infectious Diseases, ed. 3. New York, Churchill Livingstone, 1990, with permission.

mation is accompanied by minute or gross ulceration, followed by diarrhea. This may eventually lead to systemic dissemination with some organisms. The subsequent fluid secretion is probably due to a multifactorial process involving inflammatory processes and enterotoxin production (32).

Salmonella typhi, Yersinia, and some *Campylobacter* species produce systemic illness with or without diarrhea. These organisms appear to penetrate intact intestinal mucosa and multiply in the lymphatics and reticuloendothelial cells (4, 29, 31). Prostaglandins may be involved in the production of diarrhea mediated by some organisms. As *Salmonella* invade the gastrointestinal mucosal wall, stimulation of prostaglandins and the adenyl cyclase–cyclic AMP system result in the fluid secretion that is commonly seen in these infections (7, 29, 33).

A summary of the organisms associated with each type of infection according to their pathogenic mechanism is listed in Table 65.2.

Electrolyte Depletion

In addition to increased fluid secretion caused by the pathogenic mechanisms described above, these infectious processes result in a disregulation of sodium and bicarbonate homeostasis and electrolyte losses. In the parietal cell, H_2CO_3 dissociates into hydrogen and bicarbonate. The bicarbonate is secreted into the intestine along with sodium, and the hydrogen is reabsorbed into the blood. In the diarrheal process the sodium loss increases, thus causing a concomitant increase in bicarbonate loss into the intestine. This allows more hydrogen to be reabsorbed into the blood, resulting in systemic metabolic acidosis. Potassium loss increases secondary to interference with reabsorption or to activation of the aldosterone system as a result of hyponatremia or hypovolemia.

CLINICAL PRESENTATION

The clinical manifestations of gastrointestinal infections correlate well with the response expected from the specific mechanism of bacterial invasion. Diarrhea is present in all types of GE, except in some cases caused by penetrating organisms such as *S. typhi, Yersinia,* and some species of *Campylobacter.* Fecal leukocytes can be seen in all cases except those caused by noninvasive/noninflammatory processes such as ETEC and *Salmonella* (Table 65.2). The clinical picture for viral enteritis most closely resembles that of the enterotoxin-mediated diarrhea. Fever is usually present in all types of infectious GE and can range from low-grade (enterotoxin) to higher, more serious fevers (invasive and penetrating). Organisms that penetrate intact gastrointestinal membranes tend to produce infectious processes with more systemic symptoms such as vasculitic rashes, arthritis, and bacteremia (16, 20).

Since many of these bacteria cause symptoms that resemble other noninfectious diarrheal illnesses, an appropriate diagnostic approach is important.

A careful history, including recent travel, antibiotic use, family or other contact illnesses, weight loss, underlying diseases, and appearance and quantity of stool, can provide clues to the etiology. Some of this information is organized by causative agent and listed in Table 65.3. Actual examination of a stool specimen for blood, mucus, and leukocytes is preferable to a description of the stool by the patient. A stool culture can be very valuable in diagnosis, although a laboratory may not always be available. Culture technique is critical in the isolation of many enteric bacteria, since some require special media and procedures. Physical assessment of the patient for signs of dehydration and other abnormalities helps to determine the therapeutic approach. The pharmacist should know when other diagnostic procedures, such as radiologic or endoscopic evaluations, are necessary and refer patients quickly to the appropriate medical source. Information on the differential diagnosis of infectious and noninfectious diarrhea can be found elsewhere (4).

TREATMENT
Fluid and Electrolyte Therapy

The mainstay of treatment for any type of infectious diarrhea is fluid and electrolyte replacement. There are two treatment goals in managing patients with fluid losses due

Table 65.3.
Features of Gastroenteritis

	Norwalk Virus	Rotavirus	*Shigella sonnei*	Other *Shigella* spp.	*Salmonella*	ETEC	EIEC	*Campylobacter*	*Yersinia*
Stool	Clear	Clear, brown	Clear	Bloody	Green, brown	Clear	Bloody	Bloody	Pale, green
WBCs	—	—	—	++	−/+	−	++	++	+
Volume	Variable	Large	Large	Small	Moderate	Large	Small	Moderate–large	Small–moderate
Incubation Period (days)	1–2	1–3	1–3	1–2	1–2	1–3	1–3	1–7	4–10
Duration (days)	1–2	5–8	2–3	7–14	3–7	5–10	5–10	2–3	7–14

[a] From Reale EO, Enteric infections. In Herfindal ET, Hirshman JL (eds): Clinical Pharmacy and Therapeutics. ed. 3. Baltimore, Williams & Wilkins, 1983, pp 205–207.

to GE. Rehydration, or fluid-deficit replacement, is the aggressive reversal of existent dehydration, based on calculated and ongoing losses. Maintenance therapy is the ongoing replacement of fluids and electrolytes after the patient has been rehydrated. Fluid may be given by the oral or intravenous route, depending on the severity of losses and the patient's ability to maintain oral intake. If the patient's intake is less than output, intravenous therapy is recommended. Severe dehydration manifested as oliguria or anuria, thirst, dry mucous membranes, lethargy, hypotension, and sunken fontanel (infants) often requires intravenous therapy, in whole or in part. Infants and geriatric patients become dehydrated more rapidly than older children or adults. Infants most often require hospitalization and intravenous rehydration.

The volume of fluid administered depends on the size of the individual, stool losses, degree of dehydration, and the presence of fever. Severely dehydrated patients may require a 10- to 20-ml/kg bolus of normal saline initially.

The type of fluid administered is determined by the electrolyte loss and the need for caloric support. Fluids should contain carbohydrate as an energy source to prevent hypoglycemia, particularly in infants. The electrolyte content of diarrheal stools varies greatly, depending on age, food intake, type of infectious organism, and stool volume. Stool and serum electrolyte content assist in determining replacement needs.

The interpretation of serum concentrations and the treatment of electrolyte imbalances are discussed in Chapter 8. Generally, an intravenous solution of dextrose 5% with 0.25 or 0.5 normal saline meets the needs of most patients with mild-to-moderate diarrheal losses, provided their serum sodium is in the range of 130 to 150 mmol/liter (mEq/liter).

Potassium supplementation should be withheld until urination is present to avoid hyperkalemia. An intravenous solution of KCl of 20 to 40 mEq/liter should maintain adequate serum potassium levels after replacement of deficits is complete. Correction of metabolic acidosis with sodium bicarbonate is usually unnecessary unless the bicarbonate deficit is severe.

Oral fluid and electrolyte therapy has been used ex-

Table 65.4.
Products for Oral Rehydration and Maintenance[a]

	Carbohydrate	Electrolyte (mMol/liter)			
		Na+	K+	Cl−	Base
Pedialyte RS[b]	Glucose	75	20	65	30
Pedialyte	Glucose	45	20	30	30
Infalyte	Glucose	50	20	40	30
Gatorade	Glucose/sucrose	23	3	17	3
Orange juice	Glucose/fructose	0.4	50	—	50
Apple juice	Glucose/fructose	0.4	30	—	—
Grape juice	Glucose/fructose	0.5	30	—	32

[a] Adapted from Reale EO: Enteric infections. In Herfindal ET, Hirshman JL (eds): Clinical Pharmacy and Therapeutics, ed. 3. Baltimore, Williams & Wilkins, 1983, pp 205–207.

[b] Suitable for oral rehydration therapy.

tensively in countries where diarrhea is endemic. In these countries and in the United States, oral rehydration and electrolyte replacement have been accomplished even in severely dehydrated infants and children (34, 35). The United Nations Childrens Fund (UNICEF), World Health Organization (WHO), and the American Academy of Pediatrics recommend oral rehydration as the cornerstone in their child-survival efforts to treat dehydration caused by severe enteritis in infants (36, 37). Oral therapy may prevent the need for hospitalization for mildly to moderately dehydrated patients and is a helpful adjunct to intravenous therapy. Commercial products made specifically for oral rehydration are available, although many household products are suitable and are less expensive (Table 65.4). Household products high in one electrolyte should be alternated with those high in others to provide a balanced electrolyte repletion process. If the taste of these products is offensive to nauseated patients, commercially available electrolyte solutions may be more effective. WHO has recommended a formula for the aggressive oral rehydration therapy required for patients with cholera (35). Modifications of this formula can be prepared in the home and used in patients with severe acute diarrhea. A solution containing a half-teaspoon of salt and 8 teaspoons of sugar in 1 liter of water is an easy-to-make rehydration fluid that should be available in most settings. However, this formula would not be adequate to treat hypokalemia and acidosis, because of a lack of potassium and base (38). A solution containing 4 level teaspoons of sugar, ¾ teaspoon salt, and 1 teaspoon sodium bicarbonate in 1 cup of orange juice can be mixed in 1 liter (1.05 quarts) of water. This solution contains some potassium and base from the orange juice and sodium bicarbonate, and may be better for patients with hypokalemia. If hypertonicity is of concern (e.g., with children), the solution should be given with water ad lib or the salt content arbitrarily reduced (38). Free water alone should always be avoided, since this may result in hyponatremia. Patients should avoid making these solutions to taste, as too much sugar and/or salt may be added, resulting in potentially serious adverse reactions.

The carbohydrates in available oral solutions are glucose, sucrose, or fructose. In addition to providing an energy substrate, glucose facilitates the transport of water and sodium across the cell membrane during its absorption, thus reducing stool losses. Fructose transport is not linked to sodium transport, usually resulting in a less effective response. Sucrose, which must be hydrolyzed by intestinal mucosal disaccharidases to glucose and fructose, is effective except in cases of full-purging diarrhea (34).

Although the past standard of practice has been to withhold food until diarrhea is resolved, more recent evaluations have demonstrated that early food intake does not have an adverse effect on the duration or severity of diarrheal illness and is routinely advised (35, 40). Drinks or foods containing caffeine or lactose should be avoided, since they may prolong diarrhea or add to the fluid and electrolyte imbalance (34). A more conservative approach is to administer soft foods (banana, cereal, applesauce, toast, or salted crackers), breast milk, or half-strength formula once the diarrhea begins to resolve. Staple foods, such as rice, wheat, potatoes, and lentils, are being investigated to determine if they can be used as the feeding component of oral rehydration therapy (38). In general, food or formula should be advanced as tolerated.

Other Supportive Therapy

The value of antidiarrheal agents in treatment of infectious GE depends on the particular product, the infectious agent, and the age of the patient. Antidiarrheals such as tincture of opium, loperamide, and diphenoxylate-atropine are considered safe and may reduce the frequency of stool in some types of acute, self-limiting GE in adults and older children. However, agents that slow gastrointestinal motility may actually increase the duration and severity of illness because of the increase in bacterial contact time with the mucosa, especially if the pathogenesis of infection is mucosal invasion. In general, compounds that decrease peristaltic activity should not be given to patients with diar-

rhea who also describe tenesmus, a symptom that is thought to indicate the presence of active gastrointestinal inflammation.

Diphenoxylate-atropine should be avoided in young children, particularly those less than 2 years old (41). This age group may be more sensitive to the toxic effects of atropine and may experience atropinism with normal doses.

Kaolin-pectin suspension aids in the production of firmer stools, but does not reduce water loss (41). Bismuth subsalicylate (BSS) inhibits fluid secretion caused by *E. coli* in a regimen of 60 ml every half hour up to a maximum of 480 ml/day (43). This dose reduces the number of unformed stools in patients with mild-to-moderate traveler's diarrhea. There is some in vitro evidence that BSS may have bacteriostatic or bacteriocidal activity, which would explain the decreased recovery of pathogens from the stools of patients taking BSS. Additionally, the compound exhibits an antisecretory effect by increasing net water absorption in intestinal fluid and may inhibit the activity of the toxins associated with *E. coli* (44).

The use of *Lactobacillus* to recolonize the intestinal tract was not effective in preventing or altering diarrheal illness in experimentally induced ETEC diarrhea (44, 45).

Nonsteroidal antiinflammatory agents, such as indomethacin and aspirin, have shown some promise in controlling the fluid and electrolyte loss of acute diarrheal illness. This may be due to their ability to inhibit the products of arachadonic acid metabolism which affect intestinal transport of fluid and electrolytes, through an inhibition of cyclooxygenase activity (46). The exact role of these agents in the routine treatment of infectious GE remains to be elucidated.

Antimicrobial Therapy

There are no effective antimicrobial agents available for viral GE. The use of antibiotics to treat bacterial GE depends on the infecting organism, the severity and chronicity of the infectious process, and the effectiveness of the antibiotic in reducing the severity or carrier state of the illness. Since many of the GE infections experienced by ambulatory patients are self-limiting, antibiotic therapy is usually not recommended unless the infection is severe or disseminated, or the patient is chronically symptomatic or debilitated.

Antimicrobial Resistance

A major factor in the prevalence of multiresistant strains of pathogenic organisms is the indiscriminate use of antibiotics in humans and animals. The use of antibiotics is clearly related to the development of plasmid-mediated resistance in microorganisms, especially if concentrations are suboptimal. Multiresistant *Salmonella, Shigella,* and

ETEC have been associated with epidemics in developing countries (47, 48). *Shigella* strains resistant to commonly used agents vary from 7 to 87% for ampicillin, from 11 to 91% for tetracycline, and from 0 to 55% for trimethoprim-sulfamethoxazole, depending on the year or country of origin (47). Resistant *Salmonella* strains vary from 3 to 81% for ampicillin, from 8 to 48% for tetracycline, from 0 to 65% for chloramphenicol, and from 0 to 76% for trimethoprim-sulfamethoxazole (47). ETEC has also demonstrated variable rates of resistance to ampicillin, tetracycline, and trimethoprim-sulfamethoxazole (47). To minimize the development of resistant strains of bacteria, antibiotics must be carefully chosen, based on susceptibility testing and the severity of the condition.

Antibiotics of Choice

The usefulness of antibacterial agents in treating patients with infectious GE depends on the organism involved and how quickly therapy is initiated. Depending on the bacteria involved, they can decrease the duration of the illness or the duration of excretion of the pathogen in the stool. Antibiotics appear to be of most value in *Shigella*, ETEC, and *Campylobacter* infections, and the least value in *Salmonella* or *Yersinia* GE. They may be of some value in *Pseudomonas*, *Aeromonas*, noncholera *Vibrio* or *Plesiomonas* infections in certain patients. Table 65.5 lists the drug of choice by etiologic agent for those infections in which antibiotic therapy is considered most appropriate. Table 65.6 lists the usual drug dose, side effects, and monitoring parameters by drug entity.

Ampicillin has been evaluated for use in *Shigella*, *Salmonella*, and *E. coli* GE. It is very effective in GE caused by *Shigella* ampicillin-sensitive strains only. In fact, prior to the mid-1970s, oral ampicillin was considered the drug of choice for GE caused by *Shigella*. More than half of the *Shigella* strains currently encountered, however, are resistant to ampicillin. Oral ampicillin was found to not significantly affect the duration or severity of diarrhea or

the duration of fever for non–*S. typhi* GE (49, 50). One study, however, reported that parenteral ampicillin decreased the excretion of *Salmonella* in the stool, compared with placebo and oral ampicillin (51). Ampicillin may still be useful in systemic or disseminated infections caused by susceptible *Salmonella*. These infections appear to be more common in infants less than 3 months of age. EPEC and EIEC have been treated with some success with oral ampicillin, although placebo-controlled clinical trials are limited.

Tetracycline has been used successfully to treat GE caused by *Shigella* and ETEC. A single oral dose of 2.5 g of tetracycline hydrochloride (stosstherapy) is effective therapy for *Shigella* GE in adult patients (52). One group of investigators suggest that single-dose therapy may be effective in patients infected with *Shigella* that demonstrate in vitro resistance to tetracycline (52). The usual dose in adult patients is 500 mg every 6 hr for 5 days to treat GE caused by tetracycline-susceptible *Shigella*. Treatment with tetracycline shortened the mean duration of diarrhea in patients with ETEC, compared with placebo (53). The drug also significantly decreased the excretion of the organism in the feces. When treating patients with ETEC, doxycycline in a dose of 100 mg daily is usually given. Some evidence suggests that there are an increasing number of tetracycline-resistant ETEC in parts of Asia and Central America (54).

Tetracycline should not be given to pregnant women or children under 12 years old because of the potential for unwanted permanent staining of the teeth. These compounds are also associated with photosensitivity reactions, probably because of accumulation of the drug in the skin. This reaction classically occurs with demeclocycline and may be seen with doxycycline because of its use in traveler's diarrhea (ETEC-associated).

Chloramphenicol has been used to treat systemic *Salmonella* infections caused by susceptible strains, primarily in patients allergic to penicillin. This compound is associated with bone marrow suppression, both dose-related and idiosyncratic. If chloramphenicol is used, judicious monitoring of reticulocyte, red, and white cell counts as well as hematocrit and platelet counts is necessary to limit toxicity. Serum chloramphenicol drug concentrations should be less than 25 µg/ml. This may reduce the probability of dose-related bone marrow suppression.

Trimethoprim-sulfamethoxazole (TMP/SMX) has emerged as an important drug for treating bacterial GE. It is currently considered the drug of choice for GE caused by strains of *Shigella* with unknown susceptibility (54), ETEC (traveler's diarrhea) (52), and *Aeromonas/Plesiomonas* (21). TMP/SMX has been shown to be as effective as ampicillin in reducing the duration of diarrhea, fever, and fecal excretion of *Shigella* in GE caused by this organism (55, 56). It is also effective in GE caused by am-

Table 65.5.
Antibiotics of Choice for Bacterial Gastroenteritis

Causative Agent	Drug of Choice[a]	Alternative Drugs[a]
Shigella	TMP/SMX	TCN, Amp or Cipro
ETEC	TMP/SMX	Cipro or Doxy
EPEC (neonates)	AGS	—
EIEC	Amp	TMP/SMX
Campylobacter	Erythro	Cipro or TCN
Pseudomonas	AGS	—
Aeromonas/Plesiomonas	TMP/SMX	TCN, AGS or Cipro
Vibrio	TMP/SMX	Cipro or TCN

[a] TMP/SMX, trimethoprim/sulfamethoxazole; TCN, tetracycline hydrochloride; Amp, ampicillin; Doxy, doxycycline; Erythro, erythromycin; Clinda, clindamycin; AGS, oral aminoglycoside; Cipro, ciprofloxacin.

Table 65.6.
Antibiotic Dosing/Monitoring Data

Drug	Dose	Adverse Effects	Monitoring Parameters
Ampicillin	Adult: 500 mg, q6h, or 50–100 mg/ kg/day Children: 50–200 mg/kg/day	7.7% incidence of rashes, both hypersensitive and nonhypersensitive (macular, measles-like rash); diarrhea and nausea are common but usually not serious	Skin changes: usual onset of rash, 4–5 days into therapy; gastrointestinal: assess changes in symptoms despite cure of infection
Trimethoprim/ sulfamethoxazole (TMP/SMX), Cotrimoxazole	Adult: TMP/SMX, 160/800 mg, q12h Children >6 weeks: TMP/SMX, 5/ 25 mg/kg, q12h	6–8% overall incidence of side effects; megaloblastic anemia rare, usually reversible; bone marrow toxicity more common with high doses or renal failure; 1–8% incidence of rashes, probably due to SMX; Stevens-Johnson syndrome rare, due to SMX; TMP safety in pregnancy not established; increase in incidence of adverse effects in patients with AIDS	Megaloblastic anemia: peripheral smear and/or RBC indices; bone marrow toxicity: CBC, platelet count periodically
Tetracycline HCl	Adults: 250–500 mg, q.i.d. Children: >12 years: 25–30 mg/kg divided, q.i.d.	True hypersensitivity rare; nausea, vomiting, epigastric pain commonly reported; photosensitivity occurs most with demeclocycline; antianabolic effect aggravates uremia	Gastrointestinal: assess changes in symptoms despite cure of infection; photosensitivity: apply sunscreen and use sunglasses
Doxycycline	Adults: 100 mg daily Children >12 years: 4.4 mg/kg/day in 2 doses for 1st day, followed by 2.2 mg/kg in 2 doses	Dental and bone effects: permanent staining of teeth least likely with doxycycline; hematologic reactions rare; hepatotoxicity rare, results in fatty infiltration of the liver	Hematological reactions: CBC platelet count occasionally
Erythromycin	Adult: 250–500 mg q.i.d. Children: 30–50 mg/kg/day divided q.i.d.	Rash rare; nausea, vomiting, abdominal cramping 14–62%, dose related; hepatotoxicity: cholestatic jaundice (estolate most, ethyl succinate least), reversible; ototoxicity with high parenteral doses; drug interactions: interferes with hepatic metabolism of the theophylline, cyclosporine and warfarin; increases bioavailability of digoxin	Gastrointestinal: assess changes in symptoms despite cure of infection; hepatic reactions: monitor liver function tests occasionally; drug interactions: monitor serum theophylline, cyclosporine and digoxin levels, monitor PT to assess warfarin pharmacodynamics
Chloramphenicol	Adults: 500 mg q.i.d. Children: 25–100 mg/kg/day in 4 divided doses	Skin reactions rare; nausea, vomiting, diarrhea; aplastic anemia: 1 in 500–100,000 patients treated, irreversible; bone marrow suppression dose-related; gray syndrome, usually only infants and children; drug interactions: inhibits metabolism of tolbutamide, phenytoin and dicumarol	Bone marrow effects: reticulocyte count, CBC hematocrit weekly, serum drug levels with dosage adjustment
Ciprofloxacin	Adult: 500 mg b.i.d. Children: not recommended	Nausea, vomiting or diarrhea (7.8%); dizziness, headache, tremors, restlessness (3.3%) may cause elevations in theophylline concentrations; crystalluria with high doses (>100 mg/ day)	Theophylline levels; hydration status

picillin-resistant *Shigella*. If therapy is begun early (after the third loose stool) in the course of GE caused by ETEC (traveler's diarrhea), TMP/SMX has been shown to significantly shorten the duration of diarrhea, decrease the mean number of loose stools, and curtail the fecal excretion of the organism (57). TMP/SMX is more useful than doxycycline in traveler's diarrhea because it does not cause photosensitivity as consistently as tetracyclines. TMP/SMX also appears to be useful in treating GE caused by EIEC, although no placebo-controlled studies have been reported to confirm this impression (54). TMP/SMX may cause rash, vomiting, fever, Stevens-Johnson syndrome, hemolytic anemia, and bone marrow suppression manifested by thrombocytopenia, leukopenia, or agranulocytosis. Because most of this compound is excreted unchanged by tubular secretion in the kidney, the dose should be reduced in patients with severe renal dysfunction.

Erythromycin is considered the drug of choice for treating infectious GE caused by *C. jejuni*, even though few studies have shown any effect of treatment on the clinical course of the disease when compared with placebo. Several studies, however, have shown a significant decrease in the fecal excretion of the organism (58, 59). A study in children, which compared erythromycin with placebo, demonstrated that erythromycin-treated patients had a significantly shorter duration of diarrhea and curtailed excretion of the pathogen when treated within 3 days of the onset of illness (60). These investigators stressed the need to institute therapy early in the course of illness to achieve the best clinical response. The drug is usually given orally; however, it may need to be given intravenously in cases of disseminated disease. One of the major adverse effects of the erythromycin compounds is gastrointestinal intolerance, usually manifested by nausea and abdominal cramping. Surprisingly, these adverse effects may also be seen when these compounds are given intravenously. Reversible cholestatic jaundice has been seen in patients treated primarily with the estolate salt of the drug, although it has been reported with the ethylsuccinate and stearate forms as well. Liver function studies should be monitored in patients receiving all salt forms of this compound if therapy is to be used long-term.

The aminoglycoside compounds have been studied in pediatric patients with EPEC gastrointestinal infections. A short course (3 days) has been shown to produce the same clinical response as the usually recommended long course (10 days) (61). The oral use of these compounds seems to represent one of the only options for treating serious GE caused by *Pseudomonas* species. Whereas these compounds are highly polar and not appreciably absorbed from the gastrointestinal tract in patients with intact membranes, caution should be used in patients in whom the integrity of the gastrointestinal lining is known to be compromised. Absorption in this situation may occur, resulting in detectable systemic drug concentrations. The aminoglycosides are known to be nephro- and ototoxic. If these compounds are given for systemic disease, dose adjustments based on renal function must be made. Serum drug concentrations and renal function parameters must be monitored.

Quinolone compounds are becoming widely accepted as useful agents to eradicate the most common organisms causing GE. Nalidixic acid, in a dose of 55 mg/kg/day in four divided doses, appears useful in treating multiply-resistant *Shigella*, *Salmonella*, ETEC, and *Campylobacter* infections (62–64). Ciprofloxacin and norfloxacin have

been successfully used to treat patients with salmonellosis, including those with bacteremia (65, 66). Unlike other agents used to treat *Salmonella* GE, the quinolone agents shorten the course of clinical disease and decrease the excretion of organisms in the stool (66). Because of the high incidence of sulfa adverse reactions in patients with AIDS, quinolones may be preferable to SMX/TMP in the treatment of GE in AIDS patients. These agents offer the additional advantage of empiric coverage of *Campylobacter*, a common pathogen causing GE in patients with AIDS (67). The common dosages of ciprofloxacin, norfloxacin, and ofloxacin appear to be 500 to 750 mg, 400 mg, and 200 mg, orally twice daily, respectively. These agents are not approved for use in children, because of arthopathy in immature animals, although the clinical importance of this toxicity is not known (68). As clinical experience using these quinolone compounds continues to be compiled, they may indeed become the drugs of choice for many gastrointestinal infections.

Several other antimicrobials are being investigated for their in vitro activity against *Salmonella* organisms. The agents being tested include the newer cephalosporin agents, amoxicillin-clavulanic acid, aztreonam, and imipenem (66, 69). Clinical studies must be done to define the role of these agents in treating GE.

CONCLUSION

Gastroenteritis may be a mild self-limiting disease or a severe life-threatening disease in susceptible persons such as infants, the elderly, and the immunocompromised. Fluid and electrolyte therapy is the most important treatment, and intravenous administration may be required in severe cases. Antimotility agents may provide symptomatic relief in mild-to-moderate disease. Antibiotics should be chosen carefully, based upon results of cultures and sensitivity testing. The widespread inappropriate use of antibiotics in gastroenteritis has led to resistant organisms.

REFERENCES

1. Monson TP: Pediatric viral gastroenteritis. Am Fam Physician 34:95–99, 1986.
2. Bennett JV, Holmberg SD, Rogers MF, et al.: Infectious and parasitic diseases. Am J Prev Med 3 (suppl):102, 1987.
3. Barnett B: Viral gastroenteritis. Med Clin North Am 67:1031–1058, 1983.
4. Mandell GL, Douglas RG, Bennett JE: Principles and Practice of Infectious Diseases. ed. 3. New York: Churchill Livingstone, 1990, ch 83, 86.
5. Tednesco J: Pseudomembranous colitis: pathogenesis and therapy. Med Clin North Am 66:655–664, 1982.
6. Brandt CD, Kim HW, Rodriquez WU, et al.: Rotavirus gastroenteritis and weather. J Clin Microbial 16:478–482, 1982.
7. Plotkin GR, Kluge RM, Waldman RH: Gastroenteritis: etiology, pathophysiology and clinical manifestations. Medicine 58:95–114, 1979.
8. Albert MJ: Enteric adenoviruses, brief review. Arch Virology 88:1–17, 1986.

9. Ashley CR, Caul EO, Paver WK: Astro-virus associated gastroenteritis in children. J Clin Pathol 31:939–941, 1978.

10. Clarke SKR, Caul EO, Egglestone SL: The human enteric coronaviruses. Postgrad Med J 55:135–137, 1979.

11. Ryan CA, Wickels MK, Hargrett-Bean NT, et al.: Massive outbreak of antimicrobial-resistant salmonellosis traced to pasteurized milk. JAMA 259:2103–2107, 1988.

12. Sun M: Illinois traces course of salmonella outbreak. Science 228:972, 1985.

13. Anon: Annual Summary—1988. MMWR 38:3, 1980.

14. St. Louis ME, Morse DL, Potter ME, et al.: The emergence of grade A eggs as a major source of *Salmonella enteritidis* infections. JAMA 259:2103–2107, 1988.

15. Skirrow MB: *Campylobacter* enteritis in dogs and cats: a new "zoonosis." Vet Res Commun 5:13, 1981.

16. Blaser MJ, Wells JG, Feldman RA, et al.: *Campylobacter* enteritis in the United States. A multicenter study. Ann Intern Med 98:360–365, 1983.

17. Speelman P, Struelens MJ, Sanvai SC, et al.: Detection of *Campylobacter jejuni* and other potential pathogens in traveler's diarrhea in Bangladesh. Scand J Gastroenterol S84:19–23, 1983.

18. Schlages TA, Guerrant RL: Seven possible mechanisms for *Escherichia coli* diarrhiea. Infect Dis Clin North Am 2:607–624, 1988.

19. Karmali MA: Bacterial diarrhea: an update. Diag Med May, 12–19, 1985.

20. Vantrappen G, Geboes K, Ponette E: *Yersinia* enteritis. Med Clin North Am 66:639–653, 1982.

21. Holmberg SD, Farmer JJ: *Aeromonas hydrophilia* and *Plesiomonas shigelloides* as causes of intestinal infections. Rev Infect Dis 6:633–639, 1984.

22. Gracey M, Burke V, Robinson J: *Aeromonas*-associated gastroenteritis. Lancet 2:1304–1306, 1982.

23. Holmberg SD, Schell WL, Fanning GR, et al.: *Aeromonas* intestinal infections in the United States. Ann Intern Med 105:683–689, 1986.

24. Holmberg SD: Vibrosis and aeromonas. Infect Dis Clin North Am 80:336–338, 1988.

25. Johnston JM, Becker SF, McFarland LM: Gastroenteritis in patients with stool isolates of vibrio vulniticus. Am J Med 80:336–338, 1986.

26. Telzak EE, Zeig Greenberg MS, et al.: Diabetes mellitus—a newly described risk factor for infection from salmonella enteritidis. J Infect Dis 164:538–541, 1991.

27. Blacklow NR, Cukor G: Viral gastroenteritis. N Engl J Med 304:397–406, 1981.

28. Carpenter CCI: Pathogenesis of secretory diarrheas. Med Clin North Am 66:597–610, 1982.

29. Goldberg MB, Rubin RH: The spectrum of salmonella infection. Infect Dis Clin North Am 2:571–598, 1988.

30. DuPont HL: *Shigella*. Infect Dis Clin North Am 2:599–605, 1988.

31. Black RE, Slome S: *Yersinia enterocolitica*. Infect Dis Clin North Am 2:625–639, 1988.

32. Gianella RA: Pathogenesis of acute bacterial diarrheal disorders. Annu Rev Med 32:341–357, 1981.

33. Rachmilewitz D: Prostaglandins and diarrhea. Dig Dis Sci 25:897–898, 1980.

34. Banwell JG: Treatment of traveler's diarrhea: fluid and dietary management. Rev Infect Dis 8:S182–S187, 1986.

35. Mahalamabis D, Mersan MH, Barua D: Oral rehydration therapy—recent advances. World Health Forum 2:245–2249, 1981.

36. Mauer AM, Dweck HS, Finberg L, et al.: American Academy of Pediatrics' committee on nutrition: Use of oral fluid therapy and part treatment feeding following enteritis in children in a developed country. Pediatrics 75:358–361, 1985.

37. Anon: The state of the worlds children 1990. Oxford United Kingdom: Oxford University Press for UNICEF, 1990.

38. Avery ME, Snyder JD: Oral therapy for acute diarrhea: the underused simple solution. N Engl J Med 323:891–894, 1990.

39. Guerrant RL, Principles and syndromes of enteric infection. In Mandell GL, Douglas RG, Bennett JE (eds): Principles and Practice of Infectious Diseases, ed. 3. New York, Churchill Livingstone, p 847, 1990.

40. Brown KH, MacLean WC Jr: Nutritional management of acute diarrhea: an appraisal of the alternatives. Pediatrics 73:119–125, 1984.

41. Rosenstein G, Freeman M, Standard AL, et al.: Warning: the use of Lomotil in children. Pediatrics 51:132–133, 1973.

42. Portnog BL, DuPont HL, Pruitt D, et al.: Antidiarrheal agents in the treatment of acute diarrhea in children. JAMA 236:844–846, 1976.

43. Ericsson CD, DuPont HL, Johnson PC: Nonantibiotic therapy for travelers' diarrhea. Rev Infect Dis 8:S202–S206, 1986.

44. Steffen R, Heusser R, DuPont HL: Prevention of travelers' diarrhea by nonantibiotic drugs. Rev Infect Dis 8:S151–S159, 1986.

45. Clements ML, Levine MM, Black RE, et al.: *Lactobacillus* prophylaxis for diarrhea due to enterotoxigenic *E. coli*. Antimicrob Agents Chemother 2:104–108, 1981.

46. Donowitz M, Wicks J, Sharp GW: Drug therapy for diarrheal diseases: a look ahead. Rev Infect Dis 8:S188–S201, 1986.

47. Murray BE: Resistance of *Shigella*, *Salmonella*, and other selected enteric pathogens to antimicrobial agents. Rev Infect Dis 8:S172–S181, 1986.

48. WHO Scientific Working Group: Enteric infections due to *Campylobacter*, *Yersinia*, *Salmonella* and *Shigella*. Bull WHO 58:519–537, 1980.

49. Kazemi M, Gumpert TG, Marks MI: A controlled trial comparing sulfamethoxazole-trimethoprim, ampicillin and no therapy in the treatment of *Salmonella* gastroenteritis in children. J Pediatr 83:646–650, 1973.

50. Nelson JD, Kusmiesz H, Jackson LH, et al.: Treatment of *Salmonella* gastroenteritis with ampicillin, amoxicillin or placebo. Pediatrics 65:1125–1130, 1980.

51. Garcia de Olarte D, Trujallo H, Aqudelo N, et al.: Treatment of diarrhea in malnourished infants and children. Am J Dis Child 127:379–388, 1979.

52. Pickering LK, DuPont HL, Olarte J: Single-dose tetracycline for shigellosis in adults. JAMA 239:853–854, 1978.

53. Merson MLT, Sack RB, Islam S, et al. Disease due to enterotoxigenic *Escherichia coli* in Bangladeshi adults: clinical aspects and controlled trial of tetracycline. J Infect Dis 141:702–711, 1980.

54. Levine MM: Antimicrobial therapy for infectious diarrhea. Rev Infect Dis 8:S207–S216, 1986.

55. Chang MJ, Dunkle LM, Reken DV, et al.: Trimethoprim-sulfamethoxazole compared to ampicillin in the treatment of shigellosis. Pediatrics 59:726–729, 1977.

56. Nelson JD, Kusmiesz H, Jackson LH: Comparison of trimethoprim-sulfamethoxazole and ampicillin therapy for shigellosis in ambulatory patients. J Pediatr 89:491–493, 1976.

57. Blake RE, Levine MM, Clements ML, et al.: Treatment of experimentally induced enterotoxigenic *Escherichia coli* diarrhea with trimethoprim, trimethoprim-sulfamethoxazole or placebo. Rev Infect Dis 4:540–545, 1982.

58. Robins-Browne RM, Mackenjee MKR, Bodasing MN, et al.: Treatment of *Campylobacter*-associated enteritis with erythromycin. Am J Dis Child 137:282–285, 1983.

59. Pai CH, Gillis F, Tuomanen E, et al.: Erythromycin in the treatment of *Campylobacter* enteritis in children. Am J Dis Child 137:286–288, 1983.

60. Salazar-Lindo E, Sack RB, Chea-Woo E, et al.: Early treatment with erythromycin of *Campylobacter jejuni*-associated dysentery in children. J Pediatr 109:355–362, 1986.

61. Nelson JD: Duration of neomycin therapy for enteropathogenic *Escherichia coli* diarrheal disease: a comparative study of 113 cases. Pediatrics 48:248–258, 1971.

62. Haltalin KC, Nelson JD, Kusimiesz HT: Comparative efficacy of nalidixic acid and ampicillin for severe shigellosis. Arch Dis Child 48:305–312, 1973.

63. Pichler HET, Diridl B, Strickler K, et al.: Clinical efficacy of ciprofloxacin compared with placebo in bacterial diarrhea. Am J Med 82:329–332, 1987.

64. Ericsson CD, Johnson PC, DuPont HL, et al.: Ciprofloxacin or trimethoprim/sulfamethoxazole as initial treatment for travelers' diarrhea. Ann Intern Med 106:216–220, 1987.

65. Bennish ML, Salam MA, Haider R, et al.: Therapy for shigellosis II. Randomized double-blind comparison of ciprofloxacin and ampicillin. J Infect Dis 162:711–716, 1990.

66. Asperilla MO, Smego RA Jr, Scott LK: Quinolone antibiotics in the treatment of *Salmonella* infection. Rev Infect Dis 12:873–898, 1990.

67. Lopez AP, Gorbach SL: Diarrhea in AIDS. Infect Dis Clin North Am 2:705–718, 1988.

68. Schliter G: Ciprofloxacin: review of potential toxicologic effects. Am J Med 82 (suppl 4A):91–93, 1987.

69. Cherubin CE, Eng RHK, Smith SM, et al.: Cephalosporin therapy for salmonellosis, questions efficacy and cross resistance with ampicillin. Arch Intern Med 146:2149–2152, 1986.

CHAPTER 66
INFECTIVE ENDOCARDITIS

STEVEN L. BARRIERE, Pharm.D., F.C.C.P. and DEBRA KALMAN, Pharm.D.

Endocarditis is, by strict definition, an infection of the inner lining of the heart and the mucosa that underlies it. However, the term refers most commonly to an infection of a heart valve. The heart wall, papillary muscles, and chordae tendineae can be involved in the infection, but the complications and clinical manifestations arise from the involvement of the tricuspid, mitral, or aortic valves.

Subacute disease is an indolent infection that may produce signs and symptoms over periods as long as several months before a diagnosis is made. Acute infection is of rapid onset, with fulminant symptoms. Classically, patients with subacute disease had all of the "typical" manifestations of the disease (see below); however, the diagnosis is now suspected in any febrile illness of unclear etiology, so that progression to chronicity is becoming less common.

ANATOMY

As mentioned above the tissues involved in endocarditis are primarily the tricuspid, mitral, and aortic valves; the valve of the pulmonary artery is rarely infected. The tricuspid valve is a common site of infection in intravenous drug users. The mitral and aortic valves are also involved in this group of patients, and damage to these valves lead to more severe hemodynamic alterations than tricuspid disease.

The sites of the lesions are the atrial surfaces of the mitral and tricuspid valves and the ventricular surfaces of the aortic and pulmonic valves. Lesions of the chordae, atrial or ventricular walls, and the pulmonary artery or aorta are all considered satellite infections to the primary valvular involvement (1).

There has been a significant trend in recent years toward an increase in the age of patient with endocarditis. This is at least partly due to marked decreases in the prevalence of rheumatic heart disease, the longevity of persons in modern society, and increasing numbers of older patients with prosthetic cardiac valves (2). This has also led to a recognition of additional forms of heart disease that predispose to the development of endocarditis (2).

PATHOPHYSIOLOGY

Four factors are necessary in the pathogenesis of the infection: (*a*) a previously damaged cardiac valve, (*b*) a platelet-fibrin thrombus, (*c*) bacteremia, and (*d*) bacterial adherence (1). In patients with endocarditis, the mitral valve is involved in 66 to 86%, the aortic valve in 45 to 55%, tricuspid valve in 5 to 20%, and pulmonic valve in only 1% (3, 4). Correlating the pressure gradient across these valves with the relative frequency of infection makes a strong argument for mechanical stress as an important factor in the pathogenesis of endocarditis. Similarly, the hemodynamic alterations that occur across an incompetent valve result in abnormal "jets" of blood that may damage the endocardium and provide a locus for infection. This change in hemodynamics also creates a low-pressure "sink," which sets up an additional site for infection, as illustrated by the Venturi model (Fig. 66.1). A bacterial aerosol (bacteremia) flows from the high-pressure source (left ventricle) through the narrowed orifice (incompetent mitral valve) into the low-pressure area (left atrium). The development of vegetations just distal to the orifice, has been demonstrated with this model. Vegetations in endocarditis are most commonly found on the low-pressure side of the valve (1).

Once the endothelial surface of the valve is traumatized by the jet effects, collagen is exposed, and a sterile platelet-fibrin thrombus is formed. This is referred to as nonbacterial thrombotic endocarditis (NBTE) (1).

The next critical factor in the pathogenesis of the infection is bacteremia. The microorganism is delivered to the valve surface by the bloodstream. The ability of the organisms to adhere to the valve surface correlates directly with their ability to produce endocarditis (2). This process is complex, but has been associated with bacterial dextran production, among other factors (1).

ETIOLOGY

Infection due to viridans streptococci has declined over the last 3 decades. Half or more of all cases of endocarditis were due to these organisms 30 years ago. Now approximately one-fourth to one-third are caused by these streptococci (2–4). Enterococci are the causative pathogens in approximately 6 to 10% of cases, and other streptococci account for 10 to 15% of cases. Staphylococci account for 20 to 35% of all cases, particularly in intravenous drug users (5, 6). Gram-negative bacteria such as *Serratia marcescens* and *Pseudomonas aeruginosa* have been reported to be responsible for as many as 11% of cases (7, 8), again, frequently occurring in habitual IV drug users. Nearly 20% of cases of endocarditis involving prosthetic valves are due

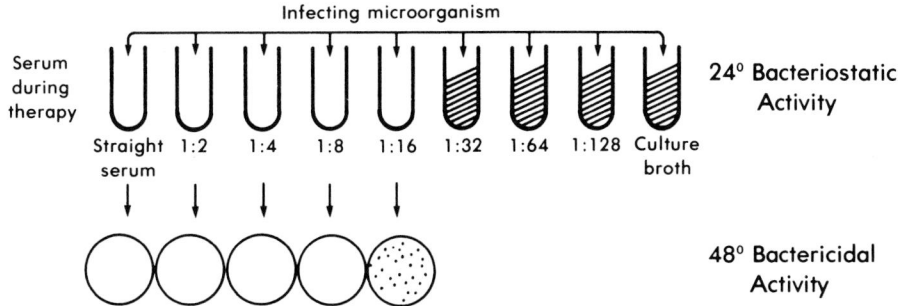

Figure 66.1. The Venturi model. (Modified from Rodbard, S: Blood velocity and endocarditis. Circulation 27:18, 1963.

to Gram-negative bacilli (2, 4). Fungi, particularly, *Candida albicans*, are seen in 5% of cases or less (3–7).

Intravenous drug users develop endocarditis more frequently than the general population, probably because of frequent nonsterile intravenous injections. The bacteriology of endocarditis in this population is composed of staphylococci (50 to 60%), streptococci (15%), and Gram-negative bacilli and fungi (25 to 35%). Anaerobes and other organisms produce only a few cases of disease in this population.

The other group of patients who are at special risk to developing endocarditis are those who have prosthetic cardiac valves. Prosthetic valve endocarditis (PVE) occurring within the first 2 months after surgery (early PVE) is caused by organisms introduced during surgery. The most frequently cultured organisms are staphylococci, especially coagulase-negative staphylococci. Infections occurring beyond 2 months (late PVE) are caused by the same organisms that produce diseases on native valves (i.e., primarily streptococci). Fungi are also a concern in these patients. Endocarditis is especially devastating in these patients since fatal complications can occur quickly (9, 10).

BACTEREMIA

Infecting organisms must reach the cardiac tissues by means of the general circulation. Bacteremia and fungemia are the initiating events in the genesis of the actual infection (as noted above).

Viridans streptococci, nonenterococcal group D streptococci, and other facultative organisms are normal flora of the nasopharynx. *Streptococcus faecalis* (*Enterococcus faecalis*) and Gram-negative bacilli usually arise from the urinary or gastrointestinal tracts. Staphylococci are quite often found on the skin. Fungi may arise from the bowel, as can certain Gram-negative and anaerobic organisms. Fungi may also colonize certain areas of skin, and thus gain entrance to the circulation via intravenous catheters.

Staphyloccal bacteremia and its management is enmeshed in a good deal of controversy. Iannini and Crossley (11) reported on 29 patients with no previous evidence of endocarditis who developed *Staphylococcus aureus* bacteremia associated with a removable focus of infection—usually an intravenous catheter. The patients were treated for only 10 to 21 days with appropriate antibiotics and none developed endocarditis. This suggests that early recognition of the problem and prompt therapy for a short duration prevents the development of endocarditis. Watanakunakorn and Baird reviewed 21 similar patients in whom bacteremia with *S. aureus* developed secondary to an intravenous device (12). They found that without therapy, endocarditis developed in 8 patients (38%), and they felt that endocarditis had been established by the time bacteremia was detected. Levine et al. (7) have noted that bacteremia in narcotic addicts in the absence of endocarditis was associated with primary skin and soft tissue infection or infection at some other site. It seems reasonable, based upon the limited information available, to treat staphylococcal bacteremia caused by a removable focus with appropriate therapy for 2 to 3 weeks, while monitoring for signs of endocarditis.

Endocarditis has been described following bacteremias arising from genitourinary infection and the use of an oral irrigation device. In addition, transient bacteremias, with the potential for producing endocarditis, have been described following tooth extraction, periodontal surgery, liver biopsy, endoscopy or sigmoidoscopy, and manipulations of the genitourinary tract (Table 66.1).

DIAGNOSIS AND CLINICAL FEATURES

The classical signs and symptoms of endocarditis such as Osler's nodes, Janeway lesions, clubbing of the fingers, splinter hemorrhages, and retinal lesions, are all seen infrequently in modern clinical medicine (3, 4). The primary reason for this is the high index of suspicion for the disease in a patient with fever of unknown etiology, leading to early diagnosis. The most common signs and symptoms are a heart murmur or a change in a previously noted murmur, fever, embolic episodes, splenomegaly, skin manifestations (primarily petechiae), weakness, dyspnea, sweats, anorexia, weight loss, malaise, and cough (3). These

Table 66.1.
Incidence and Types of Bacteremia

Procedure	Incidence of Bacteremia (%)	Organisms
Dental extraction	30–80	Streptococci Diphtherioids *S. epidermidis*
Periodontal surgery	80–90	As above Anaerobes
Tooth brushing, oral irrigation	25–50	Streptococci Staphylococci
Tonsillectomy	30–40	Streptococci
Upper GI endoscopy	10	Streptococci Staphylococci Diphtheroids
Lower GI endoscopy (sigmoidoscopy)	5–10	Enterococci Gram-negative bacilli *Bacteroides*
Liver biopsy	3–13	Streptococci Staphylococci Gram-negative bacilli
Cystoscopy, urethral dilation, etc.	20–80	Gram-negative bacilli Enterococci

are not present in 100% of cases, but the most crucial criterion for the diagnosis of the disease is positive blood cultures.

The bacteremia of endocarditis is qualitatively continuous, but quantitatively variable. Negative blood cultures may be due to uremia, poor bacteriologic technique, fastidious organisms (e.g., *Cardiobacterium hominis, Eikenella corrodens*) nonbacterial disease (e.g., Q fever, fungi, viruses), or prior antibiotic therapy (13, 14). The number of blood cultures necessary to establish or exclude the diagnosis has been determined to be at least three and perhaps as many as five. In practice, three cultures taken over a 24-hr period, in a patient who is not critically ill, should produce a very high yield. In acutely ill patients, 2 to 3 samples of blood should be taken form different sites, rapidly, before starting antibiotic therapy.

Most of the classic signs and symptoms are due to either emboli from the infected endocardium or local vasculitis. Subacute disease is characterized by one or more of the classic signs or symptoms, but acute disease may often have hemorrhage, embolus, or metastatic infection (meninges, eye, kidneys). Echocardiography is sometimes useful in detecting vegetations on valve leaflets, especially in patients with symptoms suggestive of endocarditis but negative blood cultures. This procedure is more useful in assessing valvular competence in candidates for valve replacement. Transesophageal echocardiography (TEE) is a new procedure commonly used to locate vegetations on a heart valve in a patient who previously had a nondiagnostic transthoracic echocardiogram. TEE is felt to be a more sensitive procedure.

The laboratory parameters (other than cultures) used to establish the diagnosis of endocarditis are elevated titers of rheumatoid factor; increased erythrocyte sedimentation rate; normochromic, normocytic anemia; and a decline in renal function with hematuria.

All of the above and a history consistent with risk factors compatible with endocarditis, put the disease at the top of the list of possible diagnoses. Risk factors associated with the development of endocarditis include intravenous drug abuse, underlying heart disease, or the presence of an indwelling prosthetic device.

Serologic techniques to diagnose staphylococcal endocarditis (i.e., detection of antibodies to various staphylococcal components) have been tested for many years with inconclusive results. Despite recent improvements in methodology, false-positive and false-negative results may confound the clinical findings. Therefore, their use at the present time is not recommended.

Endocarditis in intravenous drug users is frequently heralded by neurologic dysfunction or pulmonary emboli (7). This may misdirect the efforts toward a diagnosis, which again points to the importance of obtaining sufficient blood cultures in the febrile patient with a history of symptoms compatible with endocarditis.

TREATMENT

The cure of infective endocarditis requires the *sustained* application of antimicrobial agents that are capable of *killing* the organisms causing the infection.

As mentioned previously, the sequestration of the infecting organisms within valvular vegetation protects them from antibodies and macrophages, and in addition, results in slowed microbial metabolism. This slowed replication leads to relative insusceptibility to many antibiotics and requires that the organisms be killed by the antibiotics used (15). This has been proven clinically by the failure of bacteriostatic antibiotics such as the tetracyclines, erythromycin, and chloramphenicol to cure endocarditis. This relative impermeability of antibiotics and slowed microbial replication also require the use of prolonged antimicrobial therapy.

The bactericidal or fungicidal activity of the patient's serum during therapy should be assessed in infections caused by more resistant organisms (enterococci, Gram-negative bacilli, fungi, and in some cases, staphylococci) or if treatment with oral antibiotics is to be used after a shortened course of parenteral therapy. Bactericidal activity should be no less than 1:8 dilutions of serum (15) (Fig. 66.2). This has been found to correlate with good results in the therapy of endocarditis and other infectious diseases. However, it has been demonstrated recently that peak titers of 1:64 or above and trough titers of 1:32 or more are associated with 100% bacteriologic cure rates (16). Titers of 1:8 were predictive of success 93 and 97.5%

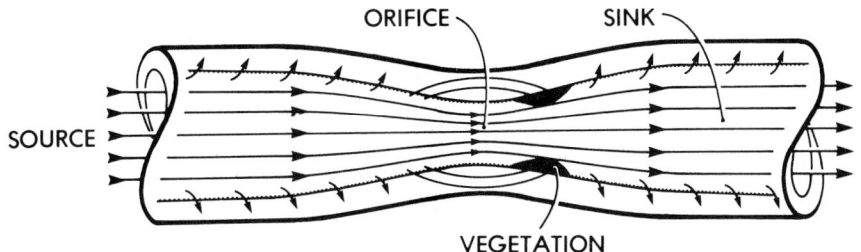

Figure 66.2. Serum dilution.

of the time, for peak and trough, respectively. This study also revealed that the serum bactericidal titer test could not predict either bacteriologic failure or clinical outcome.

Empiric therapy is often instituted before the results of culture and sensitivity tests are known, especially in patients who are acutely ill. The choice of empiric therapy is based upon the history, the physical examination, and the course of the disease. For example, an elderly man with evidence of chronic disease and a history of enterococcal urinary tract infections should be treated for enterococcal endocarditis. Likewise, an IV drug user with acute disease should be treated for staphylococcal, enterococcal, and Gram-negative endocarditis until culture results are obtained.

Table 66.2 lists drugs of first choice and alternative drugs for the treatment of the most common causes of endocarditis.

Most streptococci (except enterococci) are highly susceptible to penicillin G or ampicillin, and therapy with either of these drugs alone is adequate in nearly all cases (17–19). Abundant glycocalyx production by viridans streptococci has been associated with delayed antimicrobial sterilization in the rabbit model of endocarditis. The addition of clindamycin to such a model was studied by Dall and colleagues (20). They found that clindamycin decreased glycocalyx production, which may allow better antimicrobial penetration into the infected vegetation. Unfortunately, the use of clindamycin is limited because it is bacteriostatic. The potential exists for its use in combination therapy, but human studies are necessary before this use can be recommended. Dextranase has also been found to augment the effect of penicillin in vitro by decreasing glycocalyx production, but its clinical utility is unknown (21).

Therapy for 2 weeks, rather than the usual 4, has been evaluated and found to be effective as long as the combination of penicillin and streptomycin is used (17, 22). This regimen is cost-beneficial, but it may be more toxic because of the aminoglycoside. This regimen should not be used in the elderly, patients in shock, those with PVE or extracardiac foci of infection, or those infected with less susceptible streptococci (18). Nonenterococcal streptococci may be less sensitive to penicillin G (minimal inhibitory concentration (MIC) equal to or more than 0.1 mg/liter) and should be treated with penicillin G or ampicillin plus an aminoglycoside (streptomycin or gentamicin) (18, 23). Group D streptococci include *Enterococcus fecalis* and *Streptococcus bovis*. The latter organism is usually highly susceptible to penicillin G. The enterococcus, however, is only moderately susceptible (MIC = 1 to 2 mg/liter), and therapy with a penicillin alone has resulted in a high failure rate. Addition of an aminoglycoside results in synergistic killing of the organism in vitro and produces improved cure rates (23–25). In vitro, approximately 20 to 40% of enterococci are highly resistant to streptomycin (MIC equal to or more than 1000 mg/ml). These organisms are not killed in vitro by the penicillin-streptomycin combination and frequently not by penicillin-tobramycin, but the combination of penicillin and gentamicin is routinely bactericidal (23, 24). Combinations of penicillinase-resistant penicillins or cephalosporins plus an aminoglycoside, although sometimes shown to provide in vitro killing of enterococci, have not demonstrated this effect in vivo. Gentamicin is recommended over streptomycin in combination with a penicillin when high-level resistance is found. High-level gentamicin-resistance has recently been described in enterococci, and rarely, in viridans streptococci (26). These organisms are not killed by the penicillin/gentamicin combination. The clinical meaning of this high-level resistance is unclear, but it may result in less effective therapy.

In penicillin-allergic patients, vancomycin or a cephalosporin (except in enterococcal infection) are acceptable alternatives. The addition of an aminoglycoside to vancomycin in the management of enterococcal infection is necessary (23). A cephalosporin should probably not be given to a patient with a history of an IgE-mediated, immediate reaction to penicillin.

S. aureus is nearly always resistant to penicillin G necessitating the use of a β-lactamase-resistant antibiotic (e.g., isoxazolyl penicillins or cephalosporins).

Staphylococcal endocarditis is best treated with a penicillinase-resistant penicillin. Oxacillin or nafcillin appear to be significantly less toxic than methicillin. Ampicillin combined with sulbactam has proven in vitro coverage of *S. aureus* and has been used with success in *S. aureus*

Table 66.2.
Antimicrobial Therapy for Endocarditis

Organism	Regimen(s) of Choice	Daily Dosage	Alternatives	Daily Dosage	Comments
Streptococci (penicillin MIC < 0.1 µg/ml)	1. Penicillin G, aqueous × 4 weeks OR	200–300,000 µ/kg IV	Cephalosporin[b]	CZ: 75 mg/kg IV CP: 150–200 mg/kg IV	Choice of regiment should be dictated by severity of disease and patient's predisposition to aminoglycoside toxicity (i.e., elderly, renal dysfunction, underlying 8th nerve impairment); preferred regimen is no. 2; infection caused by organisms that are less susceptible or not killed by penicillin alone (tolerant) should be treated with combination therapy
		As above	Vancomycin	25–30 mg/kg IV	
	2. Penicillin G, aqueous × 4 weeks PLUS Aminoglycoside[a] × 2 weeks	S: 15 mg/kg (max 1 g/day i.m.) G: 3 mg/kg i.m./IV 1.2 million units q.6 hr i.m.			
	3. Procaine Pen G × 2 weeks PLUS Streptomycin × 2 weeks	As above			
Enterococci (S. faecalis and others)	Penicillin G, aqueous OR Ampicillin × 4–6 weeks PLUS Aminoglycoside × 4–6 weeks	300,000 µ/kg IV 150–200 mg/kg G: 3–4 mg/kg IV/i.m. S: 15 mg/kg (max: 1 g/day i.m.)	Vancomycin PLUS Aminoglycoside	25–30 mg/kg IV Same	Many isolates are not killed by vancomycin alone and require addition of aminoglycoside; cephalosporins are not effective in the treatment of enterococcal infection, even in combination with an aminoglycoside; gentamicin is the preferred aminoglycoside, esp vs S-resistant strains
Staphylococcus aureus	Nafcillin OR Oxacillin × 4–6 weeks	150–200 mg/kg IV	Cephalosporin[b] Vancomycin	As above As above	"Tolerant" strains require addition of aminoglycoside or rifampin for bactericidal effect; clinical significance of tolerance remains unknown
Staphylococcus epidermidis	Native valve: Same as for S. aureus Prosthetic valve: Vancomycin PLUS Aminoglycoside × 6 weeks OR Rifampin	25–30 mg/kg IV As above 600 mg/day	None		Most cases of S. epidermidis infections are on prosthetic valves
Enterobacteriaceae	Aminoglycoside[a] PLUS Cephalosporin[c]	G/T: 5–6 mg/kg IV A: 15 mg/kg IV 100–150 mg/kg IV	Trimethoprim-sulfamethoxazole Aztreonam	10 mg/kg (TMP) IV 100 mg/kg IV	Surgery is often required for cure; combination therapy is preferred since there is little experience with newer agents alone in the treatment of endocarditis; duration of therapy is probably at least 4 weeks
Pseudomonas aeruginosa	Aminoglycoside[a] PLUS a Penicillin[d] OR Ceftazidime	As above 250–300 mg/kg IV 100 mg/kg IV	Aztreonam Imipenem Ciprofloxacin	As above 60 mg/kg IV 800 mg IV 1500–2000 mg PO	
Anaerobes (B. fragilis)	Metronidazole	30 mg/kg IV	Imipenem	As above	Traditional agents for anaerobic infection (clindamycin, chloramphenicol) are bacteriostatic; newer penicillins (piperacillin, mezlocillin) and β-lactamase-inhibitor combinations may be bactericidal
Fungi (Candida, Aspergillus)	Amphotericin B × 6–8 weeks	0.5–1 mg/kg IV	None		Some Candida spp. are killed synergistically by addition of flucytosine or rifampin to amphotericin B; newer agents such as fluconazole and itraconazole have not been tested

[a] Streptomycin (S), gentamicin (G), amikacin (A), or tobramycin (T).
[b] Cephalothin/cephapirin (CP) or cefazolin (CZ).
[c] Cefotaxime or ceftizoxime.
[d] Mezlocillin, piperacillin, or ticarcillin.
[e] Ceftazidime.

infections other than endocarditis. The efficacy of ampicillin/sulbactam versus oxacillin for experimental endocarditis caused by β-lactamase-hyperproducing *S. aureus* has been evaluated (27). These authors suggest that ampicillin/sulbactam was inferior to oxacillin, but was effective in treating the infection. More studies must be carried out before the routine use of ampicillin/sulbactam in *S. aureus* endocarditis can be recommended.

First-generation cephalosporins such as cefazolin are as effective as penicillinase-resistant penicillins. Failures reported when cefazolin has been used to treat *S. aureus* endocarditis may be due to the relative instability of cefazolin to certain types of staphylococcal β-lactamases (28–30). Therefore, it must be used with caution in this patient population. Cephalothin is more β-lactamase stable and may be a more suitable alternative. Newer second- and third-generation cephalosporins are less active in vitro against staphylococci, and although they are very β-lactamase stable, should not be used.

Patients with immediate hypersensitivity reactions to β-lactams or who are infected with methicillin-resistant staphylococci should receive vancomycin (31). Questions have been raised about the efficacy of vancomycin compared with penicillinase-resistant penicillins when treating *S. aureus* endocarditis. Small and co-workers treated four IV drug abusers with vancomycin for *S. aureus* endocarditis (32). Two patients had recurrence of positive blood cultures 2 days after completing a 4-week course of vancomycin. Two other patients were cured only after modification of their regimens because of persisting bacteremia after 7 to 16 days of therapy. Time-kill studies performed with nafcillin and vancomycin for 10 isolates of *S. aureus* showed that vancomycin was less rapidly bactericidal than nafcillin. Based on such data, vancomycin should only be used when absolutely indicated.

Another therapeutic attempt to improve in vivo effectiveness of the therapy of *S. aureus* endocarditis has been the addition of gentamicin to a penicillinase-resistant penicillin. This has been effective in an animal model and in scattered case reports. A large multicenter study was performed to assess the benefit of adding gentamicin to nafcillin, compared with nafcillin alone. The results indicated that although the duration of bacteremia was shorter with the combination therapy, the overall cure rate was no different in the two groups (23, 31). However, these patients were predominantly young IV drug users, in whom endocarditis (almost always a tricuspid valve infection) appears to be easier to treat. An additional smaller study reported similar results (33). Each case must be evaluated by determination of clinical response and bactericidal activity to determine if the addition of aminoglycoside is necessary (31). The mortality rate of this infection in patients over 50 years of age is very high and these patients should be treated aggressively with large doses of oxacillin/nafcillin or vancomycin. The addition of an aminoglycoside should be weighed against the potential toxicity in an older patient.

Rifampin also has excellent in vitro activity against staphylococci and may be considered for addition to β-lactam or vancomycin regimens to enhance bactericidal activity (34). However, in vitro and experimental antagonism has been reported (31). Despite reports of successful treatment of staphylococcal endocarditis with clindamycin, it is imperative that bactericidal activity be demonstrated before embarking on therapy with this agent, since several reports of failure and the development of resistance have been published.

There have been studies assessing the efficacy of ciprofloxacin for treating *S. aureus* endocarditis. Results have been promising, but rapid emergence of resistance does occur, and the addition of another agent such as rifampin is highly recommended.

Staphylococcus epidermidis is often resistant to the semisynthetic penicillins. Infections due to these organisms, especially on prosthetic valves, should be treated with vancomycin plus either an aminoglycoside or rifampin (9, 21). Teicoplanin and daptomycin are new antibiotics currently under investigation for the treatment of Gram-positive infections. They have an antibacterial spectrum similar to that of vancomycin but longer half-lives, allowing once-daily administration. Several studies have evaluated the use of teicoplanin and daptomycin for the treatment of Gram-positive endocarditis. Early studies using relatively low doses were disappointing, since several failures occurred (35, 36). It was found that the high serum protein binding of the drugs limited their in vivo bactericidal activity (37–39). Studies with higher doses have been conducted, and in general, they have been effective and the drugs were reasonably well tolerated. However, development of resistance during therapy has been noted by Kaatz et al., particularly in patients with a high bacterial inoculum (40), which raises concerns about the utility of teicoplanin and daptomycin for the treatment of endocarditis.

The treatment of other forms of endocarditis is less well established. Infections due to Gram-negative bacilli, fungi, and anaerobes are extremely difficult to cure with antimicrobial therapy alone (23) and often require surgical intervention to repair the valve or replace the infected valve with a prosthesis. The prime indications for surgery are the development of emboli, impending heart failure, persistent bacteremia, fungal infection, pericarditis, or relapse following "adequate" therapy (41).

Should a prosthetic valve become infected, as is often the case when surgery is performed on IV drug users who continue to inject drugs intravenously, the mortality rate is very high. Sterilization of the prosthesis is difficult, and prolonged combination therapy is indicated (9, 10, 23).

Failure of the valve may lead to rapid heart failure and death.

Gram-negative bacillary endocarditis should be treated with bactericidal antibiotics to which the infecting organisms are sensitive. Unfortunately, the most common organisms found in this category are not the relatively antibiotic-sensitive *E. coli* or *Proteus mirabilis*, but rather *Serratia marcescens* and *Pseudomonas aeruginosa*. Both of these organisms are relatively insensitive to most antibiotics and many isolates of *Serratia* have become resistant to all antibiotics except amikacin, ciprofloxacin, and trimethoprim-sulfamethoxazole (TMP/SMX).

The empiric treatment of Gram-negative endocarditis should include an aminoglycoside in maximum dosage in combination with a β-lactam compound (23).

Newer cephalosporins (third generation), new penicillins (piperacillin, mezlocillin), ciprofloxacin, and imipenem may provide bactericidal therapy for endocarditis caused by *S. marcescens* and *P. aeruginosa*. To date, little clinical experience has been gained with these agents in the management of endocarditis.

TMP/SMX is a valuable antimicrobial for the treatment of many extraurinary infections including endocarditis. Bactericidal activity of the patients' serum must be assured, however. Endocarditis caused by *Pseudomonas cepacia* has been treated effectively with TMP/SMX, sometimes in combination with polymyxin B.

Ciprofloxacin has been used to treat Gram-negative endocarditis (42). It was as efficacious alone as when given with azlocillin in experimental endocarditis (43). The major disadvantage is the emergence of resistance, as seen with Gram-positive infections. One solution may be to combine ciprofloxacin with another agent such as a broad-spectrum penicillin or cephalosporin (44).

In an area with a high percentage of Gram-negative bacilli resistant to gentamicin, amikacin may be the empiric aminoglycoside of choice, since most Gram-negative bacilli retain sensitivity to it.

Anaerobic Gram-negative organisms such as *Bacteroides* spp. present a special problem.

Carbenicillin, in doses of 400 to 500 mg per kg daily has been shown to be effective in the treatment of *Bacteroides fragilis* endocarditis. Most other anaerobic organisms are highly susceptible to penicillin G. Metronidazole has also been shown to be highly bactericidal in vitro against *B. fragilis*, and isolated reports have shown it to be effective in treating anaerobic infections other than endocarditis (45). Experience in the treatment of endocarditis is needed to verify this efficacy. Cefoxitin, cefotetan, imipenem, ampicillin/sulbactam, and ticarcillin-clavulanate are also active in vitro against *B. fragilis* and should be considered (46).

Fungal endocarditis is virtually impossible to cure without surgery, and even with optimal therapy, the mortality rate is very high. This is probably due to the invasiveness of the organisms, the large vegetations produced on the valve, the absence of fungicidal activity often found with amphotericin B, and the negligible penetration of the antifungal agent into the vegetation. The mainstay of therapy is amphotericin B given for prolonged period of time. Therapy given two to three times a week on an outpatient basis has been recommended to suppress the infection and possibly achieve a cure with long-term treatment. Dosage should be tailored to the patient's tolerance. The addition of 5-fluorocytosine (5 FC) for the treatment of candidal infections should be based upon in vitro sensitivity and the assessment of fungicidal activity of the patient's serum. 5 FC is hemotoxic, however, which is manifested primarily in the presence of renal failure, often a result of amphotericin B therapy. The toxicities include agranulocytosis and hepatic necrosis. Fluconazole is a newly approved imidazole with in vitro activity against many fungi, including *Candida albicans*, *Cryptococcus*, and *Histoplasma* (47). There is potential for it to be used in fungal endocarditis but no studies to support this use. One must note however, that failures have been seen when used for *Candida* fungemia. Newer imidazoles under investigation may prove to be very useful in fungal endocarditis.

Coxiella burnetii, the agent of Q fever, can produce endocarditis. The treatment is long-term tetracycline therapy, 2.0 g per day orally. This disease carries a very poor prognosis.

Prosthetic valve replacement is becoming more widespread because of advances in surgical and life-support techniques. Along with this has come an increase in infections involving these valves (PVE). The mortality rate from this infection has been reported to be as high as 90%, depending upon the onset and types of organisms, with an overall mortality figure approaching 70%.

The greatest mortality in PVE is associated with an onset within the first few months after surgery, with Gram-negative bacillary, fungal, and *S. aureus* infections, with aortic valve involvement, and the presence of CHF (9, 10). As mentioned previously, the most common infecting organisms are staphylococci (40 to 50%) and streptococci (30 to 40%).

Therapy with antibiotics alone has resulted in a cure rate of approximately 40%, but many patients have required replacement of the infected prosthesis to achieve cures. Parenteral antibiotics should be used for a minimum of 6 weeks in endocarditis occurring on natural valves. Early replacement of infected prostheses should be considered in all patients except those with uncomplicated streptococcal or mitral valve PVE (9, 41).

COMPLICATIONS

Complications in infective endocarditis are due to the disease, the antibiotics used, or both. The overall mortality for *all* forms of infective endocarditis is approximately 25 to 30%. However, the mortality ranges from 10 to 15% in penicillin-sensitive streptococcal endocarditis to 90% or more in fungal infection. A poor prognosis is associated with old age, serious underlying cardiac or other disease, aortic or mitral valve involvement, infection of a prosthetic valve, presence of emboli, and infection with Gram-negative bacilli or fungi.

Patients with subacute disease may develop renal insufficiency. This may be due to one or more of several factors: nephrotoxicity of antimicrobials, metastatic abscess within the kidney from infected emboli (predominantly staphylococcal infection), infarction of the kidney from compromised blood flow caused by aseptic emboli, or immune-complex nephritis caused by deposition of immunoglobulins and complement on the glomerular basement membrane.

Involvement of the central nervous system occurs in nearly one-third of all patients with endocarditis. The predominant manifestations are stroke and hemorrhage. Less common are meningitis, toxic encephalopathy, mononeuritis, convulsions, and visual impairment. The visual impairment is usually due to emboli or infarction, but may be caused by secondary endophthalmitis, which may rapidly progress to loss of the eye.

The most common complications of endocarditis involve the lung (pulmonary emboli) and congestive heart failure from valvular insufficiency.

Valve replacement is indicated for many intractable complications of endocarditis. These include severe heart failure, an infecting organism that is resistant to available antimicrobials, and instability of an infected prosthetic valve (48). Other indications for surgery must be considered in light of the individual clinical situation (48).

PREVENTION OF ENDOCARDITIS

Bacteremia from most sources is usually transient and nearly always inconsequential in the normal individual. However, in the patient with congenital or acquired heart disease or a prosthetic valve, any bacteremia may lead to endocarditis. In assessing the risk of a bacteremia to an individual patient, important considerations are the incidence of bacteremia with a given procedure (Table 66.1). The most likely organisms, the type of cardiac abnormality, and perhaps, the concentration of the bacteria in the bloodstream are important, although data are lacking on this latter point. In general, Gram-positive cocci infect congenital defects or acquired valvular diseases, while Gram-negative aerobic bacilli and fungi are common pathogens in prosthetic valve infection. It has been estimated that as much as 15% of all cases of endocarditis are related to dental surgical procedures (49). In a recent survey of failures of endocarditis prophylaxis, over 90% of the cases occurred after a dental procedure, and 75% were caused by viridans streptococci (50).

General measures to reduce the risk of bacteremia are to avoid manipulation or instrumentation of infected areas, avoid procedures that may traumatize mucous membranes usually colonized with a normal flora (e.g., mouth), and avoid intravenous catheterization with plastic devices. Topical antiseptic agents do not decrease the incidence of bacteremia during dental procedures.

Only indirect evidence from animal studies demonstrates the effect of prophylactic antibiotics in bacteremia-producing procedures. No controlled trials are available, and the recommended regimens are derived from experiments in the rabbit model. In the aforementioned survey only 12% of patients received prophylactic regimens consistent with the American Heart Association (AHA) recommendations (50). However, in 63% of the failures, the infecting organism was susceptible to the prophylactic regimen used. Despite this, the AHA recommends the use of prophylactic antimicrobials prior to, during, and after a procedure likely to produce a bacteremia (51). These include all dental procedures likely to induce gingival bleeding, tonsillectomy/adenoidectomy, surgical procedures or biopsy involving respiratory mucosa, bronchoscopy, incision and drainage of infected tissue, and various genitourinary and gastrointestinal procedures. Table 66.3 lists cardiac conditions for which prophylaxis is recommended and those where it is not felt to be necessary (51).

Table 66.3.
Cardiac Conditions[a]

Endocarditis prophylaxis recommended:
  Prosthetic cardiac valves (including bioprosthetic and homograft valves)
  Most congenital cardiac malformations
  Surgically constructed systemic-pulmonary shunts
  Rheumatic and other acquired valvular dysfunction
  Idiopathic hypertrophic subaortic stenosis (IHSS)
  Previous history of bacterial endocarditis, even in the absence of heart disease
  Mitral valve prolapse with insufficiency[b]
  Hypertrophic cardiomyopathy
Endocarditis prophylaxis not recommended:
  Isolated secundum atrial septal defect
  Secundum atrial septal defect repaired without a patch 6 or more months earlier
  Patient ductus arteriosus ligated and divided 6 or more months earlier
  Postoperative coronary artery bypass graft (CABG) surgery
  Mitral valve prolapse without regurgitation
  Previous rheumatic fever without valvular dysfunction

---

[a] This table lists common conditions but is not meant to be all-inclusive.
[b] Definitive data to provide guidance in management of patients with mitral valve prolapse are particularly limited. It is clear that in general such patients are at low risk of development of endocarditis, but the risk-benefit ratio of prophylaxis in mitral valve prolapse is uncertain.

The AHA guidelines for prophylaxis are summarized in Tables 66.4 and 66.5 (52).

Recommendations for cardiac surgery are to direct short-term (2 days or less) prophylaxis against staphylococci, with a penicillinase-resistant penicillin or a first-generation cephalosporin. Vancomycin should be considered in institutions where methicilin-resistant staphylococci are prevalent. Prophylaxis is not indicated for "clean" surgeries such as thyroidectomies.

CONCLUSION

Endocarditis is a potentially life-threatening infection that requires early recognition and aggressive treatment for successful management (53). Organisms causing the disease have become progressively more difficult to treat, and combinations of antibiotics are frequently used to achieve synergistic batericidal effects. Infections due to pathogens such as the enterococcus and coagulase-negative staphy-

Table 66.4.
Summary of Recommended Antibiotic Regimens for Dental/Respiratory Tract Procedures[a]

Standard Regimen	
For dental procedures that cause gingival bleeding and oral respiratory tract surgery	Penicillin V 2.0 g orally 1 hr before, then 1.0 g 6 hours later; or amoxicillin 3 g orally 1 hr before then 1.5 g 6 hr later; for patients unable to take oral medications, 2 million units of aqueous penicillin G or ampicillin 2 g IV or i.m., 30–60 min before a procedure and one-half the dose 6 hours later may be substituted
Special Regimens	
Parenteral regimen for use when maximal protection desired e.g., for patients with prosthetic valves	Ampicillin 2.0 g i.m. or IV plus gentamicin 1.5 mg/kg i.m. or IV, one-half hr before procedure followed by 1.0 g oral penicillin V or amoxicillin 6 hr later; alternatively, the parenteral regimen may be repeated once 8 hr later
Oral regimen for penicillin-allergic patients	Erythromycin 1.0 g or clindamycin 300 mg 2 hr before, then one-half the dose 6 hours later
Parenteral regimen for penicillin-allergic patients	Vancomycin 1.0 g IV slowly over 1 hr starting 1 hr before; no repeat dose is necessary OR Clindamycin 300 mg IV 30 min before and 150 mg IV or p.o. 6 hr later

[a] Pediatric doses: ampicillin 50 mg/kg per dose; erythromycin 20 mg/kg for first dose then 10 mg/kg; gentamicin 2.0 mg/kg per dose; penicillin V full adult dose if over 60 lb (27 kg), one-half adult dose if under 60 lb (27 kg); aqueous penicillin G 50,000 units/kg (25,000 units kg for follow-up); vancomycin 20 mg/kg per dose; clindamycin 10 mg/kg. The intervals between doses are the same as for adults. Total doses should not exceed adult doses.

Table 66.5.
Summary of Recommended Regimens for Gastrointestinal Genitourinary Procedures[a]

Standard Regimen	
For genitourinary/ gastrointestinal tract procedures	Ampicillin 2.0 g i.m. or IV plus gentamicin 1.5 mg/kg i.m. or IV given one-half to 1 hr before procedure; followed by amoxicillin 1.5 g given orally 6 hr later; alternatively, the parenteral regimen may be repeated once 8 hr after the initial dose
Special Regimens	
Oral regimen for minor or repetitive procedures in low-risk patients	Amoxicillin 3.0 g orally 1 hr before procedure and 1.5 g 6 hr later
Penicillin-allergic patients	Vancomycin 1.0 g IV slowly over one hour, plus gentamicin 1.5 mg/kg i.m. or IV given 1 hr before procedure; may be repeated once 8–12 hr later

[a] Pediatric doses: ampicillin 50 mg/kg per dose; gentamicin 2.0 mg/kg per dose; amoxicillin 50 mg/kg per dose; vancomycin 20 mg/kg per dose. The intervals between doses are the same as for adults. Totals doses should not exceed adult doses.

lococci will increase in prevalence with the aging of the population at risk. Surgical removal of the infected valve is often necessary to achieve cure in cases of Gram-negative bacillary and fungal infection. Newer antimicrobials such as third-generation cephalosporins, imipenem, and aztreonam may have a role in replacing aminoglycosides for the treatment of Gram-negative infections, but further experience is needed. Prevention of infection is best achieved by recognition of patients at risk, identification of clinical situations likely to produce bacteremia, and use of the recommended prophylactic regimens.

REFERENCES

1. Sullam PM, Drake TA, Sande MA: Pathogenesis of endocarditis. Am J Med 78(6B):110–115, 1985.
2. Kaye D: Changing pattern of infective endocarditis. Am J Med 78(6B):157–162, 1985.
3. Von Reyn CF, Levy BS, Arbeit RD, Friedland G, Crumpacker CS: Infective endocarditis: Analysis based on strict case definitions. Ann Intern Med 94:505, 1981.
4. Kaplan EL, Rich H, Gersony W, Manning J: A collaborative study of infective endocarditis in the 1970's: emphasis on infections in patients who have undergone cardiovascular surgery. Circulation 59:327, 1979.
5. Hubbell G, Cheitlin MD, Rapaport E: Presentation, management, and follow-up evaluation of infective endocarditis in drug addicts. Am Heart J 102:85, 1981.
6. Chambers HF, Korzeniowski OM, Sande MA, et al.: *Staphyloccocus aureus* endocarditis: clinical manifestations in addicts and non-addicts. Medicine 62:170–177, 1983.
7. Levine DP, Crane LR, Zervos MJ: Bacteremia in narcotic addicts at the Detroit Medical Center. II. Infective endocarditis: a prospective comparative study. Rev Infect Dis 8:374–396, 1986.

8. Cohen PS, Maguire JJ, Weinstein L: Infective endocarditis caused by gram-negative bacteria: a review of the literature, 1945–77. Prog Cardiovasc Dis 22:205–242, 1980.

9. Karchmer AW, Archer GL, Dismukes WE: *Staphylococcus epidermidis* causing prosthetic valve endocarditis: microbiologic and clinical observations as guides to therapy. Ann Intern Med 98:447–455, 1983.

10. Wilson WR, Danielson GK, Giuliani ER, Geraci JE: Prosthetic valve endocarditis. Mayo Clin Proc 57:155, 1982.

11. Iannini PB, Crossley K: Therapy of *S. aureus* bacteremia associated with a removable focus of infection. Ann Intern Med 38:281, 1976.

12. Watanakunakorn C, Baird IM: *Staphylococcus aureus* bacteremia and endocarditis associated with a removable infected intravenous device. Am J Med 63:253, 1977.

13. Van Scoy RE: Culture-negative endocarditis. Mayo Clin Proc 57:149, 1982.

14. Pazin GJ, Saul S, Thompson ME: Blood culture positivity: suppression by outpatient antibiotic therapy in patients with bacterial endocarditis. Arch Intern Med 142:263, 1982.

15. Wilson WR, Nichols DR, Thompson RL, Giuliani ER, Geraci JE: Infective endocarditis: therapeutic considerations. Am Heart J 100:689, 1980.

16. Weinstein MP, Stratton CW, Ackley A, et al.: Multicenter collaborative evaluation of a standardized serum bactericial test as a prognostic indicator in infective endocarditis. Am J Med 78:262–269, 1985.

17. Wilson WR, Geraci JE: Treatment of streptococcal infective endocarditis. Am J Med 78(6B):128–137, 1985.

18. Bisno AL, Dismukes WE, Durack DT, Kaplan EL, Karchmer AW, Kaye D, Sande MA, Sanford JP, Wilson WR: Treatment of infective endocarditis due to viridans streptococci. Circulation 63:730A, 1981.

19. Tuazon CU, Gill V, Gill F: Streptococcal endocarditis: single vs combination therapy and role of various species. Rev Infect Dis 8:54–60, 1986.

20. Dall L, Keilhofner M, Herndon B, Barnes W, Lane J: Clindamycin effect on glycocalyx production in experimental viridans streptococcal endocarditis. J Infect Dis 161:1221–1224, 1990.

21. Dall L, Barnes WG, Lane JW, Mills J: Enzymatic modification of glycocalyx in the treatment of experimental endocarditis due to viridans streptococci. J Infect Dis 156:736–740, 1987.

22. Wilson WR, Thompson RL, Wildowske CJ, Washington JA, Giuliani ER, Geraci JE: Short term therapy for streptococcal infective endocarditis—combined intramuscular administration of penicillin and streptomycin. JAMA 245:360, 1981.

23. Sande MA, Schild WM: Combination antibiotic therapy of bacterial endocarditis. Ann Intern Med 92:390, 1980.

24. Wilson WR, Wilkowske CJ, Wright AJ, et al.: Treatment of streptomycin-susceptible and streptomycin-resistant enterococcal endocarditis. Ann Intern Med 100:816–823, 1984.

25. Herzstein J, Ryan JL, Mangi RJ, et al.: Optimal therapy for enterococcal endocarditis. Am J Med 76:186–191, 1984.

26. Patterson JE, Masecar BL, Zervos MJ: Characterization and comparison of two penicillinase-producing strains of *Streptococcus (Enterococcus) faecalis*. Antimicrob Agents Chemother 32:122–124, 1988.

27. Thauvin-Eliopoulos C, Rice LB, Eliopoulos GM, Moellering RC Jr: Efficacy of oxacillin and ampicillin-sulbactam combination in experimental endocarditis caused by β-lactamase hyper-producing *Staphylococcus aureus*. Antimicrob Agents Chemother 34(5):728–732, 1990.

28. Bryant RE, Alford RH: Unsuccessful treatment of staphylococcal endocarditis with cefazolin. JAMA 237:569–570, 1977.

29. Sabath LD: Reappraisal of the antistaphylococcal activities of first-generation (narrow-spectrum) and second-generation (expanded-spectrum) cephalosporins. Antimicrob Agents Chemother 33(4):407–411, 1989.

30. Kernodle DS, Classen DC, Burke JP, Kaiser AB: Failure of Cephalosporins to prevent *Staphylococcus aureus* surgical wound infections. JAMA 263(7):961–966, 1990.

31. Karchmer AW: Staphyloccocal endocarditis. Laboratory and clinical basis for antibiotic therapy. Am J Med 78(6B):116–127, 1985.

32. Small PM, Chambers HF: Vancomycin for *Staphylococcus aureus* endocarditis in intravenous drug abusers. Antimicrob Agents Chemother 34(6):1227–1231, 1990.

33. Abrams B, Sklaver A, Hoffman T, Greenman R: Single or combination therapy of staphylococcal endocarditis in intravenous drug abusers. Ann Intern Med 90:789, 1979.

34. Massanari RM, Donta ST: The efficacy of rifampin as adjunctive therapy in selected cases of staphylococcal endocarditis. Chest 73:371, 1978.

35. Hirschel B: Early termination of a prospective, randomized trial comparing teicoplanin and flucloxacillin for treating severe staphylococcal infections. J Infect Dis 155(2):187–190, 1987.

36. Glucpczynski Y, Lagast H, Vander Auwera P, et al.: Clinical evaluation of teicoplanin for therapy of severe infections caused by Gram-positive bacteria. Antimicrob Agents Chemother 29:52–71, 1986.

37. Stratton CW, Weeks LS: Effect of human serum on the bactericidal activity of daptomycin and vancomycin against staphyloccocal and enterococcal isolates as determined by time-kill kinetic studies. Diagn Microbiol Infect Dis 13:245–252, 1990.

38. Rowland M: Clinical pharmacokinetics of teicoplanin. Clin Pharmacokinet 18(3):184–209, 1990.

39. Gilbert DN, Wood CA, Bracis R, Kimbrough RC: Prospective randomized double-blind clinical comparison of teicoplanin vs vancomycin for *S. aureus* left sided valve endocarditis and endarteritis. Abstract 1988 ICAAC.

40. Kaatz GW, Seo SM, Dorman NJ, Lerner SA: Emergence of teicoplanin resistance during therapy of *Staphylococcus aureus* endocarditis. J Infect Dis 162:103–108, 1990.

41. Dinubile MJ: Surgery in active endocarditis. Ann Intern Med 96:650, 1982.

42. Gudiol F, Cabellos C, Pallares R, Linares J, Ariza J: Intravenous ciprofloxacin therapy in severe infections. Am J Med 87(suppl 5A):221–224, 1989.

43. Thauvin CL, Lecomte F, LeBoete I, Grise G, Lemeland JF: Efficacy of ciprofloxacin alone and in combination with azlocillin in experimental endocarditis due to *Pseudomonas aeruginosa*. Infection 17:31–40, 1989.

44. Eliopoulos GM, Eliopoulos CT: Ciprofloxacin in combination with other antimicrobials. Am J Med 87(suppl 5A):17–21, 1989.

45. Brogden RN, Heel RC, Speight TM, Avery GS: Metronidazole in anaerobic infections: a review of its activity, pharmacokinetics, and therapeutic use. Drugs 16:387, 1978.

46. Owens WE, Finegold SM: Comparative in vitro susceptibilities of anaerobic bacteria to cefmenoxime, cefotetan, and *N*-formimidoyl thienamycin. Antimicrob Agents Chemother 23:626–629, 1983.

47. Odds FC, Cheesman SL, Abbbot AB: Antifungal effects of fluconazole (UK 49858), a new triazole. J Antimicrob Chemother 18:473–478, 1986.

48. Alsip SG, Blackstone EH, Kirklin JW, Cobbs CG: Indications for cardiac surgery in patients with active infective endocarditis. Am J Med 78(6B):138–148, 1985.

49. Conte JE Jr: Prophylaxis of endocarditis during surgical and dental procedures. West J Med 133:141, 1980.

50. Durack DT: Current issues in prevention of infective endocarditis. Am J Med 78(6B):149–156, 1985.
51. Shulman ST, Amren DP, Bisno AL, et al.: Prevention of bacterial endocarditis. Circulation 70:1123A–1127A, 1984.
52. Dajani AS, Bisno AL, Chjung KJ, Durack MB, Freed M, Geraber MA, Karchmer AW, Millard HD, Rahimtoola S, Shulman ST, Watanakunakorn C, Taubert K: Prevention of bacterial endocarditis—

recommendations by the American Heart Association. JAMA 264:2919–2922, 1990.
53. Scheld WM, Sande MA: Endocarditis and intravascular infection. In Mandell GA, Douglas RG, Bennett JE (eds): Principles and Practice of Infectious Diseases, ed. 3. New York, John Wiley & Sons, ch 56, 1990.

CHAPTER 67

CENTRAL NERVOUS SYSTEM INFECTIONS

DONALD P. ALEXANDER, Pharm.D.

Meningitis is generally defined as an inflammation of the membranes of the brain or spinal cord (meninges). This is distinguished from encephalitis, which is inflammation of the brain tissue itself. Brain abscess is defined as a focal intracranial suppuration in brain tissue. Cerebrospinal fluid (CSF) shunt infection and subdural empyema are not discussed in this chapter. The reader is referred to excellent recently published reviews on these topics (1–3). Further general reviews on meningitis and brain abscess are available and should also be consulted (4–9).

ETIOLOGY

The most commonly encountered organisms producing meningitis and brain abscess are listed in Table 67.1. They are listed in an approximate order of frequency of occurrence, and the categories are divided into age-related and history-related incidence. Neonatal meningitis is most commonly caused by a group B streptococci, *Escherichia coli*, and *Listeria monocytogenes* (5, 10, 11). Other Gram-negative organisms causing neonatal meningitis include *Proteus* species, *Klebsiella-Enterobacter*, and *Pseudomonas*. Staphylococci and *Streptococcus pneumoniae* together account for about 10% of the cases. Infection with *Mycobacterium tuberculosis* is dealt with in Chapter 62.

Haemophilus influenzae type b, *Neisseria meningitidis*, and *S. pneumoniae* are responsible for 95% of cases of meningitis in children over 2 months of age (6). *H. influenzae* is usually the most common pathogen seen in patients between the ages of 2 months and 4 to 5 years. After 4 to 5 years of age the incidence of *H. influenzae* meningitis decreases and *N. meningitidis* (meningococcus) and *S. pneumoniae* (pneumococcus) become the most common pathogens causing meningitis (6, 10).

In adults, meningococcus and pneumococcus are the major pathogens causing meningitis (10, 12). In adults under 40 years of age without a prior history of trauma, meningococcus is more frequently reported, and after 40 years of age pneumococcus is the most frequent cause. Staphylococci infrequently cause acute spontaneous meningitis in this age group.

In adults over 60 years of age, the incidence of meningitis caused by Gram-negative bacilli and *Listeria* again begins to increase, but the pneumococcus remains an important pathogen (10, 12–14).

Meningitis following trauma is caused by a variety of bacteria, most commonly the pneumococcus in closed skull fracture and Enterobacteriaceae or staphylococci in penetrating injuries (2). Postsurgical meningitis nearly always follows procedures performed directly on the central nervous system (CNS). The most commonly encountered bacteria in this setting are Gram-negative bacilli: *Klebsiella*, *Enterobacter*, *E. coli*, *Serratia*, and *Pseudomonas*. Staphylococci are occasionally causative agents (15).

Fungal meningitis may be roughly divided into two groups for etiologic purposes: (*a*) disease in a normal (nonimmunocompromised) host and (*b*) infection in the immunocompromised patient. Fungal CNS infection in otherwise normal patients is most often seen in disseminated coccidioidomycosis and in infection with *Cryptococcus neoformans*. Fungal meningitis in the compromised host is primarily due to *C. neoformans*, *Candida* sp., and *Aspergillus* sp. However, there is much overlap between these two groups (16, 17).

Viral infections of the central nervous system are quite common. Most cases are self-limited and mild to moderate in severity. However severe viral meningoencephalitis is caused by the herpes simplex virus in the neonate and the immunocompromised host (18, 19).

The agents causing brain abscess are many and varied, and most individual abscesses are polymicrobial. Aerobic and anaerobic streptococci and anaerobic Gram-negative bacilli are the most common causes of abscess in patients without a history of trauma or surgery. Trauma predisposes to infection with staphylococci, aerobic Gram-negative bacilli, and streptococci. *Nocardia asteroides* may produce brain abscess as a manifestation of disseminated infection.

EPIDEMIOLOGY

The overall incidence of bacterial meningitis in the United States has remained approximately the same for decades, with approximately 2.7 persons per 100,000 population affected (20). This figure does not reflect the age-related disparity in incidence: 0.04% of cases occur in neonates (1 case per 2500 live births), 15% occur in infants under 1 to 2 months of age, 20 to 25% of cases occur between the ages of 2 and 12 months, and 40% of cases occur in children and adolescents 1 to 15 years of age. Meningitis is therefore mostly a pediatric problem. There is no racial predilection and only a slightly greater prevalence of males over females. Acute bacterial meningitis acquired in the hospital has been estimated to account for between 6 and 9% of all cases reported (15).

Table 67.1.
Common Pathogens in CNS Infections[a]

Bacterial meningitis	
Premature infants and neonates (up to 2 mo)	*E. coli*
	Group B streptococci
	Listeria monocytogenes
	Other Enterobacteriaceae
	Streptococcus faecalis
	Staphylococci
	Streptococcus pneumoniae
Infants and children (2 mo to 10 y)	*Haemophilus influenzae*
	Neisseria meningitidis
	S. pneumoniae
Adults	*S. pneumoniae*
	N. meningitidis
	Staphylococci
Elderly (over 60 years of age)	*S. pneumoniae*
	Enterobacteriaceae
	Listeria monocytogenes
Associated with trauma or surgery	*S. pneumoniae*
	Staphylococcus aureus
	Enterobacteriaceae
Fungal meningitis	
"Normal" host	*Cryptococcus neoformans*
	Coccidioides immitis
Immunocompromised host	*C. neoformans*
	C. immitus
	Candida albicans
	Aspergillus spp.
Viral meningoencephalitis[b]	
Neonates	*Herpes simplex*
Immunocompromised host	*Herpes zoster*
Brain abscess	
General	Streptococci
	Mixed anaerobes
	Enterobacteriaceae
Associated with trauma or surgery	*S. aureus*
	Mixed anaerobes
	Enterobacteriaceae
Immunocompromised host	*Nocardia asteroides*

[a] In approximate order.
[b] Many viruses can produce "aseptic" meningitis, but herpes virus is listed here as the only treatable cause.

PATHOGENESIS

Meningitis is most common in the very young and the elderly populations. In the neonate, the host defenses against infection are not well developed, and there are deficiencies in the function of leukocytes and complement. Immunoglobulin (Ig) deficiency of IgA and IgM may also be present at birth and result from the lack of placental transfer from the mother. Lower levels of immunoglobulins and slightly depressed leukocyte function in the elderly contribute to a decreased resistance to infection. Splenectomy, diabetes mellitus, and alcoholism increase the risk of infection because of defective leukocyte function. Individuals with altered cellular immunity from severe underlying disease or immunosuppressive therapy are also at a higher risk for developing meningitis.

A critical series of steps are now known to occur leading to the initiation of bacterial meningitis. These steps include (*a*) host acquisition of a new organism, usually by nasopharyngeal colonization; (*b*) translocation of the organism through the local mucosal tissue; (*c*) bacteremia with intravascular survival; (*d*) meningeal invasion; (*e*) bacterial survival and replication within the CNS; and (*f*) production of subarachnoid space (SAS) inflammation (21). The mechanism of bacterial mucosal attachment to the nasopharynx and translocation through local tissue are currently not fully understood. Microbial virulence factors, such as a specific outer membrane capsule that protects the organism and the presence of specialized cell surface components, are recognized to mediate the attachment and perhaps facilitate the translocation of certain bacterial strains known to cause meningitis.

After crossing the mucosal tissue barrier the organisms gain access to the bloodstream and are transported to distant tissue sites. Intravascular survival occurs largely because of bacterial encapsulation, which resists phagocytic elimination and bactericidal activity of the classical complement pathway. Bacteremia is an important factor predisposing individuals to meningitis. Bacteria may also reach the CSF by spread from contiguous tissues or by direct implantation. Otitis media, sinusitis, dental infections, and mastoiditis are predisposing conditions in meningitis. Direct implantation of bacteria by trauma or neurosurgical procedures represents only a small percentage of the cases of meningitis. How bacteria invade the CNS is still unknown, but recent information suggests that the choroid plexus and the cerebral microvasculature are likely sites of bacterial invasion. Brain abscess not induced by trauma or surgery usually results from hematogenous seeding.

Local immune defense within the SAS is minimal and permits the rapid and largely unchecked growth of the offending agents, resulting in a large bacterial inoculum within the SAS. Opsonic and bactericidal activity within the SAS are low to absent before the opening of the blood-brain barrier (BBB) and therefore render little help to local defense. The presence and amount of endotoxin in the CSF correlates with the degree of meningeal inflammation. Specific components of bacterial cell walls are the primary stimulus responsible for inducing meningeal inflammation. Although the actual cell wall components differ between Gram-positive (peptidoglycan layers or polymers of techoic acid) and Gram-negative bacteria (lipopolysaccharide, LPS), these components are strong inducers of inflammation and result in similar clinical signs and symptoms in patients. Techoic acid polymers and LPS are released when bacterial cells are killed or lysed. The initiation of bactericidal antibiotic therapy is recognized to cause a rapid and marked release of these mediators (LPS and techoic acid polymers), heightening the inflammatory response in the CNS, which may be ultimately responsible for the long-term neurologic sequelae found in patients recovering from meningitis.

Locally produced cytokines are responsible for or contribute to the inflammatory response in the CNS. Tissue necrosis factor (TNF) and interleukin-1 (IL-1) are two cytokines produced locally within the CNS and are known to be potent mediators of the inflammatory response. Elevated concentrations of IL-1 and TNF are found in the CSF of neonates, infants, and children with bacterial meningitis. TNF is not found in appreciable quantities in individuals with viral-induced meningitis, although IL-1 concentrations may be present. Neurologic sequelae are recognized in individuals who have markedly elevated concentrations of cytokines in their CSF. Significant neurologic sequelae are found in individuals when concentrations of IL-1 in the CSF exceed 500 pg/ml at the time of diagnosis. These data suggest that one or both of these cytokines are involved in the initial events of meningitis and possibly responsible for events leading to the increased permeability of the BBB. Other inflammatory mediators such as platelet-activating factor (PAF), arachidonic acid metabolites (prostaglandin E), and other interleukins may contribute to the meningeal inflammation, but their exact role remains unclear (22).

The relative contribution of the individual neutrophil and the resultant CSF neutrophil pleocytosis of the host response in purulent CSF remains unclear.

The severe inflammatory response present in the SAS results in both vasogenic and cytotoxic forms of cerebral edema, altered dynamics of CSF flow, resulting in outflow resistance and increased CSF pressure, altered brain metabolism, and decreased cerebrovascular blood flow. The interaction of all of the above-mentioned inflammatory mediators and regulatory abnormalities for a sufficient duration leads to significant neuronal injury and eventual brain damage.

DIAGNOSIS AND CLINICAL FEATURES

The clinical course of meningitis may be acute or subacute, depending on whether the signs and symptoms have been present for less than or more than 24 hr. In the acute presentation (approximately 10% of cases), the signs and symptoms are usually present for less than 24 hr and are rapidly progressive. The etiology is usually bacterial; *S. pneumoniae* or *N. meningitidis* are most common. The patient's prognosis is inversely related to the length of time from the onset of symptoms until presentation for medical care. In the subacute presentation (approximately 75% of cases) the signs and symptoms are present for 1 to 7 days before evaluation and may be caused by different viruses, fungi, or bacteria.

Signs and symptoms are usually nonspecific and may vary in different age groups. In neonates and infants under 1 year of age, the symptoms are often absent or very nonspecific. The most common clinical findings are lethargy, irritability, poor feeding, respiratory distress, cyanosis, or hypothermia. Because these findings are nonspecific, the infection may go unrecognized until irreversible brain damage has occurred. It is therefore important to identify recognized risk factors for the development of meningitis in this age group: prolonged labor, premature rupture of fetal membranes, peripartum maternal infection, or any neonatal or infant infection.

In infants over 1 year of age, older children, and adults, the symptoms are more indicative of meningeal inflammation. Fever and altered mental status are the most common findings. Other symptoms, including nausea, vomiting, headache, and photophobia, reflect increased intracranial pressure or cerebral inflammation. Neurologic signs vary, and convulsions or coma occur in approximately one-third of patients. Nuchal rigidity is a classic finding that results from meningeal inflammation. Helpful clues include Brudzinski's sign (neck flexion producing knee and hip flexion) or Kernig's sign (pain and difficulty in raising the extended leg).

The clinical presentation of patients with brain abscess usually includes headache and an altered mental state of consciousness that varies from lethargy, irritability, and confusion to coma. Focal neurologic signs may be due to an expanding intracranial mass, and depending on the location in the brain, the presentation may vary from indolent to rapidly progressive.

The etiologic agent causing meningeal inflammation cannot be determined from the patient's clinical presentation. A careful history and physical examination should be performed. If a mass lesion in the CNS is not a concern, a lumbar puncture should be performed to obtain information that includes: CSF pressure and appearance, cell count and differential, glucose and protein levels, Gram stain, and culture. Table 67.2 lists the common parameters of the CSF that are altered in various forms of meningitis. It must be emphasized that these are only general principles and the use of the numbers in this table cannot be absolute (e.g., the CSF white cell count may be less than 500 in bacterial meningitis, or may not be predominantly polymorphonuclear (PMN), or the glucose CSF/serum ratio may be normal).

A repeat lumbar puncture within 12 to 72 hr may be helpful in circumstances where patients with symptoms of meningeal inflammation have normal CSF parameters, or to distinguish bacterial from aseptic (viral) meningitis. Early viral infection may show a predominantly neutrophilic white blood cell count that soon changes to mononuclear cells.

The clinical presentation and CSF findings may be consistent with meningitis, but the diagnosis is confirmed by laboratory culture of the causative organism. However,

Table 67.2.
Cerebrospinal Fluid (CSF) Findings in Meningitis

	Appearance	WBC[a]	Type[b]	Protein	Glucose Ratio CSF/Serum
Bacterial	Turbid	500 or more	PMN	Elevated	50%
Fungal	Clear	10–500	MN	Elevated	Variable
Viral	Clear	10–500	MN	Normal or elevated	50%

[a] WBC, white blood cell count; [10^6/liter(mm^{-3})].

[b] PMN, polymorphonuclear; MN, mononuclear including lymphocytes and/or monocytes.

the CSF culture may not always be positive, particularly if antibiotics were administered prior to the lumbar puncture. It has been estimated that approximately 50% of all children with bacterial meningitis under the age of 5 years received some form of antibiotic therapy prior to the lumber puncture (23). This practice does not appreciably alter the CSF findings in Table 67.2, but it will frequently lead to negative Gram-stain and culture results.

Standard laboratory analysis of the CSF does not always provide definitive information about the presence or absence of meningitis or nature of the causative agent. A few additional laboratory tests may be helpful in the differential diagnosis of bacterial meningitis, especially when the CSF culture and Gram stain are negative. These include (a) CSF lactate concentration, which may differentiate bacterial from viral meningitis; (b) limulus amebocyte lysate assay, which may detect the presence of Gram-negative endotoxin; (c) counterimmunoelectrophoresis (CIE), latex agglutination, and enzyme-linked immunosorbant assay (ELISA), which may detect minute quantities of bacterial antigen; and (d) C-reactive protein in the CSF, which helps to differentiate bacterial from aseptic causes of meningitis.

Fungi are occasionally cultured from the CSF. The detection of fungal antigen (e.g., cryptococcal) or antibody (e.g., coccidioidomycosis) in the CSF is often essential to the diagnosis of these causative agents.

Herpesvirus encephalitis usually presents with diffuse neurologic findings and nonspecific CSF findings and usually requires a brain biopsy for diagnosis.

The diagnosis of brain abscess is complicated by a number of factors. Routine laboratory tests are usually not helpful (e.g., 20 to 40% of patients have normal white blood cell counts). A lumbar puncture is occasionally mildly abnormal and nonspecific. Gram stain and culture of the CSF are usually negative, unless the abscess has ruptured into the subarachnoid space or ventricles. Lumbar puncture is contraindicated in the presence of increased intracranial pressure or if a mass lesion is suspected. Computerized axial tomography (CT scan), or magnetic resonance imaging (MRI) are diagnostic aids used to detect brain abscesses.

COMPLICATIONS

The complications of bacterial meningitis include brain abscess, lateral sinus thrombosis, cerebral thrombophlebitis, and subdural empyema. Generalized or focal convulsions, septic shock and disseminated intravascular coagulation may occur, especially in meningococcemia. The severe inflammatory response in the CNS results in cerebral edema, altered dynamics of CSF flow, altered brain metabolism, and decreased cerebrovascular blood flow. These factors may lead to an elevated CSF pressure resulting in cortical necrosis and brain infarction progressing to herniation and eventually death.

Neurologic sequelae such as mental retardation, hydrocephalus, permanent seizure disorders, aparesis, ataxia, deafness, pychosis, and blindness occur frequently as a result of neonatal and childhood meningitis. Generally infections with H. influenzae and the pneumococcus carry the poorest prognosis with respect to neurologic sequelae at 1 month and at 1 year or longer (approximately 25 to 50% and 14%, respectively) (24, 25). The degree of neurologic sequelae may be related to the size of the bacterial inoculum or antigen load in the CSF that causes the intense inflammatory response.

The results of treatment of herpes simplex encephalitis with adenine arabinoside or acyclovir have shown that neurologic sequelae are present in approximately 50% of survivors (26).

Approximately one-third of patients with brain abscess have some residual neurologic disability.

TREATMENT

The effective treatment of CNS infections largely depends upon (a) attaining and maintaining adequate antibiotic concentrations in the CSF or brain extracellular fluid (ECF); (b) the microbiologic activity of the antibiotic while in the CNS; (c) reducing or moderating the inflammatory response within the CNS; and (d) effectively managing the complications resulting from the infection.

The blood, CSF, and brain are three different compartments that intercommunicate and maintain the homeostasis of the CNS (27). These three compartments are separated functionally and anatomically by three barriers;

the blood-brain ECF barrier, the blood-CSF barrier, and the CSF-brain ECF barrier. Traditionally, what is recognized as the blood-brain barrier (BBB) can be functionally and anatomically explained as two separate barriers (the blood-brain ECF barrier and blood-CSF barrier). Physiologically, both of these barriers contain capillaries whose cellular wall structure differs from that of capillaries elsewhere in the body in that the junctions between the cells are closely spaced (tight junctions). Functionally, these barriers require substances to pass through the cellular wall rather than between the cells. Because of this requirement, the physical properties of each antibiotic determine how well it passes from the blood into the brain ECF or CSF. Once the antibiotic has gained access to the brain ECF or CSF, equilibration between these compartments occurs relatively quickly.

The physical properties of a drug govern its penetration into the CNS and include (a) the relative affinity for lipid or water (degree of ionization and the relative lipid solubility of the unionized form); (b) the relative affinity for serum plasma proteins (only the free fraction would be expected to penetrate the CNS barrier); and (c) carrier-mediated transport (usually unimportant for antibiotics). The degree of ionization of a drug depends upon its characteristics at plasma pH. The ionized form of the drug has an increased affinity for plasma water, and it is the unionized form that is available to cross cellular membranes. The lipid solubility of the unionized form of the drug is determined by the relative affinity of that drug for lipid or water. Therefore, for a drug to readily penetrate into the CNS, three properties are important: low ionization at plasma pH, higher affinity for lipid than water, and low protein binding (28) (Table 67.3).

The failure of many drugs to reach detectable levels in the CSF, despite their ability to penetrate the barriers, is due to the rapid clearance of the drug from the CSF. Most drugs are removed by bulk flow through the arachnoid villi. The high turnover rate of the CSF prevents accumulation of these drugs in the CNS. Active transport of various organic acids and bases has also been demonstrated. This mechanism is similar to the secretory action that occurs in the kidney. Many penicillins and cephalosporins have been shown to have some degree of tubular secretion that contributes to their elimination. Probenecid decreases the renal excretion of these antibiotics as well as the elimination of these antibiotics from the CSF, resulting in higher measured levels.

There are conditions (infection, tumors, chemicals, etc.) that impair these normal physiologic mechanisms and increase the BBB permeability. Many drugs do not penetrate into the CSF in patients with normal intact meninges but do cross readily when the meninges are inflamed. This is true for most antibiotics. For example, penicillin is not detectable in the CSF of animals or humans with

Table 67.3.
Cerebrospinal Fluid (CSF) Penetration of Various Antibiotics during Meningitis

Adequate CSF penetration with systemic therapy alone
  Penicillin G
  Ampicillin/amoxicillin
  Methicillin/nafcillin
  Mezlocillin/piperacillin
  Cefotaxime/ceftriaxone
  Ceftizoxime/ceftazidime
  Cefuroxime/moxalactam
  Imipenem/aztreonam
  Ticarcillin
  Chloramphenicol
  Sulfonamides
  Trimethoprim
  Flucytosine/fluconazole
  Metronidazole
  Rifampin
  Ciprofloxacin/pefloxacin

Limited CSF penetration and/or requiring CSF instillation
  Carbenicillin (40 mg)[a]
  Vancomycin (20 mg)
  Amphotericin B (0.25–0.5 mg)[b]
  Miconazole (20 mg)
  Streptomycin (20–40 mg)
  Gentamicin/tobramycin (4–8 mg)
  Kanamycin/amikacin (10–20 mg)
  Erythromycin (3–10 mg)
  Ketoconazole/itraconazole[c]
  Polymixin B[c] (2.5–5 mg)
  Clindamycin[c]
  Cephalothin/cephalordine[c]
  Cefazolin/cefamandole[c]
  Cefoxitin/cefoperazone[c,d]
  Tetracyclines[c]

[a] Usual daily intrathecal or intraventricular dose.
[b] Diluted with CSF and given intrathecally (lumbar or intraventricular) or use a hyperbaric solution of 10% dextrose given intralumbar.
[c] Limited use because of poor penetration or lack of bactericidal/fungicidal activity.
[d] Unreliable CSF penetration.

normal meninges. During meningitis both the CSF barrier and the clearance mechanisms are usually altered. As the meningitis resolves, the permeability to drugs is reduced, and the clearance mechanisms begin to work more efficiently.

Once the antibiotic penetrates into the CSF, it must be microbiologically active. A better understanding of the CSF environment and in vitro susceptibility testing should provide information to make a more rational selection of an antibiotic. Infections of the CSF occur in an area of impaired host resistance. Low levels of CSF complement have been found in patients with meningitis, together with reduced bactericidal and opsonic activity (29). In addition, normal CSF contains only low concentrations of immunoglobulins, and an intact BBB impedes the entrance of peripheral white blood cells to the site of infection. Therefore, antibiotics that actually kill the organism (bactericidal) rather than just inhibit their growth (bacteriostatic) are required.

Concentrations of antibiotics in the CSF which are similar to or just exceed the minimum inhibitory concentration (MIC) of the infecting organism often result in bacteriologic failures (30, 31). Peak drug concentrations in the CSF should exceed the minimum bactericidal concentrations (MBC) by severalfold to produce bacterial killing. However, the size of the bacterial inoculum, the use of broth instead of CSF as the growth medium for in vitro susceptibility testing, and the altered pH of the CSF may markedly influence the activity of antibiotics. The aminoglycosides are an excellent example. The bactericidal activity of the aminoglycosides decreases when the pH decreases. The MBC of *E. coli* for gentamicin at a pH of 7.35 is 1 μg/ml and increases to 8 μg/ml when the pH is

changed to 7.0 (as may occur in meningitis). Recent experience suggests that concentrations 10 to 30 times the MBC are necessary to achieve bacterial killing in vivo (32). This may be impossible with aminoglycosides, because of the narrow therapeutic-toxic ratio. Also, the use of antibiotic concentrations far above what may be attained in the CSF to determine the in vitro susceptibility of the microorganism may be misleading.

The need for prompt antimicrobial therapy is emphasized by the rate of mortality within hours in patients with an acute presentation of meningitis. In this situation, it is not appropriate to wait for culture results to initiate therapy. After the patient history, physical examination, and collection of specimens for appropriate laboratory tests, the patient should be started on intravenous antibiotics. The choice of empiric therapy should be based upon the patient's age, history, and any specific underlying diseases

Table 67.4.
Empiric Antibiotic Therapy in Bacterial Meningitis

Age	Drug	Dose (mg/kg/day)	Usual Interval (hr)	Route
Neonate (up to 2 months old)	1. Ampicillin *or*	100–200	8–12	IV
	Penicillin *plus*	100,000–200,000 U	8–12	IV
	Aminoglycoside[a,b] *or*	5–7.5 (1 mg/day)	8–12	IV
			24	IT[c]
	2. Cefotaxime	100–150	6–8	IV
	Ceftriaxone	80–100	12–24	IV
	Ceftizoxime	100–150	6–8	IV
	Ceftazidime	60–90	8–12	IV
	Cefuroxime	200–240	8	IV
	Vancomycin	20–30	8–12	IV
	Nafcillin	100–200	8–12	IV
Infants and children (2 months to 10 years)	Ampicillin *and*	200–300	6	IV
	Chloramphenicol *or*	75–100	6	IV/PO
	Cefotaxime	150–200	6	IV
	Ceftriaxone	80–100	12–24	IV
	Cefuroxime	200–240	8	IV
	Penicillin	250,000–400,000 U	4–6	IV
Adolescents and adults (> 10 years)	Penicillin *or*	200,000–300,000 U	4–6	IV
	Ampicillin *or*	200–300	6	IV
	Ceftriaxone	80–100	12–24	IV
	Cefotaxime	150–200	6	IV
	Ceftazidime	125–150	8	IV
Associated with trauma or surgery (any age)	1. Penicillin *plus*	200,000–300,000 U	4–6	IV
	Nafcillin *plus*	150–200	4–6	IV
	Aminoglycoside[b] *or*	5–6 (4–8 mg/day)	8	IV
			24	IT[a]
		neonates 5–7.5 (1 mg/day)	8–12	IV
	2. Cefotaxime	150–200	6–8	IV
	Ceftriaxone	100	12	IV
	Ceftazidime	150	8	IV
	Vancomycin (penicillin allergy)	20–30 (20 mg/day)	8–12	IV
			24	IT[a]

[a] If enterococci are cultured use gentamicin.
[b] Gentamicin/tobramycin/amikacin: (amikacin 15–20 mg/kg/day every 12 hr for infants <7 day, 20–30 mg/kg/day for older children; 5 mg/day intrathecally in infants, 10–20 mg/day for adults).
[c] IT, Intrathecal (preferably intraventricular).

and tailored further by the results of the CSF Gram stain. Once the culture results are known and the antimicrobial sensitivities have been performed, more specific antibiotic therapy can be initiated (Table 67.4). Full doses of antibiotics should be administered for the entire course of therapy. As the patient responds, meningeal inflammation decreases, which results in decreased antibiotic penetration in the CSF. Reduction in the antibiotic dose as the patient responds has been correlated with a relapse of the infection.

A repeat lumbar puncture is usually performed 24 to 48 hr after beginning therapy, to monitor the clinical and bacteriologic response of the patient. CSF Gram stain and culture should be negative for bacteria. Occasionally Gram stains and cultures remain positive. If so, a parameningeal focus should be investigated. In enteric Gram-negative bacillary meningitis, Gram stain and culture may remain positive for several days. Persistence of Gram-negative bacteria in the CSF is often associated with ventriculitis.

The optimal duration of antibiotic therapy for meningitis is not known but should be based upon the individual patient's positive response to therapy. Current guidelines for the treatment of meningococcal, H. influenzae, and pneumococcal meningitis require treatment for a minimum of 7 days, 7 to 10 days, and 10 days, respectively. More serious cases of Gram-negative bacillary meningitis may require 3 or more weeks of therapy. Treatment of fungal meningitis may require long-term therapy (3 to 6 months or longer). The duration of treatment for brain abscess is usually 4 to 6 weeks of systemic antibiotic therapy after surgical drainage of the abscess.

NEONATAL MENINGITIS

The antibiotics of choice for E. coli meningitis have traditionally been ampicillin plus an aminoglycoside in the doses listed in Table 67.4 for a minimum of 14 days. The use of intraventricular aminoglycoside is controversial. The newer cephalosporins (cefotaxime, ceftriaxone, and ceftazidime) have been very effective in treating this form of meningitis. Most of these drugs have adequate penetration into the CNS, and all have exceptional activity against E. coli. The newer agents should provide effective therapy without requiring multiple intrathecal or intraventricular injections of aminoglycoside. Table 67.4 lists the commonly used drugs and their doses.

Group B streptococci are usually less sensitive to penicillin than other streptococci, therefore penicillin G must be given in doses of 100,000 to 200,000 units/kg/day in divided doses every 8 to 12 hr for 14 days. Ampicillin may be substituted for penicillin G, even though the organism is slightly less susceptible. Several of the newer cephalosporins (cefotaxime, cefuroxime, ceftriaxone, ceftizoxime) are very active against group B streptococci. Imipenem is also active against group B streptococci. Moxalactam, cef-

tazidime, and aztreonam display little to no antibacterial activity against gram-positive bacteria, including group B streptococci, and should not be considered for the treatment of this form of meningitis. Empiric therapy with a combination of penicillin or ampicillin plus a third-generation cephalosporin will provide adequate coverage for meningitis caused by group B streptococci and E. coli. In the penicillin-allergic patient with documented group B streptococcal meningitis, chloramphenicol may be used as an alternative antibiotic.

Meningitis caused by other Enterobacteriaceae such as Proteus species and the Klebsiella-Enterobacter-Serratia group has usually required an aminoglycoside administered both systemically and intrathecally. If these organisms are sensitive to the newer cephalosporins, these antibiotics may be the best alternative to treat this serious form of meningitis. For more resistant organisms, such as Serratia marcesens and Pseudomonas aeruginosa, an aminoglycoside alone or in combination with a penicillin (ticarcillin, piperacillin, or mezlocillin) or a newer cephalosporin (ceftazidime) should be used, depending upon the sensitivities of the pathogen. Amikacin may be required and should be dosed at 15 mg/kg/day for infants under 7 days of age, and 22.5 mg/kg/day for older infants. If intrathecal or intraventricular administration of aminoglycosides is required, doses are listed in Table 67.4. Therapy should continue for a minimum of 2 weeks, preferably 3 weeks or longer.

Appropriate therapy for Listeria meningitis is ampicillin or penicillin intravenously for 14 days. The addition of the aminoglycoside to the regimen depends upon the clinical response of the patient. In the penicillin allergic patient, trimethoprim/sulfamethoxazole should be used. A dose of 10 mg/kg/day of trimethoprim in the fixed combination should be effective.

CHILDHOOD AND ADULT MENINGITIS

Haemophilus influenzae type b is the most common cause of childhood meningitis. Because of the frequency of ampicillin-resistant organisms, both ampicillin and chloramphenicol have traditionally been initiated pending sensitivities of the organism. Once these sensitivities are known, definitive therapy can be continued and one of the antibiotics discontinued. Therapy should be continued for a minimum of 7 days. Chloramphenicol should never be given by intramuscular injection because of the poor absorption. Oral absorption produces excellent serum concentrations and may be considered after the initial few days of intravenous therapy. In the penicillin-allergic patient, chloramphenicol is generally the accepted alternative agent. The newer cephalosporins (cefotaxime, ceftriaxone, ceftazidime) have excellent activity against H. influenzae and are effective agents in the treatment of meningitis. These agents are being used in many clinical situations as drugs of first choice for the treatment of meningitis in children 2 months to 10 years of age. The choice of cephalosporin in this setting may be justified because of the frequency of β-lactamase-producing *H. influenzae*, which has required the empiric use of two antibiotics.

Meningitis due to *Streptococcus pneumoniae* or *Neisseria meningitidis* should be treated with intravenous penicillin G. Doses are listed in Table 67.4. Treatment should be given for 7 to 10 days. In the penicillin-allergic patient, chloramphenicol is a useful alternative. The newer cephalosporins do not offer any advantage over penicillin. Because of the poor Gram-positive activity of moxalactam, ceftazidime, and aztreonam, these agents should not be considered for therapy of pneumococcal meningitis.

Staphylococcal meningitis is nearly always caused by *S. aureus* and therefore seldom responds to penicillin G, because most strains are resistant. The therapy of choice is a penicillinase-resistant penicillin. The choice is nafcillin over methicillin, because nafcillin is considerably less nephrotoxic. Oxacillin would be an acceptable alternative. Appropriate doses are 150 to 200 mg/kg/day intravenously for 14 days. These doses achieve therapeutic concentrations in the CSF of patients with staphylococcal meningitis. Vancomycin is the drug of choice for meningeal infections due to methicillin-resistant staphylococci and may be used as an alternative therapy for patients allergic to penicillin. Older cephalosporins should not be used because of poor CSF penetration, the newer cephalosporins should not be considered because of generally poor antibacterial activity against Gram-positive bacteria, and chloramphenicol should not be considered because of poor bactericidal activity against staphylococci. Experience with the use of imipenem is limited.

Enterococcal (*S. faecalis*) meningitis is uncommon, and the organism is difficult to kill because of its relative insensitivity to penicillins. A combination of a penicillin (penicillin G or ampicillin) plus an aminoglycoside (gentamicin or streptomycin) is the therapy of choice. The intrathecal use of an aminoglycoside may not always be necessary to treat this infection, and careful clinical monitoring during the first 48 to 72 hr dictates this decision. Doses are listed in Tables 67.3 and 67.4. In patients allergic to penicillin, vancomycin may be used alone or in combination with an aminoglycoside, and intrathecal vancomycin may be required. Doses are listed in Tables 67.3 and 67.4. The cephalosporins do not have activity against the enterococcus and should not be used to treat this form of meningitis.

The most common fungi causing meningitis are *Cryptococcus*, *Coccidioides*, and *Candida*. Primary therapy of each of these infections is treated in approximately the same manner. Cryptococcal meningitis is treated with intravenous amphotericin B in doses up to 0.5 mg/kg/day with or without flucytosine. Intrathecal therapy with amphotericin B is usually unnecessary and is only given when there has been an inadequate clinical response with intravenous therapy. Flucytosine has been studied in this infection. Patients who received both drugs did slightly better clinically, but they also suffered more frequent and severe adverse reactions caused by flucytosine (33). Thus, flucytosine should be reserved for situations in which patients do not improve adequately on amphotericin B alone. The patients should be treated until the CSF cryptococcal antigen titers are negative. In patients who have recurrences of the infection, especially those with AIDS, chronic suppressive therapy may be needed. Fluconazole in doses of 100 to 200 mg/day has been shown to be highly effective in preventing recurrent cryptococcal infection and is lower in side effects than conventional chronic suppressive therapy with weekly infusions of amphotericin B (34).

Coccidioidomycosis is more difficult to treat, since the organisms are less sensitive to amphotericin B and are completely resistant to flucytosine (35). The systemic dose of amphotericin B must be increased to 0.75 to 1.0 mg/kg/day; daily to every-other-day intrathecal, or preferably, intracisternal or intraventricular injection of 0.25 to 0.5 mg is necessary. As with cryptococcosis, the course of this disease tends to be relapsing, and amphotericin B must be given until the coccidioides antibody in the CSF is reduced by more than fourfold. This may require 3 to 6 months of therapy. Outpatient amphotericin B therapy, given three times a week, is preferred in many situations.

Intravenous miconazole is effective in some cases; the dose is 25 to 30 mg/kg/day intravenously, with or without 20 mg/day intrathecally. There have been several reports of failure of miconazole, and it should only be used as an alternative. Ketoconazole, an imidazole antibiotic, is active against various fungi including *Coccidioides*. The concentration of ketoconazole found in CSF after oral dosing is low and depends upon the degree of BBB inflammation. Experience with the use of ketoconazole in the treatment of fungal meningitis is limited, and it is not recommended at this time. Fluconazole, a triazole antifungal antibiotic, has good CSF penetration and has demonstrated therapeutic effectiveness in the treatment of this disease, but the total experience with this drug is also very limited at this time.

Candidal meningitis is unusual, and many reported cases have resolved spontaneously (16, 36). Nevertheless, appropriate treatment seems to be the same as for cryptococcal meningitis.

The treatment of herpesvirus meningitis has been unsuccessful until recently. Previous therapy included cytosine arabinoside (ara-C) and idoxuridine, which only produced severe toxicity. Clinical trials have demonstrated the efficacy of adenine arabinoside (vidarabine) and acyclovir in the treatment of neonatal and adult herpes simplex encephalitis and disseminated herpes zoster infection in the immunocompromised patient (26). Unfortunately, although survival was definitely increased in patients given these drugs, severe morbidity was common. Therapy must be instituted early in the course of the disease (within 48 to 72 hr) to be of any benefit. The dose of vidarabine is 15 mg/kg/day and of acyclovir if 30 mg/kg/day in a single daily infusion for 5 days; if clinical response occurs, therapy is continued for 10 to 14 days. Acyclovir has become the agent of first choice because of the large fluid requirements necessary in the administration of vidarabine.

CONTROVERSIES IN ANTIBIOTIC THERAPY

Chloramphenicol

Chloramphenicol penetrates well into the CSF in concentrations ranging from 35 to 45% of serum concentrations, and it is frequently used in the treatment of meningitis. Bactericidal activity is required for effective treatment of meningitis. Chloramphenicol has been shown to be bactericidal against *H. influenzae*, *S. pneumoniae*, and *N. meningitidis*. Treatment of meningitis caused by these organisms with chloramphenicol usually results in eradication of the organisms from the CSF. Treatment of Gram-negative meningitis with chloramphenicol is controversial. Most Gram-negative organisms are only inhibited by chloramphenicol and are not killed until very large concentrations are achieved. Reports of treatments failures with the development of bacterial resistance during therapy are common (14). There is also evidence that the combination of chloramphenicol and an aminoglycoside may be less effective than an aminoglycoside alone (32). This information would suggest that chloramphenicol should be used in cases of meningitis where the antibiotic is known to be bactericidal. Chloramphenicol may be used in Gram-negative meningitis if the susceptibility (MBC) of the organism to choramphenicol is known.

Aminoglycosides

The aminoglycosides do not diffuse readily from the blood into the CSF. Little antibiotic passes through the uninflamed meninges, but during periods of inflammation up to 30% of serum concentrations can be found in the CSF. However, the amount of antibiotic present does not result in a consistently bactericidal effect because of the acid pH of infected CSF. Because of variable penetration and inconsistent bactericidal effect, direct instillation into the subarachnoid space (SAS) is required.

The CSF is formed in the third and fourth ventricles and is circulated from the ventricles in two directions: (*a*) ascending to the lateral SAS and bathing the cerebral hemispheres and (*b*) descending through the SAS to the spinal cord. If an antibiotic is placed into the SAS by lumbar injection, the normal physiology of CSF flow would pre-

clude its entrance into the ventricles. Direct instillation into the ventricles does provide drug concentrations throughout the entire SAS.

Considerable controversy surrounds the benefit of intrathecal aminoglycosides in treatment neonatal Gram-negative meningitis (37). In 1976, the Neonatal Meningitis Cooperative Study Group investigated the treatment of neonatal meningitis with and without the intralumbar instillation of gentamicin added to intravenous therapy. The results showed no benefit from intralumbar gentamicin over systemic therapy alone. A large percentage of the neonates were found to have ventriculitis, which was thought to have contributed to the lack of effect.

In 1980, a second Neonatal Meningitis Cooperative Study Group investigated the intraventricular use of gentamicin in the treatment of Gram-negative meningitis. In this study, there was a higher death rate in the group receiving intraventricular gentamicin plus systemic therapy versus those receiving systemic therapy alone. The increased mortality experienced in this group may have been caused by repeated percutaneous intraventricular injections. A controlled clinical trial of the intraventricular use of amikacin instilled into a Rickman reservoir did not substantiate the second Neonatal Cooperative Study Group's findings. In fact, all of the neonatal deaths occurred in the group that received systemic antibiotics alone. From these data, the role of intraventricular aminoglycoside therapy for treatment of neonatal Gram-negative meningitis and ventriculitis remains unclear. Further analysis of the CSF samples from the last Neonatal Cooperative Study Group's investigation demonstrated high concentrations of inflammatory cytokines in the CSF following the administration of intraventricular aminoglycosides (38). The production and release of these inflammatory cytokines is believed to be the direct result of a rapid bactericidal effect by the antibiotic, releasing bacterial endotoxin within the CSF. The high morbidity and poor outcome of the previously treated neonates may have been caused by the excessive inflammatory reaction and not be a direct effect of the drug. In adults, the use of intraventricular aminoglycosides reduces the mortality of Gram-negative meningitis.

When using the aminoglycoside to treat meningitis the following points apply: (*a*) these agents penetrate variability into the CSF, (*b*) the amount of antibiotic that passes into the CSF may not be consistently bactericidal, (*c*) direct instillation into the CSF is usually required to reach bactericidal concentrations, (*d*) intralumbar instillation provides drug levels to all areas except the ventricles, (*e*) ventriculitis is common in Gram-negative meningitis, and (*f*) repeated direct drug administration into the ventricles should be done through a reservoir.

Cephalosporins

Cephalothin should not be used to treat patients with meningitis (30). Poor penetration, minimal antibacterial activity, and toxicity of cephaloridine led to the widespread avoidance of cephalosporin antibiotics in the treatment of meningitis. Cefamandole demonstrates moderate CSF penetration and greater antibacterial activity than earlier cephalosporins. Treatment failures and the development of resistance during therapy have discouraged its use for treating meningitis. Cefoxitin, a cephamycin, penetrates moderately well into the CSF and also has greater antibacterial activity than earlier cephalosporins. Probenecid is usually required when cefoxitin is used, to increase the CSF concentrations (39). However, cefoxitin has limited utility and should only be considered in cases of meningitis caused by highly susceptible organisms. The newer cephalosporins penetrate moderately well into the CSF during meningitis. Because these drugs have excellent antibacterial activity against most Enterobacteriacae, their use in Gram-negative meningitis may be of great importance in the management of this serious infection. Although these antibiotics have increased Gram-negative activity, their activity against most Gram-positive organisms is markedly decreased. This is especially important in meningitis caused by group B streptococci, S. pneumoniae, S. aureus, and Listeria monocytogenes. Cefuroxime, cefotaxime, ceftizoxime, and ceftriaxone have been used with success in the treatment of meningitis caused by group B streptococci, S. pneumoniae, and S. aureus. These agents should not be used to treat meningitis caused by Listeria monocytogenes. Moxalactam and ceftazidime should not be used to treat Gram-positive meningitis. In addition, the activity of these antibiotics against most Pseudomonas is limited, because many strains have minimum bactericidal concentrations that are not readily attainable in the CSF. Ceftazidime has been used in a limited number of cases of pseudomonal meningitis with some success (40, 41).

Successful single-drug therapy has been documented in meningitis caused by susceptible organisms. However, these new agents will not totally replace the use of the aminoglycosides in the treatment of Gram-negative meningitis. Also, because of the decreased Gram-positive activity of many of the agents, these drugs should not be used alone for empiric therapy. Imipenem and aztreonam have been used in a limited number of cases but show promise as effective therapy of Gram-negative meningitis.

BRAIN ABSCESS

Unlike meningitis, the key to the successful treatment of brain abscess is surgery. Drainage of the abscess not only allows clinical cure, but provides accurate identification of the infecting organism(s), since CSF laboratory findings are often normal in patients with brain abscess. The importance of surgery is demonstrated by the study of Black et al., who found adequate concentrations of antibiotics in excised abscesses, but viable organisms could still be cultured (42).

Since the abscesses are often polymicrobial, a combination of antibiotics, especially penicillin G plus chloramphenicol, is usually employed. Metronidazole can be considered a good alternative to chloramphenicol. Metronidazole enters abscess fluid effectively and is active against obligate anaerobes. If the culture results reveal aerobic Gram-negative bacilli, therapy should include a third-generation cephalosporin or an aminoglycoside. If the culture results reveal staphylococci, therapy should include a penicillinase-resistant penicillin or vancomycin in an penicillin-allergic patient. These agents should be given in doses similar to those used in the treatment of meningitis. Table 67.5 lists the drugs and doses used in the treatment of brain abscess. Therapy should be prolonged (at least) 4 weeks following surgical removal or evacuation of the abscess. Nocardia asteroides produces brain abscess primarily in the immunocompromised patient and should be treated with a sulfonamide (preferably sulfadiazine) in a dose of 100 to 150 mg/kg/day for an extended period of time (a minimum of 3 to 6 months is usually required) (43). Trimethoprim-sulfamethoxazole in a dose of 10/50 mg/kg/day has also been effective. Other possible alternatives are a combination of erythromycin and ampicillin in high doses or perhaps minocycline. These alternatives are inferior to the sulfonamides, and there is little experience with them in the treatment of brain abscess.

NONANTIBIOTIC TREATMENT

Supportive therapy should be used only as an adjunct to appropriate antibiotic therapy. Shock should be managed with fluids and vasopressors. Cerebral edema and hydocephalus should be managed quickly with mannitol or a ventricular shunt. The general use of corticosteroids to reduce cerebral edema caused by meningitis has been controversial. Studies in animals with experimental meningitis have recently shown that corticosteroids reverse the development of brain edema by preventing increases in brain water content and by moderating the increases in CSF pressure (44). These effects were produced when either methylprednisolone or dexamethasone were administered early in the treatment course after the infection was established. With the recent characterization and understanding of the mechanisms of the inflammatory reaction generated with the SAS during meningitis, interest in the early use of high-dose corticosteroids has again been generated. High-dose corticosteroids have been shown to reduce the production and release of cytokines in the CNS, interleukin-1β (IL-1β), and tissue necrosis factor (TNF), in both animal and human studies (45, 46). In addition, the administration of high-dose corticosteroids has markedly reduced the amount of meningeal inflammation when given prior to the administration of effective bactericidal antibiotics. The concentrations of the inflammatory mediators were not substantially influenced when the steroids

Table 67.5.
Empiric Therapy for Brain Abscess

	Drug	Dose (mg/kg/day)	Usual Interval (hr)	Route
Unassociated with trauma or surgery	1. Penicillin *or*	200,000–300,000 U	4–6	IV
	2. Ampicillin *plus*	200–300	4–6	IV
	Chloramphenicol[a] *or*	40–60	6	IV
	Metronidazole[a]	30–40	6–8	IV
Associated with trauma or surgery	1. Nafcillin	150–200	4–6	IV
	Penicillin allergy			
	Vancomycin *plus*	20–30	8–12	IV
	Chloramphenicol[a]	40–60	6	IV
	2. Penicillin *plus*	200,000–300,000 U	4–6	IV
	Metronidazole *plus*	30–40	6–8	IV
	Aminoglycoside[b,c]	4–6	8	IV
	3. Third-generation cephalosporin[d]	(see Table 67.4)		IV

[a] Oral therapy may be given subsequent to initial intravenous therapy.
[b] Gentamicin/tobramycin/amikacin (amikacin: 15 mg/kg/day every 8 hr).
[c] Enterococcus—use gentamicin.
[d] If susceptible.

were given after the start of bactericidal antibiotics, suggesting a salutory role for steroid use preceding endotoxin-stimulated release of inflammatory cytokines (46, 47). The use of high doses of dexamethasone (0.6 mg/kg/day given for 4 days every 6 hr) prior to the administration of antibiotics in children with meningitis caused by *H. influenzae* has shown a significant reduction in neurologic complications and long-term hearing loss (48, 49). The beneficial effects seen in this study have led to the current recommendation to administer dexamethasone 0.6 mg/kg/day for 4 days prior to or concomitant with the first dose of antibiotic in patients who are mildly to severely ill, and over 2 months of age being treated for *H. influenzae* meningitis (50). High-dose corticosteroids may also be helpful for *S. pneumoniae* and *N. meningitidis* meningitis, but this is not yet known. It is unclear whether short-course corticosteroids will be beneficial in adults with mild-to-moderate illness, but its use is recommended in patients who are severely ill with an abnormal mental status. Additional data are needed to clarify the role of high-dose corticosteroids in the treatment of bacterial meningitis. Treatment failures have been cited in patients treated with prolonged courses of corticosteroids (51, 52). The proposed mechanisms for this detrimental effect was that corticosteroids decreased BBB inflammation, resulting in reduced antibiotic penetration. The short-term use of high-dose corticosteroids, early in the treatment course, does not appear to adversely influence the successful treatment of these patients.

Patients who receive high-dose corticosteroids are at risk of gastrointestinal bleeding, and monitoring of hemoglobin concentrations and examination of the stool for occult blood should be routine. It is unclear at the current time whether the bleeding is caused by the corticosteroid administration or by the stress of CNS involvement as is seen in cases of head trauma.

PREVENTION

Antibiotics (sulfonamides, minocycline, and rifampin), and meningococcal vaccines are effective in the prevention of meningococcal disease (53). The most common types of meningococci known to cause disease in the United States are serogroups B, C, and Y, and W-135. Group A is frequently associated with epidemics in other parts of the world. Group A, group C, and quadrivalent polysaccharide (A, C, Y, W-135) vaccines are currently available in the United States. Serogroup B is not sufficiently immunogenic to produce a reliable antibody response. The increased incidence of serogroup Y in the last few years has stimulated interest in evaluating the group Y capsular polysaccharide as vaccine material. Confirmation of the effectiveness of serogroup A vaccine has been found in children 3 months of age and older, but the serogroup C vaccines do not appear to be effective in children under 2 years of age. (See Chapter 59, "Immunizations.")

Serogroup B strains currently cause most infections in the United States, most frequently infants. Serogroup C strains account for about one-third of the cases, and approximately 70% of these cases occur in persons over 2 years of age. Secondary cases of infection occur more frequently in household contacts of the person with the primary infection than in the general population. Since most secondary cases occur within 2 weeks after the primary case, protection should be provided promptly. The Centers for Disease Control (CDC) have provided an algorithm for meningococcal prophylaxis (Fig. 67.1) (54).

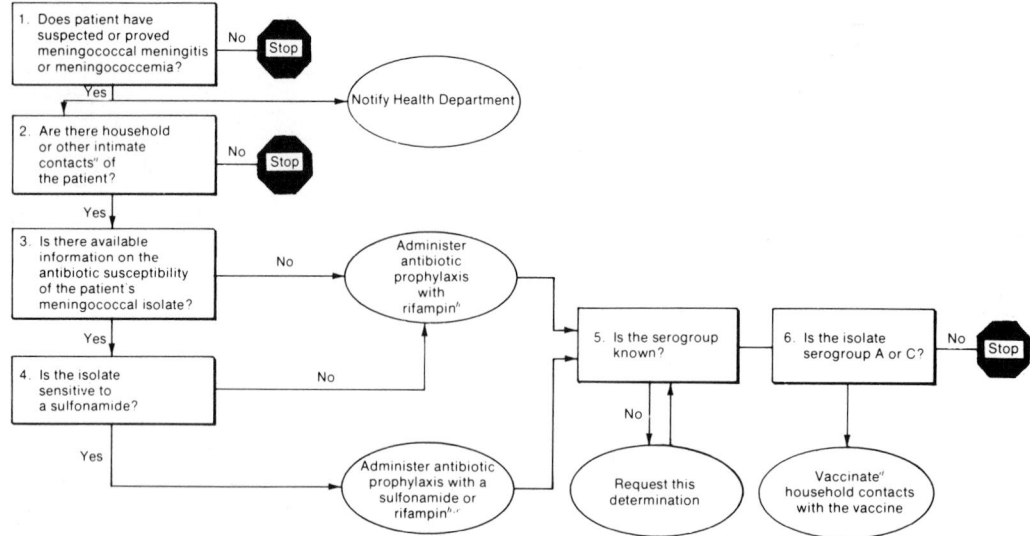

^{a} Intimate contact is defined as direct exposure to oral secretions of patients (such as through mouth-to-mouth resuscitation or kissing).

^{b} Dosage regimen is 2 days of 600 mg twice daily for adults; 10 mg/kg twice daily for children 1 to 12 years of age; and 5 mg/kg twice daily for children less than 1 year.

^{c} Dosage regimen is 2 days of sulfisoxazole or sulfadiazine 1 g twice daily for adults; 500 mg twice daily for children 1 to 12 years of age; and 500 mg once daily for children less than 1 year.

^{d} Group A and C vaccines are administered as a single 50-μg injection.

Figure 67.1. Algorithm for administration meningococcal prophylaxis. (From Jacobson JA, Fraser DW: A simplified approach to meningococcal disease prophylaxis. JAMA 236:1053, 1976. Copyright 1976, American Medical Association.)

Sulfonamides have been used classically in prophylaxis and treatment of meningococcal infection. Their use has declined because of the changing patterns of resistance of the serogroups. Twenty-five percent of strains submitted to the CDC are sulfonamide-resistant. Because of the lack of oropharyngeal penetration of penicillin, these drugs are unsuitable for prophylaxis. Minocycline and rifampin are effective in eradicating the carrier state and reducing the secondary attack rate of meningococcal infection. Minocycline is associated with an unacceptably high rate of vestibular toxicity; therefore, rifampin is the drug of choice for prophylaxis.

The pneumococcal vaccine was developed to prevent infection caused by the 23 pneumococcal serotypes most commonly encountered. The vaccine is recommended for individuals who are at increased risk of developing pneumococcal infections only if they are capable of producing antibody response to the vaccine. The vaccine is poorly immunogenic in children under 2 years of age (55). Only limited data are available on the effectiveness of the use of pneumococcal vaccine in the prevention of CNS infections. (See Chapter 59, "Immunizations".) Since secondary cases of pneumococcal meningitis have not been reported, antimicrobial prophylaxis of family and household contacts is not required. The exact role of pneumococcal vaccine is still not well defined.

Active immunization against *H. influenzae* type b has the greatest potential to prevent a large number of *H. influenzae* infections including CNS infections. Currently there are four commercially available vaccines: (*a*) purified capsular polysaccharide, PRP; (*b*) polyribosylribitol phosphate–diphtheria toxoid conjugate, PRP-D; (*c*) polyribosylribitol phosphate–outer membrane protein conjugate, PRP-OMP; and (*d*) *Haemophilus* b oligosaccharide conjugate, Hboc (56). The first commercially available vaccine, PRP, was marketed in 1985. PRP induced sufficient immunogenic responses in children 24 months of age or older, and early indicators correlated this response with protection against invasive disease. Children under 24 months of age showed variable responses to the vaccine, and children under 6 months of age demonstrated little or no response. Soon after the widespread distribution and administration of this vaccine to children 18 to 24 months of age, an unacceptably high rate of failure began to be reported. The use of this vaccine is considered to be of marginal public benefit because of the poor immunogenicity in children under 24 months of age, a high failure rate, and the variability in reported efficacy.

Subsequently, vaccines using protein carrier molecules attached to the polysaccharide component were developed. These vaccines show a markedly improved immunogenic response over the PRP vaccine, especially in younger children, and demonstrate booster responses upon repeated administration. Four conjugate vaccines have been developed, but only three are currently licensed for commercial use: PRP-D, PRP-OMP, and Hboc. All three vaccines have demonstrated efficacies of 85 to 95% in children 15 to 60 months of age. Each of the vaccines demonstrates a booster effect upon additional administered doses. Both the PRP-OMP and Hboc vaccines have been shown to produce sufficient antibody responses in infants as young as 2 months of age. Although both vaccines are currently licensed for use in this infant population, the number of doses required to induce a sufficient antibody response varies between the two vaccines. The PRP-OMP vaccine is licensed to be administered in a two-dose primary immunization schedule for (a) infants 2 to 4 months of age, whose doses should be scheduled 2 months apart with a booster dose at 12 months of age, (b) infants 5 to 10 months of age, not previously vaccinated, who should receive 2 doses of vaccine scheduled 2 months apart with a booster dose at 12 months, (c) children 11 to 14 months of age, not previously vaccinated, who should receive 2 doses scheduled 2 months apart, and (d) children 15 to 60 months, not previously vaccinated, who should receive one dose of vaccine and do not require a booster dose (57). The Hboc vaccine is licensed to be administered in a three-dose immunization schedule for (a) infants 2 to 6 months of age, whose doses should be scheduled 2 months apart (2, 4, and 6 months), (b) infants 7 to 11 months, not previously vaccinated, who should receive 2 doses of vaccine scheduled 2 months apart, (c) children 12 to 14 months of age, not previously vaccinated, who should receive a single dose of vaccine with a booster dose administered at 15 months, and (d) children 15 to 60 months of age, who should receive a single dose and do not require a booster dose (58). The Immunization Practice Advisory Committee and the American Academy of Pediatrics additionally recommend the following:

1. Children immunized with PRP-D, Hboc, or PRP-OMP at 15 months of age or older need not be reimmunized.
2. Any of the H. influenzae type b conjugate vaccines may be administered simultaneously with polio vaccines (IPV or OPV), measles-mumps-rubella vaccines, or diphtheria-tetanus-pertussis vaccines, although not all combinations have been studied.
3. Children who have experienced H. influenzae type b disease before 24 months of age should receive a dose of an H. influenzae type b conjugate vaccine, because the disease may not have rendered them immune. The vaccine should be administered at least 2 months after illness and after the child has reached at least 15 months of age (56).

Each of the conjugate vaccines has demonstrated a low side-effect profile consisting mainly of local reactions that are mild and well tolerated. (See Chapter 59, "Immunizations".)

Young children, under 6 years old, with known exposure to children who have documented, invasive H. influenzae infections, are at increased risk for developing serious infections caused by this organism. The exposure may occur in individual households or in other closed settings such as nursery schools or day-care centers. Nasopharyngeal colonization results from personal exposure to droplets or respiratory secretions of individuals who are colonized or infected with this organism. Antibiotic prophylaxis interrupts the transmission of the organism by eradicating the carrier state. Ampicillin, cefaclor, erythromycin-sulfisoxazole, and trimethoprim-sulfamethoxazole have not been successful in eradicating the H. influenzae carrier state. Rifampin has been used with success in some closed populations. Therefore, the current recommendations for prophylaxis are:

1. Rifampin prophylaxis should be given to all contacts of the index case (adults and children) in households where there are other children under 4 years of age. The dose of rifampin is 20 mg/kg/day (maximum of 600 mg/day) given once daily for 4 days.
2. Other closed communities such as nursery schools and day-care centers should be considered a "household." The routine use of rifampin prophylaxis in these populations remains controversial. The current recommendations of the American Academy of Pediatrics is to provide rifampin prophylaxis to this population when at least two concurrent cases occur among attendees.
3. Children recovering from serious H. influenzae infections often carry the organisms in their nasopharynx despite appropriate systemic antibiotic therapy. Thus prior to discharge, all children with invasive disease who have young siblings at home should receive rifampin prophylaxis to avoid introduction of the organism into their households (59).

Prophylaxis may fail to reduce the incidence of secondary disease because some carriers within the "household" group remain untreated because of poor medication compliance or contraindications to the use of rifampin.

For patients who cannot take the commercially available capsules, the capsule contents may be emptied and mixed with a small amount of applesauce or jelly prior to administration. Alternatively, a 1% suspension may be compounded. Four 300-mg or eight 150-mg (total of 1200 mg) capsules may be emptied and mixed with 20 ml of Syrup NF and then further diluted with 100 ml of Syrup NF. The resulting preparation contains rifampin 10 mg/ml. The suspension should be stored in an amber bottle, at room temperature or in the refrigerator, labeled with a maximum 4-week expiration date. Currently, only limited data exist on the stability of this preparation (60).

PROGNOSIS

The overall mortality rate for treated bacterial meningitis is about 10 to 20%. This incidence may vary depending upon the organism; meningococcal meningitis (without sepsis) and meningitis due to *H. influenzae* carry a better prognosis than pneumococcal or Gram-negative bacillary meningitis, where 20 to 40% of patients die as a result of the infection. Case fatality ratios continue to be the highest in neonates and elderly. Fungal meningitis due to *C. immitis* is ultimately a fatal disease in 100% of patients despite treatment, but the use of amphotericin B and perhaps the newer imidazole or triazole antifungal agents may prolong survival for months to years.

Statistical analysis of clinical parameters demonstrates a significant risk of death or major morbidity in patients younger than 1 year of age or older than 40 years, those with predisposing illness, those presenting with neurologic deficits, or patients in shock with positive blood cultures. Other findings such as low CSF leukocyte counts, markedly elevated CSF protein, very low CSF glucose concentration, and a delay in diagnosis may or may not predict morbidity or mortality.

CONCLUSION

Because meningitis produces a great deal of concern and anxiety in the lay public, the clinician should allay many of these fears and refer patients who do need medical attention or prophylactic antibiotics.

When treating bacterial meningitis, it should be remembered that early diagnosis and the prompt institution of appropriate antibiotic therapy may be life-saving in many instances. A clear understanding of the mechanisms of action, pharmacology, dose, and side effects of antibiotics useful in treating meningitis is necessary for successful treatment.

REFERENCES

1. Kaufman BA, Tunkel AR, Pryor JC, et al.: Meningitis in the neurosurgical patient. Infect Dis Clin North Am 4:677–701, 1990.
2. Tenney JH: Bacterial infections of the central nervous system in neurosurgery. Neurol Clin 4:91–114, 1986.
3. Silverberg AL, DeNubile MJ: Subdural empyema and crainial epidural abscess. Med Clin North Am 69:361–374, 1985.
4. McGee ZA, Baringer JR, Acute meningitis. In Mandell GL, Douglas RD Jr, Bennett JE (eds): Principles and Practice of Infectious Diseases. New York, Churchill Livingstone, 1990, pp 741–755.
5. Overturf GD: Pyogenic bacterial infections of the CNS. Neurol Clin 4:69–90, 1986.
6. Saez-Llorens X, MacCracken GH Jr: Bacterial meningitis in neonates and children. Infect Dis Clin North Am 4:623–644, 1990.
7. Wispelwey B, Scheld WM: Brain abscess. Clin Neuropharmacol 10:483–510, 1987.
8. Chun CH, Johnson, Hofstetter M, et al.: Brain abscess: a study of 45 consecutive cases. Medicine 65:415–431, 1986.
9. Sabetta JR, Andriole VT: Cyptococcal infection of the central nervous system. Med Clin North Am 69:333–344, 1985.
10. Schlech WF III, Ward JI, Band JD, et al.: Bacterial meningitis in the United States, 1978 through 1981. JAMA 253:1749–1754, 1985.
11. McSwiggan DA: Neonatal and perineal infection: routes of transmission and prevention. J Antimicrob Chemother 5(suppl A):1–12, 1979.
12. Wispelwey B, Tunkel AR, Scheld WM: Bacterial meningitis in adults. Infect Dis Clin North Am 4:645–658, 1990.
13. Roos KL: Meningitis as it presents in the elderly: diagnosis and care. Geriatrics 45:63–75, 1990.
14. Cherubin CE, Marr JS, Sierra MF, Becker S: Listeria and Gram-negative bacillary meningitis in New York City, 1972–1979, Am J Med 71:199–209, 1981.
15. Hodges GR, Perkins RL: Hospital-associated bacterial meningitis. Am J Med Sci 271:335–341, 1976.
16. Salaki JS, Louria DB, Chmel H: Fungal yeast infections of the central nervous system: a clinical review. Medicine 63:108–132, 1984.
17. Tressler CB, Sugar AM: Fungal meningitis. Infect Dis Clin North Am 4:789–808, 1990.
18. Nahamias AJ, Roizman B: Infection with herpes simplex 1 and 2. N Engl J Med 289:667–674, 719–725, 781–789, 1973.
19. Bergstrom T, Vahlne A, Alestig K, et al.: Primary and recurrent herpes simplex virus type 2-induced meningitis. J Infect Dis 162:322–330, 1990.
20. Anon: Bacterial meningitis and meningococcemia—United States, 1978. MMWR 28:277–279, 1979.
21. Tunkel AR, Wispelwey B, Scheld WM: Bacterial meningitis: recent advances in pathophysiology and treatment. Ann Intern Med 112:610–623, 1990.
22. Saez-Llorens X, Ramilo O, Mustafa MM, et al.: Molecular pathophysiology of bacterial meningitis: current concepts and therapeutic implications. J Pediatr 116:671–684, 1990.
23. Lewin EB: Partially treated meningitis. Am J Dis Child 128:145–148, 1974.
24. Pomeroy SL, Holmes SJ, Dodge PR, Feigin RD: Seizures and other neurologic sequelae of bacterial meningitis in children. N Engl J Med 323:1651–1657, 1990.
25. Taylor HG, Mills EL, Ciampi A, et al.: The sequelae of *Haemophilus influenzae* meningitis in school-age children. N Engl J Med 323:1657–1663, 1990.
26. Whitley RJ, Alford CA, Hirsch MS, et al. and the NIAID Collaborative Antiviral Study Group: Vidarabine versus acyclovir therapy in herpes simplex encephalitis. N Engl J Med 314:114–149, 1986.
27. Pollay M, Roberts PA: Blood-brain barrier: a definition of normal and altered function. Neurosurgery 6:675–685, 1980.
28. Allison RR, Stach PE: Intrathecal drug therapy. Drug Intell Clin Pharm 12:347–359, 1978.
29. Simberkoff MS, Moldover NH, Rahal JJ: Absence of detectable bactericidal and opsonic activities in normal and infected human cerebrospinal fluids. J Lab Clin Med 95:362–372, 1980.
30. Landesman SH, Corrado ML, Shah PM, et al.: Past and current roles for cephalosporin antibiotics in treatment of meningitis: emphasis on use in Gram-negative bacillary meningitis. Am J Med 71:693–703, 1981.
31. Sande MA: Antibiotic therapy of bacterial meningitis: lessons we've learned. Am J Med 71:507–510, 1981.
32. Strausbaugh LJ, Sande MA: Factors influencing the therapy of experimental *Proteus mirabilis* meningitis in rabbits. J Infect Dis 137:251–260, 1978.
33. Bennett JE, Dismukes WE, Duma RJ, et al.: A comparison of amphotericin B alone and combined with flucytosine in the treatment of cryptococcal meningitis. N Engl J Med 301:126–131, 1979.
34. Bozzette SA, Larsen RA, Chiu J, et al.: A placebo-controlled trial of maintenance therapy with fluconazole after treatment of cryptococcal meningitis in the acquired immunodeficiency syndrome. N Engl J Med 324:580–584, 1991.
35. Bouza E, Dreyer JS, Hewitt WL: Coccidioidal meningitis: an analysis of thirty-one cases and review of the literature. Medicine 60:139–172, 1981.
36. Bayer AS, Edwards JE, Seidel JS, et al.: Candida meningitis: report

of seven cases and review of the literature. Medicine 55:477–486, 1976.

37. Swartz MN: Intraventricular use of aminoglycosides in the treatment of Gram-negative bacillary meningitis: conflicting views. J Infect Dis 143:293–296, 1981.

38. Mustafa MM, Mertsola J, Ramilo O, et al.: Increased endotoxin and interleukin-1β concentrations in cerebrospinal fluid of infants with coliform meningitis and ventriculitis associated with intraventricular gentamicin therapy. J Infect Dis 160:891–895, 1989.

39. Dacey RG, Sande MA: Effect of probenicid on cerebrospinal fluid concentrations of penicillin and cephalosporin derivatives. Antimicrob Agents Chemother 6:437–441, 1974.

40. Fong IW, Tomkins KB: Review of Pseudomonas aeruginosa meningitis with special emphasis on treatment with ceftazidime. Rev Infect Dis 7:604–612, 1985.

41. Rodriquez WJ, Khan WN, Cocchetto DM, et al.: Treatment of Pseudomonas meningitis with ceftazidime with or without concurrent therapy. Pediatr Infect Dis J 9:83–87, 1990.

42. Black P, Graybill JR, Charache P: Penetration of brain abscess by systemically administered antibiotics. J Neurosurg 38:705–709, 1973.

42. Palmer DL, Harvey RL, Wheeler JK: Diagnostic and therapeutic considerations in Nocardia asteroides infection. Medicine 53:391–401, 1974.

44. Tauber MG, Khayam-Bashi H, Sande MA: Effects of ampicillin and corticosteroids on brain water content, cerebrospinal fluid pressure, and cerebrospinal fluid lactate levels in experimental pneumococcal meningitis. J Infect Dis 151:528–534, 1985.

45. Mustafa MM, Ramilo O, Mertsola, et al.: Modulation of inflammation and cachectin activity in relation to treatment of experimental Hemophilus influenzae type b meningitis. J Infect Dis 160:818–825, 1989.

46. Waagner DC, Hoyt MJ, Finitzo T, McCracken GH: Administration of dexamethasone before antibiotic therapy for bacterial meningitis. (Abstract No. 1). Presented to the 29th Interscience Conference on Antimicrobial Agents and Chemotherapy, Houston TX, Sept 1989, p 101.

47. Arditi M, Ables L, Yogev R: Cerebrospinal fluid endotoxin levels in children with H. influenzae meningitis before and after administration of intravenous ceftriaxone. J Infect Dis 160:1005–1011, 1989.

48. Level MH, Freij BJ, Syrogiannopoulos GA, et al.: Dexamethasone therapy for bacterial meningitis: results of two double-blind, placebo-controlled trials. N Engl J Med 319:964–971, 1988.

49. Odio CM, Faingezicht I, Paris M, et al.: The beneficial effects of early dexamethasone administration in infants and children with bacterial meningitis. N Engl J Med 324:1525–1531, 1991.

50. Committee on Infectious Diseases, American Academy of Pediatrics: Dexamethasone therapy for bacterial meningitis in infants and children. Pediatrics 86:130–133, 1990.

51. Harbin GL, Hodges GR: Corticosteroids as adjunctive therapy for acute bacterial meningitis. South Med J 72:977–980, 1979.

52. Brady MT, Kaplan SL, Taber LH: Association between persistence of pneumococcal meningitis and dexamethasone administration. J Pediatr 99:924–926, 1981.

53. Public Health Service Advisory Committee on Immunization Practices: Meningococcal polysaccharide vaccines. Ann Intern Med 89:949–950, 1978.

54. Jacobson JA, Fraser DW: A simplified approach to meningococcal disease prophylaxis. JAMA 236:1053–1054, 1976.

55. Schwartz JS: Pneumococcal vaccine: clinical efficacy and effectiveness. Ann Intern Med 96:208–220, 1982.

56. Committee on Iinfectious Diseases, American Academy of Pediatrics: Haemophilus influenzae type b conjugate vaccines: Immunization of children at 15 months of age. Pediatrics 86:794–796, 1990.

57. CDC: Food and Drug Administration approval of use of Haemophilus b conjugate vaccine for infants. MMWR 39:698–699, 1990.

58. CDC: Food and Drug Administration approval of a Haemophilus b conjugate vaccine for infants. MMWR 39:925–926, 1990.

59. Committee on Infectious Diseases, American Academy of Pediatrics. In Peter G (ed): Haemophilus influenzae Infections. Evanston, IL, American Academy of Pediatrics, 1988, p 204.

60. Committee on Extemporaneous Formulations: Handbook on Extemporaneous Formulations. Bethesda, MD: American Society of Hospital Pharmacists, 1987, p 43.

CHAPTER 68

BONE AND JOINT INFECTIONS

MARTIN L. JOB, Pharm.D., M.A. and HEWITT W. MATTHEWS, Ph.D.

Osteomyelitis and septic arthritis are the principal infections of the bones and joints. They involve separate infectious entities with specific etiologies, pathogenesis, and treatment. Both of these infections require prompt and accurate diagnosis to prevent serious tissue destruction and permanent bone damage and deformity. In contrast to other arthritic diseases, proper diagnosis and treatment can usually result in a cure. The discussion in this chapter is limited to only those infections of bacterial origin.

OSTEOMYELITIS

Osteomyelitis is a term most commonly associated with bacterial infections of the bone, although other causative organisms such as viruses and fungi have also been isolated. Despite the advent of modern antimicrobial therapy, expanded imaging, and newer orthopaedic techniques, osteomyelitis continues to pose a diagnostic and therapeutic challenge. Furthermore, more aggressive procedures such as hip replacement, bone grafting, other reconstructive surgeries, and radiation therapy, as well as intravenous drug abuse, have contributed to the complexity of this disease. Controversy remains about the appropriate antibiotic treatment and its duration.

Classification and Epidemiology

The classification of osteomyelitis depends upon the source of bacterial spread to the bone. Other variables such as precipitating factors and the age of the patient usually dictate which bones are involved. Osteomyelitis is usually divided into three principal categories: hematogenous, contiguous, and contiguous with vascular insufficiency (Table 68.1). These can be acute or chronic, depending on the onset of symptoms and the duration of the clinical manifestations.

Hematogenous osteomyelitis refers to infections whose source of contamination is the bloodstream. The disease is commonly seen in children and young adults below the age of 20 years but has been reported with increasing frequency in adults over 50 years of age. Hematogenous osteomyelitis accounts for approximately 20% of all bone infections (1, 2). Hematogenous spread of infection of the bone frequently involves a bacterial embolus from a distant focus (3).

Contiguous osteomyelitis refers to infections in which contamination of the bone arises with contact from a nearby infected tissue or from direct inoculation from an exogenous source. Unlike hematogenous osteomyelitis, contiguous osteomyelitis is most predominant in adults, particularly those over the age of 50, and accounts for most cases of osteomyelitis (1).

Osteomyelitis resulting from contiguous spread may also occur in the presence of vascular insufficiency. These patients are generally older (between 50 and 70 years old) and have underlying diseases that contribute to their vascular insufficiency. Similarly, these infections also develop as an extension of an existing localized infection. Because this type of osteomyelitis often involves various bones and different bacterial etiologies, its therapy generally differs from that of other types of osteomyelitis (4).

The term *chronic osteomyelitis* remains somewhat confusing, and in some cases, without a satisfactory definition. It is often described as an extension of the acute form of bone infection that has either been misdiagnosed or treated inappropriately. Although the causative organism in this situation may be similar to those in the acute process, the medical management is more difficult and challenging.

Etiology

The most common etiologic agents for osteomyelitis are shown in Table 68.2. *Staphylococcus aureus* is the most common pathogen implicated in hematogenous osteomyelitis. It is isolated in 60 to 90% of cases in children (5). Other organisms such as *Streptococcus pyogenes*, *Streptococcus pneumoniae*, and *Escherichia coli* have been isolated. *Haemophilus influenzae* is a common pathogen in young infants, particularly under the age of 5 (6). Group B streptococci and *E. coli* are common pathogens associated with osteomyelitis during the neonatal period (7). Unusual organisms such as fungi, mycobacteria, other Enterobacteriaceae species, and *Pseudomonas aeruginosa* have been isolated.

In adults, *S. aureus* is also the most common causative organism and is isolated in over 60% of cases of acute hematogenous osteomyelitis. Enterobacteriaceae have been isolated in 30% of cases, and streptococci have been isolated in less than 10%. Other organisms such as fungi, *P. aeruginosa*, enterococci, and *Salmonella* spp. have also been isolated but rarely cause hematogenous osteomyelitis in adults (8).

Table 68.1.
Major Types of Osteomyelitis[a]

	Hematogenous	Contiguous	Contiguous with Vascular Insufficiency
Age distribution	1–20 years, >50 years	>50 years	>50 years
Bones involved	Long bones, vertebrae	Femur, tibia, skull, mandible	Feet, toes
Major clinical findings	Initial episode	Initial episode	Initial and recurrent episodes
	Fever	Fever	Pain
	Local tenderness	Erythema	Swelling
	Local swelling	Swelling	Erythema
	Limitation of motion	Sinus	Drainage
	Recurrent episodes	Recurrent episodes	Ulceration
	Drainage	Drainage	
		Sinus	

[a] Modified from Norden CW, Osteomyelitis. In Mandell GL, Douglas RG, Bennett JE (eds): Principles and Practice of Infectious Diseases, ed. 3. New York, John Wiley & Sons, 1990, pp 922–930.

Table 68.2.
Common Etiologies and Empiric Antibiotic Therapy for the Treatment of Bacterial Osteomyelitis

Age Group	Likely Organisms	Antibiotics of Choice (Dose, Route, and Frequency of Administration)
Neonates (<4 weeks)	S. aureus Group B streptococcus E. coli	Nafcillin 40 mg/kg/day i.m. q. 12 hr or oxacillin 50 mg/kg/day IV q. 12 hr plus gentamicin 5 mg/kg/day IV q. 12 hr or First-generation cephalosporin (e.g., cephalothin or cefazolin 40 mg/kg/day IV q. 12 hr
Infants and children (1 month to 5 years)	S. aureus Group A streptococcus H. influenzae	Cefuroxime 100 mg/kg/day IV q. 8 hr or cefotaxime or ceftizoxime 100–150 mg/kg/day IV q. 8 hr
Children and adolescents (6–16 years)	S. aureus Group A streptococcus	Nafcillin or oxacillin 50–100 mg/kg/day IV q. 6 hr or first-generation cephalosporin (e.g., cephalothin 50–150 mg/kg/day IV q. 6 hr or cefazolin 50–150 mg/kg/day IV q. 8 hr)
Adults (>16 years)	S. aureus Nonenterococcal streptococcus Enterobacteriaceae Enterococci[a] P. aeruginosa[b] Anaerobes[c]	Nafcillin or oxacillin 50–100 mg/kg/day IV q. 6 hr or first-generation cephalosporin (e.g., cephalothin 50–150 mg/kg/day IV q. 8 hr) plus an aminoglycoside (e.g., gentamicin or tobramycin 5 mg/kg/day IV q. 8 hr or amikacin 15 mg/kg/day IV q. 8 hr) or Monotherapy with cefotaxime or ceftizoxime 100–150 mg/kg/day q. 8 hr

[a] If enterococci are cultured, use ampicillin 2 g IV q. 6 hr plus an aminoglycoside; in penicillin-allergic patient use vancomycin 0.5–1 g IV q. 6–12 hr plus an aminoglycoside.
[b] For P. aeruginosa, use an antipseudomonal penicillin (e.g., mezlocillin 4 g IV q. 6 hr or piperacillin 3 g IV q. 4 hr) or ceftazidime 2–3 g IV q. 8 hr or cefoperazone 1–2 IV q. 12 hr plus an aminoglycoside.
[c] For anaerobes other than B. fragilis, use penicillin G 2,000,000 U IV q. 4 hr. If B. fragilis is suspected, use clindamycin 900 mg IV q. 8 hr or cefoxitin 2 g IV q. 6 hr or metronidazole 500 mg IV q. 6 hr.

For the contiguous form of osteomyelitis, S. aureus continues to remain the dominant pathogen, appearing in approximately 60% of cases. The bacteriologic profile for this infection, however, differs from that of hematogenous osteomyelitis by the involvement of multiple organisms such as Proteus spp., Streptococcus spp., E. coli, and Staphylococcus epidermidis (2).

Polymicrobial infections account for 5% of cases of acute hematogenous osteomyelitis and 30 to 60% of chronic osteomyelitis (9). Anaerobes such as Bacteroides fragilis, Bacteroides spp., Fusobacterium, Clostridium,

and microaerophilic cocci are now being reported as significant pathogens in osteomyelitis (10).

Risk Factors

Risk factors that favor the development of osteomyelitis are outlined in Table 68.3. Identification and knowledge of these factors can aid in the early diagnosis and perhaps prevention of these infections.

Bacteremia, as previously stated, is the most important risk factor for the development of acute hematogenous osteomyelitis. Since most blood-borne infections originate

Table 68.3.
Common Risk Factors Associated with the Development of Osteomyelitis

Hematogenous	Contiguous	Contiguous with Vascular Insufficiency
Bacteremic foci	Direct inoculation	Diabetes mellitus
Noninvasive	Penetrating trauma	Peripheral vascular disease
Acute pharyngitis	Gunshot wounds	Pressure sores
Minor laceration	Open reduction of fracture	
Cellutitis	Orthopaedic procedures	
Cutaneous abscesses	Diagnostic procedures	
Sickle cell anemia	Animal bites	
Respiratory infections	Puncture wounds	
Invasive	Adjacent foci	
Intravenous catheters	Surgery	
Heel sticks	Postoperative wound infections	
Intravenous drug abusers	Soft tissue infections	
Hemodialysis		
Nonpenetrating trauma		

from a source, identification of risk factors associated with the promotion of bacteremia must be considered. For example, septic foci associated with acute pharyngitis, minor lacerations, cellulitis, and cutaneous abscesses have been implicated as sources of bacteremia in children with acute osteomyelitis (3). Nonpenetrating trauma is common in children with acute hematogenous osteomyelitis (11). As many as 30% of children with this infection have experienced minor injury within 2 weeks prior to the onset of the disease. Invasive procedures such as umbilical catheters, frequent heel sticks, and complicated delivery are associated with bacteremia in neonates (11, 12). Certain underlying diseases such as sickle cell anemia and related hemoglobinopathies have been associated with osteomyelitis due to *Salmonella* species. Respiratory infections are a focus of infection in 12 to 26% of cases (11).

Although hematogenous osteomyelitis is less common in adults, a number of risk factors are associated with bacteremic spread in this population. These include patients with intravenous catheters who are receiving total parenteral nutrition or chemotherapy, patients undergoing hemodialysis, and intravenous drug abusers (11). Certain underlying diseases such as infections of the urinary tract, respiratory tract, and soft tissue are associated with vertebral osteomyelitis in adults (5).

Infection of the bone by nonhematogenous spread by evolve from either direct inoculation or contiguous spread from an adjacent focus. Direct inoculation can occur from a variety of sources, such as penetrating trauma from gunshot wounds, open reduction of fractures, orthopaedic and diagnostic procedures, animal bites, and puncture wounds. The latter occur commonly in the foot and are associated with *P. aeruginosa*. Contiguous spread from an adjacent soft tissue infection is the most important risk for osteomyelitis in adults. Foci for bone infections in this situation

include soft tissue infections close to the bone, as in the case of osteomyelitis of the mastoid bone, which can originate from malignant external otitis media or other paranasal sinus infections. Osteomyelitis of the mandible has also been observed in patients with poor oral hygiene or chronic infections of the teeth. Postoperative wound infections following orthopaedic correction of the skeleton, neurosurgery, median sternotomy, and oral surgery are major contiguous sources of osteomyelitis. These risk factors differ from penetrating trauma in the sequence in which the skeletal infection develops (11).

Diabetes mellitus and severe atherosclerosis are the most common risk factors in patients with vascular insufficiency. These conditions often predispose patients to chronic draining ulcers and cellulitis of the feet and toes and promote the development of osteomyelitis. Pressure sores in chronically debilitated bedridden patients are also a major risk factor (13). Osteomyelitis should be suspected when decubiti fail to respond to standard antibiotic therapy and debridement.

Any situation such as misdiagnosis, inadequate surgical drainage, or inappropriate treatment would be considered a risk factor for chronic osteomyelitis.

Pathophysiology and Clinical Manifestations

Several unanswered questions remain in pathogenesis of osteomyelitis. For example, what is the significance of prior injury, acute injury, or trauma to the actual development of osteomyelitis? In addition, it is unclear why certain pathogens, such as *S. aureus* appear to have a greater affinity for bone and what factors enhance its ability to invade osseus tissue (14).

In acute hematogenous osteomyelitis in children, the long tubular, rapidly growing bones such as the femur, tibia, and humerus are predominantly affected. The in-

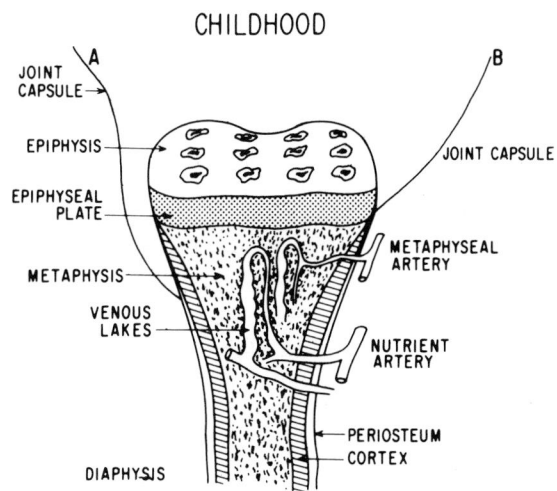

CHILDHOOD

JOINT CAPSULE
EPIPHYSIS
EPIPHYSEAL PLATE
METAPHYSIS
VENOUS LAKES

A
B
JOINT CAPSULE
METAPHYSEAL ARTERY
NUTRIENT ARTERY
PERIOSTEUM
CORTEX
DIAPHYSIS

Figure 68.1. Major structures of the bones of a child. (From Gutman LT: Acute, subacute, and chronic osteomyelitis and pyogenic arthritis in children. Curr Probl Pediatr 15(12):1–72, 1985. Copyright 1985. Chicago: Year Book Medical Publishers; reproduced with permission.)

fectious process usually begins in the sinusoidal veins in the metaphyseal region of the bone. The anatomic features and vascular structure favor the growth of microorganisms in this site, since these capillaries lack phagocytic lining cells (Fig. 68.1). Also, capillary blood flow in this region is slower and more turbulent. Following invasion of the pathogen, a typical inflammatory response ensues. Bacterial and neutrophilic enzymes are released, which contribute to breakdown of the bone, removal of calcium, and eventual necrosis. In addition, the cortical section of the bone and the metaphyses are much thinner in children than in adults, and there is less adherence of the periosteum to the underlying cortex of the bone. This situation favors the extension of the suppurative process from the metaphysis through the cortex and into the periosteum, resulting in the accumulation of pus in the subperiosteal space. Pressure can build up, causing ischemia to the nutrient artery and eventual necrosis of the bone (15).

This has been the traditional explanation for the pathogenesis of acute hematogenous osteomyelitis in children. Recent research using an avian model, which closely resembles human disease, suggests that this explanation may not be accurate. In this model, bacteria attach to the exposed growth-plate cartilaginous matrix adjacent to the extending tips of the metaphyseal vessels. The bacteria proliferate, resulting in vascular occlusion and abscess formation. The bacteria can become enclosed in a slime-like substance composed of extracellular complex sugars referred to as glycocalyx, which can act as a barrier and prevent natural host defenses or antibiotics from reaching the bacteria. This would at least refute the concept of sluggish

blood flow as the principle explanation for bacterial deposition (14, 16).

Since bacteremia is the major source of infection in acute hematogenous osteomyelitis, patients occasionally have signs and symptoms of acute sepsis, with fever being the most common sign. The fever may be accompanied by chills, muscle aches, headache, nausea, and vomiting. In the case of the staphylococcal osteomyelitis, the incidence of sepsis is quite high, occurring in 56 to 73% of cases. Moderate fever, often the only symptom, may occur along with pain, swelling, tenderness, or suppuration at the involved site (3, 7). In about one-third of cases of hematogenous osteomyelitis, a subacute form of the infection occurs, in which the child may have only mild muscular pain and no systemic findings (17).

In adults, the vertebrae appear to be the most common site of involvement for acute hematogenous osteomyelitis. This is due to the abundantly vascularized flat bone that is adjacent to the cartilage, as well as the persistent marrow cavity. Patients often experience fever, malaise, chills, back pain, and stiffness. Although symptoms may be more vague in contrast to children and may only consist of pain, local suppuration is uncommon (5).

In osteomyelitis resulting from contiguous spread, almost any bone in the body may be involved. Infections in this situation are most predominant in those bones that are more prone to fracture or open reduction, such as the femur or tibia. Other bones that are frequently involved include the skull and mandible. Osteomyelitis to the sternum has been associated with median sternotomy incision. Major symptoms are generally confined to the infected adjacent tissues and usually present as pain, tenderness, swelling, and redness. Fever may be present during the initial episode. During recurrent infections, systemic symptoms may be absent, and sinus formation and drainage are the predominant clinical findings.

Chronic osteomyelitis involves advanced bone destruction and necrosis secondary to the continued inflammatory process. The common characteristics for all types of chronic osteomyelitis are vascular thrombosis and vascular or necrotic bone, referred to as a sequestrum, which provides a bacterial milieu for persistence of the infection and perpetuation of the inflammatory process. This results in eventual vascular thrombosis and further development of necrotic bone (11). In addition, glycocalyx formation acts as a barrier to hormonal and cellular host defenses as well as enhancing the attachment of microorganisms to the bone or foreign bodies (16). Several conditions have been proposed as criteria for defining chronic osteomyelitis. These include findings such as (a) abnormal or radiological evidence of infection for 6 weeks or longer, (b) radiological evidence of sequestrum formation, (c) bone infections associated with vascular insufficiency or foreign bodies, and (d) persistence of infection or relapse following treatment.

The presence of any one of these findings constitutes chronic osteomyelitis (18).

Diagnosis and Laboratory Findings

Several laboratory findings may be useful in the diagnosis of osteomyelitis. Positive identification of the infecting pathogen is one of the most important diagnostic aids and is useful for selecting appropriate antibiotic therapy. In untreated acute hematogenous osteomyelitis, positive blood cultures occur in approximately 60 to 75% of cases (15). However, isolation of organisms from other tissues or fluids may contribute to the diagnosis.

In chronic osteomyelitis, blood cultures are rarely studied. In the case where tissue and blood cultures are negative, direct subperiosteal or metaphyseal needle aspiration is required for a definitive diagnosis. Subsequent evaluation of a Gram-stained specimen is useful for initiating therapy (7).

Culture diagnosis of osteomyelitis from contiguous spread or vascular insufficiency may be more complex. Since infection occurs from a contiguous abscess, cellulitis, or penetration to the overlying skin, specimens obtained from subcutaneous or other surrounding tissues must be evaluated. These may be obtained either by direct needle biopsy or during surgical debridement. Caution should be exercised when evaluating culture specimens obtained from superficially draining sinus tracts. The results in this case may be misleading and not indicative of the actual pathogen of the site of infection (8).

Roentgenologic changes may not be evident until at least 10 to 14 days after the onset of clinical illnesses. However, radiographic signs indicating changes in the deep tissues, as evidenced by a loss of normally defined planes between the muscles, may be present during early stages of the disease (7). Therefore, early x-rays only show changes of the adjacent tissue and not of the bone.

Radionuclide imaging or bone scan using technetium pyrophosphate–labeled compounds may reveal indirect evidence of osteomyelitis. A fixed quantity of an intravenous radioactive compound is administered, and the skeletal system, of the patient is imaged or scanned approximately 2 to 4 hr later. The scan is repeated in 24 hr. The ratio of uptake is determined between the two scanning intervals. This is often referred to as the "four-phase" bone scan. This enables the clinician to distinguish osteomyelitis from cellulitis, since technetium will disappear more rapidly from the soft tissue than from bone (19). Abnormal findings are related to the enhanced ability of the inflamed tissues to take up the labeled compound because of increased blood flow in the infected areas. However, technetium scanning is not specific for infections and may be positive in other inflammatory processes such as trauma, tumor, or arthritis. Magnetic resonant imaging (MRI) and computer-assisted tomography (CT scan) may be helpful in the diagnosis of chronic osteomyelitis.

Gallium-67 citrate is a more selective imaging radionuclide. The outcome of gallium scanning is directly related to the ability of the polymorphonuclear leukocyte to take up the radioactive compound. Since leukocytes concentrate at the site of bacterial infection, an abnormal finding or "hot spot" would be detected in the area of the infected bone. Gallium scans are quite useful in detecting acute osteomyelitis in the very early stages of the disease when conventional x-rays are of limited value or if the technetium scan yields negative results (20). Gallium scanning should not be used routinely in children because of the higher levels of radiation. However, it is an excellent test to distinguish early acute osteomyelitis from septic arthritis or when the technetium studies are normal (1, 15).

Other clinical laboratory observations that are of diagnostic importance include leukocytosis and elevated erythrocyte sedimentation rate (ESR). The white blood cell count may be normal in 40 to 75% of patients during initial examination for acute osteomyelitis. The ESR is generally normal in the early stages of the disease, but it will progressively rise as infection persists. In some cases the ESR can reach values more than 100 mm/hr. This test is most useful in the diagnosis of chronic osteomyelitis (7).

In recent years, serologic tests to detect techoic acid antibodies have been used in the diagnosis of acute osteomyelitis caused by *S. aureus*. The cell wall structure of *S. aureus* is comprised of three major components: peptidoglycan, techoic acid, and protein A. Techoic acid, the largest component, accounts for as much as 40% by weight of the total cell wall. During severe *S. aureus* infections, antibodies directed against the techoic acid antigenic portions of the wall are formed. These antibodies can be detected by counterimmunoelectrophoresis and gel diffusion techniques (21).

Medical Management

Since the treatment of osteomyelitis involves a protracted commitment to antibiotic therapy, careful evaluation and diagnosis are of paramount importance. Early diagnosis precludes serious damage to the tissue and avoids complications associated with recurrent or chronic bone infections.

The diagnosis and subsequent choice of therapy may be difficult, particularly in the early stages of the disease. Many of the clinical manifestations, such as white blood cell count, x-rays, and radionuclide scans, may be within normal limits. Furthermore, blood cultures may be positive in only 50% of cases, and superficial sinus drainage cultures may not be reliable. Therefore, antibiotic therapy, particularly during the initial phase of treatment, is largely empiric and is based predominantly on patient factors such as age, history prior to onset of symptoms, site of infection, and other underlying risk factors. The clinician must evaluate all these parameters and come to some reasonable conclusion about the most likely causative organism.

Antibiotic Therapy

S. aureus is the predominant organism in most cases of hematogenous osteomyelitis, and it is prudent to include an antibiotic that is capable of eradicating this organism. The penicillinase-resistant penicillins such as nafcillin and oxacillin are useful antistaphylococcal agents. These antibiotics are bactericidal and relatively inexpensive. They have the disadvantage that neither agent is effective against *E. coli*, a common cause of neonatal osteomyelitis. Therefore, the use of an aminoglycoside in conjunction with a penicillinase-resistant penicillin is a more appropriate choice for empiric therapy in the newborn (7). Other disadvantages of penicillins are frequent administration and severe anaphylaxis and allergic reactions such as fevers, rash, and neutrophenia (7).

First-generation cephalosporins such as cephalothin or cefazolin have relatively few adverse effects and are effective alternatives in most penicillin-allergic patients. These agents have the advantage of retaining excellent activity against *S. aureus* while providing adequate coverage against *E. coli*. Cefazolin has an added advantage in that it may be administered on an 8-hr basis (6).

Selected second-generation cephalosporins such as cefuroxime and cefamandole have antistaphylococcal activity similar to that of first-generation cephalosporins (22). In addition, these agents possess extended Gram-negative coverage, particularly against *H. influenzae*, and therefore may be useful as empiric therapy in children with hematogenous osteomyelitis when this organism is suspected (6). Hypoprothrombinemia and bleeding are associated with cefamandole and may limit the usefulness of this agent for prolonged therapy. These effects are related to the presence of the 3-methylthiotetrazole (3-MTT) side chain. This functional group interferes with the γ-carboxylation of glutamic acid that is necessary in the vitamin K–dependent step in the synthesis of prothrombin by the liver (23). Cefonicid, a long-acting second-generation cephalosporin, has been used in the treatment of acute osteomyelitis. Because of its long half-life, cefonicid can be administered once a day either intravenously or intramuscularly, which makes this agent particularly useful and cost-effective for outpatient therapy (22). Clinical data are limited, however, regarding the use of this drug for osteomyelitis in children.

Third-generation cephalosporins such as cefatoxime and ceftizoxime retain good activity against *S. aureus* and are effective in osteomyelitis caused by this organism (24). Traditionally these agents are more costly and less active against *S. aureus* than first-generation cephalosporins. A

recent study suggests that cefotaxime may be the most active third-generation cephalosporin against *S. aureus*, with minimum inhibitory concentrations approaching those of the first-generation cephalosporins. This activity has been related to the synergistic effect of its active metabolite, desacetylcefotaxime (25). Since this antibiotic possesses excellent activity against common Gram-negative organisms such as Enterobacteriaceae and *H. influenzae*, it is useful for empiric therapy for these pathogens, especially in cases of contiguous-spread osteomyelitis (26).

For patients allergic to β-lactam antibiotics, clindamycin is an effective alternative to nafcillin or methicillin in the treatment of staphylococcal osteomyelitis (27, 28). In patients who are allergic to β-lactam antibiotics and cannot tolerate clindamycin, vancomycin is the acceptable alternative for treating osteomyelitis secondary to staphylococci (29). Much attention has been focused on the side-effect profile of vancomycin, specifically its nephrotoxicity. It appears that the current overall prevalence of nephrotoxicity is low compared with previous experiences (30). This decrease in nephrototoxicity may be related to the development of a more purified product (31).

Strains of methicillin-resistant *S. aureus* (MRSA) have recently emerged as pathogens in osteomyelitis. Although cephalosporins may appear to be sensitive using disk-diffusion methods, the organism is generally resistant to this group when tested by microdilution techniques. Therefore, vancomycin remains the only acceptable effective antibiotic for the treatment of osteomyelitis due to MRSA (32).

Osteomyelitis arising from contiguous spread is similar to hematogenous osteomyelitis is that *S. aureus* remains the predominant organism. However, it is not unusual that bone infections in this category involve multiple or mixed infections etiologies. Organisms such as *P. aeruginosa* and *Proteus* species are also frequently isolated (8). Under these circumstances, an aminoglycoside should be empirically added to the traditional antistaphylococcal agent until culture reports can be obtained. Once the organism has been identified, the antibiotic regimen can be adjusted based on the sensitivities.

The prolonged use of aminoglycoside therapy may cause nephrotoxicity, particularly in the elderly or diabetic patient. Broad-spectrum β-lactam antibiotics such as cefotaxime, ceftizoxime, ceftazidime, and imipenem/cilastatin have been suggested as agents for monotherapy in the treatment of mixed-etiology bone infections (24). Cefotaxime and ceftizoxime are considered the most active against *S. aureus* and they are also quite active against common Enterobacteriaceae. However, neither agent is appreciably effective against *P. aeruginosa*. Ceftazidime is less active against *S. aureus*, but it is the most active cephalosporin against *P. aeruginosa*. Cefotaxime, ceftizoxime, and ceftazidime are associated with a low side-effect profile. Cefoperazone is another third-generation cephalosporin that has activity against *P. aeruginosa*, but it possesses the 3-MTT side chain and has been associated with hypoprothrombinemia and bleeding. Cefoperazone also has a relatively high degree of biliary tract excretion, which accounts for the high rate of diarrhea associated with its use (23). Imipenem is a carbapenem agent that structurally resembles the β-lactam antibiotics. The drug is very active against most Gram-positive and Gram-negative organisms, including *P. aeruginosa* and anaerobes, although resistance by *Pseudomonas* to imipenem has developed. Imipenem is more costly than previously mentioned agents (24).

Anaerobic bacteria have been isolated in both acute hematogenous and tissue-spread osteomyelitis. Acute hematogenous osteomyelitis as a result of anaerobic bacteremia is relatively uncommon and is responsible for about a third of the cases of anaerobic osteomyelitis. Intraabdominal infections are often a source of anaerobic bacteremia. Chronic osteomyelitis related to prior trauma is considered one of the most common forms of anaerobic osteomyelitis of the long bones. These infections may be of mixed anaerobic and aerobic etiologies. Chronic anaerobic osteomyelitis has also been associated with implantation and infection of prosthetic devices. The most common form of chronic anaerobic osteomyelitis is that related to underlying peripheral vascular disease. This syndrome is almost always associated with long-standing diabetes and nondiabetics with severe peripheral vascular disease. The small bones of the feet are most commonly involved, and there is generally a small ulcer surrounding the affected area. Anaerobic osteomyelitis of the mandibles or cranial or facial bones has been reported. The relatively high concentration of anaerobic bacteria from the oral cavity is responsible for these infections.

The clinical presentation of anaerobic osteomyelitis is similar to those of aerobic disease. Certain signs such as foul-smelling sinus tract drainage, bone biopsy or purulence as well as the presence of gas on x-ray, multiple pleomorphic organisms on Gram-stain, or negative aerobic cultures may be clues (33). Penicillin G remains the most active agent against anaerobic bacteria other than *B. fragilis*. For infections caused by *B. fragilis*, clindamycin and metronidazole remain highly effective agents. Clindamycin is also very active against *S. aureus* and has good penetration of osseous tissue. Other agents, such as cefoxitin, mezlocillin, and piperacillin, although less active against *B. fragilis* than the former compounds, are effective in the treatment of anaerobic infections. Chloramphenicol, which also remains quite active against anaerobes, including *B. fragilis*, may be used as an alternative (34); however, its potential adverse effect on the hematopoietic system precludes its use as a first-line agent in this type of infection.

Antibiotic therapy for bacterial osteomyelitis is summarized in Table 68.2.

Oral Antibiotic Therapy

In an attempt to reduce hospital stay and costs, there have been numerous clinical trials with oral antibiotic therapy in the treatment of osteomyelitis (35). The therapy was usually initiated with a parenteral antibiotic and then completed with the appropriate oral agent. Aggressive monitoring of the patient included measurements of the ESR, roentgenologic evaluation, and complete blood counts. In some cases, patients underwent surgical drainage when the initial bone aspirate contained purulent material. Antibiotic serum bactericidal titers were also used as a monitoring parameter and were associated with successful outcomes of therapy. Two-fold serial dilutions of the patient's own antibiotic-containing serum is tested against a known inoculum of the infecting organism. Favorable outcomes were seen when bactericidal levels were achieved at titers above 1:8. If the patient's bactericidal concentration was lower, the antibiotic dose was increased to provide the appropriate titer. Serum bactericidal titers have been studied most often in patients receiving oral antibiotic therapy following a brief initial course of parenteral therapy (36).

Overall, these studies clearly indicate that the treatment of acute osteomyelitis with an initial brief period of parenteral therapy followed by appropriate oral therapy and aggressive patient monitoring is effective. Although these initial studies are encouraging, several limitations must be considered before embarking on oral therapy. For example, in almost all cases the patients involved were children with acute staphylococcal osteomyelitis of recent onset. There was positive identification of the pathogen, and aggressive monitoring was employed. Surgical intervention was performed when needed. Compliance was enforced to ensure proper antibiotic consumption and to avoid relapse or failure. This is most critical to prevent exacerbation and the evolution of a chronic infection or permanent bone destruction.

In many cases of osteomyelitis, the infecting organism is not identifiable, nor is the onset of symptoms recent. In the past, the availability of an appropriate oral agent against a variety of Gram-negative organisms was limited. However, data regarding newer quinolone antibiotics such as ciprofloxacin indicate that these agents may be useful for oral therapy in the treatment of Gram-negative osteomyelitis, including that due to *P. aeruginosa* (37). Recent data suggest that ciprofloxacin given at a dose of 750 mg twice a day was well tolerated and achieved clinical success rates similar to those of conventional intravenous therapy in the treatment of osteomyelitis (38). In summary, it appears that oral therapy can only be applied to certain types of osteomyelitis and is influenced by restricted criteria such as recent onset of illness, positive identification of the organism, aggressive monitoring, availability of suitable oral agent, and good patient compliance (39, 40).

Combination Therapy

Although combination antibiotic therapy has been used with success in selected infections, this approach has not been adequately evaluated in the treatment of osteomyelitis for acute hematogenous osteomyelitis. Single-agent therapy is effective in the treatment of the most common pathogens, although there have been isolated cases where gentamicin was added in combination with cefazolin for the treatment of resistant *S. aureus* (6). At least one report deals with the combination of vancomycin and tobramycin in a small number of patients for the treatment of polymicrobial osteomyelitis, including MRSA. Outcomes were similar in both groups but a higher prevalence of nephrotoxicity was reported in the patients treated with vancomycin plus tobramycin (32). For contiguous-spread osteomyelitis, traditional empiric therapy has been the combination of a β-lactam antibiotic and an aminoglycoside.

Data on the role of newer β-lactam antibiotics as monotherapy have been impressive. Reviews of patient cases suggest that ceftazidime is effective as monotherapy for the treatment of serious Gram-negative bacillary osteomyelitis (41). Furthermore, evaluations of large numbers of clinical trials suggest that β-lactam antibiotics, particularly third-generation cephalosporins, are effective as monotherapy for osteomyelitis caused by susceptible organisms, with appropriate surgical debridement (42). Resistance to *P. aeruginosa*, however, has emerged against ceftazidime and imipenem. This creates reason for concern and suggests that combination with an aminoglycoside be used for this pathogen (24).

Preliminary reports dealing with the use of oral rifampin in combination with parenteral penicillinase-resistant penicillin for the treatment of chronic staphylococcal osteomyelitis have been encouraging. It should be noted that bacterial responses were considerably better than the clinical response. Failures were due to inadequate surgical debridement or to polymicrobial infection (43). Rifampin has been shown to act synergistically with antistaphylococcal agents when used in combination (42).

Duration of Therapy

The optimal length of therapy for the treatment of osteomyelitis has not been adequately defined. One controlled study reported a significantly higher percentage of failures when patients received parenteral antibiotics for 3 weeks or less than when therapy continued for more than 3 weeks. The addition of oral antibiotics did not appear to influence the outcome of therapy (44). The current standard is to treat the infection for a minimum of 4 weeks with high-dose parenteral therapy. Most clinicians prefer to use the amelioration of clinical signs and the normalization of laboratory parameters such as white blood cell count and ESR in determining the precise length of therapy (7).

The length of treatment for chronic osteomyelitis is even less well defined since infections in this situation may involve significant necrosis of the bone and accumulation of sequestra. Current recommendations include at least 4 to 6 weeks of parenteral therapy followed by 2 months of oral therapy (1). These guidelines were developed from patients with chronic staphylococcal osteomyelitis and may not be appropriate for infections with Gram-negative etiologies. In a more recent study, most patients evaluated who were diagnosed with chronic osteomyelitis were cured following 3 months of appropriate intravenous antibiotic therapy (45).

Home Antibiotic Therapy

With the advent of diagnosis-related groups (DRGs) and the emphasis on medical cost containment, the self-administration of antibiotics on an outpatient basis has emerged as a viable alternative to hospitalization in the long-term treatment of selected infectious diseases such as endocarditis and osteomyelitis (46). Home healthcare agencies, developed as either private corporations or hospital-based services, have flourished into a profitable industry.

In most cases, patients receive a brief course of antibiotic therapy, usually 10 to 14 days, while in the hospital. During this time, patients are observed for untoward effects and overall tolerance to the regimen. Once clinically stable, home patients are selected based on the reliability of their home environment to provide safe and adequate care. Patients should also have other family or home members willing to learn and assume the responsibilities of home drug administration. Drugs are administered through a peripheral venous access such as intermittent needle therapy (INT), a central catheter such as a peripheral intravenous central catheter (PICC line), or directly through a Hickman-Broviac catheter. The INT administration has a disadvantage in that the needle must be replaced every 3 days. Also, patients often complain of local pain and inflammation. Central catheters generally remain in place for the duration of therapy. Hickman-Broviac catheters have the disadvantage of usually requiring minor surgery and general anesthesia for insertion. Home patients generally receive several doses of prepackaged antibiotics. Ambulatory patients return to the hospital on a weekly or twice-weekly basis for their drug supply, while drugs are delivered to debilitated patients by the home-healthcare pharmacist team. The intravenous catheter care is provided by the community health nursing program. The pharmacist has both dispensing and drug-monitoring responsibilities. Hospital-based distribution of home antibiotics is an efficacious, safe, and cost-effective alternative to prolonged hospitalization in the treatment of osteomyelitis (46).

Antibiotic Bone Concentrations

Numerous studies have been done on antibiotic penetration into normal and infected bone. Antibiotic bone concentrations have been determined by assaying aliquots of solutions containing bone fragments that have been agitated in an appropriate buffer at an optimal pH. Unfortunately, data from these studies vary considerably and have produced conflicting recommendations about which agents are appropriate. Factors such as time of sample collection, extraction techniques, methods of assay, and source of specimen (whether normal or osteomyelitic bone) have all contributed to the confusion.

In the most recent analysis, antibiotic bone concentrations were evaluated in animal model bones by comparing the permeation of antibiotics into bone to an isotope with a known capillary diffusion characteristic, such as sucrose or strontium (47). This procedure was performed in both normal and osteolytic bone. The antibiotics tested included cephalothin, cefazolin, cefamandole, moxalactam, cephradine, penicillin G, and the aminoglycosides gentamicin, tobramycin, and netilmicin. Permeability was expressed as a ratio of the antibiotic agent to the isotope. In addition, volume of distribution techniques were used to determine the distribution of the various antibiotics within the fluid spaces of normal and osteomyelitic bone.

The results of the study showed that all β-lactam antibiotics tested were able to permeate capillary membranes of normal and osteomyelitic bones. Similar results were observed in the aminoglycoside group, with tobramycin and netilmicin exhibiting slightly higher diffusion ratios than gentamicin. The proposed mechanism suggests that these agents crossed capillary membranes by simple passive diffusion as well as other processes (47).

The volumes of distribution for the β-lactam antibiotics were similar to those of the isotope in both normal and osteolytic bone, and drug distribution occurred in the plasma and interstitial fluid space of osseous tissue. The volumes of distribution of aminoglycosides were observed to be larger than that of the control agent in normal bone. In osteolytic bone, gentamicin and netilmicin distribution was similar to that of sucrose in the exchangeable water space, whereas tobramycin exceeded the control by more than 150% in the exchangeable water space. This agent was highly concentrated in one or more spaces of the bone.

Concomitant serum concentrations were measured at steady-state and were shown to be similar to those of the interstitial fluid space in the osseous tissue. This indicated that serum concentrations are an adequate reflection of bone fluid concentrations (47). Serum and bone levels of β-lactam antibiotics were examined in patients with chronic osteomyelitis following debridement, and despite adequate serum concentrations, there was only minimal penetration into the necrotic bone (48).

In summary, it appears that common β-lactam antibiotics and aminoglycosides are capable of penetrating and distributing into both normal and osteolytic bone, although high-dose therapy is often employed. Serum concentrations appear to be an adequate measurement of interstitial bone concentrations. Penetration into necrotic bone appears to be minimal.

Other Treatment Modalities

LOCAL ANTIBIOTIC THERAPY

Although systemic antibiotic therapy seems to be the mainstay in the treatment of osteomyelitis, several disadvantages exist, particularly in the chronic form of this disease. These include potential side effects following prolonged therapy, questionable penetration of antibiotics into necrotic or ischemic tissue, and protracted hospitalization. As a result, a number of new techniques have been developed providing direct local application of antibiotics.

Gentamicin-impregnated polymethylmethacrylate (PMMA) beads have been used extensively in the United Kingdom but only on a limited basis in United States. The drug is marketed in Europe under the trade name of Septopal. In this system, the PMMA bead serves as a carrier for the gentamicin. Each bead contains 7.5 mg of gentamicin sulfate. The beads may be used individually for packing empty voids following surgery or strung on a multifilament stainless steel wire in the form of chains for direct attachment to the bones. The chains consist of 10, 30, or 60 beads. The beads remain in the body for approximately 14 days and provide slow release of gentamicin to the surrounding tissues at a rate of 400 to 600 μg/bead/day. Impregnated PMMA beads have the advantage of providing high local antibiotic tissue levels with minimal serum concentrations. In addition, systemic antibiotics are generally not required, reducing the need for extensive nursing care and decreasing the duration of hospital stay. Unfortunately, the use of PMMA beads is not without limitations and disadvantages. These include strict mandatory patient immobilization and bed rest. Also, the introduction of another foreign body may lead to local inflammation and the possibility of reinfection. Finally, an additional surgical procedure is required to remove the beads and chains (49).

The use of antibiotic-impregnated plaster of Paris pellets has been advocated by others in place of PMMA beads. This method is relatively simple and inexpensive to prepare and the pellets are spontaneously reabsorbed, thus eliminating the need for additional implanted devices (50). Both methods lack objective experiments to substantiate their safety and efficacy.

Another method has been the direct instillation of antibacterial solutions, usually iodophor, through a closed continuous-suction irrigation system. This is often used in cases of chronic osteomyelitis or in large areas of avascular tissue. Although this system is popular, it requires a considerable amount of monitoring by the nursing staff as well as the risk of secondary infection through the drains. As in the case of the beads and pellets, suction irrigation also lacks the documentation of well-controlled clinical studies. The use of PMMA beads appears to be easier than the continuous-drainage method (1, 50).

HYPERBARIC OXYGEN THERAPY

Much attention is currently being focused on the use of hyperbaric oxygen therapy in the treatment of chronic osteomyelitis. In this method, patients are placed in a monoplace hyperbaric chamber where they are subjected to oxygen pressures greater than those at sea level, usually 2 atmospheres. The duration of therapy ranges from 90 min to 2 hr, depending on the level of refractoriness of the chronic osteomyelitis and the subsequent results of each treatment. As many as 60 treatments may be used for a single patient.

Clinical studies have documented that intermittent short-term, high-dose oxygen inhalation has been associated with increased vascularity as well as enhancing both bone and soft tissue healing in ischemic tissue. In addition, hyperbaric oxygen is effective in controlling infections caused by anaerobes and microphilic bacteria. Common osteomyelitic organisms such as *S. aureus* and *P. aeruginosa*, however, are sensitive only at pressures unsafe for human exposure. Effectiveness of hyperbaric oxygen for these organisms is postulated to be related to the enhancement of leukocyte bactericidal activity by elevating intermedullary oxygen tension. Hearing and sight impairment are the major risks involved in the use of hyperbaric oxygen. These effects are reversible. Also, hyperbaric oxygen therapy is expensive. Hyperbaric oxygen should be used only as adjunctive therapy when there is either slow or no response to traditional medical management (51, 52).

SURGICAL INTERVENTION

A few controlled studies have evaluated the effectiveness of surgery in the management of osteomyelitis. Difficulties revolve around inabilities to control variability of local operating conditions, types of surgery, and patient factors. As a result, surgical intervention is largely empiric and is based on accepted experiential concepts rather than scientific documentation (8).

In most cases of acute hematogenous osteomyelitis, surgical intervention is generally not required other than as a necessary diagnostic procedure. However, some cases do not respond to pharmacologic management, and surgical intervention is required either for exploration or for drainage of an abscess (15).

In the treatment of contiguous-spread osteomyelitis, surgical intervention may be required to drain abscesses and close fistula tracts. In the case of chronic osteomyelitis, surgery is almost certainly required to excise necrotic bone and remove sequestra. Patients often require skin or muscle flaps to close overlying skin or fill empty cavities (53).

The decision to remove external fixation devices in an area of infected bone depends on whether union of the bone has been accomplished. If bone union occurs, infection can be treated in the presence of the device. However, if the union fails, most authorities agree that the removal of the fixation device is warranted (8). A summary of the medical management of osteomyelitis is presented in Figure 68.2.

Prognosis

Favorable prognosis depends largely on the type of osteomyelitis and whether the appropriate medical interventions are implemented as soon as possible after the onset of symptoms. Under these circumstances, it appears that acute osteomyelitis is associated with the best overall prognosis, carrying approximately 80% cure rate when parenteral antibiotics are maintained for more than 4 weeks and appropriate surgical intervention is used. Similar results are also seen in children who receive initial parenteral antibiotics followed by an appropriate oral agent if the peak bactericidal levels are maintained above 1:8 (36).

In the case of chronic osteomyelitis, the prognosis is substantially less favorable. Success rates vary from study to study depending on the criteria, such as healing of drained sinuses or changes in laboratory parameters. Original observations in the management of chronic osteomyelitis have defined a success rate as high as 90% and as low as 20%. Later studies have shown that proper surgical debridement of dead bone and sequestra along with appropriate antibiotic treatment may increase the follow-up success rate to 50%. Patients in whom surgery was contraindicated or was unsuccessful may require long-term suppressive antibiotics to control their infections (42).

Conclusion

Osteomyelitis is a serious infection of the bone, which when left untreated can result in significant bone loss and deformity. Infection can be transmitted directly via the bloodstream or spread from adjacent tissue. Most cases are caused by *S. aureus*, although other pathogens such as Enterobacteriaceae, *P. aeruginosa*, and anaerobes have also been isolated. The medical management of osteomyelitis involves a comprehensive clinical assessment of patient factors, culture material, roentgenologic studies,

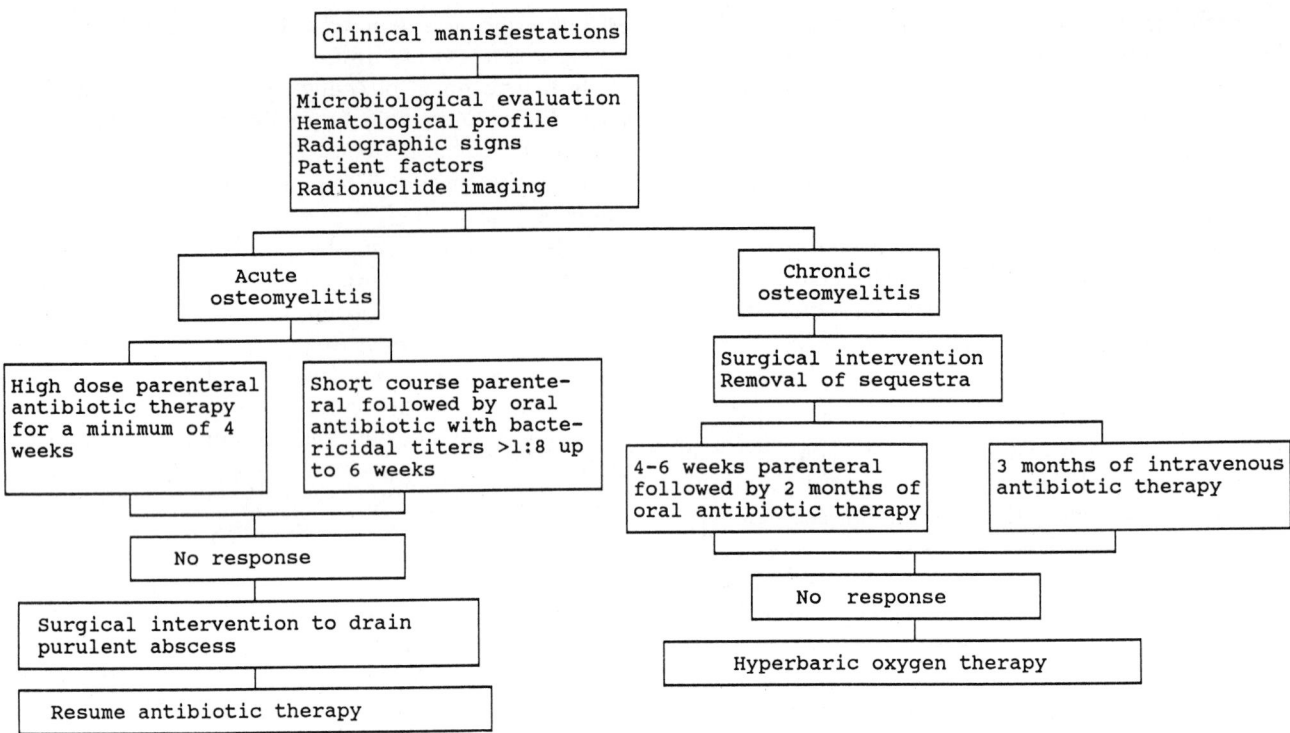

Figure 68.2. Algorithm for the management of bacterial osteomyelitis.

complete blood counts, and appropriate antimicrobial therapy. Most β-lactam and aminoglycoside antibiotics penetrate normal and osteomyelitic bone adequately but do not penetrate necrotic bone. Most cases of the acute form can be treated with monotherapy for a total of 4 to 6 weeks and are associated with a favorable prognosis. Select patients can be treated successfully with oral antibiotics with aggressive monitoring and forced compliance. Chronic osteomyelitis may require several months of treatment with intravenous and oral antibiotics and is associated with a less favorable prognosis. Some patients may require surgical intervention to remove necrotic bone fragments. Hyperbaric oxygen has been demonstrated to be a useful adjunct to antimicrobial therapy in some refractory patients. The administration of antibiotics at home has been shown to be a safe and cost-effective alternative to prolonged hospitalization.

INFECTIOUS ARTHRITIS

Infectious arthritis and *septic arthritis* are interchangeable terms used to describe inflammatory reactions of the joint space, synovium, synovial fluid, and articular cartilage following invasion by a variety of microorganisms. Infectious arthritis constitutes a medical emergency requiring immediate treatment to prevent permanent damage to the joint. Bacteria are the most common cause of joint infections, but fungi, viruses, and chlamydia have also been

isolated. This discussion deals exclusively with bacterial arthritis.

Etiology

The bacteria causing infectious arthritis are primarily age dependent. The most common bacteria isolated from children and adults of varying ages are outlined in Table 68.4. *S. aureus* is the most common organism isolated in newborns. Group B streptocci and Enterobacteriaceae, especially *E. coli*, have also been isolated and may be important pathogens. *H. influenzae* is the predominant pathogen in infants and children under 5 years of age, followed by *S. aureus* and streptococci, but it is virtually absent in late childhood and adolescence (54, 55). *S. aureus* and group A streptococci are the most common pathogens in the latter two age groups. Occasionally Gram-negative bacteria have also been isolated in this age group (55). *Neisseria gonorrhoeae* is the predominant organism in sexually active young adults, and *S. aureus* is the most common pathogen in the overall adult population, especially in patients with underlying illnesses such as rheumatoid arthritis, diabetes mellitus, and malignancy (56). Gram-negative bacilli such as *E. coli, Proteus mirabilis,* and *P. aeruginosa* have also been identified as major pathogens in infectious arthritis in adults (8, 38). Other bacteria isolated include streptococci, *Neisseria meningitidis,* and anaerobes (38, 54). *Staphylococcus epidermidis* is the most

Table 68.4.
Common Etiologies and Empiric Antibiotic Therapy for the Treatment of Infectious Arthritis

Age Group	Likely Organisms	Antibiotics of Choice (Dose, Route, and Frequency of Administration)
Neonates (<4 weeks)	S. aureus Group B streptococcus Enterobacteriaceae	Nafcillin 40 mg/kg/day IV q. 12 hr or oxacillin 50 mg/kg/day IV q. 12 hr or first-generation cephalosporin (e.g., cephalothin or cefazolin 40 mg/kg/day IV q. 12 hr) plus gentamicin 5.0 mg/kg/day IV q. 12 hr
Infants and children (1 month to 5 years)	H. influenzae S. aureus Streptococcus species[a]	Cefuroxime 100 mg/kg/day IV q. 8 hr or cefotaxime or ceftizoxime 100–150 mg/kg/day IV q. 8 hr
Children and adolescents (5–16 years)	S. aureus Group A streptococcus Occasionally Gram-negative bacteria	Nafcillin or oxacillin 50–100 mg/kg/day IV q. 6 hr or first-generation cephalosporin (i.e., cephalothin–150 mg/kg/day IV q. 8 hr) *plus* gentamicin 5 mg/kg/day IV q. 8 hr
Sexually active adults	N. gonorrhoeae	Penicillin G, 12,000,000 U/day or ceftriaxone 1 g qd
Adults with underlying illness, immunosuppressed	S. aureus Enterobacteriaceae P. aeruginosa[b] Streptococcus species	Nafcillin or oxacillin 50–100 mg/kg/day IV q. 6 hr or first-generation cephalosporin (e.g., cephalothin–150 mg/kg/day IV q. 6 hr or cefazolin 50–150 mg/kg/day IV q. 8 hr) plus gentamicin 5 mg/kg/day IV q. 8 hr)

[a] Includes S. pneumoniae, Group A and B streptococci.
[b] Ceftazidine 2–3 g IV q. 8 hr or piperacillin or mezlocillin 300 mg/kg/day IV plus tobramycin 5 mg/kg/day IV.

Table 68.5.
Risk Factors Associated with the Development of Infectious Arthritis

Corticosteroid therapy	Osteoarthritis
Diabetes mellitus	Intravenous drug abuse
Rheumatoid arthritis	Hematologic malignancies
Gout	Extra-articular foci of infection

common pathogen isolated in prostatic joint infections (57).

Risk Factors

Bacteremia is generally considered to be the most important predisposing factor, since hematogenous spread from a distant foci represents the most common mechanism for joint infections (56). A number of additional risk factors may also predispose a patient to infectious arthritis (Table 68.5). Identification of these risk factors can also assist in the diagnosis. For example, adults with previous joint damage, such as from rheumatoid arthritis, osteoarthritis, gout, and recent joint trauma, appear to be at high risk for infectious arthritis (56). Patients with chronic illness such as diabetes mellitus and serious underlying diseases such as malignancy are more vulnerable to septic arthritis. Also included in this group are patients with an impaired immune defense system. This situation may develop either through direct immunosuppressive therapy, such as from systemic or intra-articular corticosteroid, or from primary malignancy such as lymphoma (56, 58). Infections in these patients are usually associated with Gram-negative bacilli. Intravenous drug abusers have a high rate of infections caused by P. aeruginosa or Serratia species (56).

Extra-articular foci of infections can also predispose patients to joint infections. For example, cutaneous infections can result in bacteremic spread of S. aureus or Streptococcus pyogenes. Similarly, patients with pulmonary infections may be at risk for bacteremic spread of S. pneumoniae to the joint. Genitourinary and gastrointestinal tract infections have also been associated with Gram-negative septic arthritis (57). Infectious arthritis resulting from direct inoculation is rare and occurs mostly in patients with prostatic joints or those receiving steroid injections (8).

In infants and children, the underdeveloped immune system and lack of antibody response probably contributes to the predominance of H. influenzae joint infections below the age of 5 (55). Bacteremic spread from extra-articular sites can also predispose children to joint infections. Meningitis, pharyngitis, and cutaneous infections are included as the most common source of septic foci in children (55).

Pathophysiology

Microorganisms generally make their way to the joint via bacteremic spread from a distant focus. Infectious arthritis rarely begins from a contiguous focus as in the case of osteomyelitis. Ninety percent of cases involve only a single joint; in such cases the knee is most commonly involved, followed by the hip. Other joints involved include the sternoclavicular, shoulder, and sacroiliac (39).

Infectious arthritis rarely develops from direct inoculation, such as from injury or surgical procedures. Once the organism reaches the joint, factors that favor the penetration of the organism into the synovium are not completely understood but may include status of the patient's immune defense system, previous joint injury, or presence of other forms of arthritis. Special properties and virulence of the microorganism may also play a role, as in the case of Gram-positive cocci and *N. gonorrhoeae*, which have a particular affinity for bone and joint tissue and are frequent causes of infectious arthritis (58).

Once the organism invades the joint, the initial lesion usually develops in the microvasculature of the synovial membrane (Fig. 68.3). At this site the bacteria proliferate, releasing their toxic factors. A typical inflammatory response develops from subsequent formation of antigen-antibody complexes, complement activation, and phagocytic cell stimulation. During the latter process lysosomal enzymes are released, resulting in the formation of microabscesses that eventually extend into the synovial tissue and joint space. Intra-articular pressure increases, which enhances synovia and capsular erosion. The continued inflammatory process may lead to destruction of the cartilage and invasion of the adjacent bone, causing osteomyelitis (58).

Clinical Manifestations and Diagnosis

Septic arthritis generally presents as monarticular pain, swelling, and redness, which is sometimes associated with fever and chills. The patient has substantial limitation in the range of motion in the joint as a result of the swelling and tenderness (Table 68.6). There is a diffuse periarticular tenderness, and an effusion can be demonstrated in 90% of cases. These symptoms may be minimal or less

pronounced in the case of the more deeply situated joints, such as the hip, shoulder, sacroiliac, or intervertebral joints (39). Children with infectious arthritis of the hip can present with fever, apprehension, and irritability. The child assumes a position that enhances comfort to the affected joint. There is usually limited spontaneous motion in the affected extremity, referred to as *pseudo-paralysis* (55). In gonococcal arthritis, patients have systemic symptoms such as fever and skin lesion. Gonococcal arthritis is usually disseminated and polyarticulate, with sterile effusions occurring in 50% of the cases. Two-thirds of patients with gonococcal arthritis also have symptoms of tenosynovitis, an inflammation of the tendon sheath (39).

Rapid microbiologic assessment of the synovial fluid is the most useful diagnostic procedure in the evaluation of septic arthritis. Any patient who has a tender, swollen joint with limited motion accompanied by signs of infection should undergo immediate joint aspiration and drainage. A delay in this procedure can result in permanent destruction of the joint and bone, particularly in children. A Gram-stain of the aspirated fluid yields a presumptive diagnosis in 30% of cases in children and 50 to 60% of cases overall (7, 39), although recently, culture diagnosis was reported to be positive in over 84% of cases in children (55). Chemical evaluation of the joint leukocyte count can be useful in distinguishing septic arthritis from other causes of inflammatory joint reaction such as gout, pseudogout, rheumatoid arthritis, rheumatic fever, and Reiter's syndrome. Synovial leukocyte counts in infectious arthritis are much

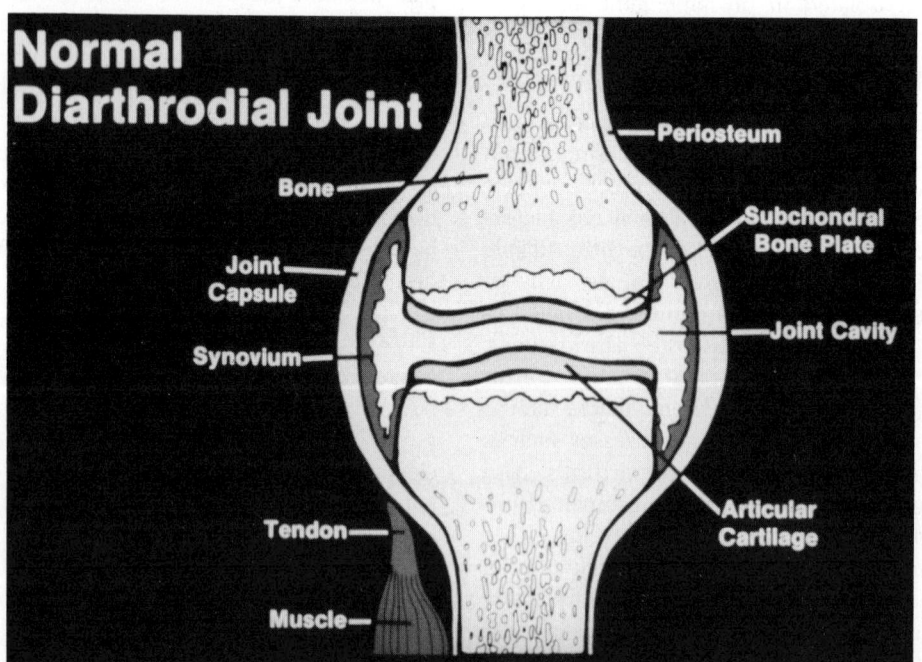

Figure 68.3.   Major structures of the joint. (From the Arthritis Teaching Slide Collection, copyright 1980. Used by permission of the Arthritis Foundation.)

Table 68.6
Clinical Symptoms of Infectious Arthritis

Monoarticular pain	Gonococcal syndrome
Swelling and redness in the joint	Fever
Fever	Skin lesions
Chills	Tenosynovitis
Limitation in joint range of motion	

higher than those from the previously mentioned conditions (59).

Evaluation of blood cultures may yield positive results in 30% of children and 10 to 60% of adults (39). Positive blood cultures for gonococci are not as reliable, occurring in less than 20% of the cases. *N. gonorrhoeae*, however, may be recovered from other infectious sites, such as the pharynx, genitourinary tract, and rectum, in 80% of cases of septic arthritis (39). The ESR and peripheral white blood cell count are usually elevated and contribute to the diagnosis (7).

Early roentgenologic evaluation of the joint is generally nonspecific, showing only joint effusion or soft tissue swelling. Radionuclide imaging, such as technetium-99 and gallium-67 citrate scanning, is also used in the diagnosis of septic arthritis. As in osteomyelitis, the technetium-99 scan may be positive for inflammatory reactions as a result of noninfectious etiologies. In this situation, the gallium scan may be more diagnostic (15). Furthermore, technetium-99 scans can remain positive for weeks to months following septic arthritis, whereas the gallium scan generally reverts to normal following successful treatment (39).

Medical Management

Appropriate medical management of septic arthritis involves a comprehensive approach of microbiologic assessment, antibiotic therapy, and aspiration and immobilization of the joint. Prompt installation of these measures will avoid destruction of the cartilage and permanent disabling damage to the joint.

Initial microbiologic evaluations should include a Gram stain to determine the morphology of the organism before definitive culture results can be obtained. If the Gram stain and cultures cannot be performed, empiric therapy should begin, using factors such as age, clinical manifestations, and underlying disease states.

An algorithm summarizing the medical management of infectious arthritis is presented in Figure 68.4.

Antibiotic Therapy

For newborns under 1 month of age, empiric therapy should begin with a penicillinase-resistant penicillin or a first-generation cephalosporin (Table 68.4). Gentamicin should be added to the regimen because Enterobacteri-

aceae may also be suspected pathogens (39, 60). For infants and young children, a second-generation cephalosporin such as cefuroxime is an excellent choice for empiric therapy. This agent is active against the two most predominant pathogens, *S. aureus* and *H. influenzae*, including β-lactase-producing strains (6, 7).

For older children and adolescents, *S. aureus* and group A streptococci have been most commonly isolated. *H. influenzae*, Enterobacteriaceae, and *N. gonorrhoeae* have also been isolated occasionally but are rare. Initial therapy with a penicillinase-resistant penicillin or a first-generation cephalosporin in combination with gentamicin is appropriate (7, 60).

For sexually active healthy adults, a trial of penicillin therapy is warranted, since *N. gonorrhoeae* is the most likely pathogen. The Centers for Disease Control (CDC) currently recommends the use of ceftriaxone at a dose of 1-g a day for 7 days for the treatment of disseminated gonococcal infection (61). Clinical improvement should be evident within 48 to 72 hr (39).

In the elderly population both Gram-positive and Gram-negative organisms, including *P. aeruginosa*, have been isolated. A reliable Gram-stain is the most valuable diagnostic tool for empiric therapy. If Gram-positive cocci are identified, a penicillinase-resistant penicillin or a first-generation cephalosporin is appropriate. When Gram-negative bacilli are suspected or identified, therapy should include an antipseudomonal penicillin or cephalosporin in combination with an aminoglycoside. For elderly patients who are immunocompromised or have an underlying illness, empiric antistaphylococcal therapy may be warranted in addition to antipseudomonal therapy until cultures can be obtained (39, 60).

Successful treatment of infectious arthritis is contingent upon the ability of the antibiotic to adequately penetrate the joint space and achieve sufficient synovial antibacterial levels. In general, penicillins and cephalosporin penetrate easily into joint fluid and achieve synovial concentrations similar to those measured in the serum. This is in contrast to certain antibiotic agents such as aminoglycosides, whose activity is decreased in joint fluid despite achieving adequate serum concentrations. This poor activity is related to the low pH and to the presence of purulent material in the synovium, both of which reduce antibacterial activity of this group of agents. One must be cautious, therefore, when interpreting in vitro aminoglycoside minimum inhibitory concentration of data since this test is normally performed in a pH 7.34. For these reasons, β-lactam antibiotics are considered to be the first-line agents for treating infections of the joint (8, 39). Although there are no documented clinical data, it is recommended that joint fluid bactericidal levels should be maintained above 1:8 dilution (60).

To ensure adequate treatment, high-dose parenteral

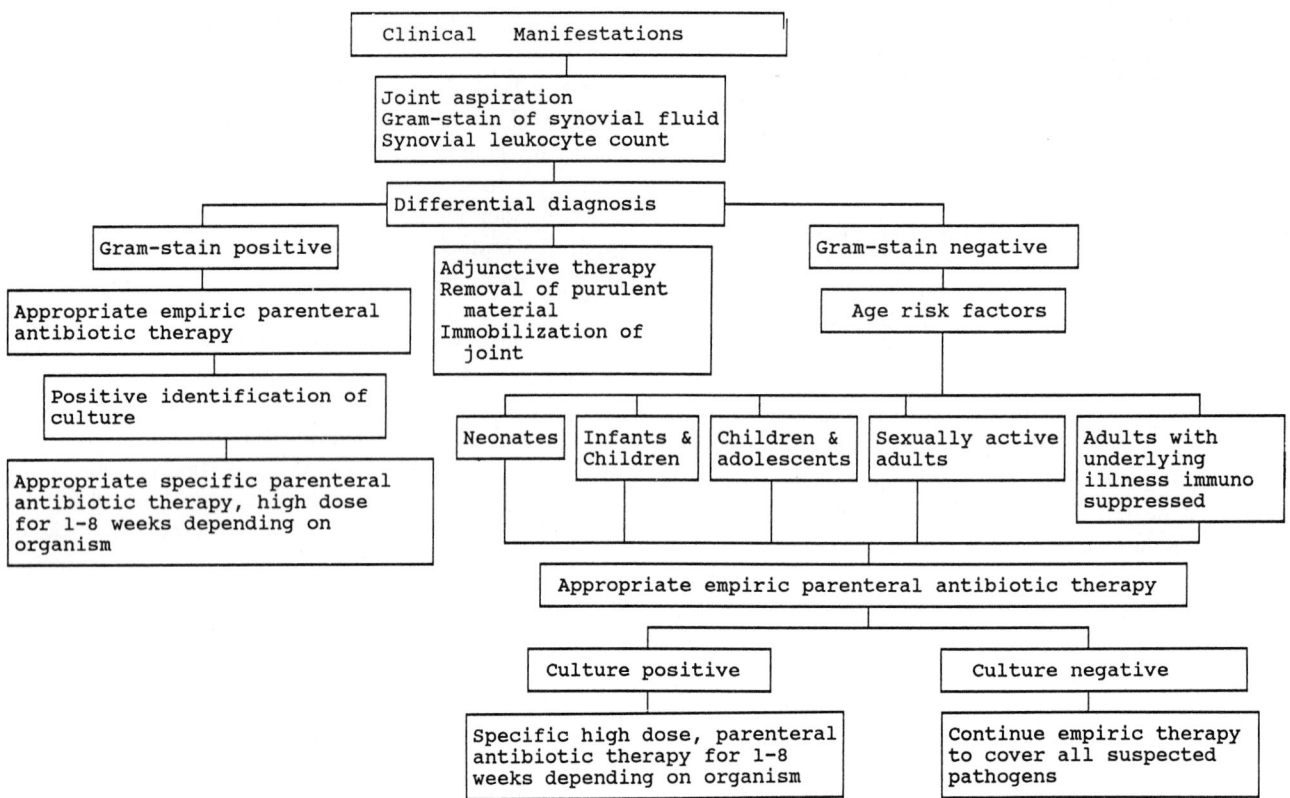

Figure 68.4. Algorithm for the management of infectious arthritis.

antibiotics should be administered for a minimum of 14 days, although the precise length of therapy usually depends on the organism being treated. For example, streptococci generally require no more than 2 weeks of therapy, whereas staphylococci and Gram-negative organisms should be treated for at least 4 weeks. *P. aeruginosa* may require as much as 6 to 8 weeks of therapy in adults. Gonorrheal arthritis responds quite well to penicillin G therapy and can be treated in as little as 1 week. Direct instillation of antibiotics into the joint space is not recommended because it can result in a chemical synovitis (56, 58).

Oral antibiotics have been used successfully without recurrence in the treatment of septic arthritis. As in osteomyelitis, oral antibiotics can provide less costly treatment and are more convenient for the patient. Only oral antibiotics that have adequate absorption to provide bactericidal concentrations should be considered. Similarly, patient compliance and follow-up are of paramount importance (35).

Adjunctive Therapy

In addition to antibiotic therapy, closed-needle aspiration of the synovium, arthrocentesis, is indicated as adjunctive therapy. The removal of purulent material containing harmful enzymes and bacterial toxins not only reduces the risk of further damage to cartilage but also improves the

activity of certain antibiotics, such as the aminoglycosides (56). Aspiration of the joint may be performed as few as two to three times for each infection or as often as twice a day for up to 7 to 10 days (39). Closed-needle aspiration is generally preferred over surgical drainage. However, in septic arthritis of the hip, needle aspiration is often anatomically difficult to perform and in some cases the purulent material is too thick to pass through the standard aspiration needle (8).

Immobilization of the joint also plays a key factor in successful treatment by helping to decrease inflammation, relieve pain, and reduce the risk of further damage. Larger weight-bearing joints may require splints or traction for initial immobilization. When the inflammation subsides, the patient may begin slow passive movements to prevent permanent disability or contracture. Use of weight-bearing joints is only recommended when all signs of the inflammatory process have ceased and no effusion is observed (56, 60). A summary of the medical management of infectious arthritis is presented in Figure 68.4.

Prognosis

The overall prognosis for septic arthritis is generally favorable. Nongonococcal septic arthritis has been associated with a mortality rate of 10%. Most deaths occur in patients with underlying risk factors such as sepsis, rheumatoid arthritis, and malignancy. Functional impairment or continuation of infection has been reported in as many as 25 to 33% of children and adults.

The successful outcome of the infection is usually contingent upon several factors. For example, in children the prognosis is correlated with several parameters such as the particular joint involved, type of organism, adequate drainage, appropriate antibiotic coverage, and time of initiation of treatment relative to the onset of symptoms. Infections of the hip are associated with the highest rate of sequelae, and the impaired mobility in these cases may not be evident until months or years later. The patient may display limitation in motion, joint fusion, deformity, and limb shortening. *S. aureus* infection has the greatest propensity for chronic problems (56).

The delay in seeking appropriate medical care has often been cited as a major predictor for long-term morbidity, although this prognostic indicator has recently been challenged in children (55). In adults, the outcome of treatment is considerably poorer when therapy is initiated more than 1 week after onset, when the offending organism is not eradicated from the joint fluid within 4 to 5 days, and where patients are over the age of 60 (39). This further emphasizes the need for rapid diagnosis and immediate treatment (8). Other determinants for unsuccessful therapy include the presence of underlying diseases, such as diabetes, immunocompromised host, and prior joint disease (39).

Conclusion

Infectious arthritis is a serious infection of the joint and surrounding tissue requiring immediate treatment to prevent permanent damage. Most infections are transmitted through the blood from a distant focus. Patients with previous joint damage, such as from rheumatoid arthritis, osteoarthritis, gout, and trauma, also appear to be at risk. The most common causative organism is *S. aureus*, although other pathogens such as Enterobacteriaceae, *P. aeruginosa*, and *N. gonorrhoeae* have also been isolated. Treatment of infectious arthritis involves prompt aspiration of the joint fluid, rapid identification of the organism, and appropriate antibiotic therapy. Most antimicrobial agents achieve therapeutic concentrations in joint space. The duration of therapy can range from 7 to 21 days, depending on the offending pathogen. Further needle aspiration may be required during therapy. Immobilization of the joint is recommended to prevent the risk of further damage to the joint and surrounding cartilage. Infectious arthritis retains an overall favorable prognosis when the appropriate medical management is provided.

REFERENCES

1. Norden CW, Osteomyelitis. In Mandell GL, Douglas RG, Bennett JE (eds): Principles and Practice of Infectious Diseases, ed. 3. New York, John Wiley & Sons, 1990, pp 922–930.

2. Waldvogel FA, Medoff C, Swartz M: Osteomyelitis: a review of clinical fractures, therapeutic considerations, and unusual aspects. N Engl J Med 282:198–206, 1970.

3. Anderson JR, Scobie WG, Watt B: The treatment of acute osteomyelitis in children: a 10-year experience. J Antimicrob Chemother 7(suppl A):43–50, 1981.

4. Kerstein lMD: Osteomyelitis associated with vascular insufficiency. Curr Ther Res Clin Exp 16:306–310, 1974.

5. Waldvogel FA, Vasey H: Osteomyelitis: the past decade. N Engl J Med 303:360–370, 1980.

6. Wilbur RB: β-Lactam therapy for osteomyelitis and septic arthritis. Scand J Infect Dis 42(suppl):155–168, 1984.

7. Jackson MA, Nelson JD: Etiology and medical management of acute suppurative bone and joint infections in pediatric patients. J Pediatr Orthop 2:313–323, 1982.

8. Waldvogel FA: Treatment of osteomyelitis and septic arthritis. Bull NY Acad Med 58:733–749, 1982.

9. Pichichero ME: Polymicrobial osteomyelitis. Report of three cases and review of the literature. Rev Infect Dis 4(1):86–89, 1982.

10. Nakata MM, Lewis RP: Anaerobic bacteria in bone and joint infections. Rev Infect Dis 6(1):S165–169, 1984.

11. Wald ER: Risk factors for osteomyelitis. Am J Med 78(suppl 6B) 206–212, 1985.

12. Puczynski MS, Dvonch VM, Menendez CE: Osteomyelitis of the great toe secondary to phlebotomy. Clin Orthop 190:239–240, 1985.

13. Sugarman B, Hawes S, Musher DM, et al.: Osteomyelitis beneath pressure sores. Ann Intern Med 143:683–688, 1983.

14. Norden CW: Lessons learned from animal models of osteomyelitis. Rev Infect Dis 10:103–110, 1988.

15. Gutman L: Acute, subacute and chronic osteomyelitis and pyogenic arthritis in children. Curr Probl Pediat 15(12):1–72, 1985.

16. Marrie TJ, Costerton JW: Mode of growth of bacterial pathogens in chronic polymicrobial human osteomyelitis. J Clin Microbiol 22:924–933, 1985.

17. Roberts JM, Drummond JS, Breed AL, et al.: Subacute hematogenous osteomyelitis in children: a retrospective study. J Pediatr Orthop 2:249–254, 1982.

18. Braun TL, Lorber B, Chronic osteomyelitis. In Schlossberg D (ed): Orthopedic Infections. New York, Springer-Verlag, 1988, pp 9–20.

19. Israel O, Gips S, Jerushalmi J, et al.: Osteomyelitis and soft tissue infection: differential diagnosis with 24 hr/ratio of Tc-m MDP uptake. Radiology 163:725–726, 1987.

20. Schwauker DS, Park HM, Mock BH, et al.: Evaluation of complicating osteomyelitis with Tc-99m MDP, IN-111 granulocytes and GA-67 citrate. J Nucl Med 25:849–853, 1984.

21. Tauzon CU: Teichoic acid antibodies in osteomyelitis and septic arthritis acaused by *Staphylococcus aureus*. J Bone Joint Surg 64(A):762–765, 1982.

22. Tartalgione TA, Pold RE: Review of the new second-generation cephalosporins: cefonocid, ceforanide, and ceruroxime. Drug Intell Clin Pharm 19:188–198, 1985.

23. Norrby SR: Adverse reactions and interactions with newer cephalosporins and cephamycin antibiotics. Med Toxicol 1:32–46, 1986.

24. Gentry LD: Role for newer β-lactam antibiotics in the treatment of osteomyelitis. Am J Med 78(suppl 6A):134–139, 1985.

25. Stratton CW, Kernodle DS, Eades SO, et al.: Evaluation of cefotaxime alone and in combination with desacetyl cefotaxime against strains of *Staphylococcus aureus* that produce variants of staphylococcal β-lactase. Diagn Microbiol Infect Dis 12:57–65, 1989.

26. Barriere SL, Flaherty JF: Third-generation cephalosporins: a critical evaluation. Clin Pharm 33:351–373, 1984.

27. Glover SC, Padfield C, McKendrick MW, et al.: Acute osteomyelitis in a district general hospital. Lancet 1:609–611, 1982.

28. Kaplan SL, Mason EO, Feigin RD: Clindamycin versus nafcillin or methicillin in the treatment of *Staphylococcus aureus* osteomyelitis in children. South Med J 75:138–143, 1982.

29. Cunha BA, Ristuccia AM: Clinical usefulness of vancomycin. Clin Pharm 2:417–424, 1983.

30. Mellor JA, Kingdom J, Cafferkey M: Vancomycin toxicity: a prospective study. J Antimicrob Chemother 15:773–780, 1985.

31. Anon: New preparations of vancomycin. Med Lett 28:121–122, 1986.

32. Sheftel TG, Mader JT, Pennick JJ: Methicillin-resistant *Staphylococcus aureus* osteomyelitis, Clin Orthop 198:231–239, 1985.

33. Mathisen GE: Bone and Joint Infections. In Finegold SM, George WL (eds): Anaerobic Infections in Humans. San Diego, Academic Press, 1989, pp 507–527.

34. Templeton WC, Wawrukiewicz A, Melo JC: Anaerobic osteomyelitis of long bone. Rev Infect Dis 692–712, 1983.

35. Black J, Hunt HL, Godley PJ, et al.: Oral antimicrobial therapy for adults with osteomyelitis or septic arthritis. J Infect Dis 155:968–972, 1987.

36. Prober CG, Yeager AS: Use of the serum bactericidal titer to assess the adequacy of oral antibiotic therapy in the treatment of acute hematogenous osteomyelitis. J Pediatr 95:131–135, 1979.

37. Arcieri G, Griffith E, Gruenwald G, et al.: Ciprofloxacin: an update on clinical experience. Am J Med 82(suppl 4A):381–386, 1987.

38. Gentry LD, Rodriquez GG: Oral ciprofloxacin compared with parenterel antibiotics in the treatment of osteomyelitis. Antimicrob Agents Chemother 34:40–43, 1990.

39. Dickie AS: Current concepts in the management of infections in bones and joints. Drugs 32:458–475, 1986.

40. Armstrong EP, Rush DR: Treatment of osteomyelitis. Clin Pharm 2:213–224, 1983.

41. Bach MC, Cocchetto DM: Ceftazidime as single-agent therapy for Gram-negative aerobic bacillary osteomyelitis. Antimicrob Agents Chemother 31:1605–1608, 1987.

42. Gentry LO: Antibiotic therapy for osteomyelitis. In Norden CW, (ed): Inf Dis Clin of North Am. Philadelphia: WB Saunders 4(3):499, 1990.

43. Norden CN, Fierer J, Bryant RE: Chronic staphylococcal osteomyelitis: treatment regimens containing rifampin. Rev Infect Dis 5:S495–501, 1983.

44. Dich VQ, Nelson JD, Holtelin KC: Osteomyelitis in infants and children. Am J Dis Child 129:1273–1278, 1975.

45. Wagner DK, Collier BD, Rytel MW: Long term intravenous antibiotic therapy in chronic osteomyelitis. Arch Intern Med 145:1073–1078, 1985.

46. Smego RA, Gainer BR: Home intravenous antimicrobial therapy provided by community hospital and a university hospital. Am J Hosp Pharm 42:2185–2189, 1985.

47. Fitzgerald RH: Antibiotic distribution in normal and osteomyelitic bone. Orthop Clin North Am 15:537–545, 1984.

48. Perry HP, Ritterbusch JK, Burdge RE, et al.: Cefamandole levels in serum and necrotic bone. Clin Orthop 15:537–545, 1984.

49. Marcinko DE: Gentamicin-impregnated PMMA beads: an introduction and review. J Foot Surg 424:116–121, 1985.

50. Mackey D, Vailet A, Debeaulmont D: Antibiotic loaded plaster of Paris pellets. Clin Orthop 167:263–268, 1982.

51. Herman DS: Hyperbaric oxygen therapy and its role in the treatment of chronic osteomyelitis: a preliminary report involving refractory osteomyelitis in the foot. J Foot Surg 24:293–300, 1985.

52. Mader JT, Adams KR, Wallace WR, et al.: Hyperbaric oxygen as adjunctive therapy for osteomyelitis. In Norden CW (ed): Inf Dis Clin North Am Philadelphia: W. B. Saunders, 4(3):433, 1990.

53. Fitzgerald RH, Rutle PE, Arnold PG, et al.: Local muscle flaps in the treatment of chronic osteomyelitis. J Bone Joint Surg 67:175–185, 1985.

54. Speiser JC, Moore TL, Osborn TG: Changing trends in pediatric septic arthritis. Semin Arthritis Rheum 15:132–138, 1985.

55. Shaw BA, Kasser JR: Acute septic arthritis in infancy and childhood. Clin Orthop 257:212–225, 1990.

56. Norman DC, Yoshikawa TT: Responding to septic arthritis. Geriatrics 38:83–91, 1983.

57. Inman RD, Gallegos KV, Brause BD, et al.: Clinical and microbiological features of prosthetic joint infections. Am J Med 77:47–53, 1984.

58. Freeland AE, Senter BC: Septic arthritis and osteomyelitis. Hand Clin 5:533–552, 1989.

59. Krey PR, Bailen DA: Synovial fluid leukocytosis—a study of extremes Am J Med 67:436–442, 1972.

60. LeFrock JL, Kannangara DW: Treatment of infectious arthritis. Am Fam Physican 30:252–257, 1984.

61. Anon: Sexually transmitted diseases treatment guidelines. MMWR (No 5–8):1–43, 1989.

CHAPTER 69

SEXUALLY TRANSMITTED DISEASES

MICHAEL N. DUDLEY, Pharm.D. and KATHLEEN K. GRAHAM, Pharm.D.

Sexually transmitted diseases (STDs) continue to be a major concern for public health. In the period from 1979 to 1986, more than 50 disease syndromes (excluding AIDS) accounted for over 13 million cases and 7000 deaths annually. The costs of treating pelvic inflammatory disease (a complication of gonorrhea) alone and its sequelae has been estimated to exceed 2.6 billion dollars annually.

In 1979, several objectives relating to the control of sexually transmitted diseases to be achieved by 1990 were established by the U.S. Public Health Service; some of these goals were (a) the reported incidence of gonorrhea should be 280 cases/100,000 persons; (b) the incidence of primary and secondary syphilis should be reduced to 7 cases per 100,000 persons per year; (c) the incidence of congenital syphilis should be reduced to 1.5 cases/100,000 births per year and the incidence of gonococcal pelvic inflammatory disease (PID) should be reduced to 60 cases per 100,000 women (1). It is of interest to assess the progress made toward these objectives as we enter the decade of the 1990s.

The incidence of gonorrhea increased in epidemic proportions from 1966 to 1975 from approximately 350,000 to 1 million cases/year; it then plateaued through 1981, and has gradually declined to approximately 800,000 per year (1). The decline in incidence has primarily been observed in white, middle- and upper-middle-class women and homosexual men (resulting from changes in sexual practices caused by the risk of AIDS), whereas the rate among poor urban minorities has remained stable. A factor further complicating control of the disease has been the dramatic increase in the incidence of gonorrhea due to antibiotic-resistant strains from 1985 to the present (1–3). Gonococci now account for <50% of all cases of PID; however, monitoring of all cases still indicates that the 1990 goal will be met (1).

The incidence of primary and secondary syphilis declined between 1982 and 1986. This decline followed a rapid rise occurring between 1977 and 1982 and likely represents changes in trends in homosexual activity and implementation of "safe sex" practices (1, 3). However, in 1987 there was an alarming increase in the number of reported cases (approximately a 20% increase); this increase was largely in black women and men. The incidence of congenital syphilis also increased steadily between 1982 and 1988. The recent increase in cases of primary and secondary syphilis in adults is expected to further increase the incidence of congenital syphilis (4).

These recent changes in the epidemiology of STDs indicate that only objectives related to control of gonorrhea and PID were likely to be met. However, since the formulation of the objectives, recognition and characterization of several new causative agents of STDs occurred. For example, during the 15-year period from 1966 to 1981, patient visits to private practitioners for the treatment of genital herpes infections increased ninefold; data from the United Kingdom over a similar period indicate the prevalence of the disease is increasing at a rate of 12%/year (1, 3). The high prevalence of infection is evident in all populations of society; antibody prevalence rates against the herpes simplex 2 virus have been as high as 80% in female prostitutes, 46% in homosexual men, and 25% in all of adults of middle to higher socioeconomic status (1, 5). The human immunodeficiency virus (HIV) has become recognized as a major STD, with much counseling directed to preventing transmission of this agent.

The epidemiology of another relatively new virus, the genital human papillomavirus (HPV) is similar to that of genital herpes, except its magnitude is nearly threefold higher and its key consequence is cervical dysplasia (6). This virus is most prevalent in women aged 20 to 24 years (6).

INFECTIOUS URETHRITIS

The major cause of sexually transmitted urethritis is *Neisseria gonorrhoeae*; however, urethritis due to several other pathogens is now more frequent than gonorrhea (7). Nongonococcal urethritis (NGU) is most commonly caused by the obligate intracellular parasite, *Chlamydia trachomatis*. Up to 50% of all cases of NGU are related to infection with *C. trachomatis*. The primary organism associated with chlamydia-negative NGU is *Ureaplasma urealyticum*. Other less common infectious causes of NGU include *Trichomonas vaginalis*, herpes simplex virus, *Candida albicans*, and a newly described organism, *Mycoplasma genitalum*. Postgonococcal urethritis (PGU) refers to NGU that develops 1 to 3 weeks after treatment for gonococcal urethritis in male patients. PGU is usually secondary to a dual infection with gonorrhea and one of the etiologic agents of NGU, primarily *C. trachomatis* and follows antimicrobial therapy that eradicates the gonococci but not the *Chlamydia*.

Neisseria gonorrhoeae, the causative agent of gonorrhea, is a Gram-negative diplococcus. Since the introduction of penicillin and tetracycline over 40 years ago, there has been an increase in gonococcal antimicrobial resistance in the United States. The incidence of infections due to both penicillinase-producing *N. gonorrhoeae* (PPNG) and chromosomally mediated–resistant *N. gonorrhoeae* (CMRNG) has increased steadily over the past decade. A recent survey indicated that 21% of isolates collected between 1987 and 1988 were resistant to penicillin, tetracycline, cefoxitin, or spectinomycin. These trends have recently had a major impact on antibiotic selection for the treatment of gonococcal infections.

Pathogenesis

Most cases of NGU are not associated with major morbidity and are generally limited to the genitourinary tract. However, untreated chlamydial infections can cause complications such as epididymitis, urethral strictures, salpingitis, and venerally acquired Reiter's syndrome. Proctitis in homosexual men and women who practice receptive anal intercourse is also a manifestation of infection. *Chlamydia* also is an important cause of neonatal inclusion conjunctivitis and pneumonia in infants exposed to the organism from an infected cervix. Approximately 50% of infants born to mothers with *C. trachomatis* infection of the cervix develop inclusion conjunctivitis, and 10 to 20% of infants may develop pneumonia. The onset of the conjunctivitis is during the second and third weeks of life, and the pneumonia occurs during the second and third months of life.

The symptoms of gonococcal urethritis and NGU are very much alike. However, gonorrhea tends to present abruptly, whereas NGU often has a less acute onset, with symptoms increasing over several days. Gonorrhea is also more commonly associated with a combination of urethral discharge and dysuria, whereas the appearance of one without the other is seen more frequently with NGU. In addition, the discharge of gonorrhea tends to be more purulent and that of NGU more mucoid (7).

The clinical features of gonorrhea can vary, depending on the site of inoculation, the age and sex of the patient, the duration of infection, and whether or not the disease has disseminated systemically. In heterosexual men, gonorrhea typically presents as an anterior urethritis with a spontaneous purulent urethral exudate, dysuria, and polyuria. These symptoms generally appear 2 to 7 days after exposure to an infected source. Complications such as epididymitis, prostatitis, and infection of the paraurethral glands and adjacent soft tissues are rare since the advent of antibiotic therapy. Untreated gonococcal infection may cause urethral stricture. In addition to the urethra, gonococcal infection in homosexual men may involve the anal canal and pharynx (7).

In women the clinical picture is extremely diverse. Common sites from which gonococci can be isolated include the endocervical canal, urethra, anal canal, and pharynx. Although the disease can frequently remain asymptomatic, gonorrhea in women may present as urethritis with dysuria, urgency, frequency, pyuria, and sometimes hematuria. Lower genital tract symptoms may resolve within a few weeks; however, the patient may remain an asymptomatic carrier of the organism. If the infection spreads to the upper genital tract, salpingitis can develop, which may lead to fibrosis and scarring of the fallopian tubes and result in sterility. Extension of the infection from the vagina and endocervix to the endometrium, fallopian tubes, and contiguous structures can also cause pelvic inflammatory disease (PID). PID is characterized by lower abdominal pain (usually, but not always, bilateral), cervical motion tenderness, and adnexal tenderness. Urinary symptoms may also be present in PID. In addition to *N. gonorrhoeae*, etiologic agents of PID include *C. trachomatis*, anaerobes such as *Bacteroides fragilis*, and facultative Gram-negative bacilli such as *Escherichia coli* (8).

Infants exposed to gonococci in utero, at birth, or during the postpartum period may develop gonococcal ophthalmia neonatorum, a destructive conjunctivitis that was a common cause of blindness before the introduction of antibiotics. Infants may also develop systemic illness such as septicemia or arthritis.

Disseminated gonococcal disease is the leading cause of acute septic arthritis in adults. Initially the illness is characterized by polyarticular arthralgias and skin lesions. The disease is more common in women and often occurs at the first menstruation following local infection. Because of antibiotics, other complications of disseminated gonococcal disease such as endocarditis, meningitis, and perihepititis are now relatively uncommon.

Diagnosis

One cannot accurately distinguish between NGU and gonorrhea solely on clinical grounds. In addition, the two pathogens most commonly associated with NGU (*C. trachomatis* and *U. urealyticum*) cannot be cultured by routine laboratory procedures. Consequently, the diagnosis of NGU has traditionally been one of exclusion and is based on the absence of typical intracellular Gram-negative diplococci on Gram stain of the patient's urethral discharge that has evidence of urethritis (four or more polymorphonuclear leukocytes). Recently, test kits have become available to detect *C. trachomatis* without requiring cell culture.

The Gram stain of urethral or endocervical exudate is considered diagnostic of gonorrhea when the characteristic Gram-negative diplococci are seen within leukocytes. The specificity and sensitivity of these findings in men exceeds 90% (9). However, the sensitivity of microscopic examination in women is only 65%, making it more difficult to establish a diagnosis (10). The results of Gram stains of cervical discharge are often negative when the cultures are positive, and nearly 20% of the smears interpreted as positive do not have corresponding positive cultures. Therefore, to confirm the diagnosis in men and to establish it in women, cultures for *N. gonorrhoeae* are necessary. A modified Thayer-Martin (MTM) medium is the most useful for culturing the gonococcus from areas that are colonized by mixed bacterial flora, such as the endocervix, rectum, and pharynx. MTM medium contains antibiotics that selectively inhibit most other organisms. In all women and in homosexual men suspected of being infected with *N. gonorrhoeae*, it is also suggested that cultures be obtained from the rectum because this may be the only site from which the organism is recovered.

Treatment

Recent guidelines for the treatment of NGU and gonococcal infections are predicated on the prevalence of infections caused by *C. trachomatis*, the increase in resistant strains of *N. gonorrhoeae*, and the availability of new antimicrobials. Table 69.1 summarizes the current Centers for Disease Control (CDC) recommendations (11).

NONGONOCOCCAL URETHRITIS

Chlamydia trachomatis and *U. urealyticum*, the most common pathogens associated with NGU are both sensitive to tetracycline and erythromycin; *C. trachomatis* is also susceptible to sulfonamides. Because it is difficult to routinely distinguish between these two organisms, an antimicrobial regimen effective against both *C. trachomatis* and *U. urealyticum* should be used for the treatment of NGU. Therefore, either oral doxycycline (100 mg twice daily) or tetracycline (500 mg, 4 times daily for 7 days). Acceptable alternatives are erythromycin base or ethylsuccinate, and ofloxacin 400 mg b.i.d. Ciprofloxacin in doses as high as 2 g per day is inferior to doxycycline (12). Erythromycin, (not the estolate, since hepatotoxicity may occur) and not tetracycline, should be used in pregnant women, and in children who are 8 years old or younger. To reduce the risk of reinfection, concurrent treatment of sexual partners is suggested. If the patient's signs and symptoms of urethritis do not improve after adequate treatment of them and their partners, further investigation to rule out less common causes of NGU, such as tetracycline-resistant *U. urealyticum*, is warranted. Oral erythromycin syrup (50 mg/kg/day in four divided doses) should be used to treat chlamydial conjunctivitis of the newborn and chlamydial pneumonia of infancy. Therapy should be continued for 2 weeks. Also, parents of newborn infants with chlamydial infection should be treated with a tetracycline or erythromycin regimen recommended for adults.

GONORRHEA

There are three important considerations in the treatment of most forms of gonorrhea: (*a*) the possibility of a coexisting chlamydial infection (which has been documented in up to 45% of gonorrhea cases when adequate tissue cultures are performed) (11); (*b*) the increase in penicillin/tetracycline-resistant *N. gonorrhoeae*; and (*c*) patient compliance, which may be a problem with multiple-day tetracycline/doxycycline regimens formerly recommended for the treatment of *N. gonorrhoeae*. Consequently, the revised CDC STD Treatment Guidelines recommend for treatment of uncomplicated gonorrhea that a single dose, 250 mg i.m. of ceftriaxone be administered with a 7-day course of doxycycline therapy for *Chlamydia*. Alternatives for patients who cannot take ceftriaxone include spectinomycin 2 g i.m. as a single dose and ciprofloxacin 500 mg orally once (both regimens followed by a 7-day course of doxycycline). Quinolones are contraindicated during pregnancy and in children 16 years old or younger. Spectinomycin should not be administered for the treatment of pharyngeal gonorrhea because of the risk of treatment failure. Amoxicillin is no longer recommended for treatment of gonococcal infections, unless the infecting organism is proven to be penicillin-sensitive (11).

Patients with disseminated gonococcal infection (arthritis/dermatitis) should be hospitalized and should receive ceftriaxone 1 g i.m. or IV every 24 hr or spectinomycin 2 g i.m. every 12 hr until symptoms resolve; then they may be discharged on oral therapy (i.e., cefuroxime axetil 500 mg twice daily) to complete 1 week of therapy (11). Following culture and sensitivity testing, patients with documented penicillin-sensitive *N. gonorrhoeae* may complete therapy with ampicillin 1 g every 6 hr IV followed by oral amoxicillin.

The pharmacokinetic determinants for a cure by penicillin of gonococcal urethritis have been published by Jaffe et al. (13). Their studies of experimentally induced gonococcal urethritis in volunteer male prisoners demonstrated that a cure by penicillin was best predicted by regimens that produced serum penicillin concentrations that remained three to four times the minimum inhibitory concentration of *N. gonorrhoeae* to penicillin for 7 to 10 hr. Therefore, long-acting forms of penicillin (such as benzathine penicillin G) should not be used in the treatment of penicillin-sensitive gonorrhea, since adequate serum concentrations cannot be achieved. In addition, parenteral first-generation cephalosporins have not been shown to be efficacious in the treatment of *N. gonorrhoeae*. Second- and third-generation parenteral cephalosporins such as cefoxitin, cefuroxime, cefotaxime, cefonicid, and ceftizoxime are more active than first-generation cephalosporins against *N. gonorrhoeae*. In addition, the monobactams such as aztreonam are relatively stable to the action of many lactamases (14). Although these agents appear to be equally effective for most penicillin-resistant gonococcal infections, both in vitro and in vivo, clinical studies have demonstrated that increased penicillin resistance in

Table 69.1.

Recommended Drug Regimens for the Treatment of Gonorrhea, Nongonococcal Urethritis, and Chlamydial Infections[a,b]

Diagnosis	Drugs	Dose	Route	Regimen	Alternatives/Comments
NGU	Doxycycline or	100 mg	p.o.	Twice daily for 7 days	Erythromycin base or stearate 500 mg orally (or ethylsuccinate 800 mg orally) 4 times a day for 7 days; suggested in pregnancy and children 8 years old and younger
	Tetracycline	500 mg	p.o.	4 times a day for 7 days	
LGV	Doxycycline or	100 mg	p.o.	21 days	
	Tetracycline	500 mg	p.o.	21 days	
Neonatal chlamydial conjunctivitis or pneumonia	Erythromycin syrup	50 mg/kg/day	p.o.	Given in 4 divided doses for 14 days	Therapy should be continued for an additional 1–2 weeks if inclusion conjunctivitis recurs after stopping therapy
Uncomplicated gonorrhea[c]	Ceftriaxone	250 mg	i.m.	Single dose	Spectinomycin 2 g × 1 can be given for significant penicillin allergy; it should not be administered for pharyngeal gonorrhea due to risk of treatment failure
	Ciprofloxacin[d]	500 mg	p.o.	Single dose	Quinolones are contraindicated in pregnancy and in children 16 years old or younger
	Cefuroxime axetil	1 g	p.o.	Single dose	
Proven penicillin-sensitive	Amoxicillin	3 g	p.o.	Single dose with 1 g probenecid	
Disseminated gonorrhea[c]	Ceftriaxone or	1 g	i.m. or IV	Once a day	24–48 hr after all symptoms resolve may complete 7-day course with oral cefuroxime axetil 500 mg 2 times a day or Augmentin 500 mg 3 times a day or if not pregnant ciprofloxacin 500 mg 2 times a day; spectinomycin 2 g i.m. twice daily is an alternative in patients with a significant penicillin allergy
	Ceftizoxime or	1 g	IV	3 times daily	
	Cefotaxime	1 g	IV	3 times daily	
Proven penicillin-sensitive	Ampicillin	1 g	IV	4 times daily	24–48 hr after all symptoms resolve may complete 7-day course with oral amoxicillin 500 mg 3 times a day.
PID (hospitalized patient)	Doxycycline	100 mg	IV	Twice daily (for at least 2 days, then continue same dose orally to complete 10–14 days total therapy	Many specialists recommend all patients be hospitalized; because compliance is unpredictable, special consideration should be given to hospitalizing adolescents; all parenteral regimens should be given for 48 hr after patient improves, then oral treatment can be continued for a total of a 10- to 14-day course
	plus Cefoxitin or	2.0 g	IV	4 times daily for at least 2 days	
	Cefotetan or	2.0 g	IV	2 times daily for at least 2 days	
	Clindamycin	900 mg	IV	3 times daily for at least 2 days can continue 450 mg orally 5 times daily to complete 10–14 days total therapy.	
	plus gentamicin	2.0 mg/kg followed by 1.5 mg/kg	IV	Maintenance dose given every 8 hr for at least 2 days in patients with normal renal function	
PID (outpatient)	Cefoxitin or	2.0 g	i.m.	Single dose with 1.0 g probenecid	
	Ceftriaxone each followed by	250 mg	i.m.	Single dose	Tetracycline 500 mg 4 times a day orally may be substituted for doxycycline but is less active against certain anaerobes
	doxycycline	100 mg	p.o.	Twice daily for 10–14 days	
Gonococcal ophthalmia neonatorum	Ceftriaxone	50 mg/kg	IV or i.m.	Single dose	Not to exceed 125 mg; caution in hyperbilirubinemic infants, especially premature *infants*

[a] Adapted from 1989 STD Treatment Guidelines. MMWR 38(S-8):1, 1989.

[b] Abbreviations: PID, pelvic inflammatory disease; NGU, nongonococcal urethritis.

[c] Except for homosexual men, patients should also receive 7 days of tetracycline, doxycycline, or erythromycin therapy as outlined under NGU because of possible coexistent chlamydial infection.

[d] Other quinolones including norfloxacin 800 mg, ofloxacin 400 mg are also effective.

CMRNG may correlate with increased resistance to second- and third-generation cephalosporins as well as tetracycline. Consequently, close monitoring of clinical outcomes and surveillance of in vitro resistance is necessary to evaluate these agents in the treatment of gonorrhea.

Other agents that are being studied for the treatment of PPNG infections include compounds such as clavulanic acid and sulbactam, which inhibit β-lactamases by irreversible binding of β-lactam enzymes and act synergistically against PPNG when combined with penicillin or ampicillin (15, 16). However, in vitro studies indicate that these agents do not exert an important effect on non-PPNG (CMRNG).

The quinolone derivatives such as oral norfloxacin, ciprofloxacin, and ofloxacin have been used successfully in the treatment of uncomplicated gonorrhea due to PPNG (17–19). However, neither *C. trachomatis* or *U. urealyticum* are susceptible to norfloxacin, and chlamydial infections have not responded as well to ciprofloxacin therapy, even in doses as high as 2 g daily (12, 20). Ofloxacin in contrast is active against both PPNG and chlamydia and has received FDA approval for both indications. Ofloxacin may be considered a single-drug alternative to ceftriaxone and doxycline for patients who cannot tolerate penicillin, tetracycline, or erythromycin. For acute uncomplicated gonorrhea, ofloxacin 400 mg is recommended as a single dose, and for cervicitis/urethritis due to *C. trachomatis* and *N. gonorrhoeae*, ofloxacin 300 mg twice daily is recommended for 7 days.

Because treatment failure of ceftriaxone/doxycycline is rare, a follow-up culture ("test-of-cure") following this regimen is not essential. Because there is less long-term experience with the newer alternative agents, such as the quinolones, it is recommended that follow-up cultures be obtained 4 to 7 days after therapy. Infection that occurs after a course of treatment is most often reinfection rather than treatment failure, which indicates a need for improved sex-partner referral and patient education (11). All patients who are being treated for gonorrhea should also be tested for syphilis and should be offered confidential counseling and testing for HIV infection (11). Patients who are seronegative and without any clinical signs of syphilis ("incubating syphilis") will most likely be cured by any of the above regimens except spectinomycin and the quinolones. Patients who have documented syphilis should be treated appropriately for the disease, as described in the next section, in addition to treatment for gonorrhea.

PELVIC INFLAMMATORY DISEASE

The treatment of choice for PID is not clearly established, because no one agent is active against the numerous pathogens (i.e., *N. gonorrhoeae*, *C. trachomatis*, aerobic Gram-negative rods, anaerobes, group B streptococci, and mycoplasmas) associated with this syndrome.

The major goal of antibiotic therapy is to prevent sterility. Hospitalization is recommended when at all possible, particularly if the diagnosis is uncertain, the patient is unstable or adolescent, or has not responded to outpatient therapy, or is expected not to be able to comply with a 72-hr follow-up. For hospitalized patients, a combination of doxycycline (100 mg intravenously twice daily) plus cefoxitin (2 g intravenously, four times daily) or cefotetan 2 g IV every 12 hr should be used for at least 4 days, and at least 48 hr after the patient improves. Doxycycline may then be continued orally (100 mg twice daily) for a total of 10 to 14 days of therapy. As an alternative regimen, a combination of intravenous clindamycin (600 mg, four times daily) and gentamicin or tobramycin (2 mg/kg followed by 1.5 mg/kg every 8 hr in patients with normal renal function) should be administered. After at least 4 days and at least 48 hr after the patient improves, intravenous therapy can be stopped and oral clindamycin (450 mg, four times daily) continued to complete 10 to 14 days of therapy. For ambulatory patients, an initial one-time dose of cefoxitin (2 g intramuscularly), should be administered in combination with a 1-g dose of oral probenecid. Alternatively, a single dose of ceftriaxone (250 mg intramuscularly) is also appropriate and does not require concurrent probenecid. After an initial dose with any of these regimens, therapy should be continued with oral doxycycline (100 gm twice daily) for a total of 10 to 14 days. Although tetracycline may be used, doxycycline is more active against certain anaerobes and is the preferred agent. Treatment with penicillin, ampicillin, amoxicillin, or a cephalosporin alone is not recommended. All male sex partners of patients with PID should be examined for sexually transmitted organisms and treated with a regimen effective against both uncomplicated gonococcal and chlamydial infection. Removal of an intrauterine device (IUD) is recommended soon after the initiation of antimicrobial therapy, although the exact effect of removal on the acute response is not known (11).

OPHTHALMIA NEONATORUM

Gonococcal ophthalmia is a potentially serious infection that may cause blindness as well as systemic gonococcal disease. Consequently instillation of a prophylactic agent into the eye is recommended for all infants, regardless of the method of delivery. The most common method of prophylaxis for years was instilling 1% silver nitrate drops into the conjunctival sac of each eye immediately after birth. However, since silver nitrate can cause a chemical conjunctivitis and does not prevent chlamydial disease, either erythromycin (0.5%) or tetracycline (1%) ophthalmic ointment can be instilled as an alternative. All three regimens are equally effective, although there is a 2% failure rate. Therefore, full-term infants born to women with untreated gonorrhea should receive a single i.m. or IV injection of ceftriaxone 50 mg/kg not to exceed 125 mg. Infants with documented gonococcal ophthalmia require hospitalization and systemic antibiotic therapy. Ceftriaxone 25 to 50 mg/kg/day IV or i.m. as a single dose should be given for 7 days (11). Topical antibiotic preparations are not required if appropriate parenteral therapy is given. Patients who fail to respond to therapy may have a simultaneous infection with *C. trachomatis*.

SYPHILIS

Syphilis is a complex systemic illness caused by the spirochete *Treponema pallidum* (21–23). Humans are the only natural hosts of the organism. Although almost always contracted sexually, syphilis may develop as a congenital infection contracted in utero, through nonsexual personal contact, or rarely from blood transfusions, since *T. pallidum* cannot survive more than 48 hr under conditions of blood-bank storage. The organism is readily killed by numerous physical and chemical disinfecting agents, including heat, desiccation, soaps, and detergents.

Pathogenesis

Syphilis is transmitted by direct contact with an active lesion, which is often teeming with spirochetes. The concentration of organisms in lesions is approximately $10^7/g$ of tissue. The spirochete penetrates intact epithelium or abraded skin, from where it enters local lymphatics and the bloodstream. Almost any organ in the body can be invaded, including the central nervous system. Although *T. pallidum* is present systemically within hours of exposure, initially there is no clinical or serologic evidence of disease. The incubation period may range from 3 to 90 days, during which time the patient is asymptomatic and noninfectious. Spirochetes multiply at the site of inoculation and clinical lesions are formed.

Primary Syphilis. The first clinical sign, or primary stage of syphilis, is the development of a chancre at the site of treponemal inoculation approximately 3 weeks after initial exposure. Chancres are usually located on external genitalia, where they are painless unless secondarily infected. Lesions in the anal canal and perianal area have been noted more frequently in homosexual males. Genital chancres in women can be missed because of their location in the vagina or on the cervix, where they may resemble a cervical erosion or even an ulcerating carcinoma. Chancres usually heal spontaneously within 2 to 6 weeks.

Secondary Syphilis. The secondary stage of syphilis develops around 2 to 12 weeks after contact. Most organs of the body can be involved, but the diagnosis is often suggested by lesions on the skin and mucous membranes. The dermatologic manifestations usually begin on the trunk and proximal extremities as pink macular lesions. Macules and papules are also often found on the palms of the hand

and soles of the feet. Lesions can develop on mucous membranes such as the lips, oral cavity, and glans penis. These lesions are painless, slightly raised gray plaques surrounded by a red periphery and are highly infectious. Systemic manifestations of secondary syphilis include fever, headache, anorexia, malaise, and a generalized lymphadenopathy.

Latent Syphilis. Untreated disease will progress to a phase during which there are no clinical manifestations, known as latent syphilis. Early latent syphilis is the period within the first 4 years following infection during which relapse of symptoms associated with earlier stages of the disease may occur, and the patient is considered infectious. Mucocutaneous relapses are the most common form. After this time, in the late latent phase, relapse seldom occurs and the patient is considered to be noninfectious. However, during this late-latent phase, a pregnant woman can infect her fetus in utero, and an infection can also be transmitted by blood transfusions. The latent stage of syphilis may extend for the patient's lifetime or be followed up by late, or tertiary syphilis. Late syphilis can affect a variety of organ systems, including the cardiovascular system, skin and skeletal structures, and the central nervous system.

Neurosyphilis. Asymptomatic neurosyphilis occurs in 10 to 30% of untreated patients. These patients have no clinical signs of neurosyphilis but do have one or more cerebrospinal fluid (CSF) abnormalities, including pleocytosis, elevated protein level, decreased glucose concentration, or a positive nontreponemal antigen test. Treatment of asymptomatic neurosyphilis can prevent symptomatic disease.

The clinical manifestations of symptomatic neurosyphilis can take a variety of forms. Meningovascular syphilis is an inflammatory process that becomes clinically evident 10 years after the initial infection. It may present as a stroke in younger individuals, producing hemiparesis, aphasia, and visual disturbances. Both generalized and focal seizures can also occur. Appropriate therapy will halt progression of the condition. Parenchymatous neurosyphilis is a degenerative disorder that includes general paresis and tabes dorsalis. Both generally occur 15 to 20 years after primary infection. General paresis, now uncommon, presents clinically as dementia, manifested by memory loss, speaking defects, impaired judgment, and rarely, delusions. If untreated, paresis progresses to paralysis and further mental and physical deterioration. Death occurs within 3 to 4 years. Tabes dorsalis (locomotor ataxia) is characterized by ataxia with a wide-based gait, bladder disturbances, impotence, and "lighting" (sharp, jabbing) pains, usually in the legs. Although uncommon, optic atrophy may occur and often accompanies tabes. Without treatment, the condition leads to progressive blindness.

Late Syphilis. In late syphilis, aortitis with aortic insufficiency affects the thoracic aorta, and occasionally its branches. The disease does not become evident clinically until 10 years or more after the primary infection. Aneurysms may develop and rupture into the pericardium, pleural space, or bronchial tree. Antibiotic therapy has made caradiovascular syphilis an extremely rare entity in the United States.

Late benign syphilis is characterized by a gumma that develops 3 to 7 years after initial infection. Gummas are granulomatous lesions that usually arise in the skeletal system, skin, and mucocutaneous tissues. They can also develop in organs such as the stomach, liver, heart, and brain. Gummas respond dramatically to appropriate antibiotic therapy.

Congenital Syphilis. Infection of the fetus in utero can occur in any untreated pregnant woman but is most likely to occur in the early stages of infection. Treatment of the mother during the first 4 months of pregnancy greatly reduces the risk that the fetus will be infected. Infection can result in late abortion, stillbirth, neonatal death, neonatal disease, or latent infection.

Early congenital syphilis is often manifested by a rhinitis, which is followed by a diffuse maculopapular rash with widespread sloughing of the epithelium. There may be a generalized osteochondritis and perichondritis that could lead to areas of bone destruction. The liver is often involved. Neonatal death is usually secondary to liver failure, pneumonia, or pulmonary hemorrhage. Congenital syphilis may progress to a latent phase if the untreated child survives. It can occur as late as 30 years after birth, with optic atrophy and eighth nerve deafness. Other later characteristics of latent congenital syphilis include arthropathy and bilateral knee effusions, as well as noted, widely spread peg-shaped upper central incisors (Hutchinsons's teeth). Neurosyphilis may also develop.

Syphilis in HIV-infected Patients. Recent surveys suggest that HIV-infected patients with syphilis may present difficulties in diagnosis and have a different course of the disease, and that standard treatment may be inadequate. Neurosyphilis has been reported to occur earlier, as well as after treatment with standard doses of benazthine penicillin G (see below) (24). Other unusual complications including early gumma formation, ophthalmologic involvement, and other sequelae have been reported (24). There is some evidence that there may be an altered serologic response to treatment (24). Currently, the CDC has no separate guidelines for management of infection in these patients.

Diagnosis

Darkfield microscopic examination of material from chancres, condyloma, or mucous patches for organisms with the characteristic morphology and motility of *T. pallidum* is the most direct method for establishing the diagnosis of the early stages of syphilis. Darkfield examination of ma-

terial from the oral cavity is less reliable, since *T. microdentium*, a nonpathogenic spirochete found in normal mouth flora, is morphologically indistinguishable from *T. pallidum*.

Two types of serologic tests are used for the diagnosis of syphilis. One group of tests measures the nonspecific antibody directed against tissue-treponemal proteins (reagin) and are termed nontreponemal tests. The other type of tests measures the specific antitreponemal antibody. The most common antitreponemal antibody test performed is the FTA-abs (fluorescent treponemal antibody absorbent test). The principle use of this test is in confirming the diagnosis of syphilis. Although it has long been felt that the FTA-abs remained positive for life in a patient, recent study shows that up to one-fourth of patients may have nonreactive FTA-abs tests by 36 months after treatment (25). However, the FTA-abs test is not helpful in assessing the acute response to therapy.

The Venereal Disease Research Laboratory (VDRL) slide flocculation test and rapid plasma reagin (RPR) agglutination test are commonly used nontreponemal reaginic tests. In contrast to the FTA-abs test, these tests measure serum reagin titers and thus can be used to evaluate therapy. Titers should become nonreactive within 1 year after treatment for primary syphilis and within 2 years after treatment of secondary syphilis. Most patients with late syphilis should have a negative test by the fifth year after therapy. Titer response does not appear to be affected by sex, age, race, or sexual orientation (25).

Treatment

Parenteral penicillin G still remains the treatment of choice for all stages of syphilis (Table 69.2). Patients with early syphilis (primary, secondary, or latent syphilis of less than 1-year duration) should receive a single intramuscular dose of benzathine penicillin G, 2.4 million units. For patients who are allergic to penicillin, oral tetracycline (500 mg, four times a day) for 15 days is recommended. A similar regimen of oral erythromycin should be administered to patients who cannot tolerate tetracycline. The efficacy of other β-lactam, fluoroquinolone, or macrolide antibiotics has not been established.

Tetracycline should not be given to pregnant women. Pregnant patients who are allergic to penicillin should be given erythromycin in doses appropriate for the stage of syphilis as recommended for nonpregnant patients (Table 69.2). Infants born to mothers treated with erythromycin during pregnancy for early syphilis should be treated with penicillin.

For syphilis of more than 1-year duration (late benign syphilis, cardiovascular syphilis), 2.4 million units of benzathine penicillin given intramuscularly once a week for 3 successive weeks is the regimen of choice. Patients allergic to penicillin should be treated with oral tetracycline or

Table 69.2.
Recommended Drug Regimens for the Treatment of Syphilis[a]

Diagnosis	Drugs	Dose	Route	Regimen	Alternatives/Comments
Early syphilis (primary, secondary, and latent syphilis of <1-year duration)	Benzathine penicillin G	2.4 million units	i.m.	Single dose	For penicillin-allergic patients: tetracycline 500 mg orally, 4 times daily for 15 days; erythromycin 500 mg orally, 4 times daily for 15 days, may be given to patients who cannot tolerate tetracycline, or patients who are pregnant and have a documented penicillin allergy
Late syphilis (latent syphilis of >1-year duration, cardiovascular syphilis)	Benzathine penicillin G	2.4 million units	i.m.	Once weekly for 3 weeks	For penicillin-allergic patients; tetracycline 500 mg orally, 4 times daily for 30 days; erythromycin 500 mg orally, 4 times daily for 30 days, may be given to patients who cannot tolerate tetracycline, or patients who are pregnant and have a documented penicillin allergy
Neurosyphilis	Aqueous crystalline penicillin G followed by benzathine	12–24 million units/ day	IV	2–4 million units every 4 hr for 10 days	Regimens employing benzathine penicillin in standard doses or APPG in doses less than 2.4 million units/day do not consistently provide treponemicidal levels of penicillin in the CSF
	penicillin G or	2.4 million units	i.m.	Once weekly for 3 weeks	
	APPG followed by benzathine penicillin G or	2.4 million units	i.m.	Once daily with probenecid (500 mg, 4 times daily) for 10 days	
	Benzathine penicillin G	2.4 million units	i.m.	Once weekly for 3 weeks	
		2.4 million units	i.m.	Once weekly for 3 weeks	
Congenital syphilis	Aqueous crystalline penicillin G or	50,000 units/kg/day	IV/i.m.	Divided in 2 doses for minimum of 10 days	Asymptomatic infants with normal CSF findings may be treated with a single dose of benzathine penicillin, 50,000 units/kg i.m.
	APPG	50,000 units/kg/day	i.m.	Daily for minimum of 10 days	

[a] Adapted from Anon: 1989 STD treatment guidelines. MMWR 38(S-8):1, 1989.

erythromycin in daily doses recommended for early syphilis, but should continue therapy for a total of 30 days.

The CDC currently recommends three potentially effective regimens for the treatment of neurosyphilis, including the same benzathine penicillin dosage schedule suggested for syphilis of more than 1-year duration (11, 24). However, regimens employing benzathine penicillin or aqueous procaine penicillin G (APPG) in daily doses of less than 2.4 million units do not consistently produce tre-

ponemicidal levels of penicillin in the CSF, and treatment failures have been reported. Therefore therapy with intravenous aqueous crystalline penicillin G (2 to 4 million units every 4 hr for 10 days) should precede the benzathine penicillin regimen. Alternatively, a 10-day course of APPG (2.4 million units intramuscularly daily) plus oral probenecid (500 mg, four times a day) may be given before administering the benzathine penicillin.

If the mother has been adequately treated with a penicillin regimen during pregnancy, the risk of congenital syphilis is small, and treatment is not necessary if follow-up can be ensured. If not, and the infant is asymptomatic, a single intramuscular dose of benzathine penicillin should be administered. However, if neurosyphilis cannot be excluded, a regimen of either aqueous crystalline penicillin G (50,000 units/kg intramuscularly or intravenously daily in two divided doses) or APPG (50,000 units/kg intramuscularly daily) should be administered for a minimum of 10 days.

The Jarisch-Herxheimer reaction is a systemic reaction occurring within a few hours of antibiotic therapy, especially with penicillin. It is a self-limiting condition that usually lasts for 12 to 24 hr and consists of fever, chills, myalgias, hypotension, and sore throat. The reaction is more common in patients treated for secondary syphilis, where the intensity of the mucocutaneous lesions may increase. The reaction is not an allergic reaction to penicillin, but is believed to be associated with release of an endotoxin or a nonendotoxin heat-stable pyrogen from the spirochetes (26). Symptoms resolve spontaneously but may be managed with antipyretics.

LYMPHOGRANULOMA VENEREUM

Lymphogranuloma venereum (LGV) is caused by *C. trachomatis*, the same organism responsible for the majority of cases of nongonococcal urethritis. Only *C. trachomatis* serotypes L_1, L_2, and L_3 produce LGV; these serotypes have been shown to be more invasive in animal models than in humans. Infection is usually acquired by sexual exposure, but laboratory or formite transmission is possible.

Clinical Presentation

LGV resembles syphilis in that infection may occur in three stages. Three days to 3 weeks after exposure, a 2 to 3-mm evanescent vesicle appears at the site of inoculation. In men, the primary lesion is usually found on the penis. The primary lesion may be found in the vagina, cervix, or labia of women. This lesion is painless and usually resolves within 2 to 3 days. The transient, nonthreatening nature of the lesion rarely results in patients seeking medical assistance; this lesion is noted in only 24 to 40% of cases, mostly men. The secondary stage of LGV usually presents 2 to 6 weeks after exposure. From the site of initial inoculation, organisms spread to the regional lymph nodes through lymphatic channels. Penile infection results in the development of enlarged, painful inguinal lymph nodes (bubo). Unilateral bubo formation is usually seen, but up to one-third of patients may have bilateral disease. Lymphadenopathy is usually painful, resulting in the patient seeking medical assistance. The location of lymphadenopathy in women depends on whether the primary lesion is

drained by lymphatics to the inguinal, obturator, iliac, or deep iliac lymph nodes. Patients may be systemically ill with fevers, chills, myalgias, arthralgias, and gastrointestinal complaints. Laboratory studies show an elevated or normal white blood cell count, elevated erythrocyte sedimentation rate (ESR), and occasionally elevated liver function test results. When left untreated, infection may progress to involve the entire chain of lymph nodes. These nodes may eventually coalesce to form large, fluctuant, suppurative masses. The areas may enlarge and rupture spontaneously, forming multiple fistulous tracts.

Late complications of untreated LGV include progressive, infiltrative and ulcerative lesions of the genitalia. Fibrosis and scarring may occlude lymph drainage, resulting in the formation of lymphorrhoids or genital elephantiasis.

Up to 25% of patients with LGV present with anorectal complaints, particularly women and homosexual men. These patients complain of a rectal discharge of blood, mucus, and pus; rectal pain may be present or absent initially. Rectal strictures with accompanying constipation or tenesmus develop in many patients.

Diagnosis

LGV must be differentiated from genital herpes, syphilis, and chancroid. The diagnosis of LGV in men is usually based upon the clinical presentation of inguinal adenopathy. LGV is less easily diagnosed in women. Isolation of *C. trachomatis* from aspirated bubo pus is possible in approximately 30% of cases when there is clinical and serologic evidence of LGV. Culturing the organism requires special techniques not routinely available in most laboratories. Detection of antichlamydial antibody by microimmunofluorescence (MIF) or enzyme-linked immunosorbent assay (ELISA) appears to be sensitive and more specific than the CF test.

Treatment

There have been no significant advances in the treatment of LGV during the past 3 decades. Management of LGV includes antimicrobial therapy against *C. trachomatis*, and when indicated, surgery for drainage of the buboes or complications due to chronic infections. Fluctuant buboes should be aspirated periodically to prevent spontaneous rupture and fistula formation. Incision and drainage are unnecessary and are discouraged because of the possible formation of sinus tracts.

The impact of antimicrobial chemotherapy on the course of LGV is poorly studied. Most authors claim that all patients "get better" with whatever drug they use. Since the growth cycle of chlamydia is approximately 48 hr, prolonged antimicrobial therapy would be expected to be necessary for clinical response. Response to antimicrobial therapy in the early inguinal phase appears to be better than the response of chronic infections. Antimicrobial therapy probably has the greatest effect on the relief of constitutional symptoms.

A course of oral tetracycline 500 mg, four times daily for at least 2 weeks, is recommended for therapy (11). Alternative agents that would be expected to be effective but have not undergone clinical study include doxycycline (100 mg twice a day), erythromycin (500 mg four times daily), or sulfamethoxazole (1 g twice daily). Multiple courses may be necessary in chronic or complicated cases. The development of buboes at another site or an increase in the size of existing undrained buboes shortly after initiating antimicrobial therapy does not connote antibiotic failure. Response to therapy is usually evaluated by the patient's clinical response. Serial CF titers are not reliable as a monitoring parameter.

HERPES GENITALIS

The herpes simplex virus (HSV), is a double-stranded DNA virus belonging to the Herpetoviridae family of viruses. In the past, herpesviruses have been separated based on clinical and epidemiologic patterns, although certain biochemical differences exist. Herpes simplex type 1 (HSV-1) is usually associated with infection "above the waist" (i.e., labialis, keratitis, and encephalitis in adults), and herpes simplex type 2 (HSV-2) is usually associated with infections "below the waist" acquired through genital contact. Oral-genital contact has likely contributed to the increasing incidence of oral HSV-2 and genital HSV-1 infections.

Pathogenesis

Genital herpes infections are usually acquired through contact with an infected symptomatic lesion, although the virus can be excreted by asymptomatic individuals. After inoculation, the virus replicates locally in epithelial cells, resulting in cell lysis and an inflammatory response. When the virus is acquired via genital contact, it ascends intra-axonally through peripheral nerves to sacral ganglia. Here the virus remains repressed until reactivated. Recurrence occurs when the virus becomes reactivated and replicates within the ganglia. Newly formed virus then migrates through an intra-axonal pathway to nerve endings to form new lesions (5).

The risk of development of genital herpes in a woman following exposure to an infected man has been estimated to be greater than 80% (27). After exposure to the virus, an incubation period of 2 to 20 days (mean approximately 6 days) precedes the onset of symptoms (5, 27, 28). The first occurrence of genital herpes infections may be described as primary or nonprimary. A patient has a primary genital infection when there is no previous history of any infection by HSV. Nonprimary herpes genital infection occurs when a patient has no previous history of genital HSV infection, but has had a prior HSV infection at another site (i.e., labialis, keratitis). The distinction between primary and nonprimary infection is important, since prior HSV-1 exposure (i.e., labialis) may prevent the acquisition of symptomatic genital HSV-1 infection, but further data are required (5). However, it is not known whether prior HSV-1 exposure prevents HSV-2 disease.

Signs and Symptoms

Prior to the appearance of herpetic lesions, patients may experience local prodromal syndromes of mild aching, itching, paresthesia, or burning at the affected site. Following these symptoms, erythema (without induration) ensues with the development of papules, and ultimately, 1- to 2-mm vesicles. These vesicles may number as many as 20 in primary infections. In men, these lesions are usually found on the penile shaft or glans of the penis. Women may have lesions on the lower legs, thighs, vulva, perineum, buttocks, cervix, or vagina. These vesicles eventually rupture, forming erosions that crust over and heal. The time to healing of initial primary lesions is usually 2 to 3 weeks but they may persist for up to 6 weeks (5, 28, 29). The time for healing is generally shorter in men than women (approximately 3 days less). Pain and excretion of virus lasts for approximately 11 days (5, 28). Other symptoms may include urethral or vaginal discharge, perianal pain, or dysuria. These symptoms tend to be of shorter duration (10 to 14 days) (5, 28, 29).

Primary perianal and anal infection with HSV-2 has been reported, particularly in homosexual men and heterosexual women who engage in anorectal intercourse. Symptoms include rectal pain, tenesmus, itching, constipation, and rectal discharge.

Studies have shown that initial genital herpes infection in patients with previous HSV infection (usually due to HSV-1) are milder, with more rapid resolution of symptoms and lesions than is observed in patients with no history of prior HSV infection (5). Following the initial genital infection, virus is shed for approximately 10 days; however, the duration of viral shedding has been shown to vary from 3 to 33 days, depending on the frequency of follow-up cultures.

One of the most intriguing yet frustrating aspects of genital HSV infection is the tendency for recurrence in nearly all patients. In men, more than two-thirds of all cases recur within the first year after initial presentation (5). One study reported that recurrence in women was lower than that in men; however, some recurrences may occur on the cervix and are asymptomatic, thereby going undetected. Recurrence is more likely and frequent in patients with genital infections due to HSV-2. Various factors have been implicated as causes for recurrence, including fever, emotional or physical stress, trauma, increased sexual activity, and menstruation. Studies in animal models of herpes infections have identified ultraviolet light, immunosuppression, and trauma to infected ganglia as precipitating factors (5). Prospective studies of newly infected patients over 3 years failed to show a decrease in the frequency of recurrence.

Recurrent genital herpes lesions tend to develop in the vicinity of the initial infections. Patients experience a prodrome similar to that of the first infection. The important difference between initial and recurrent infection is that the course of recurrent HSV infection is milder and of shorter duration. The duration of pain averaged 4 to 5 days. Herpetic lesions tend to be less numerous, and most heal in approximately 10 days. The virus is shed from recurrent lesions for only 3 to 4 days; it has been suggested that all recurrent lesions are culture-negative after 10 days (5).

There is considerable controversy about the association of genital HSV infection and neoplasms of the female genital tract. Although many studies are fraught with methodologic problems, several available retrospective studies have suggested that genital HSV infection may be involved in the later development of cervical cancer. Some studies have demonstrated HSV-2 DNA-binding proteins within the cells of lesions diagnosed as squamous cell carcinoma. Clearly, prospective study of the role of genital HSV infection and the development of neoplastic disease in women is necessary.

Maternal genital herpes infection has been associated with spontaneous abortion, premature delivery, and congenital malformations. These complications occur predominantly when infection is acquired during the first 20 weeks of gestation. Disseminated HSV infection in the neonate is associated with a 60% fatality rate, with more than 50% of survivors having neurologic sequelae. Disseminated infection in the mother has been associated with a mortality exceeding 50%. Neonatal infection presumably occurs during either vaginal delivery in mothers with active lesions or ascending infections from the maternal genital tract after fetal membranes have ruptured, and has also been associated with use of fetal monitor scalp electrodes. Neonatal infection may also be acquired by contact with nongenital sources (e.g., nosocomial infection from nursery personnel).

Pregnant women with a history of genital herpes infection should have cultures obtained after 34 weeks of gestation to assess the need for cesarean section. In neonates with evidence of disseminated infection, early institution of intravenous vidarabine or acyclovir appears to decrease the morbidity and mortality associated with HSV infection.

Diagnosis

HSV infection must be differentiated from other sexually transmitted diseases, including syphilis, LGV, and chancroid. Isolation of HSV by tissue culture of vesicles (ideally 24- to 48-hr old) remains the most definitive form of diagnosis; this can usually be accomplished within 48 to 96 hr after processing of specimens (5). Microscopic examination of scrapings from lesions using Giemsa or Wright's stain (Tzanck test) may be used to show the characteristic cellular morphology of HSV infection. However, these tests are frequently associated with false-negative results. Serologic tests for detecting antibodies to HSV are helpful only in primary infections, since antibody titers remain relatively unchanged during recurrent disease. In addition, antibodies may cross-react with both HSV-1 and HSV-2 because of antigenic similarities. In view of the limited availability and reliability of laboratory methods of diagnosis, genital HSV infections are usually diagnosed based on the history and clinical presentation.

Treatment

Effective therapy of genital HSV infection has become possible during the past decade with the development of acyclovir. The goals of therapy are to (a) decrease the severity and duration of the symptoms of active infection, (b) decrease the frequency of recurrence, and (c) decrease the duration of viral shedding from herpetic lesions (i.e., a true "antiviral effect"). The clinical and virologic courses of untreated primary and recurrent genital HSV infection are variables that must be controlled or analyzed to determine the efficacy of antiviral therapy. Table 69.3 summarizes some aspects of the infection to consider when evaluating or designing studies for treating genital HSV infection.

Several regimens with photodynamic inactivators, immunostimulants, vaccines, and topical surfactants (30) have been studied. Many evaluations were conducted in uncontrolled or poorly controlled clinical trials. However when these therapies have been evaluated in controlled clinical trials, they have been found to be of no benefit.

Acyclovir

Acyclovir is currently available as a 5% topical ointment, oral capsules, and as an intravenous formation. Table 69.4 summarizes the efficacy of the three formulations of acyclovir in the treatment of primary and recurrent genital herpes infection. In first episodes of genital herpes infections, acyclovir reduces the duration of viral shedding. The decrease in the duration of clinical symptoms (e.g., duration of pain, time to healing) is most dramatic with the systemic preparations (oral or intravenous) but still is measurable with the topical preparation. This observation is consistent with the known pathogenesis of infection. None of the preparations of acyclovir has any effect on the frequency or the time to the first recurrent episode.

The current CDC recommendation for the treatment of a primary infection is oral acyclovir at a dose of 200 mg five times daily for 7 to 10 days (11). Therapy should be initiated within 6 days of onset of lesions to obtain maximum results. Intravenous therapy should be reserved for

patients with severe symptoms or complications necessitating hospitalization because the response in most patients is not significantly different from that observed with oral therapy.

In view of the shorter and somewhat milder course of recurrent episodes of genital herpes, the effect of acyclovir on the course of a recurrent episode is less impressive. Reduction in the virologic and clinical course is limited to approximately 1 to 2 days with both the oral and topical preparations (Table 69.4). In view of the short course of untreated recurrent infection, a patient-initiated regimen might be expected to be more effective; however, controlled studies have demonstrated only slightly enhanced efficacy in patient-initiated (versus physician-initiated) regimens (27). Since the benefit of oral acyclovir therapy is small (but measurable), treatment of recurrent episodes should be limited to those with severe symptoms where therapy can be initiated within 2 days of onset of signs and symptoms (31).

The modest effects of acyclovir therapy on recurrent genital herpes infection have prompted several studies of prophylaxis/suppressive therapy using doses of 200 mg two to five times daily or 400 mg twice daily in patients with frequently recurrent genital herpes. Results of these studies show that up to 85% of patients remain completely free of recurrences during treatment, with an overall 75% reduction in recurrences in patients with more than 6 recurrent episodes per year. In patients with "breakthrough" recurrences, symptoms are often milder and of a shorter duration than those observed in patients not receiving prophylaxis. In addition, there appears to be a lower frequency of recurrences following cessation of prolonged prophylaxis (32). Suppression of recurrent genital herpes infection is recommended for patients in whom recurrences are frequent (more than six per year) with severe symptoms (11, 31, 32). The dose should be 200 mg four times daily and may be titrated upward or downward (e.g., to 200 to 400 mg b.i.d.) if there are no recurrences. Prophylaxis should be continued only for a period of up to 1 year, after which patients should remain off therapy and be allowed

Table 69.3.
Aspects of the Natural History of Genital Herpes Simplex Virus (HSV) Infection to Consider for Proper Trial Design and Evaluation of Therapeutic Regimens[a]

Considerations for evaluating the effect of therapy on severity and duration of symptoms of active infection
1. Difficulty in determining if formation of new lesions on therapy represent additional viral replication in ganglia or skin
2. Difference in clinical course between "wet" skin lesions and "dry" skin lesions
3. Necessity for rapid institution of therapy to evaluate the effects on symptoms, especially in recurrent infections
4. Difficulty in defining "healing," especially in women with intravaginal or cervical infection
5. Pronounced interpatient and intersex variability in clinical course on recurrent infection
Considerations for evaluating the effect of therapy on recurrence rates
1. Differences between the propensities of HSV-1 and HSV-2 to cause recurrent infection
2. Difference between men and women in the frequency of recurrence
Considerations for evaluating the effect of therapy on virus shedding from lesions
1. Necessity for rapid institution of therapy in recurrent disease to determine effect since period of virus shedding in untreated infections is brief
2. Pronounced interpatient variability in virologic course of recurrent disease

[a] From Dudley MN, McCloskey WW, Sexually transmitted diseases. In Herfindal ET, Gourley DR, Hart LL (eds): Clinical Pharmacy and Therapeutics, ed. 4. Baltimore, Williams & Wilkins, pp 808–826, 1988.

Table 69.4.
Efficacy of Various Preparations of Acyclovir in the Treatment of First Episode and Recurrent Herpes Genitalis[a]

Description	Route	Dose and Duration	Usual Decrease (in days) in Duration of		
			Viral Shedding	Duration of Pain	Time of Healing
First episode	5% topical	Apply to area 6 times daily × 7 days	3–6	2–3	4–5
	Oral	200 mg 5 times daily × 5–10 days	8–12	4–5	5–7
	i.v.	250mg/m^2 q 8 h × 5–7 days	7–11	4	7–12
Recurrent	5% topical	Apply to area 6 times daily × 7 days	<1	1–2	1
	Oral	200 mg 5 times daily × 5 days	1	<1	1–2

[a] Adapted from Straus SE (moderator): Herpes simplex virus infection: biology, treatment, and prevention. Ann Intern Med 103:404, 1985.

to experience a few recurrences to establish whether the patient's recurrence rate has changed, as might be expected with the variable course of the disease.

Other potential uses of prophylactic acyclovir include perioperative prophylaxis in patients with past infection undergoing surgery involving the lumbar vertebrae in whom reactivation of HSV infection may be undesirable. Another potential use would be as short-term suppressive therapy in pregnant women with recurrent herpes genitalis; the safety of acyclovir in pregnancy is not proven.

Acyclovir is well-tolerated when used in the treatment of initial or recurrent episodes of genital herpes and in suppressive therapy; long-term safety with prolonged suppressive therapy seems to be equally well-tolerated. One concern that has been raised with acyclovir treatment, particularly with prophylaxis of recurrent disease, has been the possible selection of resistant viral strains. Acyclovir-resistant herpes simplex viruses isolated have alterations of deficiencies in thymidine kinase, an enzyme necessary for the activation of the drug, or changes in DNA polymerase. Studies in animal models of infection show that herpes simplex strains that are deficient in thymidine kinase appear to be less virulent and often cannot establish latency. These strains do appear to be capable of producing infection in humans. Acyclovir-resistant strains of HSV have been most problematic in immunocompromised patients, particularly patients with the acquired immunodeficiency syndrome (AIDS) (33). Infections in patients unresponsive to acyclovir are best managed with foscarnet, but not vidarabine (34).

Supportive Measures

Symptomatic therapy attempts to reduce the discomfort associated with active herpetic lesions. Analgesics (narcotic and nonnarcotic) may be useful in reducing neuralgic pain and dysuria. Sitz or colloidal oatmeal baths may provide some relief. Topical lidocaine and warm air from hair dryers may also decrease the pain. Topical steroids should be avoided because they appear to be of no therapeutic benefit and could lead to secondary bacterial infections of the herpetic lesions.

One of the greatest concerns in the management of patients with genital HSV is overcoming the social problems and stigma concerning the disease. Many patients are unable to continue or initiate interpersonal relationships because of the fear of having a chronic, transmissible infectious disease. The availability of prophylaxis/suppressive therapy has been useful in resolving these concerns. The patient should be educated about the chronicity of the disease and must understand that sexual abstinence is necessary when active lesions are present. Women should be advised of the possible link between genital HSV infection and cervical cancer and told to have regular Papanicolaou (PAP) smear examinations.

HUMAN PAPILLOMA VIRUS (HPV) INFECTION
(See also Chapter 86, "Gynecologic Disorders.")

Condyloma acuminata or genital warts are sexually transmitted infections caused by the human papilloma virus (HPV), a member of the papovavirus family. Genital wart infections are increasing in prevalence and are among the three most common sexually transmitted diseases (STDs) diagnosed in patients attending STD clinics (35). Until the past decade, genital warts were considered to be benign skin lesions, however now there is increasing evidence that HPV are associated with the development of genital epithelial malignancies from dysplasias to squamous cell carcinoma. Currently, 57 different types of HPV have been identified. About one-quarter of these are commonly found in the genital tract (36). Some HPV types appear to have a degree of oncogenic potential, and under certain conditions, perhaps with the influence of cofactors such as cigarette smoking, may contribute directly to the development of overt malignancy (3). In an attempt to determine HPV transmission rates, Oriel studied 88 sexual contacts of patients with genital warts and found that 53 (60%) developed warts following a mean time after exposure of 2.8 months (range 3 weeks to 8 months).

Clinical Presentation. The clinical manifestations of HPV infection can be categorized as either overt or subclinical. The overt or grossly visible genital warts can be further subdivided into hyperplastic, sessile, or pigmented papules (37). The hyperplastic warts, the most common overt warts, are classic condyloma acuminata, which appear as raised, flesh-colored, pink, or hyperpigmented papules with pointed (accuminate) projections. Sessile warts are flat condyloma-like lesions with minimal elevation and a smooth surface, and pigmented papules, the least common, are pigmented sessile warts.

Subclinical infections are also known as flat condylomas. Subclinical infections can be found in the cervix, vagina, vulva, penis, and anus, the most common sites being the cervix and vagina. These lesions are not readily apparent to the eye. To visualize these lesions, application of a 3 to 5% acetic acid solution onto the site results in a shiny white plaque with distinct borders. While most overt and subclinical genital wart infections are asymptomatic, reported symptoms include itching, tenderness, bleeding, and irritation.

Diagnosis. In addition to clinical observations, other diagnostic methods of HPV infection include histologic identification of cells with koilocytes (pathognomonic for HPV infection), electron microscopy, and newer techniques such as immunocytochemistry, DNA hybridization, and polymerase chain reaction (PCR). These new techniques vary in sensitivity, specificity, and clinical utility. The only laboratory test widely available to clinicians is histology; however, recently a limited number of test kits for immunocytochemistry and DNA hybridization have become commercially available.

Treatment. The ultimate goal of treatment is to eradicate all HPV infection and corresponding risk of malignancy. Unfortunately, no therapy to date has been able to eradicate HPV from underlying and adjacent tissue, as seen by high relapse rates, nor has it been proven that treatment eliminates the risk of malignancy. Nevertheless, therapy should be offered to patients in an attempt to eliminate condylomata, reduce symptoms, reduce relapse, and prevent transmission of HPV to uninfected individuals (6). Ideally, therapy should be nontoxic, rapid, pain-free, and inexpensive. No currently available therapy for genital HPV infection fulfills these criteria (38).

Most clinical studies of the treatment of genital warts have concentrated on the treatment of overt genital warts using disappearance of visual warts as an end point of therapy. This end point cannot be used in subclinical disease. Now that subclinical disease and its association with malignancy has been recognized, researchers are beginning to use diagnostic techniques such as histology and DNA hybridization to evaluate therapeutic outcome in subclinical infection. Most therapy of HPV genital warts has been aimed at direct destruction of the lesions using podophyllin, cryotherapy, laser therapy, and interferon.

Podophyllin

Podophyllin is a plant resin that inhibits mitosis and leads to subsequent cell death. Podophyllin is given in a 10 to 25% solution in compound tincture of benzoin. The total volume of podophyllin should be limited to <0.5 ml per treatment session, and it should be thoroughly washed off in 1 to 4 hr (11). Most patients require several applications to eradicate all condyloma. The efficacy of podophyllin varies greatly, which may be due in part to varying concentrations of podophyllin among batches. Clinical trials have demonstrated cure rates with podophyllin ranging from 22 to 77%, with recurrence rates as high as 74% (38). Adverse reactions seen with podophyllin include local erythema, tenderness, itching, burning, pain, swelling, and superficial erosions. Since systemic toxicity and fetal demise have been reported, use in pregnancy is contraindicated (38). Podophyllin remains the most common therapy for genital warts in public STD clinics because of its convenience and low cost.

Cryotherapy

Cryotherapy involves rapid freezing of the wart with either nitrous oxide or liquid nitrogen in one or more freeze-thaw cycles. After two or three weekly sessions, warts usu-

ally disappear. The rates of complete clearance of genital warts with cryotherapy range from 63 to 88%, with recurrence rates of 21 to 39% (38). Cryotherapy was compared with podophyllin in 572 patients, resulting in elimination of warts in 79% of cryotherapy-treated patients and 52% of podophyllin-treated patients (39). The cryotherapy-treated patients required fewer treatments to eradicate the lesions, and adverse effects in both groups were minimal.

Laser Therapy

Carbon dioxide laser therapy converts light energy into heat energy within the cells, resulting in vaporization of the infected tissue with preservation of surrounding healthy tissue. Laser treatment is expensive and involves an experienced operator, general anesthesia, and often 1 to 3 days of postoperative hospitalization. Complete clearance of visible genital warts with a single laser procedure has been achieved in 31 to 91% of patients, with recurrence in 3 to 95% of patients (38). Adverse effects of laser therapy include a painful healing process and scar formation.

Interferon

Interferons (α, β, and γ) are a group of glycoproteins with antiviral, immunomodulatory, and antiproliferative activities. Interferon can be used to treat both symptomatic and asymptomatic HPV infection. The clinical efficacy of topical, intralesional, and systemic interferon therapy has been studied. Due to the variability in study design, dosing regimens, duration of therapy, and patient selection, the data are difficult to evaluate. Topical interferon therapy has resulted in visual clearance of warts in 33 to 100% of patients with a 0 to 100% recurrence rate and no adverse effects. Intralesional therapy has resulted in visual clearance of warts in 8 to 62% of patients with a 0 to 33% recurrence rate (38). Adverse effects commonly encountered with intralesional interferon include systemic effects such as fever, headache, myalgia, and chills, which can be reduced by acetaminophen at the time of injection (6). Systemic interferon is given by the subcutaneous or intramuscular routes. Visual clearance rates range from 0 to 82%, but systemic adverse reactions were common. Adverse reactions were recorded in 4 studies of systemic interferon, resulting in discontinuance of treatment or dose reduction in 45 (29%) of 157 patients (38). Currently, only intralesional interferon has been approved by the FDA for the treatment of condyloma acuminatum involving the external surfaces of the genital and perianal areas, but this therapy is expensive.

The Centers for Disease Control (CDC) recommends cryotherapy as the therapy of choice for external genital and perianal warts because it is nontoxic and inexpensive.

Podophyllin is an alternative, and interferon is not recommended because of high cost and toxicity. The carbon dioxide laser should be reserved for patients with extensive warts, particularly those who have not responded to cryotherapy (11). The CDC further recommends that patients with anogenital warts be made aware that they are contagious to uninfected sex partners and that condoms should be used to reduce transmission. It is also recommended that all women with anogenital warts have an annual Pap smear.

CONCLUSION

One of the most important aspects in the control of STDs is patient education about transmission and the need for treatment. The AIDS epidemic, with recognition of the risks for acquisition with certain high-risk sexual practices, has fostered a new awareness of disease transmission. Formal educational programs at the local and national levels have created a greater awareness. Over the past decade, condoms have moved from "under the pharmacy counter" to prominent store displays. Discussion of proper use, storage, and type is important to minimize the risk of disease transmission and acquisition.

STDs are among the few infectious diseases for which extensive recommendations for treatment are provided. In many cases (e.g., gonococcal urethritis), several alternatives are available. The pharmacist may assist in the assessment of the advantages, disadvantages, and cost-effectiveness of several regimens.

The ultimate answers to the control of STDs are education and therapeutics. New therapeutic agents that may be developed include vaccines for widespread use for prevention of herpes simplex virus and gonorrhea. All healthcare providers can participate in the dissemination of accurate information about prevention of all STDs.

REFERENCES

1. Anon: Progress toward achieving the 1990 objectives for the nation for sexually transmitted diseases. MMWR 39:53–57, 1990.
2. Judson FN: Gonorrhea. Med Clin North Am 74:1353–1365, 1990.
3. Cates W Jr: Epidemiology and control of sexually transmitted diseases: strategic evaluation. Infect Dis Clin North Am 1:1–23, 1987.
4. Anon: Syphilis. MMWR 40:314–316, 1991.
5. Corey L, Spear DG: Infections with herpes simplex virus (parts 1 and 2). N Engl J Med 314:686–691; 749–757, 1986.
6. Brown DR and Fife KH: Human papillomavirus infection of the genital tract. Med Clin North Am 74:1455–1485, 1990.
7. Rein M: Urethritis. In Mandell GL, Douglas RG, Bennett JE (eds): Principles and Practice of Infectious Diseases. ed. 3. New York, Churchill Livingstone, pp 942–952, 1990.
8. Ledger W: Infections of the female pelvis. In Mandell GL, Douglas RG, Bennett JE (eds): Principles and Practice of Infectious Diseases. ed. 3. New York, Churchill Livingstone, pp 965–970, 1990.
9. Jacobs NF Jr, Kraus SJ: Gonococcal and nongonococcal urethritis in men: clinical and laboratory differentiation. Ann Intern Med 82:7–17, 1975.
10. Eschenback DA, Buchanan TM, Pollock HM, et al.: Polymicrobial etiology of acute pelvic inflammatory disease. N Engl J Med 293:166–171, 1975.
11. Anon: 1989 STD treatment guidelines. MMWR 38(S-8):1, 1989.
12. Hooton TM, Rogers ER, Medina TG, et al.: Ciprofloxacin compared with doxycycline for nongonococcal urethritis: in effectiveness against Chlamydia trachomatis due to relapsing infection. JAMA 264:1418–1421, 1990.
13. Jaffe HW, Schroeter AL, Reynolds GM, et al.: Pharmacokinetic determinants of penicillin cure of gonococcal urethritis. Antimicrob Agents Chemother 15:587–591, 1979.
14. Miller LK, Sanchez PL, Berg SW, et al.: Effectiveness of aztreonam, a new monobactam antibiotic, against penicillin-resistant gonococci. J Infect Dis 148:612, 1983
15. Foulds G, Stankewich JP, Marshall DC, et al.: Pharmacokinetics of sulbactam in humans. Antimicrob Agents Chemother 23:692–699, 1983.
16. Plouffe JF: Treatment of infections caused by ampicillin-resistant pathogens with a combination of ampicillin and CP-45, 899. Antimicrob Agents Chemother 21:519–520, 1982.
17. Crider SR, Colby SD, Miller LK, et al.: Treatment of penicillin-resistant Neisseria gonorrhoeae with oral norfloxacin. N Engl J Med 311:137–140, 1984.
18. Scott GR, McMillan A, Young H: Ciprofloxacin versus ampicillin and probenecid in the treatment of uncomplicated gonorrhea in men. J Antimicrob Chemother 20:117–121, 1987.
19. Lutz FB Jr: Single-dose efficacy of ofloxacin in uncomplicated gonorrhea. Am J Med 87(suppl 6c):69s–74s, 1989.
20. Aznar J, Caballero MC, Lozano MC, et al.: Activities of new quinolone derivatives against genital pathogens. Antimicrob Agents Chemother 27:76–78, 1985.
21. Tramont EC: Treponema pallidum (syphilis). In Mandell GL, Douglas RG, Bennett JE (eds): Principles and Practice of Infectious Diseases. ed. 3. New York, Churchill Livingstone, pp 1794–1808, 1990.
22. Wooldridge WE: Syphilis: a new visit from an old enemy. Postgrad Med 84:193–202, 1991.
23. Kirchner JT: Syphilis: an STD on the increase. Am Fam Pract 44:843–854, 1991.
24. Zenker PN, Rolfs RT: Treatment of syphilis, 1989. Rev Infect Dis 12:s590–s690, 1990.
25. Romanowski B, Sutherland R, Fick GM, et al.: Serologic response to treatment of infectious syphilis. Ann Intern Med 114:1005–1007, 1991.
26. Young EJ, Weingarten NM, Baughn RE, et al.: Studies on the pathogenesis of the Jarisch-Herxheimer reaction. J Infect Dis 146:606–615, 1982.
27. Straus SE (moderator): Herpes simplex virus infection: biology, treatment, and prevention. Ann Intern Med 103:404–419, 1985.
28. Cory L, Adams HG, Brown ZA, Holmes KK: Genital herpes simplex virus infection: clinical manifestations, course, and complications. Ann Intern Med 98:958–972, 1983.
29. Arbesfeld DM, Thomas I: Cutaneous herpes simplex virus infection. Am Fam Pract 43:1655–1664, 1991.
30. Dudley MN, McCloskey WW: Sexually transmitted diseases. In Herfindal ET, Gourley DR, Hart LL (eds): Clinical Pharmacy and Therapeutics, ed. 4. Baltimore, Williams & Wilkins, pp 808–826, 1988.
31. Stone KM, Whittington WL: Treatment of genital herpes. Rev Infect Dis 12(suppl 6):S610–S619, 1990.
32. Mindel A: Prophylaxis for genital herpes: should it be used routinely? Drugs 41:319–325, 1991.
33. Hirsch MS, Schooley RT: Resistance to antiviral drugs: the end of the innocence. N Engl J Med 320:313, 314, 1989.

34. Safrin S, Crumpacker C, Chatis P, et al.: A controlled trial comparing foscarnet with vidarabine for acyclovir-resistant mucocutaneous herpes simplex in the acquired immunodeficiency syndrome. N Engl J Med 325:551–555, 1991.

35. Kirby P, Corey L: Genital human papillomavirus infections. Infect Dis Clin North Am 1:123–143, 1987.

36. Roman A, Fife KH: Human papillomaviruses: are we ready to type? Clin Microbiol Rev 2:166–190, 1989.

37. Oriel JD: Natural history of genital warts. Br J Vener Dis 47:1, 1971.

38. Kraus ST, Stone KM: Management of genital infection caused by human papillomavirus. Rev Infect Dis 12(suppl 6):S620–S632, 1990.

39. Bashi SA: Cryotherapy versus podophyllin in the treatment of genital warts. Int J Dermatol 24:535–536, 1985.

CHAPTER 70

ACQUIRED IMMUNODEFICIENCY SYNDROME (AIDS)

JOAN E. KAPUSNIK-UNER, Pharm.D.

Acquired immunodeficiency syndrome (AIDS) is the result of infection with human immunodeficiency virus (HIV). The effects of HIV on the body's host defense mechanisms are gradual and become profound, rendering the patient susceptible to other infectious diseases and cancers. Various symptoms have been identified that are specifically related to infection with HIV (e.g., flu-like syndrome, dementia, and thrombocytopenia). However, the vast majority of signs and symptoms are from opportunistic infections and cancers that manifest after immunosuppression with HIV. AIDS was first recognized in mid-1981 when an unusual cluster of patients was reported as having *Pneumocystis carinii* pneumonia (PCP). Therapeutic advances against HIV have been unprecedented; the syndrome was recognized in 1981, the virus isolated and identified in 1983, and antiretroviral therapy was FDA-approved in 1987.

ETIOLOGY AND PATHOGENESIS

HIV is an RNA retrovirus with subgroups HIV-1 and HIV-2. HIV-1, the more common isolate, has been more extensively studied. HIV is known to be transmitted only by direct inoculation with infected blood, body fluids, or secretions. Transmission occurs during intimate sexual contact, by direct exposure to contaminated blood, bodily secretions, or blood-products, and by direct in utero transmission. Infection with HIV results in selective defects in immune function. The most prominent feature in the immunopathogenesis of HIV infection is the depletion of the CD_4 (helper, inducer) subset of T lymphocytes. B cell dysfunction is also described in patients with HIV infection.

The outer envelope of HIV includes a critical structure known as gp120, which interacts with CD_4 cell receptor molecules. These receptors are also found on other cells throughout the body, thus widespread HIV binding can occur. Many cytopathic mechanisms have been proposed and observed, but a clearer picture of disease pathogenesis remains to be elucidated.

INCIDENCE/OCCURRENCE

The Public Health Service has estimated that 1.0 to 1.5 million persons are infected with HIV, whereas the Centers for Disease Control estimates only 1.0 million persons are currently infected in the United States (1). AIDS/HIV statistics world-wide are very difficult to determine because of low reporting, even in endemic areas such as Africa, and because of the different definitions for AIDS. Since 1981 more than 100,000 persons have been reported to have died from AIDS. The greatest impact has been in males age 25 to 44 years, where AIDS has become the number two cause of death, second only to unintentional injury deaths (2). Only 10% of AIDS deaths have been in women, and <2% in children under 5 years of age.

High-risk populations identified in the United States include homosexual and bisexual men who are sexually active, intravenous drug users (IVDUs), recipients of blood or blood products before HIV-screening and testing were routinely employed, and infants born to HIV-infected mothers. Elsewhere in the world, heterosexual transmission of HIV through intercourse is the major risk factor. Many experts feel that widespread education on "safe-sex" and selective education of IVDUs on avoiding "needle-sharing" will have a major impact on disease transmission. Importantly, this educational effort must cross all age, gender, cultural, and ethnic borders to truly affect the future incidence of HIV infection and not just change AIDS epidemiology.

DIAGNOSIS

Infection with HIV can be thought of as a continuum of clinical conditions, ranging from asymptomatic infection to AIDS, the most severe manifestation of this disease. The Centers for Disease Control (CDC) has published criteria for diagnosing, reporting, and surveillance (Table 70.1) (3). These criteria are expecting to change again in 1992 to include more persons as having AIDS. Objective data including laboratory tests and findings from physical examinations are useful in the diagnosis. The T lymphocyte defect in patients may be assessed and characterized by the ratio of CD_4 (helper, inducer) to CD_8 (suppressor, cytotoxic) cells, the normal ratio being 2 to 1. In HIV infection this ratio inverts, with CD_8 cells predominating. The absolute number of CD_4 cells is also useful for monitoring disease progression, with a normal number of CD_4 cells being in the range of 500 to 1100/mm^3.

Table 70.1.
Summary of the CDC 1987 Case Definition for AIDS[a]

I. Individuals[b] without laboratory evidence of HIV infection
   Indicator disease diagnosed definitively[c]
   1. Candidiasis of the esophagus, trachea, bronchi, or lungs
   2. Extrapulmonary cryptococcosis
   3. Cryptosporidiosis with diarrhea persisting >1 month
   4. Cytomegalovirus disease of an organ other than the liver, spleen, or lymph nodes in a patient >1 month of age
   5. Persistent herpes simplex virus (HSV) mucocutaneous ulcers (>1 month duration); or HSV bronchitis, pneumonitis, or esophagitis of any duration in a patient >1 month of age
   6. Kaposi's sarcoma affecting a patient <60 years of age
   7. Lymphoma of the brain (primary) affecting a patient <60 years of age
   8. Lymphoid interstitial pneumonia and/or pulmonary lymphoid hyperplasia (LIP/PLH complex) affecting a child <13 years of age
   9. Disseminated *Mycobacterium avium* complex (MAC) or *Mycobacterium kansasii* disease (to a site other than, or in addition to lungs, skin, or cevical/hilar lymph nodes)
   10. *Pneumocystis carinii* pneumonia (PCP)
   11. Progressive multifocal leukoencephalopathy (PML)
   12. Toxoplasmosis of the brain affecting a patient >1 month of age
II. Individuals[d] with laboratory evidence for HIV infection
   Indicator diseases diagnosed definitively[c]
   1. Multiple or recurrent bacterial infections[e] affecting a child <13 years of age
   2. Disseminated coccidioidomycosis (at a site other than or in addition to lungs or cervical/hilar lymph nodes)
   3. HIV encephalopathy
   4. Disseminated histoplasmosis (at a site other than or in addition to lungs or cervical/hilar lymph nodes)
   5. Isosporiasis with diarrhea persisting >1 month
   6. Kaposi's sarcoma at any age
   7. Lymphoma of the brain (primary) at any age
   8. Other non-Hodgkin's lymphoma of B cell or unknown immunologic phenotype following specific histological types
   9. Disseminated mycobacterial disease (except caused by *M. tuberculosis*) at a site other than or in addition to lungs, skin, or cervical/hilar lymph nodes
   10. Extrapulmonary *Mycobacterium tuberculosis* (may be in addition to concurrent pulmonary involvement)
   11. Recurrent *Salmonella* (nontyphi) septicemia
   12. HIV wasting syndrome (emaciation, "slim disease")
III. Individuals[b] with laboratory evidence against HIV infection
   1. *Pneumocystis carinii* pneumonia
   2. T helper/inducer (CD4) lymphocyte count <400/mm^3 plus any other of the diseases indicative of AIDS listed above in I.

---

[a] From Centers for Disease Control: Revision of the CDC serveillance case definition for acquired immunodeficiency syndrome.
[b] Individuals without causes of immunodeficiency that disqualify diseases as indicators of AIDS.
[c] Diagnosis made by appropriate microscopic, histologic, or cytologic examination or by culture techniques.
[d] Regardless of the presence of other causes of immunodeficiency.
[e] Infections of the bone or joint, septicemia, pneumonia, meningitis, and abscess of an internal organ or body cavity (except otitis media or mucosal abscesses).

Antibodies against HIV are detectable by various serologic testing methods. Antibody testing is the most widespread method of determining HIV infection, though false-positive and false-negative results often occur. HIV-antibody testing is usually done first with the ELISA method (enzyme-linked immunosorbent assay), and positive results are confirmed with a second procedure, the western blot method. False-negative serologic results might occur when a patient is newly infected and sufficient time has not elapsed for antibody production and detection or when patients are very ill and are unable to produce antibodies. HIV culture techniques are used in many research studies, but they are not available for routine clinical diagnoses. Financial considerations, as well as high false-negative rates make such tests impractical. The newest test to gain favor is the serologic test for detection of the HIV p24 antigen. When this antigen is detected in a specimen (e.g., blood or cerebrospinal fluid), it is interpreted to mean that active viral replication is occurring. The p24 viral marker differs from antibody detection in two ways: (*a*) only low concentrations of antigen are detectable (picogram concentrations) and (*b*) antigen-antibody immune complexes that form are not measurable with antigen-testing methods. During initial HIV infection, p24 antigenemia usually precedes antibody seroconversion by 2 to 3 weeks, and thus can be used as an early diagnostic methods.

CLINICAL FINDINGS

Persons who are asymptomatic with HIV infection, may remain so for many years, especially if antiretroviral therapy is instituted early. The reasons for disease progression and for unpredictable rates of progression are not well understood. AIDS-related complex (ARC) is an array of mild-to-moderate symptoms that are observed early in HIV infection. Symptoms include persistent fevers, night sweats, weight loss, headaches, lymphadenopathy, rashes, diarrhea, thrush, and hematologic abnormalities. All of these symptoms are nonspecific. With further progression of HIV infection and immunosuppression, patients have opportunistic infections and neoplasms.

The diagnosis of AIDS is made during the most advanced stage of HIV infection. The current CDC case definition of AIDS was published in 1987 and includes several categories of potential AIDS diagnoses (2). AIDS is diagnosed when specific infectious diseases or neoplasms are present (i.e., Kaposi's sarcoma (KS), *Pneumocystis carinii* pneumonia (PCP), cryptococcal meningitis, *Candida* esophagitis, *Toxoplasma* encephalitis, and disseminated atypical mycobacterial infection), which are rare illnesses otherwise. These are the so-called AIDS-indicator diseases. A second category of AIDS diagnoses include patients with known positive HIV-antibody test results, who additionally have a severe episode or unusual presentation of other infections (e.g., disseminated *Mycobacterium tuberculosis*, histoplasmosis or, coccidioidomycosis), severe wasting (Slim's disease), or dementia (HIV encephalopathy). The new proposal for AIDS include a category for patients with CD_4 cells $<200/mm^3$, independent of other symptoms.

MEDICAL TREATMENT WITH ANTIRETROVIRAL THERAPY

Zidovudine

It has been challenging to select and evaluate therapies for patients with the various stages of HIV infection. Definitions for cure and failure have been especially difficult to establish. Success is not defined by the usual virologic or microbiologic cures nor by complete resolution of clinical signs and symptoms. Treatment success is measured by parameters such as decreased mortality, improved functional status (Karnofsky's performance status), restoration of neurologic function, or a lower frequency of opportunistic infections (OIs). These improves outcomes may be achieved in most patients by the administration of an antiretroviral agent along with appropriate antimicrobial therapy for OIs. Currently, zidovudine (AZT, Retrovir) is the best studied antiretroviral agent that has been shown to be effective in controlled studies (4–6). However, progression of disease and death can occur while on AZT therapy.

AZT is a thymidine analog that is triphosphorylated by cellular kinases to become the active drug moiety. Because of the structural similarity to thymidine triphosphate, zidovudine triphosphate is used as a substrate by the viral RNA-dependent DNA polymerase, reverse transcriptase. Zidovudine triphosphate is integrated into the DNA where its 3'-azido groups prevent formation of the normal 5'–3'phosphodiester linkages. AZT thus acts as a chain terminator of viral DNA synthesis.

In early 1987 the 6-month follow-up data from a placebo-controlled study reported AZT to be effective in the management of two adult HIV-infection subpopulations (7): (*a*) AIDs patients with confirmed *Pneumocystis carinii* pneumonia and (*b*) advanced ARC patients with an absolute CD_4 count $<200/mm^3$. In this initial study the probability of survival was improved for post-PCP and ARC patients in the AZT group, versus the placebo group, and there was a significantly decreased probability of developing opportunistic infections. The results of this study were reviewed, and FDA approval for AZT was given in March 1987. The initial dosage recommendation was "full-dose" therapy of 200 mg (two 100-mg capsules) every 4 hr around-the-clock (1200 mg/day).

Adverse reactions were common in the initial placebo-controlled study with 84% and 72% of patients in AZT versus placebo groups, respectively, reporting at least one adverse event (Table 70.2) (8). Weakness, headache, diar-

Table 70.2.
Comparision of Observed Adverse Effects from a Controlled Study—Placebo versus "Full-Dose" Zidovudine

Adverse Effect	Number of Patients (%)		P^a
	Placebo ($n = 135$)	Zidovudine ($n = 143$)	
Nausea	25 (18)	66 (46)	.001
Myalgia	3 (2)	11 (8)	.043
Insomnia	1 (1)	7 (5)	.043
Anemia (<7.5 g/100 ml)	6 (4)	35 (24)	<.001
Neutropenia (<500/mm³)	3 (2)	23 (16)	<.001

^{a} By Cochran-Mantel-Haenszel method.

rhea, abdominal pain, and fever were symptoms that occurred commonly in both study groups. Nausea, myalgia, and insomnia were the only adverse experiences that were reported with significantly greater frequency in the AZT group. Headaches occurred at the same frequency, but were more severe in the AZT-treated patients. Macrocytosis developed within weeks in most patients on AZT. By week 6, anemia with hemoglobin levels of less than 75 g/liter (7.5 g/dl) developed in 24.5% and 4.4% of AZT and placebo patients, respectively (P < 0.001). Neutropenia (< 500 cells/mm³) occurred in 16.1% of AZT versus 2.2% of placebo patients (P < .001). Leukopenia and neutropenia were most marked in the patients with low CD_4 counts and AIDS upon study entry. Thirty-one percent of AZT versus 11% of placebo patients received transfusions during the study period (P < .05). Additionally, multiple transfusions were required in 21% of AZT patients compared with only 4% in placebo groups. Overall, platelet counts increased to a greater extent in patients receiving AZT than those on placebo.

Administration of exogenous recombinant erythropoietin (EPO) has been reported to improve the outcome of AZT-induced anemia (9). Erythropoietin is a glycoprotein growth factor produced by cells adjacent to the proximal renal tubules in response to hypoxemia (10). In the bone marrow, erythropoietin stimulates erythrocyte maturation, thus increasing the oxygen-carrying capacity of blood, resulting also in improvement in symptoms from the anemic state. In a randomized, double-blind, placebo-controlled trial of 63 AIDS patients receiving concomitant AZT, 29 patients received EPO 100 units/kg three times per week. Results revealed that both the number of patients needing transfusions and the number of transfusions per patient decreased for EPO recipients, versus placebo. EPO response was most effective in patients with ≤500 IU/liter baseline endogenous erythropoietin concentration. These patients had a greater rise in hematocrit values when given EPO. Recommendations for widespread use of EPO in patients on AZT do not appear to be appropriate. EPO is however a useful therapeutic modality to be initiated on a case-by-case basis when antiretroviral therapy has been modified but transfusion-dependent anemia persists.

Since 1987 there have been other important advances in our knowledge about the rationale use of AZT. A dose-comparison study was done in 524 post-PCP AIDs patients who were randomized to receive one of two AZT treatment regimens (11). One group received "standard therapy" (1500 mg/day), and the other was given an initial dosage of 1200 mg/day for 1 month followed by 100 mg every 4 hr (600 mg/day). Results revealed that both groups had comparable survival rates and frequencies of opportunistic infections. The "low-dose," 600 mg/day, regimen was, however, associated with a significantly lower incidence of hematologic toxicities. Results from this study and others using the lower AZT dosage have made 600 mg/day the new standard of care. It is not known how effective this regimen is for the treatment of HIV-encephalopathy (dementia). Additionally, patients with HIV-associated thrombocytopenia may require more than 600 mg/day of AZT for stabilization of their platelet counts (12).

Volberding et al. in 1990 published a collaborative study that reported the efficacy of AZT in patients with asymptomatic HIV infection (13). Analysis of the data has shown that patients with a CD_4 count $\leq500/mm^3$ benefit from AZT therapy. Of the 1338 participants followed for 2 years, 33 cases of AIDs were diagnosed in the placebo control group, as compared to 11 and 14 cases in AZT groups—500 mg/day and 1500 mg/day, respectively. Success was defined as a significant reduction in the rate of disease progression in both the low (500 mg/day) dose groups. Data from another recent pilot study suggests that as little as 300 mg/day of AZT may be efficacious in certain patients with HIV-infection (14). This regimen needs further study before it is routinely recommended.

Delayed AZT treatment is also known to be beneficial (15). Patients who crossed-over to AZT after the initial placebo phase did not have poorer survival rates than patients only receiving AZT. However, the survival time was improved over that of patients who received only placebo and died before being cross-over. Delayed treatment patients ($n = 102$) had 78.8% (12 month) and 64.6% (18 month) survival rates; whereas AZT patients ($n = 144$) had 84.5% (12 month), 68.12% (18 month) and 57.6% (21 month) survival rates.

General recommendations for adults infected with HIV are that persons without an AIDS diagnosis are to be started on AZT when their CD_4 count is approximately 500/mm^3 (plus or minus 100). Optimally, two consecutive counts below 500 should be obtained, at least 1 week apart, before initiating therapy. No laboratory marker other than CD_4 count is necessary in deciding when to initiate AZT therapy. A summary of AZT dosage recommendations for

Table 70.3.
Zidovudine Dosage Recommendations for Various Stages of Infection with Human Immunodeficiency Virus (HIV)

HIV Patient Group	Dosage Regimen
Adults asymptomatic HIV	
Persons with CD_4 count $\leq500/mm^3$ (q8h dosing also used)	(500 mg/day) 100 mg q5h while awake
Adults symptomatic	
AIDS and symptomatic HIV (q8h dosing also utilized)	(500 mg–600 mg/day) 100 mg q4h
HIV-induced thrombocytopenia	(500 mg–600 mg/day)
HIN-induced dementia[a] (titrate dose to patient response)	(600–1200 mg/day)
Children (>3 months–12 years)	
AIDS or HIV-symptomatic	180 mg/m² q6h
Children (>3 months–12 years)	
HIV-asymptomatic with laboratory values consistent with HIV infection	180 mg/m² q6h
Children (<3 months)	Per Treatment IND/institutional protocols

[a] It is not known what doage regimen is *most* effective for improving the neurologic dysfunction associated with HIV infection.

various ages and stages of HIV infection is given in Table 70.3.

Another important advance in the treatment of HIV infection came when the FDA accounted the sanctioning of AZT Treatment IND Protocols for children with advanced HIV infection. This action made the drug more widely available to this important HIV-infected patient population. Results from a study of 88 children (ages 4 months to 11 years) given oral AZT 180 mg/m³ q6h reported clinical, immunologic, and virologic improvements (16).

Other Antiretroviral Therapies

Other investigational antiretroviral agents are currently under study (17). Nucleoside analogs, such as didanosine (DDI, Videx) and zalcitabine (dideoxycytidine, DDC, Hivid) are being studied through expanded access programs designed to make the drug available to patients who are intolerant to, or have failed AZT. DDI was approved by the FDA in October 1991. Other controlled comparison studies with AZT are also underway. Two phase I studies of DDI in adults with AIDS or ARC have been published. One reported significant decreases in p24 antigen levels and increases in CD_4 cell counts in 37 patients receiving drug b.i.d. over a dose range of 0.4 to 66 mg/kg/day (18). Fifty percent of patients reported an increase in energy or an improved sense of well-being, 50% had significant weight gain, approximately 25% had both weight gain and subjective improvement. Unfortunately, dose-related efficacy outcomes could not be established. Evaluation of safety in this study revealed DDI to be a well-tolerated drug with an estimated maximum tolerated dosage of 12 mg/kg/day. There were however dose-limiting side effects: peripheral neuropathy and fatal pancreatitis. Also, asymptomatic elevations of amylase, liver enzyme, and uric acid levels were observed frequently. Impressive was the lack of hematologic toxicity, compared with that observed historically from AZT. In a second phase I study using q.d. dosing of oral DDI 1.6–30.4 mg/kg/day efficacy was also reported (19). Preliminary studies in children were ongoing and show DDI to be a safe and effective drug (20).

Human pharmacokinetic data are limited but DDI is reported to cross the blood-brain barrier, with CSF concentrations found to be 21% of serum concentrations (21). DDI is 50% renally eliminated. DDI's active metabolite, DDATP, has a long serum and intracellular half-life (12 to 24 hr).

Zalcitabine (DDC) is also under study (22), but expanded access has somewhat lagged behind DDI because DDC in early studies caused severe periperal neuropathy. Drug approval is projected to be in 1992. Phase I studies reviewed 5 parenteral and oral dosage regimens in 20 patients (23). Surrogate markers, p24 antigen and CD_4 counts have been monitored in DDC studies, both showing improvements with therapy. The majority of patients did, however, experience a reversible painful peripheral neuropathy after 6 to 14 weeks of treatment. Also, an alternating regimen of DDC and AZT appeared efficacious and warrants further investigation.

Dideoxycytidine (DDC, Hivid) is currently available as oral tablets at two dosages, 0.375 mg p.o. t.i.d. and 0.75 mg p.o. t.i.d. Patients are randomized to either group after entry into the compassionate-use or open-label protocols. In phase I/II studies DDC was given to hundreds of patients and was found to result in a significant decrease in p24 antigen levels. Combination therapy with AZT and DDC is also promising (24). Preliminary reports in 56 patients with advanced HIV disease reveal the combination to be well tolerated and produced greater improvements in surrogate markers, CD_4 count and p24 antigen levels.

Other drugs that have shown antiretroviral activity are being studied but are further behind in the drug-development process. The T lymphocyte cell surface glycoprotein CD_4 has been shown to be the cellular receptor for HIV envelope-glycoprotein gp120. It is felt that soluble CD_4 might exert antiretroviral activity by blocking HIV adsorption to cell surfaces. Soluble CD_4 has been produced by recombinant DNA techniques and is in phase I studies. Trichosanthin (GLQ223, compound Q) is an exciting anti-HIV compound because of its unique ability to inhibit HIV replication in infected T cells and also chronically infected macrophages/monocytes. This drug has been reported to improve p24 antigen levels in 10 to 16 patients after 3 parenteral dosages given at various times over 21 days (25). Side effects included mild and reversible myalgias, hypoalbuminemia, and delayed fevers. Most worrisome was that 6 of 51 patients developed dementia at 36 to 60 hr after drug administration. Two patients progressed to coma that reversed within 12 hr with dexamethasone therapy. Studies are ongoing with this agent, using oral and parenteral formulations.

Single-agent therapy with other investigational antiretroviral drugs has not been as successful (e.g., suramin, oral dextran sulfate, ampligen, HPA-23, AL 721, interferon, and ribavirin). However, in vitro and in vivo studies with even newer compounds with antiretroviral activity continue to be pursued (e.g., TIBO benzodiapine compounds, foscarnet, imuthiol, D4T, castanospermine, rifabutin, and inosine pranobex). It is likely that the most effective therapy for HIV infection will involve using a combination of antiretroviral drugs and immunomodulators. Advantages such as synergy might be expected from certain combination therapies as well as reduced toxicity from cycling drug therapies.

PREVENTION MEASURES

Information is theoretically the best preventative measure. Educational programs in the community and schools are critical for teaching the facts about the risk of transmission and the consequences of exposure to HIV. Opinions differ on what age children should receive what kind of information and counseling on "safe-sex," but few would dispute that safe-sex is critical. Pharmacists do and should continue to play an important role in this educational effort. Condom use is advocated as the major protective measure for stopping transmission of HIV. Condoms are sold in many settings, but probably most are purchased in pharmacies. The additional use of nonoxynol-9 spermicidal preparations during intercourse has added anti-HIV efficacy and is therefore highly recommended. Many women in the United States are unaware they are at risk for HIV infection, and HIV-infected women often remain undiagnosed until the onset of AIDS. Recurrent, refractory candidal infections (vaginal and other) may be the first sign of immunosuppression from HIV. Medical referral for such patients, which is encouraged by the pharmacist, may lead to earlier detection of HIV. Pharmacists should therefore actively distribute prepared materials (available from the CDC, Public Health Service, and other agencies) about high-risk activities, safe-sex, condom use, early signs of HIV, and how-and-where to get HIV testing/counseling. As healthcare professionals, being informed on the current issues and facts surrounding HIV infection is mandatory for pharmacists.

OCCUPATIONAL EXPOSURE TO HIV

The AIDs epidemic has also led to concern about potential occupational exposure to HIV. The rate of infection after accidental exposure from "needle-stick" injuries was estimated to be 0.4%. The implementation of universal infection control precautions may reduce the incidence of occupational exposures, but it will not entirely eliminate the risk of infection with HIV from accidental inoculation. Healthcare institutions and employee health services are faced with the difficult decision of whether or not to empirically give postexposure AZT prophylaxis. Two programs that described institution-specific policies and procedures on this matter have been reported in detail (26). A dosage regimen of 200 mg p.o. 5x/day for 1 month has been suggested, but many persons are not able to tolerate this regimen and doses are adjusted accordingly. Further data are being collected in a multicenter study to help answer the question of AZT efficacy under these circumstances. Recommendations also have been proposed by the CDC for preventing transmission of HIV to patients during exposure-prone invasive procedures.

COMPLICATIONS—KAPOSI'S SARCOMA (KS)

In addition to opportunistic infections, HIV-infected persons are also at high risk for developing certain cancers. KS is an endothelial neoplasm of either capillary or lymphatic origin and is the most commonly observed neoplasm in patients with HIV infection (28). A diagnosis of KS actually classifies a patient as having AIDs by CDC criteria. Local treatments of KS skin lesions include liquid nitrogen or intralesion vinblastine, as well as systemic therapy with antineoplastic drugs (e.g., vincristine, adriamycin, or bleomycin). The addition of AZT to the regimen of KS patients has improved their outcomes greatly. Immunomodulating compounds such as α-interferon have also been somewhat effective in the treatment of Kaposi's sarcoma.

AZT and α-interferon have been given in combination and have shown an antitumor effect as well. A dose-escalation of α-interferon plus AZT was conducted as an open, nonrandomized trial in patients with KS (29). The ability of patients to tolerate the interferon was directly related to their dose of AZT. The three oral AZT regimens studied were 250 mg q4h, 100 mg q4h, and 50 mg q4h. At a minimum of 6 weeks after starting AZT, patients were given daily subcutaneous dosages of interferon, which was initiated at 5 million units (MU) per day, increasing every 2 weeks to a maximum tolerated dose or to 35 MU/day. Only patients receiving the 50 mg q4h regimen of AZT were able to tolerate more than 15 MU/day of interferon. At the two higher AZT dosages, neutropenia, thrombocytopenia, and hepatic dysfunction were the primary toxicities. Of the 22 patients who received a stable dose of both drugs for 12 weeks, 11 patients had a complete or partial antitumor response, and 9 showed an anti-HIV effect, as measured by converting to either HIV culture-negative ($n = 6$) or p24 antigen-negative ($n = 3$). Further studies are underway with new agents and with combination treatments that will hopefully improve therapy outcomes for patients with KS.

COMPLICATIONS—OPPORTUNISTIC INFECTIONS ASSOCIATED WITH HIV DISEASE
Principles of Treatment

HIV attacks various cellular components of the immune system which are necessary host defenses in the fight against pathogen invasion and clinical infectious diseases. The resultant immunodeficiency predisposes the HIV-infected patient to a wide variety of so-called opportunistic infections (OIs). The treatment of OIs in AIDS patients may consist of multiple-drug antimicrobial therapy, including antibacterial agents, antifungal agents, antiparasitic agents, antiviral agents, and antimycobacterial agents. Table 70.4 contains a list of commonly observed opportunistic infections in HIV-infected patients and their treatments, which are discussed below.

Patients with HIV infection should be evaluated and monitored continuously for the degree of immunosuppression. A complete blood count with differential, CD_4 count, and anergy skin testing may be used to assess immune status. The severity of HIV infection, in addition to the severity of the OI may dictate the type and duration of treatment. A comprehensive treatment regimen for a given opportunistic infection may be divided into three distinct stages, and any and all stages of therapy may be appropriate for a given patient. The three stages are primary antimicrobial prophylaxis, acute treatment, and secondary prophylaxis. Primary antimicrobial prophylaxis is therapy given before development of a clinical infection. This may or may not be instituted before the patient's exposure to the pathogen. Thus two distinct situations are possible for

Table 70.4.
Opportuinistic Infections Commonly Observed in HIV-Infected Patients

Infection	Pathogen
Fungal	
PCP	*Pneumocystis carinii*
Cryptococcal meningitis	*Cryptococcus neoformans*
Oral/pharyngeal candidiasis	*Candida albicans*
Parasitic	
Toxoplasma encephalitis	*Toxoplasma gondii*
Cryptosporidial diarrhea	*Cryptosporidium*
Viral	
CMV retinitis	Cytomegalovirus
Progressive herpes infections	Herpes simplex types I & II
Shingles or herpes zoster infection	Varicella zoster virus
Mycobacterial	
Tuberculosis	*Mycobacterium tuberculosis*
Disseminated atypical mycobacterial	*Mycobacterium avium* complex

primary prophylaxis: antibiotics are started before contact with the potential pathogen or antibiotics are given after exposure to the potential pathogen but before development of clinical disease. The latter usually applies in AIDS patients. For example, primary prophylaxis is instituted for prevention of tuberculosis or PCP when an individual patient's risk of developing an acute infection is imminent, based on an assessment of their immune status. Specific criteria exist for initiating PCP prophylaxis when the CD_4 count is $<200/mm^3$.

The next stage of therapy is the acute treatment of an OI. When available, such therapy should consist when possible of *bactericidal* antimicrobial agents, as would be given in an immunocompromised cancer patient. Unfortunately, this is not possible nor practical for some of the OIs encountered in AIDS patients, such as toxomplasmosis, where oral sulfadiazine and pyrimethamine are presently the therapy of choice. *Combination regimens* are often used because of their additive or synergistic effects. Also, adequate drug penetration to the multiple sites of infection may be improved when more than one antimicrobial agent is used. Unfortunately, patients with HIV infection are generally much less tolerant to drugs, and they experience adverse effects with greater frequency and intensity. Thus, combination regimens are not always advisable (e.g., flucytosine with amphotericin B for cryptococcal meningitis).

The duration of acute treatment of opportunistic infections in patients with AIDS may be guided by experience from other patient groups as well as by individual patient response. However, in general therapy is more prolonged than for other patients. The goal of acute treatment may be only to reverse most of the signs and symptoms of infection and to bring patients back to their baseline level of health.

The last stage of antimicrobial therapy is the secondary prophylaxis regimen, which is instituted after the completion of acute treatment. The goal of maintenance therapy or secondary prophylaxis is to prevent future relapses or recurrences of clinical diseases. It may be very prolonged, possibly for a patient's entire lifetime, such as in the case of cryptococcal meningitis which has a high recurrence rate (30).

Pneumocystis carinii Pneumonia (PCP)

Pneumocystis carinii, newly reclassified as a fungus based on RNA sequencing data, is commonly observed to be part of human respiratory tract normal flora. Clinical infection with *Pneumocystis carinii* occurs in situations of host immune suppression (e.g., cancer or organ transplantation). Infection involving the lung is most common, and it is well described. In the 1980s, AIDS became the most common underlying immune disorder predisposing individuals to PCP. PCP occurs in more than 60% of AIDs patients in

the United States, with PCP being the AIDS case-defining diagnosis for most.

PCP is often an insidious infection in the HIV-infected patient, and therapy is almost always complicated by adverse drug reactions. Because PCP develops in 80 to 90% of AIDS patients, primary prophylaxis is recommended in HIV-infected persons with profound immunosuppression. Such treatment is recommended in patients with a CD_4 count of approximately 200 cell/mm^3. This preventative measure may in part be responsible for the improvement most recently observed in the long-term survival of AIDS patients.

The most frequent symptoms of acute PCP are shortness of breath, dyspnea, fever, and cough. An elevated serum lactate dehydrogenase (LDH) level and a chest x-ray with diffuse interstitial markings may indicate this pneumonia. Although patients with PCP often complain of cough, they rarely produce sputum. Patients may need to inhale a mist of hypertonic saline produced by an ultrasonic nebulizer to induce sputum. Currently, *Pneumocystis carinii* culture techniques are only reliable in the research setting, and the diagnosis of this infection depends upon obtaining an adequate sputum specimen for staining and microscopic examination. Giemsa and silver staining procedures are performed.

After diagnosis or just before (24 to 48 hr) sputum induction, patients may start acute treatment (Table 70.5). Any of the listed drug therapies is likely to be successful if the patient's pulmonary dysfunction is mild and no other OIs are present. Also, patients with PCP who have been on AZT for at least 6 weeks prior to diagnosis appear to have a better prognosis. Trimethoprim/sulfamethoxazole (T/S) is considered by most experts to be the drug of choice for PCP, unless the patient has an important history of drug intolerance or allergy. Either the oral or parenteral route of administration may be used, as the bioavailability of T/S is close to 100%. Parenteral therapy is recommended only if the patient has evidence of gastrointestinal intolerance or suspected malabsorption, or when the patient is too ill for oral medications. Parenteral T/S is usually selected as empiric therapy for the hospitalized patient, and oral therapy is used after improvement and stabilization occur. Therapy is given for a total of 14 to 21 days. Adverse reactions from T/S occur in most patients but require drug discontinuation in ≤50% of patients. Nausea and vomiting are often a problem, but it may be minimized by dividing the appropriate total daily dosage into small doses given at more frequent intervals (i.e., q6h administration). Hyponatremia and fluid overload may also be managed by administering more concentrated T/S solutions and by using diluents other than D5W (31). Other adverse reactions from T/S include hematologic toxicities (anemia, neutropenia, and thrombocytopenia), rashes, and liver transaminase enzyme elevation. T/S-induced adverse

Table 70.5.
Drug Therapy for Acute Treatment and Prophylaxis of *Pneumocystis carinii* Pneumonia

Therapy	Dosage	Route
Drug		
Trimethoprim(T)/sulfamethoxazole(S)	15–20 mg(T)/kg/day divided q6–8h	IV or p.o.
Pentamidine isethionate	3–4 mg/kg/day; q.d.	IV
Trimethoprim & dapsone	15–20 mg(T)/kg/day & 100 mg(D)/day	p.o.
Clindamycin & primaquine[a]	? 450–600 mg(C) q.i.d. & 15 mg(P) base q.d.	IV/p.o.
		p.o.
Diflornithine[a]	? 100 mg/kg q6h	IV
Trimetrexate[a] (add leukovorin rescue)	?45 mg/m^2 q24h (20 mg/m^2 q6h)	IV/p.o.
Prophylaxis		
Trimethoprim/sulfamethoxazole	One double strength tablet (160(T)/800(S)) q24h (q.o.d. and 3×/wk also studied)	p.o.
Dapsone[b]	50–100 mg q24h (q.o.d. 2–3×/wk also being studied)	p.o.
Pentamidine-aerosol	300 mg q. month	Respigard Nebulizer

[a] Considered salvage therapy with this investigational agent.
[b] Therapy remains to be evaluated in a controlled study.

reactions, for the most part, are readily reversible upon drug discontinuation.

T/S was compared with pentamidine in a prospective, randomized study of AIDS patients with PCP. There was no statistical difference in efficacies or frequencies of adverse reactions (32). The adverse reaction profile of pentamidine is potentially more serious and more often irreversible. Adverse reactions from pentamidine include nephrotoxicity, elevation of liver transaminase enzymes, hypocalcemia, hypoglycemia, pancreatitis followed by hyperglycemia and insulin-dependent diabetes mellitus, infusion-related hypotension, and thrombocytopenia (33).

The frequency of side effects from T/S in AIDS patients is not always minimized by dose-reduction, but therapy was better tolerated in one study when trimethoprim serum concentrations were monitored carefully and were maintained between 5 and 8 μg/ml (34). It is generally felt that a lower trimethoprim dose (15 mg/kg/day) may result in less toxicity to the various organ systems involved (e.g., bone marrow, liver, kidneys).

Therapeutic alternatives to T/S and pentamidine include the oral regimen of dapsone plus trimethoprim, which is as efficacious as T/S and less toxic in mild-to-moderately ill patients (35). In another study dapsone alone was not as effective as T/S (36). If a patient fails to improve on initial therapy, a switch is often made to parenteral pentamidine, or steroids can be added to the regimen (37). "Salvage therapy" for PCP or treatment with experimental regimens such as trimetrexate (38), difluormethylornithine (39), clindamycin plus pyrimethamine or BW566 (an investigational hydroxyquinone) might also be considered.

The administration of corticosteroids with antimicrobial therapy has improved outcomes in select patients with PCP (40, 41). Adults or children (over 13 years old) with documented or suspected PCP complicating HIV infection should be given corticosteroids if they have moderate a severe pulmonary dysfunction, defined as an arterial oxygen pressure <70 mm Hg or an arterial-alveolar gradient >35 mm Hg. Early treatment with corticosteroids reduces the risk of respiratory failure and death from PCP. In studies revealing these beneficial effects of adjunctive corticosteroids, steroid therapy was begun early, within 24 to 72 hr of initiating antipneumocystis therapy. The corticosteroid regimen currently recommended is: days 1 through 5—40 mg p.o. prednisone q12h; days 6 through 10—40 mg p.o. prednisone q.d.; days 11 through 21—20 mg p.o. prednisone q.d. (42).

PCP Prophylaxis

All patients who have had an episode of PCP should receive secondary prophylaxis. The same regimens recommended for primary prophylaxis of PCP can be considered for secondary prophylaxis. Either prophylaxis regimen, once begun, should be continued indefinitely (Table 70.5). The CDC has published guidelines for two acceptable prophylaxis regimens: oral T/S (160 mg/800 mg) given twice daily along with leukovorin (folinic acid) 5 mg once daily or aerosol pentamidine 300 mg administered once every four weeks (43). The "leukovorin rescue" is considered necessary by some experts to reduce the hematologic toxicity of this chronic T/S prophylactic regimen. Leukovorin has not been proven to be useful, but in this setting is thought to help reverse the effects of T/S on eucaryotic (host) cells. Ongoing studies may answer the question of leukovorin efficacy. Lower doses of T/S are also being recommended (e.g., one double-strength tablet q.d., given 3 to 7 times/week), which may obviate the need for leukovorin.

In patients (n = 60) with Kaposi's sarcoma a safety

and efficacy study was performed with T/S as primary prophylaxis (44). The study ran for a minimum of 24 months. The 160 mg (T)/800 mg (S) regimen administered twice daily was compared with placebo. T/S was observed to prevent or delay an initial episode of PCP. No patient (0/30) developed PCP while receiving T/S, compared with an increase of 53% in the placebo group (16 of 30). Eighteen patients (60%) in the T/S group died during the study, compared with 28 patients (93%) in the control group. Importantly, no patient in the T/S group died of PCP. Adverse reactions were observed in 50% of patients receiving T/S, only 5 (17%) of whom had to discontinue therapy because of severe erythroderma or neutropenia and fever. Of these 5 patients, PCP developed in 80% (4/5) within 5 months of discontinuing prophylaxis.

Aerosol pentamidine is currently the only FDA-approved prophylaxis regimen, but it may be less efficacious, as well as being economically and logistically more difficult to provide to patients. Long-term studies must compare the efficacy of oral regimens with aerosol pentamidine. The most common adverse effects reported during aerosol treatments are cough, and less frequently, wheezing. Systemic side effects (as discussed under acute treatment) have been reported but are rare after aerosol pentamidine administration. Other potential limitations of aerosol pentamidine include lack of protection against extrapulmonary disease and direct pulmonary toxicity, such as bronchospasm or pneumothorax. Recent case reports have verified disseminated *Pneumocystis carinii* infection in patients during aerosol pentamidine prophylaxis. These data and other preliminary reports suggest that aerosol pentamidine may not be the optimal prophylaxis regimen, that systemic regimens are superior. Since neither T/S nor aerosol pentamidine are known to be safe in pregnancy, neither are routinely recommended for HIV-infected, pregnant women.

Cryptococcal Meningitis

Disseminated cryptococcal infection and meningitis can occur in persons without immunodeficiency; however, the most serious cryptococcal infections are observed in those with defects in immune function. In two retrospective studies, cryptococcosis was the first-diagnosed opportunistic infection in 52% to 62% of AIDS patients (45, 46). Meningitis is the most common manifestation of cryptococcosis in AIDS patients; the lungs are usually spared, unless a simultaneous pulmonary infection occurs. The CSF glucose concentration, protein concentration, and cell count are frequently normal, although glucose levels have also been reported under 2.8 mmole/liter (50 mg/dl). Analysis of the CSF usually reveals positive results with India-ink staining, culture, and antigen-titer testing. The most common symptoms in AIDS patients with cryptococcal meningitis have been headache and fever. Other

symptoms of meningitis including nausea and vomiting, photophobia, malaise, stiff neck, focal neurologic abnormalities, mental status changes, seizures, papilledema, and flame hemorrhages of the retina occur less commonly.

Patients should ideally receive combination antifungal therapy, which includes amphotericin B (0.3 to 0.7 mg/kg/day as tolerated) plus (100 mg/kg/day) flucytosine (Ancobon; 5-fluorocytosine; 5-FC). Before amphotericin B, cryptococcal meningitis was a uniformly fatal disease; now intravenous amphotericin B is the standard therapy. The decision to add 5-FC depends mostly on the patient's baseline bone marrow status, because 5-FC suppresses the bone marrow. Toxicities observed include leukopenia (20%) and thrombocytopenia (10%); other side effects including diarrhea and rash have been reported in 8% of patients. There also has been some success with fluconazole in initial treatment of cryptococcal meningitis, but this therapy is not currently widely recommended at present (47). Fluconazole is considered by most to be an effective alternative to amphotericin only in patients who are at low risk for treatment failure (48). Optimal fluconazole doses are currently under study.

Because fluconazole is available for patients who have not responded to amphotericin B, the use of intrathecal amphotericin B has diminished dramatically. Intrathecal administration of amphotericin B previously was reserved for seriously ill patients who relapsed or were experiencing irreversible amphotericin-induced nephrotoxicity. Morbidity from intrathecal administration includes Omaya reservoir-associated complications as well as fever, pain, tinnitus, headache, and chemical ventriculitis.

5-FC is well absorbed after oral administration (76 to 79%) and distributes well into most body fluid and tissues, including the CSF. Unlike amphotericin, 5-FC is almost exclusively eliminated as unchanged drug by the kidneys, with a mean elimination half-life of 4 hr. It does not cause nephrotoxicity. Patients with renal failure do require dosage adjustment. General recommendations in the past were to maintain a therapeutic "peak" concentration between 50 and 100 μg/ml. However, these concentrations may not be as well tolerated in AIDS patients.

"Amphoterrible," a commonly used name for amphotericin B, has the potential for serious side effects, which may be related to drug administration or to more chronic end organ–associated adverse reactions. Infusion-related toxicities can usually be managed, and therapy can be continued. These may include fever, hypotension, chills, myalgias, nausea, and vomiting. Because of the seriousness of these toxicities patients must be closely monitored. If symptoms persist, premedication or treatment may be necessary with IV fluids, meperidine, diphenhydramine, aspirin, or acetaminophen. Infusion-related thrombophlebitis may be ameliorated by adding heparin (500 to 1000 units) and hydrocortisone (15 to 25 mg) to the IV. The infusion rate may also be slowed, but this is not always effective. Infusion-related shaking chills or rigors may improve with administration of meperidine.

The more chronic toxicities from amphotericin, such as hematologic effects include normochromic, normocytic anemia and thrombocytopenia. Nephrotoxicity from amphotericin B is not preventable nor is it predictable. Reported nephrotoxic effects include renal arteriolar vasoconstriction associated with a decreased glomerular filtration rate, tubular degeneration, nephrocalcinosis, decreased tubular concentrating ability, and renal tubular aciosis with potassium wasting. Sodium-loading has diminished nephrotoxicity in animal models, but adequate hydration with normal saline ≥2 liters/day is recommended in humans. Dosage adjustment (every-other-day) may also help to minimize impending renal toxicity.

Although the overall treatment response rate for AIDS patients with cryptococcal meningitis is similar to that observed for other populations, the infection does not appear to be eradicated. A marked relapse rate of at least 40% has been noted in AIDS patients, which suggests that secondary prophylaxis or suppressive therapy is necessary. Suppressive therapy with fluconazole 100 to 200 mg p.o. q.d. is currently suggested (49), though some patients may require higher doses.

Oral/Pharyngeal Candidiasis

Oropharyngeal candidiasis (thrush) is the most common fungal infection reported in AIDS patients. Infection usually causes mild inflammation and local discomfort, but it does not become invasive with symptomatic fungemia. Fungal throat-swab cultures have been studied as a screening test, but they are not useful because *Candida* species are common commensal oropharyngeal and pulmonary flora.

Topical treatment, even for the more symptomatic cases of thrush is usually adequate. Initial therapy with nystatin or clotrimazole is recommended. There is no proven benefit to combined topical regimens. To be most successful, treatment should not be on an "as needed" (p.r.n.) schedule. For thrush, it is recommended that one clotrimazole troche 10 mg be given four to five times daily until clinical resolution of signs and symptoms. The dose of nystatin suspension is 100,000 to 1,500,000 units, "swish and swallow," q 4 to 6 hr. Nystatin may also be administered topically by instructing the patient to suck on a vaginal tablet (100,000 units per tablet) three to four times daily. The slow dissolution of the vaginal tablet may actually provide more drug-contact time. Compliance may be an important issue with nystatin suspension because it has a bitter taste even though it contains sucrose; clotrimazole troches and nystatin pastilles are more palatable and are "sugar-free." Troches/lozenges should be dissolved slowly in the mouth, not swallowed whole. Chlorhexidine

gluconate 0.12% oral rinse solution has been very effective for HIV-related periodontal disease and has efficacy against oral thrush. Systemic antifungal therapy with ketoconazole or fluconazole is generally not warranted for thrush. Intermittent, short courses of ketoconazole 200 mg p.o. q.d. may be useful in patients with more resistant infection.

Esophageal candidiasis can occur without preceding symptoms of thrush and usually presents with difficulty or pain on swallowing. Other symptoms may include anorexia, nausea, fevers, and GI upset. The diagnosis of esophageal candidiasis is usually made by endoscopic examination. Systemic therapy is indicated for this fungal infection with most patients responding to ketoconazole 200 to 600 mg p.o. q.d. Patients should be told to take the ketoconazole with meals, as it is most soluble in an acid environment (100 gastric pH); thus dissolution and absorption increases when it is taken with food. Potential drug-drug interactions that are clinically significant includes medications that decrease ketoconazole bioavailability (e.g., antacids and H_2-antagonists).

Nausea and vomiting are the most commonly observed adverse reactions associated with ketoconazole therapy, but they can be minimized by taking the medication with food. Asymptomatic elevation of liver enzymes occurs in 5 to 10% of patients and does not seem to be a dose-related. Serious hepatic damage and death have occurred, but are uncommon, with a prevalence of approximately 1 in 15,000 persons. Parenteral therapy with amphotericin B is usually not warranted unless fungemia occurs as well or if the patient has difficulty swallowing oral medications. Fluconazole therapy can also be considered in ketoconazole-resistant infection or when ketoconazole toxicity or bioavailability problems occur (50). Currently there are no data on using fluconazole for prophylaxis or suppression therapy of esophageal candidiasis.

Toxoplasmosis

Toxoplasmosis in AIDS patients presents predominantly as encephalitis. Most patients are believed to have disease reactivation rather than new primary infection (51). On physical examination the predominant signs are focal neurological findings, and many patients also have a change in mental status, seizures, and fever. For most patients with HIV infection, toxoplasmosis is not their first OI. A lumbar puncture done in these patients reveals a mononuclear pleocytosis with an elevated protein and a normal or low glucose concentration. CT scans are recommended for diagnosis and monitoring and also to guide brain biopsy or excision. Currently, many centers are treating patients with clinical and radiographic findings suggestive of CNS toxoplasmosis without biopsy confirmation. Demonstration of tachyzoite forms, but not cysts, in tissue secretions or smears of body fluid (e.g., brain biopsy tissue or CSF) establishes the diagnosis of acute toxoplasma infection.

The overall prognosis of AIDS patients with *Toxoplasma* encephalitis poor (52). Median survival following initiation of therapy may be as poor as 4 months. Patients with good mentation upon diagnosis have longer survival time than patients in poorer condition (i.e., stuporous). Serological tests have limited value when making the diagnosis because of the high prevalence of positive antibody titers. CSF antibody titers are equally "useful."

Initial therapy with pyrimethamine plus sulfadiazine or trisulfapyrimidines (sulfamerazine, sulfamethazine, and sulfadiazine; "triple sulfa") is recommended. Optimal doses of these agents have not been determined; however efficacy is reported for AIDS patients receiving 50 to 100 mg q.d. pyrimethamine and 1.0 to 2.0 g q.i.d. sulfadiazine. The serum elimination half-life of pyrimethamine has been estimated to be approximately 100 hr, but issues of inter-patient pharmacokinetic variability, patient compliance, and GI intolerance have influenced most practitioners to administer this drug once daily.

Toxicity attributable to pyrimethamine or sulfonamide therapy has been reported in as many as 60% of individuals. Reversible leukopenia, thrombocytopenia, and rash are the most common adverse reactions. Crystalluria occurs in patients whose fluid intake is inadequate because this sulfonamide is not very water soluble (compared with sulfamethoxazole and sulfisoxazole). Folinic acid (leukovorin) is usually added because it is necessary to reverse their dose-related bone marrow suppressive effects. Dosages range from 5 to 15 mg/day, as "rescue treatment." Folinic acid does not antagonize the antiparasitic activity of pyrimethamine. This is not true for folic acid, which should not be administered during treatment with folate-antagonist drugs.

AIDS patients with toxoplasmosis should receive secondary prophylaxis or posttreatment suppressive therapy because of the high recurrence rates. Pyrimethamine plus sulfadiazine should be given indefinitely at a dosage that keeps patients stable, 25 to 50 mg pyrimethamine with 500 mg to 1.0 g q.i.d. sulfadiazine. Primary prophylaxis of toxoplasmosis is currently being studied.

Alternatives to sulfathiazine are being hotly pursued because of the high adverse reaction rate in AIDS patients. Clindamycin has been studies in the animal model of *Toxoplasma* encephalitis with good success (53). These data, case reports, and a recent randomized trial suggest that clindamycin has a role in the treatment of toxoplasmic encephalitis (54–56). Acute treatment with doses of clindamycin 1200 mg I.V. q.i.d. used to treat CNS toxoplasmosis are much higher than those used to treat bacterial infections, but they have generally been well tolerated. Six weeks of acute treatment followed by lower oral dosages (300 q6h or 450 q8h) are recommended along with pyr-

imethamine. Experimental agents are also being further investigated (e.g., BW566, piritrexim, roxithromycin, and azithromycin).

Cryptosporidial Diarrhea

Prior to the AIDS epidemic, only rare cases of cryptosporidial diarrhea were reported in humans, most of whom were immunocompromised hosts or animal handlers. This infection is postulated by some to be a sexually transmitted disease with AIDS patients human-to-human transmission of this infection, presumably by the oral-fecal route (57). The oral-fecal route also contributes to the transmission if poor hygiene is practiced. Symptoms of cryptosporidiosis include epigastric cramping pain, nausea, vomiting, anorexia, weight loss and diarrhea. The diarrhea may wax and wane but can be severely debilitating. The consequences may include malabsorption, electrolyte imbalance, and malnutrition. Treatment is predominantly supportive therapy with fluids and electrolytes. The diarrhea may be controlled somewhat by using bulk agents and antidiarrheals. No antimicrobial therapy to date has been shown to be effective. Research efforts have been impeded by the inability to grow the organism in vitro. Published reports describe the lack of efficacy of various agents including oral spiramycin, clindamycin, furazolidone, and quinine. Studies are ongoing with modest preliminary results using intravenous spiramycin, azithromycin diclazuril, paromomycin, and hyperimmune bovine colostrum.

Herpes Viral Infections: Cytomegalovirus Retinitis

Retinitis due to cytomegalovirus (CMV) may be the initial manifestation of AIDs, but it usually is not end-stage opportunistic infection. CMV retinitis, like CMV infection of any other organ system, may signify a profound immune deficiency of the host and may result in unilateral or bilateral blindness. CMV infection is common in normal hosts, with has many as 50% of persons being seropositive by adulthood in many parts of the world. The initial infection in most hosts does not result in acute clinical infection. CMV is the most common cause of congenital and perinatal infection causing morbidity in neonates. These infections are the primary disease in such patients, whereas in organ transplant recipients, for the most part, morbidity and mortality result from recurrences of latent infection. Treatment of CMV infections with antiviral agents had been unsuccessful until the mid-1980s when ganciclovir (Cytovene; DHPG) became available. In 1991, the FDA approved phosphonoformate (Foscarnet, Foscavir), which has shown in vitro activity against CMV and other herpesviruses in vivo efficacy.

CMV is a herpesvirus, and like herpes simplex, it can cause acute, latent, and chronic persistent infection. Subclinical CMV infection is reported in most HIV-infected persons as evidenced by serologic testing. It is as infrequent cause of serious life-threatening infection in AIDs patients (5.7% retinitis and 2.2% gastrointestinal infection) (58). CMV infection of the lung is also reported frequently, but the lung is thought to be a reservoir for CMV, and the virus commonly coexists in the lung with other pathogens. The role that CMV plays in clinical infection (pneumonia) is not always clear, and it should not always be treated.

The diagnosis of CMV retinitis is usually based on ophthalmologic examination. Patients complain of unilateral peripheral vision loss and eye findings include white fluffy patches of retinal opacifications and retinal hemorrhage. The histologic verification of this diagnosis is difficult and is rarely pursued. Isolation of the virus from the blood or urine constitutes important confirmatory data in patients with eye findings.

Empiric treatment of CMV retinitis is parenteral therapy with ganciclovir 2.5 mg/kg IV q8h or 5 mg/kg IV q12h (at least 7.5 mg/kg/day) for 10 days to 4 weeks. During this acute, or so-called induction phase of therapy, the patient is monitored closely for disease progression. An indefinite maintenance regimen (5 mg/kg/day) is necessary to prevent bilateral disease and blindness (59). For ease of administration and to minimize toxicity, this maintenance regimen is often given only Monday through Friday. The intraocular penetration of ganciclovir is generally adequate for effective concentrations and cure. Intravitreous ganciclovir administration has been useful in a few patients on AZT with neutropenia who cannot tolerate intravenous ganciclovir because of its predictable neutropenia. Rarely is it necessary to administer intravitreous ganciclovir, though the procedure is well tolerated (60). The role of colony-stimulating factors, G-CSF and GM-CSF, remains to be elucidated for patients with disease- or drug-induced neutropenias who need intravenous ganciclovir for treatment of CMV infection. Recent AIDS Clinical Trials Group data suggest that foscarnet is perhaps the best alternative in patients who cannot tolerate full-dose ganciclovir while remaining on antiretroviral therapy. For prophylaxis and chronic suppression, oral ganciclovir (currently under investigation) will be very important in CMV infection treatment.

Adverse effects from ganciclovir include bone marrow toxicity, specifically neutropenia, which is usually reversible but may be more problematic in patients receiving other bone marrow suppressants (e.g., zidovudine, pyrimethamine, trimethoprim/sulfamethoxazole). Significant neutropenia and anemia has been reported in 30 to 80% of patients (61, 62). Toxicity appears to be somewhat dose- and/or duration-dependent, so regimens may be altered to minimize neutropenia before therapy must be discontinued. Ganciclovir is eliminated by the kidneys, so dosage

alterations are also necessary in patients with renal insufficiency (63).

Foscarnet (phosphonoformate, Foscavir) is an antiviral drug with broad-spectrum activity, including activity against HIV and herpesviruses. The parenteral formulation of the drug has been used to treat severe herpetic infections including acyclovir-resistant strains in the immunocompromised transplant patients, and more recently was FDA-approved for treatment of CMV retinitis in AIDS patients (64). Recent data from ACTG trial suggests that foscarnet therapy prolonged survival of patients with CMV retinitis, compared with ganciclovir. This observation remains to be confirmed in a study designed to look at survival as an endpoint. A topical formulation of foscarnet is also under study. Like other agents against CMV, phosphonoformate cannot eradicate the infection, but only suppresses viral replication. Consequently, relapses of the CMV infection are common after discontinuation of acute therapy (as they are with ganciclovir). Initial induction therapy with foscarnet (90 mg/kg/day) is administered by intermittent infusion divided q8h IV until disease stabilization or improvement, approximately 2 weeks. Efficacy was reported in one study for 9 of 10 patients with CMV retinitis receiving this regimen (65). Maintenance therapy 60 mg/kg/day for 7 days of the week is also recommended, but efficacy data are not complete. Toxicities relating to drug infusions such as abnormalities in calcium, magnesium, and phosphorus concentrations are commonly observed. Nephrotoxicity from intermittent-infusion regimens is also reported but is less serious than earlier reports from continuous infusions. Because of these potential side effects it is recommended that patients be well hydrated and receive foscarnet via an infusion pump over hours. Foscarnet is eliminated by the kidneys, so dosage adjustments must be made for renal insufficiency. Foscarnet may prove to be a valuable alternative to ganciclovir in the treatment of serious CMV infections, but its potential toxicities and logistics of administration of hurdles to overcome in each patient.

Other Herpesvirus Infections

Many patients with HIV infection have severe, recurrent outbreaks of herpes simplex virus (HSV) infection. The CDC definition of AIDS includes chronic, progressive, or disseminated infection with HSV. Patients with HIV infection other have severe and refractory herpes zoster infections or shingles, which are recrudescent infections with varicella-zoster virus (VZV). In one report of 112 homosexual men with herpes zoster infections an analysis indicated a cumulative incidence of AIDS of 22.8% within 2 years after the herpes zoster episode (66). It was concluded that herpes zoster infection is a predictor of AIDS in persons also in an HIV high-risk group.

Acyclovir remains first-line therapy for HSV-1, HSV-

2, and VZV infections, however the dose should be titrated in patients with HIV, based upon clinical response. Acute treatment of HSV-2 infections in 200 mg p.o. 5x/day, for 7 to 10 days or longer if needed. Treatment should continue until all vesicular lesions crust or epithelialize, and symptoms resolve. When multiple recurrences occur, suppressive therapy should be considered (200 mg t.i.d. or 400 mg b.i.d.). Primary drug resistance to acyclovir has been documented, but rarely is problematic. Acyclovir-resistant HSV have emerged after several courses of acyclovir, and treatment with foscarnet has been successful. Foscarnet has also been useful in the treatment of acyclovir-resistant varicella-zoster virus infection (67).

Atypical Mycobacterial Infection

Mycobacterium avium-intracellulare complex (MAC) is a commonly encountered group of environmental contaminants. MAC is present in dust, dirt, and the water supply. Before AIDS was described, human disease with MAC was infrequent. Most cases were pulmonary infections in patients with preexisting pulmonary disease, and they rarely disseminated. Since the recognition of AIDs and immunosuppression with HIV, disseminated disease with MAC has been described with increasing frequency (68). The epidemic of disseminated MAC is concurrent with the AIDS epidemic. A major risk factor for this infection appears to be the level of HIV-induced immunosuppression and CD_4 cell count (this infection is rare in patients with counts >100/mm^3). The pathogenesis of this disease is not well understood. Symptoms of infection include fevers, night sweats, weight loss, diarrhea, pancytopenia, and hepatosplenomegaly with liver enzyme level elevation. Blood cultures and bone marrow aspirate cultures are often positive. Cultures from nonsterile sites (e.g., sputum) are also often positive, but this result cannot be distinguished from colonization by MAC.

Atypical mycobacteria are known to be more intrinsically drug-resistant than *Mycobacterium tuberculosis*. Serotype strains of MAC that cause infection in AIDS patients are also more drug resistant (69). In vivo study results have been modest. In one small study, patients who received at least 4 weeks of therapy had objective improvement described as bacterial counts declining by more than 30-fold during the period of treatment. Treatment was with multiple drugs, including amikacin 7.5 mg/kg/day (for a maximum of 4 weeks), plus ethambutol 15 mg/kg/day (maximum 1000 mg), plus ciprofloxacin 750 mg b.i.d., and rifampin 10 mg/kg/day (maximum 600 mg) (70). In patients who completed 12 weeks of therapy, blood cultures reverted to negative for 3, had reduced counts in 5, and had increased counts in 2. A reduction in clinical symptoms was reported by patients, although some patients experienced serious adverse reactions to antimycobacterial therapy (i.e., hepatitis and nausea). In another study of 67

patients mycobacteremia persisted despite treatment with multiple-drug regimens (ansamycin, clofazamine, and ethionamide or ethambutol) (71). Clarithromycin (Biaxin) a new macrolide antibiotic, has recently been FDA-approved and is bringing new hope in the treatment of MAC disease. Controlled studies are needed, but initial case reports are encouraging. No known therapy has been shown to prolong survival in AIDS patients with disseminated MAC infection. Further study on disease pathogenesis, in vitro culture-susceptibility techniques, and drug therapy is needed.

Mycobacterium tuberculosis infection

The most common mycobacterial infections in HIV-positive persons are with MAC, but infections caused by *M. tuberculosis* are much more likely to be cured. Because the CD_4 cells and macrophages play a central role in host antimycobaterial defenses, dysfunction or depletion of these cells by HIV disease places persons at risk for disease reactivation or at higher risk of acquiring primary infection (72). The incidence of tuberculosis in AIDs patients is disproportionately high, almost 500 times the incidence observed in the general population. Also, extrapulmonary forms of the infection are more likely to occur, including lymphatic and disseminated-miliary disease (73). Patients with tuberculosis may have pulmonary symptoms and radiographic lung infiltrates in any lung zone often associated with mediastinal or hilar lymphadenopathy. Specimens (e.g., sputum, blood, urine, or bone marrow) should be obtained for acid-fast staining and culture of *Mycobacterium* before instituting therapy. Tuberculin skin testing (PPD) can also be helpful in making the diagnosis, especially if a previous negative test result is known. False-negative results often occur, even when skin tests are placed properly, because of profound immunosuppression. This anergic response can be confirmed by placing controls with the PPD skin test.

Infection control measures with respiratory precautions should be instituted as soon as a patient is suspected of having pulmonary tuberculosis. Multiple-drug chemotherapy should be started after adequate specimens are obtained for acid-fast staining and culture. Most patients respond well to standard oral therapy with isoniazid 300 mg/day, rifampin 600 mg q.d. and ethambutol 15 to 25 mg/kg/day and/or pyrazinamide 20 to 30 mg/kg/day. Both ethambutol and pyrazinamide are recommended if INH-resistance is suspected. They must be administered only for the first 2 months of therapy, when cultures are pending to assess isoniazid susceptibility. The appropriate duration of therapy in HIV-infected persons is unknown, but it must be longer than the standard 9 months of therapy. A minimum of 9 months is recommended, with at least 6 months of therapy after documented culture-negative conversion. If isoniazid and rifampin are not included in the

Table 70.6.
Summary—Therapy Schedule/Monitoring Guidelines for Antimicrobial Treatments in Patients with HIV-Infection

Therapy	Monitor
Antiretroviral	
Zidovudine	CBC, platelets, CPK, anorexia,
500–600 mg/day	LFTs, N/V/HA, fatigue
Didanosine	Diarrhea, amylase, seizures,
150–300 mg (tablets) b.i.d.	triglyceride, uric acid,
	peripheral neuropathy
Dideoxycytidine	Peripheral neuropathy, seizures,
0.375–0.75 mg t.i.d.	amylase
Antipneumocystis	
Trimethoprim/sulfamethoxazole	Renal & liver function, fever/rash,
15–20 mg/kg/day TMP	CBC, hyponatremia, N/V
component (divide q8–6 as	
tolerated)	
Pentamidine (intravenous)	Renal & liver function,
3–4 mg/kg/day (one dose over	hypotension, CBC, glucose,
>1 hr)	metallic taste
Dapsone & trimethoprim	G6PD status, WBC, LFTs, rash
15–20 mg/kg/day TMP plus	
100 mg/day dapsone	
Aerosol pentamidine	Cough, bronchospasm, metallic
300 mg/month (for prophylaxis	taste
only)	
Anticryptococcal	
Amphotericin B	Renal function; CBC, K, Mg,
approx. 0.7 mg/kg/day	platelets, phlebitis
Fluconazole	Renal & hepatic function,
≥400 mg/day	platelets, neutrophils
200 mg/day maintenance	
Antitoxoplasmosis	
Sulfadiazine/pyrimethamine	Rash/fever, crystalluria, CBC,
1–2 q q6h/50–75 mg q.d.	platelets
Clindamycin/pyrimethamine	N/V/D, CBC, rash, *C. difficle*
900 mg(C) q6h/50–75 mg(P)	colitis
q.d.	
Anticytomegalovirus	
Gancyclovir (DHPG)	Neutropenia
induction 7.5–10 mg/kg (divide	
q12h)	
maintenance 5 mg/kg/day;	
5×/wk	
Foscarnet	CA, PO4, Mg, phlebitis, renal
induction 90 mg/kg/day (divide	function, CBC
t.i.d.)	
maintenance 60 mg/kg/day;	
7×/wk	

treatment regimen because of drug intolerance or resistance, therapy should be prolonged to ≥18 months, with a minimum of 12 months after culture-negative conversion.

Drug monitoring for adverse reactions to antimycobacterial agents can be difficult because of multiorgan system toxicities. Patients with HIV infection are commonly on various other agents that cause similar toxicities, such as liver toxicity rash or bone marrow suppression. Rarely

must therapy for *M. tuberculosis* be interrupted, if it is carefully monitored.

CONCLUSIONS

In summary, HIV disease is a continuum of clinical conditions, ranging from an asymptomatic state to AIDS. The early institution of antiretroviral therapy with zidovudine has increased the survival of patients and therefore is recommended in all HIV antibody-positive persons who have CD_4 cell counts ≤500/mm^3. Hematologic toxicity from AZT has been a limiting factor in the widespread use of this therapy. Ongoing studies are evaluating other antiretroviral agents, such as didanosive and DDC. Optimal therapy has yet to be described, though monotherapy is probably not the answer. Combination or sequential antiretroviral regimens are being studied for efficacy and may be less toxic. Regimens that contain immunomodulators (e.g., α-interferon) may also improve the efficacy for HIV infection and OIs. Vaccine development will help to fight this battle. The successful treatment of opportunistic infections in AIDS patients remains a challenge. Table 70-6 has a summary of therapies and monitoring parameters that are commonly used in AIDS patients. Treatment with standard therapies is routinely disrupted by adverse drug reactions and side effects. Primary and secondary prophylaxis regimens are recommended for various infections in an attempt to decrease the incidence of acute and recurrent disease.

REFERENCES

1. Centers for Disease Control: HIV prevalence estimates and AIDS case projections for the United States: report based upon a workshop. MMWR 39(RR-16):1–31, 1990.
2. Centers for Disease Control: Mortality attributable to HIV infection/AIDS—United States, 1981–1990. MMWR 40:41–44, 1991.
3. Centers for Disease Control: Revision of the CDC surveillance case definition for acquired immunodeficiency syndrome. MMWR 36(suppl 1S):3S–15S, 1987.
4. Langtry HD, Campoli-Richards DM: Zidovudine: a review of its pharmacodynamics and pharmacokinetic properties and therapeutic efficacy. Drugs 37:408–450, 1989.
5. Morse GD, Lechner JL, Santora JA, Rozek SL: Zidovudine update: 1990. Ann Pharmacother 24:754–760, 1990.
6. Yarchoan R, Mitsuya H, Myers CE, Broder S: Clinical pharmacology of 3'-azido-2',3'-dideoxythymidine (zidovudine) and related dideoxynucleosides. N Engl J Med 321:726–738, 1989.
7. Fischl MA, Richman DD, Grieco MH, et al.: The efficacy of azidothymidine (AZT) in the treatment of patients with AIDS and AIDS-related complex. N Engl J Med 317:185–191, 1987.
8. Richman DD, Fischl MA, Grieco MH, et al.: The toxicity of azidothymidine (AZT) in the treatment of patients with AIDS and AIDS-related complex. N Engl J Med 317:192–197, 1987.
9. Fischl M, Galpin JE, Levine JD, et al.: Recombinant human erythropoietin for patients with AIDs treated with zidovudine. N Engl J Med 322:1488–1493, 1990.
10. Erslev AJ: Erythropoietin. N Engl J Med 324:1339–1344, 1991.
11. Fischl MA, Parker CB, Pettinelli C, et al.: A randomized controlled trial of a reduced daily dose of zidovudine in patients with the ac-

quired immunodeficiency syndrome. N Engl J Med 323:1009–1014, 1990.

12. The Swiss Group for Clinical Studies on the Acquired Immunode- ficiency Syndrome: Zidovudine for the treatment of thrombocyto- penia associated with human immunodeficiency virus (HIV). Ann Intern Med 109:718–721, 1988.

13. Volberding PA, Lagakos SW, Koch MA, et al.: Zidovudine in asymp- tomatic human immunodeficiency virus infection. N Engl J Med 322:941–949, 1990.

14. Collier AC, Bozzette S, Coombs RW, et al.: A pilot study of low- dose zidovudine in human immunodeficiency virus infection. N Engl J Med 323:1015–1021, 1990.

15. Fischl MA, Richman DD, Causey DM et al.: Prolonged zidovudine therapy in patients with AIDS and advanced AIDS-related complex. JAMA 262:2405–2410, 1989.

16. McKinney RE, Maha MA, Connor EM, et al.: A multicenter trial of oral zidovudine in children with advanced human immunodeficiency virus disease. N Engl J Med 324:1018–1025, 1991.

17. Sandstrom E: Antiviral therapy in human immunodeficiency virus infection. Drugs 38:417–450, 1989.

18. Lambert JS, Seidlin M, Reichman RC, et al.: 2′,3′-dideoxyinosine (DDI) in patients with the acquired immunodeficiency syndrome or AIDS-related complex. N Engl J Med 322:1333–1340, 1990.

19. Cooley TP, Kunches LM, Saunders CA, et al.: Once-daily admin- istration of 2′,3′-dideoxyinosine (DDI) in patients with the acquired immunodeficiency syndrome or AIDS-related complex. N Engl J Med 322:1340–1345, 1990.

20. Butler KM, Husson RN, Balis FM, et al.: Dideoxyinosine in children with symptomatic human immunodeficiency virus infection. N Engl J Med 324:137–144, 1991.

21. Hartman NR, Yarchoan R, Pluda JM, Thomas RV, Marczyk KS, Broder S, Joghns DG: Pharmacokinetics of 2′,3′-dideoxyadenosine and 2′,3′-dideoxyinosine in patients with severe human immuno- deficiency virus infection. Clin Pharmacol Ther 47:647–654, 1990.

22. Jeffries OJ: The antiviral activity of dideoxycytidine, J Antimicrob Chemother 23(suppl A):29–34, 1989.

23. Yarchoan R, Thomas RV, Allain JP, et al.: Phase I studies of 2′,3′- dideoxycytidine in severe human immunodeficiency virus infection as a single agent and alternating with zidovudine (AZT). Lancet 2:76– 81, 1988.

24. Meng TC, Fischl MA, Boota AM, et al.: Combination therapy with zidovudine and dideoxycytidine in patients with advanced human immunodeficiency virus infection. Ann Intern Med 116:13–20, 1992.

25. Waite LA, Levin AS, Starrett BA, et al.: Trichosanthin treatment of HIV disease. Abstract S.B.466, vol 3, p 202, Sixth International Con- ference on AIDS, San Francisco, California, June 20–24, 1990.

26. Henderson DK, Gerberding JL: Prophylactic zidovudine after oc- cupational exposure to the human immunodeficiency virus: an in- terim analysis. J Infect Dis 160:321–327, 1989.

27. Centers for Disease Control: Recommendations for preventing trans- mission of human immunodeficiency virus and hepatitis B to patients during exposure-prone invasive procedures. MMWR 40:1, 1991.

28. Safai B, Johnson KG, Myskowski PL, et al.: The natural history of Kaposi's sarcoma in the acquired immunodeficiency syndrome. Ann Intern Med 103:744–750, 1985.

29. Kovacs JA, Deyton L, Davey R, et al.: Combined zidovudine and interferon-α therapy in patients with Kaposi's sarcoma and the ac- quired immunodeficiency syndrome. Ann Intern Med 111:280–287, 1989.

30. Chuck SL, Sande MA: Infectious with Cryptococcus neoformans in the acquired immunodeficiency syndrome. N Engl J Med 321:794– 799, 1989.

31. Jarosinski PF, Kennedy PE, Gallelli JF: Stability of concentrated trimethoprim-sulfamethoxazole admixtures. Am J Hosp Pharm 46:732–737, 1989.

32. Wharton M, Coleman DL, Wofsy CB, et al.: Trimethoprim-sulfa- methoxazole for Pneumocystis carinii pneumonia in the acquired immunodeficiency syndrome. Ann Intern Med 105:37–44, 1986.

33. Kapusnik JE, Mills J, Pentamidine. In Peterson, PK, Verhof J (eds): Antimicrobial Agents Annual III. Austerdam, Elsevier Science Pub- lishers BV, 1988, ch 27, pp 299–311.

34. Sattler FR, Cowan R, Nielsen DM, Ruskin J: Trimethoprim-sulfa- methoxazole compared with pentamidine for treatment of Pneu- mocystis carinii pneumonia in the immunodeficiency syndrome. Ann Intern Med 109:280–287, 1988.

35. Medina I, Mills J, Leounf G, et al.: Oral therapy for Pneumocystis carinii pneumonia in the acquired immunodeficiency syndrome. N Engl J Med 323:776–782, 1990.

36. Mills J, Leoung G, Medina I, et al.: Dapsone treatment of Pneu- mocystis carinii pneumonia in the acquired immunodeficiency syn- drome. Antimicrob Agents Chemother 32:1057–1060, 1988.

37. MacFadden DK, Hyland RH, Inouye T, et al.: Corticosteroids as adjunctive therapy in treatment of Pneumocystis carinii pneumonia in patients with acquired immunodeficiency syndrome. Lancet 1:1477–1479, 1987.

38. Allegra CJ, Chabner BA, Tuazon Cu, et al.: Trimetrexate for the treatment of Pneumocystis carinii pneumonia in patients with the acquired immunodeficiency syndrome. N Engl J Med 317:978–983, 1987.

39. Sahai J, Berry AJ: Eflornithine for the treatment of Pneumocystis carinii pneumonia in patients with the acquired immunodeficiency syndrome: a preliminary review. Pharmacother 9:29–33, 1989.

40. Gagnon S, Boota AM, Fischl MA, et al.: Corticosteroids as adjuvant therapy for severe Pneumocystis carinii pneumonia in the acquired immunodeficiency syndrome. N Engl J Med 323:1444–1450, 1190.

41. Bozzette SA, Sattler FR, Chiu J, et al.: A controlled trial of early adjuvant treatment with corticosteroids for Pneumocystis carinii pneumonia in the acquired immunodeficiency syndrome. N Engl J Med 323:1451–1457, 1990.

42. The National Institutes of Health–University of California Expert Panel for Corticosteroids as Adjuvant Therapy for Pneumocystis Pneumonia: Special report—consensus statement on the use of cor- ticosteroids as adjuvant therapy for Pneumocystis carinii pneumonia in the acquired immunodeficiency syndrome. N Engl J Med 323:1500–1504, 1990.

43. Centers for Disease Control: Guidelines for prophylaxis against Pneu- mocystis carinii pneumonia for persons with human immunodefi- ciency virus. MMWR 38:1–9, 1989.

44. Fischl MA, Dickinson GM, La Voie L: Safety and efficacy of sul- famethoxazole and trimethoprim chemoprophylaxis for Pneumocystis carinii pneumonia in AIDS. JAMA 259:1185–1189, 1988.

45. Zuger A, Louie E, Holzman RS, Simberkoff MS, Rahal JJ: Cryp- tococcal disease in patients with acquired immunodeficiency syn- drome. Ann Intern Med 104:234, 1986.

46. Kovak JA, Kovacs AA, Polis M, et al.: Cryptococcosis in the acquired immunodeficiency syndrome. Ann Intern Med 103:533, 1985.

47. Larsen RA, Leal MAE, Chan LS: Fluconazole compared with am- photericin B plus flucytosine for cryptococcal meningitis in AIDS. Ann Intern Med 113:183–187, 1990.

48. Saag MS, Powderly WG, Cloud GA, et al.: Comparison of ampho- tericin B with fluconazole in the treatment of acute AIDS-associated cryptococcal meningitis. N Engl J Med 326:83, 1992.

49. Bozzette SA, Larsen RA, Chiu J, et al.: A placebo-controlled trial of maintenance therapy with fluconazole after treatment of cryptococ- cal meningitis in the acquired immunodeficiency syndrome. N Engl J Med 324:580–584, 1991.

50. Robinson PA, Knirsch AK, Joseph JA: Fluconazole for life-threat- ening fungal infections in patients who cannot be treated with con- ventional antifungal agents. Infect Dis 12:S349–S363, 1990.

51. Wong B, Gold JWM, Brown AE, et al.: Central-nervous-system toxoplasmosis in homosexual men and parenteral drug abusers. Ann Intern Med 100:36, 1984.

52. Haverkos HW: Assessment of therapy for *Toxoplasma* encephalitis. Am J Med 82:907, 1987.

53. Hofflin JM, Remington JS: Clindamycin in a murine model of toxoplasmic encephalitis. Antimicrob Agents Chemother 31:492, 1987.

54. Dannemann B, McCutchan JA, Israelski D, et al.: Treatment of toxoplasmic encephalitis in patients with AIDS. Ann Intern Med 116:33, 1992.

55. Westblom TU, Belshe RB: Clindamycin therapy of cerebral toxoplasmosis in an AIDS patient. Scand J Infect Dis 20:561, 1988.

56. Snider WD, Simpson DM, Nielsen S, et al.: Neurologic complications of acquired immunodeficiency syndrome: analysis of 50 patients. Ann Neruol 14:403–418, 1983.

57. Koch KL, Phillips DJ, Aber RC, Current WL: Cryptosporidiosis in hospital personnel. Ann Intern Med 102:593, 1985.

58. Jacobson MA, Mills J: Serious cytomegalovirus disease in the acquired immunodeficiency syndrome (AIDS): Ann Intern Med 108:585–594, 1988.

59. Buhles WC Jr, Mastre BJ, Tinker AJ, et al.: Ganciclovir treatment of life-threatening cytomegalovirus infection: experience in 314 immunocompromised patients. Infect Dis 10(suppl 3):S4595–506, 1988.

60. Faulds D, Heel RC: Ganciclovir. Drugs 39:597–638, 1990.

61. Fletch CV, Balfour HH Jr: Evaluation of ganciclovir for cytomegalovirus disease. Drug Intell Clin Pharm 23:5–12, 1989.

62. Hochster H, Dieterich D, Bozzette S, et al. and the AIDS Clinical Trials Group: Toxicity of combined ganciclovir and zidovudine for cytomegalovirus disease associated with AIDS. Ann Intern Med 113:111–117, 1990.

63. Fletcher CV, Sawchuck R, Chinnock B, de Miranda P, Balfour HH Jr: Human pharmacokinetics of the antiviral drug DHPG. Clin Pharmacol Ther 40:281–286, 1986.

64. Minor JR, Baltz JK: Foscarnet sodium. DICP, Ann Pharmacol 25:41–47, 1991.

65. Jacobson MA, O'Donnell JJ, Mills J: Foscarnet treatment of cytomegalovirus retinitis in patients with the acquired immunodeficiency syndrome. Antimicrob Agents Chemother 33:736–741, 1989.

66. Melbye M, Grossman RJ, Goedert JJ, et al.: Risk of AIDS after herpes zoster. Lancet 1:728–730, 1987.

67. Safrin S, Berger TG, Gilson I, et al.: Foscarnet therapy in five patients with AIDS and acyclovir-resistant varicella-zoster virus infection. Ann Intern Med 115:19–21, 1991.

68. Greene JB, Sidhu GS, Lewin S, et al.: *Mycobacterium avium-intracellulare*: a cause of disseminated life-threatening infection in homosexuals and drug abusers. Ann Intern Med 97:539–546, 1982.

69. Horsburgh CR, Cohn DL, Roberts RB, et al.: *Mycobacterium avium–M. intracellulare* isolates from patients with or without acquired immunodeficiency syndrome. Antimicrob Agents Chemother 30:955–957, 1986.

70. Chiu J, Nussbaum J, Bozzette S, et al.: Treatment of disseminated *Mycobacterium avium* complex infection in AIDS with amikacin, ethambutol, rifampin, and ciprofloxacin. Ann Intern Med 113:358–361, 1990.

71. Hawkins CC, Gold JWM, Whimbey E, et al.: *Mycobacterium avium* complex infections in patients with the acquired immunodeficiency syndrome. Ann Intern Med 105:184–188, 1986.

72. Barnes PF, Bloch AB, Davidson PT, Snider DE Jr: Tuberculosis in patients with human immunodeficiency virus infection. N Engl J Med 324:1644–1650, 1991.

73. Centers for Disease Control: Diagnosis and management of mycobacterial infection and disease in persons with human immunodeficiency virus infection. Ann Intern Med 106:254–256, 1987.

CHAPTER 71

MYCOTIC AND PARASITIC INFECTIONS

PETER J. S. KOO, Pharm.D.

MYCOTIC INFECTIONS

Mycotic infections can be classified into superficial and systemic. These fungi usually cause infection in man as a result of accident or opportunism. Except for a few dermatophytes these fungi do not require the human for the propagation of the species. Dermatophytes do not invade living tissue, but they survive on the dead tissue structures of the stratum corneum of the skin, the hair, and the nails, and they depend on man-to-man or object-to-man transmission. These dermatophytes exist as saprophytes and can be found anywhere in the world.

Fungi causing systemic infections are almost always soil saprophytes with the ability to adapt to a host and therefore cause disease. These fungi are usually dimorphic; they can either grow in the soil as mycelial forms that are responsible for spore production or as budding yeast while in a host. Infection is usually acquired by inhalation of the airborne spores. These dimorphic fungi are generally restricted to distinctive geographic environments. Subclinical infections of the population in these endemic areas are common.

Another important category of fungal infection is caused by the opportunistic fungi. These organisms are generally not infective to the normal healthy host. However, they produce disease in the host who is compromised due to acquired immunodeficiency syndrome (AIDS), diabetes, neoplastic disease, or immunosuppression from drugs. Tissue response varies greatly from no response to pyogenic or granulomatous reactions. These fungi are committed mycelial forms and are not restricted to a particular geographic area.

Subcutaneous mycoses usually occur through trauma to the host. They have some ability to adapt to dimorphism. Clinically, they cause diseases known as chromomycosis and mycetoma. They are diverse varieties of soil organisms. In the tissue these organism form grains, granules, and sclerotic bodies. Infections develop slowly and so is recovery. Most of these subcutaneous mycotic organisms are confined to limited geographic areas.

SYSTEMIC MYCOSES

Aspergillosis (1–4)

Aspergillosis is a group of diseases caused by a mycotic organism from the genus *Aspergillus*. *Aspergillus fumigatus* is a primary offending organism in opportunistic infections in humans. Other *Aspergillus* species such as *A.*

terreus and *A. flavus*, have also being associated with opportunistic infections. *Aspergillus* usually infects the pulmonary system of the human host, but extrapulmonary systemic infection involving the major organs and the central nervous system can also occur. *Aspergillus* is an important pathogen in patients with AIDS and after organ transplant surgeries where immunosuppressants are frequently used. On rare occasions *Aspergillus* also causes mycetoma, subcutaneous granuloma, and other superficial mycotic infections.

Aspergillus species are ubiquitous in nature, commonly found in the soil, decaying vegetation, and in moist environments like other "molds." Their spores are readily airborne, available for infection, and pose a constant threat as an infective organism in debilitated or immunocompromised individuals.

CLINICAL FEATURES

Aspergillus bronchitis or pneumonia can mimic infections caused by other organisms. This bronchitis often develops into a chronic state if it is ineffectively treated or relapses. Allergic asthmatic attacks can occur because of *Aspergillus* growing in the bronchiole lumen and mucous plugs. Chronic allergic aspergillosis can lead to irreversible pulmonary tissue destruction. Invasive aspergillosis can occur in debilitated, neutropenic, or other immunocompromised patients and can present as a generalized systemic infection, that can be rapidly fatal if left untreated.

DIAGNOSIS (5, 6)

The diagnosis of aspergillosis is based on the isolation of the fungus from the sputum or mucous plugs from a patient has clinical symptoms of pulmonary infection. The isolation of *Aspergillus* from a known lesion of tuberculosis, bronchiectasis, or cancer presents a serious complication. Eosinophilia, allergic bronchitis, and the isolation of *Aspergillus* from the mucous plug or a positive intradermal skin test to *Aspergillus* should make a definitive diagnosis. Eosinophilia is not always seen in the pediatric population, and therefore makes the diagnosis in the pediatric patient is more difficult. The serum precipitin test is an useful aid in the diagnosis, but is not absolute.

TREATMENT (Table 71.1)

Endobronchial aspergillosis is only treated with bronchodilators and improved bronchopulmonary toilet. How-

Table 71.1.
Treatment of Mycotic Infections

Amphotericin B[257–270]
Indications: (see text)
  Aspergillosis, blastomycosis, candidiasis, coccidioidomycosis, crypto-
    coccosis, histoplasmosis
Dose: adult and child
  Intravenous: 0.6 mg/kg to 1.0 mg/kg per day given intravenously for
    disseminating systemic mycosis
  Intrathecal or intraventricular: 0.5 mg–1.0 mg in 10 ml of spinal fluid
    every other day
Side effects
  Immediate side effects including nausea, vomiting, anorexia, headache,
    myalgias, and arthralgia occur in 20 to 90% of amphotericin B re-
    cipients. Many measures have been formulated to combat these
    common side effects, but only hydrocortisone 25 mg IV at the be-
    ginning of the amphotericin B infusion has been shown to be ef-
    fective in a controlled trial. Thrombophelebitis at the infusion site
    develops in 70% of patients with prolonged therapy. The severity
    of the thrombophlebitis might be reduced by the addition of 500–
    1000 units of heparin to 500–1000 ml of the amphotericin B infusion
    solution. Controlled studies are lacking to support this procedure.
    Renal toxicity is a serious complication of amphotericin B therapy.
    Hypokalemia, renal tubular acidosis, and decrease in glomerular fil-
    tration rate (GFR) have been described. These toxicities are usually
    reversible, unless the total amphotericin B dose exceeds 4–5 g. Side
    effects from intrathecal administration of amphotericin B may in-
    clude headache, vomiting, paresthesias, arachnoiditis, and nerve pal-
    sies. Intrathecal corticosteroids may reduce inflammatory reactions,
    although their efficacy has not been proven.
Fluconazole[271–279]
Indications: (see text)
  Blastomycosis, candidiasis, coccidioidomycosis, cryptococcosis, histo-
    plasmosis
Dose
  Adult: 100–200 mg daily, administered orally or intravenously; doses
    such as 400 mg daily have also been used in patients with fungal
    meningitis
  Child: 6–12 mg/kg daily administered orally or intravenously
Side effects
  Elevations in liver transaminase levels are seen in approximately 3%
    of patients. The most frequent side effects are associated with the
    gastrointestinal tract. Other rare adverse effects such as hypokale-
    mia, CNS toxicity, and hepatocellular necrosis have also been re-
    ported. Fluconazole can produce clinically important drug inter-
    actions with tolbutamine, glyburide glipizide, warfarin, rifampin,
    cyclospore, and phenytoin. These drug interactions are due to en-
    zyme-inhibition by fluconazole.

Flucytosine[280–284]
Indications: (see text)
  Aspergillosis, candidiasis, cryptococcosis
Dose: adult and child: 100–200 mg/kg/day given orally in four divided
  doses
Side effects
  Frequent side effects include nausea, vomiting diarrhea, and head-
    aches. Less frequent side effects may include vertigo, sedation, hal-
    lucinations, confusion, and on rare occasions, bone marrow supres-
    sion and hepatotoxicity. Most of these reported hematological
    adverse reactions are associated with renal failure, although many
    renal failure patients have received flucytosine without complica-
    tions.
Ketoconazole[285–289]
Indications: (see text)
  Cryptococcosis, histoplasmosis, candidiasis, blastomycoses, coccidioi-
    domycosis
Dose
  Adult: An oral dose of 400 mg given once daily for at least 6 months
    when deep or systemic fungal infections are involved
  Child over 2 years of age: 6.6 mg/kg once daily for at least 6 months
    when deep or systemic mycotic infections are involved
Side effects
  Nausea and vomiting are the most common and are dose-dependent.
    Other side effects such as abdominal pain, headaches, pruritus, con-
    stipation, diarrhea, dysmenorrhea, anxiety, gynecomastia, infertility,
    and hypoadrenalism have also been reported. Ketoconazole is a po-
    tent cytochrome P-450 inhibitor and therefore can cause various
    drug interactions.
Miconazole[290]
Indications: (see text)
  Blastomycosis, coccidioidomycosis, cryptococcosis, histoplasmosis,
    nonsystemic candidiasis
Dose: Adult and child over 1 year of age
  Intravenous: 30–60 mg/kg/day IV in 3 divided doses. The manufacturer
    recommends not to exceed 15 mg/kg per infusion dose. In children,
    a daily total of 20–40 mg/kg is usually sufficient
  Intrathecal or intraventricular: 20 mg/day in 5% dextrose is used for
    intrathecal instillation in adults
Side effects
  Peripheral vein thrombophlebitis has been reported in 29–38% of pa-
    tients. Occasionally pruritus, nausea, fever, chill, vomiting, hyper-
    lipidemia, hyponatremia, and skin eruptions are reported. Rare side
    effects such as anemia, thrombocytosis, and anaphylaxis have oc-
    curred. Arachnoiditis has been reported after intrathecal miconazole
    instillation.

ever, pulmonary aspergillomas can lead to exsanguinating hemoptysis and require surgical intervention. Systemic *Aspergillus* infection requires appropriate antifungal therapy as well as reduction or discontinuation of immunosuppressive therapy.

Amphotericin B is the primary agent used for the treatment of systemic aspergillosis. However, combinations of amphotericin B with flucytosine and or rifampin have also been used (7–9).

Meningeal *Aspergillus* infection requires intraventricular or intrathecal administrations of amphotericin B.

Blastomycosis

Blastomycosis is a mycotic disease caused by the organism *Blastomyces dermatitidis*, which frequently involves the lungs and can disseminate to the skin and other internal organs (10–13). The lesions caused by this organism are granulomatous like those of tuberculosis. Blastomycosis was first thought to occur only on the American continent, however recent information indicates that it also occurs on the other continents. Unlike *Histoplasma* or *Coccidioides*, *Blastomyces* is not ubiquitous except where occasional outbreaks occur (14).

CLINICAL FEATURES

The clinical presentation of blastomycosis is similar to that of tuberculosis. Systemic dissemination is usually a result of primary pulmonary infection. The lesions produced by *Blastomyces* are granulomatous-pyogenic, with multiple abscesses containing polymorphonuclear leukocytic infiltrations. Cutaneous involvement first appears as a papule or pustule, but then extends to form chronic nonpainful ulcers. Usually these ulcers do not produce any local reaction or lymphadenopathy. Systemic infection and the cutaneous lesions almost always result from the dissemination of a primary pulmonary infection (15, 16). Systemic blastomycosis can involve the bone and solid organs. This is of particular importance in recipients of solid organ transplantation, because immunosuppressive therapy often leads to devastating complications including fungal infection. Although blastomycosis is an infrequent pathogen, systemic infection with blastomycosis can be life-threatening (17). Bone and joint involvement is one of the common complication of systemic blastomycosis and often presents with minimal or no symptoms (18).

DIAGNOSIS

The diagnosis of blastomycosis is based upon finding the characteristic budding mycoses within the cells of the lesions, pus, or sputum. Serological tests, skin tests, and complement fixation tests are of limited value, because the serological tests cross-react with histoplasmosis, and the skin and complement fixation test results are often negative, even with active disease. Often the mycotic lesions are mistaken for neoplastic disease.

TREATMENT (Table 71.1)

The treatment of choice for blastomycosis is amphotericin B. Other agents such as miconazole and hydroxystilbamidine also have some activity against this infection (19, 20), but the toxicity of hydroxystilbamidine and the high frequency of relapse have limited its usefulness. Ketoconazole for non-life-threatening, nonmeningeal blastomycosis infections in non-immunocompromised is 89% effective when treatment lasts 6 months (21–23). However, the success rate for ketoconazole in the treatment of blastomycosis in the immunocompromised patient is much worse than that of amphotericin B (24). Other imidazole drugs such as itraconazole and fluconazole also have shown some promise in the treatment of this infection, however, clinical data are still very limited (25, 26).

Meningeal infection may require high-dose systemic amphotericin B as well as intrathecal or intraventricular administration of amphotericin B or miconazole.

Candidiasis

Candidiasis is an infection by *Candida albicans* which is normally found in the alimentary tract and vagina of normal healthy individuals (27). *Candida* infections are generally opportunistic, appearing after the weakening of the host's defenses by some other cause such as AIDS, diabetes, neoplastic disease, immunosuppressive therapy, broad-spectrum antibiotics, or surgical stress. Prolonged indwelling catheters and peritoneal dialysis can also predispose the individual to opportunistic *Candida* infection (28–30).

CLINICAL FEATURES

Candida albicans is frequently present in the gastrointestinal tracts of both normal healthy individuals and patients with candidiasis. Therefore, it is sometimes difficult to diagnose candidiasis based on *Candida* isolates alone. *Candida* infections can be systemic as well as cutaneous. The most common cutaneous infection is *Candida* dermatitis involving the moist skin areas such the axilla, gluteal folds, perineal folds, and the folds beneath the breast. Mucous membrane infections involving the vagina and the oral cavity can cause discomfort for the infected host and generally respond well to local antifungal therapy. Oral candidiasis and esophagitis are especially troublesome in immunosuppressed patients and in AIDS patients. Oral candidiasis in these patients often indicates *Candida* esophagitis (31), which can result in perforation and hemorrhage if left untreated or treated inadequately (32). Systemic infections may involve the bladder, lungs, liver, and meninges.

TREATMENT (Table 71.1)

Candida dermatitis and mucocutaneous infections can be treated effectively with nystatin, clotrimazole, miconazole, ketoconazole, butoconazole, tioconazole, and terconazole (33–36). Often in patients with AIDS or those who are undergoing chemotherapy, prophylactic therapy may be necessary, because of frequent relapses (37). Nystatin suspension and clotrimazole troches twice daily are equally efficacious in suppressing oral *Candida* overgrowth (38). Systemic infections require treatment with more active agents such as amphotericin B and flucytosine. Flucytosine is generally not used alone for systemic candidiasis, because the organism can rapidly develop resistance to this drug. Flucytosine is more commonly used in combination with amphotericin B (39). Since flucytosine can produce myelosuppression, it must be used cautiously in patients who are immunodeficient. Both ketoconazole and fluconazole are effective in treating oralpharyngeal candidiasis and mild *Candida* esophagitis and in suppressing thrush, however, in AIDS patients with severe esophagitis or systemic *Candida* infections amphotericin B remains the drug of choice (40). Ketoconazole-resistant *Candida* esophagitis has been described in an AIDS patient (41).

Meningeal candidal infection may require administration of amphotericin B intraventricularly or intrathecally (42, 43).

Coccidioidomycosis

Coccidioidomycosis is also known as San Joaquin Valley fever, valley fever, and Posada-Wernicke disease. It is an infection caused by the organism *Coccidioides immitis*, a dimorphic fungus that grows in the soil and in culture media as a mold that reproduces by arthrospores. In tissues and under special conditions of culture, it grows spherical cells that reproduce by endospore formation. This disease is endemic in the arid areas of United States, Mexico, Honduras, Guatemala, Venezuela, Bolivia, Paraguay, and Argentina, and dusty formites from endemic areas can also transmit infections elsewhere (44). This infection can present as acute, self-limiting, primary pulmonary infection or as a malignant disseminating systemic infection after inhalation of the infective dust-borne *Coccidioides immitis* arthrospores. *Coccidioides immitis* has been isolated from pulmonary lesions in various animals in endemic areas, but there is no evidence of direct animal-to-man or man-to-man transmission. The incidence of primary infection appears to be the highest during the dry summer and autumn months.

CLINICAL FEATURES

The primary infection may be entirely asymptomatic or resemble an acute influenza with fever, chills, cough, and pleuritic pain with effusions. In most cases, recovery occurs within 2 to 3 weeks without sequelae, leaving only a thin-walled cavity or fibrotic calcification of the pulmonary lesions. However, about 5% of patients develop sensitivity to the organism that may appear as erythema nodosum, a complication that occurs most frequently in white women and rarely in black men. This form of the disease is known as San Joaquin Valley fever or valley fever. These infections are accompanied by an initial leukocytosis with a normal differential count and later followed by lymphocytosis, monocytosis, and eosinophilia.

The rare secondary or progressive coccidioidal granulomatous disease is characterized by lung lesions and single or aggregated abscesses throughout the body, especially in subcutaneous tissues, skin, bone, peritoneum, testes, thyroid, and the central nervous system. Coccidioidal meningitis occurs in approximately one-third of patients with disseminated disease, and it resembles tuber-

culous meningitis. These disseminated complications occur 10 times more frequently in blacks and Filipinos than in Caucasians.

DIAGNOSIS

The diagnosis is based upon demonstration of the organism by microscopic examination of the sputum or by culture. Reactivity to a skin test with 1:100 coccidioidin appears within 2 to 3 days after the onset of symptoms, but it may be delayed up to 3 weeks. A positive skin test result does not necessarily indicate active disease, but rather, past infection. Precipitin and complement-fixation test results are usually positive within the first 3 weeks of clinical disease. Serial skin and serological tests may be necessary to confirm a recent infection. However, the absence of an antibody response does not rule out disease in light of impaired cellular immunity such as in AIDS. There is usually an increase in titer of the complement-fixation test with disseminating disease, and the complement-fixation test is not affected by skin testing (45–49).

TREATMENT (Table 71.1)

Primary pulmonary coccidioidal infection usually does not require treatment; healing occurs spontaneously without complications. Systemic infections require antifungal therapy. The most active antifungal agent is amphotericin B (50, 51), but other agents such as miconazole and amphotericin methyl ester have also been used with some success (52–54). More recently, treatment with ketoconazole, fluconazole, and itraconazole has produced encouraging clinical results, but clinical trials comparing these with the standard amphotericin B therapy are still needed (55–64). The later agents have lower nephrotoxicity than amphotericin B. Coccidioidomycosis of the meninges may require intrathecal or intraventricular administration of amphotericin B or miconazole (65). Although high-dose oral ketoconazole or fluconazole produces appreciable CSF levels, experience with their use in CNS infection is very limited (66–72).

Cryptococcosis

Cryptococcosis is also known as torulosis, European blastomycosis, and Busse-Buschke's disease. It usually presents as a subacute or chronic meningoencephalitis. Infection of the lung, kidney, prostate, bone, or liver can also occur without local symptoms. The skin may show acneform lesions, ulcers, or subcutaneous tumor-like masses filled with gelatinous material. In the central nervous system cryptococcus may produce a variety of pathologic changes that include meningitis, granulomas in the meninges, endarteritis, infarcts, areas of softening, and destruction of nerve tissue. Cryptococcal meningitis may present as headaches and a change in personality or a variety of changes in mental status. Cryptococcosis is currently infecting about 5% of AIDS patients (73–78). Cryptococcal infection in an AIDS patient may not have significant symptoms in spite of advanced disease. Cryptococcosis is caused by the fungus *Cryptococcus neoformans*, which is widely distributed in nature in all parts of the world. This infectious agent has been isolated from the soil, from old pigeon nests, and from pigeon droppings. It is transmitted by inhalation of the infectious fungi.

CLINICAL FEATURES

The clinical presentation of cryptococcosis resembles that of tuberculosis. It is a systemic disease that often presents as meningitis with cutaneous manifestations. Lung infections are usually accompanied by a cough and some signs of chronic bronchitis with peribronchial involvement that may be confused with pulmonary tuberculosis. A low-grade fever with generalized malaise and weight loss are also frequent. The onset of central nervous system involvement is insidious, although occasionally sudden, with fever, headache, and vomiting, and an associated increase in cerebral spinal fluid pressure and monocytosis.

DIAGNOSIS

The diagnosis is based on microscopic isolation of the cryptococcal fungi from the infected tissue, spinal fluid, sputum, or the gelatinous content of a subcutaneous mass. The fungi are characteristically in an encapsulated budding form. The diagnosis can also be based on culture or histopathology. Sputum cultures may be positive for only 20% of the pulmonary cryptococcal infections. Increased CSF pressure, pleocytosis, and a low glucose concentration are often seen in cryptococcal meningitis.

TREATMENT (Table 71.1)

Amphotericin B therapy is usually required, and treatment failures can occur. Flucytosine alone is not recommended, because of the high failure rate. Itraconazole and fluconazole have also shown some promise in the treatment of deep tissue and meningeal cryptococcosis (80, 81), but large-scale studies are needed to confirm these preliminary findings. The combination of amphotericin B and flucytosine remains the treatment of choice for meningeal cryptococcosis, and the existing data appears to indicate that it is superior to either of the two agents alone or fluconazole (82–85). Miconazole has had varied success in treating cryptococcal infection, although experience with this drug is still very limited (86). Ketoconazole has shown success in treating nonmeningeal cryptococcosis (87, 88).

Cryptococcal meningitis may require intraventricular or intrathecal administration of amphotericin B or miconazole in addition to the intravenous regimen (89–92).

Histoplasmosis

Histoplasmosis, also known as reticuloendothelial cytomycosis, cave disease, and Darling's disease is caused by the fungus *Histoplasma capsulatum*. *H. capsulatum* is a soil saprophyte that prefers moist and moderate temperature environments. Often droppings from chickens, pigeons, blackbirds, and bats support its growth. With the exception of bats these animals are not infected by the fungi. Areas of infection are common over much of the Americas, Europe, eastern Asia, and Australia. *H. capsulatum* has been isolated from the soil and from numerous animals. Infection in man occurs by inhalation of the infectious soil-borne spores, and there is no evidence for man- or animal-to-man transmission (93). Clinical disease is infrequent; histoplasmin hypersensitivity occurs in as much as 80% of a population, which indicates previous infection. Infections caused by *Histoplasma* are most prevalent in parts of the eastern and central U.S.A. Prevalence increases from childhood to 30 years of age (94).

CLINICAL FEATURES (95–97)

Primary pulmonary infection may be asymptomatic, detectable only by acquired hypersensitivity to histoplasmin, or simulate a mild respiratory illness with general malaise, weakness, fever, chest pains, and cough. Erythema multiform and erythema nodosum may occur. Recovery is usually spontaneous, with residual, multiple, scattered lung calcifications that can be detected by x-ray. Secondary disseminated disease often resembles miliary tuberculosis, and symptoms may include unexplained fever, anemia, patchy pneumonia, hepatitis, endocarditis, pericarditis, meningitis, or mucosal ulcerations (98, 99). Secondary infection occurs from hematogenous spread from the primary site. Much of the damage caused by secondary infection is the result of periorgan vasculitis. Adrenal insufficiency is common in secondary disseminated infections but is usually asymptomatic. Dissemination occurs more frequently in individuals who are receiving immunosuppressive therapy, patients with AIDS, and individuals over 54 years of age (100, 101). Central nervous system involvement occurs in 10 to 20% of patients with disseminated histoplasmosis. Recently, rare infections of the colon have also been reported in HIV-infected patients (102).

DIAGNOSIS

The clinical diagnosis can be based on finding the fungus in Giemsa's or Wright's stained smears of the ulcer exudate, bone marrow, sputum, or blood (103). Final identification is based on cultures that demonstrate the typical *H. capsulatum* colonies and spores. Antihistoplasma antibody serum titer tests are available, but recent positive skin test results with histoplasmin can induce false-positive results, and the serological tests can cross-react with other mycoses (104). Cultures for *Histoplasma* are disappointing, because in noncavitary infections cultures are rarely positive, and they require 2 to 4 weeks for identification. The complement fixation test may prove to be of value in detecting *Histoplasma* infections (105, 106).

TREATMENT (Table 70.1)

Amphotericin B is the antifungal drug of choice. It is very effective against acute disseminated histoplasma infection, but with chronic disease the organism may persist in the cavitary lesions. Fluconazole, ketoconazole, and miconazole have had some success in treating disseminated histoplasmosis, but the number of cases are very limited (107–109).

PARASITIC INFECTIONS

Parasites infect humans in all regions of the world, but there is a particularly high prevalence in areas with mild climates and poor sanitation. In those underdeveloped regions, there is an abundance of species and infected-host reservoirs. Many of these parasites require special environment conditions for both reproduction and survival. Other parasites may require an intermediary host for transmission and completion of their life cycle. These intermediary hosts gain access to humans, because of inadequate preventive measures or hard-to-change cultural habits in these endemic areas. In contrast to the more developed countries in the temperate zones where degenerative, cardiovascular, and malignant diseases are the major causes of disability and death, the underdeveloped countries have to deal with diseases that afflict their young. Infections and malnutrition are sometimes so severe that 40 to 50% of the population may die before reaching the age of 50. Eating habits can also determine the incidence of parasitic infection. The practice of eating raw or partially cooked foods increases the risk of getting a parasitic infection.

Parasitic infections are not always limited to the endemic areas. Infections are frequently observed in the migrant population or in travelers, who acquire their infection in endemic areas. Thus, healthcare practitioners outside the tropics and subtropics must also have adequate knowledge of the diagnosis and treatment of parasitic diseases.

Enterobiasis (110–112)

Enterobiasis (pinworm, threadworm, or seatworm) infection is an infection of the human gastrointestinal tract by *Enterobius vermicularis*. It is one of the most common parasitic infections in temperate and well-sanitized areas today. In the United States, 5 to 15% of the general population is estimated to harbor this helminth. The highest prevalence is in school-age children, followed by children of preschool age and mothers of infected children. The infection rate is lowest among adults. Infection can be transmitted directly by oral-fecal contact or indirectly through clothing, bedding, food, or dust contaminated with viable eggs. Since this parasitic infection is readily transmitted from individual to individual, it is entirely possible that every member of the household is infected (113).

CLINICAL FEATURES (114–118)

Pinworm infection may be asymptomatic, but the most frequent symptom is intense pruritus ani produced by the migrating female helminth and the presence of eggs. This intense pruritus ani may cause secondary dermatitis, eczema, and bacterial infection from the host's constant scratching. Parasitic vulvovaginitis and urinary tract infection due to enterobiasis may occur in young girls (119, 120). Rare infections of the peritoneal cavity and the female genital tract may also occur (121–126). Behavioral changes, including inattention, irritability, and lack of cooperation, can occur in children infected with pinworm.

DIAGNOSIS

Stool examination for pinworm infection is of little value, since adult worms are only occasionally found in heavy infections, but the *Enterobius* eggs are almost always present in the perianal areas. The most satisfactory method of diagnosing pinworm infection is by the use of a perianal swab made of a wooden tongue blade and clear transparent tape. The tape is then placed on a glass slide and examined under a microscope for *Enterobius* ova. The swabs should be used in the morning before bathing and defecation. The eosinophil count is usually normal in enterobiasis. Other household members should also be screened for enterobial infection.

TREATMENT (127–132) (Table 71.2)

Numerous anthelmintics are available for the treatment of *Enterobius* infection, among them are mebendazole, albendazole, piperazine citrate, pyrantel pamoate, pyrvinium pamoate, and thiabendazole. Besides medical management of pinworm infection with pharmacological agents, treatment should also include prevention of reinfection and screening of the other household members. Personal hygiene and adequate sanitary facilities are important in the prevention of pinworm infection. The therapeutic agent of choice for the management of enterobiasis is mebendazole, because it is easy to give and has minimal side effects. Usually a single-dose treatment is adequate, but it should be repeated in 2 weeks to prevent reinfection.

Ascariasis (133–138)

Ascariasis (roundworm) infection is an infection of the human gastrointestinal tract by *Ascaris lumbricoides*. As-

Table 71.2.
Treatment of Helminthic Infections

Enterobiasis
Mebendazole (Vermox) (291–293)
Dose: adult and child over 2 years of age
  A single dose of 100 mg and repeat in 2 weeks
Side effects
  Occasional abdominal cramps and diarrhea have been reported. Rarely
  it can cause leukopenia.

Piperazine citrate (Antepar) (294)
Dose: adult and child:
  65 mg/kg not to exceed 2.5 g daily for 7 days and repeat in 2 weeks
Side effects (295, 296)
  Occasionally can cause nausea, vomiting, diarrhea, abdominal cramps,
  and headaches. On rare occasions it can cause transient vertigo,
  incoordination, muscle weakness, lethargy, erythema multiforme,
  urticaria, and visual disturbances. It can also exacerbate underlying
  seizure disorders and cause other CNS toxicity, especially in patients
  with renal dysfunction.

Pyrantel pamoate (Antiminth) (297, 298)
Dose: adult and child
  A single dose of 11 mg/kg not to exceed 1 g and repeat in 2 weeks
Side effects
  Occasionally causes abdominal cramps, diarrhea, dizziness, headaches,
  rash, and fever. A transient rise in AST has been reported.

Pyrvinium pamoate (Povan) (see text)
Dose: adult and child
  A single dose of 5 mg/kg not to exceed 250 mg and repeat in 2 weeks
Side effects
  Pyrvinium pamoate turns the stool red and can stain clothing. Occa-
  sionally it can cause nausea, vomiting, and diarrhea. Pyrvinium pam-
  oate can also cause photosensitivity on rare instances.

Thiabendazole (Mintezol) (see text)
Dose: adult and child
  25 mg/kg twice daily not to exceed 3.0 g per day for 1 day only and
  repeat in 2 weeks
Side effects
  Side effects include anorexia, headache, nausea, vomiting, and dizziness. On rare occasions it can also cause fever, chills, urticaria, and
  pruritis.

Ascariasis
Mebendazole (Vermox) (299, 300)
Dose: adult and child:
  100 mg orally twice daily for 3 days
Side effects (301)
  Abdominal cramps and diarrhea have been reported and occasionally
  it can cause leukopenia.

Piperazine citrate (Antepar) (see text)
Dose: adult and child
  75 mg/kg orally once daily not to exceed 3.5 g per day for 2 consecutive
  days
Side effects
  Adverse reactions can include nausea, vomiting, diarrhea, abdominal
  cramps, and headaches. Muscle weakness, vertigo, incoordination,
  lethargy, urticaria, erythema multiforme, and visual disturbance also
  rarely occur. In patients with renal dysfunction, CNS toxicities can
  occur as well.

Pyrantel pamoate (Antiminth) (see text)
Dose: adult and child
  A single dose of 11 mg/kg not to exceed 1 g
Side effects
  Abdominal cramps, diarrhea, headache, dizziness, rash, and fever can
  occasionally occur. Transient increases in AST have been reported.

Thiabendazole (Mintezol) (see text)
Dose: adult and child
  25 mg/kg orally twice daily not to exceed 3.0 g per day for 1 day and
  repeat in 2 weeks
Side effects
  Occasional side effects include anorexia, headache, nausea, vomiting,
  and dizziness. In rare instances pruritis, fever, chills, and urticaria
  can occur.

Trichuriasis (302–304)
Mebendazole (Vermox) (305–307)
Dose: adult and child over 2 years of age
  100 mg daily twice daily for 3 days is the treatment of choice
Side effects
  Generally well tolerated, but occasional abdominal cramps and diar-
  rhea can occur. On rare instances leukopenia can also occur.

caris infection occurs worldwide, with the highest incidence in the tropics. In the United States this disease is
most prevalent in the southern states among preschool and
early school-aged children. Approximately 4 million people
in the United States and one fourth of all the world population are believed to be infected by this parasite (139,
140). Ascariasis is transmitted via ingestion of food or soil
contaminated with feces containing viable *Ascaris* eggs
(141). Direct man-to-man transmission does not occur because the eggs require a minimum soil incubation of 2
weeks.

CLINICAL FEATURES

Symptoms caused by ascariasis are often vague and variable or absent. However, children with a heavy parasitic
burden may have symptoms of abdominal pain, vomiting,
sleep disturbance, intestinal obstruction, and malnutrition
(142–144). Individuals who ingest large numbers of *Ascaris* eggs may develop fever, cough, ascaris pneumonitis,
and prominent eosinophilia secondary to the large number
of migrating larvae. Other rare but more serious complications include appendicitis, intestinal perforation, obstruction of hepatic, pancreatic, or common bile ducts and
aspiration of the worm (145–150).

DIAGNOSIS

The diagnosis is made based upon demonstration of *Ascaris* ova in the stool or the recovery of a passed adult
worm. On occasion the diagnosis is made upon visualizing
the adult worm in the intestine by x-ray with or without

contrasting material. Administrating barium can increase the x-ray visualization of the adult worm after the barium is passed, because the barium is adsorbed onto the surface of the *Ascaris* and sometimes stored in their alimentary canal (151).

TREATMENT (Table 71.2)

Treatment of ascariasis involves treatment of the disease and prophylaxis. Several drugs are available for the treatment of ascariasis, among them are mebendazole, albendazole, piperazine citrate, and pyrantel pamoate. These agents have replaced some of the older and more toxic agents. Pyrantel pamoate is the treatment of choice, but mebendazole, albendazole, and piperazine citrate are also extremely effective in eradicating this intestinal parasite. Mebendazole and piperazine citrate should be used with some caution in children under 2 years old or in patients with seizure disorders. Prophylaxis against ascariasis should include good hygiene, especially with respect to proper disposal of human feces, and prevention of ingestion of contaminated soil. The time-honored method of fasting before treatment and purging after treatment has proved to be unnecessary. Unless the patient has total intestinal *Ascaris* obstruction, these pharmacological agents are effective in eradicating the worm and symptoms. It is quite common to see an increase in abdominal symptoms prior to the expulsion of the *Ascaris*.

Trichuriasis (152, 153)

Trichuriasis (whipworm or trichocephaliasis) is an infection of the large intestinal tract of the human by the parasite *Trichurus trichiura*. Trichuriasis has a geographic distribution like that of ascariasis. It is quite common for a patient to have ascariasis and trichuriasis simultaneously. The prevalence of trichuriasis is highest among young children in the tropics. In the United States approximately 2.2 million individuals are estimated to have trichuriasis. Among them, more than 40% are children. Trichuriasis is transmitted via ingestion of soil contaminated with feces containing viable eggs. Direct man-to-man transmission usually does not occur because the eggs require a minimum of 10 days in the soil to mature.

CLINICAL FEATURES (154–157)

Trichurus infections usually produce no clinical symptoms unless a large worm burden is present. Severe infestation of *Trichurus* can produce symptoms including dysentary, mucoid stools, abdominal cramps, weight loss, prolapsed rectum, and malnutrition. Moderate eosinophilia and stool Charcot-Leyden crystals may also be found.

DIAGNOSIS (158)

The diagnosis depends upon recovery of *Trichurus* eggs from the stool or visualizing the adult worms through sig-

moidoscopy or colonscopy. Three stool samples should be collected on alternate days and preserved in P.V.A. (polyvinyl alcohol fixative) for shipment or laboratory analysis. This method of stool sampling allows screening for other concurrent parasitic infection as well.

TREATMENT (159, 160) (Table 71.2)

Mebendazole is the drug of choice for the treatment of trichuriasis, although other agents such as albendazole and thiabendazole may also work. Thiabendazole is not recommended for use during pregnancy. Mebendazole should be used with caution in children under 2 years old and during pregnancy. Mild trichuriasis is usually self-limiting and requires no treatment, but it may be a source of infection for other family members and contacts.

Treatment of trichuriasis should also include screening of all household members and playmates (when children are involved). Follow-up stool-screening of the patient and other household members will ensure eradication of the parasite. However, the most important treatment is improved hygiene and fecal disposal.

Amebiasis (161–170)

Amebiasis (amebic dysentary, amebic colitis, or amebic enteritis) refers specifically to an infection of the human host by the protozoan *Entamoeba histolytica*. Amebiasis occurs in temperate areas worldwide. The *E. histolytica* cysts passed in the stool or immediately infective, and man-to-man transmission can occur. Unlike the cysts, the motile trophozoites are not infective because they are easily destroyed by stomach acid after ingestion. The most common mode of transmission of amebiasis is from person to person. The asymptomatic cyst-passer is an important source of infection, especially if the individual is involved in food preparation. Other modes of transmission may involve a contaminated water source, houseflies, cockroaches, and sexual contact. The exact incidence of amebiasis is not known, but the prevalence is highest in areas of poor water quality or poor sanitation. Amebiasis also has a relatively high incidence among the homosexual population.

CLINICAL FEATURES (171–178)

The clinical manifestations of amebiasis vary greatly, depending upon the site infected. The most common site of amebic infection is the intestine. Infected individuals may have mild diarrhea, bloody dysentary, or no symptoms at all. Thus, amebiasis is known as the great imitator. Amebiasis can also disseminate to other organs such as the liver, lungs, and brain. The most frequent extraintestinal organ involved is the liver. Liver abscesses may occur many years after the primary intestinal infestation; therefore, liver involvement should be treated at the time of treating the intestinal amebiasis. The factors that determine the virulence of amebiasis are poorly understood, but some evidence indicates that the pathogenesis of the disease requires the presence of symbiotic bacteria.

DIAGNOSIS (179–193)

The stools from a patient with suspected amebiasis should be examined over a period of 7 to 10 days. If direct on-location examination of the stool is not possible, the stool specimens should be preserved in P.V.A. fixative for transport and future examination. The stool should be passed into the container directly or onto paper and then transferred to the container with wooden sticks. The specimens collected during sigmoidoscopy examination may also be examined. The most difficult part of making a correct diagnosis is laboratory interpretation errors. A positive stool finding is the only indisputable evidence for diagnosing intraluminal amebiasis. However, the indirect hemagglutination (I.H.A.) test for amebiasis is valuable for diagnosis of extraluminal amebiasis. The usefulness of this test is limited by its inability to differentiate currently active extraluminal amebiasis from old dormant extraluminal amebic infection. An I.H.A. titer above 1:512 is a reasonably good indicator of recent extraluminal infection. Less than 50% of patients with hepatic amebiasis have a positive stool examination result, while 95 to 100% of them will have a positive I.H.A. titer above 1:128. Liver function tests are generally not very helpful in detecting hepatic amebiasis because 75% of these patients have normal liver function test results. However, a radioisotope scan is of value if an amebic abscess is present. When stool examinations are performed correctly, 90% of the intestinal amebiasis cases can be accurately diagnosed by three formed and one purged sample, and a 95% accuracy level can be achieved from six samples taken from patients with diarrhea. Diarrhea can be induced by giving the patient magnesium sulfate.

TREATMENT (194–206) (Table 71.3)

The treatment of amebiasis is not a clearly defined as that of the other parasitic infections. The currently available drug treatment of amebiasis remains less than optimal, and opinions among the experts are divergent. This confusion is compounded by the toxicities of some of the most active drugs. Because there are increasing numbers of reports of treatment failures after using a single agent for amebic dysentary, the therapeutic regimen is now comprised of two active agents, one for the intestinal amebiasis and the other for the possible extraluminal infection. It is necessary to repeat the stool examination 6 months after treatment to confirm total eradication of the organism.

Since no single drug is adequate in curing both types of amebiasis, a luminal and extraluminal amebicide must be employed for patients with only intestinal or hepatic amebic infection. The combination of metronidazole followed by diloxanide furoate or paromomycin is generally well tolerated and adequate for this purpose, but other drug combinations can also be used. These regimens are generally not recommended during pregnancy because of the possible teratogenicity and fetal toxicity. Other agents used for treating amebiasis include chloroquine phosphate and iodoquinol. Although emetine and emetine hydrochloride have been used very effectively for treatment of extraluminal amebic infections in the past, Cardiotoxicity limits their current use. Sterilization of contaminated water by boiling or treating with iodine or household bleach kills the amebic cysts.

Scabies (207–213)

Scabies (itch mite, or seven-year itch) belong to the family of *Sarcoptidae* itch mites. Scabies infections occur most frequently when overcrowding and poor sanitation exist. It also appears to be cyclic. Scabies mites are most readily spread through close bodily contact for prolonged periods of time. Only the female mite is implicated in transmission, and she can survive apart from the host for 2 to 3 days. She is activated by warmth and perspiration of the skin and burrows into the stratum corneum. The mite will live for approximately 2 months in the host and lay a total of several hundred eggs during her lifespan. The incubation period is 3 to 4 days for the eggs, and 10 to 12 days for the larval stage. Fortunately for the human host only 1% of eggs hatch successfully.

CLINICAL FEATURES (214, 215)

Most clinical symptoms are caused by the female mite moving through the burrows. She leaves secretions and excreta that elicit erythema, edema, and severe itching. The most common parts of the body infested by scabies mite include the arms, hands, feet, and especially in the skin folds, but other areas such as the belt line, scrotum, penis, and the skin around the nipples in women can also be infected. The most severe form of scabies is often seen in immunocompromised patients, where crusty scabs may cover the entire body. This type of severe scabies infestation has been called *crusted scabies* or *Norwegian scabies*.

DIAGNOSIS (216–219)

The diagnosis of scabies is made based on clinical presentation of intestine pruritus with associated burrow lesions measuring 1 to 10 mm in length. The distribution of excoriation marks can help with the diagnosis, but are not conclusive. Skin scrapings of suspicious areas may contain mites or eggs when examined under the microscope, and a positive finding is diagnostic of scabies.

Table 71.3.
Treatment of Protozoal Infections

Amebiasis (308–312)
Intestinal amebiasis:
Diiodohydroxyquin (various)
Dose
  Adult: 650 mg orally 3 times daily for 20 days
  Child: 40 mg/kg orally in 3 divided doses daily, not to exceed 2 g per day, for 20 days
Side effects
  Occasional abdominal cramps, diarrhea, weakness, rash, acne, pruritis ani, optic atrophy, and blindness in children with prolonged exposure. Diiodohydroxyquin may cause deafness in children from prenatal exposure, and it should be avoided during pregnancy.

Diloxanide furoate (Furamide)
Dose
  Adult: 500 mg taken orally 3 times daily for 10 days
  Child: 20 mg/kg/day given in 3 divided doses daily, not to exceed 1.5 g per day, for 10 days
Side effects
  Frequently causes flatulence and other gastrointestinal symptoms such as cramps, diarrhea, vomiting, and nausea. Occasional urticaria has also been reported.

Metronidazole (Flagyl) (see text)
Dose
  Adult: 750 mg taken orally 3 times daily for 10 days
  Child: 50 mg/kg/day given in 3 divided doses daily, not to exceed 2250 mg per day, for 10 days
Side effects (see text)
  Metronidazole at amebicidal doses may exhibit disulfiram-like side effects when alcohol is taken. Other side effects may include occasional anorexia, nausea, vomiting, diarrhea, flatulence, blurred vision, headaches, confusion, disorientation, depression, and a metallic taste in the mouth. Leukopenia may occur. Recently, metronidazole has been reported to be carcinogenic in rodents and mutagenic in bacteria; therefore this drug is relatively contraindicated for at least the first trimester of pregnancy.

Paromomycin (Humatin)
Dose: adult and child
  25–30 mg/kg/day orally in 3 divided doses, not to exceed 2.0 g per day, for 10 days
Side effects
  Gastrointestinal disturbances including nausea, vomiting, diarrhea, and abdominal cramps are most common. These side effects are frequently associated with doses in excess of 2.0 g as a total daily dose. On rare occasions, eighth-nerve damage and nephrotoxicity can also occur, since paromomycin is an aminoglycoside.

Extraintestinal amebiasis
Chloroquine (Aralen) (see text)
Dose
  Adult: 600 mg of base (1 g of chloroquine phosphate) taken orally once daily, for 2 to 3 weeks
  Child: 10 mg base (16.67 mg of chloroquine phosphate) per kilogram per day, not to exceed 300 mg base (500 mg of chloroquine phosphate) given orally once daily, for 2 to 3 weeks
Side effects
  Nausea, vomiting, rashes, corneal opacity, alopecia, muscle weakness, and exfoliative dermatitis have been occasionally observed. Rare blood dyscrasias and deafness can also occur.

Metronidazole (Flagyl) (see text)
Dose
  Adult: 750 mg taken orally 3 times daily for 10 days, or 2.0 g taken orally once daily for 3 days. These two regimens are equally effective.
  Child: 50 mg/kg/day given in 3 divided doses, not to exceed 2250 mg per day, for 10 days
Side effects
  Metronidazole may have effects similar to disulfiram when taken with alcohol. Other side effects include nausea, vomiting, diarrhea, anorexia, flatulence, blurred vision, headaches, confusion, disorientation, and depression. Leukopenia has also been observed in some patients. Metronidazole is relatively contraindicated during the first trimester of pregnancy because of recent reports of mutagenicity and carcinogenicity in bacteria and rodents, respectively.

TREATMENT (220–228) (Table 71.4)

Good personal hygiene is the foremost treatment for scabies infections, and reinfection is common when infested clothing or bedding is used. Treatment should include laundering of all clothing, especially bedclothes, treating all household contacts, and application of scabicides after a thorough bath. The scabicides used include (γ)-benzene hexachloride, crotamiton, benzyl benzoate, sulfur ointment, and 5% permethrin. Permethrin is considered by some experts as the drug of choice. Even after adequate treatment, the itching may persist for days, which should not be construed as a sign of reinfection, superinfection, or treatment failure. Overtreatment is common and can lead to toxicity with (γ)-benzene hexachloride. A second course of treatment is necessary at 7 to 10 days after the initial course in only less than 5% of the cases. (γ)-Benzene hexachloride use should be discouraged in infants, young children, and pregnant women. Sulfur ointment can be

the alternative agent for these patients. Sulfur ointment has an unpleasant odor, and it will stain clothing. Permethrin 5% is often used in the treatment of (γ)-benzene-hexachloride-resistant scabies, and it has been used successfully in place of crotamiton in children.

Pediculosis (229–234)

Pediculus (human lice) belongs to the family of Pediculidae, and three species that infest man. These species are (*a*) *Pediculus humanus corporis/humanus*, body lice; (*b*) *Pediculus humanus capitis*, head lice; and (*c*) *Phthirus pubis*, crab or pubic lice.

Pediculus humanis corporis/humanus (Body Lice)

Like the other ectoparasites, body lice are cosmopolitan in distribution. This species has been implicated in the transmission of diseases such as relapsing fever, trench

Table 71.4.
Treatment of Human Lice and Scabies

SCABIES
% (γ)-Benzene hexachloride (see text)
Cream or lotion
Directions
  Warm bath at night
  Apply lotion or cream with soft brush from neck down
  Allow application to dry
  Repeat application of lotion or cream in the morning
  Second warm bath in the evening
  This 24-hr procedure may be repeated in 4–7 days
Cautions
  Avoid overtreatment
  Symptoms may persist for 1 month after adequate treatment
  Avoid use of GBH on face or urethral meatus

Crotamiton 10% (see text)
Cream or lotion
Directions
  Warm bath at night
  Apply lotion or cream from neck down thoroughly in a massage motion
  Reapply lotion or cream in 24 hr
  Second warm bath 48 hr after the second application
Cautions
  Avoid the head, grossly inflamed areas, or excoriated areas

Permethrin 5% (see text)
Cream
No reported adverse effects on animal reproductive systems or teratogenicity, effects on humans are not known
Directions
  Warm bath at night
  Apply cream from the head to the bottoms of feet, and leaving it on for 8 hr
  Throughly wash entire body
Cautions
  Itching and erythema may increase transiently after initial application of permethrin in some patients
  May produce burning or tingling sensation after application

Sulfur ointment (see text)
2.5%, 5%, 10% in petrolatum
This is the preferred treatment in infants, young children, and pregnant women
Directions
  Warm bath at night
  Apply ointment over entire body from neck down nightly for 3 consecutive nights
  Final bath 24 hr after final application
Cautions
  Avoid the head
  The ointment will stain clothing
  The ointment has an unpleasant sulfur odor

Benzyl benzoate 25% (see text)
Solution
Directions
  Warm bath at night
  Apply solution by hand or spray over body from neck down for 3 consecutive nights
  Final bath 24 hr after last application
Cautions
  Avoid the head

BODY LICE
1% (γ)-Benzene hexachloride (see text)
Shampoo
Directions
  Sterilize clothing, bedding by laundering and hot drying, dry cleaning, or ironing
  Use 1 ounce of shampoo for adult (less for children) and lather trunk and extremities for at least 4 min, then rinse thoroughly
  Repeat procedure in 7 days

Cautions
  Same as in the treatment for scabies

1% Malathion or 0.2% pyrethrins or 0.3% allethrin with 1:10 piperonyl butoxide in an inert dusting powder
Directions
(This procedure is used in cases of heavy infestation or where cleaning facility is not available)
  Dust body and clothing with duster or a sifter can
  Pay special attention to seams and insides of the clothing
Cautions
  Avoid excessive use of the dust
  Avoid inhalation of dust or contamination of foods

HEAD AND CRAB LICE (see text)
0.5% Malathion
Solution in 78% alcohol
Directions
  Clean and wash affected area
  Apply solution to hair until the underlying skin is moist
  Leave solution on for 8 hr
  Rinse off solution and comb out nits and dead lice with a fine-tooth comb
Cautions
  This solution contains 78% alcohol and is a flammable hazard; avoid open flames or dryers before rinsing off solution
  Malathion has an unpleasant sulfur odor

1% Permethrin
Cream
Directions
  Clean and wash affected area
  Massage liberal quantities of solution into hair for at least 1 min
  Rinse area thoroughly and comb out nits and dead lice with a fine-tooth comb 10 min after application (although not necessary)
  May repeat procedure in 5 days if condition persists
Caution
  May cause local pruritis or irritation upon application of the cream. Local irritation and erythema occur in 1.2% of patients

1% (γ)-Benzene hexachloride
Shampoo
Directions
  Clean and wash affected areas well
  Apply 1 ounce of shampoo for adult (proportionally less for children) and work into hair for at least 4 min
  Thoroughly rinse out shampoo and remove nits with a fine-tooth comb
  Procedure may be repeated in 7–10 days
  Sterilize bedding and clothing used within the past 7 days
Cautions
  Same as in the treatment of scabies

Pyrethrins 0.16%, piperonyl butoxide 2.0%, and deodorized kerosene 5.0%
Liquid or gel
Directions
  Clean and wash affected area
  Massage liberal quantities of solution into hair for at least 1 min
  Rinse area thoroughly and comb out nits and dead lice with a fine-tooth comb within 10 min after application
  May repeat procedure in 24 hr
Cautions
  Avoid face and excessive contact with solution

Physostigmine 2.0% or ammoniated mercury 2.0% or ophthalmic petrolatum
Ointment
Used primarily for treatment of eye-lash infestations
Directions
  For infestation involving eye-lashes one of these ointments may be applied twice daily for 7–10 days
Cautions
  Avoid excessive use

fever, and epidemic typhus (235, 236). Body lice are most commonly found in the seams of clothing where tight contact with the body occurs, especially in areas of the axilla, perineum, belt line, neck, and shoulders. The female louse has a life-span of 3 to 4 weeks and can lay up to 300 eggs during this time. The eggs hatch in 11 to 13 days, depending on conditions, and mature to adults in 10 to 20 days. The adult parasite feeds 2 to 3 times daily. The adult and the eggs can survive without the host for up to a month. Body lice are transmitted through direct contact with a louse-infested individual, bedding, or clothing.

CLINICAL FEATURES OF BODY LICE

Most of the clinical symptoms are caused by the adult louse feeding on the host daily by digging through the skin with its claws and sucking the blood. The saliva and excreta produce the intense itching and irritation. Together, they produce the classic clinical presentation.

DIAGNOSIS OF BODY LICE

The diagnosis is based on the intense itching, excoriation, and infection from the scratching and finding the adult louse or the eggs in the seams of the clothing from the suspected infested individual.

TREATMENT OF BODY LICE (237–238) (Table 71.4)

Since communal infections are common, treatment must include all members of the household or group and sterilization of all possible vehicles of transmission such as clothing, bedding, and cosmetic objects. The most effective method of sterilization in endemic areas is the application of insecticide-containing dusting powders. The agents used to treat body lice include (γ)-benzene hexachloride, permethrin, malathion, carbaryl, and mobam. Malathion and (γ)-benzene hexachloride can be used in as a 1% dusting powder in treating outbreaks of infestations, but now there are reports of strains of pediculi that are resistant to them. Treatment with (γ)-benzene hexachloride must be repeated in 7 to 10 days, because it is not ovicidal. (γ)-Benzene hexachloride should be used with caution on infants, children, and pregnant women. Bedding and clothing should be washed in hot water or dry-cleaned. Secondary bacterial infections often accompany body lice infestation as a result of poor hygiene and excoriation, and these secondary infections may require appropriate antibiotic therapy.

Pediculus humanus capitis (Head Lice)

Head lice are similar to body lice in geographic distribution. These organisms are typically found on the hair located around the back of the head and ears. The adult female has a life-span of 33 to 40 days, and can lay 50 to 100 eggs, which she attaches individually to a hair shaft with a cement substance. The eggs hatch in 1 to 3 weeks, reach maturity in 10 to 20 days. As with body lice, the adult head louse can survive without a host for up to 10 days. The infestation is communicated by shared hats, combs, brushes, and towels and by direct contact.

CLINICAL FEATURES OF HEAD LICE

Pruritis is a cardinal clinical symptom, and excoriation frequently leads to impetigo and pyoderma.

DIAGNOSIS OF HEAD LICE

The itching and the sequelae of scratching usually cause the patient to seek medical help. The diagnosis of head lice is made when adult lice or nits are found.

TREATMENT OF HEAD LICE (Table 71.4)

Treatment of head lice involves cleaning and washing affected areas of the scalp and applying the pediculocide such as (γ)-benzene hexachloride, malathion, permethrin, or pyrethrins. Permethrin 1% cream is 95 to 98% effective with just a single application (249–255). Systemic absorption of such a short-term permethrin application is not known, but it is detectable in hair for several days after a single 10-min application. The nits must be physically removed with a fine-tooth comb (256), because they are attached to the hair shaft by a cement-like substance. Resistance to (γ)-benzene hexachloride has been reported, but there are no reported cases of resistance to malathion or carbaryl. Both malathion and carbaryl will kill not only the adult lice, but the nymphs and eggs as well. A second application is a must when (γ)-benzene hexachloride is used, and it may be necessary with the other agents if the infestation is severe.

Secondary impetigo and pyoderma will require appropriate antibiotic therapy.

Phthirus pubis (Pubic Lice or Crabs)

The pubic louse is also distributed worldwide. These organisms infest primarily the pubic hairs, but not to the exclusion of other areas. Infestation of the eye-lashes and other hairy areas can also occur. The life-span of the female louse is about 20 to 30 days, and she can produce approximately 50 eggs during this period. The eggs hatch in approximately 1 week, and develop into mature adults in 15 to 17 days. The adult crab louse can live for a maximum of 42 hr without feeding, and the eggs can stay viable for up to a month under ideal conditions. The route of transmission is almost always sexual contact, but in rare circumstances, transmission can occur by sharing bedding, underwear, or other objects.

CLINICAL FEATURES OF PUBIC LICE OR CRABS

Pruritis and the host's inflammatory response to the crab louse saliva and excreta at the site of feeding accounts for most of the clinical symptoms. Secondary infection can occur as a result of scratching and excoriation. The crab lice are usually confined to the pubic regions, but occasional infestation of other hairy areas such as the axilla, eye-lashes, beards, and chest also occurs, resulting in irritation and inflammation.

DIAGNOSIS OF PUBIC LICE OR CRABS

The diagnosis of crab louse infestation is based on the clinical symptoms, distribution of the feeding sites of the pubic lice, and the isolation of either the adult louse or the eggs that are cemented to the hair shaft.

TREATMENT OF PUBIC LICE OR CRABS (TABLE 71.4)

Treatment of crab louse infestation is very similar to the treatment of head lice. It requires cleaning and washing the affected areas and application of a delousing agent. Since crab lice is a sexually transmitted infestation, the treatment must also include sexual partners. The delousing agents used include (γ)-benzene hexachloride, pyrethrin, and physostigmine or ammoniated mercury for eye-lash involvement. No resistance to the treatment has been reported.

CONCLUSION

Parasitic diseases constitute the major cause of death in less developed areas of the world, where sanitation is inadequate or poor. The clinical presentation of these parasitic infections may vary, depending upon the host's immune system and the parasitic burden. When treating parasitic infections, one must also treat the cause of the parasitic infection by improving the sanitation of the endemic areas. Preventive measures such as purifying the drinking water and eating only cooked vegetables will reduce the risk of getting parasitic infections.

Superficial mycotic infections rarely cause serious systemic disease, and a successful treatment often includes the prevention of reinfection, even after the initial infection is successfully treated. Systemic mycotic infections often result from accidental exposure, and they frequently have only limited clinical symptoms or disease in a healthy individual. However, when a host's immune system is suppressed because of disease (e.g., AIDS) or immunosuppressant drugs, these fungi, such as *Histoplasma, Blastomyces, Coccidioides,* and *Candida,* can become opportunistic infective organisms. Opportunistic mycotic infections in immunocompromised individuals require more aggressive therapy. Even with appropriate treatment these individuals can often have relapses and require prolonged drug therapy.

REFERENCES

1. Zeluff BJ: Fungal pneumonia in transplant recipients. Semin Respir Infect 5(1):80–89, 1990.

2. Armstrong D: Problems in management of opportunistic fungal diseases. Rev Infect Dis 11(suppl 7):S1591–1599, 1989.

3. Stein DK, Sugar AM: Fungal infections in the immunocompromised host. Diagn Microbiol Infect Dis 12(4 suppl):221A–228S, 1989.

4. Brems JJ, Hiatt JR, Klein AS, et al.: Disseminated aspergillosis complicating orthotopic liver transplantation for fulminant hepatic failure refractory to corticosteroid therapy. Transplantation 46(3):479–481, 1988.

5. Paty E, De Blic D, Scheinmann, P, et al., [Sosinophilic lung in children] Le poumon eosinophile chez l'enfant. Arch Fr Pediatr 1986 43(4):243–248.

6. Simmonds EJ, Littlewood JM, Evans EG, et al.: Cystic fibrosis and allergic bronchopulmonary aspergillosis. Arch Dis Child 1990 65(5):507–511.

7. Atkinson GW, Israel HI: 5-Flurocytosine treatment of meningeal and pulmonary aspergillosis. Am J Med 55:496–504, 1973.

8. Ribner B et al.: Combination amphotericin B–rifampin therapy for pulmonary aspergillosis in a leukemic patient. Chest 70:681–683, 1976.

9. Kitahara M, Seth VK, Medoff G, Kobayashi GS: Activity of amphotericin B, 5-fluorocytosine, and rifampin against six clincal isolates of *Aspergillus.* Antimicrob Agents Chemother 9:915–919, 1976.

10. McKenzie R, Khakoo R: Blastomycosis of the esophagus presenting with gastrointestinal bleeding. Gastroenterology 88(5 Pt 1):1271–1273, 1985.

11. George AL Jr, et al.: Blastomycosis presenting as monoarticular arthritis. The role of synovial fluid cytology. Arthritis Rheum 28(5):516–521, 1985.

12. Houston MC, et al.: Necrotizing arteritis associated with blastomycosis. South Med J. 79(4):519–520, 1986.

13. Barnes L: A case of fungating skin tumors in a young man. North American blastomycosis. Arch Dermatol 122(6):713, 715–716, 1986.

14. Klein BS, et al.: Isolation of *Blastomyces dermatitidis* in soil associated with a large outbreak of blastomycosis in Wisconsin. N Engl J Med 314(9):529–534, 1986.

15. Sarosi GA, Davies SF: Blastomycosis. Compr Ther 12(4):P31–37, 1986.

16. Zinman HM, Read SE: Blastomycosis presenting as a neck abscess. Pediatr Infect Dis 5(4):491–492, 1986.

17. Hii JH, Legault L, DeVeber G, et al.: Successful treatment of systemic blastomycosis with high-dose ketoconazole in a renal transplant recipient. Am J Kidney Dis 15(6):595–597, 1990.

18. MacDonald PB, Black GB, MacKinzie R, et al.: Orthopaedic manifestations of blastomycosis. J Bone Joint Surg [Am] 72(6):860–864, 1990.

19. Wade TR, et al.: Intravenous miconazole therapy of mycotic infections. Arch Intern Med 139:784–786, 1979.

20. Rose HD, Varkey B: Miconazole treatment of relapsed pulmonary blastomycosis. Am Rev Respir Dis 118:403–408, 1978.

21. National Institute of Allergy and Infectious Diseases Mycoses Study Group: Treatment of blastomycosis and histoplasmosis with ketoconazole. Results of a prospective randomized clinical trial. Ann Intern Med 103(6(Pt 1)):861–872, 1985.

22. McManus EJ, Jones JM: The use of ketoconazole in the treatment of blastomycosis. Am Rev Respir Dis 133(1):141–143, 1986.

23. Bradsher RW, et al.: Ketoconazole therapy for endemic blastomycosis. Ann Intern Med 103(6(Pt 1)):872–879, 1985.

24. Greene NB, et al.: Failure of ketoconazole in an immunosuppressed patient with pulmonary blastomycosis. Chest 88(4):640–641, 1985.

25. Steck WD: Blastomycosis. Dermatol Clin 7(2):241–250, 1989.

26. Grant SM, Clissoid SP: Itraconazole. A review of its pharmacody-

namic and pharmacokinetic properties, and therapeutic use in superficial and systemic mycoses. Drugs 1989 37(3):310–344, 1989.

27. Utz JP: Chemotherapy of the systemic mycoses. Symposium on antimicrobial therapy. Med Clin North Am 66:221–233, 1982.

28. Torres-Rojas JR, et al.: Candidal suppurative peripheral thrombophlebitis. Ann Intern Med 96:431–435, 1982.

29. Tchekmedyian NS, et al.: Special studies of the Hickman catheter of a patient with recurrent bacteremia and candidemia. Am J Med Sci 291(6):P419–424, 1986.

30. Cheng IK, Fang GX, Chan TM, et al.: Fungal peritonitis complicating peritoneal dialysis: report of 27 cases and review of treatment. Q J Med 71(165):407–416, 1989.

31. Tavitian A, et al.: Oral candidiasis as a marker for esophageal candidiasis in the acquired immunodeficiency syndrome. Ann Intern Med 104(1):54–55, 1986.

32. Pitlik SD, et al.: Human cryptosporidiosis: spectrum of disease. Arch Intern Med 142:2269–2275, 1983.

33. Stein GE, et al.: Single-dose tioconazole compared with 3-day clotrimazole treatment in vulvovaginal candidiasis. Antimicrob Agents Chemother 29(6):969–971, 1986.

34. Balbi C, et al.: Treatment with ketoconazole in diabetic patients with vaginal candidiasis. Drugs Exp Clin Res 12(5):413–414, 1986.

35. Cohen J: Antifungal chemotherapy. Lancet. II:532–537, 1982.

36. Montagnani A, et al.: Ketoconazole treatment of chronic mucocutaneous candidiasis. Drugs Exp Clin Res 12(5):409–412, 1986.

37. Meyers JD: Fungal infections in bone marrow transplant patients. Semin Oncol 17(3 suppl 6):10–13, 1990.

38. Owens NJ, et al.: Prophylasix of oral candidiasis with clotrimazole troches. Arch Intern Med 144:290–293, 1984.

39. Edwards JE Jr, et al.: Severe candidal infections: clinical perspective, immune defense mechanisms, and current concepts of therapy. Ann Intern Med 89:91–106, 1978.

40. Young LS: Management of opportunistic infections complicating the acquired immunodeficiency syndrome. Med Clin North Am 70(3):677–692, 1986.

41. Tavitian A, et al.: Ketoconazole-resistant *Candida* esophagitis in patients with acquired immunodeficiency syndrome. Gastroenterology. 90(2):443–445, 1986.

42. Kauffman CA, Jones PG.: Candidiasis. A diagnostic and therapeutic challenge. Postgrad Med 80(1):129–134, 1986.

43. Bodey GP: Fungal infection and fever of unknown origin in neutropenic patients. Am J Med 80(5C):112–119, 1986.

44. Schwarz J: Comparative epidemiology of four deep mycoses—a review. Mykosen 29(1):5–9, 1986.

45. Hicks MJ, et al.: The prevalence of cellular immunity to coccidioidomycosis in a highly endemic area. West J Med 144(4):425–428, 1986.

46. Kaufman L, et al.: Comparison and diagnostic value of the coccidioidin heat-stable (HS and tube precipitin) antigens in immunodiffusion. J Clin Microbiol 22(4):515–518, 1985.

47. Laboratory diagnosis of mycotic and specific fungal infections. Medical Section of the American Lung Association. Am Rev Respir Dis 132(6):1373–1379, 1985.

48. Ampel NM, Wieden MA, Galgiani JN: Coccidioidomycosis: clinical update. Rev Infect Dis 11(6):897–911, 1989.

49. Hobbs ER: Coccidioidomycosis. Dermatol Clin 7(2):227–239, 1989.

50. Drutz DJ: Amphotericin B in the treatment of coccidioidomycosis. Drugs 26(4):337–346, 1983.

51. Furio MM, Wordell CJ: Treatment of infectious complications of acquired immunodeficiency syndrome. Clin Pharm 4(5):539–554, 1985.

52. Hoeprich PD, et al.: The methyl ester of amphotericin B: evolution to therapy in man. Proceedings and Abstracts of the 16th. Inter-

53. Stranz MH: Micronazole. Drug Intell Clin Pharm 15:86–95–1980.

54. Stevens DA: Miconazole in the treatment of coccidioidomycosis. Drugs 26(4):347–354, 1983.

55. Craven PC, et al.: High-dose ketoconazole for treatment of fungal infection of the central nervous system. Ann Intern Med 98:160–167, 1983.

56. Dismukes WE, et al.: "Treatment of Systemic Mycoses with Ketoconazole: Emphasis on Toxicity and Clinical Response in 52 Patients". Ann Intern Med 98:13–20, 1983.

57. Galgiani JN: Ketoconazole in the treatment of coccidioidomycosis. Drugs 26(4):355–363, 1983.

58. Stevens DA, et al.: Experience with ketoconazole in three major manifestations of progressive coccidioidomycosis. Am J Med 74(1B):58–63, 1983.

59. Dismukes WE, et al.: Treatment of systemic mycoses with ketoconazole: emphasis on toxicity and clinical response in 52 patients. National Institute of Allergy and Infectious Diseases Collabortive Antifungal Study. Ann Intern Med 98(1):13–20, 1983.

60. Graybill JR, et al.: Ketoconazole therapy for systemic fungal infections: inadequacy of standard dosage regimens. Am Rev Respir Dis 126(1):171–174, 1982.

61. DeFelice R, et al.: Ketoconazole treatment of nonprimary coccidioidomycosis. Evaluation of 60 patients during three years of study. Am J Med 72(4):681–687, 1982.

62. Knoper SR, Galgiani JN: Systemic fungal infections: diagnosis and treatment. I. Coccidioidomycosis. Infect Dis Clin North Am 2(4):861–875, 1988.

63. Tucker RM, Williams PL, Arathoon EG, et al.: Pharmacokinetics of fluconazole in cerebrospinal fluid and serum in human coccidioidal meningitis. Antimicrob Agents Chemother 32(3):369–373, 1988.

64. Tucker RM, Denning DN, Dupont B, et al.: Itraconazole therapy for chronic coccidioidal meningitis. Ann Intern Med 112(2):108–112, 1990.

65. Levy RM, et al.: Neurological manifestations of the acquired immunodeficiency syndrome (AIDS): experience at UCSF and review of the literature. J Neurosurg 62(4):475–495, 1985.

66. Craven PC, et al.: High-dose ketoconazole for treatment of fungal infections of the central nervous system. Ann Intern Med 98(2):160–167, 1983.

67. Hume AL, Kerkering TM: Ketoconazole. Drug Intell Clin Pharm 17(3):169–174, 1983.

68. Catanzaro A, et al.: Treatment of coccidioidomycosis with ketoconazole: an evaluation utilizing a new scoring system. Am J Med 74(1B):64–69, 1983.

69. Graybill JR: Potential and problems with ketoconazole. Am J Med 74(1B):86–90, 1983.

70. Varkey B: Oral antifungal therapy. Current status of ketoconazole. Postgrad Med 73(1):52–53, 1983.

71. Goodpasture HC, et al.: Treatment of central nervous system fungal infection with ketoconazole. Arch Intern Med 145(5):879–880, 1985.

72. Tucker RM, Galgiani JN, Denning DW, et al.: Treatment of coccidioidal meningitis with fluconazole. Rev Infect Dis 12(suppl 3):S380–389, 1990.

73. Lyons RW, Andriole VT: Fungal infections of the CNS. Neruol Clin 4(1):159–170, 1986.

74. Pippard MJ, et al.: Acquired immunodeficiency with disseminated cryptococcosis. Arch Dis Child 61(3):289–291, 1986.

75. Eng RH, et al.: Cryptoccal infections in patients with acquired immune deficiency syndrome. Am J Med 81(1):19–23, 1986.

76. Ricciardi DD, et al.: Cryptococcal arthritis in a patient with acquired

immune deficiency syndrome. Case report and review of the literature. J Rheumatol. 13(2):455–458, 1986.

77. Holmes GP, Noble RC: Three fungal infections in an AIDS patient. J Ky Med Assoc 84(5):225–226, 1986.

78. Zuger A, et al.: Cryptococcal disease in patients with the acquired immunodeficiency syndrome. Diagnostic features and outcome of treatment. Ann Intern Med 104(2):234–240, 1986.

79. Nelson MR, et al.: The value of serum cryptococcal antigen in the diagnosis of cryptococcal infection in patients infected with the human immunodeficiency virus. J Infect 21(2):175–181, 1990.

80. Sugar AM, et al.: Overview: treatment of cryptococcal meningitis. Rev Infect Dis 12(suppl 3):S338–348, 1990.

81. Viviani MA, Tortorano AM, Pagano A, et al.: European experience with itraconazole in systemic mycoses. J Am Acad Dermatol 23(3 Pt 2):587–593, 1990.

82. Bennett JE, et al.: A comparison of amphotericin B alone and combined with flucytosine in the treatment of cryptococcal meningitis. N Engl J Med 301:126–131, 1979.

83. Sahai J: Management of cryptococcal meningitis in patients with AIDS. Clin Pharm 1988 7(7):528–535, 1988.

84. Cohen J: Antifungal chemotherapy. Lancet II:532–537, 1982.

85. Larsen RA, Leal MA, Chan LS, et al.: Fluconazole compared with amphotericin B plus flucytosine for cryptococcal meningitis in AIDS. A randomized trial. Ann Intern Med 113(3):183–187, 1990.

86. Young RC, et al.: Fungemia in patients with compromised host resistance: a study of 70 cases. Ann Intern Med 80:605–612, 1974.

87. Dismukes WE, et al.: Treatment of systemic mycoses with ketoconazole: emphasis on toxicity and clinical response in 52 patients. National Institute of Allergy and Infectious Diseases Collaborative Antifungal Study. Ann Intern Med 98(1):13–20, 1983.

88. Difonzo EM, et al.: Therapeutic experience with ketoconazole. Drugs Exp Clin Res 12(5):397–403, 1986.

89. Weinstein L, Jacoby I: Successful treatment of cerebral cryptococcoma and meningitis with miconazole. Ann Intern 93:569–571, 1980.

90. Graybill JR, Levine MB: Successful treatment of Cryptococcus meningitis with ventricular miconazole. Arch Intern Med 138:814–816, 1978.

91. Polsky B, et al.: Intraventricular therapy of cryptococcal meningitis via a subcutaneous reservoir. Am J Med 81(1):24–28, 1986.

92. Sugar AM, Stern JJ, Dupont B: Overview: treatment of cryptococcal meningitis. Rev Infect Dis 12(suppl 3):S338–348, 1990.

93. Schwarz J: Comparative epidemiology of four deep mycoses—a review. Mykosen 29(1):5–9, 1986.

94. Wheat LJ, et al.: Diagnosis of disseminated histoplasmosis by detection of Histoplasma capsulatum antigen in serum and urine specimens. N Engl J Med 314(2):83–88, 1986.

95. Wheat LJ, Baheiger BE, Sathapatayavongs B, et al.: Histoplasma capsulatum infections of the central nervous system. A clinical review. Medicine 69(4):244–260, 1990.

96. Powderly WG: Fungal infections in patients infected with HIV, Mo Med 87(6):348–350, 1990.

97. Hiltbrand JB, McGuirt WF: Oropharyngeal histoplasmosis. South Med J 83(2):227–231, 1990.

98. Hankey GJ, Gulland DL: Disseminated histoplasmosis. Aust NZ J Med 16(1):66–86, 1986.

99. Samuel J, Wolff L: Oto-laryngeal histoplasmosis. J Laryngol Otol 100(5):587–593, 1986.

100. Dreizen S, et al.: Unusual mucocutaneous infections in immunosuppressed patients with leukemia—expansion of an earlier study. Postgrad Med 79(4):287–294, 1986.

101. Wheat LJ, et al.: Risk factors for disseminated or fatal histoplasmosis. Ann Intern Med 96:159–163, 1982.

102. Graham BD, McKinsey DS, Drik MR, et al.: Colonic histoplasmosis

103. OHara M: Histopathologic diagnosis of fungal diseases. Infect Control 7(2):78–84, 1986.

104. Wheat J, et al.: Evaluation of cross-reactions in Histoplasma capsulatum serologic tests. J Clin Microbiol 23(3):493–499, 1986.

105. Wheat J, et al.: The diagnostic laboratory tests of histoplasmosis analyses of experience in a large urban outbreak. Ann Intern Med 97:680–685, 1982.

106. Armstrong D: Empiric therapy for the immunocompromised host. Rev Infect Dis 13(suppl 9):5763–5769, 1991.

107. Hawkins SS, et al.: Progressive disseminated histoplasmosis: favorable response to ketoconazole. Ann Intern Med 95:446–449, 1981.

108. Wade TR, et al. Intravenous Miconazole Therapy of Mycotic Infections. Arch Intern Med 139:784–786, 1979.

109. Kobayashi GS, Travis SJ, Medoff G, et al.: Comparison of fluconazole with amphotericin B in treatment of histoplasmosis in normal and immunosuppressed mice. Rev Infect Dis 12(suppl 3):S291–239, 1990.

110. Benenson AS: Control of Communicable Diseases in Man, Ed. 12. An official Report of the American Public Health Association, 1975.

111. Chan CT: Enterobiasis among schoolchildren in Macao. Southeast Asian J Trop Med Public Health 16(4):549–553, 1985.

112. Libbus MK: Enterobiasis. Nurse Pract 8(8):17–18, 1983.

113. Saxena KK, et al.: Family infection in enterobiasis. Indian Journal of Pediatrics, 1988 55(4):627–630, 1988.

114. Cram EB: Studies on oxyuriasis XXVII. Summary and conclusion. Am J Dis Child 65:46–59, 1943.

115. Johnston TS: Diagnosis and treatment of five parasites. Drug Intell Clin Pharm 15:103–110, 1981.

116. Royer A, et al.: Pinworm infestation in children; the problem and its treatment. Can Med Assoc J 86:60–65, 1962.

117. Blumenthal DS. Current Concept. Intestinal Nematodes in the United States. N Engl J Med 297:1437–1439, 1978.

118. Markell EK. Intestinal nematode infections. Pediatr Clin North Am 32(4):971–986, 1985.

119. Simon RD: Pinworm infestation and urinary tract infection in young girls. Am J Dis Child 128:21–22, 1974.

120. Sachdev YV, et al.: Enterobius vermicularis infestation and secondary enuresis. J Urol 113:143–144, 1975.

121. Beckman EN, Holland JB: Ovarian enterobiasis—a proposed pathogenesis. Am J Trop Med Hyg 30(1):74–76, 1981.

122. Snow P, Cartwrit G: Enterobius in an unusual location [letter] JAMA 240:2046, 1978.

123. Bak M, Bodo M: Vaginal enterobiasis [letter]. Acta Cytol (Baltimore) 26(2):264–265, 1982.

124. McDonald GSA, et al.: Ectopic Enterobius vermicularis. Gut 13:621–626, 1972.

125. Brook STJ Jr, et al.: Pelvic granuloma due to Enterobius vermicularis. JAMA 179:492–494, 1962.

126. Knuth KR, et al.: Pinworm infestation of the genital tract. Am Fam Physician, 38(5):127–130, 1988.

127. Bambalo TS, et al.: Treatment of enterobiasis with pyrantel pamoate. Am J Trop Med Hyg 18:50–52, 1969.

128. Miller MJ, et al.: Mebendazole, an effective anthelmitic for trichuriasis and enterobiasis. JAMA, 230:1412–1414, 1974.

129. Beck JN: Treatment of pinworm infections with reduced single dose of pyrvinium pamoate. JAMA 189:511, 1964.

130. Brown HW, et al.: Treatment of enterobiasis and ascariasis with piperazine. JAMA 161:515, 1956.

131. Jagota SC: Albendazole, a broad-spectrum anthelminthic, in the treatment of nematode and cestode infection: a multicenter study in 480 patients. Clin Ther 8(2):226–231, 1986.

132. Anthelmintic Study Group on Enterobiasis: A comparative evalu-

in acquired immunodeficiency syndrome. Report of two cases. Dis Colon Rectum 34(2):185–190, 1991.

ation of mebendazole, piperazine and pyrantel in threadworm infection. Indian Pediatr 21(8):623–628, 1984.

133. Most H: Office management of common intestinal parasites. Drug Ther 3:39–45, 1973.

134. Arfaa F: Selective primary health care: strategies for control of disease in the developing world. XII. Ascariasis and trichuriasis. Rev Infect Dis 6(3):364–373, 1984.

135. Marsden PD: The treatment and control of parasitic diseases. Rev Infect Dis 4(4):885–890, 1982.

136. Nwanyanwu OC, Moore JS, Adams ED: Parasitic infections in Asian refugess in Fort Worth. Tex Med 85(12):42–45, 1989.

137. Bonar S, Burrell M, West B, et al.: Recurrent cholangitis secondary to oriental cholangiohepatitis. J Clin Gastroenterol 11(4):464–468, 1989.

138. Tankhiwale SR, et al.: Single dose therapy of ascariasis—a randomized comparison of mebendazole and pyrantel. J Commun Dis 21(1):71–74, 1989.

139. Warren KS. Helminthic disease endemic in the United States. Am J Trop Med Hyg 23:723–730, 1974.

140. Schultz MG: The surveillance of parasitic diseases in the United States. Am J Trop Med Hyg 23:744–751, 1974.

141. Raisanen S, et al.: Epidemic ascariasis—evidence of transmission by imported vegetables. Scand J Prim Health Care 3(3):189–191, 1985.

142. Tripathy K, et al.: Effects of Ascaris infection on human nutrition. Am J Trop Med Hyg 20:212–218, 1971.

143. Gupta MC: Intestinal parasitoses & malnutrition. Trop Gastroenterol. 6(4):175–187, 1985.

144. Blumenthal DS, et al.: Effects of Ascaris infection on nutritional status in children. Am J Trop Med Hyg 25:682–690, 1976.

145. Hamadto HA, et al.: Relation between intestinal parasitosis and appendicitis. J Egypt Soc Parasitol 16(1):111–116, 1986.

146. Radin DR, Vachon LA: CT findings in biliary and pancreatic ascariasis. J Comput Assist Tomogr, 10(3):508–509, 1986.

147. Baird JK, et al.: Fatal human ascariasis following secondary massive infection. Am J Trop Med Hyg 35(2):314–318, 1986.

148. Bambirra EA, et al.: Tumoral form of ascariasis: report of a case. J Trop Med Hyg 88(4):273–276, 1985.

149. Jenkins MO, et al.: Intestinal obstruction due to ascariasis: report of thirty-one cases. Pediatrics 13:419–425, 1954.

150. Katz Y, et al.: Intestinal obstruction due to Ascaris lumbricoides mimicking intussusception. Dis Colon Rectum 28(4):267–269, 1985.

151. Arene FO, Akabogu OA: Intestinal parasitic infections in pre-school children in the Niger Delta. J Hyg Epidemiol Microbiol Immunol 30(1):99–102, 1986.

152. Croll NA, Ghadirian E: Wormy persons: contributions to the nature and patterns of overdispersion with Ascaris lumbricoides, Ancylostoma duodenale, Necator americanus and Trichuris trichiura. Trop Geogr Med 33(3):241–248, 1981.

153. Annan A, et al.: An investigation of the prevalence of intestinal parasites in pre-school children in Ghana. Parasitology, 92(Pt 1):209–217, 1986.

154. Jung RC, et al.: Clinical observations on Trichocephalus trichiuras (whipworm) infestation in Children. Pediatrics 8:548–557, 1952.

155. Layrisse M, et al.: Blood loss due to infections with Trichuris trichuria. Am J Trop Med Hyg 16:613–619, 1967.

156. Lotero H, et al.: Gastrointestinal blood loss in Trichuris infection. Am J Trop Med Hyg 23:1203–1204, 1974.

157. Cooper ES, Bundy DA, MacDonald TT, et al.: Growth suppression in the Trichuris Dysentary Synrome. Eur J Clin Nutr 44(4):285–291, 1990.

158. Melvin DM, et al.: Laboratory Procedures for the Diagnosis of Intestinal Parasites. (DHEW Publication no. [CDC] 75-8282), Atlanta: Centers for Disease Control, 1974.

159. Bundy DA, et al.: Population dynamics and chemotherapeutic control of Trichuris trichiura infection of children in Jamacia and St. Lucia. Trans R Soc Trop Med Hyg, 79(6):759–764, 1985.

160. Bundy DA, et al.: Rate of expulsion of Trichuris trichiura with multiple and single dose regimens of albendazole. Trans R Soc Trop Med Hyg 79(5):641–644, 1985.

161. Brooks JL, Kozarek RM: Amebic colitis. Preventing morbidity and mortality from fulminant disease. Postgrad Med 78(1):267–274, 1985.

162. Martinez-Palomo A, Martinez-Baez M: Selective primary health care: strategies for control of disease in the developing world. X. Amebiasis. Rev Infect Dis 5(6):1093–1102, 1983.

163. Judson FN: Sexually transmitted viral hepatitis and enteric pathogens. Urol Clin North Am 11(1):177–185, 1984.

164. Kean BH: Venereal amebiasis. NY State J Med 76:930–931, 1976.

165. Mildvan D, et al.: Venereal transmission of enteric pathogens in male homosexuals. JAMA, 238:1387, 1977.

166. Schmerin MJ, et al. Amebiasis. An increasing problem among homosexuals in New York City. JAMA 238:1387, 1977.

167. Irani D, McGavran MH: Amebiasis: still present and lethal in Texas. Tex Med 82(5):34–36, 1986.

168. Steffen R: Epidemiologic studies of travelers' diarrhea, severe gastrointestinal infections, and cholera. Rev Infect Dis 8(suppl 2):S122–130, 1986.

169. Krogstad DJ, et al.: Amebiasis: epidemiologic studies in the United States, 1971–1974. Ann Int Med 88:89–97, 1978.

170. Ma P, Visvesvara GS, Martinez AJ, et al.: Naegleria and Acanthamoeba infections: review. Reviews of Infectious Diseases 12(3):490–513, 1990.

171. Jones RW: Amoebic liver abscess presenting thirty-two years after acute amoebic dysentary. Proc Soc Med 68:593–595, 1975.

172. Seidel J: Primary amebic meningoencephalitis. Pediatr Clin North Am 32(4):881–892, 1985.

173. Greenstein AJ, et al.: Amebic liver abscess: a study of 11 cases compared with a series of 38 patients with pyogenic liver abscess. Am J Gastroenterol 80(6):472–478, 1985.

174. Del-Campo C, Del-Campo M: Thoracic complications of amebiasis. Can J Surg 25(2):119–121, 1982.

175. Bia FJ, Barry M: Parasitic infections of the central nervous system. Neurol Clin 4(1):171–206, 1986.

176. Mirelman D, et al.: Entamoeba histolytica: effect of growth conditions and bacterial associates on isoenzyme patterns and virulence. Exp Parasitol 62(1):142–148, 1986.

177. Salata RA, Ravdin JI. Review of the human immune mechanisms directed against Entamoeba histolytica. Rev Infect Dis 8(2):261–271, 1986.

178. Guerrant RL: Amebiasis: introduction, current status, and research questions. Rev Infect Dis 8(2):218–227, 1986.

179. Juniper K Jr, et al. Serologic diagnosis of amebiasis. Am J Trop Med Hyg 21:157–168, 1972.

180. Kessel JG, et al.: Indirect hemagglutination and complement fixation tests in amebiasis. Am J Trop Med Hyg 14:540–555, 1951.

181. Krupp IM: Antibody response in intestinal and extraintestinal amebiasis. Am J Trop Med Hyg 19:57–62, 1970.

182. Khan AH, Das SR: Rapid micro-IHA test with FACL-SRBCs in serodiagnosis of amoebiasis. Indian J Med Res 83:377–379, 1986.

183. Healy GR: Immunologic tools in the diagnosis of amebiasis: epidemiology in the United States. Rev Infect Dis 8(2):239–246, 1986.

184. Walsh JA: Problems in recognition and diagnosis of amebiasis: estimation of the global magnitude of morbidity and mortality. Rev Infect Dis 9—2):228–238, 1986.

185. Salata RA, et al.: Patients treated for amebic liver abscess develop cell-mediated immune responses effective in vitro against Entamoeba histolytica. J Immunol 136(7):2633–2639, 1986.

186. Krupp IM, et al.: Comparative study of the antibody response in amebiasis: persistence after successful treatment. Am J Trop Med Hyg 20:421–424, 1971.

187. Healy GR, et al.: Use of the indirect hemagglutination test in some studies of seroepidemiology of amebiasis in the Western Hemisphere. Health Lab Sci 7:109–116, 1970.

188. Healy GR: The use and limitations to the indirect hemagglutination test in the diagnosis of intestinal amebiasis. Health Lab Sci 5:174–179, 1968.

189. Ravdin JI: Pathogenesis of disease caused by *Entamoeba histolytica*: studies of adherence, secreted toxins, and contact-dependent cytolysis. Rev Infect Dis 8(2):247–260, 1986.

190. Kagan IG: Serologic diagnosis of parasitic diseases. N Engl J Med 282:685–686, 1970.

191. Kim CW: The diagnosis of parasitic diseases. Prog Clin Pathol 6:267–288, 1975.

192. Sexton DJ, et al.: Amebiasis in a Mental Institution: Serologic and Epidemiologic Studies. Am J Epidemiol 100:414–423, 1974.

193. Korelitz BI: When should we look for amebae in patients with inflammatory bowel disease? J Clin Gastroenterol 11(4):373–375, 1989.

194. Campbell WC: The chemotherapy of parasitic infections. J Parasitol 72(1):45–61, 1986.

195. Ferrante A: Amphotericin B doses for primary amoebic meningoencephalitis [letter]. Lancet 2(8497):35–36, 1986.

196. Abuabara SF, et al.: Amebic liver abscess. Arch Surg 117(2):239–244, 1982.

197. Culbertson CG: Amebic meningoencephalitis. Antibiot Chemother, 30:28–53, 1981.

198. Ellis CJ: Antiparasitic agents in pregnancy. Clin Obstet Gynaecol 13(2):269–275, 1986.

199. Barrett-Connor E: Amebiasis, today, in the United States. West J Med 114:1–6, 1971.

200. Powell SJ: Therapy of Amebiasis. Bull NY Acad Med Ser 2, 47:469–477, 1971.

201. Oakley GP: The neurotoxicity of the halogenated hydroxyquinolines, JAMA 225:395–397, 1973.

202. Behrens MM: Optic atrophy in children after diiodohydroxyquin therapy, JAMA 228:693, 1974.

203. Coher HG, et al.: Comparison of metronidazole and chloroquin for the treatment of amebic liver abscess. Gastroenterology 69:35–41, 1975.

204. Anon: Is Flagyl dangerous? Med Lett Drug Ther 17:53–54, 1975.

205. Tsar SH: Experience in the therapy of amebic liver abscesses on Taiwan. Am J Trop Med Hyg 22:24–29, 1973.

206. Thoren K, Hakansson C, Beagstrom T, et al.: Treatment of asymptomatic amebiasis in homosexual men. Clinical trials with metronidazole, tinidazole, and diloxanide furoate. Sex Transm Dis 17(2):72–74, 1990.

207. Orkin M: Resurgence of Scabies. JAMA 217:593, 1971.

208. Parlette HL: Scabietic infestations of man. Cutis 16:47, 1975.

209. Currier RW: Lice & scabies control. Iowa Med 76(2):80,82, 1986.

210. Crissey JT: Scabies and pediculosis pubis. Urol Clin North Am 11(1):171–176, 1984.

211. Gurevitch AW: Scabies and lice. Pediatr Clin North Am 32(4):987–1018, 1985.

212. Wolf R, et al.: Norwegian-type scabies mimicking contact dermatitis in an immunosuppressed patient. Postgrad Med 78(1):228–230, 1985.

213. Honig PJ: Arthropod bites, stings, and infestations: their prevention and treatment. Pediatr Dermatol 3(3):189–197, 1986.

214. Richey HK, et al.: Scabies: diagnosis and management. Hosp Pract [Off] 21(2):124A–124C,124H,124K–124L passim, 1986.

215. Mellanby K: The development of symptoms. Parasitic infection and immunity in human scabies. Parasitology 35:197, 1944.

216. Oakes RC, et al.: Atopic dermatitis. A review of diagnosis, pathogenesis, and management. Clin Pediatr (Phila), 22(7):467–475, 1983.

217. Minster J: Nursing management of patients with scabies and lice. Nurs Clin North Am 15(4):747–756, 1980.

218. Buntin DM: Cutaneous features of sexually transmitted diseases. Recognition and treatment. Postgrad Med 78(7):121–128, 1985.

219. Fragola LA Jr, Watson PE: Common groin eruptions: diagnosis and treatment. Postgrad Med, 69(5):159–163, 166–169, 172, 1981.

220. Taplin D, et al.: A comparative trial of three treatment schedules for the eradication of scabies. J Am Acad Dermatol 9(4):550–554, 1983.

221. Taplin D, et al.: Eradication of scabies with a single treatment schedule. J Am Acad Dermatol 9(4):546–550, 1983.

222. Burgess I, et al.: Aqueous malathion 0.5% as a scabicide: clinical trial. Br Med J [Clin Res], 292(6529):1172, 1986.

223. Moberg SA, et al.: An epidemic of scabies with unusual features and treatment resistance in a nursing home. J Am Acad Dermatol 11(2 Pt 1):242–244, 1984.

224. Shacter B: Treatment of scabies and pediculosis with lindane preparations: an evaluation. J Am Acad Dermatol 5(5):517–527, 1981.

225. Amer M, et al.: Treatment of scabies: preliminary report. Int J Dermatol 20(4):289–290, 1981.

226. Permethrin for scabies. Med Lett Drugs Ther 32(813):21–22, 1990.

227. Taplin D, Meinking TL, Chen JA, et al.: Comparison of crotamiton 10% cream (Eurax) and permethrin 5% cream (Elimite) for the treatment of scabies in children. Pediatr Dermatol 7(1):67–73, 1990.

228. Bourgeois M, et al.: Mercury intoxication after topical application of a metallic mercury ointment. Dermatologica, 172(1):48–51, 1986.

229. NuHall G: The Biology of *Pediculus humanus*. Parasitology 10:80, 1917.

230. Gratz NG: The Current Status of Louse Infestations Throughout the World. The Control of Lice and Louse-Borne Diseases. Proc. of the Int. Symp. on Control of Lice and Louse-Borne Diseases. Washington, D.C.: Pan American Health Organization, 20037:23, 1973.

231. Nuttall G: The biology of *Phthirus Pubis*. Parasitology, 10:383, 1918.

232. Orkin M. Treatment of today's scabies and pediculosis. JAMA 236:1136, 1976.

233. Couch JM, et al.: Diagnosing and treating *Phthirus pubis palperbrarum*. Surv Ophthalmol, 26(4):219–225, 1982.

234. Monheit BM, Norris MM: Is combing the answer to headlice? J Sch Health 56(4):158–159, 1986.

235. Geigy R: Relapsing fevers. In Wienman D, Ristie M (eds): Infectious Blood Diseases of Man and Animals, vol 2. New York, Academic Press, 1968, pp 175–216.

236. Zolrodovskii PF, Golinevich EH: Wolhynian on five-day fever. In The Rickettsial Diseases. 2nd Edition, Pergoman Press, London, 1960;630.

237. Maibach HI: Therapeutic Agents for Human Skin Infections. JAMA 230:759, 1974.

238. Meinking TL, et al.: Comparative efficacy of treatments for pediculosis capitis infestations. Arch Dermatol 122(3):267–271, 1986.

239. Honig PJ: Arthropod bites, stings, and infestations: their prevention and treatment. Pediatr Dermatol 3(3):189–197, 1986.

240. Zesch A, et al.: Demonstration of the percutaneous resorption of a lipophilic pesticide and its possible storage in the human body. Arch Dermatol Res 273(1–2):43–49, 1982.

241. Feldman RJ: Percutaneous penetration of some pesticides and herbicides in man. Tox Applied P'col 28:126, 1974.

242. Council on Pharmacy and Chemistry: Toxic effects of technical benzene hexachloride and its isomers. JAMA 147:571, 1951.

243. Joslin EF: Fatal Case of Lindane Poisoning. Nat Assoc of Coroners, Proc of 1958 Symposium.

244. Rajan U: Treatment of head lice infestation with benzyl benzoate and pyrethrum. Singapore Med J, 16:297, 1975.

245. Kawaaheh MA: Eradication of a large scabies outbreak using community-wide health education. Am J Public Health, 66:564, 1976.

246. Brandenburg K, et al.: 1% permethrin cream rinse vs 1% lindane shampoo in treatinmtnr pediculosis capitis. Am J Dis Child 140(9):894–896, 1986.

247. Donaldson RJ, Logie S: Comparative trial of shampoos for treatment of head infestation. J R Soc Health 106(2):39–40, 1986.

248. Wohlfahrt DJ: Fatal paraquat poisonings after skin absorption. Med J Aust 1(12)512–513, 1982.

249. Bowerman JG, Gomez MP, Austin RD, et al.: Comparative study of permethrin 1% creame rinse and lindane shampoo for the treatment of head lice. Pediatr Infect Dis J 6(3):252–255, 1987.

250. Taplin D, et al.: Permethrin 1% creme rinse for the treatment of *Pediculus humanus* var *capitis* infestation. Pediatr Dermatol 3(4):344–348, 1986.

251. Permethrin for head lice. Med Lett Drugs Ther 28(722):89–90, 1986.

252. Brandenburg K, et al.: 1% permethrin cream rinse vs 1% lindane shampoo in treating pediculosis capitis. Am J Dis Child 140(9):894–896, 1986.

253. Edling C, et al.: New methods for applying synthetic pyrethroids when planting conifer seedlings: symptoms and exposure relationships. Ann Occup Hyg 29(3):421–427, 1985.

254. Ares-Mazas E, et al.: The efficacy of permethrin lotion in pediculosis capitis. Int J Dermatol 24(9):603–605, 1985.

255. Flannigan SA, Tucker SB: Variation in cutaneous sensation between synthetic pyrethroid insecticides. Contact Dermatitis 13(3):140–147, 1985.

256. Monheit BM, Norris MM: Is combing the answer to headlice? J Sch Health 56(4):158–159, 1986.

257. Schaffner A, Frick PG: The effect of ketoconazole on amphotericin B in a model of disseminated aspergillosis. J Infect Dis 151(5):902–910, 1985.

258. Gardner ML, Godley PJ, Wasam SM: Sodium loading treatment for amphotericin B–induced nephrotoxicity. DICP 24(10):940–946, 1990.

259. Starke JR, Mason EO Jr, Kramer WG, et al.: Pharmacokinetics of amphotericin B in infants and children. J Infect Dis Apr; 155(4):766–776, 1987.

260. Koren G, Lou A, Klein J, et al.: Pharmacokinetics and adverse effects of amphotericin B in infants and children. J Pediatr 113(3):559–563, 1988.

261. Benson JM, Nahata MC: Clinical use of systemic antifungal agents. Clin Pharm 7(6):424–438, 1988.

262. Douglas J, Healy, J: Nephrotoxic effects of amphotericin B, including renal tubular acidosis. Am J Med 46:154–162, 1989.

263. Saag MS, Dismukes WE: Treatment of histoplasmosis and blastomycosis. Chest 93(4):848–851, 1988.

264. Miller H, Bates J: Amphotericin-B toxicity: a follow-up report of 53 patients. Ann Intern Med 71:1089–1095, 1969.

265. Maddux MS, Barriere SL: A review of complications of amphotericin-B therapy: recommendations for prevention and management. Drug Intell Clin Pharm 14:177–181, 1980.

266. Barton CH, et al.: Renal magnesium wasting associated with amphotericin B therapy. Am J Med 77(3):471–474, 1984.

267. Harrison HR, et al.: Amphotericin B and imidazole therapy for coccidioidal meningitis in children. Pediatr Infect Dis 2(3):216–221, 1983.

268. Butler WP, Kaufer GI: Primary cutaneous cryptococcosis successfully treated with outpatient amphotericin B and 5-fluorocytosine. NITA, 8(4):295–297, 1985.

269. Meade RH III: Drug therapy review: clinical pharmacology and therapeutic use of antimycotic drugs. Am J Hosp Pharm 36:1326–1344, 1979.

270. Fisher MA, Talbot GH, Maislin G, et al.: Risk factors for amphotericin B–associated nephrotoxicity. Am J Med 87(5):547–552, 1989.

271. Viscoli C, Castagnola E, Fioredda F, et al.: Fluconazole in the treatment of candidiasis in immunocompromised children. Antimicrob Agents Chemother 35(2):365–367, 1991.

272. Blum RA, Wilton JH, Hilligoss DM, et al.: Effect of fluconazole on the disposition of phenytoin. Clin Pharmactol Ther 49(4):420–425, 1991.

273. Gill SK: Clinical aspects of HIV and AIDS. AIDS Care 2(4):359–361, 1990.

274. Galgiani JN, Ampel NM: *Coccidioides immitis* in patients with human immunodeficiency virus infections. Semin Respir Infect 5(2):151–154, 1990.

275. Denning DW, Follansbee SE, Scolaro M, et al.: Pulmonary aspergillosis in the acquired immunodeficiency syndrome. N Engl J Med 324(10):654–662, 1991.

276. Sugar AM: Treatment of fungal infections in patients infected with the human immunodeficiency virus. Pharmacotherapy 10(6(Pt 3):154S–158S, 1990.

277. Pasko MT, Piscitelli SC, Van Slooten AD, et al.: Fluconazole: a new triazole antifungal agent. DICP 24(9):860–867, 1990.

278. Bozzette SA, Larsen RA, Chiu J, et al.: A placebo-controlled trial of maintenance therapy with fluconazole after treatment of cryptococcal meningitis in the acquired immunodeficiency syndrome. California Collaborative Treatment Group. N Engl J Med 324(9):580–584, 1991.

279. Kowalsky SF, Dixon DM: A new antifungal agent. Clin Pharm 10:179–194, 1991.

280. Bennett JE: Flucytosine. Ann Intern Med 86:319–322, 1977.

281. Meyer R, Axelrod JL: Fatal asplatic anemia resulting from flucytosine. JAMA 224:1573, 1974.

282. Kitahara M, et al.: Activity of amphotericin B, 5-fluorocytosine, and rifampin against six clinical isolates of *Aspergillus*. Antimicrob Agents Chemother 9:915–919, 1976.

283. Steer PL, et al.: 5-Fluorocytosine: oral antifungal compound, Ann Intern Med 76:15–22, 1972.

284. van't Wout JW, Novakova F, Verhagen CH, et al.: The efficacy of itraconazole against systemic fungal infections in neutropenic patients: a randomized comparative study with amphotericin B. J Infect 22(1):45–52, 1991.

285. Gradon JD, Sepkowitz DV: Massive hepatic enlargement with fatty change associated with ketoconazole. DICP 24(12):1175–1176, 1990.

286. Caselli D, et al.: Antifungal chemoprophylaxis in cancer children: a prospective randomized controlled study. Microbiologica Oct; 13(4):347–351, 1990.

287. Walsh TJ, Rubin M, Hathorn J, et al.: Amphotericin B vs high-dose ketoconazole for empirical antifungal therapy among febrile, granulocytopenic cancer patients. A prospective, randomized study. Arch Intern Med Apr; 151(4):765–770, 1991.

288. Hii JH, Legault L, DeVeber G, et al.: Successful treatment of systemic blastomycosis with high-dose ketoconazole in a renal transplant recipient. Am J Kidney Dis 15(6):595–597, 1990.

289. Milliken ST, Powles RL: Antifungal prophylaxis in bone marrow transplantation. Rev Infect Dis 12(suppl 3):S374–379, 1990.

290. Wiley JM, Smith N, Leventhal BG, et al.: Invasive fungal disease in pediatric acute leukemia patients with fever and neutropenia

during induction chemotherapy: a multivariate analysis of risk factors. J Clin Oncol 8(2):280–286, 1990.

291. Keystone JS, Murdoch JK: Mebendazole. Ann Intern Med 91:582–586, 1979.

292. Pena C, et al.: Mebendazole, an effective broad-spectrum anthelmintic. Am J Trop Hyg 22:592–595, 1973.

293. el Kalla S, Menon NS: Mebendazole poisoning in infancy. Ann Trop Paediatr 10(3):313–314, 1990.

294. Swartzwelder JC, et al.: The use of piperazine for the treatment of human helminthiases. Gastroenterology 33:87–96, 1957.

295. Belloni C, et al.: Neurotoxic side-effects of piperazine. Lancet 2:369, 1967.

296. Miller CG, et al.: Neurotoxic side-effects of piperazine. Lancet 1:895, 1971.

297. Desowitz RS, et al.: Anthelmintic activity of pyrantel pamoate. Am J Trop Med Hyg 19:775–778, 1970.

298. Vallarejos VM, et al.: Experience with the anthelmintic pyrantel pamoate. Am J Trop Med Hyg 20:842–845, 1971.

299. Feldmeier H, et al.: Flubendazole versus mebendazole in intestinal helminthic infections. Acta Trop (Basel) 39(2):185–189, 1982.

300. Abadi K: Single dose mebendazole therapy for soil-transmitted nematodes. Am J Trop Med Hyg 34(1):129–133, 1985.

301. Katz M: Adverse metabolic effects of antiparasitic drugs. Rev Infect Dis 4(4):768–770.

302. Varma TK, Shinghal TN, Saxena M, et al.: Studies on the comparative efficacy of mebendazole, flubendazole and niclosamide against human tapeworm infection. Indian J Public Health 34(3):163–168, 1990.

303. Walden J: Parasitic diseases. Other roundworms. *Trichuris*, hookworm, and *Strongyloides*. Prim Care 18(1):53–74, 1991.

304. Upatham ES, Viyanant V, Brockelman WY, et al.: Prevalence, incidence, intensity and associated morbidity of intestinal helminths in south Thailand. Int J Pharasitol Apr; 19(2):217–228, 1989.

305. Sargent RG, et al.: A clinical evaluation of mebendazole in the treatment of trichuriasis. Am J Trop Med Hyg 23:375–377, 1974.

306. Wagner ED, et al.: Morphologically altered eggs of *Trichuris trichiura* following treatment with mebendazole. Am J Med Hyg 23:154–157, 1974.

307. Wagner ED, et al.: In vivo effects of a new anthelmintic mebendazole (R-17,635) on the eggs of *Trichuris trichiura* and hookworm. Am J Trop Med Hyg 23:151–153, 1974.

308. Krogstad, DJ, et al.: Amebiasis. N Engl J Med 298:262–265, 1978.

309. Rees PH: Amoebiasis—*Entamoeba histolytica* infections: a review. East Afr Med J 63(1):81–84, 1986.

310. Viswanathan R, et al.: An ameboma—lest we forget. J Indian Med Assoc 84(1):18–20, 1986.

311. Most H: Treatment of common parasitic infections of man encountered in the United States. N Engl J Med 287:698–702, 1972.

312. Levine GI: Sexually transmitted parasite diseases. Clin Off Pract 18(1):101–108, 1991.

CHAPTER 72

SURGICAL INFECTIONS AND ANTIBIOTIC PROPHYLAXIS

LYNDA S. WELAGE, Pharm.D.

Despite advances in medical technology and an extensive antibiotic armamentarium, infections contribute significantly to postoperative morbidity and mortality. Although, the incidence of wound infections has been reported to be approximately 4.9%, the actual risk of developing a postoperative infection depends on numerous factors and has been reported to range from 0 to 40%, depending on the surgical procedure performed (1, 2). In 1980, Cruse and Foord reported that surgical wound infections prolonged hospital stay by 10.1 days on average (1). Based on this, one may conclude that wound infections clearly have a significant economic impact on our healthcare system, and thus, great strides are undertaken to prevent such infections. Prophylactic antibiotics, one such intervention, have been shown in numerous situations to prevent the development of postoperative wound infections. In fact, the prophylactic use of antimicrobial agents accounts for approximately 30% of the total hospital use of antibiotics (3).

In general, surgical infections are considered to be related to either the surgical site or to a distant site, such as respiratory tract, urinary tract, or blood stream. The primary goal of antimicrobial surgical prophylaxis is to prevent infections that occur at or around the surgical site (i.e., infections that relate directly to the surgery). "Prophylaxis" implies that the agent is administered prior to suppuration or invasive infection (4). Thus, antimicrobial surgical prophylaxis is aimed at preventing the development of infection rather than treating an established process.

Following a surgical procedure, an infection may develop at the surgical incision or among the structures that are manipulated or exposed. The latter type of infection is often referred to as a deep infection. A wound infection is somewhat difficult to define, since cultures may be sterile even when the wound is definitely infected (5). Conversely, bacteria may sometimes colonize the surgical site and thus be recovered upon culture, although the wound is not infected. The signs and symptoms of a wound infection depend on the infecting organism and the tissue involved. The classic presentation usually involves a red, inflamed incision from which pus may be draining. However, wound infections may present as a more indolent

process in which an abscess is later diagnosed. The infection may be readily apparent before a patient's discharge, but in as many as 10% of cases, the wound infection is diagnosed following discharge (5).

BASIC PRINCIPLES OF PROPHYLAXIS

Risk of Infection

In general, infection results either from abnormalities in host defenses or a host overwhelmed by a large or highly virulent bacterial load (6). Factors associated with increased bacterial contamination, increased bacterial virulence, or decreased host resistance promote the development of infection.

Despite the use of sterile technique intraoperatively, bacteria can easily be recovered from the operative field during most surgical procedures (7, 8). Bacterial contamination may result from exogenous sources, including the operative team, instruments, or environment, or from endogenous sources such as the patient's skin or various bacteria-containing viscera (e.g., respiratory, gastrointestinal, genitourinary tracts) (5, 6, 8, 9). An ad hoc committee to the National Research Council developed a classification scheme for endogenous surgical wound contamination (Table 72.1): clean, clean-contaminated, contaminated, and dirty (8). As contamination increases, the risk of infection also increases. The infection rate averages less than 5% for clean surgery, 8 to 11% for clean-contaminated, 15 to 20% for contaminated, and 28 to 40% for dirty procedures (1, 2, 8). This classification system is frequently used in the hospital setting, but there is marked variability in the infection rates among various procedures within a given classification. For example, in one large surveillance program the infection rate for clean procedures ranged from 1.9% for patients undergoing herniorrhaphy to 18.9% for patients undergoing radical mastectomy (8).

Numerous guidelines and procedures have been developed to attempt to minimize exogenous sources of bacteria (5, 6, 9). To decrease the number of bacteria on the surgeon's hands, scrubbing them with either an iodophor preparation or a hexachlorophene product is recommended. However, since hands can not be completely sterilized by scrubbing, surgical gloves should be changed if they become torn or punctured during the procedure.

Table 72.1.
Classification of Surgical Wounds

Clean	Wounds in which the gastrointestinal, respiratory, or urinary tract are not entered; no inflamation is present and there is no break in aseptic technique; a primary closure is usually performed, and drains are rarely employed (e.g., cardiac, vascular, orthopaedic procedures)
Clean-contaminated	Wounds in which a bacterial colonized tract (oropharyngeal, respiratory, gastrointestinal, genitourinary tracts) is entered without significant spillage or mechanical drainage; clean wounds may also fall into this category when a minor break in aseptic technique occurs during procedure (e.g., colorectal, vaginal, genitourinary procedures)
Contaminated	Wounds with acute inflammation but no pus formation or cases of a major break in sterile technique or gross spillage of gastrointestinal contents
Dirty	Performed viscus wounds with pus, old traumatic wounds (>4 hr), or wounds containing foreign bodies or devitalized tissue; wounds in which organisms are present in ordinarily sterile tissue or there is evidence of active infection (e.g., perforated colonic diverticulum)

Gowns worn by the staff in the operating room may also be a source of bacteria, and attempts should be made to avoid contamination. Instruments may become contaminated with the patient's body fluids during a procedure. If the instruments come in contact with contaminating bacteria, new instruments should be used to complete the procedure. Excessive traffic in and out of the operating room and/or poor ventilation may also provide exogenous sources of bacteria.

Endogenous contamination is the primary source of bacteria, except for procedures that are classified as "clean." As previously stated, endogenous sources of bacteria include the patient's skin and bacteria-containing tracts, including the respiratory tract, genitourinary tract, and gastrointestinal tract. Methods to minimize the number of organisms on the patient's skin include preoperative shower with hexachlorophene or chlorhexidine, avoiding hair removal unless it will interfere with the procedure, preparing the operative site with a soap followed with a "degerming" agent, and demarcating the surgical field with a surgical drape (5, 6, 9, 10).

The longer the surgery, the greater the likelihood that the patient will develop a postoperative wound infection (8). This may in part be explained by a greater amount of bacterial contamination (endogenous and exogenous) occurring over time. Other possible explanations include: wound cells may be damaged by drying and instruments, increased numbers of sutures and/or electrocoagulation may reduce local resistance, or greater blood loss may lead to a decrease in the patient's level of resistance (5, 8).

Several bacteria possess properties that promote their ability to invade and subsequently cause infection. Some bacteria (*Klebsiella*, pneumococcus) have surface capsules that inhibit phagocytosis and thus contribute to their pathogenicity (6). Other bacteria produce endotoxins or exotoxins that promote cellular destruction. Bacteria may also provide a synergistic environment that facilitates the further propagation of other bacteria.

A patient may suffer a large amount of bacterial contamination during a surgical procedure without developing an infection. Conversely, an individual with minimal contamination may develop a severe wound infection. The discrepancy is explained by the individual's host defense mechanisms. An infection develops when the host defenses cannot handle the amount of contamination. A variety of factors may interfere with a patient's ability to resist infection, and a detailed discussion of risk factors and impaired host defense mechanisms is beyond the scope of this chapter. Patient factors that increase the risk of infection include advanced age, malnutrition, immunodeficiency, obesity, diabetes mellitus, uremia, advanced malignancy, prematurity, leukemia, traumatic injury, burn, and shock (5, 6, 8, 11). If possible, interventions prior to surgery should be aimed at correcting these disorders. Patients who have an infection at a distant site (pre- and/or postoperatively) have approximately a 3-fold greater risk of developing a postoperative wound infection (8). The use of steroids, antimetabolites, and anticancer agents has also been associated with an increased risk of infection (5, 6, 8, 11). Therefore, unnecessary use of these agents should be avoided in the surgical patient. The longer the patient is in the hospital prior to the surgical procedure, the greater the likelihood of a postoperative wound infection. The increased risk of infection appears to be independent of concurrent diseases and is probably explained by the fact that patients become colonized with hospital-acquired bacteria (5, 8).

If devitalized tissue and/or a foreign body is present, the risk of developing a postoperative infection is increased dramatically (6). Studies have demonstrated that in traumatic wounds in healthy subjects, bacterial contamination with more than 10^5 organisms is required to produce infection (12). The bacterial inoculum needed to produce infection is decreased dramatically in the presence of devitalized tissue and/or foreign bodies. Foreign bodies that are not removed may decrease the minimal infective dose 10,000-fold or more. Hematomas, seromas, or dead spaces also promote bacterial localization and growth (6).

Other factors that may contribute to the risk of developing a postoperative wound infection include the surgeon's skill and the use of an open drainage system such as a Penrose drain (8, 13). Farber et al. (13) demonstrated that the rate of development of postoperative wound infections was inversely proportional to the logarithmic fre-

Table 72.2.
General Risk Factors For Surgical Wound Infections

Break in sterile technique	Obesity
Burn	Prematurity
Diabetes mellitus	Presence of devitalized tissue/
Drugs (steroids, antimetabolites,	foreign body
anticancer agents)	Prolonged preoperative stay
Duration of surgery	Remote infection
Elderly	Shock
Immunodeficiency	Surgical skill level
Leukemia	Surgical wound class (degree of
Malignancy	contamination)
Malnutrition	Trauma

quency with which the operation was performed. Therefore, a higher incidence of infection may be seen in hospitals that perform only a limited number of operations.

Whether or not a given patient should receive antimicrobial surgical prophylaxis is a complex decision that involves assessment of the patient's risk of developing a postoperative wound infection (Table 72.2). In general, antimicrobial prophylaxis should be used when (a) there is an increased frequency of infection for a given procedure, (b) the development of infection may have catastrophic consequences, or (c) the patient has decreased resistance to infection (14). Thus, a relatively healthy patient who is undergoing a clean surgical procedure such as carotid endarterectomy, which is associated with an extremely low risk of infection, may not need antimicrobial prophylaxis. Conversely, a patient undergoing a clean procedure in which a prosthetic device will be implanted may be a candidate for prophylaxis, even though the incidence of infection is usually low. Infections involving prosthetic devices (e.g., heart valves and endocarditis) can have devastating consequences for the patient, and the decision to use prophylactic antibodies in this case is based in part on the consequences of a postoperative infection. Finally, patients with impaired host defenses and/or those shown to be at increased risk of infection may warrant antimicrobial prophylaxis.

Choice of Antimicrobial Regimen

The selection of a given antimicrobial regimen should be based in part on the presumed pathogens that may be encountered during the surgical procedure. Overall, the most commonly isolated pathogens from surgical wound infections include *Staphylococcus aureus*, *Enterococcus* spp., *Escherichia coli*, *Pseudomonas aeruginosa*, *Staphylococcus epidermidis*, and *Enterobacter* spp. (15). In 1984, *Bacteroides* spp. accounted for approximately 3.7% of the bacterial isolates from infected surgical wounds. Other anaerobes such as *Clostridium perfringens*, or *Peptostreptococcus* may also cause wound infections; however, the

precise frequency of anaerobic wound infections is difficult to determine because of problems associated with the isolation of anaerobes (5). As shown in Table 72.3, the pathogens responsible for postoperative wound infections vary considerably, depending on the microflora of the body cavity encountered during the procedure (10). It is unnecessary to use an antimicrobial agent with activity against all organisms that could be encountered during the procedure. Antibiotic selection should be based on the agent's microbiologic activity against the most likely pathogens. Agents with broad-spectrum activity, such as the third-generation cephalosporins, have not been shown to be superior to the first-generation cephalosporins in preventing wound infections (16).

In addition to considering the agent's spectrum of microbiological activity, one must also consider the agent's cost and its potential to produce toxicity. Although relatively short courses of antibiotics are used for surgical prophylaxis, the agents are not without the potential for toxicity. Most commonly reported adverse reactions with prophylactic antimicrobial regimens include allergic re-

Table 72.3.
Common Pathogens in Surgical Wounds, Based on Operative Procedure[a]

Procedure	Organism
Gastrointestinal	
Oral, esophageal	Viridans streptococci, *S. aureus*, Gram-negative aerobes, oral anaerobes
Gastroduodenal[b]	Viridans streptococci, *E. coli*, oral anaerobes
Biliary tract[b]	*E. coli*, *Klebsiella* spp., *Proteus* spp., enterococcus
Colorectal	*E. coli*, other Enterobacteriaceae, enterococci, *Bacteroides* spp., *Clostridium* spp.
Obstetrics and gynecology	
Vaginal hysterectomy	*S. aureus*, streptococci including engterococci, *E. coli*, anaerobes (predominantly *Provetella* spp.)
Abdominal hysterectomy	*E. coli*, *Staphylococcus* spp.
Cesarean section	Anaerobes (*Provetella* spp., *B. fragilis*, peptostreptococci), streptococci, *E. coli*
Abortion	*N. gonorrhoeae*, *C. trachomatis*, β-hemolytic streptococci, *S. aureus*, *E. coli*, anaerobes.
Neurosurgery	*S. aureus*, *S. epidermidis*
Cardiothoracic/vascular	*S. aureus*, *S. epidermidis*
Orthopaedic	*S. aureus*, *S. epidermidis*
Genitourinary	*E. coli*, *Klebsiella* spp., *Pseudomonas aeruginosa*, enterococci

[a] Compiled from information in references 10, 11, 27, 33–35, 42, 44, 46–49, 51.
[b] Under normal conditions the stomach and biliary tract are sterile environments. The bacteria listed apply only to high-risk patients.

actions and pseudomembranous colitis (17–20). It is also important to remember that antibiotic usage may promote the emergence of resistant strains of bacteria (21). Based on the ability of antibiotics to promote bacterial resistance, the widespread, haphazard, prolonged use of broad-spectrum antibiotics for surgical prophylaxis should be discouraged.

Timing of Antimicrobial Administration

The time of administration of the antimicrobial agent is crucial to ensuring therapeutic serum concentrations and thus efficacy. Historically, antibiotics were initiated following the surgical procedure and were shown to be of no benefit in preventing postoperative wound infections (2). In a series of animal investigations, Miles and Burke demonstrated that there was a well-defined window in which antimicrobial agents could be administered to minimize the development of wound infection (22, 23). To be effective, the antibiotics had to be present when the infective lesion originated. If the antibiotics were administered more than 3 hr after bacterial contamination they were ineffective. This "effective window" for administration of prophylactic antibiotics was subsequently confirmed in patients by Stone and colleagues (24). These investigators demonstrated that the incidence of wound infection following gastric, biliary, or colonic surgery was reduced dramatically if antibiotics were instituted prior to the operation. Antibiotics that were initiated following surgery were ineffective; the infection rate for patients receiving only postoperative antibiotics was similar to that observed for patients who did not receive prophylactic antibiotics. Based on the results from these studies, antimicrobial prophylaxis should be initiated immediately prior to the surgical procedure. It is currently recommended that intravenous antibiotics be administered at the induction of anesthesia or within 60 min of the surgical incision (25). The antibiotic should not be ordered on an "on call" basis. The time between administration of the "on call" antibiotic and the actual incision can be quite long and may result in subtherapeutic antibiotic concentrations during the procedure (26).

Route of Administration

For surgical prophylaxis, antibiotics have been administered by a variety routes including topical, rectal, oral, intravenous, and intramuscular. The route used depends on physician preference and the type of procedure performed. Since a major goal of antimicrobial prophylaxis is to ensure therapeutic serum and tissue concentrations, intravenous and intramuscular routes of administration are frequently used.

Oral antibiotics are useful, however, in preventing postoperative wound infections following colorectal pro-

cedures. The antibiotics (classically erythromycin and neomycin) are given the day before the procedure, which leads to a decrease in the gastrointestinal luminal concentration of bacteria (27). Oral antibiotics and intravenous antibiotics are equally efficacious to for prophylaxis of colorectal procedures (10, 11). Based on their efficacy, ease of administration, and low cost, oral antibiotics are frequently used for these procedures. In general, the oral route is not recommended for other surgical procedures because of the possibility of impaired absorption during the procedure.

Topical antibiotics may be placed directly in the wound during the operative procedure. Only a limited number of trials adequately assess the efficacy of topical antibiotics in preventing wound infections, as compared with parenteral agents (28). Potential disadvantages of topical antimicrobial prophylaxis include (a) administration of the agent usually follows bacterial contamination, (b) the antibiotics may not reach remote sites of the wound, (c) they may be systemically absorbed, (d) they may not provide therapeutic serum concentrations, and (e) they may promote the development of adhesions (29).

With the exception of colorectal procedures, the intravenous route of administration is usually preferred because it ensures bioavailability and is relatively easy to administer immediately prior to the procedure. The intramuscular route provides adequate concentrations and is efficacious, but it may be associated with patient discomfort (30).

Duration of Administration

As previously stated, antimicrobial concentrations must be present at the time of the bacterial contamination. However, major controversy exists as to whether or not these agents should be continued postoperatively. Stone and colleagues (31) demonstrated that continued antibiotic administration for 5 days postoperatively did not influence the rate of infection. Currently, antimicrobial surgical prophylaxis is frequently continued postoperatively for 24 to 48 hr. However, several studies demonstrate that a single intravenous preoperative dose is effective in preventing postoperative wound infections following several procedures, including biliary tract procedures, colorectal operations, cesarean sections, transurethral procedures, and hysterectomies (32). Physicians frequently cite the presence of catheters and or drains as reasons for continuing antimicrobial prophylaxis postoperatively. Further studies are needed to clarify the optimal duration of antimicrobial prophylaxis in these cases. Prolonged antimicrobial prophylaxis may theoretically promote bacterial resistance. In addition, prolonged prophylaxis can have substantial economic impact for an institution. Based on the potential hazards of prolonged therapy, antimicrobial prophylaxis should be continued for the shortest possible duration.

Single-dose prophylaxis should be encouraged whenever possible.

It is important to point out that the duration of the surgical procedure should be considered when deciding whether or not a single preoperative dose will be sufficient. Antimicrobial agents that have a short half-life may not provide adequate concentrations throughout prolonged procedures, which may lead to an increased incidence of infection (32). If an agent with a short half-life is used for a prolonged surgical procedure, repeated dosing intraoperatively may be warranted. Alternatively, an agent with a longer half-life may be used as a single preoperative dose.

SURGICAL PROCEDURES: USE OF ANTIBIOTIC PROPHYLAXIS

Numerous studies have examined the efficacy of various antibiotics in the prevention of wound infections following all types of surgical procedures. However, many of the trials have multiple design flaws and/or limited sample sizes. The discussion below outlines the principles that must be considered in selecting an antimicrobial agent for a given surgical procedure. The intent is not to provide an exhaustive review of all trials and all agents tested; rather one should glean the principles of prophylaxis from the description below.

Gastroduodenal Surgery

Gastric surgery is considered a clean procedure; however, the rate of infection depends on the operation performed as well as inherent patient risk factors. Normally, gastric acidity maintains the sterile environment within the stomach. Factors including achlorhydria (age-, disease-, or drug-induced), delayed motility, gastric carcinoma, gastric ulcer, and gastric hemorrhage are associated with increased bacterial colonization and risk for infection (33–35). Prophylactic antibiotics have been shown effective in decreasing the incidence of postoperative wound infections following gastric surgery in these high-risk patients (10, 11, 33–35). Other patient risk factors that may alter the patient's resistance should also be considered when deciding whether or not a given patient should receive a prophylactic agent.

The most common infecting organisms are those that reside within the gastric lumen, including mouth flora (viridans streptococci, oral anaerobes) and occasionally bowel flora such as E. coli (33, 34). In addition, skin flora such as S. aureus are potential pathogens following gastroduodenal procedures. Based on the most likely pathogens encountered during gastric procedures, cefazolin is commonly used for surgical prophylaxis (39).

Biliary Surgery

Like the stomach, the biliary tree is normally a sterile environment. The incidence of wound infection is increased dramatically if the biliary tract contains bacteria. Chetlin and Elliott (36) demonstrated that bactobilia occurred in 33% of patients undergoing biliary procedures, and infectious complications were 40 times more common in these patients than in those with negative bile cultures. Risk factors associated with bactobilia include acute cholecystitis, common duct stones with or without jaundice, and age greater than 70 years (36). Based on the presence or absence of the forementioned risk factors, a patient can be placed in a high- or low-risk group for the development of postoperative wound infections. Patients who are considered to be at high risk should receive antimicrobial prophylaxis.

The most commonly isolated pathogens from the biliary tract include E. coli, Klebsiella, enterococci and Proteus spp. (10, 11, 33, 35, 36). S. aureus and anaerobic organisms are less frequently isolated. Agents such as cefazolin or trimethoprim-sulfamethoxazole, which have activity against the presumed pathogens, have been shown to be effective in preventing wound infections following biliary tract procedures (33, 35). Keighley et al. (37) compared the efficacy of an agent that undergoes minimal biliary excretion (gentamicin) to one that is excreted predominantly in the bile (rifamide) in preventing postoperative wound infections following biliary procedures. The incidence of postoperative infection (compared with a placebo control) was reduced only with the gentamicin regimen. These investigators concluded that high biliary excretion is not a requirement for an agent to be effective in preventing infections following biliary tract procedures and that adequate serum concentrations are important for success. In addition, agents such as cefamandole or cefoperazone, which undergo extensive biliary excretion, have not been shown to be superior to cefazolin. Meijer and co-workers (38) performed a meta-analysis of the clinical trials assessing the efficacy of antibiotic prophylaxis in biliary tract surgery. The analyses revealed that wound infection rates were not significantly different among the various classes of cephalosporins (i.e., first- versus second- versus third-generation cephalosporin). In addition, single-dose prophylaxis provided a similar degree of efficacy as multiple-dose regimens.

Colorectal Surgery

The colon harbors numerous pathogens and therefore the risk for infection is high, ranging from 10 to 20% (2). Wound infections following colorectal procedures are frequently polymicrobial, with potential pathogens including E. coli, Bacteroides spp., Clostridia spp., enterococci, and other Enterbacteriaceae (33, 35). Antimicrobial regimens that have microbiological activity against both aerobic and anaerobic organisms are effective in preventing postoperative wound infections (10, 11, 33, 35).

Preoperative mechanical cleansing of the bowel with

whole-bowel irrigants, enemas, and or cathartics effectively reduces the fecal content of the bowel and are routine prior to colorectal surgery. However, the concentration of organisms within the luminal fluid remains unchanged (39).

Oral antibiotics given prior to surgery may decrease the concentration of microorganisms within the gut lumen. Bartlett and colleagues demonstrated that the concentration of bacteria in the colon was reduced by approximately 10^5 colony forming units (cfu) per ml with preoperative oral antimicrobial prophylaxis (40). Based on this principle, oral antibiotics (erythromycin plus neomycin, metronidazole alone, metronidazole plus neomycin, metronidazole plus kanamycin, kanamycin plus erythromycin or doxycycline) have been used successfully as prophylactic antibiotics for colorectal procedures (10, 11, 27, 33, 35, 41). The most commonly employed regimen in the United States is erythromycin plus neomycin. Following bowel preparation, 1 g of each of the antibiotics is administered 9, 17, and 18 hr prior to the surgical procedure (27). A potential limitation of this regimen, is patient compliance. Patients may complain of gastrointestinal discomfort and or an inability to ingest the numerous tablets.

The efficacy of intravenous antibiotics in preventing wound infections following colorectal procedures has also been well documented. Antimicrobial regimens that possess strictly aerobic activity have not been consistently proven to be efficacious (35). Similarly, regimens that possess only anaerobic activity are associated with a reduction in the infection rate but not to the level achieved when the regimen has activity against both aerobic and anaerobic organisms. Second-generation cephalosporins with activity against *B. fragilis* are commonly used effective prophylactic agents for colorectal procedures.

The concomitant administration of oral and parenteral antibiotics is a common practice. However, data supporting such practice are lacking. Condon et al. (41) demonstrated that the rate of infection for 1128 patients undergoing colorectal surgery was 7.8% in patients receiving oral antibiotics and 5.7% in those receiving oral and parenteral antibiotics; this was not significantly different.

Due to the high risk for bacterial contamination during colorectal procedures, antimicrobial prophylaxis is clearly indicated. Both oral and intravenous antibiotics have been shown to be effective. The route of administration selected is based to a large degree on physician preference.

Obstetrics and Gynecology

The value of antimicrobial surgical prophylaxis in obstetrical and gynecological procedures depends on the procedure performed. Contamination of the operative site with vaginal microflora occurs during a vaginal hysterectomy and antimicrobial prophylaxis is therefore considered to be beneficial.

The routine use of antimicrobial prophylaxis for abdominal hysterectomies is controversial. Since abdominal hysterectomies do not involve opening the vagina, the surgical site is not exposed to bacterial contamination with vaginal flora (42). Well-defined risk factors for infection following abdominal hysterectomies do not exist; obesity and old age have been suggested as possible risk factors. The decision about whether or not a given patient should receive antimicrobial prophylaxis prior to an abdominal hysterectomy should be based on the patient's risk for infection as well as the infection rate for the procedure at the given institution.

Prophylactic antibiotics are also indicated in patients who are at high risk for infection following cesarean section (10, 11, 33, 35). Based on conflicting reports, the precise identification of risk factors for infection following cesarean section is difficult. Patients undergoing primary cesarean section or patients with premature rupture of the membranes (PROM) for >6 hr prior to delivery are considered to be at high risk for postoperative infection. Other potential risk factors for postoperative endometritis and or febrile morbidity include the duration of labor, number of vaginal examinations, number of rectal examinations, parity, skill of the obstetrician, anemia, and obesity (33, 35). The routine use of antibiotics for prophylaxis of abortive procedures is greatly debated. Risk factors for postoperative infection following abortion include the presence of cervical gonorrhea or chlamydial infection at the time of the procedure, history of pelvic inflammatory disease or gonorrhea, multiple sexual partners (>2) in nulliparous women, and gestational age (42).

Vaginal secretions contain numerous aerobic and anaerobic organisms; approximately 10^7 to 10^8 aerobes per ml and 10^8 to 10^9 anaerobes per ml (42). Lactobacilli, peptostreptococci, staphylococci, streptococci, diphtheroids, and anaerobes belonging to the *Provetella* spp. (formerly referred to as *Bacteroides melaninogenicus* and *oralis* group) (10, 11, 42). Approximately, 10% of healthy women harbor *B. fragilis* and Enterobacteriaceae within their vaginal secretions (42). Postoperative vaginal cuff infections are usually polymicrobic, with *S. aureus*, streptococci including enterococci, *E. coli*, and anaerobes being common pathogens. *E. coli*, and *Staphylococcus* spp. are the most likely pathogens to cause wound infections following abdominal hysterectomies (10, 11, 33, 35, 42). Contamination of the operative wound with vaginal flora may occur during a cesarean section. Anaerobic organisms are the primary pathogens responsible for endometritis following a cesarean section. However, other vaginal flora (*E. coli*, streptococci) may also cause infection. Pathogens responsible for causing infections following abortive procedures include *N. gonorrhoeae*, *Chlamydia trachomatis*, anaerobes, β-hemolytic streptococci, and *E. coli*. The incidence of infection following an abortion is dramatically increased if the patient is infected with *N. gonorrhoeae* or *C. trachomatis* at the time of the procedure.

Cefazolin has been shown to be an effective prophylactic agent for hysterectomies (vaginal and abdominal) as well as cesarean sections (10, 11, 33, 35, 42). Based on the efficacy of cefazolin and other narrow-spectrum agents (penicillin), it does not appear necessary to use antibiotics that possess activity against all possible bacterial species (42). Supporting this concept further, second- and third-generation cephalosporins have been shown to be effective in preventing postoperative infections following hysterectomies but have not been proven superior to first-generation cephalosporins (10). Based on the possibility of *B. fragilis*, some physicians prefer to use agents such as cefoxitin, cefotetan, or cefazolin. Institutional specific infection patterns can be reviewed to assess the appropriateness of this decision. Cefazolin or ampicillin are the preferred agents for prophylaxis for cesarean sections (10, 33, 35). To minimize fetal exposure to the antibiotic, the agent should be administered after the umbilical cord is clamped. If antimicrobial prophylaxis is to be used for abortive procedures, agents such as tetracycline, penicillin, and metronidazole appear to be effective in preventing postoperative pelvic infections (35, 42).

Neurosurgery

Neurosurgical operations are categorized as clean procedures, with an average infection rate under 3.0%. However, the risk of infection is highly dependent on the procedure performed. Tenney and co-workers (43) demonstrated that deep wound infections occurred more frequently after craniotomies (4.3%) than after spinal procedures (0.9%). A high rate of infection (11%) was also seen for patients who underwent reoperation for recurrent gliomas. Based on these findings, high-risk patients such as those undergoing prolonged surgical operations, tumor resections, and or implantation of prosthetic devices or foreign bodies, may potentially benefit from antimicrobial prophylaxis.

The primary source of bacterial contamination during neurosurgical procedures is exogenous bacteria. The most common pathogens include *S. aureus* and *S. epidermidis* (11, 44). Young and Lawner (45) demonstrated a 74% reduction in infection rate when patients were administered cefazolin and gentamicin for surgical prophylaxis. Oxacillin and clindamycin are also effective in reducing the incidence of postoperative wound infections following neurosurgical procedures (33, 35, 46).

Antimicrobial prophylaxis cannot be recommended for all neurosurgical procedures. Prophylaxis may be warranted for prolonged high-risk procedures (craniotomies, implantation of foreign bodies) or high-risk patients. Selection of the agent should be based on the susceptibility profile for the most likely pathogens within the given institution.

Cardiothoracic and Vascular Surgery

The incidence of postoperative wound infection following cardiothoracic and or vascular procedures is low (less than 5%). The decision as to whether or not antimicrobial prophylaxis is indicated is therefore based on whether or not the infection is associated with catastrophic consequences or the patient has decreased host resistance. Antimicrobial prophylaxis is frequently used when prosthetic devices such as heart valves or vascular grafts are inserted.

Patients undergoing cardiac valve replacement are at risk for endocarditis. Due to the potential morbidity and mortality associated with prosthetic valve endocarditis, antimicrobial prophylaxis prior to cardiac valve replacement has become standard practice. The use of antimicrobial prophylaxis for cardiac bypass surgery is controversial. Although, Fong and McKee demonstrated that methicillin significantly decreased postoperative infections (compared with placebo), some authors still believe that the low incidence of serious infection following the procedure does not justify the widespread use of prophylactic antibiotics (47, 48). Other investigators assert that the infections that occur following coronary artery bypass (e.g., mediastinitis, sternal osteomyelitis) are serious and potentially life-threatening, and the seriousness of these infections justifies the routine use of prophylactic antimicrobial agents (49). Potential risk factors for postoperative sternal or mediastinal wound infection include obesity, diabetes mellitus, preoperative hospital stay exceeding 5 days, and cigarette smoking (50). In addition, Platt et al. (51) demonstrated that patients who had lower atrial appendage antibiotic concentrations had a higher incidence of infection. Based on this, one may postulate that the low antimicrobial tissue concentrations during a surgical procedure may be another risk factor for postoperative infection.

S. aureus and *S. epidermidis* are the most common pathogens responsible for cardiothoracic and or vascular postoperative wound infection. Based on these potential pathogens, cefazolin, cefamandole, cefuroxime, and vancomycin are commonly used agents for surgical prophylaxis (52). Hospital-specific resistance patterns should be taken into consideration when selecting an agent. Although short-course (2 days) and even single-dose antimicrobial prophylaxis with ceftriaxone has been shown to be effective in preventing postoperative wound infections, the duration of prophylaxis remains somewhat controversial. In a 1988 survey of 51 hospitals, antimicrobial prophylaxis was usually continued until all chest tubes and/or intravenous lines were removed (52). The benefit of prolonged prophylaxis (>48 hr) has not been proven in this population and therefore should be discouraged.

Orthopaedic Surgery

Although orthopaedic surgeries are classified as clean procedures, the actual incidence of wound infections following orthopaedic procedures is highly variable, ranging from 0.7 to 9%, depending on the procedure performed (44). Antimicrobial prophylaxis is only indicated for implantation of a prosthetic device or foreign material or procedures that are excessively long (10, 44). Since infections associated with prosthetic devices are difficult to treat and may necessitate the removal of the device, antimicrobial prophylaxis is considered justifiable, based on the complications associated with a possible infection. Wound infections following orthopaedic procedures are caused predominantly by staphylococcal species and therefore, cefazolin is frequently the agent of choice for prophylaxis of orthopaedic procedures. Individual hospital resistance patterns should be considered and if methicillin-resistant *S. aureus* is prevalent, vancomycin may be an alternative prophylactic agent (10).

CONCLUSION

Antimicrobial prophylaxis is effective in decreasing the risk of postoperative wound infection following several elective surgical procedures. Whether or not a given patient should receive antimicrobial prophylaxis is a complex decision, based on the risk for bacterial contamination and the patient's level of resistance (Table 72.2). In addition, specific risk factors for certain surgical procedures (e.g., biliary tract, gastroduodenal, cesarean section) facilitate the identification of high-risk patients who have a greater risk of postoperative wound infection (Table 72.4). Although orthopaedic, cardiothoracic, and vascular procedures are frequently associated with a low incidence of postoperative wound infection, prophylaxis is indicated in patients in whom a prosthetic device or foreign material is to be im-

Table 72.4.
Specific Risk Factors Based on the Surgical Procedure

Gastroduodenal	Achlorhydria, delayed motility, gastric carcinoma, gastric ulcer, gastric hemorrhage
Biliary tract	Acute cholecystitis, common duct stones with or without jaundice, age >70 years
Cesarean section	Primary cesarean section, premature rupture of the membranes for >6 hr
Abortion	Gonococcal or chlamydial infection, multiple sexual partners (>2) in nulliparous women, gestational age
Cardiothoracic, vascular, orthopaedic, and neurosurgery	Implantation of prosthetic device or foreign material, duration of surgery prolonged

Table 72.5.
Antimicrobial Prophylaxis for Surgical Procedure

Procedure	Recommended Agent[a,b,c]
Gastroduodenal[d]	Cefazolin
Biliary tract[d]	Cefazolin
Colorectal	Neomycin + erythromycin or Cefoxitin, cefotetan, cefmetazole
Vaginal/abdominal hysterectomy	Cefazolin
Cesarean section	Cefazolin or ampicillin
Neurosurgery	Cefazolin
Orthopaedic	Cefazolin

[a] Agents should be administered 30–60 min prior to the incision or at induction of anesthesia; exceptions: 1) oral erythromycin plus neomycin should be given 9, 17, and 18 hours prior to the procedure, 2) antimicrobial prophylaxis is administered after the umbilical cord is clamped during cesarean sections.
[b] General dosage regimens: cefazolin 1 g IV, neomycin 1 g plus erythromycin 1 g, cefoxitin 2 g IV, cefotetan 1–2 g IV, cefmetazole 1–2 g IV, ampicillin 1 g IV, doxycycline 0.1 g, vancomycin 1 g IV, gentamicin 1.5 mg/kg IV, clindamycin 300–600 mg IV.
[c] Antimicrobial prophylaxis should be continued for the shortest possible duration. Single-dose prophylaxis is effective for many procedures. The reader is referred to the text for greater detail.
[d] Prophylaxis recommended only for high-risk patients.

Table 72.6.
Principles of Antimicrobial Surgical Prophylaxis

1. Antimicrobial prophylaxis should be used when the risk of infection is high, when the consequences of infection could be devastating, or when the patient has decreased resistance.
2. The selection of the antimicrobial agent should be based on the "most likely" pathogens at the surgical site.
3. The antimicrobial agent should be administered *prior* to the procedure (e.g., intravenous administration may be given at induction of anesthesia.)
4. The continuation of antibiotics postoperatively >24 hr should be discouraged. Single-dose prophylaxis has been shown to be effective for many surgical procedures.

planted. Overall, when deciding whether or not antimicrobial prophylaxis should be employed, one must weigh the risk of infection (incidence and severity) against the potential pros and cons of antimicrobial prophylaxis.

If antimicrobial agents are used for surgical prophylaxis, the selection of antibiotic should be based on the most likely pathogens at the surgical site (Table 72.3). The agent should be administered intravenously either at induction of anesthesia or within 30 to 60 min prior to the incision. Alternatively, oral antimicrobial agents (erythromycin 1 g and neomycin 1 g given 9, 17, and 18 hr prior to surgery) are effective in decreasing the risk of postoperative infection associated with colorectal procedures. Table 72.5 outlines specific recommendations for antimicrobial prophylaxis of selected surgical procedures. Based on potential toxicity (e.g., promote bacterial resistance, adverse reactions, cost) antimicrobial prophylaxis should be discontinued as soon as possible after the procedure (e.g., single dose or <24 hr postoperatively). Antimicrobial prophylaxis is based on several key principles (Table 72.6) that facilitate the identification of high-risk patients and the selection of agent and provide guidelines for the appropriate use of antimicrobial prophylaxis. Understanding these basic principles allows one to design optimal antimicrobial regimens that are aimed at preventing postoperative wound infections and thus decreasing morbidity, mortality, and hospital costs.

REFERENCES

1. Cruse PJE, Foord R: The epidemiology of wound infection. Surg Clin North Am 60:27–40, 1980.
2. Conte JE, Jacob LS, Polk HC: Antibiotic Prophylaxis in Surgery. Philadelphia: JB Lippincott, 1984.
3. Shapiro M, Townsend TR, Rosner B, et al.: Use of antimicrobial drugs in general hospitals: patterns of prophylaxis. N Engl J Med 301:351–355, 1979.
4. Sandusky WR: Use of prophylactic antibiotics in surgical patients. Surg Clin North Am 60:83–92, 1980.
5. Cruse JE, Wound infections: epidemiology and clinical characteristics. In Howard RJ, Simmons RL: Surgical Infectious Diseases, ed. 2. East Norwalk, CT, Appleton & Lange, 1988, pp 319–329.
6. Alexander JW, Surgical infections and choice of antibiotics. In Sabiston DC: Textbook of Surgery: The Biological Basis of Modern Surgical Practice, ed. 13. Philadelphia, WB Saunders, 1986, pp 259–283.
7. Culbertson WR, Altemeier WA, Gonzalez LL, et al.: Studies on the epidemiology of postoperative infection of clean operative wounds. Ann Surg 154:599–610, 1961.
8. Ad Hoc Committee of the Committee on Trauma, Division of Medical Sciences, National Academy of Sciences–National Research Council: Postoperative wound infections: the influence of ultraviolet irradiation of the operating room and various other factors. Ann Surg 160(suppl 2):23, 1964.
9. Polk HC, Simpson CJ, Simmons BP, et al.: Guidelines for prevention of surgical wound infection. Arch Surg 118:1213–1217, 1983.
10. Burnakis TG: Surgical antimicrobial prophylaxis: principles and guidelines. Pharmacotherapy 4:249–271, 1984.
11. DiPiro JT, Bivins BA, Record RM, et al.: The prophylactic use of antimicrobials in surgery. Curr Probl Surg 20:69–132, 1983.
12. Elek SD: Experimental stapylococcal infections in the skin of man. Ann NY Acad Sci 65:85–92, 1965.
13. Farber BF, Kaiser DL, Wenzel RP: Relation between surgical volume and incidence of postoperative wound infection. N Engl J Med 305:200–205, 1981.
14. Lewis RT: Antibiotic prophylaxis in surgery. Can J Surg 24:561–566, 1981.
15. Horan TC, White JW, Jarvis Wr, et al.: Nosocomial infection surveillance, 1984. MMWR 35(155):1755–2955, 1986.
16. DiPiro JT, Bowden TA, Hooks VH: Prophylactic parenteral cephalosporins in surgery: Are the newer agents better? JAMA 252:3277–3279, 1984.
17. Block BS, Mercer LJ, Ismail MA, et al.: Clostridium difficile–associated diarrhea follows perioperative prophylaxis with cefoxitin. Am J Obstet Gynecol 153:835–838, 1985.
18. Cannon SR, Dyson PHP, Sanderson PJ: Pseudomembranous colitis associated with antibiotic prophylaxis in orthopaedic surgery. J Bone Joint Surg 70B:600–602, 1988.
19. Dajee H, Laks H, Miller J, Oren R: Profound hypotension from rapid vancomycin administration during cardiac operation. J Thorac Cardiovasc Surg 87:145–146, 1984.
20. Odio C, Mohs E, Sklar FH, et al.: Adverse reactions to vancomycin used as prophylaxis for CSF shunt procedures. Am J Dis Child 138:17–19, 1984.
21. Moellering RC: Interaction between antimicrobial consumption and selection of resistant bacterial strains. Scand J Infect Dis Suppl 70:18–24, 1990.
22. Miles AA, Miles EM, Burke J: The value and duration of defence reactions of the skin to the primary lodgement of bacteria. Br J Exp Pathol 38:79–96, 1957.
23. Burke JF: The effective period of preventive antibiotic action in experimental incisions and dermal lesions. Surgery 50:161–168, 1961.
24. Stone HH, Hooper CA, Kolb LD, et al.: Antibiotic prophylaxis in gastric, biliary and colonic surgery. Ann Surg 184:443–452, 1976.
25. Nichols RL: Use of prophylactic antibodies in surgical practice. Am J Med 70:686–682, 1981.
26. Nix DE, DiPiro JT, Bowden TA, et al.: Cephalosporins for surgical prophylaxis: Computer projections of intraoperative availability. South Med J 78:962–966, 1985.
27. Nichols RL, Briodo P, Condon RE, et al.: Effect of preoperative neomycin-erythromycin intestinal preparation on the incidence of infectious complications following colon surgery. Ann Surg 178:453–462, 1973.
28. Roth RM, Gleckman RA, Gantz NM, et al.: Antibiotic irrigations: a plea for controlled clinical trials. Pharmacotherapy 5:222–227, 1985.
29. Rappaport WD, Holcomb M, Valente J, et al.: Antibiotic irrigation and the formation of intraabdominal adhesions. Am J Surg 158:435–437, 1989.
30. Alexander JW, Alexander NS: The influence of route of administration on wound fluid concentration of prophylactic antibiotics. J Trauma 16:488–495, 1978.
31. Stone HS, Haney BB, Kolb LD, et al.: Prophylactic and preventive antibiotic therapy: Timing, duration and economics. Ann Surg 189:691–698, 1979.
32. DePiro JT, Cheung RPF, Bowden TA, et al.: Single dose systemic antibiotic prophylaxis of surgical wound infections. Am J Surg 152:552–559, 1986.
33. DiPiro JT, Record KE, Schanzenbach KS, et al.: Antimicrobial prophylaxis in surgery: Part 1. Am J Hosp Pharm 38:320–334, 1981.
34. Nichols RL, Webb WR, Jones JW, et al.: Efficacy of antibiotic prophylaxis in high risk gastroduodenal operations. Am J Surg 143:94–98, 1982.
35. Guglielmo BJ, Hohn DC, Koo PJ, et al.: Antibiotic prophylaxis in surgical procedures: a critical analysis of the literature. Arch Surg 118:943–955, 1983.
36. Chetlin SH, Elliott DW: Biliary bacteremia. Arch Surg 102:303–307, 1971.
37. Keighley MRB, Drysdale RB, Quoraishi AH, et al.: Antibiotics in biliary disease: the relative importance of antibiotic concentrations in the bile and serum. Gut 17:495–500, 1976.
38. Meijer WS, Schmitz PIM, Jeekel J: Meta-analysis of randomized, controlled clinical trials of antibiotic prophylaxis in biliary tract surgery. Br J Surg 77:283–290, 1990.
39. Arabi Y, Bimock F, Burdon DW, et al.: Influence of bowel preparation and antimicrobials on colonic microflora. Br J Surg 65:555–559, 1978.
40. Bartlett JG, Condon RE, Gorbach SL, et al.: Veterans administration cooperative study on bowel preparation for elective colorectal operations. Ann Surg 188:249–254, 1978.
41. Condon RE, Bartlett JG, Greenlee H, et al.: Efficacy of oral and systemic antibiotic prophylaxis in colorectal operations. Arch Surg 118:496–502, 1983.
42. Houang ET: Antibiotic prophylaxis in hysterectomy and induced abortion: a review of the evidence. Drugs 41:19–37, 1991.

43. Tenney JH, Viahov D, Saloman M, et al.: Wide variation in the risk of wound infection following clean neurosurgery. J Neurosurg 62:243–247, 1985.

44. DiPiro JT, Record KE, Schazenback KS, et al.: Antimicrobial prophylaxis in surgery: part 2. Am J Hosp Pharm 38:487–494, 1981.

45. Young RF, Lawner PM: Perioperative antibiotic prophylaxis for prevention of postoperative neurosurgical infections. J Neurosurg 66:701–705, 1987.

46. Djindjian M, Lepresle E, Homs JB: Antibiotic prophylaxis during prolonged clean neurosurgery. J Neurosurg 73:383–386, 1990.

47. Fong IW, Baker CB, McKee DC: The value of prophylactic antibiotics in aorta-coronary bypass operations. J Thorac Cardiovasc Surg 78:908–913, 1979.

48. Hirschmann JV, Inui TS: Antimicrobial prophylaxis: a critique of recent trials. Rev Infect Dis 2(1):1–23, 1990.

49. Ariano RE, Zhandel GG: Antimicrobial prophylaxis in coronary bypass surgery: A critical appraisal. DICP Ann Pharmacother 25:478–484, 1991.

50. Nagachinta T, Stephens M, Reitz B, et al.: Risk factors for surgical-wound infection following cardiac surgery. J Infect Dis 156(6):967–973, 1987.

51. Platt R, Munoz A, Stella J, et al.: Antibiotic prophylaxis for cardiovascular surgery: Efficacy with coronary artery bypass. Ann Intern Med 101:770–774, 1984.

52. Woods M, LeBlanc K, Gersema L: Antibiotic prophylaxis in cardiothoracic surgery: results of a second survey. Hosp Pharm 25:641–643, 1990.

CHAPTER 73

INFECTIONS IN THE IMMUNOSUPPRESSED PATIENT

WILLIAM J. MCINTYRE, Pharm.D. and MICHAEL D. PARR, Pharm.D.

The human immune system serves many functions including homeostasis, surveillance, and defense. Defects in the host defense can lead to a wide variety of infectious complications. This chapter reviews specific defects in the immune system and the infectious complications associated with them. This chapter primarily discusses the treatment of infection in neutropenic patients. However, a number of the principles and treatments discussed in the section on neutropenia can also be applied to other immunocompromised patients. Discussion of acquired immune deficiency syndrome (AIDS) and the associated opportunistic infections is covered in another chapter in this text.

DEFECTS IN THE IMMUNE SYSTEM

Immunodeficiency or immunosuppression occurs in patients as a result of either inherited or acquired disorders of the immune system. Inherited disorders are usually diagnosed shortly after birth and include diseases such as severe combined immune deficiency syndrome (SCIDS) and agammaglobulinemia. Acquired disorders can occur at any time in a patient's life and are induced by chemotherapy, immunosuppressive agents (e.g., azathioprine, cyclosporine, and corticosteroids), radiation, or viral infection (e.g., AIDS). The severity of the immunodeficiency varies in both inherited and acquired disorders. The types of infections seen in these patients are directly related to the severity of the deficiency. An immunocompromised state is created by defects in the immune system. Defects can be seen in four components of the immune system: granulocytes, complement synthesis and antibody formation, cellular immunity, and mucocutaneous barriers (1, 2). Alterations in any of these four components can give rise to specific types of infections.

Effects upon the granulocytes can either be quantitative or functional. Antineoplastic agents can inhibit granulocyte formation and cause severe neutropenia. A number of investigators have correlated the incidence of infection with the total granulocyte count, also referred to as the absolute neutrophil count (ANC). A patient's total granulocyte count can be determined by multiplying the percentage of circulating granulocytes (mature granulocytes plus band forms) obtained from a white blood cell (WBC) differential by the total WBC count. Patients whose total granulocyte count falls below 1×10^9/liter (1000 cells per cubic millimeter (mm^3)) are termed neutropenic or granulocytopenic. As the total granulocyte count falls below 1×10^9/liter (1000 cells per mm^3), the rate of infection increases. When the total number of granulocytes falls below 0.1×10^9/liter (100 cells per mm^3), approximately 100% of the patients will develop an infection (3). Granulocytopenic patients are particularly susceptible to infections by bacteria. The duration of granulocytopenia also has a profound effect on the rate of infectious mortality because the longer the patient is granulocytopenic the greater the risk of infection by organisms that are resistant to traditional antibiotic therapy. Granulocytes can also have functional abnormalities that are inherited or caused by certain chemotherapeutic drugs, such as asparaginase and the vinca alkaloids. These functional abnormalities modify the granulocytes' ability to migrate and phagocytose bacteria, thus increasing the patient's susceptibility to infection.

Defects in complement synthesis and antibody production can occur due to chemotherapy and often lead to recurrent pneumonia and sepsis from organisms, such as *Streptococcus pneumoniae*. The increase in infection is caused by a loss of opsonization of bacteria, which is a function performed by complement and antibodies. Opsonization describes the ability of antibodies or complement to cover a particle or cell, thereby enhancing its phagocytosis. The cellular immune system consists primarily of macrophages and T cell lymphocytes, in which subsets of the T cells protect against certain types of infection. Cellular immunity provides protection against certain types of infections including fungal, viral, and protozoal. Impairment of cellular immunity is seen in patients who receive immunosuppressive agents (e.g., the corticosteroids, cyclosporine) or have certain types of cancer (e.g., Hodgkin's lymphoma).

The loss of mucocutaneous barriers offers a way for the pathogen to gain access to the host's internal organs. Mucocutaneous barriers can be broken down by a number of medical devices, procedures, and drugs, such as central venous catheters, Foley catheters, endotracheal tubes, or chemotherapy. In addition the mucociliary mechanism of the lung can be diminished, inhibiting clearance of organisms from the bronchopulmonary tree (1).

In the immunocompromised host, a number of the above mechanisms can be affected at the same time. Cancer patients, for example, may develop chemotherapy-induced neutropenia and in addition have chemotherapy-induced mucositis, resulting in ulceration of the gastrointestinal tract. This may predispose the patient to Gram-negative infection. Also, prolonged treatment with antineoplastic agents can affect not only granulocytes but cellular immunity as well. This increases the risk of developing an opportunistic fungal or viral infection. Therefore defects in the immune system in most immunocompromised patients cannot be thought of as a single deficit of the immune system.

The specific deficit in the immune system determines the likely infective organisms and therefore the appropriate antimicrobial therapy. The most severely compromised patients are those receiving bone marrow transplantation and children with SCIDS. By far the largest group of immunosuppressed patients are those receiving antineoplastic agents for malignancy. Once neutropenia develops, these patients are highly susceptible to infection. If a fever develops in these patients, it is a medical emergency because they may die within 48 to 72 hr if the appropriate antibiotics are not initiated immediately.

TREATMENT OF NEUTROPENIC PATIENTS

Over the past 20 years, great strides have been made in the treatment of infections in neutropenic patients. Even though the initial morbidity and mortality from infection have diminished substantially, infection is still the leading cause of death in cancer patients (Table 73.1) (4). The reasons for this are not completely clear, but with improvement in antibiotic therapy, the treatment of cancer has been refined, and chemotherapeutic regimens are becoming much more aggressive. Therefore, more patients are developing neutropenia for a longer period of time. As stated previously, the longer patients are granulocytopenic, the greater are their chances of developing a fatal infection. Investigators have also shown that the more advanced the cancer, the greater the chance the patient will

Table 73.1.
Causes of Death in Neutropenic Patients

Complication	Percentage of Patients with Findings
Infection	35
Hemorrhage	27
Progression of cancer	18
Miscellaneous	20
Renal insufficiency	
Myocardial infarction	
Carcinoma meningitis	
Acute pulmonary edema	

Table 73.2.
Outcome of Infection in the Febrile Neutropenic Patient

Evidence of Infection	Percentage of Patients with Findings
Documented infection	60
Microbiologically documented infection with bacteremia	20
Microbiologically documented infection without bacteremia	20
Clinically documented infection	20
Fever of undetermined origin	20
Fever of noninfectious origin (e.g., blood product, medication)	20

die of an infection (4). Fungal organisms are becoming increasingly implicated as the cause of infections and death in the neutropenic patient. In one study up to 58% of the cancer patients autopsied had pathologic signs of an invasive fungal infection (5). Fungal infections are often more difficult to eradicate than bacterial infections.

BACTERIAL INFECTIONS

Diagnosing an infection in a granulocytopenic patient can be difficult because the classical signs of infection (e.g., redness, swelling, tenderness, heat) are absent due to the lack of granulocytes. Often the only sign of infection is fever. The situation is further complicated by the administration of blood products and medications that can precipitate fever in neutropenic patients. This frequently means that antibiotics are initiated without any documented evidence of infection. In actuality, infection is only documented in approximately 60% of the neutropenic patients presenting with fever (Table 73.2) (1). In 80% of the infections documented by culture, the infecting organism is either a Gram-negative or Gram-positive bacterium. The common organisms infecting granulocytopenic patients include *Pseudomonas aeruginosa*, *Escherichia coli*, *Klebsiella pneumoniae*, *Staphylococcus aureus*, and *Staphylococcus epidermidis*. The other 20% of positive cultures can be fungal, viral, or protozoal. Twenty years ago, before the release of methicillin, most infecting bacterial organisms were Gram-positive. Subsequently, Gram-negative organisms became the primary cause of infection in neutropenic patients. In general, the pattern appears to be changing again, and infection by *P. aeruginosa* is dropping and infection by Gram-positive organisms is increasing (3). *S. epidermidis* is becoming a major pathogen because of central venous catheters (e.g., Hickman catheters) used in cancer patients (6, 7). The increased incidence of infection by *S. epidermidis* is important because this organism is often resistant to methicillin. The main point is that the primary group of organisms causing infections in this patient population is always changing. It is therefore extremely important for

Table 73.3.
Source of Infection in a Neutropenic Patient

Oral cavity
Trachea, bronchus, or lungs
Intestine and esophagus
Nose and sinuses
Intravenous catheter sites

pharmacists to know the primary pathogens in the neutropenic population at their institutions (7, 8).

The sources for infection in neutropenic patients are primarily the gastrointestinal tract (i.e., normal flora from the mouth and alimentary canal) and the respiratory tract (Table 73.3). Pizzo and Schimpff (9) demonstrated that 80% of infections arise from organisms that colonize the patient. However 50% of these organisms were acquired in the hospital, and therefore, they may be resistant to a number of different antibiotics. It would appear from the above data that surveillance cultures (cultures employed to monitor colonization) would supply beneficial information on appropriate antibiotic treatment. However, one investigation has shown that routine surveillance cultures are not cost-effective (10). Surveillance cultures are of limited value because (*a*) no one site of colonization is consistently predictive for the offending pathogen, (*b*) other potential pathogens are usually cultured at the same time, (*c*) useful cultures are usually obtained after initiation of antibiotics, and (*d*) the current practice of using broad-spectrum combinations (5) covers the vast majority of potential pathogens in the neutropenic host (10). Therefore, surveillance cultures should not be used to monitor colonization of patients.

Antibacterial Therapy

When granulocytopenic patients develop a fever, a careful physical examination should be performed to locate any possible source of infection. The patient's medication and transfusion records should be checked to insure that the fever is not related to either of these potential causes. If antibiotic therapy is instituted, the patient must be cultured extensively. Culture specimens should be obtained from sputum, urine, throat, and blood. A duplicate set of blood cultures should be obtained if a patient has a central venous catheter (i.e., one set from the central venous catheter and one set from a peripheral venipuncture). Any area that appears to be infected, such as a venipuncture site or bone marrow aspiration site, should also be cultured. After the appropriate cultures have been collected, antibiotic therapy should be initiated immediately to prevent early mortality from infection. Antibiotic therapy will be empiric and designed to cover the most common pathogens seen

at the institution. Antibiotic therapy in the febrile neutropenic patient has traditionally used combination therapy with either two or three drug regimens. However with the introduction of the new broad-spectrum third-generation cephalosporins (e.g., cefoperazone and ceftazidime) and the carbapenems (imipenem/cilastatin), investigators are again beginning to study possible use of single-agent therapy. In selecting empiric therapy three principles should always be followed. First, the antibiotic or antibiotics must be administered in the maximum prescribed dose. Next, broad-spectrum therapy should be selected whether the clinician decides to administer single or combination therapy. Finally the antibiotic(s) chosen must take into account the resistance patterns of the institution (6).

Many antibiotic combinations have been investigated in the treatment of infections in the neutropenic patient. Antibiotic combinations fall into four categories:

1. Antipseudomonal β-lactam plus an aminoglycoside;
2. Semisynthetic penicillin plus a third-generation cephalosporin (double β-lactam);
3. Third-generation antipseudomonal cephalosporin or carbapenem (monotherapy);
4. Vancomycin added to any of the above regimens.

The selection of antibiotic combination therapy should take into account the three principles mentioned above, as well as other factors, including presence and rapidity of bactericidal activity, efficacy in the neutropenic patient, pharmacokinetics of the antibiotics, potential for synergy between the antibiotics, and toxic effects (6) Table 73.4 lists a number of studies investigating the treatment of infections in the granulocytopenic patient. In general, early morbidity and mortality are seen from Gram-negative

Table 73.4.
Antibiotic Combinations Studied in the Neutropenic Patient

Drugs	Overall Responses (%)	Reference
Semisynthetic penicillins and aminoglycosides		
Carbenicillin-gentamicin	83	(11)
Ticarcillin-amikacin	80	(12)
Ticarcillin-gentamicin	97	(13)
Third-generation cephalosporin-aminoglycoside		
Moxalactam-amikacin	83	(12)
Ceftazidime-tobramycin	71	(14)
Cefoperazone-amikacin	88	(15)
Semisynthetic penicillins and third-generation cephalosporins		
Piperacillin-moxalactam	77	(16)
Ticarcillin-moxalactam	65	(17)
Miscellaneous combinations		
Piperacillin-vancomycin	72	(18)
Cotrimoxazole-ticarcillin	77	(19)

organisms and not Gram-positive organisms, therefore, most regimens initially cover Gram-negative bacteria (8). When reviewing the literature, it becomes obvious that most antibiotic studies demonstrate a 65 to 97% overall response rate when appropriate antibiotic combinations are used. Therefore, Table 73.4 is not a list of the "ideal" combinations but a reference point for comparing antibiotic combinations.

When combination antibiotic regimens are used, the antibiotics included should be synergistic and the organism should be susceptible to at least two of the antibiotics for the patient to receive the maximum benefit from the combination regimen. Klastersky (20) demonstrated that if the two antibiotics used in a regimen showed synergy to the organism cultured from a neutropenic patient, the cure rate of the infection was 80%. If the antibiotics used were not synergistic, the cure rate was only 49%. The benefit of synergism is that the organism is usually killed by two different mechanisms (20). Studies have also shown that if antibiotic combinations are administered and the antibiotics used are both active against the cultured organism (but not necessarily synergistic), the response rate is better than that with regimens in which only one of the antibiotics is active (21, 22).

Bactericidal activity of the antibiotics is also important. Bactericidal activity can be measured by drawing peak serum samples of the antibiotics administered and performing serial dilutions of the serum, which is then cultured with the infecting organism from the patient. A peak bactericidal serum titer of 1:16 or greater correlated with a favorable clinical response in 87% of the infected neutropenic patients (22). Trough bacterial serum titers provided no additional information.

Some investigators have challenged the need for an aminoglycoside as part of the combination regimen. In one study, addition of an aminoglycoside to an antipseudomonal penicillin had no advantage over the antipseudomonal penicillin alone (23). It is also important to note that aminoglycosides have been found to be less effective in neutropenic patients (24). Finally, if aminoglycosides are used in an antibacterial regimen, peak and trough levels of the aminoglycoside should be monitored regularly. Concentrations of gentamicin or tobramycin that should be attained in this patient population are between 6 to 8 μg/ml for the peak level and between 1 to 2 μg/ml for the trough level (25).

With the introduction of the third-generation cephalosporins, renewed interest developed for monotherapy (single-agent therapy) in the treatment of infections in neutropenic patients. Good results have been obtained in trials with monotherapy. The third-generation cephalosporins provide broad coverage against Gram-negative bacteria, attain high bactericidal concentrations in the serum, and many have long plasma half-lives. The benefits

Table 73.5.
Single-Agent Antibiotic Therapy Studies in Neutropenic Patients

Drug	Average Dose	Overall Response (%)	Reference
Ceftazidime	2 g q. 8 hr	95	(25)
Ceftazidime	2 g q. 8 hr	60	(14)
Cefoperazone	6 g q. 12 hr	77	(15)
Moxalactam	1.5 g q. 8 hr	80	(75)
Imipenem/cilastatin	500 mg q. 6 hr	74	(76)

of single-agent therapy in the neutropenic patient include: avoiding nephrotoxicity because aminoglycosides are not being used, giving patients less intravenous fluid, and less costly therapy than the traditional combination therapy. However, single-agent therapy does have some drawbacks. With single-agent therapy, the infecting organism must be covered by the antibiotic being used. If not, the patient has no antibiotic coverage. Second, the beneficial effects of synergism cannot be utilized. Finally, the third-generation cephalosporins have gaps in their coverage (i.e., Gram-positive organisms). Table 73.5 lists some of the studies that have investigated single-agent therapy. In all of these studies, the investigators recommended either close monitoring of the patient for treatment failures or the addition of a second agent initially for Gram-positive coverage. Therefore, at the present time, single-agent therapy is not recommended without close observation of the patient. These regimens may require early modification. It is recommended that monotherapy be limited to patients with ANC of 0.5 to 1 $\times$ 10^9/liter (500 to 1000/mm^3) experiencing short periods of neutropenia (26).

Antifungal Therapy

The incidence of fungal infection increases dramatically in patients with prolonged granulocytopenia (1, 36). The most common infecting fungus is *Candida albicans*, however, *Aspergillus*, *Torulopsis*, and *Cryptococcus* species can also be seen. Although prolonged granulocytopenia is the major risk factor for the development of fungal infection, broad-spectrum antibiotic and corticosteroid therapy can influence the development of fungal infection. One of the major problems in the treatment of fungal infections is diagnosis of the disease. Fungi can be cultured from a number of different sites and fluids from the body, including nares, throat, sputum, and stool. Often, culturing fungi from these sites or fluids represents only colonization. A true diagnosis of fungal infection can be made only when the culture is obtained from a sterile site or by histology (37). In addition, no good serologic tests for the diagnosis of fungal infections currently exist (37). The lack of good diagnostic tests would not be important if there were an effective and safe antifungal agent available. This, unfortunately, is not the case. The most efficacious antifungal agent available is amphotericin B. However, the possibility of severe side effects makes many clinicians somewhat reluctant to use amphotericin B as empiric therapy.

Amphotericin B has excellent activity against *C. albicans* but limited efficacy against *Aspergillus* and *Cryptococcus*. The dose of amphotericin is 0.5 to 1.0 mg per kilogram of body weight per day. The manufacturer of amphotericin B recommends that a test dose of 1 mg be administered and followed by slow titration up to the calculated maintenance dose, to limit adverse reactions. However, in neutropenic patients with a documented fungal infection the dose should be escalated rapidly to the maintenance dose. If febrile neutropenic patients do not respond to antibacterial agents within 4 to 7 days and no evidence of bacterial infection is documented, amphotericin B therapy should be initiated (37). Early initiation of amphotericin B may decrease the risk of invasive fungal disease (8). The duration of amphotericin B therapy depends on whether a positive diagnosis of a fungal infection has been made. The patient with a verified fungal infection should receive a total of 2 to 3 g of amphotericin B. If no positive diagnosis of a fungal infection has been made, the drug may be stopped when the total neutrophil count is above 0.5×10^9/liter (500 cells per mm^3) (37).

Amphotericin B side effects can fall into two categories—immediate and dose-related. Immediate side effects include fever, chills, and rigors. Patients receiving amphotericin B can be pretreated with acetaminophen, diphenhydramine, and hydrocortisone in an attempt to eliminate the immediate symptoms. Often pretreatment is not effective, and the patient must endure the side effects. Long-term adverse effects from amphotericin B include renal toxicity and bone marrow suppression. Patients who develop renal toxicity due to amphotericin B lose large amounts of potassium and magnesium. If renal failure does develop, it is usually reversible once the drug has been discontinued.

Ketoconazole is an oral antifungal agent with good activity against *C. albicans* (38). An imidazole derivative, ketoconazole is only effective against fungal organisms in a growth phase. Ketoconazole is only indicated for superficial *Candida* infection and should never be prescribed when an invasive process is suspected or diagnosed. Side effects include adrenal suppression and hepatotoxicity. The usual dose of ketoconazole is 200 to 400 mg every day. Ketoconazole requires an acid environment for absorption.

Fluconazole is the first of a new class of broad-spectrum bis-triazole antifungal agents. The fungistatic activity of fluconazole inhibits fungal P-450 sterol C-14 α-demeth-ylation resulting in an accumulation of 14α-methyl sterols in the fungi. Fluconazole is currently approved for use in oropharyngeal candidiasis, systemic candidal infections, and cryptococcal meningitis. Its role in the treatment of neutropenic patients remains to be defined. However because of its lack of toxicity, compared with amphotericin B, it is promising. The usual dose for systemic candidiasis is 400 mg the first day, followed by 200 mg every day for 4 weeks. For esophageal candidiasis, the dose is 200 mg the first day followed by 100 mg every day for 2 weeks. Because fluconazole is eliminated by the kidneys, doses must be adjusted in renal insufficiency. The use of fluconazole in cryptococcal meningitis is discussed in the chapter on AIDS.

Aspergillus rarely causes infection in the immunocompetent patient. In an immunosuppressed patient, the organism is pathogenic and can cause systemic infection. Patients acquire the organism by inhalation of *Aspergillus* spores dispersed in the air. Since *Aspergillus* is normally present in the soil, the air may be seeded with fungal spores in areas near excavation or construction. The infection occurs primarily in two sites of the body: the sinuses and the lungs. The risk factors for infection include prolonged granulocytopenia and acute or chronic graft versus host disease. Aspergillosis actually is a rare disease, and it is extremely difficult to treat (29). Treatment of the infection must be extremely aggressive, with resection of the infected area if possible, followed by amphotericin B. Frequently *Aspergillus* is only moderately sensitive to amphotericin B, therefore, drugs like rifampin or flucytosine can be added to possibly increase the response to amphotericin B (39). There have been no in vivo studies demonstrating a benefit from the addition of these medications (39).

Antiviral Therapy

Viral infections can be seen in patients with acute leukemia rendered neutropenic by aggressive chemotherapy, but the infections occur more frequently in organ transplant patients (e.g., kidney, heart, liver, and bone marrow). Patients receiving organ transplants may be severely immunosuppressed to prevent rejection of the transplanted organ. Viruses are responsible for up to 33% of deaths in the transplant population (40). The mortality from viral infection (particularly from cytomegalovirus infection (CMV)) is extremely high in bone marrow transplant patients (41). Viral infection can be either a primary infection in which the host was infected for the first time or a reactivated infection where the virus has been harbored in a nerve (herpes) or in a WBC (CMV). The main goal of treatment of viral infections is to prevent the spread of the virus systemically (i.e., to the brain, lungs, gastrointestinal tract, etc.). At no time during immunosuppression should a patient received live or attenuated viral vaccines, since such vaccines may result in viral infection in these patients.

Herpesvirus infections can be caused by either type I or type II viruses. In the immunocompromised host, approximately 85% of the infections affect the oral cavity, with the other 15% involving the genital area (41). An oral herpes infection is usually diffuse and can be extremely painful, preventing the patient from taking in adequate oral nutrition. The herpetic lesion can serve as a focus for bacterial infections (42). Herpes infections frequently occur within the first 17 days after the initiation of chemotherapy in bone marrow transplant patients (40).

Today the treatment of choice for herpesvirus infections is acyclovir (40, 42). Acyclovir has significantly reduced herpes infections as the cause of death in bone marrow transplant patients (41). Acyclovir is a prodrug that is metabolized by viral thymidine kinase. The metabolized drug is a potent inhibitor of herpes simplex and varicella zoster DNA polymerases. Acyclovir has been shown to be highly effective in the treatment of herpes in a number of different studies (42, 44). The dose used in the treatment of herpes simplex is 5 mg per kilogram of body weight every 8 hr (or 250 mg per m^2 every 8 hr). Acyclovir has few side effects. The alkaline nature of the drug can cause a thrombophlebitis in peripheral veins. Good urine output should be maintained to prevent crystallization of the drug in the renal tubules. The dose of acyclovir should be adjusted in renal failure. Topical acyclovir alone should not be prescribed in widespread disease because of an increased risk of disseminated viral disease (40).

Varicella-zoster, a communicable virus, causes chickenpox in childhood as a primary disease. In immunosuppressed patients the virus is reactivated and initially occurs along a dermatomal pattern. Disseminated varicella can cause pneumonia, encephalitis, hepatitis, and pancreatitis. In an investigation of children receiving chemotherapy for malignancies who subsequently developed a varicella infection, 32% progressed to disseminated disease and 7% died of the infection (42). The greatest risk of developing disseminated varicella occurred in patients whose total granulocyte count was below 0.5×10^9/liter (500 cells/mm^3). Children with malignancies, immunosuppressed patients, and bone marrow transplantation patients who are exposed to a child with chickenpox should receive passive immunization with zoster immune globulin (ZIG). The dose of ZIG is based on the patient's body weight and the titer to varicella in the serum. Varicella zoster can be treated with either vidarabine or acyclovir. Vidarabine has been shown to be effective in the treatment of zoster if it is initiated within 72 hr of the onset of symptoms (45). The dose of vidarabine is 10 mg per kilogram of body weight a day given over 12 hr. However, the side effects of vidarabine, such as gastrointestinal distress, megaloblastic anemia, hallucinations, and seizures, have limited

its clinical usefulness. The treatment of choice for varicella zoster is acyclovir; it has demonstrated efficacy in the treatment of zoster (46, 47). The best results are seen when the drug is administered early in the course of the disease (47). The dose of acyclovir in the treatment of a varicella infection is higher than in a herpetic infection (10 mg per kilogram of body weight every 8 hr, 500 mg/m^2 every 8 hr).

Cytomegalovirus is an opportunistic virus that causes few symptoms in an immunocompetent patient (42) but becomes a serious pathogen in immunosuppressed patients. CMV in the bone marrow transplant population is responsible for 15 to 20% of all deaths. Infection from CMV can cause pneumonia, retinitis, hepatitis, and bone marrow suppression (42). The disease can be primary or can be caused by reactivation of the virus. The infection also can be transmitted by a blood transfusion that has CMV harbored in WBCs (40, 42, 48). Infection in the lungs is usually the most severe form. Patients with CMV pneumonia present with fever, dyspnea, and a nonproductive cough. On chest x-ray the infection appears as an interstitial pneumonia with bilateral infiltrates. Respiratory function deteriorates rapidly, and the patients die of respiratory failure.

Presently there is no proven-effective treatment for CMV pneumonitis. A number of antiviral medications have been tried to treat the disease including vidarabine, acyclovir, and interferon, but none of these drugs have demonstrated efficacy in controlling the infection (42, 49). Studies with ganciclovir (DHPG) have been conducted in bone marrow transplant patients with documented CMV pneumonia (50). Despite good in vitro activity against CMV, ganciclovir did not change the outcome of the disease. Ganciclovir when used in combination with immunoglobulin has been reported to increase survival (51). Ganciclovir may be useful in the treatment of pneumonia in less immunocompromised patients (i.e., AIDS and renal transplant patients) (52) and in patients who have CMV infections in organs other than the lung (e.g., liver, GI tract).

The Epstein-Barr virus has been associated with pneumonia and leukopenia in the immunosuppressed patient population. Lymphoma development has also been correlated with the Epstein-Barr virus in bone marrow transplant patients receiving bone marrow that has been T cell–depleted by monoclonal antibodies (41). High-dose acyclovir and α-interferon have been used to treat the infection (42).

Prophylaxis in Neutropenic Patients

Prophylactic antibiotics and procedures have been beneficial in certain neutropenic patient populations. Theoretically the number of infections in all neutropenic patients could be reduced, because 80% of the documented infections arise from bacterial and fungal flora (9). Therefore, if organisms colonizing a patient are decreased or completely eliminated, the infection rate in these patients could be reduced. If a prophylactic regimen were effective, morbidity and mortality would also be reduced. In addition, complications from systemic antibiotics would be decreased because patients would not require antibiotics as often. Techniques that can be used to decrease the rate of infection include (*a*) bolstering the host defense mechanisms, (*b*) reducing damage to natural body barriers, (*c*) reducing the acquisition of new organisms from the environment, and (*d*) suppressing the potential pathogenic organisms currently colonizing the patient (9). The benefits of these techniques, however, have only been shown in patients with prolonged neutropenia.

The first three techniques are measures used in the general care of the patient. Procedures to enhance host defenses include proper nutrition, use of immunostimulants, and resolution of neutropenia as rapidly as possible. The most important aspect of bolstering the host defense is proper nutrition. A patient with good nutritional intake has an improved response to stress and infection.

Protection of natural barriers helps limit access of potential pathogens to the systemic circulation. Limiting the number of venipunctures and bone marrow aspirations will decrease the number of breaks in the skin. Invasive procedures such as urinary catheterization should be avoided to prevent colonization. Healthcare personnel and visitors should wash their hands thoroughly each time they enter a patient's room to help prevent the transfer of organisms from patient to patient. Attention to these general aspects of infection control can help reduce infectious complications in the neutropenic patient.

A technique that can decrease the rate of infection by more than 50% is protected-environment isolation (54). Protective isolation involves the use of laminar-airflow rooms and total microbial suppression. Laminar-airflow rooms use high-efficiency particulate air filters (e.g., Hepa filters) to remove bacteria, fungi, and spores from the air. It is combined with good housekeeping methods and food and beverages with low microbial content (cooked meats and no fresh fruits or vegetables) to decrease exposure to pathogens. Patients in protective isolation also receive total microbial suppression, which includes both antibacterial and antifungal prophylaxis. Topical antiinfective cleaners are applied to decontaminate the skin, and oral nonabsorbable antibiotics are given to clean the gut. Nonabsorbable antibiotics used include vancomycin (500 mg) and gentamicin (160 mg) given orally three to four times a day (55). Fungal prophylaxis is discussed later in the chapter.

The above regimen of protective-environment isolation does decrease the rate of infection in neutropenic patients, but it also has some major drawbacks. First is patient compliance; patients in this protected environment are not allowed to leave their rooms during the period of neutropenia (which can last 2 months or longer). These isolation techniques thus place a great deal of psychological stress on the patient and decrease compliance. The nonabsorbable antibiotic regimens that are used are not very palatable, and compliance after several weeks is poor. In addition, patients who stop taking the oral antibiotic can colonize with organisms that are resistant to many antibiotics, and they become infected with these resistant organisms (9). Finally, facilities for protective isolation are expensive, and many hospitals cannot afford these techniques.

An alternative method of microbial prophylaxis, called selective decontamination, involves the use of antimicrobial agents to selectively suppress Gram-negative organisms. Selective decontamination involves a concept of colonization resistance which states that anaerobic bacteria provide protection in the gastrointestinal tract from colonization with pathogenic bacteria, and if the anaerobic bacteria are killed off, colonization with pathogenic organisms will occur. Therefore, if antibacterial agents are given orally that suppress Gram-negative organisms, but leave anaerobic flora intact, colonization with more virulent organism should not be seen. The two antimicrobial agents that have been administered as selective decontaminants are cotrimoxazole and nalidixic acid. Cotrimoxazole has been studied the most for this effect. Results from the various studies have been somewhat contradictory. The dose of cotrimoxazole in studies investigating selective decontamination ranges from one single-strength tablet to one double-strength tablet orally 2 to 3 times a day. From the studies performed, cotrimoxazole appears to decrease the rate of infection in patients who are neutropenic for a prolonged period of time (more than 7 days) (32, 56–59). Patients with short-term neutropenia do not realize any benefits from cotrimoxazole prophylaxis (60). Cotrimoxazole has been compared with nalidixic acid in antibacterial prophylaxis (61). Both of the therapies were efficacious, but the investigator found disadvantages with both. Both the cotrimoxazole and the nalidixic acid group produced resistant organisms that colonized the gastrointestinal tract and could have led to suprainfection. The primary disadvantage of cotrimoxazole is the possible inhibition of WBC production, which in turn could prolong the neutropenia. In several studies the period of neutropenia was longer than that of the control group (35). Ciprofloxacin has been shown to be an effective alternative to cotrimoxazole (62). However, increased fungal overgrowth is a concern (63). In summary, it appears that both total microbial decontamination and selective decontamination are effective in decreasing the incidence of infections when used appropriately, but they should only be administered to patients who are expected to have a prolonged neutropenic episode (9, 26, 54, 64).

Antifungal Prophylaxis

Antifungal agents are administered prophylactically to decrease the incidence of superficial fungal infections and fungal colonization caused by *Candida albicans*. The agents used include nystatin suspension (15 ml orally four times a day), clotrimazole troches (10 mg orally five times a day), and ketoconazole (200 to 400 mg orally once a day). One of these medications is usually combined with an antibacterial prophylactic regimen to give broad-spectrum coverage of both fungal and bacterial organisms. All of these drugs are efficacious in the treatment of superficial fungal infection and suppression of *Candida* in the GI tract, but both nystatin suspension and clotrimazole troches can cause nausea and vomiting. Ketoconazole may be more effective than nystatin, but in a comparison study there was an increase in colonization by *Torulopsis* (64). Therefore, the selection of an antifungal prophylactic agent should be made according to the patient's preference.

Antiviral Prophylaxis

Antiviral prophylaxis is aimed primarily at the herpes simplex virus and CMV. In both cases antiviral prophylaxis should only be administered to patients who are going to be severely immunosuppressed (i.e., acute leukemic patients undergoing induction therapy and bone marrow transplant patients). The prophylactic antiviral of choice for herpes simplex virus is acyclovir (65, 66). Acyclovir is given at the same dose used for treatment, 5 mk/kg every 8 hr. The use of prophylactic medication in the prevention of CMV infection is very controversial. In several studies, large doses of intravenous immunoglobulins have been administered to bone marrow transplant patients to prevent CMV pneumonitis (67, 68). The intravenous immunoglobulins were primarily prepared by the investigator laboratory by pooling CMV-positive plasma with extremely high titers to CMV (67). The result showed a decreased incidence of CMV pneumonia. Only one commercially available product has been investigated at this time (Gamimune; Cutter Laboratory), and the study showed a decrease in severity of the CMV pneumonia but no decrease in the occurrence rate of CMV pneumonia (62). There is the additional problem of the cost for the therapy. The dose administered in the Winston study was 1000 mg per kilogram of body weight every week for 100 days. The cost for a single dose of Gamimune at this dosing schedule is over $2000. Therefore, administration of this medication is limited to high-risk populations (e.g., bone marrow transplant patients).

Prophylaxis against *Pneumocystis carinii*

Pneumocystis carinii is a protozoan that can cause opportunistic infections in immunosuppressed patients. Infected patients develop pneumonia and respiratory failure. Studies have demonstrated that one double-strength cotrimoxazole tablet twice a day twice weekly can prevent development of this infection in severely suppressed patients.

Role of Colony-stimulating Factors in Neutropenia

The introduction of the colony-stimulating factors, granulocyte-macrophage colony-stimulating factor (GM-CSF) and granulocyte colony-stimulating factor (G-CSF), may have significant impact on the course of neutropenia, although the roles of these agents in the treatment of chemotherapy-induced neutropenia and BMT still remain to be clearly defined. Early clinical trials with these agents show promise.

The colony-stimulating factors exert their effect by causing leukocyte precursors to multiply and mature at a faster rate. Specifically, GM-CSF produces an increase in granulocytes, monocytes, and eosinophils. G-CSF affects the precursors of the neutrophil linage. In addition, administration of these agents may cause the release of other stimulating factors that may directly or indirectly affect other cell lines, such as erythrocytes and platelets. GM-CSF has caused an inhibition of neutrophil migration. It is unclear what clinical importance this has on the effectiveness of this agent. G-CSF does not appear to produce this effect.

The use of GM-CSF has been studied in graft failure in BMT patients (53). In a dose-escalation trial in allogenic and autologous transplant patients, GM-CSF was administered in doses of 60 to 100 $\mu g/m^2$/day to patients who failed to achieve an ANC of 0.100×10^9/liter (100/mm³) by day 28 posttransplant or day 21 posttransplant in patients with life-threatening infections. Nine of the 15 allogenic and 11 of the 21 autologous patients responded to treatment. Treatment failures were associated with marrow cellularity under 5% in the allogenic group. In the autologous group, none of the patients who received purged marrow responded. It is important to note that no patient with myelogenous leukemia relapsed and there was no increase in the incidence of graft versus host disease, which has been theorized.

GM-CSF has also been studied in patients with myelodysplastic syndromes and aplastic anemia. In one study, GM-CSF was administered to eight patients with myelodysplastic syndrome. Increases were seen in granulocytes, eosinophils, and monocytes. No increase was seen in leukemic blast during treatment or leukemic acceleration. In a clinical trial studying the use of G-CSF postchemotherapy, G-CSF in doses of 10 to 30 $\mu g/kg$/day during the first cycle of chemotherapy resulted in fewer days of neutropenia, fewer days on antibiotics, and a lower incidence of and less severe mucositis, compared with the control, cycle two. It was also noted that 100% of the patients were eligible to receive their scheduled day of chemotherapy while receiving G-CSF, compared with 40% of those not receiving G-CSF.

Side effects associated with the use of these agents in patients undergoing BMT or being treated for chemotherapy-induced neutropenia included bone and muscle pain and headache and chest discomfort. The frequency of bone pain is proportional to the dose. Nonsteroidal antiinflammatory agents have been reported to relieve this effect. Other reported side effects are pericarditis, thrombophlebitis, elevated liver transaminase levels, and rash.

Monoclonal antibodies directed against Gram-negative endotoxin and cytokines that play a role in the systemic reactions in Gram-negative bacteremia have had promising results in reducing the mortality associated with sepsis (78, 79). In patients with Gram-negative sepsis, mortality was reduced from 57% to 33% in patients treated with Ha-A1, a human monoclonal antibody that binds to Gram-negative endotoxin (79). No improvement was seen in patients with non-Gram-negative-induced sepsis. In the neutropenic rat model, monoclonal antibody to tumor necrosis factor improved survival from 67% to 100% in animals injected with lethal doses of *Pseudomonas*. Although the early trials remain promising, the role of monoclonal antibodies in treatment of the neutropenic patient is unclear.

The efficacy and safety of administering granulocyte transfusions therapeutically and prophylactically in neutropenic patients has been investigated. Therapeutic granulocyte transfusions have demonstrated some benefit in neutropenic patients with documented infection (33). Studies looking at the potential benefits of administering granulocytes prophylactically have shown no advantage in the groups receiving transfusions (34, 35), and in one study the granulocyte group did slightly worse (35). Adverse reactions seen from the transfusions, such as pulmonary infiltrates, increased incidence of cytomegalovirus infections, and cross-matching problems, also limit the use of this therapy. Therefore, at the present time, granulocyte transfusion should only be administered to patients with documented infection that is not responding to appropriate antibiotic therapy (33).

DURATION OF THERAPY

The duration of antibiotic therapy in a neutropenic patient is a topic of debate in the literature. If a patient's neutropenia and fever resolve during treatment with antibiotic(s), the antibiotic(s) can be discontinued 7 days after the febrile episode. The controversy involves patients who are still neutropenic 7 days after defervescing. A study performed by Pizzo et al. (27) investigated the duration of antibiotic therapy in this patient population. Neutropenic patients were randomized either to continue antibiotics after being afebrile for 7 days or to have their antibiotics discontinued. The patients in the group that continued to

receive antibiotic therapy developed no further infectious complications. However, in the group in which antibiotics were discontinued, 41% of the patients were restarted on antibiotics within 2 days because of recurrence of fever and/or clinical signs of infection. No suprainfections occurred in the group that continued to receive antibiotics. Some clinicians still feel that antibiotics should be discontinued after the patient has been afebrile for several days because of the possibility of suprainfection (6). Factors that must be considered in the decision to stop antibiotics in a still-neutropenic patient are the degree of neutropenia, existing sources of infection (mucositis), and the stability of the patient (26).

Patients whose fever persists for more than 3 days should be reevaluated (26). Possible considerations include resistance to current regimens, inadequate doses of antibiotics, and nonbacterial causes (26). Evidence of progressive disease suggests the need to reassess the current antibiotic regimen; if vancomycin was not a part of the initial regimen, it should be added. Persistent fever after 1 week of therapy usually dictates the addition of antifungal therapy. Antifungal therapy should be continued for 2 weeks, and if no locus for a fungal infection is found, antifungal therapy may be stopped. Empiric use of antiviral therapy is usually only recommended if evidence of viral disease exists (26). Should fever persist despite the addition of amphotericin B, anaerobic coverage should be considered.

In patients with persistent fever and pulmonary infiltrates while on broad-spectrum antibiotics, other opportunistic infections must be considered (77). In addition to *Aspergillus*, pulmonary infiltrates may be caused by other fungi such as *Zygomycetes, Cryptococcus*, and *Histoplasma* (77). Other potential pathogens include mycobacteria, *Chlamydia, Nocardia, Legionella*, and *Pneumocystis*. Bronchoalveolar lavage may help delineate the causative organism, although open lung biopsy may be necessary. Table 73.6 contains a listing of pathogens in the immunecompromised patient and appropriate antibiotic therapy.

In culture-positive patients, antibiotic therapy may be targeted against the cultured organism. However, broad-spectrum coverage should be maintained because of the possibility of a mixed infection. Culture-positive patients should receive a 10- to 14-day course of appropriate antibiotic therapy.

MONITORING THERAPY

In monitoring a neutropenic patient, the clinician should focus first on the status of the patients neutropenia and establishing the identity of the infecting organism. The second task is monitoring the patient for drug side-effects and toxicities and making the appropriate adjustments in therapy.

Once the initial workup is complete and empiric ther-

Table 73.6.
Medications to Treat Infections in Immunosuppressed Patients[a]

Organism	Drug	Dosing Regimens
Mycobacterial infection		
Mycobacterium avium-intracellulare	Isoniazid	300 mg orally daily
	Rifampin	600 mg orally daily
	Ethambutol hydrochloride	25 mg/kg/day orally for 6 weeks then 15 mg/kg/day
	Streptomycin	0.75–2.0 g daily i.m. for 2 months then 2–3 times a week
	Capreomycin	1 g i.m. daily
	Ethionamide	500–1000 mg orally daily in 1–3 divided doses
	Cycloserine	750–1000 mg orally daily in 2–4 divided doses
	Pyridoxine hydrochloride	100 mg orally daily
	Pyrazinamide	25 mg/kg/day orally
Resistant *M. avium-intracellulare*	Ansamycin	150–300 mg orally daily
	Clofazimine	300 mg orally daily in 3 divided doses
	Cotrimoxazole (TMP-SMZ)	Oral: 20 mg/kg/day TMP + 100 mg/kg/day SMZ in 4 divided doses
		Intravenous: 15 mg/kg/day TMP + 75 mg/kg/day SMZ in 4 divided doses
	Pentamidine isoethionate	4 mg/kg/day i.m. or IV
Toxoplasma gondii	Sulfadiazine	1 g orally 4 times daily
	Pyrimethamine	25 mg orally daily
Giardia lamblia	Pyrimethamine	25 mg orally daily
	Quinacrine hydrochloride	100 mg orally 3 times daily
	Metronidazole	250–500 mg orally 3 times daily
Isospora belli	Cotrimoxazole	Trimethoprim 160 mg/sulfamethoxazole 800 mg orally, 4 times daily
Cryptosporidium muris	Spiramycin	1 g orally 3–4 times daily
Fungal infections		
Candida albicans		
Oral thrush	Nystatin	500,000 units swish in mouth 4–6 times daily
	Clotrimazole	10 mg troche 5 times daily
Esophagitis	Ketoconazole	400 mg orally daily
	Fluconazole	200 mg, 100 mg daily IV or p.o.
Transient fungemia	Amphotericin B	0.3 mg/kg/day IV
Disseminated disease with or without pneumonia	Amphotericin B	0.6 mg/kg/day IV
Cryptococcus neoformans		
Meningeal	Amphotericin B plus	0.3 mg/kg/day IV
	Flucytosine	150 mg/kg/day orally in 4 divided doses
	Fluconazole	400 mg, then 200 mg daily IV or p.o.
Nonmeningeal	Ketoconazole	400 mg orally daily
Histoplasm capsulatum	Amphotericin B	0.6 mg/kg/day IV
Petriellidium boydii	Miconazole	600 mg intravenously every 8 hr
Aspergillus	Amphotericin B or	0.6 mg/kg/day IV
	Amphotericin B plus	0.3 mg/kg/day IV
	Flucytosine	150 mg/kg/day orally in 4 divided doses
Coccidioides immitis	Amphotericin B	0.6 mg/kg/day IV
	Ketoconazole	400 mg orally daily (for the treatment failures)
Chlamydia pneumoniae	Tetracycline	500 mg q.i.d. for 10–14 days
Nocardia asteroides	Sulfonamides	1 g every 4 hours

[a] Adapted from Furio MM, Wordell CJ: Treatment of infectious complications of acquired immunodeficiency syndrome. Clin Pharm 4:539–554, 1985.

apy is started, the clinician should focus on identifying the causative organism and monitoring the status of the patient for signs of a worsening condition or sepsis. As stated earlier, granulocytopenic patients may not have typical symptoms of infection. The patient must be watched carefully for subtle signs of changes in status. Complaints of fatigue or changes in mood or mental status may be the only signals of a deteriorating condition. Vital signs must be monitored carefully for signs of sepsis, such as increased heart rate, increased respiratory rate, and decreased blood pressure. The neutropenia should be accessed daily by obtaining complete blood counts with differential. Attempts to identify the causative organism must be pursued rigorously. Daily blood cultures have been advocated.

Side effects from antibiotic therapy in the granulocytopenic patient relate to the antibiotic(s) chosen. Because these patients are on a number of different antibiotics that have additive side effects or interact with their disease, the clinician must pay close attention to certain side effects. Nephrotoxicity can be seen as a result of an aminoglycoside. Studies investigating the incidence of nephrotoxicity from aminoglycosides in these patients show ranges between 0 and 15% (28–30). The incidence of nephrotoxicity may be higher when aminoglycosides are combined with other nephrotoxic drugs such as cephalothin (30), amphotericin B, and vancomycin. Ototoxicity may also occur with aminoglycosides, and the incidence ranges from 6.2% to 17% (28, 31). Patients receiving semisynthetic penicillins often lose large amounts of potassium in the urine during therapy because of the potassium-wasting effect of the penicillin. Additional potassium and magnesium can be lost if the patient is receiving amphotericin B. Thus, serum potassium and magnesium levels should be monitored closely in patients prone to potassium wasting. Cotrimoxazole (generic name for sulfamethoxazole-trimethoprim combinations) to treat infection in neutropenic patients may inhibit granulopoiesis and increase the duration of granulocytopenia (32). Finally, combination antibiotic therapy along with the administration of amphotericin B and acyclovir can substantially increase the amount of fluid a patient is receiving. This increase in fluid is due to the additional diluent that is required to administer the drug intravenously. The result is volume overload and edema.

Prognosis

The prognosis for immunosuppressed patients without correction of their underlying disease or removal of the causative agent is poor. In most cases the patient remains immunocompromised and has recurrent bouts of infection.

CONCLUSION

The treatment of infections in the immunocompromised host is difficult and requires close monitoring of any signs or symptoms of infection. Patients must be treated aggressively and promptly to prevent morbidity and mortality from the infections. Gram-negative infections are still the most frequently encountered. However, the incidence of Gram-positive infections is on the rise once again. The importance of knowing the trends at the individual institution cannot be overemphasized. Initial treatment remains empiric. Monotherapy is increasing in popularity, but combination therapy still remains the standard of practice. In patients who remain febrile, the use of antifungal therapy is indicated. The use of colony-stimulating factors and monoclonal antibodies shows promise for the future. However their roles need to be further delineated. The guidelines expressed in this chapter are empiric; each patient must be treated on an individual basis.

REFERENCES

1. Schimpff SC: Overview of empiric antibiotic therapy for the febrile neutropenic patient. Rev Infect Dis 7:S734–S740, 1985.
2. Cone LA, Woodard D, Heim NA: Clinical experience in the diagnosis and treatment of infection in the compromised host. Clin Ther 4(suppl):45–53, 1981.
3. Pizzo PA: Granulocytopenia and cancer therapy. Cancer 54:2649–2661, 1984.
4. Schlier JP, Weerts D, Klastersky J: Causes of death in febrile granulocytopenic cancer patients receiving empiric antibiotic therapy. Eur J Cancer Clin Oncol 20:55–60, 1984.
5. Armstrong D, Young LS, Meyer JD, et al.: Infectious complications of neoplastic disease. Med Clin North Am 55:729–745, 1971.
6. Bodey GP: Antibiotics in patients with neutropenia. Arch Intern Med 144:1845–1851, 1984.
7. Wade JC, Schimpff SC, Newman KA, et al.: Staphylococcus epidermidis: an increasing cause of infection in patients with granulocytopenia. Ann Intern Med 97:503–508, 1982.
8. Klastersky J: Management of infection in granulocytopenic patients. J Antimicrob Chem Ther 12:102–104, 1983.
9. Pizzo PA, Schimpff SC: Strategies for the prevention of infection in the myelosuppressed or immunosuppressed cancer patients. Cancer Treat Rep 67:223–233, 1983.
10. Kramer BS, Pizzo PA, Robichaud KJ: Role of serial microbiologic surveillance and clinical evaluation in the management of cancer patients with fever and granulocytopenia. Am J Med 72:561–568, 1982.
11. Lau WK, Young LS, Black RE, et al.: Comparative efficacy and toxicity of amikacin/carbenicillin versus gentamicin/carbenicillin in leukopenic patients: a randomized prospective trial. Am J Med 62:959–966, 1977.
12. DeJongh CA, Wade JC, Schimpff SC, et al.: Empiric antibiotic therapy for suspected infection in granulocytopenic cancer patients. A comparison between the combination of moxalactam plus amikacin and ticarcillin plus amikacin. Am J Med 73:89–96, 1982.
13. Love LJ, Schimpff SC, Hahan DM, et al.: Randomized trial of empiric antibiotic therapy with ticarcillin in combination with gentamicin, amikacin or netilmicin in febrile patients with granulocytopenia and cancer. Am J Med 66:603–610, 1979.
14. Fainstein V, Bodey GP, Bolivar ER, et al.: A randomized study of ceftazidime compared to ceftazidime and tobramycin for the treatment of infection in cancer patients. J Antimicrob Chemother 12(suppl A):101–110, 1983.
15. Piccart M, Klastersky J, Lagast MH, et al.: Single-drug versus combination empirical therapy for Gram-negative bacillary infections in

febrile cancer patients with and without granulocytopenia. Antimicrob Agents and Chemother 26:870–875, 1984.

16. Wintson DJ, Baines RC, Ho WC, et al.: Moxalactam plus piperacillin versus moxalactam plus amkacin in febrile granulocytopenic patients. Am J Med 77:442–450, 1984.

17. Fainstein V, Bodey GP, Bolivar R, et al.: Moxalactam plus ticarcillin or tobramycin for treatment of febrile episodes in neutropenic cancer patients. Arch Intern Med 144:1766–1770, 1984.

18. Jade AL, Bolivar R, Fainstein V, et al.: Piperacillin plus vancomycin in the therapy of febrile episodes in cancer patients. Antimicro Agent Chemother 26:295–299, 1984.

19. Keating MJ, Lawson R, Grose W, et al.: Combination therapy with ticarcillin and sulfamethoxazole-trimethoprim for infection in patients with cancer. Arch Intern Med 141:926–930, 1981.

20. Klastersky J: Treatment of severe infections in patients with cancer. The role of new acyl-penicillins. Arch Intern Med 142:1984–1987, 1982.

21. Young LS: Use of aminoglycoside in immunocompromised patients. Am J Med 79(suppl A):21–27, 1985.

22. Sculier JP, Klastersky J: Significance of serum bactericidal activity in Gram negative bacillary bacteremia in patients with and without granulocytopenia. Am J Med 76:429–435, 1984.

23. Bodey GP, Fainstein V, Rolston K, Elting L: Empiric therapy for the granulocytopenic patient.

24. Bodey GP: Aminoglycoside use in the compromised host. In Whelton A Neu HC (eds): The Aminoglycosides. New York, Marcel Dekker, 1982, pp 557–583.

25. Pizzo PA, Hathorn JW, Hiemenz J, et al.: A randomized trial comparing ceftazidime alone or combination antibiotic therapy in cancer patients with fever and neutropenia. N Engl J Med 315:552–558, 1986.

26. Hughes WT, Armstrong D, Bodey GB, Feld R, et al.: Guidelines for the use of antimicrobial agents in neutropenic patients with unexplained fever. J Infect Dis 161:381–396, 1990.

27. Pizzo PA, Robichaud KJ, Gill FA, et al.: Duration of empiric antibiotic therapy in granulocytopenic patients with cancer. Am J Med 67:194–200, 1979.

28. Finley RS, Fortner CL, DeJongh CA, et al.: Comparison of standard versus pharmacokinetically adjusted amikacin dosing in granulocytic cancer patients. Antimicrob Agents Chemother 22:193–197, 1982.

29. Feld R, Rachlis A, Tuffnell PG, et al.: Empiric therapy for infections in patients with granulocytopenia. Continuous V interrupted infusion of tobramycin plus cefamandole. Arch Intern Med 144:1005–1010, 1984.

30. Wade JC, Schimpff SC, Wiernik PH: Antibiotic combination—associated nephrotoxicity in granulocytopenic patients with cancer. Arch Intern Med 141:1789–1793, 1981.

31. Bender JF, Fortner CL, Schimpff SC, et al.: Comparative auditory antibiotics in leukopenic patients. Am J Hosp Pharm 36:1083–1087, 1979.

32. Gualtieri RJ, Donowitz GR, Kaiser DL, et al.: Double-blind randomized study of prophylactic trimethoprim/sulfumethoxazole in granulocytopenic patients with hematologic malignancies. Am J Med 74:934–940, 1983.

33. Young LS: Prophylactic granulocytes in the neutropenic host. Ann Intern Med 96:240–241, 1982.

34. Winston DJ, Ho WG, Gale RP: Therapeutic granulocyte transfusion for documented infections. Ann Intern Med 97:509–519, 1982.

35. Strauss RG, Connett JE, Gale RP, et al.: A controlled trial of prophylactic granulocyte transfusions during initial induction chemotherapy for acute myelogenous leukemia. N Engl J Med 305:597–603.

36. Gerson SL, Talbot GH, Hurwitz S, et al.: Prolonged granulocytopenia: the major risk factor for invasive pulmonary aspergillosis in patient with acute leukemia. Ann Intern Med 100:345–351, 1984.

37. Cohen J: Empirical antifungal therapy in neutropenic patients. J Antimicrob Chemother 13:409–411, 1984.

38. Meunier-Carpentier F: Treatment of mycoses in cancer patients. Am J Med 74(suppl):74–78, 1983.

39. Schubert MM, Peterson DE, Meyers JD, et al.: Head and neck aspergillosis in patients undergoing bone marrow transplantation. Cancer 57:1092–1096, 1986.

40. Prentice HG, Hann IM: Antiviral therapy in the immunocompromised patient. Brit Med Bull 41:367–373, 1985.

41. Burns WH, Saral R: Opportunistic viral infections. Brit Med Bull 41:46–49, 1985.

42. Wong KK, Hirsch MS: Herpes virus infections in patients with neoplastic disease, diagnosis and therapy. Am J Med 76:464–478, 1984.

43. Straus SE, Smith HA, Brickman C, et al.: Acyclovir for chronic mucocutaneous herpes simplex virus infection in immunosuppressed patients. Ann Intern Med 96:270–277, 1982.

44. Wade JC, Newton B, McLaren C, et al.: Intravenous acyclovir to treat mucocutaneous herpes simplex virus infection after bone marrow transplantation. Ann Intern Med 96:265–269, 1982.

45. Whitley RJ, Soong SJ, Dolin R, et al.: Early vidarabine therapy to control the complications of herpes zoster in immunosuppressed patients. N Engl J Med 307:971–975, 1982.

46. Balfour HH, Bean B, Laskin OL, et al.: Acyclovir halts progression of herpes zoster in immunocompromised patients. N Engl J Med 308:1448–1453, 1983.

47. Balfour HH, McMonigal KA, Bean B: Acyclovir therapy of varicella-zoster virus infections in immunocompromised patients. J Antimicrob Chemother 12(suppl B):169–179, 1983.

48. Skinhj P, Anderson HK, Moller J, et al.: Cytomegalovirus infection after bone marrow transplantation: relation of pneumonia to postgrafting immunosuppressive treatment. J Med Virol 14:91–99, 1984.

49. Meyer JD, Wade JC, McGuffin RW, et al.: The use of acyclovir for cytomegalovirus infections in the immunocompromised host. J Antimicrob Chemother 12(suppl B):181–193, 1983.

50. Shepp DH, Dandliker PS, Miranda P, et al.: Activity of 9-[2-hydroxy-1-(hydroxymethyl)ethoxymethyl]guanine in the treatment of cytomegalovirus pneumonia. Ann Intern Med 103:368–373, 1985.

51. Emamual D, Cunningham I, Jules-Elysee K, et al.: Cytomegalovirus pneumonia after bone marrow transplantation successfully treated with the combination of ganciclovir and high dose intravenous immune globulin. Ann Intern Med 109:777–782, 1988.

52. Bach MC, Bagwell SP, Knapp NP, et al.: 9(1,3-dihydroxy-2-propoxymethyl)guanine for cytomegalovirus infection in patients with the acquired immunodeficiency syndrome. Ann Intern Med 103:381–382, 1985.

53. Nemunaitis J, Singer JW, Buckner D, Durnam D: Use of recombinant human granulocyte-macrophage colony-stimulating factor in graft failure after bone marrow transplantation. Blood 76(1):245–253, 1990.

54. Schimpff SC: Infection prevention during profound granulocytopenia. New approaches to alimentary canal microbial suppression. Ann Intern Med 93:358–361, 1980.

55. Malarme M, Meunier-Carpentier F, Klastersky J: Vancomycin plus gentamicin and cotrimoxazole for prevention of infections in neutropenic cancer patients (a comparative, placebo-controlled pilot study). Eur J Cancer Clin Oncol 17:1315–1322, 1981.

56. Kauffman CA, Liepman MK, Bergman AG: Trimethoprim/sulfamethoxazole prophylaxis in neutropenic patients. Am J Med 74:599–607, 1983.

57. Riben PD, Louie TJ, Lank BA, et al.: Reduction in mortality from Gram negative sepsis in neutropenic patients receiving trimethoprim/sulfamethoxazole therapy. Cancer 51:1587–1592, 1983.

58. Wade JC, Schimpff SC, Hargadon MT, et al.: A comparison of trimethoprim/sulfamethoxazole plus nystatin with gentamicin plus nys-

tatin in the prevention of infections in acute leukemia. N Engl J Med 304:1057–1062, 1981.

59. Martino P, Venditti M, Concetta M, et al.: Co-trimoxazole prophylaxis in patients with leukemia and prolonged granulocytopenia. Am J Med Sci 287:7–9, 1984.

60. Weiser B, Lange M, Fialk MA, et al.: Prophylactic trimethoprim-sulfamethoxazole during consolidation chemotherapy for acute leukemia: a controlled trial. Ann Intern Med 95:436–438, 1981.

61. Wade JC, deJongh CA, Newman KA, et al.: Selective antimicrobial modulation as prophylaxis against infection during granulocytopenia: trimethoprim-sulfamethoxazole vs. nalidixic acid. J Infect Dis 147:624–633, 1983.

62. Dekker A, Rozenberg-Arska M, Verhoef J: Infection prophylaxis in acute leukemia: a comparison of ciprofloxacin with trimethoprim-sulfamethoxazole and colistin. Ann Intern Med 106:7–12, 1987.

63. Denning D, Flulle HH, Hellriegel KP: Chemoprophylaxis of bacterial infection in granulocytopenic patients. Okolologie 19:57–58, 1987.

64. Shepp DH, Klosterman A, Siegel MS, et al.: Comparative trial of ketoconazole and nystatin for prevention of fungal infection in neutropenic patients treated in a protective environment. J Infect Dis 152:1257–1263, 1985.

65. Hann IM, Prentice HG, Blacklock HA, et al.: Acyclovir prophylaxis against herpes virus infections in severely immunocompromised patients: randomized double blind trial. Brit Med J 287:384–388, 1983.

66. Prentice HG: Use of acyclovir for prophylaxis of herpes infections in severely immunocompromised patients. J Antimicro Chemother 12(suppl B):153–159, 1983.

67. Condie RM, O'Reilly RJ: Prevention of cytomegalovirus pneumonia with high-dose intravenous, hyperimmune; native, unmodified cytomegalovirus globulin. Am J Med 76(suppl):134–141, 1984.

68. Winton DJ, Ho WG, Lin CH, et al.: Intravenous immunoglobulin for modification of cytomegalovirus infection associated with bone marrow transplantation. Am J Med 76(suppl):128–133, 1984.

69. Purdy BD, Plaisance KI: Infection with the human immunodeficiency virus: epidemiology, pathogenesis, transmission, diagnosis, and manifestations. Am J Hosp Pharm 46:1185–1209, 1989.

70. Furio MM, Wordell CJ: Treatment of infections complications of acquired immunodeficiency syndrome. Clin Pharm 4:539–554, 1985.

71. Armstrong D, Gold JW, Dryjanski J, et al.: Treatment of infections in patients with the acquired immunodeficiency syndrome. Ann Intern Med 103:738–743, 1985.

72. Gordin FM, Simon GL, Wafsy CB, et al.: Adverse reactions to trimethoprim-sulfamethoxazole in patients with the acquired immunodeficiency syndrome. Ann Intern Med 100:495–499, 1984.

73. Small CB, Harris CA, Friedland GH, et al.: The treatment of Pneumocystis carinii pneumonia in acquired immunodeficiency syndrome. Arch Intern Med 145:837–840, 1985.

74. Pinching AJ: The acquired immune deficiency syndrome with special reference to tuberculosis. Tubercle 68:65–69, 1987.

75. Stambaugh JE, McAdams J: The efficacy and safety of moxalactam in the treatment of acute bacterial infections in immunosuppressed patient with cancer. Curr Ther Res 31:864–871, 1982.

76. Mortimer J, Miller S, Black D, Kowk K, Kirby WM: Comparison of cefoperazone and mezlocillin with imipenem as empiric therapy in febrile neutropenic cancer patients. Am J Med 85(suppl):21–30, 1988.

77. Pizzo PA: Evaluation of fever in the patient with cancer. Eur J Cancer Clin Oncol 25(suppl):9–16, 1989.

78. Opal SM, Cross AS, Kelly NM, et al.: Efficacy of monoclonal antibody directed against tumor necrosis factor in protecting neutropenic rats form lethal infection with Pseudomonas areuginosa. J Infect Dis 161(6):1148–1152, 1990.

79. Ziegler EJ, Fisher CJ, Sprung CL, et al.: Treatment of Gram negative bactermia and septic shock with HA-1A human monoclonal antibody against endotoxin. N Engl J Med 324:429–436, 1991.

CHAPTER 74

BACTEREMIA AND SEPSIS

PEGGY L. CARVER, Pharm.D.

Bacteremia refers to the presence of bacteria in the bloodstream. *Sepsis* refers to the physiologic alterations and clinical consequences of the presence of bacteria or their toxic byproducts in the bloodstream or tissues (1–3). These toxic byproducts are thought to be endotoxins from Gram-negative bacteria or the peptidoglycan/teichoic acid complex found in Gram-positive organisms (4). It is important to recognize that sepsis can occur in the absence of positive blood cultures; a presumptive diagnosis of sepsis is often made on the basis of physical and laboratory data (4). *Sepsis syndrome* refers to sepsis with evidence of altered organ perfusion, which is expressed as tachycardia, altered temperature, and evidence of inadequate organ perfusion. Sepsis can progress to *septic shock*, defined as the sepsis syndrome with hypotension (systolic blood pressure <90 mm Hg, or a decrease from baseline systolic blood pressure >40 mm Hg) despite the use of appropriate antimicrobial therapy and circulatory support. Septic shock results when peripheral circulatory failure with inadequate tissue perfusion is present (5).

Although endotoxin is found only in Gram-negative bacterial cell walls, virtually any bacteria can produce the clinical signs and symptoms characteristic of systemic sepsis (6). However, the association of severe infection with circulatory failure, hypotension, and decreased tissue perfusion is most frequently associated with Gram-negative bacteria. Gram-positive bacteria more frequently cause metastatic suppurative complications, because of their ability to adhere to endothelial cells and matrix substances such as heart valves, bones, joints, and viscera. This chapter focuses primarily on Gram-negative sepsis and septic shock.

EPIDEMIOLOGY OF GRAM-NEGATIVE SEPSIS

Osler noted in 1892 that the "organisms of suppuration" were responsible for the clinical picture of septicemia. As early as 1971, animal studies demonstrated that bacteria do not need to be viable in order to produce hypotension when injected intravenously. Later studies reported that a "tumor-necrotizing polysaccharide" derived from *Serratia marcescens* produced severe and prolonged hypotension in animals. In the late 1940s, the hypotensive properties of pyrogens were exploited in the treatment of malignant hypertension (1, 7).

Despite the widespread availability of potent, broad-spectrum antibiotics in recent years, the frequency of Gram-negative sepsis has risen almost exponentially since the introduction of penicillin and tetracycline in the early 1950s. While it is tempting to ascribe the recent surge in Gram-negative infections solely to the proliferation of antibiotics, a variety of additional factors have contributed to the dramatic increase. Advances in antimicrobial therapy were paralleled by advances in medical technology and surgical techniques, which have resulted in increased numbers of elderly patients, and those with cancer, renal failure, congestive heart failure, or diabetes mellitus (6). In addition, immunosuppression from disease or drug therapy, the use of invasive medical devices such as venous or urinary catheters, and mechanical ventilators have all contributed to an increased risk of Gram-negative sepsis (1, 7).

The morbidity and mortality associated with sepsis and septic shock are high; approximately two-thirds of patients die, generally as a result of the progressive failure of one or more vital organs (8). The incidence of Gram-negative sepsis is difficult to determine precisely, but it appears to range from 70,000 to 500,000 cases/year, with mortality ranging from 5 to 20% in patients who do not develop shock. Among patients developing sepsis with concomitant shock, the mortality can be as high as 90% (1, 8, 9). In the United States, approximately 60,000 to 80,000 deaths per year are attributable to Gram-negative sepsis (3, 7). A recent study by Bone et al. (10) reported an overall mortality due to sepsis of 26%. Mortality was 13% in patients without shock, and 43% in those who developed shock after admission. Mortality in patients with bacteremia (27%) was not significantly different from that in those without (23%).

A variety of factors affect the outcome of Gram-negative sepsis (Table 74.1), including the severity of underlying disease(s) or the presence of neutropenia, diabetes, alcoholic cirrhosis, renal or respiratory failure, or hypogammaglobulinemia. The complications of sepsis present at onset of therapy, the appropriateness of antimicrobial therapy, the interval before initiation of therapy, and patient age are also important factors influencing outcome (11).

ETIOLOGY OF SEPSIS

The major pathogens that cause Gram-negative sepsis include enteric bacteria such as *Escherichia coli*, *Klebsiella* spp., *Enterobacter* spp., and *Proteus* spp. and *Pseudo-*

Table 74.1.
Factors Affecting the Outcome of Gram-Negative Sepsis[a]

Severity of disease
Underlying disease(s)
   Neutropenia
   Diabetes
   Alcoholic cirrhosis
   Renal failure
   Respiratory failure
   Hypogammaglobulinemia
Complications of sepsis present at onset of therapy
Appropriateness of antimicrobial therapy
Polymicrobial bacteremia
Source of infection
Interval before initiation of therapy
Patient age

[a] Adapted from Young LS, Gram-negative sepsis. In Mandell GL, Douglas RB Jr, Bennett JE (eds): Principles and Practice of Infectious Diseases, ed. 3. New York, Churchill Livingstone, 1990, pp 611–636.

monas aeruginosa, which is a ubiquitous member of the flora of most hospitals (12, 13).

The gastrointestinal tract serves as the most obvious reservoir for Gram-negative bacteria, particularly *E. coli*, which constitutes the largest proportion of aerobic Gram-negative bacteria. "Normal" host flora such as enteric bacteria may extend beyond normal sites of colonization because of the administration of antimicrobial agents, the presence of neutropenia, the severity of illness, or the loss of natural protective barriers such as skin, cough reflex, and gastrointestinal tract mucosa (4, 12).

Although community-acquired Gram-negative bacteremia and sepsis usually arise from endogenous flora of the genital, urinary, or biliary tree, hospitalized patients may acquire the flora of the hospital setting. Unfortunately, the fecal flora of hospitalized patients or those who have previously received extensive courses of antimicrobial therapy frequently contains resistant strains of bacteria. Although the prevalence of *P. aeruginosa* in healthy subjects or in hospital personnel is usually <10%, fecal carriage is increased fivefold in debilitated patients and in those receiving broad-spectrum antimicrobial therapy. In 1976, the National Nosocomial Infections Surveillance survey organized by the Centers for Disease Control reported that between 49 and 56% of all bacteremias were caused by Enterobacteriaceae and *P. aeruginosa*. Gram-negative rod bacteremias outnumbered all other causes of bacteremia (15). *E. coli* remains the most common Gram-negative pathogen isolated from patients with sepsis and bacteremia, and *Klebsiella pneumoniae* the second most common. However, it is noteworthy that *P. aeruginosa* is consistently associated with the highest case fatality ratio of all bacteremic infections. This high mortality may result from its frequent association with patients with extensive burns and the neutropenic host. The 1984 survey confirmed the overall importance of Gram-negative but also reported the resurgence of Gram-positive bacteria as causes of bacteremia (16).

PATHOPHYSIOLOGY OF SEPTIC SHOCK

Knowledge of the components of the Gram-negative bacterial cell wall is important in understanding the pathogenesis and therapy of sepsis and septic shock. The three major components of the outer membrane of Gram-negative organisms are protein, lipid, and lipopolysaccharide (LPS). LPS, often referred to as endotoxin, is most often shed from dead bacteria but can also be shed from live bacteria. When released into the bloodstream or tissues of animals or humans, LPS acts as an antigen (1, 7, 17). LPS consists of three main regions (Fig. 74.1). The first region, known as the *O antigen*, is a long-chain polysaccharide with great antigenic diversity among different species of Gram-negative bacteria. The *core* region has less antigenic diversity. The third major region, *lipid A*, is very similar in aerobic and anaerobic Gram-negative bacilli. Lipid A is composed of a disaccharide and six long-chain fatty acids and is highly immunoreactive. Consequently, current immunotherapy for Gram-negative sepsis has focused on antibodies to lipid A, as its structure is common to all Gram-negative bacteria. Animal studies have demonstrated that LPS or any of its components can produce the clinical picture of sepsis; however, most of the effects are thought to be attributable to the lipid A moiety. Although LPS (endotoxin) initiates the cascade of biologic mediators known as cytokines, which ultimately result in the clinical syndrome of sepsis and septic shock, it has little or no direct effect on tissues. Minute quantities of LPS (a few micrograms per ml of blood) can trigger the septic cascade (18).

Endotoxin stimulates a complex cascade of physiological effects (Table 74.2 and Fig. 74.2), many of which are overlapping and even contradictory at times. However, LPS is not unique to Gram-negative organisms. The cell walls of certain Gram-positive bacteria contain an M protein that produces physiological effects similar to those seen following administration of endotoxin (7). Through activation of both the classical and alternative complement pathways, endotoxin causes the migration of neutrophils and other inflammatory cells into tissues, which are vital for phagocytosis and lysis of bacteria. However, neutrophils can in turn release toxic oxygen radicals and proteases, which can result in the destruction of tissues.

The release of endotoxin activates Hageman factor (factor XII), which in turn activates the intrinsic clotting cascade, resulting in the conversion of fibrinogen to fibrin, with subsequent clotting. Uncontrolled activation of coagulation results in thrombosis and consumption of platelets and clotting factors II, V, and VIII; this frequently results in the clinical end point of disseminated intravascular coagulation (DIC) (1, 7).

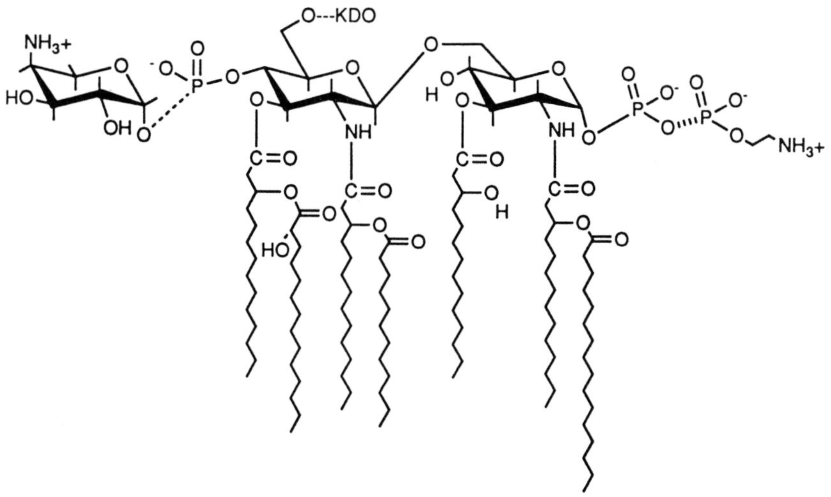

Figure 74.1. Structure of Lipopolysaccharide (Endotoxin). (Courtesy of R. Woodward, Ph.D., University of Michigan College of Pharmacy.)

Table 74.2.
Systemic Effects of Endotoxin[a]

Cardiovascular effects
  Vasoconstriction/vasodilation
  Increases vascular permeability
  Release of myocardial depressant factor
Stimulation of immune system
  Lymphocyte activation (via interleukin-1)
  Stimulation of B cells to produce antibodies
  Activation of macrophages
  Stimulates release of colony-stimulating factors
  Activation of complement factors (via the alternative pathway)
Effects on coagulation system
  Activation of tissue-plasminogen activator or plasminogen-activator inhibitors
  Activation of Hageman factor
Effects on organs
  Direct hepatotoxic effects
  Gastrointestinal disturbances
    Stress ulceration
    Enterocolitis

[a] Adapted from Young LS, Gram-negative sepsis. In Mandell GL, Douglas RB Jr, Bennett JE (eds): Principles and Practice of Infectious Diseases, ed. 3. New York, Churchill Livingstone, 1990, pp 611–636.

Endotoxin also stimulates the production of tumor-necrosis factor (TNF) or "cachectin" and interleukin-1 (IL-1) by macrophages and monocytes. TNF and IL-1 in turn stimulates inflammatory and other cells to secrete a cascade of secondary mediators, including prostaglandins, leukotrienes, interferons, platelet-activating factor, endorphins, and colony-stimulating factors. TNF and IL-1 are referred to as "endogenous pyrogens" because of their ability to produce fever (18–22).

TNF appears to be the major mediator of the clinical picture observed in Gram-negative sepsis. However, other infectious processes such as parasitic infections can result in the release of TNF. Thus, identification of TNF is not specific for Gram-negative infection. However, methods that block TNF suppress much of the process observed clinically in patients with sepsis. Supportive evidence for the role of TNF includes both animal and human data. In patients with meningococcemia, high levels of free TNF are associated with increased mortality. The administration of endotoxin to animals or human volunteers leads to release of TNF. Mice that are genetically unresponsive to endotoxin also lack the ability to produce TNF from their macrophages. Similarly, administration of purified, recombinant TNF to animals or human volunteers results in clinical findings that mimic those found in sepsis, and administration of antibodies directed against TNF increases survival (7, 18, 19, 21).

Through this complex and interwoven series of physiologic mediators, endotoxin ultimately produces alterations in virtually every organ system. Endotoxin causes the release of a myocardial-depressant factor, which leads to impaired ventricular function (23). Release of inflammatory mediators results in vasoconstriction, vasodilation, and leakage of vascular fluids and proteins into tissues. Bronchoconstriction can result from the endotoxin-stimulated release of inflammatory mediators. Direct pulmonary damage by activated leukocytes frequently results in development of the adult respiratory distress syndrome (ARDS). Renal dysfunction with oliguria occurs, due to vasospasm of the renal arteries, hypovolemia resulting from the leakage of vascular fluid, and alterations in clotting factors (1).

CLINICAL PRESENTATION OF SEPSIS

The clinical definitions of sepsis and sepsis syndrome are not clearly defined because of the numerous biological mediators and their complex interrelationships integral to

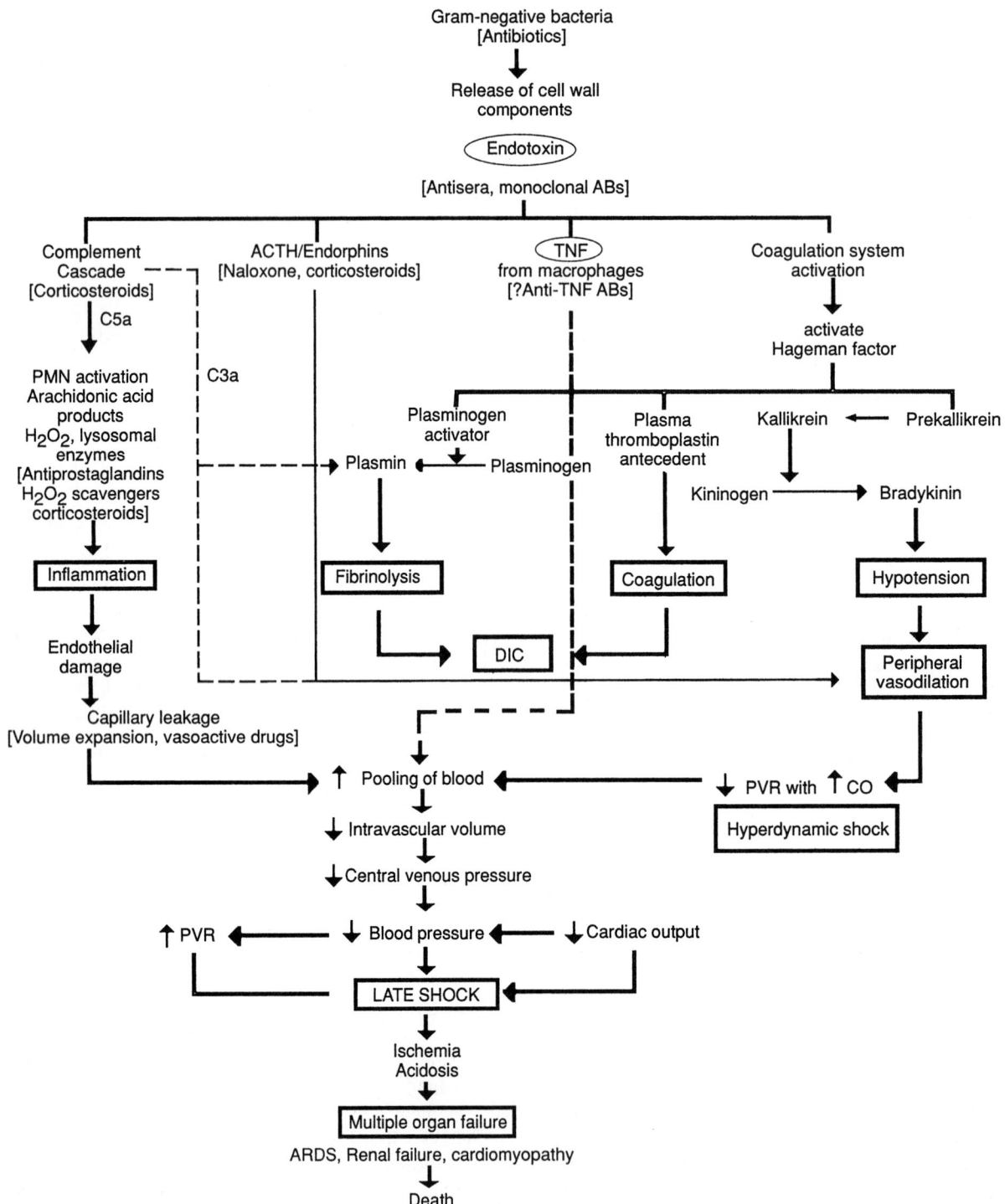

Figure 74.2.   Clinical Consequences of Endotoxin.

Table 74.3.
Early (Warm) versus Late (Cold) Septic Shock

Hyperdynamic Early or "Warm" Septic Shock	Hypodynamic Late or "Cold" Septic Shock
High CO[a]	Low CO
Low SVR[b]	High SVR
High O$_2$ consumption	Low O$_2$ consumption
Respiratory alkalosis	Respiratory acidosis
Warm, dry skin	Cold skin
Hypotension	Hypotension
Oliguria	Oliguria

[a] CO, cardiac output.
[b] SVR, systemic vascular resistance.

the development of sepsis. The clinical picture of sepsis varies widely, due to the sometimes opposing effects of endotoxin-stimulated mediators, the time at which sepsis is detected, and the amount of exposure to endotoxin (5, 24, 25).

The clinical presentation of Gram-negative sepsis usually includes fever or hypothermia, tachypnea, hyperglycemia (in diabetics), tachycardia, leukocytosis, and lactic acidosis. In general, the clinical picture of sepsis can be described as two different states (Table 74.3). The *hyperdynamic stage* of sepsis, often referred to as "early" or "warm" shock, is characterized by an elevated temperature, an increased respiratory rate and cardiac output, high oxygen consumption, respiratory alkalosis, warm dry skin, and oliguria (defined as a urine output of <20 ml/hr). Despite low systemic vascular resistance (SVR), blood pressure generally remains near normal. In many patients, transient hypotension and oliguria may respond to a fluid challenge. A change in mental status may also be observed; although lethargy or obtundation is most commonly noted, patients may become agitated or combative (12). As this hyperdynamic state continues, complement-mediated agglutination of leukocytes and capillary damage results in severe leakage of capillary contents into surrounding tissue. As intravascular volume decreases, patients progress to late or "cold" hyperdynamic shock, in which blood pressure falls, systemic vascular resistance increases, and cardiac output decreases. The decreased cardiac output results from the increase in peripheral vascular resistance and the production of cardiac depressants (4). There are some differences in the hemodynamic parameters observed in sepsis due to Gram-negative and Gram-positive bacteria. The cardiac rate and cardiac index are significantly lower in patients with Gram-negative sepsis, perhaps because of the release of vasoactive substances early in the course of Gram-negative bacteremia (23). The net result of these physiological events is decreased tissue perfusion, respiratory acidosis, and subsequent organ failure.

If not reversed, cold shock can rapidly result in multiple organ failure and ultimately death (22).

DIAGNOSIS OF SEPSIS AND SEPSIS SYNDROME

Criteria for the diagnosis of sepsis syndrome are crucial for identifying patients at risk for progression to septic shock. Currently, the most widely accepted criteria are those developed by Bone et al. (10). These criteria include fever, hypothermia, increased heart and respiratory rates, evidence of infection at any site, and clinical or laboratory signs of inadequate organ perfusion (e.g., hypoxemia, altered cerebral perfusion, lactic acidosis, or oliguria). It is important to note that positive blood cultures are not included in these criteria, as bacteremia is present in only about 45% of patients with sepsis (Table 74.4).

Although ideally one would like to document the presence of endotoxin in the bloodstream of patients with suspected Gram-negative sepsis, it has not been possible to consistently document the presence of endotoxin in bacteremic subjects. Several factors may account for this discrepancy. First, available assays are either too insensitive (the epinephrine skin test in rabbits) or demonstrate a variety of false-positive and false-negative reactions (the limulus lysate gelatin reaction). Although the limulus lysate test is sensitive to nanogram or picogram quantities of endotoxin, it is difficult to standardize the biological activity and to maintain contaminant-free reagents. In addition, fresh human serum appears to contain factors that detoxify or inactivate endotoxin.

A variety of other factors are often predictive but not diagnostic of the development of septic shock, including altered mental status, the development of leukopenia or thrombocytopenia, decreased urine output, and elevated serum lactate levels.

PROPHYLAXIS AND THERAPY OF GRAM-NEGATIVE SEPSIS

Clearly, it is imperative to avoid the development of sepsis or septic shock in patients at risk. Measures to reduce the

Table 74.4.
Criteria for Sepsis Syndrome[a]

Clinical evidence of infection
Rectal temperature >101°F or <96°F
Tachycardia (>90 beats/min)
Tachypnea (>20 spontaneous breaths/min)
At least one of the following
    Altered mental status
    Hypoxemia (PaO$_2$ <72 torr on room air)
    Elevated plasma lactate
    Oliguria (urine output <30 ml or 0.5 ml/kg for at least 1 hr)

[a] Adapted from Veterans Administration Systemic Sepsis Cooperative Study Group: Effect of high-dose glucocorticoid therapy on mortality in patients with clinical signs of systemic sepsis. N Engl J Med 317:659–665, 1987.

risk of developing sepsis include avoiding the indiscriminant use of antimicrobial agents or medical devices, particularly indwelling urinary catheters and mechanical ventilators. Maintenance of adequate nutritional status may also help decrease the risk of developing sepsis (1).

A variety of measures has been employed in an effort to decrease the incidence of bacteremia and sepsis, including the use of prophylactic topical or systemic antibiotics, active or passive immunization, granulocyte transfusions, and protective environments (7). Topical application of silver nitrate, silver sulfadiazine, or sulfamylon to burned skin reduces the incidence of burn wound sepsis secondary to *P. aeruginosa*. Suppression of aerobic Gram-negative fecal flora has been accomplished in a variety of patient populations, including cancer, transplant, and ICU patients, with one or more of the following oral administered antibiotics: aminoglycosides, polymixin B, colistin (polymixin E), vancomycin, nystatin, trimethoprim-sulfamethoxazole, norfloxacin, ciprofloxacin, and ofloxacin. Most regimens containing oral nonabsorbable antibiotics (e.g., vancomycin/polymixin/gentamicin) are unpalatable and involve multiple daily dosages; consequently, patient compliance is poor and the desired therapeutic benefit is not achieved. The use of systemically available agents such as trimethoprim-sulfamethoxazole or oral fluoroquinolones has resulted in a significant decrease in the number of Gram-negative infections in susceptible patients (14).

Once sepsis develops, however, early intervention is crucial to minimize the risk of further progression to septic shock. The treatment of sepsis depends on early suspicion of infection; support of metabolic, cardiac, and pulmonary function; aggressive antimicrobial therapy; reversal of the underlying causes of infection; and immunotherapy. Ironically, the use of antimicrobial agents can actually worsen sepsis initially, due to release of LPS from killed bacteria. Administration of a single intravenous dose of gentamicin to animals inoculated with *E. coli* results in a 4- to 20-fold increase in the levels of circulating endotoxin as compared with animals who do not receive antimicrobial therapy (7).

In most patients, blood cultures are negative or unavailable at the time antimicrobial therapy is initiated. The choice of antimicrobial therapy must be dictated by the suspected identity of causative pathogens. Therefore, an agent with a wide spectrum of activity, including Gram-negatives, staphylococci, and streptococci is generally recommended. Antimicrobial coverage of Gram-negative bacteria should include potentially resistant pathogens such as *P. aeruginosa* and *Enterobacter* species, particularly in patients with nosocomial (hospital-acquired) infections. In addition, the susceptibility patterns of the individual institution or community must also be considered. For example, if methicillin-resistant *Staphylococcus aureus* or *Staphylococcus epidermidis* are frequently isolated path-

ogens, the addition of vancomycin to the therapeutic regimen should be considered. The site of infection may assist the clinician in compiling the list of potential pathogens. For example, if the suspected source of infection is the lungs, the microbiology of recent sputum cultures should be considered. In patients with an intraabdominal source of infection, Enterobacteriaceae and anaerobes (including *Bacteroides fragilis*) should be covered (26).

Each patient must be evaluated carefully prior to initiating antimicrobial therapy, to optimize therapy. Although single-agent therapy may be used, frequently, a combination of antibiotics is used to cover a wide range of suspected pathogens. The choice of antibiotics often includes a β-lactam with antipseudomonal activity plus an aminoglycoside. Several supporting arguments for the use of combination therapy have been forwarded: (*a*) combination therapy allows coverage of a broad range of pathogens, (*b*) the use of two agents may prevent the emergence of resistance due to bacterial subpopulations that are resistant to one or the other agent, and (*c*) certain antimicrobial agents (e.g., penicillins plus aminoglycosides) provide synergistic activity when used in combination. However, no single antimicrobial regimen can be recommended over another at this time, because of the wide range of bacteria and susceptibility patterns encountered at various institutions. In addition, few well-controlled, comparative trials in humans compare the efficacies and toxicities of these agents.

Regardless of the antimicrobial therapy selected for empiric or initial therapy, the clinician must adjust individual doses and agents according to the patients' clinical status and response to therapy. As sepsis develops, deterioration of hepatic and renal function may develop rapidly, necessitating major dosage adjustments in the patients' therapeutic regimen. As the results of culture and sensitivity testing of blood, sputum, urine, and other specimens become available, antimicrobial therapy should be adjusted appropriately. The average duration of therapy for the treatment of Gram-negative sepsis in normal hosts is 10 to 14 days. However, longer therapy may be required in neutropenic or otherwise immunocompromised patients. Treatment should continue until the patient has remained afebrile for a minimum of 4 to 7 days, with an increasing neutrophil count and evidence of resolving infection at the source of the bacteremia (7).

The benefits of cardiovascular and pulmonary support with fluid resuscitation, pressors, mechanical ventilation, and hemodynamic monitoring are greater when used in the early stages of sepsis than whey they are initiated in the late stages. Patients are more likely to respond to fluid resuscitation that is initiated prior to the development of hypotension. Volume expansion is generally accomplished using crystalloid solutions (5% dextrose in water or saline) or colloid solutions such as fresh frozen plasma, albumin, hetastarch, or dextran preparations (23).

Although norepinephrine or epinephrine were used traditionally for hemodynamic support in septic patients, they have been largely replaced by isoproterenol, dopamine, and dobutamine, which enhance peripheral tissue perfusion and have a positive inotropic effect. Norepinephrine causes peripheral vasoconstriction and may cause tissue necrosis if extravasation occurs around the infusion site. The addition of low doses of dopamine (2 to 25 μg/kg/min) allows maintenance of adequate urine output. Dopamine causes vasodilatation of renal, coronary, and cerebral blood flow, while increasing systolic blood pressure and heart rate. Careful hemodynamic monitoring allows appropriate modification of therapy (23, 27).

Although total parenteral nutrition (TPN) is clearly an important therapeutic addition to the management of sepsis, there are a number of unresolved issues regarding its use. The use of branched-chain amino acids to improve outcome and reduce mortality in this population remains controversial (26).

Until recently, there was considerable controversy about the use of corticosteroids as adjunctive therapy for the treatment of sepsis (7, 28, 29). Corticosteroids possess a wide range of metabolic, antiinflammatory, and immunosuppressive effects. Although early, well-controlled, prospective studies demonstrated that relatively low dosages of corticosteroids (up to 1 mg/kg of betamethasone) failed to demonstrate a therapeutic benefit in patients with sepsis, the use of larger dosages have been advocated by many investigators (30). Several studies reported therapeutic benefit with doses of 30 mg/kg of methylprednisolone or 2 mg/kg of dexamethasone (28). Although a transient, "early" increased survival was noted, overall mortality at the conclusion of the study was similar in both groups, but the incidence of superinfections was higher in the steroid-treated group. Two recent, large, controlled clinical trials reported that the addition of methylprednisolone to standard antimicrobial therapy in the treatment of sepsis did not decrease mortality, as compared with placebo (2, 31). As observed in earlier studies, corticosteroid therapy may have been detrimental in some patients. The higher mortality in the steroid-treated group at 14 days was attributed to the higher rate of secondary infections in this group. On the basis of these studies, large doses of corticosteroids cannot be recommended as adjunctive therapy for sepsis.

A variety of other agents have been advocated as adjunctive therapy for the treatment of Gram-negative sepsis, including heparin, granulocyte transfusions, diuretics, naloxone, phenothiazines, cyclooxygenase inhibitors, and pentoxyphylline. However, at this time, no controlled studies support the clinical use of any of these agents in humans (7).

Immunotherapy of Gram-negative Sepsis

Both active and passive immunity have been used in the treatment of Gram-negative sepsis. Passive immunity in the form of intravenous gamma globulin (polyclonal IgG) has been utilized in the past, but there are insufficient data to warrant its widespread use in the treatment of sepsis (1). Polyclonal antiserum is produced by antigenic stimulation of animals, rabbits, goats, or horses. A clinical trial using intravenous IgG failed to demonstrate a beneficial effect in the treatment of sepsis (32).

The development of monoclonal antibodies for the treatment of Gram-negative sepsis is the most recent extension of work initially performed with J5 antiserum by Dr. Elizabeth Ziegler and colleagues at the University of California, San Diego in the 1970s. J5 antiserum was obtained by vaccinating human volunteers with a heat-killed strain of *E. coli* J5. J5 is a mutant strain that produces LPS without the variable polysaccharide (O antigen) side chain. J5 antiserum contains antibodies to the core LPS region of the Gram-negative bacterial cell wall. Antiserum was harvested approximately 2 weeks later, at the time of peak antibody response. In a large, multicenter, double-blind trial, J5 antisera reduced overall morbidity as well as mortality in patients with positive blood cultures who were also hypotensive or in profound shock. The mortality in 103 bacteremic subjects randomized to J5 antiserum was 22%, compared with 39% mortality in 109 patients randomized to placebo. Even more significant differences were noted in the reversal of profound shock. Antiserum did not significantly affect survival in patients with neutropenia or cancer (33). Baumgartner and colleagues (34) successfully used J5 immune serum as prophylaxis for Gram-negative sepsis in high-risk surgical patients. However, in a more recent study by Calandra and colleagues (35), intravenous administration of anti-J5 IgG was unsuccessful in reducing the mortality of Gram-negative septic shock.

Several limitations to antiserum therapy preclude its widespread clinical use. Since antiserum comes from pooled sera from many different human donors, it is costly to produce and difficult to control variability in the concentration of antibody. Vaccinating serum donors with J5 is associated with mild toxicity, and there is no booster response, so each person can donate only once. The limited spectrum of immunoreactivity prevents a vaccine developed against one Gram-negative bacteria to work against a different Gram-negative bacteria. The risk of transmitting blood-borne infections to patients is also a concern.

Addressing these problems led to the use of monoclonal antibodies (MAbs), which could be manufactured in large quantity with consistent biological activity and minimal contamination. Currently, investigators are working on agents that are targeted at one of two sites in the sepsis cascade. Agents targeted at LPS are designed to neutralize its activity in the blood or to prevent the LPS-stimulated activation of neutrophils. These agents are targeted only at Gram-negative bacteria. Gram-positive bacteria do not contain LPS. A second group of agents is designed to interrupt the cytokine-mediated immune response to sepsis (17, 28, 46).

Monoclonal Antibody Technology

In 1975, Kohler and Milstein developed a methodology for the production of virtually unlimited quantities of specific antibodies (immunoglobulins) by the use of hybridoma technology (36–38). Normally, B lymphocytes cannot survive for prolonged periods of time in tissue cell cultures. The fusion of B lymphocytes with human or mouse myeloma cells results in a *hybridoma* that retains the immortality of the myeloma cell with the antibody-producing ability of the B lymphocyte. The B lymphocytes are selected from those stimulated after injection of the desired antigen into a mouse. The hybrid cells can be cloned to produce multiple copies of the hybridoma (37, 39), which can each produce monoclonal antibodies targeted at the desired epitope of the antigen. *Monoclonal antibodies* are immunoglobulins (antibodies) produced by a clonal population of lymphocytes that bind to a single unique target site on the antigen (36, 39). A variety of techniques are used to produce large quantities of the desired monoclonal antibody. Tissue cell culture techniques can generally produce only limited quantities, although newer techniques using tiny porous spheres bathed in a nutrient media have resulted in larger harvests. Injection of the hybridoma into the mouse peritoneum results in the development of ascitic fluid containing 10 to 100 times the antibody concentration obtainable by conventional tissue culture techniques. Before in vivo use, a variety of purity, contamination, stability, and activity tests must be conducted (40, 41).

Monoclonal antibody technology avoids many of the problems associated with the production and administration of antisera or vaccines. A more detailed discussion of monoclonal antibody technology is beyond the scope of this chapter. The interested reader is referred to several excellent reviews for further information (37, 40–43).

In 1985, investigators developed a monoclonal immunoglobulin M (IgM) that binds specifically to the lipid A domain of LPS. Two products have reached clinical trials at this time (Table 74.5). HA-1A is a human monoclonal antibody, while E5 is a mouse-derived monoclonal antibody. Mouse-derived monoclonal antibodies are easier to produce since stable hybridomas are easier to develop. The mouse-derived monoclonal antibody has a shorter half-life in serum than the human-derived product (Table 74.6).

The efficacy and safety of HA-1A was evaluated in a randomized, double-blind trial in patients with sepsis and a presumed diagnosis of Gram-negative infection (44). Patients were administered either a single intravenous 100-mg dose of HA-1A (in 3.5 g of albumin) or placebo (3.5 g of albumin). All patients received appropriate antimicrobial therapy and supportive care as deemed necessary by their physicians. Of 543 patients entered into the study, 200 (37%) had documented Gram-negative bacteremia. There was no significant improvement in survival in patients *without* documented Gram-negative bacteremia or in the group of all patients receiving HA-1A, as compared with placebo. However, in the group of patients with bacteremia *or* bacteremia and shock upon entry into the study, HA-1A therapy significantly decreased overall mortality.

In in vitro studies, E5 reacts with the lipid A component of all clinically important Gram-negative bacteria. The efficacy and safety of E5 in reducing the mortality of Gram-negative sepsis was recently examined in a large, multicenter, double-blind, randomized, placebo-controlled trial in 486 patients (45). Patients were administered either 2 mg/kg of E5 (with a second dose administered 24 hr later) or placebo. Mortality was studied over a 30-day period after administration of the monoclonal antibody. There was no significant difference in survival between bacteremic and nonbacteremic patients with confirmed Gram-negative sepsis. However, E5 therapy significantly reduced mortality (P = .01), and resolution of organ failure was more frequent (P = .05) in patients with Gram-negative sepsis who were *not* in shock at the time of study entry. Four (0.1%) reversible allergic reactions were observed among 247 patients administered E5.

At this time (November 1991), HA-1A and E5 monoclonal antibodies are under review by the FDA and may be released within the next 6 to 12 months. However, there are a number of unresolved issues regarding the use of monoclonal antibodies. It is difficult to assess the comparative efficacy of these products because of differences in entry criteria and methods of data analysis. The optimal timing of doses has not been firmly established: would earlier administration be more beneficial? Would later administration provide the same efficacy as doses administered at an earlier time? There are safety concerns about the administration of mouse-derived monoclonal antibodies. Investigators are concerned about the development of human antimouse antibodies (HAMA) following repeated dosages of mouse-derived monoclonal antibodies, which might result in severe allergic reactions or in antibody titers that might limit further therapeutic effects (42). The expected high cost (>$4000 per dose) of these agents imposes severe burdens upon the healthcare system. Clearly, further studies are necessary to clarify the patient population that will optimally benefit from these therapies and the comparative efficacies of available agents. A better understanding of the pathophysiology of sepsis will allow the

Table 74.5.
Entry Criteria for HA-1A and E5 Trials for the Use of Endotoxin in the Treatment of Gram-negative Sepsis[a]

HA-1A	E5

Temperature >101 or <96°F
Tachycardia >90 beats/min
Tachypnea (RR >20 or the need for mechanical ventilation)
plus
Either:
  Hypotension (SBP <90 mm Hg or a sustained decrease in BP)
Two of the following signs of toxicity
  Unexplained metabolic acidosis
  Arterial hypoxemia
  Acute renal failure
  Coagulopathy
  Sudden decrease in mental acuity
  Unexplained metabolic acidosis
  Cardiac index >4 liters and SVR <800
	Two or more of the following within 24 h
	  Temperature >38 or <35°C
	  Leukocyte count >12,000/mm³ or <3,000/mm³ or >20% immature forms
	  Positive blood culture for gram-negative bacteria within 48 hr
	  Known or suspected site of Gram-negative infection
	and one or more of the following criteria
	  Hypotension (SBP <90 or acute drop of 30 mm Hg
	  Unexplained metabolic acidosis
	  Decreased SVR (SVR <800)
	  Tachypnea (RR >20 or min ventilation >10 liter/min if on mechanical ventilation)
	or otherwise unexplained organ dysfunction:
	  Renal failure
	  Respiratory failure
	  Altered mentation
	  Coagulopathy

[a] Adapted from Ziegler EJ, Fisher CJ, Sprung CL, et al.: Treatment of Gram-negative bacteremia and septic shock with HA-1A human monoclonal antibody against endotoxin. N Engl J Med 324(7):429–436, 1991; and Greenman RL, Schein RMH, Martin MA, et al.: A controlled clinical trial of E5 negative sepsis. JAMA 266(8):1097–1102, 1991.

Table 74.6.
Pharmacokinetics of HA-1A and E5[a]

	HA-1A	E5
Dose studied	100 mg	0–7.5 mg/kg
VD_{ss}[b]	48.2 ± 14.2 ml/kg	3.74–8.15 liter
Clearance (ml/kg/hr)	2.9 ± 1.7	1.38–9
Half-life (hr)	16.2 ± 10.7	10.24
C_{max} (μg/ml)	33.2 ± 9.4	37
C_{24hr} (μg/ml)	9.1 ± 6.4	5

[a] From Ziegler EJ, Fisher CJ, Sprung CL, et al.: Treatment of Gram-negative bacteremia and septic shock with HA-1A human monoclonal antibody against endotoxin. N Engl J Med 324(7):429–436, 1991; and Greenman RL, Schein RMH, Martin MA, et al.: A controlled clinical trial of E5 negative sepsis. JAMA 266(8):1097–1102, 1991.

development of more specific diagnostic criteria for this devastating complication of Gram-negative infection.

Studies are currently underway to assess the efficacy of monoclonal antibodies directed at TNF and other biological mediators in the treatment of sepsis.

CONCLUSION

The use of potent, broad-spectrum antibodies, fluid resuscitation, and vasoactive agents has not improved the mortality from sepsis. It is hoped that the introduction of monoclonal antibodies to Gram-negative bacteria will result in a decreased mortality. The development of better laboratory methods and clinical criteria for the early detection of sepsis may also assist in the identification of both patients at risk of sepsis and those who will most benefit from these costly therapies.

REFERENCES

1. DiPiro JT: Pathophysiology and treatment of Gram-negative sepsis. Am J Hosp Pharm 47(suppl3):S6–10, 1990.
2. Veterans Administration Systemic Sepsis Cooperative Study Group: Effect of high-dose glucocorticoid therapy on mortality in patients with clinical signs of systemic sepsis. N Engl J Med 317:659–665, 1987.
3. Dudley MN: Overview of Gram-negative sepsis. Am J Hosp Pharm 47(suppl 3):S3–5, 1990.
4. Sheagren JN, Shock syndromes related to sepsis. In Wyngaarden JB, Smith LH Jr (eds): Cecil Textbook of Medicine. Philadelphia, WB Saunders, ed. 18. 1988, pp 1538–1541.
5. Bone RC: Sepsis, the sepsis syndrome, multi-organ failure: a plea for comparable definitions. Ann Intern Med 114(4):332–333, 1991.
6. Young LS, Martin WJ, Meyer RD, et al.: Gram-negative rod bacteremia: microbiologic, immunologic and therapeutic considerations. Ann Intern Med 86:456–471, 1977.
7. Young LS, Gram-negative sepsis. In Mandell GL, Douglas RB Jr, Bennett JE, (eds): Principles and Practice of Infectious Diseases, ed. 3. New York, Churchill Livingstone, 1990, p 611–636.
8. Centers for Disease Control: Increase in national hospital discharge survey rates for septicemia—United States, 1979–1987. JAMA 263:937–938, 1990.
9. Cooper GS, Havlir DS, Shlaes DM, et al.: Polymicrobial bacteremia in the late 1980s: predictors of outcome and review of the literature. Medicine (Baltimore) 69(2):114–123, 1990.
10. Bone RC, Fisher CJ Jr, Clemmer TP, et al.: Sepsis syndrome: a valid clinical entity. Crit Care Med 17:389–393, 1989.
11. Gatell JM, Trilla A, Latorre X, et al.: Nosocomial bacteremia in a large Spanish teaching hospital: analysis of factors influencing prognosis. Rev Infect Dis 10:203–210, 1988.
12. Parillo JE, Parker MM, Natanson C, et al.: Septic shock in humans: advances in the understanding of pathogenesis, cardiovascular dysfunction, and therapy. Ann Intern Med 113:227–242, 1990.
13. Chmel H: Role of monoclonal antibody therapy in the treatment of infectious disease. Am J Hosp Pharm 47(3):S11–15, 1990.

14. Reidy JJ, Ramsay G: Clinical trials of selective decontamination of the digestive tract: review. Crit Care Med 18(12):1449–1456, 1990.

15. Centers for Disease Control: National nosocomial infectious study report, annual summary 1976. 1978, p. 1.

16. Centers for Disease Control: Nosocomial infection surveillance 1984. CDC surveillance summary. MMWR 35:19–29, 1986.

17. Dunn DL: Antibody immunotherapy of Gram-negative bacterial sepsis. Pharmacotherapy 7(2):S31–35, 1987.

18. Beutler B, Cerami P: The common mediator of shock, cachexia, and tumor necrosis. Adv Immunol 42:213–231, 1988.

19. Grunfeld C, Palladino MA Jr: Tumor necrosis factor: immunologic, antitumor, metabolic, and cardiovascular activities. Adv Intern Med 35:45–71, 1990.

20. Tracey KJ, Lowry SF: The role of cytokine mediators in septic shock. Adv Surg 23:21–56, 1990.

21. Tracey KJ, Lowry SF, Cerami A: Cachectin/TNF-α in septic shock and septic adult respiratory distress syndrome. Am Rev Respir Dis 138(6):1377–1379, 1988.

22. Fong Y, Lowry SF: Tumor necrosis factor in the pathophysiology of infection and sepsis. Clin Immunol Immunopathol 55(2):157–170, 1990.

23. Snell RJ, Parrillo JE: Cardiovascular dysfunction in septic shock. Chest 99(4):1000–1009, 1991.

24. Sprung C: Definitions of sepsis—have we reached a consensus? Crit Care Med 19(7):849–851, 1991.

25. Bone RC: Let's agree on terminology:definitions of sepsis. Crit Care Med 19(7):973–976, 1991.

26. Luce JM: Pathogenesis and management of septic shock. Chest 91(6):883–888, 1987.

27. Smith TE, Forgacs P: Haemodynamic interventions and therapy in septic shock. Drugs 24:75–82, 1982.

28. Schumer W: Steroids in the treatment of clinical septic shock. Ann Surg 184:333, 1976.

29. Nicholson DP: Review of corticosteroid treatment in sepsis and septic shock: pro or con. Crit Care Clin 5(1):151–155, 1989.

30. Klastersky J, Cappel R, Debusscher L: Effectiveness of betamethasone in management of severe infections. N Engl J Med 284:1248, 1971.

31. Bone RC, Fisher CJ Jr, Clemmer TP, et al.: A controlled clinical trial of high-dose methylprednisolone in the treatment of severe sepsis and septic shock. N Engl J Med 317:653–658, 1987.

32. McCabe WR, DeMaria A Jr, Berberich H, et al.: Immunization with rough mutants of *Salmonella minnesota*: protective activity of IgM and IgG antibody to the R595 (Re chemotype) mutant. J Infect Dis 158:291–300, 1988.

33. Ziegler EJ, McCutchan JA, Fierer J, et al.: Treatment of Gram-negative bacteremia and shock with human antiserum to a mutant *Escherichia coli*. N Engl J Med 307;1225–1230, 1982.

34. Baumgartner JD, McCutchan JA, Fierer J, et al.: Prevention of Gram-negative shock and death in surgical patients by antibody to endotoxin core glycolipid. Lancet 2:59–63, 1985.

35. Calandra T, Glauser MP, Schellekens J, et al.: Treatment of Gram-negative septic shock with human IgG antibody to *Escherichia coli* J5: a prospective, double-blind, randomized trial. J Infect Dis 158:312–319, 1988.

36. Milstein C: Monoclonal antibodies. Sci Am 243(4):66–76, 1980.

37. Kung PC, Goldstein G, Reinherz EL, et al.: Monoclonal antibodies defining distinctive human T-cell surface antigens. Science 206:24–79, 1979.

38. Kohler G, Milstein C: Continuous cultures of fused cells secreting antibody of predefined specificity. Nature 256:495–497, 1975.

39. Morrison SL: Genetically engineered (chimeric) antibodies. Hosp Pract 24(10):65–80, 1989.

40. Tami JA, Parr MD, Brown SA, et al.: Monoclonal antibody technology. Am J Hosp Pharm 43:2816–2825, 1986.

41. Bogard WC, Dean RT, Deo Y, et al.: Practical considerations in the production, purification, and formulation of monoclonal antibodies for immunoscintigraphy and immunotherapy. Semin Nucl Med 19:202–220, 1989.

42. Kwok K, Monoclonal antibodies. In Koeller J, Tami J, (eds): Concepts in Immunology and Immunotherapeutics. Bethesda, MD, American Society of Hospital Pharmacists, 1990, pp 345–409.

43. Young LS: Monoclonal antibodies: Technology and application to Gram-negative infections. Infection 12:303–308, 1984.

44. Ziegler EJ, Fisher CJ, Sprung CL, et al.: Treatment of Gram-negative bacteremia and septic shock with HA-1A human monoclonal antibody against endotoxin. N Engl J Med 324(7):429–436, 1991.

45. Greenman RL, Schein RMH, Martin MA, et al.: A controlled clinical trial of E5 murine monoclonal IgM antibody to endotoxin in the treatment of Gram-negative sepsis. JAMA 266(8):1097–1102, 1991.

CHAPTER 75

LEUKEMIAS: ACUTE AND CHRONIC

WILLIAM R. CROM, Pharm.D. and CLINTON F. STEWART, Pharm.D.

The leukemias are a group of neoplastic diseases of the blood-forming cells of the bone marrow, which result in proliferation and accumulation of immature and generally defective blood cells in both the bloodstream and the bone marrow (1). The involved cells are usually leukocytes, but several different forms of the disease may be manifested, depending on which leukocyte cell line is involved (Fig. 75.1). The leukemias are universally fatal if untreated, usually because of complications resulting from the leukemic infiltration of the bone marrow and replacement of normal hematopoietic precursor cells. These fatal complications are usually hemorrhage and infection (1). The natural history of untreated leukemia has led to the classifications of "acute" and "chronic" leukemia, referring to the rapidity of death, with average survival for untreated acute leukemia of about 3 months. Patients with chronic leukemia generally have more differentiated types of malignant cells and survive without treatment somewhat longer. However, with modern therapy, many patients with "acute" leukemia may survive for several years even if they eventually succumb to the disease, and indeed, for these patients leukemia is a chronic disease.

ACUTE LEUKEMIAS

Acute leukemia is classified by the predominant cell type involved. Because of significant differences in age distribution, responses to treatment, and prognosis, the acute leukemias are commonly divided into acute lymphocytic leukemia (ALL) and acute nonlymphocytic leukemia (ANLL). ANLL can be further divided into additional subtypes, depending on the cell line involved (Figs. 75.1 and 75.2): myelocytic, myelomonocytic, monocytic, promyelocytic, erythrocytic, and several other very rare types. However, because response to treatment is similar for all of these relatively uncommon types of leukemia, they are generally treated in the same fashion and referred to collectively as ANLL. In this chapter, ALL and ANLL are discussed separately with regard to pathophysiology, treatment, and prognosis.

Epidemiology and Etiology

Approximately 23,500 new cases of acute leukemia are identified each year in the United States, according to the NCI's Surveillance, Epidemiology, and End Results (SEER) program (2). About 18,100 Americans die each year from leukemia. Overall, leukemias and lymphomas account for about 7% of all new cancer cases and about 8% of cancer deaths (2).

The causes of acute leukemias are generally not known. Viruses have been shown to produce some types of leukemia in animals (e.g., feline leukemia), and the Epstein-Barr virus has been implicated as the causative agent of African Burkitt's lymphoma as well as some types of nasopharyngeal carcinoma (3). Currently, attention is being focused on the isolation of the human T cell leukemia virus (HTLV) from a human lymphoma. Individuals who have previously been exposed to radiation, with or without antineoplastic drugs, are also at greater risk of developing leukemia. In addition, numerous genetic derangements (particularly Down's syndrome) have been associated with a higher incidence of acute leukemia. However, in most cases in both children and adults, the cause of leukemia cannot be identified, and probably numerous factors interact to result in the malignant condition.

Despite differences in appearance and clinical behavior, all hematologic neoplasms have in common the fact that they are clonal, i.e., all cells of the malignant population in a given patient are derived from a single mutant precursor cell (4). The neoplastic clones have two important features in comparison with normal cells. First, they appear to possess an advantage over normal hematopoietic clones that results in growth of the malignant population at the expense of normal cells. Secondly, there is an imbalance between proliferation and differentiation. Most malignant populations are made up of poorly differentiated cell types that ordinarily would not proliferate or be found in the bloodstream in large numbers. However, the malignant transformation of these cells results in immature cell types that proliferate but do not further differentiate.

It is useful to review the normal production of cellular blood elements. As shown in Figure 75.1, all lymphoid and hemopoietic blood cells are derived from a small population of pluripotent stem cells. These stem cells have virtually unlimited potential for self-renewal and are capable of responding to physiologic needs by inducing production of progenitor cells committed to mature separately into

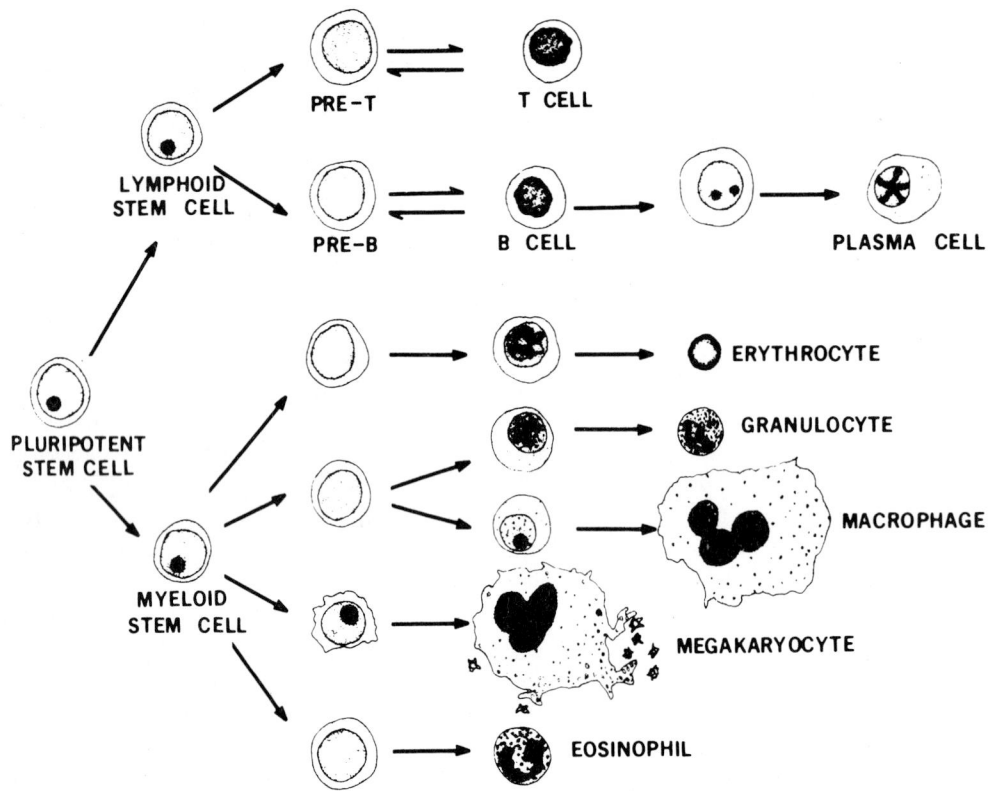

Figure 75.1. A schematic model of hematopoiesis showing clonal derivation of mature lymphoid and hemic cells from a pluripotent stem cell. (Reprinted with permission from Altman AJ, Schwartz AD: Malignant Diseases of Infancy, Childhood and Adolescence. Philadelphia: WB Saunders, 1983.)

lymphoid cells, erythroid cells, megakaryocytes, granulocytes, and monocytes. As maturation proceeds in the various cellular lineages, proliferative capacity becomes progressively restricted until eventually it is lost completely. Therefore, mature cells must be continually replaced as they complete their life cycles. Various stimulatory factors, such as erythropoietin, thrombopoietin, and colony-stimulating factors regulate the proliferation and differentiation of committed precursor cells, derived from the pluripotent stem cells. Leukemia cells do not undergo terminal differentiation and thus do not lose their proliferative potential. The leukemic cell population continues to expand, and normal bone marrow elements may be "crowded out," resulting in the characteristic signs of bone marrow failure that generally bring patients to medical attention.

Classifications of Acute Leukemia

Acute leukemia is classified by the cell of origin. However, additional classifications of leukemia have been developed to further identify differences in the clinical course, response to treatment, and prognosis of various types of acute leukemia. An important development introduced in the 1970s is the French-American-British (FAB) system

of nomenclature that is now widely used to classify the morphologic subgroups of acute leukemias (5). The FAB system is summarized in Table 75.1.

In addition to the FAB system, both immunologic and biochemical markers are used to classify and identify subtypes of leukemia cells. Immunologic "markers" refer to the surface immunoglobulin (SIg) found on the cell membrane of malignant leukocytes or to their cytoplasmic immunoglobulins (CIg). As normal cells undergo differentiation, these markers change and may be used to determine the degree of differentiation achieved by the malignant cell line. This permits identification of the type of cell involved and leads to further classification. The prognosis of various subgroups of ALL is discussed below.

Biochemical markers refer to altered concentrations of intracellular enzymes, which may be found in various forms of leukemia. Terminal deoxynucleotidyl transferase (TdT) is an intracellular enzyme that is generally not detected in mature lymphocytes but is found in most patients with ALL, excluding those with the B cell subtype. It may also be found in up to 5% of ANLL cases. Myeloperoxidase and Sudan black stain, on the other hand, are positive predominantly in cases of nonlymphocytic leukemia. The periodic acid–Schiff (PAS) reaction is positive in ALL and

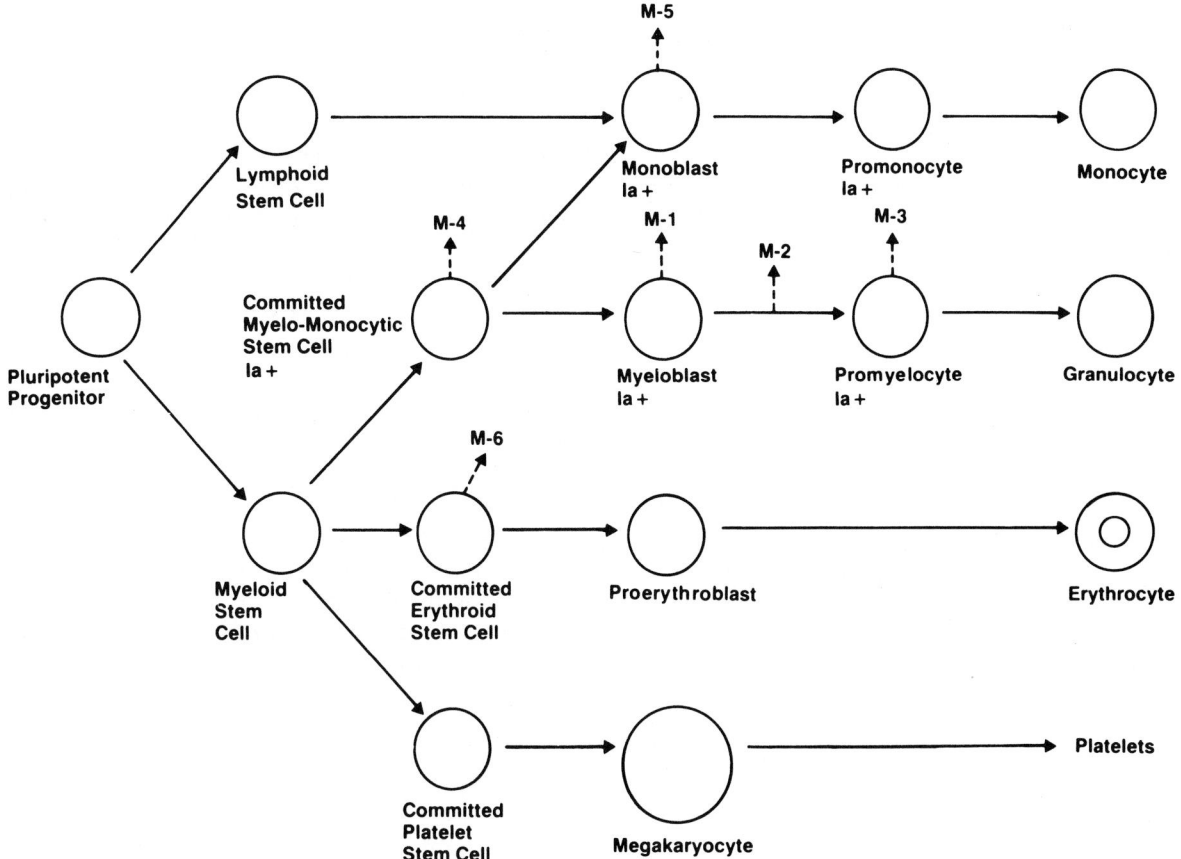

Figure 75.2. Myeloid differentiation and relationship to FAB classification of AML. *M-1*, undifferentiated myeloid; *M-2*, early (?) differentiated myeloid; *M-3*, promyelocytic; *M-4*, myelomonocytic; *M-5*, monocytic; *M-6*, erythroleukemia. (Reprinted with permission from Fernbach DJ: Natural History of Acute Leukemia. In Sutow WW, Fernbach DJ, Vietti TJ (eds): Clinical Pediatric Oncology, ed. 3. St. Louis, CV Mosby, 1984, pp 332–337.)

Table 75.1.
The French-American-British (FAB) Cooperative Group Classification of Acute Leukemias

FAB Designation	Common Terms (Abbreviations) for Leukemic Subgroups	Predominating Cell Type
L1	Acute lymphocytic leukemia Childhood (ALL)	Microlymphoblasts
L2	Acute lymphocytic leukemia, adult (ALL)	Mixed lymphoblasts, prolymphoblasts
L3	Burkitt's-type leukemia	Lymphocytes
M1	Acute myelocytic leukemia, undifferentiated; acute myelogenous, acute granulocytic	Myeloblasts
M2	Acute myelocytic leukemia, differentiated	Mixed myeloblasts, promyelocytes
M3	Acute progranulocytic leukemia	Hypergranular promyelocytes
M4	Acute myelomonocytic leukemia (AMML)	Mixed myelocytes, monocytes
M5	Acute monocytic leukemia (AMOL)	Monocytes
M6	Erythroleukemia	Mixed erythroblasts, erythrocytes, myelocytes
M7	Megakaryoblastic leukemia	

is useful in differentiating it from ANLL (6). In actual practice, the classification of a particular case of acute leukemia is based on the combination of morphology and immunologic and biochemical studies. These studies generally correlate with one another and are used to confirm the suspected classification of any particular case. (Figures 75.2 and 75.3 show the correlation between FAB classification, immunologic markers, and biochemical markers for subgroups of ALL and ANLL, respectively.

Clinical Presentation and Diagnosis

The initial symptoms of acute leukemia differ very little for ALL and ANLL. The complaints that most often bring patients to medical attention are fever, pallor, purpura, and pain (6). These symptoms result from bone marrow failure. Anemia occurs because of inadequate erythrocyte production, infections are due to inadequate neutrophil production, and bleeding is due to inadequate platelet production. In addition, infiltration of leukemia cells into the liver, spleen, or lymph nodes may result in hepatosplenomegaly, lymphadenopathy, and bone and joint pain. The

frequency of presenting complaints among patients with ALL are listed in Table 75.2. These complaints may be present for a few days or even a few weeks; rarely, there may be a history of these symptoms for several months prior to diagnosis. The most common symptom at diagnosis is fever, occurring in about 60% of patients. Although patients may be neutropenic at diagnosis, fever appears to be due to the leukemia itself, since 70% of these patients become afebrile within 72 hr of beginning induction chemotherapy but without being treated with antibiotics (7). Nevertheless, empiric antibiotic therapy is usually instituted in febrile, neutropenic leukemia patients at diagnosis, since the risk of serious systemic infections in such patients cannot be ignored.

Newly diagnosed patients with leukemia may have a total white blood cell (WBC) count that is markedly elevated, normal, or markedly depressed. A very high circulating WBC count is associated with a poorer prognosis, but even in these patients, most of the white cells in the circulation are immature blast forms that are incapable of mounting a response to bacterial infections. Therefore, at

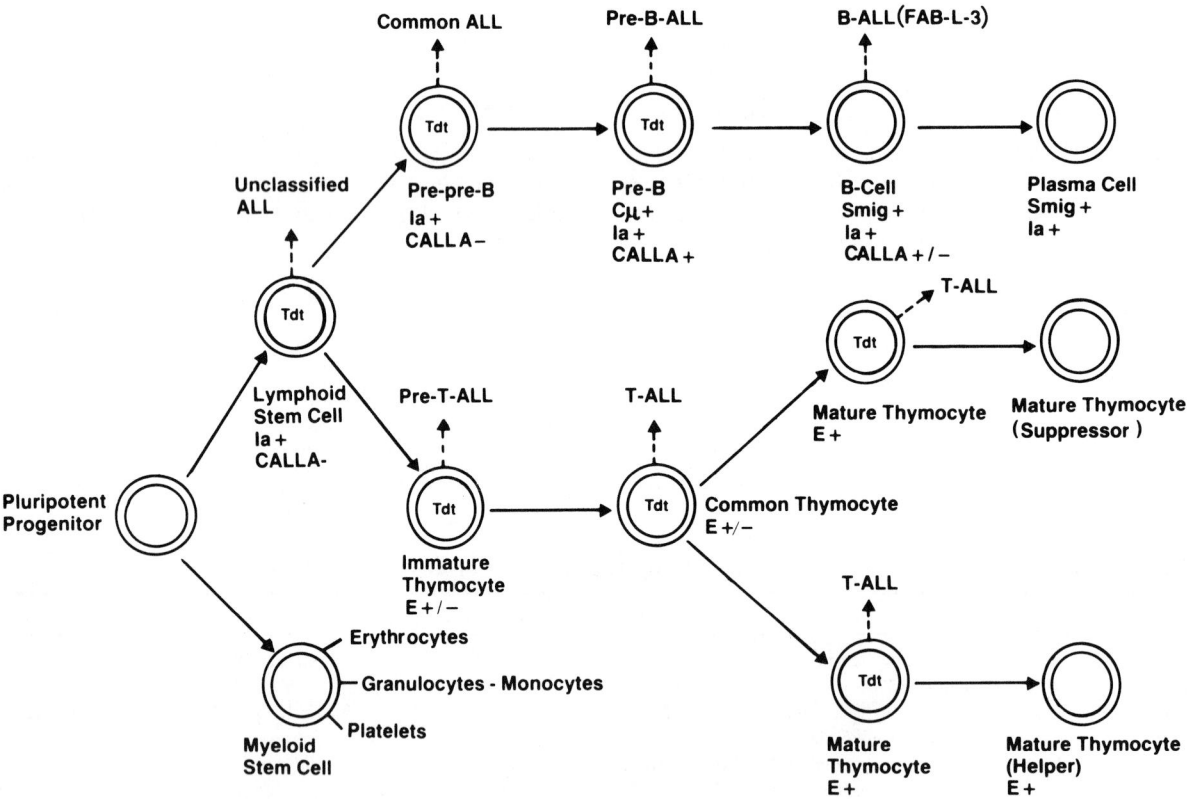

Figure 75.3. Lymphoid differentiation and relationship to ALL. *Ia*, Immune-related antigen; *CALLA*, common acute lymphocytic leukemia antigen; *Cμ*, cytoplasmic in heavy chain; *Smig*, surface membrane immunoglobulin; *E*, sheep erythrocyte rosette; *Tdt*, terminal deoxynucleotidyl transferase. L1 and L2 FAB cannot be differentiated by this schema. Lymphoblastic leuke-

mias other than B cell may be L1 or L2 in appearance. (Reprinted with permission from Fernbach DJ: Natural History of Acute Leukemia. In Sutow WW, Fernbach DJ, Vietti TJ (eds): Clinical Pediatric Oncology, ed. 3. St. Louis, CV Mosby, 1984, pp 332–337.)

**Table 75.2.
Frequency of the More
Common Presenting
Complaints among Children
with ALL**

Finding	Percent
Fever	61
Pallor	55
Hemorrhage	52
Anorexia	33
Fatigue	30
Bone pain	23
Abdominal pain	19
Joint pain	15
Lymphadenopathy	15
Weight loss	13

diagnosis most patients with leukemia are at an increased risk of opportunistic infections.

The diagnosis of acute leukemia is not usually difficult to establish. A bone marrow aspirate is performed to allow examination of the cellular elements of the bone marrow. It is often hypercellular, with 60 to 100% blast cells. A minimum of 25% blast cells is considered adequate to establish the diagnosis of acute leukemia, but most commonly this is an all-or-none diagnosis, and the pattern is obvious. Abnormal cells found in the peripheral blood may be suspicious for acute leukemia, but they are usually not considered to be diagnostic, because bizarre mononuclear cells may be seen in the blood of patients with viral illnesses. If blasts or other unidentified cells are seen in the peripheral blood, the diagnosis must be confirmed by a bone marrow examination.

Principles of Therapy

The modern cure-oriented approach to the treatment of any malignant condition usually involves some combination of surgery, radiation, and chemotherapy. Although surgery is the primary treatment of solid tumors, it is impossible to surgically remove tumor tissue in leukemia, and therefore surgery has a minor supportive role.

Radiation therapy has a more important role in leukemia, but it is not used alone as a curative modality. It is the primary treatment of either occult or overt central nervous system (CNS) leukemia. High-dose radiotherapy is also used to obliterate functional bone marrow as part of the preparation for bone marrow transplants. It may also be used in individual cases to reduce the size of an infiltrative leukemic mass, particularly where functional impairment of an organ or joint is involved.

DRUG THERAPY

Drug therapy remains the primary modality for the treatment of acute leukemias. Beginning with the use of ami-

nopterin in childhood ALL in 1948 (9), additional effective agents have been identified and introduced into routine clinical use. The mechanisms of action and common toxicities of the drugs routinely used to treat acute leukemia today are summarized in Table 75.3. This table includes investigational agents effective in the treatment of acute leukemia.

For all phases of leukemia, drugs used in combination are superior to single agents. The rationale for combination therapy is that several effective agents with different mechanisms of action are more likely to destroy different subpopulations of leukemia cells and reduce the potential for development of drug resistance. The practical problem in the design of clinical treatment programs is to use the optimal number of agents in the most effective dosages and sequence. Several principles guide the use of combination chemotherapy for malignant diseases: (a) each of the drugs used should have demonstrated single-agent activity against the tumor; (b) the drugs should have different mechanisms of action; (c) the drugs used should have minimally overlapping toxicities; and (d) the maximal optimal doses should be used, scheduled with respect to specific tumor cell kinetics.

The optimal use of anticancer drugs is limited by our incomplete understanding of their mechanisms of action, mechanisms of resistance to them, and their interactions. In addition, our understanding of the biology of tumors and the factors that control their growth is rudimentary. Current research directed at elucidating the cellular mechanisms that govern both the reproduction of malignant cells and their response to anticancer drugs is expected to improve our use of the drugs currently available, as well as lead to the development of new agents.

BONE MARROW TRANSPLANTATION

Bone marrow transplantation is a relatively new treatment modality that has an important role in the treatment of ANLL, particularly during first remission. Transplantation has also been useful in producing cures in patients with ALL who have relapsed and receive a transplant during their second remission. This procedure requires that the patient receive total body irradiation with or without high-dose drug therapy (cyclophosphamide, busulfan, and etoposide have all been used) to kill residual leukemia cells and produce irreversible bone marrow suppression. Bone marrow is obtained from an HLA-matched donor (allogeneic), an identical twin (syngeneic), or from the patient in remission (autologous). New approaches to autologous marrow transplants involve the use of monoclonal antibodies to "clean up" marrow and remove residual leukemia cells. Bone marrow is harvested from the iliac crest of the donor and then intravenously infused into the patient. Engraftment usually occurs in about 2 weeks.

Bone marrow transplants have a number of potential

Table 75.3.
Principle Toxicities and Clinical Indications for Drugs Used to Treat Leukemia

Drug	Principal Toxicities		Indications
	Acute	Delayed	
Plant alkaloids			
Etoposide	Nausea and vomiting; hypotension with rapid administration	Bone marrow depression; alopecia	ANLL
Teniposide	Nausea and vomiting; hypotension with rapid administration	Bone marrow depression; alopecia	ALL
Vincristine	Local reaction with extravasation	Peripheral neuropathy; alopecia; constipation	ALL (remission induction)
Antimetabolites			
Cytarabine	Nausea, vomiting, diarrhea	Bone marrow depression; megaloblastosis; oral ulceration	ALL, ANLL
Mercaptopurine	Occasional nausea and vomiting	Bone marrow depression; liver damage	ALL (continuation therapy)
Methotrexate	Nausea; diarrhea (usually mild)	Bone marrow depression; oral and gastrointestinal ulceration; nephrotoxicity (high doses); hepatic cirrhosis (low-dose); pulmonary infiltration	ALL (intrathecal, low doses orally or IV, high doses IV)
Thioguanine	Occasional nausea and vomiting 1 or 2 days after administration	Bone marrow depression	ANLL
Antibiotics			
Daunorubicin	Nausea and vomiting; diarrhea; local reactions at infiltration site; red urine, 1 or 2 days after administration	Bone marrow depression; cardiotoxicity; stomatitis; alopecia	ANLL, ALL
Doxorubicin	Nausea and vomiting; diarrhea; local reactions at infiltration site; red urine, 1 or 2 days after administration	Bone marrow depression; cardiotoxicity; stomatitis; alopecia; potentiation of radiation	ALL, ANLL
Alkylating agents			
Cyclophosphamide	Nausea and vomiting	Bone marrow depression; immunosupression; alopecia; hemorrhagic cystitis; sterility	ALL, ANLL
Miscellaneous			
Asparaginase	Nausea and vomiting; fever; anaphylaxis	Hepatotoxicity; hyperglycemia; pancreatitis; abdominal pain; coagulation defects; CNS depression	ALL

hazards. First, there is a risk that the transplant will not engraft. To reduce this possibility, the patient is treated with glucocorticoids, cyclosporine, or both to inhibit proliferation of T lymphocytes that cause transplant rejection. Secondly, there is the risk of infection as a result of immunosuppression. Viral and fungal infections are especially common and difficult to treat.

A third complication is graft-versus-host disease (GVHD), which may be either acute or chronic. GVHD results from T lymphocytes in the donor marrow reacting against host tissue, particularly skin, liver, and the gastrointestinal tract. Acute GVHD occurs in 30 to 60% of allogeneic transplants and develops 1 to 3 months following transplantation (8). The incidence increases with the age of the patient, and it is fatal in up to 50% of cases. To prevent GVHD, patients are treated with high-dose corticosteroids, antithymocyte globulin, and cyclosporine. Chronic GVHD usually develops more than 6 months after

transplantation and consists of immune-related immunodeficiency syndromes. Viral and fungal infections may occur, particularly interstitial pneumonitis (caused by *Pneumocystis carinii* or cytomegalovirus and other viruses), which may occur in 25 to 60% of patients.

Acute Lymphocytic Leukemia

ALL is the most common malignancy of childhood, but it is quite rare in persons over 15 years of age. The incidence in children is about 2.5 per 100,000, and it is slightly higher in boys than girls (2). There is also a higher incidence of leukemia in children with various genetic abnormalities, particularly Down's syndrome.

Childhood ALL represents one of the success stories of recent years in cancer treatment. Long-term survival in children receiving modern therapy is at least 50%, and for children with favorable prognostic factors, it may be considerably higher. In addition, the approaches used to develop optimal therapy for childhood ALL provide a useful model for the development of curative therapy for other human malignancies. Several distinct phases of therapy, each with a specific rationale, have been developed, and current efforts to improve the cure rate of ALL have focused on refining and optimizing therapy for each of these phases.

INDUCTION THERAPY

Complete remission, which is defined as the complete eradication of all detectable disease, is achieved in 90 to 95% of ALL patients with modern drug therapy. Patients in complete remission have no clinical evidence of leukemia and may lead relatively normal lives while in remission. However at diagnosis, 10^{10} to 10^{12} leukemia cells may be present, and although remission induction therapy eradicates up to 99.9% of the malignant cells, patients in remission may have as many as 10^8 clinically undetectable leukemia cells in their bodies. Therefore, a substantial number of cells remains to be eliminated after patients achieve a complete clinical remission.

The objectives of initial remission induction are to (a) eradicate as many leukemia cells as possible, within the limits of biologic tolerance; and, (b) reestablish normal hematopoiesis and general good health. "Standard" remission induction therapy generally consists of 2 or more drugs. Prednisone and vincristine are almost always used, and this combination produces a complete remission in more than 90% of patients. However, the value of remission treatment cannot be assessed only by the remission rate, because it is now known that each phase of therapy can influence the others. The initial treatment also influences the duration of remission, and addition of a third agent, either asparaginase or an anthracycline (daunorubicin or doxorubicin), appears to increase the fraction of patients who remain in continuous complete remission (CCR) and are eventually cured (10–12). Therefore, induction regimens generally include at least three drugs, prednisone, vincristine, and either asparaginase or an anthracycline.

Recently, more intensive induction regimens have been used (13). Although the fraction of patients achieving a complete remission is not increased, more intense therapy results in an increased initial cell kill and an improved cure rate. The induction regimen used at one major institution is shown in Table 75.4.

CONSOLIDATION THERAPY

Consolidation therapy refers to a period of intensive therapy administered after achievement of complete remission. The purpose of consolidation therapy is to secure the complete remission by eradicating as many of the remaining leukemic cells as possible, within the limits of biologic

tolerance. Consolidation therapy may consist of different combinations of agents or may consist of repeated courses of the regimen used to achieve the initial clinical remission. Not all treatment schemes for ALL include a distinct consolidation phase.

CENTRAL NERVOUS SYSTEM THERAPY

An important site of initial relapse in patients who achieve a complete remission is the CNS. Up to 60% of patients have their initial reappearance of malignant blast cells in the CNS (14), probably because of poor penetration across the blood-brain barrier by the drugs used to induce remission. Presence of the CNS as a "pharmacologic sanctuary" for ALL led to the development of CNS "prophylaxis" as a standard component of treatment for this disease. Proposed by George and Pinkel in the 1960s (15), CNS therapy has reduced the CNS relapse rate to less than 10% (14). The mainstay of CNS therapy has been cranial irradiation, either with spinal irradiation or intrathecal methotrexate. The dose originally used was 2400 rads delivered over 2 to 3 weeks, but more recently it has been shown that 1800 rads provides adequate treatment with less toxicity and morbidity (16). Intrathecal methotrexate has been used with success in place of spinal irradiation, resulting in less myelosuppression and fewer growth abnormalities (17). Dosages of intrathecal medication are based on age, rather than body weight or surface area (18). The usual dose for all patients over 3 years of age is 12 mg (19). Cytarabine (at a dosage of 36 mg), hydrocortisone (at a dosage of 24 mg), or both may be added to methotrexate to further improve the effectiveness of CNS therapy.

Another approach to CNS treatment is the use of high-dose methotrexate intravenously, without irradiation (20). This therapy consists of methotrexate in dosages of 500 mg/m² or more, infused over 24 hr. The long infusion time is intended to improve penetration of methotrexate across the blood-brain barrier. Although cerebrospinal fluid (CSF) methotrexate concentrations are typically only 1% or less of the concurrent plasma concentrations (21), use of high-dose methotrexate allows prolonged high plasma concentrations to achieve cytocidal methotrexate concentrations in the CSF. Leucovorin "rescue" is then administered to prevent excessive and intolerable toxicity to normal tissues. High-dose intravenous methotrexate may be combined with intrathecal methotrexate to further boost CSF concentrations. Doses as high as 33.6 g/m² have been used (22) to achieve CSF concentrations of 10 μM from intravenous methotrexate alone. However, no improvement in overall survival has been shown as a result of using this approach. In general, high-dose methotrexate may result in a slightly higher CNS relapse rate than cranial irradiation with intrathecal methotrexate (23), but overall disease-free survival does not appear to be different. This

Table 75.4.
Induction Therapy Schema for Acute Lymphocytic Leukemia

Agent	Dosage and Route	No. of Doses	Schedule
Prednisone	40 mg/m^2 daily p.o.	28	Days 1 through 28
Vincristine	1.5 mg/m^2 IV (2.0 mg maximum)	4	Days 1, 8, 15, 22
Daunomycin	25 mg/m^2 IV	2 (or 3)[a]	Days 2 and 8 ($\pm$ day 15)[a]
Asparaginase	10,000 Units/m^2 i.m.	6 (or 9)[a]	Days 3, 4, 6, 8, 10, 12 ($\pm$ days 15, 17, 19)[a]
Teniposide	200 mg/m^2 IV	3	Days 22, 25, 29
Cytarabine	300 mg/m^2 IV	3	Days 22, 25, 29
Methotrexate/hydrocortisone/cytarabine	12 mg i.t.	3	Days 2, 22, 43
	24 mg i.t.		
	36 mg i.t.		

[a] Patients with definite residual lymphoblasts in bone marrow aspirates on day 15 receive three additonal doses of daunomycin and asparaginase. Another bone marrow aspirate is then performed on day 22 in these patients to assess the antileukemic response. A final bone marrow aspirate is performed on day 43 to document complete remission status.

suggests that high-dose methotrexate may improve control of disease in the bone marrow as well. In addition, cranial irradiation results in more significant CNS toxicities compared to high-dose methotrexate.

The optimal dosage of high-dose methotrexate in the treatment of ALL has not been defined. One study (24) has identified a relationship between plasma methotrexate concentration and the probability of relapse. Patients received 15 courses of methotrexate, 1000 mg/m^2, given as a 200 mg/m^2 loading dose, followed by 800 mg/m^2 over 24 hr. This therapy was delivered as CNS therapy and during the first 75 weeks of continuation therapy. Patients who achieved steady-state plasma concentrations above 16 μM for at least half their courses were more likely to remain in complete continuous remission than patients whose plasma concentrations were lower. The variability in plasma concentrations was due solely to interpatient differences in drug elimination, since all patients were treated with identical methotrexate dosages. This study provides insight into how best to use methotrexate in ALL and offers guidance in selecting a dosage of methotrexate that will yield optimal cytotoxic exposure and the most efficacious results. A rationale for prospective pharmacokinetic monitoring of high-dose methotrexate to improve its therapeutic benefit in ALL patients is also presented by this study.

CONTINUATION (MAINTENANCE) THERAPY

In patients who have achieved a complete remission, only a small proportion (perhaps 15%) will be long-term survivors if no additional therapy is administered (25). Continuation, or maintenance, therapy appears to be necessary to eradicate the remaining leukemia cells that are undetectable during remission. The growth fraction of leukemia cells is relatively small, and the cell-cycle time is fairly long. Therefore, at any given time only a small fraction of the total number of leukemia cells is susceptible to the effects of most anticancer drugs, which are cell-cycle phase-specific agents. Hence, a prolonged period of exposure to anticancer drugs is necessary to further reduce the malignant population. Most commonly, continuation therapy has consisted of a two-drug combination of mercaptopurine and methotrexate (25). Mercaptopurine is given orally in dosages of 50 to 90 mg/m^2/day, and methotrexate is given orally, intravenously, or intramuscularly at dosages of 15 to 30 mg/m^2/week.

The optimal duration of continuation therapy is not known, and current guidelines are based on empiric trial-and-error approaches. Most treatment programs use a duration of 2 to 6 years for continuation therapy. In determining the length of continuation therapy, the risk of off-therapy relapses must be considered in comparison with the risks of undesirable toxic effects of the therapy. Therapy may be stopped after 30 months of continuous complete remission or at least 12 months of continuous remission after an isolated nonmedullary relapse (CNS or testes). Results of several large long-term studies indicate that 70% of patients who have therapy electively stopped in this fashion will remain disease-free and be long-term survivors (25).

Although continuation therapy is well tolerated, an important problem with current approaches is on-therapy relapses. A substantial fraction (perhaps 40%) of patients relapse during the continuation phase of therapy, presumably as a result of the development of resistant disease. In addition, continuation therapy is immunosuppressive and associated with the risk of opportunistic infections. Therefore, alternative strategies have been used both to overcome the development of resistance and to reduce the risk of infections and other complications.

Approaches to prevent bone marrow relapse during remission have included increasing the number of drugs administered during remission, periodic repetition of the agents used to induce the initial remission (referred to as "reinforcement" pulses), and intermittent rather than continuous chemotherapy. Use of more than two agents simultaneously does not appear to improve the rate of disease-free survival, but it does increase the toxicity of the therapy (26).

One approach to the continuation therapy of ALL is rotational use of non-cross-resistant anticancer drugs early in therapy. This concept is based on the somatic mutation theory of Luria and Delbrück (27) and its further development by Goldie and Coldman (28, 29). This hypothesis states that intense early therapy and sequential or rotational use of multiple non-cross-resistant agents during continuation therapy will reduce the likelihood of the emergence of a drug-resistant subpopulation of leukemia cells. Bone marrow relapses while on continuation therapy account for the largest fraction of patients who succumb to ALL, and this is undoubtedly due to the development of resistance, either by mutation or selection, to the methotrexate-mercaptopurine combination usually administered during this phase of therapy. The rationale for administering additional non-cross-resistant agents during continuation therapy is to reduce the opportunity for resistance to the primary combination to be manifested. Therefore, other effective agents such as etoposide, cyclophosphamide, cytarabine, teniposide, or additional anthracyclines may be administered during continuation therapy, in addition to the more customary methotrexate and mercaptopurine. However, the negative aspect is the increase in toxicity that may be encountered with some of these other agents. Since up to 50% of patients may be cured with the relatively well-tolerated methotrexate-mercaptopurine combination, additional more toxic drugs during continuation therapy may result only in more morbidity for patients who may be cured with less aggressive therapy. This dilemma points out the need to develop a better understanding of the various subtypes of ALL and significant prognostic factors, to more readily identify those patients who would be expected to do well with less intense therapy.

PROGNOSTIC FACTORS

Numerous variables have been identified that are associated with the likely prognosis for ALL. These factors are used in much the same way that staging is used for solid tumors, to give patients and families some indication of the likely outcome of treatment and to develop treatment plans appropriate for the type of disease. Some of the most widely-recognized factors are listed in Table 75.5. Age at diagnosis is important, with children under 2 years old and those over 10 years of age having a higher mortality rate with current standard therapy. Several studies have shown that boys have a slightly greater risk of relapse than girls, even after accounting for nonmedullary relapses in the testes, which apparently act as a pharmacologic sanctuary

Table 75.5.
Adverse Prognostic Factors at Diagnosis of ALL

Age
  <2 years, >10 years
Sex
  Male
Race
  Nonwhite
Physical findings
  Hepatosplenomegaly
  Lymphadenopathy
  Mediastinal mass (on chest roentgenogram)
  Lymphoblasts in CNS
Hematologic findings
  Elevated WBC count
  Elevated hemoglobin
  Decreased platelets
FAB morphology
  L2, L3
Immunologic markers
  T cell or B cell leukemia
Cytogenetics
  DNA index <1.16
  Translocations
  Philadelphia chromosome

from systemic anticancer drugs. WBC count at diagnosis is universally recognized as an important prognostic factor, since higher WBC counts represent a greater tumor burden and are associated with a poorer outcome. T cell and B cell leukemias, identified by their characteristic SIgs, have a poorer prognosis than leukemia expressing other SIgs. Many series have shown that nonwhite patients may have a poorer prognosis, although there has been speculation that this may be due at least partly to socioeconomic factors that may cause delays in diagnosis and treatment. A thymic or mediastinal mass on chest roentgenograms is a high-risk feature, although this is often associated with T cell disease. Patients with lymphoblasts detectable in the CSF at diagnosis have a poorer prognosis.

More recently, genetic characteristics have also been recognized as having prognostic significance. Leukemic clones with more than 53 chromosomes or a ratio of DNA content greater than 1.15 times normal (sometimes referred to as the "DNA index") are more responsive to treatment, and patients with this disease have a better prognosis (30). Cytogenetic studies have shown that leukemia clones that exhibit various types of translocations result in a poorer prognosis.

It is important to note that these risk factors often cosegregate; patients with T cell leukemia often have a high WBC count, for example. Therefore, none of these factors should be regarded as having completely independent prognostic value, and any treatment plan that uses these factors to individualize therapy should consider how these factors interact and correlate with one another. Most comprehensive treatment programs for ALL, such as cooperative group studies, use sophisticated multivariate mathematical models to assign patients to risk groups for whom treatment is individualized. These models are based on statistical analysis of current treatment results and often include several prognostic factors. It appears highly likely that as our understanding of the molecular biology of leukemia improves, the genetically oriented prognostic factors will gradually replace the more traditional clinical factors in assigning risk categories and designing treatment regimens. On the other hand, any prognostic factor is important relative only to the treatment currently used. If a major new treatment advance is developed, all currently used prognostic factors could lose their predictive value.

Acute Nonlymphocytic Leukemia

ANLL differs in many respects from ALL, particularly with regard to its age distribution and prognosis. While ALL is primarily a childhood disease, ANLL is primarily a disease of adults. In addition, in both children and adults, it has proven much more resistant to treatment, and in order to achieve a cure, most patients require much more intense, toxic, and myelosuppressive therapy than that required for ALL. The most successful treatment programs available today result in cure rates of no more than about one-third of all patients with ANLL. In addition, the more intense therapy results in greater morbidity and mortality, particularly in older patients, which may limit the amount of effective therapy that can be administered. Bone marrow transplants have a better-established role in the treatment of ANLL for those who have an acceptably matched donor.

Although early attempts to treat ANLL used the same drugs that had been found to be successful in ALL, the two groups of diseases are quite different in their biologic characteristics and their responses to therapy. The two most effective agents in the treatment of ANLL are cytarabine and daunorubicin. Almost all current treatment protocols administer 5 to 10 days of cytarabine by continuous infusion. Daunorubicin is administered daily for 2 or 3 days, either prior to cytarabine or simultaneously at the beginning of the cytarabine continuous infusion. This combination results in complete remissions in up to 75% of patients (31–33). However, the challenge in the treatment of ANLL is to maintain remission. Most patients who relapse do so because of resistant disease in the bone marrow; isolated extramedullary relapses are uncommon. In addition, relapses generally occur earlier than with ALL, during the first year following diagnosis. Therefore, most current treatment regimens have emphasized early intense therapy, but use a shorter duration of therapy, relative to ALL. Other drugs that may be used in the treatment of ANLL are etoposide, thioguanine, and the investigational

agents 5-azacytidine, amsacrine, and 2-chlorodeoxyadenosine.

Treatment of the CNS is of lesser importance in ANLL, since the primary reason for treatment failure is bone marrow relapse. Although lymphoblasts are found in the CSF more frequently in ANLL than in ALL, treatment of the CNS is often limited to intrathecal drugs, with irradiation administered at the end of therapy to patients with CNS disease at diagnosis. CNS treatment delivered earlier has no effect on disease-free survival, because of the inadequacy of systemic therapy and bone marrow relapses. Intrathecal therapy usually consists of methotrexate, cytarabine, and hydrocortisone.

Splenectomy has been evaluated as a treatment for ANLL and has shown no substantial therapeutic benefit and had little impact on the clinical course of the disease (34).

With the limitations of current therapy, the most promising new treatment modality available to ANLL patients is bone marrow transplant. The optimal time for a transplant is as soon as possible after achieving a clinical remission. This procedure is complicated by the occurrence of both acute and chronic GVHD, and only a limited number of ANLL patients (25 to 40%) have compatible bone marrow donors. Therefore, bone marrow transplants do not offer a universal cure for this disease.

PROGNOSTIC FACTORS

Prognostic factors for ANLL are less well-defined than for ALL, primarily because the overall survival is much poorer. Nevertheless, a number of variables have been identified that are associated with either a poor likelihood of achieving a clinical remission or a short duration of remission. These factors are summarized in Table 75.6. Variables associated with a poor prognosis are advancing age, the presence of a hemorrhage or significant infection (particularly in adults), hepatosplenomegaly, and a prolonged symptomatic interval preceding diagnosis. Like ALL, patients with a high WBC count have a poorer prognosis. In addition, the degree of bone marrow involvement, the presence of Auer rods, and elevated serum lysozyme concentrations carry a poor prognosis. Cytogenetic studies have not identified specific abnormalities that are associated with a poor prognosis, but all abnormal karyotypes are unfavorable, including presence of the Philadelphia chromosome (a classic marker for chronic myelocytic leukemia).

Supportive Therapy

The improving prognosis of acute leukemias is due in large part to the advancements in supportive care that have occurred over the past 10 years. Deaths during induction therapy caused by hemorrhage, infections, and metabolic

Table 75.6.
Adverse Prognostic Factors at Diagnosis of ANLL

Age
  >60 years
Sex
  Male
Symptomatic preleukemic interval
Treatment-induced leukemia
  Following treatment for Hodgkin's disease or other malignancy
Physical findings
  Hepatosplenomegaly
  Significant infection or hemorrhage
  Leukemia cells in the CNS
Hematologic findings
  Elevated WBC count
  Decreased hemoglobin
  Severe thrombocytopenia
  Marrow infiltration >75%
FAB morphology
  M5
Cytogenetics
  All abnormal karyotypes
  Philadelphia chromosome

derangements have been reduced as a consequence of the improved ability to manage these complications. In addition, deaths during remission caused by opportunistic infections are less frequent today, and certain types of lethal infections, notably *Pneumocystis carinii* pneumonia, have been virtually eradicated from the leukemia patient population. Use of central venous catheters has also simplified the delivery of complicated chemotherapy regimens, although these devices are associated with numerous complications of their own. The use of parenteral nutritional support has also been important in the management of these patients. All of these factors have permitted the routine use of more intense therapies in an attempt to develop effective, curative therapy for acute leukemia.

Infection in the immunosuppressed granulocytopenic cancer patients remains an important cause of morbidity and mortality. The risk of life-threatening septicemia or pneumonia increases dramatically as the patient's granulocyte count decreases and the duration of the granulocytopenia increases (35). Since immunosuppressed patients are unable to mount a response to infectious organisms, common clinical signs of infection (leukocytosis, purulence) may be absent. Therefore, fever is of supreme importance in diagnosing infections in the granulocytopenic patient, and the presence of fever in such patients should be regarded as a medical emergency. Infections that are not promptly treated progress rapidly, and death from septicemia or pneumonia may occur in a few hours. Prompt institution of empiric broad-spectrum antibiotic coverage prevents mortality in most cases.

A potentially lethal opportunistic infection for immunosuppressed patients is *Pneumocystis carinii* pneumonia. This organism is ordinarily innocuous and is found virtually everywhere in the environment. However, in immunosuppressed cancer patients, who are not necessarily granulocytopenic, this organism can produce a potentially fatal infection, and in the past it has been a major cause of death during remission for ALL patients. Low daily doses of cotrimoxazole (trimethoprim/sulfamethoxazole) administered prophylactically during remission prevented this infection in virtually all immunosuppressed ALL patients (36). Equally efficacious protection can be achieved by administering this combination for only 3 consecutive days each week (37). This reduced exposure has the advantage of fewer adverse effects, primarily the occurrence of systemic mycoses. Although neutropenia has been reported as an unwanted consequence of prophylaxis with cotrimoxazole in some studies, no difference in neutropenia was detected in this study.

Hyperuricemia is a complication of the initial antileukemic therapy in some patients, particularly those with a very high initial WBC count. A very brisk response to induction therapy results in massive cell death and the release of intracellular nucleoproteins into the circulation. The purine by-products of these nucleoproteins are metabolized by xanthine oxidase to uric acid, which in high concentrations can produce obstructive urate nephropathy. Administration of allopurinol, a xanthine oxidase inhibitor, prevents the production of uric acid and the development of nephropathy. In addition, vigorous hydration and urinary alkalinization (to increase the solubility of uric acid) should be instituted in patients with an initial high WBC count.

Because of bone marrow suppressive effects of both the disease and its therapy, most patients need extensive support with blood products, including platelet, erythrocyte, and occasionally, granulocyte transfusions. Hemorrhages, particularly, are a cause of significant morbidity and mortality in leukemia patients, and the ability to collect platelets from either whole blood or by plasmapheresis is essential in the modern therapy of leukemia. The hematocrit may be decreased as a result of decreased erythrocyte production, and packed red blood cells may be required to maintain the hematocrit at adequate levels. Granulocyte transfusions have no apparent role in the prevention of infection but may be effective in treating documented sepsis along with antibiotic therapy. However, because of the cost of preparing granulocyte transfusions, the very short life-span of transfused granulocytes in the patient, and the serious side effects of granulocyte transfusions, this procedure is usually reserved for only the most gravely ill patients.

The availability and clinical application of recombinant human hematopoietic growth factors may alter the management of infectious complications of acute leukemia in the future. Currently two such products have been approved by the FDA and are commercially available: filgrastim or granulocyte colony-stimulating factor (G-CSF) and sargramostim or yeast-produced granulocyte-macrophage colony-stimulating factor (GM-CSF). These two factors differ in their target progenitor cells. G-CSF stimulates the proliferation, maturation, and functional integrity of primarily neutrophils, whereas GM-CSF stimulates not only neutrophils, but may also stimulate eosinophils. G-CSF has been shown to reduce the number of infectious complications, days of hospitalization, and antibiotic usage associated with a number of anticancer drug regimens (38). It is currently approved for use as an adjunct for myelosuppressive chemotherapy regimens in patients with nonmyeloid malignancies. GM-CSF, on the other hand, is approved only for acceleration of granulocyte recovery in patients with non-Hodgkin's lymphoma, Hodgkin's disease, and acute lymphocytic leukemia undergoing autologous bone marrow transplantation. Neither product is approved for use in ANLL or other myeloid malignancies, because of the possibility that they may stimulate leukemic cell growth.

The administration of CSFs in conjunction with antineoplastic drugs has the potential to decrease the morbidity and mortality of standard dose chemotherapy. Of more importance, however, may be the possibility that they will permit the administration of higher, more frequent, and intensive (and potentially more curative) dosages of antineoplastic drugs. Studies are currently underway to evaluate the potential benefits, as well as adverse effects, of CSFs in ALL.

Disseminated intravascular coagulation (DIC) is an occasional but life-threatening complication of ANLL, particularly for patients with progranulocytic leukemia, and it results in severe hemorrhages. It is characterized by thrombocytopenia, hypofibrinogenemia, decreased factor V levels, and increased levels of fibrin split products.

Conclusions

Tremendous advances have been made in the treatment of the acute leukemias over the past 10 years, and the successes that have been achieved in the treatment of childhood ALL serve as a model for treatment of other human malignancies. Today acute leukemias are potentially curable diseases in many patients, and considerable prolongation of useful and productive life can be achieved for many others. Current research efforts in immunology and molecular biology are likely to lead to powerful new treatments.

CHRONIC LEUKEMIAS

Compared with acute leukemia, the leukemia cells of patients with chronic leukemia are generally mature, differentiated cells that because of unregulated growth result in an elevated white blood cell count. Chronic myelogenous leukemia (CML) and chronic lymphocytic leukemia (CLL) are the two most prevalent categories of chronic leukemia.

Clinical Presentation and Diagnosis

The clinical presentation and diagnosis for patients with CML and CLL are similar. Generally nonspecific signs and symptoms bring the patient with chronic leukemia to the physician. Some patients have symptoms of anemia, splenomegaly, or bleeding; however, an increasing proportion of patients are identified as a result of blood tests during a routine physical examination. Both the clinical presentation and the course of chronic leukemia are highly variable. The earliest clinical manifestations include insidious onset of fatigue and reduced exercise tolerance, weight loss, or abdominal discomfort or distention from organomegaly. The spleen, liver, and lymph nodes are often enlarged; occasionally, nodular skin infiltrates or other cutaneous lesions occur. Bone marrow aspirate and biopsy may be used to establish a diagnosis of chronic leukemia or to evaluate the need for therapy. Red blood cell counts are usually reduced at diagnosis because of bone marrow infiltration by leukemic white blood cells. Platelet counts are usually normal in patients with CLL, and thrombocytosis may be observed in 40% of cases of CML, although bleeding abnormalities rarely occur in chronic leukemia.

Chronic Myeloid Leukemia (CML)

CML is a clonal myeloproliferative disorder that accounts for 15 to 20% of all adult leukemias and has an annual incidence of approximately 1 per 105,000 of the population (2). CML is a disease that affects middle-aged adults with a median age of onset of 45 years. Although there is a slight male predominance (male:female ratio of 1.3:1), the course of the disease is similar regardless of sex. Ionizing radiation and heavy occupational exposure to benzene have been associated with an increased incidence of CML (39). However, neither radiation nor chemical exposure can explain the observed incidence of CML.

CML is the first malignancy that has been consistently associated with a specific acquired chromosomal abnormality, the Philadelphia chromosome (Ph) (40). The Ph chromosome is an acquired abnormality that can be found in the hematopoietic cells of all lineages and their committed progenitors in nearly 95% of patients with CML. The Ph chromosome results from a translocation of genetic material between chromosomes 9 and 22 (41). For the translocation to occur, breaks in each chromosome must occur. The break on chromosome 22 occurs in a restricted region termed the breakpoint cluster region (bcr). The break on chromosome 9 occurs within a large region of 200 kb at the 5' end of a cellular oncogene (c-abl). During formation of Ph, the c-abl oncogene is translocated to the bcr region of chromosome 22, creating a novel fusion gene that encodes for a protein of molecular weight 210 kDa (P210) (42). This protein is unique to CML and has elevated levels of tyrosine kinase activity. The P210 may play a central role in the pathogenesis of the chronic phase of CML and may provide additional insights into strategies to kill leukemic cells and spare normal hematopoietic cells.

CML is characterized by at least two phases, chronic and acute. During the chronic phase, an excessive proliferation of myeloid cells occurs without loss of their capacity to differentiate. This is followed by an acute phase, or the blast crisis, which is characterized by an uncontrolled proliferation of immature myeloid or lymphoid cells with a loss of cellular differentiation. Blast crisis has the appearance of an aggressive acute leukemia, and most patients will die of their disease within 6 months. Often, the transition from the chronic phase to the blast crisis occurs somewhat insidiously, and this intermediate phase is often referred to as the accelerated phase (43).

The highly variable course of CML has been recognized by investigators for many years. Discrimination among "good-risk" patients (i.e., Ph patients in chronic phase of CML) at diagnosis would be of great value clin-

ically. It would allow the clinician to stratify patients in clinical trails, select patients for high-risk or investigational therapy, and compare patients in different series. A variety of disease features and patient characteristics have been shown statistically to be associated with long-term survival in CML. Multivariate analysis of these factors has generated a Cox model with four variables, age, spleen size, platelet count, and percentage of circulating blasts (44). Based on these data patients can be divided into poor, average, and good risk groups, with median duration for the chronic phase of 2.5, 3.5, and 5 years, respectively. The use of this model requires confirmation in prospective studies.

The two major goals of therapy for CML are to delay the onset of blast crisis and control signs and symptoms associated with the disease. The overall treatment of patients with CML is summarized as an algorithm in Figure 75.4. The best approach to treating the patient with CML is to eradicate the Ph leukemic clone. At present no systemic therapy has been shown to consistently eradicate the Ph clone or to increase the probability of surviving without leukemia for 5 years, or "cure" CML. However, HLA-identical sibling donor bone marrow transplantation performed early in the chronic phase has lead to an actuarial probability of surviving without leukemia of 55% at 5 years, or "cure" (45). Given the present therapy for

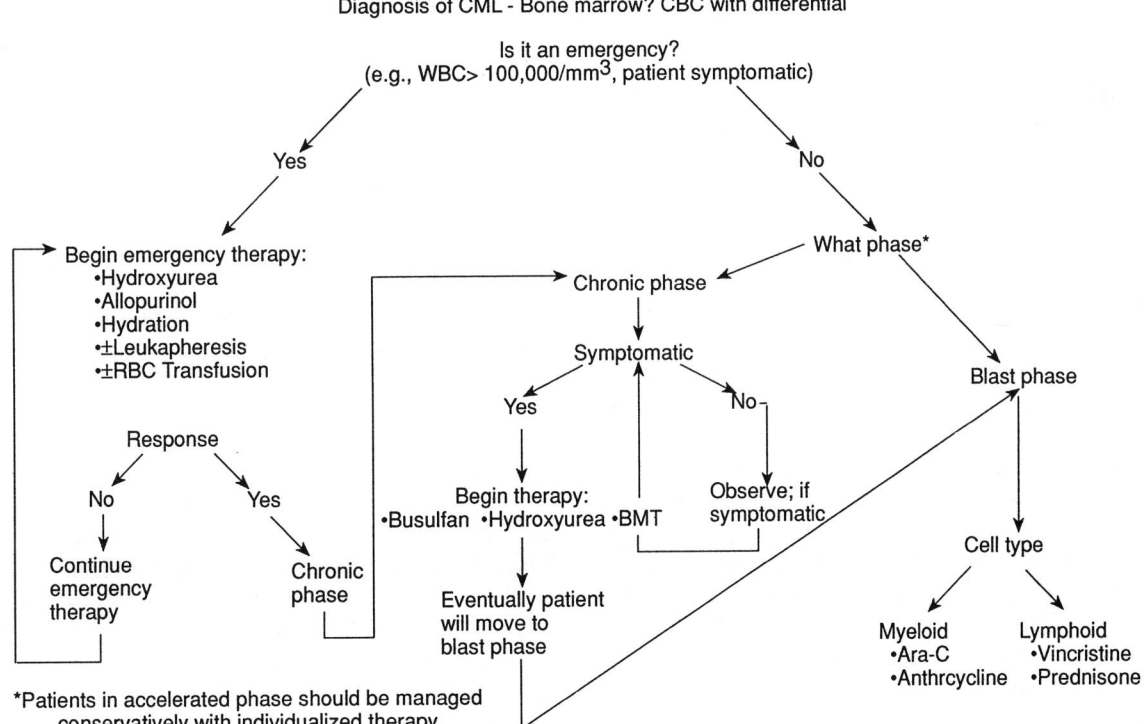

Figure 75.4.   Treatment algorithm for chronic myelocytic leukemia.

treatment of CML, it is likely that a patient may respond or achieve a "clinical remission" (i.e., normalization of blood counts and control of signs and symptoms), but Ph-positive cells may still persist in the bone marrow.

The role of splenectomy in patients with CML is unclear. No convincing data have shown that splenectomy prolongs the chronic phase of CML, increases survival, or enhances the response to chemotherapy (46). Splenectomy is generally reserved for patients who exhibit a hematologic response to chemotherapy but retain symptomatic splenomegaly or those who develop excessive thrombocytopenia with chemotherapy. Splenic radiotherapy provides palliative relief but is rarely used since one controlled study demonstrated shorter survival with splenic irradiation than with chemotherapy (47).

Leukapheresis, although tedious for the patient and time-consuming for the technical staff, is useful when chemotherapy is relatively contraindicated (e.g., pregnancy) or in emergency therapy of hyperleukocytosis. It has also been reported to be useful in obtaining adequate material for cryopreservation for subsequent autografting (48).

No convincing evidence exists to prove that maintenance of the white blood cell count within a "normal" range results in significant prolongation of the chronic phase or of survival. The initiation of therapy based solely on an arbitrary WBC count [e.g., $>50 \times 10^9$/liter ($>50,000$/mm^3)] is unjustified. Patients with CML may experience a periodic (usually every 2 months) fluctuation of the WBC count; thus, a period of observation is often warranted prior to initiating treatment. Whenever the patient with CML becomes symptomatic and cytotoxic therapy is considered, allopurinol 300 mg orally per day should be given for at least 3 to 5 days before therapy to prevent urate nephropathy. Currently therapy for the chronic phase of CML consists of a single agent, usually an alkylating agent such as busulfan or hydroxyurea.

Busulfan was one of the first chemotherapeutic agents used with success to treat CML (49), and it is still the drug of choice for intermittent therapy. Therapy is usually begun with 4 to 6 mg/day (up to 12 mg/day) of busulfan orally until the WBC has decreased to 20 to 30 $\times 10^9$/liter (20,000 to 30,000/mm^3). Busulfan affects primarily the hematologic stem cells and has a prolonged duration of effect; thus blood counts must be carefully monitored to avoid life-threatening neutropenia. If the WBC count exceeds 50 $\times 10^9$/liter (50,000/mm^3) and the patient is symptomatic, busulfan may be restarted. In some instances, pulse-dosing of busulfan (50 to 150 mg every 2 to 4 weeks) may be used to control WBC count. Toxicities related to busulfan therapy include pulmonary fibrosis, marrow hyperplasia, and a clinical picture resembling Addison's disease (46). The cumulative dose of busulfan in the first year of therapy has been shown to have prognostic importance,

since patients who receive higher doses of busulfan have a shorter survival (50). Currently, many transplant centers recommend that patients likely to receive a bone marrow transplant not receive busulfan as cytotoxic chemotherapy, because of the increased complications associated with patients receiving busulfan prior to transplant.

Hydroxyurea is an alternative to busulfan, especially when rapid reduction of white cell and platelet counts is desired (as in emergency situations of hyperleukocytosis). Hydroxyurea therapy is started with 500 mg to 2 g per day orally in divided doses. After a "clinical remission" is achieved, maintenance dosing (i.e., 20 mg/kg) is recommended to keep the WBC count between 10 to 20 $\times 10^9$/liter (10,000 to 20,000/mm^3). Hydroxyurea is usually well tolerated, and infrequent side effects include gastrointestinal symptoms, rashes, and headaches. Patients who have received busulfan as therapy for the chronic phase of CML have a higher incidence of complications associated with bone marrow transplantation. Accordingly most bone marrow transplant centers recommend that patients who might undergo bone marrow transplantation receive hydroxyurea as therapy for chronic phase CML. Other drugs with clear activity in CML include 6-mercaptopurine, 6-thioguanine, melphalan, and dibromomannitol.

Recently, recombinant human α- and γ-interferon have been investigated to determine their activity in CML. In one study, 57 patients in the chronic phase of CML were treated with recombinant human interferon-α2a, 5 $\times 10^6$ IU/m^2 IM per day (51). Of the 33 patients receiving therapy within 12 months of diagnosis, approximately 70% had a complete hematologic remission, and 42% had Ph chromosome suppression. In another study, 59 previously untreated CML patients were administered recombinant human interferon-α2b, 2 to 5 $\times 10^6$ IU/m^2 three times a week (52). After therapy for a median of 11 weeks, complete hematologic response was noted in 40 of 59 patients (68%). A dose-response relationship was noted with nine patients obtaining a response after the interferon-α2b dose was increased from 2 to 5 $\times 10^6$ IU/m^2 three times a week. In contrast to the results from studies of recombinant interferon-α2, recombinant interferon-γ has shown activity controlling symptoms and suppressing the Ph chromosome, but to a lesser extent. Interferon-γ has shown activity in patients who are resistant to interferon-α2, and patients resistant to interferon-γ have responded to interferon-α2. This is consistent with the known different mechanisms of actions and binding to different cell surface receptors. Toxicities of interferon therapy are generally mild and rarely dose-limiting. Early toxicities consist of fever, chills, and a flu-like syndrome. Serious side effects occurred in less than 10% and included anorexia and weight loss, neurotoxicity with Parkinsonian-like symptoms, immune-mediated thrombocytopenia, and other rare complications (e.g., hypothyroidism, cardiac and renal abnormalities).

Use of the interferons to treat chronic-phase CML promises to be an active area of investigation for the present and future. Important considerations for the use of interferon to treat chronic-phase CML include the slow response to therapy, requiring months for the optimal response. Early studies suggest a dose-response relationship for interferon in chronic-phase CML, suggesting that if a response is not seen at one dosage, the dosage should be escalated to either unacceptable toxicity or hematologic response. Finally, as studies are published, it will be important to identify prognostic factors for subgroups that have a better response. Currently, studies are ongoing to evaluate combined modality (chemotherapy and interferon) approach to treating chronic-phase CML. Preliminary results are encouraging, but the exact role of interferons in treating CML remains to be defined.

A number of aggressive chemotherapy regimens have been investigated for their ability to eradicate the Ph chromosome and postpone the onset of blast crisis. Although these regimens may have a slightly longer median survival than single-agent therapy, they are often associated with significant morbidity related to myelosuppression. The critical question left to be answered is when the increased length of survival is worth the increased morbidity.

Accelerated-phase CML is a loosely defined stage characterized by increased maturation arrest, proliferation, and resistance to therapy. The clinical management of the accelerated phase differs from that of the blastic phase. Many patients in the accelerated phase of CML may have a relatively indolent disease process, and conservative management is recommended (53). The therapeutic strategy should be tailored to the needs of each patient. The results of chemotherapy to treat blast-phase CML have been disappointing, even when very aggressive combination regimens are used (Table 75.7).

Although a number of regimens induce a complete hematologic response in patients with chronic-phase CML, inevitably the disease evolves into a terminal blast-crisis phase. The cellular morphology of CML blast crisis is generally myeloid (70%), but approximately 30% of patients have blasts with lymphoid characteristics such as terminal deoxynucleotidyl transferase (TdT) activity, common acute lymphoblastic leukemia antigen expression, and immunoglobulin gene rearrangements indicating a level of differentiation similar to that of pre-B-cells (54). A major advance in the therapy of blast crisis is the recognition that 50 to 60% of patients with lymphoid blast crisis respond to a regimen of vincristine and prednisone (vincristine 2 mg IV each week and prednisone usually 60 mg/m² orally daily) (55). Most clinicians agree that treatment should be continued at least 2 or 3 weeks before the patient is considered a treatment failure. The duration of remission is

Table 75.7.

Treatment of Blast-Crisis Phase in Chronic Myelogenous Leukemia

Chemotherapy Regimen[a]	# Pts	Blast Morphology	CR (%)	PR (%)	Reference
VCR/Pred	22	9 Lymphoid	56	0	(55)
		11 Myeloid	27	0	
	52	18 Lymphoid	50	0	(78)
		34 Myeloid	18	0	
	42	14 Lymphoid	71	21	(79)
		28 Myeloid	7	14	
	21	11 Lymphoid	67	0	(54)
		10 Myeloid	0	0	
TRAMPCOL	19	Not specified	42	47	(80)
HDARAC	21	Not specified	24	13	(81)
5-AZA/VP-16	27	Not specified	4	56	(82)
Plica/HU	9	3 Lymphoid	100	NR	(56)
		6 Myeloid	33	NR	

[a] VCR, vincristine; Pred, prednisone; TRAMPCOL, 6-thioguanine, danorubicin, cytarbine, methotrexate, prednisone, cyclophosamide, vincristine, L-asparaginase; HDARAC, high-dose Ara-C, cytarbine; VP-16, etoposide; 5-AZA, 5-azacytidine; Plica, plicamycin, HU, hydroxyurea.

often brief (usually 5 to 7 months, with less than 20% alive at 1 year), and maintenance therapy is usually ineffective.

Patients with myeloid blast crisis receive therapy similar to that used in patients with acute nonlymphocytic leukemia. Results from clinical trials evaluating the role of this therapy in myeloid blast-crisis CML have demonstrated a complete response rate under 30%, with median survival in responders being 6 months, compared with 2 months for patients who do not respond to therapy. Recently, another approach to treating myeloid blast crisis was proposed in which drugs with documented in vitro differentiating activity were used. In this approach, drugs were used to cause leukemia cells to differentiate into more mature stages. Specifically, six of nine patients treated with a combination of plicamycin and hydroxyurea had complete remissions, some of which were prolonged (up to 83 weeks) (56).

Although not essential to long-term survival, eradication of the leukemic clone provides the best opportunity for a patient with CML to be cured, and bone marrow transplantation theoretically provides this opportunity. The probability of long-term survival (i.e., 3-year survival) following allogenic bone marrow transplantation in chronic phase CML is 50 to 60%. In this approach intensive marrow ablative therapy is used to eradicate the Ph chromosome, and then normal hematopoiesis is restored with cells from a matched normal donor. The major side effects of this treatment approach are graft versus host disease (only in allogenic BMT) and interstitial pneumonitis. Studies suggest that the length of time from diagnosis to transplant affects the outcome (57). As many as 70% of the patients receiving a transplant within the first year after diagnosis will be long-term survivors. If the transplant is delayed 1 to 3 years, the percentage long-term survivors decreases to 40 to 50%; however, this potential benefit must be weighed against the possible risks of such a procedure and the fact that many patients can be maintained with relatively nontoxic chemotherapy in the chronic phase for months before the onset of acute phase.

In addition to the length of time from diagnosis, disease phase also affects the outcome of bone marrow transplantation. The probability of long-term survival for patients transplanted in the accelerated phase is 15 to 28%, and for patients in blast crisis long-term survival is 14 to 16% (58).

The prospects for the future for the patient with CML are much brighter, but many questions remain. It is unlikely that currently available cytotoxic therapy will contribute significantly to prolongation of life for patients with CML. Thus, the use of other therapy such as the biological response modifiers (e.g., interferon, hematopoietic growth factors), differentiating agents (plicamycin and ara-C), and combination therapy hold the promise for increased long-term survival. Questions about bone marrow transplantation remain to be answered and include timing of transplant and by what method. Autotransplants are an option for patients lacking a suitable donor, but many questions remain about the role of this modality (59). Answers to all these questions will provide prognostic variables that clinicians will use prospectively to decide upon the timing and nature of appropriate therapy for the patient with CML.

Chronic Lymphocytic Leukemia

Chronic lymphocytic leukemias are a diverse collection of B and T cell disorders that are characterized by uncontrolled growth of mature-appearing, yet functionally deficient lymphocytes. These disorders exhibit variability in clinical presentation, natural history, and response to therapy. Approximately 95% of cases of CLL are a clonal disorder of the B lymphocyte, although T cell CLL occurs in approximately 5% of cases.

CLL is the most common leukemia in the United States, with an annual incidence of 1.8 to 3 per 100,000 population (60). However, in the 55 to 59 year range the overall age-adjusted incidence increases to 5.2 per 100,000, and 30.4 per 100,000 in the 80 to 84 year range. Like CML, CLL occurs more often in men than women (2:1 to 3:1), but no racial difference in occurrence has been reported. In contrast to CML, no characteristic chromosomal abnormality is currently known for CLL.

CLL cells are probably an expansion of minor subclones of B cells that are normally present (61). CLL B cells are characterized by weak expression of SIg, lack of C3b receptors, and rosette formation with mouse erythrocytes. Approximately 90% of cases express CD5, a 67-

Kd surface protein previously believed to be a pan-T antigen, but now known to occur on small numbers of B cells normally located at the edge of the germinal center of lymph nodes in various organs (62). CD5$^+$ cells are found in other immunologic disorders and may be a target for biologic therapy. Patients with CLL progressively lose humoral immune function and become increasingly susceptible to systemic infections that are predominantly bacterial and commonly involve the respiratory tract (63). Immunologic defects identified in CLL include increased numbers of T cells and reversal of the CD4/CD8 ratio, abnormal response to mitogens, decreased helper and cytotoxic activity, excessive suppressor activity, depressed production of interleukin-2 (IL-2) by peripheral blood T cells, and decreased natural killer cell activity (64). It has been suggested that the excessive suppressor activity may limit the immunoglobulin response of residual normal B cells in CLL, eventually leading to hypogammaglobulinemia seen in as many as 75% of patients with CLL. Neutropenia from aggressive cytotoxic therapy combined with hypogammaglobulinemia are important factors responsible for increased susceptibility to infection in patients with CLL.

Parenteral γ-globulin therapy has been recommended to prevent infection in patients with CLL who are hypogammaglobulinemic (65). Prospective trials will be required before routine use of this expensive therapeutic modality can be routinely advocated for recurrent infections. Pneumococcal polysaccharide vaccines are probably not useful in patients with CLL, since many are unable to adequately respond to an antigen challenge, and a defect in complement activation may also contribute to this increased susceptibility to infections.

A major problem in the clinical management of a patient with CLL is to determine the optimal therapeutic strategy for each patient (66). This is further complicated by the highly variable course of CLL. Many patients are older (i.e., median age of onset 60 years), have only increased WBC count or asymptomatic lymphadenopathy or splenomegaly, and have no other complicating medical factors. These patients may require no therapy, and it is improbable they will die from leukemia. Compared with these patients are the patients with a rapid, progressive course (median survival <2 years). Finally, most patients fall into an intermediate group who do well for several years without therapy but eventually require specific therapy. To answer the question of "When does one begin therapy?" a staging system to identify potential prognostic factors would be helpful (67). The Rai classification is the most widely used and provides a clinically relevant staging system (68). Other staging systems receiving acceptance include the Binet system (69) and one proposed by the International Workshop of Chronic Lymphocytic Leukemia which integrated the Rai and the Binet systems (70).

Table 75.8.
Clinical Staging Criteria Used in Rai and Binet Procedures

Stage	Description
Rai system	
0	• Lymphocytosis only [>15 × 10⁹/liter (15 × 10³/mm³)]
I	• Lymphocytosis + lymphadenopathy
II	• Lymphocytosis + splenomegaly
III	• Lymphocytosis + hemoglobin <110 g/liter (11 g/dl)
IV	• Lymphocytosis + platelets <100 × 10⁹/liter (100 × 10³/mm³)
Binet system	
A	• Lymphocytosis [>15 × 10⁹/liter (15 × 10³/mm³)] plus <3 involved lymph nodes
B	• Lymphocytosis plus 3 or more involved lymph nodes
C	• Lymphocytosis plus hemoglobin <100 g/liter (10 g/dl) and platelets <100 × 10⁹/liter (100 × 10³/mm³)

Summarized in Table 75.8 are the Rai and Binet staging systems. Current approaches to staging the patient with CLL have several limitations, including failure to resolve the heterogeneity between patients with intermediate stage and prognosis, inability to identify the patient with low-stage disease who requires therapy, and lack of the use of cytogenetic and molecular biology variables.

The absolute lymphocyte count, the lymphocyte doubling time, and the pattern of bone marrow involvement has been used to predict survival (71). However, clinical stage has consistently been the most important prognostic factor in CLL. Patients with low-stage disease usually will die from causes unrelated to their disease (e.g., cardiac disease), whereas most patients with advanced disease die from disease-related causes (e.g., infection).

Progress in the management of patients with CLL has been exceedingly slow, and conventional treatment for patients who require therapy has remained relatively unchanged over the past two decades. When making treatment decisions in patients with CLL, both the aim of therapy and its potential risks and benefits must be carefully considered. Prolonging survival while maintaining quality of life is the most important aim in the therapy for CLL.

Although splenectomy has been useful in the management of hemolytic anemia, thrombocytopenia, pancytopenia, and painful splenomegaly, there is no curative role for splenectomy in CLL. Leukapheresis also may be beneficial in select patients unresponsive to traditional therapy.

Total body irradiation has been reported to improve symptoms, physical signs, peripheral blood counts, and bone marrow infiltration in a study of selected patients with advanced disease; however, because of the toxic effects observed and the specialized nature of this treatment modality, total body irradiation has limited usefulness in the management of CLL. Local radiation provides palliative relief for enlarged lymph nodes or bone lesions, and splenic radiation is useful to provide relief from painful splenomegaly, progressive lymphocytosis, anemia, and thrombocytopenia.

The traditional approach has been to delay therapy for patients with Rai stages O and I, or Binet stage A, in contrast to patients with Rai stages III-IV, or Binet stage C who are started on therapy. Patients with Rai stage II, or Binet B, are usually treated if they have evidence of active disease (e.g., weight loss >10%, night sweats, high tumor burden with splenomegaly or lymphadenopathy).

Alkylators are currently the foundation of chemotherapy for CLL, and chlorambucil is the most active and best-tolerated alkylator. Chlorambucil is administered at a dose of 6 to 14 mg orally daily, and blood counts and symptoms are checked weekly. Once the signs and symptoms leading to therapy (e.g., splenomegaly) have diminished, the dose can be decreased by 50%, and once the patient is stable the drug is discontinued altogether. No maintenance therapy is necessary. Recent studies have shown that pulse therapy with chlorambucil (i.e., 15 mg/m² every 2 weeks) has equal efficacy, with possibly reduced myelosuppression (72). The overall response rate is approximately 70%, regardless of the method of administration of chlorambucil, but only 10% are complete responses. Cyclophosphamide (100 to 200 mg orally daily) is an acceptable alternative to chlorambucil therapy, or it may be used in patients who have failed chlorambucil therapy, since cross-resistance has not been demonstrated.

Prednisone (30 to 60 mg orally daily) has been used as a single agent, particularly in patients with autoimmune hemolytic anemia or immune thrombocytopenia. However, prednisone has been used more often in combination with an alkylator, such as chlorambucil, and this combination is considered by many to be the treatment of choice.

Many intensive combination chemotherapy regimens have been evaluated in treating CLL. Most of the studies evaluating these intensive regimens have been uncontrolled and had small populations. However, recent results suggest that the combination regimen cyclophosphamide, adriamycin, vincristine, and prednisone (CHOP) in patients with advanced disease (Rai stage III, IV, Binet stage C) shows a survival advantage over cyclophosphamide, vincristine, and prednisone (COP) (73). This observation will require confirmation before it can be considered standard therapy.

Recently three purine analogs, fludarabine monophosphate, deoxycoformycin, and 2-chlorodeoxyadenosine have shown activity in patients with CLL refractory to traditional alkylator therapy. Fludarabine, the most extensively studied of these, has shown a 55 to 60% complete plus partial response rate in previously treated patients (74). More recent studies have shown an overall response rate of 79% in previously untreated CLL (75). Fludarabine combined with prednisone did not alter the response rate seen with fludarabine alone. However, most of these patients had failed prior prednisone-containing regimens, and studies are ongoing now in patients not previously treated with prednisone to determine whether adding it to fludarabine does improve response. In general, characteristics that have been reported to be associated with improved response rate with fludarabine include younger age, earlier disease stage, low white blood cell count, and normal serum albumin. Studies have shown that deoxycoformycin and 2-chlorodeoxyadenosine both have activity in treating CLL, and studies are ongoing to determine their exact role in therapy.

Eight patients, with varying stages of CLL, have received allogeneic bone marrow transplants, and seven have had durable remissions lasting from 5 to 48 months following the procedure (76). Multimodality preparative therapy with autologous bone marrow rescue using purged or unpurged marrow collected and stored while the patient was in complete remission is a therapeutic option for patients under 60 years old. One disappointing aspect of bone marrow transplantation thus far has been the failure to return to normal immune function or normal immunoglobulin levels, even in patients achieving a complete remission. This finding raises the potential for the selective use of biologic agents to reconstitute immune function.

Biological therapies to treat CLL have been used with limited success. α-Interferon has shown modest activity in previously untreated patients with early stage disease (77). Since CLL cells have characteristic membrane antigens, monoclonal antibody therapy with anti-CD5 (also known as T101) has been studied. Thus far, results have been disappointing, with responses to antibodies either alone or conjugated with immunotoxins infrequent or short-lived. The use of other antibodies (e.g., anti-B4, CD19) and conjugated immunotoxins may offer interest to this biologic approach to treating CLL.

Conclusions

The importance of the therapy of chronic leukemia lies in the fact that many of the drugs used to treat it are used orally and are dispensed on an outpatient basis. Pharmacists can counsel patients on correct usage and monitor therapy. The pharmacist should always keep current with the advances in basic sciences, which provide the basis for new and innovative therapy, and what is involved in monitoring therapy for those patients. Also pharmacists should be aware of the new advances that occur in supportive therapy, especially the use of intravenous immunoglobulin

for the prevention of infection. Increased understanding of the biology of chronic leukemia gained through the disciplines of molecular biology and immunology will translate directly to improved therapy for the patient with chronic leukemia.

REFERENCES

1. Clarkson B, The acute leukemias. In Thorn GW, Adams RD, Braunwald E, Isselbacher KJ, Petersdorf RG: Harrison's Principles of Internal Medicine, ed. 8. New York, McGraw-Hill, 1977, pp 1767–1777.
2. Anon: Cancer facts and figures—1990. American Cancer Society, 1990.
3. Gallo RD, Wong-Staal F: Retroviruses as etiologic agents of some animal and human leukemias and lymphomas and as tools for elucidating the molecular mechanism of leukemogenesis. Blood 60:545–556, 1982.
4. Altman AJ, Schwartz AD: Malignant Diseases of Infancy, Childhood and Adolescence. Philadelphia: WB Saunders, 1983, pp 187–238.
5. Bennett JM, Catovsky D, Daniel M-T, et al.: Proposals for the classifications of the acute leukemias; French-American-British (FAB) co-operative group. Br J Haematol 33:451–458, 1976.
6. Fernbach DJ: Natural history of acute leukemia. In Sutow WW, Fernbach DJ, Vietti TJ: Clinical Pediatric Oncology, ed. 3. St. Louis, CV Mosby, 1984, pp 332–377.
7. Freeman AI, Pantazopoulos N, DeCastro L, et al.: Infections in children with acute leukemia. Med Pediatr Oncol 1:67–73, 1975.
8. Champlin RE, Gale RG: Role of bone marrow transplantation in the treatment of hematologic malignancies and solid tumors: critical review of syngeneic, autologous, and allogeneic transplants. Cancer Treat Rep 68:145–161, 1984.
9. Farber S, Diamond LK, Mercer RD, et al.: Temporary remissions in acute leukemia in children produced by folic antagonist 4-amethopteroylglutamic acid (aminopterin). N Engl J Med 238:787–793, 1948.
10. Jacquillat C, Weil M, Gemon MF, et al.: Combination therapy in 130 patients with acute lymphoblastic leukemia (protocol 06 LA 66-Paris). Cancer Res 33:3278, 1973.
11. Ortega JA, Nesbit ME Jr, Donaldson MH, et al.: L-Asparaginase, vincristine and prednisone for induction of the first remission in acute lymphocytic leukemia. Cancer Res 37:535, 1977.
12. Sackman JF, Pavlovsky S, Penalver JA, et al.: Evaluation of induction of remission, intensification and central nervous system prophylactic treatment in acute lymphoblastic leukemia. Cancer 34:418, 1974.
13. Rivera GK, Raimondi SC, Hancock ML, et al.: Improved outcome in childhood acute lymphoblastic leukaemia with reinforced early treatment and rotational combination chemotherapy. Lancet 337:61–66, 1991.
14. Aur RJA, Simone JV, Hustu HO, et al.: A comparative study of central nervous system irradiation and intensive chemotherapy early in remission of childhood acute lymphocytic leukemia. Cancer 29:381, 1972.
15. George P, Pinkel D: CNS radiation in children with acute lymphocytic leukemia in remission (abstract). Proc Am Assoc Cancer Res 6:22, 1965.
16. Nesbit ME, Robison LL, Littman PS, et al.: Presymptomatic central nervous system therapy in previously untreated childhood acute lymphoblastic leukaemia: comparison of 1800 rad and 2400 rad. A report for Children's Cancer Study Group. Lancet 1:461, 1981.
17. Aur RJA, Hustu HO, Verzosa MS, et al.: Comparison of two methods of preventing central nervous system leukemia. Blood 42:349, 1973.
18. Bleyer WA, Coccia PF, Sather HN, et al.: Reduction in central ner-

vous system leukemia with a pharmacokinetically derived intrathecal methotrexate dosage regimen. J Clin Oncol 1:317–325, 1983.

19. Bleyer WA: Clinical pharmacology of intrathecal methotrexate. II. An improved dosage regimen derived from age-related pharmacokinetics. Cancer Treat Rep 61:1419–1425, 1977.

20. Freeman AI, Weinberg V, Brecher ML, et al.: Comparison of intermediate-dose methotrexate with cranial irradiation for the postinduction treatment of acute lymphocytic leukemia in children. N Engl J Med 308:477–484, 1983.

21. Evans WE, Crom WR, Yalowich JC, Methotrexate. In Evans WE, Schentag JJ, Jusko WJ: Applied Pharmacokinetics; Principles of Therapeutic Drug Monitoring, ed. 2. Spokane, Applied Therapeutics, 1986, pp 1009–1056.

22. Balis FM, Savitch JL, Bleyer WA, et al.: Remission induction of meningeal leukemia with high-dose intravenous methotrexate. J Clin Oncol 3:485–489, 1985.

23. Freeman AI, Weinberg VE, Brecher ML, et al.: Comparison of intermediate-dose methotrexate with cranial irradiation for the postinduction treatment of acute lymphocytic leukemia in children. N Engl J Med 308:477–484, 1983.

24. Evans WE, Crom WR, Abromowitch M, et al.: Clinical pharmacodynamics of high-dose methotrexate in acute lymphocytic leukemia; identification of a relation between concentration and effect. N Engl J Med 314:471–477, 1986.

25. Simone JV, Rivera G, Management of acute leukemia. In Sutow WW, Fernbach DJ, Vietti TJ: Clinical Pediatric Oncology, ed. 3. St. Louis, CV Mosby, 1984, pp 378–402.

26. Aur RJA, Simone JV, Verzosa JS, et al.: Childhood acute lymphocytic leukemia: study VIII. Cancer 42:2123, 1978.

27. Luria SE, Delbrück M: Genetics 28:491–511, 1943.

28. Goldie JH and Coldman AJ: A mathematical model for relating the drug sensitivity of tumors to their spontaneous mutation rate. Cancer Treat Rep 63:1727–1733, 1979.

29. Goldie JH, Coldman AJ, Gudauskas GA: Rationale for the use of alternating non-cross-resistant chemotherapy. Cancer Treat Rep 66:439–449, 1982.

30. Williams DL, Tsiatis A, Brodeur GM, et al.: Prognostic importance of chromosome number in 136 untreated children with acute lymphoblastic leukemia. Blood 60:864–871, 1982.

31. Lister TA, Rohatiner AZS: The treatment of acute myelogenous leukemia in adults. Semin Hematol 19:172–192, 1982.

32. Gale RP: Advances in the treatment of acute myelogenous leukemia. N Engl J Med 300:1189–1199, 1979.

33. Gale RP, Foon KA, Cline M, et al.: Intensive chemotherapy for acute myelogenous leukemia. Ann Intern Med 94:753–757, 1981.

34. Dahl G, Kalwinsky D, Kumar M, et al.: A randomized trial of splenectomy in childhood acute nonlymphocytic leukemia (ANLL) (abstract). Proc Am Assoc Cancer Res and Am Soc Clin Oncol 22:480, 1981.

35. Schimpff SC: Therapy of infection in patients with granulocytopenia. Med Clin North Am 61:1101–1118, 1977.

36. Hughes WT, Kuhn S, Chaudhary S, et al.: Successful chemoprophylaxis for Pneumocystis carinii pneumonitis. N Engl J Med 297:1419–1426, 1977.

37. Hughes WT, Rivera GK, Schell MJ, et al.: Successful intermittent chemoprophylaxis for Pneymocystis carinii pneumonitis. N Engl J Med 316:1627–1632, 1987.

38. Balmer CM: Clinical use of biologic response modifiers in cancer treatment: an overview. Part II. Colony-stimulating factors and interleukin-2. Drug Intell Clin Pharm 25:490–498, 1991.

39. Bottomley RH, Aetiology and epidemiology. In Shaw MT (ed): Chronic Granulocytic Leukemia, ed. 1. London, Praeger, 1982.

40. Nowell RC, Hungerford DA: A minute chromosome in human chronic granulocytic leukemia. Science 132:1497, 1960.

41. Rowley JD: A new consistent chromosomal abnormality in chronic myelogenous leukemia identified by quinacrine fluorescence and Giemsa staining. Nature 243:290–293, 1973.

42. Fialkow PJ, Singer JW, Chronic leukemias. In DeVita V, Helling S, Rosenberg S, (eds): Cancer, Principles and Practice of Oncology, ed. 3. Philadelphia, JB Lippincott, 1988.

43. Spiers ASD: Metamorphosis of chronic granulocytic leukemia: Diagnosis, classification and management. Br J Haematol 41:1–7, 1979.

44. Sokal JE, Baccarani M, Russo D, Tura S: Staging and prognosis in chronic myelogenous leukemia. Semin Hematol 25:49–61, 1988.

45. Goldman JM, Gale RP, Horowitz MM, et al.: Bone marrow transplantation for chronic myelogenous leukemia in chronic phase. Increased risk of relapse associated with T-cell depletion. Ann Intern Med 108:806–814, 1988.

46. Council of Medical Research for Working Party in therapeutic Trials and Leukaemia: Randomized trial of splenectomy in Ph[1]-positive chronic granulocytic leukaemia including an analysis of prognostic features. Br J Haematol 154:415, 1983.

47. Medical Research Council: Chronic granulocytic leukemia: comparison of radiotherapy and busulfan therapy. Br Med J 1:210, 1968.

48. Lowenthal RM, Buskard NA, Goldman JM, et al.: Intensive leukapheresis as initial therapy for chronic granulocytic leukemia. Blood 46:835–844, 1975.

49. Galton DAG: Myeleran in chronic myeloid leukaemia. Lancet 1:208, 1953.

50. Wareham NJ, Johnson SA, Goldman JM: Relationship of the duration of chronic phase in chronic granulocytic leukaemia to the need for treatment during the first year after diagnosis. Cancer Chemother Pharmacol 8:205, 1982.

51. Talpaz M, Kantarjian HM, McCredie K, et al.: Hematologic remission and cytogenetic improvement induced by recombinant human interferon alpha A in chronic myelogenous leukemia. N Engl J Med 314:1065–1069, 1986.

52. Morra E, Alimena G, Liberati AM, et al.: Recombinant alpha 2 interferon (r-IFNα2) in the treatment of chronic myelogenous leukemia (CML). Proc Am Soc Clin Oncol 6:145, 1987.

53. Spiers ASD: Chronic granulocytic leukemia. Med Clin North Am 68:713–727, 1984.

54. Griffin JDG, Todd RF, Ritz J, et al.: Differentiation patterns in the blast phase of chronic myeloid leukemia. Blood 61:85, 1983.

55. Marks SM, Baltimore D, McCaffrey R.: Terminal transferase as a predictor of initial responsiveness to vincristine and prednisone in blastic chronic myelogenous leukemia. N Engl J Med 298:812, 1978.

56. Koller CA, Miller DM.: Preliminary observations on the therapy of the myeloid blast phase of chronic granulocytic leukemia with plicamycin and hydroxyurea. N Engl J Med 315:1433–1438, 1986.

57. Applebaum FR: Marrow transplantation for hematologic malignancies: A brief review of current status and future prospects. Semin Hematol 25:16–22, 1988.

58. Champlin RE, Goldman JM, Gale RP: Bone marrow transplantation in chronic myelogenous leukemia. Semin Hematol 25:74–80, 1988.

59. Butturini A, Keating A, Goldman J, Gale RP: Autotransplants in chronic myelogenous leukemia: strategies and results. Lancet 335:1255–1258, 1990.

60. Surveillance Epidemiology End Results Incidence and Mortality Data: 1973–1977, NCI Monograph 57, p 10. Bethesda, MD, National Cancer Institute, 1981.

61. Freedman AS, Boyd AW, Bieber FR, et al.: Normal cellular counterparts of B-cell chronic lymphocytic leukemia. Blood 70:418–427, 1987.

62. Foon KA, Schroff RW, Bunn RA, et al.: Effects of monoclonal antibody therapy in patients with chronic lymphocytic leukemia. Blood 64:1085–1093, 1984.

63. Chapel HM, Bunch C: Mechanisms of infection in chronic lymphocytic leukemia. Semin Hematol 24:291–296, 1987.

64. Burton JD, Weitz CH, Kay NE: Malignant chronic lymphocytic leukemia B-cells elaborate soluble factors that down-regulate T-cells and NK function. Am J Hematol 30:61–67, 1989.

65. Cooperative Group for the Study of Immunoglobumin in Chronic Lymphocytic Leukemia: Intravenous immunoglobulin for the prevention of infection in chronic lymphocytic leukemia. N Engl J Med 319:902–907, 1988.

66. Mughal TI, Goldman JM: Chronic leukaemias: can they be cured? Part II: chronic lymphocytic leukaemia. Br J Clin Pract 43:353–356, 1989.

67. Foon KA, Gale RP: Staging and therapy of chronic lymphocytic leukemia. Semin Hematol 24:264–274, 1987.

68. Rai KR, Sawitsky A, Cronkite EP, et al.: Clinical staging of chronic lymphocytic leukemia. Blood 46:219–234. 1975.

69. Binet JL, Auquier A, Dighiero G, et al.: A new prognostic classification of chronic lymphocytic leukemia derived from a multivariate survival analysis. Cancer 48:198–206, 1981.

70. International Workshop on CLL: Proposal for a revised prognostic staging system. Br J Haematol 48:365–368, 1981.

71. Rai KR, Montserrat E: Prognostic factors in chronic lymphocytic leukemia. Semin Hematol 24:252–256, 1987.

72. Knospe WH, Loeb V, Huguley CM: Bi-weekly chlorambucil treatment of chronic lymphocytic leukemia. Cancer 33:555–562, 1974.

73. French Cooperative Group on Chronic Lymphocytic Leukemia: Long-term results of the CHOP regimen in stage C chronic lymphocytic leukemia. Br J Haematol 73:334–340, 1989.

74. Keating MJ, Kantarjian H, Talpaz M, et al.: Fludarabine: A new agent with major activity against chronic lymphocytic leukemia. Blood 74:19–25, 1989.

75. Keating MJ, Kantarjian H, Talpaz M, et al.: Results of therapy in previously treated (PT) and untreated (UNT) chronic lymphocytic leukemia (abstract). Blood 72(suppl 1):207a, 1988.

76. Michallet M, Corront B, Hollard D, Gratwohl A, Domingo A, Burnett S: Allogeneic bone marrow transplantation in chronic lymphocytic leukemia: report from the European Cooperative Group for bone marrow transplantation (8 cases). Nouv Rev Fr Hematol 30:467–470, 1988.

77. Rozman C, Montserrat E: Chronic lymphocytic leukaemia: when and how to treat. Blut 59:467–474, 1989.

78. Rosenthal S, Canellos GP, Whang-Peng J, Gralnick HR: Blast crisis of chronic granulocytic leukemia. Morphologic variants and therapeutic implications. Am J Med 63:542–547, 1977.

79. Janossy G, Woodruff RK, Pipard MJ, et al.: Relation of "lymphoid" phenotype and response to chemotherapy incorporating vincristing-prednisolone in the acute phase of Ph[1] positive leukemia. Cancer 43:426–434, 1979.

80. Spiers ASD, Goldman JM, Catovsky D, Costello C, Buskard NA, Galton DAG: Multiple-drug chemotherapy for acute leukemia. The TRAMPCOL regimen: results in 86 patients. Cancer 40:20–29, 1977.

81. Iacoboni SJ, Plunkett W, Kantarjian HM, et al.: High-dose cytosine arabinoside: treatment and cellular pharmacology of chronic myelogenous leukemia blast crisis. J Clin Oncol 4:1079–1088, 1986.

82. Schiffer CA, deBellis R, Kasdorf H, Wiernik PH: Treatment of blast crisis of chronic myelogenous leukemia with 5-azacytidine and VP16-213. Cancer Treat Rep 66:267–271, 1982.

CHAPTER 76

MALIGNANT LYMPHOMAS

REBECCA S. FINLEY, Pharm.D., M.S. and CLARENCE L. FORTNER, M.S.

The lymphoreticular system constitutes the anatomic basis of both cellular and humoral immunity. Lymphocytes are the principal cellular component of the lymphoreticular system and are widely distributed in the body both singly and in aggregated centers (most commonly the lymph nodes). Reticulum cells and cells of the monocyte-macrophage series are also included in this system. Lymphoid cells originate in the bone marrow, undergo differentiation, and migrate by way of the blood and lymphatic vessels to populate the other lymphoreticular tissues (Fig. 76.1). T lymphocytes are processed through the thymus gland and are responsible for cell-mediated immunity. T lymphocytes are the predominant lymphocytes in peripheral blood and occupy the deep cortex of the lymph nodes. B lymphocytes are derived from the bone marrow and confer humoral immunity. B lymphocytes constitute only 10 to 15% of circulating lymphocytes and predominate in the follicles of the lymph nodes.

Lymphoreticular malignancies may manifest in either the bone marrow and peripheral blood or in one of the centers of aggregation (Fig. 76.2). When they present as extramedullary tumors arising primarily in the lymph nodes or other sites, these tumors are referred to as malignant lymphomas; when the bone marrow is the major site of the disease, they are classified as leukemias. Malignant lymphomas are generally separated into Hodgkin's disease and non-Hodgkin's lymphomas (NHLs). The term "non-Hodgkin's lymphomas" represents multiple diseases with diverse morphologic and clinical features.

Most lymphomas can be classified by their cellular origin. The precise cellular origin of Hodgkin's disease has not yet been firmly established. It has been suggested that it is derived from an immature lymphoid stage of development that undergoes malignant transformation prior to B or T cell differentiation and that the different subtypes of Hodgkin's disease arise from different lymphoid progenitor cell lines (1, 2). In adults, most NHLs are derived from B lymphocytes, with only about 15% of T cell origin in developed countries such as the United States (3).

For unexplained reasons, the incidence of lymphomas in the U.S. appears to be rising. The American Cancer Society estimated that during 1992 there will be 7400 new cases of Hodgkin's disease and 41,000 new cases of NHL diagnosed, with 1,500 and 19,400 deaths attributed to each disease (4). The incidence of NHL increases steadily from childhood to age 80, and it is more common in males than females (5). Hodgkin's disease exhibits a bimodal incidence curve, with the first peak occurring in the late 20s, after which there is a decline in incidence until about age 45. After age 45, the incidence increases steadily with age. Hodgkin's disease is also more common in males than in females (6).

The etiology of malignant lymphomas is largely unknown. A potential infectious etiology of Hodgkin's disease has been suggested. The Epstein-Barr virus (EBV) has been indirectly associated with the disease in several ways. First, there has been a small, but consistent increased risk of Hodgkin's disease among persons who have had infectious mononucleosis (7–9). Also, many Hodgkin's disease patients have elevated titers of antibody against the EBV, and a recent study reported elevated levels of antibodies to antigens associated with EBV (10–12). EBV has also been detected in Hodgkin's disease biopsy specimens (13, 14). It is not clear whether EBV has a direct role in the development of Hodgkin's disease or whether EBV infection is a result of a decreased immune competency that is linked to the pathogenesis of Hodgkin's disease (12). Epidemiologic studies have also reported clustering of patients with Hodgkin's disease in a high school (15, 16). Overall, there is insufficient evidence to support the hypothesis that Hodgkin's disease is transmitted by person-to-person contact.

Patients with primary immunodeficiency diseases (e.g., Wiscott-Aldrich syndrome, ataxia-teleangectasia) and those receiving chronic immunosuppressive therapy (e.g., renal and cardiac transplant, chronic renal disease, inflammatory bowel disease, systemic lupus erythematosus) appear to have an increased risk of NHL (3, 17, 18). Other diseases that may predispose to the development of lymphomas include Klinefelter's syndrome, sarcoidosis, and Sjögren syndrome (3). Many cases of lymphomas have been reported in patients with the acquired immunodeficiency syndrome (AIDS) (19). Ionizing radiation may induce lymphomas, as evidenced by the increased incidence in survivors of Hiroshima and patients irradiated for ankylosing spondylitis (3, 20).

The only documented viral associations of lymphomas have been that of Burkitt's lymphoma in Africans with the EBV and the human T cell leukemia virus (HTLV-I) in adult T cell leukemia/lymphoma (21, 22).

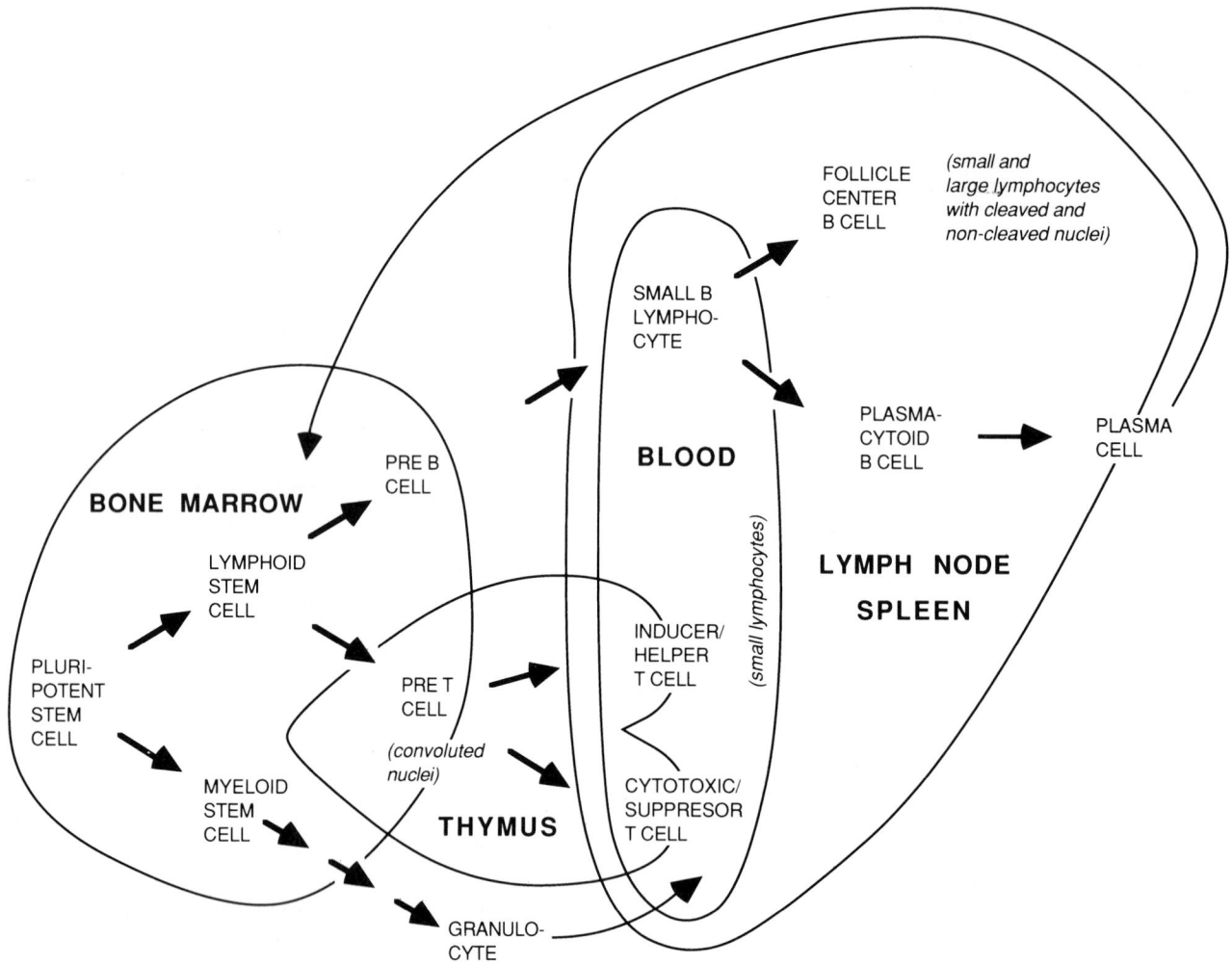

Figure 76.1. Tissue distribution of lymphocytes. (From Aisenberg AC: Cell lineage in lymphoproliferative disease. Am J Med 76:680, 1983, with permission.)

PATHOLOGY

The diagnosis and classification of malignant lymphoma can be made only by biopsy and histopathologic examination under a light microscope.

A biopsy specimen of Hodgkin's disease reveals a heterogeneous cellular population of normal-appearing lymphocytes, eosinophils, plasma cells, and Reed-Sternberg cells. These Reed-Sternberg (R-S) cells, the characteristic malignant cells of Hodgkin's disease, are multinucleated giant cells that are usually necessary to make a pathologic diagnosis. A mononuclear variant of the R-S cell, sometimes called the Hodgkin's disease cell, is also seen in some biopsy specimens (2). The histopathology of Hodgkin's disease is divided according to the Rye classification into four major subgroups (Table 76.1) (23). This classification has been widely accepted because of its simplicity, and in the past, it provided a crude correlation with prognosis, but the availability of highly curative treatments has dimin-

ished this importance (24). The lymphocyte-predominant, mixed-cellularity and lymphocyte-depleted histologies can be differentiated from one another by the increased frequency of R-S cells (25). The nodular sclerosis histology is characterized by bands of collagen that partly or completely divide the lymphoid tissue into nodules.

The lymphocyte-predominant histology is characterized by a cellular proliferation of benign-appearing lymphocytes, and at least three important subtypes exist (26). It is more common in men and most often occurs in patients under 35 years. Most patients have clinically localized disease and are asymptomatic. The prognosis is usually favorable.

The mixed-cellularity subtype contains a proportion of neoplastic cells intermediate between the lymphocyte-predominant and lymphocyte-depleted histologies. This type is also more common in older patients and in men. Patients may present in any clinical stage and often experience sys-

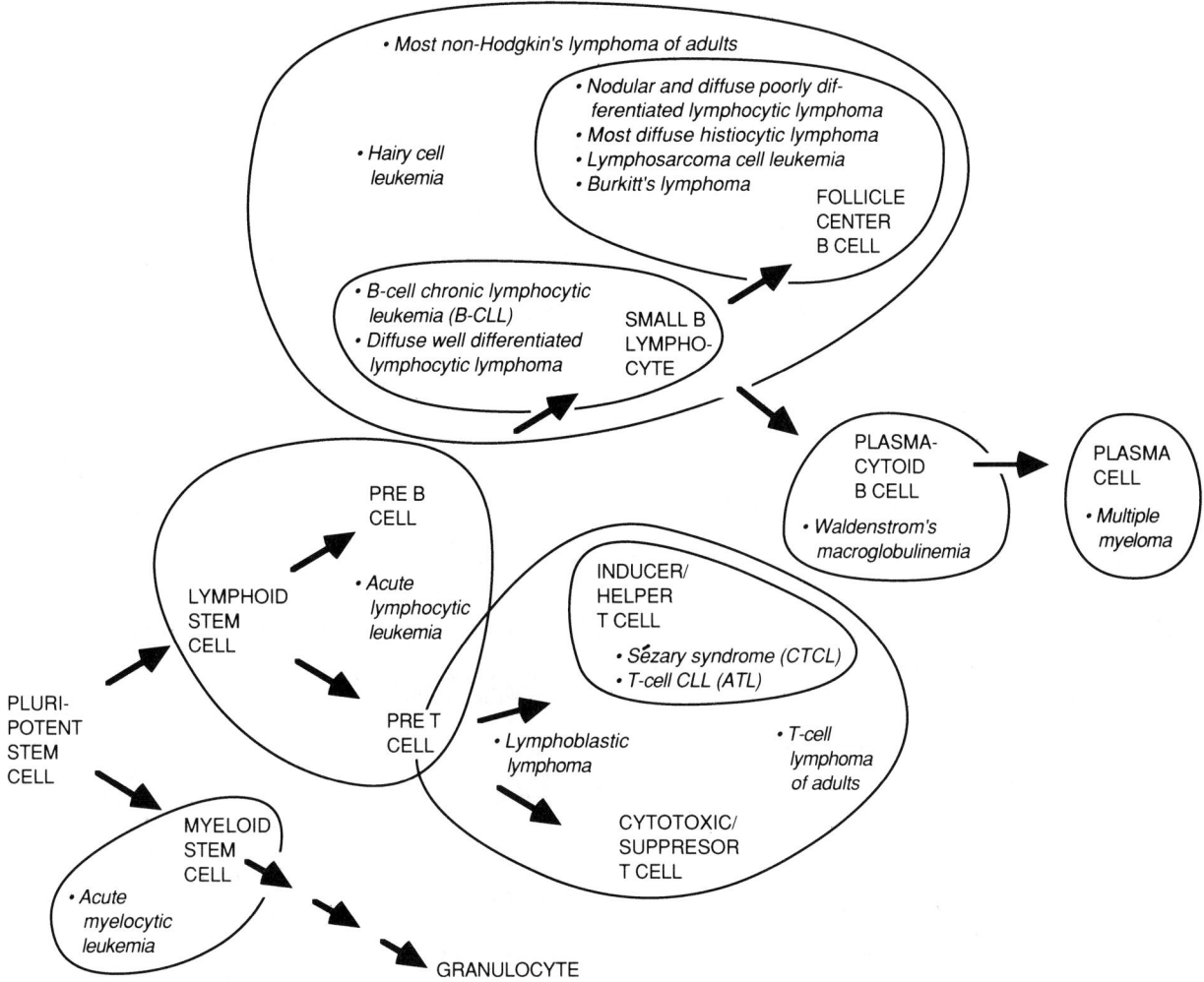

Figure 76.2. Cell lineage in lymphoproliferative disease. (From Aisenberg AC: Cell lineage in lympho-proliferative disease. Am J Med 76:682, 1983, with permission.)

temic symptoms. This histology carries an intermediate prognosis.

Lymphocyte-depleted Hodgkin's disease is characterized by a predominance of abnormal and R-S cells, with a relative paucity of lymphocytes. This subtype is most commonly seen in older patients, who often have symptomatic and disseminated disease. This is also the most common type of Hodgkin's disease seen in patients with AIDS.

Nodular-sclerosing Hodgkin's disease is more commonly found in women and most frequently occurs in adolescents and young adults. It is associated with a good prognosis, especially in localized disease.

The classification of NHLs is based on the cellular origin and immunologic characteristics of the malignant cells. Six different histologic classification systems have been used in recent years. The number of classifications used reflects the difficulties encountered in the morphologic characterization of these neoplasms. The most commonly used system in the United States is the Rappaport System (Table 76.2). This system categorizes lymphomas on the basis of morphology (diffuse, nodular), cell type (lymphocytic, "histiocytic," or mixed), and degree of differentiation. The nodular (or follicular) lymphomas localize to the follicular centers within normal lymph nodes and express characteristics of the B lymphocyte (29). Diffuse lymphomas are a more heterogeneous group of disorders, representing mixtures of both B cell and T cell neoplasms. Although the Rappaport system has provided useful distinctions in prognosis between the more indolent nodular lymphomas and the more aggressive diffuse lymphomas, it has been criticized for several reasons. Most criticism has centered around the recognition that many "histiocytic" lymphomas (based solely on morphology)

Table 76.1.
Rye Classification of Histologic Subtypes Found in Hodgkin's Disease

1. Lymphocyte predominance
   A. Lymphocytic and/or histiocytic diffuse: sinusoids of lymph nodes become filled with lymphocytic cells and general normal architecture of the lymph node becomes obscured; this picture does not occur uniformly throughout the node and normal foci may be found; the lymph node capsule is not invaded by lymphocytes in early stages of the disease
   B. Nodular proliferative type: this form differs little from the diffuse form except for the tendency of the lymphocytic cells to be placed into poorly defined large and closely arranged nodules
2. Nodular sclerosis
   This tissue type is characterized by formation of bands of connective tissue which intercommunicate and separate the cellular and necrotic areas into islands
3. Mixed cellularity
   Presents a picture between lymphocyte predominance and lymphocyte depleted and characterized by having a variable number of lymphocytes and the presence of neutrophils, eosinophils and plasma cells
4. Lymphocyte depleted
   A. Diffuse fibrosis: characterized by widespread disorderly fibrosis with depletion of lymphoid cells and eventually of all other cellular elements
   B. Reticular type: lesions in this category have no significant characteristics other than a predominance of Reed-Sternberg cells to distinguish them from other diffuse, fibrotic, mixed, or even nodular sclerotic lesions

have been shown by ultrastructural and immunologic techniques to be neoplasms of large transformed lymphocytes, and in fact, true histiocytic lymphomas are rare.

In recent years many attempts have been made to develop a new classification system that will integrate the information derived from the Rappaport system with the evolving knowledge of the functional classification of lymphocytes. From 1976 to 1980 the National Cancer Institute sponsored a multiinstitutional study in which 12 pathologists evaluated the reproducibility and comparability of the six major classification systems. It was concluded that although each of the systems had particular merits, none was clearly superior to the others. These pathologists reached a consensus (Working Formation of Non-Hodgkin's Lymphomas) to group lymphomas according to biologic aggressiveness, or grade (28).

The major groups (low-, intermediate-, and high-grade) of the Working Formulation are based primarily upon differences in survival. As in the Rappaport system, the presence of a follicular or nodular pattern remains an important prognostic indicator. These tumors are usually not rapidly proliferating, and their course is often indolent. However, they can disseminate throughout the lymphoid system and present with stage III or IV disease. Slightly less than half of the NHLs are composed of follicular his-

tologies. The natural history of some follicular lymphomas is progression to a diffuse pattern (where the lymphoma diffusely replaces the normal follicular architecture of the lymph node) as well as a shift from the small, relatively slowly proliferating cells to large, more rapidly proliferating cells. The large-cell lymphomas are composed of both B and T cell neoplasms, and although they are aggressive (they spread rapidly), they are potentially curable with intensive chemotherapy. Although the natural history of small-cell lymphomas is less aggressive than that of large cell-lymphomas (patients with low-grade lymphomas may survive for long periods of time without therapy), they are seldom completely cured with chemotherapy.

Although the large-cell lymphomas usually progress rapidly if not treated and the small-cell lymphomas gen-

Table 76.2.
Comparison of the Rappaport and "Working Formulation" Classifications for Non-Hodgkin's Lymphomas

Rappaport (27)	"Working Formulation" (28)
	Low-grade malignancy
Lymphocytic, well-differentiated	A. Malignant lymphoma: small lymphocytic consistent with chronic leukemia; plasmacytoid
Nodular (follicular) lymphocytic, poorly differentiated	B. Malignant lymphoma: follicular, predominantly small cleaved by diffuse areas; sclerosis
Nodular (follicular) mixed lymphocytic and histiocytic	C. Malignant lymphoma: follicular mixed, small cleaved and large cell sclerosis
	Intermediate-grade malignancy
Nodular (follicular) histiocytic	D. Malignant lymphoma: follicular, predominantly large-cell diffuse areas sclerosis
Diffuse lymphocytic, poorly differentiated	E. Malignant lymphoma: diffuse small cleaved cell sclerosis
Diffuse mixed, lymphocytic and histiocytic	F. Malignant lymphoma: diffuse mixed, small and large cell sclerosis, epithelioid cell component
Diffuse histiocytic (with or without sclerosis)	G. Malignant lymphoma: diffuse large cell cleaved cell, noncleaved cell sclerosis
	High-grade malignancy
Diffuse histiocytic (with or without sclerosis)	H. Malignant lymphoma: large cell, immunoblastic plasma cytoid clear cell polymorphous epithelioid cell component
Lymphoblastic (with or without convoluted cells)	I. Malignant lymphoma: lymphoblastic convoluted cell, nonconvoluted cell
Diffuse, undifferentiated (Burkitt's and non-Burkitt's type)	J. Malignant lymphoma: small cleaved, Burkitt's tumor; follicular areas
	K. Miscellaneous: composite mycosis fungoides, histiocytic, extramedullary plasmacytoma

erally have a more indolent course, Burkitt's lymphoma, which is composed of noncleaved small cells, is an exception to this principle and carries a poor prognosis. Burkitt's lymphoma is of B lymphocyte origin and has been recognized as a clinicopathologic entity for many years. In the United States, Burkitt's lymphoma accounts for less than 5% of NHL. Although a definite association of Burkitt's lymphoma in African children with EBV has been established, EBV-positive tumors are rare in Americans.

T cell NHL are far less common than B cell lymphomas, especially in adults. Tumors of differentiated T cells frequently arise in the lymph nodes and skin (e.g., mycosis fungoides and Sézary syndrome) or may be widespread (i.e., T cell leukemia). The cellular appearance of T cell malignancies varies and may include cytologic types ranging from small, atypical lymphoid cells to large and often convoluted lymphoid cells. Mycosis fungoides, a cutaneous T cell lymphoma, is characterized by proliferation of mature T cells (helper or inducer cells). Its prognosis is related to the stage of the disease, with most patients having a chronic course. The Sézary syndrome is closely related to mycosis fungoides and generally represents a leukemic phase.

Lymphoblastic lymphoma represents less than 10% of NHLs and is closely related to T cell acute lymphoblastic leukemia. It is more common in adolescents and young adults, and without very aggressive treatment, it has a poor prognosis. About one-half of lymphoblastic lymphomas are characterized morphologically by convoluted nuclear configurations.

PRESENTATION AND NATURAL HISTORY

Most patients with malignant lymphomas have superficial lymphadenopathy. Although superficial lymphadenopathy in adults is most frequently related to an acute infectious process, discrete hard lymph nodes, particularly if they are fixed or matted, should be biopsied. The cervical nodes are the most common site of presentation in Hodgkin's disease (65 to 80%), but this presentation is less common in NHL (30 to 40%). Twenty to 35% of patients with NHL have disease only outside the lymph nodes. Most of these lymphomas exhibit a diffuse histologic pattern. The most commonly involved extranodal site is the head and neck area, followed by the gastrointestinal tract. Other primary extranodal sites include the skin, central nervous system, liver, lung, testes, and bone marrow. When bone marrow involvement occurs, half of the patients show variable degrees of blood invasion (30).

Hodgkin's disease is believed to be unifocal in origin, probably beginning with a single cervical or retroperitoneal lymph node. Spread occurs to adjacent nodes via lymph channels and either by direct extension into adjacent organs or by blood vessel invasion with dissemination to the spleen, bone marrow, liver, bone, and other organs.

Lymph node involvement begins with a few malignant cells surrounded by normal lymphocytes. As the disease progresses, there is a tendency toward a worsening of the histology, with depletion of normal lymphocytes, an increased number of malignant cells, destruction of the lymph node architecture, and onset of symptoms. Effective therapy may interrupt this progression.

In NHL, with disease initially confined to the lymph nodes, there is a tendency to spread to contiguous lymphatic sites or occasionally, to adjacent extranodal sites. In contrast to Hodgkin's disease, NHL spreads more rapidly to distant nodal and extranodal sites via the blood stream, similar to the metastatic dissemination of many other tumors. Presentation of NHL depends on the histology of the disease. Low-grade NHL may initially present with slowly progressive, nontender peripheral lymphadenopathy that may wax and wane spontaneously, while intermediate- and high-grade NHL generally progress steadily.

In rare cases, Hodgkin's disease may present with massive mediastinal adenopathy causing superior vena cava obstruction with headache; congestion of the face; subcutaneous edema involving face, neck, and thorax; and cough and dyspnea (see "Complications" below). Lymphoblastic lymphoma may also present with mediastinal adenopathy, which may also produce vena cava obstruction. NHL, and less commonly Hodgkin's disease, may present with massive retroperitoneal adenopathy that may obstruct the ureters or the inferior vena cava, giving rise to ascites and edema in the lower extremities.

An initial presentation 20% of lymphocytes with NHL and 30 to 40% of patients with Hodgkin's disease experience systemic or constitutional symptoms (fever, night sweats, weight loss, and pruritus). These symptoms may develop about the same time as the lymph node enlargement or may occasionally precede the detection of adenopathy. These symptoms generally subside rapidly with treatment, and their appearance at any time in the course of the disease represents an unfavorable prognostic sign. In patients with Hodgkin's disease, the frequency of systemic symptoms increases with the stage of disease and unfavorable histology.

Lymphomas Associated with the Acquired Immunodeficiency Syndrome

Since the AIDS epidemic began in 1981, the number of reports of lymphoma in patients with AIDS and the AIDS-related complex (ARC) has steadily increased. Currently, about 5% of AIDS patients have been diagnosed with lymphoma (31). This is not unexpected because various other immunodeficiency disorders have also been associated with an increased incidence of lymphomas (3, 17, 18). Non-Hodgkin's lymphomas of several histologic types, including Burkitt's lymphoma (32), immunoblastic lymphoma (33), and lymphoblastic lymphoma (34) as well as

Hodgkin's disease (35), have been reported in patients with AIDS (19); however, most patients have had high-grade, B cell lymphomas. Early reports indicated that many of these lymphomas presented at advanced stages, with unusual clinical features including prodromal manifestations, a high frequency of extranodal and central nervous system involvement, and an unusually poor prognosis with respect to the histologic subtypes (19). In 1985, the Centers for Disease Control (CDC) amended its case definition of AIDS to include patients with high-grade, B cell non-Hodgkin's lymphoma and documented HIV infection (36).

In a series of NHLs in 90 homosexual men, 62% of the lymphomas were high grade, 29% were immediate grade and 7% were low grade (19). In 46% of these patients, the diagnosis of AIDS preceded the recognition of the lymphoma, and an additional 15% of patients developed AIDS following the diagnosis of the lymphoma. All but 2 of these patients had extranodal involvement. Thirty-eight patients (42%) had involvement of the central nervous system, and 30 patients (33%) had bone marrow involvement. These frequencies are far in excess of that expected in de novo NHL. The response to treatment and survival in this series was poor in comparison with treatment results in other patients with similar types of lymphoma. Many other reports have now confirmed that the lymphomas in AIDS are highly aggressive and frequently involve extranodal sites including the CNS, gastrointestinal tract, bone marrow, liver, lung, rectum, heart, bile duct, and pleura (35). It has been estimated that up to 25% of HIV-associated NHL are confined to only the CNS.

DIAGNOSIS AND STAGING

Decisions about appropriate therapy for a patient with a lymphoma depend upon the correct morphologic diagnosis and accurate assessment of the extent of disease. Diagnosis of malignant lymphoma requires histopathologic confirmation of lymph node biopsy. When lymphadenopathy is present, one or more complete nodes must be excised. Needle biopsies are generally not adequate. When primary extranodal lymphoma presents with regional or distant adenopathy, both sites should be examined histologically to ensure a correct diagnosis. When the primary disease is only extranodal in certain sites (e.g., stomach, breast, testicle), a diagnosis of carcinoma is often made on clinical grounds, and NHL is discovered from the surgical pathology.

Staging systems have been developed to facilitate therapeutic planning and communication of data about the natural history of the disease and treatment outcomes. The Ann Arbor staging system (Table 76.3) was developed for use in Hodgkin's disease, but it has also been used for staging NHL. In Hodgkin's disease this system has been reproducible and predictive of response to therapy. The

Table 76.3.
Ann Arbor Classification for the Staging of Hodgkin's Disease[a]

Stage I: Disease involvement of a single contiguous lymph node region (I) or of a single localized extralymphatic organ or site (I_E) on the same side of the diaphragm

Stage II: Disease involvement of two or more contiguous lymph node regions on the same side of the diaphragm (II) or localized involvement of an extralymphatic organ or site and of one or more lymph node regions on the same side of the diaphragm (II_E); an optional recommendation is that the number of node regions involved be indicated by a subscript (e.g., II_3)

Stage III: Disease involvement of lymph node regions on both sides of the diaphragm (III), which may also be accompanied by localized involvement of an extralymphatic organ or site (III_E) or by involvement of the spleen (III_S), or both (III_{SE})

Stage IV: Diffuse or disseminated disease involvement of one or more extralymphatic organs or tissues with or without associated lymph node enlargement. The extralymphatic sites of involvement should be identified by symbols.

[a] Each stage is subdivided into A (asymptomatic) and B (symptomatic). Symptoms are (a) weight loss greater than 10% of body weight, (b) unexplained fever with temperature above 38°C (100.4°F), and (c) night sweats.

Ann Arbor Classification is divided into four stages, and each stage is further subdivided into A (asymptomatic) and B (symptomatic) groups. As the disease progresses from stage I to stage IV, the prognosis becomes worse. The presence of symptoms (designated B) confers a worse prognosis. The clinical symptoms associated with Hodgkin's disease are general rather than specific; they are unexplained weight loss of more than 10% of the body weight, unexplained fever with temperature above 38°C (100.4°F), and night sweats. A patient may experience additional symptoms such as pruritus or alcohol-induced pain, but they generally do not correlate with the severity of disease and are not considered in the staging evaluation.

In patients in whom localized extranodal disease is contiguous to involved lymph nodes (often in the lungs or vertebrae adjacent to involved lymph nodes), staging is based on the appropriate lymph node involvement followed by the subscript "E," which denotes direct extension. These patients have a more favorable prognosis than those with clearly disseminated (stage IV) disease. In general, the "E" designation is used in patients with extranodal disease so limited in extent and location that it can be easily irradiated.

The diaphragm has key significance in the staging of Hodgkin's disease. It is the reference point from which the extent (or stage) of Hodgkin's disease is measured. If the disease is confined to lymph nodes on only one side (above or below) of the diaphragm, the disease is considered to be localized, and the prognosis is generally better than if the disease were more disseminated and present on both sides of the diaphragm.

Table 76.4.
Staging Procedures for Hodgkin's Disease and Non-Hodgkin's Lymphomas

Required procedures
1. Detailed history with special attention to the presence (and duration) or absence of systemic symptoms (i.e., fever, unexplained sweating, unexplained weight loss)
2. Careful physical examination with special attention to all lymph node areas
3. Adequate surgical biopsy review by an experienced hemopathologist
4. Routine laboratory tests including complete blood count, erythrosedimentation rate, liver and renal function tests, serum uric acid
5. Radiologic examination of the chest, gastrointestinal tract, and skeletal system of any areas of bone tenderness
6. Bilateral bone marrow biopsy
7. Computed tomography (CT) scan of chest
8. Abdominal computed tomography scan

Procedures necessary under certain circumstances
1. Bilateral lower extremity lymphography
2. Exploratory laparotomy and splenectomy

Procedures necessary for accurate clinical staging of Hodgkin's disease are listed in Table 76.4. A detailed patient history is obtained, making note of the presence or absence of symptoms, and a thorough physical examination must be performed, giving particular attention to areas of bone tenderness and the size of the liver and spleen. Laboratory tests and procedures that are conducted are designed to detect any clinical abnormality that may implicate a specific organ or organ system invaded by Hodgkin's disease. Further pathologic staging is then necessary to definitively diagnose Hodgkin's disease is tissues that have been implicated by the clinical staging procedures. Pathologic staging involves biopsy and microscopic examination of the suspicious tissue. More aggressive staging techniques have included exploratory laparotomy and splenectomy. In the past, these procedures have made tremendous contributions in staging accuracy and knowledge of the natural history of Hodgkin's disease; however, the role of staging laparotomy is under reevaluation, and computerized tomography (CT) and magnetic resonance imaging (MRI) are now the most commonly used procedures for evaluation of the abdomen. Current recommendations specify that laparotomy should be performed only if management decisions depend upon the identification of abdominal disease, and in some of these situations, laparoscopy combined with needle marrow biopsies may substitute for this procedure. Laparotomy is of most value in identifying patients eligible for treatment with radiation therapy alone (i.e., patients with negative laparotomy results). If systemic chemotherapy is already considered essential to the patient's management, based on noninvasive studies, then staging laparotomy becomes superfluous. Although the overall morbidity is low, laparotomy plus splenectomy increases the risk of sepsis from encapsulated

organisms (i.e., *Streptococcus pneumoniae*, *Haemophilus influenzae*), varicella zoster infection, and bowel obstruction resulting from adhesions among the intestinal loops. Therefore, the decision to perform such a staging procedure must be carefully weighed, especially because a CT or MRI scan is easy to administer and noninvasive.

The distribution of Hodgkin's disease (at initial diagnosis) is stage I, 13%; stage II, 38%; stage III, 35%; and stage IV, 14% (37). Data collected over the years have revealed some interesting statistics regarding the correlation of the clinical stage of Hodgkin's disease with histologic tissue type. Patients with the lymphocyte-predominant variety have a strong association with clinical stages I and II, whereas the lymphocyte-depleted variety is seen mainly in patients with clinical stages III and IV. The mixed-cellularity variety occurs in all clinical stages of the disease, without any strong correlations. The nodular-sclerosis variety is seen primarily in patients with clinical stage II disease and is the one histologic subtype that presents with a distinctive anatomical pattern of distribution, namely, a predilection to involve the lower cervical lymph nodes and mediastinum (38). The lymphocyte-predominant, lymphocyte-depleted, and mixed-cellularity types exhibit a variable propensity for anatomical involvement when compared within the same clinical stage.

Non-Hodgkins Lymphoma

Non-Hodgkin's lymphomas are not as predictable in their patterns of involvement, nor do they reflect discrete changes in their prognosis with changes in stages, as seen with Hodgkin's disease. In spite of these limitations, the Ann Arbor staging system has been widely used in defining patient groups in clinical trials, and it will continue to be used until a more satisfactory system is developed (39). In contrast to those with Hodgkin's disease, patients with NHL are more likely to have disseminated disease, so local therapeutic options such as surgery and radiation therapy are less commonly used. Therapeutic options in NHL are more likely to be limited by the advanced age or concomitant illnesses of the patient. Because of the divergent clinical features of patients with NHL, no rigid or routine staging plan is appropriate for all patients. Many of the staging procedures used in Hodgkin's disease (Table 76.4) are used for the NHLs, although they are less applicable because of the high prevalence of extranodal disease. These staging procedures should be considered carefully with regard to the histologic subtype, the individual patient, and the anticipated and available therapy. Extensive staging procedures should be reserved for clinical trials or for patients in whom a specific therapeutic alternative, such as radiation therapy, is available.

As in Hodgkin's disease, a thorough physical examination and routine laboratory tests are aimed at the detection of potential sites of involvement. Although the bone marrow is frequently involved in NHL, peripheral blood abnormalities are uncommon. Bilateral bone marrow aspirations and biopsies are generally indicated in follicular lymphomas or clinically advanced diffuse histologies. The frequency of bone marrow involvement ranges from 5 to 15% in patients with diffuse "histiocytic" lymphoma (DHL) to 55 to 85% of patients with nodular, poorly differentiated lymphoma (NPDL). Although relatively uncommon in DHL, bone marrow involvement may predict central nervous system involvement, and patients with this finding should receive a lumbar puncture with examination of the cerebrospinal fluid.

Gastrointestinal studies are indicated in patients with abdominal symptoms or masses and in patients with nasopharyngeal lymphomas, to obtain prognostic information, to plan therapy, and to establish involvement or impending obstruction of the gastrointestinal or genitourinary tract. Although lymphangiography has been widely used for assessment of retroperitoneal and intraabdominal disease, computed tomography scanning has replaced this procedure to a large extent. As in Hodgkin's disease, there is no justification for routine staging laparotomy, and this procedure should be used only when it will influence management decisions.

TREATMENT

The treatment of malignant lymphomas centers mainly around radiation therapy and chemotherapy. Surgery, although useful in the management of many other malignancies, does not play a major role in the therapy of lymphomas. Today the only roles for surgery in lymphomas are (a) initial staging and diagnostic procedures; (b) relief of obstruction related to localized lymph node enlargement not responding to therapy; (c) management of a gastrointestinal lymphoma, to reduce the rate of perforation or hemorrhage; and (d) management of complications of lymphomas, such as hypersplenism.

Lymphomas were recognized early as being very responsive to radiation therapy, and until the end of the 1960s, radiation therapy was the only successful modality that could, under appropriate circumstances, achieve cure in some malignant lymphomas. Although radiation therapy has been used since the early 1900s, it was not until the 1950s, the era of megavolt radiation (using ^{60}Co and linear accelerators), that the use of large fields, exposing entire lymph node chains to radiation in the range of 3500 to 4000 rads ("rad" stands for radiation absorbed dose and equals 100 ergs/g tissue) was possible. With these advances in technique, the therapeutic results of patients with all types of lymphomas have improved progressively.

Radiation therapy essentially has the same effect on cellular biochemistry as do the alkylating agents used in chemotherapy. Deoxyribonucleic acid (DNA) replication is prevented by interfering with cross-links necessary to maintain the double-helix DNA molecule. Proliferating tissue, characteristic of malignancies, is especially radiosensitive because of its constant DNA production necessary for cell division. The epithelial lining of the gastrointestinal tract is also rapidly dividing tissue and frequently encountered side effects with radiation therapy are radiation-induced pharyngitis, esophagitis, and gastroenteritis. The rapid production of cells in the bone marrow makes this site very susceptible to radiation-induced bone marrow suppression. It is therefore important that vital, uninvolved organs and viscera be shielded during radiation therapy to minimize radiation-induced toxicities.

Possible radiation fields used for the treatment of lymphomas are described in Table 76.5 and Figure 76.3.

The use of drugs in the management of neoplastic diseases was developed after the end of World War II, and lymphomas, and leukemias were among the first tumors to respond to such chemotherapy. In general, with single-agent chemotherapy, the complete response rate has rarely exceeded 20 to 30%, so the treatment of lymphomas relies upon the use of drug combinations. Combination chemotherapy uses drugs with different mechanisms of action that attack proliferating cells at different stages of cell replication.

Although the great majority of cytotoxic drugs can produce objective response in lymphomas, it was only in 1970 with the four-drug regimen known as MOPP (mechlorethamine, vincristine, procarbazine, and prednisone) that DeVita et al. showed that chemotherapy could induce a

Table 76.5.
Radiation Therapy Fields Used in the Management of Lymphomas

Mantle: Encompasses mediastinal, hilar, and bilateral supraclavicular, infraclavicular, cervical, and axillary node chains, with lead shields shaped to lungs, heart, and spinal cord

Inverted-Y: Encompasses splenic or splenic pedicle, para-aortic, iliac, inguinal, and femoral node chains, with lead shields for rectum and bladder, iliac and upper femoral bone marrow, and "gap" at junction with mantle fields

Para-aortic/hepatic: Encompasses splenic hilar and para-aortic node chains and entire right lobe of liver, usually joined across another "gap" by a separate pelvic field

Waldeyer: Encompasses preauricular nodes and lymphatic tissues of Waldeyer's ring when clinically involved or when adenopathy is present in high cervical nodes.

Total nodal: Encompasses all lymph node regions above the diaphragm (cervical, supra- and infraclavicular, axillary, mediastinal) and all lymph node regions below the diaphragm (periaortic, retroperitoneal, inguinal, and splenic regions

Subtotal nodal: Encompasses the mantle plus para-aortic, spleen and pedicle fields

Involved field: Encompasses only the known involved sites

Extended field: Encompasses known involved sites plus contiguous uninvolved regions

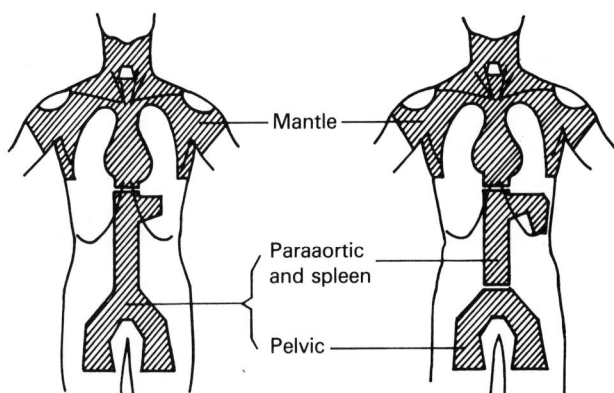

Figure 76.3. "Mantle" and "Inverted Y" radiation fields used in the management of lymphomas. (From Rosenberg S, Kaplan HS: Hodgkin's disease and other malignant lymphomas. Calif Med 113(4):23–38, 1970, with permission.)

Table 76.6.
Criteria for Treatment Response

Complete remission (CR): Disappearance of all signs and symptoms of the disease; includes the return to normal of all previously abnormal parameters and a negative second biopsy of known involved extranodal sites

Partial remission (PR): A reduction of more than 50% in the product of the longest perpendicular diameters of all measurable lesions

Minimal response (MR) or no change: A reduction of less than 50% in the product of the longest perpendicular diameters of all measurable lesions

Treatment failure (TF): Increase in size of any lesion and/or appearance of new lesion(s)

high rate of complete remission in advanced Hodgkin's disease (40). Later, the ability of chemotherapy to produce long-term remissions (compatible with cure) in Hodgkin's disease and certain NHL histologies was confirmed.

After radiation therapy or chemotherapy has been administered to a patient with lymphoma, the patient's response to treatment must be assessed to evaluate both its efficacy and its duration. Standard criteria are generally used for the objective evaluation of treatment response (Table 76.6) so that various therapies may be compared in a consistent manner. Objective reduction of the disease manifestations usually begins within the first month after the start of treatment. However, this depends on the histologic type of lymphoma and is usually more rapid in Hodgkin's disease than in NHL.

Selection of the appropriate type of therapy depends upon confirmation of the histologic subtype and the extent of the disease, as well as any patient-specific factors (e.g., age, concomitant illness) that may influence the patient's ability to withstand treatment. With few exceptions, the initial approach to management of malignant lymphomas

must have curative intent, regardless of disease extent and histologic type.

Hodgkin's Disease

EARLY STAGE (I, II, III$_A$)

Stage I and II are very amenable to radical radiation therapy (i.e., high doses of radiation with curative intent), because the disease is present in a few well-defined, focal areas, not disseminated, and can be effectively treated with radiation therapy (41). Treatment may be limited to the known involved sites (involved field, IF), given to only the known involved sites plus contiguous uninvolved regions (extended field, EF), or delivered to all major lymphoid regions (total nodal irradiation, TNI). It is generally recommended that local tumor masses receive "boost therapy" to a minimum dose of 4000 to 4400 rads, whereas apparently uninvolved areas treated for subclinical disease appear to be controlled adequately with doses of 3000 to 3500 rads. One hundred fifty to 220 rads/day are usually administered 5 days each week, so the duration of treatment is 4 to 6 weeks.

Using either TNI of subtotal nodal irradiation (sTNI), the 5-year relapse-free survival rate (which is often equated to cure) in patients with stages I and II is 75 to 90%. If only the IF is irradiated, the response rate has been poorer (38%) than with TNI, although overall survival was comparable at 5 years (90%) because most patients who relapse after radiation respond to chemotherapy (42). sTNI is not associated with significantly more toxicity than IF, although it dramatically improves relapse-free survival; therefore this technique is generally the standard approach for stages I and II. Systemic symptoms, age, histologic subtype, and limited extranodal extension do not appear to affect the prognosis of stage I and II patients treated with radiation (43). The presence of a large mediastinal mass does appear to adversely affect relapse-free survival when treated with radiation therapy alone (44). Therefore, some investigators advocate the use of chemotherapy plus local irradiation initially, whereas others believe that chemotherapy should be reserved for those who do relapse following radiation (37).

Some evidence indicates that treatment of early-stage disease with chemotherapy alone is at least as effective as radiation therapy. When patients with stages I$_B$, II$_A$, or III$_A$ disease were randomized to receive either radiation or MOPP chemotherapy, Longo et al. reported a CR rate of 96% in each arm of the study. At a median follow-up of 7.5 years, 35% of patients in the radiation group and 13% of patients who received MOPP therapy had relapsed. The projected 10-year disease-free survival for radiation therapy patients is 60%, versus 86% for MOPP-treated patients (p = .009), although overall survival was not significantly different (45). Chemotherapy has certain advantages. Systemic chemotherapy eliminates the need for the patient to undergo a laparotomy or splenectomy and the associated morbidity. However, the acute toxicities associated with chemotherapy may be worse than those associated with radiation. Further follow-up of this and similar trials is necessary to assess late and chronic treatment-related side effects.

For patients with stage III$_A$ disease the 5-year relapse-free survival when treated with radiation alone is only 35 to 66%, although overall survival ranges from 80 to 92% at 5 years, emphasizing the effectiveness of salvage treatment (37). Currently, it is believed that radiation therapy alone is inadequate in stage III$_A$ and that combination chemotherapy is the treatment of choice (46). Several clinical studies have reported improved relapse-free survival with the use of chemotherapy plus radiation (47–49). Other studies suggest that combined modality therapy is not superior to chemotherapy alone (50, 51). In addition, combined modality therapy is associated with more toxicity (52).

STAGES III$_B$ AND IV

Chemotherapy with or without radiation therapy is the treatment of choice for patients with stage III$_B$ or IV Hodgkin's disease. Stage IV disease is not well suited for radiation therapy, since sites of the disease in this stage may be so numerous and diffuse that localized radiation cannot be effectively carried out. Parenchymal organs cannot tolerate curative doses of radiation, and the presence of Hodgkin's disease in these areas precludes the use of radical radiation. Stage IV disease is therefore treated primarily with systemic chemotherapy, which has access to all sites of disease. "Spot" radiation is also used in stage IV disease for palliative treatment to anatomical areas of disease involvement not responding to chemotherapy and causing pain, tenderness, or obstruction.

A drug combination that has been very successful in obtaining the induction of remissions in Hodgkin's disease is MOPP (mechlorethamine or Mustargen, vincristine or Oncovin, prednisone, and procarbazine). Pioneered by DeVita et al. (40). MOPP therapy has endured and is considered by many to be a valuable front-line chemotherapy for Hodgkin's disease (53, 54) (Table 76.7). After 20 years of experience with this regimen at the NCI, 159 of 198 patients (80%) achieved a complete remission, with 54% of these patients remaining disease-free at 20 years. MOPP therapy is given in cycles that repeat every 28 days. Patients should receive a minimum of six complete cycles of therapy at maximally tolerated doses. When they are considered to be in complete remission, which must be determined by appropriate restaging, two more cycles of chemotherapy should be given. Once complete remission has been achieved, there is no real advantage in prolonging treat-

Table 76.7.
MOPP Regimen with Dosing Adjustments

Mechlorethamine	6 mg/m^2 IV	Days 1 and 8
Vincristine (Oncovin)	1.4 mg/m^2 IV	Days 1 and 8
Procarbazine	100 mg/m^2 p.o.	Days 1 through 4
Prednisone[a]	40 mg/m^2 p.o.	Days 1 through 14, cycles 1 and 4 only
	Repeat cycle every 4 weeks	
	Six cycles minimum	

WBC Count	Platelet Count	Dose Adjustment
≥4000/mm^3	100,000/mm^3	100% all drugs
3000–4000/mm^3	100,000/mm^3	100% vincristine, 50% procarbazine and mechlorethamine
2000–3000/mm^3	50,000–100,000/mm^3	100% vincristine, 25% procarbazine and mechlorethamine
1000–2000/mm^3	50,000/mm^3	50% vincristine, 25% procarbazine and mechlorethamine
<1000/mm^3	50,000/mm^3	No therapy

[a] No dosage adjustment required.

ment or administering any type of maintenance therapy. Similar chemotherapy regimens have yielded comparative results and toxicities (Table 76.8). In addition to MOPP and MOPP derivatives, other novel combination chemotherapy regimens have shown similar efficacy when used as first-line therapy. Bonadonna et al. first described the ABVD regimen (doxorubicin or Adriamycin, bleomycin, vinblastine, and dacarbazine) (Table 76.8) in patients who had relapsed following MOPP (55). Following their positive results, they undertook a prospective study to evaluate MOPP versus MOPP alternating with ABVD.

Goldie and Coldman proposed that during treatment malignant cells may mutate and become resistant to therapy (60). The use of alternating, non-cross-resistant chemotherapy regimens has been suggested as a possible means of improving the complete response rate and lengthening the median duration of disease-free survival by exposing tumor cells to an increased number of cytotoxic drugs. This strategy offers the possibility of reducing treatment failures caused by overgrowth of singly, doubly or even multidrug-resistant phenotypes. The ABVD regimen consists of drugs that are individually non-cross-resistant with the agents in the MOPP regimen. This combination has demonstrated a complete response rate as high as the MOPP regimen and has been proven to be effective in patients resistant to MOPP therapy. In a randomized study of patients with advanced Hodgkin's disease, alternating monthly cycles of MOPP and ABVD (MOPP/ABVD) were compared with MOPP therapy

Table 76.8.
Other Combination Chemotherapy Regimens Used in Hodgkin's Disease

Acronym	Agents	Dose (mg/m^2)	Treatment Days	Frequency of Cycles	Reference
ABVD	Doxorubicin	25	1, 15	Every 28 days	(55)
	Bleomycin	10	1, 15		
	Vinblastine	6	1, 15		
	Dacarbazine	375	1, 15		
MVPP	Mechlorethamine	6	1, 8	Every 28 days	(56)
	Vinblastine	10	1, 8, 15		
	Procarbazine	100	1–15		
	Prednisolone	40	1–15		
MVVPP	Mechlorethamine	0.4 mg/kg	1	Every 57 days	(57)
	Vincristine	1.4 (max 2 mg)	1, 8, 15		
	Vinblastine	6	22, 29, 36		
	Prednisone	40	1–22, then taper		
	Procarbazine	100	22–43		
MOPP/APB	Mechlorethamine	6	1	Every 28 days	(58)
	Vincristine	1.4 (max 2 mg)	1		
	Prednisone	40	1–14		
	Procarbazine	100	1–7		
	Doxorubicin	35	8		
	Bleomycin	10	8		
	Vinblastine	6	8		
EVA	Etoposide	100	1–3	Every 28 days	(59)
	Vinblastine	6	1		
	Doxorubicin	50	1		

alone. The rates of complete response (89 versus 74%) and 8-year relapse-free survival (73 versus 45%) were superior for the MOPP/ABVD regimen, with a similar incidence of serious toxicities (61, 62).

Klimo and Connors reported the results of a similar hybrid regimen (MOPP/ABVD) (Table 76.8), which administered 7 drugs in single monthly cycles. This regimen omitted the dacarbazine and increased the dose of doxorubicin from 25 mg/m^2 to 35 mg/m^2, and 13% of patients also received some local radiation therapy. The complete response rate was 97.5%, and at a median follow-up of 3.5 years, the overall survival rate was 93.5% and the relapse-free survival was 90.5% (58). Recently, Glick et al. reported a complete response rate of 81% and a 22-month relapse-free survival of 80% using this hybrid regimen (63).

Another promising regimen recently described includes etoposide, vinblastine or vincristine, and doxorubicin (EVA). In patients who have previously relapsed following MOPP or are MOPP-resistant, a 41% complete response rate and a 2-year failure-free survival rate of 38% has been reported (59). This regimen incorporated yet another active agent, etoposide (64), into the treatment of Hodgkin's disease. This regimen has the potential advantage of fewer emetogenic complications and less pulmonary toxicity than many of the other second-line regimens.

Over the past 25 years, it has become apparent that several factors influence the overall long-term response to Hodgkin's disease therapies. Factors that have a negative impact on potential cure include age (>40 years), stage of disease, number of extranodal sites, and constitutional symptoms (65–67). After chemotherapy is initiated, the rate of tumor regression and the dose intensity (i.e., amount of drug administered per unit time) also appear to influence the duration of response and survival (54, 68). Review of outcome data has shown that the best overall results are seen in patient subsets who received chemotherapy at closest to the intended dose and schedule (without dosage attenuation or delay between cycles) (25). The dose-intensities of the mechlorethamine, procarbazine, and vincristine have each been suggested to correlate with outcome in MOPP or MOPP-derivative regimens (54, 62, 68–72). For example, although the original MOPP regimen includes 1.4 mg/m^2 of vincristine, many clinicians have limited each dose to a maximum of 2 mg. Using full doses is associated with significant neurotoxicity, but no patient was permanently disabled if a sliding-scale dose, taking into account the patient's symptoms, was used to adjust the dose. Conversely, no study using the 2-mg dose maximum has shown results as good as those with the original regimen, and retrospective analyses have shown that the dose of vincristine does make an impact on treatment results (46).

The most common dose-limiting toxicity of many of the other drugs used in Hodgkin's disease regimens is myelosuppression. Therefore the use of colony-stimulating factors in combination with chemotherapy regimens may allow for higher dosage intensity to be tolerated.

Chemotherapy such as the MOPP or ABVD regimens is also appropriate therapy for patients whose Hodgkin's disease relapses after radiation therapy (53, 73). DeVita et al. reported that 94% of patients whose disease recurred following local irradiation achieved a complete remission with MOPP therapy (53).

The optimal management for patients who relapse following primary chemotherapy (e.g., MOPP) or for those failing initial chemotherapy is not clearly established. At the NCI, 59% of 32 patients who relapsed after MOPP achieved a complete remission when retreated with MOPP therapy. Patients whose first complete remission was longer than 1 year were more likely to achieve a second complete remission. The duration of the second remission was also longer in patients whose initial remission was longer than 1 year (74). Overall, about 35% of patients who relapse after initial chemotherapy-induced complete remission have a long-term disease-free survival (25).

A number of other antineoplastic agents, including doxorubicin, carmustine, lomustine, vinblastine, dacarbazine, and bleomycin, have demonstrated important activity in Hodgkin's disease. These agents have been assembled in various combinations (Table 76.8). Patients resistant to MOPP should receive one of the established non-cross-resistant regimens. The most widely used regimen in this situation has been the ABVD regimen, which produced complete remissions in 60% of 54 MOPP-resistant patients with a 17-month median disease-free survival (53). In relapsed patients who initially received ABVD, retreatment with ABVD may be difficult because of the risks of cumulative doxorubicin cardiotoxicity and bleomycin pulmonary toxicity.

Patients who fail first-line therapy are much less likely to respond to other conventional therapies (55). Even if such patients do achieve a complete remission with second-line therapy, it is likely to be of only brief duration. The use of high-dose chemotherapy with allogeneic or autologous bone marrow transplant may offer better chances of long-term survival (75, 76). With this treatment approach, the complete response rate is generally about 50%, and 30 to 40% of patients appear to have a long remission (>2 years) (77–81). Best treatment results are seen in patients with low tumor volumes, good performance status, and chemotherapy-sensitive disease (i.e., showing some indication of tumor response prior to BMT). Clinical trials have reported 8 to 20% treatment-related deaths. Many of these deaths and other treatment morbidities are associated with the profound myelosuppression prior to

bone marrow engraftment. Numerous trials using colony-stimulating factors have now reported accelerated myeloid recovery, fewer febrile days, and shorter hospitalizations (82, 83).

Non-Hodgkin's Lymphoma

The management for non-Hodgkin's lymphomas depends upon many factors, including the age of the patient, presence of concomitant disease, and the stage and histologic subgroup of the primary disease.

LOW-GRADE NHL

Fewer than 10% of patients with favorable prognosis (low grade) histologies (Table 76.2) have localized disease (i.e., stage I or II). Local or regional radiation therapy is generally very effective in achieving disease control in the irradiated areas (84). If patients relapse following radiation therapy, it is usually in unirradiated nodal or extranodal sites. However, because of the indolent nature of this disease asymptomatic patients may not require immediate therapy.

Over 50% to 75% of patients with low-grade lymphomas have stage III or IV disease at initial diagnosis (85, 86). Treatment options for patients with favorable histologies and advanced disease include total nodal irradiation, total body irradiation, single-agent chemotherapy, and combination chemotherapy. Radiation therapy alone (TLI) appears to be most effective in patients with fewer than 5 sites of disease involvement, no systemic symptoms, and small tumor masses (less than 10 cm); however, patients may continue to relapse for up to 10 years following therapy (87).

A number of agents, including mechlorethamine, melphalan, chlorambucil, cyclophosphamide, vincristine, vinblastine, doxorubicin, carmustine, and etoposide have activity in the follicular lymphomas. Although complete response rates as high as 65% have been reported with several of these agents, and the duration of relapse-free survival may be up to 50 months, this type of therapy is not considered to be curative (88, 89). In an attempt to improve on the results observed with single-agent therapy, a number of combination chemotherapy regimens have been developed. Initially, one of the most widely used regimens was the CVP (cyclophosphamide, vincristine, and prednisone) regimen (Table 76.9). Although studies with this regimen suggested higher complete response rates than with single-agent therapy, the overall disease-free survival and survival were not significantly altered. In response to this information, a number of more aggressive regimens (with and without radiation therapy) have been investigated. Trials using regimens such as CHOP-bleo, CMOPP, M-BACOD, COPP, and carmustine, cyclophos-

Table 76.9.
Combination Chemotherapy Regimens Utilized in Non-Hodgkin's Lymphoma

Acronym	Agents	Dose (mg/m^2)	Treatment Days	Frequency of Cycles	Reference
C-MOPP or COPP	Cyclophosphamide	650	1, 8	Every 28 days	(90)
	Vincristine	1.4 (max 2 mg)	1, 8		
	Procarbazine	100	1–14		
	Prednisone	100	1–14		
CVP	Cyclophosphamide	400	1–5	Every 21 days	(91)
	Vincristine	1.4 (max 2 mg)	1		
	Prednisone	100	1–5		
CHOP	Cyclophosphamide	750	1	Every 21 days	(92)
	Doxorubicin	50	1		
	Vincristine	1.4 (max 2 mg)	1		
	Prednisone	100	1–5		
CHOP-bleo	Same as above plus bleomycin	15	1, 5		(93)
M-BACOD	Methotrexate	3000	14	Every 28 days	(94)
	Bleomycin	4	1		
	Doxorubicin	45	1		
	Cyclophosphamide	600	1		
	Vincristine	1	1		
	Dexamethasone	6	1–5		
	Leucovorin				
MACOP-B	Methotrexate	400	8, 36, 64	Only one cycle is given	(95)
	Doxorubicin	50	1, 15, 29, 43, 57, 71		
	Cyclophosphamide	350	1, 15, 29, 43, 57, 71		
	Vincristine	1.4	8, 22, 36, 50, 64, 78		
	Bleomycin	10	22, 50, 78		
	Prednisone	75 (total)	1–63, taper 64–78		
ProMACE	Prednisone	60	1–14		(96)
	Methotrexate	500	15		
	Doxorubicin	25	1, 8		
	Cyclophosphamide	650	1, 8		
	Etoposide	120	1, 8		
ProMACE-CytaBOM	Cyclophosphamide	650	1	Every 21 days	(98)
	Doxorubicin	25	1		
	Etoposide	120	1		
	Prednisone	60	1–15		
	Cytarabine	300	8		
	Bleomycin	5	8		
	Vincristine	1.4	8		
	Methotrexate	120	8		
	Leucovorin	25 q. 6	9		

phamide, and vincristine plus dexamethasone have now reported higher long-term disease-free survival rates (93, 99–101). Overall survival has not been improved, but this is probably due to the long survival (median >8 years) observed even in patients who do not achieve a CR. Patients who do not achieve CR often receive various palliative therapies for many years. A longer duration of disease-free survival is almost certainly associated with a better quality of life for the patient and fewer treatment-related side effects. Unfortunately, many patients with low-grade lymphomas still cannot be cured with currently available treatment.

Another approach to managing asymptomatic patients with advanced disease is to delay therapy until the disease progresses. This approach is appealing, especially in older patients who are less likely to tolerate the side effects of chemotherapy. However, recent data support therapy at initial diagnosis. Young et al. reported similar survival durations but higher complete response rates and disease-free survival rates in patients receiving therapy at diagnosis (102). The ProMace-MOPP regimen followed by TLI has reported a CR rate of 78%, with over 80% of these patients still in CR at 4 years.

Patients with these indolent lymphomas usually

undergo multiple-treatment regimens and inevitable relapse after varying durations of response. Such patients eventually die of unrelated causes, toxicity of the therapy, progressive disease, or transition to a more aggressive type of lymphoma.

The follicular low-grade NHL have shown responsiveness to α-interferon. In an NCI-sponsored trial, 13 (4 complete responses, 9 partial responses) of 24 patients responded to a regimen of 50 million units/m^2 given three times weekly. The responses included both lymph node and extranodal disease. The median duration of response was 8 months (103). Other dosages and schedules as well as combination therapy with cytotoxic drugs or other biological agents (e.g., monoclonal antibodies) are under investigation).

INTERMEDIATE-AND HIGH-GRADE NHL

Patients with stage I intermediate-grade or high-grade histologies may often be managed with radiation therapy. Patients with contiguous stage II disease may be also treated with radiation therapy, whereas noncontiguous stage II disease requires systemic chemotherapy. In some patients, combined radiation and chemotherapy may improve overall survival (104).

For most patients with stage II disease and for all patients with stages III and IV of intermediate and high-grade histologies, systemic chemotherapy is required. Although a number of single agents are active in these diseases, few patients achieve complete remission, and the duration of response is usually short (105). However, the prognosis of many of these histologies has improved with the use of intensive combination chemotherapy. Unlike the indolent follicular histologies, patients with these more aggressive histologies may succumb to their disease rapidly, unless they respond to therapy.

Advances observed in the management of Hodgkin's disease prompted the use of combination therapy in the aggressive NHLs. C-MOPP or COPP (cyclophosphamide substituted for the mechlorethamine in the MOPP regimen) (Table 76.9) was one of the first regimens that demonstrated that long-term relapse-free survival and possibly even cure could be achieved in patients with diffuse histiocytic lymphoma (Rappaport classification). With this regimen about 40% of patients achieved a complete response, and all but one of the complete responders remained disease-free 26 to 105 months after therapy. With the intent of increasing the percentage of long-term, disease-free survivors, a number of other regimens have been used in clinical trials (Table 76.9). These regimens have used other active agents such as doxorubicin, bleomycin, cytarabine, and methotrexate.

In addition to combining active drugs, many regimens have also used innovative approaches to scheduling in an attempt to maximize response while maintaining accept-

able degrees of toxicity. Examples of such regimens include the M-BACOD and the ProMACE combinations, in which the relatively nonmyelosuppressive high-dose methotrexate is given between the myelosuppressive agents to prevent regrowth of the lymphoma between cycles of treatment. A 75% CR rate was reported for M-BACOD, and initial projections are that 55 to 60% of patients would be cured (94). The MACOP-B regimen includes weekly administration of active agents for 12 weeks, with myelosuppressive and nonmyelosuppressive intravenous agents given on alternating weeks. The reported complete response rate with this regimen is 84%, with a predicted median duration of response of more than 2 years. This initial evidence suggests that this regimen is as effective as other regimens, although it can be administered in one-half the time or less (95). Other regimens have also reported CR rates exceeding 80%, and it has been estimated that approximately 70% of patients who achieve a CR are cured of the disease (97). The success of these and similar regimens is thought to be related to the use of high doses of many drugs early in the treatment course.

Encouraging early results using an alternating non-cross-resistant regimen prompted investigators at the NCI to develop several such regimens, including ProMACE-MOPP and ProMACE-CytaBOM, which maximize dose-intensity and tumor exposure to a large number of active drugs early in the treatment course. The NCI's ProMACE-MOPP uses alternating cycles of ProMACE and MOPP, with the patients' rate of response determining how many cycles of each they will receive. ProMACE primary induction therapy is given until complete remission is achieved or the rate of response slows. At that time MOPP therapy is given for the same number of cycles. If the patient is in complete remission, late intensification with the same number of ProMACE cycles is given. Although this therapy has been quite toxic, the results have been excellent, even in patients with poor prognostic factors (106). ProMACE-CytaBOM used 8 drugs given over 17 weeks. When compared in a randomized trial, ProMACE-CytaBOM produced a higher CR rate (86% versus 74%) and survival than ProMACE-MOPP (98).

In these aggressive lymphomas, only patients who achieve a complete response will have a long, disease-free survival. Factors that appear to adversely affect the ability to attain a complete response include advanced stage of the disease, the presence of systemic symptoms, bone marrow or liver involvement, gastrointestinal masses greater than 10 cm in diameter, a hemoglobin of less than 12 g/dl, and a lactate dehydrogenase level above 250 units (107). Other factors that may also adversely affect the prognosis include more than 3 sites of disease involvement, advanced age, or a slow rate of response to initial therapy (108). Variability in response rates to similar regimens in different clinical trials may be due to a different mix of prognostic factors in the patient population. If patients with poor prognostic factors do attain a complete remission, then overall survival does not appear to be compromised.

Patients with NHLs who respond to chemotherapy should receive a minimum of six courses of therapy. If they appear to be in clinical complete remission after pathologic restaging, two more cycles of chemotherapy should be given. Although the aggressive treatment regimens are effective, they also produce serious side effects. In patients experiencing toxicity it is often tempting to prolong the interval between courses of therapy to allow more recovery time. However, the specified schedule must be adhered to, whenever possible, to produce the best results. In many cases, prolongation by even 1 week may be associated with rapid tumor regrowth. Few clinical trials have directly addressed the significance of dose-intensity in the aggressive lymphomas; however, a recent meta-analysis of 22 studies suggested that dose-intensity may correlate with remission rate in advanced-stage intermediate-grade lymphoma (111).

Maintenance chemotherapy following a complete response does not appear to prolong survival in most types of NHL, but it is indicated in patients with lymphoblastic lymphoma and Burkitt's lymphoma. Patients with bone marrow involvement (leukemia-like), lymphoblastic lymphoma, and Burkitt's lymphoma may benefit from prophylactic intrathecal methotrexate, if they did not receive high-dose methotrexate as part of their systemic therapy.

Patients who are not responsive to initial chemotherapy or who relapse in less than 1 year should be given non-cross-resistant regimens. However, the results of salvage treatments for NHLs are far less encouraging than those described for Hodgkin's disease. Patients whose initial remission exceeds 1 year may benefit from retreatment with the original regimen, but patients who relapse after chemotherapy-induced CR have very little chance of long-term disease-free survival (i.e., cure) with conventional chemotherapy regimens.

The use of high-dose chemotherapy with or without total body irradiation combined with autologous or allogeneic bone marrow transplant may offer an improved prognosis for some subsets of NHL patients (112, 113). The patients most likely to derive benefit from this type of therapy are those who achieve a CR following salvage chemotherapy, those who only achieve a PR following initial chemotherapy, and those with poor prognostic features who achieve a CR following initial chemotherapy. When used as salvage therapy in patients who have relapsed or had disease refractory to first-line therapy, CR rates of 40 to 60% have been reported, with 15 to 20% long-term survivors (114–116).

OTHER NHL

Lymphoblastic lymphomas (T cell type) generally occur in adolescent and young adult males. These patients are more likely to have bone marrow, mediastinal, and central nervous system involvement than those with other lymphomas. Regimens similar to those used to treat acute lymphoblastic leukemia with central nervous system prophylaxis and maintenance chemotherapy have given encouraging results.

Three other relatively rare intermediate histologies (Rappaport) are nodular "histiocytic" lymphoma (NH), diffuse mixed lymphoma (DML), and diffuse poorly differentiated lymphoma (DPDL). Aggressive chemotherapy regimens in these diseases have produced complete response rates in the range of 40 to 60%, with median durations of response of 20 to 40 months. However, of this group, only NH is known to be cured with chemotherapy.

Systemic chemotherapy is the treatment of choice for Burkitt's lymphoma. Surgical reduction of the tumor prior to chemotherapy may improve the outcome, because the overall prognosis of the disease is directly proportional to the volume of the tumor (109). Although aggressive chemotherapy regimens have achieved durable systemic remissions, many patients have relapses in the central nervous system. Therefore, such regimens should be augmented with intermittent intrathecal methotrexate or cytarabine prophylaxis. Initial chemotherapy must contain high doses of cyclophosphamide, and commonly used regimens also use vincristine, doxorubicin, prednisone, and high-dose methotrexate. Regimens such as these are producing 2-year disease-free survival rates in the range of 50 to 70% (110).

There are five well-established treatment modalities for mycosis fungoides and Sézary syndrome: (a) topical therapy with mechlorethamine, (b) photochemotherapy with psoralen and ultraviolet light, (c) electron-beam therapy to the whole body, (d) systemic chemotherapy, and (e) α-interferon. Patients with disease limited to plaque lesions (without erythroderma or other tissue involvement) generally respond well to topical mechlorethamine or photochemotherapy, but most patients experience relapse within a few years. Electron-beam irradiation also produces complete responses in most patients with only plaque lesions and in some patients with more extensive disease, although relapse generally occurs within 3 years. Systemic chemotherapy is reserved for patients with disease that has spread to other organs. Combination chemotherapy regimens used in mycosis fungoides are similar to those used in other NHL. Although these regimens produce complete responses in about 25% of patients, the duration of response is usually brief (3).

Treatment of HIV-Associated Lymphomas

Patients with AIDS-related lymphomas have a much poorer prognosis than individuals with similar histologies who are not infected with the HIV. Within the AIDS-associated lymphoma group, patients with poor Karnofsky performance status, a history of AIDS prior to the diagnosis of lymphoma, bone marrow involvement, other extranodal involvement, or a CD4 cell count under 100/dl have all been reported to have a shorter survival (117, 118).

Due to the aggressiveness and extent of these lymphomas, intensive chemotherapy regimens similar to those used in intermediate and high-grade non-HIV lymphoma have been used. Complete response rates have been somewhat less than those reported for those regimens in the non-HIV population, but several investigators have reported significant complete response rates (>50%) (119–122). Complete response rates have been highest in patients without the poor prognostic factors mentioned above. Despite these encouraging responses, many investigators have reported median survivals of less than 1 year (118, 119, 121, 122) with patients either dying from AIDS-related complications (e.g., opportunistic infections), treatment toxicity, or recurrent disease.

The high incidence of treatment-related complications and mortality has led to the use of less intensive regimens. The AIDS Clinical Trials Groups reported the results of a low-dose m-BACOD regimen with CNS and *Pneumocystis carinii* prophylaxis followed by zidovudine. Forty-six percent of 42 patients achieved a complete response, and at the time of publication the median duration of complete response exceeded 14 months (123). A subsequent follow-up study demonstrated that higher dosages of chemotherapy could be administered in combination with granulocyte-macrophage colony-stimulating factor (124).

Evidence suggests that patients without poor prognostic signs and who are able to tolerate combination chemotherapy and achieve a complete response may experience a 1- to 2-year disease-free survival. Unfortunately, with currently available therapeutic options, few patients attain a long-term disease-free survival. Therefore, less intensive (lower-dose) regimens that are associated with fewer complications and comparable response and survival outcomes are reasonable at this time.

COMPLICATIONS

Patients with malignant lymphomas may experience a wide variety of complications, which may be secondary to either the disease or the therapy (Table 76.10). Although many of the disease-related complications have been reduced or eliminated through the use of more effective therapies, the use of more aggressive treatment regimens has resulted in more treatment-related complications. Additionally, the increased cure rate for Hodgkin's disease and many of the NHLs has stimulated concern about late and long-term treatment-associated toxicities.

Many disease-related complications result from infiltration or obstruction of organs, tissues, or blood vessels by the lymphoma. Rapidly growing lymphomas (e.g., nodular sclerosing Hodgkin's disease, lymphoblastic lym-

Table 76.10.
Serious Complications Associated with Malignant Lymphomas

Disease-related
  Superior vena cava obstruction
  Spinal cord compression
  Central nervous system infiltration
  Renal failure
  Immunologic abnormalities
  Pleural effusion
  Hemolytic anemia
Treatment-related
  Chemotherapy-related
    Granulocytopenia and infection
    Tumor lysis syndrome
    Gonadal injury/sterility
    Secondary leukemia
    Organ damage secondary to specific agents
  Radiation therapy–related
    Tumor lysis syndrome
    Pneumonitis
    Pericarditis
    Hypothyroidism

phoma) may produce obstruction of the superior vena cava. Patients with this complication frequently have shortness of breath; swelling of the face, neck, and upper extremities; headache; and sensations of choking. Occurrence of superior vena cava syndrome should be considered an oncologic emergency. Therapy must often be initiated before a tissue diagnosis is made (if this is the initial presentation of the lymphoma) and includes immediate radiation therapy to the mass, diuretics, and combination chemotherapy.

Lymphoma masses may occasionally cause compression of the spinal cord. Initially, this is generally more common in Hodgkin's disease than in NHL, however, it is more common overall in relapsed or refractory NHL and HIV-associated lymphomas. The most common presenting symptom is central back pain. As the degree of compression progresses, other neurologic symptoms develop (e.g., motor dysfunction, parasthesias, incontinence), and paraplegia may result if not treated. Appropriate therapy depends upon the extent of compression. If detected early enough, chemotherapy and/or radiation therapy may elicit rapid improvement. In some more advanced spinal cord compressions, emergency surgery (laminectomy) followed by radiation therapy may be required. Corticosteroids are also used to prevent edema or promote its resolution. These agents may have a direct oncolytic effect as well (125).

Some lymphomas (mostly diffuse NHL with bone marrow involvement) may infiltrate the central nervous system and develop meningeal seeding (leptomeningeal involvement). Signs of this complication include headache, nausea, vomiting, and lethargy. Confirmation of meningeal involvement is made by examination of the cerebrospinal fluid, and treatment includes corticosteroids and intrathecal chemotherapy agents (e.g., methotrexate, cytarabine) and radiation therapy. Intracerebral lymphomas may also occur, but these are generally primary tumors (now most commonly seen in HIV patients) and not complications of other systemic disease.

Renal failure in patients with lymphoma may be due to infiltration of the kidneys or obstruction of the ureters by the lymphoma. Infiltration of the kidneys is usually treated with systemic therapy (although low-dose, local radiation therapy may occasionally be used), and ureteral obstruction may be treated with local radiation therapy combined with systemic chemotherapy.

As would be anticipated from the nature of the disease, immunologic abnormalities occur commonly in patients with malignant lymphomas. Abnormalities in delayed hypersensitivity, particularly cutaneous anergy, develop with extensive involvement of lymphatic tissues or severe lymphocytopenia. Depressed cell-mediated immunity (T lymphocyte) is associated with a high risk of opportunistic infections, including tuberculosis, salmonellosis, toxoplasmosis, and herpes zoster. This is particularly true in patients with Hodgkin's disease. In some cases, infection may precede diagnosis of the disease (126). Furthermore, patients may continue to have an underlying T cell function deficit that persists after they are in remission (127). Radiation and chemotherapy also contribute to decreased immunologic functions and subsequent infectious complication.

Granulocytopenia secondary to myelosuppressive chemotherapy also predisposes patients to serious infections. Gram-negative bacilli (i.e., *Escherichia coli*, *Klebsiella pneumoniae*, *Pseudomonas aeruginosa*) and Gram-positive cocci (*Staphylococcus aureus* and *Staphylococcus epidermidis*) are the most common pathogens responsible for infections during granulocytopenia. As chemotherapy regimens have become more aggressive, especially those used in NHL, the degree and duration of granulocytopenia have increased, placing more patients at risk of infectious complications.

Acute and chronic toxicities associated with the administration of combination chemotherapy are determined by the individual agents included in the treatment regimen. In addition to myelosuppression, these toxicities may include nausea and vomiting, mucositis, neurotoxicity, cardiotoxicity, skin changes, and pulmonary toxicity. Many of these toxicities are avoidable or reversible if the clinician(s) managing the patient are familiar with the agents being used and their associated risks. The major long-term complications of chemotherapy of lymphomas are sterility and the risk of second malignancies.

Testicular function in adult men is particularly susceptible to injury by many chemotherapeutic agents. The MOPP regimen has been reported to cause azoospermia and germinal aplasia in more than 80% of men receiving this regimen (128). Although chemotherapy-associated azoospermia is generally persistent, recovery may be observed in a small portion of patients several years after the cessation of therapy. A comparison of the MOPP and ABVD regimens revealed that azoospermia occurred in 100% of MOPP-treated men but in only 15 to 35% of those receiving ABVD therapy. In addition, spermatogenesis almost always recovered in the ABVD-treated men (128, 130). This information may be important in planning treatment for young men with Hodgkin's disease who are concerned about preservation of fertility following treatment.

Gonadal injury also occurs in women following combination chemotherapy. Ovarian failure is associated with arrest of follicular maturation or frank destruction of ova and follicles. Unlike the profound effects of the MOPP regimen on testicular function, it appears to produce ovarian dysfunction and amenorrhea in only 40 to 50% of women (74, 131). Ovarian injury from MOPP therapy is correlated with age at treatment, with older patients (over age 35) much more likely to experience persistent amenorrhea (132). Persistent amenorrhea also appears to be less common following ABVD therapy than following MOPP therapy (129).

The potential of second malignancies, particularly acute nonlymphocytic leukemia, is a well-documented complication associated with Hodgkin's disease and/or its therapy. Several studies have provided convincing evidence that the risk of leukemia varies markedly with the form of therapy for Hodgkin's disease. Secondary leukemias appear to occur largely in patients who have received MOPP with or without radiotherapy, and the 10-year cumulative risk of such patients is between 5 and 10% (133–136). Leukemia has usually developed between 3 and 10 years after initiation of treatment for Hodgkin's disease, and most patients have been in complete remission of the Hodgkin's disease when the leukemia develops (133). Patients with Hodgkin's disease are also at increased risk of developing NHL. Non-Hodgkin's lymphomas apparently occur more frequently after combined radiation and chemotherapy (137). Patients with Hodgkin's disease may also have a slightly increased risk of developing solid tumors (133, 136). In particular, excess lung cancer risk has been observed in patients who received radiation therapy (in the irradiated field) (136). Patients treated for NHL also have an increased risk of developing acute nonlymphocytic leukemia, and the intensity of therapy appears to be correlated with the likelihood of developing a secondary leukemia (133).

Complications following radiation therapy are largely related to the field that has been irradiated, although fatigue generally occurs in most patients. Nausea, vomiting, mucositis/esophagitis, diarrhea, and anorexia commonly occur following abdominal radiation, while dryness of the mouth and throat, dysphagia, alteration in taste, and increased dental caries may occur following irradiation of the head and neck regions. Bone marrow depression may occur during abdominal-pelvic irradiation and may require interruption of treatment. In addition to these acute side effects, long-term complications may pose more serious problems. Long-term effects are usually related to the volume of normal tissue that has been irradiated, the total dose given, and the size of the daily dose administered. They include radiation pneumonitis, pericarditis, nephritis, hepatitis, growth retardation (in children), and hypothyroidism.

CONCLUSION

The lymphomas are malignant disorders that originate from lymphoreticular cells. These disorders may disseminate via contiguous lymphatics or the blood stream to other lymph nodes and other organ systems. Malignant lymphomas are generally separated into Hodgkin's disease and non-Hodgkin's lymphomas, but the term *non-Hodgkin's lymphomas* represents multiple diseases with diverse morphologic and clinical features. The prognosis and treatment of each lymphoma are related to the histopathology and the anatomic extent of disease as determined by staging procedures. Most lymphomas are sensitive to radiation therapy as well as many chemotherapeutic agents. Combination chemotherapy regimens are now successful in curing many patients with Hodgkin's disease and high-grade non-Hodgkin's lymphomas. In addition, many other patients experience a significant prolongation of disease-free survival following chemotherapy. It is likely that high-dose chemotherapy with bone marrow transplantation and biological response modifiers (e.g., interferon) will assume a much more prominent role in the management of lymphomas.

Management of patients with lymphomas requires not only an understanding of the disease process and its appropriate therapy but also an understanding of the variety of complications that may arise secondary to the disease or its therapy. These complications include opportunistic infections, obstruction by the tumor, secondary malignancies, and chemotherapy-associated toxicities. Anticipation and appropriate management of these complications can greatly reduce the overall morbidity experienced by the patient.

REFERENCES

1. Diehl V, vonKalle C, Fonatsch C, et al.: The cell origin in Hodgkin's disease. Semin Oncol 17:660–672, 1990.
2. Slivnick DJ, Nawrocki JF, Fisher RI: Immunology and cellular biology of Hodgkin's disease. Hematol Oncol Clin North Am 3:205–220, 1989.
3. DeVita VT, Jaffe ES, Mauch P, Longo DL, Lymphocytic lymphomas. In DeVita VT, Hellman S, Rosenberg SA (eds): Cancer. Principles and Practice of Oncology, ed. 3. Philadelphia, JB Lippincott, 1989, p 1741.
4. American Cancer Society: Facts and Figures, 1992. New York, American Cancer Society, 1992.
5. Cantor KP, Fraumeni JF: Distribution of non-Hodgkin's lymphoma in the United States between 1950 and 1975. Cancer Res 40:2645–2652, 1980.
6. MacMahon B: Epidemiological evidence of the nature of Hodgkin's disease. Cancer 10:1045–1054, 1957.
7. Miller RW, Beebe GW: Infectious mononucleosis and the empirical risk of cancer. J NCI 50:315–321, 1973.
8. Connolly RR, Chistene BW: A cohort study of cancer following infectious mononucleosis. Cancer Res 34:1172–1178, 1974.
9. Rosdahl N, Larsen SO, Clemmensen J: Hodgkin's disease in patients with previous mononucleosis, 30 years experience. Br Med J 2:253–256, 1974.
10. Gottlieb-Stematsky T, Vonsover A, Ramot B, et al.: Antibodies to Epstein-Barr virus in patients with Hodgkin's disease and leukemia. Cancer 36:1640–1645, 1975.
11. Evans AS, Gutensohn NM: A population-based case-control study of EBV and other viral antibodies among persons with Hodgkin's disease and their siblings. Int J Cancer 34:149–157, 1984.
12. Mueller N, Evans A, Harris NL, et al.: Hodgkin's disease and Epstein-Barr virus. Altered antibody pattern before diagnosis. N Engl J Med 320:689–695, 1989.
13. Staal SP, Ambinder R, Beschorner WE, et al.: A survey of Epstein-Barr Virus DNA in lymphoid tissue. Frequent detection in Hodgkin's disease. Am J Clin Pathol 91:1–5, 1989.
14. Weiss L, Movahed LA, Warnke RA, et al.: Detection of Epstein-Barr viral genomes in Reed-Sternberg cells of Hodgkin's disease. N Engl J Med 320:502–506, 1989.
15. Vianna NJ, Greenwald P, Davies JNP: Extended epidemic of Hodgkin's disease in patients with previous mononucleosis, 30 years experience. Br Med J 2:253–256, 1974.
16. Vianna JH, Dolan AK: Epidemiological evidence for transmission of Hodgkin's disease. N Engl J Med 289:499–502, 1973.
17. Penn I: The incidence of malignancies in transplant recipients. Transplant Proc 7:323, 1975.
18. Matas AJ, Hertel BF, Rosai J, et al.: Post-transplant malignant lymphoma. Distinctive morphologic features related to its pathogenesis. Am J Med 61:716, 1976.
19. Ziegler JL, Beckstead JA, Volberding PA, et al.: Non-Hodgkins lymphoma in 90 homosexual men. Relation to generalized lymphadenopathy and the acquired immunodeficiency syndrome. N Engl J Med 311:565–570, 1984.
20. Anderson RE, Nishiyama H, Yohei I, Kenzo T, Nobukazo O: Pathogenesis of radiation related leukemia and lymphoma. Speculations based primarily on experience of Hiroshima and Nagasaki. Lancet 1:1060–1062, 1972.
21. Reedman BM, Klein G: Cellular localization of an Epstein-Barr virus (EBV)–associated complement fixing antigen in producer and nonproducer lymphoblastoid cell lines. Int J Cancer 11:499–520, 1973.
22. Blattner WA, Gibbs WN, Saxinger C, et al.: Human T-cell leukaemia/lymphoma virus-lymphomareticular neoplasia in Jamaica. Lancet 2:61–64, 1983.
23. Lukes RJ, Butler JJ, Hicks ED: Natural history of Hodgkin's disease as related to its pathologic picture. Cancer 42:1039–1045, 1978.
24. Parker BA, Green MR, Hodgkin's disease. In Moosa AR, Schimpff SC, Robson MC (eds): Comprehensive Textbook of Oncology, ed. 2. Baltimore, Williams & Wilkins, 1991, p 1257.

25. Hellman S, Jaffe ES, DeVita VT, Hodgkin's disease. In DeVita VT, Hellman S, Rosenberg SA (eds): Cancer. Principles and Practice of Oncology, ed. 3. Philadelphia, JB Lippincott, 1989, p 1969–1741.

26. Poppema S, Kaiserling E, Lennert K: Nodular paragranuloma and progressively transformed germinal centers: ultrastructural and immunohistologic findings. Virchows Arch (Cell Pathol) 31:211–225, 1979.

27. Rappaport H, Tumors of the hematopoietic system. In Atlas of Tumor Pathology, Sec III, Fasc 8. Washington D.C., Armed Forces Institute of Pathology, 1966.

28. Anon: National Cancer Institute sponsored study of classification of non-Hodgkin's lymphomas: Summary and description of a working formulation for clinical usage. Cancer 49:2112–2135, 1982.

29. Jaffe ES, Shevach EM, Frank MM: Nodular lymphoma: Evidence for origin from follicular B lymphocytes. N Engl J Med 290:813–819, 1976.

30. Foucar K: Incidence and patterns of bone marrow and blood involvement by lymphoma in relationship to the Lukes-Collins classification. Blood 54:1417–1422, 1979.

31. Levine AM: Epidemiology, clinical characteristics, and management of AIDS-related lymphomas. Hematol Oncol Clin North Am 5:331–342, 1991.

32. Ziegler JL, Drew WL, Miner RC, et al.: Outbreak of Burkitt's-like lymphoma in homosexual men. Lancet 2:631–633, 1982.

33. Snider WD, Simpson DM, Aronyk KE, Nielson SL: Primary lymphoma of the nervous system associated with acquired immunodeficiency syndrome. (letter) N Engl J Med 308:45, 1983.

34. Ciobanu N, Adreeff M, Safai B, Koziner B, Mertelsmann R: Lymphoblastic neoplasia in a homosexual patient with Kaposi's sarcoma. Ann Intern Med 98:151–155, 1983.

35. Ioachim HL, Cooper MC, Hellman GC: Lymphomas in men at high risk for acquired immune deficiency syndrome. Cancer 56:2831–2842, 1985.

36. Centers for Disease Control: Revision of the case definition of acquired immunodeficiency syndrome for national reporting—United States. MMWR 34:373–375, 1985.

37. Portlock CS: Hodgkin's disease. Med Clin North Am 68:629–740, 1984.

38. Berard C, Thomas LB, Axtell LM: The relationship of histopathological subtype to clinical stage of Hodgkin's disease of diagnosis. Cancer Res 31:1776, 1971.

39. Haller DG: Non-Hodgkin's lymphoma. Med Clin North Am 68:741–756, 1984.

40. DeVita VT, Serpick A, Carbone P: Combination chemotherapy in the treatment of advanced Hodgkin's disease. Ann Intern Med 73:881–895, 1970.

41. Hoppe RT: Radiation therapy in the treatment of Hodgkin's disease. Semin Oncol 7:56–66, 1980.

42. Gladstein E: Radiation in Hodgkin's disease: past achievements and future progress. Cancer 39:837–842, 1977.

43. Hoppe RT, Coleman CN, Cox RS, et al.: The management of stage I-II Hodgkin's disease with irradiation alone or combined modality therapy: the Stanford experience. Blood 59:455–465, 1982.

44. Mauch P, Goodman R, Hellman S: The significance of mediastinal involvement in early stage Hodgkin's disease. Cancer 42:1039–1045, 1978.

45. Longo DL, Glatstein E, Duffy PL, et al.: Radiation therapy versus combination chemotherapy in the treatment of early-stage Hodgkin's disease: seven year results of a prospective randomized trial. J Clin Oncol 9:906–917, 1991.

46. Longo DL: The use of chemotherapy in the treatment of Hodgkin's disease. Semin Oncol 17:716–735, 1990.

47. Stein RS, Golomb HS, Wiernik PH, et al.: Anatomic substages of stage IIIA Hodgkin's disease: followup of a collaborative study. Cancer Treat Rep 66:733–741, 1982.

48. Hoppe RT, Cox RS, Rosenberg SA, et al.: Prognostic factors in pathologic stage III Hodgkin's disease. Cancer Treat Rep 66:743–749, 1982.

49. Mouch PM, Rosenthal DS, Canellos GP, et al.: Improved survival for stage IIIA and IIIB Hodgkin's disease patients treated with combined radiation therapy (RT) and chemotherapy. Proc Am Soc Clin Oncol 2:213, 1983.

50. Lister TA, Dorreen MS, Faux M, et al.: Treatment of stage III$_A$ Hodgkin's disease. J Clin Oncol 1:745–749, 1983.

51. Crowther D, Wagstaff J, Deaken D, et al.: A randomized study comparing chemotherapy alone and chemotherapy followed by radiotherapy in patients with pathologically staged III$_A$ Hodgkin's disease. J Clin Oncol 2:892–897, 1984.

52. Brookman MA, Longo DL: Concomitant illness in patients treated for Hodgkin's disease. Cancer Treat Rev 13:77–111, 1986.

53. DeVita VT, Simon RM, Hubbard SM, et al.: Curability of advanced Hodgkin's disease with chemotherapy: long-term follow up of MOPP treated patients at NCI. Ann Intern Med 92:587–595, 1980.

54. Longo DL, Young RC, Wesley M, et al.: Twenty years of MOPP therapy for Hodgkin's disease. J Clin Oncol 4:1295–1306, 1986.

55. Harker WG, Kushlan P, Rosenberg SA: Combination chemotherapy for advanced Hodgkin's disease after failure of MOPP: ABVD and B-CAVe. Ann Intern Med 101:440–446, 1984.

56. Nicholson WM, Beard MEJ, Crowther D, et al.: Combination chemotherapy in generalized Hodgkin's disease. Br Med J 3:7–10, 1976.

57. Farber LR, Prosnitz LR, Cadman EC, et al.: Curative potential of combined modality therapy for advanced Hodgkin's disease. Cancer 46:1590–1597, 1980.

58. Klimo P, Connors JM: An update on the Vancouver experience in the management of advanced Hodgkin's disease treated with the MOPP/ABV hybrid program. Semin Hematol 25:34–40, 1988.

59. Canellos GP, Anderson BA, Peterson BA, Gottlieb AJ: EVA: etoposide, vinblastine, doxorubicin (adriamycin)—an effective regimen for the treatment of Hodgkin's disease in relapse following MOPP. A study of the Cancer and Leukemia Group B. Proc Am Soc Clin Oncol 10:273, 1991.

60. Goldie JH, Coldman AJ: A mathematical model for relating the drug sensitivity of tumors to their spontaneous mutation rate. Cancer Treat Rep 63:1727–1733, 1979.

61. Santoro A, Bonadonna G, Bonfante V, et al.: Alternating drug combinations in the treatment of advanced Hodgkin's disease. N Engl J Med 306:770–775, 1982.

62. Bonadonna G, Valgussa P, Santoro A: Alternating non-cross-resistant combination chemotherapy or MOPP in stage IV Hodgkin's disease. Ann Intern Med 104:739–746, 1986.

63. Glick J, Tsiatis A, Schilsky R, et al.: A randomized phase III trial of MOPP/ABV hybrid vs. sequential MOPP-ABVD in advanced Hodgkin's disease: preliminary results of the intergroup trial. Proc Am Soc Clin Oncol 10:271, 1991. Abstract

64. Taylor RE, McElwin TJ, Barrett A, et al.: Etoposide as a single agent in relapsed advanced lymphomas—a phase II study. Cancer Chemother Pharmacol 7:175–177, 1982.

65. Oliver IN, Wolf MM, Cruickshank D, et al.: Nitrogen mustard, vincristine, procarbazine, and prednisolone for relapse after radiation in Hodgkin's disease. Cancer 62:233–239, 1988.

66. Pillai GN, Hagemeister RB, Valasquez WS, et al.: Prognostic factors for stage IV Hodgkin's disease treated with MOPP, with or without bleomycin. Cancer 55:691–697, 1985.

67. Wagstaff J, Gregory WM, Swindell R, et al.: Prognostic factors for survival in stage III$_B$ and IV Hodgkin's disease: a multivariate analysis comparing two specialist treatment centres. Br J Cancer 58:487–492, 1988.

68. Carde P, MacKintosh FR, Rosenberg SA: A dose and time response

analysis of the treatment of Hodgkin's disease with MOPP chemotherapy. J Clin Oncol 1:146–153, 1983.

69. Canellos GP: Can MOPP be replaced in the treatment of advanced Hodgkin's disease? Semin Oncol 17(suppl 2):2–6, 1990.

70. Levis A, Vitolo U, CioccaVasina MA, et al.: Predictive value of the early response to chemotherapy in high-risk stages II and II Hodgkin's disease. Cancer 60:1713–1719, 1987.

71. Green JA, Dawson AA, Fell LF, et al.: Measurement of drug dosage intensity in MVPP therapy in Hodgkin's disease. Br J Clin Pharmacol 9:511–514, 1980.

72. Van Rijswijk RE, Haanen C, Dekker AW, et al.: Dose intensity of MOPP chemotherapy and survival in Hodgkin's disease. J Clin Oncol 7:1776–1782, 1989.

73. Santoro A, Viviana S, Villarreal CJ, et al.: Salvage chemotherapy in Hodgkin's disease irradiation failures: superiority of doxorubicin-containing regimens over MOPP. Cancer Treat Rep 70:343–348, 1986.

74. Fisher RI, DeVita VT, Hubbard SM, et al.: Prolonged disease-free survival in Hodgkin's disease with MOPP reinduction after first relapse. Ann Intern Med 90:761–763, 1979.

75. Vose JM, Bierman PJ, Armitage JO: Hodgkin's disease: the role of bone marrow transplantation. Semin Oncol 17:749–757, 1990.

76. Williams SF, Bitran JD: The role of high-dose therapy and autologous bone marrow reinfusion in the treatment of Hodgkin's disease. Hematol Oncol Clin North Am 3:319–329, 1989.

77. Jagannath S, Armitage JO, Dicke KA, et al.: Prognostic factors for response and survival after high-dose cyclophosphamide, carmustine, and etoposide with autologous bone marrow transplantation. J Clin Oncol 7:179–185, 1989.

78. Carella AM, Congiu AM, Gaozza E, et al.: High-dose chemotherapy with autologous bone marrow transplantation in 50 advanced resistant Hodgkin's disease patients: an Italian Study Group report. J Clin Oncol 6:1411–1416, 1988.

79. Gribben JG, Linch DC, Singer CRJ, et al.: Successful treatment of refractory Hodgkin's disease by high-dose combination chemotherapy and autologous bone marrow transplantation. Blood 73:340–344, 1989.

80. Goldstone AH: EBMT experience of autologous BMT (ABMT) in non-Hodgkin's lymphoma and Hodgkin's disease. Bone Marrow Transplant 1(suppl):289–292, 1986.

81. Phillips GL, Solff SN, Herzig RH, et al.: Treatment of progressive Hodgkin's disease with intensive chemoradiotherapy and autologous bone marrow transplantation. Blood 73:2086–2092, 1989.

82. Taylor K McD, Jagannath S, Spinolo JA, et al.: Recombinant human granulocyte colony-stimulating factor hastens recovery after high-dose chemotherapy and autologous bone marrow transplantation in Hodgkin's disease. J Clin Oncol 7:791–799, 1989.

83. Nemunaitis J, Singer JW, Buchner CD, et al.: Use of recombinant human granulocyte-macrophage colony-stimulating factor in autologous marrow transplantation for lymphoid malignancies. Blood 72:834–836, 1988.

84. Portlock CS: Management of the low-grade non-Hodgkin's lymphomas. Semin Oncol 17:51–59, 1990.

85. Chabner BA, Johnson RE, Young R, et al.: Sequential non-surgical and surgical staging of non-Hodgkin's lymphomas. Ann Intern Med 85:149–154, 1976.

86. Rosenberg SA: Validity of Ann Arbor staging of the non-Hodgkin's lymphomas. Cancer Treat Rep 61:1023–1027, 1977.

87. Paryani SB, Hoppe RT, Cos RS, et al.: The role of radiation therapy in the management of stage III follicular lymphomas. J Clin Oncol 2:841–848, 1984.

88. Portlock CS: Management of the indolent non-Hodgkin's lymphomas. Semin Oncol 7:292–301, 1980.

89. Hoppe RT, Kushlan P, Kaplan HS, et al.: The treatment of advanced stage favorable histology non-Hodgkin's lymphoma: a preliminary report of a randomized trial comparing single agent chemotherapy, combination chemotherapy, and whole body irradiation. Blood 58:592–598, 1981.

90. DeVita VT, Canellos GP, Chabner BA, et al.: Advanced diffuse histiocytic lymphoma, a potentially curable disease. Results with combination chemotherapy. Lancet 1:248–250, 1975.

91. Portlock CS, Rosenberg SA: Chemotherapy of the non-Hodgkin's lymphomas: the Stanford experience. Cancer Treat Rep 61:1049–1055, 1977.

92. Armitage JO, Dick FR, Corder MP, et al.: Predicting therapeutic outcome in patients with diffuse histiocytic lymphoma treated with cyclophosphamide, adriamycin, vincristine, and prednisone (CHOP). Cancer 50:1695–1702, 1982.

93. Merchant N, McLaughlin P, Fuller L, et al.: Follicular (nodular) mixed lymphoma: a review of 65 cases. Proc Am Soc Clin Oncol 3:249, 1984. Abstract

94. Skarin AT, Canellos GP, Rosenthal DS, et al.: Improved prognosis of diffuse histiocytic and undifferentiated lymphoma by use of high dose methotrexate alternating with standard agents. (M-BACOD). J Clin Oncol 1:91–98, 1983.

95. Klimo P, Connors JM: MACOP-B chemotherapy for the treatment of diffuse large-cell lymphoma. Ann Intern Med 102:596–602, 1985.

96. Urba WJ, Duffy PL, Longo DL: Treatment of patients with aggressive lymphomas: an overview. J NCI Monographs 10:29–37, 1990.

97. Fisher RI, DeVita VT, Hubbard SM: Diffuse aggressive lymphomas: increased survival after alternating flexible sequences of ProMACE and MOPP chemotherapy. Ann Intern Med 98:304–309, 1983.

98. Longo DL, DeVita VT, Duffy PL, et al.: Superiority of ProMACE-CytaBOM over ProMACE-MOPP in the treatment of advanced diffuse aggressive lymphoma: results of a prospective randomized trial. J Clin Oncol 9:25–38, 1991.

99. Anderson KC, Skarin AT, Rosenthal DS, et al.: Combination chemotherapy for advanced non-Hodgkin's lymphomas other than diffuse histiocytic or undifferentiated histologies. Cancer Treat Rep 68:1343–1348, 1984.

100. Case DC: Comparison of M-2 protocol with COP in patients with nodular lymphoma. Oncology 41:159, 1984.

101. Ezdinli EZ, Anderson JR, Melvin F, et al.: Moderate versus aggressive chemotherapy of nodular lymphocytic poorly differentiated lymphoma. J Clin Oncol 3:769–775, 1985.

102. Young RC, Longo DL, Gladstein E, et al.: The treatment of indolent lymphomas: watchful waiting versus aggressive combined modality treatment. Semin Hematol 25:11–16, 1988.

103. Foon KA, Sherwin SA, Abrams PG: Treatment of advanced non-Hodgkin's lymphoma with recombinant leukocyte A interferon. N Engl J Med 311:1148–1152, 1984.

104. Longo DL, Glatstein E, Duffey P, et al.: Treatment of localized aggressive lymphomas with combination chemotherapy followed by involved-field radiation therapy. J Clin Oncol 7:1295–1302, 1989.

105. Jones SE, Rosenberg SA, Kaplan ES, et al.: Non-Hodgkin's lymphomas: single agent chemotherapy. Cancer 43:417–425, 1972.

106. Fisher RI, DeVita VT, Hubbard SM, et al.: Diffuse aggressive lymphomas: increased survival after alternating flexible sequences of ProMACE and MOPP chemotherapy. Ann Intern Med 98:304–309, 1983.

107. Fisher RI, Hubbard SM, DeVita VT, et al.: Factors predicting long-term survival in diffuse mixed, histiocytic, or undifferentiated lymphoma. Blood 58:45–50, 1981.

108. Vose JM, Armitage JO, Weisenburger DD, et al.: The importance

of age in survival of patients treated with chemotherapy for diffuse large-cell lymphoma—rapidly responding patients have more durable remissions. J Clin Oncol 4:160–164, 1986.

109. Magrath I, Lee YJ, Anderson T, et al.: Prognostic factors in Burkitt's lymphoma: importance of total tumor burden. Cancer 45:1507–1515, 1980.

110. Ziegler JL: Burkitt's lymphoma. N Engl J Med 305:735–745, 1981.

111. Meyer RM, Hryniuk WM, Goodyear MDE: The role of dose intensity in determining outcome in intermediate-grade non-Hodgkin's lymphoma. J Clin Oncol 9:339–347, 1991.

112. Kessinger A, Nademanee A, Forman SJ, Armitage JO: Autologous bone marrow transplantation for Hodgkin's and non-Hodgkin's lymphoma. Hematol Oncol Clin North Am 4:577–587, 1990.

113. Williams SF: The role of bone marrow transplantation in the non-Hodgkin's lymphomas. Semin Oncol 17:88–95, 1990.

114. Phillips GL, Herzig RH, Lazarus HM, et al.: Treatment of resistant malignant lymphoma with cyclophosphamide, total body irradiation, and transplantation of cryopreserved autologous marrow. N Engl J Med 310:1557–1561, 1984.

115. Armitage JO, Gingrich RD, Klassen LW, et al.: Trial of high-dose cytarabine, cyclophosphamide, total-body irradiation, and autologous marrow transplantation for refractory lymphoma. Cancer Treat Rep 70:871–875, 1986.

116. Takvoran T, Canellos GP, Ritz J, et al.: Prolonged disease free survival after autologous bone marrow transplantation in patients with non-Hodgkin's lymphoma with a poor prognosis. N Engl J Med 316:1499–1505, 1987.

117. Levine AM, Loureiro C, Sullivan-Halley J, et al.: HIV-related lymphoma: prognostic factors predictive of survival. Blood 1988:72:247a, 1988.

118. Kaplan LD, Abrams DI, Feigal E, et al.: AIDS-associated non-Hodgkin's lymphoma in San Francisco. JAMA 261:719–724, 1989.

119. Gill PS, Levine AM, Krailo M, et al.: AIDS-related malignant lymphoma: results of prospective treatment trials. J Clin Oncol 5:1322–1328, 1987.

120. Bermudez MA, Grant KM, Rodvien R, Mendes F: Non-Hodgkin's lymphoma in a population with or at risk for acquired immunodeficiency syndrome: indications for intensive chemotherapy. Am J Med 86:71–76, 1989.

121. Knowles DM, Chamulak GA, Subar M, et al.: Lymphoid neoplasia associated with the acquired immunodeficiency syndrome (AIDS). Ann Intern Med 108:744–753, 1988.

122. Lowenthal DA, Straus DJ, Campbell SW, et al.: AIDS-related lymphoid neoplasia. Cancer 61:2325–2337, 1988.

123. Levine AM, Wernz JC, Kaplan L, et al.: Low dose chemotherapy with central nervous system prophylaxis and zidovudine maintenance with AIDS-related lymphoma: a multi-institutional trial. Blood 74:897a, 1989.

124. Walsh C, Wernz J, Laubenstein L, et al.: Phase I study of M-BACOD and GM-CSF in AIDS-associated non-Hodgkin's lymphoma: preliminary results. Blood 74:466a, 1989.

125. Posner JB, Howieson J, Cvitkovic E: "Disappearing" spinal cord compression: oncolytic effect of glucocorticoids (and other chemotherapeutic agents) on epidural metastases. Ann Neurol 2:409–413, 1977.

126. Hohl RJ, Schilsky RL: Nonmalignant complications of therapy for Hodgkin's disease. Hematol Oncol Clin North Am 3:331–343, 1989.

127. Vanhaelan CPJ, Fisher RI: Increased sensitivity of T cells to regulation by normal suppressor cells persists in long-term survivors with Hodgkin's disease. Am J Med 72:385–390, 1982.

128. Schilsky RL, Sherins RJ. Adverse effects of treatment: gonadal dysfunction. In DeVita VT, Hellman S, Rosenberg SM: Cancer Principles and Practice of Oncology, ed. 2. Philadelphia, JG Lippincott, 1985, p 2032.

129. Santoro A, Viviani S, Zucali R, et al.: Comparative results and toxicity of MOPP vs ABVD combined with radiotherapy in PS IIB, III Hodgkin's disease. Proc Am Soc Clin Oncol 2:223, 1983.

130. Bonadonna G, Santoro A: ABVD chemotherapy in the treatment of Hodgkin's disease. Cancer Treat Rev 9:21–35, 1982.

131. Chapman RM, Sutcliff SB, Malpas JS: Cytotoxic-induced ovarian failure in women with Hodgkin's disease. I. Hormone function. JAMA 242:1877–1881, 1979.

132. Schilsky RL, Serins RJ, Hubbard SM, et al.: Long term follow up of ovarian function in women treated with MOPP chemotherapy for Hodgkin's disease. Am J Med 71:552–556, 1981.

133. Li FP: Adverse effects of treatment: second cancers. In DeVita VT, Hellman S, Rosenberg SA: Cancer Principles and Practice of Oncology, ed. 2. Philadelphia, JB Lippincott, 1985, p 2040.

134. Pedersen-Bjergaard J, Larsen SO: Incidence of acute nonlymphocytic leukemia, preleukemia, and acute myeloproliferative syndrome up to 10 years after treatment of Hodgkin's disease. N Engl J Med 307:965–971, 1982.

135. Coltman CA, Dixon DO: Second malignancies complicating Hodgkin's disease: a Southwest Oncology Group 10-year follow-up. Cancer Treat Rep 66:1023–1033, 1982.

136. VanLeeuwen FE, Somers R, Taal BG, et al.: Increased risk of lung cancer, non-Hodgkin's lymphoma and leukemia following Hodgkin's disease. J Clin Oncol 7:1046–1058, 1989.

137. Krikorian JG, Burke JS, Rosenberg SA, et al.: Occurrence of non-Hodgkin's lymphoma after therapy for Hodgkin's disease. N Engl J Med 300:452–458, 1979.

CHAPTER 77

BREAST CANCER

SUZANNE M. FIELDS, Pharm.D. and JIM M. KOELLER, M.S.

Approximately 175,900 new cases of breast cancer will be diagnosed in the United States during 1991 and the incidence rate continues to rise by about 1% a year (1). The disease occurs primarily in women, and one out of every 9 American women can expect to be diagnosed with breast cancer during her lifetime. Women under the age of 30 are rarely diagnosed with breast cancer, but the incidence rate increases dramatically after the age of 30 and plateaus around the age of 50. Less than 1% ($\approx$900 cases) of the cases diagnosed annually occur in men, but the prognosis is generally poorer for male patients. Although public awareness and early detection of breast cancer have significantly increased over the past 40 years, the mortality rate from the disease has changed very little. An estimated 44,800 people will die with breast cancer in 1991. Breast cancer is the second most common cause of cancer death in women, surpassed only recently by lung cancer. Conflicting reports in the literature have created a great deal of controversy about the appropriate clinical management of particular patient subsets, such as women with node-negative disease or postmenopausal women with node-positive disease. Resolution of these controversies will require the willingness of both physicians and patients to participate in randomized, controlled clinical trials.

ETIOLOGY

The etiology of breast cancer is unknown, but several predisposing factors for the disease have been determined. These factors can be divided into three major categories: genetic, endocrine, and environmental factors (Table 77.1).

Women who have a first-degree relative (e.g., mother and/or sister) with breast cancer have a twofold to three-fold increased risk of developing breast cancer (2, 3). This risk may be increased further if more than one first-degree relative is diagnosed with the disease, the relative is young at the time of diagnosis, or the relative presents with bilateral breast cancer (4). Women with endometrial, ovarian, or colon cancer may also have an increased risk of developing breast cancer because of the transmission of an autosomal dominant trait for the disease (2). Patients who have this family cancer syndrome are frequently diagnosed at an earlier age, and the disease is often bilateral. Finally, women who have a personal history of breast cancer have a higher probability than the average woman of developing primary breast cancer in the contralateral breast (3).

Patients with benign breast disease have an increased risk of developing breast cancer if they have proliferative lesions with atypical hyperplasia (2, 3). Their risk is increased further if there is also a positive family history for breast cancer. Patients in these higher risk groups may warrant close monitoring for breast cancer development, but other patients with benign breast disease (e.g., fibro-cystic or "lumpy breast") should be treated like the general population. Both endogenous and exogenous hormones have also been associated with an increased risk for breast cancer. The incidence of breast cancer appears to correlate with prolonged high levels of estrogen in the bloodstream, which would occur in women with long menstrual histories. As a result, women with early menarche (age <12) or late menopause (age >55) are at higher risk for the development of breast cancer (5, 6). Nulliparous women are also at a greater risk for breast cancer than parous women. However, the age at which a woman experiences her first full-term pregnancy also influences her risk of developing breast cancer. A first full-term pregnancy after the age of 35 increases the risk for breast cancer, because of hormonal changes and latent breast tissue differentiation that occur during pregnancy, particularly the first pregnancy (3, 5). Theoretically, increasing the number of menstrual cycles with either oral contraceptive use or postmenopausal hormone-replacement therapy could be associated with an increased risk of breast cancer. However, the studies that have been published in this area to date still show some conflicting results. Most studies have been conducted retrospectively with numerous hormone preparations and have shown no relation between oral contraceptives and breast cancer.

In a recently published meta-analysis of the case-control studies available in the literature through 1989, a positive trend in the risk of breast cancer was noted among premenopausal women who used oral contraceptives for an extended period prior to their first term pregnancy (7). Several studies have also suggested an increased risk of breast cancer in women taking oral contraceptives during the perimenopausal period (5). Prolonged duration of postmenopausal hormone-replacement therapy has also been associated with an increased risk of breast cancer in studies conducted in both Europe and the United States (8). Additional large prospective studies will be required

Table 77.1.
Risk Factors for Breast Cancer Development

Personal history of breast cancer
Family history of breast cancer in first-degree relatives
Proliferative benign breast disease
Early menarche, late menopause
Nulliparity
First pregnancy after age 35 years
Exogenous estrogens (postmenopausal, oral contraceptives)
Obesity
Dietary factors—alcohol, high-fat diet
Radiation
Endometrial, ovarian, or colon cancer

to determine the true association between exogenous estrogen administration and the risk of breast cancer.

Based on the incidence rates of breast cancer in various countries, it would appear that environmental factors contribute to the development of breast cancer in women. Western countries, such as the United States, have high breast cancer rates, while countries like Japan have a low incidence of the disease. Furthermore, when people migrate from Japan to the United States they acquire the higher incidence rates of their new environment (9). The difference in breast cancer rates is thought to be partially due to dietary differences between the two populations, specifically the amount of fat that is consumed in the diet. Data obtained from several large studies have failed to show a direct correlation between high-fat diets and the risk of breast cancer. However, there does appear to be a connection between elevated estrogen levels and diets high in fat content. Therefore, a diet consisting of <30% fat is recommended. Obesity has also been associated with increased estrogen levels, but it has only been directly associated with an increased risk of breast cancer in postmenopausal women (2, 9). Women who are physically active during adolescence and young adulthood may also have a decreased risk of developing breast cancer, possibly due to infrequent or irregular menstrual cycles and maintaining a lean body weight (10). The combination of these factors probably contributes to the development of breast cancer in many women.

Several prospective and case-control studies have consistently demonstrated a positive correlation between alcohol consumption and the risk of breast cancer. These studies are somewhat difficult to compare because the amount and type of alcohol consumed has varied with each study (11). However, a meta-analysis of 16 studies conducted in 1988 did uncover a dose-response relationship between alcohol consumption and breast cancer risk (12). The combined data indicate that women who consume two drinks per day have a 40 to 70% increased risk for breast cancer over women who did not drink at all.

Survivors of the atomic bomb blasts during World War II have experienced an increased incidence of breast cancer because of radiation exposure (3, 11). Similar breast cancer incidence rates have also been reported in women treated with radiation for mastitis and women receiving multiple fluoroscopies for the treatment of tuberculosis. There is a 10- to 15-year latency period between radiation exposure and tumor development, and women over 40 years of age at the time of exposure appear to experience little or no increased risk for breast cancer. Some physicians have expressed concern about the use of repeated screening mammographies in women, due to the link between radiation exposure and breast cancer. However, the amount of radiation a woman is exposed to during a mammogram is extremely low, and there have been no case reports to date of breast cancer development secondary to mammography screening.

BREAST ANATOMY AND TUMOR DEVELOPMENT

Human breast tissue is composed primarily of connective tissue and fat. There is also an elaborate duct system within the breasts that is used during lactation. Breast tissue has an abundant blood supply and an extensive lymphatic network. Lymphatic drainage of the mammary tissues flows into the axillary, interpectoral, and internal mammary lymph nodes. This is important because breast cancer commonly spreads via the lymphatic system, and metastatic disease is frequently discovered in the regional lymph nodes at the time of diagnosis (Fig. 77.1).

A woman's breast tissue and glands begin to develop around the time of puberty, due to the influence and interaction of sex hormones. However, the amount of breast development occurring at puberty is limited, and most occurs during the first pregnancy. The large amounts of estrogen and progesterone produced by the ovaries during pregnancy stimulate rapid growth and terminal differentiation of immature breast tissue. A delay in the terminal differentiation of breast tissue until a later age may help explain why women who become pregnant for the first time after the age of 35 have an increased risk for breast cancer development, as immature cells are more susceptible to cycling estrogen effects and estrogens are known to initiate tumor growth (13).

The development of breast cancer occurs when breast cells lose their normal differentiation and proliferation controls. The proliferation of these abnormal, or tumor cells, is influenced by various hormones and growth factors (Fig. 77.2). There is now strong evidence to suggest that estrogen directly and indirectly stimulates the growth of tumor cells (14). Furthermore, numerous growth factors that also play a role in tumor development are secreted by the breast cancer cells themselves. These factors can be classified as either autocrine (if they stimulate their own growth) or paracrine (if they have an effect on other cells).

Figure 77.1. Breast tissue drainage and its relationship to tumor metastases. (From Copeland EM III, Bland KI: The breast. In Sabiston DC Jr (ed): Essentials of Surgery. WB Saunders, Philadelphia, 1987, with permission.)

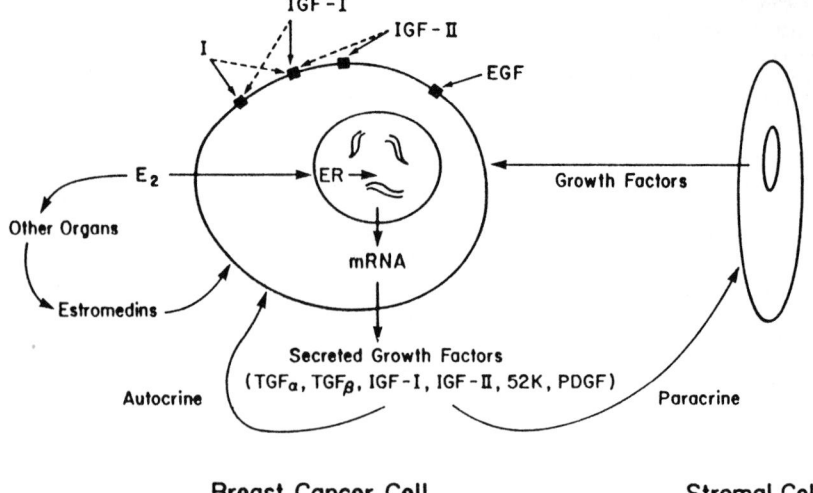

Breast Cancer Cell   **Stromal Cell**

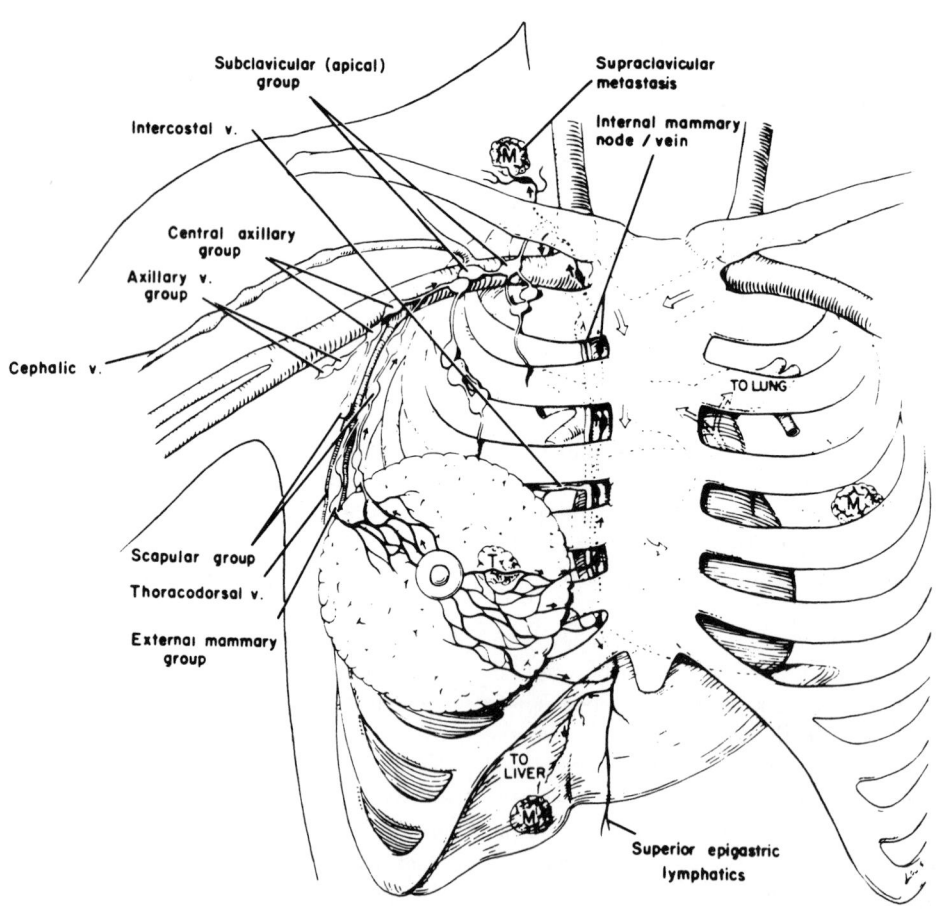

Figure 77.2. Proposed schema for breast cancer cell development. (From Osborne CK, Arteaga CL: Autocrine and paracrine growth regulation of breast cancer: clinical implications. Breast Cancer Res Treat 15:3–11, 1990, with permission.)

Examples of the autocrine growth factors include transforming growth factor-α (TGF-α) and insulin-like growth factors I and II (IGF-I and IGF-II). Transforming growth factor-β (TGF-β), platelet-derived growth factor (PDGF), and procathepsin D (52K protein) are all paracrine growth factors. The exact mechanism of tumor development is not completely understood presently, but tremendous progress has been made in this area in the past few years with the discovery of the autocrine and paracrine growth factors. Furthermore, the mechanism of action of several of the hormonal agents used for the treatment of breast cancer involves alteration of the growth factors involved in tumor development.

DETECTION AND DIAGNOSIS

Early detection of breast cancer is critical because patients with limited-stage disease have a better prognosis. Three screening techniques have been shown to be effective for breast cancer detection—breast self-examination (BSE), physical examination by a physician, and mammography.

A large majority of breast cancers are discovered by patients themselves during regular breast self-examination. Breast self-examination is a simple procedure that should be performed by all women on a monthly basis. In a prospective study involving over 200 women diagnosed with breast cancer, Huguley et al. demonstrated that women who performed breast self-examinations had a better prognosis than women who did not do self-examinations [15]. Women conducting self-examinations were generally diagnosed with earlier stage disease and had a higher 5-year survival rate (76.7% vs. 60.9%) than women not performing self-examinations. Numerous confounders could account for 25% of the excess breast cancer in the nonexaminers, and more limited disease among the self-examiners could account for 50% of the remaining survival difference. As a result, a 5 to 6% survival difference between the two groups could be attributed to breast self-examinations. Currently, the American Cancer Society recommends that all women perform monthly breast self-examinations and numerous educational brochures are available to aid women in this procedure. However, for breast self-examination to be an effective screening tool, women must conduct thorough monthly examinations.

A physical examination conducted by a trained physician is also an important screening technique for breast cancer detection. The American Cancer Society recommends that women over the age of 40 have a yearly physical examination by their physician. Although mammography is more sensitive for detecting small breast tumors than physical examination, approximately 10% of palpable masses are missed by mammography [16]. Therefore, it is critical that both physical examinations and screening mammography be performed. When the two procedures are used together, it is estimated that over 90 + % of diagnosed breast cancers are detected [17].

The importance of physical examination and mammography as screening tools to detect breast cancer has been confirmed with two large, randomized, prospective clinical trials—The Health Insurance Plan of Greater New York (HIP) and the Breast Cancer Detection Demonstration Project (BCDDP). The HIP study randomized 31,000 women between the ages of 40 and 64 to receive an initial screening examination plus mammography with three annual follow-up screenings [18]. The matched control group for the study consisted of 31,000 additional women who received only routine medical care. At the 5-year analysis, a 38% reduction in breast cancer mortality was noted in the patients receiving annual physical examinations and mammography, compared with the control group. Furthermore, the reduction in mortality has persisted throughout 18 years of follow-up and remains at 23% [19]. The BCDDP enrolled 280,000 women between the ages of 35 and 72 at centers throughout the United States who were screened with physical examination and mammography [20]. The women were also instructed about breast self-examination and were encouraged to perform monthly examinations. There were 4443 breast cancers diagnosed during the study period, and approximately one-third of these were <1 cm in size at the time of diagnosis. Furthermore, more than 80% of the cancers detected had no axillary nodal involvement at the time of detection. The BCDDP further supported the use of screening mammography since ≈42% of the tumors were detected by mammography alone. When the data were initially analyzed at the 5-year follow-up point, there was some question about whether women under 50 benefited from screening mammograms. However, the final analysis conducted after 10 years of follow-up demonstrated that screening for breast cancer with mammography is effective in younger women as well as older women [21]. As a result of this study, the American Cancer Society recommended that all women receive a baseline mammography between the ages of 35 and 40 years. These guidelines are currently being changed, based on more recent data. In the new guidelines, yearly monitoring for women between the ages of 40 and 49 is suggested. The current American Cancer Society guidelines for breast cancer detection are listed in Table 77.2.

Approximately 90% of breast masses are detected by the patients themselves, through either breast self-examination or accidental contact [2]. Breast cancer masses tend to be painless, solitary, unilateral, hard, irregular, or nonmobile. Patients may also present with skin changes, nipple discharge, or axillary lymphadenopathy. Any woman with suspected benign or malignant breast disease should have mammography. Furthermore, any breast mass that is suggestive of malignancy by mammography or on physical

Table 77.2.
American Cancer Society Guidelines for Breast Cancer Detection

Age Group (years)	Screening Recommendation
20–39	Monthly breast self-examination
	Breast physical examination every 3 years
	Baseline mammogram at age 35–39 years
40–49	Monthly breast self-examination
	Yearly breast physical examination
	Mammogram every 2 years
>50	Monthly breast self-examination
	Yearly breast physical examination and mammogram

Table 77.3.
TNM Staging System for Breast Cancer

Stage	Tumor Size (T)	Nodal Involvement (N)	Metastases (M)
0	T_{is}[a]	Negative axillary nodes	None
I	≤2 cm	Negative axillary nodes	None
II	>2 cm ≤5 cm	Positive axillary nodes	None
III	>5 cm or any size with skin or chest wall fixation	Positive axillary nodes	None
IV	Any size	Any involvement	Present

[a] T_{is}, carcinoma in situ.

examination should be biopsied by either fine-needle aspiration, core-needle biopsy, incisional biopsy, or excisional biopsy. While needle aspirations and core biopsies do provide enough evidence for a histologic diagnosis of breast cancer, they do not delineate the size of the tumor or allow for estrogen receptor determination of the tumor (17).

STAGING

The TNM classification system is the most commonly accepted staging system for breast cancer. Tumor size (T) is described on a scale of 0–4 based on characteristics of the primary tumor. Extent of lymph node involvement (N), based on location and palpability and the presence or absence of distant metastases (M), are also included in the system. In the management of breast cancer, the ipsilateral axillary, internal mammary, and pectoral nodes are all considered to be regional spread of the disease. Involvement of any other lymph nodes, however, is considered distant metastases. Table 77.3 summarizes the TNM staging system utilized for breast cancer.

PROGNOSTIC FACTORS

The natural history of breast cancer varies greatly between patients. Some patients have extremely aggressive disease

that progresses rapidly, while others are diagnosed with disease that follows a more indolent course. Due to these variations, the ability to predict which patients have a better disease prognosis is extremely important. Table 77.4 lists the prognostic factors that have been determined in breast cancer patients to date.

The single most important prognostic factor at the time of diagnosis is the extent of axillary lymph node involvement. Numerous studies have confirmed the significance of nodal involvement for predicting disease recurrence and survival. The number of affected nodes is inversely related to disease recurrence (22). Only 25 to 30% of patients with negative lymph nodes will have disease recurrence at 10 years (23). This recurrence rate increases to 55 to 65% when 1 to 3 nodes are involved, and 80 to 90% in patients with four or more positive nodes. Tumor size at the time of diagnosis is also an important prognostic factor for breast cancer (23, 24). Although large tumors have a greater tendency to metastasize to axillary lymph nodes, tumor size is also an independent predictor for breast cancer recurrence (Table 77.5). A third important prognostic factor is estrogen and progesterone receptor status. Laboratory assays for the determination of estrogen receptor content in tumors were originally developed in an attempt to predict tumor response to hormonal therapy. However, in 1977 Knight and his colleagues recognized the prognostic importance of estrogen receptor (ER) status by demonstrating a higher rate of disease recurrence in pa-

Table 77.4.
Prognostic Factors in Breast Cancer

Tumor size
Extent of nodal involvement
Extrogen and progesterone receptor status
Patient age
Menopausal status
Histologic grade
Cell proliferation indices
Oncogene and growth-factor-receptor expression
Estrogen-regulated proteins

Table 77.5.
Ten-Year Survival (%) Related to Primary Tumor Size (cm) and Level of Axillary Involvement[a]

Axillary Status	Size of Primary Lesion (cm)		
	<2	2–5	>5
Negative	92	76	44
Positive	68	51	31

[a] Adapted from Henderson CI, Harris JR, Kinne DW, et al.: Cancer of the breast. In DeVita VT, Hellman S, Rosenberg S (eds): Cancer, Principles & Practice of Oncology. Philadelphia, JB Lippincott, 1989, p 1209.

tients with ER-negative tumors (23, 25). Furthermore, in patients with node-positive disease, the presence of progesterone receptors in tumor tissue is indicative of an improved disease-free survival compared with patients without progesterone receptors.

The rate of tumor cell proliferation also has prognostic significance in breast cancer recurrence. Rate of cell proliferation can be determined using either the tritiated-thymidine labeling index (TLI) or DNA flow cytometry, which determines the percentage of tumor cells actively dividing in the S-phase of the cell cycle. Both techniques indicate that patients with rapidly proliferating tumors have a decreased disease-free survival, compared with patients with slowly proliferating tumors (26, 27). Additionally, flow cytometry can detect abnormal DNA content, or aneuploidy, in breast cancer cells. Patients with aneuploid tumors also appear to have a decreased disease-free survival (27). Increased levels of the HER-2/neu oncogene, a protein that promotes tumor cell development, have also been correlated with decreased disease-free and overall survival in patients with node-positive disease (28). A final important prognostic factor is the level of cathepsin D in breast cancer cells. Cathepsin D is a protease that promotes tumor cell growth and possibly disease metastasis. In women with node-negative disease, high levels of cathepsin D have been associated with a decreased disease-free and overall survival (29).

Predicting disease recurrence in patients with breast cancer is a difficult task, especially in patients with negative nodal involvement at the time of diagnosis. The ability to determine prognostic factors for disease recurrence would be extremely useful clinically, as patients with a poor prognosis could be treated more aggressively initially in an attempt to prolong survival.

TREATMENT OF BREAST CANCER
Early-Stage Breast Cancer

Approximately 75 to 80% of women diagnosed with breast cancer will have stage I or II disease at the time of diagnosis. In the past, the primary treatment for breast cancer was a radical mastectomy. The goal of this treatment was to remove the breast underlying tissues and regional lymph nodes. However, more recent data suggest that a modified radical mastectomy, which spares the pectoralis muscles and some high axillary lymph nodes, was as effective in the treatment of primary disease as a radical mastectomy (30). Furthermore, at the NIH Consensus Conference in June 1990, it was determined that breast conservation treatment is acceptable therapy for most women with stage I or II disease, based on survival rates obtained from several randomized clinical trials (31, 32). Breast conservation treatment is defined as lumpectomy or partial mastectomy accompanied by axillary node dissection and followed by radiation therapy. Although the

local recurrence rate in women receiving breast conservation treatment is low (10 to 30%), the use of adjuvant chemotherapy or hormonal therapy may help further reduce this recurrence rate.

Adjuvant therapy is chemotherapy or hormonal therapy that is administered in an attempt to treat the residual micrometastatic disease that remains following surgery. In May 1988, the National Cancer Institute issued a clinical alert to physicians concerning the use of adjuvant hormonal or cytotoxic chemotherapy in the treatment of women with node-negative breast cancer (stage I) (33). This alert was issued because of the results of four randomized clinical trials using adjuvant therapy in node-negative breast cancer patients (34–37). Although the treatment regimens used in the four trials were different, all demonstrated a statistically significant increase in disease-free survival in patients with node-negative disease (Table 77.6). However, overall survival was not prolonged significantly in any of these studies. Because the differences in disease-free survival between treated and untreated patients were relatively small and the disease-free survival in patients receiving no adjuvant therapy is 70 to 90%, many physicians question whether all patients with node-negative disease should receive adjuvant therapy (39). Furthermore, both the acute and delayed toxicities and the cost-effectiveness of the therapy must be considered. The direct cost of treating all patients with node-negative disease may considerably outweigh the benefits achieved in disease-free survival ($338,174,200 per year to achieve a disease-free survival advantage in approximately 5000 patients) (39). Furthermore, indirect costs in the form of drug toxicities and decreased quality of life during therapy are difficult to quantitate, but they should be included when weighing the risks and benefits of adjuvant therapy. Acute toxicities, such as nausea, vomiting, mucositis, and myelosuppression did result in patient death in a small percentage of patients in the randomized clinical trials. Long-term toxicities in the form of secondary malignancies (i.e., leukemia following alkylating agents and endometrial cancers following tamoxifen therapy), venous and arterial thrombosis, and congestive heart failure secondary to anthracycline administration were not addressed because of the relatively short follow-up period. These delayed toxicities are increasingly important when the survival benefits associated with adjuvant therapy are minimal or nonexistent (40). Until the data from these four and other clinical trials mature, the recommended treatment for stage I breast cancer will remain controversial. Due to the discrepancies in the data collected to date, physicians are encouraged to enroll their newly diagnosed patients in large, prospectively randomized clinical trials. Outside the clinical trial setting, the decision to treat node-negative breast cancer with chemotherapy or hormonal therapy must be made on an individual basis. The presence or

Table 77.6.
Clinical Trials of Adjuvant Therapy for Node-negative Breast Cancer

Trial	No. Patients	Treatment Regimen	Disease-free Survival Treated (%) vs. Control (%)		P Value	Reference
Ludwig V	1275	CMF × 1 month[a]	77	73	.04	(36)
Intergroup	406	CMFP × 6 months[b]	84	69	.0001	(34)
NSABP B13	679	MF × 12 months[c]	80	71	.003	(35)
NSABP B14	2644	TAM × 5 years[d]	83	77	<.00001	(36)

[a] Cyclophosphamide 400 mg/m^2 IV days 1 and 8; methotrexate 40 mg/m^2 IV days 1 and 8; fluorouracil 600 mg/m^2 days 1 and 8 (leucovorin 15 mg IV/p.o. days 1 and 8 was also given to 69% of patients).
[b] Cyclophosphamide 100 mg/m^2 p.o. days 1–14 ; methotrexate 40 mg/m^2 IV days 1 and 8; fluorouracil 600 mg/m^2 IV days 1 and 8; prednisone 40 mg/m^2 p.o. days 1–14.
[c] Methotrexate 100 mg/m^2 IV days 1 and 8; fluorouracil 600 mg/m^2 IV days 1 and 8 (leucovorin 10 mg/m^2 p.o. q6h × 6 doses).
[d] Tamoxifen 10 mg p.o. b.i.d.

absence of prognostic factors and the patient's desire to receive treatment should influence the physician's final judgment concerning adjuvant therapy. For example, a woman with a small primary tumor (<2 cm) that possesses estrogen receptors and is diploid with a low S-phase fraction may be encouraged not to receive adjuvant therapy but to undergo close medical observation. Continued research in the area of adjuvant therapy for node-negative breast cancer is clearly warranted.

The management of stage II breast cancer (tumor <5 cm with positive nodal involvement) is more straightforward, based on the results of more than 100 randomized trials using systemic adjuvant therapy. Although the results of the individual trials are often contradictory, a meta-analysis of many of the trials combined indicates that systemic adjuvant therapy can prolong disease-free and overall survival in stage II breast cancer (41). This analysis involved 61 trials in which 28,896 women were enrolled. Several conclusions concerning various patient subsets can be drawn from the pooled data.

There were 31 trials in which systemic adjuvant chemotherapy (both single-agent and combination regimens) were compared with no-adjuvant therapy (41). An overall reduction in the odds of death as a result of treatment in patients receiving adjuvant chemotherapy was 14%, regardless of patient age and treatment regimen. When analyzed by patient age, the reduction in the annual odds of death was significantly greater in women under the age of 50 (22%) compared with older patients. No significant survival benefit was demonstrated with adjuvant chemotherapy in women ≥50 years of age. Furthermore, the use of combination chemotherapy regimens appeared to be more effective than single-agent regimens, and prolonged treatment with chemotherapy (>6 months) had no survival advantage over short-term therapy.

While combination chemotherapy regimens have proven to be more effective than single-agent therapy, the optimal combination regimen has not been determined. Numerous drug combinations were used in the various

clinical trials, but the combination of cyclophosphamide, methotrexate, and fluorouracil (CMF) has been studied most extensively. However, doxorubicin has demonstrated the most activity of all drugs as single-agent therapy in phase II clinical trials in breast cancer and has produced increased response rates when used in combination-chemotherapy regimens (42). To determine whether doxorubicin should be included in standard combination-chemotherapy regimens used for breast cancer, a direct comparison between CMF and a similar regimen containing doxorubicin must be conducted. Furthermore, the effect of the addition of tamoxifen to standard combination-chemotherapy regimens in the treatment of premenopausal women also remains to be determined.

The overview analysis also contained 28 trials involving adjuvant therapy with oral tamoxifen (41). The primary benefit of adjuvant tamoxifen therapy was seen in post-menopausal patients over the age of 50 years. This patient population experienced a 20% decrease in mortality with adjuvant tamoxifen therapy. Premenopausal patients also experienced a decrease in mortality, although not as great as in the postmenopausal patients. However, the number of young women in the trial receiving single-agent tamoxifen therapy was small, so these results are difficult to interpret. The data also suggest that various doses of tamoxifen (20, 30, or 40 mg) are equally effective and that prolonged drug administration may be more effective (i.e., 2 years versus 1 year). Further trials must be conducted to determine the optimal use of tamoxifen as systemic adjuvant therapy for breast cancer. Other questions concerning the long-term benefits and side effects of tamoxifen therapy must also be addressed.

Tamoxifen is a weak estrogen that has both estrogenic and antiestrogenic effects. Its primary mechanism of action in breast cancer involves binding of the estrogen receptor, followed by inhibition of tumor cell growth (43). Because the antitumor activity of tamoxifen is cytostatic rather than cytotoxic, the potential use of tamoxifen as chemosuppressive therapy against the development of breast cancer is being considered. If the drug is to be used in this setting or as long-term adjuvant therapy in early stage disease, then the benefits of therapy must outweigh the risks. Fortunately, the acute toxicities associated with tamoxifen therapy are minimal and include nausea, hot flashes, mild edema, and vaginitis. Tamoxifen also has several favorable long-term effects due to its estrogenic activity on tissues other than breast. For example, tamoxifen significantly decreased total cholesterol and low-density lipoprotein cholesterol levels in postmenopausal women receiving 2 years of adjuvant therapy for node-negative breast cancer (44). Plasma high-density lipoprotein levels were also increased, resulting in lipoprotein profiles that are favorable for the prevention of coronary heart disease and artherosclerosis. Laboratory data have also suggested that tamoxifen may retard bone resorption secondary to its estrogenic activity (43, 45). Although several small studies have supported this finding, large controlled trials evaluating the effect of tamoxifen on bone mineral density must be conducted (46).

Long-term tamoxifen administration may also be associated with minimal side effects. Due to its effects on coagulation factors, tamoxifen has been reported to cause thrombophlebitis in some patients (43, 45). The development of thrombophlebitis in women participating in clinical trials has been minimal to date. Presently, the most concerning side effect reported with long-term tamoxifen therapy in the occurrence of endometrial cancer. Scattered reports have appeared in the literature over the years of the development of endometrial cancer following tamoxifen administration (47). Furthermore, in a large, randomized study conducted in Scandinavia, women receiving tamoxifen had a relative risk for the development of uterine cancer that was 6.4 times greater than the patients in the control group (48). More randomized, prospective clinical trials must be conducted to determine the safety of long-term tamoxifen therapy. However these trials will require large numbers of patients and extensive follow-up. As a result, they may not be feasible.

In summary, the management of stage II breast cancer depends primarily upon patient age and estrogen receptor status. All premenopausal women should be treated with 6 months of adjuvant systemic chemotherapy, regardless of their estrogen-receptor status. The most commonly used adjuvant regimen is CMF. The effectiveness of hormonal therapy combined with chemotherapy remains to be established in this patient population. In postmenopausal estrogen-receptor positive patients, adjuvant endocrine therapy in the form of oral tamoxifen is the treatment of choice. Current recommendations are to administer tamoxifen in a dose of 20 mg daily for a minimum of 2 years. Postmenopausal estrogen-receptor-negative patients form the only patient subset in which treatment remains undetermined. Adjuvant systemic chemotherapy has proven beneficial in this patient subset, but it remains investigational at this time. The combination of adjuvant chemotherapy and endocrine therapy may also prove to be beneficial, but it is considered investigational. However, optimal therapy has not been determined for any patient subset, and all patients should be encouraged to participate in clinical trials.

Locally Advanced Disease

Patients diagnosed with locally advanced breast cancer (stage III disease) have tumors >5 cm or direct tumor involvement of the skin or underlying chest wall. These patients also have extensive lymph node involvement. Due to the bulk of disease at the time of diagnosis, surgical management is generally not feasible. Furthermore, standard treatment modalities are minimally effective resulting in very poor survival in these patients. In an attempt to improve the overall survival rate in women with locally advanced disease, researchers began to use combined modality therapy. Radiation therapy, systemic chemotherapy, and surgery have all been used in various regimens in randomized clinical trials. Neoadjuvant therapy involves the use of chemotherapy before surgery, to decrease the size of the tumor and improve resectability (49). Other advantages of neoadjuvant chemotherapy include earlier treatment of micrometastatic disease, intact tumor vasculature resulting in improved drug delivery, the ability to determine tumor responsiveness to chemotherapy in vivo, and the ability to customize postsurgical systemic therapy based on this response. Following neoadjuvant chemotherapy, patients may receive radiation therapy, surgery alone, or a combination of the two modalities. However, the local control rates achieved in studies using the combination of surgery and radiation therapy following chemotherapy are greater than the control rates obtained with either modality alone (49). When all three modalities are combined, more than 90% of patients with locally advanced breast cancer are disease-free following treatment, and many will remain disease-free for up to 3 to 5 years. Many questions remain to be answered about the use of combined modality therapy in patients with stage III disease at diagnosis. Some of these questions include: (*a*) Which combined treatment regimen is the most effective?; (*b*) How many courses of neoadjuvant therapy should be administered prior to surgery?; (*c*) Which drugs should be used for neoadjuvant therapy?; and (*d*) Should patients also receive systemic adjuvant therapy (either chemotherapy or endocrine therapy) postoperatively? Randomized clinical trials designed to answer some of these questions are currently being conducted, and results remain to be determined.

Metastatic Breast Cancer

Radiation therapy, hormonal therapy, and chemotherapy have all been used in the treatment of metastatic breast cancer to palliate the patient and possibly prolong survival. Because "cure" is not the primary goal of therapy at this point, the easiest, least toxic treatment that can provide the best possible response is generally preferred. Breast cancer can metastasize to virtually any site, but the most common sites include bone, lung, pleura, liver, soft tissue, and the central nervous system. The choice of therapy for metastatic disease is based on the site of disease involvement and the presence or absence of certain patient characteristics (2, 50). For example, patients who experience a longer disease-free survival (≥2 years), have disease that is primarily located in bone or soft tissue, have responded to primary endocrine therapy, and are late premenopausal or postmenopausal will most likely respond to endocrine therapy. The most important factor predicting response to hormonal therapy, however, is the presence of estrogen and progesterone receptors on tumor tissues. Fifty to 60% of ER-positive patients and 75 to 85% of ER- and PR-positive patients have a chance of responding to hormonal therapy, while those with no hormone receptors have a 90% chance of failure with hormone therapy (2). Chemotherapeutic drugs are most commonly used as palliative therapy in patients who would not be expected to respond to hormonal therapy (i.e., patients with rapidly progressive lung, liver, or bone marrow disease) or patients who have failed to respond to initial treatment with endocrine therapy (50). Radiation therapy is primarily used to control symptomatic disease such as bone metastases, metastatic brain lesions, and spinal cord compressions. Both brain and spinal cord metastases seldom respond to chemotherapy and hormonal manipulations but do respond somewhat to irradiation.

The most common endocrine therapies used in the management of metastatic breast cancer are listed in Table 77.7. Basically, the response rates to all types of endocrine

therapy are equivalent, so it would be prudent to begin therapy with the least toxic agent. If a patient fails to respond to initial hormonal therapy or progresses during therapy following an initial response, an alternative hormonal manipulation should be attempted, as multiple responses may occur. The median duration of response to the first attempt at hormonal manipulation is usually in the range of 9 to 12 months, and the duration of any subsequent responses is generally shorter (51). Figure 77.3 contains the schema for the hormonal management of both premenopausal and postmenopausal women with metastatic breast cancer.

Ovarian ablation (oophorectomy) via surgery or radiation has been used primarily in the treatment of premenopausal women with metastatic breast cancer, and it produced response rates of 30 to 45% (52). Surgery that has a mortality rate of <5%, is generally preferred over radiation, because of the possible latent side effects of radiation therapy. Although oophorectomy was used as first-line therapy for metastatic disease in premenopausal women in the past, the development of pharmacologic agents that block estrogen binding or produce medical castration has resulted in drug therapy as first-line treatment. Administration of oral tamoxifen therapy or luteinizing-hormone releasing hormone (LHRH) analogs suppresses ovarian estrogen production in premenopausal women (53). However, tamoxifen does not completely antagonize estrogen production, and menses will continue to occur. Furthermore, women who fail initial tamoxifen therapy may respond to an oophorectomy, indicating that ovarian ablation with tamoxifen may not be complete (2, 53). Following an initial stimulation of ovarian hormone production, the LHRH analogs down-regulate the luteinizing-hormone-releasing factor (LHRH) receptors, resulting in ablation of ovarian hormone production that is re-

Table 77.7.
Endocrine Therapies Used for Metastatic Breast Cancer

Class	Drug	Dose	Side Effects
Antiestrogen	Tamoxifen	10–20 mg p.o. b.i.d.	Disease flare, hot flashes, nausea, vomiting, edema
LHRH analogs	Leuprolide	7.5 mg s.q. q28d	Amenorrhea, hot flashes, occasional nausea
	Goserelin	3.6 mg s.q. q28d	
Progestins	Medroxyprogesterone acetate	400–1000 mg i.m. qwk	Weight gain, hot flashes, vaginal bleeding
	Megestrol acetate	40 mg p.o. q.i.d.	
Aromatase inhibitors	Aminoglutethimide	250 mg p.o. b.i.d. × 2 weeks then q.i.d. with hydrocortisone 40 mg/day	Lethargy, rash, postural dizziness, ataxia, nystagmus
Estrogens	Diethylstilbestrol	5 mg p.o. t.i.d.	Nausea/vomiting, fluid retention, hot flashes, anorexia, thromboembolism, hepatic dysfunction
	Ethinylestradiol	1 mg p.o. t.i.d.	
	Conjugated estrogens	2.5 mg p.o. t.i.d.	
Androgens	Fluoxymesterone	10 mg p.o. b.i.d.	Deepening voice, alopecia, hirsutism, facial/truncal acne, fluid retention, menstrual irregularities, cholestatic jaundice

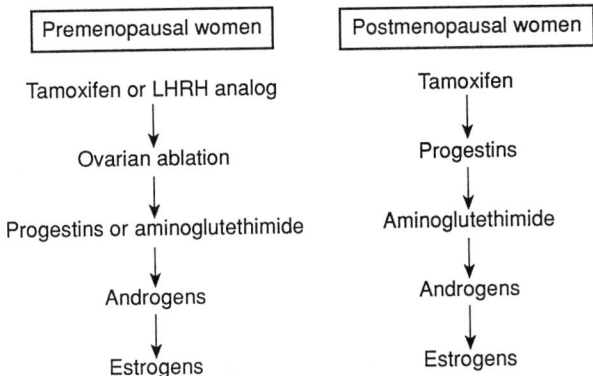

Figure 77.3. Hormonal management of metastatic breast cancer. If a patient does not respond to hormonal therapy at any point in the schema, combination chemotherapy should be used.

versible upon drug discontinuation. Unfortunately, the rate at which sex hormones decline following LHRH administration is much slower than the rate of decline following surgery (1 month versus 2–7 days) (54). Several studies support the use of LHRH analogs in premenopausal women with metastatic breast cancer. The largest study, conducted by Kaufmann and colleagues, used depot goserelin administered subcutaneously every 28 days. An overall response rate of 45% was obtained, with estrogen-receptor-positive patients responding more frequently (55). Currently, the LHRH analogs commercially available include leuprolide (Lupron) and goserelin (Zoladex). Both of these agents are administered subcutaneously as depot injections every 4 weeks and are associated with minimal side effects including amenorrhea, hot flushes, and occasional nausea. Further studies using oophorectomy, tamoxifen, or LHRH analogs as first-line therapy in premenopausal patients with metastatic breast cancer are necessary to determine the definitive choice for initial therapy. Combination endocrine therapy with tamoxifen plus an LHRH analog is also under investigation (54). The rationale behind this combination is that tamoxifen interferes with peripheral estradiol production while the LHRH analog interferes with ovarian estradiol production. Various other endocrine combinations are also being studied (56). In postmenopausal women, tamoxifen therapy appears to be the first-line treatment of choice due to ease of administration and lack of serious side effects. Comparative trials between tamoxifen and other forms of endocrine therapy (i.e., estrogen, progestins, and androgens) have not demonstrated superiority of tamoxifen, based on clinical response, but the toxicity profiles do support the use of tamoxifen initially over other therapies (56). However, progestins may be an alternative to first-line therapy with tamoxifen. Approximately 35 to 50% of patients who respond initially to tamoxifen therapy experience a response to second-line hormonal therapy (53). The choice

of second- and third-line endocrine therapy is currently based on toxicity, cost, and ease of administration rather than response, because of the comparable response rates between agents. The recommended doses, routes of administration, and side effects reported with the endocrine therapies used for metastatic breast cancer are listed in Table 77.7. Currently several randomized trials are being conducted with high-dose megestrol acetate therapy (800 to 1600 mg/day) in an attempt to increase response rates (57). In a large study conducted by Muss and colleagues, high-dose megestrol acetate produced a higher overall response rate (27% versus 10%) and increased median survival (22.4 versus 6.5 months), when compared with standard dose therapy (58). The most commonly reported toxicity with the high-dose regimen was weight gain, with 43% of the patients gaining more than 20 pounds. While weight gain may be beneficial in some cachectic cancer patients, it may also be distressing psychologically for some women. Five major cardiovascular events were also reported during therapy with megestrol acetate. Further studies must be conducted to determine the appropriate role of high-dose megestrol acetate in the treatment of metastatic breast cancer.

Manipulation of hormone levels via oophorectomy, adrenalectomy, and hypophysectomy have fallen somewhat out of favor as therapy for metastatic breast cancer, because of the morbidity and mortality associated with them. Furthermore, the ability to manipulate hormones pharmacologically with decreased costs and toxicities has resulted in increased usage of endocrine therapy for the treatment of metastatic disease. Because the various endocrine therapies produce similar response rates, the choice of therapy should be based on convenience, toxicity, and cost. First-line hormonal therapy should be administered for at least 6 to 8 weeks before disease response is assessed. Following initiation of therapy, some patients may experience a flare (or worsening) of their disease that may or may not be accompanied by hypercalcemia. Therapy may need to be withheld or decreased during this initial period, but treatment can usually continue. Furthermore, 5 to 10% of patients may actually experience regression of their tumor when therapy is withdrawn (51). Clinical trials using combination endocrine therapy or the combination of hormonal therapy and cytotoxic chemotherapy are required before their utility in the management of metastatic disease can be determined.

Patients with rapidly progressive disease and those who do not fulfill the criteria for treatment with endocrine therapy should receive chemotherapy initially. Patients who fail to respond to endocrine therapy should also be treated with chemotherapy. The chemotherapeutic agents that have demonstrated activity in the treatment of breast cancer include doxorubicin, cyclophosphamide, 5-fluorouracil, methotrexate, mitoxantrone, vinblastine, mitomycin C,

Table 77.8.
Combination Chemotherapy Regimens Used in the Treatment of Breast Cancer

Regimen	Drug	Dose
CMFVP "Cooper Regimen"	Cyclophosphamide	2 mg/kg/day p.o.
	Methotrexate	0.7 mg/kg/wk IV × 8 wk
	5-Fluorouracil	12 mg/kg/wk IV × 8 wk then q.o. wk
	Vincristine	35 µg/kg/wk IV × 4–5 wk
	Prednisone	0.75 mg/kg/day reduced by 50% q10d to 5 mg/day × 3 wk
CMF ± P	Cyclophosphamide	100 mg/m^2/day p.o. days 1–14
	Methotrexate	40 mg/m^2 IV days 1 and 8
	5-Fluorouracil	600 mg/m^2 IV days 1 and 8
	Prednisone	40 mg/m^2 p.o. days 1–14
CAF^a	Cyclophosphamide	400–500 mg/m^2 IV day 1
	Doxorubicin	40–50 mg/m^2 IV day 1
	5-Flourouracil	400–500 mg/m^2 IV days 1 and 8
CA	Cyclophosphamide	200 mg/m^2 p.o. days 3–6
	Doxorubicin	40 mg/m^2 IV day 1

^{a} Mitoxantrone 10 mg/m^2 IV day 1 may be substituted for doxorubicin in this regimen.

Table 77.9.
Toxicities of Commonly Used Antineoplastic Agents

Drug	Toxicity
Cyclophosphamide	Myelosuppression, nausea/vomiting, alopecia, hemorrhagic cystitis, stomatitis
Methotrexate	Myelosuppression, mucositis, diarrhea, nausea/vomiting, hepatic dysfunction, nephrotoxicity
5-Fluorouracil	Myelosuppression, mucositis, alopecia, nausea/vomiting, skin hyperpigmentation, chest pain, cerebellar ataxia
Vincristine	Neurotoxicity, constipation, alopecia
Doxorubicin	Myelosuppression, nausea/vomiting, alopecia, stomatitis, radiation recall, skin necrosis following extravasation, cardiotoxicity (occurs more frequently with cumulative doses ≥550 mg/ml^2)
Mitoxantrone	Myelosuppression, nausea/vomiting, alopecia, mucositis, urine discoloration

thiotepa, and melphalan. The objective response rates reported with these drugs as single-agent therapy range from 20 to 40% (50, 59, 60). However, higher response rates (50 to 80%) have been obtained with combination chemotherapy regimens versus single-agent therapy in the treatment of metastatic breast cancer. The chemotherapy regimens most frequently used and the common toxicities associated with the drugs in these regimens are listed in Tables 77.8 and 77.9. Because palliation is the goal of systemic chemotherapy for metastatic disease and quality of life is important, the toxicities and ease of administration of the various regimens should be considered when choosing a treatment regimen. For example, although mitoxantrone is slightly less active than doxorubicin in the management of breast cancer, its use should be considered for patients in whom drug toxicity is a problem, because of the decreased toxicity profile of mitoxantrone (61).

The choice of an initial combination-chemotherapy regimen may be a difficult one. Although regimens containing doxorubicin produce slightly higher response rates than regimens without, doxorubicin-containing regimens may not be the treatment of choice. The reason for this is that patients with disease refractory to doxorubicin therapy are extremely difficult to treat. If women receive the combination of cyclophosphamide, methotrexate, and fluorouracil (CMF) as adjuvant therapy or as first-line therapy for metastatic disease, they may respond to a doxorubicin-containing regimen upon disease progression (50). The development of chemotherapeutic agents that are non-cross-resistant with doxorubicin would be beneficial in this treatment setting. Other issues that remain to be determined in the management of metastatic disease with systemic chemotherapy include the optimal duration of treatment and the standard combination regimen of choice. The use of combination chemotherapy and hormonal therapy is also being investigated for the treatment of metastatic disease.

Future Directions

Although progress has been made in the treatment of breast cancer, further improvements in therapy are essential. Current avenues of research include new methods of administration for commercially available drugs and the development of new drugs. Continuous-infusion therapy and the use of liposome-encapsulated doxorubicin are two ways in which researchers are attempting to decrease the toxicities and increase the efficacy of doxorubicin administration (62, 63). Intraarterial administration of chemotherapy is also being investigated in the management of locally advanced breast cancer, to increase local control of the disease (64). The search for synergistic drug combinations using conventional agents in an attempt to increase response rates and overall survival is also being conducted. Furthermore, new therapeutic agents such as vindesine (a vinca alkaloid), bisantrene (an anthraquinone), epirubicin (an anthracycline), and toremifine (a hormonal agent) are currently being investigated in clinical trials and have demonstrated important activity in the treatment of breast cancer (62).

High-dose chemotherapy intensification with or without autologous bone marrow support is also being investigated for the treatment of relapsed breast cancer. Many antineoplastic agents show a linear relationship between dose and tumor response, but the toxic effects of the drug on the marrow limit the dose that can be administered. Prior to intensification therapy with autologus bone marrow support, patients are usually treated with intensive induction chemotherapy for their disease. Various treatment regimens have been used as induction therapy, and patients who exhibit stable or responsive disease will undergo a transplant as intensification therapy (65, 66). Various preparative regimens including single agents or combinations of drugs with or without total body irradiation have been used prior to bone marrow transplantation (67). These regimens have produced overall response rates ranging from 60 to 97% in patients with refractory metastatic breast cancer (67–69). In an attempt to overcome drug resistance with the possibility of less toxicity, some investigators are also using double high-dose therapy (tandem transplants) with non-cross-resistant preparative regimens. Complete response rates of 23 to 55% have been reported with these regimens, and toxicity does not appear to be increased with the second cycle of therapy (70, 71). The treatment-related mortality is approximately 10%. The availability of the recombinant human colony-stimulating factors (i.e., granulocyte colony-stimulating factor (GCSF) and granulocyte-macrophage colony-stimulating factor (GM-CSF) may help to reduce the morbidity and mortality associated with both high-dose chemotherapy alone and high-dose chemotherapy with autologous bone marrow transplantation (66, 67). Overall response rates ranging from 61% to 97% have been reported in women undergoing bone marrow transplant for refractory metastatic breast cancer (68–71). Response durations in these patients have ranged from months to as long as 6 years, but the follow-up period for most patients is minimal, and long-term survival remains to be determined. The precise role of bone marrow transplantation in the management of advanced breast cancer awaits the results of further clinical trails.

SUMMARY

The incidence of breast cancer continues to rise by approximately 1% every year. Public awareness and early detection of breast cancer have increased significantly over the past 40 years. Furthermore, the recent determination of important prognostic factors for breast cancer recurrence are helpful clinically in the determination of disease management. Appropriate clinical management of particular patient subsets has been established with the help of numerous clinical trials, but the standard treatment of some patients subsets remains to be determined. This will require willingness of both physicians and patients to participate in randomized, controlled clinical trials. Additionally, the development of new antineoplastic agents with activity in breast cancer and continued research in the area of dose intensification will hopefully help decrease the mortality rate of breast cancer, as it has changed very little over the years.

REFERENCES

1. Boring CC, Squires TS, Tong T: Cancer Statistics, 1991. CA 41:19–36, 1991.
2. Hutchins L, Broadwater R Jr, Lang N, Maners A, Bowie M, Westbrook KC: Breast cancer. DM 35:63–125, 1990.
3. Henderson IC, Harris JR, Kinne DW, Hellman S, Cancer of the breast. In DeVita VT Jr, Hellman S, Rosenberg SA (eds): Cancer Principles and Practice of Oncology. Philadelphia, JB Lippincott, 1989, pp 1197–1268.
4. Anderson DE: A genetic study of human breast cancer. J Natl Cancer Inst 48:1029–1034, 1972.
5. Henderson DE: Endogenous and exogenous endocrine factors. Hematol Oncol Clin North Am 3:577–598, 1989.
6. Jawed Iqbal M, Taylor W: Hormonal and reproductive factors—new evidence. In Stoll BA (ed): Women at High Risk to Breast Cancer. Dordvecht, Kluwer Academic Publishers, 1989, pp 41–46.
7. Romieu I, Berlin JA, Colditz G: Oral contraceptives and breast cancer. Review and meta-analysis. Cancer 66:2253–2263, 1990.
8. Hulka BS: Hormone-replacement therapy and the risk of breast cancer. CA 40:289–296, 1990.
9. London S, Willett W: Diet and the risk of breast cancer. Hematol Oncol Clin North Am 3:559–576, 1989.
10. Frisch RE, Wyshank G, Albright NL, et al.: Lower prevalence of breast cancer and other cancers of the reproductive system among former college athletes compared to nonathletes. Br J Med 52:885–891, 1985.
11. Kelsey JL, Berkowitz GS: Breast cancer epidemiology. Cancer Res 48:5615–5623, 1988.
12. Longnecker MP, Berlin JA, Orza MJ, et al.: A meta-analysis of alcohol consumption in relation to risk of breast cancer. JAMA 260:652–656, 1988.
13. Pike MC, Krailo MD, Henderson DE, et al.: Hormonal risk factors, breast tissue age and age-incidence of breast cancer. Nature 303:676–770, 1983.
14. Osborne CK, Arteaga CL: Autocrine and paracrine growth regulation of breast cancer: clinical implications. Breast Cancer Res Treat 15:3–11, 1990.
15. Huguley CM, Brown RL, Greenberg RS, Clark WS: Breast self-examination and survival from breast cancer. Cancer 62:1389–1396, 1988.
16. Kopans DB, Breast cancer detection, diagnosis, and radiation therapy. In Rich MA, Hager JC, Keydar I (eds): Breast Cancer: Progress in Biology, Clinical Management, and Prevention. Boston, Kluwer Academic Publishers, 1989, pp 71–84.
17. Stockdale FE, Breast cancer. In Rubenstein E, Federman DD (eds): Scientific American Medicine. New York, Scientific American, 1990, pp 1–16.
18. Shapiro S, Strax P, Venet L: Periodic breast cancer screening in reducing mortality from breast cancer. JAMA 215:1777–1785, 1971.
19. Shapiro S, Venet W, Strax P, et al., Current results of the breast cancer screening randomized trial: The Health Insurance Plan of Greater New York study. In Day NE, Miller AB (eds): Screening for Breast Cancer. Toronto, Hans Huber, 1988, pp 3–15.
20. Baker LH: Breast cancer detection demonstration project: five-year summary report. CA 32:194–225, 1982.
21. Seidman H, Gelb SK, Silverberg E, LaVerda N, Lubera JA: Survival experience in The Breast Cancer Detection Demonstration Project. CA 37:258–290, 1987.
22. McGuire WL, Clark GM: Prognosis in breast cancer. Recent Results Cancer Res 115:170–174, 1989.

23. Osborne CK: Prognostic factors in breast cancer. Princ Pract Oncol Updates 4:1–11, 1990.

24. Merkel DE, Osborne CK: Prognostic factors in breast cancer. Hematol Oncol Clin North Am 3:641–652, 1989.

25. Clark GM, McGuire WL: Steroid receptors and other prognostic factors in primary breast cancer. Semin Oncol 15(suppl 1);20–25, 1988.

26. Silverstrini R, Daidone MG, Valagussa P, et al.: ³H-Thymidine labeling index as a prognostic indicator in node-positive breast cancer. J Clin Oncol 8:1321–1326, 1990.

27. Clark GM, Dressler LG, Owens MA: Prediction of relapse or survival in patients with node-negative breast cancer by DNA flow cytometry. N Engl J Med 320:627–633, 1989.

28. Tandon AK, Clark GM, Chamness GC, Ullrich A, McGuire WL: HER-2/neu oncogene protein and prognosis in breast cancer. J Clin Oncol 7:1120–1128, 1989.

29. Tandon AK, Clark GM, Chamness GC, Chirgwin JM, McGuire WL: Cathepsin D and prognosis in breast cancer. N Engl J Med 322:297–302, 1990.

30. Crile G, Jr: Results of conservative treatment of breast cancer at ten and 15 years. Ann Surg 181:26–30, 1975.

31. Treatment of early-stage breast cancer. NIH Consensus Dev Conf Consensus Statement 1990 June 18–31;8(6).

32. Harris JR, Recht A, Connolly J, et al: Conservative surgery and radiotherapy for early breast cancer. Cancer 66:1427–1438, 1990.

33. Anon: Clinical alert from the National Cancer Institute. Br Cancer Res Treat 12:3–5, 1988.

34. Mansour EG, Gray R, Shatila AH, et al.: Efficacy of adjuvant chemotherapy in high-risk node-negative breast cancer. An intergroup study. N Engl J Med 320:485–490, 1989.

35. Fisher B, Redmond C, Dimitrov NV, et al.: A randomized clinical trial evaluating sequential methotrexate and fluorouracil in the treatment of patients with node-negative breast cancer who have estrogen-receptor-negative tumors. N Engl J Med 320:473–478, 1989.

36. Fisher B, Costantino J, Redmond C, et al.: A randomized clinical trial evaluating tamoxifen in the treatment of patients with node-negative breast cancer who have estrogen-receptor-positive tumors. N Engl J Med 320:479–484, 1989.

37. Ludwig Breast Cancer Study Group: Prolonged disease-free survival after one course of perioperative adjuvant chemotherapy for node-negative breast cancer. N Engl J Med 320:491–496, 1989.

38. Hayes DF, Henderson IC: Adjuvant therapy for node-negative breast cancer patients. Adv Oncol 6:8–18, 1990.

39. McGuire WL: Adjuvant treatment of node-negative breast cancer. (editorial) N Engl J Med 320:525–527, 1989.

40. Henderson IC, Hayes DF, Parker LM, et al.: Adjuvant systemic therapy for patients with node-negative tumors. Cancer 65:2132–2147, 1990.

41. Early Breast Cancer Trialists' Collaborative Group: Effects of adjuvant tamoxifen and of cytotoxic therapy on mortality in early breast cancer: An overview of 61 randomized trials among 28,896 women. N Engl J Med 319:1681–1692, 1988.

42. Henderson IC: Adjuvant systemic therapy: state of the art, 1989. Br Cancer Res Treat 14:3–22, 1989.

43. Love RR: Tamoxifen therapy in primary breast cancer: biology, efficacy, and side effects. J Clin Oncol 7:803–815, 1989.

44. Love RR, Newcomb PA, Wiebe DA, et al.: Effects of tamoxifen therapy on lipid and lipoprotein levels in post-menopausal patients with node-negative breast cancer. J Natl Cancer Inst 82:1327–1332, 1990.

45. Love RR: Prospects for antiestrogen chemoprevention of breast cancer. J Natl Cancer Inst 82:18–21, 1990.

46. Fornander T, Rutgrist LE, Siöberg HE, Blomqvist L, Mattsson A, Glas U: Long-term adjuvant tamoxifen in early breast cancer: Effect on bone mineral density in post-menopausal women. J Clin Oncol 8:1019–1034, 1990.

47. Gusberg SB: Tamoxifen for breast cancer: associated endometrial cancer (editorial). Cancer 65:1463–1464, 1990.

48. Fornander T, Cedermark B, Mattsson A, et al.: Adjuvant tamoxifen in early breast cancer: occurrence of new primary cancers. Lancet 1:117–120, 1989.

49. Hortobagyi GN: Comprehensive management of locally advanced breast cancer. Cancer 66:1387–1391, 1990.

50. Henderson IC, Garber JE, Breitmeyer JB, Hayes DF, Harris JR: Comprehensive management of disseminated breast cancer. Cancer 66:1439–1448, 1990.

51. Buzdar AU: Current status of endocrine treatment of carcinoma of the breast. Semin Surg Oncol 6:77–82, 1990.

52. Schacter LP, Rozencweig M, Canetta R, Kelley S, Nicaise C, Smaldone L: Overview of hormonal therapy in advanced breast cancer. Semin Oncol 17(suppl 9):38–46, 1990.

53. Santen RJ, Manni I, Harvey H, Redmond C: Endocrine treatment of breast cancer in women. Endocr Rev 11:221–265, 1990.

54. Nicholson RI, Walker KJ, Walker RF, et al.: Review of the endocrine actions of lutenizing hormone-releasing hormone analogues in pre-menopausal women with breast cancer. Horm Res 32(suppl 1):198–201, 1989.

55. Kaufmann M, Jonat W, Kleeberg U, et al.: Goserelin, a depot gonadotrophin-releasing hormone agonist in the treatment of pre-menopausal patients with metastatic breast cancer. J Clin Oncol 7:1113–1119, 1989.

56. Pritchard KI, Sutherland DJA: The use of endocrine therapy. Hematol Oncol Clin North Am 3:765–805, 1989.

57. Abrams JS, Parnes H, Aisner J: Current status of high-dose progestins in breast cancer. Semin Oncol 17(suppl 9):68–72, 1990.

58. Muss HB, Case LD, Capizzi RL, et al.: High versus standard-dose megestrol acetate in women with advanced breast cancer: a phase III trial of the Piedmont Oncology Association. J Clin Oncol 8:1797–1805, 1990.

59. Garber JE, Henderson IC: The use of chemotherapy in metastatic breast cancer. Hematol Oncol Clin North Am 3:807–821, 1989.

60. Buzdar AU: Chemotherapeutic approaches to advanced breast cancer. Semin Oncol 15(suppl 4):65–70, 1988.

61. Henderson IC, Allegra JC, Woodcock T, et al.: Randomized clinical trial comparing mitoxantrone with doxorubicin in previously treated patients with metastatic breast cancer. J Clin Oncol 7:560–571, 1989.

62. Valagussa P, Brambilla C, Bonnadonna G, Chemotherapy of advanced disease. In Hoogstraten B, Burn I, Bloom JHG (eds): UICC Current Treatment of Cancer: Breast Cancer. Berlin, Springer-Verlag, 1989, pp 233–256.

63. Treat J, Greenspan A, Forst D, et al.: Antitumor activity of liposome-encapsulated doxorubicin in advanced breast cancer: Phase II study. J Natl Cancer Inst 82:1706–1710, 1990.

64. Stephens FO: Intraarterial induction chemotherapy in locally advanced stage III breast cancer. Cancer 66:645–650, 1990.

65. Frei II E, Antman K, Teicher B, Eder P, Schnipper L: Bone marrow autotransplantation for solid tumor-prospects. J Clin Oncol 7:515–526, 1989.

66. Jones RB, Shpall EJ, Shogan J, et al.: The Duke AFM Program: intensive induction chemotherapy for metastatic breast cancer. Cancer 66:431–436, 1990.

67. Antman K, Bearman SI, Davidson N, et al., Dose intensive therapy in breast cancer: current status. In Champlin RE, Gale RP (eds): New Strategies in Bone Marrow Transplantation. New York, Wiley-Liss, 1991, pp 423–436.

68. Jones RB, Shpall EJ, Ross M, Bast R, Affronti M, Peters WP: AFM induction chemotherapy, followed by intensive alkylating agent consolidation with autologous bone marrow support (ABMS) for ad-

vanced breast cancer. Current results. Proc ASCO 9:9(#30), 1990 (abstract).

69. Peters WP, Shpall EJ, Jones RB, Ross M: High-dose combination cyclophosphamide (CPA), cisplatin (CDDP) and carmustine (BCNU) with bone marrow support as initial treatment for metastatic breast cancer: three-six year follow-up. Proc ASCO 9:10(#31), 1990 (abstract).

70. Wallerstein, R Jr, Spitzer G, Dunphy F, et al.: A phase II study of mitoxantrone, etoposide, and thiotepa with autologous marrow support for patients with relapsed breast cancer. J Clin Oncol 8:1782–1788, 1990.

71. Dunphy FR, Sptizer G, Buzdar AU, et al.: Treatment of estrogen receptor-negative or hormonally refractory breast cancer with double high-dose chemotherapy intensification and bone marrow support. J Clin Oncol 8:1207–1216, 1990.

72. Gianni AM, Bregni M, Siena S, et al.: Recombinant human granulocyte-macrophage colony-stimulating factor reduced hematologic toxicity and widens clinical applicability of high-dose cyclophosphamide treatment in breast cancer and non-Hodgkin's lymphoma. J Clin Oncol 8:768–778, 1990.

73. Brandt SJ, Peters WP, Atwater SK, et al.: Effect of recombinant human granulocyte-macrophage colony-stimulating factor on hematopoietic reconstitution after high-dose chemotherapy and autologous bone marrow transplantation. N Engl J Med 318:869–876, 1988.

CHAPTER 78

LIVER TUMORS

ROBERT J. STAGG, Pharm.D.

Liver tumors are classified as either primary tumors arising from the hepatobiliary system or secondary tumors metastasizing to the liver from a site elsewhere in the body. As a group, liver tumors represent one of the most common malignancies in the world. Due to the vital bodily functions of the liver, tumors involving this organ often govern the survival of a patient, even in the presence of tumor at other sites. Hepatic malignancies, both primary and metastatic, account for about 20% of cancer deaths in the United States. Primary and metastatic liver tumors will be discussed separately, as they have distinct biological and clinical features.

LIVER ANATOMY

The liver is a wedge-shaped organ that is suspended from the diaphram and lies in the right upper quadrant of the abdomen (Fig. 78.1). The liver is comprised of 3 lobes: the right lobe, which is the largest; the left lobe; and the caudate lobe, which is the smallest and is located on the dorsal aspect of the liver. The right lobe is further subdivided into the anterior and posterior segments, while the left lobe is subdivided into the medial and lateral segments.

The liver has a dual blood supply, coming from both the portal vein and the hepatic artery. Normal liver parenchyma receives most of its blood supply from the portal vein, while hepatic tumors receive most of their blood supply from the hepatic artery (1). Several of the modalities used in the treatment of liver tumors attempt to exploit this finding. The blood from both the portal vein and the hepatic artery is drained from the liver by the hepatic vein, which returns it to the inferior vena cava. The inferior vena cava lies in a groove on the dorsal aspect of liver. Each segment of the liver has its own biliary system, which join intrahepatically to form the right and left hepatic ducts and then unite as they exit the liver to form the common bile duct. The hepatic artery enters and the portal vein and bile duct exit the liver at the hilum, in a region known as the porta hepatis.

PRIMARY LIVER TUMORS

Table 78.1 lists the different types of benign and malignant primary liver tumors.

Benign Primary Liver Tumors

Infantile hemangioendothelioma is a vascular tumor that occurs in the first 6 months of life. Asymptomatic patients require no treatment, as spontaneous regression of the mass usually occurs within 1 year. However, some patients have symptomatic hepatomegaly and congestive heart failure secondary to arteriovenous shunting. These patients should be managed medically with diuretics and inotropic agents. If medical management is unsuccessful, symptoms may be controlled with steroids, radiotherapy, hepatic arterial ligation (2), or embolization. Surgical resection is usually not feasible because of the large size of the tumor.

Cavernous hemangioma is a hypervascular tumor that most commonly occurs in adults in their fourth, fifth, and sixth decades of life. It is the most common benign tumor of the liver, occurring in up to 7% of the population. Hemangiomas increase in size during pregnancy and with estrogen administration. Thus, estrogens should be avoided in these patients. Hemangiomas are usually asymptomatic and most often merely found incidentally at autopsy. Occasionally patients have symptoms, including right upper quadrant pain, abdominal mass, and vomiting. Only severely symptomatic patients and those having lesions larger than 10 centimeters are at risk for intraperitoneal hemorrhage and should be treated. Therapeutic modalities that have been used include steroids, radiation, hepatic arterial ligation, embolization, and surgical resection (3). Surgical resection is the treatment of choice.

Hepatic adenoma occurs primarily in young women of childbearing age and usually presents as a large solitary mass in the liver. Oral contraceptives, anabolic steroids, and type 1 glycogen storage disease have been implicated in the etiology of hepatic adenoma (4). Although benign, surgical resection is frequently performed because of the propensity of this tumor to rupture. There is no role for radiation or chemotherapy in the management of this disease. Oral contraceptives should be strictly avoided in all patients with a history of resected or unresected hepatic adenoma.

Focal nodular hyperplasia occurs more often in females and presents as an asymptomatic hepatic mass. The etiology of focal nodular hyperplasia is largely unknown. Oral contraceptives have been reported to play a possible role in the etiology of this tumor, although recent evidence seems to refute this (4). Surgical resection is generally not indicated, as this tumor rarely ruptures or causes complications.

Malignant Primary Liver Tumors

Hepatocellular carcinoma is the most prevalent malignant tumor of the liver, and it is the major focus of this section.

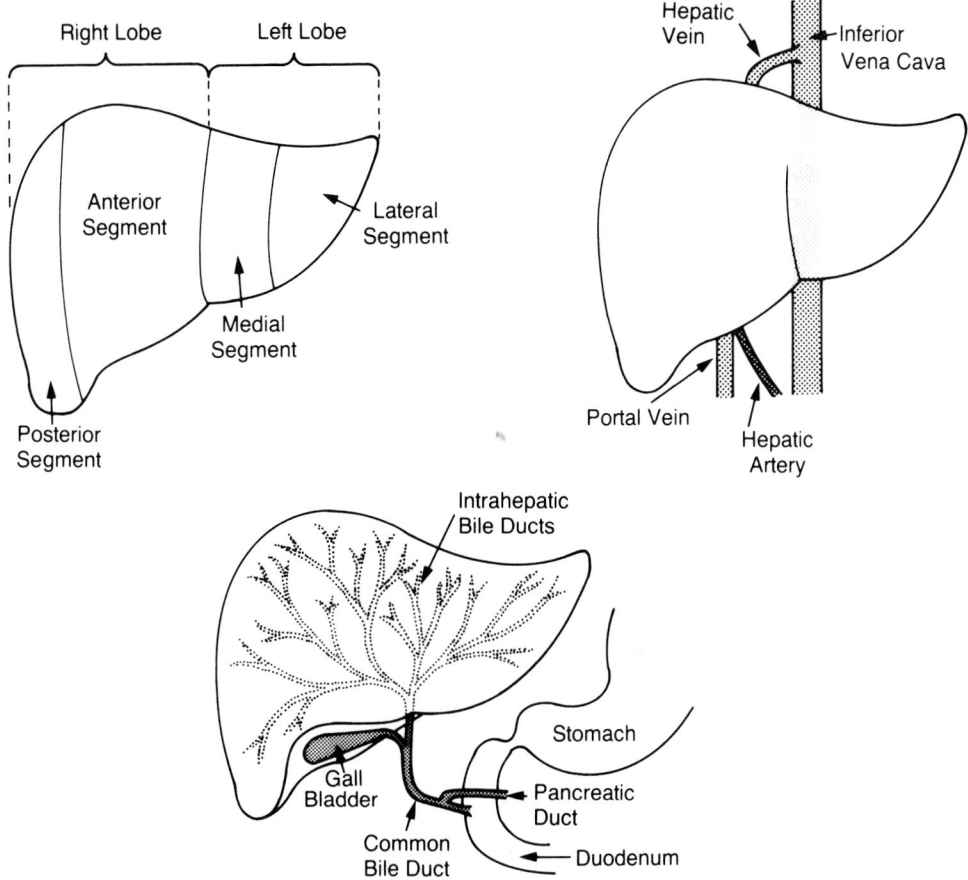

Figure 78.1. *Left*, Right and left hepatic lobes. *Center*, Hepatobiliary system. *Right*, Hepatic blood supply.

Table 78.1.
Primary Liver Cancers

Benign	Malignant
Infantile hemangioendothelioma	Hepatocellular carcinoma
Cavernous hemangioma	Hepatoblastoma
Hepatic cell adenoma	Intrahepatic cholangiocarcinoma
Focal nodular hyperplasia	Angiosarcoma
	Epithelioid
	hemangioendothelioma
	Undifferentiated sarcoma

Other primary malignant tumors occur uncommonly but warrant mention. Hepatoblastoma, the most common primary malignant liver tumor in children, usually occurs in the first 2 to 3 years of life and almost never occurs in children older than 6 years. It sometimes occurs in conjunction with congenital anomalies, such as tetralogy of Fallot, persistent ductus arteriosis, or extrahepatic biliary atresia. Hepatoblastoma most often presents as an asymptomatic solitary mass and is usually discovered by the child's parents or by the pediatrician on routine physical examination. Approximately 30 to 50% of patients with

hepatoblastoma are cured by surgical resection (5). Preoperative chemotherapy or radiation may reduce tumor bulk, allowing removal of originally unresectable disease (6). Systemic chemotherapy for patients having unresectable primaries and those having metastatic disease has been minimally effective (7).

Intrahepatic cholangiocarcinoma is a tumor that arises from the intrahepatic bile ducts and is the second most frequently occurring malignant primary tumor of the liver. Rarely, liver tumors are found on pathologic examination to be mixtures of cholangiocarcinoma and hepatocellular carcinoma. Intrahepatic cholangiocarcinoma may arise from a peripheral bile duct or a major intrahepatic duct and has a low tendency to metastasize. The median survival of untreated patients is approximately 6.5 months, although patients having small peripheral tumors may survive much longer. Surgical resection is occasionally curative and should be performed whenever possible. A partial response rate of 31% has been reported with intravenous chemotherapy using 5-fluorouracil, mitomycin, and doxorubicin (8). Responses have also been observed with intra-arterial chemotherapy (9). A new treatment using anti-CEA (carcinoembryonic antigen) antibodies to selectively deliver radiotherapy to the tumor produced a 33%

response rate in 37 patients with intra-hepatic cholangiocarcinoma (10). Further investigation of this treatment is required to determine what if any role it will play in the management of this tumor.

Angiosarcoma, although uncommon, is the most frequent sarcoma of the liver. It is a rapidly growing tumor that is often accompanied by thrombocytopenia. Approximately 40% of cases are associated with exposure to a carcinogen, specifically, thorium oxide (thorotrast), vinyl chloride, arsenic, radium, androgenic steroids, birth control pills, and diethylstilbesterol (11). Resection offers the only potential for cure and is the treatment of choice whenever feasible. Radiation and chemotherapy both produce partial responses in some patients with unresectable lesions, although the experience with these modalities is limited (11).

Epithelioid hemangioendothelioma is a rare hypervascular tumor of the liver (12). It occurs primarily in women and appears to be causally related to oral contraceptive use. Epithelioid hemangioendothelioma causes hepatic fibrosis and frequently infiltrates the hepatic and portal veins. Clinically, it often resembles Budd-Chiari syndrome (portal vein thrombosus). Various treatments have been used including liver transplantation, partial hepatectomy, chemotherapy, and radiation.

Undifferentiated (enbryonal) sarcoma of the liver describes a group of very rare pediatric sarcomas of the liver that defy categorization as they lack cellular differentiation (13). They are usually rapidly fatal, although cures have been reported with surgical resection. Radiation and chemotherapy have both been used in the treatment of unresectable lesions and metastatic disease. However, the true efficacy of these modalities is unknown because of the low incidence of these tumors.

Hepatocellular Carcinoma

Hepatocellular carcinoma (HCC), also referred to as hepatoma, accounts for 40% of childhood and 90% of adult malignant primary tumors of the liver. It occurs more frequently in males than in females. HCC is uncommon before the age of 40 years and increases in frequency thereafter, with the peak incidence occurring in the sixth decade of life. HCC is relatively uncommon in the United States with about 4000 to 5000 cases diagnosed annually (14). However, it is one of the most prevalent cancers in Asia, Africa, and the South Pacific Islands. In some parts of Asia, HCC is so prevalent that population screening is advocated. With an estimated worldwide annual incidence of up to 1,200,000 cases, HCC is thought to be the world's most prevalent noncutaneous malignancy. HCC has a fatality ratio of 0.92 and accounts for 30 to 40% of all cancer deaths in those countries with high incidences.

ETIOLOGY

HCC occurs most frequently in the presence of a preexisting liver injury. In the United States, approximately 50% of patients with HCC have diffuse cirrhosis (15). Alcoholic cirrhosis, postnecrotic cirrhosis, and cirrhosis secondary to hemochromatosis all appear to predispose patients to HCC. Primary biliary cirrhosis, chronic active autoimmune cirrhosis, and the cirrhosis associated with Wilson's disease do not appear to be predisposing diseases. It is estimated that about 5% of all patients having cirrhosis will eventually develop HCC.

The most important etiologic factor in the development of HCC worldwide is exposure to the hepatitis B virus (16). Epidemiologic studies have revealed an unusually high incidence of HCC in patients residing in regions where hepatitis B is endemic. Two theories to explain this predisposing relationship have been proposed. The first, is that the development of HCC is secondary to the liver injury (postnecrotic cirrhosis) caused by the hepatitis B infection. The second theory hypothesizes that the viral DNA is incorporated into the host DNA and that the altered genome causes malignant transformation of the cell years later. Whatever the mechanism, about 80% of cases of HCC worldwide are thought to be attributable to prior host infection with the hepatitis B virus. Assuming this is so, the hepatitis B virus ranks in importance with tobacco as a human carcinogen. The availability of hepatitis B vaccines (Hepatovax-B and Recombivax HB, Merck, Sharp & Dohme, West Point, PA) offers a potential means for preventing this tumor (17). Suspicion that hepatitis C might also play a role in the etiology of HCC led investigators to test the serum of patients with HCC for antibodies to this virus. While two studies have shown antibodies to hepatitis C in a high percentage of patients with HCC, it remains unclear what if any role hepatitis C plays in the etiology of HCC (18). There is no evidence that hepatitis A predisposes patients to develop HCC.

Aflatoxins, a group of mycotoxins produced by *Aspergillus flavus*, have also been implicated as a cause of HCC (19). Aflatoxins are found on several foodstuffs consumed in large quantities in those parts of the world having a high incidence of HCC. These foodstuffs include peanuts, rice, soybeans, corn, wheat, bread, milk, and cheese. Aflatoxins produce HCC in 100% of some susceptible animal species, while other species are completely unaffected.

There appears to be a possible association between oral contraceptives and the development of HCC (20). However, the number of cases of HCC that are caused by oral contraceptives is small. In addition, there have been at least 3 reports of HCC occurring in men taking androgens (21). It remains unclear whether patients taking steroids are at increased risk for developing HCC.

PATHOLOGY

HCC is a soft grayish white to bright yellow tumor that is usually not encapsulated. Occasionally, encapsulated HCC is found in older patients, and it is a slower growing, less invasive tumor than typical HCC (22). Three major cate-

Table 78.2.
Histologic Variants of
Hepatocellular Carcinoma

Hepatic or trabecular
Pleomorphic
Adenoid or acinar
Sclerosing
Giant cell
Clear cell
Fibrolamellar
Mixed

gories of HCC have been described, based on macroscopic appearance. The most common type is the nodular form in which the liver is studded with tumor. The second type is the massive form, which presents as a large single mass and may be associated with satellite lesions. The last type is the diffuse form, which is the rarest and presents as finely scattered tumor throughout the liver. The diffuse form always occurs in association with cirrhosis.

Eight different histologic subgroups of HCC have been identified, based on the microscopic appearance of the tumor (Table 78.2). The hepatic variant, also called the trabecular variant, is the most common. The fibrolamellar variant is noteworthy, as it is typically solitary and has a better prognosis than ordinary HCC (23). It occurs primarily in women between the ages of 15 and 30 years and is not associated with cirrhosis. The clear cell variant may also be associated with a prognosis that is better than typical HCC.

HCC often infiltrates the diaphragm and invades the intrahepatic portal veins. Less often the tumor invades the hepatic vein or bile duct. Frequently, regional lymph nodes are involved with tumor, but unless this occurs in the porta hepatis, such involvement usually does not alter the patient's clinical course. At autopsy, about 40 to 50% of patients with HCC are found to have distant metastases. The lung is the most common site of metastases, although almost any region can be involved. The presence of metastatic disease rarely alters the patient's outcome, as the hepatic tumor usually determines the duration of survival.

CLINICAL PRESENTATION

Unfortunately, HCC usually does not produce symptoms until there is advanced disease. The most common presenting symptom is abdominal pain. Other symptoms occurring in at least 50% of patients include abdominal distension, fatigue, anorexia, weight loss, and fevers. On examination, virtually all patients have hepatomegaly. Less often, patients are found to have ascites, edema, and/or jaundice. Rarely, patients have bleeding esophageal varices (often a preterminal event). Spontaneous rupture of the tumor with intraperitoneal hemorrhage is an infrequent

presenting symptom in North American patients, but has been reported in up to 20% of Asian and African patients.

Many laboratory abnormalities may be present in the patient with HCC. The hepatic transaminase and alkaline phosphatase levels are elevated in almost all patients, while the bilirubin level is elevated in up to 50% of patients. Due to the decreased synthetic ability of the liver and the cachectic state of patients, the albumin level is often decreased and the prothrombin and partial thromboplastin times may be increased. A mild anemia and a reactive leukocytosis frequently occur. Rarely, erythrocytosis is present in patients having HCC with underlying cirrhosis.

Hypoglycemia occurs in two distinct patient populations with HCC. The first are patients with good performance statuses who have an acquired form of glycogen storage disease, secondary to their tumor, with reduced hepatocellular levels of glucose-6-phosphatase and a phosphorylase required for the breakdown of glycogen. The second group are terminal patients in whom hepatic gluconeogenesis is impaired.

Approximately one-third of patients have high serum cholesterol levels. Hypertriglyceridemia has also been reported. Lastly, some patients have hypercalcemia due to either bone metastases or a parathormone-like substance produced by the tumor.

DIAGNOSIS

The diagnostic workup of a patient suspected of having HCC usually proceeds from the physician's clinical suspicion to laboratory tests, to noninvasive radiologic studies, and eventually, to tissue biopsy. The clinician usually first suspects HCC when the patient complains of right upper quadrant pain or an enlarged liver is detected on physical examination. These findings are even more suspicious in a patient with a prior history of hepatitis B or cirrhosis.

Laboratory tests may be helpful in the diagnosis, but most are nonspecific. The most useful laboratory test in diagnosing HCC is the α-fetoprotein level. α-Fetoprotein is a glycoprotein synthesized by fetal liver, fetal intestine, and yolk sac cells. Levels are very high in both the pregnant female and the fetus prior to birth and fall to adult levels of less than 10 ng/ml after delivery. α-Fetoprotein levels are elevated in about 75 to 90% of patients having HCC (24). While levels are elevated in a few other malignant disorders, the frequency of elevated levels in patients with HCC makes this a useful initial test. When elevated, the α-fetoprotein level can also be used to follow the clinical course of patients: it falls with response to therapy and rises with disease progression. Ferritin levels are elevated in patients with HCC. However, they are also elevated in most patients with uncomplicated cirrhosis, and thus this lacks specificity (25). In addition, ferritin levels do not correlate with therapeutic response as does α-fetoprotein.

Several radiologic tests may be used to confirm the presence of a hepatic mass. Arteriography may be used to assist in the diagnosis when other radiographic techniques fail. On arteriographic examination, HCC typically has a dilated feeding artery with a hypervascular tumor bed. Radionuclide liver-spleen scanning was once the preferred technique for imaging liver tumors, but it is now rarely used because of its relative lack of sensitivity and its inability to image the rest of the abdomen. Standard ultrasound is inexpensive and is associated with no morbidity, but it is also rarely used because abdominal gas interferes with scanning and may obscure lesions. Computerized axial tomography and magnetic resonance imaging are the standard imaging techniques for visualizing liver tumors. While these two methods are more expensive, they often provide a superior image and allow examination of the entire abdomen. The most sensitive radiographic technique for detecting hepatic lesions is intraoperative ultrasound. This procedure should be performed whenever hepatic resection is contemplated, as it is more sensitive for detecting lesions than even the surgeon's visual and tactile inspection of the liver (26).

All of these radiographic techniques are useful for documenting the presence of a hepatic mass and/or following the clinical course after the diagnosis is confirmed and therapy has been instituted. However, by themselves they do not provide a definitive diagnosis. This requires pathologic examination of a tissue specimen. Tissue specimens may be obtained by percutaneous biopsy, peritoneoscopy with directed needle biopsy, or open biopsy at laparotomy.

PROGNOSIS

HCC is an aggressive tumor that usually carries a grave prognosis. The reported median survival in untreated patients from the time of diagnosis varies from 3 to 6 months. Several factors appear to be of prognostic importance (Table 78.3) (27). The most important of these is the resectability of the tumor. As is discussed at length in the treatment section, surgical resection offers the only potential cure for HCC.

The performance status of a patient has been shown to be of prognostic importance, as patients who are ambulatory generally survive longer than those who are bedridden. The amount of tumor in the liver at the time of presentation is inversely related to the duration of survival. Additionally, the location of the tumor(s) within the liver can alter outcome. Patients with lesions near the porta hepatis may deteriorate rapidly, since a small increase in tumor volume may cause compression of the inferior vena cava, portal vein, hepatic artery, and/or bile duct, leading to subsequent ascite, edema, and/or jaundice.

The patient's baseline liver function is important: patients with normal liver function test results, bilirubin and albumin levels, prothrombin and partial thromboplastin times, without ascites or signs of portal hypertension have the best prognosis. Patients with the fibrolamellar variant

Table 78.3.
Prognostic Variables in Patients with Hepatocellular Carcinoma

Factor	Favorable	Unfavorable
Resectability	Yes	No
Liver function	Normal LFTs	Abnormal LFTs
	Bilirubin <36 μmol/liter	Bilirubin >36 μmol/liter
	Normal albumin	Hypoalbuminemia
	Normal PT, PTT	Abnormal PT, PTT
	No ascites	Ascites
	No portal hypertension	Portal hypertension
Metastases	No	Yes
Performance status	Ambulatory	Bedridden
Age	<45 years	>45 years
Sex	Female	Male
Country	North American	African, Asian
Histology	Fribrolamellar variant	Nodular
	Clear cell variant (?)	Massive
	Encapsulated tumor	Diffuse
Cirrhosis	No	Yes

or an encapsulated tumor and probably those with the clear cell variant generally survive longer. Although metastatic disease itself rarely determines outcome, its presence suggests a more aggressive tumor and is associated with a shorter survival.

Other important prognostic factors include the patients age, sex, country of origin, and the presence or absence of cirrhosis. Patients under 45 years of age have a better prognosis than those over 45, and female patients survive longer than their male counterparts. For reasons not completely understood, South African blacks with HCC have a shorter survival than North Americans. Lastly, patients with otherwise normal livers survive longer and respond better to chemotherapy than those with cirrhosis.

TREATMENT

Several modalities have been used, either alone or in combination, in the treatment of HCC. These treatments include surgical resection, radiotherapy, hormonal therapy, intravenous chemotherapy, intra-arterial chemotherapy, hepatic arterial ligation, embolization, chemoembolization, cryosurgery, and percutaneous alcohol injection.

Surgical Resection. Surgical resection of HCC is the only modality that offers a potential for cure. Partial hepatic resection has an operative mortality of 4 to 27%, and therefore should only be attempted with curative intent when the tumor is confined to the liver and all of the macroscopic tumor can be safely resected (27–35). This is usually only feasible when the lesions are confined to one lobe of the liver, allowing removal by either a wedge resection, a segmentectomy, or a right or left hepatectomy. Occasionally,

Table 78.4.
Results of Surgical Resection for Hepatocellular Carcinoma

Author/Year	Number of Patients	Perioperative Mortality (%)	5-Year Survival (%)	Reference
Okuda/1980	222	27	12	(27)
Adson/1981	230	—	30	(28)
Huguet/1985	42	24	15	(29)
Nagao/1986	94	20	25	(30)
Lin/1987	225	8	18	(31)
Chen/1989	120	4	32[a]	(32)
Toshihara/1990	119	15	33	(33)
Choi/1990	174	13	15	(34)
Yamanaka/1990	128	—	54	(35)

[a] 4-Year survival.

the tumor can be resected even if it involves both lobes by removing 3 of the 4 segments of the liver (trisegmentectomy). Following resection, an otherwise normal liver regenerates rapidly, returning to its normal size in about 6 to 8 weeks. Patients with underlying cirrhosis are not good candidates for extensive hepatic resections, as cirrhotic livers have poor regenerative capability.

Preoperatively, one-third of HCC appears to be resectable by radiographic examination, but of those only about one-third are resectable at surgery. Table 78.4 summarizes the results with surgical resection for HCC. The 5-year survival rates for patients who have undergone a potentially curative resection range from 12 to 33%. Approximately 20% of the 5-year survivors die of recurrent disease, thus about 10 to 25% of resected patients are cured.

Liver transplantation has been performed in patients having locally confined, but unresectable HCC (36, 37). The results have been discouraging; about 75% of patients surviving transplantation develop recurrent tumor within 1 to 3 years posttransplant. However, two small subgroups of patients with HCC have more encouraging survival rates following transplantation. Patients undergoing liver transplant for a nonmalignant indication who are incidentally found to have a small HCC at the time of transplantation and those with the fibrolamellar variant of HCC have a 50 to 70% 5-year survival (37). Thus, for these two small subgroups of patients with HCC, liver transplantation appears to be an appropriate modality. For the remainder of patients with HCC, liver transplantation remains experimental.

Radiotherapy. External-beam radiation is of limited benefit in the management of HCC because of the inherent intolerance of normal liver tissue to radiation. Doses in excess of 3000 cGy to the liver produce radiation hepatitis in a significant fraction of patients (38). Some partial responses to external beam radiation alone at doses of 2000

to 3000 cGy fractionated over 7 to 10 days have been reported, although survival did not appear to be appreciably altered (39). A few trials have suggested that radiotherapy may be more effective when combined with chemotherapy, as response rates of 35 to 46% have been reported (40).

Recently, radiolabeled antibodies have been used to treat HCC (41). Since HCC often produces ferritin, polyclonal antibodies to ferritin, labeled with iodine-131, have been administered to patients in an attempt to target the radiation to the tumor. These antibodies plus radiosensitizing doses of chemotherapy produced a response rate of 48% in 105 patients. Most of the patients who responded to treatment had non-α-fetoprotein-secreting HCC. The toxicity was limited primarily to thrombocytopenia. Further investigation of this modality is necessary to determine what, if any, role radiolabeled antibodies should play in the treatment of HCC.

Hormonal Therapy. Some HCCs are estrogen-receptor-positive, much like many breast cancers (42). Based upon this finding, small series of patients have been treated with megesterol acetate or tamoxifen citrate (42–43). While responses have been observed with both agents, hormonal therapy is felt to have limited activity and is rarely used in the treatment of HCC.

Intravenous Chemotherapy. Intravenous chemotherapy is of limited benefit in altering the natural history of HCC. However, it is usually the only treatment option for patients with widely metastatic disease. The experience with single-agent chemotherapy is summarized in Table 78.5. The agent most extensively studied has been doxorubicin in doses of 20 to 75 mg/m^2 administered intravenously every 21 days (44–52). It has shown the most reproducible activity, with response rates ranging from 9 to 32%. The median survivals reported in these trials ranged from 4 to 15 months. Two similar agents, mitoxantrone and 4′epidoxorubicin, appear to have activity comparable to that of doxorubicin (53–57).

5-Fluorouracil has been administered both orally (46, 58–59) and intravenously (59–61) to patients with HCC. By both routes, the response rates have been low. Amsacrine, dichloromethotrexate, etoposide, cisplatin, and α-interferon have all produced occasional responses, but the overall activity of these agents has been low (48, 62–71). Thus, the activity of a single-agent chemotherapy for the treatment of HCC is limited. Various combination regimens have been tested, but they have not improved upon the results obtained with single-agent therapy.

Intra-arterial Chemotherapy. Because of the discouraging results obtained with intravenous chemotherapy, investigators have administered chemotherapeutic agents directly into the hepatic artery in an attempt to increase the total drug exposure (concentration versus time) at the tumor site, and thus, enhance the efficacy (72, 73). The

Table 78.5.
Results of Single-Agent Intravenous Chemotherapy for Hepatocellular Carcinoma

Drug	Number of Patients	Partial Responses	Response Rate (%)	Reference
Doxorubicin	41	6/41	(15)	(44)
	44	14/44	(32)	(45)
	57	9/57	(16)	(46)
	74	22/74	(30)	(47)
	28	8/28	(29)	(48)
	35	3/35	(9)	(49)
	52	6/52	(11)	(50)
	45	11/45	(24)	(51)
	109	11/109	(10)	(52)
	485	90/485	(19)	
Mitoxantrone	22	6/22	(27)	(53)
	20	0/20	(0)	(54)
	42	6/42	(14)	
4'-Epidoxorubicin	18	3/18	(17)	(55)
	13	3/13	(23)	(56)
	33	3/33	(9)	(57)
5-Fluorouracil	12	6/12	(50)	(58)
	48	0/48	(0)	(46)
	21	0/21	(0)	(59)
	10	1/10	(10)	(60)
	8	0/8	(0)	(61)
	99	7/99	(7)	
Amsacrine	23	3/23	(13)	(62)
	16	0/16	(0)	(63)
	20	1/20	(5)	(64)
	35	1/35	(3)	(65)
	94	5/95	(5)	
Dichloromethotrexate	14	0/14	(0)	(66)
	7	3/7	(43)	(67)
	21	3/21	(14)	
Etoposide	24	3/24	(13)	(68)
	38	7/38	(18)	(48)
	62	10/62	(16)	
Cisplatin	13	1/13	(8)	(69)
	29	1/29	(3)	(70)
	42	2/42	(5)	
Interferon	28	2/28	(7)	(71)
	25	2/25	(8)	(72)
	53	4/53	(8)	

and doxorubicin have rapid total body clearances and high hepatic extractions. Therefore, the intra-arterial administration of these drugs results in a substantial increase in drug exposure at the tumor site and a decrease in systemic exposure. Conversely, cisplatin and mitomycin C have relatively slow total body clearances and low hepatic extractions. Thus, the intra-arterial administration of these agents produces fewer dramatic changes in the tumor and less systemic drug exposure.

In the past, the most common technique for administering hepatic arterial chemotherapy involved radiographically placing a transcutaneous catheter into the common hepatic artery via either the femoral or brachial artery. This can be successfully accomplished in about 80% of patients, but it is associated with several complications including catheter migration, drug misperfusion, infection, catheter thrombosis, hepatic arterial thrombosis, and arterial emboli. To avoid catheter migration, transcutaneous catheters may be surgically secured into the hepatic artery. However, with this approach the difficulties of a transcutaneous catheter remain.

The advent of totally implanted ports and pumps in the early 1980s made the administration of long-term ambulatory hepatic arterial chemotherapy feasible. Implantable ports are surgically placed into a subcutaneous pocket, and the catheter is inserted into the ligated gastroduodenal artery, with the tip at the hepatic artery. Implanted ports are optimal for bolus administration of chemotherapy. However, continuous-infusion chemotherapy with implanted ports requires the use of an external pump and is technically cumbersome. Totally implanted pumps allow the administration of continuous-infusion hepatic arterial chemotherapy in the ambulatory setting (Fig. 78.2). Table 78.7 lists the characteristics of the various constant-flow and programmable implantable infusion pumps available to deliver intra-arterial chemotherapy. All of the devices have a drug chamber that is filled by percutaneously passing a needle into the inlet septum and injecting the next course of therapy. In addition, the pumps have a side port that may be used for bolus administration of chemotherapy. The pump, like the port, is implanted in a subcuta-

drug exposure is most dramatically increased when the agent being administered has a rapid total body clearance, as intra-arterial infusion enables the drug to be delivered in a high concentration to the tumor prior to its elimination from the body. An additional benefit is derived from intra-arterial administration when the agent administered has a high hepatic extraction. The high first-pass extraction of the drug by the liver leads to a lower systemic drug exposure (than with intravenous administration), and thus, the patient experiences fewer adverse effects. Table 78.6 lists the total body clearances and hepatic extractions of those chemotherapeutic agents commonly used to treat hepatic malignancies (74–79). Floxuridine, 5-fluorouracil,

Table 78.6.
Total Body Clearances and Hepatic Extractions of Drugs Administered by Hepatic Intra-Arterial Infusion

Drug	Total Body Clearance (ml/min)	Hepatic Extraction Ratio (%)	Reference
Floxuridine	4800	95	(57)
Doxorubicin	2000	50	(58)
5-Fluorouracil	1000	80	(59, 60)
Cisplatin	600	24	(61)
Mitomycin C	575	10	(62)

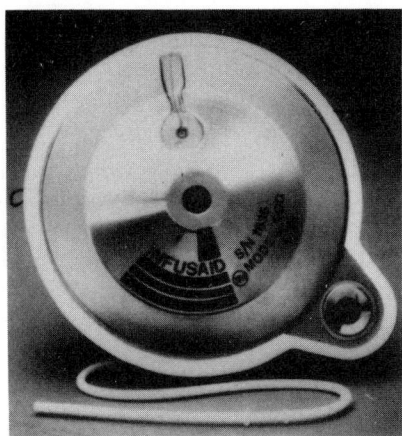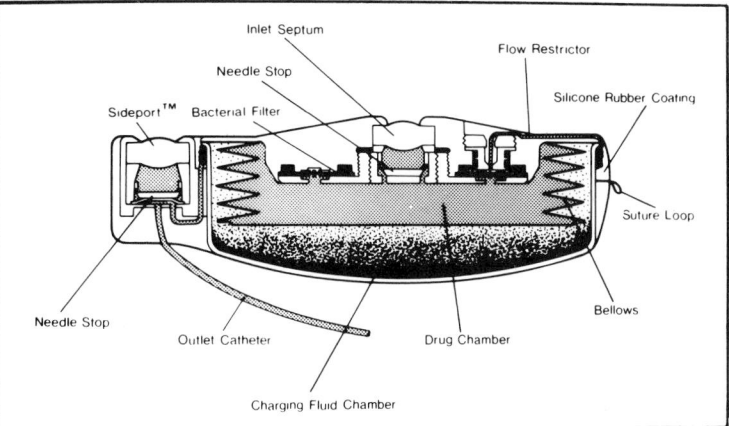

Figure 78.2. *Left*, Shiley-Infusaid (Norwood, MA) implantable pump. *Right*, Cross-section of implantable pump.

Table 78.7.
Implantable Pumps

Device	Diameter	Weight	Volume	Flow Rate	Side Port	Battery	Alarms	Cost
Constant flow								
Infusaid (Model 400) Single catheter	87 mm	208 g	50 ml	1–10 ml/day	Yes	No	No	$4795
Infusaid (Model 400) Double catheter	87 mm	229 g	50 ml	1–10 ml/day	Two	No	No	$5495
Infusaid (Model 600)	63 mm	100 g	23 ml	0.7 or 1.4 ml/day	Yes	No	No	$4795
Therex	77 mm	136 g	30 ml	0.5–2 ml/day	Yes	No	No	$3000
Programmable								
Infusaid (Model 1000)	9.0 cm	226 g	25 ml	0–12 ml/day	Yes	Yes	No	Unknown
Medtronics	7.0 cm	185 g	18 ml	0.1–21 ml/day	Optional	Yes	Occlusion Low battery	$6900

neous pocket created in the abdominal wall, and the catheter is placed in the ligated gastroduodenal artery with the tip at the hepatic artery.

Table 78.8 summarizes the clinical results with single-agent hepatic arterial chemotherapy in the treatment of HCC. While the clinical trials are few in number and have small patient samples, the response rates are higher than those reported with intravenous chemotherapy. Single-agent intra-arterial floxuridine administered via implanted pump produces responses in approximately 55% of patients (80, 61). Due to the high first-pass hepatic extraction of floxuridine, intra-arterial infusions do not produce systemic toxicity. However, hepatobiliary toxicity has been reported, including biliary sclerosis and cholecystitis (88). Biliary sclerosis is a potentially serious toxicity that probably results from perfusion of the bile duct with high con-

centrations of floxuridine (88). Serious biliary toxicity can be prevented with appropriate dosage adjustments and careful monitoring. Prophylactic cholecystectomy is recommended if repeated courses of hepatic intra-arterial floxuridine are to be administered. Additionally, gastritis and gastroduodenal ulcers have been reported. This is a result of drug misperfusion into the gastroduodenal blood supply and can be prevented by surgically ligating the arterial feeders to the stomach and duodenum arising from the hepatic artery. While 5-fluorouracil has not been tested extensively as a single agent in the United States, results from Japan suggest that it may have similar activity to floxuridine when administered intra-arterially for HCC (81). Doxorubicin also appears to have enhanced activity when infused intra-arterially, with responses of 40 to 50% (47, 81–85). Mitomycin C has been reported to have significant

Table 78.8.
Results of Single-Agent Intra-Arterial Chemotherapy for Hepatocellular Carcinoma

Drug	Number of Patients	Partial Responses	Response Rate (%)	Reference
Floxuridine	16	9	56	(61)
	28	15	54	(80)
	44	24	55	
Fluorouracil	9	2	22	(81)
Doxorubicin	10	4	40	(47)
	4	2	50	(82)
	13	6	46	(83)
	2	1	50	(84)
	6	3	50	(85)
	19	8	42	(81)
	44	20	45	
Cisplatin	16	3	19	(86)
Mitoxantrone	22	6	27	(87)

efficacy when administered intra-arterially. However, detailed response data is unavailable (25). Lastly, hepatic intra-arterial cisplatin and mitoxantrone have produced some responses in patients with HCC (86–87).

High response rates have also been reported with combination intra-arterial chemotherapy. Responses were observed in 8/15 (53%) patients receiving an intra-arterial combination of mitomycin C, 5-fluorouracil, vinblastine, vincristine, and doxorubicin (89) and 8/12 (67%) patients receiving floxuridine, doxorubicin, and mitomycin C (90). It remains unclear whether combination intra-arterial chemotherapy is superior to single-agent treatment.

In an attempt to augment the efficacy of intra-arterial chemotherapy, suspensions of antineoplastic agents in the lipid lymphographic agent, lipiodol, have been administered (91). Lipiodol, when injected into the hepatic artery, has been found to remain selectively in liver tumors long after its infusion. On the basis of this finding, lipiodolized chemotherapeutic agents have been administered in an attempt to promote the selective uptake of the drug by the tumor. While the experience with hepatic intra-arterial lipiodolized anticancer agents is limited, the early results are interesting and warrant further research.

Hepatic Artery Ligation. Surgical ligation of the hepatic artery has been performed in patients having HCC without significant extrahepatic involvement in an attempt to produce tumor necrosis secondary to ischemia. This approach has been used as a single modality as well as in combination with chemotherapy (92–93). Responses with hepatic arterial ligation are often transient because extrahepatic collateral arteries develop rapidly, reperfusing the tumor (94). The procedure is generally well tolerated with pain, fevers, and elevated hepatic enzyme levels being the principle adverse effects. Rarely, hepatic arterial ligation causes hepatic necrosis leading to death. Patients with severely com-

promised hepatic function or portal vein thrombosis should not undergo this procedure. Hepatic artery ligation has recently fallen out of favor as an initial treatment because permanent loss of the hepatic artery precludes its use for other liver-directed therapies (i.e., intra-arterial chemotherapy, embolization, or chemoembolization). However, ligation of the hepatic artery may be used successfully to stop bleeding in patients with hemoperitoneum from a ruptured HCC (95).

Embolization and Chemoembolization. Two related modalities, embolization and chemoembolization, have recently been used to treat HCC. Embolization of HCC involves radiographic placement of a transcutaneous catheter into the hepatic artery and injection of a substance that occludes the arterial blood flow at the capillary level and produces tumor ischemia. Small particles have been commonly used for embolization including, Angiostat (5 × 75 microns) (Target Therapeutics, Los Angeles, CA), Gelfoam powder (40 to 60 microns) or cubes (1 to 3 millimeters) (Upjohn, Kalamazoo, MI), and Ivalon particles (150 to 500 microns) (Unipoint Lab, High Point, NC). Ethibloc (Ethicon, Hamburg, Germany), a viscous substance that solidifies after injection, has also been used. Embolization with Angiostat or Gelfoam produces a transient occlusion, while Ivalon and Ethibloc causes a permanent blockage of the tumor capillary bed. Compared with hepatic arterial ligation, embolization offers the advantages of being nonsurgical and associated with the development of fewer collateral arteries. In one study, responses with embolization were reported in 6 of 9 patients with HCC who had failed hepatic arterial chemotherapy (96). In Japan, 120 patients with HCC were treated with Gelfoam embolization and 90% responded with survival rates of 44, 29, and 15% at 1, 2, and 3 years after treatment, respectively (97).

Chemoembolization combines the tumor ischemia produced by embolization with prolonged, high, local concentrations of chemotherapy within the tumor. This is accomplished by either preparing special embolizing microspheres that contain the chemotherapeutic agent or mixing concentrated chemotherapy with the embolizing substance. In two studies, biodegradable albumin microspheres containing mitomycin C were used to embolize patients with HCC, and responses were observed in 7 of 7 patients and 15 of 20 patients (98, 99). Chemoembolization with Gelfoam and doxorubicin, mitomycin C, and cisplatin produced responses in 12 of 50 patients, using standard response criteria (100). However, 70% of patients showed evidence of liquifaction necrosis on CT scan. Both embolization and chemoembolization are generally well tolerated with liver pain, fever, and elevated liver function test results being the primary adverse effects, although these tend to be more severe with chemoembolization. Rare cases of acute renal failure and necrosis of the bile ducts and/or gallbladder have been reported. Additionally, if the embolization particles are inadvertently injected into an area other than the tumor capillary bed, necrosis of that region may result.

Cryosurgery and Percutaneous Alcohol Injection. Two new techniques being explored in the treatment of HCC are cryosurgery and percutaneous alcohol injection. Cryosurgery is performed by exposing the hepatic tumor through a right upper abdominal incision. A liquid nitrogen cryoprobe is then placed on the tumor surface until freezing of the mass is accomplished. Although only limited investigation of cryosurgery has occurred, encouraging survival rates have been reported for patients with small tumors of less than 5 centimeters (101). Similarly, ethanol has been injected percutaneously under ultrasound guidance directly into small HCCs to produce coagulation necrosis. In one study of percutaneous alcohol injection, 35 patients with HCC having tumors less than 5 centimeters in size had an 80% 3-year survival (102). The preliminary work with both of these modalities suggests that their potential role may be in the treatment of patients with small HCCs who are not surgical resection candidates by virtue of their underlying liver disease. In these patients, either modality could be used to cytoreduce the tumor, while sparing the liver parenchyma from injury.

SECONDARY LIVER TUMORS

Metastases to the liver may occur from virtually any malignancy. Of all the organs in the body, the liver is the most common site of blood-borne metastases. In an autopsy series of 9497 cancer patients, 8055 (84.8%) had metastatic disease, and 4444 (46.8%) had liver metastases (103). Liver metastases may be the only site of metastatic disease or part of a more widely metastatic process. Hepatic metastases occur most frequently in patients with primary tumors originating in organs drained by the portal vein, including tumors of the stomach, small intestine, colon, pancreas, gallbladder, and extrahepatic biliary tract. However, some malignancies such as breast cancer, lymphomas, testicular cancer, and ocular melanoma, which arise in organs having other sources of venous drainage (nonportal), are also associated with a high incidence of liver metastases.

The factors contributing to the high incidence of liver metastases in cancer patients are complex and not completely understood. On an ultrastructural level, the sinusoidal fenestrations of the liver may be more permeable to metastatic cells than the capillary endothelium of other organs. Also, the liver has relatively little connective tissue, which in other organs may act as a physical barrier to metastatic cells. From a physiologic standpoint, the liver, as the organ that "filters" the blood, may inherently be more efficient than other organs at removing metastatic cells from the blood. Lastly, in patients with tumors originating in organs drained by the portal circulation, the liver is the first organ encountered by the metastatic cells after their release into the bloodstream, and thus, is the organ presented with the highest burden of metastatic cells. The remainder of the discussion on liver metastases focuses on colorectal cancer, as it is by far the most common tumor that metastasizes to the liver.

Colorectal Carcinoma Metastatic to the Liver

CLINICAL PRESENTATION

At the time of diagnosis, about 30 to 40% of patients with colorectal cancer have distant metastases. The liver is the most common site of metastatic involvement, followed by the lung. Often the diagnosis of liver metastases is made incidentally at surgery in patients without antecedent signs or symptoms suggestive of hepatic involvement or during routine follow-up. The most frequent complaints in patients with symptomatic liver metastases include abdominal pain and distension, anorexia, weight loss, fatigue, jaundice, and/or unexplained fever.

DIAGNOSIS

The diagnosis of liver metastases generally proceeds from the physical examination to laboratory tests, to radiographic imaging, and often, to tissue biopsy. The most common finding on physical examination is hepatomegaly. In patients with advanced hepatic metastases, the tumor may occlude the bile duct, portal vein, and/or inferior vena cava, resulting in jaundice, portal hypertension (ascites, esophageal varices), and/or lower extremity edema, respectively.

Approximately 60% of patients with hepatic metastases have elevated levels of serum glutamic-pyruvate transaminase (ALT), serum glutamic-oxaloacetic transaminase (AST), lactic dehydrogenase (LDH), and/or alkaline phosphatase (AP) (104). Additionally, serum bilirubin levels are often elevated in patients with advanced hepatic metastases. The greater the extent of liver involvement, the more likely these test results will be elevated. No single liver enzyme is superior to the others for detecting liver metastases. While hepatic enzyme level elevations are somewhat useful in identifying patients who may have liver metastases, elevations can occur in patients without liver metastases, and thus these tests lack specificity.

Another laboratory test that is helpful in diagnosing colorectal cancer is the carcinoembryonic antigen (CEA) level. CEA is a glycoprotein that is produced in small amounts by normal columnar epithelial cells (normal value <4 ng/ml). The serum CEA is elevated in 60 to 90% of patients with colorectal cancer metastatic to the liver. While colorectal cancer at any site may produce CEA, levels greater than 20 ng/ml are most frequently associated with liver metastases (105–106). Approximately, 70% of patients with colorectal cancer metastatic to the liver have elevated CEA levels (106). However, since CEA levels are elevated in a variety of other malignant and nonmalignant conditions, this lacks diagnostic specificity. Thus, its major role lies in screening patients for recurrent disease and monitoring patients known to have metastases who are receiving treatment: the level tends to fall with tumor regression and to rise with disease progression.

Several radiographic techniques are helpful in diagnosing liver metastases (107, 108). Ultrasound has the advantages of being inexpensive and not exposing the patient to radiation. However, intestinal gas, excessive fat, and overlying ribs can interfere with imaging. Thus, small lesions may be undetected. Radionuclide liver-spleen scanning using technetium sulfur colloid is easy to perform, but it is associated with high false-positive and false-negative results, is unable to image extrahepatic tumor, and often does not detect lesions smaller than 2 centimeters. Computerized tomography and magnetic resonance imaging are the two preferred radiographic techniques for detecting liver metastases. While these methods are more expensive, they more accurately detect small lesions, they are more reproducible, and they allow simultaneous imaging of the rest of the abdomen. Lastly, intraoperative ultrasound is the most sensitive method of detecting liver metastases and is especially useful if surgical resection is contemplated.

Tissue biopsy to confirm the presence of liver metastases is usually unnecessary in colorectal cancer patients, since the data from the patient history, physical examination, laboratory tests, and radiographic studies are sufficient to make an accurate diagnosis. If a tissue specimen is required to confirm the diagnosis, it may be obtained by percutaneous biopsy, peritoneoscopy with needle-directed biopsy, or open biopsy at laparotomy.

PROGNOSIS

In general, colorectal cancer metastatic to the liver carries a poor prognosis. By far the most important prognostic factor is the resectability of the hepatic metastases. Surgical resection is the only potentially curative modality for liver metastases, and it should be performed whenever possible.

The most important factor in patients with unresectable tumor is the extent of hepatic involvement (109). The survival in untreated patients ranges from 2 to 22 months (median, 8 months). Patients with the smallest amount of tumor survive the longest. Another important factor is the degree of histologic differentiation. Patients with well-differentiated tumors survive longer than those with poorly differentiated tumors (110). In addition, patients with poor performance statuses, significant weight loss, low albumin levels, ascites, elevated hepatic enzyme levels, and/or bilirubin levels have a shortened survival.

TREATMENT

Several modalities have been used either singly or in combination in the treatment of colorectal cancer metastatic to the liver: surgical resection, radiotherapy, hepatic arterial ligation, and hepatic intra-arterial chemotherapy. The following is a discussion of the results obtained with these treatments.

Surgical Resection. Surgical resection is the only modality that offers a potential cure for patients with colorectal cancer metastatic to the liver, and thus it should be performed when technically feasible in patients with 4 or fewer metastases. Unfortunately, this is only feasible in 10 to 20% of patients. Recent results with surgical resection of liver metastases from colorectal cancer are summarized in Table 78.9 (111–119). The operative mortality in these series ranges from 0 to 14%. The percentage surviving 1 year, 3 years, and 5 years after resection is approximately 90, 45, and 30%, respectively. Patients with solitary metastases (114), those without extrahepatic disease (114), those who are female (114), those with synchronous metastases (compared with those who develop metachronous metastases) (116, 117), those with clear margins of resection (118), and those whose primary originated in the colon (compared to the rectum) (119) survive longer following resection.

Radiotherapy. External-beam radiation plays a limited role in the management of liver metastases from colorectal cancer because of the inherent radiosensitivity of the liver. As mentioned earlier, life-time doses above 3000 rads are associated with a high incidence of radiation hepatitis (38). Fractionated doses of 1800 to 2400 rads can provide pain relief for patients with symptomatic metastases. However, radiotherapy has not prolonged survival (119). Additionally, radiotherapy has been used in combination with chemotherapy, although it is unclear whether the outcome is superior to that obtained with chemotherapy alone (120).

Table 78.9.
Results of Surgical Resection for Colorectal Cancer Metastatic to the Liver

Author	Number of Patients	Operative Mortality (%)	Survival (%)			Reference
			1 year	3 year	5 year	
Marrow/1982	29	—	—	—	27	(111)
Rajpal/1982	34	11.8	84	42	—	(112)
Iwatsuki/1983	24	0	—	—	52	(113)
Adson/1984	141	4	—	—	25	(114)
Steele/1984	30	6.6	90	—	30	(115)
Fortner/1984	65	7	89	57	—	(116)
Petrelli/1985	36	14	—	32	—	(117)
Nordlinger/1987	80	5	—	41	25	(118)
Hughes/1989	800	—	—	—	32	(119)

Hepatic Arterial Ligation. As with HCC, ligation of the hepatic artery has been performed in patients with liver metastases from colorectal cancer in an attempt to produced tumor necrosis secondary to ischemia (121). Symptomatic improvement is observed in some patients following hepatic arterial ligation, but it is usually transient. In addition, ligation of the hepatic artery prevents its future use for other liver-directed therapies, such as intra-arterial chemotherapy.

Intravenous Chemotherapy. Systemic chemotherapy is of limited benefit in the treatment of patients with colorectal cancer metastatic to the liver (122). The agents having activity include 5-fluorouracil, mitomycin C, and the nitrosoureas (methyl-CCNU, BCNU, CCNU). Intravenous 5-fluorouracil is the most commonly used agent, producing partial responses in about 15 to 20% of patients. Coadministering leucovorin with 5-fluorouracil appears to increase the response rate to about 30 to 35%, but it also enhances toxicity (123). The most common side effects of intravenous 5-fluorouracil are nausea, vomiting, stomatitis, diarrhea, and myelosuppression. Mitomycin C administered in doses of 10 to 15 mg/m² every 6 to 8 weeks also produces partial responses in about 15 to 20% of patients. However, cumulative myelosuppression makes continued administration difficult (122), so mitomycin C is usually reserved for patients who fail 5-fluorouracil. While methyl-CCNU has activity similar to that of 5-fluorouracil and mitomycin C, it is not available in the United States because of its excessive toxicity and carcinogenicity (124). While the experience with the other nitrosoureas (BCNU, CCNU) in the management of metastatic colorectal cancer is limited, these agents probably have activity similar to that of methyl-CCNU.

Intra-arterial Chemotherapy. Hepatic intra-arterial chemotherapy has been widely used in the treatment of colorectal cancer metastatic to the liver (for a complete discussion of the rationale of intra-arterial chemotherapy the reader is referred to the section earlier in this chapter on intra-arterial chemotherapy for the treatment of hepatocellular carcinoma). Table 78.10 summarizes the results with single-agent hepatic intra-arterial chemotherapy. The most commonly administered agent has been floxuridine, primarily because it is available in a convenient formulation for use in implantable pumps. It has produced partial responses ranging from 29 to 88% of patients and median survival times ranging from 13 to 26 months (125–131). However, single-agent hepatic intra-arterial floxuridine is associated with a high incidence of hepatobiliary toxicity. 5-Fluorouracil has also been administered by hepatic intra-arterial infusion, with responses ranging from 34 to 67% and median survivals of 9 to 12 months (132–136). The lower solubility of 5-fluorouracil (relative to floxuridine) prevents its use in the implantable pump and requires external pumps with radiographically placed per-

Table 78.10.
Results of Single-Agent Intra-Arterial Chemotherapy for Colorectal Cancer Metastatic to the Liver

Drug	Number of Patients	Response Rate (%)	Median Survival (months)	Reference
Floxuridine	81	88	26	(125)
	93	80	20	(126)
	77	83	13	(127)
	17	29	13	(128)
	24	73	22	(129)
	41	37	—	(130)
	14	36	—	(131)
5-Fluorouracil	52	67	—	(132)
	369	55	—	(133)
	24	50	9	(134)
	30	34	10	(135)
	30	57	11.9	(136)

Table 78.11.
Results of Combination Intra-Arterial Chemotherapy for Colorectal Cancer Metastatic to the Liver

Drugs	Number of Patients	Response Rate (%)	Median Survival (months)	Reference
Floxuridine & 5-fluorouracil	52	81	—	(114)
	48	54	—	(137)
	64	50	22	(138)
Floxuridine & mitomycin C	12	83	15	(139)
	40	20	14	(140)
Floxuridine & dichloromethotrexate	13	69	20	(140)
5-Fluorouracil & mitomycin C	20	55	8	(141)
	30	50	11	(142)
Floxuridine & cisplatin & mitomycin	29	52	12	(143)
Floxuridine & mitomycin C & BCNU	36	70	12	(144)
5-Fluorouracil & adriamycin & mitomycin	23	35	22	(145)

cutaneous catheters to administer the drug. This approach limits the frequency and duration of treatment, making it difficult to compare the results with intra-arterial floxuridine administered by the implantable pump.

To improve upon the results obtained with single-agent intra-arterial chemotherapy, various combinations regimens have been tried (Table 78.11). Unfortunately, the results have been similar to those with single-agent therapy. The response rates have ranged from 20 to 83% and the median survival times from 8 to 22 months (114, 137–145). However, one combination regimen using floxuridine and 5-fluorouracil may offer an advantage over other regimens, as it appears to be associated with fewer treatment-limiting toxicities (138).

Four phase III trials of intravenous versus intra-arterial chemotherapy have been conducted (146–149). All 4 studies reported statistically significant higher response rates for the intra-arterial arm, but in 3 of the 4 studies, survival between the two arms was not significantly different. However, two of the large randomized trials (146–147) allowed patients who failed intravenous therapy to cross over and receive intra-arterial treatment, thus confounding the analysis of survival. A definitive non-cross-over, randomized trial of the intra-arterial versus intravenous therapy must be conducted to determine whether the higher response rates obtained with intra-arterial therapy translate into a survival advantage.

CONCLUSION

Liver tumors are a diverse group of malignancies that occur in the hepatobiliary system. They can be divided into primary tumors originating from the hepatobiliary system and secondary tumor metastasizing to the liver from neoplasms elsewhere in the body. The most prevalent primary malignancy of the liver is hepatocellular carcinoma, also referred to as hepatoma, and the most common cause of hepatic metastases is colorectal cancer. Malignant tumors of the liver, both primary and metastatic, are potentially curable only when complete surgical removal of all of the tumor is feasible. Unfortunately, complete resection is only possible in about 10% of patients, and of those patients, only about 30% are cured. Thus, most patients have incurable hepatic malignancies. Several therapies have been used to treat unresectable liver tumors. Radiotherapy has been used but is of limited benefit because of the inherent intolerance of the normal liver tissue to radiation. Systemic chemotherapy is commonly used, but it produces partial response in only 15 to 35% of patients. More encouraging results have recently been obtained with liver-directed therapies such as hepatic intra-arterial chemotherapy and chemoembolization. Further research is required to develop more efficacious therapies for liver tumors.

REFERENCES

1. Bierman HR, Byron RL Jr, Kelly LH, Grady A: Studies on the blood supply of tumors in man: III. Vascular patterns of the liver by hepatic arteriography in vivo. JNCI 12:107–227, 1951.
2. Nguyen L, Shandling B, Ein S, Stephens C: Hepatic hemangiomas in childhood: medical management or surgical management? J Pediatr Surg 17:576–579, 1982.
3. Hobbs KE: Hepatic hemangiomas. World J Surg 14:468–471, 1990.
4. Nichols FC, van Heerden JA, Weiland LH: Benign liver tumors. Surg Clin North Am 69:297–314, 1989.
5. Exelby PR, Filler RM, Grosfield JL: Liver tumors in children: in particular reference to hepatoblastoma and hepatocellular carci-

noma. American Academy of Pediatric Surgical Section Survey, 1974. J Pediatr Surg 10:329–337, 1975.
6. Takayama T, Makuuchi M, Takayasu K, et al.: Resection after intraarterial chemotherapy of a hepatoblastoma originating in the cuadate lobe. Surgery 107:231–235, 1990.
7. Tan Am, Tan CL, Phua KB, et al.: Chemotherapy for hepatoblastoma in children. Ann Acad Med Singapore 19:286–289, 1990.
8. Harvey JH, Smith FP, Schein PS: 5-Fluorouracil, mitomycin, and doxorubicin (FAM) in carcinoma of the biliary tract. J Clin Oncol 2:1245–1248, 1984.
9. Smith GW, Bukowski RM, Hewlett JS, Groppe CW: Hepatic artery infusion of 5-fluorouracil and mitomycin C in cholangiocarcinoma and gallbladder carcinoma. Cancer 54:1513–1516, 1984.
10. Stillwagon GR, Order SE, Klein JL, et al.: Multi-modality treatment of primary nonresectable intra-hepatic cholangiocarcinoma with 131-I anti-CEA. A Radiation Oncology Group Study. Int. J Radiat Oncol Biol Phys 13:687–695, 1987.
11. Locker GY, Doroshow JG, Zwelling LA, et al.: The clinical features of hepatic angiosarcoma—A report of four cases and a review of the English literature. Medicine 58:48–64, 1979.
12. Dean PJ, Haggett RC, O'Hara CJ: Malignant epithelioid hemangioendothelioma of the liver in young women. Relationship to oral contraceptive use. Am J Surg Pathol 9:695–704, 1985.
13. Stocker JT, Ishak KG: Undifferentiated (embryonal) sarcoma of the liver. Report of 31 cases. Cancer 42:336–348, 1978.
14. Silverberg E, Lubera J: Cancer Statistics, 1990. CA: A Journal for Clinicians 40:9–26, 1990.
15. Moertel CG, The liver. In Holland JF, Frei E III (eds): Cancer Medicine. Philadelphia, Lea & Febiger, 1973, pp 1541–1547.
16. Popper G, Gerber MA, Thung SN: The relation of hepatocellular carcinoma to infection with hepatitis B and related viruses in man and animals. Hepatology 2:1S–9S, 1982.
17. Blumberg BS, London WT: Hepatitis B virus and the prevention of primary hepatocellular carcinoma. N Engl J Med 304:782–784, 1981.
18. Johnson PJ, Williams R: Hepatitis C antibodies and hepatocellular carcinoma: New clues or a false trial? JNCI 82:986–987.
19. Enwonwu CO: The role of dietary aflatoxin in the genesis of hepatocellular carcinoma in developing countries. Lancet 2:956–958, 1984.
20. Palmer JR, Rosenberg L, Kaufmann DW, et al.: Oral contraceptive use and liver cancer. Am J Epidemiol 130:878–882, 1989.
21. Farrell GC, Uren RF, Perkins RW, Joshua DE, Baird PJ, Kronenberg H: Androgen induced hepatoma. Lancet 1:430–431, 1975.
22. Okuda K, Musha H, Nakajima Y, et al.: Clinicopathologic features of encapsulated hepatocellular carcinoma: a study of 26 cases. Cancer 40:1240–1245, 1977.
23. Ruffin MT: Fibrolamellar hepatoma. Am J Gastroenterol 85:577–581, 1990.
24. Waldmann TA, McIntire KR: The use of radioimmunoassay for α-fetoprotein in the diagnosis of malignancy. Cancer 34:1510–1515, 1974.
25. Okuda K, Ohtsuki T, Obata H: Natural history of hepatocellular carcinoma and prognosis in relation to treatment. Study of 850 patients. Cancer 56:918–928, 1985.
26. Salminen PM, Hockerstedt K, Edgren J, et al.: Intraoperative ultrasound as an aid to surgical strategy in liver tumor. Acta Chir Scand 156:329–332, 1990.
27. Okuda K and The Liver Tumor Study Group of Japan: Primary liver cancers in Japan. Cancer 45:2663–2669, 1980.
28. Adson MA, Weiland LH: Resection of primary solid hepatic tumors. Am J Surg 141:18–21, 1981.
29. Huguet C, Nordlinger B, Vacher B, Parc R, Halami F, Loygue J: Surgical resection of hepatocellular carcinoma. Retrospective study of 42 cases. Gastroenterol Clin Biol 9:244–249, 1985.

30. Nagao T, Inque S, Gato S, et al.: Hepatic resection for hepatocellular carcinoma. Ann Surg 205:33–40, 1987.

31. Lin TY, Lee CS, Chen KM, et al.: Role of surgery in the treatment of primary carcinoma of the liver: a 31 year experience. Br J Surg 74:839–842, 1987.

32. Chen MF, Hwang TL, Jeng CB, et al.: Hepatic resection in 120 patients with hepatocellular carcinoma. Arch Surg 124:1025–1028, 1989.

33. Toshihara T, Sugioka A, Veda M, et al.: Hepatic resection for hepatocellular carcinoma. Surgery 107:511–520, 1990.

34. Choi TK, Edward CS, Fan ST, et al.: Results of surgical resection for hepatocellular carcinoma. Hepatogastroenterology 37:172–173, 1990.

35. Yamanaka N, Okamoto E, Toyosaka A, et al.: Prognostic factors after hepatectomy for hepatocellular carcinoma. Hepatogastroenterology 37:172–173, 1990.

36. Iwatsuki S, Gordon RD, Shaw BW, Starzi TE: Role of liver transplantation in cancer therapy. Ann Surg 202:401–497, 1985.

37. Jenkins RL, Pinson CW, Stone MD: Experience with transplantation in the treatment of liver cancer. Cancer Chemother Pharmacol 23:104–109, 1989.

38. Ingold JA, Reed GB, Kaplan HS, Bagshw MA: Radiation hepatitis. Am J Roentgenol 93:200–208, 1965.

39. Phillips R, Murikama K: Primary neoplasms of the liver. Results of radiation therapy. Cancer 4:714–720, 1960.

40. Volberding PA, Friedman MA, Phillips TL: Hepatoma treated with intra-arterial polychemotherapy plus whole liver radiation. Proc Am Soc Clin Oncol 21:418, 1980.

41. Stizmann JV, Order SE: Immunoradiotherapy for primary nonresectable hepatocellular carcinoma. Surg Clin North Am 69:393–400, 1989.

42. Friedman MA, Demanes DJ, Hoffman PG: Hepatomas: hormone receptors and therapy. Am J Med 73:362–366, 1982.

43. Paliard P, Clement G, Saez S, Chabel J, Partensky C: Treatment of hepatocellular carcinoma with tamoxifen (letter). Gastroenterol Clin Biol 8:680–681, 1984.

44. Vogel CL, Bayley AC, Brockes RJ: A phase II study of adriamycin in patients with hepatocellular carcinoma from Zambia and the United States. Cancer 39:1923–1929, 1977.

45. Johnson PJ, Williams R, Thomas H, Sherlock S, Murray-Lyon IM: Induction of remission in hepatocellular carcinoma with doxorubicin. Lancet 1:1006–1009, 1978.

46. Falkson G, Lavin P, Moertel CG, Pretorious FJ, Carbone PP: Chemotherapy studies in primary liver cancer: a prospective randomized clinical trial. Cancer 42:2149–2156, 1978.

47. Olweny CLM, Katongole-Mbidde E, Bahendeka S, Otim D, Mugerwa J, Kyalwazi SK: Further evidence in treating patients with hepatocellular carcinoma in Uganda. Cancer 46:2717–2722, 1980.

48. Melia WM, Johnson PJ, Williams R: Induction remission in hepatocellular carcinoma: a comparison of VP-16 with adriamycin. Cancer 51:206–210, 1983.

49. Yang P, Sheu J, Chen D, et al., Systemic chemotherapy of hepatocellular carcinoma with adriamycin alone and FAM regimen. In Ogawa M (ed): Chemotherapy of Hepatic Tumors. Tokyo, Elsevier, 1984, pp 41–47.

50. Chlebowski RT, Brezechwa-Adjukiewicz A, Cowdon A, et al.: Doxorubicin for hepatocellular carcinoma: clinical and pharmacokinetic results. Cancer Treat Rep 68:487–491, 1984.

51. Choi TK, Lee NW, Wong J, et al.: Chemotherapy for advanced hepatocellular carcinoma—adriamycin versus quadruple chemotherapy. Cancer 53:401–405, 1984.

52. Sciarrino E, Simonetti RG, Moli SL, et al.: Adriamycin treatment for hepatocellular carcinoma: experience with 109 patients. Cancer 56:2751–2755, 1985.

53. Dunk AA, Scott SC, Johnson PJ, et al.: Mitozantrone as single agent therapy in hepatocellular carcinoma: a phase II study. J Hepatol 1:395–404, 1985.

54. Lai KH, Tsai YT, Lee SD, et al.: Phase II study of mitoxantrone in unresectable primary hepatocellular carcinoma following hepatitis B infection. Cancer Chemother Pharmacol 23:54–56, 1989.

55. Hochster HS, Green MD, Speyer J, et al.: 4'Epidoxorubicin (epirubicin) activity in hepatocellular carcinoma. J Clin Oncol 3:1525–1540, 1985.

56. Tan YO, Lim F: 4'Epidoxorubicin as a single agent in advanced primary hepatocellular carcinoma—a preliminary experience. Ann Acad Med Singapore 15:169–171, 1986.

57. Shiu W, Leung N, Li M, et al.: The efficacy of high dose 4'epidoxorubicin in hepatocellular carcinoma. Jpn J Clin Oncol 18:235–237, 1988.

58. Kennedy PS, Lehane DE, Smith FE, Lane M: Oral fluorouracil therapy of hepatoma. Cancer 39:1930–1935, 1977.

59. Link JS, Bateman JR, Paroly WS, Durkin WJ, Peters RL: 5-Fluorouracil in hepatocellular carcinoma: report of 21 cases. Cancer 39:1936–1939, 1977.

60. Davis HL, Ramirez H, Ansfield FJ: Adenocarcinomas of the stomach, pancreas, liver, and biliary tracts: Survival of 328 patients treated with fluoropyrimidine therapy. Cancer 33:193–197, 1974.

61. Al-Sarraf M, Go TS, Kithier K, Vaitkevicius VK: Primary liver cancer: a review of the clinical features, blood groups, serum enzymes, therapy and survival of 65 cases. Cancer 33:574–582, 1974.

62. Bukowski RM, Legna S, Saidi J, Eyre HJ, O'Bryan R: Phase II trial of M-AMSA in hepatocellular carcinoma: a Southwest Oncology Group Study. Cancer Treat Rep 66:1651–1652, 1982.

63. Cheng E, Lightdale C, Young C, Yagoda A, Fortner J, Golbey R: Phase II trial of (m-AMSA) 4'-9 (acridinylamino)-methane-sulfonm-aniside in primary liver cancer. Am Clin Oncol 6:211–213, 1983.

64. Amrein PC, Richards F, Coleman M, et al.: Phase II trial of Amsacrine in patients with hepatoma: a Cancer and Leukemia Group B study. Can Treat Rep 68:923–924, 1984.

65. Falkson G, Coetzer B, Klaasen DJ: A phase II study of m-AMSA in patients witih primary liver cancer. Cancer Chemother Pharmacol 6:127–129, 1981.

66. Vogel CL, Adamson RH, DeVita VT, Johns DG, Kyalwazi SK: Preliminary clinical trials of dichloromethotrexate (NSC-29630) in hepatocellular carcinoma. Cancer Chemother Rep 56:249–258, 1972.

67. Tester WJ, Donehower RS, Eddy JL, Myers CE, Ihde DC: Evaluation of weekly escalating doses of dichloromethotrexate in patients with hepatocellular carcinoma and other solid tumors. Cancer Chemother Pharmacol 8:305–310, 1982.

68. Cavalli F, Rosencweig M, Renard J, Goldhirsch A, Hansen HH: A phase II study of oral VP-16-213 in patients with hepatocellular carcinoma. Proc Am Soc Clin Oncol 22:457, 1981.

69. Melia WM, Westaby D, Williams R: Diaminodichloride platinum (cis-platinum) in treatment of hepatocellular carcinoma. Clin Oncol 7:275–280, 1981.

70. Anon: A prospective trial of recombinant human interferon 2B in previously untreated patients with hepatocellular carcinoma—The Gastrointestinal Tumor Study Group. Cancer 66:135–139, 1990.

71. Lai LL, Wu PL, Lok AS, et al.: Recombinant α-2 interferon is superior to doxorubicin for inoperable hepatocellular carcinoma: a prospective randomized trial. Br J Cancer 60:928–933, 1989.

72. Eckman WW, Patlak CS, Fenstermacher JD: A critical evaluation of the principles governing the advantages of intra-arterial infusions. J Pharmacokinet Biopharm 2:257–285, 1974.

73. Chen HG, Gross JF: Intra-arterial infusion of anticancer drugs: Theoretical aspects of drug delivery and review of responses. Cancer Treat Rep 64:31–40, 1980.

74. Ensminger WS, Rosowsky A, Raso V, et al.: A clinical pharmacologic

evaluation of hepatic arterial infusions of 5-fluoro-2'-deoxyuridine and 5-fluorouracil. Cancer Res 38:3784–3792, 1978.

75. Garnick MB, Ensminger WD, Israel M: A clinical pharmacologic evaluation of hepatic arterial infusion of adriamycin. Cancer Res 39:4105–4110, 1979.

76. Fraile RJ, Baker LH, Buroker TR, Horwitz J, Vaitkevicius VK: Pharmacokinetics of 5-flourouracil administered orally, by rapid intravenous and by slow infusion. Cancer Res 40:2223–2228, 1980.

77. Ensminger W, Stetson P, Gyves J, et al.: Dependence of hepatic arterial fluorouracil pharmacokinetics on dose, route and duration of infusion. Proc Am Soc Clin Oncol 2:25, 1983.

78. Campbell TN, Howell SB, Pfeifle CE, Wung WE, Bookstein J: Clinical pharmacokinetics of intraarterial cisplatin in humans. J Clin Oncol 12:755–762, 1983.

79. Gyves JI, Ensminger W, Stetson P, et al.: Clinical pharmacology of mitomycin C by hepatic arterial infusion. Proc Am Soc Clin Oncol 2:25, 1983.

80. Wellwood JM, Cady B, Oberfield RA: Treatment of primary liver cancer: response on regional chemotherapy. Clin Oncol 5:25–31, 1979.

81. Doci A, Bignami P, Bozzetti F, et al.: Intrahepatic chemotherapy for unresectable hepatocellular carcinoma. Cancer 61:1983–1987.

82. Bern MM, McDermott W, Cady B: Intraarterial hepatic infusion and intravenous adriamycin for treatment of hepatocellular carcinoma: a clinical and pharmacology report. Cancer 42:399–406, 1978.

83. Urist MM, Balch CM: Intra-arterial chemotherapy for hepatoma using adriamycin administered via an implantable infusion pump. Proc Am Soc Clin Oncol 3:146, 1983.

84. Shepherd FA, Evans WK, Fine S, Blackstein ME, Mullis B: Hepatic arterial infusion of mitoxantrone and adriamycin in the treatment of primary hepatocellular carcinoma. Proc Am Soc Clin Oncol 4:95, 1985.

85. Ukeka H, Kuroda S, Ohnoshi T, et al.: Intraarterial adriamycin for patients with hepatocellular carcinoma and metastatic carcinoma. Gan To Kagaku Ryoho 11:2579–2584, 1984.

86. Cheng E, Watson RC, Fortner J, Kemeny N, Golbey R: Regional intraarterial infusion of cisplatin in primary liver cancer. Proc Am Soc Clin Oncol 1:179, 1982.

87. Shepard FA, Evans WK, Blackstein ME, et al.: Hepatic arterial infusion of mitoxantrone in the treatment of primary hepatocellular carcinoma. J Clin Oncol 5:635–640, 1987.

88. Hohn DC, Melnick J, Stagg RJ, et al.: Biliary sclerosis in patients receiving hepatic arterial infusions of floxuridine. J Clin Oncol 3:98–102, 1985.

89. Douglas CC: Prolongation of survival with periodic percutaneous multidrug arterial infusions in patients with primary and metastatic gastrointestinal carcinoma to the liver. Proc Am Soc Clin Oncol 21:416, 1980.

90. Patt YZ, Chuang VP, Wallace S, Benjamin RS, Fuqua R, Mavligit GM: Hepatic artery chemotherapy and occlusion for palliation of primary hepatocellular and unknown primary neoplasms in the liver. Cancer 51:1359–1363, 1983.

91. Katagiri Y, Mabuchi K, Itakura T, et al.: Adriamycin-Lipiodol suspension for IA chemotherapy of hepatocellular carcinoma. Cancer Chemother Pharmacol 23:238–242, 1989.

92. Lee YT, Irwin L: Hepatic artery ligation and adriamycin infusion chemotherapy for hepatoma. Cancer 41:1245–1255, 1978.

93. Nagasue N, Inokuchi K, Kobayashi M, Saku M: Serum α-fetoprotein levels after hepatic artery ligation and postoperative chemotherapy: correlation with clinical status in patients with hepatocellular carcinoma. Cancer 40:615–618, 1977.

94. Charnsangavej C, Chuang VP, Wallace S, Soo CS, Bowers T: Angiographic classification of hepatic arterial collaterals. Radiology 144:485–494, 1982.

95. Chearanai O, Plengvanit U, Asavanich C, Damrongsak D, Sindhvananda K, Boonyapisit S: Spontaneous rupture of primary hepatoma: report of 63 cases with particular reference to the pathogenesis and rationale treatment by hepatic artery ligation. Cancer 51:1532–1536, 1983.

96. Wallace S, Charnsangavej C, Carrasco H, Bechtel W: Infusion-embolization. Cancer 54:2751–2765, 1984.

97. Yamada R, Sato M, Kawabata M, et al.: Hepatic artery embolization in 120 patientss with unresectable hepatoma. Radiology 148:397–401, 1983.

98. Fujimoto S, Miyazaki M, Endoh F, Takahashi O, Okui K, Morimoto Y: Biodegradable mitomycin C microspheres given intra-arterially for operable hepatic cancer. Cancer 56:2404–2410, 1985.

99. Ohnishi K, Tsuchiya S, Nakayama T, et al.: Arterial chemoembolization of hepatocellular carcinoma with mitomycin C microcapsules. Radiology 152:51–55, 1984.

100. Venook A, Stagg R, Lewis B, et al.: Chemoembolization for hepatocellular carcinoma. J Clin Oncol 8:1108–1114, 1990.

101. Zhou X, Tang Z, Yu Y, et al.: Clinical evaluation of cryosurgery in the treatment of primary liver cancer. Cancer 61:1889–1892, 1988.

102. Livraghi T, Vettori C: Percutaneous ethanol injection therapy of hepatoma. Cardiovasc Intervent Radiol 13:146–152, 1990.

103. Weiss L, Gilbert HA (eds): Liver Metastases. Boston: GK Hall Medical Publishing, 1982.

104. Beck PR, Belfield A, Spooner RJ, Blumgart LH, Wood CB: Serum enzyme elevations in colorectal cancer. Cancer 43:1772–1776, 1979.

105. Kemeny MM, Sugarbaker PH, Smith TJ, et al.: A prospective analysis of laboratory tests and imaging studies to detect hepatic lesions. Ann Surg 195:163–167, 1982.

106. Szymendera JJ, Nowacki MP, Szawlowski AW, Kaminska JA: Predictive value of plasma CEA levels: preoperative and postoperative monitoring of patients with colorectal carcinoma. Dis Colon Rectum 25:46–52, 1982.

107. Funven P, Makuuchi M, Takayasu K, Moriyama N, Yamasaki S, Hasegawa H: Preoperative imaging of liver metastases. Comparison of angiography, CT scan, and ultrasound. Ann Surg 202:573–579, 1985.

108. Schreve RH, Terpstra OT, Ausema L, Lameris JS, van Seijen AJ, Jeekel J: Detection liver metastases. A prospective study comparing liver enzymes, scintigraphy, ultrasonography, and computed tomography. Br J Surg 71:947–949, 1984.

109. Pettavel J, Morgenthaler F: Protracted arterial chemotherapy of liver tumors: an experience of 107 cases over a 12-year period. Prog Clin Cancer 7:217–233, 1978.

110. Goslin R, Steele G, Zamcheck N, Mayer R, Macintyre J: Factors influencing survival in patients with hepatic matastases from adenocarcinoma of the colon or rectum. Dis Colon Rectum 25:749–754, 1982.

111. Morrow CE, Grage TB, Sutherland DE, Najarian JS: Hepatic resection for secondary neoplasms. Surgery 92:610–614, 1982.

112. Rajpal S, Dasmahapatra, Ledesma EJ, Mittelman A: Extensive resections of isolated metastasis from carcinoma of the colon and rectum. Surg Gynecol Obstet 155:813–816, 1982.

113. Iwatsuki S, Shaw BW, Starzl TE: Experience with 150 liver resections. Ann Surg 197:247–259, 1983.

114. Adson MA, van Heerden JA, Adson MH, Wagner JS, Ilstrap DM: Resection of hepatic metastases from colorectal cancer. Arch Surg 119:647–651, 1984.

115. Steele G, Osteen RT, Wilson RE, Brooks DC, Mayer RJ, Zamcheck N, Ravikumar TS: Patterns of failure after surgical resection of large liver tumors. Am J Surg 147:554–559, 1984.

116. Fortner JG, Silva JS, Golbey RB, Cox EB, Maclean BJ: Multivariate analysis of a personal series of 247 consecutive patients with liver metastases from colorectal cancer. Ann Surg 199:306–316, 1984.

117. Pettrelli NJ, Nambisan RN, Herrera L, Mittelman A: Hepatic resection for isolated metastasis from colorectal carcinoma. Am J Surg 149:205–209, 1985.
118. Nordlinger BN, Quilichinis M, Pac R, et al.: Hepatic resection for colorectal liver metastases. Ann Surg 205:256–263, 1987.
119. Hughes K, Schilel J, Sugerbaker P, et al.: Surgery for colorectal cancer metastatic to the liver. Surg Clin North Am 69:339–359, 1989.
119. Borgelt BB, Gelber R, Brady LW, et al.: The palliation of hepatic metastases: Results of Radiation Therapy Oncology Group pilot study. Int J Radiat Oncol Biol Phys 7:587–591, 1981.
120. Barone RM, Byfield JE, Goldfarb PB, Frankel S, Ginn C, Greer S: Intra-arterial chemotherapy using an implantable infusion pump and liver irradiation for the treatment of hepatic metastases. Cancer 50:850–862, 1982.
121. Evans JT: Hepatic artery ligation in hepatic metastases from colon and rectal malignancies. Dis Colon Rectum 22:370, 1979.
122. Moertel CG: Chemotherapy of gastrointestinal cancer. N Engl J Med 299:1049–1052, 1978.
123. Machover D, Goldschmidt E, Chollet P, et al.: Treatment of advanced colorectal and gastric adenocarcinoma with 5-fluorouracil and high-dose folinic acid. J Clin Oncol 4:685–696, 1986.
124. Boice JD, Greene MH, Killen JY, et al.: Leukemia and preleukemia after adjuvant treatment of gastrointestinal cancer with semustine (methyl-CCNU). N Engl J Med 309:1079–1084, 1983.
125. Balch CM, Urist MM, Soong SJ, McGregor M: A prospective phase II clinical trial of continuous FUDR regional chemotherapy for colorectal metastases to the liver using a totally implantable pump. Ann Surg 198:567–573, 1983.
126. Niederhuber JE, Ensminger W, Gyves J, Thrall J, Walker S, Cozzi E: Regional chemotherapy of colorectal cancer metastatic to the liver. Cancer 53:1336–1343, 1984.
127. Reed ML, Vaitkevicius VK, Al-Sarraf M, et al.: The practicality of chronic hepatic artery infusion therapy of primary and metastatic hepatic malignancies: ten-year results in 124 patients in a prospective protocol. Cancer 47:402–409, 1981.
128. Weiss GR, Garnick MB, Osteen RT, et al.: Long-term hepatic arterial infusion of 5-fluorodeoxyuridine for liver metastases using an implantable infusion pump. J Clin Oncol 1:337–344, 1983.
129. Kemeny MM, Goldberg DA, Browning S, Metter GE, Miner PJ, Terz JJ: Experience with continuous regional chemotherapy and hepatic resection as treatment of hepatic metastases from colorectal primaries. A prospective randomized study. Cancer 55:1265–1270, 1985.
130. Kemeny N, Daly J, Oderman P, Shike M, Chun H, Petroni G, Geller N: Hepatic artery pump infusion: toxicity and results in patients with metastatic colorectal carcinoma. J Clin Oncol 2:595–600, 1984.
131. Riether RD, Khubchandani IT, Sheets JA, Stasik JJ, Rosen L: A prospective study of continuous hepatic perfusion with implantable pump. Dis Colon Rectum 28:24–26, 1985.
132. Tandon RN, Bunnell IL, Cooper RG: The treatment of metastatic carcinoma of the liver by the percutaneous selective hepatic artery infusion of 5-fluorouracil. Surgery 73:118–121, 1973.
133. Ansfield FJ, Ramirez G: The clinical results of 5-flourouracil intra-hepatic arterial infusion in 528 patients with metastatic cancer to the liver. Prog Clin Cancer 7:201–206, 1978.
134. Petrek JA, Minton JP: Treatment of hepatic metastases by percutaneous hepatic arterial infusion. Cancer 43:2182–2188, 1979.
135. Grage TB, Vassilopoulos PP, Shingleton WW, et al.: Results of a prospective randomized study of hepatic arterial infusion with 5-fluorouracil versus intravenous 5-fluorouracil in patients with hepatic metastases from colorectal origin. Surgery 86:550–555, 1979.
136. Berger M: Hepatic infusion for metastatic colorectal cancer in a community hospital setting (Abstract). Proc Am Soc Clin Oncol 22:456, 1981.
137. Oberfield RA, McCafferey JA, Polio J, Clouse ME, Hamilton T: Prolonged and continuous percutaneous intra-arterial hepatic infusion chemotherapy in advanced metastatic liver adenocarcinoma from colorectal primary. Cancer 44:414–423, 1979.
138. Stagg RJ, Venook AP, Chase JL, et al.: Alternating hepatic intra-arterial FUDR and 5-FU; a less toxic regimen for the treatment of colorectal cancer metastatic to the liver. JNCI 83:423–428, 1991.
139. Patt Y, Mavligit GM, Chaung VP, et al.: Percutaneous hepatic arterial infusion (HAI) of mitomycin C and floxuridine (FUDR): an effective treatment for metastatic colorectal cancer to the liver. Cancer 46:261–265, 1980.
140. Shepard KV, Levin B, Karl RC, et al.: Therapy for metastatic colorectal cancer with hepatic artery infusion chemotherapy using a subcutaneous implanted pump. J Clin Oncol 3:161–169, 1985.
141. Hatfield AK, Kammer BA, Danley RA, Miller AG, Houston JG, Harder L: Intermittent hepatic artery perfusions for symptomatic metastatic colon carcinoma (Abstract). Proc Am Soc Clin Oncol 1:102, 1982.
142. Theodors A, Bukowski RM, Lavery I, Hewlett JS, Livingston RB, Buonocore E: Hepatic artery infusion with 5-fluorouracil and mitomycin-C in metastatic colorectal carcinoma phase II study. Med Pediatr Oncol 10:463–470, 1982.
143. Patt YZ, Boddie AW Jr, Charnsangavej C, Ajani JA, Wallace S, Soski M, Claghorn L, Mavligit GM: Hepatic arterial infusion with floxuridine and cisplatin: overriding importance of antitumor effect versus degree of tumor burden as determinants of survival among patients with colorectal cancer. J Clin Oncol 4:1356–1364, 1986.
144. Cohen AM, Schaeffer N, Higgins J: Treatment of metastatic colorectal cancer with hepatic arterial combination chemotherapy. Cancer 57:1115–1117, 1986.
145. Wils J, Schlangen J, Naus A: Phase II study of hepatic artery infusion with 5-fluorouracil, adriamycin, and mitomycin C (FAM) in liver metastases from colorectal carcinoma. Cancer Chemother Pharmacol 13:215–217, 1984.
146. Hohn DC, Stagg RJ, Friedman MA, et al.: A randomized trial of continuous intravenous versus hepatic intra-arterial floxuridine in patients with colorectal cancer metastatic to the liver: The Northern California Oncology Group Trial. J Clin Oncol 1989:1646–1654, 1989.
147. Kemeny N, Daly JM, Reichman B, et al.: Intrahepatic or systemic infusion of fluorodeoxyuridine in patient with liver metastases from colorectal carcinoma. Ann Intern Med 107:459–465, 1987.
148. Chang AE, Schneider PD, Sugarbaker PH, et al.: A prospective randomized trial of regional versus systemic continuous 5-fluorodeoxyuridine chemotherapy in the treatment of colorectal liver metastases. Ann Surg 6:685–693, 1987.
149. Martin JK, O'Connell MJ, Wieand HS, et al.: Intra-arterial floxuridine versus systemic fluorouracil for hepatic metastases from colorectal colorectal cancer. A randomized trial. Arch Surg 125:1022–1027, 1990.

CHAPTER 79

GASTROINTESTINAL CANCER

GREGORY V. STAJICH, Pharm.D. and RAVI P. SARMA, M.D., F.A.C.P.

Cancers of the gastrointestinal tract (esophagus, stomach, large intestine, and rectum) represent a major health problem throughout the world. The morbidity and mortality from these malignancies are shown in Table 79.1. The first-line therapy is often surgery. For localized tumors, complete resection results in a modest increase in survival. Results from these trials have prompted the addition of radiotherapy and chemotherapy regimens to improve survival rate. Combinations using different treatment modalities have not yet made significant improvements. Therefore, most of the new directions toward an effective cure have been aimed at an earlier diagnosis. This is accomplished through regular proctosigmoidoscopy and stool tests for occult blood.

ESOPHAGEAL CANCER

Approximately 8% of all gastrointestinal cancer deaths in the United States are caused by carcinoma of the esophagus. The American Cancer Society estimates that 10,600 new cases will be diagnosed in 1990 (1).

Worldwide, there is a more striking geographic variation in the incidence of esophageal cancer than any other malignant neoplasm. It occurs frequently within a so-called Asian esophageal cancer belt, which extends from the southern shore of the Caspian Sea on the west to northern China on the east and encompasses parts of Iran, Soviet Central Asia, Afghanistan, Siberia, and Mongolia (2). In some of the areas, such as north China, the disease has been relatively common for generations. In addition, there are marked variations in incidence in populations situated only a few kilometers apart. For most of Europe, rates of esophageal cancer are low, except for certain areas in France where the disease is a major problem among males (3). Cancer of the esophagus is virtually unknown in western and northern Africa, but it is common in regions of southern and eastern Africa, where the disease represents one-fifth to almost one-half of all registered cancers.

In North America, the incidence of esophageal cancer in blacks is at least three times that in whites. The disease is now considered to be one of the most common types of cancer among blacks (4). There is considerable geographic variation, with rates for white and nonwhite males being highest in the Northeast, increasing markedly with urbanization. Among women the rate of esophageal cancer was highest in the South, particularly in rural areas (5).

The cancer is more common in men (sex ratio 4:1) and appears most frequently after 50 years of age (1).

Etiology

No one set of factors can explain the cause of esophageal carcinoma. In North America and Western Europe, the major risk factors for esophageal cancer are excessive alcoholic consumption and a long-standing history of cigarette smoking, accounting for approximately 80 to 90% of the cases each year. The relative risk increases with the amount and type of alcoholic beverage consumed or the tobacco used. Consumption of whiskey seems to be linked to a higher incidence than intake of wine and beer. The combined exposure to alcohol and tobacco has a synergistic effect on relative risk. Alcohol itself does not appear to be a direct carcinogen, but it can increase the risk of esophageal cancer in smokers (6).

Among extrinsic risk factors, the relationship between carcinoma of the esophagus and heat burns has been known for some time. Heat trauma is associated with the ingestion of hot foods and/or beverages. The mechanism involved in the risk of esophageal carcinoma from heat burns is similar to that of chemical burns produced by highly alcoholic beverages. Both heat burns and alcohol increase esophageal mucosal cell turnover, thereby increasing exposure to carcinogens, such as those in cigarette smoke (7). Additional extrinsic risk factors that are inhaled or ingested include nitrates, smoked opiates, and pickled vegetables, as well as mucosal injury from physical insults such as ingestion of lye, asbestos, and radiation-induced strictures (8).

Intrinsic disorders associated with the possible development of esophageal carcinoma include achalasia, reflux esophagitis, and hiatal hernia, and the risk has been estimated to be approximately 7% in persons with Barrett esophagus (9). Other etiological factors associated with esophageal cancer include malnutrition and dietary deficiency of molybdenum, zinc, or vitamin A. Individuals who have undergone partial gastrectomy appear to be at a high risk of developing esophageal carcinoma. In one study conducted between 1965 and 1983, 12 of 129 gastrectomy patients eventually developed esophageal carcinoma (10). No genetic factors are known to influence the development of esophageal carcinoma.

Table 79.1.
New Cases and Deaths of Cancer of the Gastrointestinal Tract, United States, 1990[a]

Site	Total	Male	Female
Estimated New Cases by Sex for All Sites			
Esophagus	10,600	7,400	3,200
Stomach	23,200	13,900	9,300
Small intestine	2,800	1,500	1,300
Large intestine	110,000	52,000	58,000
Rectum	45,000	24,000	21,000
Estimated Cancer Deaths by Sex for All Sites			
Esophagus	9,500	7,000	2,500
Stomach	13,700	8,300	5,400
Small intestine	900	500	400
Large intestine	53,300	26,000	27,300
Rectum	7,600	4,000	3,600

[a] Adapted from Silverberg E, Boring CC, Squires TS: Cancer Statistics. CA 40: 9–26, 1990.

Pathology

The esophagus is susceptible to various types of malignant neoplasms. Squamous cell carcinoma, which arises from the esophageal mucosa, accounts for over 90% of all esophageal cancers. Adenocarcinoma is less common, accounting for 0.8% to 8% of esophageal malignancies (11).

In general, 15% of the malignancies occur in the upper third of the esophagus, 50% in the middle third, and 35% in the lower third. The natural history of esophageal cancer can be divided into four phases: initial, developing, overt, and terminal. The initial or precancerous phase covers a period up to 20 years or more. The first observed changes are mild-to-moderate hyperplasia of esophageal basal epithelial mucosal cells, eventually progressing to dysplasia. The next phase involves the development of in situ cancer. This phase is clinically latent and may remain so for a long time. The rapidly progressing overt phase begins when the in situ malignancy breaks through the basement membrane. The final or terminal phase is usually very short. In this phase, the cancer is extensive, inoperable, and has distant metastases.

Carcinoma of the esophagus is usually invasive by the time of discovery, and metastases begin early in the course of the disease. Lymphatic dissemination also begins early because of the rich submucosal lymphatic network of the esophagus. Sites invaded depend upon the location of the neoplasm in the esophagus. Neoplasms in the upper third of the esophagus may invade the larynx, trachea, and soft tissues of the neck. Those in the middle third may invade the respiratory tract or invade and perforate the aorta. Neoplasms in the lower third may invade the mediastinum, diaphragm, and gastric cardia.

Metastases by the hematogenous route are common in patients with advanced cancer of the esophagus. Approximately a third of patients have demonstrable distant metastases on admission. The liver is the most frequent site of visceral involvement. Other involved sites are the lungs and pleura, bones, kidneys, omentum and peritoneum, and adrenals. Local and regional invasion is the cause of death far more frequently than distant metastases.

Screening and Diagnosis

Chinese studies have demonstrated that mass screening programs are quite successful in identifying the early stages of esophageal cancers (12). In most cases, early diagnosis is associated with high resection and cure rates. In the United States and other low-risk countries, the incidence of esophageal cancer is too low to justify mass screening, except for those predisposed to esophageal cancer (13).

Methods used to detect cancer early include abrasive cytology (balloon method), fiberoptic endoscopy with guided forceps biopsy, and brush cytology. Early esophageal carcinoma can be difficult to detect by endoscopy alone. The ratio of detected invasive cancer to early cancer of the esophagus is 10 times less than that of gastric cancer. However, flexible fiberoptic endoscopy, coupled with biopsy and brush cytology is reported to have a sensitivity approaching 100% for squamous cell carcinoma (11).

Patients who are symptomatic are usually first tested with a barium esophagogram. A follow-up esophagoscopy and biopsy are indicated. Computed tomography (CT) scan is an important addition to the diagnostic workup of esophageal cancer. The cross-sectional CT image allows detection of direct invasion or the presence of metastatic disease often not detectable with other diagnostic techniques.

Staging

An accurate staging is important in determining the appropriate therapy. The TNM staging system recommended by the American Joint Committee on Cancer (Table 79.2) is used in denoting the extent of the disease.

Clinical Manifestations

Approximately 90% of patients with esophageal cancer present with mild complaints related to swallowing and weight loss (14). Frequently encountered symptoms include pain on swallowing (odynophagia) and burning, or delay in the passage of food through the esophagus. The symptoms can be intermittent and evolve over a period of months to several years. Approximately 10% of patients have no symptoms if the lesion is limited to the mucosa and submucosa.

The early symptoms of esophageal cancer should be

Table 79.2.
Esophageal Primary Tumor and Metastasis Classification by the American Joint Committee for Cancer[a]

Primary tumor (T)

T_0	No evidence of primary tumor
T_{is}	Carcinoma in situ
T_1	Neoplasm involving 5 cm or less of esophageal length; no obstruction, no circumferential involvement, and without extraesophageal spread
T_2	Neoplasm more than 5 cm without extraesophageal spread; or a neoplasm of any size producing obstruction, or involving entire circumference of the esophagus
T_3	Neoplasm that presents evidence of extraesophageal spread

Node involvement (N)

N_x	Not assessed
N_0	No clinically palpable nodes
N_1	Movable, unilateral palpable nodes
N_2	Movable, bilateral, palpable nodes
N_3	Fixed nodes

Distant metastases (M)

M_x	Not assessed
M_0	No evidence of distant metastases
M_1	Distant metastases present

Stage grouping

Stage I	T_1, N_0, M_0; or T_1, N_x, M_0
Stage II	T_2, N_0, M_0; or T_2, N_x, M_0
Stage III	Any T_3; or any N_1; or any M_1

[a] Adapted from Beahrs OH, Myers MH (eds): Manual for Staging of Cancer. Philadelphia, JB Lippincott, 1983, p 67.

differentiated from symptoms associated with chronic pharyngitis and esophagitis, which are also common in cancer of the esophagus. Patients with chronic pharyngitis or esophagitis present with an obstructive or boring sensation in the hypopharynx and upper retrosternal region, which occurs when the patient is not eating. However, the symptoms of early esophageal cancer occur only upon swallowing food.

The classic symptom during the late stages of esophageal cancer is dysphagia. Dysphagia is usually intermittent at first, eventually becoming persistent. Temporary partial relief is common, possibly due to partial necrosis and sloughing of the obstructing neoplasm. As the esophageal lumen progressively narrows, there is a gradual decrease in the oral intake of food, leading to weight loss. As a result, the physical appearance of patients with esophageal cancer frequently gives evidence of a serious nutritional deficit. Additional common problems encountered by patients with esophageal cancer are

1. Pain in the chest, neck, and abdomen;
2. Cough due to regurgitation of food or because of a bronchoesophageal fistula;
3. Vocal cord paralysis, tracheal compression, airway obstruction, pneumonitis, and lung abscess;
4. Progressive production of tenacious mucus;
5. Fetid odor due to fermentation of food in the esophagus;
6. Jaundice, ascites, hepatic coma due to secondary liver involvement.

Patients may present with one or more of the above problems as the chief complaint.

Prognosis

After staging, patients are usually divided into two treatment groups. Those with local regional disease in whom the disease is still potentially curable and those with extensive disease, (metastatic disease outside of the local regional area or invasion of the airway) in whom currently available therapy is solely toward control of symptoms. Despite advances in surgical techniques and radiation therapy, the prognosis for esophageal cancer remains dismal. Fewer than 10% can expect to live beyond 5 years. These survival figures have remained virtually unchanged over the past three decades (1). Features that appear to be the most significant in survival are size of the neoplasm, local invasion, and metastases. When the malignant change is confined to the mucosa, the 5-year survival reaches 90% (15). The higher the lesion, the graver the prognosis, because of injury to the neighboring structures rather than to the neoplasm itself. The causes of death in most patients with esophageal cancer are cachexia, tracheoesophageal or esophageal-aortic fistulas, mediastinitis, and distant metastases.

Treatment

The most common treatment of esophageal cancer is surgery, either alone or in combination with radiation therapy. Even early in the diagnosis of the disease, when the tumor is limited to a regional area, the outlook for most patients remains bleak. For a patient with a nonresectable primary lesion or metastic disease, the addition of chemotherapy has met with limited success. This has prompted a number of investigators to use a multimodality approach in an attempt to improve local control or cure rate, or to provide substantial palliation. The discussion of treatment will be confined to the epidermoid cell type, since 90 to 95% of esophageal cancers are of this cell type.

Surgery

Surgery is the mainstay of therapy for the treatment of esophageal cancer when the tumor is potentially resectable. In addition, surgery is used for local tumor control, palliation of symptoms, and accurate staging. It is the consensus among surgeons that tumors that arise in the lower one-third of the esophagus are most amenable to surgical resection and cure. The preferred procedure is radical esophagectomy with esophagogastrostomy, which allows for removal of gastric and celiac nodes. Of those who undergo resection and removal of all macroscopic disease, 5-year survival rates range from 8 to 22% (16). Even in patients with metastic disease, unresectable tumors with obstruction, and tracheoesophageal fistula, surgery may prolong and improve the quality of life, allowing the patient to swallow food and saliva without difficulty. Complications of surgery include strictures, anastomotic leaks, respiratory failure, pulmonary embolism, and sepsis. All of these problems contribute to a high perioperative mortality (10 to 40%). The 5-year survival rate from surgery approaches 20% for most surgical series (11, 15).

Radiation Therapy

Radiation therapy affords a less invasive and traumatic approach to the treatment of esophageal cancer and is the most common treatment for nonresectable tumors. Generally, radiation is preferable to surgery for tumors that arise in the upper two-thirds of the esophagus. Gross tumor is generally treated with the usual dose of 5000 to 6000 rads over a 4- to 6-week period. Radiation therapy can also be used for palliative purposes in tumors that are inoperable or unresectable. Palliative doses are generally in the range of 5000 rads. When radiation is given, dysphagia improves beginning in 10 to 14 days, in approximately 50 to 75% of patients (17).

Curative results for carcinoma of the esophagus using radiation alone remain poor. A retrospective study of 49 trials reviewing the results of treatment of 8489 patients receiving 5500 to 6000 rads of external-beam radiation showed 5-year survival rates that were nearly identical to the survival rate of patients treated with surgery (18). Although there was less morbidity with radiation, less satisfactory palliation of obstructive symptoms was reported. Complications from radiation therapy include esophagitis, tracheoesophageal fistula, pulmonary fibrosis, paracarditis, and myelosuppression.

Cobalt teletherapy and megavoltage energy machines such as linear accelerators, together with sophisticated imagery now permit the precise delivery of high-dose radiation.

PREOPERATIVE RADIATION THERAPY

As part of a curative treatment approach to carcinoma of the esophagus, radiation therapy is often used preoperatively. The rationale for this combination is that radiation can reduce tumor bulk, and in some cases increase resectability rates. Preoperative radiation may also be important in suppressing microscopic disease in regional lymph nodes, which may be undetected and not removed by the surgery. Surgery 2 to 6 weeks later provides for a more extensive visualization of the esophagus. Long-term survival from preoperative radiation correlates with the extent of tumor destruction seen in the operative specimen. A study found 44% 2-year and 28% 5-year survival rates when preoperative radiation showed extensive tumor destruction (19). In general, the disappearance of tumor is an important goal in preoperative radiation, and most long-term survivors come from the groups whose tumor was nearly or completely eradicated by radiation.

POSTOPERATIVE RADIATION THERAPY

Postoperative radiation is used when there are positive surgical margins or lymph node involvement. If an exploratory laparotomy reveals an unresectable carcinoma, radiation is given with a palliative intent. In the latter situation, during the operation the surgeon can also place radiopaque clips around the tumor, thus providing the radiotherapist a more accurate way of directing treatment to the involved area. The dose of radiation is usually 4000 to 5000 rads. Additionally, it may also be effective in controlling implantation or seeding of tumor cells, which may have occurred at the time of the operation.

Chemotherapy

Most patients with esophageal cancer have regional or distant metastases at diagnosis. The rationale for using chemotherapy before and after surgery for esophageal carcinoma is similar to that described for the use of pre- and postoperative radiation. In addition, chemotherapy has the potential to eradicate microscopic distant metastases. Single-agent chemotherapy trials of many agents have shown only minimal degrees of activity. Agents known to be active include cisplatin, vindesine, 5-fluorouracil (5-FU) (with response rate reported to be higher with infusion than with bolus), methotrexate, and bleomycin (20–21). Bleomycin is often incorporated in a number of protocols because of its relative lack of myelosuppression. However, potentially fatal pulmonary toxicity can develop, especially if combined with radiation therapy (22). Almost all responses seen with single-agent therapy are partial, and they are usually brief in duration. Data from these single-agent studies have shown modest activity that might be improved in combination regimens. Most of the combination-therapy regimes are cisplatin-based (Table 79.3). Because cisplatin-based combination chemotherapy produced tumor regression in nearly one-third of patients, but was associated with considerable toxicity, there has been interest in a second-generation platinum analog, carboplatin. Although significantly less toxic than cisplatin, carboplatin was less active and therefore, does not appear to be a substitute for cisplatin in this disease (22, 24). In clinical trials reported since 1987, cisplatin-based combination chemotherapy has been associated with response rates between 17 and 76% and a survival of 4 to 8 months (25, 26).

Table 79.3.
Combination Chemotherapy (Pooled) for Carcinoma of the Esophagus[a]

Regimen	Protocol	Recycle Every	Response Rate[b] (%)	Duration (months)
DDP[c] + Bleo + VIN	DDP = 50 mg/m², day 1 Bleo = 15 mg/m², day 1 VIN = 3 mg/m², weekly	3 weeks	47	7
DDP + DOX + 5FU	DDP = 75 mg/m², day 1 DOX = 30 mg/m², day 1 5FU = 600 mg/m², day 1 & 8	29 days	33	9
DDP + VIN + MGBG	DDP = 100 mg/m², day 2 VIN = 1.6 mg/m², days 1–4 MGBG = 500 mg/m², days 1 & 14	29 days	41	3
DDP + Bleo	DDP = 20 mg/m², day × 8 Bleo = 10 mg, infusion day 1–8		17.4	6
DDP + MTX + Bleo	DDP = 50 mg/m², day 4 Bleo = 10U, i.m., weekly	3 weeks	32	5.5

[a] Data adapted from Lichter AL, Roth JA: Carcinoma of the esophagus, Symposia. Proc Am Soc Clin Oncol 9:51–72, 1989.
[b] Includes partial and complete responses.
[c] Abbreviations: DDP, cisplatin; 5FU, fluorouracil; DOX, doxorubicin; MCBG, mitoguazone; Bleo, bleomycin; VIN, vindesine; MTX, methotrexate.

Multimodality Treatment

Surgery, radiation, and chemotherapy, either alone or in combination, have not had a major impact on the treatment of esophageal cancer. Randomized treatment protocols now in use combine multiagent chemotherapy and radiation therapy at the time of diagnosis, prior to attempting resection, and additional drug treatment is administered following surgery. An intergroup trial between the Eastern Cooperative Oncology Group (ECOG) and the Radiation Therapy Oncology Group (RTOG) is attempting to answer the validity of the multimodality treatment approach.

A study in which patients treated with neoadjuvant chemotherapy, surgery, and radiation reported a 5-year survival rate of 36% for the 47 resected patients, with median survival of 23.7 months (27). Other studies have reported similar encouraging results with combination of chemotherapy, given either preoperatively or postoperatively, with radiation (28, 29). It is hoped that within the next few years the role of combined multimodality therapy in the management of carcinoma of the esophagus will be clarified. The synergy between 5-FU and α-interferon is currently in phase II trials (30). This treatment regimen shows significant activity in esophageal carcinoma, and it can be given as an outpatient regimen. However, until doses and scheduling are optimized, further studies are warranted.

GASTRIC CANCER

The incidence of stomach cancer is decreasing dramatically in the United States. It now ranks sixth as a cause of death in patients with cancer. Approximately 20,000 new cases are expected to occur in 1990 (1). The mean age at the time of diagnosis of gastric cancer is 55 years. It is twice as common in men as in women.

However, cancer of the stomach remains a major worldwide health problem, with marked variability in incidence, depending on the geographic area, race, diet, heredity, and gender. This suggests that gastric cancer has a multiplicity of etiologies. High-risk countries such as Japan, Costa Rica, and Iceland have approximately five to seven times the death rate of low-risk countries such as the United States, Australia, and New Zealand (31). Although no etiological factors have been clearly defined, diet has been studied intensely. For instance, the hypertonic salted and pickled fish and vegetable diet of Japan and the high consumption of smoked salmon and trout in Iceland have been implicated as being mutagenic (32). There is speculation that long-term ingestion of high concentrations of nitrates from these diets, which are converted to nitrites and carcinogenic nitrosamines may promote gastric carcinogenesis. Vitamin C possibly blocks the formation of these mutagens in the stomach and may play a role in prevention (33). The incidence of gastric cancer has been decreasing in the United States since 1930, when it was the most frequent cause of cancer death. The declining incidence of stomach cancer has been attributed to the wide availability of refrigeration, thereby decreasing the need for salt and nitrate as preservatives.

Predisposing factors that enhance the risk for developing gastric cancer may be environmental and have a genetic element in pathogenesis (Table 79.4). First-generation immigrants from countries with high gastric rates continue to be at high risk, compared with their offspring

Table 79.4.
Factors Associated with Cancer of the Stomach[a]

Low Cancer Rate	High Cancer Rate
Not related to gastric cancer patients	Relatives of gastric patients
Blood group O	Blood group A
Females	Males
Younger patients	Older patients
Meat-eating population	Dried or salted fish-eating population
Bland diet	Salty or spicy diet
High vitamin C intake	Low vitamin C intake
Normal gastric secretions	Atrophic gastritis, achlorhydria
Japanese born and living in USA	Japanese born and living in Japan
White	Black

[a] From Ramming KP, Haskell CM, Stomach cancer. In Haskell CM (ed): Cancer Treatment, ed. 3. Philadelphia, WB Saunders, 1990, with permission.

born in the new country. Therefore, it has been postulated that the decreased incidence of gastric cancer in the second-generation offspring in American-born persons of Japanese descent may be related to dietary differences in dried fish mutagens and increased consumption of vegetables and fruits high in vitamin C (34). Another factor in the pathogenesis of the disease is that family members of patients with gastric cancer, as well as individuals with blood group A, are at a higher risk of developing the disease than individuals with blood group O. There is an increased risk of gastric cancer in pernicious anemia, atrophic gastritis, gastric polyps, or achlorhydria. No direct association has been found between duodenal ulcers and gastric cancer. The concerns with the long-term use of H_2 antagonists in the treatment of gastric ulcers indicates that these drugs, in producing hypochlorhydria, may have a carcinogenic potential (35). At present, the risks from these agents appear to be minimal. However, it should serve to caution against indiscriminate use for treatment in patients with undiagnosed gastric lesions or complaints.

Pathology

Adenocarcinomas constitute 95% of the malignant neoplasms of the stomach, although benign pseudolymphomas, lymphomas, sarcomas, and other rare tumors have been described (36). The site where a malignancy develops depends upon the integrity of the mucosal lining or of coexisting stomach disorders. Most tumors arise in the antrum or lower third of the stomach. If gastric atrophy is present, the tumor develops in the upper section of the stomach. The lesser curvature of the stomach is involved most often, followed by the anterior or posterior walls. The greater curvature is least affected by malignancy.

Stomach cancer and other gastrointestinal cancers may spread by similar routes. These include: (a) direct invasion into either the esophagus, omentum, liver, spleen, pancreas, or adjacent viscera; (b) spread via the lymphatics, or (c) hematogenous spread, where they can metastasize to bone, liver, lungs, and brain.

Additionally, spillage of malignant cells, either from the surface or lumen of the stomach at the time of an operative procedure, may initiate the metastatic process.

Screening and Diagnosis

Researchers in high-risk areas such as Japan, South America, and Eastern Europe have for some time conducted mass fluoroscopy screening for detection of gastric cancer. These screening studies show that gastric cancer can be detected early, while the prognosis is still good.

In the United States, the first diagnostic technique used involves barium-roentgenographic studies. However, several problems can be encountered with this technique. A major problem is differentiating benign from malignant ulcers. Another problem is that early gastric lesions may not be seen unless carefully performed air-contrast techniques are used (37). If the barium x-ray is positive, it is followed by endoscopy, which is considered to be the best overall method for diagnosing gastric cancer. The endoscope not only allows viewing, but it also has biopsy channels that enable easy collection of material for histologic and cytologic study. The CT scan is being used increasingly to identify metastases.

Carcinoembryonic antigen (CEA) activity has been detected in gastric juice and plasma of patients with gastric cancer, but the test is of little initial diagnostic value. Plasma CEA levels more than likely would be negative in early gastric cancer. However, CEA may be elevated in 15 to 30% of patients with more advanced cancer or suggest recurrence of carcinoma (38).

Staging

Staging of the patient with gastric cancer is based on the clinical extent of the disease as demonstrated by both the physical examination and roentgenographic and endoscopic studies. The extent of spread is a major factor to consider when selecting a therapeutic course and determining the prognosis of gastric carcinoma. The American Joint Committee recommends the use of the TNM classification for gastric carcinoma (Table 79.5).

Clinical Manifestations

Gastric cancer most often presents when the tumor has reached an advanced stage. By this time there is involvement of lymph nodes, and distant metastases may be present. Vague abdominal discomfort is the most common initial symptom. Other symptoms include early satiety, weakness, weight loss, and change in bowel habits. Iron deficiency anemia is quite common. Seventy-five percent of patients with gastric carcinoma present with guaiac-pos-

Table 79.5.
TNM Classification of Stomach Neoplasms by the American Joint Committee on Cancer[a]

Primary tumor (T)

T_x	Minimum requirements to assess the primary tumor cannot be met
T_0	No evidence of primary tumor
T_{is}	Tumor limited to mucosa
T_1	Tumor limited to mucosa or mucosa and submucosa regardless of its extent (or location)
T_2	Tumor involves the mucosa and the submucosa (including the muscularis propria), and extends to or into the serosa but does not penetrate through the serosa
T_3	Tumor penetrates through the serosa without invading contiguous structures
T_{4a}	Tumor penetrates through serosa and involves immediately adjacent tissues
T_{4b}	Tumor penetrates through the serosa and involves the adjacent organs

Nodal involvement (N)

N_x	Minimum requirements to assess the regional nodes cannot be met
N_0	No metastases to regional lymph nodes
N_1	Involvement of perigastric lymph nodes within 3 cm of the primary tumor
N_2	Involvement of the regional lymph nodes more than 3 cm from the primary tumor
N_3	Involvement of other intra-abdominal lymph nodes

Distant metastasis (M)

M_x	Minimum requirements to assess the presence of distant metastasis cannot be met
M_0	No (known) distant metastasis
M_1	Distant metastasis present

Stage grouping

Stage 0	T_{is}, N_0, M_0
Stage I	T_1, N_0, M_0
Stage II	T_2, T_3, N_0, M_0
Stage III	T_1–T_3, N_1, N_2, M_0
	T_{4a}, N_0–N_2; M_0
Stage IV	T_1–T_3, N_3, M_0
	T_{4b}, any N, M_0
	Any T, any N, M_1

[a] Adapted from Beahrs OH, Myers MH (eds): Manual for Staging of Cancer. Philadelphia, JB Lippincott, 1983, p 67.

itive stools. The duration of symptoms before patients seek medical attention may vary, but averages 6 months. Symptoms of several years duration are not uncommon. In early gastric cancer the disease is usually asymptomatic, but patients may present with "new" indigestion or they may suddenly be aware of food entering their stomach after eating. Pain resembling symptoms of duodenal ulcer has been reported in over 75% of patients by the time the diagnosis of stomach cancer is confirmed (39, 40). Unlike a duodenal ulcer, the pain usually is not relieved by food or antacids. The physical signs that suggest advanced disease include palpable supraclavicular lymph nodes, palpable ovarian mass, hepatomegaly, abdominal mass, ascites, jaundice, and cachexia. Patients with suspected gastric cancer should have a careful evaluation of the liver, with liver function tests, bilirubin, alkaline phosphase, LDH, ALT, and CT scan of the liver.

Prognosis

The prognosis for gastric cancer in the United States continues to be grim, with an overall 5-year survival of 8 to 12% (36, 41). However, the prognosis can be somewhat variable, depending upon the extent of the malignancy and the physical condition of the patient. Important prognostic factors are the depth of invasion through the gastric wall, the spread of lymph nodes, and the presence of distant metastases.

Surgery

In 1881 Theodore Billroth performed the first successful gastrectomy. Since that time surgical removal of all visible tumor has remained the only curative treatment of malignancies of the stomach.

Subtotal gastrectomy appears to be preferred by most surgeons in patients with localized gastric carcinoma (stages I and II). In this procedure, over three-fourths of the stomach, omentum, duodenum, and regional lymph nodes are excised. Total gastrectomies have shown an increase in operative mortality and side effects and failed to demonstrate a better 5-year survival rate than subtotal gastrectomies (42). There was also a relationship between the progression and location of the tumor and postoperative survival time. The survival rate declined from 85% if the tumor was confined to the mucosa to 50% if involvement included penetration into or through serosa (stage III), and was further reduced to 15% if metastatic spread to perigastric lymph nodes had occurred (stage IV). Because of the poor prognosis of stages III and IV gastric cancer, multimodality treatments are being investigated.

Radiation

Most clinicians believe that radiation therapy is ineffective as curative treatment for gastric carcinomas. Tumors of gastric origin are relatively radiation-resistant. A radiation dose of 4000 to 5000 rads over a 4- to 5-week period generally exceeds the tolerance of most normal organs in this region. Thus the role of radiation therapy has been limited to palliation of pain and adjuvant therapy in combination with surgery and chemotherapy.

Chemotherapy

In the treatment of locally advanced, nonresectable disease, several agents have activity against gastric cancer. The fluorinated pyrimidines, particularly (5-FU) were some of the first agents studied, and they produced a response in 20 to 25% of patients with advanced disease (36, 41). Other agents with activity included doxorubicin (Adrimycin), mitomycin (Mutamycin), the nitrosoureas—primarily BCNU (Carmustine), methyl-CCNU (Semustine), and *cis*-platinum (Platinol). However, response rates from single agents are generally under 30%. In addition, methyl-CCNU is now only commercially available for investigational use, because of long-term toxicities that include leukemia and renal toxicity.

Combination of these agents show increased response rates over single-drug therapy. For the past two decades, the regimen initially reported by MacDonald as the FAM regimen (5-FU, doxorubicin, mitomycin) was preferred by most oncologists (43). This protocol incorporated the three drugs with the highest single-drug activity in gastric cancer and produced a 30 to 35% response rate. Over the past decade, a multitude of drug permutations have been investigated in randomized and nonrandomized studies for locally advanced and technically unresectable gastric carcinoma. Most regimens now use some combination of 5-FU or etoposide. The experience with combination chemotherapy is summarized in Table 79.6. The results from these studies have confirmed that gastric carcinoma is chemosensitive. The high remission rate (50%) and long median survival time (> 1 year) achieved with ELF (etoposide, doxorubicin, cisplatin) and EAP (etoposide, leucovorin, 5-FU) plus good patient tolerability offer the best chance for improving the prognosis (44). Currently EAP is the regimen preferred by most oncologists.

Adjuvant Therapy

In an effort to improve upon the modest success attained from individual treatment modalities, a number of controlled trials conducted in the United States and Japan have reported minimal survival advantages for patients treated with postsurgical adjuvant chemotherapy. The Gastrointestinal Tumor Study Group (GITSG) reported a significant survival advantage at 4 years for gastric cancer patients treated with 5-FU and methyl-CCNU within 6 weeks of gastrectomy, compared with randomized control patients who received no chemotherapy (45). However, a similar adjuvant study conducted by the Veterans Administration Surgical Oncology Group (VASOG) that used lower doses of these agents showed no benefit (46). The Japanese Research Society for Gastric Cancer (JRSGC) using similar protocols, has reported response rates well in excess of 50% (47). Much of the JRSGC success is due to public education and earlier detection of tumor and initiation of adjuvant therapy. In Japan, adjuvant chemotherapy is administered almost immediately after surgery, so the entire adjuvant program may be completed by the time the patient leaves the hospital following surgery. In the United States adjuvant chemotherapy does not even begin until 3 to 6 weeks postoperatively, to allow adequate time for wounds and anastomoses to heal. In a prospectively randomized trial conducted by the Eastern Oncology Research Treatment Center (EORTC), patients with advanced gastric cancer were randomized to FAM and FAMTX regimens. The median survival of all eligible patients was 40 weeks in the FAMTX arm, versus 29 weeks in the FAM arm. Also the 5-year survival was significantly different, 38 versus 17% respectively. The toxicities in both arms were comparable although there was a cumulative hematologic toxicity in patients treated with FAM and not in those treated with FAMTX. The EORTC has recommended that FAMTX be considered standard treatment for a surgical adjuvant program after curative resection for gastric cancer (48).

CANCER OF THE LARGE BOWEL

Colorectal carcinoma is one of the most frequent malignant diseases afflicting Western civilization. In 1990, 110,000 new cases were estimated, and more than 53,300 Americans were expected to die of the disease (1). This is surpassed only by malignancies of the lung. Although the incidence is slowly rising, the death rate in females has decreased for unknown reasons. The peak incidence of the

Table 79.6.
Results with the More Frequently Used Combinations in Advanced Gastric Cancer[a]

	Regimen	Response Rate[b] (%)	Median Survival (Months)
F	Fluorouracil	33	6–8
A	Doxorubicin		
M	Mitomycin		
F	Fluorouracil	43	6–8
A	Doxorubicin		
B	Bleomycin		
F	Fluorouracil	36	6–13
A	Doxorubicin		
P	Cisplatin		
F	Fluorouracil	43	8
A	Doxorubicin		
MTX	Methotrexate		
E	Etoposide	56	9–18
A	Doxorubicin		
P	Cisplatin		
E	Etoposide	52	11
L	Leucovorin		
F	Fluorouracil		

[a] Adapted from Wilke H, Preusser P, Fink U, et al.: New developments in the treatment of gastric carcinoma. Semin Oncol 17(suppl 2):61–70, 1990.
[b] Includes partial and complete responses.

disease generally occurs after the age of 60. Before 1950, the occurrence of the disease was greater among whites than blacks, but since that time, colorectal cancer has risen among blacks so that rates are equal for both races. The urban rates tend to be slightly higher than rates for rural areas (49). Current research emphasis has been directed toward prevention, screening, and early diagnosis and treatment of colorectal cancer.

Colorectal cancer is more common in the Western world than in underdeveloped countries (50). While genetic susceptibility, and longer life expectancy may contribute to the higher incidence seen in the United States, it appears that dietary habits, the so-called Western diet, play a major role in the development of colorectal cancer (51, 52). Individuals at greatest risk of developing colorectal cancer have diets that are high in fats and red meat, with inadequate intake of foods rich in fiber, such as cereals, vegetables, and fruits. The hypothesis is based on studies from low-incidence countries such as Japan, where fat provides only 12% of the total caloric intake, and Africa where the diet is rich in fiber. In high-risk countries such as the United States, fat intake represents 40 to 44% of caloric intake (53).

The exact role of fats and red meat in the development of colorectal cancer is not known. Diets high in fat and red meat possibly increase the population of certain intestinal bacteria capable of producing enzymes such as β-glucoronidase and azoreductase. These enzymes metabolize acid and neutral sterols to carcinogens and cocarcinogens by increasing the amount of bile acid and cholesterol metabolized in the feces. There is a high correlation between colon cancer mortality and the intake of animal protein (54, 55). The breakdown of red meat protein produces tryptophan metabolites, phenols, and nitrosamines that appear to have carcinogenic effects. The relationship of red meat and fat to colorectal cancer is not accepted by all investigators. The reason for the apparent inconsistency relates to studies involving Mormons who are not vegetarians, but have as low an incidence of colon cancer as Seventh-Day Adventists, who are vegetarians (56). Western diets contain numerous carcinogens, procarcinogens, and mutagens. The time interval from exposure to known or unknown carcinogens and diagnosis of cancer is usually several decades.

Fiber might be involved in decreasing the risk of colorectal cancer. Since all dietary fibers are not the same, some studies are attempting to relate specific types of fiber to their effect on the incidence of colorectal cancer. Evidence suggests that any benefit accruing from a high-fiber diet might be indirect, caused by a secondary restriction of caloric intake (57). Therefore, the mechanical effects of fiber may be of little or no consequence. Additional factors that may minimize the risk of colorectal cancer include diets rich in vitamin A, ascorbic acid, and selenium (58).

Genetic susceptibility may be a significant factor. Genetic syndromes that predispose patients to colorectal cancer are familial polyposis and its variants, Gardner's syndrome, hereditary adenocarcinomatosis, and juvenile polyposis. Malignant transformation occurs over a period of time in these high-risk patients. Prophylactic colectomy has been recommended for these patients. The inflammatory bowel diseases, ulcerative colitis and Crohn's disease, are additional risk factors. Patients with Crohn's disease have a higher incidence of colorectal cancer than the general population, although the risk is much lower than in patients with chronic ulcerative colitis (59). The offspring of patients with a particularly strong family history of colorectal cancer should be part of an intensive surveillance program. Beginning by age 25, annual examination of the stool for occult blood, and colonoscopy or a barium enema once every 3 years are recommended (60).

Pathology

More than 95% of primary colorectal cancers are adenocarcinomas. These colorectal adenocarcinomas are not evenly distributed throughout the bowel. The frequency decreases from the ascending (16%), through the transverse and splenic flexure (8%), to the descending (6%), followed by a sharp rise in the sigmoid and rectum (70%) (61). Most of these lesions are located in the distal segment and appear in various sizes and shapes. The size of the lesion ranges from a few millimeters to several centimeters.

Colorectal cancer is usually either left-sided or right-sided. The early neoplasm on the left side appears as a small elevated button or as a small polypoid mass. Within 1 to 2 years, the lesion totally encircles the affected part of the lumen. Eventually a "napkin-ring" constriction develops, followed by ulceration in the middle of the ring. Malignant lesions in the right colon have a beginning similar to those in the left side, but their pattern of progression tends to differ. Most often they become bulky, cauliflower-like masses or large, irregular spreading papillomatous plaques, extending into the lumen. As a result, they are much less likely to cause obstruction, compared with the "napkin-ring" lesion.

Colorectal adenocarcinomas tend to remain superficial for a long time, slowly invading the deeper layers of the intestinal wall. As the lesion progresses, there is extension through the bowel wall into the pericolonic fat. In addition to direct extension to adjacent organs, the cancer also disseminates via lymphatic and hematogenous routes to the liver or lungs.

Screening and Diagnosis

The American Cancer Society recommends several procedures for early detection of colorectal cancer for asymptomatic individuals.

1. Men and women over 50 years of age should have a stool guaiac-type test every year.
2. Men and women over 50 years of age, after having two initial annual negative examinations, should have a sigmoidoscopic examination every 3 to 5 years.
3. Men and women over 40 years of age should have a digital examination of the rectum every year.
4. Individuals with a family history of colorectal cancer should undergo the above examinations a decade earlier.

The stool-blood guaiac test (Hemoccult test) is a relatively simple and inexpensive procedure that detects the presence of blood in the stool. The sensitivity of the test has been reported at 0.2 μg Hb/100 g of stool (62). Although the test is not specific for colorectal malignancies, it is useful in identifying blood originating from both benign or malignant growths in the GI tract. Since the guaiac test is triggered by peroxidase activity, some commonly ingested foods can interfere with the test results. In general, some uncooked fruits and vegetables such as horseradish, turnips, and bananas have peroxidase activity that can produce false-positive results, while ascorbic acid (in doses greater than 1 g), an oxidation inhibitor, may produce a false-negative result (62). It is important to stress that colorectal cancer and polyps may bleed intermittently, therefore a negative test does not definitely rule out cancer. All positive tests require a more extensive evaluation.

Usually the first specialized test performed is sigmoidoscopy. The instrument can visualize about one-third of colorectal neoplasia. If a mass is discovered, the examination is not complete without a biopsy from two to four different places in the tumor mass. If the lesion is ulcerated, specimens should be taken from the rolled edges of the crater.

A barium enema is used to rule out a large-bowel neoplasm if the patient's history suggests colorectal pathology. The barium enema is needed even when sigmoidoscopy is positive, because the procedure helps to further characterize the neoplasm. Both the single-contrast and double-contrast methods are used. Colonoscopy is extremely valuable for preoperative definition of many colon lesions. This procedure is especially important because a small percentage of colon cancers coexist with a second malignancy somewhere within the large bowel. Some of these polyps are less than 1 cm in diameter and difficult to see by barium enema evaluation alone.

The CEA assay has proved to be useful in the prognosis for colorectal carcinoma. A low or normal preoperative level does not guarantee a localized neoplasm. However, a marked elevation in plasma CEA denotes widespread metastases, especially to the liver. Monitoring the CEA level provides an indirect measure of tumor response to various treatment modalities, although this practice is controversial (63, 64).

Two other levels are increased on colorectal malignancies and are related to tumor bulk. Serum carbohydrate antigen (CA19-9) and β-2 microglobulin levels have been suggested to be a more reliable tumor marker than CEA (65).

Staging

The staging of colorectal carcinoma has been complicated by the fact that it has evolved over half a century, and various authors have developed systems that use the same descriptions to represent different stages. The Dukes' staging system, which was introduced in 1930, is often used today for its simplicity. In this system, malignancies of the large bowel are separated into three groups. Modifications were made in 1949 and by Astler and Coller in 1954 to reflect finer levels of penetration and nodal mestases, and they have been extended to include the colon as well as the rectum. A revised, 1987 combined American Joint Committee on Cancer (ATCC) and the International Union Against Cancer (UIAC) have proposed staging systems using the TNM classification (66). Today, the current system has expanded Dukes' categories to more than six and have given the categories more pragmatic value (Table 79.7).

Clinical Manifestations

The signs and symptoms of colorectal cancer are often subtle and nonspecific. However, the visible presence of blood in the stool, abdominal pain, and changes in bowel habits prompt patients to seek medical attention. The presence and severity of symptoms vary with the portion of the bowel involved and the extent of the disease. Tumors of the right colon usually do not produce a change in bowel habits, although occasionally diarrhea may occur. The lesions frequently ulcerate, producing a chronic blood loss that is diluted in the stool, giving rise to a normal-appearing but guaiac-positive stool. Patients may experience symptoms of iron deficiency anemia (fatigue, dizziness). Tumors located in the transverse or left colon are more likely to be associated with changes in bowel habits and abdominal pain. As the stool passes into this area, constipation from the narrowing lumen may lead to diarrhea. The so-called napkin-ring lesion in the left colon tends to produce intermittent pain, with the patient often complaining of gas cramps. The presence of gross blood in the stool is more common in left colon (50 to 80%) than cancer of the right colon (30%) (61). Cancers that arise in the rectosigmoid are associated with bright red blood and tenesmus. The passage of bright red blood may be mistakenly attributed to hemorrhoids.

Weight loss and fever are also nonacute symptoms of colorectal cancer. About half of patients report a weight loss, but it is almost never the sole manifestations of colorectal cancer. The presence of fever is unclear but may be related to infectious involvement by tumor penetration into adjacent organs (67).

Table 79.7.
Modifications of the Dukes Classification Staging System[a]

Dukes original (1932)

A	Cancer limited to the bowel wall
B	Extension of growth into extrarectal tissues
C	Metastases to regional lymph nodes

Modified Astler-Coller (MAC) (1954)

A	Limited to mucosa (carcinoma in situ)
B_1	Penetration of muscularis mucosae
B_2	Penetration through muscularis propria
C_1	B_1 with positive nodes
C_2	B_2 with positive nodes

AJCC/UIAC staging classification of colorectal cancer (1987)

T	The primary tumor		N	Regional lymph nodes
TX	Primary tumor cannot be assessed		Nx	Regional nodes cannot be assessed
T0	No evidence of primary tumor		N0	No regional lymph node metastasis
Tis	Carcinoma in situ		N1	Metastasis in 1 to 3 pericolic or perirectal lymph nodes
T1	Tumor invades submucosa		N2	Metastasis in 4 or more pericolic or perirectal lymph nodes
T2	Tumor invades muscularis propria		N3	Metastasis in any lymph node along the course of a named vascular trunk
T3	Tumor invades through muscularis proporia into subserosa or into nonperitonealized pericolic or perirectal tissues		M	Distant metastasis
T4	Tumor perforates the visceral peritoneum or directly invades other organs or structures		MX	Minimum requirements to assess the presence of distant metastasis cannot be met
			M0	No distant metastasis
			M1	Distant metastasis

Staging and prognosis of colorectal cancer

Stage	Dukes	MAC	TNM	Description	5-Year Survival (1960s and 1970s)
I	A	A	T1NoMo	Involves submucosa	90%
		B_1	T2NoMo	Invades muscularis	
II	B	B_2	T3NoMo	Invades thru the muscularis proporia, into the serosa/pericolic fat	85%
			T4No-Mo	Invades into peritoneal cavity/neighboring organs	70–75%
		B_3	T4No-Mo		35–65%
III	C	C_1	T2N1-Mo	1–3 nodes positive	35–65%
			T2N2-Mo	>3 nodes positive	
		C_2	T3/4N1/N2Mo		
		C_3	T4N1/N2Mo		
IV	D		-M1	Distant metastases	<5%

[a] Adapted from International Union Against Cancer. In Hermanek P, Sobin LH (eds): TNM Classification of Malignant Tumors, ed. 4. New York: Springer-Verlag, 1987.

Prognosis

The prognosis for patients with colorectal cancer is closely associated with the depth of tumor penetration into the bowel wall, regional lymph involvement, and distant metastases. The 5-year survival based on the Dukes' classification of colorectal cancer was 80% when the tumor was confined to bowel mucosa (stage A) to less than 5% when distant metastases (stage D) were present (50). The prognostic importance of lymph node metastases is also critical. Studies show a 5-year survival of 49% with no lymph node involvement, 24% when there are 1 to 5 positive nodes, 9% with 6 to 15 positive nodes, and 0% with 16 or more positive nodes (68, 69). In contrast to the prognosis for patients with most other solid tumors, the size of the primary neoplasm appears to have little relationship to prognosis. However, location of the primary lesion can influence the prognosis in nearly every major surgical series. The poorest outlook is almost entirely associated with cancer of the distal section of the rectum. The malignancy spreads both to hypogastric lymph nodes along the pelvic side walls and to mesorectal lymph nodes along the superior hemorrhoidal artery. As a result, surgical removal of the affected tissues is rarely possible.

Extraintestinal organ involvement has a negative impact upon the prognosis for colorectal cancer. Hepatic metastases from colorectal cancer are a major cause of increased morbidity and mortality. The median survival time, from the time of diagnosis of the metastatic colon cancer to the liver was 146 days, with 9.5% surviving more than 10 months (61, 70). Survival time is similar in patients with hepatic metastases from rectal cancer. Survival rates are also decreased if the patient has any of the following: elevated serum lactic dehydrogenase (LDH); bilirubin; aspartate aminotransferase (AST); CEA; and decreased albumin levels. Although these tests are relatively nonspecific, the levels usually signify liver metastases in patients with colorectal cancer. A report of a 10-year, time-trend, case-control study reported that individuals in whom colorectal cancer develops share the same level of serum cholesterol as the general population initially. But during the 10 years preceding the cancer demonstrate a decline in serum cholesterol that is opposite to the rising level seen with age in the general population (71).

Surgery

The primary curative procedure for patients with the disease in stages I, II, or III (Dukes' A, B, and C) is surgical resection of the bowel (72). The aim of surgery is to remove the cancer-containing segment of the intestine, as well as adequate margins of grossly uninvolved intestine and surrounding adjacent lymphatics. The degree of success is directly related to the extent to which the tumor has disseminated by the time of the procedure. Continual improvement in earlier detection of tumors and improvement in surgical technique have resulted in declining operative infection and mortality rate (73). The specific surgical procedure used depends upon the location of the malignancy and its corresponding lymphatic drainage. Some surgeons strongly recommend wide removal of the involved segment to include lymphatic drainage. The standard procedures for right colon tumors (e.g., malignancies of the cecum and ascending colon) is right hemicolectomy; for left-sided tumors (e.g., malignancies of the transverse descending and sigmoid); it is a left hemicolectomy. In malignancies in the upper portion of the rectum an anterior resection and reanastomosis is performed. Below this site an anteroposterior resection and colostomy become necessary.

Radiation

Carcinomas arising in the rectum are associated with a local recurrence rate far higher than that observed with colon tumors; approximately 25% of the patients with stage B2 rectal tumors and close to 50% of individuals with stage C rectal lesions may be expected to experience pelvic recurrences after surgery alone (72). Therefore, adjuvant radiation therapy was introduced to remove tumor cells of the rectum that were located in surgically inaccessible tissue.

In the adjuvant use of radiation therapy for resectable adenocarcinomas of the rectum, both preoperative and postoperative treatment appears to be appropriate. The goal of preoperative radiation therapy is to decrease the dissemination of tumor cells at surgery. A study performed by the VASOG randomized 700 patients to be treated preoperatively with 2000 to 2500 rads 2 weeks prior to surgery or to be treated with surgical resection alone (74). In the preoperative group, significant differences were shown in decreasing the local failure rate and improving 5-year survival, compared with surgical resection alone. Postoperative radiation therapy is used for patients at high risk for local recurrence (e.g., those with transmural invasion, nodal metastases, and direct invasion of adjacent organs). An interim report from GITSG has shown the 4-year disease-free survival was 43% in patients treated with surgery alone, 48% in those treated with postoperative chemotherapy, 65% in patients receiving adjuvant postoperative radiation therapy, and 68% in those treated with all three modalities (75). In patients who could not tolerate a major surgical procedure or who had a tumor that was unresectable, newer techniques such as intraoperative electron-beam radiation therapy have been described (76, 77). Patients are able to receive direct maximum doses (5000 rads) to the malignant area, while minimizing damage to adjacent sensitive bowels.

For palliative purposes, radiation therapy of the rectosigmoid area is best for controlling pain, bleeding, and tenesmus. Although only a small portion of patients are cured, some objective symptomatic benefit is achieved in almost 85% of patients undergoing some form of radiation therapy (61).

Chemotherapy

Colorectal cancer is extremely resistant to most chemotherapic agents. Various approaches have been studied using systemic or regional infusions of chemotherapy in the treatment of colorectal cancer. The pharmacologic characteristics of the agents used the in treatment of colorectal cancer are listed in Table 79.8. Numerous phase II trials have examined the activity of single agents and various drug combinations, but none of these protocols proved to be superior to 5-FU alone (61).

SINGLE-AGENT CHEMOTHERAPY

In 1957, the fluorinated pyrimidine 5-FU was introduced as an antineoplastic agent for disseminated colon and rectal

Table 79.8.

Pharmacologic Characteristics of the Antineoplastic Agents Used in the Treatment of Gastrointestinal Cancer

Drug/Trade Name/ Manufacturer	Product Available	Pharmacokinetics	Toxicity	Comments
Bleomycin sulfate (Bleo) Blenoxane Bristol-Myers	Vial: 15 IU = 15 mg powder	$T_{1/2}$: biphasic; α 10–20 min, 1.5–2.5 hr Renal excretion; 60% active drug	Acute: fever, chills, anaphylaxis ($\approx$1% in lymphoma) Chronic: pulmonary fibrosis, dermatologic effects (increased keratin, hyperpigmentation, nail ridging, desquamation), alopecia, stomatitis	Initial 1–2 IU test dose recommended Maximum cummulative lifetime dose is 400 IU Increased pulmonary toxicity with renal failure or recent prior cisplatin
Cisplatin (DDP) Platinol Bristol-Myers	Vial: 10, 50 mg powder	$T_{1/2}$: biphasic; 25–79 min, 58–73 hr Rapid plasma clearance; 10% detected in 1 hr Renal excretion; 25% in 24 hr	Acute: nausea & vomiting (severe & persistent), anaphylaxis (rare), hypomagnesemia Chronic: myelosuppression (nadir: 10–14 days), nephrotoxicity, ototoxicity, peripheral neuropathy, delayed nausea & vomiting, color blindness	Pre- & posthydration to maintain urine output Pretreat with antiemetics Monitor SCr, urine output, magnesium Avoid concurrent nephrotoxic drugs
Doxorubicin hydrochloride (DOX) Adriamycin Adria	Vial: 10, 20, 50 mg red powder with 50 & 100 mg lactose	$T_{1/2}$: biphasic; 1.1 hr, 17 hr Hepatic metabolism; active & inactive compounds Primary biliary excretion Renal excretion; 10% unchanged in 24 hr	Acute: nausea & vomiting, diarrhea, pericarditis, cardiac arrhythmia, erythema or hives, streaking along injection vein, anaphylaxis Chronic: myelosuppression (nadir: 14 days), alopecia, GI effects (stomatitis, ulceration), cardiotoxicity (dose-limiting)	Vesicant: pain & necrosis if extravasated Caution in liver & cardiac dysfunction Decrease dose with increased bilirubin Weekly dosing & continuous infusion may reduce cardiac toxicity Decrease cumulative dose with prior mediastinal radiation therapy or cardiomyopathy Maximum cumulative lifetime dose is 450–550 mg/m²
Etoposide (VP-16-213) VePesid Bristol-Myers	Vial: 100 mg/5 ml Capsule: 50 mg, pink	$T_{1/2}$: biphasic; 1.5, 7 hr Partial p.o. absorption (50%) CSF level 5% of plasma level Renal excretion; 60% unchanged in 72 hr Fecal excretion; 2–16% in 72 hr	Acute: nausea & vomiting, hypotension, anaphylaxis, fever, muscle cramps Chronic: myelosuppression nadir: 7–14 days), alopecia	Infuse slowly (<60–90 min)
Floxuridine (FUDR, fluorodeoxyuridine) FUDR Roche	Vial: 500 mg white powder	Rapid conversion to 5-FU (IV) Hepatic extraction; 95% (IA) 80% (IV)	Acute: nausea & vomiting, diarrhea (IV) Chronic: myelosuppression (nadir: 7–14 days), GI effects, biliary sclerosis, (increased alkaline phosphatase); IV: ulcer, enteritis, abdominal cramps, stomatitis, keratitis, diarrhea	D/C at first sign of biliary sclerosis, intractable nausea & vomiting, GI bleeding
5-Fluorouracil (5-FU) Adrucil Adria Flourouracil Roche Efudex Roche Fluoriplex Herbert	Ampule: 500 mg/10 ml Vial: 500 mg/10 ml Topical cream: 5% Efudex, 1% Fuoroplex Topical solution: 2%, 5% Efudex, 1% Fluoroplex	$T_{1/2}$: 5–20 min Hepatic extraction; 80% maximum (dose rate dependent) Enters effusion, CFS Renal excretion; 10–15% unchanged in 6 hr	Acute: nausea & vomiting, diarrhea Chronic: myelosuppression (nadir 7–14 days), GI effects (stomatitis, ulcer), rash, hyperpigmentation, alopecia, cerebral ataxia, conjunctivitis, dry eyes	Decrease dose in hepatic or renal dysfunction D/C at first sign of intractable nausea & vomiting or GI bleeding

(continued)

Table 79.8. *(Continued)*

Drug/Trade Name/ Manufacturer	Product Available	Pharmacokinetics	Toxicity	Comments
Levamisole Ergamisol Janssen	Tablet: 50 mg	Rapidly absorbed from GI tract Metabolized in liver Excreted urine, feces Elimination is 95% complete within 2 days after dose	Acute: nausea, vomiting, dizziness, confusion, metallic taste Chronic: flu-like symptoms, convulsions, agranulocytosis, rash	
Leucovorin (citrovorum factor, folinic acid) Wellcovorin Burroughs Wellcome Leucovorin calcium Lederle	Tablet: 5 mg Oral solution: 60 mg/60 ml Ampule: 3 mg/1 ml, 5 mg/ 1 ml, 25 mg/5 ml Vial: 50 mg powder with 45 mg NaCl	Absorption: p.o. $\leq$25 mg, 100%; 50 mg, 75%; 75 mg, 50%; i.m., 90%	Acute: allergic sensitization	Rescue if 24-hr serum MTX level >5 $\times$ 10^{-7}M Injectable form can be given orally May counteract bone marrow toxicity from trimethoprim & sulfa drugs
Methotrexate (MTX) Folex Adria Mexate Bristol-Myers Methotrexate Lederle	Tablet: 2.5 mg Vial: 5 mg/2 ml, 50 mg/ 2 ml Powder: 20, 25, 50, 100, 200, & 250 mg	$T_{1/2}$: IV: triphasic 0.45, 2, 14 hr, increases in renal failure, effusions, bowel obstruction Bioavailability: p.o. <30 mg/m^2 = 80%; >50 mg/m^2 = 20–50% Renal excretion; 50–80% unchanged in 24 hr	Acute: nausea & vomiting (uncommon), neurotoxicity with I.T. administration (headache, quadriplegia) Chronic: myelosuppression (nadir: 7–10 days), GI effects (ulcer, stomatitis, diarrhea), hepatotoxicity, nephrotoxicity with high dose)	Monitor serum MTX concentration: 24 hr (1 $\times$ 10^{-6} M); 48 hr (1 $\times$ 10^{-8}M) Continue leucovorin until serum MTX level <5 $\times$ 10^{-8}M Force diuresis & urinary alkalization with high-dose MTX Leucovorin should be prescribed at the same time as high-dose MTX Drug interaction: probenecid, salicylates, sulfonamides, penicillins, nonsteroidal antiinflammatory drugs increase MTX toxicity; avoid use in patients with poor renal function, ascites, or pleural effusions
Mitomycin C (MMC) Mutamycin Bristol-Myers	Vial: 5, 20 mg powder with 10, 40 mg mannitol	$T_{1/2}$: biphasic; 8.2, 52 min Renal excretion; 6 to 10% unchanged	Acute: nausea & vomiting (moderate), fever Chronic: myelosuppression especially platelets (nadir: 28 days), pulmonary fibrosis, alopecia, diarrhea, mucositis, hemolytic uremic syndrome	Vesicant: pain & tissue necrosis if extravasated Monitor renal function
Vindesine sulfate (VID) Eldisine Lilly	Vial: 5 mg lyophilized powder	$T_{1/2}$: triphasic; 2, 54, 1400 min Hepatic metabolism (incomplete) Biliary excretion Renal excretion; approximately 19% unchanged in 84 hr (nausea, vomiting, stomatitis, mucositis, constipation, paralytic, ileus, diarrhea)	Acute: local pain, phlebitis, jaw pain Chronic: myelosuppression (nadir: 11 days), neurotoxicity (paresthesia, hyporeflexia, muscle weakness, abdominal cramps, tremor, urinary retention), GI effects	Vesicant: pain & tissue necrosis if extravasated Decrease dose with increased bilirubin

[a] Adapted from Cancer Chemotherapeutic Agents, American Cancer Society, 87-25M-No. 3443.

cancer, and it was found to be capable of inducing tumor regressions in a small but consistent portion of patients. Unfortunately, this did not translate into improvement in survival (78). In the early trials, a loading dose (15 mg/kg/day) intravenous (IV) 5-FU as a bolus daily for 5 days followed by four half-doses (7.5 mg/kg/day) on alternate days. This protocol produces substantial toxic effects including nausea, vomiting, and stomatitis in 50 to 90% of patients and severe myelosuppression in more than 70%. Maximum depression of white blood cell count usually occurred within 7 to 14 days, with recovery by 20 to 30 days (79). The response rates for 5-FU have generally been around 20%, with the medium duration of response about 5 months.

Research has identified 5-FU as an antimetabolite with major cytotoxicity occurring in the S phase of the cell cycle. Because of the very short plasma half-life of 5-FU (11 min) the limited efficacy of bolus administrated in colorectal cancer was supported by in vitro studies using human tumor stem cell assays (80). Based on this theoretical consideration of a profound schedule-dependency for 5-FU cytotoxicity, a number of researchers explored continuous infusion schedules to optimize the administration of the drug. A large phase III trial randomized patients with advanced, measurable colorectal cancer between IV 5-FU (300 mg/m^2/day) via a battery-operated pump for 12 weeks and 5-FU (500 mg/m^2) administered as a daily IV bolus for 5 consecutive days every 5 weeks (81). The study reported a significant difference in response rate (30 vs 7%) in favor of 5-FU infusion. In addition, less myelosuppression was reported with the continuous infusion; although more gastrointestinal toxicity developed. Currently, trials are underway using this schedule of administration with drug escalation in an effort to further improve response rates.

Administration of the active metabolite of 5-FU, 5-floxuridine (5-FUDR), through intra-arterial infusion has been achieved with development of an implantable, constant-infusion pump (Infusaid). However, prolonged infusion of 5-FUDR has led to gastritis, chemical hepatitis (50%), and jaundice in more than 20% of treated patients (82). Infusional chemotherapy has not proved to be superior to systemic chemotherapy, although many phase I and II are studies in progress.

COMBINATION CHEMOTHERAPY

The modest response rates produced by single-agent chemotherapy prompted researchers to study various combinations during the past 3 decades with hopes of improving response rates, but again no increase in survival has been seen. During this period, the combinations that generated the most interest were methyl-CCNU plus derivatives of 5-FU or methyl-CCNU/vincristine (Oncovin)/5-FU. Response rates were generally 20% or less, regard-

less of the multidrug regimen studied. In these studies, response rates above 30% were not consistently reproducible by other investigators (83, 84). The ECOG conducted numerous studies using various combinations and omission of 5-FU. From these trials it was concluded that combination chemotherapy was no more effective than single-agent 5-FU in the treatment of colorectal cancer. This conclusion was ultimately supported by the findings of several university and national cooperative group studies (61, 85).

The lack of novel drugs for colorectal cancer has encouraged researchers to enhance the cytotoxic effect of 5-FU through biochemical modulation. In the late 1970s, a schedule-dependent cytoxic synergism between methotrexate (MTX) and 5-FU had been described (86). Preliminary reports suggest that response rates between 30 and 40% can be achieved, however recent trials have been unable to confirm this (85). More recently, trials with folinic acid (leucovorin) have been encouraging. Leucovorin increases the ability of 5-FU to inhibit thymidylate synthase, which is an essential factor in colon cancer cell replication (87).

In a randomized study involving 429 patients the North Central Cancer Treatment Group (NCCTG) used six different treatment regimens to study the effectiveness of various ways in which the use of 5-FU might be enhanced in the treatment of colorectal cancer (88). The study showed a significant improvement in the response rates with 5-FU plus high- and low-dosage leucovorin. In addition, a significant improvement in quality of life, performance status, and nutritional status was observed. It appears that the modulation of 5-FU with leucovorin represents a significant step in the treatment of metastatic colorectal carcinoma. Small trials with recombinant α-2a-interferon (rIFNα-2a) are reporting a marked enhancement of the cytotoxicity with the combination of 5-FU (89, 90). The regimen demonstrates activity against disseminated colorectal cancer, however further trials are needed to confirm this activity and to determine the optimal conditions for combing 5-FU and rIFNα-2a.

Adjuvant Therapy

Current studies have centered on the role of postoperative chemotherapy administered to patients following the resection of stage B or C colorectal cancer. Although innumerable trials had been conducted by many cooperative oncology groups, the precise role of chemotherapy following surgery remains unclear. The failure of chemotherapy to provide significant response rates with sustained disease-free remissions against colorectal cancer has prompted investigators to seek alternative treatment strategies. Adjuvant trials with nonspecific immunostimulants, bacillus Calmette-Guevin (BCG) or its methanol-extractable residue (MER) alone or in combination with chemotherapy failed to demonstrate any survival advantage, when compared with a nontreatment group (91).

Another area of considerable interest has involved levamisole, an old antiparasitic widely used for treatment of ascariasis in animals. Levamisole can stimulate immune responses, particularly depressed T cell activity, resulting in increased antibody formation as well as increased delayed hypersensitivity and increased phagocytosis (92). In a randomized trial by the NCCTG, the use of levamisole in combination with 5-FU produced a significant reduction in recurrence rates and increased disease-free period, when compared with untreated controls in Dukes' C cancer (93). Toxicity with levamisole consisted of mild nausea with occasional dermatitis or leukopenia, and occasional CNS side effects including seizures may be seen. In 1990, a panel convened by the National Cancer Institute recommended that this two-drug adjuvant regimen be regarded as the standard for patients with disease involving regional lymph nodes or extension into nearby tissues or any organs without spread to lymph nodes (Dukes' C colon cancer). In addition, this regimen should serve as the control arm in future studies.

CONCLUSION

Although recent developments in the treatment of gastrointestinal cancer are encouraging, satisfactory response rates and prolonged remission periods have still eluded researchers. In most cases, surgery remains the only curative modality, but radiation and chemotherapy are useful in palliative roles and as adjuvants.

Emphasis is now placed on prevention and screening for colorectal cancer, particularly those individuals who are at risk or have genetic predisposition. In the meantime, investigators continue to search for new, effective antineoplastic agents and chemical modulators to improve drug efficacy. Although the role and benefits of immunotherapy remain to be identified, the accumulating experience with levamisole combined with 5-FU should provide more insight into this type of treatment. This decade should provide more answers to the pathogenesis and treatment of gastrointestinal cancer.

REFERENCES

1. Silverberg E, Boring CC, Squires TS: Cancer Statistics. CA 40:9–26, 1990.
2. Ying-Kai W, Guo-jun H, Ling-fang S, et al.: Progress in the study and surgical treatment of cancer of the esophagus in China. 1940–1980. J Thorac Cardiovas Surg 84:325–333, 1982.
3. Tuyns AJ, Masse G: Cancer of the esophagus: an incidence study in Ille-et-Valaine. Int'l J Epid 4:55–59, 1975.
4. Rogers EL, Goldking L, Goldkind SF: Increasing frequency of esophageal cancer among black male veterans. Cancer 49:610–618, 1982.
5. Fraumeni JF Jr, Blot WJ: Geographic variation in esophageal cancer mortality in the United States. J Chronic Dis 30:759–767, 1977.
6. Schottenfeld D: Epidemiology of cancer of the esophagus. Semin Oncol 11:91–100, 1984.
7. Ziegler BG: Alcohol-nutrient interactions in cancer etiology. Cancer 58 (suppl 8):1942–1948, 1986.
8. Dowlatshahi K, Mobarhan S. Diet and environment in the etiology of esophageal carcinoma. In Levin B, Riddell RH, (eds): Frontiers in Gastrointestinal Cancer. New York, Elsevier, pp 1–73, 1984.
9. Sjogren RW Jr, Johnson LF: Barrett's esophagus: a review. Am J Med 74:313–320, 1983.
10. Maeta M, Shigemesa K, Hideo A, et al.: Esophageal carcinoma developed after gastrectomy, Surgery 99:87–91, 1986.
11. Rosenberg JC, Lichter AS, Leichman LP, et al., Cancer of the esophagus, In DeVita VT Jr, Hellman S, Rosenberg SA (eds): Cancer Principles and Practice of Oncology, ed. 3. Philadelphia, JB Lippincott, pp 725–754, 1989.
12. Qui SL, Yang GR: Precursor lesions of esophageal cancer in high-risk populations in Henan Province, China. Cancer 62:551–557, 1988.
13. Lightdale CJ, Winawer SJ: Screening diagnosis and staging of esophageal cancer. Semin Oncol 11:101–112, 1984.
14. Bruckstein AH: Dysphagia. Am Fam Physician 39:147–156, 1989.
15. Nabeya K, Markers of cancer risk in the esophagus and surveillance of high risk groups. In Sherlock P, Morson BC, Barbara L, et al. (eds): Precancerous Lesions of the Gastrointestinal Tract. New York, Raven Press, pp 71–86, 1983.
16. Skinner DB: Surgical treatments for esophageal carcinoma. Semin Oncol 11:135–143, 1984.
17. Marsh JC: Management of cancer of the esophagus. Curr Conc Oncol 8:15–22, 1986.
18. Earlam R, Cunha-Melo JR: Oesophageal squamous cell carcinoma: II. A critical review of radiotherapy. Br J Surg 67:457–468, 1980.
19. Morita K, Takagi I, Watanabe M, et al.: Relationship between the radiologic features of esophageal cancer and the local control by radiation therapy. Cancer 55:2668–2678, 1985.
20. Advani SH, Saiha TK, Swrcop S, et al.: Anterior chemotherapy in esophageal cancer. Cancer 56:1502–1506, 1985.
21. Kelsen D: Chemotherapy of esophageal cancer. Semin Oncol 11:159–168, 1984.
22. Weiss RB, Muggia FM: Cytoxic drug-induced pulmonary disease. Am J Med 68:259–266, 1980.
23. Sternberg C, Kelsen D, Heelan R, et al.: Phase II trial of carboplatin in esophageal cancer. Cancer Treat Rep 69:1305–1306, 1985.
24. Einzig A, Kelsen D, Magill G, et al.: Phase II trial of carboplatin adenocarcinomas of the upper gastrointestinal tract. Cancer Treat Rep 69:1453–1454, 1985.
25. Coonley C, Bains M, Kelsen DP, et al.: Cisplatin-bleomycin in the treatment of esophageal carcinoma: a final report. Cancer 54:2351–2355, 1984.
26. Kies M, Rose S, Tsans T, et al.: Cisplatin and 5-fluorouracil in the primary management of squamous esophageal cancer. Cancer 60:2156–2160, 1987.
27. Carey RW, Hilgenberg AD, Grillo HC, et al.: Esophageal carcinoma: Long term follow-up of patients treated by neoadjuvant chemotherapy, surgery and possible postoperative radiation and/or chemotherapy. Proc Am Soc Clin Oncol 9:(abstr 404), 1990.
28. Bidoli P, Spinazze S, Valente M, et al.: Combined chemotherapy, radiotherapy with and without esophagectomy in squamous cell cancer of the esophagus. Proc Am Soc Clin Oncol 9:(abstr 424), 1990.
29. Forastiere AA, Orringer MB, Perez-Tamayo C, et al.: Concurrent chemotherapy and radiation therapy followed by transhiatal esophagectomy for local-regional cancer of the esophagus. J Clin Oncol 8:119–127, 1990.
30. Strack M, Wadler S, Lyver A, et al.: Phase II trial of fluorouracil and recombinant alpha-2 α-interferon in patients with advanced carcinoma of the esophagus. Proc Am Soc Clin Oncol 9:(abstr 462), 1990.

31. Stroehlein JR, Ajani JA, Gastric carcinoma. In Bayless TM, (ed): Current Therapy in Gastroenterology and Liver Disease, vol 2. Toronto, Philadelphia, BS Decker, pp 120–123, 1986.

32. Correa P: Clinical implications of recent developments in gastric cancer pathology and epidemiology. Semin Oncol 12:2–10, 1985.

33. Block G, Menkes M, Ascorbic acid in cancer prevention, In Moon TE, Micozzi MS (eds): Nutrition and Cancer Prevention. New York, Marcel Dekker, pp 341–388, 1989.

34. Correa P, Cuello C, Fajardo LF: Diet and gastric cancer: nutrition survey in a high-risk area. JNCI 70:673–679, 1983.

35. Langman MJS: Antisecretory drugs and gastric cancer. Br J Med 290:1850–1852, 1985.

36. Ramming KP, Haskell CM, Stomach cancer. In Haskell CM (ed): Cancer Treatment, ed. 3. Philadelphia, WB Saunders, pp 217–229, 1990.

37. Amberg JR, Juhl JH, The stomach and duodenum. In Juhl JH, Crummy AB (eds): Essentials of Radiologic Imaging, ed. 5. Philadelphia, JB Lippincott, pp 525–537, 1987.

38. Ellis DJ, Spevis C, Kingston RD, et al.: Carcinoembryonic antigen levels in advanced gastric carcinoma. Cancer 42:623–625, 1978.

39. Cassell R, Robinson JO: Cancer of the stomach: a review of 854 patients. Br J Surg 63:603–607, 1976.

40. Oleochyle AS: Gastric carcinoma: a critical review of 243 cases. Am J Gastroenterol 70:25–45, 1978.

41. MacDonald JS, Steele G, Gunderson LL: Cancer of the stomach. In DeVita VTR Jr, Hellman S, Rosenberg SA (eds): Cancer Principles and Practices of Oncology, ed. 3. Philadelphia, JB Lippincott, pp 765–799, 1989.

42. Green HR, O'Toole, Slonium D, et al.: Increasing incidence and excellent survival of patients with early gastric cancer. Am J Med 85:658–661, 1988.

43. MacDonald JS, Schein PS, Wooley PV, et al.: 5-Fluorouracil, doxorubicin, and mitomycin (FAM) combination-chemotherapy for advanced gastric cancer. Ann Intern Med 93:533–536, 1980.

44. Wilke H, Preusser P, Fink U, et al.: New developments in the treatment of gastric carcinoma. Semin Oncol 17(suppl 2):61–70, 1990.

45. The Gastrointestinal Tumor Study Group: Controlled trial of adjuvant chemotherapy following curative resection for gastric cancer. Cancer 49:1116–1122, 1982.

46. Higgens GA Jr, Amadeo JH, Smith DE, et al.: Efficacy of prolonged intermittent therapy with combined 5-FU and methyl-CCNU following resection for gastric carcinoma: a Veterans Administration Surgical Oncology Group report. Cancer 52:1105–1112, 1983.

47. Kajitani T, Mina K: Treatment results of stomach carcinoma in Japan 1963–1966. In WHO—CC Monograph No. 2. Statistics by the Japanese Research Society for Gastric Cancer. Tokyo, WHO Collaborating Center for Evaluation of Methods of Diagnosis and Treatment of Stomach Cancer, 1979.

48. Wils J, Klein HD, Bleiberg H, et al.: FAMTX: a step ahead in the treatment of advanced gastric cancer. Proc Am Soc Clin Oncol 9:(abstr 392), 1990.

49. Jansson B: Geographic mappings of colorectal cancer rate: a retrospect of studies, 1974–1984. Cancer Detect Prev 3:341–348, 1985.

50. Bruckstein AH: Update on colorectal cancer. Postgrad Med 86:83–92, 1989.

51. Zaride DG: Environmental etiology of large bowel cancer. JNCI 70:389–400, 1983.

52. Executive Summary of the Report of the Committee on Diet, Nutrition and Cancer: Diet, nutrition, and cancer. Cancer Res 43:3018–3023, 1983.

53. Gregor O, Toma R, Prasova F: Gastrointestinal cancer and nutrition. Gut 10:1031–1039, 1969.

54. Jenkins DJ, Jenkins AL, Rao AV, et al.: Cancer risk: possible protective role of high carbohydrate high fiber diets. Am J Gastroenterol 81:931–935, 1986.

55. Kolonel L: Fat and colon cancer: how firm is the epidemiologic evidence? Am J Clin Nutr 45(suppl 1):336–341, 1987.

56. West DW, Lyon JL, Gardner JW: Cancer risk factors: an analysis of Utah Mormans and non-Mormans. JNCI 65:1083–1095, 1980.

57. Trock B, Lanza E, Greenwald P: Dietary, fiber, vegetables, and colon cancer: critical review and meta-analysis of the epidemiologic evidence. JNCI 82:650–661, 1990.

58. Kok FJ, DeBruijn AM, Hofman A, et al.: Is selenium a risk factor for cancer in men only? Am J Epidemiol 125:12–16, 1987.

59. Olson HW, Lawrence WA, Snook CW, et al.: Review of recurrent polyps and cancer in 500 patients with initial coloscopy for polyps. Dis Colon Rectum 31:222–227, 1988.

60. Russin SZ, Lipkin M, Winawer SJ: Inherited colon cancer: clinical implications. Am J Gastroenterol 72:448–457, 1979.

61. Cohen AM, Shank B, Friedman MA, Colorectal cancer. In DeVita VT Jr, Hellman S, Rosenberg SA (eds): Cancer Principles and Practices of Oncology, ed. 3. Philadelphia, JB Lippincott, pp 895–964, 1989.

62. Gnavck R, Macrae FA, Aleisher M: How to perform the fecal occult blood test. CA—A Cancer J for Clinicians 34:134–147, 1983.

63. Fletcher RH: Carcinomembryonic antigen. Ann Intern Med 104:66–73, 1986.

64. Minton JP, Hoehn JL, Gerber DM, et al.: Results of a 400-patient carcinoembryonic antigen second-look colorectal cancer study. Cancer 55:1284–1290, 1985.

65. Klein B, Klein T, Figer A, et al.: Serum β-2-microglobulin in colon cancer pts; a sensitive indicator of tumor bulk. Proc Am Soc Clin Oncol 9:(abstr 483), 1990.

66. NIH Consensus Conference: Adjuvant therapy for patients with colon and rectal cancer. JAMA 264:1444–1450, 1990.

67. Fry RD, Fleshman JW, Kodner IJ: Cancer of the colon and rectum. Clin Symp 41:2–32, 1989.

68. Malcolm W, Olson RM, Perencevich NP, et al.: Patterns of recurrence following curative resection and adenocarcinoma of the colon and rectum. Cancer 45:2969–2974, 1980.

69. The Gastrointestinal Tumor Study Group: Adjuvant therapy of colon cancer—results of a prospectively randomized trial. N Engl J Med 310:737–743, 1984.

70. Schein PS, Levin B, Neoplasms of the colon. In Calabresi P, Schein P, Rosenburg SA (eds): Medical Oncology: Basic Principles and Clinical Management of Cancer, ed. 1. New York, Macmillan, pp 884–915, 1985.

71. Winawer SJ, Fiehinger BJ, Buchalter J, et al.: Declining serum cholesterol levels prior to diagnosis of colon cancer. JAMA 263:2083–2085, 1990.

72. Mendenhall MW, Million RR, Pfaff WW: Patterns of recurrence in adenocarcinoma of the rectum and rectosigmoid treated with surgery alone: implications in treatment planning with adjuvant radiation therapy. Int J Radiat Oncol Biol Phys 9:977–985, 1983.

73. Sugarbaker PH, Coslew S: Influence of surgical techniques on survival in patients with colorectal cancer: a review. Dis Colon Rectum 25:545–557, 1982.

74. Higgins GA, Conn JH, Jordan PH Jr, et al.: Preoperative radiotherapy for colorectal cancer. Ann Surg 181:624–631, 1975.

75. Mittleman A, Holyoke PRM, Moertel CG, et al., Adjuvant chemotherapy and radiotherapy following rectal surgery: an interim report from the Gastrointestinal Tumor Study Group (GITSG). In Salmon SE, Jones SE (eds): Adjuvant Therapy of Cancer. New York, Grune & Stratton, vol III, pp 547–557, 1981.

76. Mellow MH: Endoscopic laser therapy as an alternative to palliative surgery for adenocarcinoma of the rectum—comparison of costs and complications. Gastrointest Endosc 35:283–287, 1989.

77. Buchi KN: Endoscopic laser surgery in the colon and rectum. Dis Colon Rectum 31:739–745, 1988.

78. Heidelberger C: Fluoroinated pyrimides, a new class of tumor inhibitory compound. Nature 179:663–669, 1957.

79. Moertel CG: Clinical management of advanced gastrointestinal cancer. Cancer 36:675–682, 1975.

80. Drewinko B, Tang LY: Cellular basis for the inefficiency of 5-FU in human colon carcinoma. Cancer Treat Rep 69:1391–1398, 1985.

81. Lokich JJ, Ahlgren JD, Gullo JJ, etal.: A prospective randomized comparison of continuous infusion fluorouracil with a conventional bolus schedule in metastatic colorectal carcinoma: a mid-Atlanta oncology program study. J Clin Oncol 7:425–432, 1989.

82. Kemeny N, Daly J, Oderman P, et al.: Hepatic artery pump infusion toxicity and results in patients with metastatic colorectal carcinoma. J Clin Oncol 2:595–600, 1984.

83. Engstrom PF, MacIntyre JM, Douglass HO: Combination chemotherapy containing semustine (MeCCNU) in patients with advanced colorectal cancer previously treated with 5-fluorouracil (5-FU). Am J Clin Oncol 6:175–180, 1983.

84. Engstrom PF, MacIntyre JM, Douglass HO, et al.: Combination chemotherapy of advanced colorectal cancer utilizing 5-fluorouracil, semustine, decarbazine, vincristine, and hydroxyurea: a phase II trial by the Eastern Cooperative Oncology Group. Cancer, 49:1555–1560, 1982.

85. Valone FH, Friedman MA, Wittlinger PS, et al.: Treatment of patients with advanced colorectal carcinomas with fluorouracil alone, high dose leucovorin plus fluorouracil, and leucovorin: a randomized trial of the northern California oncology group. J Clin Oncol 7:1427–1436, 1989.

86. Bertino JR, Sawicki WL, Lindquist CA, et al.: Schedule-dependent antitumor effects of methotrexate and 5-fluorouracil. Cancer Res 37:327–328, 1977.

87. Santi DV, McHenry CS, Sommer H: Mechanism of interaction of thymidylate synthetase with 5-fluorodeoxyuridylate. Biochemistry 13:471–481, 1974.

88. Poon MA, O'Connell MJ, Moertel CG, et al.: Biochemical modulation of fluorouracil: evidence of significant improvement of survival and quality of life in advanced colorectal carcinoma. J Clin Oncol 7:1407–1418, 1989.

89. Huberman M, Bering H, Tessitore J, et al.: 5-Fluorouracil plus recombinant α-interferon in advanced colorectal cancer. Proc Am Soc Clin Oncol 9:(abstr 448), 1990.

90. Walder S, Schwartz EL, Goldman M, et al.: Fluorouracil and recombinant α-2a-interferon: an active regimen against advanced colorectal carcinoma. J Clin Oncol 7:1769–1775, 1989.

91. Wolmark N, Fisher B, Rockette H, et al.: Postoperative adjuvant chemotherapy or BCG for colon cancer. Results from NSABP protocol C-01. JNCI 80:30–36, 1988.

92. Anon: Levamisole with fluorouracil for colon cancer. Med Letter 31:89–90, 1989.

93. Laurie JA, Moertel CG, Fleming TR, et al.: Surgical adjuvant therapy of large bowel carcinoma; an evaluation of levamisole and the combination of levamisole and 5-fluorouracil. The North Central Cancer Treatment Group and the Mayo Clinic. J Clin Oncol 7:1447–1456, 1989.

CHAPTER 80

LUNG CANCER

BETTY J. CHAFFEE, Pharm.D.

Lung cancer is one of the most frequently occurring malignancies in the United States (1). It is the second most commonly occurring tumor in men, ranks number three among women, and is the most frequent cause of cancer-related deaths in both sexes. Although there is not yet a standard treatment for lung cancer, antineoplastic chemotherapy has become important in the treatment of this disease in recent years (2).

ETIOLOGY AND EPIDEMIOLOGY

The major cause of lung cancer is cigarette smoking; it is estimated to be the cause of 80% of all cases. Smoking filtered cigarettes appears to put individuals at a lower risk for lung cancer than smoking nonfiltered cigarettes (3), but the risk is still significantly higher than for nonsmokers. Other risk factors associated with the development of lung cancer include asbestos exposure (especially in combination with cigarette smoking), air pollution, exposure to uranium and certain other metals, and exposure to certain chemicals (3). Exposure to environmental radon has recently been shown to increase the risk of lung cancer (4), and it appears likely that passive inhalation of cigarette smoke also may increase the risk (5). Chronic inflammatory lung diseases, including interstital fibrosis, scleroderma, and tuberculosis, have also been associated with the development of lung cancer (3). Additionally, recent epidemiologic studies have begun to identify a potential genetic susceptibility that increases the risk of developing lung cancer is certain individuals who are exposed to carcinogens (i.e., cigarette smoke) (6, 7).

The risk of lung cancer is relatively low in individuals under the age of 35. The risk increases dramatically at that point, and peaks between the ages of 55 and 65. The male:female ratio is presently slightly lower than 2:1 and is decreasing rapidly (1).

SUBTYPES OF LUNG CANCER

The World Health Organization (WHO) has defined four major histologic subtypes of lung cancer (Table 80.1). The pathologic behavior of small-cell lung cancer (SCLC) is quite different from that of non-small-cell lung cancer (NSCLC). Although the pathologic behavior of each NSCLC subtype is somewhat unique, it has become increasingly apparent that most of these differences in disease course are not as distinct as was previously thought (5).

Squamous cell carcinoma accounts for approximately 32% of all cases of lung cancer. This type of tumor grows slowly, usually in the hilar or perihilar region. It tends to grow into the bronchial lumen, producing bronchial obstruction with associated pneumonitis early in the disease course, but it is unlikely to metastasize early. Squamous cell carcinoma is the most likely of all subtypes to present as a superior sulcus (Pancoast) tumor. This designation is given to a tumor located in the apex of the lung, which grows by local extension to involve the eighth cervical and first thoracic nerves, resulting in a one-sided Horner's syndrome (ptosis, meiosis, anhydrosis) and often, severe pain.

Adenocarinoma presently accounts for approximately 31% of all lung cancer cases and accounts for over 50% of cases in women. This tumor consists of cells that grow to form recognizable gland-like structures. Unlike squamous cell lung tumors, adenocarcinomas are more often peripheral and tend to invade the overlying pleura. Adenocarcinoma is the most widely metastatic of all lung tumor types and metastasizes most frequently to the contralateral lung, liver, bone, kidney, and central nervous system.

Large-cell carcinoma accounts for about 16% of lung cancer cases, and is recognized as an undifferentiated cell with an abundance of cytoplasm. Large-cell carcinoma most often presents peripherally, like adenocarcinoma, but is a large, subpleural tumor with necrotic or cavitary surfaces. Large-cell lung carcinoma metastasizes early, with predilection for mediastinal lymph nodes, pleura, adrenal glands, bone, and the central nervous system.

Small-cell carcinoma represents approximately 20% of lung cancer cases. This type of tumor consists of lymphocyte-like cells with a small amount of cytoplasm. In early stages, SCLC appears as a submucosal infiltrate, then becomes a hilar or perihilar mass that may progress to bronchial obstruction later in the disease course, secondary either to tumor compression of bronchi or tumor within bronchi. Metastatic disease occurs very early, with spread of disease to regional and abdominal lymph nodes, lung, liver, adrenal glands, bone, bone marrow, and the central nervous system. It is now accepted that SCLC is a systemic disease that is microscopically metastatic is nearly all patients at the time of diagnosis.

DIAGNOSIS AND STAGING

Tissue diagnosis and staging of suspected lung carcinoma are extremely important procedures, because treatment

1360

and prognosis depend on both histologic subtype and extent of disease. Tissue diagnosis is most often made by fiberoptic bronchoscopy with biopsy of suspicious lesions. In most cases, it is possible to make a diagnosis based on sputum cytology or examination of bronchial washings or brushings. Sites of disease spread, such as bone marrow, pleural effusion, liver nodules, bone lesions, or enlarged supraclavicular or mediastinal lymph nodes can be examined to make a tissue diagnosis when the primary tumor is inaccessible. When all other methods have proven inadequate, percutaneous, transthoracic, fine-needle biopsy, or exploratory thoracotomy are last resort diagnostic techniques.

Staging of lung carcinoma follows the tissue diagnosis. Staging of NSCLC is currently performed using the revised tumor-node-metastasis (TNM) classification system, known as the International System for Staging Lung Cancer (8). Tumor size is denoted by the letter T, with a subscript of x, 1, 2, 3, or 4 (Table 80.2). Progression of the disease to nodes is denoted by the letter N, with a subscript of 0, 1, 2, or 3, and metastatic spread of disease is denoted by the letter M, with a subscript of 0 or 1 to describe the absence of presence, respectively, of metastatic disease.

Table 80.1.
Histopathologic Subtypes of Lung Cancer

Non-small-cell types
   Adenocarcinoma
   Large cell carcinoma
   Squamous cell (epidermoid) carcinoma
Small cell carcinoma

Table 80.2.
TNM Classification for Non-Small-Cell Lung Cancer[a]

Tumor
T_x: positive cytology
T_{is}: carcinoma in situ
T_1: <3 cm, no invasion
T_2: >3 cm, extension to hilar region
T_3: tumor of any size with extension to chest wall, diaphragm, pleura, or pericardium
T_4: tumor of any size with invasion of mediastinum or involving heart, vertebral body, great vessels, trachea, esophagus, or carina, or presence of effusion.
Node
N_1: peribronchial/ipsilateral hilar nodes
N_2: ipsilateral mediastinal/subcarinal nodes
N_3: contralateral mediastinal or hilar/scalene/supraclavicular nodes
Metastasis
M_0: absent
M_1: present

[a] From Mountain CR: A new international staging system for lung cancer. Chest 89(suppl 4):225–233, 1986, with permission.

Table 80.3.
Staging System for Non-Small-Cell Lung Cancer[a]

Occult disease	$T_x N_0 M_0$
Stage 0	T_{is}
Stage I	$T_1 N_0 M_0$
Stage II	$T_1 N_1 M_0$
	$T_2 N_1 M_0$
Stage IIIa	$T_3 N_0 M_0$
	$T_3 N_1 M_0$
	$T_{1-3} N_2 M_0$
Stage IIIb	$T_{any} N_3 M_0$
	$T_4 N_{any} M_0$
Stage IV	$T_{any} N_{any} M_1$

[a] From Mountain CR: A new international staging system for lung cancer. Chest 89(suppl 4):225–233, 1986, with permission.

The TNM categories are then grouped together into five major prognostic categories, or stages (Table 80.3).

The staging of SCLC does not generally follow the TNM classification. Because SCLC is thought to be a systemic disease in nearly all cases, it is classified into two major categories: (*a*) limited disease, defined as disease confined to one hemithorax, mediastinum, and supraclavicular nodes; and (*b*) extensive disease, defined as disease outside these bounds (3).

Staging of lung carcinoma is performed by a series of tests. Most important is the chest radiograph, which shows the location and size of the tumor. Fiberoptic bronchoscopy can further define these characteristics. Computed tomography (CT scan) of the chest must be performed to determine the extent of nodal involvement. CT scans are also useful in the evaluation of common metastatic sites in the upper abdomen, such as the liver and adrenal glands. A thorough history from and careful physical examination of the patient, along with routine laboratory tests, are performed to determine the presence or absence of metastatic disease. Any abnormalities identified by this process should be investigated.

TREATMENT OF LUNG CARCINOMA

Although the WHO recognizes four histologic subtypes of lung cancer, at the present time treatment is based on only two categories: NSCLC and SCLC. NSCLC includes squamous cell carcinoma, large-cell carcinoma, and adenocarcinoma and differs from SCLC in that non-small-cell tumors are relatively slow growing, slow to metastasize, and less responsive to chemotherapy and radiation therapy than small-cell tumors. NSCLC can be treated successfully as a localized disease in many patients, whereas SCLC must be treated as a systemic disease in nearly all patients.

Evaluation of antineoplastic chemotherapy in the

treatment of lung cancer is difficult. Early trials of chemotherapeutic agents in the treatment of lung carcinoma often did not separate response rates to NSCLC from those in SCLC, and it has since become apparent that response rates with chemotherapy are, in general, much higher in SCLC. The criteria for response were often not specified or were much less strict than the criteria of today. Performance status of the patients, extent of disease, and prior treatment, all of which are now known to affect outcome of treatment, were very often not reported. For these reasons, comparisons between studies are often difficult or impossible, and response rates and survival may differ widely between studies.

Non-Small-Cell Lung Carcinoma

SURGICAL TREATMENT

Definitive resection of the tumor is without question the treatment of choice for NSCLC when possible. In stage I NSCLC, resection results in a 60 to 70% 5-year survival rate, and the 5-year survival rate is even higher in patients with $T_1N_0M_0$ (70 to 80%), compared with $T_2N_0M_0$ (50 to 60%). Stage II NSCLC is less amenable to surgical treatment, with a 5-year survival rate of 40 to 50% for squamous cell carcinoma and 30 to 40% for large-cell and adenocarcinoma (5). Surgical resection of stage IIIa NSCLC results in about 15 to 20% and 10% 5-year survival rates for squamous cell and large-cell/adenocarcinoma, respectively (5).

Unfortunately, only about 30% of patients with NSCLC are surgical candidates, as a result of either extent of disease or concurrent medical problems. In the other 70% of patients and in resected patients who develop recurrent disease, other methods of treatment must be considered.

RADIATION THERAPY

Radiation therapy has been studied extensively in the treatment of NSCLC. It is used both as primary treatment and as an adjunct to surgery. As primary treatment, radiation therapy has been administered with curative intent in patients with resectable tumors who are unable to tolerate a surgical procedure for other medical reasons. When used in this fashion, radiation therapy has resulted in a 5-year survival rate of 21 to 23% (2, 9). In patients who are not surgical candidates because of extent of disease, radiation therapy given with intention of cure has resulted in 5-year survival rates of 3 to 10% (2, 5).

Postoperative radiation therapy has been shown to be of potential benefit only to patients who are found to have stage III $N_{1,2}M_0$ disease when surgically staged. In one study, a 26% 5-year survival rate was achieved in patients who received radiation therapy to the chest after the discovery of positive mediastinal nodes at surgery, whereas

the 5-year survival rate is similar patients who did not receive radiation therapy in other studies was much lower (2). Another study, however, showed that while local recurrence was decreased in patients who received postoperative radiation therapy, the overall survival was similar to that in patients who did not receive immediate postoperative radiation (10).

Preoperative radiation therapy is used in the management of patients with superior sulcus tumors and marginally resectable tumors. A 22 to 29% 5-year survival rate has been reported in patients with superior sulcus tumors treated preoperatively with radiation (2). However, the superiority of the combination of radiation and surgery compared with either radiation or surgery alone has been questioned (9, 11). No definitive evidence is currently available to answer this question (5). Preoperative radiation given in an attempt to increase the resectability of marginally resectable tumors, although advocated in the past, has not been shown to improve the survival of patients in randomized or uncontrolled trials (2, 9, 11). Thus, the issue of preoperative radiation therapy remains unresolved.

CHEMOTHERAPY

Until recently, chemotherapeutic agents had not shown encouraging results in NSCLC. Initial trials showed response rates of less than 10% for most single agents. A number of agents showed initially promising results (2, 12, 13); however, the results were much less encouraging when patients with SCLC were excluded from the analysis. More recently, some newer antineoplastic agents have been found to be active in NSCLC (14, 15). Table 80.4 lists the antineoplastic agents with significant activity in NSCLC, as well as a number of agents that have traditionally been used for the treatment of this disease. Thus far, no single agent has been shown to affect survival when used alone (2, 13–15). For this reason, and because great advances have been made in the treatment of other neoplastic diseases with the use of combination chemotherapy, most research in NSCLC is now being done with combination chemotherapy.

Table 80.5 lists some of the more commonly used combinations that have shown relatively reproducible response rates in patients with NSCLC. These regimens may vary widely between institutions in terms of both dose and dosing interval, because studies have not delineated the optimum regimen for any of the combinations. In addition, no one combination has been consistently better than the others in producing responses in NSCLC (13, 16–18). Examples of initial dose regimens are provided in Table 80.5; the initial dose regimen may be modified for subsequent courses when the patient experiences expected or unexpected side effects or complications.

Major side effects of antineoplastic agents commonly

Table 80.4.
Antineoplastic Agents Active in the Treatment of NSCLC[a]

Active Single Agents	Other Commonly Used Agents
Cisplatin	Bleomycin
Ifosfamide	CCNU
Etoposide	Cyclophosphamide
Mitomycin C	Dacarbazine
Vinblastine	Doxorubicin
Vindesine	5-Fluorouracil
	Mechlorethamine
	Procarbazine
	Vincristine

[a] From information in Zeinrich ES, Baker RR, Ettinger DS, et al.: New frontiers in the treatment of lung cancer. CRC Crit Rev Oncol Hematol 3:279–308, 1985; Cohen MG, Perevokchikova NI, Single agents chemotherapy of lung cancer. In Muggia F, Rozenweig M (eds): Lung Cancer: Progress in Therapeutic Research. New York, Raven Press, 1979, p 343; Hoffman PC, Bitran JD, Golomb HM: Chemotherapy of metastatic non-small cell bronchiogenic carcinoma. Semin Oncol 10:111–122, 1983; Johnson DH: Chemotherapy for unresectable non-small cell lung cancer. Semin Oncol 17(suppl 7):20–29, 1990; Gralla RJ: New directions in non-small cell lung cancer. Semin Oncol 17(suppl 7):14–19, 1990; and Muggia FM, Blum RH, Foreman JD: Role of chemotherapy in the treatment of lung cancer: evolving strategies for non-small cell histologies. Int J Radiat Oncol Biol Phys 10:137–145, 1984.

used in the treatment of both NSCLC and SCLC are found in Table 80.6. Knowledge of these side effects makes it possible to tailor chemotherapy combinations to the patient. A choice can be made between two effective combinations with different toxicities. For example, a patient with chronic congestive heart failure would be at a very high risk of morbidity or mortality if doxorubicin cardiotoxicity were to occur, and therefore should ideally be treated with a combination of agents not containing doxorubicin. Similarly, a patient with a history of kidney dysfunction would be at a very high risk of further kidney damage if cisplatin or methotrexate were administered, and therefore should ideally be treated with a combination not containing either of these nephrotoxic agents.

The current research emphasis in the treatment of NSCLC is on finding combinations of antineoplastic agents that will produce reliable response rates. Combinations containing cisplatin, a vinca alkaloid, and/or etoposide, have been widely used with high and reproducible response rates, and they are the focus of much of the research currently being conducted in NSCLC (14). Important information to be gained from this research includes optimal drug combinations, as well as optimal doses of the individual agents used (15). In addition, some data suggest that older agents that are ineffective as single agents may provide synergism when used with active single agents (14, 15).

Research is also being focused on the optimal use of chemotherapy in NSCLC. Several investigators have studied the efficacy of chemotherapy in prolonging survival in patients with metastatic or localized, inoperable NSCLC. Although some data suggest that survival is prolonged with chemotherapy, other studies have shown no effect (14). In addition, no attempt has been made to assess the quality of life in patients who received chemotherapy (14). At this time, no clear indication for chemotherapy in stage III or IV NSCLC has been found.

Additionally, the role of chemotherapy in combination with radiation and/or surgical resection is currently under study. Trials of neoadjuvant and adjuvant chemotherapy in patients with localized disease are currently being conducted, as well as trials of neoadjuvant and adjuvant radiation therapy (14). Chemotherapy and radiation therapy in combination with surgery are also being tested (14).

Obviously, chemotherapeutic approaches to the treatment of NSCLC are still experimental. However, because of the potential increase in survival for patients who respond to treatment, all eligible patients should be offered the option of chemotherapy, or, ideally, the opportunity to participate in a clinical trial. Increases in survival time, although significant, have not been as impressive in NSCLC as in other neoplastic diseases, rarely amounting to 8 to 20 months.

Small-Cell Lung Carcinoma

NONPHARMACOLOGIC TREATMENT

SCLC is considered a systemic disease at initial diagnosis. Local treatment has not produced impressive results in this disease. Surgery alone has little effect on survival because of the rapid occurrence of metastatic disease even after complete resection of the primary tumor. Radiation therapy, on the other hand, has been shown to prolong survival from 2 to 4 months to 10 months in patients with limited disease, but these patients also eventually succumb to metastatic disease (2).

CHEMOTHERAPY

Chemotherapy has now been accepted as standard treatment for SCLC, in both limited and extensive disease, because of its ability to prolong survival significantly, even in patients with extensive disease. Table 80.7 contains a list of drugs that have been shown to have activity as single agents in the treatment of SCLC (2, 19–21). As in NSCLC, although single agents induce responses in SCLC, they have had little effect on survival because of the rapid occurrence of metastatic disease.

Combination chemotherapy has been extensively investigated in the treatment of SCLC. A number of different regimens have become standard treatment of SCLC in some hospitals. Some of the more common combinations are listed in Table 80.8, along with initial dose regimens. The etoposide-containing regimens, especially the combination of cisplatin and etoposide, are currently the

Table 80.5.
Combination Chemotherapeutic Regimens Used in the Treatment of NSCLC

Regimen		Initial Doses	Response Rate (%)
CAP	CTX	400–600 mg/m^2 IV day 1 ⎫	22–48
	DXR	40 mg/m^2 IV day 1 ⎬ q. 4–6 weeks	
	DDP	40–120 mg/m^2 IV day 1 ⎭	
FAM	5-FU	600 mg/m^2 IV days 1, 8, 29, 36 ⎫	33–36
	DXR	30 mg/m^2 IV days 1, 29 ⎬ q. 56 days	
	Mito	10 mg/m^2 IV day 1 ⎭	
CAMP	CTX	300 mg/m^2 IV days 1, 8 ⎫	15–44
	DXR	20 mg/m^2 IV days 1, 8 ⎬	
	MTX	15 mg/m^2 IV days 1, 8 ⎬ q. 29 days	
	PCBZ	100 mg/m^2 p.o. days 1–10 ⎭	
COMB	CTX	800–1000 mg/m^2 IV day 1 q. 4–6 weeks	23
	VCR	0.5–1.0 mg/m^2 IV twice/week × 6–24 weeks	
	MeCCNU	100 mg/m^2 p.o. day 1 q. 4–6 weeks	
	Bleo	7.5–30 mg IV twice/week × 6–24 weeks	
PACE	DDP	50–60 mg/m^2 IV in 1–3 doses ⎫	29–46
	DXR	30 mg/m^2 IV days 1, 22 ⎬	
	CTX	300 mg/m^2 IV days 1, 22 ⎬ q. 6 weeks	
	VDS	3 mg/m^2 IV days 1, 15, 22, 36 ⎭	
BACON	Bleo	30 units IV day 1 weekly × 6	21–45
	DXR	40 mg/m^2 IV day 1 q. 4 weeks	
	CCNU	65 mg/m^2 p.o. day 1 q. 8 weeks	
	VCR	0.75–1.0 mg IV day 1 weekly × 6	
	NM	8 mg/m^2 IV day 1 q. 4 weeks	
MACC	MTX	30–40 mg/m^2 IV day 1 ⎫	12–50
	DXR	30–40 mg/m^2 IV day 1 ⎬	
	CTX	400 mg/m^2 IV day 1 ⎬ q. 3 weeks	
	CCNU	30 mg/m^2 p.o. day 1 ⎭	
DDP/VP16	DDP	60–100 mg/m^2 IV day 1 ⎫ q. 3 weeks	28–41
	VP16	100–120 mg/m^2 IV days 1, 2, 3 ⎭	
DDP/VBL	DDP	120 mg/m^2 IV days 1, 28 then q. 6 weeks	39–60
	VBL	8 mg/m^2 IV days 1, 14, 28 then q. 3 weeks	
DDP/VDS	DDP	60–120 mg/m^2 IV days 1, 29 then q. 6 weeks	40–46
	VDS	3 mg/m^2 IV q. week × 7 then q. 2 weeks	

[a] Information from Zeinrich ES, Baker RR, Ettinger DS, et al.: New frontiers in the treatment of lung cancer. CRC Crit Rev Oncol Hematol 3:279–308, 1985; Hoffman PC, Bitran JD, Golomb HM: Chemotherapy of metastatic non-small cell bronchogenic carcinoma. Semin Oncol 10:111–122, 1983; and Gralla RJ, Wittes RE, Casper ES, et al. Chemotherapy of non-small cell lung cancer: clinical trials at Memorial Sloan-Kettering Cancer Center. World J Surg 5:667–673, 1981.

[b] Abbreviations: CTX, cyclophosphamide; DXR, doxorubicin; DDP, cisplatin; 5-FU, fluorouracil; Mito, mitomycin C; MTX, methotrexate; PCBZ, procarbazine; VCR, vincristine; MeCCNU, semustine; Bleo, bleomycin; VP16, etoposide; NM, mechlorethamine; VBL, vinblastine; VDS, vindesine; CCNU, lomustine

most widely used. As for NSCLC, the initial dose and dosing intervals vary for a given combination because none has been shown to be superior. Doses may be adjusted if a patient experiences side effects from the chemotherapy. Side effects of antineoplastic agents are listed in Table 80.6.

With most combination regimens, objective responses are seen in over 70% of patients with SCLC, with complete response in over 50% of patients with limited disease and 25% of patients with extensive disease (2, 22–24). The median survival of patients treated with combination chemotherapy is 12 to 18 months for limited disease and 8 to 12 months for extensive disease. No major break-throughs have been made in the study of combination chemotherapy for SCLC in the past few years.

Several promising avenues are presently being pursued in the treatment of SCLC. Current studies are investigating optimal drug doses, the optimal number of drugs used in combination, duration of treatment, alternating non-cross-resistant regimens, and the use of chemotherapy combined with radiation therapy or surgery. There are indications that intensive doses of antineoplastic agents induce greater responses and prolong survival more than lower doses (19–21). It has been suggested that intensive dosing of two antineoplastic agents may be as effective as or more effective than lower doses of three or more agents.

Table 80.6.

Major Toxicities of Antineoplastic Agents Used in the Treatment of Lung Carcinoma

Agent[a]	Toxicity[b]	Comments
Bleo	Anaphylaxis (A)	
	Skin toxicity (C)	
	Pneumonitis (C)	More frequent as cumulative dose increases; may present as reversible pneumonitis or irreversible pulmonary fibrosis
DDP	N/V (A)	Frequently severe, requires aggressive antiemetics
	Nephrotoxicity (A, C)	May present as acute renal failure (reversible) or as a cumulative decrease in renal function; hypomagnesemia is a common finding; can usually be prevented with aggressive hydration
	Neurotoxicity (C)	May present as peripheral neuropathy or hearing loss
CTX	BMS, alopecia (A)	
	Sterile cystitis (A, C)	May present after one or multiple doses; dysuria, frequency, hematuria are common symptoms; can usually be prevented with adequate hydration
DXR	Stomatitis, BMS, alopecia (A)	
	Vesicant reactions (A)	
	Cardiomyopathy (C)	More frequent as cumulative dose increases; presents as congestive heart failure; can be medically managed; may be reversible in some cases
VP16	BMS, alopecia (A)	
5-FU	BMS (A)	
	Stomatitis, gastritis proctitis (A)	May be dose-limiting
IFOS	BMS, alopecia (A)	
	Sterile cystitis	Similar to cystitis resulting from CTX; can be prevented with hydration and with the use of MESNA
CCNU	BMS (A)	Delayed nadir
	Alopecia (A)	
NM	BMS (A)	
	Vesicant reactions (A)	
MTX	BMS (A)	
	Stomatitis (A)	
	Nephrotoxicity (A)	Usually presents as acute renal failure; can be prevented with adequate hydration and urine alkalinization
	Hepatotoxicity (A, C)	More common with high-dose or continuous low-dose therapy
Mito	BMS (A)	Delayed nadir
	Vesicant reaction (A)	
PCBZ	BMS (A)	Delayed nadir
MeCCNU	BMS (A)	Delayed nadir
VBL	BMS (A)	
	Vesicant reaction (A)	
VCR	Neurotoxicity (A, C)	May present with initial constipation/paralytic ileus, progressing to peripheral neuropathy and motor neuropathy, which are dose-limiting
	Vesicant reaction (A)	
VDS	BMS (A)	
	Neurotoxicity (A, C)	Similar to vincristine
	Vesicant reaction (A)	

[a] See Table 80.5 for key to abbreviations.

[b] A, acute toxicity; C, cumulative toxicity; N/V, nausea and vomiting; BMS, bone marrow suppression.

The magnitude of the dose that will increase therapeutic efficacy without significantly increasing toxicity is still in question for many agents. Moderately intensive doses of three or more chemotherapeutic agents are being investigated in an attempt to produce maximal response with minimal treatment-related morbidity and mortality. Additionally, the availability of colony-stimulating factors (CSFs) may allow the administration of much more intensive doses of antineoplastic agents without the profound, life-threatening bone marrow suppression commonly seen now. Studies currently underway will define the doses of chemotherapy that can be used safely in combination with CSFs (25).

The optimal duration of treatment of SCLC with antineoplastic agents is another unresolved issue. A common approach at some institutions have been to administer chemotherapy for 12 months or until the disease relapses. Most patients who achieve remission, however, do so between the 6th and 12th week of treatment. An uncontrolled study in which chemotherapy was continued for only 12 weeks reported survival equal to other studies in which chemotherapy was continued for a much longer period. Other studies, however, suggest that survival may be improved when maintenance chemotherapy is continued in patients who respond initially, although quality of life may be compromised (26). The available data suggest that 6 to 12 months of chemotherapy is adequate for most patients (21, 25, 26).

An interesting and recent approach to the treatment of SCLC is the use of non-cross-resistant chemotherapy regimens. This approach is based on the theory that relapse of SCLC is due to mutation of neoplastic cells toward resistance to chemotherapeutic agents. Because of this theory and because tumors that progress during combination chemotherapy often respond to a combination of other antineoplastic agents, it has been suggested that initial therapy should include alternating combinations of non-cross-resistant agents (27). Randomized trials published to date have shown increased response rates and/or an increased response duration, but no survival benefit has thus far been shown. One study reported a modest survival benefit from alternating cisplatin-etoposide (DDP/VP16) and cyclophosphamide-doxorubicin-vincristine (CAV), compared with CAV alone (28). Some common alternating regimens are shown in Table 80.9.

Another theory about the treatment of SCLC is that neoplastic cells become decreasingly sensitive to antineoplastic agents as the tumor size decreases (19). If this is the case, then doses of chemotherapeutic agents should be intensified after tumor response has been induced. This method of chemotherapy administration in known as "late intensification" or "consolidation." Several trials testing this method of drug administration have been reported, one of which showed significant improvement in the survival rate in patients who received late intensification compared with those who did not. Other trials have shown no benefit (19). This method of treatment is still under investigation (25, 29).

The role of radiation therapy in the treatment of SCLC

Table 80.7.
Chemotherapeutic Drugs Active as Single Agents in the Treatment of SCLC

Carmustine	Lomustine
Cisplatin	Mechlorethamine
Cyclophosphamide	Methotrexate
Doxorubicin	Procarbazine
Etoposide	Vincristine
Ifosfamide	Vindesine

Information from Zeinrich ES, Baker RR, Ettinger DS, et al.: New frontiers in the treatment of lung cancer. CRC Crit Rev Oncol Hematol 3:279–308, 1985; Greco FA, Johnson DH, Hainsworth JD; et al.: Chemotherapy of small cell lung cancer. Semin Oncol 12(suppl 6):31–37, 1985; Ihde DC: Current status of therapy for small cell carcinoma of the lung. Cancer 54:2722–2728, 1984; and Mortsyn GE, Ihde DC, Lichter AS, et al.: Small cell lung cancer 1973–1983: early progress and recent obstacles. J Radiat Oncol Biol Phys 10:515–539, 1984.

Table 80.8.
Combination Chemotherapeutic Regimens Used in the Treatment of SCLC[a]

Regimen	Agents	Initial Doses	Response Rate (%)
CMC	CTX	500–1000 mg/m^2 IV days 1, 22	45–90
	MTX	10–15 mg/m^2 p.o. twice/week × 5 weeks	
	CCNU	100 mg/m^2 p.o. day 1	
CAV	CTX	750–1200 mg/m^2 IV day 1	62–72
	DXR	40–70 mg/m^2 IV day 1 } q. 3 weeks	
	VCR	1 mg/m^2 (max 2 mg) IV day 1	
CAVP16	CTX	1000 mg/m^2 IV day 1 } q. 3 weeks	82–90
	DXR	45 mg/m^2 IV day 1	
	VP16	50 mg/m^2 IV days 1–5	
DDP/VP16	DDP	60–100 mg/m^2 IV day 1 } q. 3 weeks	76–95
	VP16	100–120 mg/m^2 IV days 1, 2, 3	
CAV/VP16	CTX	1000 mg/m^2 IV day 1	74
	DXR	50 mg/m^2 IV day 1 } q. 3 weeks	
	VCR	1.4 mg/m^2 (max 2 mg) IV day 1	
	VP16	125 mg/m^2 IV day 1	

[a] Information from Zeinrich ES, Baker RR, Ettinger DS, et al.: New frontiers in the treatment of lung cancer. CRC Crit Rev Oncol Hematol 3:279–308, 1985; Evans WK, Feld R, Osoba D, et al.: VP16 alone and in combination with cisplatin in previously treated patients with small cell lung cancer. Cancer 53:1461–1466, 1984; Lowenbraun S, Birch R, Buchanan R, et al.: Combination chemotherapy in small cell carcinoma. Cancer 54:2344–2350, 1984; and Klastersky J, Sculier JP, Dumont JP, et al.: Combination chemotherapy with adriamycin, etoposide, and cyclophosphamide for small cell carcinoma of the lung. Cancer 56:71–75, 1985.

Table 80.9.
Non-Cross-Resistant Alternating Combination Chemotherapeutic Regimens Used in the Treatment of SCLC[a]

Regimen	Response Rate (%)
CMC-VAP	94
CMC (described in Table 80.7) alternating with VCR/DXR/PCBZ	
CAV-VP16/DDP	95
CAV (described in Table 80.7) alternating with VP16/DDP	

[a] Data from Zeinrich ES, Baker RR, Ettinger DS, et al.: New frontiers in the treatment of lung cancer. CRC Crit Rev Oncol Hematol 3:279–308, 1985; and Natale RB, Shank B, Hilris BS, et al.: Combination cyclophosphamide, adriamycin, and vincristine rapidly alternating with combination cisplatin and VP16 in treatment of small cell lung cancer. Am J Med 79:303–308, 1985.

has not yet been established, but it is currently being widely investigated. Because relapse of SCLC often occurs at the primary site, a number of studies have looked at the addition of chest radiation to systemic chemotherapy, with the hope of decreasing the frequency of local relapse, thereby increasing survival. Two randomized trials designed to answer this question have been published (30, 31). Both showed a significant survival benefit for patients with limited-stage SCLC treated with combination chemotherapy and radiation to the primary site. Treatment-related toxicity was increased with the combination but was acceptable. Recent data suggest that concurrent administration of radiation therapy and chemotherapy is more effective in prolonging survival than chemotherapy followed by radiation therapy (29, 32). Research continues in this area.

Surgical resection of the primary site has also been studied as a means of increasing survival when used in combination with systemic chemotherapy. Some investigators have reported excellent results with resection alone (33), and research is continuing into the combination of surgical resection and chemotherapeutic treatment.

Prophylactic cranial irradiation (PCI) has reduced the rate of relapse of SCLC in the brain from 20 to 6% (34). Although PCI does not affect survival, it is standard treatment in most institutions for patients achieving complete response from systemic chemotherapy, because it decreases the morbidity that occurs with relapse of SCLC in the brain. Unfortunately, studies in which a few patients were long-term survivors noted that PCI may cause late neurologic toxicity (21, 35, 36). Administration of PCI during systemic chemotherapy may increase the risk of neurological toxicity, and it has been suggested that research is necessary to delineate the optimal time for administration of PCI (36).

SCLC is a common, rapidly progressive, and fatal disease. However, combination chemotherapy has prolonged

survival from an average of 2 to 4 months without treatment to 12 to 24 months with treatment. A recent report documented a 5% 10-year survival rate in patients with this disease (37).

CONCLUSION

Lung cancer is one of the most frequently occurring malignancies in the United States. Treatment of both NSCLC and SCLC involves surgery, radiotherapy, and chemotherapy. Localized NSCLC can be successfully treated with surgery or radiotherapy, and cures are common. Disseminated NSCLC and SCLC must be treated with systemic chemotherapy, and long-term survival is much more difficult to achieve.

Research in NSCLC is being directed largely at identifying active antineoplastic agents. Marginal increases in survival rates have been possible with some combinations of antineoplastic agents. SCLC is much more sensitive to chemotherapy than NSCLC and survival times have been prolonged in patients with SCLC with the use of chemotherapy. Research in the treatment of SCLC includes combination chemotherapy, alternating non-cross-resistant chemotherapy, and the use of radiation or surgery in combination with chemotherapy.

REFERENCES

1. Anon: 1991 Cancer Facts & Figures. New York, American Cancer Society, 1991.
2. Zeinrich ES, Baker RR, Ettinger DS, et al.: New frontiers in the treatment of lung cancer. CRC Crit Rev Oncol Hematol 3:279–308, 1985.
3. Van Houtte P, Salazar OM, Phillips EC, et al.: Lung cancer. In Rubin P (ed): Clinical Oncology for Medical Students and Physicians. New York, American Cancer Society, 1983, p 142.
4. Hart BL, Mettler FA, Harley NH: Radon: Is it a problem? Radiology 172:593–599, 1989.
5. Minna JD, Pass H, Glatstein E, et al., Cancer of the lung. In De Vita VT, Hellman S, Rosenberg SA (eds): Cancer: Principles and Practice of Oncology, ed. 3. Philadelphia, JB Lippincott, 1989, pp 591–705.
6. Ooi WL, Elston RC, Chen VW, et al.: Increased familial risk for lung cancer. JNCI 76:217–222, 1986.
7. Lynch HT, Kimberling WJ, Markvicka SE, et al.: Genetics and smoking-associated cancers: a study of 485 families. Cancer 57:1640–1646, 1986.
8. Mountain CR: A new international staging system for lung cancer. Chest 89(suppl 4):225–233, 1986.
9. Cox JD, Byhardt RW, Komaki R: The role of radiotherapy in squamous, large cell, and adenocarcinoma of the lung. Semin Oncol 10:81–94, 1983.
10. The Lung Cancer Study Group, et al.: Effects of postoperative mediastinal radiation on completely resected stage II and stage III epidermoid cancer of the lung. N Engl J Med 315:1377–1381, 1986.
11. Mountain CR, Hermes KE, Management implications of surgical staging studies. In Muggia F, Rozenweig M (eds): Lung Cancer: Progress in Therapeutic Research. New York, Raven Press, 1979, p 233.
12. Cohen MG, Perevokchikova NI, Single agents chemotherapy of lung

cancer. In Muggia F, Rozenweig M (eds): Lung Cancer: Progress in Therapeutic Research. New York, Raven Press, 1979, p 343.

13. Hoffman PC, Bitran JD, Golomb HM: Chemotherapy of metastatic non-small cell bronchogenic carcinoma. Semin Oncol 10:111–122, 1983.

14. Johnson DH: Chemotherapy for unresectable non-small cell lung cancer. Semin Oncol 17(suppl 7):20–29, 1990.

15. Gralla RJ: New directions in non-small cell lung cancer. Semin Oncol 17(suppl 7):14–19, 1990.

16. Muggia FM, Blum RH, Foreman JD: Role of chemotherapy in the treatment of lung cancer: evolving strategies for non-small cell histologies. Int J Radiat Oncol Biol Phys 10:137–145, 1984.

17. Klastersky J, Sculier JP: Chemotherapy of non-small cell lung cancer. Semin Oncol 12(suppl 6):39–48, 1985.

18. Gralla RJ, Wittes RE, Casper ES, et al.: Chemotherapy of non-small cell lung cancer: clinical trials at Memorial Sloan-Kettering Cancer Center. World J Surg 5:667–673, 1981.

19. Greco FA, Johnson DH, Hainsworth JD, et al.: Chemotherapy of small cell lung cancer. Semin Oncol 12(suppl 6):31–37, 1985.

20. Ihde DC: Current status of therapy for small cell carcinoma of the lung. Cancer 54:2722–2728, 1984.

21. Mortsyn GE, Ihde DC, Lichter AS, et al.: Small cell lung cancer 1973–1983: early progress and recent obstacles. J Radiat Oncol Biol Phys 10:515–539, 1984.

22. Evans WK, Feld R, Osoba D, et al.: VP16 alone and in combination with cisplatin in previously treated patients with small cell lung cancer. Cancer 53:1461–1466, 1984.

23. Lowenbraun S, Birch R, Buchanan R, et al.: Combination chemotherapy in small cell lung carcinoma. Cancer 54:2344–2350, 1984.

24. Klastersky J, Sculier JP, Dumont JP, et al.: Combination chemotherapy with adriamycin, etoposide, and cyclophosphamide for small cell carcinoma of the lung. Cancer 56:71–75, 1985.

25. Kristjansen PEG, Hansen HH: Management of small cell lung cancer: a summary of the third international association for the study of lung cancer workshop on small cell lung cancer. JNCI 82:263–266, 1990.

26. Spiro SG, Souhami RL: Duration of chemotherapy in small cell lung cancer. Thorax 45:1–2, 1990.

27. Natale RB, Shank B, Hilris BS, et al.: Combination cyclophosphamide, adriamycin, and vincristine rapidly alternating with combination cisplatin and VP16 in treatment of small cell lung cancer. Am J Med 79:303–308, 1985.

28. Evans WK, Feld R, Murray N, et al.: Superiority of alternating non-cross-resistant chemotherapy in extensive small cell lung cancer. Ann Intern Med 107:451–458, 1987.

29. McCracken JD, Janaki LM, Crowley JJ, et al.: Concurrent chemotherapy/radiotherapy for limited small-cell lung carcinoma: a Southwest Oncology Group study. J Clin Oncol 8:892–898, 1990.

30. Bunn PA, Lichter AS, Makuch RW, et al.: Chemotherapy alone or chemotherapy with chest radiation therapy in limited stage small cell lung cancer. Ann Intern Med 106:655–662, 1987.

31. Perry MC, Eaton WL, Propert KJ, et al.: Chemotherapy with or without radiation therapy in limited small-cell carcinoma of the lung. N Engl J Med 316:912–918, 1987.

32. Turrisi AT: Limited small cell lung cancer—the role of radiotherapy. Oncology 2:19–28, 1988.

33. Shields TW, Higgins GA, Matthews MJ, et al.: Surgical resection in the management of small cell carcinoma of the lung. J Thorac Cardiovasc Surg 84:481–488, 1982.

34. Bleehen NM, Bunn PA, Cox JD, et al.: Role of radiation therapy in small cell anaplastic carcinoma of the lung. Cancer Treat Rep 67:11–19, 1983.

35. Johnson BE, Ihde DC, Bunn PA, et al.: Patients with small-cell lung cancer treated with combination chemotherapy with or without irradiation. Ann Intern Med 103:430–438, 1985.

36. Turrisi AT: Brain irradiation and systemic chemotherapy for small-cell lung cancer: dangerous liaisons? J Clin Oncol 8:196–199, 1990.

37. Johnson BE, Grayson J, Makuch RW, et al.: Ten-year survival of patients with small-cell lung cancer treated with combination chemotherapy with or without irradiation. J Clin Oncol 8:396–401, 1990.

CHAPTER 81

PROSTATE CANCER

JOHN D. HIRSH, Pharm.D. and ROWENA N. SCHWARTZ, Pharm.D.

Prostate cancer is the most commonly diagnosed cancer in males, based on 1991 estimates from the National Cancer Institute's Surveillance, Epidemiology and End Results (SEER) program (1). In 1991, the number of new cases first diagnosed in the United States is estimated at 122,000, which represents a 15% increase from the preceding year. In recent years, the incidence of prostate cancer has increased steadily due primarily to the aging of the population and possibly due to improved diagnosis, and this trend is expected to continue. Prostate cancer ranks behind lung cancer as the most common cause of death in males.

RISK FACTORS AND EPIDEMIOLOGY

Little is known about the etiology of prostate cancer. Epidemiologic studies have detected trends and identified potential risk factors. Prostate cancer is clearly a disease of the elderly, with the incidence increasing continuously with increasing age. More than 80% of cases are diagnosed in men over the age of 65 years (1). Prostate cancer is most common in North America and Northern Europe, and is seen less frequently in Asian countries, South America, Central America, and Africa (1, 2). Black Americans have the highest incidence rate in the world. It is difficult to distinctly separate race as a risk factor from environment, culture, and/or diet. For example, the incidence of carcinoma of the prostate in second-generation Japanese-Americans is between that of Japanese and American men (3, 4). A number of case-controlled studies have implicated dietary animal fat as a risk factor. One study found that men drinking only whole milk had a two-fold risk of developing prostate cancer, compared with men drinking low-fat milk or not drinking milk (5). However, sufficient evidence does not yet exist to warrant a formal public health recommendation. Studies involving other possible etiologic risk factors such as hormones, heredity, marital status, sexual activity, viruses, and nonmalignant prostatic disease have yielded conflicting information.

ANATOMY AND HISTOLOGY

The prostate gland is a solid organ made up of glandular and nonglandular elements, including a fibromuscular element containing blood and lymphatic vessels, and nerves. The prostate gland is located between the base of the bladder and the urogenital diaphragm. The prostate produces seminal fluid that is released through ejaculatory ducts into the prostatic urethra, which is surrounded by the prostate gland.

The prostate is divided into anatomic regions that differ histologically and biologically (3, 6). These regions are the central, transition, and peripheral zones. The great majority of prostatic cancers are adenocarcinomas that arise from the prostatic acini in the peripheral zone. Prostatic tissues obtained at biopsy are histologically graded by several systems. In general, patients with glandular tumor tissue that more closely resembles normal tissue (well-differentiated) have a better prognosis than those with significant changes in glandular tissue (poorly differentiated). Recently, a pattern of histologic changes termed *prostatic intraepithelial neoplasia* (PIN) was identified in prostatic tissue that is felt to be premalignant (7). While therapy is not indicated, regular and long-term follow-up is appropriate.

PATHOPHYSIOLOGY

The growth of prostate cancer depends on stimulation by androgen, specifically dihydrotestosterone (DHT). The influence of the endocrine system on prostate cell growth are shown in Figure 81.1). The exact mechanism of androgen utilization by prostate cells is unknown. In the adult male prostate, cell growth is mediated through the intracellular production of DHT, 95% of which is derived from testosterone produced in the testis. Testosterone secretion is controlled by the hypothalamic-pituitary-gonadal axis. The hypothalamus releases luteinizing-hormone-releasing hormone (LHRH) in a pulsatile manner that stimulates the pituitary to release luteinizing hormone (LH). LH stimulates the Leydig cells in the testis to produce testosterone. Testosterone is transported into the prostate cell, where it is enzymatically converted to DHT. DHT interacts with cytoplasmic receptors. The DHT-receptor complex is translocated into the nucleus where it triggers protein synthesis that influences cell growth. The remaining 5% of androgens, dihydroepiandrosterone (DHEA) and androstenedione, is secreted from the adrenal gland. The importance of adrenal androgens in modulating normal and malignant prostate cell growth remains undefined.

Feedback inhibition of further LH and testosterone production is mediated through negative feedback of testosterone on the pituitary and hypothalamus. Increased circulating levels of estrogens also inhibit LH release. Ad-

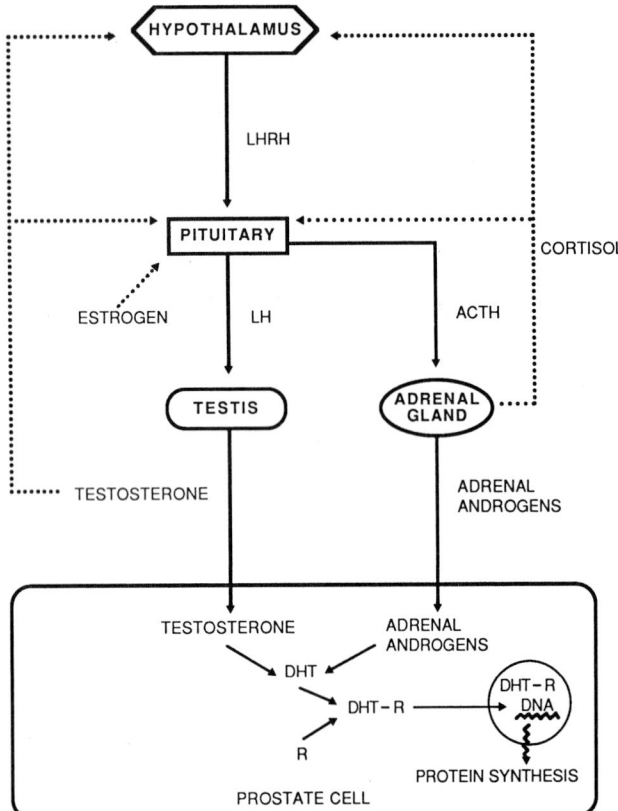

Figure 81.1. Influences of endocrine system on prostate cell growth. (→), negative feedback; *LHRH*, luteinizing hormone-releasing hormone; *ACTH*, adrenicocorticotropic hormone; *LH*, luteinizing hormone; *DHT*, dihydrotestosterone; *R*, receptor.

renal secretion of androgens is inhibited by negative feedback of cortisol on the pituitary to decrease release of adrenocorticotropic hormone (ACTH).

On the basis of a rat tumor model, it is believed that prostate cancers are made up of a heterogeneous population of cells that differ in their sensitivity to androgen stimulation. One clone of cells may be androgen-dependent while another clone of cells is relatively androgen-insensitive. The relative preponderance of particular cell types would influence the response to hormonal treatment. The measurement of prostate cell hormone receptors to predict tumor hormone responsiveness has not been clinically useful. The inability to achieve clinical "cures" with hormonal therapy may be explained by the killing of hormone-sensitive cells, leaving a resistant, hormone-insensitive population. It is possible that androgen-independent growth factors exist that influence the growth of the hormone-insensitive cell population (8).

PATTERNS OF SPREAD

Prostate cancer spreads by direct local invasion, or more distantly, through lymphatic and vascular vessels. Initially,

the tumor spreads from the periphery of the gland into the center. The fibrous connective tissue and smooth muscle capsule surrounding the gland serve as initial barriers to disease spread. As the tumor spreads, it penetrates through the capsule and can invade the neck of the bladder and the distal ureters, causing ureteral obstruction.

Tumor cells can invade lymphatic channels within the glandular structure of the prostate cell, commonly causing lymph node metastases. Lymph node involvement is associated with increased tumor size and more undifferentiated histology.

Hematogenous tumor spread results most commonly in bone metastases, which are present in approximately 85% of end-stage patients with prostate cancer (9). The most common sites of bony metastasis, in decreasing order of frequency, are the axial skeleton, lumbar spine, proximal femur, pelvis, thoracic spine, ribs, sternum, skull, and humerus. Spinal cord compression may occur with resultant lower extremity paralysis. The most common sites of visceral metastases are the liver, lungs, and adrenal glands.

SIGNS AND SYMPTOMS

Patients in early stages of localized, potentially curable disease are often asymptomatic. As prostate cancer begins to advance locally, several nonspecific symptoms may be present. These symptoms may mimic those seen with benign prostatic hyperplasia. Bladder outlet obstruction may cause urinary hesitancy, dribbling, frequency, nocturia, and incomplete bladder emptying. Cystitis and microscopic or macroscopic hematuria may also be present.

Patients with advanced disease may present with bone pain and back stiffness that could result in pathologic fracture, or if ignored, spinal cord compression. Most patients have significant pain that limits normal activity. The incidence of spinal cord compression in prostate cancer ranges from 1 to 10% and must be treated as an emergency (10). Ureteral obstruction is common and may cause anuria, uremia, and symptoms of bladder outlet obstruction. Other signs and symptoms include lymphadenopathy, weight loss, anemia, lower extremity edema secondary to pelvic lymph node metastases blocking venous return, rectal obstruction, and generalized bleeding secondary to coagulation defects.

DIAGNOSIS AND STAGING

Patient history, digital rectal examination (DRE), and biopsy are the traditional backbone of diagnosis. Prostate-specific antigen (PSA) and transrectal ultrasound (TRUS) are newer modalities that are useful in early detection (11). PSA is a tumor marker produced exclusively by normal and neoplastic prostate ductal epithelium and secreted into the glandular lumen. PSA is elevated in 30 to 50% of patients with benign prostatic hyperplasia. A key to an early diagnosis is a high index of suspicion based on patient history and DRE. Palpable nodules must be confirmed by biopsy, since approximately 50% of palpable prostatic nodules are carcinoma. DRE should be performed annually in men 50 years of age and older. The American Cancer Society recommends annual DRE in men 40 years of age or older for early detection of colon cancer. Catalona and colleagues found that the combination of the measurement of the serum PSA concentration and DRE, with TRUS performed in patients with abnormal findings, provides a better method (lower error rate) than DRE alone (11). TRUS may also be useful in evaluating high-risk patients and those with PIN (1, 3, 12). Currently, the primary use of TRUS is to guide prostatic biopsy. PSA is also used as a method of following disease in patients with prostate cancer.

Prognosis and treatment depend on the determination of extent of disease. Several staging systems have been used to describe the extent of disease. The two most commonly used staging systems are the American Urological System (A–D) and the TNM (tumor-node-metastases) classification (see Table 81.1) (13). Prior to 1987, two different TNM systems were used by the American Joint Committee on Cancer (AJCC) and the International Union Against Cancer (UICC). The use of consistent staging systems would facilitate the comparison of study results and clinical decision making. In 1987, the TNM classification was updated and adopted by both the AJCC and UICC. Unfortunately, changes in the TNM classification system have been met with controversy by some cooperative study groups that still use the previous TNM system (14). When reviewing prostate cancer studies, the differences in the staging systems should be kept in mind.

Staging is most often based on clinical data using multiple modalities such as physical examination, laboratory data, radiographic studies and TRUS (see Table 81.2). First, the extent of local spread is assessed. TRUS is a relatively new method that is useful in determining extracapsular penetration. The use of DRE, TRUS, and serum PSA together may increase the correlation of clinical staging to pathologic diagnosis (3). The serum PSA level increases with advancing clinical stage and is proportional to the estimated tumor volume. Since PSA levels are nonspecific, a biopsy should be done to rule out carcinoma in patients with an elevated serum PSA but a negative DRE. Transrectal magnetic resonance imaging (MRI) has recently been studied and shows promise in the early diagnosis of prostate cancer (15). Flow cytometry is being evaluated as a supplemental method to predict tumor progression (3). Tumor grade and stage appear to correlate with diploid, tetraploid, and aneuploid DNA content.

When definitive treatment is considered, studies should be done to detect distant metastases. Radionuclide bone scans are the most sensitive procedure to detect dis-

Table 81.1.
Staging Classification Systems

American Urological Association			TNM	
A	Incidental carcinoma	T0	No evidence of primary tumor
A1	Focal	T1a	3 or fewer microscopic foci
A2	Diffuse	T1b	More than 3 microscopic foci
B	Confined to prostate	T2	Tumor present clinically or grossly limited to gland
B1	Small, discrete nodule	T2a	Tumor 1.5 cm or less in greatest dimension, normal tissues on at least 3 sides
B2	Large or multiple nodules	T2b	Tumor > 1.5 cm in greatest dimension or in more than 1 lobe
C	Localized to periprostatic area	T3	Tumor invades prostatic apex, into or beyond capsule, bladder neck, or seminal vesicle; not fixed
C1	No involvement of seminal vesicles	T4	Tumor fixed or invades adjacent structures other than those listed in T3
C2	Involvement of seminal vesicles		
D	Metastatic disease	N1	Metastasis in single lymph node, 2 cm or less in greatest dimension
D1	Pelvic lymph node metastases	N2	Metastasis in single lymph node, > 2 cm but < 5 cm in greatest dimension
D2	Bone of distant lymph node or organ or soft tissue metastases	N3	Metastasis in lymph node > 5 cm in greatest dimension
		M1	Distant metastases

tant bone metastases. An elevated serum alkaline phosphatase level provides supportive evidence of bone involvement. Chest x-rays are used to detect soft tissue metastases and should be done in all patients. PSA may be useful in these patients.

If the workup for distant bone metastases is negative, then it is important to evaluate lymphatic spread to determine the appropriate therapeutic approach. Lymphangiography is the most commonly used noninvasive method, but it is limited by a high false-negative rate. A fine-needle aspiration should be performed to histologically confirm a positive noninvasive study. CT scanning and MRI offer

Table 81.2.
Staging Modalities

	TNM Stage	A–D Stage	Staging Modality
Local extent	T_0–T_4	A, B, C	Digital rectal examination
			Transrectal ultrasound
			Prostate-specific antigen
			Cystoscopy
			IVP
			Flow cytometry
Lymph node	N	D	Pelvic lymphadenopathy
			Lymphangiography
			CT scan
			MRI
Distant Metastases	M	D	Radionuclide bone scan
			Bone x-ray
			Serum alkaline phosphatase
			Chest x-ray

Table 81.3.
Relative 5-Year Survival Rates (%)[a]

Year	Relative 5-Year Survival Rates	
	White	Black
1960–1963	50	35
1970–1973	63	55
1974–1976	67	58
1977–1980	72	62
1981–1986	75	62

[a] Adapted from Boring CC, Squires TS, Tong T: Cancer statistics, 1991. CA 41:19–36, 1991.

no significant advantages over lymphangiography. Since clinical staging does not always reflect the "true" stage, surgical pelvic lymphadenectomy is indicated in patients with apparently localized disease (stage A_2, B_1, and B_2).

PROGNOSIS

Over the past 30 years the relative 5-year survival rate for prostate cancer has increased significantly (Table 81.3) (1). This increase has become statistically significant in recent years, probably because of improvements in early detection and the treatment of early-stage disease rather than improvements in the treatment of advanced disease. The survival of white patients has been consistently greater than that of black patients. This may be because black patients are more often diagnosed with advanced disease. Major prognostic factors include clinical stage, the degree of histological tumor differentiation, and the underlying biologic behavior of the tumor. For example the observed 3-year survival rate for local disease is 83%; regional disease, 67%; and distant disease, 42% (16). In patients with metastatic disease, the extent of disease on the bone scan, performance status at initiation of therapy, and pretreat-

ment serum testosterone levels are important variables in determining progression-free survival (17, 18). Patients with higher pretreatment serum testosterone levels have longer survival following androgen-deprivation therapy.

TREATMENT

Treatment Overview

Treatment of prostate cancer, like most solid malignancies, depends upon the extent of disease. Patients with clinically silent, well-differentiated, local adenocarcinoma that are discovered incidentally during a transurethral resection or a needle biopsy (stage A1) require no treatment because of the usual slow progression of disease to advanced stages (19). In patients with clinical or pathologic evidence of metastatic disease (stage D) at the time of diagnosis, androgen deprivation is accepted as a preferred treatment, but controversy exists about the appropriate time to initiate endocrine therapy (20), the role of chemotherapy, and the use of concomitant radiation. The treatment of patients with stage A2, B, or C disease remains controversial (Table 81.4).

Surgery

Radical prostatectomy is a therapeutic option when the tumor is confined to the prostate, with the largest optimal volume of tumor that is amenable to surgical cure being approximately 1 to 4 centimeters (21). The anatomical location of the prostate makes this procedure technically difficult, and historically it is associated with a high incidence of postsurgical impotence and incontinence. Improved surgical techniques and the development of a nerve-sparing radical retropubic prostatectomy has resulted in increased preservation of postsurgical sexual function and a resultant increase in enthusiasm for total proctectomy to control localized prostatic cancer (stages A2 and B) (22). Surgery is also an option for the rapid reduction of serum androgens. (See "Hormonal Manipulation.")

Table 81.4.
Treatment of Prostate Cancer

Stage	Management Options
A1	Observation
A2, B	Radical prostatectomy (nerve-sparing procedure)
	Interstitial irradiation + staging lymphadenectomy
	External irradiation
C	External-beam irradiation
D	Radiation therapy—palliation
	Hormonal manipulations
	Chemotherapy
	Combination hormonal manipulations/chemotherapy

Radiation

Interstitial and external irradiation with iodine-125 and gold-198 have been used in patients with tumor confined to the prostate who are not candidates for surgical resection. Complications of radiation include impotence, proctitis, and cystitis. Additionally, radiation has been used in patients following radical proctectomy when residual disease is evident by positive margins in the surgical specimens or microscopic areas of lymph node metastases are discovered at surgery (23). Local radiation therapy is also used for palliation for painful bony metastatic disease and for prophylactic breast irradiation to prevent the pain and discomfort of gynecomastia associated with various endocrine therapies (24).

Pharmacotherapy

HORMONAL MANIPULATION

The premise for manipulation of the hormonal environment for prostate cancer management is based on reports first published in 1941 by Huggins and associates (25). Their report indicated that prostatic carcinoma cells retain some characteristics of normal prostatic epithelium. Additionally, all known types of adult prostatic epithelium appear to atrophy when androgenic stimulation is reduced. Huggins and colleagues, and later, other investigators (26) demonstrated that when the level of circulating androgen was decreased in patients with prostate cancer following orchiectomy or receiving supplemental estrogen therapy, a concurrent relief of symptoms and a reduction in serum acid phosphatase resulted. Currently, there are four strategies to manipulate the androgenic environment in the adult male including: ablation of androgen sources, inhibition of luteinizing hormone release, inhibition of androgen action, and inhibition of androgen synthesis.

Pharmacologic inhibition of androgens and the effects of androgens can be accomplished by a variety of mechanisms. Indirect suppression of testicular androgen production can be accomplished pharmacologically from estrogens, progestational agents, and luteinizing-hormone-releasing-hormone (LHRH) agonists. Agents that directly suppress testicular and adrenal androgen synthesis are available and include aminoglutethimide, ketoconazole, and spironolactone. The effects of androgens can be blocked pharmacologically at the end organ by the antiandrogens flutamide and cyproterone acetate. A combination of these approaches may lead to a more complete suppression of the effect of androgens.

Surgical Ablation. While orchiectomy rapidly reduces serum androgen levels to castration levels (<50 mg/dl), surgery is not an option in all patients because of advanced age at diagnosis, concomitant disease, and/or patient preference. Adverse effects associated with orchiectomy include nausea, vomiting, breast tenderness, gynecomastia,

impotence, and psychological disturbances. While adrenalectomy and hypophysectomy can further reduce circulating androgens, these procedures are associated with high mortality rates and are now infrequently performed.

Estrogen Therapy. The primary effect of exogenous estrogen in prostate cancer is thought to be a suppression of pituitary luteinizing-hormone release and a subsequent reduction in testosterone synthesis. The fall in serum testosterone occurs within the first week of therapy. Estrogens have been shown to also have a direct inhibitory effect on the synthesis of androgens and on the prostatic epithelial cells. Diethylstilbestrol (DES), a synthetic, nonsteroidal estrogen is the most commonly used form of estrogen therapy. A variety of other estrogen products have been used including ethinyl estradiol, conjugated estrogens, chlorotrianisene (TACE), and polyestradiol phosphate. These agents have demonstrated efficacy but have shown no therapeutic advantage over DES.

In a series of randomized trials, the Veterans Administration Cooperative Urologic Research Group (VACURG) compared the role of estrogen therapy to orchiectomy in patients with locally advanced or metastatic prostate cancer. In the initial trial, DES 5 mg/day, orchiectomy, or a combination of orchiectomy and DES 5 mg/day were compared with a placebo group (27). For patients with locally advanced disease, there was an increased risk of death from cardiovascular complications in patients treated with estrogens. Patients with distant metastases had similar overall survival rates regardless of treatment.

In the second VACURG trial, DES given at doses of 0.2 mg, 1 mg, or 5 mg daily was compared with placebo in patients with advanced disease (28, 29). DES 1 mg and 5 mg daily both reduced cancer-related deaths, compared with DES 0.2 mg, although excessive cardiovascular deaths were again noted in the patients treated with DES 5 mg. DES 5 mg daily significantly decreased acid phosphatase and testosterone levels, although clinical responses were similar in patients treated with DES 1 mg and 5 mg. DES 1 mg daily did not completely suppress serum testosterone to castration level. This trial confirmed the hazards of DES 5 mg per day. This cardiovascular risk appears to be greatest in men over 75 years of age with a previous history of cardiovascular disease. Other potential cardiovascular risk factors may include S-T segment depression during exercise and increased luteinizing hormone levels (30). Nausea, vomiting, and gynecomastia was also seen in the estrogen-treated patients.

From the results of this trial the current recommended dose of DES in the treatment of prostate cancer is 3 mg daily given in three divided doses to achieve castration levels of testosterone and minimize cardiovascular risk. This dose is between the 1-mg and 5-mg doses used in the second VACURG study. The choice between orchiectomy and estrogens as primary therapy requires consideration of the relative advantages and disadvantages of each and patient preference. There is no evidence of benefit for the concurrent or sequential use of orchiectomy and estrogen therapy. Initiating hormonal treatment in patients with asymptomatic metastatic disease is controversial (20).

LHRH Analogs. Potent LHRH analogs given in higher than physiologic doses or as a continuous infusion produce an inhibition of gonadotropin release and subsequent inhibition of testosterone production through a down-regulation of receptors in the pituitary and the testes (31). After an initial surge of LH and testosterone during the first week of drug administration, LH and testosterone decline to castration level by 2 to 4 weeks of continual therapy. The initial surge of LH and testosterone may exacerbate symptoms of disease and disease-related bone pain. LHRH agonists should be used with caution in patients with spinal metastasis and/or urinary obstruction.

Leuprolide was the first LHRH analog approved for use in the United States for the management of advanced prostate cancer. Initial phase I and II studies showed no statistically significant difference in efficacy between daily 1-mg and 10-mg subcutaneous doses (32). Common side effects included loss of libido, impotence, and hot flashes. In subsequent randomized studies, leuprolide 1 mg/day given subcutaneously was compared with DES 3 mg/day given orally (33). Median times to disease progression were not significantly different. As expected, the side-effects profile of each therapy was different. Patients treated with DES more commonly experienced painful gynecomastia, nausea, vomiting, edema, and thromboembolism compared with patients treated with leuprolide. The leuprolide treatment group reported a higher incidence of hot flashes. These studies indicate that an LHRH agonist may be a suitable alternative to estrogen therapy, but they are significantly more expensive.

Goserelin was the second LHRH agonist to be FDA-approved. Goserelin is available in a depot formulation containing the active drug in a biodegradable, sustained-release copolymer (34). The drug is administered by subcutaneous injection. The active drug is continuously released from the formulation over a 4-week period.

Although LHRH agonists have demonstrated the ability to decrease the production of testosterone, there may be a significant initial increase in androgen production that may cause disease progression. To prevent the problems associated with LHRH agonist-induced disease flare, LHRH agonists have been combined with antiandrogens (flutamide, cyproterone acetate). This combination is an attempt to further exploit the therapeutic effects of testosterone ablation and to minimize the clinical effects of the initial testosterone surge associated with LHRH monotherapy. Additionally this combination may decrease disease progression secondary to incomplete androgen blockade seen with LHRH agonists when used alone. Leuprolide has been combined in vitro and in vivo with antiandrogen agents such as flutamide (35) and cyproterone acetate (36). In one controlled trial, patients with disseminated, previously untreated prostate cancer were treated with a combination of leuprolide 1 mg daily given subcutaneously and flutamide 250 mg three times daily given orally or randomized to a combination of lueprolide and placebo (37). Patients in the leuprolide and flutamide combination group demonstrated a longer progression-free survival and an increase in the median length of survival. This treatment benefit is greatest in patients with minimal disease. A similar approach with the combination of goserelin 3.6 mg subcutaneously every 4 weeks and flutamide demonstrated similar patient survival and a small advantage in delayed time to objective disease progression, as compared with orchiectomy alone (38).

Progestational Agents. Progestational agents such as megestrol acetate, progesterone, and medroxyprogesterone acetate act by suppressing pituitary LH release, directly interfering with hormonal synthesis, and acting as an antiandrogen in prostate tissue (32). Although these agents have been studied clinically in the treatment of advanced prostate cancer (39), their use has been limited because of a reported rise in testosterone levels seen after prolonged use (40).

Miscellaneous Agents. Aminoglutethimide has been shown to inhibit the synthesis of all adrenal steroids, and therefore it leads to a reduction of serum testosterone. Aminoglutethimide, when administered with corticosteroid replacement, has been shown to produce remission in patients with prostate cancer who have previously relapsed after orchiectomy (41). Despite reports of success, aminoglutethimide is not used routinely in the management of prostate cancer. It has been reported that corticosteroids alone can reduce plasma androgen levels in orchiectomised men, and therefore the effects of aminoglutethimide are in question. Additionally, because of the inhibitory effects of aminoglutethimide on the adrenal gland, the side-effect profile of aminoglutethimide is undesirable relative to other available endocrine treatment modalities. Lastly, plasma androgen concentrations may increase in patients treated with this agent.

Ketoconazole, a substituted imidazole developed as an antifungal antibiotic, has been shown to suppress testicular and adrenal steroidogenesis through inhibition of P-450-dependent enzymes (42). Doses of ketoconazole above 400 mg have been shown to reduce serum testosterone and cortisol concentrations for 8 to 12 hr (43). Ketoconazole has been used in the treatment of advanced hormone-refractory prostate cancer (44, 45) and in previously untreated patients (45). Objective and subjective responses have been demonstrated in both settings. Adverse effects have limited the use of this agent and include gastrointestinal intolerance, hepatotoxicity, and hypoadrenalism.

The role of hormonal manipulation in the management of advanced prostate cancer is firmly established. The choice of approach or agent depends on a variety of patient factors including concurrent medical problems/risks, compliance, preference, and financial considerations. Although the LHRH analogs in the depot formulation provide an assured drug delivery in a noncompliant patient, the relative cost compared with DES may not make this a first-line approach in some patients. Conversely, the cardiovascular risks associated with estrogen therapy may preclude this as an option for some patients with concurrent heart disease. Additionally, as disease progresses through one form of hormonal manipulation, the wide variety of agents allows clinicians to modify therapy as required by patient course.

CYTOTOXIC THERAPY

The role of cytotoxic chemotherapy in the management of prostate cancer is unclear and has been reported to have little benefit (47, 48). A variety of factors contribute to the conflicting reported responses and the disappointing results of chemotherapy treatment. These include patient and disease characteristics and the methods used to measure disease response.

Since prostate cancer is primarily a disease of the elderly, concurrent medical problems and diseases play an important role in treatment choices and treatment outcomes. Men diagnosed with carcinoma of the prostate die from a wide variety of causes during the course of the disease, which may be unrelated to the malignancy. Additionally, concurrent medical problems such as cardiovascular disease or osteoblastic bone involvement of the cancer may lower the patients' ability to tolerate chemotherapy-related adverse effects. Since the clinical course of prostate cancer is variable and patients often die of unrelated medical problems, survival is often a poor criterion of therapeutic efficacy of prostate cancer therapy.

The lack of consistent response criteria has been identified as a problem with earlier clinical trials evaluating chemotherapy in prostate cancer. The assessment of the true role of chemotherapy has been difficult because of the lack of consistent criteria in the past. With the more structured criteria, hopefully current and future trials will better define the role of cytotoxic agents.

Currently, there are a variety of potentially useful strategies for chemotherapy in the management of patients with prostate cancer. However, no chemotherapy treatment approach has demonstrated a survival advantage. Therapy has included single-agent chemotherapy, combination-chemotherapy regimens, and combination chemotherapy with other treatment modalities such as surgery, radiation, hormonal manipulations, and most re-

Table 81.5.
Chemotherapy Used in
Treatment of Prostate Cancer

Doxorubicin
Mitoxantrone
Cisplatin
Cyclophosphamide
5-Fluorouracil
Methotrexate
Estradiol + chlormethine
Hydroxyurea
Melphalan
Vincristine
Bleomycin
Mitomycin
Streptozocin

cently, biologic-response modifiers. Additionally, the appropriate timing of chemotherapy in the course of disease also requires further investigation. Since prostate cancer is a disease responsive to hormonal manipulations, at this time chemotherapy is often reserved for patients with extensive disease unresponsive to endocrine manipulation or those who have escaped control after primary hormone therapy.

Single agents that have shown response rates above 20% are listed in Table 81.5. The most active agents appear to be doxorubicin and the alkylating agents such as cisplatin and cyclophosphamide.

Stable response and objective tumor responses are similar for patients receiving single-agent or combination chemotherapy. Randomized clinical trials have failed to demonstrate any superiority of combination chemotherapy to single-agent therapy. An analysis of the prospective, randomized clinical trials in the English literature concluded that there is no firm evidence to support the use of any chemotherapeutic agent as a standard against new treatments (49). Chemotherapy should be used in the setting of a controlled clinical trial to help gain information about the place of chemotherapy in the treatment of prostate cancer.

Hormonal Priming. A possible reason for the lack of response of prostate cancer to chemotherapy is the prolonged doubling time of advanced prostate cancer cells causing resistance to cytotoxic therapy. Treatment of patients with androgens prior to chemotherapy has been tried in an attempt to induce cancer cells into the cell cycle (50). Some potential problems with androgen priming have included reports of an initial tumor flare involving severe pain, tumor growth and resultant spinal cord compression.

COMBINATION THERAPY: CHEMOTHERAPY AND HORMONAL

A potential cause of tumor resistance to endocrine manipulation includes the heterogeneity of the tumor cell population. The concurrent use of cytotoxic and endocrine therapy, the use of hormone-cytotoxic conjugates or the sequencing of chemotherapy followed by hormonal therapy are strategies to overcome the heterogeneity of the tumor.

Estramustine is a nitrogen mustard covalently bound to estradiol. It is unclear if the main effect from this agent was from the hormone, the alkylating agent or the combination.

BIOLOGICAL-RESPONSE MODIFIERS

Biological-response modifiers (BRM) may prove to be potentially useful when given alone or in combination with other agents (48). Possible applications include the use of growth factors to reduce bone marrow suppression for patients receiving chemotherapy, the use of immunotherapy for antitumor effect, and the use of recombinant interferons to potentiate or to modify the expression of corticosteroid/hormone receptors on tumor cells. As with chemotherapy, the role of the various biological-response modifiers must be further explored to identify the clinical application in the management of patients with prostate cancer.

CONCLUSIONS

Currently, any hope for improvements in patient survival depend on improving the early detection of prostate cancer. Unfortunately, the pharmacotherapeutic management of prostate cancer remains palliative. An increasing number of hormonal therapy options have become available during recent years. While these options have not been shown to improve patient survival, therapy choices to meet individual patient needs have increased. The role of antineoplastic therapy and other modalitites remains an enigma. Additional studies using consistent assessment criteria are needed to determine any additional role for these agents.

REFERENCES

1. Boring CC, Squires TS, Tong T: Cancer statistics, 1991. CA 41:19–36, 1991.
2. Zaridze DG, Boyle P: Cancer of the prostate: epidemiology and aetiology. Br J Urol 59:493–502, 1987.
3. Drago JR: The role of new modalities in the early detection and diagnosis of prostate cancer. CA 39:326–336, 1989.
4. Smith JA, Middleton RG: Clinical Management of Prostatic Cancer. Chicago: Year Book Medical Publishers, 1987, ch 1, 2.
5. Mettlin C, Selenskas S, Natarajan N, et al.: β-Carotene and animal fats and their relationship to prostate cancer risk. Cancer 64:605–612, 1989.
6. McNeal JE, Bostwick DG, Anatomy of the prostate: implications for disease. In Bostwick DG: Pathology of the Prostate. New York, Churchill Livingstone, 1990, pp 3–5.
7. Bostwick DG: Prostatic intraepithelial neoplasia (PIN). Urology (suppl) 34:16–22, 1989.
8. Matuo Y, Nishi N, Wada F, Prostatic growth factor (PGF). In Karr JP, Yamanaka H: Prostate Cancer. The Second Tokyo Symposium, New York, Elsevier, 1989, p 45.
9. Gross JS: Current management modalities for prostate cancer. Geriatrics 45:60–68, 1990.
10. Surya BV, Provet JA: Manifestations of advanced prostate cancer: prognosis and treatment. J Urol 142:921–928, 1989.
11. Catalona WJ, Smith DS, Ratliff TL, et al.: Measurement of prostate-specific antigen in serum as a screening test for prostate cancer. N Engl J Med 324:1156–1161, 1991.
12. Lee F, Torp-Pederson ST, Siders DB: The role of transrectal ultrasound in the early detection of prostate cancer. CA 39:337–360, 1989.
13. Anon: Genitourinary sites. Prostate. In American Joint Committee on Cancer: Manual for Staging of Cancer, ed. 3. Philadelphia, JB Lippincott, 1988, p 177.
14. Schroder FH, Cooper EH, Debruyne MJ, et al.: TNM classification of genitourinary tumors 1987—position of the EORTC genitourinary group. Br J Urol 62:502–510, 1988.
15. Gittes RF: Carcinoma of the prostate. N Engl J Med 324:236–245, 1991.
16. Menck HR, Garfinkel L, Dodd GD: Preliminary report of the national cancer data base. CA 41:7–18, 1991.
17. Soloway MS: The importance of prognostic factors in advanced prostate cancer. Cancer 66:1017–1021, 1990.
18. Chodak GW, Vogelzang NJ, Caplan RJ, et al.: Independent prognostic factors in patient with metastatic (stage D2) prostate cancer. JAMA 265:618–621, 1991.
19. Byar DP: Veterans Administration Cooperative Urological Research Group: survival of patients with incidentally found microscopic cancer of the prostate: results of a clinical trial with conservative treatment. J Urol 108:908–913, 1972.
20. Grayhack JT, Keeler TC, Kozlowski JM: Carcinoma of the prostate: hormonal therapy. Cancer 60:589–601, 1987.
21. Perez CA, Fair WR, Ihde DC, Carcinoma of the prostate. In Devita VT, Hellman S, Rosenberg SA: Cancer Principles and Practice of Oncology. Philadelphia, JB Lippincott, 1989, pp 1023–1058.
22. Walsh PC, Preservation of sexual function and the surgical treatment of prostatic cancer: an anatomic surgical approach. In DeVita VT, Hellman S, Rosenberg SA (eds): Important Advances in Oncology 1988. Philadelphia, JB Lippincott, 1988.
23. Pilepich MV, Walz BJ, Baglan RJ: Postoperative irradiation in carcinoma of the prostate. Int J Radiat Oncol Biol Phys 10:1869–1873, 1984.
24. Corvalan JG, Gill WM, Egleston TA, et al.: Irradiation of the male breast to prevent hormone produced gynecomastia. Am J Roentgenol Radiat Ther Nucl Med 106:839–840, 1969.
25. Huggins C, Hodges CV: Studies on prostatic cancer: 1. The effect of castration, of estrogen and of androgen injection on serum phosphatases in metastatic carcinoma of the prostate. Cancer Res 1:293–297, 1941.
26. Nesbit RM, Baum WC: Endocrine control of prostatic carcinoma: clinical and statistical survey of 1818 cases. JAMA 143:1317–1320, 1950.
27. Veterans Administration Cooperative Urologic Research Group: Carcinoma of the prostate: treatment comparisons. J Urol 98:516–522, 1967.
28. Bayr DP: The VACURG studies of cancer of the prostate. Cancer 32:1126–1130, 1973.
29. Blackard CE: The VACURG studies of carcinoma of the prostate: a review. Cancer Chemother 59:225–227, 1975.
30. Henriksson P, Edhag O, Eriksson A, Johansson SE: Patients at high risk of cardiovascular complications in oestrogen treatment of prostatic cancer. Br J Urol 63:186–190, 1989.
31. Eisenberger MA, O'Dwyer PJ, Friedman: Gonadotropin hormone-

releasing hormone analogues: a new therapeutic approach for prostatic carcinoma. J Clin Oncol 4:414–424, 1986.

32. Schmidt JD, Johnson DC, Scott WW, et al.: The National Prostatic Cancer Project. Chemotherapy of advanced prostatic cancer, evaluation of response parameters. Urology 7:602–610, 1976.

33. The Leuprolide Study Group: Leuprolide versus diethylstilbesterol for metastatic prostate cancer. N Engl J Med 311:1281–1286, 1984.

34. Peeling WB: Phase II studies to compare goserelin (zoladex) with orchiectomy and with diethylstilbesterol in treatment of prostatic carcinoma. Urology (suppl) 23:45–52, 1989.

35. Labrie F, Dupont A, Belanger A, et al.: Simultaneous administration of pure antiandrogens, a combination necessary for the use of luteinizing hormone-releasing hormone agonists in the treatment of prostate cancer. Proc Natl Acad Sci 81:3861–3863, 1984.

36. Schulze H, Senge T: Influence of different types of antiandrogens on luteinizing hormone-releasing hormone analogue-induced testosterone surge in patients with metastatic carcinoma of the prostate. J Urol 144:934–941, 1990.

37. Crawford ED, Eisenberger MA, McLeod DG, et al.: A controlled trial of leuprolide with and without flutamide in prostatic carcinoma. N Engl J Med 321:419–424, 1989.

38. Iversen P, Suciu S, Sylvester R, et al.: Zoladex and fluamide versus orchiectomy in the treatment of advanced prostatic cancer: a combined analysis of two european studies, EORTC 30853 and DAP-ROCA 86. Cancer 66(suppl):1067–1073, 1990.

39. Bonomi P, Pessis D, Bunting N, et al.: Megestrol acetate used as promary hormonal therapy in stage D prostatic cancer. Semin Oncol 12:36–39, 1985.

40. Geller J, Albert J, Yen SSC: Treatment of advanced cancer of prostate with megestrol acetate. Urology 12:537–541, 1987.

41. Shaw MA, Nicholls PJ, Smith HJ: Aminoglutethimide and ketoconozole: historical perspectives and future prospects. J Steroid Biochem 31:137–146, 1988.

42. Loose DS, Kan PB, Hirst MA, et al.: Ketoconozole blocks adrenal steroidogenesis by inhibiting cytochrome P450–dependent enzymes. J Clin Invest 71:1495–1499, 1983.

43. Trachtenberg J, Halpern N, Pont A: Ketoconozole: a novel and rapid treatment for advanced prostatic cancer. J Urol 130:152–153, 1983.

44. Trump DL, Havlin KH, Messing EM, et al.: High-dose ketoconazole in advanced hormone-refractory prostate cancer: endocrinologic and clinical effects. J Clin Oncol 7:1093–1098, 1989.

45. Juberlirer SJ, Hogan T: High dose ketoconazole for the treatment of hormone refractory metastatic prostate carcinoma: 16 cases and review of the literature. J Urol 142:89–91, 1989.

46. Trachtenberg J: Ketoconazole therapy in advanced prostatic cancer. J Urol 132:61–63, 1984.

47. Raghavan D: Non-hormone chemotherapy for prostate cancer: principles of treatment and application to the testing of new drugs. Semin Oncol 15:371–389, 1988.

48. Chisholm GD: Chemotherapy for prostate cancer: present concerns and future considerations. Drugs 39:331–336, 1990.

49. Eisenberger MA, Abrams JS: Chemotherapy for prostatic carcinoma. Semin Urol 4:303–310, 1988.

50. Manni A, Santen R, Boucher AE, et al.: Androgen priming and chemotherapy in advanced prostate cancer: interim analysis of an ongoing randomized trials. Anticancer Res 6:309–314, 1986.

CHAPTER 82

PANCREATIC CANCER

JUDY L. CHASE, Pharm.D.

Pancreatic cancer is one of the greatest challenges faced by today's oncologists. In the United States pancreatic cancer is the fourth most common cause of cancer death. Only 1% of patients survive 5 years (1). In addition to the very high mortality rate, this disease is associated with morbidity secondary to the pain, malnutrition, and obstruction of the gastrointestinal or biliary tract that may occur. The only possible cure is surgical resection at an early stage, when the tumor is small and localized to the pancreas. Even in these patients the 3-year survival rate is only 15% (2). For most patients who present with advanced disease the indications for therapy are rather uncertain, and treatments that will improve survival are still being sought.

EPIDEMIOLOGY

Pancreatic cancer is a relatively rare malignancy, with approximately 28,200 new cases diagnosed in the United States in 1991 (1). The incidence has increased over the last several decades, probably as a result of an increased awareness of the disease and advances in diagnostic technology. However, the incidence and mortality have been relatively stable since 1970, except for black women whose rates have increased slightly.

It is mainly a disease of the elderly, with the median age at the time of diagnosis being 69 years; however, it may occur in young adults. There is a slight male preponderance in the incidence, which appears to vary, depending on the age of the patient at the time of diagnosis. In patients under 40 years of age, the male to female ratio is 3:1. This ratio gradually equalizes as the age of the patient increases, so that the ratio becomes 1:1 by age of diagnosis of 80 years (3). In the United States the incidence has increased in female native American Indians, black men, and in both sexes of Spanish descent. The incidence is higher in urban than in rural areas and higher in industrialized nations, implying that environmental factors play a role in the etiology. Countries with a high incidence include New Zealand, Australia, Poland, Scotland, Sweden, and certain areas of Canada. Japan and China have a low incidence compared with the U.S.; however the incidence rises rapidly in groups who immigrate to countries of high incidence.

Approximately 25,200 deaths/year in the United States are attributed to pancreatic cancer, making it the fourth most common cause of cancer death, behind lung, breast, and colorectal cancers (1). The median survival from the time of diagnosis for all patients with pancreatic cancer is 6 months, making it one of the most aggressive solid tumors (2). Most patients die of the disease and its complications such as malnutrition, gastrointestinal obstruction, and liver failure.

ETIOLOGY

Many dietary and environmental factors have been implicated as possible etiologic factors in the development of pancreatic cancer, but definite causal relationships have not been established in all cases. Employees of petroleum and chemical industries appear to be at especially high risk. Workers exposed to industrial solvents or petroleum products for more than 10 years have up to a 5-fold increase in incidence of pancreatic cancer. Cigarette smoking appears to be associated with a 2- to 3-fold increase in incidence of the disease (4, 5). Some studies have suggested an association between chronic pancreatitis, alcohol, or coffee consumption and the development of pancreatic cancer, but these findings have not been confirmed.

Approximately 15% of patients diagnosed with pancreatic cancer have a history of diabetes mellitus, implying a causal relationship between diabetes mellitus and the development of pancreatic cancer (6). However, in more than half of these patients the onset of clinical diabetes preceded the diagnosis of pancreatic cancer by only a few months. This suggests that the cancer may cause the pancreatic endocrine (insulin) insufficiency. Diabetes presenting many months to years before the diagnosis of pancreatic cancer would be better evidence for a etiologic correlation.

PATHOPHYSIOLOGY

The pancreas lies transversely in the posterior part of the upper abdomen. The head of the pancreas is on the right side of the abdomen and rests against the curve of the duodenum. The body of the pancreas lies beneath the stomach, and the tail of the pancreas extends across the abdomen to the left side. The pancreas is virtually surrounded by other organs in the upper abdomen. However, unlike other organs, it cannot be palpated because of its posterior position. Because of its position and large functional reserve, symptoms of pancreatic disease, including cancer, often do not appear until the disorder is far advanced.

The pancreas is both an endocrine and exocrine organ. Most tumors (95%) occur in the exocrine portion. Tumors of the endocrine portion are usually benign. Malignant tumors may arise from pancreatic ductal epithelial cells, acinar cells, connective tissue, or lymphatic tissue. Histologically, ductal adenocarcinoma accounts for more than 80% of all pancreatic malignancies. The head of the pancreas is the site for approximately 70% of all pancreatic tumors, with 20% occurring in the body, and 10% in the tail (2).

On gross examination, tumors of the pancreas usually appear hard, gritty, and whitish. The surrounding tissue often displays evidence of chronic pancreatitis. Tumors in the head of the pancreas are usually less than 5 cm in diameter, often associated with pancreatic and common bile duct obstruction, invasion, ulceration, and obstruction of the adjacent duodenum, and portal vein or superior mesentary artery obstruction. Tumors occurring in the tail of the pancreas are usually larger (5 to 10 cm) at the time of diagnosis and associated with splenic vein obstruction.

Early subclinical metastases are characteristic of pancreatic cancer. Less than 20% of patients have disease confined to the pancreas at the time of diagnosis. Forty percent of patients have locally advanced (regional lymph nodes, adjacent organs) disease and more than 40% have distant metastases at diagnosis.

CLINICAL PRESENTATION

The early symptoms of pancreatic cancer tend to be very nonspecific and insidious in onset, thus making the early diagnosis of the disease difficult. Approximately 80 to 90% of patients have advanced disease at the time of diagnosis. Pain in the upper abdomen is the single most common presenting symptom and is usually the reason patients seek medical attention. The pain often mimics the pain associated with peptic ulcer disease, and thus it is often misdiagnosed. Other common presenting symptoms include nausea, anorexia, weight loss, and weakness. Gastrointestinal bleeding is commonly associated with tumors in the head of the pancreas, but it is rare in tumors of the body or tail. As most tumors arise in the ductal system, biliary obstruction is common. Obstructive jaundice occurs in approximately 50% of all patients with pancreatic cancer and in up to 90% of patients with tumors in the head of the pancreas. Splanchnic nerve invasion may lead to gastrointestinal motility problems, mechanical obstruction, and severe pain. Gastrointestinal obstruction may occur secondary to local tumor invasion.

Pancreatic cancer may spread by direct invasion of surrounding tissues or by metastasizing to distant sites. Direct invasion into the abdominal lymph nodes, liver, and gastroduodenum is often present at diagnosis. In addition, pancreatic cancer commonly metastasizes to the perito-

neum and less frequently to the lungs, liver, adrenals, kidney, bone, and brain (2).

DIAGNOSIS

Since the symptoms of pancreatic cancer tend to be nonspecific and often attributed to other medical conditions, it takes a high index of suspicion on the part of the physician to make an accurate and timely diagnosis. Pancreatic cancer should be included in the differential diagnosis of any patient presenting with unexplained jaundice, pancreatitis, weight loss, and/or nonspecific upper abdominal or back pain. The goal of the evaluation in a patient with suspected pancreatic cancer is to establish the presence/absence of a primary tumor, and if present to determine the extent of local and metastatic disease. The diagnostic evaluation usually begins with a physical examination to establish clinical correlations such as jaundice, weight loss, palpable mass, ascites, or metastatic disease. Blood tests are obtained to help evaluate jaundice, liver function tests, and pancreatic serum enzyme levels. Serum enzyme levels such as amylase, lipase, alkaline phosphatase, leucine aminopeptidase, and pancreatic ribonuclease may be elevated in patients with pancreatic cancer. If the tumor involves the liver, levels of lactic dehydrogenase and the transaminases may also be elevated.

The diagnostic workup continues with noninvasive radiologic studies, then proceeds to more invasive radiologic and endoscopic procedures, and eventually to tissue biopsy. Ultrasonography of the upper abdomen is commonly used as an initial screening examination in patients suspected of having pancreatic cancer. It has the advantages of being noninvasive and relatively inexpensive, but the diagnostic yield is often limited. Computed tomography (CT) continues to be the mainstay for diagnosis, as it provides evaluation of the extent of disease (local and metastatic) and determination of resectability in patients with presumed pancreatic cancer. The most common findings on CT scan include an enlarged pancreas, a pancreatic mass, dilatation of the biliary and pancreatic ducts, hepatic metastases, and retroperitoneal lymphadenopathy. While more expensive than ultrasonography, the CT scan offers the advantages of producing superior images and allowing visualization of the entire abdomen. More invasive procedures to aid in the diagnosis of pancreatic cancer include endoscopic retrograde cholangiopancreatography (ERCP), transhepatic cholangiography, and arteriography of the pancreas. These procedures are used to visualize the pancreas, biliary tree, and vasculature.

Once a suspected pancreatic mass is identified, additional radiologic and endoscopic tests may be required to determine the extent of disease (local versus metastatic) and the surgical resectability of the tumor, if localized. If the tumor is considered unresectable or if metastatic disease is present, then histologic diagnosis should be obtained by direct fine-needle biopsy of the pancreas or percutaneous biopsy of a liver metastasis. If the tumor is considered to be possibly resectable and the patient is a surgical candidate, then the patient should be scheduled for an exploratory laparotomy. At surgery, biopsies of the pancreas, lymph nodes, and liver are obtained to confirm the diagnosis and extent of disease.

A variety of biologic substances identified in the serum of patients with pancreatic cancer may be considered tumor markers. Tumor markers are important because, depending on their sensitivity and specificity, they may aid in the differential diagnosis, identify favorable/unfavorable prognostic groups, and assist in the clinical follow-up of tumor response in patients with poorly measurable disease. At the current time, a number of potential markers have been identified, including carcinoembryonic antigen (CEA), tumor-associated carbohydrate antigen (CA 19-9), CA 125 antigen, and monoclonal antibody products (DU-PAN-2, SPAN-1). CEA is elevated in approximately 50% of patients with pancreatic cancer, but it is also elevated in many other benign and malignant gastrointestinal diseases. CA 19-9 is elevated in approximately 80% of patients with pancreatic cancer and appears to be more sensitive than CEA (7). CA 125 is elevated in less than 50% of patients with pancreatic cancer and will probably not be very clinically useful. DU-PAN-2 appears to be quite specific for identifying and following patients with pancreatic cancer, but it may also be elevated in patients with other gastrointestinal malignancies or diseases (8). Further investigation into the development of more specific and sensitive tumor markers in pancreatic cancer is required before they will be considered to be consistently clinically useful.

STAGING/PROGNOSIS

The staging system used for pancreatic cancer is based on the extent of the primary tumor, regional lymph nodes, and metastatic disease (9). The TNM staging system is presented in Table 82.1. The tumor status (T) is defined by the degree of tumor extension through the pancreatic capsule; nodal status (N) by the presence of regional lymph node involvement; and metastatic status (M) is defined by the presence of distant nodal, peritoneal, or visceral disease. The surgical staging classification based on the TNM system is defined as follows: stage I disease is localized to the pancreas and is surgically resectable; stage II disease is locally advanced and not surgically resectable; stage III disease involves the regional lymph nodes; and stage IV disease has metastatic spread. Obviously, patients with stage I disease have the best prognosis and are the only patients in which the disease is curable. Unfortunately, less than 15% of patients have stage I disease at the time of presentation. Most patients present with advanced disease (stages II, III, IV) and are considered unresectable and

Table 82.1.
TMN Staging System for Pancreatic Cancer

T1	No direct extension of the primary tumor beyond the pancreas
T2	Limited direct extension to duodenum, bile ducts, or stomach
T3	Advanced direct extension (not surgically resectable)
TX	Direct extension of tumor not assessed
N0	Regional lymph nodes not involved
N1	Regional lymph nodes involved
NX	Regional lymph nodes not assessed
M0	No known distant metastases
M1	Distant metastases present
MX	Distant metastases not assessed
Stage 1	T1–2, N0, M0: No direct extension or limited extension of tumor with no regional nodal involvement
Stage 2	T3, N0, M0: Direct extension of tumor into adjacent tissue with no lymph node involvement
Stage 3	T1–3, N1, M0: Regional lymph node involvement with or without direct tumor extension, but without distant metastases
Stage 4	T1–3, N0–1, M1: Distant metastases present

uncurable. These patients have a very poor prognosis, with less than 10% of them surviving 1 year after diagnosis.

TREATMENT

Surgery, radiation therapy, and chemotherapy are treatment options for patients with pancreatic cancer. Since most patients present with advanced-stage disease and only those with localized (resectable) disease may be potentially cured by surgical resection, the great majority of patients require palliative treatment. Unfortunately, the treatment options for this large percentage of patients have not changed the outcome in recent years.

Localized, Resectable Disease (Stage I)

Cancer of the pancreas usually presents in advanced stages with local invasion into vital structures. This makes curative surgery an option for only a small number of patients. In addition, laparotomy often reveals that the pancreatic malignancy is more advanced than was apparent on preoperative studies. Therefore, many patients thought to have the potential of being cured by surgical resection may receive only pallative operations at the time of surgery. For patients who are deemed resectable at the time of surgery, a Whipple procedure is usually performed. This operation involves the en bloc removal of the distal stomach and duodenum, the first portion of the jejunum, and the head and part of the body of the pancreas. A surgical alternative is a total pancreatectomy, which may have the advantage of preventing local recurrence. However, there are disadvantages, such as pancreatic exocrine insufficiency and permanent diabetes mellitus requiring lifelong replacement therapy. Regardless of the surgical procedure performed, it is currently recommended that patients receive postoperative (adjuvant) treatment with radiation plus chemotherapy (5-fluorouracil). Radiation therapy involves 180 to 200 cGy given daily for 5 days, followed by a 1-week rest, and then repeated for another 5-day course. The 5-fluorouracil (5-FU) is given as an intravenous bolus dose of 500 mg/m^2 on the first 3 days of each radiation course and then continued on a weekly schedule starting 1 month after the completion of the radiation treatments. This postoperative adjuvant therapy appears to increase the disease-free survival, compared with patients who receive no adjuvant therapy (10–13).

Localized, Unresectable Disease (Stages II and III)

Patients who fall into this category may be treated with a palliative surgical bypass procedure, depending on physician judgement. These palliative procedures (choledochojejunostomy or cholecystojejunostomy) are performed to treat obstructive jaundice and real or impending gastric outlet obstruction.

These operations do not prolong survival, but they usually improve the quality of life for these patients. In addition to palliative bypass surgery, these patients should be offered combined-modality therapy (radiation and chemotherapy). Based on the results of a Gastrointestinal Tumor Study Group trial completed in 1988, patients with locally unresectable pancreatic cancer who receive combined modality therapy (radiation and chemotherapy) have a prolonged survival compared with patients who receive radiation therapy alone (14). The optimal combined-modality treatment is yet to be determined. No multidrug plus radiation combination has been proven to be superior to 5-FU alone plus radiation, and therefore none can be recommended. Many types of investigational radiation therapy techniques are currently being tested including, intraoperative electron-beam irradiation, high-energy particle-beam irradiation, and interstitial implantation of I-125 (15–18). Currently, a major research focus is the use of preoperative radiation plus chemotherapy (neoadjuvant) to maximize tumor shrinkage and hopefully increase the resectability rates. Hopefully these newer radiation therapies will improve local control, but further investigation is needed. Currently there is no standard of practice; therefore, as an alternative to external-beam irradiation plus 5-FU, these patients may be entered into investigative clinical trials.

Metastatic Disease (Stage IV)

For patients with metastatic pancreatic cancer, systemic chemotherapy is the only treatment option. Radiation therapy may be used to help provide some symptomatic palliation, but the mainstay of treatment is chemotherapy. Unfortunately, only a small number of patients benefit from chemotherapy. The most active single agents include

Table 82.2.
Combination Chemotherapy Regimens for Pancreatic Cancer

FAM	5-Fluorouracil 600 mg/m^2 IV bolus days 1, 8, 29, and 36
	Doxorubicin 30 mg/m^2 IV bolus days 1 and 29
	Mitomycin C 10 mg/m^2 IV bolus day 1
	Repeat cycle every 6–8 weeks
SMF	Streptozocin 1 g/m^2 IV over 1–2 hr days 1, 8, 29, and 36
	Mitomycin C 10 mg/m^2 IV bolus day 1
	5-Fluorouracil 600 mg/m^2 IV bolus days 1, 8, 29, and 36
	Repeat cycle every 6–8 weeks

5-FU, doxorubicin, mitomycin C, streptozocin, ifosphamide, and methyl-CCNU. Only 10 to 30% of patients respond to these agents, and the responses rarely last more than 2 or 3 months (2). Many investigational agents are currently being studied, but only a few have shown response rates above 10% (epirubicin, neocarzinostatin) (19). To improve on the dismal results obtained with single-agent chemotherapy, combination chemotherapy has been used. Regimens such as FAM (5-FU, doxorubicin, mitomycin C) and SMF (streptozocin, mitomycin C, 5-FU) are outlined in Table 82.2. These regimens produced initial response rates of approximately 40%; however, subsequent trials have not confirmed the initial response rates. Response rates with these combination regimens have ranged from 2 to 40%, with a median of 20% (20). This is not substantially different from the results seen with single-agent 5-FU. Currently, no combination-chemotherapy regimen appears to be consistently superior to any other in the treatment of advanced pancreatic cancer, and there is little support for combination chemotherapy over 5-FU used as a single agent. The only chemotherapy regimen that appears to be superior to 5-FU alone is 5-FU plus leucovorin (21). The leucovorin acts as a biochemical modulator, making 5-FU more active. A variety of treatment schedules exist for administration of 5-FU and leucovorin, ranging from bolus administration to continuous infusion (Table 82.3). Which administration schedule is superior is yet to be determined. As with many other gastrointestinal cancers, the addition of leucovorin to 5-FU appears to increase response rates. Whether an increase in survival can be demonstrated remains to be documented. At the present time there is no standard therapy for patients with metastatic pancreatic cancer. Therefore, it is recommended that patients receive chemotherapy as part of a clinical trial whenever possible. Alternatively, for patients ineligible for or those who refuse clinical trials, 5-FU plus leucovorin appears to be the most reasonable choice.

SUPPORTIVE CARE

The presenting symptoms of pancreatic cancer almost always include nausea, vomiting, anorexia, weight loss, weak-

Table 82.3.
5-Fluorouracil plus Leucovorin Administration Schedules

Daily bolus schedule
Leucovorin 20 mg/m²/day × 5 days, IV over 2 hr
5-FU 375–425 mg/m²/day × 5 days, IV over 15 min, give 1 hr after the start of the leucovorin infusion
Repeat every 28 days
Weekly bolus schedule
Leucovorin 20–500 mg/m² IV over 10–15 min
5-FU 600 mg/m² IV over 10–15 min following leucovorin
Repeat weekly
Bolus schedule
Leucovorin 50–100 mg/m² IV over 10–15 min
5-FU 30 mg/kg IV over 10–15 min, 1 hr after leucovorin
Repeat every 2–4 weeks as tolerated
Continuous-infusion schedule
Leucovorin 20 mg/m²/day IV over 24 hr
5-FU 500–600 mg/m²/day IV over 24 hr
Repeat daily for 4–7 days every 28 days

---

ness, and pain. The clinical course is characterized by clinical wasting and pain, with survival usually measured in weeks to months. Given this scenario, supportive care of the patient with pancreatic cancer often becomes more important than treatment of the primary disease. Supportive care for this patient population includes but is not limited to pain control, nutritional support, and control of gastrointestinal symptoms (nausea, vomiting, constipation, gastrointestinal obstruction, etc.).

Pain

Almost all patients with pancreatic cancer experience moderate-to-severe pain during the course of their illness (22). The pathogenesis for the pain associated with pancreatic cancer is not completely understood. Etiologies may include (a) pain induced by nerves being stretched by bulky tumor mass as they pass through the retroperitoneum and over the swollen pancreas; (b) direct invasion of the autonomic and/or somatic sensory nerves by tumor; or (c) obstruction of pancreatic and/or biliary ducts by tumor, causing ductal distention and pain. The pain syndromes may overlap and be exacerbated by gastrointestinal symptoms such as the reduced bowel motility or obstruction commonly seen in these patients. Therefore, one of the first steps in pain control is recognizing the type of pain syndrome and all of the possible contributing factors. Maintaining adequate bowel function by controlling diarrhea or constipation will help decrease abdominal symptoms. Similarly, a gastrostomy or jejunostomy may provide significant relief of symptoms in patients with upper gastrointestinal obstruction.

The pancreas and surrounding structures are innervated by both somatic and visceral nerves, making pancreatic pain complex. The predominant type of pain in

pancreatic cancer is chronic, but acute pain from surgery, procedures, treatment, and/or intermittent biliary obstruction may be superimposed. The treatment of pain secondary to pancreatic cancer involves use of pharmacologic, surgical, radiologic, and neurolytic modalities. Since most of the pain associated with pancreatic cancer is secondary to the presence of tumor, the use of tumor ablative therapy should decrease pain. Unfortunately, as discussed earlier, the use of surgery, radiation, and chemotherapy has been of only limited benefit in the treatment of this disease and in the reduction of pain. Therefore, since we can not control the etiology of the pain we are often left with providing symptomatic treatment.

Analgesic drugs are the mainstay of cancer pain control. The classes of analgesics used include nonnarcotic analgesics, narcotic analgesics, and adjuvant agents (amitriptyline, carbamazepine, antihistamines, steroids, etc.). Successful application of the analgesic agents requires a full understanding of the pharmacology and pharmacokinetics, as well as the narcotic dose equivalencies. Consideration of the selection of the appropriate drug for the type and intensity of pain, regularly scheduled drug administration for chronic pain with provision for "rescue" medication for breakthrough pain, and route of administration is essential. Because of the high incidence of severe pain and gastrointestinal dysfunction in this population, parenteral drug administration is often required. Continuous infusion or intermittent administration may be accomplished in the outpatient setting by teaching self-administration or with the assistance of home-care agencies.

Many of the pain syndromes associated with pancreatic cancer are visceral, with stimuli being transmitted via the celiac plexus (24). The celiac plexus is composed of afferent and efferent fibers from T5 through T12 of the sympathetic ganglia. It innervates most of the upper abdomen, including the stomach, pancreas, liver, spleen, kidneys, and small and large bowel. Therefore, interruption of the afferent pain input by means of a celiac plexus block is a potentially effective means of controlling this visceral pain. A celiac plexus block can be performed via the percutaneous route or during surgery. This procedure is often used when pharmacologic agents have failed to adequately control the pain. After needle placement into the celiac plexus is verified, a block is accomplished by injection of a neurolytic solution, such as 50 to 100% alcohol. Approximately 85% of patients receiving celiac blocks have excellent results (significant reduction in pain), allowing a decrease in the use of pharmacologic analgesic agents (25). Complications from celiac plexus blocks performed by an experienced practitioner are minimal. Hypotension and transient back pain occur in almost all patients and should be expected. Most other complications are a result of incorrect needle placement and range from leg and chest pain to paralysis.

External-beam or intraoperative radiation therapy may also be used to reduce the pain associated with pancreatic cancer. Approximately 50% of patients experience significant pain relief within 1 to 2 weeks of treatment with these techniques. However, high doses of external-beam irradiation are required, which may cause damage to other organs, and intraoperative radiation is still considered investigational and is only available at limited medical centers in the United States.

Other procedures used in an effort to decrease the pain associated with pancreatic cancer include surgical vagotomy or splanchnicectomy. The reported experience with these procedures is too small to determine their role in the management of pancreatic cancer pain.

Nutritional Support

Weight loss and malnutrition are common in patients with pancreatic cancer, and nutritional supplementation with enteral or intravenous products may be required. Patients with gastrointestinal obstruction may require total parenteral nutrition until the obstruction can be corrected or bypassed surgically. Many patients require enteral supplementation with high-calorie products that may be given orally or by using a feeding tube. Please refer to Chapter 11, "Parenteral and Enteral Nutrition" for further recommendations.

Many patients with pancreatic cancer experience diarrhea and steatorrhea, which further hampers nutritional status. The reduction in pancreatic enzymes secondary to surgical procedures or the presence of tumor predisposes patients to malabsorption. Pancreatic enzyme replacements should be prescribed. Pancreatin and pancrelipase are substances containing amylase, lipase, and protease, which are obtained from the pancreas of the hog (Cotazym, Pancrease, Ku-Zyme, Entolase, Zymase, Viokase, Creon, Ilozyme, Festal). The dosage of these agents must be individualized, based on eating frequency and patient response. The usual initial dosage is 1 to 3 capsules or tablets before each meal or snack. The dose may be increased as necessary until symptomatic improvement occurs. Further variation in dosing requirements exists secondary to the susceptibility of these agents to acid-peptic inactivation in the stomach and duodenum. Concomitant administration of antacids or histamine (H2)-receptor antagonists (cimetidine, rantidine) may be used to decrease the inactivation of enzymes.

Another pancreatic insufficiency problem is blood glucose control secondary to reduced insulin production. This is most common in patients who have undergone pancreatic resection or total pancreatectomy. Insulin requirements must be individualized, but typically, patients will require a morning dose of NPH insulin (plus or minus some regular insulin) as well as a sliding scale of insulin that maintains mild hyperglycemia (26). Mild hypergly-cemia prevents sudden drops in serum glucose. Patients must be taught to monitor their blood glucose and administer/adjust their own insulin.

CONCLUSIONS

Pancreatic cancer is a relatively rare, but highly lethal disease resulting in the death of over 95% of patients within 5 years of diagnosis. The symptoms of this disease are vague and often attributed to more benign conditions, allowing the disease to progress to advanced stages prior to diagnosis. Only patients with very early disease are potentially curable, and the treatment of choice is surgical resection plus adjuvant radiation and chemotherapy. Effective treatments for advanced disease are still being sought. As there is no consistently effective treatment for advanced disease, these patients should be entered into clinical trials whenever possible. Since most patients experience progressive deterioration, supportive care often becomes the mainstay of therapy. Patients often require supportive care that includes control of gastrointestinal symptoms (nausea, vomiting, diarrhea, constipation, obstruction), pain control, and nutrition/metabolic support.

REFERENCES

1. Boring CC, Squires TS, Tong T: Cancer Statistics 1991. CA—A Cancer Journal for Clinicians 41:19–36, 1991.
2. Brennan MF, Kinsella T, Friedman M, Cancer of the pancreas. In De Vita VT: Cancer Principles and Practice of Oncology. Philadelphia, JB Lippincott, 1989, pp 800–835.
3. Fontham ET, Correa P: Epidemiology of pancreatic cancer. Surg Clin North Am 69:551–567, 1989.
4. Mack TM, Yu M, Hanisch R, et al.: Pancreas cancer and smoking, beverage consumption, and past medical history. JNCI 76:49–60, 1986.
5. Olsen GW, Mandel JS, Gibson RW, et al.: A case-control study of pancreatic cancer and cigarettes, alcohol, coffee and diet. Am J Public Health 79:1016–1019, 1989.
6. Karmody A, Kyle J: The association between carcinoma of the pancreas and diabetes mellitus. Br J Surg 56:362–364, 1969.
7. Steinberg W: The clinical utility of the CA 19-9 tumor associated antigen. Am J Gastroenterol 85:350–355, 1990.
8. Kiriyama S, Hayakawa T, Kondo T, et al.: Usefulness of a new tumor marker, Span-1, for the diagnosis of pancreatic cancer. Cancer 65:1557–1561, 1990.
9. Beahrs OH (ed): American Joint Committee on Cancer, Manual for Staging of Cancer, ed. 3. Philadelphia: JB Lippincott, 1988, p 109.
10. Wiley AL: Pancreatic Cancer. New York: Masson Publishing, 1980, p 107.
11. Tepper J, Nardi G, Suit H: Carcinoma of the pancreas: review of MGH experience from 1963–1973. Cancer 37:1519–1524, 1976.
12. Gastrointestinal Tumor Study Group: Pancreatic cancer adjuvant combined radiation and chemotherapy following curative resection. Arch Surg 120:899–903, 1985.
13. Gastrointestinal Tumor Study Group: Further experience of effective adjuvant combined radiation and chemotherapy following curative resection of pancreatic cancer. Cancer 59:2006–2010, 1987.
14. Gastrointestinal Tumor Study Group: Treatment of locally unresectable carcinoma of the pancreas: comparison of combined modality therapy (chemotherapy plus radiotherapy) to chemotherapy alone. JNCI 80:751–755, 1988.

15. Whittington R, Solin L, Mohiuddin M, et al.: Multimodality therapy of localized unresectable pancreatic adenocarcinoma. Cancer 54:1991–1998, 1984.

16. Dobelbower RR, Merrick H, Ahuja R, et al.: 125I interstitial implant, precision high-dose external beam therapy and 5-FU for unresectable adenocarcinoma of pancreas and extrahepatic biliary tree. Cancer 58:2185–2195, 1986.

17. Roldan GE, Gunderson L, Nagorney D, et al.: External beam versus intraoperative and external beam irradiation for locally advanced pancreatic cancer. Cancer 61:1110–1116, 1988.

18. Bagne FR, Dobelbower RR, Milligan AJ, et al.: Treatment of cancer of the pancreas by intraoperative electron beam therapy: physical and biological aspects. Int J Radiat Oncol Biol Phys 16:231–242, 1989.

19. Cersosimo RJ, Hong WK: Epirubicin: a review of the pharmacology, clinical activity, and adverse effects of an adriamycin analogue. J Clin Oncol 4:425–439, 1986.

20. Haskell CM, Selch MT, Ramming KP, Exocrine Pancreas. In Haskell CM: Cancer Treatment, ed. 3. Philadelphia, WB Saunders, 1991, p 259.

21. Bruckner HW, Crown J, McKenna A, et al.: Leucovorin and 5-fluorouracil as a treatment for disseminated cancer of the pancreas and unknown primary tumors. Cancer Res 48:5570–5572, 1988.

22. Ventafridda GV, Caraceni AT, Sbanotto AM, et al.: Pain treatment in cancer of the pancreas. Eur J Surg Oncol 16:1–6, 1990.

23. Foley KM: Pain syndromes and pharmacologic management of pancreatic cancer pain. J Pain Symptom Manage 3:176–187, 1988.

24. Saltzburg D, Foley K: Management of pain in pancreatic cancer. Surg Clin North Am 69:629–649, 1989.

25. Brown DL, Moore DC: The use of neurolytic celiac plexus block for pancreatic cancer: anatomy and technique. J Pain Symptom Manage 3:206–209, 1988.

26. Spross JA, Manolatos A, Thorpe M: Pancreatic cancer: nursing challenges. Semin Oncol Nurs 4:274–284, 1988.

CHAPTER 83

GYNECOLOGICAL CANCER

KEVIN M. RODONDI, Pharm.D.

It was estimated that in 1990 there were approximately 72,000 new cases of gynecological cancers and 23,500 deaths associated with this disease. Gynecological cancers are the fourth most common cause of cancer death in women, preceded by lung, breast, and colorectal cancers (1). The specific gynecological cancers include: vulvar, vaginal, cervical, endometrial, ovarian, and gestational trophoblastic neoplasia. This chapter focuses on the three most common gynecological cancers: ovarian, endometrial and cervical.

OVARIAN CANCER

Ovarian cancer is the fifth most common cause of cancer death in women in the United States and is the leading cause of gynecological cancer death in women. In 1990 there were an estimated 20,500 new cases of ovarian cancer and 12,400 deaths attributed to ovarian cancer in the United States (1). Epithelial ovarian cancer is the most common, representing approximately 80 to 90% of cases; the remainder are germ cell cancers. Epithelial ovarian cancers occur most frequently in adult white women and are more common after menarche, with a peak incidence in the 45- to 70-year age range. Germ cell tumors are more frequent in the nonwhite population and are primarily seen in children and young women (2–4).

Epithelial Ovarian Cancer

ETIOLOGY

The highest rates of ovarian cancer are found in industrialized countries. The exception is Japan, which has one of the lowest rates of ovarian cancer in the world. Environmental factors appear to play a role, since Japanese women migrating to the United States have an increased risk of ovarian cancer, which approaches the rate of white women in the United States by the second generation (3). A number of possible risk factors have been associated with epithelial ovarian cancer, but no clear etiology has been identified. Possible risk factors include nulliparity or low parity; ovulation not suppressed by pregnancy, lactation, or oral contraceptives; familial history of ovarian cancer; and exposure of the ovaries to industrial by-products such as talc through introduction into the vagina and retrograde flow through the reproductive tract to the peritoneal cavity (2, 3).

PATHOLOGY

Epithelial tumors disseminate by surface shedding, by lymphatic spread, or rarely, by hematogenous spread. Ovarian cancer originates and grows in the ovary and invades the ovarian capsule. After invading the capsule, the tumor sheds cells into the intraperitoneal cavity, where they are carried by the peritoneal fluid to sites on the peritoneal surfaces to form micrometastases. The micrometastases continue to shed cells into the peritoneum, increasing the spread of disease. Free-floating tumor cells are removed from the peritoneal cavity by lymphatic channels in the diaphragm. Blockage of the lymphatics of the diaphragm can result in malignant ascites. Common sites of tumor spread include the diaphragm, peritoneum, omentum, bowel surfaces, and retroperitoneal lymph nodes. Although disease is usually confined to the peritoneum, metastases to distant organs can also occur (3, 4).

SCREENING AND DIAGNOSIS

Early ovarian cancer is usually asymptomatic or associated with vague complaints such as nausea and lower abdominal discomfort, which are often dismissed or treated symptomatically. When symptoms do develop, they are usually a sign of advanced disease. Because the ovaries are in a spacious peritoneal cavity, the tumor can grow considerably before producing symptoms of pain or pressure. Pain is usually nonspecific, and there may also be discomfort from compression of the bladder or rectum. It is therefore essential that women with abdominal symptoms have a thorough physical and pelvic examination, especially perimenopausal and postmenopausal women who have other risk factors for ovarian cancer.

Tumor markers that could detect early ovarian cancer would be invaluable, since most disease is diagnosed only when it has already advanced. CA-125 is currently the most valuable marker for ovarian cancer; however, it is a nonspecific indicator and is associated with a significant number of false-negatives in early disease. For these reasons, it is not a useful screening tool for the diagnosis of ovarian cancer. Nonetheless, CA-125 does correlate with the stage and extent of disease, and elevated CA-125 levels are useful in monitoring the response to therapy. A persistent elevation of CA-125 after treatment in patients with a history of ovarian cancer is usually an indication of residual disease; however, the CA-125 level can be normal in the presence of residual disease (3, 4).

PROGNOSIS

The most significant prognostic indicators for women with ovarian cancer are the stage of the disease at the time of surgery, the amount of residual disease following initial debulking surgery, and the histologic grade of disease. Survival decreases with more advanced stages, with 5-year survival ranging from up to 80% in stage I disease to 5 to 10% in stage IV disease. The response to chemotherapy in advanced ovarian cancer is greater in patients that have minimal residual disease as a result of optimal resection at the time of surgery. Patients with well-differentiated tumor (grade 1) or moderately well differentiated tumor (grade 2) have significantly higher 5-year survival rates than patients with poorly differentiated tumors (grade 3) (3). Tumors that fall into the histological class of "low malignant potential" account for approximately 15% of all ovarian tumors and have a favorable prognosis regardless of the stage of disease (5).

TREATMENT

Surgery. Ovarian cancer requires surgery for proper staging of the disease using a system according to the International Federation of Gynecology and Obstetrics (FIGO) listed in Table 83.1. Patients undergo a thorough exploratory laparotomy that includes a careful inspection and palpation of the entire intra-abdominal space for evidence of macroscopic disease. All tumor is surgically removed when possible. If macroscopic disease is not found, a careful search for microscopic disease is undertaken, including abdominal washings and multiple biopsies. Improper staging of ovarian malignancies can affect subsequent treatment decisions and response to therapy. Treatment options after surgery are summarized in Table 83.2.

Stage I. Surgery for the removal of the primary tumor is sufficient for the treatment of stages Ia and Ib, grade 1 ovarian malignancies. Patients will undergo a thorough staging laparotomy and an abdominal hysterectomy and bilateral salpingo-oophorectomy. The uterus and contralateral ovary can be preserved in women with stage Ia disease who desire to preserve fertility. Patients with more poorly differentiated tumor (grade 3) or those who have stage Ic disease will require additional therapy with either chemotherapy, intra-abdominal radiation therapy with ^{32}P, or whole abdominal radiation therapy.

Advanced Disease. Patients with advanced disease at the time of the staging laparotomy should undergo cytoreductive surgery to remove as much of the primary tumor and metastases as possible to improve the response to subsequent chemotherapy. If removal of all of the metastases is not possible, the goal is to reduce the tumor burden to an optimal level (overall tumor dimensions <1.5 to 2.0 cm). A decision tree for treatment of advanced disease after initial surgery is outlined in Figure 83.1.

Second-look operations are performed in patients who

Table 83.1.
FIGO Stage for Primary Carcinoma of the Ovary

Stage I	Growth limited to the ovaries
Stage Ia	Growth limited to one ovary; no ascites; no tumor on the external surface; capsule intact
Stage Ib	Growth limited to both ovaries; no ascites; no tumor on the external surfaces; capsules intact
Stage Ic[a]	Tumor either stage Ia or Ib but with tumor on the surface of one or both ovaries; or with capsule ruptured; or with ascites present containing malignant cells or with positive peritoneal washings
Stage II	Growth involving one or both ovaries with pelvic extension
Stage IIa	Extension and/or metastases to the uterus and/or tubes
Stage IIb	Extension to other pelvic tissues
Stage IIc[a]	Tumor either stage IIa or IIb, but with tumor on the surface of one or both ovaries; or with capsule(s) ruptured; or with ascites present containing malignant cells or with positive peritoneal washings
Stage III	Tumor involving one or both ovaries with peritoneal implants outside the pelvis and/or positive retroperitoneal or inguinal nodes; superficial liver metastasis equals stage III; tumor is limited to the true pelvis, but with histologically proven malignant extension to small bowel or omentum
Stage IIIa	Tumor grossly limited to the true pelvis with negative nodes but with histologically confirmed microscopic seeding of abdominal peritoneal surfaces
Stage IIIb	Tumor of one or both ovaries with histologically confirmed implants of abdominal peritoneal surfaces, none exceeding 2 cm in diameter; nodes negative
Stage IIIc	Abdominal implants >2 cm in diameter and/or positive retroperitoneal or inguinal nodes
Stage IV	Growth involving one or both ovaries with distant metastasis; if pleural effusion is present there must be positive cytologic test results; parenchymal liver metastasis equals stage IV

[a] In order to evaluate the impact on prognosis of the different criteria for alloting cases to stage Ic or IIc, it would be of value to know if rupture of the capsule was 1) spontaneous or 2) caused by the surgeon; and if the source of the malignant cells detected was 1) peritoneal washings or 2) ascites.

have undergone primary surgery and subsequent chemotherapy and have no clinical evidence of disease. This procedure is used to evaluate the patient's response to initial therapy and to determine if therapy should be discontinued in patients who have no pathological evidence of disease. However, because second-line or salvage therapies in patients with persistent ovarian malignancies have not yet demonstrated an improvement in overall survival, second-look operations should be reserved for a research setting (6, 7).

Radiation Therapy. There is evidence that radiation therapy can permanently eradicate tumor deposits in patients with residual ovarian cancer. The objective of radiation therapy is to achieve tumoricidal doses to eradicate tumor deposits while preventing damage to sensitive tissues and organs in the abdominal cavity. The amount of

Table 83.2.
Treatment for Ovarian Cancer after Debulking/Staging Surgery

Stage	Treatment[a]
Ia or Ib, grade 1	No further treatment
Ia or Ib, grades 2, 3	Single-agent chemotherapy
Ic	Intraperitoneal ^{32}P radiation therapy, or total abdominal and pelvic radiation therapy, or combination chemotherapy
Stage II with postsurgical residual disease <2 cm	Systemic chemotherapy, or total abdominal and pelvic radiation therapy, or intraperitoneal ^{32}P radiation therapy
Stage II with postsurgical residual disease >2 cm	Combination chemotherapy (CP, or CC, or CAP)
Stage III with postsurgical residual disease <2 cm	Combination chemotherapy (CP, or CC, or CAP, or H-CAP, or clinical trials), or total abdominal and pelvic radiation
Stage III with postsurgical residual disease >2 cm	Combination chemotherapy (CP, or CC, or H-CAP, or clinical trials)
Stage IV	Combination chemotherapy (CP, or CC, or H-CAP, or clinical trials), intraperitoneal chemotherapy under investigation
Recurrent or refractory	Palliative surgery, single-agent salvage chemotherapy (ifosfamide, hexamethylmelamine, carboplatin, taxol), or clinical trials

[a] Abbreviations: CC, cyclophosphamide and cisplatin; CP, cyclophosphamide and carboplatin; CAP, cyclophosphamide, cisplatin, and doxorubicin; H-CAP, hexamethylmelamine, cyclophosphamide, doxorubicin, and cisplatin.

radiation required depends on tumor size. The tumoricidal dose for large tumors is approximately 5000 to 6000 cGy. Tumors <2 cm probably require doses in the range of 4500 to 5000 cGy. Lower doses may be used for microscopic ovarian carcinoma. The total dose of radiation is fractionated into multiple doses delivered over a period of approximately 30 days (4).

The acute adverse effects of radiation therapy in the treatment of ovarian carcinoma include diarrhea, nausea, vomiting, and weight loss. Radiation enteritis is the most common dose-related complication of radiation therapy. Gastrointestinal symptoms usually subside a few weeks after completion of therapy. However, diarrhea can persist for months afterwards. Radiation-induced hepatitis and nephritis can occur with doses exceeding 2500 cGy, especially if precautions have not been taken to minimize organ exposure during treatment. Radiation may cause bone marrow suppression, with a reduction in peripheral blood counts that return to normal after cessation of therapy. However, irradiated bone marrow can remain impaired for extended periods, which should be considered

for patients who may subsequently receive myelosuppressive chemotherapeutic agents (4).

Radioactive ^{32}P. Radioactive phosphorus (^{32}P), or chromic phosphate, is a radioisotope that emits beta particles with a penetration range of 3 to 5 mm. The intraperitoneal instillation of ^{32}P may sterilize microscopic peritoneal implants of tumor tissue, but it cannot treat larger tumors effectively. The usual dose of ^{32}P is 20 to 24 mCi diluted in 1 to 1.5 liters of saline and instilled into the peritoneal cavity. The most common complication of therapy is small-bowel obstruction and stenosis (3, 4).

Chemotherapy: *Initial Therapy.* With the recent introduction of more active agents, chemotherapy has become the most common form of treatment for advanced epithelial ovarian carcinoma. Alkylating agents have been studied extensively, and melphalan, cyclophosphamide, chlorambucil, and thiotepa have demonstrated similar response rates. Doxorubicin as a first-line agent has a response rate of approximately 30%. Cisplatin is one of the most active agents against ovarian cancer, with overall response rates of 25 to 40% when used as a single agent.

Selected combination regimens used in the treatment of ovarian cancer are described in Table 83.3. The standard chemotherapeutic regimen of choice for patients with advanced disease has been a two-drug combination of cisplatin and cyclophosphamide (CP) (8, 9). There appears to be a clinically relevant dose-response relationship with cisplatin over a range of 25 to 100 mg/m^2. It has not been determined if the dose-response relationship continues with doses above 100 mg/m^2, and dose-limiting peripheral neuropathy with cisplatin prevents studies at higher doses (10, 11).

Carboplatin is a second-generation platinum compound that has a dose-limiting toxicity of myelosuppression and is less nephrotoxic and emetogenic than cisplatin. Carboplatin can be administered without the hydration required for cisplatin. Studies have demonstrated that carboplatin at a dose of 400 mg/m^2 is therapeutically equivalent to cisplatin 100 mg/m^2. Initial studies comparing the substitution of carboplatin for cisplatin in the treatment of ovarian cancer have demonstrated similar response rates when given at equivalent doses (12, 13).

Patients who do not respond to an initial regimen containing cisplatin or carboplatin or who have bulky residual disease will not benefit from additional therapy with platinum compounds. These patients should be entered into clinical trials or given salvage therapy. Promising second-line agents under investigation include taxol (14), hexamethylmelamine (4), and ifosfamide (15). Therapy with these agents is outlined in Table 83.4.

A second-look laparotomy in a research setting can be useful to determine the need for additional therapy. Patients with a pathologically confirmed complete remission after initial platinum-based therapy should be observed for

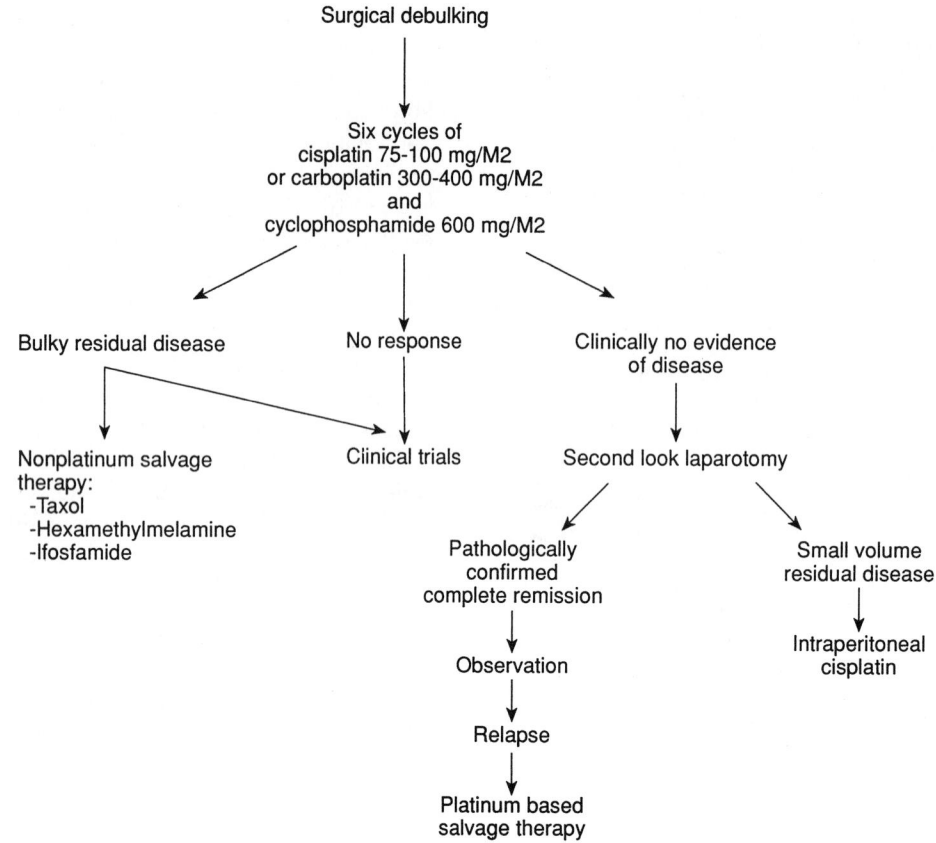

Figure 83.1.   Management of advanced stage ovarian cancer. (Reprinted with permission from Ozols RF:
New approaches to management of ovarian cancer. Adv Oncol 6:9–17, 1990.)

recurrence. If disease recurs in these patients, they should be given additional platinum-based therapy, since resistance does not develop in patients who initially respond to the platinum compounds (16). Patients who have small-volume residual disease at the time of second-look laparotomy can be given intraperitoneal cisplatin treatment (17).

Intraperitoneal Chemotherapy. Ovarian cancer usually remains confined to the peritoneal cavity throughout the disease course, and patients usually die of intra-abdominal carcinomatosis. Intraperitoneal chemotherapy was selected as a potential treatment for ovarian cancer because of the theoretical advantage of obtaining extremely high concentrations of chemotherapeutic agents at the site of the tumor, while minimizing systemic exposure to the drug. Optimal agents for intraperitoneal therapy have a low peritoneal clearance and a high systemic clearance, which prolongs contact time at the tumor site and minimizes systemic toxicity. Drugs that lend themselves to intraperitoneal therapy have a high molecular weight and low lipid solubility, achieve concentrations in the peritoneal cavity that are cytotoxic to the tumor, and are minimally toxic to the peritoneum (4, 17).

Intraperitoneal chemotherapy involves the instillation of chemotherapeutic agents into the peritoneal cavity through a specialized catheter and peritoneal-access device. The chemotherapeutic agent is usually diluted into 1.5 to 2 liters of fluid to achieve adequate distribution throughout the cavity. The fluid is instilled over 30 to 60 min and removed after a dwell-time of approximately 6 hr. The most common complications are peritonitis and catheter failure. Peritonitis is due to irritation from the drug or from infection, usually with *Staphylococcus epidermidis* or *Staphylococcus aureus* (17).

Intraperitoneal chemotherapy in ovarian cancer has been performed for a number of years, and multiple phase II studies have established numerous drugs that can be given intraperitoneally, including cytarabine, fluorouracil, methotrexate, cisplatin, carboplatin, etoposide, mitoxantrone, and α-interferon. However, there is no good evidence that intraperitoneal therapy can improve survival. Studies to date have established that intraperitoneal therapy (*a*) is technically feasible using technologically advanced catheter devices and has an acceptable complication rate; (*b*) leads to significantly higher drug concentrations in the peritoneum; (*c*) is less effective in patients with bulky disease (>2 cm); and (d) can achieve an objective response in 30% of previously treated patients with small-volume disease (18).

Germ Tumors

Germ cell tumors are relatively uncommon but aggressive tumors that occur more commonly in childhood and adolescence. These tumors are staged like epithelial tumors. There are a number of types of germ cell tumors, based

Table 83.3.
Selected Regimens for Ovarian Cancer

Epithelial Cell

AP	Doxorubicin 50–60 mg/m² IV day 1
	Cisplatin 50–60 mg/m² IV day 1
	Repeat cycle every 21 days
CAP (PAC)	Cisplatin 50 mg/m² IV day 1
	Doxorubicin 50 mg/m² day 1
	Cyclophosphamide 500 mg/m² day 1
	Repeat cycle every 21 days × 8 cycles
CDC	Carboplatin 300 mg/m² IV day 1
	Doxorubicin 40 mg/m² IV day 1
	Cyclophosphamide 500 mg/m² day 1
	Repeat cycle every 28 days
CHAP	Cyclophosphamide 300–500 mg/m² IV day 1
	Hexamethylmelamine 150 mg/m² p.o. days 1–7
	Doxorubicin 30–50 mg/m² IV day 1
	Cisplatin 50–60 mg/m² day 1
	Repeat cycle every 28 days
CP	Cyclophosphamide 1000 mg/m² IV day 1
	Cisplatin 50–60 mg/m² IV day 1
	Repeat cycle every 21 days
Hexa-CAF	Hexamethylmelamine 150 mg/m² p.o. days 1–14
	Cyclophosphamide 150 mg/m² p.o. days 1–14
	Methotrexate 40 mg/m² IV days 1 and 8
	Flurouracil 600 mg/m² IV days 1 and 8

Germ Cell

VAC	Vincristine 1.2–1.5 mg/m² (maximum 2 mg) IV weekly for 10–12 weeks, or every 2 weeks for 12 doses
	Dactinomycin 0.3–0.4 mg/m² IV days 1–5
	Cyclophosphamide 150 mg/m² IV days 1 and 8

on cellular classifications, with dysgerminomas and endometrial sinus tumors being the most common (3). Surgery and radiation are the treatments of choice in early disease, unless an attempt is being made to preserve fertility in the patient. In advanced disease, chemotherapy with VAC (vincristine/dactinomycin/cyclophosphamide) is usually used, but bleomycin-containing regimes such as PVB (cisplatin/vinblastine/bleomycin) or BEP (bleomycin/etoposide/cisplatin) may be more effective in some cases.

CERVICAL CANCER
Etiology

Cancer of the cervix is the third most frequent of the female genital cancers, with an estimated 13,500 new cases in 1990 and 6000 deaths (1). Cervical cancer is one of the only gynecological cancers that can be prevented by an inexpensive mass-screening program for detection of preinvasive lesions and early intervention in the disease process. The peak incidence of cervical cancer is between 48 and 55 years of age, with most invasive cancers occurring after age 35 (19, 20).

The frequency of cervical cancer is greater in women from a lower socioeconomic status, women who begin sexual intercourse at an earlier age, women with multiple sexual partners, and those who smoke (19, 20). The human papillomavirus (HPV) has been associated with the development of cervical cancer. Although chemical agents have not been identified as increasing the incidence of cervical cancer, the use of diethylstilbesterol (DES) in pregnant women has resulted in an increased incidence of carcinoma of the cervix and vagina in their daughters (19–21).

Pathology

Cervical carcinoma begins at the squamous-columnar junctions between the endocervical canal and cervix. The precursor lesion is dysplasia or carcinoma in situ (cervical intraepithelial neoplasia (CIN), which can become invasive cancer. Progression from dysplasia or CIN to invasive disease can be quite long, with 30 to 70% of untreated patients developing invasive carcinoma over a 10-year period.

Table 83.4.
Nonplatinum Salvage Therapy for Advanced Ovarian Cancer

Drug	Dose	Response % (patients)[a]	Reference
Hexamethylmelamine	40 mg p.o. daily on days 1–14; off days 15–28; repeat cycle	CR 15% (8/52)	(26)
Taxol	100–250 mg/m² IV over 24 hr; repeat every 22 days	PR 28% (11/40)	(27)
		CR 3% (1/40)	
Ifosfamide	1.5 g/m²/day × 5 days; repeat every 4 weeks	PR 7% (3/41)	(15)
		CR 12% (5/41)	

[a] PR, partial response (>50% reduction in tumor size); CR, complete response (disappearance of disease).

When the tumor becomes invasive, it breaks through the basement membrane into underlying tissue. In addition to local invasion, tumor spread can occur through the lymphatics or bloodstream, which can cause a distant metastasis. However, cervical cancer usually progresses in a predictable manner, and tumor dissemination is generally a function of the extent of local tumor invasion (19, 20).

Most cervical cancer is of the squamous cell type (90%), with the remainder being adenocarcinoma. There are three types of gross cervical lesions: endophytic, exophytic, and excavating or ulcerative lesions. Endophytic lesions are located within the endocervical canal of a normal-appearing cervix. Exophytic lesions are cauliflower-like, are friable, and bleed easily. These lesions may become large enough to distend the cervix, creating "barrel-shaped lesions." Ulcerative lesions are necrotic areas that erode and replace the cervix and upper vagina. They are associated with a purulent discharge and local infection (20).

Screening and Diagnosis

The woman with preinvasive disease is usually asymptomatic and is diagnosed by cytologic screening using Papanicolaou smears (Pap smears) taken during a routine pelvic examination. Routine screening has resulted in a decline in mortality from cervical cancer. Asymptomatic women 20 years of age and older and those under 20 years of age who are sexually active should have cytologic screening for 2 consecutive years and at least one screening every 3 years until age 65. Women who have multiple sexual partners, are multiparous, or began sexual activity at an early age are at higher risk and should have a yearly screening test. Routine cytologic testing is performed by many clinicians during routine annual pelvic examination (19, 21).

If dysplastic or malignant cells are discovered during screening, a visual examination using colposcopy and biopsy is recommended to further define possible disease. The staging of cervical cancer is based on clinical findings and follows the FIGO classification scheme outlined in Table 83.5.

Clinical Manifestations

Initial symptoms of early invasive disease include a watery, blood-tinged discharge. The bleeding is intermittent and may appear as postcoital spotting. As the lesion progresses the bleeding can become more pronounced. Flank or leg pain, dysuria, and rectal bleeding are symptoms of advanced disease and usually indicate pelvic metastases.

Prognosis

The major factors influencing prognosis are stage, volume and grade of tumor, histologic type, lymphatic spread and

Table 83.5.
FIGO Stage for Invasive Carcinoma of the Cervix

Stage 0	Carcinoma in situ, intraepithelial carcinoma
Stage I	Carcinoma confined to the cervix (extension to the corpus should be disregarded)
Stage Ia	Preclinical carcinomas of the cervix (diangosed only by microscopy)
Stage Ia1	Minimal microscopically evident stromal invasion
Stage Ia2	Lesions detected microscopically that can be measured, showing no more than a 5 mm depth of invasion when taken from the base of the epithelium and no more than 7 mm of horizontal spread
Stage Ib	Lesions of greater dimensions than stage Ia2 whether seen clinically or not
Stage II	Involvement of the vagina, but not the lower third, or infiltration of the parametria, but not out to the side wall
Stage IIa	Involvement of the vagina, but no evidence of parametrial involvement
Stage IIb	Infiltration of the parametria but not out to the side wall
Stage III	Involvement of the lower third of the vagina or extension to the pelvic side wall; all cases with hydronephrosis or nonfunctioning kidney unless known to be from another cause
Stage IIIa	Involvement of the lower third of the vagina, but not out to the pelvic side wall
Stage IIIb	Involvement of one or both parametria out to the side wall or hydronephrosis or nonfunctioning kidney
Stage IV	Extension beyond the true pelvis
Stage IVa	Involvement of the mucosa of the bladder or rectum
Stage IVb	Distant metastasis

vascular invasion. The 5-year survival rates range from 65 to 90% for stage I disease (70 to 75% for adenocarcinoma) to less than 15% for stage IV disease. Patients with adenocarcinomas tend to have a less favorable prognosis than patients with squamous cell carcinoma of the same stage.

Treatment

Surgery and radiotherapy are equally effective in early disease. Surgery may be preferred in younger patients to preserve reproductive function and avoid vaginal atrophy and stenosis. The utility of adjuvant chemotherapy in advanced disease has not been established, and most chemotherapeutic agents have limited activity in cervical cancer (19, 20).

CHEMOTHERAPY

Because surgery and radiation are effective initial treatments for cervical cancer, chemotherapy has not been studied extensively. Agents that have been used in the treatment of cervical cancer are listed in Table 83.6. Cisplatin is the single agent with the best documented activity against cervical cancer. Combination regimens have not

Table 83.6.
Single-Agent Chemotherapy in Cervical Cancer[a]

Drug	Overall Response (%)
Alkylating agents	
Cyclophosphamide	14
Chlorambucil	25
Ifosfamide	30
Antimetabolites	
5-Fluorouracil	20
Methotrexate	16
Mitotic inhibitors	
Vincristine	23
Antitumor antibiotics	
Doxorubicin	10
Bleomycin	10
Platinum compounds	
Cisplatin	40
Carboplatin	28

[a] Modified from Hoskins WJ, Perez C, Young RC, Gynecological tumors. In Devita VT, Hellman S, Rosenberg S: Cancer Principles and Practice of Oncology, ed. 3. Philadelphia, JB Lippincott, 1989, pp 1099–1161.

demonstrated an improvement in survival over single-agent therapy (19).

Intra-arterial chemotherapy has also been studied because of the isolated blood supply to the area of tumor burden. However, results have not demonstrated an improvement in outcome (19). Hydroxyurea has been studied as a radiosensitizer to improve the tumor-killing effect of radiation (22). Limited study results are encouraging, and other radiosensitizing agents (e.g., cisplatin) are being investigated.

ENDOMETRIAL CANCER
Etiology

Endometrial cancer is the most common gynecologic malignancy in the United States, representing more than half of the new cases of gynecologic cancers diagnosed annually. Although the incidence is high, the mortality of the disease is low, representing less than 2% of cancer deaths in women. Early diagnosis is probably responsible for the low mortality of the disease (23, 24).

The endometrium is a complex tissue responsive to endogenous and exogenous fluctuations in hormonal balance. Conjugated-estrogen therapy for the symptomatic control of menopausal symptoms without concommitant progesterone therapy (unopposed estrogen use) has been associated with an increased risk of endometrial cancer. This resulted in a warning letter to physicians from the Food and Drug Administration in 1976 (24). Other risk factors include excessive endogenous estrogen, nulliparity, obesity, diabetes, early menarche, and late menopause

(23). Recent evidence also suggests that the antiestrogen tamoxifen used in the adjuvant therapy for patients with early breast cancer can increase the risk of endometrial cancer (25). Endometrial cancer is uncommon in a women with normal menstrual cycles, presumably due to the cyclic exposure of the endometrium to progesterone. The use of a combination oral contraceptive may protect against the development of endometrial cancer (23).

Diagnosis and Clinical Manifestations

Abnormal uterine bleeding is a clearly recognizable symptom of endometrial cancer that allows early detection. Most endometrial cancers are detected early, with 95% being grade 1 or 2 adenocarcinomas (25). Diagnosis is made with a thorough physical examination to determine the tumor location and size in addition to direct cytologic sampling of the endometrium. If the tumor is advanced, additional procedures will be necessary to determine if metastases are present. Metastatic spread occurs in a characteristic pattern, and metastases can be found in the pelvic and para-aortic lymph nodes. Distant metastases can occur in the lungs, inguinal and supraclavicular nodes, liver, bones, brain, and vagina. The staging of endometrial cancer follows the FIGO classification scheme outlined in Table 83.7.

Prognosis

Endometrial cancer is highly curable, especially when diagnosed early. Stages 0 and I localized disease have a 5-year survival rate of 100% and 75 to 100%, respectively. Survival decreases as the cancer spreads outside the endometrium. The 5-year survival ranges from 60% for stage II disease to 5% for stage IV disease.

Treatment

Patients with localized disease can be adequately treated with surgery alone. Standard therapy is either hysterec-

Table 83.7.
FIGO Staging for Endometrial Carcinoma

Stage 0	Atypical hyperplasia or carcinoma in situ
Stage Ia	Tumor limited to the endometrium
Stage Ib	Invasion of $<\frac{1}{2}$ of the myometrium
Stage Ic	Invasion to $>\frac{1}{2}$ of the myometrium
Stage IIa	Endocervical glandular involvement only
Stage IIb	Cervical stromal invasion
Stage IIIa	Tumor invades serosa, adnexa, and/or positive peritoneal cytology
Stage IIIb	Vaginal metastases
Stage IIIc	Metastases to pelvic and/or para-aortic lymph nodes
Stage IVa	Tumor invasion of bladder and/or bowel mucosa
Stage IVb	Distant metastases, including intra-abdominal and/or inguinal lymph nodes

tomy or hysterectomy with adjuvant radiation therapy, depending on the histologic grade and location of the tumor. Standard therapy is usually inadequate for patients with regional or distant metastases and these patients are rarely curable.

HORMONAL THERAPY

Progestational agents have played a role in the treatment of endometrial cancer for over 20 years. Recent studies reveal an expected response of approximately 20%, but overall survival is brief. Agents that have been studied alone and in combination include medroxyprogesterone acetate, hydroxyprogesterone caproate, oxyprogesterone caproate, megesterol acetate, methyl-hydroxyprogesterone acetate, and progesterone. The antiestrogen agent tamoxifen has also been used as single-agent therapy or in combination with progestational agents. There have been no studies to compare progestational agents. Progestational agents appear to be more effective in tumors that have estrogen and progesterone cellular receptors, and the lack of receptors is an indicator of poor response to hormonal therapy (24).

CYTOTOXIC CHEMOTHERAPY

Chemotherapy is most commonly used as salvage therapy in patients with advanced disease who have failed hormonal therapy. Although many agents have been used, only several agents have been studied in sufficient numbers of patients to determine efficacy. Doxorubicin appears to have the best activity, with responses of up to 25%. Cisplatin or carboplatin also have reproducible activity, with overall responses ranging from 4 to 15%. Combination chemotherapy does not appear to have any advantage over doxorubicin alone (24). In general, there is limited information on the efficacy of chemotherapeutic agents in advanced endometrial cancer, and patients with advanced disease should be referred into clinical trials.

SUMMARY

Endometrial, cervical, and ovarian cancers are the most commonly occurring gynecological cancers. Although endometrial cancer is the most common, it is also the most curable, because of early detection of the disease. Conversely, ovarian cancer has the lowest incidence of the three, yet it is the leading cause of gynecological cancer deaths, since it is usually not detected until the disease has advanced. Improvements in the management of gynecological cancer have centered around early diagnosis versus innovative treatment. Surgery is still the treatment of choice in early disease. However, new uses of chemotherapeutic agents have improved the outcome in patients with advanced disease (Table 83.8).

Table 83.8.
Commonly Used Chemotherapeutic Agents in Gynecological Cancers

Drug	Dose	Dose Adjustment	Toxicity	Comments
Cisplatin	50–100 mg/m^2 IV	Reduce or avoid if CrCl <50 ml/min	Nephrotoxicty, peripheral neuropathy, ototoxicity	May potentiate other nephrotoxic drugs; nephrotoxicity can be reduced with hydration; causes severe nausea/vomiting
Carboplatin	300–400 mg/m^2 IV	Thrombocytopenia,[a] renal dysfunction	Myelosuppression	Does not require hydration like cisplatin and can be given easily in outpatient setting
Cyclophosphamide	500–1000 mg/m^2 IV		Hemorrhagic cystitis, myelosuppression	Hydration will reduce hemorrhagic cystitis
Ifosfamide	1200–1500 mg/m^2/day × 5 day with MESNA		Hemorrhagic cystitis, myelosuppression	Hemorrhagic cystitis common at doses >1 g if not administered with MESNA
Doxorubicin	30–60 mg/m^2	Elevated bilirubin	Cardiac	Vesicant; cardiac toxicity is cumulative and is more common at doses >550 mg/m^2 or less with chest radiation, other cardiotoxic drugs, or older patients
Hexamethylmelamine	150–260 mg/m^2/day p.o. for 14 or 21 days in a 28-day cycle	Unresponsive N/V, myelosuppression, neuropathy	Nausea and vomiting, peripheral neuropathy	Toxicities more common at initially studied high-dose continuous regimens, less pronounced with intermittent regimens
Taxol	110–150 mg/m^2 IV by 24-hr cont. infusion	Hematologic toxicity	Neutropenia, hypersensitivity	Investigational drug from yew tree; in short supply; hypersensitivity may be due to cremophor vehicle

[a] Two dosage-adjustment formulas for carboplatin have been suggested: the Calvert model (28), based on the desired area under the curve (AUC), and the Egorin model (29), based on the desired degree of thrombocytopenia.

REFERENCES

1. Silverberg E, Boring CC, Squire TS: Cancer statistics 1990. CA 40:9–26, 1990.
2. Yoder L: The epidemiology of ovarian cancer: a review. Oncol Nurs For 17:411–415, 1990.
3. Eriksson JH, Walczak JR: Ovarian cancer. Sem Oncol Nurs 6;214–217, 1990.
4. Young RC, Fuks A, Hoskins WJ, Cancer of the ovary. In Devita VT, Hellman S, Rosenberg S: Cancer Principles and Practice of Oncology, ed. 3. Philadelphia, JB Lippincott, 1989, pp 1162–1196.
5. Barnhill DR, O'Connor DM: Management of ovarian neoplasms of low malignant potential. Oncology 5:21–26, 1991.
6. Ho AG, Beller U, Speyer JL, et al.: A reassessment of the role of second-look laparotomy in advanced ovarian cancer. J Clin Oncol 5:1316–1321, 1987.
7. Young RC: A second-look at second-look laparotomy. J Clin Ontol 5:1311–1313, 1989.
8. Neijt JP, ten Bokkel Huinink WW, van der Burg MEL, et al.: Randomised trial comparing two combination chemotherapy regimens (CHAP-5 v CP) in advanced ovarian carcinoma. J Clin Oncol 5:8,1157–1168, 1987.
9. Omura GA, Bundy BA, Berek JS, et al.: Randomized trial of cyclophosphamide plus cisplatin with or without doxorubicin in ovarian carcinoma: a Gynecologic Oncology Group study. J Clin Oncol 7:4, 457–565, 1989.
10. Levin L, Hryniuk WM: Dose intensity analysis of chemotherapy regimens in ovarian carcinoma. J Clin Oncol 5:5, 756–767, 1978.
11. Ozols RF: New approaches to management of ovarian cancer. Adv Oncol 6:9–17, 1990.
12. Alberts D, Breen S, Hannigan E, et al.: Improved efficacy of carboplatin/cyclophosphamide vs cisplatin/CPA: preliminary report of a phase III randomized trial in stages III–IV suboptimal ovarian cancer. Proc Am Soc Clin Oncol 8:588, 1989.
13. Conte PF, Bruzzone M, Carino F, et al.: Carboplatin, doxorubicin, and cyclophosphamide versus cisplatin, doxorubicin, and cyclophosphamide: a randomized trial in stage III–IV epithelial ovarian carcinoma. J Clin Oncol 9:658–663, 1991.
14. Rowinsky EK, Cazenave LA, Donehower R: Taxol: a novel investigational antimicrotubule agent. JNCI 82:1247–1259, 1990.
15. Sutton CP, Blessing JA, Jomesley HD, et al.: Phase II trial of ifosfamide and mesna in advanced ovarian cancer: A Gynecologic Oncology Group study. J Clin Oncol 7:1672–1676, 1989.
16. Markman M, Rothman R, Hakes T, et al.: Second-line platinum therapy in patients with ovarian cancer previously treated with cisplatin. J Clin Oncol 9:389–393, 1991.
17. McClay EF, Howell SB: A review: intraperitoneal cisplatin in the management of patients with ovarian cancer. Gynecol Oncol 36:1–6, 1990.
18. Ozols RF: Intraperitoneal therapy in ovarian cancer: time's up (editorial). J Clin Oncol 9:197–199, 1991.
19. Hoskins WJ, Perez C, Young RC, Gynecological tumors. In Devita VT, Hellman S, Rosenberg S: Cancer Principles and Practice of Oncology, ed. 3. Philadelphia, JB Lippincott, 1989, pp 1099–1161.
20. Thompson LJ: Cancer of the cervix. Semin Oncol Nurs 6:190–197, 1990.
21. Anon: Cervical cancer (commentary). Oncology 4:121–126, 1990.
22. Vokes EE, Weichselbaum RR: Concomitant chemoradiotherapy: rationale and clinical experience in patients with solid tumors. J Clin Oncol 8:911–934, 1990.
23. Hubbard JL, Holcombe JK: Cancer of the endometrium. Semin Oncol Nurs 6:206–213, 1990.
24. Moore TD, Phillips PH, Nerenstone SR, Cheson BD: Systemic treatment of advanced and recurrent endometrial carcinoma: current status and future directions. J Clin Oncol 9:1071–1088, 1991.
25. Gurpide E: Endometrial cancer: biochemical and clinical correlates. JNCI 83:405–416, 1991.
26. Mannetta A, MacNeill C, Lyter J, et al.: Hexamethylmelamine for advanced ovarian cancer. Proc Am Soc Clin Oncol 8:833, 1989.
27. McGuire WP, Rowinsky EK, Rosenshein NB, et al.: Taxol: a unique antineoplastic agent with significant activity in advanced ovarian epitheleal neoplasms. Ann Intern Med 111:273–279, 1989.
28. Calvert AH, Newell DR, Gumbrell LA, et al.: Carboplatin dosage: prospective evaluation of a single formula based on renal function. J Clin Oncol 7:1748–1756, 1989.
29. Egorin MJ, Van Echo DA, Olman LA, et al.: Prospective validation of a pharmacologically based dosing scheme for the *cis*-diamminedichloroplatinum(II) analogue diamminecyclobutanedicarboxylatoplatinum. Cancer Res 45:6502–6506, 1985.

CHAPTER 84

PEDIATRIC AND NEONATAL THERAPY

ROBERT H. LEVIN, Pharm.D.

Pediatrics deals with humans from birth through adolescence, with specific terminology for different age groups (Table 84.1). Within pediatrics, there are as many medical specialities as there are in adult internal medicine.

Neonates, infants, and children require unique considerations, since age-related differences in physiology alter the pharmacokinetics of many drugs. In infants, particularly in neonates, differences in drug absorption, distribution, excretion, metabolism, and sensitivity affect the use and dosing of drugs. Pediatric dosing also involves various methods of calculating doses and consideration of appropriate drug formulations. The child's family or caretakers must be included in any discussion of medical treatment that involves the administration of drugs to the child. The issue of compliance with therapeutic regimens rests on the willingness of others to assist in the child's medical care.

Healthy growth and development of children are the major focuses for "Well Baby" clinics. During visits to the clinics, the parents are informed about proper nutrition, breast feeding, maternal diet, and drugs to be avoided. The feeding of synthetic infant formulas, baby foods, and table foods are also discussed. Diseases are prevented by proper nutrition and the use of prophylactic agents such as immunizations. The advantages and possible adverse effects of each immunization are thoroughly discussed.

DRUG THERAPY FACTORS
Drug Absorption

Drugs are most frequently administered to children by the oral route. Neonates have the potential for altered drug absorption as a result of decreased production of gastric acid that also reduces gastric emptying time. Neonates have a relative achlorhydria. Those drugs that are absorbed in the stomach, by remaining in the stomach for an additional 6 to 8 hr, may have enhanced effects as a result of increased absorption. Although gastric acid production increases and the pH decreases rapidly over the first 24 hr of life, levels of gastric acid equivalent to those of an adult are not reached until the child is about 1 year old. This causes a decreased absorption of acidic drugs such as aspirin. As the neonate matures into infancy, the gastrointestinal transit time increases, so that sustained-re-

lease drug products pass through the intestine very quickly. For example, in case of Theodur Sprinkles only about 50% of the drug is absorbed in children under 5 years old. The hydrolytic enzyme system of the newborn or infant may not be sufficient for absorption of certain drugs. Infants under 6 months old lack the hydrolytic enzyme to split palmitic acid from chloramphenicol palmitate, which prevents its absorption. Oral phenytoin may also be inadequately absorbed in infants under 6 months old, necessitating doses greater than usual (15 to 20 mg/kg/day) to produce therapeutic serum levels (1). Finally, conditions such as diarrhea markedly decrease the absorption of orally administered drugs.

The rectal route is used more frequently in young children than in adults, since children frequently have difficulty swallowing medications. No specific physiologic differences influence rectal absorption of medication in children; however, problems have been documented with certain suppository dosage forms. Outdated suppositories or those exposed to air may have erratic melting characteristics that cause decreased and unpredictable drug absorption. Appropriate therapeutic responses occur with suppositories of aspirin, acetaminophen, prochlorperazine, promethazine, glycerin, and others. An aqueous retention enema of theophylline is available and should be used instead of suppositories if rectal administration is necessary.

Ointments, lotions, and creams are commonly used for topical treatment of localized skin lesions that usually occur in the diaper area in infants and on the trunk, limbs, and face in children. A number of factors should be considered before selecting a topical agent. Infants, in contrast to older children, have a proportionally larger skin surface area that is capable of absorbing more topical drugs, especially if the drugs are applied to the groin and face. Inflammation increases the amount of drug absorbed, as does the occlusion that occurs with plastic-coated diapers. An infant's skin is very sensitive, so a number of chemicals frequently cause local irritation (e.g., parabens, methylsalicyclate).

The parenteral route, frequently used in hospitalized children, is seldom needed for medication administration in ambulatory children, except for immunizations or insulin administration to diabetics. Infants have a small mus-

**Table 84.1.
Pediatric Definitions**

Category	Age
Premature	<38 weeks gestation
Newborn, neonate	Birth to 1 month old
Infant, baby	1–24 months
Young child	1–5 years
Older child	6–12 years
Adolescent	13–18 years

**Table 84.2.
Percentages of Body Water**[a]

Age (Weight)	Extracellular Water (%)	Intracellular Water (%)	Total Body Water (%)
Premature baby (1.5 kg)	60	40	83
Full-term baby (3.5 kg)	56	44	74
5-month-old (7.0 kg)	50	50	60
1-year-old (10.0 kg)	40	60	59
Adult male	40	60	60

[a] Developmental changes from birth to adulthood. The extracellular and intracellular water are expressed as a percentage of total body weight. Total body water is expressed as a percentage of body weight. Data from Friis-Hansen B: Body composition during growth. Pediatrics 47:264, 1971.

cle mass, and intramuscular injections must be given in the lateral thigh rather than the arm or buttock. Absorption from intramuscular sites in neonates is slower and more erratic because of the smaller muscle mass and blood supply. Therefore, in neonates, the intravenous route is preferred. In neonates, infants, and young children, the accurate and timely administration of doses is particularly important. This requires precise dose calculation, measurement, and delivery. Microinfusion devices must deliver small volumes of fluids and medications accurately and safely. These neonatal microinfusion devices deliver intravenous fluid or medication in increments of tenths of a milliliter and have safeguards against uncontrolled free flow of fluid (2, 3).

Drug Distribution

Most drugs are primarily distributed into the aqueous portion of the body. The body weight of neonates is about 75% water; therefore, the volume of distribution of many drugs is increased. For example, the volume of distribution of theophylline in a neonate is approximately 1 liter/kg compared to 0.48 liter/kg in a 6-year-old. In addition, the total body water of neonates is 56% extracellular fluid, and many drugs are primarily distributed in total body water. Body water composition gradually falls to 40% extracellular and 60% intracellular water and 60% total body water by 1 year of age (Table 84.2) (4). Many drugs are less avidly

bound to plasma proteins in neonates, and plasma protein concentrations are also lower in neonates. This produces a higher unbound fraction of drugs such as phenytoin and sulfasoxizole, leading to an increased clearance and decreased half-life. A higher unbound fraction can also lead to increased toxicity. Thus phenytoin, which is normally 90% protein-bound, may be only 70% bound in neonates or premature infants. Serum levels of phenytoin are reported as total phenytoin levels, so that a level of 10 mg/liter (90% protein bound) really means that the unbound active level of the drug is 1 mg/liter while with 70% binding, the unbound level is 3 mg/liter, and there is the possibility of toxic effects.

Drug Metabolism

Liver metabolism is the predominant method for drug transformation. Liver enzymes are present at birth and are stimulated to proliferate by the buildup of endogenous substrate. Each of the enzyme systems matures at a different rate, but there are sufficient enzymes at 3 days postpartum, in a full-term infant, to adequately metabolize endogenous substrates. Bilirubin requires metabolism through the glucuronyl transferase pathway. This pathway matures slowly, so that by 1 to 2 weeks of neonatal age, it is capable of glucuronidating exogenous substances. At this time drugs dependent on this pathway can be safely used. If chloramphenicol were to be given to an infant under 1 week old, at the usual dose for children of 100 mg/kg/day, the drug would accumulate and cause cardiovascular collapse and cyanosis, "gray baby syndrome" (5). If required, chloramphenicol in a dose of 25 mg/kg/day can be used in the first week of neonatal life (6–8).

Bilirubin itself can be toxic to the newborn. The unconjugated, protein-bound fraction of bilirubin crosses into the brain very readily. When serum bilirubin levels reach 12 to 20 mg/dl, bilirubin will cross the blood-brain barrier and cause a yellow staining of the brain called kernicterus. Kernicterus may progress to irreversible brain damage and death when bilirubin levels are greater than 21 mg/dl. Irreversible brain damage can also occur at lower bilirubin serum levels of 12 to 20 mg/dl, if drugs such as sulfasoxizole, aspirin, or caffeine are given to the neonate. These drugs displace bilirubin from albumin and allow it to pass into the brain. Bilirubin levels over 12 mg/dl are usually treated by placing the infant under fluorescent lights. The light metabolizes the bilirubin in the skin to harmless metabolites, which are then excreted by the kidney. Other forms of treatment are phenobarbital, which induces liver enzymes, or exchange blood transfusions.

Drug Excretion

Both metabolized and unmetabolized drugs are excreted by the kidneys. Drugs are also excreted through the gas-

Table 84.3.
Age-Dependent Half-Life of Antibiotics in Serum

Age Group (Days Old)	Carbenicillin[a]		Penicillin[b]	
	Number of Patients	Average Half-Life (hr)	Number of Patients (Average Age in Days)	Average Half-Life (hr)
1–3	13	5.7	—	—
4–7	23	4.2	7 (3.7)	3.21
8–14	13	3.4	13 (9.5)	1.74
15–21	2	2.2	6 (18.5)	1.4
22–45	4	1.5	—	—

[a] Data from Nelson JD, McCracken GM: Clinical pharmacology of carbenicillin and gentamicin in the neonate and comparative efficacy with ampicillin and gentamicin. Pediatrics 52:801, 1973.
[b] Data from McCracken GH, Ginsberg C, et al.: Clinical pharmacology of penicillin in newborn infants. J Pediatr 82:692, 1973.

trointestinal tract, lungs, and sweat glands. With most drugs, these latter pathways are of only limited importance. Neonatal kidney function matures rapidly. At birth, a full-term newborn has approximately 33% of the glomerular filtration rate and renal tubular excretion capacity of an adult. This capacity is about 15% or less in premature infants. The capacity to excrete a solute load quickly increases in the first few weeks of life to about 50% of adult levels at 1 month of age. This change is reflected in the decreasing half-lives of penicillin and carbenicillin in neonates (Table 84.3). Doses of drugs that depend to a large degree on renal excretion (e.g., aminoglycosides and penicillins) must therefore be adjusted for the neonate. For example, gentamicin is given every 12 hr in the 1-week-old and every 8 hr in the 2- to 4-week-old neonate. Because of the rapidly changing characteristics of the newborn, drug-level monitoring should be used for adminoglycosides. Doses should be based on the neonate's age and weight. Drugs for normal infants and older children are administered in the usual therapeutic doses, with no adjustment needed for renal function. At about 9 to 12 months of age, the infant kidney is functioning at adult levels.

Drug Sensitivity

Neonates and infants are more sensitive to the effects of many drugs because of the immaturity of their organs. The central nervous system matures slowly and reaches adult levels at about 8 years of age. Because of this and the increased permeability of the blood-brain barrier, the neonate appears to be especially sensitive to the depressant effects of drugs such as phenobarbital, morphine sulfate, chloral hydrate, meprobamate, and chlopromazine. Codeine and meperidine do not produce this exaggerated effect in neonates.

The cardiovascular system usually functions adequately in the neonate and infant except in times of stress, when exaggerated responses may occur. General anesthetics may cause cardiovascular depression. Diuretics or antihypertensives in normal doses may induce severe hypotension.

Table 84.4.
Drugs Causing Hyperthermia[a]

Drug	Comment
Salicylates[b] Aspirin Sodium salicylate Methyl salicylate Diflunisal	Increase temperature with toxicity and cause sweating and dehydration
Nonsteroidal antiinflammatory agents[b] Ibuprofen, naproxen	Increase temperature with toxic doses
Indomethacin Mefenamic acid Piroxicam	
Dinitrophenols Herbicides, fungicides Nitrophenols Miscellaneous pesticides Insecticides	Increase temperature up to 2 days after heavy exposure, whether inhaled, ingested, or by skin contact
Anticholinergics Atropine Scopolamine Belladonna Benztropine Propantheline	High temperature can result from large doses or repeated therapeutic doses
Sympathomimetics Amphetamine and congeners Ephedrine Epnephrine Propylhexedrine inhalers Cocaine	Large doses cause chills and fever
Para-aminophenols[b] Acetaminophen	Large doses cause sweating and chills and probably fever
Antihistamines Diphenhaydramine Hydroxyzine	Large doses cause fever
Boric acid	Large doses cause fever
Thyroid preparations Leuothyroxine	Large doses cause fever
Alcohol[b]	Large doses cause fever
Antipsychotics[b] Phenothiazines Chlorpromazine	Overdoses cause fever
Tricyclic antidepressants Amitryptyline	
Others MAO inhibitors Haloperidol	
Phencyclidine (PCP)	Overdoses cause fever

[a] Adapted from Levin RH, Maltz HE, Fluid balance in drug therapy. In Waechter EH, Blake JB (eds): Nursing Care of Children, ed. 9. Philadelphia, JB Lippincott, 1976, p 102.
[b] Also causes hypothermia (see Table 84.5).

The temperature-regulating system is unstable and immature in the neonate and infant. Many drugs cause wide fluctuations in temperature and have exaggerated responses in neonates and infants. Drugs in therapeutic doses that normally lower temperature, such as aspirin and acetaminophen, can also raise the temperature when taken in toxic doses (Tables 84.4 and 84.5). The skin, in addition to its immature thermal regulatory ability, increased permeability, and large surface area, is also more sensitive to drugs. This drug sensitivity may be either allergic or toxic and may occur throughout infancy and childhood. Allergic reactions are the most common and may be of the immediate-onset type, such as urticaria, angioneurotic edema, and anaphylaxis, or of the delayed-onset types such as erythema multiforme or a fixed drug eruption. These drug-induced reactions mimic skin eruption caused by other processes. The most common drugs leading to skin reactions in pediatrics are sulfonamides, tetracyclines, penicillins, isoniazid, cephalosporins, barbiturates, phenytoin, chloral hydrate, phenothiazines, narcotics, aspirin, indomethacin, iodides, griseofulvin, and topical antihistamines. There are a number of other adverse drug effects that occur in children; (a) growth suppression with tetracycline and corticosteroids; (b) sexual precocity with androgens; (c) neurotoxicity with hexachloraphene; (d) prepubertal effects with levodopa; (e) intracranial hypertension with corticosteroids, naldixic acid, vitamins A and D, and nitrofurantoin; (f) jaundice with novobiocin, sulfonamides, and vitamin K; and (g) a bulging fontanel and tooth staining with tetracycline (9).

Dosing

Children are not small adults. Doses for neonates must be tailored to their age, weight, and decreased liver and kidney function. Doses given on a milligram per kilogram basis that have established efficacy in neonates, infants, and children can be found in a number of sources (10, 11). Drugs that are very toxic, such as cancer chemotherapeutic agents, should be, for better accuracy, dosed on a milligram per square meter basis. Body surface area takes into account the child's height and weight and is especially useful for children who are not normal for their age in either height or weight. If necessary, the body surface area can be calculated from a child's height and weight, or a suitable monogram can be used (Fig. 84.1). If a dose for a drug cannot be found in appropriate texts or current publications, the drug may not be suitable for pediatric use. This should be evaluated carefully before any dose is calculated. There are many formulas to calculate doses by the child's weight, age, body surface area, or height; however, they are all inaccurate and should not be used.

Compliance

Most compliance studies of adult ambulatory patients reveal that 50 to 70% of patients fail to complete a course of therapy. In addition, 90% of patients make at least some error in taking their medication, such as a missed dose or a dose taken at the incorrect time. In pediatrics, similar compliance problems occur. Very ill children are often unwilling to take medications. Becker et al. (12) studied mothers whose children had otitis media and were treated with oral penicillin. Mothers who were the most diligent in completing drug therapy had the following traits: (a) they were concerned about the child's health and current illness, (b) they felt that the illness was a major threat to

Table 84.5.
Drugs Causing Hypothermia[a]

Drug	Comment
Salicylates[b]	Lower fever in therapeutic doses
Aspirin	
Sodium salicylate	
Methyl salicylate (oil of wintergreen)	
Diffunisal	
Nonsteroidal antiinflammatory agents[b]	Decrease temperature with therapeutic doses
Ibuprofen, naproxen	
Indomethacin	
Mefenamic acid	
Piroxicam	
Para-aminophenol[b]	Therapeutic doses will lower fever
Acetaminophen	
Phenylbutazone	Usually used for arthritis and gout but can be used to lower temperature
Indomethacin	
Colchicine	
Chlorpromazine[b]	Lower fever
Other phenothiazines also	
Cholinergic agents	Large dose or repeated small doses cause profuse sweating and cold extremities
Physostigmine	
Pilocarpine	
Neostigmine	
Topical agents	Local cooling causes lower temperature
Water	
Alcohol[b]	
Volatile oils	
Menthol	
Sedative hypnotics	Overdoses decrease fever, causes sympatholytic syndrome
Barbiturates	
Alcohol	
Benzodiazepines	
Diazepam	
Opiates	Overdoses decrease fever by causing sympatholytic syndrome
Clonidine	Overdoses decrease fever by causing sympatholytic syndrome
Hypoglycemic agents	Overdoses decrease fever
Tolbutamide	

[a] Adapted from Levin RH, Maltz HE, Fluid balance in drug therapy. In Waechter EH, Blake JB (eds): Nursing Care of Children, ed. 9. Philadelphia, JB Lippincott, 1976, p 102.

[b] Also causes hyperthermia (see Table 84.4).

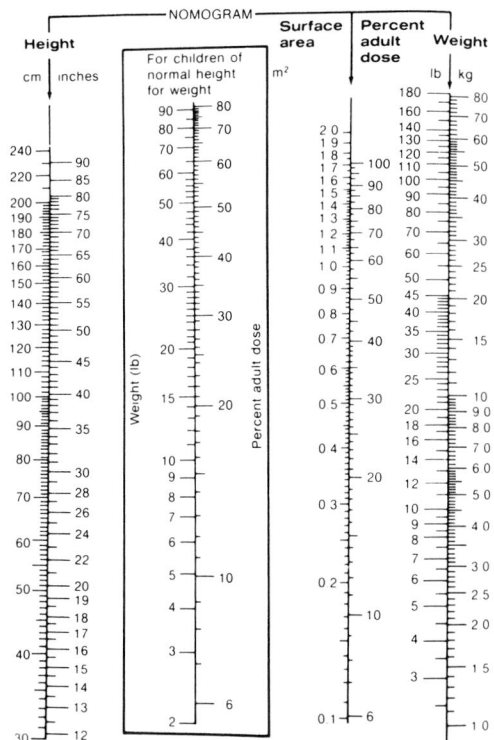

Figure 84.1. Pediatric drug therapy nomogram. (From Kegel SM, Singer MI, Critical care of infants and children after the neonatal period. In Zschoche DA (ed): Mosley's Comprehensive Review of Critical Care. St. Louis, CV Mosby, 1976. Modified from Nelson WE: Textbook of Pediatrics, ed. 8. Philadelphia, WB Saunders, 1964.)

the child's health and welfare, (c) they had confidence in the child's physician and the prescribed medication, (d) they had a more satisfactory experience with their pediatric clinic, (e) they actively endeavored to keep the child healthy and prevent future illness, and (f) they were better able to manage the problems of everyday life. In contrast, mothers who complied less well with the medication regimen had attitudes opposite to the above. Additionally, these latter mothers thought their health was bad and were more concerned with their own health problems than the health problems of their child. To achieve maximum success with medication regimens, therefore, healthcare personnel should emphasize and reinforce those traits that lead to increased compliance. Mattar et al. (13) reported that by emphasizing verbal and written patient instructions and providing calibrated measuring devices and calendars, pharmacists were able to achieve compliance levels of 51% in a cohort of 33 patients being treated with antibiotics for otitis media. In comparison, only 8.5% of 200 control patients were compliant.

Drugs that are taken only once or twice a day, are easy to swallow and palatable, and are easy to use, carry, and

store should increase compliance. The person giving medications should approach the child firmly but gently. A provocative, angry, or punishing attitude will increase the child's hostility and defensive medication-avoidance behavior. This adversary behavior affects compliance and interferes with good relationships, even in adolescents. The adolescent has all the compliance considerations of the child plus those of the adult; therefore, adolescents must be knowledgeable about and in control of their medications.

INFANT NUTRITION

Human breast milk is the most healthy and complete food for the full-term infant. It should be the only source of nutrition for infants up to 6 months of age (14, 15). Breast-feeding is usually supplemented with food in the child over 6 months old. In the United States, of those infants who are breast-fed, over 50% of infants are breast-fed until at least 3 months of age. This decreases to 25% of 6-month-old infants, and less than 5% of 9- to 12-month-old infants are still breast-feeding. In some cultures, however, children at 4 to 6 years of age are still breast-feeding to gain needed protein. There are advantages to breast-feeding: it is less expensive than infant formula, the breast is an antiseptic environment, and breast milk has proteins of better biologic value, curds that are easier to digest, more easily absorbed fat, immunoglobulins, lysozymes, antistreptococcal enzymes, complement, lactoferrin and macrophages that decrease infections.

Infants in the United States who breast-feed have a lower incidence of gastrointestinal disease, respiratory disease, otitis media, and allergies (16). There is also mounting evidence that breast-feeding is somewhat protective against developing obesity, allergy, arteriosclerosis, cystic fibrosis, celiac disease, early onset diabetes and other metabolic disorders in adulthood (17). There are also advantages for the mother: it enhances postpartum recovery, it returns women to their prepartum weight quicker, and it enhances maternal-infant bonding (14).

There are disadvantages to breast-feeding. The mother must want to nurse for it to be satisfactory and rewarding for her and the infant. The breasts must be prepared for nursing during the last trimester of pregnancy. Sometimes pain, inconvenience, engorgement, minor infections, and inflammation are associated with breast-feeding. The mother should have an adequate diet and must be careful about taking drugs that are excreted into breast milk. The mother should not breast-feed if she has active, untreated tuberculosis, breast cancer, or a serious infection. In many cases, active support and encouragement by healthcare personnel overcome most, if not all, of the maternal apprehension about breast-feeding. The maternal use of medications can be carefully planned to least affect the breast-feeding infant.

Normal Breast Physiology

The breast is composed of glandular, fibrous, and adipose tissue and rests on a bed of connective tissue. The glandular tissue is composed of 15 to 20 lobes, arranged radially around the nipple. Strands of fibrous tissue connect the lobes, and adipose tissue occupies the space between and around the lobes. Each lobe is divided into several lobules and connected by aveolar tissue, blood vessels, and ducts (Fig. 84.2a) (18). Each lobule contains a small lactiferous duct. Eventually, these lactiferous ducts unite and form a single main canal for each lobe. These 15 to 20 main canals each become dilated and form a reservoir (sinus lactiferous) for milk storage and finally merge and pass through the nipple.

The functioning part of the breast is the alveoli or acini (sacs) in the lobule (Fig. 84.2b). It is in the acini that milk is produced and secreted into the lactiferous ducts. Drugs cross from the blood in the capillary beds through the acini epithelium and into the lactiferous ducts.

Normal Composition of Milk

The composition of milk is determined by the mammary gland, with little or no external control (19, 20). The milk occurs in three forms: colostrum, transitional, and mature milk. Colostrum, which serves as a precursor of milk, may be expressed from the breasts as early as the fourth month of pregnancy, but it usually appears after parturition. It is scanty the first few days after birth, becomes well-established on the third or fourth day, and usually continues for no more than 5 days. It has, however, been known to continue for as long as 10 days. Colostrum is a transudate consisting primarily of serum albumin (3 to 5%) and cast-off epithelium (colostrum corpuscles) that has undergone fatty degeneration. It has a higher specific gravity than mature milk (1.030 to 1.060 compared with 1.026 to 1.036) and also a higher average pH (7.7 compared with 6.8). It is richer in vitamin A, sodium, potassium, and other minerals but lower in sugar and fat. Colostrum is quickly modified by the mammary gland into transitional milk.

Transitional milk is produced within the first week of breast-feeding. It usually lasts for a few weeks, during which time a moderate increase in fat and sugar and gradual decrease in proteins and minerals occurs. Milk finally matures near the end of the first month of lactation.

Mature milk has between 0.9 and 1.6% protein, 2 to 6% fat, and 6.5 to 8% lactose. The composition of milk at the beginning of a feeding is highest in protein and lowest in fat. This is reversed toward the end of the feeding. The effect of this on the excretion of drugs is unknown.

Once established, mature milk varies little in composition (19, 20). If the mother has adequate nutritional intake, her diet can be quite varied without affecting milk composition or volume. A deficiency in maternal diet will first cause a decrease in the quantity of milk but will not

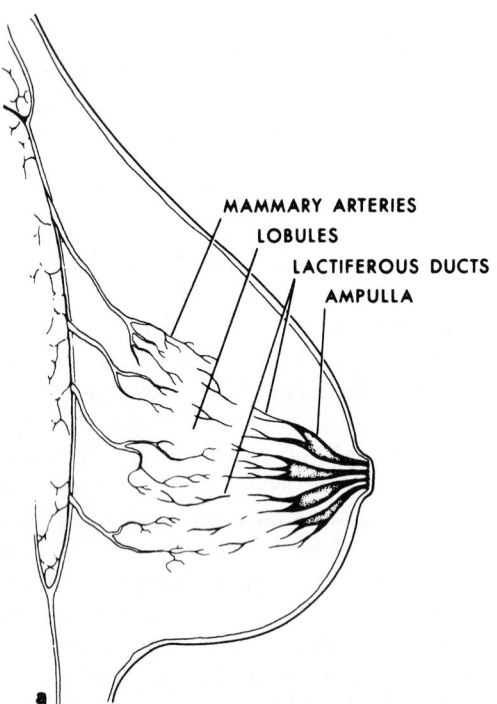

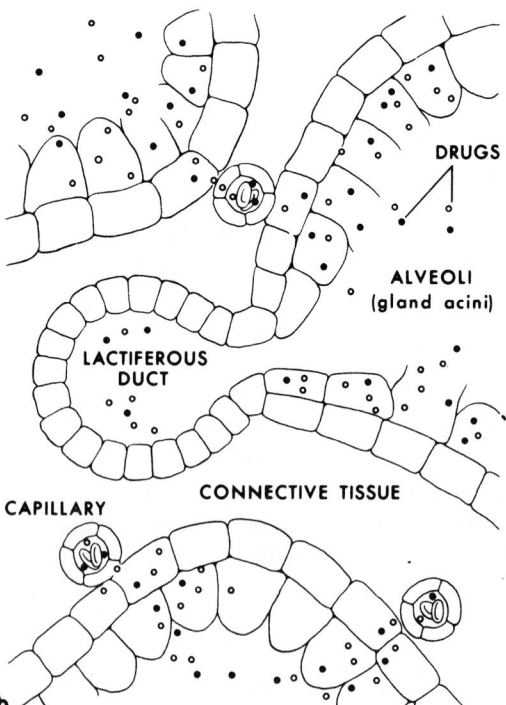

Figure 84.2. *A*, Cross-section of breast. *B*, Magnified cross-section of lobule depicting drugs entering alveoli from capillaries.

(Adapted from Arena J: Contamination of the ideal food. Nutr Today 5:2, 1970.)

affect milk composition unless the mother's tissue stores are depleted. A decreased water intake will cause maternal thirst before it affects milk production.

Control of Milk Production

The initiation and maintenance of milk production has not been adequately studied; however, the evidence regarding physiologic and endocrine factors in lactation is better understood now (16). Lactation usually begins at birth or shortly thereafter. The inhibition of lactation during pregnancy is assumed to be the result of the high estrogen or progesterone levels. The effects of estrogen on milk secretion are dose-dependent. At low endogenous levels occurring postpartum, milk secretion occurs, whereas lactation is inhibited by high doses of estrogens (diethylstilbestrol or parental estrogens given postpartum). In most women, low-dose oral contraceptives do not decrease lactation, even when given immediately postpartum (21). Estrogens may work partly by affecting prolactin (lactogenic factor), which is secreted from the anterior pituitary.

Prolactin is presently under extensive investigation in an effort to delineate its true role during pregnancy and lactation (16). During pregnancy, prolactin, estrogen, progesterone, and human growth hormone stimulate breast development. There are high concentrations of prolactin during pregnancy and breast-feeding, but low concentrations after birth in the absence of breast-feeding. If breast-feeding is successful and unrestricted, the high levels of prolactin have been reported to be contraceptive (22). This contraceptive effect is seen only in certain societies and has not been observed in the U.S.A., where formula supplements are frequently given.

The posterior pituitary, in addition to the anterior pituitary, is involved in and stimulated by an infant breast-feeding. The release of oxytocin by the posterior pituitary initiates the "letdown" reflex. Oxytocin stimulates the expression of ejection of milk from the breast, the letdown reflex, whereas prolactin stimulates milk production. The letdown reflex is responsive to other internal and external factors. The actions and sounds associated with nursing can initiate this reflex. In contrast, distractions such as fright, pain, and emotional distress can inhibit milk expression. It is hypothesized that the high levels of the catecholamines, adrenaline and norepinephrine produced in such circumstances cause a vasoconstriction in the mammary circulation that prevents oxytocin from reaching the contractile cells (16). Excessive doses of medications that also release endogenous catecholamines (e.g., amphetamines and most decongestants) many interfere with milk secretion.

Quantity of Milk Produced

The quantity of milk produced depends upon the demands of the infant. If the infant's demand is increasing, milk

Table 84.6.
Quantities of Milk Ingested

Amount at Each Feeding[a] (ml)	Age (weeks)
20–45	1
30–90	2
40–140	4
60–150	6
75–165	12
90–175	16
120–225	24

[a] Feedings are usually every 3–4 hr; quantity consumed depends on infant's weight.

supply will adjust accordingly within 2 days and vice versa. The actual secretion of milk is a discontinuous process. During feeding there is increased milk secretion as a result of the depletion of milk stores. In all probability, drugs are excreted into milk in larger amounts when the milk is being actively secreted. To derive the total quantity of drug ingested (measured as milligrams per deciliter), it is necessary to know the quantity of milk ingested by the infant. This depends on the age and weight of the infant (Table 84.6). See Chapter 88, "Drugs in Pregnancy and Lactation," for a discussion of drugs excreted in breast milk.

If women cannot breast-feed, prepared infant formulas are the best substitute and are covered in Chapter 85, "Pediatric and Neonatal Nutrition."

Infants who are over 6 months old usually do not require the standard formulas with 20 cal/oz, so a reduced 16-cal/oz formula such as Advance was developed. Cow's milk plus baby food also provides adequate nutrition for this age group. If cow's milk is used, the daily intake should be kept to 1 quart or less. More than 1 quart/day can lead to milk intolerance, diarrhea, and iron-deficiency anemia secondary to the large intake of protein, which may cause an enteropathy. Reducing the intake of milk to less than a quart and supplementing with iron-rich infant food resolves the enteropathy and its sequelae. The infant foods used should be those with the least possible added salt, sugar, and monosodium glutamate (MSG). These substances are added to improve the taste for increased adult acceptability. The added sodium and MSG have been casually implicated in predisposing susceptible infants to developing hypertension as adults (23). The inclusion of MSG in infant food seems unwarranted. The added sugar may predispose infants to obesity by increasing the total number of fat cells.

The daily intake of infant foods for the 6-month-old should consist of two or more servings of meat, four or more servings of vegetables, one or more servings of citrus fruits, and four or more servings of bread or cereal. The size of each serving should increase as the child grows. The use of infant foods may start as early as 2 to 3 months of age, with cereals, and then the addition of vegetables,

Table 84.7.
Causes of Fever of Unknown Origin (FUOs)

Causes	Age <6 Years (%)	Age 6–14 Years (%)	Age >14 Years (%)
Infections	65	38	36
Neoplastic diseases	8	4	19
Autoimmune diseases	8	23	13
Miscellaneous	13	17	25
Undiagnosed (FUOs)	6	18	7

fruits, and meats as tolerated. Junior foods, which contain small chunks of solid food, are usually begun at 8 to 12 months of age. Adult table food is usually begun at 1 year of age. If the child receives a normal, varied diet that contains the required nutrients, no added supplements are needed. Giving a normal child additional vitamins and minerals adds nothing to health and is an unneeded expense. Vitamins and minerals should only be used if nutritional deficiencies have been documented.

FEVERS IN CHILDREN
Etiology

One of the most common symptoms of illness is fever, which is a mechanism for fighting infection. It is one of the most common childhood complaints, and it is important to separate mild febrile disease from a serious infection. The cause of mild fevers in children are usually upper (URIs) and lower (LRIs) respiratory infections caused by assorted viruses, including influenza. Bacterial infections causing otitis media, sore throat, urinary tract infections, or respiratory infections also quite commonly cause fever.

Complications

Children who are at the greatest risk for complications from a febrile illness and who must be watched carefully if they develop a sudden fever, are those that are (*a*) under 2 months of age with temperature over 38°C, (*b*) those 6 to 24 months old with temperature over 40°C, or (*c*) any child with a temperature over 41°C. Children under 2 months old do not manifest the usual signs and symptoms of systemic disease, for example, fever or inflammation, and it is therefore very difficult to diagnose serious disease in these infants before it becomes life-threatening. Children between 6 and 24 months with a fever have a high risk of having been infected with either *Streptococcus pneumoniae* or *Haemophilus influenzae*. Children at any age with high fevers (above 41°C) are at great risk of having severe systemic bacterial sepsis or meningitis.

Children who have prolonged undiagnosed fevers (>38°C) for more than 2 weeks in duration are classified as having a fever of unknown origin (FUO). There are a number of causes of FUOs, as depicted in Table 84.7.

These unexplained fevers require a much more extensive workup and are generally much more serious. Most fevers are caused by infections. Neoplastic disease is the least common cause of fever in the 6- to 14-year-olds.

Treatment

Fever does not have to be treated pharmacologically unless it is causing morbidity or is debilitating for the patient. Fevers should be treated if the patient is irritable, very sick, delirious, or has shaking chills or seizures. In bacterial infections, the fever decreases as the child recovers and provides a convenient monitoring parameter for the efficacy of antibiotics.

The two most commonly used antipyretic analgesics for treating fevers in children are aspirin and acetaminophen. The analgesic/antipyretic dose is the same on a milligram-for-milligram basis for both agents. The usual oral or rectal dose is 5 to 10 mg/kg/dose (about 65 mg/kg/day) given every 4 to 6 hr. If one agent at the maximum dose is not effective for lowering temperature, both agents can be used, alternating doses every 2 hr. This avoids doubling the dose of either agent and causing toxicity. The toxicities of these agents are different. Aspirin causes more toxicity in children under 2 years old, and in overdoses leads to fluid, electrolyte, and acid-base imbalances. Acetaminophen, generally thought to be less toxic, may in high doses cause hepatic toxicity (24, 25).

Caution is needed when treating fevers or pain with analgesics in children or adolescents under 19 years old with flu or varicella infections. Acetaminophen is the analgesic of choice because of the risk of developing Reye's syndrome. The syndrome usually starts in a patient recovering from the illness, who suddenly starts vomiting and deteriorates rapidly. Some patients may get better slowly, but many go on to develop symptoms that consist of metabolic encephalopathy associated with hepatic failure. Although it is a rare disease, 204 cases were reported in 1984 and none in 1989 in the United States (26). Most cases of Reye's syndrome occur in children between 6 and 18 years of age. Reye's syndrome may occur in children whether or not they have taken aspirin during their antecedent illness, but aspirin seems to increase the chances for developing this syndrome, possibly by altering the immune system of susceptible children, and therefore, increasing the virulence of infection. It may also predispose the child to metabolic complications by acting as an additional insult (27–31).

The treatment consists of fluid and electrolyte therapy for the patient's metabolic requirements and mannitol and other agents to reduce cerebral edema. Vitamin K, barbiturates, hypothemia, or corticosteroids may also be used. The mortality rate is between 20 and 40%, and permanent brain damage may occur in those who survive (32).

The FDA now requires a warning on all aspirin-containing products: "Children and teenagers should not use this medicine (aspirin) for chickenpox or flu symptoms before a doctor is consulted about Reyes syndrome, a rare but serious illness." Patients and parents should be alerted to this warning.

CONCLUSION

Health maintenance and disease prevention, including proper nutrition and an immunization program, are important aspects of the practice of pediatrics. Certain illnesses such as upper respiratory viral infections, otitis media, infantile diarrhea, and other febrile diseases are so common that all children can be expected to suffer several episodes before they are 6 years old.

Proper therapy instituted quickly can prevent these minor diseases from becoming more serious. Although many of these pediatric diseases are treated in the same way as they are in adults, neonates, infants, and children have unique characteristics that call for additional knowledge of drug therapy. Considerations in drug therapy in pediatrics include the influence of normal growth and development on drug absorption, distribution, and elimination, as well as dosage formulation to facilitate compliance.

REFERENCES

1. Watson PD, Powell JR, Mimaki T, Anticonvulsant usage. In Jaffe ST (ed): Pediatric Pharmacology and Therapeutics—Principles in Practice. New York, Grune & Stratton, 1980, pp 195–212.
2. Zenk KE: Drug use in neonates. U.S. Pharmacist 11:H2–H20, 1986.
3. Zenk KE: Special delivery: delivering IV antibiotics to children. Nursing 86 16:50–52, 1986.
4. Friis-Hansen B: Body composition during growth. Pediatrics 47:264, 1971.
5. Nelson JD: Antimicrobial drugs. In Jaffe SJ (ed): Pediatric Pharmacology and Therapeutics—Principles in Practice. New York, Grune & Stratton, 1980, pp 187–198.
6. Nelson JD, McCracken GM: Clinical pharmacology of carbencillin and gentamicin in the neonate and comparative efficacy with ampicillin and gentamicin. Pediatrics 52:801, 1973.
7. McCracken CH, Ginsberg C, Nelson JD, et al.: Clinical pharmacology of penicillin in newborn infants. J Pediatr 82:692, 1973.
8. Levin RH, Maltz HE, Fluid balance in drug therapy. In Waechter EH, Blake JB (eds): Nursing Care of Children, ed. 9. Philadelphia, JB Lippincott, 1976, p 102.
9. Tatro DA, Adverse drug reactions in children. In Pagliaro LA, Levin

10. Zenk KE, Neonatal and pediatric dosing. In Pagliaro LA, Levin RH (eds): Problems in Pediatric Drug Therapy. Hamilton, IL: Drug Intelligence Publications, 1979.
11. Levin RH, Zenk KE, Medication table. In Rudolph AM (ed): Pediatrics, ed. 18. Norwalk, CT, Appleton-Century-Crofts, 1987.
12. Becker MH, Drachman RH, Kirscht JP: Predicting mothers' compliance with pediatric medical regimens. J Pediatr 81:843, 1972.
13. Mattar ME, Markello J, Jaffe SJ: Pharmaceutical factors affecting pediatric compliance. Pediatrics 55:101, 1975.
14. Lawrence RA: Breastfeeding: A guide for the medical profession, ed. 3. St. Louis, CV Mosby, 1989, p 12.
15. Barness LA: Bases of weaning recommendations, J of Pediatrics. Supplement on Dietary Patterns and Nutrient Intake of U.S. Infants. 117:S84–85, 1990.
16. Chen Y, Yu s, Li Wx: Artifical feeding and hospitalization in the first 18 months of life. Pediatrics 81:52, 1988.
17. Lawrence RA: Breastfeeding and medical disease. Med Clin North Am 73:583–603, 1989.
18. Arena J: Contamination of the ideal food. Nutr Today 5:2, 1970.
19. Holt LE, Feeding techniques and diets. In Barnett HL (ed): Pediatrics, ed. 15. New York, Meredith Corp. 1972, p 148.
20. Jelliffe DB, Jelliffe EFP: The volume and composition of human milk in poorly nourished communities—a review. Am J Clin Nutr 31:492, 1978.
21. Gambrell R: Immediate postpartum oral contraception. Obstet Gynecol 36:101, 1970.
22. Jelliffe DB, Jelliffe EFP: Lactation, conception and the nutrition of the nursing mother and child. J Pediatr 81:829, 1972.
23. Committee on Nutrition: Sodium Intake by Infants in the United States. Evanston IL: American Academy of Pediatrics, 1979.
24. APHA Project Staff: Handbook of Non-prescription Drugs, ed. 7. Washington, D.C. American Pharmaceutical Association, 1982, p 123.
25. Anon: Aspirin or paracetamol. Lancet 2:287, 1981.
26. Centers for Disease Control: Summary of notifiable diseases, United States 1989. MMWR 38 (54), 1990.
27. Anon: Salicylate labeling may change because of Reye's syndrome. FDA Drug Bull 12:9, 1982.
28. Waldman RJ, Hall WN, McGee M, et al.: Aspirin as a risk factor in Reye's syndrome. JAMA 247:3089, 1982.
29. Halpin TJ, Holtzhauer FJ, Campbell RJ, et al.: Reye's syndrome and medication use. JAMA 248:687, 1982.
30. Starko KM, Ray CGJ, Dominguez LB, et al.: Reye's syndrome and salicylate use. Pediatrics 66:859, 1980.
31. Hurwitz ES, Barrett MJ, Bregman D, et al.: Public Health Service Study on Reye's Syndrome and Medications. N Engl J Med 313:849, 1985.
32. Rudolph AM: Pediatrics, ed. 18. Norwalk, CT, Appleton-Century Crofts, 1987.

CHAPTER 85

PEDIATRIC AND NEONATAL NUTRITION

CHRISTINE A. MOWATT-LARSSEN, Pharm.D., EMILY B. COCHRAN, Pharm.D., MICHAEL L. CHRISTENSEN, Pharm.D., STEPHANIE J. PHELPS, Pharm.D., and RICHARD A. HELMS, Pharm.D.

Adequate nutrition is necessary throughout life to maintain body structure and integrity. Pediatric patients require additional nutrients to meet the demands of growth and development. Failure to provide essential nutrients can result in serious sequelae, including growth retardation, impairment of the immune system, and neurological deficits. The premature neonate presents a unique nutritional challenge to the clinician, since transition to the extrauterine environment is made before the fetus is fully developed. With increased prematurity, there is a decreased lean body mass, decreased fat stores, decreased micronutrient and mineral stores, and organ system immaturity, which affect the approach to nutrition support in these patients.

During the past 20 years, important advances have been made in our understanding of nutrient requirements in children. Preterm and term infants who are unable to tolerate breast milk may receive a number of enteral formulas that meet their specialized nutrient requirements. Likewise, there are a number of commercially available enteral formulas to meet the nutritional requirements of older children and adolescents. The most significant advancement in the nutritional care of the high-risk neonate has been the development of parenteral nutrition. Although the first report of the successful use of total parenteral nutrition in an infant occurred almost 50 years ago, only in the last 20 years has parenteral nutrition been widely used. Hospitalized and ambulatory children with a variety of surgical or medical conditions have been successfully nourished using parenteral nutrition. During the past 2 decades, our understanding of macronutrient and micronutrient requirements has rapidly expanded. Practitioners are now able to individualize various nutrients with the parenteral nutrition solution based on age, weight, nutritional status, and disease.

NUTRITIONAL ASSESSMENT AND MONITORING

While similar nutritional assessment techniques (1–5) are used in both children and adults (see Chapter 11, "Parenteral and Enteral Nutrition"), children require unique consideration for almost all parameters assessed.

Weight

All pediatric patients receiving parenteral nutrition should have their weight measured on a daily basis, unless medically prohibited. The addition or deletion of clothes, wound dressings, or arm boards used to stabilize an intravenous line can alter the apparent weight, making interpretation of daily fluctuations difficult. Significant variation in weight can also be seen when different scales are used. Assessment of weight gain should be made over several days, since daily weight change may be related to factors other than increases in lean body mass.

Intake and Output

Intake and output should be carefully assessed and summarized daily. A patient's intake consists of maintenance fluids, blood products, and fluid used in the delivery of medications and flushes. Output includes urine, stool, nasogastric or gastrostomy tube drainage, emesis, blood loss, ventriculostomy drainage, and wound drainage. In an infant, urine and stool losses can be approximated by weighing diapers before and after elimination. If possible, urine and stool volumes should be recorded separately. Evaluation of daily weight in conjunction with daily assessment of total intake and output will aid in the evaluation of fluid balance.

Growth Charts

Growth charts derived from large populations of pediatric patients in the United States allow an individual child to be compared graphically to age-related standards for height, weight, and head circumference (6). Growth-chart information should be used as a preliminary assessment of nutritional status and may often assist the practitioner in identifying nutrition deficits and in differentiating between acute and chronic malnutrition (7). A weight below the population standard may indicate acute malnutrition, while a weight and height below the population standard may suggest chronic malnutrition (7). After initial measurements have been made and values plotted on growth curves, periodic assessment of weight and height allow the chart to be used for longitudinal assessment of growth and response to nutritional support (8).

Anthropometric Measurements

Anthropometric measurements can be an effective means of monitoring response to nutritional support in children (8). Age-related nomograms have been developed for arm circumference and triceps skinfold using American children from 10 states (9). Using this nomogram, Frisancho calculated age-related percentiles for arm muscle area, arm muscle diameter, and arm muscle circumference (10). Subscapular skinfold standards have also been developed using British children (11). To minimize variability between consecutive measurements, the same trained individual, same site of measurement, and same caliper type should be used to assess a given patient.

Visceral Proteins

Serum albumin, transferrin, transthyretin (prealbumin), and retinol-binding protein are the primary visceral protein markers used in nutritional assessment (12–16). While the half-lives of visceral proteins in children are similar to those in adults, the age-related normal serum concentrations are lower for younger patients. Transthyretin and retinol-binding protein concentrations increase following nutritional support in otherwise healthy appropriate-for-gestational-age infants (17) and premature infants (18). Likewise, these markers increase in critically ill, malnourished infants receiving nutrition support (19). Recently, a simplified, inexpensive nephelometric prealbumin kit (PAB, Beckman Instruments, Inc., Brea, CA) was introduced. The commercial availability of this micronized assay technology may increase the clinical use of transthyretin measurements in pediatric patients.

Urine Studies

A 24-hr urine collection is used to determine total nitrogen output and to calculate nitrogen balance ([total nitrogen in] − [total nitrogen out]). Nitrogen balance studies are used routinely in adults to assess adequate provision of protein and energy. Although nitrogen balance studies are relatively easy and noninvasive to perform in older children, problems exist with similar studies in neonates and infants (20). To collect urine for 24 hr in an uncatheterized pediatric patient, a urine collection bag must be placed around the genital area with an adhesive and remain affixed securely for 24 hr. Collection bags that do not fit adequately, adhesives that do not stick properly, skin breakdown under the adhesive, and stool contamination of the collected urine lead to inaccurate results. When a 24-hr urine collection is impractical, a 6-hr urine collection has been proposed as an alternative means of estimating nitrogen losses for nitrogen-balance calculation (21). Despite the difficulties encountered with urine collections in neonates and infants, skilled nursing care and accurate intake and output records enable the clinician to make a reasonable estimate of urinary nitrogen excretion. Other indirect methods for estimating lean body mass have been used including urinary 3-methylhistidine and creatinine excretion (22, 23).

Immune Function

Assessments of immune function may be less helpful in assessing the nutritional status of children than of adults. The lack of an immunologic response to a specific challenge may not indicate malnutrition but may be secondary to immaturity or a lack of antigenic experience (24, 25). Only 12% of healthy infants under 7 months of age exhibited a delayed hypersensitivity response to an intradermal *Candida* skin test, while 80% of infants above 7 months of age had a positive response (25). Helms et al. noted improved lymphocyte function and enhanced expression of T-cell populations in malnourished infants receiving short-term parenteral nutrition (8, 26). Immune system maturation in neonates and premature infants dictates their immune response and must be considered when interpreting immune function studies.

FLUID REQUIREMENTS

Fluid needs are based on water losses from skin and respiration, urine and stool output, water accumulation in newly formed tissues, and water production from the oxidation of carbohydrate (27, 28). Evaporative skin losses are related directly to the body surface area and the quality of the skin as a barrier. The body surface area per unit weight is greater in children than adults, resulting in greater fluid requirements per unit weight in children. Fluid requirements are 90 to 100 ml per 100 calories in children (29), and decrease to 45 ml per 100 calories in adults. Maintenance fluid requirements for term infants and children can be calculated from the equations described by Holliday and Segar (Table 85.1) (30).

Fluid requirements may be altered by immaturity, activity, environment, or pathology (27, 31, 32). During gestation, the percentage of total body weight as water and the percentage of body water as extracellular fluid decrease in the fetus. Following birth, the extracellular fluid volume contracts, and a diuresis occurs that results in weight loss (27, 33, 34). With increasing prematurity, the percentage of extracellular fluid is increased; therefore, the percentage of total body weight loss is increased (31). Organ immaturity and greater body surface area per unit weight in

Table 85.1.
Daily Maintenance Fluid Requirement for Term Infants and Children[a]

Weight	Fluid
Up to 10 kg	100 ml/kg[b]
>10 to 20 kg	1000 ml + 50 ml/kg for every kg >10 kg
>20 kg	1500 ml + 20 ml/kg for every kg >20 kg

[a] Adapted from Holliday MA, Segar WE: The maintenance need for water in parenteral fluid therapy. Pediatrics 19:823–832, 1957.
[b] Preterm infants may require 120–150 ml/kg.

Table 85.2.
Range of Electrolyte Composition (mEq/liter) of
Gastrointestinal Secretions

Secretion	Na$^+$	K$^+$	Cl$^-$	HCO$_3^-$
Saliva	35–60	10–20	15–35	50
Gastric	10–115	5–35	10–150	0
Pancreatic	115–155	5–10	55–110	70–90
Bile	130–165	5–15	80–120	35–50
Midjejunum	70–125	5–30	70–135	10–20
Ileostomy	90–140	5–30	60–135	15–50
Diarrhea	25–50	35–60	20–40	35–45

the preterm neonate results in increased sensible and insensible water losses. The skin and subcutaneous tissue are thinner and more permeable in the preterm infant, resulting in increased evaporative losses (35). In addition, these infants are likely to be under radiant warmers or require ultraviolet light for treatment of neonatal jaundice, which may further increase evaporative water losses (36, 37). Renal immaturity may result in an inability to excrete a concentrated urine, which will increase the fluid volume that preterm neonates require (38, 39). Renal function matures with increasing postconceptional age; thus, the ability of neonates to regulate water metabolism should improve with time (40). Certain diseases in the preterm neonate have been associated with excessive fluid intakes, including bronchopulmonary dysplasia (41), necrotizing enterocolitis (42), intraventricular hemorrhage (43), and a patent ductus arteriosus (44).

Like adults, children with congenital cardiac or renal anomalies, increased intracranial pressure, syndrome of inappropriate secretion of antidiuretic hormone (SIADH), or pulmonary edema may require varying degrees of fluid restriction. Conversely, patients with excessive fluid losses (i.e., fever, diarrhea or increased stool or ostomy output, vomiting, burn or wound exudate, fistula drainage, or patients under radiant warmers or ultraviolet lights) require additional fluids to compensate for these losses. These outputs should be replaced with fluids that are equivalent in volume and electrolyte composition (Table 85.2).

PARENTERAL NUTRITION
Administration

Numerous venous access sites have been used for the infusion of parenteral nutrition solutions. Peripheral catheters are generally placed in the dorsum of the foot or hand, and scalp veins may be used in small infants and children with limited vascular access. Peripheral access limits the composition of the parenteral nutrition solution. As the solution tonicity increases, infusion complications such as phlebitis and infiltration become important considerations. An important problem with peripheral infu-

sion is infiltration of the fluid into the interstitial tissue, an expected event but usually relatively benign. However, infants and small children who have limited extravascular tissue space and who may not be able to communicate pain adequately are at risk for the development of serious sequelae secondary to infiltration. Phelps and Helms described risk factors for infiltration in children (45).

In practice, the final osmolality for peripherally infused solutions is similar to that used for adults, but dextrose concentration is usually higher (10 to 12.5%) and amino acid concentration lower (2 to 3%). Although peripheral solutions are considerably less hypertonic than central venous solutions (850 mOsm/liter vs 1800 mOsm/liter), they are still potentially harmful to tissue should infiltration occur. Calcium and potassium, two known irritants, should not be administered in peripheral solutions at concentrations exceeding 6 to 10 mEq/liter or 40 to 60 mEq/liter, respectively. Several techniques have been used to prolong survival of peripheral venous catheters in children, including the concomitant infusion of intravenous fat emulsion and the addition of heparin 1 U/ml parenteral nutrition solution.

Peripheral parenteral nutrition can be used successfully in pediatric patients who are relatively well-nourished and require parenteral nutrition for less than 14 days. Fifty to 75 kcal/kg/day and 2 to 3 g/kg/day of protein can be provided by this route, if fluids are not restricted.

Children that require extended periods of parenteral nutrition, due to prolonged alimentary tract dysfunction, should have a central venous catheter placed surgically. The most common and convenient site for placement is the superior vena cava, with the catheter tip lying at the superior vena cave–right atrial junction (Fig. 85.1). A chest radiograph is obtained immediately after insertion to verify that the catheter is appropriately placed.

The most frequently used central venous catheters for long-term access are the Broviac or Hickman catheters. A Dacron cuff, which is part of both catheters, is placed subcutaneously near the exit site and stimulates the formation of a fibrous adhesion that anchors the catheter and prevents migration of pathogenic organisms from the skin surface to the central circulation. Totally implantable vascular-access devices are now used in pediatric patients who require long-term central venous access. Compared with external catheters, implantable access devices require less maintenance, are less noticeable, impose fewer restrictions on patient activity, and have a lower infection rate (46, 47). A Huber needle is required for insertion through the skin into the port. Careful care of the skin over the port is essential if infectious complications associated with needle insertion are to be avoided.

Composition of Parenteral Nutrition Solutions
Typically, parenteral nutrition solutions contain 2 to 5% amino acids, 10 to 25% dextrose, and electrolytes, vitamins,

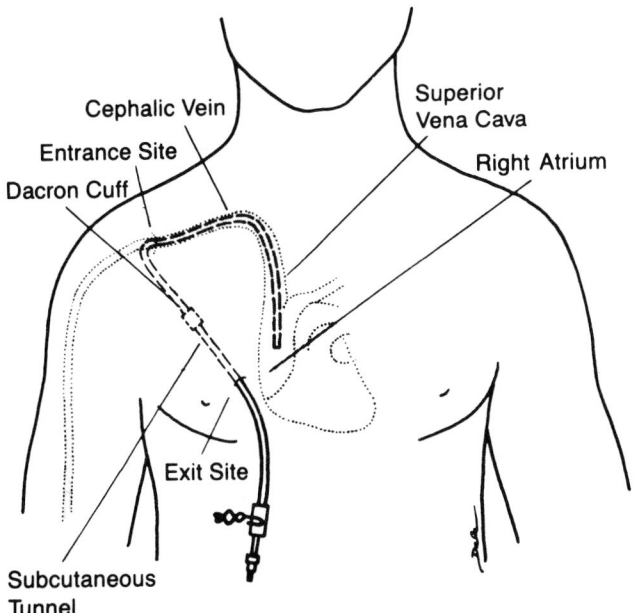

Figure 85.1. Placement of central venous catheter.

and minerals in amounts sufficient to meet the patient's daily requirements (Table 85.3). Intravenous fat emulsions (10 or 20%) offer a concentrated source of calories and are used as a source of essential fatty acids. The proportion of calories from each of the major nutrients should approach the percentages in the average enteral diet: 50 to 60% carbohydrate, 30 to 40% fat (higher percentage fat in neonatal and infant diet), and 10 to 15% protein. Providing a balanced formula reduces the risk of toxicities or complications associated with excessive or inadequate administration of any nutrient. In some institutions, the fat emulsion is added directly to the parenteral nutrition solution, referred to as a total nutrient admixture (TNA) or three-in-one (48). The use of TNAs in pediatrics is subject to several compositional limitations including pH changes that alter calcium and phosphorous solubility and lipid particle instability resulting from a high calcium concentration. In addition, a 0.22-micron filter cannot be used with TNAs.

Protein Requirements

Approximately 20 years ago, protein hydrolysates were used parenterally; however, these products were associated with hyperammonemia, compositional variability, occasional allergic reactions, and poor nitrogen utilization (49). Early crystalline amino acid products were also associated with metabolic acidosis that occurred secondary to the use of hydrochloride salt forms of several amino acids and hyperammonemia that resulted from inadequate arginine at least one formulation. Today, crystalline amino acid formulations are the source for nitrogen in parenteral

nutrition solutions. Compositional inadequacies in standard amino acid formulations have led investigators to consider the development of an "ideal" amino acid formulation for pediatric patients (50).

Parenteral protein requirements in children are determined by age, development, and coexisting disease. Although protein requirements in the premature infant and the catabolic older child are still areas of intense research, sufficient experience permits general recommendations about protein requirements in the pediatric patient. Guidelines for protein needs can be found in Table 85.4.

The preterm infant and neonate require not only quantitatively greater protein intake than the older child or adult but also qualitatively different amino acids for optimal growth and development (50). Cysteine, taurine, tyrosine, and histidine have all been described as condi-

Table 85.3.
Typical Peripheral and Central Line Solutions Used in Infants and Children (per liter)

	Dextroxe 10% Solutions for Peripheral Use		Dextrose 25% Solutions for Central Use	
Solution name[a]	CPF 3%	IPF 2.4%	CCF 3%	ICF 2.4%
Amino acid (g)	30[b]	24[c]	30[b]	24[c]
Dextrose (g)	100	100	250	250
Electrolytes				
Sodium	51 mEq	38.5 mEq	51 mEq	38.5 mEq
Potassium	20 mEq	20 mEq	20 mEq	20 mEq
Chloride	51 mEq	38.5 mEq	51 mEq	38.5 mEq
Acetate	12 mEq	8.2 mEq	12 mEq	8.2 mEq
Phosphate	5.5 mmol	8 mmol	5.5 mmol	8 mmol
Calcium	6 mEq	10 mEq	8 mEq	25 mEq
Magnesium	3 mEq	4 mEq	3 mEq	4 mEq
PTE[d]	NR[e]	3 ml	2 ml	3 ml
Selenium	NR	30 μg	20 μg	30 μg
Multivitamin[f]				

[a] CPF, child (≥12 kg) peripheral formula; IPF, infant peripheral formula; CCF, child central formula; ICF, infant central formula.
[b] Standard crystalline amino acid formulation.
[c] Pediatric crystalline amino acid formulation (L-cysteine HCl at 40 mg/g protein (admixed at dispensing).
[d] Pediatric trace element solution, per ml: 1 mg Zn, 100 μg Cu, 25 μg Mn, 1 μg Cr.
[e] NR, none required for short-term administration.
[f] Pediatric multivitamin (see dosing recommendations with vitamin section).

Table 85.4.
Parenteral Protein Requirements (g/kg/day)

Preterm	2.5–3.0
Infant/neonate	2.0–2.5
Infant	1.5–2.0
Preschool/school-age	1.0–1.5
Adolescent	0.8–1.5
Adult	0.8–1.0

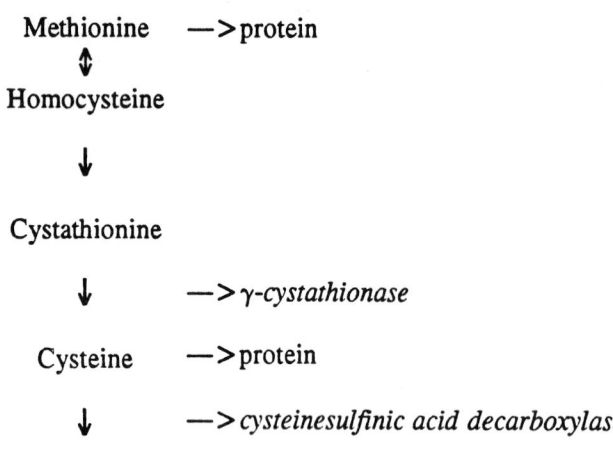

Figure 85.2. Metabolic pathway for the conversion of methionine to cysteine and taurine.

tionally essential amino acids for preterm infants and neonates. Enzyme immaturity in the metabolic conversion of methionine to cysteine and cysteine to taurine renders the latter two amino acids essential (Fig. 85.2). Similar enzymatic immaturity may limit the synthesis of tyrosine from phenylalanine as well as the synthesis of histidine.

Plasma amino acids are in active equilibrium with metabolically active cells and are directly affected by the quantity and quality of the protein infused (49, 51). In preterm infants and neonates receiving parenteral nutrition, achieving plasma amino acid concentrations similar to those found in neonates 2 to 3 hr after human milk feeding has been associated with ideal growth and appears to be a better plasma amino acid target range than concentrations found in cord or fetal blood (52). Avoiding amino acid concentrations above or below the normal range results in better protein anabolism, and perhaps reduces parenteral nutrition–related toxicities (53, 54).

The differences in amino acid need and the aberrant plasma amino acid concentrations described above have led to the development of pediatric-specific formulations. Two pediatric-specific amino acid products (i.e., Aminosyn-PF; Abbott Laboratories, Chicago, IL and TrophAmine; McGaw, Inc., Irvine, CA) are available for use in parenteral nutrition solutions in the United States. These products vary from standard amino acid formulations in that they contain less methionine and glycine and have added or admixed the dicarboxylic amino acids (aspartate, glutamate), taurine, cysteine, and tyrosine (as N-acetyl-L-tyrosine in TrophAmine) (Table 85.5). The two pediatric-specific formulations marketed in the United States vary from each other notably in their contents of methionine and tyrosine (lower in Aminosyn-PF) and taurine (lower in TrophAmine).

The use of the pediatric-specific amino acid formulations in preterm infants has resulted in nitrogen balance and weight gain similar to that occurring during intrauterine growth (50, 53). Use of TrophAmine in term neonates and older infants has resulted in appropriate-for-age weight gain and nitrogen retention (55). Pediatric-specific amino acid formulations may provide adequate growth, even when infants receive protein, and more notably, calorie intakes that are below previously described norms (56, 57). This is likely the result of optimal plasma availability of amino acids for anabolism.

Parenteral protein requirements of the older child can be met using a standard crystalline amino acid formulation. Some incremental increases in protein intake, over those found in Table 85.4, may be required for the severely catabolic patient. Adequate concurrent monitoring is essential for patient- or disease-specific adjustments in protein intake.

Caloric Requirements

Unlike the adult who requires nonprotein calories for basal metabolic demands, activity, and maintenance of body temperature; children also require calories for growth and development. The most elegant work depicting global and

Table 85.5.
Comparison of Parenteral Amino Acid Products

Amino Acid	Composition (mole %)				
	Aminosyn	FreAmine III	Travesol (8.5%)	Aminosyn-PF	TrophAmine (6%)
L-Isoleucine	6.4	6.3	4.1	7.4	8.2
L-Leucine	8.4	8.4	5.3	11.6	14.1
L-Lysine	5.7	6.0	3.5	5.9	7.3
L-Methionine	3.1	4.3	4.3	1.5	2.9
L-Phenylalanine	3.1	4.1	4.2	3.3	3.9
L-Tryptophan	0.9	0.9	1.0	1.1	1.3
L-Threonine	5.1	4.0	4.0	5.5	4.6
L-Valine	8.0	6.8	4.4	7.1	8.8
L-Arginine	6.6	6.6	5.5	9.1	9.2
L-Histidine	2.3	2.2	2.5	2.6	4.1
L-Alanine	16.8	9.6	26.0	10.1	7.9
L-Proline	8.7	11.7	4.1	9.1	7.8
Glycine	19.9	22.5	30.8	6.6	6.4
L-Serine	4.7	6.8	0	6.1	4.8
L-Tyrosine	0.3	0	0.2	0.4	0.5
N-Acetyl-L-tyrosine[a]	0	0	0	0	1.2
L-Glutamic acid	0	0	0	7.2	4.5
L-Aspartic acid	0	0	0	5.1	3.1
L-Cysteine[b]	0	0	0	0	0.4
Taurine	0	0	0	0.7	0.3
Total	100.0	100.2	99.9	100.4	101.3

[a] As tyrosine equivalents.
[b] Admixed to Aminosyn-PF, TrophAmine.

Table 85.6.
Parenteral Calorie Requirements (kcal/kg/day)

Preterm infant/neonate	85–130
Infant	90–120
1–6 years	75–90
7–12 years	50–75
13–18 years	30–50
Adult	25–35

compartmental energy needs in preterm infants used indirect calorimetry (58). Enterally fed low-birth-weight infants had global energy requirements of 150 kcal/kg/day. Approximately 18 kcal/kg/day were lost in stool; thus, 132 kcal/kg/day were required for metabolizable energy. Of these 132 kcal/kg/day, basal metabolism required 63 kcal/kg/day, activity required 4 kcal/kg/day, and the remaining 65 kcal/kg/day were required for growth.

Parenteral caloric requirements for optimal growth of the preterm infant and neonate range from 85 to 135 kcal/kg/day (59, 60). Lower calorie and adequate protein intakes are associated with positive nitrogen balance and modest weight gain (57, 60). Caloric requirements (per kilogram body weight) decrease during the first year of life and continue to fall until adult needs are approached (Table 85.6). As with protein requirements, the recommendations for caloric intake are merely guidelines for the practitioner. Assessment of clinical outcome, including weight gain, height or length, nitrogen balance, visceral and somatic protein measurements, and achievement of developmental milestones, should dictate substrate delivery.

Carbohydrate. Dextrose is used almost exclusively as the carbohydrate calorie source in children. Neonates, particularly premature neonates, are less glucose-tolerant and are at risk for developing hyperglycemic-induced hyperosmolar coma and intraventricular hemorrhage (61). Thus, initial parenteral nutrition solutions should be limited to 5 g/kg/day of dextrose and be advanced slowly by no more than 3 g/kg/day with close monitoring of serum glucose. Older infants and children can initially receive approximately 10 g/kg/day of dextrose. Doses may be increased by 5 g/kg every 12 to 24 hr to a maximum of 30 to 35 g/kg/day, if the patient has a central venous catheter and is glucose-tolerant. Dextrose concentrations should be advanced slowly in individuals receiving corticosteroids, since hyperglycemia may develop even when dextrose intake is low.

Fat. As in adults, infusion of fat emulsion prevents or reverses essential fatty acid deficiency (EFAD); provides a concentrated, isotonic source of calories; provides a more physiologic "diet"; and prolongs survival time of peripheral

intravenous lines in patients receiving parenteral nutrition. Fat emulsion products are compared in Table 85.7.

Fat emulsion should be initiated at an intake not exceeding 0.5 g/kg/day in premature neonates. Term infants and infants older than 1 month can usually be started at 1 g/kg/day. If serum triglyceride or free fatty acid levels are within normal limits, fat emulsion can be increased by 0.25 g/kg/day to a maximum of 3 g/kg/day in preterm neonates and by 0.5 to 1 g/kg/day to a maximum of 4 g/kg/day in term and older infants (62). Ideally, fat emulsion should be given continuously over 24 hr to promote clearance from the circulation. Unlike adults, biochemical evidence of EFAD (a triene to tetraene ratio above 0.4) (63, 64) may be evident after a few days of no fat intake in preterm neonates (Fig. 85.3). While linolenic acid does not reverse EFAD as linoleic acid does, current evidence suggests that linoleic acid may also be essential (65).

Neonates, particularly premature neonates, frequently develop physiologic jaundice and hyperbilirubinemia because of their inability to conjugate bilirubin. When the serum bilirubin concentrations exceed 18 to 20 mg/dl, kernicterus, defined as the deposition of unconjugated bilirubin in brain cells, may occur. Fatty acids and bilirubin bind competitively to albumin; thus, bilirubin can be displaced from high-affinity albumin binding sites by free fatty acids. This displacement results in increased unconjugated bilirubin concentrations and an increased risk of kernicterus. Andrew et al. found that the molar ratio of serum free fatty acid to albumin must exceed 6 for bilirubin to be displaced from high-affinity binding sites on albumin (66). Furthermore, an in vitro study found that Intralipid

Table 85.7.
Composition of 10% Fat Emulsions[a]

Ingredient or Characteristic	Liposyn II (Abbott Laboratories)	Liposyn III (Abbott Laboratories)	Intralipid (Clintec Nutrition)
Source			
Soybean oil (%)	5	10	10
Safflower oil (%)	5	—	—
Fatty acid distribution			
Linoleic acid (%)	65.8	54.5	50
Oleic acid (%)	17.7	22.4	26
Palmitic acid (%)	8.8	10.5	10
Linolenic acid (%)	4.2	8.3	9
Stearic acid (%)	3.4	4.2	3.5
Egg yolk phospholipids (%)	1.2	1.2	1.2
Glycerin (%)	2.5	2.5	2.25
Calories (per ml)	1.1	1.1	1.1

[a] In 20% fat emulsions, the oil sources are the same for each product but the amounts are doubled, resulting in a lower phospholipid to triglyceride ratio and a 2 kcal/ml concentration.

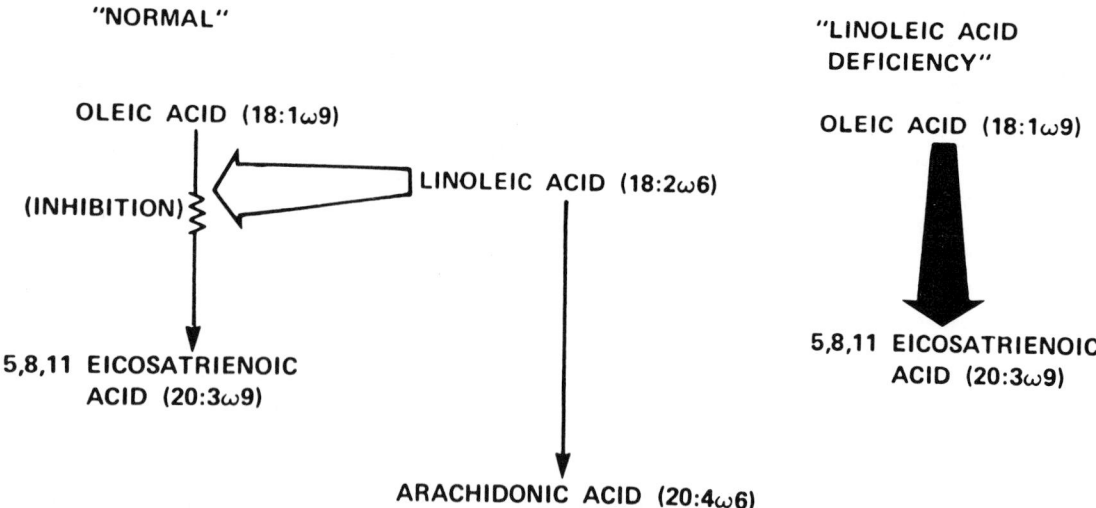

Figure 85.3. Essential fatty acid deficiency. Under "normal" conditions the *large blank arrow* indicates linoleic acid's inhibition of the oleic acid conversion to 5,8,11 eicosatrienoic acid. During linoleic acid deficiency the *dark arrow* depicts enzymatic elongation and desaturation of oleic acid to form abnormal 5,8,11 eicosatrienoic acid, resulting in a greater triene to tetraene ratio.

Liposyn enhanced the reserve capacity for the binding of bilirubin to albumin (67). Therefore, hyperbilirubinemia alone should not absolutely restrict the use of intravenous fat emulsion, and provision of 2 to 4% of the total daily caloric requirements as fat emulsion to prevent EFAD should not present a problem.

The effects of fat emulsion on immune function are controversial. Both in vitro incubation of white blood cells with fat emulsion and in vivo infusion of fat emulsion inhibit leukocyte chemotaxis, phagocytosis, bacteriocidal capacity, and lymphoproliferation (68–71). Others have found no effect of fat emulsion on immune function (24, 72, 73). There have also been several reports of restorative and augmentative effects of fat emulsion on immune function (24, 74). These conflicting findings are probably secondary to the complexities (duration of exposure, lipid concentration and composition, responding cell-type, etc.) of fatty acid and fatty acid metabolite interactions with immunoreactive cells. The conservative use of parenteral lipids is suggested in patients with sepsis.

The use of fat emulsion in neonates with pulmonary compromise is also controversial. Because fat emboli were found in pulmonary capillaries during postmortem examinations of neonates who received Intralipid, the infusion of fat emulsion in neonates with respiratory compromise was postulated to alter pulmonary function. Schroder et al. (75) found no pulmonary fat accumulation in infants given Intralipid when the lungs were fixed in situ immediately after death. These authors attributed the previous findings to artifact, which occurred secondary to a delay in the fixation of the lung after death. Pereira et al. found that appropriate-for-gestational-age neonates under 1 week of age with respiratory distress syndrome who received fat emulsion had lower PO_2 values than age-related neonates who received no Intralipid (76). Although infants received a large dose of fat emulsion (i.e., Intralipid 1 g/kg over 4 hr), the PO_2 did not correlate with elevations in serum triglyceride. Brans and co-workers found that oxygen diffusion in the lungs of premature neonates was not affected by infusion of Intralipid up to 4 g/kg/day over 24 hr (77). Therefore, to avoid excessive fat concentrations in the circulation and potential changes in pulmonary microcirculation that may result in a lowering of PO_2, the total daily dose of fat emulsion should be infused over 24 hr whenever possible.

ELECTROLYTE AND MINERAL REQUIREMENTS

The reader is referred to Chapter 8 for a discussion of electrolytes and minerals. As with adults, factors such as hydration, cardiovascular status, renal function, and concurrent medications, should be considered when determining electrolyte requirements in children. Additional considerations in pediatric patients include varying electrolyte needs with age and organ maturity. The phlebotomy technique used to obtain the sample can also be important, since hemolysis can be a problem with heel or fingersticks and result in the reporting of erroneously high potassium concentrations.

The daily maintenance electrolyte requirements for neonates, infants, and children are listed in Table 85.8 (78–80). Patients with excessive body fluid losses should receive replacement fluid with comparable electrolyte contents (Table 85.2). Replacement fluids are delivered most efficiently as a separate intravenous infusion.

Amino acid solutions also contain various amounts of anions and cations, which should be considered when de-

Table 85.8.
Daily Electrolyte Requirements (mEq/kg/day)

	Preterm and Term Infants	Infants (>1 year old) and Children
Sodium	2–8	2–5
Potassium[a]	1.4–10	2–3
Chloride	1.1–5	2–3
Magnesium	0.25–0.6	0.25–0.5
Calcium	2.5–3.5	1–2
Phosphate[b]	1.3–1.5	0.5–1.0

[a] Reflects patients receiving diuretics.
[b] Units are mmol/kg/day.

Table 85.9.
Electrolyte Content of Commercially Available Amino Acid Products (mEq/liter)

	g/100 ml	Ac	Cl	Na	Phos[a]	pH
TrophAmine	6	56	<3	5		5–6
	10	97	<3	5		5–6
Aminosyn-PF	7	32.5		3.4		5–6.5
	10	46		3.4		5–6.5
Aminosyn	7	105		5.4		4.5–6
	10	148		5.4		4.5–6
Aminosyn II	7	50.3		31.3		5–6.5
	10	71.8		45.3		5–6.5
Novamine	15	151				5.2–6.0
FreAmine III	8.5	72	<3	10	10	6.5
	10	89	<3	10	10	6.5
Travasol	8.5	45	34			6–8
	10	60	40			6–8
Cysteine HCl	5		6.3			

[a] Units are mmol/liter.

termining anion distribution (Table 85.9). L-Cysteine HCl provides additional chloride (6.3 mEq/g) to parenteral nutrition solutions.

Sodium

Premature infants have functionally immature kidneys that allow excessive urinary sodium losses (81). Sodium requirements in these infants may be as high as 8 mEq/kg/day. When determining an individual's sodium needs, other potential sources of sodium, such as flushes, continuous infusion of normal saline through arterial lines, or antibiotics as sodium salts should be considered.

Frequent causes of abnormal serum sodium concentrations in the pediatric population are vomiting and diarrhea. Patients receiving diuretics or those with certain renal disorders (e.g., renal tubular acidosis) have increased urinary sodium losses and often require additional sodium. Parenteral nutrition solutions high in sodium may be desirable in closed head injury patients to increase serum osmolality and ultimately decrease intracranial pressure.

Specific types of malignancies, pulmonary diseases, central nervous system disorders, and drugs (e.g., vincristine, carbamazepine, cyclophosphamide, barbiturates) may cause hyponatremia secondary to the syndrome of inappropriate antidiuretic hormone (SIADH).

Potassium

Potassium requirements vary from 1.4 to 10 mEq/kg/day, depending on organ maturity, presence of disease, and medications. Critically ill preterm infants may have increased potassium requirements secondary to increased urinary losses resulting from elevated plasma aldosterone concentrations, increased prostaglandin synthesis, or drug therapy.

Peripheral intravenous delivery of potassium is irritating to vessels, may be painful to the patient, and should be limited to about 40 mEq/liter for solutions infused peripherally. Patients with central venous access can receive solutions with more potassium, but the maximum rate of potassium delivery should not exceed 0.5 mEq/kg/hr. Patients receiving 0.5 mEq/kg/hr should be monitored by electrocardiogram, since cardiac arrhythmias may develop when potassium is infused rapidly (82, 83). In adults, potassium chloride solutions have been administrated centrally at 20 mEq/hr without adverse effects (84).

Neonatal serum samples are often hemolyzed because they are obtained by heel puncture, which may require considerable squeezing to obtain an adequate blood volume. Hemolysis releases intracellular potassium, causing an apparent elevation in serum potassium concentration. When hyperkalemia is noted in an asymptomatic patient, the phlebotomy method should be reviewed, and the potassium serum concentration validated by venipuncture before aggressive treatment is undertaken.

Although several factors affect potassium homeostasis (e.g., acid-base status, insulin, glucocorticoids, aldosterone, catecholamines), the ultimate determinants of potassium balance are gastrointestinal and renal potassium excretion. Vomiting, diarrhea, and draining fistulas are the primary causes of extrarenal potassium loss. Metabolic alkalosis secondary to gastrointestinal losses of hydrogen ion may also result in hypokalemia. Diuretic therapy, amphotericin, and cisplatin are frequent causes of drug-associated hypokalemia. Other drugs such as the aminoglycosides and penicillins (85) also promote renal potassium excretion. If hypokalemia is refractory to potassium supplementation, a magnesium depletion may coexist. In this situation, the magnesium must be repleted before serum potassium concentrations will respond to supplementation. Since potassium is the principal intracellular cation, it is difficult to estimate the extent of potassium depletion by extracellular serum concentrations; therefore, frequent serum monitoring is necessary until repletion occurs.

Phosphorus

Phosphate functions as a cofactor in multiple enzyme systems necessary for the metabolism of protein, carbohydrate, and fat, and is required for production of the high-energy bonds of adenosine triphosphate (ATP). Therapeutic refeeding of a severely malnourished patient has been associated with severe hypophosphatemia caused by total body phosphate depletion and increased intracellular shifting of phosphate during refeeding (86). Hypophosphatemia may also occur secondary to hyperparathyroidism (increased urinary phosphate excretion) or respiratory alkalosis (intracellular phosphate shifting). Phosphate, in addition to calcium, is particularly important in bone development and maturation, which is an important concern in pediatric patients. Phosphorus content, as the phosphate ion, in parenteral nutrition solutions is limited by solubility factors (see calcium discussion). Most parenteral nutrition solutions are able to deliver 1 to 1.5 mmol/kg/day of phosphate in patients who are not fluid-restricted. Since phosphate exists in two valence states that fluctuate with changing physiologic pH, phosphate requirements are usually described in millimoles or milligrams, not milliequivalents. The use of milliequivalents does not reflect the concentration of phosphorus in solution and may lead to dosing errors. The following conversion may be helpful: 1 mmol phosphate = 31 mg elemental phosphorus. Intravenous phosphate salt preparations provide 3 mmol/ml of phosphate and 4 mEq of sodium or 4.4 mEq/ml of potassium.

Calcium

Calcium, the most abundant mineral in the body, is important in maintaining the functional integrity of cellular membranes, neuromuscular activity, regulation of various endocrine and exocrine secretory activities, blood coagulation, and bone development and maturation. In newborns, 98% of total body calcium is present in bone. Approximately 40% of total serum calcium is bound to serum proteins, and 80 to 90% of this calcium is bound to albumin. Variations in the serum protein concentration and serum pH will proportionately alter protein-bound and total serum calcium concentrations.

Parathyroid hormone (PTH) and calcitonin respond inversely to acute changes in calcium and magnesium serum concentrations. Acute increases in these cations cause a decrease in PTH production and an increase in calcitonin production. Likewise, an acute decrease in calcium concentration causes an increase in PTH concentration and a decrease in calcitonin, resulting in the release of calcium from bone. Therefore, serum calcium concentrations may not be sensitive or specific indicators of the adequacy of calcium intake.

Infants with DiGeorge syndrome are born without parathyroid glands and may have severe hypocalcemia.

Neonatal hypocalcemia is a risk factor of maternal diabetes and may be related to decreased parathyroid responsiveness (87). The severity and prevalence of hypocalcemia is directly related to the severity of maternal diabetes. Because hypomagnesemia may contribute to a resistant hypocalcemia, serum magnesium should be monitored in patients unresponsive to calcium supplementation (87).

Pediatric patients require substantial amounts of calcium and phosphorous to support rapid skeletal bone development and maturation. Premature infants have the greatest risk for developing osteopenia, rickets, and spontaneous fractures. Premature infants require 5 to 7.5 mEq/kg/day of elemental calcium to accrete bone in utero rates. No parenteral or enteral formula can meet this estimated need. Additionally, premature infants have secondary diseases such as bronchopulmonary dysplasia and congenital heart disease that require fluid restriction and diuretic therapy. Fluid restriction further limits the amounts of calcium and phosphate that can be provided in the same solution, while diuretics enhance the excretion of calcium (88). The alternation of calcium- and phosphate-containing parenteral nutrition solutions over 12-hr infusion periods has been investigated, but it resulted in undesirable fluctuations in the corresponding serum concentrations (89). Others have focused on delivery of calcium and phosphate in a physiologic ratio (1.7:1 [mg:mg]) to promote retention of these minerals in premature infants (90). Patients suspected of having osteopenia and rachitic changes should be evaluated by roentgenograms or radiographic densitometry (91).

The delivery of adequate calcium and phosphorus in infants is limited by the solubility of these ions in solution. The solubility of calcium and phosphate in parenteral nutrition solution is affected by pH, temperature, calcium salt, sequence of calcium and phosphate salt addition to the solution, and the final concentrations of calcium and phosphate. Calcium may react with phosphate to form monobasic or dibasic calcium phosphate, depending on pH. At low pHs, the predominant form of calcium phosphate is monobasic, which is quite soluble. As the pH rises, more dibasic phosphate becomes available to bind with calcium, and precipitation occurs more easily (92). Aminosyn-PF and TrophAmine have a low pH, and therefore, improved calcium and phosphate solubility (93). The addition of cysteine HCl further decreases the pH, allowing increased calcium and phosphate supplementation (94). Elevated temperature also increases the likelihood of calcium phosphate precipitation. For example, infants in isolettes or those receiving ultraviolet light therapy have warmer environmental temperatures, causing calcium and phosphate to precipitate near the infant in the intravenous line. Less precipitation occurs with the gluconate than with the chloride salt; thus, calcium supplementation in parenteral nutrition solutions is generally done with calcium gluconate (95). In some cases, precipitation has occurred within the catheter as the infusing solution was warmed by the patient's body temperature. When compounding the solution, the addition and mixing of phosphate early in the process and the addition of calcium last will minimize precipitation (96).

Magnesium

Magnesium, the second most common intracellular cation, is necessary for numerous enzymatic reactions involving energy storage and utilization. Extracellular magnesium is used during neuromuscular transmission and is required for cardiovascular tone. Approximately 2% of the body's total magnesium is present in the extracellular compartment, while 98% is found intracellularly, primarily in bone.

Magnesium balance and serum magnesium concentration are largely determined by renal magnesium excretion, which is primarily regulated by the glomerular filtration rate, tubular reabsorption, and PTH. When necessary, the kidney can conserve or increase urinary magnesium excretion, depending on the body's magnesium stores (97).

Hypomagnesemia is often present in infants with DiGeorge syndrome and those born to diabetic mothers. Neonatal hepatitis and congenital biliary atresia are commonly associated with hypomagnesemia (98). Since magnesium is absorbed in the proximal jejunum, patients that undergo intestinal resection are at risk for developing hypomagnesemia. Similarly, patients with extensive diarrheal or ileostomy fluid losses may have increased magnesium losses. Diuretics, amphotericin, cyclosporine, and cisplatin increase urinary magnesium losses and may contribute to hypomagnesemia. Magnesium depletion may precipitate refractory hypokalemia or hypocalcemia (99). Patients with suspected magnesium depletion should have serum concentrations monitored to evaluate replacement and response.

VITAMINS

The guidelines for the Recommended Dietary Allowances (RDAs) of vitamins are based upon oral vitamin delivery in healthy infants and children. Parenteral multivitamin preparations are sensitive to pH, light, and temperature. Additionally, vitamins may interact with each other or leach onto the plastic matrix of administration sets, thus decreasing bioavailability (96). All of these factors result in a parenteral multivitamin preparation with greater amounts of vitamins than may be required by the infant or child.

The Food and Drug Administration (FDA) currently recommends that infants weighing less than 1 kg receive daily 30% (1.5 ml) of a single full dose (5 ml) and infants weighing 1 to 3 kg receive daily 65% (3.25 ml) of a single

full dose. Infants and children weighing 3 kg or more up to 11 years of age should receive the full single-dose vial (5 ml) daily. The pediatric multivitamin product has been tested primarily in medically stable infants and children receiving parenteral nutrition and is effective in maintaining acceptable vitamin serum concentrations (80).

Research in preterm infants has demonstrated that the pediatric multivitamin preparation does not adequately maintain all vitamin concentrations in the desired range. Greene et al. have recently suggested dosing the pediatric multivitamin product in preterm infants at 2 ml/kg/day, with the maximum of 5 ml/day to address the increased concentrations of the water-soluble vitamins resulting from the manufacturer's recommended dose (80). In addition, the current pediatric multivitamin formulation contains polysorbate 80, an emulsifier, that may have some safety concerns in premature infants (80). Because of apparent altered vitamin requirements and possible impaired metabolism of the emulsifier, it has been proposed that a separate intravenous multivitamin product be developed specifically for preterm infants (80).

Children over 11 years old should receive the adult multivitamin product. This preparation differs from the pediatric product in that vitamin D concentration is lower and there is no vitamin K. The remaining 10 vitamins are present in greater amounts in the adult product to address the RDA for adults.

TRACE ELEMENTS

The trace elements constitute less than 0.01% of human body weight. Despite their low body content, trace elements have an important role in biochemical processes and in growth and development. Zinc, copper, manganese, and chromium have been identified as essential and are all included in various trace-element preparations. There has been minimal research conducted to define pediatric trace-element requirements, hence reports of deficiency currently guide the recommended intravenous doses. Because individual manufacturer's preparations contain varying amounts of each trace element, the package insert should be consulted for individual dosing information.

Premature neonates have low body stores of trace elements, which puts them at increased risk of developing deficiencies. Patients with persistent diarrhea or excessive ostomy outputs have increased zinc losses in these body fluids and thus may require additional supplementation. Patients with exterior biliary drainage or jejunostomies may have increased copper losses, resulting in increased requirements. Selenium deficiency has been reported to result in cardiomyopathy and skeletal muscle myopathy and is recommended to be supplemented at 2 µg/kg/day (80). In pediatric patients receiving long-term parenteral nutrition, molybdenum is recommended at 0.25 µg/kg/day (80). Selenium, chromium, and molybdenum are excreted primarily by the kidneys; thus patients with renal insufficiency should be supplemented at lower doses or not at all, depending on their trace element status and degree of renal impairment. Copper and manganese are excreted into bile, and patients with severe liver disease, including cholestasis, should not receive these trace elements (80). Each trace element is available as a single-entity product for patients requiring an individualized approach to supplementation.

PARENTERAL NUTRITION COMPLICATIONS

Parenteral nutrition is a technically complex method of delivering nutrients that bypasses normal digestive and absorptive processes. Parenteral nutrition provides the most basic form of nutrients and introduces them directly into the bloodstream. Frequently, these solutions are infused into the superior vena cava through a catheter that is surgically placed (Fig. 85.1). Because of the nature of the solutions and catheters and the direct link to the bloodstream, there are inherent risks for a variety of technical, metabolic, and infectious complications.

Technical

Patients who require parenteral nutrition for relatively long periods of time generally have central venous catheters placed specifically for this purpose. In small infants and children with limited or difficult peripheral vascular access, a central venous catheter may be required, even if parenteral nutrition is necessary for only a short time (100). Placement of a central venous catheter requires a surgical procedure usually performed while the patient is under general anesthesia. Complications have occurred at the time of catheter placement including pneumothorax, vein or cardiac perforation, chylothorax, and hemorrhagic bleeding (101). Following catheter placement, cracks have occurred in the hub or the line. Cracks in the hub or on the proximal (exposed) portion of the catheter may often be repaired, but catheter removal may be necessary.

Parenteral nutrition solutions may extravasate into the thoracic or pericardial cavity. Solutions that are inadvertently infused through extravasated or infiltrated catheters will be resorbed, in time, after the infusion is discontinued. Extravasation may result in hypoglycemia caused by the abrupt discontinuation of the infusion of concentrated dextrose solution into the central circulation. In addition, extravasation may cause pleural or pericardial effusion with respiratory and cardiac decompensation.

Accidental removal or migration out of the desired position can also occur (102) and may be related specifically to the type of catheter (103). Broviac or Hickman-type silastic catheters are tunneled and anchored by fibrin adhering to the cuff. Therefore, these catheters are less likely to migrate out of position or be accidentally removed

than Teflon catheters that are placed percutaneously (Fig. 85.1).

Catheters located in the right atrium may stimulate dysrhythmias by coming in contact with nodal tissue. The dysrhythmias may be resolved by pulling the catheter back a short distance so there is no contact.

Catheters may become occluded due to fibrin formation (104) or precipitates (105). In many instances, the catheter that is not completely occluded can be managed pharmacologically (106, 107). Urokinase or streptokinase may be effective in dissolving fibrin that partially occludes a catheter. Catheters that are partially occluded by precipitates, such as calcium and phosphate, may be recannulated by decreasing the pH inside the catheter with the instillation of 0.1 N HCl in the catheter (106). Other agents such as ethanol may be used to dissolve soaps that develop with total-nutrient admixtures (107).

For patients requiring short-term parenteral nutrition, more dilute parenteral nutrition solutions may be infused through peripheral veins (see "Administration"). Concomitant infusion of fat emulsion with the dextrose and amino acid solution has been shown to increase the length of time to infiltration in infants receiving peripherally infused parenteral nutrition. Peripheral infusion of parenteral nutrition solutions may cause phlebitis. Infiltration or extravasation of parenteral nutrition solutions can result in localized swelling and edema, which may progress to necrosis. The infiltrated site can be treated with hyaluronidase injections to increase the rate of solution absorption and decrease potential tissue damage.

Metabolic

Metabolic complications can include electrolyte and mineral abnormalities, aberrant plasma amino acid patterns, osteoporosis, micronutrient deficiencies, cholestasis, hypersensitivity reactions, acid-base abnormalities, and alterations in pulmonary and immunologic function (108). Many of these complications have been reviewed earlier, but several important metabolic complications with a significant impact on pediatric patients require special focus.

Hepatic. Cholestasis associated with parenteral nutrition is a well-documented problem. Its occurrence is inversely related to the maturity of the infant, and directly related to the length of parenteral nutrition and enteral fasting (109). The etiology of cholestasis is complex. Investigators have proposed that competition between certain amino acids and bile salts for uptake into the hepatocyte may be a possible cause. Additionally, the enhanced production of secondary bile salts (110) and the provision of excessive calories and protein (111) may contribute to the development of cholestasis. Patients who are at risk for developing parenteral nutrition–associated cholestasis may also have experienced septic episodes, hepatitis, and other diseases or insults known to contribute to the development of cholestasis. Thus, the diagnosis of parenteral nutrition–associated cholestasis is one of exclusion. Cholestasis associated with parenteral nutrition is generally not recognized by alterations in liver function tests before 10 days of parenteral nutrition. Early markers include the enzymes 5′ nucleotidase and γ-glutamyl transferase (γGT) and direct bilirubin concentration (112). Cholestasis generally resolves when the parenteral nutrition is discontinued. In many cases, this cannot be done, and the infant must continue to receive parenteral nutrition. In these infants, initiation of small-volume enteral feeding for gut stimulation is probably the most important intervention. Offering the patient a protein- and calorie-free period by weaning the parenteral nutrition solution may be beneficial. Phenobarbital, a choleretic agent, has not been successful in the treatment of parenteral nutrition–associated cholestasis (113). Cholecystokinin has been proposed as a useful agent to promote bile flow and potentially treat cholestasis, but there is insufficient experience to recommend its use for this purpose (114). Finally, the use of pediatric-specific amino acid formulations should be considered. As mentioned, a more balanced and complete formula should result in adequate substrate availability, reducing the risk for amino acid excess or deficiency and promoting normal hepatic function.

Bone Disease. High serum, urine, and bone aluminum concentrations have been associated with metabolic bone disease in patients receiving long-term parenteral nutrition. Parenteral nutrition solutions have several possible sources of aluminum contamination including calcium and phosphate salts, albumin, and heparin. Aluminum has been reported to accumulate in the bones of premature infants receiving parenteral nutrition. The contribution of aluminum to metabolic bone disease is difficult to delineate because premature infants receiving parenteral nutrition have multiple causitive factors. Aluminum can not be disproved as a contributing factor in metabolic bone disease; therefore, it is recommended that the aluminum content of parenteral nutrition solutions be minimized (use of salts lower in aluminum), especially in preterm infants and long-term parenteral nutrition patients (115, 116).

Other Complications. Hypersensitivity reactions have been described for dextrose/amino acid and fat emulsion components of parenteral nutrition. Anaphylaxis has been attributed to the amino acid solutions, (117) vitamin preparation, (117, 118) magnesium sulfate, (117) fat emulsion, (119) iron, and soybean oil (120). In addition, bradycardia (121) and diarrhea (122) have been associated with fat emulsion infusions.

A variety of hematologic abnormalities have been reported in patients receiving parenteral nutrition. Thrombocytopenia has been related to fat emulsion infusions and appears to be dose-related (123). In contrast, an increased peripheral platelet count has also been described in pre-term neonates on parenteral nutrition (124). Parenteral nutrition–associated eosinophilia (124) occurs with greater frequency in premature neonates and appears to be self-limiting. Hemolysis may be associated with parenteral nutrition regimens that fail to provide sufficient antioxidant (vitamin E) or antioxidant cofactors (selenium) (125). This may result in inadequate free radical scavengers, causing peroxidation of red blood cell membranes or other tissues. Evidence of intravascular hemolysis has been reported with rapid infusion of Intralipid in adults (126, 127).

Impairment of immune function has been described with deficiency or insufficiency of a variety of micronutrients including zinc, (128) selenium, pyridoxine and pantothenic acid, (129, 130) vitamin E, (131, 132) vitamins A and D, (131) arginine, (133) and glutamine (134).

Infectious

Infection is a serious complication associated with central venous catheters and may be a blood-borne, exit-site or tunnel-tract infection. Because the central venous catheter provides direct access between the outside environment and the central circulation, the risk for introducing microorganisms into the bloodstream is significant unless aseptic technique protocols are strictly followed. Studies in pediatric patients receiving long-term parenteral nutrition show that the incidence of catheter-related sepsis ranges from 42 to 57% (135). Premature neonates have a greater risk for infection because of their immature immune systems. Because of problems with venous access in small children, central venous catheters are used for multiple purposes, increasing their risk for infection. Bowel disease in infants increases the potential for bacteria normally present in the gastrointestinal tract to cross the intestinal lumen and enter the bloodstream, a process called gut bacterial translocation. Bacteria entering the bloodstream by translocation or hematogenous spread from another infection site may adhere to the fibrous material of the catheter and begin to grow and proliferate. Common organisms cultured from patients with catheter-related infections are listed in Table 85.10.

Ideally, infected catheters should be removed and a new catheter placed in a different site after the infection

Table 85.10.
Microorganisms Frequently Cultured from Central Venous Catheters

Staphylococcus epidermidis	31–32%
Streptococcal species	11–12%
Staphylococcus aureus	11–26%
Gram-negative rods	20–63%
Fungi	0–5%
Other	6%

is resolved. In pediatric patients, however, sites for catheter placement are limited by difficulties in central venous access, and the decision to remove a central line in a patient who depends on this route for hydration and nutrition must be made with considerable forethought.

If the patient with catheter-related sepsis continues to require central venous access, antimicrobial therapy may be used to treat the infection without removing the catheter. Studies have shown that 55 to 89% of catheter-related infections can be successfully treated in situ with the administration of appropriate antibiotics (136, 137). The appropriate dosage of the antimicrobial agent(s) should be infused through the infected catheter. In addition, antibiotics can be instilled and allowed to reside in the catheter for varying lengths of time. Daily blood cultures are obtained through the catheter and from a peripheral site to ensure that the microorganism is being eradicated (136, 137).

The body recognizes indwelling central venous catheters as foreign. Fibrin is deposited around the outside of the line and can also accumulate inside the lumen of the catheter, particularly if the line is used for blood withdrawal (104). Microorganisms may be harbored within the fibrin, providing a nidus for infection. Even appropriate microbial therapy may not penetrate through the fibrin web and eradicate microorganisms residing inside. While urokinase, streptokinase, and possibly HCl can dissolve the fibrin within the catheter lumen, it is less likely that fibrin on the outside of the catheter lumen will be affected. It has been suggested that monthly treatment of central lines with urokinase decreases the number of central line infections. However, dissolution of a fibrin sheath that is harboring a large number of microorganisms will release these microorganisms into the bloodstream. The resultant bacteremia may result in an acute septic event or seed distant infection sites requiring concurrent evaluation and possible antimicrobial therapy.

The catheter exit site or tunnel tract may also become infected. Local antibiotic therapy may not be sufficient to treat exit-site infections, and systemic antimicrobial therapy may be required. Tunnel-tract infections should be treated with systemic antibiotics. In both cases, care should be taken with dressing changes and the central line dressing change protocol should be followed strictly. While the exit site or tunnel is infected, the central line dressing may require more frequent changing.

ENTERAL NUTRITION
Infant Formulas

The Recommended Dietary Allowance (RDA) provides guidelines for the provision of nutrients in infant formulas. The RDA is defined as the level of intake of essential nutrients that is judged by the Food and Nutrition Board, on the basis of scientific knowledge, to be adequate to

Table 85.11.
Recommended Dietary Allowances (RDA) for Energy Intake[a]

	Kcal/kg
Infants	
Birth–6 months	108
>6–12 months	98
>1–3 years	102
4–6 years	90
7–10 years	70
Males	
11–14 years	55
Females	
11–14 years	47

[a] Adapted from Recommended Dietary Allowances, ed. 10. Washington, D.C., National Academy of Sciences, 1989.

Table 85.12.
Recommended Dietary Allowances (RDA) for Protein[a,b]

	g/kg
Infants	
Birth–6 months	2.2
>6–12 months	1.6
>1–3 years	1.2
4–6 years	1.1
7–10 years	1.0
Males	
11–14 years	1.0
Females	
11–14 years	1.0

[a] Adapted from Recommended Dietary Allowances, ed. 10. Washington, D.C., National Academy of Sciences, 1989.
[b] Standard protein—human milk.

meet known nutrient needs of healthy persons (138). The RDAs are estimates that exceed the requirements of most healthy infants and children. Therefore, they do not provide guidelines for premature infants and may not provide adequate allowances for infants and children during disease or drug therapy. The RDA requirements of energy and protein for healthy infants and children are listed in Tables 85.11 and 85.12, respectively. Energy required for growth is greatest during the newborn period. Then, as infants grow, their total caloric requirement increases, but because of the increasing body size, the proportion of kilocalories per kilogram decreases. From infancy to childhood, the protein-requirement curve falls off more sharply than the energy-requirement curve. This reflects an increase in activity (requiring energy) and a decrease in

Table 85.13.
Recommended Dietary Allowances (RDA) for Vitamins[a]

	Fat-soluble Vitamins				Water-soluble Vitamins						
	Vitamin A (μg)	Vitamin D (μg)	Vitamin E (mg)	Vitamin K (μg)	Vitamin C (mg)	Thiamin (mg)	Riboflavin (mg)	Niacin (mg)	Vitamin B_6 (mg)	Folate (μg)	Vitamin B_{12} (μg)
Infants											
Birth–6 months	375	7.5	3	5	30	0.3	0.4	5	0.3	25	0.3
>6–12 months	375	10	4	10	35	0.4	0.5	6	0.6	35	0.5
>1–3 years	400	10	6	15	40	0.7	0.8	9	1.0	50	0.7
4–6 years	500	10	7	20	45	0.9	1.1	12	1.1	75	1.0
7–10 years	700	10	7	30	45	1.0	1.2	13	1.4	100	1.4
Males											
11–14 years	1000	10	10	45	50	1.3	1.5	17	1.7	150	2.0
Females											
11–14 years	800	10	8	45	50	1.1	1.3	15	1.4	150	2.0

[a] Adapted from Recommended Dietary Allowances, ed. 10. Washington, D.C., National Academy of Sciences, 1989.

Table 85.14.
Recommended Dietary Allowances (RDA) for Minerals[a]

	Calcium (mg)	Phosphorus (mg)	Magnesium (mg)	Iron (mg)	Zinc (mg)	Selenium (μg)
Birth	400	300	40	6	5	10
>6 months	600	500	60	10	5	15
>1 year	800	800	80	10	10	20
4–6 years	800	800	120	10	10	20
7–10 years	800	800	170	10	10	30
Male 11–14 years	1200	1200	270	12	15	40
Female 11–14 years	1200	1200	280	15	12	45

[a] Adapted from Recommended Dietary Allowances, ed. 10. Washington, D.C., National Academy of Sciences, 1989.

growth rates (requiring protein). Carbohydrate and fat contribute approximately equally to the energy needs in infants and children.

The RDA requirements for vitamin and minerals in infants and children are listed in Tables 85.13 and 85.14, respectively. While infant formulas contain vitamins and minerals, it is important to determine whether their total daily intake delivers the recommended amounts. Often, premature infants require additional vitamin supplementation with an infant multivitamin liquid preparation (139). Critically ill patients may also require additional supplementation.

The nutrient distribution in standard dilution infant formulas available for infants under 1 year of age reflects their distribution in human milk. Therefore, there is minimal variation in composition among these products (Table 85.15A). Preferably, infant formulas should have an osmotic load similar to that of human milk (277 to 303 mosm/kg), to avoid diarrhea induced by a high osmotic load.

Concentrated commercial formulas are available to meet the needs of infants with premature gastrointestinal tracts (Table 85.15) (140). Protein, carbohydrate, and fat components require less complex digestive processes. The protein content in these formulas is primarily whey, which forms smaller curds and are more digestible. In addition, whey protein has an amino acid composition high in cysteine and low in tyrosine, making it more desirable for the premature infant with immature enzymatic pathways. Lactose is the carbohydrate found in human milk, however, low lactase activity is found in the intestinal mucosa of premature infants. Lactose content of preterm formulas has been limited to 40 to 50% of the available carbohydrate. The remaining carbohydrate is provided in the form of maltodextrins or "corn syrup," which is a mixture of mono-, oligo-, and polysaccharides. The mixture of carbohydrates enhances utilization by relying on multiple digestive and absorptive pathways. Premature infants are frequently unable to digest long-chain triglycerides (LCT) because of reduced bile acid pool size and decreased pancreatic lipase activity. Thus, 13 to 50% of fat in these formulas is provided as medium-chain triglycerides (MCT). MCT are easily absorbed and do not require bile acids for solubilization. MCT oil does not provide essential fatty acids, thus a portion of fat must be supplied as LCT.

Table 85.15.
Infant Formulas[a]

	kcal/ oz	Sources			Content/100 ml							
		Carbohydrate	Protein	Fat	Carbohydrate (g)	Protein (g)	Fat (g)	Na[a] (mEq)	K (mEq)	mg Ca/ mg P	Fe (mg)	mOsm/ kg H₂O
Standard dilution												
Enfamil with iron	20	Lactose	Reduced mineral whey and nonfat milk solids	Coconut and soybean oil	6.9	1.5	3.7	0.78	1.8	46/31	1.3	300
Similac with iron	20	Lactose	Nonfat milk	Soybean and coconut oil	7.1	1.5	3.6	0.81	1.8	50/39	1.2	300
Concentrated, premature												
Similac Special Care	24	Lactose, corn solids	Nonfat milk, whey protein concentrate	MCT (from coconut), soybean and coconut oil	8.5	2.1	4.3	1.7	2.9	144/72	1.8	300
Premature Enfamil	24	Corn syrup solids, lactose	Demineralized whey, nonfat milk solids	MCT (from coconut), soybean and coconut oil	8.9	2.4	4.1	1.3	2.1	132/67	1.5	300
Preemie SMA	24	Maltodextrins	Nonfat milk, whey	MCT (from coconut), safflower and soybean oil	8.4	1.9	4.3	1.3	1.9	72/40	0.3	280

[a] Infant formula content changes are possible. The authors suggest referring to the most recent publication of product literature or consulting clinical dietetics for product information.

Three specialized infant formulas (Nutramigen, Pregestimil, Alimentum) are available for easy protein digestion (Table 85.16). The protein component is cow's milk that has undergone partial acid-hydrolysis resulting in free amino acids and peptides of varying size. These formulas may be appropriate for infants with intestinal resection, cow's milk allergy, or other protein allergic sensitivities (i.e., human milk). The formulas are very similar in content except for the fat component. While Nutramigen contains 100% of its fat content as LCT, Pregestimil and Alimentum contain MCT oil and may be more appropriate for infants with steatorrhea or those with short bowel syndrome who malabsorb fat. Portagen, a formula with 86% of its fat content as MCT is available for infants with significant steatorrhea, which may occur with cystic fibrosis, pancreatic insufficiency, or intestinal resection (Table 85.16). Portagen has been used in patients with chylothorax to reduce lipid transport through the lymphatic system and thereby reduce the outflow of chyle.

Formulas are also available for infants with disaccharidase deficiency or specific types of carbohydrate intolerance (i.e., lactose- and sucrose-free formulas). All of these formulas contain hypoallergenic soy protein and are also indicated if cow's milk allergy is suspected (i.e., Isomil, Isomil SF, Nursoy, Prosobee; Table 85.15B). Low renal-solute formulas (e.g., PM 60/40 and SMA) contain approximately half the sodium of other specialized formulas and are indicated when the infant's status requires low sodium intake (Table 85.16). Although these formulas have a whey protein to casein protein concentration of approximately 60 to 40% (more like human milk), the carbohydrate content is solely lactose, which means if these are used in premature infants they may experience intolerance.

Infant formulas are available as ready-to-feed unit-of-use or multiple-use containers, concentrated liquids, or dry powders. Prior to feeding, infant formula should be stored in a cool, dry place, since temperature extremes can cause irreversible physical changes. The ready-to-feed solutions should not be diluted before feeding unless the physician prescribes a dilute formula. The concentrated liquid and dry powder formulas require reconstitution prior to infant feeding. Instructions for the amount of water to be added are provided on each container. Regular tap water that meets federal drinking water standards is acceptable for reconstituting infant formula. However, in certain situations the physician may suggest sterilization of tap water before reconstitution. Because salts are added to chemically softened water, it should not be used to reconstitute infant formula. Commercially prepared sterile water is not necessary for formula preparation at home.

Infant formula preparation should take place in a clean area, using clean utensils. The individual preparing the formula should have clean hands and use good technique, to avoid contaminating the formula during reconstitution.

Immediately after reconstitution of concentrated formula or opening a ready-to-feed multiple-use container,

Table 85.16.
Specialized Infant Formulas[a]

	kcal/ oz	Sources			Content/100 ml							
		Carbohydrate	Protein	Fat	Carbohydrate (g)	Protein (g)	Fat (g)	Na (mEq)	K (mEq)	mg Ca/ mg P	Fe (mg)	mOsm/ kg H₂O
Nutramigen	20	Corn syrup solids and glucose polymers	Casein hydrolysate, amino acid premix	Corn oil	8.9	1.9	2.6	1.4	1.9	63/42	1.3	320
Pregestimil	20	Corn syrup solids, modified corn starch	Casein hydrolysate, cystine tyrosine, tryptophan, taurine, and carnitine	Corn, MCT (from coconut), and safflower oil	6.9	1.9	3.7	1.1	1.9	63/42	1.3	320
Alimentum	20	Sucrose and modified tapioca starch	Casein hydrolysate	MCT (from coconut), and safflower oil	6.8	1.8	3.7	1.3	2.0	70/50	1.2	370
Portagen	20	Corn syrup solids, sucrose, and citrates	Sodium caseinate	MCT (from coconut), corn oil, and soybean oil	7.7	2.3	3.2	1.6	2.1	63/47	1.3	236
Isomil	20	Corn syrup and sucrose, Isomil SF contains 100% glucose polymers	Soy protein isolate	Soybean and coconut oils	6.7	1.8	3.6	1.3	1.8	70/50	1.2	240
Nursoy	20	Sucrose	Soy protein isolate	Safflower, coconut, oleo, and soybean oil	6.8	2.1	3.5	0.87	1.8	60/42	1.1	296
ProSobee	20	Corn syrup solids and glucose polymers	Soy protein isolate	Coconut, soybean, and corn oil	6.7	2.0	3.5	1.0	2.1	63/49	1.3	180
SMA	20	Lactose	Nonfat milk, reduced mineral whey	Oleo, coconut, soybean, and safflower oil	7.1	1.5	3.5	0.64	1.4	42/28	1.2	300
Similac PM 60/40	20	Lactose	Whey protein concentrate, sodium caseinate	Soy and coconut oil	6.8	1.6	3.7	0.70	1.5	37/19	0.15	260

[a] Infant formula content changes are possible. The authors suggest referring to the most recent publication of product literature or consulting clinical dietetics for product information.

the portion required for an individual feeding should be put in an appropriate bottle for feeding and the remainder stored in a clean container in the refrigerator. After the infant has begun feeding, any formula left in the bottle after 2 hr should be discarded. Reconstituted formula can be stored in the refrigerator for up to 24 hr.

Smaller infants should be fed formula that is not cooler than room temperature and may prefer warmed formula. Older infants do not require warmed formula but may prefer it. The bottle with the required amount of formula for a single feeding can be warmed with warm, running tap water. If a bottle warmer is used, electric warmers are preferred over water-containing warmers because of the potential for bacterial contamination of the water contained in the warmer. Microwaves should never be used to warm infant formula because hot spots can develop throughout the formula and may burn the infant. In addition, the excessive heat can physically alter the formula and degrade nutrients.

Other additives can be admixed with the infant formula. Carbohydrate (e.g., polycose) or fat (e.g., medium-chain triglycerides) can be added to formula to enhance calorie content. The manufacturers recommend that medications not be added to infant formula because of potential drug-nutrient interactions.

After the initial opening, formula powder can be covered and stored in a cool, dry place for up to 4 weeks in the original container. Refrigeration is not necessary. However, opened liquid formula (ready-to-feed or concentrate) should be stored in the original container in the refrigerator and may be used for up to 48 hr after opening. Reconstituted formula no longer in the original container should be discarded if not used within 24 hr.

Oral electrolyte solutions, Pedialyte, Resol and Ricelyte, are available for maintenance of fluid and electrolyte balance during mild-to-moderate diarrhea (Table 85.17). Rehydrolyte was formulated for infants with moderate-to-severe diarrhea.

Table 85.17.
Infant Electrolyte Solutions (mEq/liter)

	kcal	Na$^+$	K$^+$	Cl$^-$	Citrate
Rehydralyte	100	75	20	65	30
Pedialyte	100	45	20	35	30
Resol^a	83	50	20	50	34
Ricelyte	126	50	25	45	34

^{a} Additionally contains Ca^{2+} 4 mEq/liter; phosphate 5mM/liter and Mg^{2+} 4 mEq/liter.

Administration

Common feeding routes in sick infants and children are similar to those for adults and include nasogastic, gastrostomy, and transpyloric jejunal feeding routes. Indications for continuous tube feedings include prematurity (< 34 weeks gestational age), short-term coma, hypermetabolic state, and initiation of feedings after severe diarrhea. Patients fed by the oral or nasogastric route who have gastroesophageal reflux or intractable vomiting are at risk for aspiration. Intestinal perforation may occur with long-term therapy or by malposition of the feeding tube. Gastrostomy-tube feeding is indicated in patients with upper gastrointestinal tract anomalies (cleft palate, esophageal atresia), esophageal injury, or tracheoesophageal fistula. Infants and children requiring prolonged tube feeding, such as patients with long-term coma or severe cardiac, neurologic, or respiratory disease, should be considered for gastrostomy-tube placement. This route of administration facilitates intermittent bolus feeding, which is especially desirable in the patient receiving long-term feedings. Gastrostomy-tube feeding may be undesirable in infants and children with GER, delayed gastric emptying, or intractable vomiting. Transpyloric jejunal feeding tubes are used most frequently in infants and children with gastrointestinal anomalies or delayed gastric motility or after upper gastrointestinal surgery. Continuous or intermittent jejunal feedings may also be used in pediatric patients with short gut syndrome requiring long-term tube feedings. Complications with jejunal feeding include malabsorption and bowel perforation (139).

After the appropriate formula is chosen, the feeding is delivered continuously or on an intermittent basis (e.g., every 3 hr) and advanced as tolerated. Often the patient's feeding history and close monitoring of tolerance guides the practitioner in determining the rate of feeding advancement. Diarrhea is the most frequent form of intolerance. In patients being fed by the oral, nasogastric, or gastrostomy route, gastric residuals or decant volumes are also used to assess feeding tolerance. Patients demonstrating intolerance (either diarrhea or increased gastric residuals) may require a different formula or further gastrointestinal evaluation. Patients may receive supplemental parenteral nutrition with enteral nutrition until most of their nutrient requirements are met by the enteral route.

CONCLUSION

In this chapter the reader has been apprised of the uniqueness of pediatric nutritional needs and the limitations of assessment techniques used in children. As has been stated so often, children are not small adults and therefore, should not be treated as small adults. Children (particularly neonates and infants) require quantitatively and qualitatively different nutrients than adults. Failure to address these unique substrate requirements can result in abnormal growth and development. They are also vulnerable to nutritionally induced physical and neurologic deficits that can be irreversible if they occur during rapid, substrate-dependent development.

REFERENCES

1. Costa G: Determination of nutritional needs. Cancer Res 37:2419–2424, 1977.
2. Merritt RJ, Blackburn GL, Nutritional assessment and metabolic response to illness of the hospitalized child. In Suskind RM (ed): Textbook of pediatric nutrition. New York, Raven Press, 1981, p 285.
3. Grant JP, Custer PG, Thurlow J: Current techniques of nutritional assessment. Surg Clin North Am 61:437–463, 1981.
4. Morriss FH: Trace minerals. Semin Perinatol 3:369–379, 1979.
5. Kerner JA, Sunshine P: Parenteral alimentation. Semin Perinatol 3:417–434, 1979.
6. Hamill PVV, Drizd TA, Johnson CL, et al.: Physical growth: National Center for Health Statistics percentiles. Am J Clin Nutr 32:607–629, 1979.
7. Waterlow JC: Some aspects of childhood malnutrition as a public health problem. Br Med J 4:88–90, 1974.
8. Helms RA, Miller JL, Burckart GJ, et al.: Clinical outcome as assessed by anthropometric parameters, albumin and cellular immune function in high-risk infants receiving total parenteral nutrition. J Pediatr Surg 18:564–569, 1983.
9. Gurney JM, Jelliffe DB: Arm anthropometry in nutritional assessment: nomogram for rapid calculation of muscle circumference and cross-sectional muscle and fat areas. Am J Clin Nutr 26:912–915, 1973.
10. Frisancho AR: Triceps skin fold and upper arm muscle size norms for assessment of nutritional status. Am J Clin Nutr 27:1052–1058, 1974.
11. Tanner JM, Whitehouse RH: Revised standards for triceps and subscapular skinfolds in British children. Arch Dis Child 50:142–145, 1975.
12. Ingenbleek Y, van den Schrieck H, de Nayer P, et al.: Albumin, transferrin, and the thyroxine-binding prealbumin/retinol binding protein (TBPA-RBP) complex in assessment of malnutrition. Clin Chim Acta 63:61–67, 1975.
13. Rothschild MA, Oratz M, Schreiber SS: Albumin synthesis. N Engl J Med 286:748–757, 1972.
14. Awai M, Brown EB: Studies of the metabolism of I^{131}-labeled human transferrin. J Lab Clin Med 61:363–396, 1963.
15. Oppenheimer JH, Surks MI, Bernstein G, et al.: Metabolism of I-131 labeled thyroxine binding prealbumin in man. Science 149:748–751, 1965.
16. Peterson PA: Demonstration in serum of two physiological forms

of the human retinol-binding protein. Eur J Clin Invest 1:437–444, 1971.

17. Giacoia GP, Watson S, West K: Rapid turnover transport proteins, plasma albumin, and growth in low birth weight infants. JPEN J Parenter Enteral Nutr 8:367–370, 1984.

18. Moskowitz SR, Pereira G, Spitzer A, et al.: Prealbumin as a biochemical marker of nutritional adequacy in premature infants. J Pediatr 102:749–753, 1983.

19. Helms RA, Dickerson RN, Ebbert ML, et al.: Retinol-binding protein and prealbumin: useful measures of protein repletion in critically ill, malnourished infants. J Pediatr Gastroenterol Nutr 5:586–592, 1986.

20. Heird WC, Winters RW: Total parenteral nutrition. J Pediatr 86:2–16, 1975.

21. Lopez AM, Wolfsdorf J, Raszynski A, et al.: Estimation of nitrogen balance based on a six-hour urine collection in infants. JPEN J Parenter Enteral Nutr 10:517–518, 1986.

22. Seashore JH, Huszar GB, Davis EM: Urinary 3-methylhistidine excretion and nitrogen balance in healthy and stressed premature infants. J Pediatr Surg 15:400–404, 1980.

23. Forbes GB, Bruining GJ: Urinary creatinine excretion and lean body mass. Am J Clin Nutr 29:1359–1366, 1976.

24. Lawton AR, Cooper MD, Ontogeny of immunity. In Stiehm ER, Bulginiti VA (eds): Immunologic Disorders in Infants and Children. Philadelphia, WB Saunders, 1980, p 36.

25. Shannon DC, Johnson G, Rosen FS, et al.: Cellular reactivity to Candida albicans antigen. N Engl J Med 275:690–693, 1966.

26. Helms RA, Herrod HG, Burckart GJ, et al.: E-Rosette formation, total T-cells and lymphocyte transformation in infants receiving intravenous safflower oil emulsion. JPEN J Parenter Enteral Nutr 7:541–545, 1983.

27. Costarino A, Baumgart S: Modern fluid and electrolyte management of the critically ill premature infant. Pediatr Clin North Am 33:153–178, 1986.

28. Heeley AM, Talbot NB: Insensible water losses per day by hospitalized infants and children. Am J Dis Child 90:251–256, 1955.

29. Levine SZ, Wheatlye MA: Respiratory metabolism in infancy and in childhood; daily heat production in infants, predictions based on insensible loss of weight compared with direct measurements. Am J Dis Child 51:1300–1323, 1936.

30. Holliday MA, Segar WE: The maintenance need for water in parenteral fluid therapy. Pediatrics 19:823–832, 1957.

31. Bell EF, Oh W: Fluid and electrolyte balance in very low birth weight infants. Clin Perinatol 6:139–150, 1979.

32. Perkin RM, Levin DL: Common fluid and electrolyte problems in the pediatric intensive care unit. Pediatr Clin North Am 27:567–586, 1980.

33. Friis-Hansen B: Body water compartments in children: changes during growth and related changes in body composition. Pediatrics 28:169–181, 1961.

34. Kagan BM, Stanincova V, Felix NS, et al.: Body composition of premature infants: relation to nutrition. Am J Clin Nutr 25:1153–1164, 1972.

35. Stuart HC, Sobel EH: The thickness of the skin and subcutaneous tissue by age and sex in childhood. J Pediatr 28:637–647, 1946.

36. Williams PR, Oh W: Effects of radiant warmer on insensible water loss in newborn infants. Am J Dis Child 128:511–514, 1974.

37. Jones RWA, Rochefort MJ, Baum JD: Increased insensible water loss in newborn infants nursed under radiant heaters. Br Med J 2:1347–1350, 1976.

38. McCance RA, Maylor NJB, Widdowson EM: The response of infants to a large dose of water. Arch Dis Child 29:104–109, 1954.

39. Leake RD, Zakuddin S, Trygstad CW, et al.: The effects of large volume intravenous fluid infusion on neonatal renal function. J Pediatr 89:968–972, 1976.

40. Arant BS Jr: Developmental patterns of renal functional maturation compared in the human neonate. J Pediatr 92:705–712, 1978.

41. Van Marter LJ, Leviton A, Allred EN, et al.: Hydration during the first days of life and the risk of bronchopulmonary dysplasia in low birth weight infants. J Pediatr 116:942–949, 1990.

42. Goldman HI: Feeding and necrotizing enterocolitis. Am J Dis Child 134:553–555, 1980.

43. Goldberg RN, Chung D, Goldman SL, et al.: The association of rapid volume expansion and intraventricular hemorrhage in the preterm infant. J Pediatr 96:1060–1063, 1980.

44. Bell EF, Warburton D, Stonestreet BS, et al.: Effect of fluid administration on the development of symptomatic patent ductus arteriosus and congestive heart failure in premature infants. N Engl J Med 302:598–604, 1980.

45. Phelps SJ, Helms RA: Risk factors affecting infiltration of peripheral venous lines in infants. J Pediatr 111:384–389, 1987.

46. Wurzel CL, Halom K, Feldman JG, et al.: Infection rates of Brovac-Hickman catheters and implantable venous devices. Am J Dis Child 142:536–540, 1988.

47. Mirro J, Rao B, Kuman M, et al.: A comparison of placement techniques and complications of externalized catheters and implantable port use in children with cancer. J Pediatr Surg 25:120–124, 1990.

48. Rollins CJ, Elsberry VA, Pollack KA, et al.: Three-in-one parenteral nutrition: a safe and economical method of nutritional support for infants. JPEN J Parenter Enteral Nutr 14:290–294, 1990.

49. Steginck LD, Baker GL: Infusion of protein hydrolysates in the newborn infant: plasma amino acid concentrations. J Pediatr 78:595–602, 1971.

50. Helms RA, Christensen ML, Mauer EC, Storm MC: Comparison of pediatric versus standard amino acid formulation in preterm neonates requiring parenteral nutrition. J Pediatr 110:466–470, 1987.

51. Anderson TL, Muttart CR, Bilber MA, et al.: A controlled trial of glucose versus glucose and amino acids in premature infants. J Pediatr 94:947–951, 1979.

52. Polberger SKT, Axelsson IE, Raiha NCR: Amino acid concentrations in plasma and urine in very low birth weight infants fed protein-unenriched or human milk protein-enriched human milk. Pediatrics 86:909–915, 1990.

53. Heird WC, May W, Helms RA, et al.: Pediatric parenteral amino acid mixture in low birth weight infants. Pediatrics 81:41–50, 1988.

54. Helms RA, Christensen ML, Storn MC: Outcome in infants receiving a pediatric amino acid formulation. Clin Res 33:272A, 1985.

55. Heird WC, Dell RB, Helms RA, et al.: Amino acid mixture designed to maintain normal plasma amino acid patterns in infants and children requiring parenteral nutrition. Pediatrics 80:401–408, 1987.

56. Duffy B, Gunn T, Collinge J, et al.: The effect of varying protein quality and energy intake on the nitrogen metabolism of parenterally fed very low birthweight (< 1600 g) infants. Pediatr Res 15:1040–1044, 1981.

57. Chessman K, Johnson M, Fernandes E, Helms R: Changing parenteral substrate requirements in neonates receiving a pediatric amino acid formulation. JPEN J Parenter Enteral Nutr 12:105, 1988. (abstract)

58. Reichman BL, Chessex P, Putet G, et al.: Partition of energy metabolism and energy cost of growth in the very low-birth-weight infant. Pediatrics 69:446–451, 1982.

59. Kerner JA Jr, Caloric requirement. In Kerner JA Jr (ed): Manual of Pediatric Parenteral Nutrition. New York, John Wiley & Sons, 1983, p 63.

60. Zlotkin SH, Bryan MH, Anderson GH: Intravenous nitrogen and energy intakes required to duplicate in utero nitrogen accretion in prematurely born human infants. J Pediatr 99:115–120, 1981.

61. Thomas DB: Hyperosmolality and intraventricular haemorrhage in premature babies. Acta Paediatr Scand 65:429–432, 1976.

62. Committee on Nutrition, American Academy of Pediatrics: Commentary on parenteral nutrition. Pediatrics 71:547–552, 1983.

63. Press M, Kikuchi H, Shimoyana J, et al.: Diagnosis and treatment of essential fatty acid deficiency in man. Br Med J 2:247–250, 1974.

64. Pelham LD: Rational use of intravenous fat emulsions. Am J Hosp Pharm 38:198–208, 1981.

65. Bivins BA, Bell RM, Rapp RP, et al.: Linoleic acid versus linolenic acid: what is essential. JPEN J Parenter Enteral Nutr 7:473–478, 1983.

66. Andrew G, Chan G, Schiff D: Lipid metabolism in the neonate: II. The effect of Intralipid on bilirubin binding in vitro and in vivo. J Pediatr 88:279–284, 1976.

67. Burckart GJ, Whitington PF, Helms RA: The effect of two intravenous fat emulsions and their components on bilirubin to albumin. Am J Clin Nutr 36:521–526, 1982.

68. Nordenstrom J, Jarstrand C, Wiernick A: Decreased chemotactic and random migration of leukocytes during Intralipid infusion. Am J Clin Nutr 32:2416–2422, 1979.

69. Tovan JA, Mahour GH, Miller SW, et al.: Endotoxin clearances after Intralipid infusion. J Pediatr Surg 11:23, 1976.

70. Jarstrand C, Berghem L, Lahnborg G: Human granulocyte and reticuloendothelial system function during Intralipid infusion. JPEN J Parenter Enteral Nutr 2:663–670, 1978.

71. Ladisch S, Poplark DG, Blaese RM: Inhibition of human lymphoproliferation by intravenous lipid emulsion. Clin Immunol Immunopathol 25:196–202, 1982.

72. Palmbald J, Brostrom O, Lahnborg G, et al.: Neutrophil functions during total parenteral nutrition and Intralipid infusion. Am J Clin Nutr 35:1430–1436, 1982.

73. Strunk RC, Murrow BW, Thilo E, et al.: Normal macrophage function in infants receiving Intralipid by low-dose intermittent administration. J Pediatr 106:640–645, 1985.

74. Escudier EF, Escudier BJ, Henry-Amar MC, et al.: Effects of infused Intralipids on neutrophil chemotaxis during total parenteral nutrition. JPEN J Parenter Enteral Nutr 10:596–598, 1986.

75. Schroder H, Paust H, Schmidt R: Pulmonary fat embolism after Intralipid therapy—a postmortem artefact? Acta Paediatr Scand 73:461–464, 1984.

76. Pereira GR, Fox WW, Stanley CA, et al.: Decreased oxygenation and hyperlipemia during intravenous fat infusions in premature infants. Pediatrics 66:26–30, 1980.

77. Brans YW, Dutton EB, Andrew DS, et al.: Fat emulsion tolerance in very low birth weight neonates: effect on diffusion of oxygen in the lungs and on blood pH. Pediatrics 78:79–84, 1986.

78. Arnold WC: Parenteral nutrition, and fluid and electrolyte therapy. Pediatr Clin North Am 37:449–461, 1990.

79. Lorch V, Lay SA: Parenteral alimentation in the neonate. Pediatr Clin North Am 24:547–556, 1977.

80. Greene HL, Hambidge KM, Schanler R, et al.: Guidelines for the use of vitamins, trace elements, calcium, magnesium, and phosphorus in infants and children receiving total parenteral nutrition: report of the Subcommittee on Pediatr Parenteral Nutrient Requirements from the Committee on Clinical Practice Issues of The American Society for Clinical Nutrition. Am J Clin Nutr 48:1324–1342, 1988.

81. Sulyok E, Varga F, Gyory E, et al.: Postnatal development of renal sodium handling in premature infants. J Pediatr 95:787–792, 1979.

82. Schaber DE, Uden DL, Stone FM, et al.: Intravenous KCl supplementation in pediatric cardiac surgical patients. Pediatr Cardiol 6:25–28, 1985.

83. Benitz WE, Tatro SS: The Pediatric Drug Handbook. Chicago: Year Book Medical Publishers, 1988, p 330.

84. Kruse JA, Carlson RW: Rapid correction of hypokalemia using concentrated intravenous potassium chloride infusions. Arch Intern Med 150:613–617, 1990.

85. Stapleton FB, Nelson B, Vats TS, et al.: Hypokalemia associated with antibiotic treatment. Am J Dis Child 130:1104–1108, 1976.

86. Solomon SM, Kirby DF: The refeeding syndrome: a review. JPEN J Parenter Enteral Nutr 14:90–97, 1990.

87. Tsang RC, Donovan EF, Steichen JJ: Calcium physiology and pathology in the neonate. Pediatr Clin North Am 23:611–626, 1976.

88. Vileisis RA: Furosemide effect on mineral status of parenterally nourished premature neonates with chronic lung disease. Pediatrics 85:316–322, 1990.

89. Kimura S, Nose O, Seino Y, et al.: Effects of alternate and simultaneous administrations of calcium and phosphorous on calcium metabolism in children receiving total parenteral nutrition. JPEN J Parenter Enteral Nutr 10:513–516, 1986.

90. Pelegano JF, Rowe JC, Carey DE, et al.: Simultaneous infusion of calcium and phosphorus in parenteral nutrition for premature infants: use of physiologic calcium/phosphorus ratio. J Pediatr 114:115–119, 1989.

91. Lyon AJ, Hawkes DJ, Doran M, et al.: Bone mineralization in preterm infants measured by dual energy radiographic densitometry. Arch Dis Child 64:919–923, 1989.

92. Eggert LD, Rusho WJ, MacKay MW, et al.: Calcium and phosphorus compatibility in parenteral nutrition solutions for neonates. Am J Hosp Pharm 39:49–53, 1982.

93. Lenz GT, Mikrut BA: Calcium and phosphate solubility in neonatal parenteral nutrient solutions containing Aminosyn-PF or TrophAmine. Am J Hosp Pharm 45:2367–2371, 1988.

94. Schmidt GL, Baumgartner TG, Fischlschweiger W, et al.: Cost containment using cysteine HCl acidification to increase calcium/phosphate solubility in hyperalimentation solutions. JPEN J Parenter Enteral Nutr 10:203–207, 1986.

95. Henry RS, Jurgens RW Jr, Sturgeon R, et al.: Compatibility of calcium chloride and calcium gluconate with sodium phosphate in a mixed TPN solution. Am J Hosp Pharm 37:673–674, 1980.

96. Niemiec PW Jr, Vanderveen TW: Compatibility considerations in parenteral nutrient solutions. Am J Hosp Pharm 41:893–911, 1984.

97. Schrier RQ: Renal and Electrolyte Disorders. Boston: Little, Brown & Co, 1986, ch 7.

98. Tsang RC: Neonatal magnesium disturbances. Am J Dis Child 124:282–293, 1972.

99. Whang R, Aikawa JK: Magnesium deficiency and refractoriness to potassium repletion. J Chron Dis 30:65–68, 1977.

100. Eichelberger MR, Rous PG, Hoelzer D, et al.: Percutaneous subclavian venous catheters in neonates and children. J Pediatr Surg 16:547–552, 1981.

101. Ruggiero RP, Caruso G: Chylothorax—a complication of subclavian vein catheterization. JPEN J Parenter Enteral Nutr 9:750–753, 1985.

102. Gutcher G, Cutz E: Complications of parenteral nutrition. Semin Perinatol 10:196–207, 1986.

103. Welch GW, McKell DW, Silverstein P, et al.: The role of catheter composition in the development of thrombophlebitis. Surg Gynecol Obstet 138:421–424, 1974.

104. Hoshal VL, Ause RG, Hoskins PA: Fibrin sleeve formation on indwelling subclavian central venous catheters. Arch Surg 102:353–358, 1971.

105. Breaux CW Jr, Duke D, Georgeson KE, et al.: Calcium phosphate crystal occlusion of central venous catheters used for total parenteral nutrition in infants and children: prevention and treatment. 22:829–832, 1987.

106. Duffy LF, Kerzner B, Gebus V, et al.: Treatment of central venous catheter occlusions with hydrochloric acid. J Pediatr 114:102–104, 1989.

107. Pennington CR, Pithie AD: Ethanol lock in the management of catheter occlusion. JPEN J Parenter Enteral Nutr 11:507–508, 1987.

108. Baker SS, Dwyer E, Queen P: Metabolic derangements in children requiring parenteral nutrition. JPEN J Parenter Enteral Nutr 10:279–281, 1986.

109. Black DD, Suttle EA, Whitington PF, et al.: The effect of short-term total parenteral nutrition on hepatic function in the human neonate: a prospective randomized study demonstrating alteration of the hepatic canalicular function. J Pediatr 99:445–449, 1981.

110. Farrell MK, Balistren WF, Sucky FY: Serum-sulfated lithocholate as an indicator of cholestasis during parenteral nutrition in infants and children. JPEN J Parenter Enteral Nutr 6:30–33, 1982.

111. Whitington PF: Cholestasis associated with total parenteral nutrition in infants. Hepatology 5:693, 1985.

112. Beale EF, Nelson RM, Bucciarelli RL, et al.: Intrahepatic cholestasis associated with parenteral nutrition in premature infants. Pediatrics 64:342–347, 1979.

113. Gleghorn EE, Merritt RJ, Subramanian N, et al.: Phenobarbital does not prevent total parenteral-associated cholestasis in noninfected infants. JPEN J Parenter Enteral Nutr 10:282–283, 1986.

114. Doty JE, Pitt HA, Porter-Fink V, et al.: Cholecystokinin prophylaxis of parenteral nutrition-induced gallbladder disease. Ann Surg 201:76–80, 1985.

115. Koo WWK, Kaplan LA, Horn J, et al.: Aluminum in parenteral nutrition solution—sources and possible alternatives. JPEN J Parenter Enteral Nutr 10:591–595, 1986.

116. Klein GL, Alfrey AC, Shike N, et al.: Parenteral drug products containing aluminum as an ingredient or a contaminent: response to FDA notice of intent. Am J Clin Nutr 53:399–402, 1991.

117. Pomeranz S, Gimmon Z, Zvi AB, et al.: Parenteral-nutrition-induced anaphylaxis. JPEN J Parenter Enteral Nutr 11:314–315, 1987.

118. Bullock L, Etchason E, Fitzgerald JF, et al.: Case report of an allergic reaction to parenteral nutrition in a pediatric patient. JPEN J Parenter Enteral Nutr 14:98–100, 1990.

119. Kamath KR, Berry A, Cummins G: Acute hypersensitivity reaction to Intralipid. N Engl J Med 304:360, 1981.

120. Hiyama DT, Griggs B, Mittman RF, et al.: Hypersensitivity following lipid emulsion infusion in an adult patient. JPEN J Parenter Enteral Nutr 13:318–320, 1989.

121. Sternberg A, Gruenevald T, Duetsch AA, et al.: Intralipid-induced transient sinus bradycardia. N Engl J Med 304:422–423, 1981.

122. Connon JJ: Diarrhea possibly caused by total parenteral nutrition. N Engl J Med 301:273–274, 1979.

123. Campbell AN, Freedman MH, Pendharz PI, et al.: Bleeding disorder from the "fat overload" syndrome. JPEN J Parenter Enteral Nutr 8:447–449, 1984.

124. Bhat AM, Scanlon JW: The pattern of eosinophilia in premature infants. J Pediatr 98:612–616, 1981.

125. Rotruck JT, Pope AL, Ganther HE, et al.: Selenium: biochemical role as a component of gluthathione perioxidase. Science 179:588–590, 1973.

126. Marks LM, Patel N, Kurtides ES: Hematologic abnormalities associated with intravenous lipid therapy. Am J Gastroenterol 73:490–495, 1980.

127. McGrath KM, Zalcberg JR, Slonim J: Intralipid induced haemolysis. Br J Haematol 50:376–378, 1982.

128. Golden MHN, Harland PAEG, Golden BE, et al.: Zinc and immunocompetence in protein-energy malnutrition. Lancet 1:1226–1227, 1978.

129. Hodges RE, Bean WB, Ohlson MA, et al.: Factors affecting human antibody response V. Combined deficiencies of pantothenic acid and pyridoxine. Am J Clin Nutr 11:187–199, 1962.

130. Axelrod AE: Immune process in vitamin deficiency states. Am J Clin Nutr 24:265–271, 1971.

131. Kinsella JE, Lokesh B, Broughton S, et al.: Dietary polyunsaturated fatty acids and eicosanoids: potential effects on the modulation of inflammatory and immune cells: an overview. Nutrition 6:24–44, 1990.

132. Meydani SN, Yogeeswaran G, Liu S, et al.: Fish oil and tocopherol-induced changes in natural killer cell-mediated cytotoxicity and PGE_2 synthesis in young and old mice. J Nutr 118:1245–1252, 1988.

133. Barbul A, Sisto DA, Waserkurg HL, et al.: Arginine stimulates lymphocyte immune response in healthy human beings. Surgery 90:244–251, 1981.

134. Burke DJ, Alverdy JC, Aoys E, et al.: Glutamine-supplemented total parenteral nutrition improves gut immune function. Arch Surg 124:1396–1399, 1989.

135. Vargas JH, Ament ME, Berquist WE: Long-term home parenteral nutrition in pediatrics. Ten years of experience in 102 patients. J Pediatr Gastroenterol Nutr 6:24–37, 1987.

136. Flynn PM, Shenep JL, Stokes DC, et al.: In situ management of confirmed central venous catheter-related bacteremia. Pediatr Infect Dis J 6:729–734, 1987.

137. Hartman GE, Shochat SJ: Management of septic complications associated with Silastic catheters in childhood malignancy. Pediatr Infect Dis J 6:1042–1047, 1987.

138. National Research Council: Recommended Dietary Allowances, ed. 10. Washington, D.C.: National Academy Press, 1989, ch 3–9.

139. Rombeau JL, Caldwell MD: Clinical Nutrition—Enteral and Tube Feeding. Philadelphia: WB Saunders, 1990, ch 18.

140. American Academy of Pediatrics, Committee on Nutrition. Nutritional needs of low-birth-weight infants. Pediatrics 75:976–986, 1985.

CHAPTER 86

GYNECOLOGIC DISORDERS

RONALD J. RUGGIERO, Pharm.D.

Disorders of the female reproductive tract result in many gynecologic complaints and problems. In addition to the need for contraceptive measures, discussed in Chapter 87, dysmenorrhea, the premenstrual syndrome, endometriosis, vaginitis, venereal warts, and estrogen replacement therapy for hot flushes, atrophic vaginitis, and the prevention of estrogen deficiency-induced osteoporosis require rational drug management.

Teratogenicity should be considered when treating a woman with childbearing potential, and women who are taking potentially teratogenic drugs must be using an effective method of contraception.

DYSMENORRHEA

It is estimated that 30 to 50% of the 35 million women of childbearing age in the United States are affected by painful menstrual periods or dysmenorrhea, and 10 to 15% of those women are incapacitated for 1 to 3 days each month. Dysmenorrhea is the greatest single cause of absenteeism from school and work among young women (1). The cost for the estimated 600 million work hours lost annually in the United States is approximately 2 billion dollars (2).

Primary dysmenorrhea occurs during ovulatory cycles, and unlike secondary dysmenorrhea, it has no detectable pelvic pathology such as adhesions on the reproductive organs.

The chief symptom that most women experience is spasmodic pain of the lower abdomen that may radiate to the back and along the thighs. The pain is accompanied by one or more of the following systemic symptoms in more than 50% of the patients: nausea and vomiting (89%), fatigue (85%), diarrhea (60%), lower backache (60%), and headache (45%). The duration is usually 48 to 72 hr, with the pain starting a few hours before or just after the onset of menstrual flow (3).

The etiology of these symptoms is related to the pharmacologic actions of prostaglandin E2 (PGE2) and prostaglandin F2α (PGF2α), which are formed from the phospholipids of dead cell membranes in the menstruating uterus. PGE2 causes disaggregation of platelets and is a vasodilator, while PGF2α mediates or potentiates pain sensations and stimulates smooth muscle contraction (1). Additionally, estrogens can stimulate synthesis and/or re-

lease of PGF2α and vasopressin (VP), which cause uterine hyperactivity. For this reason, progestin-dominant combination oral contraceptives are often used to alleviate dysmenorrhea (4).

The goal of therapy for primary dysmenorrhea is to avoid the lower abdominal spasmodic pains and other prostaglandin-induced effects. The efficacy of such therapy is monitored solely by the subjective responses of the patient.

Table 86.1 lists drug therapy regimens currently used for primary dysmenorrhea, including nonsteroidal antiinflammatory drugs (NSAIDs) and combination oral contraceptives (COCs).

Clinically there is no way to predict whether a certain NSAID will give maximal benefit to any given patient, based on current data in the literature. Few direct comparisons of one NSAID to another have been done. Even though most studies show superiority of the active drug over placebo, no single NSAID has been found to be superior, although some studies give mefenamic acid a slight edge. The initial selection should be tried for at least 2 to 4 cycles. If therapy is unsuccessful, some patients may still respond to another NSAID class, and NSAIDs are successful in 77 to 80% of dysmenorrhea patients. Ibuprofen, naproxen, or naproxen sodium are the usual initial choices, with mefenamic acid being reserved for more difficult cases.

Patients should be told that the NSAIDs need not be taken until the onset of symptoms, since the half-life of prostaglandins is only minutes. With the short-term use of NSAIDs for dysmenorrhea, side effects are infrequent and usually mild. Gastrointestinal irritation is best avoided by taking the NSAIDs with food or milk. Other NSAIDs such as aspirin should not be taken with the NSAIDs listed in Table 86.1, because they may greatly enhance their effect and toxicities such as peptic ulceration, liver damage, and renal damage. Patients with allergies to aspirin, especially anaphylactic reactions, should be cautioned to never take NSAIDs in prescription or over-the-counter preparations.

COCs relieve dysmenorrhea in 90% of patients, probably by a reduction in the amount of endometrium formed and consequently the amount of prostaglandins formed. Compliance with the COC is essential for maintenance of anovulatory cycles.

Table 86.1.
Drug Therapy of Primary Dysmenorrhea

Drug	Usual Dose
NSAIDS	
Acetic Acids	
Indomethacin	25 mg p.o. t.i.d.
Tolmetin	400 mg p.o. t.i.d.
Sulindac	200 mg p.o. q. 4–6 h.
Fenamates	
Mefenamic Acid[a] (CDOC)[b]	500 mg p.o. stat, then 250 mg q. 6 h.
Meclofenamate	100 mg p.o. stat, then 50–100 mg q. 6 h.
Oxicams	
Piroxicam	20 mg p.o. daily
Proprionic acids	
Ibuprofen[a] (CDOC)	400 mg p.o. q. 4 h.
Naproxen[a] (CDOC)	500 mg p.o. stat, then 250 mg q. 6–8 h.
Naproxen sodium[a] (CDOC)	550 mg p.o. stat, then 275 mg q. 6–8 h.
Ketoprofen[a] (CDOC)	50 mg p.o. t.i.d.
Salicylic acids	
Diflunisal	1000 mg p.o. stat, then 500 mg q. 12 h.
Combination oral contraceptives (28-day cycle pack, progestin dominant)	1 daily
α-Adrenergic agonists[c]	
Clonidine	0.1 mg p.o. t.i.d.

[a] FDA-approved for primary dysmenorrhea.
[b] CDOC, clinical drug of choice: (a) No single NSAID has proven superiority-proprionic acids often used initially; (b) NSAIDs may be ineffective in 20–30% of patients; (c) COCs may be ineffective in 10% of patients.
[c] Only preliminary data available, therefore last therapeutic choice.

Since NSAIDs do not relieve pain in 20 to 30% of patients with dysmenorrhea and COCs do not relieve pain in 10% of patients, another cause of dysmenorrhea has been proposed: excessive stimulation of the uterus by the adrenergic nervous system. In a recent report of four patients who failed on either NSAIDs or COCs, the α-adrenergic agonist clonidine in a dose of 0.1 mg three times daily worked very well (5). Clonidine may therefore be useful as the last-alternative therapy, although large, well-controlled studies are needed to confirm its efficacy in primary dysmenorrhea.

PREMENSTRUAL SYNDROME

It is estimated that 30 to 50% of menstruating women experience symptoms of the premenstrual syndrome (PMS), with 20 to 30% reporting moderate to severe symptoms. Absenteeism due to PMS is costly, since 60% of women are in the work force today.

Unlike primary dysmenorrhea, PMS lacks a consensus definition. The most widely accepted definition states that the following criteria be met to document PMS (6):

1. The signs and/or symptoms must occur cyclically and recur to some degree in the luteal phase (i.e., after ovulation) of the menstrual cycle. They are usually present to some degree each cycle.
2. During the follicular phase (i.e., prior to ovulation), the patient should be free of symptoms. There must be at least 7 symptom-free days in each cycle. Most patients do not have symptoms for several days after the onset of menses until near ovulation.
3. The combination of distressing physical, psychologic, and/or behavioral changes is of sufficient severity to result in deterioration of interpersonal relationships and/or interfere with normal activities.

Table 86.2 lists many of the commonly reported chief symptoms of PMS. The etiology of PMS remains as elusive as the definition and the myriad of symptoms attributed to this disorder.

The goal of drug therapy is to alleviate the symptoms of PMS. Monitoring the efficacy of such therapy depends largely on the subjective responses of the patient and on the observations of persons close to her and her healthcare providers.

Table 86.3 lists the current drug therapy regimens of PMS. The lack of consistent definition and the paucity of carefully designed drug studies of PMS have led to less than satisfactory treatment (7). Complicating the study results is the fact that placebo responses have been as high as 60 to 80% in many studies. No one drug has been shown to be superior or satisfactory for the long-term treatment of PMS. The studies available are not very helpful in choosing appropriate therapy. Most case reports and uncontrolled clinical trials describe beneficial effects for the agent being studied. However, the same agent's therapeutic benefit is frequently lacking when a placebo-con-

Table 86.2.
Symptoms of PMS[a]

Psychologic[b]	Somatic[b]
Anxiety	Abdominal bloating
Depression	Edema
Irritability	Weight gain
Wide mood swings	Constipation
Increased appetite	Hot flashes
Aggression	Breast pain
Lethargy or fatigue	Headache
Forgetfulness/reduced concentration	Acne
Sleep disorders	Rhinitis
Phobias	Palpitations

[a] Adapted from Chihal HJ: Premenstrual syndrome: an update for the clinician. Obstet Gynecol Clin North Am 17(2):457–479, 1990.
[b] In approximate order of frequency of occurrence.

Table 86.3.
Effectiveness of the Current Drug Therapy of PMS[a]

Drug	Average Dose/Regimen	Average Patient Improvement[b] (%)
Spironolactone (CDOC)[c]	25 mg p.o. q.i.d. days 14–28	0–80
Various COCs (28s) (CDOC)	one p.o. daily days 1–28	0–29
Pyridoxine (CDOC)	50–500 mg p.o. days 1–28	0–76
Lithium	200 mg p.o. q.i.d. days 1–28	0–60
Mefenamic acid	500 mg p.o. t.i.d. days 14–28	0–92
Oil of evening primrose	3 g p.o. day 15 to menses	0–60
Progesterone suppositories (8) (CDOC)	200–400 mg p.v. days 14–28	0–60
Bromocriptine	1.25–2.5 mg p.o. b.i.d. day 14 to menses	0–80
Alprazolam[d] (9)	0.25–5.0 mg p.o. daily (Average 2.25 mg)	75
Clonidine	17 µg/kg/day p.o.	100
GnRH agonist (D-Trp6-Pro-9-NEt-GnRH[e] (10)	50 µg s.c. daily × 90 days	100[f]

[a] Data from True BL, Goodner SM, Burns EA: Review of the etiology and treatment of premenstrual syndrome. Drug Intell Clin Pharm 19:714–722, 1985; Harrison W, Sharpe L, Endicott J: Treatment of premenstrual symptoms. Gen Hosp Psychiatry 7:54–65, 1985; and Smith S, Shiff I: The premenstrual syndrome—diagnosis and management. Fertil Steril 52(4):527–543, 1989.

[b] Study results vary greatly.

[c] CDOC, clinical drug of choice. In the treatment of PMS, the CDOCs are most often tried, although none are satisfactory for long-term improvement of symptoms and the studies available are not helpful in choosing therapy.

[d] Addictive quality of alprazolam is a main drawback and many PMS patients have a history of substance dependence, depression, and other psychiatric disorders (9).

[e] Effective for short term. Whether prolonged therapy would be safe and effective or even necessary remains to be determined. The only worrisome side effect is a substantial decrease in estradiol that could, with long-term use, lead to osteoporosis. The cost of GnRH agonists such as leuprolide and nafarelin is prohibitive unless they are used as a last resort.

[f] Small (8 patients) but well-controlled double-blind cross-over study.

trolled clinical trial is performed, as is the case with various forms of progesterone (13). Because of this, most clinicians use stress-reduction classes, counseling, and exercise programs with drug therapy.

Patients must understand the empirical nature of the various therapies and realize that some patients have responded very well to any given drug, ancillary treatment, or combination of treatments.

Recently, both the somatic and psychologic symptoms of PMS were attenuated by "medical ovariectomy" using daily administration of the gonadotropin-releasing hormone (GnRH) agonist D-TrP6-Pro9-NEt-GnRH to a small, carefully selected group of patients (10). This lends support to the theory that cyclical fluctuations in ovarian steroids are involved in the regulation of neuropeptides, which in turn modulate mood and behavior (11).

Some authors believe that 80% of patients with PMS can be treated with education, stress reduction, and dietary modifications without drugs (12, 14). Some are also studying alprazolam because of its anxiolytic and antidepressant effects during the symptomatic premenstrual days, but they must worry about its addiction liability. Alprazolam, GnRH agonists, and clonidine must be considered the last choices of therapy until larger, well-controlled studies confirm their efficacy in PMS. Until that time, the clinical drugs of choice (CDOCs) will remain spironolactone, various COCs, pyridoxine, and progesterone in appropriately selected patients.

Progesterone, in various forms, has been the most commonly prescribed therapy for PMS for several decades and yet is the most controversial. For example, uncontrolled clinical trials have consistently demonstrated that progesterone suppositories are an effective treatment for PMS, and they are the basis for the widespread use of progesterone therapy in the United States. Unfortunately, progesterone deficiency has never been proven to be a cause for PMS, and most controlled clinical trials have failed to demonstrate the superiority of progesterone therapy over placebo (13). Advocates of progesterone therapy seem unwilling to accept unfavorable clinical trial data because they have very few alternative agents to offer their PMS patients.

ENDOMETRIOSIS

Possibly 5 to 15% of all premenopausal women have endometriosis to some degree. It is a common abnormal pelvic finding in women over 25 years of age and may be found in 40 to 50% of women who undergo surgery for the diagnosis and treatment of infertility. The average age at diagnosis is 28 years, and 75% of women with endometriosis are between 24 and 50 years old (15).

Endometriosis is a disorder in which there are islands of endometrium in extrauterine locations which exhibit the histologic and hormonal responsiveness of native endometrium. Cyclic change in these islands of endometrium is associated with menstrual-like bleeding and resultant localized inflammation (15).

Endometriosis most commonly occurs within the pelvis, on or within the ovaries, on the peritoneum, or beneath the serosa of pelvic viscera. Extrapelvic endometriosis, which occurs less frequently, involves location outside the genital tract such as the bowel, rectum, appendix, umbilicus, scars, pleura, lung, kidney, ureter, bladder, and nerves (16).

The most frequent symptoms of genital tract endometriosis are secondary dysmenorrhea and pelvic pain, dyspareunia, menstrual irregularities, and infertility. Depending on the location of the extrapelvic endometriosis, the symptoms and signs vary. Interestingly, the severity of the disease does not directly correlate with the severity of the symptoms (17).

The etiology of endometriosis, most widely accepted, involves retrograde menstruation. This has been recently supported by findings that (a) retrograde menstruation is a common (90%) event in menstruating women with patent fallopian tubes and (b) the anatomic distribution of endometriosis found at laparoscopy is consistent with retrograde menstruation. It has also been suggested that endometrial cells may successfully implant only in women with alterations in cell-mediated immunity and that such translocated cells may receive a stimulus for ectopic implantation and growth from activated macrophages (18). There are at least four other possible causes of endometriosis: (a) ectopic functioning endometrium may develop as a result of atypical development of germinal epithelium, since various parts of the pelvic peritoneum are embryologically derived from totipotential coelomic epithelial cell elements; (b) metastases of normal endometrium via uterine lymphatic vessels; (c) hematogenous spread via blood vessels to distant sites; or (d) cell rests of Muellerian epithelium develop into functioning ectopic endometrial implants.

The goals of drug therapy of endometriosis are to ameliorate pain and to correct menstrual irregularities and infertility by the suppression of ectopic endometrial implants.

Danazol (Table 86.4) was the first hormonal agent approved by the Food and Drug Administration for the treatment of endometriosis. Although called an "antigonadotropin," its mechanism of action is much more complex in that it inhibits gonadotropin surge, inhibits the action of steroidogenic enzymes, and interacts with androgen and progesterone receptors (19).

Amenorrhea occurs with doses of 200 to 800 mg per day without significantly decreasing circulating levels of

Table 86.4.
Danazol Therapy for Endometriosis[a]

CDOC?[b]		
Dose[c]	Moderate-to-severe symptoms	400 mg p.o. b.i.d.
	Mild symptoms	100–200 mg p.o. b.i.d.

Side Effect	Percentage	Side Effect	Percentage
Weight gain	85	Decreased libido	20
Muscle cramps	52	Nausea	17
Flushing	42	Headache	17
Mood changes	38	Dizziness	10
Seborrhea	37	Insomnia	10
Depression	32	Rash	8
Sweating	32	Increasing libido	8
Edema	28	Deepening voice	7
Change in appetite	28	Increased LDL	
Acne	27	Decreased HDL	
Fatigue	25	Increased hepatic enzymes	
Hirsutism	21	Fetal masculinization	
Decreased breast size	48		

[a] Data from Metzger DA, Luciano AA: Hormonal therapy of endometriosis. Obstet Gynecol Clin North Am 16(1):105–121, 1989.
[b] CDOC, clinical drug of choice. Although approved for the treatment of endometriosis, the many side effects and the availability of newer, less troublesome therapies may have displaced danazol in this disorder.
[c] It is essential that therapy continue uninterrupted for 3 to 6 months, but it may be extended to 9 months if necessary. The dose may be adjusted to patient response.
Note: Cost to patient: 200 mg/day = $75.00 per month; 400 mg/day = $143.00 per month; 800 mg/day = $234.00 per month.

gonadotropins or estrogens. The manufacturer recommends use of a nonhormonal method of contraception because ovulation may occur and further warns that use of danazol during pregnancy can result in androgenic effects on the fetus. To date, these have been limited to clitoral hypertrophy and labial fusion of the external genitalia in the female fetus. The manufacturer further recommends that therapy should begin during menstruation or after a reliable pregnancy test.

Table 86.4, Danazol Therapy for Endometriosis, lists the average dose, duration and side effects of danazol.

Continuous progestational therapy with medroxyprogesterone acetate (MPA) by mouth is becoming popular because of its low cost and generally well tolerated side effects, compared with danazol. Although depot–medroxyprogesterone acetate (DMPA) is available, oral administration may be preferable in the patient desiring to get pregnant because of the well-documented prolonged anovulatory effect of DMPA. At a daily oral dose of 50 mg for 4 months, MPA did not adversely alter serum concentrations of lipids or lipoproteins (19). Table 86.5 lists average dose, duration, and side effects of MPA.

The inability of danazol to achieve complete ovarian suppression and its high frequency of side effects led to efforts to develop agents more effective against steroidogenesis. Long-acting gonadotropin-releasing hormone agonists (GnRH-a) create a temporary and readily reversible "medical oophorectomy" and are currently the best therapy next to actual oophorectomy in the treatment of endometriosis. Endogenous GnRH is normally released in a circadian pattern every 60 to 90 min in the follicular phase. Down-regulation of the pituitary occurs if the peptide is given continuously or as a long-acting synthetic agonist analog. Although GnRH-a can be administered intravenously intramuscularly, subcutaneously, intranasally, in-

Table 86.6.
Gonadotropin-releasing Hormone Agonist (GnRH-a) Therapy for Endometriosis[a]

GnRH-a	Dosage Regimen/Route	Duration
Nafarelin (CDOC)[b]	200 μg in one nostril in the morning, 200 μg in the other nostril in the evening[c]	6 months
Buserelin	300 μg intranasally 3 times daily	6 months
Leuprolide	0.5 mg subcutaneously daily	6 months
Leprolide (CDOC)[d]	3.75 mg (depot) monthly	6 months

GnRH-a Side Effects	
Hot flashes	Decreases libido
Vaginal dryness	Decreased bone mineral content

[a] Data from Metzger DA, Luciano AA: Hormornal therapy of endometriosis. Obstet Gynecol Clin North Am 16(1): 105–121, 1989; and Erickson LD, Ory SJ: GnRH analogues in the treatment of endometriosis. Obstet Gynecol Clin North Am 16(1):123–145, 1989.
[b] CDOC, clinical drug of choice.
[c] If amenorrhea does not occur after 2 months of treatment use 1 spray (200 μg) into both nostrils in the morning and evening (total = 800 μg daily). Treatment should begin between days 2 and 4 of menses and not last for more than 6 months, since safety data for retreatment are not available. Do not use topical nasal decongestants until 30 min after dosing. The manufacturer suggests use of a nonhormonal (barrier) method of contraception since the drug is Pregnancy Category X, having induced major malformations in 4/80 rat fetuses at 7 times the maximum human dose.
Note: Cost to patient: 400 μg/day = $289.00 per month; 800 μg/day = $571.00 per month.
[d] CDOC, clinical drug of choice. Depot leuprolide has the advantage of avoidance of compliance with daily injections or twice daily nasal sprays.
Note: Cost to patient: 0.5 mg/day = $194.00 per month; 3.75 mg = $260.00 per month.

travaginally, or rectally, only subcutaneous once-daily doses, intramuscular monthly doses of depot forms, or twice-daily nasal sprays are currently used in the United States. Both depot–leuprolide acetate and intranasal nafarelin acetate have been approved for the treatment of endometriosis by the Food and Drug Administration at this time. Table 86.6 lists average dosages, routes, duration, and side effects for GnRH-a preparations.

After 6 months of therapy, nafarelin decreased total vertebral bone mass by a mean of 5.9%. Six months after completion of treatment the total vertebral mass was still 1.4% below pretreatment levels. For this reason and because safety data for retreatment are not available, the manufacturer suggests bone density studies before retreating.

It is not clear which of the above hormonal therapies is the most efficacious therapy for symptomatic endometriosis (19). Depot leuprolide has the advantage of avoiding compliance problems, with daily injections or twice-daily nasal spraying.

Although the above hormonal therapies have proved effective in relieving pain and combating the histologic

Table 86.5.
Medroxyprogesterone Acetate Therapy for Endometriosis[a]

Dose: 30–50 mg p.o. daily[b]	
Side Effect	Percentage
Amenorrhea	70
Weight gain	60
Edema, bloating	60
Dysfunctional bleeding	20
Anxiety, irritability	20
Cyclic bleeding	10
Depression	5

[a] Data from Metzger DA, Luciano AA: Hormonal therapy of endometriosis. Obstet Gynecol Clin North Am 16(1):105–121, 1989.
[b] Cost to patient: 30 mg daily = $31.00 per month; 50 mg daily = $48.00 per month.

manifestations of endometriosis, currently no clear evidence validates the efficacy of any medical approach in treating infertility (19).

Finally, the role of low-dose combination oral contraceptives (LDCOCs) in preventing endometriosis, in limiting progression of established disease, or in minimizing the risk of recurrence following hormonal and/or surgical therapy has not been clarified. Only the lowest possible dose of estrogen should be used (19). The cost to the patient is only $20 per month.

VAGINITIS (VULVOVAGINITIS)

At least one-third of all women of childbearing age currently have one or more vulvovaginal infections. The chief symptoms are varying degrees of vaginal discharge, itching, and burning. The fears, shame, physical discomfort, esthetic revulsions, psychosexual problems, and embarrassments experienced as a result of vulvovaginal infections cause more unhappiness than any other gynecologic disorder, and the cost of treatment is substantial (21).

Basic Physiology and Flora

Normally, women of childbearing age have a thick, protective epithelium that is maintained by estrogen. A pH of 4.5 to 5.5 is maintained by the normal flora, a mixture of aerobic and anaerobic bacteria that break down epithelial cell carbohydrates, particularly glycogen, to lactic acid. The flora often includes clostridia, anaerobic streptococci (peptostreptococcus), aerobic group, D and β-hemolytic streptococci, coliforms, and sometimes *Listeria*, in addition to the normally present Doderlein's bacilli (*Lactobacillus* species). If lactobacilli are suppressed by antibiotic drugs, yeasts or various bacteria normally present may become pathogenic by increasing in numbers and causing irritation and inflammation. After menopause, lactobacilli diminish and a mixed flora predominates; the pH changes from acid to neutral or alkaline, which along with a thinning of the vaginal epithelium and a reduction of cervical mucus, leads to increased vaginal infections and atrophic vaginitis. Normally, cervical mucus has antibacterial activity and contains lysozyme. In some women the vaginal introitus contains a heavy flora similar to that of the perineum and perianal area, which may predispose them to recurrent urinary tract infections. Table 86.7 includes the vulvovaginitide. Herpes genitalis is discussed in Chapter 69.

Nonspecific Vaginosis

A toxonomic controversy is responsible for the many etiologies and names proposed for nonspecific vaginosis. The former names given the disease, "*Haemophilus* vaginitis," "*Corynebacterium* vaginitis," and "*Gardnerella* vaginitis," reflected the suspected bacterial cause. Now, nonspecific

Table 86.7.

Prevalence of Various Vulvovaginitides in 1000 Consecutive Patients with Lower Genital Tract Infections (Gonorrhea and Syphilis Excluded)[a]

Disorder	Incidence Number	Percentage	Percentage with One or More Other Pathogens[b]
Nonspecific vaginosis	425	42.5	23.3
Vaginal candidosis	373	37.3	17.7
Trichomoniasis	142	14.2	37.7
Herpes genitalis	94	9.4	16.4
Condylomata acuminata	72	7.2	55.6

[a] Adapted from Gardner HL, Infectious vulvovaginitis. In Monif GR (ed): Infectious Diseases in Obstetrics and Gynecology, ed. 2. Philadelphia, Harper & Row, 1982, p 515.
[b] One patient had five infections simultaneously, 2 had four, and 126 had two. Incidence and numbers of simultaneous infections depend on the patient population studied.

vaginosis is the preferred name, pointing to the vagina as one of the body sites in which normally colonizing bacteria may become pathogenic.

Normally, lactobacilli, the predominant vaginal organism, control the growth of anaerobes and other bacteria by producing hydrogen peroxide. If hydrogen peroxide is produced in very low levels, the mixed anaerobic and aerobic vaginal flora become free to proliferate 10- to 10,000-fold and grow *Gardnerella vaginalis*, which is normally present in 40 to 60% of women. *Gardnerella* vaginalis produces amino acids. Anaerobes produce enzymes that cleave these amino acids and form amines that increase the vaginal pH and cause epithelial shedding that produces a discharge. Thus a vicious cycle starts in which an elevated pH decreases lactobacilli, anaerobes predominate, and extremely high numbers of *G. vaginalis* are present (22).

The chief symptom of bacterial vaginosis is vaginal discharge with a characteristic foul "fish" odor that worsens after intercourse because of a shift to alkaline pH in the vagina. This discharge is grey and homogeneous and frequently coats the labia. Minimal vulvovaginal itching and burning may occur.

There are four criteria to diagnose nonspecific vaginosis:

1. Homogeneous vaginal discharge;
2. pH > 4.5;
3. "Clue cells" (a squamous epithelial cell whose border contains adherent *G. vaginalis*);
4. Positive "sniff" test (10% potassium hydroxide added to discharge releases the rotten fish odor of amines).

The goal of drug treatment of nonspecific vaginosis is to restore the normal vaginal flora and alleviate the minimal vulvar itching and burning, the grey homogeneous discharge, and the "fishy" odor. Monitoring the efficacy of the drug therapy does not necessitate reexamination of the patient unless symptoms persist.

Clearly, metronidazole is the CDOC and therefore the initial choice for nonspecific vaginosis in nonpregnant women. Metronidazole, although given an approximate Pregnancy Category of B by the manufacturer, should not be used in pregnancy because of its observed mutagenicity in bacteria and carcinogenicity in animal models. In pregnancy, recent studies suggest that nonspecific vaginosis may be a factor in premature rupture of membranes and premature delivery, but they need substantiation. Until such studies have been conducted, routine treatment appears to be unnecessary or optional. Since metronidazole is contraindicated in the first trimester and its safety in the rest of pregnancy is still in question, treatment with clindamycin 300 mg orally twice daily for 7 days is recommended (23). Ampicillin, amoxicillin, or cephradine are acceptable alternatives and can be used in pregnant patients.

No clinical counterpart of nonspecific vaginosis is recognized in the male, and treatment of the male sex partner has not been shown to be beneficial for the patient or the male partner (23).

Patients should be instructed to abstain from intercourse while taking the drug or to use condoms. It is absolutely essential to complete the full course of drug therapy because symptoms may disappear before there is bacteriologic cure.

The current drug therapies for nonspecific vaginosis are summarized in Table 86.8.

Vaginal Candidosis

Candida albicans in 90 to 95% of cases and *Candida glabrata* in 5 to 10% of cases are colonized in the female genital tract and bowel and do not produce symptoms. Because of this, the former terms "candidiasis" or "moniliasis" have been replaced with the term "vaginal candidosis."

Table 86.8.
Drug Treatment of Nonspecific Vaginosis[a]

Drug	Dose/Regimen
Metronidazole (CDOC)[b]	500 mg p.o. b.i.d. for 7 days (23)
Clindamycin (CDOC)[c]	300 mg p.o. b.i.d. for 7 days (23)
Ampicillin	500 mg p.o. q.i.d. for 7 days (21)
Amoxacillin	500 mg p.o. t.i.d. for 7 days (21)
Cephradine	250 mg p.o. q.i.d. for 7 days (21)
Tetracycline	500 mg p.o. q.i.d. for 7 days (21)

[a] Many authorities do not recommend treatment of asymptomatic infection. Treatment of the male sex partner has not been shown to be beneficial for the patient or the male partner.
[b] CDOC, clinical drug of choice; metronidazole is clearly the best treatment.
[c] CDOC, clinical drug of choice; recommended in pregnancy and as an alternative to metronidazole.

Predisposing factors to vaginal candidosis include (21):

1. Pregnancy and "pseudopregnancy" from oral contraceptives by:
   a. Increased vaginal glycogen from estrogens;
   b. Vaginal thinning from progestins;
   c. Altered sugar metabolism;
   d. Sexual habits (i.e., anal, followed by vaginal intercourse);
   e. Increased *Candida* colonization (but not infection).
2. Antibiotic therapy by:
   a. Increased candidal colonization by suppressing bacterial competition in the genital tract and bowel;
   b. Reduced phagocytosis of *Candida*;
   c. Direct growth stimulation of Candida.
3. Diabetes mellitus, if poorly controlled, by increased glucose secretions or alterations in the immune system.

The chief symptoms of vaginal candidosis are severe itching of the vulva, vagina, or both and meatal dysuria. The vulvitis symptoms are normally aggravated by tight clothing.

There are three criteria for the diagnosis of vaginal candidiasis:

1. Thick, white, curd-like secretions;
2. pH 3.8 to 5.0.
3. Long thread-like fibers of mycelia with tiny buds of conidia attached when one or two drops of 10% potassium hydroxide are added to a vaginal exudate slide (KOH preparation).

Nickerson's medium is infrequently used to confirm the diagnosis before the treatments summarized in Table 86.9 are instituted.

The goal of drug treatment of vaginal candidosis is to restore normal vaginal flora and thereby alleviate the vulvar erythema; the fungal patches; the severe itching and burning of the vagina, vulva, or both; and the white, dry, curd-like vaginal discharge. Alleviation of symptoms is evidence of efficacy, and reexamination of the patient is unnecessary unless symptoms persist.

Of all the drug therapies of vaginal candidosis, only nystatin is fungistatic and is therefore no longer recommended (23). *Candida glabrata* is best treated with gentian violet.

Patient compliance improves as the duration of therapy decreases. Fortunately, the 3-day therapies listed in Table 86.9 are approximately as effective as the 7-day therapies. Single-day therapies should only be used in mild or early cases, and recently many experts have recommended that 1-day therapy not be used at all (23).

Patients should understand that strict regimen compliance is necessary, that creams are usually preferable to tablets or suppositories since some cream can be applied to the perineum, and that treatment should always be continued through menses, if it occurs, and when vaginal contraceptives are used. The patient should also be instructed to report any new vaginal irritation, since vaginal irritation

Table 86.9.
Drug Treatment of Vaginal Candidosis

Drug/Dose	Regimen
Seven-day therapy	
Clotrimazole 1% vag cr (CDOC)[a]	App 1 p.v. h.s. × 7
Clotrimazole 100-mg vag tabs	Tab 1 p.v. h.s. × 7
Miconazole nitrate 2% vag cr	App 1 p.v. h.s. × 7
Miconazole nitrate 100-mg vag supp	Supp 1 p.v. h.s. × 7
Terconazole 0.4% vag cr	App 1 p.v. h.s. × 7
Tioconazole 80-mg supp	Supp 1 p.v. h.s. × 7
Three-day therapy[b]	
Butoconazole Nitrate 2% vag cr	App 1 p.v. h.s. × 3
Clotrimazole 1% vag cr	App 1 p.v. b.i.d. × 3
Clotrimazole 100-mg vag tabs	Tab 2 p.v. h.s. × 3
Econazole 150-mg vag tabs	Tab 1 p.v. h.s. × 3
Miconazole nitrate 2% vag cr	App 1 p.v. b.i.d. × 3
Miconazole nitrate 200-mg vag supp	Supp 1 p.v. h.s. × 3
Terconazole 80-mg vag supp	Supp 1 p.v. h.s. × 3
One-day therapy[c]	
Clotrimazole 500-mg vag tab[d]	Tab 1 p.v. h.s. × 1
Tioconazole 6.5% vag oint	App 1 p.v. h.s. × 1
Miscellaneous therapies	
Ketoconazole 200-mg oral tab[e]	Tab 1 p.o. b.i.d. × 3 days
Gentian Violet Tampons[f] 5 mg	Tampon 1 p.v. one to two times daily for 3–4 hr for 12 days

[a] CDOC, clinical drug of choice is any of the 7-day therapies.

[b] Three-day therapies are as efficacious as 7-day therapies except for pregnant, diabetic, or corticosteroid-using women. For these conditions use only 7-day therapy.

[c] One-day therapy is only good for mild or early cases. Three- and 7-day therapies are superior. In general, 1-day therapy is not recommended because of poor efficacy (23).

[d] Single dose serves as a vaginal depot for at least 3 days (24).

[e] Should be the last treatment of choice for recurrent or persistent cases. The drug is hepatotoxic and is contraindicated in pregnancy because of known teratogenic effects in rats, manifested as limb deformities.

[f] Best treatment for *Candida glabrata*; Caution: purple staining.

Note: If any first course fails, reconfirm diagnosis with microscopic examination and treat with an alternate drug.

Note: Treatment of pregnant patients can use any of the above medications (23) except ketoconazole.

Note: Nystatis Vag Tabs 100,000 units are intentionally omitted from this table because they are only fungistatic; all of the other therapies are fungicidal (23).

in 0 to 6.6% of patients has been reported with miconazole > tioconazole > butoconazole > econazole > clotrimazole > nystatin. Irritation may necessitate changing the drug therapy. Terconazole use has been reported to cause headaches in 26% of patients. When gentian violet is used the patient should be advised of its permanent purple staining characteristics.

Recurrent Vaginal Candidosis

Recurrent vaginal candidosis may be due to:

1. Intestinal reservoir: Up to 100% correlation has been found between simultaneous infestations of *C. albicans* in the vaginal and fecal material. A persistent intestinal reservoir may

recolonize the perianal area and lead to recurrent infection (25).

2. Sexual transmission: Unequivocal proof that a colonized penis may transmit *C. albicans* is lacking, even though circumstantial evidence shows that 5 to 25% of male partners of infected females may asymptomatically carry yeast, usually in the coronal sulcus. Some clinicians advocate treatment of the male for 7 days with a cream from Table 86.9 (25).

3. Therapy failure: *Candida* blastospores invade intact epithelial cells in the superficial layers of the vaginal mucosa to a depth of several layers and may reemerge weeks or months later when the epithelial cells are normally shed. Approximately 20 to 50% of women clinically responding by culture to standard antifungal therapy are culture-positive within 30 days (25).

Therefore, for recurrent vaginal candidosis the following regimens may be employed.

1. For nonpregnant women:
   a. Ketoconazole 200-mg oral tablets one orally twice daily for 3 days (26).
   b. Optionally treat male partners with a topical cream from Table 86.9 for 7 days.
2. For pregnant women:
   a. Nystatin 500,000-unit oral tablets one orally three times daily for 14 days, plus
   b. Clotrimazole 1% vaginal cream applied once vaginally at bedtime for 14 days.
   c. Optionally treat the male with topical antifungal creams from Table 86.9 for 14 days.

The 1989 STD Treatment Guidelines state that systemic therapy is usually not indicated and that patients with frequent unexplained infections should be evaluated for predisposing conditions (especially HIV infection) and should be referred to an expert for care (23).

Trichomonas Vaginitis

Trichomoniasis is a disease of the vagina and the lower urinary tract of men and women. Sexual transmission is well recognized, although transmission by communal fomites, toilet splash, gloves, and instruments may rarely occur. Transmission to newborns of untreated mothers also occurs, and the child will require treatment. Male partners should be treated simultaneously, since 80% may be culture-positive (21).

The chief symptoms of *Trichomonas* vaginitis are variable, ranging from a mild yellow-green or grey vaginal discharge, to a moderate malodorous discharge, to itching, burning, discharge with odor, to intermenstrual or postcoital bleeding. Dysuria is present in at least 10% of patients.

There are four diagnostic parameters:

1. Thick or thin white, yellow, green, or grey malodorous discharge;
2. pH 5.0 to 7.5;
3. Highly motile, pear-shaped, unicellular *Trichomonas vagi-*

Table 86.10.
Drug Treatment of *Trichomonas* Vaginitis[a]

A. Metronidazole CDOC 500-mg tabs: 4 p.o. in a single dose
B. Metronidazole 500 mg b.i.d. for 7 days
  1. Male sex partners of infected women should be treated with regimen A or B.
  2. Asymptomatic women should be treated with regimen A or B.
  3. If failure occurs with either regimen, the patient should be treated with metronidazole 500 mg twice daily for 7 days.
  4. If repeated failure occurs, the patient should be treated with a single 2-g dose of metronidazole daily for 3 to 5 days.
  5. Cases in which there are additional culture-documented treatment failure in which reinfection has been excluded should be managed in consultation with an expert who can determine the susceptibility of *Trichomonas vaginalis* to metronidazole.
  6. Metronidazole is contraindicated in the first trimester of pregnancy, and its safety in the rest of pregnancy is not established. However, no other adequate therapy exists. For patients with severe symptoms after the first trimester, treatment with 2 g of metronidazole in a single dose is suggested.
  7. For lactating women, use regimen A, interrupting breast feeding for at least 24 hr after therapy.

[a] From Anon: 1989. Sexually transmitted diseases treatment guidelines. MMWR 38(S-8):1–43, 1989.

nalis seen on saline-mount microscopy (a flagellated protozoan about twice the size of a white blood cell);
4. "Strawberry" vagina or cervix (seen in only about 10% of patients) caused by swollen papillae projecting through vaginal secretions.

The goal of drug treatment of *Trichomonas* vaginitis is to restore the normal vaginal flora and thereby alleviate the vaginal itching, burning, and the malodorous yellow-green or grey discharge. Reexamination is only necessary when symptoms persist.

Table 86.10 summarizes current treatment of *Trichomonas* vaginitis in primary and recurrent cases. Unfortunately, only metronidazole is adequately effective and is therefore CDOC. Since 80% of male partners may be culture-positive, they must be treated simultaneously.

Patient education should include discussion of the necessity of strict compliance with the simultaneous treatment for both partners and the use of condoms until the regimens are completed. A metallic taste in the mouth and brown urine may occur, and patients taking metronidazole should avoid the consumption of alcohol because of the possibility of a disulfiram-type reaction.

GENITAL AND ANAL WARTS (CONDYLOMATA ACCUMINATA)

Approximately 60% of sexual partners of individuals with condylomata acuminata develop genital or anal warts, with an average incubation period of 2 to 3 months. The typical lesions in women are found most often in the fourchette and on the labia, and less commonly, on other parts of the

vulva, perineum, and anus. In addition, cervical warts are common. During pregnancy, genital warts tend to enlarge and grow more rapidly, taking on a cauliflower appearance. They may involve both the labia and vagina, rather than the perianal area, and may render vaginal delivery difficult. The causative agent is the human papillomavirus (HPV). A decade ago, genital and anal warts were thought to be trivial lesions of little importance. Today, they are recognized as one of the most important of the sexually transmitted diseases because of a 460% increase in 15 years in the United States. There is an estimated 2% incidence of flat condyloma of the cervix of all women of childbearing age. These data suggest that genital and anal warts are being encountered as often as herpes genitalis and gonorrhea (27).

Under certain circumstances some types of HPV (most commonly types 16, 18, and 31) have been found to be strongly associated with genital dysplasia and carcinoma. Fortunately, exophytic genital warts are most frequently caused by HPV types 6 and 11. However, a biopsy is needed in all instances of atypical, pigmented, or persistent warts. All women with anogenital warts should have a yearly pap smear (23).

The chief symptom reported by patients is an occasional itching of the lesions. The diagnosis is made by the presence of verrucose growths, usually on the vulva or genital area, and a positive sexual history.

The goals of drug treatment of genital and anal warts is to destroy the HPV-infected tissue, prevent recurrence and sexual transmission, and possibly prevent the sequellae of squamous cell genital cancer. Unfortunately, no therapy has been shown to eradicate HPV. HPV has been demonstrated in adjacent tissue after laser treatment of HPV-associated cervical intraepithelial neoplasia and after attempts to eliminate subclinical HPV by extensive laser vaporization of the anogenital area. Therefore, the goal of treatment is not the eradication of HPV (23). Sex partners should be examined for evidence of warts and treated as needed.

The CDOC at this time for vaginal and cervical warts is 5-fluorouracil (Table 86.11), along with the treatment and patient instructions for other genital and anal warts. Cryotherapy, electrosurgery, carbon dioxide laser therapy, and surgery are normally used for persistent, recurrent, or extensive infestations of genital and anal warts.

Treatments include cytotoxic, destructive, immunologic, and surgical methods. The cytotoxic treatment regimens with podophyllin or 5-fluorouracil and the destructive treatment with trichloroacetic acid are covered in Table 86.11.

Cryotherapy with liquid nitrogen or dry ice, electrosurgery, and carbon dioxide lasers (28) are other useful destructive treatments. Shave- and scissor-excision of

Table 86.11.
Drug Treatment of Genital or Anal Warts (Condylomata Accuminata)[a,b]

Trichloroacetic acids 80–90% (CDOC)[c]
1. Apply skin protectant[d] to surrounding tissues.
2. Treatment is adequate if a white color develops 30–60 sec later
3. Patient will experience a sharp, burning pain for 15–30 min.

Podophyllin 10–25% in compound tincture of benzoin
1. Apply skin protectant[d] to surrounding tissues.
2. Apply <0.5 ml per treatment; treat <10 cm².
3. Wash off thoroughly in 1–4 hr.
4. If four applications fail, other treatments are indicated.
5. Not for extensive lesions or pregnancy; podophyllin is absorbed and is toxic.

Podofilox 0.5% topical solutions
1. Apply skin protectant[d] to surrounding tissues.
2. Apply with cotton-tipped applicator twice daily morning and evening (every 12 hr) for 3 consecutive days, then withold use for 4 consecutive days. This 1-week cycle of treatment may be repeated up to four times until there is no visible wart tissue. If there is incomplete response after 4 treatment weeks, alternative treatment should be considered since the safety and effectiveness of more than 4 treatment weeks have not been established.
3. Treatment should be limited to less than 10 cm² of wart tissue and to no more than 0.5 ml of the solution per day.
4. Systemic absorption studies did not result in detectable serum levels. However, it should only be used in pregnancy if trichloroaqcetic acid therapy fails.

5-Fluorouracil cream 5% (28) (CDOC)
1. Only for vaginal/cervical/penile warts.
2. Female: Insert ½ vaginal applicator (2.5 g) p.v. h.s. for 5 days. Male: Apply 1–2 nights weekly to entire penis; avoid the urethra; therapy is for 3 months; apply a tissue between underside of penis and scrotum and wear a jockstrap to keep penis in place.
3. Female to apply a skin protectant[d] to vulva and urethra h.s. and a.m. after washing external genitalia.
4. Avoid during pregnancy, since 5-FU may be teratogenic.

---

[a] Information from Anon: 1989 Sexually transmitted diseases treatment guidelines. MMWR 38(S-8):1–43, 1989; and Lynch PJ: Condylomata acuminata (anogenital warts). Clin Obstet Gynecol 28:142–151, 1985 (except podofilox).
[b] Condoms shoud be used until warts disappear.
[c] CDOC, clinical drug of choice.
[d] Zinc oxide ointment 20%, silicone cream, or silver sulfadiazine 1% cream.

---

larger lesions are acceptable surgical methods. Interferon immunotherapy is currently under study (29).

ESTROGEN REPLACEMENT THERAPY

The female climacteric is a clinical epoch secondary to the physiologic depletion of ovarian follicles. Menopause refers to the cessation of menses. A patient is postmenopausal after 1 year of amenorrhea. Statistics indicate that by age 51.1, the average age of menopause, a woman can expect to live another 28 years. Therefore, more than 32 million women in the United States 51.1 years of age and older can expect to live 40% of their lives in a state of estrogen deficiency. The consequences of this estrogen deficiency include vasomotor instability, atrophic vaginitis, and osteoporosis.

Vasomotor Symptoms

Approximately 80% of women within the first year of ovarian failure or castration experience hot flushes that are caused by a decrease in the tone of arterioles, resulting in an increased blood flow to the skin with a rise in skin temperature. Hot flushes appear to be synchronous with increased hypothalamic release of GnRH. Since GnRH neurons are close to the centers that regulate temperature in the intact hypothalamus, it is likely that α-adrenergic stimulation of GnRH release concomitantly stimulates these centers. Although the symptoms may last for at least 5 years for 70% of this group, homeostatic adjustments eventually occur. The most likely explanation of why all women do not experience hot flushes seems to be varying amounts of endogenous estradiol (5 to 20 μg/day versus 50 to 300 μg/day before menopause) produced in the liver and adipose tissue. Obese women may produce twice as much estradiol as slender women.

The chief vasomotor symptoms reported by patients are described as "hot flushes" or "hot flashes" occurring over the anterior part of the body, especially the chest, neck, and face. An episode usually lasts only a few minutes, and it is commonly precipitated by anxiety or excitement. The vasomotor symptoms vary considerably in duration, frequency, and severity. One variation, "night sweats," is experienced by some patients, who usually describe awakening at night covered in perspiration and throwing off the bed covers.

It is estimated that following physiologic menopause, 15% of patients seek treatment for vasomotor symptoms; 50% of reproductive-age women undergoing castration request treatment. The vasomotor symptoms themselves are not thought to be harmful, but they indicate an estrogen deficiency and are usually treated upon request. The lowest dosage of estrogen to reduce the vasomotor symptoms to a tolerable level should be used and reevaluated every 6 months. Reduced symptoms during the drug-free evaluation period are found within 2 to 5 years of menopause. Clinically, there is no reasonable means to follow the response to treatment other than subjective symptomatic improvement.

All potential patients for estrogen therapy should undergo a baseline evaluation, including pelvic examination, cytology, breast examination, blood pressure, and a thorough history, to rule out the following contraindications:

1. Active thrombophlebitis or thromboembolic disorders (or history thereof); (*Note*: Women on estrogen replacement therapy have not been reported to have an increased risk of thrombophlebitis and/or thromboembolic disease. However, there is insufficient information regarding women who have had previous thromboembolic disease.)
2. Cerebrovascular accident (or history thereof);
3. Coronary artery disease (or history thereof);

Table 86.12.
Treatment of Hot Flushes and Equivalent ERT Regimen[a]

Generic Name	Equivalent Regimen
Conjugated estrogens (CDOC)[b]	0.625 mg p.o. × 25 day/month[c]
Estropipate	0.625 mg p.o. × 25 day/month[c]
Ethinyl estradiol	0.2 mg p.o. × 25 day/month[c]
17β-Estradiol	0.5 mg × 25 day/month[c]
17β-Estradiol (transdermal)	0.05 mg patch to skin b.i.w.[d]
Medroxyprogesterone acetate	20 mg p.o. daily[e]
Clonidine	0.2 mg p.o. b.i.d.[f]

[a] With all ERT regimens add medroxyprogesterone acetate 2.5–10 mg 10–13 days/month to prevent endometrial hyperplasia and possible malignancy in all women who have not had their uterus removed.

[b] CDOC, clinical drug of choice; conjugated estrogens are the initial choice because of the extensive literature on their use.

[c] Over 80% of ERT patients in the United States are given conjugated estrogens. Little in the literature supports the advantage of one preparation over another if equivalent doses are used.

[d] 75% effective, similar to oral ERT; up to 20% minor skin irritation (29).

[e] Mechanism unknown; >70% effective; not an approved use; may be used when estrogens are contraindicated; about one-third of women with intact uteri may have vaginal bleeding. Progestins will not prevent vaginal atrophy and may not prevent osteoporosis (30).

[f] α-Adrenergic agonist; <50% effective; dry mouth and sedation limit usefulness; not an approved use; more studies needed; last choice (31).

4. Known or suspected carcinoma of the breast (or history thereof);
5. Known or suspected estrogen-dependent neoplasia (or history thereof);
6. Benign or malignant liver tumor (or history thereof);
7. Known impaired liver function at the present time;
8. Any undiagnosed vaginal bleeding.

Patient education should include the major adverse estrogen effects as well as instructions about the importance of yearly physical examinations repeating the baseline parameters. Patients should also be warned of the cardiovascular and neoplastic liabilities of smoking, which with estrogens may contribute to these disorders, although this has not been established in the literature.

Recommended therapies for vasomotor symptoms and equivalent estrogen replacement therapy (ERT) doses and regimens appear in Table 86.12.

Vaginal Atrophy, Atrophic Vaginitis, and Dysuria

Postmenopausal estrogen deficiency leads to a thinning of the vaginal epithelium, a decreased blood supply, dryness, and a change to a neutral or alkaline pH that predisposes to infection.

The chief symptoms are vaginal discharge secondary to infection, complaints of painful intercourse (dyspareunia) due to dryness, and dysuria. Estrogens increase the vascularity and epithelial proliferation of the vagina, allowing greater lubrication, increased protection from vaginitis, and reduced vaginal trauma from coitus. The in-creased vascularity resulting from estrogen therapy is associated with increased blood flow through the periurethral venous plexus leading to small increases in periurethral pressure occasionally sufficient to correct urinary stress incontinence.

The goals of therapy are to eliminate the atrophy, dysuria, and predisposition to vaginal infections caused by estrogen deficiency.

The atrophy and dysuria can be treated with equal effectiveness by either systemic or vaginally applied estrogen. However the response to conjugated-estrogen cream may be lost after 14 days because of tissue cornification or down-regulation of the estrogen receptors. This can be overcome by stopping treatment for 7 to 14 days and restarting using 0.1 mg daily rather than the 1.25 to 2.5 mg dose recommended by the manufacturer (32). For this reason the systemic effects and topical response may be erratic. Conjugated estrogens, estropipate, and estradiol vaginal creams contain 0.625 mg/g, 1.25 mg/g, and 0.1 mg/g, respectively, and supply applicators graduated from 1 to 4 g. A full applicator of dienestrol cream 0.01% is approximately equal to 1g of the others.

The CDOC is conjugated-estrogen vaginal cream, since most clinical data concern its use. Patient instructions and warnings are basically the same as with oral estrogens, since systemic estrogen levels may be reached. Most experts recommend the addition of 10 to 13 days of medroxyprogesterone acetate 2.5 to 10 mg daily in women with intact uteri to prevent endometrial hyperplasia and possible malignancy. Current recommended treatments for vaginal atrophy and dysuria are listed in Table 86.13.

Osteoporosis Secondary to Estrogen Deficiency

Conservatively, osteoporosis secondary to estrogen deficiency may be responsible for 100,000 wrist fractures and

Table 86.13.
Currently Recommended Treatments for Vaginal Atrophy and Dysuria[a,b]

Generic Name	Regimen
Conjugated estrogen cream 0.625 mg/g (CDOC)[c]	0.2–1 g p.v. daily × 10, then b.i.w.-t.i.w.
Estropipate cream 1.25 mg/g	0.2–1 g p.v. daily × 10, then b.i.w.-t.i.w.
17β-Estradiol cream 0.1 mg/g	0.2–1 g p.v. daily × 10, then b.i.w.-t.i.w.
Dienestrol cream 0.01%	0.2–1 applicatorful daily × 10, then b.i.w.-t.i.w.

[a] These regimens are extrapolated from Dyer GI, Townsend PT: Dose related changes in vaginal cytology after topical conjugated equine oestrogens. Br Med J 284:789, 1982, and differ from the manufacturer's recommendations.

[b] Most experts recommend cyclic addition of 10–13 days of progestin monthly if the uterus is present to prevent endometrial hyperplasia and possible malignancy.

[c] (CDOC), clinical drug of choice.

250,000 hip fractures annually in the United States. The acute-care cost may total $3 billion following the hip fractures, and the mortality may be as high as 15 to 30%, or 27,000 to 60,000 deaths/year, for the year following a hip fracture, usually due to complications such as pneumonia, pulmonary embolism, or congestive heart failure. An additional 40,000 patients will require prolonged institutionalization (33), which helps bring the annual total of direct and indirect costs to $7 billion (34).

In women, maximal mineral content in cortical bone of the radius occurs in the mid-30s, and it declines 3%/decade until menopause, 9%/decade until age 75, and 3%/decade thereafter, with as much as 66% skeletal loss by age 80. Of women over 60, 25% have spinal compression fractures, causing much pain and debilitation; by age 75, this figure reaches as high as 50% (33).

Since patients prone to osteoporosis cannot be predicted, all women who are postmenopausal or lack ovarian function or ovaries should receive ERT, when not contraindicated, soon after the diagnosis of estrogen deficiency. An exception to this may be black women, who have a greater bone mass and higher calcitonin levels than nonblack women, leading to a low risk for osteoporosis. Pure black women may only need ERT for premature surgical menopause, hot flushes, atrophic vaginitis, or estrogen-deficiency dysuria.

A decline in circulating estrogens enhances calcium efflux from bone mineral stores and increases the serum concentration of ionized calcium. This suppresses secretion of parathyroid hormone (PTH), which in turn, reduces the synthesis of 1,25-dihydroxyvitamin D_3 by the renal tubular cells. The lowered concentration of 1,25-dihydroxyvitamin D_3 causes a decrease in the intestinal absorption of calcium. Studies of PTH and vitamin D have not demonstrated a consistent relationship between their levels and osteoporosis. However, calcitonin secretion declines progressively with age and estrogen deficiency. Calcitonin inhibits bone resorption and is known to be increased with ERT. Therefore, there may be beneficial effects on bone due to estrogens at nonestrogen or estrogen receptor sites.

PREVENTION OF OSTEOPOROSIS

The risks associated with hormonal therapy and the need for lifelong ERT to prevent osteoporosis have made both patients and practitioners hesitant to use ERT.

The association of endometrial cancer with ERT exists because it is well known that estrogens stimulate the growth of the endometrium and that the resultant proliferation can potentially progress to atypical hyperplasia and adenocarcinoma. However, the highest incidence of cancer is usually in users of estrogens not opposed by progestins, the lowest incidence in users of estrogen and progestin combination therapy, and intermediate incidence is in women not taking estrogens or progestins. Progestins decrease estrogen receptors in endometrial cells and induce estradiol dehydrogenase and isocitrate activity, which are the mechanisms whereby these cells metabolize estrogens (35).

Since the likelihood of developing breast cancer is higher than that of endometrial cancer in all women, and breast cancer has a less desirable outcome, it is comforting at this time to find that there is no evidence that estrogens increase the risk of breast cancer, and that progestin added to ERT significantly reduced the risk of mammary malignancy in at least one study (35). Because breast cells are not cyclically shed by the action of progesterone, the protective mechanism most likely operates at the intracellular level through changes in receptors. Therefore, according to this study, progestins should be given even to those women who have had a hysterectomy, for 10 to 13 days each month, whenever they are prescribed estrogen therapy (35). Many experts disagree with this practice.

In general, epidemiologic data from case-control and cohort studies have suggested that postmenopausal estrogen confers a moderate degree of protection from coronary artery disease, with reductions in overall mortality rates for acute myocardial infarction in comparison with nonestrogen-users (36).

ROLE OF CALCIUM INTAKE

Healthy postmenopausal women whose usual daily elemental calcium dietary intake is less than 400 mg lose mineral from the spine at a greater rate than women whose intake is higher. In a recent study, in women who had undergone menopause 5 or fewer years earlier, bone loss from the spine was rapid and was not affected by supplementation with 500 mg of elemental calcium daily in addition to their normal lower than 400 mg or 400 to 650 mg daily dietary intake. In women who had been postmenopausal for 6 years or more given placebo, bone loss was less rapid in those normally taking 400 to 650 mg. None of the women had used estrogen, glucocorticoids, or other medications known to affect calcium or bone metabolism within the past year in this double-blind, placebo-controlled, randomized trial to determine the effect of calcium on bone loss from the spine, femoral neck, and radius. During the 2-year study, those with the lower calcium intake maintained bone density at the femoral neck and radius but not the spine when treated with calcium carbonate. Although it has not been a consistent finding, increased rates of bone loss have been reported to occur for 2 to 5 years after menopause. Therefore, the authors conclude, since the median daily intake of calcium in women over 44 years of age in the United States is known to be 475 mg, healthy postmenopausal women whose usual dietary calcium intake is low should be urged to increase their calcium intake to 800 mg per day, the current recommended daily allowance (37), to limit bone loss (38).

Table 86.14.
Oral Calcium Supplementation[a]

Generic Preparation	%Ca²⁺	Tablet Size (mg Ca²⁺/Tab)	#/Day to Supply 1 g	Cost/Day[b] ($)
Calcium carbonate (CDOC)[c]	40	650 (260)	4	0.48
Dibasic calcium PO₄	23	500 (115)	9	0.47
Calcium lactate	13	650 (84.5)	12	0.49
Calcium gluconate	9	650 (58.5)	17	0.44

[a] Adapted from Bauwens SF, Drinka PJ, Boh L: Pathogenesis and management of primary osteoporosis. Clin Pharm 5:639–659, 1986.
[b] Based on average wholesale price, 1990 Redbook.
[c] CDOC, clinical drug of choice.

Although calcium citrate malate was more bioavailable and shown to be more effective than calcium carbonate in the study cited above, it is not available commercially at this time (38). For those requiring calcium supplementation, calcium carbonate is usually the easiest calcium source to take since it contains the most elemental calcium per tablet. It should be taken with meals to assure adequate stomach acid secretion to facilitate absorption (39).

The main adverse effects of calcium supplementation are constipation in the elderly and possible kidney stone formation in those predisposed individuals who take at least 2000 mg of elemental calcium daily.

Dairy products are the best food source of calcium, with 8 oz of skim or whole milk containing roughly 300 mg of elemental calcium, 8 oz of yogurt having roughly 345 mg, 1 oz of cheese having 211 mg, and 8 oz of ice cream having 200 mg (39). Dietary sources may be supplemented with oral calcium salts (Table 86.14).

CURRENT DRUG THERAPIES TO PREVENT ESTROGEN-DEFICIENCY OSTEOPOROSIS

The minimum effective dose of estrogen to prevent bone loss is conjugated estrogens 0.625 mg or the equivalent (40). Combining 1500 mg elemental calcium per day and 0.3 mg conjugated estrogen produced an actual increase in vertebral trabecular mass over 2 years in one study (41). For those unable to tolerate estrogens, progestins alone may be used since there is some evidence that they decrease bone turnover. Giving 150 mg of depo-medroxyprogesterone acetate intramuscularly monthly has been suggested, although this has not been clearly established (42). (*Note*: The original article incorrectly states that 150 mg was given days 1 through 25 monthly). The 21 patients given 150 mg of depo-medroxyprogesterone acetate intramuscularly once monthly had significantly lowered urinary calcium/creatinine, and hydroxyproline/creatinine ratios that were similar to those of the 22 patients who received oral conjugated-estrogens 0.625 mg days 1

through 25 of each month. Unfortunately, the number of study patients was small and the study duration was only 3 months, so the study must be verified with larger numbers of patients participating for a much longer time.

In a 3-year prospective study of 200 perimenopausal women suffering from various menopausal symptoms, the 100 women who were given a triphasic oral contraceptive containing levonorgestrel and ethinyl estradiol were cleared of their various menopausal symptoms within 6 months, with no adverse effects on liver function tests, blood glucose, blood pressure, or coagulation factors, and with marked improvement in plasma lipids. At 3 years, the controls showed a loss of about 6% of bone mass, when compared to pretreatment levels, while the drug group did not lose bone mass, even though both groups averaged 1000 mg daily elemental calcium intake (43). However, with these triphasics, the average daily intake of ethinyl estradiol is 32 mg compared with the 20 mg normal ERT dose.

The results of a recent study show that intermittent cyclical therapy with oral etidronate is effective in reversing the progressive loss of vertebral bone that occurs in postmenopausal osteoporosis (44). Continuous, high doses of etidronate may lead to the impairment of bone mineralization and the cessation of bone remodeling.

Therefore, to reduce bone resorption through the inhibition of osteoclastic activity, 400 mg of oral etidronate per day was given, after a 4 hr fast in the afternoon, with water for 2 weeks, since the average oral absorption is only 3% of the dose when fasting, followed by a 13-week period in which no drugs were taken. While on etidronate, 500 mg of elemental calcium and 400 units of vitamin D supplements were taken in the morning. The 15-week cycles were repeated 10 times for a total of 150 weeks, resulting in small but significant increases in the bone mineral content of vertebrae, and after approximately 1 year of treatment, a stabilization in the progression of spinal deformity and a significant decrease in the rate of new vertebral fractures. Because of the long remodeling cycle in osteoporosis, the effects of antiresorptive agents such as etidronate are not likely to be fully appreciated during the first year of therapy. Oral etidronate is well tolerated, and no significant side effects were noted during the study.

Recently, nasal salmon calcitonin 100 IU in the morning and 100 IU in the evening has been studied for the treatment of established osteoporosis in a 1-year double-blind, placebo-controlled study (45). Further bone loss was prevented with no side effects. The patients also received 500 mg of elemental calcium daily.

Finally, two questions remain unanswered about transdermal 17-β estradiol: (*a*) Will osteoporosis be prevented? and (*b*) Will the favorable lipid patterns seen with oral ERT be seen?

Preliminary data on osteoporosis comes from a 2-year

prospective study of 20 women using an estradiol transdermal system releasing 0.05 mg of estradiol per day for 3 weeks, with the addition of a variety of progestins for the last 10 days of the hormonal cycle. The study was conducted for 24 months with 24 patients as controls. The vertebral mass of the control patients, measured by dual photon absorptiometry, decreased significantly (-4.3%) ($p < .001$), while treated women had a net gain of 5.4% ($p < .001$) (54). These data, although encouraging, need verification with larger number of patients enrolled in studies for much longer times (46).

Long-term studies evaluating the effect of transdermal 17-β estradiol on serum lipids are yet to be completed. One 24-week study found a significant increase in HDL cholesterol and reductions in both total serum cholesterol and LDL levels in 10 patients using a patch that released 0.1 mg of estradiol per day every day of the month (47). Larger numbers of patients using this therapy for a much longer duration are needed to verify this study and also the use of much more sophisticated lipoprotein determinations such as HDL_2 subtractions.

The onset of symptoms of osteoporosis is insidious, and the condition leads to wrist fractures and painful spinal vertebral fractures in patients in their 60s and hip fractures in patients in their 70s.

The goals of therapy with ERT are to prevent menopausal symptoms, vaginal atrophy, dysuria secondary to estrogen deficiency, and osteoporosis. All patients should be instructed to do monthly self-breast examinations, and report any lumps or retractions discovered as well as any signs of jaundice, such as yellowing of the skin or sclera. Finally, any irregular noncyclical bleeding should be reported since it may indicate neoplastic changes in the genital tract. Postmenopausal patients may have withdrawal bleeding when on cyclical regimens of estrogen and progestin (see Table 86.15), as long as they have intact uteri.

There are 3 reasons for adding progestin to ERT therapy: (a) to reduce the risk of estrogen-induced irregular bleeding, endometrial hyperplasia, and carcinoma; (b) to protect against breast carcinoma; and (c) to enhance the effect on bone conservation. Unfortunately, unequivocal data showing that progestins favorably modify the response of the breast and the skeleton to estrogens are lacking and endometrial protection remains the only well-substantiated reason for adding progestin to estrogen regimens (48).

When used sequentially for 10 to 13 days per month, endometrial protection should occur for most patients with medroxyprogesterone acetate 10 mg, or norethindrone or norethindrone acetate 0.7 to 1.0 mg, or dl-norgestrel 150 µg, or micronized progesterone 300 mg (48).

Many patients experience some unwanted progestational effects: breast tenderness, bloating, edema, abdominal cramping, anxiety, irritability, and depression. The C-19-nortestosterone derivatives such as norgestrel, norethindrone, or norethindrone acetate possess some androgenic activity and thus tend to be associated with acne and

Table 86.15.
Current Regimens to Prevent Estrogen Deficiency Osteoporosis

Drug	Regimen	Reference
1. Conjugated estrogens or equivalent[a] (CDOC)[b]	0.625 mg daily days 1–25 per month	(40) (see Table 86.12)
PLUS		
Medroxyprogesterone acetate or equivalent[c] (CDOC)	2.5–10 mg days 13–16 through 25 each month	(50, 51)
2. Conjugated estrogens or equivalent[a]	0.3 mg days 1 through 25 each month	(41)
PLUS		
Medroxyprogesterone acetate or equivalent	2.5–10 mg days 13–16 through 25 each month	(50, 51)
AND		
Daily elemental calcium intake	1500 mg daily	(41)
3. Conjugated estrogens or equivalent[a,b]	0.625 mg daily	(48)
PLUS		
Medroxyprogesterone acetate or equivalent[c,d]	2.5–5.0 mg daily	(48)
3. Depomedroxyprogesterone acetate[e]	150 mg intramuscularly monthly	(42)
4. Levonorgestrel plus ethinyl estradiol triphasic oral contraceptive[f]	daily days 1 through 21 each month	(43)

[a] 97% of women with intact uteri will experience withdrawal bleeding with this regimen until age 60, and 60% of those age 60–65 will experience withdrawal bleeding (48).

[b] CDOC, clinical drug of choice.

[c] Norethindrone or norethindrone acetate 0.7–1 mg; dl-norgestrel 150 µg; micronized oral progesterone 150 mg twice daily (48). Further studies are ongoing to find optimal doses of all progestins (50, 51).

[d] There is no convincing proof that continuous/combined therapy reduces progestin-induced problems as compared with sequential regimens (48).

[e] Depo-medroxyprogesterone acetate usually may be used where estrogens are contraindicated. Etidronate (44), nasal salmon calcitonin (45), and calcium carbonate alone (38) may also be of benefit for patients who cannot use estrogens.

[f] Needs further study and should be last choice.

greasy skin and hair. The C-21 derivatives such as medroxyprogesterone acetate are less androgenic and are more likely to be associated with depression and anxiety (48).

Oral micronized progesterone while an attractive alternative has a significant first-pass hepatic metabolism and therefore requires large doses and twice-daily administration. Progesterone 200 to 300 mg per day causes drowsiness in approximately 30% of patients (48).

Probably the greatest benefit of ERT is reduction of the risk of death from cardiovascular disease, even in women normally considered to be at high risk from obesity, previous angina, or hypertension (49). It is feared that the addition of a progestin may negate the beneficial estrogen effects and possibly increase the risk of cardiovascular disease. Therefore, the minimum dose of progestin for endometrial protection should be prescribed (48).

There is also no proof that continuous/combined therapy of estrogen with progestin on a daily basis reduces the progestin-induced problems, as compared with sequential regimens. Additionally, there is a high incidence of vaginal bleeding in 18 to 58% of patients in 12 studies reported so far. With unopposed estrogen regimens, approximately 25% of patients experience regular withdrawal bleeding during each cycle of ERT. With sequential therapies, regular bleeding occurs in about 85% of patients, appearing as a light, predictable bleeding lasting 4 to 5 days. Over time, the bleeding often becomes lighter and shorter, and in some patients amenorrhea develops (48).

Table 86.15 summarizes current ERT regimens to prevent osteoporosis.

CONCLUSION

The pharmacotherapies of gynecologic disorders afford varying degrees of clinical efficacy. For example, prostaglandin inhibitors are very successful in the treatment of primary dysmenorrhea. At the other end of the spectrum is the success of the pharmacotherapy of the premenstrual syndrome, which also lacks precise definition. Somewhere in between lies the success of the pharmacotherapies of endometriosis, the vulvovaginitides, and the disorders resulting from estrogen deficiency.

Three major clinical dilemmas result from these pharmacotherapies. First, the adequate treatment of the premenstrual syndrome remains elusive. Second, the validity and safety of long-term estrogen replacement with or without progestin opposition for the prevention of osteoporosis needs further study. Finally, although not unique to gynecology, the dilemma of the teratogenic potential of all pharmacotherapies must be continually evaluated and re-evaluated in women in their reproductive years.

REFERENCES

1. Smith RP: Drug therapy for dysmenorrhea. IMJ 169:22–25, 1986.
2. Dawood MY: Dysmenorrhea. Clin Obstet Gynecol 33(1):168–178, 1990.
3. Anon: Dysmenorrhea. ACOG Tech Bull 68:1–5, 1983.
4. Ekstrom P, Juchnicka E, Laudanski T, et al.: Effect of an oral contraceptive in primary dysmenorrhea—changes in uterine activity and reactivity to agonists. Contraception 40(1):39–47, 1989.
5. Kleber HD, Kosten TR: Use of clonidine for dysmenorrhea in four patients. Psychosomatics 26:539–546, 1985.
6. Chihal HJ: Premenstrual syndrome: an update for the clinician. Obstet Gynecol Clin North Am 17(2):457–479, 1990.
7. Smith MA, Youngkin EQ: Managing the premenstrual syndrome. Clin Pharm 5:788–797, 1986.
8. Maddocks S, Hahn P, Moller F, et al.: A double-blind placebo controlled trial of progesterone vaginal suppositories in the treatment of premenstrual syndrome. Am J Obstet Gynecol 154:573–581, 1986.
9. Smith S, Rinehart JS, Ruddock VE: Treatment of premenstrual syndrome with alprazolam: results of a double-blind, placebo-controlled, randomized crossover clinical trial. Obstet Gynecol 70(1):37–43, 1987.
10. Muse KN, Cetel NS, Futterman LA, et al.: The premenstrual syndrome: effects of "medical ovariectomy." N Engl J Med 311:1345–1349, 1984.
11. True BL, Goodner SM, Burns EA: Review of the etiology and treatment of premenstrual syndrome. Drug Intell Clin Pharm 19:714–722, 1985.
12. Harrison W, Sharpe L, Endicott J: Treatment of premenstrual symptoms. Gen Hosp Psychiatry 7:54–65, 1985.
13. Smith S, Schiff I: The premenstrual syndrome—diagnosis and management. Fertil Steril 52(4):527–543, 1989.
14. Pariser SF, Stern SL, Shank ML, et al.: Premenstrual syndrome: concerns, controversies and treatment. Am J Obstet Gynecol 153:599–604, 1985.
15. Anon: Management of endometriosis. ACOG Tech Bull 85:830–835, 1985.
16. Markham SM, Carpenter SE, Rock JA: Extrapelvic endometriosis. Obstet Gynecol Clin North Am 16(1):193–219, 1989.
17. Galle PC: Clinical presentation and diagnosis of endometriosis. Obstet Gynecol Clin North Am 16(1):29–41, 1989.
18. Guzick DS: Clinical epidemiology of endometriosis and infertility. Obstet Gynecol Clin North Am 16(1):43–59, 1989.
19. Metzger DA, Luciano AA: Hormonal therapy of endometriosis. Obstet Gynecol Clin North Am 16(1):105–121, 1989.
20. Erickson LD, Ory SJ: GnRH analogues in the treatment of endometriosis. Obstet Gynecol Clin North Am 16(1):123–145, 1989.
21. Gardner HL, Infectious vulvovaginitis. In Monif GR (ed): Infectious Diseases in Obstetrics and Gynecology, ed. 2. Philadelphia, Harper & Row, 1982, p 515.
22. Sweet RL: Importance of differential diagnosis in acute vaginitis. Am J Obstet Gynecol 152:945–947, 1985.
23. Anon: 1989 Sexually transmitted diseases treatment guidelines. MMWR 38(S-8):1–43, 1989.
24. Ritter W: Pharmacokinetic fundamentals of vaginal treatment with clotrimazole. Am J Obstet Gynecol 152:945–947, 1985.
25. Sobel JD: Epidemiology and pathogenesis of recurrent vulvovaginal candidiasis. Am J Obstet Gynecol 152:924–934, 1985.
26. Fregoso-Duenas F: Ketoconazole in vulvovaginal candidosis. Rev Infect Dis 2:620–624, 1980.
27. Lynch PJ: Condylomata acuminata (anogenital warts). Clin Obstet Gynecol 28:142–151, 1985.
28. Ferenczy A: Comparison of 5-fluorouracil and CO_2 laser for treatment of vaginal condylomata. Obstet Gynecol 64:773–778, 1984.
29. Place VA, Powers M, Darley PE, et al.: A double-blind comparative study of Estraderm and Premarin in the amelioration of postmenopausal symptoms. Am J Obstet Gynecol 152:1092–1099, 1985.
30. Schiff I, Tulchinsky D, Cramer D, et al.: Oral medroxyprogesterone in the treatment of postmenopausal symptoms. JAMA 244:1443–1445, 1980.

31. Laufer LR, Erlik Y, Meldrum DR, et al.: Effect of clonidine on hot flashes in postmenopausal women. Obstet Gynecol 60:583–586, 1982.

32. Dyer GI, Townsend PT: Dose related changes in vaginal cytology after topiocal conjugated equine oestrogens. Br Med J 284:789, 1982.

33. DeFazio J, Speroff L: Estrogen replacement therapy: current thinking and practice. Geriatrics 40:32–48, 1985.

34. Anon: Osteoporosis. ACOG Tech Bull 118:1–5, 1988.

35. Gambrell RD: Cancer and the use of estrogens. Int J Fertil 31:112–122, 1986.

36. Henderson BE, Ross RK, Paganini-Hill A, et al.: Estrogen use and cardiovascular disease. Am J Obstet Gynecol 154:1181–1186, 1986.

37. Anon: Recommended Dietary Allowances, ed. 10. Washington, D.C., National Academy Press, 1989, p 180.

38. Dawson-Hughes B, Dallal GE, Krall EA, et al.: A controlled trial of the effect of calcium supplementation on bone density in postmenopausal women. N Engl J Med 323:878–883, 1990.

39. Bauwens SF, Drinka PJ, Boh L: Pathogenesis and management of primary osteoporosis. Clin Pharm 5:639–659, 1986.

40. Lindsay R, Hart M, Clark DM: The minimum effective dose of estrogen for the prevention of postmenopausal bone loss. Obstet Gynecol 63:759–763, 1984.

41. Gordan GS, Gennant HK: The aging skeleton. Clin Geriatr Med 1:95–118, 1985.

42. Lobo RA, McCormick W, Singer F, et al.: Depo-medroxyprogesterone acetate compared with conjugated estrogens for the treatment of postmenopausal women. Obstet Gynecol 63:1–5, 1984.

43. Shargil AA: Hormone replacement therapy in perimenopausal women on a triphasic contraceptive compound: a three year prospective study. Int J Fertil 30:15–28, 1985.

44. Storm T, Thamsborg G, Steiniche T, et al.: Effect of intermittent cyclical etidronate therapy on bone mass and fracture rate in women with postmenopausal osteoporosis. N Engl J Med 322:1265–1271, 1990.

45. Overgaard K, Riis BJ, Christiansen C, et al: Nasal calcitonin for the treatment of established osteoporosis. Clin Endocrinol 30:435–442, 1989.

46. Ribot C, Tremollieres JM, Louvet JP, et al.: Preventive effects of transdermal administration of 17-beta-estradiol on postmenopausal bone loss: a 2-year prospective study. Obstet Gynecol 75 (suppl):42–25, 1990.

47. Stanczyk FZ, Shoupe D, Nunez V, et al.: A randomized comparison of nonoral estradiol delivery in postmenopausal women. Am J Obstet Gynecol 159:1540–1546, 1988.

48. Whitehead MI, Hillard TC, Crook D: The role and use of progestogens. Obstet Gynecol 75(suppl):59–76, 1990.

49. Henderson BE, Ross RK, Paganini-Hill A: Estrogen use and cardiovascular disease. J Reprod Med 30(suppl):814–820, 1985.

50. Gambrell RD: Clinical use of progestins in the menopausal patient. J Reprod Med 27:531–538, 1982.

51. Lane G, Siddle NC, Ryder TA, et al.: Is Provera the ideal progestogen for addition to postmenopausal estrogen therapy? Fertil Steril 45:345–352, 1986.

CHAPTER 87

CONTRACEPTION AND INFERTILITY

JANET M. CARMICHAEL, Pharm.D.

HORMONAL BIRTH CONTROL

The use of female sex hormones to prevent the development of the female egg was suggested as early as 1940, but it was not until 1956, after the discovery of norethynodrel, that field trials were begun on what we now know as birth control pills ("the pill"). In 1960, the U.S. Food and Drug Administration (FDA) first approved the use of the combination pill. Today about 60 million women worldwide, 13 million in the United States, use oral contraceptive products. Almost one-fourth of American women 15 to 44 years of age take oral contraceptives. Despite widespread adverse publicity, the pill remains a safe and acceptable contraceptive method for many women. The popularity of the pill undoubtedly relates to both its theoretical and use effectiveness (Table 87.1). To understand the many aspects of hormonal birth control, it is necessary to review the physiology of the menstrual cycle and the development of estrogens and progestins used in contraceptive products.

Menstrual Cycle

The average menstrual cycle (Fig. 87.1) lasts 28 days. Several organ systems are involved in this cycle. The changes that occur at the ovaries during this 28-day cycle can be divided into three phases: follicular, ovulatory, and luteal.

The follicular phase occupies about the first 14 days of the cycle. At the beginning of this phase, several follicles, each containing an oocyte, begin to enlarge in response to pituitary follicle-stimulating hormone (FSH). After 5 to 6 days, one of the follicles begins to develop more rapidly. The granulosa cells of this follicle multiply, and under the influence of pituitary luteinizing hormone (LH), synthesize and release estrogens from the ovary at an increasing rate. The estrogens appear to inhibit FSH before midcycle (a negative-feedback inhibition system); however, the high level and rate of increase of estrogens stimulates a surge of FSH and LH at the end of this phase, which in turn causes final-stage growth and rupture of the ovum (ovulation).

The ovulatory phase ordinarily occurs at midcycle, on day 14 or 15. At the time of ovulation, the granulosa cells of the follicle begin to secrete progesterone.

The luteal phase follows. Under the influence of LH, the ruptured follicle fills with blood and the surrounding theca and granulosa cells proliferate and replace the blood to form the corpus luteum. The cells of this structure pro-

duce estrogens and progesterone for the remainder of the cycle unless pregnancy occurs. If pregnancy does not occur during this cycle, the corpus luteum begins to degenerate and ceases hormone production. This drop in serum level of estrogens and progesterone results in endometrial shedding (menstruation) and the beginning of a new cycle. If pregnancy does occur, the corpus luteum remains active because it is stimulated by human chorionic gonadotropin (hCG) derived from the developing placenta; thus maintaining the high levels of progesterone and estrogen necessary for pregnancy.

The changes that occur in the uterus over the 28-day cycle can also be divided into three phases.

1. The menstrual phase starts on day 1 of the menstrual cycle with the sloughing of the old endometrium and the onset of vaginal bleeding. This phase lasts 3 to 6 days.
2. The proliferative phase is a period of growth of the endometrial lining lasting from day 6 to day 14. Estrogens from the developing follicles are responsible for the growth as well as for the growth of uterine glands and the proliferation of uterine vessels.
3. The secretory phase is primarily under the influence of progesterone. During this phase, the endometrium becomes thicker and is held in place, the uterine glands branch, and the secretory function of these glands begins. The endometrium would be prepared for implantation if pregnancy occurred.

Estrogens

The major natural estrogens produced by women are estradiol, estrone, and estriol. Estradiol is the major secretory product of the ovary. Some estrone is also produced in the ovary, although most of it (and estriol) is formed in the liver from estradiol or converted in the peripheral tissues.

Several synthetic estrogens have been manufactured. Compared with natural estrogens, synthetic estrogens have increased biopotency when administered orally. Only two synthetic estrogens are used in all of the various oral contraceptives on the U.S. market—ethinyl estradiol and mestranol. Ethinyl estradiol is estradiol with an ethinyl group an the 17α position. Mestranol, in addition, has a methyl group at the 3α position (Fig. 87.2).

Mestranol is metabolized in the liver to ethinyl estradiol. The amount and extent of this metabolism may vary from patient to patient. Strictly speaking, mestranol is slightly less potent than the same weight of ethinyl estra-

Table 87.1.
Contraceptive Effectiveness: First Year Failure Rates[a]

Method	Theoretical Effectiveness (%) (Used Correctly and Consistently During 1 Year)	Typical Effectiveness (%) (Average U.S. Failure Rate During 1 Year)
Oral contraceptives		
Combined	0.1	3
Progestin only	0.5	2
Injectable medroxyprogesterone acetate	0.3	0.3
Intrauterine devices		6
Progesterone T	2.0	
Copper T 380A	0.8	
Diaphragm with spermicide	3	18
Cervical cap with spermicide	5	18
Condom	2	12
Sponge	5–8	18–28
Spermicide	3	21
Tubal sterilization	0.4	0.4
Vasectomy	0.4	0.4
Fertility awareness[b]	2–20	24
Chance (sexually active)	90	90

[a] Data from Hatcher RA, Guest F, Stewart FH, Stewart GK et al.: Contraceptive Technology, 1988–89, ed. 14. New York: Irvington Publishers Inc., 1988; Trussel J, Kost K: Stud Fam Plann, 18:237, 1987; and Sivin I, Schmidt F. Contraception, 36:55, 1987.

[b] Basal body temperature, cervical mucus, calendar, and "rhythm."

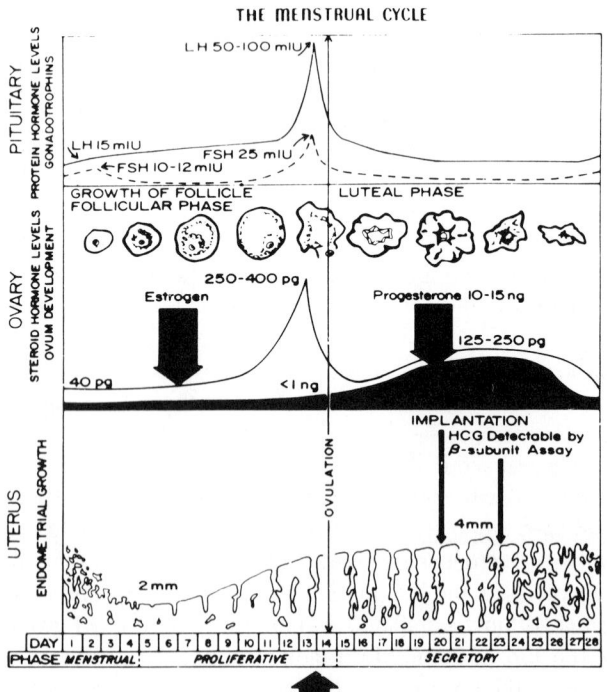

Figure 87.1 The menstrual cycle. (From Hatcher RA: Contraceptive Technology, 1980–1981. New York: Irvington Publishers Inc., 1980.)

ESTRADIOL

ETHINYL ESTRADIOL

MESTRANOL

Figure 87.2 Configuration of the major estrogens.

Table 87.2.
Pharmacokinetics of Oral Contraceptive Steroids

Steroid	$t\frac{1}{2}$ (hr)	Range of First Pass (%)	Range of Bioavailability (%)
Ethinyl estradiol	10.0	56–62	38–48
Norethindrone	7.5	27–53	47–73[a]
Levonorgestrel	11.4	≈0	≈100[b]

[a] Wide ranges of oral bioavailability have been reported for norethindrone due to intersubject variability of first-pass metabolism.

[b] In contrast to norethindrone, levonorgestrel is not subject to first-pass extraction by the liver and results in virtually 100% bioavailability. This consistent absorption may be significant to reduce breakthrough bleeding and drug interaction in products containing levonorgestrel.

diol. Although there is some argument about the exact equivalence of these two estrogens, for practical purposes they can be considered to be nearly equally potent. The difficulty may result from the plasma kinetics of ethinyl estradiol. Ethinyl estradiol undergoes extensive first-pass hepatic metabolism, which can result in considerable patient-to-patient variation in plasma and urine steroid concentrations (Table 87.2).

Progestins

Progesterone is the most important natural progestin and also serves as a precursor to the estrogens, androgens, and adrenocortical steroids. Progesterone is rapidly absorbed following parenteral administration, but is poorly absorbed when given orally. Its half-life in plasma is from 3 to 90 min. As is the case with estrogens, it is partially stored in body fat and is almost completely metabolized in one passage through the liver. To overcome these problems, synthetic progestins were developed for use in oral contraceptives.

The four synthetic progestins available in U.S. oral contraceptives are 19-norandrogens derived from testosterone (Fig. 87.3). There are fundamentally two types of progestins: (a) those that contain or are metabolized to norethisterone and (b) those that contain norgestrel. Norethindrone acetate and ethynodiol diacetate are effective in vivo after they have been metabolized to norethisterone and therefore can be considered part of the norethisterone family. Acetylation does confer different pharmacokinetic properties such as a longer half-life to norethindrone. In addition, metabolic effects of these agents are altered by this chemical change. However, based on the ability to inhibit ovulation in clinical practice, any of the norethindrone group are microgram for microgram, equipotent. The minimum contraceptive dose of norethindrone is approximately 350 μg. Wide ranges of oral bioavailability have been reported for norethindrone because of intersubject variability of first-pass metabolism.

As first introduced, norgestrel was a mixture of d- and l-isomers. It has since been recognized that activity rests entirely with the levo form. Original products still contain the racemic norgestrel, but newer products contain half the amount of levonorgestrel. The minimum contraceptive

dose of levonorgestrel is approximately 30 μg. Thus norgestrel is 5 to 10 times as potent and levonorgestrel is 10 to 20 times as potent as similar doses of norethindrone. In contrast to norethindrone, levonorgestrel is not subject to first-pass extraction by the liver and results in virtually 100% bioavailability. This consistent absorption may help reduce the level of breakthrough bleeding and drug interactions in products containing levonogestrel, in some patients (Table 87.2).

The "Pill"

Two basic types of preparations are available for use as oral contraceptives: (a) the combination pill and (b) the mini-pill. Combination oral contraceptives (COCs) are subdivided into fixed combination (monophasic), biphasic, and triphasic products. Monophasic contraceptive pills contain a fixed ratio of estrogen and progestin given daily for 21 days, beginning on day 5 of the menstrual cycle.

Biphasic products contain a fixed dose of estrogen (days 1 to 21) with a lower progestin dose on days 1 to 10 than on days 11 to 21. Only one such product is available on the U.S. market. Three triphasic products are currently available in the U.S. In the triphasic pills, progestin is given throughout the cycle, the dose being increased only at midcycle in one and again in the last 7 to 10 days in the other two products. Note that the dose of estrogen is fixed in two products and increased at midcycle in the third (Table 87.3).

The triphasic pills are a response to the evidence that the safest combined oral contraceptive would use the lowest possible dose of both synthetic steroids. In Triphasil, for example, the progestin intake is 39% less than that in the lowest COC containing levonorgestrel. However, several fixed-dose monophasic formulations currently marketed have a lower total dose of norethindrone than the triphasic formulation containing norethindrone. Since the triphasic products have relative estrogen dominance and progestin deficiency, estrogen-related side effects can be expected to predominate (Table 87.3). However, women with cardiovascular or metabolic abnormalities would be excellent candidates for these products.

Three manufacturers of high-dose (greater than 50 μg estrogen) COCs have discontinued distribution of these products as oral contraceptives. Enovid 5 and 10 mg, Ortho-Novum 2 mg, and Norinyl 2 mg are available for treatment of endometriosis, hypermenorrhea, and cycle withdrawal bleeding only. The use of COCs with less than 50 μg of estrogen are associated with very low pregnancy rates, similar to those of the discontinued products, and a significantly lower incidence of serious adverse effects.

Menstrual bleeding usually begins 1 to 4 days after cessation of a cycle of COCs. The patient then resumes the same dosage exactly 7 days after the last pill. Twenty-

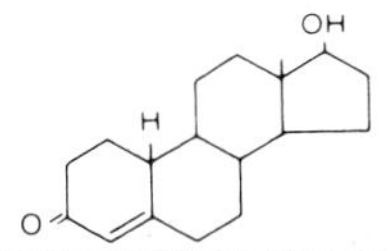

19 NORTESTOSTERONE

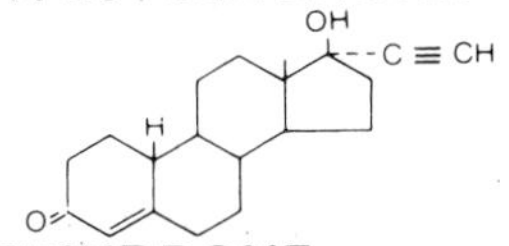

NORETHINDRONE

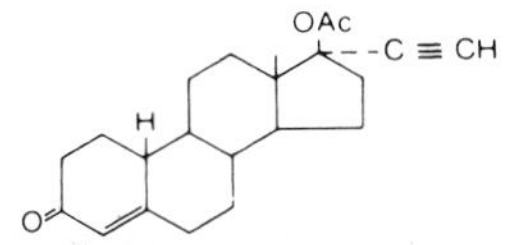

NORETHINDRONE ACETATE

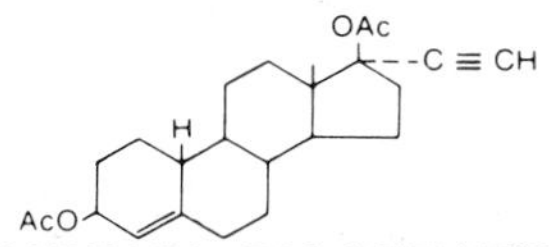

ETHYNODIOL DIACETATE

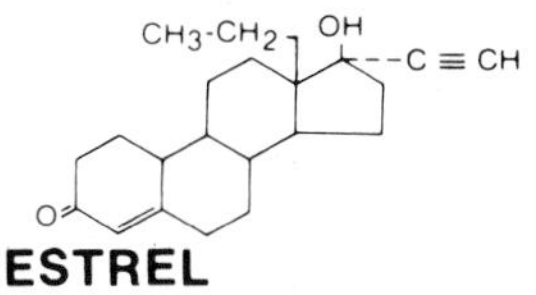

NORGESTREL

Figure 87.3 Configuration of the synthetic progestins.

Table 87.3.
Oral Contraceptive Activity[a]

Trade Name	Combined Estrogen Potency[b]	Progestin Potency[c]	Androgenic Potency[d]	Trade Name	Combined Estrogen Potency[b]	Progestin Potency[c]	Androgenic Potency[d]
Fixed-Combination Contraceptives				*Biphasic Combination Contraceptives*			
>50 μg of estrogen				Nelova 10/11 and			
Enovid-5 mg	240	1.3	0.00	Ortho-Novum 10/11			
50 μg of estrogen				(day 1–10)	42	0.5	0.17
Demulen 1/50	26	1.4	0.21	(day 11–21)	38	1.0	0.34
Ovral	42	1.3	0.79				
Ovcon-50	50°	1.0	0.34	*Triphasic Combination Contraceptives*			
Genora 1/50	32	1.0	0.34				
Nelova 1/50M	32	1.0	0.34	Ortho-Novum 7/7/7			
Norethin 1/50M	32	1.0	0.34	(day 1–7)	42°	0.5	0.17
Norinyl 1 + 50	32	1.0	0.34	(day 8–14)	40°	0.75	0.26
Ortho-Novum 1/50	32	1.0	0.34	(day 15–21)	38°	1.0	0.34
Norlestrin 2.5/50	16	2.7	1.31	Tri-Norinyl			
Norlestrin 1/50	39	1.2	0.52	(day 1–7)	42°	0.5	0.17
<50 μg of estrogen				(day 8–16)	38°	1.0	0.34
Demulen 1/35	19	1.4	0.21	(day 17–21)	42°	0.5	0.17
Genora 1/35	38	1.0	0.34	Tri-Levlen and			
Gynex 1/35E	38	1.0	0.34	Triphasil			
N.E.E.	38	1.0	0.34	(day 1–6)	25°	0.27	0.16
Nelova 1/35E	38	1.0	0.34	(day 7–11)	33°	0.4	0.24
Norcept-E 1/35	38	1.0	0.34	(day 12–21)	25°	0.67	0.40
Norethin 1/35E	38	1.0	0.34				
Norinyl 1/35	38	1.0	0.34	*Progestin-only Contraceptives*			
Ortho-Novum 1/35	38	1.0	0.34	Micronor	1	0.12	0.12
Brevicon	42	0.5	0.17	Nor-Q.D.	1	0.12	0.12
Gynex 0.5/35E	42	0.5	0.17	Ovrette	0	0.08	0.12
Modicon	42	0.5	0.17				
Nelova 0.5/35E	42	0.5	0.17				
Ovcon-35	40°	0.4	0.14				
Lo-Ovral	25	0.8	0.47				
Levlen	25	0.8	0.47				
Nordette	25	0.8	0.47				
Loestrin 1.5/30	14	1.7	0.79				
Loestrin 1/20	13	1.2	0.52				

[a] Adapted from Dickey RP: Managing Contraceptive Pill Patients, ed. 4. Durant, OK: Creative Infomatics Inc., 1986.
[b] Micrograms of ethinyl estradiol equivalents per day (derived from mouse uterine epithelial assays).
[c] Milligrams of norethindrone equivalents per day (derived from the induction of glycogen vacuoles in human endometrium).
[d] Milligrams of methyl testosterone equivalents per 28 days (derived from rat ventral prostate assay).
° Estimate.

eight-day pills have placebo or iron tablets to mark these 7 days for the patient.

The combination pill is effective for several reasons. First, ovulation is inhibited by the negative-feedback inhibition that estrogens have on the hypothalamus, with the subsequent suppression of FSH and LH production. Progestogens in sufficient doses inhibit ovulation through suppression of the preovulatory LH surge. Without FSH and LH, the ovarian follicle fails to grow and ovulation does not occur. The combination products inhibit ovulation by a synergistic action of estrogen and progestogen at the level of the hypothalamus. Nevertheless, in combination products containing 50 μg or less of estrogen,

ovulation is probably suppressed only 95 to 98% of the time (2). The 99 + % efficacy of these agents must be attributed to synergy with the progestin. Progestins alone may inhibit ovulation via a subtle alteration in hypothalamic-pituitary-ovarian function and midcycle changes in FSH and LH levels. Additional nonovulatory mechanisms may also add to the effectiveness of the pill. Second, progestins cause thick, tenacious cervical mucus that is very resistant to sperm migration and reduces sperm survival. Third, progestins alter fallopian tube secretions, thereby indirectly affecting the motility of the ovum and sperm. Fourth, an atrophic endometrium often results from this dose of progestins. Implantation of the blastocyst is not satisfactory in an atrophic endometrium. All these effects combine to make the combination pill the most popular and effective oral contraceptive on the market.

The second type of oral contraceptive is the mini-pill. Progestin only is given for 28 days continuously. These pills contain a smaller amount of progestin than most combination pills and no estrogen (Table 87.3). Although ovulation may be inhibited in some women, approximately 40% of women will ovulate consistently, 40% will have anovulatory cycles, and the other 20% will ovulate sporadically (2). The aforementioned progestin effects contribute to the effectiveness of the mini-pill. It is less effective than combination oral contraceptive products, especially if one or more tablets are missed. However, the mini-pill may be a good choice in lactating women or patients who are unable to take estrogens. Estrogen-related side effects that may indicate a need to switch to mini-pills include hypertension, chloasma, cycle weight gain, nausea, and headache.

SIDE EFFECTS

Oral Contraceptives and Cardiovascular Disease

The first serious side effects that were attributed to oral contraceptive agents related to the cardiovascular system. A critique of the epidemiologic studies on oral contraceptives and the occurrence of venous thromboembolism, stroke, myocardial infarction, and cardiovascular death is presented elsewhere. COC use has been shown to cause certain thromboembolic phenomena. Based on scientific weakness and bias in this literature, the debate on the link of COCs to CVD will no doubt continue. The use of low-dose COCs is clearly seen as a positive influence on the decline of these cardiovascular complications.

On the venous side of the circulation, very good evidence exists that increasing doses of estrogen increase the risk of venous thromboembolism. Most recent epidemiologic data would support thrombosis not atherosclerosis as the cause of increased cardiovascular disease in COC users. However, hypertension, impaired glucose tolerance, and hyperlipidemia are three of the major atherogenic risk factors believed to influence the occurrence of cardiovascular disease. Oral contraceptives worsen these risk factors to some degree in almost all women and become important in women with underlying disease or those who have specific susceptibility. Although laboratory values may remain within normal limits, the whole distribution of these risk factors is shifted upward. It remains to be seen whether these changes will have an effect on cardiovascular mortality.

Hypertension

There seems to be no doubt that a small rise in blood pressure occurs in most patients taking oral contraceptives

containing at least 50 μg of estrogen and 1 to 4 mg progestin (4, 5). This rise in blood pressure occurs in previously normotensive women and aggravates existing hypertension. The average increase varies with age, becoming substantial in women about 35 or older. The time of onset and extent of increase varies between individuals. The hypertensive effect may increase with duration of oral contraceptive use (6). It has been estimated that 5% of oral contraceptive users develop frank hypertension within 5 years. This is an incidence three to six times that of nonusers (7, 8). In addition to producing overt hypertension in some women, oral contraceptives elevate pressure to some extent in almost all women (9) (on the average 1 mm Hg diastolic, 5 mm Hg systolic). These effects may take 6 to 12 months to manifest.

The risk of hypertension seems to be much lower when low-dose formulations are used. One study showed no effect of oral contraceptive agents or pretreatment blood pressures in women with either preexisting hypertension or in those who had previously normal blood pressure (10). However, another study (11) showed small but significant increases in both systolic and diastolic blood pressures in women who were taking a combination of 30 μg of ethinylestradiol with either 150 μg levonorgestrol or 2 mg of ethynodiol diacetate. This study also showed no effect on blood pressure from progestogen-only contraceptive agents.

This information has several important implications for patients follow-up. Emphasis should be placed on women 35 years old or older, smokers, those with a history of hypertension, and patients on COCs with higher doses of estrogen. The mechanism of COC-associated hypertension appears to be complex. Whereas an estrogen or a progesten alone had no effect on the occurrence of hypertension, if an estrogen is given with a progestin, there is an increased risk of hypertension. In addition, ethinyl estradiol increases the hepatic production of angiotensinogen in a dose-dependent fashion, thus increasing peripheral resistance. Although these are primarily estrogen effects, progestins may have a synergistic effect because a direct relationship between the amount of norethindrone acetate in COCs and hypertension has been reported (14).

Hypertension associated with birth control pills is reversible. After discontinuing oral contraceptives, the return to normal blood pressure may take from 3 to 4 months. The patient's blood pressure should be monitored at the initiation of oral contraceptive therapy and periodically thereafter. If a large rise in blood pressure is detected, oral contraceptives should be discontinued.

Lipid Metabolism

Estrogens appear to stimulate a significant increase in fasting serum triglyceride levels (15). Very rarely, hyperlipidemic crisis with pancreatitis has been reported and must be attributed to the estrogen in these products (16). Certain progestins in COCs oppose this action of estrogen and lower triglyceride levels (17). Ethynodiol diacetate, however, does not have this antiestrogenic action but instead may be synergistic, to increase triglycerides (18).

Much more interest has been focused on low-density lipoprotein (LDL) cholesterol because of the positive correlation between it and the risk of coronary heart disease. The inverse relationship between high-density lipoprotein (HDL) cholesterol and coronary heart disease risk has received even more attention. Thus, COCs that simultaneously elevate LDL and decrease HDL cause the most concern. Although lipid levels generally remain within normal limits, it is likely that all COCs elevate LDL-cholesterol to some extent in all users, and certain formulations do so to a marked degree. While estrogens raise HDL-cholesterol levels, progestins lower HDL-cholesterol levels. Combination oral contraceptive products containing the more potent progestins (i.e., norgestrel) cause the most adverse changes (18, 19). The potency of estrogen and the potency and type of progestin in COCs have important effects on lipoprotein lipids in women and may be responsible for an increased risk of arteriosclerotic disease. For these reasons, progestin-dominant COCs should be prescribed with caution in women with known risk factors for cardiovascular disease. Many of the newer products have been formulated to minimize these changes in LDL- and HDL-cholesterol by the use of less potent progestins, norethindrone being the most popular.

Carbohydrate Metabolism

Women taking most combination oral contraceptives show a mild worsening of glucose tolerance curves [an average serum glucose increase of 0.6 mmol/liter (11 mg/dl) in 1 hr]. Many normal women have shown elevations in plasma insulin response to glucose and worsening of prediabetic-type responses. Patients with established diabetes on older, high-dose COCs showed a worsening of carbohydrate intolerance. It would appear that these changes are due to the progestin components of oral contraceptives, because estrogens do not affect carbohydrate metabolism (20). Recent studies show that low-dose COCs do not change glucose tolerance (21). Given adequate supervision, low-dose COCs may be used safely in patients with insulin-dependent and gestational diabetes.

Myocardial Infarction and Stroke

Although the above effects of oral contraceptives on blood pressure, carbohydrates, and lipid metabolism may appear minor from a clinical standpoint, from an epidemiologic viewpoint this combination of atherogenic factors may have serious implications. A direct link between altered metabolism and increased mortality and morbidity is largely hypothetical. Much debate continues on the exact relationship of COCs and the risk of myocardial infarction (MI) and stroke. Early data showed that risks seem to increase substantially with age and the presence of such risk factors as smoking more than 15 cigarettes daily, preexisting hypercholesterolemia, diabetes mellitus, or hypertension (22, 23). Overall, oral contraceptives were found to multiply the effects of age and other risk factors for MI and stroke, rather than just add to them (23). Because cigarette smoking is far more prevalent among women of reproductive age than any of these other risk factors, it becomes by far the most important factor.

These epidemiologic studies were published in the late 1970s, and so the data were based on women who took only COC formulations with 50 μg or more of estrogens. More recent analysis of new data on low-dose products concludes that there is no increased risk of myocardial infarction among former users of oral contraceptives (24). Analysis of data from 1977 to 1982 in 65,000 women, 15 to 44 years of age, showed that no myocardial infarctions and only one stroke occurred in COC users during this 6-year period (25, 26). Only healthy users and controls were enrolled, but smokers were not excluded. In this study there was a steadily increasing percentage of women using formulations of COCs containing less than 50 μg of estrogen. The risk ratio for stroke among users of COCs was 0.9, but the risk of venous thrombosis remained significantly increased, as compared with controls. During the 6-year study, there were eleven deaths due to cardiovascular disease; all in the women who were not using oral contraceptives (27). It is important to note that women with medical illnesses likely to increase risk, such as hypertension and diabetes were excluded from the analysis in both groups, which may explain the absence of an increased risk of serious cardiovascular disease. A large British cohort study has confirmed these results (28), showing a relative risk of MI among current users of COCs = 0.87.

In addition, recent epidemiologic studies indicate no increased risk of MI among former COC users (29, 30). The Nurses Health Study (30), prospectively studied 119,061 women 30 to 55 years of age in 1976. During 8 years of follow-up, there was no evidence to suggest an increase in the risk of cardiovascular disease among users of COC, even with prolonged previous use.

Because of the early epidemiologic data, COCs are not generally prescribed for women over the age of 35. However, recent data indicate that the use of COCs containing less than 50 μg of estrogen in healthy, nonsmoking women up to the age of 45 is not associated with an increased risk of serious cardiovascular disease. The American College of Obstetrics and Gynecology has recently stated that healthy nonsmoking women 35 to 44 years of age can continue to use COCs. However, COCs should not be used in women with preexisting systemic disease that may affect the cardiovascular system (e.g., hypertension, diabetes, hyperlipidemia) or by women over 35 years of age who smoke.

Venous Thromboembolic Disease

Combination oral contraceptives have been found to increase the risks of venous thromboembolic disease (deep vein thrombosis and/or pulmonary embolism) during the first month of oral contraceptive use (27). This effect remains constant regardless of the duration of use, past use, presence of obesity, or cigarette smoking. After discontinuation of therapy, this risk seems to decline within 1 month to the level found among women who have never used the drug (31).

The most reliable source of information regarding the magnitude of risks for overt venous thromboembolic disease comes from two British cohort studies that began in 1968 (32, 33). The relative risk of thromboembolic disease in current users, compared with nonusers, was found to be approximately 3 times for idopathic superficial venous thrombosis, in the range of 4 to 11 times for deep vein thrombosis or pulmonary embolism, and in the range of 1.5 to 6 times for venous thrombosis or pulmonary embolism in women with conditions that predispose to the development of thromboembolic disease. It must be kept in mind that COCs during this time contained more than 50 μg of estrogen.

Although oral contraceptives have been shown to increase the risk of death from thromboembolic disease, this effect is very rare. During over 450,000 women years of follow-up, these studies observed only 5 fatalities from venous thromboembolic disease.

It is the estrogen component that increases the risk of thromboembolic disease. Furthermore, this effect appears to be dose-related, as evidenced by a drop of one-half to two-thirds in fatal or nonfatal pulmonary embolism when the dose of mestranol or ethinyl estradiol was reduced from 100 to 150 μg to 50 to 80 μg/tablet (28). Because most COCs prescribed today contain less than 50 μg of estrogen, it is not surprising that this problem is seen less frequently now.

Oral contraceptives appear to cause structural and histochemical vascular changes in veins and arteries (34). A large number of changes in blood coagulation have been noted, including an increase in platelet stickiness, a possible elevation of platelet count, a rise in prothrombin, and an increase in factors VII, VIII, IX, and X (35, 36).

The amount of antithrombin III, an enzyme that inactivates thrombin, is nearly normal in women using oral contraceptives. However, antithrombin III *activity* is substantially decreased (37). In addition, oral contraceptives containing 75 to 150 μg of mestranol or ethinyl estradiol decrease antithrombin III activity to a greater extent than do oral contraceptives containing only 50 μg (38).

Progestins, in the low-dose pills, play some role in this effect because antithrombin III activity is reduced significantly in patients who are taking COCs that contain 30 μg of ethinyl estradiol and a member of the norethindrone family, but there is no significant change in activity in women taking 30 μg ethinyl estradiol and levonorgestrel, whether in a fixed dose or as a triphasic preparation (39).

Antithrombin III levels are lower in nonuser women of blood types A, B, and AB (especially type A) than in women of blood type O. This may account for the increase in risk from idiopathic deep venous thromboembolic disease among users and nonoral contraceptive users of blood types A, B, or AB.

Tumorigenic Aspects

Because the normal breast is hormone-dependent, women who use oral contraceptive tablets may develop some mammary abnormalities. The relationship between the consumption of oral contraceptives and the development of breast disease is by no means a simple one. Oral contraceptives reduce two common benign forms of breast disease, fibroadenoma and fibrocystic disease.

To date most studies have found no overall increase in the risk of breast cancer in oral contraceptive users. One dissenting study (40) reported an increased risk of breast cancer only with long-term use in women who began using "high-progestin potency" pills before age 25. Their findings contradict most published data, including two large important studies (41, 42). These results provided no grounds for concern about the risk of breast cancer in relation to COC use, either overall or in relation to particular hormone components. However, certain existing breast cancers may be worsened by the estrogen in oral contraceptive preparations. In spite of widespread oral contraceptive use and extensive observation, no increased incidence of cancer has been observed.

A summary of COC risk factors for cancer of the ovary, endometrium, breast, and uterine cervix is reviewed in Table 87.4 (43).

Hepatomas may occur in women taking oral contraceptives. A wide array of different types of benign liver tumors have been reported, the most common of which are focal nodular hyperplasia and liver cell adenomas. If we compare cases of focal nodular before and after COCs became available, there is little or no change with respect to incidence, age, range, location, or microscopic features of this lesion. One important difference, however, is noted. Before oral contraceptives, no serious hemorrhages had been reported. Since the introduction of oral contraceptives, this tumor is sometimes fatal, with death usually due to sudden hepatic rupture and hemorrhage.

There has been an increase, however, in the incidence

Table 87.4.
Cancer Risks and Oral Contraceptive Use: Summary of Recent Evidence for Cancer of the Ovary, Endometrium, Breast, and Uterine Cervix

Disease	Estimated Relative Risk[a]	Risk with Duration of Use	Comments
Ovarian cancer	0.4–0.8	Decreased	Overall protective effect, especially epithelial type; most notable in nulliparous; effect after 6 months of use
Endometrial cancer	0.4–0.6	Decreased (especially with decreased progestogen content)	Protective; most notable in nulliparous; effect after 1 year of use
Breast cancer	0.9–1.3	No trend	Possibly no increased risk; effect less certain
Cervical cancer	1.1–1.3	? Increased (data conflicting)	Possible slight increase but influence of sexual activity, cigarettes, cytologic screening yet to be defined

[a] Relative risk estimate: ratio of number of observations in cases and that in control subjects.

of a formerly rare liver cell adenoma. Numerous cases of this adenoma, which was rarely reported before 1960, have now been reported. Risk is increased by age, duration of use, and dose of steroid.

It is generally agreed that the risk of developing a hepatoma is equally shared with the use of products containing mestranol and ethinyl estradiol. There should be increased clinician and patient awareness of the possibility of this tumor in women with a long history of oral contraceptive use, and the abdomen should be carefully palpated to detect small masses when evaluating an oral contraceptive user.

Breakthrough Bleeding

Spotting or midcycle bleeding is a common occurrence among pill users. Patients may expect some degree of breakthrough bleeding the first several months of contraceptive use until the body becomes accustomed to the synthetic hormones. If spotting continues after 3 months of use, the dose of estrogen or progestogen can be adjusted. If spotting occurs before midcycle, the estrogen component should be increased. If spotting occurs after midcycle, the progestogen potency should be increased. These changes should be made while keeping in mind the hormone potency of the product the patient is now taking.

Gallbladder Disease

Use of oral contraceptives was originally thought to increase the incidence of gallstones and cholecystitis at least twofold. Estrogens alter the composition of the bile. It has been suggested that a rise in cholesterol saturation of gallbladder bile may account for the increase in gallbladder disease. With a decrease in estrogen content, these effects may be less common. One large retrospective cohort study showed the risk ratio for gallbladder disease in users to be 1.14, which achieved statistical significance (44). Among users of COCs with less than 50 μg of estrogen, the risk ratio was 0.97.

Depression

The incidence of depression among oral contraceptive users is approximately 5 to 6%. The symptoms noted include lethargy, loss of libido, irritability, and crying. Because of the lack of well-controlled trials and the underlying prevalence of depression in this patient population, much controversy exists as to the etiology. Proponents of a biochemical theory offer evidence that brain amine metabolism is altered as a result of any abnormal tryptophan metabolism. An increased requirement for vitamin B6 by pyridoxine-deficient oral contraceptive users was found. Supplementation relieved the symptoms of depression (45).

Breast-Feeding

The World Health Organization (WHO) studied the effects of hormonal contraception on milk in women who breast-feed their children (46). Since estrogen inhibits the action of prolactin in breast tissue receptors, milk production is thought to be related to the amount of estrogen in the COC. Women who took COCs had a 42% reduction in milk volume at 18 weeks of treatment. There was a decline in volume starting at 6 weeks. No effect was seen at 6 weeks in mini-pill users, but at 18 weeks a 12% reduction in volume occurred. Women using nonhormonal techniques had a 6% reduction in milk volume at 18 weeks.

Although specific nutrients, mainly protein, fat, and calcium, were decreased in some women using COCs, no differences in the growth of the infants in any treatment group were noted. The WHO concluded that although COCs containing 30 μg of estrogen do cause some reduction in milk volume, there are no adverse effects on infant growth. Some constituents of COCs are transferred to the infant. Although these are metabolized rapidly by the infant and, currently, there is no reason to believe that they cause harm, long-term studies have not been reported.

Drug Interactions

Evidence indicates that certain drugs may impair the efficacy of COCs. The converse is also true; COCs may modify the action of other drugs. Mechanisms thought to be responsible for these interactions include:

1. Interference with the amount of steroids absorbed or reabsorbed through enterohepatic circulation of steroid metabolites;
2. Stimulating or depressing hepatic metabolism;
3. Displacement of contraceptive steroids from their biologic receptor site;
4. Opposing steroid action by some physiologic effect.

Gastroenteritis has long been associated with decreased gastrointestinal (GI) transit time and steroid absorption. Because ethinyl estradiol conjugates are excreted in the bile and may be broken down by gut bacteria in the colon to liberate active hormone, which can then be reabsorbed, anything that increases GI motility (i.e., diarrhea, laxatives) could reduce circulating concentrations of oral contraceptives. Likewise, ampicillin or other antibiotics such as tetracycline or cotrimoxazole may eliminate the gut microflora necessary for this enterohepatic circulation. Although not substantiated by detailed study in humans, numerous well-documented clinical reports have appeared of pregnancies in women who have missed no COCs but who took an antibiotic agent. From a practical point of view, not many women are at risk of this interaction, but if antibiotics are prescribed for oral contraceptive users, especially during days 1 to 14, barrier concentration should be added for the remainder of the cycle.

The most clinically significant drug interactions occur with other drugs that are metabolized by the same hepatic microsomal pathway as estrogen. Case reports of failure of COCs have appeared in women taking phenytoin, primidone, barbiturates, carbamazepine, ethosuximide, rifampin, and griseofulvin (47). Conversely, estrogens are inhibitors of hepatic microsomal enzymes and may slow the metabolism of other drugs (Table 87.5). In addition, sex hormone–binding globulin (SHBG) binds common progestins with high affinity. It has been shown that SHBG capacity to bind is significantly increased in women taking anticonvulsants. This would decrease free levels of progestins and decrease the efficacy of oral contraceptives. It has been suggested that a young woman who wishes to use a COC and is receiving treatment for a seizure disorder should take one of the preparations with 30 µg of estrogen. If breakthrough bleeding occurs, then an additional dose of a 20-µg estrogen should be added (48). Valproic acid has not been associated with apparent oral contraceptive failure. If clinically appropriate for seizure control, use of valproic acid may be considered in women needing maximal assurance of contraception.

Table 87.5.
Combination Oral Contraceptive (COC) Drug Interactions[a]

Increase COC concentrations	*Decrease COC concentrations*
Ascorbic acid	Antibiotic agents
Acetaminophen	Barbiturates
	Phenytoin
	Primidone
	Carbamazepine
	Griseofulvin
	Rifampin
Have their concentrations increased by COC	*Have their concentrations decreased by COC*
Alprazolam	Acetaminophen
Antipyrine	Clofibrate
Caffeine	Lorazepam
Chlordiazepoxide	Morphine
Corticosteroids	Oxazepam
Diazepam	Temazepam
Imipramine	
Metoprolol	
Nitrazepam	
Theophylline	
Triazolam	
Vitamin A	
Vitamin D	

[a] Adapted from Shenfield GM: Drug interactions with oral contraceptive preparations. Med J Aust 144:205–211, 1986.

COCs increase the concentration of certain clotting factors, and it is not surprising that COCs have have been reported to reduce the efficacy of anticoagulants. In general women should not be taking these two preparations together. Likewise, high-dose COCs may cause impaired glucose tolerance in some patients. Use of a low-estrogen COC or another method of contraception may be necessary for these patients.

Other Side Effects

Previously, tests that monitored thyroid function were affected by oral contraceptives. Thyroid function was not changed; the laboratory tests used to measure thyroid function were changed. Estrogens increase the thyroid-binding globulin, therefore tests that are used to measure thyroid function such as protein-bound iodine thyroxine, T-4 by column, and T-4 by Murphy Pattee (total T-4) will have elevated results, and triiodothyronine (T-3) resin uptake will be decreased. These tests are not used as frequently now. To accurately assess thyroid function in COC users, a free T-4 should be done (see Chapter 16 "Thyroid and Parathyroid Disorders"). Abnormal thyroid values return to normal 2 to 4 weeks after the discontinuation of oral contraceptives.

Nausea and vomiting appear to be related to the estrogen dose of oral contraceptives. It is a common side effect that may decrease with continued use. Pharmacokinetic data suggest that most estrogen is absorbed within 2 hr after oral administration. It would be wise to repeat the dose if vomiting occurs during the absorption period. Management of pill-associated nausea includes (a) use of low-dose estrogen-containing oral contraceptives, (b) reassurance if temporary nausea can be tolerated, and (c) taking the pill at bedtime so the patient will be asleep during peak serum concentrations.

Weight gain with oral contraceptives has been divided into two categories: persistent weight gain and cyclic weight gain. Persistent acyclic weight gain is thought to be secondary to the anabolic testosterone-like progestogen increase in appetite or decrease in activity. Cyclic weight gain, on the other hand, is thought to be an estrogen-related side effect, secondary to water retention.

An increase in the frequency of headache (both tension and migraine) has been noted with oral contraceptive use. Because headaches are common among all women of reproductive age and because of poor literature documentation, it is difficult to determine the etiology of birth control pill–associated headaches. There is evidence that falling estrogen levels may incite the cerebrovascular system to respond by producing migraine headaches. Patients who develop migraine (vascular headaches) while taking oral contraceptives should discontinue the pill (see Chapter 47 "Headache").

Increased corneal sensitivity, particularly contact lens discomfort, has been noted in about 1:5 women who take oral contraceptives (49). Changes in corneal curvature and decreased tear secretion have been blamed for this side effect in oral contraceptive users and pregnant patients. A variety of ocular changes have been attributed to the pill, ranging from retinal vascular accidents to decreases in visual acuity and color changes (50). However, repeated prospective and retrospective studies failed to find a correlation between the use of birth control pills and many of these abnormalities, which are found normally in a population of women of reproductive age. However, caution should be exerted in prescribing oral contraceptives to women with known ophthalmologic disorders.

Erythema nodosum, erythema multiforme, and urticaria are hypersensitivity reactions that are occasionally seen with oral contraceptive therapy. They are rare events, occurring in at most 1:1000 users. Oral contraceptives should be discontinued at once. This reaction usually is attributed to the progestin component of the pill, and it seems to regress when patients are taken off the pill (6).

Oral contraceptives have been rarely associated with flare-ups of systemic lupus erythematosus (SLE) (51). However, it is more common to see SLE and antinuclear antibody (ANA) tests turn positive in patients using oral contraceptive drugs and revert to negative on discontinuation. The importance of this is unknown.

Megaloblastic anemia has been reported in oral contraceptive users for two reasons: (a) a relative folic acid deficiency, which may exist because of increased binding of folic acid and (b) (rarely) a decrease in serum vitamin B_{12}. It is likely that oral contraceptives contribute to, but do not produce, this anemia in otherwise healthy women, and it responds to appropriate replacement therapy. Other vitamin deficiencies have been reported. The most marked are in the water soluble vitamins: thiamine (B_1), riboflavin (B_2), pyridoxine (B_6), cobalamin (B_{12}), and ascorbic acid (C).

Fewer women on oral contraceptives have iron deficiency anemia. This probably reflects a decrease in menstrual flow secondary to the use of oral contraceptives, with subsequent increases in serum iron and iron-binding capacity.

Other side effects that have been attributed to the pill include acne, chloasma (skin hyperpigmentation), abnormal hair growth, changes in libido, breast tenderness, galactorrhea, postpill amenorrhea, photosensitivity, exacerbation of acute intermittent porphyria, exacerbation of Wilson's disease, and ischemic colitis. Some of these side effects have been attributed to a particular component of birth control pills, or lack thereof, and are listed in Table 87.6.

Table 87.6.
Side Effects That May Require Adjustment of the Estrogen/Progestogen Balance

Estrogen excess	Progestogen excess
Nausea, bloating	Increased appetite
Cervical mucorrhea, polyposis	Persistent weight gain
Hypermenorrhea	Tiredness, fatigue
Hyperpigmentation	Hypomenorrhea
Uterine or leg cramps	Acne, oily scalp
Hypertension	Hair loss
Migraine headache	Depression
Breast tenderness	Hirsutism
Dizziness, vertigo	Breast regression
Cyclic weight gain	Changes in libido
Fibroid growth	
Cervical eversion	
Estrogen deficiency	Progestogen deficiency
Irritability, nervousness	Late breakthrough bleeding
Early and/or midcycle	Amenorrhea
breakthrough bleeding	Hypermenorrhea
Increased spotting	Weight loss
Hot flashes	
Hypomenorrhea	
Amenorrhea	
Dyspareunia	

Table 87.7.
Contraindications to Oral Contraceptive Use

Absolute contraindications
  Estrogen-dependent neoplasm
  Impaired liver function or past history of cholestatic jaundice
  Deep vein thrombosis, pulmonary embolism, stroke, or history of thromboembolic disorders
  Previous myocardial infarction
  Pregnancy
  Undiagnosed abnormal genital bleeding

Relative contraindications
  Diabetes mellitus
  Hypertension or history of hypertension during pregnancy
  Migraine headaches
  Depression
  Glaucoma
  Systemic lupus erythematosus
  Acute intermittent porphyria
  Epilepsy
  Smoking
  Obesity

ASSOCIATED BENEFITS OF ORAL CONTRACEPTIVE USE

Noncontraceptive benefits associated with COCs also are of note. In addition to the decrease in endometrial and ovarian cancer previously noted, there is a decline in the risk of rheumatoid arthritis, pelvic inflammatory disease, ectopic pregnancy, functional ovarian cysts, acne, dysmenorrhea, and morbidity and mortality associated with pregnancy and childbirth. It has been estimated that the use of COCs will prevent 1 to 7 million requests for abortions annually (52).

CONTRAINDICATIONS TO ORAL CONTRACEPTIVE USE

The absolute and relative contraindications for the use of oral contraceptives are listed in Table 87.7.

SELECTION OF AN ORAL CONTRACEPTIVE PRODUCT

When selecting a combination oral contraceptive product for a patient, there are several very important considerations:

1. The product should contain the lowest effective dose of estrogen and progestin. Nearly all patients do well on products containing 35 μg or less of estrogen.
2. The product should have the minimum side effects acceptable to the patient.
3. Any problems or concomitant diseases that the patient has should be considered and minimized if possible.
4. An effort should be made to discontinue oral contraceptives by age 45, since the incidence of side effects increases greatly after this point. Women with preexisting systemic disease that

may affect the cardiovascular system or smokers should discontinue use at 35 years of age.

It is important to understand that oral contraceptives play the role of temporary contraception in family planning, to be used for delaying the first birth and spacing children. Once the family is complete, surgical sterilization is the safest.

In addition to the above criteria, it is important to have an understanding of the relative estrogen and progestogen potencies of oral contraceptive products. These potencies reflect the total amount of estrogen and progestogen as well as the effects they have on each other. (Table 87.3).

Table 87.8 lists the common products on the U.S. market and their relative estrogenic and progestogenic potencies. Because of the large number of products available, it is important to be able to recommend a more or less potent product when an estrogen- or progestogen-related side effect occurs.

The ovarian and the uterine cycles are superimposed for 28 days to form the menstrual cycle. When estrogens and progestins in the form of oral contraceptive pills are added to this cycle, an attempt is made to alter the ovarian cycle without affecting the uterine cycle. However, since these synthetic agents are not identical to the naturally produced hormones, some changes from the "normal" are likely to occur (i.e., a decrease in menstrual flow, occasional spotting, or a missed period). A woman relies on her normal menstrual bleeding as a sign to indicate that she is not pregnant. If pregnancy has been ruled out, the patient should be reassured if concern is expressed over the above changes.

RISK-BENEFIT RATIO

For the first time in history, normal, healthy people are taking a potent medication over a long period of time. It is increasingly important to discuss the risk of this therapy with the patient, especially when the lay press, which is read most by women, tends to emphasize these risks. Perhaps some perspective can be gained if the risks of taking oral contraceptives are compared with other common risks of mortality (Fig. 87.4).

MISSED PILLS

As a practical matter, it is important to know what to tell patients when birth control pills are missed. Certain information should be obtained before any advice is given:

1. What oral contraceptive product is the patient taking?
2. How long has the patient been taking oral contraceptives?
3. On which days of the menstrual cycle were the pill(s) missed?
4. How many pills were missed?

Ovulation is not always suppressed in products con-

Table 87.8.
Oral Contraceptives Available in the United States

Trade Name	Manufacturer	Estrogen	(μg)	Progestin	(mg)
		Fixed-Combination Contraceptives			
>50 μg of estrogen					
Enovid 5 mg	Searle	mestranol	75	norethynodrel	5.0
50 μg of estrogen					
Demulen 1/50	Searle	ethinyl estradiol	50	ethynodiol diacetate	1.0
Ovral	Wyeth	ethinyl estradiol	50	norgestrel	0.5
Ovcon-50	Mead Johnson	ethinyl estradiol	50	norethindrone	1.0
Genora 1/50	Rugby	ethinyl estradiol	50	norethindrone	1.0
Nelova 1/50M	Warner Chilcott	ethinyl estradiol	50	norethindrone	1.0
Norethin 1/50M	Searle	ethinyl estradiol	50	norethindrone	1.0
Norinyl 1 + 50	Syntex	mestranol	50	norethindrone	1.0
Ortho-Novum 1/50	Ortho	mestranol	50	norethindrone	1.0
Norlestrin 2.5/50	Parke-Davis	ethinyl estradiol	50	norethindrone acetate	2.5
Norlestrin 1/50	Parke-Davis	ethinyl estradiol	50	norethindrone acetate	1.0
<50 μg of estrogen					
Demulen 1/35	Searle	ethinyl estradiol	35	ethynodiol diacetate	1.0
Genora 1/35	Rugby	ethinyl estradiol	35	norethindrone	1.0
Gynex 1/35E	Searle	ethinyl estradiol	35	norethindrone	1.0
N.E.E.	MetroMed	ethinyl estradiol	35	norethindrone	1.0
Nelova	Warner Chilcott	ethinyl estradiol	35	norethindrone	1.0
Norcept-E 1/35	Gyno Pharma	ethinyl estradiol	35	norethindrone	1.0
Norethin 1/35E	Searle	ethinyl estradiol	35	norethindrone	1.0
Norinyl 1/35	Syntex	ethinyl estradiol	35	norethindrone	1.0
Ortho-Novum 1/35	Ortho	ethinyl estradiol	35	norethindrone	1.0
Brevicon	Syntex	ethinyl estradiol	35	norethindrone	0.5
Gynex 0.5/35E	Searle	ethinyl estradiol	35	norethindrone	0.5
Modicon	Ortho	ethinyl estradiol	35	norethindrone	0.5
Nelova 0.5/35E	Warner Chilcott	ethinyl estradiol	35	norethindrone	0.5
Ovcon-35	Mead Johnson	ethinyl estradiol	35	norethindrone	0.4
Lo-Ovral	Wyeth	ethinyl estradiol	30	norgestrel	0.3
Levlen	Berlex	ethinyl estradiol	30	levonorgestrel	0.15
Nordette	Wyeth	ethinyl estradiol	30	levonorgestrel	0.15
Loestrin 1.5/30	Parke-Davis	ethinyl estradiol	30	norethindrone acetate	1.5
Loestrin 1/20	Parke-Davis	ethinyl estradiol	20	norethindrone acetate	1.0
		Biphasic Combination Contraceptives			
Nelova 10/11 and	Warner Chilcott				
Ortho-Novum 10/11	Ortho				
(day 1–10)		ethinyl estradiol	35	norethindrone	0.5
(day 11–21)		ethinyl estradiol	35	norethindrone	1.0
		Triphasic Combination Contraceptives			
Ortho-Novum 7/7/7	Ortho				
(day 1–7)		ethinyl estradiol	35	norethindrone	0.5
(day 8–14)		ethinyl estradiol	35	norethindrone	0.75
(day 15–21)		ethinyl estradiol	35	norethindrone	1.0
Tri-Norinyl	Syntex				
(day 1–7)		ethinyl estradiol	35	norethindrone	0.5
(day 8–16)		ethinyl estradiol	35	norethindrone	1.0
(day 17–21)		ethinyl estradiol	35	norethindrone	0.5
Tri-Levlen and	Berlex				
Triphasil	Wyeth				
(day 1–6)		ethinyl estradiol	30	levonorgestrel	0.05
(day 7–11)		ethinyl estradiol	40	levonorgestrel	0.075
(day 12–21)		ethinyl estradiol	30	levonorgestrel	0.125
		Progestin-only Contraceptives			
Micronor	Ortho			norethindrone	0.35
Nor-Q.D.	Syntex			norethindrone	0.35
Ovrette	Wyeth			norgestrel	0.075

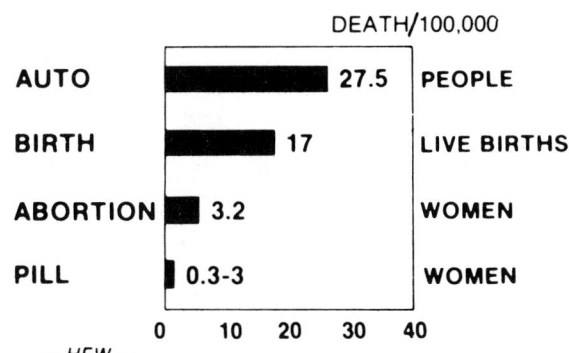

Figure 87.4 Relative risks of mortality of various causes.

taining low-dose estrogen. The more estrogen and progestin in a product, the more reliable it will be, at the expense of having more side effects. One missed pill would be of less consequence in a patient taking a high-dose product than for a patient taking a low-dose pill. In addition, the progestin content of the low-dose pill contributes to the contraceptive effect and must be present daily.

Modest fluctuations in the levels of FSH and LH among pill users have been observed. This might indicate that follicular development may proceed to a greater extent in some women, resulting in more breakthrough ovulation. Because women who have taken oral contraceptives for a long period of time have ovaries in a semidormant state, they are less likely to experience breakthrough ovulation as a result of a missed pill. On the other hand, women who are short-term oral contraceptive users are more likely to have mature follicles ready for ovulation; they may be more affected by a missed pill or by missing the usual dosing time by several hours. Oral contraceptives should be taken at the same time each day.

Contrary to popular belief, missing pills at midcycle is not the greatest risk. A high level of hormones early in the cycle is necessary at the level of the hypothalamus for suppression of FSH and LH. Therefore, missing pill number 2, for example, would be more likely to result in a pregnancy than missing pill number 20.

Many clinicians believe that if a patient misses one pill, that missed pill should be taken as soon as it is remembered: the next day's pill should be taken at the regular time (two pills may be taken at the same time). If two consecutive pills are missed, the medication should be doubled for the following 2 consecutive days. Barrier methods of contraception should be started immediately and used for the rest of the cycle.

The above information should be evaluated with care. If for example, a patient has been taking a product that contains 50 μg of estrogen for 3 years and missed pill 18, she probably would not get pregnant. On the other hand,

if a patient misses pills 2 and 3 of her second pack of 20-μg pills, she is likely to ovulate.

The triphasic oral contraceptives introduce an even smaller margin of error. Basal concentrations of FSH and LH are only partially depressed during the last 3 days of therapy, producing less inhibition than standard COCs. Ovulation is effectively inhibited, but after missed doses, FSH and LH concentrations recover more quickly. Excellent reviews on managing contraceptive pill patients have appeared elsewhere (1, 2, 53).

"MORNING-AFTER" PILLS

The implantation of the blastocyte is inhibited by high doses of estrogen. Synthetic, natural, and conjugated estrogens have been administered as "morning-after" pills. Therapy is not recommended for routine use, but rather for cases of rape, incest, or mechanical contraceptive failure near midcycle. The interval between conception and implantation is approximately 6 days. When high-risk unprotected intercourse has occurred, it is important to begin therapy within 72 hr.

In the 1960s and early 1970s, high doses of diethylstilbestrol (DES) 25 to 50 mg/day or ethinylestradiol 0.5 to 5 mg/day for 5 days was used as "morning-after" therapy. Nausea and vomiting are complications of this high-dose estrogen therapy.

Although DES is an effective postcoital contraceptive agent, failures can occur. Cases of vaginal adenosis, vaginal adenocarcinoma, and cervical adenocarcinoma in young female offspring of women who took DES during pregnancy have been reported. This teratogenic effect of DES appears to occur at the ninth week of pregnancy (54). Thus, no evidence of teratogenicity has been demonstrated in association with the failure of postcoital estrogens. However, abortion should be a first consideration if these agents fail.

Today, the most popular regimen is 100 μg ethinyl estradiol and 1 mg norgestrel (i.e., two Ovral tablets) initially, repeated after 12 hr. The patient should experience withdrawal bleeding within 10 days of administration. Again, treatment must be initiated within 72 hr of exposure. Experience with 1300 treatment cycles with this regimen indicates a failure rate of 1.6% (55).

SUBDERMAL IMPLANTS

A new method of delivering contraceptive progestogen was recently approved by the FDA. Norplant contains levonorgestrel in six silicone rods about 1 ⅓ inches long. A small incision under local anesthesia is required to insert, in a fanlike arrangement, the device in the upper arm. The steroid is released at a relatively constant rate and provides effective contraception for 5 years. The annual pregnancy rate is less than 1% in women who weigh less than 150 pounds. The removal of the capsules also requires an incision and local anesthesia, but fertility returns to normal promptly after removal. As with other contraceptives containing progestin only, the main side effect is irregular bleeding. About 15% of patients have the Norplant removed because of bleeding.

OTHER HORMONE CONTRACEPTIVES

Several countries are testing a new progestin in COC products—norgestimate (NGM). NGM in a dose of 250 µg is combined with ethinyl estradiol (EE) 35 µg in a new COC. NGM is relatively free of androgenic activity, producing a more natural menstrual pattern and a positive impact on lipoprotein metabolism. NGM/EE products have consistently produced significant increases in HDL and concommitant improvement in LDL/HDL ratios (56).

Another device that has received extensive testing is a silicone rubber vaginal ring that releases 20 µg of levonorgestrel per 24 hr. Pregnancy rates are 3.6 per 100 women years. The principle reasons for discontinuation are menstrual disturbances, vaginal symptoms, and repeated expulsion of the ring.

THE "SHOT"

Medroxyprogesterone acetate (MPA) has been used in other countries around the world as an injectable contraceptive agent. The drug suppresses the preovulatory surge of LH and thus inhibits ovulation. It also produces the progestin mucus changes and endometrial growth changes discussed earlier.

The dose of MPA is 150 mg intramuscularly every 90 days. Women using this form of contraceptive experience very irregular menstrual bleeding patterns. Amenorrhea is to be expected 2 to 12 months after beginning use of the medication. The average length of time for return of fertility after discontinuation of this drug is about 8 to 10 months.

The same contraindications exist for MPA as for the "pill," although it is not presently known if thromboembolic disorders increase as a result of MPA use. Concern for possible carcinogenicity has prevented the marketing of this product in the United States.

Mifepristone (RU 486)

Mifepristone is a 19-norsteroid analog used in France and China to induce an abortion. Treatment with this drug early in pregnancy leads to detachment and expulsion of the products of conception. The drug has a high affinity for progesterone and glucocorticoid receptors, and to a lesser extent, to androgen receptors. It also stimulates the synthesis of prostaglandins. Both prostaglandins and withdrawal of progesterone stimulate uterine contractility.

The drug is administered orally alone or in combination with a small dose of prostaglandin analog administered by vaginal suppository or intramuscularly. Clinical studies have shown that 400 to 800 mg of mifepristone alone, either in divided doses or as a single 600-mg dose, can terminate early pregnancy in approximately 85% of cases. The incidence of complete abortion increases to about 95% when combined with a dose of prostaglandin.

Bleeding begins 1 to 2 days after treatment and lasts 1 to 2 weeks. Crampy abdominal pain occurs in most patients for a few hours after administration.

MECHANICAL BIRTH CONTROL

The four common mechanical birth control devices are the intrauterine device, diaphragm, condom, and foam. The efficacy of these products in theory and in use can be seen in Table 87.1.

Intrauterine Device

The idea of inserting a foreign body into the uterus to prevent pregnancy is not new. Many years ago natural fibers such as silkworm gut as well as stones and wires containing silver and copper were used as intrauterine contraceptive devices. After World War II, man-made fibers and various types of polythene were available and were molded in many ways as intrauterine devices (IUDs). The copper-containing IUD regained popularity in the 1960s, and an IUD that slowly releases progesterone was an innovative development of the 1970s. All but two IUDs have been voluntarily withdrawn by the manufacturers from the U.S. market. Makers cite increased litigation costs as reasons for discontinuing their products. Progestasert (Alza), is a T-shaped unit containing a reservoir of 38 mg progesterone with barium sulfate dispersed in silicone oil. This device is associated with less blood loss and a lower frequency of primary dysmenorrhea as a result of the progesterone. It is recommended the Progestasert be replaced yearly. The copper T 380A (ParaGard-Gynomed) is a copper-containing IUD. The T 380A is believed to be the most effective IUD in current use, particularly for women over age 25. The National Association of Family Planning Doctors has proposed that copper-containing IUDs need not be generally changed more often than every 5 years.

The mechanism of action of an IUD is still unclear. Ovulation seems to be unimpaired in the presence of an IUD. All the postulated mechanisms of action are at the level of the uterus. It is possible any or all of the following mechanisms may be operative.

1. Changes in tubal motility and uterine motility produced by the IUD have been shown in animal studies. The ovum, normally fertilized in the fallopian tube, may be propelled through the genital tract too rapidly for proper implantation to occur. It is questionable whether this effect occurs in humans.

2. The stretching or distortion of the uterus by these devices may have a contraceptive effect. However, most of the newer devices have been designed to avoid this distention. It has also been postulated that a mechanical dislodging of the implanted blastocyst may occur; however, most experts believe they interfere with fertilization.

3. The presence of the device results in the mobilization of polymorphonuclear leukocytes into the endometrium. The local inflammatory response causes the release of prostaglandins and may increase phagocytic activity against sperm and blastocysts.

4. For devices containing copper it is thought that copper increases the inflammatory reaction, decreases the viability of sperm, and impairs ovum transport.

Theoretically, the IUD is about 97 to 99% effective. Its use effectiveness is approximately the same, since very little compliance is required on the part of the patient.

The only absolute contraindications for the insertion of an IUD in a normal healthy woman are active pelvic infection and pregnancy. However, a number of complications may follow insertion. For instance, there may be an increase in the amount of menstrual flow as well as pain associated with the IUD, particularly for the first several months following IUD insertion. This increased blood loss may cause anemia in some patients. Spotting may also occur. Moreover, all types of IUD may be expelled through the cervix. Obviously, the device can be of no value when it is absent. Patients should be taught to check for the IUD string in the vagina to ensure that the device is in place. Uterine perforation is most likely to occur at the time of insertion. However, IUDs may gradually work their way through the uterine wall and may need to be removed from the abdominal cavity by use of laparoscopic procedures.

Most serious complications from IUDs are related to infections, including sepsis and in some cases death. IUD use is associated with about a threefold increased incidence of developing acute salpingitis (pelvic inflammatory disease or PID) in comparison with users of oral contraceptives and diaphragms. The Dalkon Shield was withdrawn from the market after several deaths from septic spontaneous abortions. If pregnancy occurs with an IUD in place, there is a threefold increased risk of spontaneous abortion and a 10-fold increased risk of ectopic pregnancy.

Diaphragm

The diaphragm ranges in diameter from 55 to 100 mm. It is inserted into the vagina and blocks the opening to the uterus. The diaphragm must be fitted by a clinician and should be refitted if the woman delivers a baby, aborts, or gains or loses 10 lb or more.

It was thought that the mechanical barrier of the diaphragm would prevent sperm migration into the uterus; however, it has been shown that the diaphragm moves about during coitus (2). Therefore, its primary mechanism is to hold the spermicidal agent near the cervical os. The diaphragm should not be used without spermicidal jelly or cream. These agents also aid insertion because of their lubrication properties.

At least a teaspoonful of spermicidal jelly or cream should be spread around the inside of the rim before insertion. It takes 6 to 8 hr for the spermicidal agent to work. Therefore, the diaphragm must remain in place at least 8 hr. Another applicatorful of spermicide should be inserted in the vagina, leaving the diaphragm in place, before each subsequent coitus.

The key to successful diaphragm use is motivation. Many clinicians fail to recognize the diaphragm as a viable contraceptive alternative. However, because of its mechanical action, it represents a method of contraception practically devoid of side effects.

Cervical Cap

There has been a resurgence of interest in a barrier method, smaller than a diaphragm, that fits over the cervix, called a cervical cap. The Prentif is now available in the U.S. It should be used with spermicide but can be left in place 48 hr without adding more spermicide. The cap is manufactured in four sizes and may be more difficult to fit for both the provider and user than the diaphragm. Pregnancy rates are similar to other barrier methods. Because of concern about possible adverse effects of the cap on cervical tissue, they should be used only by women with normal Pap smears. Smears should be checked after the first 3 months of cap use and annually thereafter.

Condom

Condoms are latex rubber sheaths that are worn over an erect penis during coitus. This mechanical barrier prevents transmission of the male semen into the vagina. Although pregnancy rates are higher than in users of COCs, barrier methods are effective in preventing the transmission of venereal disease, including AIDS, from either partner. Several in vitro studies have demonstrated that condoms prevent the transmission of viruses, specifically the herpes virus and human immunodeficiency virus (HIV) as well as the *Chlamydia trachomatis*, bacteria and gonorrheal infections, frequent causes of salpingitis.

Condoms are marketed rolled or unrolled, lubricated or unlubricated, and ribbed, and may have reservoir ends to collect the semen. When the condom is put on, one-half inch of empty space should be left at the tip if the condom does not have a reservoir end. A condom should be used only once.

Petroleum jelly should never be used to lubricate a condom (this causes the latex to deteriorate). K-Y jelly, contraceptive foam, or saliva are good lubricants.

Spermicidal Agents

Contraceptive foam is marketed in an aerosol can or bottle with an applicator or as a tablet. The foam is the medium that holds the spermicidal agent against the cervical os. Nonoxynol-9 is the spermicidal agent used in most of these over-the-counter (OTC) preparations. Two full applicators of foam should be inserted high in the vagina no earlier than 30 min before each ejaculation. Spermicides also reduce the frequency of clinical infections with sexually transmitted diseases, both bacterial and viral.

Although contraceptive foam is fairly effective alone, it can be used in conjunction with a diaphragm or condom to produce a very effective method of birth control. Vaginal spermicides marketed to be used with a diaphragm are usually less potent, having a different consistency but the same active ingredient.

If a particular brand of foam is irritating to either partner, the couple should try another brand. Foam is often confused with "feminine hygiene" products. To confuse the issue further, a variety of other insertable spermicides are marketed. There are tablets that are supposed to foam, creams and jellies that are supposed to spread, and suppositories that are supposed to melt; sometimes they do not.

Douching may force sperm into the uterus and is not recommended for at least 8 hr after intercourse when using a diaphragm or foam for contraception. These products should not be used during pregnancy. The literature is not conclusive, although there have been case reports of birth defects following the use of spermicides during pregnancy. These studies were probably flawed by recall bias. Several well-designed recent studies have shown no increased risk of congenital malformations in newborns (57) or spontaneous abortuses (58) of women who conceived while using spermicides.

Contraceptive Sponge

The most popular form for a vaginal spermicide is a disposable, polyurethane foam sponge, slightly thicker and smaller than a diaphragm with a ribbon loop for removal. The sponge is impregnated with nonoxynol-9 and can be left in place about 24 hr. The spermicide must be activated before insertion by adding 1 ounce of water to the sponge. It has been shown that parous women have the highest failure rates with this method.

A few cases of toxic shock syndrome (TSS) have been reported in users of the sponge, but the role of this contraceptive device as a causative agent is not clearly defined. If symptoms of TSS develop, the sponge should be removed immediately, and the patient's symptoms reported to a physician.

Toxic Shock Syndrome

Billions of tampons have been produced and used by millions of women throughout the world over the past several decades. In the last several years, a circumstantial relationship has existed between the use of tampons and several disease entities.

The first cases of TSS were described in 1978 (59). Since then a wide variety of clinical symptoms have been described. TSS generally affects previously healthy young women of childbearing age during an otherwise normal menstrual period. It usually begins with a sudden high fever (greater than 102°F) and may be accompanied by severe headache, sore throat, vomiting, and diarrhea. Progressive hypotension may proceed to shock. Palmar erythema is frequent, and a diffuse sunburn-like rash has been described. A nonpurulent conjunctivitis is described at the disease onset, and a superficial desquamation of skin on the palms and soles often follows within 2 to 3 weeks of the onset of the disease.

TSS is associated with the use of highly absorbant tampons and the contraceptive sponge as well as with the isolation of coagulase-positive *Staphylococcus aureus* from the vagina or from focal infections of infected patients. The presence of exotoxin from an *S. aureus* infection could certainly account for the number of clinical symptoms identified with this disease. Clinicians should be aware of the possibility of TSS in any menstruating woman with sudden onset of a febrile illness. Prompt removal of tampons, as well as symptomatic treatment including support of blood pressure, may be critical. Use of β-lactamase-resistant penicillins has been shown to lower risk of the recurrence (60). In addition, patients with TSS should be instructed to permanently discontinue the use of tampons. The incidence of TSS has fallen in the last several years and may relate to a decrease in the degree of absorption of marketed tampons.

INFERTILITY

Infertility has been labeled "epidemic" in the United States, with at least 15% (4.5 million couples) experiencing some degree of infertility (61). Over three-quarter million prescriptions were filled for infertility drugs in 1984, and an upward trend is expected to continue as more couples seek medical advice for infertility.

Primary infertility is present when there is no proof of pregnancy ever occurring, and secondary infertility exists when after having given birth previously to a viable fetus, a woman does not become pregnant again in a 1-year period of regular, unprotected intercourse. The spontaneous cure rate for primary infertility is of note. Twenty-five percent of couples desiring pregnancy will conceive without medical intervention in the first month. By 6 months, this will rise to 60%. By the end of a year, 88% of couples desiring a pregnancy will have conceived. Of the remaining 12%, approximately 10% (1 in 10) will conceive during the next year (62).

Infertility is a symptom with many causes. In general,

35% of infertility is a problem solely of the female; another 35% is a problem solely with the male. In about 25% of cases a problem is found in both members of the couple. Only about 3.5% of infertility is unexplained when a thorough evaluation of both partners has been done (61).

Many known causes for infertility in the male and female can be successfully treated with medical or surgical techniques. It has been estimated that between 20 and 50% of all infertile women are anovulatory or ovulate inconsistently (oligoovulation). Progress in understanding normal and abnormal menstrual physiology has led to the development of effective modalities for the induction of ovulation. Improvement in the treatment of ovulatory dysfunction has been one of the most successful therapeutic advances in gynecologic endocrinology in the last 2 decades. Currently, women whose infertility is caused by anovulation or oligoovulation have the highest chance of being treated successfully.

Female Reproductive System

The delicate balance in the hypothalamic-pituitary-ovarian axis and its feedback controls on normal follicular maturation are important to understanding the use of fertility agents. During menses, the hypothalamus responds to low levels of circulating estrogen with the production and release of GnRH. GnRH causes the anterior pituitary to release FSH and LH. Throughout the cycle, FSH levels fluctuate via a negative-feedback system involving estrogen (estradiol e-2); LH levels fluctuate by both positive and negative feedback systems involving estrogen and by the negative feedback of progesterone during the luteal phase (Fig. 87.5). This complex mechanism is exquisitely sensitive to alterations in any or all components. Breakdown in the ovulatory process can be grouped by the source of malfunction of the system.

Once ovulation is suspected, fertilization can occur within 12 to 24 hr. The easiest and most inexpensive method to detect whether, and perhaps when, ovulation occurs is to chart basal body temperature (BBT). To use this method, only a special BBT thermometer and temperature charts (Fig. 87.6) are needed. A woman should take her temperature immediately upon waking and before any activity, even before leaving the bed. The BBT usually shows a distinct, biphasic pattern with an elevation during the postovulatory phase of the cycle. This elevated temperature has been attributed to the thermogenic effect of progesterone.

There appears to be no difference if the thermometer is placed orally, rectally, or vaginally, as long as it is inserted at least 5 cm and the location is consistent (63). In addition, the hour of waking should be recorded, because variation in time may affect results (64). Endometrial biopsy showing histologic findings characteristic of the luteal phase or a single measurement of serum progesterone or urinary

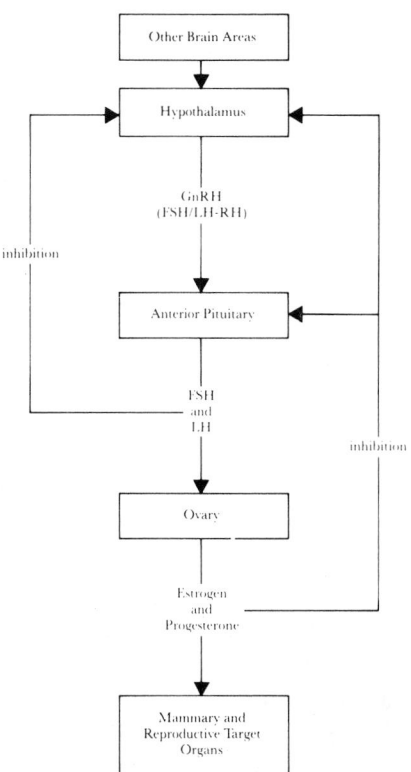

Figure 87.5 Feedback system in the hypothalamic-pituitary-ovarian axis.

pregnanediol at midluteal phase is also used to document ovulation. The problem with these methods of predicting the most fertile time is that they occur after ovulation.

Luteinizing hormone (LH) urine tests are OTC products available to aid in documenting ovulation. These tests take advantage of the LH surge just prior to the ovulatory phase. Diluted urine is processed so that monoclonal antibodies selectively bind to LH in the urine. An enzyme-linked immunoassay indicates the amount of LH bound to the monoclonal antibodies via a change in color intensity. A darker color on the test, as compared with a color chart that is provided, indicates the surge in LH. Ovulation is expected in the 36 hr after such a color change.

A variety of ovulation test kits are available and contain a series of 5 to 9 urine tests that take 4 min to 1 hr each morning to perform, depending on the test. During the testing period, urine is tested daily. If there is a color change or if the color change is darker than the surge guide, then the LH surge has occurred.

Conditions such as endometriosis, ovarian cysts, hyperthyroidum, and the onset of menapause can cause high LH levels that are not due to ovulation. Drugs such as the menatropins, danazol, steroids, and initial treatment with GnRH analogs can produce a false-positive result. If LH testing is required in these circumstances, serum radioimmune assay techniques can be used.

Figure 87.6 Sample basal body temperature chart. (From Carmichael JM: Pharmacologic Treatment of Infertility. Randolph, MA: Serono Laboratories, 1986.)

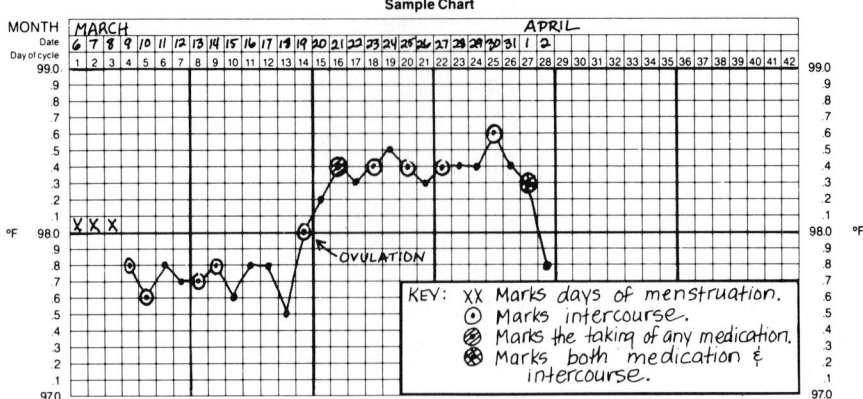

Patient Selection for Fertility Drugs

Once anovulation has been determined, certain prerequisites must be met to ensure a safe and successful outcome with fertility drug use. Serum prolactin and androgen levels should be determined, because hyperprolactinemia can be found in approximately 15% of women with anovulation, and its discovery alters the therapy required. In addition, increased androgen levels may be found in 35% of these patients. A variety of therapeutic drugs have been associated with increased serum prolactin levels, including phenothiazines, tricyclic antidepressants, meprobamate, haloperidol, methyldopa, and isoniazid (65). Hypothyroidism and a pituitary tumor may also cause hyperprolactinemia. When these secondary conditions have been excluded, idiopathic hyperprolactinemia is treated with bromocriptine 1.25 to 7.5 mg daily, taken with meals to decrease GI intolerance. The drug should be discontinued as soon as a positive pregnancy test is obtained (Fig. 87.7).

In addition to hyperprolactinemia, adrenal and thyroid disorders as causes of anovulation should be diagnosed and treated. Ovaries capable of responding to endogenous gonadotropin secretions are a prerequisite to clomiphene therapy. A simple functional test of follicular activity involves the induction of withdrawal bleeding by progesterone administration. Upon successful induction of withdrawal bleeding, indicating unopposed estrogen stimulation, ovulation induction with clomiphene citrate is indicated.

CLOMIPHENE CITRATE

It has been approximately 40 years since the synthesis of clomiphene citrate (Serophene and Clomid). Despite a cumulative bibliography approaching 8000 publications, the mechanism(s) and site(s) of action of clomiphene are still unclear (66). This knowledge gap is particularly striking in view of the widespread and highly successful use of clomiphene worldwide.

Clomiphene citrate (CC) is a weak estrogen that is capable of blocking the effects of more potent estrogens (such as estradiol) (67), thus producing a mixed agonist/antagonistic effect. Clomiphene is capable of interacting with a variety of estrogen-dependent tissues, including the hypothalamic-pituitary unit, ovary, endometrium, cervical mucus-producing glands, and vaginal mucosa.

Current concepts favor the notion that the ability of clomiphene to initiate an ovulatory sequence is due primarily, and perhaps exclusively, to its ability to interact with estrogen receptors at the level of the hypothalamus. Its administration results in release of GnRH, FSH, and LH. Adashi (66) suggests that the overall effects of clomiphene may reflect not only the action on the hypothalamus, but the sum of its direct effects on the estrogen-dependent tissue at the hypothalamic, pituitary, and ovarian levels.

The result at the hypothalamic level is that, in the presence of clomiphene, estradiol is incapable of exerting its negative feedback on GnRH. Thus, clomiphene will enhance FSH and LH release. This mechanism is also applicable in the male hypothalamus, since the negative-feedback inhibitory effect of testosterone on GnRH secretion is produced after metabolism of testosterone to an estrogen in hypothalamic cells. In women, the drug is of no value in patients with primary pituitary or ovarian failure and is useful only in patients with hypothalamic dysfunction.

Treatment with clomiphene is begun with a dose of 50 mg daily for 5 days beginning on the fifth day following spontaneous or induced bleeding (administration of a progestin, usually oral MPA (Provera) to induce bleeding in an amenorrheic woman, although not essential, offers a convenient starting point for the cycle). If ovulation occurs, as measured by BBT or urine tests for LH, without pregnancy, the same dose of clomiphene is repeated in the next treatment course. In the absence of ovulation, the daily dose should be increased to 100 mg given as a single daily dose for 5 days.

Most patients who respond do so during the first

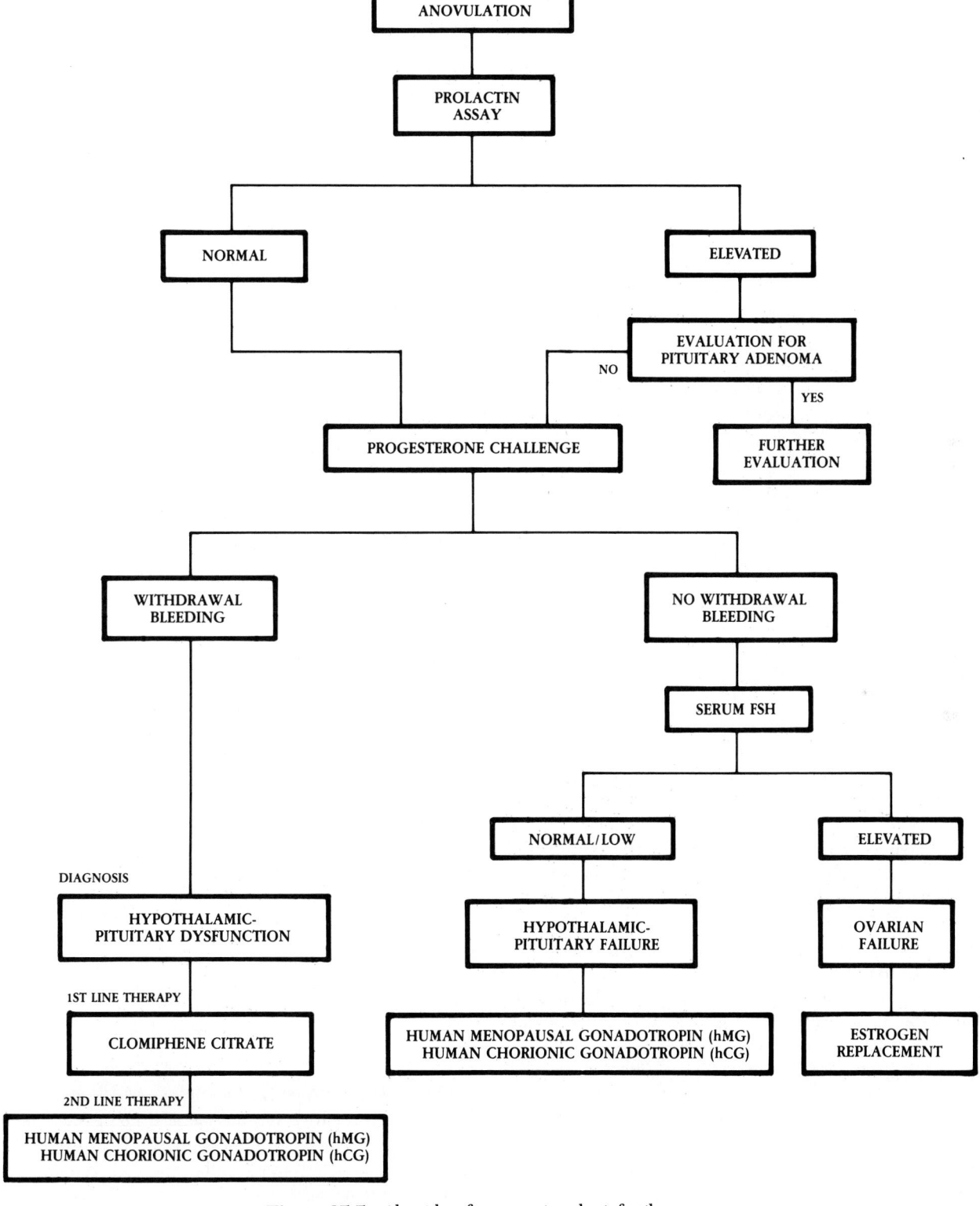

Figure 87.7 Algorithm for managing the infertile woman.

course of therapy. Three courses constitute an adequate therapeutic trial for achievement of a pregnancy. The failure to achieve a pregnancy may be due to anovulation or, on occasion, the antiestrogenic effect of clomiphene on cervical mucus. At the time of ovulation, cervical mucus becomes thin and watery under the influence of estrogen. The thinner the mucus, the more elastic. This elastic quality is known as spinnbarkheit, and the micelles of the mucus arrange in such a fashion that sperm migration is optimal. Clomiphene behaves as an antiestrogen on cervical mucus. Therefore, if clomiphene has been administered over a long period of time without pregnancy occurring, the end-organ effect of clomiphene may be seen as an inadequate cervical mucus, an inadequate function of the corpus luteum, or an inadequate response of the lining of the uterus. After 6 to 8 months of clomiphene treatment, reevaluation should be undertaken. In addition, infertility of the male partner should be reconsidered (68).

To obtain optimal results, clomiphene therapy should be carefully monitored by the following:

1. Urine tests for LH or BBT;
2. Pelvic examination each cycle to rule out ovarian enlargement and pregnancy;
3. Sperm cervical mucus penetration test to evaluate cervical mucus and sperm transport and survival;
4. Serum progesterone and/or endometrial biopsy to assess ovulation, if indicated.

Ovulation and Pregnancy Rates following Clomiphene Therapy

Ovulation rates range between 62 and 83%. Pregnancy rates range from 25 to 56%. It is important to counsel patients about side effects of clomiphene. The most common symptom, occurring in approximately 21% of patients, is ovarian enlargement with simultaneous growth of multiple follicles and abdominal pelvic discomfort from excessive GnRH, FSH, and LH secretion. Menopause-like symptoms of hot flushes occur in 11% of patients as an antiestrogenic effect. A variety of other minor and reversible side effects include nausea/vomiting, breast discomfort, visual symptoms, headache, heavy menses, mental depression, nervousness, insomnia, and weight gain. Many women complain that their cycles lengthen on clomiphene. Clomiphene administration mimics the normal cycle from day 1. If one counts the first day of clomiphene administration as day 1, then ovulation is expected about day 13 to 15 and menses, day 28. However, because clomiphene was begun day 5, the normal cycle of CC is actually 33 days long.

The frequency of multiple births with adequate patient selection and monitoring is 10% or less (67).

Hypothalamic-Pituitary Failure

When clomiphene alone is unsuccessful in inducing ovulation, it is often administered in combination with other agents. Human menopausal gonadotropin (hMG) in conjunction with hCG is used to stimulate ovulation in women who do not ovulate but have potentially functional ovaries. In males, hMG and hCG treatment can stimulate spermatogenesis in patients with gonadotropin deficiency. Both endocrine and gametogenic function can be restored by this treatment.

Gonadotropins isolated from human postmenopausal urine (hMG-menotropin-Pergonal) are supplied as lyophilized powder in vials containing 75 IU of FSH and 75 IU of LH. It is dissolved in normal saline before use and injected intramuscularly. The preparation has predominantly FSH-like activity and stimulates ovarian follicle development in women and spermatogenesis in men. In both sexes, it must be used with hCG (which has LH activity). hCG (Profasi-HP (Serono), A.P.L. (Ayerst), Antuitrin-S (Parke-Davis), and others) is used to trigger ovulation of the primed follicle, to maintain the corpus luteum in women, and to permit testosterone production from Leydig cells in men.

The dose of hMG and the duration of treatment cannot be decided in advance and must be adjusted individually. Sensitivity to gonadotropins varies widely among patients and even in the same individual from cycle to cycle. Therefore, the amount of hMG must be carefully monitored and adjusted in each cycle. Brown et al. (69) reported a ninefold range for FSH doses among 45 patients treated.

Although varying doses are reported in the literature, the following dose is recommended by the manufacturers:

1. *First treatment:* One ampule each day (75 IU FSH, 75 IU LH), administered intramuscularly, for 9 to 12 days, followed by hCG 10,000 U, 1 day after the last dose of hMG. The intramuscular injection of 10,000 U hCG results in an initial blood level 20 times higher than the maximal value of LH peak during spontaneous ovulation. The $t_{1/2B} = 23.9$ hr, enabling persistent levels for several days to induce ovulation and maintain the corpus luteum for 14 days.
2. *Second treatment:* If there is evidence of ovulation after the first treatment but no pregnancy, the dosing regimen is repeated at least two more times before increasing the dose. If there is no evidence of ovulation after the first treatment, the dose of hMG is increased to 150 IU FSH, 150 IU LH for 9 to 12 days, followed by 10,000 U of hCG 1 day after the last dose of hMG. 150 IU of FSH/LH has proven to be the most effective dose. If evidence of ovulation is present, but pregnancy does not ensue, the same dose is repeated for two more courses.

Since gonadotropin induction of ovulation is sometimes associated with serious medical complications, including overstimulation of the ovaries, it is vital that monitoring be conducted. In hMG therapy, estrogen levels are higher than in normal cycles because more than one follicle is stimulated, and each follicle secretes estrogen. The character of cervical mucus changes under the influence of estrogen. In the past, before the availability of laboratory support, clinicians tended to monitor gonadotropin therapy by physical signs: observation of the appearance and volume of cervical mucus, spinnbarkheit, ferning of cervical mucus, and vaginal cytology. Cervical mucus examination has been carefully evaluated by combining various measurements into a composite "cervical score." Although effective to a point, further increases in plasma estrogen concentration do not cause a proportional increase in cervical mucus secretion. The clinician may, therefore, be misled and either give hCG prematurely or delay hCG and continue hMG to the point of hyperstimulation of the ovary. For these reasons, the combination of pelvic examinations with the above clinical indices, although important, is insufficient if used alone. In combination with serum or urinary estradiol levels and ultrasonography, these indices provide an ideal means for monitoring the growth and development of follicles, timing the hCG administration, and minimizing the risk of hyperstimulation.

Because of the expense of monitoring, determination of estrogen levels may be postponed until the cervical score reaches 8 or more, provided that abnormal cervical factors have been excluded previously. Treatment is continued with hMG until the effective daily dose that causes a significant and steady estrogen rise is achieved. If total urinary estrogen excretion is less than 100 μg in 24 hr, or the estradiol excretion less than 50 μg in 24 hr prior to hCG administration, the hyperstimulation syndrome is less likely to occur. Serum estradiol levels in the range of 2936 to 5500 pmol/liter (800 to 1500 pg/ml) usually indicate an ovulatory surge. Sonographic visualization can discriminate between single and multiple follicular growth. These measurements may aid in the interpretation of estrogen levels. Evidence is accumulating that follicles with diameters greater than 16 mm will be most likely to ovulate when hCG is administered. Therefore, ultrasonic visualization is important to determine these sizes. If numerous large follicles are observed on ultrasound, hCG can be withheld to reduce the risk of multiple births.

In a group of 723 patients with hypothalamic-pituitary dysfunction who failed to ovulate or conceive on clomiphene therapy, hMG treatment led to a pregnancy rate of 21.4% (70). Although the frequencies of ovulation and pregnancy are similar to those reported for clomiphene, the frequency of multiple births is 20%, and the estimate of early spontaneous abortion is 25% (67).

There is no evidence of teratogenicity with hMG/hCG. Side effects include hyperstimulation syndrome (bloating, abdominal pain, ovarian enlargement, ascites from excessive fluid escaping from multiple rupturing follicles, hypovolemia, and possible shock). In addition, rupturing of an ovarian cyst (hemoperitoneum), fever, and arterial thrombosis (due to elevated estradiol levels) may occur.

GnRH

A promising new avenue for treatment of primary hypothalamic amenorrhea and infertility are GnRH analogs. Normal release of GnRH from the hypothalamus is pulsatile. When given to induce ovulation, administration of the drug must also be pulsatile; otherwise GnRH would initially stimulate release of gonadotropins, but with continued use, would become inhibitory (see endometriosis and prostate cancer treatment). Normal pituitary and ovarian function are required for the drug to act. Gonadorelin acetate (Lutrepulse) is a synthetic decapeptide identical in amino acid sequence to GnRH approved for this use. Gonadrelin is rapidly broken down to inactive peptide fragments that are excreted in the urine ($t_{1/2a}$ = 10 min, $t_{1/2b}$ = 10 to 40 min).

Pulses of gonadorelin are injected intravenously through a catheter, usually into a forearm vein, using a reservoir and pump, available from the manufacturer, which can be worn under clothing. Initial dose is 5 μg every 90 min for 21 days or until ovulation occurs. If pregnancy occurs, the drug may be continued for up to 2 additional weeks to maintain the corpus luteum. The cannula and IV site should be changed every 48 hr. Multiple follicular stimulation should be monitored by ultrasound. If ovulation does not occur after 3 cycles of treatment, doses can be increased to a maximum of 30 μg.

Adverse effects include infection and inflammation of the infusion site. Hyperstimulation with sudden ovarian enlargement is unlikely because pulsatile administration preserves the ovarian-pituitary feedback mechanism. Multiple pregnancies have occurred in 12% of women who became pregnant with gonadorelin. Cutaneous hypersensitivity and anaphylaxis have occurred.

In anovulatory women, with abnormal or absent GnRH secretion, gonadorelin can induce ovulation. The manufacturer reports that among 44 women with primary hypothalamic amenorrhea treated with pulsatile IV doses of the drug, 41 ovulated and 24 (62%) of 39 patients desiring pregnancy became pregnant.

In vitro Fertilization

The technologies for treatment of infertility with in vitro fertilization (IVF) are only 10 to 15 years old. Early success was obtained when one oocyte was obtained at the time of ovum aspiration. However, various methods of ovarian hyperstimulation have been used, allowing more than one embryo to be transferred at a time to the uterus.

The combination of clomiphene citrate and hMG (menotropins) was used by most workers in IVF, however some groups had considerable success using hMG alone (71). Subsequently pure follicle-stimulating hormone (FSH) was used (Metrodin) instead of hMG, but the results did not seem to be further improved.

All these methods of hyperstimulation are complicated

by premature luteinization of the follicle or the occurrence of an endogenous LH surge in up to 20% of patients treated. Patients who receive either pure FSH or hMG require luteal-phase support. Patients (except those with an endogenous LH surge) also may require hCG at the time of follicle maturity.

More recently, the GnRH agonists have been used to produce pituitary suppression and thus prevent the onset of the endogenous LH surge (72). The GnRH agonist is given immediately prior to the initial injection of hMG. An increase in gonadotropin occurs, and most groups have reported more oocytes being obtained. However, significant ovarian hyperstimulation has been noted in some patients.

CONCLUSION

The therapeutic management of management of common gynecologic problems, contraception, infertility, endometriosis, and toxic shock syndrome requires an understanding of the female reproductive system with its delicate balance of hormonal-axis regulation and feedback control. Knowledge of the pharmacologic effects of the different components of oral contraceptives and fertility agents allow us to effectively tailor specific products for selected patients as well as identify patients in whom such therapy is contraindicated.

REFERENCES

1. Dickey RP: Managing Contraceptive Pill Patients, ed. 4. Durant, OK: Creative Infomatics Inc., 1986.
2. Hatcher RA, Guest F, Stewart GK, Stewart FS, et al.: Contraceptive Technology, 1988–89, ed. 14. New York: Irvington Publishers, 1988.
3. Realini JP, Goldzieher JW: Oral contraceptives and cardiovascular disease: a critique of the epidemiologic studies. Am J Obstet Gynecol 152:729–798, 1985.
4. Crane MG, Harris JJ, Winston W III: Hypertension, oral contraceptive agents and conjugated estrogens. Ann Intern Med 74:13, 1971.
5. Goodlin RC, Waechter V: Oral contraceptives and blood pressure. Lancet 1:1262, 1969.
6. Royal College of General Practitioners' Oral Contraception Study: Oral Contraceptives and Health. New York: Pitman & Sons, 1974.
7. Ramcharan S, Pellegran FA, Hoag E, The occurrence and cause of hypertensive disease in users and non-users of oral contraceptive drugs. In Fregley MJ, Fregley MS (eds): Oral Contraceptives and High Blood Pressure. Gainesville, FL, Dolphin Press, 1974, p 1.
8. Fisch IR, Frank J: Oral contraceptives and blood pressure. JAMA 237:2499, 1977.
9. Kunin CM, McCormack RC, Abernathy JR: Oral contraceptives and blood pressure. Arch Intern Med 123:362, 1969.
10. Tsai CC, Williamson HO, Kirkland BH, et al.: Low-dose oral contraception and blood pressure in women with a past history of elevated blood pressure. Am J Obstet Gynecol 151:28–32, 1985.
11. Wilson ESB, Cruickshank J, McMaster M, Weir RJ: A prospective controlled study of the effect on blood pressure of contraceptive preparations containing different types and dosages of progestogen. Br J Obstet Gynecol 91:1254–1260, 1984.
12. Saruta T, Saade GA, Kaplan NM: A possible mechanism for hypertension induced by oral contraceptives. Arch Intern Med 126:621, 1970.
13. Laragh JH, Sealey JE, Ledingham JG, et al.: Oral contraceptives: renin, aldosterone, and high blood pressure. JAMA 201:918, 1967.
14. Anon: Effect on hypertension and benign breast disease of progestogen component in combined oral contraceptives: Royal College of General Practitioners' Oral Contraception Study. Lancet 1:624, 1977.
15. Hazzard WR, Spiger MJ, Bagdale JD, et al.: Studies on the mechanism of increased plasma triglyceride levels induced by oral contraceptives. N Engl J Med 280:471–474, 1969.
16. Davidoff F, Tishler S, Rosoff C: Marked hyperlipidemia and pancreatitis associated with oral contraceptive therapy. N Engl J Med 289:552, 1973.
17. Donde UM, Virkar K: The effect of combination and low-dose progestogen oral contraceptives on serum lipids. Fertil Steril 26:62–67, 1975.
18. Wahl P, Walden C, Knopp R, et al.: Effect of estrogen/progestin potency on lipid/lipoprotein cholesterol. N Engl J Med 308:862–867, 1983.
19. Bradley DB, Wingerd J, Petti DB, et al.: Serum high-density lipoprotein cholesterol in women using oral contraceptive estrogens and progestins. N Engl J Med 299:17, 1978.
20. Spellacy W: Carbohydrate metabolism during treatment with progestogen and low-dose oral contraceptives. Am J Obstet Gynecol 142:732–734, 1982.
21. Duffy TJ, Ray R: Oral contraceptive use: prospective follow-up of women with suspected glucose intolerance. Contraception 3:197–208, 1984.
22. Mann JI, Doll R, Thorogood M, et al.: Risk factors for myocardial infarction in young women. Br J Prev Soc Med 30:94, 1976.
23. Collaborative Group for the Study of Stroke in Young Women: Oral contraceptives and stroke in young women: associated risk factors. JAMA 231:718, 1975.
24. Mishell DR: Contraception. N Engl J Med 320:777–787, 1989.
25. Porter JB, Hunter JR, Jick H, Stergachis A: Oral contraceptives and nonfatal vascular disease—recent experience. Obstet Gynecol 59:299–302, 1982.
26. Porter JB, Hunter JR, Jick H, Stergachis A: Oral contraceptives and nonfatal vascular disease. Obstet Gynecol 66:1–4, 1985.
27. Porter JB, Jick H, Walker AM: Mortality among oral contraceptive users. Obstet Gynecol 70:29–32, 1987.
28. Mant D, Villard-Mackintosh L, Vessey MP, Yeates D: Myocardial infarction and angina pectoris in young women. J Epidemiol Community Health 41:215–219, 1987.
29. Layde PM, Ory HW, Schlesselman JJ: The risk of myocardial infarction in former users of oral contraceptives. Fam Plann Perspect 14:78–80, 1982.
30. Stampfer MJ, Willett WC, Colditz GA, Speizer FE, Hennekens CH: A prospective study of past use of oral contraceptive agents and risk of cardiovascular disease. N Engl J Med 319:1313–1317, 1988.
31. Anon: Oral contraceptives and venous thromboembolic disease, surgically confirmed gallbladder disease, and breast tumors: report from the Boston Collaborative Drug Surveillance Programe. Lancet 1:1399, 1973.
32. Anon: Oral contraceptives, venous thrombosis, and varicose veins: Royal College of General Practitioners' Oral Contraceptive Study. J R Coll Gen Pract 28:393, 1978.
33. Vessey MP, McPherson K, Yeates D: Mortality in oral contraceptive users. Lancet 1:549, 1981.
34. Irey NS, Manion WC, Taylor HB: Vascular lesions in women taking oral contraceptives. Arch Pathol 89:1, 1970.
35. Caspery EA, Peberdy M: Oral contraception and blood platelet adhesiveness. Lancet 1:1142, 1965.

36. Howie PW, Mallinson AC, Prentice CRM, et al.: Effect of combined estrogen-progestogen oral contraceptives on antiplasmin and antithrombolic activity. Lancet 2:1329, 1970.

37. Peterson C, Kelly R, Minard B, et al.: Antithrombin III: comparison of functional and immunologic assay. Am J Clin Pathol 69:500, 1978.

38. Conard J, Samama M, Salomon Y: Antithrombin III and the oestrogen content of combined oestrogen-progestagen contraceptives. Lancet 2:1148, 1972.

39. Bonnar J, Sabra A, Comparative data on the effects of low-dose oral contraceptives on coagulation. In Elstein M (ed): Update on Triphasic Oral Contraception. Amsterdam, Excerpta Medica 1983, pp 9–19.

40. Pike MC, Henderson BE, Krarlo MD, et al.: Breast cancer in young women and use of oral contraceptives: possible modifying effect of formulation and age at use. Lancet 2:926–929, 1983.

41. Centers for Disease Control Cancer and Steroid Hormone Study: Long term oral contraceptive use and the risk of breast cancer. JAMA 249:1591–1595, 1983.

42. Schlesselman JJ: Cancer of the breast and reproductive tract in relation to use of oral contraceptives. Contraception 40:1–38, 1989.

43. Khoo SK: Cancer risks and the contraceptive pill. What is the evidence after nearly 25 years of use? Med J Aust 144:185–190, 1986.

44. Strom BL, Tamragouri RN, Morse ML, et al.: Oral contraceptives and other risk factors for gall bladder disease. Clin Pharmacol Ther 39:335–341, 1986.

45. Adams PW, Wynn V, Rose DP, et al.: Effect of pyridoxine hydrochloride (vitamin B-6) upon depression associated with oral contraception. Lancet 1:897, 1973.

46. WHO Special Programme of Research, Development and Research Training in Human Reproduction. Task Force on Oral Contraceptives: Effects of hormonal contraceptives on milk volume and infant growth. Contraception 30:505–522, 1984.

47. D'Arcy PF: Drug interactions with oral contraceptives. Drug Intell Clin Pharm 20:353–362, 1986.

58. Anon: Drugs, oral contraceptives and pregnancy (editorial). N Z Med J 92:200, 1980.

49. Smith MB: A quantitative estimate of ocular iatrogenic disease in humans. J Am Optom Assoc 45:751, 1974.

50. Wood JR: Ocular complications of oral contraceptives. Ophthalmic Semin 2:371, 1977.

51. Chapel TA, Burns RE: Oral contraceptives and exacerbation of lupus erythematosus. Am J Obstet Gynecol 110:366, 1971.

52. Magendotz HB: Oral contraceptives. Collected Letter of the International Correspondence Society of Obstetricians and Gynecologists 22:170, 1981.

53. Smith MA, Youngkin EQ: Current perspectives on combination oral contraceptives. Clin Pharm 3:485–522, 1984.

54. Ostergard DR: DES-related vaginal lesions. Clin Obstet Gynecol 24:379, 1981.

55. Yuzpe AA, Smith RP, Rademaker AW: A multi-center clinical investigation employing ethinyl estradiol combined with D,L-norgestrol as a post-coital contraceptive agent. Fertil Steril 37:508, 1982.

56. Corson SL: Efficacy and clinical profile of a new oral contraceptive containing norgesimate. U.S. Clinical Trials. Acta Obstet Gynecol Scand Suppl 152:25–31, 1990.

57. Louik C, Mitchell AA, Werle MM, Hanson JW, Shaprio S: Maternal exposure to spermicides in relation to certain birth defects. N Engl J Med 317:474–478, 1987.

58. Strobino B, Kline J, Lai A, Stein Z, Sussec M, Warburton D: Vaginal spermicides and spontaneous abortion of known karyotype. Am J Epidemiol 123:431–443, 1986.

59. Todd J, Fishaut M, Kapral F, et al.: Toxic-shock syndrome associated with phage-group I staphylococci. Lancet 2:1116, 1978.

60. Friedrich EG: Tampon effects on vaginal health. Clin Obstet Gynecol 24:395, 1981.

61. Schreiner WE: Labhart's Textbook of Endocrinology. Berlin: Springer-Verlag, 1974, p 511.

62. Corson SL: Conquering Infertility. Norwalk, CT: Appleton-Century-Crofts, 1982, p 3.

63. Abrams RM, Rayston JP: Some properties of rectum and vagina as sites for basal body temperature measurements. Fertil Steril 35:313–316, 1981.

64. Rayston JP, Abrams RM, Higgins MP, et al.: The adjustment of basal body temperature measurements to allow for time of waking. Br J Obstet Gynecol 87:1123–1127, 1980.

65. Olive DL, Hammond CB: Evaluation of the anovulatory patient. Postgrad Med 77:205–216, 1985.

66. Adashi EY: Clomiphene citrate: mechanism(s) and site(s) of action—a hypothesis revisited. Fertil Steril 42:331–334, 1984.

67. Rahwan RG: Antiabortifacient and fertility-inducing drugs. Am J Pharm Educ 49:86–94, 1985.

68. Thorneycroft IH: Current status of ovulation induction with clomiphene citrate. Fertil Steril 41:806–808, 1984.

69. Brown JB, Evans JH, Adey FD, et al.: Factors involved in the induction of fertile ovulations with human gonadotropins. J Obstet Gynaecol Br Commonw 76:289, 1969.

70. Lunenfeld B, Romen Y, Blankenship J: Current Problems in Obstetrics and Gynecology: Ovulation Induction. Chicago: Year Book, 1982, vol 5, p 55.

71. Johnston WIH, Lopata A, Pepperell RJ, The use of in vitro fertilization in the infertile couple. In Pepperell RJ, Hudson B, Wood C, (eds): The Infertile Couple, ed. 2. Edinburgh, Churchill Livingston, 263–312, 1987.

72. MacLachlan V, Besanko M, O'Shea F: A controlled study of luteinizing hormone-releasing hormone agonist (Buserelin) for the induction of folliculogenesis before in vitro fertilization. N Engl J Med 320:1233–1237, 1989.

CHAPTER 88

DRUGS IN PREGNANCY AND LACTATION

KELLIE D. MCQUEEN, Pharm.D.

A pregnant woman may take up to 11 different medications during her pregnancy (1, 2). Symptoms commonly treated include pain, nausea and vomiting, gastrointestinal upset, edema, and the common cold. Conditions such as diabetes mellitus, infections, or hypertension may also require treatment. It is estimated that 35 to 100% of pregnant women have taken some type of drug during pregnancy (3–5). Many of these drugs are taken without medical supervision and may be taken immediately after conception, before the woman knows she is pregnant.

The administration of drugs to a pregnant female generates many concerns for the clinician and patient. Most drugs ingested by the gravida reach the fetus. The risk of causing congenital defects must, therefore, be weighed against the benefit of treating the woman. Out of nearly 1000 drugs that have been evaluated for teratogenic potential, only around 30 are proven teratogens. Examples of these are listed in Table 88.1. A teratogen is an agent that is present during critical periods of development and is able to produce a congenital defect. The term congenital defect refers to major and minor malformations, either in structures or function, which deviate from the norm. Cleft palate, behavioral variations, and latent defects such as vaginal carcinoma in offspring of women treated with diethylstibesterol while pregnant provide examples. It is difficult to prove without doubt the teratogenicity of most drugs. The reason behind this becomes evident in the process of evaluating the literature.

DOCUMENTING TERATOGENICITY/LITERATURE EVALUATION

Since the tragedy of the defects caused by thalidomide, the United States Food and Drug Administration (FDA) has required since the early 1960s, that before becoming commercially available, all medications must be tested for teratogenicity on animals. This can provide some knowledge of the teratogenic risk of drugs in humans. If defects have been demonstrated in several animal species, then a causal association should at least be made to the same defect when demonstrated in humans. However, there are several limitations to animal studies. First of all, differences exist in the teratogenicity of a drug between species. For example, thalidomide causes malformations in rabbits and humans, but not in rodents. The drug was not known to be teratogenic in humans until a number of infants were born with important defects and the cause was traced back

to in utero thalidomide exposure. Other drugs, such as steroids, have been shown to be teratogenic in animals, but at therapeutic doses, have not been shown to produce important malformations in humans. Secondly, the pharmacokinetic properties of a drug vary between species and among the same species. Rates of absorption, biotransformation, maternal elimination, and the extent of placental transfer vary and may produce inconsistent results. Also, animals may react differently to environmental factors than humans, which may also impact on the susceptibility to a teratogen. Clearly, it is very difficult to extrapolate animal data to humans.

Unfortunately, most human data are anecdotal, uncontrolled, and considerably flawed. Few epidemiologic studies have been done. The Collaborative Perinatal Project is best known and was performed from 1959 to 1965. It collected data on a cohort of 50,282 mother-child pairs to investigate the teratogenic role of drugs. Twelve centers in the United States participated. The rates of various birth defects in infants of drug-exposed women were compared to those of infants in non-drug-exposed women. The published results can serve as a useful reference for many individual cases (6). Even among well-controlled studies, collecting teratologic information is complicated, and the data must be carefully evaluated. Many studies and reports lack uniform definitions of malformations and diagnostic criteria. Investigator objectivity is difficult to ensure in epidemiologic studies, but it must be maintained. Similar to other medical illnesses, the incidence of many drug-induced birth defects may vary depending upon demographic data. Results can be biased if a study population is significantly unbalanced in regards to its race, geographic location, genetic makeup, or diet. Similarly, bias may arise if the observer is aware of confounding elements in the study. Diseases or viruses, for example, may directly or indirectly be responsible for defects. If these influences are not noted by the investigator, false inferences could be made. Such biases can be controlled by altering the study design or by using certain forms of statistical analysis. Statistics play an additional role in limiting biases by determining the probability that the outcome was due to chance. Furthermore, many studies exclude the reporting of certain types of malformations (e.g., stillbirths or spontaneous abortions). Most reporting concentrates on major anatomic abnormalities detected at birth. Minor abnormalities are often omitted, and follow-up studies to detect

Table 88.1.
Drugs Known or Suspected to Be Teratogenic in Humans[a]

Androgenic hormones
Busulfan
Coumarin derivatives
Cyclophosphamide
Diethylstilbestrol
Etretinate
Isotretinoin
Lithium
Methimazole
Penicillamine
Phenytoin
Trimethadione
Tetracyclines (particularly during weeks 24–26)
Thalidomide
Valproic acid

[a] Adapted from Anon, Congenital malformations and inherited disorders. In Cunningham FG, MacDonald PC, Gant NF (eds): William's Obstetrics. Norwalk, CT, Appleton & Lange, 1989, p 561.

Table 88.2.
Key Principles of Teratogens[a]

1. The susceptibility of an embryo to a teratogen depends upon the developmental stage at which the agent is applied.
2. Each teratogen acts on a particular aspect of cellular metabolism. Different teratogenic agents, therefore, tend to produce different effects, although acting at the same period of embryonic development and on the same system.
3. The genotype influences to a degree the reaction to a teratogen.
4. An agent capable of causing malformations also usually causes an increase in embryonic mortality.
5. A teratogen need not be deleterious to the maternal organism.

[a] Adapted from Wilson JG: Experimental studies on congenital malformations. J Chron Dis 10:111–114, 1959.

abnormalities in later life are rare. Also, maternal reporting of drugs taken during pregnancy is generally not accurate. Drugs actually taken may not be accounted for by the mother, nor the correct dose or timing of ingestion (4). Mothers of infants with birth defects tend to have more accurate reporting than those of normal infants (7).

The consequence of these limitations is that information specific to the case at hand is not always available. The certainty with which one can predict the precise teratogenic potential of a drug in any one patient is limited. Yet, several factors help determine the sensitivity to teratogenesis. Key factors described previously by Wilson and outlined in Table 88.2 (8). Most important is the time during fetal development in which the conceptus was exposed to the agent. Knowing the developmental stage when insult was applied can aid in predicting the possible

defect. From fertilization to implantation of the ovum, days 0 to 14, most dangerous agents either prevent implantation of the conceptus or have no harmful effect at all. The most sensitive period is from implantation to the end of organogenesis. Exposure to agents in this period, days 18 through 60, may damage developing organs. A classic example is thalidomide, which produces distinct deficits in limbs with exposure 21 to 40 days after conception. During the fetal period, the time after 8 weeks to birth, morphologic changes may occur as the developmental and growth phases continue. This includes maturation of the brain. When a type of defect can occur anytime during pregnancy (e.g., pyloric stenosis or various genital defects), an investigation into drug exposures throughout gestation must be made. Another example is the behavioral abnormalities that can result from alcohol ingested during pregnancy.

Other factors that influence the outcome and association of possible insult from drugs in utero include: the nature of the agent and the mechanism by which it causes the defect, the maternal and the fetal metabolism of the drug, the dose, duration of exposure, species, and genetic makeup. The extent to which the drug crosses the placenta is also a factor. Most drugs cross the placenta, primarily by simple diffusion, although other processes such as active transport play a role. Drugs with molecular weights below 600, high lipid solubility, low protein binding, and those that are nonionized readily cross the placenta (3, 9–11). When determining the risk of exposure to the fetus, in addition to the few available studies and reports and the pharmacokinetic and pharmacodynamic properties of the drug, the clinician may also consider other sources of information.

There are two systems that rate the teratogenic risk of drugs. TERIS is an computer data-base resource. It evaluates the chance of harm that could occur to the fetus if the mother takes a medication. It is based on published studies, standard teratology references, and clinical experience. The most commonly used drugs in the outpatient setting are evaluated. Ratings for agents under conventional therapeutic settings are described by teratologists as "none," "minimal," "small," "moderate," "high," and "undetermined." The system relies primarily on human data and is designed to assess risk; it is not designed to provide therapeutic guidance (12).

In 1979, the FDA devised a system that determines the teratogenic risk of drugs by considering the quality data from animal and human studies (13). In contrast to TERIS, the FDA system also considers the benefits of therapy to the patient and any perinatal risks. Thus, this system may provide some therapeutic guidance for the clinician. It does not denote a rating for all drugs, however. A description of the FDA risk factors is presented in Table 88.3. In determining whether the risk of therapy exceeds

Table 88.3.
FDA Ratings

A: Controlled studies show no risk. Adequate, well-controlled studies in pregnant women have failed to demonstrate risk to the fetus.

B: No evidence of risk in humans. Either animal findings show risk, but human findings do not; or, if no adequate human studies have been done, animal findings are negative.

C: Risk cannot be ruled out. Human studies are lacking, and animal studies are either positive for fetal risk, or lacking as well. However, potential benefits may justify the potential risk.

D: Positive evidence of risk. Investigational or postmarketing data show risk to the fetus. Nevertheless, potential benefits may outweigh the potential risk.

X: Contraindicated in pregnancy. Studies in animals or human, or investigational or postmarketing reports have shown fetal risk that clearly outweighs any possible benefit to the patient.

the benefit, the FDA has defined five categories: A, B, C, D, or X. Although the A category is considered the safest, some drugs with A, B, C, or even D ratings are commonly used in pregnant women. β-Blockers are in the C category, while multivitamins are in the A classification. Category D is generally reserved for drugs that have no safer alternatives. Phenytoin is rated D. Only category X denotes that the drug is contraindicated and that there is no reason to risk using the drug in pregnancy. Isotretinoin or conjugated estrogens are examples of this group. Any rating system should be used in conjunction with a complete history and physical examination of the patient.

Taking any medication while pregnant involves some degree of risk. An estimation should be made of whether the risk of teratogenesis from drug exposure exceeds the 3 to 6% baseline malformation rate. If it does not, then although birth defects may still occur, there is no known increased risk with drug therapy. This concept is useful in patient counseling.

ETIOLOGY/INCIDENCE

Approximately 3% of infants are born with major congenital malformations. This baseline incidence rate does not include minor malformations or defects that are manifested in later life, such as anomalies of internal organs or behavioral or growth deficiencies. These abnormalities have been thought to double the prevalence of birth defects to 6%. Etiologies of malformations may be classified into three main categories: (*a*) unknown factors, (*b*) genetic origin, and (*c*) environmental influences (11, 14). Most defects (65%) are due to unknown factors. These include polygenic or multifactorial causes or spontaneous errors of development. Genetic influences include chromosomal abnormalities, mutant genes, and autosomal genetic diseases. These account for up to 20% of all congenital malformations. Environmental factors can include diabetes mellitus, poor nutritional status, maternal infec-

tions with rubella or cytomegalovirus, toxoplasmosis, syphilis, or other infections. These factors account for nearly 10% of all malformations (11, 14, 15). Chemicals, drugs, and drug metabolites are estimated to account for roughly 3% of all defects. This 3% incidence rate may be greater, depending upon the methods used to collect and interpret data.

The pathogenesis of birth defects may be divided into four different categories: deformation, disruption, dysplasia, and malformation. Abnormalities may be further classified into five subcategories, depending upon their relationship to each other: single-system defects, complexes, syndromes, associations, or sequences. The discussion of these mechanisms is beyond the scope of this chapter. The reader is referred to a review by Aase (16). A group of abnormalities that develop in a consistent pattern is called a syndrome. Common syndromes due to drug exposure are discussed briefly.

SYNDROMES

The fetal alcohol syndrome (FAS) is estimated to occur an average of three live births per 1000 (17). It is characterized by defects of the central nervous system, craniofacial abnormalities, and growth and mental deficiencies. Most affected infants are born with hypotonia, poor coordination, decreased adipose tissue, low birth weight, shorter length, a myoplastic maxilla, and shortened and upturned nose. Many demonstrate hyperactivity in childhood. Mental retardation is the most significant consequence (11, 18, 19). Infants may experience alcohol withdrawal symptoms such as irritability, tremors, abdominal distention, or opisthotonos. Withdrawal may occur with or without the physical disfigurements of FAS (20, 21). These defects vary in extent and severity. Nearly 20 to 30% of alcoholic women have infants with complete FAS, and 50 to 70% have infants with partial expression of the syndrome (15).

FAS is caused by ethanol or its metabolites. Investigation into the effects of acetaldehyde has been conducted but the exact relationship between this by-product of ethanol and FAS is yet unclear. Additional maternal factors that may contribute to expression of the syndrome include poor nutrition, smoking, drug abuse, inadequate prenatal care, and low socioeconomic status. The effects are dose-related, but the amount of ethanol that may be ingested without causing abnormalities is unknown. Two drinks per day (30 ml of absolute alcohol) has been related to lower birth weights. Moderate consumption (more than 30 ml of absolute alcohol) has been associated with decreased birth weight, spontaneous abortion, and impaired motor and mental development. As many as six hard drinks (around 75 to 90 ml of absolute alcohol) per day carries a major risk for severe complications and possibly stillbirth. The complete FAS is associated with alcoholic women who consume more than four drinks (60 ml of absolute alcohol) per day (14, 22). More research is needed to clearly understand the effects of moderate- or low-level alcohol consumption. Pregnant women should be informed of the dangers of alcohol and realize that a safe level of consumption is not known. Neither is it clear which phase of development is most susceptible to damage; women should thus avoid alcohol when trying to conceive. Women should also avoid antitussive medications with alcohol, if possible. Over-the-counter products can contain as much as 25% alcohol. Cough medications with no alcohol are available and are preferred.

The fetal warfarin syndrome is another recognizable syndrome. It is estimated to occur in 10 to 25% of infants exposed to coumarin derivatives in the first trimester, particularly around the sixth to ninth gestational week. The syndrome is characterized primarily by nasal hypoplasia and stippling of uncalcified epiphyses. Limb defects, low birth weight, and severe upper airway obstruction may also occur. In the second and third trimester, exposure to coumadin is likely to produce central nervous system defects and hemorrhage (11, 14, 18, 23, 24).

The fetal hydantoin syndrome is associated with anticonvulsant therapy. Although generally related to phenytoin, FHS is not specific for any one anticonvulsant and may be seen with phenytoin, phenobarbital, carbamazepine, or a combination of these agents (25). Defects may include mental retardation, limb and craniofacial abnormalities such as cleft lip and/or cleft palate, and physical growth defects. Short neck, umbilical or inguinal hernia, strabismus, or hirsutism rarely occur (18, 26). There is a 5 to 10% risk for a fetus exposed to phenytoin to develop most of these abnormalities; while a one-in-three risk exists for only partial expression of the syndrome (18, 27). Some investigators have cited up to a 15% incidence of abnormalities similar to FHS in untreated epileptic women (28). Hence, the exact etiology of FHS is unknown. While epilepsy itself may be the cause, folic acid deficiency, maternal toxicity from the drug, or fetal genotype are other possible mechanisms. Causation may also be related to fetal exposure to the drug or its metabolites. Phenytoin and carbamazepine are oxidized in the liver by the enzyme epoxide hydrolase, resulting in epoxide metabolites. These metabolites have a high affinity for binding to fetal proteins, which may result in developmental defects (27, 29, 30). Recently, investigators have measured epoxide hydrolase activity of amniocytes to predict which infants might be at risk for FHS (27).

CAFFEINE/SMOKING

Certain substances frequently used in daily life are not perceived as drugs or deterrents to health by many people. Two of the most commonly used substances are caffeine and cigarettes. If used in pregnancy, they may produce adverse fetal effects. The pregnant women should be informed of possible complications that may result from smoking or ingesting caffeine.

Caffeine

Caffeine is found in coffee, cola drinks, tea, cocoa, analgesics, and some other nonprescription products such as cold remedies, diet aids, and stimulants. The caffeine content varies greatly in these products. On average, 5 ounces of coffee can have 30 to 180 mg of caffeine; decaffeinated coffee (6 ounces), 3 to 5 mg; 12 ounces of cola drinks, 36 to 90 mg; 1 ounce baking chocolate, 26 mg; and 1 ounce milk chocolate, 6 mg of caffeine. Stimulant products can have 100 to 200 mg of caffeine, while over-the-counter appetite suppressants contain up to 120 mg.

An estimated 80% of women are exposed to caffeine during the first trimester. This potent CNS stimulant crosses the placenta. The teratogenicity associated with caffeine in animals is dose-related. Caffeine has not been shown to be a major teratogen in humans, however (9). Some investigators have shown no association between caffeine consumption and the occurrence of congenital malformation, others have demonstrated complications in pregnancy. These latter studies have shown that over 150 mg/day of caffeine (moderate to heavy intake) increased the risk of late second and third trimester spontaneous abortions. Others have shown that six to eight cups/day of brewed coffee increased the incidence of low-birth-weight infants, miscarriages, prematurity, and stillbirths. These findings may be influenced by confounding variables. Heavy caffeine users also tend to smoke, have a high alcohol intake, and are of low socioeconomic status. Difficulty in becoming pregnant may be related to recent caffeine intake. The relative risk increases as the number of beverages over three cups of brewed coffee per day increases. The association of low-to-moderate caffeine intake and congenital defects or complications in pregnancy are yet to be proven. Reduced birth weight, spontaneous abortions, and difficulty in becoming pregnant may be associated with high caffeine intake (over 100 to 150 mg per day) (31–33). Further research is needed to clarify other effects of high doses of caffeine. While moderate intake is probably safe, women should use caffeine sparingly, if at all, while pregnant.

Smoking

Maternal smoking is one of the few known preventable causes of perinatal morbidity and mortality. Women of childbearing age are the fastest growing population of smokers in the country today. The adverse effects of smoking on the fetus have been well documented. Fetal, neonatal, and infant mortality is increased, birth weight and length decreased, gestation shortened, and frequency of fetal breathing movements is reduced. Complications of pregnancy also may occur such as: abruptio placentae, premature rupture of membranes, amnionitis, and placenta previa. Changes in uterine and placental oxygenation or blood flow may be the cause of infant death, prematurity, or spontaneous abortions. Complications in infancy and childhood may present as deficits in long-term physical growth or intellectual and behavioral performance (19, 20, 34, 35). The effect on the placenta, uterus, fetus, and infant are dose-related. Light smoking (less than one pack per day) was found to increase fetal death rate by 20% and heavy smoking (one or more packs per day) to increase the risk by 35% (20). Similarly, the more cigarettes smoked per day, the lower the birth weight. Almost half of low-birth-weight infants are born to pregnant women who smoke (35). According to the Surgeon General's 1990 Report on smoking cessation, women who quit smoking within the first 3 to 4 months of pregnancy or before pregnancy reduce their risk of having a low-birth-weight baby to that of women who never smoked. Smoking cessation during pregnancy may also decrease the incidence of perinatal deaths and preterm deliveries. Birth weight may not be improved if a woman simply cuts down on the number of cigarettes smoked while pregnant (36). Pregnant women who smoke should be informed of the adverse health effects not only to themselves but also their fetus. A primary target population for this education is women who have not completed high school. They are most likely to continue smoking while pregnant. All women should be encouraged to quit smoking while pregnant, and smoking cessation programs designed for pregnant women may be beneficial.

SPECIFIC CONDITIONS

Treating a pregnant woman requires consideration of the potential risks and benefits. One of the first questions to ask is whether the mother's condition demands drug therapy. Many times, nonpharmacologic approaches can be effective. Therapy is usually appropriate if the untreated maternal condition will increase fetal morbidity or mortality. However, the risk of adverse effects occurring from drug exposure in utero must be evaluated. Many times these risks are unknown.

Nausea and Vomiting

Nausea and vomiting are common during pregnancy, occurring in up to 80% of patients, and may be mild to severe (37). Nausea and vomiting in pregnancy (NVP) is distinguished from hyperemesis gravidarum, the term used to identify severe nausea and vomiting. Hyperemesis gravidarum consists of intractable vomiting leading to electrolyte imbalance, maternal weight loss, altered nutritional status, and at times, end-organ or neurologic damage. Hy-

peremesis gravidarum occurs in about one case per 1000 births and requires hospitalization (37).

Symptoms of NVP are usually experienced during the first 14 to 16 weeks of pregnancy. Around 8% of women in one study reported suffering before the first missed menstrual period (38). Nausea and vomiting may last throughout the second trimester. "Morning sickness" is experienced in nearly 80% of women, and most women report nausea and vomiting throughout the entire day (38, 39). Nausea alone in the first trimester is experienced by many women. Nearly 83% of women take some form of medication for symptom relief (38).

The etiology of NVP includes several possibilities. Natural pregnancy-related changes in the endocrine system, hypersensitivities to proteins or antigens common in pregnancy, or toxic and metabolic mechanisms may all play a role. Psychosomatic reasons and unpleasant odors or sights may also contribute (37, 40). Treatment is chosen with consideration to the teratogenic risk of the antiemetic agents. The goal of therapy is to eliminate the symptoms.

Mild-to-moderate nausea and vomiting can usually be managed by nonpharmacologic measures. The patient can be instructed to eat small, frequent meals. High-carbohydrate meals, crackers, or high-protein snacks during the day and before bedtime may also be helpful. Spicy foods and noxious odors should be avoided, and many patients find relief by lying down.

If drug therapy is required, meclizine is a reasonable drug of choice because it is associated with low teratogenic risk. Daily doses of 25 to 50 mg by mouth are usually effective. Dimenhydrate 50 to 100 mg orally every 4 hr or 50 mg i.m./IV every 3 to 4 hr is an alternative. If symptoms are not controlled, phenothiazines, when used in low doses for a reasonable duration of time, are generally considered safe in pregnancy. The potential for adverse effects is low, but these agents should be reserved as second-line agents (40, 41). Promethazine 50 mg per day given orally or intramuscularly in two to four divided doses may be effective. Alternatively, prochlorperazine 5 to 10 mg orally or i.m. three to four times daily may be given. If NVP persists, metoclopramide 5 to 10 mg orally three times daily or 5 to 10 mg i.m./IV three times daily may be more effective than prochlorperazine. Metoclopramide appears to be safe in pregnancy. No congenital defects or other fetal or newborn complications due to therapy have been reported. The drug has been used as early as 7 to 10 weeks of gestation and in doses of up to 60 mg per day. Droperidol is not commonly used as an antiemetic in pregnant patients, but some have used it during labor as a sedative without documenting adverse effects. Others have briefly stated their experience with the drug throughout gestation (25).

The demand for pyridoxine is increased during pregnancy, and women may develop a deficiency of this vitamin. This generally does not occur until the second or third trimester. Pyridoxine deficiency has been thought to cause NVP. However, this would not explain symptoms that occur with normal pyridoxine levels. For many years, studies have been conducted with pyridoxine, but they have not been well designed or controlled, and the efficacy of pyridoxine in eliminating symptoms has not been proven (41, 42). Doses of 10 to 30 mg per day have been safely administered to pregnant women for NVP. Dietary supplementation of pyridoxine is recommended during pregnancy to prevent deficiencies.

Pyridoxine 10 mg was one ingredient in Bendectin, the only product ever approved by the FDA for NVP in the first trimester. This product also contained doxylamine succinate 10 mg, and up until 1976, 10 mg of dicyclomine. The latter ingredient was discontinued in the product marketed in the Untied States, because of suspected ineffectiveness. Doxylamine is currently available in over-the-counter sleep aids. Bendectin came under considerable scrutiny because of case reports describing malformations in infants exposed to the drug in utero, for example congenital heart defects, limb abnormalities, and neural-tube defects. Despite these case reports, in epidemiologic studies conducted in slightly over 6000 patients, no evidence of an increased risk of teratogenicity was documented. However, in 1984 the manufacturer encountered high costs in litigation and requested physicians to stop prescribing the drug. Even though there was confidence in the safety profile of Bendectin, the product was voluntarily removed from the market because of the expense of legal cases (40).

Asthma

Asthma is the most common obstructive lung disease in pregnancy, occurring in 0.4 to 1.3% of pregnant women (43). The effect of pregnancy on asthma is variable. The condition may improve, decline, or go unaltered. There is an increased frequency of maternal and fetal morbidity and mortality when asthma is not adequately treated during pregnancy. Perinatal mortality, hyperemesis, preeclampsia, hemorrhage, and increased rate of prematurity may be more frequent in pregnant asthmatics than in normal controls (43–45). If asthma is controlled, infants are born with no greater risk for congenital abnormalities than the general population (43, 44, 46). Complications could be due to the disease or the drug therapy. The benefits in treating the pregnant asthmatic support the administration of drugs to these patients (44, 47). The goal of therapy and the drugs used are similar to those for nonpregnant patients.

Mild and infrequent asthmatic episodes may be treated with inhaled β-agonists. Subcutaneous injections or oral administration of sympathomimetic agents is possible, but systemic adverse effects are lessened by using aerosolized therapy. The use of selective β₂-agonists also lessens adverse effects such as cardiac abnormalities or tremor. All β-sympathomimetics may cause fetal and maternal tachycardia, maternal hyperglycemia or hypotension, or neonatal hypoglycemia. Terbutaline is used as a tocolytic. The inhibition of labor at term when the drug is used for asthma, may require that terbutaline be discontinued. Metaproterenol is used routinely in pregnant women. Albuterol, isoetharine, terbutaline, and isoproterenol are possible alternatives (48–51). An association of minor congenital malformations with first-trimester use of sympathomimetics has been suggested, but the benefits of therapy generally outweigh risks. Patients should be informed to monitor for adverse effects and to not overuse the inhaler. A dose of two puffs every 4 to 6 hr is usually adequate for most inhalers.

Methylxanthines may be used in patients requiring continuous bronchodilator therapy. Theophylline may be used in conjunction with inhalation therapy for long-term control. Theophylline or aminophylline should be carefully administered, to maintain nontoxic maternal serum concentrations. These agents cross the placenta, and adverse fetal effects include jitteriness, cardiac arrhythmias, hypoglycemia, vomiting, tachycardia, and feeding difficulties. If steroids are indicated, they should not be withheld (46). Prednisolone or prednisone may be used for oral therapy. Doses needed to control attacks can be administered and then tapered slowly over several days to the lowest effective dose. Every-other-day dosing is optimal if continued steroid treatment is indicated. Case reports describe infants exposed to prednisone through gestation being born with congenital cataracts and immunosuppression. The association has not been supported by other studies, however. No evidence has confirmed that prednisone increases fetal mortality or morbidity, and the risk of prednisone to the fetus and newborn is considered to be low. Methylprednisolone or hydrocortisone are adequate if IV steroid administration is needed. Inhaled beclomethasone has been used in pregnant patients and provides the advantages of topical therapy (51). Defects perhaps associated with beclomethasone such as low birth weight, prematurity, and cardiac malformations have been documented in some reports. Due to various confounding elements, the association was unclear. Triamcinolone is also available, but less information is available about the safety of this drug in pregnant women, compared with beclomethasone.

Cromolyn sodium is indicated for the prevention of asthmatic attacks. It is administered via inhalation; therefore, significant concentrations of the drug are not achieved in the plasma. It is unknown whether cromolyn crosses the placenta. There has been no evidence proving an association between this drug and congenital defects. Cromolyn has been used without adverse maternal or fetal outcomes (44–46, 50, 51).

Ipratropium is an anticholinergic marketed for relief of asthma attacks. Little is known about the safety of the drug in pregnant women. Since the systemic absorption of the drug is small, adverse effects would be expected to be minimal.

Status asthmaticus is experienced in nearly 0.2% of pregnant women (44). This is a life-threatening condition, and treatment is the same for pregnant and nonpregnant patients.

Hypertension

Hypertension complicates about 7% of all pregnancies. Preeclampsia/eclampsia or chronic hypertension affect most of these patients (52–54). Hypertension contributes significantly to maternal and perinatal morbidity and mortality (52, 55). Complications may include intrauterine growth retardation, placental insufficiency or abruptio, and preterm labor and delivery. The fetus can be deprived of oxygen and nutrients if the hypertension is severe enough to diminish the uteroplacental blood flow. The incidence of these complications increases in direct proportion to increased maternal blood pressure.

Risk factors for developing hypertension during pregnancy include the primigravidae, women over 35 years, a family history or previous history of preeclampsia, black women, a low socioeconomic status, poor nutritional state, diabetes, obesity, or twinning (55, 56). The need to treat is determined by considering the individual patient, complicating factors, maximum blood pressure recorded, and stage of gestation. The risk-benefit ratio of therapy must also be considered. While the benefits of treating mild hypertensive pregnant patients is controversial, severe hypertension (170/180 mm Hg) requires treatment to reduce fetal and maternal morbidity and mortality.

Few well-controlled, well-designed studies have been conducted to determine the optimal antihypertensive regimen for the pregnant patient. Nondrug therapy is preferred if possible. Such measures include bed rest, relaxation techniques, limited physical activity, abstinence from smoking or drinking alcohol, and proper nutrition. If antihypertensive medications are indicated, unlike the step-care approach used in nonpregnant patients, agents with the most available information regarding their use in pregnancy are preferred. However, it may be appropriate for some women who have been controlled on antihypertensive medications before conception, to continue their drug regimen throughout gestation. The recommendations are not standard, but some propose that continuing β-blocker or diuretic therapy during pregnancy is acceptable (57).

If therapy is initiated during gestation, methyldopa has been used most frequently. Methyldopa readily crosses the placenta, and only rare adverse effects have been documented in the newborn. It is the only antihypertensive with data on long-term effects in offspring exposed to the drug in utero. Normal mental and physical development for up to 7 years has been reported (52). Methyldopa may be given at a dose of 250 mg two or three times daily. An alternative centrally acting agent is clonidine. Although not used as extensively in pregnancy as methyldopa, clonidine has been effective in severe hypertension in late pregnancy. No reports of congenital defects have been associated with clonidine use in late gestation. However, it offers little to no therapeutic advantage over methyldopa. Hydralazine, 10 to 25 mg orally two or three times daily, is usually preferred as an alternative to methyldopa for long-term antihypertensive therapy in pregnancy.

In cases where neither methyldopa or hydralazine are appropriate, propranolol or metoprolol are viable alternatives. β-Blockers, including propranolol, atenolol, metoprolol, and labetalol, have been used in pregnancy for various indications. Effects on the fetus and mother vary among these agents because of their differences in pharmacodynamic and pharmacokinetic profiles. Experience with atenolol, labetalol, and metoprolol in the first trimester is limited. These drugs cross the placenta and may block the β-receptors in the fetus, causing a decrease in heart rate reactivity. Thus, the fetus exposed to the drug near delivery, should be monitored for 24 to 72 hr after birth for signs of β-blocking activity. β-Blockers have not been found to induce premature labor or, when used in second and third trimesters, produce congenital malformations. Unlike methyldopa, no long-term follow-up studies past 1 year have been conducted for any of the β-blockers. β-Blockers are considered to be relatively safe in pregnancy, and propranolol or metoprolol are commonly favored. Propranolol has been effective in doses of 80 to 140 mg/day; the lower dose being associated with fewer adverse effects. Hypoglycemia, lower birth weights, bradycardia, and respiratory depression are some of the adverse effects that have been reported in newborns. Metoprolol has been found to be safe at doses of 100 mg/day, and it has been shown to reduce perinatal mortality in one report (58). Atenolol may be given in daily doses of 50 to 100 mg. Reduced birth weight has been reported; however, 1-year follow-up studies have noted normal growth and development in exposed offspring (59, 60). Atenolol has been used primarily in late pregnancy. Labetalol has not been used extensively, but many favor this drug in the pregnant patient. It may be less likely to decrease cardiac output and uteroplacental flow due to the α- and β-blocking activities it possesses. Doses of 400 to 800 mg/day have been used. Newborns may have transient hypotension, but most infants do not appear to be adversely affected (61, 62).

Limited information is available on calcium-channel blockers in pregnancy. In animal studies, nifedipine has been associated with fetal hypoxemia, acidosis, and decreased uterine blood flow (25). Nifedipine has been used in only a small number of patients in the second or third trimesters, and some women have delivered healthy infants. Until further studies are completed to evaluate the safety of nifedipine, the drug is not recommended for general use in pregnancy. Nifedipine may increase the neuromuscular-blockade properties of magnesium sulfate. The combination of these drugs should be avoided.

Angiotension I converting enzyme inhibitors are not recommended as antihypertensive agents in pregnant patients. Severe renal compromise and fatal anuria have been reported. Captopril and enalapril may result in fetal renal failure by inhibiting the production of angiotensin II. Stillbirths in animal studies and severe neonatal hypotension in humans has been reported. Captopril has been used in multiple-drug regimens where defects have been documented, although the cause of injury has not been proven. Because other antihypertensive medications are much safer, captopril and enalapril should not be used in pregnancy. If they are required in refractory or special cases, the mother should be closely monitored (54).

The use of diuretics in pregnant hypertensives is controversial (52). The main concern about diuretic use is their effect on the volume status of the patient. Diuretics cause a decrease in plasma and extracellular fluid volume, decrease in cardiac output, and decreased perfusion of the placenta and uterus. This may cause problems in a women with previously contracted fluid volumes and preeclampsia. The necessary expansion of fluids during pregnancy may be counteracted by diuretic therapy, but this remains to be proven. Thiazides and loop diuretics have been used in the first trimester. Adverse fetal and neonatal effects with thiazide use in later pregnancy have included hypoglycemia, electrolyte imbalances, thrombocytopenia, decreased birth weight, and increased perinatal mortality. Decreased maternal weight gain may also result. Though diuretic therapy maybe indicated in some clinical situations (e.g., pulmonary edema), normal blood pressure can usually be achieved with other agents. Thiazide and loop diuretics are not, therefore, first-line drugs of choice for initiating antihypertensive therapy during pregnancy. Some clinicians recommend that women continue diuretic therapy throughout pregnancy, if blood pressure control was achieved with a diuretic before conception (57).

Hydralazine has been used most commonly to control acute exacerbations and severe hypertension in pregnancy. Information on the use of the drug in all three trimesters is available. Hydralazine use has not been clearly associated with congenital defects, and it has been used safely in combination with other antihypertensives such as β-blockers. Patients may experience tachycardia, flushing, or palpitations. In general, hydralazine appears to be safe in pregnant women. Doses should be carefully administered to avoid maternal hypotension or fetal distress. An alternative vasodilator such as nitroprusside has been used for life-threatening hypertensive emergencies. Nitroprusside

crosses the placenta. Thus, the fetus is sensitive to cyanide toxicity, which can result with extensive nitroprusside therapy. The dose of nitroprusside should be monitored closely in pregnant women. Diazoxide is best replaced with drugs for which more information is available (54).

Epilepsy

Less than 1% of pregnancies are complicated by seizure disorders (63). Pregnant epileptics have a better than 90% chance of having a normal child, but the risk for congenital malformations and mental retardation in offspring of epileptics is twice that of the normal population (64, 65). Increased rates of stillbirths may occur with status epilepticus. Fetal harm is a possibility in pregnant epileptics for several reasons. Seizures can produce hypoxia and acidosis, which can be damaging, and adverse effects from antiepileptic drugs may indirectly cause harm. The genetic or biochemical makeup of the epileptic parent may also be a factor. The importance of anyone of these factors is unclear, because most patients have confounding factors. However, drug therapy has been associated with an increase in congenital defects.

Pregnancy improves the seizure control of nearly one-fourth of all pregnant epileptics. Similarly, one-fourth of patients have a worsening of their disorder. Uncontrolled seizures are dangerous to the mother and the fetus. The benefit of treatment generally outweighs the risk (65). When drug therapy is required, the lowest effective dose should always be used. Single-agent therapy is also best, if possible. In addition, the clinician should be aware that the pharmacokinetic profile of anticonvulsant medications is altered in pregnancy. Volume of distribution and renal and hepatic clearance are increased. Gastrointestinal absorption and protein binding are decreased (64). During the postpartum period, the pharmacokinetic parameters return to normal. Thus, serum concentrations should be monitored throughout pregnancy and at least up to the sixth week postpartum.

Phenytoin is teratogenic in animals and may produce adverse effects in the fetus and newborn, and effects may be evident in childhood. The fetal hydantoin syndrome, discussed earlier, may be expressed. Hemorrhage has been reported in newborns and may be fatal. The bleeding is thought to be caused by a deficiency in vitamin K–dependent clotting factors or phenytoin-induced thrombocytopenia. Although further research is needed to determine the best means of prevention and treatment, some clinicians recommend the administration of vitamin K to the mother in the late stages of pregnancy (65). Phenytoin has been linked with various tumors in children whose mothers took the drug while pregnant. Offspring should be monitored throughout childhood for any carcinogeneic effects of the drug. In summary, although the adverse effects can be serious, phenytoin should not be withheld if required for seizure control. Maternal supplementation with vitamin K prior to delivery should be considered. Phenytoin serum concentrations should be carefully monitored. Because phenytoin can induce folic acid deficiency, administration of folic acid throughout gestation is usually recommended. Despite available information on the safety of other anticonvulsants, patients adequately controlled on phenytoin should, in general, not be switched to other drugs (64, 65).

Phenobarbital is considered by some to be the anticonvulsant of choice in pregnant epileptics. Minor abnormalities have been associated with its use in the gravida. As with phenytoin, neonatal hemorrhage shortly after delivery, partial expression of the fetal hydantoin syndrome, and maternal folic acid deficiency may occur. Unlike phenytoin, phenobarbital may cause neonatal addiction and withdrawal symptoms such as hyperactivity and feeding problems. Withdrawal symptoms generally occur within 1 week of delivery. In this case, parents should be advised to monitor for these symptoms and to not blame themselves for the behavior of the baby or for poor parenting skills. The newborn may require treatment for withdrawal symptoms.

Other anticonvulsant medications are available to the clinician. Ethosuximide is considered the drug of choice in petit mal epilepsy in pregnancy (63). Documentation on the use of this agent in pregnant women is limited, however. Carbamazepine has been used in the pregnant epileptic as monotherapy and in combination therapy with phenobarbital or phenytoin. Carbamazepine readily crosses the placenta and has been associated with minor abnormalities including craniofacial defects, fingernail hypoplasia, and developmental delay (66, 67). A pattern of abnormalities similar to the fetal hydantoin syndrome has been noted with carbamazepine therapy. The use of this drug in pregnancy is not without risk to the fetus. Valproic acid is contraindicated in pregnancy. It has been linked with neural tube defects in 1 to 2% of exposures. Minor and major cardiovascular and craniofacial malformations have occurred, as have deficiencies in mental and physical development and meningomyelocele (63).

Diabetes Mellitus

The risk of congenital abnormalities is three times greater in pregnant diabetics than in the nondiabetic pregnant population. Similarly, major abnormalities are six times more likely to occur in the diabetic population. These anomalies are important, since 20 to 50% of perinatal deaths of offspring from diabetic women are caused by birth defects. Evidence suggests that these birth defects are due to inadequate metabolic control and poor control of blood sugar levels. In fact, euglycemic control of the maternal blood sugar levels is essential in decreasing the incidence of perinatal mortality and morbidity. Maternal

hyperglycemia during the period of organogenesis is thought to be associated with an increased incidence of congenital abnormalities. This may explain why gestational diabetics have a lower risk of congenital abnormalities than overt diabetics. The onset of gestational diabetes does not occur until around the 24th week. Therefore, in the gestational diabetic, early in pregnancy, the maternal blood sugar and glycosolated hemoglobin levels are normal, and the fetus has an increased chance of normal development. The incidence of perinatal mortality has decreased dramatically over the last several years, to around 6.5%. This is largely due to tighter control of maternal blood sugar levels. Maternal risk factors for high perinatal mortality include pyelonephritis, diabetic ketoacidosis, hypertension, vascular disease, and lack of antenatal care. Diabetic ketoacidosis can occur at lower glucose concentrations than in the nonpregnant diabetic. Ketoacidosis is associated with a 50% perinatal mortality rate, and patients should be carefully monitored to prevent this from developing.

Diabetes mellitus during pregnancy is commonly categorized by the White classification (68). This system has been used for many years and classifies patients based on the presence of vascular disease, the age of onset, and the duration of diabetes mellitus in the patient. The goal of therapy in the pregnant diabetic is to achieve normalization of the blood sugar and avoid extreme fluctuations in insulin and glucose plasma concentrations. Throughout gestation, the amount of insulin required varies for insulin-dependent diabetics. During the first 24 weeks of gestation, the fetus receives its required nutrients from the mother; the transport of which can lead to maternal hypoglycemia. The mother generally requires less insulin during this part of the pregnancy. However, in the late second and third trimesters, the demand for insulin increases. This is due, in part, to an increase in placental hormones that are diabetogenic. After delivery, the amount of insulin needed by the mother is similar to that required before conception.

If at all possible, a diabetic woman who wishes to become pregnant should carefully plan conception. Proper obstetric management includes an evaluation of the woman for complicating risk factors including retinopathy, renal impairment, and vascular disease or a history of problems with previous pregnancies. Tight control of blood sugar levels before conception is key in the planning process. Patients may be asked to achieve a glycosolated hemoglobin level below 8.5% before attempting to conceive. In any case, a pregnancy test should be performed soon after the patient misses her first menstrual period. Because of the risk to the fetus of hyperglycemia, a pregnant woman should be tested for gestational diabetes around the 22nd to 26th week. If the diagnosis is not made at this time, glucose concentrations should be remeasured in the 32nd week. After a diagnosis of diabetes, patient education is important. Although nutritional needs increase in pregnancy diet and exercise regimens similar to those for the nonpregnant diabetic should be taught to the patient. If diet fails to control blood sugar levels, insulin is indicated. Oral hypoglycemic agents are not recommended in pregnancy. They may induce insulin secretion from the fetal pancreas and lead to fetal hypoglycemia. As mentioned previously, insulin amounts vary during gestation. A mix of intermediate-acting and short-acting insulins is generally most effective. NPH and regular can be given in a regimen specific to the patient's needs. Multiple daily injections are usually required to achieve euglycemia. Patients must monitor their glucose concentration at home. The best control dictates that the blood sugar level should be checked four to eight times daily. Measurements may be taken before breakfast, 2 hr after each meal, and at bedtime. In some patients, once effective control is adequately demonstrated, the blood glucose level should be checked twice daily. Patients should be instructed to check their glucose concentration anytime they feel that it is high or low. Fasting plasma glucose concentrations near 100 mg/100 ml and postprandial concentrations of less than 120 mg/100 ml have been recommended (69). Maternal glucose concentrations must be carefully controlled during labor and delivery. The newborn also needs monitoring after delivery, to ensure normal glucose concentrations.

Anticoagulation

Coagulation disorders affect 0.2 to 0.4% of pregnant women (70). Anticoagulants may be taken for a variety of indications including thrombophlebitis, thromboembolic disease, and valvular heart prostheses (71). The high reduction of antepartum mortality rates from 13 to 1% in women with thromboembolic disease supports treatment of the pregnant patient with anticoagulant therapy (70).

The anticoagulant of choice for the pregnant patient is heparin. It does not cross the placenta and has not been associated with congenital defects. Heparin may be used for short-term anticoagulation at doses of 5000 units subcutaneously every 12 hr, with little risk to the mother and fetus. The main risk to the mother in this setting is bleeding. Long-term therapy (over 6 months) poses the risk of maternal thrombocytopenia or osteoporosis. An advantage to heparin is that any bleeding that occurs can be readily reversed by protamine sulfate. Coumarin derivatives are well-known teratogens that may produce abnormalities such as embryopathy, particularly in the first trimester (as mentioned previously). Central nervous system defects are most likely to be seen with second- or third-trimester exposure. Hemorrhage can result from exposure in these same trimesters. Problematic deliveries may be complicated with hemorrhage. Both of these effects may produce serious long-term disabilities such as blindness (11, 14, 18, 19, 23, 24). Exposure to warfarin throughout pregnancy has been associated with abnormalities of the facies, skeletal system, and limbs. Stillbirths, spontaneous abortion, mental retardation, and impairment of physical growth are also possible effects. Coumarin derivatives carry great risk to the fetus and should be avoided during pregnancy, particularly in the first and third trimesters.

Gastroesophageal Reflux Disease (GERD)

Nearly 80% of pregnant patients complain of heartburn. This is generally described as a burning sensation in the substernal or epigastric region, which may radiate to the back or neck. The etiology of heartburn in pregnancy is not clearly understood. During pregnancy there is increased pressure from the uterus onto the stomach, particularly during the third trimester, and progesterone is thought to relax lower esophogeal sphincter tone. A decrease in gastrointestinal motility may also play a role. Patients generally do not experience any serious sequelae from GERD, and the symptoms can usually be managed conservatively.

Nonpharmacological therapy should be tried initially. A diet low in fat is recommended. Patients should also avoid irritating substances such as coffee, spicy foods, orange juice, tomato juice, or peppermint. Relief is generally obtained by eating small, frequent meals and avoiding any food intake immediately before bedtime. Patients should avoid lying down immediately after eating during the day. Elevating the head of the bed is sometimes effective. Antacids provide relief for most patients. Products containing aluminum hydroxide, magnesium hydroxide, or magnesium trisilicate in tablet or liquid form may be used. Products with combinations of these ingredients are also safe and effective for most patients. If doses of 15 to 30 ml as needed do not relieve symptoms, dosing every 1 to 3 hr after meals and before bedtime may be effective. Patients with problems related to sodium retention should use low-sodium-containing antacids. Drugs used in the nonpregnant patient to manipulate the lower esophogeal sphincter tone are not currently recommended for pregnant patients. Sodium bicarbonate, histamine 2–antagonists, bethanechol, and metoclopramide are better replaced with antacids (72).

Constipation

Pregnant patients commonly complain of straining, decreased frequency of bowel movement, pain during defecation, and rectal bleeding. Etiologies of constipation in pregnancy are similar to the nonpregnant state, but an increased pressure on the colon, increased intestinal transit time, or increased colonic absorption of sodium, potassium, and water are other possible causes (73). Treatment is also similar to that of the nonpregnant patient. Patients should first increase the amount of fiber in their diet. Their daily water intake should be sufficient. Exercise and stress-reduction techniques also help in attaining regularity.

Bulk laxatives may be recommended to patients. These products contain active ingredients such as tragarcanth, acacia, and agar, or a type of cellulose. Psyllium is readily available and is safe and effective at doses of 1 to 2 tablespoons, once or twice daily. An alternative agent is magnesium hydroxide. Stool softeners may also be used. Docusate sodium or dioctyl sulfosuccinate 100 to 200 mg daily generally provides relief. Mineral oil should be avoided in pregnant women because of possible interference with lipid soluble vitamins. Strong laxatives and enemas are not recommended during pregnancy.

Common Cold

The common cold frequently affects pregnant women whose resistance is weakened. The virus causing the common cold has not been shown to be teratogenic. Most problems associated with the common cold are the symptoms; they can be intolerable. Patients may complain of watery eyes and nose, cough, sneezing, and congestion. Although many products are available, the patient should be informed that treatment is not curative. If at all possible, medication therapy should be avoided. To limit drug exposure further, combination products should not be used when the patient can be treated with only one active component of the product.

If the patient's most bothersome symptom requires an antihistamine, both chlorpheniramine and triprolidine have been used commonly in pregnancy. A significantly increased relative risk of birth defects has been documented with brompheniramine use in the first trimester, and this drug is not generally recommended.

Sympathomimetic amines are useful in patients needing a decongestant. Minor malformations have been documented with first-trimester use of this class of drugs. In many patients it is difficult to determine whether the drug, the disease, the virus, or other drugs caused the defect. However, use of this class of drugs is not without risk. Pseudoephedrine has not been associated with adverse outcomes. Phenylpropanolamine in the first trimester should be avoided, and epinephrine has been associated with increased incidence of birth defects. Phenylephrine is most frequently used as a topical nasal decongestant. Topical application is advantageous in limiting systemic exposure and toxicity. Oxymetazoline is a longer-acting topical product that may also be used in pregnancy. Xylometazoline and ephedrine have not been associated with birth defects.

Antitussives or expectorants that may be used in pregnant women include dextromethorphan, guaifenesin, and cetylpyridinium. There is no documented increased risk associated with these agents. Iodides, including saturated solution of potassium iodine, are contraindicated in pregnancy, as they may induce goiter in the fetus. Cough syrups and elixirs customarily contain some kind of sedative, sugar, and alcohol. Pregnant women should avoid products with these extra ingredients. The fetal alcohol syndrome was reported in one case where a woman abused cough medicine (74).

DRUGS IN LACTATION

Since the 1970s, the incidence of women who breast-feed has increased. This increase has been most evident and easily documented among well-educated, white, married, older women of above average income (75). Rates of women who breast-feed vary from 25 to 75%, depending on geographic location, employment, socioeconomic status, education, and time from delivery. By the year 2000, the national health objective is to have 75% of women breast-feeding at hospital discharge and 50% at 6 months postpartum. Achieving a high rate of breast-fed infants is especially important in areas with insufficient medical care, where nutrition and sanitation are poor. Breast-feeding was once commonly replaced with manufactured formulas for various reasons. Although formulas are indicated under some conditions, there is no duplication for human milk. It is specific for humans and provides among many things, the total nutritional needs of the growing infant.

Knowing the importance of breast-feeding is basic in the overall management of the patient. Human milk provides several benefits to the infant that cannot be duplicated by other means. Nutrients are balanced and sufficient to the growing infant and are delivered consistently throughout each day as the baby nurses. Healthy infants are ready to suckle at birth. Nurslings are provided with unsurpassed protection against immunologic disorders and infections, and protection against diseases, such as those of the gastrointestinal and respiratory systems. Comparisons between bottle-fed and breast-fed babies show that the latter have lower incidences of metabolic disorders, heart disease, obesity, and allergies, and that a unique psychologic bond is developed between infant and mother. In addition, nursing enhances the maternal physiologic recovery from childbirth as body weight and hormones return to prepregnant levels (76, 77).

If a nursing woman requires drug therapy, numerous interrelated factors should be considered to ensure that the therapy is rational and safe to both mother and child. Consideration must be given to the amount of drug excreted into the milk and the amount ingested by the infant. The pharmacologic handling of the drug by the mother is a primary factor involving evaluation of the complete dosage regimen including drug, dose and route of administration, and the mother's ability to absorb, metabolize, and eliminate the drug. A second factor involves the milk produced. Depending upon the quantity of milk produced, the amount of drug available for the infant to ingest will also vary. Human milk is primarily water, but also contains fat, lactose, and protein. The composition of the milk influences the extent to which a drug crosses into it. The contents of milk varies between individuals and even within the same individual; however, the pH of human milk is generally near 7.0. Thus, drug distributes into the milk not only in relation to its water and fat content, but also to its pH. The physicochemical properties of the drug are a third factor to consider. Distribution of a drug into breast milk primarily occurs by passive diffusion. Other mechanisms such as carrier-mediated and active transport (and possibly reabsorption) also play a role. Transport into the milk is largely determined by the pK_a of the drug. The lipid and water solubility, molecular weight, and extent of protein binding also influence transport across membranes. Large molecules, such as heparin, will not pass into the milk. Ionized drugs and those highly bound to plasma proteins (such as warfarin) will not pass either. Acidic drugs do not enter the milk to an important extent. Finally, the infant must be considered. How much drug the infant consumes is influenced not only by the factors described above but also by the amount of milk ingested by the infant. Nursing times must be known. If the baby nurses when the drug has reached peak concentrations in the milk, the amount ingested will be much greater than if nursing occurred just before the mother took a dose.

The information on drugs in lactation has several limitations. It consists primarily of case reports citing individual accounts of drug concentrations measured in breast milk. Many clinicians have also documented adverse effects that they have seen infants experience because of drug exposure via breast milk. Animal studies have been conducted, but this information is not always applicable to the human situation. The composition of milk varies between species, as does the pharmacokinetic handling and dosing of drugs. In many human studies, the pharmacokinetic properties of the drug are rarely taken into consideration when milk concentrations are determined. The peak concentration of the drug in breast milk may occur much later than that in the plasma. Also, most concentrations are determined after a single dose, and the timing in relation to the dose or stage of breast-feeding is not stated. Thus, it is difficult to estimate the actual amount of drug accumulated in the milk and ingested by the infant. Another weakness in the literature is that studies include very few patients. Also, drug companies have published little to no data on the distribution of their drug into breast milk. They are not required by law to research this topic and find the methods of doing so expensive and logistically difficult. Unpublished information may be obtained from the companies, but it may not be of clinical use and it should be carefully evaluated for accuracy (78).

The goals of therapy in a lactating woman are to treat

Table 88.4.
Drugs Contraindicated During Breast-feeding[a]

Amphetamine	Cocaine
Bromocriptine	Cyclosporine
Cyclophosphamide	Ergotamine
Heroin	Marijuana
Lithium	Methotrexate
Phencyclidine	

[a] Adapted from Anon: Transfer of drugs and other chemicals into human milk. American Academy of Pediatrics. Pediatric 84(5):924–936, 1989.

Table 88.5.
Drugs That May Suppress Lactation[a]

Androgens	Bromocriptine
Clomiphene citrate	Thiazide diuretics
Monoamine oxidase inhibitors	Levodopa
Ergot derivatives	High-dose pyridoxine

[a] Adapted from Anon: Transfer of drugs and other chemicals into human milk. American Academy of Pediatrics. Pediatric 84(5):924–936, 1989.

the underlying disorder, avoid drug exposure and adverse effects in the nursing infant, and to continue breast-feeding. Drug therapy should rarely interrupt breast-feeding. In addition to estimating the amount of drug in the milk and the amount ingested by the infant, modifications can usually be made so that the goals of therapy can be achieved (76, 77).

In choosing a drug to administer, consider the safety profile of the agent in the infant. There may be an alternative drug that is safer for newborns. For example, acetaminophen is preferred over aspirin for analgesia because of the possibility of salicylism in the infant. The American Academy of Pediatrics Committee on Drugs has identified drugs that they consider to be contraindicated during breast-feeding because of symptoms produced in the infant (79). These drugs are listed in Table 88.4. Drugs that inhibit lactation are included in Table 88.5.

Altering the patient's drug regimen may be another option. Nursing should be avoided when the drug reaches peak concentrations in the milk and plasma. The mother should be instructed to nurse immediately before taking the medication, if at all possible. If the mother takes the medication and feeds frequently, these two activities should be spaced as far as possible from one another. Taking the medication just before the infant sleeps may be helpful, if sleeping patterns can be identified. In certain cases, the mother may need to discontinue breast-feeding for a limited time. She can pump her breasts before beginning drug therapy, and the milk can be stored and administered to the infant while the medication is being me-

Table 88.6.
Effect of Various Drugs during Breast-feeding[a]

Drugs whose effect on nursing infants is unknown but may be of concern

Diazepam	Desipramine
Lorazepam	Doxepin
Amitryptilline	Imipramine
Amoxapine	Trazodone
Haloperidol	Chlorpromazine
Chloramphenicol	Chlorprothixene
Metronidazole	

Drugs that have caused significant effects on some nursing infants and should be given to nursing mothers with caution

Aspirin	Phenobarbital
Sulfasalazine	Clemastine
Primidone	

[a] Adapted from Anon: Transfer of drugs and other chemicals into human milk. American Academy of Pediatrics. Pediatrics 84(5):924–936, 1989.

tabolized and eliminated from the mother's body. Breast-feeding can resume once the drug is cleared. This is recommended with metronidazole. Rapidly eliminated drugs lessen the time that the mother will need to give stored milk to her infant. Similarly, drugs with a short half-life will be more rapidly eliminated by the baby. Nursing infants must be closely monitored. The parents should be instructed to monitor for possible adverse effects such as abnormal growth or sleeping patterns, or restlessness. Sleepiness may commonly be seen when anticonvulsant medications are given to a mother. It maybe necessary to monitor milk and serum concentrations.

In summary, breast-feeding provides unsurpassed benefits to both mother and child. If drug therapy is indicated, many interrelated factors influence the extent to which the drug passes into the mild and is ingested by the infant. These factors include the mother, the milk, the drug, and the infant. While most drugs enter the milk to some extent, several interventions can decrease the adverse effects of the drug in the infant and yet not interrupt breast-feeding. In addition, the Academy of Pediatrics has identified drugs whose effects on nursing infants is unknown but may be of concern and those which should be given to nursing mothers with caution (79). These are presented in Table 88.6.

SUMMARY

Pregnancy is a symptom-producing condition. Pain, heartburn, nausea and vomiting, and constipation are among the possible symptoms that may require treatment. Some women need drug therapy for chronic diseases that existed before the pregnancy, such as diabetes mellitus or hypertension. What is unique in the pregnant patient is the need to consider the effect of the ingested drug on the developing fetus. Most drugs taken by the mother will reach the fetus to some extent. It is important to assess whether the risk of a congenital defect from drug exposure exceeds the risk of a defect occurring without drug exposure. The estimated baseline rate of infants born with congenital malformations is 3%, which may rise to 6% if minor malformations are included. It is difficult to assess with total confidence the exact probability of a drug causing damage to the fetus. Information available from the literature is limited, partly because of the logistic problems of data capture and analysis associated with this type of research. Anecdotal information composes most of the literature. One of the most important factors to consider in assessing risk to the fetus is the time during pregnancy of the fetal drug exposure. In addition, if a maternal disease is left untreated, it may adversely affect perinatal or even maternal morbidity or mortality. No drug taken during any stage of pregnancy is without risk. The mother must be well informed about drug therapy in pregnancy so that she and her physician can make an educated decision.

This communication is also important after a baby is born. Breast-feeding provides unsurpassed nutrition for the infant. Yet, many drugs distribute into breast milk and are ingested by the nursling. Whether or not the mother needs medication is the first question. If drug therapy is indicated, then a drug with a low milk-to-plasma ratio should be chosen. Drugs with a short half-life are preferable to long-acting medications. The mother may need to schedule taking the drug around the breast-feeding. The child should be monitored for adverse effects of ingested medication. Educating and communicating with the mother is vital in ensuring proper care of both mother and baby.

REFERENCES

1. Doering PL, Stewart RB: The extent and character of drug consumption during pregnancy. JAMA 239:843–846, 1978.
2. Rudd CC, Brazy GE: Drugs in the perinatal period: implications for the preterm infant. Pediatrics 14(20):30–37, 1988.
3. Anon, Congenital malformations and inherited disorders. In Cunningham FG, MacDonald PC, Gant NF (eds): Williams's Obstetrics. Norwalk, CT, Appleton & Lange, 1989, p 561.
4. Bodendorfer TW, Briggs GG, Gunning JE: Obtaining drug exposure histories during pregnancy. Am J Obstet Gynecol 135:490–494, 1979.
5. Bonati M, Bortolus R, Marchetti F, Romero M, Tognoni G: Drug use in pregnancy: an overview of epidemiological (drug utilization) studies. Eur J Clin Pharmacol 38:325–328, 1990.
6. Heinonen OP, Slone D, Shapiro S (eds): Birth defects and drugs in pregnancy. Littleton, MA: PSG Publishing, 1977.
7. Werler MM, Pober BR, Nelson K, Holmes LB: Reporting accuracy among mothers of malformed and nonmalformed infants. Am J Epidemiol 129:415–421, 1989.
8. Wilson JG: Experimental studies on congenital malformations. J Chron Dis 10:111–114, 1959.

9. Hill LM, Kleinberg F: Effects of drugs and chemicals on the fetus and newborn, Part I. Mayo Clin Proc 59:707–716, 1984.

10. Shephard TH. Teratogenicity of therapeutic agents. Curr Probl Pediatr 10(2):3–43, 1979.

11. Dicke JM. Teratology: principles and practice. Med Clin North Am 73(3):567–582, 1989.

12. Friedman JM, Little BB, Brent RL, Cordero JF, Hanson JW, Shepard TH: Potential human teratogenicity of frequently prescribed drugs. Obstet Gynecol 75:594–599, 1990.

13. Anon: Fed Regist 44:37434–37467, 1980.

14. Beckman DA, Brent RL: Mechanisms of teratogenesis. Annu Rev Pharmacol Toxicol 24:483–500, 1984.

15. Kalter H, Warkany J: Congenital malformations, etiological factors and their role in prevention. N Engl J Med 308(8):424–431, 1983.

16. Aase JM, Principles of normal and abnormal embryogenesis. In Aase JM (ed): Diagnostic Dysmorphology. New York, Plenum, 1990, p 5.

17. Clarren SK, Smith DW: The fetal alcohol syndrome. N Engl J Med 298(19):1063–1067, 1978.

18. Jones KL: Smith's Recognizable Patterns of Human Malformations. Philadelphia: WB Saunders, 1983, p 491.

19. Hill LM, Kleinberg F: Effects of drugs and chemicals in the fetus and newborn, Part II. Mayo Clin Proc 59:755–765, 1984.

20. Hill LM, Stern L: Drugs in pregnancy: effects on the fetus and newborn. Drugs 17:182–197, 1979.

21. Coles CA, Smith IE, Fernhoff PM, Falek A: Neonatal ethanol withdrawal: characteristics in clinically normal, nondysmorphic neonates. J Pediatr 105:445–451, 1984.

22. Barrison IG, Waterson EF, Murray-Lyon IM: Adverse effects of alcohol in pregnancy. Br J Addiction 80:11–25, 1985.

23. Shaul WL, Hall JG: Multiple congenital anomalies associated with oral anticoagulants. Am J Obstet Gynecol 127:191–198, 1977.

24. Briggs GG, Freeman RK, Yaffe SJ: Drugs in Pregnancy and Lactation. Baltimore: Williams & Wilkins, 1990, p 158.

25. Donaldson JO: Neurological complications. In Burrows GN, Ferris TF (eds): Medical Complications during Pregnancy. Philadelphia, WB Saunders,1988, p 485.

26. Hanson JW: Teratogen update: fetal hydantoin effects. Teratology 33:349–353, 1986.

27. Buehler BA, Delimont D, Van Waes M, Finnel RH. Prenatal prediction of risk of the fetal hydantoin syndrome. N Engl J Med 322(22):1567–1572, 1990.

28. Hanson JW, Buehler BA: Fetal hydantoin syndrome: current status. J Pediatr 101(5):816–818, 1982.

29. Kaneko S, Otani K, Fukushima Y, Ogawa Y, Nomura Y, Ono T, et al.: Teratogenicity of antiepileptic drugs: analysis of possible risk factors. Epilepsia 29(4):459–467, 1988.

30. Lindhout D, Hoppener RJ, Meinardi H: Teratogenicity of antiepileptic drug combinations with special emphasis on epoxication. Epilepsia 25(1):77–83, 1984.

31. Johnson TRB, Niebyl JR: Caffeine in Pregnancy. In Niebyl JR (ed): Drug Use in Pregnancy. Philadelphia, Lea & Febiger, 1988, pp 231–233.

32. Wilcox A, Weinberg C, Baird D. Caffeinated beverages and decreased fertility. Lancet 2:1453–1456, 1988.

33. Kalter H, Warkany J: Congenital malformations, Part II. N Engl J Med 308(9):491–497, 1983.

34. Olsen J, Pereira A, Olsen SF: Does material tobacco smoking modify the effect of alcohol on fetal growth? Am J Public Health 181:69–73, 1991.

35. Berkowitz GS: Smoking and Pregnancy. In Niebyl JR (ed): Drug Use in Pregnancy. Philadelphia, Lea & Febiger, 1988, pp 173–191.

36. Centers for Disease Control: The Surgeon General's 1990 Report on The Health Benefits of Smoking Cessation (Executive Summary). MMWR 39(No. RR-12), 1990.

37. Walters WAW: The management of nausea and vomiting during pregnancy. Med J Aust 147:290–291, 1987.

38. Vellacott ID, Cooke EJA, James CE: Nausea and vomiting in early pregnancy. Int J Gynecol Obstet 27:57–62, 1988.

39. DiIorio C: The management of nausea and vomiting in pregnancy. Nurs Pract 13(5):23–28, 1988.

40. Niebyl JR, Maxwell KD: Treatment of nausea and vomiting of pregnancy. In Niebyl JR (ed): Drug Use in Pregnancy. Philadelphia, Lea & Febiger, 1988, pp 11–19.

41. Leathem AM: Safety and efficacy of antiemetics used to treat nausea and vomiting in pregnancy. Clin Pharm 5:660–668, 1986.

42. Weinstein BB, Wohl Z, Mitchell GJ, Sustendal GF: Oral administration of pyridoxine hydrochloride in the treatment of nausea and vomiting of pregnancy. Am J Obstet Gynecol 47:389–394, 1944.

43. Weinberger SE, Weiss ST, Pulmonary disease. In Burrow GN, Ferris TF: Medical Complications during Pregnancy. Philadelphia, WB Saunders, 1988, p 448.

44. Schwartz DB: Medical disorders in pregnancy. Emerg Med Clin North Am 5(3):509–528, 1987.

45. DiMarco AF: Asthma in the pregnancy patient: a review. Ann Allergy 62(6):527–533, 1989.

46. Noble PW, Lavee AE, Jacobs MM: Respiratory disease in pregnancy. Obstet Gynecol Clin North Am 15(2):391–423, 1988.

47. Steinius-Aarniala B, Piirila P, Teramo K: Asthma and pregnancy: perspective study of 198 pregnancies. Thorax 43:12–18, 1988.

48. Schatz M, Zeiger RS, Harden KM, Hoffman Cp, Forsythe AB, Chilinger LM, et al.: The safety of inhaled β-agonist bronchodilators during pregnancy. J Allergy Clin Immunol 82:686–695, 1988.

49. Romero R, Lockwood C: The use of anti-asthmatic drugs in pregnancy. In Niebyl JR (ed): Drug Use in Pregnancy. Philadelphia, Lea & Febiger, 1988, pp 67–82.

50. Huff RW: Asthma in pregnancy. Med Clin North Am 73(3):653–659, 1989.

51. Greenberger PA, Patterson R: Management of asthma during pregnancy. N Engl J Med 312(14):897–902, 1985.

52. Drayer JI, Zegarelli EC: Hypertension and pregnancy. Cardiovasc Clin 19(3):97–111, 1989.

53. Schoenfeld A, Segal J, Freidman S, Hirsch M, Oradia J: Adverse reactions to antihypertensive drugs in pregnancy. Obstet Gynecol Surv 41(2):67–73, 1986.

54. Doany W, Brinkman CR III: Antihypertension drugs in pregnancy. Clin Perinatol 14(4):783–805, 1987.

55. Liauw PCY: The management of hypertension in pregnancy. Sing Med J 30:590–596, 1989.

56. Repke JT: Pharmacologic management of hypertension in pregnancy. In Niebyl JR (ed): Drug Use in Pregnancy. Philadelphia, Lea & Febiger, 1988, pp 55–65.

57. Feinberg LE, Hypertension and preeclampsia. In Abrams RS, Wexler P (eds): Medical Care of the Pregnant Patient. Boston, Little, Brown, 1983, pp 161–182.

58. Rubin PC: Current concepts: β-blockers in pregnancy. N Engl J Med 305:11323–11326, 1981.

59. Dubois D, Peticolas J, Temperville B, Klepper A: Treatment with atenolol of hypertension in pregnancy. Drugs 25(suppl 2):215–218, 1983.

60. Rubin PC, Butters L, Clark DM, Reynolds B, Sumner DJ, Steedman D, et al.: Placebo-controlled trial of atenolol in treatment of pregnancy-associated hypertension. Lancet 1:431–434, 1983.

61. Frishman WH, Chesner M: Beta-adrenergic blockers in pregnancy. Am Heart J 115:147–152, 1988.

62. Pickles CJ, Symonds EM, Broughton Pipkin F: The fetal outcome in a randomized trial of labetalol versus placebo in pregnancy-induced hypertension. Br J Obstet Gynecol 96:38–43, 1989.

63. Scialli AR: Anticonvulsants in pregnancy. In Niebyl JR (ed): Drug Use in Pregnancy. Phildelphia, Lea & Febiger, 1988, pp 45–54.

64. Anon: Anticonvulsants and pregnancy. American Academy of Pediatrics Committee on Drugs. Prediatrics 63:331–333, 1979.

65. Patterson RM: Seizure disorders in pregnancy. Med Clin North Am 73(3):661–665, 1989.

66. Janz D: Antiepileptic drugs and pregnancy: altered utilization patterns and teratogenesis. Epilepsia 23(suppl):S53–S63, 1982.

67. Jones KL, Lacro RV, Johnson KA, Adams J: Pattern of malformations in the children of women treated with carbamazepine during pregnancy. N Engl J Med 320:1661–1666, 1989.

68. Hare JW, White P: Gestational diabetes and the White classification. Diabetes Care 3:394–398, 1980.

69. Coustan DR, Felig P, Diabetes mellitus. In Burrow GN, Ferris TF (eds): Medical Complications during Pregnancy. Philadelphia, WB Saunders, 1988, pp 34–64.

70. Goldberg E, Anticoagulants in pregnancy. In Niebyl JR (ed): Drug Use in Pregnancy. Philadelphia, Lea & Febiger, 1988, pp 83–88.

71. Hall JG, Pauli RM, Wilson KM: Maternal and fetal sequelae of anticoagulation during pregnancy. Am J Med 68:122–140, 1980.

72. Key TC, Gastrointestinal diseases. In Creasy RK, Resnik R (eds): Maternal-Fetal Medicine: Principles and Practice. Philadelphia, WB Saunders, 1989, pp 1032–1046.

73. Parry E, Shields R, Turnbull AC: The effect of pregnancy on colonic absorption of sodium, potassium and water. Br J Obstet Gynecol 77:616–620, 1970.

74. Chasnoff IJ, Diggs G, Schnoll SH: Fetal alcohol effects and maternal cough syrup abuse. Am J Dis Child 135:968–974, 1981.

75. MacGowan RJ, MacGowan CA, Serdula MK, Lane M, Joesoef RM, Cook FH: Breast-feeding among women attending women, infants, and children clinics in Georgia, 1987. Pediatr 87(3):361–366, 1991.

76. Lawrence RA: Breastfeeding and medical disease. Med Clin North Am 73(3):583–603, 1989.

77. Berlin CM Jr: Drugs and chemicals: exposure of the nursing mother. Pediatr Clin North Am 36(5):1089–1097, 1989.

78. Anderson PO: Drugs and breastfeeding. Drug Intell Clin Pharm 11:208–223, 1977.

79. Anon: Transfer of drugs and other chemicals into human milk. American Academy of Pediatrics. Pediatrics 84(5):924–936, 1989.

CHAPTER 89

ALZHEIMER'S DISEASE

DARLENE FUJIMOTO, Pharm.D. and SAM K. SHIMOMURA, Pharm.D.

The most common cause of dementia is a primary cerebral disorder called Alzheimer's disease or primary dementia of the Alzheimer's type, which was first described in 1907 by a neuropsychiatrist, Alois Alzheimer. Alzheimer's disease is recognized as a syndrome of clinical features characterized by a decline of memory and other cognitive functions in comparison with the patient's previous level of function (1). Alzheimer's disease has an insidious onset, is progressive, and is differentiated by the exclusion of other diseases that would account for the cognitive deterioration and personality changes. Disturbances in memory are the hallmark of this disease, but other cognitive areas such as language use, visual-spatial perception, the ability to learn, solve problems, think abstractly and make judgments are also affected (2).

EPIDEMIOLOGY

Alzheimer's disease is responsible for about 55% of cases of dementia and afflicts approximately 2 to 4 million people in the United States. A recent study found that 10.3% of the population over 65 has Alzheimer's disease. The prevalence increases with age: for those 65 to 74 years of age, it is 3.0%; 75 to 84 years of age, 18.7%; and among those over 85 years, 47.2% (3). It is estimated that over 50% of nursing home patients have dementia. It also appears to occur slightly more frequently in women than in men (2). More than 100,000 people die of Alzheimer's disease each year, making it the fourth most prevalent cause of death in adults after heart disease, cancer, and stroke (4).

ETIOLOGY

Although the dementia syndrome may be caused by over 60 disorders, most cases are due to Alzheimer's disease followed by multiinfarct dementia or a combination of the two. Other important causes of dementia include infections, neurodegenerative disorders, toxins, and metabolic disorders (Table 89.1). The cause of up to 5% of cases of dementia remains unknown. The risk factors for Alzheimer's dementia include advancing age and sex (women more than men), a history of serious head trauma, thyroid disease, and Down's syndrome. Approximately one-third of Alzheimer's patients appear to have a genetic link (5).

Alzheimer's disease is thought to be correlated with diminished neuron function and a decrease in neurotransmitters. The major biochemical abnormality observed in Alzheimer's disease is a 40 to 90% decrease in the enzyme choline acetyltransferase in the cerebral cortex and hippocampus. The deficiency of this enzyme causes decreased synthesis of acetylcholine in the brain. The loss of acetyltransferase in the brain appears to begin within the first year of onset of the symptoms of dementia, and there seems to be a strong correlation between the degree of enzyme reduction and the decline of mental status scores. Trials with precursors of acetylcholine such as choline or lecithin have predictably not demonstrated improvement in mental status, since Alzheimer's disease patients lack acetyltransferase and are unable to convert the precursors to acetylcholine. On the other hand, drugs such as physostigmine, which block acetylcholinesterase and therefore decrease the catabolism of acetylcholine, have had limited success. This type of drug would only be effective when acetylcholine is still being formed by the remaining cholinergic neurons.

Acetylcholine is the primary neurotransmitter deficit associated with Alzheimer's disease, but other neurotransmitters have been implicated. For example, somatostatin is often deficient in patients with Alzheimer's disease, as are the number of somatostatin receptors. There is also a study that reports a decrease in corticotropin-releasing factor (6). Variable losses in the amount of norepinephrine, the biosynthetic enzyme dopamine β-hydroxylase, and serotonin cells have been studied, but no consistent correlations have been shown with Alzheimer's disease.

PATHOGENESIS

From brain autopsy studies, Alzheimer's disease patients have been found to have cortical atrophy, a significant loss of neurons, an increase in neuritic plaques, and a high density of neurofibrillary tangles (Fig. 89.1). Neurofibrillary tangles are abnormal neurons containing bundles of filamentous structures in the cytoplasm. These filaments are wound around each other in a helical fashion. Neuritic plaques are small spheres with an amyloid protein core surrounded by degenerating nerve terminals. Two amyloid proteins, β-amyloid protein and paired helical filament protein are present in those hallmark lesions and may be

Table 89.1.
Causes of Dementia Syndrome[a]

Psychiatic disorders	Metabolic diseases	Intracranial conditions
Depression	Renal failure	Hydrocephalus
Delirium	Fluid and electrolyte imbalances	Brain tumor
Paranoid states	Hypoglycemia	Multiinfarct dementia (stroke)
Schizophrenia	Hyperglycemia	Degenerative neurological disorders
Trauma	Hypothyroidism	Alzheimer's disease
Subdural hematoma	Hyperthyroidism	Pick's disease
Dementia pugilistica	Hepatic failure	Huntington's chorea
Drugs and toxins	Addison's disease	Parkinson's disease
Antidepressants	Cushing's syndrome	Cardiovascular
Lithium carbonate	Hypopituitarism	Congestive heart failure
Anticholinergics	Severe anemia	Arrhythmia
Alcohol	Hypoxia and anoxia	Vascular occlusion
Benzodiazepines	Infections	Nutritional disorders
Barbiturates	AIDS	Vitamin B_{12} deficiency
Propranolol	Neurosyphilis	Folate deficiency
Methyldopa	Meningitis	Collagen vascular disorders
Reserpine	Tuberculosis	Systemic lupus erythematosus
Heavy metal poisoning	Pneumonia	Temporal arteritis
Organophosphates	Creutzfeldt-Jakob (slow-virus) dementia	

[a] Table represents a partial list.

Figure 89.1. Neurofibrillary degeneration (*arrows*) within Sommer's sector of the hippocampus. Bielschowsky silver impregnation, ×360.

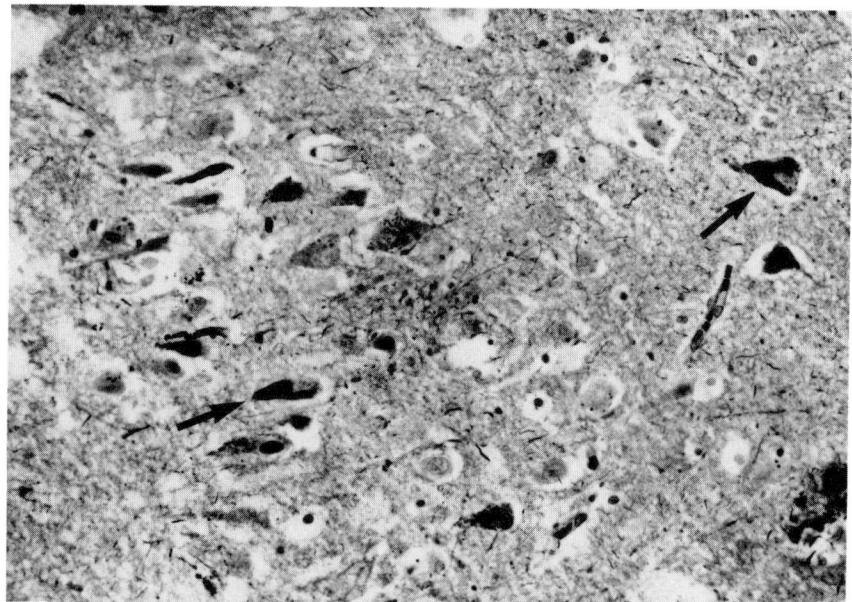

linked to the cause of Alzheimer's disease (7). In autopsy studies, the degree of plaque formation has been highly correlated with the degree of clinical impairment observed when the patient was alive.

SIGNS AND SYMPTOMS

To help clarify discussions of the disease, the progression of Alzheimer's disease is divided into three stages. The first stage, or mild Alzheimer's disease is characterized by signs of minimal memory impairment, especially in recall of recent events. The onset of symptoms is often overlooked as a natural progression of aging. The loss of choline acetyltransferase begins within the first year of the onset of symptoms in these patients (8). Patients may express concern about forgetfulness but do not display a clear memory deficit during clinical interview. There may be some disorientation, impaired concentration, and anxiety, all of which are fairly nonspecific symptoms. Judgment is relatively intact and the capacity for independent living remains.

In the second stage, or moderate Alzheimer's disease, memory impairment progresses, and deficits of the early stage become more pronounced. There is decreased performance in demanding employment or social situations; co-workers notice poor performance at work, and friends and co-workers may become aware of deficits before the patient does. Blunting of emotions and apathy are common. Judgment and the capacity for abstract thinking and calculation begin to wane or are lost. Patients have difficulty finding words and names. The prevalence of agitation can increase with disease progression. Psychotic symptoms such as hallucinations, delusions, and paranoia may become more prevalent toward the end of this stage. Patients often become disoriented, lost, or wander, and independent living becomes hazardous.

In the final stage, or severe Alzheimer's disease, there is a disturbance of practically all intellectual function. Patients are disoriented and incapacitated. Activities of daily living are so impaired that independent living is impossible. There are marked neurologic deficits and often increased muscle tone and akinesia, resulting in a slow, unsteady gait. There is emotional disinhibition with a loss of former personality traits. Patients cannot recognize relatives or remember their own names. They eventually become bedfast, incontinent of bowel and bladder, and suffer progressive wasting of functions. Death is usually the result of pneumonia or other infections.

From onset of symptoms, the life-span of a patient with Alzheimer's disease ranges from 2 to over 20 years. The average life-span after onset is about 7 years.

DIAGNOSIS AND CLINICAL FINDINGS

The National Institute of Neurological and Communicative Disorders and Stroke and the Alzheimer's Disease and Related Disorders Association (now known as the Alzheimer's Association) established a group to refine the diagnosis of Alzheimer's disease in 1984 (9). The work group's criteria are compatible with DSM-III-R (Table 89.2). NINCDS/ADRDA Criteria for Clinical Diagnosis of Alzheimer's disease (Table 89.3) are used as a standard for clinical and research diagnosis. With these criteria, the accuracy rate for diagnosis has increased from less than 50% to at least 90%.

There is a definite need to accurately identify any treatable or reversible causes of dementia. A thorough history and an extensive battery of tests should be performed, not to diagnose Alzheimer's disease, but to eliminate these other causes (Table 89.4). Diagnostic errors are often made because of the failure to recognize depression or pseudodementia, as a cause of memory loss and other symptoms associated with Alzheimer's disease. Depression is a potentially treatable illness that must be distinguished

Table 89.2.
DSM-IIIR Criteria for Alzheimer's Disease (Primary Degenerative Dementia)[a]

Dementia
> Demonstrable evidence of impairment in short- and long-term memory.
> At least one of the following:
> 1. Impairment in abstract thinking (e.g., inability to find similarities and differences between related words, difficulty in defining words and concepts)
> 2. Impaired judgment (inability to make reasonable plans to deal with interpersonal, family, and job-related problems and issues)
> 3. Other disturbances of higher cortical function (e.g., aphasia, apraxia, agnosia, and "constructional difficulty"
> 4. Personality change
> The impairment or disturbances significantly interferes with work or usual social activities or relationships with others
> The impairment or disturbances does not occur exclusively during the course of delirium
> Either of the following:
> 1. There is evidence from the history, physical examination, or laboratory tests of a specific organic factor (or factors) judged to be etiologically related to the disturbance
> 2. In the absence of such evidence, an etiologic organic factor can be presumed if the disturbance cannot be accounted for by any nonorganic mental disorder (e.g., major depression accounting for cognitive impairment)
Insidious onset with uniformly progressive deteriorating course
Exclusion of all other specific causes of dementia by history, physical examination, and laboratory tests

[a] From American Psychiatric Association Diagnostic and Statistical Manual of Mental Disorders, IIIR, Washington, D.C., 1987.

from Alzheimer's disease. Mental status examinations and psychometric testing are important in the clinical identification of depression versus dementia.

Drugs often cause delirium or exacerbate an existing organic dementia. Although delirium tends to have a more abrupt onset and fluctuating course, its presentation may mimic dementia syndrome. Any medication the patient is taking should be evaluated for its ability to cause memory problems and confusion. The elderly use many medicines high in anticholinergic side effects and are very susceptible to the delirium they might cause. Stopping the use of any unnecessary medications or changing the selection of medication to decrease side effects may be a vital therapeutic intervention.

TREATMENT

Although there are no truly successful treatments to be discussed in the drug therapy of Alzheimer's disease, it is important to be acquainted with the wide variety of drug therapies that have been tried over the years and their purported rationales. The families of Alzheimer's disease patients are often desperate to find a cure and will turn to unproven and often expensive treatment modalities.

Table 89.3.
NINCDS/ADRDA Criteria for Clinical Diagnosis of Alzheimer's Disease*a*

Criteria for the clinical diagnosis of *probable* Alzheimer's disease include
  Dementia established by clinical examination and documented by the
    Mini-Mental State Examination, Blessed Dementia Scale, or some
    similar examination and confirmed by neuropsychologic tests
  Deficits in two or more areas of cognition
  Progressive worsening of memory and other cognitive functions
  No disturbance of consciousness
  Onset between ages 40 and 90, most often after age 65
  Absence of systemic disorders or other brain diseases that could ac-
    count for the progressive deficits in memory and cognition
The diagnosis of *probable* Alzheimer's disease is supported by
  Progressive deterioration of specific cognitive functions such as lan-
    guage (aphasia), motor skills (apraxia), and perception (agnosia)
  Impaired activities of daily living and altered patterns of behavior
  Family history of similar disorders, particularly if confirmed neuro-
    pathologically
  Laboratory results as follows: normal lumbar puncture as evaluated by
    standard techniques; normal pattern or nonspecific changes in EEG,
    such as increased slow-wave activity; and evidence of cerebral atro-
    phy on CT with progression documented by serial observation
Other Clinical features consistent with the diagnosis of *probable* Alz-
  heimer's disease, after exclusion of causes of dementia other than Alz-
  heimer's disease, include
Plateaus in the course of progression of the illness
Associated symptoms of depression, insomnia, incontinence, delusions,
  illusions, hallucinations, sexual disorders, weight loss, and cata-
  strophic verbal, emotional, or physical outbursts
Other neurologic abnormalities in some patients especially with more
  advanced disease and including motor signs such as increased muscle
  tone, myoclonus, or gait disorder
Seizures in advanced disease
CT normal for age
	Features that make the diagnosis of *probable* Alzheimer's disease un-
	  certain or unlikely include
	  Sudden, apoplectic onset
	  Focal neurologic findings such as hemiparesis, sensory loss, visual field
	    deficits, and incoordination early in the course of the illness
	  Seizures or gait disturbances at the onset or very early in the course
	    of the illness
	Clinical diagnosis of *possible* Alzheimer's disease
	  May be made on the basis of the dementia syndrome, in the absence
	    of other neurologic, psychiatric, or systemic disorders sufficient to
	    cause dementia and in the presence of variations in the onset, pre-
	    sentation, or clinical course
	  May be made in the presence of a second systemic or brain disorder
	    sufficient to produce dementia, which is not considered to be *the*
	    cause of the dementia
	  Should be used in research studies when a single, gradually progressive,
	    severe cognitive deficit is identified in the absence of another iden-
	    tifiable cause
	Criteria for diagnosis of *definite* Alzheimer's disease are
	  The clinical criteria for probable Alzheimer's disease
	  Histopathologic evidence obtained from a biopsy or autopsy
	Classification of Alzheimer's disease for research purposes should specify
	  features that may differentiate subtypes of the disorder, such as
	  Familial occurrence
	  Onset before age 65
	  Presence of trisomy 21
	  Coexistence of other relevant conditions, such as Parkinson's disease

a NINCDS, National Institute of Neurological and Communicative Disorders and Stroke; ADRDA, Alzheimer's Disease and Related Disorders Association.

General guidelines for treating Alzheimer's patients are outlined in Table 89.5. Patients and caregivers must be guided by well-informed professionals.

There are two basic divisions of Alzheimer's drug treatment. The first, and most often used, is *symptomatic* drugs that are palliative and help control unwanted behaviors and maintain patient functioning. The armamentarium consists primarily of psychotropic agents. The other division is *therapeutic*. These agents are used to stop or reverse the disease process and are largely experimental.

Symptomatic Treatments

During the course of Alzheimer's disease, patients experience memory dysfunction, progressive loss of cognitive ability, difficulties in the use of language, and lack of emotional control that often results in disorientation, confusion, agitation, disruption of the sleep-wake cycle and personality changes. Psychotropic medicines are very often needed to help alleviate some of these symptoms as the disease progresses. All psychotropics should be used with caution; those low in anticholinergic side effects are pref-

erable. They should be started at low doses and titrated according to therapeutic response and side effects (Table 89.6).

ANTIDEPRESSANTS

Early stages of Alzheimer's disease are often accompanied by depressive symptoms, which may respond to drug therapy. Resolution of depression results in improvement of mood, functional abilities, and possibly cognitive faculties (10). All patients with dementia should be carefully evaluated for depression. Depressive symptoms such as agitation, memory loss, and insomnia can easily be confused with dementia. A therapeutic trial of antidepressants can be effective in treating a masked depression whose symptoms often mimic Alzheimer's disease. In general, antidepressants should be chosen for Alzheimer's disease patients as for any other depressed patient, by side-effect profiles and a trial for response. Low doses of nortriptyline or trazodone given once or twice a day are often beneficial. Sedating antidepressants can also be used for their calming

Table 89.4.
Diagnosis of Dementia

History—from patient, relative, close associates
Mental status examination (especially mild and moderate stages)
Physical examination including vital signs
Neurologic examination
CT scan/magnetic resonance imaging
Laboratory tests
    Thyroid function tests (T_4, T_3RU, TSH)
    Serum B_{12}
    Folic acid
    CBC with RBC indices
    Syphilis serology (VDRL, FTA/MHATP)
    Glucose
    BUN/creatinine
    Calcium/phosphorus
    Albumin
    Electrolytes
    Alkaline phosphatase
    Sedimentation rate
Optional/suggested procedures and tests:
    Chest x-ray
    Electrocardiogram
    Electroencephalogram
    Lumbar puncture
    Urinalysis
    Drug screens/levels

Table 89.5.
Guidelines for Treatment of Patients with Alzheimer's Disease

1. The differential diagnosis of cognitive impairment is imperative prior to treatment. Rigorously pursue the diagnosis of any treatable states that may cause dementia; especially consider depression.
2. Avoid any unnecessary use of medications. Alzheimer's disease patients have little reserve capacity against toxicities and are therefore more prone to adverse effects.
3. Individualize therapy. Each patient exhibits different behavioral and cognitive manifestations of the disease. Optimum dosages of medications used in Alzheimer's disease have not be established. Dosages must be individually titrated and monitored. Also consider that, because of the progressive nature of the disease, therapy should not be static and must be reevaluated and changed accordingly.
4. Carefully monitor patients on medications. The effects seen are usually moderate or may only manifest as a slowing of decline rather than improvement in function. Adverse effects are frequent; also note other medications (e.g., cardiac, nonsteroidal antiinflammatory, antihypertensive) may exacerbate mental decline.
5. Always be cognizant of the fact that medications all have toxicities that may cause or unmask the very problems they are trying to treat.
6. Discontinue ineffective or unnecessary medications.

Table 89.6.
Representative Starting Doses of Psychotropic Medications Used with Alzheimers's Disease Patients

Antidepressants	
Nortriptyline (Pamelor)	10 mg b.i.d.-t.i.d.
Trazodone (Desyrel)	25 mg q.d.-b.i.d.
Desipramine (Norpramin)	10 mg b.i.d.-t.i.d.
Penelzine (Nardil)	15 mg b.i.d.
Fluoxetine (Prozac)	20 mg q.o.d.
Anxiolytics	
Lorazepam (Ativan)	0.5 mg b.i.d.
Alprazolam (Xanax)	0.25 mg b.i.d.-t.i.d.
Oxazepam (Serax)	10 mg b.i.d.-t.i.d.
Buspirone (Buspar)	5 mg b.i.d.-t.i.d.
Neuroleptics	
Thioridazine (Mellaril)	10 mg q.d.-b.i.d.
Haloperidol (Haldol)	0.5 mg q.d.-b.i.d.
Thiothixene (Navane)	1.0 mg q.d.-b.i.d.
Hypnotics	
Triazolam (Halcion)	0.125 mg q.d.
Temazepam (Restoril)	15 mg q.d.
Chloral hydrate (Noctec)	250–500 mg q.d.

effects to help decrease excessive excitation and agitation. A bedtime dose may alleviate symptoms of insomnia.

The clinical symptoms of Alzheimer's disease have been correlated in neurochemical studies to deficits of acetylcholine in the brain. Some clinicians are therefore wary of using drugs with anticholinergic properties to treat these patients because of the possibility of exacerbating memory impairment and cognitive decline. In most cases, antidepressants are beneficial, and with proper titration and monitoring they can be safely recommended.

In depressed Alzheimer's disease patients who do not respond to tricyclic antidepressants and other standard antidepressants or those who suffer troublesome side effects, the use of monoamine oxidase inhibitors (MAOIs) should be considered. The enzyme monoamine oxidase (MAO) has been shown to increase with age, and demented patients may have even higher levels of MAO than age-matched controls (11). MAOIs do not adversely affect memory and cognitive function like tricyclics; unfortunately postural hypotension and the possibility of hypertensive crisis can limit their usefulness in these patients.

HYPNOTICS

Insomnia is a common complaint in the elderly, and sleep disturbances are more frequent in patients with dementia. Sleep difficulties often distress patients and can lead to exhaustion of caregivers. Sleep disturbance can be manifested by patients being awake at night, pacing, trying to go outside, or searching for lost items. Hypnotics should be avoided if at all possible because of their widespread central nervous system depressant effects. Regulating patients' schedules, keeping them active during the day, and preventing daytime napping all help to decrease insomnia. When a hypnotic is absolutely necessary, the lowest dose for the shortest duration should be used. The short-acting benzodiazepines (triazolam 0.125 mg, temazepam 15 mg) are often helpful, but they should be used judiciously because they can increase confusion and memory impairment, worsen depressive symptoms, and aggravate most other cognitive symptoms occurring in Alzheimer's disease. Longer half-life benzodiazepines should be avoided because of their tendency to accumulate and cause oversedation. Chloral hydrate in low doses (250 mg to 1 g) has been used with benefit. Chloral hydrate has many adverse side effects and more drug interactions than benzodiazepines, and as with the benzodiazepines, caution should be taken because this drug can also exacerbate symptoms of Alzheimer's disease. Diphenhydramine, an antihistamine, has been used for its moderate sedating properties, but it also has anticholinergic effects that may increase confusion. Because of its limited efficacy and potential side effects it is not recommended. It is important to minimize the constant use of hypnotics. The efficacy of long-term, routine use of hypnotics has not been proven. Maintaining daytime activity and giving other sedating medications at bedtime and "as needed" hypnotics can sufficiently control insomnia.

ANXIOLYTICS

Anxiety frequently affects patients with memory loss. The elderly often manifest their anxiety in somatic form such as agitation, motor restlessness, and insomnia. The judicious use of benzodiazepines or neuroleptics in treating these symptoms has been successful. Short half-life benzodiazepines in low doses given once or twice a day are often useful. The use of benzodiazepines for anxiety is limited by side effects. They act on the central nervous system to produce confusion, drowsiness, and amnesia, which mimics and confounds Alzheimer's disease. They also can cause gait instability and have been correlated with an increased frequency of falls.

NEUROLEPTICS

Neuroleptics are indicated for the treatment of psychotic symptoms such as hallucinations, paranoia, and severe agitation, which are stressful to the patient or interfere with the daily care of the patients. Neuroleptics do not affect higher cortical functions such as memory, judgment, and problem solving. No single neuroleptic emerges as a superior agent. The high-potency antipsychotics (haloperidol, fluphenazine) leave the patient prone to extrapyramidal side effects such as pseudoparkinsonism and tardive dyskinesia. Low-potency (chlorpromazine, thioridazine) agents are anticholinergic and have cardiovascular side ef-

fects. The adverse effects may further impair the remaining physical and cognitive functions of Alzheimer's disease patients. Movement may be decreased, hypotension may cause falling, and sedation may exacerbate confusion. Low doses (e.g., haloperidol 0.5 to 1 mg) given once or twice a day are usually sufficient. A late afternoon or early evening dose may lessen daytime sedation and decrease "sundowning" (a phenomenon of agitation and confusion worsening in the evening).

Benefits of psychotropic medications are variable, and responses to agents are highly individual and limited by adverse effects. Psychotropics are useful and can improve behavior and functioning, easing the burden of care. The efficacy of neuroleptics in controlling agitation is modest at best. Neuroleptics have potentially severe and permanent side effects and their use should be minimized. Strict monitoring is imperative to prevent more harm than benefit from the use of these medications. Developing literature has suggested alternative drugs for uncontrollable agitation such as carbamazepine and trazodone; benefits have been shown, but studies are preliminary and include only a small population of patients.

Because the disease is progressive, therapy should be evaluated at least every 6 months to ensure that the fewest drugs are being used in the lowest effective doses. Tapering psychotropic medications in stabilized patients at regular intervals is effective in assessing the need for continued drug therapy. Families and caregivers should be counseled. They must understand that psychotropic medications may improve some symptoms but will not improve dementia or prevent further deterioration of function. The caregivers' understanding of the disease process and the effects of drug therapy often lessens the use of medication.

Therapeutic Treatments

Therapeutic drugs are believed to slow or reverse defects that might contribute to brain failure in Alzheimer's disease patients. Most therapeutic treatments are investigational. Pharmacologic investigations of drug therapy present several vexing problems:

1. *Patient selection is variable.* Alzheimer's disease is a diagnosis of exclusion. Definitive diagnosis by biopsy at this time is unwarranted, and autopsy is the only sure means of conclusively identifying the cause of this clinical syndrome. Misdiagnosis is possible. Study patients are probably heterogeneous, with some patients having combinations of diseases (e.g., Alzheimer's disease, multinfarct dementia, Parkinson's disease) that further cloud their diagnosis and complicate treatment.
2. *Evaluation of drug therapy is complicated.* Cognition and behavior are difficult to monitor empirically. There are no standardized testing procedures for monitoring the wide range of deficits and symptoms occurring with this disease.
3. *Alzheimer's disease is a multisymptom disease.* Various phys-

ical, cortical changes, and neurotransmitter deficits have been correlated with the disease. When Alzheimer's disease is further characterized, treatment will probably consist of a combination of therapies. Drug therapy will probably affect the balance of cholinergic and other neurotransmitter systems because of the multiple neurochemical abnormalities and brain functions affected.

METABOLIC ENHANCERS

Hydergine (ergoloid mesylates) is the only drug with a Food and Drug Administration (FDA) approved indication for use in the cognitive decline of the elderly. It was originally thought that the beneficial effect of the ergoloid mesylates was the result of cerebral vasodilation. This is no longer believed to be the mechanism of benefit, because Alzheimer's disease patients have not been shown to have greatly decreased cerebral blood flow. In fact, by dilating normal arteries in the brain and periphery, blood may be shunted away from ischemic areas. Ergoloid mesylates are now classified as metabolic enhancers. Their proposed mechanisms are to increase certain enzymes, alter glucose and oxygen utilization, and act as α-adrenoreceptor blockers and as serotonin and dopamine agonists. How the pharmacologic effects are related to clinical efficacy is uncertain (12). They are purported to stabilize and possibly slow the mental decline of Alzheimer's disease.

Studies show some improvement in behavioral variables that include mood, attention, and performance of specific tasks when given early in the course of dementia, which may be related to a mild antidepressant effect. Once the disease has progressed and there is serious cognitive impairment, little effect is expected. Ergoloid mesylates can usually be safely administered with mild and occasional adverse effects of gastrointestinal upset and bradycardia.

Optimum doses for Alzheimer's disease patients have not been established. However, most recent studies have used 6 mg/day or more, which is above the FDA-recommended dosage of 3 mg/day. Liquid capsules are recommended because of their higher bioavailability (approximately 12% more bioavailable than the tablet). A drug trial during mild or early moderate stages of Alzheimer's disease may be beneficial and should last at least 6 months. If no benefit is seen or if symptoms of the disease progress, the drug should be discontinued.

The efficacy and dosage of ergoloid mesylates are still questionable. Despite a preponderance of studies showing positive effects, the favorable results are not consistent from one study to another and tend to be more statistically significant than medically important.

CHOLINERGIC AGENTS

At present the cholinergic deficit hypothesis provides a viable explanation of the memory impairment that occurs in Alzheimer's disease, but it does not account for all the clinical deficits that occur in this type of dementia. Neurochemical studies of Alzheimer's disease patients have shown a deficiency of the neurotransmitter acetylcholine and the enzyme responsible for its synthesis, choline acetyltransferase. A positive correlation has been reported between the degree of cognitive impairment in Alzheimer's disease patients and decreases in choline acetyltransferase and acetylcholine (13). Comparisons between Alzheimer's disease patients and age-matched controls have demonstrated neuronal losses in the nucleus basalis of Meynert, an area thought to provide cholinergic input to the cortex and a major cholinergic pathway leading from the septum to the hippocampus, a structure critical to normal memory function (14).

Several pharmacologic efforts to augment cholinergic activity have focused on (*a*) increasing acetylcholine synthesis and release, (*b*) limiting acetylcholine breakdown by inhibiting acetylcholinesterase, and (*c*) directly stimulating acetylcholine receptors (15).

Agents such as choline and lecithin (phosphytidylcholine) serve as precursors to acetylcholine, and large amounts have been shown to increase acetylcholine concentrations in the brain. Lecithin raises plasma choline levels and does not produce the foul odor that occurs with choline administration. Clinical trials of choline and lecithin have not shown convincing evidence that these substances alone improve cognition in Alzheimer's disease patients. Increasing substrate may not result in increased acetylcholine synthesis. This is probably because the enzyme choline acetyltransferase, required for the synthesis of acetylcholine, is depleted in Alzheimer's disease.

An alternative approach has been to add an agent that facilitates cholinergic neurotransmission. Piracetam, classified as a nootropic agent, is a cyclic derivative of γ-aminobutyric acid (GABA) that enhances the firing rate of the presynaptic neurons. Additionally, it is thought to have an effect as a neuronal metabolic enhancer that may augment the uptake of choline and increase the release of acetylcholine. Studies suggest that piracetam in combination with acetylcholine precursors may benefit a subgroup of patients who have some functionally intact cholinergic neurons (16).

Cholinesterase inhibitors (physostigmine, tacrine) increase the amount of available acetylcholine in the synaptic cleft by limiting its breakdown. Physostigmine is a centrally active acetylcholinesterase inhibitor that prevents the enzymatic hydrolysis of acetylcholine released in the synapse. It has been administered both intravenously and orally with some success. In human studies, physostigmine has been shown to have a therapeutic window. It enhances memory in a narrow, low-dose range; at higher doses physostigmine can actually impair memory. Therefore individual doses must first be tested for each subject using the drug. Intravenous doses have shown statistically significant, moderate, and transient improvements in visual recognition memory tests (17). Although several studies corroborate improvements (18), clinical applicability is more difficult to prove, and physostigmine use is limited by the short duration of action and adverse side effects such as nausea, vomiting, diarrhea, dizziness, and headache. Oral physostigmine has resulted in modest improvements in cognitive areas, some selective memory tests, and overall functioning in certain patients (19). Variability of the responses to oral physostigmine is due to differences in drug absorption and penetration into the central nervous systems of individual patients (20).

Tacrine (tetrahydroaminoacridine or THA), a centrally active anticholinesterase with a longer duration of action than physostigmine, has shown encouraging results as a palliative treatment in Alzheimer's disease (21). However, concern over hepatotoxicity have dimmed the early optimistic reports. There has been a high prevalence (30%) of abnormal liver function tests, which usually return to normal with decreases in doses or discontinuance of drug therapy. A few occurrences of liver necrosis and jaundice have been reported. The data available on tacrine remain inconclusive (22).

There appears to be no further loss of muscarinic receptors in Alzheimer's disease patients beyond that found with normal aging (23). Bethanecol, an acetycholine-like agonist, given by intracranial infusion resulted in clinical improvement in some patients (24). These drug trials are all preliminary, with testing completed on small sample populations. When improvements occurred they were in no way dramatic, and the memory of demented patients remained impaired. Cholinergic agents are limited by their toxicities including liver impairment and seizures, short half-lives, and difficult administration. It is also hypothesized that acetylcholine is released in a pulsatile fashion and that replacement by infusion may not be physiologically equivalent, limiting therapeutic benefits.

The minimal benefits, systemic side effects, and difficulty of administration presently limit the applicability of most cholinergic treatments. It is still to be determined if any or all of these cholinergic mechanisms are involved in the cognitive impairment of Alzheimer's disease patients. Ultimately, treatments using these pharmacologic strategies may have to be used in combination, with regimens individualized for each patient.

Although evidence supports the cholinergic hypothesis of memory and cognitive function, it is highly unlikely that this impairment is the sole disorder occurring in Alzheimer's disease. Alzheimer's disease probably results from a combination of neuronal changes (such as decreases in protein synthesis, production of abnormal proteins, and impaired energy production) and neurotransmitter deficits in the brain. With advancing knowledge of the etiology of Alzheimer's disease, new therapies can be developed. The list of pharmacologic efforts to treat Alzheimer's disease are based on various theories, and the list of therapies tried continues to expand. Table 89.7 lists several of these agents. Most outcomes of these trials are moderately positive at best, and there is yet no clinically useful pharmacologic agent for the treatment of Alzheimer's disease. Ultimately therapy will probably consist of a combination of medications based on etiology and symptoms. The optimum therapy will prevent or reverse the disease process itself.

Environment

Besides pharmacotherapy, a comprehensive plan should include adequate nutrition, correction of sensory deficits (e.g., glasses, hearing aids), and attention to the social environment. A stable, comfortable environment will minimize the strain of decreasing mental capacities and lessen confusion. Patients should be stimulated and helped to function, but choices, which may overwhelm and confuse them, should be limited. Labeling items with names, and laying out one change of clothes will help maintain the patient's ability to perform activities of daily living. Alterations in surroundings such as room changes should be minimized. Physical and psychosocial stressors such as minor surgery, bereavement, or institutionalization, can and often will aggravate intellectual deficits in a demented patient. Within reason, familiar furnishings, diet, and routines should be maintained.

Caregiver training is important. Caregivers must understand the limitations of the patient's cognition and how that affects their behaviors. Patients are often confused and cannot process what is going on around them. A lot of the interactions between patients and caregivers can be modified to best suit the patient and prevent or minimize incidents that might lead to agitation and difficulty in caring for the patient.

Family Support

The treatment plan should provide adequate emotional support for family members and those providing most patient care. Referring the family to the local branch of the Alzheimer's Association and to books such as the *Thirty-Six Hour Day* (25) is often as valuable as any current drug therapy. Relatives of Alzheimer's disease patients who are experiencing changes in the patient's cognitive abilities and personality and in their relationship with the Alzheimer's disease patient grieve for their own sense of loss (26). Families must be educated about the disease and expectations of therapy. There are no medical cures, and the disease waxes and wanes but is progressive. Often a rational presentation of the disease will allay fears, allow sensible expectations, and enhance the family's ability to provide sup-

Table 89.7.
Drugs Tried in the Treatment of Alzheimer's Disease

Drug	Rationale for Use/Mode of Action	Evaluation
Metabolic enhancer		
Ergoloid mysylates	Metabolic enhancer	Modest, but statistically significant effect of clinical symptoms, possibly due to mood elevation
Nootropic agents		
Piracetam	Enhance brain metabolism	Controlled clinical studies show equivocal results, limited clinical utility; response may improve when given with precursors (e.g., lecithin)
Vasodilators		
Cyclandelate	Enhanced blood flow to the brain	Limited clinical efficacy; AD is not correlated with a decrease in blood flow; may actually be detrimental by shunting blood from diseased tissue
Isoxsuprine		
Psychostimulants		
Methylphenidate	Central nervous system stimulants	No sound evidence of therapeutic benefit; may be of limited value in treating symptoms of fatigue, motor retardation, depressed mood
Pemoline		
Pentylenetetrazol		
Anesthetic		
Procaine hydrochloride (Gerovital H3)	Mild CNS stimulant with local anesthetic action; weak MAO inhibitor	May have mild mood-elevating effects; not approved by FDA for dementia
Precursors to acetylcholine		
Choline chloride	Increase amount of ACh in plasma	Most clinical trials conclude not effective alone
Lecithin		
Acetylcholinersterase inhibitors		
Tacrine	Prevent breakdown of ACh	Mostly clinically modest effects on selected cognitive measures
Physostigmine		
ACh-like agonists		
Bethanecol	Muscarinic agonists	Some subjective improvement reported

port to the patient without the use of medications. It must always be remembered that all drugs have toxicities and many may exacerbate the symptoms they are given to treat. Medications are often used to maintain patients in the home. Caregivers must understand the dangers of over-medication and the need to administer medications only as directed. Families and caregivers closest to the patients should be included in therapeutic decisions and often provide the best monitoring information available.

Because of the lack of nursing home beds and their high costs, alternative care will become even more important in the future. Patients in early stages of Alzheimer's disease need education and counseling. They are often responsible for their own drug therapy. When family members become involved in care, their understanding of drug therapy and the ability to comply with regimens should be evaluated. Care for the caregivers is often as important as care of the patient. Remember that an aging spouse may be on the borderline of competency and the added burden of caring for a demented mate may be too much for that person to properly handle. When the caregiver gives out, the care system suffers. Social services provide some aid with home care. Day-care services are offered by various local agencies and provide different levels of supervision and activities for Alzheimer patients. Day-care is especially important in providing much needed respite for the caregivers at home. Eventually most patients will become incapacitated, suffering from aggression, wandering, and incontinence and will often require long-term care placement.

Conclusion

Alzheimer's disease is a complex, progressive, degenerative disorder with no known cure. All potentially reversible causes of dementia should be excluded or treated before a diagnosis of Alzheimer's disease is made. Management includes supportive care and control of detrimental symptoms. The goals of therapy are to maintain the most appropriate level of care and to keep the patient as functional as possible for as long as possible.

REFERENCES

1. Huppert FA, Tym E: Clinical and neuropsychological assessment of dementia. Br Med Bull 42:11–18, 1986.
2. Katzman R: Alzheimer's disease. N Engl J Med 314:964–973, 1986.
3. Evans DA, Funkenstein HH, Albert MS, et al.: Prevalence of Alzheimer's disease in a community population of older persons: higher than previously reported. JAMA 262:2551–2556, 1989.
4. Katzman R: The prevalence and malignancy of Alzheimer's disease, a major killer. Arch Neurol 33:217–218, 1976.

5. Fox JH, Heston LL, Terry RD: Zeroing in on Alzheimer's disease. Patient Care 20:68–91, 1986.

6. Bissette G, Reynolds GP, Kilts CD, et al.: Corticotropin-releasing factor-like immunoreactivity in senile dementia of the Alzheimer type: reduced cortical and striatal concentrations. JAMA 254:3067–3069, 1985.

7. Caputo CB, Salama AI: The amyloid proteins of Alzheimer's disease as potential targets for drug therapy. Neurobiol Aging, 10(5):451–461, 1989.

8. Francis PT, Palmer AM, Sims NR, et al.: Neurochemical studies of early-onset Alzheimer's disease. N Engl J Med 313:7–11, 1985.

9. McKhann G, Drachman D, Folstein M, et al.: Clinical diagnosis of Alzheimer's disease. Neurology 34:939–944, 1984.

10. Reifler BS, Larson E, Teri L, et al.: Dementia of the Alzheimer's type and depression. J Am Geriatr Soc 34:855–859, 1986.

11. Gottfried CG, Adolfsson R, Aquilonius SM, et al.: Biochemical changes in dementia disorders of Alzheimer type (AD/SDAT). Neurobiol Aging 4:261–271, 1983.

12. Hollister LE, Yesavage J: Ergoloid mesylates for senile dementias: unanswered questions. Ann Intern Med 100:894–898, 1984.

13. Bartus RT, Dean RL, Beer B, et al.: The cholinergic hypothesis of geriatric memory dysfunction. Science 217:408–414, 1982.

14. Davis BM, Mohs RC, Greenwald BS, et al.: Clinical studies of the cholinergic deficit in Alzheimer's disease 1. Neurochemical and neuroendocrine studies. J Am Geriatr Soc 33:741–748, 1985.

15. Hollander E, Mohs RC, Davis KL: Cholinergic approaches to the treatment of Alzheimer's disease. Br Med Bull 42:97–100, 1986.

16. Schneck MK, Nootropics. In Reisberg B: Alzheimer's Disease, New York, The Free Press, 1983, p 362.

17. Davis KL, Mohs RC: Enhancement of memory processes in Alzheimer's disease with multiple dose intravenous physostigmine. Am J Psychol 139:1421–1424, 1982.

18. Christie JE, Shering A, Ferguson J, et al.: Physostigmine and arecoline effects of intravenous infusions in Alzheimer presenile dementia. Br J Psychol 138:46–50, 1981.

19. Thal LJ, Masur DM, Blau AD, et al.: Chronic oral physostigmine without lecithin improves memory in Alzheimer's disease. J Am Geriatr Soc 37:42–48, 1989.

20. Hollander E, Mohs RC, Davis KL: Cholinergic approaches to the treatment of Alzheimer's disease. Br Med Bull 42:97–100, 1986.

21. Summer WK, Majovski LV, Marsh GM, et al.: Oral tetrahydroaminoacridine in long-term treatment of senile dementia, Alzheimer type. N Engl J Med 315:1241–1245, 1986.

22. Gamzu ER, Thal LJ, Davis KL: Therapeutic trials using tacrine and other cholinesterase inhibitors. Adv Neurol 51:241–245, 1990.

23. Bartus RT, Dean RL, Beer B, et al.: The cholinergic hypothesis of geriatric memory dysfunction. Science 217:408–414, 1982.

24. Harbaugh RE, Roberts DW, Coombs DW, et al.: Preliminary report: Intracranial cholinergic drug infusion in patients with Alzheimer's disease. Neurosurgery 15:514–518, 1984.

25. Mace NL, Rabins PV: The 36 Hour Day. Baltimore: Johns Hopkin's University Press, 1981.

26. Howell M: Caretakers' views on responsibilities for the care of the demented elderly. J Am Geriatr Soc 32:657–660, 1984.

CHAPTER 90

GERIATRIC DRUG THERAPY

ROBERT J. ANDERSON, Pharm.D. and SUSAN W. MILLER, Pharm.D.

Over 27 million people in the United States are more than 65 years of age. Although they represent only 12% of the population, the geriatric segment consumes 30% of all prescription medications and 40% of all nonprescription medications. They occupy over 30% of all hospital beds and virtually all nursing home beds. By the year 2000, it is projected that 17% of the U.S. population will be over the age of 65 years; the 75- to 84-year-old age group will increase by 60% and the very old, those over the age of 85 will increase by 100%. These demographic changes will continue to have a major impact on both manpower and healthcare expenditures.

Prescription medications are used to manage chronic diseases, especially in the aging population. They help maintain functional capacities, control pain, and keep the elderly out of nursing homes. Despite these potentials, 23% of nursing home admissions can be attributed primarily to patients' inability to manage their medications at home (1), and up to 9% of hospital admissions of patients above the age of 65 are attributable to adverse drug reactions (2). The elderly have more ailments and consequently must take more drugs than younger people. This increases their chances for drug interactions or noncompliance. Some geriatric patients have mental confusion and memory loss related to age, disease, or drugs.

Adverse drug reactions (ADRs) occur much more often in elderly patients than in those under age 60 (Table 90.1). The higher rate of ADRs has been correlated both with age and with the number of drugs taken (3, 4), although number of drugs is clearly the most important single factor. In one study (5), iatrogenic disease, mostly ADRs, more than doubled the duration of the hospitalization. Careful drug-therapy monitoring of the elderly patient by the pharmacist can have a major favorable impact on reducing both the costs of healthcare and the incidence of ADRs. Adverse drug effects may present atypically in geriatric patients. The presentation may be subtle and is often confused with disease progression or concomitant drug therapy.

AGE-RELATED PHYSIOLOGIC AND PHARMACOLOGIC CHANGES

In most cases, clinical response, both therapeutic and toxic, is directly related to the average plasma concentration of the drug. It has been estimated that 70 to 80% of ADRs in the elderly are dose-related pharmacokinetic changes and thus may be prevented. The aging process alone can markedly influence drug response by interfering with the fraction of drug absorbed (f), the plasma drug half-life ($T\frac{1}{2}$), the volume of drug distribution in the body (Vd), and the metabolic and renal clearance from the body (Cl). By knowing which drugs are affected by age-related pharmacokinetic changes, the proper dose and dosing interval can be better estimated. It should be remembered that results of pharmacokinetic studies may differ in healthy-elderly and sick-elderly populations. In addition to alterations in drug kinetics, age can also influence the pharmacologic response of drugs.

Physiologic Changes Influencing Drug Absorption

Both formulation and inherent drug properties (e.g., polarity, solubility, ionization) and patient variables (e.g., gastric pH and emptying time) can influence the rate and in some cases the extent of drug absorbed. It is common for a geriatric patient to be unable to swallow a tablet or capsule. It is frequently necessary to use a liquid dosage form or crush the tablet for administration with food or via a nasogastric tube. In general, extended-release, enteric-coated and sublingual products should not be crushed because of changes in absorption, half-life, and toxicity. For example, crushing removes the protective coating of pentoxifylline, causing patient discomfort, and crushing may cause dumping of large doses of time-release medications. In some situations such as with theophylline preparations, a potential for toxicity exists.

Age-related physiologic changes in the gastrointestinal tract include elevated gastric pH, delayed gastric emptying time, and decreases in both gastrointestinal motility and intestinal blood flow. The decrease in stomach pH lowers response to clorazepate by interfering with its acid-dependent hydrolysis to its active metabolite desmethyldiazepam (6).

The delay in gastric emptying allows (a) more contact time in the stomach for potentially ulcerogenic drugs such as the nonsteroidal antiinflammatory drugs (NSAIDs); (b) a higher frequency of antacid drug interactions, providing more chance for binding; (c) increased absorption of poorly soluble drugs; (d) a higher frequency of diarrhea due to incomplete absorption; and (e) a delay in onset of action of the weakly basic CNS drugs. A threefold increase in levodopa availability in the elderly was thought to be caused by slower gastric emptying, which allowed in-

Table 90.1.
Reasons For High Frequencies of ADRs In Elderly

- Multiple chronic diseases requiring treatment with potent medications
- Several physicians (specialists) prescribing therapy independently
- Inappropriate identification of ADRs
- Patients not complying with prescribed medications or self-medicating inappropriately
- Inadequate patient education on prescribed and over-the-counter (OTC) drugs
- Age-related physiological changes that alter drug kinetics and pharmacological responses to the prescribed medication

creased degradation by dopa decarboxylase to dopamine (7).

Age influences the active transport mechanisms involved in the absorption of sugars (galactose), vitamins (thiamin, folic acid), and minerals (calcium, iron). Because of these changes in absorption and because the elderly often do not consume a balanced diet for economic reasons, the use of a multivitamin/mineral supplement may be indicated. Age-related physiologic changes alone do not seem to influence the passive transport mechanisms by which most drugs are absorbed.

Drugs have reduced bioavailability because of incomplete absorption or first-pass metabolism. Drugs with poor water solubility are likely candidates for incomplete absorption.

Bioavailability problems have been reported with many drugs and the issue of generic substitution is especially important to the geriatric patient because drug costs are so vital to this population (9). It has been suggested that generic substitution not be mandated with certain critically ill patients, those with certain diseases, or those receiving certain drugs (10). Indiscriminate switching among generic products should be avoided, especially for drugs in critical therapeutic categories and for drugs prescribed for debilitated patients. Studies have demonstrated wide bioavailability differences in various brands of generic tolbutamide (8), phenytoin, prednisone, furosemide, and digoxin.

Selected drugs with a high intrinsic clearance in the liver are metabolized during their passage from the portal vein through the liver to the systemic circulation, thus reducing their bioavailability (Fig. 90.1). Elderly patients have collateral circulation that shunts incoming blood directly into the hepatic vein, bypassing the liver and increasing drug bioavailability (11). The bioavailabilities of propranolol, labetalol (12), and verapamil (13) are increased, presumably by a decrease in first-pass metabolism. Other drugs that undergo first-pass metabolism and which may be influenced by age are included in Table 90.2.

Although the total amount of drug absorbed is affected

for only a few drugs, age-related physiologic changes can alter the rate of absorption, resulting in an erratic and sometimes inconsistent pharmacologic response. Physiologic changes and diseases such as acute congestive heart failure often necessitate the use of the intravenous route of administration because of incomplete absorption via the oral and intramuscular (i.m.) routes. There is also a decrease in absorption of i.m.-administered drugs in bedridden elderly patients, probably because of changes in regional blood flow.

Physiologic Changes Influencing Drug Distribution

Age can also change the distribution of the drug to the target organ. Although total protein is unaffected, the plasma albumin portion can decrease with age. Albumin acts as a drug carrier, binding the drug until it is needed. If albumin is decreased, there will be a compensatory increase in active, or unbound, drug. In addition to age, disease states such as cirrhosis, renal failure, and malnutrition can lower albumin levels. The other binding protein, α-l-glycoprotein, does not appear to be affected by age.

Increased blood levels of naproxen, diflunisal, salicylate, acetazolamide, and valproate have been found in the elderly, presumably as a result of this decrease in albumin protein binding (14). Increased blood levels of NSAIDs may be responsible for the reported higher rate of gastric bleeding from peptic ulcers (15).

Decreased protein binding is also seen with phenytoin, but the drug is cleared from the plasma and system more rapidly as a result of an increase in the fraction of free phenytoin in the blood (16). Seizure control is expected to be seen at lower measured drug levels. In the case of meperidine, there is a decrease in binding to red blood cells with increased age (17), thus increasing the amount of free drug available in the patient. Although higher therapeutic effects of some drugs may be beneficial, the accompanying risks of toxicity are unacceptable in the geriatric patient. Doses of most highly protein-bound drugs (greater than 90% protein-bound) should be reduced and increased slowly if there is evidence of decreased albumin. If several highly protein-bound drugs are used together, the chance of the patient suffering a drug interaction increases.

Changes in the ratio of lean body weight to fat can also alter drug distribution and thus pharmacologic response. In the elderly patient, total body water is decreased and total body fat is increased. These changes influence the onset and duration of action of highly tissue-bound drugs such as digoxin and water-soluble drugs such as alcohol, lithium, or morphine. The dosages of most water-soluble drugs are based on an estimation of lean body weight (Table 90.3). If actual weight is less than estimated

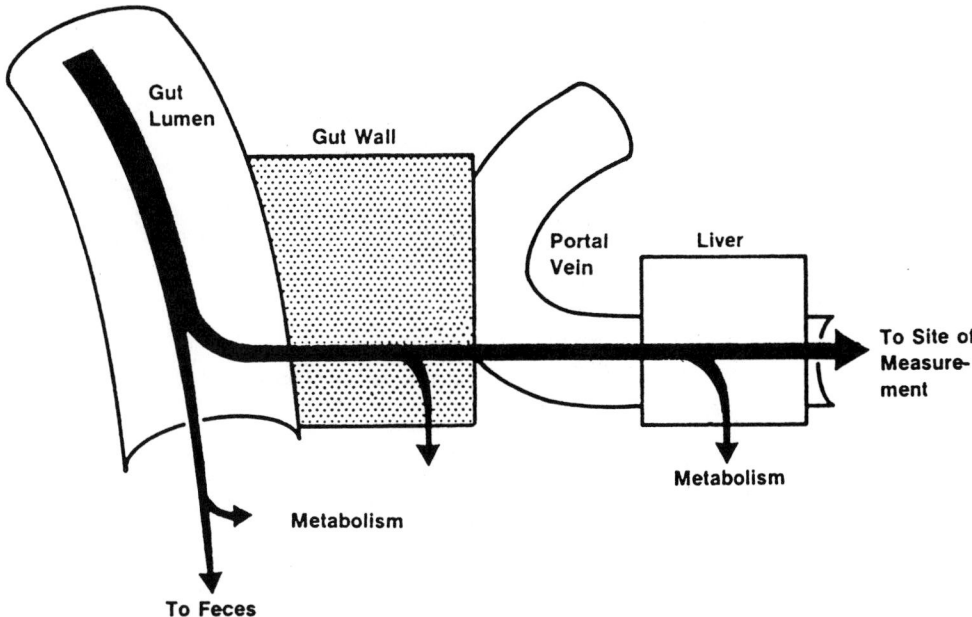

Figure 90.1. The loss of drug as it first passes through the gut wall and the liver during the absorption process is known as the first-pass effect. (Reprinted with permission, from Rowland M, Tozer TN: Clinical Pharmacokinetics: Concepts and Applications, ed. 2. Philadelphia, Lea & Febiger. 1989.

Table 90.2.
Representative Drugs Showing Low Oral Availability Due to Extensive First-Pass Hepatic Elimination[a]

Alprenolol	Methylphenidate
Amitriptyline	Metoprolol
Despiramine	Morphine
Dextropropoxyphene	Nifedipine
Dihydroergotamine	Nitroglycerin
Diltiazem	Pentazocine
5-Fluorouracil	Propranolol
Hydralazine	Salicylamide
Labetolol	Verapamil
6-Mercaptopurine	

[a] Adapted from Pond SM, Tozer TN: First-pass elimination: basic concepts and clinical consequences. Clin Pharmacokinet 9:1–25, 1984.

Table 90.3.
Estimation of Lean Body Weight[a]

Males = 50 kg + 2.3 (inches in height >5′)
Females = 45 kg + 2.3 (inches in height >5′)

[a] Adapted from Devine, B: Gentamicin therapy. Drug Intell Clin Pharm 8:650–655, 1974.

Table 90.4.
Examples of Fat-Soluble Drugs

Antidepressants
Barbiturates
Benzodiazepines
Calcium-channel blockers
Phenothiazines

lean body weight, the actual weight should be used in dosage calculations.

Between the ages of 18 and 85 years, total body fat increases in both females and males; lean body mass eventually decreases in both groups as well. With age, the volume of distribution of lipophilic drugs increases as a result of a decrease in total body weight, diminished protein binding, and an increase in the fat to lean muscle ratio. Fat-soluble drugs (Table 90.4) may have delayed onset of action and accumulate in adipose tissue, prolonging their action sometimes to the level of toxicity.

Physiologic Changes Influencing Drug Elimination

Drugs are primarily cleared from the body by metabolism in the liver, excretion by the kidneys, or by some combination of the two. A decrease in total body clearance results in higher average plasma drug concentrations and an enhanced pharmacologic response, which could lead to toxicity.

Liver metabolism is highly dependent on blood flow. From 25 to 65 years of age, there is a significant decrease in liver blood flow. In the presence of congestive heart failure, hepatic blood flow is further compromised. With drugs that are highly dependent on liver metabolism such as most β-blockers, lidocaine, or the narcotic analgesics, the decrease in liver clearance could increase the plasma concentration to toxic levels.

In addition to alterations of hepatic blood flow, age influences the hepatic clearance rate by causing changes in the intrinsic activity of selected liver enzymes. This has been shown in the oxidative or phase I metabolism enzyme pathway. Common drugs using this pathway influenced by age include selected benzodiazepines such as diazepam, chlordiazepoxide, clorazepate, and prazepam. Enzymatic demethylation of amitriptyline (18), imipramine (19), thioridazine (20), and theophylline (21) is also decreased in the elderly.

Drugs that undergo phase II enzymatic biotransformation (e.g., oxazepam, lorazepam, and temazepam) do not appear to be adversely affected by age and are preferred for use in the elderly. Drug metabolism can also be affected at all ages by genetics, smoking, diet, sex, other drugs, and diseases. Unlike renal function, no accurate laboratory tests directly measure liver function for drug-dosing adjustment. Nonspecific tests to monitor liver function include alanine aminotransferase (ALT) and plasma albumin levels and prothrombin time.

Age-related physiologic changes in the kidney influence drug elimination and response in the geriatric patient more than those in the liver. Between the ages of 20 and 90 years, the glomerular filtration rate may decrease as much as 50%, with an average decline of 35%. The serum creatinine level is frequently used to monitor kidney function, but this test is of limited usefulness in monitoring the glomerular filtration rate of the geriatric patient. Significant elevations do not occur unless most kidney function has deteriorated. The production of creatinine, which depends upon muscle mass, is decreased in the elderly; therefore, an apparently normal serum creatinine level in a geriatric patient may not be a valid predictor of drug elimination. Blood urea nitrogen (BUN) concentration is also not useful because it can be affected by hydration status, diet, and blood loss.

The most accurate estimation of glomerular filtration rate in the elderly population is the creatinine clearance (Cl cr), which correlates well with both the glomerular filtration rate and tubular secretion. Creatinine clearance can be estimated by a standard equation (Table 90.5) developed by Cockroft and Gault (22), which takes into consideration age, patient body weight, and serum creatinine in patients with stabilized renal function. This equation underestimates renal function in female patients, and it has been recommended that adjustments for lower muscle mass in elderly females are not necessary (23). It is important to remember that even this mathematical equation is simply an estimate of an individual's actual renal func-

Table 90.5.
Estimation of Creatinine Clearance[a]

$$\text{Cl}_{cr}^{b} \text{ (Male)} = \frac{\text{Lean body weight (kg)} \times (140 - \text{Age in yrs})}{\text{Serum creatinine} \times 72}$$

$$\text{Cl}_{cr}^{b} \text{ (Female)} = 0.85 \times \text{Cl}_{cr} \text{ (Male)}$$

[a] From Cockroft DW, Gault MH: Prediction of creatinine clearance from serum creatinine. Nephron 16:31–41, 1976.
[b] In ml/min.

Table 90.6.
Examples of Drugs Primarily Excreted by the Kidney

Acetazolamide	Cimetidine
Amantadine	Digoxin
Aminoglycoside antibiotics	Disopyramide
Cephalosporins	Lithium
Chlorpropamide	Procainamide

tion. This estimate appears to be less accurate in the very old geriatric population, those over the age of 85.

Dosages of renally excreted drugs should be adjusted if the patient has lost more than 30% of kidney function. If clearance is less than 30 ml/min, major dosage adjustments are necessary to avoid drug toxicity. Drugs with low therapeutic-toxic ratios, which are excreted primarily unchanged by the kidneys may be found in Table 90.6.

Age-related Pharmacodynamic Changes Influencing Drug Response

With increasing age, there is an increased intolerance to drugs as a result of altered pharmacodynamic response at the target organ. Altered response may be due to depletion of neurotransmitters, the presence of disease, or physiologic changes. With aging, there is evidence of a depletion of acetylcholine, dopamine, and serotonin levels, a decrease in the enzymatic degradation of monoamine oxidase, an impaired baroreceptor response to blood pressure changes, a decreased responsiveness to β-adrenergic receptors, and increased pain tolerance.

Altered end-organ sensitivity may result in an exaggerated pharmacologic response, as seen with the barbiturates and benzodiazepines, or diminished pharmacologic response, as seen with the β-blockers, β-agonists, and calcium-channel blockers. Other drug classes affected include the narcotic analgesics, antihypertensive agents, antiparkinson drugs, phenothiazines, and antidepressants. The frequency and irreversibility of tardive dyskinesia are increased in the elderly, which may be due to age related imbalances in neurotransmitters (24). Dosing adjustments are often necessary, since many of these same drugs are also influenced by age-related physiologic changes, especially drug distribution and elimination. The net effect in an individual patient is often difficult to predict. For example, elderly patients have an increased bioavailability of β-blockers but decreased responsiveness at the receptor site level. Another example is that the inotropic effect of theophylline is increased with age, but the bronchodilator effect is decreased (25).

Verapamil is an example of a racemic drug with S and R enantiomers in a fixed ratio in its formation, each of which exhibit different pharmacokinetic and pharmacodynamic properties. Aging may influence this ration of S/R enantiomers by decreasing their hepatic or renal clearance, resulting in an altered pharmacologic response. This may explain why toxicity with verapamil sometimes occurs at therapeutic plasma concentrations or why elderly patients appear to be more sensitive to normal therapeutic doses. This may also prove to be an important factor in the generic bioequivalence issue with verapamil as well as many other drugs.

CHANGES IN LABORATORY VALUES

The compilation of normal laboratory values in the elderly is complicated by latent or overt disease, multisystem disease, physiologic and anatomic changes associated with aging, and the effect of diet and malnutrition or many laboratory factors. Laboratory screening in the elderly should be limited to those tests related to the suspected clinical disease, and organ profiling is therefore the method of choice. Test profiles should be established aiming at the investigation of thyroid dysfunction, liver failure, myocardial and congestive cardiac failure, renal failure, renal disease, bone disease, and nutritional disorders.

It appears that the ranges of common biochemical tests results in the elderly are not very different from those in younger patients, with few exceptions. In interpreting laboratory test findings, it is important to know whether the results should be modified for age. Automated procedures show a 5 to 10% incidence of abnormal values in all patients, and some studies have shown abnormal values in 15% of the elderly. Some of these abnormalities may be attributed to aging processes such as decline in renal function or impaired glucose tolerance.

When determining therapy for elderly diabetics, age-related glucose tolerance becomes a factor. Due to the increasing hyperglycemia with age, (approximately 0.11 mmol/liter) increase in fasting glucose level and 5 to 10 mg/dl (0.28 to 0.56 mmol/liter) increase in the 2-hour postprandial glucose level with each decade over age 50, the diagnostic criteria for diabetes mellitus in an elderly patient require a random blood glucose level of more than 200 mg/dl (11 mmol/liter) or two fasting blood glucose levels of more than 140 mg/dl (7.78 mmol/liter) (26). A negative urinary glucose determination does not necessary correlate with a normal blood glucose; thus, urine testing has limited usefulness in monitoring disease activity in el-

derly patients. Blood glucose measurements provide the best index of control because of the increased renal threshold for glucose, which occurs with advancing age.

CARDIOVASCULAR DISEASES

With a high incidence of heart disease in the elderly, including hypertension, congestive heart failure, angina pectoris, and the cardiac arrhythmias, the elderly patient is often maintained on more than one therapeutic agent. These drugs often have a narrow therapeutic-toxic index, and their use can add to the increased incidence of ADRs in elderly patients.

HYPERTENSION

According to the Framingham study (27) over one-third of all patients over age 65 have an abnormal systolic blood pressure (>160 mm Hg) and/or an abnormal diastolic blood pressure (>90 mm Hg). The incidence of hypertension and the risk of cardiovascular complications are even higher in both elderly black males and females. An elevated systolic pressure has been demonstrated to be as valid a predictor as a diastolic pressure for coronary artery disease, stroke, left ventricular hypertrophy, and congestive heart failure (28).

According to the Framingham study, the overall mortality rate in men between ages 65 and 74 whose systolic pressure is higher than 160 mm Hg is twice that of men in the same age group whose pressure is less than 130 mm Hg. Each 10 mm Hg rise in systolic pressure increases the frequency of stroke by 30% (29). A blood pressure of 180/90 mm Hg causes an increase on the workload of an already compromised heart.

Several studies strongly suggest that treatment to reduce the blood pressure in the elderly is as effective in reducing disease complications as in the younger population of patients. In the classic VA Cooperative Study, the incidence of cardiovascular complications was reduced from 63 to 29% in patients over the age of 59 (30). In 1979, the Hypertension Detection and Follow-up Study demonstrated a 16.3% decrease in mortality in the treatment group of patients between the ages of 60 and 69 (31). The Australian National Blood Pressure Study confirmed that both cardiovascular morbidity and mortality were reduced in the elderly, even with mild diastolic hypertension (32). The European Working Party Study of Hypertension in the Elderly (33) has demonstrated the feasibility and effectiveness of lowering blood pressure; with a prolonged potassium-sparing diuretic alone, 85% of patients responded with a 25/10 mm Hg reduction in blood pressure. A follow-up study indicated that the main benefits of treatment in mild and moderate hypertensives were a reduction in fatal myocardial infarctions, severe heart failure, and stroke (34).

Aging produces several hemodynamic changes that may influence the choice of drug, such as an increase in peripheral vascular resistance and a decrease in renal blood flow, plasma volume, plasma renin, aldosterone, and cardiac output. A decline in the baroreceptor reflex response also occurs. The interplay of stroke volume and heart rate determines the cardiac output. Until recently, it was widely accepted that cardiac output decreased with age. Newer studies have shown that with increasing age, cardiac output at rest may be either unchanged or decreased (35). Drugs that can further reduce the perfusion to the myocardium, such as the β-blockers, should be used cautiously, at reduced doses, and with small incremental increases in doses. With a significant 50% increase in peripheral vascular resistance (36), drugs that reduce peripheral vascular resistance may have an enhanced pharmacologic response in older patients.

If treatment for hypertension is indicated, the end points of therapy must be realistic. Blood pressure should be lowered to within a range of 130 to 160 mm Hg systolic and 80 to 100 mm Hg diastolic, without causing side effects. Therapy should be reevaluated every 6 to 12 months because blood pressure may decrease with age as a result of the progression of atherosclerotic disease. Aggressive treatment often results in severe orthostasis, leading to falls and subsequent bone fractures. Additional complications of aggressive therapy are cognitive dysfunction resulting from hypoperfusion to the brain or drug side effects of antihypertensive drugs.

Antihypertensive Agents

With age-related declines in renal function, the choice and dosage of a diuretic is important. Since older patients have a decreased plasma volume and lower levels of aldosterone, aggressive diuretic therapy to reduce the blood pressure is generally not indicated. The recommendation is to start with a small initial dose of hydrochlorothiazide (6.25 to 12.5 mg) or its equivalent, with a maximum dose of 12.5 mg twice daily. If diuretic therapy is overzealous or water intake is reduced, the elderly patient is at risk of dehydration because of a diminished renal concentrating ability. With electrolyte disturbances, the elderly may be more susceptible to sudden death from ventricular arrhythmias, especially in the presence of left ventricular hypertrophy.

With a creatinine clearance of less than 30 ml/min, furosemide, bumetanide, or metolazone are recommended, since thiazide drugs will be ineffective. Diuretic combinations with a potassium-sparing agent can be useful, but hyperkalemia may develop from reduced potassium excretion, the concurrent use of potassium supplements, or concurrent use of angiotensin-converting enzyme (ACE) inhibitors.

The calcium-channel blockers are being used increasingly in the geriatric patient for the treatment of hypertension as well as other cardiac and noncardiac disorders. With increasing age, there is evidence of a decrease in total body clearance of both verapamil and its active metabolites because of impaired renal elimination (13). The metabolism of verapamil can be altered by congestive heart failure, liver disease, and concomitant use of cimetidine. Verapamil interferes with the tubular secretion of digoxin, sometimes leading to toxic levels (37). Caution should also be exercised with the combination of verapamil and the β-blockers because of their additive negative inotropic and chronotropic effects.

Both young and elderly patients show a decrease in metabolism and an increase in plasma half-life of diltiazem administered chronically. There is an increased incidence of edema, but the more serious effects on myocardial function do not occur (38). Increases in both bioavailability (39) and plasma half-life (40) have been demonstrated for nifedipine. Orthostatis is the rate-limiting side-effect with the use of nifedipine. Nicardipine has been shown to be safe and effective in elderly hypertensives, even though both absorption and plasma levels are increased (41).

Calcium-channel blockers have been shown to decrease blood pressure as effectively as hydrochlorothiazide, β-blockers, or sympathetic inhibitors in elderly hypertensives but with fewer side effects and no adverse metabolic reactions. Patients over the age of 60 years may have a more pronounced blood-pressure-lowering response to calcium antagonists (95%) than middle-aged (50%) or younger (28%) hypertensive patients (42). Dosage adjustment is prudent with all these drugs, since the elderly are more susceptible to the side effects.

Captopril and other ACE inhibitors reduce blood pressure in elderly hypertensive patients by reducing peripheral vascular resistance through non-renin-related mechanisms (43). The ACE inhibitors are also well tolerated in the elderly without adverse metabolic effects, though renal function must be monitored. Elderly patients with cardiac failure have been reported to be more susceptible to reduced renal clearance and drug accumulation with lisinopril (44).

For propranolol, both single-dose (45) and multiple-dose studies (46) indicate a two- to threefold increase in average peak plasma levels of the drug in older patients, as a result of changes in first-pass metabolism. Similar findings have been reported with metoprolol and labetalol. Patients over the age of 60 are twice as likely to suffer an ADR involving β-blockers than patients under 50 years of age (47). Many life-threatening reactions have occurred during the first 4 hr of therapy, even with the use of low doses. It would appear that the starting dose of propranolol in the geriatric patient should not exceed 20 mg/day. With the longer-acting β-blockers such as metoprolol, nadolol, and betaxolol, a once-daily dose is usually sufficient.

Despite increases in bioavailability, β-blockers are generally less effective in elderly hypertensives (20%) than in younger hypertensives (90%) because of decreases in β-receptor sensitivity and decreased plasma renin (48). These drugs may also cause an undesirable decrease in cardiac output and an increase in peripheral resistance. Both propranolol and metoprolol are relatively highly lipophilic, and thus they may cause more unwanted CNS side effects in elderly hypertensive.

When selecting a β-blocker for use in the geriatric patient, the choice of a long-acting water-soluble agent such as nadolol or atenolol may minimize the occurrence of side effects and maximize patient compliance. Labetalol may be an alternative choice. Studies have shown that labetalol, with its α-blocking activity, is effective as an antihypertensive in reducing peripheral vascular resistance and is well tolerated in the elderly, without adversely compromising cardiac output. A reduction in clearance in the elderly is the justification for starting with a lower dose (49).

Diminished baroreceptor sensitivity has been demonstrated in hypertensive patients over the age of 60. There is evidence that a 20 mm Hg or greater drop in blood pressure occurs in one-fourth of normal elderly patients undergoing positional changes, without antihypertensive drugs. Drugs that interfere with the baroreceptor reflex, such as adrenergic-blocking agents, should be used cautiously because of the increased risk of falls and fractures. Clonidine and methyldopa can be used as second-line agents with diuretics if lower dosages are prescribed to minimize bothersome side effects. Guanethidine should be avoided in geriatric patients because of its dramatic effect of postural hypotension. Reserpine is not recommended for use in geriatrics because it has a high rate of CNS side effects, notably depression, caused by its effect on reducing brain serotonin levels, which are often decreased with age. In general, starting doses of antihypertensives are reduced by one-third to one-half, with slow titration until desired patient response is reached.

CONGESTIVE HEART FAILURE

Although the incidence and prevalence of congestive heart failure (CHF) increase exponentially with age, the risk and benefit of several therapeutic modalities remain unassessed. In view of the high incidence of toxicity associated with digoxin therapy in the elderly population, it may be wise to initiate therapy with vasodilators and/or diuretics in older patients who are in sinus rhythm.

Digoxin

In patients between the ages of 60 and 80, the renal clearance of digoxin is reduced approximately 50% by age-related changes in renal function. The half-life of digoxin is twice the normal value in young, healthy patients. In calculating the digitalizing dose, the total dose should be based on lean body weight, not actual weight. Both the digitalizing dose and the maintenance dose are influenced by impaired renal function. This decrease in renal elimination may partially account for a high prevalence of digoxin toxicity in the elderly population. Unless the immediate inotropic effects of digoxin are needed (as in the case of acute congestive heart failure), most geriatric patients can be treated with daily maintenance doses rather than risk toxicity with the administration of a loading dose. Peak therapeutic response will be delayed 2 to 3 weeks because of the long half-life of digoxin.

Classic digoxin toxicity may not be present in the elderly. Instead of nausea and vomiting, the patient may experience anorexia and weight loss; instead of haloes and color vision changes, the patient may complain of hazy or muddy vision. Although commonly seen in physician orders, ("hold dose if pulse less than 60"), bradycardia may not be a sensitive indicator of digoxin toxicity. Suspected toxicity should be confirmed by electrocardiograms and digoxin plasma levels.

Long-term maintenance digoxin is not always necessary. Studies (50, 51) have shown that over 80% of elderly patients could be safely withdrawn from digoxin if there was no evidence of heart failure and if the heart was in normal sinus rhythm. Successful discontinuation was more likely if the plasma digoxin blood level was below 0.8 ng/ml. Based on the widespread and often undocumented use of this drug with a narrow therapeutic-toxic index, a digoxin-free trial should be recommended to the physician in patients at risk for an ADR who are asymptomatic. Signs of atrial fibrillation or symptoms of congestive heart failure should be monitored if withdrawal from digoxin is attempted in the hospital or nursing home.

Due to concerns about toxicity with digoxin, there is a trend toward the use of ACE inhibitors in geriatric patients with congestive heart failure. ACE inhibitors have been shown to be more effective in prolonging survival than digoxin, with fewer side effects, in patients with severe CHF (52). Captopril is also more effective in improving exercise time and functional class in mild and moderate CHF than digoxin in patients maintained on diuretic therapy, though decreasing mortality has not been shown. Hypotension was the only major side effect reported (53).

Quinidine can displace digoxin from tissue stores as well as interfere with its tubular secretion, thus increasing the digoxin effect, which can be seen as early as 24 hr after starting quinidine, with the peak effect seen at steady-state levels 5 days after initiating therapy. A reduction in the digoxin dose may be indicated when therapy with quinidine is initiated. If long-term therapy is necessary with these drugs, a digoxin blood level should be determined

5 days after starting quinidine, to adjust the maintenance dose.

ANGINA PECTORIS

β-Blockers, calcium-channel blockers and nitrates used alone or in combination remain the cornerstone of therapy for angina pectoris.

Nitrates in oral, sublingual, topical, and intravenous formulations are used in the treatment of both angina pectoris and congestive heart failure because of their effects on coronary vasodilation and in reducing preload on the myocardium. There are increases in plasma half-life and volume of distribution with nitrates, producing a severe drop in blood pressure (54). Nitroglycerin ointment is preferred over the nitroglycerin patch because of ease in dose titration and less chance of developing drug tolerance (55). If a nitroglycerin patch is used, a nitrate-free period is recommended, to prevent development of nitrate tolerance (56).

In patients with ischemic heart disease, abrupt withdrawal of β-blockers can increase the risk of myocardial infarction or cardiac arrhythmias, because of sympathetic sensitivity. In these patients, drug therapy should be tapered over 14 days. The combination of these agents with sympathetic inhibitors, such as clonidine or methyldopa, is discouraged because of unopposed α-vasoconstriction upon withdrawal, therapy increasing catecholamine response.

CARDIAC ARRHYTHMIAS

The benefits of treatment of selected atrial and ventricular arrhythmias must outweigh the risks of drug toxicity—especially the development of proarrhythmias. Due to changes in liver and renal clearance, the geriatric patient is at higher risk of drug toxicity.

Antiarrhythmic Drugs

For quinidine, age-related changes can decrease both hepatic and renal clearance and cause a 33% increase in plasma half-life and antiarrhythmic response (57); active metabolites can also accumulate, contributing to both pharmacologic and toxic effects. To account for these changes, a reduction in dose or an increase in dosing interval is indicated. Instead of the standard dose of 300 mg every 6 hr, the recommendation may be 300 mg every 8 hr, or 200 mg every 6 hr. The sustained-release products are generally not recommended for use in the elderly because of a decreased bioavailability, due in part to alterations in first-pass hepatic metabolism. Plasma concentrations of quinidine can be increased if concurrent congestive heart failure is present.

Procainamide has an active metabolite (N-acetylprocainamide or NAPA) that is 100% excreted unchanged by the kidney. Drug accumulation may result in hypotension and heart block. Dosage recommendations for the geriatric patients are 250 to 375 mg of procainamide every 4 to 6 hr. Blood levels should be maintained in the 4 to 8 μg/ml range, remembering that the NAPA metabolite also possesses important antiarrythmic activity. Congestive heart failure further compromises drug clearance.

Lidocaine is metabolized in the liver, and a decrease in perfusion will alter drug kinetics. Decreases in plasma clearance occur with age as a result of a decrease in cardiac output or in the presence of congestive heart failure or liver disease. If any of these risk factors are present, the patient may experience toxicity exhibited as CNS depression, hypotension, or convulsions at standard intravenous bolus doses (100 to 105 mg) or at a conservative infusion rate of 20 μg/kg per min (58). Low-dose boluses (75 mg) of lidocaine repeated at longer intervals (30 to 60 min) may be necessary for the patient with severe heart failure and/or liver disease. Repeated bouts of premature ventricular depolarizations may be seen in the first 24 hr, despite lidocaine infusion, because of the delay in reaching a steady-state blood level.

The rate of ADRs associated with lidocaine in patients over the age of 70 is twice that of those under 50 years of age (59). Most of these reactions occur during the initial 2 days of therapy. Additional risk factors include weight loss, myocardial infarction, and congestive heart failure, which decrease cardiac output and drug clearance. Mexiletine and tocainide are oral antiarrhythmic agents. Since mexiletine is less dependent on elimination by the kidneys than tocainide, it may be the preferred "oral lidocaine" maintenance drug in the elderly.

Disopyramide is primarily excreted by the kidney, with 50% excreted unchanged and 30% as metabolites, some of which have antiarrhythmic activity. Disopyramide may induce mild heart failure as a result of a profound negative inotropic effect (60). This drug should be used with caution in patients with a history of heart failure and in those being maintained on β-blockers. Elderly patients are more sensitive to the anticholinergic effects of urinary retention and bladder atony. A reduced dose is often necessary because of age- or disease-related decreases in renal function or increased pharmacologic sensitivity.

CENTRAL NERVOUS SYSTEM DRUGS

Age-related pharmacokinetic and pharmacologic changes in geriatric patients alter the response to drugs that affect the central nervous system (CNS). Many drugs routinely prescribed for geriatric patients have either a therapeutic or an adverse effect on the CNS. Careful monitoring of these agents is required to differentiate among drug effectiveness, adverse effects, or progression of the disease.

Table 90.7.
Anxiolytics and Sedative Hypnotics

Drug	Drug Half-Life (hr)	Usual Maximum Daily Dosage (µg) for Age 65 & Over
Benzodiazepines		
Alprazolam	12–15	2
Chlordiazepoxide	5–30	40
Chlorazepate	30–100	30
Clonazepam	18–50	1.5
Diazepam	20–80	20
Halazepam	14	80
Lorazepam	10–20	3
Oxazepam	5–20	60
Prazepam	30–100	30
Nonbenzodiazepines		
Buspirone	2–11	30
Meprobamate	6–48	Not recommended
Antihistamines		
Diphenhydramine	12	50
Hydroxyzine	3+ in the elderly	100

Sedative-Hypnotics

As many as half of patients over the age of 50 report insomnia, and hypnotic drug use increases with age. In a survey of nursing home patients, 40 to 50% of the patients reviewed received a sedative-hypnotic or anxiolytic prescription on a regular basis (61). A general guideline for dosing the sedative-hypnotics in geriatrics is to start with one-third to one-half the usual recommended starting dose, or for sedatives, increase the time interval between doses. Repeat doses of hypnotics, that are ordered because of a lack of expected response, should be avoided to prevent overmedication, additive side effects, and hypersomnolence (Table 90.7).

Benzodiazepines

The agents prescribed most often as sedative-hypnotics are the benzodiazepines. Geriatric patients are more sensitive to the cortical depressant effect of the benzodiazepines and can appear to be demented, depressed, or both as a result of chronic intoxication. In general, benzodiazepines are effective in reducing sleep latency, but chronic or repeat use is not indicated in older patients. When used on a regular basis in the elderly, benzodiazepines can cause toxicity including dependence, hangover effect, dysphoria, and withdrawal effects.

A withdrawal syndrome, usually mild but potentially severe, ranging from tremors and agitation to rebound insomnia, psychosis, or convulsions, can occur following the abrupt cessation of benzodiazepine therapy. The severity of the withdrawal syndrome depends upon the dose and duration of therapy, and the appearance of the withdrawal reaction is correlated with a drop in the plasma benzodiazepine level. Rebound insomnia occurs following withdrawal of nightly doses of most benzodiazepines and may be more severe and begin earlier following use of the short-acting agents. Active metabolites of benzodiazepines may be present in the plasma for days or weeks so that if rebound insomnia occurs, it can be seen for as long as 10 to 20 days after withdrawal of the drug (62).

Although anterograde amnesia has been reported with most benzodiazepines (63), the risk may be higher with short-acting agents such as lorazepam and triazolam. As a result of reported reactions to benzodiazepines, it has been recommended that anterograde amnesia be listed as a potential risk for triazolam and possibly temazepam, lorazepam, and flurazepam use (64).

These drugs are also associated with residual cognitive deficits in geriatric patients. The increased risk of hip fracture has been directly correlated with the use of long-acting benzodiazepines; users of short half-life benzodiazepines had no significantly increased risk, compared with controls (65).

In selecting a particular benzodiazepine for an elderly patient, considerations should include specific symptoms and needs (i.e., sleep latency, sleep maintenance, and/or early morning wakening) and the metabolic pathway. In elderly patients, the benzodiazepines that may be preferable include oxazepam, lorazepam, and temazepam. Triazolam may be used, but with extreme caution and in very low doses. (For dosing information, see Table 90.7.)

Benzodiazepines are also useful as anxiolytic agents in elderly patients when specific target symptoms have been identified for treatment. The same considerations of half-life and metabolism apply when the agents are used as anxiolytics.

Buspirone

Buspirone, a new nonbenzodiazepine anxiolytic, may also be useful in the treatment of behavioral symptoms in the cognitively impaired. This drug is as effective as diazepam, clorazepate, or lorazepam and is more effective than placebo for the treatment of generalized anxiety disorders. However, patients who have previously taken benzodiazepines are less likely to respond to buspirone than those who have not. There is evidence that the pharmacokinetics of buspirone are not significantly different in the elderly, with only severe hepatic or renal insufficiency resulting in a reduction in clearance. Most anxious patients who have taken buspirone even for long periods (more than 3 months) report few side effects, and there is a low rate of discontinuation due to side effects. Buspirone does not impair daytime wakefulness or performance, interfere with cognitive function, cause drowsiness, or add to the depressant effect of other drugs acting on the CNS. Thus, it may be an effective alternative to benzodiazepines in relieving the symptoms of anxiety. It will be interesting to see if it proves to be any more effective than benzodiazepines for the treatment of behavioral symptoms in elderly demented patients. Buspirone does not require dosage alteration in the healthy elderly (66) (Table 90.7).

Chloral hydrate is an effective hypnotic agent in the geriatric patient in a dose of 250 to 500 mg at bedtime. However, tolerance develops in as little as 1 week if the drug is used on a routine daily basis. Diphenhydramine is good for occasional use in the geriatric patient as a sedative in a dose of 25 to 50 mg at bedtime. Anticholinergic delirium or worsening of the patient's cognitive state can occur if the drug is used too frequently, in excessive doses, or with other drugs that have anticholinergic activity.

The barbiturates are extremely lipid soluble and can produce excessive sedation and paradoxical excitement in elderly patients, especially in patients with increased body fat stores. This latter reaction can range from mild restlessness, in which case the dose of the hypnotic should not be increased, to frank psychosis that should not be treated with phenothiazines. For these reasons, barbiturates should not be used in the elderly, and the practice of combining a hypnotic and a sedative at bedtime should be discouraged.

Neuroleptics

The neuroleptics or antipsychotics are useful for treatment of psychoses and severe behavioral manifestations of the dementias. Behavioral symptoms commonly associated with dementia include impaired cognitive functioning, anxiety, agitation, paranoia, hallucinations, and combativeness. These symptoms are disturbing to both the patient and the caregiver. The phenothiazines have prominent sedative, cardiovascular, anticholinergic, and neurologic side effects that are often seen in the elderly, probably as a result of a decreased ability of the liver enzymes to metabolize the drugs to inactive metabolites and altered receptor sensitivity. Usual starting doses of antipsychotics should be one-quarter to one-third those commonly prescribed for younger adults. The dosage should be gradually increased, according to the clinical response of the patient. Initially, drugs may be given in divided doses or a single small dose with "as needed orders" for repeating the dose to determine the lowest effective dose and to minimize side effects. Maximum doses should also be one-fourth those recommended in younger patients (Table 90.8).

The low-potency phenothiazines such as chlorpromazine and thioridazine are more likely to cause sedation, orthostatic hypotension, tachyarrhythmias, loss of ocular accommodation, constipation, urinary retention, and other anticholinergic effects. The high-potency phenothiazines such as trifluoperazine and thiothixene, in addition to the butyrophenone derivative haloperidol, cause a higher frequency of extrapyramidal symptoms. Low-dose haloperidol is frequently used because of a low incidence of both CNS and cardiovascular side effects.

Extrapyramidal symptoms occur in 50% of all patients on phenothiazines between the ages of 60 and 80 years (67), and 90% of these reactions occur within the first 10 weeks of therapy. These acute side effects can be minimized by using the lowest effective dose or they may be effectively treated with antiparkinson agents such as benzotropine or diphenhydramine. After 3 months of continuous therapy, most patients can be withdrawn from the antiparkinson agents without a recurrence of extrapyramidal symptoms. Antiparkinson agents should not be used prophylactically because use of these agents may expose the patient to additive anticholinergic effects in addition to mild confusion, nightmares, and increased forgetfulness. The rate of tardive dyskinesia can be minimized by proper use of antiparkinsonism drugs, adjusting maintenance doses of phenothiazines to the lowest effective levels, avoiding large bedtime doses, and using drug holidays for patients.

Drug holidays are recommended for use in patients

Table 90.8.
Side Effects/Adverse Effects and Dosage Information for Antipsychotics

Type of Antipsychotic	Common Side Effects[a]				Starting Dosage for Elderly Patients (mg/day)	Recommended Max Dosage for Elderly Patients (mg/day)
	S	A	EPS	H		
Chlorpromazine	3+	2+	2+	3+	10–20	400–800
Thioridazine	3+	3+	1+	3+	10–20	200–400
Trifluoperazine	1+	1+	3+	1+	1–2	20–40
Perphenazine	1+	1+	3+	1+	2–4	16–32
Fluphenazine	1+	1+	4+	1+	1–2.5	10–20
Thiothixene	1+	1+	3+	1+	2–3	15–30
Haloperidol	1+	±	4+	1+	0.75–5	15–50
Loxapine	1+	1+	3+	1+	6–10	60–125

[a] Degree of effect: 0, none; 1+, slight,; 2+, moderate; 3+, high; 4+, very high; ±, not well documented. Abbreviations: S, sedation; A, anticholinergic; EPS, extrapyramidal symptoms; H, orthostatic hypotension.

receiving antipsychotics for extended periods of time. Drug holidays are accomplished by withholding the drug from the patient for 1 to 3 consecutive days a week. These drug-free intervals reduce the total amount of drug ingested by the patient and lessen the occurrence of serious side effects. Drug holidays can help identify medication that is either unnecessary or inappropriate. Studies involving drug holidays have shown that no serious complications resulted from the use of one or two drug-free days in long-term-care patients (68, 69). Drug-free periods in geriatric patients could compensate for increased drug sensitivity by reducing drug accumulation, and they allow the practitioner to evaluate the patient's responsiveness and drug therapy requirements. An additional benefit to drug holidays is the cost savings for the patient.

A recent multicenter study showed that the atypical antipsychotic agent, clozapine, was significantly superior to chlorpromazine in treatment-resistant chronic schizophrenic patients (70). The value of clozapine in demented patients is not known and although clozapine is relatively free of extrapyramidal reactions, there is a serious risk of agranulocytosis.

Patients with dementia who are experiencing sundowning, an acute confusional state occurring at dusk, generally obtain the best therapeutic effects from the low-dose, sedating neuroleptics such as chlorpromazine or thioridazine. The dose should be given 1 to 2 hr prior to the expected time of agitation to allow therapeutic levels to accumulate and take advantage of the side effects of sedation. An alternative treatment for sundowning is the use of physical restraints, but their use should be for short periods of time to avoid patient injury.

There is no effective treatment at present for Alzheimer's disease, although several drugs are presently in clinical trials. Hydergine, a combination of ergoloid mesylates is the only approved medication for Alzheimer's disease, but despite widespread use, its efficacy remains to be established. A recent study was conducted with a liquid-capsule formulation of the drug, reported to have greater bioavailability. The dose studied was 1 mg p.o. three times daily. Although the medication was shown to be safe and well tolerated, it was ineffective in the Alzheimer's disease patients in the study (71). Currently, several agents are undergoing investigation for effectiveness in treatment of Alzheimer's disease. Among the more promising agents are tetrahydroaminoacridine (THA) and the calcium-channel blockers such as nimodipine.

Antidepressants

Depression is common among geriatric patients, occurring in as many as 10 to 15% of the population. The diagnosis of depression should be made only after a thorough history and physical examination. Depression in an older patient may not resemble that of younger patients, and it may be atypical, first presenting as cognitive impairment, or it could be iatrogenic. Three categories of elderly patients tend to respond poorly to all heterocyclic antidepressants: those not truly clinically depressed, those whose depression is long-standing and resistant to previous therapy, and those with concomitant psychotic or delusional symptoms.

In the treatment of depression, the tricyclic secondary amines (despiramine and nortriptyline) are as efficacious as the tertiary amines (imipramine and amitriptyline), but the secondary amines have lessened anticholinergic, cardiovascular, and sedating side effects, which is desirable in the apathetic, withdrawn, or depressed elderly patient. For agitated, depressed patients, more-sedating antidepressants such as amitriptyline, doxepin, or maprotiline may offer some advantage. Two new antidepressants are trazadone and fluoxetine. Trazodone lacks anticholinergic side effects but is sedating and can cause hypotension. It is recommended as a second-choice antidepressant for elderly patients who have not responded to desipramine or nortriptyline (72). Fluoxetine lacks anticholinergic effects and lacks cardiotoxicity at therapeutic doses, yet anorexia and weight loss have been reported. It is effective in treating depression in the elderly, but its very long elimination half-life may be dangerous for this population (73).

Geriatric patients require lower initial doses and gradual titration of maintenance doses of heterocyclic antidepressants because they metabolize and excrete these drugs more slowly. With nortriptyline there are no changes in drug kinetics with age (74), but there is tremendous interpatient variability in drug dose, requiring careful titration and perhaps monitoring of plasma levels. Therapeutic plasma levels of imipramine, desipramine, and nortriptyline correlate with therapeutic effect. For nortriptyline, the therapeutic level in geriatric patients is between 50 and 150 ng/ml, and for imipramine and desipramine, the therapeutic level should be at least 200 ng/ml. Plasma levels should be used in selected patients as guidelines for dosing, and patient response should be closely monitored.

Antidepressants should generally be given in divided doses to avoid the sudden rise in blood levels that may result in increased side effects if the total dose were administered at one time. Large, single, daily doses at bedtime should be avoided in the elderly, especially in patients with cardiovascular disease. The patient with insomnia and depression or the patient who cannot tolerate the anticholinergic side effects should be given a larger dose (⅔ of total daily dose) at bedtime to take advantage of the sedative properties. For most antidepressant drugs, the low initial dose can be increased every 3 to 4 days to gradually achieve a total dosage of 75 to 150 mg/day (Table 90.9). The final dose depends on the clinical response and on the appearance and severity of side effects.

The most commonly seen ADRs of the antidepressants

Table 90.9.
Side Effects/Adverse Effects and Dosage Information for Antidepressants

Type of Antidepressant	Common Side Effects[a]				Drug Half-Life (hr)	Starting Dosage for Elderly Patients (mg/day)	Recommended Dosage for Elderly (mg/day)
	A	S	H	C			
Nortriptyline	2+	2+	1+	2+	18–93	10	30–50
Desipramine	1+	1+	1+	3+	14–62	20	25–150
Doxepin	2+	3+	2+	2+	6–19	25	25–150
Amitriptyline	4+	3+	2+	3+	10–50	20	50–150
Imipramine	2+	2+	3+	4+	6–28	30	50–150
Trimipramine	2+	3+	2+	3+	7–30	25	50–150
Protriptyline	3+	1+	1+	4+	55–198	5	15–20
Amoxapine	1+	2+	1+	2+	8	50	50–150
Maprotiline	1+	2+	1+	3+	21–51	25	50–150
Trazodone	1+	2+	2+	1+	4–9	50	100–400
Fluoxetine	±	±	±	1+	24–72	20	20–40
Bupropion	±	0	0	0	10–20	150	150–450

[a] Degree of drug effect: 0, none; 1+, slight; 2+, moderate; 3+, high; 4+, very high; ±, not well documented. Abbreviations: A, anticholinergic; S, sedation; H, orthostatic hypotension; C, cardiac effects.

Table 90.10.
Major Risk Factors for Noncompliance

Chronic disease or long-term therapy
Use of multiple pharmacies
Psychiatric illness
Multiple physicians
Multiple drugs
Multiple doses

are peripheral anticholinergic effects, central anticholinergic effects, cardiovascular effects, and lowering of the seizure threshold. The peripheral anticholinergic effects such as blurred vision, urinary retention, tachycardia, and constipation are usually present, but transient. The central anticholinergic effects are toxic delirium, confusion, disorientation, visual and auditory hallucinations, and disorganized thoughts. The postural hypotension that may develop is caused by relaxation of the vascular smooth muscle. This may be especially dangerous because it imposes the risk of cerebrovascular insufficiency, falls, and injuries in the elderly patient. Elderly patients are especially susceptible to orthostatic hypotension when suddenly arising from recumbent or seated positions. Blood pressure readings are recommended before initiating antidepressant therapy. The selection of an antidepressant agent for use in a geriatric patient should based on the degree and frequency of side effects for a particular agent (Table 90.10).

Lithium

In recent years unipolar depression and recurrent bipolar disorder, lithium carbonate (300 to 900 mg daily) may be prescribed prophylactically. Lithium is primarily indicated for the treatment of mania, but elderly depressed patients who cannot tolerate antidepressant therapy may respond to lithium, either alone or in combination. Side effects and toxicity are more likely in elderly patients, and occur at lower blood levels than in younger adults. The recommended starting daily doses for elderly patients should be one-half to one-third less than those in younger patients (75) (150 to 300 mg), and the therapeutic blood level should be maintained between 0.4 and 0.7 meq/liter.

Anticonvulsants

The use of anticonvulsant agents in geriatric patients must take into consideration their toxicity. The potential for CNS and cardiovascular toxicity and drug interactions increases in elderly patients with underlying illnesses or decreased organ reserves and those who are taking multiple drugs. All of the anticonvulsant agents produce dose-related CNS toxicity: impaired cognition, agitation, and involuntary movement disorders. Phenytoin, carbamazepine, and phenobarbital are the drugs most likely to be used in the geriatric patient. Single-agent therapy is recommended because of a safe side-effect profile. Plasma drug levels should be monitored to achieve optimal doses for seizure prevention with the least toxicity.

Phenytoin has several characteristics that make its dosing susceptible to age changes: narrow therapeutic range, extensive liver metabolism, and a high degree of protein binding. In patients with hypoalbuminemia, the unbound (free) fraction of phenytoin is increased. Clinicians must always consider altered protein binding and whether the fraction of free drug is altered when interpreting or establishing desired plasma drug concentrations. Low plasma protein concentrations decrease the concentration of bound drug, but generally not that of the free drug; therefore, the fraction of free drug concentration increases as plasma protein concentration decreases. In the clinical situation, a patient with a low serum albumin and an apparently low plasma phenytoin concentration still has a therapeutically acceptable plasma drug concentration (when adjusted for low serum albumin).

In a study of nursing-home patients (76), no loss of seizure control for patients taking once-daily phenytoin (200 to 300 mg) was noted when this regimen was compared with the standard dose of 100 mg three times a day. No evidence of toxicity or side effects was reported. The data suggest that extended-release phenytoin sodium administered to geriatric patients as a single daily dose provides adequate seizure control without increased toxicity or side effects.

Phenobarbital is not recommended for seizure control in the elderly because of the fear of excessive sedation or paradoxical excitation. Administration of the daily dose at bedtime avoids most of the sedation; however tolerance to the sedation develops within a few weeks. If a paradoxical response is seen, an alternate drug may be substituted. Phenobarbital may be the preferred drug for stroke patients who have had a seizure because it is believed to have beneficial effects of hypoxia and ischemic brain tissue. Respiratory depression is not a problem with ordinary doses, but combinations with alcohol or other CNS drugs such as benzodiazepines may depress the respiratory center.

The psychomotor depression that can complicate the use of phenytoin and phenobarbital dose not occur with carbamazepine. Carbamazepine may have beneficial psychotropic effects, especially in brain-damaged patients. Aplastic anemia is a rare but serious side effect of carbamazepine. A CBC determination, including platelets, reticulocyte count and serum iron concentration should be done prior to the initiation of therapy, every 2 weeks for the first 2 months, then every 3 to 6 months for the duration of therapy. Other adverse reactions usually reported with high doses include hyponatremia (SIADH), diplopia, and ataxia. Initial dosing of carbamazepine in the geriatric patient should be with 100 mg to 200 mg every 12 hr, with subsequent adjustments being made slowly to minimize gastrointestinal side effects. The dosage should achieve the lowest effective blood levels between 4 and 12 μg/ml. Ataxia often occurs at subtherapeutic levels and cannot be used as an indicator of toxicity.

Analgesics

Although it is unclear how age affects clinical pain, there is no doubt that age influences the analgesic effect of drugs. The type of pain should be fully assessed before initiating treatment. Older patients may suffer from acute pain, a biological indicator of a problem requiring treatment, or from chronic pain, which is defined as pain persisting beyond the usual course of an acute disease or beyond a reasonable time for an injury to heal. Chronic pain often mimics depression, with accompanying symptoms of insomnia, eating disturbances, and loss of interest in usual activities.

Geriatric patients are significantly more sensitive to the pain-relieving effect of narcotics because of alteration of receptors, changes in plasma protein binding and decreased clearance of these agents (77). These changes allow narcotics to be more effective in small doses in geriatric patients than in younger patients. One study (78) demonstrated that in patients 70 years of age, the duration of pain relief at 4 hr was identical at doses of 8 mg and 16 mg of morphine, although the incidence of side effects was higher in the high-dose group.

The elderly, as a group, are more likely to develop narcotic side effects of constipation, respiratory depression, cough suppression, and clouding of mental functions. These side effects may occur at lower doses than in younger patients. Constipation can be serious in the elderly patient, and it can be prevented or treated by minimizing the narcotic dose or frequency of administration, using a high-bulk diet, increasing the fluid intake, or increasing the activity level.

No evidence currently supports the choice of one narcotic over another on the basis of age alone. The dose of narcotic analgesics in the geriatric patient should be gradually increased until the patient obtains pain relief for at least 4 hr. It should be administered before the pain occurs to avoid anticipatory anxiety and behavioral reinforcement of drug use, especially in terminally ill patients with chronic pain.

Analgesic Adjuvants

The total dose of narcotic can be decreased by concomitant use of nonnarcotic analgesics, nonsteroidal antiinflammatory drugs (NSAIDs), and other analgesic adjuvants. If adjuvants are used, additive side effects may occur.

Antidepressants that affect the serotonergic system, such as trazodone, amitriptyline, doxepin, and imipramine have documented analgesic properties. In patients with chronic pain, the drugs provide analgesia, may alleviate depression, and aid in reestablishing disturbed sleep patterns (79). Low doses are recommended initially (10 to 25 mg at bedtime), with 25-mg increases weekly until the desired effect is achieve. Analgesic effects are seen at lower doses than antidepressant effects, and the therapeutic trial should last 4 to 6 weeks. Other effective adjuvant analgesics include anticonvulsants, neuroleptics, anxiolytic sedatives, and steroids (81).

Nonsteroidal Antiinflammatory Drugs (NSAIDs)

NSAIDs should be used with caution in the geriatric patient because of their side effects. Most of the toxicity from the NSAIDs is dose-related, and cumulative toxicity is rarely a problem. The risk of serious hematologic reactions is extremely low. CNS toxicity may include delirium, hallucinations, melancholia, agitation, lethargy, or even seizures. These symptoms usually resolve within 48 hr of stopping the therapy (80).

GI complaints are the predominant adverse effect caused by NSAIDs. Through inhibition of the protective effects of GI prostaglandins, all NSAIDs can cause GI side effects. The studies support a high rate of asymptomatic GI pathology with all NSAIDs, a low frequency of serious adverse GI effects, no difference in risk between young and elderly patients, but a greater morbidity from adverse effects in elderly patients (81). Patients at risk for renal adverse effects from NSAIDs include those with renal disease, heart failure, cirrhosis with ascites, volume depletion, and diuretic use (82). Signs and symptoms of drug-induced renal dysfunction include increased blood urea nitrogen, serum creatinine and potassium levels, increased body weight (due to edema), decreased urinary output, and a worsening of congestive heart failure. Monitoring weight, laboratory values, and vital signs is essential.

Antimicrobial Agents

Toxicities of the aminoglycoside antibiotics include both nephrotoxicity and ototoxicity that can be irreversible if not recognized early. In the elderly, ototoxicity may be difficult to determine because of a previous hearing impairment. Standard doses and therapy beyond 10 days are to be discouraged and the serum creatinine level should be closely monitored for evidence of renal tubular damage. Other risk factors for toxicity include sustained high blood levels (i.e., trough levels greater than 2 mg/100 ml for gentamicin), concurrent administration of some cephalosporins or high-dose loop diuretics, and a relative state of dehydration.

One study (83) suggests that tobramycin is the preferred aminoglycoside in the elderly because of lower rate of clinical nephrotoxicity than with gentamicin. Other clinical studies suggest no difference, with gentamicin being the most cost-effective agent, especially if drug levels are monitored and adjusted properly. Other less toxic agents, including the newer cephalosporins and fluoroquinolones may reduce the need for aminoglycoside antibiotics in the elderly. Most cephalosporins are eliminated unchanged in the kidney, so reduced drug clearance produces longer antimicrobial activity. Although this class of drugs has a high safety profile, a reduction in dosing interval may be indicated if renal function is decreased in the elderly.

Vancomycin is used in the hospital to treat or protect against methicillin-resistant *Staphylococcus aureus*. In elderly patients, a decrease in total body clearance coupled with an increase in volume of distribution as a result of increased drug tissue binding, resulted in a 70% increase in plasma half-life of vancomycin, from 7.24 to 12.14 hr (84).

The fluoroquinolones, such as ciprofloxacin and norfloxacin, are widely used, especially in the nursing home population. Their use has increased because they are bactericidal and have a broad spectrum of activity against common pathogens in the urinary and respiratory tracts. Appropriate use may limit patient exposure to more toxic antimicrobials or more costly combinations and may shorten patient stay in the hospital or allow the patient to receive treatment in the long-term care facility. These drugs are generally not effective against pneumococcus, group A streptococci, or anaerobes.

Enhanced absorption and bioavailability of ciprofloxacin can result from changes in gastric emptying, first-pass metabolism, or reduced renal clearance with age (85). Antacids can reduce absorption, so administration times should be specified. The effect of age on renal elimination of the active metabolites of ciprofloxacin must be studied. Doses should be reduced or dosage intervals extended to every 12 hr to compensate for these pharmacokinetic changes in absorption and clearance, which vary among the various fluoroquinolone drugs.

Ciprofloxacin can inhibit the metabolism of theophylline, caffeine, NSAIDs, warfarin, phenytoin, and cyclosporine (86), requiring dosage adjustment or closer monitoring for toxicity. Norfloxacin does not appear to inhibit drug metabolism and may be preferred in the elderly patient on multiple-drug therapy. Inappropriate long-term use of all antibiotics should be discouraged, to minimize the development of bacterial resistance.

One study in elderly males suggests that the number of slow acetylators increases with age. This may interfere with the metabolism of isoniazid. With isoniazid, the frequency of drug-induced toxic hepatitis is increased in patients over the age of 50. Current recommendations from the Centers for Disease Control state that prophylactic use of isoniazid should be avoided in patients over 35 years of age, unless the risk of active tuberculosis outweighs the risk of hepatotoxicity. Examples of patients at risk include recent converters, positive reactors, or immunosuppressed patients. Liver disease, alcohol intake history and diet are additional risk factors for the incidence of drug-induced hepatitis. For elderly patients who are recent converters, the risk of contracting tuberculosis is greater than the risk of hepatitis (87). Prodromal symptoms of hepatitis are anorexia, nausea, and vomiting. These should be monitored, and if they occur when liver enzyme activity is five times baseline, the drug should be discontinued.

Mortality from pneumococcal pneumonia and influenza epidemics is very high in the elderly. Elderly patients respond with antibody formation to the polyvalent pneumococcal vaccine like a younger population (88). Recommendations now are to immunize high-risk elderly patients every 6 years rather than once a lifetime. A favorable antibody response is likewise elicited from an annual influenza vaccine, with an efficacy of 70 to 80% against the influenza strains of the season. It usually takes 4 to 8 weeks to elicit a full antibody response, so vaccinations must be made before the anticipated flu season. Most elderly patients with chronic disease should be immunized with both pneumococcal and an annual influenza vaccine.

During the first 48 hr of symptoms in a flu epidemic, high-risk, nonimmunized elderly patients may be given chemoprophylaxis with 200 mg per day of amantadine, and even symptomatic immunized elderly patients may benefit from treatment. Chemoprophylaxis only protects against influenza A, which is responsible for 80% of all cases. CNS side effects such as hallucinations are common with amantadine, especially in patients with reduced renal function.

Bronchodilators

The clearance of theophylline can be reduced in congestive heart failure, liver disease, and chronic respiratory disease as well as by concurrent therapy with cimetidine, erythromycin, and ciprofloxacin. Decreased clearance can lead to a higher frequency of drug-induced cardiac arrhythmias. Reports conflict on whether age alone can alter theophylline clearance (89). It appears that the loading dose of IV aminophylline (5 to 6 mg/kg infused slowly over 20 min) can be safely administered, regardless of risk factors. The maintenance infusion dose for the elderly, based on lean body weight, is 0.4 mg/kg/hr (90). If liver disease or severe congestive heart failure is present, this rate should be further reduced. No specific guidelines exist for dosage adjustment of oral theophylline products, but a dosage decrease of 33% (12 to 14 mg/kg/day) is reasonable if other factors are present, especially in nonsmokers. Blood levels (samples for determination drawn 2 hr after dose for peak, prior to the next dose for trough) should be maintained in the 7.5 to 15 mg/100ml range to optimize benefits and minimize side effects, because toxicity may occur at blood concentrations at the lower end of the therapeutic range (91). Ipratropium bromide or inhaled β-agonists may be better choices for therapy of COPD in elderly patients because of the adverse effects and costly monitoring necessary with theophylline usage (92).

H-2 Receptor Antagonists and Sucralfate

The bioavailability of cimetidine increases with age (93), most likely because of decreased hepatic clearance. Cimetidine is a potent inhibitor of the hepatic microsomal oxidase system, which is responsible for the high frequency of drug interactions occurring with this agent. Reversible confusional states have occasionally occurred following administration of cimetidine to geriatric and/or severely ill patients (those with renal and/or hepatic insufficiency).

The symptoms of mental confusion may range from agitation to paranoia to delusions. These changes occur 5 days after initiating therapy and are reversible 36 hr after the drug is discontinued. The recommended oral dose of cimetidine should be reduced by 33 to 50% to between 600 and 900 mg per day for the acute phase of treatment rather than the standard 800 to 1200 mg per day. The prophylactic or maintenance dose for cimetidine is 400 mg at bedtime.

Ranitidine undergoes variable metabolism as well as renal excretion of the unchanged parent drug. A recent study (94) reported an increase in the plasma concentration of ranitidine in the elderly that could lead to side effects (e.g., confusion) similar to those seen with cimetidine. With renal dysfunction, (a creatinine clearance time of less than 50 ml/min), a 150-mg daily dose may be sufficient for both active treatment and prophylaxis. Because of its different chemical structure, fewer drug interactions are reported with ranitidine than with cimetidine. The efficacy, as measured by ulcer healing and relapse rates, and the incidence of side effects is the same in elderly and younger patients (95). Famotidine only requires dose or interval adjustment in severe renal impairment (96), and nizatidine appears to be handled much like ranitidine.

Constipation is the common side effect of sucralfate, a basic aluminum salt used for the treatment or prevention of ulcers. In the elderly patient with reduced renal function and on chronic therapy, sucralfate may produce a hypophosphatemia or an accumulation of aluminum. Long-term prophylaxis, defined as longer than 12 months, should be reevaluated with all antiulcer agents, especially in patients experiencing side effects or on multiple potentially interacting drugs.

Antineoplastic Drugs

With age-related depression of the immune system, the elderly patient is more susceptible to the development of solid tumors, lymphomas, and leukemias. A review of the medical literature indicates that certain neoplastic diseases or the drugs used to treat them may alter drug pharmacokinetics (97). In the case of a patient with metastatic cancer, hepatic involvement could further alter the hepatic metabolism of prescribed drugs.

A decrease in the absorption of procarbazine may be a reason for a refractoriness in elderly patients with Hodgkin's disease. A defective transport in folate across the cell membranes may be responsible for the decrease in absorption seen with methotrexate and leucovorin. This may result in reduced efficacy of the leucovorin rescue procedure in patients on high doses of methotrexate. Efficient liver metabolism is needed to activate metabolites of cyclophosphamide and decarbazine or to inactivate toxic parent drugs such as BCNU or metabolites of CCU. Elderly patients are more susceptible to drug toxicities involving the hematopoietic system, GI tract, heart, and nervous system because of drug accumulation or altered pharmacologic response.

An intact kidney is needed for renal elimination of methotrexate, bleomycin, and cisplatinum. To avoid drugs toxicity, dosage alterations are necessary. The incidence and severity of myelotoxicity in elderly female patients with advanced cancer of the breast was reduced with no decrease in efficacy when the dose was adjusted to creatinine clearance time (99). In the future, the combination of individualized dosing of antineoplastics and drug administration based on circadian cycles may minimize or delay drug toxicity and allow better response from prolonged treatment with first-line drugs.

Oral Hypoglycemics and Insulin

There has always been a controversy as to whether tight control of the disease will delay or prevent the vascular complications of diabetes. In the geriatric patient, hypoglycemia should be avoided, while also avoiding marked symptomatic hyperglycemia. Aggressive therapy may result in severe hypoglycemia and subsequent changes in mental status. Older patients may also exhibit a blunted response to hypoglycemia, which may mask the signs and symptoms of the condition. In general, plasma glucose concentrations should be lowered to as near normal as possible without subjecting the patient to the risk of frequent or profound hypoglycemia.

Treatment of the geriatric diabetic patient differs little from that of the younger patient, including diet, exercise, oral hypoglycemic agents, and insulin. With increasing age, the pancreas may be less able to secrete insulin when stimulated. Advantages of oral hypoglycemics for treatment of non-insulin-dependent mellitus in the geriatric patient include ease of administration, effectiveness in lowering glucose levels, relative safety, and decreased need for precise meal timing. Disadvantages are the risk of development of hypoglycemia, decreased efficacy over time, interactions with other drugs, altered metabolism and excretion in geriatric patients, and rarity of euglycemia.

In elderly patients who may have declining renal function or sporadic timing of meals, a shorter-acting first-generation sulfonylurea agent such as tolbutamide, which is metabolized in the liver, is safer than a longer-acting agent such as chlorpromide, which can accumulate because of decreased renal elimination. Overall, the frequency of side effects with chlorpropramide is twice that of other oral hypoglycemic agents. In general, oral hypoglycemic doses are reduced or dosing intervals increased based on clinical response and age or disease-related changes in the liver or kidney. The second-generation agents such as glyburide and glipizide are increasingly being used due to their single daily dosing, liver metabolism, and favorable side-effect profile. The pharmacokinetics of glipizide were shown to be similar in healthy and diabetic elderly patients, compared with a younger population, so dosage alteration is not necessary (99). Patients maintained on oral hypoglycemics should be rechallenged annually with drug withdrawal to determine if continued use or a lower dose is necessary.

Insulin should be used in geriatric patients when blood glucose fails to respond to diet alone or to oral sulfonylureas (fasting plasma glucose level under 150 mg/dl) and in the 10% of the geriatric diabetics who have type I diabetes mellitus. Frequently, satisfactory control can be achieved with a single daily injection of intermediate-acting insulin such as NPH or Lente. As the maintenance of euglycemia becomes increasingly difficult, split-dose insulin (two-thirds of the dose in the morning and one-third in the early evening) may be required.

Anticoagulants

Sensitivity to warfarin may increase in the elderly because of a greater inhibition of vitamin K–dependent synthesis. Recommendations for warfarin include reducing the average daily dose by 30 to 40%. Elderly females have been reported to be more susceptible to the bleeding complications of heparin (100). However, no age-related relationship exists between plasma heparin concentration and its anticoagulant effect (101), so increased bleeding complications would be due to altered pharmacologic response at the receptor site. Hematuria and prothrombin (PT) and partial thromboplastin times (PTT), are sensitive parameters to monitor for potential heparin or warfarin toxicity.

Glaucoma Therapy

Acetazolamide is a carbonic anhydrase inhibitor that is used in the pharmacologic management of open-angle glaucoma. It is highly protein bound and eliminated from the body solely by renal excretion. In one study (102), 55% of elderly glaucoma patients showed toxicity at commonly prescribed doses, manifested as an acute hyperchloremic metabolic acidosis. The high frequency of adverse effects is due to an age-related decrease in renal clearance, which requires dosage adjustments and careful electrolyte monitoring (103). For these reasons, topical agents such as pilocarpine, timolol, and the other β-blockers should be the first choice of therapy for glaucoma. When using topical ocular therapy, patients should be carefully monitored for adverse effects that could result from systemic absorption of the drug. Of the topical agents, the β-blockers may be the best choice because of once- or twice-daily dosing and the lack of adverse effects that are common with pilocarpine.

PHARMACIST-INITIATED DRUG REGIMEN REVIEWS

Federal regulations implemented in 1974 and expanded in 1987 require pharmacists to provide monthly drug-regimen review in long-term care facilities. These reviews identify potential drug problems within facilities. They have been shown to decrease polypharmacy, minimize duplicate therapy, prevent drug interactions, reduce inappropriate use of drugs, insure appropriate monitoring of drug therapy, and reduce drug costs.

Compliance in the Elderly

Compliance is defined as the extent to which a patient's behavior coincides with a prescriber's planned medical regimen. Noncompliance with drug therapy occurs in one-third to one-half of elderly patients (104). Most of the time they are taking too little medication (105). Although the elderly population is at risk for noncompliance because of the number of drugs that they are prescribed, studies have failed to prove that older patients, as a group, are less compliant than the general population (106). Poor communication with health professionals and declining cognitive function are major reasons for noncompliance. Pharmacists must make a special effort to counsel these high-risk patients by providing both verbal reinforcement and written instructions, to assure an understanding of why the drug was prescribed, its use, the proper administration time consistent with their lifestyle, and common side effects. On refill visits to the pharmacy, questions related to side effects and serious adverse reactions should be asked by the pharmacist. Eliminating unnecessary or duplicative therapy and simplifying the regimen help minimize adverse drug reactions and maximize compliance. Healthcare professionals should be aware of the major risk factors for noncompliance and assess each patient for their presence (Table 90.10).

Above all, communication should be encouraged among those involved in patient care—the patient, the physician, and the pharmacist. Pharmaceutical care is now defined as the responsible provision of drug therapy for the purpose of achieving definite outcomes that improve a patient's quality of life. Indications and realistic goals of therapy must be clearly identified in the patient medical record. The professional responsibilities of the pharmacist include assuring the appropriate use of each drug prescribed and monitoring for its efficacy and toxicity. Drugs of choice and dosage adjustments must be individualized for each geriatric patient.

To minimize drug interactions and serious adverse reactions causing costly and unnecessary hospitalizations, the number of drugs on the patient profile should be minimized. The frequency of administration of "as needed" drugs should be reviewed monthly and may provide clues to signs of drug toxicity; the necessity of these "as needed" drugs should be reassessed quarterly. In-service programs for the nursing staff can help the pharmacist carrying out these drug therapy monitoring responsibilities.

CONCLUSION

The increasing number of geriatric patients represents many opportunities for healthcare professionals, and an understanding of the age-related physiologic and pathologic changes is essential for the provision of quality medical care. The potential for drug-related problems in the geriatric population is established, and all healthcare professionals, including pharmacists, need to be aware of this potential when designing and monitoring drug therapy.

REFERENCES

1. Green LW, Mullen PD, Stainbrook GL: Programs to reduce drug errors in the elderly: direct and indirect evidence from patient education. J Geriatr Drug Ther 1:3–18, 1986.
2. Nolan L, O'Malley K: Prescribing for the elderly Part I: sensitivity of the elderly to adverse drug reactions. J Am Geriatr Soc 36:142–149, 1988.
3. Williamson J, Chopin JM: Adverse reactions to prescribed drugs in the elderly: a multicenter investigation. Age Aging 9:73–80, 1980.
4. Michocki RJ, Lamy PP: A "risk" approach to adverse drug reactions. J Am Geriatr Soc 36:79–81, 1988.
5. Steel K, Gertman PM, Crescenzi C, et al.: Iatrogenic illness on a general medical service in a unversity hospital. N Engl J Med 304(11):638–642, 1981.
6. Ochs, HR, Greenblatt DJ, Allen MD, et al.: Effect of age and Billroth gastrectomy on absorption of desmethyldiazepam from clorazepate, Clin Pharmacol Ther 26:449–456, 1979.
7. Evans MA, Triggs EJ, Broe GA, et al.: L-Dopa in the elderly parkinsonian patient, Eur J Clin Pharmacol 17:215–221, 1980.
8. Tuttle CB, Mayersohn M, Walker GC: Biological availability and urinary excretion of oral tolbutamide formulations in man. Can J Pharm Sci 8:31, 1974.
9. Miller SW, Strom JG: Drug-product selection: implications for the geriatric patient. Consul Pharm 5:30–37, 1990.
10. Lamy PP: Critical patients, critical drugs, critical diseases. Maryland Pharm 61:22–25, 1985.
11. Gugler R, Lain P, Azarnoff DL: Effect of portocaval shunt on the disposition of drugs with and without first pass effect. J Pharmacol Exp Ther 195:416–423, 1975.
12. Kelly JG, McGarry K, O'Malley K, et al.: Bioavailability of labetalol increases with age. Br J Clin Pharmacol 14:304–305, 1982.
13. Storstein L, Larsen A, Saevareid L: Pharmacokinetics of calcium channel blockers in patients with renal insufficiency and in geriatric patients. Acta Med Scand 681(suppl. 1):25–30, 1984.
14. Wallace SM, Verbeek RO: Plasma protein binding of drugs in the elderly. Clin Pharmacokinet 12:41–72, 1987.
15. Somerville K, Faulkner G, Langman M: Non-steroidal anti-inflammatory drugs and bleeding peptic ulcer. Lancet 1:462–464, 1986.
16. Hayes MJ, Langman MJS, Short AH: Changes in drug metabolism with increasing age. Br J Clin Pharmacol 2:73–79, 1975.
17. Mather LE, Tucker GT, Pflug AE, et al.: Meperidine kinetics in man. Clin Pharmacol Ther 17:21–30, 1975.
18. Dawling S, Lynn K, Rosser R, Braithwaite R: Nortriptyline metabolism in chronic renal failure: metabolic elimination. Clin Pharm Ther 32:322–329, 1982.
19. Abernathy DR, Greenblatt DJ, Shader RI: Imipramine and desipramine disposition in the elderly. J Pharm Exp Ther 232:183–188, 1985.
20. Cohen BM, Sommer BR: Metabolism in thioridazine in the elderly. J Clin Psychopharmacol 8:336–339, 1988.
21. Antal EJ, Kramer PA, Mercik SA, Chapron DJ, Lawson IR: The-

ophylline pharmacokinetics in advanced age. Br J Clin Pharmcol 12:637–645, 1981.

22. Cockroft DW, Gault MH: Prediction of creatinine clearance from serum creatinine. Nephron 16:31–41, 1976.

23. Friedman JR, Norman DC, Yoshikawa TT: Correlation of estimated renal function parameters versus 24-hour creatinine clearance in ambulatory elderly. J Am Geriatr Soc 37:145–149, 1989.

24. Smith JM, Baldessarini RJ: Changes in prevalence, severity, and recovery in tardive dyskinesia with age. Arch Gen Psychiatry 37:1368–1373, 1980.

25. Feely J, Cloakley D: Altered pharmacodynamics in the elderly. Clin Geriatr Med 6(2)269–283, 1990.

26. Morley JE, Mooradian AD, Rosenthal MJ, et al.: Diabetes mellitus in elderly patients is it different? Am J Med 83:533–544, 1987.

27. Kannell WB, Gordon T (eds.): The Framingham Study: An Epidemiologic Investigation of Cardiovascular Disease. Washington, D.C.: U.S. Government Printing Office, 1974.

28. Kannell WB, Gordon T, Schwartz MJ: Systolic vs. diastolic blood pressure and risk of coronary heart disease. The Framingham Study. Am J Cardiol 27:335–346, 1971.

29. Kannel WB, Wolf PA, McGee DL, et al.: Systolic blood pressure, arterial rigidity and risk of stroke: The Framingham Study. JAMA 245:1225–1229, 1981.

30. Veterans Administration Cooperative Study on Antihypertensive Agents: Effects of treatment on morbidity in hypertension. III. Influence of age on diastolic pressure and prior cardiovascular disease; further analysis of side effects. Circulation 45:991–1004, 1972.

31. Hypertension, Detection and Follow-up Program Cooperative Group: Five year findings of the hypertension detection and follow-up program II. Mortality by race, sex and age. JAMA 242:2572–2577, 1979.

32. Anon: The Australian Therapeutic Trial in Mild Hypertension. Lancet 2:1261–1267, 1980.

33. Amery A, Berthaux P, Birkenhager W, et al.: Antihypertensive therapy in patients above age 60: Fourth interim report in the European Working Party on high blood pressure in the elderly. Clin Sci Mol Med 55(suppl 4)S263–270, 1978.

34. Amery A, Birkenhager W, Brixko P, et al.: Mortality and morbidity results from the European Working Party on high blood pressure in the elderly trial. Lancet 1:1349–1354, 1985.

35. Lakatta EG and Gerstenblith G, Alterations in circulatory function. In Hazzard WR, Andres R, et al. (eds): Principles of Geriatric Medicine and Gerontology. McGraw-Hill, New York, 1990.

36. Terasawa F, Kuramoto K, Ying LH, et al.: The study of the hemodynamics in old hypertensive patients. Acta Gerontol Jap 56:47, 1972.

37. Pederson KE, Dorph-Pederson A, Hvidt S, et al.: Digoxin-verapamil interaction. Clin Pharmacol Ther 30:311–316, 1981.

38. Abernethy DR, Montamat SC: Acute and chronic studies of diltiazem in elderly versus young hypertensive patients, Am J Cardiol 60(17):116I–120I, 1987.

39. Robertson DR, Waller DG, Renwick AG, et al.: Age-related changes in the pharmacokinetics and pharmacodynamics of nifedipine. Br J Clin Pharmacol 25(3):297–305, 1988.

40. Scott M, Castleden CM, Adam HR, et al.: The effect of aging on the disposition of nifedipine and atenolol. Br J Clin Pharmacol 25(3):289–296, 1988.

41. Forette F, McClaran J, Hervy MP, et al.: Nicardipine in elderly patients with hypertension: a review of experience in France. Am Heart J 117(1):256–261, 1989.

42. Kiowski W, Bahler FR, Fadayomi MO, et al.: Age, race, blood pressure and renin: predictors for antihypertensive treatment with calcium antagonists. Am J Cardiol 56:81H–85H, 1985.

43. Zuzman RM: Renin and non-renin mediated antihypertensive actions of converting enzyme inhibitors. Kidney Int 25:969, 1984.

44. Guatam PC, Vargas E, Lye, M: The pharmacokinetics of lisinopril in healthy young and elderly subject and in elderly patients with cardiac failure. J Pharm Pharmacol 39(11)929–931, 1987.

45. Casteleden CM, Kaye CM, Parson RL: The effect of age on plasma levels of propranolol and practolol in man. Br J Clin Pharmacol 2:303–306, 1975.

46. Castleden CM, George CF: The effect of aging on the hepatic clearance of propranolol. Br J Clin Pharmacol 7:49–54, 1979.

47. Greenblatt DJ, Koch-Weser J: Adverse reactions to propranolol in hospitalized medical patients. Am Heart J 86:478–484, 1973.

48. Butler FR, Burkhart F, Lutold BE, et al.: Antihypertensive beta-blocking action as related to renin and age. Am J Cardiol 36:653, 1975.

49. Abernethy DR, Schwartz JB, Plachetka JR, et al.: Comparison in young and elderly patients of pharmacodynamics and disposition of labetalol in systemic hypertension. Am J Cardiol 60(8):697–702, 1987.

50. Fleb JL, Gottlieb SJ, Lakatta EG: Is digoxin really important in treatment of compensated heart failure? Am J Med 73:244–249, 1982.

51. Gheorghiade M, Beller GA: Effects of discontinuing maintenance digoxin therapy in patients with ischemic heart disease and congestive heart failure in sinus rhythm. Am J Cardiol 51:1243, 1983.

52. Consensus Trial Study Group: Effects of enalapril on mortality in severe congestive heart failure. Results of the Cooperative North Scandinavian Survival Study (Consensus). N Engl J Med 316:1429–1435, 1987.

53. The Captopril-Digoxin Multicenter Research Group: Comparative effects of therapy with captopril and digoxin in patients with mild and moderate congestive heart failure. JAMA 259:539–544, 1988.

54. Alpert JS: Nitrate therapy in the elderly. Am J Cardiol 65(21):230–270, 1990.

55. Jordan R, Seth L, Casebolt P, et al.: Rapidly developing tolerance to transdermal nitroglycerin in congestive heart failure. Ann Intern Med 104:294–298, 1986.

56. Cowan JC, Bourke JP, Reid DS, et al.: Prevention of tolerance to nitroglycerine patches by over-night removal. Am J Cardiol 60:271–275, 1987.

57. Ochs HR, Greenblatt DJ, Woo E, et al.: Reduced quinidine clearance in elderly persons. Am J Cardiol 42:481–485, 1978.

58. Thomson PD, Melman KL, Richardson JA, et al.: Lidocaine pharmacokinetics in advanced heart failure, liver disease and renal failure in humans. Ann Intern Med 78:499–508, 1973.

59. Pfeifer HJ, Greenblatt DJ, Koch-Weser J: Clinical use and toxicity of intravenous lidocaine. Am Heart J 92:168–173, 1976.

60. Podrid P, Schoeneberger A, Lawn B: Congestive heart failure caused by oral disopyramide. N Engl J Med 302:614–617, 1980.

61. Stewart RB, May FE, Moore MT, Hale WE: Changing patterns of psychotropic drug use in the elderly: A five-year update. Drug Intell Clin Pharm 23:610–613, 1989.

62. Preskorn SH, Denner LJ: Benzodiazepines and withdrawal psychosis. JAMA 237:36–38, 1977.

63. Lister RG: The amnesic action of benzodiazepines in man. Neurosci Biobehav Rev 9:87–94, 1985.

64. Gillin JC, Byerley WF: The diagnosis and management of insomnia. N Engl J Med 322:239–248, 1990.

65. Ray WA, Griffin MR, Downey W: Benzodiazepines of long and short elimination half-life and the risk of hip fracture. JAMA 262:3303–3307, 1989.

66. Gammans RE, Westrick ML, Shea JP, et al.: Pharmacokinetics of buspirone in elderly subjects. J Clin Pharmacol 29(1):72–78, 1989.

67. Inoue F: Adverse reactions to antipsychotic drugs. Drug Intel Clin Pharm 13:198–207, 1979.

68. Simonson W, Schaeffer K, Williams R: Assessing the impact of a drug-holiday program. Consult Pharm 1:203–209, 1986.

69. Napoli JFX: Assessing a long-term care drug holiday program. Consult Pharm 3:457–461, 1988.

70. Kane JM, Honigfeld G, Singer J, et al.: Clozapine for the treatment-resistant schizophrenia: a double-blind comparison with chlorpromazine. Arch Gen Psychiatry 45:789–796, 1988.

71. Thompson TL, Filley CM, Mitchell WD, et al.: Lack of efficacy of hydergine in patients with Alzheimer's disease. N Engl J Med 323(7):445–448, 1990.

72. Plotkin DA, Gerson SC, Jairrh, LF, Antidepressant drug therapy in the elderly. In Meltzer HY (ed): Psychopharmacology: The Third Generation of Progress. New York, Raven Press, pp 1149–1158, 1987.

73. Feighner JP, Bayer WF, Meredith CH, et al.: An overview of fluoxetine in geriatric depression. Br J Psychiatry 153(suppl 3):105–108, 1988.

74. Katz IR, Simpson GM, Jethanandani V: Steady state pharmacokinetics of nortriptyline in the frail elderly. Neuropharmacology 2(3):229–236, 1989.

75. Hardy BG, Shulman KI, Mackenzie SE, et al.: Pharmacokinetics of lithium in the elderly. J Clin Psychopharmacol 7:153–158, 1987.

76. Clark BG: Phenytoin once-daily dosing in geriatric patients. Drug Intell Clin Pharm 19:584, 1985.

77. Foley KM, Inturisi CE: Analgesic drug therapy in cancer pain: principles and practice. Med Clin North Am 71:207, 1987.

78. Kaiko RF, Wallenstein SL, Rogers AG, et al.: Narcotics in the elderly. Med Clin North Am 66:1079–1089, 1982.

79. Wall RT: Use of analgesics in the elderly: Clin Geriatr Med 6:345–369, 1990.

80. Iobat WJ, Bridger CR, Regan-Smith MG: Antirheumatic agents: CNS toxicity and its avoidance. Geriatrics 44:95, 1989.

81. Murphy MD, Brater DC: Nonsteroidal anti-inflammatory drugs. Clin Geriatr Med 6(2):365–397, 1990.

82. Blackshear J, Davidson M, Stillman M. Identification of risk factors for renal insufficiency from nonsteroidal antiinflammatory drugs. Arch Intern Med 143:1130–1134, 1983.

83. Kumin GD: Clinical nephrotoxicity of tobramycin and gentamicin. JAMA 244:1808–1810, 1980.

84. Cutler NR, Narang PK, Lesko LJ, et al.: Vancomycin disposition: the importance of age. Clin Pharmacol Ther 366:803–810, 1984.

85. Ljungberg B, Nilsson-Ethie I: Pharmacokinetics of ciprofloxacin in the elderly: increased oral bioavailability and reduced renal clearance. Eur J Clin Microbial Infect Dis 8(6)515–520, 1989.

86. Davey PG: Overview of drug interactions with the quinolones. J Antimicrob Chemother 22(suppl C)97–107, 1988.

87. Stead WW, To T, Harrison RW, et al.: "Benefit-risk considerations in preventive treatment for tuberculosis in elderly persons". Ann Intern Med 107:843–845, 1987.

88. Ammann AJ, Schiffman G, Austrian R: The antibody responses to pneumococcal capsular polysaccharides in aged individuals. Proc Soc Exp Biol Med 164:321, 1980.

89. Jackson SH, Wiffen JK, Johnston A, et al.: The relationship between clearance of theophylline and age within the adult range. Eur J Clin Pharmacol 29:177–179, 1985.

90. Nielson-Kudsk F, Magnussen I, Jakobsen P: Pharmacokinetics of theophylline in elderly patients. Acta Pharmacol Toxicol 42:226–234, 1978.

91. Klein JJ, Lefkowitz MS, Spector SL, et al.: Relationship between serum theophylline levels and pulmonary function before and after inhaled beta-agonist in stable asthmatics. Am Rev Respir Dis 127:413, 1983.

92. Adelman AM, Daly MP, Michocki RJ: Alternate drugs. Clin Geriatr Med 6(2):423–444, 1990.

93. Redolfi A, Borgogelli E, Lodola E: Blood level of cimetidine in relation to age. Eur J Clin Pharmacol 15:257–261, 1979.

94. Greene DS, Szego PL, Anslow JA, et al.: The effect of age on ranitidine pharmacokinetics. Clin Pharmacol Ther 39:300–305, 1986.

95. Mills R, Begun JM, Holland CE, et al.: Ranitidine for duodenal ulcer disease in the elderly: a retrospective review of four multicenter trials. J Geriatr Soc 3(2):43–56, 1989.

96. Lin JH, Chremos AN, Yeh KL, et al.: Effects of age and chronic renal failure on the urinary excretion kinetics of famotidine in man. Eur J Clin Pharmacol 34(1)41–46, 1988.

97. Balducci L, Parker M, Sexton W, et al.: Pharmacology of antineoplastic agents in the elderly patient. Semin Oncol 16(1):76–84, 1989.

98. Gelman RS, Taylor SG: Cyclophosphamide, methotrexate and 5-fluorouracil chemotherapy in women more than 65 years old with advanced breast cancer: the elimination of age trends in toxicity by using doses bases on creatinine clearance. J Clin Oncol 2:1406–1414, 1984.

99. Kradjan WA, Kobayashi KA, Bauer LA, et al.: Glipizide pharmacokinetics: effects of age, diabetes and multiple dosing. J Clin Pharmacol 29:1121–1127, 1989.

100. Jick H, Slone D, Borda IT, et al.: Efficacy and toxicity of heparin in relation to age and sex. N Engl J Med 279:284–286, 1968.

101. Whitfield LR, Schentag JJ, Levy G: Relationship between concentration and anticoagulant effect of heparin in plasma of hospitalized patients: magnitude of predictability of interindividual differences. Clin Pharmacol Ther 32:503–516, 1982.

102. Heller I, Halevy J, Cohen S, et al.: Significant metabolic acidosis induced by acetazolamide. Arch Intern Med 145:1815–1817, 1985.

103. Chapron DJ, Gomolin IH, Sweeney KR: Acetazolamide blood concentrations are excessive in the elderly: propensity for acidosis and relationship to renal function. J Clin Pharmacol 29:348–353, 1989.

104. Morrow D, Leirer V, Sheikh J: Adherence and medication instructions: review and recommendations. J Am Geriatr Soc 36:1147–1160, 1988.

105. Cooper JK, Love DW, Raffoul PR: Intentional prescription nonadherence (noncompliance) by the elderly. J Am Geriatr Soc 30:329–333, 1982.

106. Montamat SC, Cusack BJ, Vestal RE: Management of drug therapy in the elderly. N Engl J Med 321;303–309, 1989.

CHAPTER 91

CRITICAL CARE THERAPEUTICS

DONALD L. KENDZIERSKI, Pharm.D. and LOUISE G. KENDZIERSKI, Pharm.D.

Treating a patient in an intensive care unit is a demanding endeavor. Patients have multiple medical problems complicating their presentation and course in the ICU. The drug therapy of these patients may be complex, requiring multiple interventions, modifications, and alternatives. This challenges the clinician's expertise in drug selection, dosing, and patient monitoring. Unfortunately, the scope of critical care is too broad to be covered in a single chapter. The management of diabetic ketoacidosis, myocardial infarction, respiratory failure from asthma or COPD, burns, status epilepticus and delerium tremens is discussed in previous chapters. Select diseases are presented because of diverse drug therapy and the need to intervene quickly to prevent death or significant morbidity.

SEPTIC SHOCK

Bacterial sepsis and septic shock are major causes of morbidity and mortality in hospitalized patients. There may be as many as 400,000 cases of sepsis, 200,000 cases of septic shock, and 100,000 deaths per year from the disease (1). The precise incidence is unknown because many patients may have clinical evidence of sepsis without an organism being isolated from the blood.

Sepsis can be defined as a severe infection caused by the invasion of microorganisms (bacteria, fungi, etc.) and their toxins in the bloodstream. *Septic shock* encompasses the hemodynamic and metabolic consequences of the infection, including circulatory failure, hypotension, and inadequate tissue perfusion. Some of the risk factors for developing sepsis include surgical procedures, mechanical ventilation, immunosuppressive drugs, invasive devices (e.g., intravascular catheters), and antimicrobial resistance (1).

Pathophysiology of Septic Shock

Septic shock begins with the introduction of blood-borne bacteria from localized sites such as the skin, respiratory tract, urinary tract, gastrointestinal tract, and mucous membranes. Common pathogens in the septic process are Gram-negative organisms such as *Escherichia, Klebsiella, Enterobacter, Serratia, Proteus,* and *Pseudomonas* species. However, any organism, including Gram-positive bacteria and various fungi, may produce the various manifestations of sepsis. The Gram-negative rods invade the bloodstream and release toxic substances called *endotoxins*.

Gram-negative endotoxin is a product of the bacterial cell wall. The bacteria have an outer cell-wall membrane consisting of 3 major components: transmembrane protein, lipid, and lipopolysaccharide. The lipid-A moiety of the lipopolysaccharide molecule appears to produce the endotoxic effects seen in septic shock (2). The lipopolysaccharide molecule also triggers a cascade of biological mediators important in septic shock (2).

To initiate the process, endotoxin stimulates monocytes and macrophages to produce tumor necrosis factor and interleukin-1, two primary mediators. These mediators then cause synthesis and release of prostaglandins, leukotrienes, myocardial-depressant factor, interferons, platelet-activating factor, endorphins, and colony-stimulating factors. The physiologic effects exerted by some of these mediators are listed in Table 91.1.

Clinical Manifestations of Septic Shock

Early recognition of the signs and symptoms of sepsis and septic shock are essential for treating this disease promptly and effectively. The clinical manifestations of sepsis are vary, depending upon when the diagnosis is made (Table 91.2).

Fever is the most frequent manifestation of sepsis, mediated by the release of pyrogenic substances from the microorganism or the host. The fever is usually accompanied by tachypnea, tachycardia, and chills. Tachypnea causes hyperventilation and respiratory alkalosis. While most septic patients are febrile, normothermia or even hypothermia may be present. Hypothermia is seen most commonly in the very young, very old, or debilitated patients (3). The mortality tends to be higher in patients who are hypothermic during the initial 24 hr (4).

Alterations in mental status are important clinical findings in sepsis. They range from mild disorientation, confusion, lethargy, and obtundation to combativeness or agitation. Although the pathogenesis of the altered mental status remains controversial, hypoxia, hypotension, electrolyte disturbances, decreased cerebral blood flow, and altered amino acid metabolism may play a role (4).

Cardiovascular and pulmonary manifestations of sepsis

and septic shock must be recognized early to ensure appropriate treatment. Classically, shock has been described in terms of "warm shock" in the vasodilated, hyperdynamic patient and "cold shock" in the vasoconstricted patient. However, the clinical findings are best understood when the process is viewed as a temporal sequence of preshock, early shock, and late shock (Table 91.3).

The preshock phase of sepsis is characterized by a normal blood pressure with a decrease in the systemic vascular resistance and an increase in the cardiac output. The most common acid-base abnormality is a marked respiratory alkalosis, usually with an arterial carbon dioxide pressure less than or equal to 30 mm Hg. Patients at this stage have blood pressure that is responsive to intravenous fluids and adequate tissue perfusion with warm extremities. As the syndrome progresses to the early shock phase, blood pressure and systemic vascular resistance decrease. At this point, the cardiac output continues to be elevated to compensate for the falling systemic vascular resistance. How-

ever, this increase in cardiac output is insufficient to maintain adequate tissue perfusion pressures, and the shock state ensues. In the late stage of shock there is a profound decrease in blood pressure and the systemic vascular resistance may rise due to α-adrenergic compensatory responses. The cardiac output falls, and a severe metabolic acidosis is present. At this stage the patient has refractory hypotension and acidosis, which usually results in death.

The earliest pulmonary responses to sepsis are tachypnea, hyperventilation, and respiratory alkalosis. As sepsis advances, the patient experiences respiratory muscle fatigue, hypoxia, and respiratory acidosis, usually requiring mechanical ventilation. In addition, endotoxin and various mediators of sepsis may produce acute changes in pulmonary capillary permeability, leading to the development of the adult respiratory distress syndrome (ARDS). ARDS is among the most devastating complications of sepsis. ARDS is characterized by refractory hypoxemia and pulmonary edema. The exudation of fluid and protein into the pulmonary interstitium is secondary to increased capillary permeability and may result in alveolar collapse. The net result is perfusion of unventilated alveoli, leading to severe hypoxemia and respiratory failure.

Leukocytosis with an increase in immature cells is one of the main hematologic findings in sepsis. These changes result from demargination and release of less mature neutrophils from the bone marrow. However, overwhelming bacteremia may produce profound neutropenia in the very young, the elderly, or the chronically debilitated patient. Thrombocytopenia, with or without coagulation abnormalities, is also common.

Coagulation abnormalities may include prolonged prothrombin or partial thromboplastin times or disseminated intravascular coagulation (DIC). DIC is characterized by intravascular thrombin generation and fibrin deposition, consumption of clotting factors and platelets, and secondary fibrinolysis. Laboratory abnormalities include thrombocytopenia, prolonged prothrombin time, elevated fibrin-fibrinogen degradation products, and decreased levels of fibrinogen and coagulation factors V and VIII. This syndrome is triggered by endotoxin and may result in hemorrhagic and/or thrombotic complications.

Common renal manifestations of sepsis include azo-

Table 91.1.
Physiologic Effects of Endotoxin

Vasoconstriction
Vasodilation
Tissue destruction
Inflammatory response
Febrile response
Disseminated intravascular coagulation
Increased vascular permeability

Table 91.2.
Manifestations of Sepsis

Hyperthermia	Thrombocytopenia
Hypothermia	Hypoprothrombinemia
Chills	Hypofibrinogenemia
Hyperventilation	Metabolic acidosis
Altered mental status	Pulmonary edema
Bleeding	Oliguria/anuria
Cyanosis	Jaundice
Hypotension	

Table 91.3.
Hemodynamic Alterations in Sepsis

Parameter	Preshock	Early Shock	Late Shock
Blood pressure	Normal or decreased	Decreased	Decreased
Systemic vascular resistance	Decreased	Decreased	Normal or increased
Cardiac output	Normal or increased	Increased	Decreased
Responsiveness to volume administration	+ + + +	+ +	—
Acid-base abnormality	Respiratory alkalosis	Mixed respiratory alkalosis/metabolic acidosis	Metabolic acidosis

temia, oliguria, and proteinuria. The degree of injury may range from a mild nephropathy to acute renal failure. In shock, these findings usually result from acute tubular necrosis, a condition in which the urinary sediment contains tubular epithelial cells and coarse granular casts. The etiology of acute tubular necrosis in sepsis is not certain, but it is likely that hypotension and/or volume depletion are involved.

Gastrointestinal manifestations of sepsis include hepatic dysfunction, stress ulceration, and gastrointestinal bleeding (4). The liver dysfunction usually presents as an increase in transaminase enzyme levels or cholestatic jaundice. Abnormal laboratory values present in cholestatic jaundice include elevated alkaline phosphatase and serum bilirubin levels. Sepsis also predisposes patients to upper gastrointestinal tract bleeding. When patients develop a severe infection, most will develop 1- to 2-mm erosions of the stomach and/or duodenum (5). Factors contributing to stress ulceration include an alteration in mucosal blood flow, hypoxia of gastric mucosal cells, release of mucosal lysozyme, and disruption of the gastric mucosal barrier (3).

Treatment of Septic Shock

When sepsis occurs, early and rapid intervention is vital to prevent complications and death. A number of measures must be instituted simultaneously, including supporting the cardiovascular, pulmonary, and metabolic systems, obtaining cultures, and initiating appropriate antimicrobial therapy.

The most important therapy in the initial management of patients with septic shock is adequate volume support with hemodynamic monitoring because of ongoing capillary leakage.

A number of solutions are readily available to expand intravascular volume, including crystalloids (normal saline, Ringer's lactate), colloids (albumin, hetastarch), and various blood products. Although Ringer's lactate contains 27 mEq/liter of lactate, it does not potentiate lactic acidosis associated with shock (6). The optimal type of volume replacement is controversial. Most clinicians feel that crystalloids are appropriate for initial volume replacement and that colloids may be used later for patients requiring large amounts of fluid.

Administration of a fluid challenge is the most common approach to fluid resuscitation. It is important to remember that each patient responds differently and close monitoring is essential. A fluid challenge consists of 500 ml to 1 liter of fluid administered over 30 min to patients without a history of congestive heart failure and 250 ml over 30 min to those with a history of congestive heart failure. (See Chapter 8, "Fluid and Electrolyte Therapy and Acid-Base Balance.")

The distribution of crystalloid solutions depends upon the colloid oncotic pressures and hydrostatic pressures in-

side and outside the vascular space. When administered to a normal adult, 25% of the infused volume remains in the intravascular space after 1 hr (7). In critically ill patients, 20% or less may be retained in the intravascular space (7). Administration of crystalloid solutions in septic shock must be carefully controlled and monitored. Peripheral and pulmonary edema are potential side effects from excessive use. Overall, these solutions are inexpensive, readily available, easily stored, and effective in correcting extracellular volume and electrolyte deficits.

For major volume resuscitation, albumin and hetastarch are also effective in restoring hemodynamic stability in shock patients. A 500-ml infusion of 5% albumin increases the intravascular space by 450 to 500 ml, and approximately 90% remains in the vascular space after two hours. With Hetastarch, maximal plasma expansion occurs several minutes after the end of the infusion and is slightly in excess of the volume infused. Effective plasma volume expansion may persist for 24 hr or longer. Hetastarch is usually less costly than albumin, but both are substantially more expensive than crystalloids. (See Chapter 8, "Fluid and Electrolyte Therapy and Acid-Base Balance.")

GUIDELINES FOR INSTITUTING EMPIRIC ANTIMICROBIAL THERAPY IN SEPTIC SHOCK

One of the most crucial aspects in the management of septic shock is the rapid institution of antimicrobial therapy. To select a rational and comprehensive antimicrobial regimen, a number of factors must be considered.

Defining the Most Likely Organisms. Two important factors in determining the most likely organisms involved in the infection are the immunocompetence of the patient and the source of the infection. As shown in Table 91.4, certain pathogens are associated with certain underlying diseases or host defense abnormalities. Specific microorganisms also have a characteristic portal of entry, which may give important clues as to the site of infection (Table 91.5). Finally, the history of the present illness is invaluable in identifying the most likely source of infection.

Choosing an Antibiotic Regimen. When choosing an antibiotic regimen, empiric therapy should be broad enough to cover the most likely pathogens for the clinical setting. For example, if there is an uncertainty whether the pathogen is Gram-negative or Gram-positive, coverage must be considered for both. In general, the more acutely ill the patient, the broader the regimen tends to be.

To ensure adequate penetration, antibiotic choices should have good distribution to the portal of entry or site of infection at the doses clinically employed. In addition, the route of administration should involve as few variables as possible. The intravenous route of administration is almost always preferred in hemodynamically compromised patients.

For serious Gram-negative rod infections, most cli-

Table 91.4.
Pathogens Associated with Host Defense Abnormalities

Host Defense Abnormality	Pathogens
Agammaglobulinemia	*Streptococcus pneumoniae*
	Neisseria meningitidis
	Haemophilus influenzae
Complement deficiency	*Streptococcus pneumoniae*
	Streptococcus pyogenes
	Staphylococcus aureus
	Neisseria meningitidis
	Neisseria gonorrhoeae
	Haemophilus influenzae
	Escherichia coli
	Klebsiella spp.
	Serratia spp.
	Enterobacter spp.
	Pseudomonas spp.
Splenectomy	*Streptococcus pneumoniae*
	Haemophilus influenzae
	Neisseria meningitidis
Granulocytopenia	*Escherichia coli*
	Pseudomonas aeruginosa
	Klebsiella spp.
	Serratia spp.
	Enterobacter spp.
	Staphylococcus aureus
	Staphylococcus epidermidis
	Candida spp.

nicians use a combination of bactericidal agents (2). There are several advantages to this mode of therapy. The use of two agents may prevent the emergence of resistance by eliminating small subpopulations that are resistant to one of the agents in the combination (2). In addition, some antibiotic combinations may have additive or synergistic activity, often resulting in enhanced bactericidal activity (2). Examples of empiric antibiotic regimens are outlined in Table 91.6.

The duration of treatment in normal hosts with Gram-negative sepsis is 10 to 14 days; however, this may be extended if the patient has persistent infection. Neutropenic patients should be treated until they are normothermic (minimum of 4 to 7 days), the infection resolves, and the neutrophil count is rising and in excess of 0.5×10^9/liter (500/mm^3) (2).

Patient Monitoring. Although an antimicrobial regimen has been chosen, it is still vital to obtain the results of culture and sensitivity tests. The clinician can then optimize the antibiotic regimen based upon these data. The patient must also be monitored closely for response within a reasonable time. Changing the antibiotic regimen without good reason or making too many changes makes patient evaluations difficult. Finally, identifying alternative regimens is important if an inadequate therapeutic re-

sponse occurs or adverse effects develop. Deciding on alternative agents involves knowing which organisms the initial regimen does not cover, the body compartments that are not being penetrated, and potential toxicities. If the patient is experiencing severe adverse effects, an agent with similar coverage but without the same toxic potential may be used as a replacement.

Table 91.5.
Pathogens Associated with Portal of Entry

Portal of Entry	Pathogens
Genitourinary tract	*Escherichia coli*
	Klebsiella spp.
	Enterobacter spp.
	Serratia spp.
	Proteus spp.
	Pseudomonas spp.
	Streptococcus faecalis
Respiratory tract	*Streptococcus pneumoniae*
	Haemophilus influenzae
	Staphylococcus aureus
	Escherichia coli
	Klebsiella pneumoniae
	Gram-positive and Gram-negative anaerobes
	Pseudomonas spp.
Biliary tract	*Escherichia coli*
	Klebsiella spp.
	Enterobacter spp.
Bowel	*Escherichia coli*
	Klebsiella spp.
	Enterobacter spp.
	Serratia spp.
	Gram-positive and Gram-negative anaerobes
	Streptococcus faecalis

Table 91.6.
Suggested Antibiotic Regimens in Septic Patients

Portal of Entry	Antibiotic Regimen
Genitourinary tract	Ampicillin with or without aminoglycoside OR third-generation cephalosporin
Lung—community-acquired	Penicillin G
Lung—hospital-acquired	Antipseudomonal penicillin, aztreonam, imipenem, ticarcillin with clavulanic acid with or without aminoglycoside; ceftazidime
Intraabdominal—biliary source	Third-generation cephalosporin OR clindamycin or metronidazole with an aminoglycoside
Intraabdominal—bowel source	Metronidazole or clindamycin with an aminoglycoside plus ampicillin
Febrile neutropenic patient	Antipseudomonal penicillin plus an aminoglycoside, ceftazidime

Table 91.7.
Inotropic Agents[a]

Drug	Dose	MAP	PCWP	SVR	CO
Dopamine	1–20 μg/kg/min	0/ ↑	0/ ↑	0/ ↑	↑
Dobutamine	2.5–15 μg/kg/min	0/ ↓	↓	0	↑
Norepinephrine	2–10 μg/min	↑	↑	↑	↑ /0

[a] MAP, mean arterial pressure; PCWP, pulmonary capillary wedge pressure; SVR, systemic vascular resistance; CO, cardiac output; ↑, increased; ↓, decreased; 0, no change.

Table 91.8.
Effects of Dopamine

Infusion Rate	Effects
0.5–2.0 μg/kg/min	Dopaminergic-receptor stimulation
5–10 μg/kg/min	β-receptor stimulation
10–20 μg/kg/min	α- and β-receptor stimulation
≥20 μg/kg/min	α-receptor stimulation predominates

VASOACTIVE AGENTS

The patient in septic shock is often hypotensive or has evidence of hypoperfusion despite volume resuscitation. In this case, a vasopressor and/or inotropic agent may be necessary. The agents most commonly used in septic shock are discussed below, and a summary of doses and effects appear in Table 91.7.

Dopamine. Dopamine is the immediate precursor in the synthesis of norepinephrine. Dopamine has complex direct and indirect sympathomimetic effects. The hemodynamic effects of dopamine are largely a result of a direct effect upon α, β, and dopaminergic receptors. Also, dopamine releases norepinephrine from endogenous storage sites. Dopamine acts upon specific dopaminergic receptors in the renal, mesenteric, coronary, and intracerebral vascular beds to cause vasodilation. Dopamine has dose-dependent inotropic, chronotropic, and vasoactive properties (Table 91.8).

At doses of 0.5 to 2 μg/kg/min, dopamine stimulates dopaminergic receptors in the renal vascular beds, producing increases in renal blood flow, glomerular filtration rate, and urine output. As cardiac output improves with higher doses, renal function may improve further. With infusion rates of 2 to 5 μg/kg/min in normal subjects, dopamine increases cardiac output and contractility with little change in heart rate, blood pressure, or systemic vascular resistance. Doses up to 10 μg/kg/min result in a further increase in cardiac output, with small increases in heart rate and blood pressure. With infusion rates in excess of 10 μg/kg/min, dopamine stimulates α-adrenergic receptors. The resultant hemodynamic effects include increases in systemic vascular resistance and mean arterial pressure and vasoconstriction of the renal vasculature. Do-

pamine also constricts capacitance vessels, which may raise pulmonary capillary wedge pressure or preload.

An intravenous infusion of dopamine has a rapid onset of action and a half-life of approximately 1 min. Steady state is achieved within 5 min. Dopamine is metabolized in the liver by catechol-*o*-methyltransferase (COMT) and monoamine oxidase (MAO). Side effects of dopamine include nausea, vomiting, headache, tachyarrhythmias, angina/myocardial ischemia, hypertension, and profound vasoconstriction (gangrene).

Dopamine is one of the initial vasoactive agents used in septic shock patient because it increases systemic vascular resistance and blood pressure. In addition, dopamine increases urine blood flow and cardiac output, both of which may be persistently depressed after volume replacement. Dopamine should be initiated at 5 μg/kg/min and titrated upward depending upon blood pressure, heart rate, and perfusion of the kidneys, brain, and extremities. While specific end points vary in each patient, a mean arterial pressure of 60 to 70 mm Hg, a urine output above 0.5 ml/kg/hr, warm extremities, and a responsive patient are desirable. Most patients respond to less than 20 μg/kg/minute of dopamine, but some may require higher infusion rates.

Norepinephrine. Norepinephrine is a neurotransmitter of the sympathetic nervous system and the biosynthetic precursor of epinephrine. The major indication for norepinephrine is elevation of blood pressure in hypotensive patients who have failed to respond to adequate volume resuscitation and other less potent inotropes such as dopamine. The drug acts predominantly by α-adrenergic receptor stimulation, causing vasoconstriction and increases in preload and afterload. Norepinephrine is also a potent β₁-agonist with minimal β₂ effects. At doses above 2.5 μg/min, hemodynamic effects include an increase in blood pressure, systemic vascular resistance, mean arterial pressure, preload, and myocardial oxygen demand. Norepinephrine causes vasoconstriction and decreased blood flow to the renal vasculature, pulmonary vessels, skin, and skeletal muscle. Norepinephrine stimulates β₁-adrenergic receptors in the heart, producing a positive inotropic effect. Cardiac output may decrease with prolonged use or with high doses, because of the potent vasoconstrictive effects on capacitance and resistance vessels.

After intravenous administration, a pressor response occurs rapidly, and the drug has an average half-life of 2 to 2.5 min. Norepinephrine is metabolized by COMT and MAO. Side effects may be severe and include headache, angina, peripheral and organ ischemia, skin necrosis, palpitations, and decreased urine output. Norepinephrine is usually initiated as an intravenous infusion of 2 μg/min and titrated to blood pressure response. The dosage range is 2 to 10 μg/min.

Dobutamine. Dobutamine is a synthetic sympathomimetic drug and a derivative of isoproterenol. Dobutamine has a high affinity for β_1-adrenergic receptors, which gives it relatively selective inotropic activity. In therapeutic doses, dobutamine also has mild β_2- and α_1-adrenergic agonist effects. Unlike dopamine, dobutamine does not release endogenous norepinephrine nor does it stimulate renal dopamine receptors. The β_1-adrenergic effects of dobutamine result in increased myocardial contractility, stroke volume, and cardiac output. The increase in cardiac output causes a reflex reduction in systemic vascular resistance, but the net effect upon blood pressure is minimal. Heart rate is usually not changed substantially, and dobutamine tends to be less arrhythmogenic than dopamine. In general, dobutamine also lowers central venous and pulmonary wedge pressure (preload), with little effect on pulmonary vascular resistance. Although it lacks a selective renal vascular effect, dobutamine enhances urine output by improving cardiac output and renal perfusion. Dobutamine has inotropic action equal to or greater than that of dopamine.

Following intravenous administration, dobutamine has an onset of action of 2 min, with the peak effect occurring in 10 min. The plasma half-life is approximately 10 min. Dobutamine is metabolized in the liver by COMT and by conjugation with glucuronic acid. The adverse effects of dobutamine include nausea, vomiting, dyspnea, headache, angina, tachycardia, and ventricular ectopy.

Dobutamine may be used with dopamine in septic shock patients. Once fluids are administered and the blood pressure is stabilized with dopamine, patients may have a persistently depressed cardiac output and an elevated pulmonary artery wedge pressure. Dobutamine is effective in improving cardiac output and left ventricular contractility while decreasing the pulmonary artery wedge pressure. The result is effective inotropic support necessary to maintain an adequate perfusion pressure. Dobutamine may also be administered as an inotropic agent prior to dopamine if hypotension is not severe. A typical starting dose of dobutamine is 2.5 μg/kg/min titrated to 15 μg/kg/min to achieve the desired hemodynamic response.

Although all three vasoactive agents are commonly used, controlled studies have not clearly established which drug is the most useful in treating septic shock. A reasonable approach is to use dopamine initially because of its favorable effects on blood pressure and contractility. Dobutamine may then be added to augment the positive inotropic effects of dopamine. Finally, norepinephrine is used for patients who do not exhibit an adequate blood pressure response to dopamine or dopamine/dobutamine combination. The choice of monitoring parameters depends upon what organ systems are being affected by the shock state (Table 91.9). It is helpful to identify the clinical presentation of the shock state and observe for progression

Table 91.9.
Monitoring Parameters for Septic Shock

Vital signs	Blood pressure
	Heart rate
	Temperature
	Respiratory rate
	Fluid intake
	Urine output, NG output
	Wound drainage
Physical examination	Skin temperature
	Perfusion of extremities
	Mental status
Hemodynamic parameters	Cardiac output/index
	Stroke volume index
	Pulmonary capillary wedge pressure
	Systemic vascular resistance
	Stroke work index
	Oxygen delivery
Laboratory examination	Arterial pH, pO_2, pCO_2
	Arterial oxygen saturation
	Serum Na^+, K^+, Cl^-, $[HCO_3]^-$
	Serum creatinine, BUN
	WBC count, WBC differential
	Platelet count
	Prothrombin time
	AST, ALT, LDH, albumin
Microbiologic examination	Gram stain of body fluids
	Culture of body fluids

or regression of those findings during or after the infusion of these vasoactive inotropes.

ALTERNATIVE TREATMENT MODALITIES

Corticosteroids. There has been controversy for many years over the efficacy of high-dose corticosteroids as adjunct therapy in septic shock. Corticosteroids have a variety of metabolic, antiinflammatory, and immunosuppressive effects that theoretically may be beneficial in septic shock. Short-term administration often results in defervescence, thus leading to a clinical impression of improvement (8–10). Recently, three large clinical trials have failed to confirm the beneficial effect of corticosteroids in septic shock (8–10). In fact, in selected patients, their use may have contributed to secondary infections. In view of these findings, large doses of corticosteroids cannot be recommended routinely as adjunctive therapy in septic shock.

Naloxone. Naloxone, a pure opiate antagonist, has been shown to block the endorphins that produce hypotension. However, the exact role of naloxone in managing septic patients is unclear, because evidence of beneficial effects in humans is lacking. Clear guidelines for dosage recommendations or duration of therapy are not available.

Nonsteroidal Antiinflammatory Agents. Nonsteroidal antiinflammatory drugs (NSAIDs) may decrease the production of several mediators of sepsis, including prostaglandins and thromboxane. These agents have been effective in some animal models, but current data in humans are lacking.

Immunotherapy. Other treatment modalities that are still in the investigational stage include antiserum to endotoxin, intravenous gamma globulin (polyclonal IgG), and monoclonal antibodies directed against lipopolysaccharides from Gram-negative bacteria. (See Chapter 74, "Bacteremia and Sepsis.") Immunotherapy will undoubtedly continue to be an important possibility for treating septic shock in future years.

Summary

Septic shock is a serious syndrome that carries a high mortality in the intensive care setting. Early recognition and prompt therapy with adequate fluids, appropriate antibiotics, and if necessary, vasoactive agents are essential to achieve a positive outcome. Ongoing research in the area of immunology appears promising and may eventually increase the survival from this devastating syndrome.

ADULT RESPIRATORY DISTRESS SYNDROME

The adult respiratory distress syndrome (ARDS) is a severe form of respiratory failure affecting more than 150,000 patients each year and is a frequent cause of respiratory failure in medical and surgical patients (11). However, ARDS is associated with a number of clinical disorders (Table 91.10). Common clinical disorders associated with ARDS are the sepsis syndrome and aspiration of gastric contents (12).

The principle symptom of ARDS is dyspnea. Additional findings include pulmonary edema, hypoxemia, decreased lung distensibility (compliance), decreased lung volumes, and increased pulmonary vascular resistance (12). ARDS has a rapid onset, occurring within 6 to 24 hr in most patients at risk (12).

Pathophysiology

The pathophysiology of ARDS involves several interrelated processes (Table 91.11). A number of agents have been

Table 91.10.
Clinical Disorders Associated with ARDS

Infection	Trauma
Sepsis syndrome	Burns
Severe pneumonia	Fractures
Shock	Pulmonary contusion
Septic	Near drowning
Hypovolemic	Disseminated intravascular
Aspiration of gastric contents	coagulation
Cardiopulmonary bypass	Acute pancreatitis
Multiple transfusions	Drug overdose
Oxygen toxicity	Acetylsalicylic acid
	Heroin

Table 91.11.
Pathophysiology of ARDS

Increased vascular permeability
Intrapulmonary shunting of blood flow
Increased pulmonary vascular resistance

Table 91.12.
Mediators of ARDS

Exogenous	Bacterial endotoxin
Endogenous	Complement
	Cytokines
	Leukotrienes
	Prostaglandins
	Platelet-activating factor
Cellular macrophages	Monocytes
	Neutrophils

implicated as mediators of ARDS (Table 91.12). Bacterial endotoxin initiates a complex cascade of complement activation and release of endogenous mediators. Endogenous mediators (tumor necrosis factor, prostaglandins, leucotrienes) released by monocytes and macrophages cause neutrophil sequestration in the lung and other organs (13). Neutrophils are the source of toxic oxygen radicals and lysosomal enzymes that cause widespread damage to the pulmonary vascular endothelium. Increased vascular permeability to fluid and protein causes severe pulmonary edema (14). Increased lung water decreases lung distensibility (compliance) and lung volumes and produces alveolar collapse.

Pulmonary vascular endothelial damage causes diffuse thromboembolism, vasoconstriction, and destruction of the pulmonary capillary bed (14). This causes alterations in pulmonary blood flow. Pulmonary blood flow may be distributed to nonfunctional or poorly functional alveolar units. Mismatch of pulmonary blood flow and alveolar ventilation further impairs gas exchange.

Combined effects of pulmonary vascular damage and hypoxic pulmonary vasoconstriction cause a marked increase in pulmonary vascular resistance and pulmonary artery pressure. This abrupt increase in right ventricular afterload may result in right ventricular dysfunction or indirectly impair left ventricular function.

Areas of alveolar edema, alveolar hemorrhage, and alveolar collapse may be perfused by blood from the right side of the heart. This defect is intrapulmonary shunting. Blood is not oxygenated because defective alveolar units cannot exchange gas, and unoxygenated blood is returned to the systemic circulation. Intrapulmonary shunts produce severe systemic hypoxemia that cannot be supported by the administration of oxygen-enriched gas.

Table 91.13.
Organ System Effects of ARDS

Organ System	Manifestations
Cardiac dysfunction	Cardiac index <2.0 liter/min/m^2
	Mean arterial pressure <60 mm Hg
	Ventricular fibrillation or asystole
Renal dysfunction	Urine output <600 ml/24 hr
	Serum creatinine >176.8 μmol/liter (2.0 mg/dl)
GI dysfunction	Ileus, malabsorption, hemorrhage, pancreatitis
CNS dysfunction	Confusion, agitation, seizures, coma
Hematologic dysfunction	Thrombocytopenia
	Leucopenia
	Hypofibrinogenemia
Hepatic dysfunction	Hyperbilirubinemia
	Elevated prothrombin time
	Decreased serum albumin

Table 91.14.
Factors Affecting Oxygen Delivery and Consumption

Parameter	Factors
Oxygen delivery	Cardiac output
	Hemoglobin concentration
	Oxygen saturation of hemoglobin
Oxygen consumption	Metabolic rate
	Body temperature

ARDS may also be an early manifestation of a more generalized loss of vascular autoregulation (11). This causes tissue oxygen utilization to be directly dependent on the oxygen delivery. Fluctuations in cardiac output, hemoglobin levels, or hemoglobin oxygen saturation cause marked alterations in tissue oxygenation, resulting in systemic organ system dysfunction. The major organ systems affected in ARDS are listed in Table 91.13.

General Principles of Therapy

The general therapeutics principle of ARDS is maintenance of oxygen delivery while minimizing oxygen consumption (13) (Table 91.14). Organ system dysfunction or the presence of systemic lactate levels indicate that oxygen delivery is inadequate to meet tissue oxygen requirements. Increasing hemoglobin oxygen saturation, cardiac output, or hemoglobin levels increases oxygen delivery. Additionally, interventions are aimed at decreasing tissue oxygen demand.

Improvement of hemoglobin oxygen saturation through intubation and mechanical ventilation is the mainstay therapy. The goal of mechanical ventilation is to assure adequate oxygenation and carbon dioxide elimination (15). Unfortunately, the administration of high oxygen concentrations (above 50%) has limited effect on oxygenation in ARDS. Furthermore, high oxygen concentrations may cause oxygen toxicity and additional lung damage. Support of oxygenation is accomplished through use of positive end-expiratory pressure (PEEP) or continuous positive airway pressure (CPAP). These modalities are delivered through a mechanical ventilator and are designed to maintain a positive pressure within the lung during inspiration, expiration, and at rest. Maintenance of a positive pressure during all phases of the respiratory cycle restores lung volume, recruits collapsed alveoli, improves lung compliance, and decreases intrapulmonary shunting (16).

Although quite beneficial in supporting gas exchange in ARDS, PEEP/CPAP may have deleterious effects. PEEP/CPAP decreases venous return to the heart and may decrease cardiac output, compromising oxygen delivery to the tissues (17–19). Additionally, PEEP/CPAP may cause alveolar rupture, resulting in gas being forced into the mediastinum (pneumomediastinum), subcutaneous tissue (subcutaneous emphysema), or the pleural space (tension pneumothorax). Because of these adverse effects, PEEP/CPAP is usually applied in small increments of 3 to 5 cm H$_2$O pressure with close monitoring of the patient's hemodynamic state and gas exchange (16). The least amount of PEEP/CPAP is administered to reduce the oxygen concentration in the inspired gas to below 50% while maintaining an arterial PO$_2$ above 60 mmHg.

The cardiac output must be maintained in a patient with ARDS to assure that oxygen delivery is adequate to meet tissue oxygen needs. If a patient is volume-depleted or has limited cardiac reserve, the application of small amounts of PEEP/CPAP may cause a fall in preload. There is a profound decrease in cardiac output, manifested by hypotension, poor tissue perfusion, and decreased tissue oxygen delivery (19). Volume replacement is commonly administered to treat the fall in cardiac output.

Monitoring of fluid therapy may be done with a Swan-Ganz catheter, because excessive volume administration may further increase extravascular lung water. Since the Swan-Ganz catheter lies within the chest, the pressures it measures may be altered by PEEP/CPAP. Thus, the pulmonary capillary wedge pressure (PCWP) may not totally reflect the left ventricular filling pressure or be an accurate index of the left ventricular preload (19). Therefore, fluid challenges may be given as they result in an increase in the cardiac output, the PCWP does not increase excessively or gas exchange deteriorate (19, 20).

In ARDS, alterations in the vascular permeability of the lung make the choice of a volume expander difficult. Crystalloid solutions increase intravascular volumes transiently and may increase lung water if excessively administered. Packed red blood cells (PRBCs) increase intravascular volume and increase the oxygen-carrying capacity of the blood by increasing the hemoglobin concentration. Unfortunately, PRBC administration carries the risk of hepatitis. Additionally, PRBC administration will increase blood viscosity and right ventricular afterload (21). These effects may decrease cardiac output (22). Therefore, PRBCs should be reserved for patients whose hematocrit is below 0.30 (30%) (19). Administration of colloid solutions (albumin, hetastarch, dextran) to increase intravascular colloid osmotic pressure has not been consistently demonstrated to decrease lung water and improve gas exchange (23–25). The colloid will not stay in the intravascular compartment because of alterations in vascular permeability (23–25). Fluid administration in ARDS must proceed with caution and careful patient assessment. Excessive increases in PCWP should be avoided, and the PCWP should be maintained at the lowest level that allows adequate cardiac output and tissue perfusion. If gas exchange deteriorates or the cardiac output remains inadequate after volume administration, then inotropic agents are indicated or a reduction in PEEP/CPAP should be attempted.

Inotropic agents will support a depressed cardiac output due to PEEP/CPAP. Dopamine and dobutamine increase cardiac output and oxygen delivery in ARDS (26). However, dopamine increases the PCWP (26, 27) while dobutamine decreases the PCWP (26). If the patient is hypotensive due to a low systemic vascular resistance, dopamine is the preferred agent despite its effects on PCWP. Dopamine is administered as an intravenous infusion of 5 μg/kg/min and titrated in 2.5 to 5.0 μg/kg/min increments. Effects on PCWP, cardiac output, blood pressure, organ perfusion, and gas exchange are closely monitored during dopamine infusions.

Dobutamine has been recommended in ARDS because of its beneficial effects on PCWP (19). Unfortunately, dobutamine will not result in a significant increase in blood pressure if the patient is hypotensive because of low systemic vascular resistance.

Nitroglycerin and nitroprusside are vasodilators used to lower PCWP and improve cardiac output. However, these agents have potential disadvantages in ARDS. Nitroprusside and nitroglycerin administration causes poorly ventilated areas of the lung to receive more blood flow (19). The change in pulmonary blood flow distribution increases perfusion through intrapulmonary shunts and worsens gas exchange. Additionally, these agents may reduce systemic blood pressure unless carefully administered (23, 28, 29).

Correction of body temperature elevations may allow stabilization of oxygen demand. Because a fever will increase cellular oxygen demand, acetaminophen 325 to 650 mg every 4 to 6 hr should be used to lower a patient's temperature to 37°C (15). The daily dose of acetaminophen should not exceed 2.4 g/day and should be avoided in patients with liver dysfunction. NSAIDs should be avoided because of the risk of reducing renal blood flow in some patients (15). Patients with contraindications to acetaminophen or not responding to antipyretic agents may be treated with cooling blankets.

Judicious use of sedative agents is useful in agitated patients. Agitation greatly increases tissue oxygen consumption, causing it to exceed oxygen delivery. Administration of sedatives is beneficial in decreasing tissue oxygen consumption to a level that can be supported by oxygen delivery. However, care must be taken to assure that the agitation is not due to the effects of hypoxemia, pain, or a metabolic abnormality (e.g., hypoglycemia, hyponatremia).

Pharmacologic Therapy of ARDS

A number of therapies directed against the pathophysiology of ARDS have been studied. Corticosteroids inhibit complement activation and production of tumor necrosis factor, prostaglandins, and leukotrienes (30). Large doses of corticosteroids have reversed the permeability defect in patients with ARDS and septic shock (31). However, clinical trials revealed that corticosteroids did not affect mortality when administered to patients with sepsis syndrome or septic shock (10, 32), prevent ARDS, or hasten the reversal of established ARDS (33).

Prostaglandin E_1 inhibits macrophage activation and neutrophil chemotaxis and prevents release of toxic oxygen radicals from neutrophils (30). Clinical trials in patients with ARDS have shown improvement in oxygenation (34) and peripheral oxygen delivery (35). However, the use of prostaglandin E_1 did not improve the mortality in patients with ARDS (34, 35).

Surfactant is a lipid protein complex that lowers alveolar surface tension, improves lung compliance, and prevents alveolar collapse at low lung volumes (30). In neonatal respiratory distress syndrome caused by surfactant deficiency, the prophylactic administration of surfactant improved oxygenation, decreased complications due to mechanical ventilation, and decreased mortality (36). In patients with established neonatal respiratory distress syndrome, improved oxygenation and mortality followed the administration of surfactant (37, 38). The role of surfactant administration in ARDS has yet to be determined.

Endotoxin and tumor necrosis factor initiate a cascade of events leading to septic shock and ARDS (30). Antibodies to endotoxin have been shown to improve survival in patients with sepsis and septic shock (39). Antibodies to tumor necrosis factor may prevent the development of shock, respiratory failure, and hemodynamic changes of sepsis (40). While these interventions may offer a means to interrupt the disease process, their effect on the incidence or outcome of ARDS is unknown.

Summary

ARDS is a severe lung disease that requires mechanical ventilation to support lung function. While a number of pharmacologic interventions have been studied in ARDS, management consists of mechanical ventilation with PEEP/CPAP until the defect in gas exchange abates. Fluid administration and inotropic support are used to treat decreases in oxygen delivery caused by the use of PEEP/CPAP.

HYPERTENSIVE EMERGENCY

With the improvement in antihypertensive therapy over the last decade, the incidence of hypertensive emergency is quite low. Currently, less than 1% of hypertensive patients progress to a hypertensive emergency (41). A hypertensive emergency is defined as a severe elevation in blood pressure, generally considered to be above 120 to 130 mm Hg diastolic, with the presence of acute or ongoing end-organ damage. The seriousness of the clinical situation is determined by the association between the blood pressure and the evidence of end-organ damage, not the absolute blood pressure value. A true hypertensive emergency can be life-threatening and requires prompt reduction of blood pressure within minutes to 1 hr. This is accomplished by intravenous drug therapy in an intensive care setting.

A hypertensive emergency occurs most commonly in patients with a history of hypertension who are either noncompliant with their medications or are receiving inadequate therapy. A hypertensive emergency is precipitated by an abrupt increase in systemic vascular resistance resulting from increased levels of vasoconstrictive substances such as norepinephrine, angiotensin II, and vasopressin (42). Due to high arteriolar pressure, these patients also experience vascular smooth muscle damage and some loss of arteriolar autoregulation. It is the combination of hypertension and this loss of arteriolar autoregulation that may lead to end-organ damage.

The signs and symptoms of hypertensive emergency (Table 91.15) are diverse and result from damage to specific organ systems such as the central nervous system, heart, kidney, and eyes.

The central nervous system manifestations of a hypertensive emergency are known collectively as hypertensive encephalopathy. Hypertensive encephalopathy is thought to be caused by cerebral edema resulting from a loss of cerebral blood-flow autoregulation (43). The manifestations may present solely as a headache or may be accompanied by dizziness, nausea, vomiting, anorexia, and visual disturbances. More severe and progressive clinical features include papilledema, mental confusion, agitation or lethargy, nystagmus, and occasionally transient focal neurologic deficits, seizures, and reversible blindness. The neurologic syndrome usually resolves a few hours after blood pressure reduction. Other severe CNS consequences include cerebral infarction, intracerebral hemorrhage, and subarachnoid hemorrhage.

Table 91.15.
Manifestations of Hypertensive Emergency

Organ System	Manifestation
CNS	Encephalopathy
	Cerebral infarction
	Intracranial hemorrhage
Cardiovascular	Angina
	Myocardial infarction
	Aortic dissection
	Congestive heart failure
Renal	Hematuria
	Proteinuria
	Azotemia
	Oliguria
Ocular	Blurred vision
	Retinal hemorrhage
	Retinal exudates
	Papilledema
	Temporary blindness

The major cardiovascular complications that occur in a hypertensive emergency are angina or myocardial infarction, congestive heart failure, and aortic dissection. Angina may occur as a result of both atherosclerotic coronary artery disease and an acute increase in myocardial oxygen demand caused by the increase in systemic vascular resistance (afterload). Typical signs and symptoms of angina include chest pain, shortness of breath, and ischemic changes on electrocardiogram. If the ischemia is severe enough, myocardial infarction may ensue. Severe hypertension may also precipitate congestive heart failure. The patient may have shortness of breath, pulmonary edema, and an S_3 gallop. Finally, the impact of high pressures and shearing forces on an abnormal vessel may cause dissection. Dissection of the aorta occurs when the inner layer, the intima, is interrupted, allowing blood entry and separation of its layers. The patient may complain of severe diffuse chest pain in the back, chest, or abdomen, and have mediastinal widening on chest x-ray.

Renal manifestations of severe hypertension include hematuria, proteinuria, azotemia, and oliguria. Patients whose previous renal function was not severely impaired usually recover following blood pressure control.

Ocular symptoms of hypertensive emergency are blurred vision and transient or reversible blindness. These symptoms are associated with the funduscopic findings of retinal hemorrhages, exudates, and papilledema.

Drug Therapy and Hypertensive Emergency

Because of the high risk of irreversible organ damage or death, immediate, aggressive antihypertensive therapy is indicated in a hypertensive emergency. The goal of initial treatment is not to achieve normotension, but to reduce arterial pressure in a controlled manner to a range of 100 to 110 mm Hg diastolic or a mean arterial pressure of 120 mm Hg (44). This can be achieved over a period of several minutes to several hours, depending upon the clinical situation. Precipitous reductions in blood pressure to normotensive or hypotensive levels should be avoided because of the risk of end-organ ischemia or infarction. The target level of 100 to 110 mm Hg diastolic appears to be the lower limit of the autoregulatory range of blood pressure for patients with a history of uncontrolled hypertension. Cerebral blood flow may be compromised below this level. The blood pressure should be maintained at target levels for several days, and then a normal blood pressure can be achieved over an extended period of time.

Even though there is no "ideal" drug to treat a hypertensive emergency, certain characteristics are desirable. For example, the drug should allow a controlled reduction in blood pressure as opposed to a precipitous drop. The agent should also have a rapid onset and short duration of action. These qualities are important in achieving rapid blood pressure reduction and in quickly reversing undesirable effects. Moreover, the drug should also have a good dose-response curve, a favorable therapeutic index, and minimal side effects. Finally, the agent should be easy to administer and monitor (44). The antihypertensive agents that share many of these characteristics can be classified into two categories according to their mechanism of action: direct vasodilators and sympathetic inhibitors (Table 91.16).

DIRECT VASODILATORS

Nitroprusside. Nitroprusside is currently the most potent and consistently effective agent for the treatment of a hypertensive emergency. Nitroprusside is a direct-acting in-travenous vasodilator that dilates both venous and arterial vessels. A mild tachycardia usually occurs as a result of this vasodilation. These effects are particularly advantageous for the patient whose hypertension is complicated by congestive heart failure or myocardial ischemia. Its onset is immediate, and the antihypertensive effect disappears within 2 to 5 min after discontinuation. This rapid action allows the blood pressure to be lowered to desired levels over approximately 20 to 40 min. The use of nitroprusside necessitates an infusion pump, careful nursing supervision, and preferably intraarterial blood pressure monitoring.

Nitroprusside reacts rapidly with sulfhydryl groups in the blood and tissue to produce free cyanide ions, which are converted to thiocyanate in the liver. Thiocyanate is then excreted primarily by the kidneys. Cyanide toxicity has been reported rarely in patients with severe hepatic disease or poor hepatic perfusion (45). The risk of thiocyanate toxicity increases when nitroprusside is infused for more than 24 to 48 hr, especially if renal function is impaired. At moderate dosages (2 to 5 µg/kg/min), toxic levels can occur in 7 to 14 days in patients with normal renal function and in 3 to 6 days with severe renal disease (46). Toxicity is reflected by serum levels above 1.7 mmol/liter (10 mg/dl), and the signs and symptoms include nausea, psychosis, hyperreflexia, confusion, weakness, tinnitus, seizures, and coma. Adverse effects of the parent drug include headache, nausea, vomiting, dizziness, muscular twitching, and fatigue. The recommended starting dose for a continuous infusion of nitroprusside is 0.25 to 0.5 µg/kg/min titrated to a maximum dose of 10 µg/kg/min. **Diazoxide.** Diazoxide is a potent, rapid-acting hypotensive agent closely related to the thiazide group of drugs.

Table 91.16.
Drugs for Hypertensive Emergencies

Drug	Mechanism of Action	Onset/Duration	Dose/Administration	Adverse Effects
Direct vasodilators				
Nitroprusside	Arteriolar and venous vasodilator	Immediate/3–5 min	0.5–10 µg/kg/min via continuous infusion	Hypotension, nausea, vomiting, thiocyanate toxicity
Diazoxide	Arteriolar vasodilator	1–5 min/4–24 hr	IV bolus: 50–150 mg every 5 min Infusion: 7.5–30 mg/min	Hypotension, tachycardia, sodium retention, hyperglycemia
Nitroglycerin	Venous and arteriolar vasodilator	1–2 min/3–5 min	5–100 µg/min via continuous infusion	Nausea, vomiting, headache
Hydralazine	Arteriolar vasodilator	10–30 min/2–4 hr	IM: 10–50 mg OR IV: 10–20 mg q. 4–6 hr	Nausea, vomiting, headache, tachycardia, hypotension
Sympatholytics				
Labetolol	α- and β-receptor blocker	<5 min/≥6 hr	20–80 mg IVP q. 10 min to maximum of 300 mg, 0.5–2.0 mg/min via continuous infusion	Nausea, vomiting, hypotension, heart block, bronchospasm, precipitation of CHF
Trimethaphan	Ganglionic blocker	1–5 min/10 min	0.5–5.0 mg/min via continuous infusion	Blurred vison, urinary retention, ileus, hypotension

The hypotensive action is mediated through a direct relaxation of arterioles, reducing peripheral vascular resistance. As arterial pressure decreases, sympathetic reflex responses are activated, resulting in cardiac stimulation and increased heart rate, stroke volume, and cardiac output. The onset of an intravenous bolus begins within 1 min, with the maximal effect occurring in 2 to 5 min. The duration of action can be up to 24 hr (range 3 to 15 hr).

Diazoxide is usually administered as several intravenous bolus injections of 1 to 3 mg/kg (50 to 150 mg) every 5 to 15 min, up to a maximum dose of 600 mg. It can also be given as a slow infusion of 7.5 to 30 mg/min to achieve the desired blood pressure reduction.

Advantages of diazoxide include its rapid onset and ease of administration. However, it also causes reflex tachycardia, which can precipitate or worsen anginal symptoms in patients with coronary artery disease. Achieving a controlled reduction in blood pressure is more difficult than with nitroprusside, and precipitous drops in blood pressure have occurred following intravenous injection. Diazoxide also causes significant sodium and water retention, which could be deleterious to a patient with congestive heart failure and pulmonary edema. Concomitant administration of an intravenous diuretic agent is recommended. Other adverse effects include nausea, vomiting, weakness, flushing, hyperglycemia, and hyperuricemia.

Nitroglycerin. Nitroglycerin is a direct-acting vasodilator that acts predominantly on venous capacitance vessels. When large doses are given, arteriolar dilation also occurs. Nitroglycerin also dilates coronary blood vessels and improves perfusion to ischemic areas in the myocardium. The drug is useful in acute hypertension developing before, during, or after coronary artery bypass surgery.

The onset of nitroglycerin is 1 to 2 min, with a 3 to 5 min duration of action. An intravenous infusion of nitroglycerin is started at 3 to 5 μg/min and titrated to blood pressure response (usual range 5 to 100 μg/min). Adverse effects include nausea, vomiting, headache, tolerance (with prolonged use), and worsening of angina.

Hydralazine. Hydralazine reduces total peripheral resistance through relaxation of arterial smooth muscle. The vasodilation is accompanied by a reflex tachycardia with increased stroke volume, cardiac output, and myocardial oxygen demand. These effects pose a risk to patients with underlying coronary artery disease. Hydralazine is not used frequently to treat hypertensive emergencies because it is not consistently effective and the antihypertensive response is less predictable than with other parenteral agents. Hydralazine administered intravenously or intramuscularly has an onset of 10 to 30 min and a duration of 2 to 4 hr. Typical dosages are 10 to 50 mg IM or 10 to 20 mg IV given every hour until a response is seen. A maintenance dose is then given every 4 to 6 hr. The most com-

mon adverse effects of hydralazine are nausea, vomiting, tachycardia, palpitations, dizziness, and weakness.

SYMPATHETIC INHIBITORS

Labetalol. Labetalol is a rapid-acting antihypertensive agent with combined α- and β-adrenergic blocking activity. These pharmacologic effects result in reduction in peripheral vascular resistance (afterload), blood pressure, and heart rate, with virtually no change in resting cardiac output and stroke volume. These effects are advantageous in patients with coronary artery disease, angina, or acute myocardial infarction (when cardiac performance is not impaired), or following acute vascular surgical procedures. Labetalol has a rapid onset of 5 min or less, and the blood pressure effects may persist for 6 hr or longer. The drug is eliminated by glucuronidation in the liver, with less than 5% of the dose excreted unchanged in the urine in 24 hr.

When treating hypertensive emergencies, labetalol may be administered by repeated bolus injections or by continuous infusion. The initial dose for bolus administration is 20 mg over 2 min followed by repeated injections of 40 to 80 mg at 10-min intervals to a total dose of 300 mg. A controlled, smooth reduction in blood pressure can also be achieved by a continuous infusion of 0.5 to 2 mg/min titrated to response or cumulative dose of 300 mg.

Labetalol is available orally, which allows easy conversion from intravenous to oral therapy. Side effects seen with labetalol include orthostatic hypotension, nausea, vomiting, parasthesias, dizziness, flushing, and headaches. Because of its nonspecific β-blocking effects, labetalol is contraindicated in asthma, severe decompensated congestive heart failure, second- or third-degree heart block, or significant bradycardia.

Trimethaphan. Trimethaphan is a short-acting ganglionic blocking agent that inhibits both sympathetic and parasympathetic activity, resulting in both arteriolar and venous dilation. Trimethaphan is used to treat acute dissection of the aorta, because of its ability to reduce preload, cardiac output, and the velocity of left ventricular ejection. However, trimethaphan is also an alternative agent for other types of hypertensive emergencies. Trimethaphan is administered by continuous infusion, with a usual dosage range of 0.5 to 5 mg/min (up to 10 mg/min), and has a rapid onset of 1 to 5 min with a duration of 10 min. The administration of trimethaphan requires constant intra-arterial blood pressure monitoring. Tachyphylaxis to this agent may to occur after 24 to 48 hr when large doses are used. Significant adverse effects include orthostatic hypotension, ileus, urinary retention, dry mouth, and visual impairment.

DIURETIC THERAPY

Many clinicians today use diuretic agents as adjunct therapy in the treatment of hypertensive emergencies. However, most patients who have severe hypertension tend to be volume-depleted because of an associated pressure diuresis (47). Diuretic administration in this circumstance may cause further volume depletion, increasing systemic vascular resistance and worsening the hypertension. Fluid replacement with isotonic saline may be indicated in severely volume-depleted patients to control the blood pressure and improve organ perfusion. Thus, diuretic agents should not be used routinely unless there is clinical evidence that the patient is fluid-overloaded.

Summary

A hypertensive emergency can be a life-threatening circumstance that requires prompt recognition, appropriate intravenous drug therapy, and continuous monitoring in an intensive care setting. To allow healing of end-organ damage and maintenance of adequate organ perfusion, a potent, rapid-acting intravenous agent should be used. This agent should allow a controlled, stepwise reduction of blood pressure to the target goal, at which time the patient may be converted to oral therapy.

INTRACRANIAL HYPERTENSION

Elevations in intracranial pressure (ICP) may have severe consequences for patients, depending upon the cause of the increased ICP, the pathophysiology, and the magnitude of the elevation. Elevations in ICP may be caused by head trauma, brain tumors, intracerebral or subarachnoid hemorrhage, Reye's syndrome, and toxic or viral encephalopathies (48). In addition, elevations in ICP are commonly associated with head trauma and may account for one-half of deaths due to closed head trauma (48). The mortality associated with intracranial hypertension depends upon the magnitude of the rise in ICP. Elevations from the normal ICP of 0 to 10 torr to 40 torr are associated with a 65% mortality, and elevations of ICP to 60 torr are associated with a 100% mortality (48).

Pathophysiology

The normal cranial contents include brain tissue, cerebrospinal fluid (CSF), and blood. The brain accounts for approximately 80% of the intracranial volume, while the CSF and blood comprise 10%. In addition, the brain itself is approximately 80% water. Because of this composition, none of the three compartments is compressible. Therefore, an increase in the volume of one compartment must be at the expense of volume normally taken up by one of the other two compartments. Elevations in ICP exert deleterious effects through displacement of brain tissue or through alterations in cerebral blood flow. Depending upon the affected area, displacement of brain tissue around or through bony structures results in extensive neuronal damage and gives rise to a number of herniation syndromes. Alterations in cerebral blood flow may result in an area of focal or diffuse cerebral ischemia.

Perfusion of the brain is determined by the cerebral perfusion pressure. The cerebral perfusion pressure (CPP) depends on the relationship between the mean arterial pressure (MAP) and the ICP according to the following relationship:

$$CPP = MAP - ICP$$

The CPP may be decreased by a decrease in the MAP or an increase in the ICP.

The normal CPP is above 50 torr. A decrease in the CPP below 50 torr decreases cerebral blood flow and may result in focal or global ischemia. A decrease in the CPP to 20 torr results in cessation of cerebral blood flow and cerebral anoxia (49).

The manifestations of an increased ICP depend upon the magnitude of the elevation, the presence of cerebral ischemia, or the development of a herniation syndrome. Symptoms include headache, diplopia, vomiting, decreased visual acuity, and slowed mentation. Signs include papilledema, bradycardia, posturing, hypertension, and fixed unresponsive pupils (49).

Principles of Therapy

The goal of therapy for elevations of ICP depends upon the cause of the elevation. Surgical treatment is indicated for removable masses. The immediate goal of medical management is to reduce the total volume of cranial contents. This may be accomplished by reducing the volume of any compartment without compromising cerebral blood flow. In situations where the ICP is elevated, small alterations in the volume of the intracranial compartments may markedly reduce the ICP while maintaining cerebral blood flow. Elevated ICP should be controlled until the underlying condition is identified and corrected. Treatment usually commences when the ICP increases to 20 torr or greater.

The initial treatment of an elevated ICP involves elevating the patient's head 15 to 20° and restricting fluid intake to less than 1000 ml/day. Intravenous solutions containing dextrose only (dextrose 5% in water) should be avoided because the additional free water may contribute to edema of the brain (50). Although intravenous fluid therapy must be individualized to the patient's serum electrolytes, serum osmolality, volume status, and ICP, the intravenous fluid should consist of a balanced salt solution. Patients should be quieted and prevented from excessive involuntary movements or straining, as this may further increase the ICP. Morphine and midazolam help calm the patient, but the clinician must carefully assess the benefits and risks of such interventions. These agents may depress the level of consciousness and make assessment of the patient's neurologic status more difficult.

The most rapid means of reducing ICP is through removal of small volumes of cerebral spinal fluid (48). This may be accomplished after placement of a catheter into one of the ventricles of the brain. This catheter may allow intracranial pressure monitoring and removal of aliquots of cerebrospinal fluid. Removal of 1 to 2 ml of cerebrospinal fluid may cause a marked reduction in ICP (48). The removal of cerebrospinal fluid may be repeated as necessary when the ICP increases.

The cerebral vasculature is very sensitive to changes in arterial pCO_2. The cerebral vasculature constricts or dilates with decreases or increases in the arterial pCO_2. Cerebral blood flow decreases by 2 to 3% for each 1 mm Hg decrease in the arterial pCO_2. Therefore, hyperventilating the patient until the arterial pCO_2 reaches 20 to 25 mm Hg may reduce an elevated ICP by as much as 50%. Hyperventilation may reduce the ICP within 10 min. However, these effects are also short-lived, diminishing within 24 to 48 hr. Any further reduction in ICP with an arterial pCO_2 of less than 20 mm Hg is minimal (49). Excessive cerebral vasoconstriction may result in cerebral hypoxia. While useful for rapid reductions in ICP, hyperventilation requires intubation and mechanical ventilation to maintain an appropriate arterial pCO_2. Hyperventilation should be discontinued slowly. Rapid discontinuation will cause rapid changes in arterial pCO_2 and may cause a rapid rise in ICP. Although effective, hyperventilation has not been demonstrated to alter the mortality associated with rises in ICP. Therefore, it should be considered a temporizing measure until more definitive interventions are instituted.

OSMOTIC AGENTS

Given the high water content of the brain and the characteristics of the blood-brain barrier, agents that increase the osmolality of the blood will lower the ICP. This increase in the blood osmolality relative to the brain tissue results in the movement of water out of this tissue down an osmotic gradient. Osmotic agents can reduce the water content of normal brain tissue only when the blood-brain barrier is intact. Any alteration in this barrier due to ischemia will result in a loss of effectiveness.

Mannitol is the osmotic agent most commonly used to lower elevated ICP (49). The intravenous dose of mannitol is 0.25 to 2.0 g/kg administered over 10 to 60 min (49). Mannitol lowers ICP within 20 min of administration. More rapid administration results in a greater reduction in ICP (49). Mannitol's duration of action depends on the size of the dose and the cumulative number of doses given. In general, mannitol should be readministered every 4 to 6 hr or as indicated by an increase in the ICP. Since mannitol is an osmotic diuretic, its administration may cause significant diuresis. This limits the effectiveness of mannitol in lowering ICP because the drug is cleared rapidly through the kidneys. Moreover, fluid and electrolyte im-

balance may occur, with the development of volume depletion, hypokalemia, and hypernatremia. Caution should be exercised during mannitol administration to avoid the development of systemic hyperosmolality. Serum osmolality should be measured 2 to 4 times daily and be maintained below 320 mOsm/kg (49). Mannitol should be used cautiously in patients with underlying renal or cardiac disease.

Glycerol is another osmotic agent that lowers ICP and increases cerebral blood flow. An intravenous dose of 0.5 to 1.0 g/kg is administered at 0.3 g/min and repeated every 4 to 8 hr (49). Alternatively, glycerol may be administered as a continuous infusion at a rate of 0.3 to 1.0 g/kg/hr (49). Unfortunately, an intravenous preparation of glycerol is not available in this country. However, glycerol may be administered orally. The oral dose is 0.5 to 1.0 g/kg every 4 hr (49). Although the oral regimen is effective in lowering the ICP, the onset of action is approximately 30 min. The most common adverse effects of oral glycerol are nausea, vomiting, and diarrhea. Dehydration, hypokalemia, and hypernatremia can also occur. As with mannitol, the serum osmolality should be measured 2 to 4 times a day during glycerol administration and maintained below than 320 mOsm/kg. Glycerol should be used cautiously in patients with underlying renal or cardiac disease.

LOOP DIURETICS

The use of furosemide in association with osmotic diuretics causes a slightly greater reduction in ICP and prolongs the duration of the ICP reduction (49). The mechanism of action of furosemide in lowering ICP is not clear. Proposed mechanisms include a reduction in water and ion permeability of the blood-brain barrier, inhibition of cerebrospinal fluid formation, and increased osmolality due to the diuretic-induced water loss. Recommended doses of furosemide are 0.5 to 1.0 mg/kg administered intravenously after the osmotic diuretic (49). Use of mannitol or glycerol in combination with furosemide requires careful attention and monitoring for excessive volume depletion, hypokalemia, hypernatremia, hyponatremia, and hypochloremia.

CORTICOSTEROIDS

Dexamethasone therapy is effective in lowering ICP in select settings. Alterations in the permeability of the brain capillary endothelial cells from solid tumors are the most responsive to the effects of corticosteroids (51). Dexamethasone is also administered in conjunction with antituberculous agents in the therapy of tuberculosis meningitis. Corticosteroids are of little value when elevated ICP is a result of stroke, intracerebral hematoma, or head injury (48). The optimal dose of dexamethasone has not been well established. Two recommended regimens consist of giving an initial dose of 10 mg intravenously followed by 4 mg every 4 to 6 hr or 100 to 400 mg daily for 1 to 3 days followed by 4 mg every 6 hr (49). Unlike hyperventilation or osmotic therapy, which have rapid onsets of action, the effects of dexamethasone on ICP become evident 12 to 24 hr after the initiation of therapy. Once control of the ICP has been attained, the dose of dexamethasone may be tapered. Since the tapering regimen must be individualized, the patient must be followed closely for recurrence of signs or symptoms of increased ICP.

The adverse effects of dexamethasone are similar to those seen with high-dose corticosteroid therapy: increased susceptibility to infection, hyperglycemia, and gastrointestinal upset. If dexamethasone therapy is continued for prolonged periods, muscle wasting, weight gain, pituitary-hypothalamic-adrenal axis suppression, and cushingoid features may develop.

BARBITURATE THERAPY

Barbiturate derivatives have been used to control intracranial hypertension resistant to conventional therapy in cases of head injury, Reye's syndrome, focal or global cerebral ischemia, and anoxia. The mechanism of barbiturate action in lowering an elevated ICP is poorly understood. Possible mechanisms include increased cerebral vascular resistance, decreased cerebral metabolic requirements, and inactivation of free radicals (49). Increased cerebral vascular resistance decreases cerebral blood flow, cerebral blood volume, and the ICP. Decreased cerebral metabolism decreases energy and oxygen requirements of the brain. Elimination of oxygen free radicals may prevent permanent neuronal damage from these entities.

Pentobarbital is the barbiturate derivative most frequently used in the management of elevated ICP. Pentobarbital is administered intravenously as a 3 to 10 mg/kg loading dose over 30 min to 3 hr (48). Typical maintenance doses of pentobarbital are 1.5 to 2.0 mg/kg intravenously every 1 to 2 hr or an infusion of 0.5 to 3.0 mg/kg/hr (48, 49). The dosage of pentobarbital is then adjusted to maintain the ICP below 25 torr or serum blood levels between 110 and 177 μmol/liter (25 and 40 mg/dl) (48, 49). Pentobarbital use requires close monitoring to prevent the development of adverse effects. Serum blood levels should be measured every 24 to 48 hr. Pentobarbital levels above 18 μmol/liter (4 mg/dl) may cause hypotension (48). Serum drug levels above 22 μmol/liter (5 mg/dl) may cause severe suppression of activity in the cortical, respiratory, and vasomotor centers (49). Depression of the respiratory center results in hypercapnia and hypoxemia unless the patient is intubated and mechanically ventilated.

Summary

Intracranial hypertension is a severe, life-threatening consequence of acute neurologic events, systemic diseases, or tumors of the brain. Therapy to lower the ICP should be instituted immediately. Patients may require more than one modality to lower their ICP. Therapy is individualized on the basis of the underlying disease causing intracranial hypertension, signs and symptoms, and any other systemic diseases. Patients require close monitoring to prevent adverse effects from the interventions to lower ICP.

MANAGEMENT OF PAIN, ANXIETY AND AGITATION

Intensive care units can be stressful and frightening places for patients. This environment often promotes extreme anxiety, paranoia, and agitation for the patient, especially those who are intubated. Physical causes of anxiety and agitation include pain, hypoxia, hypercapnia, delirium tremens, acute hepatic or uremic encephalopathy, and various electrolyte disorders. Since such pain, anxiety, or combativeness may actually be deleterious to the patient's condition, pharmacologic intervention with drugs such as opiates, benzodiazepines, and neuromuscular blockers is an important aspect of intensive care.

Pain Management

NARCOTICS (Table 91.17)

Opiate narcotics, particularly morphine, codeine, meperidine, and fentanyl, are commonly used in intensive care settings for their analgesic and sedative effects. Intermittent intravenous injection is the preferred route of administration, as intramuscular injections produce unpredictable drug concentrations. Short-acting narcotics (e.g., fentanyl) are usually given continuously, to maintain effective analgesia. In general, opiates exhibit a mild negative inotropic and chronotropic effect as well as vasodilatory effects. Vasodilation usually results in decreased right ventricular filling pressures and decreased left ventricular end-diastolic pressure, which may be beneficial in patients with congestive heart failure and pulmonary edema. A potential disadvantage of opiates is their direct depressive effect on the respiratory center. Narcotics may also release histamine, which may be deleterious in patients with asthma. Other side effects common to opiates include drowsiness, euphoria, cough suppression, nausea, vomiting, and decreased gastrointestinal motility. Opiates also potentiate the cardiovascular and respiratory depressant effects of sedative and hypnotic drugs.

Morphine sulfate is probably the most widely used of all narcotic analgesic/sedatives. In appropriate doses, morphine is an extremely effective analgesic and anxiolytic. Morphine can be easily titrated to the patient's response, and the effects are rapidly reversed with a narcotic antagonist. Dosage requirements vary immensely, but a typical morphine dose is 2 to 5 mg given intravenously every 1 to 2 hr. Meperidine and codeine are similar to morphine in

Table 91.17.
Characteristics of Narcotic Derivatives

Drug	Equivalent Dose (mg)	Analgesic Dose	Peak Effects	Duration of Analgesia
Codeine inj.	120	15–60 mg q. 4–6 hr	15–30 min (s.c.)	4–6 hr
Fentanyl inj.	0.1	Load: 50–500 µg	2–3 min (IV)	30–60 min
		Infusion: 50–500 µg/hr		
Meperidine inj.	100	50–150 mg q. 3–4 hr IVP or i.m.	10 min (i.m.)	2–4 hr
Morphine inj.	20	2–15 mg q. 1–4 hr IVP	15–20 min (IV)	4–6 hr
		Infusion: 0.8–10 mg/hr		

Table 91.18.
Benzodiazepine Derivatives

Drug	IV Dose	Onset of Sedation (min)	Duration of Sedation (hr)	Half-life (hr)
Diazepam	1–10 mg q. 1–4 hr	1–5	0.25–1	20–50
Lorazepam	1–2 mg q. 3–4 hr	1–5	6–8	10–20
Midazolam	Load: 1–10 mg	1–5	2–6	1.5–12.3
	Infusion: 2–7 mg/hr			

effect but are used for less intense pain management. Compared with morphine, meperidine tends to be somewhat shorter-acting.

Fentanyl is a synthetic opioid that is 100 to 150 times more potent than morphine. Fentanyl is more rapid acting (1 to 2 min) but has a shorter duration of action (30 to 40 min). This allows immediate control of pain in the intensive care setting. Compared with morphine and meperidine, fentanyl produces minimal histamine release and has less effect on cardiovascular hemodynamics. Because fentanyl is a more effective analgesic than sedative, it is often used in combination with a benzodiazepine for sedative effects.

Management of Anxiety and Agitation

BENZODIAZEPINES (Table 91.18)

Benzodiazepines have been used for the treatment of anxiety in the critically ill patient for many years. Benzodiazepines act as sedatives, anxiolytics, anticonvulsants, hypnotics, and skeletal muscle relaxants. These agents are useful in intensive care units because of their minimal effects on the cardiovascular system, autonomic nervous system, and respiratory drive. However, combined with other intravenous sedative hypnotics or analgesics, they may cause severe respiratory and circulatory depression. Other pharmacologic effects include central nervous system depression, ranging from light sedation to coma, and anterograde amnesia. Benzodiazepines are rapidly effective by the intravenous route and are widely distributed into body tissues, including the blood-brain barrier.

Diazepam, lorazepam, and midazolam are the most commonly used benzodiazepines in the critical care setting. In general, they are metabolized in the liver and excreted in the urine. Prolonged elimination may occur in geriatric patients and in those with liver disease. Benzodiazepines can easily be titrated to effect and offer a wide margin of safety.

Diazepam is erratically absorbed if given intramuscularly, thus the intravenous route is preferred. However, hypotension and respiratory depression can occur if administration is too rapid. Lorazepam has less effect on respiratory and cardiovascular centers than other benzodiazepines. The sedative and anxiolytic effects are somewhat longer than those of diazepam and chlordiazepoxide, lasting from 6 to 8 hr.

Midazolam is a very short-acting benzodiazepine that is becoming quite popular in intensive care units. The sedative effect is three to four times that of diazepam. Midazolam has a short half-life (1.5 to 3.5 hr), which allows easy dosage titration with boluses or continuous infusion. Upon discontinuation, the recovery time is very short. Adverse effects include apnea and respiratory arrest, which occurs most commonly in the elderly, debilitated, and those with pulmonary disease. Small doses should be given very slowly in these patients. Hypotension and bradycardia have also occurred when midazolam was used as premedication for short-term procedures.

ANTIPSYCHOTICS/NEUROLEPTICS

Other agents often used as sedatives/anxiolytics include the phenothiazines and the butyrophenones. Chlorpromazine is a potent phenothiazine antipsychotic agent that possesses significant sedative properties. It is most useful in sedating the agitated patient who has difficulty discerning reality. Chlorpromazine can compound the central nervous system depressive effects of benzodiazepines, and it may also cause hypotension. The drug is given intramuscularly at a starting dose of 25 to 50 mg every 4 to 6 hr. Haloperidol is a butyrophenone neuroleptic agent that is useful for agitation related to psychosis. Haloperidol produces less sedation than chlorpromazine and has little effect on cardiovascular hemodynamics. The drug is usually given intramuscularly, (dosage range 0.5 to 10 mg, depending upon severity of agitation) with peak levels occurring within 10 to 20 min and peak response in 30 to 40 min. Although not an FDA-approved route of administration, haloperidol has been given intravenously in the ICU setting. Side effects include acute dystonic reactions, severe extrapyramidal reactions, and neuroleptic malignant syndrome.

ANTIHISTAMINES

Diphenhydramine and hydroxyzine are antihistamine agents that produce sedative effects. These agents are particularly useful in patients in whom the respiratory depressive effects of benzodiazepines are contraindicated. Diphenhydramine is usually given in a dose of 25 to 50 mg IV, i.m. or p.o. Effects of an IV dose are seen within 15 min and may persist for 4 to 6 hr. Hydroxyzine has a similar onset and duration and is administered orally or by intramuscular injection. Hydroxyzine is often used concomitantly with opiates to relieve anxiety. The major side effect of these agents is a dry mouth.

NEUROMUSCULAR BLOCKING AGENTS

Many patients in intensive care units are mechanically ventilated because of respiratory failure. These intubated patients often become uncomfortable, extremely agitated, and may "fight" the ventilator, i.e., they have spontaneous respirations that oppose the ventilator, compromising ventilation and oxygenation. If sedation is inadequate to achieve control, neuromuscular blockers are used to paralyze the patient and facilitate ventilation. Patients who undergo paralysis are not necessarily asleep and require adequate sedation and analgesia as adjunct therapy.

Neuromuscular blockers commonly used in critical care are pancuronium, vecuronium, and atracurium. These agents are nondepolarizing neuromuscular blockers. Nondepolarizing agents compete with acetylcholine for receptor-binding sites at the neuromuscular junction, inhibit acetylcholine binding, and prevent depolarization. Ultimately, the drugs produce a controlled, prolonged paralysis.

There is very limited information on the pharmacodynamics and pharmacokinetics of neuromuscular blockers in intubated ICU patients. The onset of effect of these agents depends largely upon blood flow to the muscle tissue, which depends upon cardiac output. The duration of paralysis depends upon the dose and frequency of administration, renal and hepatic function, and the presence of active metabolites. In general, the first signs of neuromuscular blockade occur within 2 min of an intravenous dose, and maximal effects occur in 3 to 6 min. The drugs as a class have the potential to block acetylcholine recep-

Table 91.19.
Pharmacokinetics of Skeletal Muscle Relaxants

Drug	Half-life (min)	Onset (min)	Duration (min)	Elimination	Equivalent Dose (mg)
Pancuronium	120	2–5	90	Renal	0.33
Vecuronium	65	2–5	25–40	Biliary	0.25
Atracurium	20	2–5	35–45	Plasma esterase	1.0

tors of the heart, producing an increase in heart rate. However, these effects tend to be dose-and drug-related. Neuromuscular blockers may also cause histamine release with resultant hypotension and bronchospasm. Vecuronium is 1 to 1.5 times more potent than pancuronium, and atracurium is 25 to 30% less potent.

Pharmacokinetics (Table 91.19). Approximately 30 to 40% of a dose of pancuronium is excreted by the kidneys, with 11% eliminated via the biliary tract. The remaining drug is metabolized in the liver. One metabolite, 3-hydroxypancuronium, is pharmacologically active. Vecuronium undergoes hydrolysis in the liver to two active metabolites that are excreted via the biliary tract. Renal elimination accounts for 15 to 25% of a dose. Atracurium undergoes rapid metabolism via Hofmann elimination and nonspecific blood esterases. The product of the degradation is laudanosine, a weakly active compound that may have seizure potential. Atracurium and its metabolites are excreted in the urine and in feces via biliary elimination (30 to 50%).

Adverse Effects. The most common adverse effects of neuromuscular blockers include hemodynamic changes, histamine release, and neuromuscular effects. The adverse cardiovascular effects include tachycardia and elevated blood pressure. These effects are related to the activity of the drugs on cholinergic receptors of the autonomic ganglia and the adrenal medulla and occur most commonly with pancuronium, followed by vecuronium and atracurium. All neuromuscular blockers can cause histamine release, resulting in bronchospasm, vasodilation, transient hypotension, and cutaneous flushing. Skeletal muscle weakness and disuse atrophy occur when these agents are administered for prolonged periods. Prolonged paralysis has been reported with all three agents. Full recovery of muscle use may take from weeks to months.

Guidelines for Selection and Dosing. Neuromuscular blockers are administered intravenously in critically ill patients. This route ensures a rapid onset of action and easy dose adjustment. Selection of a neuromuscular blocker should be based upon the pharmacokinetic and pharmacodynamic differences among the available agents. Since pancuronium and vecuronium have an intermediate duration of action, they are administered intravenously every

Table 91.20.
Doses of Skeletal Muscle Relaxants

Drug	Intermittant Dosing	Continuous Infusion
Pancuronium	0.06–0.1 mg/kg q. 1–3 hr	Load: 0.04–0.1 mg/kg Maintenance: 0.06–0.1 mg/kg/hr
Vecuronium	0.1–0.2 mg/kg q.h.	Load: 0.08–0.1 mg/kg Maintenance: 0.05–0.1 mg/kg/hr
Atracurium	Not recommended	Load: 0.3–0.5 mg/kg Maintenance: 0.4–1.0 mg/kg/hr

1 to 3 hr or as a continuous infusion. Atracurium is commonly administered as a continuous infusion. Dosing for all three drugs is described in Table 91.20.

Special Patient Populations: Renal dysfunction. Pancuronium and its metabolites will accumulate in patients with renal dysfunction, and the duration of effect is prolonged (52). Consequently, the dose should be adjusted to the degree of renal insufficiency. The excretion of vecuronium and atracurium is much less affected by altered renal function during short-term use. However, there have been several reports of vecuronium and its metabolites accumulating during long-term infusion (53–55). This accumulation can result in prolonged paralysis and recovery time. Atracurium may also be used in patients with renal insufficiency or failure, because it is unlikely to accumulate. The potential accumulation and effects of its metabolite, laudanosine, need further investigation.

Special Patient Populations: Hepatic Dysfunction. Since pancuronium is metabolized in the liver and excreted via the biliary tract, the clearance may be reduced and the half-life prolonged in liver dysfunction. Similarly, the pharmacokinetics of vecuronium are altered in liver disease because of its high biliary excretion (30 to 50%). Atracurium, on the other hand, does not depend upon hepatic function for metabolism and can be given in liver failure without dose adjustment.

Summary

The patient with pain, anxiety, or agitation is a challenge for caregivers in the intensive care setting. Fortunately, effective drugs like opiates, benzodiazepines, and neuromuscular blocking agents help to alleviate these situations and ultimately facilitate the patient's recovery.

Conclusion

Critical care therapeutics represents a diverse set of challenges for members of the healthcare team. Management of critically ill patients requires a detailed understanding of disease pathophysiology, pharmacology, and therapeutics. Patients require multiple interventions, and drug regimens may require constant modification because of a rapidly changing clinical state.

These demands underscore the usefulness of a team approach to manage these patients. Pharmacists are in a unique position to render valuable aid in drug selection, dosing, monitoring, and evaluation of drug-induced disease. Furthermore, the growing understanding of disease pathophysiology with advances in biotechnology and drug product development may cause the development and use of new drug products. These agents may substantially modify the pathophysiologic processes of critically ill patients and impact significantly on patient morbidity and mortality. The role of the pharmacist will expand greatly as more becomes known about the use, effect, disposition, and monitoring of drug therapy in critically ill patients.

REFERENCES

1. Parillo JL, Septic shock in humans: clinical evaluation, pathophysiology, and therapeutic approach. In Shoemaker WC, Thompson WL, Holbrook P, et al.: Textbook of Critical Care, ed. 2. Philadelphia: WB Saunders, 1989, pp 1006–1023.
2. Mandell GL, Douglas RG Jr, Bennett JE: Principles and Practice of Infectious Disease, ed. 3. New York: Churchill Livingstone, 1990, ch 59.
3. Harris RL, Musher DM, Bloom K, et al.: Manifestations of sepsis. Arch Intern Med 147:1895, 1987.
4. Kreger BE, Craven DE, McCabe WR: Gram-negative bacteremia. Reevaluation of clinical features and treatment in 612 patients. Am J Med 68:344–355, 1980.
5. Lucas CE, Sugawa C, Riddle J, et al.: Natural history and surgical dilemma of 'stress' gastric bleeding. Arch Surg 102:266–273, 1971.
6. Trinkle JK, Rush BF, Eiseman B: Metabolism of lactate following major blood loss. Surgery 63:782–787, 1968.
7. Hauser CJ, Shoemaker WC, Turpin I: Oxygen transport responses to colloids and crystalloids in critically ill surgical patients. Surg Gynecol Obstet 150:811–817, 1980.
8. Sprung CL, Caralis PV, Marcial E, et al.: The effects of high-dose corticosteroids in patients with septic shock: a prospective, controlled study. N Engl J Med 311:1137–1143, 1984.
9. Bone RC, Fisher CJ Jr, Clemmer TP, Slotman GJ, Metz CA, Balk RA: A controlled clinical trial of high-dose methylprednisolone in the treatment of severe sepsis and septic shock. N Engl J Med 317:653–658, 1987.
10. Hinshaw L, Peduzzi P, Young E, et al.: Effect of high-dose glucocorticoid therapy on mortality in patients with clinical signs of systemic sepsis. The Veterans Administration Systemic Sepsis Cooperative Study Group. N Engl J Med 317:659–665, 1987.
11. Dorinsky PM, Gadik JE: Multiple organ failure. Clin Chest Med 11:581–591, 1990.

12. Matthay MA: The adult respiratory distress syndrome. Definition and prognosis. Clin Chest Med 11:575–580, 1990.

13. Rinald JE, Christman JW: Mechanisms and mediators of the adult respiratory distress syndrome. Clin Chest Med 11:621–632, 1990.

14. Tomashefsky JF: Pulmonary pathology of the adult respiratory distress syndrome. Clin Chest Med 11:593–619, 1990.

15. Schumacker PT, Samsel RW: Oxygen supply and consumption in the adult respiratory distress syndrome. Clin Chest Med 11:715–722, 1990.

16. Stoller JK, Kacmarek RM: Ventilatory strategies in the management of the adult respiratory distress syndrome. Clin Chest Med 11:755–772, 1991.

17. Dhainaut JF, Devaux JY, Monsallier JF, et al.: Mechanisms of decreased left ventricular preload during continuous positive pressure ventilation in ARDS. Chest 90:74–80, 1991.

18. Fewell JE, Abendschein Dr, Carlson CJ, et al.: Mechanism of decrease right and left ventricular end-diastolic volumes during continuous positive pressure ventilation in dogs. Circ Res 47:467–472, 1980.

19. Broaddus VC, Berthiaume Y, Biondi JW, et al.: Hemodynamic management of the adult respiratory distress syndrome. J Intensive Care Med 2:190–213, 1987.

20. Jardin F, Gurdijan F, Fouilladieu JL, et al.: Pulmonary and systemic haemodynamic disorders in the adult respiratory distress syndrome. Intensive Care Med 5:127–133, 1979.

21. Agarwa JB, Paltoo R, Palmer WH: Relative viscosity of blood at varying hematocrits in pulmonary circulation. J Appl Physiol 29:866–871, 1970.

22. Murray JF, Gold P, Johnson BL: The circulatory effects of hematocrit variations in normovolemic and hypervolemic dogs. J Clin Invest 42:1150–1159, 1963.

23. Prewitt RM, McCarthy J, Wood LDH: Treatment of acute low pressure pulmonary edema in dogs. Relative effects of hydrostatic and oncotic pressure, nitroprusside and positive end-expiratory pressure. J Clin Invest 1967:409–418, 1963.

24. Staub NC: Pulmonary edema. Physiologic approaches to management. Chest 74:559–564, 1978.

25. Nanjo S, Bhattacharya J, Staub NC: Concentrated albumin does not affect lung edema formation after acid instillation in the dog. Am Rev Resp Dis 128:884–889, 1983.

26. Molloy WD, Ducas J, Dobson K, et al.: Hemodynamic management in clinical acute hypoxemic respiratory failure: dopamine vs. dobutamine. Chest 89:636–640, 1986.

27. Molloy WD, Dobson K, Girling L, et al.: Effects of dopamine in cardiopulmonary function and left ventricular volumes in patients with acute respiratory failure. Am Rev Resp Dis 130:396–399, 1984.

28. Wood LDH, Prewitt RM: Cardiovascular management in acute hypoxemic respiratory failure. Am J Cardiol 47:963–972, 1981.

29. Prewitt RM, Raizen M, Ghignone M, et al.: Effects of increased hematocrit (viscous load) on right ventricular function in canine acute respiratory failure. Am Rev Resp Dis 129:A98, 1984.

30. Goldstein G, Luce JM: Pharmacologic treatment of the adult respiratory distress syndrome. Clin Chest Med 11:773–787, 1990.

31. Sibbald WJ, Anderson RA, Reid B, et al.: Alveolar-capillary permeability in ARDS. Effect of high dose corticosteroid therapy. Chest 78:133–142, 1981.

32. Bone RE, Fishcer CJ, Clemmer TP, et al.: A controlled clinical trial of high dose methylprednisolone in the treatment of severe sepsis and septic shock. N Engl J Med 317:653–658, 1987.

33. Bernard GR, Luce JM, Sprung J, et al.: High dose corticosteroids with the adult respiratory distress syndrome. N Engl J Med 317:1565–1570, 1987.

34. Holcraft JW, Vassar MJ, Weber CJ: Prostaglandin E_1 and survival in patients with the adult respiratory distress syndrome. Ann Surg 203:371–378, 1986.

35. Bone RC, Slotman G, Maunder R, et al.: Randomized double-blind, multicenter study of prostaglandin E_1 in patients with the adult respiratory distress syndrome. Chest 96:114–119, 1989.

36. Merritt TA, Hullman JM, Bloom BT, et al.: Prophylactic treatment of very premature infants with human surfactant. N Engl J Med 315:785–790, 1986.

37. Horbar JD, Gold FR, Sutherland JM, et al.: A multicenter randomized, placebo controlled trial of surfactant therapy for respiratory distress syndrome. N Engl J Med 320:959–965, 1989.

38. Collaborative European Multicenter Study Group: Surfactant replacement therapy for severe neonatal respiratory distress syndrome: an international randomized clinical trial. Pediatrics 82:683–691, 1988.

39. Ziegler EJ, McCrutchen JA, Fierer J, et al.: Treatment of gram negative bacteremia and shock with human antiserum to a mutant *Escherichia coli*. N Engl J Med 307:1225–1230, 1982.

40. Tracy KJ, Fong Y, Hesse DG, et al.: Anti-cachetin TNF monoclonal antibodies prevent septic shock during lethal bacteremia. Nature 333:662–664, 1982.

41. Ledingham J: Management of hypertensive crisis. Hypertension 5 (suppl III):114, 1983.

42. Kincaid-Smith P: Understanding malignant hypertension. Aust NZ J Med 11(suppl I): 64–68, 1981.

43. Skinhoj E, Strandgaard S: Pathogenesis of hypertensive encephalopathy. Lancet 1:461, 1973.

44. Garcia JY Jr, Vidt DG: Current management of hypertensive emergencies. Drugs 34:263–278, 1987.

45. Vesey CJ, Cole PV, Simpson PJ: Cyanide and thiocyanate concentrations following sodium nitroprusside infusion in man. Br J Anaesth 48:651, 1976.

46. Sculz V: Clinical pharmacokinetics of nitroprusside, cyanide, thiosulphate, and thiocyanate. Clin Pharmacokinet 9:239, 1984.

47. Houston M: Hypertensive emergencies and urgencies: pathophysiology and clinical aspects. Am Heart J 111:205–210, 1986.

48. McGillicuddy JE: Cerebral protection: pathophysiology and treatment of increased intracranial pressure. Chest 87:85–93, 1985.

49. Woster PS, LeBlanc K: Management of elevated intracranial pressure. Clin Pharm 9:762–772, 1990.

50. Lehman LB: Intracranial pressure monitoring and treatment: a contemporary view. Ann Emerg Med 19:295–303, 1990.

51. Fishman RA: Brain edema. N Engl J Med 293:706–711, 1975.

52. Vandenbrom RHG, Wierda JMKH: Pancuronium bromide in the intensive care unit: a case of overdose. Anesthesiology 69:996–997, 1988.

53. Segredo, Matthay MA, Sharma ML, et al.: Prolonged neuromuscular blockade after long-term administration of vecuronium in two critically ill patients. Anesthesiology 72:566–570, 1990.

54. Darrah WC, Johnston JR, Mirakhur RK: Vecuronium infusions for prolonged muscle relaxation in the intensive care unit. Crit Care Med 17:1297–1300, 1989.

55. Lyman DP, Cronnelly R, Arden J, et al.: The pharmacodynamics and pharmacokinetics of vecuronium in patients with and without renal failure. Anesthesiology 65:A296, 1986. Abstract.

CHAPTER 92

TRANSPLANTATION

THERESA A. SALAZAR, Pharm.D. and FRANCESCA T. AWEEKA, Pharm.D.

Transplantation of the kidney, liver, and heart has revolutionized the treatment of patients with end-stage renal, hepatic, or cardiac disease, and for the treatment of diabetes, pancreas transplantation is gaining acceptance. Though surgical techniques for organ transplantation have been available since the early 1900s, successful transplantation has a relatively recent history due to the delayed development of effective immunosuppressive protocols used to prevent rejection (Table 92.1) (1, 2). The first attempt to transplant a human kidney was made without antirejection therapy by the Russian surgeon Voronoy in 1933 and over the next 2 decades several more unsuccessful surgeries took place. In 1954 a successful kidney transplant procedure took place between monozygotic twins. Without the possibility of rejection, this procedure demonstrated that normal health could be restored in a transplant recipient in the absence of rejection. Pharmacologic immunosuppressive therapy for transplantation was first introduced in 1962, after it was discovered that azathioprine suppresses the immune response. Shortly thereafter, azathioprine and prednisone were incorporated into immunosuppressive protocols, and an increasing number of successful kidney transplant procedures followed. The first successful liver and heart transplants took place in 1967.

In the 1970s, advances were made in histocompatibility (tissue) matching, organ preservation, and antilymphocyte sera therapy that led to further success in transplanted allograft survival. (See Table 92.2 for definitions of graft terminology). Tissue typing established that close donor and recipient matching could be obtained, and the progress made on the development of new immunosuppressive drugs revolutionized transplantation. More recently, cyclosporine and the new monoclonal antibodies have become available for both the prevention and treatment of rejection episodes. With the introduction of cyclosporine in 1981, the 1-year kidney allograft survival in cadaver transplant recipients rose from 53 to 80%. The new immunosuppressive agents and the progress made in perfecting surgical techniques has resulted in the increased use and success of transplant procedures for patients with end-stage organ disease and disorders such as diabetes mellitus. Kidney, heart, liver, and even pancreas and lung transplantation have become a dominant activity of some surgical services at major medical centers throughout the United States, and it is now properly characterized as dramatic, life-saving, and one of the few true cures for disease treatment.

IMMUNOBIOLOGY OF TRANSPLANTATION

The immune system is a highly complex system that scientists have only recently begun to understand. Much of the research has resulted from the increasing role of organ transplantation and the need for effective immunosuppressive therapy designed to suppress the rejection process. Tissue-matching techniques have been developed to identify appropriate donor-recipient matches. Studies in histocompatibility and studies with the new monoclonal antibodies and other immunosuppressive agents have provided a better understanding of how the various cells and proteins of the immune system work together to respond to foreign tissue. Histocompatibility testing characterizes the tissue surface antigens specific for both the donor and the recipient, and though not without some limitations, this helps to predict the likelihood of the donor developing

Table 92.1.
Historical Overview of Transplantation[a]

1905	Development of vascular suture techniques
1933	First human kidney transplant attempted
1954	First successful human kidney transplant
1960	Development of tissue typing begins
1962	Azathioprine used as a single immunosuppressive agent
1963	First human liver transplant attempted
1963	Steroids and azathioprine shown to have synergistic immunosuppressive effects
1966	First human segmental pancreas transplant attempted
1966	Antilymphocyte globulin used clinically as adjunctive immunosuppressive therapy
1967	First successful human liver transplant
1967	First successful human orthotopic heart transplant
1968	First human heart-lung transplant attempted
1970	Cyclophosphamide tried as a substitute for azathioprine
1974	First clinical heterotopic heart transplant
1978	Clinical trials of cyclosporine initiated
1982	First successful human heart-lung transplant
1983	Cyclosporine approved by FDA
1983	Clinical trials of muromonab CD3 (Orthoclone OKT3) initiated
1987	Orthoclone OKT3 approved by FDA
1989	Clinical trials of FK506 and animal trials of rapamycin initiated
1990	Clinical trials of RS-61443 initiated

[a] Adapted from Pifarre R, Sullivan H, Montoya A, et al.: Cardiac transplantation. Cardiol Clin 7:183–194, 1989; and Flye M, History of transplantation. In Flye M: Principles of Organ Transplantation. Philadelphia, WB Saunders, 1989, pp 1–17.

an immune response to most transplanted allografts. The basis of this technology is summarized, and the major components of the immune system, the mechanisms behind allograft rejection, and its clinical presentations are reviewed.

HLA System

Transplanted tissues are rejected due to immunologic responses directed at donor antigens on the transplanted allograft. All mammalian species show evidence of a single chromosome region that encodes for the major tissue sur-

Table 92.2.
General Graft Terminology

Current Nomenclature	Past Nomenclature	Definition
Autograft	Autograft	A transplant of tissue or organ taken from the recipient
Syngraft	Isograft	A transplant of tissue or organ taken from a genetically identical donor such as monozygotic twins
Allograft	Homograft	A transplant of tissue or organ taken from a genetically different donor of the same species
Xenograft	Heterograft	A transplant of tissue or organ taken from a donor belonging to a different species.
Heterotopic transplant		The recipient's native organ is left in place and the donor organ is grafted into an ectopic position or site
Orthotopic transplant		The recipient's native organ is removed and the donor organ is placed with normal or near-normal anatomic reconstruction

face antigens (3), and in humans these antigens were originally named HLA for human leukocyte antigen. They are glycoproteins that are collectively referred to as the major histocompatibility complex (MCH). The genes for the major histocompatibility complex are located on the short arm of chromosome 6 (Fig. 92.1).

There are at least five defined HLA loci on chromosome 6: HLA-A, HLA-B, HLA-C, HLA-DR, and the HLA-D region (4). Each locus can express many variations of each gene (alleles), which produce distinct glycoproteins or antigens for a given individual (e.g., at least 32 different types of HLA-B antigens have been identified).

The antigens that make up the major histocompatibility complex are grouped into two classes: HLA class I and HLA class II (4–6). Class I antigens, i.e., HLA-A, -B, and -C are present on the plasma membranes of most nucleated cells in the body, including the T and B cells, platelets, and cells of the heart, kidney, and liver. They are the primary targets for cytotoxic T lymphocytes and are easily detected serologically from peripheral blood lymphocytes (5). Class I antigens are remarkable for their extreme genetic polymorphism, which makes it very difficult to obtain matches for transplantation between unrelated persons. Class II antigens (i.e., HLA-DP, -DQ, and -DR,) are less well characterized and have a restricted distribution. They are normally found on B lymphocytes, activated T cells, macrophages, vascular endothelium, and some epithelial cells and are detected serologically from the isolation and purification of B lymphocytes (5).

Histocompatibility testing of the donor and recipient is used to minimize donor-specific immune responses to a transplanted organ, although the overall benefits of close tissue matching for patients managed with potent immunosuppression is controversial. Theoretically, the more antigens that match, the less likely rejection is to occur. A donor and recipient are considered HLA identical when

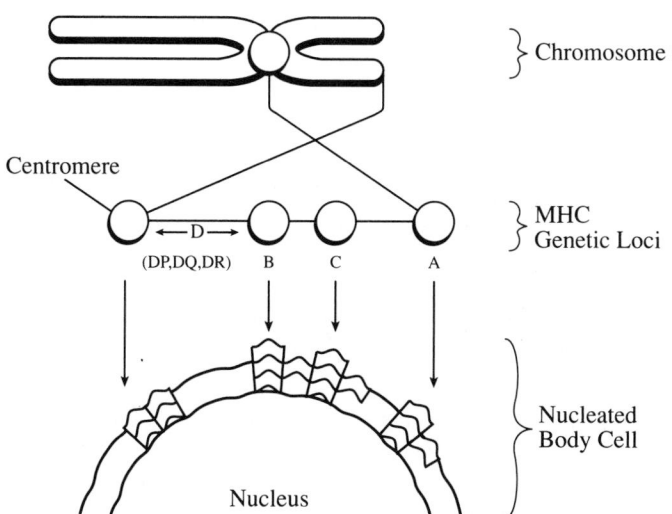

Figure 92.1. The human major histocompatibility complex (MHC). Genetic loci designated *A*, *B*, and *C* encode class I MHC (HLA) antigens. Genetic region designated D contains at least three subloci, *DR*, *DQ*, and *DP*, encoding for class II MHC (HLA) antigens. (Adapted with permission of Kluwer Academic Publishers.)

all detectable antigens are the same. Though it remains unclear, some studies suggest that HLA-DR antigen mismatching is more closely linked to rejection episodes than class I antigen mismatching (7).

Immune System

Acquired immunity is the body's genetic mechanism designed to ward off invasions by foreign substances or organisms (antigens). The immune response is the result of a complex cascade that results in the formation of antibodies (immunoglobulins) and sensitized cells (lymphocytes) that take part in specific humoral or cell-mediated responses to antigenic stimuli (Fig. 92.2). Humoral immunity is mediated by serum antibodies produced by B cells, whereas cellular immunity depends upon T cells. When presented with a foreign antigen, the immune response is initiated, and immature B lymphocytes are stimulated to proliferate and differentiate into lymphoblasts. These cells ultimately mature into the plasma cells that produce the antibodies secreted into the lymphatic circulation and the blood. The antibodies primarily target the graft endothelium and bind to the foreign antigens (e.g., donor histocompatibility antigens). Then in conjunction with the complement system, they cause cell destruction by agglutination, precipitation, opsonization, and cell lysis. Macrophages and T lymphocytes help regulate this arm of the immune system and can augment or suppress the degree to which B lymphocytes produce antibodies.

Cell-mediated immunity is initiated by a T lymphocyte response directed against specific foreign substances or organisms that are viewed as invader antigens. T lymphocytes are classified according to their functions as effector cells or regulators. Cytotoxic T cells are effector cells that function as killer cells. They can cause cellular lysis and death of specific antigen-bearing cells. They recognize transplanted tissues as foreign invading substances and are the lymphocytes mainly responsible for graft rejection.

The T lymphocytes that modulate the cytotoxic effect by regulating the proliferation and maturation of cytotoxic T cells are classified as regulator cells. They are the T helper and T suppressor cells. The T helper cells are stimulated by macrophages to produce the lymphokine interleukin-2 (IL-2, T cell growth factor), an important regulatory protein of the immune system. IL-2 stimulates the proliferation of other T helper cells as well as the differentiation of mature cytotoxic T cells. Stimulated T helper cells also produce other regulatory lymphokines such as γ-interferon, macrophage inhibitory factor, and B cell growth factor. Conversely, the T suppressor cell provides a feedback mechanism that inhibits the growth and function of T helper cells and suppresses antibody production from plasma cells.

When antigens from the donor graft elicit a response from the recipient's immune system, the sequence of events that ensues can be subdivided into afferent and efferent arms. During the afferent arm of the immune response the antigens from the donor graft are recognized by the recipient's circulating T lymphocytes and the early stages of the immune response are initiated. The efferent arm begins when the recipient's immune system mounts a response against the graft with infiltration of lymphoid and phagocytic cells into the allograft tissue (8).

Rejection

Allograft rejection is a complex mixture of cellular and inflammatory responses triggered by histocompatibility antigens on the donor allograft. Host cytotoxic effects directed against the cells of the transplanted organ or severe nonspecific inflammatory responses result in structural and functional alterations within the grafted organ (9, 10). Rejection of organ allografts is divided into three categories, hyperacute, acute, and chronic, as described in Table 92.3 (4), with the descriptions relating to the onset of graft function deterioration and the immunological mediators most likely to be responsible for the rejection process (4, 8).

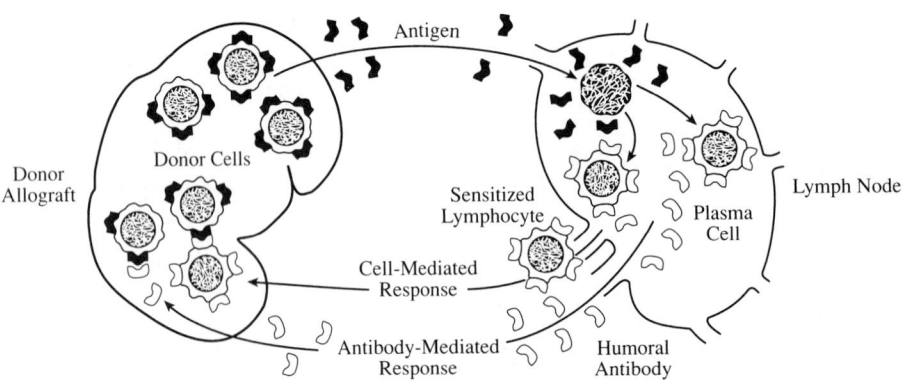

Figure 92.2. Schematic representation of an allograft undergoing rejection. (Modified from JAMA 1987; 258:2993–3000 figure 22-4a copyright 1987, American Medical Association, with permission.)

Table 92.3.
Types of Rejection Reactions

Type	Time after Transplantation	Probable Mediators
Hyperacute	Minutes to 1–5 days	Preformed lymphocytoxic antibodies
Acute	Weeks to months	Newly developed antibodies, delayed-type hypersensitivity of helper and inducer T lymphocytes
Chronic	Months to years	T lymphocytes and donor-specific anibody response directed at allograft vasculature

Clinically, hyperacute rejection occurs within minutes to hours following vascularization of the graft, most commonly while the patient is still in the operating room. It is caused by cytotoxic antibodies that have been preformed in response to ABO blood group antigens, vascular endothelial antigens, and histocompatibility antigens. Hyperacute rejection progresses rapidly, resulting in the obstruction of blood vessels and ischemia. It is an irreversible process, unresponsive to antirejection therapy and requiring immediate removal of the transplanted organ. Hyperacute rejection occurs less frequently in the liver than in other allograft organs, for reasons that remain unclear (11, 12). The overall incidence of hyperacute rejection for all solid organ allografts has been reduced to less than 1% by the use of pretransplantation antidonor lymphocyte–toxic antibody assays (13, 14).

Acute rejection is both cell- and antibody-mediated, and it involves both helper and inducer T lymphocytes. These lymphocytes gradually become sensitized by antigens released from the donor allograft. This leads to injury or destruction of certain epithelial structures of the transplanted allograft, e.g., monocytes in the heart, renal tubules in the kidney, and the bile duct epithelium of the liver. Acute rejection occurs most frequently between the first week and the first few months following transplantation, but it may occur within a few days or as late as years after transplantation (8). The diagnosis of acute rejection depends on the particular organ transplanted and is generally based on clinical and laboratory findings (see "Diagnosis of Rejection" and Table 92.4). Acute rejection is usually reversible, especially if treated early.

Chronic rejection presents as the gradual but progressive impairment of allograft function in the absence of other specific disease. However, for some solid organs such as liver, organ function may remain intact until late in the chronic rejection process. This form of rejection is most likely caused by organ ischemia resulting from the narrowing and occlusion of arteries (and bile ducts in liver allografts) by graft arteriosclerosis (15, 16). Although the immune mechanisms are unclear, chronic rejection is antibody-mediated and can result in foam cell deposition in the walls of medium-sized arteries, leading to arteriosclerotic lesions in the graft (17, 18). Graft arteriosclerosis was first described in cardiac transplant patients, but all organ allografts may develop this vascular disease. Typically, chronic rejection does not occur before 6 months to 1 year after transplantation. Accelerated graft coronary arterosclerosis due to chronic rejection can be detected on coronary arteriogram in 40% of cardiac recipients by 2.5 years following cardiac transplantation (19, 20). In one recent series, chronic rejection in kidney transplant patients was reported to be the major cause of allograft loss 2 years beyond transplantation (21). Chronic rejection is essentially irreversible with currently available antirejection therapy.

Diagnosis of Rejection

Transplant patients are at their highest risk for developing acute cellular rejection during the first 3 months following transplantation. Later occurrences are less common, unless immunosuppressive therapy has been withdrawn or the patient develops a serious viral infection. Allograft recipients experiencing rejection are often febrile and have marked malaise, with body temperatures ranging from 38 to 39.5° C. Tenderness and swelling of the graft and leukocytosis are also common symptoms. Specific clinical and physiologic features of allograft rejection differ with each type of organ transplanted (Table 92.4). The differential diagnosis often includes infection as well as rejection and therefore symptoms must be evaluated in view of other physical and laboratory findings.

Clinical signs of rejection of the heart are usually absent unless rejection is prolonged or severe. The transplanted heart is denervated, so angina and chest pain are not present. The most common subjective complaints include shortness of breath, decreased exercise tolerance, and dyspnea on exertion. Asymptomatic ECG changes, S_3 heart sounds, hypotension, tachycardia, and congestive heart failure are also common. The diagnosis of acute cardiac rejection is determined by endomyocardial biopsy (EMB). Routine biopsies are performed weekly during the early postoperative period, and then at less frequent but regular intervals (1, 22). Histologic changes detected on biopsy, which are consistent with rejection, include diffuse mononuclear infiltrates.

Acute rejection following renal transplantation is characterized by a rise in serum creatinine concentration (increase >26.5 µmol/liter (0.3 mg/dl)), decreased urine output, and enlargement and tenderness of the allograft. Other symptoms may include malaise, fever, leukocytosis, hypertension, and edema of the lower extremities. Unilateral leg edema on the side of the transplanted kidney

Table 92.4.
Signs and Symptoms of Rejection Related to Specific Transplanted Organ

Organ	Clinical Signs	Laboratory Signs	Ref
Heart	Fever, lethargy, weakness, SOB, DOE, hypotension, tachycardia, atrial flutter, ventricular arrhythmias	Leukocytosis, endomyocardial biopsy positive for mononuclear infiltrates	(1, 22)
Kidney	Fever, graft tenderness and swelling, decrease in urine output, malaise, hypertension, weight gain, edema	Scr increase of >26 μmol/liter above baseline, increased BUN, leukocytosis, renal biopsy positive for lymphocytic infiltration	(25, 38, 39)
Liver	Fever, lethargy, change in color or quantity of bile in patients with biliary T-tube, graft tenderness and swelling, back pain, anorexia, ileus, tachycardia; in severe rejection: jaundice, ascites, overt encephalopathy	Abnormal LFTs, rapid rise in GGTP, increased serum bilirubin, increased alkaline phosphatase, increased serum transaminase, core-needle biopsy positive for mononuclear cell infiltrate with evidence of tissue damage	(24, 241)
Pancreas	Fever, graft tenderness and swelling, abdominal pain, ileus, malaise	FBS >11 mmol/liter, leukocytosis, human C-peptide <0.7 ng/ml, urinary amylase levels <167 μkat/liter (bladder anastomosis)	(25, 26, 38)

is common and is attributed to lymphatic obstruction by the enlarged kidney. Acute rejection in renal transplantation must be differentiated from cyclosporine-induced nephrotoxicity, renal artery or vein stenosis, and CMV infection. Renal biopsy is one of the most useful tools for confirming allograft rejection, and the predominate histological findings include lymphocytic infiltration and tissue damage within the interstitium (10, 23).

Signs of acute hepatic rejection include abnormal liver function test results, fever, ileus, ascites, abdominal pain, and jaundice. An increase in serum γ-glutamyl transpeptidase (GGTP) activity is an early but nonspecific indicator of acute rejection. Increases in bilirubin, alkaline phosphatase, and amyloid A protein levels may also occur, along with a change in the color and quantity of bile. The diagnosis of rejection can be confirmed by core-needle biopsy whose histologic findings include mononuclear portal inflammatory cell infiltrates with evidence of tissue damage. Intraoperative liver biopsies are obtained at the time of transplantation for later comparison with routine serial biopsies (12, 24).

Following pancreas transplantation, allograft function is monitored by measuring serum glucose and amylase levels as well as urinary amylase levels in those patients with bladder anastomosis (see "Surgical Procedures"). A presumptive diagnosis of acute rejection may be based on a 25% increase over baseline in fasting or postprandial glucose levels. Serum amylase levels are usually normal in the functioning pancreatic graft, so a sudden increase in serum amylase followed by hyperglycemia suggests acute rejection. Clinical symptoms of rejection are often absent and are nonspecific. In patients who have received both a transplanted pancreas and kidney, diagnoses of rejection often depends on renal function tests. Biopsy is not routinely performed in pancreas transplantation, since this requires a surgical procedure (25–27).

Rejection Treatment

The overall goal for treatment of acute rejection is to minimize the intensity of the immune response toward the transplanted organ. Episodes of moderate-to-severe rejection are usually treated in the hospital, while mild episodes may be treated on an outpatient basis.

The treatment of acute rejection episodes usually involves steroid pulses (bursts of high doses) or a recycling of steroids (resumption of induction doses). Although the exact protocols vary between transplant centers the general practice is to increase the dose for 3 to 7 days and then taper to the maintenance or prerejection dose. The usual treatment is methylprednisolone 1 to 2 g per day for 3 days or until there is evidence of improved allograft function. Lower doses of 2 to 4 mg/kg/day have also been effective.

If the rejection is not controlled with high-dose steroids, treatment with antilymphocyte globulin (ALG) or orthoclone CD3 (OKT3) may be initiated. ALG is dosed at 10 to 20 mg/kg for 7 doses, and OKT3 is dosed at 5 mg for 7 to 14 days. It is believed that ALG is most effective when used for acute rejection occurring within the first weeks following transplantation (172, 227). (See "Specific Immunosuppressive Agents.")

SURGICAL CONSIDERATIONS

The criteria used for selecting an appropriate transplant recipient can vary widely between transplant centers and often depend on the experience of the center and donor organ availability. Kidney transplantation has become so common that the guidelines now used for selecting a recipient are far less limiting than those used 10 to 20 years ago. Recipients may now be over 60 years old and have underlying diseases that were previously considered contraindications for transplantation (e.g., diabetes). The contraindications to liver and heart transplantation surgery have diminished over the years, especially when compared with life-threatening nature of end-stage hepatic and cardiac disease.

An important factor that limits the number of transplant procedures is the inadequate supply of donor organs. Currently, more than 13,000 patients with kidney disease, 1000 with severe cardiac disease, and 500 with liver disease are on the United Network Organ Sharing (UNOS) list awaiting an appropriate donor. Unfortunately, approximately 30% of potential donor organs are made available for transplantation. New approaches have been implemented by some states to increase this percentage. Since 1988 most states have implemented a "routine inquiry" law requiring administrators to inform families of deceased persons that organs can be made available for transplantation. Once a suitable donor is identified, the UNOS coordinates the selection of an appropriate recipient(s). A complicated scoring system is used by the UNOS computer for patients awaiting transplantation around the country.

Operative Procedures

The surgical techniques used for transplantation may influence the therapeutic management of patients posttransplantation. Therefore, a brief overview of the procedures used for heart, kidney, liver, and pancreas transplantation will be presented, including the site of organ implantation and the major arterial and venous anastomoses. The descriptions are not extracted from any one specific protocol, and the reader is directed to more extensive reviews (28–39).

HEART

Orthotopic transplantation is the most common procedure used for the heart. At the time of surgery, the patient is placed on cardiopulmonary bypass to maintain adequate circulation throughout the surgical procedure. Once the patient is stable, the native heart is removed (cardiectomy), leaving most of both atria and septum in place. Implantation of the donor heart is performed by anastomosis of the left atrium of the heart to the residual left atrial wall of the recipient, followed by joining of the right atrial wall and atrial septum. The main pulmonary artery is then connected to the ascending aorta (Fig. 92.3).

Following implantation, recovery of cardiac function may require 40 to 60 min of bypass support as the patient is slowly "weaned" and cardiac circulation is restored. The transplanted heart is denervated and therefore relies on circulating catecholamines for normal function (1, 28–30).

KIDNEY

In kidney transplantation, the transplanted allograft can be from either a cadaver or a living related donor. In most cases, the native kidneys of the recipient remain in place. The donor kidney may be implanted in either iliac fossa, however the right is the site of choice. The hypogastric, common iliac, external iliac, or internal iliac artery is used for the arterial anastomotic site, and the common or external iliac vein for the venous anastomosis (Fig. 92.4).

Revascularization of the new kidney takes about 30 min, with the production of urine often beginning immediately. With proper circulation intact, anastomosis of the ureter can begin. Reconstruction of the urinary tract is frequently done by passing the donor ureter through the recipient's posterior bladder wall. The ureter is then joined to the bladder mucosa (ureteroneocystostomy). Alternatively, the ureter may be connected directly to the

Figure 92.3. Completed heart transplant with sites of major surgical anastomoses. (Modified from Heart and heart-lung transplantation. Ed J Wallwork. 1989, Philadelphia, WB Saunders, with permission.)

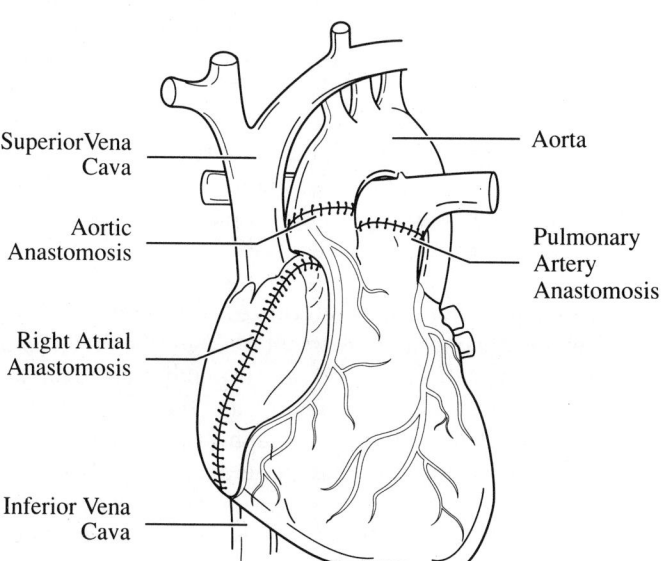

Superior Vena Cava

Aorta

Aortic Anastomosis

Pulmonary Artery Anastomosis

Right Atrial Anastomosis

Inferior Vena Cava

Figure 92.4. Completed kidney transplant into right iliac fossa with sites of major surgical anastomoses. (Adapted with permission of Mosby Year Book.)

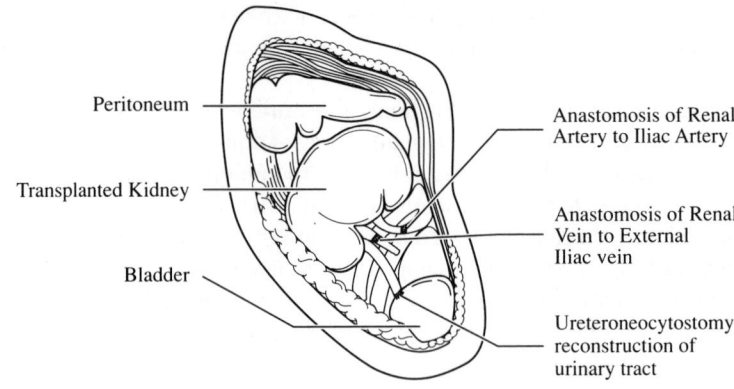

Peritoneum

Transplanted Kidney

Bladder

Anastomosis of Renal Artery to Iliac Artery

Anastomosis of Renal Vein to External Iliac vein

Ureteroneocytostomy reconstruction of urinary tract

dome of the bladder without passage through the bladder wall (31–33).

LIVER

In orthotopic liver transplantation, the length of time between harvesting the donor liver and transplantation is of major concern because of the poor viability of the transplanted organ. Prior to the development of new storage solutions, the ischemic time limit for a harvested liver was 6 to 10 hr. This critical time limit has recently been increased to 20 hr. Due to these time restrictions, surgery is performed on the recipient prior to the arrival of the donor organ. The donor and recipient are generally matched for liver size (± 20%), since insertion of an excessively large liver would lead to splinting of the diaphragm and pulmonary complications (34–37).

Once the donor liver arrives, the diseased liver of the recipient is removed intact and implantation of the donor liver begins. This involves four major vascular and one biliary surgical anastomoses. Vascular sites of anastomosis include the hepatic artery, inferior and superior vena cavae, and the portal vein (Fig. 92.5). When liver function has resumed, anastomosis of the biliary tract is carried out by connecting the donor and recipient's common ducts over a drainage tube (T-tube). Use of a system to divert circulation during the transplant operation (veno-venous bypass) remains controversial because of such risks as pulmonary embolism, nerve damage, or lymphoceles (35).

PANCREAS

In pancreas transplantation the native pancreas is left in place (heterotopic procedure). Pancreas transplants may be either segmental (tail and body) or whole organ. Segmental grafts are commonly placed extra- or intraperitoneally in the pelvis, with vascular anastomosis to the iliac vessels. The whole organ graft is obtained as a bloc dissection and includes the pancreas, spleen, and a long duodenal segment. It is placed intraperitoneally where the exudates of the pancreas can be absorbed by the highly

vascular peritoneum. Placed into the right iliac fossa, the arterial supply of the graft is anastomosed to the common iliac artery, and its venous drainage is anastomosed to the common iliac vein (Fig. 92.6). The exocrine duct is often drained into the bladder for urinary excretion of pancreatic enzymes (25, 38, 39).

PRINCIPLES OF IMMUNOSUPPRESSION

Immunosuppressive therapy is necessary in transplantation to blunt the body's immune response to foreign antigens on the transplanted allograft. Ideally, an immunosuppressant should specifically inhibit the cells responsible for the allograft rejection process, affecting only the lymphocyte subsets directed against donor-specific alloantigens. Unfortunately, the development of drugs with this specificity has been difficult. The immunosuppressive agents used in transplantation today interfere directly with one or more steps in the immune response (Fig. 92.7). The two tenets of current immunosuppressive therapy are to prevent rejection and avoid infection, and these two objectives are in constant conflict. The clinical challenge is to balance the doses of immunosuppressive agents so that the optimal immunosuppression is achieved and the risk of infection is minimized. This is not a static process, but rather an ongoing process that requires constant monitoring and adjustment in accord with the clinical course of each patient. Although the dose of immunosuppressive agents may be tapered with time, the transplant recipient must continue to use them indefinitely. Withdrawal of immunosuppression, except in the case of homozygous twin transplant recipient, almost inevitably leads to allograft rejection.

Immunosuppressive protocols exist for both rejection prophylaxis and for the treatment of established rejection. The specifics of the protocols vary, depending on the organ transplanted, the transplant center, and the collective clinical data available at the time. Prophylactic regimens usually include an induction phase, where relatively high doses of immunosuppressive agents are administered early posttransplant, and a maintenance phase, where lower doses

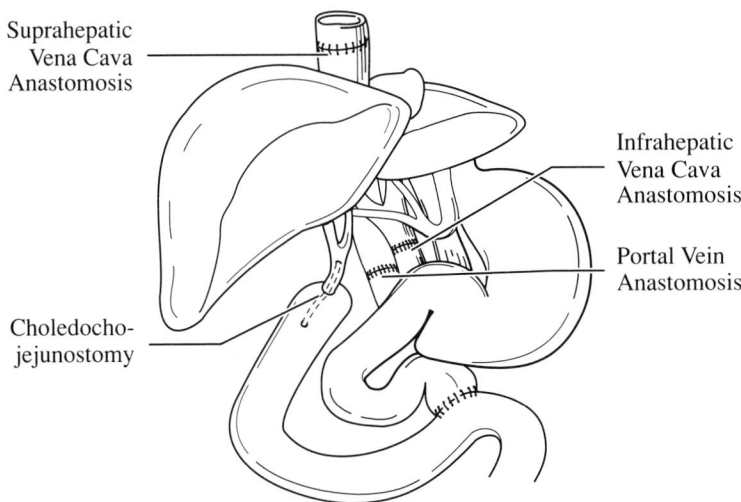

Figure 92.5. Completed liver transplant with sites of major surgical anastomoses. (Adapted with permission of Mosby Year Book.)

Suprahepatic Vena Cava Anastomosis

Infrahepatic Vena Cava Anastomosis

Portal Vein Anastomosis

Choledocho-jejunostomy

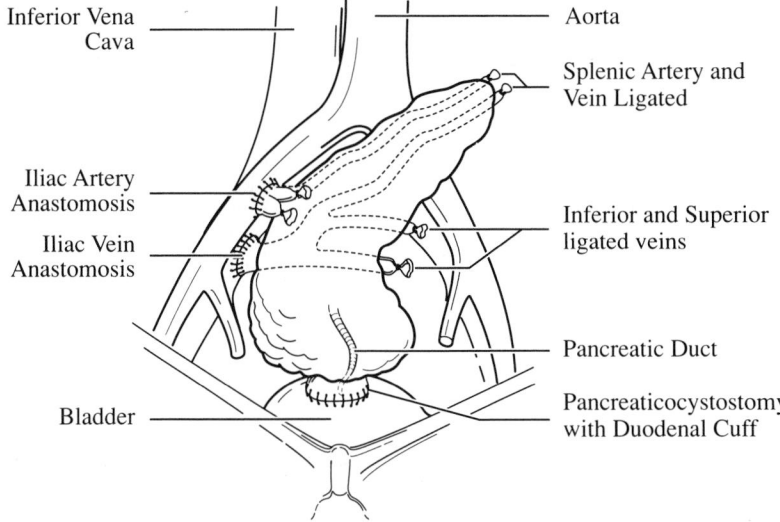

Figure 92.6. Completed whole pancreas transplant with sites of major surgical anastomoses. (Adapted with permission of Mosby Year Book.)

Inferior Vena Cava

Aorta

Splenic Artery and Vein Ligated

Iliac Artery Anastomosis

Iliac Vein Anastomosis

Inferior and Superior ligated veins

Pancreatic Duct

Pancreaticocystostomy with Duodenal Cuff

Bladder

of immunosuppressants are adequate because the risk of rejection decreases with time. Most maintenance regimens include at least two agents (cyclosporine and either prednisone or azathioprine) or three agents (cyclosporine, azathioprine, and prednisone) used at lower doses. Table 92.5 lists some immunosuppression protocols for rejection prophylaxis currently in use. Various immunosuppressive protocols for the treatment of established rejection have also been developed. Rejection regimens may include high-dose steroids (e.g., intravenous prednisolone) or antilymphocyte preparations (e.g., antilymphocyte globulin, muromonab CD3). Table 92.6 summarizes the agents used most frequently in immunosuppressive therapy.

SPECIFIC IMMUNOSUPPRESSIVE AGENTS
Corticosteroids

Corticosteroids such as prednisone or methylprednisolone are part of most immunosuppressive protocols for organ transplantation. They have been an important component of immunosuppressive therapy since the early days of transplantation and are used routinely for both the prevention and treatment of allograft rejection. Currently, prednisone, prednisolone, and methylprednisolone are used most often in clinical transplantation.

Prednisone and prednisolone are often used interchangeably, with prednisolone considered to be the pharmacologically active moiety. For oral maintenance immunosuppression, prednisone is preferred in the United States, while prednisolone is used exclusively by many European transplant centers. For the treatment of rejection, both intravenous methylprednisolone or prednisolone and high-dose oral prednisone have been used successfully.

Corticosteroids such as prednisone have been shown to inhibit the inductive phase of cytotoxic T cells by decreasing the production of important immunomodulating proteins such as IL-1 and IL-2, which results in diminished

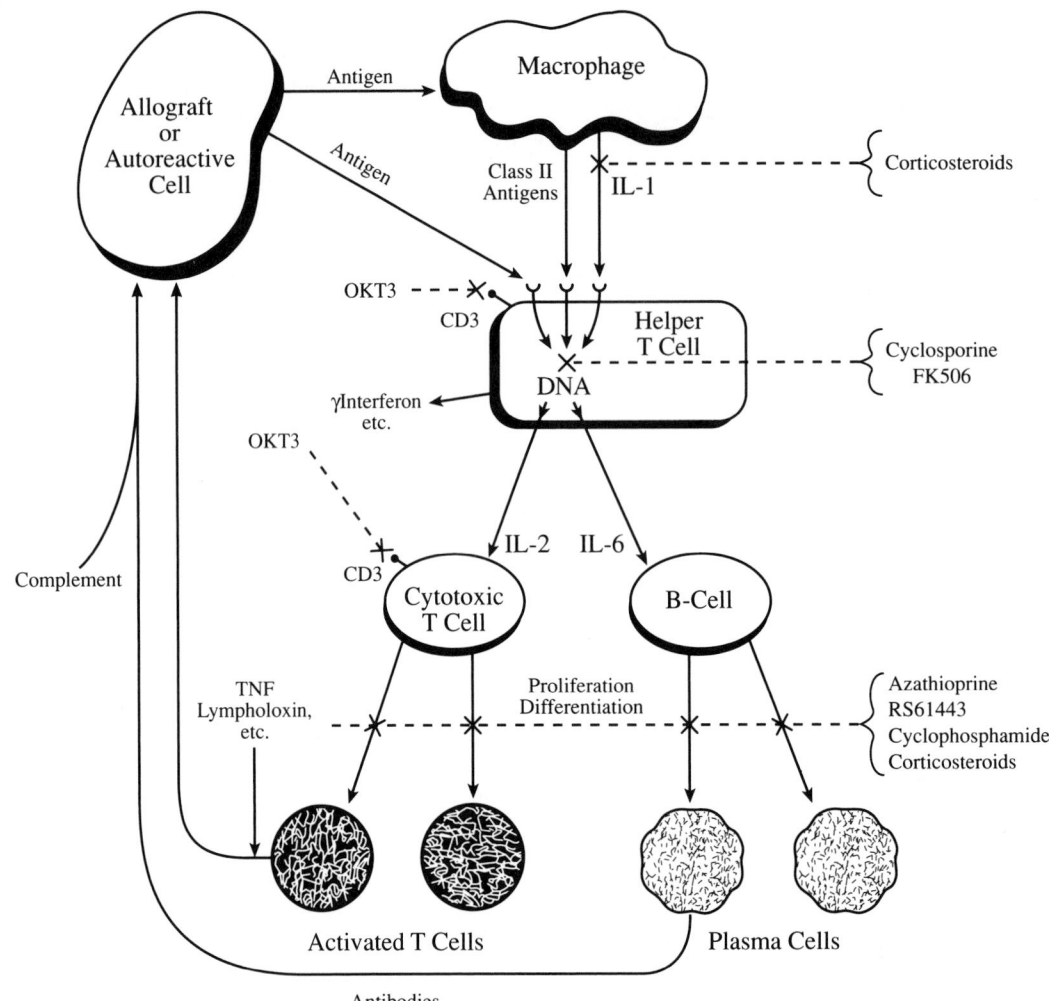

Figure 92.7. Schematic representation summarizing the mechanism of action of immunosuppressive agents. (Modified from RE Handschumacher: Immunosuppressive Agents. In Goodman and Gillmans's The Pharmacological Basis of Thera- peutics, ed. 8. edited by AG Gillman, TW Rall, AS Nies, P Taylor. Copyright (c) 1990, Pergamon Press, Inc. Reprinted with per- mission Macmillan Publishing Company.)

T lymphocyte proliferative response to alloantigens. The production of γ–interferon by T cells is also decreased (40– 42). In addition, high-dose rejection therapy can decrease the expression of HLA antigens and β-2 microglobulins on peripheral blood lymphocytes. The immunogenicity of transplanted organs is thereby decreased (42, 43).

The dose of corticosteroids used in organ transplan- tation is empirical, and dosage adjustments are based on both therapeutic and toxic clinical responses. Though ther- apy is not routinely monitored by plasma levels, the phar- macokinetics of the corticosteroids are complex, with changes occurring in various disease states (e.g., renal dys- function) (Table 92.7, 44–47).

Immunosuppressive protocols vary widely from one transplant center to another and depend on the organ transplanted. Due to the widespread use of cyclosporine, steroid doses are currently lower than those used previ- ously. Transplant protocols use prednisone doses ranging from 20 to 140 mg/day initially. These doses are usually tapered to maintenance doses of 5 to 30 mg/day approx- imately 3 months posttransplantation. Maintenance doses starting at 12 to 18 months range from 5 to 10 mg/day. A typical protocol includes high-dose prednisone (200 mg/ day orally) at the time of transplant followed by a rapid taper over 5 days to 20 mg/day. Others start with a pred- nisone dose of 30 mg/day orally that is slowly tapered to 7.5 to 15 mg/day at 12 to 18 months.

Corticosteroid protocols for the treatment of trans- plant rejection episodes vary, but doses of approximately 5 to 10 mg/kg of prednisolone or methylprednisolone ad- ministered for 3 days are routinely used. Steroid-resistant rejection can be treated with more-potent agents such as

Table 92.5.
Examples of Immunosuppression Protocols for Rejection Prophylaxis[a,b]

Heart Transplant Protocols

Example A

Drug	Day	Dose
MePred	Day 0	500 mg IV
	Day 1	125 mg IV q8h × 3 doses
AZA	Day 0–4	2–3 mg/kg IV or p.o.
	Day 5+	1.5–2 mg/kg/day adjust dose to maintain WBC >4.5
CSA	Day 0	4–10 mg/kg p.o.
	Day 1	3–5 mg/kg IV q12h plus 1–2 mg/kg continuous infusion (day 1–3)
	Day 2	1 mg/kg-day p.o. q12h
	Day 3	5–6 mg/kg-day p.o.
	Day 4+	Titrate dose to trough whole blood HPLC levels of 300 ng/ml

Example B

Drug	Day	Dose
MePred	Day 0	500 mg intraop
	Day 1	125 mg IV q8h × 3 doses
AZA	Day 0	4 mg/kg p.o.
	Day 2+	2 mg/kg/day p.o. or IV (keep WBC >4.5)
OKT3	Day 2–16	5 mg IV q.d. with HC 1 mg/kg
Pred	Day 1	0.25mg/kg/day
	Day 5–14	1 mg/kg/day for 7 days, then tapered
	Day 14–21	off over 2 weeks
CSA	Day 13+	2mg/kg q12h, titrate dose to trough serum RIA levels of 100–300 ng/ml serum, RIA

Example C

Drug	Day	Dose
MALG	Day 0–9	15 mg/kg/day IV
MePred	Day 0	1 g IV intraop
	Day 1	100 mg IV b.i.d.
CSA	Day 1–30	5–2.5 mg/kg/day based on Scr; once Scr and BUN stable adjust dose by to achieve whole blood HPLC levels of 300 ng/ml for the first month, 100–250 ng/ml during the first year, and 100–150 ng/ml thereafter
	Day 60+	
AZA	Day 9+	1 mg/kg/day, adjusted to 2 mg/kg/day as tolerated for WBC >4

Kidney Transplant Protocols

Example D

Drug	Day	Dose
MePred	Day 0	1 g in OR
CSA	Day 0	7 mg/kg
	Day 1	4 mg/kg IV
	Day 2–7	14 mg/kg/day p.o.
	Day 8–14	12 mg/kg/day p.o.
	Day 15+	10 mg/kg/day p.o., adjust dose to maintain TDX whole blood levels 200–250 ng/ml during months 1 to 6 and 100–125 ng/ml after 7 months
Pred	Day 1–14	140 mg/day, taper dose to 20 mg/day
	Week 3–52	20 mg/day, taper dose to 7.5 mg/day
	Week 53+	7.5 mg q.o.d., most patients are converted to q.o.d. at 1 year

Example E

Drug	Day	Dose
Pred	Day 0	2 mg/kg
	Day 1+	0.5 mg/kg
AZA	Day 0	4 mg/kg
	Day 1+	1 mg/kg
MALG	Day 1–7	20 mg/kg IV
CSA	Day 5–13	10 mg/kg/day p.o. if Scr >221
	Day 14–45	8 mg/kg/day p.o.
	Day 45+	6 mg/kg/day p.o.

Example F

Drug	Day	Dose
AZA	Day 0	3 mg/kg
	Day 1–5	2.5 mg/kg/day
Pred	Day 0–2	1 mg/kg/day
	Day 3–5	0.75 mg/kg/day
	Day 6–11	0.6 mg/kg/day
	Day 12–17	0.5 mg/kg/day
	Day 18–28	0.4 mg/kg/day
	Week 5+	0.3 mg/kg/day, taper dose to 0.15 mg/kg/day
CSA	Day 1+	8 mg/kg/day

(continued)

Table 92.5. (Continued)

Liver Transplant Protocols

Example G

Drug	Day	Dose
MePred	Day 1	1 mg/kg IV
CSA	Day 1+	3 mg/kg/day as a continuous infusion Start p.o. once bowel function returns; adjust dose to maintain trough whole blood HPLC levels 200–300 ng/ml Usual dose 5–15 mg/kg/day
Pred	Day 1+	2 mg/kg/day IV; start p.o. once bowel function returns Taper dose to 0.1 mg/kg/day by 3 to 6 months posttransplant
AZA	Day 1+	1.5 mg/kg/day IV; start once bowel function returns, adjust dose to maintain WBC >3

Example H

Drug	Day	Dose
HC	Day 0	1 g intraop
AZA	Day 0	2 mg/kg/day IV
	Day 1–7	2 mg/kg/day IV or p.o.
	Day 8+	Taper off over 1–2 days
MePred	Day 0	50 mg
	Day 1–5	50 mg q6h × 1 day, 40 mg Q6h × 1 day, then continue to taper
	Day 2–5	by 40 mg/day until DC
CSA	Day 0	10 mg/kg p.o. or 2 mg/kg IV
	Day 1+	1–2 mg/kg q8–12h (DC IV when T-tube clamped). Adjust dose to maintain whole blood RIA levels 250–400 ng/ml for 1.5 months, then 200 ng/ml for 1.5–2 months, then 200 ng/ml
Predlon	Day 6–59	10 mg q12h
	Day 60+	15 mg q.d. × 4 months, then 12.5 mg q.d. × 6 months, then 10 mg q.d.

Example I

Drug	Day	Dose
MePred	Day 0+	1.5 mg/kg/day tapered by 10 mg/day to 0.25 mg/kg/day
CSA	Day 0–10	4 mg/kg IV divided b.i.d.
	Day 11–90	12 mg/kg p.o. beginning when T-tubed is clamped
	Month 4+	Reduce daily dose by 50 mg now and again in 6 months if no rejection; adjust dose to maintain 12-hr serum trough TDX levels at 200–300 ng/ml
Pred	Day 5+	Switch to p.o. dose equivalent to IV MePred dose; reduce dose by 5 mg each year to a minimum of 7.5 mg/day; consider q.o.d. dosing for severe side effects

Pancreas Transplant Protocols

Example J

Drug	Day	Dose
ALG/ATG	Day 1	0.5 g IV
	Day 2–4	0.7–1.2 g IV
	Day 5+	1.5 g IV (dose adjusted to WBC and platelet count)
MePred	Day 0–2	1 g/day IV
CSA	Day 0–3	4 mg/kg IV over 24 h
	Day 4+	4 mg/kg/day p.o. in doses
Predlon	Day 1–3	1 mg/kg/day
	Day 4–5	0.8 mg/kg/day
	Day 6	0.6 mg/kg/day
	Day 7+	0.5 mg/kg/day
AZA	Day 1	2–5 mg/kg/day
	Day 2+	1–2.5 mg/kg/day

Example K

Drug	Day	Dose
OKT3 or MALG	Day 0–14	5 mg/kg/day
	Day 0–14	20 mg/kg/day
CSA	Day 0	14 mg/kg preop
	Day 0–5	3 mg/kg/day IV postop
	Day 6+	8 mg/kg/day p.o., adjust dose to maintain whole blood HPLC levels of 200 ng/ml
AZA	Day 0–2	5 mg/kg preop and 5 mg/kg/day postop
	Day 3–5	4 mg/kg/day
	Day 6–8	3 mg/kg/day
	Day 9+	2.5 mg/kg/day
Pred	Day 0	1 mg/kg preop and postop
	Day 1–2	2 mg/kg/day
	Day 3–17	1.75 mg/kg/day, taper dose by 0.25 mg/kg every 2 days to a dose of 0.75 mg/kg/day
	Day 18+	0.6 mg/kg/day, taper dose by 0.05 mg/kg to achieve a dose of 0.3 mg/kg/day by 1 year

Example L

Drug	Day	Dose
MePred	Day 0	3 mg/kg
	Day 1	2 mg/kg
	Day 2	1 mg/kg
AZA	Day 0	5 mg/kg preop
	Day 1+	2 mg/kg/day IV or p.o.
	Month 6+	1–1.5 mg/kg/day; adjust dose downward to maintain WBC >4
CSA	Month 1–6	Boost dosage to obtain induction whole blood HPLC levels of 200–250 ng/ml
	Month 7+	Adjust dose to maintain whole blood HPLC levels of 100–150 ng/ml

a Data taken from Burdine J, Fischel R, Bolman R: Cardiac transplantation. Crit Care Clin 6:927–945, 1990; Toledo-Pereyra L, Dewan S, Mittal V, et al.: Clinical pancreas transplantation: complete review of eight years experience. Ann Surg 55:576–581, 1989; Walker AM, Funch DP, Birmann BM: Transplant Protocols. Chestnut Hill, MA: Epidemiology Resources, 1990; Stock PG, Payne WD: Liver transplantation. Crit Care Clin 6:911–925, 1990; and Bolman RM, Saffitz J: Early postoperative care of the cardiac transplantation patient: routine considerations and immunosuppressive therapy. Prog Card Dis 33:137–148, 1990.

b Abbreviations: MALG, Minnesota antilymphocyte globulin; MePred, methylprednisolone; CSA, cyclosporine; Pred, prednisone; AZA, azathioprine; Predlon, prednisolone; OKT3, muromonab CD3; HC, hydrocortisone; ALG/ATG, antilymphocyte/antithymocyte globulin.

Table 92.6.
Summary of Immunosuppressive Agents

Agent	Primary Mechanism of Action	Usual Dose	Adverse Effects	Comments
Corticosteroids	Blocks synthesis or response to IL-2, IL-1, prostaglandins and γ-interferon; reduces T cell proliferative reponse to specific antigens	Initial prednisone: 0.5–2 mg/kg/day p.o. Maintenance prednisone: 0.1–0.2 mg/kg/day p.o.	Suppression of adrenal function, hypertension, fluid retention, hyperglycemia, psychosis, delayed wound healing, osteoporosis, cataracts	Administer with food or milk to minimize GI side effects
Azathioprine	Antimetabolite, acts during proliferative cycle of effector T or B lymphocytes to block DNA and RNA synthesis in response to antigenic stimulation	Initial: 1–4 mg/kg/day p.o. or IV at the time of surgery Maintenance: 1–3 mg/kg/day	Leukopenia, megaloblastic anemia, nausea, vomiting, anorexia, diarrhea, drug fever, rash, alopecia; incidences of hepatotoxicity and pancreatitis also reported	Tablets may be administered with or after meals to minimize GI side effects; protect IV solutions from light; the IV dose is usually the same as the oral dose
Cyclosporine	Inhibits T helper cell activity by decreasing IL-2 production, interacts with cytosolic protein cyclophylin	Initial: 0.5–5 mg/kg/day IV or 10–15 mg/kg/day p.o. Maintenance: 2–5 mg/kg/day p.o., adjust dose based on measured trough levels and adverse reactions	Nephrotoxity, hypertension, nausea, vomiting, hyperkalemia, hypomagnesemia, hepatotoxicity, tremors, parathesias, hirsutism, gingival hyperplasia	IV dose is approximately ⅓ of oral dose; administer IV dose as slow infusion (over 2–24 hr); glass containers should be used for administration of both IV and oral solutions; oral solution has 12.5% and IV solution has 32.9% alcohol; do not refrigerate cyclosporine
Cyclophosphamide	Suppresses DNA synthesis, inhibits early activation and proliferation of B and T cells	1–2 mg/kg/day	Leukopenia, thrombocytopenia, nausea, vomiting, alopecia, hemorrhagic cystitis	Ample fluid intake and frequent voiding help to prevent the development of hemorrhagic cystitis
Antilymphocyte globulin (ALG)	Depletion of circulating T and B lymphocytes	10–20 mg/kg IV for 5–21 days	Fever, chills, leukopenia, thrombocytopenia, hematuria, nausea, vomiting, rash, arthralgia, myalgia, hypotension; anaphylaxis and serum sickness also reported	Administer as slow IV infusion (approx. 8 hr) through a central line using a 5.0-micron filter; avoid D_5W as diluent; may cause protein aggregation
Muromonab CD3	Immediately decreases circulating T cells; interferes with antigen recognition by binding to CD3 cell surface	5 mg/day for 5–14 days	Fever, chills, tremor, headache, diarrhea, cramping, nausea, vomiting, hypotension, pulmonary edema	Administer undiluted over approx. 1 min; the solution should first be filtered through a 0.22-micron filter; do not mix with other solutions; use with extreme caution in patients with a recent history of fluid overload

antilymphocyte globulin (ALG) or monoclonal antibodies (e.g., muromonab CD3). Many clinicians prefer dosing steroids on a weight basis because of the large variability in patient size.

Adverse effects associated with corticosteroid use include fluid retention, growth retardation, delayed wound healing, hyperglycemia, and mental status changes. Long-term steroid use can lead to abnormalities such as osteoporosis and adrenal insufficiency (41). In addition, transplant patients requiring long-term steroid therapy are at increased risk for infection. To minimize steroid toxicity, alternative-day regimens are sometimes used for stable transplant patients. The full spectrum of steroid side effects is discussed in Chapter 15, "Adrenocortical Dysfunction and Clinical Use of Steroids."

Azathioprine

Azathioprine is a cytotoxic derivative of 6-mercaptopurine (6-MP). It was first synthesized in the early 1950s and was intended to be a slow-release prodrug of 6-MP (48) but it was found to have a superior therapeutic index for immunosuppression. First used for organ transplantation in 1962 (49), it has become a mainstay of immunosuppressive therapy. Azathioprine becomes active after it is metabolized to 6-MP and further converted to active 6-thioguanine nucleotides (50). These metabolites act by inhibiting early immune responses during the proliferative cycle of effector T or B lymphocytes (51). Intracellularly, they are incorporated into DNA, where they inhibit purine nucleotide synthesis and metabolism, and later, the synthesis and function of RNA (52, 53). Although azathioprine is

Table 92.7.
Pharmacokinetic Parameters for Immunosuppressive Agents

Drug	Cl (ml/min/kg)	Vd (liter/kg)	$T_{1/2}$ (hr)	F (%)	Protein Binding (%)	Elimination Route	Ref
Prednisolone/ Prednisone	1.6–2.8[a]	0.3–0.7	2.2	85–99	70–95[a]	Hepatic metabolism; concentration-dependent kinetics; renal excretion of metabolites 7–15% excreted unchanged in urine	(44–47)
Azathioprine	0.81[b]	0.8	0.2 (6MP: 0.5–1)	60	Unknown	Primarily metabolized to active 6-mercaptopurine (6MP)	(54, 55)
Cyclosporine	4–13	3.5	6–13	<0.5–89 (ave. 28%)	>96	Extensively metabolized to active and inactive metabolites	(75, 92, 93)
Cyclophosphamide	1–1.5	0.6	4–15	75	12–14	Hepatic metabolism to active and inactive metabolites; 5–10% excreted unchanged in the urine	(190–193)

[a] Concentration dependent.
[b] Based on weight of 70 kg.

useful in preventing the onset of acute rejection, it has little or no value in the treatment of ongoing rejection.

Azathioprine is readily absorbed from the gastrointestinal tract after oral administration and is rapidly removed from the blood. The pharmacokinetic parameters for azathioprine are summarized in Table 92.7 (54, 55). Azathioprine and 6-MP are rapidly metabolized in vivo with the ultimate end product being 6-thiouric acid (6-TU). Renal dysfunction does not impair the overall elimination of azathioprine or 6-MP (51). Although it is known that the elimination of 6-TU is delayed in the presence of renal dysfunction, the clinical importance of this remains unclear.

The principle toxic effects of azathioprine are related to bone marrow suppression. Leukopenia is the most common manifestation although other hematologic disorders such as thrombocytopenia and megaloblastic anemia may occur. These hematologic effects appear to be dose-related and may be worse in renal transplant patients experiencing rejection (56–58). Careful monitoring of CBC and dosage adjustment based on WBC are necessary. Other adverse effects include pruritis, dermatitis, fever, myopathy, alopecia, and pancreatitis. Gastrointestinal disturbances such as nausea, vomiting, and diarrhea may also occur, but they are most frequent in patients who are receiving large doses of azathioprine and may be avoided by giving the drug in divided doses or with meals. Drug-induced hepatitis has been reported as a late complication of azathioprine therapy. It is manifested as a low-grade jaundice with an increase in serum transaminases and bilirubin levels (56, 59, 60). This toxicity is usually reversible upon discontinuation of the drug.

The potential drug interaction of allopurinol and azathioprine is clinically very important. By inhibiting xanthine oxidase, allopurinol prevents the metabolic formation of 6-TU and therefore markedly prolongs the durations of action of azathioprine and 6-MP. Concomitant use of allopurinol without a reduction in azathioprine dose can therefore exacerbate the adverse effects of azathioprine (61). Doses of azathioprine should be reduced by 25 to 50% to prevent this complication.

Azathioprine is used in conjunction with other immunosuppressive agents for the prevention of solid organ rejection. It is usually administered on a continuous basis, since withholding the drug in the early posttransplant period has led to transplant rejection (62). Azathioprine is commonly given in standard doses of 1 to 4 mg/kg at the time of surgery and then orally in doses of 1 to 3 mg/kg posttransplantation. Doses are adjusted based on the white blood cell count. A white blood cell count of 3.0 to 5.0 10^9/liter (3000/mm^3) has been used as a parameter for decreasing the azathioprine dose. When dose reductions are necessary, improvement in neutropenia usually occurs after 3 to 5 days. Other causes of neutropenia should also be considered (e.g., cytomegalovirus infection). Some clinicians use lower doses in renal disease because of the increased bone marrow suppression in patients with renal impairment. This may be due to accumulation of potentially toxic metabolites (63–65).

Oral azathioprine is available in 50-mg tablets and may be administered as a single dose or in divided doses. In its parenteral form it is available in 100-mg vials. Intravenous infusions are administered over 30 to 60 min.

Cyclosporine

Cyclosporine (CSA) is a lipophilic 11-amino-acid cyclic peptide that is the major metabolite of the fungus, *Tolypocladium inflatum* (66). It was discovered in 1972 from a soil sample containing the fungus and was shown to have immunosuppressive properties in 1976 (67). Clinical studies using cyclosporine in bone marrow and renal transplantation began in 1978. Since that time, the success rate for all forms of transplantation has increased dramatically. The 1-year cadaver renal allograft survival rate increased from 53 to 80% following the introduction of cyclosporine, resulting from a decreased frequency and severity of rejection episodes. The 1-year graft survival rate for liver transplants has increased from 60 to 80%. While most immunosuppressive agents have bone marrow suppressive properties, cyclosporine does not. Instead it induces a selective, nonmyelotoxic immunosuppression, and because of this it has revolutionized immunosuppression for organ and tissue transplantation.

MECHANISM OF ACTION

Cyclosporine causes immunosuppression by preventing early steps in the autoimmune response that normally follow antigen recognition. It causes the T cells to remain in the resting phase of the cell cycle. Thus disabled, the T cells cannot transform and release lymphokines that normally would induce and mount an immune response (68–70). The effect of cyclosporine on T cell function is believed to involve two primary mechanisms. First, it interacts with a cytosolic protein (cyclophillin) that blocks T cell signal transduction processes and therefore T cell activity. Secondly, it reduces the production of a number of important regulatory proteins of the immune system. Cyclosporine inhibits the macrophage production of IL-1, a lymphokine necessary for T cell activation (8). It reduces the production and release of IL-2 from T helper cells by decreasing mRNA synthesis (71), and this impairs the continuous activation and proliferation of T helper and T cytotoxic cells. Additional effects of cyclosporine may include deactivation of antibody production from B cells through the inhibition of B cell growth factor; the reduction of cidal activity due to the inhibition of γ-interferon, a macrophage activating factor that causes enhanced cidal activity; and the suppression of granulocyte colony-stimulating factor production in the bone marrow (8). Cyclosporine spares suppressor T cells and appears to prevent rather than suppress the rejection process (72, 73). This plus the fact that it is also thought to lack activity against mature cytotoxic T cells makes it essentially ineffective in the treatment of rejection (74).

PHARMACOKINETICS

After oral administration, cyclosporine absorption is slow and incomplete. Peak concentrations may occur at various times, with one study reporting the time to peak (tp) range from 1 to 8 hr postdose (mean, 3.8 hr) (75). The reported bioavailability also varies widely from <5% to 89% (mean, 28%). Duration of therapy can be a factor, with the bioavailability increasing three- to fivefold over a 3-month period from the time of transplantation (76). The reason

Table 92.8.
Factors Altering Cyclosporine Kinetics[a]

Factor	Total Body Clearance	Gastrointestinal Absorption	Ref
Diarrhea	↔	↓	(83–85)
Bile deficit	↔	↓	(86)
Food intake	↔/↑	↑	(77, 79)
Liver failure	↓	↓	(87, 88, 91)
Cigarette smoking	↑	↔	(89)
Age			
Pediatric	↑	↔	(88, 90)
Old age	↓	↔	(91)

[a] Symbols: ↑, increase; ↓, decrease; ↔, no change.

for this is unknown. A number of factors can affect cyclosporine absorption (Table 92.8). Diet may be a factor, with one study reporting enhanced absorption of cyclosporine administered with high-fat meals (77). Cyclosporine solution is commonly mixed in beverages such as milk, chocolate milk, and orange juice before administration, and these liquids do not seem to reduce its bioavailability (75). Cyclosporine is a lipophilic drug that requires bile for its absorption. Therefore, factors causing bile deficits (e.g., biliary diversions or cholestasis in liver transplant patients) will decrease cyclosporine absorption (71, 78). Absorption may also be reduced in patients with liver disease, postoperative ileus, gastroparesis, and diarrhea (73, 75, 79).

Cyclosporine distributes widely in the body, with an average volume of distribution of 3.5 liter/kg. The liver accounts for most of the body stores of cyclosporine, but it can also be found in fat, blood, kidney, heart, lung, and pancreas (80). In blood, 58% of cyclosporine is bound to erythrocytes (81, 82). The drug in plasma is approximately 80% bound to plasma lipoproteins. Since the lipoprotein profile may be significantly altered in patients with hepatic and renal dysfunction, a change in cyclosporine binding capacity may occur.

Cyclosporine undergoes extensive metabolism via the hepatic cytochrome P-450 system to at least 21 metabolites. Less than 1% of cyclosporine is excreted unchanged in the urine. The clearance of cyclosporine in patients with normal renal and hepatic function ranges from 4 to 13 ml/min/kg. This clearance rate is similar in stable renal and liver transplant recipients (75). In patients with cirrhosis, cyclosporine clearance decreases to an average of 2.8 ml/min/kg. Since higher cyclosporine concentrations have been measured in these patients, dosing adjustments may be necessary. In patients with impaired renal function, the clearance of cyclosporine remains within the range observed in normal patients (6.2 ml/min/kg), so no dosing adjustments are necessary (80). Factors that may affect cyclosporine clearance are summarized in Table 92.8 (79,

83–91). The mean elimination half-life of cyclosporine ranges from 6 to 13 hr in patients with normal renal and hepatic function. The pharmacokinetics of cyclosporine are summarized in Table 92.7 (75, 92, 93).

The clinical importance of the metabolites of cyclosporine remains controversial (94, 95). Some reports have suggested that up to six identified metabolites possess some immunosuppressive activity (78, 96–100). Metabolites 1, 17, 18, and 21 are usually found in detectable concentrations in the blood of cyclosporine patients (using high-pressure liquid chromatography). The reported activity of metabolite 17 ranges between 8 and 20%, compared with cyclosporine (99, 101, 102). Other metabolites have been associated with neurotoxicity and nephrotoxicity (103). Biliary excretion accounts for 10 to 40% of the elimination of cyclosporine metabolites. Enterohepatic recirculation of these metabolites may explain a biphasic immunosuppressive response observed following cyclosporine administration (104, 105).

DRUG-LEVEL MONITORING

The monitoring of cyclosporine concentrations is an important part of the postoperative management of transplantation because the cyclosporine level does not correlate well with the administered dose (80). This is due to the large degree of inter- and intraindividual variability in cyclosporine pharmacokinetics (107). In addition, many significant drug-drug and drug-disease interactions make a priori dose predictions hazardous and unreliable. Cyclosporine drug-level monitoring helps guide the dosage adjustments necessary to maintain therapeutic concentrations and helps minimize toxicity. Compliance can also be monitored in this way.

Currently clinicians are faced with a choice of measuring cyclosporine concentrations in plasma or whole blood using three different assay procedures: high-pressure liquid chromatography (HPLC), radioimmunoassay (RIA), and fluorescence-polarization immunoassay (FPIA). HPLC is a specific method that can measure cyclosporine and/or its metabolites separately (108–110). Because of the specificity of HPLC, many believe that this method can better monitor cyclosporine immunosuppressive activity. Traditional HPLC methods require large sample volumes, technical expertise, expensive equipment, and 6 to 24 hr to analyze samples. However, new rapid techniques may overcome these disadvantages. HPLC is the preferred method of analysis for pharmacologic and clinical research in cyclosporine metabolism and pharmacokinetic determinations.

Two types of RIA procedures for measuring cyclosporine are available: RIA polyclonal antibody procedure and a newer RIA monoclonal antibody procedure (80, 111). The polyclonal assay procedure is nonspecific, cross-reacting with cyclosporine metabolites and measuring concentrations 2 to 4 times higher than those measured by HPLC. The new monoclonal antibody–based assay is specific for the parent cyclosporine compound and yields results similar to those measured by HPLC (112). RIA has a low operational cost, a quick turn-around time (compared with HPLC), and is readily available in most clinical laboratories. Some prefer the nonspecific RIA method because they believe that cyclosporine metabolites contribute significantly to the activity and toxicity of cyclosporine.

Another assay method based on the FPIA has recently been developed (113–115). Like RIA, FPIA has low specificity for cyclosporine, and in fact, FPIA cross-reacts with a larger number of cyclosporine metabolites than RIA. Concentrations obtained with FPIA are approximately 25% higher than those measured with RIA (116). FPIA is simpler and safer (no radioactivity as with RIA); it has a relatively quick turnaround time, and a large sample load may be analyzed. This procedure may offer a viable alternative to the RIA procedure in the clinical monitoring of cyclosporine.

The relative distribution of cyclosporine between red blood cells and plasma depends on the temperature, the hematocrit, and the lipoprotein composition of the plasma (81, 82, 117, 118). At temperatures below 37°C, cyclosporine distributes more readily out of the red blood cells and into the plasma. Therefore, when measuring cyclosporine in plasma, it is essential that samples be maintained at 37°C both prior to and during centrifugation to assure that cyclosporine distribution is equivalent to that occurring in vivo. Currently, whole blood is used most frequently for cyclosporine measurement (80).

Cyclosporine has a narrow therapeutic index, and unfortunately the therapeutic range for cyclosporine has been difficult to establish. The widespread use of various analytical procedures and different biological fluids has contributed to the relative lack of correlation between cyclosporine concentrations and clinical response. The dose-response relationship is further confounded by the changing pharmacokinetics of cyclosporine with time, the variability in patients' development of tolerance, and the additive or synergistic effects of immunosuppressive combinations. Since cyclosporine is used in recipients of different organ transplants and to prevent different pathologic disorders (graft rejection vs. graft versus host disease), the minimum concentration to prevent rejection may be different, even if the same assay technique is used (119). Although there is no agreement about the optimal trough levels of cyclosporine in transplant recipients, trough concentrations in the range of 150 to 400 ng/ml using RIA (monoclonal) in whole blood, and 100 to 300 ng/ml using HPLC in whole blood are generally considered to be the therapeutic range (120, 121). Concentrations at the high end of the therapeutic range are usually required during immunosuppression induction, whereas

Table 92.9.
Cyclosporine Trough Concentration Ranges for Various Assay Methods[a]

Assay Method	Specific for Parent CSA	Reported Concentrations Ranges[b] (ng/ml)	
		Whole Blood	Serum/plasma
RIA, specific monoclonal	Yes	150–400	50–125
RIA, polyclonal	No	200–600	50–300
FPIA	No	100–600	150–300
HPLC	Yes	100–300	

[a] Data taken from references 120, 122–125.
[b] Specific target concentrations depend upon the organ transplanted, the time from transplantation, and the transplant center. Specific ranges used by individual transplant centers are generally narrower.

lower concentrations are adequate during maintenance therapy (122). Table 92.9 summarizes target cyclosporine concentrations for various assay methods (120, 122–125). Although the occurrence of side effects is not clearly related to trough concentrations, cyclosporine concentrations above 700 ng/ml (RIA) have been associated with toxicity.

DRUG INTERACTIONS

Drug interactions with cyclosporine have been reviewed extensively (88, 126–128). Although many of these reports are anecdotal, some cases have been substantiated by clinical experience and controlled studies. Drugs that interact with cyclosporine generally interfere with the metabolism of cyclosporine by affecting the cytochrome P-450 enzyme system. Cyclosporine metabolism is increased and its concentration lowered by drugs such as phenytoin, phenobarbital, valproic acid, carbamazepine, and rifampin, which induce the cytochrome P-450 enzyme system. On the other hand, drugs that inhibit the cytochrome P-450 enzyme system or compete for metabolism cause cyclosporine concentrations to increase. Drugs such as ketoconazole, erythromycin, verapamil, and diltiazem have been reported to inhibit metabolism. Alterations in intestinal absorption of cyclosporine may also account for changes in concentrations. Tables 92.10 and 92.11 summarize substantiated cyclosporine drug interactions (129–176).

Besides pharmacokinetic interactions, other drugs may potentiate the nephrotoxicity of cyclosporine. Some drugs that may have this effect include aminoglycosides, amphotericin B, trimethoprim-sulfamethoxazole, cephalosporins, and indomethacin (163, 165, 177–180). Concomitant use of these drugs with cyclosporine requires careful monitoring of renal function. If renal toxicity occurs, renal function usually returns to baseline upon discontinuation of these agents (75).

TOXICITY PROFILE

Cyclosporine is associated with numerous side effects, the most common and clinically important of which is nephrotoxicity. It has been shown to occur in 50 to 70% of renal transplant patients, and approximately the same incidence has occurred following heart and liver transplantation (181–183). Acute reversible nephrotoxicity is often related to high cyclosporine trough concentrations. The effects of cyclosporine nephrotoxicity are dose- and patient-dependent and involve a reduction in glomerular filtration rate. The clinical presentation is a rise in serum creatinine level or a decrease in creatinine clearance time, often with oligouria, hyperkalemia, and decreased renal blood flow. In kidney transplant patients it is often difficult to differentiate cyclosporine-induced nephrotoxicity from allograft rejection. Cyclosporine nephrotoxicity is suspected when patients have concentrations above 300 ng/ml (whole blood, RIA) and a gradual increase in serum creatinine level.

Hepatotoxicity, another serious adverse effect of cyclosporine, occurs in 4 to 7% of allograft recipients. It is characterized by a rise in serum bilirubin (>34 μmol/liter (>2 mg/100 ml)), increased serum transaminases (AST and ALT), alkaline phosphatase, and total bilirubin levels (184–187). In liver transplant patients, the changes in liver enzymes make it difficult to rule out toxicity or rejection. These effects appear to be dose-dependent and reversible with dosage reduction.

Other side effects attributable to cyclosporine are hypertension, gingival hyperplasia, hirsutism, hypomagnesemia, and a variety of neurologic syndromes such as tremor, paresthesias, confusion, and seizures (71).

DOSING

Cyclosporine is administered following organ transplantation according to protocols that differ between institutions. Doses vary widely and range from 6 to 30 mg/kg. The dose varies with the organ transplanted and the use of concomitant immunosuppressive therapy. Initial doses of 10 to 15 mg/kg are commonly used and are subsequently titrated downward based on drug levels, immunologic parameters, and indices of graft function. The maintenance dose is usually 5 to 10 mg/kg/day. Some centers have successfully tapered the dose as low as 3 mg/kg/day in selected renal transplant patients.

Cyclosporine is available as an oral solution of 100 mg/ml in an olive oil and alcohol base, 25-mg and 100-mg gelatin capsules, and a parenteral solution of 250 mg/5 ml vial for dilution.

Cyclosporine doses should be administered on a consistent schedule with respect to time of day and meals. To make cyclosporine oral solution more palatable, it may be diluted with milk, chocolate milk, or orange juice, preferably at room temperature. If necessary, cyclosporine oral

Table 92.10.
Drug Interactions With Cyclosporine (CSA)[a]

Drug	Proposed Mechanism	Ref
Drugs increasing CSA concentrations		
Diltiazem	Inhibition of CSA metabolism	(138, 146–149)
Erythromycin	Inhibition of CSA metabolism and biliary excretion, increased CSA absorption	(138–145)
Ketoconazole	Inhibition of CSA metabolism	(129–138)
Metoclopromide	Increased CSA absorption	(150)
Methyltestosterone	Inhibition of CSA metabolism	(151)
Nicardipine	Inhibition of CSA metabolism	(152–154)
Oral contraceptives/danazol	Inhibition of CSA metabolism	(138, 155–159)
Verapamil	Inhibition of CSA metabolism	(160–162)
Drugs decreasing CSA concentrations		
Carbamazepine	Induction of CSA metabolism	(163–165)
Isoniazid	Induction of CSA metabolism	(166, 167)
Nafcillin	Induction of CSA metabolism	(168)
Octreotide	Alters intestinal absorption of CSA	(169, 170)
Phenobarbital	Induction of CSA metabolism	(171)
Phenytoin	Induction of CSA metabolism, reduced CSA absorption	(171–174)
Rifampin	Induction of CSA metabolism	(166, 167, 175, 176)

[a] Substantial interactions based on three or more patient case reports.

Table 92.11.
Miscellaneous Cyclosporine Interactions

Drug	Effect	Ref
Disulfiram, metronidazole, moxalactam	Possible disulfiram-like reaction due to alcohol content of cyclosporine solution	(242, 243)
Lovastatin	Increased incidence of myopathy	(244–246)
Methylprednisolone (high-dose)	Convulsions	(247, 248)
Minoxidil	Additive hirsuitism	(24)
Nifedipine	Increased gingival hyperplasia	(249)
Potassium-sparing diuretics, potassium supplements	Possible hyperkalemia	(243, 250)
Verapamil	Enhanced immunosuppression	(162)

solution may be put directly into a nasogastric (NG) tube via the measuring pipette and then flushed with water.

Parenteral cyclosporine solutions should be prepared by diluting 1 ml of drug in 20 to 100 ml 0.9% NaCl or D_5W and be given by slow IV infusion over 2 to 24 hours. Intravenous cyclosporine is administered when the patient is unable to tolerate p.o. or NG administration. IV doses are administered at approximately one-third the oral dose.

Cyclophosphamide

Cyclophosphamide is an alkylating agent most commonly used as a cancer chemotherapeutic agent. It has been used as an immunosuppressive agent in renal transplant recipients when azathioprine had to be withdrawn because of heptatotoxicity (188). However, since cyclophosphamide has no therapeutic advantage over azathioprine and its overall toxicity profile is more severe, its use in transplantation has been limited. Cyclophosphamide must be converted in the liver to activated alkylating metabolites. The immunosuppressive activity of these metabolites is due to cross-linking of DNA strands with subsequent reductions in the metabolic and proliferative capacities of both B and T lymphocytes (189). The pharmacokinetic parameters for cyclophosphamide are summarized in Table 92.7 (190–193).

Cyclophosphamide can cause profound leukopenia, thrombocytopenia, and severe gastrointestinal abnormalities. Nausea and vomiting are common, and alopecia occurs frequently. Hemorrhagic cystitis due to renally eliminated active metabolites of cyclophosphamide may occur. Cyclophosphamide has been associated with a high potential for inducing sterility, especially for 3 to 6 months after drug administration. Rare side effects such as cardiomyopathy associated with high-dose use, hepatotoxicity, and interstitial pneumonitis may also occur (194).

The dose of cyclophosphamide used in renal transplantation ranges from 0.25 to 2 mg/kg. The drug is primarily metabolized, but some cytotoxic metabolites may accumulate in renal failure. It is therefore recommended that the dose be empirically decreased in renal failure (Clcr <10 ml/min). Dosing adjustments should be based on clinical response and signs of toxicity. Since hepatic disease can cause a reduction in the conversion of cyclophosphamide to its active metabolites, the dose should be titrated in these patients. Hematologic monitoring similar to that used with azathioprine is necessary, with a decreased platelet count being an important indication of toxicity.

Cyclophosphamide is available in both intravenous and oral forms. Oral cyclophosphamide is available in 50-mg and 25-mg tablets.

ANTILYMPHOCYTE GLOBULIN

The experimental use of heterologous antilymphocyte preparations began over 25 years ago. Lymphocyte globulin was first used in clinical transplantation in 1966. Since then various antilymphocyte preparations have been used extensively in clinical transplantation. Antilymphocyte preparations are produced by injecting human lymphoid cells into a laboratory animal (horse, rabbit, or goat) that produces antibodies to the foreign antigen. The animal serum is then separated and purified to yield antilymphocyte globulin (ALG) or antithymocyte globulin (ATG). On occasion, the unseparated serum is used directly as antilymphocyte serum (ALS). A variety of antilymphocyte globulin preparations are available. ATGAM, an equine ATG, is commercially available, but the supply of this preparation has been erratic. For this reason Minnesota ALG (MALG) is preferred by many centers.

ALG administration causes a profound decrease in the number of circulating T cells, and a decrease in their proliferative function results. The mechanism of action of ALG is not precisely known. It most likely involves a complex formation of ALG with circulating T and B cells, opsonization, phagocytosis, and removal by the reticluloendothelial system (RES).

Adverse effects of ALG include fever and chills, which are most often associated with the first dose of the drug. These are frequently managed by administration of acetaminophen, diphenhydramine, and steroids prior to ALG administration. Other reported adverse effects include thrombocytopenia, hematuria, nausea, vomiting, diarrhea, myalgia, arthralgia, rash, and pruritis. Anaphylaxis is rare, but when it occurs immediate discontinuation is required with general supportive care. In general, acute side effects are less frequent and severe than those accompanying administration of muromonab CD3 (OKT3), a monoclonal antibody with similar indications. Prolonged use of ALG can produce profound immunosuppression and should be avoided; it is associated with an increase in opportunistic infections such as herpes simplex virus and cytomegalovirus (195, 196). Since ALG exerts its effect primarily by decreasing circulating T cells, the daily monitoring of T cells could be used as a guide in determining the appropriate dose. Although not widely accepted, suppression of the T cell fraction to less than 10% of circulating lymphocytes has been used as an indicator of a satisfactory response (188).

Antilymphocyte globulin has been used for both induction and antirejection therapy. In induction, ALG has been used prior to cyclosporine as temporary maintenance therapy to minimize cyclosporine-induced nephrotoxicity and postoperative tubular necrosis (196). Because of the high costs associated with ALG use, some clinicians use cyclosporine immediately for induction and reserve ALG for the treatment of steroid-resistant rejection (48).

ALG is administered by slow infusion over 4 to 6 hr via a central vein. Injection of ALG through a peripheral vein is contraindicated by a severe risk of thrombophlebitis and thrombosis. For immunosuppressive induction and the treatment of allograft rejection, the recommended dose of ALG ranges from 10 to 20 mg/kg daily. Duration of therapy may range from 5 to 21 days, depending on the indication and clinical response of the patient, but usually is 7 days.

Muromonab CD3 (OKT3)

The agent muromonab CD3 (OKT3) is a murine-derivative monoclonal antibody that has been shown to be effective in the treatment of allograft rejection. OKT3 does not affect the nonspecific host defense system. OKT3 is an IgG_{2a} antibody specifically directed against the T3 (CD3) complex on the surface of mature T lymphocytes. In the body, OKT3 may act in three different ways (188, 197). Initially, OKT3 coats the circulating T lymphocytes, causing an immediate decrease in their number due to opsonization. Destruction by phagocytes follows, and subsequent removal by the reticuloendothelial system (RES) occurs in the liver and spleen. Then OKT3 is thought to modulate the T lymphocyte antigen receptor–CD3 complex of circulating lymphocytes, which results in the production of T lymphocytes that are immunologically nonfunctional without further depletion of the T lymphocyte population. OKT3 also inhibits T lymphocyte antigen recognition by simply blocking the receptor itself.

OKT3 has been shown to be highly effective in the treatment of acute rejection, including steroid-resistant acute rejection. Most studies have been conducted in patients undergoing kidney transplantation, but promising results have also been demonstrated in liver and heart transplantation (197, 198). In clinical practice the overall reversal rate is 81% in kidney transplants, about 70% in liver transplants (199, 200), 90% in heart transplants (201, 202), and 62.5% in pancreas transplants. Although OKT3 has been generally limited to treatment of acute rejection, a growing number of transplant centers are using it in induction therapy in renal transplant recipients with oliguria from acute tubular necrosis (196).

The recommended dose of OKT3 is 5 mg intravenous daily for 5 to 14 days. In patients weighing less than 30 kg, the dose may be decreased to 2.5 mg. The initial side effects of OKT3 are similar to those of ALG. They include high fever, shaking chills, headache, rigors, and hypotension. Acetaminophen and diphenhydramine are often given prior to the daily dose of OKT3 to lessen the fever and chills. In patients with fluid overload, a pulmonary edema–type response may occur. For this reason, OKT3 administration is not advised for patients whose body weight has increased more than 3% during the week before therapy. Other side effects associated with OKT3 include tremor, seizure, nausea, vomiting, diarrhea, thrombocytopenia, and leukopenia. In rare cases, OKT3 causes aseptic meningitis that is manifested by fever, severe headache, and seizures. Patients frequently develop reactive anti-OKT3 antibodies that, over time, may lead to tachyphylaxis and neutralization of the murine antibody OKT3. This may result in an allergic response when this agent is used more than once (197). Anti-OKT3 antibody titers $\geq$ 1:1000 may render the drug ineffective for subsequent administrations (203).

OKT3 is available as 5 mg/5 ml vials. The vials should be refrigerated until ready for use.

Investigational Immunosuppressive Agents

FK 506

FK 506 is a recently discovered immunosuppressive agent obtained from cultures of a new strain of bacteria, *Streptomyces tsukubaensis* (204, 205). It is a macrolide that is approximately 100 times more potent than cyclosporine as an immunosuppressive agent. Although it has a totally different molecular structure, its immunosuppressive properties are similar to those of cyclosporine, and it too induces a selective nonmyelotoxic immunosuppression. Unlike cyclosporine which was discovered by accident, the discovery of FK 506 is the result of an aggressive search for naturally occurring immunosuppressive and chemotherapeutic agents (206, 207).

Based on in vitro and in vivo studies, FK 506 (like cyclosporine) inhibits the production of IL-2 and other lymphokines in T lymphocytes. Like the effects of cyclosporine, inhibition of the expression of IL-2 receptors and interaction with a distinct cytosolic protein may play a role in the immunosuppressive effects of FK 506 (208, 209). A limited number of clinical studies have shown FK-506 to be effective for preventing allograft rejection. Studies using the drug as salvage therapy for liver transplant recipients who experienced rejection with conventional immunosuppression have shown a 1-year survival rate of 90%; kidney transplant recipients with complex and difficult clinical histories had a reported 1-year graft survival rate of 80% (210, 211). Though the optimum dose for FK 506 has not been established, a dose of 0.075 mg/kg IV every 12 hr is commonly used (infused over 4 hr), followed by oral doses of 0.15 mg/kg every 12 hr. Some centers use lower doses. Oral doses are adjusted according to whole blood or plasma measurements and clinical response.

Following oral dosing, the time to reach peak concentrations for FK 506 varies from 1 to 4 hr, with the oral bioavailability averaging 27%. The drug distributes extensively into tissues (average Vd of 20 liter/kg), and the half-life averages 9 hr (212). FK 506 is extensively metabolized, with less than 1% eliminated in the urine unchanged. The concentration of FK 506 in plasma is also temperature-dependent, requiring separation of the plasma at 37°C for accurate measurement (212).

Early animal studies demonstrated synergism between FK 506 and other immunosuppressive agents (208). However, combined administration of FK 506 with cyclosporine, as well as FK 506 administration to patients with nephrotoxicity due to prior cyclosporine usage has led to deterioration in renal function (213, 214). The adverse reactions of FK 506 were worse following intravenous administration than with oral administration (211, 215). Commonly reported side effects are nausea, vomiting, headaches, insomnia, tremors in the upper extremities, and hyperthesias of the feet (210, 211, 213). FK 506 causes a pattern of nephrotoxicity that appears to be similar to that reported for cyclosporine (214). Hyperkalemia has been reported in 35% of the patients following treatment (210, 213). Hair loss has also been reported. In patients receiving cyclosporine and FK 506 concomitantly, the half-life of cyclosporine increased from 6 to 15 hr to 26 to 74 hr (212).

RS-61443

RS-61443 is the first immunosuppressive agent that is believed to suppress both cellular- and antibody-mediated responses of the immune system (216). It is a semisynthetic derivative of the active component, mycophenolic acid (MPA), which has been chemically altered to improve its oral absorption (217). MPA has been shown to have antifungal, antibacterial, antiviral, and immunosuppressive properties, and has been used for the treatment of psoriasis on a compassionate basis for the last decade (216, 218, 219).

MPA is a well-characterized inhibitor of de novo purine synthesis. Following oral administration, RS-61443 is rapidly hydrolyzed to liberate MPA, which selectively inhibits two enzymes (inosine monophosphate dehydrogenase and guanosine monophosphate synthetase) important for the synthesis of guanosine monophosphate. Since T and B cells cannot use the salvage biosynthesis pathway, they must depend on the de novo pathway for purine synthesis. Deprived of it, their proliferative responses to antigens and mitogens do not take place (220, 221).

Clinical studies are underway to evaluate the use of this compound in solid organ transplantation in humans. Studies in animals have reported prolonged allograft survival when RS-61443 is used alone or in combination with other immunosuppressive agents (216, 220–222).

Following oral administration, RS-61443 is readily absorbed from the stomach, reaching peak plasma levels 1 hr after dosing, followed by a rapid decline in levels over 10 to 12 hr (222). The active MPA is metabolized in the liver to the inactive MPA-glucuronide (MPAG). Studies in mice reveal extremely high levels of MPAG in the bile, suggesting that bile is an important pathway for elimination (216).

Ongoing clinical trials are underway to determine optimal RS-61443 dosages. At average doses of 20 mg/kg/day, renal, liver or bone marrow toxicity has not been observed (216). Adverse reactions reported in patients receiving large doses of MPA (approximately 3000 mg/day) for psoriasis are primarily gastrointestinal (nausea, abdominal cramps, diarrhea, vomiting) and general malaise (218, 223).

RAPAMYCIN

Rapamycin is a lipophilic macrolide with both antifungal and antitumor properties (224). Rapamycin has shown potent immunosuppressive activity in animal models of transplantation. It is currently undergoing human clinical trials.

Rapamycin is a structural analog of FK 506, but it suppresses T and B cell function differently by inhibiting the proliferation of T lymphocytes (225). Rapamycin is a stronger inhibitor of T cell proliferation than cyclosporine, and unlike cyclosporine is cell-cycle independent. Combined rapamycin and cyclosporine work synergistically to inhibit T lymphocyte proliferation. Unfortunately, rapamycin acts antagonistically with FK 506 by competing for an important cellular binding site (226).

POSTTRANSPLANT MANAGEMENT

Hypertension

Hypertension is a common cardiovascular complication posttransplantation. While hypertension may be present in some patients prior to transplantation, the reported incidence of arterial hypertension posttransplantation is 42 to 100% in renal transplant recipients, 60 to 90% in heart transplant recipients, and 31 to 64% in liver transplant recipients (22, 24, 254). The causes are multifactorial and may be related to an underlying disease state, volume expansion due to steroid therapy, late or chronic rejection, or immunosuppressive therapy (prednisone or cyclosporine). Hypomagnesemia and the dose of cyclosporine may contribute to the severity of hypertension (228). Lowering the dose of cyclosporine may decrease the severity, but the occurrence is not always prevented.

As with the management of nontransplant patients with chronic hypertension, dietary sodium restriction and weight control are important for proper management of hypertension following transplantation. If needed, antihypertensive drug therapy should follow the step-care approach used in patients with essential hypertension. Antihypertensive drugs used in the treatment of posttransplant hypertension include loop diuretics (furosemide), β-blockers (propranolol, metoprolol, atenolol), calcium-channel blockers (nifedipine, verapamil, diltiazem), or angiotensin-converting-enzyme inhibitors (captopril, enalopril). Since many antihypertensive agents can alter cyclosporine pharmacokinetics, alterations of this therapy require close monitoring of cyclosporine blood levels.

Infection

Infection is another common posttransplantation complication. Most of the infections that occur early in the posttransplant period are bacterial. Heart transplant recipients frequently develop infection due to Gram-positive bacteria. Sternal wound infections in this population can be particularly difficult to treat. Urinary tract infections occur commonly in renal allograft patients, with E. coli being the most common pathogen. Liver transplant recipients may develop more serious infections including pneumonia and abdominal abcess caused by Gram-negative, anaerobic, or staphylococcal bacteria. As the postoperative course continues, viral (cytomegalovirus and herpes), fungal (Candida, Aspergillus), and protozoal (PCP) infections become more prevalent (22, 24, 229).

The incidence of mild CMV infection after solid organ transplantation is approximately 50 to 75%, whereas the incidence of serious CMV infection is approximately 10 to 30%. High-dose steroids and use of ALG to treat rejection have been associated with a higher incidence and severity of CMV infections. Though data are limited, one study reports that prophylactic oral acyclovir (800 mg QID) helps minimize the incidence of CMV infection (230).

Parasitic infections are usually Pneumonocystis carinii pneumonia (PCP) and toxoplasmosis. Prophylaxis with oral trimethoprim-sulfamethoxazole (TMP-SMZ) has resulted in a significant decrease in the incidence of PCP after solid organ transplantation (231, 232). The most frequently used regimen is oral TMP-SMZ twice daily three times per week. In renal transplant recipients, TMP-SMZ is also used to prevent urinary tract infections and possible pyelonephritis, since most renal transplant ureters reflux urine.

Two common fungal infections, caused by Candida and Aspergillus, occur in approximately 20% of transplant recipients. Candida infections are most frequent and range from mild, mucocutaneous infections to disseminated disease. Oral antifungal prophylaxis with nystatin or clotrimazole may reduce the incidence of fungal infections. Use of ketoconazole or fluconazole for antifungal prophylaxis or treatment of infection requires diligent cyclosporine drug level monitoring, since significant increases in cyclosporine concentrations can occur (Table 92.10).

The American Heart Association has guidelines and recommendations for antibiotic prophylaxis of patients undergoing various surgical procedures likely to produce bacteremia. Many transplant centers advocate following similar guidelines for their transplant patients perioperatively.

Patient Education

Patient compliance with the immunosuppressive drug regimen is one of the key factors in long-term graft survival (233–238). The incidence of noncompliance with medications and follow-up care in transplant recipients has been reported to be 15–18% (233, 234). The consequences of noncompliance have been severe. Reportedly, 28% of graft loss beyond 2 years has been due to noncompliance (21), and 91% of noncompliant kidney transplant patients either lost the graft or died (233).

Posttransplant patients are often managed with 6 to 12 medications per day, which may involve as many as 28 individual doses daily (239). Patients must become skilled at self-medicating a potentially complicated medication regimen, as well as trained to recognize the signs and symptoms of adverse drug effects, toxicity, and organ rejection. Patients ultimately need to become conscientious, self-reliant, and responsible for their regimens without the aid of family or friends. Self-medication teaching should be nonthreatening and easy to follow. Given the diversity of patient lifestyles, cultures, learning rates, and concerns, the teaching should be tailored to suit each patient's unique circumstance.

Patients should be given detailed information about each medication they are receiving. This information should include which medications should not be taken together, what to do if doses are forgotten or missed, and when to contact their physician. Patients should be advised not to take any medications, including common over-the-counter medications, without first consulting with their primary healthcare provider.

SUMMARY

The prevention of allograft rejection depends on a precise therapeutic regimen whose close therapeutic monitoring is essential. Due to the toxicities associated with this regimen's immunosuppressive agents, the monitoring of such parameters as drug concentrations (e.g., cyclosporine), platelet counts, and white blood cell counts is used to minimize complications. In addition, the potential drug interactions of these compounds must be considered when managing other medical problems in these patients.

Solid organ transplantation is now a common therapeutic modality for patients with end-stage organ failure, and the use of new immunosuppressive agents has resulted in excellent success rates for many transplant procedures.

The literature is full of reports on the benefits of transplantation to the quality of life for these patients, and much has been written to point out that the cost justifies the means (255–260). However, drugs that affect only the immunologic components of rejection are still needed, and as such compounds become available, greater improvement in graft and patient survival will result.

REFERENCES

1. Pifarre R, Sullivan H, Montoya A, et al.: Cardiac transplantation. Cardiol Clin 7:183–194, 1989.
2. Flye M, History of transplantation. In Flye M: Principles of Organ Transplantation. Philadelphia, WB Saunders, 1989, pp 1–17.
3. Monaco A: Development of clinical immunosuppression for organ transplantation. Jpn J Surg 18:119–130, 1988.
4. Kirkpatrick CH: Transplantation immunology. JAMA 258:2993–3000, 1987.
5. Chapel H, Haeney M: Essentials of Clinical Immunology, ed. 2. Palo Alto: Blackwell Scientific Publications, 1988, pp 12–15.
6. Tami JA, Parr MD, Thompson JS: The immune system. Am J Hosp Pharm 43:2483–2493, 1986.
7. Morris P, Fuggle S, Ting A, et al.: HLA and organ transplantation. Br Med J 43:184–202, 1987.
8. Thomson A, Sewell H, Rejection, the immune response, and the influence of cyclosporin A. In Catto G: Clinical transplantation: Current Practice and Future Prospects. Norwell, MA, MTP Press, 1987, pp 134–154.
9. Solinger A: Organ transplantation and the immune response. Med Clin North Am 69:565–583, 1985.
10. Rao K: Mechanism, pathophysiology, diagnosis, and management of renal transplant rejection. Med Clin North Am 74:1039–1057, 1990.
11. Snover DC, Liver transplantation. In Sale GE: The Pathology of Organ Transplantation. Stoneham, Butterworths, 1990.
12. Demetris A: The pathology of liver transplantation. Prog Liver Dis 9:687–709, 1990.
13. Sibley R, Payne W: Morphologic findings in the renal allograft biopsy. Semin Nephrol 5:294, 1985.
14. Gordon R, Iwatsuki S, Esquive C, et al.: Liver transplantation across ABO blood groups. Surgery 100:342–348, 1986.
15. Foegh M: Chronic rejection-graft arteriosclerosis. Transplant Proc 22:119–122, 1990.
16. Brunt E, Pathology of transplanted organs. In Flye M: Principles of Organ Transplantation. Philadelphia, WB Saunders, 1989, pp 105–134.
17. Cabrol C, Gandjbakhch I, Pavie A, et al.: Current problems in cardiac transplantation. Biomed Pharmacother 43:87–92, 1989.
18. Hayry P, Renkonen R, Leszcynski D, et al.: Local events in graft rejection. Transplant Proc 21:3716–3720, 1989.
19. Schroeder J, Hunt S: Cardiac transplantation: Where are we? N Engl J Med 315:961–962, 1986.
20. Billingham ME, Cardiac transplantation. In Sale GE: The Pathology of Organ Transplantation. Stoneham, Butterworths, 1990.
21. Dunn J, Golden D, Van Buren C, et al.: Causes of graft loss beyond two years in cyclosporine era. Transplantation 49:349–353, 1990.
22. Burdine J, Fischel R, Bolman R: Cardiac transplantation. Crit Care Clin 6:927–945, 1990.
23. Sanfilippo F, Renal transplantation. In Sale GE: The Pathology of Organ Transplantation. Stoneham, Butterworths, 1990.
24. Shaw B, Stratta R, Donovan J, et al.: Postoperative care after liver transplantation. Semin Liver Dis 9:202–230, 1989.
25. Cook D, Sasaki T: Current status of pancreas transplantation. West J Med 150:309–313, 1989.

26. Toledo-Pereyra L, Dewan S, Mittal V, et al.: Clinical pancreas transplantation: complete review of eight years experience. Am Surg 55:576–581, 1989.

27. Sibley RK, Pancreas transplantation. In Sale GE: The Pathology of Organ Transplantation. Stoneham, Butterworths, 1990.

28. Barnhart G, Lower R, Cardiac transplantation. In Cerilli G: Organ Transplantation and Replacement. St. Louis, JB Lippincott, 1988, pp 493–510.

29. McGregor C, Cardiac and cardiopulmonary transplantation. In Catto G: Clinical transplantation: Current Practice and Future Prospects. Norwell, MTP Press, 1987, pp 211–231.

30. Macdonald SN, Naucke NA, Heart transplantation. In Smith SL: Tissue and Organ Transplantation: Implications for Professional Nursing Practice. St. Louis, Mosby-Yearbook, 1990, pp 210–244.

31. Engeset J, Youngson G, Surgical aspects of renal transplantation. In Catto G: Clinical Transplantation: Current Practice and Future Prospects. Norwell, MTP Press, 1987, pp 31–55.

32. Lee H. Technical aspects of renal transplantation. In Cerilli G: Organ Transplantation and Replacement. St. Louis, JB Lippincott, 1988, pp 337–348.

33. Perryman JP, Stillerman PU. Kidney transplantation. In Smith SL: Tissue and Organ Transplantation: Implications for Professional Nursing Practice. St. Louis, Mosby-Yearbook, 1990, pp 176–209.

34. Starzl T, Demetris A, Van Thiel D: Liver transplantation (part 1). N Engl J Med 321:1014–1022, 1989.

35. Roberts J, Forsmark C, Lake J, et al.: Liver transplantation today. Annu Rev Med 40:287–303, 1989.

36. Munoz S, Friedman L: Liver transplantation. Med Clin North Am 73:1011–1039, 1989.

37. Smith SL, Ciferni M, Liver transplantation. In Smith SL: Tissue and Organ Transplantation: Implications for Professional Nursing Practice. St. Louis, Mosby-Yearbook, 1990, pp 273–300.

38. Sutherland D, Goetz F, Najarian J: Current status of transplantation of the pancreas. Adv Surg 20:303–340, 1987.

39. Wills B, Post L, Pancreas transplantation. In Smith SL: Tissue and Organ Transplantation: Implications for Professional Nursing Practice. St. Louis, Mosby-Yearbook, 1990, pp 301–311.

40. Goodwin J, Durgaprasadarao A, Sierakowski S, et al.: Mechanism of action of glucocorticosteroids. J Clin Invest 77:1244–1250, 1986.

41. Haynes RJ, Adrenocorticotropic hormone; adrenocortical steroids and their synthetic analogs; inhibitors of the synthesis and actions of adrenocortical hormones. In Goodman Gillman A, Rall T, Nies A, Taylor P: Goodman and Gillman's The Pharmacological Basis of Therapeutics, ed. 8. New York, Pergamon Press, 1990, pp 1431–1462.

42. Cupps T, Fauci A: Corticosteroid-mediated immunoregulation in man. Immunol Rev 65:113–155, 1982.

43. Dupont E, Wybran J, Toussaint C: Corticosteroids and organ transplantation. Transplantation 37:331–335, 1984.

44. Gambertoglio J, Frey F, Holford N, et al.: Prednisone and prednisolone bioavailability in renal transplant patients. Kidney Int 21:621–626, 1982.

45. Uribe M, Summerskill W, Go V: Comparative serum prednisone and prednisolone concentrations following administration to patients with chronic active liver disease. Clin Pharmacokinet 7:452–459, 1982.

46. Uribe M, Go V: Corticosteroid pharmacokinetics in liver disease. Clin Pharmacokinet 4:233–240, 1979.

47. Uribe M, Schalm S, Summerskill W, Go V: Oral prednisone for chronic active liver disease: dose responses and bioavailability studies. Gut 19:1131–1135, 1978.

48. Chan G, Gruber S, Skjei K, et al.: Principles of immunosuppression. Crit Care Clin 6:841–891, 1990.

49. Murray J, Merrill J, Harrison J, et al.: Prolonged survival of human kidney homografts by immunosuppressive drug therapy. N Engl J Med 268:1315–1323, 1963.

50. Ahmed A, Mory R: Azathioprine. Int J Dermatol 20:461–467, 1981.

51. Chan G, Canafax D, Johnson C: The therapeutic use of azathioprine in renal transplantation. Pharmacotherapy 7:165–177, 1987.

52. Elion G: Biochemistry and pharmacology of purine analogues. Fed Proc 26:898–904, 1967.

53. Tidd D, Paterson A: Distinction between inhibition of purine nucleotide synthesis and the delayed cytotoxic reaction of 6-mercaptopurine. Cancer Res 34:733–737, 1974.

54. Ding T, Gambertoglio J, Amend J, et al.: Azathioprine bioavailability and pharmacokinetics in kidney transplant patients. Clin Pharmacol Ther 27:250, 1980.

55. Lin S, Jessup K, Floyd M, et al.: Quantitation of plasma azathioprine and 6-MP levels in renal transplant patients. Transplantation 29:290–294, 1980.

56. Soko J, Arunas S: Liver disease in renal transplant patients. Am J Med 64:139–146, 1978.

57. Delphin E: Principles of immunosuppression. Surg Clin North Am 12:283–298, 1979.

58. Bach J, Dardenne M: The metabolism of azathioprine in renal failure. Transplant 12:253–259, 1971.

59. Berne T, Chaterjee S, Craig J, et al.: Hepatic dysfunction in recipients of renal allografts. Surg Gynecol Obstet 141:171–175, 1975.

60. Zarday Z, Veith F, Giliedman M, et al.: Irreversible liver damage after azathioprine. JAMA 222:690–691, 1972.

61. Kirkman R, Strom T, Weir M, et al.: Late mortality and morbidity in recipients of long-term renal allografts. Transplantation 34:347–352, 1982.

62. Oncevski A, Rostoker G, Buisson C: Is long-term triple-drug therapy required for maintaining kidney allograft tolerance? Effect of azathioprine withdrawal at 3 months post-transplantation. Transplant Proc 21:1625–1626, 1989.

63. Lennard L, Brown C, Fox M, et al.: Azathioprine metabolism in kidney transplant recipients. Br J Clin Pharm 18:693–700, 1984.

64. Winlkelstein A: The effects of azathioprine and 6MP on immunity. J Immunopharmacol 1:429–454, 1979.

65. Gamelli R, Foster R: Increased azathioprine toxicity after ureteral ligation and nephrectomy. Surg Forum 29:358–359, 1978.

66. Borel J, Kis Z: The discovery and develoment of cyclosporine (Sandimmune). Transplant Proc 23:1867–1874, 1991.

67. Borel J: Comparative study of in vitro and in vivo drug effects on cell mediated cytotoxicity. Immunology 31:631–641, 1976.

68. Borel J: Pharmacology of cyclosporine (Sandimmune): Pharmacological properties in vivo. Pharmacol Rev 41:259–371, 1989.

69. Hess A, Turschka P, Santos G: Effect of cyclosporin A on human lymphocyte response in vitro. J Immunol 128:355–359, 1982.

70. Larsson E: Cyclosporin A and dexamethasone suppress T cell response by selectively acting at distinct sites of the triggering process. J Immunol 124:2828–2833, 1980.

71. Kahan B: Cyclosporine. N Engl J Med 321:1725–1738, 1989.

72. Cohen D, Loertscher R, Rubin M, et al.: Cyclosporine: A new immunosuppressive agent for organ transplantation. Ann Intern Med 101:667–682, 1984.

73. Tilney N, Strom T, Chemical manipulation of the immune responses. In Cerilli G: Organ Transplantation and Replacement. Philadelphia, JB Lippincott, 1988, pp 118–136.

74. Lillehoj H, Malek T, Shevach E: Differential effect of cyclosporin A on the expression of T and B lymphocytes activation antigens. J Immunol 133:244–250, 1984.

75. Ptachcinski R, Venkataramanan R, Burckart G: Clinical pharmacokinetics of cyclosporine. Clin Pharmacokinet 11:107–132, 1986.

76. Kahan B, Reid M, Newburger J: Pharmacokinetics of cyclosporine in human renal transplantation. Transplant Proc 15:446–453, 1983.

77. Gupta S, Benet L: High fat meals increase the clearance of cyclosporine. Pharmaceut Res 7:46–48, 1990.

78. Frey F: Pharmacokinetic determinants of cyclosporine and prednisone in renal transplant patients (clinical conference). Kidney Int 39:1034–1050, 1991.

79. Ptachcinski R, Venkataramanan R, Rosenthal J, et al.: The effect of food on cyclosporine absorption. Transplant 40:174–176, 1985.

80. National Academy of Clinical Biochemistry/American Association for Clinical Chemistry: Critical issues in cyclosporine monitoring: Report of the task force on cyclosporine monitoring. Clin Chem 33:1269–1288, 1987.

81. Niederberger W, Lemaire M, Maurer G, et al.: Distribution and binding of cyclosporine in blood and tissues. Transplant Proc 15(suppl 1):2419–2421, 1983.

82. LeMaire M, Tillement J: Role of lipoproteins and erythrocytes in the in vitro binding and distribution of cyclosporin A in the blood. J Pharmacol 34:715–718, 1982.

83. Roberts R, Sketris I, Abraham I, et al.: Cyclosporine absorption in two patients with short-bowel syndrome. Drug Intell Clin Pharm 22:570–572, 1988.

84. Atkinson K, Britton K, Palul P, et al.: Detrimental effect of intestinal disease on absorption of orally administered cyclosporine. Transplant Proc 15(suppl 1):2446–2449, 1983.

85. Atkinson K, Biggs J, Britton K, et al.: Oral administration of cyclosporin A for recipients of allogenic marrow transplants: implications of clinical gut dysfunction. Br J Haematol 56:223–231, 1984.

86. Mehta M, Venkataramanan R, Burckart G, et al.: Effect of bile on cyclosporine absorption in liver transplant patients. Br J Clin Pharmacol 25:579–584, 1988.

87. Venkataramanan R, Starzl T, Ptachcinski R, et al.: Cyclosporine kinetics in liver disease. Clin Pharmacol Ther 37:234–239, 1985.

88. Venkataramanan R, Habucky K, Burckart G: Clinical pharmacokinetics in organ transplantation. Clin Pharmacokinet 16:134–161, 1989.

89. Lake K: Cyclosporine drug interactions: a review. Cardiac Surg 2:617–630, 1988.

90. Yee G, Lennon T, Gmar D, et al.: Effect of age on cyclosporine kinetics in marrow transplant recipients. Transplant Proc 19:1704–1705, 1987.

91. Kahan B, Kramer B, Wideman C, et al.: Demographic factors affecting the pharmacokinetics of cyclosporine estimated by radioimmunoassay. Transplant 41:459–463, 1986.

92. Burckart G, et al.: Cyclosporine absorption following orthotopic liver transplantation. J Clin Pharmacol 26:647–651, 1986.

93. Venkataramanan R, et al.: Cyclosporine bioavailability in liver disease. Drug Intell Clin Pharm 19(abs):451, 1985.

94. Wallemacq P, Lhoest G, Latinne D, et al.: Isolation, characterization and in vitro activity of cyclosporine A metabolites. Transplant Proc 21:906–910, 1989.

95. Combalbert J, Fabre J, Fabre G, et al.: Metabolism of cyclosporine A. IV. Purification and identification of the rifampin-inducible human liver cytochrome P450 enzyme (cyclosporine A oxidase) as a product of P450IIIA gene subfamily. Drug Metab Dispos 17:197–207, 1989.

96. Freed B, Rosano T, Quick C, et al.: In vitro immunosuppressive properties of cyclosporine metabolites. Transplantation 43:123–127, 1987.

97. Hartmann N, Trimble L, Vederas J, et al.: An acid metabolite of cyclosporine. Biochem Biophys Res Comm 133:964–971, 1985.

98. Rosano T, Freed B, Cerilli J, et al.: Immunosuppressive metabolites of cyclosporine in the blood of renal allograft recipients. Transplantation 42:262–267, 1986.

99. Ryffel B, Hiestrand P, Foxwell B, et al.: Nephrotoxic and immunosuppressive potentials of cyclosporine metabolites in rats. Transplant Proc 18:41–45, 1986.

100. Schlitt H, Christians U, Wonigeit K, et al.: Immunosuppressive activity of cyclosporine metabolites in vitro. Transplant Proc 19:4248–4251, 1987.

101. Schlitt H, Christians U, Bleck J, et al.: Contribution of cyclosporine metabolites to immunosuppression in liver transplanted patients with severe graft dysfunction. Transplant Int 4:38–44, 1991.

102. Fahr A, Hiestand P, Ryffel B: Studies on the biologic activities of Sandimmun metabolites in humans and in animal models: review and original experiments. Transplant Proc 3:1116–1124, 1990.

103. Sewing K-F, Christians, U, Kohlhaw K, et al.: Biologic activity of cyclosporine metabolites. Transplant Proc 22:1129–1134, 1990.

104. Rodighiero V: Therapeutic drug monitoring of cyclosporine. Practical applications and limitations. Clin Pharmacokinet 16:23–37, 1989.

105. Wood A, Maurer G, Neiderberger W, et al.: Cyclosporine: pharmacokinetics, metabolism, and drug interactions. Transplant Proc 15:2409–2412, 1983.

106. Venkataramanan R, Ptachcinski R, Burckart G, et al.: The clearance of cyclosporine by hemodialysis. J Clin Pharmacol 24:528–531, 1984.

107. LeMaire M, Fahr A, Maurer G: Pharmacokinetics of cyclosporine: inter- and intra-individual variations and metabolic pathways. Transplant Proc 22:1110–1112, 1990.

108. Sawchuk R, Cartier L: Liquid chromatographic determination of cyclosporine A in blood and plasma. Clin Chem 27:1368–1371, 1981.

109. Speck R, Frey F, Frey B: Cyclosporine kinetics in renal transplant patients as assessed by high-performance liquid chromotography and radioimmunoassay using monoclonal and polyclonal antibodies. Transplant 47:802–806, 1989.

110. Gupta S, Benet L: HPLC measurement of cyclosporine in blood, plasma, and urine and simultaneous measurement of its four metabolites in blood. J Liq Chromatog 1989:1451–1462, 1989.

111. Donatsch P, Abisch E, Homberger M, et al.: A radioimmunoassay to measure cyclosporine A in plasma and serum samples. J Immunoassay 2:19–32, 1981.

112. Schran H, Rossano T, Hassell A, et al.: Determination of cyclosporine concentrations with monoclonal antibodies. Clin Chem 33:2225–2229, 1987.

113. Hooks M, Millikan W, Henderson J, et al.: Comparison of whole-blood cyclosporine levels measured by radioimmunoassay and fluorescence polarization in patients post orthotopic liver transplant. Ther Drug Monit 11:304–309, 1989.

114. Vandenbroucke AC: Evaluation of the TDx method for cyclosporine and a comparison of CYCLO-Trac RIA in renal transplant patients. Clin Biochem 21:307–309, 1988.

115. Sanghvi A, Warren D, Seltman H, et al.: Abbott's fluorescence polarization immunoassay for cyclosporine and metabolites compared with the Sandoz "Sandimmune" RIA. Clin Chem 34:1904–1906, 1988.

116. Schroeder T, Pesce A, Hasan F, et al.: Comparison of Abbott TDx fluorescence polarization immunoassay, Sandoz radioimmunoassay, and high-performance liquid chromatography methods for the assay of serum cyclosporine. Transplant Proc 20(suppl):345–347, 1988.

117. Lensmeyer GL, Wiebe DA, Carlson IH: Distribution of cyclosporine A metabolites among plasma and cells in whole blood: effect of temperature, hematocrit, and metabolite concentration. Clin Chem 35:56–63, 1989.

118. Wenk M, Follath F: Temperature dependency of apparent cyclosporine A concentrations in plasma. Clin Chem 29:1965, 1983.

119. Burckart G, Canafax D, Yee G: Cyclosporine monitoring. Drug Intell Clin Pharm 20:649–652, 1986.

120. Keown P: Therapeutic monitoring of cyclosporine by Sandoz's RIA, Cyclotrac and TDx methods. Transplant Immun lett 5:8–9, 1988.

121. Ptachcinski R, Burckart G, Venkataramanan R: Cyclosporine. Drug Intell Clin Pharm 19:90–100, 1985.

122. Keown P: Optimizing cyclosporine therapy: dose, levels, and monitoring. Transplant Proc 20(2)(suppl 2):382–389, 1988.

123. Kahan B, Grevel J: Optimization of cyclosporine therapy in renal transplantation by a pharmacokinetic strategy. Transplantation 46:631–644, 1988.

124. Faynor S, Moyer T, Sterioff S: Laboratory medicine: therapeutic drug monitoring of cyclosporine. Mayo Clin Proc 59:571–572, 1984.

125. Burkle W: Cyclosporine pharmacokinetics and blood level monitoring. Drug Intell Clin Pharm 19:101–105, 1985.

126. Wadhwa N, Schroeder T, Pesce A, et al.: Cyclosporine drug interactions: a review. Ther Drug Monit 9:399–406, 1987.

127. Yee G, McGuire T: Pharmacokinetics drug interactions with cyclosporin (Part II). Clin Pharmacokinet 19:400–415, 1990.

128. Yee G, McGuire T: Pharmacokinetic drug interactions with cyclosporin (Part I). Clin Pharmacokinet 19:319–332, 1990.

129. Lokiec F, Poirier O, Gluckman E, et al.: Pharmacokinetic study of cyclosporine A. In Touraine J, Gluckman E, Griscelli C (eds): Bone Marrow Transplantation in Europe II. Amsterdam, Excerpta Medica, 1981, pp 160–164.

130. Ferguson R, Sutherland D, Simmons R, et al.: Ketoconazole, cyclosporine metabolism and renal transplantation. Lancet ii:882–883, 1982.

131. Dieperink H, Moller J: Ketoconazole and cyclosporine. Lancet ii:1217, 1982.

132. Morgenstern G, Powles R, Robinson B, et al.: Cyclosporine interaction with ketoconazole and melphalan. Lancet ii:1342, 1982.

133. Daneshmend T: Ketoconazole-cyclosporine interaction. Lancet i:1342–1343, 1982.

134. White D, Blatchford N, Canwenbergh G: Cyclosporine and ketoconazole. Transplantation 37:214–215, 1984.

135. Gumbleton M, Brown J, Hawksworth G, et al.: The possible relationship between hepatic drug metabolism and ketoconazole enhancement of cyclosporine nephrotoxicity. Transplantation 40:454–455, 1985.

136. Anderson J, Blaschke T: Ketoconazole inhibits cyclosporine metabolism in vivo in mice. J Pharmacol Exp Ther 236:671–674, 1986.

137. Dieperink H, Kemp E, Leyssac P, et al.: Ketoconazole and cyclosporine A: combined effects on rat renal function and on serum and tissue cyclosporine A concentration. Clin Nephrol 25(suppl 1):S137–S143, 1986.

138. Henricsson S, Lindholm A: Inhibition of cyclosporine metabolism by other drugs in vitro. Transplant Proc 20:569–571, 1988.

139. Whiting P, Simpson J, Thomson A: Nephrotoxicity of cyclosporine in combination with aminoglycoside and cephalosporin antibiotics. Transplant Proc 15(2)(suppl 1):702–705, 1983.

140. Ptachcinski R, Carpenter B, Burckart G, et al.: Effect of erythromycin on cyclosporine levels. N Engl J Med 313:1416–1417, 1985.

141. Kohan D: Possible interaction between cyclosporine and erythromycin. N Engl J Med 314:448, 1986.

142. Gonwa T, Ngheim D, Schulak J, et al.: Erythromycin and cyclosporine. Transplantation 41:797–799, 1986.

143. Martell R, Heinrichs D, Stiller C, et al.: The effect of erythromycin in patients treated with cyclosporine. Ann Intern Med 104:660–661, 1986.

144. Gupta S, Bakran A, Johnson W, et al.: Erythromycin enhances the absorption of cyclosporine. Br J Clin Pharm 25:401–402, 1988.

145. Wadhwa N, Schroeder T, O'Flaherty E, et al.: Interaction between erythromycin and cyclosporine in a kidney and pancreas allograft recipient. Ther Drug Monit 9:123–125, 1987.

146. Pochet J, Pirson Y: Cyclosporine-diltiazem interaction. Lancet ii:979, 1986.

147. Grino J, Sebate I, Castelao A, et al.: Influence of diltiazem on cyclosporine clearance. Lancet i:1387, 1986.

148. Neumayer H, Wagner K: Dilitiazem and economic use of cyclosporine. Lancet ii:523, 1986.

149. Wagner K, Henkel M, Heinemeyer G, et al.: Interaction of calcium blockers and cyclosporine. Transplant Proc 20:561–568, 1988.

150. Wadhwa N, Schroeder T, O'Flaherty E, et al.: The effect of oral metoclopramide on the absorption of cyclosporine. Transplantation 43:211, 1987.

151. Moller B, Ekelund B: Toxicity of cyclosporine during treatment with androgens. N Engl J Med 312:1416, 1985.

152. Cantarovick M, Hiesse C, Lockiec F, et al.: Confirmation of the interaction between cyclosporine and the calcium channel blocker nicardipine in renal transplant patients. Clin Nephrol 28:190–1103, 1987.

153. Bourbigot B, Guiserix J, Aixiau J, et al.: Nicardipine increases cyclosporine blood levels. Lancet i:1447, 1986.

154. Kessler M, Netter P, Renoult E, et al.: Influence of nicardipine on renal function and plasma cyclosporine in renal transplant patients. Clin Pharmacol 36:637–638, 1989.

155. Deray G, LeHoang P, Cacoub P, et al.: Oral contraceptive interaction with cyclosporine. Lancet i:158–159, 1987.

156. Koneru B, Hartner C, Iwatsuki S, et al.: Effect of danazol on cyclosporine pharmacokinetics. Transplantation 45:1001, 1988.

157. Ross W, Roberts D, Griffin P, et al.: Cyclosporine interaction with danazol and norethisterone. Lancet ii:330, 1986.

158. Schroder O, Schmitz N, Kayser W, et al.: Increased cyclosporine levels with simultaneous danazol treatment. Dtsch Med Wochenschr 111:602–603, 1986.

159. Maurer G: Metabolism of cyclosporine, Transplant Proc 17(suppl 1):19–26, 1985.

160. Lindholm A, Henricsson S: Verapamil inhibits cyclosporine metabolism. Lancet i:1262–1263, 1987.

161. McMillen M, Tesi R, Baumgarten W, et al.: Potentiation of cyclosporine by verapamil in vitro. Transplantation 40:444–445, 1985.

162. Tesi R, Hong J, Butt K, et al.: In vivo potentiations of cyclosporine immunosuppression by calcium antagonists. Xth Inter Cong Transplant 27:2, 1986.

163. Termeer A, Hoitsma A, Koene R: Severe nephrotoxicity caused by the combined used of gentamicin and cyclosporine in renal allograft recipients. Transplantation 42:220–221, 1986.

164. Lele P, Peterson P, Yang S, et al.: Cyclosporine and tegretol—another drug interaction. Kidney Int 27:344, 1985.

165. Gluckman E, Devergie A, Lokiec F, et al.: Role of immunosuppressive drugs for prevention of graft-v-host disease after HLA matched bone marrow transplantation. Transplant Proc 19(suppl 7):61–65, 1987.

166. Langhoff E, Madsen S: Rapid metabolism of cyclosporine and prednisone in kidney transplant patients on tuberculostatic treatment. Lancet ii:1031, 1983.

167. Coward R, Raftery A, Brown C: Cyclosporine and antituberculous therapy. Lancet i:1342–1343, 1985.

168. Veremis S, Maddox M, Pollak R, et al.: Subtherapeutic cyclosporine concentrations during nafcillin therapy. Transplantation 43:913–915, 1987.

169. Rosenberg L, Dafoe D, Schwartz R, et al.: Administration of somatostatin analog (SMS 201-995) in the treatment of a fistula occurring after pancreas transplant: interference with cyclosporine immunosuppression. Transplant 43:764–766, 1987.

170. Landgraf R, Landgraf-Leurs M, Nusser J, et al.: Effect of somatostatin analog (SM5201-995) on cyclosporine levels. Transplantation 44:724–725, 1987.

171. Carstensen H, Jacobsen N, Dreperink H: Interaction between cyclosporine A and phenobarbital. Br J Clin Pharm 21:550, 1986.

172. Keown P, Stiller C: Control of rejection of transplanted organs. Adv Intern Med 31:17–46, 1986.

173. Freeman D, Laupacis A, Keown P, et al.: Evaluation of cyclosporine-phenytoin interaction with observation on cyclosporine metabolites. Br J Clin Pharm 18:887, 1984.

174. Rowland M, Gupta S: Cyclosporine-phenytoin interaction: reevaluation using metabolite data. Br J Clin Pharm 24:329–334, 1987.

175. Allen R, Hunnisett A, Morris P: Cyclosporine and rifampicin in renal transplantation. Lancet i:980, 1985.

176. Cassidy M, Van Zyl-Smit R, Pascoe M, et al.: Effect of rifampicin on cyclosporine A. Blood levels in a renal transplant recipient. Nephron 41:207–208, 1985.

177. Hows J, Palmer S, Want S, et al.: Serum levels of cyclosporine A and nephrotoxicity in bone marrow transplant patients. Lancet ii:145–146, 1981.

178. Tutschka PJ, Beschorner W, Hess A, et al.: Cyclosporine-A to prevent graft-versus-host disease. A pilot study in 22 patients receiving allogenic marrow transplants. Blood 61:318–325, 1983.

179. Kennedy M, Deeg H, Siegal M, et al.: Acute renal toxicity with combined use of amphotericin B and cyclosporine after marrow transplantation. Transplantation 35:211–215, 1983.

180. Gluckman E, Devergie A, Poirier O, et al.: Use of cyclosporine as prophylaxis of graft-vs-host disease after human allogenic bone marrow transplantation: report of 38 patients. Transplant Proc 15(suppl 1):2628–2633, 1983.

181. Klintmalm G, Iwatsuki S, Starzl T: Nephrotoxicity of cyclosporine A in liver and kidney transplant patients. Lancet 1:470–471, 1981.

182. Hamilton D, Calne R, Evans D, et al.: Effects of long-term cyclosporine A on renal function. Lancet 1:1218–1219, 1981.

183. Shulman H, Striker G, Deeg H, et al.: Nephrotoxicity of cyclosporine A after allogenic marrow transplantation. N Engl J Med 305:1392–1395, 1981.

184. Klintmalm G, Iwatsuki S, Starzl T: Cyclosporine A hepatotoxicity in 66 renal allograft recipients. Transplantation 32:488–499, 1981.

185. Rodger R, Turney J, Haines I, et al.: Cyclosporine and liver function in renal allograft patients. Transplant Proc 15(suppl 1):2754–2756, 1983.

186. Schade R, Gugliemi D, Van Theil D, et al.: Cholestasis in heart transplant recipients treated with cyclosporine. Transplant Proc 15(suppl 1):2757–2760, 1983.

187. Atkinson K, Biggs J, Dodds A, et al.: Cyclosporine-associated hepatotoxicity after allogenic marrow transplantation in man: differentiation from other causes of posttransplant liver disease. Transplant Proc 15(suppl 1):2761–2767, 1983.

188. Flye M. Immunosuppressive therapy. In Flye M: Principles of Organ Transplantation. Philadelphia, WB Saunders, 1989, pp 155–175.

189. Colvin M. The alkylating agents. In Chaner B: Pharmacologic Principles of Cancer Treatment. Philadelphia, WB Saunders, 1982, pp 276–308.

190. Bagley C, Bostick F, De Vita V: Clinical pharmacology of cyclophosphamide. Cancer Res 33:226–233, 1973.

191. Juma F, Rogers H, Trounce J: Pharmacokinetics of cyclophosphamide and alkylating activity in man after intravenous and oral administration. Br J Clin Pharmacol 8:209–217, 1979.

192. Juma F, Rogers H, Trounce J: The effect of renal insufficiency on the pharmacokinetics of cyclophosphamide and some of its metabolites. Eur J Clin Pharmacol 19:443–451, 1981.

193. Wang L, Lee C, Majeske B, Marbury T: Clearance and recovery calculations in hemodialysis: application to plasma, red blood cell and dialysate measurements for cyclophosphamide. Clin Pharmacol Ther 29:365–372, 1981.

194. Calabresi P, Chabner B, Antineoplastic agents I. Alkylating agents. In Goodman Gillman A, Rall T, Nies A, Taylor P (eds): Goodman and Gillman's The Pharmacological Basis of Therapeutics, ed. 8. New York, Pergamon Press, 1990, pp 1209–1222.

195. Monaco A: Antilymphocyte globulin: a clinical transplantation research opportunity. J Kidney Dis 2:67–78, 1982.

196. Sankary H, Williams J, Immunosuppression and liver transplantation. In Williams J: Hepatic Transplantation. Philadelphia, WB Saunders, 1990, pp 165–179.

197. Hooks MA, Wade CS, Millikan WJ: Muromonab CD-3: a review of its pharmacology, pharmacokinetics, and clinical use in transplantation. Pharmacotherapy 11:26–37, 1991.

198. Canafax D, Draxler C: Monoclonal antilymphocyte antibody (OKT3) treatment of acute renal allograft rejection. Pharmacother 7:121–124, 1987.

199. Gordon R, Tzakis A, Iwatsuki S, et al.: Experience with Orthoclone OKT-3 monoclonal antibody in liver transplantation. Am J Kidney Dis 11:141–144, 1988.

200. Starzl T, Fung J: Orthoclone OKT-3 in the treatment of allografts rejected under cyclosporine-steroid therapy. Transplant Proc 18:934–941, 1986.

201. Gilbert E, Elswirth C, Renlund D, et al.: Use of Orthoclone OKT-3 monoclonal antibodies in cardiac transplantation: early experience with rejection prophylaxis and treatment of refractory rejection. Transplant Proc 19(suppl 2):45–53, 1987.

202. Kremer A, Barnes L, Hirsch R, et al.: Orthoclone OKT-3 monoclonal antibody reversal of hepatic and cardiac rejection unresponsive to conventional immunosuppressive treatments. Transplant Proc 19(suppl 1):54–57, 1987.

203. Schroeder T, First M, Mansour M, et al.: Antimurine antibody formation following OKT3 therapy. Transplantation 49:48–51, 1990.

204. Starzl T, Fung J: Transplantation. JAMA 263:2686–2687, 1990.

205. Thomson A, Woo J: Immunosuppressive properties of FK-506 and rapamycin. Lancet ii:443–444, 1989.

206. Thomson A: FK 506-How much potential? Immunol Today 10:6–10, 1989.

207. Goto T, Kino T, Hatanaka H, et al.: Discovery of FK-506, a novel immunosuppressant isolated from *Streptomyces tsukubaensis*. Transplant Proc 19(suppl 6):4–8, 1987.

208. Morris R, Hoyt E, Murphy M, et al.: Immunopharmacology of FK 506. Transplant Proc 21:1042–1044, 1989.

209. Thomas J, Matthews C, Carroll R, et al.: The immunosuppressive action of FK 506. Transplantation 49:390–396, 1990.

210. Fung J, Todo S, Jain A, et al.: Conversion from cyclosporine to FK 506 in liver allograft recipients with cyclosporine-related complications. Transplant Proc 22(suppl 1):6–12, 1990.

211. Starzl T, Fung J, Jordan M, et al.: Kidney transplantation under FK 506. JAMA 264(1):63–67, 1990.

212. Venkataramanan R, J ain E, Cardoff V, et al.: Pharmacokinetics of FK 506: preclinical and clinical studies. Transplant Proc 22(suppl 1):52–56, 1990.

213. Fung J, Todo S, Tzakis A, et al.: Conversion of liver allograft recipients from cyclosporine to FK 506—based on immunosuppression: benefits and pitfalls. Transplant Proc 23:14–21, 1991.

214. McCauley J, Fung J, Jain A, et al.: The effects of FK 506 upon renal function after lever transplantation. Transplant Proc 22:17–20, 1990.

215. Shapiro R, Fung J, Jain A, et al.: The side effects of FK 506. Transplant Proc 22(suppl 1):35–36, 1991.

216. Platz K, Eckhoff D, Hullett D, et al.: RS-61443 studies: review and proposal. Transplant Proc 23(suppl 2):33–35, 1991.

217. Nelson P, Eugui E, Wang C, et al.: Synthesis and immunosuppressive activity of some side-chain variants of mycophenolic acid. J Med Chem 33:833–838, 1990.

218. Epinette W, Parker C, Jones E, et al.: Mycophenolic acid for psoriasis. J Am Acad Dermatol 17:962–971, 1987.

219. Goldsmith M: Researchers follow varied molecular paths toward better control of organ rejection. JAMA 263:1184, 1990.

220. Morris R, Hoyt E, Wang J: RS-61443 (RS) is a novel and specific inhibitor of T and B cell purine synthesis that induces transplant tolerance, reverses acute rejection and prolongs xenograft survival. J Heart Transplant 9:62, 1990.

221. Morris R, Hoyt E, Murphy M, et al.: Mycophenolic acid morpholinoethylester (RS-61443) is a new immunosuppressive that prevents and halts heart allograft rejection by selective inhibition of T- and B-cell purine synthesis. Transplant Proc 22:1659–1662, 1990.

222. Platz K, Sollinger H, Hullett D, et al.: RS-61443 a new, potent immunosuppressive agent. Transplant 51:27–31, 1991.

223. Lynch W, Roenigk H Jr: Mycophenolic acid for psoriasis. Arch Dermatol 113:1203–1208, 1977.

224. Calne R, Collier D, Lim S, et al.: Rapamycin for immunosuppression in organ allografting. Lancet ii:227, 1989.

225. Kimball P, Kerman R, Kahan B: Rapamycin and cyclosporine produce synergistic but nonidentical mechanisms of immunosuppression. Transplant Proc 23:1027–1028, 1991.

226. Sigal N, Siekierka J: Inhibition of human T-cell activation by FK 506, rapamycin, and cyclosporine A. Transplant Proc 23(suppl 2):1–5, 1991.

227. Howard R, Condi R, Sutherland D, et al.: The use of antilymphoblast globulin in the treatment of renal allograft rejection. Transplant Proc 13:473–474, 1981.

228. June C, Thompson C, Kennedy M, et al.: Correlation of hypomagnesemia with the onset of cyclosporine-associated hypertension in renal transplant patients. Transplantation 41:47–51, 1986.

229. Vernon W, Sollinger H: Management of combined pancreaticorenal allograft recipients. Transplant Man 1:3–4, 13–14, 1990.

230. Balfour H, Chace B, Stapleton J: A randomized, placebo-controlled trial of oral acyclovir for the prevention of cytomegalovirus disease in recipients of renal allografts. N Engl J Med 320:1381–1383, 1989.

231. Higgens R, Bloom S, Hopkins J, et al.: The risks and benefits of low-dose cotrimoxazole prophylaxis for Pneumocystis pneumonia in renal transplantation. Transplantation 47:558–560, 1989.

232. Hughes W, Rivera G, Schell M, et al.: Successful intermitten chemoprophylaxis for Pneumocystis carinii pneumonitis. N Engl J Med 316:1627–1632, 1987.

233. Schweizer R, Rovelli M, Palmieri D, et al.: Noncompliance in organ transplant recipients. Transplantation 49:374–377, 1990.

234. Christopherson L: Cardiac transplantation: a psychological perspective. Circulation 75:57–62, 1987.

235. Surman O: Psychiatric aspects of organ transplantation. Am J Psychiatry 146:8:972–982, 1989.

236. Dressler D: Psychosocial effects of cardiac transplantation. J Intensive Care Med 6:126–134, 1991.

237. White M, Ketefian S, Starr A, et al.: Stress, coping, and quality of life in adult kidney transplant recipients. ANNA Journal 17:421–430, 1990.

238. Rodriguez A, Diaz M, Colon A, et al.: Psychosocial profile of noncompliant transplant patients. Transplant Proc 23:1807–1809, 1991,

239. Salazar T: Self medication instruction utilizing a heart transplant patient medication manual. Am Soc Hosp Pharm 47:P-65D(abstract), 1990.

240. Didlake R, Dreyfus R, Kerman C, et al.: Patient noncompliance: a major cause of late graft failure in cyclosporine-treated renal transplants. Transplant Proc 20(suppl 3):63–69, 1988.

241. Starzl T, Demetris A: Liver transplantation: a 31-year perspective part II. Curr Prob Surg March:27:117–178, 1990.

242. Cockburn I: Cyclosporine A: a clinical evaluation of drug interactions. Transplant Proc 18(suppl 5):50–55, 1986.

243. Hansten P: Cyclosporine interactions. Drug Interact News 4:29–31, 1984.

244. East C, Alizvizatos P, Grundy S, et al.: Rhabdomyolysis in patients receiving lovastatin after cardiac transplantation. N Engl J Med 318:47–48, 1988.

245. Norman D, Illingworth D, Munson J, et al.: Myolysis and acute renal failure in a heart transplant recipient receiving lovastatin. N Engl J Med 318:46–47, 1988.

246. Tobert J: Rhabdomyolysis in patients receiving lovastatin after cardiac transplantation. N Engl J Med 318:47–48 Letter, 1988.

247. Durrant S, Chipping P, Palmer S, et al.: Cyclosporine A, methylprednisolone, and convulsions. Lancet ii:829–830, 1982.

248. Boogaerts M, Zachee P, Verwilghen R: Cyclosporine, methylprednisolone, and convulsions. Lancet ii:1216–1217, 1982.

249. Slavin J, Taylor J: Cyclosporine, nifedipine, and gingival hyperplasia. Lancet ii:739, 1987.

250. Gerson B: Cyclosporine controversies. Ther Drug Monit 7:669–686, 1987.

251. Walker AM, Funch DP, Birmann BM: Transplant Protocols. Chestnut Hill, MA, Epidemiology Resources, 1990.

252. Stock PG, Payne WD: Liver transplantation. Crit Care Clin 6:911–925, 1990.

253. Bolman RM, Saffitz J: Early postoperative care of the cardiac transplantation patient: routine considerations and immunosuppressive therapy. Prog Card Dis 33:137–148, 1990.

254. Munoz SJ, Vlasses PH, Boullata JI, et al.: Elevated arterial blood pressure in survivors of liver transplantation and treated with cyclosporine and corticosteroids. Transplant Proc 20(suppl 3):23–37, 1988.

255. Simmons RG, Abress L, Anderson CR: Quality of life after kidney transplantation. Transplant 45:415–421, 1988.

256. Showstack J, Katz P, Amend W, et al.: The effect of cyclosporine on the use of hospital resources of kidney transplantation. N Engl J Med 312:1086–1092, 1989.

257. Canafax DM, Gruber SA, Chan GLC, et al.: The pharmacoeconomics of renal transplantation: increased drug costs with decreased hospitalization costs. Pharmacotherapy 10:105–110, 1990.

258. Evans, RW: The socioeconomics of organ transplantation. Transplant Proc 17(suppl 4):129–136, 1985.

259. Simon DG: A cost-effectiveness analysis of cyclosporine in cadaveric kidney transplantation. Med Decis Making 6:199–207, 1986.

260. Manninen DL, Evans RW, The cost and outcomes of kidney transplantation according to initial immunosuppressive drug protocol. In Teraski P (ed): Clinical Transplants 1987. Los Angeles, UCLA Press, 1987, pp 269–275.

INDEX

Page numbers in italics denote figures; those followed by "t" denote tables.